Harrison's
PRINCIPLES OF INTERNAL MEDICINE

EDITORS OF PREVIOUS EDITIONS

T. R. Harrison, Editor-in-Chief, Editions 1, 2, 3, 4, 5

W. R. Resnik, Editor, Editions 1, 2, 3, 4, 5

M. M. Wintrobe, Editor, Editions 1, 2, 3, 4, 5
            Editor-in-Chief, Editions 6, 7

G. W. Thorn, Editor, Editions 1, 2, 3, 4, 5, 6, 7
            Editor-in-Chief, Edition 8

R. D. Adams, Editor, Editions 2, 3, 4, 5, 6, 7, 8, 9, 10

P. B. Beeson, Editor, Editions 1, 2

I. L. Bennett, Jr., Editor, Editions 3, 4, 5, 6

E. Braunwald, Editor, Editions 6, 7, 8, 9, 10

K. J. Isselbacher, Editor, Editions 6, 7, 8, 10
            Editor-in-Chief, Edition 9

R. G. Petersdorf, Editor, Editions 6, 7, 8, 9
            Editor-in-Chief, Edition 10

J. D. Wilson, Editor, Editions 9, 10

J. B. Martin, Editor, Edition 10

Harrison's
PRINCIPLES OF INTERNAL MEDICINE
Eleventh Edition

Editors

EUGENE BRAUNWALD, A.B., M.D., M.A. (Hon.), M.D. (Hon.)   Hersey Professor of the Theory and Practice of Physic and Herrman Ludwig Blumgart Professor of Medicine, Harvard Medical School; Chairman, Department of Medicine, Brigham and Women's and Beth Israel Hospitals, Boston

KURT J. ISSELBACHER, A.B., M.D. Mallinckrodt Professor of Medicine, Harvard Medical School; Physician and Chief, Gastrointestinal Unit, Massachusetts General Hospital, Boston

ROBERT G. PETERSDORF, A.B., M.D., M.A. (Hon.), D.Sc. (Hon.), M.D. (Hon.), L.H.D. (Hon.) Professor of Medicine, Dean and Vice Chancellor, Health Sciences, University of California School of Medicine, San Diego, La Jolla

JEAN D. WILSON, M.D. Professor of Internal Medicine, The University of Texas Southwestern Medical School, Dallas

JOSEPH B. MARTIN, M.D., Ph.D., F.R.C.P.(C), M.A. (Hon.)   Julieanne Dorn Professor of Neurology, Harvard Medical School; Chief, Neurology Service, Massachusetts General Hospital, Boston

ANTHONY S. FAUCI, M.D. Chief, Laboratory of Immunoregulation and Director, National Institute of Allergy and Infectious Diseases, National Institutes of Health, Bethesda

gotá
exico
São Paulo

McGRAW-HILL B

Harrison's
Principles of Internal Medicine

1 2 3 4 5 6 7 8 9 0   DOW DOW   8 9 8 7 6

Foreign Editions
FRENCH (Eleventh Edition)—Flammarion, © 1988 (est.)
GERMAN (Tenth Edition)—Schwabe and Company, Ltd., © 1986
GREEK (Tenth Edition)—Parissianos, © 1986
ITALIAN (Eleventh Edition)—McGraw-Hill Libri Italia S.r.l. © 1987 (est.)
JAPANESE (Tenth Edition)—Hirokawa, © 1985
PORTUGUESE (Eleventh Edition)—Editora Guanabara Koogan, S.A., © 1987 (est.)
SPANISH (Tenth Edition)—Libros McGraw-Hill de Mexico, S.A., © 1986

This book was set in Times Roman by Monotype Composition Company.
The editors were J. Dereck Jeffers, Eileen J. Scott, and Mariapaz Ramos-Englis
The indexer was Philip James; the production supervisor was Ave McCracken; the cover was designed by Edward R. Schultheis
R. R. Donnelley & Sons Company was printer and binder.

Library of Congress Cataloging-in-Publication Data

Principles of internal medicine.
  Harrison's principles of internal medicine.

  Also issued in 2 v.
  Includes bibliographies and index.
  1. Internal medicine. I. Harrison, Tinsley Randolph, Date. II. Braunwald, Eugene, Date.
III. Title. [DNLM: 1. Internal Medicine. WB 115 P957]
RC46.P895   1987   616   86-14383
ISBN 0-07-007261-2 (1-vol. ed.)
ISBN 0-07-079454-5 (2-vol. ed. : set)

ABBREVIATED CONTENTS

CONTENTS

**PART SEVEN
DISORDERS OF THE GASTROINTESTINAL
SYSTEM**

Section 1: Disorders of the alimentary tract

Section 2: Hepatobiliary disease

Section 3: Disorders of the pancreas

**PART EIGHT
DISORDERS OF THE IMMUNE SYSTEM,
CONNECTIVE TISSUE, AND JOINTS**

Section 1: Disorders of the immune system

PART TWELVE
DISORDERS OF THE CENTRAL AND PERIPHERAL NERVOUS SYSTEM

Section 1: Disorders of the central nervous system

Section 2: Disease of nerve and muscle

PART THIRTEEN
PSYCHIATRY

Section 1: Psychiatric disorders

Section 2: Alcoholism and drug dependency

LIST OF CONTRIBUTORS

RAYMOND D. ADAMS, B.A., M.A., M.D., M.A. (Hon.), D.Sc. (Hon.), M.D. (Hon.)
Bullard Professor of Neuropathology, Emeritus, Harvard Medical School; Consultant Neurologist and formerly Chief of Neurology Service, Massachusetts General Hospital; Emeritus Director, Eunice K. Shriver Research Center, Boston; Médicin Adjoint, L'Hôpital Cantonale de Lausanne, Lausanne

JOHN W. ADAMSON, M.D.
Professor of Medicine and Head, Division of Hematology, Department of Medicine, University of Washington School of Medicine, Seattle

ELLIOT ALPERT, M.D.
Professor of Medicine and Chief, Division of Gastroenterology, Baylor College of Medicine, Houston

JOSEPH S. ALPERT, M.D.
Professor of Medicine, University of Massachusetts Medical School; Director, Division of Cardiovascular Medicine, University of Massachusetts Medical Center, Worcester

ROBERT J. ANDERSON, M.D.
Associate Professor of Medicine, University of Colorado Health Sciences Center, Denver

JACK P. ANTEL, M.D.
Associate Professor of Neurology, University of Chicago Pritzker School of Medicine, Chicago

BARRY G. W. ARNASON, M.D.
Professor and Chairman, Department of Neurology, University of Chicago Pritzker School of Medicine, Chicago

PAUL M. ARNOW, M.D.
Associate Professor of Medicine, Section of Infectious Disease, University of Chicago Hospital and Clinics, Chicago

ARTHUR K. ASBURY, M.D.
Ruth Wagner Van Meter and J. Ray Van Meter Professor of Neurology, University of Pennsylvania School of Medicine and Hospital of the University of Pennsylvania, Philadelphia

K. FRANK AUSTEN, M.D.
Theodore B. Bayles Professor of Medicine, Harvard Medical School; Physician-in-Chief, Robert B. Brigham Division and Chairman, Department of Rheumatology and Immunology, Brigham and Women's Hospital, Boston

ROBERT AUSTRIAN, M.D., D.Sc. (Hon.)
John Herr Musser Professor and Chairman, Department of Research Medicine, University of Pennsylvania School of Medicine, Philadelphia

BERNARD M. BABIOR, M.D., Ph.D.
Head, Division of Biochemistry, Department of Basic and Clinical Research, Scripps Clinic and Research Foundation, La Jolla

JEFFREY P. BAKER, M.D., F.R.C.P. (C)
Assistant Professor of Medicine, University of Toronto; Consultant Staff Gastroenterologist, Toronto Western Hospital, Toronto

M. FLINT BEAL, M.D.
Assistant Professor, Harvard Medical School; Assistant Neurologist, Massachusetts General Hospital, Boston

HARRY N. BEATY, M.D.
Professor of Medicine and Dean, Northwestern University Medical School, Chicago

ARTHUR L. BEAUDET, M.D.
Investigator, Howard Hughes Medical Institute; Professor of Pediatrics and Cell Biology, Baylor College of Medicine, Houston

JOHN E. BENNETT, M.D.
Head, Clinical Mycology Section, National Institute of Allergy and Infectious Diseases, National Institutes of Health, Bethesda

JEFFREY D. BERNHARD, M.D.
Assistant Professor of Medicine, Director, Division of Dermatology, and Director of Phototherapy Center, Department of Medicine, University of Massachusetts Medical Center, Worcester

EDWIN L. BIERMAN, M.D.
Professor of Medicine and Chief, Division of Metabolism, Endocrinology, and Nutrition, University of Washington School of Medicine, Seattle

ALAN B. BISNO, M.D.
Professor of Medicine and Chief, Division of Infectious Diseases, University of Tennessee Center for the Health Sciences, Memphis

HENRY R. BOURNE, M.D.
Chairman, Department of Pharmacology, School of Medicine, University of California, San Francisco

WALTER G. BRADLEY, D.M., F.R.C.P.
Chairman and Professor of Neurology, University of Vermont College of Medicine; Chairman, Department of Neurology, University Health Center, Burlington

DAVID L. BRAFF, M.D.
Associate Professor, Department of Psychiatry, School of Medicine, University of California at San Diego; Director, Psychiatric Inpatient Services, U.C.S.D. Medical Center, San Diego

EUGENE BRAUNWALD, A.B., M.D., M.A. (Hon.), M.D. (Hon.)
Hersey Professor of the Theory and Practice of Physic and Herrman Ludwig Blumgart Professor of Medicine, Harvard Medical School; Chairman, Department of Medicine, Brigham and Women's and Beth Israel Hospitals, Boston

BARRY M. BRENNER, B.S., M.D., M.A. (Hon.)
Samuel A. Levine Professor of Medicine, Harvard Medical School; Senior Physician and Director, Renal Division, Brigham and Women's Hospital, Boston

KAREN THATCHER BRITTON, M.D., Ph.D.
Assistant Professor of Psychiatry, School of Medicine, University of California at San Diego, La Jolla

SAMUEL BRODER, M.D.
Associate Director, Clinical Oncology Program, Division of Cancer Treatment and Deputy Clinical Director, National Cancer Institute, National Institutes of Health, Bethesda

MICHAEL S. BROWN, M.D.
Paul J. Thomas Professor, Department of Molecular Genetics, The University of Texas Health Science Center, Dallas

H. FRANKLIN BUNN, M.D.
Professor of Medicine, Harvard Medical School; Senior Physician and Director, Hematology Research, Brigham and Women's Hospital; Investigator, Howard Hughes Medical Institute, Boston

JOHN R. BURTON, M.D.
Associate Professor of Medicine, Johns Hopkins University School of Medicine; Deputy Director of Department of Medicine, Director of Division of Geriatric Medicine, Francis Scott Key Medical Center, Baltimore

ALFRED E. BUXTON, M.D.
Assistant Professor of Medicine, University of Pennsylvania School of Medicine; Director, Cardiac Electrophysiology Laboratory, Hospital of the University of Pennsylvania, Philadelphia

CHARLES B. CARPENTER, M.D.
Professor of Medicine, Harvard Medical School; Senior Physician, Brigham and Women's Hospital, Boston

CHARLES C. J. CARPENTER, M.D.
Professor of Medicine, Brown University; Physician-in-Chief, The Miriam Hospital, Providence

BRUCE R. CARR, M.D.
Associate Professor, Department of Obstetrics and Gynecology and Cecil and Ida Green Center for Reproductive Biology Sciences, The University of Texas Health Science Center, Dallas

EDWIN CASSEM, M.D.
Associate Professor of Psychiatry, Harvard Medical School; Chief, Psychiatric Consultation–Liason Service, Massachusetts General Hospital, Boston

RICHARD CHAMPLIN, M.D.
Associate Professor of Medicine and Director, Leukemia/Bone Marrow Transplant Service, School of Medicine, University of California at Los Angeles

KEITH H. CHIAPPA, M.D.
Assistant Professor of Neurology, Harvard Medical School; Director, EEG and Evoked Potentials Unit of the Clinical Neurophysiology Laboratory and Department of Neurology, Massachusetts General Hospital, Boston

WALLACE A. CLYDE, Jr., M.D.
Professor of Pediatrics and Microbiology, University of North Carolina School of Medicine, Chapel Hill

FREDRIC L. COE, M.D.
Professor of Medicine and Physiology and Chief, Nephrology Program, University of Chicago Pritzker School of Medicine, Chicago

ALAN S. COHEN, M.D.
Chief of Medicine and Director, Thorndike Memorial Laboratory, Boston City Hospital; Conrad Wesselhoeft Professor of Medicine, Boston University School of Medicine, Boston

HARVEY R. COLTEN, M.D.
Professor and Chairman, Department of Pediatrics, Washington University School of Medicine, St. Louis

WILSON S. COLUCCI, M.D.
Assistant Professor of Medicine, Harvard Medical School; Associate Physician, Brigham and Women's Hospital, Boston

PATRICIA C. COME, M.D.
Assistant Professor of Medicine, Harvard Medical School; Director, Noninvasive Cardiovascular Diagnostic Laboratory, Beth Israel Hospital, Boston

MAX D. COOPER, M.D.
Professor of Pediatrics and Microbiology, Cellular Immunobiology Unit, The University of Alabama in Birmingham, Birmingham

RICHARD A. COOPER, M.D.
Dean and Professor of Medicine, Medical College of Wisconsin, Milwaukee

LAWRENCE COREY, M.D.
Professor of Laboratory Medicine and Microbiology and Adjunct Professor of Medicine and Pediatrics, University of Washington School of Medicine, Seattle

RONALD G. CRYSTAL, M.D.
Chief, Pulmonary Branch, National Heart, Lung and Blood Institute, National Institutes of Health, Bethesda

JOHN J. CUSH, M.D.
Fellow in Rheumatology, Department of Internal Medicine, The University of Texas Health Science Center, Dallas

DAVID C. DALE, M.D.
Professor of Medicine and Dean, University of Washington School of Medicine, Seattle

JAMES E. DALEN, M.D.
Professor and Chairman, Department of Medicine, University of Massachusetts Medical School; Physician-in-Chief, University of Massachusetts Hospital, Worcester

THOMAS M. DANIEL, M.D.
Professor of Medicine, Case Western Reserve University School of Medicine; Physician, University Hospitals of Cleveland, Cleveland

GILBERT H. DANIELS, M.D.
Associate Professor of Medicine, Thyroid Unit, Massachusetts General Hospital, Boston

ROBERT B. DAROFF, M.D.
Gilbert W. Humphrey Professor and Chairman, Case Western Reserve University School of Medicine, Director, Department of Neurology, University Hospitals of Cleveland; Neurology Service, Cleveland Veterans Administration Medical Center, Cleveland

JOHN R. DAVID, M.D.
Professor of Medicine, Harvard Medical School; Chief, Division of Tropical Medicine, Robert B. Brigham Division of Brigham and Women's Hospital; John LaPorte Given Professor and Chairman, Department of Tropical Public Health, Harvard School of Public Health, Boston

G. ROBERT DeLONG, M.D.
Assistant Professor of Neurology, Harvard Medical School; Associate Neurologist and Associate Pediatrician, Massachusetts General Hospital, Boston

VINCENT T. DeVITA, Jr., M.D.
Director, National Cancer Institute, National Institutes of Health, Bethesda

MARC A. DICHTER, M.D., Ph.D.
Professor of Neurology, University of Pennsylvania School of Medicine, Philadelphia

JULES L. DIENSTAG, M.D.
Associate Professor of Medicine, Harvard Medical School; Assistant Physician, Massachusetts General Hospital, Boston

ROBERT G. DLUHY, M.D.
Associate Professor of Medicine, Harvard Medical School; Associate Program Director of the Clinical Research Center, Brigham and Women's Hospital, Boston

RAPHAEL DOLIN, M.D.
Professor of Medicine and Head, Infectious Diseases Unit, University of Rochester School of Medicine and Dentistry, Rochester

ANDREW G. ENGEL, M.D.
Professor of Neurology, Mayo Medical School; Department of Neurology, Mayo Clinic, Rochester

KENNETH H. FALCHUK, M.D.
Associate Professor of Medicine, Harvard Medical School; Brigham and Women's Hospital, Boston

ANTHONY S. FAUCI, M.D.
Chief, Laboratory of Immunoregulation and Director, National Institute of Allergy and Infectious Diseases, National Institutes of Health, Bethesda

MURRAY J. FAVUS, M.D.
Associate Professor of Medicine, University of Chicago Pritzker School of Medicine, Chicago

RALPH D. FEIGIN, M.D.
Professor and Chairman, Department of Pediatrics, Baylor College of Medicine; Physician-in-Chief, Texas Children's Hospital, Houston

BERNARD N. FIELDS, M.D.
Adele Lehman Professor and Chairman, Department of Microbiology and Molecular Genetics, Harvard Medical School; Professor of Medicine, Division of Infectious Diseases, Brigham and Women's Hospital, Boston

ALFRED P. FISHMAN, M.D.
William Maul Measey Professor of Medicine, University of Pennsylvania; Director, Cardiovascular-Pulmonary Division, Hospital of the University of Pennsylvania, Philadelphia

THOMAS B. FITZPATRICK, M.D., Ph.D.
Edward Wigglesworth Professor of Dermatology and Chairman, Department of Dermatology, Harvard Medical School; Chief, Dermatology Service, Massachusetts General Hospital, Boston

DANIEL W. FOSTER, M.D.
Professor of Internal Medicine, The University of Texas Health Science Center, Dallas

MICHAEL M. FRANK, M.D.
Chief, Laboratory of Clinical Investigation and Clinical Director, National Institute of Allergy and Infectious Diseases, National Institutes of Health, Bethesda

STANLEY D. FREEDMAN, M.D.
Head, Division of Infectious Diseases, Scripps Clinic and Research Foundation; Associate Clinical Professor of Medicine, University of California at San Diego, La Jolla

LAURENCE S. FRIEDMAN, M.D.
Assistant Professor of Medicine, Jefferson Medical College and Thomas Jefferson University Hospital, Philadelphia

PAUL A. FRIEDMAN, M.D.
Associate Professor of Medicine and Pharmacology, Harvard Medical School; Associate Physician, Beth Israel Hospital, Boston

WILLIAM F. FRIEDMAN, M.D.
J. H. Nicholson Professor of Pediatrics and Executive Chairman, Department of Pediatrics, Los Angeles Medical Center, University of California, Los Angeles

LAWRENCE A. FROHMAN, M.D.
Professor of Medicine, Director of Division of Endocrinology and Metabolism, University of Cincinnati College of Medicine, Cincinnati

JOHN I. GALLIN, M.D.
Scientific Director, National Institute of Allergy and Infectious Diseases, National Institutes of Health, Bethesda

ROBERT C. GALLO, M.D.
Chief, Laboratory of Tumor Cell Biology, Division of Cancer Treatment, National Cancer Institute, National Institutes of Health, Bethesda

PIERCE GARDNER, M.D.
Professor of Medicine and Pediatrics, University of Chicago Pritzker School of Medicine; Director, Infectious Diseases Training Program, University of Chicago Medical Center, Chicago

MARC B. GARNICK M.D.
Associate Professor of Medicine, Dana-Farber Cancer Institute, Harvard Medical School; Associate Physician, Brigham and Women's Hospital, Boston

JAMES L. GERMAN III, M.D.
Professor (Genetics), Department of Pediatrics, Cornell University Medical College; Senior Investigator and Director, Laboratory of Human Genetics, The New York Blood Center, New York

ELOISE R. GIBLETT, M.D.
Research Professor of Medicine, University of Washington School of Medicine; Executive Director, Puget Sound Blood Center, Seattle

BRUCE C. GILLILAND, M.D.
Professor of Medicine and Laboratory Medicine, University of Washington School of Medicine; Chief of Medicine, Pacific Medical Center, Seattle

J. CHRISTIAN GILLIN, M.D.
Professor of Psychiatry, University of California at San Diego, La Jolla

SID GILMAN, M.D.
Professor and Chairman, Department of Neurology, The University of Michigan Medical Center, Ann Arbor

RICHARD J. GLASSOCK, M.D.
Professor of Medicine, School of Medicine, University of California at Los Angeles; Chairman, Department of Medicine, Harbor-UCLA Medical Center, Torrance

ROBERT M. GLICKMAN, M.D.
Samuel Bard Professor of Medicine, Columbia University College of Physicians and Surgeons; Director, Medical Service, Presbyterian Hospital, New York

DAVID W. GOLDE, M.D.
Professor of Medicine and Chief, Division of Hematology/Oncology, School of Medicine, University of California at Los Angeles, Los Angeles

STEPHEN E. GOLDFINGER, M.D.
Associate Professor of Medicine and Associate Dean of Continuing Education, Harvard Medical School; Physician, Gastrointestinal Unit, Massachusetts General Hospital, Boston

PAUL GOLDHABER, D.D.S.
Dean and Professor of Periodontology, Harvard School of Dental Medicine, Boston

LEE GOLDMAN, M.D.
Associate Professor of Medicine, Harvard Medical School; Assistant Physician-in-Chief, Brigham and Women's Hospital, Boston

JOSEPH L. GOLDSTEIN, M.D.
Paul J. Thomas Professor and Chairman, Department of Molecular Genetics, The University of Texas Health Science Center, Dallas

RAJ K. GOYAL, M.D.
Rabb Professor of Medicine, Harvard Medical School; Chief, Division of Gastroenterology, Beth Israel Hospital, Boston

JOHN W. GRAEF, M.D.
Assistant Clinical Professor, Harvard Medical School; Director, The Lead/Toxicology Clinic, The Children's Hospital, Boston

IGOR GRANT, M.D.
Professor of Psychiatry, School of Medicine, University of California at San Diego, La Jolla

HARRY B. GREENBERG, M.D.
Associate Professor of Medicine, Department of Medicine, Stanford University Medical School; Palo Alto Veterans Administration Medical Center, Palo Alto

NORTON J. GREENBERGER, M.D.
Peter T. Bohan Professor and Chairman, Department of Medicine, University of Kansas School of Medicine, Kansas City

JAMES E. GRIFFIN III, M.D.
Associate Professor of Internal Medicine, The University of Texas Health Science Center, Dallas

ROBERT C. GRIGGS, M.D.
Professor of Neurology and Medicine, University of Rochester School of Medicine and Dentistry, University of Rochester Medical Center, Rochester

JOHN H. GROWDON, M.D.
Associate Professor of Neurology, Harvard Medical School; Associate Neurologist, Massachusetts General Hospital, Boston

RICHARD L. GUERRANT, M.D.
Professor of Medicine and Head, Division of Geographic Medicine, University of Virginia School of Medicine, Charlottesville

BEVRA HANNAHS HAHN, M.D.
Professor of Medicine and Chief of Rheumatology, University of California, Los Angeles

ROBERT I. HANDIN, M.D.
Associate Professor of Medicine, Harvard Medical School; Director, Hematology Division, Brigham and Women's Hospital, Boston

H. HUNTER HANDSFIELD, M.D.
Director, Sexually Transmitted Disease Control Program, Seattle-King County Department of Public Health; Associate Professor of Medicine, University of Washington School of Medicine, Seattle

JAMES P. HARNISCH, M.D.
Clinical Associate Professor of Medicine, University of Washington School of Medicine; Chief of Dermatology, Pacific Medical Center, Seattle

DONALD H. HARTER, M.D.
Benjamin and Virginia T. Boshes Professor of Neurology and Chairman, Department of Neurology, Northwestern University Medical School; Chairman, Department of Neurology, Northwestern Memorial Hospital, Chicago

BARTON F. HAYNES, M.D.
Associate Professor of Medicine and Assistant Professor of Microbiology and Immunology, Duke University School of Medicine, Durham

HARLEY A. HAYNES, M.D.
Associate Professor of Dermatology, Harvard Medical School; Director, Dermatology Division, Department of Medicine, Brigham and Women's Hospital; Chief, Dermatology, West Roxbury Veterans Administration Hospital, Boston

WILLIAM R. HAZZARD, M.D.
Professor and Chair, Department of Medicine, Bowman-Gray School of Medicine, Wake Forest University; Chief of Medicine, North Carolina Baptist Hospital, Winston-Salem

STEVEN C. HEBERT, M.D.
Assistant Professor of Medicine, Harvard Medical School; Associate Physician, Brigham and Women's Hospital, Boston

FRED J. HENDLER, M.D., Ph.D.
Assistant Professor of Internal Medicine, Division of Hematology/Oncology, The University of Texas Health Science Center, Dallas

JANE ELLEN HENNEY, M.D.
Associate Vice Chancellor and Associate Professor of Medicine, Division of Clinical Oncology, Department of Medicine, University of Kansas Medical Center, Kansas City

RAYMOND L. HINTZ, M.D.
Professor of Pediatrics and Head, Division of Pediatric Endocrinology, Stanford University School of Medicine, Stanford

MARTIN S. HIRSCH, M.D.
Associate Professor, Harvard Medical School; Associate Physician, Infectious Disease Unit, Massachusetts General Hospital, Boston

JAN V. HIRSCHMANN, M.D.
Assistant Chief, Medical Service, Seattle Veterans Administration Medical Center; Associate Professor of Medicine, University of Washington School of Medicine, Seattle

FRED HOCHBERG, M.D.
Associate Professor of Neurology, Harvard Medical School; Associate Neurologist, Massachusetts General Hospital, Boston

PAUL D. HOEPRICH, M.D.
Professor of Medicine and Chief, Section of Medical Mycology, Department of Internal Medicine, Division of Infectious and Immunologic Diseases, School of Medicine, University of California, Davis

JOHN H. HOLBROOK, M.D.
Associate Professor of Medicine, Division of General Internal Medicine, Department of Medicine, University of Utah Medical Center, Salt Lake City

MICHAEL F. HOLICK, M.D., Ph.D.
Professor of Physiology and Nutrition and Director of Vitamin D and Bone Metabolism Laboratory, U.S. Department of Agriculture/Human Nutrition Research Center, Tufts University, Boston

NORMAN K. HOLLENBERG, M.D.
Professor of Radiology, Harvard Medical School; Physician, Brigham and Women's Hospital, Boston

KING K. HOLMES, M.D., Ph.D.
Professor and Vice Chairman, Department of Medicine, University of Washington School of Medicine; Chief of Medicine, Harborview Medical Center, Seattle

THOMAS M. HOSTETTER, M.D.
Associate Professor of Medicine, University of Minnesota School of Medicine; Director, Division of Renal Diseases, University Hospital, Minneapolis

LEIGHTON Y. HUEY, M.D.
Associate Professor of Psychiatry, University of California at San Diego; Chief of Psychiatry Service, San Diego Veterans Administration Medical Center, San Diego

GARY W. HUNNINGHAKE, M.D.
Professor of Internal Medicine and Director, Pulmonary Division, University of Iowa College of Medicine, Iowa City

SIDNEY H. INGBAR, M.D., D.Sc.
William Bosworth Castle Professor of Medicine, Harvard Medical School; Director, Thorndike Laboratory, Beth Israel Hospital, Boston

ROLAND H. INGRAM, Jr., M.D.
Parker B. Francis Professor of Medicine, Harvard Medical School; Director, Respiratory Division, Brigham and Women's Hospital, Boston

KURT J. ISSELBACHER, A.B., M.D.
Mallinckrodt Professor of Medicine, Harvard Medical School; Physician and Chief, Gastrointestinal Unit, Massachusetts General Hospital, Boston

KHURSHEED N. JEEJEEBHOY, M.B.B.S., Ph.D., F.R.C.P. (Lond.), F.R.C.P. (Edin.), F.R.C.P. (C).
Professor of Medicine, University of Toronto; Director, Division of Gastroenterology, Toronto General Hospital, Toronto

MARK E. JOSEPHSON, M.D.
Professor of Medicine, University of Pennsylvania School of Medicine; Chief, Cardiovascular Section, Hospital of the University of Pennsylvania, Philadelphia

LEWIS L. JUDD, M.D.
Professor and Chairman, Department of Psychiatry, School of Medicine, University of California at San Diego, La Jolla

DENNIS L. KASPER, M.D.
Professor of Medicine, Harvard Medical School; Chief, Division of Infectious Diseases, Beth Israel Hospital; Associate Director, Channing Laboratory, Brigham and Women's Hospital, Boston

SATISH KATHPALIA, M.D.
Assistant Professor of Medicine, University of Chicago Pritzker School of Medicine; Attending Physician, Michael Reese Hospital and Medical Center, Chicago

DONALD KAYE, M.D., F.A.C.P.
Professor and Chairman, Department of Medicine, Medical College of Pennsylvania; Chief of Medicine, Hospital of the Medical College of Pennsylvania, Philadelphia

WILLIAM N. KELLEY, M.D.
John G. Searle Professor and Chairman, Department of Internal Medicine, University of Michigan Medical School, Ann Arbor

PHILIP KIRBY, M.D.
Instructor in Medicine, Division of Dermatology, University of Washington School of Medicine, Seattle

J. PHILLIP KISTLER, M.D.
Associate Professor of Neurology, Harvard Medical School; Associate Neurologist, Massachusetts General Hospital, Boston

RAYMOND S. KOFF, M.D.
Professor of Medicine, Boston University School of Medicine; Chief of Hepatology Section, Boston University Medical Center; Chief of Medicine, Framingham Union Hospital, Framingham

WILLIAM J. KOVACS, M.D.
Assistant Professor of Medicine, Division of Endocrinology, Vanderbilt University School of Medicine, Nashville

STEPHEN M. KRANE, M.D.
Professor of Medicine, Harvard Medical School; Physician and Chief, Arthritis Unit, Massachusetts General Hospital, Boston

J. THOMAS LaMONT, M.D.
Professor of Medicine, Boston University Medical Center; Chief, Gastrointestinal Section, University Hospital, Boston

LEWIS LANDSBERG, M.D.
Professor of Medicine, Harvard Medical School; Director, Division of Endocrinology and Metabolism, Beth Israel Hospital, Boston

H. CLIFFORD LANE, M.D.
Senior Investigator, Laboratory of Immunoregulation and Deputy Clinical Director, National Institute of Allergy and Infectious Diseases, National Institutes of Health, Bethesda

THOMAS J. LAWLEY, M.D.
Senior Investigator, Dermatology Branch, National Cancer Institute, National Institutes of Health, Bethesda

ALEXANDER R. LAWTON, M.D.
Professor of Pediatrics and Microbiology, Division of Pediatric Immunology, Vanderbilt University School of Medicine, Nashville

J. MICHAEL LAZARUS, M.D.
Associate Professor of Medicine, Harvard Medical School; Physician, Brigham and Women's Hospital, Boston

NORMAN G. LEVINSKY, M.D.
Wade Professor and Chairman, Division of Medicine, Boston University School of Medicine; Physician-in-Chief and Director, Evans Memorial Department of Clinical Research, University Hospital, Boston

PETER E. LIPSKY, M.D.
Professor of Internal Medicine and Microbiology and Chief, Division of Immunologic and Rheumatologic Diseases, Department of Internal Medicine; Director, Harold C. Simmons Arthritis Research Center, The University of Texas Health Science Center, Dallas

RICHARD M. LOCKSLEY, M.D.
Assistant Professor of Medicine, University of San Francisco; Chief of Infectious Diseases, University of San Francisco Medical Center, Moffitt-Long Hospital, San Francisco

DAN L. LONGO, M.D.
Associate Director, Biological Response Modifiers Program, Division of Biology and Diagnosis, National Cancer Institute-Frederick Cancer Research Facility, Frederick

FREDERICK H. LOVEJOY, JR., M.D.
Associate Professor, Harvard Medical School; Associate Physician-in-Chief, The Children's Hospital; Director, Massachusetts Poison Control System, Boston

SHEILA A. LUKEHART, Ph.D.
Research Assistant Professor, Division of Infectious Diseases, University of Washington School of Medicine, Seattle

WALTER C. MacDONALD, M.D.
Chairman, GI Tumor Group, Cancer Control Agency of British Columbia, Vancouver

RAYMOND MACIEWICZ, M.D.
Assistant Professor of Neurology, Harvard Medical School; Assistant Neurologist, Massachusetts General Hospital, Boston

HENRY J. MANKIN, M.D.
Edith M. Ashley Professor of Orthopedic Surgery, Harvard Medical School; Chief, Orthopedic Services, Massachusetts General Hospital, Boston

FRANCIS E. MARCHLINSKI, M.D.
Assistant Professor of Medicine, University of Pennsylvania School of Medicine; Director, Arrhythmia Evaluation Center, Hospital of the University of Pennsylvania, Philadelphia

JOSEPH B. MARTIN, M.D., Ph.D., F.R.C.P. (C), M.A. (Hon.)
Julieanne Dorn Professor of Neurology, Harvard Medical School; Chief, Neurology Service, Massachusetts General Hospital, Boston

HENRY MASUR, M.D.
Deputy Chief, Critical Care Medicine, Clinical Center, National Institutes of Health, Bethesda

ROGER J. MAY, M.D.
Instructor in Medicine, Harvard Medical School; Assistant in Medicine, Beth Israel Hospital, Boston

E.R. McFADDEN, JR., M.D.
Argyl J. Beams Professor of Medicine and Director, Asthma and Allergic Disease Center, Case Western Reserve University, Cleveland

JAMES E. McGUIGAN, M.D.
Chairman, Department of Medicine, University of Florida College of Medicine, Gainesville

RIMA McLEOD, M.D.
Associate Professor of Medicine, University of Chicago Pritzker School of Medicine; Attending Physician, Michael Reese Hospital and Medical Center, Chicago

MARK S. McPHEE, M.D.
Clinical Associate Professor of Medicine and Director, Gastrointestinal Endoscopy Unit, University of Kansas, Kansas City

NANCY K. MELLO, Ph.D.
Professor of Psychology, Department of Psychiatry, Harvard Medical School; Co-Director, Alcohol and Drug Abuse Research Center, McLean Hospital, Belmont

JERRY R. MENDELL, M.D.
Professor of Neurology, Ohio State University College of Medicine, Columbus

JOHN MENDELSOHN, M.D.
Chairman, Department of Medicine and Head, Division of Medical Oncology, Memorial Sloan-Kettering Cancer Center; Professor of Medicine, Cornell University Medical College, New York

JACK H. MENDELSON, M.D.
Professor of Psychiatry, Harvard Medical School; Co-Director, Alcohol and Drug Abuse Research Center, McLean Hospital, Belmont

URS A. MEYER, M.D.
Professor of Pharmacology and Chairman, Department of Pharmacology, Biocenter of the University of Basel, Basel, Switzerland

MARTIN C. MIHM, JR., M.D.
Professor of Pathology, Harvard Medical School; Chief, Dermatopathology Unit, Massachusetts General Hospital, Boston

EDGAR L. MILFORD, M.D.
Assistant Professor of Medicine, Harvard Medical School; Associate Physician, Brigham and Women's Hospital, Boston

MYRON MILLER, M.D.
Professor of Medicine, State University of New York Upstate Medical Center; Chief of Gerontology, Veterans Administration Medical Center, Syracuse

RICHARD A. MILLER, M.D.
Assistant Professor of Medicine, University of Washington School of Medicine; Division of Infectious Diseases, Pacific Medical Center, Seattle

JOHN D. MINNA, M.D.
Chief, NCI-Navy Medical Oncology Branch, National Cancer Institute, National Institutes of Health; Professor of Medicine, Uniformed Services University for the Health Sciences, Naval Hospital, Bethesda

JAY P. MOHR, M.D.
Sciarra Professor of Clinical Neurology, College of Physicians and Surgeons of Columbia University Neurological Institute, New York

KENNETH M. MOSER, M.D.
Professor of Medicine, School of Medicine, University of California at San Diego; Director, Pulmonary and Critical Care Division, U.C.S.D. Medical Center, San Diego

ARNOLD M. MOSES, M.D.
Professor of Medicine and Director, Clinical Research Center, State University of New York Upstate Medical Center; Chief, Endocrinology Section, Veterans Administration Medical Center, Syracuse

DAVID B. MOSHER, M.D.
Clinical Instructor in Dermatology, Harvard Medical School; Assistant in Dermatology, Massachusetts General Hospital, Boston

HARALAMPOS M. MOUTSOPOULOS, M.D., F.A.C.P.
Professor and Head of Medicine, Medical School, University of Ioannina, Ioannina, Greece

FREDERICK M. MURPHY, M.D.
Fellow in Neonatology, Baylor School of Medicine, Houston

JOHN F. MURRAY, M.D., D.Sc. (Hon.)
Professor of Medicine, University of California at San Francisco; Chief, Chest Service, San Francisco General Hospital, San Francisco

ROBERT J. MYERBURG, M.D.
Professor of Medicine and Physiology and Director, Division of Cardiology, University of Miami Medical Center, Miami

THEODORE E. NASH, M.D.
Senior Scientist, Laboratory of Parasitic Diseases, National Institute of Allergy and Infectious Diseases, National Institutes of Health, Bethesda

PAUL NEIMAN, M.D.
Professor of Medicine, University of Washington School of Medicine; Member and Associate Director for Basic Sciences, Fred Hutchinson Cancer Research Center, Seattle

HAROLD C. NEU, M.D.
Professor of Medicine and Pharmacology and Chief, Division of Infectious Diseases, College of Physicians and Surgeons, Columbia University, New York

JOHN A. OATES, M.D.
Professor and Chairman, Department of Medicine, Vanderbilt University School of Medicine; Physician-in-Chief, Vanderbilt University Hospital, Nashville

JERROLD M. OLEFSKY, M.D.
Professor of Medicine and Head, Division of Endocrinology and Metabolism, School of Medicine, University of California at San Diego, La Jolla

ROBERT A. O'ROURKE, M.D.
Charles Conrad and Anna Sahm Brown Professor of Medicine, University of Texas; Director, Division of Cardiovascular Diseases, The University of Texas Health Science Center, San Antonio

THOMAS D. PALELLA, M.D.
Assistant Professor of Internal Medicine, Division of Rheumatology, University of Michigan Medical School, Ann Arbor

DARWIN L. PALMER, M.D.
Professor of Medicine and Chief, Division of Infectious Disease, University of New Mexico School of Medicine; Chief, Infectious Disease Section, Veterans Administration Medical Center, Albuquerque

JOHN A. PARRISH, M.D.
Professor of Dermatology, Harvard Medical School; Director, Wellman Research Laboratory, Massachusetts General Hospital, Boston

A. WILLIAM PASCULLE, D.Sc.
Associate Professor of Pathology, University of Pittsburgh School of Medicine; Associate Director of Microbiology, Presbyterian-University Hospital, Pittsburgh

RICHARD C. PASTERNAK, M.D.
Assistant Professor of Medicine, Harvard Medical School; Assistant Physician and Director, Coronary Care Unit, Beth Israel Hospital, Boston

MADHUKAR A. PATHAK, M.S., Ph.D.
Senior Associate in Dermatology, Harvard Medical School; Dermatology Service, Massachusetts General Hospital, Boston

RICHARD D. PEARSON, M.D.
Associate Professor of Medicine and Pathology, Division of Geographic Medicine, University of Virginia School of Medicine, Charlottesville

LAWRENCE L. PELLETIER, Jr., M.D.
Professor of Medicine, University of Kansas School of Medicine; Chief, Medical Service, Wichita Veterans Administration Medical Center, Wichita

PETER L. PERINE, M.D., M.P.H.
Professor and Director, Division of Tropical Public Health and Professor of Medicine, Uniformed Services University of the Health Sciences School of Medicine, Bethesda

ROBERT G. PETERSDORF, M.D., M.A. (Hon.), D.Sc. (Hon.), M.D. (Hon.), L.H.D. (Hon.)
Dean and Professor of Medicine and Vice Chancellor, Health Sciences, School of Medicine, University of California at San Diego, La Jolla

KIRK L. PETERSON, M.D.
Professor of Medicine, University of California at San Diego; Director, Cardiology Service, U.C.S.D. Medical Center, San Diego

JAMES J. PLORDE, M.D.
Professor, Departments of Medicine and Laboratory Medicine and Chief, Clinical Microbiology Laboratory, Veterans Administration Medical Center, Seattle

FRANCIS ALLAN PLUMMER, M.D., F.R.C.P. (C)
Assistant Professor, Departments of Medicine and Medical Microbiology and Division of Community Medicine, University of Manitoba, Winnipeg

DANIEL K. PODOLSKY, M.D.
Associate Professor of Medicine, Harvard Medical School; Assistant Physician, Gastrointestinal Unit, Massachusetts General Hospital, Boston

JOHN T. POTTS, Jr., M.D.
Jackson Professor of Clinical Medicine, Harvard Medical School; Chief of the General Medical Service, Massachusetts General Hospital, Boston

LAWRIE W. POWELL, M.D.
Professor of Medicine, University of Queensland; Physician, Royal Brisbane Hospital, Brisbane, Australia

DARWIN J. PROCKOP, M.D., Ph.D.
Professor and Chairman, Department of Biochemistry, Jefferson Medical College of Thomas Jefferson University; Director, Department of Biochemistry, Jefferson Institute of Molecular Medicine, Philadelphia

AMY PRUITT, M.D.
Assistant Professor of Neurology, Harvard Medical School; Associate Neurologist, Massachusetts General Hospital, Boston

PAUL G. RAMSEY, M.D.
Associate Professor of Medicine, Department of Medicine, University of Washington School of Medicine, Seattle

JOEL M. RAPPEPORT, M.D.
Associate Professor of Medicine, Harvard Medical School; Physician, Brigham and Women's Hospital, Boston

C. GEORGE RAY, M.D.
Professor of Pathology and Pediatrics and Chief, Clinical Virology-Serology and Pediatrics Infectious Diseases Sections, University of Arizona College of Medicine, Tucson

PETER REICH, M.D.
Professor of Psychiatry, Harvard Medical School; Chief of Psychiatry, Brigham and Women's Hospital, Boston

RICHARD C. REICHMAN, M.D.
Associate Professor of Medicine, Infectious Diseases Unit, University of Rochester School of Medicine and Dentistry, Rochester

JACK S. REMINGTON, M.D.
Chairman, Department of Immunology and Infectious Diseases, Research Institute, Palo Alto Medical Foundation; Professor of Medicine, Division of Infectious Diseases, Stanford University School of Medicine, Palo Alto

EDWARD P. RICHARDSON, Jr., M.D.
Bullard Professor of Neuropathology, Harvard Medical School; Neurologist, Massachusetts General Hospital, Boston

HAL B. RICHERSON, M.D.
Professor of Internal Medicine and Director, Allergy-Immunology Division, University of Iowa College of Medicine, Iowa City

JAMES M. RICHTER, M.D.
Assistant Professor of Medicine, Harvard Medical School, Assistant Physician, Gastrointestinal Unit, Massachusetts General Hospital, Boston

CRAIG RISCH, M.D.
Associate Professor of Psychiatry, School of Medicine, University of California at San Diego, La Jolla

L. JACKSON ROBERTS II, M.D.
Associate Professor of Medicine, Pharmacology, and Clinical Pharmacology, Vanderbilt University School of Medicine, Nashville

R. PAUL ROBERTSON, M.D.
Professor of Medicine, Director of Clinical Research Center, and Director, Diabetes Center, University of Minnesota, Minneapolis

ALLAN R. RONALD, M.D.
H.F. Sellers Professor and Chairman, Department of Medicine, University of Manitoba; Physician-in-Chief, Department of Medicine, Health Sciences Centre, Winnipeg

RICHARD K. ROOT, M.D.
Professor and Chairman, Department of Medicine, University of California, San Francisco

ALLAN H. ROPPER, M.D.
Associate Professor of Neurology, Harvard Medical School; Director of Neurological/Neurosurgical Intensive Care Unit and Assistant Neurologist, Massachusetts General Hospital, Boston

LEON E. ROSENBERG, M.D.
Dean and C.N.H. Long Professor of Human Genetics, Medicine, and Pediatrics, Yale University School of Medicine, New Haven

MICHAEL ROSENBLATT, M.D.
Vice President for Biological Research, Merck, Sharp and Dohme Research Laboratories, West Point

JOHN ROSS, Jr., M.D.
Professor of Medicine and Head, Division of Cardiology, School of Medicine, University of California at San Diego; Attending Physician, U.C.S.D. Medical Center, San Diego

ARTHUR H. RUBENSTEIN, M.D.
Professor and Chairman, Department of Medicine, University of Chicago Pritzker School of Medicine, Chicago

CYRUS E. RUBIN, M.D.
Professor of Medicine and Adjunct Professor of Pathology, Division of Gastroenterology, University of Washington School of Medicine, Seattle

DANIEL RUDMAN, M.D.
Chief, Geriatric Medicine Division and Chief of Staff, Veterans Administration Medical Center; Professor of Medicine, University Health Science Center, Chicago Medical School, Chicago

ARTHUR I. SAGALOWSKY, M.D.
Associate Professor of Urology and Surgical Director of Renal Transplantation, The University of Texas Health Science Center, Dallas

JAY P. SANFORD, M.D.
Professor of Medicine and Dean, F. Edward Hebert School of Medicine; President, Uniformed Services University of the Health Sciences, Bethesda

DENNIS R. SCHABERG, M.D.
Associate Professor of Medicine, University of Michigan, Ann Arbor

ANDREW I. SCHAFER, M.D.
Assistant Professor of Medicine, Harvard Medical School; Associate Physician, Brigham and Women's Hospital, Boston

I. HERBERT SCHEINBERG, M.D.
Professor of Medicine and Head, Division of Genetic Medicine, Albert Einstein College of Medicine; Attending Physician, Hospital of the Albert Einstein College of Medicine, New York

ALAN L. SCHILLER, M.D.
Associate Professor of Pathology, Harvard Medical School; Associate Pathologist and Chief, Autopsy Pathology and Bone Laboratory, Massachusetts General Hospital, Boston

RUDI SCHMID, M.D.
Professor of Medicine and Dean, School of Medicine, University of California, San Francisco

R. NEIL SCHIMKE, M.D.
Professor of Pediatrics and Internal Medicine and Director, Division of Metabolism, Endocrinology, and Genetics, The University of Kansas College of Health Sciences, Kansas City

ROBERT T. SCHOOLEY, M.D.
Assistant Professor of Medicine, Harvard Medical School; Massachusetts General Hospital, Boston

ROBERT W. SCHRIER, M.D.
Professor and Chairman, Department of Medicine, University of Colorado School of Medicine, Denver

MARC A. SCHUCKIT, M.D.
Professor of Psychiatry, School of Medicine, University of California at San Diego; Director, Alcohol Research Center, San Diego Veterans Administration Medical Center, San Diego

WILLIAM J. SCHWARTZ, M.D.
Assistant Professor of Neurology, Harvard Medical School; Assistant Neurologist, Massachusetts General Hospital, Boston

DAVID S. SEGAL, Ph.D.
Professor of Psychiatry, School of Medicine, University of California at San Diego, La Jolla

JULIAN L. SEIFTER, M.D.
Assistant Professor of Medicine, Harvard Medical School; Associate Physician, Brigham and Women's Hospital, Boston

ANDREW P. SELWYN, M.D.
Associate Professor of Medicine, Harvard Medical School; Director, Cardiac Catheterization Laboratory, Brigham and Women's Hospital, Boston

BHAGWAN T. SHAHANI, M.B., B.S.
Associate Professor of Neurology, Harvard Medical School; Associate Neurologist, Massachusetts General Hospital, Boston

GORDON C. SHARP, M.D.
Professor of Medicine and Pathology and Director, Division of Rheumatology, University of Missouri-Columbia School of Medicine, Columbia

ELIZABETH M. SHORT, M.D.
Director, Division of Biomedical Research and Faculty Development, American Association of Medical Colleges, Washington, DC

WILLIAM SILEN, M.D.
Johnson and Johnson Professor of Surgery, Harvard Medical School; Surgeon-in-Chief, Department of Surgery, Beth Israel Hospital, Boston

FRED E. SILVERSTEIN, M.D.
Associate Professor of Medicine, Division of Gastroenterology, University of Washington School of Medicine, Seattle

JAMES B. SNOW, JR., M.D.
Professor and Chairman, Department of Otorhinolaryngology and Human Communication, University of Pennsylvania School of Medicine, Philadelphia

BURTON E. SOBEL, M.D.
Lewin Professor of Medicine, Washington University School of Medicine; Director, Cardiovascular Division, Barnes Hospital, St. Louis

ARTHUR J. SOBER, M.D.
Associate Professor of Dermatology, Harvard Medical School; Associate Dermatologist, Massachusetts General Hospital, Boston

FRANK E. SPEIZER, M.D.
Professor of Medicine, Harvard Medical School; Director, Occupational and Environmental Health Center, Brigham and Women's Hospital, Boston

JOHN W. STAKES, M.D.
Instructor in Neurology, Harvard Medical School; Assistant Neurologist, Massachusetts General Hospital, Boston

WALTER E. STAMM, M.D.
Professor of Medicine, University of Washington School of Medicine; Head, Division of Infectious Disease, Harborview Medical Center, Seattle

ALLEN C. STEERE, M.D.
Associate Professor of Medicine, Yale University School of Medicine, New Haven

KARI STEFANSSON, M.D.
Assistant Professor of Neurology and Pathology (Neuropathology), University of Chicago Pritzker School of Medicine, Chicago

GENE H. STOLLERMAN, M.D.
Professor of Medicine, Boston University School of Medicine; Attending Physician, University Hospital, Boston

D. E. STRANDNESS, JR., M.D.
Professor of Surgery, University of Washington School of Medicine; University Hospital, Seattle

DAVID H. P. STREETEN, M.B., D. Phil, F.R.C.P.
Professor of Medicine and Head, Section of Endocrinology, State University of New York Upstate Medical Center, Syracuse

E. DONNALL THOMAS, M.D.
Professor, Department of Medicine, University of Washington School of Medicine; Associate Director for Clinical Programs, Fred Hutchinson Cancer Research Center, Seattle

GENNARO M. TISI, M.D.
Professor of Medicine, Pulmonary and Critical Care Division, School of Medicine, University of California at San Diego; U.C.S.D. Medical Center, San Diego

PHILLIP P. TOSKES, M.D.
Professor of Medicine and Director, Division of Gastroenterology, Hepatology, and Nutrition, University of Florida College of Medicine; Veterans Administration Medical Center, Gainesville

MARVIN TURCK, M.D.
Professor of Medicine and Associate Dean, University of Washington School of Medicine; Medical Director, Harborview Medical Center, Seattle

KENNETH L. TYLER, M.D.
Assistant Professor of Neurology, Harvard Medical School; Clinical Assistant in Neurology, Massachusetts General Hospital, Boston

JOHN E. ULTMANN, M.D.
Professor of Medicine, Department of Medicine; Director, University of Chicago, Cancer Research Center; Dean for Research and Development, Division of the Biological Sciences, University of Chicago Pritzker School of Medicine, Chicago

MAURICE VICTOR, M.D.
Professor of Neurology, Case Western Reserve University School of Medicine; Director, Neurology Service, Cleveland Metropolitan General Hospital, Cleveland

JAMES F. WALLACE, M.D.
Professor of Medicine, University of Washington School of Medicine; Associate Physician-in-Chief, University Hospital, Seattle

PATRICK C. WALSH, M.D.
David Hall McConnell Professor and Director, Department of Urology, The Johns Hopkins University School of Medicine; Urologist-in-Chief, James Buchanan Brady Urological Institute, The Johns Hopkins Hospital, Baltimore

PETER D. WALZER, M.D.
Associate Professor of Medicine, University of Cincinnati College of Medicine; Chief, Infectious Diseases Section, Cincinnati Veterans Administration Medical Center, Cincinnati

JACK R. WANDS, M.D.
Associate Professor of Medicine, Harvard Medical School; Associate Physician, Gastrointestinal Unit, Massachusetts General Hospital, Boston

LOUIS WEINSTEIN, M.D., Ph.D., Sc.D. (Hon.)
Lecturer in Medicine, Harvard Medical School; Senior Consultant in Medicine, Brigham and Women's Hospital, Boston

JOHN B. WEST, M.D., Ph.D., D.Sc., F.R.C.P., F.R.A.C.P.
Professor of Medicine and Physiology, School of Medicine, University of California at San Diego; Physician, U.C.S.D. Medical Center, San Diego

NICHOLAS J. WHITE, M.D., M.R.C.P
Tropical Medicine Unit, Nuffield Department of Clinical Medicine, Oxford University, England; Faculty of Tropical Medicine, Mahidol University, Bangkok, Thailand

RICHARD J. WHITLEY, M.D.
Professor of Pediatrics and Microbiology, School of Medicine, University of Alabama in Birmingham, Birmingham

GRANT R. WILKINSON, M.D.
Professor of Pharmacology, Vanderbilt University School of Medicine, Nashville

GORDON H. WILLIAMS, M.D.
Professor of Medicine, Harvard Medical School; Chief, Endocrinology-Hypertension Division, Brigham and Women's Hospital, Boston

JEAN D. WILSON, M.D.
Professor of Internal Medicine, The University of Texas Health Science Center, Dallas

SHELDON M. WOLFF, M.D.
Endicott Professor and Chairman, Department of Medicine, Tufts University School of Medicine; Physician-in-Chief, New England Medical Center, Boston

ALASTAIR J. J. WOOD, M.D., M.B., Ch.B., M.R.C.P.
Associate Professor of Medicine and Associate Professor of Pharmacology, Vanderbilt University School of Medicine; Attending Physician, Vanderbilt University Hospital, Nashville

THEODORE E. WOODWARD, B.S., M.D., D.Sc. (Hon.)
Professor of Medicine Emeritus, University of Maryland School of Medicine; Distinguished Physician; Veterans Administration Hospital, Baltimore

SHIRLEY H. WRAY, M.D., Ph.D., F.R.C.P.
Associate Professor of Neurology, Harvard Medical School; Director, Unit for Neurovisual Disorders, Department of Neurology, Massachusetts General Hospital, Boston

JOSHUA WYNNE, M.D.
Professor of Internal Medicine and Chief, Division of Cardiology, Wayne State University School of Medicine; Chief, Section of Cardiology, Harper-Grace Hospitals, Detroit

JAMES B. YOUNG, M.D.
Professor of Medicine, Harvard Medical School; Associate Physician, Beth Israel Hospital, Boston

ROBERT R. YOUNG, M.D.
Professor of Neurology, Harvard Medical School; Neurologist and Director, Clinical Neurophysiology Laboratory, Massachusetts General Hospital, Boston

PREFACE

In this, the eleventh edition of *Harrison's Principles of Internal Medicine*, the editors have attempted to incorporate the latest advances in the biology, pathophysiology, diagnosis, and treatment of disease. The objective has been to provide appropriate bridges between the basic sciences and clinical medicine and to emphasize those advances in biomedical research which are of clinical importance, while retaining those facts which, while not new, remain clinically useful.

In adherence to the principles of those who founded the book, Part One, "Cardinal Manifestations of Disease," remains a mainstay of this edition. Its 54 chapters form a comprehensive introduction to clinical medicine with an emphasis on the pathophysiology of disease and the mechanisms of symptoms. The chapters in Part Two, "Biologic Considerations in the Approach to Clinical Medicine," focus on disorders which usually affect multiple organ systems, including genetic diseases, immune disturbances, disorders of nutrition, neoplasia, and geriatric medicine. In this section the interface between the "new biology" and clinical medicine receives major emphasis. These multisystem disorders are then followed, in Part Three, by a predominantly etiologically oriented section on infections, while the diseases of the major organ systems are discussed in the remaining ten parts of the book.

The eleventh edition also pays close attention to updated and current references. Although space constraints require that references be kept to a modest number, the editors have made particular efforts to include papers that were published in 1984, 1985, and even 1986. Although this has required omission of some important older papers, these almost always appear in the bibliographies of the newer ones. The reverse is, of course, not the case and hence our effort to keep the references up-to-date.

Cognizant of the current requirements for continuing education for licensure and relicensure, as well as the emphasis on certification and recertification, a revision of the *PreTest Self-Assessment and Review* appears in conjunction with this edition. *PreTest Self-Assessment and Review* consists of several hundred questions based upon the textbook, along with answers and explanations for the answers.

The rapid developments in clinical medicine and in the basic sciences on which it rests have mandated more extensive changes in the preparation of this edition of *Harrison's* than of any other edition.

Although we cannot highlight in this short preface all of the new and extensively updated parts of the eleventh edition, we would like to call the reader's attention to several of these:

• A new chapter attempts to demonstrate how rigorous quantitative methods may be applied in clinical reasoning and decision making.

• The genetics section has been reorganized and expanded to emphasize the relevance of molecular genetics to medicine in general and of oncogenes to the understanding of neoplasia.

• The endocrinology and metabolism section contains new comprehensive chapters on neuroendocrine and anterior pituitary disease, on disorders of growth, and on hereditable disorders of connective tissue. The chapter on diabetes mellitus has been extensively revised to take into account advances in the nosology and etiology of the disease. The section on disorders of bone and mineral metabolism has been extensively revised and contains a new chapter on hypercalcemic and hypocalcemic disorders.

• The autonomic nervous system is recognized to play a key role in many disease states, and drugs which affect this system are of increasing importance in many areas of clinical medicine. The normal and abnormal physiology and the pharmacology of this system are discussed in an expanded chapter.

• In the area of infectious diseases, more than a third of the chapters are new. Among these, the following are of particular importance: The chapter on *infections in the compromised host* has been completely revised and includes the most current understanding

of the mechanisms of host defenses and their relationship to protection from infectious disease. The significance of *skin rashes* in infections is covered both in the text and in the expanded color atlas. There is an extensive update on *antibiotics,* including agents that are still under investigation, but are likely to become available in the near future; there is a new chapter on *antiviral chemotherapy.* In view of the growing importance of *sexually transmitted diseases,* there is considerable expansion of these chapters. The section on *virology* has been entirely revamped, with particular emphasis on the molecular biology of viral diseases. The chapters on cytomegalovirus infection and Epstein-Barr virus infection include the most current understanding of the relationship of these infections to modulation of the immune system. The chapter on *Pneumocystis carinii pneumonia* has been revised, particularly with regard to the newly appreciated importance of this infection in patients with AIDS. New chapters on *schistosomiasis* and such new parasitic pathogens as *cryptosporidiosis* have been added. An extensive and up-to-date description of Lyme arthritis is provided.

• The major advances in cardiology that are emphasized in new or radically revised chapters include noninvasive methods of cardiac examination, electrophysiologic approaches to the diagnosis and treatment of cardiac arrhythmias, percutaneous transluminal angioplasty, and thrombolytic treatment of acute myocardial infarction.

• There has been considerable progress in understanding the pathogenesis and management of cystic fibrosis, hypersensitivity pneumonitis, and interstitial lung disease. The section on respiratory disease includes new chapters on these important disorders.

• Major revisions have been made in the gastrointestinal section with special emphasis on gastrointestinal endoscopy. New color plates of the appropriate endoscopic findings of various gastrointestinal disorders are included.

• The entire section on liver diseases has undergone major revision with a totally new chapter on viral as well as on drug-induced hepatitis, including the approach to the diagnosis of non-A, non-B hepatitis and the delta agent. Similarly, the important area of cirrhosis has also been revised. There is a new chapter on liver transplantation.

• The sections on disorders of the immune system and disorders of immune-mediated injury have been rewritten almost completely. These chapters now represent the most updated understanding of the relationship between aberrancies of immune function and immune-mediated diseases. Of particular note is the chapter on the acquired immunodeficiency syndrome which provides an in-depth understanding of all aspects of this syndrome. Also of note in this section is the much expanded chapter on the vasculitic syndromes. This chapter provides a coherent organization of these complex diseases and a better understanding of pathogenesis as well as the most modern approaches toward therapy.

• In the section on hematology there are new chapters on the anemias due to bone marrow failure and bone marrow transplantation. The chapters on platelets and blood coagulation are completely new with a new author for this important section. The chapter on enlargement of lymph nodes and spleen has been expanded to include a detailed description of the multiple mechanisms of lymph node and spleen enlargement, while the chapter on disorders of the phagocytic cells includes the most updated understanding of the metabolism of functional capabilities of phagocytic cells.

• The rapid advances in oncology are reflected in new chapters on the basic principles of neoplasia, carcinoma of the ovary and testis, the endocrine manifestations of neoplasia, and neurologic manifestations of neoplastic disorders. The chapter on the human T-lymphotropic virus is a comprehensive and authoritative treatise on the role of these important retroviruses in human diseases, an observation which has only recently been made and which has important potential implications in understanding the role of viruses in neoplastic as well as nonneoplastic diseases. The new chapter on the leukemias includes the modern classification of these important disorders.

● The neurology section, long a key component of *Harrison's*, has undergone substantial change. There are new chapters on acute and chronic pain, on dizziness and vertigo, ataxia and disorders of equilibrium and gait, the peripheral neuropathies, cerebrovascular diseases, and brain trauma. A radically revised chapter on the degenerative diseases of the nervous system with particular focus on Alzheimer's disease and Parkinson's disease brings the latest information about the neurochemistry, neuropathology, and management of these important disorders.

● The entire section on psychiatry has been rewritten and represents a major addition to this edition.

One of the strengths of *Harrison's* has been the close-knit relationships among the editors. Dr. Joseph Martin, the Julieanne Dorn Professor of Neurology at Harvard Medical School and Chief of the Neurological Services of the Massachusetts General Hospital, worked together with his distinguished predecessor, Dr. Raymond D. Adams on the tenth edition. With the latter's retirement from the textbook, Dr. Martin assumed sole editorial responsibility for the sections on neurology, myology, and psychiatry in the eleventh edition. He has been an important addition to the editorial group.

The editors warmly welcome Dr. Anthony S. Fauci, Director of the National Institute of Allergy and Infectious Diseases and Chief of its Laboratory of Immunoregulation, to *Harrison's*. Dr. Fauci is one of the leading clinical immunologists in the world. He has made a profound contribution to this edition with his expertise in this critically important area of biology and his ability to describe its impact on many areas of internal medicine.

We also wish to express our appreciation to our many associates and colleagues who, as experts in their fields, have helped us with constructive and valuable criticisms of the chapters in the eleventh edition. We wish to thank the following for many helpful suggestions: Drs. Stuart Aaronson, Raymond D. Adams, John W. Adamson, John F. Alksne, Ronald J. Anderson, Elliott M. Antman, Gust H. Bardy, Robert C. Bast, John E. Bennett, David Bilheimer, Harry G. Bluestein, Neil Breslau, Oscar L. Bronsther, Michael S. Brown, Robert H. Brown, George P. Canellos, Antonino Catanzaro, Bayard D. Catherwood, Bruce A. Chabner, Robert M. Chanock, Harold A. Chapman, Thomas N. Chase, William W. Chin, Mario Chojkier, Charles G. Cochrane, David I. Cohen, Steven E. Come, Rex William Cowdry, Clyde S. Crumpacker, Gilbert H. Daniels, Charles E. Davis, David M. Dawson, Leonard J. Deftos, Thomas L. Delbanco, Robert O. Dillman, Robert G. Dluhy, William P. Docken, Jeffrey M. Drazen, David M. Eddy, Leonard Ellman, Arthur S. Elstein, Darrell D. Fanestil, Alvan R. Feinstein, Mark Feldman, Joshua Fierer, Brian

G. Firth, Daniel W. Foster, Fred H. Frankel, Lawrence S. Friedman, Paul A. Friedman, Peter Friedman, Theodore Friedmann, Gary R. Fujimoto, Harris H. Funkenstein, Ary L. Goldberger, Joseph L. Goldstein, John L. Gollan, Harvey H. Gralnick, Mark R. Green, James E. Griffin, Robert C. Griggs, Richard H. Haas, Ivan R. Harwood, Fred Hendler, Martin S. Hirsch, Stephen B. Howell, Gary W. Hunninghake, Jon I. Isenberg, Stephen P. James, Kenneth Lee Jones, Lewis L. Judd, Albert Z. Kapikian, Dennis L. Kasper, Barrett Katz, Robert Katzman, Robert S. Kauffman, Martin J. Kelly, Anthony L. Komaroff, Conrad V. Kufta, Randi Y. Leavitt, Mark Leshin, Ronald Levy, Matthew H. Liang, Markku Linnoila, John D. Loeser, Kenneth Luskey, Paula Macrae, John A. Mannick, Lawrence F. Marshall, Henry Masur, J. Allen McCutchan, Henry F. McFarland, Dale E. McFarlin, George R. Merriam, Edgar L. Milford, Brian R. Murphy, James R. Nelson, Anne Nicholson-Weller, Michael R. Oxman, Charles Y. C. Pak, Alan G. Palestine, Sebastian Palmeri, Alfred F. Parisi, Joseph E. Parillo, Stephen G. Pauker, Alan S. Pearlman, James E. Pennington, Candace B. Pert, Marion Peters, Kirk L. Peterson, Willy F. Piessens, Richard Platt, Robert M. Post, William Z. Potter, Joe W. Ramsdell, Samuel I. Rapaport, Peter Reich, Michael Ronthal, Richard K. Root, Allan H. Ropper, Saul W. Rosen, David S. Rosenthal, John F. Rothrock, Daniel Rotrosen, John W. Rowe, John D. Rutherford, John E. Salvaggio, Martin A. Samuels, Stephen Scharfstein, Joseph D. Schmidt, Brian Schmitt, Edward L. Schneider, Lowell E. Schnipper, Peter H. Schur, John D. Schwankhaus, William J. Schwartz, Dennis J. Selkoe, Larry J. Shapiro, Clifford W. Shults, Cecelia M. Smith, Stephen A. Spector, Frank E. Speizer, Stephen E. Straus, Michael R. Swenson, Raymond Taetle, Ira B. Tager, Michael D. Tharp, David E. Trentham, Jerry S. Trier, H. Richard Tyler, Athol J. Ware, Steven E. Weinberger, Michael E. Weinblatt, Michael H. Weisman, Peter F. Weller, Alison Wichman, Robert F. Wilkens, Shirley H. Wray, Neal S. Young, Randall K. Young, Robert C. Young, Robert R. Young, and Elizabeth J. Ziegler.

This book could not have been edited without the dedicated help of our coworkers in the editorial offices of the individual editors. We are especially indebted to Patricia A. Clougherty, Patricia E. DeLosh, Lourdes C. Felix, Hilda Gardner, Brenda Hennis, Mary Jackson, Ann C. London, Lucy Renzi, Darlene Reynolds, Janice Stearns, and Michéle M. Stewart.

Finally, we need to say a word of thanks to our colleagues at McGraw-Hill, Dereck Jeffers, Executive Editor, and Eileen Scott, Development Editor. They formed a most effective team who gave the editors constant encouragement, and were of enormous help in the countless efforts involved in bringing this complex effort to fruition.

THE EDITORS

Harrison's
PRINCIPLES
OF INTERNAL
MEDICINE

Harrison's
PRINCIPLES OF INTERNAL MEDICINE

Eleventh Edition

VOLUME 1

**PART ONE
THROUGH
PART FOUR**

1 THE PRACTICE OF MEDICINE

THE EDITORS

WHAT IS EXPECTED OF THE PHYSICIAN The practice of medicine combines both science and art. The role of science in medicine is clear. Technology based on science is the foundation for the solution to many clinical problems; the dazzling advances in biochemical methodology and in biophysical imaging techniques that allow access to the remotest recesses of the body are the products of science. So too are the therapeutic maneuvers which increasingly are a major part of medical practice. Yet skill in the most sophisticated application of laboratory technology or the use of the latest therapeutic modality alone does not make a good physician. The ability to extract from a mass of contradictory physical signs and from the crowded computer printouts of laboratory data those items that are of crucial significance, to know in a difficult case whether to "treat" or to "watch," to determine when a clinical clue is worth pursuing or when to dismiss it as a "red herring," and to estimate in any given patient whether a proposed treatment entails a greater risk than the disease are all involved in the decisions which the clinician, skilled in the practice of medicine, must make many times each day. This combination of medical knowledge, intuition, and judgment is termed the *art of medicine*. It is as necessary to the practice of medicine as a sound scientific base.

However much the knowledge base of medicine has expanded and will continue to expand, the fundamental commitment of the physician to the care of the patient remains unaltered. The editors of the first edition of *Harrison's Principles of Internal Medicine* put it so eloquently that their words bear repeating:

Tact, sympathy and understanding are expected of the physician, for the patient is no mere collection of symptoms, signs, disordered functions, damaged organs, and disturbed emotions. He is human, fearful, and hopeful, seeking relief, help and reassurance. To the physician, as to the anthropologist, nothing human is strange or repulsive. The misanthrope may become a smart diagnostician of organic disease, but he can scarcely hope to succeed as a physician. The true physician has a Shakespearean breadth of interest in the wise and the foolish, the proud and the humble, the stoic hero and the whining rogue. He cares for people.

THE PATIENT-PHYSICIAN RELATIONSHIP It may be trite to emphasize that physicians need to approach patients not as "cases" or "diseases" but as individuals whose problems all too often transcend the complaints which bring them to the doctor. Most patients are anxious and frightened. Often they go to great ends to convince themselves that illness does not exist, or unconsciously they set up elaborate defenses to divert attention from the real problem that they perceive to be serious or life-threatening. Some patients use illness to gain attention or to serve as a crutch to extricate themselves from an emotionally stressful situation; some even feign physical illness. Whatever the patient's attitude, the physician needs to consider the terrain in which an illness occurs—in terms not only of the patients themselves but also of their families and social backgrounds. All too often medical workups and records fail to include essential information

about the patient's origins, schooling, job, home and family, hopes and fears. Without this knowledge it is difficult for the physician to gain rapport with the patient or to develop insight into the patient's illness. Such a relationship must be based on thorough knowledge of the patient and on mutual trust and the ability to communicate with one another.

The direct, one-to-one patient-physician relationship which traditionally has characterized the practice of medicine is changing, primarily because of the changing setting in which medicine is being practiced. Often the management of the individual patient requires the active participation of a variety of trained professional personnel as well as several physicians. In most instances, health care is a team effort. The patient can benefit greatly from such collaboration, but it is the duty of the primary physician to guide the patient through an illness. To carry out this increasingly difficult task, this physician must have some familiarity with the techniques, skills, and objectives of specialist physicians as well as colleagues in the fields allied to medicine. In giving the patient an opportunity to receive all the benefits of the important advances of science, the primary physician must, in the last analysis, retain responsibility for the major decisions concerning diagnosis and treatment.

Increasingly, patients are being cared for by groups of physicians, clinics, hospitals, and health-maintenance organizations (HMOs) rather than by individual independent practitioners. There are many potential advantages in the use of such organized medical groups, but there are also potential drawbacks, the chief of which is a loss of identity of the physician who is primarily and continuously responsible for the patient. It is essential, even in the group setting, that each patient have a physician who has an overview of the patient's problems and who maintains familiarity with the patient's reaction to his or her illness, to the drugs given, and to the challenges of daily living. Moreover, because a number of physicians may, at any one time, contribute to the care of a particular patient, accurate and detailed medical records are essential to good patient care.

In the United States in particular, but to a progressively greater extent throughout the world, the modern hospital poses a particularly intimidating environment for most patients. Lying in a bed surrounded by air jets, buttons, and lights; invaded by tubes and wires; beset by the numerous members of the health care team—nurses, nurses' aides, physicians' assistants, social workers, technologists, physical therapists, medical students, house officers, attending and consulting physicians, and many others; transported to special laboratories and x-ray chambers replete with machines with blinking lights and strange sounds, it is little wonder that patients lose their sense of reality. In fact, the patient's physician is often the only tenuous link between the patient and the real world. A strong personal relationship with the physician is essential in order to sustain the patient in such a stressful situation.

Many influences in contemporary society have the potential of leading to the impersonalization of medical care. Some of these have been mentioned already and include (1) vigorous efforts to reduce the escalating costs of health care; (2) the increasing reliance on technologic advances and computerization for many aspects of diagnosis and treatment; (3) the increased geographic mobility of both patients and physicians; (4) the growing number of "closed-system" arrangements, such as health maintenance organizations, in which the patient has little if any choice in selecting a physician; (5) the need for more than a single physician to be involved in the care of most patients who are seriously ill; and (6) an increasing reliance by patients on legal means to express their disappointments with the health care system (i.e., by malpractice litigation). Given these changes in the medical care system, maintaining the humanistic aspects of medical care and the humanistic qualities of the physician is a particular challenge. It is now more important than ever that the physician consider each patient to be a unique individual deserving of humane treatment, regardless of personal or financial circumstances.

The American Board of Internal Medicine has defined humanistic qualities as encompassing integrity, respect, and compassion. Availability, the expression of sincere concern, the willingness to take the time to explain all aspects of the patient's illness, and an attitude of being nonjudgmental with patients who have lifestyles, attitudes, and values which are different from the physician's own and which he or she may in some instances even find repugnant are just a few of the characteristics of the humane physician. Every physician will, at times, be challenged by patients who evoke strongly negative (and occasionally strongly positive) emotional responses. Physicians should be alert to their own reactions to such patients and situations and consciously monitor and control their behavior so that the patients' best interests remain the principal motivation for their actions at all times.

The famous statement of Dr. Francis Peabody is even more relevant today than when delivered more than a half century ago:

The significance of the intimate personal relationship between physician and patient cannot be too strongly emphasized, for in an extraordinarily large number of cases both the diagnosis and treatment are directly dependent on it. One of the essential qualities of the clinician is interest in humanity, for the secret of the care of the patient is in caring for the patient.

CLINICAL SKILLS   History taking   The written history of an illness should embody all the facts of medical significance in the life of the patient. If the history is recorded in chronologic order, recent events should be given the most attention. Likewise, if a problem-oriented approach is used, the problems that are clinically dominant should be listed first. Ideally, the narration of symptoms or problems should be in the patient's own words. However, few patients have sufficient powers of observation or recall to give a history without some guidance from the physician, who must be careful not to suggest the answers to the questions being posed. Often a symptom which has concerned a patient has little significance, while a seemingly minor complaint may be of considerable importance. Therefore, the physician must be constantly alert to the possibility that any event related by the patient, however trivial or apparently remote, may be the key to the solution of the medical problem.

An informative history is more than an orderly listing of symptoms. Something is always gained by listening to patients and noting the way in which they talk about their symptoms. Inflections of voice, facial expression, and attitude may betray important clues to the meaning of the symptoms to the patient. In listening to the history, the physician discovers not only something about the disease but also something about the patient.

With experience, the pitfalls of history taking become apparent. What patients relate for the most part consists of subjective phenomena colored by past experience. Patients obviously differ widely in their responses to the same stimuli and in their coping mechanisms. Their attitudes are variably influenced by fear of disability and death and by concern over the consequences of their illness to their families. Sometimes the accuracy of the history is affected by language or sociologic barriers, by failing intellectual powers which interfere with recall, or by disorders of consciousness that make them unaware of their illness. It is not surprising, then, that even the most careful physician may at times despair of collecting factual data and be forced to proceed with evidence that represents little more than an approximation of the truth. It is in obtaining the history that the

physician's skill, knowledge, and experience are most clearly in evidence.

The family history serves several functions. First, in rare single-gene defects a positive family history of a similarly affected individual or a history of consanguinity may have important diagnostic implications. Second, in diseases of multifactorial etiology that have a familial aggregation, it may be possible to identify patients at risk for disease and to intervene prior to development of overt manifestations. For example, recent weight gain is a more ominous development in a woman who has a family history of diabetes than in one who does not. In certain situations the family history has major implications for preventive medicine. When a diagnosis of a hereditary condition known to predispose to cancer is made, it is the physician's obligation to follow up this possibility carefully in the patient, to survey the family, and to educate them about the need for long-term follow-up.

However accurate and complete, the medical history does much more than provide facts of critical importance. The very act of taking the history provides the physician with the opportunity to establish or enhance the unique bond that is the basis for the critically important patient-physician relationship. An effort should be made to place the patient at ease, regardless of the circumstances of the encounter. The patient should, at some point, have the opportunity to tell his or her own story of the illness without frequent interruption and, when appropriate, should receive expression of interest, encouragement, and empathy from the physician. It is often enlightening to develop an appreciation of the patient's own perception of the illness and the patient's expectations of the physician and the medical care system. The patient's financial status, at least as it relates to the ability to pay for the costs of care, should also be discussed. The confidentiality of the patient-physician relationship should be emphasized, and the patient should be given the opportunity to identify those aspects of the history which he or she wishes not to be disclosed to anyone else.

Physical examination   Physical signs are the objective and verifiable marks of disease and represent solid, indisputable facts. Their significance is enhanced when they confirm a functional or structural change already suggested by the patient's history. At times, the physical signs may be the only evidence of disease, especially when the history has been inconsistent, confused, or lacking altogether.

The physical examination should be performed methodically and thoroughly, with due regard for the patient's comfort and modesty. Although attention has often been directed by the history to the diseased organ or part of the body, the examination must extend from head to toe in an objective search for abnormalities. Unless the examination procedure is systematic, important parts of it may be omitted, an error which is common even among the most skilled clinicians. The results of the examination, like the details of the history, should be recorded at the time they are elicited, not hours later when they are subject to the distortions of memory. Many inaccuracies stem from the careless practice of writing or dictating notes long after the examination has been concluded. Skill in physical diagnosis is acquired with experience, but it is not merely technique that determines success in eliciting signs. The detection of a few scattered petechiae, a faint diastolic murmur, or a small mass in the abdomen is not a question of keener eyes and ears or more sensitive fingers but of a mind prepared to be alert to these findings. Skill in physical diagnosis reflects a way of thinking more than a way of doing. Physical findings are subject to change. Just because the examination is normal on one occasion does not guarantee that this will be the case on subsequent examinations. It is important, therefore, to repeat pertinent parts of the physical examination as long as the clinical situation warrants.

Laboratory tests   The marked increase in the number and availability of laboratory tests has inevitably resulted in increasing reliance being placed on knowledge gained from these studies in the solution of clinical problems. It is essential, however, to bear in mind the limitations of such procedures, which by virtue of their impersonal quality and complexity often gain an aura of authority regardless of the fallibility of the tests themselves, of the individuals doing or interpreting them, or of their instruments. More importantly, the accumulation of laboratory data cannot relieve the physician from the responsibility of careful observation and study of the patient. Physicians also must weigh carefully the hazards and the expense involved in the laboratory procedures they order. Moreover, laboratory tests are rarely ordered and reported singly. Rather, they are produced as "batteries." Some laboratories now perform batteries of 24 and even 40 tests. The various combinations of laboratory tests are often useful. For example, they may provide the clue to such nonspecific symptoms as generalized weakness and increased fatigability by revealing abnormalities of hepatic function together with elevated levels of serum IgG which, in turn, would suggest the diagnosis of chronic liver disease. Sometimes a single abnormality, such as an elevated serum calcium, points to a specific disease, such as hyperparathyroidism.

The thoughtful use of screening tests should not be confused with indiscriminate laboratory testing. The use of screening tests is based on the fact that a group of laboratory determinations can be carried out conveniently on a single specimen of blood at relatively low cost. Biochemical measurements, together with simple laboratory examinations such as blood count, urinalysis, and sedimentation rate, often provide the major clue to the presence of a pathologic process. At the same time the physican must learn to evaluate occasional abnormalities among the screening tests that may not necessarily connote significant disease. There is nothing more wasteful and unproductive than an in-depth workup following a report of an isolated laboratory abnormality in a patient who is otherwise well. Among the more than 40 tests that are performed on many patients, one is often slightly abnormal. If there is no clinical suspicion of an underlying illness, the test is ordinarily repeated to ensure that the abnormality does not represent a laboratory error. If the abnormality is confirmed it is important to distinguish a minor one (less than two standard deviations) from a major one (more than two standard deviations). Even in the case of the latter, the decision of whether to proceed with further workup is a test of the physician's clinical judgment.

Newer imaging techniques The last decade and a half have seen the arrival of ultrasonography, a variety of isotopic scans that employ new isotopes to visualize organs heretofore inaccessible, computerized tomography with its varying permutations, and magnetic resonance imaging. Aside from opening up new diagnostic vistas, this new, highly sophisticated technology benefits patients because it has frequently supplanted invasive techniques which require surgical biopsy or the insertion of tubes, wires, or catheters into the body—procedures which are often painful and sometimes risky. While the enthusiasm for noninvasive technology is understandably justified, all too often the results have not been validated properly before they are disseminated as clinical dogma. Moreover, the expense entailed in performing these imaging tests is often substantial and is not always considered when ordering them. There is no question that a tool like computerized tomography has led to a reassessment of the problem of adrenal tumors, just as routine measurement of calcium caused a redefinition of hyperparathyroidism. The principles being espoused here are simply to use these examinations judiciously, preferably in lieu of, not in addition to, the invasive maneuvers they are meant to replace.

THE DIAGNOSIS OF DISEASE Accurate diagnosis requires, first of all, the collection of accurate data. But much more is required in making a diagnosis. Each item of data must be interpreted in the light of what is known about the structure and function of the involved organ(s). Knowledge of anatomy, physiology, and biochemistry must be combined into a plausible pathophysiologic mechanism.

Clinical diagnosis requires both aspects of logic—analysis and synthesis—and the more difficult the clinical problem, the more important is a logical approach to it. Such an approach requires that the physician list carefully each problem suggested by the patient's symptoms and physical and laboratory findings and seek answers to each. Most physicians attempt consciously or unconsciously to fit a given problem into one of a series of syndromes. *The syndrome is a group of symptoms and signs of disordered function, related to one another by means of some anatomic, physiologic, or biochemical peculiarity*. It embodies a hypothesis concerning the deranged function of an organ, organ system, or tissue. Congestive heart failure, Cushing's syndrome, and dementia are examples. In congestive heart failure dyspnea, orthopnea, cyanosis, dependent edema, engorged neck veins, pleural effusion, rales, and hepatomegaly are known to be connected by a single pathophysiologic mechanism—insufficiency of the cardiac pump mechanism. In Cushing's syndrome the moon facies, hypertension, diabetes, and osteoporosis are the recognized effects of excess glucocorticoids acting on many target organs. In dementia, deterioration of memory, incoherent thinking, impaired language functions, visual-spatial disorientation, and faulty judgment are related to destruction of the association areas of the cerebrum.

A syndrome usually does not identify the precise cause of an illness, but it greatly narrows the number of possibilities and often suggests certain special clinical and laboratory studies. The derangements of each organ system in humans are reducible to a relatively small number of syndromes. The diagnosis is simplified greatly if a clinical problem conforms neatly to a well-defined syndrome, because only a few diseases need to be considered in the differential diagnosis. In contrast, the search for the cause of an illness that does not conform to a syndrome is more difficult because a much greater number of diseases have to be sought. Even here an orderly approach which proceeds from symptom to sign to laboratory findings will result in the diagnosis most of the time.

CARING FOR THE PATIENT The care of the patient begins with the development of a personal relationship between the patient and the physician. In the absence of a sense of trust and confidence on the part of the patient, the effectiveness of most therapeutic measures is diminished. In many instances, when there is confidence in the physician, reassurance is the best treatment and is all that is needed. Likewise, in those cases which do not lend themselves to easy solutions or for which no effective treatment is available, a feeling on the part of the patient that the physician is doing all that is possible is one of the most important therapeutic measures that can be provided. An important aspect of clinical decision making and patient care involves the "quality of life," a subjective assessment of what each patient values most. Such an assessment requires detailed, sometimes intimate knowledge of the patient, which can usually be obtained only through deliberate, unhurried, and often repeated conversation. In situations where complete freedom from signs and symptoms of disease is impossible, maximization of the quality of life becomes the major goal of therapy.

Drug therapy With each succeeding year, more drugs are released, every one with the hope and the promise that it is an improvement over its predecessor. Although the pharmaceutical industry must be given most of the credit for advances in drug therapy, it is also true that many new drugs have only a marginal advantage over the agents they are aimed to replace. The barrage of new information with which practitioners are deluged does little to provide a clear picture of clinical pharmacology; on the contrary, to most physicians new drugs are confusing. With some exceptions, however, the approach to a new drug should be one of caution. Unless the new agent is established beyond doubt to be a real advance, it is wiser to use well-tested and well-established agents which are not only efficacious but whose safety has been well-established.

Iatrogenic disorders An iatrogenic disorder occurs when the deleterious effects of a procedure or drug produce pathology independent of the condition for which the drug is given. No matter what the clinical situation, it is the responsibility of the physician to use new and powerful therapeutic measures wisely, with due regard to their action, potential dangers, and cost. Every medical procedure, whether diagnostic or therapeutic, has the potential for harm, but it would be impossible to afford the patient all the benefits of modern scientific medicine if reasonable steps in diagnosis and therapy were withheld because of possible risks. "Reasonable" implies that the physician has weighed the pros and cons of a procedure and has concluded on rational grounds that it is advisable or essential for the relief of discomfort or the cure or amelioration of disease. For example, the use of glucocorticoids to arrest progressive disseminated lupus erythematosus may produce Cushing's syndrome. In this instance, the benefits usually exceed the untoward side effects. However, much harm can result when the deleterious effects of a procedure or a drug exceed any possible advantages that might have been anticipated. Examples include the dangerous or fatal drug reactions that occasionally follow the use of antibiotics given for trivial respiratory infections, the gastric hemorrhage or perforation caused by glucocorticoid administration for mild arthritis, or the occurrence of fatal hepatitis that may follow needless transfusions of blood or plasma.

But the harm that a physician can do to a patient is not limited to the imprudent use of medication. Equally important are ill-considered or unjustified remarks. Many a patient has developed a cardiac neurosis because the physician ventured a grave prognosis on the basis of a misinterpreted electrocardiogram. Not only the treatment itself but the physician's words and behavior are capable of causing injury.

The physician must never become so absorbed in the disease as to forget the patient who is its victim. As the science of medicine advances, it is all too easy to become so fascinated by the manifestations of disease that the ailing person's fears and concerns about job and family, the cost of medical care, and the specter of economic insecurity are disregarded. Treatment of a patient consists of more than the dispassionate confrontation of a disease. It embodies also the exercise of warmth, compassion, and understanding.

Informed consent   In an era of rapidly advancing technology, patients will require diagnostic and therapeutic procedures that are painful and that pose some risk. These include all surgical procedures, e.g., biopsies of tissues, radiographic maneuvers involving the insertion of catheters, endoscopy, and many others. In most American hospitals and clinics, patients undergoing such procedures are required to sign a form consenting to them. More important, however, is the notion that the patient must understand clearly the risk entailed in these procedures; this is the definition of *informed consent*. It is incumbent upon the physician to explain to the patient, in a clearly understandable fashion, the procedures which he or she faces. By doing this conscientiously much of the dread of the unknown that is inherent in hospitalization will be mitigated.

Accountability   Throughout the world physicians, once licensed to practice medicine, have not had to account for their actions except to their peers. In the United States, however, during the past decade and a half, there have been increasing demands for physicians to account for the way in which they practice medicine by meeting certain standards prescribed by federal and state governments. Hospitalized patients whose health care is reimbursed by the government (Medicare and Medicaid) and other third parties have been subjected to utilization review. This means that the physician must defend the cause for and duration of a patient's hospitalization if it falls outside certain "average" standards. In some instances a second opinion is necessary before a patient can be admitted to the hospital for elective surgery. The purpose of these regulations is to contain spiraling health care costs. It is likely that this type of review will be extended to all phases of medical practice and will inevitably alter the practice of medicine.

Physicians also may be expected to give account of their continuing competence by mandatory continuing education, patient record audit,

recertification by examination, or relicensure. While these measures probably enhance the physician's factual knowledge, there is no evidence that they have a similar effect on the quality of practice.

Cost-effectiveness in medical care   As the cost of medical care continues to rise, it has become necessary to establish stringent priorities in the expenditure of health care dollars. In some instances, preventive measures offer the greatest return per dollar; outstanding examples include vaccination, immunization, reduction in accidents and occupational hazards, and improved environmental control. The cost of "newborn screening" for metabolic diseases is being evaluated. For example, the detection of phenylketonuria by screening of large populations may result in a net saving of many thousands of dollars.

As resources become more and more constrained, it will be necessary to weigh the justifiability of performing prohibitively costly operations that provide only a limited life expectancy against the pressing need for more primary care for those persons who do not have adequate access to medical services. At the level of the individual patient it is important to minimize costly hospital admissions as far as possible, if total health care is to be provided at an expense which most can afford. This, of course, implies and depends upon a close cooperative effort between patients, their physicians, their employers, third-party carriers, and government, along with constant surveillance of those types of procedures which can be conducted safely and effectively on an ambulatory basis. Equally important in reducing total health care expenditures is the need for individual physicians to monitor carefully both the cost and effectiveness of the drugs they prescribe. In the last analysis the medical profession should provide leadership and guidance to the public in matters of cost control, and the medical profession must take this responsibility seriously without being or seeming to be self-serving. It is important, however, that these significant socioeconomic aspects of health care delivery not be permitted to interfere with the concern of physicians for the welfare of their patients. The patient must be able to rely on the individual physician as his or her principal advocate in matters of health care.

Research and teaching   The title "doctor" is derived from the Latin *docere*, "to teach," and the physician should share information and medical knowledge with others and be willing to teach what he or she has learned to colleagues as well as to students of medicine and related professions. The practice of medicine is dependent on the sum total of medical knowledge, which in turn is based on an unending chain of scientific discovery, clinical observation, analysis, and interpretation. Advances in medicine depend on the acquisition of new information, i.e., on research, which must often involve patients; improved medical care requires the transmission of this information. As part of broader societal responsibilities, the physician should encourage patients to participate in ethical and properly approved clinical investigations if they do not impose undue hazard, discomfort, or inconvenience.

Incurability and death   No problem is more distressing than that presented by the patient with an incurable disease, particularly when premature death is inevitable. What should the patient and family be told, what measures should be taken to maintain life, and how is death to be defined?

Although some would argue otherwise, there is no ironclad rule that the patient must be told "everything," even if the patient is an adult and the head of a family. How much the patient is told should depend upon the patient's ability and capacity to deal with the possibility of imminent death; often this capacity grows with time and, whenever possible, gradual rather than abrupt disclosure is the best strategy. This decision may also take into consideration the patient's religious beliefs, financial and business affairs, and to some extent the wishes of the family. The patient must be given an opportunity to talk with the physician and ask questions. Patients may find it easier to share their feelings about death with their physician, who is likely to be more objective and less emotional than family members.

One thing is certain; it is not for you to don the black cap and, assuming the judicial function, take hope away from any patient . . . hope that comes to us all.

William Osler

Even when the patient directly inquires, "Doctor, am I dying?" the physician must attempt to determine whether this is a request for information, a demand for reassurance, or even an expression of hostility. Most would agree that only open communication between the patient and the physician can resolve these questions and guide the physician in what to say and how to say it.

The physician should provide or arrange for emotional, physical, and spiritual support, and must be compassionate, unhurried, and open. Pain should be adequately controlled, human dignity maintained, and isolation from family avoided. The last two in particular tend to be overlooked in hospitals, where the intrusion of life-sustaining apparatus can so easily detract from attention to the whole person and concentrate instead on the life-threatening disease. The physician must also prepare to deal with guilt feelings on the part of the family when a member becomes gravely or hopelessly ill. It is important for the doctor to reassure the family that everything possible has been done.

The President's Committee for the Study of Ethical Problems in Medicine defined death as (1) irreversible cessation of circulatory and respiratory function, or (2) irreversible cessation of all functions of the entire brain, including the brain stem. Clinical and electroencephalographic criteria are at hand which permit the reliable diagnosis of cerebral death. According to the criteria adopted by the staff of the Massachusetts General Hospital and the Harvard Committee on Brain Death, death occurs when all signs of receptivity and responsivity are absent, including all brainstem reflexes (pupillary reactions, ocular movement, blinking, swallowing, breathing), and the electroencephalogram is isoelectric. Occasionally, intoxications and metabolic disorders may simulate this state; hence the diagnosis requires expert evaluation. Under the aforementioned circumstances, to continue with heroic, highly costly supportive measures merely for the purpose of preserving cardiac function is against the best interests of patient, family, and society. In such instances, the dilemma of continuing care could be avoided if the medical profession, in accord with social sanction, can be brought to redefine life and death by these criteria.

A practice which has proved acceptable in many settings is as follows:

1 The diagnosis of brain death, based on the above criteria, should be corroborated by another physician and confirmed by clinical examination and EEG, repeated one or more times.
2 The family should be informed of the irreversibility of brain function but should not be requested to ratify the decision of whether the medical treatment should be discontinued. An exception to this limited decision-making power of the family might apply where the patient has directed the family that he or she wishes them to make the decision.
3 The physician, after consultation with a professional colleague, may withdraw supportive measures, assuming that nothing more can be offered. This interpretation is in general agreement with that of most religions.
4 The possibility that such patients may become sources of organs for grafting should not enter into the aforementioned decisions, although prior to the cessation of heart action the family may be asked whether this would be their wish, or the family may suggest that organs be used for this purpose.

"Do not resuscitate" orders and cessation of therapy When carried out in a timely and expert manner, cardiopulmonary resuscitation is often useful in the prevention of sudden, unexpected death. However, unless there are reasons to the contrary it should not ordinarily be carried out when it merely prolongs life in a patient with terminal, incurable disease. The decision not to resuscitate a patient and decisions about the intensity of therapy and, indeed, whether or not treatment is to be delivered at all to patients who are

incurably and terminally ill must be reviewed frequently and must take into consideration any unexpected changes in the patient's condition. These decisions must take into account both the underlying medical condition and the wishes of the patient or if these cannot or have not been ascertained directly, those of a close relative or other surrogate who can be relied upon to transmit the patient's feelings and to be guided by the patient's best interests. Legal rulings, reflecting societal views, increasingly support the view that medical interventions of any kind which only sustain biologic functions in the hopelessly ill are futile and unnecessary gestures.

The issues involving death and dying are among the most difficult in medicine. In approaching them rationally and consistently, the physician must combine the art of medicine with the science.

2 QUANTITATIVE ASPECTS OF CLINICAL REASONING

LEE GOLDMAN

The process of clinical reasoning is poorly understood but is based upon factors such as experience and learning, inductive and deductive reasoning, interpretation of evidence that itself varies in reproducibility and validity, and intuition that often is difficult to define. In an effort to improve clinical reasoning, a number of attempts have been made to analyze quantitatively the many factors involved, including defining the cognitive approaches that clinicians apply to difficult problems, devising computerized decision support systems that are designed to emulate certain features of decision making, and applying decision theory to understand how judgments should be reached. While each of these approaches has advanced the understanding of the diagnostic process, all have practical and/or theoretical problems that limit their direct applicability to the care of the individual patient.

Nevertheless, these preliminary attempts to apply the rigor and logic inherent in the quantitative method have provided significant insights into the process by which clinical reasoning is accomplished, have identified ways in which the process may be improved, and have made it possible to minimize certain features of the workup that are not cost-effective. Thus, while clinical reasoning cannot be reduced to probabilities or numbers, attempts at quantitative analysis of the process may improve the ways in which the problems of individual patients are approached and solved.

In a simplified model, quantitative clinical reasoning includes five phases. It begins with an investigation of the chief complaint through key questions that are included in the history of the present illness (Table 2-1). These questions are supplemented by the past medical history and by a physical examination that emphasizes detailed investigation of potential key organ systems. In the second phase, the physician may select an array of diagnostic tests, each with its own accuracy and usefulness for investigating the possibilities raised in the differential diagnosis. Since each test costs something, and some entail discomfort and risk as well, the physician must ask whether the history and physical examination are sufficiently diagnostic before ordering tests. Third, the clinical data must be integrated with test results to estimate the likelihood of conditions in the differential diagnosis. Fourth, the comparative risks and benefits of

TABLE 2-1 Phases of clinical reasoning and decision making

1 Investigation of the complaint by means of clinical examination (history and physical examination)
2 Ordering of diagnostic tests, each with its own intrinsic accuracy and usefulness
3 Integration of clinical findings with test results to assess diagnostic probabilities
4 Weighing of comparative risks and benefits of alternative courses of action
5 Determination of patient's preferences and development of a therapeutic plan

further diagnostic and therapeutic options must be weighed to reach a recommendation for the patient. Finally, this recommendation is presented to the patient, and after appropriate discussion of the options, a therapeutic plan is initiated. Each of the five steps in this simplified model of the clinical reasoning process can be analyzed individually.

HISTORY AND PHYSICAL EXAMINATION It originally had been assumed that physicians begin investigating a patient's chief complaint by obtaining a comprehensive history, which includes many if not most of the questions included in a full review of systems, and by performing an all-inclusive physical examination. However, experienced clinicians begin to form hypotheses based on the chief complaint and on the responses to initial questioning, and they ask further questions in a sequence that allows them to evaluate the initial hypotheses and, if necessary, shorten or amend the list of possibilities. Only a limited number of diagnostic hypotheses can be entertained at any one time, and information is used to build a case for or against the most likely. In such a way, high-priority questions are selected from the almost limitless number that might be asked, and these specific questions are incorporated into the history of the present illness. Often, a key response, such as a history of melena, will be selected, a list of potential explanations for it will be formulated, and this list will then be trimmed, based on the response to more probing questions, so that a principal diagnosis can be selected and then tested. This process, termed *iterative hypothesis testing*, is an efficient approach to diagnosis and is preferable to attempts to gather every conceivable piece of information prior to formulating a differential diagnosis.

Advocacy of iterative hypothesis testing does not argue against the need for a systematic, thorough, and complete history of the present illness, past medical history, review of systems, family history, social history, and physical examination. For example, if a patient presents with abdominal pain, the physician may gather information regarding its location and quality as well as the factors that precipitate and/or relieve it. The physician then asks questions relating to the diagnoses that may be suspected based on the response to the initial questions. If the pain is suggestive of pancreatitis, the clinician might ask about alcohol intake, the use of thiazide diuretics or glucocorticosteroids, symptoms suggestive of concomitant gallbladder disease, a family history of pancreatitis, and questions aimed at uncovering the possibility of a posterior penetrating ulcer. Alternatively, if the discomfort seems more typical of reflux esophagitis, a different sequence of questions would be triggered. The use of iterative hypothesis testing encourages the physician to elicit detailed information in high-yield areas, without forgoing a systematic and thorough approach to the patient. Findings on the history and physical examination should influence each other. The history focuses the physical examination on certain organs, and findings on physical examination should encourage more detailed review of certain systems.

As physicians proceed through this reasoning process with both the history and physical examination, a variety of issues may influence the accuracy of the decision-making process. First is the potential for some historical information to be poorly reproducible, either because the patient's responses vary or because different physicians ask questions differently or vary in the way they interpret the answers. For example, in one study, two physicians' estimates of functional cardiac class agreed only about half of the time. When a subjective scale was replaced by a more specific series of precisely worded questions, both reproducibility and validity improved significantly, although some patients still gave frankly conflicting responses to the same question when asked by different interviewers on the same day. The careful use of clear, and when possible, precise questions can increase the reproducibility and validity of the medical history, but still cannot eliminate all variability.

When assessing the reproducibility of findings on the physical examination, two observers frequently agree that an uncommon abnormality such as an enlarged spleen is not present but agree less often when one of them thinks that it is present in a patient in whom it would not usually be expected. This principle can best be demonstrated by understanding that some agreement always occurs by chance, and the likelihood of chance agreement is higher if the finding is either very common or very uncommon. For example, if two physicians each consider 90 percent of patients to be abnormal in some manner, such as having a systolic heart murmur, they will agree 81 percent of the time by chance alone. In some studies of the reproducibility of common signs and symptoms, such as whether or not a liver was enlarged, actual agreement rates have not been substantially better than chance. Disagreement rates may be reduced by emphasizing physical examination skills during medical training, by looking for other correlative physical findings, and by learning how physical findings correlate with the results of diagnostic tests. Therefore, when a clinician notes an unexpected and somewhat subjective abnormality for which there may be a high rate of interobserver disagreement, such as an unexpectedly enlarged spleen, other abnormalities that may often be associated with it, such as hepatomegaly or lymphadenopathy, should be sought to increase the likelihood that the spleen would be expected to be abnormal. In some situations, ordering a diagnostic test, such as a liver and spleen scan, to assess the finding more objectively should be considered if the test is sufficiently reliable.

These comments about the factors that limit the reproducibility and validity of the medical history and physical examination do not denigrate their critical importance in clinical reasoning. Rather, they emphasize that care and diligence in the application of these skills are necessary.

When physicians use the history and the physical examination to arrive at a diagnosis, they are rarely certain of it. Therefore, it would be better to assess the likelihood of the diagnosis in terms of probabilities. All too frequently, this probability is not expressed as an actual percentage but rather in such terms as "nearly always," "commonly," "sometimes," or "rarely." Since different physicians may assign different probabilities to the same terms, these imprecise words frequently lead to major misunderstandings among physicians or between the physician and the patient. Physicians should be as rigorous and quantitative as possible in their assessments, and when feasible, a quantitative expression of probability should be used. For example, rather than saying that it is unlikely that a radiographic pattern is indicative of a carcinoma of the colon, it would be preferable, if possible, to provide a more precise indication of the probability of carcinoma with this radiographic pattern. A 10 to 15 percent probability of carcinoma may be interpreted as "unlikely," but from a clinical perspective usually warrants further evaluation because of the serious consequences of missing a potentially resectable tumor.

Although such quantitative estimates would be desirable, they usually are not available in practice. Even experienced physicians often are unable to estimate accurately the likelihood of particular conditions. There is a tendency to overestimate the likelihood of relatively uncommon conditions, and physicians are especially poor at quantifying probabilities that are very high or very low. For example, a physician may not know whether the probability of bacterial meningitis or of another disease that could be diagnosed by a lumbar puncture in a patient with a severe headache is 1 in 20 or 1 in 200. In both situations, the probability is low, but the decision as to whether a lumbar puncture should be performed may depend on this estimate.

Since the establishment of valid diagnostic probabilities is a cornerstone to clinical reasoning, accumulated clinical experience, often in the form of computerized data banks, has been used to generate statistical approaches for improving diagnostic predictions. In such research, it is common to identify factors that have a univariate correlation with the diagnosis in question. Then, these univariate correlates may be included in a multivariate analysis to determine which of them are significant independent predictors of the diagnosis.

Some analyses may identify the important predictive factors and then assign them "weights," which can be transformed to calculate a probability. Alternatively, the analysis may result in a limited number of categories of patients, each with a discrete probability of the diagnosis.

These quantitative approaches to the estimation of various diagnostic probabilities, which are often termed "prediction rules," are especially helpful if they are in a format that is readily usable by the clinician and if they have been validated prospectively on a sufficient number and spectrum of patients. For example, by carefully defining the key historical questions and findings on physical examination that might predict the causes of common acute complaints observed in ambulatory patients, algorithms have been devised to guide nonphysicians on the ordering of diagnostic tests and the need for an examination by a physician; nonphysicians aided by these algorithms, and working under the general supervision of a physician, can provide care that is less costly and as effective as that provided by unaided physicians.

For such prediction rules to be useful to the clinician, they must be derived from relevant patient populations and use tests that are reproducible and readily available, so that the results can be extrapolated to local medical practice. Since only a minority of published prediction rules have adhered to rigid criteria as to the number and spectrum of patients examined and their prospective validation, most are not yet suitable for routine clinical application. Furthermore, many prediction rules cannot evaluate the probability of each of the diagnoses or outcomes that the clinician must consider.

As was emphasized in Chap. 1, the history and physical examination have other important purposes. They allow the physician to evaluate the emotional status of the patient and to understand how the present problems fit into the context of the patient's social and family life, and they encourage the development in the patient of confidence in the physician, which is so necessary for reaching an agreement on the coming plan of action.

DIAGNOSTIC TESTS: INDICATIONS, ACCURACY, AND USEFULNESS A diagnostic test should be ordered for specified clinical indications, be sufficiently accurate to be efficacious for such indications, and be the least expensive and/or risky of the available efficacious tests. No diagnostic test is totally accurate, and physicians often have difficulty interpreting test results. It is therefore critical to understand several commonly used terms in test analysis and epidemiology, including prevalence, sensitivity, specificity, positive predictive value, and negative predictive value (Table 2-2).

Although reports of the accuracies of diagnostic tests are commonly expressed in terms of positive and negative predictive values, these calculated values are dependent on the prevalence of the disease in the population being studied (Table 2-3). A test with a particular sensitivity and specificity has different positive and negative predictive values when used in groups that have different prevalences of disease. For example, a mildly abnormal alkaline phosphatase level in a young adult with a known lymphoma suggests hepatic involvement by the tumor, i.e., it is likely to be a *true positive*, while the same alkaline phosphatase level as part of a routine screening battery of blood tests in an asymptomatic person of the same age is unlikely to be due to tumor, i.e., in this setting it is more likely to be a *false positive*.

Although the sensitivity and specificity of a test do not depend on the prevalence (or percentage of patients being tested who have the disease), they do depend on the spectrum of patients in whom the test is being evaluated. For example, a technetium pyrophosphate scintiscan for diagnosing myocardial infarction (Chap. 179) will appear to have a nearly perfect sensitivity and specificity if the diseased population has a history typical of myocardial infarction, electrocardiographic changes of transmural infarction, and clear-cut elevations of the MB isoenzyme of creatine kinase (CK) and the nondiseased population is composed of normal medical students. If, however, without changing the prevalence of disease in the population being tested, the spectrum of the diseased and nondiseased patients is altered by including patients with other characteristics, i.e., if the population of patients with myocardial infarction were composed principally of those with non-Q-wave infarctions and small or borderline elevations of CK-MB, while the population without acute infarction included patients with old infarcts and unstable angina pectoris, the sensitivity and specificity might change dramatically. In the latter situation, the sensitivity and specificity of the technetium pyrophosphate scintiscan are not only lower than in the first example, because the spectrum of diseased and nondiseased patients has been changed, but, more importantly, they are so low that the test has little clinical value. This example also demonstrates the methodologic problems encountered when applying data from one study to a different type of patient or when pooling data from studies of different subsets of patients.

In some situations, uncertainty about the sensitivity and specificity of the test in the type of patient being assessed may limit its clinical value. Since the physician rarely knows (or can know) the population on which every test which is ordered has been standardized, the results provide information that is far less decisive than usually thought. Furthermore, it may be quite difficult to distinguish random laboratory errors from test results that might be falsely positive or negative because of coexistence of a process that can affect the test, such as the finding of an elevated level of CK in a patient who has undergone strenuous exercise and is being evaluated for chest pain.

Because no single value or cutoff point of an individual test can be expected to have both a perfect sensitivity and a perfect specificity, it is often necessary to determine which value or cutoff point is the most appropriate to guide decision making. A graph (Fig. 2-1) of the test's *receiver operating characteristic curve*, which displays the inevitable trade-off between emphasizing a high sensitivity, such as defining an exercise electrocardiogram as abnormal if it shows ≥ 0.5 mm of ST-segment depression, versus emphasizing a high specificity, such as defining an exercise electrocardiogram as abnormal only if it shows ≥ 2.0 mm of ST-segment depression, can help the clinician understand the implications of various definitions of a "positive" test result. Such a graph demonstrates that different definitions of

TABLE 2-2   Definitions of commonly used terms in epidemiology and decision making

Test result	Disease state	
	Present	Absent
Positive	a (true positive)	b (false positive)
Negative	c (false negative)	d (true negative)

Prevalence (prior probability)	=	$(a+c)/(a+b+c+d)$	= all patients with the disease/all patients tested
Sensitivity	=	$a/(a+c)$	= true-positive test results/all patients with the disease
Specificity	=	$d/(b+d)$	= true-negative test results/all patients without the disease
False-negative rate	=	$c/(a+c)$	= false-negative test results/all patients with the disease
False-positive rate	=	$b/(b+d)$	= false-positive test results/all patients without the disease
Positive predictive value	=	$a/(a+b)$	= true-positive test results/all positive test results
Negative predictive value	=	$d/(c+d)$	= true-negative test results/all patients with negative results
Overall accuracy	=	$(a+d)/(a+b+c+d)$	= true-positive + true-negative test results/all tests

FIGURE 2-1 *The inherent trade-off between sensitivity and specificity. For any diagnostic test, an increase in sensitivity will be associated with a decline in specificity. The closer this curve comes to the upper-left-hand corner, the more useful the test; the closer to the broken line, the less useful it is. When deciding on the cutoff between normal versus abnormal, one must determine what sensitivity and specificity are most useful clinically.*

normal versus abnormal may be appropriate depending on whether one wishes to rule in the disease with a test result that has a high specificity or to exclude the disease with a test result that has a high sensitivity. Different tests may have different sensitivities and specificities, and better tests may have both a higher sensitivity and a higher specificity than poorer tests.

One example of a sensitive test is an M-mode echocardiogram to exclude severe aortic stenosis in adults: the sensitivity of the test for aortic stenosis is close to 100 percent, and a normal aortic valve echogram virtually excludes the diagnosis of severe aortic stenosis in the adult. Unfortunately, this sensitive test is not very specific, and many patients who have abnormal aortic valves on echocardiogram do not have severe aortic stenosis and require further testing (e.g., with Doppler echocardiography and perhaps cardiac catheterization) to establish the diagnosis (Chap. 187). A common example of a reasonably specific test would be an electrocardiogram to diagnose acute myocardial infarction. While the precise specificity depends on

the spectrum of patients being tested, the presence of new ST-segment elevations exceeding 1.0 mm in two or more adjacent leads in patients who present to an emergency room with prolonged acute chest pain consistent with myocardial ischemia is sufficiently specific, i.e., sufficiently unlikely to be a false positive, that admission to an intensive care unit is virtually always recommended. However, this test is not sensitive, and if admission to the unit were restricted to patients with this electrocardiographic finding, almost half of patients with myocardial infarctions presenting to hospital emergency rooms would be missed.

To optimize the clinical value of a diagnostic test, it is helpful to obtain local experience with it; oftentimes, its value will differ from that reported in the literature. Reports of the efficacy of a test should emphasize its accuracy when compared to an independent standard, and the test must be evaluated in a spectrum of patients with varying severities of the disease in question and in patients who have conditions that are part of the same differential diagnosis. The reproducibility of the test should be known, and the "normal limits" of the test should be clear and appropriate. In some instances, the test or procedure required to establish the validity of a diagnostic test is so risky that only a skewed sample of patients are included in a study, as, for example, in the analysis of the usefulness of the abdominal CT scan in patients with suspected pancreatic carcinoma. If patients with "negative" CT scan results never come to laparotomy or postmortem examination, neither the sensitivity nor specificity of the CT scan for pancreatic carcinoma can be assessed. In such situations, an estimated value of the diagnostic test may be inaccurate because it has not been validated.

INTEGRATION OF CLINICAL DATA AND TEST RESULTS Although, as we have seen, neither clinical data nor test results may be entirely accurate, the integration of the two can lead to better diagnostic predictions than either alone. By knowing the probability that the patient has a particular condition before a test is performed (the prior, or pretest, probability), and by knowing the sensitivity and the specificity of the test, the posttest probability can be calculated. A common mathematical technique for integrating clinical data and a test result is the odds-likelihood form of Bayesian analysis (Table 2-4). A pretest probability can be expressed as odds (as in a horse race for example) and multiplied by the likelihood ratio (which is the sensitivity of the test divided by 1 minus the specificity of the test) to yield the posttest odds, which may be transformed back into a posttest probability. This approach can be employed in any situation in which the physician can use clinical findings to estimate a pretest

TABLE 2-3 How the positive and negative predictive values of the same test vary depending on the prior probability of disease

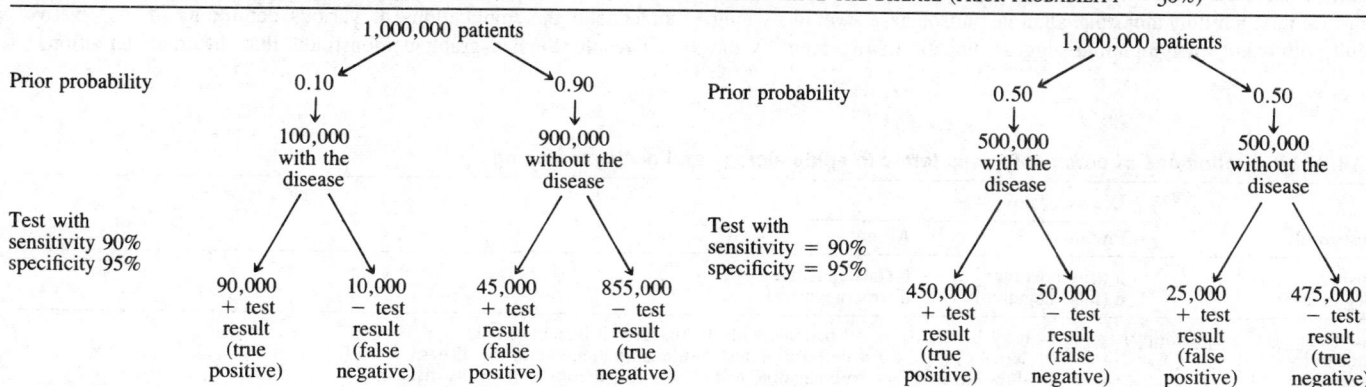

INTERPRETATION OF THE TEST RESULT WHEN 10% OF THE PATIENTS BEING TESTED HAVE THE DISEASE (PRIOR PROBABILITY = 10%)

INTERPRETATION OF THE TEST RESULT WHEN 50% OF THE PATIENTS BEING TESTED HAVE THE DISEASE (PRIOR PROBABILITY = 50%)

1,000,000 patients

Prior probability   0.10   0.90

100,000 with the disease   900,000 without the disease

Test with sensitivity 90% specificity 95%

90,000 + test result (true positive)   10,000 – test result (false negative)   45,000 + test result (false positive)   855,000 – test result (true negative)

1,000,000 patients

Prior probability   0.50   0.50

500,000 with the disease   500,000 without the disease

Test with sensitivity = 90% specificity = 95%

450,000 + test result (true positive)   50,000 – test result (false negative)   25,000 + test result (false positive)   475,000 – test result (true negative)

The probability of disease in a patient with a positive test result (positive predictive value) = 90,000/135,000 = 67%
The probability of no disease in a patient with a negative test result (negative predictive value) = 855,000/865,000 = 99%

The probability of disease in a patient with a positive test result (positive predictive value) = 450,000/475,000 = 95%
The probability of no disease in a patient with a negative test result (negative predictive value) = 475,000/525,000 = 90%

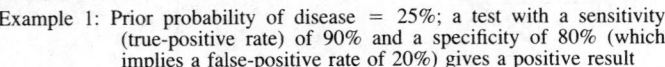

TABLE 2-4 Example of the use of Bayesian analysis to integrate the pretest probability with the test result to calculate a posttest probability

Example 1: Prior probability of disease = 25%; a test with a sensitivity (true-positive rate) of 90% and a specificity of 80% (which implies a false-positive rate of 20%) gives a positive result

Example 2: Same pretest probability and test, but now the test gives a negative result. Here the true-negative rate would be 80% and the false negative rate (which is 1 − sensitivity) would be 10%.

Clinical data
↓
Prior probability → prior odds

25%   1:3

$$\frac{0.90}{0.20} \xleftarrow{\quad} \frac{\text{sensitivity*}}{(1-\text{specificity})\dagger} \leftarrow \text{positive test}$$

Posttest odds

$$(1:3) \times \frac{0.90}{0.20} = 4.5:3$$

Posttest probability

$$\frac{4.5}{7.5} = 60\%$$

Clinical data
↓
Prior probability → prior odds

25%   1:3

$$\frac{0.10}{0.80} \xleftarrow{\quad} \frac{(1-\text{sensitivity})\ddagger}{\text{specificity}\S} \leftarrow \text{negative test}$$

Posttest odds

$$(1:3) \times \frac{0.10}{0.80} = 0.125:3 = 1:24$$

Posttest probability

$$\frac{1}{25} = 4\%$$

---

* *Sensitivity = probability of a positive test result in a patient with the disease*
† *(1 − Specificity) = probability of a positive test result in a patient without the disease*

‡ *(1 − Sensitivity) = probability of a negative test result in a patient with the disease*
§ *Specificity = probability of a negative test result in a patient without the disease*

diagnostic probability and integrate this with the result as well as the sensitivity and specificity of the diagnostic test. Many clinical situations may be so complex that it is not practical to estimate the prior probabilities of all likely diagnoses or to know the sensitivities and specificities of each of the tests that might be performed individually or in sequence. Nevertheless, attempts in this direction will stimulate critical thinking, expose uncertainties, and generate ideas for original investigations or a review of past experiences to facilitate the application of Bayesian analysis to the integration of clinical data and laboratory tests.

The results of Bayesian analyses often can be expressed in graphic form, such as the value of exercise electrocardiograms for predicting the presence of coronary artery disease (Fig. 2-2; also see Chap. 189). This series of curves also demonstrates how to consider a test whose result may be in the "gray zone" rather than clearly positive or clearly negative.

One of the key assumptions inherent in most such analyses is that the correlation between the pretest probability and the test result is no greater than expected by chance. If the diagnostic test simply duplicates information that has already been obtained by the clinical examination, it will not have any additional benefit for predicting whether or not the disease is present. For example, in trying to determine whether or not a patient with carcinoma of the colon has hepatic metastases, the finding of jaundice on physical examination should be a strong predictor. The degree of hyperbilirubinemia can also be measured, but the bilirubin level in a patient with clinical jaundice does not add substantial *independent* information to that obtained by a careful physical examination. When integrating a diagnostic test with clinical information, such a test is helpful only when it adds incremental information to what can be inferred based on the history and physical examination and on prior less costly or less risky diagnostic tests. If a diagnostic test (such as a retrograde cholangiogram in the patient with hyperbilirubinemia) provides information that cannot be inferred directly, it is less likely that its results are associated with pretest probabilities to an extent greater than would be expected by chance.

A diagnostic test has an impact on the evaluation of a specific patient only if it changes the diagnostic probability to the extent that the new probability dictates a change in the diagnostic strategy or therapeutic plans or if the test serves as part of a sequence of tests that moves the probability across such a threshold. An example is a patient suspected of having a pulmonary embolism, with an estimated probability of 50 percent based on clinical data alone. A "low probability" pulmonary ventilation-perfusion scan may reduce the probability of pulmonary embolism, but if the goal is to exclude pulmonary embolism with the highest possible degree of certainty, a pulmonary angiogram would be required (Chap. 211).

Because diagnostic tests oftentimes do not provide important new information even when their results are accurate, several questions should be considered in deciding when to order diagnostic tests. First, how likely is the disease in question? Second, what would be the clinical consequences if the diagnosis were missed or if the patient were mistakenly treated for a disease that is not present? Third, what is the likelihood that the diagnostic test will change the probability sufficiently to have an effect on either diagnosis or therapy? The physician should consider the probabilities, the risks, the likelihood and costs of obtaining new information, and the adverse consequences of delay, because observation and follow-up are always among the available diagnostic options.

COMPARING RISKS AND BENEFITS: DECISION ANALYSIS Inherent in the concept that probabilities can guide decision making is the assumption that one can arrive at a reasonable threshold by knowing the relative risks (or costs) and benefits of various options and deciding at what probability this ratio changes to favor an alternative strategy. Decision analysis is an organized process for evaluating such situations and identifies the key issues and problems.

One problem with applying decision-analysis techniques to difficult clinical problems is that the decision analysis is no better than the data on which it is based. In some instances, an attempted decision analysis of a complex clinical problem may yield no more information than that the critical data required for the analysis are missing and that more research in the field needs to be performed. In addition, when clinicians are uncertain about diagnostic or therapeutic strategies, formal analyses may indicate that the differences in outcome among various strategies are very small. In such cases, the formal analysis may have such inherent error that it is not dependable. Even when decision analysis is potentially helpful, it may not be feasible to complete the detailed estimations and calculations within the time constraints of bedside decision making. Nevertheless, the value of the analytic approach to decision making is that it integrates available data, mandates rigorous thinking, and exposes areas of uncertainty or ignorance.

Decision analysis depicts graphically two types of issues in the decision making process: first, the decisions (or choices) available to the physician and second, the probabilities of all of the events that may result from each decision. To illustrate how this process works, a decision analysis of whether to biopsy the brain, treat, or wait in suspected herpes encephalitis (Chap. 136) may be considered. Figure 2-3 depicts the decision tree for this problem. The square box or

FIGURE 2-2 *How the exercise tolerance test affects the probability of coronary artery disease. The prior, or before-test, probability of coronary artery disease (CAD) will be modified by the result of the exercise electrocardiogram to yield a posterior, or after-test, probability of CAD. Note that the finding of <1 mm of ST depression will reduce the probability of CAD, whereas ≥1 mm of ST depression will increase the probability. For example, if a patient with a before-test probability of CAD of 90 percent, which is about the probability in a middle-aged man with very typical anginal symptoms, had 2 to 2.49 mm of ST depression of exercise testing, the after-test probability of CAD would be 99.5 percent. In contrast the same exercise test result in a.* *patient with 30 percent before-test probability of CAD, which is about what one would expect in a patient with atypical anginal symptoms, would yield an after-test probability of about 90 percent. In an asymptomatic patient, with a before-test probability of about 5 percent, the same exercise test result would yield an after-test probability of 53 percent. Thus, the same test yields different after-test probabilities in patients with different before-test probabilities. (Adapted, with permission of the New England Journal of Medicine, from RD Rifkin, WB Hood: Bayesian analysis of electrocardiographic exercise stress testing. N Engl J Med 297:684, 1977.)*

"node" labeled A indicates a decision that the physician must make. The circular nodes, labeled B through I, indicate where different outcomes, each of which has an estimatable probability, could occur. In this analysis, the initial choices were to treat with vidarabine (a relatively toxic drug), not to treat with vidarabine, or to perform a brain biopsy and use its results to guide the treatment decision. The use of vidarabine may or may not result in complications of therapy, and a biopsy itself may or may not be associated with a complication.

Each of the possible outcomes for a patient is typically assigned a "utility," which is the relative preference for the outcome, where 1.0 is a perfect outcome and 0 is the worst possible outcome. Each terminal branch of the decision tree is assigned the utility corresponding to its outcome, and the "expected value" of each terminal branch is calculated by multiplying its probability by its utility. To calculate the "expected value" of each of the three possible courses of action (see Fig. 2-3, node A), the expected values of each of the terminal branches that originate from it would be summed. The preferred course of action is the one which, when all possible outcomes are considered, yields the highest expected value, which is the sum of the product of the probability multiplied by the utility for each of its possible outcomes.

In performing any decision analysis, the relevant probabilities

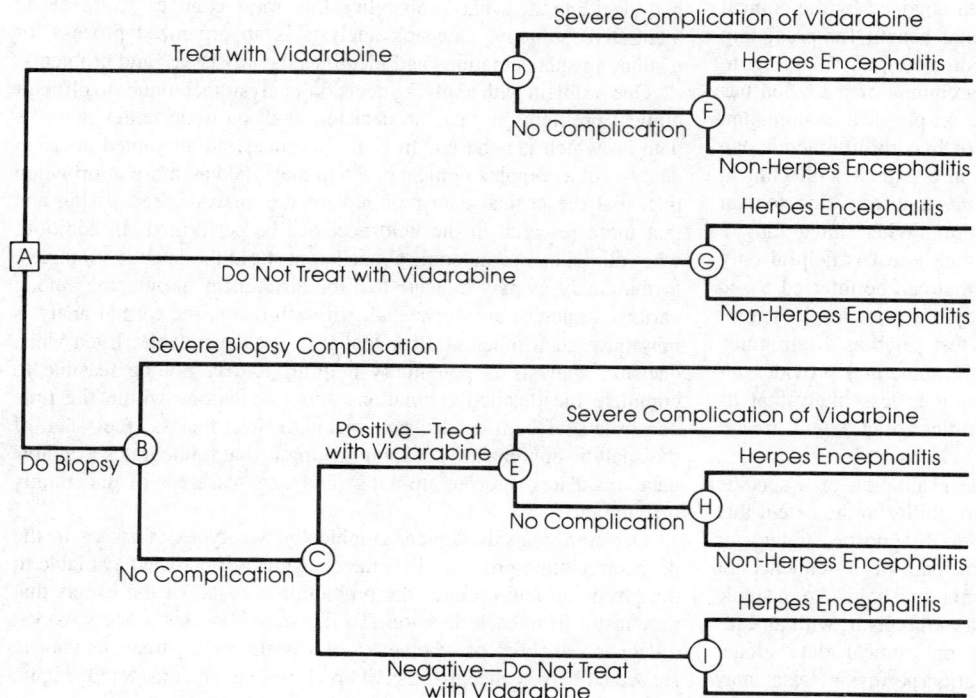

FIGURE 2-3 *Decision tree for diagnosis and treatment of suspected herpes simplex encephalitis. The square node represents the decision point, and the round nodes denote chance events. See text for details. (Reprinted with permission from M Barza, SG Pauker, The decision to biopsy, treat, or wait in suspected herpes encephalitis, Ann Intern Med 92:644, 1980.)*

must be known or estimated, a process that sometimes requires guesswork. Next, utilities could be assigned to each of these outcomes. A major practical limitation of decision analysis is the subjective judgment often required to estimate utilities. It is also difficult to adjust future years of life for their quality in any numerical fashion, for example, in considering how drug toxicity or the disability resulting from disease or treatment lowers the quality of future years of life.

The results and usefulness of a decision analysis depend on the probabilities and utilities that are used in the calculation, and it is imperative for decision analyses to include a *sensitivity analysis*, in which various estimates for each probability are included in the analysis to determine if the conclusions would be changed. For example, in the analysis in Fig. 2-3, some range of probabilities must be assumed for vidarabine toxicity, for serious complications of brain biopsy, and for the likelihood of false-positive or false-negative biopsy results. The authors of this particular analysis concluded that waiting, i.e., neither treating nor performing a biopsy, was the preferable course of action when the likelihood of herpes encephalitis is less than 3 percent. At probabilities between 3 and 42 percent, the analysis favored brain biopsy, but at probabilities above 42 percent, it favored immediate treatment with vidarabine. However, it is uncommon for any patient to have substantially greater than a 42 percent probability of herpes encephalitis, and hence it would be unusual for empiric vidarabine treatment ever to be preferred over brain biopsy. The authors demonstrated that these conclusions did not change when they varied the assumptions about the probabilities of several relevant events. If the conclusions of an analysis were altered by relatively minor changes in the assumptions on which it was based, the analysis would not be sufficiently reliable to become the basis for decision making.

Decision analysis sometimes demonstrates a clear and dramatic advantage with one particular option. In other circumstances, there may be little difference between two options; either option may be reasonable, or secondary issues that cannot be taken into account in the formal analysis, such as the patient's feelings about taking risks or the recent local experience with particular interventions, should be the final determinants in the decision. Physicians who perform a decision analysis therefore must determine the probabilities of each of the possible events by reviewing the pertinent patient experience at their own institution or practice, or by reviewing the pertinent literature. Even when the outcome of the analysis seems clear, the physician or the patient may believe that the situation in question is an exception to the rule. Furthermore, even the best analyses, like all clinical intuition, are based on assumptions that may be open to debate.

In the preceding example, the management of an individual patient with possible herpes encephalitis, decision analysis indicated the preferred strategy in terms of outcome but did not consider the costs at which such benefits might be achieved. In determining health policy, a formal cost-effectiveness analysis can be performed to determine how many dollars must be spent to achieve a unit of benefit, often defined as a life saved, a year of life saved, or a quality-adjusted year of life saved, in which the years are adjusted to take into account the quality of life during that time. For example, 1 year of in-center hemodialysis can be estimated to cost about $35,000 in 1986 dollars; this figure includes only the direct medical costs and not indirect costs related to issues such as time lost or travel, or any benefits in terms of a patient's ability to work. In some situations, the ability of the patient to maintain gainful employment may offset some or all of the direct medical expenses.

Although many analyses are now expressed in terms of cost-effectiveness, where dollars spent are compared to lives or years of life gained, some studies have utilized cost-benefit analyses in which a dollar value is placed on the life that is saved. For example, an analysis of the rubella vaccination, which attempted to place a dollar value on the vaccine's ability to prevent the congenital rubella syndrome and the resulting expenses, concluded that the optimal national policy would be to vaccinate all females at age 12.

ETHICS AND PATIENT INPUT In both quantitative and nonquantitative clinical reasoning, the physician must consider ethical issues as well as the patient's values and preferences. While a detailed discussion of these issues is beyond the scope of this chapter, it is important to emphasize that patients' preferences for alternate therapies may not agree with the preferences that the physicians propose on the basis of their own clinical judgment or the results of a decision-analysis approach. For example, many patients with carcinoma of the larynx may prefer radiation therapy, with a lower cure rate but a higher likelihood of maintaining speech, to extirpative surgery. It is imperative that physicians assess those characteristics of life that the patient prizes most (the elusive "quality of life") prior to basing controversial decisions solely on quantitative approaches, the physicians' own subjective impressions of the likely medical benefits, their own personal preferences, or their assumptions about the patient's preferences. Therefore, the final plan should reflect an agreement between a well-informed patient and a sympathetic physician who has detailed knowledge of the relevant medical issues and of the impact of the various possible outcomes on the specific patient.

REFERENCES

ELSTEIN AS et al: *Medical Problem Solving. An Analysis of Clinical Reasoning.* Cambridge, Harvard University, 1978

GOLDMAN L et al: Comparative reproducibility and validity of systems for assessing cardiovascular functional class: Advantages of a new specific activity scale. Circulation 64:1227, 1981

GREENFIELD S et al: Efficiency and cost of primary care by nurses and physician assistants. N Engl J Med 298:305, 1978

MCNEIL BJ et al: Speech and survival: Trade offs between quality and quantity of life in laryngeal cancer. N Engl J Med 305:982, 1981

RANSOHOFF DF, FEINSTEIN AR: Problems of spectrum and bias in evaluating the efficacy of diagnostic tests. N Engl J Med 299:926, 1978

ROBERTS SD et al: Cost-effective care of end-stage renal disease: A billion dollar question. Ann Intern Med 92:243, 1980

SCHOENBAUM SC et al: Benefit-cost analysis of rubella vaccination policy. N Engl J Med 294:303, 1976

WEINSTEIN MC, FINEBERG HV: *Clinical Decision Analysis.* Philadelphia, Saunders, 1980

section 1 Pain

3 PAIN: PATHOPHYSIOLOGY AND MANAGEMENT

RAYMOND MACIEWICZ / JOSEPH B. MARTIN

Pain is the most common symptom of disease. Although the nature, location, and etiology of pain differ in each case, approximately half of all patients who visit a physician have a primary complaint of pain. For most patients, correct treatment of a self-evident, limited disease process (such as a broken bone) alleviates the pain. In many, however, the symptom of pain itself must be carefully assessed and evaluated to interpret its significance and to establish an approach for its treatment. In some patients uncontrolled pain continues as a major problem. The cost of medical treatment of patients with chronic pain is in excess of $50 billion annually, and low back pain alone accounts for the loss of 100 million work days each year. Chronic pain is therefore not only a difficult medical management problem but also an issue of major social concern.

The evaluation of the patient with pain is frequently complex, partially because pain is a perception rather than a sensation. A person's physical state, past experience, and anticipation all influence the way a given sensory input is interpreted. For example, soldiers and athletes may deny pain despite an acute injury, while certain patients with chronic pain may continue to suffer despite the lack of an obvious nociceptive stimulus. Our knowledge of pain and most of our treatments for it focus on decreasing the nociceptive sensory input; however, a patient's interpretation of a sensation, the affective reaction, and the behavioral response are equally important factors that deserve the physician's careful attention.

ORGANIZATION OF PAIN PATHWAYS Nociceptive afferents
Sensory stimuli of potentially tissue-damaging intensity activate free nerve endings in skin, underlying tissue, and viscera. Nociceptive signals are conveyed to the spinal cord by unmyelinated and small myelinated sensory axons. In humans, stimulation of individual small sensory axons can evoke the report of pain in the area of skin supplied by that fiber, clearly demonstrating that under certain conditions even single axons can transmit activity that is interpreted as "pain" by the brain.

Many unmyelinated nociceptive afferents exhibit "polymodal" responses. Such fibers can be activated by intense mechanical stimulation, potentially tissue-damaging thermal stimulation, and chemical stimulation by substances injected into skin. Any intense stimulus applied to normal skin can produce a "triple response" that consists of a red flush at the site of stimulation, a surrounding red flare due to arterial dilatation, and local edema caused by increased vascular permeability. Many substances likely play an important role in this response. Some of these agents are released by damaged tissue (potassium, histamine, serotonin, prostaglandins), while others enter from the circulation (bradykinin) or come from local nerve endings themselves (substance P). Certain of these substances also activate free nerve endings, and their long-lasting effects may partially explain the hypersensitivity of the skin that often follows a noxious stimulus.

Dorsal horn Sensory fibers extend distally and proximally from cells located in the segmental dorsal root ganglia. Nociceptive afferents enter the spinal cord through the dorsal root to terminate on dorsal horn neurons (Fig. 3-1A). Many of the fine afferents ending in these regions contain neuropeptides, including substance P, cholecystokinin, and somatostatin. There is increasing evidence that these peptides play an important role in normal sensory transmission. Chemical destruction of substance P fibers in animals produces analgesia in certain tests for pain and there is also a marked decrease in substance P terminal staining in the dorsal horn in patients with congenital neuropathies that are associated with decreased sensitivity to pain.

The spinal dorsal horn can be divided into a series of layers based on cell morphology and arrangement. Neurons that process nociceptive information are found in several of these layers. The output neurons that project to brainstem and thalamus are found principally in layers I and V, zones where many small-caliber afferents terminate. The axons of these dorsal horn neurons form a crossed pathway that ascends in the ventrolateral quadrant of the spinal cord, the spinothalamic tract.

Spinothalamic system The axons of nociceptive dorsal horn neurons that form the spinothalamic tracts terminate in several brainstem and thalamic nuclei. The spinothalamic tract can be divided conceptually into two systems based on these connections: a direct spinothalamic system that carries sensory discriminative information about pain to thalamic levels, and a phylogenetically older spinoreticulothalamic system that terminates more diffusely in brainstem reticular nuclei.

The direct spinothalamic system that ends in the thalamus may be important for the conscious perception of nociceptive sensations. This system terminates in an orderly fashion within the *nucleus ventralis posterolateralis* (VPL). The terminal field of the spinothalamic tract in VPL overlaps the dorsal column–medial lemniscal input that relays light touch and joint sensation. The organized pattern of terminations and the convergence of light touch and pain information within VPL may be important for perception of the sensory discriminative aspects of pain, including the location, nature, and intensity of a noxious input. Consistent with this view, cells in VPL project principally to primary somatosensory cortex.

The more diffuse spinoreticulothalamic system may mediate aspects of the autonomic and affective reactions to pain. Ascending spinoreticular fibers terminate at several levels of the brainstem reticular formation, forming part of a polysynaptic system that terminates in the medial thalamic nuclei (*nucleus centralis lateralis* and *nucleus parafascicularis*). Cells throughout the spinoreticulothalamic system have large, bilateral sensory receptive fields that can include the entire body surface. These cells often respond best to noxious sensory input. Such cells are unlikely to be important for sensory discrimination or localization; they probably are important for arousal or orientation to a painful stimulus.

Under normal conditions, there appears to be a balance between the precise, specific information channeled through VPL and the more generalized alerting effects mediated through the medial thalamus. Clinical disorders that partially destroy the lateral thalamus including VPL can result in a syndrome of continuous, burning pain involving the contralateral side of the body (the thalamic syndrome of Déjerine and Roussy); the pain frequently has an exaggerated emotional or autonomic component. This condition may be due to an unrestricted flow of sensory information through the medial thalamus which is interpreted as pain by the brain. The fact that in some patients surgical lesions of the medial thalamus may relieve this type of continuous central pain is consistent with this idea.

Descending analgesic pathways In addition to the major ascending pain pathways outlined above, the brain contains powerful descending circuits that suppress nociceptive inputs (Fig. 3-1*B*). In animals, electrical stimulation of the midbrain periaqueductal gray region can produce generalized analgesia without other obvious sensory or motor responses. A similar system may exist in humans, as stimulation of the nearby periventricular gray is reported to relieve clinical pain. This effect appears to be at least partly mediated at the spinal level, since it can be blocked in animals by cutting pathways that carry descending projections from the brainstem to the dorsal horn. However, few periaqueductal gray cells project directly to the spinal cord. Instead, the descending pathway important for analgesia appears to first synapse in the midline raphe nuclei of the medulla (principally *nucleus raphe magnus*). Raphe neurons in turn project to the spinal cord where they inhibit the nociceptive response of dorsal horn neurons. This descending system can potentially gate the flow of nociceptive information from the level of the first synapse in the dorsal horn.

The periaqueductal gray region, the medullary raphe, and the dorsal horn all contain a high density of endogenous opiate peptides and opiate receptors. Systemic narcotic analgesics may in part work by activating the descending analgesia system at these sites. High densities of opiate receptors are also found in the medial thalamus and limbic forebrain; these structures may play an additional, important role in the analgesic response to, and the addictive potential of, systemically administered narcotics.

Biogenic amines represent another class of neurotransmitters found in the descending pathways that modulate nociception. Serotonin is contained in many of the raphe neurons that end in the dorsal horn, and some serotonergic axon terminals end directly on spinothalamic tract neurons. A major descending inhibitory pathway containing norepinephrine also arises in the *nucleus locus coeruleus* of the pons; this system appears to inhibit the nociceptive responses of dorsal horn neurons by an alpha-adrenergic mechanism. Drugs that potentiate the central effects of biogenic amines, such as the tricyclic antidepressants, may therefore be effective analgesic adjuvants that work by enhancing the effects of these descending pathways.

EVALUATION OF THE PATIENT WITH PAIN Somatic pain Pain usually occurs when a potentially tissue-damaging stimulus excites peripheral nociceptive afferents. When a noxious stimulus activates receptors in skin, muscle, or joint, the somatic pain that results is usually well-localized and easily described by the patient (see Table 3-1). In contrast, pain of visceral origin is often poorly localized and may be referred to an area of skin supplied by the same sensory roots that innervate the diseased visceral organ. For example, myocardial pain activates visceral afferents terminating in the upper four thoracic segments of the spinal cord. This nociceptive information converges on the same neurons that receive cutaneous input from the T1 to T4 dermatomes, and the reported pain is frequently referred to this region of otherwise normal skin or underlying tissue. Visceral pain originating in the gallbladder or kidney will similarly refer pain to the corresponding dermatome.

Both cutaneous and visceral pain are common experiences and do not always signal a disease process. The somatic pain resulting from a new injury or illness is therefore generally familiar to the patient and described in the context of prior similar pains. Somatic pain due to activation of normal nociceptive mechanisms is usually effectively relieved by a brief course of an appropriate analgesic.

Neuropathic pain Pain can also result from injury to, or chronic changes in, peripheral or central somatosensory pathways. This may be due to the induced abnormal pattern of afferent neuronal activity that reaches the dorsal horn and more central structures. Damage to sensory pathways may also decrease the inhibitory controls that are normally activated by a peripheral input. Neuropathic pain that follows damage to sensory pathways can develop and persist without a demonstrable primary nociceptive stimulus. In contrast to most somatic pain, neuropathic pain is frequently poorly localized. The patient often uses unusual terms to describe the pain, emphasizing the distinction between perception of normal somatic pains and neuropathic sensations (Table 3-1).

The sensory symptoms in neuropathic pain can be either focal or

FIGURE 3-1 *A. Ascending nociceptive pathways. The direct spinothalamic tract terminates in the nucleus ventroposterolateralis (VPL). The indirect, spinoreticulothalamic pathway relays through the brainstem reticular formation and ends in nuclei of the medial and intralaminar thalamus [nuclei parafascicularis (Pfc) and centralis lateralis (CL)]. B. Descending analgesia pathways. Periaqueductal gray neurons project to nucleus raphe magnus. A descending projection from raphe magnus inhibits the nociceptive responses of dorsal horn neurons. A separate inhibitory pathway from the nucleus locus coeruleus also directly ends in dorsal horn.*

THALAMUS

CL

VPL

Pfc

Reticulo-Thalamic System

Spinothalamic System

Dorsolateral Fasciculus

Periaqueductal Gray Region

MIDBRAIN

Locus Coeruleus

PONS

Raphe Magnus

MEDULLA

SPINAL CORD

A   B

more generalized. Trauma or irritation to a peripheral nerve may result in a *neuralgia,* which is defined as pain in the distribution of a single nerve; the pain is often (but not always) accompanied by signs of nerve dysfunction, such as sensory loss or weakness of muscles innervated by the nerve. Frequently the pain consists of a background spontaneous burning or aching sensation (*dysesthesia*) that can be associated with paroxysmal jabs of sharp pain within the affected region. Despite an elevated sensory detection threshold, patients will often have an exaggerated response to a nociceptive stimulus (*hyperalgesia*) or to touch (*hyperesthesia*) or perceive a non-nociceptive stimulus as painful (*allodynia*). These terms for altered hypersensitivity to sensory stimuli are commonly grouped under the term *hyperpathia.*

In some forms of neuralgia (such as trigeminal neuralgia) paroxysmal, lancinating pain predominates without other signs of nerve dysfunction. In contrast, *causalgia* following nerve injury is characterized by a continuous, severe burning pain, allodynia, and evident sympathetic dysfunction. Pain can also be a feature of more generalized neuropathies associated with the degeneration of small caliber axons. In such cases there can be multiple locations for the pain as well as a variety of types of pain. In diffuse sensory or sensorimotor neuropathies, the pain is usually symmetric and distal, affecting the feet and, with progression, the hands. As with more focal neuralgias, the pain often consists of a spontaneous aching or burning sensation with superimposed paroxysmal jabs of pain. Allodynia and hyperalgesia are common features during acute, painful phases of the disease.

Pain may also be a debilitating symptom following damage to central somatosensory pathways. Lesions of the ascending somatosensory pathways at the level of the cord, brainstem, thalamus, or cortex can result in a syndrome of continuous spontaneous pain that is referred to the periphery, often with superimposed sensory abnormalities as discussed above.

Psychological aspects of pain   In certain pain patients, particularly those with chronic pain, there is often little correlation between the severity of active disease and the amount of pain behavior. Social and psychological factors may be important dimensions that exacerbate and perpetuate pain complaints in such patients. An appraisal by a psychiatrist or a psychologist should therefore be part of the complete evaluation of most patients with persistent pain complaints. Psychological tests, including the Minnesota Multiphasic Personality Profile, can form an important part of this evaluation.

Several categories of psychological diagnoses can be associated with chronic pain syndromes. The two most common presentations are patients with depression and patients with somatoform disorders.

DEPRESSION   Depressive symptoms are common in patients with chronic pain, and depressive illness is found in approximately 30 percent. Many pain patients deny depression and do not show a depressed affect. In such patients vegetative signs of insomnia, diminished libido, and lack of energy may be present.

The relationship between pain and depression is complex. The pain threshold is lowered in clinically depressed patients, and pain is a common complaint among patients with primary depression. Patients with pain associated with chronic somatic disease also frequently develop depressive symptoms. However, the incidence of depression defined by strict clinical criteria is not clearly different in chronic pain patients when compared to medically ill patients without pain.

In an effort to delineate more clearly the relationship between pain and depression, a subgroup of chronic pain patients with a "pain-prone" disorder has been described. Such patients tend to have a hypochondriacal preoccupation with their pain. The pain is often continuous in nature and obscure in origin. Associated with the pain complaint, the patient may have depressive symptoms of insomnia, fatigue, and despair. Pain-prone individuals have developmental histories characterized by stress and unmet dependency needs. There may be a family history of depression, alcoholism, or physical abuse. Before the onset of their pain, however, such

TABLE 3-1   Characteristics of somatic and neuropathic pain

SOMATIC PAIN

1 Nociceptive stimulus usually evident.
2 Pain is usually well localized; visceral pain may be referred.
3 Pain is similar to other somatic pains in the patient's experience.
4 Pain is relieved by anti-inflammatory or narcotic analgesics.

NEUROPATHIC PAIN

1 No obvious nociceptive stimulus.
2 Pain is often poorly localized.
3 Pain is unusual, dissimilar from somatic pain.
4 Pain is only partially relieved by narcotic analgesics.

individuals have an idealized view of themselves and their family relations, denying conflicts. They may also have compulsive work records and hold several jobs. Chronic pain in this group of individuals may be associated in part with unresolved personal or interpersonal conflicts.

Consistent with the association of pain and depression, antidepressant drugs can stabilize the sleep pattern and improve the dysphoric symptoms of patients with chronic pain. There is often a reduction in the intensity of reported pain that may be associated with a decrease in the requirement for analgesics. Antidepressants may therefore have an important role in the management of chronic pain, although it is still uncertain whether these drugs act primarily to potentiate analgesics or to relieve subclinical depression.

SOMATOFORM DISORDERS   Patients with somatoform disorders have symptoms that suggest an organic disease but have no evidence of a physical disorder that might explain these symptoms. The heading "somatoform disorders" includes patients with somatization disorder, conversion disorder, hypochondriasis, or psychogenic pain disorder. Although symptoms of chronic pain are often part of the presentation of a somatoform disorder, patients with this diagnosis are not clinically depressed and do not usually respond to antidepressants. However, such patients seek out doctors and undergo repetitive tests to evaluate vague complaints. A variety of analgesics, anxiolytics, and muscle relaxants are usually prescribed with little or no benefit. Surgical procedures are often performed for pain relief without success.

Patients with somatoform disorders need frequent reassurance that their pain is benign; the management of these conditions is therefore primarily supportive. These patients should have careful follow-up from a small number of care givers to minimize unnecessary tests and reduce the amount of medication prescribed. In this group of patients diagnosing new pains that signal true organic pathology can be a clinical challenge.

MANAGEMENT OF PATIENTS WITH PAIN   Acute somatic pain is usually effectively treated with nonnarcotic analgesic agents which decrease pain without causing an alteration in the level of consciousness (Table 3-2). Aspirin, 300 to 600 mg, or acetaminophen, 600 mg, orally every 4 h is often effective. Other nonsteroidal anti-inflammatory agents, including phenacetin, naproxen, sulindac, or ibuprofen, may be used; however, there is little evidence that these agents are clearly better than the less expensive analgesics aspirin and acetaminophen. All nonsteroidal anti-inflammatory drugs have side effects of gastrointestinal irritation and may cause allergic reactions. The side effects of aspirin, particularly dyspepsia, gastrointestinal bleeding, and inhibition of platelet aggregation, are not observed with acetaminophen; however, acetaminophen does not have anti-inflammatory properties. Aspirin and acetaminophen in combination are not more effective than either one alone, but either in combination with codeine is more effective than codeine alone.

Narcotic analgesics are usually required for relief of severe pain. In general, patients should be treated with only one narcotic agent at a time, and therapy should be begun with an intermediate strength narcotic such as codeine, 30 mg every 4 to 6 h. In oral doses, codeine is relatively safe, potent, and well tolerated. However, if codeine,

TABLE 3-2 Drugs used to relieve pain

NONNARCOTIC ANALGESICS: EQUIVALENT DOSES AND INTERVALS

Generic Name	Dose, mg	Interval
Aspirin	750–1250	q 3 h
Phenacetin	750–1000	q 3 h
Acetaminophen	600–800	q 3 h
Phenylbutazone	200–400	q 4 h
Indomethacin	50–75	q 4 h
Ibuprofen	200–400	q 4 h
Naproxen	250–500	q 4 h
Nefopam	60–120	q 4 h

NARCOTIC ANALGESICS COMPARED TO 10 MG MORPHINE SULFATE (MS)

Generic Name	IM Dose, mg	PO dose, mg	Differences from MS
Oxymorphine	1	6	None
Hydromorphine	1.5	7.5	Shorter acting
Levorphanol	2	4	Good PO-IM potency
Heroin	4		Short-acting
Methadone	10	20	Good PO-IM potency
Morphine	10	60	
Oxycodone	15	30	Short-acting
Meperidine	75	300	None
Pentazocine	60	180	Agonist-antagonist
Codeine	130	200	More toxic

ANTICONVULSANTS

Generic Name	PO Dose, mg	Interval
Phenytoin	100	q 6–8 h
Carbamazepine	200	q 6 h
Clonazepam	1	q 6 h

ANTIDEPRESSANTS

Generic name	PO Dose, mg	Range, mg/day
Doxepin	200	75–400
Amitriptyline	150	75–300
Imipramine	200	75–400
Nortriptyline	100	40–150
Desipramine	150	75–300
Amoxapine	200	75–300
Trazodone	150	50–600

60 mg orally every 4 h, fails to provide relief, then it should be discontinued in favor of a higher potency narcotic, such as morphine or meperidine in the appropriate dosage and frequency. Increasing doses of codeine well above the recommended range will increase the frequency of side effects without clearly adding to its analgesic effectiveness.

Patients with pain due to evident organic disease are frequently treated with parenteral narcotic analgesics such as morphine or meperidine on an "every 6 h when necessary" basis. Effective analgesia from such drugs usually lasts only 2 to 3 h, allowing the patient to reexperience pain before the next dose. Analgesics given on a when necessary basis are also rarely administered as frequently as ordered, resulting in periods of inadequate analgesia; this produces a situation that reinforces "pain behavior," potentially delaying recovery. Inadequate analgesia in postoperative patients reduces the tidal volume due to splinting and delays patient mobilization. When indicated, narcotic analgesics should be given frequently enough and in high enough doses to alleviate pain. Pain medication should be offered the patient on a routine rather than a when necessary basis, with the understanding that the patient can refuse the drug if the level of analgesia is sufficient. Changes in analgesic doses and the need to taper narcotics as the acute phase of pain passes should be understood by the patient.

Chronic diseases usually cause recurrent bouts of acute pain rather than continuous discomfort. The management of acute painful exacerbations should be the same as the treatment of any new, acute pain. Analgesics should be available to the patient when pain is present, with the understanding between patient and physician that the drugs will be discontinued as the acute episode subsides.

Patients with terminal diseases such as metastatic cancer often suffer from continuous or recurrent acute pain. In such patients, tolerance to medications becomes an important factor. Increasing doses of narcotic analgesics may be necessary in such patients to maintain satisfactory analgesia, although the underlying disease process remains essentially unchanged. As the narcotic dose is increased, the frequency of side effects including sedation, dysphoric reactions, and constipation may also increase. In selected patients with terminal disease, morphine injections through spinal epidural or intrathecal catheters can provide substantial analgesia with potentially few side effects. For most patients, however, a change in drug, dose, or the addition of an adjuvant analgesic can often improve pain relief while minimizing adverse reactions.

Management of neuropathic pain Neuropathic pain is often a chronic disabling condition that can involve pathophysiologic changes at many levels of the nervous system. The medical management of neuropathic pain is disappointing, however, and patients rarely achieve substantial, lasting improvement with any single therapy. For patients with neuropathic pain, conventional analgesics are only rarely effective. The search for improved forms of treatment in such patients has resulted in a number of approaches.

ANTICONVULSANTS   In patients with neuropathic pain with little or no evidence of sympathetic dysfunction, anticonvulsants and antidepressant drugs are frequently prescribed, although there is only limited evidence that such medications are effective.

Phenytoin, carbamazepine, or clonazepam may be helpful in certain patients with painful neuropathies or neuralgias. Anticonvulsants are particularly effective in treating the sharp, lancinating pains associated with focal neuralgias such as trigeminal neuralgia. They are less effective for the more constant dull, burning sensations that are a major component of conditions such as postherpetic neuralgia or diabetic neuropathy.

ANTISYMPATHETIC AGENTS   In some patients, traumatic neuralgias can present with spontaneous burning pain and evidence of sympathetic dysfunction in the affected limb. This condition is termed *causalgia* and may be a distinct form of sympathetic dystrophy. Associated with the sensory changes in causalgia are disturbances in the sympathetic innervation of the affected limb. Sympathectomy by either surgery or local anesthetic block frequently relieves the pain in causalgia, and in the opinion of a number of authors pain relief by sympathetic block is an essential part of the diagnosis.

When pain relief follows a sympathetic block, treatment with intravenous regional or systemic antisympathetic drugs such as guanethidine may provide sustained relief in some patients.

TRICYCLIC ANTIDEPRESSANTS   Antidepressant drugs are frequently used to treat pain following peripheral nerve injury. Tricyclic iminodibenzyl derivatives are the most commonly used drugs. Their pharmacologic effects include facilitation of monoamine transmission by inhibition of transmitter reuptake at the synapse and changes in pre- and postsynaptic adrenergic receptor sensitivity. The important site of action of tricyclic antidepressants for pain relief is not clear. However, they may act to potentiate the brainstem inhibition of nociceptive transmission at the level of the dorsal horn. Tricyclic antidepressants also have major effects on ascending monoaminergic systems that project into the forebrain. It seems probable that these ascending systems are also important in pain perception, although how antidepressant drugs influence sensory pathways at the level of the thalamus and cortex remains speculative.

TRANSCUTANEOUS ELECTRICAL NERVE STIMULATION (TENS)   Electrical stimulation with a TENS unit applied to the painful region or over the proximal nerve may provide substantial pain relief in patients with painful nerve injuries. However, the duration of the effect is usually limited to the period of stimulation. After a period of days to months, in many patients the analgesic response to TENS habituates, and electrical stimulation may actually worsen the patient's pain.

Management of chronic pain Unrelieved pain that has continued to be a major, disabling condition for a minimum of 6 months is usually referred to as "chronic" pain. Patients with chronic pain often present special problems in evaluation and management.

When patients with long-standing chronic pain are seen for a new evaluation, they often have unrealistic expectations of the physician. Frequently they state that none of their prior physicians was competent and that this is their last hope for relief from their suffering. A detailed medical history will often reveal poor compliance with previous treatment recommendations made by other physicians.

To avoid another treatment failure, the chronic pain patient should be evaluated by a multidisciplinary group of specialists skilled in managing chronic pain complaints. The specialists composing this group may vary, depending on the nature of the pain complaint and the resources available at an institution. At a minimum, however, a patient should receive a medical, psychological, neurologic, and physical therapy evaluation. A group approach avoids potential confrontation between patient and physician that may stall progress; it also enhances the credibility of the treatment group, increasing the likelihood of patient compliance. The goal of this evaluation is to establish a treatment plan with specific objectives. Each objective should be accomplished according to a timetable mutually agreed on by the patient and the treatment team.

In general, three main goals should be emphasized. First, drug treatment should be simplified and minimized. In many chronic pain patients, common analgesics and muscle relaxants are only minimally effective. The patient therefore tends to increase the dosage in the hope of enhancing pain relief. With the patient's understanding, the number of medications should be reduced by eliminating redundant or ineffective drugs. The dosages of the remaining medications should then be decreased systematically to a point where the patient is taking only drugs that have a definite beneficial effect with minimal side effects.

The second goal of therapy is to assist the patient in developing a better understanding of the pain and the factors that exacerbate it. The psychological significance of the pain and its relationship to developmental or interpersonal factors may be worth exploring with individual patients. Antidepressant medications also have a role in the management of affective symptoms in certain chronic pain patients.

The third goal of therapy should be to increase mobilization and functional ability. Under the direction of a specialist in rehabilitation medicine, a program of physical treatments for pain relief (TENS, massage, etc.) should be coupled with an exercise program to increase pain-free movement. Realistic timetables should be set for a return to self-care and independent function.

Social and interpersonal factors may perseverate pain; certain chronic pain patients are therefore refractory to treatment on an outpatient basis. Admission to an in-patient multidisciplinary pain treatment facility can provide an opportunity for an intensive program of evaluation and treatment of such patients. Standards for such in-patient units have been established by the Committee on Standards of Pain Treatment Facilities of the American Pain Society. Studies of the effectiveness of pain treatment units demonstrate a decreased report of pain, decreased drug use, and increased functional ability in the majority of patients completing this type of program. However, the ultimate success of such programs depends on maintained functional improvement in patients over long periods following discharge. Careful follow-up and reevaluation of successfully managed chronic pain patients, as with all medical patients, becomes a priority.

REFERENCES

ARONOFF GM: Psychological aspects of nonmalignant chronic pain, in *Evaluation and Treatment of Chronic Pain*, GM Aronoff (ed). Baltimore, Urban and Schwarzenberg, 1985

ASBURY A, FIELDS HL: Pain due to peripheral nerve damage: An hypothesis. Neurology 34:1587–1590, 1984

BASBAUM AI, FIELDS HL: Endogenous pain control systems: Brainstem spinal pathways and endorphin circuitry. Ann Rev Neurosci 7:309–338, 1984

BLUMER D, HEILBRONN: Chronic pain as a variant of depressive disease. J Nerv Ment Dis 170:381–406, 1982

FIELDS HL: Pain II: New approaches to management. Ann Neurol 9:101, 1981

HACKETT TP: The pain patient: Evaluation and treatment, in *Massachusetts General Hospital Handbook of General Hospital Psychiatry*, TP Hackett (ed). pp 41–63, 1978

HANNINGTON-KIFF JG: Antisympathetic drugs in limbs. In *Textbook of Pain*, PD Wall, R Melzack (ed). Edinburgh, Churchill Livingstone, 1983

MACIEWICZ R, FIELDS HL: Pain pathways, in *Diseases of the Nervous System*, A Asbury, G McKann (ed). London, Saunders, 1986

SWEET WH, POLETTI CE: Causalgia, in *Evaluation and Treatment of Chronic Pain*, GM Aronoff (ed). Baltimore, Urban and Schwarzenberg, 1985

TASKER RR: Deafferentation, in *Textbook of Pain*, P Wall (ed). Edinburgh, Churchill Livingstone, 1984, pp 119–132

TAUB A, COLLINS WF: Observations on the treatment of denervation dysesthesia with psychotropic drugs: Postherpetic neuralgia, anesthesia dolorosa, peripheral neuropathy, in *Advances in Neurology*, JJ Bonica (ed). New York, Raven, 1974, pp 309–315

WHITE JC, SWEET WH: *Pain and the Neurosurgeon—A Forty Year's Experience*. Springfield, Illinois, Charles C Thomas, 1969

YAKSH TL, HAMMOND DL: Peripheral and central substrates involved in the rostrad transmission of nociceptive information. Pain 13:1–85, 1982

4   CHEST DISCOMFORT AND PALPITATION

EUGENE BRAUNWALD

CHEST DISCOMFORT

Chest discomfort is one of the most frequent complaints for which patients seek medical attention; the potential benefit (or harm) resulting from the proper (or improper) assessment and management of the patient with this complaint is enormous. An incorrect diagnosis of a potentially hazardous condition such as angina pectoris is likely to have harmful psychologic and economic consequences and may lead to unnecessary complex procedures, such as cardiac catheterization and coronary arteriography, while failure to recognize a serious disorder, such as ischemic heart disease or mediastinal tumor, may result in the dangerous delay of much-needed treatment. There is little relation between the severity of chest discomfort and the gravity of its cause. Therefore, a frequent problem in patients who complain of chest discomfort or pain is distinguishing trivial disorders from coronary artery disease and other serious disorders.

The radiation of pain arising in the thoracic viscera can usually be explained in terms of the known facts concerning nerve supply (Chap. 3). One occasionally sees a patient with extension of discomfort to a location which cannot be logically explained. In most instances, such a person will be found to have more than one disorder capable of causing chest discomfort. The presence of one condition may affect the radiation of the pain produced by the other disorder. For example, when the discomfort of transient myocardial ischemia, i.e., angina pectoris, extends to the back or abdomen, the patient may be found to have also a significant degree of spinal arthritis or an upper abdominal disorder, such as hiatus hernia, disease of the gallbladder, pancreatitis, or peptic ulcer. Pain impulses which enter one cord segment may spill over and excite nearby cord segments. In this manner, the pain of myocardial ischemia may be referred to the epigastrium in a patient with chronic cholecystitis.

It should not be assumed that the presence of an objective abnormality, such as a hiatus hernia or an electrocardiographic abnormality, necessarily means that an *atypical* chest pain arises in the stomach or the heart. Such an assumption is justified only if a careful clinical examination, if necessary supported by appropriate laboratory tests, indicates that the behavior of the discomfort is compatible with the site of origin suggested by the objective finding.

THE LEFT-ARM MYTH There is a long tradition, widely accepted by physicians and nonphysicians alike, that discomfort in the left arm, especially when appearing in conjunction with chest discomfort, has a unique and ominous significance as being almost certain evidence of the presence of ischemic heart disease. This is a myth that has neither theoretic nor clinical foundation. Impulses from somatic structures, such as the skin, and visceral structures, such as the esophagus and heart, converge on a common pool of neurons in the posterior horn of the spinal cord. Their origin may be confused by the cerebral cortex. Also, stimulation of one of the thoracic nerves that also innervates the heart by, for example, protrusion of an intervertebral disk, may be misinterpreted as pain originating from the heart.

From a theoretic standpoint, *any* disorder involving the deep afferent fibers of the left upper thoracic region should be capable of causing discomfort in the chest, the left arm, or both areas. Hence almost any condition capable of causing chest discomfort may induce radiation to the left arm. Such localization is common not only in patients with coronary disease but also in those with numerous other types of chest pain. Although discomfort due to myocardial ischemia most frequently is substernal, radiates down the ulnar aspect of the left arm (Chap. 189), and is pressing and constricting in nature, the location, radiation, and quality of the discomfort are of less diagnostic significance than its behavior in terms of the conditions which induce it and relieve it.

Most persons also believe that cardiac pain is situated in the region of the left breast, and therefore left inframammary pain is one of the common symptoms that brings the patient to seek medical advice. It differs radically from the discomfort due to myocardial ischemia, i.e., angina pectoris. The left inframammary discomfort is either a momentary, sharp and lancinating pain, or a long-lasting, dull ache, occasionally accentuated by sharp stabs. Relief of non-anginal discomfort is often sudden, or occurs slowly and after prolonged rest, and may not be temporally related to nitroglycerin administration. In contrast to angina pectoris, such precordial pain usually has *no* relationship to exertion, may be accompanied by tenderness over the precordium and is frequently observed in patients who are tense, easily fatigued, unusually anxious, or psychoneurotic. Angina pectoris, on the other hand, is usually described as a *discomfort* rather than frank *pain* in the chest and is characteristically substernal rather than precordial. It is further characterized on page 19.

DISCOMFORT DUE TO MYOCARDIAL ISCHEMIA   Physiologic considerations of the coronary circulation

Discomfort due to myocardial ischemia occurs when the oxygen supply to the heart is deficient in relation to the oxygen need. The oxygen consumption of this organ is closely related to the physiologic effort made during contraction. It is dependent primarily on three factors: (1) the tension developed by the myocardium, (2) the contractile (inotropic) state of the myocardium, and (3) the heart rate. When these three factors remain relatively constant, an elevation of stroke volume produces an efficient type of response because it leads to an increase in the external work of the heart (i.e., in the product of cardiac output and arterial pressure) with little accompanying augmentation of myocardial oxygen requirements. Thus, a rise in flow load (unless it raises intraventricular wall tension markedly by increasing preload substantially) causes less increment in myocardial oxygen consumption than does a comparable increase in cardiac work brought about by elevation either of pressure or of heart rate. The net effects of the changes in these hemodynamic variables depend not on oxygen need alone, but rather on the balance between the demand for and the supply of oxygen. The heart is always active, and the coronary venous blood is normally much more desaturated than that draining other areas of the body. Thus the removal of more oxygen from each unit of blood, which is one of the adjustments commonly utilized by exercising skeletal muscle, is already employed in the heart in the basal state. Therefore, the heart must rely primarily on an increase in the coronary blood flow for obtaining additional oxygen.

The blood flow through the coronary arteries is directly proportional to the pressure gradient between the aorta and the ventricular myocardium during systole and the ventricular cavity during diastole, but is also proportional to the fourth power of the radius of the coronary arteries. Thus a relatively slight alteration in coronary diameter below a critical level of coronary luminal diameter can produce a large change in coronary flow, provided that other factors remain constant. Coronary blood flow occurs primarily during diastole, when it is unopposed by systolic myocardial compression of the coronary vessels. Coronary flow is regulated primarily by myocardial oxygen needs, probably through the release of vasodilator metabolites, such as adenosine, and through variations in myocardial P_{O_2}. Control of the lumen of the coronary arterial bed through autonomic nerves and by hydraulic factors constitute additional important mechanisms of regulation of coronary blood flow.

When the epicardial coronary arteries are narrowed critically (>70 percent stenosis of the luminal diameter), the intramyocardial coronary arterioles dilate in an effort to maintain total coronary blood flow at a level that will avert myocardial ischemia at rest. Further dilatation which normally occurs during exercise is therefore not possible. Thus, any condition in which increased heart rate, arterial pressure, or myocardial contractility occurs in the presence of coronary obstruction tends to precipitate anginal attacks by increasing myocardial oxygen needs in the face of a fixed supply. Bradycardia, when not severe, usually has the opposite effects, and this apparently explains the rarity of angina in patients with complete heart block, even when this disorder is associated with coronary disease.

Causes of myocardial ischemia   By far the most frequent underlying cause is organic narrowing of the coronary arteries secondary to coronary atherosclerosis. A *dynamic* component of increased coronary vascular resistance, secondary to spasm of the major epicardial vessels, often near an atherosclerotic placque, or to constriction of smaller coronary arterioles is present in many, perhaps the majority, of patients with chronic angina pectoris. Less frequently, narrowing of the coronary orifices due to syphilitic aortitis or to distortion by an aortic dissection may be responsible. There is no evidence that systemic arterial constriction or increased cardiac contractile activity (rise in heart rate or blood pressure, or increase in contractility due to liberation of catecholamines or adrenergic activity) due to emotion can precipitate angina unless there is also narrowing of the coronary vessels.

Aside from conditions which narrow the lumen of the coronary arteries, the only other frequent causes of myocardial ischemia are disorders, such as aortic stenosis and/or regurgitation (Chap. 187), which cause a marked disproportion between the perfusion pressure and the heart's oxygen requirements. Under such conditions the rise in left ventricular systolic pressure is not, as in hypertensive states, balanced by a corresponding elevation of aortic perfusion pressure.

An increase in heart rate is especially harmful in patients with coronary atherosclerosis and with aortic stenosis, because on the one hand it increases myocardial oxygen needs, and on the other it shortens diastole more than systole and thereby decreases the total available perfusion time per minute.

Patients with marked *right ventricular hypertension* may have exertional pain which is quite similar to that of the common type of angina. It is likely that this discomfort results from relative ischemia of the right ventricle brought about by the increased oxygen needs and by the elevated intramural resistance, with reduction of the normally large systolic pressure gradient which perfuses this chamber. Angina is common in patients with *syphilitic aortitis,* in whom the relative roles of aortic regurgitation and of coronary ostial narrowing are difficult to assess. The importance of tachycardia, decline in arterial pressure, thyrotoxicosis, or diminution in arterial oxygen content (such as occurs in anemia or arterial hypoxia) in the production of myocardial hypoxia will be apparent from the above discussion. However, these are precipitating and aggravating factors rather than the underlying cause of angina; as already noted, the latter is, in almost all instances, coronary arterial narrowing.

Effects of myocardial ischemia   A common manifestation of ischemia is *anginal discomfort*, considered in some detail in Chap. 189. Usually it is described as a heavy pressure or squeezing, a sensation of strangling or constriction in the chest, a "burning" or "heavy feeling," or difficulty in breathing, and it occurs particularly on walking, especially after meals, on cold days, against a wind or uphill. Typically it develops gradually during exertion, after heavy meals, and with anger, excitement, frustration, and other emotional states; it is not precipitated by coughing or respiratory movements or other motion. When angina is induced by walking, it forces the patient to stop or to reduce speed; it is characteristically relieved by rest and nitroglycerin. The exact mechanism of the stimulus for anginal discomfort is still unknown, but it is probably related to an accumulation of metabolites within the heart muscle. Angina occurs most typically in the substernal region, anteriorly across the midthorax; it may radiate to or rarely occur alone in the interscapular region, in the arms, shoulders, teeth, and abdomen. It rarely radiates to below the umbilicus or to the back of the neck or the occiput. The more severe the attack, the greater the radiation from the substernal areas to the left arm, especially its ulnar aspect.

Myocardial infarction is usually associated with a discomfort similar in quality and distribution to that of angina but of longer duration (usually 30 min) and of sufficient intensity that it qualifies as true *pain*. In contrast to angina, the pain of myocardial infarction is not relieved by rest or by coronary dilator drugs and may require large doses of narcotics. It may be accompanied by diaphoresis, nausea, and hypotension (Chap. 190).

A second effect of myocardial ischemia consists of *electrocardiographic changes* (Chaps. 178, 189, and 190). Many patients with angina have normal tracings between attacks, and the record may even remain normal during the episode of pain. However, depression of the ST segments, caused by myocardial ischemia, typically occurs during exertion and is accompanied by anginal discomfort; moreover, electrocardiographic evidence of myocardial ischemia may occur at rest and with or without accompanying chest discomfort. The finding of flat or downsloping ST-segment depressions of 0.1 mV or greater during an attack of pain, with a return to normal after the pain subsides, strongly suggests that the pain is anginal in origin. The value and limitation of electrocardiographic changes occurring after exercise in the diagnosis of angina pectoris are discussed in Chap. 189.

A third effect of myocardial ischemia is impairment of *myocardial contraction*. The left ventricular end-diastolic and pulmonary vascular pressures may rise during anginal attacks, particularly if they are prolonged and are caused, presumably, by the decreased contractility and reduced distensibility of the ischemic areas. A fourth heart sound is also frequently heard during the anginal episode; paradoxic pulsations may be evident on palpation of the precordium and can be recorded by apex cardiography. Two-dimensional echocardiography or left ventricular angiography carried out during myocardial ischemia often reveals left ventricular dysfunction, i.e., hypokinesis or akinesis (Chap. 179) in the territory of the obstructed vessel(s).

Another characteristic effect of myocardial ischemia is liability to sudden death (Chap. 30). This may never occur, despite thousands of anginal episodes. However, it may supervene early in the disease and even in the first attack. The usual mechanism is probably ischemia-induced ventricular fibrillation, but occasionally sudden death may be due to ventricular standstill in patients with impaired atrioventricular conduction.

PAIN DUE TO IRRITATION OF SEROUS MEMBRANES OR JOINTS Pericarditis

The visceral surface of the pericardium ordinarily is insensitive to pain, as is the parietal surface, except in its lower portion, which has a relatively small number of pain fibers carried in the phrenic nerves. The pain associated with pericarditis is believed to be due to inflammation of the adjacent parietal pleura. These observations explain why noninfectious pericarditis (e.g., that associated with uremia and with myocardial infarction) and cardiac tamponade with relatively mild inflammation are usually painless or accompanied by only mild pain, whereas infectious pericarditis, being nearly always more intense and spreading to the neighboring pleura, is usually associated with pain having some pleuritic features, i.e.,

it is aggravated by breathing, coughing, etc. Since the central part of the diaphragm receives its sensory supply from the phrenic nerve (which arises from the third to fifth cervical segments of the spinal cord), pain arising from the lower parietal pericardium and central tendon of the diaphragm is felt characteristically at the tip of the shoulder, the adjoining trapezius ridge, and the neck. Involvement of the more lateral part of the diaphragmatic pleura, supplied by branches from the sixth to ninth intercostal nerves, causes pain not only in the anterior part of the chest but also in the upper part of the abdomen or corresponding region of the back, sometimes simulating the pain of acute cholecystitis or pancreatitis.

Pericarditis causes two distinct types of pain (Chap. 194). The commonest is pleuritic pain, related to respiratory movements and aggravated by cough and/or deep inspiration. It is sometimes brought on by swallowing, because the esophagus lies just beyond the posterior portion of the heart and is often altered by a change of bodily position, becoming sharper and more left-sided in the supine position and reduced when the patient sits upright, leaning forward. It is frequently referred to the neck and lasts longer than the pain of angina pectoris. This type of pain is due to the pleuritic component of infectious pleuropericarditis.

The second form of pericardial pain is the steady, crushing substernal pain which mimics that of acute myocardial infarction. The mechanism of this steady substernal pain is not certain, but it may arise from marked inflammation of the relatively sensitive inner parietal surface of the pericardium, or from irritated afferent cardiac nerve fibers lying in the periadventitial layers of the superficial coronary arteries. Occasionally both types of pain may be present simultaneously.

The painful syndromes which may follow trauma to or operations on the heart (i.e., the postcardiotomy syndrome) or myocardial infarction are discussed in later chapters (Chaps. 190 and 194). Such pain often but not always arises in the pericardium.

Pleural pain is very common; it generally results from stretching of inflamed parietal pleura and may be identical in character with that of pericarditis. It occurs in fibrinous pleurisy, as well as when pneumonic processes reach the periphery of the lung. Pneumothorax and tumors involving the pleural space may also irritate the parietal pleura and cause pleural pain; the latter is sharp, knifelike, superficial in quality, and its aggravation by each breath and by coughing distinguishes it from the deep, dull, relatively steady pain of myocardial ischemia.

The pain resulting from *pulmonary embolism* may resemble that of acute myocardial infarction, and in massive embolism it is located substernally. In patients with smaller emboli the pain is located more laterally, is pleuritic in nature, and may be associated with hemoptysis (Chap. 211). Massive pulmonary emboli and other causes of acute pulmonary hypertension may cause severe, persistent substernal pain, presumably due to distention of the pulmonary artery. The pain of *mediastinal emphysema* (Chap. 214) may be intense and sharp and may radiate from the substernal region to the shoulders; often a distinct crepitus is heard. The pain associated with *mediastinitis* and *mediastinal tumors* usually resembles that of pleuritis but is more likely to be maximal in the substernal region, and the associated feeling of constriction or oppression may cause confusion with myocardial infarction. The pain due to *acute dissection of the aorta* or to an expanding aortic aneurysm results from stimulation of the adventitia; it is usually extremely severe, is localized to the center of the chest, lasts for hours, and requires unusually large amounts of analgesics for relief. It often radiates into the back but is not aggravated by changes in position or respiration (Chap. 197).

The *costochondral and chondrosternal articulations* are the commonest sites of anterior chest pain. Objective signs in the form of swelling (Tietze's syndrome), redness, and heat are rare, but sharply localized tenderness is common. The pain may be darting and lasting for only a few seconds, or a dull ache enduring for hours or days. An associated feeling of tightness due to muscle spasm (see below) is frequent. When the discomfort persists for a few days only, a story of minor trauma or of some unaccustomed physical effort can often be obtained. *Pressure on the chondrosternal and costochondral junctions is an essential part of the examination of every patient with chest pain* and will reproduce the pain arising from these tissues. A large percentage of patients with costochondral pain, especially those who also have minor and innocent T-wave alterations, are erroneously labeled as having coronary disease, sometimes with dire consequences. Pain in the xiphoid (xiphodynia) can also be reproduced by pressure on the xiphisternum.

Pain secondary to *subacromial bursitis* and *arthritis of the shoulder and spine* may be precipitated by exercise of the local area but not by general exertion. It may be brought about by passive movement of the involved area as well as by coughing. Other forms of chest pain include the "precordial catch," which may be associated with poor posture and characteristically lasts only a few seconds. Myofascitis of the pectoral muscle or biceps tendonitis may be confused with angina pectoris but may be reproduced by squeezing the pectoral muscles or the head of the biceps.

PAIN DUE TO TISSUE DISRUPTION Rupture or tear of a structure may give rise to pain that sets in abruptly and reaches its peak of intensity almost instantly. Such a story should arouse the suspicion of aortic dissection, pneumothorax, mediastinal emphysema, a cervical disk syndrome, or rupture of the esophagus. However, the patient may be too ill to recall the precise circumstances, or the pain may be atypical and increase gradually in severity. Likewise, other and more benign conditions, such as a slipped costal cartilage or an intercostal muscle cramp, may also produce pain with an abrupt onset.

CLINICAL ASPECTS OF THE COMMONER CAUSES OF CHEST PAIN The more serious causes of chest pain such as myocardial ischemia, aortic dissection, pericarditis, and disorders of the pleura, esophagus, stomach, duodenum, and pancreas are considered in the appropriate chapters dealing with these problems.

Pain arising in the chest wall or upper extremity This may develop as a result of muscle or ligament strains brought on by unaccustomed exercise and felt in the costochondral or chondrosternal junctions or in the chest wall muscles. Other causes are *osteoarthritis* of the dorsal or thoracic spine and *ruptured cervical disks*. Pain in the left upper extremity and precordium may be due to compression of portions of the brachial plexus by a cervical rib or by spasm and shortening of the scalenus anticus muscle secondary to high fixation of the ribs and sternum. Finally, pains in the upper extremity (shoulder-hand syndrome) and in the pectoral muscles may, through unknown mechanisms, occur in patients following myocardial infarction.

Pain arising in the chest wall or shoulder girdles or arms is usually recognized by the presence of localized tenderness of the affected area and the clear relation between pain and motion. Deep breathing, turning or twisting of the chest, and movements of the shoulder girdle and arm may elicit and duplicate the pain of which the patient complains. The pain may be very brief, lasting only a few seconds, or full and aching and enduring for hours. The duration is, therefore, likely to be either longer or shorter than untreated angina pectoris, which usually lasts for only a few minutes.

These skeletal pains often have a sharp or sticking quality. In addition, there is frequently a feeling of tightness, which is probably due to associated spasm of intercostal or pectoral muscles. This may produce the "morning stiffness" seen in so many skeletal disorders. The discomfort is unaffected by nitroglycerin but often is abolished by infiltration of the painful areas with procaine. When chest wall pain is of recent origin and follows trauma, strain, or some unusual activity involving the pectoral muscles, it presents no problem in diagnosis. However, since both disorders are common, long-standing skeletal pain is frequent in persons who also have angina pectoris. This coexistence of the two different types of chest pain in the same patient is frequently confusing because in the patient's mind the anginal needle may be hidden in the skeletal haystack. Thus every middle-aged or elderly patient who has long-standing anterior chest

wall pain merits careful study for the presence of ischemic heart disease.

The confusion created by the presence of innocent skeletal pain impairs the reliability of the history and is probably the commonest cause of errors—both positive and negative—in the diagnosis of angina pectoris. It may be necessary also to learn by direct observation whether exercise alone or postprandial exertion is capable of producing the pain. Repeated tests may be required, comparing the relative effects of preceding placebos and nitroglycerin on the amount of exertion required to induce the pain. When the history is inconclusive, the exercise electrocardiogram, or in patients with equivocal or nondiagnostic tests, the exercise stress test with thallium scintigraphy (Chap. 179), may furnish useful information concerning the existence of myocardial ischemia. In rare instances coronary arteriography may be required.

Esophageal pain This usually presents as deep thoracic pain; it results from chemical (acid) irritation of the esophageal mucosa secondary to acid reflux or from spasm of the esophageal muscle and characteristically follows deglutition. The sudden relief of pain by one or two swallows of food or water suggests esophageal pain. Accompanying dysphagia, regurgitation of undigested food, and weight loss direct attention to the esophagus (see Chaps. 32 and 234). The Bernstein acid perfusion test, in which an attempt is made to reproduce the pain by infusing 0.1 *M* HCl into the esophagus, is helpful in establishing acid gastric reflux into the esophagus as the cause of pain. Esophageal manometry and measurement of lower esophageal sphincter pressure, sometimes with ergonovine stimulation, are useful in identifying esophageal spasm as the origin of the pain.

Emotional disorders These are also common causes of chest pain. Usually, the discomfort is experienced as a sense of "tightness," sometimes called "aching," and occasionally it may be sufficiently severe as to be designated a pain of considerable magnitude. Since the discomfort has almost always the additional quality of tightness or constriction, and is often localized at least in part beneath the sternum, it is not surprising that this type of discomfort is frequently confused with that of myocardial ischemia. Ordinarily, it lasts for a half hour or more and may persist for a day or less with slow fluctuation of intensity. The association with fatigue or emotional strain is usually clear, although this may not be recognized by the patient until called to his or her attention. The pain probably develops through unconscious and prolonged increase of muscle tone, perhaps enhanced by accompanying hyperventilation (by causing a contraction of the chest wall muscles similar to the painful tetany of the extremities). When the hyperventilation and/or the associated adrenergic effect due to anxiety also causes innocent changes in the T waves and ST segments, the confusion with coronary disease is strengthened. However, the long duration of the pain, the lack of any relation to exertion but association rather with fatigue or tension, and the usually periodic occurrence on successive days without any limitation of capacity for exercise usually make the differentiation from ischemic pain quite clear.

Other causes of chest pain The several *abdominal disorders* which may at times mimic anginal pain may usually be suspected from the history, which, as in esophageal pain, ordinarily indicates some relationship to swallowing, eating, belching, etc. Pain resulting from gastric or duodenal ulcer (Chap. 235) is epigastric or substernal, commences about 1 to $1\frac{1}{2}$ h after meals, and is usually promptly relieved by antacids or milk. The gastrointestinal roentgenogram is of crucial significance, and roentgenographic examination is also often helpful in differentiating biliary, gastrointestinal, aortic, pulmonary, and skeletal disease pain from angina pectoris. The demonstration of the presence of a coexistent abdominal disorder such as a hiatus hernia does not constitute proof that the chest pain of which the patient complains is due to this. Such disorders are frequently asymptomatic and are not at all uncommon in patients who also have angina pectoris.

Substernal discomfort also frequently occurs in the presence of *tracheobronchitis;* it is described as a burning sensation accentuated by coughing. A variety of *disorders involving the breast,* including inflammatory breast disease, benign and malignant tumors, as well as mastodynia, are common causes of thoracic pain. The localization in the breast and superficial swelling and tenderness of this organ are of diagnostic importance. A number of other causes of thoracic pain or discomfort including spinal arthritis, herpes zoster, anterior scalene and hyperabduction syndromes, compression of the cervical roots, malignant disease of the ribs, while less common, can usually be readily recognized after appropriate observation.

APPROACH TO THE PATIENT WITH CHEST DISCOMFORT Most persons with this complaint will fall into one of two general groups. The first consists of persons with prolonged and often severe pain without obvious initiating factors. Such persons will frequently be seriously ill. The problem is that of differentiating such serious conditions as myocardial infarction, aortic dissection, and pulmonary embolism from each other and from less grave causes. In some such instances, a careful history and physical examination will provide significant clues, which can then be followed up by appropriate laboratory tests [electrocardiogram, serum enzymes, various forms of diagnostic imaging] which will commonly provide the correct answer.

The second group of patients comprises those who have brief episodes of pain and are otherwise in apparently excellent health. Here, the resting electrocardiogram will rarely supply decisive information, but records taken during or immediately after exercise or pain will often reveal characteristic changes (Chap. 189). Radionuclide scintigraphy at rest and during exercise (Chap. 179) is often helpful as well. However, in many instances it is the study of the subjective phenomenon, i.e., of the pain itself, that will lead to the diagnosis. Of the several methods of investigation which are available for such patients, three are of cardinal importance.

A detailed and *meticulous history* of the behavior of the pain is the most important method. The location, radiation, quality, intensity, and duration of the episodes are important. Even more so is the story of the aggravating and alleviating factors. A history of sharp aggravation by breathing, coughing, or other respiratory movements will usually point toward the pleura and pericardium or mediastinum as the site, although chest wall pain is likewise affected by respiratory motions. Similarly, a pain which regularly appears on rapid walking and vanishes within a few minutes upon standing still suggests the diagnosis of angina pectoris, although a similar story will occasionally be obtained from patients with skeletal disorders.

When the history is inconclusive, the *study of the patient at the time of the spontaneous episode* will often supply crucial information. For example, the electrocardiogram, which may be normal both at rest and even during or after exercise in the absence of pain, will occasionally demonstrate striking changes when recorded during an anginal episode. Similarly, radiographic study of the esophagus or of the stomach may show no evidence of cardiospasm or of hiatal hernia except when the observation is made during the pain.

The third method of study represents the *attempt to produce and alleviate the pain at will.* This procedure is necessary only when doubt exists following the history or when needed for psychotherapeutic purposes. Thus the demonstration that a localized pain, which can be reproduced by pressure on the chest, is completely relieved by local infiltration with procaine will often be of conclusive importance in convincing the patient that the heart is not the site. When the pain is precipitated by intravenous injections of ergonovine and this is accompanied by electrocardiographic ST-segment elevations and coronary spasm on arteriography, the diagnosis of Prinzmetal's angina can be made.

When, as is often the case, the history is atypical, the correct diagnosis of angina pectoris may be aided by noting the response to nitroglycerin. Relief of pain after its sublingual administration does not necessarily prove that there is a cause-and-effect relationship. It is necessary to be certain that the pain vanishes more rapidly (usually within 5 min) and more completely when the drug is used than when it is not employed. A false-negative impression concerning the effect of nitroglycerin may be the result of the use of a deteriorated preparation which has been exposed to light. In doubtful instances, repeated exercise tests, with and without preceding administration of nitroglycerin, may be necessary. The demonstration that the time required for a given exercise to produce pain is consistently and considerably longer when it is undertaken within a few minutes after a sublingual nitroglycerin pill than after a placebo may, in some instances, represent powerful clinical evidence for the recognition of angina pectoris. A completely negative response to such repeated tests constitutes powerful evidence against angina. Angina is rarely relieved within a few seconds of lying down, nor is angina suddenly precipitated by stooping forward.

In patients in whom the question of whether there is coronary disease cannot be resolved despite the aforementioned clinical and laboratory tests, including exercise electrocardiography (Chap. 178) and nuclear scintigraphy (Chap. 179), cardiac catheterization and coronary arteriography may be required. A useful stress test that can be carried out at the time of catheterization is to elevate the heart rate in stepwise fashion by electrical pacing; the development of ST-segment depressions on the electrocardiogram and the reproduction of the pain support the diagnosis of myocardial ischemia. Coronary arteriography will show critical (more than 70 percent) reduction of the luminal diameter in at least one major vessel in patients with obstructive coronary artery disease (Chaps. 180 and 189).

PALPITATION

Palpitation is a common, disagreeable symptom which may be defined as an awareness of the beating of the heart, an awareness most commonly brought about by a change in the heart's rhythm or rate or by an augmentation of its contractility. Palpitation is not pathognomonic of any particular group of disorders; indeed, often it signifies not a primary physical disorder but rather a psychological disturbance. Even when it occurs as a more or less prominent complaint, the diagnosis of the underlying disease is made largely on the basis of other associated symptoms and data. Nevertheless, palpitation is frequently of considerable importance in the minds of patients, who fear that it may indicate heart disease. Concern is all the more pronounced in patients who have been told that they *may* have heart disease; to them palpitation may seem to be an omen of impending disaster. Since the resulting anxiety may be associated with increased activity of the autonomic nervous system, with consequent increases of the cardiac rate and rhythm and the vigor of contraction, the patient's awareness of these changes may then lead to a vicious cycle, which may ultimately be responsible for incapacitation.

Palpitation may be described by the patient in various terms, such as "pounding," "fluttering," "flopping," and "skipping," and in most cases it will be obvious that the complaint is of a sensation of disturbed heartbeat. The sensitivity to alterations in cardiac activity among different individuals varies widely. Some patients seem to be unaware of the most serious and chaotic dysrhythmias; others are seriously troubled by an occasional extrasystole. Patients with anxiety states often exhibit a lowered threshold at which disorders of rate and rhythm result in palpitation. The awareness of the heartbeat also tends to be more common at night and during introspective moments, but is less marked during activity. Patients with organic heart disease and chronic disorders of cardiac rate, rhythm, or stroke volume tend to accommodate to these abnormalities and are often less sensitive than normal persons to such events. Persistent tachycardia and/or atrial fibrillation may not be accompanied by continuous palpitation, in contrast to a sudden, brief alteration in cardiac rate or rhythm which often causes considerable subjective discomfort. Palpitation is particularly prominent when the precipitating cause for increased heart rate or contractility or arrhythmia is recent, transient, and episodic. Conversely, in emotionally well-adjusted individuals palpitation becomes progressively less disconcerting as the cause (e.g., anemia, frequent extrasystoles, complete atrioventricular block) persists.

PATHOGENESIS OF PALPITATION   Under ordinary circumstances the rhythmic heartbeat is imperceptible to the healthy individual of placid or even average temperament. Palpitation may be experienced by normal persons who have engaged in strenuous physical effort or have been aroused emotionally or sexually. This type of palpitation is physiologic and represents the normal awareness of an overactive heart—i.e., a heart that is beating at a rapid rate and with an increased contractility. Palpitation due to overactivity of the heart may also occur in certain pathologic states, e.g., fever, acute or severe anemia, or thyrotoxicosis.

When palpitation is heavy and regular, it is usually caused by an augmented stroke volume, and it should raise the question of aortic regurgitation or of a variety of hyperkinetic circulatory states (anemia, arteriovenous fistula, thyrotoxicosis, and the so-called idiopathic hyperkinetic heart syndrome). It may also occur immediately after the onset of cardiac slowing, as with the sudden development of complete atrioventricular block, or upon the conversion from atrial fibrillation to sinus rhythm. Unusual movements of the heart within the thorax are also frequently the mechanism of palpitation. Thus, the ectopic beat and/or the compensatory pause may be appreciated, since both are associated with alterations in cardiac motion.

IMPORTANT CAUSES OF PALPITATION   See also Chap. 184.

Extrasystoles   In most cases the diagnosis will be suggested by the patient's story. The premature contraction and postpremature beat are often described as a "flopping," or the patient may say that it feels as if "the heart were turning over." The pause following the premature contraction may be felt as an actual cessation of the heartbeat. The first ventricular contraction succeeding the pause may be felt as an unusually vigorous beat and will be described as "pounding" or "thudding."

When extrasystoles are numerous, clinical differentiation from atrial fibrillation can be made by any procedure that will bring about a definite increase in the ventricular rate; at increasingly rapid heart rates, the extrasystoles usually diminish in frequency and then disappear, whereas the ventricular irregularity of atrial fibrillation increases.

Ectopic tachycardias   These conditions, which are considered in detail in Chap. 184, are common and medically important causes of palpitation. Ventricular tachycardia, one of the most serious arrhythmias, rarely is manifested as palpitation; this may be related to the abnormal sequence, and hence impaired coordination and vigor, of ventricular contraction. If the patient is seen between attacks, the diagnosis of ectopic tachycardia and its type will have to depend on the history, but the precise diagnosis can be made only when an electrocardiogram and observations on the effect of carotid sinus pressure are made during the episode. The mode of onset and offset gives the most important lead in distinguishing sinus from one of the various forms of ectopic tachycardias; sinus tachycardia commences and ceases over the course of minutes or seconds, but not instantaneously as is characteristic of ectopic rhythms. Continuous ambulatory (Holter) electrocardiography and asking the patient to record the time of onset and cessation of the palpitations in a diary are extremely helpful in determining the cause of this symptom.

Other causes   These include thyrotoxicosis (Chap. 324), hypoglycemia (Chap. 329), pheochromocytoma (Chap. 326), fever (Chap. 9), and drugs. The relationship between the development of palpitation and the use of tobacco, coffee, tea, alcohol, epinephrine, ephedrine, aminophylline, atropine, or thyroid extract is usually obvious.

Palpitation as a manifestation of the anxiety state   Persons who are healthy physically and well adjusted emotionally may have palpitation under certain circumstances. During or immediately after vigorous physical exertion or during sudden emotional tension, palpitation is common and is usually associated with sinus tachycardia. In poorly conditioned persons without organic heart disease, the sinus tachycardia of exercise may be excessive and associated with palpitation.

In some persons, palpitation may be one of the outstanding manifestations of an episode of acute anxiety. In others the palpitation may, with other symptoms, represent prolonged anxiety neurosis or a lifelong disorder characterized by volatile autonomic function. Whether these illnesses are simply an expression of a chronic, deep-seated anxiety state superimposed on a normal autonomic nervous system or whether they depend on instability of the autonomic nervous system is not clear. At any rate, the clinical significance of the differentiation between the transitory and the enduring forms is that the former is often dissipated by firm reassurance from the physician, whereas the latter is usually resistant even to the most thorough and expert psychiatric care. In the latter case, the patient must be treated with most carefully planned psychological support and tranquilizing medications. This chronic form of palpitation is known by various names such as *Da Costa's syndrome, soldier's heart, effort syndrome, irritable heart, neurocirculatory asthenia,* and *functional cardiovascular disease.* Aside from palpitation, the chief symptoms are those of an anxiety state.

Physical examination usually reveals the typical findings of the hyperkinetic syndrome. These include a left parasternal lift, a precordial or apical systolic murmur, a wide pulse pressure, rapidly rising pulse, and excessive perspiration. The electrocardiogram may display minor depressions of the ST junction and inversion of T waves and so occasionally lead to a mistaken diagnosis of coronary disease; this is particularly likely to occur when these findings are associated with complaints by the patients of an aching feeling of substernal tightness, commonly present in emotional stress. The presence of any kind of organic disease is one of the commonest causes of the underlying anxiety which frequently precipitates this functional syndrome. Thus, even when a patient presents undoubted objective evidence of organic cardiac disease, the possibility that a superimposed anxiety state may be responsible for the symptoms described above should be considered. Palpitation associated with organic cardiac disease is nearly always accompanied by arrhythmia or tachycardia, whereas the symptom may exist with regular rhythm and with a heart rate of 80 beats per minute or less in patients with the anxiety state. An anxiety state, in contrast to heart disease, causes a sighing type of dyspnea. Also pain localized to the apex, either brief and lancinating in character or lasting for hours or days and

TABLE 4-1 Items to be covered in history

Does the palpitation occur:	If so, suspect:
As isolated "jumps" or "skips"?	Extrasystoles
In attacks, known to be of abrupt beginning, with a heart rate of 120 beats per minute or over, with regular or irregular rhythm?	Paroxysmal rapid heart action
Independent of exercise or excitement adequate to account for the symptom?	Atrial fibrillation, atrial flutter, thyrotoxicosis, anemia, febrile states, hypoglycemia, anxiety state
In attacks developing rapidly though not absolutely abruptly, unrelated to exertion or excitement?	Hemorrhage, hypoglycemia, tumor of the adrenal medulla
In conjunction with the taking of drugs?	Tobacco, coffee, tea, alcohol, epinephrine, ephedrine, aminophylline, atropine, thyroid extract, monoamine oxidase inhibitors
On standing?	Postural hypotension
In middle-aged women, in conjunction with flushes and sweats?	Menopausal syndrome
When the rate is known to be normal and the rhythm regular?	Anxiety state

accompanied by hyperesthesia, is due usually to an anxiety state, not to structural cardiac disease. Giddiness due to this syndrome can usually be reproduced by hyperventilation or by change from the recumbent to the erect posture.

The *treatment* of the anxiety state with palpitation is difficult and depends on removal of the cause. In many instances a thorough examination of the heart and a statement that it is normal will suffice. Instructions to take more rather than less physical exercise will reinforce these statements. When the anxiety state is a manifestation of chronic anxiety neurosis or related emotional disorder, the symptoms are more likely to persist.

Table 4-1 summarizes the main points of information to be ascertained in the history in elucidating the significance of palpitation. The recording of an ambulatory electrocardiogram and the precise temporal correlation of the cardiac rate and rhythm with the presence of palpitation are extremely useful in the identification or exclusion of an arrhythmia if the symptom does not occur when the patient is under direct observation. The effectiveness of antiarrhythmia treatment can also be assessed objectively in this manner, without the necessity of relying only on the patient's subjective symptoms. Beta-adrenergic blockade with propranolol, beginning with 40 mg per day in divided doses, and ranging as high as 400 mg per day, can be extremely effective in patients with palpitation and sinus rhythm or sinus tachycardia.

One point merits special emphasis. *As a rule palpitation produces anxiety and fear out of all proportion to its seriousness.* When the cause has been accurately determined and its significance explained to patients, their concern is often ameliorated and may disappear entirely.

REFERENCES

ARESKOG NH, TIBBLING L (eds): Differential diagnostic aspects of chest pain. Acta Med Scand (suppl):644, 1980
BRAUNWALD E: Control of myocardial oxygen consumption: Physiologic and clinical considerations. Am J Cardiol 27:416, 1971
CHRISTIE LG et al: Systematic approach to evaluation of angina-like chest pain: Pathophysiology and clinical testing with emphasis on objective documentation of myocardial ischemia. Am Heart J 102:897, 1981
COHN PF, BRAUNWALD E: Chronic ischemic heart disease, in *Heart Disease,* 2d ed, E Braunwald (ed). Philadelphia, Saunders, 1984, chap 39, p 1334
CONSTANT J: The clinical diagnosis of nonanginal chest pain: The differentiation of angina from nonanginal chest pain by history. Clin Cardiol 6:11, 1983
DEMEESTER et al: Esophageal function in patients with angina-type chest pain and normal coronary angiograms. Ann Surg 196:488, 1982
DRESSLER W: *Clinical Aids in Cardiac Diagnosis.* New York, Grune & Stratton, 1970
GOLDSCHLAGER N: Use of the treadmill test in the diagnosis of coronary artery disease in patients with chest pain. Ann Intern Med 97:383, 1982
HURST JW et al: The history: Past events and symptoms related to cardiovascular disease, in *The Heart,* 6th ed, JW Hurst (ed). New York, McGraw-Hill, 1986, p 113
LEVENE DL: *Chest Pain.* Philadelphia, Lea & Febiger, 1977, p 203
PATTERSON DR: Diffuse esophageal spasm in patients with undiagnosed chest pain. J Clin Gastroenterol 4:415, 1982

5   ABDOMINAL PAIN

WILLIAM SILEN

The correct interpretation of acute abdominal pain is one of the most challenging demands made of any physician. Since proper therapy often requires urgent action, the luxury of the leisurely approach suitable for the study of other conditions is frequently denied. Few other clinical situations demand greater experience and judgment, because the most catastrophic of events may be forecast by the subtlest of symptoms and signs. Nowhere in medicine is a meticulously executed, detailed history and physical examination of greater importance. The etiologic classification in Table 5-1, although not complete, forms a useful frame of reference for the evaluation of patients with abdominal pain.

The diagnosis of "acute or surgical abdomen" so often heard in

TABLE 5-1   Some important causes of abdominal pain

I Pain originating in the abdomen
  A Parietal peritoneal inflammation
    1 Bacterial contamination, e.g., perforated appendix, pelvic inflammatory disease
    2 Chemical irritation, e.g., perforated ulcer, pancreatitis, mittelschmerz
  B Mechanical obstruction of hollow viscera
    1 Obstruction of the small or large intestine
    2 Obstruction of the biliary tree
    3 Obstruction of the ureter
  C Vascular disturbances
    1 Embolism or thrombosis
    2 Vascular rupture
    3 Pressure or torsional occlusion
    4 Sickle cell anemia
  D Abdominal wall
    1 Distortion or traction of mesentery
    2 Trauma or infection of muscles
  E Distention of visceral surfaces, e.g., hepatic or renal capsules
II Pain referred from extraabdominal sources
  A Thorax, e.g., pneumonia, referred pain from coronary occlusion
  B Spine, e.g., radiculitis from arthritis
  C Genitalia, e.g., torsion of the testicle
III Metabolic causes
  A Exogenous
    1 Black widow spider bite
    2 Lead poisoning and others
  B Endogenous
    1 Uremia
    2 Diabetic ketoacidosis
    3 Porphyria
    4 Allergic factors (C'1 esterase inhibitor deficiency)
IV Neurogenic causes
  A Organic
    1 Tabes dorsalis
    2 Herpes zoster
    3 Causalgia and others
  B Functional

emergency wards is not an acceptable one because of its often misleading and erroneous connotation. The most obvious of "acute abdomens" may not require operative intervention, and the mildest of abdominal pains may herald the onset of an urgently correctable lesion. Any patient with abdominal pain of recent onset requires early and thorough evaluation with specific attempts at accurate diagnosis.

SOME MECHANISMS OF PAIN ORIGINATING IN THE ABDOMEN
Inflammation of the parietal peritoneum
The pain of parietal peritoneal inflammation is steady and aching in character and is located directly over the inflamed area, its exact reference being possible because it is transmitted by overlapping somatic nerves supplying the parietal peritoneum. The intensity of the pain is dependent upon the type and amount of foreign substance to which the peritoneal surfaces are exposed in a given period of time. For example, the sudden release into the peritoneal cavity of a small quantity of *sterile* acid gastric juice causes much more pain than the same amount of grossly contaminated neutral fecal material. Enzymatically active pancreatic juice incites more pain and inflammation than does the same amount of sterile bile containing no potent enzymes. Blood and urine are often so bland as to go undetected if exposure of the peritoneum has not been sudden and massive. In the case of bacterial contamination, such as in pelvic inflammatory disease, the pain is frequently of low intensity early in the illness until bacterial multiplication has caused the elaboration of irritating substances.

So important is the rate at which the irritating material is applied to the peritoneum that cases of perforated peptic ulcer may be associated with entirely different clinical pictures dependent only upon the rapidity with which the gastric juice enters the peritoneal cavity.

The pain of peritoneal inflammation is invariably accentuated by pressure or changes in tension of the peritoneum, whether produced by palpation or by movement, as in coughing or sneezing. Consequently, the patient with peritonitis lies quietly in bed, preferring to avoid motion, in contrast to the patient with colic, who may writhe incessantly.

Another of the characteristic features of peritoneal irritation is tonic reflex spasm of the abdominal musculature, localized to the involved body segment. The intensity of the tonic muscle spasm accompanying peritoneal inflammation is dependent upon the location of the inflammatory process, the rate at which it develops, and the integrity of the nervous system. Spasm over a perforated retrocecal appendix or perforated ulcer into the lesser peritoneal sac may be minimal or absent because of the protective effect of overlying viscera. As in pain of peritoneal inflammation, a slowly developing process often greatly attenuates the degree of muscle spasm. Catastrophic abdominal emergencies such as a perforated ulcer have been repeatedly associated with minimal or occasionally no detectable pain or muscle spasm in obtunded, seriously ill, debilitated elderly patients or in psychotic patients.

Obstruction of hollow viscera The pain of obstruction of hollow abdominal viscera is classically described as intermittent, or colicky. Yet the lack of a truly cramping character should not be misleading, because distention of a hollow viscus may produce steady pain with only very occasional exacerbations. Although not nearly as well localized as the pain of parietal peritoneal inflammation, some useful generalities can be made concerning its distribution.

The colicky pain of obstruction of small intestine is usually periumbilical or supraumbilical and is poorly localized. As the intestine becomes progressively dilated with loss of muscular tone, the colicky nature of the pain may become less apparent. With superimposed strangulating obstruction, pain may spread in the lower lumbar region if there is traction on the root of the mesentery. The colicky pain of colonic obstruction is of lesser intensity than that of the small intestine and is often located in the infraumbilical area. Lumbar radiation of pain is common in colonic obstruction.

Sudden distention of the biliary tree produces a steady rather than colicky type of pain; hence the term *biliary colic* is misleading. Acute distention of the gallbladder usually causes pain in the right upper quadrant with radiation to the right posterior region of the thorax or to the tip of the right scapula, and distention of the common bile duct is often associated with pain in the epigastrium radiating to the upper part of the lumbar region. Considerable variation is common, however, so that differentiation between these may be impossible. The typical subscapular pain or lumbar radiation is frequently absent. Gradual dilatation of the biliary tree as in carcinoma of the head of the pancreas may cause no pain or only a mild aching sensation in the epigastrium or right upper quadrant. The pain of distention of the pancreatic ducts is similar to that described for distention of the common bile duct but in addition is very frequently accentuated by recumbency and relieved by the upright position.

Obstruction of the urinary bladder results in dull suprapubic pain, usually low in intensity. Restlessness without specific complaint of pain may be the only sign of a distended bladder in an obtunded patient. In contrast, acute obstruction of the intravesicular portion of the ureter is characterized by severe suprapubic and flank pain which radiates to the penis, scrotum, or inner aspect of the upper region of the thigh. Obstruction of the ureteropelvic junction is felt as pain in the costovertebral angle, whereas obstruction of the remainder of the ureter is associated with flank pain, which often extends into the corresponding side of the abdomen.

Vascular disturbances A frequent misconception, despite abundant experience to the contrary, is that pain associated with intraabdominal vascular disturbances is sudden and catastrophic in nature. The pain of embolism or thrombosis of the superior mesenteric artery or that of impending rupture of an abdominal aortic aneurysm certainly may be severe and diffuse. Yet just as frequently, the patient with occlusion of the superior mesenteric artery has only mild continuous diffuse pain for 2 or 3 days before vascular collapse or findings of peritoneal inflammation appear. The early, seemingly insignificant discomfort is caused by hyperperistalsis rather than peritoneal inflammation. Indeed, absence of tenderness and rigidity in the presence of continuous, diffuse pain in a patient likely to have vascular disease is quite characteristic of occlusion of the superior mesenteric artery. Abdominal pain with radiation to the sacral region, flank, or genitalia should always signal the possible presence of a rupturing abdominal aortic aneurysm. This pain may persist over a period of several days before rupture and collapse occur.

Abdominal wall Pain arising from the abdominal wall is usually constant and aching. Movement and pressure accentuate the discomfort and muscle spasm. In the case of hematoma of the rectus sheath, now most frequently encountered in association with anticoagulant therapy, a mass may be present in the lower quadrants of the abdomen. Simultaneous involvement of muscles in other parts of the body usually serves to differentiate myositis of the abdominal wall from an intraabdominal process which might cause pain in the same region.

REFERRED PAIN IN ABDOMINAL DISEASES Pain referred to the abdomen from the thorax, spine, or genitalia may prove a vexing problem in differential diagnosis, because diseases of the upper part of the abdominal cavity such as acute cholecystitis, perforated ulcer, or subphrenic abscesses are frequently associated with intrathoracic complications. A most important, yet often forgotten, dictum is that the possibility of intrathoracic disease must be considered in every patient with abdominal pain, especially if the pain is in the upper part of the abdomen. Systematic questioning and examination directed toward detecting the presence or absence of myocardial or pulmonary infarction, pneumonia, pericarditis, or esophageal disease (the intrathoracic diseases which most often masquerade as abdominal emergencies) will often provide sufficient clues to establish the proper diagnosis. Diaphragmatic pleuritis resulting from pneumonia or pulmonary infarction may cause pain in the right upper quadrant and pain in the supraclavicular area, the latter radiation to be sharply distinguished from the referred subscapular pain caused by acute distention of the extrahepatic biliary tree. The ultimate decision as to the origin of abdominal pain may require deliberate and planned observation over a period of several hours, during which time repeated questioning and examination will provide the proper explanation.

Referred pain of thoracic origin is often accompanied by splinting of the involved hemithorax with respiratory lag and decrease in excursion more marked than that seen in the presence of intraabdominal disease. In addition, apparent abdominal muscle spasm caused by referred pain will diminish during the inspiratory phase of respiration, whereas it is persistent throughout both respiratory phases if it is of abdominal origin. Palpation over the area of referred pain in the abdomen also does not usually accentuate the pain and in many instances actually seems to relieve it. The frequent coexistence of thoracic and abdominal disease may be misleading and confusing, so that differentiation might be difficult or impossible. For example, the patient with known biliary tract disease often has epigastric pain during myocardial infarction, or biliary colic may be referred to the precordium or left shoulder in a patient who has suffered previously from angina pectoris. For the explanation of the radiation of pain to a previously diseased area, see Chap. 3.

Referred pain from the spine, which usually involves compression or irritation of nerve roots, is characteristically intensified by certain motions such as cough, sneeze, or strain and is associated with hyperesthesia over the involved dermatomes. Pain referred to the abdomen from the testicles or seminal vesicles is generally accentuated by the slightest pressure on either of these organs. The abdominal discomfort is of dull aching character and is poorly localized.

METABOLIC ABDOMINAL CRISES Pain of metabolic origin may simulate almost any other type of intraabdominal disease. Here several mechanisms may be at work. In certain instances, such as hyperlipemia, the metabolic disease itself may be accompanied by an intraabdominal process such as pancreatitis, which can lead to unnecessary laparotomy unless recognized. C′1 esterase deficiency associated with angioneurotic edema is also often associated with episodes of severe abdominal pain. Whenever the cause of abdominal pain is obscure, a metabolic origin must always be considered. Abdominal pain is also the hallmark of familial Mediterranean fever (Chap. 271).

The problem of differential diagnosis is often not readily resolved. The pain of porphyria and of lead colic usually is difficult to distinguish from that of intestinal obstruction, because severe hyperperistalsis is a prominent feature of both. The pain of uremia or diabetes is nonspecific, and the pain and tenderness frequently shift in location and intensity. Diabetic acidosis may be precipitated by acute appendicitis or intestinal obstruction, so that if prompt resolution of the abdominal pain does not result from correction of the metabolic abnormalities, an underlying organic problem should be suspected. Black widow spider bites produce intense pain and rigidity of the abdominal muscles and of the back, an area infrequently involved in disease of intraabdominal origin.

NEUROGENIC CAUSES Causalgic pain may occur in diseases which injure nerves of sensory type. It has a burning character and is usually limited to the distribution of a given peripheral nerve. Normal stimuli such as touch or change in temperature may be transformed into this type of pain, which is also frequently present in a patient at rest. A helpful finding is the demonstration that cutaneous pain spots are now irregularly spaced, and this may be the only indication of an old nerve lesion underlying causalgic pain. Even though the pain may be precipitated by gentle palpation, rigidity of the abdominal muscles is absent, and the respirations are not disturbed. Distention of the abdomen is uncommon, and the pain has no relationship to the intake of food.

Pain arising from spinal nerves or roots comes and goes suddenly and is of a lancinating type (see Chap. 7). It may be caused by herpes zoster, impingement by arthritis, tumors, herniated nucleus pulposus, diabetes, or syphilis. Again, it is not associated with food intake, abdominal distention, or changes in respiration. Severe muscle spasm, as in the gastric crises of tabes dorsalis, is common but is either relieved or is not accentuated by abdominal palpation. The pain is made worse by movement of the spine and is usually confined to a few dermatome segments. Hyperesthesia is very common.

Psychogenic pain conforms to none of the aforementioned patterns of disease. Here the mechanism is hard to define. The most common problem is the hysterical adolescent or young woman who develops abdominal pain; she frequently loses an appendix and other organs because of it. Ovulation or some other natural event that causes brief mild abdominal discomfort may sometimes be experienced as an abdominal catastrophe.

Psychogenic pain varies enormously in type and location but usually has no relation to meals. It is often at its onset markedly accentuated during the night. Nausea and vomiting are rarely observed, although occasionally the patient reports these symptoms. Spasm is seldom induced in the abdominal musculature and if present does not persist, especially if the attention of the patient can be distracted. Persistent localized tenderness is rare, and if found, the muscle spasm in the area is inconsistent and often absent. Restriction of the depth of respiration is the most common respiratory abnormality, but this is in the nature of a smothering or choking sensation and is part of an anxiety state (see Chap. 11). It occurs in the absence of thoracic splinting or change in the respiratory rate.

APPROACH TO THE PATIENT WITH ABDOMINAL PAIN There are few abdominal conditions which require such urgent operative intervention that an orderly approach need be abandoned, no matter how ill the patient. Only those patients with exsanguinating hemorrhage must be rushed to the operating room immediately, but in such instances only a few minutes are required to assess the critical nature of the problem. Under these circumstances, all obstacles must be swept aside, adequate access for intravenous fluid replacement obtained, and the operation begun. Many patients of this type have

died in the radiology department or the emergency room while awaiting such unnecessary examinations as electrocardiograms or films of the abdomen. *There are no contraindications to operation when massive hemorrhage is present.* Although exceedingly important, this situation fortunately is relatively rare.

Nothing will supplant an orderly, painstakingly *detailed history,* which is far more valuable than any laboratory or roentgenologic examination. This kind of history is laborious and time-consuming, making it not especially popular even though a reasonably accurate diagnosis can be made on the basis of the history alone in the majority of cases. In cases of *acute* abdominal pain, a diagnosis is readily established in most instances, whereas success is not so frequently achieved in patients with *chronic* pain. Since the irritable bowel syndrome is one of the most common causes of abdominal pain, the possibility of this diagnosis must always be kept in mind (see Chap. 239). The *chronological sequence of events* in the patient's history is often more important than emphasis on the location of pain. If the examiner is sufficiently open-minded and unhurried, asks the proper questions, and listens, the patient will often provide the diagnosis. Careful attention should be paid to the extraabdominal regions which may be responsible for abdominal pain. An accurate menstrual history in a female patient is essential. Narcotics or analgesics should be withheld until a definitive diagnosis or a definitive plan has been formulated, because these agents often make it more difficult to secure and to interpret the history and physical findings.

In the examination, simple critical inspection of the patient, e.g., of facies, position in bed, and respiratory activity, may provide valuable clues. The amount of information to be gleaned is directly proportional to the *gentleness* and thoroughness of the examiner. Once a patient with peritoneal inflammation has been examined in a brusque manner, accurate assessment by the next examiner becomes almost impossible. For example, eliciting rebound tenderness by sudden release of a deeply palpating hand in a patient with suspected peritonitis is cruel and unnecessary. The same information can be obtained by gentle percussion of the abdomen (rebound tenderness on a miniature scale), a maneuver which can be far more precise and localizing. Asking the patient to cough will elicit true rebound tenderness without the need for placing a hand on the abdomen. Furthermore, the brusque demonstration of rebound tenderness will startle and induce protective spasm in a nervous or worried patient in whom true rebound tenderness is not present. A palpable gallbladder will be missed if palpation is so brusque that voluntary muscle spasm becomes superimposed upon involuntary muscular rigidity.

As in history taking, there is no substitute for sufficient time spent in the examination. It is important to remember that abdominal signs may be minimal but nevertheless, if accompanied by consistent symptoms, may be exceptionally meaningful when carefully assessed. Signs may be virtually or actually totally absent in cases of pelvic peritonitis, so that careful *pelvic and rectal examinations are mandatory in every patient with abdominal pain.* The presence of tenderness on pelvic or rectal examination in the absence of other abdominal signs must not lead the examiner to exclude such important operative indications as perforated appendicitis, diverticulitis, twisted ovarian cyst, and many others.

Much attention has been paid to the presence or absence of peristaltic sounds, their quality, and their frequency. Auscultation of the abdomen is probably one of the least rewarding aspects of the physical examination of a patient with abdominal pain. Severe catastrophes, such as strangulating small-intestinal obstruction or perforated appendicitis, may occur in the presence of normal peristalsis. Conversely, when the proximal part of the intestine above an obstruction becomes markedly distended and edematous, peristaltic sounds may lose the characteristics of borborygmi and become weak or absent even when peritonitis is not present. It is usually the severe chemical peritonitis of sudden onset which is associated with the truly silent abdomen. Assessment of the patient's state of hydration is important. The hematocrit and urinalysis permit an accurate estimate of the severity of dehydration, so that adequate replacement can be carried out.

Laboratory examinations may be of enormous value in the assessment of the patient with abdominal pain, yet with but a few exceptions they rarely establish a diagnosis. Leukocytosis should never be the single deciding factor as to whether or not operation is indicated. A white blood cell count greater than 20,000 per cubic millimeter may be observed with perforation of a viscus, but pancreatitis, acute cholecystitis, pelvic inflammatory disease, and intestinal infarction may be associated with marked leukocytosis. A normal white blood cell count is by no means rare in cases of perforation of abdominal viscera. The diagnosis of anemia may be more helpful than the white blood cell count, especially when combined with the history.

The urinalysis is also of great value in indicating to some degree the state of hydration or to rule out severe renal disease, diabetes, or urinary infection. Determination of the blood urea nitrogen, blood sugar, and serum bilirubin levels may also be helpful. The serum amylase determination is overrated, since in carefully controlled series of patients with proven pancreatitis where the determination has been done within the first 72 h, amylase was less than 200 Somogyi units in one-third of the cases, between 200 and 500 in another one-third of the cases, and greater than 500 in one-third. Since many diseases other than pancreatitis, e.g., perforated ulcer, strangulating intestinal obstruction, and acute cholecystitis, may be associated with very marked increase in the serum amylase, great care must be exercised in denying an operation to a patient solely on the basis of an elevated serum amylase level. The determination of the serum lipase may have a somewhat greater accuracy than the serum amylase.

Peritoneal lavage is a safe and effective diagnostic maneuver in patients with acute abdominal pain. It is of special value in patients with blunt trauma to the abdomen in whom evaluation of the abdomen may be difficult because of other multiple injuries to the spine, pelvis, or ribs and in whom blood in the peritoneal cavity produces only a very mild peritoneal reaction. The gallbladder is the only organ which may continue to seep fluid following accidental perforation, so that the region of this organ must be assiduously avoided. Determination of the pH of the aspirated fluid to ascertain the site of a perforation is misleading, because even highly acid gastric juice is rapidly buffered by peritoneal exudate.

Plain and upright or lateral decubitus roentgenograms of the abdomen may be of the greatest value. They are usually unnecessary in patients with acute appendicitis or strangulated external hernias. However, in cases of intestinal obstruction, perforated ulcer, and a variety of other conditions, films may be diagnostic. During a search for free air, the patient should be kept in the decubitus or upright position for at least 10 min before the appropriate film is taken lest a small pneumoperitoneum be missed. In rare instances, barium or water-soluble medium examination of the upper part of the gastrointestinal tract may demonstrate partial intestinal obstruction which may elude diagnosis by other means. If there is any question of obstruction of the colon, oral administration of barium sulfate should be avoided. On the other hand, barium enema is of inestimable value in cases of colonic obstruction and should be used with greater frequency where the possibility of perforation does not exist. Ultrasound recently has proved to be useful in detecting an enlarged gallbladder or pancreas, the presence of gallstones, or a localized collection of fluid or pus. Radioisotopic scans (HIDA) may help differentiate acute cholecystitis from acute pancreatitis.

Sometimes, even under the best of circumstances with all available auxiliary aids and with the greatest of clinical skill, a definitive diagnosis cannot be established at the time of the initial examination. Nevertheless, despite lack of a clear anatomic diagnosis it may be abundantly clear to an experienced and thoughtful physician and surgeon that on clinical grounds alone operation is indicated. Should that decision be questionable, watchful waiting with repeated questioning and examination will often elucidate the true nature of the illness and indicate the proper course of action.

REFERENCES

DE DOMBAL FT: Acute abdominal pain. Scand J Gastroenterol (Suppl) 14:29, 1979
LEE PWR: The plain x-ray in the acute abdomen: A surgeon's evaluation. Br J Surg 63:763, 1976
LEEK BF: Abdominal and pelvic visceral receptors. Br Med Bull 33:163, 1977
SILEN W: *Cope's Early Diagnosis of the Acute Abdomen*, 16th ed. London, Oxford Press, 1983
STANILAND JR et al: Clinical presentation of acute abdomen: Study of 600 patients. Br Med J 2:393, 1972
VALMAN HB: Acute abdominal pain. Br Med J 282:1858, 1981

6 HEADACHE

RAYMOND D. ADAMS / JOSEPH B. MARTIN

The term *headache* should encompass all aches and pains located in the head, but in common language its application is restricted to unpleasant sensations in the region of the cranial vault. Facial, pharyngeal, laryngeal, and cervical pain are described in Chaps. 7 and 352. (See also Table 6-1.)

Headache represents one of the most frequent human discomforts. Its significance is often abstruse, for it may signal serious disease or represent only tension or fatigue. Fortunately, in most instances it reflects the latter, and only exceptionally does it warn of an intracranial abnormality. But it is this dual significance, the benign and the potentially malignant, that should keep the physician on the alert. Systematic approach to the headache problem necessitates a broad knowledge of medical and surgical diseases of which it is a symptom and a clinical methodology which leaves none of the common and treatable causes unexplored.

GENERAL CONSIDERATIONS The quality, location, duration, and time course of the headache and conditions which produce, exacerbate, or relieve it should be carefully reviewed. Unfortunately, except in special circumstances such as temporal arteritis, physical examination of the head itself is seldom useful.

The patient is rarely helpful in describing the *quality* of cephalic pain. In fact persistent questioning on that point occasions surprise, for the patient usually assumes that the word *headache* conveys adequate information about the nature of the discomfort. Most headaches are dull, deeply located, and of aching character. Occasionally superficial burning or stinging pain localized to the skin is reported. The patient may make allusion to tightness, pressure, or a bursting feeling, terms which may give clues to muscular tension or psychologic state.

Queries about the *intensity* of the pain are seldom of value since they reflect more the patient's attitude toward the condition than the true severity. The stoical person tends to minimize discomfort, whereas the neurotic or depressed patient dramatizes it. Degree of incapacity is a better index. A severe migraine attack seldom allows performance of the day's work. The pain which awakens the patient from sleep at night, or prevents sleep, is also more likely to have a demonstrable organic basis. As a rule, the most intense cranial pains are those that accompany subarachnoid hemorrhage and meningitis, which have grave implications, or migraine and paroxysmal nocturnal *cluster* headaches, which are benign.

Data regarding *location* of the headache are often informative. If the source is in extracranial structures, as is usually the case, the correspondence with the site of the pain is fairly precise. Inflammation of an extracranial artery causes pain localized to the site of the vessel. Lesions of paranasal sinuses, teeth, eyes, and upper cervical vertebrae induce a less sharply localized pain, but one that is still referred in a regional distribution that is fairly constant. Intracranial lesions in the posterior fossa cause pain in the occipital-nuchal region, homolateral if the lesion is one-sided. Supratentorial lesions induce frontotemporal pains, again homolateral to the lesion if it is on one side. But localization can also be very uninformative or misleading. Ear pain, for example, although it may mean disease in the ear, more often is referred from other regions such as the neck, and eye pain may be referred to the occiput or cervical spine.

Duration and *time-intensity curve* of headaches both during the attack itself and in their life profile are most useful. The headache of bacterial meningitis or subarachnoid hemorrhage occurs usually in single attacks over a period of days. Single, brief, momentary (1 to 2 s) pains in the cranium (icepick-like headaches) are common but uninterpretable and rarely indicate serious underlying disease. Migraine of the classic type has its onset in the early morning hours or daytime, reaches its peak of severity in a half hour or so, lasts, unless treated, for several hours up to 1 to 2 days, is often accompanied by nausea or vomiting, and is terminated by sleep. A frequency of more than a single attack every few weeks is exceptional. A migraine patient having several attacks per week usually proves to have a combination of migraine and tension headaches. In contrast to this is the nightly occurrence (2 to 3 h after onset of sleep) over a period of several weeks to months of the rapidly peaking, nonthrobbing orbital or supraorbital pain of cluster headache, which tends to dissipate within an hour. The headache of intracranial tumor characteristically can occur at any time of day or night, can interrupt sleep, varies in intensity, and lasts a few minutes to hours. The natural history is one of increasing frequency and intensity over a period of months. Tension headache, once commenced, may persist continuously for weeks or months, often waxing and waning from hour to hour or day to day.

Headache that bears a more or less constant relationship to certain biologic events and also to physical environmental changes may prove to be informative. Premenstrual headaches, most typically of migrainous or tension type, may occur as part of the premenstrual syndrome; they usually vanish after the first day of vaginal bleeding. The headaches of cervical arthritis are most typically intense after a period of inactivity, and the first movements in the morning are both difficult and painful. Hypertensive headaches, like those of cerebral tumor, tend to occur on waking in the morning, but, as with all vascular headaches, excitement and tension may provoke them. Headache from infection of nasal sinuses may appear, with clocklike regularity, upon awakening and in midmorning, and is characteristically worsened by stooping and jarring of the head. Eyestrain headaches naturally follow prolonged use of the eyes, as in reading, peering for a long time against glaring headlights in traffic, or watching a movie. Atmospheric cold may evoke pain in the so-called fibrositic or nodular headache or when the underlying condition is arthritic or neuralgic. Anger, excitement, or irritation may initiate common migraine in certain disposed persons; this is more typical of common migraine than of the classic type. Change of position, stooping, straining, cough, and sexual intercourse are each known to produce a special type of headache, described below. Exertional headaches, another well-known type, are usually benign (only 1 in 10 will have an intracranial lesion) and disappear within weeks to months.

PAIN-SENSITIVE STRUCTURES OF THE HEAD Understanding of headache has been greatly augmented by observations made during surgery of pain-sensitive structures. The following are sensitive to mechanical stimulation: (1) skin, subcutaneous tissue, muscles, arteries, and periosteum of skull; (2) tissues of the eye, ear, and nasal and sinus cavities; (3) intracranial venous sinuses and their tributary veins; (4) parts of the dura at the base of the brain and the arteries within the dura mater and pia-arachnoid; and (5) the trigeminal, glossopharyngeal, vagus, and first three cervical nerves. Interestingly, pain is practically the only sensation produced by stimulation of these structures. The bony skull, much of the pia-arachnoid and dura, and the parenchyma of the brain lack sensitivity.

Sensory stimuli from the head are conveyed to the central nervous system via the trigeminal nerves for structures above the tentorium in the anterior and middle fossae of the skull, and the first three

cervical nerves for those in the posterior fossa and infradural structures. The ninth and tenth cranial nerves supply part of the posterior fossa and refer the pain to the ear and throat. The pain of intracranial disease is commonly referred to a part of the cranium lying within the areas supplied by these nerves. There may be associated local tenderness of the scalp at the site of reference. Dental or jaw pain may also have cranial reference. The pain of disease in other parts of the body is not referred to the head, although it may initiate headache by other means.

Headache can occur as a result of (1) distention, traction, or dilatation of intracranial or extracranial arteries, (2) traction or displacement of large intracranial veins or of their dural envelope, (3) compression, traction, or inflammation of cranial and spinal nerves, (4) voluntary or involuntary spasm, inflammation, and trauma to cranial and cervical muscles, and (5) meningeal irritation and raised intracranial pressure. More specifically, intracranial mass lesions cause headache only if they deform, displace, or exert traction on vessels, dural structures, or cranial nerves at the base of the brain, and this may happen long before intracranial pressure rises. Raised intracranial pressure causes headache in a bioccipital or bifrontal distribution which is rapidly relieved by lumbar puncture and lowering of the cerebrospinal fluid (CSF) pressure.

Dilatation of the extracranial, temporal, and intracranial *arteries* with stretching of surrounding sensitive structures is believed to be the mechanism of most of the pain of migraine. Extracranial, temporal, and occipital arteries, when involved in giant cell arteritis (cranial or ''temporal'' arteritis), a disease which usually afflicts individuals over 50 years of age, give rise to headache of dull aching and throbbing type, at first localized and then more diffuse. Characteristically it is severe and persistent over a period of weeks or months. The offending artery, strangely, is not always tender to pressure, yet section of it, as in biopsy, may relieve the pain (Chap. 269). Evolving atherosclerotic thrombosis of internal carotid, anterior, and middle cerebral arteries is sometimes accompanied by pain in the forehead or temple; with vertebral artery thrombosis the pain is postauricular, and basilar artery thrombosis causes referred pain in the occiput and sometimes the forehead.

In *infection or blockage of paranasal sinuses*, pain is usually felt over the antrum or in the forehead; with the *ethmoid* and *sphenoid sinuses*, the pain localizes around the eyes on one or both sides or in the vertex. Usually it is associated with tenderness of the skin in the same distribution. The pain may have two remarkable properties: (1) When throbbing, it may be abolished by compressing the carotid artery on the same side. (2) It tends to recur and subside at the same hours, i.e., on awakening, with gradual disappearance when the person is upright, and coming again in the late morning hours. The time relations are believed to yield information concerning the mechanism; morning pain is ascribed to the sinuses filling at night, and its relief on arising to emptying after the erect posture has been assumed. Stooping, blowing the nose, and jarring the head intensify the pain; and inhalant sympathomimetic drugs such as phenylephrine, which reduce swelling and congestion, tend to relieve the pain. Sinus pain may persist after all purulent secretions have disappeared, probably because of persistent blockage of the draining orifices eliciting a vacuum or suction effect on the sinus wall (*vacuum sinus headaches*). The condition is relieved when aeration is restored. During air flights both earache and sinus headache tend to occur on descent, when the relative pressure in the blocked viscus falls.

Headache of ocular origin is usually located in the orbit, forehead, or temple, and has a steady, aching quality which may follow prolonged use of the eyes in close work. Ocular muscle imbalance, hyperopia, astigmatism, and impaired convergence and accommodation may give rise to sustained contraction of extraocular as well as frontal, temporal, and even occipital muscles. Raised intraocular pressure in acute glaucoma or iridocyclitis causes steady, aching pain felt in the eye. When intense, it may radiate throughout the distribution of the ophthalmic division of the trigeminal nerve. The pain of diabetic third nerve palsy, intracranial aneurysm, pituitary tumor,

TABLE 6-1 Common types of headache

Type	Site	Age and sex	Clinical characteristics	Diurnal pattern	Life profile
Common migraine	Frontotemporal Uni- or bilateral	Children, young to middle-aged adults, both sexes, female > male	Throbbing and/or dull ache; worse behind one eye or ear, nausea or vomiting Becomes generalized	Upon awakening or later in day Duration: hours to 1–2 days	Irregular interval, weeks to months Tends to disappear in middle age and during pregnancy
Classic migraine	Same as above	Same as above	Same as above; visual prodrome common.	Same as above	Same as above
Cluster, histamine headache, or migrainous neuralgia	Orbital Temporal Unilateral	Adolescent and adult males (80–90%)	Intense, nonthrobbing pain	Usually nocturnal; occurs one or more hours after falling asleep Rarely diurnal	Nightly for several weeks to months (cluster) Recurrence: years later
Tension headaches	Generalized	Children, adolescents, and adults, both sexes	Pressure (nonthrobbing); tightness Aching	Continuous, variable intensity, for weeks and months	One or more periods of months to years
Meningeal irritation (meningitis, subarachnoid hemorrhage)	Generalized	Any age, both sexes	Intense, steady deep pain, may be worse in neck	Duration: days to a week or more	Single episode
Brain tumor	(See text)	Any age, both sexes	Variable in intensity May awaken patient Steady pain	Lasts minutes to hours; increasing severity	Once in a lifetime: weeks to months
Temporal arteritis	Unilateral, temporal, or occipital	Over 50 years, either sex	Persistent burning, aching	Continuous or intermittent	Persists for weeks to a few months

SOURCE: *After J Patten, Neurological Differential Diagnosis, London, Harold Starke, Springer-Verlag, 1977.*

cavernous sinus thrombosis, and Raeder's paratrigeminal syndrome is often referred to the eye.

The *headaches accompanying disease of ligaments, muscles, and apophyseal joints* in the upper part of the spine, which are referred to occipital and upper cervical regions, are difficult to separate from the more common muscular contraction (tension) headaches. Such referred pains are especially frequent in middle and late adult life in patients with rheumatoid arthritis and cervical spondylosis and tend also to occur after whiplash injuries to the neck. If the pain is articular or synovial in origin, the first movements after being still for some hours are both stiff and painful. In fact, evocation of pain by active and passive motion of the spine should indicate traumatic or other disease of movable parts. The pain of *myofibrositis*, evidenced by tender nodules near the cranial insertion of cervical and other muscles, is more obscure. There are no pathologic data as to the nature of these vaguely palpable lesions, and it is uncertain whether the pain actually arises in them. They may represent only the deep tenderness felt in the region of referred pain or the involuntary secondary protective spasm of muscles. Characteristically, the pain is steady (nonthrobbing) and spreads from one to both sides of the head. Exposure to cold or draft may precipitate it. Though severe at times, it seldom prevents sleep. Massage of muscles and heat have unpredictable effects but relieve the pain in some cases.

The *headache of meningeal irritation* (infection or hemorrhage) is acute in onset, severe, generalized, deep-seated, constant, especially intense at the base of the skull, and associated with stiffness of neck on bending forward. Dilatation and congestion of inflamed meningeal vessels are likely the main cause of the pain.

Lumbar puncture headache is characterized by a steady occipital-nuchal or bifrontal pain that comes on a few minutes after arising from a recumbent position and is relieved within a few minutes by lying down. Its cause is persistent leakage of CSF into the lumbar

tissues through the needle site. The CSF pressure is low. The headache is usually increased by compression of the jugular veins and is unaffected by digital obliteration of one carotid artery. It is probable that in the upright position a low intraspinal and negative intracranial pressure exerts traction on dural attachments and dural sinuses by caudal displacement of the brain. Understandably, then, headache following cisternal puncture is rare. As soon as the leakage of CSF stops and CSF pressure is gradually restored (usually from a few days up to a week or so), the headache disappears. "Spontaneous" low-pressure headache may also follow a sneeze or strain, presumably because of rupture of the spinal arachnoid along a nerve root.

The mechanism of the *throbbing or steady headache which accompanies febrile illnesses*, located in frontal or occipital regions or generalized, is probably vascular. It is much like histamine headache in being relieved on one side by carotid artery compression and on both sides by jugular vein compression or the subarachnoid injection of saline solution. It is increased by shaking the head. It seems probable that the meningeal vessels pulsate unduly and stretch pain-sensitive structures around the base of the brain. In certain cases, however, the pain may be lessened by compression of temporal arteries, and in these cases a component of the headache seems to be derived from the walls of extracranial arteries, as in migraine.

The so-called *tension headaches* of patients with anxiety states and depression are allegedly due to chronic spasm of cranial and cervical muscles. Combinations of the tension and vascular headaches give rise to the "mixed headaches" so common in many patients.

PRINCIPAL CLINICAL VARIETIES OF HEADACHE Usually there is no difficulty in diagnosing the headache of glaucoma, purulent sinusitis, bacterial meningitis, and brain tumor, and a fuller account of these special headaches will be found where these diseases are described in other sections of the book. It is when headache is

Provoking factors	Associated features	Treatment
Bright light, noise, tension, alcohol Dark room and sleep relieve Scalp sensitive Pressure helps	Nausea in some cases	Ergot preparation at onset Phenergan in established phase Inderal and Bellergal Methysergide for prevention
Same as above	Blindness and scintillating lights Unilateral numbness Disturbed speech Vertigo Confusion	Same as above
Alcohol in some	Lacrimation, congested eye	Ergot preparation at bedtime Amitriptyline and lithium carbonate for prevention
Fatigue and nervous strain	Depression, nervousness, anxiety, insomnia	Antianxiety and antidepressant drugs
None	Neck stiff on forward bending Kernig and Brudzinski signs	For meningitis or bleeding (see text)
None Sometimes position	Papilledema Vomiting Slow mentation	Corticosteroids Mannitol Glycerol Treatment of tumor
Scalp sensitive Tender arteries	Intermittent or permanent loss of sight Rheumatic myalgia Fever	Corticosteroid therapy

chronic, recurrent, and unattended by other important signs of disease that the physician faces one of the most difficult medical problems.

The types of headache subsequently described should then be considered.

Migraine The term *migraine* refers to periodic, hemicranial, throbbing headaches often accompanied by nausea and vomiting which usually begin in childhood, adolescence, or early adult life and recur in diminishing number and intensity during advancing years. Migraine is frequent, with a prevalence of 20 to 30 percent in the population. Women are affected three times as often as men. There is a tendency for the headaches to occur during the period of premenstrual tension and fluid retention and to decrease during pregnancy. The immediate family history is positive for migraine in over 60 percent of cases. Migraine or vascular headaches present in one of four clinical patterns: (1) classic migraine, (2) common migraine, (3) complicated migraine, and (4) cluster headache.

Classic migraine begins with a prodrome of prominent neurologic symptoms such as visual scintillations, dazzling zigzag lines (fortification spectra), photophobia and spreading scotomas, or dizziness and tinnitus. Classic migraine may be heralded hours before the attack by premonitory symptoms, most commonly a feeling of elation, excessive energy, thirst, a craving for sweet foods, or drowsiness. At other times, there may be a slowing of mentation or a feeling of impending doom or of depression, or there may be no warning whatsoever. The disturbance of vision that commences the attack may be followed by homonymous hemianopic field defects; sometimes they are bilateral, and even total blindness may rarely occur.

In *common migraine* there is an unheralded onset of headache, often with nausea and sometimes vomiting, following the same temporal pattern but without the antecedent neurologic symptoms.

Both of these headache syndromes respond to ergot preparations, if administered early in the attack. A genetic basis is suggested by history of headaches in near relatives in over 50 percent of cases.

Complicated migraine refers to headaches accompanied by neurologic symptoms that may either precede or accompany the headache. Numbness and tingling of the lips, face, hand, and leg on one side may occur, sometimes in combination with an aphasic disorder. The arm and leg may become weak or paralyzed on one side, mimicking a stroke. The numbness or weakness spreads from one part of the body to another slowly over a period of minutes. Full recovery usually occurs. However, permanent deficits consisting of hemianopia (lesion in distribution of the posterior cerebral artery), hemiplegia or hemianesthesia (lesion in territory of middle cerebral artery), or ophthalmoplegia (usually third nerve lesion) may occur.

Several other neurologic syndromes have been delineated in association with complicated migraine. Bickerstaff first called attention to *basilar migraine,* in which the visual disorder and paresthesias are bilateral and are accompanied by confusion, stupor, rarely coma, aggressive outbursts, vertigo, diplopia, and dysarthria. While the full syndrome is infrequent, partial basilar syndromes are found in some 30 percent of children with migraine. Alternating hemiplegias in children have also been attributed to basilar migraine but could as well be due to alternating involvement of the middle cerebral arteries.

It is also recognized that neurologic syndromes may occur due to migraine which are not followed by headache. In children, abdominal pain and vomiting, sometimes cyclical, may occur without headache as the sole expression of migraine; the same is true of some cases of paroxysmal vertigo in children. Such *migraine equivalents* may be manifest as pain localized in the thorax, pelvis, or extremities; bouts of fever; paroxysmal vertigo; transient disturbances in mood (psychic equivalents). The first neurologic syndrome due to migraine may occur in late adult life in a person not previously known to have migraine. Fisher refers to these as *transient migrainous accompaniments* to distinguish them from transient cerebral ischemic attacks (TIAs).

Cluster headache, also called paroxysmal nocturnal cephalalgia, migrainous neuralgia, histamine headache, and Horton's syndrome, has a fourfold higher incidence in men than in women. It is characterized by constant, unilateral orbital pain, with onset usually within 2 or 3 h after falling asleep. It tends to occur during the phase of rapid eye movement (REM) sleep. The pain is intense and steady (nonthrobbing) with lacrimation, blocked nostril, then rhinorrhea, and sometimes miosis, ptosis, flush, and edema of cheek, all lasting approximately an hour or two. It tends to recur nightly for several weeks or a few months (hence the term *cluster*), followed by complete freedom for years. The pain of a given attack may leave as rapidly as it began. Clusters may recur over the years, being possibly more likely in times of stress, prolonged strain, overwork, and with upsetting emotional experiences. Episodes of cluster headache lasting 2 to 3 weeks may recur several times over a lifetime. Often the pain involves the same orbit in each cluster. Occasionally alcohol, nitroglycerin, or tyramine-containing foods precipitate an attack. Rarely, the condition may occur in daytime and may not cluster but continue for years. The picture is so characteristic that its presentation is diagnostic, though to those unfamiliar with it the possibility of a carotid aneurysm, hemangioma, brain tumor, or sinusitis may be suggested.

The relationship of the cluster headache to migraine remains conjectural. A portion of the cases have a background of migraine, which led to the earlier postulation of migrainous neuralgia, but the majority do not.

MECHANISM AND PATHOPHYSIOLOGY A satisfactory theory of the pathophysiology of migraine has eluded clinical investigators. Certain facts appear indisputable; the symptoms of migraine are associated with changes in cerebral blood flow, presumably secondary to changes in vessel caliber; the prodromal phase with neurologic symptoms is accompanied by arteriolar constriction and decreased cerebral blood flow beginning most often in the posterior part of the brain; the decrease in cerebral blood flow in migraine proceeds at a rate of about 2 mm/min, resembling the spreading depression originally described by Leão, which is characterized by a transient self-propagating perturbation of brain electrical activity followed by hypoperfusion. Less certain is the assumption that the headache that follows is due to vascular dilatation, since direct measurements of cerebral blood flow during the headache phase fail to show significant increases. In the studies reported by Lauritzen and coworkers regional cerebral blood flow, measured by xenon 133, showed oligemic regions of cortex during migraine attacks with diminished reactivity to carbon dioxide, suggesting an abnormality of vessel responses. Between attacks of migraine, patients had normal regulation of brain circulation.

The factors that elicit these changes in cerebral blood flow are unknown. Two general hypotheses about the cause of migraine have emerged. The first is that it is due to a central nervous system neurovascular disorder that triggers alterations in vasomotor regulation. The premonitory symptoms of changes in mood, appetite, and thirst have led some to consider a central hypothalamic disorder to be the cause. The second considers migraine to be a systemic metabolic disregulation with attacks elicited secondary to intravascular events associated with changes in serotonin metabolism. Changes in platelet serotonin levels, shown to fall during the attack, accompanied by increased urinary excretion of serotonin and of 5-hydroxyindole-acetic acid support the contention that migraine is a systemic disorder. Further support for a role of serotonin comes from observations that reserpine, which triggers serotonin release, causes migraine in some patients and that antiserotonin drugs, like methysergide, show some success in its treatment. However, there is difficulty in understanding how changes in intravascular serotonin, which has little direct effect on vessel contraction, can induce the changes of migraine. Lance considers the mechanism of migraine to involve changes in biogenic amine or neuropeptide neurotransmitters in the central nervous system, associated with or followed by platelet release reactions. Recent work has focused on the neurotransmitters found in nerve fibers that innervate cerebral blood vessels. Moskowitz has demonstrated that cerebral vessels are innervated by nerves that contain substance P, a peptide important for pain transmission (see Chap. 3) and also thought to be capable of eliciting local tissue reactions resembling inflammation. Other neuropeptides found in cerebral blood vessels and known to affect vascular tone include vasoactive intestinal polypeptide, neurotensin, and neuropeptide Y.

There is persistent debate concerning factors that trigger the migraine attacks. Dietary factors are likely important in some patients. Monro and coworkers identified sensitivity to milk and wheat products in patients with severe refractory migraine. Many patients learn to avoid alcohol (particularly red wine), chocolate, coffee, tea, or other agents with pharmacologically active ingredients. How these substances elicit the attacks is unknown. Some patients describe exposure to sunlight, exercise, tension, or the use of oral contraceptives as increasing the frequency and severity of migraine.

DIFFERENTIAL DIAGNOSIS   Classic migraine usually causes no difficulty in diagnosis. Difficulties arise from two sources: (1) ignorance of the fact that a progressively unfolding neurologic syndrome may be migrainous in origin, and (2) lack of appreciation that the neurologic disorder may occur without headache.

The neurologic symptoms of the migraine syndrome may resemble focal epilepsy, the clinical picture of a vascular malformation such as an angioma or aneurysm, or some other vascular disease such as a thrombotic or embolic stroke. The pace of the neurologic symptoms of migraine, rather than their character, reliably distinguishes them from epilepsy. The clinical profile of the aura of epilepsy is measured in seconds, for it depends on spreading neural excitation, in contrast to the slow progression of migraine, which is based on spreading depression of nervous tissue. Nevertheless, there are instances where episodes of coma with electroencephalogram (EEG) abnormality may be either migraine or epilepsy. Furthermore, a seizure is often followed by a generalized headache.

Ophthalmoplegic migraine always suggests a carotid aneurysm,

and carotid arteriography may be necessary to exclude it. Despite many claims that vascular malformations may cause hemicranial pain occurring invariably on the same side of the head (unlike migraine), larger series of cases have shown this only rarely to be the case. Focal epilepsy, protracted headache, stiff neck and bloody CSF, a persistent neurologic deficit, and cranial bruit are indicative of a vascular type of headache associated with angioma or aneurysm. Only in the earlier stages, when periodic throbbing headache is the sole symptom, are these conditions confused with true migraine.

Tension headache   The tension headache is usually bilateral, often with diffuse extension over the top of the cranium. Occipital-nuchal or bifrontal localization is common. Although the sensation may be described as pain, close questioning may uncover other sensations, viz., fullness, tightness, or pressure (as if the head is surrounded by a band or in a vise), on which waves of aching pain are superimposed. The onset of a given attack is more gradual than in migraine and not infrequently a throbbing "vascular" type of headache is described. Tension headache may occur acutely under conditions of emotional duress or intense worry and lasts for hours or a day or two. More often it persists unremittingly for weeks or months. In fact, this is the only type of headache that exhibits the peculiarity of being absolutely continuous day and night for long periods of time. Although sleep may be possible, whenever the patient awakens, the headache is present; a common feature is the finding that analgesic remedies have relatively little effect in alleviating the pain. In contrast to migraine, in which pain is periodic and lifelong, with tendency to lessen in late adult years, tension headache occurs more often in middle age and may persist for many years.

It is unlikely that the origin of the pain is sustained muscle activity, since electromyographic (EMG) investigations show no changes in forehead or neck muscles. On the other hand, elicitation of headache after administration of amyl nitrite, a vasodilator, in about 50 percent of patients suggests a vascular contribution to the pain. Histamine can also cause headaches in these patients.

It is a common experience for both tension headache and common migraine to coexist in the same patient. The management of such patients may require therapy of both types of headache.

Psychologic studies of groups of patients with tension headaches have revealed prominent symptoms of depression, anxiety, and in some hypochrondriasis. Kudrow records that 65 percent of depressed patients have this type of headache and that over 60 percent of his patients with tension headaches were depressed.

Headache of angioma and aneurysm   The temporal profile of any given attack shows the onset to be sudden or very acute, with the pain reaching a peak within minutes. Neurologic disturbances such as defects in vision, unilateral numbness, weakness, or aphasia may precede or occur after the onset of headache and outlast it. Should hemorrhage occur, the headache is often extremely severe and localizes in the occiput and neck, lasting many days in association with stiff neck. A cranial or cervical bruit and the presence of blood in the CSF establish the diagnosis. The claim that vascular malformations may give rise to migraine is probably untenable. Statistical data show migraine to be no more frequent in this group of patients than in the general population. Vascular lesions may exist for long periods of time without headache, or headache may develop many years after other manifestations such as epilepsy and hemiplegia (see Chap. 343).

Traumatic headaches   Severe, chronic, continuous, or intermittent headaches often associated with giddiness, vertigo, or tinnitus appear as the cardinal symptoms of the posttraumatic syndrome. The cause of the headache is unknown, but it is a clear-cut disorder unrelated in most instances to medicolegal issues of compensation. *Posttraumatic dysautonomic cephalalgia* is a term given by Vijayan and Dreyfus to severe, episodic, throbbing, unilateral headaches accompanied by ipsilateral mydriasis and excessive facial sweating. The condition follows injury to the neck in the region of the carotid sheath. It was postulated that the sympathetic nervous supply of the cranium had been disinhibited, and there was clinical and pharmacologic evidence of sympathetic dysfunction (see Chap. 344).

Headache and dizziness of fluctuating severity, followed by drowsiness, stupor, coma, and hemiparesis, are the usual manifestations of *chronic subdural hematoma*. The head injury may have been minor and forgotten by patient and family. The headaches are deep-seated, steady, unilateral or generalized, and respond to the usual analgesic drugs. The typical attack profile of the headache and other symptoms is one of increasing frequency and severity over several weeks or months. Diagnosis is established by computerized tomography (CT) scan and arteriography (see Chap. 344).

Headaches of brain tumor Headache is the outstanding symptom of cerebral tumor. Unfortunately, the quality of the pain has no specific feature. It tends to be deep-seated, nonthrobbing (or throbbing), and aching or bursting. Attacks last a few minutes to an hour or more and occur once or many times during the day. Activity and, frequently, change in the position of the head may provoke pain, while rest in bed diminishes its frequency. Nocturnal awakening because of pain, although typical, is by no means diagnostic. Unexpected forceful (projectile) vomiting may punctuate the illness in its later stages. As the tumor grows, the pain becomes more frequent and severe; it sometimes is nearly continuous terminally. If unilateral, the headache is homolateral to the tumor in 9 out of 10 patients. Supratentorial tumors are felt anterior to the interauricular circumference of the skull; posterior fossa tumors behind this line. Bifrontal and bioccipital headache, coming on after unilateral headache, signifies the development of increased intracranial pressure.

Headaches related to medical disorders Experienced physicians are aware of many conditions in which headache figures as a dominant symptom. These include fevers of any cause, carbon monoxide exposure, chronic lung disease with hypercapnia (headaches often nocturnal), hypothyroidism, Cushing's syndrome, withdrawal of corticosteroid medication, chronic nitrite or ergot exposure, occasionally Addison's disease, aldosterone-producing adrenal tumors, use of contraceptive medications, acute rises in blood pressure, e.g., from pheochromocytoma, and acute anemia with hemoglobin below 10 g. Hypertension per se is an uncommon cause of headache.

Unusual types of headache Sharp, jabbing pains in the head (icepick-like pains) last a second or two, and have no clinical significance. They are reported in up to 3 percent of the normal population and in 46 percent of migrainous patients. The pain is usually felt in the temporal or orbital region.

Cough and exertional headache or headache brought on by stooping follows the initiating action by a few seconds and lasts a minute or two. Usually no explanation is apparent, but exceptionally it occurs in patients with arteriovenous malformations, Paget's disease of the skull, Arnold-Chiari malformation, or an intracranial tumor. In a series of 103 patients followed for 3 years or longer by Rooke only 10 developed neurologic signs. The mechanism of this headache may be venous distention, for jugular compression has induced it in some of our patients. Lance has described a generalized headache that begins suddenly during coitus usually at the time of orgasm. It may last minutes or hours. Most of his 21 patients were males.

Erythrocyanotic headache is a rare form of generalized throbbing headache which occurs in conjunction with flushing of the face and hands and numbness of the fingers (erythromelalgia). The condition has been reported in association with (a) mastocytosis (infiltration of tissues with mast cells, which elaborate histamine, heparin, and serotonin); (b) carcinoid tumors; (c) some tumors of pancreatic islets; (d) pheochromocytoma.

HEADACHE AND FACIAL PAIN   The facial neuralgias are discussed in Chap. 352 (see Table 6-2).

APPROACH TO THE PATIENT WITH HEADACHE Obviously very different possibilities are raised by a patient who presents for the first time with severe headache and a patient who has had recurrent headache over a period of years. The chances of uncovering the cause in the first instance are much greater than in the second and in the former the underlying conditions (meningitis, subarachnoid hemorrhage, epidural or subdural hematoma, glaucoma, and purulent sinusitis) often are more serious. In general, severe, persistent headache with stiff neck and fever means meningitis, and the same combination without fever, subarachnoid hemorrhage. A lumbar puncture is mandatory. Acute persistent headache over a period of hours or days may occur in systemic infections such as influenza (febrile) or as a manifestation of an acute tension state. If there is a diagnosable febrile disease and no stiffness of the neck, lumbar puncture may be deferred. The first attack of migraine may also present in this way, but of course there is no fever.

In searching for the cause of recurrent headache one should investigate the status of cardiovascular and renal systems by blood pressure and urine examination, eyes by fundoscopy, intraocular pressure, and refraction, the sinuses by transillumination and x-rays, the cranial arteries by palpation (and biopsy?), the cervical spine by the effect of passive movement of the head and x-rays, the nervous system by neurologic examination, and psychic function by mental status.

Hypertension is frequent in the general population and is not often a cause of recurrent headaches. Severe hypertension with diastolic blood pressures of over 110 mmHg may be associated with headache. If headache is severe and frequent, the possibilities of underlying anxiety or tension state or a common migraine syndrome should be considered.

The adolescent with daily frontal headaches represents a special type of problem. Often the relationship of the headaches to eyestrain is unclear, and refraction of the eyes and new eyeglasses do not relieve the condition. Anxiety or tension is probably a factor in such cases, but it is difficult to be certain of a causal relationship. Some of the most persistent and inexplicable headaches, which have led to a survey by a battery of diagnostic procedures for tumor, have proved in the end to be associated with endogenous depression.

Equally puzzling is the somber, tense adult whose primary complaint is headache, or the migrainous person who in late life or at menopause begins to have daily headaches. Here it becomes important to assess mental status along the lines suggested in Chaps. 11 and 23, looking for evidences of anxiety, depression, and hypochondriasis. The quality and persistence of the headache are suggestive of the possibility of psychiatric illness. Sometimes a direct question as to the patient's idea of what is the matter may elicit suspicion and fear of brain tumor. Antidepressant drugs given as an empirical test may relieve the headache, thus clarifying the diagnosis.

The most worrisome type of patient is the one who has headache of increasing frequency and severity over a period of months or a year or so. Since an intracranial mass lesion (tumor, abscess, subdural hematoma) is a leading possibility, a complete neurologic survey, including careful inspection of optic discs, CT scan, and electroencephalogram, should be performed.

Every person over 50 to 55 years with severe headache of some few days' or weeks' duration should be considered as possibly having cranial arteritis (see Chap. 269). The overall incidence in patients over 50 years is 1 in 750; that of polymyalgia rheumatica in the same age group is 1 in 200. Women are more often affected than men (4:1), and there is an associated polymyalgia in 25 percent of cases. Conversely, in 50 percent of polymyalgia rheumatica patients there is a cranial arteritis. Increased sedimentation rate, fever, and anemia may occur. The findings of a thickened, tender temporal artery and claudication of jaw muscles from involvement of facial arteries are important. The disease may cause blindness and/or ophthalmoplegia but rarely involves intracranial arteries. Arterial biopsy and response to corticosteroids establish the diagnosis.

TREATMENT The most important steps in the treatment of headache are those measures which uncover and remove the underlying disease or functional disturbance.

For the *common everyday headache* due to fatigue, acute stress, or excessive use of alcohol and tobacco, the physician advises

TABLE 6-2 Types of facial pain

Types	Site	Clinical characteristics	Aggravating-relieving factors	Diseases	Treatment
Trigeminal neuralgia (tic douloureux)	Second to third division of trigeminal nerve, unilateral	Men : women = 1:3 Over 50 years Paroxysms (10–30 s) of stabbing, burning pain Trigger points, intermittent ache No sensory or motor paralysis	Touching face, chewing, smiling, talking, blowing nose	Idiopathic If in young adults unilateral or bilateral, multiple sclerosis Vascular anomaly Tumor of fifth cranial nerve	Carbamazepine (Tegretol) Phenytoin Radiofrequency lesion of ganglion
Atypical facial neuralgia	Unilateral or bilateral	Predominantly female 30–50 years Continuous intolerable pain Mainly maxillary areas	None	Depressive and anxiety states Hysteria Idiopathic	Antidepressant and antianxiety medication
Supraorbital ciliary, infraorbital, sphenopalatine neuralgias	Unilateral in eye, cheek, ear, neck	Persistent, aching pain	Occasional nasal obstruction	Idiopathic Paranasal sinus disease	Decongestant nasal medication ?Nerve section and injection
Postzoster neuralgia	Unilateral Any one of trigeminal divisions	History of zoster Aching, burning pain; jabs of pain Paresthesia, slight sensory loss Dermal scars	Contact, movement	Herpes zoster	Carbamazepine and phenytoin and antidepressants
Costen's syndrome	Unilateral, near temporomandibular joints	Elderly females Severe aching pain, intensified by chewing Tenderness over joints Malocclusion	Chewing, pressure over temporomandibular joint	Loss of teeth, rheumatoid arthritis	Bite correction and surgery
Tolosa-Hunt syndrome	Unilateral, mainly orbital	Intense sharp, aching pain; associated ophthalmoplegias of varying degree Pupil inequality, sensory loss	None	?Arteritis and granulomatous lesions	Corticosteroids
Raeder's paratrigeminal syndrome	Unilateral, frontotemporal and maxilla	Intense sharp, aching pain Pupil inequality, sensory loss	None	Tumors, granulomatous lesions, injuries	Depends on type of lesion

SOURCE: *After J Patten, Neurological Differential Diagnosis, London, Harold Starke, Springer-Verlag, 1977.*

avoidance of the offending activity or agent, and symptomatic therapy in the form of aspirin, 0.6 g, or acetaminophen, 0.6 g, given every 6 to 8 h. Chronic headaches falling into the common migraine or tension category are much more difficult to manage. Analgesics may alleviate the pain, but rarely abolish it. Patients commonly self-administer four to eight tablets daily for years despite acknowledging minimal benefit. Such headaches often respond to amitriptyline given in gradually increased doses to 100 to 150 mg preferably administered as a single bedtime dose. *Premenstrual headache,* if troublesome, can usually be helped by the use of a diuretic compound for the week preceding the menstrual period and a mixture of mild analgesic and sedative medications (aspirin or acetaminophen, 0.6 g, and barbiturate). If the headaches are severe and incapacitating, they should be treated as common migraine.

Migraine may require no treatment at all, other than an explanation of its nature to the patient and a reassurance that it will do no harm. Some patients know, or allege to know, that certain factors induce attacks, and these should be avoided. In some patients alcoholic drinks, particularly red wine, are invariably followed by a migraine. Others claim reduction of attacks of headache by an elimination diet, correction of refractive error, or by psychotherapy. Biofeedback can reduce the number of migraine attacks in some patients, and practiced relaxation is beneficial in others.

Drugs used for treatment of migraine can be separated into agents used for the acute attack and those administered for prophylaxis. Patients who experience more than two or three severe attacks each month should be considered for preventive treatment. Treatment of the neurologic aura of migraine is rarely required or possible because

of its brevity. If the deficits are lasting, inhalation of an ampul of amyl nitrite can be tried as a preventive measure; it should be used at the first premonition of the attack. The time to initiate treatment of the oncoming headache is during the neurologic disorder. If many of the headaches are mild, the patient may already have learned that 0.6 g aspirin or acetaminophen will control the pain. A combination of analgesic and soporific medicine such as Fiorinal or Bellergal may be helpful. If severe disabling attacks are expected, they too may respond to simple analgesic medication and rest in a quiet, darkened room. Some patients find relieve with ergot preparations given orally, 1 to 3 mg held under the tongue until dissolved, or ergotamine tartrate, 0.25 mg by intravenous injection. These treatments if given early will abort a classic migraine attack in 80 to 90 percent of patients. Sometimes the combination of caffeine, 100 mg with 1 mg ergotamine, is preferred. It may be taken in the form of a tablet (two at the onset of headache and a third in half an hour) or as a rectal suppository (2 mg ergotamine and 100 mg caffeine) if vomiting prevents oral administration.

Because of the danger of prolonged vascular spasm in patients who have vascular disease or are pregnant, ergot preparations must be used cautiously, if at all. Even in healthy individuals more than 10 to 15 mg ergotamine per week is risky, for it may in itself produce headache. Hakkareinen et al. report that tolfenamic acid, an anti-inflammatory agent that blocks prostaglandin receptors in oral doses of 200 mg, was found to be as effective as ergotamine tartrate. For the frequent atypical migraine headaches, some of which respond poorly to ergot, one should prescribe a preparation containing 150 mg aspirin, 160 mg phenacetin, and dextroamphetamine sulfate,

5 mg, with phenobarbital, 30 mg. This can be repeated once or twice in a severe attack. Once the headache has become intense (after 30 min), ergot is of little help, and one must resort to codeine sulfate, 30 mg, or meperidine, 50 mg, as the only means of terminating the pain. If sleep customarily terminates headache, 50 mg of promethazine orally is helpful; it also relieves vomiting.

In individuals with frequent migrainous attacks (more than one to three a month), efforts at prevention are worthwhile. Some success has been obtained with preparations of ergot, 0.5 mg, atropine, 0.3 mg, and phenobarbital, 15 mg, two or three times a day for a few weeks. Propranolol, 40 mg three times a day, has been effective in reducing the frequency and intensity of attacks in approximately two-thirds of cases. For the most severe forms of the disorder, methysergide in a dose of 6 to 8 mg per day given for several weeks or months has proved to be most promising in reducing the frequency of or abolishing attacks. The main adverse effect has been retroperitoneal and pulmonary fibrosis; this complication has been reported in several dozen cases when the patient has been treated continuously for more than 6 months. Discontinuing treatment for 1 month out of every 6 has greatly reduced the incidence of this complication. Recently, claims have been made for pizotifen (a histamine- and serotonin-blocking agent), for amitriptyline, apart from its antidepressant action, for phenelzine, a monoamine oxidase inhibitor, and for calcium channel blockers. Severe attacks of migraine lasting for several days or even weeks have been treated successfully with chlorpromazine in large doses of 50 to 100 mg daily. Prednisone in divided doses of 20 mg three or four times a day is also effective in some severe cases.

All experienced physicians appreciate the importance of helping patients rearrange their schedules so as to control the tensions and hard-driving ways of living so often a feature of many migrainous patients. There is no one way of accomplishing this, but in general, long and costly psychotherapy has not been helpful, or at least one can say there are no substantial data as to its value.

Cluster headaches have proved to be most resistant to treatment. One capsule of Cafergot or 1.0 mg of ergotamine tartrate at bedtime is most widely recommended. However, if the headaches are frequent, severe, and diurnal as well as nocturnal, the intake of ergot may reach dangerous levels. Success has also been claimed for amitriptyline, 25 to 100 mg three times a day, and methysergide, 6 to 8 mg per day, as means of interrupting a cluster. Lance recommends prednisone, 40 mg daily for 5 days then reduced to an amount necessary to control headaches. Lithium carbonate in an initial dose of 250 mg three times a day is said to give relief in 80 to 90 percent of cases. Histamine desensitization, originally proposed by Horton, has been little used in recent years because of inconsistent results. In rare cases of persistent cluster headaches lasting for 10 to 20 years spectacular success has been obtained by indomethacin.

Hypertensive headaches respond to agents which lower blood pressure and relieve muscle tension. Chlorothiazide, 250 to 500 mg twice a day, and methyldopa, 250 to 500 mg per day, when combined with a small amount of phenobarbital, 15 mg three times a day, or propranolol, 40 mg three times a day, have given satisfactory results. Meprobamate, 200 mg three times a day, or chlordiazepoxide hydrochloride, 5 mg three times a day, may be administered in place of phenobarbital.

The *muscle tension headaches* respond best to massage, relaxation, and a combination of drugs which relieve depression (e.g., amitriptyline or imipramine) and anxiety (e.g., meprobamate and chlordiazepoxide hydrochloride). Pain-relieving medicine of non-habit-forming type (e.g., aspirin and propoxyphene hydrochloride) should be added when throbbing headache is present. Stronger analgesic medication (codeine or meperidine hydrochloride) should be avoided. Psychotherapy may be helpful in this group of patients.

The headache of the *posttraumatic syndrome* requires supportive psychotherapy in the form of reassurance and frequent explanation of its benign and transient nature, a program of increasing physical activity, and drugs which allay anxiety and depression. However, the tricyclic antidepressants are generally less effective than in the mixed tension and throbbing headaches of anxious depressions. Tender scars from scalp laceration may be novocainized repeatedly (subcutaneous injection of 5 mL of 1% procaine) with some degree of success. Settlement of litigation as soon as possible works to the patient's advantage.

Heat, massage, salicylates, and indomethacin or phenylbutazone usually effect some improvement in those arthritic diseases of the cervical spine which are associated with cervicocranial pain (see Chaps. 263 and 274). A soft collar and traction may be beneficial.

Corticosteroid therapy is indicated in *cranial arteritis* to prevent disastrous blindness by occlusion of the ophthalmic arteries, which occurs in 50 percent of untreated patients. Prednisone should be given in full doses (40 to 60 mg per day) for at least a month and continued until all symptoms and laboratory abnormalities have disappeared. The headaches of cranial tumor often respond promptly to large doses of corticosteroids.

In conclusion, it is well to mention the importance of general hygienic measures. Young physicians in particular are apt to seek a specific therapy for each headache syndrome and give little thought to the general health of the patient. We have observed that most of the recurrent and chronic headaches are likely to be more severe and disabling whenever the patient becomes nervous, sick, and tired. A well-rounded diet, adequate rest, a reasonable amount of physical exercise, and a balanced view of the sources of daily anxieties and how to cope with them should be the goal of all therapeutic programs.

REFERENCES

APPENZELLER O: *Pathogenesis and Treatment of Headache.* New York, Spectrum, 1976

BICKERSTAFF ER: Basilar artery migraine. Lancet 1:15, 1961

BOGDUK N, LANCE JW: Pain and pain syndrome including headache, in *Current Neurology,* SF Appel (ed). New York, Wiley, 1981, vol 3, chap 14

CAVINESS VS, O'BRIEN P: Headache. N Engl J Med 302:446, 1980

COUCH JR, HASSANEIM RS: Platelet aggregability in migraine. Neurology 27:843, 1977

CRITCHLEY M et al (eds): *Advances in Neurology,* vol. 33: *Headache: Physiopathological and Clinical Aspects.* New York, Raven Press, 1982

DIAMOND S: Prolonged benign exertional headache. Headache 22:96, 1982

EHYAI A, FENICHEL GM: Natural history of acute confusional migraine. Arch Neurol 35:368, 1978

FISHER CM: Transient migrainous accompaniments of late onset. Stroke 10:96, 1979

GELMERS HJ: Nimodipine, a new calcium antagonist, in the prophylactic treatment of migraine. *Headache* 23(3):106, 1983

HAKKAREINEN H et al: Tolfenamic acid is as effective as ergotamine during migraine attacks. Lancet 2:326, 1979

HOCKADAY JM: Basilar migraine in children. Dev Med Child Neurol 21:455, 1979

KAYAN A, HOOD JD: Neuro-otological manifestations of migraine. Brain 107:1123, 1984

LAKE A, RAINEY J, PAPSDORF JD: Biofeedback and rational-emotive therapy in the management of migraine headache. Appl Behav Anal 12:127, 1979

LANCE JW: Headache. Ann Neurol 10:1, 1981

———: Headaches related to sexual activity. J Neurol Neurosurg Psychiat 39:1226, 1976

MOSKOWITZ M: Neurobiology of vascular head pain. Ann Neurol 16:157, 1984

OLESON J et al: Focal hyperemia followed by spreading oligemia in classic migraine. Ann Neurol 9:344, 1981

PEROUTKA J: The pharmacology of calcium channel antagonists: Novel class of anti-migraine agents? Headache 23:278, 1983

RASKIN NH, SCHWARTZ RK: Icepick-like pain. Neurology 29:550, 1979

VIJAYAN N, DREYFUS PM: Posttraumatic dysautonomic cephalalgia: Clinical observations and treatment. Arch Neurol 32:649, 1976

VINKEN PJ, BRUYN GW (eds): *Handbook of Clinical Neurology,* vol 5: *Headache and Cranial Neuralgias.* Amsterdam, North-Holland, 1968.

7 PAIN IN THE BACK AND NECK

HENRY J. MANKIN / RAYMOND D. ADAMS

ANATOMY AND PHYSIOLOGY OF THE LOWER PART OF THE BACK

The bony spine is a complex structure, anatomically divisible into two parts. The anterior part consists of a series of cylindrical vertebral bodies connected to one another by the intervertebral disks and held together by the anterior and posterior longitudinal ligaments. The posterior part consists of more delicate elements that extend from the vertebral body as pedicles and broaden posteriorly to form laminae, which together with ligamentous structures form the vertebral canal. The posterior elements are joined to adjacent vertebrae by two small facetal synovial joints which allow a range of motion (Fig. 7-1). Stout transverse and spinous bony processes project laterally and posteriorly and serve as the attachments of muscles which move, support, and protect the vertebral column. The stability of the spine depends on two types of support: that provided by the bony articulations (principally by the diskal joints and the synovial articulations of the posterior elements) and a second type provided by the ligamentous (passive) and muscular (active) supporting structures. The ligamentous structures are quite strong, but because neither they nor the vertebral body–disk complexes have sufficient integral strength to resist the enormous forces acting on the column during even simple movements, voluntary and reflex contractions of the sacrospinalis, abdominal, gluteal, psoas, and hamstring muscles afford most of the stability.

The vertebral and paravertebral structures derive their innervation from the recurrent branches of the spinal nerves. Pain endings and fibers have been demonstrated in the ligaments, muscles, periosteum of bone, outer layers of annulus fibrosus, and synovium of the articular facets. The sensory fibers from these structures and the sacroiliac and lumbosacral joints join to form the sinovertebral nerves which pass via the recurrent branches of the spinal nerves of the first sacral and the fifth to first lumbar vertebrae into the gray matter of the corresponding segments of the spinal cord. Efferent fibers emerge from these segments and extend to the muscles through the same nerves.

The parts of the back that possess the greatest freedom of movement, and hence are most frequently subject to injury, are the lumbar and cervical regions. In addition to the voluntary motions required for bending, twisting, and other movements, many actions of the spine are reflex in nature and are the basis of posture.

FIGURE 7-1 *Left: Superior view of a stripped lumbar vertebra. Right: Lateral view of two articulated lumbar vertebrae. B = body; SC = spinal canal; IVF = intervertebral foramen; IF = inferior articular facet; SF = superior articular facet; P = pedicle; TP = transverse process; SP = spinous process; L = lamina. (Adapted from DB Levine, in Arthritis and Allied Conditions: A Textbook of Rheumatology, 10th ed, DJ McCarty (ed), Philadelphia, Lea & Febiger, 1985.)*

GENERAL CLINICAL CONSIDERATIONS

TYPES OF LOW BACK PAIN   Four types of pain may be differentiated: local, referred, radicular, and that arising from secondary (protective) muscular spasm.

Local pain is caused by any pathologic process which impinges upon or irritates sensory endings. Involvement of structures which contain no sensory endings is painless. The central, medullary portion of the vertebral body may be destroyed by tumor, for example, without evocation of pain, whereas cortical fractures, or tears and distortions of the periosteum, synovial membranes, muscles, annulus fibrosus, and ligaments are often exquisitely painful. Although painful states are often accompanied by swelling of the affected tissues, this may not be apparent if a deep structure of the back is the site of disease. Local pain is often described as steady but may be intermittent, varying considerably with position or activity. The pain may be sharp or dull and although often diffuse is always felt in or near the affected part of the spine. Reflex splinting of the spine segments by paravertebral muscles is frequently noted, and certain movements or postures that alter the position of the injured tissues aggravate the pain. Firm pressure or percussion upon superficial structures in the region involved usually evokes tenderness, which is of aid in identifying the site of the abnormality.

Referred pain is of two types: that projected from the spine into regions lying within the area of the lumbar and upper sacral dermatomes and that projected from the pelvic and abdominal viscera to the spine. Pain due to diseases of the upper part of the lumbar spine is usually referred to the anterior aspects of the thighs and legs; that from the lower lumbar and sacral segments is referred to the gluteal regions, posterior thighs, calves, and sometimes feet. Pain of this type, although of deep, aching quality and rather diffuse, tends at times to be superficially projected. In general the referred pain parallels in intensity the local pain in the back. In other words, maneuvers which alter local pain have a similar effect on referred pain, though not with such precision and immediacy as in radicular, or "root," pain. Referred pain may be confused with pain from visceral disease, but the latter is usually described as "deep" and tends to radiate from the abdomen through to the back. Also, visceral pain is usually unaffected by movement of the spine, does not improve with recumbency, and may be modified by the activity of the involved viscus.

Radicular, or "root," *pain* has some of the characteristics of referred pain but differs in its greater intensity, distal radiation, circumscription to the territory of a root, and the factors which excite it. The mechanism is distortion, stretching, irritation, or compression of a spinal root, most often central to the intervertebral foramen. Although the pain itself is often dull or aching, various maneuvers which increase the irritation of the root may greatly intensify the pain, eliciting a lancinating quality. Nearly always the radiation of pain is from a central position near the spine to some part of the lower extremity. Cough, sneeze, and strain are characteristically evocative maneuvers; but since they may also jar or move the spine, they may aggravate local pain as well. Any motion which stretches the nerve, e.g., forward bending with the knees extended or "straight-leg raising," in disease of the lower part of the lumbar spine excites radicular pain; jugular vein compression, which raises intraspinal pressure and may cause a shift in the position of or pressure on the root, may have a similar effect. The fourth and fifth lumbar and first sacral roots, which form the sciatic nerve, cause pain which extends mainly down the posterior aspects of thigh, the postero- and anterolateral aspects of the leg, and into the foot, in the distribution of this nerve—so called sciatica. Tingling, paresthesias, and numbness or sensory impairment of the skin, soreness of the skin, and tenderness along the nerve usually accompany radicular pain. Reflex loss, weakness, atrophy, fascicular twitching, and occasionally stasis edema may occur if motor fibers of the anterior root are involved.

Pain resulting from muscular spasm is usually mentioned in relation to local pain. Muscle spasm may be associated with many disorders of the spine and can produce significant distortions of the normal posture. Chronic tension in muscles may give rise to a dull and sometimes cramping ache. One can in this instance feel the tautness of the sacrospinalis and gluteal muscles and demonstrate by palpation that the pain is localized to these structures.

Other pains often of undetermined origin are sometimes described by patients with chronic disease of the lower part of the back. In the legs, drawing, pulling, cramping sensations (without involuntary muscle spasm), tearing, throbbing, or jabbing pains, or feelings of burning or coldness are difficult to interpret and, like paresthesias and numbness, should always suggest the possibility of nerve or root disease.

In addition to assessing the character and location of the pain, one should determine the factors which aggravate and relieve it, its constancy, and its relationship to recumbency and such stereotypical movements and maneuvers as forward bending, cough, sneeze, and strain. Frequently the most important lead comes from the knowledge of the mode of onset and circumstances which initiated the pain. Inasmuch as many painful afflictions of the back are the result of injury incurred during work or in an accident, the possibility of exaggeration or prolongation of pain for purposes of compensation or other personal reasons, or because of hysteria or malingering, must always be kept in mind.

EXAMINATION OF THE LOWER PART OF THE BACK

Inspection of the normal spine shows a dorsal kyphosis and lumbar lordosis in the sagittal plane, which in some individuals may be exaggerated (swayback). In spinal disorders, one should observe the spine closely for excessive curvature, flattening of the normal lumbar arch, presence of a gibbus (a short, sharp, kyphotic angulation usually indicative of a fracture or congenital abnormality), pelvic tilt or obliquity, or asymmetry of the paravertebral or gluteal musculature. In severe sciatica, one may observe abnormalities of posture of the affected leg, presumably to reduce tension on the irritated part.

The spine, hips, and legs should be observed during certain motions. No advantage accrues from trying to find out how much the patient can be hurt. Instead, it is much more important to determine when and under what conditions the pain commences. One looks for limitation of the natural motions of the patient while he or she is disrobing, standing, and reclining. When standing, the motion of forward bending normally produces flattening and reversal of the lumbar lordotic curve and exaggeration of the dorsal curve. With lesions of the lumbosacral region which involve the posterior ligaments, articular facets, or sacrospinalis muscle and with ruptured lumbar disks, protective reflexes prevent stretching of these structures. As a consequence, the sacrospinalis muscles remain taut and limit motion in the lumbar part of the spine. Forward bending then occurs at the hips and at the lumbar-thoracic junction. With disease of the lumbosacral joints and spinal roots, the patient bends in such a way as to avoid tensing the hamstring muscles and putting undue leverage upon the pelvis. In unilateral "sciatica," with its increased curvature toward the side of the lesion, lumbar and lumbosacral motions are splinted, and bending is mainly at the hips; at a certain point the knee on the affected side is flexed to relieve hamstring spasm and tilting of the pelvis occurs to slacken the lumbosacral roots and sciatic nerve.

In unilateral ligamentous or muscular strain, bending to the opposite side aggravates the pain by stretching the damaged tissues. Moreover, in lateral disk lesions, bending of the spine toward the side of the lesion is restricted. In diseases of the lower part of the spine, flexion while sitting with the hips and knees flexed can normally be performed easily, even to the point of bringing the knees in contact with the chest. The reason is that knee flexion relaxes the tightened hamstring muscles and also relieves stretch of the sciatic nerve.

With lumbosacral lesions and sciatica, passive lumbar flexion in the supine position causes little pain and is not limited as long as the hamstrings are relaxed and there is no stretching of the sciatic nerve. With lumbosacral and lumbar spine disease (e.g., arthritis), passive flexion of the hips is free, whereas flexion of the lumbar spine may be impeded and painful. Passive straight-leg raising (possible in most normal individuals up to 80 to 90° except in those who have unusually tight hamstrings), like forward bending in the standing posture with the legs straight, places the sciatic nerve and its roots under tension, thereby producing pain. It may also cause an anterior rotation of the pelvis around a transverse axis, increasing stress on the lumbosacral joint, and thus causing pain if this segment is arthritic or otherwise impaired. Consequently, in diseases of the lumbosacral joints and lumbosacral roots, this movement is limited on the affected side and to a lesser extent on the opposite side. Lasègue's sign (pain and limitation of movement during flexion of the hip when the knee is extended) is a useful test of this condition. Straight-leg raising of the opposite leg may also cause contralateral pain but of lesser degree and is believed by some to be a sign of a more extensive lesion, such as an extruded disk fragment, rather than a simple prolapse or protrusion. It is important to remember, however, that the evoked pain is always referred to the diseased side, no matter which leg is flexed.

Hyperextension is best performed with the patient standing or lying prone. If the condition causing back pain is acute, it may be difficult to extend the spine in the standing position. A patient with lumbosacral strain or disk disease can usually extend or hyperextend the spine without aggravation of pain. If the lesion is in the upper lumbar segments or if an active inflammatory process or fracture of the vertebral body or posterior elements is present, hyperextension may be markedly limited.

Palpation and percussion of the spine are the last steps in the examination. It is preferable to palpate first those regions which are the least likely to evoke pain. At all times the examiner should know what structures are being palpated (see Fig. 7-2). Localized tenderness

FIGURE 7-2   *(1) Costovertebral angle. (2) Spinous process and interspinous ligament. (3) Region of the articular fifth lumbar to the first sacral facet. (4) Dorsum of sacrum. (5) Region of iliac crest. (6) Iliolumbar angle. (7) Spinous processes of fifth lumbar to first sacral vertebrae (tenderness = faulty posture or occasionally spina bifida occulta). (8) Region between posterior superior and posterior inferior spines. Sacroiliac ligaments (tenderness = sacroiliac sprain, often tender with fifth lumbar to first sacral disk). (9) Sacrococcygeal junction (tenderness = sacrococcygeal injury, i.e., sprain or fracture). (10) Region of sacrosciatic notch (tenderness = fourth to fifth lumbar disk rupture and sacroiliac sprain). (11) Sciatic nerve trunk (tenderness = ruptured lumbar disk or sciatic nerve lesion).*

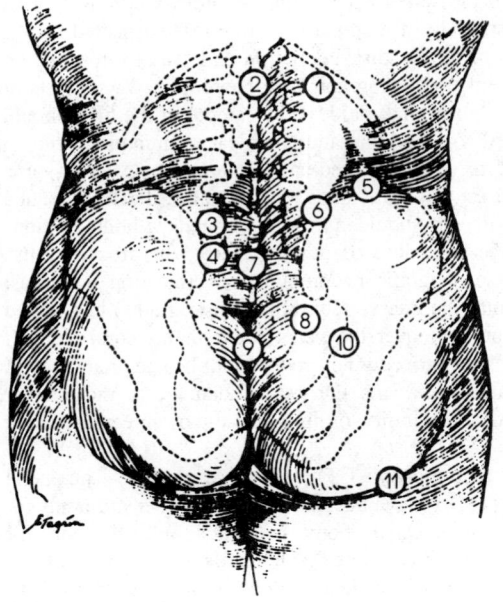

is seldom pronounced in disease of the spine because the involved structures are so deep that they rarely give rise to surface tenderness. Mild superficial and poorly localized tenderness signifies only a disease process within the affected segment of the body, i.e., dermatome.

Tenderness over the costovertebral angle often indicates renal disease, adrenal disease, or an injury to the transverse processes of the first or second lumbar vertebra. Hypersensitivity on palpation of the transverse processes of the other lumbar vertebrae as well as the overlying sacrospinalis muscles may signify fracture of the transverse process or a strain of muscle attachments. Tenderness of a spinous process or aggravation of pain by the jarring of gentle percussion may be nonspecific but frequently indicates the presence of a disk lesion at the site deep to it, inflammation (as in disk space infection), or fracture. Tenderness in the region of the articular facets between the fifth lumbar and first sacral vertebrae is consistent with disease of a lumbosacral disk [Fig. 7-2 (3)]. It is also frequent in rheumatoid arthritis.

In palpation of the spinous processes, it is important to note any deviation in the lateral plane (this may be indicative of fracture or arthritis) or in the anteroposterior plane. A "step-off" forward displacement of the spinous process may be an important clue to a spondylolisthesis, one segment below the displaced level.

Abdominal, rectal, and pelvic examination and assessment of the status of the peripheral vascular system are important parts of the examination of the patient with complaints in the lower back and should not be omitted. They may provide evidence for vascular, visceral, neoplastic, or inflammatory disorders which may extend to the spine or cause pain to be referred to this region.

Finally, a careful neurologic examination should be performed, with special attention given to motor, reflex, and sensory changes (see "Protrusion of Lumbar Intervertebral Disks," below), particularly in the lower extremities.

SPECIAL LABORATORY PROCEDURES   Useful laboratory tests, depending on the nature of the problem and the circumstances, include a complete blood count, erythrocyte sedimentation rate (especially helpful in screening for infection or myeloma), measurement of serum calcium, phosphorus, alkaline phosphatase, acid phosphatase (the last mentioned is of importance if one suspects metastatic carcinoma from the prostate), protein electrophoresis, immunoglobulin electrophoresis, and tests for rheumatoid. Roentgenograms of the lumbar part of the spine should be taken in every case of low back pain and sciatica in the anteroposterior, lateral, and oblique planes. Special spot views or stereoscopic or laminographic films may provide further information in certain cases. Bone scans are of aid in revealing some fractures and neoplastic and inflammatory lesions.

Examination of the spinal canal with a contrast medium is often of great value, especially if a spinal cord tumor is suspected or if a patient is thought to have a disk herniation and fails to improve on a conservative regimen. Myelography can be combined with tests of dynamics of the cerebrospinal fluid, and a sample of the fluid should always be removed for cytologic and chemical examination prior to the instillation of the contrast medium (Pantopaque, Myodil, or a water-soluble contrast medium). Injection and removal of Pantopaque require special skill and should not be attempted without previous experience with the procedure. If done properly, the procedure has a very low incidence of significant complications. Injection of contrast medium directly into the intervertebral disk (diskograms) has waxed and waned in popularity over the years and remains controversial. The technique of this procedure is more complicated than that of myelographic examination, and the risk of damage to the disk or nerve roots and the possibility of introduction of infection is not inconsiderable.

Computerized tomography (CT) and more recently, magnetic resonance imaging (MRI) have become very valuable instruments for the study of the spinal canal, bony segments, and adjacent soft tissues. CT, particularly if combined with instillation of water-soluble contrast media, provides excellent definition of a narrow canal,

destructive lesions of the vertebral bodies and posterior elements, presence of a paravertebral soft tissue mass, and by appropriate computerized reconstruction techniques can also identify disk herniations, sometimes with greater accuracy than the myelogram. Even without radiopaque material in the canal, the reconstructed CT scans have a high resolution and provide a noninvasive method of study of disk disease with a relatively low level of radiation.

Confirmation of proximal motor and sensory nerve and root disease can be obtained by nerve conduction studies, H and F responses, and electromyography (see Chap. 354).

PRINCIPAL CONDITIONS WHICH GIVE RISE TO DISABLING PAIN IN THE LOWER PART OF THE BACK

CONGENITAL ANOMALIES OF THE LUMBAR SPINE   One of the most common disorders is a failure of fusion of the laminae of the neural arch (spina bifida) of one or several of the lumbar vertebrae or of the sacrum. Hypertrichosis or hyperpigmentation in the sacral area may betray the condition, but in most patients the spine defect remains entirely occult until disclosed by x-ray. The anomaly has greater potentiality for pain if accompanied by malformation of vertebral joints. Usually the pain is induced by injury. Other congenital anomalies that affect the lower lumbar vertebrae such as asymmetrical facetal joints, abnormalities of the transverse processes, sacralization of the fifth lumbar vertebra (in which L5 is firmly fixed to the sacrum), or lumbarization of the first sacral vertebra (in which the first sacral resembles a sixth lumbar) are rarely the cause of specific symptomatology.

Spondylolysis consists of a bony defect probably caused by trauma to a congenitally abnormal segment in the pars interarticularis (a segment near the junction of the pedicle with the lamina) of the lower lumbar area. The defect is best visualized on oblique projections. In some individuals the defect is bilateral. Under the circumstance of single or multiple injuries, the vertebral body, pedicle, and superior articular facet move anteriorly, leaving the posterior elements behind. This latter abnormality, known as *spondylolisthesis,* usually results in symptoms. The patient complains of pain in the low back radiating into the thighs, and there is limitation of motion. Often tenderness is elicited near the segment which has "slipped" forward (most often L5 on S1 or occasionally L4 on L5), and one can feel a "step" on deep palpation of the posterior elements. The pelvis is sometimes rotated and hip flexion limited by hamstring spasm; a variety of neurologic deficits indicative of radiculopathy complete the clinical syndrome. In exceptionally severe degrees of spondylolisthesis the trunk may be shortened and the abdomen protuberant, both the result of the extreme forward displacement of L5 on S1.

TRAUMATIC AFFLICTIONS OF THE LOWER PART OF THE BACK Trauma constitutes the most frequent cause of low back pain. In severe acute injuries, the examining physician must be careful to avoid further damage. In tests of mobility, all movements must be kept to a minimum until a diagnosis has been made and adequate measures have been instituted for the proper care of the patient. A patient complaining of back pain and inability to move the legs may have a fractured spine. The neck should not be flexed, nor should the patient be allowed to sit up. (See Chap. 353 for further discussion of spinal cord injury.)

Sprains, strains, and derangements   The terms lumbosacral *sprain* and *strain* are often used loosely by physicians, and do not clearly relate to a known anatomic lesion. The authors prefer the term *low back derangement* or *strain* for minor, self-limited injuries usually associated with lifting a heavy object, a fall, or a sudden deceleration as may occur in an automobile accident. Occasionally, these syndromes are more chronic in nature, suggesting that diskal or arthritic factors may play a role. The patients with low back derangement are often acutely discomfited and may assume unusual postures related to spasm of the sacrospinalis muscles. The pain is usually confined to the lower back and is almost invariably relieved by rest within a few days. More extensive or longer lasting problems, formerly classified as sacroiliac strain or sprain are now known to be due to disk disease in most instances (see below).

Vertebral fractures   Most fractures of the lumbar vertebral body are the result of flexion injuries and consist of anterior wedging or compression. With more severe trauma the patient may sustain a fracture dislocation, "bursting" fracture, or asymmetrical fracture involving not only the body but the posterior elements. The initiating trauma which causes fractures of the vertebrae is usually a fall from a height (in which case the calcanei may also be fractured) or may result from an automobile accident or other violence. When fractures occur with minimal trauma (or spontaneously), the bone is presumed to have been previously weakened by some pathologic process. Most of the time, particularly in older individuals, the cause of such an event is idiopathic osteoporosis, but there are many other underlying systemic disorders such as osteomalacia, hyperparathyroidism, hyperthyroidism, multiple myeloma, metastatic carcinoma, and a large number of local conditions that may play a role in weakening the vertebral body. Spasm of the lower lumbar muscles, limitation of motion of the lumbar section of the spine, and the roentgenographic appearance of the damaged lumbar segment (with or without neurologic abnormalities) are the basis of clinical diagnosis. The pain is usually immediate, though occasionally it may be delayed in onset for a few days. The patient may develop a mild paralytic ileus or urinary retention during the acute period.

Fractures of the transverse processes are almost always associated with tearing of the paravertebral muscles, principally the psoas. They may cause significant retroperitoneal hemorrhage resulting in a marked depression in hematocrit and, in extensive fractures, hypovolemic shock. Such injuries may be diagnosed by the finding of deep tenderness at the site of the injury, local muscle spasm on one side, and limitation of all movements which stretch the lumbar muscles. Radiologic evidence including bone scans, body CT, or MRI scanning provides the final confirmation. Fractures of multiple transverse processes, although seemingly trivial, should be the object of considerable concern, and the patient should be carefully watched for internal hemorrhage.

Protrusion of lumbar intervertebral disks   This condition is the major cause of severe and chronic or recurrent low back and leg pain. It is most likely to occur between the fifth lumbar and first sacral vertebrae, and, with lessening frequency, between the fourth and fifth lumbar, the third and fourth lumbar, the second and third lumbar, and rarely, between the first and second lumbar vertebrae. Rare in the thoracic portion of the spine, it is next most frequent between the sixth and seventh and fifth and sixth cervical vertebrae. The cause is usually a flexion injury, but in many cases no trauma is recalled. Degeneration of the posterior longitudinal ligaments and the annulus fibrosus, which occurs in most adults of middle and advanced years, may have taken place silently or have been manifested by mild, recurrent lumbar ache. A sneeze, lurch, or other trivial movement may then cause the nucleus pulposus to prolapse, pushing the frayed and weakened annulus posteriorly. In more severe cases of disk disease, the nucleus may protrude through the annulus or become extruded to lie as a free fragment in the vertebral canal.

The fully developed syndrome of ruptured lumbar intervertebral disk consists of backache, abnormal posture, and limitation of motion of the spine (particularly flexion). Nerve root involvement is indicated by radicular pain, sensory disturbances (paresthesias, hyper- and hyposensitivity in dermatome pattern), coarse twitching and fasciculation, muscle spasms, and impairment of a tendon reflex. Motor abnormalities (weakness and muscle atrophy) may also occur but are usually less prominent than the pain and sensory disorder. Since herniation of the intervertebral lumbar disks most often occurs between the fourth and fifth lumbar vertebrae and the fifth lumbar and first sacral vertebrae with irritation and compression of the fifth lumbar

and first sacral roots, respectively, it is important to recognize the clinical characteristics of lesions of these two roots. *Lesions of the fifth lumbar root* produce pain in the region of the hip, groin, posterolateral thigh, lateral calf to the external malleolus, dorsal surface of the foot, and the first or second and third toes. Paresthesias may be in the entire territory or only in the distal parts of these territories. The tenderness is in the lateral gluteal region and near the head of the fibula. Weakness, if present, involves the extensor of the great toe and less often of the foot. The knee and ankle reflexes are seldom altered, although occasionally the ankle jerk is moderately depressed. Walking on the heels may be more difficult, because of weakness of dorsiflexion of the foot, and more uncomfortable than walking on the toes. In *lesions of the first sacral root* the pain is felt in the midgluteal region, posterior part of the thigh, posterior region of the calf to the heel, and the plantar surface of the foot and fourth and fifth toes. Tenderness is most pronounced over the midgluteal region (sacroiliac joint), posterior thigh area, and calf. Rarely it may be referred to the rectum, testicles, or labia. Paresthesias and sensory loss are mainly in the lower leg and outer toes, and weakness, if present, involves the flexor muscles of the foot and toes, abductors of the toes, and hamstring muscles. The ankle reflex is diminished or absent in the majority of cases. Walking on the toes is more difficult, because of weakness of plantar flexors, and more uncomfortable than walking on the heel. With lesions of either root there may be limitation of straight-leg raising during the acute, painful stages.

Degeneration of the intervertebral disk without frank extrusion of a fragment of disk tissue may give rise to low back pain, or the disk may herniate into the adjacent vertebral body, giving rise to a Schmorl's node, usually visualized by x-ray. Such cases often show no signs of nerve root involvement though the back pain may be referred to the thigh and leg.

The rarer *lesions of the fourth and third lumbar roots* give rise to pain in the anterior part of the thigh and knee, with corresponding sensory loss. The knee jerk is diminished or abolished. An inverted Lasègue sign (pain with hypertension of the limb in relation to the trunk, best elicited with the patient in the prone position) is positive when the third lumbar root is affected.

The lumbar disk syndromes are usually unilateral. Only with massive derangements of the disk or the extrusion of a large, free fragment into the canal do bilateral symptoms and signs occur, and these may sometimes be associated with paralysis of the sphincters. The pain may be mild or severe. All or part of the above syndrome may be present. There may be back pain with little or no leg pain, and occasionally the patient experiences leg pain with little or no discomfort in the back. The rupture of multiple lumbar or lumbar and cervical disks is not infrequent, suggesting a diffuse disorder of the connective tissue of the disks, including both the annulus fibrosus and the nucleus pulposus.

When all components of the syndrome are present, the diagnosis is easy; when only one part is present (particularly backache), it may be difficult, especially if there has not been a clearly remembered initiating traumatic event. Since similar symptoms may occur without demonstrable disk rupture, other diagnostic procedures are required. Plain roentgenograms usually show no abnormality or at most a narrowing of the intervertebral space, sometimes more on the side of the rupture. Traction spurs, which are indicative of disk degeneration, may be present; in extreme cases, there may be a "vacuum" disk sign, in which a gas-density shadow is present in the intervertebral space, usually on lateral roentgenogram. Frequently, however, one must resort to Pantopaque or soluble contrast media myelography, which in most cases will reveal an indentation of the lumbar subarachnoid space or deformity of the root sleeve. Occasionally, with large lesions there is a complete interruption of the flow of contrast material. In some patients, CT with or without contrast material may show the disk herniation clearly even when it is small or laterally placed. A small ruptured disk may not show any abnormality in the CT scan or myelogram, especially at the fifth lumbar to first sacral level where there is a large space between the spinal canal and dura. Some clinics use diskograms (opaque material is injected directly into the disk) to reveal any evidence of extrusion, but the procedure is risky, and the results are difficult to interpret. The electromyogram is helpful in showing denervation of paravertebral and leg muscles (see Chap. 354). The protein level of the cerebrospinal fluid may be elevated in some instances.

Tumor of the spinal canal, epidural or intradural, may produce a syndrome similar to that of ruptured disk (see Chap. 353).

OTHER CAUSES OF LOW BACK PAIN AND SCIATICA   A large experience with lumbar back pain, gluteal neuralgia, and sciatica in a medical referral center has impressed the authors with the sizable number of patients whose symptoms cannot be ascribed to a ruptured disk. Often the patients have had an operation for diskogenic disease with or without attempted fusion of the lumbar vertebrae, but the pain has not remitted. The indications for the original surgery may have been questionable; only a disk bulge ("hard disk") without definite neurologic signs. To explain these chronic pain states a number of new pathologic entities, some of uncertain status, have been introduced. Entrapment of one or more nerve roots may be the consequence not only of a disk but also of spondylotic spurs with variable stenosis of the lateral recess and intervertebral canal, hypertrophy of apophyseal facets, or "spinal arachnoiditis."

Spondylotic spurs and stenosis of the lateral recess and intervertebral foramen have been distinguished clinically from ruptured disk. The pain involves one or both legs on standing and walking and is relieved by squatting or lying down. In the 35 cases reported by Mikhael et al. motor, reflex, and sensory changes were present. Radiologically, there was stenosis at one vertebral level. Most often the superior facet at L5 had narrowed the lateral recess at the upper border of the pedicle, compressing the L5 root and sometimes S1, as well. By polytomography the lateral recess was seen to be reduced to less than 3 mm. A more proper designation for this condition is *unilateral spondylosis,* and in some instances *spondylolysis.* In this condition, the adjacent articular capsule may suffer injury and add direct and referred pain to a radicular syndrome (see below and Chap. 353 for further discussion of the lumbar stenosis or claudication syndrome).

The *unilateral facet syndrome* is closely related. Reynolds et al. have reported 22 cases in which a lumbar monoradiculopathy had simulated that of a ruptured disk: 16 had an L5 radiculopathy, 3 an S1 radiculopathy, and 3 an L4 radiculopathy. Coexisting back pain was present in 15 of the cases. No disk rupture was found by myelography. At operation the spinal root was compressed against the floor or roof of the intervertebral canal by an enlarged superior or inferior facet. Foraminotomy and facetectomy relieved the symptoms in 12 of the 15 operated cases. Denervation of the lumbar facets by radiofrequency electrodes (percutaneous rhizolysis) of nerves supplying the zygoapophyseal joints has been utilized by Collier, who obtained relief of the patients' symptoms in 35 of 122 cases. But there is doubt as to whether the favorable results were due to the rhizolysis or to some other factor.

In some cases myelography has revealed a loculated, cystlike expansion of the perineurial sheath. It may extend beyond the intervertebral canal. Multiple cervical or lumbar spinal nerves may be involved. There are numerous surgical reports of relief of radicular pain and other symptoms by opening the cysts. The authors find it difficult to evaluate the results.

Lumbar adhesive arachnoiditis with radiculopathy is receiving increasing attention. This is an ambiguous entity in which patients after multiple lumbar operations and myelograms are left with backache and leg pain in combination with motor, sensory, and reflex changes. The arachnoidal membrane is thickened and opaque, adherent to dura, and tightly bound to pia and roots. The contrast medium during myelography does not fill the root sheaths and tends to be irregularly loculated. According to a British survey lumbar arachnoiditis was found in only 80 of 7600 myelograms, but judging from the American literature it is much more frequent. In our case material,

disk rupture, multiple Pantopaque myelograms, operative procedures, infection, and subarachnoid hemorrhage, in various combinations, are factors which favor its development. Treatment is unsatisfactory; lysis of adhesions and intrathecal steroid therapy have been of no value.

In patients with persistent chronic low back pain and sciatica after failed disk surgery, or due to spondylitic spurs, spondylolysis, facetal joint degeneration, or arachnoiditis, some surgeons have attributed the disability in part, at least, to "instability" of the lumbar segments and the perpetuation of the pain to excessive or abnormal movements of the lumbar vertebral segments. For such patients spinal fusion is occasionally advocated and can in certain circumstances provide a measure of relief. A posterior arthrodesis of the fourth and fifth lumbar segments to the sacrum may reduce motion at these parts and decrease pressure on the nerve roots associated with abnormal movements. More often than not, however, the patient continues to have pain (although often reduced in degree), and the procedure should not be regarded as a panacea. The authors rarely advocate such an operative intervention, unless clear anatomic evidence exists for a mechanical problem which could be alleviated by stabilization of the spine.

ARTHRITIS   Arthritis of the spine is a major cause of backache, cervical pain, and occipital headache.

Osteoarthritis (see also Chap. 274)   This more frequent type of osteoarthritic spinal disease occurs usually in later life and may involve any part of the spine. It is most prevalent in the cervical and lumbar regions, however, and the exact location determines the localization of the symptoms. Patients often complain of pain centered in the spine which is increased by motion and is almost invariably associated with complaints of stiffness and limitation of motion. There is a notable absence of systemic symptoms such as fatigue, malaise, and fever, and the pain usually can be relieved by rest. The severity of the symptoms often bears little relation to the radiologic findings; pain may be present when there are minimal findings on an x-ray, and, conversely, marked osteophytic overgrowth with spur formation, ridging, and bridging of vertebrae can be seen in asymptomatic patients in middle and later life. Osteoarthropathic changes in the cervical spine and to a lesser extent in the lumbar spine may by their location compress roots or even the cauda equina or spinal cord, giving rise to the spondylitic form of myelopathy (see Chaps. 353 and 354).

Multiple spondylitic caudal radiculopathy (SCR) is another variant of hypertrophic arthritis. A congenital smallness of the lumbar canal, especially at the L4 to L5 level, renders the individual susceptible to either a rupture of an intervertebral disk or arthrosis. The latter condition further narrows the anteroposterior diameter of the canal and leads to compression of lumbosacral roots and even to a block of the spinal canal. The roots are actually caught between the posterior surface of the vertebral body and the ligamentum flavum posterolaterally. Lumbosacral pains are followed by weakening of the lower legs, impairment of ankle and knee reflexes, and numbness and paresthesia in the feet and legs. Extension of the lumbar spine during walking and standing produces or aggravates the neurologic symptoms, and flexion relieves them. The clinical picture and its intermittency correspond to the so-called intermittent claudication of the spinal cord. The diagnosis may be suspected on the basis of history and radiographic findings but may be confirmed by myelography, CT, or MRI scan, which will demonstrate the narrowed lumbar canal. Decompression of the spinal canal relieves the symptoms in a considerable proportion of the cases but should be approached with caution since it may lead to instability, necessitating an arthrodesis. SCR is the lumbar equivalent of spondylitic cervical myelopathy (SCM), described below. SCR is a cauda equina syndrome, and its differential diagnosis is discussed in Chap. 353.

Rheumatoid arthritis and ankylosing spondylitis (see also Chaps. 263 and 267)   Arthritic disease of the spine takes two distinct forms, ankylosing spondylitis (the more common) and rheumatoid arthritis.

Patients with *ankylosing spondylitis* (also called Marie-Strümpell arthritis) are usually young men who complain of mild to moderate pain which early in the course of the disease is centered in the back and on occasion radiates to the back of the thighs. The symptoms may be vague at first (tired back, "catches" up and down the back, sore back) and the diagnosis may be overlooked for a considerable period. Although the pain is often intermittent, the finding of limitation of movement is constant and progressive and over a period of time tends to dominate the picture. Early in the course, this finding is described as "morning stiffness" or increasing stiffness after periods of inactivity, and may be present long before radiologic changes are manifest. Limitation of chest expansion, tenderness over the sternum, and decreased motion and flexion contractures of the hips may also be present early in the course. The radiologic hallmarks of the disease are destruction and subsequent obliteration of the sacroiliac joints, development of syndesmophytes on the margins of the vertebral bodies, followed by bridging by bone to produce the characteristic "bamboo spine." The entire spine becomes immobilized, often in a flexed position, and usually the pain then subsides. Patterns of restricted movement, indistinguishable from those of ankylosing spondylitis, may accompany Reiter's syndrome, psoriatic arthritis, and chronic inflammatory bowel diseases. Patients with these disorders rarely show the joint manifestations of peripheral rheumatoid arthritis, and seldom do they display involvement of the hips or knees. The rheumatoid factor is usually absent, but the sedimentation rate is often rapid, and many of the patients are found to have an HLA-B27 antigen.

Occasionally ankylosing spondylitis is complicated by progressively destructive vertebral lesions. This complication should be suspected whenever the pain returns, after a period of quiescence, or becomes localized. The etiology of these lesions is not known, but they may represent an exaggerated healing response to fracture or excessive production of fibrous inflammatory tissues. Rarely they may result in collapse of a segment of the spine and compression of the spinal cord. Another complication of severe ankylosing spondylitis is bilateral ankylosis of the ribs to the spine, which, coupled with a decrease in the height of axial thoracic structures, causes marked impairment of respiratory function.

Spinal rheumatoid arthritis tends to be localized to the cervical apophyseal joints and atlantoaxial articulation; the pain, stiffness, and limitation of motion are then in the neck and back of the head. Unlike ankylosing spondylitis, rheumatoid arthritis is rarely confined to the spine, and it does not lead to significant degrees of intervertebral bridging. Because of major affection of other joints, the diagnosis is relatively easy to make, but significant involvement of the neck may be overlooked. In the advanced stages of the disease, one or several of the vertebrae may be displaced anteriorly, or a synovitis of the atlantoaxial joint may damage the transverse ligament of the atlas, resulting in forward displacement of the atlas on the axis, i.e., atlantoaxial subluxation. In either instance serious and even life-threatening compression of the spinal cord may occur gradually or suddenly (see Chaps. 263 and 353). Lateral roentgenograms in flexion and extension, performed cautiously, are necessary to visualize dislocation or subluxation.

OTHER DESTRUCTIVE DISEASES   Neoplastic, infectious, and metabolic diseases   Metastatic carcinoma (breast, lung, prostate, thyroid, kidney, gastrointestinal tract), multiple myeloma, and non-Hodgkin's and Hodgkin's lymphomas are the malignant tumors which most frequently involve the spine. Since the primary site may be overlooked or asymptomatic, the presenting complaint in such patients may be pain in the back. The pain tends to be constant and dull, and is often unrelieved by rest. Indeed, it may be worse at night. Radiographic changes may be absent early in the disease, but when they appear, usually are manifest as destructive lesions in one or several vertebral bodies with little or limited involvement of the disk space, even in the face of a compression fracture. A ^{99m}Tc diphosphonate bone scan is helpful in demonstrating "hot spots," indicating areas of increased blood flow and reactive bone formation associated with destructive, inflammatory, or arthritic lesions. It should be noted, however, that myeloma and sometimes metastatic thyroid carcinoma may fail to show increased activity on a bone scan.

Infection of the vertebral column is usually the result of pyogenic organisms (staphylococci or coliform bacilli) or tubercle bacilli and is often diffcult to distinguish on the basis of clinical findings. Patients complain of pain in the back of subacute or chronic nature that is exacerbated by motion but not materially relieved by rest. There is limitation of motion, tenderness over the spine of the involved segments, and pain with jarring of the spine, such as occurs with walking on the heels. Usually, these patients are afebrile and often do not have a leukocytosis although the erythrocyte sedimentation rate is almost invariably elevated. Radiographs may demonstrate narrowing of a disk space with erosion and destruction of the two adjacent vertebrae. A paravertebral soft tissue mass may be present, indicating an abscess, which may in the case of tuberculosis drain spontaneously, at sites quite remote from the vertebral column. In addition to a bone scan, a gallium scan is sometimes helpful in identifying a soft tissue inflammatory or infectious lesion even when overt bone destruction is not visible in x-rays.

Special mention should be made of the spinal *epidural abscess* (usually staphylococcal), which necessitates urgent surgical treatment. The symptoms are a localized pain, occurring spontaneously, aggravated by percussion and palpation. The patient is febrile and usually has severe radicular complaints, often bilateral, progressing rapidly to a flaccid paraplegia (see Chaps. 340 and 353).

In so-called metabolic bone diseases (osteoporosis or osteomalacia) a considerable degree of loss of bone substance may occur without any symptoms whatsoever. Many patients with such conditions do, however, complain of aching in the lumbar or thoracic area. This is most likly to occur following an injury, sometimes of trivial degree, which leads to collapse or wedging of a vertebra. Certain movements greatly enhance the pain, and certain positions relieve it. One or more spinal roots may be involved. Paget's disease of the spine is nearly always painless but may lead to compression of the spinal cord or roots because of encroachment on the canal or foramina by the pagetoid bone. The recognition of these bone disorders is discussed in some detail elsewhere (Chaps. 337 and 338).

In general, patients thought to have neoplastic, infectious, or metabolic disease of the spine should be thoroughly evaluated by means of radiographs, bone scans, CT scans, and appropriate laboratory studies (see above).

REFERRED PAIN FROM VISCERAL DISEASE   The pain of disease of the pelvic, abdominal, or thoracic viscera is often felt in the region of the spine; i.e., it is referred to the posterior parts of the spinal segment which innervates the diseased organ. Occasionally back pain may be the first and only sign. The general rule is that pelvic diseases are referred to the sacral region, lower abdominal diseases to the lumbar region (centering around the second to fourth lumbar vertebrae), and upper abdominal diseases to the lower thoracic spine (eighth thoracic to the first and second lumbar vertebrae). Characteristically there are no local signs or stiffness of the back, and motion is of full range without augmentation of the pain. However, some positions, e.g., flexion of the lumbar area of the spine in the lateral recumbent position, may be more comfortable than others.

Low thoracic and upper lumbar pain in abdominal disease   Peptic ulceration or tumor of the wall of the stomach and of the duodenum most typically induces pain in the epigastrium (see Chaps. 235 and 255); but if the posterior wall is involved, and particularly if there is retroperitoneal extension, the pain may be felt in the region of the spine. The pain may be central in location or more intense on one side, or it may be felt in both locations. If very intense, it may seem to encircle the body. It tends to retain the characteristics of pain from the affected organ; e.g., if due to peptic ulceration, it appears about 2 h after a meal and is relieved by food and antacids.

Diseases of the pancreas (peptic ulceration with extension to the pancreas, cholecystitis with pancreatitis, cyst, or tumor) are apt to cause pain in the back, being more to the right of the spine if the head of the pancreas is involved and to the left if the body and tail are implicated.

Diseases of retroperitoneal structures, e.g., lymphomas, sarcomas, and carcinomas, may evoke pain in this part of the spine with some tendency toward radiation to the lower part of the abdomen, groin, and anterior thighs. A secondary tumor of the iliopsoas region on one side often produces a unilateral lumbar ache with radiation toward the groin and labia or testicle; there may also be signs of involvement of the upper lumbar spinal roots. An aneurysm of the abdominal aorta may induce pain which is localized to this region of the spine but may be felt higher or lower, depending on the location of the lesion.

The sudden appearance of obscure lumbar pain in a patient receiving anticoagulants should arouse the suspicion of retroperitoneal bleeding.

Lumbar pain with lower abdominal diseases Inflammatory diseases of segments of the colon (colitis, diverticulitis) or tumor of the colon cause pain which may be felt in the lower part of the abdomen between the umbilicus and pubis, in the midlumbar region, or in both places. If very intense, the pain may have a beltlike distribution around the body. A lesion in the transverse colon or first part of the descending colon may be central or left-sided, and its level of reference to the back is to the second to third lumbar vertebrae. If the sigmoid colon is implicated, the pain is lower, in the upper sacral region and anteriorly in the midline suprapubic region or left lower quadrant of the abdomen.

Sacral pain in pelvic (urologic and gynecologic) diseases The pelvis is seldom the site of a disease which causes obscure low back pain although gynecologic disorders may manifest themselves in this manner. Of painful pelvic lesions less than a third are due to inflammatory disease; other more hypothetical entities, such as relaxation of uterine supporting structures, retroversion of uterus, pelvic varicosities, and adnexal edema, have been largely discredited. Recently, diagnostic laparoscopy has been recommended as a valuable supplement to rectal and pelvic examinations, sigmoidoscopy, and intravenous pyelography. The importance of psychiatric illness in the majority of undiagnosed cases has been stressed.

Menstrual pain itself may be felt in the sacral region. It is rather poorly localized, tends to radiate down the legs, and is of a crampy nature. The most important source of chronic back pain from the pelvic organs, however, is the uterosacral ligaments. Endometriosis or carcinoma of the uterus (body or cervix) may invade these structures, while malposition of the uterus may pull on them. The pain is localized centrally in the sacrum below the lumbosacral joint but may be more on one side. In endometriosis the pain begins during the premenstrual phase and often continues until it merges with menstrual pain. Malposition of the uterus (retroversion, descensus, and prolapse) is thought by some to lead to sacral pain, especially after the patient has been standing for several hours. One may observe the effect of postural influences here as when a fibroma of the uterus pulls on the uterosacral ligaments. Carcinomatous pain due to involvement of nerve plexuses is continuous and becomes progressively more severe; it tends to be more intense at night. The primary lesion may be inconspicuous, being overlooked upon pelvic examination. Papanicolaou smears, pyelogram, and CT scan are the most useful diagnostic procedures. X-ray therapy of these tumors may produce sacral pain consequent to necrosis of tissue and injury to nerve roots. Low back pain with radiation into one or both thighs is a common phenomenon during the last weeks of pregnancy.

Chronic prostatitis, evidenced by prostatic discharge, burning and frequency of urination, and slight reduction in sexual potency, may be attended by a nagging sacral ache; it may be mainly on one side, with radiation into one leg if the seminal vesicle is involved on that side. Carcinoma of the prostate with metastases to the lower part of the spine is another more common cause of sacral or lumbar pain. It may be present without urinary frequency or burning. Spinal nerves may be infiltrated by tumor cells, or the spinal cord itself may be compressed if the epidural space is invaded. The diagnosis is established by rectal examination, roentgenograms and bone scans of the spine, and measurement of acid phosphatase (particularly the prostatic phosphatase fraction). Lesions of the bladder and testes are usually not accompanied by back pain. When the kidney is the site of disease, the pain is ipsilateral, being felt in the flank or lumbar region.

Visceral derangements of whatever type may intensify the pain of arthritis, and the presence of arthritis may alter the distribution of visceral pain. With disease of the spine in the lumbosacral region, for example, distention of the ampulla of the sigmoid by feces or a bout of colitis may aggravate the arthritic pain. In patients with arthritis of the cervical or thoracic spine the pain of myocardial ischemia may radiate to the back.

OBSCURE TYPES OF LOW BACK PAIN AND THE QUESTION OF PSYCHIATRIC DISEASE The practitioner is frequently consulted by persons who complain of low back pain of obscure origin. Usually the disorder is benign in nature and results from some minor derangement, muscular strain, or diskal prolapse. This is particularly true for those lesions which are of acute onset, aggravated by motion, and relieved by rest. Considerably more difficult are patients with chronic pain, especially those who have had prior back surgery or chronic visceral disease, or those who have severe and progressive pain in which neoplasia or infection is considered.

Even when exhaustive studies have been performed, there remains a group of patients in whom no anatomic or pathologic lesion can be found. These patients generally fall into two categories: those with postural back pain and those with psychiatric illness.

Postural back pain Many slender asthenic individuals and some obese middle-aged individuals have discomfort in the back. Their backs ache much of the time, and the pain interferes with effective work. The physical examination is negative except for slack musculature and poor posture. The pain is diffuse in the mid or low region of the back and characteristically is relieved by bed rest and induced by the maintenance of a particular posture over a period of time. Pain in the neck and between the shoulder blades is a common complaint among thin, tense, active women and seems to be related to taut trapezius muscles.

Psychiatric illness Low back pain may be encountered in compensation hysteria and malingering, in anxiety or neurocirculatory asthenia (formerly called neurasthenia), in depression and hypochondriasis, and in many nervous persons whose symptoms and complaints do not fall within any category of psychiatric illness. It is probably correct to assume that pain in the back in such patients usually signifies diseases of the spine and adjacent structures, and one should always search for a specific cause. However, even when organic factors are found, the pain may be exaggerated, prolonged, or woven into a pattern of invalidism or disability because of coexistent psychological factors. This is especially true when there is the possibility of secondary gain (notably compensation).

PAIN IN THE NECK AND SHOULDER

It is useful to distinguish three major categories of painful disease—of the spine, brachial plexus (thoracic outlet), and shoulder. Although pain in these three regions of the body may overlap, the patient usually can indicate the site of origin. Pain arising from the cervical spine is felt in the neck and back of the head (though it may often be projected to the shoulder and arm), is evoked or enhanced by certain movements or positions of the neck, and is accompanied by tenderness and limitation of motions of the neck. Similarly, pain resulting from abnormalities of the thoracic outlet is experienced in and around the shoulder in the supraclavicular region, or between the shoulders; is induced by the performance of certain tasks and by certain positions; and is associated with tenderness of structures above the clavicle. There may be a palpable abnormality above the clavicle (aneurysms of the subclavian artery, tumor, cervical rib). The combination of circulatory symptoms and signs referable to the lower part of the brachial plexus, manifested in the hand by obliteration of pulse when the patient holds a full breath with the head tilted back or turned (Adson's test), unilateral Raynaud's phenomenon, trophic changes in the fingers, and sensory loss over the ulnar side of the hand with or without interosseous atrophy complete the clinical picture. Roentgenograms showing a cervical rib, deformed thoracic outlet, or superior sulcus tumor of the lung (Pancoast's syndrome) corroborate disease in this location. Electromyography and conduction studies along the plexus from points stimulated above and below the clavicle, and studies of arterial and venous circulation (venograms, noninvasive Doppler techniques) are especially helpful in evaluating this problem.

Pain localized to the shoulder region, often worse at night, associated with tenderness and aggravated by abduction, internal rotation, and extension points toward a lesion of the tendinous structures about the shoulder. Most often these are in the form of a tendonitis or bursitis (sometimes calcific) usually affecting the supraspinatus tendon and the adjacent subdeltoid bursa; occasionally the lesion is more extensive and consists of a rupture of the rotator cuff, in which case the patient may have weakness on abduction and forward flexion. In some such patients there is an adhesive capsulitis, leading to profound limitation of motion, designated as a "frozen shoulder." Shoulder pain may radiate into the arm or hand, but the sensory, motor, and reflex changes which indicate disease of nerve roots, plexus, or peripheral nerves are absent.

Osteoarthritis of the cervical part of the spine may cause pains which radiate into the back of the head, shoulders, and arms on one or both sides of the thorax. Coincident involvement of nerve roots is manifested by paresthesias, sensory loss, weakness, or deep tendon reflex change. Should bony ridges form in the spinal canal (spondylosis) the spinal cord may be compressed (see Chap. 353). A myelogram or CT scan may reveal the degree of encroachment on the spinal canal (narrowing of the canal to less than 11 mm in the anteroposterior diameter) at the level at which the spinal cord is affected. The authors have experienced difficulty in distinguishing spondylosis with or without disk rupture and spinal cord compression from primary neurologic diseases (syringomyelia, amyotrophic lateral sclerosis, or tumor) with an unrelated osteoarthritis of the cervical portion of the spine, particularly at the fifth to sixth and sixth to seventh cervical vertebrae, where the disk spaces are often narrowed in the adult. A combination of anxiety with osteoarthritis of the cervical part of the spine or a painful injury to ligaments and muscles after an accident in which the neck is forcibly extended and flexed (e.g., "whiplash" injury to spine) may be a difficult diagnostic problem, particularly if in the course of the injury a cerebral concussion has occurred. If the pain is persistent and limited to the neck, the problem will sometimes prove to have been due to disruption of a disk, but it is often complicated by psychological factors.

RUPTURED CERVICAL DISKS   One of the commonest causes of neck, shoulder, and arm pain is disk herniation in the lower cervical region. As with rupture of the lumbar disks, the complete syndrome includes the disorder of spinal function and evidence of neural involvement. It may develop after trauma either major or minor (sudden hyperextension of the neck, diving, forceful manipulations, etc.). Virtually every patient exhibits an abnormality in range of motion of the neck (limitation and pain). Hyperextension is the movement that most consistently aggravates the pain, although one occasionally sees patients whose principal limitation is in flexion. Rotation and lateral movements are often moderately restricted by pain. With laterally situated disk lesions between the fifth and sixth cervical vertebrae, the symptoms and signs are referred to the sixth cervical roots. The full syndrome is characterized by pain felt at the trapezius ridge, tip of the shoulder, anterior upper part of the arm, radial forearm, and often in the thumb; paresthesias and sensory impairment or hypersensitivity in the same regions; tenderness in the

area above the spine of the scapula and in the supraclavicular and biceps regions; weakness in flexion of the forearm; diminished to absent biceps and supinator reflexes (triceps retained or exaggerated). When the protruded disk lies between the sixth and seventh cervical vertebrae, the seventh cervical root is involved. Under these circumstances, in the patient with the complete syndrome, the pain is in the region of the shoulder blade, pectoral region and medial axilla, posterolateral upper arm, elbow and dorsal forearm, index and middle fingers, or all the fingers; tenderness is most pronounced over the medial aspect of the shoulder blade opposite the third to fourth thoracic spinous processes, in the supraclavicular area and triceps region; paresthesias and sensory loss are most pronounced in the second and third fingers or tips of all the fingers; weakness is seen in extension of the forearm, in the extension of the wrist, and in the hand grip; the triceps reflex is diminished to absent, and the biceps and supinator reflexes are preserved. Either of these syndromes may be incomplete in that only one of several of the typical findings (e.g., pain) is present. Usually the patient states that cough, sneeze, and downward pressure on the head in the hyperextension position exacerbate pain and traction (even manual) tends to relieve it.

Unlike lumbar disks, the cervical ones, if large and centrally situated, may result in compression of the spinal cord (central disk, all the cord; paracentral disk, part of the cord). The central disk is often nearly painless, and the cord syndrome may simulate a degenerative disease (amyotrophic lateral sclerosis, combined system disease). A common error is to fail to think of a ruptured disk in the cervical region in patients with obscure symptoms in the legs. The diagnosis of ruptured cervical disk should be confirmed by the same laboratory procedures that were mentioned under "Spondylosis," above.

OTHER CONDITIONS   Metastases to the cervical spine are fortunately less common than to other parts of the vertebral column. They are frequently painful and the cause of disordered root function. Compression fractures or extension of the tumor posteriorly may lead to rapid development of quadriplegia.

Shoulder injuries (rotator cuff), subacromial or subdeltoid bursitis, the frozen shoulder (periarthritis or capsulitis), tendonitis, and arthritis may develop in patients who are otherwise well, but these conditions are also frequent in hemiplegics or in individuals suffering from coronary heart disease. The pain is often severe and extends toward the neck and down the arm into the hand. The dorsum of the latter may tingle without other signs of nerve involvement. Vasomotor and arthropathic changes also may occur in the hand (shoulder-hand syndrome, reflex dystrophy), and after a time, osteoporosis and atrophy of cutaneous and subcutaneous structures occur (Sudeck's atrophy or Sudeck-Leriche syndrome). These conditions fall more within the province of orthopedics than of medicine and are not discussed here in detail. The physician, however, must know that they can often be prevented by proper exercises (Chap. 198).

The *carpal tunnel syndrome,* with paresthesias and numbness in palmar distribution of the median nerve and aching pain which extends up into the forearm, may be mistaken for disease of the shoulder or neck. Similarly, other less common forms of nerve entrapment may involve the ulnar, radial, or median nerves and lead to a mistaken diagnosis of brachial plexus lesion or cervical syndrome. Electromyography and conduction studies are especially helpful in such conditions (Chap. 354).

MANAGEMENT OF BACK AND NECK PAIN

Without doubt the preventive aspects of back pain are important. There would be far fewer back problems if adults kept their trunk muscles in optimal condition by regular exercise such as swimming, bicycle riding, walking briskly, running, or calisthenic programs. A regular exercise program to strengthen abdominal and paraspinal muscles is frequently very beneficial for patients with chronic low back discomfort. Morning is the ideal time since the back of the older adult tends to stiffen during the night because of inactivity. This happens regardless of whether a bed board or a stiff mattress is used. Sleeping with back hyperextended and sitting for long times in an overstuffed chair or a badly designed auto seat commonly cause difficulties for the patient with low back problems. It is estimated that pressures between disks are increased 200 percent by changing from a recumbent to a standing position and by 400 percent by sitting slumped in an easy chair. Correct sitting posture lessens this. Long trips in a car or plane without change in position put maximal strain on disk and ligamentous structures in the spine. Lifting from a position of flexed trunk, as in removing a suitcase from the trunk of a car, is dangerous (always lift with the object close to the body). Sudden strenuous activity without conditioning and warm-up also is likely to cause trouble to disks and their ligamentous envelopes (the commonest sources of back pain); certain families seem disposed.

Muscular and ligamentous strains and minor disk prolapses are usually self-limited, responding to simple measures in a relatively short period of time. The basic principle of therapy is rest in a recumbent position for several days to weeks. When weight bearing is resumed, a light lumbosacral support is usually helpful in continuing the immobilization until the patient is restored to full health. Physical measures such as heat, cold, diathermy, or massage are of limited value; of considerably greater importance are active exercises to both reduce the spasm and improve muscle tone. Analgesic medication should be given liberally during the first few days: codeine, 30 mg, and aspirin, 0.6 g, or pentazocine, 50 mg, propoxyphene, 65 mg, or meperidine, 50 mg. Muscle relaxants are often a valuable adjunct, particularly in that such drugs as diazepam, 8 to 40 mg in divided doses may make bed rest more tolerable. If an inflammatory component is suspected, indomethacin, 75 mg per day (in divided doses), or ibuprofen, 600 mg 3 or 4 times daily, may be helpful.

In the treatment of an acute or chronic rupture of a lumbar or cervical disk, complete bed rest is essential, at least initially, and strong analgesic medication may be required. Traction is of little value in lumbar disk disease, and it is best to permit the patient to find the most comfortable position. Cervical traction with a halter may be of considerable benefit to patients with cervical disk syndrome. It can be administered with the patient in recumbency, or after sufficient improvement to allow ambulation, can be performed intermittently in the erect position using special equipment. During the recumbent phase of treatment of lumbar disk disease, exercises to reduce spasm, muscle relaxants, and anti-inflammatory agents as described above may be of considerable value. After 2 to 3 weeks in bed, the patient can be allowed to slowly resume activities, usually with the protection of a brace or light spinal support. Exercise programs designed to increase the strength of the abdominal and paraspinal muscles are helpful at this point. The patient may suffer some minor recurrence of the pain but be able to carry on his or her usual activities, and eventually most individuals will recover. If the pain and neurologic findings do not disappear on prolonged, conservative management, or if the patient suffers frequently recurring acute episodes, surgical management may be indicated. This should always be preceded by a myelogram and a computerized reconstructed body scan to localize the lesion (and rule out the presence of intra- or extradural tumors). The surgical procedure most often indicated is a hemilaminectomy with excision of the disk involved. Arthrodesis of the involved segments is indicated only in cases in which there is extraordinary instability usually related to an anatomic abnormality (such as spondylolysis) or in the cervical region when an extensive laminectomy has rendered the spine unstable. The results of conservative management of so-called sciatica cases in the controlled study of Coxhead et al. was approximately 80 percent improved at the end of 4 weeks, regardless of whether traction, exercises, manipulation, or corset, or some combination thereof, was used.

Over the past two decades, orthopedists and neurosurgeons have performed several trials of intradiskal administration of the enzyme chymopapain in the treatment of disk disease. The theoretical advantages of such a technique are clear; if the lesion can be sharply localized by myelography and diskography and the disk space injected with this potent proteoglycanolytic agent, the patient should get relief of localized back and radicular pain within a short period of time and be spared the risk, disability, and prolonged convalescence of an operative procedure. It has become apparent during these trials, however, that the use of this agent is not always effective; and, more importantly, its use is not without some rather spectacular complications which are not entirely predictable and may seriously threaten the patient's well-being. A small but significant number of patients develop an anaphylactoid response to the agent and many experience severe spasms of the low back and legs immediately after the procedure. Of greater concern is a very small number of patients who have developed an irreversible transverse myelitis or other major neurologic problems following the procedure. Although the authors have not encountered these complications, we currently do not advocate the procedure except in individuals in whom the pain fails to respond to conservative management and for whom open surgery is contraindicated.

Spondylosis of the cervical spine, if painful, is helped by bed rest and traction; if signs of spinal cord involvement are present, a collar to limit movement may lead to improvement. Decompressive laminectomy or anterior fusion is reserved for severe instances of the disease with advancing neurologic symptoms. The shoulder-hand syndrome may benefit from stellate ganglion blocks or ganglionectomy, but the basic treatment is physiotherapy, with or without prednisone, and surgical procedures are used only as measures of last resort.

The management of patients with thoracic outlet syndrome is complex and requires first a careful study to be certain that the cause of the lesion is really a mechanical encroachment of the brachial plexus in the interspace between the clavicle and first rib. Exercises to reduce the tension in this region are mainly designed to strengthen the clavicular musculature and improve posture, thus opening the outlet. Many patients benefit from change of work circumstances, and for women with pendulous breasts, a better designed brassiere is sometimes helpful. Nonsteroidal anti-inflammatory agents are sometimes beneficial, as are muscle relaxants such as diazepam. In the event that the patient's difficulties are intractable or the root compression causes neurologic deficits, exploration of the anterior scalene triangle with resection of the first rib is advocated with usually excellent results.

REFERENCES

Armstrong JR: *Lumbar Disc Lesions*, 3d ed. Baltimore, Williams & Wilkins, 1965

Bogduk N: The innervation of the lumbar spine. Spine 8:286, 1983

Brady LP et al: An evaluation of the electromyogram in the diagnosis of lumbar disk lesion. J Bone Joint Surg 51A:539, 1969

Chevetz NI et al: Recognition of lumbar disk herniation with NMR. Am J Radiol 141:1153, 1983

Collier B: Treatment for lumbar sciatic pain in posterior articular lumbar joint syndrome. Anesthesia 34:202, 1979

Coxhead CE et al: Multicenter trial of physiotherapy in the management of sciatic symptoms. Lancet 1:1065, 1981

Edeiken J, Pitt MJ: The radiologic diagnoses of disk disease. Orthop Clin North Am 2:405, 1971

Friedenberg AB, Miller WT: Degenerative disk disease of the cervical spine. J Bone Joint Surg 45A:1171, 1963

Grabias SL, Mankin HJ: Pain in lower back. Bull Rheum Dis 30:1040, 1980

Mikhael MH et al: Neurologic evaluation of lateral recess syndrome. Radiology 140:97, 1981

Murphy RW: Nerve roots and spinal nerves in degenerative disk disease. Clin Orthop 129:46, 1977

Naylor A: The changes in the human intervertebral disk in degeneration and nuclear prolapse. Orthop Clin North Am 2:343, 1971

Raskin SP: Computerized tomographic findings in lumbar disk disease. Orthopedics 5:419, 1981

Reynolds AV et al: Lumbar monoradiculopathy due to unilateral facet hypertrophy. Neurosurgery 10:480, 1982

Rothman RC, Simeone F: *Lumbar Disc Disease*. Philadelphia, Saunders, 1975, pp 443–458

Williams AL et al: Computed tomography in the diagnosis of herniated nucleus pulposus. Radiology 135:95, 1980

Wilson ES, Brill RF: Spinal stenosis: The narrow lumbar canal syndrome. Clin Orthop 122:244, 1977

section 2 Alterations in body temperature

8 DISTURBANCES OF HEAT REGULATION

ROBERT G. PETERSDORF / RICHARD K. ROOT

CONTROL OF BODY TEMPERATURE In health, the body temperature of humans is maintained within a narrow range despite extremes in environmental conditions and physical activity. This is also true for most birds and mammals, and such animals are termed *homeothermic,* or warm-blooded. An almost invariable accompaniment of systemic illness is a disturbance in temperature regulation, usually an abnormal elevation, or *fever*. In fact, fever is such a sensitive and reliable indicator of the presence of disease that thermometry is probably the commonest clinical procedure in use. Even in the absence of a frank febrile response, interference with heat regulation by disease is evident. This may take the form of flushing, pallor, sweating, shivering, and abnormal sensations of cold or warmth, or it may consist of erratic fluctuations of body temperature within normal limits when a patient is at bed rest.

Heat production The major source of basal heat production is through thyroid thermogenesis and the action of adenosine triphosphatase (ATPase) on the sodium pump of all membranes. The muscles are most important in promoting increased heat production through increased shivering. Heat production by muscle is of particular importance because the quantity can be varied according to the need. In most circumstances this variation consists of small increases and decreases in the number of nerve impulses to the muscles, causing inapparent tensing or relaxing. When, however, there is a strong stimulus for heat production, muscle activity may increase to the point of shivering, or even to a generalized rigor. During digestion of food, gastrointestinal production of heat is significant.

Heat loss Heat is lost from the body in several ways. Small amounts are used in warming food or drink and in the evaporation of moisture from the respiratory tract. Most heat is lost from the surface of the body by *convection,* i.e., the transfer of heat to a fluid medium. Heat loss by convection depends on the existence of a temperature gradient between the body surface and the ambient air. A second mechanism for heat loss is *radiation,* which may be defined as an exchange of electromagnetic energy between the body and the radiant environment. *Evaporation* is the third major mechanism for dissipating heat and is particularly important when the ambient temperature exceeds that of the body, or when core temperatures are increased by vigorous exercise.

The principal method of regulating heat loss is by varying the volume of blood flowing to the surface of the body. A rich circulation in the skin and subcutaneous tissues carries heat to the surface, where it can escape. In addition, sweating increases heat loss by providing water to be vaporized. The sweat, or eccrine, glands are under the control of the sympathetic nerves which, in this instance, mediate cholinergic stimuli. Heat loss by sweating may be tremendous, and as much as 1 liter per hour of sweat may be evaporated. The amount of heat loss through sweating is also dependent upon the humidity in the air. The greater the humidity, the less the ability to lose heat through sweat.

When there is need for conservation of heat, adrenergic autonomic stimuli cause a sharp reduction in the blood flow to the surface. This causes vasoconstriction and transforms the skin and subcutaneous tissue into layers of insulation.

Heat transfer within the body This depends upon *conduction,* i.e., the transfer of heat between adjacent organs, and upon *circulatory convection,* which is governed by bulk movement of body fluids and which is responsible for the transfer of heat between the cells and the bloodstream. It is useful, although oversimplified, to visualize the body as a central core at uniform temperatures surrounded by an insulating shell. The role of the shell as a mediator for heat conservation and heat loss is determined in part by its blood supply and by vasoconstriction or vasodilatation. Although insulation is relatively uniform throughout the body, some parts, such as the digits, are particularly susceptible to cold because of the increased surface-to-volume ratio. Moreover, blood that reaches the digits has already been cooled on the way. Insulation may be enhanced by the addition of clothing.

Neural control of temperature The control of body temperature, integrating the various physical and chemical processes for heat production or heat loss, is a function of cerebral centers located in the hypothalamus. A high-decerebrate animal has a normal temperature if the hypothalamus is left intact. On the other hand, an animal whose brainstem has been sectioned loses ability to control body temperature, which consequently tends to vary with the environment, a condition referred to as *poikilothermia*. Animal experiments suggest that the preoptic anterior hypothalamus and some centers in the spinal cord have neurons which respond directly to local temperature and act as a sensor for internal temperature. This function is distinct from the integrative function which responds to temperature-sensitive structures all over the body.

FACTORS AFFECTING NEURAL CONTROL OF TEMPERATURE The temperature-regulating system is a negative feedback control system, and possesses three elements essential to such a system: (1) receptors which sense the existing central temperatures; (2) effector mechanisms, consisting of the vasomotor, sudomotor, and metabolic effectors; and (3) integrative structures which determine whether the existing temperature is too high or too low and which activate the appropriate motor response. It is a negative feedback system because a rise in central temperature initiates mechanisms for losing heat while a fall in central temperature activates mechanisms for heat production and heat conservation. The activation of these effector responses is governed by a central integrative mechanism which may be compared with a thermostat and which responds to a variety of stimuli, such as the sensory impulses engendered in flushing or sweating, behavioral impulses, exercise, endocrine influences, and probably the temperature of the blood circulating through the hypothalamic centers. In a sense all these stimuli reset the thermostat, thereby activating compensatory heat loss or heat conservation mechanisms.

A classic example of the endocrine influence on temperature is the effect of menstruation. The mean body temperature of women is higher during the second half of the menstrual cycle than it is between the onset of menstruation and the time of ovulation. The sensations of intense heat followed by diaphoresis that characterize the vasomotor instability experienced by some women at the menopause are undoubtedly the result of endocrine imbalance. The activation of the adrenal medulla in response to cold is another example of the relationship between the endocrine system and the thermoregulatory apparatus.

Normal body temperature It is not practical to designate an exact upper level of normal body temperature because there are small differences among normal persons. There are rare individuals whose temperatures are always elevated slightly above accepted "normal" levels, and there is considerable variation in temperature in a given individual. In general, however, it is safe to regard an oral temperature above 99°F (37.2°C) in a person at bed rest as probable indication of disease. The temperature may be as low as 96.5°F (35.8°C) in healthy persons. Rectal temperature is usually 0.5 to 1.0°F higher than oral temperature. In very hot weather the body temperature may be elevated by 0.5 or even 1.0°F.

There is a distinct diurnal variation in body temperature in healthy human beings. Oral readings of 97°F (36.1°C) are relatively common on arising in the morning. Body temperature rises steadily through the day, reaches a peak of 99°F (37.2°C) or greater between 6 P.M. and 10 P.M., and then drops slowly to reach a minimum at 2 A.M. to 4 A.M. Although it has been postulated that this diurnal variation is dependent upon increasing activity during the day and rest at night, the pattern is not reversed in individuals who work at night and sleep during the day for long periods of time. The febrile patterns of most human diseases also tend to follow this normal diurnal pattern. Fevers tend to be higher, to "spike," in the evening, and many patients with febrile disease have relatively normal temperatures in the early morning hours.

Body temperature is more labile in young children, and transient elevations after relatively slight exertion in warm weather are frequently observed in them.

Severe or prolonged exercise can produce considerable elevation in body temperature. For example, marathon runners often have temperatures between 103.2 and 105.8°F (39 and 41°C). Although this marked increase in temperature with exercise tends to be balanced by compensatory cutaneous vasodilatation, resulting in loss of heat, and hyperventilation, these compensatory mechanisms may fail, leading to hyperpyrexia and, if uncontrolled, to heat stroke. Many of the adverse effects of long-distance running can be prevented by holding races only if the ambient temperature is below 82°F (27.8°C), preferably in the early morning or early evening, and by ensuring ample fluid intake both before and during a race.

Disordered thermoregulation In exercise, there is a temporary imbalance between heat production and heat loss with prompt reestablishment of normal temperatures at rest due to continuing activation of heat loss mechanisms. In fact, in prolonged exercise, cutaneous vasodilatation in response to an increase in central body temperature stops in order to preserve central temperature. Less adaptation occurs in fever because once a stable body temperature is reached, heat production equals heat loss, but both are greater than in the basal state. Cutaneous blood flow plays a greater role in controlling heat production and heat loss in fever than does sweating. At the beginning of fever, the body temperature as sensed by the thermoreceptors is low and the individual responds physiologically as if he or she were cold. *Heat production* is increased by shivering, and *heat loss* is decreased by vasoconstriction. These events explain the sensation of cold or chills that characterizes the beginning of fever. Conversely, when the cause of fever is removed, the temperature returns to normal, and the individual responds as if warm. Cutaneous vasodilatation, sweating, and inhibition of shivering are the compensatory responses.

Deviations of 5°F (approximately 3.5°C) from the normal body temperature do not interfere appreciably with most bodily functions. Convulsions are common at temperatures higher than 106°F (41.1°C) in children, and irreversible brain damage, presumably due to protein denaturation (impairment of normal enzymic functions), is common when temperatures of 108°F (42.2°C) are reached. Fortunately, when hyperthermia reaches dangerous levels, the mechanisms for heat loss are suddenly activated; consequently, oral temperatures above 106°F (41.1°C) are relatively rare in humans. Conversely, when temperatures are lowered to 91°F (32.8°C), loss of consciousness occurs; at 86°F (30°C) poikilothermia sets in, and between 83 and 84°F (28.5°C)

slow atrial fibrillation supervenes. Ventricular fibrillation occurs at extremely hypothermic temperatures.

The systemic symptoms accompanying deviations in temperature are poorly understood. For example at temperatures of 102°F (39°C) many patients have malaise, drowsiness, weakness, and generalized aches and pains. Many others, however, feel entirely well. Why some individuals are able to tolerate fever so well while others become markedly ill remains an enigma. Perhaps the inciting stimulus rather than fever per se is the major determinant of systemic complaints. The macrophage product, endogenous pyrogen/interleukin-1 (IL-1), may also play a role in the systemic symptoms accompanying fever.

DISEASES OF THE NERVOUS SYSTEM Disease of the regulatory centers in the hypothalamus may affect body temperature. Cases have been observed in which there was destruction of the centers controlling heat-conserving mechanisms, with resulting hypothermia. More commonly, cerebral lesions are manifested by hyperthermia; this may occur with tumors, degenerative diseases, vascular accidents, particularly cerebral hemorrhage, or infections involving the hypothalamus, such as encephalitis. All these may result in loss of neurons and gliosis. Central fever is accompanied by lack of a diurnal variation, absence of sweating, resistance to antipyretic drugs, excessive response to external cooling, and loss of consciousness.

There are several diseases, of which heat stroke is the cardinal example, in which the central mechanisms for cooling suddenly fail and the patient ceases to sweat, despite the fact that his or her temperature is rising. Some of the highest temperatures ever observed in human beings [112 to 113°F (44.4°C)] have been in cases of heat stroke. A temperature higher than 114°F (45.6°C) is probably not compatible with life.

INCREASED HEAT PRODUCTION Patients with thyrotoxicosis show exaggerated heat production, and their temperature is often 1 to 2°F above the normal range.

IMPAIRMENT OF HEAT LOSS Patients with *congestive heart failure* often have an elevation of body temperature between 0.5 and 1.5°F. Perhaps this elevation is caused by impairment of heat dissipation as a result of diminished cardiac output, decline in cutaneous blood flow (with increasing insulation of the central temperature core), the insulating effect of edema, and the increased heat production incident to the muscular activity of dyspnea. On the other hand, patients with congestive heart failure are likely to have other causes of fever, such as venous thrombosis, pulmonary embolism and infarction, myocardial infarction, pneumonia, and urinary tract infection. However, since slight fever is so regularly present even in the absence of such complications, the circulatory disturbance may be responsible.

Patients with skin disorders such as *ichthyosis* and *congenital absence of sweat glands* may have fever in a warm environment because of inability to lose heat from the surface of the body. Individuals with congenitally absent sweat glands lack the ability of active cutaneous vasodilatation and hence are unable to dissipate heat by at least two mechanisms. Drugs which impair sweating, such as atropine, scopolamine, phenothiazines, monoamine oxidase inhibitors, glutethimide, lysergic acid diethylamide (LSD), amphetamines, and inhalation anesthetics, may result in elevated temperatures.

Patients with severe burns tend to be hyperthermic, probably because occlusive dressings interfere with heat loss despite large areas of denuded skin; they are also hypermetabolic, and heat production is increased.

PATHOGENESIS OF FEVER Fever may be produced by many stimuli, including bacteria and their endotoxins; viruses; yeasts; spirochetes; immune reactions; hormonal substances, exemplified by progesterone; drugs; and synthetic polynucleotides like poly I:poly C. These substances, which have been termed collectively *exogenous pyrogens,* are both diverse and complex. It has been postulated that they act through an intermediary substance termed *endogenous pyrogen* (EP). Most of the knowledge concerning EP has come from work in experimental animals.

EP is now known to be identical to interleukin-1 (IL-1), a product of monocytes and macrophages which initiates many of the reactions termed collectively the "acute phase response." EP/IL-1 is a polypeptide of about 15,000 molecular weight that is synthesized in response to exogenous pyrogens. In addition to temperature-regulating centers in the anterior hypothalamus, other targets for EP/IL-1 include B and T lymphocytes, myeloid cells in the bone marrow, mature neutrophils, fibroblasts, striated muscle, hepatocytes, and cerebral neurons responsible for slow-wave sleep signals. The action of EP/IL-1 at each of these sites is quite different and with some targets involves an intermediate role for specific prostaglandin metabolites.

When EP/IL-1 engages thermosensitive neurons in the preoptic region of the hypothalamus, an abrupt increase in muscular heat production (rigors) occurs, accompanied by decreased heat loss (cutaneous vasoconstriction, and "goose flesh," i.e., "chills"). The core body temperature increases until a higher stable point is reached in the balance between heat production and heat loss. The temperature of the blood bathing the hypothalamus is equivalent to the new "set point."

Within the hypothalamus EP/IL-1 appears to act by inducing the synthesis of prostaglandins of the E series using arachidonate released from target cell membranes. In particular, prostaglandin E_1 (PGE_1) activates heat generating and conserving mechanisms by inducing synthesis of cyclic adenyl monophosphate (cyclic AMP). The precise chemical events remain to be elucidated; however, the antipyretic actions of aspirin and nonsteroidal anti-inflammatory drugs can be ascribed to their inhibition of cyclooxygenase and resultant blockade of PGE_1 and PGE_2 synthesis. Glucocorticoids are antipyretic through more complex mechanisms including inhibition of EP/IL-1 production peripherally and arachidonate release centrally. Fever contrasts with hyperthermia of other causes in which there is no resetting of the central thermostat by EP/IL-1; core temperatures are increased because heat loss mechanisms fail to balance heat production.

EP/IL-1 plays a key role in initiating the immune response by activating helper/inducer T cells to synthesize the polypeptide interleukin-2 (IL-2), which causes clonal expansion of responding T cells. Furthermore, T-cell mitogenesis in response to IL-2 is enhanced at febrile temperatures reaching an optimum at 103.1°F (39.5°C). By this means, fever induction appears to exert a positive feedback in the specific immune response. B-cell proliferation and specific antibody production are also enhanced by IL-1.

EP/IL-1 mobilizes myeloid cells from marrow storage pools, has chemotactic activity for neutrophils and monocytes and induces lysosomal discharge in neutrophils. It also stimulates neutrophil microbicidal oxidative metabolism. Hence, key nonspecific inflammatory mechanisms which can eradicate microorganisms are promoted by the action of EP/IL-1.

Other less well defined actions of EP/IL-1 appear to contribute to antimicrobial and protective mechanisms during infection. These include induction of hypoferremia and a fall in plasma zinc concentrations. Iron is an essential growth factor for many microorganisms. Hepatic synthesis of acute phase proteins is augmented. These include complement factors and C-reactive protein, which may participate directly in antimicrobial events as well as haptoglobin, ceruloplasmin, certain protease inhibitors, fibrinogen, and serum amyloid A protein. The precise role of many of these proteins in host defense requires elucidation, but some, at least, have the capacity to regulate inflammatory mechanisms triggered during infection.

EP/IL-1 mobilizes amino acids from muscle through a proteolytic mechanism mediated by cyclooxygenase and PGE_1. Mobilization can be inhibited by cyclooxygenase inhibitors and presumably functions to supply amino acids as nutrients for other cells. PGE_1 production and muscle degradation are enhanced at febrile body temperatures, indicative of a positive feedback in this event as there is for stimulation of immune responses. Muscle wasting in febrile states can be profound and lead to weight loss of up to a kilogram per day. Myalgias experienced during fever are relieved by aspirin and other antipyretics and may reflect inhibition of muscle catabolism by lysosomal proteases.

EP/IL-1 activates fibroblasts to synthesize collagen. This presumably contributes to tissue reparative responses during infection. Production of IL-1 at local sites may contribute to site-specific inflammatory processes such as joint injury in rheumatoid arthritis, periodontal disease, and even sunburn (ultraviolet-induced keratinocyte production of IL-1).

Finally, EP/IL-1 contained and released by astrocytes in the brain may not only cause fever during cerebral hemorrhage but activates slow-wave sleep–inducing neurons. The drowsiness and prolonged sleep characteristic of febrile illnesses may have their basis in the action of EP/IL-1 and serve as additional protective mechanisms.

Both fever and specific events mediated by the fever-producing molecule EP/IL-1 have a broad and highly integrated role in the characteristic responses to infection and/or acute inflammation. Some of these responses may be viewed as protective, whereas others contribute to deleterious symptoms and signs. Given this complexity it is not surprising that conflict surrounds the need to treat fever with antipyretics or by other means. While symptomatology might be relieved, the cost could be interference with normally protective mechanisms including the specific immune response and the mobilization of nutrients necessary to promote a successful recovery.

DISORDERS ASSOCIATED WITH HIGH TEMPERATURES Heat syndromes
Four clinical syndromes are associated with high environmental temperature: *heat cramps, heat exhaustion, exertional heat injury,* and *heat stroke.* Although each of these entities may be separated from the other on clinical grounds, there is considerable overlap between them, and they may be considered as a series of syndromes along a single spectrum. The incidence of heat syndromes is unknown, but during an ordinary summer about 200 cases of heat stroke are reported. During the heat wave of June 1984, there was a 35 percent increase in mortality in New York City almost exclusively due to a rise in deaths in elderly persons living at home. Heat syndromes occur primarily at elevated temperatures (>90°F) and at high relative humidities (>60%); and elderly individuals, those with mental illness or alcoholism or who receive antipsychotic drugs, diuretics, and anticholinergics, or those who reside in poorly ventilated places without air conditioning are most susceptible. Heat syndromes are especially prevalent during the first days of a heat wave before effective acclimatization can occur. Prophylaxis by augmenting fluid intake prior to exposure and by ensuring that susceptible individuals, particularly the elderly or the very young, wear light clothing, take frequent cool baths, remain in a cool environment, and avoid strenuous physical activity can help prevent the full-blown syndrome, especially heat stroke.

ACCLIMATIZATION The basic mechanism by which humans accommodate to excessive temperatures is unknown. Acclimatization does not increase the threshold for sweating. However, sweating is the most effective natural means of combating heat stress and can occur with little or no change in the core temperature of the body. As long as sweating continues, humans can withstand remarkably high temperatures, provided water and sodium chloride, the most important physiologic constituents of sweat, are replaced. The concentration of sodium chloride varies between that of interstitial fluid and very low concentrations and the ability to secrete sweat with low sodium chloride content, as well as to increase the quantity of sweat, is a major mechanism for the conservation of salt in hot weather. Dilatation of the peripheral blood vessels in an attempt to dissipate heat is another major way for the body to acclimatize to hot temperatures. Other alterations include a decrease in total circulating blood volume, a decrease in renal blood flow, an increase of antidiuretic hormone (ADH) as well as aldosterone, a decrease in urine sodium, and an increase in respiratory and pulse rates. Ordinarily, acclimatization takes from 4 to 7 days. The hyperaldosteronism may result in potassium loss, which may be aggravated by replacement of sodium without concomitant repletion of potassium. Initially there is an increase in cardiac output but as heat stress persists, venous return diminishes and heart failure may occur. If environmental temperatures in excess of the body's temperature persist, heat is retained and hyperpyrexia develops.

HEAT CRAMPS Heat cramps, called "miner's cramps" and "stoker's cramps," are the most benign heat syndrome. Cramps are characterized by painful spasms of the voluntary muscles and usually follow strenuous exercise. In general, only individuals in good physical condition develop this syndrome. External temperatures need not exceed the body temperature, and direct exposure to the sun is not necessary. The body temperature is usually not elevated. Muscle cramps usually occur after excessive sweating and may even be precipitated by strenuous exercise in cold environments in untrained persons heavily clothed. Muscles of the extremities bear the brunt of physical activity and hence show the highest incidence of cramps. Physical examination of the patient is normal between the paroxysms. Examination of the blood reveals a concentration of the formed elements and a decreased sodium chloride concentration. Excretion of these ions in the urine is characteristically low. Treatment consists of sodium chloride; cessation of cramps with replacement of sodium chloride and water is striking and supports the hypothesis that the cause of heat cramps is depletion of these essential electrolytes. Occasionally cramps involve the abdominal musculature, mimicking an intraabdominal emergency. Such patients have had mistaken exploratory surgery performed, often with disastrous results. Replacement of saline prior to surgery would have obviated such operations.

HEAT EXHAUSTION Heat prostration, or heat collapse, is probably the most common heat syndrome. It represents a failure of the cardiovascular responses to high external temperatures and is particularly common in elderly individuals who are receiving diuretics. Weakness, vertigo, headache, anorexia, nausea, vomiting, the urge to defecate, and faintness may precede collapse. Heat collapse occurs in both physically active and sedentary individuals. The onset is usually sudden and the duration of collapse brief. During the acute stage, the patient looks ashen-gray. The skin is cold and clammy. The pupils are dilated. The blood pressure may be low and the pulse pressure elevated. Since prostration develops before exposure to heat is prolonged, body temperature is subnormal or normal. The duration of exposure and the extent to which sweat is lost determine the degree of hemoconcentration. Treatment consists of removal of the patient to a cool area and placing him or her in the recumbent position. Spontaneous recovery then usually takes place. Intravenous administration of saline solution or whole blood is necessary only rarely. Although the pathogenetic mechanism of heat prostration is not primarily a depletion of water and salt, it is likely that maintenance of these electrolytes will prevent heat prostration in individuals exposed to high temperatures.

EXERTIONAL HEAT INJURY This syndrome occurs in individuals who are exerting themselves in hot ambient temperatures (about 80°F) when the relative humidity is high. It is particularly common in runners who enter races with insufficient acclimatization, inadequate conditioning, or improper hydration (before and during the race). Obesity, age, and previous heat stroke are contributing predisposing factors. In contrast to classic heat stroke, individuals with exertional heat injury usually sweat freely, and their temperatures are lower (102 to 104°F as opposed to 106°F and higher in heat stroke). Symptoms consist of headache, piloerection (gooseflesh) on the chest and upper arms, chills, overbreathing, nausea, vomiting, muscle cramps, ataxia, unsteady gait, and incoherent speech. In some individuals, loss of consciousness occurs. Physical examination shows tachycardia, hypotension, and evidence of low peripheral resistance. Laboratory data show hemoconcentration, hypernatremia, abnormal liver and muscle enzymes, hypocalcemia, hypophosphatemia, and, in some instances, hypoglycemia. An occasional patient has thrombocytopenia, hemolysis, disseminated intravascular coagulation, rhabdomyolysis, myoglobinuria, and acute tubular necrosis. Injury to the vascular endothelium may be widespread and contribute to these manifestations as well as organ failure. These severe complications can be avoided by prompt treatment, which consists of placing the victim under wet cold sheets to lower core temperature to 100.4°F (38°C) as quickly as possible, massaging the extremities to improve blood flow from the core to the periphery, and infusing fluids consisting primarily of hypotonic glucose-saline. Patients should be hospitalized for 36 h of observation.

Exertional heat injury can be prevented by (1) running races early in the morning (before 8 A.M.) when the temperature and humidity are likely to be low, (2) educating runners to enter a race well hydrated by drinking 300 mL of water 10 min before a race and 250 mL every 3 to 4 km (salt and glucose solutions should be avoided), (3) placing aid stations at 5-km intervals, (4) instructing runners not to increase their pace after most of the race has been run, and (5) avoiding alcohol before a race.

HEAT STROKE Heat hyperpyrexia, heat stroke, or sunstroke is most common in elderly individuals with preexisting chronic disease. Among these are arteriosclerosis and congestive heart failure, particularly when patients receive diuretics. Other predisposing factors include diabetes mellitus, alcoholism, the use of anticholinergic drugs, and skin disorders in which it may be difficult to lose heat such as ectodermal dysplasia, congenital absence of the sweat glands, or severe scleroderma. Heat stroke is also common in military recruits undergoing basic training, and in an occasional long-distance runner. The mechanism for heat stroke is not known. Although most patients with heat stroke cease sweating, in some sweating is preserved. The vasoconstriction that accompanies heat stroke prevents dissipation of heat from the core, but whether this vasoconstriction is cause or effect is not clear. Direct exposure to the sun is not a necessary prerequisite.

There may be few premonitory symptoms of heat stroke, and loss of consciousness may be the first sign. Other patients may complain of headache, vertigo, faintness, abdominal distress, confusion, or hyperpnea. Delirium may develop in more severe cases.

Pyrexia and prostration are the significant findings on physical examination. A rectal temperature greater than 106°F (41.1°C) is common and internal body temperatures as high as 112 to 113°F (44.4°C) have been recorded. The skin is hot and dry, and, in most cases, sweating is absent. The pulse rate is increased, and respirations are rapid and weak. The blood pressure is usually low. The muscles are flaccid, and tendon reflexes may be diminished. Lethargy, stupor, or coma, depending on the severity, is present. Shock is common in fatal cases.

Examination of the blood and urine may show few abnormalities. Hemoconcentration is common. Leukocytosis is characteristic as are proteinuria, cylindruria, and an elevation in BUN. There is usually a respiratory alkalosis which is followed by a metabolic acidosis. Lactacidemia is common. Serum potassium is normal or low and there are usually hypocalcemia and hypophosphatemia. The electrocardiogram may show, in addition to tachycardia and sinus arrhythmia, flattening and subsequent inversion of the T wave and depression of the ST segment. Diffuse myocardial necrosis with ECG evidence of myocardial infarction has been reported. Other major laboratory abnormalities include thrombocytopenia; prolonged bleeding, clotting, and prothrombin times; afibrinogenemia and fibrinolysis; and disseminated intravascular coagulation. All these may be responsible for diffuse bleeding. Liver damage is common; it appears 24 to 36 h after admission and is characterized by clinically apparent jaundice and, often, by abnormalities in hepatocellular enzymes. Renal failure is a common complication of heat stroke.

Patients with heat stroke may die within a few hours after being discovered, or may die of complications such as acute renal failure. However, a number of patients will die several weeks after the acute episode, usually of myocardial infarction, heart failure, renal failure, bronchopneumonia, or complicating bacteremia. In them autopsy may show extensive parenchymal damage to various organs, either from hyperpyrexia per se or from petechial hemorrhages in the brain, heart, kidneys, or liver.

Heat stroke requires heroic emergency measures. Time is most important. The patient should be placed in a cool place with adequate circulation of fresh air and with most of the clothing removed. Because the pathogenesis of heat stroke involves failure of the heat-regulating mechanism with cessation of sweating, external means of heat dissipation must be employed. The most effective measure is to immerse the patient in an ice-water bath, and there is no effective substitute for this seemingly drastic treatment. An ice-water bath does not induce shock or stimulate significant cutaneous vasoconstriction. The bath should be given with a minimum of delay. The patient should be watched constantly by a nurse or physician and the rectal temperature monitored. The bath may be discontinued when the rectal temperature falls below 101°F (38.3°C), but treatment should be resumed if there is a febrile rebound. Compared with immersion in ice water, other forms of therapy are less effective, but covering the patient with cold wet towels under a fan may be satisfactory if a bath is not available. After the bath the patient should be placed in a cool, well-ventilated room. Massage of the skin should be employed along with cooling because it stimulates return of the cool peripheral blood to the overheated brain and viscera and aids acceleration of heat loss. The patient should be well hydrated with hypotonic crystalloid solutions. Phenothiazine may be helpful in reducing shivering. Stimulants such as epinephrine and narcotics are contraindicated. A Swan-Ganz catheter should be inserted, and urinary output needs to be monitored. Prompt ice-bath cooling, massage of the limbs, and vigorous hydration, along with establishment of a proper airway, avoidance of aspiration, treating coma and convulsions, and watching for arrhythmia, will lead to survival of most patients, particularly if they are young and were previously well. Unfortunately, the poor, ill, and elderly who are often not discovered until heat hyperpyrexia has been present for some hours have a much less favorable outcome. Both dehydration and heart failure must be avoided. Fresh blood should be given in case of bleeding, and clear-cut evidence of disseminated intravascular coagulation calls for heparin (7500 units per hour). Persistent oliguria is an indication for early dialysis.

Malignant hyperthermia ETIOLOGY Malignant hyperthermia (MH) consists of a group of inherited disorders that are characterized by a rapid increase in temperature to 102.2 to 107.6°F (39 to 42°C) in response to inhalational anesthetics such as halothane, methoxyflurane, cyclopropane, and ethyl ether or muscle relaxants, notably succinylcholine. In one form of the disease where the mechanism of inheritance is autosomal dominant, the individuals are normal between attacks although about 50 percent have an elevation in creatine phosphokinase (CPK), and in 90 percent, muscle from susceptible individuals contracts on exposure to concentrations of caffeine, halothane, or hexamethonium that cause only minimal changes in normal muscle. A second recessive form occurs in young boys and, less commonly, girls, with a number of congenital abnormalities including short stature, undescended testes, lumbar lordosis, thoracic kyphosis, pectus carinatum, webbed neck, winged scapulae, small chin, low-set ears, and an antimongoloid obliquity of the palpebral fissures. This form is called the *King syndrome*. MH has also been described in several other myopathies including myotonia congenita, central core disease, and Duchenne's muscular dystrophy. The incidence of the autosomal dominant form is 1:50,000 to 1:100,000.

PATHOGENESIS The triggering anesthetic releases calcium from the membrane of the muscle cell's sarcoplasmic reticulum, which is defective in storing this ion. The result is a sudden increase in myoplasmic calcium. The calcium activates myosin ATPase, which converts adenosine triphosphate (ATP) to adenosine diphosphate, phosphate, and heat. There are also inhibition of tropanin, uncoupling of oxidative phosphorylation, activation of phosphorylase kinase, and increased glycolysis. Muscular contraction occurs and it, as well as the chemical events, leads to production of heat.

MANIFESTATIONS Existence of malignant hyperthermia can be suspected if less relaxation is noted during induction of anesthesia and muscle fasciculations become evident when succinylcholine is given. In some patients trismus during intubation is the first sign of a muscle disorder. Although the elevation in temperature is the result of muscular contraction, it may rise very rapidly, and if the temperature is not monitored, the first signs may be a hot skin and tachycardia or a cardiac arrhythmia. In addition to the high fever, there is muscle rigidity, hypotension, and mottled cyanosis.

Early laboratory abnormalities include respiratory and metabolic acidosis, hyperkalemia and hypermagnesemia, and elevation in blood lactate and pyruvate. Late complications include massive skeletal muscle swelling, pulmonary edema, disseminated intravascular coagulation, and acute renal failure.

TREATMENT Malignant hyperthermia is a medical emergency. Surgery must be interrupted and the patient cooled with ice. One hundred percent oxygen should be given, along with sodium bicarbonate, to combat the severe metabolic acidosis. A diuresis should be induced with fluids and diuretics to reduce myoglobinemia and hyperkalemia. Specific treatment consists of dantrolene sodium, 1 mg/kg, by rapid intravenous infusion. The drug should be continued until symptoms have begun to subside or up to a maximum single dose of 10 mg/kg. The regimen can be repeated if symptoms recur. Procainamide to combat arrhythmias, in dosage of 0.5 to 1 (mg/kg)/min with ECG monitoring, should be administered as well.

PREVENTION Because of the tendency of this syndrome to run in families, its detection is essential. This can be achieved by monitoring the temperature of all patients under anesthesia; the best way to avert it altogether is to take a thorough family history. Examining patients preoperatively is often not helpful because between attacks persons susceptible to malignant hyperthermia may be entirely normal. Some have increased muscle bulk, some have localized areas of muscle weakness, some have spontaneous muscle cramps, and a few have generalized muscle weakness. In some of these patients, the CPK is elevated, but in many this test is entirely normal. Prophylactic dantrolene orally has not been successful in preventing MH. In susceptible patients, surgery should be performed under spinal, epidural, or regional anesthesia. If this is not possible, a combination of Pentothal and diazepam is probably safest. Phosphorylase A and adenylate cyclase are elevated in muscles of MH patients and along with their increased contractility provide useful biochemical markers of MH.

Neuroleptic malignant syndrome (NMS) This syndrome is characterized by muscular rigidity, hyperthermia, altered consciousness, and autonomic dysfunction. Rigidity and akinesia develop concomitantly with fever as high as 106°F (41°C). Consciousness fluctuates from alertness to coma. Autonomic dysfunction is manifested by tachycardia, labile blood pressure, profuse sweating, dyspnea, and incontinence. Laboratory abnormalities consist of leukocytosis (15,000 to 30,000) and elevation in CPK. The syndrome occurs after use of potent neuroleptics in therapeutic doses. Most cases have been reported after haloperidol, thiothixene, or piperazine phenothiazine. Young adult males predominate. The NMS lasts 5 to 10 days after administration of oral neuroleptics is discontinued, and longer after depot injection. The overall mortality is 20 percent and fatalities have occurred as late as 30 days after onset and have been due to renal failure or arrhythmias. Although the etiology of NMS is unknown, its similarity to malignant hyperthermia is striking, and the fact that MH has occurred in the wake of neuroleptic drugs strengthens the hypothesis that NMS may be a variant of MH. No specific treatment for NMS has been described, although dantrolene sodium may be worth trying if supportive measures, cooling, and drug withdrawal do not result in improvement.

DISORDERS ASSOCIATED WITH LOW TEMPERATURES Cold acclimatization
The state of increased resistance to cold injury is the result of exposure to a cold but tolerable environment. Adaptive responses consist of circulatory adjustments protecting the temperatures of exposed portions of the body, metabolic adaptation providing

greater heat production to compensate for increased heat loss, and behavioral and neural adaptations minimizing either the actual cold stress or the discomfort resulting from physiologically tolerable hypothermia. In contrast with heat acclimatization, it is not possible to delineate adaptive physiologic changes to cold. Nevertheless, primitive people live at zero temperatures wearing little or no clothing; pain perception is less in persons, such as fishermen, who work periodically with their hands in ice water; and military personnel shiver less during cold exposure after training in the Arctic. Adaptation may take place either by shivering, with production of excess heat, or, as is the case with Australian aborigines, by a drop of internal temperature with only minimal shivering.

Hypothermia Although far less common than is elevation in temperature, hypothermia is of considerable importance because it can represent a medical emergency which lends itself to treatment.

ACCIDENTAL HYPOTHERMIA This is a well-known complication of exposure and has been reported frequently during the winter months. It usually occurs in elderly or inebriated individuals after prolonged exposure, not necessarily to excessively low external temperatures. It is true, however, that both of these groups detect low temperatures less well than normal. The diagnosis of hypothermia may prove elusive because *clinical thermometers do not record temperatures below 95°F (35°C). Whenever a patient presents with a temperature below this level, the true temperature should be determined with an incubator thermometer or a thermocouple.* Accidental hypothermia has been found in association with myxedema, pituitary insufficiency, Addison's disease, hypoglycemia, cerebrovascular disease, Wernicke's encephalopathy, myocardial infarction, cirrhosis, pancreatitis, and ingestion of drugs or alcohol. For example, it is not uncommon to find a derelict in a railroad yard or under a bridge following an alcoholic debauch with a temperature between 85 and 90°F (28.5 and 32.3°C) or lower. These patients usually appear cold and pale and, when their temperatures are very low, give the appearance of having rigor mortis, so stiff is their musculature. Patients with temperatures less than 80°F (26.7°C) are usually unconscious. The pupils are usually miotic, respirations tend to be shallow and slow, there is bradycardia, and most patients are hypotensive. Generalized edema is often present. When the temperature falls below 77°F (25°C), coma, areflexia, and lack of pupillary response are present. Laboratory data tend to show hemoconcentration, mild azotemia, and metabolic acidosis. The acidosis is due to lactacidemia which is, in part, a result of hypoxemia in peripheral tissues. At cold temperatures, the hemoglobin dissociation curve is shifted to the left, and there is decreased unloading of oxygen in the peripheral tissues. Some patients have hypoglycemia while others have hyperglycemia. Thyroid function tests may give results typical of myxedema. Some patients have elevations in serum amylase, and a few show pancreatitis at autopsy. The electrocardiogram is distorted by muscular tremors and may show bradycardia or slow atrial fibrillation and a characteristic J wave (occurring at the junction of the QRS complex and ST segment). Other arrythmias are common; ventricular fibrillation is usually a terminal event. The mortality rate is five times higher in people over 75.

Hypothermia is a medical emergency, and therapy should be instituted at once. The following steps are indicated:

1 An airway must be established and maintained, and the patient should be well oxygenated. Warmed oxygen may be helpful.
2 Blood gases should be monitored; they should be corrected for temperature.
3 Blood volume should be expanded with glucose and saline, low-molecular-weight dextran, or albumin. Maintenance of blood volume is necessary to prevent the infarctions which have been a hallmark in fatal cases and to avert "rewarming shock."
4 Because of the tendency to arrythmias, serum potassium should be monitored carefully; a transvenous pacemaker may be indicated.
5 Sodium bicarbonate should be given if pH is less than 7.25.
6 Although external rewarming with blankets or placing the patient

in a warm room is appropriate in patients with mild hypothermia, patients who are moderately hypothermic require reestablishment of core temperature. This can be done effectively by placing the patient in a warm bath or a Hubbard tank at 104 to 108°F (40 to 42°C). This maneuver must be carried out cautiously; physiologic monitoring may be difficult, and if an arrhythmia occurs, resuscitation is hampered. Nevertheless, external warming tends to dilate the constricted peripheral blood vessels and to divert blood from the visceral organs. In severely hypothermic patients, this may result in rewarming shock and does not lead to sufficient restoration of the core temperature to warm the myocardium sufficiently to make it responsive to antiarrhythmic agents. In this situation hemodialysis, during which the blood is warmed externally, or peritoneal dialysis, during which the dialysate is warmed to 98.6°F (37°C), are the methods of choice. It is particularly important to rewarm the myocardium because in cases of ventricular fibrillation defibrillation will not be successful until myocardial temperature is raised to near normal levels.
7 There is a tendency for these patients to develop pneumonia, which should be treated promptly with antibiotics.
8 Finally, resuscitative efforts should be vigorous and prolonged despite the poor prognosis which is related primarily to the advanced age and associated debilitating disease of these patients. In younger individuals, some remarkable rescues have been recorded; one young woman was resuscitated even after her temperature had dropped to 69°F (20.6°C). *Authorities agree that hypothermia victims without vital signs (prolonged asystole) should not be pronounced dead until they have been rewarmed to 96.8°F (36°C) and remain unresponsive to CPR at that temperature.*

HYPOTHERMIA SECONDARY TO ACUTE ILLNESS There is a group of patients who develop moderate hypothermia in association with acute diseases including congestive heart failure, uremia, diabetes mellitus, drug overdose, acute respiratory failure, and hypoglycemia. These patients are generally elderly and upon admission to the hospital are found to have temperatures of 92 to 93.9°F (33.3 to 34.4°C). They also have a severe metabolic acidosis, due to increased production of lactic acid, and cardiac arrhythmias. Most of these patients are comatose. This entity differs from accidental hypothermia only in the absence of exposure; these cases have all occurred at normal ambient temperatures. The mechanism appears to be an acute failure of thermoregulation; shivering did not occur in any of these patients. Usually these patients have been rewarmed within a few hours by means of an alcohol-circulating blanket. Upon return to normal temperature, cardiac arrythmias, which were present in most of these patients, responded to treatment, and the sensorium returned to normal. With the exception that core rewarming is established by external means, other facets of therapy should follow the steps outlined above. In addition, treatment of the underlying disease such as diabetes with insulin, uremia with dialysis, or congestive heart failure with appropriate cardiac drugs and diuretics is essential. The prognosis is good provided the syndrome is recognized early and treatment is instituted at once.

IMMERSION HYPOTHERMIA Responses to cold-water immersion may be classified as (1) stimulatory, with deep body temperature normal to 95°F (35°C); (2) depressant, with deep body temperature 95 to 86°F (35 to 30°C); and (3) critical, with deep body temperature 86 to 77°F (30 to 25°C).

The long-distance swimmer is able to maintain a normal body temperature for periods of 15 to 25 h or more in water that may plunge skin temperature to 59°F (15°C) or lower, which is some 28°F below deep body temperature, lending support to the concept of a body core insulated by a body shell. The vasoconstriction operative in cold water greatly reduces heat loss. However, there is great individual variability in heat loss in cold water. The relatively obese swimmer may maintain a normal rectal temperature for 2 h without shivering in 61°F (16°C) water. A lean person under the same conditions, despite violent shivering, may experience a fall in rectal temperature of several degrees and become incapacitated from the rigor. In hypersensitive persons, immersion in cold water may be followed by vascular spasm, vomiting, and syncope.

Other compensatory responses include bradycardia, a slight rise in blood pressure, and an early rise in rectal temperature followed by a fall. At 86°F (30°C), atrial fibrillation is common.

Rewarming in warm water has been recommended as the treatment of immersion hypothermia. In severe cases, hemodialysis or peritoneal dialysis should be instituted.

Local cold injuries MECHANISMS OF FREEZING INJURY These can be divided into phenomena which affect cells and extracellular fluids (direct effects) and those which disrupt the function of organized tissues and the integrity of the circulation (indirect effects).

When tissue freezes, ice crystals form and, concomitantly, solutes in the residual liquid become concentrated. The physical dislocation during slow freezing is extreme. Ice crystals many times the size of individual cells form but only in the extracellular spaces. Large ice crystals can develop between cells in soft tissue without producing irreversible injury as long as the percentage of water frozen does not exceed a critical amount. A major source of damage to living cells during freezing and thawing appears to be the strong salt solutions which develop during formation and dissolution of ice; changes in the proportions of lipids and phospholipids in the cell membrane are also of great importance.

The fulminating vascular reaction and stasis which supervene are associated with production of histamine-like substances which increase the permeability of the capillary bed. Within blood vessels, cellular elements aggregate. Irreversible occlusion of small blood vessels by cell masses has been demonstrated in thawed tissue following freezing injury. The damaged frozen tissue simulates tissue damage produced by burns.

MANIFESTATIONS The mildest form of cold injury is called *frostnip* and tends to occur in organs farthest removed from the core of the body such as the earlobes, nose, cheeks, fingers and toes, and hands and feet. It can be prevented by warm clothing and treated with simple rewarming. More consequential local cold injuries may be divided into freezing (frostbite) and nonfreezing (immersion-foot) injuries. The two types may be observed in the same extremity or in different extremities in the same individual. The diagnosis of freezing versus nonfreezing injury generally can be made on the basis of history and clinical manifestations.

Immersion foot is an entity observed in shipwreck survivors or in soldiers (trench foot) whose feet have been wet but not freezing cold for prolonged periods. There is primarily injury to nerve and muscle tissue, but no gross or irreparable pathologic changes occur in blood vessels and skin. The clinical picture reflects primary hypoxic trauma giving rise to three clearly recognizable conditions: (1) *ischemia*, denoted by a pale, pulseless extremity; (2) *hyperemia*, characterized by a bounding pulsatile circulation in red, swollen, painful feet; and (3) the *posthyperemic* or recovery period. The initial cold-induced vasoconstriction, increased blood viscosity, and impaired oxygen transport in the ischemic state are aggravated by such factors as malnutrition, general hypothermia, dehydration, and trauma from relatively fixed, pendant extremities. The problem of rewarming is critical in these patients during the stage of ischemia, when overheating of tissue may lead to gangrene. In the state of hyperemia, the red, swollen feet require judicious cooling. Severe cases may show muscular weakness, atrophy, ulceration, and gangrene of superficial areas. Sensitivity to cold and pain on weight bearing, which may cause discomfort for many years, are sequelae even of milder injuries.

Frostbite stands in contrast with immersion foot because the blood vessels may be severely and irreparably injured, the circulation of blood ceases, and the vascular bed of the frozen tissue is occluded by agglutinated cell aggregates and thrombi. The cutaneous injury consists in part of separation of the epidermal-dermal interface. Early, the intravascular clumping is reversible. However, with the passage of time, clumped red blood cells within vessels in injured tissue lose their morphologic identity and take on the appearance of a homogenous, hyalinaceous plug. It has been shown in some, but not all, experimental studies that much of the intravascular aggregation following freezing injury can be reversed and microcirculatory perfusion improved if low-molecular-weight dextran is given intravenously shortly after injury, but the data in humans are less convincing. Frostbitten tissues unfortunately are often neglected and with thawing become macerated; if this is the situation, the method of rewarming is not important. The method of rewarming has been a matter of controversy. It seems most rational to warm the core of the body before treating the local area of frostbite. Following restoration of the core temperature to normal, warming of a frostbitten limb should begin in water at 50 to 59°F (10 to 15°C), which is then increased 9°F (5°C) every 5 min to a maximum of 104°F (40°C).

Once the frostbitten limb has been rewarmed, treatment should be conservative and consists of bed rest, elevation of the injured part, tetanus toxoid administration, and use of antibiotics if infection is present; early drainage of blebs and bullae; daily washes with chlorhexidine or an iodophor; and early institution of physiotherapy. Alcohol and cigarettes are strongly contraindicated. Surgical amputation and reconstruction is usually not necessary. Regional sympathectomy performed 24 to 48 h after thawing has not been of value in acute frostbite although it has prevented some late complications, and recurrent episodes of cold injury in individuals who have been reexposed. The effect of regional sympathectomy is probably due to ablation of persistent vasospasm and to restoration of cold perception. Intraarterial reserpine has effects similar to sympathectomy.

Some patients with frostbite have residua consisting of excessive sweating, pain, cold feet, numbness, abnormal color, and pain in the joints. The symptoms are generally worse in the winter and following exposure to cold. These patients also often show abnormal nails, discoloration and pigmentation, hyperhydrosis, and, by x-ray, osteoporosis and cystic defects near the joints. These abnormalities tend to be milder in patients who have had sympathetic blockade. Most cold injuries are preventable by graded exposure to cold, as well as appropriate clothing in freezing temperatures.

REFERENCES

Temperature regulation

ATKINS E: Fever: The old and the new. J Infect Dis 149:339, 1984

BARACOS V et al: Stimulation of muscle protein degradation and prostaglandin E₂ release by leukocytic pyrogen (interleukin-1): A mechanism for increased degradation of muscle during fever. N Engl J Med 308:553, 1983

BULLEN JJ: The significance of iron in infection. Rev Infect Dis 3:1127, 1981

DINARELLO CA: Interleukin-1 and the pathogenesis of the acute phase response. N Engl J Med 311:1413, 1984

———: Interleukin 1. Rev Infect Dis 6:41, 1984

KREUGER JM et al: Sleep promoting effects of endogenous pyrogen (interleukin-1). Am J Physiol (in press)

Heat injury

BRITT BA: Etiology and pathophysiology of malignant hyperthermia. Fed Proc 38:44, 1979

CLOWES GHA JR, O'DONNEL TF JR: Current concepts: Heat stroke. N Engl J Med 291:564, 1974

COSTRINI AM et al: Cardiovascular and metabolic manifestations of heat stroke and severe heat exhaustion. Am J Med 66:296, 1979

DOWNEY GP et al: Neuroleptic malignant syndrome. Patient with unique clinical and physiologic features. Am J Med 77:338, 1984

GRONERT GA: Malignant hyperthermia. Anesthesiology 53:395, 1980

HANSON PG, ZIMMERMAN SW: Exertional heat stroke in novice runners. JAMA 242:159, 1979

MCPHERSON EW, TAYLOR CA JR: The King syndrome: Malignant hyperthermia, myopathy and multiple anomalies. Am J Med Genet 8:159, 1981

SHIBOLET S et al: Heat stroke: A review. Aviat Space Environ Med 47:280, 1976

SPRUNG CL et al: The metabolic and respiratory alterations of heat stroke. Arch Intern Med 140:665, 1980

WILLNER JH et al: Increased myophosphorylase A in malignant hyperthermia. N Engl J Med 303:138, 1980

——— et al: High skeletal muscle adenylate cyclase in malignant hyperthermia. J Clin Invest 68:1119, 1981

WYNDHAM CH: Heat stroke and hyperthermia in marathon runners. Ann NY Acad Sci 301:128, 1977

Cold injury

Bouwman DL et al: Early sympathetic blockade for frostbite—Is it of value? J Trauma 20:744, 1980

Gage AM: Frostbite. Trauma and Emergency Med 7:25, 1981

MacLean D et al: Metabolic aspects of spontaneous recovery in accidental hypothermia and hypothermic myxedema. Q J Med (n.s.) 43:371, 1974

Southwick FS, Dalglish PH Jr: Recovery after prolonged asystolic cardiac arrest in profound hypothermia. JAMA 243:1250, 1980

Vaughn PB: Local cold injury—Menace to military operations: A review. Military Med 143:305, 1980

Whittle JL, Bates JH: Thermoregulatory failure secondary to acute illness: Complications and treatment. Arch Intern Med 139:418, 1979

Wickstrom P et al: Accidental hypothermia. Am J Surg 131:622, 1976

9   CHILLS AND FEVER

ROBERT G. PETERSDORF / RICHARD K. ROOT

Omitting disorders which may involve cerebral thermoregulatory centers directly, such as brain tumors, intracranial hemorrhage or thrombosis, or heat stroke, the following disease states may be accompanied by fever:

1 All *infections*, whether caused by bacteria, rickettsias, chlamydia, viruses, or parasites, can cause fever.

2 *Mechanical trauma*, e.g., a crushing injury, frequently gives rise to fever lasting 1 or 2 days. Not infrequently, however, complicating infection sets in.

3 Many *neoplastic diseases* are associated with fever. In most patients, fever in patients with cancer is related to obstruction or infection produced by the tumor. In some solid tumors, however, fever may be due to the tumor per se, particularly following metastasis to the liver. Tumors which are associated with fever include hypernephroma, carcinoma of the pancreas, lung, or bone, and hepatoma. In tumors of the reticuloendothelial system, including Hodgkin's disease, non-Hodgkin's lymphoma, acute leukemias, and malignant histiocytosis, fever may be one of the prominent early manifestations. The production of endogenous pyrogen/interleukin-1 (EP/IL-1) by these tumors is responsible for fever production.

4 *Hematopoietic disorders*, e.g., acute hemolytic episodes, may be characterized by pyrexia.

5 *Vascular accidents* of any magnitude, e.g., myocardial, pulmonary, and cerebral infarctions, nearly always cause fever.

6 *Diseases due to immune mechanisms* are often febrile. These include the connective tissue diseases, drug fevers, and fever due to other immunologic abnormalities.

7 Certain *acute metabolic disorders*, such as gout, porphyria, hypertriglyceridemia, Fabry's disease, and Addisonian or thyroid crises, sometimes are associated with fever. The pathogenesis varies from activation of the inflammatory response (EP/IL-1 production) to alterations in thermogenesis and heat regulation (hyperthyroidism).

ACCOMPANIMENTS OF FEVER   Systemic symptoms   The perception of fever by patients varies enormously. Some persons can tell with considerable accuracy whether their body temperatures are elevated; others with chronic febrile illnesses (e.g., patients with tuberculosis) may be wholly unaware of body temperature as high as 103°F (39.4°C). Often, patients may pay no attention to fever because of other unpleasant symptoms such as headache and pleuritic pain. Pain in the back, generalized myalgias, and arthralgia without arthritis are commonly associated with fever. Whether these symptoms reflect the presence of an infectious agent or are merely a manifestation of IL-1 activity is not clear (see Chap. 8).

Chills   Abrupt onset of fever with a *chill* or *rigor* is characteristic of some diseases and, in the absence of antipyretic drugs, rare in others. Although repeated rigors are typical of pyogenic infection

with bacteremia, a similar pattern of fever may occur in noninfectious diseases such as lymphoma. It is important to differentiate a true chill, which is accompanied by teeth chattering and bed shaking, from the chilly sensation which occurs in almost all fevers, particularly those in viral infections. In some instances, however, a true rigor occurs in viremia. Chills may be evoked or perpetuated by the intermittent administration of aspirin or other antipyretics. These agents may cause a sharp depression in temperature, which is followed by compensatory involuntary muscular contractions, i.e., a chill. This unpleasant side effect of antipyretic drugs can be averted by administering these agents no less frequently than every 3 h, around the clock, rather than by prescribing them only for elevations in temperature above a certain level.

Herpes labialis   So-called fever blisters result from activation of latent herpes simplex virus infection by elevations in temperature. For reasons which are obscure, fever blisters are common in pneumococcal infections, streptococcosis, malaria, meningococcemia, and rickettsioses but are rare in mycoplasma pneumonia, tuberculosis, brucellosis, smallpox, and typhoid.

Delirium   This may result from elevation of body temperature and is particularly common in patients with alcoholism, cerebrovascular disease, or senility.

Convulsions   Some febrile children, especially those with a family history of epilepsy, develop seizures with fever. Febrile convulsions do not, in general, reflect serious cerebral disease.

CLINICAL IMPORTANCE OF FEVER   The temperature is a simple, objective, and accurate indicator of a physiologic state and is much less subject to external and psychogenic stimuli than the other vital signs, such as pulse, respiratory rate, and blood pressure. For these reasons, determination of the body temperature assists in estimating the severity of an illness, its course and duration, and the effect of therapy, or even in deciding whether a person has an organic illness.

Benefit of fever   There are a few infections of humans in which pyrexia appears definitely to be beneficial to the host, such as neurosyphilis, some forms of chronic arthritis, and widespread cancer. Certain other diseases, such as uveitis and rheumatoid arthritis, sometimes improve after fever therapy. Specific immune responses are accelerated at febrile body temperatures, as are catabolic processes involving mobilization of amino acids from muscle. These events are mediated by EP/IL-1 and may involve synthesis of prostaglandins of the E series. In humans, the benefits of fever on other host defense mechanisms other than the multiple actions of EP/IL-1 (see Chap. 8) are not as apparent as in cold-blooded animals. In these species higher ambient temperatures augment the acute inflammatory response. Minor increases in phagocytosis and chemotaxis by human polymorphonuclear leukocytes have been observed at febrile incubation temperatures. Aged and debilitated patients with infection may have little or no fever, and this is generally interpreted as a bad prognostic sign.

Detrimental aspects of fever   Fever accelerates many metabolic processes and is accompanied by EP/IL-1–mediated muscle wasting and weight loss. The work and the rate of the heart are increased. Sweating aggravates loss of salt and water. There may be discomfort due to headache, photophobia, general malaise, or an unpleasant sensation of warmth. Fever may precipitate seizures in epileptic patients. The rigors and profuse sweats of hectic fevers are particularly unpleasant for the patient. In elderly individuals with overt or potential cardiac or cerebral vascular disease, fever may be particularly deleterious.

MANAGEMENT OF FEVER   Since fever ordinarily does little harm, imposes no great discomfort, and may have benefits to host defense mechanisms, antipyretic drugs are rarely essential to patient welfare and may obfuscate the effect of a specific therapeutic agent or of the natural course of the disease. There are situations, however, in which lowering of the body temperature is of vital importance; e.g., heat stroke, postoperative hyperthermia, delirium due to hyperpyrexia, epileptic seizures, or shock associated with fever and heart failure. Under these circumstances lowering the temperature is indicated. Cooling blankets which can be set at hypothermic temperatures are a highly effective means for external cooling. Alternatively, sponging the body surface with cool saline solution or the application of cool compresses to the skin and forehead may be employed. There is no advantage in sponging with alcohol, which, because of its pungent odor, makes some patients ill. When high internal temperature is combined with cutaneous vasoconstriction, as in heat stroke or postoperative hyperthermia, the cooling measures should be combined with massage of the skin in order to bring blood to the surface, where it may be cooled. Immediate immersion in a tub of ice water should be considered a lifesaving emergency procedure in patients with heat stroke if the internal body temperature is in excess of 108°F (42.2°C). If cooling blankets are available, they are preferable to immersion in ice in most instances.

Antipyretic drugs, such as aspirin (0.3 to 0.6 g) or acetaminophen (0.5 g), are often employed in lowering temperature, particularly if patients are uncomfortable or if fever poses a high risk to them, as is the case in patients with heart failure, febrile seizures (usually children), head injury, mental disorders, or pregnancy. Antipyretics are sometimes associated with unpleasant diaphoresis, an alarming fall in blood pressure, and the subsequent return of fever occasionally accompanied by a chill. These can be mitigated by enforcing a liberal fluid intake and by administering the drugs regularly and frequently at 2- to 3-h intervals. Although glucocorticosteroids are also potent antipyretics, they must be used with caution because of their tendency to precipitate abrupt falls in temperature accompanied by hypotension. The capacity of these drugs to mask other manifestations of infection also constitutes a relative contraindication to their use. In contrast to other antipyretics, glucocorticoids inhibit EP/IL-1 production and may thereby diminish beneficial actions induced by this molecule (see Chap. 8).

The discomfort of a rigor can be alleviated in many patients by the intravenous injection of calcium salts. This procedure will stop the shivering and chilliness but has no influence on the ultimate height of the fever. Severe disruptive rigors sometimes need to be abolished with morphine sulfate (10 to 15 mg subcutaneously) or with parenteral chlorpromazine.

DIAGNOSTIC CONSIDERATIONS IN FEVER   In many illnesses fever is the most prominent and often the only manifestation of disease. It is not an indication of any particular type of disease; rather it should be considered a reaction to injury comparable with an elevated leukocyte count or a rapid erythrocyte sedimentation rate.

Definitions of fever   Fever is classically described as intermittent, remittent, sustained, or relapsing. In *intermittent fever* the temperature falls to normal each day. When the variation between the peak and the nadir is very large, the fever is called *hectic* or *septic*. Intermittent fevers are characteristic in pyogenic infections, particularly abscesses, lymphomas, and miliary tuberculosis. In *remittent fever* the temperature falls each day but does not return to normal. Most fevers are remittent, and this type of febrile response is not characteristic of any disease. A *sustained fever* is characterized by persistent elevation without significant diurnal variation. It is exemplified by the fever of untreated typhoid or typhus. With *relapsing fever* short febrile periods occur between one or several days of normal temperature. Examples of relapsing fever are the following:

Malaria (see Chap. 154) had vanished from the United States almost completely, but for several years Vietnam war veterans constituted an important and sizable reservoir of this infection, as do other persons recently arrived from foreign countries. It is most unusual, however, for malaria to recur after a symptom-free interval of 1 year or more. Febrile bouts recur at 2- or 3-day intervals, or more irregularly in falciparum infections, depending on the maturation cycle of the parasite. The diagnosis depends on demonstration of the parasites in the blood.

Relapsing fever (see Chap. 126) occurs in the southwest part of the United States, as far east as Texas, the Pacific Northwest, and in many other parts of the world. The recurrences are related to the cyclic development of parasites. Diagnosis is by demonstration of the spirochetal organisms in stained films of the blood.

Rat-bite fever (see Chap. 125) is brought about by two agents— *Spirillum minus* and *Streptobacillus moniliformis*, both transmitted by the bite of a rat. Both may cause an illness characterized by periodic exacerbations of fever. The clue to the diagnosis depends on obtaining a history of rat bite 1 to 10 weeks prior to the onset of symptoms. The cause can be established by appropriate laboratory procedures.

Localized *pyogenic infections* in rare instances give rise to periodic bouts of fever separated by afebrile and relatively symptom-free intervals. The so-called Charcot's intermittent biliary fever, i.e., cholangitis with biliary obstruction due to stones, is an example. *Urinary tract infection*, with episodes of ureteral obstruction due to small stones or inspissated pus, can also cause recurrent fever.

A few patients with Hodgkin's disease at some time have so-called Pel-Ebstein fever—bouts of fever lasting 3 to 10 days, separated by afebrile and asymptomatic periods of 3 to 10 days. These cycles may be repeated regularly over a period of several months. In rare instances this periodicity of the fever has been sufficiently striking to suggest the correct diagnosis before lymphadenopathy or spleno-megaly became evident. However, relapsing fevers indistinguishable from Pel-Ebstein fever usually have causes other than Hodgkin's disease.

Epidemiology of fever   The diagnosis of febrile illnesses must take into consideration the context of the epidemiologic setting. For example, an acute febrile illness in southeast Asia or Africa is probably due to one of the arboviruses (see Chap. 143) or malaria (see Chap. 154); in a college student in the United States it may result from infectious mononucleosis or some other viral infection; and in an octogenarian following prostatectomy it is probably an indication of urinary tract infection, wound infection, pulmonary infarction, or aspiration pneumonia. In children, infections are more likely to be responsible for prolonged fevers than in adults. Likewise, travelers returning from short trips to foreign countries are much more likely to have febrile illnesses indigenous to their home than to the foreign country they have visited. Patients whose host defenses are altered by malignancy, cytotoxic or steroid therapy, or congenital or acquired immune deficiency are much more likely to have unusual infections as a cause for fever than are normal hosts.

Rare versus common diseases   Most of the time fever is a manifestation of a common disease, and fever associated with a pulmonary infiltrate is much more likely to be due to pneumococcal than to *Pneumocystis* pneumonia. Failure to appreciate this cardinal principle has led to many prolonged and futile diagnostic workups.

Febrile illnesses of short duration   Acute febrile illnesses of less than 2 weeks' duration are common in medical practice. In many instances they run their course, progressing to complete recovery, and a precise diagnosis is not made. In most instances, however, it is safe to assume that the illness is of infectious origin. Although short febrile illnesses may be noninfectious (e.g., allergic fevers due to drugs, thromboembolic disease, hemolytic crises, or gout), these are decidedly in the minority.

Most undiagnosed acute febrile infectious diseases are probably viral and remain undiagnosed because diagnostic methods are un-available, cumbersome, or not cost-effective. It is not practical to carry out tests needed to identify all the known viruses, and, furthermore, there must be a considerable number of still unidentified viruses pathogenic for humans. In bacterial infections, on the other hand, laboratory diagnosis is simpler, and these infections are often rapidly controlled with chemotherapy.

The following characteristics, though not restricted solely to acute infections, are highly suggestive that infection is present:

1 Abrupt onset

2 High fever, i.e., 102 to 105°F (38.9 to 40.6°C), with or without chills

3 Respiratory symptoms—sore throat, coryza, cough

4 Severe malaise, with muscle or joint pain, photophobia, pain on movement of the eyes, headache

5 Nausea, vomiting, or diarrhea

6 Acute enlargement of lymph nodes or spleen

7 Meningeal signs, with or without spinal fluid pleocytosis

8 Leukocyte count above 12,000 or below 5000 per cubic millimeter

9 Dysuria, frequency, and flank pain

None of the symptoms or signs listed is encountered only in infection. Many of these features could be seen in acute leukemia or in disseminated lupus erythematosus. Nevertheless, in a given instance of acute febrile illness with some of or all the manifestations listed, the probabilities strongly favor infection, and the patient may be given reasonable reassurance that he or she will probably recover in a week or two, regardless of a precise diagnosis.

It is desirable, of course, to establish an accurate diagnosis, and whatever steps are practicable in the circumstances to establish the cause should be taken. Cultures of the throat, blood, urine, or feces should be obtained before institution of antibacterial chemotherapy. Skin and/or serologic tests should be carried out when indicated.

There is a tendency to rely immediately and excessively on the laboratory in ascertaining the cause of fever. In many instances, a thorough history and a complete and, if necessary, repeated physical examination, along with a complete blood count (CBC), urinalysis, and sedimentation rate will provide the answer. Often a little patience, in the form of watchful waiting, before plunging into an expensive and extensive laboratory workup, will lead to the diagnosis.

Prolonged febrile illnesses Some of the knottiest problems in medicine are found in cases of prolonged fever in which the diagnosis remains obscure for weeks or even months. Eventually, however, the true nature of the illness usually reveals itself, since a disease which causes injury sufficient to evoke temperature elevations to 101°F (38.3°C) or higher for several weeks does not often subside without leaving some clue as to its nature. The elucidation of problems of this sort calls for skillful application of all diagnostic methods—careful history, thorough physical examination, and the carefully considered use of laboratory examinations and imaging techniques.

FEVER OF UNKNOWN ORIGIN In some patients fever becomes the dominant sign or symptom in a patient's illness, and when its cause escapes detection, it is defined as fever of unknown origin (FUO). It is appropriate to use this term only in patients who have elevations in temperature [>101°F (38.3°C)] for a prolonged period (at least 2, and preferably 3, weeks) and in whom the diagnosis cannot be made during at least 1 week of intensive study. These rigid criteria eliminate from this diagnostic category patients with common bacterial or viral infections, those in whom the diagnosis is obvious, and those whose fever is due to a sequential occurrence of etiologically unrelated diseases. An example is a patient who is febrile following a myocardial infarction, who then develops thrombophlebitis that is associated with fever, and in whom this is followed by multiple pulmonary emboli, also a febrile disease. Much of the confusion in the literature concerning causes of FUO is due to failure to define the criteria employed in classifying patients who have had fever of unknown origin.

DISEASES CAUSING PROLONGED FEVERS Table 9-1 lists some of the diseases responsible for prolonged fever. Some of these disorders must initially be considered to be FUO; in others the diagnosis comes to mind readily.

Infections Infections occupy a less prominent position among causes of prolonged fever now than formerly because of the common practice of administering antibiotics to any patient in whom fever persists for more than a few days. Consequently, many infections are eradicated by more or less "blind" therapy without accurate determination of

their nature or location. In the 1950s, patients with infections comprised about 40 percent of patients with FUO, but in a comparable series collected in the 1970s this figure had fallen to 32 percent, while neoplasms had risen from 20 to 33 percent. Many of these infections are relatively resistant to rapid eradication by host defenses (e.g., localized pyogenic infections or intracellular infections), which allows them to pursue a chronic or subacute course.

ABSCESSES (see Chap. 87) Abscesses are the most common form of infection presenting as FUO and are important because they can be cured with early diagnosis and treatment, while failure to make the diagnosis may eventuate fatally. These abscesses usually arise in the abdomen or pelvis including the subphrenic space, the liver or spleen, or a ruptured diverticulum or appendix. Ultrasonography, liver-spleen scan, or CT scan should provide the diagnosis in most instances. Laparotomy is usually necessary to confirm the diagnosis and to achieve cure.

MYCOBACTERIAL INFECTIONS Although less common than formerly, mycobacterial infections, such as tuberculosis (see Chap. 119) and, less commonly, atypical mycobacterial infections (see Chap. 121), cause FUO. These infections are more common among blacks, native Americans, southeast Asians, and individuals from outside the United States. In patients with the acquired immunodeficiency syndrome, disseminated infection due to Mycobacterium-avium-intracellulare (MAI) is a common preterminal event. Most of these infections are extrapulmonary and involve the bones, lymph nodes, genital or urinary organs, peritoneum, or liver. Extrapulmonary or miliary tuberculosis may not be detectable by x-ray until late in the course. Many of these patients are debilitated and have overwhelming disease. Despite this, the diagnosis, which is usually made by biopsy of lymph nodes or involved tissue, is essential because patients with Mycobacterium tuberculosis infection respond well to treatment, particularly with bactericidal drugs such as isoniazid and rifampin. In contrast, infection with MAI is often resistant to treatment.

RENAL INFECTIONS Ordinary pyelonephritis is rarely accompanied by prolonged fever; if pyrexia occurs in these patients, intrarenal or extrarenal obstruction should be considered. Ureteral obstruction by either a mass of leukocytes or renal epithelium, as in papillary necrosis, may be accompanied by prolonged fever. Prostatic abscess should be considered in males. These patients may not have dysuria or rectal pain. Occasionally, focal pyelonephritis may cause prolonged fever.

OTHER BACTERIAL INFECTIONS These include sinusitis, vertebral osteomyelitis (usually occurring in association with chronic bacteriuria, and most easily diagnosed by bone scan), infected intravenous or intraarterial catheters, and retroperitoneal infection such as aneurysms that have become filled with organizing clot and debris that have become secondarily infected. Enteric pathogens (including Escherichia coli, Bacteroides, and Salmonella) have been isolated frequently from patients with such infections. Surgery is mandatory for both diagnosis and therapy. In addition, some patients with dissecting aneurysms have fever without superimposed infections.

BACTERIAL ENDOCARDITIS Perhaps because of a high index of suspicion, the ubiquitous use of blood cultures, and the indiscriminate use of antibiotics, which must cure some patients, bacterial endocarditis has become a rare cause of FUO. Similarly, bacteremia due to Neisseria, Salmonella, and Brucella rarely causes FUO, but must be considered in the proper epidemiologic setting.

IATROGENIC INFECTIONS These include catheter infections, infected arteriovenous fistulas, and sometimes ordinary wound infections in obscure locations. Usually, their cure requires removal of a foreign body in addition to antimicrobial therapy. Infection of intravascular grafts constitutes a particularly difficult management problem which may give rise to prolonged bacteremia.

VIRAL, RICKETTSIAL, AND CHLAMYDIAL INFECTIONS These are rarely the cause of prolonged fevers, but occasionally patients with Epstein-

TABLE 9-1 Common disease entities in the United States causing prolonged fever

I Infections
  A Granulomatous infections
    1 Tuberculosis
    2 Deep-seated fungus infections
    3 Atypical mycobacterial infections
  B Pyogenic infections
    1 Upper abdominal infections
      a Cholecystitis (stone), empyema of gallbladder
      b Cholangitis
      c Liver abscess
      d Lesser sac abscess
      e Subphrenic abscess
      f Splenic abscess
    2 Lower abdominal infections
      a Diverticulitis (± abscess)
      b Appendicitis
    3 Pelvic inflammatory disease
    4 Urinary tract infections
      a Pyelonephritis (rare)
      b Intrarenal abscess
      c Perinephric abscess
      d Ureteral obstruction
      e Prostatic abscess
    5 Sinusitis
    6 Osteomyelitis
  C Intravascular infections
    1 Bacterial endocarditis (acute and subacute)
    2 Intravascular catheter infections
  D Bacteremias without overt primary focus
    1 Meningococcemia
    2 Gonococcemia
    3 Vibriosis
    4 Listeriosis
    5 Brucellosis
    6 Coliform bacteremia in patients with cirrhosis
  E Viral, rickettsial, and chlamydial infections
    1 Infectious mononucleosis
    2 Cytomegalovirus
    3 Hepatitis
    4 Group B coxsackievirus diseases
    5 Q fever (including endocarditis)
    6 Psittacosis
  F Parasitic diseases
    1 Amebiasis
    2 Malaria
    3 Trichinosis
  G Spirochetal infections
    1 Leptospirosis
    2 Relapsing fever
II Neoplasms
  A Solid (localized)
    1 Kidney
    2 Lung
    3 Pancreas
    4 Liver
    5 Large bowel
    6 Atrial myxoma
  B Metastatic
    1 From gastrointestinal tract
    2 From lung, kidneys, bone, cervix, ovary
    3 Melanoma
    4 Sarcoma
  C Tumors of the reticuloendothelial system
    1 Hodgkin's disease
    2 Non-Hodgkin's lymphoma
    3 Malignant histiocytosis
    4 Immunoblastic lymphadenopathy
    5 Lymphomatoid granulomatosis
    6 Mucocutaneous lymph node syndrome (children)
III Connective tissue disease
  A Rheumatic fever
  B Systemic lupus erythematosus
  C Rheumatoid arthritis (particularly Still's disease)
  D Giant cell arteritis (polymyalgia rheumatica)
  E Hypersensitivity vasculitis
  F Periarteritis nodosa
  G Wegener's granulomatosis
  H Panaortitis
IV Granulomatus diseases
  A Crohn's disease (regional enteritis)
  B Granulomatous hepatitis
  C Sarcoidosis
  D Erythema nodosum
V Miscellaneous
  A Drug fever
  B Pulmonary emboli
  C Thyroiditis
  D Hemolytic states
  E Cryptic trauma with bleeding into enclosed spaces (hematomas)
  F Dissecting aneurysm (with or without infection)
  G Whipple's disease
VI Metabolic and inherited diseases
  A Familial Mediterranean fever
  B Hypertriglyceridemia and hypercholesterolemia
  C Fabry's disease
VII Psychogenic fevers
  A Habitual hyperthermia
  B Factitious fever
VIII Periodic fevers (e.g., cyclic neutropenia)
IX Thermoregulatory disorders
X Undiagnosed
  A Resolved
    1 Without treatment
    2 With antibiotics
    3 With anti-inflammatory drugs
  B Recurrent
    1 Suppressed with steroids

Barr or cytomegalovirus infections may have febrile illnesses, which are often characterized by spontaneous remissions and exacerbations. Cytomegalovirus (with or without *Pneumocystis*) is becoming a progressively more common cause of prolonged fever in immunocompromised hosts. In them, it should not pose a diagnostic problem, but an infectious mononucleosis–like syndrome or postperfusion fever in otherwise healthy patients may be difficult diagnostic dilemmas. Since these patients are generally not very ill and improve spontaneously, they should not be subjected to prolonged, expensive FUO workups. *Psittacosis* may look much like typhoid fever, and *Q-fever endocarditis* has been a particularly puzzling and lethal illness that must be treated both with antibiotics and valve replacement.

PARASITIC DISEASES   Amebiasis can present as an FUO, either in the form of diffuse hepatitis or liver abscess. The diagnosis of malaria demands a history of recent exposure.

Neoplasms HODGKIN'S DISEASE   Fever may be the principal symptom and only objective finding early in the course of Hodgkin's disease, especially because patients with this disease who present with FUO may have only intraabdominal or retroperitoneal disease or involvement of the bone marrow. The diagnosis is usually made by biopsy or staging laparotomy. It is important to arrive at the diagnosis early because, with proper chemotherapy, prolonged remissions and even cure may be achieved.

LYMPHOMA-LIKE SYNDROMES   Several disease entities have been described which are clinically and histologically similar to non-Hodgkin's lymphoma but which may have a better prognosis or respond differently to steroids and antitumor agents. Among these entities, all of which may present as FUOs, are immunoblastic lymphadenopathy, lymphadenoid granulomatosis, acute megakaryocytic myelosis, and, in children, the mucocutaneous lymph node syndrome (Kawasaki's disease). These diseases are discussed more fully in Chap. 55.

NON-HODGKIN'S LYMPHOMA   These illnesses usually present with fever, nonspecific symptoms, and lymphadenopathy which the patient recognizes. Hepatosplenomegaly and bone pain and tenderness are common. The laboratory findings usually consist of anemia, leukocytosis, and atypical lymphocytosis. The diagnosis is usually made by lymph node biopsy, but biopsies can be mistaken for reactive hyperplasia or atypical lymphocytic infiltrates, at least initially. Improvements in chemotherapy have led to prolonged remissions.

MALIGNANT HISTIOCYTOSIS   This is a rare infiltrative disease secondary to malignant proliferation of cutaneous Langerhans cells. A poor prognosis presenting with fever, wasting, generalized lymphadenopathy, and hepatosplenomegaly is characteristic. The bone marrow, lung, and skin may also be involved by this rapidly progressing illness. There tends to be anemia, leukopenia, and thrombocytopenia, or a combination of the three. Biopsied tissue is often difficult to diagnose definitively but a rapidly progressive febrile illness, and the presence of large, malignant, primitive reticuloendothelial cells with histiocytic predominance and erythrophagocytosis should yield the answer.

LEUKEMIAS   It is not uncommon for acute leukemia to be mistaken for acute infection at the onset. The acute leukemias are nearly always accompanied by fever, sometimes as high as 105°F (40.6°C). The diagnosis is characteristically delayed by the absence of blast cells in the blood or bone marrow. However, the patients are usually anemic and leukopenic and often have been labeled as having preleukemia. Chronic lymphatic or granulocytic leukemia may be characterized by fever, but such fever is usually due to concomitant infection. Because of the typical changes in circulating leukocytes, fever does not often cause a diagnostic problem. Before it is assumed that fever in a patient with leukemia is due to the blood dyscrasia, infection must be ruled out by appropriate tests and cultures, and attempts to treat the "most likely" pathogen must be made.

SOLID TUMORS   An invariable feature of solid tumors causing FUO is the presence of metastatic cancer in the abdomen. These patients are usually older; the diagnosis is characteristically made by laparotomy which is directed to the proper location on the basis of history, physical examination, and noninvasive studies. The sites of the primary vary widely and include the kidney, liver, pancreas, stomach, pleura, lung, and bowel. Not surprisingly, survival is short.

ATRIAL MYXOMA   Patients with changing heart murmurs, peripheral embolic phenomena, and joint pains are usually suspected of having bacterial endocarditis, rheumatic fever, or occasionally some other connective tissue disease. In the face of persistence of these symptoms and signs without a positive diagnosis, two-dimensional echocardiography and, if the echocardiogram is positive, angiography should be performed with the possibility that an atrial myxoma may be responsible.

Connective tissue disease   RHEUMATIC FEVER   Perhaps because of the common use of immunologic diagnostic tests, connective tissue diseases now form a smaller part of FUO series. The incidence of rheumatic fever in North America and Europe has decreased dramatically. Systemic lupus erythematosus often presents with fever, but is usually diagnosed promptly.

RHEUMATOID ARTHRITIS   In its classic form, this disease is not difficult to recognize, but in certain patients who initially have FUO, arthritis is absent early in the course of the illness; these patients have primarily fever, hepatosplenomegaly, lymphadenopathy, evanescent rashes, anemia, and leukocytosis. Joint changes do not appear until late in the disease. This disease usually occurs in young adults and may be considered the adult counterpart of juvenile rheumatoid disease. The diagnosis is made usually only after prolonged observation, in part because serologic tests for rheumatoid disease are characteristically negative. The prognosis is generally good, and patients respond well to aspirin, nonsteroidal anti-inflammatory drugs, or steroids. Arthritis and a characteristic skin rash (erythema chronicum migrans) caused by infection with *Borrelia burgdorferi* (Lyme disease) may cause confusion in the diagnosis (see Chap. 278).

GIANT CELL ARTERITIS (POLYMYALGIA RHEUMATICA)   This is a disease of elderly persons, who complain of fever, headache, and pain in the muscles and joints. Overt arthritis is unusual. At times, fever is the only symptom, and there are no abnormal physical findings. The sedimentation rate tends to be very rapid, and there may be anemia, leukocytosis, or eosinophilia. Occasionally, the temporal or occipital arteries are inflamed and tender, but usually they are normal. In either instance, the diagnosis can be made by temporal artery biopsy. There may be accompanying visual defects or blindness because of involvement of the retinal artery. This disease responds extremely well to low doses of steroids, which may be used as a therapeutic trial.

OTHER CONNECTIVE TISSUE DISEASES   These include classical periarteritis nodosa, with or without hepatitis B infection, a disease that involves small and medium-sized arteries as well as the aorta and its main branches (see Chap. 269).

Granulomatous diseases   SARCOIDOSIS   Ordinarily, fever is not characteristic of sarcoidosis, but it is prominent in a minority of cases, especially those characterized by arthralgia, hilar lymphadenopathy, and cutaneous lesions resembling erythema nodosum, or in those with extensive hepatic lesions. The diagnosis is suggested by lymphoid enlargement, ocular lesions, and hyperglobulinemia and is clinched by biopsy of skin, lymph nodes, muscle, and liver. Serum angiotensin–converting enzyme activity is increased (see Chap. 270). The diagnosis may be obfuscated by the presence of erythema nodosum or other vascular rashes long before granulomas are found.

REGIONAL ENTERITIS   Inflammatory lesions of the large and small intestine rarely present as FUO, but an occasional patient who has only fever, abdominal pain, recurrent bouts of diarrhea, or subtle changes in bowel habits which may indicate low-grade obstruction will be found to have regional enteritis. Likewise, Whipple's disease may make itself known by fever, without arthritis or malabsorption.

GRANULOMATOUS HEPATITIS   This disease of unknown etiology is a relatively common cause of FUO. It is probably a manifestation of hypersensitivity, although the responsible antigens are rarely identified. Liver biopsy typically shows noncaseating granulomas. Specific diseases which can cause this reaction must be excluded and include tuberculosis, Hodgkin's disease, histoplasmosis, sarcoidosis, drug reactions, primary biliary cirrhosis, and schistosomiasis, to name only some. The fever generally subsides spontaneously over a period of weeks or months. Sometimes defervescence can be achieved with anti-inflammatory drugs or steroids, but because the diagnosis of tuberculosis cannot be ruled out completely, patients to whom steroid therapy is given should also be given antituberculous medication.

Miscellaneous causes of fever   DRUG FEVER   This is an important cause of cryptic fever; a careful history of drug intake should be taken in every patient with unexplained fever. Fever due to allergy to one of the antibiotics may become superimposed on the fever of the infection for which the drug was given, resulting in a very confused picture. Often, fever is due to common drugs, including sulfonamides, bromides, arsenicals, iodides, thiouracils, barbiturates, and laxatives, especially those containing phenolphthalein. Any questions of drug fever can be resolved rapidly by discontinuing all medications. The diagnosis can be further substantiated by giving a test dose of the drug after fever has subsided, but this may result in a very unpleasant or even dangerous reaction.

MULTIPLE PULMONARY EMBOLI   Multiple pulmonary emboli are decreasing as a cause of FUO; in fact, in one series, they were overdiagnosed. Nevertheless, symptomless thrombosis of deep calf or pelvic veins may cause prolonged febrile illness either because of the thrombophlebitis or as a result of repeated small pulmonary emboli. These emboli may not be manifested by pleuritic pain or hemoptysis, but cough, dyspnea, and vague thoracic discomfort are likely to be present. Lung scans and venography should reveal the diagnosis. Sometimes these patients present with a nephrotic syndrome due to renal vein thrombosis. Pelvic thrombophlebitis with or without pulmonary emboli is an important cause of FUO in postpartum patients.

HEMOLYTIC EPISODES   Most hemolytic diseases are characterized by bouts of fever, and acute hemolytic crises may give rise to shaking chills and marked elevations of temperature. The difficulty sometimes encountered in differentiating sickle cell disease from acute rheumatic fever is well known. The presence of these hemolytic disorders is suggested by the more rapid development of anemia than occurs in other febrile illnesses and by the usual accompaniment of reticulocytosis and jaundice. Fever is not characteristic of severe anemia due to external blood loss or of the anemia of uremia.

CRYPTIC HEMATOMAS   Accumulation of old blood in closed spaces, for instance, at sites of remote trauma, particularly in the perisplenic area, in the pericardium, or in the retroperitoneal area, particularly in patients receiving anticoagulants, has resulted in prolonged fever. The diagnosis is important because evacuation of the clot is often curative. Fever often accompanies intraluminal dissection of the aorta.

NONSPECIFIC PERICARDITIS   Occasionally, this entity escapes diagnosis and presents as an FUO.

FAMILIAL MEDITERRANEAN FEVER (see Chap. 271)   Either the disease is decreasing in incidence, or it is being recognized more readily.

THERMOREGULATORY DISORDERS   Rare patients have fever due to an abnormality in their temperature-regulating mechanism. They may be febrile without any other cause or may have exaggerated responses in temperature during the course of other fever-producing diseases. The diagnosis is made by exclusion. Some patients have responded to chlorpromazine.

Psychogenic fever   HABITUAL HYPERTHERMIA   Not infrequently, a patient, while not appearing acutely ill, has been subject to elevation of body temperature above the "normal" range level, i.e., temperatures in the range of 99.0 to 100.5°F (37.2 to 38°C). Prolonged low-grade fever may be a manifestation of serious illness, or it may be a matter of no real consequence. Possibly there are some persons whose "normal" temperatures are in this range. However, there is no certain way of identifying such individuals. The possibilities to be considered in such cases vary considerably according to the age groups concerned. A special problem termed *habitual hyperthermia* is encountered in young females. The patient may have temperatures ranging from 99.0 to 100.5°F (37.2 to 38.0°C) regularly or intermittently for years and also usually has a variety of complaints characteristic of psychoneurosis, such as fatigability, insomnia, bowel distress, vague aches, and headache. Prolonged careful study and observation fail to reveal evidence of organic disease. Unfortunately, many of these people go from physician to physician and are subjected to a variety of unpleasant, expensive, and even harmful tests, treatments, and operations. The diagnosis of this syndrome can be made with reasonable certainty after a suitable period of observation and study, and if the patient can be convinced of its validity, a real service will have been rendered.

In a patient past middle age, even low-grade fever should always be regarded as a probable indication of organic disease. The possibilities to be considered in this age group are the same as those discussed earlier under "Prolonged Febrile Illness."

FACTITIOUS FEVER   Occasionally, patients will produce purposeful false elevations in temperature. Many of these patients are young women, who are often allied health professionals. Some are schoolchildren wishing to avoid school. They fall into two groups—one infects itself with bacteria or other contaminated materials and the second finds a way to cause the thermometer to register higher than the true temperature. If malingering is suspected, all that is necessary to prove it is to repeat the temperature determination immediately after a high reading has been obtained, with someone remaining at the bedside while the thermometer is in place. Other clues to false elevations in the temperature are a dissociation between pulse and temperature, and excessively high fevers [greater than 106°F (41.1°C) in adults] and the absence of chills, sweats, or tachycardia. These patients fall into the psychiatric diagnostic category of "borderline syndrome," a state between neurosis and psychosis, in which the prognosis is guarded. Others, mostly young girls, falsify their temperatures as a means of asking for psychiatric help and do well with psychotherapy.

Patients with FUO who remain undiagnosed   These patients divide themselves into several groups. Some have a self-limited, prolonged viral infection that resembles infectious mononucleosis, cytomegalovirus, hepatitis virus, or adenovirus infection, but in which these agents are never isolated. They recover spontaneously. Others appear to have responded to antibiotics and can be presumed to have had a cryptic bacterial infection. A third group has a steroid-responsive fever which resembles, but is not diagnostic of, immunologically mediated diseases. Some of these patients eventually no longer require steroids for suppression of fever, but some do not stay free of pyrexia or other inflammatory symptoms without steroids. An occasional elderly patient looks like an example of a superannuated juvenile rheumatoid arthritis (Still's disease).

DIAGNOSTIC PROCEDURES IN FEVER OF UNKNOWN ORIGIN

With so large a number of possibilities, it is obvious that no single plan can be outlined for the systematic study of every problem in unexplained fever. In any given patient, the history, physical examination, and, most importantly, epidemiologic setting must determine the diagnostic approach. If the features suggest infectious disease, the main dependence will be upon microbiologic methods, whereas when a person in the "cancer age group" has an obscure febrile disorder, the best chance of early diagnosis may lie in x-ray studies, scans, and biopsy.

History   Careful attention to the patient's past history and the chronologic development of symptoms may provide important leads. Places of recent residence, contact with domestic or wild animals and birds, preceding acute infectious diseases such as diarrheal illness or boils, and contact with persons with tuberculosis may provide clues to infection. Localizing symptoms may provide a lead to the affected organ system. It is important to query the patient repeatedly. All too often facts of historical importance do not come to light until several interviews have been held.

Physical examination   Careful search should be made for skin lesions and for petechial hemorrhages in the ocular fundi, conjunctivas, nail beds, and skin. The lymph nodes should be carefully palpated, with special attention given to the supraclavicular, axillary, and epitrochlear areas. The finding of a heart murmur may be important, particularly if it occurs in diastole. Detection of an abdominal mass may be the first lead to the diagnosis of neoplastic disease. Palpable enlargement of the spleen suggests infection, leukemia, or lymphoma and points away from a diagnosis of solid tumors. Enlargement of the liver and spleen suggests lymphoma, leukemia, chronic infection, or cirrhosis. A large liver without a palpable spleen points to liver abscess or metastatic cancer. The rectum and the female pelvic organs may reveal masses or abscesses; the testicles may reveal tumor or tuberculosis.

Laboratory tests   Patients with FUO are subjected to a large number of laboratory tests, often repeatedly and to excess. The following may be useful guidelines in the use of these tests.

HEMATOLOGY   These tests are often abnormal, showing anemia, leukopenia, thrombocytopenia or thrombocytosis, and elevation in the sedimentation rate. They are rarely specific. Blood smears for morphology show many abnormalities but, by virtue of the type of patient who presents with FUO, are rarely diagnostic.

CHEMISTRY   Unless specific organ dysfunction is defined, these tests are rarely useful. Even serum enzymes indicating hepatic infiltrative disease such as the alkaline phosphatase or 5'-nucleotidase may be normal in the presence of liver disease.

IMMUNOLOGIC TESTS   These are most helpful in the diagnosis of fevers caused by connective tissue disorders or, occasionally, because of secondary immune complex disease or infectious endocarditis.

MICROBIOLOGY   In the initial evaluation of prolonged fever, blood cultures are indicated. However, in no instance should more than six blood cultures (which are expensive) be performed on any one patient. Smears and cultures of pus are useful but in sick patients should not delay institution of therapy. Anaerobic cultures should be performed in all abscesses. Mycobacterial cultures continue to be the mainstay in the diagnosis of acid-fast disease. Cultures and special stains or biopsies of suspected tissues are often required to diagnose disseminated fungal infections.

SEROLOGY   Serologic testing is useful in Epstein-Barr virus and occasionally cytomegalovirus infections and in amebiasis. Routine febrile agglutinins are rarely helpful, but may reveal brucellosis.

SKIN TESTS   These are rarely helpful, due to anergy or nonspecificity for acute infection. Many patients with far-advanced neoplasia are anergic. Not all patients with disseminated tuberculosis have positive tuberculin tests. Patients with disseminated histoplasmosis are usually skin test–negative.

Imaging techniques   ROENTGENOGRAMS   Chest x-rays and, when urinary tract involvement is suspected, intravenous urograms are the most valuable films in the diagnosis of FUO. Review of earlier films, including those performed at other institutions, often turns up important clues when viewed by a fresh observer. Conversely, there is nothing to be gained by repeating earlier films that are technically satisfactory, provided such films were obtained within a reasonable period of time. Sinus and bone films are also often useful. In contrast, gastrointestinal x-rays; oral, intravenous, transhepatic, or retrograde endoscopic cholangiograms; aortograms; and lymphangiograms are helpful only if there are clues that clearly indicate the likelihood of an abnormality in the organ or organ system to be imaged.

ULTRASONOGRAPHY   This technique has come into vogue to detect abdominal, renal, retroperitoneal, or pelvic mass lesions. While both false-positive and false-negative results are common, the techniques are still evolving and with further improvement will provide relatively inexpensive, noninvasive screening for masses. It is probably the method of choice for imaging the gallbladder and biliary tree.

RADIONUCLIDE SCANS   Of all nuclide scans, the technetium sulfocolloid liver-spleen scan remains the most useful. Gallium scanning, on the other hand, is subject to many false-positive and false-negative tests and has been overrated. Indium 111 leukocyte scanning may be more reliable in the diagnosis of intraabdominal abscesses. Lung scans may reveal pulmonary emboli, and simultaneous liver and lung scans are useful in delineating subphrenic abscess. Bone scans may detect osseous metastases or osteomyelitis more readily than x-rays. Renal scans are helpful in the diagnosis of hypernephroma.

COMPUTERIZED TOMOGRAPHY (CT) SCANS   CT scans are very useful in the detection of subphrenic, abdominal, and pelvic abscesses and are the most effective method for imaging the retroperitoneum, which is often the site of the cause of FUO in the form of retroperitoneal lymph nodes, tumors, abscesses, or hematomas. CT scanning is excellent for detecting space-occupying lesions in the liver, although some feel that ultrasound is more effective for visualizing the gallbladder and biliary tree.

Biopsies   Often the best means of definitive diagnosis is a biopsy.

Bone marrow biopsy may be helpful not only in clarifying the histologic nature of the marrow but also for occasional demonstration of other disease processes such as metastatic carcinoma or granulomas and for culture. Bone marrow is one location where blind sampling is productive.

Needle biopsy of the liver, while often abnormal, has a low diagnostic yield. It may be particularly helpful in granulomatous diseases. It rarely yields the diagnosis if there are no abnormalities in liver function tests.

Biopsies of other tissues that appear abnormal on physical examination or by noninvasive imaging tests are more likely to be helpful in the diagnosis than of tissues that are biopsied blindly. These include biopsies of the lung, muscle, skin, gastrointestinal mucosa, bone, and arteries. Occasionally, "blind biopsies" of muscle or temporal artery will yield abnormalities, but even here tenderness of the affected part makes finding an abnormality much more likely.

Lymph node biopsy is helpful in the diagnosis of many diseases, including the lymphomas, metastatic cancer, tuberculosis, and mycotic infections. Inguinal nodes are notoriously unsatisfactory for biopsy and are too frequently chosen because of their easy accessibility. Axillary, cervical, and supraclavicular nodes are much more likely to yield helpful information, and the node excised need not necessarily be large.

Exploratory laparotomy   Exploratory laparotomy has been advocated as the most definitive diagnostic maneuver in FUO but is valuable only when other investigations, including history, physical examination, noninvasive imaging techniques, and laboratory data point to the abdomen as a possible source of disease. Laparotomies are most helpful in patients with solid tumors or intraabdominal abscesses. The clues to intraabdominal disease are often subtle, but they are present nonetheless. Blind exploration of the abdomen simply because the diagnosis is obscure is poor practice.

Therapeutic trials   It is common practice to give a trial of antibiotics to patients with unidentified febrile disorders. Occasionally, this kind of marksmanship is effective, but in general, blind therapy does more harm than good. Undesirable features include drug toxicity, superinfection due to resistant pathogenic bacteria, and interference with accurate diagnosis by cultural methods. Furthermore, a coincidental fall in temperature not due to therapy is likely to be interpreted as response to treatment, with the conclusion that an infectious disease is present. If therapeutic trials are instituted, they should be as specific as possible. Examples are *isoniazid* and *ethambutol* or *rifampin* for tuberculosis; *aspirin* for rheumatic fever; *metronidazole* for hepatic amebiasis; *penicillin* and *gentamicin* for enterococcal endocarditis; and *chloramphenicol* for *Salmonella* bacteremia. Relatively few trials with antibiotics will be successful; those with aspirin, nonsteroidal anti-inflammatory agents, and steroids are more likely to be effective, but these drugs should be used with caution and only in patients in whom the likelihood of connective tissue disease is high and in whom granulomas, infection, and cancer have been ruled out as definitively as possible.

Prognosis in FUO   The intelligent application of appropriate diagnostic maneuvers should provide the answer in approximately 90 percent of patients with prolonged obscure febrile illness. The mortality rate in patients with FUO is high among elderly patients, particularly since cancer is the most likely cause of the fever in this age group. Fortunately, most of the remaining patients respond to medical or surgical treatment or recover spontaneously. Of those who do come to autopsy (about 10 percent), fewer than half have had potentially curable disease.

A brief philosophy about patients with FUO   Many patients are placed in the FUO category because attending physicians overlook, disregard, or reject an obvious clue. This statement implies no malice; it simply means that physicians, being human instruments, are far from perfect. No algorithms or computers are likely to reverse this trend; moreover, even the new technology is not sufficiently sophisticated to sort out the causes of fever in these patients who often present in very atypical fashion.

In order to mitigate these human errors, clinicians have to work harder. This requires repeated histories and physical examinations, frequent chart reviews to look for the "clue" that is there but has not been appreciated, extensive discussion of the problem with colleagues, and last but not least, time spent in quiet contemplation of the clinical enigma. It does not mean yet another barrage of tests, some of which might be painful and all of which are likely to be expensive, or dousing the patient with more drugs, or, in the absence of corroborating data and as a last resort, subjecting the patient to exploratory surgery. Physicians who care for patients with FUO need to observe them, to talk to them, and to think about them. There are no substitutes for these simple clinical principles.

REFERENCES

ADUAN RP et al: Factitious fever and self-induced infection. Ann Intern Med 90:230, 1979

BUJAK JS et al: Juvenile rheumatoid arthritis present in the adult as fever of unknown origin. Medicine 52:431, 1973

DINARELLO CA, WOLFF SM: *Fever. Current Concepts.* Kalamazoo, The Upjohn Company, 1980, pp 3–38

FAUCI AS et al: The spectrum of vasculitis: Clinical pathologic, immunologic and therapeutic considerations. Ann Intern Med 89:660, 1978

GHOSE MK et al: Arteritis of the aged (giant cell arteritis) and fever of unexplained origin. Am J Med 60:429, 1976

JACOBY GA, SWARTZ MN: Fever of undetermined origin. N Engl J Med 289:1407, 1973

KLATSKIN G: Hepatic granulomata: Problems in interpretation. Mt Sinai J Med 44:798, 1977

LARSON EB et al: Fever of undetermined origin: Diagnosis and follow-up of 105 cases, 1970–1980. Medicine 61:269, 1982

MALMVALL BE et al: The clinical pictures of giant cell arteritis: Temporal arteritis, polymyalgia rheumatica and fever of unknown origin. Postgrad Med 67:141, 1980

McDOUGALL IR et al: Evaluation of ^{111}In leukocyte whole body scanning. Am J Roentgenol 133:849, 1979

McNEIL BJ et al: A prospective study of computed tomography, ultrasound and gallium imaging in patients with fever. Radiology 139:647, 1981

MITCHELL DP et al: Fever of unknown origin: Assessment of the value of percutaneous liver biopsy. Arch Intern Med 137:1001, 1977

PETERSDORF RG, BEESON PB: Fever of unexplained origin: Report of 100 cases. Medicine 40:1, 1961

QUINN MJ et al: Computed tomography of the abdomen in evaluation of patients with fever of unknown origin. Radiology 136:407, 1980

SIMON HB, WOLFF SM: Granulomatous hepatitis and prolonged fever of unknown origin: A study of 13 patients. Medicine 52:1, 1973

WOLFF SM et al: Unusual etiologies of fever and their evaluation. Ann Rev Med 26:277, 1975

section 3 Alterations in nervous system function

10 APPROACH TO THE PATIENT WITH NERVOUS SYSTEM DISEASE

JOSEPH B. MARTIN

The symptoms and signs of disordered nervous system function, to be described in the following chapters, are among the most frequent and complex in clinical medicine. Because neurologic disorders may affect higher cortical function with disturbances in language, perception, and memory, as well as produce specific symptoms referable to subcortical structures, spinal cord, peripheral nerve, or muscle, the array of symptoms experienced by the patient is numerous and diverse. Such symptoms are common, not only because diseases that primarily affect various parts of the nervous system occur frequently, but also because many systemic diseases may at one time or another cause disorders of the nervous system. A careful assessment of the character and pattern of the symptoms, their temporal profile, and associated complaints, together with a focused neurologic examination, permit a conclusion to be reached among various alternatives.

These considerations are made more complicated by the difficulties that often arise in distinguishing so-called neurologic from psychiatric diseases. In general, the neurologist has defined disease of the nervous system as any condition that produces a visible anatomic or definable biochemical lesion. However, it is now recognized that many primary neurologic disorders, which present with severe clinical manifestations, fail to show any demonstrable neuropathologic or neurochemical abnormality, even when scrutinized by the most modern techniques of neurobiology. The conditions of dystonia musculorum deformans, spasmodic torticollis, tardive dyskinesia, and Gilles de la Tourette's syndrome, for example, are considered to be neurologic disorders, yet no defined structural abnormality has been reported. The possibility that such disorders are caused by abnormalities of neurotransmitter release or of receptor function is currently viewed as likely because of their partial response to various neuropharmacologic drugs. In other disorders traditionally treated by the psychiatrist, in particular the major psychoses of schizophrenia and of manic-depressive disease, accumulated evidence based on genetic analysis, responses to neuroactive agents, and documented neuroendocrine-biochemical abnormalities suggest that these, too, are primary disorders of nervous system function. This conclusion is supported further by observations that similar psychotic symptoms can be observed in patients with readily identifiable lesions of the nervous system (chronic temporal

lobe seizures, brain tumor) or after the administration of certain drugs, such as lysergic acid or amphetamines.

Despite the importance of these areas of overlap between neurology and psychiatry, most neurologic conditions for which a patient seeks general medical care are due to readily demonstrated disease processes. It is the task of the clinician to develop a neurologic method of analysis that will result in accurate diagnosis of the site of the disorder and of its likely cause. Only then can effective approaches to management and treatment be developed.

In this volume, the sections on neurology and psychiatry are considered separately because many of the approaches to diagnosis and treatment remain distinct. In this and the chapters that follow are described the approach to neurologic and psychiatric disorders and a discussion of the manifestations of neurologic diseases as they present to the neurologist or general internist. The aim in these introductory chapters is lucid description of each of the major symptoms and signs of disordered nervous system function. Currently accepted explanations in terms of anatomy, physiology, pharmacology, and chemistry are offered. Sections on specific neurologic diseases are found in Chaps. 341 to 359 and those of psychiatric disorders in Chaps. 360 to 367.

THE NEUROLOGIC METHOD OF CLINICAL EVALUATION The strategy used in evaluating a patient with neurologic illness is to begin with the question, Where is the lesion? The first clues to answering this question appear in the history, and the examination is then "tailor-made" to clarify uncertainties or to make distinctions suggested by the history. Thus, optokinetic nystagmus might be an important part of the examination in a patient with a left hemiparesis and dressing apraxia, but irrelevant to the examination of a patient complaining of burning feet. In a patient who presents with the history of ascending paresthesia and weakness, the examination must be *directed* to deciding, among other things, if the location of the lesion is the spinal cord or a peripheral nerve. Notations regarding muscle stamina or endurance might be crucial to the examination of a patient with myasthenia gravis, as opposed to the usual tests of peak muscle power. What one does with the neurologic examination depends on what the questions are; the questions are formulated by a properly taken history.

Deciding "where the lesion is" accomplishes the task of delimiting the number of possible etiologies to a manageable, finite size. In addition, this strategy safeguards against making really tragic errors. Symptoms of recurrent vertigo, diplopia, and nystagmus should not trigger "multiple sclerosis" as an answer (etiology), but "brainstem" or "pons" (location); then a diagnosis of brainstem arteriovenous malformation will not be missed because it is not considered. The combination of optic neuritis and spastic, ataxic paraparesis should not be memorized as "multiple sclerosis"; then central nervous system syphilis and vitamin B_{12} deficiency (both treatable) will not be overlooked.

Only after the clinician decides "where the lesion is," should the question "what the lesion is" be asked.

The neurologic history   A bewildering array of clinical abnormalities require documentation and interpretation during the neurologic evaluation of a patient. The analysis becomes difficult because similar symptoms and signs may present in a patient with any of several disorders. A number of general principles relevant to obtaining a complete neurologic history are important for the physician, whether a generalist or a specialist. Careful attention to the description of the symptoms as experienced by the patient and substantiated by family members or friends permits, in many instances, an accurate localization and determination of the probable cause of the complaints even before an examination of the patient has been undertaken. Two principles should be followed. First, each complaint ought to be chased down as far as possible in an effort to delineate (before the examination) where the lesion might be or, more importantly, *to formulate a set of questions to be answered by the examination.* A patient complains of weakness of the right upper limb. What are the associated features? Is this weakness for brushing the hair or opening a twist-top can? Second, in neurology—where many of the diseases are due to *anatomically restricted* lesions—*negative* associations may be crucial. A patient with a right hemiparesis without a language deficit likely has a different lesion (and likely etiology) than a patient with a right hemiparesis and aphasia. Several of the important factors that aid greatly in defining the nature of the neurologic disorder include:

1 *Temporal course of the illness.* It is particularly important to ascertain the precise rate of appearance and progression of the symptoms experienced by the patient. A paroxysmal onset of a neurologic complaint, occurring within seconds or minutes, usually indicates a cerebrovascular lesion or a seizure. Attention to the temporal march of symptoms may help define a focal seizure, a transient cerebral ischemic attack (TIA), or the onset of a migraine. For example, the onset of sensory symptoms located in one extremity that spreads over a few seconds to adjacent portions of that extremity and then to the other limb or to the face suggests a seizure. A more gradual onset involving less discrete regions of the extremities points to the possibility of a TIA. A similar, but slower progression of sensory change occurring in a young person together with other symptoms of headache, nausea, or visual disturbance suggest migraine. In general, the march of a migraine is slower than that of seizure, and a TIA tends to be more generalized in location on the side of the body or extremities. The presence of positive sensory symptoms or motor movements suggests a seizure; in contrast, transient loss of a function (negative symptom) suggests a TIA. A stuttering onset where symptoms appear, stabilize, regress, and then progress over hours or days also suggests the presence of impending vascular ischemia. In some cases, a demyelinating process may produce new symptoms over the course of a few hours. Progressing symptoms associated with the systemic manifestation of fever, stiff neck, and altered level of consciousness or awareness suggest the possibility of an infectious process. The course of the illness over years in terms of remissions and exacerbations offers additional clues to the nature of the process. Recurrent neurologic symptoms involving any level of the neuraxis with partial or complete recovery suggest the possibility of multiple sclerosis. Slowly progressive disorders without remissions tend to be characteristic of the neurodegenerative processes that affect the nervous system.

2 *Subjective descriptions of the complaint.* It is wise for the physician to recall that patient vocabularies are limited and that symptoms are interpreted within the experience of the patient. Descriptions are highly introspective and subject to the patient's degree of intelligence and general familiarity with medical terminology. The same words often mean very different things to individual patients. For example, dizziness may be a description applied by the patient to impending syncope, to a sense of giddiness, or to true vertigo. Numbness may mean a complete loss of feeling, a positive sensation of tingling, or paralysis. Blurring of vision may be used to describe unilateral visual loss, as in amaurosis fugax, or diplopia. It is important to determine the level of understanding that the patient exhibits with respect to the complaint in order to assess accurately the precise significance of the symptom.

3 *Corroboration of the history by other close associates.* It is often useful to obtain additional information from family, friends, or observers to corroborate or expand the patient's description. Memory loss, personality change, drug abuse, excess alcohol intake, and other factors may severely impair the ability of patients to describe accurately their subjective experiences or prevent them from being completely open and forthright about the factors that have contributed to the illness. Complaints of loss of consciousness which may be due to syncope or seizures necessitate seeking details from patients and family to ascertain the exact circumstances. It is often important to recognize the major manifestations of depression and anxiety which may mask or color the presentation given by the patient. Failure to note these underlying factors which interfere with the patient's performance may result in the incorrect interpretation that a variety of complaints are actually due to structural disease of the brain.

4 *Family history.* Many neurologic disorders, particularly those presenting in childhood or early adulthood, are familial or inherited conditions. It is important to ascertain the familial frequency of occurrence of systemic diseases such as hypertension, heart disease, or stroke, which may affect the nervous system. It is essential to inquire about the possibility of consanguinity of the parents or of the existence of similar symptoms in other members of the family. These may provide clues to a propensity toward a hereditary neurologic condition. It is critical to distinguish between a *negative* family history and an *incomplete* family history. It is insufficient to simply ask, Is there any similar illness in any member of your family? A negative response to such an inquiry may mean that there is, in fact, no such illness in the patient's family, but it may also mean that the patient is unfamiliar with relatives or their medical histories. It is wise to elicit specific positive or negative data about relatives as follows: Are your parents living? If so, are they well? If not, what illness did they have and how did they die? It should always be remembered that maternity is a fact, but paternity is only an assumption.

It is also important to elicit family history data regarding all illnesses rather than just neurologic and psychiatric disorders. Many familial neurologic illnesses are associated with signs and symptoms in other systems (e.g., the phakomatoses, hepatocerebral disorders, neuroophthalmic syndromes, etc.).

5 *Medical illnesses.* Many neurologic illnesses occur in the context of systemic disorders. A history of allergy and asthma may suggest the onset of polyarteritis, with mononeuritis multiplex. Previous or current medical illnesses such as diabetes mellitus, hypertension, and abnormalities of blood lipids may be relevant to evolving symptoms that affect the nervous system. Similarly, the presence of systemic diseases that have an increased association with peripheral neuropathy should be explored. Most patients with coma in a hospital setting can be shown to have a metabolic, toxic, or infectious process.

6 *The patient's perception of the disease.* It is frequently helpful to ask patients what they perceive to be wrong. Do they have a particular fear about a disease like Alzheimer's disease, a brain tumor, or multiple sclerosis? Increasingly, patients who complain of failing memory are concerned about early symptoms of Alzheimer's disease. Patients with headaches may fear that a tumor or an impending stroke is a possibility. Patients with sensory

symptoms frequently are concerned about the possibility of multiple sclerosis. Or the patient may seek attention because a relative or friend has been diagnosed with a serious neurologic illness. More often, however, patients are concerned only about the discomfort and disability caused by a chronic headache or low back pain which persists despite repeated attempts at diagnosis and treatment.

7 *Drug use and abuse and toxin exposure.* It is essential to inquire about the history of drug use, both prescribed and illicit. Complaints of yellow vision may occur with digitalis administration. Excessive vitamin administration may lead to peripheral neuropathy, as has been recently demonstrated in the case of pyridoxine. Aminoglycoside antibiotics may exacerbate symptoms of weakness in patients with disorders of neuromuscular transmission, such as myasthenia gravis. Dizziness may be secondary to ototoxicity caused by the aminoglycosides. In eliciting a history of drug use it is often necessary to be quite specific and to use lay terminology. Most patients are, for example, unaware that over-the-counter sleeping pills, cold preparations, and diet pills are actually drugs. Alcohol, the most prevalent neurotoxin, is often not recognized as such by patients. History of environmental or industrial exposure to neurotoxins may provide the essential clue; consultation with the patient's family or employer may be required.

8 *History of malignancy.* Because malignant tumors may present with nervous system metastases or occasionally with any of several paraneoplastic syndromes, it is important to determine whether any history of malignancy exists and whether chemotherapy or radiotherapy was given. Patients with prior malignancy can present with unexpected and unusual neurologic complications.

9 *Formulating an impression of the patient.* Use the opportunity while taking the history to form an impression of the patient. Is there evidence of anxiety, depression, hypochondriasis? Are there any clues to defects of language, memory, inappropriate behavior, or secondary gain? The neurologic assessment begins as soon as the patient walks into the room and the first introduction is made.

The neurologic examination   After obtaining a complete medical and neurologic history, the physician should have reliable clues to the portions of the nervous system to be examined. By the elicitation of specific signs it is then determined whether the nervous system is affected, and, if so, to what degree and which part. The anatomic localization of the lesion assumes special significance in neurology, as certain diseases are known to affect certain regions of the nervous system and not to involve others. Recognition of a constellation of symptoms and signs (a syndrome) points to the possible existence of certain diseases and to the exclusion of others. *Anatomic diagnosis in neurology is ordinarily the most important first step in the diagnostic workup.*

A systematic neurologic examination should encompass a survey of all functions from the cerebrum to peripheral nerve and muscle, i.e., from the mental status examination to the simplest reflexes. Such a detailed examination requires the performance of a series of physical tests aimed at eliciting the functional capacities of each part of the nervous system. The examiner must acquire skills that come only from the repeated use of the same techniques and instruments on a large number of normal and abnormal individuals. Errors and serious omissions are avoided if the examination procedure is orderly and systemic, beginning with mental (cerebral) functions and continuing with cranial nerves, then with motor, reflex, and sensory functions of the arms, trunk, and legs, and finishing with an analysis of posture and gait.

The mental status is already appreciated while the history is being taken. But rather profound disorders of recent memory or of spatial organization may be missed unless specifically tested for. Faults of memory, incoherence of thought, dominating ideas, peculiarities of mood and outlook, aphasic errors, problems of articulation, and loss of insight and judgment should be sought. If abnormalities are noted, a more formal analysis of these functions is undertaken along the lines suggested in Chaps. 11, 22, 23, and 24. The function of each cranial nerve is then examined in order, beginning with olfaction (see

Chaps. 13, 14, 19, and 352). Examination of the motor system should include estimates of power of each of the major muscle groups, evidence of atrophy or fasciculation, and assessment of the tone of the musculature during passive manipulations, looking for signs of spasticity, rigidity, or hypotonia (as outlined in Chap. 15). Speed and coordination of the limbs are assessed. Next, prevailing postures and the stance and gait are evaluated (Chap. 16). The tendon reflexes are examined for evidence of increased or decreased (or absent) response or of asymmetry between right and left sides or between arms and legs. The superficial cutaneous reflexes, abdominal and plantar, are then evaluated. Touch, pain, vibration, and joint-position sense are tested as the final part of the examination (see Chap. 18).

This detailed neurologic examination is undertaken only if there are symptoms of disturbed nervous system functioning. If none are present, it suffices to do an abbreviated examination which includes evaluation only of pupils, ocular movements, optic fundi, facial movements, speech, strength of arm and leg muscles, tendon and plantar reflexes, pain and vibratory sensation in hands and feet, and gait. All of this can be completed in 3 to 5 min. The findings, even in the short examination, should be recorded in the patient's record for future reference.

Two additional points about the examination are worth noting. First, in recording observations it is important for the physician to describe what is found, rather than to apply a poorly defined medical term (i.e., "patient groans to sternal rub" rather than "obtunded"). Second, if the patient's complaint is brought out by some activity, reproduce the activity in the office. If the complaint is of dizziness when raising the right arm and turning the head to the left, have the patient do it. If pain occurs after walking two blocks, have the patient demonstrate it and repeat the examination.

Experience teaches that the neurologic examination may be normal even in patients with a serious neurologic disease, such as one which causes seizures or syncope. Or the patient may arrive in a coma with no available history, and the examination proceeds along the lines described in Chap. 21. An inadequate history may to some extent be replaced by a succession of examinations from which the course of the illness may be plotted.

The formulation of the problem and establishment of an etiologic diagnosis   The clinical data obtained from the history and the examination are assembled into one of the known syndromes and are interpreted and translated in terms of neuroanatomy and neurophysiology. From the syndrome the physician should be able to determine the anatomic localization(s) that best explains the clinical findings. The anatomic localization, mode of onset and course of illness, other medical data, and laboratory findings are then integrated. Finally, the etiologic diagnosis is reached, and therapy appropriate for the disorder is proposed.

The proper selection of laboratory tests which will assist in arriving at an anatomic, but more particularly at an etiologic, diagnosis poses another set of problems for the clinician. In Chaps. 341 and 354 are described the principal tests and when they should be used. Radiologic imaging techniques, utilizing computerized tomography (CT) scanning, and magnetic resonance imaging (MRI) have had a major impact on the neurologic assessment. It cannot be overemphasized, however, that the anatomic method of physical diagnosis should proceed together with imaging studies for localization of the site of the disorder. There are commonly great discrepancies between the findings on examination and on brain imaging which are resolved only after continued careful assessment of the patient, together with further radiologic study. Assiduous attention to the clinical method in neurology remains as important today as it ever was.

In some neurologic and in most psychiatric diseases, there are no available specific laboratory tests, so one must rely primarily on the history and physical examination. The physician must reject the tendency to label as hysterical or malingering those symptoms that are not readily interpretable.

The application of the neurologic method described above offers an assured and rational approach to the majority of neurologic diseases and conditions. Some problems seen daily in a general hospital defy solution. Sometimes, one reaches an anatomic diagnosis without being able to determine etiologic diagnosis, and one must wait patiently for further developments. Because of the irreversibility of lesions that destroy neurons, a major objective of the neurologic method is diagnosis and treatment at the earliest stage of disease or, even better, the prevention of it. For the clinical investigator the diagnosis of untreatable disease is equally important, for the identification of a disease entity is the first step in its scientific study.

REFERENCES

Adams RD, Victor M: *Principles of Neurology*, 3d ed. New York, McGraw-Hill, 1985
DeJong RN: *The Neurologic Examination*. New York, Harper and Row, 1979
Swanson PD: *Symptoms and Signs in Neurology*. Philadelphia, Lippincott, 1984

11 APPROACH TO THE PATIENT WITH MENTAL AND EMOTIONAL COMPLAINTS

EDWIN H. CASSEM

Physicians see many patients with subjective complaints that are difficult to ascribe to a given clinical disorder; fatigue, tension, nervousness, listlessness, anxiety, depression, giddiness. One patient may complain that he is constantly "on edge," another that her thoughts are being broadcast through the local television station, a third that she has lost all interest in living since the birth of her last child. With other complaints the symptom itself is somatic—dizziness, shortness of breath, unsteadiness, or pain (headache, backache, cramps), but the intensity of the complaint is out of proportion to the physical findings, if any. In such patients, it is the anxiety, tears, look of despair, or a shirt soaked in the axillary area despite a cool room that catch the physician's eye. Or perhaps use of a handkerchief to open the office door, virtual absence of eye contact, a condescending manner with secretaries, or repeated demands for analgesic prescriptions may be the clue to a clinical disorder. Strictly, these behaviors are not "complaints" and when asked about them, the patient may indignantly deny them or have a ready excuse ("The secretary made me stand there for 5 minutes"; "My infant son flushed my Demerol tablets down the toilet"). Nevertheless, such behaviors are important for the examining physician to recognize since they are often relevant to the diagnosis.

Whenever somatic complaints are vague, unexplained by the physical examination or unaccompanied by signs of emotional upset, the physician can inquire about stress. "Sometimes the wear and tear of our daily lives can produce symptoms very much like yours. Have you been under much pressure lately?" is a question which may lead to a lucid account of a recent death in the family, financial loss, or job stress that began or worsened shortly before the patient's symptoms. Often the discussion of such life stresses and emotionally generated symptoms can make the patient feel better. Such interactions are taken for granted in this chapter, since careful observation and listening are basic components of the medical examination.

When are mental and emotional disturbances "abnormal"? No person escapes stress of some sort in daily life. Anxiety or despondency may be a normal response to a threat or disappointment. Few people go through life without some idiosyncrasy of manner. Psychiatry, like the rest of medicine, does not focus on the normal. Disease is the formal object of the physician's diagnostic quest. In all clinical encounters with patients complaining of or demonstrating abnormalities of thought, feeling, or behavior, the physician's primary question

is not about "mental health" (impossible to define) but whether these symptoms and signs are manifestations of a psychiatric *disorder*.

When symptoms are vague and unexplained by the physical examination, and when the patient denies any psychological cause ("I'm not depressed; I'd be fine if I could only get rid of these headaches"), discovery of a diagnosis that explains them may be difficult. Many of these complaints are caused by common and treatable psychiatric disorders like the anxiety and affective disorders which affect 8.3 and 6 percent of American adults, respectively (Robins et al, 1984). The physician, with the mistaken notion that psychiatric diagnoses are only subjective, lack defining criteria, or are diagnoses of exclusion, may fail to include these common disorders in the differential diagnosis of patient complaints. Another common difficulty arises when the patient has an obvious disorder, such as Parkinson's disease, appropriate treatment is prescribed which leads to significant improvement in the core symptoms of rigidity and bradykinesia, yet the patient continues to complain of exhaustion, insomnia and inability to concentrate. In this case, the patient suffers from both Parkinson's disease and major depression and requires treatment for both conditions. On the other hand, this same patient could have presented to the physician with the primary complaint of exhaustion and "inability to get going." This could be misconstrued as an emotional complaint, and the diagnosis of Parkinson's disease overlooked.

This chapter formulates an approach to the diagnosis of mental, emotional, and behavioral complaints and abnormalities. The classification of such symptoms, as defined in the Diagnostic and Statistical Manual of Mental Disorders (DSM III), is organized to ascertain whether the patient's complaints and findings meet diagnostic criteria for psychiatric disorders.

THE HISTORY OF THE COMPLAINT Chapter 10 discussed the approach to the patient with nervous system disease. Examination of the patient with psychiatric symptoms or signs must be equally careful and systematic. Historical information provides the foundation for the diagnostic formulation. Five factors must be included.

Onset Was the onset of problems sudden or gradual? Did the feelings of depression follow a loss, childbirth, initiation of medication, beginning of a systemic illness (stroke, infectious mononucleosis, or malignancy), stopping a medication or illicit drug (benzodiazepine or cocaine)?

Longitudinal course Is this the first such event? Onset of clinical hypomania in a 70-year-old man, for example, with no prior history of depression or mania, strongly suggests the presence of an organic disorder. Is the symptom recurrent with remissions of normal function or has it been sustained? Recurrent paranoid episodes with remissions or fully normal function make depressive illness more likely than schizophrenia. Did the patient ever consult anyone about the symptoms? Were any treatments attempted and with what success?

Family history Do these symptoms or any other psychiatric disorder appear in the patient's family? Inquiries about depression, mania, panic attacks, phobia, alcoholism, psychosis, and epilepsy should always be solicited directly. Major depression is a familial disorder. Drugs which were successfully used to treat a first-degree relative may be specifically helpful to the patient being examined, should diagnosis prove to be similar.

Premorbid functioning Quality of function will help distinguish some disorders. The chronic schizophrenic, for example, usually has a history of poor interpersonal relations and premorbid difficulty more often than the manic-depressive patient, who may report having been successful in academic, extracurricular, athletic, and interpersonal activities before entering a sustained interval of psychiatric disorder. The patient with antisocial personality disorder always has a history of a rather dramatic constellation of disruptive behaviors (e.g., truancy, theft, vandalism, lying) before the age of 15. As with other medical conditions, these elements of past and family history may not be given willingly by the patient and must be sought from family and other professionals who have treated the patient in the past. Patients with psychiatric disorders may be unable (because of psychosis, memory impairment, or sheer lack of insight) or unwilling (because of embarrassment, wish to deceive, or fear of not being taken seriously) to provide past history.

Hypochondriasis, conversion disorders, substance abuse disorders, somatization disorder and factitious disorders are conditions in which the patient's past medical record is often the most important historical clue to the diagnosis.

Current symptoms and signs   When seen by the physician, patients demonstrate what their conditions look like in cross-sectional view. Examination may reveal a person with a major depressive episode; yet a past history of a hypomanic episode or a family history of bipolar illness may suggest that lithium will be the drug of choice. Drugs and other substances can produce severe and distressing symptoms; drug and substance use is an essential component of every history.

THE PSYCHIATRIC EXAMINATION   Since mental and emotional symptoms may be the first and even the only symptoms of a medical illness, the physician must be cautious in "jumping to conclusions." A systematic psychiatric examination is the best guarantee that a correct diagnosis will be made. The assessment of patients with psychiatric disorders is described in detail in Chaps. 360 to 367.

The general inspection of the patient should include the factors listed in Table 11-1. Although not an exhaustive list, it demonstrates that the psychiatric examination cannot be limited to inferences based on "hunches" or "intuition," but must be systematic and thorough, going beyond examination of verbal productions of the patient.

Psychiatric disorders involve five spheres; cognition, emotion, behavior, perception, and memory. Just as the internist examines organ systems sequentially—heart, lungs, liver, kidneys, etc., the psychiatrist examines thought, feeling, and behavior.

Cognition   Cognition includes orientation, level of awareness, thought, attention, language, judgment, and insight into illness. Whenever defects are found in this realm which are not due to some other medical illness, the diagnosis is usually among the neurologic disorders, including the dementias or the psychoses (see Chaps. 23 and 364). Memory evaluation is of particular importance. A patient may state "I am losing my mind," focusing specifically on an inability to remember names and details. Examination of memory may indicate that concentration and attention are primarily disordered, such that the patient performs accurately only when stimulated or even provoked. The misnomer "*pseudodementia* of depression" is often given to such a condition. Although it can be difficult at times to sort out the cognitive defects in depressed patients, major depression alone does not directly impair memory. Difficulty concentrating, along with the other diagnostic criteria for major depression, point to a diagnosis of depression. With treatment of the depression and restoration of the ability to concentrate (as well as the capacity to take interest in the topic), the "memory" defect disappears. If, on the other hand, a patient with such a complaint reveals a history of insidious, increasing difficulty with simple monetary transactions, following directions, and interpersonal relations, and examination shows some trouble naming, memory impairment, mild apraxia, and difficulty with abstraction, dementia is then highly likely. Depression and dementia can, of course, coexist. In such a case, when the depression is treated, the patient's mental functioning is noticeably improved—but any improvement in memory will be due to improvement in concentration, attentiveness, and motivation, not to improvement in recent recall, which is permanently impaired in dementia.

Emotion   Feelings can be reduced to four basic states, each with its variation of intensity: depression (sadness, grief), elation (joy, mania), anxiety (fear, panic), and anger (irritation, rage). Some persons quite accurately perceive their feelings, others seem completely out of touch with them. Facial expression, raised voice, grimacing, gritted

TABLE 11-1   General inspection of the patient

Appearance
   Dress (jewelry, colors)
   Skin (tattoos, hirsutism)
   Posture
   Grooming
Body build
   Thin (anorexic)
   Obese
Eye contact
Speech
   Quantity
   Quality (loud, articulate, fluent)
   Content (logic, ability to name)
Motor activity
   Quantity (over- or underactive)
   Quality (tic-ridden, clumsy, choreoid)
Consciousness
   Alert
   Not alert: clouded, stuporous
Mood
General cognition
Cooperativeness

teeth, a clenched fist, darting eyes, sweating, tears, and many other clues indicate not only the presence of emotion but often the general category to which it belongs. When patients put their feet on the physician's desk or repeatedly drop ashes on the carpet, they are most likely hostile—even though their response to inquiry about feelings of anger may include fervent protestations that they were unaware these behaviors might adversely affect the physician. A patient can weep profusely when mentioning the death of a spouse or parent yet deny depression. "That's all in the past" shows only the discrepancy between the subjective evaluation and the objective behavior displayed. Psychiatric disorders with disturbed emotions are commonly the affective and the anxiety disorders (Chaps. 360 and 361).

Behavior   Behavioral disturbances may be either motor or interpersonal in form. Automatisms, stereotypy, and compulsions are gross examples which usually appear in the history or examination. Examination of interpersonal behavior should include the patient's family, work, and play histories, as well as past interactions with physicians. Disorders of thought and emotion regularly interfere with these dimensions of a person's life, at least temporarily. With psychosis or severe depression patients commonly lose ability to function effectively in any of these areas. When the physician can find no disorder of thought or emotion, it is the behavioral history which may provide the clue. The patient may present such a problem as a chief complaint, like premature ejaculation. This is classified as a sexual dysfunction and can occur without any other psychiatric disorder. At other times the patient either cannot or will not specify the behavioral problem. The personality disorders may have their only manifestations in the behavioral realm. For example, after an illness the dependent personality may continue to complain of symptoms because the illness brought so much caring attention. The patient is not depressed and may appear anxious but fits no psychiatric diagnosis of anxiety disorder. Examination may show that symptoms worsen only when the spouse returns home. The patient with hypochondriasis may have a thick medical chart which documents visits to a dozen prior physicians for a variety of symptoms, but always with the fear that there is an underlying malignancy. The examinations reveal no structural pathology, so the patient seeks another opinion, genuinely convinced that cancer is present.

Perception   Disorders of perception include hallucinatory or illusory abnormalities, which can involve any of the primary sensory modalities, alone or in combination. Hearing accusatory voices when no one is present is common in psychotic depression, while hearing one's thoughts broadcast to all the other shoppers in the supermarket is more characteristic of schizophrenia. Visual hallucinations should alert the physician to the likelihood of an organic illness: temporal lobe epilepsy, alcohol withdrawal, or digitalis intoxication are examples of conditions associated with these phenomena.

Memory   Memory is the process by which information is stored by the brain for later recall. For clinical purposes it is divided into present and past memory. There is an important interaction with attention and concentration which must be considered when memory is tested. Present memory is tested by asking the patient to recall a list of items or a story. Inability to do so is commonly associated with dementia, chronic alcohol abuse, and drug abuse. Disorders of past memory are sometimes also referred to as *amnesia*. Past memory is impaired in progressive dementia, but when a patient with a normal memory complains of an amnesic episode, the cause may be either organic, as with transient global amnesia, or functional, as with a hysterical fugue episode. Such a patient typically may have disappeared, assumed a new identity, and been unable to recall the past. Psychogenic amnesia occurs when a patient has no apparent ability to recall a traumatic event, such as a sexual molestation by a parent in childhood. A patient may also lie about inability to recall a past event, which is called *malingering*. Memory can also be distorted by a number of abnormal processes. Sometimes false details may be added to a true event, as a "fish story" grows with time. Commonly seen in patients with organic brain disease is *confabulation,* in which the patient attempts to fill in memory defects by telling a plausible but false story in answer to specific questions. *Déjà vu* distorts a present new situation so that it seems to the subject to be the exact repetition of an event that occurred in the past.

FORMULATION OF THE PROBLEM   Proceeding in a manner similar to that for any nonpsychiatric symptom, the physician considers the past, present, and family history, the past medical history, the current medications, and the current examination with relevant laboratory tests, and makes a differential diagnosis. The differential diagnosis for psychiatric symptoms has two basic steps: exclusion of organic disease and psychiatric differential diagnosis. Every physician is encouraged to approach psychiatric presentations in this manner.

Exclusion of organic disease   Even when the symptoms suggest a psychiatric origin, the physician begins the differential diagnostic process by giving thought to those medical illnesses that might give rise to the constellation of symptoms and signs elicited during the patient examination. The more vague and diffuse the symptoms, the harder it is to be confident that an underlying systemic illness is not the culprit. One need only consider how dramatically disordered thought, feeling, and behavior can be in cases of severe hypoglycemia, hypertensive encephalopathy, Wernicke's encephalopathy, acute hypoxia, subarachnoid hemorrhage, meningitis, or a drug overdose. Many a hypoglycemic diabetic has been initially mistaken for a drunk because of clouded consciousness, slurred speech, and abusive behavior. The fear of the physician is that carelessness or trusting too much in clinical "intuition" might cause a premature dismissal of the symptoms without that sort of careful, systematic diagnostic thinking that insists on further history, vital signs, and laboratory tests to confirm or reject critical hypotheses. This entire textbook is devoted to equipping the physician with more comprehensive knowledge of diseases. The reminder here, however, is that systemic medical illnesses have *psychiatric* symptomatology in many cases. Syphilis has been called "the great imitator" because its manifestations are protean. When a patient with neurosyphilis presents with a manic psychosis, only the physician who includes this diagnosis in a systematic differential diagnosis will never miss it.

Psychiatric-like symptoms can be categorized as depressive, anxious, psychotic, confusional, and euphoric/irritable. The same set of symptoms can be caused by two or more diseases. Just because the patient fully meets the diagnostic criteria for major depression is no guarantee that the cause is not a prescribed drug or a disease like myxedema.

Symptoms of depression   Complaints of fatigue, weakness, insomnia, and poor concentration can be caused by many exogenous substances and endogenous diseases. Alcohol, antihypertensive medications—reserpine, alphamethyldopa, and beta-adrenergic blocking agents—and corticosteroids, are frequently implicated in causing depression. Cimetidine, more often a cause of confusion, can produce a strikingly "pure" clinical picture of depression. Use of cocaine, barbiturates, and amphetamines are often associated with a depressive syndrome. Hypothyroidism, hyperparathyroidism, Cushing's and Addison's diseases, and subcortical dementias like Huntington's and Parkinson's diseases are often *heralded* by depression. Anemia, hypo- and hyperglycemia, hyponatremia, hypercalcemia, hypokalemia, encephalitis, and an occult malignancy regularly produce symptoms of weakness and fatigue that can mistakenly be ascribed to depression. An apathetic state, mistakenly labeled by family or nursing staff as depression, can be due to frontal lobe disease or a right hemisphere stroke.

Symptoms of anxiety   Few symptoms are more challenging to the diagnostician than anxiety. The feeling state itself, in its "pure" mental denotation, is often defined by somatic symptoms: "butterflies" or a knot in the stomach, sweating, tremulousness, palpitations, flushing, breathlessness, numbness, muscular tension, pallor, dry mouth, urinary frequency. The normal diet contains caffeine and monosodium glutamate, each capable of inducing acute and, in the case of caffeine, chronic anxiety. Withdrawal from alcohol, barbiturates, meprobamate, and benzodiazepines can produce dramatic anxiety, occasionally progressing to a life-threatening medical emergency. Diseases that cause the physical symptoms of anxiety commonly frighten the patient, who may be unaware of the underlying disease. Any event or disorder causing episodic tachycardia or adrenergic arousal, such as hyperthyroidism, paroxysmal atrial tachycardia, mitral valve prolapse, pheochromocytoma, insulinoma, myocardial infarction, or hypoglycemia can produce symptoms of anxiety. Ingestion of excess thyroid medication, sympathomimetic amines, and bronchodilators like theophylline can produce tachycardia and, with it, anxiety. Pulmonary diseases causing breathlessness regularly make the patient anxious: asthma, obstructive pulmonary disease, pneumothorax, pulmonary embolism. Pulmonary edema and congestive heart failure do the same. These conditions are not often mistaken for an emotional disorder unless they are subtle—as occult, intermittent showers of pulmonary emboli may be.

Fear is the commonest emotion produced by a complex partial seizure. Carcinoid tumor, the commonest endocrine neoplasm of the digestive tract, is of special interest because its clinical episodes of flushing and tachycardia may be triggered by intense emotion. In such a case a patient may relate that anger caused the feeling of being "on fire." Patients who receive neuroleptic medications occasionally develop *akathisia,* a side effect characterized by extreme restlessness, inability to remain seated (which gives the condition its name), and a state hard to distinguish from anxious agitation. Failure to recognize this side effect may cause the physician to increase the dose of the neuroleptic, which only worsens the akathisia. Paradoxically, even though depression and anxiety are classified as two separate categories of psychiatric disorder, anxiety is one of the most common and most severe features of major depression. Unless the physician includes depression in the differential diagnosis of the symptoms of anxiety the diagnosis will be missed.

Psychosis with a clear sensorium   Psychosis generally refers to a state in which cognition is disorderd by delusions, hallucinations, or both. Schizophrenia, perhaps because it is such a dramatically disabling disorder, retains a premier position as the "hallmark" of psychotic disorders, but it is far from being their commonest cause. The more bizarre delusions are patently absurd, such as those of being controlled, of thought broadcasting, or of thought insertion. These are commonly, but by no means always, associated with schizophrenia. Manic psychosis often presents with similar bizarre delusions. Somatic delusions (that one's body is rotting or giving off a foul odor), grandiose delusions (that one has discovered the secret to world peace), paranoid delusions, and hallucinations of any kind (auditory, visual, olfactory, tactile) require a systematic differential diagnosis. All of these symptoms are commonly found in confusional states, but even when the patient is alert and fully oriented, they may be due to medical illness or exogenous agents. Amphetamine and cocaine abuse tend to produce paranoid states. L-Dopa, administered to patients with Parkinson's disease, may produce paranoid, manic, or confusional states. Lysergic acid (LSD), mescaline, phencyclidine (PCP), and other psychotomimetic agents may produce isolated hallucinations or delusions or both; PCP is particularly associated with severe confusional states marked by agitation and violence. Characteristic organic delusions are described with neurologic disorders, such as denial of blindness after bilateral occipital lobe lesions (Anton's syndrome) or the denial of hemiparesis after a parietal lobe injury. This latter lesion may be associated with the delusion that the involved side of the body has multiple limbs. Another neurologic "delusion," *reduplicative paramnesia,* is a state in which the patient is convinced that he or she is simultaneously in two different places. Such patients may be mentally clear in all other aspects. Ideas of reference, e.g., a sudden intense belief that the television news commentator is referring to oneself, may be the result of a complex partial seizure. Psychosis indistinguishable from functional psychosis can also occur with complex partial seizures.

Delusions with paranoid and depressive content are most commonly associated with depressive disorder. Other delusions, such as those occurring in elderly perons who believe they are infested by parasites and in younger persons who believe that their noses (males) or breasts (females) are too large, are classified as monosymptomatic hypochondriacal psychosis. The younger persons are exceedingly difficult to help, but the older patients with delusions of parasitosis often respond to the dopamine antagonist pimozide. Diffuse brain disease of structural (such as Alzheimer's disease) or toxic/metabolic etiology may be associated with psychotic manifestations, and it may be the psychotic manifestation that first leads to a consultation with the physician.

Hallucinations are often associated with organic conditions. Visual hallucinations ought to be considered as due to an organic etiology until proven otherwise. Alcoholic hallucinosis, as distinguished from delirium tremens, is unique in usually being *auditory,* with a paranoid theme (accusatory voices). The sensorium is clear, there is often no tremor, and it occurs during drinking, not withdrawal (see Chap. 365). It usually occurs after many years of drinking. Withdrawal from addicting substances, especially alcohol, can produce formed visual hallucinations. Formed visual hallucinations have also been reported with digoxin and pentazocine, viral encephalitis, Creutzfeldt-Jakob disease, and sensory deprivation. Macropsia, micropsia (the illusion of objects expanding or shrinking in size), formed visual hallucinations, olfactory hallucinations, déjà vu or jamais vu, and amnesic episodes are symptoms common to focal epilepsy of the temporal lobe or subcortical limbic structures.

Confusion and delirium Confusional states are defined as global dysfunctional states characterized by abnormal orientation, attention, arousal, thought, and memory (see Chap. 23). The findings may be subtle, as when a patient labeled as depressed by the family turns out on examination to have Alzheimer's disease, or dramatic, like delirium tremens. When the state is acute in onset, a toxic state is more likely to prove to be the cause. Whenever mental functions are globally impaired, medications must be considered as potential causes, due either to toxic side effects or abrupt withdrawal. Abrupt cessation of alcohol, barbiturates, meprobamate, benzodiazepines, other sedative hypnotics, and opiates regularly produce an adrenergic, hyperarousal state with symptoms of tremor, tachycardia, mydriasis, sweating, insomnia, and agitation progressing to delirium. Withdrawal of barbiturate anticonvulsants in children can cause similar acute symptoms. In the adult, abrupt withdrawal of tricyclic antidepressants can produce acute symptoms of insomnia, nightmares, gastrointestinal symptoms, and movement disorder with bradykinesia and rigidity. These symptoms are thought to be caused by "cholinergic overdrive," which results when these highly anticholinergic substances are stopped. For the same reason, sudden withdrawal of the anticholinergic neuroleptic thioridazine may cause the same symptoms. Rebound mania may occur after abrupt withdrawal of an antidepressant in

manic-depressive patients. In its most severe form it can be difficult to distinguish from delirium. Rebound mania has also been observed following sudden cessation of phenelzine, a monoamine oxidase inhibitor devoid of anticholinergic activity.

More often, confusion is caused directly by a medication prescribed for the patient. Common culprits include anticholinergic drugs (atropine, scopolamine, tricyclic antidepressants) anti-parkinsonian drugs, barbiturates, long-acting benzodiazepines, and bromides. Lithium, essential for treatment of mania or depression, in excessive doses can cause confusion. Almost every drug has been reported on occasion to cause confusion; narcotics, antiarrhythmic agents, antibiotics, digoxin and other digitalis preparations, cimetidine, beta-adrenergic blocking agents, alphamethyldopa, metrizamide, prostaglandin synthetase inhibitors, theophylline, L-dopa, bromocriptine, and clonidine have all been frequent offenders. Antineoplastic agents such as procarbazine, methotrexate, cytosine arabinoside, and occasionally vincristine and vinblastine may cause confusion or delirium. Cyclosporine, so important in protecting transplanted organs from rejection, has also produced confusion in rare cases.

Drugs of abuse, including PCP and other hallucinogens, cocaine, and amphetamines, and combinations of many drugs with alcohol must be considered when a delirious patient is brought to the emergency ward.

Delirious and confusional states are common manifestations of neurologic disorders (see Chap. 23). Trauma, cerebral hypoxia, brain tumor, complex partial status epilepticus, viral encephalitis or meningitis, and Creutzfeldt-Jakob disease may cause an acute confusional state. Acute confusional states occur commonly in demented patients hospitalized for medical illnesses.

Systemic disorders may cause similar adverse results on general mentation; hypercarbia, hypoxemia, renal failure, liver failure, and electrolyte imbalances may present first with alterations in cognition (see Chap. 349). Deficiencies of thiamine, B_{12}, folate, and niacin can produce confusional states. Endocrine disorders, hyper- and hypothyroidism, hyper- and hypoparathyroidism, Cushing's and Addison's diseases, panhypopituitarism, the disorders of glucose metabolism, systemic lupus erythematosus, and hypertensive encephalopathy can cause confusion.

Surgical procedures quite remote from the CNS can produce a setting for unexpected encephalopathy. Most common is the delirium that begins on the third or fourth day after cardiac surgery, which may last several days. No specific cause may be identified. Morbidly obese patients treated with jejunoileostomy have been reported to experience confusional states after ingesting a high carbohydrate diet, thought to be associated with elevated concentration of D-lactate in blood.

Euphoria/irritability Patients who appear "hyper"—expansive, elated, hypertalkative, egotistical, distractable, and boundlessly energetic with a decreased need for sleep—may be manifesting a lifelong personality style or be either manic or hypomanic; or they may be medically ill. If ill, the cause is either drug ingestion or brain disease. The drugs most commonly associated with manic-like symptoms are corticosteroids and ACTH, stimulants like cocaine, amphetamines, sympathomimetics, and excessive thyroid replacement substances, antidepressants and anti-parkinsonian agents.

Rarely brain tumor, ACTH-producing tumors, viral encephalitis, temporal lobe seizures, neurosyphilis, multiple sclerosis, Huntington's disease, uremia, hyperthyroidism, B_{12} deficiency, carcinoid syndrome, and dialysis dementia syndrome can cause mania. Whenever manic symptoms appear in a patient over 50 years of age who has no prior history of either mania or depression, the abnormal state is almost always "secondary" to one of the conditions listed above and not a "primary" psychiatric disorder.

Psychiatric differential diagnosis The general physician, cannot be expected to become an expert in psychiatric disorders. Some disorders, however, are so common that general physicians not only see them frequently but see more of their total number than do psychiatrists. This is most often the case, for example, with major depression. Estimates suggest that up to 60 percent of depressed patients are seen by general physicians and internists and 20 percent by psychiatrists or other mental health professionals, while 20 percent consult no professional for help with their disorder. The general physician who includes depression in the differential diagnosis is in an excellent position to recognize this disorder when it appears and to treat it appropriately.

What does this mean in practical terms? Two psychiatric disorders, major depression and panic disorder serve as examples (Chaps. 360 and 361). For purposes of brevity, we can say that to make the diagnosis of depression the physician needs to find that the patient has at least four of eight symptoms, and for the diagnosis of panic disorder four of twelve (different) symptoms. Since these are common disorders in the general population, these two symptom constellations should be known and readily available for the process of differential diagnosis. Were this the case, differential diagnosis could proceed as follows: When a patient complained of severe anxiety, restlessness, and inability to concentrate, the history, physical, and laboratory exams could be conducted to exclude any likely medical illness. At any time during this process, the physician, noting that the patient already had two (psychomotor agitation and poor concentration) of the eight symptoms of a major depressive episode, would inquire about the other six (sleep or appetite disturbance, blunted interests, decreased energy, guilt, and recurrent thoughts of death or suicide). Should the patient have four or more of these symptoms, qualifying for the diagnosis, major depression might from the outset seem the most likely diagnosis. Even so, a careful approach would mandate the quick but systematic review of illnesses capable of causing a similar symptom constellation. If confident that the patient had no such occult medical illness, the physician could treat the patient's depression.

What if this process has been carefully completed, and there remains neither medical nor psychiatric diagnosis? The term *neurotic*, or *psychoneurotic*, while descriptive of certain conflicts that patients may have, is no longer a psychiatric diagnosis. Certain other terms, like *neurasthenia, psychasthenia, neurocirculatory asthenia*, and *soldier's heart* have also been eliminated from lists of psychiatric diagnoses because more precise diagnostic categories have replaced them. Because medicine's basic activities are diagnosis and treatment, attempts to specify thought, feeling, or behavior as abnormal are valuable as long as there is an effort to make a diagnosis. Then the physician can prescribe treatment and alleviate the distress that caused the patient to seek medical help.

REFERENCES

AMERICAN PSYCHIATRIC ASSOCIATION: Diagnostic and Statistic Manual of Mental Disorders (DSM III), 3d ed, Washington, 1980

CUMMINGS JL: Organic delusions: Phenomenology, anatomical correlations, and review. Br J Psychiatr 146:184, 1985

GREDEN JF: Laboratory tests in psychiatry, in HI Kaplan, BJ Sadock (eds), *Comprehensive Textbook of Psychiatry IV*. Baltimore, Williams & Wilkins, 1985, vol II, pp 2028–2033

KAPLAN HI, SADOCK BJ: Typical signs and symptoms of psychiatric illness, HI Kaplan, BJ Sadock (eds), *Comprehensive Textbook of Psychiatry IV*. Baltimore, Williams & Wilkins, 1985, vol I, pp 499–501

LUDWIG AM: *Principles of Clinical Psychiatry*. New York, Free Press, 1980

ROBINS LN et al: Lifetime prevalence of specific psychiatric disorders in three sites. Arch Gen Psychiatry 41:949, 1984

12   FAINTNESS, SYNCOPE, AND SEIZURES

RAYMOND D. ADAMS / JOSEPH B. MARTIN

Episodic faintness, light-headedness or giddiness, and reduced alertness are frequently difficult to distinguish, tending to shade into one another. The difference between faintness and frank syncope is often only quantitative. Types of episodic weakness, such as myasthenia gravis, cataplexy, and familial periodic paralysis, which cause striking reduction of muscular strength but no impairment of consciousness, should be set apart (see Chaps. 358 and 359). Seizures, an important cause of altered consciousness, usually differ from syncope, but in some instances their distinction may be difficult. The features that distinguish seizures from syncope are discussed at the end of this chapter and in Chap. 342.

SYNCOPE AND FAINTNESS

Syncope comprises a generalized weakness of muscles, with loss of postural tone, inability to stand upright, and a loss of consciousness. The term *faintness*, in contrast, refers to lack of strength, with sensation of impending loss of consciousness. At the beginning of a syncopal attack the patient is nearly always in the upright position, either sitting or standing [the Stokes-Adams attack (see Chap. 183) is exceptional in this respect]. Usually the patient is warned of the impending faint by a sense of "feeling bad." A sense of giddiness and movement or swaying of the floor or surrounding objects ensues. The senses become confused; the patient yawns or gapes, there are spots before the eyes, vision may dim, and the ears may ring. Nausea and sometimes vomiting accompany these symptoms. There is a striking pallor or ashen gray color of the face, and very often the face and body are bathed in cold perspiration. The deliberate onset may often allow the patient time for protection against injury; a hurtful fall is exceptional. If the patient can lie down promptly, the attack may be averted without complete loss of consciousness.

The depth and duration of unconsciousness vary. Sometimes the patient is not completely oblivious of the surroundings, or there may be profound coma with complete lack of awareness and of capacity to respond. The patient may remain in this state for seconds to minutes or even as long as half an hour. Usually the patient lies motionless with skeletal muscles relaxed, but a few clonic jerks of the limbs and face may occur shortly after the beginning of the unconsciousness. Sphincter control is usually maintained. The pulse is feeble or cannot be felt; the blood pressure may be low and breathing may be almost imperceptible. Once the patient is in a horizontal position, perhaps from having fallen, gravitation no longer hinders the flow of blood to the brain. The strength of the pulse then improves, color begins to return to the face, breathing becomes quicker and deeper, and consciousness is regained. There is from this moment onward a correct perception of the environment. The patient is, nevertheless, keenly aware of physical weakness, and rising too soon may precipitate another faint. Headache and drowsiness, which, with mental confusion, are the usual sequelae of a convulsion, do not follow a syncopal attack.

ETIOLOGY   The list of causes in Table 12-1 is based on established or assumed physiologic mechanisms. The commoner types of faint are reducible to a few simple mechanisms. Syncope results from a sudden impairment of brain metabolism usually brought about by hypotension with reduction of cerebral blood flow.

Nature has provided humans with several mechanisms by which circulation adjusts to the upright posture. Approximately three-fourths of the systemic blood volume is contained in the venous bed, and any interference with venous return may lead to a reduction in cardiac output. Cerebral blood flow may still be maintained, as long as systemic arterial vasoconstriction occurs; but when this adjustment fails, serious hypotension with resultant cerebral underperfusion to less than half of normal results in syncope. Normally, the pooling of blood in the lower parts of the body is prevented by (1) pressor reflexes which induce constriction of peripheral arterioles and venules, (2) reflex acceleration of the heart by means of aortic and carotid reflexes, and (3) improvement of venous return to the heart by activity of the muscles of the limbs. Placing a normal person on a tilt table to relax the muscles and tilting upright slightly diminishes cardiac output, and allows the blood to accumulate in the legs to a slight degree. This may then be followed by a slight transitory fall in systolic arterial pressure and, in patients with defective vasomotor reflexes, may be a means of producing faints.

TYPES OF SYNCOPE   Vasovagal (vasodepressor) syncope   This syncope is the common faint that may be experienced by normal persons; it is frequently recurrent and tends to take place during emotional stress (especially in a warm, crowded room), after an injurious, shocking accident, and during pain. Mild blood loss, poor physical condition, prolonged bed rest, anemia, fever, organic heart disease, and fasting are other factors which increase the possibility of fainting in susceptible individuals. A short premonitory phase is characterized by nausea, perspiration, yawning, epigastric distress, hyperpnea, tachypnea, weakness, confusion, tachycardia, and pupillary dilatation. Physiologically, there is first a marked fall in arterial pressure and systemic vascular resistance which is most notable in the skeletal muscular beds. Cardiac output may be within normal limits but fails to exhibit the expected increase which normally occurs with hypotension. Output declines when vagal activity leads to marked bradycardia, replacing tachycardia, resulting in further lowering of arterial pressure and reduction of cerebral perfusion. Assumption of the supine posture with elevation of the legs and removal of the offending stimulus will rapidly restore consciousness.

Postural hypotension with syncope   This type of syncope affects persons who have a chronic defect in, or variable instability of, vasomotor reflexes. The fall in blood pressure on assumption of upright posture is due to a loss of vasoconstriction reflexes in resistance and capacitance vessels of the lower extremities. Though the character of the syncopal attack differs little from that of the vasovagal or vasodepressor type, the effect of posture is its cardinal feature; sudden arising from a recumbent position or standing still are the circumstances under which it is most likely to happen.

Postural syncope tends to occur under the following conditions:

1 In otherwise normal persons who for some unknown reason have defective postural reflexes (this may be familial). In such individuals fainting may occur when tilted on a table. Under such circumstances it has been found that at first the blood pressure diminishes slightly and then stabilizes at a lower level. Shortly thereafter, the compensatory reflexes suddenly fail and the arterial pressure falls precipitously.

2 In *primary autonomic insufficiency* and in the *dysautonomias*. At least three syndromes have been delineated.

a Acute or subacute dysautonomia. In this disease an otherwise healthy adult or child is afflicted over a period of a few days or weeks with a partial or complete paralysis of the parasympathetic and sympathetic nervous systems. Pupillary reflexes are lost, as are lacrimation, salivation, and sweating, and there is impotence, paresis of bladder and bowel musculature, and orthostatic hypotension. The CSF protein is increased. Sensory and motor nerve fibers are demonstrably intact, but nonmedullated autonomic ones have degenerated. Recovery occurs within a few months, possibly hastened by prednisone therapy. The disease is believed to represent a variant of acute idiopathic polyneuritis, akin to Landry-Guillain-Barré syndrome.

b Chronic postganglionic autonomic insufficiency. This is a disease of middle-aged and elderly individuals who gradually develop chronic orthostatic hypotension, sometimes in conjunction with impotence and sphincter disturbances. Upon standing for 5 to 10 min, the blood pressure decreases at least 35 mmHg and the pulse pressure narrows, both without increase in pulse rate, pallor, or nausea. Men are more often affected than women. The condition is relatively benign and seemingly irreversible.

c Chronic preganglionic autonomic insufficiency. In this condition orthostatic hypotension with variable anhidrosis, impotence, and sphincter disturbances is combined with any one of three or more disorders of the central nervous system. These include (1) tremor, extrapyramidal rigidity, and akinesia (Shy-Drager syndrome); (2)

progressive cerebellar degeneration, some instances of which are familial; and (3) a more variable extrapyramidal and cerebellar disorder (striatonigral degeneration). These syndromes lead to disability and often death within a few years. (See Chap. 350.)

The differentiation of the chronic peripheral postganglionic and central preganglionic insufficiency is based on pathologic and pharmacologic evidence. In the postganglionic type, neurons of the sympathetic ganglia degenerate, whereas in the central type, the lateral horn cells of the thoracic spinal cord degenerate. In the postganglionic peripheral type, the resting levels of norepinephrine are subnormal because of failure to release norepinephrine from postganglionic endings, and there is hypersensitivity to injected norepinephrine. In the central type, resting levels of norepinephrine are normal. On standing, unlike the reaction in the normal individual, there is little if any rise in norepinephrine levels in either type. And in both types, the levels of plasma dopamine β-hydroxylase (the enzyme that converts dopamine to norepinephrine) are subnormal.

The distinction between the various types of orthostatic hypotension has therapeutic significance. In the peripheral postgan-

TABLE 12-1   Causes of recurrent weakness, faintness, and disturbances of consciousness

I Circulatory (reduced cerebral blood flow)
  A Inadequate vasoconstrictor mechanisms
    1 Vasovagal (vasodepressor)
    2 Postural hypotension
    3 Primary autonomic insufficiency
    4 Sympathectomy (pharmacologic due to antihypertensive medications such as alphamethyldopa and hydralazine, or surgical)
    5 Diseases of central and peripheral nervous systems, including autonomic nerves (Chap. 355)
    6 Carotid sinus syncope (see also "Bradyarrhythmias," below)
    7 Hyperbradykininemia
  B Hypovolemia
    1 Blood loss—gastrointestinal hemorrhage
    2 Addison's disease
  C Mechanical reduction of venous return
    1 Valsalva maneuver
    2 Cough
    3 Micturition
    4 Atrial myxoma, ball valve thrombus
  D Reduced cardiac output
    1 Obstruction to left ventricular outflow: aortic stenosis, hypertrophic subaortic stenosis
    2 Obstruction to pulmonary flow: pulmonic stenosis, primary pulmonary hypertension, pulmonary embolism
    3 Myocardial: massive myocardial infarction with pump failure
    4 Pericardial: cardiac tamponade
  E Arrhythmias (Chaps. 183 and 184)
    1 Bradyarrhythmias
      a Atrioventricular (AV) block (second- and third-degree), with Stokes-Adams attacks
      b Ventricular asystole
      c Sinus bradycardia, sinoatrial block, sinus arrest, sick-sinus syndrome
      d Carotid sinus syncope (see also inadequate vasoconstrictor mechanisms, above)
      e Glossopharyngeal neuralgia (and other painful states)
    2 Tachyarrhythmias
      a Episodic ventricular fibrillation with or without associated bradyarrhythmias
      b Ventricular tachycardia
      c Supraventricular tachycardia without AV block
II Other causes of weakness and episodic disturbances of consciousness
  A Altered state of blood to the brain
    1 Hypoxia
    2 Anemia
    3 Diminished carbon dioxide due to hyperventilation (faintness common, syncope seldom occurs)
    4 Hypoglycemia (episodic weakness common, faintness occasional, syncope rare)
  B Cerebral
    1 Cerebrovascular disturbances (cerebral ischemic attacks, see Chap. 343)
      a Extracranial vascular insufficiency (vertebral-basilar, carotid)
      b Diffuse spasm of cerebral arterioles (hypertensive encephalopathy)
    2 Emotional disturbances, anxiety attacks, and hysterical seizures (see Chap. 11)

glionic type, the most effective treatment is 9α-fluorohydrocortisone (oral dose 0.1 to 0.2 mg per day) and salt loading to increase blood volume, supplemented by mechanical devices to prevent pooling of blood in the legs and lower trunk (g suit). However, salt together with mineralocorticoids may induce serious supine hypertension, and the dose of the drug must be adjusted for this. For the central preganglionic type, there has been greater success with use of a sympathomimetic amine such as tyramine (which releases norepinephrine from intact postganglionic endings) supplemented by a monoamine oxidase inhibitor (to prevent destruction of the amine), and possibly propranolol. Levodopa has been effective in some cases. In the postganglionic type, judicious use of phenylephrine or ephedrine may be beneficial. Initial reports of the effectiveness of indomethacin in chronic orthostatic hypotension have not been substantiated.

3 After physical deconditioning, e.g., after prolonged illness with recumbency, especially in elderly individuals with reduced muscle tone.

4 After a sympathectomy that has abolished vasopressor reflexes.

5 In diabetic, alcoholic, and other neuropathies; syringomyelia; and diseases of the nervous system which cause muscular atrophy and paralysis of vasopressor reflexes. The most common form of neurogenic orthostatic hypotension is that which accompanies diseases of the peripheral nervous system. Diabetic polyneuropathy, beriberi, amyloid polyneuropathy, and the Adie syndrome are examples. Usually the orthostatic hypotension is associated with disturbances in sweating, impotence, and sphincter difficulties. Presumably the lesion involves postganglionic, nonmedullated fibers in peripheral nerves.

6 In patients receiving antihypertensive and vasodilator drugs as well as those who may be hypovolemic because of diuretics, excessive sweating, or adrenal insufficiency.

Micturition syncope, a condition usually seen in the elderly during or after urination, particularly after arising from the recumbent position, is probably a special type of postural syncope. It has been suggested that release of intravesicular pressure causes sudden vasodilatation, augmented by standing, and that vagally mediated bradycardia is a contributory factor.

Hyperbradykininemia Deficient kinin-inactivating enzymes with apparently normal sympathetic function may result in symptoms of faintness or syncope on assumption of upright posture. Hyperbradykininemia causes arteriolar and venular dilatation giving rise to postural hypotension and syncope with tachycardia. The pathophysiology of this condition remains uncertain. Treatment with beta-receptor antagonists has been beneficial.

Syncope of cardiac origin (cardiac syncope) Cardiac syncope results from a sudden reduction in cardiac output, caused most commonly by a cardiac arrhythmia. In normal individuals slow ventricular rates, but above 35 to 40 beats per minute, and fast ones not exceeding 180 beats per minute do not reduce cerebral blood flow, especially if the person is in the supine position, but changes in pulse rate outside these limits may impair cerebral circulation and function. The upright posture, cerebrovascular disease, anemia, and coronary, myocardial, or valvular disease all reduce the tolerance to alterations in rate.

Complete atrioventricular block is the commonest arrhythmia that leads to fainting, and syncopal episodes associated with this arrhythmia are known as the Stokes-Adams-Morgagni syndrome. The etiology of disturbances in atrioventricular conduction is considered elsewhere (Chap. 183), but in patients with these attacks the block may be persistent or intermittent; it is often preceded or followed by disturbed conduction in one or two of the three fascicles through which the ventricles are normally activated, by second-degree atrioventricular block (Mobitz type II), or bifascicular or trifascicular block. When the block is complete and the pacemaker below the block fails to function, syncope occurs. A brief bout of ventricular tachycardia or

fibrillation may also be responsible for the syncopal episode (Chap. 184). Recurrent syncope due to ventricular fibrillation, characterized by a prolonged QT interval (sometimes associated with congenital deafness), has been reported; this condition may be familial or sporadic.

Stokes-Adams attacks occur usually without more than a momentary sense of weakness, the patient suddenly losing consciousness. After cardiac standstill of more than several seconds, the patient turns pale, falls unconscious, and, as in other types of fainting, may exhibit a few clonic jerks. With longer periods of asystole, the ashen gray pallor gives way to cyanosis, stertorous breathing, fixed pupils, incontinence, and bilateral Babinski signs. Prolonged confusion and neurologic signs due to cerebral ischemia may occur in some patients, and permanent impairment of mental function may result, although focal neurologic signs are rare. Cardiac faints of this type may recur several times a day. Occasionally the heart block is transitory, and the electrocardiogram taken later may not show any arrhythmia.

Less commonly, a decreased rate of discharge of the sinoatrial node leads to syncope. Recurrent attacks of tachyarrhythmias—including atrial flutter and paroxysmal atrial and ventricular tachycardia with normal AV conduction—may also suddenly reduce cardiac output to a degree sufficient to cause syncope.

In another form of cardiac syncope the heart block is reflexive and is due to irritation of the vagus nerves. Examples of this phenomenon have been observed in patients with esophageal diverticula, mediastinal tumors, gallbladder disease, carotid sinus disease, glossopharyngeal neuralgia, and pleural and pulmonary irritation. However, in these conditions reflex bradycardia is more commonly of the sinoatrial than the atrioventricular type.

Cardiac syncope may also result from *acute massive myocardial infarction,* particularly when associated with cardiogenic shock. *Aortic stenosis* often sets the stage for exertional syncope, most commonly by limiting cardiac output in the face of peripheral vasodilatation, but sometimes during exertion, with resultant myocardial and cerebral ischemia and occasionally arrhythmias. *Idiopathic hypertrophic subaortic stenosis* may also lead to exertional syncope, because of intensified obstruction and/or ventricular arrhythmias (Chap. 192). In *primary pulmonary hypertension* a relatively fixed cardiac output and bouts of acute right ventricular failure may be associated with syncope (Chap. 191). However, vagal reflexes may be involved in this condition as well as in the syncope that occurs with *pulmonary embolism.* Ball valve thrombus in the left atrium, left atrial myxoma, or thrombosis or malfunction of a prosthetic valve may produce sudden mechanical obstruction of the circulation and syncope. *Tetralogy of Fallot* is the congenital cardiac malformation most commonly responsible for syncope. In this condition systemic vasodilatation, perhaps associated with infundibular spasm, greatly increases the right-to-left shunt and produces arterial hypoxia, which leads to syncope (Chap. 185).

Carotid sinus syncope The carotid sinus is normally sensitive to stretch and gives rise to sensory impulses carried via the nerve of Hering, a branch of the glossopharyngeal nerve, to the medulla oblongata. Massage of one or both of the carotid sinuses, particularly in elderly persons, causes (1) a reflex cardiac slowing (sinus bradycardia, sinus arrest, or even atrioventricular block), the so-called vagal type of response and (2) a fall of arterial pressure without cardiac slowing, the so-called depressor type of response. Both types of carotid sinus response may coexist.

Syncope due to carotid sinus sensitivity may be initiated by turning of the head to one side, by a tight collar, or, as in a few reported cases, by shaving over the region of the sinus. But the absence of such stimuli is of no aid in diagnosis, since spontaneous attacks may occur. The attack nearly always begins when the patient is in an upright position, usually when standing. The period of unconsciousness seldom lasts longer than a few minutes. The sensorium is immediately clear when consciousness is regained. The majority of the reported cases have been in men. In a patient displaying faintness on compression of one carotid sinus, it is important to distinguish between the benign disorder (hypersensitivity of one carotid sinus) and a much more serious condition—atheromatous narrowing of the opposite carotid or of the basilar artery (see Chap. 343).

Other forms of vasovagal syncope have been described. Exceptionally intense pain of visceral origin may inhibit cardiac action through vagal stimulation, e.g., cardiac standstill during an attack of gallbladder colic, a lesion of the esophagus or mediastinum, bronchoscopy, pleural or peritoneal taps, intense vertigo from labyrinthine or vestibular disease, and needling of body cavities. Occasionally, a patient with a severe migraine attack will sustain a syncopal episode.

Vagal and glossopharyngeal neuralgia Occasionally this induces a reflex type of fainting. Again the sequence is always pain, then syncope; in this instance the pain is localized to the base of the tongue, pharynx or larynx, tonsillar area, and ear. It may be triggered by pressure at these sites. Section of the appropriate branches of the ninth or tenth cranial nerve relieves the condition. The cardiovascular effects are attributable to excitation of the dorsal motor nucleus of the vagus via collateral fibers from the nucleus of the tractus solitarius.

Tussive syncope (laryngeal vertigo) This is a rare condition that results from a paroxysm of coughing, usually in men with chronic bronchitis. After hard coughing the patient suddenly becomes weak and loses consciousness momentarily. The intrathoracic pressure becomes elevated and interferes with the venous return to the heart, as does the Valsalva maneuver (exhaling against a closed glottis).

Syncope associated with cerebrovascular disease This is usually caused by partial or complete occlusion of the large arteries in the neck. Physical activity may then critically reduce blood flow to the upper part of the brainstem, causing abrupt loss of consciousness (see Chap. 343).

PATHOPHYSIOLOGY OF SYNCOPE The loss of consciousness in each type of syncope is caused by reduction of oxygenation to those parts of the brain which subserve consciousness. During syncopal attacks, there are demonstrable reductions in cerebral blood flow, cerebral oxygen utilization, and cerebrovascular resistance. The electroencephalogram reveals high-voltage slow waves, two to five per second, coincident with the loss of consciousness. If the ischemia lasts only a few minutes, there are no lasting effects on the brain. If it persists for a longer time, it may result in necrosis of brain tissue in the border zones of perfusion between the vascular territories of the major cerebral and cerebellar arteries.

When faintness is related to reduced cerebral blood flow resulting directly from a disorder of cardiac function, there is likely to be a combination of pallor and cyanosis. When, on the other hand, the peripheral circulation is at fault, pallor is usually striking but is not accompanied by cyanosis or respiratory disturbances. When the primary disturbance lies in the cerebral circulation, the face is likely to be florid and the breathing slow and stertorous. During the attack a heart rate faster than 150 beats per minute indicates an ectopic cardiac rhythm, while a striking bradycardia (rate of less than 40 beats per minute) suggests complete heart block. In a patient with faintness or syncope attended by bradycardia, one has to distinguish that due to failure of neurogenic reflexes from that due to a cardiogenic (Stokes-Adams) attack. The electrocardiogram is decisive, but even without it, the Stokes-Adams attacks can be recognized clinically by their longer duration, by the greater constancy of the slow heart rate, by the presence of audible sounds synchronous with atrial contractions, by atrial contraction (A) waves in the jugular venous pulse, and by marked variation in intensity of the first sound, despite the regular rhythm (Chap. 183).

DIFFERENTIAL DIAGNOSIS OF CONDITIONS INVOLVING EPISODIC WEAKNESS AND FAINTNESS BUT NOT SYNCOPE
Anxiety attacks and the hyperventilation syndrome are discussed in detail in Chaps. 11 and 360. The giddiness of anxiety is frequently interpreted as a feeling of faintness without actual loss of consciousness. Such symptoms are not accompanied by facial pallor and are

not relieved by recumbency. The diagnosis is made on the basis of symptoms, and part of the attack can be reproduced by hyperventilation. Two of the mechanisms known to be involved in the attacks are reduction in carbon dioxide as the result of hyperventilation and the release of epinephrine. Hyperventilation results in hypocapnia, alkalosis, increased cerebrovascular resistance, and decreased cerebral blood flow.

Hypoglycemia, when severe, is usually traceable to a serious disease, such as a tumor of the islets of Langerhans or advanced adrenal, pituitary, or hepatic disease, or to excessive administration of insulin. The clinical picture is one of confusion or even a loss of consciousness. When mild, as is usually the case, hypoglycemia is often of the reactive type (Chap. 329), occurring 2 to 5 h after eating, and is not usually associated with a disturbance of consciousness. The diagnosis depends on the history and the documentation of reduced blood sugar during an attack.

Acute hemorrhage, usually within the gastrointestinal tract, is an occasional cause of syncope. In the absence of pain and hematemesis the cause of the weakness, faintness, or even unconsciousness may remain obscure until the passage of a black stool.

Cerebral ischemic attacks occur in some patients with arteriosclerotic narrowings or occlusion of the major arteries of the brain. The main symptoms vary from patient to patient and include dim vision, hemiparesis or sudden drop attacks, numbness of one side of the body, dizziness, and thick speech. In any one patient all attacks are of identical type and indicate a temporary deficit of function in a certain region of the brain due to inadequate circulation.

Hysterical fainting is rather frequent and usually occurs under dramatic circumstances. The attack is unattended by any outward display of anxiety. The evident lack of change in pulse and blood pressure or color of the skin and mucous membranes distinguishes it from the vasodepressor faint. The diagnosis is based on the bizarre nature of the attack in a person who exhibits the general personality and behavioral characteristics of the hysteric.

Type of onset When the attack begins over the period of a few seconds, carotid sinus syncope, postural hypotension, sudden atrioventricular block, ventricular standstill, or fibrillation is likely. When the symptoms develop gradually during a period of several minutes, hyperventilation or hypoglycemia should be considered. Onset of syncope during or immediately after exertion suggests aortic stenosis, idiopathic hypertrophic subaortic stenosis or excessive bradycardia, and, in elderly subjects, postural hypotension. Exertional syncope is seen occasionally in persons with aortic insufficiency and with severe occlusive disease of cerebral arteries. In patients with ventricular standstill or ventricular fibrillation, loss of consciousness occurs several seconds later, followed rapidly by cessation of electroencephalographic activity and then often by brief clonic muscle contractions.

Position at onset of attack Epilepsy and syncopal attacks due to hypoglycemia, hyperventilation, or heart block are likely to be independent of posture. Faintness associated with a decline in blood pressure (including carotid sinus attacks) and with ectopic tachycardia usually occurs only in the sitting or standing position, whereas faintness resulting from orthostatic hypotension is apt to set in shortly after change from the recumbent to the standing position.

Associated symptoms such as palpitation are likely to be present when the attack is due to anxiety or hyperventilation, to ectopic tachycardia, or to hypoglycemia. Numbness and tingling in the hands and face are frequent accompaniments of hyperventilation. Genuine convulsions during the attack may occasionally occur with heart block, ventricular standstill, or fibrillation. When *duration of attack* is very brief, i.e., a few seconds to a few minutes, carotid sinus syncope or one of the several forms of postural hypotension is most likely. A duration of more than a few minutes but less than an hour suggests hypoglycemia or hyperventilation.

SPECIAL METHODS OF EXAMINATION In many patients who complain of recurrent weakness or syncope but do not have a spontaneous attack while under observation, an attempt to reproduce attacks is of great assistance in diagnosis.

When hyperventilation is accompanied by faintness, the pattern of symptoms can be reproduced readily by having the subject breathe rapidly and deeply for 2 to 3 min. This test is often of therapeutic value also, because the underlying anxiety tends to be lessened when the patient learns that the symptoms can be produced and alleviated at will simply by controlling breathing.

Among other conditions in which the diagnosis is commonly clarified by reproducing the attacks are carotid sinus hypersensitivity (massage of one or the other carotid sinus), orthostatic hypotension and orthostatic tachycardia (observations of pulse rate, blood pressure, and symptoms in the recumbent and standing positions), and tussive syncope (by inducing the Valsalva maneuver). In all these instances the crucial point is not whether symptoms are produced (the procedures mentioned frequently induce symptoms in healthy persons) but whether the exact pattern of symptoms that occurs in the spontaneous attacks is reproduced in the artificial ones. Careful, continuous Holter monitoring of the electrocardiogram in the hospital or the recording of the electrocardiogram over 1 or 2 days using a portable lightweight tape recorder in an ambulatory patient may be extremely useful in identifying an arrhythmia responsible for the syncopal episode. Monitoring is most helpful if it shows that the syncopal episode is characterized by a bout of cardiac standstill, extreme bradycardia, or tachyarrhythmia.

In cases of recurrent syncope of unknown cause, the use of intracardiac electrophysiologic techniques with programmed stimulation can be helpful in determining cardiac abnormalities and in establishing effective treatment. During stimulation, up to two-thirds of such patients can be shown to have rapid ventricular tachycardia, His bundle conduction delays, atrial flutter, sick-sinus syndrome, or hypervagotonia.

The electroencephalogram may be helpful in differentiating syncope from seizures. In the interval between epileptic seizures it may show some degree of abnormality in 40 to 80 percent of cases. In the interval between syncopal attacks it should be normal.

TREATMENT   In most instances fainting is relatively benign. In dealing with patients who have fainted, the physician should think first of those causes of fainting that constitute a therapeutic emergency. Among them are massive internal hemorrhage and myocardial infarction, which may be painless, and cardiac arrhythmias. In elderly persons a sudden faint, without obvious cause, should arouse the suspicion of complete heart block, even though all findings are negative when the patient is seen.

Patients seen during the preliminary stages of fainting or after they have lost consciousness should be placed in a position which permits maximal cerebral blood flow, i.e., with head lowered between the knees, if sitting, or in the supine position. All tight clothing and other constrictions should be loosened and the head turned so that the tongue does not fall back into the throat, blocking the airway. Peripheral irritation, such as sprinkling or dashing cold water on the face and neck or the application of cold moist towels, is helpful. If the temperature is subnormal, the body should be covered with a warm blanket. Since emesis is frequent, aspiration should be prevented. The head should be turned to the side and nothing should be given by mouth until the patient has regained consciousness. Patients should not be permitted to rise until the sense of physical weakness has passed, and they should be watched carefully for a few minutes after rising.

The *prevention* of fainting depends on the mechanisms involved. In the usual vasovagal faint of adolescents, which tends to occur in periods of emotional excitement, fatigue, hunger, etc., it is enough to advise the patient to avoid such circumstances. In postural hypotension, patients should be cautioned against arising suddenly from bed. Instead, they should first exercise their legs for a few seconds, then sit on the edge of the bed and make sure they are not light-headed or dizzy before starting to walk. Sleeping with the headposts of the bed elevated on wooden blocks 8 to 12 in high and wearing snug elastic abdominal binder and elastic stockings are often helpful. Drugs of the ephedrine group may be useful if they do not cause insomnia. If there are no contraindications, a high intake of sodium chloride, which expands the extracellular fluid volume, may be beneficial.

In the syndrome of chronic orthostatic hypotension, special corticosteroid preparations (fludrocortisone acetate tablets, 0.1 to 0.2 mg per day in divided doses) have given relief in some cases. Binding of the legs (g suit) and sleeping with head and shoulders elevated are helpful.

The treatment of carotid sinus syncope involves first of all instructing the patient in measures that minimize the hazards of a fall (see below). Loose collars should be worn, and the patient should learn to turn the whole body, rather than the head alone, when looking to one side. Atropine or the ephedrine group of drugs should be used, respectively, in patients with pronounced bradycardia or hypotension during attacks. If atropine is not successful, a demand pacemaker should be inserted into the right ventricle. Radiation or surgical denervation of the carotid sinus has apparently yielded favorable results in some patients, but it is rarely necessary. Once it has been concluded that the attacks are due to a narrowing of major cerebral arteries, some of the surgical measures discussed in Chap. 343 must be considered.

The treatment of the various cardiac arrhythmias which may induce syncope is discussed in Chap. 183. The treatment of hypoglycemia will be found in Chap. 329 and of the hyperventilation syndrome and hysterical fainting in Chap. 11.

The chief hazard of a faint in most elderly persons is not the underlying disease but fracture or other trauma due to the fall. Therefore, patients subject to recurrent syncope should cover the bathroom floor and bathtub with rubber mats and should have as much of their home carpeted as is feasible. Especially important is the floor space between the bed and the bathroom, because faints are common in elderly persons when walking from bed to toilet. Outdoor walking should be on soft ground rather than hard surfaces, and the patient should avoid standing still, which is more likely than walking to induce an attack.

SEIZURES

A seizure or convulsion is defined as an abrupt alteration in cortical electrical activity manifested clinically by a change in consciousness or by a motor, sensory, or behavioral symptom. Seizures, which may be due to a variety of causes, become important in the differential diagnosis of syncope when the episode occurs with minimal or no warning and results in only a brief loss of consciousness. *Epilepsy* (discussed in Chap. 342) is the term used to describe recurrent seizures present over months or years, often with a stereotyped clinical pattern.

CLINICAL CHARACTERISTICS OF SEIZURES   A detailed account of the types of seizures, of their pathophysiology, and of their treatment is found in Chap. 342. The purpose here is to recount briefly the varieties of seizures that occur (Table 12-2), and to outline their clinical presentation, particularly with respect to their distinction from syncope. A single seizure may occur during the course of many medical illnesses; its importance derives from the fact that it signifies involvement of the central nervous system by the disease process.

Partial seizures (focal seizures)   The appearance of focal motor or sensory manifestations provides clinical documentation of the localization of the cerebral lesion. Deviation of the eyes and head to one side (aversive seizure) usually points to an irritative focus in the opposite prefrontal region. A Jacksonian seizure begins as a clonic movement in one portion of the body, often the thumb, the corner of the mouth, or the great toe, and spreads to adjacent muscular groups over a few seconds or minutes. The seizure may progress to involve the entire side or become generalized with attendant loss of consciousness.

Jacksonian seizures almost always are accompanied by an abnormal interictal EEG.

Complex partial seizures (temporal lobe or psychomotor seizures) These differ from generalized motor seizures by (1) the frequent occurrence of an aura that arises from discharges in the autonomic, visceral, and olfactory portions of the temporal lobe and limbic system; and (2) loss of awareness or contact with the environment, often associated with behavioral or complex motor movements for which the patient is amnesic after the attack. Subjective experiences of the aura include hallucinations (olfactory, gustatory, visual, or auditory), illusions (spatial distortions, shrinkage, or angulation), aberrations in cognition (déjà vu, a sense of familiarity; jamais vu, a sense of unfamiliarity; or recurrent memory), and affective changes (anxiety, fear, and, very rarely, rage). The seizure may terminate with only the subjective component or may progress to the motor phase which is often evident by repetitive motor acts like smacking the lips, swallowing, undressing, and incoherent or dysphasic speech.

The abrupt onset of complex partial seizures often indicates a disorder of the temporal lobe and its connection to the limbic system. Complete investigation in search of the cause is indicated.

Tonic-clonic (grand mal) seizure The abrupt presentation, without warning, of a generalized motor seizure is one of the commonest indications of involvement of the cerebral cortex by a disease process. Grand mal seizures usually begin with opening of the eyes and mouth, flexion and abduction of the arms, and extension of the legs. The *tonic* phase of the seizure is often heralded by contraction of the respiratory muscles resulting in a vocalization. These motor signs are followed by closure of the jaw, often with laceration of the tongue, respiratory arrest with plethora and cyanosis, and urinary, or less commonly, fecal incontinence. The tonic phase of the seizure, which usually persists for only 15 to 30 s, is followed immediately by the *clonic* phase, characterized by violent rhythmic muscular contractions affecting the whole body including the muscles of respiration. Eye movements, facial grimacing, and persistence of respiratory apnea are evident. The clonic movements subside in amplitude and frequency and the seizure terminates, usually within 1 to 2 min. Normal respiration resumes and the patient falls asleep; arousal may occur in a few minutes but lethargy, fatigue, and postseizure (postictal) confusion are common and may persist for several hours. Postictal headache is also common.

The generalized seizure occurring in the course of a major medical illness signifies involvement of the central nervous system by the disorder and requires careful assessment and investigation. Such a seizure may accompany high fever, hyponatremia, metabolic acidosis, alcohol or drug withdrawal, and renal or liver failure, indicating the presence of a *metabolic encephalopathy*, without requiring the postulation of another separate neurologic illness. The determination that a metabolic encephalopathy may be responsible is dependent upon documentation of the systemic illness and careful attention to the exclusion of an additional infectious, vascular, or neoplastic lesion in the nervous system. Central nervous system evaluation should include a careful history, a detailed neurologic examination searching for focal neurologic deficit, and, in many cases, electro-encephalography and computerized tomography (CT) scan. If infection is suspected, an examination of the cerebrospinal fluid is mandatory. Recurrent seizures (status epilepticus) indicate a serious compromise of cerebral cortical function and require vigorous treatment to prevent hypoxic damage to the brain and, following termination of the seizures, a thorough investigation of the cause.

An isolated generalized seizure occurring in an otherwise healthy, asymptomatic patient when observed by family or other bystanders is not difficult to distinguish from syncope. More difficult to assess is the circumstance of sudden loss of consciousness occurring without warning and unwitnessed by an observer or an akinetic "drop-seizure" (atypical petit mal). The latter may be indistinguishable from syncope. Postictal confusion or drowsiness, injury such as laceration of the tongue, urinary or fecal incontinence, or muscle

soreness suggests that a convulsion has occurred. One common clinical presentation is the sudden occurrence of a brief clonic seizure during a minor surgical or dental procedure. The patient is usually in a seated position and the episode is considered to be due to cerebral ischemia associated with systemic hypotension and bradycardia accompanying vasovagal syncope. There are usually only two or three clonic movements, without a prior tonic phase, and recovery is rapid without postictal symptoms. Such patients should have a neurologic examination and an EEG and, if these are normal, be treated with reassurance and not given anticonvulsants. There is no evidence to indicate an underlying cerebral lesion in such patients.

Generalized seizures may be preceded by a specific warning or *aura*, and attention to these symptoms may be important in aiding in the localization of the seizure focus and can assist in distinguishing the episode from syncope. Tingling or numbness points to involvement of the parietal lobe, and visual or auditory sensations suggest occipitotemporal localization. More complex psychological and cognitive sensations may accompany temporal lobe seizures. Such symptoms may also accompany transient cerebral ischemic attacks (see Chap. 343), but in this case the symptoms usually persist for many minutes or hours.

Absence (petit mal) seizures Absence seizures, in contrast to grand mal, are noted for their brevity and for the degree of loss of awareness accompanied by minimal motor manifestations. They are abrupt in onset and are often evident only by a stare or cessation of ongoing behavior; they may be accompanied by fluttering of the eyelids or by a few facial twitches. Full recovery occurs in 5 to 10 s, and the episode may go unnoticed by the patient, the family, or the teacher. Loss of postural tone (atonic or akinetic seizure) with falling is uncommon but when present requires distinction from syncope. The EEG is diagnostic in such cases, consisting of three-per-second spike and wave discharges. This condition, which indicates a specific generalized disorder of cerebral electrical activity, is responsive to specific drug treatments (see Chap. 342).

DIFFERENTIAL DIAGNOSIS OF SEIZURES AND SYNCOPE Syncope must be distinguished from disturbances of cerebral function, caused by a seizure. A seizure may occur day or night, regardless of the position of the patient; syncope rarely appears when the patient is recumbent, the only common exception being the Stokes-Adams attack. The patient's color may not change in seizures, though there may be cyanosis; pallor is an early and invariable finding in all types of syncope, except chronic orthostatic hypotension and hysteria, and it precedes unconsciousness. Seizures are often heralded by an aura, which is caused by a focal seizure discharge and hence has brain localizing significance. It is usually followed by rapid return to normal or by loss of consciousness. The onset of syncope is usually more deliberate and without aura. Injury from falling is frequent in a seizure and rare in syncope, for the reason that only in seizures are protective reflexes abolished instantaneously. Tonic-convulsive movements with upturning eyes are a feature of seizures and usually do not occur with syncope, although, as stated above, brief tonic clonic seizure-like activity can accompany fainting episodes. The period of unconsciousness tends to be longer in seizures than in syncope. Urinary incontinence is frequent in seizures and rare in syncope. The return of consciousness is prompt in syncope, slow after a seizure. Mental confusion, headache, and drowsiness are common sequelae of seizures; physical weakness with a clear sensorium characterizes

TABLE 12-2 Classification of seizures

I Partial or focal seizures
  A Simple partial seizures (with motor, sensory, autonomic, or psychic signs)
  B Complex partial seizures (psychomotor or temporal lobe seizures)
  C Secondary generalized partial seizures
II Primary generalized seizures
  A Tonic clonic (grand mal)
  B Absence (petit mal)
  C Myoclonic
  D Atonic or akinetic

the postsyncopal state. Repeated spells of unconsciousness in a young person at a rate of several per day or month are more suggestive of epilepsy than of syncope. No one of these points will absolutely differentiate a seizure from syncope, but taken as a group and supplemented by electroencephalograms, they provide a means of distinguishing the two conditions.

REFERENCES

CRILL WE: Neuronal mechanisms of seizure initiation, in *Antiepileptic Drugs: Mechanisms of Action*, GH Glaser et al (eds). New York, Raven Press, 1980, p 169

DAY SC: et al: Evaluation and outcome of emergency room patients with transient loss of consciousness. Am J Med 73:15, 1982

DIMARCO JP et al: Intracardiac electrophysiologic techniques in recurrent syncope of unknown cause. Ann Intern Med 95:542, 1981

ECTOR H et al: Bradycardia, ventricular pauses, syncope, and sports. Lancet 1:591, 1984

EWING DJ et al: The natural history of diabetic autonomic neuropathy. Q J Med 49:95, 1980

HICKLER R: Fainting, in *Signs and Symptoms*, 6th ed, RS Blacklow (ed). Philadelphia, Lippincott, 1977, chap 33

JOHNSON RH, SPAULDING JMK: *Disorders of the Autonomic Nervous System*. Philadelphia, Davis, 1974

KAPOOR WN et al: A prospective evaluation and follow-up of patients with syncope. N Engl J Med 309:197, 1983

LEE JE et al: Episodic unconsciousness, in *Diagnostic Approaches to Presenting Syndromes*, JA Barondess (ed). Baltimore, Williams & Wilkins, 1971, pp 133–167

POLINSKY RJ et al: Pharmacologic distinction of different orthostatic hypotension syndromes. Neurology 31:1, 1981

RICHARDS AM et al: Syncope in aortic valvular stenosis. Lancet 1:1113, 1984

SILVERSTEIN MD et al: Patients with syncope admitted to medical intensive care units. JAMA 248:1185, 1982

STREETER DHP et al: Hyperbradykininism: A new orthostatic syndrome. Lancet 2:1048, 1972

SUTHERLAND JM, EADIE MJ: *The Epilepsies*, 3d ed. Edinburgh, Churchill Livingstone, 1980

WEISSLER AM, WARREN, JV: Syncope and shock, in *The Heart*, 4th ed, JW Hurst et al (eds). New York, McGraw-Hill, 1978, p 705

WRIGHT KE JR, MCINTOSH MD: Syncope: Review of pathophysiological mechanisms. Prog Cardiovasc Dis 13:580, 1971

YOUNG RR et al: Pure pandysautonomia with recovery. Description and discussion of diagnostic criteria. Brain 98:613, 1975

13   DISTURBANCES OF VISION AND OCULAR MOVEMENTS

SHIRLEY H. WRAY

The eye, if not the window of the soul, is the mirror reflecting the body's health. No clinician can afford not to examine an organ which gives so many clues to systemic disorders, and one that is the only part of the body where vascular and neural tissue can be viewed directly.

Rose

The eye is a sensory optical organ designed to focus light on a highly photosensitive neuronal membrane, the retina. Light entering the eye passes through the cornea, aqueous humor, lens, and vitreous humor before traversing the transparent layers of the retina to reach photoreceptors in the outer nuclear layer.

The amount of light entering the lens for imaging on the retina is controlled by the iris diaphragm. Its opening, the pupil, can be constricted or dilated by the action of the muscles of the iris. At the start of the visual process light is detected by photoreceptor cells called rods and cones. These neurons contain visual pigments that enable them to capture units of light, called photons. A physiologic interaction involving both excitation and inhibition takes place at progressively more complex synaptic levels among the multiple cell types in the retina. This permits characteristics of incident light striking the eye to be analyzed in terms of spatial, luminous, spectral, and temporal functions.

Rods and cones differ in their capabilities. Rods detect light at low intensity (scotopic condition), have poor image discrimination, and do not detect color. Cones function at high light intensity (photopic condition), have good image resolution, and mediate color vision. Cones are abundant at the center of the retina, in the macula. The macula contains the thin fovea and the tiny circular foveola. The fovea lies 3 mm temporal to the margin of the optic disc. It is the site of maximum acuity (normal 20/20). Visual acuity drops off rapidly in the paramacular areas, where cone concentration drops off abruptly. Rods outnumber cones in the human retina (100 million rods to 60 million cones). They are absent in the foveola and peak in concentration at 20° from the fovea, gradually diminishing peripherally.

The distribution of the retinal ganglion cells parallels that of the cones. In the foveola a single ganglion cell connects via a bipolar cell to an individual cone, a 1:1 ratio that maximizes visual discrimination. Once the initial processing of visual information is completed by the retina, the analysis is relayed as electrical impulses from the ganglion cells through their nerve fibers in the optic nerve, to the lateral geniculate nucleus. After synaptic relay, fibers project via the geniculocalcarine pathway to the visual cortex. Visual function is classified under the terms *form sense, color sense,* and *light sense.*

FORM SENSE   Form sense in clinical practice is tested by the determination of visual acuity, a test of macular function. This should be part of any complete medical examination, regardless of symptomatology or lack thereof. The Snellen chart, commonly used for distance vision, is placed 20 feet (approximately 6 meters) away from the patient. The chart consists of letters of graduated sizes; the distance at which each size subtends an angle of 5' is indicated along the side of the chart. A patient with a corrected refractive error should wear eyeglasses for the test. The vision of a normal eye is 20/20. If the patient is able to read down only to the 20/30 line, the vision is recorded as 20/30. If the patient is unable to read even the large E at the top, he or she may be moved closer so that the distance is changed. The visual acuity may then be recorded as 10/400, for instance, if the patient is able to read this letter at 10 feet from the chart. Pinhole vision should be tested if the patient is unable to read the 20/30 line. A patient whose visual loss is secondary to a refractive error should read close to 20/20 through the pinhole because of the narrow alignment of light rays transmitted through the hole. If the pinhole fails to improve the visual acuity score, the examiner should suspect another cause for the reduced vision, such as opacities in the ocular media or macular or optic nerve disease. Visual acuity corrected by glasses or contact lenses only to 20/200 or less in both eyes or visual fields less than 10° centrally constitutes legal blindness in the United States, and the patient should be registered by the Commission for the Blind in the patient's home state.

COLOR SENSE   Many abnormalities of visual function are characterized by acquired defects in color vision. For example, red and green often cannot be distinguished, although the vision for white is normal, in some types of macular disease (due to toxic or degenerative causes), and in optic nerve disease (due to multiple sclerosis, toxins, drugs, or nutritional deficiencies, such as occurs in tobacco-alcohol amblyopia). The most commonly used quantitative tests for color sense are the polychromatic plates of Ishihara, which identify defects in red-green discrimination, and the Hardy-Rand-Ritler (HRR) figures, which are useful in detecting red-green and blue-yellow defects. Demonstration of adequate color vision is mandatory for certain jobs. Hereditary red-green and other types of inherited color blindness are reviewed in the *Manual of Ocular Diagnosis and Therapy* (see references).

LIGHT SENSE   Light sense is assessed by visual field examination. Abnormalities indicate damage to a portion of the visual pathway from the retina to the visual cortex. A conventional method of testing visual fields is called kinetic perimetry (Goldmann hemispheric perimeter), which consists of moving a target to identify points of equal sensitivity in the two fields (Anderson). The patient signals when the target is seen, indicating when it disappears and when it reappears. In this way the visual fields can be charted accurately for defects from the periphery into central or foveal fixation. Monocular confrontation visual field testing with a cotton pledget or white-headed pin compares the periphery of the patient's visual field with that of the examiner. The visual field is considered normal if the patient sees the target 90° temporally, 50° nasally, 50° upward, and 65° downward.

Each of these indices of visual function may be affected singly or in combination. Failing eyesight may thus be due to an abnormality of the refractive media of the eye, or to a lesion of the retina, the optic nerve, or those parts of the brain with which they are connected.

DISORDERS OF VISION AND THE VISUAL PATHWAY

THE CORNEA The cornea, the main refracting surface of the eye, is vulnerable to environmental hazards including exposure (direct trauma, drying, radiant and ionizing energy), infectious agents (bacteria, viruses—notably herpes simplex and herpes zoster—fungi, and parasites), and inflammation, sometimes in association with systemic dermatologic disorders such as atopic dermatitis, cicatricial pemphigoid, and erythema multiforme (Stevens-Johnson syndrome). *Keratitis* is an inflammation or infection of the cornea. It is often associated with inflammation of the iris (iritis) or of the uveal tract—the iris, ciliary body, and choroid (uveitis). Keratitis combined with uveitis or iritis is seen commonly in Reiter's disease and occasionally in Behçet's disease. Keratitis and uveitis may also occur with herpes simplex infection, in sarcoidosis (Chap. 270), and in collagen vascular diseases (Chap. 269). Metabolic disorders can also cause opacification of the cornea since the cornea can store material present in excess in the body. In hypercalcemia secondary to sarcoid (Chap. 270), hyperparathyroidism (Chap. 336), and vitamin D intoxication (Chap. 337), calcium phosphates and carbonates precipitate beneath the corneal epithelium in a plane corresponding to the interpalpebral fissure, so-called band keratopathy: cystine crystals are deposited in cystinosis (Chap. 308), cholesterol esters in hypercholesterolemia (arcus senilis) (Chap. 315), chloroquine crystals in treatment of discoid lupus, polysaccharides in Hurler's disease (Chap. 319), and copper in hepatolenticular degeneration (Kayser-Fleischer ring) (Chap. 311). Keratoplasty (transplantation) for restoration of sight may be warranted when the cornea is sufficiently scarred and/or opaque.

THE PUPIL Normal pupil size is determined by the level of light entering the eye. Slight degrees of pupil asymmetry (anisocoria) with equal pupil reflexes to light and accommodation can be normal. Pathologic anisocoria occurs with lesions of the sympathetic (Horner's syndrome) or parasympathetic (internal ophthalmoplegia) innervation of the eye. Horner's syndrome is characterized by an ipsilateral normal-reacting miotic pupil, partial ptosis, and, occasionally, impaired facial sweating. An internal ophthalmoplegia (third nerve) causes a fixed or poorly responsive dilated pupil which constricts with 1% pilocarpine eyedrops. The use of different concentrations of topical pilocarpine allows the physician to distinguish between a third nerve palsy, a drug-induced (atropine) mydriasis, and the myotonic pupil of Adie. The test is detailed in the reference by Rose.

AQUEOUS HUMOR AND GLAUCOMA Glaucoma is a condition in which elevated intraocular pressure (IOP) transmitted through the aqueous humor damages the optic nerve. Aqueous humor, formed by secretion of the epithelium of the ciliary body, functions to support metabolism of the avascular lens and cornea. The level of IOP represents a balance between the rate of aqueous humor formation and the resistance to its outflow through the trabecular meshwork to the canal of Schlemm and the aqueous veins. Glaucoma is caused in most cases by an abnormality in outflow from the anterior chamber, not from an increased rate of aqueous humor formation.

Glaucoma is the second leading cause of blindness in the United States; approximately 1 of 50 individuals over age 35 have the condition. About 1 million persons in the United States are estimated to have glaucoma without being aware of it. Detection of glaucoma is, therefore, a major public health problem; measurement of eye pressure should be part of any routine eye examination. An IOP greater than 22 mmHG (Schiötz tonometry) is abnormal, but since considerable diurnal variation of IOP may occur in patients with glaucoma, including normal values, it is important to inspect the optic disc for evidence of glaucoma. The cup usually enlarges vertically before visual field loss occurs, and asymmetry of the optic disc cup may be an early sign. With progressive glaucomatous damage to the nerve, there is loss of nerve tissue and optic atrophy develops, with changes in both contour (cupping) and color (pallor) changes in the disc.

The major types of glaucoma are open-angle, angle-closure, congenital, and secondary.

Open-angle glaucoma Open-angle glaucoma arises as a complication of chronic obstruction of aqueous humor reabsorption in the trabecular meshwork. Open-angle glaucoma is usually asymptomatic and only rarely causes ocular pain or corneal edema. Visual loss occurs first in the peripheral fields and visual acuity remains normal until late in the course of the disorder.

Diagnosis depends on measurement of elevated IOP, and direct visualization (gonioscopy) of the structures at the angle. Management consists initially of careful follow-up with repeated measurements of IOP, visual field assessment, and careful funduscopic evaluation for disc cupping.

The treatment of open-angle glaucoma is primarily medical. Cholinergic drugs (pilocarpine or carbachol) and beta-adrenergic blockers (timolol) decrease IOP after topical application. Carbonic anhydrase inhibitors (acetazolamide or methazolamide) may be beneficial.

Surgery to prevent permanent visual loss is necessary in only a minority of patients. *Laser trabeculoplasty* or creation of a fistula from the anterior chamber to the subconjunctival space are the techniques used.

Angle-closure glaucoma Angle-closure glaucoma develops when aqueous outflow is impeded by a narrow anterior chamber. Tissue in the periphery of the iris covers the trabecular meshwork, preventing egress of aqueous humor. The obstruction may occur acutely, usually in one eye. The eye is red and painful and the pupil may be dilated and nonreactive to light. Vision is impaired. Chronic angle-closure glaucoma may present with visual loss, pupillary dilation, and pain. Gonioscopy is necessary to distinguish open-angle from angle-closure glaucoma in cases with chronic or subacute onset.

Angle-closure glaucoma can be precipitated by administration of drugs to dilate the pupil. Because a narrow angle predisposes to this complication, it is important, particularly in patients over age 50, to examine the anterior chamber of the eye before pharmacologic dilation.

The treatment of acute angle-closure glaucoma is a medical emergency. Intravenous mannitol, parenteral acetazolamide, and topical pilocarpine or timolol are used to counteract the acute increase in IOP. Surgical treatment may be required after acute medical management to create a communication between the anterior and posterior chambers.

Congenital glaucoma This is a rare cause of open-angle glaucoma arising from dysgenesis of structures in the angle of the eye. It may lead to visual loss, enlargement of the eye, and corneal damage. Early recognition is important, followed by medical and surgical management.

Secondary glaucoma Secondary glaucoma can occur as a complication of a systemic disease, or result from a local disorder of the eye. Systemic diseases and drugs that may be associated with glaucoma are (1) hematologic diseases: leukemia, sickle cell disease, Waldenström's macroglobulinemia; (2) collagen diseases: ankylosing spondylitis, rheumatoid arthritis, sarcoidosis; (3) diseases of the skin:

atopic diseases (corticosteroid use), nevus of Ota; (4) infectious diseases: congenital rubella, onchocerciasis; (5) metabolic diseases: amyloidosis, Marchesani's syndrome; (6) musculoskeletal disorders: Conradi's syndrome, osteogenesis imperfecta; (7) neoplastic disease: metastases to the trabecular meshwork; (8) phacomatoses: neurofibromatosis, Sturge-Weber syndrome; (9) pulmonary diseases: asthma and emphysema (corticosteroid use); (10) renal diseases: Lowe's syndrome (aminoaciduria), Wilms's tumor, renal transplantation (corticosteroid use); (11) toxic substances: amphetamines, corticosteroids, hexamethonium, reserpine; and (12) anticholinergic drugs. Local eye disorders causing glaucoma include ocular trauma and dislocation of the lens, as occurs in homocystinuria and Marfan's syndrome.

THE LENS AND CATARACT A cataract is an opacity of the lens; the opacity may be located in the center of the lens (nuclear), in the superficial cortical region, or in the posterior subcapsular area. Cataracts may be congenital or acquired. Lens fibers opacify in response to alterations of the physical and chemical milieu within the semipermeable lens capsule.

Congenital cataracts occur in rubella, herpes simplex, syphilis, and cytomegalic inclusion disease. Acquired cataracts can result from trauma, radiation, drugs, metabolic disorders or aging (senile cataracts). Two types of cataracts are described in diabetes mellitus: metabolic (or snowflake) and senile. Snowflake cataracts are common in insulin-dependent diabetics and begin in the subcapsular region. Senile cataracts occur at an earlier age in diabetics than in control subjects and mature more rapidly. Other metabolic disorders frequently complicated by cataracts include hypocalcemia (Chap. 366), galactosemia (Chap. 314), and hypoglycemia. Cataracts located in the posterior lens occur in more than one-third of patients with myotonic dystrophy. Systemic corticosteroid treatment promotes formation of posterior subcapsular cataracts. Cataracts may also be associated with the following: (1) chromosomal disorders: Alport's syndrome, cri-du-chat syndrome, Conradi's syndrome, Crouzon's syndrome, Turner's syndrome; (2) metabolic and nutritional diseases: aminoaciduria (Lowe's syndrome), Fabry's disease, hypervitaminosis D, hypoparathyroidism, hypothyroidism, mucopolysaccharidoses, Wilson's disease; (3) infectious diseases: acquired cysticercosis, leprosy, onchocerciasis, and toxoplasmosis; (4) toxic substances: corticosteroids, haloperidol, and miotics.

Visual symptoms of cataract include glare, image blur for near visual tasks, image duplication (monocular diplopia), altered color perception, and impaired visual acuity. Cataract extraction may lead to complete visual rehabilitation.

Dislocation or subluxation of the lens (ectopia lentis) can occur in homocystinuria (Chap. 306) and in Marfan's syndrome (Chap. 319) (Fig. A4-15). Dislocation may precipitate glaucoma in these conditions.

VITREOUS HUMOR The vitreous humor undergoes significant physical and biochemical changes with aging. The commonest vitreous opacities are benign "floaters" which appear to patients as gray or black spots or elongated, irregular objects that move with eye movement. Vitreous hemorrhage usually arises from retinal vessels; it may be diffusely dispersed in the vitreous cavity. Massive hemorrhages may reduce vision severely. Vitreous hemorrhage and membrane formation are seen in diabetic retinopathy, retinal vein occlusion, sickle cell retinopathy, congenital retinal vascular anomalies, trauma, disciform macular lesions, choroidal malignant melanoma, and subarachnoid hemorrhage. Asteroid hyalitis (Benson's disease) is characterized by tiny yellow vitreous opacities containing calcium soaps (palmitate and stearate). This condition, which represents dystrophy of the vitreous, can occur in diabetics, but is also a frequent finding in patients with no known ocular disease. Vitreous opacifications can also occur in primary amyloidosis. In reticulum cell sarcoma and retinoblastoma, tumor cells may be seen floating freely in the vitreous. Vitrectomy, the most significant advance in the treatment of vitreous disease, is used to clear vitreous opacities and relieve or prevent vitreoretinal traction. Vitreous biopsy may be useful in establishing the diagnosis in suspected amyloidosis or reticulum cell sarcoma.

THE RETINA Retinal vasculopathies that are potentially blinding are associated with many major medical conditions. The severity of the arterial changes in hypertensive retinopathy, for example, correlates closely with the level of systemic hypertension. Grade I shows moderate arteriolar attenuation and a silver-wire arteriolar reflex; grade II is characterized by arteriovenous crossing defects, hard exudates, and splinter hemorrhages; grade III includes retinal edema, hemorrhages, and cotton-wool spots, the latter due to focal ischemia in the nerve fiber layer; grade IV combines all the signs of grade III plus papilledema, often with a macular star of hard exudates.

Cotton-wool spots are the hallmark of malignant hypertension, but they are also found in anemia, leukemia, collagen vascular diseases, dysproteinemia, infective endocarditis, and diabetes mellitus. They are the most common ophthalmic lesion in acquired immunodeficiency syndrome (AIDS); other retinal manifestations in AIDS may include cytomegalovirus retinitis and retinal periphlebitis.

Diabetic retinopathy is classified into two groups: (1) background retinopathy characterized by microaneurysms, hemorrhages, cotton-wool spots, hard exudates, intraretinal microvascular shunt vessels, and venous bleeding; and (2) proliferative retinopathy characterized by neovascularization and macular edema, which commonly leads to a decrease in visual acuity to 20/200 or worse. Panretinal photocoagulation is beneficial in delaying blindness in such patients.

Permanent blindness can result if the retina is infarcted due to occlusion of the central retinal artery (CRA). Funduscopic examination shows boxcar segmentation of blood flow in the retinal veins, an opaque milky white retina and a central cherry red spot due to visualization of the vascular choroid (Fig. A4-2). CRA occlusion is an ophthalmic emergency and paracentesis of aqueous humor to reduce IOP is the best method to increase blood flow. Embolization of the CRA should be suspected in cases where atheroma is present in the ipsilateral internal carotid artery, aorta, or heart. Other causes of CRA occlusion include giant cell (temporal) arteritis, arteriosclerosis, collagen vascular disease, and hyperviscosity states. Monocular transient blurring of vision (amaurosis fugax) may herald CRA occlusion and/or an impending stroke. Patients with this symptom need urgent attention (see Chaps. 343 and 352).

Venous retinopathies can also threaten vision. Central retinal vein (Fig. A4-3) and branch vein occlusion (common in hypertension) and low-pressure venous stasis retinopathy due to impaired retinal perfusion may occur in carotid occlusive disease, pulseless disease, macroglobulinemia, and polycythemia.

The systemic coagulopathies (thrombocytopenia and disseminated intravascular coagulopathy) may cause retinal hemorrhages or clotting in the submacular choriocapillaries, sometimes associated with choroidal hemorrhage and detachment of the retina. Patients complain of blurred vision due to a focal loss of vision (scotoma). Retinal vascular anomalies are rare. They include retinal telangiectasia (Coat's disease), retinal angiomatosis (von Hippel's disease, Chap. 351) and arteriovenous cirsoid aneurysm (Wyburn-Mason syndrome).

Aside from the visible vascular lesions, other alterations of the retina may also impair vision. The most important of these are detachment or tears of the retina. Retinal degeneration can take several forms:

Retinal degeneration Degeneration of the outer receptor layer and subjacent pigment epithelium occurs as a hereditary trait in retinitis pigmentosa. This condition presents with loss of night vision followed by deficits in peripheral and eventually central vision. Multisystem disorders that include retinal degeneration are abetalipoproteinemia (Bassen-Kornzweig syndrome, Chap. 355), neuronal lipofuscinosis (Batten-Mayou disease, Chap. 350), Refsum's disease Chap. 355), and the Kearns-Sayre syndrome (Chap. 357).

Degeneration of Bruch's membrane Bruch's membrane supports the layer of pigment epithelium adjacent to the rods and cones.

Degeneration results in angioid streaks (breaks) which extend from the disc to the equator. Angioid streaks signify the frequent association of widespread degenerative changes involving elastic tissue elsewhere, such as occur in pseudoxanthoma elasticum, Paget's disease, lead poisoning, and familial hyperphosphatemia.

Degeneration of the outer retinal layers This may occur as a toxic side effect of phenothiazine drugs. These drugs conjugate with the melanin of the pigment layer and should be used in the lowest therapeutic dosages possible. Central visual fields should be tested at 3-month intervals with small red and white test objects in patients receiving chronic therapy with these agents.

Degeneration of the inner retinal layers This may occur as a toxic side effect of chloroquine and hydroxychloroquine.

THE CHOROID Diseases affecting the choroid are uncommon and are discussed in the *Manual of Ocular Diagnosis and Therapy.*

THE OPTIC DISC Elevation or swelling of the optic disc occurs in papilledema (Fig. A4-4), papillitis, optic disc drusen (Fig. A4-5), infiltration of the nerve head by malignant cells, and many other conditions.

True papilledema due to axonal swelling and axoplasmic stasis is caused by elevation of the intracranial cerebrospinal fluid (CSF) pressure which is transmitted to the subarachnoid space around the optic nerves. Visual acuity is minimally affected at first except for transient visual obscurations, constriction of the visual fields, and enlargement of the blind spots (Fig. 13-1C). Vascular changes, i.e., hyperemia, venous congestion, and hemorrhage, are secondary phenomena in papilledema. As a general rule, the presence of spontaneous venous pulsations on the disc indicates that the CSF pressure is not elevated. The term *pseudopapilledema* refers to congenitally elevated discs secondary to hyaloid tissue (drusen) or hyperopia.

Papillitis is the term used to describe disc swelling associated with optic neuritis and is accompanied by early visual loss. Papillitis can occur with inflammation, demyelination of the optic nerve (multiple sclerosis, neuromyelitis optica), degeneration (Leber's optic neuropathy), malignant cell infiltration, or vascular disorders of the nerve head. It is important to distinguish this condition from *retrobulbar optic neuritis,* which is characterized by demyelinative lesions of the nerve that intitially show no abnormality in the fundus or disc. Retrobulbar neuritis causes visual loss and an afferent pupillary constriction defect in the light reflex. A comparison of the direct response of the pupil to light in each eye with that elicited indirectly (consensual response) is important to localize the side of the afferent defect. The test to determine this is sometimes called the swinging flashlight test. A Marcus Gunn pupil is a pupil that shows a better constriction to an indirect response than to direct light.

Retrobulbar optic neuritis must be differentiated from hysterical visual loss (steropsis intact, no afferent pupil defect). A history of trauma, drug abuse, toxic exposure, or alcoholism is important to the diagnosis. In young adults, with idiopathic optic neuritis (papillitis or retrobulbar), the risk of developing multiple sclerosis is approximately 30 to 40 percent (Chap. 348). In elderly patients, on the other hand, a common cause of loss of visual acuity and field defects is infarction of the optic nerve (anterior ischemic optic neuropathy) (Fig. A4-6) due to giant cell (temporal) arteritis, nonarteritic arteriosclerosis, or emboli to the posterior ciliary circulation.

Optic disc pallor (Fig. A4-7) is the sequel to most optic nerve lesions, and three etiologic processes are recognized: (1) heredofamilial optic atrophy (Fig. A4-7); (2) primary optic atrophy consequent to death of retinal ganglion cells and axons, and (3) secondary optic atrophy following papillitis and chronic papilledema.

THE CENTRAL VISUAL PATHWAY Visual disturbances can be caused by defects in the retina, optic nerve, chiasm, and tracts, lateral geniculate nucleus, geniculocalcarine path, and striate cortex of the occipital lobes. Retinal lesions cause arcuate scotomas defined as islands of impaired vision within the visual field that point directly to or emanate from the blind spot (Fig. 13-1A). Arcuate (nerve fiber

bundle) defects have a sharp border on the horizontal meridian and when extensive produce an altitudinal defect (Fig. 13-1B). Damage to the papillomacular bundle which subserves foveal visual fixation produces central (involving the fixation point) (Fig. 13-1D) or centrocecal (involving both the fixation point and the blind spot) scotomas (Fig. 13-1E). Small central scotomas in macular disease often cause distorted vision, particularly for straight lines (metamorphopsia), which aids in the distinction between a macular lesion and one in the optic nerve. A centrocecal scotoma (Fig. 13-1E) is a specific and common sign of optic nerve disease due to intrinsic (demyelinative, infiltrative, degenerative) and occasionally to extrinsic compressive lesions (aneurysms, tumor). Toxic states (methyl alcohol, quinine, and certain phenothiazine tranquilizing drugs) and nutritional disorders (tobacco-alcohol amblyopia) are characterized by relatively symmetric bilateral central or centrocecal scotomas. Progressive generalized constriction of peripheral isopters with relative sparing of central vision (Fig. 13-1G) may occur with circumferential compression by a tumor, e.g., a perioptic sheath meningioma.

FIGURE 13-1 *Types of monocular visual field loss in left eye. A. Superior arcuate scotoma (inferior nerve fiber bundle defect). B. Inferior altitudinal field defect respecting the horizontal meridian (superior nerve fiber bundle defect). C. Enlargement of the blind spot in the left eye. D. Central scotoma, normal blind spot. E. Centrocecal scotoma. F. Temporal hemianopsia respecting the vertical meridian but with involvement of central vision. G. Generalized constriction of the visual field to 2 isopters. H. Nonorganic "corkscrew" field defect to 1 isopter. (From Wray, 1985; by permission.)*

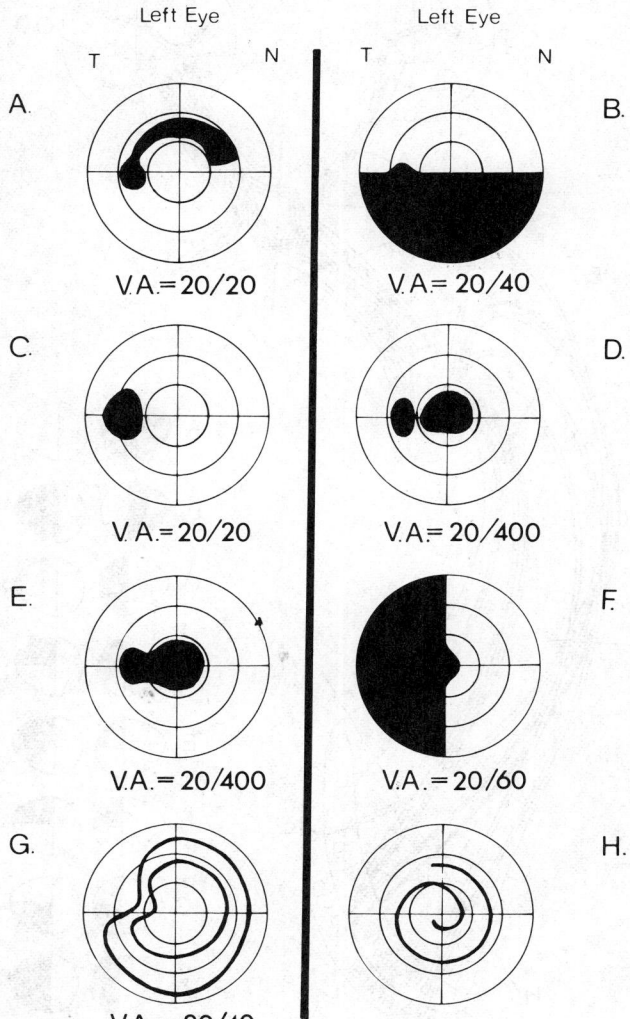

Types of Monocular Visual Field Loss

Nonorganic (hysteria, malingerer) corkscrew constriction (Fig. 13-1H) or tubular fields persist despite the distance tested. In organic defects, the outer circumference of the field loss will enlarge in a physiologic manner as the distance between the eye and the test object is increased. Hemianopsia means blindness in one-half of the visual field. The defect has a sharp border aligned to the vertical meridian (Figs. 13-1F, 13-2B, and 13-2C). Bitemporal hemianopsia (Fig. 13-2B) indicates a lesion of the decussating nasal retinal fibers

FIGURE 13-2 *Diagram showing the nerve fiber anatomy of the visual pathways from retina to occipital cortex. The effect on the fields of vision produced by lesions at various points along the optic pathway is shown on the right. A. complete blindness in left eye. B. Bitemporal hemianopsia. C. Nasal hemianopsia of left eye. D and E. Right incongruous homonymous hemianopsia. F and G. Right upper and lower homonymous quadrantanopia. H. complete right homonymous hemianopsia. Courtesy of DD Donaldson. (From Wray, 1985; by permission.)*

of the optic chiasm and is due usually to compression of the chiasm (pituitary tumor, craniopharyngioma, meningioma of the diaphragm of the sella, suprasellar aneurysm of the circle of Willis). Homonymous hemianopsia (a loss of vision in corresponding halves of the visual fields) (Fig. 13-2D to H) signifies a lesion of the visual pathway behind the chiasm and, if complete, gives no more information than that. Incomplete homonymous hemianopsia has more localizing value: if the field defects in the two eyes are identical (congruous), the lesion is likely to be in the calcarine cortex; if incongruous, the visual fibers in the optic tract or lateral geniculate nucleus or in the parietal or temporal radiations are more likely to be implicated.

In optic tract lesions, incongruous homonymous hemianopsia is characteristic. Chronic tract lesions are accompanied by an afferent pupil defect and transverse band optic atrophy in the contralateral eye. In postgeniculate lesions (Fig. 13-2B to H) the pupil reflexes are normal. Fibers from the lower quadrants of the retina extend for a variable distance into the temporal lobe; hence, lesions of this lobe may be accompanied by an homonymous upper quadrantic field defect (Fig. 13-2E to F). Parietal lobe lesions may affect the lower quadrants more than the upper (Fig. 13-2G), or cause a complete hemianopic defect due to inattention. A complete homonymous hemianopsia with splitting of the macula fibers results if the entire calcarine cortex is destroyed on one side (Fig. 13-2H). Macular sparing is frequently due to imperfect fixation. Bilateral homonymous hemianopsia results from bilateral, usually ischemic lesions of the visual cortex supplied by the posterior cerebral arteries. Permanent cortical blindness may result, and such patients may show *Anton's syndrome:* bilateral blindness, denial of blindness, normal pupil reflexes, and bilateral occipitoparietal infarcts.

Other disturbances of central vision include various types of distortion in which the perceived objects appear too small (micropsia), too large (macropsia), or askew. When bilateral, such phenomena suggest disease of the temporal lobes, in which case the visual disturbances tend to occur in attacks and may be accompanied by complex visual hallucinations, or other manifestations of temporal lobe seizures (Chap. 342).

In addition to the visual field examination, electrophysiologic techniques are valuable in the analysis of lesions of the anterior visual pathways—especially the flash electroretinogram (ERG), the pattern electroretinogram (P-ERG), and the pattern stimulus visual evoked response (VER) (see Chap. 341). The ERG measures the chain of graded electrical responses from each layer of the retina and can detect retinal disease before funduscopic changes are evident, e.g., in retinitis pigmentosa. However, the ERG is normal in diseases of the retinal ganglion cells and afferent visual pathways. The P-ERG is used as a marker of ganglion cell activity. Such activity is impaired or absent in disorders of the optic nerve secondary to retrograde ganglion cell loss (Leber's optic atrophy, demyelination). The VER is a macular dominant response recorded at the occipital pole of the cerebral cortex (Chap. 341). In the absence of retinal disease it evaluates primarily the function of the anterior visual pathways and particularly the optic nerve. The VER has been useful in establishing the diagnosis of multiple sclerosis by providing objective evidence of an optic nerve lesion even when other clinical signs of visual impairment are lacking (Chap. 348).

DISORDERS OF EYE MOVEMENT

THE ANATOMY OF EYE MOVEMENTS: THIRD, FOURTH, AND SIXTH NERVES AND CENTRAL CONNECTIONS Cranial nerves III, IV, and VI innervate the eye muscles. The oculomotor (third nerve) nuclear complex lies on either side of the midline in the rostral midbrain. It supplies five extraocular muscles including the levator muscle of the eyelid and contains the parasympathetic neurons (Edinger-Westphal nucleus) mediating pupillary constriction and accommodation. Subnuclear groups of motor neurons for individual eye muscles are anatomically distinct within the complex. Those for the medial rectus, inferior oblique, and inferior rectus are ipsilateral to the eye they innervate. The subnucleus for the superior rectus is contralateral to its muscle. The levator palpebrae superioris is innervated by a central group of cells. The motor neurons of the fourth nerve (trochlear) are continuous with the larger oculomotor complex. The left trochlear nucleus innervates the right superior oblique muscle and vice versa. The motor neurons of the sixth nerve (abducens), which innervates the ipsilateral lateral rectus muscle, lie in the abducens nuclei in the caudal pons. All three oculomotor nerves, after leaving the brainstem, pass through the cavernous sinus and enter the orbit through the superior orbital fissure. Accurate binocular vision is achieved by the associated action of individual ocular muscles which yoke the two eyes together.

Conjugate eye movements are controlled by supranuclear gaze centers and their connections. Functionally, there are five distinct supranuclear systems for gaze: *saccadic, pursuit, vergence, position maintenance fixation,* and *vestibular.* Ipsilateral *saccadic* (rapid) eye movements originate in the contralateral frontal cortical eye field (area 8), except for fovea-initiated movements occurring in response to visual stimuli, which arise from the occipitoparietal region. These frontal and occipital control centers project bilaterally to supranuclear brainstem centers, whose function is also modulated by inputs from the cerebellum and the vestibular complex. The paramedian pontine reticular formation (PPRF) acts as the brainstem center for conjugate saccadic eye movements. Simultaneous innervation of one medial rectus and the opposite lateral rectus, during horizontal gaze, is mediated through the medial longitudinal fasciculus (MLF) which connects one abducens nucleus with the contralateral medial rectus subnucleus in the oculomotor complex. Bilateral cortical input to the PPRF is required to initiate vertical saccades. The PPRF relays signals up the brainstem to the supranuclear vertical gaze center—the rostral interstitial nucleus of the medial longitudinal fasciculus (RiMLF)—located in the mesencephalon.

The cortical center for smooth *pursuit* or tracking motions of the eyes is located in the occipitoparietal region. The control is ipsilateral; i.e., the right occipitoparietal region controls smooth pursuit to the right. The control for *vergence* movements is less well understood, but the vergence neurons are known to be located in the mesencephalic reticular formation surrounding the oculomotor complex. They project to the motor neurons of the medial rectus muscle.

A brainstem center called the neural integrator is responsible for *position maintenance of fixation* (gaze-holding). This center converts eye velocity signals into eye position signals. Neurons with this dynamic property lie in the pons caudal to the abducens nucleus.

Coordination of eye movements in response to changes in gravitation and acceleration is mediated by the *vestibular system* (vestibular-ocular reflex) (see Chaps. 14 and 21). Diplopia develops if binocular fusion is impaired since images then fall on disparate (noncorresponding) parts of the two retinas. In *congenital strabismus* or squint, a muscle imbalance that results in improper alignment of the two eyes (nonparalytic strabismus) may result in the brain suppressing one image. The resulting diminished visual acuity in the nonfixing eye is called *amblyopia ex anopsia.* In *paralytic strabismus,* diplopia is due to paralysis of an eye muscle, usually secondary to a lesion of one of the third, fourth, or sixth cranial nerves.

OCULAR MUSCLE AND GAZE PALSIES   There are three types of paralysis of extraocular muscles: (1) paralysis of isolated ocular muscles, (2) paralysis of conjugate movements (gaze), and (3) mixed ocular and gaze paralysis.

Paralysis of isolated ocular muscles   Characteristic clinical disturbances result from single lesions of the third, fourth, and sixth cranial nerves. A complete third nerve lesion causes ptosis (paresis of levator palpebrae) and inability to turn the eye upward, downward, or inward; a divergent strabismus due to unopposed action of the lateral rectus muscle; a dilated nonreactive pupil (iridoplegia); and paralysis of accommodation (cycloplegia). When only the muscles

of the iris and ciliary body are paralyzed, the condition is termed *internal ophthalmoplegia.* Fourth nerve lesions (superior oblique palsy) result in extorsion of the eye and a weakness of downward gaze most marked when the eye is turned inward. Diplopia is corrected by head tilt to the opposite shoulder, which causes a compensatory intorsion of the unaffected eye.

A sixth nerve palsy results in paralysis of abduction and a convergent strabismus, owing to the unopposed action of the medial rectus muscle. With incomplete sixth nerve palsies, the patient may turn the head toward the side of the paretic muscle to overcome diplopia by compensating for the paretic lateral rectus muscle. The foregoing signs may occur with variable degrees of completeness, depending on the severity and site of the lesion or lesions.

Paralysis of conjugate gaze   The term conjugate gaze refers to the simultaneous movement of the two eyes in the same direction. An acute lesion in one frontal lobe, as occurs in infarction, may cause a transient paralysis of voluntary contralateral horizontal gaze with preservation of the full range of ocular movement elicited by doll's-head maneuver of passive head turning, or by a caloric stimulus (Chap. 21). A unilateral caudal PPRF lesion, at the level of the abducens nucleus, causes a permanent horizontal gaze palsy to the ipsilateral side and absent oculocephalic reflex movements. Lesions of the RiMLF in the rostral midbrain and/or a lesion of the posterior commissure produce a supranuclear paralysis of conjugate upward gaze and light-near dissociation of the pupils (pupils are sluggish in response to light but constrict briskly to near vision or accommodation). Occasionally, paralysis of convergence is also present. This grouping of signs, called Parinaud's syndrome, is seen in pineal region tumors, and occasionally with infarction, multiple sclerosis, or hydrocephalus. Isolated paralysis of downward gaze is rare. When it occurs, it is usually due to occlusion of a midline penetrating artery and bilateral midbrain infarction. With certain extrapyramidal degenerative disorders, e.g., Huntington's chorea and progressive supranuclear palsy, ocular movements may be limited in all directions, especially upward (Chap. 350).

Mixed gaze and ocular muscle paralyses   A combination of gaze paralysis and ocular muscle paralysis is usually a sign of mesencephalic or pontine disease. A lesion of the lower pons affecting the abducens nucleus may cause an ipsilateral horizontal saccadic palsy and sixth nerve palsy. Lesions of the MLF (internuclear ophthalmoplegia) interfere with horizontal gaze in a different way. Unilateral lesions caused by an infarct or demyelination of the MLF cause failure of full adduction of the eye. This may be observed as a complete paralysis with failure to adduct the eye past the midline, or as a mild subclinical paresis characterized by a decrease in the velocity of adducting saccades (adduction lag). In the eye contralateral to the MLF lesion, the main abnormality is abducting nystagmus: a gaze-evoked nystagmus on abduction with a slow centripetal drift toward the midline followed by rapid horizontal corrective saccades. *Skew deviation,* a vertical misalignment of the eyes, is common with unilateral internuclear ophthalmoplegia. The higher eye (hypertropia) is ipsilateral to the side of the lesion. Bilateral internuclear ophthalmoplegia caused by demyelination, tumor, infarct, or an arteriovenous malformation causes a more complete ocular motility syndrome characterized by bilateral adduction weakness, bilateral abduction nystagmus, and impaired vertical, vestibular, and pursuit eye movements. Impairment of ability to maintain vertical gaze is observed with an upbeat nystagmus on looking up and a downbeat (gaze-evoked) nystagmus on looking down. Convergence may be impaired in rostral midbrain MLF lesions.

NYSTAGMUS AND OTHER ENTITIES THAT MIMIC NYSTAGMUS
Nystagmus is a repetitive, to-and-fro movement of the eyes. The term includes two types of movements: *pendular nystagmus,* smooth sinusoidal oscillations, and *jerk nystagmus,* alternation of slow drift and corrective quick phase. Normal subjects show nystagmus in response to vestibular and optokinetic stimuli. Identification of the

cause of a patient's nystagmus requires historical information (especially drug use, alcohol) and a complete ocular motor evaluation.

Pathologic nystagmus is due to disorders of the mechanisms that maintain fixation. The vestibular, optokinetic, and pursuit systems each act to hold images steady on the retina, and a neural integrator enables the subject to hold eccentric positions of gaze. Disorders of these systems create nystagmus. The most important types of nystagmus are now discussed.

CONGENITAL NYSTAGMUS   Long-standing horizontal pendular or jerk nystagmus is characteristic. Occasionally congenital nystagmus is accompanied by anomalies of the visual pathways and impaired vision. The mechanism and site of the abnormality are unknown.

LABYRINTHINE-VESTIBULAR NYSTAGMUS   Disease of the vestibular apparatus causes constant velocity slow-phase drifts with corrective quick phases that create a "saw-tooth" jerk nystagmus (see also Chap. 14). Such unidirectional slow-phase drifts reflect an imbalance in the tonic neural activity of the vestibular nuclei. If, for example, disease occurs in one semicircular canal, there results a slow deviation of the eyes to the side of the lesion, followed by a quick corrective movement directed away from the side of the lesion. The abnormality is the slow drift to one side, but by convention the side of the nystagmus is designated by the direction of the quick corrective saccade (fast phase). Such an imbalance of vestibular tone usually causes *vertigo* and *oscillopsia* (illusory movement of the environment) (see Chap. 14). In peripheral vestibular disease, since more than one labyrinthine canal is nearly always affected, an imbalance results between inputs from individual semicircular canals, and the nystagmus is usually of mixed type. For example, in *benign positional nystagmus,* a mixed vertical-torsional nystagmus is common. In unilateral labyrinthine destruction, a mixed horizontal-torsional nystagmus occurs. Peripheral vestibular nystagmus is suppressed by fixation and exacerbated by changes in head position. With disturbances of central vestibular connections, there occurs a central imbalance between semicircular canal inputs, and disruption of ascending vestibular or cerebellar-vestibular connections. Central vestibular nystagmus may mimic nystagmus caused by disease of one semicircular canal, but purely bilateral vertical (upbeat, downbeat), torsional, or horizontal nystagmus is probably more common. This type of nystagmus is poorly suppressed by fixation, but exacerbated or induced by change in head position (Chap. 14). Three forms of labyrinthine-vestibular nystagmus are of clinical importance because of their anatomic localizing value—downbeat, upbeat, and horizontal (sidebeat) nystagmus.

Downbeat nystagmus is usually present in the primary position and is accentuated on lateral gaze. It occurs in posterior fossa anomalies such as the Arnold-Chiari malformation and basilar invagination, and in multiple sclerosis, cerebellar atrophy, hydrocephalus, metabolic disorders, familial periodic ataxia, or as a toxic side effect of anticonvulsant drugs. *Upbeat nystagmus* in the primary position occurs with lesions localized anatomically to the anterior vermis of the cerebellum. It occurs with diffuse brainstem disease (Wernicke's encephalopathy, meningitis, drug side effect). *Horizontal (sidebeat) primary position nystagmus* is usually due to peripheral vestibular disease and only rarely to a posterior fossa tumor, or Arnold-Chiari malformation.

GAZE-EVOKED NYSTAGMUS   This type of nystagmus is elicited by the eye assuming an eccentric position in the orbit. It implies a weakness in holding the eyes in the desired position due to defect in the neural integrator in the brainstem. Asymmetric but conjugate horizontal gaze–evoked nystagmus occurs with unilateral cerebellar disease and cerebello–pontine angle tumors (acoustic neuroma). A common cause is drugs (sedatives, anticonvulsants). Horizontal gaze nystagmus in which the quick phases of the adducting eye are slower than the abducting eye (dissociated nystagmus) is characteristic of internuclear ophthalmoplegia.

CONVERGENCE-RETRACTION NYSTAGMUS   This movement, stimulated by attempting to look up, is characterized by opposed adducting saccades that converge and retract the eyes. It is usually accompanied by other dorsal midbrain signs (Parinaud's syndrome).

PERIODIC ALTERNATING NYSTAGMUS   In this condition, horizontal nystagmus occurs in the primary position but reverses direction periodically, usually every 1 to 2 min. Gaze-evoked and downbeat nystagmus may accompany it. It occurs in a congenital form, with craniocervical junction anomalies, in multiple sclerosis, and with anticonvulsant intoxication. Baclofen usually abolishes the nystagmus and oscillopsia in acquired cases.

SEESAW NYSTAGMUS   The eyes show alternating movements. As one eye rises and intorts, the other falls and extorts. Seesaw nystagmus reflects an abnormality of the mesencephalic reticular nuclei including the interstitial nucleus of Cajal. It occurs with suprasellar tumors (craniopharyngioma), head trauma, and rarely with infarcts. Bitemporal hemianopsia frequently coexists.

OTHER ENTITIES THAT MIMIC NYSTAGMUS   A variety of motility disorders can mimic nystagmus. These include square-wave jerks (small horizontal saccades away from fixation and back), ocular flutter (horizontal oscillations), opsoclonus (back-to-back saccadic oscillations), superior oblique myokymia (monocular torsional-vertical movements), ocular bobbing (rapid downward deviation of the eyes with slow drift up), and ping-pong gaze (periodic horizontal deviation of the eyes changing direction every few seconds. These conditions are discussed in detail by Leigh and Zee.

This chapter began with an analogy—the eye as a mirror reflecting the body's health. It closes with an analogy that is less passive: that disturbances of vision and ocular movement are in fact diagnostic distress flags whose recognition can significantly expand the physician's understanding. Those internists who truly are alert to the signals the eye can send will not only recognize them, they will read them.

REFERENCES

ANDERSON DR: *Testing the Field of Vision.* St. Louis, Mosby, 1982

BURDE RM et al: *Clinical Decisions in Neuro-ophthalmology.* St. Louis, Mosby, 1985

COGAN D: *Ophthalmic Manifestations of Systemic Vascular Disease*, vol 3. Philadelphia, Saunders, 1974

LEIGH RJ, ZEE DS: *The Neurology of Eye Movement.* Philadelphia, Davis, 1983

PAVAN-LANGSTON D (ed): *Manual of Ocular Diagnosis and Therapy,* 2d ed. Boston, Little, Brown, 1985

ROSE CF: *The Eye in General Medicine.* London, Chapman & Hall, 1983

WALL M, WRAY SH: The one-and-a-half syndrome—a unilateral disorder of the pontine tegmentum: A study of 20 cases and a review of the literature. Neurology 33:971, 1983

WRAY SH: Neuro-ophthalmologic diseases, in *The Clinical Neurosciences*, RN Rosenberg et al (eds). New York, Churchill Livingstone, 1983

WRAY SH: Neuro-ophthalmology: Visual fields, optic nerve, and pupil, in *Manual of Ocular Diagnosis and Therapy*, 2d ed, D Pavan-Langston (ed). Boston, Little, Brown, 1985

14   DIZZINESS AND VERTIGO

ROBERT B. DAROFF

Dizziness is a common and often vexing symptom. Patients use the term to encompass a variety of sensations including those which seem semantically appropriate (e.g., lightheadedness, fainting, spinning, giddiness, etc.) as well as those which are seemingly inappropriate, such as blurred vision, blindness, headache, tingling, "walking on cotton," etc. Moreover, some patients with gait disturbances will describe their problem as "dizziness." A careful history is necessary to determine exactly what a patient who states, "Doctor, I'm dizzy," is experiencing.

After eliminating misleading sensations such as blurred vision, ''dizziness'' usually means either *faintness* (analogous to the feelings that precede syncope) or *vertigo* (an illusory sense of environmental or bodily movement). In other instances, none of these terms accurately describes a patient's symptoms, and the explanation may only become apparent when the neurologic examination reveals spasticity, parkinsonism, or other ambulation disturbances as the cause of the complaint. Operationally, dizziness is classified into four categories: (1) faintness, (2) vertigo, (3) miscellaneous head sensation, and (4) gait disturbances.

FAINTNESS   Fainting (syncope) is a loss of consciousness secondary to cerebral ischemia, more specifically ischemia to the brainstem (see Chap. 12). Prior to the actual faint, there are often prodromal symptoms (*faintness*) reflecting ischemia to a degree insufficient to impair consciousness. The sequence of symptoms is reasonably stereotyped and includes increasing lightheadedness, visual blurring proceeding to blindness, and heaviness in the lower limbs progressing to postural sway. The symptoms increase in severity until consciousness is lost or the ischemia is corrected, often by assumption of the recumbent position. True vertigo almost never occurs during the presyncopal state.

The causes of faintness are described in Chap. 12 and include the multiple etiologies of decreased cardiac output, postural (orthostatic) hypotension, and mimics such as vertebrobasilar insufficiency and seizures.

VERTIGO   Vertigo is an illusion of self- or environmental movement, most commonly a feeling of spinning, usually due to a disturbance in the vestibular system. The end organs of this system, situated in the bony labyrinths of the inner ears, consist of the three semicircular canals and the otolithic apparatus (utricle and saccule) on each side. The canals transduce angular acceleration while the otoliths transduce linear acceleration and static gravitational forces, the latter providing a sense of head position in space. The neural output of the end organs is conveyed to the vestibular nuclei in the brainstem via the eighth cranial nerves. The principal projections from the vestibular nuclei are to the nuclei of cranial nerves III, IV, and VI, the spinal cord, cerebral cortex, and cerebellum. The vestibuloocular reflex serves to maintain visual stability during head movement and depends upon direct projections from the vestibular nuclei to the sixth cranial nerve (abducens) nuclei in the pons and, via the medial longitudinal fasciculus, to the third (oculomotor) and fourth (trochlear) cranial nerve nuclei in the midbrain. These connections account for the nystagmus (to-and-fro oscillation of the eyes) which is an almost invariable accompaniment of vestibular dysfunction. The vestibulospinal pathways assist in the maintenance of postural stability. Projections to the cerebral cortex, via the thalamus, provide conscious awareness of head position and movement. The vestibular nerves and nuclei project to areas of the cerebellum (primarily the flocculus and nodulus) which modulate the vestibuloocular reflex.

The vestibular system is one of three sensory systems subserving spatial orientation and posture; the other two are the visual system (retina to occipital cortex) and the somatosensory system that conveys peripheral information from skin, joint, and muscle receptors. The three stabilizing systems overlap sufficiently to compensate (partially or completely) for each other's deficiencies. Vertigo may represent either physiologic stimulation or pathologic dysfunction in any of the three systems.

Physiologic vertigo   This occurs when (1) the brain is confronted with a mismatch among the three stabilizing systems or (2) the vestibular system is subjected to unfamiliar head movements to which it has never adapted, such as in seasickness. Intersensory mismatch explains carsickness, height vertigo, and the visual vertigo most commonly experienced during motion picture chase scenes; in the latter the visual sensation of environmental movement is unaccompanied by concomitant vestibular and somatosensory movement cues. *Space sickness*, a frequent transient effect of active head movement in the weightless zero-gravity environment, is another example of physiologic vertigo.

Pathologic vertigo   This results from lesions of the visual, somatosensory, or vestibular systems. Visual vertigo is caused by new or incorrect spectacles or by the sudden onset of an extraocular muscle paresis with diplopia; in either instance, central nervous system compensation rapidly counteracts the vertigo. Somatosensory vertigo, rare in isolation, is usually due to a peripheral neuropathy which reduces the sensory input necessary for central compensation when there is dysfunction of the vestibular or visual systems.

The most common cause of pathologic vertigo is vestibular dysfunction. The vertigo is frequently accompanied by nausea, jerk nystagmus, postural unsteadiness, and gait ataxia.

LABYRINTHINE DYSFUNCTION   This causes severe rotational or linear vertigo with the illusion of movement, whether of environment or self, directed away from the side of the lesion. The fast phases of nystagmus beat away from the lesion side, and the tendency to fall is toward the side of the lesion.

When the head is straight and immobile, the vestibular end organs generate a tonic resting firing frequency which is equal from the two sides. With any rotational acceleration, the anatomic positions of the semicircular canals on each side necessitate an increased firing rate from one and a commensurate decrease from the other. This change in neural activity is ultimately projected to the cerebral cortex where it is summed with inputs from the visual and somatosensory systems to produce the appropriate conscious sense of rotational movement. The end organs' response to deceleration continues for some time after cessation of prolonged rotation. The side with the initially increased firing rate decreases below the steady state level and the other side increases. A sense of rotation in the opposite direction is experienced; since there is no actual head movement, this illusory sensation is *vertigo*. Any disease state that changes the firing frequency of an end organ, producing unequal neural input to the brainstem and ultimately the cerebral cortex, causes vertigo. The symptom can be conceptualized as the cortex inappropriately interpreting the abnormal neural input from the brainstem as indicating actual head rotation. Transient deficits produce short-lived symptoms. With a fixed unilateral deficit, central compensatory mechanisms ultimately diminish the vertigo. Since compensation depends upon plasticity of connections between the vestibular nuclei and cerebellum, patients with brainstem or cerebellar disease have diminished adaptive capacity and symptoms may persist indefinitely. Compensation is always inadequate for severe fixed bilateral lesions despite normal cerebellar connections; these patients are symptomatic indefinitely.

Acute unilateral labyrinthine dysfunction is caused by infection, trauma, ischemia, and toxins (usually drugs or alcohol). Often, no specific etiology is uncovered and the nonspecific term *acute labyrinthitis* or, preferably, *acute peripheral vestibulopathy* is used to describe the event. It is impossible to determine whether a patient recovering from the first bout of vertigo will have recurrent episodes.

Schwannomas involving the eighth cranial nerve (*acoustic neuroma*) grow slowly and produce such a gradual reduction of labyrinthine output that central compensatory mechanisms usually prevent or minimize the vertigo; auditory symptoms of hearing loss and tinnitus are the most common manifestations. While lesions of the brainstem or cerebellum can cause acute vertigo, associated signs and symptoms permit distinction from a labyrinthine etiology (Table 14-1). Rarely, an acute lesion of the vestibulocerebellum may present with monosymptomatic vertigo indistinguishable from a labyrinthopathy.

Recurrent unilateral labyrinthine dysfunction, in association with signs and symptoms of cochlear disease (progressive hearing loss and tinnitus), is usually due to Ménière's disease. When auditory manifestations are absent, the term *vestibular neuronitis* denotes recurrent monosymptomatic vertigo. Transient ischemic attacks of the posterior cerebral circulation (vertebrobasilar insufficiency) almost never cause recurrent vertigo without concomitant motor, sensory, cranial nerve, or cerebellar signs.

Positional vertigo is precipitated by a recumbent head position, either to the right or to the left. Benign paroxysmal positional vertigo

TABLE 14-1 Differentiation of peripheral and central vertigo

Sign or symptom	Peripheral (labyrinth)	Central (brainstem or cerebellum)
Direction of associated nystagmus	Unidirectional; fast phase opposite lesion*	Bidirectional or unidirectional
Purely horizontal nystagmus without torsional component	Uncommon	Common
Vertical or purely torsional nystagmus	Never present	May be present
Visual fixation	Inhibits nystagmus and vertigo	No inhibition
Severity of vertigo	Marked	Often mild
Direction of spin	Toward fast phase	Variable
Direction of fall	Toward slow phase	Variable
Duration of symptoms	Finite (minutes, days, weeks) but recurrent	May be chronic
Tinnitus and/or deafness	Often present	Usually absent
Associated central abnormalities	None	Extremely common
Common causes	Infection (labyrinthitis), Ménière's, neuronitis, ischemia, trauma, toxin	Vascular or demyelinating disease, neoplasm, trauma

In Ménière's disease, the fast phase is variable in direction.

(BPPV) is particularly common. Although the condition may be due to head trauma, usually no precipitating factors are identified. It generally abates spontaneously after weeks or months. The vertigo and accompanying nystagmus have a distinct pattern of latency, fatigability, and habituation that differs from the less common central positional vertigo (Table 14-2) due to lesions in and around the fourth ventricle.

Position*al* must be distinguished from position*ing* vertigo. The latter is provoked by head movement rather than head position and is an invariable feature of *all* vestibulopathies, central or peripheral. Since vertigo increases with quick head movements, patients tend to hold their heads still.

Vestibular epilepsy, vertigo secondary to temporal lobe epileptic activity, is rare, and almost always intermixed with other epileptic manifestations.

Psychogenic vertigo, usually a concomitant of agoraphobia (fear of large open spaces, crowds, or leaving the safety of home), should be suspected in patients so "incapacitated" by their symptoms that they adopt a prolonged housebound status. Despite their discomfort, most patients with organic vertigo attempt to function. Vertigo should be accompanied by nystagmus; a psychogenic etiology is almost certain when nystagmus is absent during a vertiginous episode.

EVALUATION OF PATIENTS WITH PATHOLOGIC VESTIBULAR VERTIGO
The evaluation depends upon whether a central etiology is suspected (Table 14-1). If so, computerized tomography, with emphasis upon the posterior fossa, is mandatory. Such an examination is rarely helpful in cases of recurrent monosymptomatic vertigo with a normal

TABLE 14-2 Benign paroxysmal positional (BPPV) and central positional vertigo

Features	BPPV	Central
Latency*	3–40 s	None: immediate vertigo and nystagmus
Fatigability†	Yes	No
Habituation‡	Yes	No
Intensity of vertigo	Severe	Mild
Reproducibility§	Variable	Good

* Time between attaining head position and onset of symptoms.*
† *Disappearance of symptoms with maintenance of offending position.*
‡ *Lessening of symptoms with repeated trials.*
§ *Likelihood of symptom production during any examination session.*

neurologic examination. BPPV requires no investigation after the diagnosis is made (Table 14-2).

Vestibular function tests serve to (1) demonstrate an abnormality when the distinction between organic and psychogenic is uncertain, (2) establish the side of the abnormality, and (3) distinguish between peripheral and central etiologies. The standard test is electronystagmography (ENG) where warm and cold water (or air) is applied, in a prescribed fashion, to the tympanic membranes, and the slow phase velocities of the resultant nystagmus from the right and left ears are compared. A velocity decrease from one side indicates hypofunction ("canal paresis"). An inability to induce nystagmus with ice water denotes a "dead labyrinth." Some institutions have the capability of quantitatively determining various aspects of the vestibuloocular reflex using computer-driven rotational chairs and precise oculographic recording of eye movements.

Treatment of acute vertigo consists of bed rest and vestibular suppressant drugs such as antihistaminics (meclizine, dimenhydrinate, promethazine), centrally acting anticholinergics (scopolamine) or a tranquilizer with GABA-ergic effects (diazepam). If the vertigo persists beyond a few days, most authorities advise ambulation in an attempt to induce central compensatory mechanisms, despite the short-term discomfiture to the patient. Chronic vertigo of labyrinthine origin may be treated with a systematized exercise program to facilitate compensation.

Prophylactic measures to prevent recurrent vertigo are variably effective. Antihistamines are commonly utilized. Ménière's disease may respond to a low-salt diet combined with a diuretic. The unusual examples of persisting (beyond 4 to 6 weeks) BPPV respond dramatically, usually within 7 to 10 days, to a specific exercise program.

There are a variety of surgical procedures for all forms of refractory chronic or recurrent vertigo, but these are only rarely necessary.

MISCELLANEOUS HEAD SENSATIONS This designation is used, primarily for purposes of initial classification, to describe dizziness which is neither faintness nor vertigo. However, cephalic ischemia or vestibular dysfunction may be of such low intensity that the usual symptomology is not clearly identified. For example, a small decrease in blood pressure or a slight vestibular imbalance may cause sensations different than distinct faintness or vertigo but which may be identified properly during provocative testing techniques. Other causes of dizziness in this category are hyperventilation syndrome, hypoglycemia, and the somatic symptoms of a clinical depression. All these patients should have normal neurologic examinations.

GAIT DISTURBANCES Some individuals with gait disorders complain of dizziness despite the absence of vertigo or other abnormal cephalic sensations. The causes include peripheral neuropathy, myelopathy, spasticity, parkinsonian rigidity, and cerebellar ataxia. In this context, the term dizziness is being used to describe disturbed mobility. There may be associated lightheadedness, particularly with impaired sensation from the feet or poor vision; this is known as *multiple sensory defect dizziness* and occurs in elderly individuals who complain of dizziness only during ambulation. Decreased position sense (secondary to neuropathy or myelopathy) and poor vision (from cataracts or retinal degeneration) create an overreliance on the aging vestibular apparatus. A less precise, but sometimes comforting, designation is *benign dysequilibrium of aging.*

EVALUATION OF THE DIZZY PATIENT The most important diagnostic tool is a careful history focused upon the meaning of "dizziness" to the patient. Is it faintness? Is there a sensation of spinning? If either of these is affirmed, and the neurologic examination is normal, appropriate investigations for the multiple etiologies of cephalic ischemia or vestibular dysfunction are undertaken.

When the source of the dizziness is uncertain, provocative tests may be helpful. These office procedures simulate either cephalic ischemia or vestibular dysfunction. The former becomes obvious if the dizziness is duplicated during orthostatic hypotension. Further provocation involves the Valsalva maneuver, which decreases cerebral blood flow and should reproduce ischemic symptoms.

The simplest provocative test for vestibular dysfunction is rapid rotation and abrupt cessation of movement in a swivel chair. This always induces vertigo which the patient can compare to his or her symptomatic dizziness. The intense induced vertigo may be unlike the spontaneous symptoms but shortly thereafter, when the vertigo has all but subsided, a lightheadedness supervenes which may be identified as "my dizziness." When this occurs, the dizzy patient, originally classified as suffering from "miscellaneous head sensations," is now properly diagnosed as having mild vertigo secondary to a vestibulopathy.

Another technique for provoking vertigo is with caloric testing. A tympanic membrane is irrigated with cold water until vertigo is induced; the sensation is then compared to the patient's complaint. Since visual fixation inhibits the caloric response, provocative caloric testing (as distinct from the diagnostic quantitative calorics of ENG) is best performed with the eyes closed or using special spectacles which preclude visual fixation (Frenzel lenses). Patients with symptoms of positional vertigo should be appropriately tested (Table 14-2); as with provocative calorics, positional testing is more sensitive when visual fixation is eliminated.

A final provocative test, requiring the use of Frenzel lenses, is vigorous head shaking in the horizontal plane for about 10 s. If nystagmus develops after the shaking stops, even in the absence of vertigo, vestibular dysfunction is demonstrated. The maneuver can then be repeated in the vertical plane. If the provocative tests establish the dizziness as a vestibular symptom, the previously described evaluation of vestibular vertigo is undertaken.

Hyperventilation is the cause of dizziness in many anxious individuals; tingling of the hands and face may be absent. Two minutes of forced hyperventilation is indicated for patients with enigmatic dizziness and normal neurologic examinations. Similarly, depressive symptoms (which patients usually insist are "secondary" to the dizziness) must alert the examiner to a clinical depression as the *cause*, rather than the effect, of the dizziness.

Central nervous system disease can produce dizzy sensations of all types. Consequently, a neurologic examination is always required even if the history or provocative tests suggest a cardiac, peripheral vestibular, or psychogenic etiology. Any abnormality on the neurologic examination should prompt appropriate neurodiagnostic studies.

REFERENCES

Baloh RW: *Dizziness, Hearing Loss, and Tinnitus: The Essentials of Neurotology.* Philadelphia, Davis, 1984

Brandt T, Daroff RB: The multisensory physiological and pathological vertigo syndromes. Ann Neurol 7:195, 1980

Hinchcliffe FR: *Hearing and Balance in the Elderly.* New York, Churchill Livingston, 1983, section II, pp 227–488

Leigh RJ, Zee DS: *The Neurology of Eye Movements.* Philadelphia, Davis, 1984, Chaps 2 and 9

Oosterveld WJ: Vertigo—Current concepts in management. Drugs 30:275, 1985

15 PARALYSIS AND OTHER DISORDERS OF MOVEMENT

JOHN H. GROWDON / ROBERT R. YOUNG

Impairments of motor function may be subdivided into (1) paralysis due to disorders of bulbar or spinal motor neurons, (2) paralysis due to lesions of corticospinal, corticobulbar, or brainstem descending (subcorticospinal) neurons, (3) abnormalities of coordination (ataxia) due to lesions in the cerebellar system, including its inputs and outputs, (4) abnormalities of movement and posture due to disease of the extrapyramidal motor system, and (5) apraxic or nonparalytic disturbances of purposive movement due to involvement of the cerebrum. This chapter reviews those symptoms and signs which result from lesions of lower motor neurons, descending corticospinal and other tracts, and the extrapyramidal system. It also includes consideration of apraxic disorders. The cerebellar system is discussed in Chap. 16.

THE MOTOR SYSTEM

DEFINITIONS When applied to voluntary muscles, *paralysis* means loss of contraction due to interruption of one or more motor pathways from the cerebrum to the muscle fiber. In everyday medical parlance motor paralysis usually stands for either partial or complete loss of function; it is preferable to use *paresis* for slight and *paralysis* or *plegia* for severe loss of motor function. In addition to weakness, lack of facility of movement is an important functional deficit.

PARALYSIS DUE TO DISEASE OF THE LOWER MOTOR NEURONS
Each motor nerve cell, through the extensive arborization of the terminal part of its fiber, comes into contact with hundreds of muscle fibers; altogether they constitute "the motor unit." All variations in force and type of movement are determined by differences in the number and size of motor units called into activity, the frequency of their actions, and the patterns of activity in different muscles. Feeble movements recruit few units, stronger ones many more units of increasing size. Motor units involved in tonic contractions (type I) have muscle fibers rich in oxidative enzymes and mitochondria, and those involved in powerful, phasic contractions (type II) are anaerobic. When a motor neuron becomes diseased, as in progressive muscular atrophy, its axon may manifest increased irritability, and all the muscle fibers that it controls may discharge sporadically, in isolation from other units. The result of the contraction of one or several such units is a visible twitch, or *fasciculation*, which can be recorded in the electromyogram (EMG). If the motor neuron or its axon is destroyed, all the muscle fibers to which it is attached undergo a profound denervation atrophy. Individual denervated muscle fibers begin to be hypersensitive and to contract spontaneously, though they can no longer do so in response to a nerve impulse. Isolated activity of individual muscle fibers is called *fibrillation;* it is so fine that it cannot be seen through the intact skin and can be recorded only as a short-duration spike potential in the EMG. Motor nerve fibers of each anterior root intermingle with those from adjacent roots and join to form plexuses. Although the innervation of muscles is roughly according to segments of the spinal cord, each large muscle is supplied by two or more roots. In contrast, a single peripheral nerve usually provides the complete motor innervation of a muscle or group of muscles. For this reason the distribution of paralysis due to disease of the anterior horn cells or anterior roots differs from that which follows a lesion of a peripheral nerve.

Lower motor neuron paralysis is the direct result of physiologic block or destruction of anterior horn cells or their axons in anterior roots and nerves. The signs and symptoms vary according to the location of the lesion. Probably the most important question for clinical purposes is whether sensory changes coexist. The combination of flaccid, areflexic paralysis and sensory loss usually indicates involvement of mixed motor and sensory nerves or affection of both anterior and posterior roots. If sensory changes are absent, the lesion must be situated in the gray matter of the spinal cord, in the anterior roots, in a purely motor branch of a peripheral nerve, or in motor axons alone. The distinction between nuclear (spinal) and anterior root (radicular) lesions may at times be impossible to make.

All motor activity, even of the most elementary reflex type, requires the cooperation of several muscles. Analysis of a relatively simple movement, such as clenching the fist, affords some idea of the complexity of the underlying neural arrangements. In this act the primary movement is a contraction of the flexor muscles of the fingers, the flexor digitorum sublimis and profundus, the flexor pollicis longus and brevis, and the adductor pollicis brevis. These muscles act as *agonists,* or *prime movers,* in this act. In order for flexion to be smooth and forceful, finger extensor muscles (antagonists) must relax at the same rate at which the flexors contract. The muscles which flex the fingers also tend to flex the wrist; and since that weakens the grip, muscles which extend the wrist must be brought into play to prevent its flexion. The action of the wrist extensors is *synergic,* and these muscles are called synergists in this particular act. The elbow and shoulder must be stabilized by appropriate flexor and extensor muscles, which serve as *fixators.* The coordination of agonists, antagonists, synergists, and fixators involves reciprocal innervation and is managed entirely by segmental spinal mechanisms with guidance from proprioceptive input. Only the agonist movement in a voluntary act is believed to be initiated at a cortical level.

In addition, there are many basic motor activities, such as the maintenance of certain postures and stepping movements where agonists and antagonists contract simultaneously (see Chap. 16). The alternating movements of spinal stepping represent an even more elaborate type of coordination. Also, in the support of the body in an upright posture, when the limb must be as rigid as a pillar, and in shivering, the agonists and antagonists must act together. In general, the more delicate the movement, the more precise the coordination between agonist and antagonist muscles.

If all or practically all peripheral motor nerves supplying a muscle are destroyed, voluntary, postural, and reflex movements are abolished. The muscle becomes soft and yields excessively to passive stretching, a condition known as *flaccidity.* Muscle tone—the slight resistance that normal relaxed muscle offers to passive movement—is reduced (*hypotonia* or *atonia*). The denervated muscles undergo extreme atrophy, usually being reduced to 20 to 30 percent of their original bulk within 4 months. The reflex reaction of the muscle to sudden stretch, as by tapping its tendon, is lost. If only a few motor units in the muscles are affected, partial paralysis will ensue. With partial denervation, EMG evidence of fibrillations may also be obtained.

Muscle tone and tendon reflexes are known to depend on muscle spindles and the afferent fibers to which they give origin. A tap on a tendon, by stimulating muscle spindles, activates afferent neurons which transmit impulses to alpha motor neurons. The result is the familiar brief muscle contraction or tendon reflex.

PARALYSIS DUE TO DISEASE OF CORTICOSPINAL, CORTICO-BULBAR, AND SUBCORTICOSPINAL NEURONS   The corticospinal tract at the level of the medulla contains approximately 1 million

axons. Many fibers arise not only from the giant Betz cells of the motor cortex (area 4 of Brodmann) but also from the smaller Betz cells of area 4, cells of the adjacent precentral cortex (area 6), and those of the secondary motor cortex in the superior frontal convolution and postcentral cortex (areas 1, 2, 3, 5, 7). The corticospinal tract is the only direct connection from the cerebrum to the spinal cord. At the level of the internal capsule these corticospinal fibers are intermingled with many others destined to end in the striatum, globus pallidus, substantia nigra, red nucleus, and reticular substance and with others ascending from the thalamus. Fibers to the cranial nerve nuclei become separated at about the level of the midbrain, where they cross the midline to the contralateral cranial nerve nuclei. These fibers form the corticomesencephalic, corticopontine, and cortico-bulbar tracts, and since they have functions similar to those of the corticospinal tract, they may be included in the pyramidal system of motor neurons. The decussation of the corticospinal tract at the lower end of the medulla is variable. Most of the crossing fibers come to occupy a position in the posterolateral part of the lateral funiculus; a few cross to form an anterior fasciculus. A small number of fibers, 10 to 20 percent, do not cross but descend ipsilaterally as the uncrossed corticospinal tract. Exceptionally, all of them cross; rarely, none. The termination of the corticospinal tract is predominantly upon interneurons in the intermediate zone of spinal gray matter, and not more than 25 percent establish direct synaptic connection with anterior horn cells (Fig. 15-1).

The motor area of the cerebral cortex includes that part of the precentral convolution which contains Betz cells (area 4), but it also extends anteriorly into area 6 and the secondary motor area of the superior frontal convolution and posteriorly into the anterior parietal lobe, where it overlaps the sensory areas. Physiologically it is defined as the region of electrically excitable cortex from which isolated movements can be evoked by stimuli of minimal intensity. The muscle groups of the contralateral face, arm, trunk, and leg are represented in the motor cortex, those of the face being at the lower end of the precentral convolution and those of the leg in the paracentral lobule on the medial surface of the cerebral hemisphere. The parts of the body capable of the most delicate movements have, in general, the largest cortical representation. One of the functions of the motor cortex is to synthesize simple movements into an infinite variety of finely graded, highly differentiated patterns.

Corticospinal paralysis may be due to lesions in the cerebral cortex, subcortical white matter, internal capsule, brainstem, or spinal cord. Almost always much more is involved than the corticospinal,

FIGURE 15-1 *The distribution of terminations of cortical and brainstem descending pathways (dots) in the spinal intermediate zone and motor neuronal cell groups in rhesus monkey. Note that lateral brainstem pathways (arising from the magnocellular red nucleus and the ventrolateral pontine tegmentum) end on interneurons concerned principally with hand muscles. Ventromedial brainstem pathways (from the superior colliculus, interstitial nucleus of Cajal, pontine, medullary and mesencephalic medial reticular formation, and vestibular nuclei) end on interneurons concerned with trunkal and limb girdle muscles. [From HGJM Kuypers, in JE Desmedt (ed). New Developments in Electromyography and Clinical Neurophysiology, Basel, Karger, 1973, vol. 3.]*

or pyramidal, tract. The effects of a pure lesion of the corticospinal system are considerably less than are typically seen with a hemiplegia due to a vascular lesion or other cause. Where only the pyramid of the medulla is destroyed on one side, there is a remarkable degree of recovery of motor function in the contralateral arm and leg, leaving only slight spasticity, an increase in phasic myotatic or tendon reflexes, and an inverted plantar reflex (Babinski's sign). This recovery may be due to preservation of a few fibers in the pyramid or to preservation of lateral brainstem pathways, but the more important idea revealed by such cases is that complete spastic hemiplegias in humans involve interruption not only of the corticospinal tract but of other descending fibers from the cerebral cortex (corticorubral, corticostriatal, corticopallidal, corticopontine, and corticoreticular) and from the brainstem (reticulospinal, vestibulospinal, and rubrospinal). The influence of these nonpyramidal fibers not only is reflected in the degree of paralysis but also in the status of the disconnected segmental motor neurons subserving reflex, postural, and locomotory functions. It is therefore unwise to refer to spastic hemiplegia as "the pyramidal syndrome." Hemiplegic dystonia (see below) involves some dysfunction of ventromedial brainstem pathways (Fig. 15-1).

With corticospinal lesions in humans the distribution of the paralysis varies with the locale of the lesion, but there are certain common features. Paralysis due to a lesion of these upper motor neurons always involves a group of muscles, never individual muscles. Concerning whatever volitional movement remains, the maximum effort is attained more slowly than in the normal limb, fewer motor units are recruited, and the frequency of their discharge is reduced. The paralysis never involves all the muscles on one side of the body, even with a complete hemiplegia. Movements that are invariably bilateral, such as those of the eyes, jaw, pharynx, larynx, neck, thorax, and abdomen, are little if at all affected. The hand and arm muscles suffer most severely, the leg muscles next, and of the cranial musculature only the muscles of the lower part of the face and tongue are involved to any significant degree. The cortical control of all movements is to some extent bilateral. Examples that prove this are hemiplegias that worsen when the contralateral motor system is interrupted by disease. Corticospinal motor paralysis is rarely complete for any long period of time; in this respect it differs from the total and absolute paralysis due to a complete destruction or interruption of anterior horn cells and their axons. The paralyzed arm may suddenly move during yawning and stretching, and various spinal reflexes can be elicited at all times.

Acute lesions of the corticospinal and subcorticospinal motor systems, at lower levels, such as the cervical cord, may not only cause a paralysis of voluntary movement but may also abolish temporarily the spinal reflexes subserved by segments below the lesion. This condition is known as *spinal shock*. After a few days to weeks the shock disappears if the patient is otherwise healthy and gives way to a phenomenon known as *spasticity*. The latter is a feature of all lesions of the motor system at cerebral, capsular, midbrain, and pontine levels. In cerebral and brainstem lesions it does not usually appear immediately, and in exceptional cases the paralyzed limbs remain flaccid but with lively reflexes. Spasticity is related to the excessive activity of the released or disinhibited spinal motor neurons. It is defined as a motor disorder characterized by a velocity-dependent increase in tonic stretch reflexes ("muscle tone") with exaggerated tendon jerks, resulting from hyperexcitability of the stretch reflex; it is one component of the "upper motor neuron" syndrome. The postures of the arm and leg inform us that certain spinal neurons are more active than others. With supraspinal lesions, the arm is maintained in a pronated, flexed position and the leg in an adducted, extended position. Any attempts to extend the arm or flex the leg passively will encounter, after a brief free interval, a resistance which increases and then may yield (clasp-knife phenomenon). When the limb is left in the new position, the resistance reappears (lengthening and shortening reactions). Actually the clasp-knife type of spasticity is infrequent. It is more usual for combined

lesions of corticospinal and other suprasegmental tracts to produce a sustained resistance to movement. The nocifensive spinal flexion reflexes, of which Babinski's sign is a part, are also released and the cutaneomuscular abdominal and cremasteric reflexes abolished. With cerebral lesions exaggerated stretch and cutaneous reflexes can also be elicited in cranial as well as limb and trunk muscles, and when the corticospinal disorder is bilateral, there is pseudobulbar paralysis (dysarthria, dysphonia, and dysphagia with bifacial paralysis) accompanied commonly by "emotional lability." Prolonged flexor and extensor spasms occur with lesions of the spinal cord; they are due to a release of cutaneous reflexes. Retention of reflexes and spasticity in muscles weakened by a spinal lesion point to a lesion of the descending motor tracts and integrity of the segments below the level of the lesion.

Spasticity may be present when the limbs are not paralyzed but only paretic, and it is then associated with interesting abnormalities of voluntary movements. In general, all attempts by the patient to move the hemiparetic extremities appear to be hampered. Discrete movements of individual fingers and finely coordinated movements of the hand are lost. Proximal muscles are under better voluntary control. Synergies of movements eventually appear. For example, in the upper extremity a flexion synergy consisting of finger flexion, wrist flexion and pronation, elbow flexion, and shoulder elevation and abduction is produced in a slow, massive, stereotyped fashion upon attempted grasp of an object. Attempts to push with the hand result in a weaker pronation of the hand, extension or flexion of the fingers, extension of the wrist and elbow, adduction of the upper arm, and lowering of the shoulder. In the lower extremity the extensor synergy (thigh adduction, thigh and knee extension, and plantar flexion of the toes and foot) is more powerful than the flexor synergy of hip abduction, hip and knee flexion, and dorsiflexion and inversion of toes and foot. The latter part of this flexion synergy is called Strumpell's tibialis sign, which appears during attempts to elevate a paretic leg. A bias toward extensor synergy facilitates weight-bearing and walking, which are eventually achieved by nearly all hemiplegic patients. These synergies indicate that there is not only a diminution in voluntary anterior horn cell activation (the negative effect of a motor lesion), but excessive reflex and synergistic discharges in the same motor neuron pools (positive effects of the lesion). Strong-willed effort to move the paretic limb may also evoke symmetric associated (mirror) movements in the normal limb.

The neurotransmitters for excitation and inhibition of spinal motor neurons by the corticospinal, rubrospinal, vestibulospinal, and reticulospinal tracts, or by peripheral sensory afferents, have not been fully elucidated. At least five neurotransmitters—acetylcholine (ACh), noradrenaline, serotonin, glycine, and γ-aminobutyric acid (GABA)—have been identified. Some, such as ACh, are excitatory; others, like glycine and GABA, are inhibitory. But their precise localizations have not been established. Even in spasticity, where the neurons responsible for excitation of the extensor muscles of the leg and flexors of the arm are overactive, it is not known whether there is a functional excess of excitatory neurotransmitters or a deficiency of inhibitory transmitter *or both*. Current evidence indicates that drugs that decrease spasticity act at the spinal cord level to alter neurotransmitter function. Baclofen interferes with release of excitatory neurotransmitters and diazepam facilitates GABA-mediated presynaptic inhibition.

Table 15-1 shows the main differences between corticospinal and lower motor neuron syndromes.

APRAXIC OR NONPARALYTIC DISORDERS OF MOTOR FUNCTION Aside from upper and lower motor neuron paralysis with cerebral lesions, there may be loss of learned movement that can simulate paresis of a limb. This is called *apraxia;* it can be defined as a disorder of learned movement that is not due to weakness, incoordination, sensory loss, or failure to comprehend commands. Actions acquired by learning or practice depend on the formation of movement patterns, particularly gestures and those actions which involve the use of tools and instruments. Once established, they are

TABLE 15-1 Differences between paralysis due to lesions of upper versus lower motor neurons

Upper motor neuron paralysis	Lower motor neuron paralysis
Muscle groups affected diffusely, never individual muscles	Individual muscles may be affected
Atrophy slight	Atrophy pronounced, 70 to 80 percent of total bulk
Spasticity with hyperactivity of the tendon reflexes	Flaccidity and hypotonia of affected muscles with loss of tendon reflexes
Extensor plantar reflex, Babinski's sign	Plantar reflex, if present, is of normal flexor type
Fascicular twitches not produced	Fasciculations may be present
	Electromyogram reveals reduced numbers of motor units and fibrillations

remembered and may be reproduced under the proper circumstances. Any purposive act of these types may be conceived as occurring in several stages. The idea of an act must be aroused in the mind of the subject by an appropriate stimulus situation, perhaps by a spoken command to do something. In right-handed and most left-handed persons the neural mechanisms for the comprehension and formulation of an idea of an act (motor schema or image) in response to a spoken command or a verbal stimulus and its reproduction are located posteriorly at the junction of the left parietal and temporal lobes; this region (Wernicke's area) is connected with the left premotor regions for the control of the right hand and thence through the corpus callosum with the motor areas of the right cerebral hemisphere for the control of the left side. Disconnection of Wernicke's area from motor areas of the right hemisphere (most commonly by lesions of the midcorpus callosum) results in *apraxia* of left limbs when tested by response to verbal commands.

A failure to execute certain acts in the correct context while retaining the ability to carry out the individual movements upon which such acts depend is the main feature of apraxia. The most adequate clinical test of motor deficits of this type is to observe a series of self-initiated actions such as using a comb, a razor, a toothbrush, or a common tool, or gesturing, e.g., waving goodbye, saluting, shaking the fist as though angry, or blowing a kiss. These actions can be normally elicited by a command or a request to imitate the examiner. Of course, failure to follow a spoken or written request may be due to an aphasia that prevents understanding of what is asked, or an agnosia may prevent recognition of the tool or object to be used. But when these difficulties are excluded, there remains a peculiar motor deficit in which the patient appears to understand but has lost the memory of how to perform a given act, especially if it is called for in an unnatural setting. The patient may have the idea of what to do but cannot translate the idea of the sequence of movements into a precise, well-executed act. This apraxic deficit may be evident both after a spoken command and in requests to imitate the gestures of the examiner. Sometimes these two conditions may be dissociated; the patient, while not aphasic, cannot execute a spoken command but can still imitate the act if it is called forth by gesture. Also, if merely given the tool, the patient may use it properly in an automatic fashion.

DIFFERENTIAL DIAGNOSIS OF PARALYSIS The diagnostic consideration of paralysis may be simplified by the following subdivisions, which relate to the location and distribution of weakness.

Monoplegia The examination of patients who complain of weakness of one extremity often discloses an unnoticed weakness in another limb, and the condition is actually hemiplegia or paraplegia. Or instead of weakness of all the muscles in a limb, only isolated groups are found to be affected. Ataxia, sensory disturbances, or pain in an extremity will often be interpreted by the patient as weakness, as will the mechanical limitation resulting from arthritis or the rigidity of parkinsonism.

In general, the presence or absence of atrophy of muscles in a monoplegic limb can be of diagnostic help.

PARALYSIS WITH LITTLE OR NO ATROPHY Long-continued disuse of a limb may lead to atrophy, but this is usually not so marked as in diseases that denervate muscles; the tendon reflexes are normal, and the response of the muscles to electric stimulation and on EMG are unaltered.

The most frequent cause of monoplegia without muscular wasting

is a lesion of the cerebral cortex. Rarely does it occur in diseases which interrupt the corticospinal tract at the level of the internal capsule, brainstem, or spinal cord because fibers to arm and leg are very close together there. A cortical vascular lesion (thrombosis or embolus) is the commonest cause, but a discrete traumatic lesion, tumor, or abscess may have the same effect. Multiple sclerosis and spinal cord tumor, early in their course, may cause weakness of one extremity, usually the leg. Weakness due to damage to the corticospinal and subcorticospinal system is usually accompanied by spasticity, increased reflexes, and an extensor plantar reflex (Babinski's sign). However, acute diseases that destroy the motor tracts in the spinal cord may at first (for several days) reduce the tendon reflexes and cause hypotonia (*spinal shock*). This does not occur in partial or slowly evolving lesions and occurs only to minimal degree, if at all, in lesions of brainstem and cerebrum. In acute diseases affecting the lower motor neurons the tendon reflexes are always reduced or abolished, but atrophy may not appear for several weeks. Hence one must take into account the mode of onset and the duration of the disease in evaluating the tendon reflexes, muscle tone, and degree of atrophy before reaching an anatomic diagnosis.

PARALYSIS WITH MUSCULAR ATROPHY In addition to the paralysis, reduced or abolished tendon reflexes, and decreased tone, there may be visible fasciculations. The EMG shows reduced numbers of motor units (often of large size), fasciculations at rest, and fibrillations. The lesion may be in the spinal cord, spinal roots, or peripheral nerves. Its location can usually be decided by the distribution of the palsied muscles (whether the pattern is one of nerve, spinal root, or spinal cord involvement), by the associated neurologic symptoms and signs, and by special tests (cerebrospinal fluid examination, CT or magnetic resonance imaging (MRI) scans of the spine, and myelogram).

Brachial atrophic monoplegia (affecting the arm) is relatively rare, and when present, it should suggest in an infant brachial plexus trauma, in a child poliomyelitis, in an adult poliomyelitis, syringomyelia, amyotrophic lateral sclerosis, or other brachial plexus lesions. Crural monoplegia (affecting the leg) is more frequent and may be caused by any lesion of thoracic or lumbar cord, i.e., trauma, tumor, myelitis, multiple sclerosis, etc. Multiple sclerosis almost never causes atrophy, and ruptured intervertebral disk and the many varieties of neuritis rarely paralyze all or most of the muscles of a limb. Muscle dystrophy may begin in one limb, but by the time the patient is seen the typical more or less symmetric pattern of proximal limb and trunk involvement is evident. A unilateral retroperitoneal tumor may paralyze the leg by implicating the lumbosacral plexus.

Hemiplegia Loss of strength in the arm, leg, and sometimes face on one side of the body is the most frequent distribution of paralysis in humans. With rare exceptions (a few unusual cases of poliomyelitis or motor system disease) this pattern of paralysis is due to involvement of the descending motor tracts.

LOCATION OF LESION-PRODUCING HEMIPLEGIA The site or level of the lesion can usually be deduced from the associated neurologic findings. Diseases localized in the cerebral cortex, cerebral white matter (corona radiata), and internal capsule usually evoke weakness or paralysis of the face, arm, and leg on the opposite side. The occurrence of convulsive seizures or the presence of a defect in speech (aphasia), a cortical type of sensory loss (astereognosis, loss of two-point discrimination, etc.), anosognosia, or defects in the visual fields suggest a cortical or subcortical location. A pure, isolated hemiplegia affecting simultaneously the face, arm, and leg indicates a lesion in the posterior limb of the internal capsule, often a vascular lacune.

Damage to the corticospinal and corticobulbar tracts in the upper portion of the brainstem will cause paralysis of the face, arm, and leg on the opposite side. The lesion in such cases is localized by the presence of a paralysis of the muscles supplied by the oculomotor nerve on the same side as the lesion (Weber's syndrome) or other neurologic findings. With low pontine lesions an ipsilateral abducens or facial palsy is combined with a contralateral weakness or paralysis of the arm and leg (Millard-Gubler syndrome). Lesions of the lowermost part of the brainstem, i.e., in the medulla, affect the tongue and sometimes the pharynx and larynx on one side and arm and leg on the other side. These "crossed paralyses," so common in brainstem diseases, are described in Chap. 343. Ataxic hemiplegia with or without dysarthria also indicates a lesion in the contralateral basis pons.

Rarely, a homolateral hemiplegia (sparing cranial muscles) may be caused by a lesion in the lateral column of the cervical spinal cord. At this level, however, the pathologic process often induces bilateral signs, with resulting quadriparesis or quadriplegia. Homolateral paralysis, if combined with a loss of vibratory and position sense on the same side and a contralateral loss of pain and temperature (Brown-Séquard syndrome), signifies unilateral disease of the spinal cord (Chap. 353).

Muscle atrophy of minor degree often is associated with a hemiplegia but never reaches the proportions seen in diseases of the lower motor neurons. The former atrophy is largely due to disuse. When the motor cortex and adjacent parts of the parietal lobe are damaged in infancy or childhood, the normal development of the muscles and the skeletal system in the affected limbs is retarded. The palsied limbs and even the trunk on one side are small. This does not occur if the paralysis begins after the greater part of skeletal growth is attained (after puberty). In the hemiplegia due to spinal cord injury, muscles at the level of the lesion may undergo atrophy if there is associated damage to anterior horn cells or ventral roots.

CAUSES OF HEMIPLEGIA Vascular diseases of the cerebrum and brainstem exceed all others as causes of hemiplegia. Trauma (brain contusion, epidural and subdural hemorrhage) ranks second, and other diseases such as brain tumor, brain abscess and encephalitis, demyelinative diseases, and complications of meningitis, tuberculosis, and syphilis are less important.

Paraplegia Paralysis of both lower extremities may occur in diseases of the spinal cord and the spinal roots or of the peripheral nerves. Parasagittal tumors and hydrocephalus can, on occasion, cause leg weakness. If the onset is acute, it may be difficult to distinguish spinal from neural paralysis, for in any acute myelopathy spinal shock may result in abolition of reflexes and flaccidity. As a rule, in acute spinal cord diseases the paralysis affects all muscles below a given level; often, if the white matter is extensively damaged, sensory loss below a particular level (loss of pain and temperature sense—lateral spinothalamic tracts and loss of vibratory and position sense—posterior columns) is conjoined. Also, in bilateral disease of the spinal cord the bladder and bowel sphincters are paralyzed. Alterations of cerebrospinal fluid (dynamic block, increase in protein or cells) are frequent. In peripheral nerve diseases both sensory loss and motor loss tend to involve the distal muscles of the legs more than the proximal ones (an exception is acute idiopathic polyneuritis), and the sphincters are spared or only briefly deranged in function. Sensory loss, if present, is more likely to consist of distal impairment of touch, vibration, and position sense, with pain and temperature sense spared in many instances. The cerebrospinal fluid protein level may be normal or elevated. Studies of nerve conduction through spinal roots (F waves) are always abnormal.

Acute paraplegia (except that due to trauma or metastatic tumor) is relatively infrequent. Rarely it may be due to a medial pontine lesion affecting the leg fibers which are near to the midline (as in pontine infarction or central pontine myelinolysis). Spontaneous hematomyelia with bleeding from a vascular malformation (angioma, telangiectasis), thrombosis of a spinal artery with infarction (myelomalacia), and dissecting aortic aneurysm or atherosclerotic occlusion of nutrient spinal arteries arising from the aorta with resulting infarction (myelomalacia) are the commonest varieties of sudden paraplegia (or quadriplegia, if the cervical cord is involved). Postinfectious or postvaccinial myelitis, acute demyelinative myelitis (Devic's disease if the optic nerves are affected), necrotizing myelitis, and epidural abscess or hemorrhage with spinal cord compression tend to develop somewhat more slowly, over a period of hours or days, but they may have an acute onset. Poliomyelitis, in those countries where immunization is incomplete, presents as a purely motor disorder with meningitis, and must be distinguished from the other acute myelopathies.

In adult life subacute or chronic paraplegia can occur in multiple sclerosis, subacute combined degeneration, spinal cord tumor, ruptured cervical disk and cervical spondylosis, syphilitic meningomyelitis, chronic epidural infections (fungus and other granulomatous diseases), motor system disease, familial spastic paraplegia, and syringomyelia. (See Chap. 353 for discussion of these spinal cord diseases.) The several varieties of polyneuritis and polymyositis must be considered in their differential diagnosis, for they, too, may cause paraparesis. Friedreich's ataxia and familial paraplegia, progressive muscular dystrophy, and the chronic varieties of polyneuritis tend to appear during late childhood and adolescence and are slowly progressive.

Paraplegia (or paraparesis) may be due to a lesion of the leg areas of the motor cortex. Arterial (anterior cerebral arteries) or venous (superior sagittal sinus and tributary cerebral veins) distribution cerebral infarction are causes of acute paraplegia; parasagittal meningioma is a cause of asymmetric chronic paraplegia. Usually other signs such as confusion, stupor, or seizures indicate the cerebral localization, and differential diagnosis is not a problem.

Quadriplegia All that has been written about the common causes of paraplegia applies to quadriplegia except that the lesion is in the cervical rather than the thoracic or lumbar segments of the spinal cord. If it is situated in the low cervical segments and involves the anterior half of the spinal cord, as in occlusion of the anterior spinal artery, the arm paralysis may be flaccid and areflexic and the leg paralysis spastic (anterior spinal syndrome). There are only a few points of difference between the common paraplegic and quadriplegic syndromes. Repeated cerebral vascular accidents may lead to bilateral hemiplegia, usually accompanied by pseudobulbar palsy.

Isolated paralysis Paralysis of isolated muscle groups usually indicates a lesion of one or more peripheral nerves. The diagnosis of a lesion of an individual peripheral nerve is based on the presence of weakness or paralysis of the muscle or group of muscles and impairment or loss of sensation in the distribution of the nerve in question (Chap. 355). Complete transection or severe injury to a peripheral nerve is usually followed by atrophy of the muscles it innervates and by loss of their tendon reflexes. Trophic changes in the skin, nails, and subcutaneous tissue may also occur. It is of considerable importance to decide whether the lesion is only a temporary one (conduction block), or whether there has been a dissolution of axonal continuity, requiring nerve regeneration for recovery. EMG is of value here.

EXAMINATION SCHEME FOR MOTOR PARALYSIS AND APRAXIA The first step is to inspect the paralyzed limb, taking note of its posture and of the presence or absence of muscle atrophy, hypertrophy, and fascicular twitchings. Slight atrophy may be due to disuse from any cause, i.e., pain, fixation as the result of a cast, or any type of paralysis. Pronounced atrophy usually occurs only with denervation of several weeks' or months' standing. The patient is then called upon to move each muscle group, and the power and facility of movement are graded and recorded. The range of passive movement is then determined by moving all the joints. This provides information concerning alterations of muscle tone, i.e., hypotonia, spasticity, and rigidity. Dislocations, diseased joints, and ankyloses may also be revealed by these same maneuvers. The tendon reflexes are then tested. The usual routine is to try to elicit the jaw jerk (increased in pseudobulbar palsy) and the supinator, biceps, triceps, quadriceps, and Achilles tendon reflexes. Two cutaneous reflexes are then tested, the abdominal and plantar reflexes.

If there is no evidence of upper or lower motor neuron disease, but certain acts are nonetheless imperfectly performed, one should look for a disorder of postural sensibility, cerebellar incoordination, or rigidity with abnormality of posture and movement due to disease of the basal ganglia. In the absence of these disorders, the possibility of an apraxic disorder may be investigated by watching the patient's own movements and those called forth by specific command and gesture.

Hysterical paralysis may pose problems. Usually it is easily distinguished from chronic lower motor neuron disease by absence of areflexia and severe atrophy. Diagnostic difficulty arises only in certain acute cases of upper motor neuron disease that lack all the usual changes in reflexes and muscle tone. In hysterical paralysis one arm or one leg or all one side of the body may be affected. The hysterical gait is sometimes diagnostic (Chap. 16). Often there is loss of all forms of sensation (touch, pain, smell, vision, and hearing) on the paralyzed side, a group of sensory changes that is never seen in organic brain disease. The patient should be asked to move the affected limbs; the movement is seen to be slow and jerky, often with contraction of both agonist and antagonist muscles simultaneously or intermittently. Hoover's sign and Babinski's combined leg flexion test are helpful in distinguishing hysterical from organic hemiplegia. To elicit Hoover's sign, the patient, lying on the back, is asked to raise one leg from the bed against resistance; in a normal individual the back of the heel of the contralateral leg presses firmly down, and the same is true when the patient with organic hemiplegia attempts to lift the paralyzed leg. The hysteric will press down the supposedly paralyzed leg more strongly under these circumstances than when asked to do so directly. To carry out Babinski's combined leg flexion test, a patient with an organic hemiplegia is asked to sit up without using the arms; in doing this, the paralyzed or weak leg flexes at the hip and the heel is lifted from the bed, while the heel of the sound leg is pressed into the bed. This sign is absent in hysterical hemiplegia.

THE BASAL GANGLIA

The basal ganglia subserve motor functions that are distinct from those attributed to the pyramidal (corticospinal) tract. The term *extrapyramidal* underscores this distinction and calls attention to a set of neurologic illnesses caused by lesions that affect the basal ganglia. Familiar examples include Parkinson's disease, Huntington's disease, and Wilson's disease. This section reviews the basal ganglia and describes the clinical symptoms and signs that arise from their dysfunction.

ANATOMIC CONNECTIONS AND NEURONAL TRANSMITTERS IN THE BASAL GANGLIA The basal ganglia are paired subcortical masses of gray matter that form anatomically distinct nuclear groups. The major nuclei are the caudate and the putamen (which together are called the striatum), the internal and external segments of the globus pallidus, the subthalamic nucleus, and the substantia nigra (Fig. 15-2). The striatum receives afferent inputs from many sources, including the cerebral cortex, thalamic nuclei, brainstem raphe nuclei, and the substantia nigra. Cortical neurons that project to the striatum release the excitatory amino acid glutamate. Neurons that project to the striatum from the raphe nuclei synthesize and release serotonin (5-HT). Neurons in the pars compacta of the substantia nigra synthesize and release dopamine (DA), which acts as an inhibitory neurotransmitter on striatal neurons. Transmitters released by thalamic projections are unknown. The striatum contains two distinct classes of cells: local circuit neurons, whose axons do not project beyond the confines of the nucleus, and other neurons whose axons project to the globus pallidus and substantia nigra. Local circuit neurons synthesize and release acetylcholine (ACh), gamma aminobutyric acid (GABA), and neuropeptides, including somatostatin and vasoactive intestinal polypeptide. Striatal neurons that inhibit the pars reticulata of the substantia nigra release GABA, whereas those that excite the nigra release substance P (Fig. 15-3). Transmitters released in the striatal projections to the globus pallidus include GABA, the enkephalins, and substance P.

Axons that originate in the internal segment of the globus pallidus form the main efferent projection from the basal ganglia. There is a massive projection around and through the internal capsule (the ansa and fasciculus lenticularis that pass through the fields of Forel) to the ventral anterior and ventral lateral thalamus as well as to intralaminar thalamic nuclei, including the centromedian nucleus. Chemical transmitters released by this pathway are unknown. Other efferent projections from the basal ganglia include direct dopaminergic connections from the substantia nigra to regions of limbic and frontal cerebral cortex; the pars reticulata of the substantia nigra also sends a projection to thalamic nuclei and to the superior colliculus.

Recent anatomic studies have clarified the cortical distribution of ascending thalamic fibers. Ventral thalamic neurons project to premotor and motor cerebral cortices; medial thalamic nuclei project primarily to prefrontal cortex. The supplementary motor cortex receives a prominent input from the basal ganglia, including a dopaminergic projection from the substantia nigra, whereas the

FIGURE 15-2 *Simplified schematic diagram of the major neuronal connections between the basal ganglia, thalamus, and cerebral cortex. The projection from the internal segment of the globus pallidus constitutes the principal efferent pathway from the basal ganglia. Abbreviations: ext = external, int = internal, pc = pars compacta, pr = pars reticulata, cm = centromedian, va = ventroanterior, vl = ventrolateral.*

primary motor and premotor cortex receives a major input from the cerebellum. Thus there are a series of parallel loops reciprocally linking specific basal ganglionic structures and cerebral cortical regions. Although the exact mechanism whereby these various inputs are translated into coordinated volitional acts remains uncertain, it is clear that most of the basal ganglionic and cerebellar influences on the motor system are funneled through this ventral plane of thalamic nuclei. The major cerebellar output, which exits from the cerebellum through the superior cerebellar peduncle, terminates with the pallidal-thalamic fibers in the ventroanterior and ventrolateral thalamic nuclei. This region of the thalamus forms an essential link in the ascending fiber systems from both the basal ganglia and the cerebellum to the motor cortex. Despite the apparently crucial nature of these structures, lesions placed stereotactically in the ventral thalamus can abolish essential-familial tremor or the rigidity and tremor in Parkinson's disease without producing functional deficits. Ascending thalamo-cortical fibers pass through the internal capsule and cerebral white matter, so lesions in these parts or in the cortex may simultaneously affect both corticospinal and extrapyramidal systems.

Axons from some cortical neurons form the internal capsule (the corticobulbar and corticospinal tracts); these and others also project to the striatum. This forms a complete loop—from cerebral cortex to striatum, to globus pallidus, to thalamus, to cerebral cortex. Axons that originate in the centromedian nucleus of the thalamus project back to the striatum, thus completing a subcortical loop from striatum to globus pallidus, to centromedian nucleus, to striatum. There is another subcortical loop between the striatum and the substantia nigra: Dopaminergic neurons in the pars compacta of substantia nigra project to the striatum, and separate striatal neurons that release GABA and substance P send projections to the pars reticulata of the substantia nigra. There are reciprocal connections between the pars reticulata and pars compacta of the substantia nigra; the pars reticulata sends projections to ventral thalamus, superior colliculus, and brainstem reticular formation structures as well. The subthalamic nucleus receives fibers from the neocortex and from the external segment of the globus pallidus; neurons within the subthalamic nucleus form reciprocal connections with the external segment of the globus pallidus and also send axons to the internal segment of the globus pallidus and pars reticulata of the substantia nigra. The neurochemicals involved in these pathways remain unknown, although GABA has been implicated.

PHYSIOLOGY OF THE BASAL GANGLIA Recordings from neurons in the globus pallidus and substantia nigra in awake, performing primates confirm the main motor function of the basal ganglia. Cells within these regions clearly participate in the initiation of movement,

since they increase their firing rates before movement is observed clinically or detected by EMG. Discharges in the basal ganglia are related principally to contralateral rather than ipsilateral limb movements. Many neurons increase their firing rates during slow (ramp) movements, but some others discharge during more rapid (ballistic) movements. There is somatotopic localization of leg, arm, and face within the internal segment of the globus pallidus and pars reticulata of the substantia nigra. This observation provides a possible explanation for the occurrence of restricted dyskinesias: Focal dystonia and buccal-lingual-masticatory tardive dyskinesia may result from localized pallidal or nigral biochemical lesions that affect only regions with hand or face representation.

Although the basal ganglia are motor nuclei, it is not possible to identify a specific type of basal ganglia movement. Hypotheses about the function of the basal ganglia in human beings derive from correlations between clinical signs and sites of pathologic lesions in patients with extrapyramidal diseases. The basal ganglia are a constellation of nuclei centered around the globus pallidus, through which impulses are channeled to the thalamus and onward to the cerebral cortex (Fig. 15-2). Neurons in each satellite nucleus contribute excitatory and inhibitory impulses, and the sum of these influences on the main pathway from basal ganglia to thalamus and cerebral cortex, modified by the cerebellum, determine smooth motor function as expressed through the corticospinal and other descending cortical tracts. If one or more of the supporting nuclei is damaged, the sum of the impulses to the globus pallidus changes and disordered mobility can occur. Hemiballismus is the most dramatic of these; damage to the subthalamic nucleus apparently removes inhibitory influences on the substantia nigra and globus pallidus, which results in violent, involuntary, rotatory flinging movements of the contralateral arm and leg. Similarly, damage to the caudate nucleus often results in chorea, whereas the opposite phenomenon, akinesia, typically occurs when dopamine-producing cells in the substantia nigra degenerate, releasing the intact caudate nucleus from inhibition. Lesions restricted to the globus pallidus often cause flexion dystonia and impaired postural reflexes.

NEUROPHARMACOLOGY OF THE BASAL GANGLIA: GENERAL PRINCIPLES Transfer of information from one cell to another in the mammalian nervous system usually involves one or more chemicals released from the first neuron to a specific receptor site on a second neuron, thereby altering the biochemical and physical properties of the second neuron. These chemicals taken together are called neuroregulators. There are three distinct classes of neuroregulators: neurotransmitters, neuromodulators, and neurohormones. Neurotransmitters, such as the catecholamines, GABA, and ACh, are the best

FIGURE 15-3 *Schematic diagram of the excitatory and inhibitory effects of neuroregulators released by neurons in the basal ganglia pathways. The area (enclosed by dashed lines) in the striatum indicates neurons with efferent projection systems. The other striatal transmitters are present in intrinsic neurons. Plus sign (+) indicates an excitatory postsynaptic effect. Minus sign (−) indicates an inhibitory effect. Abbreviations: cm = centromedian nucleus, GABA = gamma aminobutyric acid, TRH = thyrotropin releasing hormone, va/vl = ventroanterior and ventrolateral.*

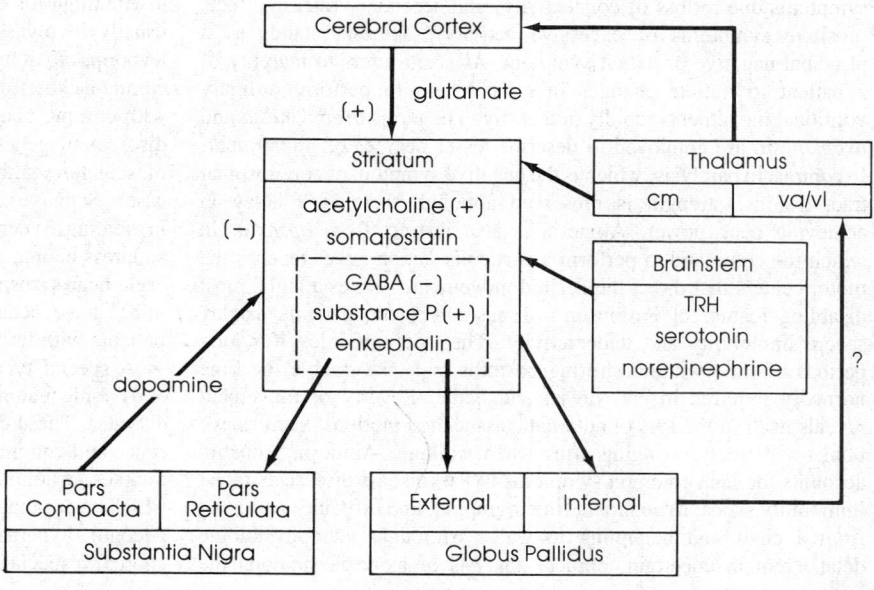

known and clinically most important class of neuroregulators. They cause short-latency, brief postsynaptic effects (e.g., depolarization) close to their point of release. Neuromodulators, such as the endorphins, somatostatin, and substance P, also exert effects close to the point of release but generally do not initiate neuronal depolarization. The neuromodulators apparently can enhance or diminish effects of the classic neurotransmitters. Many neurons that contain classic neurotransmitters also contain neuromodulator peptides. Substance P coexists within raphe neurons that synthesize 5-HT, for example, and vasoactive intestinal polypeptide coexists with ACh in many cortical cholinergic neurons. Neurohormones, such as vasopressin and angiotensin II, differ from other regulators because they are released into the bloodstream and are transported to remote receptors. Their effects are slow in onset and have a long duration of action. The distinction between the various classes of neuroregulators is not absolute. DA, for example, acts as a neurotransmitter in the caudate nucleus but is believed to act as a neurohormone in the hypothalamus.

Neuroregulators of the neurotransmitter class are the best-studied transmitters in the basal ganglia and the ones on which most drugs exert their effects. Neurotransmitters are synthesized in the presynaptic terminals of neurons and some, like the catecholamines and ACh, are stored in vesicles. Following the arrival of an electric impulse, neurotransmitters are released from the presynaptic terminal into the synaptic cleft, diffuse across the synaptic gap, and combine with specific receptor sites on the postsynaptic cell. This initiates a series of biochemical and biophysical changes; the sum of all postsynaptic excitatory and inhibitory influences determines the likelihood that a given neuron will discharge. The biogenic amines DA, norepinephrine (NE), and 5-HT are inactivated by uptake into the presynaptic terminals; ACh is inactivated by intrasynaptic hydrolysis. There are also receptor sites on the presynaptic terminal, called autoreceptors, and their stimulation generally causes a decrease in synthesis and release of the transmitter. The affinity of an autoreceptor for its neurotransmitter is often much greater than that of the postsynaptic receptor. Drugs that stimulate DA autoreceptors can be expected to decrease dopaminergic transmission and possibly be useful in the treatment of hyperkinetic movement disorders such as Huntington's disease and tardive dyskinesia. Receptors may be further subdivided based on response to pharmacologic agents. There are at least two separate populations of DA receptors, for example: Stimulation of D-1 sites activates adenylate cyclase, whereas D-2 receptor stimulation does not. The ergot alkaloid bromocriptine, used in the treatment of Parkinson's disease, stimulates D-2 but blocks D-1 receptors; most neuroleptics block D-2 receptors.

CLINICAL MANIFESTATIONS OF LESIONS OF THE BASAL GANGLIA Akinesia
When extrapyramidal diseases are analyzed along classic neurologic lines into primary functional deficits (negative symptoms due to loss of connectivity) and secondary release effects (positive symptoms of excessive activity), akinesia stands as a principal negative or deficit symptom. *Akinesia* refers to inability of a patient to initiate changes in activity and to perform ordinary volitional movements rapidly and easily. The terms *bradykinesia* and *hypokinesia* are employed to describe lesser degrees of impairment. In contrast to paralysis, which is the negative symptom of corticospinal tract lesions, strength is preserved although there is a delay in achieving peak power. Akinesia is also distinct from *apraxia,* in which the command to perform a particular action never reaches the motor centers that direct the desired movement. Akinesia is the most disabling feature of Parkinson's disease. Akinetic patients display severe immobility and underactivity. They sit motionless for long periods of time without shifting postures and take double the time normally required to eat, dress, and bathe. Poverty of movement reveals itself in the loss of automatic associated motions, such as eye blinks and freely swinging arms when walking. Akinesia probably accounts for such common symptoms in Parkinson's disease as facial immobility, vocal hypophonia, micrographia, and difficulty in arising from a chair and beginning to walk. Although pathophysiologic details remain uncertain, clinical analysis of akinesia supports the hypothesis that the basal ganglia are mainly responsible for initiation and automatic execution of learned motor plans. Neuropharmacologic evidence suggests that akinesia itself results from DA deficiency.

Rigidity *Muscle tone* is defined as the amount of resistance encountered when a relaxed limb is moved passively. In rigidity, the muscles are in continuous contraction and resistance to passive movement is constant. Rigidity secondary to extrapyramidal disorders may superficially resemble spasticity due to corticospinal tract lesions in that both produce increases in muscular tone. A few clinical guidelines provide help in distinguishing these conditions at the bedside. The distribution of increased tone often differs in rigidity and spasticity. Although rigidity is present in both flexor and extensor muscle groups, it tends to be more prominent in those that maintain a flexed posture. Rigidity is easy to detect in large muscle groups, but smaller muscles of the face, tongue, and larynx are also often affected. In contrast to rigidity, spasticity usually produces increased tone in the extensor muscles of the legs and the flexor musculature of the arms. The quality of hypertonus can also be used to distinguish the two conditions. Resistance to passive movements is constant in rigidity, accounting for terms such as "lead pipe" and "plastic" resistance. In spasticity, there may be a free interval followed classically by the clasp-knife phenomenon; muscles do not contract until they are stretched a bit, and later during stretch the augmentation in muscle tone quickly subsides. Deep tendon reflexes are normal in rigidity but increased in spastic states. Spasticity results from hyperactivity of the stretch reflex arc due to central changes but without increased sensitivity of the muscle spindle; spasticity can be abolished by sectioning posterior spinal roots. Rigidity has less relationship with hyperactivity of segmental reflex arcs and depends more upon heightened discharge of alpha motor neurons. A special type of rigidity is the cogwheel phenomenon, which is especially common in Parkinson's disease. When the hypertonic muscle is passively stretched, the resistance may be rhythmically jerky, as though the resistance of the limb were controlled by a ratchet.

Chorea Derived from the Greek word meaning "dance," chorea refers to widespread arrhythmic movements of a forcible, rapid, jerky, restless type. Choreic movements are noted for their irregularity and variability; they are generally continuous, may be simple or quite elaborate, and affect any part of the body. They may resemble voluntary movement in complexity, but they are never combined into a coordinated act unless the patient incorporates them into a deliberate movement in order to make them less noticeable. Normal volitional movements are possible because there is no paralysis, but they may be excessively quick, poorly sustained, and deformed by choreic movements. Chorea may be generalized or limited to one side of the body. Generalized chorea is the predominant involuntary movement in Huntington's disease and in rheumatic (Sydenham's) chorea, and usually involves the face, trunk, and limbs; it is often seen with levodopa toxicity in patients with Parkinson's disease. Another common choreiform disorder, tardive dyskinesia, occurs in association with chronic neuroleptic administration. Choreic movements in this disorder are generally restricted to the buccal, lingual, and mandibular musculature, although trunk and limbs may be involved in severe cases. Sedatives such as phenobarbital or a benzodiazepine are used in treating Sydenham's chorea; neuroleptics are commonly used to suppress chorea in Huntington's disease. Drugs that increase cholinergic neurotransmission, such as phosphatidylcholine and physostigmine, have been used to suppress chorea in about 30 percent of patients with tardive dyskinesia.

A special type of paroxysmal chorea, sometimes with athetosis or dystonic features, occurs sporadically, or as an autosomal dominant disorder. These disorders usually appear during childhood or adolescence and continue throughout life; patients have paroxysms that last minutes to hours. In one special subtype, the chorea is kinesogenic, which means that it may be initiated by a sudden voluntary movement. Alcohol, hypernatremia, and phenytoin may precipitate paroxysmal chorea, especially in patients who have Sydenham's chorea in childhood. In some cases, anticonvulsant drugs, including phenobarbital and clonazepam, and in other instances levodopa have prevented attacks.

Athetosis This term is from a Greek word meaning "unfixed" or "changeable." Athetosis is characterized by an inability to sustain the muscles of the fingers, toes, tongue or any other group of muscles in one position. The maintained posture is interrupted by continuous slow, purposeless movements. These are most pronounced in the digits and hands and consist of extension, pronation, flexion, and supination of the arm with alternating flexion and extension of the fingers. Athetotic movements are slower than those associated with chorea, but gradations are commonly seen and termed *choreoathetosis* when it is impossible to distinguish between the two. Generalized athetosis may be seen in children with static encephalopathy (cerebral palsy); it can also occur in Wilson's disease, in torsion dystonia, and following cerebral anoxia. Posthemiplegic athetosis is unilateral and occurs especially in children who have suffered a stroke. Patients whose athetosis is due to cerebral palsy or cerebral anoxia have variable degrees of additional motor deficit due to associated corticospinal tract disease. Discrete individual movements of the tongue, lips, and hands are often impossible, and attempts to perform such voluntary movements result in contraction of all the muscles in the limb and other parts of the body. Variable degrees of rigidity are generally associated with all forms of athetosis and may account for the slower quality of movement in this disorder in contrast to chorea. Treatment of athetosis is generally unsatisfactory, although some patients improve with the drugs used to suppress chorea and dystonia.

The dystonias Dystonia refers to abnormally increased muscular tone that causes fixed abnormal postures. Some patients with dystonia also have shifting postures resulting from irregular, forceful twisting movements that affect trunk and extremities and produce bizarre, grotesque movements and positions of the body. The mobile spasms of dystonia are similar to those of athetosis but are generally slower and involve axial (trunk) rather than appendicular (extremity) muscles. Dystonic movements increase during volitional motor activity, nervousness, and emotional stress; they diminish during relaxation and, like most extrapyramidal movement disorders, disappear completely during sleep. *Primary torsion dystonia*, formerly known as dystonia musculorum deformans, is frequently inherited as an autosomal recessive characteristic in Ashkenazic Jews and as an autosomal dominant trait in non-Jewish families. Spontaneous cases are also common. Manifestations of dystonia usually begin in the first two decades of life, but adult forms are recognized. Generalized torsion spasms can also occur in children with kernicterus and after cerebral hypoxia.

"Dystonia" is also used in another sense, to describe any fixed posture which may be the end result of a motor system disease. For example, dystonia secondary to a stroke (flexed arm and extended leg) is often called hemiplegic dystonia, and that associated with parkinsonism called flexion dystonia. In contrast to these permanent dystonic states, drugs such as the neuroleptics, and levodopa in patients with parkinsonism, can induce dystonic postures and spasms that subside once the offending medication is discontinued.

Secondary or *focal dystonias* are more common than torsion dystonia and include such disorders as spasmodic torticollis, writer's cramp, blepharospasm, spastic dystonia, and Miege's syndrome. In the focal dystonias as a group, symptoms tend to be highly localized, to remain stable, and not to spread to involve other body parts. Focal dystonias occur more frequently in adults and most often arise spontaneously without known genetic transmission or antecedent illness. Spasmodic torticollis is the most common focal dystonia. There are intermittent or continuous spasms of the sternocleidomastoid, trapezius, and other neck muscles, usually more prominent on one side than the other, that cause turning or tipping of the head. Torticollis is involuntary and cannot be inhibited, and thereby differs from habit spasm or tic. Torticollis is worse when the patient sits, stands, or walks; placing a finger to the chin or side of the jaw often alleviates the muscle imbalance. Women are affected twice as often as men; the average age of onset is 40.

Torsion dystonia is classified as an extrapyramidal disease even though no pathologic lesions have been observed in the basal ganglia or elsewhere in the brain. Development of rational therapy is further impaired by the lack of information regarding possible neurotransmitter abnormalities. Effective treatment of secondary dystonias is no more satisfactory than that of torsion dystonia. Symptomatic relief is sometimes achieved with sedatives such as the benzodiazepines and high doses of anticholinergic drugs; levodopa has been helpful in some instances. Biofeedback therapy has sometimes been beneficial but psychiatric treatment is ineffectual. When spasmodic torticollis is severe, surgical denervation of the affected muscles (C1 to C3 bilaterally and C4 on one side) has given favorable results in most patients. Blepharospasm has been successfully treated by injecting a dilute solution of botulinum toxin into periocular muscles. The toxin produces a mild neuromuscular blockade; its effect is transient and treatment must be repeated every 2 or 3 months.

Myoclonus This is a descriptive term for very brief, involuntary, random muscular contractions. Myoclonus can occur spontaneously at rest, in response to sensory stimuli, or with voluntary movements. Myoclonus may involve a single motor unit and simulate a fasciculation, or it may simultaneously involve groups of muscles that displace the limb or distort its voluntary movement. Myoclonus is a symptom that occurs in a wide variety of generalized metabolic and neurologic disorders collectively called the myoclonias. Posthypoxic intention myoclonus is a special myoclonic syndrome that occurs as a sequel to transient cerebral anoxia such as might occur, for example, during a brief cardiorespiratory arrest. Cognitive abilities are usually preserved; however, there are cerebellar signs, and voluntary movements are marred by action myoclonus involving the extremities, facial muscles, and even the voice. Action myoclonus deforms all movement and severely limits the patient's ability to eat, talk, write, or even walk. Myoclonus may also result from lipid storage disease, encephalitis, Creutzfeldt-Jakob disease, or metabolic encephalopathies due to respiratory failure, chronic renal failure, hepatic failure, or electrolyte imbalance. Posthypoxic intention myoclonus and idiopathic myoclonus may be treated with the 5-HT precursor 5-hydroxytryptophan (Fig. 15-4); alternate therapies include baclofen, clonazepam, and valproic acid.

Asterixis Quick arrhythmic movements that occur due to brief interruptions in background tonic muscular contractions are called asterixis; in a sense, asterixis may be considered as negative myoclonus. Asterixis may be observed in any voluntary muscle during contraction but is usually demonstrated clinically as a brief lapse of posture with prompt restoration during voluntary extension of the limb with dorsiflexion of the wrist or ankle. Asterixis is characterized by 50- to 200-ms silent periods in ongoing EMG activity in all muscle groups in one limb (Fig. 15-5). This results in the wrist or ankle moving down before muscular activity resumes and restores the limb to its original position. Asterixis is commonly observed bilaterally in metabolic encephalopathies, and its description in hepatic failure accounted for the original term "liver flap." Asterixis may be caused by drugs, including all anticonvulsants and the radiographic contrast agent metrizamide. Unilateral asterixis can occur after brain lesions in the distributions of the anterior or posterior cerebral arteries. The smallest brain lesion that can cause unilateral asterixis involves structures that are destroyed during stereotactic ventrolateral thalamotomy.

Hemiballismus Hemiballismus is a hyperkinetic movement disorder characterized by violent flinging motions in the arm contralateral to a lesion (usually vascular) in or near the subthalamic nucleus. The movements in ballism also have a rotary component at the shoulder and hip; there may be concomitant flexion and extension movements in the hand and foot as well. The involuntary motions persist throughout the day but generally attenuate during sleep. Strength and muscle tone may be slightly decreased in the affected extremities and

L. EXT.

L. FLEX.

L. TRI.

L. BIC.

L. ACC.

L. ACC.

A   B

FIGURE 15-4 *Recordings from the left arm of a patient with posthypoxic intention myoclonus (A) before and (B) during treatment with 5-hydroxytryptophan. In both, the arm was held out horizontally from the shoulder. The upper four traces are EMGs from wrist extensors, wrist flexors, triceps, and biceps. The lower two traces are from accelerometers at right angles to one another on the hand. The horizontal calibration is 1 s. A. The continuous,*

large, jerky movements during voluntary activity are produced by arrhythmic bursts of EMG activity interspersed with irregular periods of EMG silence. The former positive and latter negative abnormalities occurred synchronously in antagonistic muscle groups. B. Only a little irregular tremor remains, and the EMG is much more continuous. (From JH Growdon et al, Neurology 26:1135, 1976.)

FIGURE 15-5 *Asterixis recorded from the outstretched left arm of a patient with metrizamide-induced encephalopathy. The upper four EMG traces are identical to those in Fig. 15-4. The bottom trace is from an accelerometer on the dorsum of the hand. Calibration is 1 s. Note the continuous voluntary EMG interrupted at the arrow by a brief involuntary silent period in all four muscles. This silent period is followed by a lapse of posture and its jerky restitution, which is recorded by the accelerometer.*

accurate movements are impaired, but patients with hemiballismus are not paralyzed. Both experimental and clinical observations indicate that the subthalamic nucleus probably exerts a controlling influence on the globus pallidus. Damage to the subthalamic nucleus destroys this restraining influence and results in hemiballismus. The exact biochemical consequences of these lesions remain unclear, but indirect evidence suggests that there is an increase in dopaminergic tone in the remaining basal ganglia structures. Medical treatment with neuroleptic drugs given to block DA receptors are generally effective in suppressing ballismus. Surgery is reserved for refractory cases; a stereotactic lesion placed in the ipsilateral globus pallidus, thalamic fasciculus, or ventrolateral thalamus can also abolish hemiballismus and restore normal function. Although recovery can be complete, many patients are left with variable amounts of hemichorea involving the hand and foot.

Tremor This common symptom consists of a rhythmic oscillation of a part of the body around a fixed point. Tremors usually involve the distal parts of limbs; the head, tongue, or jaw; and rarely the trunk. There are several different types of tremor, and each has its own clinical setting, pathophysiology, and therapeutic requirements. Often several different tremors exist in the same patient and must be treated individually. In a general hospital, most patients who appear tremulous actually have asterixis as a manifestation of one or another metabolic encephalopathy. Tremors may be subdivided clinically according to their distribution, amplitude, and relationship to volitional movement.

Tremor at rest is a coarse tremor with an average rate of four to five beats per second. It is most often localized in one or both hands and, occasionally, in the jaw or tongue. It is frequently a feature of Parkinson's disease. It characteristically occurs when there is postural (tonic) contraction of axial and limb girdle musculature when the limb is in an attitude of repose; willed movement temporarily suppresses it (Fig. 15-6). If the proximal muscles are completely relaxed, the tremor usually disappears, but the average patient rarely achieves this state. In some cases the tremor is constant; in others it varies from time to time and may extend from one group of muscles to another as the disease progresses. In some patients with Parkinson's disease there is no tremor; in others the tremor tends to be rather gentle and more or less limited to the distal muscles, whereas in a minority of parkinsonian patients and in patients with Wilson's disease (hepatolenticular degeneration) it often has a wider range and involves proximal muscles. In many cases there is a variable degree of rigidity of a plastic type in the tremulous limb or elsewhere. Although it is a source of great embarrassment and often is deemed responsible for all of a patient's motor difficulties, this type of tremor interferes with voluntary movements surprisingly little: It is not uncommon to see a patient who has been trembling violently raise a full glass of water to the lips and drain the contents without spilling a drop. The handwriting of these patients is often small and cramped (micrographia). The gait may be of festinating type. It is the combination of tremor at rest, slowness of movement, rigidity, flexed postures without true paralysis, and postural instability that constitutes Parkinson's syndrome. Often patients with Parkinson's disease also suffer from the tremor of stage fright (one of the enhanced physiologic tremors—see below) or from essential-familial tremor. Both may be exaggerated by increased levels of catecholamines in the blood stream and may be suppressed by drugs, such as propranolol, that block beta-adrenergic receptors.

The exact pathologic anatomy of *tremor at rest* is unknown. In Parkinson's disease, the visible lesions are predominantly in the substantia nigra. In Wilson's disease, in which tremor is mixed with cerebellar ataxia, the lesions are diffuse. Elderly persons may develop resting tremor without rigidity, slowness of movement, flexed postures, or masked facies. Unlike patients with parkinsonism, individuals with this syndrome do not progress to motor disability; their tremor does not respond to anti-parkinsonian drugs. In any given case it is not predictable whether a tremor is the initial sign of Parkinson's disease. Patients with titubation and a proximal tremor at rest (rubral tremor) as a symptom of cerebellar system dysfunction can be differentiated by the presence of ataxia and dysmetria from those with Parkinson's disease.

Action tremor refers to tremors present when the limbs are active, either when maintained in a certain position, as when outstretched, or throughout voluntary movement. Tremor amplitude may increase slightly as the action of the limbs becomes more precise, but it never approaches the degree of augmentation seen with cerebellar ataxia/dysmetria. Action tremors are easily made to disappear when the limbs are relaxed. Some of the action tremors are an exaggeration of normal *physiologic tremor;* such enhanced physiologic tremors are

TABLE 15-2 Conditions that enhance physiologic tremors

HYPERADRENERGIC STATES
Anxiety
Bronchodilators and other beta agonists
Excitement
Hypoglycemia
Hyperthyroidism
Pheochromocytoma
Peripheral metabolites of levodopa
Stage fright

POSSIBLE HYPERADRENERGIC STATES
Amphetamines
Antidepressants
Withdrawal from alcohol or opiates
Xanthines in tea and coffee

STATES OF UNCERTAIN ETIOLOGY
Corticosteroid therapy
Exercise
Fatigue
Lithium therapy

extremely common. They are experienced occasionally by all normal persons as well as by patients with essential-familial tremor or Parkinson's disease. They involve the outstretched hand as well as head, lips, and tongue. In general, they are due to a hyperadrenergic state and sometimes are iatrogenic (Table 15-2). Activation of beta$_2$ receptors in muscle alters the mechanical properties of muscle, eliciting action tremor. These alterations are reflected in discharges of muscle spindle afferents which modify the timing of activity around the stretch reflex arc and serve to augment the amplitude of preexisting physiologic tremor. Only patients without functional stretch reflex arcs are immune to these tremors. Peripherally active drugs that block beta$_2$ adrenergic receptors diminish enhanced physiologic tremors. This type of tremor is seen in numerous medical, neurologic, and psychiatric diseases and is therefore more difficult to interpret than tremor at rest.

There is another, somewhat slower action tremor which may occur as the only neurologic abnormality either sporadically or in several members of a family. It is known as *essential-familial tremor* (Fig. 15-7). It may begin in childhood but usually comes on later and persists throughout adult life. It becomes a source of embarrassment because it suggests to the onlooker that the patient is nervous. A curious fact about this tremor is that one or two drinks of an alcoholic beverage may abolish it but it will become worse after the effects of

FIGURE 15-6 *Tremor at rest in a patient with Parkinson's disease. The upper two traces are surface EMG recordings from extensors and flexors of the left wrist; the lower trace is from an accelerometer attached to the left hand. The horizontal calibration denotes 1 s. Note the tremor at rest results* *from alternating contractions of antagonistic muscles at approximately 5 Hz. At the arrow, the patient is asked to dorsiflex the left wrist, and the tremor at rest disappears.*

R. EXT.

R. FLEX.

R. ACC.

FIGURE 15-7 *Action tremor in a patient with essential-familial tremor. Recordings from the right upper extremity are with the hand actively dorsiflexed; otherwise, traces are similar to Fig. 15-4. The horizontal calibration denotes 500 ms. Note that during this action tremor, bursts of EMG activity at approximately 8 Hz occur synchronously in antagonistic muscles.*

the alcohol have worn off. Essential-familial tremors are suppressed by primidone or CNS-active beta-adrenergic blocking agents such as propranolol.

Intention tremor is an ambiguous term: The abnormal movements are certainly not intentional, and the abnormality is best described as an oscillatory ataxia generated proximally rather than as tremor. True tremors tend to affect distal musculature and the movements are more rhythmic and tend to be in one plane. Cerebellar ataxia, in which the direction of abnormal movement varies from second to second, requires for its full expression the performance of an exacting, precise, willed movement. The ataxia is absent when the limbs are inactive and during the first part of a voluntary movement, but as the action continues and greater precision is demanded (e.g., in touching a target such as the patient's nose or the examiner's finger), a jerky, somewhat rhythmic interruption of forward progression, with side-to-side oscillation, appears. It continues for a fraction of a second or so after the act is completed. Such dysmetria may seriously interfere with the patient's performance of skilled acts. Sometimes the head is involved (titubation). This movement disorder invariably indicates disease of the cerebellar system including its connections. When the disease is very severe, every movement, even the lifting of a limb, results in a wide-ranging oscillation of such violence as to throw the patient off balance. This state is occasionally seen in multiple sclerosis, Wilson's disease, and vascular, traumatic, and other lesions of the tegmentum of the midbrain and subthalamus but not of the cerebellum.

Habit spasms and tics Many individuals develop habitual movements that persist unchanged throughout life. Common examples include sniffing, clearing the throat, protruding the chin, and pulling on the collar. These are called habit spasms. These individuals admit that the movements are voluntary, but that they feel compelled to make them in order to relieve tension. Habit spasms can be inhibited for a time by a willful effort but reappear when attention is diverted. In certain cases, they become so ingrained that the person is unaware of them and unable to control them. Children between 5 and 10 years of age are especially likely to have habit spasms.

Tics are characterized by stereotyped, purposeless, and irregularly repetitive movements. Gilles de la Tourette syndrome is the most common and severe form of multiple tic disorder. This syndrome is a neuropsychiatric disorder with motor and behavior abnormalities; it usually begins in the first two decades of life and affects boys four times more frequently than girls. Motor symptoms include multiple brief muscular spasms, known as convulsive tics, in the face, neck, and shoulders. Vocal tics, including grunts and barking sounds, are also common. Behavioral abnormalities include coprolalia (swearing and repeating other vile utterances) and repeating the words of others (echolalia). The cause of Tourette's syndrome is unknown, and its pathophysiology remains obscure. Treatments with neuroleptic drugs will decrease the severity and frequency of tics in 75 to 90 percent of patients with Tourette's syndrome, regardless of disease severity. The noradrenergic agonist clonidine has also been used to suppress symptoms of Tourette's syndrome.

EXAMINATION AND DIFFERENTIAL DIAGNOSIS OF EXTRAPYRAMIDAL SYNDROMES In broad terms, all of the extrapyramidal disorders should be viewed in terms of primary deficit (negative symptoms) and of the new phenomena (abnormal postures and involuntary movements) that have appeared. The positive symptoms are ascribed to release from inhibition or disequilibrium of undamaged motor parts of the nervous system. The physician must cultivate the habit of accurately observing and describing abnormalities of movement and must not be content merely to give the condition a name or to force it into some superficial category. The fully developed extrapyramidal motor syndromes can be recognized without difficulty once the physician has become familiar with the typical pictures. A mental picture of Parkinson's disease, with its slowness of movement, poverty of facial expression, tremor at rest, and rigidity, should be fixed in mind. Similarly, the gross distortions of postural abnormalities in dystonia, whether widespread in trunk muscles or involving only neck muscles as in spasmodic torticollis, should be easily recognized. Athetosis, with its instability of postures, ceaseless movements of finger and hands, and intention spasm; chorea, with its rapid and complicated movements; myoclonus, with its abrupt movements that flit over the body, are other standard syndromes. There tends to be a mild defect in the voluntary use of the affected parts in all extrapyramidal syndromes.

Early or mild forms of these conditions, like all medical diseases, may offer special difficulties in diagnosis. Cases of Parkinson's disease, seen before the appearance of tremor, are often overlooked. Uncertainty of balance and short gait (*marche à petit pas*) in the elderly is often incorrectly attributed to loss of confidence and fear of falling. Patients may complain of being nervous and restless and describe a stiffness and aching in parts of the body. Because there is no weakness or change in reflexes, the disorder may then be considered rheumatic or even psychogenic. Parkinson's disease often begins in a hemiplegic distribution, and for this reason, the illness may be misdiagnosed as cerebral thrombosis or tumor. Facial immobility, a suggestion of a limp, mild rigidity, failure of an arm to swing naturally in walking, or loss of certain movements of cooperation will help in diagnosis at this time. Every case presenting with atypical extrapyramidal symptoms should be surveyed for Wilson's disease in order to avoid missing a treatable illness. Mild or early chorea is often mistaken for simple nervousness. Observing the patient at rest as well as in action is critical to the diagnosis. There are instances, nonetheless, in which it is impossible to distinguish simple fidgets from early chorea, especially in children, and there are no laboratory tests to aid in the diagnosis. The first postural manifestations of dystonia may suggest hysteria, and it is only later when the fixity of the postural abnormality becomes apparent that accurate diagnosis is reached.

Motor disorders seldom appear in pure form, and extrapyramidal syndromes often coexist with lesions in the corticospinal tract or cerebellar systems. For example, syndromes such as progressive supranuclear palsy, olivopontocerebellar atrophy, or the Shy-Drager syndrome have many elements of Parkinson's disease but also have paralysis of voluntary eye movements, ataxia, apraxia, postural hypotension, or spasticity with bilateral Babinski signs. Wilson's disease usually displays tremor at rest, rigidity, slowness of movement, and flexion dystonia of the trunk, but exceptionally there are athetosis, dystonia, and intention tremor. Emotional or cognitive abnormalities may be the presenting signs in Wilson's disease. Hallervorden-Spatz disease may take the form of universal rigidity and flexion dystonia, but choreoathetosis is sometimes observed. In some forms of Huntington's disease, particularly with juvenile onset, rigidity replaces choreoathetosis. Corticospinal and various extrapyramidal disorders may be associated in patients with cerebral diplegia. Some of the neurodegenerative diseases in which corticospinal tract and basal ganglia lesions coexist are described in Chap. 350.

Anatomic and neuropathologic studies of the basal ganglia, coupled with biochemical analyses of neurotransmitter content and behavioral responses to neuropharmacologic agents, provide the basis for understanding disorders involving the basal ganglia and for guiding their treatment. This is most clearly seen in Parkinson's disease and Huntington's disease. In Parkinson's disease, the DA content of the striatum is depleted owing to a loss of neurons in the substantia nigra and degeneration of their axonal projection to the striatum. As a result of decreased DA release, neurons within the striatum that synthesize ACh are released from inhibition. This results in the preponderance of cholinergic neurotransmission relative to dopaminergic transmission that accounts for most of the symptoms in Parkinson's disease. Recognition of this imbalance provides the basis for rational pharmacologic treatments. According to this formulation, drugs that increase dopaminergic neurotransmission, such as levodopa or bromocriptine, would be expected to rectify the imbalance between cholinergic and dopaminergic tone. These drugs, often prescribed in combination with anticholinergic drugs, are now standard therapy in Parkinson's disease. Excess levodopa or bromocriptine in patients with Parkinson's disease may induce a wide variety of abnormal movements that result from excessive stimulation of DA receptors in the striatum. The most frequent of these is craniofacial choreoathetosis, but more generalized choreoathetosis, facial and cervical spasms, dystonic postures, and myoclonic jerks may also occur. On the other hand, administration of drugs that block DA receptors (such as the neuroleptics) or deplete DA storage (such as reserpine or tetrabenazine) may produce a parkinsonian syndrome in an otherwise normal individual.

Huntington's disease is in many ways the clinical and pharmacologic opposite of Parkinson's disease. In Huntington's disease, characterized by personality change and dementia, gait abnormality, and chorea, there is a loss of neurons within the caudate and putamen, with resultant depletion of GABA and ACh but preserved DA content. The symptoms of chorea are believed to result from relative excess of DA compared with other transmitters in the striatum; drugs that block DA receptors, such as the neuroleptics, generally suppress chorea, whereas levodopa administration increases it. Similarly, physostigmine, given to increase cholinergic neurotransmission, may suppress chorea, whereas anticholinergic drugs enhance it.

These examples of clinical pharmacology further confirm the existence of delicate balances between excitatory and inhibitory impulses in the basal ganglia. In any one patient, the variable clinical manifestations seen during therapy are due to alterations in the neurochemical environment; the anatomic lesions remain unchanged. These examples illustrate the power of neuropharmacologic therapy in basal ganglia disease and provide the basis for optimism regarding the future ability of drugs to benefit patients with extrapyramidal movement disorders.

REFERENCES

DELONG MR, GEORGOPOULOS AP: Motor functions of the basal ganglia, in *Handbook of Physiology*, Section I, *The Nervous System*, vol II: *Motor Control, Part 2*, VB Brooks (ed). Bethesda, American Physiological Society, 1981, pp 1017–1062

DELWAIDE PJ, YOUNG RR (eds): *Restorative Neurology*, vol. 1: *Clinical Neurophysiology in Spasticity*. Amsterdam, Elsevier, 1985

EMSON PC (ed): *Chemical Neuroanatomy*. New York, Raven Press, 1983

FELDMAN RG et al (eds): *Spasticity: Disordered Motor Control*. Chicago, Year Book Medical Publishers, 1980

GESCHWIND N: The apraxias: Neural mechanisms of disorders of learned movement. Am Sci 63:188, 1975

GROWDON JH, SCHEIFE RT: Medical treatment of extrapyramidal diseases, in *Update III: Harrison's Principles of Internal Medicine*, KJ Isselbacher et al (eds). New York, McGraw-Hill, 1982, pp 185–208

KUYPERS HGJM: Anatomy of the descending pathways, in *Handbook of Physiology*, Section I, *The Nervous System*, vol II: *Motor Control, Part 1*, VB Brooks (ed). Bethesda, American Physiological Society, 1981, pp 597–666

LAWRENCE DG, KUYPERS HGJM: The functional organization of the motor system in the monkey. Brain 91:1, 1968

MARSDEN CD: The mysterious motor function of the basal ganglia. Neurology 32:514, 1982

MARTIN JB: Huntington's disease: New approaches to an old problem. Neurology 34:1059, 1984

YOUNG RR, SHAHANI BT: Asterixis: One type of negative myoclonus, in *Myoclonus*, S Fahn et al (eds). New York, Raven Press, 1985, pp 12–30

YOUNG RR, DELWAIDE PJ: Drug therapy: Spasticity. N Engl J Med 304:28, 1981

16 ATAXIA AND DISORDERS OF EQUILIBRIUM AND GAIT

SID GILMAN

In the assessment of patients with neurologic disorders, it is important to inquire when taking the history about posture and gait and to examine these functions routinely as part of the neurologic examination. Abnormalities of posture and gait can result from disorders of several levels of the nervous system, and the type of abnormality observed clinically often indicates the site affected.

NEURAL STRUCTURES REQUIRED FOR STANDING AND WALKING The structures in the central nervous system that control standing and walking are the basal ganglia, a "locomotor region" in the mesencephalon, the cerebellum, and the spinal cord. The cerebral cortex doubtless is important in many aspects of standing and walking, but in experimental animals, complete removal of the cerebral cortex during the neonatal period, preserving the basal ganglia, thalamus, and lower structures, leaves stance and locomotion essentially normal. If the cerebral cortex, basal ganglia, and thalamus are removed, leaving the mesencephalon and lower brainstem intact, standing and walking are still possible. Electrical stimulation in a region of the mesencephalon termed the "locomotor region" evokes walking motions, and the speed and form of locomotion can be modified from a slow walk to a trot or gallop with changes in stimulation strength. This region receives projections from the basal ganglia, including the subthalamic and endopeduncular nuclei and the substantia nigra.

The spinal cord contains neural circuitry that coordinates the muscles for locomotion. After experimental transection of the spinal cord in the midthoracic region, the hindlimbs maintain the capacity to perform coordinated walking movements when placed on a moving treadmill. With increased treadmill speed, walking movements can switch to simultaneous movements of the hindlimbs, as in a gallop. After a high spinal transection, both the forelimbs and the hindlimbs can generate alternating movements and the sets of limbs remain coordinated. Thus, neural circuitry in the spinal cord can coordinate movements among all four limbs. The cerebellum controls many of the movements required for walking. Ablation of the cerebellum results in severe disorders of standing and walking.

In summary, walking is the result of integrated activity of the basal ganglia, mesencephalon, cerebellum, and spinal cord. Sensory inputs from movements of joints and muscle afferents provide important components for the control of walking. Without appropriate sensory feedback information, the pattern of walking is severely disrupted.

THE CEREBELLUM The cerebellum does not initiate movements, but it works closely with the motor cortex, basal ganglia, and many brainstem structures in executing a variety of movements. The cerebellum is needed to maintain proper posture and balance for walking and running; to perform fine voluntary movements such as those needed for writing, dressing, and eating; to carry out rapidly alternating and repetitive movements as in playing a musical instrument or working with a computer; and to coordinate smooth tracking movements of the eyes. The cerebellum is able to control certain properties of movements, including trajectory, velocity, and acceleration. Voluntary movements can be performed in the absence of cerebellar function, but the movements are clumsy and disorganized. The disturbances of movement from cerebellar dysfunction are termed *dyssynergia* (also *asynergia* or *ataxia*).

The cerebellum consists of a midline vermal region and two hemispheres which are attached to the medulla, pons, and midbrain by three peduncles on each side. A layer of gray matter, the cerebellar cortex, covers the cerebellar surface and encloses an internal core of white matter. Three pairs of deep cerebellar nuclei are buried within the cerebellum. From medial to lateral these consist of the fastigial, interposed (globose and emboliform), and dentate nuclei.

The cerebellum consists of three lobes. The *flocculonodular lobe*, which is the oldest part of the cerebellum phylogenetically (archicerebellum), consists of the paired flocculi and the nodulus. It receives input principally from the vestibular nuclei. The *anterior lobe*, the second oldest part (paleocerebellum), consists of vermal and paravermal structures in the anterior superior portion of the cerebellum. It receives input chiefly from the spinal cord. The *posterior lobe* is the largest and phylogenetically newest part of the cerebellum (neocerebellum) and is located between the other two lobes. The posterior lobe receives projections from the cerebral hemispheres via the pontine nuclei.

The cerebellar cortex contains three layers: an outermost *molecular layer*, a middle *Purkinje cell layer*, and an inner *granular layer*. The afferent fibers reaching the cerebellar cortex send collateral projections to the deep cerebellar nuclei and terminate either in the granule cell layer as *mossy fibers* or upon the dendrites of Purkinje cells as *climbing fibers*. Mossy fiber afferents are derived from the spinal cord, pontine nuclei, vestibular receptors and nuclei, trigeminal nuclei, reticular nuclei, and deep cerebellar nuclei. Climbing fiber afferents are derived exclusively from the inferior olive. Both mossy fiber and climbing fiber inputs are excitatory to the deep cerebellar nuclei and the cortex. Purkinje cells provide the only route for all information exiting from the cerebellar cortex and are inhibitory to the deep cerebellar and vestibular nuclei.

Projections to the cerebellum also originate in the locus coeruleus

and the raphe nuclei of the brainstem. The afferents to the cerebellum from the locus coeruleus are noradrenergic; those from the raphe nuclei are serotonergic; and both sets of afferents are inhibitory. Several amino acids have been identified as putative neurotransmitters in the cerebellum. These include glutamate, which is used by granule cells; aspartate, which is used by climbing fibers; and γ-aminobutyric acid, which is used by Purkinje cells, Golgi cells, and basket cells.

The *inferior cerebellar peduncle (restiform body)* consists chiefly of afferent fibers. The peduncle contains a single efferent tract, the fastigiobulbar tract, which projects to the vestibular nuclei and completes a vestibular circuit through the cerebellum. Afferent fibers enter the inferior cerebellar peduncle from at least six sources (Fig. 16-1): (1) fibers from the vestibular nerve and nuclei; (2) olivocerebellar fibers from the inferior olivary nuclei; (3) the dorsal spinocerebellar tract; (4) some of the fibers from the dorsal spinocerebellar tract; (5) the cuneocerebellar tract from the accessory cuneate nuclei in the medulla; and (6) reticulocerebellar fibers. *The middle cerebellar peduncle (brachium pontis)* consists almost entirely of crossed afferent fibers from the pontine nuclei in the gray substance of the basal part of the pons (pontocerebellar or transverse pontine fibers) (Fig. 16-2). The major projections to the pontine nuclei originate within the cerebral cortex. The *superior cerebellar peduncle (brachium conjunctivum)* consists principally of efferent projections from the cerebellum. Rubral, thalamic, and reticular projections arise from the dentate and interposed nuclei. Some of the fastigiobulbar tract fibers also run with the superior penduncle for a short distance before they enter the inferior cerebellar peduncle. The superior cerebellar peduncle contains afferent projections from the ventral spinocerebellar tract, a portion of the rostral spinocerebellar tract, and trigeminocerebellar projections.

Except for direct projections of Purkinje cells onto vestibular nuclei, the efferent pathways of the cerebellum begin with the deep nuclei. The fastigial nucleus sends fibers to the reticular and vestibular nuclei of the brainstem. These nuclei project into the spinal cord and are concerned with posture and balance. The interposed nuclei of each side of the cerebellum project axons through the superior cerebellar peduncle to the red nucleus of the contralateral side. The red nucleus projects into the spinal cord via the rubrospinal tract (Fig. 16-2). This tract crosses the midline and descends into the spinal cord. The origin of this pathway in the interposed nuclei and the terminal portion in the spinal cord are on the same side of the body. Both the dentate and the interposed nuclei send fibers through the superior cerebellar peduncle to the contralateral ventrolateral nucleus of the thalamus. The ventrolateral nucleus relays fibers to

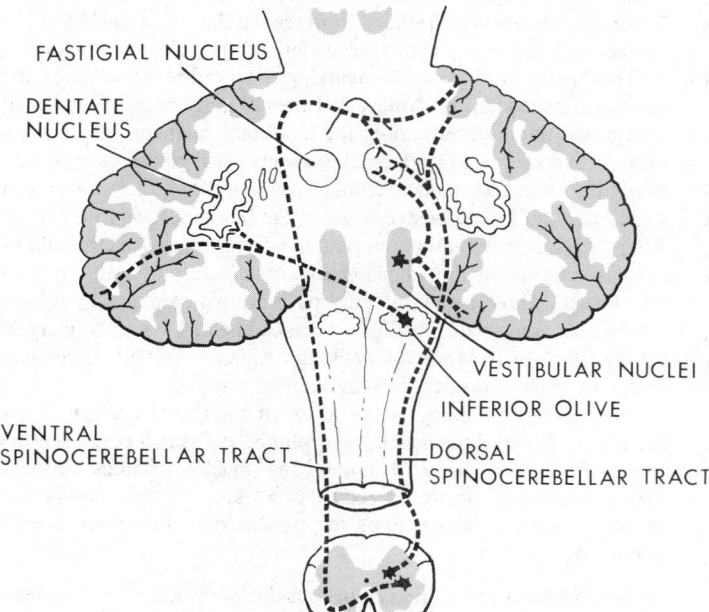

FIGURE 16-1 *The central nervous system connections of the dorsal and ventral spinocerebellar tracts, the fastigial nuclei, and the vestibular nuclei. (Adapted from S Gilman and SS Winans, in Manter & Gatz's Essentials of Clinical Neuroanatomy and Neurophysiology, 6th ed, Philadelphia, Davis Co, 1982.)*

FASTIGIAL NUCLEUS

DENTATE NUCLEUS

VESTIBULAR NUCLEI

INFERIOR OLIVE

VENTRAL SPINOCEREBELLAR TRACT

DORSAL SPINOCEREBELLAR TRACT

the motor regions of the ipsilateral frontal lobe. The thalamic endings in the cerebral cortex make connection with corticospinal neurons whose efferent fibers pass through the pyramidal tract and cross to the contralateral side of the spinal cord. Thus, the origin of the cerebellothalamocortical pathway in the dentate and interposed nuclei and its termination in the spinal cord are on the same side of the body (Fig. 16-2).

For clinical purposes, a useful method of describing the cerebellum is based upon the existence of longitudinal sagittal zones. Each half of the cerebellum is subdivided into three longitudinal strips arranged from medial to lateral, including the cerebellar cortex, underlying white matter, and deep cerebellar nuclei: (1) a midline zone consisting of the vermal region with the fastigial nucleus; (2) an intermediate zone, the paravermal region, with the interposed nuclei; and (3) a lateral zone consisting of the cerebellar hemisphere with the dentate nucleus. Lesions of the midline zone cause disorders of stance and gait, truncal ataxia and titubation, and rotated or tilted postures of the head. Lesions of the lateral zone lead to disturbances in coordinated limb movement (ataxia), dysarthria, hypotonia, nystagmus, and kinetic tremor. Lesions of the intermediate zone cause symptoms characteristic of involvement of both the midline and lateral zones.

Ataxia is the result of dysmetria and decomposition of movement. *Dysmetria* is a disturbance of the trajectory or placement of a limb during active movement in which the limb falls short of its target (*hypometria*) or extends beyond its target (*hypermetria*). *Decomposition of movement* refers to errors in the sequence and speed of the component parts of a movement. The result is a lack of speed and skill in acts requiring the smoothly coordinated activity of several muscles. Movements previously fluid and accurate become halting

and imprecise. *Ataxia* presents clinically as a disturbance in the rate and extent of an individual movement and commonly occurs from lesions of the cerebellum or of the sensory systems. Ataxia of gait consists of irregularities in the rate, length, and consistency of walking movements with veering to one side or the other.

PHYSIOLOGIC RESPONSES IMPORTANT IN STANDING AND WALKING Maintenance of the upright posture results from the actions of a number of postural reflex responses: (1) local static reactions acting on individual limbs; (2) segmental static reactions linking the extremities together; and (3) general static reactions resulting from the position of the head in space. *Local static reactions* include the stretch reflex and the positive supporting reaction. The simplest *stretch reflex* is illustrated by the muscle stretch response (deep tendon reflex), a brief muscle twitch evoked by rapid stretch of the muscle's tendon. Maintenance of muscle extension results in sustained contraction of that muscle through the stretch reflex. The *positive supporting reaction*, as elucidated in animal studies, results from a light cutaneous contact of the skin of the foot and also by proprioceptive stimulation owing to stretch of the interosseous muscles. The result of these stimuli is an extensor thrust by the limb.

The *segmental static reactions* include the crossed extension reflex and interlimb coordination. In the crossed extension reflex, application of noxious stimulation to an extremity results in flexion of that limb and simultaneous extension of the contralateral limb. With stronger stimulation, the crossed extension reflex triggered from a hindlimb can induce flexion in the contralateral forelimb and extension in the ipsilateral forelimb. Thus, the whole body moves along a diagonal path through the extended contralateral hindlimb and ipsilateral

FIGURE 16-2 *The central nervous system connections of the dentate nucleus and interposed (emboliform and globose) nuclei. (Adapted from S Gilman and SS Winans, in Manter & Gatz's Essentials of Clinical Neuroanatomy and Neurophysiology, 6th ed, Philadelphia, Davis Co, 1982.)*

forelimb, thereby removing the stimulated limb from the source of noxious stimulation. This diagonal pattern of interlimb coordination also provides postural adjustments in various situations.

The *general static reactions* consist of two general types. The first, the *tonic neck* and *labyrinthine reflexes*, function together to adjust body posture when the head moves relative to the trunk in space. The second, the *righting reflex*, is triggered by labyrinthine, neck, and visual stimuli and helps the animal to regain an upright position after a fall. The *grasp reflex* is a component of the righting reflex. Other forms of general static reactions include the placing and hopping reactions as well as adjustment of body postures during limb movements.

CLINICAL APPROACH TO DISORDERS OF EQUILIBRIUM AND GAIT When evaluating a disorder of gait, the physician should inquire whether the disturbance occurs more in the dark than in the light; whether there is any accompanying vertigo, giddiness, or lightheadedness; and whether there is pain, numbness, tingling, or other type of paresthesias of the limbs. Inquiry should search for weakness, bowel and bladder dysfunction, and limb stiffness or rigidity. The physician should ask whether there is difficulty in the initiation or termination of walking.

Examination of stance and gait is performed best in a setting in which the physician can observe the patient walk from the front, back, and sides. The patient should rise quickly from a chair, walk normally at a slow pace, then more rapidly, and then turn around. Walking should be examined on the heels, on the toes, and in tandem, placing the heel of one foot directly in front of the toes of the opposite foot, attempting to progress in a straight line. The patient should stand erect with the feet together and the head straight, first with the eyes open and then with the eyes closed to determine whether balance can be maintained (Romberg's sign). It is often helpful to observe the gait initially as the patient comes into the examining room when the patient is unaware that gait and stance are being examined.

With normal walking the body should be held erect, the head should be straight and the arms should hang loosely at the sides, each moving in rhythm with movement of the opposite leg. The shoulders and hips should be level and the arms should swing equally. The steps should be straight and equal in length. The head should not be tilted and there should be no appreciable scoliosis or lordosis. With each step the hip and knee should flex smoothly, the ankle should dorsiflex and the foot should clear the ground easily. The heel should strike the ground first and the weight of the body should be transferred successively onto the sole of the foot and then onto the toes. The head and body should rotate slightly with each step without lurching or falling movements. Each person walks in a characteristic fashion which is often familial. Some people walk with the toes turned inward, others with the toes turned outward. Some people stride with large steps and others shuffle, making small steps. A person's gait is often a reflection of personality traits and can reflect shyness and timidity or aggressiveness and self-confidence.

Hemiparesis The patient with weakness of the limbs on one side of the body from a lesion of the corticospinal tract usually develops a characteristic gait disorder. The severity of the disorder depends upon the degree of weakness and stiffness of the affected limbs. The severely hemiparetic subject will stand and walk with the affected arm adducted at the shoulder and flexed at the elbow, wrist and fingers and the affected leg stiffly extended at the hip, knee, and ankle. There is difficulty in flexing the hip and knee and dorsiflexing the ankle. Thus, the paretic leg swings outward at the hip so that the foot does not scrape the floor. The leg is held stiffly and rotates in a semicircle, first away from and then toward the trunk in a circumduction movement. Often the upper body tilts slightly to the opposite side during the leg movement. The arm on the hemiparetic side usually swings little during walking. The loss of arm swing can be an early sign of a progressive hemiparesis. A person with a mild hemiparesis may show a gait disorder similar to that of the severely

hemiparetic individual, but with a lesser degree of abnormality. In this case, a decrease in arm swing may be associated with subtle circumduction of the leg, without clear stiffness or weakness of the affected limbs.

Paraparesis Diseases of the spinal cord that affect leg function produce a characteristic gait resulting from a combination of spasticity and weakness of the lower extremities. Walking requires considerable effort and consists of slow, stiff movements at the hips and knees. The legs are usually maintained extended or slightly flexed at the hips and knees and adducted at the hips. In some people with paraparesis the legs may cross with each step, producing a scissoring motion. The steps usually are regular and short, and the patient may move the trunk from side to side, attempting to compensate for the stiff movements of the legs. The legs circumduct at the hips and the feet scrape along the floor so that the soles of the shoes become worn at the toes.

Parkinsonism Patient's with Parkinson's disease have a characteristic posture and gait. The severely affected individual stands in a posture of flexion, with the thoracic spine bent forward, the head bent downward, the arms moderately flexed at the elbows and the legs slightly flexed at the hips and knees. The patient sits or stands with striking immobility, showing a fixed facial expression with infrequent blinking and making few automatic movements of the limbs. The patient seldom crosses the legs or adjusts body posture when seated in a chair. Although the arms are held immobile, often a tremor involves the fingers and wrists at four to five cycles per second. In some people the tremor also occurs at the elbows and even at the shoulders. In advanced cases there may be drooling and a rhythmic tremor of the jaw. The patient usually gets up slowly to walk and, with walking, the trunk bends even farther forward, the arms remain immobile at the sides of the body or become further flexed and carried a bit ahead of the body. The arms fail to swing. As forward progression begins, the legs remain bent at the hips, knees, and ankles. Characteristically, the steps are short so that the feet barely clear the ground and the soles of the feet shuffle and scrape the floor. With forward locomotion the steps become successively more rapid and the patient may fall unless assisted (*festination*). If the patient is pushed forward or backward, compensatory flexion or extension movements of the trunk fail to occur and the patient is forced to make a series of propulsive or retropulsive steps.

Patients with Parkinson's disease often have great difficulty in rising from a chair or walking after standing still. The individual may initiate walking with several small steps before taking longer strides. Walking may stop involuntarily with attempts to pass through a doorway or into an elevator. Parkinsonian patients at times can walk with surprising speed and dexterity for brief intervals. In times of acute emergency, as in a fire, a person previously immobile can walk rapidly or even run briefly.

Cerebellar disease Disease of the cerebellum causes difficulty in standing without support and in walking. The disorder may result from lesions intrinsic to the cerebellum or from lesions in the connecting pathways to and from the cerebellum. The difficulty is worsened by attempts to walk with a narrow base. The affected person usually stands with the legs apart, and standing may provoke *titubation*, a coarse forward and backward tremor of the trunk. Attempting to stand with the feet together provokes swaying or falling. The instability is the same whether the eyes are open or closed. The patient walks cautiously, taking steps of varying lengths, and lurches from side to side. The patient complains of difficulty with balance, is fearful of walking without support, and may insist upon holding onto objects such as a bed or chair, moving cautiously between these objects. Frequently the individual does not need to be supported; simply touching a wall or an object in the room makes it possible to walk with a greater sense of security. When a mild gait disorder is present, walking may deteriorate with attempts to walk in tandem in a straight line. This causes the patient to lose balance and, in response, to place one foot to the side to avoid falling. With unilateral lesions of the cerebellum, balance is lost toward the side of the lesion.

When disease is restricted to the midline (vermal) portions of the cerebellum, as occurs in alcoholic cerebellar degeneration, disorders of stance and gait may develop without other signs of cerebellar dysfunction such as limb ataxia or nystagmus. In contrast, disease of the cerebellar hemispheres, either unilaterally or bilaterally, often causes marked limb ataxia and nystagmus in association with a gait disorder. With a lesion confined to one cerebellar hemisphere, ipsilateral disturbances of posture and movement commonly accompany the gait disorder. The patient usually stands with the shoulder on the side of the lesion lower than the other, and there may be an accompanying scoliosis. The limbs on the side of the cerebellar lesion show diminished resistance to passive manipulation (hypotonia). On walking the patient staggers and deviates toward the affected side. This can be demonstrated by asking the patient to walk around a chair. Rotation toward the affected side results in a fall into the chair, and rotation toward the normal side causes movement away from the chair in a spiral. The affected arm and leg show marked ataxia in tests of coordinated movement such as successively touching the patient's nose and then the examiner's finger or running the heel of the affected leg down the shin of the opposite leg.

Sensory ataxia A characteristic gait disorder results from loss of sensation in the lower extremities due to disease processes in the peripheral nerves, dorsal roots, dorsal columns of the spinal cord, or medial lemnisci. The most disabling component of the sensory disorder is the loss of joint position sense, but loss of input from muscle spindle receptors, vibration detectors, and cutaneous receptors also contributes to the disability. People with sensory ataxia are unaware of the position of the lower extremities and consequently have difficulty in both standing and walking. The patient usually stands with the legs spread widely apart. The patient remains stable if asked to stand with the feet together and the eyes open, but sways and often falls (positive Romberg's sign) when the eyes are closed. The test for Romberg's sign cannot be performed if the patient is unsteady when standing with the feet together and the eyes open, as may occur with cerebellar disease.

The patient with sensory ataxia walks with the legs spread widely apart, watching the ground carefully. The legs are lifted higher than necessary at the hips and are flung forward and outward in abrupt motions. The steps vary in length and the feet make characteristic slapping sounds as they contact the floor. The patient usually holds the body somewhat flexed at the hips, often using a cane for support. If vision is impaired or the patient attempts to walk in the dark, the gait disturbance worsens. The patient becomes unsteady and often falls when attempting to wash the face because of the temporary loss of visual compensation occurring with closure of the eyes.

Cerebral palsy This term encompasses a number of different motor abnormalities, most of them resulting from hypoxic-ischemic injury to the central nervous system in the perinatal period. The severity of the gait disturbance varies with the nature and extent of the lesion. Mild limited lesions can lead to increased deep tendon reflexes and extensor plantar responses with a slight degree of talipes equinovarus, without a clear gait disorder. More severe and extensive lesions commonly lead to bilateral hemiparesis. The patient stands and walks with a paraparetic posture and gait. The arms are adducted at the shoulders and flexed at the elbows and wrists.

Movement disorders commonly alter the gait in patients with cerebral palsy. Athetosis occurs frequently and consists of slow or moderately rapid serpentine movements of the arms and legs, with postures alternating between the extremes of flexion with supination and extension with pronation. On walking, patients with athetotic cerebral palsy show involuntary limb movements that are accompanied by rotary movements of the neck and frequent facial grimacing. The arms are usually flexed and the legs are extended, but asymmetric limb postures can occur with ambulation. For example, one arm may flex and supinate and the other may extend and pronate. Asymmetric

limb postures commonly occur as the head rotates from side to side. Usually when the chin turns to one side, the arm on that side extends and the opposite arm flexes.

Chorea Patients with choreic movements often develop a characteristic gait disorder. Chorea occurs most frequently in children with Sydenham's chorea, in adults with Huntington's disease, and occasionally in adults with Parkinson's disease treated with excessive amounts of dopamine agonist medications. Choreic movements consist of intermittent rapid movements of the face, trunk, neck, and limbs. Flexion, extension, and rotary movements of the neck occur along with grimacing movements of the face, twisting movements of the trunk and limbs, and rapid piano-playing movements of the digits. Frequently, in early chorea, flexion and extension movements of the hips occur so that the patient constantly seems to be crossing and uncrossing the legs. The patient may scowl, frown, and smile involuntarily. Walking usually accentuates the choreic movements. Sudden forward or sideward thrusting movements of the pelvis and rapid twisting movements of the trunk and limbs result in a gait that resembles a series of dance steps. The steps are usually irregular in size, and the patient has difficulty walking in a straight line. The rate of progression varies from slow to rapid owing to variability in the rate and amplitude of each step.

Dystonia This is an involuntary postural and movement disorder affecting children (dystonia musculorum deformans or torsion dystonia) and adults (dystonia of adult onset). The condition may occur sporadically without known cause, as a genetic disorder, or as part of another process such as Wilson's disease. In dystonia musculorum deformans, which commonly begins in children, the first symptom often consists of an abnormal gait. Characteristically the patient will walk with one foot inverted at the ankle, placing weight on the lateral side of the foot; as the disease progresses, this problem worsens and other postural abnormalities develop. These include elevation of one shoulder, elevation of a hip, twisted postures of the trunk, and excessive flexion of the wrist and fingers of one upper limb. Intermittent spasms of the trunk and limbs may interfere with walking. Eventually torticollis, tortipelvis, lordosis, and scoliosis may supervene. In extreme cases, the patient becomes unable to walk. Adult onset dystonia often results in a similar progression of movement disorders.

Muscular dystrophy Marked weakness of the muscles of the trunk and proximal portions of the legs causes a characteristic stance and gait. In attempting to rise from a seated position, the affected person bends forward, flexing the trunk at the hips, places the hands on the knees, and pushes the trunk upward by working the hands up the thighs. Standing occurs with exaggerated lumbar lordosis and a protuberant abdomen owing to weakness of the abdominal and paravertebral muscles. The patient walks with the legs spread widely apart and develops a waddling motion of the pelvis because of weakness of the gluteal muscles. The shoulders often slope forward, and winging of the scapulae may be seen with walking.

Frontal lobe disease Bilateral frontal lobe disease causes a characteristic gait disorder which is usually associated with dementia and frontal lobe release signs including grasp, suck, and snout reflexes. The patient characteristically stands with the feet spread widely apart and takes a first step only after a long delay. This hesitancy is followed by very small shuffling steps and then by a few steps of moderate amplitude after which time the patient freezes, unable to continue walking. The cycle then is repeated. Affected individuals usually do not show muscular weakness, abnormalities of the deep tendon reflexes, sensory changes, or extensor plantar reflex responses. Usually the patient can perform the individual limb movements required for walking if asked to mimic walking movements while lying supine. The gait disorder with frontal lobe disease is a form of apraxia, i.e., a disturbance in the performance of a motor function in the absence of weakness of the muscles required for the function.

Normal-pressure hydrocephalus Normal-pressure hydrocephalus (NPH) is a disorder characterized by dementia, gait apraxia, and urinary incontinence. Computerized axial tomography reveals large cerebral ventricles, widening of the callosal angle, and lack of filling with cerebospinal fluid of the subarachnoid space over the cerebral hemispheres. Injection of radioactive isotope into the lumbar sub-arachnoid space demonstrates pathologic reflux of the isotope into the ventricular system and inadequate penetration into the cortical subarachnoid spaces.

The gait in NPH resembles that seen in apraxia from frontal lobe disease, consisting of a series of small, shuffling steps making it appear that the feet are glued to the floor. Initiation of walking is impaired, and slow and small angular displacements of the hip, knee, and ankle joints occur along with low clearance of the foot from the floor so that the patient appears to be sliding the feet along the floor. There is continuous contraction of the antigravity muscles of the legs but low muscle activity in the calf muscles. The gait disorder in NPH is thought to result from impaired function of the frontal lobes. In about half the patients with NPH the gait is improved by surgical shunting of cerebrospinal fluid from the cerebral ventricles into the venous system.

Aging Changes in gait and difficulties with balance occur with aging. Elderly men develop forward flexion of the upper portion of the trunk with flexion of the arms and knees, decreased arm swing, and shortening of step length. Elderly women develop a waddling gait with shortening of step length. Abnormalities of gait and balance predispose the elderly to falls. About half the falls in the aged result from environmental factors, including poor illumination, stairs, and uneven or slippery surfaces. Other causes of falls include drop attacks, orthostatic hypotension, turning movements of the head, and vertigo.

Lower motor neuron disorders Diseases of the lower motor neurons or peripheral nerves characteristically cause distal limb weakness. Foot drop is a common manifestation. In the case of lower motor neuron disease, the limb weakness occurs in association with fascic-ulations and muscle atrophy. The patient usually cannot dorsiflex the foot and compensates by raising the knees higher than usual, thereby walking with a "steppage gait." If proximal muscles are affected, the gait also can take on a waddling quality.

Hysterical gait disorders Hysterical disorders of gait commonly appear in association with hysterical paralysis of one or more limbs. Usually the gait is bizarre, easily recognized as hysterical and unlike any disorder of gait evoked by organic disease. In other instances, however, hysterical gait disorders may resemble organic gait disorders and can be difficult to identify. Hysterical gait disorders can occur in men or women and can appear in youth, young adulthood, and middle age.

In hysterical hemiplegia, the patient drags the affected leg along the ground behind the body and does not circumduct the leg or use it to support the body weight. At times the hemiplegic leg may be pushed ahead of the patient and used mainly for support. The arm on the affected side often remains limp, hanging uselessly beside the body and does not develop the flexed posture commonly seen in hemiplegia from organic causes. The patient with hysterical hemi-plegia usually shows "give way" weakness. This is tested by asking the patient to make a maximum contraction of a set of muscles in an affected limb. Initially a strong contraction may occur, but as the examiner attempts to oppose the contracting muscles, the contraction suddenly gives way. Hysterical patients also commonly contract their muscles very slowly upon request, displaying great concentration and effort to evoke the contraction. Objective signs of neurologic disease are absent; the affected limbs show normal resistance to passive manipulation, the deep tendon reflexes are equal on the two sides of the body, and the plantar responses are downgoing.

In hysterical paraplegia, the patient usually walks with one or two crutches or lies in bed with the legs maintained either completely limp or stiffly extended. The term *astasia-abasia* refers to patients who cannot stand or walk but who can carry out natural movements of the limbs when lying in bed. Some patients with hysterical paraparesis walk with seeming difficulty but show normal power and coordination when lying in bed. On walking, the hysterical person clings to the bed or the furnishings of the room. If asked to walk without support the patient may lurch forward dramatically, veering from side to side at regular intervals. The patient can manage feats of extraordinary balance to avoid falling and may assume a variety of postures, walking with the legs in stiff extension, as if the legs are granite pillars, or walking with the legs in flexion and teetering from side to side. The hysterical patient may fall with walking, but only when a nearby physician or family member can catch the patient or when soft objects are available to cushion the fall. The gait disturbance is usually dramatic when an audience is present, and the patient can display remarkable agility in the rapid postural adjustments that occur.

REFERENCES

GILMAN S: Gait disorders, in *Merritt's Textbook of Neurology*, LP Rowland (ed). Philadelphia, Lea & Febiger, 1984, pp 44–48
——— et al: *Disorders of the Cerebellum*. Philadelphia, Davis, 1981
GRILLNER S: Neurobiological bases of rhythmic motor acts in vertebrates. Science 228: 143, 1985
ITO M: *The Cerebellum and Neural Control*. New York, Raven, 1984
KATZMAN R, TERRY R: *The Neurology of Aging*. Philadelphia, Davis, 1983
KNUTSSON E, LYING-TUNELL U: Gait apraxia in normal-pressure hydrocephalus: Patterns of movement and muscle activation. Neurology 35:155, 1985

17 MUSCLE PAINS, SPASMS, CRAMPS, AND EPISODIC WEAKNESS

ROBERT C. GRIGGS

Spontaneous or exercise-related discomfort from muscles or joints is usually benign and does not signal neuromuscular disease. Such symptoms may, however, provide clues to disabling disorders that too often evade diagnosis. The terms pain, spasm, and cramp are often used interchangeably by patients to describe symptoms referable to muscles. Other terms, including aching, heaviness, stiffness, and rheumatism, are also used, and usually connote less certainty about the source or localization of the discomfort. In clinical terminology, *spasm* refers to a brief, unsustained contraction of a single or multiple muscles. *Cramp* is a paroxysmal, spontaneous, prolonged, and painful contraction of one or more muscles.

SPASMS Abnormal movements of muscle may arise from abnormal electrical activity of the central nervous system mediated via the motor neuron, or occur within the muscle fiber itself. It may be difficult on clinical grounds alone to determine the precise site of origin of the abnormal motor activity. In general, movements originating in the central nervous system affect the entire side of the body, an entire limb, or a group of muscles. Central disorders may be rhythmic or intermittent; those arising in the periphery are usually random. The electroencephalogram may provide evidence for altered cortical activity in some conditions with a central nervous system etiology. The electromyogram (EMG) is less helpful because it reflects motor activity from any cause. EMG evidence of an underlying nerve disease may, however, be helpful in diagnosis (see Chap. 354) and certain abnormal muscle contractions have characteristic EMG features.

Intermittent, nonrhythmic movements of an entire limb, of the trunk, or of a portion of the face may result from cerebral seizure activity (Chap. 342) or from myoclonus (Chap. 15). Flexor and extensor spasms of an entire side or of the lower limbs result from a loss of motor inhibition within the central nervous system (Chap. 15). *Segmental myoclonus* results from focal disease within the brainstem or spinal cord that causes an abnormal discharge of groups of motor neurons. Localized vascular disease, tumor, or another lesion may be implicated.

Abnormal facial movements   *Hemifacial spasm* results from paroxysmal facial nerve activity, sometimes triggered by pressure from a tortuous blood vessel adjacent to the facial nerve as it leaves the brainstem. Hemifacial spasm commonly occurs in muscles about the eye, but may also involve or spread to the entire side of the face. Symptoms are often intermittent and intensified when patients are using facial muscles in activities such as speaking. Hemifacial spasm is painless but embarrassing, especially to individuals dealing with the public. Since it is often intensified and more severe when the patient is in stressful situations, an erroneous diagnosis of tic (habit spasm) is often made. Cerebellopontine angle lesions can occasionally produce a similar disorder. Neuroradiologic investigation is indicated in patients with facial hemispasm. Anticonvulsant medications occasionally alleviate the spasms, but surgical exploration and shielding of the facial nerve from the adjacent vessel is curative.

Facial *tics* (habit spasms) are stereotyped movements of the face such as eyeblinking, headturning, or grimacing that are under voluntary control but may be suppressed only by effort and anxiety on the part of the subject (see Chap. 15). Some tics are so frequently encountered as to be considered mannerisms, analogous to excessive clearing of the throat. The repetitious elevation of the eyebrows by frontalis muscle contraction is an example. Certain hereditary movement disorders such as Gilles de la Tourette syndrome are characterized by multiple tics (Chap. 15).

Synkinesias of the face result from aberrant regeneration of the facial nerve following facial paralysis from Bell's palsy or other facial nerve lesions. Nearly 50 percent of patients who recover from Bell's palsy display such movements; an example is *jawwinking*, where voluntary movements of the lower face elicit contraction of the orbicularis oculi muscle with eye closure.

Trigeminal neuralgia (tic douloureux) is characterized by brief, paroxysmal, lancinating pain in one side of the face (see Chap. 352). Although the portion of the nerve involved is almost exclusively sensory, the severity of the pain causes involuntary contraction of facial muscles; hence the name tic. Abnormal movements do not occur in the absence of pain.

Facial myokymia refers to a nearly continuous, fine or coarse rippling and fascicular twitching of facial muscles. Although often benign it may result from lesions of the pons such as a neoplasm or multiple sclerosis. Similar movements occur in motor neuron diseases such as amyotrophic lateral sclerosis or occasionally as an isolated, hereditary condition.

Abnormal limb movements   No movement should be visible in totally relaxed muscles. Diseases of motor neurons or their proximal axons are often associated with *fasciculations*, the spontaneous firing of an entire motor unit. Fasciculations are visible on inspection of muscle or perceived by the patient as a pulsation or quivering within muscle. Fasciculations occur at times in most normal individuals and unless weakness is present are seldom of any significance. Fasciculations are normal if observed in incompletely relaxed muscles. *Myokymia*, consisting of numerous, repetitive fasciculations, may also occur in limb muscles, giving a writhing appearance. Myokymia disappears with neuromuscular blockade, proving that the activity originates in anterior horn cells or in peripheral nerve. In patients with long-standing muscle denervation and reinnervation, motor unit size enlarges and fasciculations may be so large as to produce movement of the limbs, particularly of the fingers, a condition termed *minipolymyoclonus*. Similarly, the enlarged motor units of chronic denervation may be associated with a tremor of the fingers on extension.

Certain conditions are characterized by a compulsion to move the extremities. *Akathisia* or motor restlessness occurs in Parkinson's disease and other disorders of the basal ganglia including drug-induced movement disorders. The *restless legs syndrome* describes an uncomfortable sensation in muscles, usually in the legs and thighs, which occurs most commonly in middle-aged women. Patients feel they need to move their legs to relieve the abnormal sensation. The restless leg syndrome is frequent in uremia and may occur in other neuropathies, suggesting that the sensation is caused by an underlying neuropathy. It may also be familial and detailed study of such patients has failed to demonstrate any evidence of neuropathy. The restless sensation may be accompanied by myoclonic jerks of muscle often occurring during sleep. These myoclonic jerks are similar to the myoclonus observed in normal individuals entering REM sleep (see Chap. 20).

These forms of muscle spasm and myoclonus are somewhat similar to a group of unusual and unexplained *startle* syndromes or *hyper-ekplexias* characterized by sudden jerking of limbs or occasionally of trunk muscles. Sudden noise or touch may cause a patient to jump or to fling an extremity. Their cause is unknown.

SUSTAINED MUSCLE CONTRACTIONS   Distinguishing central from peripheral causes of sustained muscle contraction is often difficult. Abnormal muscle contractions with increased muscle tone usually result from central nervous system disease. Thus, loss or disturbance of central nervous system inhibition may lead to abnormal muscle contraction characteristic of spasticity, rigidity, or "paratonic" rigidity. In most instances there is other evidence of central nervous system disorder (Chap. 15). Diseases of the basal ganglia, presumably resulting from altered neurotransmitter release, may lead to dystonia (Chaps. 15 and 16).

Abnormal muscle contractions may also arise from repetitive depolarization of the component portions of the motor unit: the motor neuron; the peripheral axon of the neuron; the neuromuscular junction; or muscle fibers. Electrically inactive contractions may arise from disorders of the muscle contractile system.

Motor neuron disorders   *Cramp* is a term often used by patients to refer to a painful, involuntary contraction of a single muscle or a muscle group. Muscle cramps can arise from spontaneous firing of groups of anterior horn cells followed by contraction of many motor units. EMG recordings indicate that motor units fire at a rate of up to 300 per second, much higher than occurs with voluntary contraction. Cramps occur frequently in the legs in elderly patients and when severe are followed by residual tenderness and evidence of muscle fiber necrosis including elevation of serum creatine kinase. Cramps in the calf muscles are so common as to be considered normal, but more generalized cramps may be a sign of chronic disease of the motor neuron such as amyotrophic lateral sclerosis. They may be particularly troublesome during pregnancy, in patients with electrolyte disturbances (hyponatremia), and in patients on hemodialysis. When recurrent and localized to one muscle group they suggest nerve root disease. In many instances, however, it is impossible to determine the cause of cramps. Benign cramps, occurring commonly at night, may be relieved by quinine sulfate. Other causes of contractions arising from the motor neuron include *tetanus* (Chap. 99) and the *stiff-man syndrome*. In both disorders a loss of inhibitory neuronal input to anterior horn cells may result in repeated firing of motor neurons, producing severe, painful muscle contraction. A similar clinical picture may occur acutely with *strychnine poisoning*. Diazepam improves these spasms but may cause respiratory depression in doses sufficient to alleviate muscle contraction.

Peripheral nerve   *Tetany* is characterized by contractions of predominantly distal muscles, particularly in the hand (carpal spasm) and feet (pedal spasm). Laryngospasm may also occur. Tetany results from increased excitability of peripheral nerves. The muscle contractions are initially painless, but if sustained may cause muscle damage with pain. Severe tetany may involve spine musculature to produce opisthotonus. Tetany is usually caused by hypocalcemia, but may occur with hypomagnesemia or severe respiratory alkalosis (see Chap. 336). Idiopathic normocalcemic tetany, *spasmophilia*, occurs in both hereditary and sporadic forms.

Muscle MYOTONIA Repetitive depolarization of muscle cells can cause muscle contraction resulting in muscle stiffness and impaired relaxation. Myotonia is usually painless, but may disable patients by interfering with fine hand movements or by slowing ambulation. Myotonic dystrophy is the commonest disorder associated with myotonia although other manifestations of the disease such as cataracts and muscle weakness are usually more symptomatic (see Chap. 357). Myotonia congenita and paramyotonia congenita are less common, but more troublesome in terms of severity of myotonia. Myotonia is often worsened by cold and characteristically is attenuated by "warm-ups," decreasing with repeated activity. *Paradoxical myotonia* worsens with repeated activity and is characteristic of paramyotonia congenita; these patients also suffer from episodic and cold-induced weakness (Chap. 377). Impaired muscle relaxation that is electrically inactive is characteristic of the delayed relaxation of myxedema. This delay produces the characteristic "hung-up" ankle reflexes but is essentially asymptomatic.

CONTRACTURE Muscle contracture is a painful shortening of a muscle unassociated with muscle membrane depolarization. It occurs in disorders where a metabolic defect such as myophosphorylase deficiency limits the production of high-energy phosphates. Contractures are precipitated by exercise and are usually intensely painful. This use of the term *contracture* is confusing since the same word is used to describe the unrelated limitation of joint movement by shortening of muscle tendons seen in rheumatologic disorders, cerebral palsy, or chronic myopathies. Muscle rigidity from metabolic contracture can occur in the malignant hyperthermia syndrome, usually associated with general anesthesia. In the hyperthermia of the neuroleptic malignant syndrome, muscle rigidity arises from central nervous system overactivity, and intense electrical activity is present in muscle.

MUSCLE PAIN, ACHING, AND TENDERNESS

Painful muscles do not always imply muscle disease. Joint and bone disease frequently produce complaints of muscle pain and may further confuse the anatomic localization of symptoms by resulting in disuse atrophy and moderate muscle weakness. Pain from disease of overlying subcutaneous tissue or fascia and of tendons may also be referred to muscle. Additionally, disease of major peripheral nerves or of their small intramuscular branches may produce both muscle pain and weakness. Muscle pain may be a major symptom in inflammatory, metabolic, endocrine, and toxic myopathies (Chaps. 356 and 357).

Muscle trauma Vigorous activity, even in conditioned athletes may be associated with muscle and tendon tears which lead to temporary acute muscle pain, swelling, and tenderness. Rupture of muscle tendons such as the biceps or gastrocnemius muscle may produce visible muscle shortening.

The almost-pleasurable ache and fatigue of muscles after strenuous activity is separable only by degree from more severe, but still normal pain following severe, unaccustomed activity. Such symptoms are often associated with laboratory evidence of profound muscle damage including a rise in serum enzymes (creatine kinase) and widespread muscle necrosis on biopsy. Myoglobinemia and myoglobinuria may occur. Particularly likely to produce muscle pain and necrosis are certain types of exercise: brief periods of contracting a muscle while it is lengthening (eccentric contractions); and prolonged exercise such as marathon running. The point at which such symptoms become abnormal is not clear. Many patients have pain with moderate activity. Such exertional muscle pain is also characteristic of metabolic disorders of muscle including carnitine palmityl transferase deficiency and myoadenylate deaminase deficiency; deficiencies of enzymes of glycolysis are more commonly associated with contractures. The majority of patients with exertional and postexertional muscle pain do not have a definable abnormality.

Diffuse myalgias Muscle pain in the absence of muscle weakness can occur in acute infections caused by influenza and Coxsackie viruses. Fibrositis, fibromyalgia, and fibromyositis are synonyms for a disorder associated with pain and tenderness of muscle and adjacent connective tissue. Focal "trigger points" of tenderness can be identified and systemic symptoms such as fatigue, insomnia, and depression are frequently present (see Chap. 356). Although patients often identify painful swellings, histologic evaluation discloses no abnormality of muscle or connective tissue. Symptoms may respond partially to nonsteroidal anti-inflammatory agents, but the disorder tends to be chronic and unrelenting. Patients whose symptoms persist for months or years are often considered to have a psychiatric disorder, but its nature has not been defined.

Polymyalgia rheumatica occurs in patients over age 50 and is characterized by stiffness and pain in shoulder and hip musculature. Despite symptoms of pain localized to muscles, there is convincing evidence that the disease includes a proximal, inflammatory arthritis; joint effusions are often present in knees and other peripheral joints as well. Patients often develop profound disuse atrophy of muscles and complain of weakness, giving rise to a suspicion of polymyositis. However, creatine kinase levels are usually normal, and muscle biopsy shows atrophy without evidence of muscle necrosis or inflammation. The erythrocyte sedimentation rate is elevated in most patients, and giant cell arteritis may be present. Treatment with nonsteroidal anti-inflammatory agents is advocated except in patients with giant cell arteritis, for whom prednisone (50 to 100 mg daily) is recommended. Patients with polymyalgia rheumatica who fail to respond to nonsteroidal anti-inflammatory agents may require low-dose prednisone (10 to 20 mg daily). Myalgias are also frequent in other rheumatologic disorders including rheumatoid arthritis, systemic lupus erythematosus, polyarteritis nodosa, scleroderma, and the mixed connective tissue syndrome. When muscle pain occurs as an early symptom, it may erroneously suggest a primary muscle disease, and the myalgia may be due to inflammatory muscle involvement that can occur in each of these conditions (see Chap. 356). Patients with polymyositis and dermatomyositis may have myalgias, although in the majority, muscle pain is lacking or minimal (Chap. 356).

EPISODIC WEAKNESS

The term *weakness* is often used by a patient to describe a loss of stamina or decreased "energy." Even careful efforts at eliciting a history of true as opposed to subjective weakness may fail to distinguish the two conditions. The most helpful strategy is to ask the patient to identify whether a discrete loss of function has occurred and to elicit the circumstances in which symptoms are noted.

Weakness whether true or perceived may be due to disorders of the central or peripheral nervous system. Weakness from central nervous system disorders such as transient cerebral ischemia is usually associated with a change in level of consciousness or cognition, with increased muscle tone and muscle stretch reflexes, and often with alterations of sensation. Most neuromuscular causes of intermittent weakness are associated with normal mental function but with diminished muscle tone and muscle stretch reflexes. The major causes of intermittent weakness are listed in Table 17-1. Central causes are considered in Chap. 343.

EPISODIC ASTHENIA Patients who describe intermittent "weakness" as *fatigue* and loss of *stamina* suffer from asthenia, which can be separated from true weakness by the fact that patients do not lack the ability to do a task but rather the ability to perform it repetitively. Asthenia is a major problem in many patients with serious renal, hepatic, cardiac, or pulmonary disease. Examination of such patients usually confirms their ability to do all functional activities at least once, such as rising from a knee bend, climbing stairs, or rising from a chair. Fatigue is also characteristic of relatively selective damage to central nervous system descending motor tracts, in which signs of neurologic abnormality may be minimal.

Intermittent weakness due to peripheral neuromuscular disease may result from abrupt changes in peripheral nerve function; intermittent destruction of muscle; alterations of electrophysiologic properties of muscle from abnormalities of blood electrolytes; and intermittent failure of neuromuscular transmission.

FAILURE OF PERIPHERAL NERVE CONDUCTION A number of uncommon peripheral neuropathies are associated with recurrent weakness. *Hereditary liability to pressure palsies*, often termed *tomaculous* neuropathy because of the sausage-like appearance of myelin on nerve biopsy, is an autosomal dominant disorder characterized by abrupt paralysis following compression of a peripheral nerve. The paralysis is usually self-limited, lasting days to weeks. Other types of peripheral neuropathy may also predispose to the development of reversible, compressive neuropathies (see Chap. 355).

DISORDERED NEUROMUSCULAR JUNCTION TRANSMISSION *Myasthenia gravis*, particularly in its initial manifestations, is characterized by transient weakness. Cranial muscles are usually affected first, causing double vision, ptosis, dysphagia, and dysarthria. Rarely, limb weakness may herald the onset of myasthenia gravis and in the absence of cranial muscle dysfunction may escape diagnosis for months. Diurnal variation in strength is typical, and reflexes are preserved. Other, less-common defects of the neuromuscular junction such as the Eaton-Lambert syndrome may also present with intermittent weakness (see Chap. 358).

INTERMITTENT ALTERATIONS IN ELECTROLYTES Transient shifts in serum potassium are associated with profound alterations in muscle strength. Although the primary periodic paralyses (hypo- and hyperkalemic periodic paralysis) spring to mind in a patient with weakness and an abnormality in serum potassium, other causes of abnormal serum potassium more frequently result in episodic weakness (see Chap. 359). Familial periodic paralysis seldom presents after age 30; other causes are usually present in older patients. Hypokalemic periodic paralysis may occur in patients with hyperthyroidism. Episodic weakness due to hypokalemia may occur with renal or gastrointestinal potassium loss; major causes include renal tubular acidosis, diuretic-induced hypokalemia, hyperaldosteronism, Bartter's syndrome, and villous adenoma of the colon.

Hyperkalemic weakness occurs in chronic renal or adrenal insufficiency, with hyporeninemic hypoaldosteronism, and on an iatrogenic basis from injudicious administration of oral potassium preparations alone or in combination with potassium-sparing diuretics such as triamterene, amiloride, and spironolactone. The use of potassium salts as a substitute for table salt may cause hyperkalemia in patients with impaired potassium excretion.

Other electrolyte disturbances may occasionally produce intermittent weakness as the initial clinical manifestation of a severe metabolic abnormality. These include elevation or depression of serum sodium, calcium, or magnesium as well as hypophosphatemia.

METABOLIC MUSCLE DISEASE (see Chap. 347) A number of uncommon defects in glycogen and lipid utilization are associated with impaired energy production by muscle and cause intermittent weakness, usually accompanied by muscle pain. Carnitine palmityl transferase deficiency is one such condition. Other metabolic defects of muscle such as mitochondrial disorders and the purine nucleotide cycle defect, myoadenylate deaminase deficiency, may also cause episodic weakness. This latter disorder occurs in approximately 1 percent of the population but inexplicably causes symptoms in a small proportion of subjects deficient in the enzyme.

Recurrent attacks of a feeling of "weakness" often occur in patients with the *hyperventilation syndrome*; such patients are, however, of normal strength when tested. Similarly, *recurrent hypoglycemic episodes* are associated with subjective weakness though hypoglycemia is uncommon as the cause of this symptom. Central nervous system disorders infrequently cause generalized weakness without an associated alteration of consciousness. *Drop attacks* resulting from impaired blood supply to the motor pathways of the brainstem cause sudden paraparesis or quadriparesis, usually lasting only a few seconds. Patients with narcolepsy may have sudden loss of muscle strength and tone during episodes of *cataplexy*. A disorder of the reticular activating system is responsible for these episodes as well as for *sleep paralysis* that occurs as narcoleptic patients are falling asleep or awakening (see Chap. 20).

TABLE 17-1   Causes of episodic generalized weakness

Electrolyte disturbances
  Hypokalemia: Primary hyperaldosteronism (Conn's syndrome); barium poisoning; primary renal tubular acidosis; renal tubular acidosis secondary to amphotericin B or toluene abuse; juxtaglomerular apparatus hyperplasia (Bartter's syndrome); villous adenoma of colon; alcoholism; diuretics; licorice; para-aminosalicylic acid; corticosteroids
  Hyperkalemia: Addison's disease; chronic renal failure; hyporeninemic hypoaldosteronism; recurrent rhabdomyolysis
  Hypercalcemia
  Hypocalcemic tetany
  Hyponatremia
  Hypophosphatemia
  Hypermagnesemia
Neuromuscular junction disorders
  Myasthenia gravis
  Eaton-Lambert syndrome
Central nervous system causes
  Cataplexy and sleep paralysis associated with narcolepsy
  Multiple sclerosis
  Transient ischemic attacks
Disorders with only subjective weakness: hyperventilation, hypoglycemia

REFERENCES

AUGER RG et al: Hereditary form of sustained muscle activity of peripheral nerve origin causing generalized myokymia and muscle stiffness. Ann Neurol 15:13 1984

CLARK S et al: Clinical characteristics of fibrositis. II. A "blinded," controlled study using standard psychological tests. Arthritis Rheum 28:132, 1985

GRIGGS RC: The myotonic disorders and the periodic paralyses. Adv Neurol 17:143, 1977

LAYZER RB: Muscle pain, cramps and fatigue, in AG Engel, BQ Banker (eds), *Myology*. New York, McGraw-Hill, 1986

SAENZ-LOPE E et al: Hyperekplexia: A syndrome of pathological startle responses. Ann Neurol 15:36, 1985

18 NUMBNESS, TINGLING, AND OTHER ABNORMALITIES OF SENSATION

ARTHUR K. ASBURY

Normal somatic sensation is a continuous process occupying a considerable proportion of moment-to-moment nervous system activity. Little of the activity intrudes upon consciousness or exacts notice. In contrast, disordered sensation, particularly pains and paresthesias, may be highly intrusive, alarming, and tenacious and may dominate attention. Abnormalities of sensation tend to bring patients quickly to medical attention. The physician must have a framework of knowledge in order to assess abnormal sensations, estimate their likely site of origin, and recognize their implications. When abnormal sensations are perceived as painful, medical advice is even more quickly sought. For a consideration of pain, see Chap. 3.

POSITIVE AND NEGATIVE PHENOMENA It is useful to divide all abnormal sensory phenomena into two great categories, positive and negative. Positive phenomena include tingling, pins-and-needles, pricking, bandlike sensations, lightning-like shooting feelings (lancinations), aching, and knifelike, twisting, drawing, pulling, tightening, burning, searing, electrical, and raw sensations. These descriptors are frequently the actual words used by patients. Such sensations may or may not be experienced as painful. It is thought that the pathophysiologic basis of positive phenomena resides in the ectopic generation of volleys of impulses at some site of lowered neural threshold along the sensory pathways, either in peripheral or central sensory fibers. Such trains of ectopically generated afferent impulses arising from sites other than normal peripheral nerve receptors determine the quality of the abnormal sensation experienced, depending upon the number, rate, and distribution of impulses and the type and size of nerve fibers in which they arise.

Positive phenomena represent heightened activity in sensory pathways; therefore they are not in and of themselves necessarily associated with any demonstrable sensory deficit upon examination, an important point for the examiner to bear in mind.

Negative phenomena result from loss of sensory function and are characterized by numbness, or diminution or absence of feeling in a particular distribution. Negative phenomena, in contrast to positive phenomena, are accompanied by abnormal findings on sensory examination. In disorders affecting peripheral sensation, it is estimated that at least one-half of afferent fibers innervating a given site must be lost or functionless in order for sensory deficit to be demonstrated. This estimate probably varies according to how rapidly sensory fibers have lost function. If the rate of loss is slow and chronic, lack of cutaneous feeling may be difficult to demonstrate on examination, even though few sensory fibers are functioning. Rapidly evolving sensory abnormality usually evokes positive phenomena of some type and is more readily recognized by patients than insidious deafferentation. Subclinical degrees of sensory dysfunction not demonstrable on clinical sensory examination may be revealed by sensory nerve conduction studies or somatosensory cerebral evoked potentials (see Chaps. 341 and 354).

Terminology Two general types of medical terms are used to characterize abnormal sensation, those referring to symptoms of which patients complain (both positive and negative phenomena) and those describing abnormalities found on examination (only negative phenomena). *Paresthesia* and *dysesthesia* are terms used to denote positive phenomena. Paresthesia carries the implication that the abnormal sensation is perceived without an apparent stimulus; whereas dysesthesia is a more general term used to describe all types of positive sensations whether stimulus-generated or not. Abnormalities on examination are denoted by *hypesthesia* or *hypoesthesia* (reduction of cutaneous sensation to a specific type of testing such as pressure, light touch, and warm or cold stimuli), *anesthesia* (complete absence of skin sensation to the same stimuli plus pinprick), and *hypalgesia* (referring to loss of pain perception, i.e., nociception, such as the pricking quality elicited by a pin). *Hyperesthesia* connotes exaggerated perception of sensations in response to light touch or stroking of the skin. Similarly *allodynia* describes the situation in which an ordinarily nonpainful stimulus, once perceived, is experienced as painful, even excruciating. An example is elicitation of a painful sensation by application of a vibrating tuning fork. *Hyperalgesia* denotes an exaggerated response to a noxious stimulus, and *hyperpathia,* a broad term, encompasses the phenomena implied by hyperesthesia, allodynia, and hyperalgesia.

Disorders of deep sensation, arising from muscle spindles, tendons, and joints, deserve special comment. Normally these afferents subserve proprioception (position sense) and the moment-to-moment sense of the state of muscle contraction. If a significant number of these special nerve endings become denervated, the resulting manifestations include imbalance, particularly with eyes closed or in the dark, clumsiness of precision movements, and unsteadiness of gait,

all of which is referred to as *sensory ataxia* (see Chap. 16). Other findings on examination are reduced or absent joint position and vibratory sensibility in the affected limbs. Romberg's sign is positive, which means that the patient sways or topples when asked to stand with feet close together and eyes closed.

In severe states of deafferentation involving deep sensation, the patient cannot walk or stand unaided, or even sit unsupported. Continuous, sometimes wormlike involuntary movements, called *pseudoathetosis,* of the hands and arms occur, particularly with eyes closed. Such patients are severely disabled.

Normal sensation Cutaneous afferent innervation is subserved by a rich variety of receptors, both naked endings (nociceptors and thermoreceptors) and encapsulated terminals (mechanoreceptors). Each has its own set of sensitivities to specific stimuli (see Table 18-1), size and distinctness of receptive fields, and adaptational qualities. Much of the knowledge about these receptors has come from the development of techniques to study single intact nerve fibers intraneurally in alert unanesthetized human subjects. It is possible not only to record from single nerve fibers, large or small, but also to stimulate single fibers in isolation. A single impulse, whether elicited by a natural stimulus or evoked ty electrical microstimulation, in a large myelinated afferent fiber may be both perceived and localized.

Afferent fibers in peripheral nerve trunks sort themselves into topographically coherent patterns as they approach the dorsal roots and enter the dorsal horn of the spinal cord. From there, the polysynaptic projections of the smaller fibers (unmyelinated and small myelinated), which in general subserve nociception and temperature sensibility, cross and ascend in the contralateral spinothalamic tract through spinal cord, through brainstem, to the ventral posterolateral nucleus (VPL) of the thalamus, and ultimately project to the postcentral gyrus of the parietal cortex (see Chap. 3). The larger fibers which subserve tactile and position sense and kinesthesia project rostrally in the ipsilateral posterior column of the spinal cord and finally make their first synapse in the gracile or cuneate nuclei of the lower medulla (see Fig. 18-1). The second-order neuron decussates and ascends in the medial lemniscus located medially in the medulla and in the tegmentum of the pons and midbrain, and synapses in VPL. The third-order neuron projects to parietal cortex; this system is referred to as *lemniscal.*

Although the fiber types and functions which make up the spinothalamic and lemniscal systems are relatively well known, it has been found that many other fibers, particularly those associated with touch, pressure, and position sense, ascend in a diffusely distributed pattern both ipsilaterally and contralaterally in the anterolateral quadrants of the spinal cord. These anatomic facts explain why an individual with a known complete lesion of the posterior columns of the spinal cord may have little sensory deficit on examination.

EXAMINATION OF SENSATION The initial step in examination of the somatosensory system is to do the tests of primary sensation,

TABLE 18-1 Human cutaneous sensory receptors*

Receptor type	Location	Activating stimulus	Afferent nerve fiber	Sensation evoked	Central pathway
Meissner's corpuscle	S	Light pressure, once or repetitive	LM	Tapping, fluttering	Lemiscal
Merkel's disk	S	Sustained pressure	LM	Sense of pressure	
Pacinian corpuscle	D	Light touch, once or repetitive	LM	Sense of vibration	
Ruffini's ending	D	Sustained, angulated pressure	LM	None, thought to be proprioceptive	
Naked ending	S	Noxious	SM	Sharp pain	Spinothalamic
Naked ending	S	Noxious	UM	Dull pain, itch	
Naked ending	S	Thermal; 34–50°C	UM	Warmth	
Naked ending	S	Thermal, range uncertain	SM	Coldness	

* LM = large myelinated fiber; SM = small myelinated fiber; UM = unmyelinated fiber; D = deep; S = superficial.
SOURCE: *After Lindblom and Ochoa, 1986.*

TABLE 18-2 Testing primary sensation

Sense	Test device	Endings activated	Fiber size mediating	Central pathway*
Pain	Pinprick	Cutaneous nociceptors	Small	SpTh, also D
Temperature, heat	Flask with warm water	Cutaneous thermoreceptors for hot	Small	SpTh
Temperature, cold	Flask with cold water	Cutaneous thermoreceptors for cold	Small	SpTh
Touch	Cotton wisp, fine brush	Cutaneous mechanoreceptors, also naked endings	Large and small	Lem, also D and SpTh
Vibration	Tuning fork, 128 Hz	Mechanoreceptors, especially pacinian corpuscles	Large	Lem, also D
Joint position	Passive movement of specific joints	Joint capsule and tendon endings, muscle spindles	Large	Lem, also D

*D = diffuse ascending projections in ipsilateral and contralateral anteriolateral columns; SpTh = spinothalamic projection, contralateral; Lem = posterior column and lemniscal projection, ipsilateral.

which by convention include the sense of pain, touch, vibration, joint position, and thermal sensation, both hot and cold. These tests have gradually become codified through tradition, but they do appear to assess, if crudely, the major afferent functions and pathways (see Table 18-2). Testing of both primary sensation and cortical sensory function can be carried out in the office or at the bedside with a minimum of special equipment.

Some general principles pertain to the sensory examination. First, it should be remembered that the examiner is depending upon subjective patient response; therefore, discriminating responses depend upon the level of alertness, motivation, and intelligence of the patient and also upon the skill with which the examiner has made the task clear. In a stupefied or obtunded patient, the examiner is reduced to observing the briskness of withdrawal and the complexity of defensive movements of the patient in response to a pinch or other noxious stimulus. In the alert but uncooperative patient, it is often possible to get some idea of proprioceptive function by observing the patient's best performance in casually observed movements requiring balance and precision, but cutaneous sensation may be unexaminable. Second, sensory examination should not be pressed if the patient is fatigued. An abbreviated survey will suffice until a more extensive examination can be carried out in the rested patient. Third, sensory examination in a patient who has no neurologic complaints should be quite abbreviated and may consist of pin, touch, and vibration testing in the hands and feet plus evaluation of station and gait including Romberg's maneuver, which also tests the integrity of motor and cerebellar systems. Fourth, patients should be tested with their eyes closed or covered during both primary sensation and cortical sensory function examination.

Primary sensation (see Table 18-2) The sense of pain is usually tested with a pin, asking the patient to focus on the pricking or unpleasant quality of the stimulus and not just the pressure or touch sensation elicited. Areas of hypalgesia should be mapped by proceeding from the most hypalgesic zones to less affected ones (see Figs. 18-2 and 18-3).

Temperature sensation, both to hot and to cold, is probably best tested by touching the skin for a couple of seconds with a water flask filled with water of the desired temperature, using a thermometer to verify the temperature. For most purposes, it is satisfactory if a patient can identify as warm the flask which is 35 or 36°C and as cool the one which is at 28 to 32°C. Between 28 and 32°C, most individuals can distinguish temperature differences in 1°C steps. Both cold and warm should be tested because different receptors respond to each.

Touch is usually tested with a wisp of cotton or a fine camel's hair brush. In general, it is better to avoid testing touch on hairy skin because of the profusion of sensory endings which surround each hair follicle. The patients, whose eyes are covered, should be asked to say "now" each time they feel the stimulus. They may also be asked to point to the site where the stimulus was felt, although this

tests not only the sense of touch but also touch localization (see cortical sensory testing below).

Joint position testing is a measure of proprioception, one of the most important functions of the sensory system. Joint position is usually tested first in the great toe and in the fingers. Patients are asked to keep their eyes closed and to relax completely the part to be examined. In the case of the great toe, one starts with the toe in a neutral position and grasps it lightly between the thumb and the forefinger on either side of the toe (not top and bottom) and then the toe is moved a few degrees either in a dorsal or a plantar direction, and the patient is asked to say whether the movement was up or down. One must make sure that the patient understands that it is the direction of movement which is being tested and not the direction the toe is pointing when it stops. A patient with absence of position sense in the part being tested will have a 50 percent error rate because only two choices are available. Answers which are consistently greater

FIGURE 18-1 *Schematic diagram of lemniscal system which subserves proprioception and discriminative touch.*

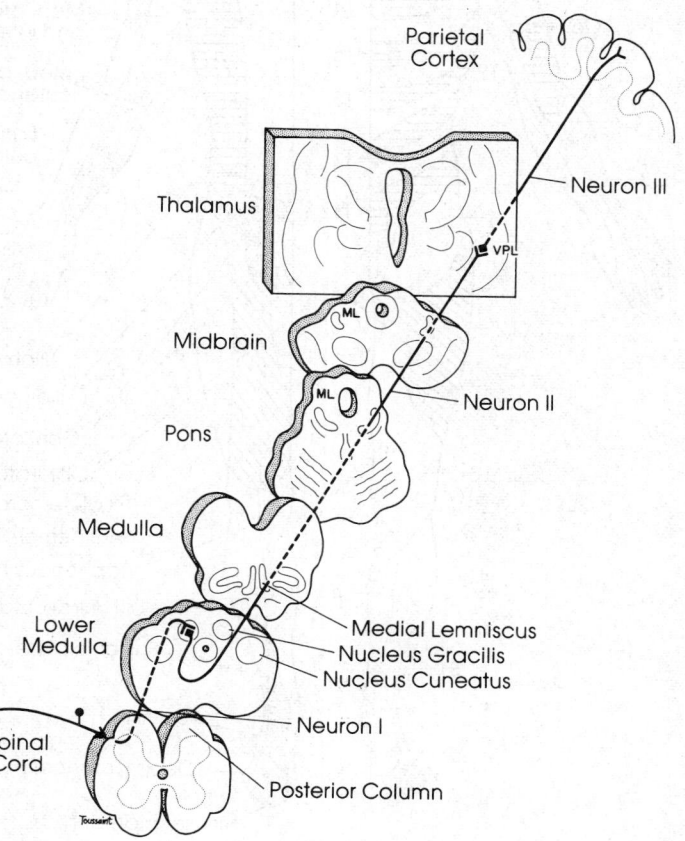

than 50 percent in error should be viewed with skepticism. If errors are made in recognizing the direction of passive movements of the toe, then passive movements of the ankle or even of the knee should be undertaken in the same way. Similarly, position sense at the proximal interphalangeal joint of the index finger may be tested, and if abnormal, other finger joints and the wrist and elbow joints should also be tested. A test of proximal joint position sense, primarily at the shoulder, can be carried out by asking the patient to bring the two index fingers together with the arms extended and the eyes closed. Normal individuals should be able to do this quite accurately with errors of a centimeter of less.

The sense of vibration is tested with a tuning fork, preferably a large one which vibrates at 128 Hz. The decay of vibration using this fork is slow enough to be of quantitative use because it requires between 15 and 20 s to decay below the threshold of perceptibility. Vibration is usually tested at bony prominences, specifically the malleoli at the ankles, the patella, the anterior iliac spine, the spinous processes of the vertebral bodies, the metacarpal-phalangeal joints (knuckles), the styloid process of the ulna, the elbow, and the acromion of the shoulder. Control sites at which to test vibration are the sternum and on the forehead. The examiner can compare the threshold at a given site for both patient and self. A crude approximation of degree of vibratory sense loss can be made by counting the seconds that the examiner can feel the sense of vibration longer than the patient. It must be clear to the patient that it is the sense of vibration and not just the pressure of the end of the tuning fork to which attention is directed.

Cortical sensation Cortical sensory testing includes two-point discrimination, touch localization, stereognosis, graphesthesia, and bilateral simultaneous stimulation, to name the most commonly used methods. Abnormalities of these sensory tests, in the presence of normal primary sensation and an alert cooperative patient, signifies a lesion of the parietal cortex or thalamocortical projections to the parietal lobe. If primary sensation is altered, it is not possible to test for these cortical discriminative functions.

Two-point discrimination is tested by special calipers whose points may be set from 2 mm to several centimeters apart and then applied simultaneously to the site to be tested. The pulp of the fingertips is a common site to test; a normal individual can distinguish about 3-mm separation of points there. One can distinguish more closely set points on the tongue and lips, but the threshold for discriminating two points may be centimeters at other sites on the body. Comparisons should always be made between analogous sites on the two sides of the body, since the deficit, with a specific parietal lesion, is likely to be hemilateral. This point holds true for all cortical sensory testing.

Touch localization is usually carried out by light pressure with the examiner's fingertip, asking the patient, whose eyes are closed, to identify the site of touch. It is usual to ask the patient to touch the same site with a fingertip. Bilateral simultaneous stimulation at

FIGURE 18-2 *Anterior view of dermatomes (left) and cutaneous areas supplied by individual peripheral nerves (right). (From MB Carpenter and J Sutin, in Human Neuroanatomy, 8th ed, Baltimore, Williams & Wilkins, 1983.)*

Ophthalmic n.
Mandibular n.
Great auricular n.
Transverse colli n.
Supraclavicular nn.
Intercostal nn.
1. Ant. cutaneous rami
2. Lat. cutaneous rami
Axillary n.
Med. brachial cutaneous and intercostobrachial nn.
Med. antebrachial cutaneous n.
Lat. antebrachial cutaneous n.
Radial n.
Median n.
Ulnar n.
Iliohypogastric n.
Ilioinguinal n.
Genitofemoral n.
Obturator n.
Lat. femoral cutaneous n.
Ant. femoral cutaneous n.
Saphenous n.
Lat. sural cutaneous n.
Superficial peroneal n.
Sural n.
Deep peroneal n.
Medial plantar n.

C2 C3 C4 C5 C6 C7 C8 T1 L1 L2 L3 L5 S1
C4 T2 T4 T6 T8 T10 T12 L1 L2 L4

analogous sites (e.g., the dorsa of both hands) can be carried out to determine whether the perception of touch is extinguished consistently on one side or the other. The phenomenon is referred to as extinction on bilateral simultaneous stimulation.

Graphesthesia means the capacity to recognize letters or numbers drawn by the examiner's fingertip on various parts of the body while the patient maintains eyes closed. The usual comparison is the palm of one hand versus the palm of the other. Numbers should be drawn large enough to occupy most of the palm. Once again, the comparison of one side to the other is of prime importance. Failure to recognize numbers or letters is termed *agraphesthesia*.

Stereognosis refers to the ability to identify common objects by palpation, recognizing their shape, texture, and size. Common standard objects are the best test objects, such as a marble, a paper clip, a small rubber ball, or coins. Patients with normal stereognosis should be able to distinguish a dime from a penny and certainly a nickel from a quarter. Patients should only be allowed to feel the object with one hand at time. If they are unable to identify it in one hand, it should be placed in the other for comparison. Individuals unable to identify common objects and coins in one hand who can do so in the other are said to have *astereognosis* of the abnormal hand. Note that the major comparison is one side of the body with the other.

Localization of sensory abnormalities   Peripheral neuropathies are generally graded, distal, and symmetric in their distribution of deficit.

Although most peripheral neuropathies are pansensory and affect all modalities of sensation, selective sensory dysfunction according to nerve fiber size may occur. In small fiber neuropathies, the hallmark is burning, painful dysesthesias with reduced pinprick and thermal sensation but with sparing of proprioception, motor function, and even deep tendon jerks. Touch is variably involved, but when spared, the sensory pattern is referred to as sensory dissociation (see below). In contrast to small fiber neuropathies, large fiber neuropathies are characterized by position sense deficit, imbalance, absent tendon jerks, variable motor dysfunction, but preservation of most cutaneous sensation and few or no dysesthesias.

Paresthesias and dysesthesias may be of either peripheral nerve or spinal cord origin, and probably can arise in the brainstem, but in every instance are thought to represent abnormal showers of impulses generated from an ectopic focus or foci. By themselves, paresthesias may not be localizable, but when accompanied by other signs of neuropathy or of myelopathy, the correct site of origin may be deduced.

Dissociated sensory deficit patterns, in which pinprick and thermal sensation is lost but touch is spared, are usually a sign of spinothalamic tract involvement in the spinal cord, especially if the deficit is unilateral and has an upper level on the torso. Bilateral spinothalamic tract involvement occurs with lesions affecting the center of the spinal cord, such as happens with expansion of the central canal in hydromyelia or syringomyelia. Sensory dissociation may also occur

FIGURE 18-3   *Posterior view of dermatomes (left) and cutaneous areas supplied by individual peripheral nerves (right). (From MB Carpenter and J Sutin, in Human Neuroanatomy, 8th ed, Baltimore, Williams & Wilkins, 1983.)*

in peripheral neuropathies in which afferent cutaneous nerve fibers of small diameter are preferentially affected. Neuropathies in which sensory dissociation may occur include leprous neuritis, hereditary sensory neuropathy, and certain cases of amyloid and diabetic polyneuropathy (see Chap. 355).

Hemisensory disturbance with tingling numbness from head to foot is usually thalamic in origin. If abrupt in onset, the thalamic lesion is likely to be due to a small stroke (lacunar infarction). Occasionally, with lesions affecting the posterolateral thalamus (VPL) or adjacent white matter, a syndrome of thalamic pain, also called Déjerine-Roussy syndrome, may ensue. This is a persistent unrelenting hemipainful state often described in dramatic terms such as "like the flesh is being torn from my limbs" or "as though that side is bathed in acid" (see Chap. 3). Harlequin patterns of sensory disturbance, in which one side of the face and the opposite side of the body are affected, localize to the lateral medulla where a small lesion may damage both the ipsilateral descending trigeminal tract and ascending spinothalamic fibers (lateral lemniscus) subserving the opposite arm, leg, and hemitorso (see "Lateral Medulla Syndrome," Chap. 343).

With lesions of the parietal lobe, either of the cortex or subjacent white matter, the most prominent symptoms are contralateral hemineglect, hemi-inattention, and a tendency not to use the opposite hand and arm. Tests of primary sensation are usually normal or minimally altered, but tests of cortical sensation are often severely abnormal (see Chap. 24). Dysesthesias or even a sense of numbness are unusual except in the special circumstance of focal sensory seizures. These are generally due to lesions in or near the postcentral gyrus. Symptoms of focal somatosensory seizures are usually combinations of numbness and tingling, but frequently additional, more complex sensations are present, such as a rushing feeling, a sense of warmth, a sense of movement without visible motion, or an unpleasantly dysesthetic quality. Duration of seizures is variable; they may be transient, lasting only seconds, or may persist for hours. Focal motor features (clonic jerking) may supervene, and seizures can become generalized with loss of consciousness. Likely sites of symptoms are unilaterally in the lips, face, digits, or foot, and symptoms may spread as in a Jacksonian march. On occasion, symptoms may occur in a symmetric bilateral fashion, for instance, in both hands; this results from involvement of the second sensory area (unilaterally) located in the rolandic area at and just above the Sylvian fissure.

REFERENCES

CULP W, OCHOA JL (eds): *Abnormal Nerves and Muscles as Impulse Generators*. Oxford University, New York, 1982

DYCK PJ et al: Detection thresholds of cutaneous sensation in humans, in PJ Dyck, PK Thomas, EH Lambert, RP Bunge (eds), *Peripheral Neuropathy*, 2d ed. Philadelphia, Saunders, 1984, pp 1103–1138

LINDBLOM U, OCHOA JL: Somatosensory function and dysfunction; in AK Asbury, GM McKhann, WI McDonald (eds), *Diseases of the Nervous System*, Philadelphia, Saunders, 1986, (in press)

MACKEL R: Single unit analysis of regenerated cutaneous afferents in man. Ann Neurol 18:165, 1985

VALLBO AB et al: Somatosensory, proprioceptive, and sympathetic activity in human peripheral nerve. Physiol Rev 59:919, 1979

19   DISTURBANCES OF SMELL, TASTE, AND HEARING

JAMES B. SNOW, JR. / JOSEPH B. MARTIN

SMELL   The sense of smell determines the flavor and palatability of food and drink. It serves along with the trigeminal system as a monitor of inhaled chemicals including dangerous substances such as natural gas, smoke, and air pollutants. Although qualitative sensations

of smell are subserved by the olfactory neuroepithelium, many substances are capable of producing somatic sensations of coolness, warmth, and irritation through the trigeminal, facial, glossopharyngeal, and vagal afferents in the nose, oral cavity, tongue, pharynx, and larynx. The sense of smell should be considered as one of several chemosensory systems since most chemical substances initiate olfactory, trigeminal, and taste perceptions.

The *olfactory neuroepithelium* is located in the superior part of the nasal cavities. It contains an orderly arrangement of bipolar olfactory receptor cells, microvillar cells, sustentacular cells, and basal cells. The dendritic process of the bipolar cell has a bulb-shaped knob or vesicle that projects into the mucous layer and bears 10 to 20 cilia. The receptor sites for odorant molecules are located on the cilia. The microvillar cells are located adjacent to the receptor cells on the surface of the neuroepithelium. The sustentacular cells, unlike their counterparts in the respiratory epithelium, are not specialized to secrete mucus. Their function is unknown. The basal cells are progenitors of other cell types in the olfactory neuroepithelium including the bipolar receptor cells. There is a regular turnover of the bipolar receptor cells, which function as the primary sensory neurons. In addition with injury to the cell body or its axon, the receptor cell is replaced by a basal cell which reestablishes a central neural connection. *Hence, these primary sensory neurons are unique among sensory systems in that they are regularly replaced and regenerate after injury.*

The unmyelinated axons of the receptor cells form the fila of the olfactory nerve, pass through the cribriform plate, and terminate within spherical masses of neuropil, termed glomeruli, in the olfactory bulb. The glomeruli are a focus of a high degree of convergence of information, since many more fibers enter than leave them. The main second-order neurons are the mitral cells. The primary dendrite of each mitral cell extends into a single glomerulus. Axons of the mitral cells project along with the axons of adjacent tufted cells to the limbic system, including the anterior olfactory nucleus, the prepiriform cortex, the periamygdaloid cortex, the olfactory tubercle, the nucleus of the lateral olfactory tract, and the corticomedial nucleus of the amygdala.

Odorants are absorbed into the mucus overlying the olfactory neuroepithelium, diffuse to the cilia, and reversibly bind to membrane receptor sites. The process causes conformational changes in the receptor proteins which induce a chain of biochemical events that results in generation of action potentials in the primary neurons. Intensity appears to be coded by the amount of firing in the afferent neurons. Indeed, a clear relationship exists in humans between psychophysical measures of intensity and the magnitude of the evoked potential from the olfactory neuroepithelium. Little is known about quality coding. Individual receptor cells are responsive to a wide range of stimuli. It is thought that more than one type of receptor site is present on each cell.

Disturbances of the sense of smell   Disturbances of the sense of smell are caused by conditions that interfere with the access of the odorant to the olfactory neuroepithelium (transport loss), injure the receptor region (sensory loss), or damage central olfactory pathways (neural loss).

Transport olfactory loss can result from swollen nasal mucous membrane in acute viral upper respiratory infections, bacterial rhinitis, sinusitis, and allergic rhinitis and with structural changes in the nasal cavity such as deviations of the nasal septum, polyps, and neoplasms. It is also likely that abnormalities of mucous secretion in which the olfactory cilia are immersed could result in a loss of olfactory sensitivity. Currently little is known about alterations in the mucous environment of the olfactory neuroepithelium.

Sensory olfactory losses are caused by destruction of the olfactory neuroepithelium by viral infections, neoplasms, the inhalation of toxic chemicals, drugs that affect cell turnover, and radiation therapy to the head. *Neural olfactory losses* occur in head trauma, with or without fracture of the base of the anterior cranial fossa or cribriform plate area, neoplasms of the anterior cranial fossa, neurosurgical procedures, administration of neurotoxic drugs, and in some congenital disorders such as Kallmann's syndrome.

From the psychophysical point of view, disturbances of the sense of smell may be categorized by either the patient's complaint or the objective sensory measurements as *total anosmia* (general anosmia)—inability to detect any qualitative olfactory sensations; *partial anosmia*—ability to detect some, but not all, qualitative olfactory sensations; *specific anosmia*—loss of ability to appreciate only one or a very limited number of odorants; *total hyposmia* (general hyposmia)—decreased sensitivity to all odorants; *partial hyposmia*—decreased sensitivity to some odorants; *dysosmia* (cacosmia or paraosmia)—distortion in the perception of an odor, that is, the perception of an unpleasant odor when a pleasant odorant is being presented or the perception of an odor when there is no odorant in the environment; *total hyperosmia* (general hyperosmia)—increased sensitivity to all odorants; *partial hyperosmia*—increased sensitivity to some odorants; and *agnosia*—inability to classify, contrast, or identify odor sensations verbally, even though the ability to distinguish between odorants or to recognize them may be normal.

CLINICAL EVALUATION   The history of the onset and development of the disturbance of the sense of smell may be of paramount importance in making an etiologic diagnosis. Unilateral anosmia is rarely a complaint. Only by separate testing of smell in each nasal cavity can it be recognized. Bilateral anosmia, on the other hand, does bring patients to medical attention. The usual complaint is of a loss of taste, because taste to a large extent depends on the volatile substances in food, and the sensation of flavor is a combination of smell and taste. The physical examination should include a complete examination of the ears, upper respiratory tract, and head and neck. A neurologic examination emphasizing the cranial nerves is essential. Computerized tomography scans of the head with enhancement is required to rule out neoplasms of the anterior cranial fossa, unsuspected fractures of the anterior cranial fossa, paranasal sinusitis, and neoplasms of the nasal cavity and paranasal sinuses.

The sensory evaluation of olfactory function is necessary for corroboration of the patient's complaint, evaluation of the efficacy of treatment, and determination of the degree of permanent impairment. The first step in the sensory evaluation is to determine the degree to which qualitative sensations are present. For this assessment, a smell identification test is used that consists of a 40-item, forced choice, microencapsulated odor, scratch-and-sniff paradigm. For example, one of the items reads, "This odor smells most like (a) chocolate, (b) banana, (c) onion, or (d) fruit punch," and the patient is instructed to answer one of the alternatives. The test is highly reliable (short-term test-retest reliability r = 0.95) and is sensitive to age and sex differences (Fig. 19-1). It is an accurate quantitative determination of the relative degree of olfactory deficit. Persons with a total loss of smell function score in the range of 7 to 19 out of 40. The average score for total anosmics is slightly higher than that expected on the basis of chance because of the inclusion of some odorants which act by trigeminal stimulation.

The second step is to establish a detection threshold for the odorant phenylethyl alcohol, using a graduated stimulus. Although the detection threshold usually agrees with the results of the smell identification test, in some instances patients who fail the smell identification test perform well on the threshold test. However, the reverse is much less common. Since the threshold test can be influenced by trigeminal and nonolfactory nerve clues, the results of the smell identification test are relied upon more heavily in the sensory evaluation.

Techniques have been developed to biopsy the olfactory neuroepithelium but in view of the widespread degeneration of the olfactory neuroepithelium and intercalation of respiratory epithelium in the olfactory area of adults with no apparent olfactory dysfunction, biopsy material must be interpreted cautiously.

DIFFERENTIAL DIAGNOSIS   At the present time there are no psychophysical methods to differentiate sensory from neural olfactory losses. Fortunately, the history of the disease provides important clues to the cause. The leading causes of olfactory disorders are head trauma and viral infections. Head trauma is a more frequent cause of anosmia in children and young adults, and viral infections are more important causes of anosmia in older adults.

Cranial trauma is followed by uni- or bilateral impairment of smell in 5 to 10 percent of cases. Frontal injuries and fractures disrupt the cribriform plate and olfactory axons which perforate it. Sometimes there is an associated cerebrospinal fluid (CSF) rhinorrhea resulting from a tearing of the dura overlying the paranasal sinuses. If the anosmia is unilateral, it is usually on the side of the CSF leak, and this fact aids in localization of the fistula. Anosmia may also follow blows to the occiput. Once traumatic anosmia develops, it is usually permanent; only about 10 percent of patients ever improve or recover. Perversion of the sense of smell may occur as a phase in the recovery process.

The occurrence of a permanent hyposmia or anosmia may follow viral infections and is called *postviral anosmia*. In this instance the sensory epithelium of the olfactory zone is destroyed by the virus and replaced by respiratory epithelial and goblet cells and scar tissue. The congenital anosmias, one type of which is associated with a

FIGURE 19-1 *Smell identification test. Scores for a group of male and female subjects 5 to 99 years in age are shown.* ●——●: *Females (n = 1158);* □-----□: *males (n = 797);* ———: *total group (n = 1955). (Reprinted with permission from RL Doty et al. Copyright 1984 by the AAAS.)*

hypothalamic defect (Kallmann's syndrome, or congenital anosmia with hypogonadotropic hypogonadism), are rare but important causes of anosmia or hyposmia. Anosmia can also occur in albinos. The receptor cells are present but hypoplastic, lack cilia, and do not project above the surrounding supporting cells.

Meningioma of the inferior frontal region is the most frequent neoplastic cause of anosmia; rarely anosmia can occur with glioma of the frontal lobe. Occasionally pituitary adenomas, craniopharyngiomas, suprasellar meningiomas, and aneurysms of the anterior part of the circle of Willis extend forward and damage olfactory structures. These tumors and hamartomas may also induce seizures with olfactory hallucinations, indicating involvement of the uncus.

Paraosmia and dysosmia, subjective distortions of olfactory perception, may occur with intranasal disease that partially impairs smell, or may represent a phase in the recovery from a neurogenic anosmia. Most paraosmic disturbances consist of disagreeable or foul odors, and they may be accompanied by distortions of taste. Dysosmia may also be a symptom in elderly patients with depression. Every article of food has an extremely unpleasant odor (cacosmia). Sensations of disagreeable taste are often noted (cacogeusia).

Olfactory hallucinations are descriptions of smelling an odor that no one else can smell. They occur in alcohol withdrawal, in which olfactory hallucinations are occasionally associated with other types of hallucinations, and in uncal seizures, which are brief and clearly related to a derangement of consciousness and other epileptic components. In other settings, olfactory hallucinations usually signify a psychiatric disease. A huge range of odors may be reported, most of them foul. Some patients perceive the smell as emanating from themselves (intrinsic); others perceive the source to be external (extrinsic). Most are associated with schizophrenia and depressive illnesses.

TREATMENT   Therapy for patients with transport olfactory losses due to allergic rhinitis, bacterial rhinitis and sinusitis, polyps, neoplasms, and structural abnormalities of the nasal cavities can be undertaken rationally and with a high chance of improvement. Allergic management, antibiotic therapy, topical and systemic corticosteroid therapy, and operations for nasal polyps, deviation of the nasal septum, and chronic hyperplastic sinusitis are frequently effective in restoring the sense of smell.

There is no treatment with demonstrated efficacy for sensorineural olfactory losses. Fortunately spontaneous recovery often occurs. Zinc and vitamin therapy are advocated by some. Profound zinc deficiency can undoubtedly result in losses and distortion of the sense of smell, but it is not a clinical problem except in very limited geographic areas. Vitamin therapy has mainly been in the form of vitamin A. The epithelial degeneration associated with vitamin A deficiency can cause anosmia, but vitamin A deficiency is not a common clinical problem in the United States. Unfortunately at the present time there are no effective therapeutic strategies for the sensorineural disorders of the sense of smell.

TASTE   Many patients with a loss of olfactory sensitivity also complain of a loss of the sense of taste. On psychophysical testing, most of these patients have normal detection thresholds for taste. Disturbances of the sense of taste are far less frequent than disturbances of the sense of smell.

The taste receptor cells are located in the taste buds, spherical groups of cells arranged like the segments of a citrus fruit. At the surface, the taste bud has a pore into which microvilli of the receptor cells project. Taste buds have a similar appearance wherever they are located. Unlike the olfactory system the receptor cell is not the primary neuron. Instead, gustatory afferent nerve fibers contact individual taste receptor cells.

The sense of taste is mediated through the facial, glossopharyngeal, and vagal nerves. The gustatory system consists of at least five receptor populations. Taste buds are located in the foliate papillae along the lateral margin of the tongue, in the fungiform papillae throughout the dorsum of the tongue, in the circumvallate papillae at the junction of the dorsum and the base of the tongue, in the

palate, and in the epiglottis. The chorda tympani branch of the facial nerve subserves taste from the lateral margin of the tongue, while the greater superficial petrosal branch of the facial nerve carries the taste afferents from the dorsum of the tongue and the palate. The lingual branch of the glossopharyngeal nerve subserves taste from the circumvallate papillae, and the internal branch of the superior laryngeal nerve of the vagus nerve contains the taste afferents from the epiglottis.

The central connections of the nerves terminate in the brainstem in the nucleus of the tractus solitarius. The fibers of the chorda tympani and greater superficial petrosal nerves go to the cephalic portion of the nucleus. The glossopharyngeal gustatory fibers go to the middle, and the superior laryngeal nerve fibers to the caudal portion of the nucleus. The central pathway from the nucleus of the tractus solitarius projects to the ipsilateral parabrachial nuclei of the pons. Two divergent pathways project from the parabrachial nuclei. One ascends to the gustatory relay in the dorsal thalamus, synapses, and continues to the cortex of the insula. There is also evidence for a direct pathway from the parabrachial nuclei to the cortex. (Olfaction and taste appear to be unique among sensory systems in that at least some fibers bypass the thalamus.) The other pathway from the parabrachial nuclei goes to the ventral forebrain including the lateral hypothalamus, substantia innominata, central nucleus of the amygdala, and the stria terminalis.

Tastants gain access to the receptor cells through the taste pore. Four classes of taste are recognized: sweet, salt, sour, and bitter. Individual gustatory afferent fibers almost always respond to a number of different chemicals. Response patterns of gustatory afferent axons can be grouped into classes based on the stimulus chemical that produces the largest response. For example, for sucrose-best response neurons, the second-best stimulus is almost always sodium chloride. The fact that individual gustatory afferent fibers respond to a large number of different chemicals led to the *across-fiber-pattern* theory of gustatory coding, while the best-stimulus analysis led to the concept of *labeled* afferents. It appears that labeled fibers are important for establishing gross quality, but the across-fiber-pattern within a best-stimulus category, and perhaps among categories, is needed for discriminating chemicals within qualities. For example, sweetness may be carried by sucrose-best neurons, but the differentiation of sucrose and fructose may require a comparison of the relative activity among sucrose-best, salt-best, and quinine-best neurons. As with olfaction and other sensory systems, intensity appears to be encoded by the quantity of neural activity.

Disturbances of the sense of taste   Disturbances of the sense of taste are caused by conditions that interfere with the access of the tastant to the receptor cells in the taste bud (transport loss), injure receptor cells (sensory loss), or damage gustatory afferent nerves and central gustatory pathways (neural loss).

Transport gustatory losses result from xerostomia due to many causes including Sjögren's syndrome, heavy metal intoxication, and bacterial colonization of the taste pore. The salivary milieu of the receptors may prove to be important to diverse causes of gustatory loss.

Sensory gustatory losses are caused by inflammatory and degenerative diseases in the oral cavity, a vast number of drugs, particularly those that interfere with cell turnover such as antithyroid and antineoplastic agents, radiation therapy to the oral cavity and pharynx, viral infections, endocrine disorders, neoplasms, and aging.

Neural olfactory losses occur with neoplasms, trauma, and operations in which the gustatory afferents are injured. Taste buds degenerate when their gustatory afferents are transected but remain when their somatosensory afferents are severed.

CLINICAL MANIFESTATIONS   From the psychophysical point of view disturbances of the sense of taste may be categorized by either the patient's complaint or the objective sensory measurements as *total ageusia*—inability to detect the qualities of sweet, salty, bitter, or sour; *partial ageusia*—ability to detect some but not all of the qualitative gustatory sensations; *specific ageusia*—inability to detect the taste quality of certain substances; *total hypoguesia*—decreased sensitivity to all tastants; *partial hypogeusia*—decreased sensitivity to some tastants; *dysgeusia*—distortion in the perception of a tastant, that is, the perception of the wrong quality when a tastant is presented or the perception of a taste when there has been no tastant ingested. Confusions of sour and bitter are common and, at times, may be semantic misunderstandings. Frequently, however, they have physiologic or pathophysiologic bases.

It may be possible to differentiate between the loss of flavor recognition in patients with olfactory losses who complain of a loss of taste as well as smell by asking if they are able to taste sweetness in sodas, saltiness in potato chips, etc.

Patients who complain of loss of taste should be evaluated psychophysically for gustatory function in addition to being evaluated for olfactory function. The first step is to perform suprathreshold whole-mouth taste testing for quality, intensity, and pleasantness perception with sucrose, citric acid, quinine hydrochloride, and sodium chloride. In the quantification of the sense of taste, detection thresholds are obtained by applying graduated dilutions to the tongue quadrants or by whole-mouth sips. Finally suprathreshold magnitude estimation may be used to shed further light on the patient's complaint. Electric taste testing (electrogustometry) lacks sufficient specificity, validity, and reliability for routine clinical taste evaluations at the present time.

Biopsy of the foliate or fungiform papillae for histopathologic study of taste buds remains experimental but holds promise of shedding light on the categorization of taste disorders.

DIFFERENTIAL DIAGNOSIS   As with olfaction, psychophysical methods for differentiating transport, sensory, and neural gustatory losses are not available. Once there is objective evidence of a disorder of taste, it is important to establish, as is done in other neurologic deficits, an anatomic diagnosis before proceeding to an etiologic diagnosis. The history of the disease often provides important clues to the cause. For example, absence of taste on the anterior two-thirds of the tongue associated with a facial paralysis indicates that the lesion is proximal to the point of junction of the chorda tympani branch with the facial nerve (near the inner ear).

TREATMENT   Therapy for gustatory losses remains limited. Artificial saliva benefits some patients with a disturbed salivary milieu. Treatment for bacterial and fungal infections of the oral cavity are appropriate and may be helpful. Withdrawal of drugs affecting cell turnover are usually helpful if the patient's general condition permits. Zinc and vitamin therapy for gustatory losses are advocated by some, but lack demonstrated efficacy. No therapeutic strategies exist for the sensorineural disorders of taste.

HEARING   Hearing occurs by air conduction and bone conduction. In air conduction, sound waves reach the ear by propagation in air, enter the external auditory canal, and set the tympanic membrane in motion, which in turn moves the malleus, incus, and stapes. Movement of the footplate of the stapes causes pressure changes in the fluid-filled inner ear eliciting a traveling wave in the basilar membrane of the cochlea. The traveling wave moves from the base to the apex of the cochlea. Hairs of the hair cells of the organ of Corti, which rests on the basilar membrane, are imbedded in the tectorial membrane and are deformed by the traveling wave. A point of maximal displacement of the basilar membrane determined by the frequency of the stimulating tone occurs with each traveling wave. High-frequency tones cause maximal displacement of the basilar membrane near the base of the cochlea. As the frequency of the stimulating tone decreases, the point of maximal displacement moves toward the apex of the cochlea. Hearing by bone conduction occurs when the sounding source, in contact with the head, results in vibration of the bones of the skull including the temporal bone, producing a traveling wave in the basilar membrane.

The deformation of the hairs of the hair cells produces several bioelectric phenomena. The cochlear microphonic, an alternating current response that faithfuly represents the frequency and intensity

of the stimulating tone, occurs about 0.5 ms prior to the eighth nerve action potential. This latency is taken as evidence for release of an as yet unidentified neurotransmitter at the hair cell and cochlear nerve dendrite interface. Each of the cochlear nerve neurons can be activated at a frequency and intensity specific for that cell. This phenomenon of the characteristic or best frequency occurs at each point of the central auditory pathway: superior olivary complex, lateral lemniscus, inferior colliculus, medial geniculate body, and auditory cortex. At low frequencies, individual auditory nerve fibers can respond more or less synchronously with the stimulating tone. At higher frequencies, phase-locking occurs so that neurons take turns in responding to particular phases of the cycle of the sound wave. Intensity is encoded by the amount of neural activity in individual neurons, the number of neurons that are active, and the specific neurons that are activated.

Disturbances of the sense of hearing   A loss of hearing can result from lesions in the external auditory canal, middle ear, inner ear, or central auditory pathways. Lesions in the external auditory canal or the middle ear cause conductive hearing losses while lesions in the inner ear or eighth nerve cause sensorineural hearing losses.

Conductive hearing losses result from obstruction of the external auditory canal by cerumen, debris and foreign bodies, swelling of the lining of the canal, and stenosis and neoplasms of the canal. Perforations of the tympanic membrane, as in chronic otitis media, disruption of the ossicular chain, as occurs with necrosis of the long process of the incus in trauma or infection, fixation of the ossicles as in otosclerosis, and fluid, scarring, or neoplasms in the middle ear also result in conductive hearing losses. *Sensory hearing losses* are due principally to damage to the hair cells of the organ of Corti caused by intense noise, viral infections, ototoxic drugs, fractures of the temporal bone, meningitis, cochlear otosclerosis, Ménière's disease, and aging. Neural hearing losses are due mainly to cerebellar angle tumors such as acoustic neurinomas, but may also result from any neoplastic, vascular, demyelinating, or degenerative disease affecting the central auditory pathways.

CLINICAL EVALUATION OF HEARING   The physical examination should evaluate the external ear canal and tympanic membrane. Careful inspection of the nose, nasopharynx, and the upper respiratory tract is indicated. The other nerves should be carefully evaluated. Conductive and sensorineural hearing losses can be differentiated by comparing the threshold of hearing by air conduction with that elicited by bone conduction. Testing the hearing by air conduction is accomplished by presenting the stimulus in air. Hearing by air conduction is affected by the patency of the external auditory canal, the efficiency of the middle ear, and the integrity of the inner ear, eighth nerve, and the central auditory pathways. Testing the hearing by bone conduction is accomplished by placing an oscillator or the stem of a vibrating tuning fork in contact with the head. Hearing by bone conduction bypasses the external auditory canal and middle ear and tests the integrity of the inner ear, eighth nerve, and central auditory pathways. If air conduction thresholds are elevated and bone conduction thresholds are in the normal range, the lesion causing hearing loss is in the external auditory canal or middle ear. If both air conduction and bone conduction thresholds are elevated, the lesion is in the inner ear, eighth nerve, or central auditory pathways. Of course, conductive and sensorineural hearing losses can coexist, in which case both the air conduction and bone conduction thresholds are elevated, but in this case, air conduction thresholds are elevated more than bone conduction thresholds.

The Weber and Rinne tuning fork tests are used to differentiate conductive from sensorineural hearing losses. Weber's test is performed by placing the stem of a vibrating tuning fork on the head in the midline and asking the patient whether the tone is heard in both ears or better in one ear than in the other. With a unilateral conductive hearing loss, the tone is perceived in the affected ear. With a unilateral sensorineural hearing loss, the tone is perceived in the unaffected ear. Rinne's test compares the ability to hear by air conduction with the ability to hear by bone conduction. The tines of a vibrating tuning fork are held near the opening of the external auditory canal and then the stem is placed on the mastoid process. The patient is asked to indicate whether the tone is louder by air conduction or bone conduction. Normally a tone is heard louder by air conduction than by bone conduction. With a conductive hearing loss, the bone conduction stimulus is perceived as louder than the air conduction stimulus. With sensorineural hearing losses, both air and bone conduction perception are reduced, but the air conduction stimulus is perceived as louder, as it is in normal hearing. The combined information from the Weber and Rinne tests permits a tentative conclusion as to whether a conductive or sensorineural hearing loss is present.

Measurement of hearing   Quantification of hearing loss is obtained with an audiometer, an electronic device that allows the presentation of specific frequencies at specific intensities to each ear by either air or bone conduction. The testing is done in a sound-attenuated chamber, and masking, usually with broad-spectrum noise, is presented to the nontest ear so that responses are based on perception from the ear under test. Frequencies from 250 to 8000 Hz are used in clinical testing. The responses are measured in decibels. A decibel (dB) is equal to 10 times the logarithm of the ratio of the acoustic power required to achieve threshold in the patient to the acoustic power required to achieve threshold in a normal hearing person. An audiogram is a plot of intensity in decibels versus frequency.

The audiometric pattern of hearing loss is often of diagnostic value. Conductive hearing losses usually have a fairly equal threshold elevation for each frequency. Conductive hearing losses with a large mass component, as is often seen in middle ear effusions, have a greater elevation of thresholds in the higher frequencies. Conductive hearing losses with a large stiffness component, as in fixation of the footplate of the stapes in early otosclerosis, have a greater elevation of thresholds in the lower frequencies. In general, sensorineural hearing losses tend to have a greater threshold elevation at each higher frequency. Interesting exceptions to this generalization are noise-induced hearing loss, in which the loss at 4000 Hz is greater than it is at higher frequencies, and in Ménière's disease, particularly in the early stages of the disease, where thresholds are elevated more in lower than in higher frequencies.

Speech audiometry provides essential additional information. The *spondee threshold*, defined as the intensity at which speech is recognized as a meaningful symbol, is obtained by presenting through an audiometer two-syllable words with an equal accent on each syllable. The intensity at which the patient can repeat 50 percent of the words correctly is the spondee threshold and usually approximates the average threshold at the speech frequencies (500, 1000, and 2000 Hz). Once the spondee threshold is determined, the discrimination ability is tested by presenting one-syllable words at 25 to 40 dB above the spondee threshold. An individual with normal hearing can repeat 90 to 100 percent of the words correctly. Likewise, individuals with a conductive hearing loss do well in discrimination testing. On the other hand, patients with a sensorineural hearing loss have a loss of discrimination attributable to the loss of peripheral analysis of sound in the inner ear or eighth nerve. With a lesion in the inner ear, the discrimination is moderately affected, usually in the 50 to 80 percent range, while with neural lesions the discrimination is severely affected, often in the 0 to 50 percent range.

The discrimination testing may then be done at higher intensities than 25 to 40 dB above the spondee threshold to determine the performance-intensity function. A deterioration in discrimination ability at higher intensities suggests a lesion in the eighth nerve or central auditory pathways.

Tympanometry measures the impedance of the middle ear to sound. A sounding source and microphone are introduced into the ear canal with an airtight seal. The amount of sound that is absorbed through the middle ear or reflected from the middle ear is measured at the microphone. In conductive hearing losses, more sound is reflected than in the normal middle ear. The pressure in the ear canal can be increased or decreased from atmospheric pressure. Normallly the middle ear is most compliant at atmospheric pressure. With a negative pressure in the middle ear as with eustachian tube obstruction, the point of maximal compliance occurs with negative pressure in the ear canal. With discontinuity of the ossicular chain, no point of maximal compliance can be obtained. Tympanometry is particularly useful in the identification and diagnosis of middle ear effusions in children.

During tympanometry, an intense tone (80 dB above the hearing threshold) elicits contraction of the stapedius muscle. The change in compliance of the middle ear with contraction of the stapedius muscle can be detected. The presence or absence of this *acoustic reflex* is important in the anatomic localization of facial nerve paralysis. The presence or absence of *acoustic reflex decay* helps differentiate sensory from neural hearing losses. In neural hearing loss, the reflex adapts or decays with time.

In order to evaluate a patient with a loss of hearing the minimum audiologic assessment should include the measurement of pure tone air and bone conduction thresholds, spondee threshold, discrimination score, performance-intensity function, tympanometry, acoustic reflexes, and acoustic reflex decay. This information provides a comprehensive screening evaluation of the whole auditory system and allows one to determine whether further differentiation of a sensory from a neural hearing loss is indicated.

In addition to these tests, testing for recruitment, the short increment sensitivity index, tone decay, Békésy audiometry, and brainstem auditory evoked responses (BAERs) help differentiate sensory from neural hearing losses. Of these, BAERs are the most powerful means of differentiating the site of sensorineural hearing loss (see Chap. 341). In response to sound, five distinct waves can be recorded with computer averaging from scalp surface electrodes. Poor or absent waveforms, abnormal latency of waves, and abnormal interwave latency are evidence of lesions in the eighth nerve and brainstem. In addition BAERs are valuable in situations in which patients cannot or will not give reliable voluntary thresholds. It also is used to monitor the integrity of the auditory nerve and brainstem intraoperatively and in determination of brain death.

CLINICAL ASSESSMENT OF A COMPLAINT OF HEARING LOSS   In evaluating patients who complain of loss of hearing, associated symptoms of tinnitus, vertigo, earache, otorrhea, and aural fullness should be sought along with a careful reconstruction of the history of evolution of the hearing deficit. A sudden onset of unilateral hearing loss, with or without tinnitus, may represent a viral infection in the inner ear. Gradual progression in a hearing deficit is common with otosclerosis, schwannoma of the acoustic nerve, or Ménière's disease. In the latter case, intermittent tinnitus and dizziness are usual. Hearing loss can occur with demyelinative lesions in the brainstem. Hearing loss is a hallmark of several genetic diseases, some with onset at birth, others occurring in children or adults (see Konigsmark for review).

Tinnitus is defined as the perception of a sound when there is no sound in the environment. It may have a buzzing, roaring, or ringing quality and may be pulsatile (synchronous with the heartbeat). Tinnitus is usually associated with a conductive or sensorineural loss of hearing. The pathophysiology of tinnitus is not well understood. The cause of the tinnitus can usually be determined by finding the cause of the associated hearing loss. Tinnitus may be the first symptom of a serious condition such as an acoustic schwannoma. Pulsatile tinnitus requires evaluation of the vascular system of the head to exclude vascular tumors such as glomus jugulare tumors, aneurysms, and stenotic lesions.

DIFFERENTIAL DIAGNOSIS   Most patients with conductive and unilateral or asymmetric sensorineural hearing losses should have CT scans of the temporal bone. Patients with sensorineural hearing losses should have the vestibular system evaluated with electronystagmography and caloric testing (see Chap. 14).

TREATMENT   Most patients with conductive hearing losses can be treated with middle ear reconstruction using procedures such as tympanoplasty after chronic otitis media and trauma, and stapedectomy for otosclerosis. Tympanostomy tubes allow the prompt return of hearing to normal in children and adults with middle ear effusions. Hearing aids are effective and well-tolerated for patients with conductive hearing losses. Patients with mild, moderate, and severe sensorineural hearing losses are regularly rehabilitated with hearing aids of varying configuration and strength. The profoundly deaf may benefit from cochlear implants.

The treatment of tinnitus is particularly problematic. The frequency range and intensity of tinnitus can often be matched with the use of an audiometer. Relief of the tinnitus may be obtained by masking it with background music. Hearing aids also are helpful in tinnitus suppression, as are tinnitus maskers, devices that present a sound to the affected ear which is more pleasant to listen to than the tinnitus. The use of a tinnitus masker is often followed by several hours of inhibition of the tinnitus.

REFERENCES

DALLOS P: *The Auditory Periphery: Biophysics and Physiology.* New York, Academic Press, 1973
DOTY RL: A review of olfactory dysfunctions in man. Am J Otolaryngol 1:57, 1979
—— et al: Smell identification ability: Changes with age. Science 226:1441, 1984
JERGER JR: *Modern Developments in Audiology*, 2d ed. New York, Academic Press, 1973
KONIGSMARK BW: Hereditary diseases of the nervous system with hearing loss, in PJ Vinken, GW Bruyn (eds), *Handbook of Clinical Neurology.* Elsevier, Amsterdam, 1975, vol 22, chap 23, pp 499–526
NAKASHIMA T et al: Structure of human fetal and adult olfactory neuroepithelium. Arch Otolaryngol 110:641, 1984
NORGREN R: The gustatory system in mammals. Am J Otolaryngol 4:234, 1983
RINTELMAN WF: *Hearing Assessment.* Baltimore, Baltimore University, 1979
SNOW JB: Sudden deafness, in MM Paprella, DA Shumrick (eds), *Otolaryngology*, 2d ed. Philadelphia, Saunders, 1980, pp 1751–1767
—— et al: Central auditory imperception. Laryngoscope 87:1450, 1977
——: Clinical problems in chemosensory distrubances. Am J Otolaryngol 4:224 1983

20 THE SLEEP-WAKE CYCLE AND DISORDERS OF SLEEP

WILLIAM J. SCHWARTZ / JOHN W. STAKES / JOSEPH B. MARTIN

The outward appearance of sleep—its passivity, relative immobility, and decreased sensitivity to external stimuli—belies an underlying organized brain activity both complex and heterogeneous. The operating characteristics and input-output relationships of physiologic systems change dramatically from wakefulness to sleep, and many systems which function normally during the day can decompensate during the night. Sleep pathology may present merely as an unrefreshing night's sleep or may masquerade as misleading symptoms of headache, lethargy, or unsatisfactory daytime performance. All these complaints must be pursued and addressed by the physician, not overlooked or pharmacologically suppressed.

Sleep length and depth vary markedly between healthy individuals. The average total sleep period is 7.5 h and ranges from 4 to 10 h. Sleep duration and organization also vary within individuals as a function of age. Total sleep time is highest in infancy, decreases to adult levels after completion of body growth, and declines with old age. Therefore, "how much sleep is enough" must be judged empirically. Sleep should be both *efficient,* resulting in few nocturnal arousals and minimal diurnal sleepiness, and *effective,* permitting maximal daytime function.

SLEEP STAGES AND CYCLES *Polysomnography,* the use of continuous recordings of brain waves (electroencephalogram, EEG), muscle electrical activity (electromyogram, EMG), and eye movements (electrooculogram, EOG), together with measurements of the respiratory rate, blood pressure, and heart rate, has provided important information about normal patterns of sleep and given clues to the nature of sleep disorders. For such studies, EEG electrodes are attached to the scalp, EOG electrodes to the skin at the outer canthus of both eyes, and EMG electrodes to the skin overlying the chin (mentalis) muscle.

The characteristic EEG pattern during wakefulness, with the eyes closed, is a sinusoidal posterior alpha rhythm of 8 to 12 Hz combined with low-voltage fast (beta) activity of mixed frequency (13 to 22 Hz). The EMG shows high-amplitude tonic activity. There are two defined states of sleep, *non-rapid eye movement* (NREM) sleep, and *rapid eye movement* (REM) sleep. NREM sleep is divided into four stages. Stage I sleep is characterized by low-voltage, mixed-frequency EEG activity, accompanied by slow eye movements recorded on the EOG. The EMG shows continuous high-amplitude discharges, which are decreased in size from those of the waking stage. Stage II sleep is represented by a moderately low-voltage EEG, interspersed with brief, generalized high-voltage discharges (K complexes), vertex waves, and low- to moderate-amplitude discharges of 12 to 15 Hz (sleep spindles). Stage III sleep consists of high-amplitude background activity of theta (5 to 7 Hz) and delta (1 to 3 Hz) slow waves, as well as K complexes and sleep spindles. Such high-voltage, slow-wave activity is present for 20 to 50 percent of the record. Stage IV sleep consists of high-voltage (75 μV or greater) delta waves present for 50 percent or more of the record. Spindles are rare. Low-voltage muscle potentials persist during each NREM sleep stage. Eye movements are infrequent or absent in stages III and IV. Delta sleep is the deepest (highest threshold to arousal) of the NREM stages.

The transition to REM sleep consists of a change in the EEG to low-voltage, fast-frequency (6 to 22 Hz) activity which resembles that seen during waking or stage I sleep. Moderately high amplitude, 3- to 5-Hz triangular-shaped waveforms (sawtooth waves) are also commonly observed. The EOG shows clusters of fast conjugate eye movements (REM activity). EMG activity becomes either totally absent or markedly suppressed, an effect due to descending inhibition of motor neurons from the brainstem reticular formation. The deep tendon and H reflexes are also absent. Upon awakening from REM sleep, subjects commonly recall vivid, hallucinatory dreams, but such cognitive activity is not restricted to this stage.

REM sleep alternates with NREM sleep approximately every 90 to 100 min, the first REM period usually occurring about 90 to 100 min after the onset of sleep. The full sequence of transition through stages I, II, III, and IV of NREM typically occurs after first going to sleep (Fig. 20-1). The sequence is then reversed through stages IV, III, and II, and REM sleep appears. A normal night's sleep consists of four to five such alternating cycles, characterized as the night progresses by an increasing duration and percentage of REM-sleep episodes. Stages III and IV occur predominantly during the first one-third of the sleep period. Stage I sleep normally occupies approximately 5 to 10 percent of total sleep, stage II about 50 percent, stage III approximately 15 percent, stage IV about 10 percent, and REM sleep approximately 20 percent.

Although NREM and REM sleep are defined by electrical recordings, they are characterized as *states* by a constellation of physiologic events. Blood pressure and heart and respiratory rates decrease during progressive stages of NREM sleep and fluctuate abruptly during REM sleep. During REM sleep, penile erections occur, effective thermoregulation is absent, and ventilatory responses to CO_2 are depressed. A number of endocrine functions are temporally associated with sleep. There is a major surge of growth hormone secretion during the first 2 h of sleep that is commonly, but not exclusively, associated with stages III and IV sleep. Adrenocorticotropic hormone (ACTH)–cortisol secretion occurs as a series of individual surges during the latter half of night sleep. Prolactin secretion in both men and women also increases during the night, especially immediately after sleep onset. Increased sleep-associated luteinizing hormone secretion has been shown to occur during puberty in boys and girls.

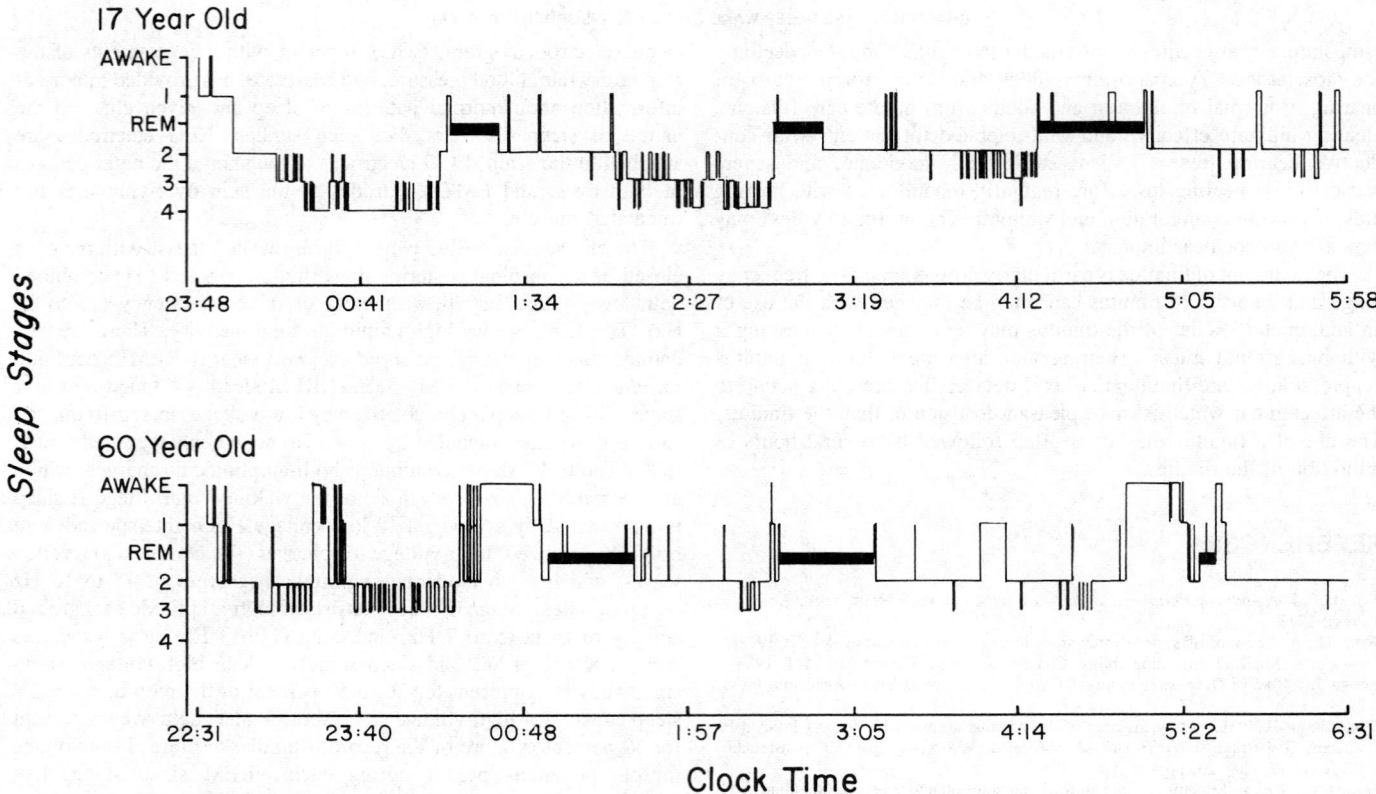

FIGURE 20-1 *Plots of the four stages of NREM sleep and REM sleep (solid bars) over the course of an entire night's sleep for a representative young (upper panel) and aged (lower panel) adult. In the elderly, there is diminished delta sleep and frequent spontaneous awakenings. Actual histograms are from the Sleep-Wake Disorders Unit, Massachusetts General Hospital.*

NEUROBIOLOGY OF SLEEP Although numerous theories have been proposed, the function(s) of sleep is unknown. Answering this question is likely to be as difficult and complex as investigating the "function" of wakefulness. The notion has emerged that NREM sleep serves some restorative, recuperative functions for the brain, although the nature, purpose, or necessity for such "rest" is unclear. REM sleep, with its intense neural activity generated independent of sensory input and uncoupled from motor output, is thought to play some as yet undefined rejuvenative role essential for the proper operation of higher neocortical activity during wakefulness.

A focus of contemporary sleep research has been to localize the brain mechanisms responsible for generating NREM-REM cycles. Especially implicated is the pontine tegmentum and the neurotransmitters norepinephrine, serotonin, and acetylcholine located in the locus coeruleus, dorsal raphe nucleus, and gigantocellular tegmental field. Over the course of development, a different neural mechanism matures to consolidate and restrict the expression of these sleep cycles to the nighttime portion of the 24-h day. An important component of this endogenous timekeeping mechanism ("circadian clock") is the suprachiasmatic nucleus of the anterior hypothalamus. The coupling of these mechanisms is unknown but has stimulated the characterization of endogenous sleep-inducing substances. This research is in its infancy, but apparent sleep-promoting peptides have been isolated from the body fluids of both sleep-deprived and sleeping animals.

An obvious approach for assessing the function of sleep is to prevent its occurrence and search for resulting deficits. Healthy adults can tolerate 10 or more days of sleep deprivation without overt medical impairment. Performance on simple, subject-paced, short-duration tasks is unaffected. There is no evidence that selective REM deprivation leads to psychological instability or psychosis. With prolonged deprivation, subjects experience increasing fatigue, irritability, lapses of attention, and diminished motivation. Performance

of tasks deteriorates, apparently due to transient and intrusive "microsleep" episodes. The frustration and difficulty of this research is epitomized by the facetious statement that the principal effect of sleep deprivation is to make people sleepy.

Recovery after prolonged sleep deprivation shows that the amount of sleep restored is not equal to the amount lost. During the first recovery sleep period the subject rapidly falls into stage IV of NREM sleep, often with "supernormal" slow waves in the EEG, and remains there at the expense of stage II sleep; REM sleep is decreased. By the second night, there is some REM sleep "rebound" which exceeds that of the predeprivation period.

SLEEP DISORDERS Disorders of sleep are common. Between 8 and 15 percent of the adult population in the United States have frequent and chronic complaints about the quality and the amount of their sleep. From 3 to 11 percent of adults use sedative-hypnotic drugs, and the percentage increases with age.

Sleep disorders can occur at any period of life. Some are peculiar to specific age groups, such as nocturnal enuresis, night terrors, and somnambulism in children and adolescents, and insomnia and hypersomnia in middle and old age. Others, such as the narcolepsy-cataplexy syndrome, may begin in childhood and persist throughout life.

The classification of sleep disorders is still evolving. Recently, a committee of the Association of Sleep Disorders Centers proposed a classification based principally on clinical symptomatology (see Table 20-1 and descriptions in references by Hauri and Weitzman).

Insomnias Insomnia, defined as want of sleep, is used popularly to indicate any impairment in duration, depth, or restorative properties of sleep. Insomnia may occur as a primary disorder; as a secondary manifestation of psychiatric illness, anxiety, drug use, or medical conditions; and in association with other disorders of sleep such as sleep apnea.

In order to understand the cause of insomnia, it is important to document the patient's sleep disturbance. A sleep log provided by the patient and observations by the bed partner of snoring, partial arousals, or kicking may suggest a more specific diagnosis. The history may determine whether sleep is disturbed by irregular sleep-wake schedules and wake-up times, afternoon naps, excessive nighttime noise or heat, self-medication by over-the-counter preparations, or consumption of alcohol, tobacco, or caffeine and its derivatives. The nature of the sleep complaint may also furnish etiologic clues. Inability to fall asleep or awakening 2 to 3 h after sleep onset may occur with the use of drugs or alcohol, painful or debilitating medical illness, periodic movements of sleep, or nonobstructive sleep apnea. Other patients go to sleep promptly and sleep well most of the night, only to awaken too early in the morning. Frequently in this category are individuals with depression or anxiety, or older persons who spontaneously go to bed and arise early in the day.

PSYCHOPHYSIOLOGIC INSOMNIA Situational insomnias are defined as lasting less than 3 weeks, usually with a suggested emotional cause. Symptoms include difficulty falling asleep, frequent arousals, or persistent early morning awakening, each contributing to feelings of chronic fatigue and irritability. Such symptoms may become persistent or worsened by worry about sleep loss. Anxiously lying awake at night and angrily trying to fall asleep, such patients often estimate 1 to 2 h sleep loss as 3 to 4 h. Such individuals may show no evidence of anxiety or depressive disorder.

Benzodiazepines are currently the hypnotic drugs of choice for the short-term management of insomnia. The effectiveness of long-term use (greater than 30 days) of any hypnotic has not been established. Flurazepam, 15 to 60 mg before going to bed, is the most frequently prescribed hypnotic in the United States. Older sedatives include chloral hydrate and barbiturates, but tolerance and withdrawal limits their use. L-Tryptophan, 1 to 5 g, has been advocated by some investigators, but its clinical effectiveness has not been conclusively demonstrated.

The widespread use of benzodiazepines as nighttime sedatives is now complicated by recognition of certain undesirable properties. First, they are mildly addictive and show cross-tolerance with each other and with alcohol. Second, rebound insomnia may occur with tolerance to or withdrawal from these agents (see below). Third, active metabolites of flurazepam and certain other benzodiazepines have biologic effects lasting 36 to 48 h (or longer in the elderly).

When psychophysiologic insomnia becomes chronic, pharmacologic therapy alone is rarely efficacious. A vicious cycle develops as the patient's conditioned arousal at bedtime and fear over sleep loss aggravate the insomnia. This can be one of the most difficult problems in office practice and requires combined psychosocial and behavioral approaches in addition to hypnotics.

INSOMNIA ASSOCIATED WITH THE AFFECTIVE PSYCHIATRIC DISORDERS The sleep abnormalities found in the affective disorders consist of chronic or recurrent inability to maintain sleep through the expected sleep period. Patients complain of persistent restlessness at night and of a tired, apathetic feeling during the day. More frequent arousal throughout the night, failure to "sleep deeply," and early morning awakening complete the clinical picture.

The affective disorders have been divided into major depressive and bipolar (manic-depressive) disorders (see Chap. 360). The sleep disorder in unipolar depression is characterized by repeated awakenings with a shortened REM latency (time from sleep onset to first episode of REM sleep) and decreased stages III and IV NREM sleep. Patients with bipolar depression also show these polysomnographic features, but they often have excessive daytime sleepiness (take naps) and have extended sleep periods at night. During periods of hypomania, partial or total sleeplessness may occur, lasting for several days.

Treatment is directed to the underlying psychiatric disorder and may include nighttime administration of tricyclic antidepressants or monoamine oxidase inhibitors. Several new nonpharmacologic treatments for depression are currently under study, including manipulation of the timing of sleep within the 24-h day. REM sleep deprivation or progressive phase advance of sleep onset have been reported to reverse the depressive phase of bipolar illness in some patients.

INSOMNIA ASSOCIATED WITH THE USE OF DRUGS AND ALCOHOL The widespread use and abuse of central nervous system depressants (hypnotic and sedative drugs, tranquilizers, or bedtime use of alcohol) is well documented and may produce an insomnia syndrome. As tolerance develops with continued use, the sleep-promoting properties of such drugs are lost, and the patient and the physician tend to increase the dosage. Specific sleep-disturbing symptoms caused by partial withdrawal can develop, even though administration of the drug is continued. The resulting early morning arousal is often misinterpreted, and dosage is increased further. In patients who regularly and chronically use hypnotic agents, sleep is interrupted by frequent awakenings lasting more than 5 min, especially during the second half of the night. Stages III and IV and REM sleep are decreased, and sleep-stage demarcations are less clear. These observations point to a considerable degree of sleep disorganization.

After rapid or acute withdrawal from hypnotic agents used chronically in high daily doses, the percentage of REM sleep greatly increases. Sleep-related periodic movements (nocturnal myoclonus) may also occur during the withdrawal period. In addition, daytime symptoms appear, including restlessness, nervousness, myalgias, and, in severe cases, drug withdrawal symptoms, including confusion, hallucinations, and grand mal convulsions. These complications are most common after barbiturate and glutethimide withdrawal, but may be seen with benzodiazepines as well. In patients who are chronic high-dose users of multiple hypnotic drugs, withdrawal should be gradual and supervised by a clinician. Many patients then show substantial improvement in both objective and subjective sleep patterns, although they may not return immediately to a fully normal sleep.

Heavy and sustained ingestion of alcohol severely disrupts sleep-stage organization. REM sleep periods are shortened and nightly awakenings occur. Acute withdrawal from alcohol in the chronic alcoholic leads to a lengthening of the latency to sleep onset, a decrease in NREM sleep, and an increase in REM sleep with shortened latency. If severe, acute toxic withdrawal syndrome (delirium tremens) may develop. In the abstaining alcoholic, abnormal sleep patterns may persist for many weeks, although normal sleep usually returns within 2 weeks.

INSOMNIA ASSOCIATED WITH SLEEP-RELATED MYOCLONUS In some patients with primary insomnia and in many with other forms of

TABLE 20-1 Classification of sleep disorders

I Insomnias: Disorders of initiating and maintaining sleep
  A Psychophysiologic—situational or persistent
  B Associated with psychiatric disorders, particularly affective disorders
  C Associated with drugs and alcohol
    1 Tolerance to or withdrawal from CNS depressants
    2 Sustained use of CNS stimulants
    3 Sustained use of or withdrawal from other drugs
    4 Chronic alcoholism
  D Associated with sleep-induced respiratory impairment
    1 Sleep apnea syndrome
    2 Alveolar hypoventilation syndrome
  E Associated with sleep-related (nocturnal) myoclonus and "restless legs"
  F Miscellaneous—other medical, toxic, or environmental conditions
II Hypersomnias: Disorders of excessive somnolence
  A Psychophysiologic—situational or persistent
  B Associated with psychiatric disorders, particularly affective disorders
  C Associated with drugs and alcohol
  D Associated with sleep-induced respiratory impairment (as in *D* above)
  E Narcolepsy-cataplexy
  F Miscellaneous—other medical, toxic, environmental, or idiopathic conditions
III Disorders of the sleep-wake schedule
  A Transient—jet lag, work shift
  B Persistent
    1 Delayed sleep phase syndrome
    2 Advanced sleep phase syndrome
    3 Non-24-h sleep-wake syndrome
IV Parasomnias: Dysfunctions associated with sleep, sleep stages, or partial arousal
  A Sleepwalking
  B Sleep terrors and dream anxiety attacks
  C Enuresis
  D Nocturnal seizures
  E Other sleep-related dysfunctions

insomnia, *periodic movements of sleep* (PMS) occur, usually during NREM sleep. The movements consist of stereotyped, repetitive dorsiflexion of the foot and big toe and sometimes flexion of the knee and hip. Movements recur every 20 to 30 s and last about 2 s each. They are to be distinguished from the common and benign "night starts" which occur at the onset of sleep. Sleep recordings indicate that PMS occur in a wide variety of sleep disorders in middle-aged persons, including narcolepsy-cataplexy, sleep apnea, and drug-dependency insomnia. The symptoms thus appear to be secondary to a chronic sleep-wake disturbance rather than representing a primary disorder. Although the neurophysiologic mechanisms responsible for PMS are unknown, modest therapeutic successes have been reported with clonazepam, 1 mg before bedtime.

In *restless legs syndrome,* the affected individual feels an irresistible urge to move the legs, generally when sitting or lying down, especially prior to sleep. There is a discomfort deep inside the calves which is alleviated by moving, exercising, or walking about. This interferes with sleep onset and may recur during the night. Usually by morning the restless legs symptoms have diminished, and the patient may be able to fall asleep. PMS is present in all cases of restless legs syndrome studied polygraphically.

MISCELLANEOUS CAUSES OF INSOMNIA   Patients with sleep apnea or hypopnea, especially the nonobstructive type, may be frequently awakened and complain of unrefreshing sleep (see below). Poor sleep may occur in persons with a debilitating or painful illness which generates more pain and restlessness as muscles relax to leave painful areas unsplinted. Medical disorders such as paroxysmal nocturnal dyspnea, nocturnal asthma, and rheumatic or gastrointestinal illness may cause insomnia.

Hypersomnias   These disorders are typified by inappropriate sleepiness leading to sleep during a time when the patient wishes to be awake. The patient complains of an irresistible urge to sleep during the day, decreased concentration, excessive yawning, and an increase in total sleep time over a 24-h period. The complaint of excessive sleep need should be distinguished from self-imposed sleep deprivation and from other symptoms of lethargy, fatigue, and apathy that commonly accompany anxiety or depression.

A classification of disorders of excessive daytime somnolence is given in Table 20-1. In clinical practice two major disorders, sleep-induced respiratory impairment and the narcolepsy-cataplexy syndrome, account for about 80 percent of patients with complaints of hypersomnia.

SLEEP-INDUCED RESPIRATORY IMPAIRMENT (THE SLEEP APNEA–HYPERSOMNIA SYNDROME)   Excessive daytime somnolence is the usual complaint. In addition, disturbing nighttime symptoms include intermittent inspiratory snoring alternating with periods of apnea lasting from 10 to 120 s. Episodes begin with increasing snoring over 20 to 60 s, culminating in a loud gasp. Brief arousal followed by a variable period of apnea recurs cyclically. In serious cases, more than 500 apneas may occur per night. The patient often talks during sleep (somniloquy) and awakens in the morning unrefreshed, still sleepy, and often with a generalized headache. Polysomnography shows that the periods of apnea may result in oxygen desaturation (often below 50% saturation), occasional bradycardia alternating with tachycardia, and cardiac arrhythmias. Stages III and IV of NREM sleep are decreased.

The ratio of men to women with the sleep apnea–hypersomnia syndrome is 20:1, and the age range is the fourth to sixth decade. Approximately two-thirds of the patients are obese. A rapid weight gain may precipitate or increase the severity of the symptoms. Hypertension and signs of right heart failure may be associated.

In *obstructive apnea,* there is absent airflow despite respiratory effort. Direct endoscopic observations of the airway during the apneic episode show that the site of obstruction is in the oral pharynx at the level of the velopharyngeal sphincter. Obstruction is caused by apposition of the lateral pharyngeal walls and by posterior movement of the base of the tongue. Narrowing of the upper airway may be

secondary to enlarged tonsils or adenoids, mandibular abnormalities, or pharyngeal soft tissue alterations in acromegaly and hypothyroid myxedema. Apnea may also result from cessation of respiratory movements (central or *nonobstructive apnea*). Neuromuscular disorders with respiratory muscle weakness have been associated with this condition. An initial nonobstructive apnea may be followed by obstruction (*mixed apnea*). Also, oxygen desaturation and arousals may be seen with a variety of other respiratory disturbances including hypopneas and partial obstructions. Each of these patterns may be present in an individual patient.

Treatment should begin with weight loss, but many individuals require tracheostomy to establish an adequate airway during sleep. Other treatments for milder forms have included tricyclic antidepressants (e.g., protriptyline HCl), oral progesterone, and continuous nasal positive airway pressure.

NARCOLEPSY-CATAPLEXY   The narcolepsy-cataplexy syndrome is characterized by recurrent episodes of irresistible daytime sleepiness associated with abnormal manifestations of REM sleep. The "sleep attacks" appear as clinically normal sleep, are characteristically brief (about 15 min), and are often precipitated by boredom, but also occur inappropriately during coitus, athletics, or while driving an automobile. Patients usually awake refreshed, and there is a refractory period of from one to a few hours before the next attack occurs. Between attacks the patient is sleepy and inattentive; waking behaviors may become automatic and interrupted by "microsleeps." This can be quantitated using a multiple sleep latency test. Nocturnal sleep is usually also disturbed by frequent awakenings.

In about 80 percent of cases, there is also a history of *cataplexy,* characterized by sudden, brief episodes of loss of muscle tone without loss of consciousness. Cataplexy is commonly triggered by an emotional event such as laughter, anger, fear, or surprise. In its most severe form, the cataplectic attack results in total flaccid paralysis (with sparing of diaphragmatic and extraocular eye muscle movements), and collapse to the floor. Less severe symptoms may consist of sagging of the jaw or head, speechlessness, or a feeling of weakening of the knees. Full recovery occurs within a minute or two, or sleep may supervene. Two other symptoms complete the clinical tetrad of the narcolepsy-cataplexy syndrome. *Sleep paralysis* is a frightening sensation of inability to move the voluntary muscles, occurring at the transition of sleep onset or at awakening. *Vivid hallucinations* (usually visual) may occur either at sleep onset (hypnagogic) or on awakening (hypnopompic).

The disorder occurs with a prevalence of 40 per 100,000 population and has a genetic predisposition. It affects men and women equally, usually begins in adolescence with daytime sleepiness, and is a lifelong illness. The condition has severe psychosocial consequences. Symptoms often pass unrecognized, and poor school performance is ascribed to laziness; in adults, accidents, job disruptions, and depression may occur.

Narcolepsy is believed to represent a disorder of the REM sleep process. Polygraphic sleep recordings show that narcoleptics frequently begin their sleep with an REM period (sleep-onset REM). The sleep attacks that occur suddenly during the waking state are often sleep-onset REM attacks, and cataplexy, with loss of muscle tone, appears to be the quiescent state of the EMG during REM sleep. Hypnagogic hallucinations and sleep paralysis are the subjective equivalents of dreaming and muscle paralysis, respectively, which occur at the waking-sleeping interphase as manifestations of the activated REM state. Animal models of this disorder have been recently described in dogs and horses.

The treatment of narcolepsy is symptomatic. Two separate classes of drugs are effective in the management of narcolepsy and cataplexy, respectively. Narcoleptics may show improvement with strategically timed naps (during lunch hour or after meals), but most require administration of central adrenergic stimulant drugs. Methylphenidate, 10 mg two to three times daily, or amphetamine sulfate, 5 to 10 mg three to four times daily, are given to sustain the patient through the most difficult periods of the day. Late afternoon or evening administration should be avoided since it may interfere with night sleep. Cataplexy responds best to imipramine or desipramine, in doses ranging from 75 to 200 mg daily. These drugs suppress REM sleep by facilitation of adrenergic transmission and inhibition of cholinergic systems. Each class of drug should be titrated separately to achieve best results for the symptoms of narcolepsy and cataplexy, respectively.

OTHER CONDITIONS ASSOCIATED WITH EXCESSIVE DAYTIME SOMNOLENCE The *Kleine-Levin syndrome* (periodic hypersomnia) is a rare disorder that first presents between the ages of 12 and 20. It is more common in men but is also described in women. Recurrent periods of hypersomnolence lasting from a few days to several weeks alternate with asymptomatic intervals of months or years.

During a bout of hypersomnolence, the patients develop a voracious appetite and may exhibit disturbances in mood, show sexual hyperactivity and exhibitionism, and have hallucinations, disorientation, and memory deficits. The condition is usually self-limited, rarely occurring beyond the fourth or fifth decade. The etiology is unknown, and no specific neuropathology has been associated, although the disorder has been postulated to be a dysfunction of limbic and hypothalamic rhythms. Rarely, cerebrospinal fluid pleocytosis has been found, which suggests that an episode of encephalitis may underlie the disorder in some cases.

Excessive somnolence is a feature of many endocrine and metabolic disorders, including uremia, liver failure, hypothyroidism (severe, with myxedema), chronic pulmonary disease (with hypercapnia), and diabetes mellitus with incipient coma or with severe hypoglycemia. Sleep-onset REM can be rarely observed following sleep deprivation or withdrawal from REM-suppressant drugs. In addition, hypersomnolence may occur in central nervous system disorders, such as a tumor in the area of the third ventricle, obstructive hydrocephalus, and meningoencephalitis. Finally, there is a category of hypersomnolence (idiopathic central nervous system hypersomnolence) for which no etiology has been identified. Such patients respond to stimulant medications. In all of the above conditions, it is important to distinguish complaints of tiredness, fatigue, and apathy secondary to metabolic, endocrine, neurologic, and pyschiatric disease from sleepiness per se.

Disorders of the sleep-wake schedule Sleep is one of many daily rhythms synchronized to the earth's 24-h geophysical cycle. Normal humans studied in controlled laboratory conditions in the absence of environmental time cues show that the endogenous length of the "free-running" circadian period for humans is approximately 25 h. Under such time-isolated conditions, the normal coupling of the rhythms of body temperature, plasma hormone levels, and sleep cycles is lost as the phase relationships between them become desynchronized.

Disorders of the circadian sleep-wake cycle are classified under two categories, transient and persistent. The transient dyssomnia of a rapid time-zone change ("jet lag") is very familiar, as is that found after an acute work-shift change. The sleep disturbance that results is due to both sleep deprivation and the circadian phase-shift change. The symptoms include an inability to sustain sleep with frequent arousals and sleepiness at inopportune clock times. Resynchronization takes several days to 2 weeks.

Persistent disorders of the sleep-wake cycle include (1) delayed sleep phase syndrome, (2) advanced sleep phase syndrome, and (3) non-24-h sleep-wake syndrome. The delayed sleep phase syndrome is a sleep disorder that can be differentiated from other forms of insomnia. Patients cannot fall asleep at the desired clock time required to meet work or study schedules; typically, they finally fall asleep at 2 to 6 A.M. However, when not required to maintain a strict schedule (e.g., weekends, holidays, and vacation periods), the patient will sleep normally if allowed to retire and awaken spontaneously. These individuals have normal sleep duration and architecture, but the *timing* of their sleep period within the 24-h day is abnormal. Such patients have been successfully treated by a progressive phase delay

of their sleep times (chronotherapy). By delaying the time of going to sleep by 3 h each day (i.e., a 27-h sleep-wake cycle) the patient's sleep can be "reset" to occur at a socially acceptable clock time.

The advanced sleep phase syndrome describes individuals with normal sleep duration and architecture but with inappropriate early sleep onset and wake times. These "early to bed, early to rise" people rarely seek medical help. The process of aging leads to a characteristic change in the timing of sleep such that older individuals spontaneously awaken earlier in the morning and become sleepy and go to sleep earlier in the evening.

The non-24-h sleep-wake (hypernychthermal) syndrome is characterized by an inability to be entrained to society's 24-h day. These individuals develop a 25- to 27-h biologic day length in spite of all social cues. Blindness or a personality disorder may predispose to this condition.

Parasomnias A number of undesirable behavioral and physiologic events occur in association with sleep or specific sleep stages. Since their etiologies and interrelationships are uncertain, they are usually listed as individual clinical entities.

SLEEPWALKING (SOMNAMBULISM) In this condition, individuals suddenly sit up in bed, walk, or carry out automatic and semipurposeful complex motor activities. Patients remain unconscious and will resist being aroused. On occasion, dangerous acts, such as climbing out a window, can occur. The episode lasts less than 15 min and is finished by returning to bed or spontaneous arousal (without dream report). Sleepwalking occurs in stage III or IV of NREM sleep. There is no evidence of seizure activity either preceding or during the episode, although clinically it must be distinguished from a nocturnal seizure disorder originating in the temporal lobes.

This condition occurs normally in children and adolescents; 15 percent of all children have one or more episodes. A small percent of children (1 to 6 percent) have frequent attacks (at times, nightly). Psychopathology may be found if the episodes begin or persist into adulthood.

SLEEP TERRORS AND DREAM ANXIETY ATTACKS Sleep terrors (pavor nocturnus, incubus) commonly occur in children. The attacks occur within the first 1 to 2 h of the night, during stage III or IV of NREM sleep. With a frightened scream, the child sits up in bed, agitated and panicked. Autonomic changes appear, including sweating, tachycardia, hyperventilation, and pupillary dilation. It may be difficult to arouse the child fully, and the attack may persist for several minutes before sleep returns. There is no report of dream imagery after the attack and no memory for the event the following morning. Night terrors are almost always benign and time-limited so that reassurance is both adequate and sufficient.

Dream anxiety attacks (nightmares) occur later in the night during REM sleep. Screams are uncommon, and arousal is rapid. Vivid hallucinatory and emotionally charged dreams are usually recounted. Recurrent nightmares may reflect underlying psychological conflicts.

SLEEP-RELATED ENURESIS Bed-wetting occurs during stage III and IV of NREM sleep, usually during the first third of the night. Primary enuresis is the persistence of bed-wetting from infancy to childhood, whereas secondary enuresis occurs after a period of successful toilet training. Both need to be distinguished from symptomatic enuresis, which is caused by a known organic lesion affecting bladder regulation. All forms need to be separated from nocturnal seizures associated with incontinence.

NOCTURNAL SEIZURES Paroxysmal abnormalities of brain electrical activity of the type seen in seizure disorders sometimes occur in epileptic patients during or shortly after the onset of sleep. Up to 25 percent of subjects with grand mal attacks have them only at night during sleep. Seizures are often accompanied by tongue biting and incontinence and by muscle soreness the following day. Other seizures may mimic somnambulism, sleep terrors, and enuresis, or may present as fragmented, unrefreshing sleep periods.

OTHER SLEEP-RELATED DYSFUNCTIONS The list of such disturbances is growing and includes bruxism, head banging (jactatio capitis nocturnus), sleep-related painful erections, cluster headaches, gastroesophageal reflux, paroxysmal nocturnal hemoglobinuria, and sleep palsies due to compression of peripheral nerves.

REFERENCES

COLEMAN R et al: Sleep-wake disorders based on a polysomnographic diagnosis. JAMA 247:997, 1982

GUILLEMINAULT C (ed): *Sleeping and Waking Disorders: Indications and Techniques.* Menlo Park, Calf, Addison-Wesley, 1981

HAURI P: *The Sleep Disorders.* Kalamazoo, Mich, Upjohn, 1977

HOBSON JA, BRAZIER MAB (eds): *The Reticular Formation Revisited.* New York, Raven, 1980

KALES A et al: Insomnia and other sleep disorders. Med Clin North Am 66:971, 1982

MCGINTY DJ, SIEGEL JM: Sleep States, in *Handbook of Behavioral Neurobiology,* vol 6, *Motivation,* E Satinoff and P Teitelbaum (eds). New York, Plenum, 1983, p 105

MOORE-EDE MC et al: Circadian timekeeping in health and disease. N Engl J Med 309:469, 530, 1983

OREM J, BARNES CD (eds): *Physiology in Sleep.* New York, Academic, 1980

ROFFWARG H: Diagnostic classification of sleep and arousal disorders. Sleep 2:1, 1979

WEITZMAN ED: Sleep and its disorders. Ann Rev Neurosci 4:381, 1981

21 COMA AND OTHER DISORDERS OF CONSCIOUSNESS

ALLAN H. ROPPER / JOSEPH B. MARTIN

Coma is a common problem in general medicine; it is estimated that up to 3 percent of admissions to the emergency ward of large municipal hospitals are due to diseases that cause a disorder of consciousness. The importance of this class of neurologic disorders points to the necessity of acquiring a systematic approach to their diagnosis and management.

The increased availability of computerized tomography (CT) has resulted in an artificial orientation to the diagnosis of coma by focusing attention on lesions that are detectable by CT (e.g., hemorrhages, tumors, or hydrocephalus). This approach, although at times expedient, is often imprudent because most coma is metabolic or toxic in origin. The physician confronted with an unresponsive patient should formulate a differential diagnosis based on the history and the clinical signs before leaving the bedside. Certain signs observed during general and neurologic examination allow the physician to decide which of several generic diseases is responsible for coma, thus limiting the diagnostic possibilities. A rational approach to the precise diagnosis and subsequent management can then be planned and clinical changes anticipated. The clinical approach must be coupled to knowledge of the pathologic entities that cause coma. This chapter describes a practical approach to coma based on the anatomy and physiology of consciousness and a consideration of the general and neurologic examination and CT.

Coma is epitomized by unresponsiveness and as such is easily recognized. The interesting and sometimes subtle distinctions made between coma, stupor, and drowsiness are largely semantic because there is no anatomic or physiologic basis for distinguishing them except as relative degrees of unresponsiveness. A narrative description of the clinical state of the patient and of responses evoked by various stimuli, precisely as they are observed at the bedside, remains the optimal way to characterize coma and related disturbances of consciousness. Such a description is preferable to summary terms such as *stupor, semicoma,* or *obtundation,* which are often ambiguous and commonly differ between observers. *Stupor,* as currently used, implies a state in which the patient can be aroused by vigorous stimuli but verbal responses are slow or absent; *semicoma* suggests a state of unsustained stirring, moaning, or agitation in response to stimulation.

Although the definition of consciousness is a psychological and philosophical matter, the distinction between *level* of consciousness, or wakefulness, and *content* of consciousness, or awareness, has physiologic significance. Wakefulness or alertness is maintained by a diffuse system of upper brainstem and thalamic neurons, the reticular activating system (RAS), and its connections to the cerebral hemispheres as a whole. Therefore, depression of either hemispheral or RAS activity may cause reduced wakefulness. Awareness is dependent on integrated and organized material thoughts, subjective experience, emotions, and mental processes, each of which resides to some extent in anatomically defined regions of the brain. The inability to maintain a coherent sequence of thoughts and actions is called *confusion* and is a disorder of content of consciousness. Reduced wakefulness often precludes evaluation of content of consciousness, but content of consciousness can be severly impaired, as in confusion, without affecting arousal. Confusion is used to describe a state of inattention, and lack of clarity in thinking. In special cases it is accompanied by illusions (misperceptions of environmental sight, sound, or touch) or hallucinations (spontaneous endogenous perceptions). Psychiatrists often use the term *delirium* for any confusion, but delirium should be reserved as a description for an agitated, hypersympathotonic, frequently hallucinatory state most often due to specific causes such as alcohol or drug withdrawal. Usually, the confused patient is subdued, not inclined to speak, and less active physically than usual. Many processes that ultimately lead to coma begin with confusion, and diagnostic considerations should address the primary problem as an alteration in the level of consciousness. Confusion alone generally indicates a metabolic derangement, although focal cerebral lesions that cause deficits in language, orientation, or memory may make the patient appear to be confused.

ANATOMIC CORRELATES OF CONSCIOUSNESS A normal level of consciousness (wakefulness) depends upon activation of the cerebral hemispheres by groups of neurons located in the brainstem RAS. Both of the cerebral hemispheres, the RAS, and the connections between them must be preserved for normal consciousness. The principal causes of coma are, therefore, (1) bilateral hemispheral damage or suppression by drugs or toxins and (2) a brainstem lesion or metabolic derangement that damages or suppresses the RAS. There is some evidence that large, purely unilateral hemispheral lesions particularly on the left may cause drowsiness (though not coma), even in the absence of damage to the opposite hemisphere or RAS.

Reticular activating system The RAS is best defined as a physiologic system, not an anatomic one. It is contained within the reticular formation, which consists of loosely grouped neurons located bilaterally in the medial tegmental gray matter of the brainstem extending from the medulla to the posterior diencephalon. These neurons have been shown in neuroanatomic studies to span long rostrocaudal distances within the reticular formation. Animal experiments and human clinical-neuropathologic observations have established that *the neurons located in the region extending from the rostral pons to the caudal diencephalon are of primary importance for maintaining wakefulness.* Lesions here that produce coma also commonly affect adjacent brainstem structures concerned with control of pupillary constriction and mechanisms for eye movements (Fig. 21-1). Abnormalities in these systems on physical examination provide signposts of brainstem damage. Lesions confined to the cerebral hemispheres do not directly affect the brainstem RAS, though secondary derangement may result from midline compression due to shifts in a cerebral hemisphere.

Brainstem RAS neurons project rostrally to the cortex, primarily via "nonspecific" thalamic relay nuclei which exert a tonic influence on the activity of the cerebral cortex. Experimental work suggests that the brainstem RAS indirectly affects the level of consciousness by suppressing the activity of the nonspecific nuclei. Electrical stimulation of the pontine and midbrain RAS desynchronizes the electroencephalogram (EEG), a pattern associated with behavioral arousal. Stimulation of the thalamic relay nuclei opposes this activity, resulting in synchronization and slowing of the EEG. The basis of behavioral arousal by environmental stimuli (somesthetic, auditory, and visual) depends on the rich innervation of the RAS by each sensory system.

The relay between the RAS and thalamic and cortical areas is accomplished by neurotransmitters. Of these, the influence of acetylcholine and norepinephrine on arousal is the best established. Cholinergic fibers connect the midbrain to other areas of the upper brainstem, thalamus, and cortex. These pathways are thought to mediate the clinical and EEG arousal observed after administration of cholinergic drugs such as physostigmine. Noradrenergic neurons in the locus coeruleus and serotonergic cells of the raphe nucleus of the pons are known to project diffusely to the cortex. Serotonin and norepinephrine subserve important functions in the regulation of the sleep-wake cycle (see Chap. 20). Their roles in arousal and coma have not been clearly established, although the alerting effects of amphetamines are likely to be mediated by catecholamine release.

Cerebral hemispheres and consciousness The specialized functions of the cerebral cortex in language, control of movement, and perception are regionalized (see Chaps. 22 to 24). In contrast, wakefulness is related in a semiquantitative way to the total mass of functioning cortex (and RAS connections) and is not focally represented in any region of the hemispheres. Hemispheral lesions may cause coma in one of three ways: (1) most commonly, bilateral, generalized hemispheral lesions or metabolic derangements such as occur in encephalitis, generalized epilepsy, drug ingestion, ischemia, and hypoglycemia interfere with awareness in a graded fashion as more cortical territory is damaged or rendered functionally inactive; (2) rarely, enlarging masses or secondary brain swelling initially confined to one side of the brain may compress the contralateral hemisphere, effectively creating bilateral hemispheral lesions; and (3) large lesions in one or both hemispheres may compress the brainstem and diencephalon causing coma indirectly by damaging the RAS. *The degree of decrease in alertness is often related to the acuteness of onset of the cortical dysfunction.*

The concept of *transtentorial herniation* with progressive brainstem compression has dominated thinking about neurologic signs in coma caused by supratentorial mass lesions. Herniation refers to displacement of brain tissue away from a mass, past a less mobile structure such as dura, and into a space that it normally does not occupy. Herniation suggests a degree of irreversibility because the tissue is

trapped in its new location. The common herniations seen at postmortem are transfalcial (under the falx in the anterior midline), transtentorial (into the tentorial opening), and cerebellar tonsillar (into the foramen magnum). Uncal transtentorial herniation, or impaction of the uncal gyrus into the cistern between the free edge of the tentorium and lateral edge of the midbrain, causes compression of the third nerve with pupillary dilation and subsequent coma due to midbrain compression. Central transtentorial herniation denotes downward movement of the diencephalon (thalamic region) through the tentorial opening in the midline and is said to be heralded by miotic pupils and drowsiness. In both cases an orderly progression of rostral to caudal compression of first the midbrain, then pons, and finally medulla leads to the sequential appearance of neurologic signs and progressively diminished alertness. However, many patients with supratentorial masses do not follow these stereotypic patterns; an orderly progression of signs from midbrain to medulla is rarely seen in catastrophic lesions where all brainstem functions are lost almost simultaneously. Furthermore, stupor typically occurs with only moderate lateral shifts at the level of the diencephalon (4 to 8 mm) before actual herniation is evident on a CT scan.

PATHOPHYSIOLOGY OF COMA The pathophysiologic basis of coma is either mechanical destruction of crucial areas of the brainstem or cerebral cortex (anatomic coma) or global disruption of brain metabolic processes (metabolic coma). Coma of metabolic origin may be produced by interruption of energy substrate delivery (hypoxia, ischemia, hypoglycemia) or by alteration of the neurophysiologic responses of neuronal membranes (drug or alcohol intoxication, epilepsy, or acute head injury).

The brain is markedly dependent on continuous blood flow and delivery of oxygen and glucose, which are consumed at rates of 3.5 mL per 100 g per minute and 5 mg per 100 g per minute, respectively. Brain stores of glucose provide energy for approximately 2 min after blood flow is interrupted, although consciousness is lost within 8 to 10 s. When hypoxia occurs simultaneously with ischemia, available glucose is exhausted more rapidly. Normal resting cerebral blood flow (CBF) is approximately 75 mL per 100 g per minute in gray matter and 30 mL per 100 g per minute in white matter (mean = 55 mL per 100 g per minute). This provides for adequate metabolic supplies with a modest safety factor to accommodate most physiologic changes. When mean CBF diminishes to 25 mL per 100 g per minute, the EEG becomes diffusely slowed (typical of metabolic encepha-

FIGURE 21-1 *Brainstem reflexes in the coma examination. Midbrain and third nerve function are tested by pupillary reaction to light, pontine function by spontaneous and reflex eye movements and corneal responses, and medullary function by respiratory and pharyngeal responses.*

Reflex conjugate, horizontal eye movements are dependent upon the medial longitudinal fasciculus (MLF) interconnecting the sixth and contralateral third nerve nuclei. Eye movements are elicited by head rotation (oculocephalic reflex) or caloric stimulation of the labyrinths (oculovestibular or vestibuloocular reflex). These reflex movements are suppressed in the awake patient by the cerebral hemispheres via their connections to the brainstem.

lopathies), and at 15 mL per 100 g per minute brain electrical activity ceases. If all other conditions such as temperature and arterial oxygenation remain normal, CBF less than 10 mL per 100 g per minute causes irrevocable brain damage.

Coma due to hyponatremia, hyperosmolarity, hypercapnia, and the encephalopathies of hepatic and renal failure are associated with a variety of metabolic derangements of neurons and astrocytes. The toxic effects of these conditions on the brain are frequently multifactorial, producing impaired energy supplies, changes in resting membrane potentials, neurotransmitter abnormalities, and in some instances morphologic changes. For example, hepatic coma may be related in part to a high brain ammonia concentration which interferes with cerebral energy metabolism and the Na^+,K^+-ATPase pump. The increased number and size of astrocytes seen in the brains of patients who die as a result of hepatic encephalopathy may contribute to neurologic symptoms. This change may be due to the need to detoxify ammonia. In addition, abnormalities of neurotransmitters have been found in experimental hepatic coma, including possible ''false'' neurotransmitters, which may act competitively at monoaminergic receptor sites.

The exact cause of the encephalopathy of renal failure is also poorly understood. Urea itself does not produce nervous system toxicity. A multifactorial cause is likely, including increased permeability of the blood-brain barrier to toxic substances such as organic acids and an increase in brain calcium or cerebrospinal fluid (CSF) phosphate content. Cellular membrane potentials change in uremia due to brain potassium shifts, but the magnitude of this effect is small and unlikely to account for neurologic symptoms. Parathyroid hormone excess may also play a part in uremic encephalopathy.

Abnormalities of osmolarity are involved in the coma and seizures caused by several medical disorders including diabetic ketoacidosis, the nonketotic hyperosmolar state, and hyponatremia. In hyperosmolarity, brain volume is reduced while hypoosmolarity leads to brain swelling. Brain water volume correlates best with level of consciousness in hyponatremic-hypoosmolar states but other factors probably also play a role. Sodium levels below 115 meq per liter are associated with coma and convulsions, depending to some extent on the rapidity with which the hyponatremia develops. Serum osmolarity is generally above 350 mosmol per liter in hyperosmolar coma.

Hypercapnia produces a diminished level of consciousness proportional to the P_{CO_2} tension in the blood and to acuteness of onset. A relationship between CSF acidosis and severity of symptoms has been established. The pathophysiology of other metabolic encephalopathies such as hypercalcemia, hypothyroidism, vitamin B_{12} deficiency, and hypothermia are incompletely understood but probably reflect multifaceted derangements of cerebral biochemistry.

Central nervous system (CNS) depressant drugs and some endogenous toxins probably produce coma by suppression of metabolic and membrane electrical activities in both the RAS and cerebral cortex. For this reason combinations of cortical and brainstem signs occur in drug overdose and other metabolic comas which may lead to a specious diagnosis of structural brainstem damage. Certain anesthetic agents have a predilection for affecting the brainstem RAS neurons out of proportion to the cortex.

Although all metabolic derangements alter neuronal electrophysiology, the disturbance of brain electrical activity most commonly encountered in clinical practice is epilepsy. Continuous, generalized electrical discharges of the cortex may be associated with coma even in the absence of epileptic motor activity. Coma following seizures (postictal state) may be due to exhaustion of energy metabolites or be secondary to locally toxic molecules produced during the seizures. Recovery from postictal unresponsiveness occurs when neuronal metabolic balance is restored. The postictal state produces a pattern of continuous, generalized slowing of the background EEG activity similar to that of metabolic encephalopathy.

PRACTICAL APPROACH TO THE COMATOSE PATIENT　The diagnosis and acute management of coma depend on understanding the pitfalls of examining the comatose patient, an interpretation of

brainstem reflexes, and on the wise use of selected diagnostic tests. Respiratory and cardiovascular problems should be attended to prior to neurologic diagnosis. The general medical evaluation, except for the vital signs and examination for nuchal rigidity, should be deferred until the neurologic evaluation has established the severity and nature of coma.

History　In many cases the cause of coma is immediately evident (e.g., trauma, cardiac arrest, and known drug ingestion). However, in the remainder, historical information about the onset of coma is often sparse. The most useful historical points, when obtainable, are (1) the circumstances and temporal profile of the onset of neurologic symptoms, (2) the precise details of preceding neurologic symptoms (weakness, headaches, seizures, dizziness, diplopia, or vomiting), (3) the use of drugs or alcohol, (4) history of liver, kidney, lung, heart, or other medical disease. Telephone calls to family and observers on the scene are an important part of the initial evaluation of coma.

PHYSICAL EXAMINATION AND GENERAL OBSERVATIONS　The temperature, pulse, respiratory rate and pattern, and blood pressure should be measured. Fever suggests systemic infection, bacterial meningitis, or a brain lesion that has disturbed the temperature-regulating centers. High body temperature, 42 to 44°C, associated with dry skin should arouse the suspicion of heat stroke. Hypothermia is observed with bodily exposure; alcoholic, barbiturate, or phenothiazine intoxication; hypoglycemia; peripheral circulatory failure; or myxedema. Hypothermia causes coma directly only when the temperature is below 31°C. Aberrant respiratory patterns commonly reflect brainstem disorders and are discussed below. A change of pulse rate combined with hyperventilation and hypertension may signal an increase in intracranial pressure. Marked hypertension occurs in patients with hypertensive encephalopathy, cerebral hemorrhage, and, at times, in those with other causes of increased intracranial pressure. Hypotension may occur in the coma of alcohol or barbiturate intoxication, internal hemorrhage, myocardial infarction, gram-negative bacillary septicemia, and Addisonian crisis. The funduscopic examination is useful in detecting subarachnoid hemorrhage (subhyaloid hemorrhages), hypertensive encephalopathy (exudates, hemorrhages, vessel-crossing changes), and increased intracranial pressure (papilledema). Generalized cutaneous petechiae suggest thrombotic thrombocytopenic purpura or a bleeding diathesis causing intracerebral hemorrhage.

General neurologic assessment　An exact description of spontaneous and elicited movements in coma is of great value in establishing the level of neurologic dysfunction. The patient's state is observed first without examiner intervention. The nature of respirations, similarity to sleep, and spontaneous movements are observed. Patients who toss about, reach up toward the face, cross the midline with an arm, cross their legs, yawn, swallow, cough, or moan are closest to being awake. Adventitious movements or postures may be subtle and must be specifically sought. For example, the only sign of seizures may be small excursion twitching of a foot, finger, or facial muscle. An outturned leg at rest or lack of restless movements on one side suggests a hemiparesis.

The terms *decorticate* and *decerebrate rigidity* or ''posturing'' have been adapted from animal experiments to describe stereotyped tonic flexor and extensor arm movements, respectively, with extension of the legs. Spontaneous flexion of the elbows and wrists and arm supination (decortication) suggest severe bilateral damage in the hemispheres above the midbrain, while extension of the elbows and wrists with pronation (decerebration) suggests damage in the midbrain or diencephalon. Arm extension with weak leg flexion or flaccid legs has been associated with lesions in the low pons. Acute lesions, however, frequently cause limb extension regardless of location, and almost all extensor posturing becomes flexor in nature as time passes, so posturing alone cannot be depended upon to make an accurate anatomic localization. Metabolic coma, especially after acute hypoxia, may produce vigorous spontaneous extensor (decerebrate) rigidity. Posturing may alternate or coexist with purposeful limb movements, usually reflecting subtotal damage to the motor system. Multifocal myoclonus is almost always an indication of metabolic disorder, particularly azotemia, or drug ingestion. The later stages of Creutzfeldt-Jakob disease may also produce coma with myoclonus that is stimulus-sensitive. In an awake, confused patient, asterixis is a certain sign of metabolic encephalopathy.

Elicited movements and level of arousal A sequence of increasingly intense stimuli is used to determine the patient's best level of arousal and the optimal motor response of each limb. If the patient is not aroused by conversational voice, shouting should be tried. Shaking the patient is attempted next, then painful pressure on the limbs. Nasal tickle with a cotton wisp is a strong arousal stimulus. Deep pressure on the knuckles or bony prominences is the preferred and humane form of noxious stimulus. Pinching the skin over the face or chest may cause unsightly ecchymoses and is rarely necessary.

Responses to noxious stimuli should be appraised critically. Abduction avoidance of a limb is a purposeful, cortically derived movement and denotes an intact corticospinal system to that limb. If abduction is present in all limbs, it is a reliable sign of only minimal motor dysfunction. Stereotyped posturing following stimulation of a limb indicates severe dysfunction of the corticospinal system. Adduction and flexion of the stimulated limbs may occur as reflex movements and do not imply an intact corticospinal system. Brief oscillatory limb movements frequently occur at the end of elicited extensor posturing excursions and should not be mistaken for seizures.

Brainstem reflexes Brainstem signs are the key to the localization of the causative lesion in coma (Fig. 21-1). As a rule, coma associated with normal brainstem function indicates widespread and bilateral hemispheral disease. The brainstem contains several intrinsic reflexes that are convenient to examine. Normal pupillary symmetry, size, shape, and reaction to light indicate intact functioning of the midbrain and efferent parasympathetic fibers of the third cranial nerve responsible for pupillary constriction. The afferent component of the light reflex utilizes the optic nerve. Pupillary reaction should be examined with a bright diffuse light and, if absent, confirmed with a magnifying lens. Excessive room lighting mutes pupillary reactivity. Equal and reactive round pupils (2.5 to 5 mm in diameter) usually exclude midbrain damage as the cause of coma. An enlarged (greater than 5 mm) and unreactive or poorly reactive pupil can result either from an intrinsic midbrain lesion (on the same side) or, more commonly, be secondary to compression of the midbrain and/or third nerve as occurs in transtentorial herniation. Unilateral pupillary enlargement usually denotes an ipsilateral mass but rarely can occur contralaterally by compression of the cerebral peduncle of the midbrain against the opposite tentorial margin. Oval and slightly eccentric pupils (corectopia) often accompany early midbrain–third nerve compression. Bilaterally dilated and unreactive pupils indicate severe midbrain damage, usually from secondary compression by transtentorial herniation or metabolically by ingestion of drugs with anticholinergic activity. The unannounced use of mydriatic eye drops by a previous examiner or direct ocular trauma may cause misleading pupillary enlargement. Reactive and bilaterally small but not pinpoint pupils (1 to 2.5 mm) are most commonly seen in metabolic encephalopathy or after deep bilateral hemispheral lesions such as hydrocephalus or thalamic hemorrhage. This has been attributed to dysfunction of sympathetic nervous system efferents emerging from the posterior hypothalamus. Profound barbiturate-induced coma may produce similar-sized pupils. Very small but reactive pupils (less than 1 mm) denote narcotic overdose but may also occur with acute, extensive bilateral pontine damage. The response to naloxone and the presence of reflex eye movements (see below) distinguishes these. The unilaterally small pupil of a Horner's syndrome is rare in coma but may occur ipsilateral to a large cerebral hemorrhage.

Eye movements are the foundation of physical diagnosis in coma because their examination permits exploration of a large portion of the rostrocaudal extent of the brainstem. The eyes are first observed by elevating the lids and noting the resting position and spontaneous movements of the globes. Horizontal divergence of the eyes at rest is normally observed in drowsiness. As patients either awaken or slip deeper into coma, the ocular axes become parallel again. An adducted eye at rest indicates lateral rectus paresis (weakness) due to a sixth nerve lesion and may indicate damage to the pons. However, sixth nerve paresis, often bilateral, occurs with increased intracranial pressure and is not a localizing sign. An abducted eye at rest indicates medial rectus paresis due to third nerve paresis. With few exceptions, vertical separation of the ocular axes, or *skew deviation,* results from pontine or cerebellar lesions. In hydrocephalus with dilatation of the third ventricle, the eye globes frequently rest below the horizontal meridian.

When spontaneous eye movements are present in coma, they generally take the form of conjugate horizontal roving. This motion exonerates the midbrain and pons and has the same meaning as normal reflex eye movements (see below). Cyclic vertical downward movements are seen in specific circumstances. "Ocular bobbing" describes a brisk conjugate downward and slow upward movement of the globes in situations in which horizontal eye movement mechanisms have been disrupted and is diagnostic of bilateral pontine damage. "Ocular dipping" is a slow downward movement followed by a faster upward movement in patients with normal reflex horizontal gaze. Dipping occurs particularly in patients with diffuse anoxic damage to the cerebral cortex and may be preceded by sustained up or down gaze. The eyes may turn down and inward in thalamic and upper midbrain lesions. Conjugate ocular deviation at rest is discussed below.

Doll's-eye, or *oculocephalic,* movements are tested by moving the head from side to side or vertically, first slowly then briskly. Reflex eye movements are evoked in the opposite direction to head turning (Fig. 21-1). These responses are mediated by brainstem mechanisms originating in the labyrinths and vestibular nuclei and cervical proprioceptors. They are normally suppressed by visual fixation mediated by the cerebral hemispheres in awake patients. The neuronal pathways for reflex horizontal eye movements require integrity of the region surrounding the sixth nerve nucleus and are yoked to the contralateral third nerve via the medial longitudinal fasciculus (MLF) (Fig. 21-1). Two disparate pieces of information can be obtained from the reflex eye movements. *First,* in coma resulting from bihemispheral disease or early metabolic or drug depression, the eyes move easily or "loosely" from side to side in a direction opposite to the direction of head turning. The ease with which the globes move toward the opposite side is a reflection of disinhibition of brainstem reflexes by damaged cerebral hemispheres. In drowsy patients, the first two or three head rotations cause opposite conjugate eye movements following which the maneuver itself usually causes arousal and the reflex movements stop. *Second,* full conjugate oculocephalic movements require integrity of the brainstem pathways extending from the high cervical spinal cord and medulla, where vestibular and proprioceptive input from head turning originates, to the midbrain, where the third nerve originates, and the MLF running between these regions. Thus, the oculocephalic maneuver is a convenient way to demonstrate the functional integrity of a large segment of brainstem pathways and to exclude a lesion in the brainstem as the cause of coma. Faulty abduction of an eye suggests a sixth nerve lesion, due either to ipsilateral pontine damage or the distant effects of increased intracranial pressure. Lack of complete adduction indicates an ipsilateral midbrain (third nerve) lesion or, alternatively, damage to the pathways mediating reflex eye movements in the MLF (i.e., internuclear ophthalmoplegia). Third nerve damage is usually associated with an enlarged pupil and horizontal ocular divergence at rest, whereas MLF destruction shows neither. Adduction of the globes is by nature more difficult to obtain with head turning than abduction, and subtle symmetric abnormalities in the doll's-eye maneuver should be interpreted with caution.

Caloric stimulation of the vestibular apparatus (*oculovestibular* or *vestibuloocular response*) is a useful adjunct to the oculocephalic test and acts as a stronger stimulus to reflex eye movements. Irrigation of the external auditory canal with ice-cold water causes convection currents in the endolymph of the labyrinths of the inner ear. With the head placed at 30° elevation from the supine position, endolymph movement is induced primarily in the horizontal semicircular canals. An intact brainstem response is indicated by tonic deviation of both eyes (lasting 30 to 120 s) to the side of cold-water irrigation. Bilateral conjugate eye movements have the same significance as full oculocephalic responses. If the cerebral hemispheres are intact, a rapid corrective conjugate movement is generated away from the side of tonic deviation. The absence of this saccadic, nystagmus-like quick phase signifies damage to the opposite cerebral hemisphere.

Conjugate ocular deviation at rest or incomplete conjugate eye movements with head turning indicates damage in the pons on the side of the gaze paresis or frontal lobe damage on the opposite side. This phenomenon may be summarized by the phrase "the eyes look toward a hemispheral lesion and away from a brainstem lesion." It is usually possible to overcome the ocular deviation associated with frontal lobe damage by brisk head turning. Seizures may also cause aversive (opposite) eye deviation with rhythmic, jerky movements to the side of gaze. On rare occasions, the eyes may turn paradoxically away from the side of a deep hemispheral lesion ("wrong-way eyes").

A major pitfall in coma diagnosis may occur when reflex eye movements are suppressed by drugs. The eyes often move with the head as it is turned as if locked in place, thus spuriously suggesting anatomic brainstem damage. Overdoses of phenytoin, tricyclic antidepressants, and barbiturates are commonly implicated as well as, on occasion, alcohol, phenothiazines, diazepam, and neuromuscular blockers such as succinylcholine. The presence of normal pupillary size and light reaction will distinguish most drug-induced coma from brainstem damage (except for pontine infarction or hemorrhage in which the pupils remain small). Both absent oculocephalic responses and dilated, fixed pupils may occur with glutethimide intoxication. Small to midposition, nonreactive pupils may also occur with very high serum levels of barbiturates or secondary to hydrocephalus (see below).

Although the *corneal reflexes* are rarely useful alone, they may corroborate eye movement abnormalities because they also depend on the integrity of pontine pathways. By touching the cornea with a wisp of cotton, a response consisting of brief bilateral lid closure may be observed. The corneal response may be lost when the afferent fifth nerve, the efferent seventh nerve, or their reflex connections within the pons are damaged. The normal efferent response is bilateral, with closure of both eyelids. Nervous system depressant drugs diminish or eliminate the corneal responses soon after the reflex eye movements become paralyzed but before the pupils become unreactive to light.

Respiration Respiratory patterns have received much attention in coma diagnosis but are of inconsistent localizing value. Shallow, slow, but well-timed regular breathing suggests metabolic or drug depression. Rapid, deep (Kussmaul) breathing usually implies metabolic acidosis but may also occur with pontomesencephalic lesions. Cheyne-Stokes respiration in its classic cyclic form, ending with a brief apneic period, signifies mild bihemispheral damage or metabolic suppression and commonly accompanies light coma. Gasps, held in inspiration, reflect bilateral lower brainstem damage and are well known as the terminal respiratory pattern of severe brain damage. In brain-dead patients, shallow respiratory-like movements with irregular, nonrepetitive back arching may be stimulated by hypercapnia or hypoxia and are probably generated by the surviving cervical spinal cord and lower medulla. Other cyclic breathing variations are not usually diagnostic of specific local lesions.

COMA-LIKE SYNDROMES AND RELATED STATES The simple observation of inability to arouse a patient characterizes most comatose states. Several syndromes, however, appear to render patients unresponsive or insensate but are considered separately because of their unusual features. The *vegetative state* occurs in patients who were earlier comatose but whose eyes have subsequently opened giving

the appearance of being awake. There may be yawning, grunting, picking with the hands, and random limb and head movements. These are associated with signs of extensive damage to both cerebral hemispheres, i.e., Babinski signs, decerebrate or decorticate posturing, absence of response to visual stimuli, and absent corrective nystagmus on vestibuloocular testing. Autonomic nervous system functions such as cardiovascular and thermoregulatory and neuroendocrine control are preserved and may be subject to periods of overactivity. The syndrome is best viewed as a severe dementia resulting from global damage to the cerebral cortex and differs somewhat from akinetic mutism (described below) because of a complete inability to respond to commands or communicate. *Akinetic mutism,* or coma vigil, refers to the appearance of a partially or fully awake patient who is immobile and silent. The state may result from hydrocephalus or may occur with masses in the region of the third ventricle or with lesions in the cingulate gyrus or other portions of both frontal lobes. *Abulia* is a mild form of akinetic mutism in which the patient is hypokinetic and slow to respond but generally gives correct answers. Lesions in the periaqueductal or low diencephalic regions may cause a similar state in which hypophonia is prominent. The *locked-in syndrome* (pseudocoma) describes patients who are awake but selectively deefferented, i.e., have no means of producing speech or limb, face, or pharyngeal movements. This results from infarction or hemorrhage of the ventral pons which transects all descending corticospinal and corticobulbar pathways but spares the RAS arousal system. Vertical eye movements and blinking are generally normal because these midbrain functions are outside the field of infarction in basilar artery thrombosis. Such movements can be used by the patient to signal to the examiner. A similar awake state simulating unresponsiveness may occur in severe cases of acute polyneuritis or myasthenia gravis as a result of total paralysis of limb and bulbar musculature. Unlike basilar artery stroke, vertical eye movements are not selectively spared in these nerve and muscle diseases.

Certain psychiatric states mimic coma because they produce apparent unresponsiveness. *Catatonia* is a generic term for peculiar motor activities associated with major psychosis. In the typical hypomobile form catatonic patients appear awake with eyes open but make no voluntary or responsive movements, though they blink spontaneously and may not appear distressed. There may be associated "waxy flexibility" in which limbs maintain their posture when lifted by the examiner. Upon recovery, such patients have full memory of events that occurred during their catatonic stupor. Patients with *pseudocoma conversion* states (trance) have signs which indicate voluntary attempts to appear comatose. They may resist eyelid elevation, blink to threat when the lids are held open, and move the eyes concomitantly with head rotation, all signs belying brain damage.

LABORATORY EXAMINATION IN COMA Four laboratory tests are used most frequently in the diagnosis of coma: chemical-toxicologic analysis of blood and urine, CT or MRI, EEG, and cerebral spinal fluid (CSF) examination.

Chemical blood determinations are routinely made to investigate metabolic, toxic, or drug-induced encephalopathies. The major metabolic aberrations encountered in clinical practice are those of electrolytes, calcium, blood urea nitrogen (BUN), glucose, and hepatic dysfunction. Toxicologic analysis is of great value in any case of coma where the diagnosis is not immediately clear. However, the presence of exogenous drugs or toxins, especially alcohol, does not ensure that other factors, particularly head trauma, may not also contribute to the clinical state.

The notion that a normal CT scan excludes anatomic lesions as the cause of coma is erroneous. Early hemisphere infarction, small brainstem lesions, encephalitis, mechanical shearing of axons as a result of closed head trauma, absent cerebral perfusion associated with brain death, sagittal sinus thrombosis, and subdural hematomas which are isodense to adjacent brain are some of the lesions which may be overlooked by CT. Nevertheless, in coma of unknown etiology, a CT scan should be obtained early in the evaluation. In those cases in which the etiology is clinically apparent, the CT provides verification and defines the extent of the lesion.

The EEG is rarely diagnostic in coma, with the occasional exceptions of coma due to ongoing clinically unrecognized seizures, herpes virus encephalitis, and Creutzfeldt-Jakob disease. Examination of the EEG does, however, provide important information about the general electrophysiologic state of the cortex, and asymmetries may point to unilateral lesions not visualized on the CT scan. The amount of background slowing of the EEG is useful for gauging and following the severity of any diffuse encephalopathy. The EEG pattern of "alpha coma" deserves separate mention. It is defined by widespread, invariant 8- to 12-Hz activity superficially resembling the normal alpha rhythm of waking, but which is unresponsive to environmental stimuli. Alpha coma results from either high pontine or diffuse cortical damage and is associated with a poor prognosis. Coma due to persistent epileptic discharges that are not clinically manifested may be revealed by EEG recordings. Normal alpha activity on the EEG may also alert the clinician to the "locked-in" syndrome. Evoked potential recordings (auditory and somatosensory) are currently under investigation as additional methods of coma diagnosis and monitoring.

Lumbar puncture is now used more judiciously than previously because the CT scan excludes intracerebral hemorrhages and most subarachnoid hemorrhages. The use of lumbar puncture in coma is limited to diagnosis of meningitis-encephalitis, occasional cases of subarachnoid hemorrhage, and cases with normal CT in which the origin of coma is obscure. If the CT is normal or unavailable and suspicion of meningeal infection or subarachnoid hemorrhage remains, then the CSF should be examined for white cells, microorganisms, and blood. Xanthochromia is documented by spinning the CSF in a large tube and comparing the supernatant to water. Yellow coloration indicates preexisting blood in the CSF and permits exclusion of a traumatic puncture. In addition, initial and final tubes should be inspected for a decrement in the number of erythrocytes, indicating traumatic puncture.

DIFFERENTIAL DIAGNOSIS OF COMA

In most instances, coma is part of an obvious medical problem such as known drug ingestion, hypoxia, stroke, trauma, or liver or kidney failure. Attention is appropriately focused on the primary illness. A complete listing of all diseases which cause coma would serve little purpose since it would not aid diagnosis. Some general rules, however, are helpful. Illnesses which cause sudden or acute coma are due to drug ingestion or to one of the catastrophic brain lesions—hemorrhage, trauma, or hypoxia. Coma which appears subacutely is usually related to preceding medical or neurologic problems, including the secondary brain swelling which surrounds a preexisting lesion. Coma diagnosis, therefore, requires familiarity with the common intracerebral catastrophies. These are described in more detail in Chap. 343, but may be summarized as follows: (1) basal ganglia and thalamic hemorrhage (acute but not instantaneous onset, vomiting, headache, hemiplegia, and characteristic eye signs); (2) subarachnoid hemorrhage (instantaneous onset, severe headache, neck stiffness, vomiting, third or sixth nerve lesions, transient loss of consciousness, or sudden coma with vigorous extensor posturing); (3) pontine hemorrhage (sudden onset, pinpoint pupils, loss of reflex eye movements and corneal responses, ocular bobbing, posturing, hyperventilation, and sweating); (4) cerebellar hemorrhage (occipital headache, vomiting, gaze paresis, and inability to stand); (5) basilar artery thrombosis (neurologic prodrome or warning spells, diplopia, dysarthria, vomiting, eye movement and corneal response abnormalities, and asymmetric limb paresis). The commonest stroke, namely, infarction in the territory of the middle cerebral artery, does not cause coma acutely. The syndrome of acute hydrocephalus causing coma may accompany many intracranial catastrophes, including subarachnoid hemorrhage, or obstructive lesions of the cerebral aqueduct in the midbrain, due to cerebellar hemorrhage, tumors, or cysts. Acute symmetric enlargement of both lateral ventricles causes headache and vomiting. Further ventricular enlargement leads to drowsiness that may progress quickly to coma, with extensor posturing of the limbs, bilateral Babinski

signs, often small (1 mm diameter) nonreactive pupils, and impaired vertical oculocephalic movements.

If the history and examination are not typical for any neurologic diagnosis, and metabolic or drug causes are excluded, then information obtained from CT may be used as outlined in Table 21-1. The neurologic examination remains preeminent because it allows localization of lesions to one or both hemispheres or to the brainstem (with the exceptions noted above). The CT scan is useful to focus the differential diagnosis, and because of its accuracy and general availability, the diagnoses which it facilitates are listed in the table. The majority of medical causes of coma are established without a CT or with the study being normal.

COMA AFTER HEAD TRAUMA Concussion is a common form of transient coma which probably results from torsion of the hemispheres about the midbrain-diencephalic junction with brief interruption of RAS function. Persistent coma after head trauma presents a more complex and serious problem. (Chap. 344).

EMERGENCY TREATMENT OF THE COMATOSE PATIENT The immediate goal in acute coma is prevention of further nervous system damage. Hypotension, hypoglycemia, hypoxia, hypercapnia, and hyperthermia should be rapidly and assiduously corrected. An oro-

---

TABLE 21-1 Approach to the differential diagnosis of coma

I Normal brainstem reflexes, no lateralizing signs
  A Anatomic lesions of hemisphere found
    1 Hydrocephalus
    2 Bilateral subdural hematomas
    3 Bilateral contusions, edema, or axonal shearing of hemispheres due to closed head trauma, subarachnoid hemorrhage
  B Bilateral hemispheral dysfunction without mass lesion (CT normal)
    1 Drug-toxin ingestion (toxicologic analysis)
    2 Endogenous metabolic encephalopathy (glucose, ammonia, calcium, osmolarity, P_{O_2}, P_{CO_2}, urea, sodium)
    3 Shock, hypertensive encephalopathy
    4 Meningitis (CSF analysis)
    5 Nonherpetic viral encephalitis (CSF analysis)
    6 Epilepsy (EEG)
    7 Reye's syndrome (ammonia, increased intracranial pressure)
    8 Fat embolism
    9 Subarachnoid hemorrhage with normal CT (CSF analysis)
    10 Acute disseminated encephalomyelitis (CSF analysis)
    11 Acute hemorrhagic leukoencephalitis
    12 Advanced Alzheimer's and Creutzfeldt-Jakob disease
II Normal brainstem reflexes (with or without unilateral compressive third nerve palsy), lateralizing motor signs (CT abnormal)
  A Unilateral mass lesion found
    1 Cerebral hemorrhage (basal ganglia, thalamus)
    2 Large infarction with surrounding brain edema
    3 Herpes virus encephalitis (temporal lobe lesion)
    4 Subdural or epidural hematoma
    5 Tumor with edema
    6 Brain abscess with edema
    7 Vasculitis with multiple infarctions
    8 Metabolic encephalopathy superimposed on preexisting focal lesions (i.e., stroke)
    9 Pituitary apoplexy
  B Asymmetric signs accompanied by diffuse hemispheral dysfunction
    1 Metabolic encephalopathies with asymmetric signs (blood chemical determinations)
    2 Isodense subdural hematoma (brain scan, angiogram)
    3 Thrombotic thrombocytopenic purpura (blood smear, platelet count)
    4 Epilepsy with focal seizures or postictal state (EEG)
III Multiple brainstem reflex abnormalities
  A Anatomic lesions in brainstem found
    1 Pontine, midbrain hemorrhage
    2 Cerebellar hemorrhage, tumor, abscess
    3 Cerebellar infarction with brainstem compression
    4 Mass in hemisphere causing advanced bilateral brainstem compression
    5 Brainstem tumor or demyelination
    6 Traumatic brainstem contusion-hemorrhage (clinical signs, auditory-evoked potentials)
  B Brainstem dysfunction without mass lesion
    1 Basilar artery thrombosis causing brainstem stroke (clinical signs, angiogram)
    2 Severe drug overdose (toxicologic analysis)
    3 Brainstem encephalitis
    4 Basilar artery migraine
    5 Brain death

pharyngeal airway is adequate to keep the pharynx open in drowsy patients who are breathing normally. Tracheal intubation is indicated if there is obvious apnea, hypoventilation, or emesis, or if the patient is liable to aspirate. Mechanical ventilation is required if the patient is apneic or hypoventilating or if there is an intracranial mass and hypocapnia is therapeutically necessary. An intravenous access is established and naloxone and dextrose administered if narcotic overdose or hypoglycemia are even remote possibilities. Thiamine is generally administered with glucose in order to prevent an exacerbation of Wernicke's encephalopathy. The veins of intravenous drug abusers may be difficult to cannulate; in such cases, naloxone can be injected sublingually through a small-gauge needle. In cases of suspected basilar thrombosis with brainstem ischemia, intravenous heparin is administered after obtaining a CT scan, keeping in mind that cerebellar and pontine hemorrhages bear some resemblance to the syndrome of basilar occlusion. Physostigmine, when used by experienced physicians with careful monitoring, may awaken patients with anticholinergic-type drug overdose, but many physicians believe that this is justified only if cardiac arrhythmias are a problem. Intravenous fluid administration should be carefully monitored in any serious acute nervous system illness because of the potential for exacerbating brain swelling. Neck injuries must not be overlooked, particularly prior to attempting the oculocephalic maneuver. Headache accompanied by fever and meningismus indicate need for examination of the CSF to diagnose meningitis, and *lumbar puncture should not be delayed while awaiting a CT scan.*

Enlargement of one pupil usually indicates secondary midbrain compression by a hemispheral mass and demands immediate reduction of intracranial pressure. Intravenous fluids are slowed to the minimum necessary to support blood pressure. Therapeutic hyperventilation is then used to achieve an arterial P_{CO_2} of 28 to 32 mmHg. This acts rapidly to reduce intracranial pressure, but the beneficial effect rarely lasts more than 2 h. Hyperosmolar therapy with mannitol may be used simultaneously with hyperventilation in critical cases, but its effects are not apparent for several minutes. It is generally best to administer mannitol before attempting to intubate a patient with suspected, impending herniation. A ventricular puncture may be necessary to decompress the intracranial compartment by removing CSF if medical measures fail. Virtually all patients who survive to arrive in an emergency room can be protected from further brain damage by these means until definitive therapy is possible. The use of high-dose barbiturates soon after cardiac arrest has not been shown in clinical studies to be beneficial, although they may still be useful in lowering intracranial pressure acutely under special circumstances.

BRAIN DEATH   Brain death results from total cessation of cerebral blood flow and global infarction of the brain at a time when cardiovascular and respiratory functions remain preserved, the latter requiring artificial support. It is the only type of irrevocable loss of brain function recognized by law as death. Many sets of roughly equivalent criteria have been advanced for the diagnosis of brain death, and it is essential to adhere to those approved locally and recognized as standard practice. Ideal criteria are ones that are simple and conducted at the bedside and which allow no chance of diagnostic error. Widespread cortical destruction is usually shown by an isoelectric EEG and unresponsiveness to the environment, midbrain damage by absent pupillary light reaction, pontine damage by absent oculovestibular and corneal reflexes, and medullary dysfunction by apnea. Some period of observation, usually 6 to 24 h, is desirable during which this state is shown to be sustained. The pupils need not be fully dilated but should not be constricted. The absence of spinal reflexes is not required since the spinal cord remains functional in many cases. The possibility of profound drug-induced or hypothermic nervous system depression should always be excluded.

The demonstration of apnea generally requires that the P_{CO_2} be high enough to stimulate respiration. This can be safely accomplished in most patients by removing the respirator and using diffusion oxygenation sustained by a tracheal cannula connected to an oxygen supply. In brain-dead patients, CO_2 tension increases approximately 2 mmHg/min during apnea. At the end of an appropriate interval, arterial P_{CO_2} should be at least above 50 mmHg (higher limits have been suggested) for the test to be valid. Large posterior fossa lesions that compress the brainstem, nervous system–depressant drugs, and profound hypothermia can simulate brain death, but adherence to recognized protocols for diagnosis will prevent these errors. Radionuclide brain scanning or cerebral angiography may be used to demonstrate the absence of cerebral blood flow in brain death. These techniques have the virtue of rapidity but are often cumbersome and expensive and have not been extensively correlated with pathologic material.

There is no implicit pressure to make the diagnosis of brain death except when organ transplantation or difficult resource allocation (intensive care) issues are involved. Although it is eminently reasonable to disconnect the respirator from a brain-dead patient after proper explanations to the family, there is no obligation to do so and some physicians prefer to await the inevitable cardiovascular failure that follows brain death if full medical support is omitted, usually within a week.

PROGNOSIS OF COMA   Interest in predicting the outcome of coma is oriented toward allocating medical resources and limiting the support of hopeless cases. To date, no collection of clinical signs except those of brain death assuredly predicts coma outcome. Children and young adults may have ominous, early clinical findings such as abnormal brainstem reflexes and yet recover. All schemes for prognosis should, therefore, be taken as only approximate indicators, and medical judgments must be conservatively tempered by other factors such as age, underlying disease, general medical condition, and the previously expressed wishes of the patient. In an attempt to collect prognostic information from large numbers of patients with head injury, a "coma scale" scoring system has been devised which empirically has predictive value in cases of brain trauma (see Chap. 344). Major points include a 95 percent death rate in patients whose pupillary reaction or reflex eye movements were absent 6 h after onset of coma, and a 91 percent death rate if the pupils were unreactive at 24 h (though 4 percent made a good recovery).

Prognostication of nontraumatic coma is more difficult because of the heterogeneity of contributing diseases. Unfavorable signs in the first hours after admission have been reported to be the absence of any two of pupillary reaction, corneal reflex, or the oculovestibular response. One day after the onset of coma, the above signs, in addition to absence of eye opening and muscle tone, predicted death or severe disability and the same signs at 3 days strengthened the prediction of a poor outcome. In many patients precise combinations of predictive signs do not occur and coma scales lose their value. The use of evoked potentials has recently been shown to aid prognostication in head-injured and postcardiac arrest patients. Bilateral absence of cortical somatosensory evoked potentials is associated with death or a vegetative state in most cases. It may be wisest to fully support all but those patients whose extreme signs convincingly suggest a poor outcome. Medical practitioners are becoming less reluctant to withdraw support from brain-dead patients as predictions become more reliable and resources more limited.

REFERENCES

FINKLESTEIN S, ROPPER A: The diagnosis of coma: Its pitfalls and limitations. Heart Lung 8:1059, 1979

FISHER CM: The neurological examination of the comatose patient. Acta Neurol Scand 45 (Suppl 6):1, 1969

IVAN L, BRUCE D: *Coma.* Springfield, Ill, Charles C Thomas, 1982

JENNET B et al: Prognosis of patients with severe head injury. Neurosurgery 4:283, 1979

LEVY D et al: Prognosis in non-traumatic coma. Ann Intern Med 94:229, 1981

PLUM F, POSNER J: *The Diagnosis of Stupor and Coma,* 3d ed. Philadelphia, Davis, 1980

ROPPER AH: Coma and acutely raised intracranial pressure, in *Diseases of the Nervous System,* A Asbury, G McKhann, I McDonald (eds). Philadelphia, Saunders, 1986

22 DISORDERS OF SPEECH AND LANGUAGE

JAY P. MOHR / RAYMOND D. ADAMS

Language and speech are fundamental both to social intercourse and to intellectual life. When disordered as a consequence of disease of the brain, the loss exceeds blindness, deafness, or paralysis in gravity.

The terms *speech* and *language* refer to complex and poorly understood activities of the cerebrum. The terms are not synonymous.

Speech involves the execution of acquired skills of the vocal, manual, auditory, and visual systems in communication. These skills include pronunciation of words; variations in stress, intonation, and melody; the production of graphic marks in the accepted spatial orientation; the auditory discrimination of spoken speech and its classification as to speaker; the visual discrimination of handwritten or printed speech; the visual search patterns involved in scanning a text; and the use of other, less specifiable behaviors. Deficiencies in these skills impede communication apart from any separate impairment in language usage; when intact, these skills suffice only for elemental communication, such as that between two individuals who speak languages unfamiliar to each other.

Language has a wider connotation and refers to the selection and serial ordering of individual words according to rules that permit a person using the speech modalities to modify the behavior of another and to express that poorly understood cerebral activity termed *thinking*. A disturbance of language usage, usually accompanied by a disturbance in speech from cerebral dysfunction, is referred to as *aphasia*, or more properly as *dysphasia*.

CEREBRAL DOMINANCE AND ITS RELATIONSHIP TO SPEECH AND HANDEDNESS

The dominant side is inferred from which eye, hand, or foot is chosen preferentially for intricate, complex acts. Such preference is more complete in some persons than in others. The reason for preference of a hand, foot, or eye depends on hereditary and anatomic factors and is partly acquired. Over 90 percent of people are right-handed. Left-handedness may be hereditary or may result from disease of the left cerebral hemisphere in early life. Handedness and cerebral dominance may fail to develop in some individuals and in certain families.

Anatomic differences exist between the dominant and the minor cerebral hemispheres. The planum temporale, a part of Wernicke's language zone, is larger in the left hemisphere in right-handed individuals. Many children are shifted at an early age from left to right (shifted sinistrals) because it is a handicap to be left-handed in a right-handed world. A disturbance in language is produced in almost all right-handers by unilateral brain damage that affects the left hemisphere. Lesions in the left cerebral hemisphere also account for most language disturbances in left-handed individuals, implying that cerebral dominance can differ for different functions.

LANGUAGE DISORDERS IN MEDICAL PRACTICE

Language disorders may be divided into four categories:

1 *Aphasia* is defined as a state in which there is a loss more or less exclusively of the production and/or comprehension of speech and language from an acquired cerebral lesion. The more limited term, dysphasia, is commonly used.
2 *Dysarthria* is a defect in articulation. These defects are pure motor disorders of the muscles of articulation in the presence of intact mental functions and may be due to flaccid or spastic paralysis, rigidity, repetitive spasms (stuttering), or ataxia.
3 *Aphonia or dysphonia* is the loss of voice due to a disease of the larynx or its innervation.
4 *Disturbances of language* occur with diseases that produce delirium and dementia (see Chap. 23). Speech is seldom lost, and language is deranged as part of a general impairment of cerebral functions.

APHASIA OR DYSPHASIA As a general orientation, most lesions that lead to aphasia occur in the perisylvian regions (frontal, temporal, and parietal) of the dominant cerebral hemisphere, i.e., the left side in right-handed individuals. The anatomic site of the lesion can usually be characterized by computerized tomography (CT scan) or magnetic resonance imaging (MRI).

Diseases of the cerebral surface gray matter produce a more significant deficit than those confined to the white matter: tumors, located largely in the white matter, usually reach a large size before causing a speech or language deficit. Infarcts or traumatic lesions of one or more centimeters in diameter are usually associated with an evanescent deficit that fades to functional insignificance within weeks or months.

Deficits due to acute lesions are most easily demonstrated in the acute phase. Improvements over weeks to months occur in all but the largest vascular lesions, but those due to tumors show progression. The site is more significant than the size of the lesion: the former determines the qualitative features of the deficit, while size determines the severity of the syndrome. Furthermore, deficits in speech function predominate in smaller lesions, while major disturbances in language are superimposed on the speech disturbance in the larger lesions.

Anteriorly placed sylvian lesions mainly disturb the acts of speaking, ranging from mutism, through impaired articulation, to disordered transitions from syllable to syllable, to abnormalities in phrasing, intonation, and melody. Lesions more posterior produce malpositioning of the tongue, lips, and other structures in the oropharynx with errors from some anticipatory syllables occurring out of sequence. Lesions grouped around the posterior sylvian fissure including the superior temporal lobe and its auditory gyri are manifested by disordered understanding of spoken words, resulting in poor repetition of speech sounds.

The language deficits that are superimposed on the speech disturbances are less well correlated with anatomic pathology. Language disturbances can be separated by pathoanatomic considerations into two large groups. Large anterior lesions involving the bulk of the frontal operculum (that region which lies above the insula) and the insula itself result in agrammatism, featuring sharply contracted sentence structure, absence of most small words, and a preservation of words serving mainly a predicative, interjectional, or substantive function. The patient may only be able to say "hi," "no," "hello" or to use simple nouns, i.e., ball, top, key. Large posterior sylvian lesions show almost the opposite, with simple speech elements missing or replaced by substitutions in which the desired response is only approximated (*paraphasias*). These latter may consist of faulty pronunciations (*literal paraphasias*) or faulty word selections (*verbal paraphasias*). Verbal paraphasias may approximate the desired word with a similarity of sound or of spelling (*formal verbal paraphasias*), such as "stock" for "stop" or by similarity of meaning (*semantic verbal paraphasias*) such as "slow" for "stop." Disturbances in understanding language, both auditory and visual speech, occur in both types of major paraphasias.

Lesions well away from the sylvian region either cause no disturbance of human communicative skills or alter them only secondarily. An example of the latter is the lesion of the anterior frontal lobes, especially the medial and orbital parts, that impairs all motor activities and often results in lack of attention and responsiveness (abulia), verging on the akinetic mute state (see Chap. 21). The speech is laconic with long pauses between utterances, and there is an inability to sustain monologue and narrative. Extensive occipital lesions impair reading and reduce the utilization of all visual, lexical stimuli. Thalamic and deep cerebral lesions impair alertness and cause fluctuating states or inattention and disorientation, thereby inducing fragmentation of words (neologisms) and phrases, and protracted uncontrollable talking (logorrhea). Strong stimulation to increase momentarily the level of awareness and altertness will show that such patients have intact language mechanisms.

The nondominant hemisphere provides the substratum for several types of behavior: motor responses of mimicry, social anticipation (smiling, handshaking, modesty reactions), and self-care (washing and feeding); avoidance behavior to noxious stimuli; and the capability of cross matching visually when presented simple words with pictures. It follows that tests which elicit these behaviors are no guide to functions of the hemisphere dominant for language.

Lesions of the frontal (motor) regions are generally believed to produce syndromes independent from those of the posterior (sensory) regions; the dysphasias can be classified as motor (Broca's) or sensory (Wernicke's) and can be further specified as subcortical, cortical, or transcortical in location. Subcortical lesions are believed to cut off the main efferent or afferent projections of the cortical "center"; cortical lesions involve the centers themselves; transcortical lesions isolate the centers from one another, i.e., a kind of "conduction" aphasia, or from other regions of the brain related to speech. These basic concepts provide a useful framework for the classification of the aphasias but are inadequate as guides to the lesions site and size.

TYPES OF APHASIA   Disturbances of speech and language can result from several abnormalities. Classifications have been based upon the predominant form, the presumed physiologic or psychological bases, and the anatomy of the underlying diseases. The classification utilized here has been formulated on the basis of the anatomic

localization and the clinical presentation (see Table 22-1). The prognoses are helpful in management, particularly in the choice of corrective measures in therapy. Aphasias may also be classified according to the severity of impediment to speech production and flow. *Fluent aphasias* are characterized by runs of well-articulated speech, of basically normal rhythm and flow, although lacking in language meaning. The defect is usually a lesion in the dominant parietal or temporal lobe. *Nonfluent aphasias* are characterized by slow, incorrectly articulated words and sentences. The lesion usually lies in the dominant frontal lobe.

Complete (global) aphasia   In complete, or global, aphasia the causative lesion destroys a large part of the speech and language areas of the major cerebral hemisphere, producing the maximal aphasic deficit and has the least chance of improvement of any aphasic syndrome. Infarction from occlusion of the left internal or the middle cerebral artery at its origin, or a large hemorrhage, major tumor, or trauma is most often responsible. In the rare instances of rapid improvement, the main cause is transitory ischemia from a fragmenting embolus, posttraumatic edema, or postconvulsive paralysis; rarely, hyperthermia, infection, or hyponatremia may transiently cause a temporary relapse of aphasia due to an old lesion.

Most patients with total aphasia say at most a few words; they do not read or write, and they understand only a few words and phrases of the speech of others. Related signs include right hemiplegia, hemianesthesia, and homonymous hemianopsia. The state of consciousness may vary from full alertness to semicoma. The alert patient

TABLE 22-1   Classification of aphasic disorders

	Anatomic location	Clinical manifestations	Etiology	Associated clinical symptoms
MAJOR SYNDROMES				
Global aphasia	Large lesion of dominant frontal, parietal, and superior temporal lobe	Minimal speech; nonfluent aphasia; comprehension poor for spoken and written language	Infarction in distribution of internal carotid or middle cerebral artery; trauma; tumor	Contralateral hemiplegia; hemisensory loss; hemianopsia
Broca's aphasia	Cortical and subcortical lesion of prefrontal and frontal regions	Nonfluent aphasia; agrammatic sentences; poor articulation; dysprosody; may be mute	Infarction in distribution of superior frontal branch middle cerebral artery; hemorrhage; tumor	Contralateral hemiparesis; minor or no sensory loss; no visual field disturbance; oral dyspraxia; cortical dysarthria; severe impairment in writing
Wernicke's aphasia (central or sensory aphasia)	Posterior perisylvian structures of the parietal and temporal lobe	Fluent speech; total incomprehension of spoken speech; inability to read or to repeat sounds or words; alexia, agraphia, paraphasia common	Infarction; distribution of lower division of middle cerebral artery; tumor; herpes simplex encephalitis	Parietal lobe sensory deficits; hemianopsia; no motor disturbance
MINOR CENTRAL APHASIA SYNDROMES				
Conduction aphasia	Upper bank of sylvian fissure; inferior parietal lobule	Paraphasia; difficulty in repetition of speech and in reading aloud; aware of deficit; adequate comprehension of written and spoken words	Embolic occlusion of posterior branches of middle cerebral artery	Contralateral hemihypesthesia or homonymous hemianopsia; abnormal optokinetic nystagmus
Mainly auditory (pure word deafness)	Lesion in superior temporal gyrus	Impaired auditory comprehension; inability to repeat a sentence or write a dictation	Infarction; tumor; abscess	Rare deafness
Mainly visual (dyslexia with dysgraphia)	Parietooccipital lesion	Visual language compromised more than auditory; cannot read or write	Infarction; tumor, lobar hemorrhage	Hemianopsia
OTHER SYNDROMES				
Pure word blindness	Left occipito-striate cortex, adjacent association cortex, and posterior corpus callosum (splenium)	Normal spoken language and writing, with inability to read	Infarction in distribution of posterior cerebral artery; tumor, lobar hemorrhage	Hemianopsia
Isolation of speech areas	Ischemic infarction in border (watershed) zones between anterior, middle and posterior cerebral artery distributions	Parrot-like speech; echolalia	Systemic hypotension or hypoxia; cardiac arrest	Decreased alertness and responsiveness; bilateral leg weakness
Amnesic-dysnomic aphasia	Deep temporal lobe lesions, parahippocampal, hippocampal gyrus	Inability to recall names of objects or parts of objects; difficulty with recent memory	Tumor; Alzheimer's disease; infarct; distribution posterior cerebral artery; herpes simplex encephalitis	Apraxia; dementia; no motor or sensory abnormalities; upper quadrantic visual field defect

may participate in common gestures of greeting, may show modesty and avoidance reactions, and is able to engage in self-help activities. The early appearance of clearly vocalized stereotyped words, such as "hi" and "yes," are often falsely encouraging signs; they may reflect the uninhibited function of the right hemisphere. With the passage of time some degree of understanding of spoken speech may be evident, and a few spoken words may emerge.

Broca's aphasia (major motor aphasia) This term is used to designate a complex syndrome, which features failure of motor aspects of speaking and writing, accompanied by agrammatism with a less obvious impairment in language comprehension. Although formerly thought to be due to a circumscribed lesion in the inferior frontal convolution (Broca's area), the syndrome is the result of a much larger lesion involving cortical and subcortical structures along the frontal and superior sylvian fissure and the insula. This·region may not be well visualized by CT scan since the tissue defect may seem to merge with the sylvian fissure.

The syndrome is most often due to embolic occlusions of the upper division of the left middle cerebral artery; major putaminal hypertensive hemorrhage, huge frontal lobe tumor or abscess, metastatic lesions, subdural hematoma, and encephalitis are less common causes.

The lesions are smaller than those causing complete aphasia and usually involve the sensorimotor rolandic region, producing an accompanying persisting hemiparesis and hemisensory syndrome. Initially, a transient ipsilateral deviation of the eyes is observed, due to the frontal infarction.

In the acute phase, the entire language mechanism appears to be inactivated, and the helplessly mute, noncommunicative, and uncomprehending patient presents the syndrome of complete or global aphasia, indistinguishable by present methods from that resulting from infarction of the whole left middle cerebral artery territory. Within weeks to years, the disorder of comprehension abates somewhat but remains detected by formal testing. The improvement in comprehension exceeds that in speaking and writing, leaving a syndrome that conforms to the traditional motor aphasia.

For a time, despite a satisfactory comprehension of spoken words and the ability to read simple commands, an apraxia of the lingual and oropharyngeal apparatus retards efforts to make purposeful or commanding movements. Imitation of the examiner's actions may be better performed than execution of acts on command, and self-initiated actions are often, but not always, normal. Certain stereotyped and simple phrases or curses are uttered more easily, such as "hi," "good morning," "how are you," and the words of popular songs may be sung surprisingly well. The patient's efforts to speak and facial expressions suggest an awareness of his or her own ineptitudes and mistakes, and an accompanying exasperation and despair are common.

As improvement occurs, particularly in the milder forms of motor aphasia, the patient is able to speak aloud to some degree. Words are enunciated slowly and laboriously. Articulation and the melody of speech (prosody) are impaired. This dysfluency takes the form of improper accent on stress on certain syllables, incorrect phrasing of words in a series and pacing of the speed of word sequences, and even a stammering quality to the uttered phrases. Speech is sparse and consists mainly of nouns, transitive verbs, and important adjectives; many of the small words (articles, prepositions, conjunctions) are omitted, giving the speech an *agrammatic* and telegraphic character. The preservation of substantive words allows the patients to communicate despite the gross mechanical and language difficulties. Once fully established, these speech impediments persist and improve only slightly despite years of therapy.

Most patients with Broca's aphasia have a correspondingly severe impairment in writing. Should their right hand be paralyzed, they cannot print with their left one; if manual mobility is spared, they fail as completely in writing out their commands or replies to questions as in speaking them. Writing from dictation is severely impaired, though letters and words can still be copied. On careful testing,

however, communication by writing is superior to that of speaking, suggesting a certain independence between these two acts as vehicles of language.

Minor motor aphasia More circumscribed focal lesions along the anterior and superior sylvian operculum and insula produce remarkably discrete effects on the mechanical elaboration of speech. The important point with minor motor aphasias is that they at first may resemble major motor aphasia except for the satisfactory understanding of spoken and written words. The prognosis for nearly full recovery is excellent. Indeed, *none of these focal lesions produces significant or lasting deficits in language usage.* However, in the acute phase the experienced listener can easily detect the error patterns in speech and, through them, discern the nature of the communicative difficulties of the sufferer, who is acutely aware of and discouraged by the deficit.

The effects of speech or focal lesions take several forms. *Broca's area infarction* involves the lower premotor cortex adjacent to the motor cortex for the oropharynx, larynx, and respiratory apparatus; the infarct interrupts skilled movements of these muscle groups, and the resultant dyspraxia in speech takes the form of impaired transitions between syllables and words and disruption of the melodic intonation of phrases (dysprosody). Involvement of this region alone is insufficient to produce the major syndrome referred to as Broca's aphasia. *Rolandic infarction* involves the sensorimotor cortex itself; either the syndrome of dysprosody occurs or speech has poor articulation and lowered volume and pitch, while a nasal quality to the voice reveals the paresis of the nasopharyngeal musculature. *Postcentral, anterior parietal infarction* is associated with errors in the positioning of the oral cavity for individual sounds, syllables, and whole words; the acoustic features of the utterance are often distorted by these malpositions of the oral cavity and strike the ear as literal paraphasias. Since they are easily produced in tests of repeating, reading aloud, and occur in conversation, the patient could be mislabeled as having "conduction" aphasia.

Lesions in the lateral parts of the dominant frontal lobe, sparing Broca's area may also cause an aphasic disorder. Usually speech output is reduced and nonfluent, and auditory comprehension is intact. Repetition of words spoken by the examiner is preserved. This condition has been called *transcortical motor aphasia*. It must be distinguished from a closely related condition in which spontaneous speech is lacking (mutism) and all motor activity is reduced (akinesia). What is lacking is the impulse to speak or to move. The causative lesions are more widespread—in the medial part of the frontal lobe, the supplementary motor area, and the cingulate gyrus.

Most such focal lesions are due to emboli to the sequential branches of the upper division of the middle cerebral artery. Deeper, larger lesions or larger emboli involving the stem of the upper division can cause several types of deficit in a single patient, making these individual distinctions less clear and blending with the major syndrome of Broca's aphasia. Facial, lingual, and sometimes brachial paresis and ideomotor dyspraxia of the face and left, nondominant limbs commonly accompany the speech disorder. Most of these syndromes recede within weeks or months.

Wernicke's aphasia (major central or sensory aphasia) This term encompasses a range of syndromes that arise from lesions of the posterior perisylvian structures or the posterior temporal, parietal, and occipital regions supplied by the lower division of the middle cerebral artery. There is disruption of the whole array of language behavior. When restricted to the temporal lobe, the main disturbance is most evident in language tasks involving words heard; and when more parietal and occipital, in words seen.

Spoken and written efforts in communication as well as in auditory and visual comprehension are affected, a combination that justifies the term *central aphasia*. The term *sensory aphasia* was formerly used to accentuate the contrast with motor (Broca's) aphasia. Instead of the difficult articulation, faulty transitions, dysmelodic speaking, and disproportionate condensation of grammatical forms that characterize Broca's aphasia, the speech of Wernicke's aphasia is fluent, hence the name *fluent aphasia*.

In severe cases, the patients utters a series of incomprehensible syllables, makes illegible marks on a page in attempts at writing, cannot be made to repeat aloud or copy correctly at sight, and treats the examiner's attempts at written and verbal communication as if they were in a wholly unfamiliar foreign language. In less severe cases, the patient can repeat aloud and copy but echoes the words heard with faulty pronunciation or copies the words in a slavish manner, imitating even the examiner's handwriting style, as though the test words were unfamiliar. The disturbance in language does not simply reflect a disturbance in hearing or in vision. In the mildest cases, the deficits are manifested in errors in word comprehension and usage. The patient may choose words that show approximation to the desired response, the words often belonging to the same functional class [i.e., *cow* for *pig*, but not *cow* for *yellow* (such errors are labeled *semantic verbal paraphasias*)]; or they may be similar in sound or shape (*formal verbal paraphasias*) such as "flee" for "tree"; there may be errors in word structure, with improper tenses, prefixes, suffixes (i.e., *beautifuling*); or other errors that resemble those of normal people unfamiliar with the language in question. Some such patients pass for normal in brief or casual conversation. In its milder form or later in the course of the illness, the speech resembles that of a person tired or distracted, and the abnormality is detected only on tests of complex language function.

CT scanning and MRI are the best methods to delineate the topography of the lesion. Arteriographic findings are an unreliable basis of correlation because the vascular occlusions, most often due to cerebral embolism, frequently fail to show the embolus because it has disintegrated or drifted distally into one or more smaller branches. Radionuclide brain scanning is useful only for the largest lesions.

Minor central aphasia syndromes In time, Wernicke's aphasia improves, and a number of lesser syndromes appear. These latter, however, may be present in comparatively pure form from the beginning, when only a small, restricted lesion involves some part of the territory of the lower division of the middle cerebral artery.

The posterior sylvian region, comprising posterosuperior temporal, opercular, supramarginal, and posterior insular gyri, appears to encompass a variety of language functions. Seemingly minor changes in size and locale of the lesion are associated with important variations in the elements of Wernicke's aphasia. Depending on the location of the lesion, language behavior dependent on auditory function (hearing spoken words, echoing sounds and speech, relating the spoken to the written word, and finally repeating and writing it) may be deranged partially or completely. The same is true of language behavior dependent upon visual function, when the left posterior parietal lobe is involved. These partial syndromes are termed conduction aphasia, pure word deafness, dyslexia with dysgraphia, and pure word blindness.

CONDUCTION APHASIA: SEPARATION OF WERNICKE'S AND BROCA'S LANGUAGE AREAS The principal abnormality resembles Wernicke's aphasia. There is the same degree of paraphasia in self-initiated speech, in repeating what is heard, and in reading aloud. However, little or no difficulty is encountered in comprehending words that are heard or seen. Because the motor regions are unaffected, no element of dysarthria or dysprosody occurs. The patient is alert and unaware of the deficit. The mistakes take the form of literal paraphasia; i.e., errors in oropharyngeal positioning produce detectably different sounds from those intended. The disorder in repeating from dictation becomes more apparent when the rate of presentation of auditory material is increased, the uttered words are polysyllabic, or when words are unfamiliar, e.g., sets of nonsense syllables. Since nouns are usually the longest words in sentences, one may gain an impression that they are specifically affected.

The lesion at autopsy is located in the cortex and subcortical white matter in the upper bank of the sylvian fissure, involving the supramarginal gyrus of the inferior parietal lobule. The posterior part

of the superior temporal region is occasionally affected. The usual cause is an embolus in the ascending parietal or posterior temporal branch of the middle cerebral artery. Deeper, larger lesions that interrupt the arcuate fasciculus connecting the temporal and frontal lobes may produce the syndrome, but usually they involve other pathways as well, giving rise to a more extensive speech deficit (Wernicke's aphasia or amnesic aphasia). However, these latter types of aphasia, as they regress, may resolve into conduction aphasia. More anterior insular lesions usually include some degree of Broca's aphasia.

PURE WORD DEAFNESS Instead of a disturbance confined to auditory comprehension, this more inclusive syndrome is the auditory form of Wernicke's aphasia. The most obvious findings are an impaired auditory comprehension and inability to repeat what is said or to write to dictation. Spoken language is less impaired but rarely normal, and occasionally the patient is initially diagnosed as having Wernicke's aphasia. By audiometric testing no hearing defect is found, or minor abnormalities appear that reveal the underlying deficit in individual cases. Ordinary sounds can be distinguished. The patient is forced to depend heavily on visual cues in understanding the remarks of others and frequently uses these cues well enough to obviate much of the difficulty. Tests that prevent the use of visual cues readily uncover the deficit. Comprehension of visually presented material such as printed matter, although not normal, is better than auditory comprehension. There may be full preservation of reading skill, in which instance one is justified in using the traditional term *pure word deafness*.

In most autopsy studies a lesion is embolic, bilateral in the superior temporal gyrus, in position to damage the primary auditory cortex in the transverse gyrus of Heschl and to impair its relation to the associated areas of the superior, posterior part of the temporal lobe. The occasional unilateral lesions are localized in this part of the major (dominant) temporal lobe and encroach on those regions whose involvement precipitates the larger syndrome of Wernicke's aphasia.

DYSLEXIA WITH DYSGRAPHIA This language disturbance is often a late sequela of the larger syndrome of Wernicke's aphasia, most evident in reading and writing. The syndrome is the visual form of Wernicke's aphasia. Errors occur in response to lexical stimuli. Auditory comprehension, while not normal, is less impaired than visual comprehension. Since conversational testing is frequently the only type of clinical evaluation in such patients, satisfactory auditory comprehension, ability to repeat aloud, and mild paraphasic errors in spontaneous speech frequently lead to a misdiagnosis of mild Wernicke's aphasia. Detailed testing of reading aloud and reading for comprehension and tests of spontaneous writing and of writing in response to dictated and visually presented material reveal a greater disturbance in these tasks and expose the syndrome.

The parietal and occipital region is usually affected. Although a discrete embolism is unusual, a small clot may pass through the more proximal territory and lodge distally. Tumors, abscess, and lobar hemorrhages usually disrupt other structures as well, and this syndrome is often a less conspicuous part of a larger clinical picture. Systemic hypotension and hypoxia may leave dyslexia with dysgraphia as a residual impairment, but more often they produce a more severe defect, described below under "Isolation of speech areas."

PURE WORD BLINDNESS In the fully developed syndrome, the victims lose the ability to read and usually to name colors. The patient is unable to name or point to a letter or word on command. However, understanding spoken language, repetition of what is heard, writing to dictation, and conversation are all intact. Because the victim may be unaware the deficit exists, the examiner is often required to test for its presence, rather than simply assume the complaint will be volunteered. In the most severe alexics, the actual letter or name responses have little connection with the presented stimuli. The response may be corrected and the defect obscured if other visual cues are available, such as the bottle on which the words Coca-Cola appear. The naming of common colors presented singly and of objects is also impaired. In lesser degrees of the affection, reading is impaired mainly in the affected visual field, producing a dyslexia for the letters on the affected side of the longer words (so-called hemidyslexia). The condition is also sometimes termed *dyslexia without dysgraphia.*

Right homonymous hemianopsia, an amnesic defect (see Chap. 23), and a hemisensory defect on the right reflect the involvement of the left occipital lobe, the left fornix and its decussation, and the left thalamus, respectively, a combination that nearly always signifies thrombosis or embolism of the left posterior cerebral artery, placing the origin of this syndrome rather remote from the main language zone supplied by the middle cerebral artery territory.

Autopsy usually demonstrates a lesion that destroys the left visual striate cortex (area 17) and visual association areas (18 and 19), as well as the connections of the right visual cortex and association areas with the temporoparietal region. This latter "disconnection" usually is due to interruption of the fibers passing through the posterior part (splenium) of the corpus callosum, which connect the visual association areas of the two hemispheres. A lesion deep in the left parietooccipital region may also prevent visual information from both occipital lobes reaching the left angular gyrus. In this case the right homonymous hemianopsia may be absent. With purely left cerebral lesions, aside from infarction, there may be a primary or secondary tumor, or, rarely, multifocal leukoencephalopathy.

Isolation of speech areas   Following prolonged hypoxia, widespread cerebral ischemia can affect the vascular anatomic border zones linking the major cerebral arteries and their distal branches on the cerebral surfaces and spread centripetally into their adjacent territories. The central fields of supply of these arteries may be spared. In the middle cerebral artery territory, this sparing leaves largely intact the sylvian region and its speech areas. With much of the rest of the brain out of action in patients who survive such episodes, the speech mechanism can be activated by spoken words. There is parrotlike repetition of words and sounds (echolalia) and similar findings which indicate that the auditory-vocal loop is functional. Scant evidence of comprehension or self-initiated conversation is present, reflecting the widespread injury outside the speech regions. The syndrome is common following cardiac arrest.

Amnesic-dysnomic aphasia   This may be a relatively early or an isolated manifestation of disease of the nervous system. The patient loses only the ability to produce names on demand, including nouns, adjectives, and other descriptive parts of speech. There are typical pauses in speech, groping for words, and substitution of another word or phrase that conveys the meaning (circumlocution). When shown a series of common objects, the patient may tell of their use instead of giving their names. The difficulty applies not only to objects seen but to the names of things heard or felt. By contrast, other verbal tasks, including recall of the names of the letters and digits, reading, writing, spelling, etc., are almost invariably preserved. That the deficit is principally one of naming is shown by the patient's correct use of the object and, usually, by an ability to point to the correct object on hearing or seeing the name. There is a tendency among patients to attribute the failure to forgetfulness or to give some other excuse for the disability, suggesting that they are not completely aware of the nature of their difficulty.

The causative lesion is usually deep in the temporal lobe, presumably interrupting connections of sensory speech areas with the hippocampal-parahippocampal regions concerned with learning and memory. Masses such as a tumor or abscess are the most frequent; as they enlarge, an upper contralateral quadrantic visual field defect or Wernicke's aphasia is added. Dysnomia may be part of the syndromes produced by occlusion of the temporal branches of the posterior cerebral artery. Alzheimer's disease may begin with a dysnomic or amnesic type of aphasia; by the time the patient's difficulty is fully recognized, other disorders of speech and indifference, apathy, and abulia are conjoined. Dysnomia may also be present in confusional states caused by metabolic, infectious, intoxicative,

or other acute medical illnesses, but then it has no certain localizing value.

The combination of dysnomia and major impairment of auditory comprehension with a remarkable retention of the ability to repeat what is heard is called *transcortical sensory aphasia.* The causative lesion spares the auditory cortex and Wernicke area and involves the inferior temporal cortices, particularly area 37.

DISORDERS OF ARTICULATION AND PHONATION   In simple dysarthria there is no abnormality of the cortical centers. Dysarthric patients are able to understand what they hear, to read, and to write, even though they are unable to utter a single intelligible word.

The highly coordinated act of speaking involves the larynx, pharynx, palate, tongue, lips, and respiratory musculature, which are innervated by the hypoglossal, vagal, facial, and phrenic nerves. Their nuclei are controlled through the corticobulbar tracts by both motor cortices and by extrapyramidal influences from the cerebellum and basal ganglia. The current of air is produced by expiration and is finely regulated by the activity of the various muscles engaged in speech. *Phonation,* or the production of vocal sounds, is a function of the larynx. Changes in the size and shape of the glottis and in the length and tension of the vocal cords are controlled by the laryngeal muscles, which transmit their vibrations to the column of air passing over the vocal cords. Sounds thus formed are modified as they pass through the nasopharynx and mouth, which act as resonators. Articulation consists of contractions of the tongue, lips, pharynx, and palate, which interrupt or alter the vocal sounds. Vowels are of laryngeal origin, as are some consonants, but the latter are formed for the most part during articulation. For instance, the consonants *m, b,* and *p* are labial; *l* and *t* are lingual; and *nk* and *ng* are nasoguttural.

Disorders of phonation prompt examination of the vocal cords, tongue, palate, and pharynx. Defects in articulation can be subdivided into paretic dysarthria; spastic and rigid dysarthria; choreic, myoclonic, and ataxic dysarthria.

Paretic dysarthria   This is due to a neural or bulbar (medullary) weakness or paralysis of the articulatory muscles (lower motor neuron paralysis). There is a special difficulty in the correct utterance of vibratives, such as *r;* the voice develops a nasal quality due to palatal weakness; as the paralysis becomes more complete, lingual and labial consonants are not pronounced. In the advanced stages, the shriveled tongue lies inert on the floor of the mouth, and the lips are relaxed and tremulous. Saliva collects in the mouth because of dysphagia and spills over the lips causing drooling. Bulbar palsy, peripheral neuropathies, and muscle diseases, including myasthenia gravis, are common causes.

Spastic and rigid dysarthria   These are more frequent than the paralytic variety. Diseases that involve the corticobulbar tracts, usually from vascular disease or motor system disease, either simultaneously or in stages, cause pseudobulbar palsy. In the past, the patient may have had a minor stroke affecting the corticobulbar fibers on one side; but since the bulbar muscles are probably represented in both motor cortices, there is no impairment in speech or swallowing from a unilateral lesion. Should another stroke then occur, involving the other corticobulbar tract and possibly the corticospinal tract at the pontine, midbrain, or capsular level, the patient becomes anarthric or dysarthric and dysphagic. Often the muscles of facial expression on both sides are weakened as well. Unlike bulbar paralysis due to lower neuron involvement, this condition entails no atrophy or fasciculation of the paralyzed muscles; the jaw jerk and other facial reflexes are exaggerated; the palatal reflexes are retained; emotional control is poor (pathologic laughter and crying); and sometimes breathing is periodic (Cheyne-Stokes). When the frontal operculum alone is involved, the speech deficit may be a pure dysarthria but usually without the impairment in emotional control. In the beginning, the patient may be totally anarthric and aphonic, but when improvement occurs or when the patient has a milder version of the same condition, speech is notably slow, thick, and indistinct, much like that of partial bulbar paralysis.

An extrapyramidal disturbance of articulation occurs in Parkinson's syndrome. The patient speaks hastily and articulates poorly, slurring over many syllables and trailing the ends of sentences. The voice is low-pitched, monotonous, and lacking in inflection; voice volume diminishes. In advanced cases speech is almost unintelligible; only whispering is possible.

In many cases of capsular hemiplegia or partially recovered Broca's aphasia, residual dysarthria may be difficult to distinguish from a pure articulatory defect.

Choreic and myoclonic dysarthria   In chorea and myoclonus, speech may also be characteristic. Unlike the defect of pseudobulbar palsy or parkinsonism, chorea and myoclonus abruptly interrupt the pronunciation of words by the abnormal movements. Grimacing and other characteristic motor signs suggest the diagnosis.

Ataxic dysarthria   This is characteristic of acute and chronic cerebellar lesions and may be observed in multiple sclerosis, Friedreich's ataxia, cerebellar atrophy, and heat stroke. The principal speech abnormality is slowness; imprecise enunciation, monotony, and unnatural, irregular separation of the syllables of words (scanning) are additional features. Coordination of speech and respiration are poor. There may not be enough breath to utter certain words, and others may be ejaculated explosively. Myoclonic jerks involving the speech musculature may be superimposed on cerebellar ataxia in a number of diseases.

APHONIA AND DYSPHONIA   Some speech disorders involve disturbances of voice. Paresis of the respiratory movements, as in poliomyelitis and acute infectious polyneuritis, or incoordination as part of extrapyramidal disease may affect the voice because insufficient air is provided for phonation and speech. Reduced volume of speech due to limited excursion of the breathing muscles is common; the patient is unable to speak above a whisper or to shout. Whispering speech is also a feature of stupor, but strong stimulation may make the voice audible.

Paresis of both vocal cords causes complete aphonia. There is no voice, and the patient can speak only in whispers. Since the vocal cords normally separate during inspiration, their failure to do so when paralyzed may result in an inspiratory stridor. If one vocal cord is paralyzed, the voice becomes hoarse, low-pitched, and rasping. Involvement of one of the tenth cranial nerves by tumor, for example, may also cause a nasal voice because the posterior nares do not close during phonation. Consonants such as *b, p, n,* and *k* are followed by escape of air into the nasal passages. The abnormality may be less pronounced in recumbency and may increase when the head is thrown forward. Hoarseness may also be due to structural changes in the vocal cords caused by cigarette smoking, chronic inflammation, polyps, etc.

Spastic dysphonia is a poorly understood neurologic disorder similar to dystonia. Many patients, middle-aged or elderly, otherwise healthy, gradually lose the ability to speak quietly and fluently. Any effort to speak results in contraction of the speech musculature so that the voice is strained and phonation is labored. The patients are not neurotic, and psychotherapy and speech therapy are ineffective. The condition differs from the stridor caused by spasm of the laryngeal muscles in tetany. It is nonprogressive but may be combined with restricted extrapyramidal disorders such as blepharospasm and spasmodic torticollis. Surgical section of the superior laryngeal nerve on one side has been found to at least partially diminish the rigidity.

CLINICAL APPROACH TO LANGUAGE DISORDERS Aphasia   In investigating aphasia, it is first necessary to enquire into the patient's native language, handedness, and previous education. Some left-handed children are trained to use their right hand for writing; therefore, one must ask which hand is used for throwing a ball; threading a needle; or using a spoon, hammer, or saw. It is important to establish that the patient is alert and can participate reliably in testing, because assessment of language depends on these factors, as does determining whether the patient has other signs of cerebral

disease such as hemiplegia, facial weakness, homonymous hemianopsia, or cortical sensory loss. When hemiplegia, hemianesthesia, and homonymous hemianopsia coexist, the aphasic disorder is usually complete or global. Such major neurologic signs are seldom associated with the less complete forms of language disorder, the posterior sylvian syndromes, or the dissociative syndromes, though one defect may exceed others. Dyspraxia of limbs and speech musculature, in response to spoken commands or to visual mimicry, is generally associated with Broca's aphasia and sometimes with Wernicke's aphasia. Bilateral or unilateral homonymous hemianopsia without motor weakness is often linked with pure word blindness (alexia or dyslexia) or to amnesic-dysnomic aphasia. Bilateral hemiplegias due to extensive frontal lesions are accompanied not infrequently by pure word muteness. The special types of aphasia—alexia, pure word deafness, etc.—are often associated with evidence of embolism to other parts of the brain or other organs.

Conversational testing permits quick assessment of the motor aspects of speech (praxis and prosody), apparent language formulation, and auditory comprehension. Disabilities in the purely motor aspects of speech suggest a motor aphasia, and this possibility can be pursued by tests of repeating from dictation and by tests of praxis of the oropharyngeal and respiratory apparatus. Disabilities in language formulation such as literal paraphasias with impaired comprehension are indicative of Wernicke's aphasia. Disorders confined to naming, generally without paraphasias, when other language functions (reading, writing, spelling, etc.) are adequate, are diagnostic of amnesic dysnomia.

When conversation shows virtually no disabilities, other tests may be revealing. Reading aloud single letters, words, and text may reveal pure word blindness, while tests of writing in this syndrome are normal. Literal and verbal paraphasic errors may appear in milder cases of Wernicke's aphasia as the patient reads aloud from text or from words in the examiner's handwriting. Similar errors occur more frequently when the patient is asked to explain the text, read aloud, or give explanations in writing. Adequacy of response channels is determined by presenting tasks that permit a response physically identical with the test stimulus, such as copying visual stimuli and repeating aloud from auditory stimuli. Inadequacy of receptive or response channels precludes further analysis of the deficit involving that channel in more complex types of tests, except in the unlikely instance that the more complex test is better performed. If reception and response channels are adequate in these initial tests, they may then be used in tests requiring all types of language function, such as writing from dictation, vocal naming of visual stimuli, matching physically dissimilar stimuli having a name in common (e.g., the word *cow* and a picture of a cow). By utilizing the same test material used in the earlier tests, direct comparison of performances in spoken naming, written naming, and matching can be compared from visual, auditory, and palpated stimuli. A performance profile can be constructed separately for each type of stimulus material tested (objects, pictures, words, letters, numbers, colors, etc.) The resultant profile can then be used to determine whether the main deficits fall across one or more input or response channels. These data provide a baseline against which later changes may be compared.

Articulatory-phonation disorders   Disturbances of articulation point to involvement of a different set of neural structures, such as the motor cortices; the corticobulbar pathways; the seventh, ninth, and tenth nuclei; the brainstem; and extrapyramidal nuclei and tracts. It may be necessary to use other neurologic findings to decide which of these are implicated. It is particularly important to distinguish between the pseudobulbar or supranuclear palsies and the bulbar palsies. The information obtained by separating these two types of dysarthria is particularly helpful in differential diagnosis.

Dysphonia should lead to an investigation of laryngeal disease, either primary or secondary to an abnormality of innervation. Inspection of the vocal cords is necessary.

TREATMENT   Except for almost pure motor defects, most patients show remarkably little concern over the sudden loss of speech. The very lesion that deprives them of speech also appears to cause a partial loss of insight into the disability. For example, in Wernicke's aphasia patients may become indignant when others cannot understand their jargon. Nonetheless, as improvement occurs, many patients become discouraged. Reassurance and a positive program of speech rehabilitation are the best ways of helping the patient at this stage.

Most aphasias are due to vascular disease of the brain, and some degree of spontaneous improvement usually occurs over days to months after the stroke. Sometimes recovery is complete within hours or days; at times not more than a few words are regained after a year or two of assiduous speech training. Nevertheless, many experts in the field believe that speech training is worthwhile.

As a rule, speech therapy is not advisable in the first few days of an aphasic illness, because one does not know how lasting it will be. Also, if a global aphasia is present, the speech therapist is helpless. Under such circumstances, it is preferable to wait until some of the language function has begun to return. Then the physician may begin to encourage and help the patient to use the function to a maximal degree. In milder aphasic disorders speech therapy can be begun as soon as the illness is stabilized. Although speech therapy has not been proved, in controlled studies, to be of benefit to recovery, its value in terms of support for the patient and the family needs to be emphasized. The methods of speech training are specialized, and it is advisable to consult an expert in this field.

There is no special treatment for the dysarthric disturbance of speech.

PROGNOSIS The outcome depends on the underlying disease and the magnitude of the lesion within the speech areas. Global aphasias lasting more than a week or two usually have a bad outcome. Seldom is there enough recovery of communicative speech to permit resumption of occupation or profession. Partial aphasias frequently improve, sometimes to a gratifying degree, if of vascular or encephalitic origin. Aphasias due to embolism, whether global or restricted, may disappear in hours to days or may persist.

REFERENCES

ALBERT ML et al: *Clinical Aspects of Dysphasia.* New York, Springer-Verlag, 1981

DAMASIO AR, GESCHWIND N: The neural basis of language. Ann Rev Neurosci 7:127, 1984

GESCHWIND N: Disconnection syndromes in animals and man. Brain 88:237, 585, 1965

KERTESZ A: *Localization in Neuropsychology.* New York, Academic, 1983

LECOURS AR et al: *Aphasiology.* London, Bailliere Tindall, 1983

MOHR JP: Broca's area and Broca's aphasia, in *Studies in Neurolinguistics,* H Whitaker (ed). New York, Academic, 1975, chap 6

———, SIDMAN M: Aphasia: Behavioral aspects, in *American Handbook of Psychiatry,* vol 4, M Reiser (ed). New York, Basic Books, 1975, pp 279–298

---

23 CONFUSION, DELIRIUM, AMNESIA, AND DEMENTIA

MAURICE VICTOR / RAYMOND D. ADAMS

All physicians must be able to assess with complete objectivity the patient's character, intellectual function, mood, memory, judgment, and other attributes of personality and behavior. Examination of these affective and cognitive functions permits the physician to reach certain conclusions regarding the patient's *mental status.* Without such data, errors will be made in evaluating the patient's history, in diagnosing the neurologic or psychiatric disease from which he or she suffers, and in conducting an appropriate therapeutic program.

DEFINITION OF TERMS

The definition of normal and abnormal states of mind is difficult because the terms used to describe these states have been given so many different meanings in both medical and nonmedical writings (see also Chap. 11). Compounding the difficulty is the fact that the pathophysiology of the confusional states, delirium, and dementia, is not fully understood, and the definitions depend on their clinical relationships, with the lack of precision which this entails. The following nomenclature, though tentative, has been found useful by the authors and will be employed throughout this textbook.

Confusion is a general term denoting an incapacity of the patient to think with customary speed and clarity. This abnormality may depend on any one of several factors or conditions. At certain stages in the evolution or devolution of stupor and coma, as indicated in Chap. 21, confusion is aligned with a disorder of conscious awareness and perception. In patients with dementia, confusion is related to a derangement of intellectual function, i.e., an inability to learn, remember, calculate, make appropriate deductions from given premises, or reason abstractly. In toxic psychosis, inattention, impairment of perception, and the intrusion of illusory and hallucinatory experiences are mainly responsible for the confusional state. Intense anxiety and other emotional experiences may temporarily interfere with coherence of thinking.

The term *delirium* is used here to denote a special type of confusional state, acute in onset and transient in nature. It is characterized by gross disorientation in the presence of heightened alertness, i.e., an increased readiness to respond to stimuli; a disorder of perception in which illusions and vivid hallucinations are prominent; and overactivity of psychomotor and autonomic nervous functions. Implicit in the definition are certain nonmedical connotations of the term—agitation, excitement, vivid dreams, and creations of the imagination. Most stuporous and many demented patients, in contrast to those with delirium, show a *reduced* state of arousal, alertness, and attentiveness; *decreased* psychomotor activity; and a *relatively slight* tendency to hallucinate. For these reasons, and also because of the particular clinical settings in which they occur, it seems worthwhile to set the delirious states apart from those of depressed consciousness on the one hand and of dementia and amnesia on the other. Such a concept is far from new. To a greater or lesser extent, the terms *symptomatic psychosis, toxic psychosis, infective-exhaustive psychosis,* and *drug, traumatic,* or *febrile delirium* all have reference to the syndrome of delirium. Each of these terms conveys the idea of an acute and transient (reversible) confusional state, occurring in a particular clinical setting and carrying a serious prognosis by virtue of adding its burden to an already serious medical illness.

It should be pointed out that not all psychiatrists agree with our distinction between delirium and other confusional states. Some, such as Lipowski and Engel and Romano, use the term *delirium* in reference to confusional states of all types. Our insistence on their separation is based on the differences in their clinical manifestations and in the clinical settings in which they occur.

The term *amnesia,* in the clinical sense, refers to the inability of the patient to remember past events, coupled with an inability to form new memories, i.e., to learn. The term presupposes an alert state of mind and ability to grasp the problem, to comprehend and use language normally, and to maintain adequate motivation. The failure is mainly one of retention, recall, and reproduction. It should be distinguished from the impairment or loss of memory that accompanies states of drowsiness and acute confusion, in which information seems never to have been adequately assimilated or registered in the first place.

The term *dementia* literally means a loss of mind and, more particularly, means a deterioration of all intellectual and cognitive functions (see above), without disturbance of consciousness, awareness, or perception. Implied in this designation is a gradual and in most instances irreversible enfeeblement of mental powers in a person who formerly possessed a normal mind. *Amentia,* by contrast, indicates a developmental failure to achieve normal intellectual capacity, i.e., mental retardation.

OBSERVABLE ASPECTS OF BEHAVIOR

The components of mentation and behavior that lend themselves to bedside examination are (1) the processes of sensation and perception; (2) the capacity for memorizing; (3) the ability to think and reason; (4) temperament, mood, and emotion; (5) initiative, impulse, and drive; and (6) insight. Of these, (1) is sensorial, (2) and (3) are cognitive, (4) is affective, and (5) is volitional or conative. Insight (6) includes all introspective observations made by patients concerning their own normal or disordered functioning. Each of these components has its objective side, expressed in behavioral responses that are produced by certain stimuli, and its subjective side, expressed in what the patient thinks and feels in relation to the stimuli.

DISTURBANCES OF PERCEPTION Perception, i.e., the processes utilized in acquiring through the senses a knowledge of the "world about" or of one's own body, involves a number of psychological mechanisms in addition to a simple awareness of the attributes of a stimulus. It includes the maintenance of attention, the selective focusing on a stimulus, the elimination of all extraneous stimuli, and the identification of the stimulus by recognizing its relationship to personal, remembered experience. The perception of a stimulus undergoes predictable types of derangement in disease affecting the cerebrum. Commonly, there is a reduction in the number of perceptions in a given unit of time and a failure to synthesize them properly and to relate them to the ongoing activities of the mind. There may be inattention or fluctuations of attention, distraction (pertinent and irrelevant stimuli have equal value), and inability to persist in an assigned task. Qualitative changes also appear, mainly in the form of sensory distortions, causing misinterpretation of sounds and objects and misidentification of persons (illusions). These changes form the basis for certain hallucinatory experiences in which the patient reports and reacts inappropriately to stimuli present in the environment. There is also an inability to perceive simultaneously all elements of a complex of stimuli, which has been referred to as a *failure of subjective reorganization*. These major disturbances in the perceptual sphere, sometimes called *clouding of the sensorium*, occur most often in deliria and other acute confusional states, but a quantitative deficiency may also become evident in amentia and in the advancing stages of dementia.

DISTURBANCES OF MEMORY Memory, the retention of learned experiences, is involved in all mental activities. It may be arbitrarily subdivided into several parts: (1) registration, which includes all that was mentioned under perception; (2) mnemonic integration and retention; (3) recall; and (4) reproduction. In severe disturbances of perception and attention there may be a complete failure of learning and consequently, of memory, because the material to be learned was never registered and assimilated. In Korsakoff's amnesic syndrome (see below), newly presented material appears to be temporarily registered but cannot be retained for more than a few minutes, and there is always an associated defect in the recall and reproduction of memories that had been formed some days, weeks, or even years before the onset of the illness (*retrograde amnesia*). Proof of the integrity of immediate memory, i.e., registration, is the ability to repeat phrases or numbers to be learned. Normal retention with failure of recall is at times a normal state ("tip of the tongue" syndrome, benign forgetfulness); when it is severe and extends to all events of past life, including personal identity, it is usually due to hysteria or malingering. Proof that the processes of registration and retention are intact under the latter circumstances comes from hypnosis and suggestion and from questioning under amobarbital or thiopental sodium narcosis, whereby the lost items are fully recalled and reproduced. Since some aspect of memory is involved to some extent in all mental processes, it becomes the most testable component of mentation and behavior.

DISTURBANCES OF THINKING Thinking, which is central to practically all intellectual activity, remains the most elusive of all mental operations. If by thinking we mean the selective ordering of symbols for problem solving and the capacity to reason and form sound judgments (the usual definition), then the working units of this type of mental activity are mainly words and numbers. The substitution of words and numbers for the objects for which they stand (symbolization) is a fundamental part of the process. The formation of these symbols into ideas or concepts and the arrangement of new and remembered ideas into certain orders or relationships, according to the rules of logic, constitute other intricate parts of thought. One test of logical thinking is problem solving—the capacity to formulate a problem into several hypotheses, to analyze critically the evidence for and against each hypothesis, and to make a correct choice. In a general way one may examine thinking for speed and efficiency, ideational content, coherence and logical relationships of ideas, quantity and quality of associations with a given idea, and the propriety of the feeling and behavior engendered by an idea.

Information concerning the thought processes and associative functions is best obtained by analyzing the patient's spontaneous verbal productions and by engaging him or her in conversation. If the patient is taciturn or mute, one may have to depend on the responses to direct questions or upon written material, e.g., letters, etc. One notes the prevailing trends of the patient's thoughts; whether the ideas are to the point, reasonable, and coherent or vague, circumstantial, tangential, and irrelevant; and whether the thought processes are shallow and fragmented. Disorders of thinking are observed regularly in deliria and other confusional states and in dementia and schizophrenia. Incoherence of thinking characterizes confusional states of all types. The patient may be excessively critical, rationalizing, and hairsplitting; this type of thinking is often manifest in depressive psychosis. Derangement of thinking may also take the form of a flight of ideas; the patient moves nimbly from one thought to another, and associations are numerous and loosely linked. This is a common feature of hypomanic or manic states. The opposite condition, poverty of ideas, is characteristic both of depression, in which it is combined with gloomy thoughts, and of dementing diseases, in which it is part of a general reduction in intellectual activity. Thinking may be distorted in such a way that patients fail to check their ideas against reality. When a belief is maintained in spite of convincing contradictory evidence, the patient is said to have a *delusion*. Delusions are common in many psychiatric illnesses, particularly manic-depressive and schizophrenic states, but may also occur in dementing illnesses and in chronic infections of the central nervous system.

DISTURBANCES OF EMOTION, MOOD, AND AFFECT The emotional life of the patient is expressed in a variety of ways. In the first place, rather marked individual differences in basic temperament are observed in otherwise normal persons; some persons are throughout life cheerful, gregarious, optimistic, and free from worry, whereas others are just the opposite. Strong emotional states such as fear and anxiety are more easily induced in some individuals than others; they are normal reactions to life situations and may be accompanied by derangements of visceral function. If disproportionate to the stimulus and persistent, they are usually manifestations of an anxiety disorder or depression. Emotional responses that are excessively labile and poorly controlled or uninhibited are a common manifestion of many cerebral diseases, particularly those involving the corticopontine and corticobulbar pathways. Such responses then constitute a part of the syndrome of pseudobulbar palsy.

Temperament, mood, and other emotional experiences are evaluated by the appearance of the patient and by verbalized accounts of his or her feelings. For these purposes some psychiatrists divide emotionality into mood and feeling (affect). By *mood* is meant the prevailing emotional state of the individual without reference to impinging stimuli. It may be cheerful or melancholic. Language, e.g., the adjectives used, and facial expressions, attitudes, postures, and speed of movement most reliably betray the patient's mood. By contrast, *feelings* (or *affect*) are said to be emotional experiences evoked by particular stimuli.

DISTURBANCES IN IMPULSE (CONATION) Impulse, that basic biologic urge, driving force, or purpose by which every organism is directed to reach its objectives, is another important and observable, though somewhat neglected, dimension of behavior. Again, one notes wide normal variations in strength of impulse to action and thought, and these individual differences are present throughout life. Many types of cerebral diseases (particularly those which involve the medial-orbital parts of the frontal lobes) cause a reduction in impulse coupled with an indifference or lack of concern about the consequences of actions. In such cases all other measurable aspects of psychic function may be normal. Pathologic lack of impulse, or *abulia*, may reach an extreme degree—to the point of mutism and immobility, a state sometimes called *akinetic mutism. Psychomotor retardation* is a lesser degree of the same state and is a feature of both cerebral disease and depression.

LOSS OF INSIGHT Insight, the state of being fully aware of the nature and degree of one's deficits, becomes manifestly impaired or abolished in all types of cerebral disease that cause complex disorders of behavior. Rarely does the patient with such a disorder seek advice or help for the illness. Instead, the family usually brings the individual to the physician. Thus, diseases which produce high-order or complex mental abnormalities not only evoke observable changes in mentation and behavior but also alter or reduce the patient's capacity for self-observation.

APPROACH TO THE PATIENT

Confronted by a patient with one of these disorders, the physician must adopt an examination technique designed to expose fully the perceptual and intellectual defect. Abnormalities of posture, movement, sensation, and reflexes cannot be relied upon for the full demonstration of the neurologic deficit, for it must be remembered that the association and limbic areas of the brain may be severely damaged without demonstrable neurologic signs of these types.

The initial assessment of the patient should include (1) a reliable history of the illness; (2) findings on mental examination, i.e., so-called mental status; (3) findings on the rest of the neurologic examination; and (4) application of special laboratory procedures, including endocrine, biochemical, and toxic studies, CT scanning or MRI imaging, lumbar puncture, electroencephalogram, and sometimes angiography.

The history should always be supplemented by information obtained from a person other than the patient. Through lack of insight, patients are often unaware of their illness; indeed, they may be ignorant even of their chief complaint. Special inquiry should be made about the patient's general behavior, social adjustment, capacity for work, personal habits, and family history.

A systemic examination of the mental status should provide answers to the following questions:

1 Insight (patient's replies to questions about the chief symptoms): What is your difficulty? Are you ill? When did your illness begin?
2 Orientation:
   a Knowledge of personal identity and present situation: What is your name? What is your occupation? Where do you live? Are you married? What are you doing now?
   b Place: What is the name of the place where you are now? How did you get here? What floor is it on? Where is the secretary's or nurses' desk or the bathroom?
   c Time: What is the date today? What day of the week is it? What is the time of day? What meals have you had? When was the last holiday?
3 Memory:
   a Remote: Tell me the names of your children and their birth dates. When were you married? What was your mother's maiden name? What was the name of your first school teacher? What jobs have you held?
   b Recent past: Tell me about your recent illness (compare with previous statements). What did you have for breakfast today? What is my name or the nurse's name? When did you see me for the first time? What tests were done yesterday? What were the headlines in the newspaper today? Give patient a simple story, oral or written, and ask her or him to recall it after 3 to 5 min.
   c Immediate recall (short-term memory): Repeat these numbers after me (give a series of three, four, five, six, seven and then eight digits at the speed of one per second). Now when I give a series of numbers, repeat them in reverse order.
   d Visual span: Show patient a picture of several objects; ask him or her to name what has been seen and note any inaccuracies.
4 General information: Ask about the names of presidents, well-known historic dates, or the names of large rivers or cities. Ask the patient to give the names of 10 fruits, 10 flowers, or 10 vegetables as quickly as possible.
5 Capacity for sustained mental activity:
   a Calculation: Test ability to add, subtract, multiply, and divide. Serial subtraction of 7s or 3s from 100 is a good test of calculation as well as of concentration.
   b Abstract thinking: See if patient can detect similarities and differences between classes of objects or explain a proverb of a fable.
6 General behavior (attitudes, general bearing, attentiveness, manner of dress, etc.):
   a Content of thought: What ideas occupy the patient's thoughts? Does the patient believe that his or her thoughts and actions are being controlled or broadcasted to others? Are there hallucinations and/or delusions? Is there a press of speech or lack of speech?
   b Mood: Do patients appear cheerful or sad? How do they feel? Are they nervous, worried, or apprehensive? What feeling is revealed through speech, attitude, and facial expression?
7 Special tests of localized cerebral functions: Tests for grasping and sucking; tests for aphasia, praxis with both hands, cortical sensory function, and visual field defects; tests of ability in drawing clock face, map of United States or Europe, floor plan of patient's house, etc.

In order to enlist the full cooperation of patients, physicians must prepare them for questions of this type. Otherwise, the patient's first reaction will be one of embarrassment or anger because of the implication that his or her mind is not sound. Reassurance that these are not tests of intelligence or of sanity is helpful.

More formal methods of examining the mental capacity of adults, such as the Wechsler Adult Intelligence Scale (WAIS), are widely available. Discrepancies between vocabulary, picture-completion, and object-assembly tests as a group (which correlate well with premorbid intelligence and are relatively resistant to dementing brain disease) and arithmetic, block design, digit span, and digit symbol tests (which decline in dementia) provide an index of deterioration. The Wechsler Memory Scale is a reliable method for quantitating the degree of impairment of retentive memory. Characteristically, in patients with Korsakoff's amnesic syndrome there is a striking discrepancy between performance on the WAIS and that on the Wechsler Memory Scale.

COMMON SYNDROMES

DELIRIUM Clinical features These are most perfectly depicted in the alcoholic patient. The symptoms usually develop over a period of 2 or 3 days. The first indications of the approaching attack are difficulty in concentrating, restless irritability, tremulousness, insomnia, and poor appetite. One or several generalized convulsions are the initial major symptom in almost 30 percent of the cases. The patient's rest becomes troubled by unpleasant and terrifying dreams or by hallucinations. There may be momentary disorientation as revealed by an occasional inappropriate remark.

These initial symptoms rapidly give way to a clinical picture which, in severe cases, is one of the most colorful and dramatic in medicine. The state of consciousness becomes altered (sensorium is "clouded") in that the patient is inattentive and unable to perceive all elements of the situation. The patient may talk incessantly and incoherently and look distressed and perplexed; the facial expression is in keeping with vague notions of being annoyed or threatened. From the patient's manner and speech content it is evident that he or she misinterprets the meaning of ordinary objects and ambient sounds and has vivid visual, auditory, and tactile hallucinations, often of a most unpleasant type. At first the patient can be brought momentarily in touch with reality and may in fact answer questions correctly, but almost at once there is a relapse into the preoccupied, confused state; the patient gives wrong answers, is unable to think coherently, and is incapable of self-orientation. Before long the patient is unable to shake off the hallucinations even for a second and does not recognize family or physician. Coarse tremor and restless movements are usually present. Sleep is impossible or occurs only in brief naps. The countenance is flushed, the pupils are dilatated, and the conjunctivas are injected; the pulse is rapid, and the temperature may be raised. There is much sweating, and the urine is scanty and of high specific gravity. The signs of overactivity of the autonomic nervous system, more than any other signs, distinguish delirium from all other confusional states.

In most patients the symptoms abate after 3 to 5 days, although in a few they may persist for several weeks. The most certain indication of the end of the attack is the occurrence of sound sleep and of lucid intervals of increasing length. Recovery is usually complete. The most severe form ends fatally in a small percentage of patients.

Delirium is subject to all degrees of variability, not only from patient to patient but in the same patient from day to day and hour to hour. The entire syndrome may be observed in one patient and only one or two components in another. In its mildest form, as so often occurs in febrile diseases, it consists of an occasional wandering of the mind and incoherence of verbal expression, interrupted by periods of lucidity. This form, lacking motor and autonomic over-activity, is sometimes referred to as a *quiet delirium* (or *hypokinetic delirium*) and is difficult to distinguish from other confusional states. Agitation and excitement resembling delirium can also occur in hepatic encephalopathy, hyponatremia, and, transiently, in hypogly-cemia.

Morbid anatomy and pathophysiology   The brains of patients who have died in delirium tremens usually show no pathologic changes of significance. Those diseases that give rise to local lesions in the brain that may cause delirium include focal embolic encephalitis, viral encephalitis, and trauma. The topography of these lesions is of particular interest. They tend to be localized in the high midbrain and subthalamus and in the temporal lobes, where they involve the reticular activating and limbic systems.

Penfield's studies of the human cortex during surgical exploration indicate the importance of the temporal lobe in producing visual, auditory, and olfactory hallucinations. With subthalamic and midbrain lesions there may be visual hallucinations that are pleasant, animated, and accompanied by good insight (the peduncular hallucinosis of Lhermitte).

The electroencephalogram in delirium may show nonfocal theta activity (5 to 7 Hz) with return to normal as the delirium clears. In other patients only low-voltage, fast activity (11 to 20 Hz) is seen, and in milder degrees of delirium there is usually no abnormality at all.

An analysis of the several conditions conducive to delirium suggests at least three different physiologic mechanisms. First, the withdrawal of alcohol, barbiturates, or other sedative-hypnotic drugs, following a period of chronic intoxication, is the most common cause of delirium. These drugs have a strong depressant effect on certain areas of the central nervous system; presumably the release and overactivity of these parts, after withdrawal of the drug, are the basis of the delirium. Second, in the case of bacterial infections, toxic encepha-lopathies, or drug-induced delirium such as occurs with atropine or scopolamine, the delirious state probably results from the direct action of the toxin or chemical agent on these same parts of the brain. Third, destructive lesions, such as those of the temporal lobes in trauma or herpes simplex encephalitis, may cause delirium by disturbing the function of these particular areas.

ACUTE CONFUSIONAL STATES ASSOCIATED WITH REDUCED ALERTNESS AND DECREASED PSYCHOMOTOR ACTIVITY   Clin-

ical features   In the most typical examples of these states, all mental functions are reduced to some degree but alertness, attentiveness, and the ability to grasp all elements of the immediate situation suffer most. In the mildest form the patient may pass for normal; only failure to recollect and reproduce happenings of the past few hours or days reveals the inadequacy of mental function. The more obviously confused patient spends much time in idleness, and what the patient does may be inappropriate. Only the more automatic acts and verbal responses are properly performed, but these may permit the examiner to obtain from the patient a number of relevant and accurate replies to questions about age, occupation, and residence. Reactions are slow and indecisive, and it is difficult for the patient to sustain a conversation. The patient may fall asleep during the interview and if left alone sleeps more hours each day than is natural. Responses tend to be rather abrupt, brief, and mechanical. Disturbances of perception are frequent, causing misinterpretation of voices, common objects, and the actions of other persons. Often one cannot discern whether the patient is hallucinating, i.e., hearing and seeing things that do not exist, or merely misinterpreting stimuli in the environment. Inadequate perception and forgetfulness result in a constant state of bewilderment. Failing to recognize the surroundings and having lost all sense of time, the patient repeats the same question and makes the same remarks over and over again. Irritability may or may not be present. Some patients are extremely suspicious, demanding, and aggressive; in fact, a paranoid trend may be the most pronounced and troublesome feature of the illness.

As the confusion deepens, conversation becomes more difficult, and at a certain stage the patient no longer notices or responds to much of what is occurring. Questions may be answered with a single word or a short phrase spoken in a soft, tremulous voice or whisper, or the patient may be mute. In its most advanced stages confusion gives way to stupor and finally to coma. As the patient improves, there may again be a stage of stupor and confusion, occurring in the reverse order. This informs us that at least one category of confusion is a manifestation of the disease processes which, in their severest form, cause coma.

In the most typical cases, this type of confusional state is readily distinguished from delirium; in others, with more than the usual degree of irritability and restlessness, one cannot fail to notice the resemblance of one to the other. Similarly, when a delirium is complicated by an illness that superimposes stupor (e.g., delirium tremens with pneumonia, meningitis, or hepatic encephalopathy), it may be difficult to distinguish the delirium from other confusional states.

When clouding of consciousness is minimal and the confusion is of insidious onset and several weeks' duration, it may mimic dementia. Lipowski has called this "reversible dementia," claiming that it is an intermediate state between delirium and dementia and still poten-tially reversible. We would classify it as a protracted confusional state.

Morbid anatomy and pathophysiology   Confusional states are so diverse and are associated with such a wide variety of diseases that one would hardly expect a common anatomy or pathophysiologic basis. In general there is a more frequent occurrence with lesions of the right (nondominant) hemisphere, especially its posterior parts. Large ischemic and other acute lesions of the parietal lobe tend to render patients underactive, apathetic, and unaware of their neurologic disabilities; disorientation and inattentiveness are often associated (see Chap. 24). Only if the lesion is large enough to cause a hemiplegia, hemisensory disorder, or homonymous hemianopsia will the focal nature of the lesion be appreciated. Infarction of the thalamus, particularly of the dominant side, is commonly associated with a confusional state with recent memory impairment. This condition may persist for days or weeks, but usually clears.

More frequently, the basis of the confusional state is an acute metabolic disease, and the pathologic changes, if detectable, are bilateral and diffuse. Hypoxia, hyperglycemia, uremia, metabolic acidosis or alkalosis, hepatic stupor, hyponatremia, and certain drug intoxications are the commonly recognized causes which are readily corroborated by appropriate biochemical analyses of blood, urine, and cerebrospinal fluid. Clues to these biochemical derangements are often provided by alterations of respiration and the presence of asterixis, myoclonus, and tremor, with preserved pupillary reflexes. Correction of the biochemical derangements may result in rapid improvements in the patient's condition. Table 23-1 is a classification of the conditions that cause delirium and confusion.

DEMENTIA The term *dementia,* in current neurologic parlance, usually denotes a clinical syndrome composed of failing memory and loss of other intellectual functions due to chronic progressive degenerative disease of the brain. Such a definition is too narrow. The syndrome of dementia is characterized not only by intellectual deterioration but also by certain behavioral abnormalities and changes in personality. Moreover, it is illogical to set apart any one constellation of cerebral symptoms on the basis of their tempo of evolution and duration. Since there are several states of dementia of multiple causation and mechanism and because chronic degeneration of neurons is only one of the many causes, it is more correct to speak of the *dementias* or the *dementing diseases.*

Another concept that requires qualification is that of dementia as a global loss, in which all intellectual functions are affected more or less equally. When the latter are carefully analyzed they are found to include several separable though related functions, such as memory, verbal facility, and the ability to deal with mathematical symbols, to perceive visuospatial relationships, and to think abstractly and solve problems. Each of these functions (except thinking) has a definable anatomy in the cerebrum and can therefore be affected individually by a disease. For example, retentive memory involves neural mechanisms located bilaterally in the inferomedial parts of the temporal lobes, and the language mechanisms lie in the para-Sylvian region of the left (dominant) hemisphere. It comes as no surprise, therefore, that the dementing illnesses may affect certain intellectual functions predominantly or in various combinations and sequences.

Another point of importance is that most dementing diseases appear during the senium and many others during late adult life. In 17 series comprising 15,000 persons over the age of 60 years, the mean incidence of moderate to severe dementia was found to be 4.8 percent. In 1983, according to Terry and Katzman, there were in the United States about 1.3 million patients with severe dementia, and an additional 2.8 million with mild to moderate intellectual impairment. Since the elderly population in the western world is increasing both in percentage of the population and in absolute numbers, the magnitude of the medical problems they will present reaches an alarming dimension. Finally, it needs to be emphasized that the dementias of the elderly are to be regarded not as merely the inevitable consequences of growing old but as age-linked diseases, some 15 percent of which are treatable (Wells, 1981).

Clinical features These clinical features are observed most commonly and prototypically in patients with Alzheimer's disease. The earliest signs of dementia may be so subtle as to escape the notice of even the most discerning physician. Often an observant relative of the patient or an employer is the first to become aware of a certain lack of initiative, irritability, loss of interest, forgetfulness, and inability to perform up to the usual standard. Later there is distrac-

tibility and inattentiveness; inability to think with accustomed clarity; reduced general comprehension; perseveration in speech, action, and thought; and defective memory, especially for recent events. Frequently, a change in mood becomes apparent, taking the form more often of apathy than of depression or elation. Excessive lability of mood may be observed, i.e,. easy fluctuation from laughter to tears on slight provocation. Lapses in social graces and conduct occur and judgment becomes impaired, early in some cases and late in others. Paranoid ideas, delusions, and sometimes hallucinations may develop. As a rule, the patient has little or no realization of these changes in behavior and lacks insight into their meaning. However, early in the disease the patient may be aware of his or her declining capacities and become depressed on this account.

As the condition progresses, particularly in the degenerative diseases, there is loss of almost all intellectual faculties. Speech and language disturbances are almost invariable. The proper word or name cannot be found. Words are misspelled. Reading and auditory comprehension fail. Later, sphincteric incontinence, reduced responsivity, and finally mutism may be added to the clinical picture. Secondary physical deterioration eventually takes place. Food intake, which may be increased in the beginning of the illness, is in the end usually limited, with resulting emaciation. Locomotion fails; voluntary movements become poorly coordinated. Any febrile illness or metabolic upset induces a marked increase in confusion and even stupor or coma, indicating the precarious state of cerebral compensation. Finally, the patient remains in bed most of the time and dies of pneumonia or some other intercurrent infection. This whole process may evolve over a period of months or years, usually the latter.

Many of the alterations of behavior are the direct result (i.e., primary symptoms) of disease of the nervous system; others are

TABLE 23-1   Classification of delirium and acute confusional states

I Delirium
  A In a medical or surgical illness (no focal or lateralizing neurologic signs; cerebrospinal fluid usually clear)
    1 Postoperative (hypoxia) and postconcussive states
    2 Febrile illness: pneumonia, typhoid fever, malaria, septicemia from streptococcus, rheumatic fever
    3 Thyrotoxicosis and ACTH intoxication (rare)
  B In neurologic disease that causes focal or lateralizing signs or changes in the cerebrospinal fluid
    1 Vascular, neoplastic, or traumatic lesions, particularly those involving the temporal lobes and upper part of the brainstem
    2 Acute bacterial and tuberculous meningitis
    3 Subarachnoid hemorrhage
    4 Viral encephalitis or meningoencephalitis, particularly herpes simplex encephalitis
  C In the abstinence states, exogenous intoxications, and postconvulsive states (signs of other medical, surgical, and neurologic illnesses absent or coincidental)
    1 Withdrawal of alcohol (delirium tremens), barbiturates, and nonbarbiturate sedative drugs following chronic intoxication
    2 Drug intoxications: amphetamine, camphor, caffeine, ergot, scopolamine, atropine, etc.
    3 Postconvulsive delirium
II Acute confusional states associated with psychomotor underactivity
  A Associated with a medical or surgical disease (no focal lateralizing neurologic signs; cerebrospinal fluid clear)
    1 Metabolic disorders: hepatic stupor, uremia, hypoxia, hypercapnea, hypoglycemia, porphyria, electrolyte imbalance
    2 Febrile illnesses
    3 Congestive heart failure, with hypoxia
    4 Postoperative and posttraumatic states
  B Associated with drug intoxication (no focal or lateralizing signs; cerebrospinal fluid clear): opiates, barbiturates and other sedatives, trihexyphenidyl, etc.
  C Associated with diseases of the nervous system (the focal or lateralizing neurologic signs and cerebrospinal fluid changes are commoner in these conditions than in delirium)
    1 Cerebral vascular disease, tumor, abscess
    2 Subdural hematoma
    3 Meningitis
    4 Encephalitis
    5 Senile or other brain disease in combination with infective fevers, drug reactions, heart failure, or other medical or surgical disease ("beclouded dementia")

secondary, i.e., they are reactions to the catastrophe of losing one's mind. For example, the dement is said to seek solitude to hide the affliction and may thus appear asocial or apathetic. Again, excessive orderliness may be an attempt to compensate for failing memory; apprehension, gloom, or irritability may reflect general dissatisfaction with a necessarily restricted life. It would appear that even in a state of fairly advanced deterioration the patient is still capable of reacting to the illness and to the persons who provide care.

Degenerative diseases may terminate in virtually complete decortication. The patient lies with eyes open but is unaware of what is happening. He or she no longer speaks or responds to spoken commands. There is no interest in food or drink, though they are swallowed if placed in the mouth. The facial and limb muscles are stiff with increased tendon reflexes and occasionally Babinski's signs are present. Grasping and sucking are prominent. The sphincters are incontinent.

Morbid anatomy and pathophysiology Dementia is usually related to obvious structural disease of the cerebrum and the diencephalon. In some, such as the Alzheimer–senile dementia complex and Pick's disease, the main process appears to be a degeneration and loss of nerve cells in the association areas of the cerebral cortex, with secondary changes in the cerebral white matter. A degeneration of neurons confined to the thalamus may also cause dementia. In others, such as Huntington's chorea and certain of the spinocerebellar and cerebral-basal ganglionic degenerations, dementia is associated with a degeneration of neurons in the putamen and caudate nuclei. Arteriosclerotic vascular disease may result in multiple foci of infarction throughout the thalami, basal ganglia, brainstem, and cerebrum with dementia. Cerebral involvement may include the motor, sensory, or visual projection areas as well as the association areas. This condition, in the relatively rare instances in which mental deterioration dominates the clinical picture, is called *multi-infarct dementia*. Trauma may cause contusions of cerebral convolutions, particularly of the inferior and anterior parts of the frontal and temporal lobes, as well as necroses and hemorrhages in the midbrain, lesions which are responsible for protracted stupor, coma, or dementia. Most diseases that produce dementia are quite extensive, and the frontal and temporal lobes are affected more often than other parts of the cerebrum.

Mechanisms other than the destruction of brain tissue may be operative in some cases. Chronic increased intracranial pressure or chronic hydrocephalus (with large ventricles the pressure may not exceed 180 mmHg), regardless of cause, is often associated with a general impairment of mental function. Gait is usually also impaired. Compression of cerebral white matter is the main factor. The compression of one or both of the cerebral hemispheres by chronic subdural hematomas may cause a widespread disturbance of cortical function. A diffuse inflammatory process is at least in part the basis for dementia in syphilis and in certain virus infections such as herpes simplex encephalitis. Lastly, several of the toxic and metabolic diseases discussed in Chaps. 349 and 350 may interfere with nervous function over a period of time and create a clinical picture similar, if not identical, to that of dementia. One must suppose that the altered biochemical environment has affected neuronal function.

Classification of dementia Not all of the diseases listed in Table 23-2 are of equal importance as causes of dementia. Some are rare. In a series of 84 patients with established presenile dementia (at less than 65 years of age) admitted to a British neurologic center, 58 percent had brain atrophy, probably of the Alzheimer type, and 10 percent had multi-infarct dementia. Because this was a primary neurologic referral hospital, the incidence of tumors was high, nearly 10 percent. Normal-pressure hydrocephalus, alcoholic dementia, Creutzfeldt-Jakob disease, Huntington's chorea, posttraumatic sequelae, and alcoholism accounted for the remaining 30 percent. In an older population (over 65 years), brain atrophy was found in approximately 80 percent and multi-infarct dementia in 15 percent (Tomlinson). Probably the statistics amassed by Wells from a survey of patients with dementia entering a university hospital are the most representative. These are presented in Table 23-3.

The degenerative diseases that cause dementia are discussed further in Chap. 350. The special features of the dementias that accompany arteriosclerotic, syphilitic, traumatic, nutritional, and metabolic diseases are discussed in the appropriate chapters.

Differential diagnosis The first task in dealing with this class of patients is to make sure that the central probem is one of progressive general deterioration of intellect and personality change. It may be necessary to examine the patient several times before one is confident of the clinical findings. In this regard, use of standardized scales for assessment of dementia, such as the Blessed scale, may be useful.

An easy mistake is to assume that mental function is normal if patients complain only of nervousness, fatigue, insomnia, or vague somatic symptoms, and to label the illnesses as psychiatric disorders. *This will be avoided if one keeps in mind that such disorders rarely begin in middle or late adult life.* A practical rule is to assume that all mental illnesses beginning during this period are due either to structural disease of the brain or to a depressive psychosis.

A mild aphasia must not be mistaken for dementia. Aphasic patients appear uncertain of themselves, and their speech may be incoherent. Furthermore, they may be anxious and depressed over this ineptitude. Careful attention to the language performance of these patients will lead to the correct diagnosis in most instances, and further observation will disclose that their behavior, except that which is related to the language disorder, is within normal limits.

Depressed patients present another type of problem. They may remark that their mental function is poor or that they are forgetful and cannot concentrate. Scrutiny of these remarks will show, however,

---

TABLE 23-2   Bedside classification of dementia

I Diseases in which dementia is usually the only evidence of neurologic or medical disease
  A Alzheimer's disease and senile dementia
  B Pick's disease
II Diseases in which dementia is associated with other neurologic signs but not with other obvious medical disease
  A Invariably associated with other neurologic signs
    1 Huntington's chorea (choreoathetosis)
    2 Leukodystrophies: Schilder's disease, adrenoleukodystrophy, metachromatic leukodystrophy, and related demyelinative diseases (spastic weakness, pseudobulbar palsy, blindness, deafness)
    3 Lipofuscinosis and other lipid storage diseases (myoclonic seizures, blindness, spasticity, cerebellar ataxia)
    4 Myoclonic epilepsy (diffuse myoclonus, generalized seizures, cerebellar ataxia)
    5 Creutzfeldt-Jakob disease (diffuse myoclonus and cerebellar ataxia)
    6 Cerebrocerebellar degeneration (cerebellar ataxia of olivopontocerebellar type and others)
    7 Cerebral-basal ganglionic degenerations (apraxia, rigidity) and supranuclear palsy (paralysis of vertical gaze, neck dystonia)
    8 Dementia with spastic paraplegia
    9 Basal ganglia calcification (idiopathic and hypoparathyroidism)
    10 Hallervorden-Spatz disease (pyramidal and extrapyramidal signs)
    11 Dementia with Parkinson's disease (tremor, rigidity, bradykinesia)
  B Often associated with other neurologic signs
    1 Cerebral arteriosclerosis and ischemic infarction
    2 Brain tumor, especially gliomas of frontal and temporal lobes and corpus callosum
    3 Brain trauma (cerebral contusions, midbrain hemorrhages, chronic subdural hematoma)
    4 Marchiafava-Bignami disease (apraxia and other frontal lobe signs)
    5 Normal-pressure hydrocephalus (nearly always with ataxia of gait and often with sphincteric incontinence)
    6 Chronic CNS infections: cryptococcosis, toxoplasmosis, dementia associated with acquired immunodeficiency syndrome (AIDS)
III Diseases in which dementia is usually associated with clinical and laboratory signs of other medical disease
  A Hypothyroidism
  B Cushing's disease
  C Nutritional deficiency states such as pellagra, the Wernicke-Korsakoff syndrome, and subacute combined degeneration of spinal cord and brain (vitamin B_{12} deficiency)
  D Neurosyphilis: general paresis and meningovascular syphilis
  E Hepatolenticular degeneration, familial and acquired
  F Chronic drug intoxication (barbiturates and other sedative drugs)

that they can actually remember details of their history and that no qualitative change in cognitive function has occurred. Their difficulty is either a lack of energy and interest or an anxiety that prevents the focusing of attention on anything except their own problems. Even during mental tests their performance may be impaired by their emotional state in much the same way as the performance of a worried student is impaired during examinations. When patients are calmed by reassurance and given more time in the performance of tests, mental function improves, indicating that intellectual deterioration has not occurred. Hypomanic patients may fail in tests of intellectual function because of restlessness and distractibility. It is helpful to remember that demented patients, except in the early phases of their illness, rarely have sufficient insight to complain of mental deterioration; those who admit to poor memory seldom realize the degree of their disability. The physician must never rely on the patient's statements concerning the efficiency of mental function and must always evaluate a poor performance on tests in the light of the emotional state and motivation at the time the test is given. Especially difficult is the mildly demented patient who is also depressed and whose CT scan shows some degree of ventricular enlargement—even to a degree that raises the question of normal-pressure hydrocephalus. Sometimes the contribution of depression can only be ascertained by an empirical trial of antidepressant drugs.

Certain metabolic or endocrine disorders, i.e., hypothyroidism, ACTH therapy, Cushing's disease, or Addison's disease, or the postpartum state may create difficulties in diagnosis because of the wide variety of clinical pictures by which they manifest themselves. Some such patients appear to be suffering from a dementia, others from an acute confusional psychosis; if mood change or delusions predominate, a manic-depressive psychosis or schizophrenia is suggested. In these conditions, some degree of confusion can usually be recognized, and on this basis one can exclude schizophrenia and manic-depressive psychosis. It is well to remember that acute onset of mental symptoms always suggests a confusional state of delirium; inasmuch as these conditions are generally reversible, they must be distinguished from the dementing diseases (see preceding sections).

Once it is decided that the patient suffers from a dementing disease, the next step is to determine, by careful physical examination, whether there are other signs or indications of neurologic or medical disease. This enables the physician to place the case in one of the three categories of the bedside classification (Table 23-2). CT scans, MRI, EEG, lumbar puncture, and toxic metabolic studies are obtained. The final step is to determine, from the total clinical picture, the particular disease within any one category. This may sometimes be difficult. If the dementia is of recent onset, complicated by the use of drugs, or associated with temporal lobe seizures or an endocrine disease, a period of observation may be required before the diagnosis can be settled. Finally, it is important to keep in mind that the correct diagnosis of treatable forms of mental disease (e.g., general paresis, subdural hematoma, brain tumor, chronic drug intoxication, normal-pressure hydrocephalus, pellagra and other deficiency states, and hypothyroidism) is of greater practical importance than the diagnosis of the untreatable ones.

SENILE DEMENTIA AND OTHER CEREBRAL DISEASES COMPLICATED BY MEDICAL OR SURGICAL ILLNESS (BECLOUDED DEMENTIA)
Many elderly patients who enter the hospital with a medical or surgical illness are mentally confused. Presumably this deterioration is determined by preexisting brain disease, in most instances senile dementia of the Alzheimer type, which may or may not have been obvious to the family before the onset of the complicating illness. Other cerebral diseases (vascular, neoplastic, or demyelinative) may have the same effect.

All the clinical features that one observes in the acute confusional states may be present. The severity varies greatly. The confusion may be reflected only in the patient's inability to relate sequentially the history of the illness, or it may be so severe that the patient is virtually *non compos mentis*.

Although almost any complicating illness may bring out the

confusion, it is particularly frequent with infectious diseases; with posttraumatic and postoperative states, notably after concussive brain injuries and the removal of cataracts (in which case the confusion is probably related to being temporarily deprived of vision); and with congestive heart failure, chronic respiratory disease, and severe anemia, especially pernicious anemia. Often it is difficult to determine which of several possible factors is responsible for the confusion, and there may be more than one. In a cardiac patient with a confusional psychosis, for example, there may be low-grade fever, a marginally reduced cerebral blood flow, intoxication with one or more drugs, marginal renal function, and water and electrolyte imbalance.

When these patients recover from their medical or surgical illness, they usually return to their premorbid state, though their shortcomings, now drawn to the attention of the family and physician, may be more obvious than before.

THE AMNESIC SYNDROME   The *amnesic syndrome, the amnestic-confabulatory syndrome,* and *Korsakoff's psychosis* are terms used interchangeably to designate a unique but common disorder of cognitive function in which memory is deranged out of all proportion to other components of mentation and behavior. It possesses two salient features which may vary in severity but are always conjoined: (1) an impaired ability to recall events and other information that had been recorded before the onset of the illness (retrograde amnesia), and (2) an impaired ability to acquire new information, i.e., to learn or to form new memories (anterograde amnesia). Other cognitive functions (particularly the capacity for concentration, spatial organization, and visual and verbal abstraction), which depend little or not at all on memory, are also impaired but to a relatively minor degree. The patient tends to lack initiative and spontaneity and is usually complacent. Ability to repeat a series of numbers or a spoken sentence (immediate memory) is intact. Recent memories are affected more than remote ones, but the extent of this varies with the nature and severity of the disease. *Confabulation,* meaning the fabrication of ready answers or the recital of fictitious experiences, is variably present. The latter is observed mainly in the acute phase of the illness.

The definition of Korsakoff's psychosis is predicated also upon the intactness of certain aspects of behavior and mental function. The patient should be alert, attentive, responsive, and capable of understanding the written and spoken word, capable of making appropriate deductions from given premises, and capable of solving such problems as can be concluded within his or her forward memory span. These "negative" features are of particular importance because they help to distinguish Korsakoff's psychosis from a number of other disorders in which the basic defect is not in retentive memory but in some

TABLE 23-3   Frequency of dementing cerebral diseases (417 patients)

	Number	Percent
Dementia of unknown cause*	199	47.7
Alcoholic dementia (Korsakoff's syndrome)	42	10.0
Multi-infarct dementia	39	9.4
Normal-pressure hydrocephalus	25	6.0
Intracranial masses	20	4.8
Huntington's chorea	12	2.9
Drug toxicity	10	2.4
Posttraumatic dementia	7	1.7
Other identified cerebral diseases (subarachnoid hemorrhage, hypo- and hyperthyroidism, encephalitis, hypoxia, pernicious anemia, etc.)	28	6.7
Pseudodementias:		5.5
Schizophrenia	5	
Depression	16	
Mania	2	
Other:		2.6
No diagnosis	7	
No dementia	4	

* *The majority of patients in this group are assumed to have Alzheimer's disease.*
SOURCE: *Wells, 1977.*

other psychological mechanism, e.g., in attention and perception (as in the delirious, confused, or stuporous patient), in recall (as in the hysterical patient), or in volition (as in the abulic patient with frontal lobe disease).

Pathologic anatomy The anatomic structures of particular importance in memory function are the diencephalon (specifically the medial portions of the medial dorsal nuclei of the thalamus) and the inferomedial portions of the temporal lobes, particularly the hippocampal formations and underlying white matter. Bilaterally placed lesions in either of these regions derange memory and learning out of all proportion to other cognitive functions, and even a unilateral lesion in the dominant thalamus or hippocampus produces the same effect to a lesser degree. It would appear that the aforementioned anatomic structures are involved in all forms of learning and integration of newly formed memories, and that they form a tenuous but vital link between the high brainstem reticular formation (the integrity of which is necessary to maintain an alert state of mind, a prerequisite for any learning) and the cerebral cortex, which is the locus for special memories, i.e., memories for words, geometric figures, numbers, and so forth.

Classification of diseases characterized by an amnesic syndrome A classification of these diseases is given in Table 23-4. Some of these amnesic syndromes are unique. For example, in *transient global amnesia,* described originally by Fisher and Adams, an elderly person (usually over 50 years) will suddenly become bewildered, being uncertain as to his or her whereabouts, the time of day, and what he or she is doing. If told, the patient quickly forgets and asks the same questions repeatedly. In contrast to the patient having a temporal lobe seizure, the patient with transient global amnesia is in contact with the environment and can reply to complex questions, read, calculate, and perform routine tasks. There is also a loss of memory for events that had occurred hours or days before the attack began. During the episode of amnesia, there is no evidence of pallor, twitching, or altered consciousness. Within a few hours the patient makes a complete recovery but is left with a gap in memory that covers the period of the attack and a short period before its onset. During the attack, an EEG may disclose minor changes in the temporal regions. An ischemic attack due to occlusive disease of the temporal branches of the posterior cerebral arteries is one postulated cause. Most patients have only a single attack and no treatment is necessary. Second, third, or several attacks may occur, however, and nothing is known about how to prevent them.

Herpes simplex encephalitis is a common cause of an amnesic state, because of its tendency to localize in the medial parts of the temporal lobes (see Chap. 347). In some patients with carcinomatosis, a limbic encephalitis of unknown etiology has been found (see Chap. 304). Some gliomas infiltrate the temporal lobes, fornices, and

TABLE 23-4 Classification of diseases characterized by an amnesic syndrome

I Amnesic syndrome of sudden onset, usually with gradual but incomplete recovery
   A Bilateral or unilateral (dominant) hippocampal infarction due to atherosclerotic-thrombotic or embolic occlusion of the posterior cerebral arteries or their inferior temporal branches
   B Trauma to the diencephalic or inferomedial temporal regions
   C Spontaneous subarachnoid hemorrhage
   D Carbon monoxide poisoning and other hypoxic states (rare)
II Amnesia of sudden onset and brief duration with full recovery
   A Temporal lobe seizures
   B Postconcussive states
   C Transient global amnesia
III Amnesic syndrome of subacute onset with varying degrees of recovery, usually leaving permanent residue
   A Wernicke-Korsakoff disease
   B Herpes simplex encephalitis
   C Tuberculous and other forms of meningitis characterized by a granulomatous exudate at the base of the brain
IV Slowly progressive amnesic states
   A Tumors involving the walls of the third ventricle and temporal lobes
   B Alzheimers disease and other degenerative disorders (early stage only)

thalamus over a period of weeks to months, resulting in a characteristic syndrome.

In many of these diseases other components of intellectual function are impaired and other neurologic disorders are conjoined. Lack of impulse—a psychomotor retardation—is the most frequent.

OTHER BEHAVIORAL DISORDERS ASSOCIATED WITH CEREBRAL DISEASE When one attempts to categorize all the patients with relatively acute or subacute disorders of mentation and behavior under the types of syndromes above, there are still a considerable number that remain difficult to classify. They present themselves as an almost infinite variety of syndromes in which the following abnormalities of function may occur: reduced or increased levels of speech, thought, and action; disorientation as to time and place; loss of initiative and lack of interest; loss of spontaneity and sense of humor; muteness and hypokinesia, resistiveness and negativism; hostility, lack of observance of social customs, and use of abusive and vulgar language; inexplicable fright, euphoria, or lack of proper concern; complaints of visual distortion or of excess sensitivity to sounds; distortions of smell and taste; inability to find the names of objects, to follow a conversation, and to think coherently; sexual indiscretion, lack of modesty, and other signs of disinhibition; seizures; and disturbances of sleep. Obviously these many symptoms do not all have the same basic significance, and the majority possess only relative localizing value. They may be associated with definite hemiparesis, hemihypesthesia, frank aphasia, or homonymous hemianopsia, but even without these lateralizing signs they point to the existence of cerebral disease.

Syndromes comprising these elements may be observed in subacute sclerosing panencephalitis, listeriosis with meningoencephalitis, Behçet's meningoencephalitis, adult toxoplasmosis, infectious mononucleosis, acute or subacute demyelinative diseases (acute or subacute recurrent multiple sclerosis), granulomatous and other forms of angiitis, gliomatosis cerebri, carcinomatosis with encephalopathy of multifocal type, multiple tumor metastases, acute and subacute bacterial endocarditis, and thrombotic thrombocytopenia. Fuller accounts of some of the cerebral symptoms enumerated above are found in chapters dealing with these diseases.

PATIENT MANAGEMENT

CARE OF THE DELIRIOUS AND CONFUSED PATIENT The primary therapeutic effort is directed to the control of the underlying medical disease. Other important objectives are to quiet the patient and protect him or her against injury. A private nurse, an attendant, or a member of the family should be with the patient at all times, if this can be arranged. Depending on the degree of the patient's activity, a locked room, screened windows, and a low bed should be arranged. It is preferable that the patient be allowed to walk about the room rather than be tied into bed, which may provoke him or her to struggle to the point of exhaustion and collapse. If less active, the patient can be kept in bed by leather wrist restraints, a restraining sheet, or a net thrown over the bed. The patient should be permitted to sit up or walk part of the day, unless this is contraindicated by the primary disease.

Any drug that can possibly be responsible for the acute confusional state or delirium should be discontinued (unless withdrawal effects are believed to underlie the illness). In these circumstances, chlordiazepoxide, chlorpromazine, and diazepam are the drugs favored by most physicians, but the older sedatives—paraldehyde and chloral hydrate—are equally safe and effective if given in full doses. Whichever drug is used should be given until natural sleep is restored. In the case of severe delirium, drugs must be used with caution. One should not attempt to suppress agitation completely; to accomplish this may require very large doses of drugs, and vital functions may then be dangerously impaired. The purpose of sedation is to blunt the agitation so that the patient does not become exhausted and nursing care is facilitated.

Confusional states related to antidepressant drugs, e.g., amitriptyline, are said to be reversed by a 2-mg dose of physostigmine.

A fluid intake and output chart should be kept, and any fluid and electrolyte deficit should be corrected. The pulse and blood pressure should be recorded at frequent intervals in anticipation of circulatory collapse. Transfusions of whole blood and vasopressor drugs may be lifesaving if shock develops.

Finally, the physician should be aware of many small therapeutic measures that may allay fear and suspicion and reduce the tendency toward hallucinations. The room should be kept dimly lighted at night, and if possible the patient should not be moved from one room to another. Every procedure should be explained in detail, even such simple ones as the taking of blood pressure or temperature. The presence of a member of the family may enable the patient to maintain contact with reality.

Most delirious patients tend to recover if they receive competent medical and nursing care. The family should be reassured on this point and must also understand that the abnormal behavior and irrational actions of the patient are not willful but rather are symptomatic of a brain disease. Once recovered, the patient will be at least partly amnesic for the period of confusion; the gap must be filled by information provided by physician and family.

MANAGEMENT OF THE PATIENT WITH DEMENTIA AND THE AMNESIC STATE These major mental derangements are clinical states of the most serious nature, and usually it is worthwhile to admit the patient to the hospital for a period of observation. The physician then has an opportunity to see the patient several times in a neutral and fairly constant hospital environment, and certain special procedures such as CT scan, MRI, lumbar puncture and EEG as well as analysis of blood for endocrine state, toxic or metabolic abnormalities, and drugs can be carried out.

Once it is established that the patient has an untreatable dementing or amnesic brain disease, a responsible member of the family should be apprised of the medical facts. The patient should be told that he or she has a neurologic condition for which rest and treatment has been prescribed; often little is accomplished by telling more. The family should be given the diagnosis and prognosis if these are sufficiently certain for this to be done. If the abnormalities are slight and circumstances are suitable, the patient should remain at home, continue customary activities, and receive appropriate medication. If the patient becomes demented while still at work, plans for occupational retirement should be carried out. In more advanced stages of disease, mental and physical enfeeblement become pronounced and institutional care should be advised. Seizures should be treated symptomatically. Nerve tonics, vitamins, and hormones are of no value in the treatment of dementia. They may, however, offer some support to the patient and family. Sometimes, stimulants in the form of dextroamphetamine, caffeine, and nicotinic acid cause transitory improvement in mental function. Undesirable restlessness, nocturnal wandering, belligerency, or anxiety may be reduced by appropriate sedative drugs. Drugs advocated for specific treatment of dementia are currently under investigation.

REFERENCES

ADAMS RD, VICTOR M: *Principles of Neurology*, 3d ed. New York, McGraw-Hill, 1985

BENSON FD, BLUMER D: *Psychiatric Aspects of Neurologic Disease*. New York, Grune & Stratton, 1975, chap 2

BLESSED, G et al: The association between quantitative measures of dementia and of senile change in the cerebral grey matter of elderly subjects. Brit J Psychiat 114:797, 1968

BUTTERS N, MILIOTIS, P: Amnesic disorders, in *Clinical Neuropsychology*, K Heilman and E Valenstein (eds). London, Oxford, 1985, pp 403–451

ENGEL GL, ROMANO J: Delirium, a syndrome of cerebral insufficiency. J Chronic Dis 9:260, 1959

FISHER CM, ADAMS RD: Episodic global amnesia. Acta Neurol Scand 40:Suppl 9, 1964

GRAFF-RADFORD, NR et al: Nonhaemorrhagic thalamic infarction: Clinical, neuropsychological and electrophysiological findings in four anatomical groups defined by computerized tomography. Brain 108:485, 1985

LIPOWSKI ZJ: *Delirium: Acute Brain Failure in Man*. Springfield, Ill., Charles C Thomas, 1980

LISHMAN WA: *Organic Psychiatry: The Psychological Consequences of Cerebral Disorders*. Oxford, Blackwell, 1978

TERRY RD, KATZMAN R: Senile dementia of the Alzheimer type. Ann Neurol 14:497, 1983

TOMLINSON BE: The pathology of dementia, in *Dementia*, CE Wells (ed). Philadelphia, Davis, 1977, chap 6

WELLS CE: *Dementia*, 2d ed. Philadelphia, Davis, 1977

WELLS CE: Treatable forms of dementia, in *Update II: Harrison's Principles of Internal Medicine*, KJ Isselbacher et al (eds). New York, McGraw-Hill, 1981

24 SYNDROMES DUE TO FOCAL CEREBRAL LESIONS

RAYMOND D. ADAMS / MAURICE VICTOR

In addition to the general syndromes described in Chap. 23, there are many others which relate to lesions of particular parts of the cerebrum. Recognition of these constitutes irrefutable evidence that all parts of the cerebrum are not functionally equivalent. Some of the symptoms and signs which make up these syndromes have the same diagnostic value as a hemiplegia, and, once identified, require the same type of clinical analysis as to cause and pathophysiologic mechanism.

These focal syndromes will be described in terms of the conventional anatomic divisions of the cerebrum, but it will be obvious that most diseases do not respect these boundaries. Hence the syndromes may overlap or occur in a number of combinations.

FRONTAL LOBES In Fig. 24-1, it is seen that the frontal lobes lie anterior to the central (rolandic) sulcus and superior to the Sylvian

FIGURE 24-1 *Diagram to show cortical areas, numbered according to the scheme of Brodmann. The speech areas are in black, the three main ones of which are 39, 41, and 45. The zone marked by vertical stripes in the superior frontal convolution is the secondary motor area which, like Broca's area 45, if stimulated causes vocal arrest. (After Handbuch der Inneren Medizin, Berlin, Springer-Verlag, 1939.)*

Calcarine Fissure

fissure. They consist of several functionally different parts, which are conventionally designated in the neurologic literature by numbers (according to the scheme devised by Brodmann) or by letters (according to the scheme of von Economo and Koskinas).

The posterior parts, areas 4 and 6 of Brodmann, are specifically related to motor function. There is also a secondary motor area in the posterior part of the superior frontal convolution. Voluntary movement in humans depends on the integrity of these areas, and lesions in them produce spastic paralysis of the contralateral face, arm, and leg. This is discussed in Chap. 15. A lesion limited more or less to the premotor area (area 6) is accompanied by a contralateral grasp reflex, and bilateral lesions are accompanied by a suck reflex. A lesion in area 8 of Brodmann interferes with the mechanism concerned with turning the head and eyes contralaterally. A lesion of the left supplementary motor area can result in mutism at its onset; in time the condition resolves to a state of transcortical motor aphasia with reduced language output with preserved repetition and naming. There may be hypokinesia of the arms, especially on the right. Lesions of the left premotor area in many instances result in a phonetic-articulatory defect (*cortical dysarthria*) and verbal perseveration. Agrammatism, with retention of ''content words'' but not of functional connecting words, is characteristic (see Chap. 22). A lesion in area 44 (Broca's area) of the dominant cerebral hemisphere, usually the left one, results in at least a temporary loss of verbal expression. Lesions of the anterior cingulate gyrus, in the acute stages, may cause a speechless, aphonic state; with recovery, speech returns through whispering and hoarseness rather than dysarthria and aphasia, according to Brown. Lesions in the medial limbic or piriform cortex (areas 23 and 24), where the mechanisms controlling respiration, circulation, and micturition are organized bilaterally, have relatively unclear clinical effects.

The remaining parts of the frontal lobes (areas 9 to 12 of Brodmann), sometimes called the *prefrontal areas,* have less specific and measurable functions. In contrast to the motor areas of the frontal lobes and other areas of the brain, stimulation of the prefrontal areas in humans has yielded a paucity of findings. Many patients with gunshot wounds of these areas have shown only mild and inconsistent abnormalities of behavior. Nevertheless, the following groups of symptoms have been observed in patients with large lesions of one or both of the frontal lobes and of the central white matter and the anterior part of the corpus callosum by which they are joined:

1 Lack of initiative and spontaneity in conjunction with diminished speech and with motor inactivity (apathetic-akinetic-abulic state). Necessary daily activities are neglected. Interpersonal social reactions are reduced and shallow.

2 Change of personality, usually expressed as lack of concern over the consequences of any action. Sometimes it may take the form of a childish excitement, an inappropriate joking and punning, a thoughtless impulsivity, an instability and superficiality of emotion, or irritability. The capacity for worry, anxiety, and depression (tortured self-concern) is reduced.

3 Slight impairment of intelligence, usually described as lack of concentration, vacillation of attention, inability to carry out planned activity, difficulty in changing from one activity to another, or perseveration. Goldstein reduced the difficulty to a loss of the capacity for abstract thinking, but the authors believe this tendency to concrete thinking to be another manifestation of abulia and perseveration. According to Luria, who views the frontal lobe as a regulating mechanism of the organism's activities, planned action is deficient with respect to steady control and goal orientation. With left frontal lesions, intelligence is reduced more (10 points on the IQ scale) than with right frontal lesions, probably because of reduced verbal skills. There is also a memory impairment, usually slight, probably because of loss of the mental strategies needed for memorization and recall.

4 Motor abnormalities such as decomposition of gait and upright stance, wide-based gait, flexed posture, and small shuffling steps, culminating in an inability to stand (Bruns' frontal lobe ataxia or

gait apraxia) accompanied by abnormal postures, reflex grasping or sucking, and incontinence of sphincters.

Some differences have been noted between the dominant (left) and right frontal lobes. In psychological tests, left frontal lesions impair verbal fluency and cause a greater degree of perseveration, and right frontal lesions impair the learning of visual spatial patterns and cause impersistence (see Hecaen and Albert, and Luria for details). From these comments it should be evident that the frontal lobes have not a unitary function, but participate in a number of interconnected functional components, each subserving a different component of behavior

TEMPORAL LOBES The boundaries of the temporal lobes are illustrated in Fig. 24-1. The Sylvian fissure separates the superior surface of each temporal lobe from the frontal lobe and anterior part of the parietal lobe. There is no definite anatomic boundary between the temporal and occipital lobes or the posterior temporal and parietal lobes. The temporal lobe includes the superior, middle, and inferior temporal, fusiform, and hippocampal convolutions and the transverse convolutions of Heschl, which are the auditory receptive area, present on the superior surface within the Sylvian fissure. The hippocampal convolution was once believed to be related to olfactory function, but now it is known that lesions here do not cause anosmia. Only the medial and anterior parts of the temporal lobes (uncal regions) are related to smell. The lower fibers of the geniculocalcarine pathway (from the inferior retina) swing in a wide arc over the temporal horn of the ventricle into the white matter of the temporal lobe en route to the occipital lobes, and lesions which interrupt them characteristically produce a contralateral upper homonymous quadrantanopsia. Hearing, localized in the superior surfaces of the temporal lobes (Heschl's gyri), is bilaterally represented, which accounts for the fact that both temporal lobes need to be affected to cause deafness. Loss of equilibrium has not been observed with temporal lobe lesions. Disease in the superior convolution of the left temporal lobe and adjacent inferior parietal lobule in right-handed individuals results in a Wernicke's aphasia. This syndrome, discussed in Chap. 22, consists of paraphasic speech or jargon aphasia and inability to read, write, repeat, or understand the meaning of spoken words.

Between the auditory and olfactory projection areas there is a large expanse of temporal lobe which subserves three specific functional systems. In the inferolateral parts (areas 20, 21, and 37) are located some of the visual-associated projections. In the superior-lateral parts (areas 22, 41, and 42) are the primary and secondary areas for acoustic perception. In the mediobasal parts are the limbic structures (amygdaloid nuclei and hippocampi) where the neural organizations for emotional and memory processes lie. Bilateral lesions of the visual parts result in cortical blindness; visual and limbic disorders contribute to the Klüver-Bucy syndrome. Bilateral hippocampal/parahippocampal lesions produce a deficit in which the patient is unable to record events and information, i.e., has a loss of memory, in both its general and specific aspects (see Chap. 23). Lastly, the temporal lobes include a large part of the limbic system, which subserves the emotional and motivational aspects of behavior and vegetative functions (''visceral brain'').

Apart from aphasia, psychological studies have shown a difference between the effects of dominant and nondominant temporal lobe lesions. With dominant lesions there is impairment in learning auditorially presented verbal material; with nondominant lesions there is a failure in learning visually presented nonverbal material. In addition, about 20 percent of patients with either a right or left lobectomy have shown an alteration of personality similar to that described after lesions in the prefrontal parts of the brain (see above).

The study of patients with uncinate epilepsy, with the characteristic dreamy state, olfactory or gustatory hallucinations, and masticatory movements, suggests that all these functions are organized through the temporal lobes. Stimulation of the posterior parts of the temporal lobes of fully conscious epileptic patients during surgical procedures has brought to light the interesting fact that complex memories and visual and auditory images, some with strong emotional content, can be aroused. Studies of the effects of stimulation of the amygdaloid nucleus, which is in the anterior and medial part of the temporal lobe, have shed additional light on this subject. Some symptoms like those of schizophrenia and mania may be evoked. Complex emotional experiences that had occurred previously may be revived. There are also remarkable autonomic effects: the blood pressure rises, pulse increases, respirations increase in frequency and depth, and the patient looks frightened. In temporal lobe epilepsy, there may be an intensification of the patient's emotional reactions, vague preoccupation with moral and religious issues, a tendency to write excessively, and sometimes aggressiveness. Ablation of the amygdaloid nuclei has eliminated uncontrollable rage reactions in psychotic patients. Hippocampal and adjacent convolutions have been excised bilaterally, with a disastrous loss of ability to learn or to establish new memories (Korsakoff psychosis).

Bilateral destruction of the temporal lobes in both humans and monkeys results in placidity, loss of visual recognition, tendency to examine objects by touch and mouthing, and hypersexuality. This is called the Klüver-Bucy syndrome.

The abnormalities consequent upon lesions of the temporal lobes may be summarized as follows:

1 Effects of unilateral disease of the dominant temporal lobe
 a Upper homonymous quadrantanopsia
 b Wernicke's aphasia
 c Impairment in tests of verbal material presented through the auditory sense
 d Dysnomia or amnesic aphasia
 e Amusia (inability to name scores and read and write music)
2 Effects of unilateral disease of nondominant temporal lobe
 a Upper homonymous quadrantanopsia
 b Inability to judge spatial relationships in rare cases
 c Impairment in tests of nonverbal visually presented material
 d Agnosia for nonlexical qualities of music
3 Effects of disease of either temporal lobe
 a Auditory illusions and hallucinations
 b Psychotic behavior (aggressivity)
4 Effects of bilateral disease
 a Korsakoff amnesic defect
 b Apathy and placidity ⎫
 c Increased sexual activity ⎬ Klüver-Bucy syndrome
 d Sham rage ⎭
 e Cortical deafness
 f Loss of other unilateral functions

PARIETAL LOBES   The postcentral convolution is the terminus of somatic sensory pathways from the opposite half of the body. However, destructive lesions here do not abolish cutaneous sensation but cause mainly a defect in sensory discrimination with variable impairment of primary sensation. In other words, the perception of painful, tactile, thermal, and vibratory stimuli is affected little or not at all, whereas stereognosis, sense of position, distinction between single and double contacts (two-point threshold), and the localization of sensory stimuli are impaired or lost (atopognosia). There is also the phenomenon of extinction, i.e., if a stimulus (tactile, painful, visual) is delivered simultaneously to both sides of the body, only the stimulus on the normal side is perceived. This type of sensory disturbance, sometimes called *cortical sensory defect,* is discussed in Chap. 18. Extensive lesions deep in the white matter of the parietal lobes produce an impairment of all forms of sensation contralaterally, and if these lesions encroach upon the uppermost part of the temporal lobe, there may be a contralateral homonymous hemianopsia, often incongruous and greater in the inferior quadrants. Lesions of the angular gyrus of the dominant hemisphere result in an inability to read (alexia).

More recent investigations have centered on the function of the parietal lobes in the perception of one's position in space, the interrelationships of objects in space, and the relationship of the various parts of the body to one another. Since the time of Babinski it has been known that patients with large lesions of the minor parietal lobe are often unaware of their hemiplegias and hemianesthesias. Babinski called this condition *anosognosia.* Related psychological disorders are lack of recognition of the left arm and leg, neglect of the left side of the body (as in dressing) and of the external space on the left side, and constructional apraxia (an inability to construct simple figures). All of these disorders may occur with left-sided lesions as well but are observed only infrequently, in part because the aphasia that occurs with lesions of the left hemisphere makes it difficult to adequately test other parietal lobe functions.

Another frequent constellation of symptoms, usually referred to as *Gerstmann's syndrome,* occurs only with lesions of the dominant parietal lobe. This consists of inability to write (agraphia), calculate (acalculia), distinguish right from left, and identify fingers (finger agnosia). This syndrome is a true *agnosia,* since it represents a defect in the formulation and use of symbolic concepts, including the significance of numbers and letters and the names of parts of the body. An ideomotor apraxia may or may not be associated. *Apraxia* and *agnosia* are discussed in Chaps. 15 and 18.

The effects of disease of the parietal lobes may be organized into three major categories:

1 Effects of unilateral disease of the parietal lobe, right or left
 a Cortical sensory syndrome and sensory extinction (or total hemianesthesia with large acute lesions of white matter)
 b In children, mild contralateral hemiparesis and hemiatrophy
 c Visual inattention or, less often, homonymous hemianopsia, and sometimes anosognosia, neglect of the opposite one-half of the body and extrapersonal space (more frequent with right than with left parietal lesions)
 d Abolition of optokinetic nystagmus to one side
2 Effects of unilateral disease of the dominant parietal lobe (left hemisphere in right-handed patients), additional phenomena
 a Disorders of language (especially alexia)
 b Gerstmann's syndrome
 c Bimanual astereognosis (tactile agnosia)
 d Bilateral apraxia of the ideomotor type
3 Effects of lesions of the nondominant parietal lobe, additional phenomena
 a Disorders of location and orientation, and constructional apraxia
 b Unawareness of paralysis (anosognosia) and misidentification of left arm and leg
 c Dressing apraxia
 d Bland mood, indifference to illness or neurologic defects

In all these lesions, if sufficiently extensive, there may be a reduction in the capacity to think clearly, inattentiveness, and impaired memory.

OCCIPITAL LOBES   The occipital lobes are the termini of the geniculocalcarine pathways and are essential for visual sensation and perception. Destructive lesions in one occipital lobe result in a contralateral homonymous hemianopsia, i.e., a loss of vision in part or all of the homonymous fields. Occasionally patients complain of changes in the form and contour of visually perceived objects (metamorphopsia), as well as illusory displacement of images from one side of the visual field to another (visual allesthesia), or of abnormal persistence of the visual image after the object has been removed (palinopsia). Visual illusions and elementary (unformed) hallucinations may also occur. Bilateral lesions cause "cortical" blindness, a state of blindness without change in optic fundi or pupillary reflexes.

Lesions in Brodmann's areas 18 and 19 of the dominant hemisphere (Fig. 24-1) cause a loss of recognition of objects presented visually, despite the ability to see, at least to some degree—a state termed *visual object agnosia.* In the classic form of this disorder, individuals with intact mental powers are unable to recognize objects visually, even though by tests of visual acuity and perimetry they appear to see sufficiently well to do so; they are able to recognize objects by tactile or other nonvisual senses. In these terms, *alexia*, or inability to read, represents a visual verbal agnosia or "word blindness." Patients can see letters and words but do not know their meaning, although they can still recognize them through tactile or auditory senses. Other types of agnosia, for recognition of faces (prosopagnosia), for a complex of objects the elements of which are perceived but not the whole (simultanagnosia), and for color, and Balint's syndrome (inability to look at and grasp an object, visual ataxia, and visual inattention) are observed with bilateral occipital lesions.

The details of these syndromes of the different lobes of the cerebrum can be found in the textbook of Adams and Victor and the monograph by Walsh.

CORPUS CALLOSUM AND THE DISCONNECTION SYNDROMES
Considerable attention has been devoted to the study of each of the two cerebral hemispheres in isolation. This is possible only when the corpus callosum, which forms a bridge between the two hemispheres, is surgically sectioned (for epilepsy) or destroyed by infarction or tumors. From these studies emerges the well-known fact that the left hemisphere is dominant in all language functions and auditory perception and the right hemisphere is superior in spatial and visual perception. Partial lesions of the corpus callosum or of the long tracts in the cerebral white matter are found to be associated with a number of interesting syndromes (commissural and intrahemispheric) which will be described below.

When the corpus callosum is sectioned by a surgical procedure or destroyed by an anterior cerebral artery occlusion (anterior four-fifths), the language and perceptual areas of the left hemisphere are isolated from the sensory and motor areas of the right hemisphere. These patients, if blindfolded, are then unable to match an object held in one hand with an identical object in the other hand. Further, they cannot match an object seen in the right half of the visual field with one in the left half. If given verbal commands, they perform correctly with the right hand but not with the left. Without vision, objects placed in the right hand are named correctly, but not those in the left. In lesions confined to the posterior fifth of the corpus callosum (splenium), only the visual part of the disconnection syndrome occurs. Occlusion of the left posterior cerebral artery provides the best examples of this. Infarction of the left occipital lobe cause a right homonymous hemianopsia, as a consequence of which all visual information needed for activating the speech areas of the left hemisphere must come from the right occipital lobe, across the splenium of the corpus callosum. If there is a lesion in the corpus callosum (or in other portions of the crossing fibers), the patient cannot read or name colors because the visual information cannot reach the left angular gyrus. There is no difficulty in copying words, though the patient cannot read what he or she has written; matching colors without naming them is done without error. Apparently the visual information for activating the left motor area crosses the corpus callosum more anteriorly. A disconnection in the anterior third of the corpus callosum, where fiber systems between the right and left premotor areas must pass, results only in failure of the left hand to obey commands, the right one performing perfectly (left-sided apraxia). The left hand can still imitate the examiner's movements or carry out the patient's intention.

There are also intrahemispheric disconnections, of which the most important are the following:

1 *Conduction aphasia* (also called *central* aphasia). The patient has fluent but paraphasic speech and writing with nearly perfect comprehension of spoken or written language. Repetition of what is heard or read is, however, severely impaired. The lesion is presumably in the arcuate fasciculus, which connects Wernicke's area with Broca's area.
2 *Pure word deafness*. Although the patient is able to hear and identify nonverbal sounds, there is a loss of ability to comprehend spoken language. The patient's speech remains normal. The defect has been attributed to a subcortical lesion, undercutting Wernicke's area.

The reader is referred to Geschwind and to Dimond for further details on the disconnection syndromes.

DIAGNOSIS AND MANAGEMENT OF PATIENTS WITH FOCAL CEREBRAL LESIONS
These involve the same principles described in Chap. 23. Special tests, mostly of the psychological type, are available for each of the focal cerebral syndromes (Walsh). The investigation and care of individual patients will, of course, also be governed by the underlying disease.

REFERENCES

ADAMS RD, VICTOR M: *Principles of Neurology*, 3d ed. New York, McGraw-Hill, 1985
BRODAL A: *Neurological Anatomy in Relation to Clinical Medicine*, 3d ed. New York, Oxford University Press, 1981
BROWN JW: Frontal lobe syndromes, in *Handbook of Clinical Neurology*, JAM Frederiks (ed). Amsterdam, Elsevier Science, 1985, vol 45, chap 3
DIMOND SJ: The disconnection syndromes, in *Modern Trends in Neurology*, D. Williams (ed). London, Butterworth, 1975
GESCHWIND N: Disconnection syndromes in animals and man. Brain 88:237, 585, 1965
HACAEN H, ALBERT ML: Disorders of mental functioning related to the frontal lobes, in *Modern Trends in Neurology*, D Williams (ed). London, Butterworth, 1975
LURIA AR: *The Working Brain: An Introduction to Neuropsychology*. New York, Basic Books (translation Penguin Books Ltd), 1973
WALSH KW: *Neuropsychology: A Clinical Approach*. London, Churchill Livingstone, 1978

section 4   Alterations in circulatory and respiratory function

25   COUGH AND HEMOPTYSIS

GENNARO M. TISI / EUGENE BRAUNWALD

COUGH

Cough, one of the most frequent cardiorespiratory symptoms, is an explosive expiration which provides a means of clearing the tracheobronchial tree of secretions and foreign bodies.

MECHANISM   Coughing may be initiated either voluntarily or reflexly. As a defensive reflex it has both afferent and efferent pathways. The *afferent limb* includes cough receptors within the sensory distribution of the trigeminal, glossopharyngeal, superior laryngeal, and vagus nerves. The *efferent limb* includes the recurrent laryngeal nerve (which causes glottic closure) and the spinal nerves (which cause contraction of the thoracic and abdominal musculature). The *sequence of a cough* includes an appropriate stimulus which initiates a deep inspiration. This is followed by glottic closure, relaxation of the diaphragm, and muscle contraction against a closed glottis so as to produce maximally positive intrathoracic and intraairway pressures.

These positive intrathoracic pressures result in a narrowing of the trachea, produced by an infolding of its more compliant posterior membrane. Once the glottis opens, the combination of a large pressure differential between the airways and the atmosphere coupled with this tracheal narrowing produces flow rates through the trachea close to the speed of sound. The shearing forces which are developed aid in the elimination of mucus and foreign materials. A tracheostomy short-circuits glottic closure and therefore decreases the effectiveness of the cough mechanism.

ETIOLOGY Cough is produced by inflammatory, mechanical, chemical, and thermal stimulation of the cough receptors. *Inflammatory* stimuli are initiated by edema and hyperemia of the respiratory mucous membranes, and by irritation from exudative processes. Such stimuli may arise either in the airways (as in laryngitis, tracheitis, bronchitis, and bronchiolitis) or in the alveoli (as in pneumonitis and lung abscess). *Mechanical* stimuli are produced by inhalation of particulate matter, such as dust particles, and by compression of the air passages and pressure or tension upon these structures. Lesions associated with airway compression may be either extramural or intramural in type. The former include aortic aneurysms, granulomas, pulmonary neoplasms, and mediastinal tumors; intramural lesions include bronchogenic carcinoma, bronchial adenoma, foreign bodies, granulomatous endobronchial involvement, and contraction of airway smooth muscle (bronchial asthma). Pressure or tension upon the air passages is usually produced by lesions associated with a decrease in pulmonary compliance. Examples of specific causes include acute and chronic interstitial fibrosis (Chap. 209), pulmonary edema, and atelectasis. *Chemical* stimuli may result from inhalation of irritant gases, including cigarette smoke and chemical fumes. Finally, *thermal* stimuli may be produced by inhalation of either very hot or cold air.

Cough is commonly associated with episodic wheezing secondary to bronchoconstriction in symptomatic patients with bronchial asthma (Chap. 202). Recent reports have drawn attention to patients with chronic, persistent cough as the *sole* presenting manifestation of bronchial asthma, ("cough asthma"). Such patients are characterized by (1) absence of a history of episodic wheezing and (2) no evidence of expiratory airflow obstruction by spirometry, but (3) hyperreactive airways (characteristic of asthma) when challenged with a cholinergic agent, methacholine.

DIAGNOSTIC EVALUATION When one is considering the above list of causes, answers to the following general questions will significantly narrow the diagnostic possibilities: Is the cough acute or chronic? Is it productive of sputum or nonproductive?

Features of the history, physical examination, chest roentgenogram, screening pulmonary function studies (static lung volumes and dynamic flow rates), and sputum examination may indicate a specific cause. The *history* may indicate specific diagnoses. Acute episodes of cough may be associated with such viral infections as acute tracheobronchitis or pneumonitis or with bacterial bronchopneumonia. Cough associated with an acute febrile episode and associated with hoarseness is usually produced by viral laryngotracheobronchitis. Postnasal drip is also a common cause of chronic cough.

The character of the cough may suggest the anatomic site of involvement: the patient with a "barking" type of cough may have epiglottal involvement, (i.e., "whooping cough" due to *Haemophilus pertussis* infection in young children), while the cough associated with tracheal or major airway involvement is often loud and "brassy." Cough associated with generalized wheezing may be produced by acute bronchospasm. The time of occurrence of a cough may indicate a specific cause: a cough which occurs selectively at night suggests congestive heart failure; one related to meals suggests a tracheoesophageal fistula, a hiatal hernia, or an esophageal diverticulum; a cough precipitated by a change in position suggests a lung abscess or a localized area of bronchiectasis. The description of sputum or secretions produced in conjunction with the cough may also be helpful: putrid sputum suggests a lung abscess; bloody sputum, bleeding (see "Hemoptysis," below); frothy and pink-tinged sputum,

pulmonary edema; mucoid and massive sputum, alveolar cell carcinoma; purulent and/or large amounts of sputum, lung abscess and bronchiectasis.

On *physical examination* the character of the auscultatory findings may suggest the site of disease: inspiratory stridor and wheezing may be present in laryngeal disease, inspiratory and expiratory rhonchi favor tracheal and major airway involvement, coarse subcrepitant inspiratory rales may indicate interstitial fibrosis and/or edema, fine crepitant rales may indicate a process such as pneumonitis or pulmonary edema, which fills the alveoli with fluid. The *chest roentgenogram* may reveal the cause of the cough; it may show an intrapulmonary mass lesion which may be either central or peripheral (Chap. 213), an alveolar filling process which may be pneumonic or nonpneumonic, an area of honeycombing and cyst formation which may indicate an area of localized bronchiectasis, or bilateral hilar adenopathy which may indicate sarcoidosis or a lymphoma.

Screening pulmonary function studies (Chap. 200) may also indicate specific diagnoses. Significant expiratory obstruction to airflow (as determined from a forced expiratory flow maneuver), coupled with a history of cough and significant sputum production, suggests that irrespective of other lesions the patient has significant bronchitis. Decreased lung volume (as determined from the static lung volumes) indicates that a restrictive type of lung disease is present—reduction of lung volumes produced by thoracic, pleural, alveolar, or interstitial disease. Finally, a careful *sputum examination* may be more enlightening than a patient's description of the character of the sputum. Examination shows whether the sputum is thin or viscid, purulent or not, foul-smelling or not, blood-tinged or not, scant or copious. In pneumococcal pneumonia the sputum has a "rusty" color, while in *Klebsiella* pneumonia it may look like "currant jelly." Gram stain and culture of the deep-cough specimen may reveal a specific bacterial, fungal, or mycoplasmal causation, while sputum cytology may result in a positive diagnosis of a pulmonary neoplasm.

Two features of cough should be highlighted: (1) A cough is often so common in the cigarette smoker as to be ignored or minimized. *Any change in the nature or character of a chronic cigarette cough should initiate immediate diagnostic evaluation, with particular attention directed to detection of bronchogenic carcinoma.* (2) Female patients are inclined to swallow sputum and not to expectorate as male patients do. This tendency may lead to the incorrect conclusion that a cough in a female patient is irritative and nonproductive.

COMPLICATIONS Three complications may be produced by the coughing mechanism: paroxysms of coughing may precipitate syncope (cough syncope, Chap. 12), and strenuous coughing may produce rupture of an emphysematous bleb and rib fractures. A potential mechanism for cough syncope includes the development of markedly positive intrathoracic and alveolar pressures which decrease venous return, producing a decrease in cardiac output and resultant syncope. Although cough fractures of the ribs may occur in otherwise normal patients, their occurrence should at least raise the possibility of pathologic fractures, which are seen in multiple myeloma, osteoporosis, and osteolytic metastases.

THERAPY Definitive treatment of cough depends on determining its precise cause and then initiating specific therapy for the underlying cause. Symptomatic therapy should be considered when the cause of the cough is idiopathic and the cough performs no useful function or represents a potential hazard to the patient. An irritative, nonproductive cough may be suppressed by an antitussive agent, such as codeine or dextromethorphan, 15 mg qid. These drugs are particularly useful in interrupting prolonged, self-perpetuating paroxysms. However, a cough productive of significant quantities of sputum should not be suppressed, since retention of sputum in the tracheobronchial tree may interfere with the distribution of ventilation, alveolar aeration, and the ability of the lung to resist infection. When secretions are tenacious and thick, adequate hydration, expectorants, and humidification of the air with an ultrasonic nebulizer may be helpful.

Ipratropium (a new class of bronchodilator with antimuscarinic actions) may prove especially useful in patients with cough asthma.

HEMOPTYSIS

For purposes of definition hemoptysis includes both blood-streaked sputum and gross hemoptysis. It is apparent that any patient with gross hemoptysis should be given appropriate diagnostic tests so that a specific cause may be found. The patient with blood-streaked sputum should also be studied unless one can be certain that this type of hemoptysis is due to a benign condition. A major pitfall in dealing with hemoptysis is to ascribe recurrent episodes to a previously established diagnosis, such as chronic bronchiectasis or bronchitis. Such an approach may result in missing a serious but potentially treatable lesion. The safest approach to a recurrent episode of hemoptysis is to treat it as if it were the initial episode and proceed with a complete diagnostic evaluation.

ETIOLOGY AND INCIDENCE Prior to embarking upon an extensive diagnostic workup of hemoptysis, it is essential to determine that the blood is in fact coming from the respiratory tract, not from the nasopharynx or gastrointestinal tract. Distinguishing hemoptysis from hematemesis is difficult at times. In hemoptysis, the prodrome is usually a tingling in the throat or a desire to cough, the blood is coughed up, and it is usually bright-red and *frothy*; in hematemesis, the prodrome includes nausea and abdominal discomfort, the blood is vomited, and it is usually *magenta* in color. Once this point is established, the diagnostic tests for hemoptysis may proceed. Although there are numerous single case reports of diseases which have been associated with hemoptysis, Table 25-1 presents the more common disorders.

The incidence of the diagnoses listed in Table 25-1 depends upon the nature of the series reported and whether one includes both gross bleeding and blood streaking of the sputum. If both types of bleeding are included, then the major causes (approximately 60 to 70 percent) are chronic bronchitis and bronchiectasis. If the definition is restricted to gross bleeding (greater than several tablespoons) then the incidence depends upon the type of series reported. Surgical series favor the incidence of mass lesions and operable lesions (carcinoma, 20 percent; localized, segmental, or lobar bronchiectasis, 30 percent). Those from centers with a large tuberculosis population favor this condition (incidence varying between 2 and 40 percent). Combined medical-surgical series include a wider representation of those lesions which present with hemoptysis (carcinoma, 20 percent; bronchiectasis, 30 percent; bronchitis, 15 percent; other inflammatory lesions including tuberculosis, 10 to 20 percent; other lesions including the vascular, traumatic, and hemorrhagic etiologies listed in Table 25-1, 10 percent). Despite the most extensive of evaluations, 5 to 15 percent of cases entailing gross hemoptysis remain undiagnosed.

TABLE 25-1 Causes of hemoptysis

1 Inflammatory
    a Bronchitis
    b Bronchiectasis
    c Tuberculosis
    d Lung abscess
    e Pneumonia, particularly *Klebsiella*
2 Neoplastic
    a Lung cancer: squamous cell, adenocarcinoma, oat cell
    b Bronchial adenoma
3 Other
    a Pulmonary thromboembolism
    b Left ventricular failure
    c Mitral stenosis
    d Traumatic, including foreign body and lung contusion
    e Primary pulmonary hypertension; arteriovenous malformation; Eisenmenger's syndrome; pulmonary vasculitis including Wegener's granulomatosis and Goodpasture's syndrome; idiopathic pulmonary hemosiderosis; and amyloid
    f Hemorrhagic diathesis including anticoagulant therapy

Two points should be highlighted with reference to diseases associated with hemoptysis: (1) *hemoptysis is rare in metastatic carcinoma to the lung*; (2) *although hemoptysis may occur at some time during the course of a viral or pneumococcal pneumonia, it is usually scanty and its occurrence should always raise the question of a more serious underlying process.*

DIAGNOSIS The *history* may suggest specific diagnoses: recurrent, chronic hemoptysis in a young, otherwise asymptomatic female favors the diagnosis of a bronchial adenoma; recurrent hemoptysis with chronic, marked sputum production associated with ring shadows, tram lines (abnormal air bronchograms), and cyst formation on the roentgenogram suggests a diagnosis of bronchiectasis; putrid sputum production suggests a lung abscess; weight loss and anorexia in a male smoker over the age of 40 raise the possibility of a bronchogenic carcinoma; a recent history of blunt trauma to the chest suggests a lung contusion; and acute pleuritic chest pain raises the possibility of pulmonary embolism with infarction or some other pleurally based lesion (lung abscess, coccidioidomycosis cavity, and vasculitis). Several findings on the *physical examination* may also suggest a specific diagnosis: a pleural friction rub suggests those diagnoses just mentioned in connection with pleuritic pain; the findings of pulmonary hypertension raise the diagnostic possibilities of primary pulmonary hypertension, mitral stenosis, recurrent or chronic thromboembolism, and Eisenmenger's syndrome; a localized wheeze over a major lobar airway suggests an intramural lesion such as a bronchogenic carcinoma or a foreign body; systemic arteriovenous communications or the presence of a murmur over the lung fields suggest the diagnosis of Osler-Rendu-Weber disease with pulmonary arteriovenous malformation; evidence of significant expiratory obstruction to airflow coupled with sputum production suggests that whatever other lesion may be present, the patient has significant bronchitis. Finally, the *chest roentgenogram* is critical to diagnosis. The presence of ring shadows favors a diagnosis of bronchiectasis; an air-fluid level, the diagnosis of a lung abscess; and a mass lesion, the diagnosis of a central or peripheral pulmonary neoplasm. A mass lesion which may cause hemoptysis should be distinguished from an area of blood pneumonitis caused by aspiration of blood into contiguous areas.

One of the most demanding diagnostic problems is the identification of the site of bleeding in a patient with normal findings on physical examination and a normal roentgenogram of the chest. A patient with hemoptysis tends to keep the bleeding side dependent. Otherwise, gravitational drainage would cause aspiration into the noninvolved dependent lung. The patient may also be able to give a history of a burning or deep pain which may localize the side of bleeding; bronchoscopy may then be useful. This procedure generally is most helpful when the bleeding is scant, and of least help when the bleeding is massive, since blood may be aspirated into contiguous airways. Such aspiration may produce alveolar filling (i.e., a "blood pneumonitis") that may obscure the etiology of the hemoptysis on the initial chest roentgenogram. Blood pneumonitis usually clears within a week, and once clearing has occurred, a repeat chest roentgenogram may disclose the origin of the hemoptysis.

Following the history and physical examination, the diagnostic approach to a patient with hemoptysis includes whatever specialized studies and procedures are required to make a specific diagnosis. The first step is to obtain a roentgenogram. Usually bronchoscopy is the procedure employed next. Rigid bronchoscopy permits visualization of the more central airways. It is of particular value when the source of bleeding is in this portion of the airway system, the degree of hemoptysis is massive, and selective endobronchial intubation is being considered. Fiberoptic bronchoscopy (Chap. 201) includes within the range of visualization airways as small as several millimeters in diameter. This endoscopic technique may provide definitive visual, biopsy, or cytologic information. Since direct visualization of more peripheral portions of the airway system is now possible, the indications for bronchography in the evaluation of hemoptysis are being modified. The principal indications for bronchography in such patients are (1) to establish the presence of localized bronchiectasis (including a sequestered lobe) and (2) to rule out the presence of more generalized bronchiectasis in a patient with localized disease who is regarded as a surgical candidate because of either repetitive hemoptysis or recurrent infections. The majority of patients with bronchiectasis have a normal chest roentgenogram. If bronchoscopy in such patients is also negative, bronchography is the only means of establishing an anatomic diagnosis of bronchiectasis. If the chest roentgenogram is abnormal, revealing either ring shadows or tram lines, a diagnosis of bronchiectasis may be made without the need for bronchography.

THERAPY Since hemoptysis is such an alarming symptom, there is a tendency to overtreat the patient. Usually hemoptysis is scant and will stop spontaneously without specific therapy. If the hemoptysis is substantial, the mainstays of therapy include keeping the patient calm, instituting complete bed rest, excluding unnecessary diagnostic procedures until the hemoptysis has begun to subside, and suppressing cough if it is present and an aggravating feature of the hemoptysis. The emergency care of such a patient demands that intubation and suctioning equipment be at the bedside. In patients in danger of asphyxiation by flooding of the lung contralateral to the site of hemorrhage, intubation by a technique which isolates the hemorrhaging lung and prevents contralateral aspiration of blood should be carried out. This can be accomplished by strategic location of a balloon catheter whose introduction into the bronchus in question is facilitated by direct visualization through a fiberoptic bronchoscope.

The management of potentially lethal massive hemoptysis remains controversial. The choice between a medical approach and surgical intervention hinges on the words *potentially lethal*. Massive hemoptysis, usually defined as greater than 600 to 800 mL in 24 h, is an alarming clinical situation in which asphyxiation due to aspiration of blood represents the principal threat to life. The choice between surgical and medical management relates most often to the anatomic basis for the massive hemoptysis. In patients with cavitary tuberculosis, anaerobic lung abscess, and lung cancer, the risk of mortality is far greater than when the cause of the hemoptysis is bronchitis or bronchiectasis. Operation may occasionally be necessary in the former, but virtually never in the latter group. In either case the initial management should include the conservative measures suggested above. With such management, spontaneous cessation of bleeding usually occurs. Surgical intervention should be considered in that small group of patients with a definable lesion on chest roentgenogram (i.e., cavitary disease, lung abscess, lung cancer) who have evidence of uncontrollable respiratory or hemodynamic compromise. If a patient is a surgical candidate, bronchoscopy should be performed to identify the specific site of bleeding. Otherwise bronchoscopy should be deferred for several days because of the tendency of this procedure to aggravate cough and thereby perpetuate the hemoptysis. Bronchial arterial catheterization and embolization are new modalities of treatment currently under evaluation for the nonsurgical control of massive hemoptysis, especially in patients with nonresectable lung cancer. Laser (neodymium YAG—yttrium aluminum garnet) therapy should also be considered as a palliative modality for massive hemoptysis in such patients.

REFERENCES

ADELMAN M et al: Cryptogenic hemoptysis: Clinical features, bronchoscopic findings, and natural history in 67 patients. Ann Intern Med 102:829, 1985

BOUSHEY HA et al: Medical staff conference: Evaluating and treating intractable cough. West J Med 143:223, 1985

CONLAN AA: Massive hemoptysis: Diagnostic and therapeutic implications. Surg Ann 17:337, 1985

CORRAO WMC et al: Chronic cough as the sole presenting manifestation of bronchial asthma. N Engl J Med 300:633, 1979

GROSS NJ et al: Anticholinergic, antimuscarinic bronchodilators. Am Rev Resp Dis 129:856, 1984

IRWIN RS et al: Persistent cough in the adult: The spectrum and frequency of causes and successful outcome of specific therapy. Am Rev Resp Dis 123:413, 1981

LEITH DE: The development of cough. Am Rev Respir Dis 131:S39, 1985

WILLIAMS MH: Management of massive hemoptysis. Pulmonary Perspectives, a publication of the American College of Chest Physicians 1:3, 1984

26 DYSPNEA AND PULMONARY EDEMA

ROLAND H. INGRAM, JR. / EUGENE BRAUNWALD

DYSPNEA

The breathing pattern is controlled by a series of higher central and peripheral mechanisms which can increase ventilation in excess of metabolic demands in conditions such as anxiety and fear, and can increase ventilation appropriate to increased metabolic demands during physical activity. A normal resting person is unaware of the act of breathing, and while he or she may become conscious of breathing during mild to moderate exertion, no discomfort is experienced. However, during and following exhausting exertion an individual may become unpleasantly aware of breathing, yet feel reasonably assured that the sensation will be transitory and is appropriate to the level of exercise. Therefore, as a cardinal symptom of diseases affecting the cardiorespiratory system, dyspnea is defined as an *abnormally uncomfortable awareness of breathing*.

Although dyspnea is not painful in the usual sense of the word, it is, like pain, involved with both the perception of a sensation and the reaction to that perception. Patients experience a number of uncomfortable sensations related to breathing and use an even larger number of verbal expressions to describe these sensations, such as "cannot get enough air," "air does not go all the way down," "smothering feeling in the chest," "tightness in the chest," "fatigue in the chest," and a "choking sensation." It may be necessary, therefore, to review meticulously the patient's history in order to ascertain whether the more abstruse descriptions do, in fact, represent dyspnea. Once it is established that a patient does have dyspnea, it is of paramount importance to define the circumstances in which it occurs and to assess associated symptoms. There are situations in which breathing appears labored but in which dyspnea does not occur. For example, the hyperventilation in association with metabolic acidemia is rarely accompanied by dyspnea. On the other hand, patients with apparently normal breathing patterns may complain of shortness of breath.

QUANTITATION OF DYSPNEA The gradation of dyspnea may usefully be based upon the amount of physical exertion required to produce the sensation. In actual practice the major functional classifications of patients with heart or lung disease are based largely on dyspnea in relation to degree of exertion. However, in assessing the severity of dyspnea, it is important to obtain a clear understanding of the patient's general physical condition, work history, and recreational habits. For example, the development of dyspnea in a trained runner upon running 2 mi may signify a more serious disturbance than a similar degree of breathlessness in a sedentary person upon running a fraction of this distance. Some patients with lung or heart disease may have such reduced capabilities due to other disease (e.g., peripheral vascular insufficiency or severe osteoarthritis of the hips or knees) that exertional dyspnea is precluded despite serious impairment of pulmonary or cardiac function.

Some patterns of dyspnea are not directly related to physical exertion. Sudden and unexpected dyspneic episodes at rest can be associated with pulmonary emboli, spontaneous pneumothorax, or anxiety. Nocturnal episodes of severe paroxysmal dyspnea are characteristic of left ventricular failure. Dyspnea upon assuming the supine posture, *orthopnea* (see below), thought to be mainly characteristic of congestive heart failure, may also occur in some patients with asthma and chronic obstruction of the airways and is a regular finding in the rare occurrence of bilateral diaphragmatic paralysis. *Trepopnea* is used to describe the unusual circumstance in which dyspnea occurs only in the left or right lateral decubitus position, most often in patients with heart disease, while *platypnea* is dyspnea which occurs only in the upright position. Both of these patterns remain to be fully explained but may be related to positional alterations in ventilation-perfusion relations (Chap. 200).

MECHANISMS OF DYSPNEA   Physicians usually relate the symptom of dyspnea to a process such as obstruction of the airways or congestive heart failure and generally proceed with further diagnostic and/or therapeutic attempts, having satisfied themselves that they understand the mechanism of the dyspnea. In fact, elucidation of the *actual* mechanism(s) of dyspnea has eluded clinical investigators.

Dyspnea occurs whenever the work of breathing is excessive. Increased force generation is required of the respiratory muscles to produce a given volume change if the chest wall or lungs are less compliant or if resistance to airflow is increased. Increased work of breathing also occurs when the ventilation is excessive for the level of activity. Although an individual is more apt to become dyspneic when the work of breathing is increased, the work theory does not account for the perceptual difference between a deep breath with a normal mechanical load and a normal-sized breath with an increased mechanical load. The work might be the same with both breaths, but the normal one with the increased load will be associated with discomfort. In fact, with respiratory loading, such as adding a resistance at the mouth, there is an increase in respiratory center output, as gauged by newer indexes, that is disproportionate to the increase in work of breathing. Hence, a more appealing theory is one that links inappropriate length to tension in the respiratory muscles. Campbell has proposed that a sense of discomfort arises when there is misalignment of the nerve spindles, which are sensing tension, in relation to muscle length. This misalignment would lead to the sensation that a person is getting an insufficient breath for the tension generated by the respiratory muscles. Such a theory is difficult to test and, if tested and proved in some circumstances, would still not explain why patients who are completely paralyzed, either by cord transections or neuromuscular blockade, experience dyspnea although aided by a mechanical ventilator. It is probable, in these circumstances, that signals from the lungs and/or airways travel via the vagus nerve to the central nervous system to account for the sensation.

In all likelihood several different mechanisms operate to different degrees in the various clinical situations in which dyspnea occurs. Perhaps, in some circumstances, dyspnea is evoked by stimulation of receptors in the upper respiratory tract; in others it may originate from receptors in the lungs, airways, respiratory muscles, or some combination of those structures. In any event, dyspnea is characterized by an excessive or abnormal activation of the respiratory centers in the brainstem. This activation comes about from stimuli transmitted from or through a variety of structures and pathways including (1) intrathoracic receptors via the vagi; (2) afferent somatic nerves, particularly from the respiratory muscles and chest wall, but also from other skeletal muscles and joints; (3) chemoreceptors in the brain, aortic and carotid bodies, and elsewhere in the circulation; (4) higher (cortical) centers; and perhaps (5) afferent fibers in the phrenic nerves. In general, there is a reasonably good correlation between the severity of dyspnea and the disturbances of pulmonary or cardiac function which are responsible.

DIFFERENTIAL DIAGNOSIS   Obstructive disease of airways   (see also Chaps. 202 and 208)   Obstruction to airflow can be present anywhere from the extrathoracic airways out to the small airways in the periphery of the lung. Large extrathoracic airway obstruction can occur acutely, as with aspiration of food or a foreign body or with angioneurotic edema of the glottis. Circumstantial evidence or testimony from witnesses should cause the physician to suspect aspiration, and an allergic history together with a few scattered hives should raise the possibility of glottic edema. The acute form of upper airway obstruction is a medical emergency. More chronic forms can occur with tumors or with fibrotic stenosis following tracheostomy or prolonged endotracheal intubation. Whether acute or chronic, the cardinal symptom is dyspnea, and the characteristic signs are stridor and retraction of the supraclavicular fossae with inspiration.

Obstruction of intrathoracic airways can occur acutely and intermittently or can be present chronically with worsening during respiratory infections. Acute intermittent obstruction with wheezing is typical of *asthma*. Chronic cough with expectoration is typical of *chronic bronchitis* and *bronchiectasis*. Most often there is a prolongation of expiration and coarse rhonchi which are generalized in chronic bronchitis and may be localized in the case of bronchiectasis. Intercurrent infection results in worsening of the cough, increased expectoration of purulent sputum, and more severe dyspnea. During such episodes the patient may complain of nocturnal paroxysms of dyspnea with wheezing relieved by cough and expectoration of sputum.

Many years of exertional dyspnea progressing to dyspnea at rest characterize the patient with predominant *emphysema* (Chap. 208). Although a parenchymal disease by definition, emphysema is invariably accompanied by obstruction of airways.

Diffuse parenchymal lung diseases (see also Chap. 209)   This category includes a large number of diseases ranging from acute pneumonia to chronic disorders such as sarcoidosis and the various forms of *pneumoconiosis*. History, physical findings, and radiographic abnormalities often provide clues to the diagnosis. The patients are often tachypneic with arterial P_{CO_2} and P_{O_2} values below normal. Exertion often further reduces the arterial P_{O_2}. Lung volumes are decreased and the lungs are stiffer, i.e., less compliant than normal.

Pulmonary vascular occlusive diseases (see also Chap. 211)   Repeated episodes of dyspnea at rest often occur with recurrent pulmonary emboli. A source for emboli, such as phlebitis of a lower extremity or the pelvis, is quite helpful in leading the physician to suspect the diagnosis. Arterial blood gases are almost invariably abnormal, but lung volumes are frequently normal or only minimally abnormal.

Diseases of the chest wall or respiratory muscles (see also Chap. 215)   The physical examination establishes the presence of a chest wall disease such as severe kyphoscoliosis, pectus excavatum, or spondylitis. Although all three of these deformities may be associated with dyspnea, only severe kyphoscoliosis regularly interferes with ventilation sufficiently to produce chronic cor pulmonale and respiratory failure. Even though vital capacity, lung volumes, and airflow rates are normal with pectus excavatum, there is some evidence that cardiac compression from the posteriorly displaced sternum interferes with diastolic filling of the ventricle during the increased demands of exercise. Hence a cardiogenic component to the dyspnea may be present in this condition.

Both weakness and paralysis of respiratory muscles can lead to respiratory failure and dyspnea (Chap. 215), but most often the signs and symptoms of the neurologic or muscular disorder are more prominently manifested in other systems.

Heart disease   In patients with cardiac disease exertional dyspnea occurs most commonly as a consequence of an elevated pulmonary capillary pressure; aside from uncommon causes such as obstructive disease of the pulmonary veins (Chap. 185), pulmonary capillary hypertension is a consequence of left atrial hypertension, which in turn may be due to left ventricular dysfunction (Chaps. 181 and 182), reduced left ventricular compliance, and mitral stenosis. The elevation of hydrostatic pressure in the pulmonary vascular bed tends to upset the Starling equilibrium (see ''Pulmonary Edema,'' below) with resulting transudation of liquid into the interstitial space, reducing the compliance of the lungs and stimulating J (juxtacapillary) receptors in the alveolar interstitial space. When prolonged, pulmonary venous hypertension results in thickening of pulmonary vessels and an increase in perivascular cells and fibrous tissue, causing a further reduction in compliance. The competition for space between vessels, airways, and increased liquid within the interstitial space compromises the lumina of small airways, increasing the airways' resistance. Diminution in compliance and an increase in airways' resistance increase the work of breathing which, to some degree, is minimized by a reduction in tidal volume which is compensated for by an increase in frequency of respiration. In severe heart disease, usually involving elevation of both pulmonary and systemic venous pressures, hydro-thorax may develop, further interfering with pulmonary function and intensifying dyspnea. In patients with heart failure and a severely diminished cardiac output, dyspnea may also be related to fatigue of the respiratory muscles as a consequence of their reduced perfusion. The metabolic acidosis characteristic of severe heart failure may play a contributory role. Dyspnea may also be associated with severe systemic and cerebral anoxia, as occurs during exertion in patients with congenital heart disease and right-to-left shunts.

Cardiac dyspnea usually begins as breathlessness on strenuous exertion and, over the course of months or years, progresses until the patient is dyspneic at rest. Occasionally, a nonproductive cough developing in the recumbent position, particularly at night, may be the first complaint.

Orthopnea, i.e., dyspnea in the recumbent position and *paroxysmal nocturnal dyspnea*, i.e., attacks of shortness of breath which usually occur at night and awaken the patient from sleep, are characteristic of more advanced forms of heart failure associated with elevations of pulmonary venous and capillary pressures and are discussed in Chap. 182. Orthopnea is the result of the alteration of gravitational forces when the recumbent position is assumed. This augmentation of intrathoracic blood volume elevates pulmonary venous and capillary pressures which increases the pulmonary closing volume (Chap. 200) and reduces the vital capacity. An additional factor associated with recumbency is the elevation of the diaphragm, which results in a lower end-expiratory lung volume. This combination of lower end-expiratory lung volume and increase in closing volume results in a significant alteration of alveolar-capillary gas exchange.

PAROXYSMAL (NOCTURNAL) DYSPNEA   Also known as *cardiac asthma*, this condition is characterized by attacks of severe shortness of breath which generally occur at night and usually awaken the patient from sleep. The attack is precipitated by stimuli which aggravate the previously existing pulmonary congestion; frequently the total blood volume is augmented at night because of the reabsorption of edema from dependent portions of the body during recumbency; the redis-tribution of blood volume which takes place results in an increase in intrathoracic blood volume and therefore produces pulmonary conges-tion. A sleeping patient can tolerate relatively severe pulmonary engorgement and may awaken only when actual pulmonary edema and bronchospasm have developed, with the feeling of suffocation and with wheezing respirations.

CHEYNE-STOKES RESPIRATION   See Chap. 182.

DIAGNOSIS   The diagnosis of cardiac dyspnea depends on the rec-ognition of heart disease on the basis of the history and physical examination. There may be a history of antecedent myocardial infarction, third and fourth heart sounds may be audible, and/or there may be evidence of left ventricular enlargement, jugular neck vein distention, and/or peripheral edema. Often there are radiographic signs of heart failure, with evidence of interstitial edema, pulmonary vascular redistribution, and accumulation of liquid in the septal planes and pleural cavity. Cardiomegaly is often present, but the overall heart size may be normal, particularly in patients with dyspnea due to acute myocardial infarction or mitral stenosis; an enlarged left atrium is usually evident in the latter condition. The electrocardiogram (Chap. 178) is rarely specific for heart disease and cannot specifically indicate whether a patient's dyspnea is caused by heart disease; however, it is rarely normal in patients with cardiac dyspnea.

Differentiation between cardiac and pulmonary dyspnea   In most patients with dyspnea there is obvious clinical evidence of disease of either heart or lungs. The dyspnea of chronic obstructive lung disease tends to develop more gradually than that of heart diseases; exceptions, of course, occur in patients with obstructive lung disease who develop an episode of infectious bronchitis, pneumonia, or pneumothorax, or an exacerbation of asthma. Like patients with cardiac dyspnea,

patients with chronic obstructive lung disease may also waken at night with dyspnea, but this is usually associated with sputum production; the dyspnea is relieved after these patients rid themselves of secretions.

The difficulty in the distinction between cardiac and pulmonary dyspnea may be compounded by the coexistence of diseases involving both organ systems. Patients with a history of chronic bronchitis or asthma who develop left ventricular failure tend to develop recurrences of bronchoconstriction and wheezing in association with bouts of paroxysmal nocturnal dyspnea and pulmonary edema. This condition, i.e., cardiac asthma, usually occurs in patients with overt clinical evidence of heart disease. Acute cardiac asthma is further differentiated from acute attacks of bronchial asthma by the presence of diaphoresis, more bubbly airway sounds, and the more common occurrence of cyanosis.

It is desirable to carry out pulmonary function testing in patients in whom the etiology of dyspnea is not clear, for these tests should be helpful in determining whether dyspnea is produced by heart disease, lung disease, abnormalities of the chest wall, or anxiety. In addition to the usual means of assessing patients for heart disease (Chap. 176), determination of the ejection fraction at rest and during exercise by radionuclide ventriculography (Chap. 179) is helpful in the differential diagnosis of dyspnea; the left ventricular ejection fraction is depressed in left ventricular failure while the right ventricular ejection fraction may be low at rest or may decline during exercise in patients with severe lung disease; both ejection fractions are normal both at rest and during exercise in dyspnea due to anxiety or malingering. Careful observation during the performance of an exercise treadmill test will often help in the identification of the patient who is malingering or whose dyspnea is secondary to anxiety. Under these circumstances the patient usually complains of severe shortness of breath but appears to be breathing either effortlessly or totally irregularly.

Anxiety neurosis   Dyspnea experienced by someone with an anxiety neurosis is a difficult symptom to evaluate. The signs and symptoms of acute and chronic hyperventilation do not serve to distinguish between anxiety neurosis and other processes, such as recurrent pulmonary emboli. Another potentially confusing situation is seen when chest pain and electrocardiographic changes accompany the hyperventilation syndrome. When present and attributable to this condition, often referred to as *neurocirculatory asthenia* (Chap. 4), the chest pain is often sharp, fleeting, and in various loci, and the electrocardiographic changes are most often seen during repolariza-tion; yet occasional ventricular ectopic activity can be seen as well. A rather extensive series of pulmonary and cardiac function tests, carried out both at rest and during exercise, may be needed to be certain that anxiety is, in fact, the cause of the dyspnea. Certain clues are helpful in leading one to suspect a psychogenic origin. Frequent sighing respirations and a bizarre, irregular breathing pattern are helpful. Often the breathing pattern returns to normal during sleep.

PULMONARY EDEMA

CARDIOGENIC PULMONARY EDEMA   An increase in pulmonary venous pressure, which results initially in the engorgement of the pulmonary vasculature, is common in most instances of dyspnea in association with congestive heart failure. The lungs become less compliant, the resistance of small airways increases, and there is an increase in lymphatic flow which apparently serves to maintain a constant pulmonary extravascular liquid volume. At this early stage there is usually mild tachypnea, and if arterial blood gases are measured, the arterial P_{O_2} and P_{CO_2} are both lowered with an increase in the alveolar-to-arterial oxygen difference. Tachypnea itself, which might result from stimulation of receptors in the pulmonary intersti-tium, apparently increases lymphatic flow by augmenting ventilator pumping of lymphatic vessels. The changes described are seen we in advance of auscultatory findings or radiographic signs pointing congestive heart failure. If sufficient both in magnitude and duration, the increase in intravascular pressure results in a net gain of liquid in the extravascular space despite further increases in lymphatic flow. It is at this point that symptoms worsen, tachypnea increases, gas exchange deteriorates further, and radiographic changes, such as Kerley B lines and loss of distinct vascular margins, are seen. Even at this intermediate stage, the capillary endothelial intercellular junctions have been shown to widen and allow passage of macromolecules into the interstices. Up to and including this stage, the edema is purely *interstitial*. Sufficient further elevations in intravascular pressure result in disruption of the tighter junctions between alveolar lining cells, and alveolar edema ensues with outpouring of liquid, which contains both red blood cells and macromolecules. At this point *alveolar edema* is present. Although originally considered an early and subtle radiographic sign of interstitial edema, recent evidence suggests that an antigravity redistribution of pulmonary blood flow occurs only after the onset of alveolar edema. With yet more severe disruption of the alveolar-capillary membrane, edematous liquid floods the alveoli and airways. At this point, full-blown clinical pulmonary edema with bilateral wet rales and rhonchi will occur, and the chest radiograph may show diffuse haziness of the lung fields with greater density in the more proximal hilar regions. Typically, the patient is anxious and perspires freely, and the sputum is frothy and blood-tinged. Gas exchange is more severely compromised with worsening hypoxia and possibly hypercapnia. Without effective treatment (Chap. 182) progressive acidemia, hypoxia, and respiratory arrest ensue.

The earlier sequence of fluid accumulation described above follows the Starling law of capillary–interstitial fluid exchange:

$$\text{Fluid accumulation} = K[(P_c - P_{IF}) - \sigma(\pi_{pl} - \pi_{IF})] - Q_{lymph}$$

where K = permeability coefficient
P_c = mean intracapillary pressure
π_{IF} = oncotic pressure of interstitial fluid
σ = reflection coefficient of macromolecules
P_{IF} = mean interstitial liquid pressure
π_{pl} = oncotic pressure of the plasma
Q_{lymph} = lymphatic flow

The pressures tending to move liquid out of the vessel are P_c and π_{IF}, which are normally more than offset by pressures tending to move liquid back into the vasculature, i.e., the algebraic sum of P_{IF} and π_{pl}. Implicit in the above equation is that lymphatic flow can increase in the case of imbalance of forces and result in no net accumulation of interstitial fluid. However, in later sequences, with opening of first the endothelial and then the alveolar intercellular junctions, the permeability and reflection coefficients change strikingly. Thus, the initial process of hemodynamic pulmonary edema is one of liquid filtration and clearance. With further increasing pressures, disruption of both the structure and the function of the alveolar-capillary membrane occurs.

NONCARDIOGENIC PULMONARY EDEMA   There are several clinical conditions which are associated with pulmonary edema based upon an imbalance of Starling forces other than through primary elevations of pulmonary capillary pressure. Although diminished plasma oncotic pressure in hypoalbuminemic states (e.g., severe liver disease, nephrotic syndrome, protein-losing enteropathy) might be expected to lead to pulmonary edema, the balance of forces normally so strongly favors resorption that even under these conditions some elevation of capillary pressure is necessary before interstitial edema develops. Increased negativity of interstitial pressure has been implicated in the genesis of unilateral pulmonary edema following rapid evacuation of a large pneumothorax. In this situation the findings are apparent only by radiography. It has been recently proposed that large negative intrapleural pressures during acute severe asthma may be associated with the development of interstitial edema. If this proposal can be supported by sufficient clinical data, then asthma would represent an additional example of edema due to increased negativity of interstitial pressure. Lymphatic blockade secondary to fibrotic and inflammatory diseases or lymphangitic carcinomatosis may lead to interstitial edema. In such instances both clinical and radiographic manifestations are dominated by the underlying disease process.

There are other conditions characterized by increases in the interstitial liquid content of the lungs which begin neither with an imbalance between intravascular and interstitial forces nor with alterations in lymphatics, but rather appear to be associated primarily with disruption of the alveolar-capillary membranes. Experimentally the prototype for such conditions is the pulmonary edema following alloxan administration. Any number of spontaneously occurring or environmental toxic insults, including diffuse pulmonary infections, aspiration, shock (particularly due to gram-negative septicemia and hemorrhagic pancreatitis, and following cardiopulmonary bypass), are associated with diffuse pulmonary edema which clearly does not have a hemodynamic origin. These conditions, which may lead to the adult respiratory distress syndrome, are discussed in Chap. 216.

Other forms of pulmonary edema   There are three forms of pulmonary edema which have not been clearly related to increased permeability, inadequate lymphatic flow, or an imbalance of Starling forces; hence their precise mechanism remains unexplained. *Narcotic overdose* is a well-recognized antecedent to pulmonary edema. Although illicit use of parenteral heroin has been the most frequent cause, parenteral and oral overdoses of legitimate preparations of morphine, methadone, and dextropropoxyphene have also been associated with pulmonary edema. Thus the earlier idea that injected impurities lead to the disorder is untenable. Available evidence suggests that there are alterations in the permeability of alveolar and capillary membranes rather than elevation of pulmonary capillary pressure.

Exposure to high altitude in association with severe physical exertion is a well-recognized setting for pulmonary edema in unacclimatized, yet otherwise healthy, persons. Recent data show that acclimatized high-altitude natives also develop this syndrome upon return to high altitude after a relatively brief sojourn at low altitudes. The syndrome is far more common in persons under the age of 25 years. The mechanism for high-altitude pulmonary edema remains obscure, and studies have been conflicting, some suggesting pulmonary venous constriction and others indicating pulmonary arteriolar constriction as the prime mechanisms. A role for hypoxia at altitude is suggested by the fact that patients respond to the administration of oxygen and/or return to lower altitudes. Hypoxia per se does not alter permeability of the alveolar-capillary membrane. Hence, increased cardiac output and pulmonary arterial pressures with exercise combined with hypoxic pulmonary arteriolar constriction, which is more prominent in young persons, may combine to make this an example of prearteriolar, high-pressure pulmonary edema.

Neurogenic pulmonary edema has been suspected in patients with central nervous system disorders and without apparent preexisting left ventricular dysfunction. Although most experimental equivalents have implicated sympathetic nervous system activity, the mechanism whereby sympathetic efferent activity leads to pulmonary edema is a matter of speculation. It is known that a massive adrenergic discharge leads to peripheral vasoconstriction with elevation of blood pressure and shifts of blood to the central circulation. In addition, it is probable that a decrease in left ventricular compliance also occurs, and both factors serve to increase left atrial pressures sufficiently to induce pulmonary edema on a hemodynamic basis. Recent experimental evidence suggests that stimulation of adrenergic receptors increases capillary permeability directly, but this effect is relatively minor as compared to the imbalance of Starling forces.

TREATMENT OF PULMONARY EDEMA   See Chap. 182.

REFERENCES

AYRES SM: Mechanism and consequences of pulmonary edema: Cardiac lung, shock lung, and principles of ventilatory therapy in adult respiratory distress syndrome. Am Heart J 103:97, 1982

FISHMAN AP, RENKIN EM (eds): *Pulmonary Edema.* Washington, DC, American Physiological Society, 1979

INGRAM RH JR, BRAUNWALD E: Pulmonary edema: Cardiogenic and noncardiogenic, in *Heart Disease*, E. Braunwald (ed). Philadelphia, Saunders, 1984, p 560

KILLIAN KJ, CAMPBELL EJM: Dyspnea and exercise. Ann Rev Physiol 45:465, 1983

MALIK AB: Mechanisms of neurogenic pulmonary edema. Circ Res 57:1, 1985

MCFADDEN ER, INGRAM RH JR: Relationship between diseases of the heart and lungs, in *Heart Disease*, E Braunwald (ed). Philadelphia, Saunders, 1984, p 1782

RASANEN J et al: Continuous positive airway pressure by face mask in acute cardiogenic pulmonary edema. Am J Cardiol 55:296, 1985

ROUSSOS C, MACKLEM PT: Disorders of the respiratory muscle function, in *Update III: Harrison's Principles of Internal Medicine*, KJ Isselbacher et al (eds). New York, McGraw-Hill, 1982, p 83

SCHOENE RB et al: High altitude pulmonary edema and exercise at 4400 meters on Mount McKinley: Effect of expiratory positive airway pressure. Chest 87:330, 1985

SNIDERMAN A et al: Pulmonary blood flow: A potential factor in the pathogenesis of pulmonary edema. J Thorac Cardiovasc Surg 87:130, 1984

SPRUNG CL et al: The spectrum of pulmonary edema: Differentiation of cardiogenic, intermediate, and noncardiogenic forms of pulmonary edema. Am Rev Resp Dis 124:718, 1981

STAUB NC: The pathogenesis of pulmonary edema. Prog Cardiovasc Dis 23:53, 1980

ZEMA MJ et al: Dyspnea: The heart or the lungs? Differentiation at bedside by use of the simple valsalva maneuver. Chest 85:59, 1984

27 CYANOSIS, HYPOXIA, AND POLYCYTHEMIA

EUGENE BRAUNWALD

CYANOSIS

Cyanosis refers to a bluish color of the skin and mucous membranes resulting from an increased amount of reduced hemoglobin, or of hemoglobin derivatives, in the small blood vessels of those areas. It is usually most marked in the lips, nail beds, ears, and malar eminences. The "red cyanosis" of polycythemia vera (Chap. 289) must be distinguished from the true cyanosis discussed here. A cherry-colored flush, rather than cyanosis, is caused by carboxyhemoglobin (Chap. 171). The degree of cyanosis is modified by the quality of cutaneous pigment, the color of the blood plasma, and the thickness of the skin, as well as by the state of the cutaneous capillaries. The accurate clinical detection of the presence and degree of cyanosis is difficult, as proved by oximetric studies. In some instances central cyanosis can be reliably detected when the arterial saturation has fallen to 85 percent; in others it may not be detected until the saturation has reached 75 percent.

The increase in the quantity of reduced hemoglobin in the cutaneous vessels which produces cyanosis may be brought about either by an increase in the quantity of venous blood in the skin as the result of dilatation of the venules and venous ends of the capillaries, or by a decrease in the oxygen saturation in the capillary blood. In general, cyanosis becomes apparent when the mean capillary concentration of reduced hemoglobin exceeds 5 g/dL. It is the *absolute* rather than the *relative* amount of reduced hemoglobin which is important in producing cyanosis. Thus, in a patient with severe anemia the relative amount of reduced hemoglobin in the venous blood may be very large when considered in relation to the total amount of hemoglobin. However, since the latter is markedly lowered, the absolute amount of reduced hemoglobin may still be small, and therefore patients with severe anemia and even marked arterial desaturation do not display cyanosis. Conversely, the higher the total hemoglobin content, the greater the tendency toward cyanosis; thus, patients with marked polycythemia tend to be cyanotic at higher levels of arterial oxygen saturation than patients with normal hematocrit values. Likewise, local passive congestion, which causes an increase in the total amount of reduced hemoglobin in the vessels in a given area, may cause cyanosis. Cyanosis also is observed when nonfunctional hemoglobin is present in the blood; as little as 1.5 g/dL methemoglobin or 0.5 g sulfhemoglobin is sufficient to produce cyanosis.

Cyanosis may be subdivided into *central* and *peripheral* categories. In the *central* type, there is arterial blood unsaturation or an abnormal hemoglobin derivative, and the mucous membranes and skin are both affected. *Peripheral* cyanosis is due to a slowing of blood flow to an area and abnormally great extraction of oxygen from normally saturated arterial blood. It results from vasoconstriction and diminished peripheral blood flow, such as occurs in cold exposure, shock, congestive failure, and peripheral vascular disease. Often, in these conditions the mucous membranes of the oral cavity or those beneath the tongue may be spared. Clinical differentiation between central and peripheral cyanosis may not always be simple, and in conditions such as cardiogenic shock with pulmonary edema there may be a mixture of both types.

DIFFERENTIAL DIAGNOSIS (See Table 27-1) **Central cyanosis** Decreased arterial oxygen saturation results from a marked reduction in the oxygen tension in the arterial blood. This may be brought about by a decline in the tension of oxygen in the inspired air without sufficient compensatory alveolar hyperventilation to maintain alveolar oxygen tension. Cyanosis does not occur in a significant degree in an ascent to an altitude of 8000 ft but is marked in a further ascent to 16,000 ft. The reason for this becomes clear on studying the *S* shape of the oxygen dissociation curve (Fig. 283-4). At 8000 ft the tension of oxygen in the inspired air is about 120 mmHg, the alveolar tension is approximately 80 mmHg, and the hemoglobin is nearly completely saturated. However, at 16,000 ft the oxygen tensions in atmospheric air and alveolar air are about 85 and 50 mmHg, respectively, and the oxygen dissociation curve shows that the arterial blood is only about 75 percent saturated. This leaves 25 percent of the hemoglobin in the reduced form, an amount likely to be associated with cyanosis in the absence of anemia. Similarly, a mutant hemoglobin with a low affinity for oxygen (Hb Kansas) causes lowered arterial oxygen saturation and resultant central cyanosis (Chap. 288).

Seriously *impaired pulmonary function,* through alveolar hypoventilation or perfusion of unventilated or poorly ventilated areas of the lung, is a common cause of central cyanosis (Chap. 200). This may occur acutely, as in extensive pneumonia or pulmonary edema, or with chronic pulmonary diseases (e.g., emphysema). In the last situation polycythemia is generally present and clubbing of the fingers may occur. However, in many types of chronic pulmonary disease

TABLE 27-1 Causes of cyanosis

I Central cyanosis
  A Decreased arterial oxygen saturation
    1 Decreased atmospheric pressure—high altitude
    2 Impaired pulmonary function
      a Alveolar hypoventilation
      b Uneven relationships between pulmonary ventilation and perfusion
      c Impaired oxygen diffusion
    3 Anatomic shunts
      a Certain types of congenital heart disease
      b Pulmonary arteriovenous fistulas
      c Multiple small intrapulmonary shunts
    4 Hemoglobin with low affinity for oxygen
  B Hemoglobin abnormalities
    1 Methemoglobinemia—hereditary, acquired
    2 Sulfhemoglobinema—acquired
    3 Carboxyhemoglobinemia (not true cyanosis)
II Peripheral cyanosis
  A Reduced cardiac output
  B Cold exposure
  C Redistribution of blood flow from extremities
  D Arterial obstruction
  E Venous obstruction

with fibrosis and obliteration of the capillary vascular bed, cyanosis does not occur because there is relatively little perfusion of underventilated areas.

Another cause of decreased arterial oxygen saturation is *shunting of systemic venous blood into the arterial circuit*. Certain forms of congenital heart disease are associated with cyanosis (Chap. 185). Since blood normally flows from a high-pressure to a low-pressure region, in order for a cardiac defect to result in a right-to-left shunt, it must ordinarily be combined with an obstructive lesion distal to the defect or with elevated pulmonary vascular resistance. The commonest congenital cardiac lesion associated with cyanosis in the adult is the combination of ventricular septal defect and pulmonary outflow tract obstruction (tetralogy of Fallot). The more severe the obstruction, the greater the degree of right-to-left shunting and resultant cyanosis. The mechanisms for the elevated pulmonary vascular resistance which may produce cyanosis in the presence of intra- and extracardiac communications without pulmonic stenosis are discussed elsewhere (Chap. 185). In patients with patent ductus arteriosus, pulmonary hypertension, and right-to-left shunt, *differential cyanosis* results; i.e., cyanosis occurs in the lower extremities but not in the upper extremities.

Pulmonary arteriovenous fistulas may be congenital or acquired, solitary or multiple, microscopic or massive. The degree of cyanosis produced by these fistulas depends upon their size and number. They occur with some frequency in hereditary hemorrhagic telangiectasia (Chap. 280). Arterial oxygen unsaturation also occurs in some patients with cirrhosis, presumably as a consequence of pulmonary arteriovenous fistulas or portal vein–pulmonary vein anastomoses.

In patients with cardiac or pulmonary right-to-left shunts, the presence and severity of cyanosis depend on the size of the shunt relative to the systemic flow as well as on the oxyhemoglobin saturation of the venous blood. In patients with central cyanosis due to arterial oxygen unsaturation, the severity of cyanosis increases with exercise. With increased extraction of oxygen from the blood by the exercising muscles, the venous blood returning to the right side of the heart is more unsaturated than at rest, and shunting of this blood or its passage through lungs incapable of normal oxygenation intensifies the cyanosis. Also, since the systemic vascular resistance normally decreases with exercise, the right-to-left shunt is augmented by exercise in patients with congenital heart disease and communications between the two sides of the heart. Secondary polycythemia occurs frequently in patients with arterial unsaturation and contributes to the cyanosis.

Cyanosis can be caused by small amounts of circulating methemoglobin and by even smaller amounts of sulfhemoglobin (Chap. 288). Although they are uncommon causes of cyanosis, these abnormal hemoglobin pigments should be sought by spectroscopy when cyanosis is not readily explained by malfunction of the circulatory or respiratory systems. Generally, clubbing does not occur with them. The diagnosis of methemoglobinemia can be suspected, if, on mixing the patient's blood in a test tube and exposing it to air, it remains brown.

Peripheral cyanosis   Probably the most common cause of peripheral cyanosis is generalized vasoconstriction resulting from exposure to cold air or water. This is a normal response. When cardiac output is low, as in severe congestive heart failure or shock, cutaneous vasoconstriction occurs as a compensatory mechanism, so that blood is diverted to more vital areas [central nervous system, heart (Chap. 182)], and intense cyanosis associated with cool extremities may result. Even though the arterial blood is normally saturated, the reduced volume flow through the skin and the reduced oxygen tension at the venous end of the capillary result in cyanosis.

Arterial obstruction to an extremity, as with an embolus, or arteriolar constriction, as in cold-induced vasospasm (Raynaud's phenomenon, Chap. 198), generally results in pallor and coldness, but there may be associated slight cyanosis. If there is venous obstruction, the extremity is usually congested and also cyanotic, and there is true stagnation of blood flow. Venous hypertension, which may be local (as in thrombophlebitis) or generalized (as in tricuspid

valve disease or constrictive pericarditis), dilates the subpapillary venous plexuses and intensifies cyanosis.

APPROACH TO THE PATIENT WITH CYANOSIS   Certain features are important in arriving at the proper cause of cyanosis:

1 The history, particularly the duration (cyanosis present since birth is usually due to congenital heart disease); possible exposure to drugs or chemicals which may produce abnormal types of hemoglobin.
2 Clinical differentiation of central as opposed to peripheral cyanosis. Objective evidence by physical or radiographic examination of disorders of the respiratory or cardiovascular systems. Massage or gentle warming of a cyanotic extremity will increase peripheral blood flow and abolish peripheral but not central cyanosis.
3 The presence or absence of clubbing of the fingers. Clubbing without cyanosis is frequent in patients with infective endocarditis and in association with ulcerative colitis, it may occasionally occur in healthy persons, and in some instances it may be occupational, e.g., in jackhammer operators. Slight cyanosis of the lips and cheeks, without clubbing of the fingers, is common in patients with well-compensated mitral stenosis and is probably due to minimal arterial hypoxia resulting from fibrotic changes in the lungs secondary to long-standing congestion combined with reduction of cardiac output (Chap. 187). The combination of cyanosis and clubbing is frequent in many patients with certain types of congenital cardiac disease and is seen occasionally in persons with pulmonary disease such as lung abscess or pulmonary arteriovenous shunts. On the other hand, peripheral cyanosis or acutely developing central cyanosis is not associated with clubbed fingers.
4 Determination of arterial blood oxygen tension or oxygen saturation, spectroscopic and other examinations of the blood for abnormal types of hemoglobin.

CLUBBING   Clubbing is the selective bullous enlargement of the distal segment of a digit due to an increase in soft tissue. It may be hereditary or idiopathic, or acquired and associated with a variety of disorders, including cyanotic heart disease, infective endocarditis, and a variety of pulmonary conditions (among them, primary and metastatic lung cancer, bronchiectasis, lung abscess, and mesothelioma), as well as with some gastrointestinal diseases (including regional enteritis, chronic ulcerative colitis, and hepatic cirrhosis). Primary lung cancer, mesothelioma, neurogenic diaphragmatic tumors, and rarely cyanotic congenital heart disease may be associated with hypertrophic osteoarthropathy, the subperiosteal formation of new bone in the distal diaphyses of the long bones of the extremities. Although the mechanism of clubbing is unclear, it appears to be secondary to a (presumably humoral) substance, which causes dilation of the vessels of the fingertip.

HYPOXIA

The fundamental purpose of the cardiorespiratory system is to deliver oxygen (and substrates) to the cells and to remove carbon dioxide (and other metabolic products) from them. Proper maintenance of this function depends on intact cardiovascular and respiratory systems and a supply of inspired gas containing adequate oxygen. Changes in oxygen and in carbon dioxide tension as well as changes in the intraerythrocytic concentration of certain *organic phosphate compounds,* especially 2,3-diphosphoglyceric acid (2,3-DPG), cause shifts in the oxygen dissociation curve. These are discussed in detail in Chap. 283 and are illustrated in Fig. 283-4. When hypoxia results as a consequence of respiratory failure, arterial P_{CO_2} usually rises (Chaps. 208 and 216), and the oxygen dissociation curve tends to be displaced to the right. Under these conditions the percentage saturation of the hemoglobin in the arterial blood at a given level of alveolar oxygen tension declines. Thus arterial hypoxia and cyanosis are likely to be more marked in proportion to the degree of depression of alveolar oxygen tension when such depression results from pulmonary disease than when the depression occurs as the result of a decline in the partial pressure of oxygen in the inspired air, in which case arterial P_{CO_2} falls and the oxygen dissociation curve is displaced to the left.

DIFFERENTIAL DIAGNOSIS Anemic hypoxia Any decrease in hemoglobin concentration is attended by a corresponding decline in the oxygen-carrying capacity. The P_{O_2} in the arterial blood remains normal, but the absolute amount of oxygen transported per unit volume of blood is diminished. As the anemic blood passes through the capillaries, and the usual amount of oxygen is removed from it, the P_{O_2} in the venous blood declines to a greater degree than would normally be the case.

Circulatory hypoxia As in anemic hypoxia, arterial P_{O_2} is normal, but venous and tissue P_{O_2} are reduced as a consequence of reduced tissue perfusion in the face of normal tissue oxygen consumption. For this reason the term *stagnant hypoxia* may be used for this condition. Generalized circulatory hypoxia occurs in heart failure (Chap. 182), and in most forms of shock (Chap. 29).

Specific organ hypoxia Decreased circulation to a specific organ resulting in localized stagnant hypoxia may be due to organic arterial or venous obstruction or may occur as a consequence of vasoconstriction. The latter may occur in the upper extremities in Raynaud's phenomenon. Reduced circulation may occur in all limbs in patients with heart failure or hypovolemic shock in an attempt to maintain adequate perfusion to more vital organs. When organic arterial obliterative disease develops, ischemic hypoxia results, with accompanying pallor. Localized hypoxia may also result from venous obstruction which results in congestion. Edema, which increases the distance through which oxygen diffuses before it reaches the cells, can also cause localized hypoxia.

Increased oxygen requirements Even if oxygen diffusion into blood perfusing the pulmonary capillary bed is unhampered and the hemoglobin is qualitatively and quantitatively normal, the P_{O_2} in venous blood (hence, capillary and tissue P_{O_2}) may be reduced if the oxygen consumption of the tissues is elevated without a corresponding increase in volume flow per unit of time. Such a situation may be encountered when fever or thyrotoxicosis occurs in patients in whom the cardiac output cannot rise normally. Under such conditions the circulation may be considered deficient relative to the metabolic requirements.

Ordinarily, the clinical picture of patients with hypoxia due to an elevated basal metabolic rate is quite different from that in other types of hypoxia; the skin is warm and flushed, owing to increased cutaneous blood flow which dissipates the excessive heat produced, and cyanosis is absent in these patients.

Exercise is a classic example of increased tissue oxygen requirements. The increased demands are normally met by several mechanisms: (1) increasing the cardiac output and ventilation and thus oxygen delivery to the tissues; (2) preferentially directing the blood to the exercising muscles and away from resting muscles (by changing vascular resistances in various circulatory beds, directly and/or reflexly); (3) increasing oxygen extraction from the delivered blood and widening the arteriovenous oxygen differences; (4) reducing the pH of the tissues and capillary blood, thereby unloading more oxygen from hemoglobin. If the capacity of these mechanisms is exceeded, then hypoxia, especially of the exercising muscles, will result.

Carbon monoxide intoxication (Chap. 171) This condition is analogous to anemic hypoxia in that the hemoglobin which is combined with the carbon monoxide (carboxyhemoglobin) is unavailable for oxygen transport. In addition, the presence of carboxyhemoglobin shifts the dissociation curve of hemoglobin to the left, so that the oxygen can be unloaded only at lower tensions. By such formation of carboxyhemoglobin a given degree of reduction in oxygen-carrying

power produces a far greater degree of tissue hypoxia than the equivalent reduction in hemoglobin due to simple anemia.

Improper oxygen utilization Cyanide (Chap. 171) and several other similarly acting poisons cause a paradoxic state in which the tissues are unable to utilize oxygen and as a consequence the venous blood tends to have a high oxygen tension. This condition has been termed *histotoxic hypoxia*. Cyanide produces cellular hypoxia by paralyzing the electron-transfer function of cytochrome oxidase so that it cannot pass electrons to oxygen, whereas diphtheria toxin is believed to inhibit the synthesis of one of the cytochromes and thus interfere with oxygen consumption and energy production by the cells involved.

EFFECTS OF HYPOXIA Changes in the central nervous system, particularly the higher centers, are especially important. Acute hypoxia produces impaired judgment, motor incoordination, and a clinical picture closely resembling that of acute alcoholism. When hypoxia is long-standing, the symptoms consist of fatigue, drowsiness, apathy, inattentiveness, delayed reaction time, and reduced work capacity. As hypoxia becomes more severe, the centers of the brainstem are affected, and death usually results from respiratory failure. With reduction of arterial oxygen tension, cerebrovascular resistance decreases and cerebral blood flow increases, which tends to reduce the cerebral hypoxia. On the other hand when the reduction of arterial P_{O_2} is accompanied by hyperventilation and diminution of P_{CO_2}, cerebrovascular resistance rises, blood flow falls, and hypoxia is enhanced. Compared with the brain, the phylogenetically older spinal cord and peripheral nerves are relatively insensitive to hypoxia. Hypoxia also causes pulmonary arterial constriction, which serves the useful function of shunting blood away from poorly ventilated areas toward better-ventilated portions of the lung. However, it has the disadvantage of causing increased pulmonary vascular resistance and an increased burden on the right ventricle.

A complex disturbance of cellular functions results from the metabolic effects of severe acute hypoxia. In liver and muscles the breakdown of the primary foodstuff, carbohydrate, normally proceeds anaerobically (i.e., without oxidation) to the stage of formation of pyruvic acid. The breakdown of pyruvate requires oxygen, and when this is deficient, increasing proportions of pyruvate are reduced to lactic acid, which cannot be broken down further (Chap. 328). Hence, there is an increase in the blood lactate, with decrease in bicarbonate and a corresponding acidosis. Under these circumstances the total energy obtained from foodstuff breakdown is greatly reduced, and the amount of energy available for continuing resynthesis of energy-rich phosphate compounds becomes inadequate, leading to a complex disturbance of cellular function.

Most of the useful respiratory response to hypoxia originates in special chemosensitive cells in the carotid and aortic bodies, although the respiratory center is also stimulated directly by oxygen lack. The resultant increase in ventilation, with loss of carbon dioxide, leads to respiratory alkalosis. On the other hand, the diffusion of additional quantities of lactic acid from the tissues into the blood tends to produce metabolic acidosis. In either case the total amount of bicarbonate, and hence the carbon dioxide–combining power, tends to be diminished.

Diminished oxygen tension in any tissue results in local vasodilatation, and the diffuse vasodilatation which occurs in generalized hypoxia causes an elevation of total cardiac output (Fig. 283-5). In patients with preexisting heart disease, particularly coronary artery disease, the combination of hypoxia and the requirements of the peripheral tissues for an increase of cardiac output may precipitate congestive heart failure. Prolonged or severe hypoxia may also impair hepatic and renal function.

One of the important mechanisms of compensation for prolonged hypoxia is an increase in the quantity of hemoglobin in the blood (Fig. 283-5). This is due not to direct stimulation of the bone marrow but to the effect of erythropoietin, which originates primarily in the kidneys. Assayable levels of erythropoietin are increased by hypoxia, and its production has been found to be regulated by the balance between tissue oxygen supply and demand.

TABLE 27-2   Differential diagnosis of erythrocytosis

ABSOLUTE (↑ RED CELL MASS)

I Autonomous erythroid proliferation (↓ EP*); polycythemia vera
II Secondary erythroid proliferation
   A Autonomous or inappropriate increase in EP
      1 Neoplasm
      2 Renal lesions
      3 Familial erythrocytosis (autosomal recessive inheritance)
   B Secondary increase in EP
      1 Hypoxia (↓ arterial P_{O_2})
         a High altitude
         b Alveolar hypoventilation
         c Pulmonary disease
         d Cardiac right-to-left shunt
      2 Abnormal hemoglobin function (normal arterial P_{O_2})
         a High-affinity variants (autosomal dominant inheritance)
         b Congenital methemoglobinemia
         c Carboxyhemoglobin (smokers')
   C Hormonal stimulus to erythropoiesis
      1 Cushing's syndrome
      2 Androgen or corticosteroid administration

RELATIVE (REDUCED PLASMA VOLUME, NORMAL RED CELL MASS)

I Dehydration
II Stress erythrocytosis

* *Erythropoietin.*
SOURCE: *Adapted from HF Bunn et al, Human Hemoglobins, Philadelphia, Saunders, 1977.*

POLYCYTHEMIA (See also Chap. 289)

The term *polycythemia* signifies an increase above the normal in the number of red blood cells in the circulating blood. This increase is usually, though not always, accompanied by a corresponding increase in the quantity of hemoglobin and in the hematocrit. The increase may or may not be associated with an increase in the total quantity of red blood cells in the body. It is important to distinguish between *absolute* polycythemia (an increase in the total red cell mass) and *relative* polycythemia, which occurs when, through loss of blood plasma, the concentration of the red cells becomes greater than normal in the circulating blood. This may be the consequence of abnormally lowered fluid intake, of the loss of plasma into the interstitial fluid, or of the marked loss of body fluids, such as occurs in persistent vomiting, severe diarrhea, copious sweating, or acidosis.

Because the term polycythemia is used loosely to refer to all

varieties of increase in the number of red corpuscles, the terms *erythrocytosis* and *erythremia* are preferred in referring to two forms of *absolute* polycythemia. Erythrocytosis denotes absolute polycythemia which occurs in response to some known stimulus (secondary polycythemia); erythremia (polycythemia vera) refers to the disease of unknown etiology (Chap. 289). An approach to the differential diagnosis of erythrocytosis should begin with a consideration of its mechanisms (Table 27-2). Erythrocytosis develops as a consequence of a variety of factors and represents a physiologic response to conditions of hypoxia.

Sojourn at high altitudes leads to defective saturation of arterial blood with oxygen and stimulates the production of more red cells. The oxygen saturation, rather than oxygen tension, appears to be the more important determinant of the erythropoietic response to chronic hypoxia (Fig. 27-1). A disorder may set in insidiously after several years of continued residence at high altitudes, leading to the development of a condition known as *chronic mountain sickness* or *seroche* (Monge's disease), which appears to be caused by the development of alveolar hypoventilation superimposed on a lowered inspired O_2 concentration. Prominent manifestations are a florid color which turns to cyanosis on mild exertion, mental torpor, fatigue, and headache. Those affected are usually in the fourth to sixth decades. Return to sea level promptly relieves the symptoms. Living at high altitudes also evokes a number of compensatory reactions which act to increase oxygen delivery to the tissues. These include hyperventilation, which reduces the oxygen gradient between ambient and alveolar air, an augmentation of pulmonary capillary blood volume, an increase of diffusing capacity, and an increase in cardiac output.

Any pulmonary disease which produces chronic hypoxia may lead to erythrocytosis. The increased blood viscosity secondary to the polycythemia elevates pulmonary arterial pressure and, combined with the elevation of pulmonary vascular resistance resulting from hypoxia, further elevates right ventricular pressure, contributing to the development or intensification of cor pulmonale (Chap. 191). The *abnormal ventilatory conditions* present in very obese individuals may cause alveolar hypoventilation and result in arterial unsaturation, erythrocytosis, hypercapnia, and somnolence (the Pickwickian syndrome, Chap. 215). This syndrome is observed less commonly in nonobese persons (sleep-apnea syndrome), in whom decreased sensitivity of the respiratory center to CO_2 may play a role (Chap. 215).

The partial shunting of blood from the pulmonary circuit, such as occurs in *congenital heart disease,* causes the most striking erythrocytosis resulting from abnormalities in the heart or lungs (Chap. 185). Erythrocyte counts as high as 13 million per cubic millimeter, which are possible only when the red corpuscles are smaller than normal, have been observed in such patients, with volumes of packed red blood cells even as high as 86 mL/dL of blood. As the polycythemia develops, there is a progressive rise in blood viscosity, which begins to rise logarithmically when the volume of packed red blood cells exceeds 55 percent. The commonest defects producing such polycythemia in the adult are tetralogy of Fallot and Eisenmenger's complex. Other conditions include transposition of the great arteries, tricuspid atresia, and persistent truncus arteriosus. The polycythemia of cyanotic congenital heart disease may lead to spontaneous thrombosis at any site, including the central nervous system. The increase in hematocrit and the sharp increase in viscosity which occur when these patients become dehydrated are particularly hazardous. This condition may also be accompanied by a variety of blood coagulation defects, including reduced fibrinogen and prothrombin concentrations, as well as thrombocytopenia. Reduction in red blood cell volume (phlebotomy with reinfusion of the plasma) is sometimes performed in severely symptomatic patients with extremely high hematocrit levels, but it must be carried out slowly and with caution. It results in a reduction of the elevated blood viscosity which improves blood flow.

The excessive use of coal-tar derivatives and other forms of chronic poisoning, by producing abnormal hemoglobin pigments such as *methemoglobin* and *sulfhemoglobin* (Chap. 288), also may cause

FIGURE 27-1 *Relationship between mean arterial oxygen saturation (percent) and the mean hemoglobin content (grams per deciliter) in healthy male residents at various altitudes. (From Hurtado, by permission of Annals of Internal Medicine.)*

erythrocytosis. Patients with abnormal hemoglobins which displace the oxygen dissociation curve to the left and interfere with oxygen unloading in the tissues stimulate the production of erythropoietin and a secondary erythrocytosis unassociated with leukocytosis or thrombocytosis (Chap. 288).

Mild erythrocytosis is sometimes found in *Cushing's syndrome* and can be produced by the administration of large amounts of adrenocortical steroids. Androgens also exert an erythropoietic effect and when administered to normal individuals can produce erythrocytosis. Especially intriguing are the instances of erythrocytosis observed in association with various *tumors* which produce erythropoietin or an erythropoietin-like substance. These have been chiefly of two varieties, *infratentorial* and *renal*. The tumors in the posterior fossa have usually been vascular (hemangioblastomas). The renal tumors have included hypernephroma, adenoma, and sarcoma. Other tumors that have been associated with erythrocytosis include uterine myoma, hepatic carcinoma, and pheochromocytoma. Erythrocytosis also has been reported in association with solitary and polycystic disease of the kidneys, with hydronephrosis, and with renal artery stenosis. However, only a small proportion of the various renal disorders mentioned above have been associated with polycythemia. Plasma erythropoietin levels have been found to be elevated in a number of these patients. Erythropoietin-like activity has been demonstrated in tumor extracts and in renal cyst fluid, and erythrocytosis has disappeared after the associated tumor was removed.

The term *stress erythrocytosis* has been applied to the polycythemia seen occasionally in very active, hard-working, middle-aged white males who are typically hypertensive and overweight and in a state of anxiety, who appear florid but who have none of the other characteristic signs of polycythemia vera—no splenomegaly or leukocytosis with immature cells in the blood. In such persons the total red blood cell mass is normal, and the plasma volume is below normal. Thus, they have an elevated hematocrit and *relative* polycythemia. *Smokers' polycythemia* is a closely related condition, but the high carboxyhemoglobin concentration may cause a small absolute increase in red cell mass which is often asssociated with a reduced plasma volume.

The *clinical features* of polycythemia include, in addition to the symptoms of the underlying condition (in the secondary forms), a characteristic "ruddy" cyanosis, dizziness, headache, epistaxes, and an increased incidence of thrombotic complications.

The *differential diagnosis* of absolute polycythemia is discussed in Chap. 289. In polycythemia vera, erythropoietin levels are usually absent, leukocyte alkaline phosphatase and vitamin B_{12} levels and platelet and total white blood cells are usually elevated, and splenomegaly is common; the bone marrow shows hyperplasia of all elements. In secondary polycythemia with hypoxia, arterial P_{CO_2} is reduced, erythropoietin levels are elevated, while levels of leukocyte alkaline phosphatase, serum vitamin B_{12}, platelet, total white blood cell, and differential counts are all normal, and the liver and spleen are not enlarged; the bone marrow shows only erythroid hyperplasia. In the absence of features of either polycythemia vera or polycythemia secondary to hypoxia or to a tumor, a hemoglobin with a high affinity for oxygen should be sought for.

REFERENCES

Doll DC, Greenberg BR: Cerebral thrombosis in smokers' polycythemia. Ann Intern Med 102:786, 1985

Erslev AJ: Erythrocytosis (sec 17, Chaps 73–75), in *Hematology*, 3d ed, WJ Williams (ed). New York, McGraw-Hill, 1983, p 673.

Hurtado A: Some clinical aspects of life at high altitudes. Ann Intern Med 53:247, 1960

Lanken PN, Fishman AP: Clubbing and hypertrophic osteoarthropathy, in *Pulmonary Diseases and Disorders*, AP Fishman (ed). New York, McGraw-Hill, 1980, p 84

Lupinetti FM et al: Pathophysiology of chronic cyanosis in a canine model. Functional and metabolic response to global ischemia. J Thorac Cardiovasc Surg 90:291, 1985

Rosenthal A, Tyler DC: Effect of red cell volume reduction or pulmonary blood flow in polycythemia of cyanotic congenital heart disease. Am J Cardiol 33:410, 1974

Smith JR, Landaw SA: Smokers' polycythemia. N Engl J Med 298:6, 1978

28 EDEMA

EUGENE BRAUNWALD

Edema is defined as an increase in the extravascular (interstitial) component of the extracellular fluid volume, which may expand by several liters before the abnormality is recognized. Therefore, a weight gain of several kilograms usually precedes overt manifestations of edema, and a similar weight loss from diuresis can be induced in a slightly edematous patient before "dry weight" is achieved. *Ascites* (Chap. 39) and *hydrothorax* refer to accumulation of excess fluid in the peritoneal and pleural cavities, respectively, and are considered to be special forms of edema. *Anasarca* refers to gross, generalized edema. Depending on its etiology and mechanism, edema may be localized or have a generalized distribution; it is recognized in its generalized form by puffiness of the face, which is most readily apparent in the periorbital areas, and by the persistence of an indentation of the skin following pressure; this is known as "pitting" edema. In its more subtle form, it may be detected by the fact that the rim of the bell of the stethoscope leaves an indentation on the skin of the chest that lasts a few minutes. One of the early symptoms a patient may note is the ring on a finger fitting more snugly than in the past, or difficulty in putting on shoes, particularly in the evening.

PATHOGENESIS (See also Chap. 41)   About one-third of the total body water is confined to the extracellular space. This compartment, in turn, is composed of the plasma volume and the interstitial space. Under ordinary circumstances the plasma volume represents about 25 percent of the extracellular space, and the remainder is interstitial fluid. The forces that regulate the disposition of fluid between these two components of the extracellular compartment are frequently referred to as the Starling forces (page 144). In general terms, the hydrostatic pressure within the vascular system and the colloid oncotic pressure in the interstitial fluid tend to promote movement of fluid from the vascular to the extravascular space. In contrast, the colloid oncotic pressure contributed by the plasma proteins and the hydrostatic pressure within the interstitial fluid, referred to as the *tissue tension,* promote a movement of fluid into the vascular compartment. As a consequence of these forces there is a movement of water and diffusible solutes from the vascular space at the arteriolar end of the capillaries. Fluid is returned from the interstitial space into the vascular system by way of the lymphatics, and unless these channels are obstructed, lymph flow tends to increase if there is net movement of fluid from the vascular compartment to the interstitium. These forces are usually balanced so that a steady state exists in the size of the intravascular and interstitial compartments, and yet a large exchange between them is permitted. However, should any one of these forces be altered significantly, a net movement of fluid from one component of the extracellular space to the other will occur.

An increase in capillary pressure may result from an increase in venous pressure due to local obstruction in venous drainage, to congestive heart failure, or rarely to the simple expansion of the vascular volume by the administration of large volumes of fluid at a rate in excess of the ability of the kidneys to excrete them. The colloid oncotic pressure of the plasma may be reduced, owing to any factor that may induce hypoalbuminemia, such as malnutrition, liver disease, loss of protein into the urine or into the gastrointestinal tract, or a severe catabolic state.

Edema may also result from damage to the capillary endothelium, which increases their permeability and permits the transfer to the interstitial compartment of fluid containing more protein than usual. Injury to the capillary walls can result from chemical, bacterial, thermal, or mechanical agents. Increased capillary permeability may also be a consequence of a hypersensitivity reaction and is characteristic of immune injury. Damage to the capillary endothelium is presumably responsible for inflammatory edema, which is nonpitting, usually localized, and accompanied by other signs of inflammation—redness, heat, and tenderness.

To formulate a hypothesis about the pathophysiology of an edematous state, it is important to discriminate between the *primary* events, such as venous or lymphatic obstruction, reduction of cardiac output, hypoalbuminemia, trapping of fluid in spaces such as the peritoneal cavity, or an increase in capillary permeability, and the predictable *secondary* consequences, which include the renal retention of salt and water. There are instances in which an abnormal positive balance of salt and water may, in fact, be the primary disturbance. In these circumstances the edema is a secondary manifestation of the generalized increase in extracellular fluid volume. These special instances are usually related to conditions characterized by an acute reduction in renal function, such as acute tubular necrosis or acute glomerulonephritis (Fig. 28-1).

These circumstances aside, a hypothesis can be advanced, which, although incomplete, leads to improved understanding of the events and enhances the perception of the pathophysiology. The basic premise is that the primary disorder concerns one or more alterations in the Starling forces so that there is a net movement of fluid from the vascular system into the interstitium or into a "third space" or from the arterial compartment of the vascular space into the chambers of the heart or into the venous circulation itself. The *effective arterial blood volume*, an as yet poorly defined parameter of the filling of the arterial tree, is reduced, and as a consequence a series of physiologic responses designed to restore it to normal are set into motion. A key element of these responses is the retention of an increment of salt and therefore of water, and in many instances this repairs the deficit of the effective arterial blood volume; often this occurs without the development of overt edema. If, however, the retention of salt and water is insufficient to restore and maintain the effective arterial blood volume, the stimuli are not dissipated, the retention of salt and water continues, and edema develops. This sequence of events is operative in dehydration and hemorrhage. Although, in these conditions there is a reduction of effective arterial blood volume and activation of the entire sequence shown on the right side of Fig. 28-1, including the diminished excretion of salt and water, edema does not occur because the net sodium and water balance is negative. In most conditions that lead to edema the mechanisms responsible for maintaining a normal effective osmolality in the body fluids operate efficiently so that sodium retention promotes thirst and secretion of the antidiuretic hormone, which, in turn, lead to the ingestion and retention of approximately 1 liter of water for each 140 mmol sodium retained. Similarly, measures that promote the loss of sodium into the urine, such as the administration of diuretics, are accompanied by the net loss of an equivalent volume of water from the body.

A reduction of cardiac output, whatever the cause, is associated with a reduction of the effective arterial blood volume as well as of renal blood flow and an elevation of the filtration fraction, i.e., the ratio of glomerular filtration rate to renal plasma flow. In severe heart failure the blood flow to the outer renal cortex, in particular, is reduced with less depression in the more central regions of the kidney, and there is a reduction in the glomerular filtration rate. This constriction of renal cortical vessels plays an important role in the retention of salt and water and in the formation of edema in heart failure. At different stages of heart failure, activation of the sympathetic nervous system or of the renin-angiotensin systems is responsible for renal vasoconstriction. Activation of the former can be counteracted by the administration of alpha-adrenergic blocking agents, a finding which indicates that the elevated renal vascular resistance in heart failure is mediated, at least in part, by sympathetic stimuli. The augmented renal blood flow and profound diuresis induced by treatment with angiotensin-converting enzyme inhibitors points to the

FIGURE 28-1 *Sequence of events leading to the formation and retention of salt and water and the development of edema. ANF, atrial natriuretic factor; ------, inhibits renal vasoconstriction.*

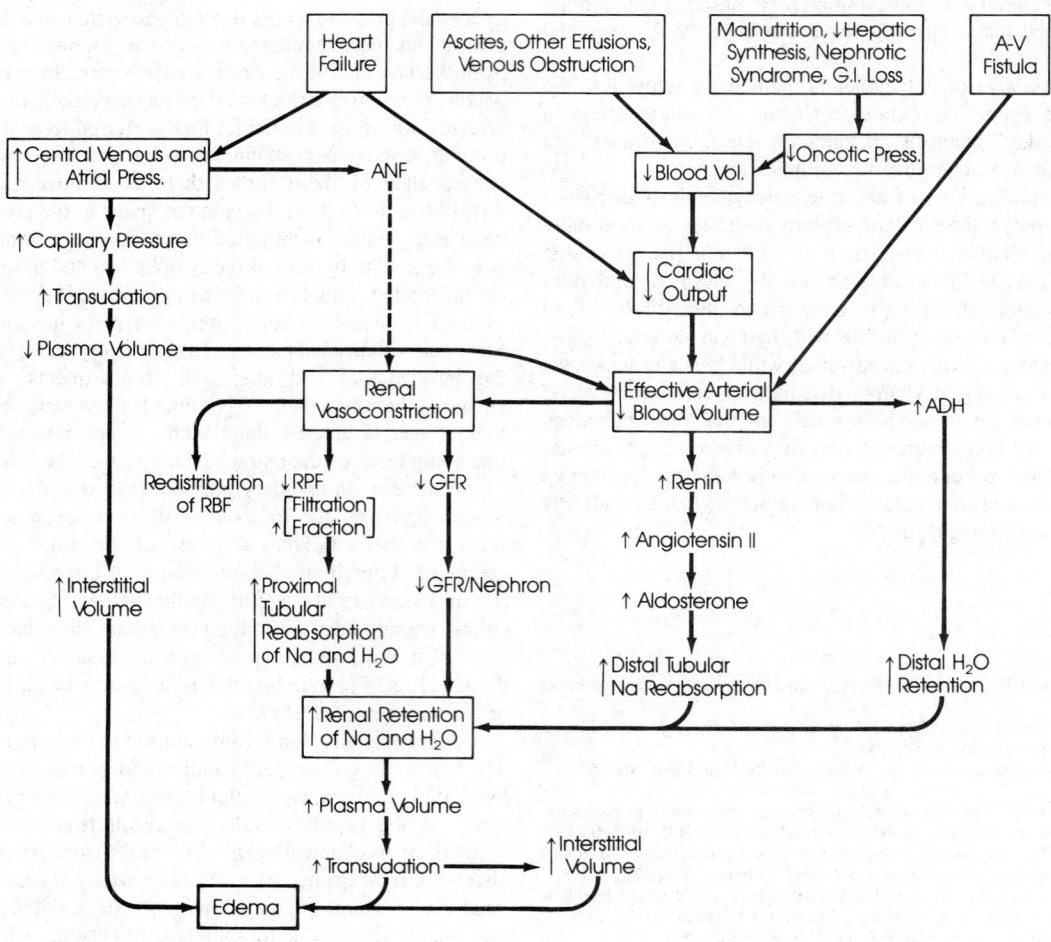

involvement of the renin-angiotensin system in the retention of salt and water in heart failure.

An increase in the tubular reabsorption of glomerular filtrate plays a principal role in the salt and water retention of heart failure. However, the precise sites(s) in the renal tubules, loops of Henle, and collecting ducts which are involved is not clear, nor have the responsible mechanism(s) been identified. Alterations in intrarenal hemodynamics appear to play a significant role. Heart failure, by augmenting renal arteriolar constriction, reduces the hydrostatic pressure and raises the colloid osmotic pressure in the peritubular capillaries, thus enhancing salt and water reabsorption in the proximal tubule. The aforementioned distribution of intrarenal blood flow characteristic of heart failure may be responsible for augmentation of sodium reabsorption in the ascending limb of the loop of Henle.

In addition, the diminished renal blood flow characteristic of states in which the effective arterial blood volume is reduced is translated by the renal juxtaglomerular cells into a signal for increased renin release (Chap. 325). The specific nature of the signal is complex. One factor involves a baroreceptor mechanism, in which reduced renal perfusion results in incomplete filling of the renal arterioles and diminished stretch of the juxtaglomerular cells, a signal that provides for the elaboration or release, or both, of renin. A second mechanism involves the macula densa; as a result of reduced glomerular filtration the sodium load reaching the distal renal tubules is reduced. This is sensed by the macula densa, which in an undefined manner signals the neighboring juxtaglomerular cells to secrete renin. A third mechanism involves the sympathetic nervous system and circulating catecholamines. Activation of the beta-adrenergic receptors in the juxtaglomerular cells stimulates renin release. These three mechanisms generally act in concert.

Renin, an enzyme with a molecular weight of about 40,000, acts on its substrate, angiotensinogen, an alpha$_2$ globulin synthesized by the liver to release angiotensin I, a decapeptide, which is broken down to angiotensin II, an octapeptide with vasoconstrictor properties. The intrarenal production of angiotensin II may also contribute to renal vasoconstriction and to the salt and water retention in heart failure. Angiotensin II also enters the circulation and stimulates the production of aldosterone by the zona glomerulosa of the adrenal cortex. In patients with heart failure, not only is aldosterone secretion elevated, but the biologic half-life of aldosterone is prolonged, which further increases the plasma level of the hormone. A depression of hepatic blood flow, particularly during exercise, secondary to a reduction in cardiac output, is responsible for the reduced hepatic catabolism of aldosterone.

Although increased quantities of aldosterone are secreted in heart failure and in other edematous states and although blockade of the action of aldosterone by spironolactone often induces a moderate diuresis in edematous states, augmented levels of aldosterone (or other mineralocorticoids) do not always promote accumulation of edema, as witnessed by the lack of striking fluid retention in most instances of primary aldosteronism (Chap. 325). Furthermore, although normal subjects retain some salt and water under the influence of a potent mineralocorticoid, such as deoxycorticosterone acetate or fludrocortisone, the accumulation is self-limiting, despite continued exposure to the steroid and to salt and water. The failure of normal subjects to accumulate large quantities of fluid is probably a consequence of an increase in glomerular filtration rate, other hemodynamic influences, and most importantly the increase in volume which promotes an increased excretion of salt that is independent of the filtered load of sodium, i.e., through the action of natriuretic substance(s). The role of aldosterone in the accumulation of fluid in edematous states may be more important because these patients are unable to repair the deficit in effective arterial blood volume.

Atrial distention and/or a sodium load cause release into the circulation of atrial natriuretic factor (ANF), a polypeptide whose active fraction contains 21 to 33 amino acids; a high-molecular-weight precursor of ANF is stored in secretory granules within atrial myocytes. Release of ANF causes (1) excretion of sodium and water by augmenting glomerular filtration rate and inhibiting release of renin and aldosterone; and (2) arteriolar and venous dilatation. Thus, ANF has the capacity to oppose sodium retention and arterial pressure elevation in states characterized by hypervolemia. There is also some evidence for the existence of a distinctly different natriuretic factor, a low-molecular-weight substance that is activated or released as a result of the expansion of the extracellular fluid and causes natriuresis by inhibiting renal sodium reabsorption through inhibiting ouabain-sensitive Na^+,K^+-ATPase. The role of this factor and of ANF in normal and pathophysiologic conditions requires clarification.

Obstruction of venous and lymphatic drainage of a limb In this condition the hydrostatic pressure in the capillary bed upstream to the obstruction increases so that more fluid than normal is transferred from the vascular to the interstitial space; since the alternate route (i.e., the lymphatic channels) is obstructed as well, this event causes an increased volume of interstitial fluid in the limb, i.e., a trapping of fluid in the extremity, at the expense of the blood volume in the remainder of the body, thereby reducing effective arterial blood volume and leading to the consequences shown in Fig. 28-1.

As fluid accumulates in the interstitium of the limb in which venous and lymphatic drainage are obstructed, tissue tension rises until it counterbalances the primary alterations in the Starling forces, at which time no further fluid accumulates in that limb. At this point the additional accumulation of fluid repairs the deficit in plasma volume, and the stimuli to retain more salt and water are dissipated. The net effect is an increase in the volume of interstitial fluid in a local area, and the secondary responses repair the plasma volume deficit incurred by the primary event. This same sequence occurs in ascites and hydrothorax in which fluid is trapped or accumulates in the interstitial space, depleting the intravascular volume and leading to secondary salt and fluid retention as already described.

Congestive heart failure (see also Chap. 182) In this disorder the defective systolic emptying of the chambers of the heart promotes an accumulation of blood in the heart and venous circulation at the expense of the arterial volume, and the aforementioned sequence of events (Fig. 28-1) is initiated. In many instances of mild heart failure, a small increment of volume may repair the volume deficit and establish a new steady state because, through the operation of Starling's law of the heart, up to a point, an increase in the volume of blood within the chambers of the heart promotes a more forceful contraction and may thereby increase the cardiac output (Fig. 181-4). However, if the cardiac disorder is more severe, retention of fluid cannot repair the deficit in effective arterial blood volume. The increment accumulates in the venous circulation, and the increase in hydrostatic pressure therein promotes the formation of edema. The formation of edema in the lungs (Chap. 26) impairs gas exchange and may induce hypoxia, which embarrasses cardiac function still further.

In addition to the sequence shown on the right-hand side of Fig. 28-1, incomplete ventricular emptying leads to an elevation of ventricular diastolic pressure. If the impairment of cardiac function involves the right ventricle, then incomplete ventricular emptying leads to an elevation of right ventricular diastolic volume and pressure; as a consequence pressures in the systemic veins and capillaries also rise, thereby augmenting transudation of fluid into the interstitial space and enhancing the likelihood of peripheral edema. The elevated systemic venous pressure is transmitted to the thoracic duct with consequent reduction of lymph drainage, further increasing edema formation. If the impairment of cardiac function involves the left ventricle, then pulmonary venous and capillary pressures rise [leading in some instances to pulmonary edema (Chap. 26)], as does pulmonary artery pressure; this in turn interferes with the systolic emptying of the right ventricle, leading to an elevation of right ventricular diastolic and central and systemic venous pressures, enhancing the likelihood of formation of systemic edema.

Nephrotic syndrome and other hypoalbuminic states (see also Chap. 223) The primary alteration in this disorder is a diminished colloid oncotic pressure due to massive losses of protein into the urine. This promotes a net movement of fluid into the interstitium, causes hypovolemia, and initiates the sequence of events described above. As long as the hypoalbuminemia is severe, the salt and water retained cannot be restrained within the vascular compartment, and hence the stimuli to retain salt and water are not abated. A similar sequence of events occurs in other conditions which lead to severe hypoalbuminemia, including severe nutritional deficiency states, protein-losing enteropathy, congenital hypoalbuminemia, and severe, chronic liver disease.

Cirrhosis (see also Chaps. 39 and 249)   The total blood volume in cirrhosis of the liver is commonly increased when the disorder is accompanied by a system of dilated venous radicles and multiple small arteriovenous fistulas. Effective systemic perfusion, the effective arterial blood volume, and the intrathoracic blood volume appear to be diminished, probably as a consequence of the passage of blood through these fistulas, as well as from the portal venous hypertension and the obstruction of the lymphatic drainage of the liver. These alterations are frequently complicated by reduced serum albumin, which reduces the effective arterial blood volume even further, leading to activation of the renin-angiotensin-aldosterone system and other salt- and water-retaining mechanisms. Initially, the excess interstitial fluid is localized preferentially behind the congested portal venous system and obstructed hepatic lymphatics, i.e., in the peritoneal cavity. In late stages of the disease, particularly when there is hypoalbuminemia, peripheral edema may also be noted.

Idiopathic edema   This syndrome, which occurs almost exclusively in women, often with psychosocial difficulties, is characterized by periodic episodes of edema, frequently accompanied by abdominal distention. Fairly large, diurnal alterations in weight occur, so that the patient may weigh several pounds more after having been in the upright posture for several hours. Such large diurnal weight changes suggest an increase in capillary permeability which appears to fluctuate in severity and is aggravated by hot weather. The fact that it occurs most commonly in women, appears to be most prominent during the premenstrual period, and may be improved by progesterone administration suggests that there may be a hormonal effect on the permeability of the vessels that permits the loss of plasma volume into the interstitial space in the upright position and that leads in turn to a contraction in plasma volume and the subsequent retention of salt and water.

The treatment of idiopathic cyclic edema includes a reduction in salt intake, education in the use of rest in the supine position for several hours each day, the wearing of elastic stockings which are put on before arising in the morning, and an attempt to understand any underlying emotional problems. The angiotensin-converting enzyme inhibitor captopril, progesterone, the dopamine receptor agonist bromocriptine, and the sympathomimetic amine dextroamphetamine have all been reported to be useful when administered to patients who do not respond to simpler measures. Diuretics are initially useful but may lose their effectiveness with continuous administration; accordingly, they should be employed sparingly, if at all.

DIFFERENTIAL DIAGNOSIS   As a rule, localized edema can be readily differentiated from generalized edema. The great majority of patients with noninflammatory generalized edema of significant degree suffer from advanced cardiac, renal, hepatic, or nutritional disorders. Consequently, the differential diagnosis of generalized edema should be directed toward implicating or excluding these several conditions.

Localized edema   Edema originating from inflammation or hypersensitivity is usually readily identified. Localized edema due to venous or lymphatic obstruction may be caused by thrombophlebitis, chronic lymphangitis, resection of regional lymph nodes, filariasis, etc. Lymphedema is particularly intractable because restriction of lymphatic flow results in increased protein concentration in the interstitial fluid, a circumstance which severely impedes removal of retained fluid.

Edema of heart failure   Evidence of heart disease, as manifested by cardiac enlargement and gallop rhythm together with evidence of cardiac failure, such as dyspnea, basilar rales, venous distention, and hepatomegaly, usually provides an indication on clinical examination of the pathogenesis of edema resulting from heart failure. Noninvasive tests such as echocardiography and radionuclide angiography may be helpful in establishing the diagnosis of heart failure (see also Chaps. 179 and 182).

Edema of the nephrotic syndrome   Massive proteinuria, (> 3.5 g per day), severe hypoalbuminemia, and in some instances hypercholesterolemia are present. This syndrome may occur during the course of a variety of kidney diseases, which include glomerulonephritis, diabetic glomerulosclerosis, and hypersensitivity reactions. A history of previous renal disease may or may not be elicited (see also Chap. 223).

Edema of acute glomerulonephritis   The edema occurring during the acute phases of glomerulonephritis is characteristically associated with hematuria, proteinuria, and hypertension. Although some evidence supports the view that the fluid retention is due to increased capillary permeability, in most instances the edema in this disease results from primary retention of sodium and water by the kidneys owing to renal insufficiency. This state differs from congestive heart failure in that it is characterized by a normal or increased cardiac output, normal or diminished circulation time, a reduction in the hematocrit, and a normal arterial–mixed venous oxygen difference. Patients commonly have evidence of pulmonary congestion on chest roentgenograms before cardiac enlargement is significant and do not develop orthopnea (see also Chap. 223).

Edema of cirrhosis   Ascites and evidence of hepatic disease (collateral venous channels, jaundice, and spider angiomas) characterize edema of hepatic origin. The ascites is frequently refractory to treatment because it collects as a result of a combination of obstruction of hepatic lymphatic drainage, portal hypertension, and hypoalbuminemia. Edema may also occur in other parts of the body in these patients as a result of hypoalbuminemia. Furthermore, the sizable accumulation of ascitic fluid may increase intraabdominal pressure and impede venous return from the lower extremities; hence, it tends to promote accumulation of edema in this region as well (see also Chap. 249).

Edema of nutritional origin   An inadequate diet over a prolonged period may produce hypoproteinemia and edema, which may be intensified by beriberi heart disease, in which multiple peripheral arteriovenous fistulas result in reduced effective perfusion and effective arterial blood volume, thereby enhancing edema formation (Chap. 193). More striking edema is commonly observed when these famished subjects are provided with an adequate diet. The ingestion of more food may increase the quantity of salt ingested, which is then retained along with water. In addition to hypoalbuminemia, hypokalemia and caloric deficits may be involved in the edema of starvation.

Other causes of edema   These include hypothyroidism in which myxedema may be located typically in the pretibial region and which may also be associated with periorbital puffiness. Exogenous hyperadrenocortism, pregnancy, and administration of estrogens and vasodilators may also all cause edema.

Distribution   The distribution of edema is an important guide to the cause. Thus, edema of one leg or of one or both arms is usually the result of venous and/or lymphatic obstruction. Edema resulting from hypoproteinemia characteristically is generalized, but it is especially evident in the very soft tissues of the eyelids and face and tends to be most pronounced in the morning because of the recumbent posture assumed during the night. Edema associated with heart failure, on the other hand, tends to be more extensive in the legs and to be accentuated in the evening, a feature also determined largely by posture. In the rare types of cardiac disease, such as tricuspid stenosis and constrictive pericarditis, in which orthopnea may be absent and the patient actually prefers the recumbent posture, the factor of gravity may be equalized and facial edema observed. Less common causes of facial edema include trichinosis, allergic reactions, and myxedema. Unilateral edema occasionally results from lesions in the central nervous system affecting the vasomotor fibers on one side of the body; paralysis also reduces lymphatic and venous drainage on the affected side.

Additional factors in diagnosis The color, thickness, and sensitivity of the skin are significant. Local tenderness and increase in temperature suggest inflammation. Local cyanosis may signify a venous obstruction. In individuals who have had repeated episodes of prolonged edema, the skin over the involved areas may be thickened, hard, and often red.

Measurement of the venous pressure is of importance in evaluating edema. Elevation in an isolated part of the body usually reflects localized venous obstruction. Generalized elevation of systemic venous pressure usually suggests the presence of congestive heart failure, although it may occur with the hypervolemia that accompanies acute renal insufficiency. Ordinarily, significant increase in venous pressure can be recognized by the level at which cervical veins collapse; in doubtful cases and for accurate recording, the central venous pressure should be measured. In patients with obstruction of the superior vena cava, edema is confined to the face, neck, and upper extremities, where the venous pressure is elevated compared with that in the lower extremities. Measurement of venous pressure in the upper extremities is also useful in patients with massive edema of the lower extremities and ascites; it is elevated when the edema is on a cardiac basis (e.g., constrictive pericarditis or tricuspid stenosis) but is normal when it is secondary to cirrhosis.

Determination of the concentration of serum proteins, and especially of serum albumin, identifies those patients in whom edema is due, at least in part, to diminished intravascular colloid oncotic pressure. The presence of proteinuria affords useful clues. The complete absence of protein in the urine is evidence against renal disease as a cause of edema. Slight to moderate proteinuria is the rule in patients with heart failure, whereas persistent massive proteinuria is usually due to the nephrotic syndrome.

APPROACH TO THE PATIENT WITH EDEMA A significant question to ask is whether the edema is localized or generalized. If it is localized, those phenomena that may be responsible should be concentrated upon. In this context, localized edema may include hydrothorax, ascites, or both, in the absence of congestive heart failure or hypoalbuminemia. Either of these collections may be a consequence of local venous or lymphatic obstruction, as in inflammatory disease or carcinoma.

If the edema is generalized, it should be determined, first, if there is hypoalbuminemia of significant degree, e.g., serum albumin concentration less than 2.5 g/dL. If there is, the history, physical examination, urinalysis, and other laboratory data will help evaluate the question of cirrhosis, severe malnutrition, protein-losing gastroenteropathy, or the nephrotic syndrome as the underlying disorder. If hypoalbuminemia is not present, it should be determined if there is evidence of congestive heart failure of a severity to promote generalized edema. Finally, it should be ascertained whether the patient has an adequate urine output, or if there is significant oliguria or even anuria. These abnormalities are discussed in Chaps. 40, 219, and 220. The major differential diagnosis in these instances is frequently the discrimination between primary renal retention of salt and water and congestive heart failure.

REFERENCES

BUCKALEW VM JR, GRUBER KA: Natriuretic hormone. Ann Rev Physiol 46:343, 1984
GOLDEN MHN: Protein deficiency, energy deficiency, and the oedema of malnutrition. Lancet 1:1261, 1982

HRICIK DE, KASSIRER JP: The nephrotic syndrome, in *Disease-A-Month,* NJ Cotsonas et al (eds). Chicago, Year Book Medical, 1982, p 5
NEEDLEMAN P et al: Atriopeptins as cardiac hormones. Hypertension 7:469, 1985
SEIFTER JL et al: Control of extracellular fluid volume and pathophysiology of edema formation, in BM Brenner, FC Rector (eds): *The Kidney,* 3d ed. Philadelphia, Saunders, 1986, p 343
SKORECKI KL, BRENNER BM: Body fluid homeostasis in congestive heart failure cirrhosis with ascites. Am J Med 72:325, 1982
STAUB NC, TAYLOR AE (eds): *Edema.* New York, Raven, 1984
STREETEN DHP: Idiopathic edema: Pathogenesis, clinical features, and treatment. Metabolism 27:353, 1978
SUZUKI H et al: Effect of the angiotensin converting enzyme inhibitor, captopril (SQ14,225), on orthostatic sodium and water retention in patients with idiopathic edema. Nephron 39:244, 1985

29 ALTERATIONS IN ARTERIAL PRESSURE AND THE SHOCK SYNDROME

EUGENE BRAUNWALD / GORDON H. WILLIAMS

CONTROL AND MEASUREMENT OF ARTERIAL PRESSURE

Arterial pressure must be maintained at levels sufficient to permit adequate perfusion of the capillary networks in the systemic vascular bed. The pressure in the central arterial bed is dependent on the product of two factors—the volume of blood ejected by the left ventricle per unit of time, i.e., the cardiac output, and the resistance to blood flow offered by the vessels in the peripheral vascular bed. The resistance of a blood vessel, in turn, varies inversely as the fourth power of its radius, and at any given level of cardiac output arterial pressure is therefore largely dependent upon the degree of constriction of the smooth muscle in the walls of the arterioles. Though resistance to flow also varies with the viscosity of the fluid and the length of the vessels, alterations in these factors are ordinarily of only secondary importance.

Cardiac output is controlled largely by factors which regulate ventricular end-diastolic volume (preload), the level of myocardial contractility, the impedance against which the left ventricle ejects (afterload), and heart rate (Chap. 181). The autonomic nervous system (Chap. 66) plays a major role in the maintenance of arterial pressure by its influences on all four determinants of cardiac output through activation of adrenergic receptors in the sinoatrial node, myocardium, smooth muscle in the walls of the arterioles, venules, and veins. The afferent limbs of the autonomic reflex arcs regulating arterial pressure acutely arise in stretch receptors in the carotid sinuses, the aortic arch, the chambers of the heart, and the lungs. Impulses are transmitted along afferent fibers in the glossopharyngeal and vagus nerves to extensive central autonomic connections in the medulla. Synapses connect not only the sympathetic and parasympathetic nuclei and efferent arcs, but also the cerebral cortex and hypothalamic nuclei which control hormonal secretion via the pituitary gland.

A rapid reduction of arterial pressure diminishes the stimulation of pressoreceptors, which in turn activates sympathetic outflow and inhibits parasympathetic activity. As a result, the vascular smooth muscle in arterioles and veins constricts, while heart rate and myocardial contractility are augmented. In addition, as arterial pressure falls, adrenal medullary secretion increases, along with the output of antidiuretic hormone (ADH), adrenocorticotropic hormone (ACTH), renin, and aldosterone; all these effects act to restore the arterial pressure to control levels. Opposite changes occur if arterial pressure is raised acutely. Thus, the operation of the pressoreceptor and a number of humoral systems normally serve to buffer the body from a variety of influences which would otherwise produce marked alterations in arterial pressure.

MEASUREMENT OF ARTERIAL PRESSURE Arterial pressure is determined clinically with a pneumatic cuff; ordinarily, this indirect method provides slight underestimation of the true arterial pressure. However, considerable error may be introduced if proper precautions are not taken in determining blood pressure by this method. The arterial pressure may be significantly underestimated if the air in the cuff is released too rapidly, especially in the presence of bradycardia or an irregular rhythm, or if inadequate inflation of the cuff does not result in complete vascular occlusion. This indirect method is most accurate when, in normal-sized adults with arm circumferences between 24 and 32 cm, a "standard adult" cuff is employed. However, when a cuff of this size is used on children or adults with unusually thin arms, blood pressure may be seriously underestimated, or conversely, it may be overestimated when employed on an arm or thigh greater than 33 cm in girth. Sphygmomanometers for adults are available in four sizes. The proper size should be employed in any given patient. Marked vasoconstriction resulting in severely attenuated limb blood flow and/or marked reductions in pulse pressure may also result in serious underestimation of arterial pressure by the auscultatory method. Under these circumstances direct intraarterial recordings may reveal a normal or even an elevated pressure, while the absence of Korotkoff sounds makes the pressure unobtainable by the indirect methods. Diastolic pressure usually corresponds closely to the disappearance (phase V) of the Korotkoff sounds, but in severe aortic regurgitation it corresponds with the muffling (phase IV) of the sounds.

THE "NORMAL" BLOOD PRESSURE The "normal" blood pressure is difficult to define. Traditional statistical approaches define

TABLE 29-1 Etiologic factors in shock

I Hypovolemia
  A External fluid losses
    1 Hemorrhage
    2 Gastrointestinal
      a Vomiting (pyloric stenosis, intestinal obstruction)
      b Diarrhea
    3 Renal
      a Diabetes mellitus
      b Diabetes insipidus
      c Excessive use of diuretics
    4 Cutaneous
      a Burns
      b Exudative lesions
      c Perspiration and insensible water loss without replacement
  B Internal sequestration
    1 Fractures
    2 Ascites (peritonitis, pancreatitis, cirrhosis)
    3 Intestinal obstruction
    4 Hemothorax
    5 Hemoperitoneum
II Cardiogenic
  A Myocardial infarction
  B Arrhythmia (paroxysmal tachycardia or fibrillation, severe bradycardia)
  C Severe congestive heart failure with low cardiac output
  D Cardiac mechanical factors
    1 Acute mitral or aortic regurgitation
    2 Rupture of interventricular septum
III Obstruction to blood flow
  A Pulmonary embolus
  B Tension pneumothorax
  C Cardiac tamponade
  D Dissecting aortic aneurysm
  E Intracardiac (ball valve thrombus, atrial myxoma)
IV Neuropathic
  A Drug induced
    1 Anesthesia
    2 Ganglion-blocking or other antihypertensive drugs
    3 "Ingestion" (barbiturates, glutethimide, phenothiazines)
  B Spinal cord injury
  C Orthostatic hypotension (primary autonomic insufficiency, peripheral neuropathies)
V Other
  A Infection
    1 Gram-negative septicemia (endotoxin)
    2 Other septicemias
  B Anaphylaxis
  C Endocrine failure (Addison's disease, myxedema)
  D Anoxia

normality on the basis of values included within two standard deviations of the mean of pressures obtained in a large population of presumably healthy individuals. However, a better definition of abnormality would be based on demonstrated deleterious effects of blood pressure levels exceeding certain limits. If such criteria are used, chronic *hypotension* would seem to occur very rarely. However, the incidence of hypertension based on casual blood pressure levels exceeding 140/90 (widely accepted as hazardous because it is associated with increased risk of cardiovascular mortality which can be reduced by therapy) is estimated to be approximately 20 percent in the adult population of the United States, the incidence in the black population exceeding that in the nonblacks by 50 to 100 percent. Even these statistics may understate the prevalence of hypertension if one accepts the validity of actuarial data indicating that longevity is shortened progressively in adults whose blood pressures exceed 100/60 (see Chap. 196).

ACUTE HYPOTENSION AND SHOCK

Hypotension and shock are not synonymous; although shock is usually associated with hypotension, a previously hypertensive patient may be in shock despite an arterial pressure within normal limits, and hypotension may occur in the absence of shock. *Shock* may be defined as a state in which there is widespread, serious reduction of tissue perfusion, which, if prolonged, leads to generalized impairment of cellular function.

CAUSES The most common clinical causes of shock are listed in Table 29-1. Since arterial pressure is dependent on the product of cardiac output and systemic vascular resistance, marked reductions in either of these variables without a compensatory elevation of the other results in systemic hypotension. Reduction of cardiac output may be due to (1) hypovolemia, with volume loss being external (e.g., hemorrhage or diarrhea) or endogenous (e.g., anaphylaxis); (2) myocardial failure (e.g., cardiogenic shock); (3) circulatory obstruction (e.g., pulmonary embolism); (4) redistribution of blood into the venous capacitance bed ("distributive shock," e.g., septic shock); and (5) reduction of peripheral vasomotor tone, caused, for example, by acute spinal cord injury, which results in reduced systemic vascular resistance and venous dilatation, the latter causing reduced venous return and cardiac output. In many patients, particularly in the late stages of shock, multiple factors are involved simultaneously regardless of the inciting event.

    Hypovolemia has been studied much more extensively than any other cause of shock; the mechanism of development is usually readily evident and well understood, and therapy, i.e., restoration of blood volume, is both simple and effective if applied before irreversible tissue damage occurs. Whether the primary insult is the external loss of blood, plasma, or water and salt or the internal sequestration of these fluids in a hollow viscus or body cavity, the general effect is similar, i.e., reduced venous return and decreased cardiac output. This leads to a set of reflex responses designed to maintain the supply of oxygen to critical organs, such as the brain and heart. However, these responses may so limit perfusion of other organs, such as the gut, as to produce necrosis. For purposes of a general discussion of shock, hemorrhagic hypovolemia will be used as the model, but the consequences of general reduced tissue perfusion are similar in other forms of shock.

Stages of hypovolemic shock Depending upon the severity and rate of development of hypovolemia, the shock syndrome may develop abruptly or evolve gradually. If the precipitating factors progress unabated, the endogenous defense mechanisms, while initially competent to maintain adequate circulation, eventually are extended beyond their capacity for compensation. The development of the shock syndrome may be thought to evolve through several stages which merge with one another. The first is the period in which the blood volume deficit is relatively minor and in which the patient may be asymptomatic. In a previously healthy individual compensation for an acute blood loss of as much as 10 percent of the normal blood volume (as with venesection of 500 mL blood from a donor) is achieved acutely by constriction of the arteriolar bed and an augmentation of heart rate, effects mediated by reflex increases in the release of norepinephrine from sympathetic nerve endings and of both norepinephrine and epinephrine from the adrenal medulla. Other responses with more gradual effects include the increased secretion of antidiuretic hormone and the activation of the renin-angiotensin-aldosterone axis (Chap. 325). Arterial pressure is maintained and cardiac output is normal, or only slightly reduced, primarily as a consequence of selective reductions of blood flow to the skin and muscle beds. Heart rate may rise and arterial pressure decline modestly when the patient assumes the erect posture. Hemorrhage may be associated with thrombocytosis, increased platelet adhesiveness, and resultant stasis in blood flow in some capillary beds.

During the second stage, with a reduction in blood volume of 15 to 25 percent, cardiac output falls markedly, even in the recumbent position, and is redistributed with larger fractions going to the liver, heart, and brain and smaller fractions to the kidney, gut, and skin. Despite intense arteriolar constriction in most vascular beds, systolic arterial pressure declines by 10 to 20 mmHg in previously normotensive individuals, although it falls proportionately less than cardiac output. Generalized venoconstriction occurs, increasing the fraction of the total blood volume in the central circulation and tending to sustain venous return. Fluid moves from the interstitial to the intravascular compartment and the hematocrit falls. There is a massive reflex adrenergic discharge accompanied by tachycardia, tachypnea, intense cutaneous vasoconstriction, pallor, cold distal extremities, diaphoresis, piloerection, oliguria, apprehension, and restlessness. The latter mental signs relate to a reduction in cerebral circulation due to decreased perfusion pressure rather than to local vasoconstriction. Angina may occur in patients who have intrinsic coronary vascular disease. Reduced availability of oxygen to tissues activates anaerobic glycolysis, plasma lactate levels rise, and a metabolic acidosis develops. Tachypnea causes a compensatory respiratory alkalosis.

Once the patient has achieved this state of maximal mobilization of compensatory mechanisms, small additional losses of blood result in the third stage characterized by rapid deterioration of the circulation, with life-threatening reductions of cardiac output, blood pressure, and tissue perfusion. The duration of this shock state, the severity of tissue anoxia, and the age and underlying physical state of the patient are of primary importance in determining the ultimate outcome. If tissue perfusion is restored rapidly, recovery may be expected. However, if shock persists, severe vasoconstriction, a compensatory mechanism which aids in the maintenance of arterial pressure, may itself become a complicating factor, and by reducing tissue perfusion even further may initiate a vicious cycle leading to an irreversible state due to widespread cellular injury. Blood flow to the brain, heart, and kidneys is further reduced, and severe ischemia of these vital organs leads to irreversible tissue damage which may result in impaired function of the organ and, eventually, death. Impaired coronary perfusion depresses cardiac function, particularly in patients with some coronary vascular obstruction, and this may lead to further lowering of cardiac output, thus perpetuating a vicious cycle. Cardiac function may also be depressed by the release of a myocardial *depressant factor* from the hypoperfused pancreas. Reduced flow to the medullary vasomotor center late in the stage of shock depresses the activity of compensatory reflexes. Anoxia, hypercapnia, and lactic acidosis result from hypoperfusion of tissues and anaerobic metabolism. These metabolic derangements ultimately result in failure of the energy-requiring active transport systems of cell membranes. The cellular high-energy phosphate reserves are depleted. The integrity of the cells is compromised, and potassium ions, intracellular lysosomal enzymes, peptides, and other vasoactive compounds are released into the circulation. The integrity of capillary membranes is disrupted, and fluid, proteins, and cellular constituents of the blood seep into the extravascular space of tissues.

In profound shock from any cause, an additional important factor which may exacerbate the status of the microcirculation is platelet aggregation and widespread disseminated intravascular coagulation (DIC, Chap. 281) in the bowel, kidney, and other organs. The resultant ischemia produced in the bowel may further complicate the circulatory compensation as a result of breakdown of the mucosal barrier, leading to entry of bacteria and toxic bacterial products into the circulation. Similar changes in the capillary network of the lungs result in interstitial and alveolar edema (noncardiogenic pulmonary edema), impaired respiratory gas transfer, and ultimately development of the adult respiratory distress syndrome (ARDS, Chap. 216), a common lethal complication of shock. Acute tubular necrosis, caused by prolonged renal hypoperfusion, may result in prolonged postshock renal insufficiency (Chap. 219). Because many bacterial substances are potent vasodilators, vasoconstrictor mechanisms may be inhibited, with a further decrease in blood pressure despite intense sympathetic activity. The release of oxygen-derived free radicals may occur during treatment and may be responsible for severe postischemic tissue injury.

Just as tissue perfusion may fall to dangerous or even fatal levels because of actual fluid losses or sequestration with diminished venous return, acute cardiac failure (cardiogenic shock) or a massive pulmonary embolus may have similar effects. Furthermore, even in the presence of a normal blood volume and cardiac function, "vasomotor collapse" due to drug-induced or neuropathic failure of sympathetic vasomotor activity can result in shock because of reduction of peripheral resistance, the pooling of blood in the venous bed, and reduction of cardiac output.

Other forms of shock   A complex form of shock may result from infection, especially gram-negative bacteremia with endotoxin release (Chap. 86). This form of shock is associated in its early stage with fever, arteriovenous shunting, low systemic vascular resistance and arterial pressure, and an elevated cardiac output, with warm, dry skin, and in its late stages with vascular pooling, diminished venous return, reduced cardiac output, and hypotension despite increased vascular resistance, and with activation of complement leading to further cell damage. In anaphylactic shock (Chap. 260), release of histamine, leukotrienes, prostaglandins, and other mediators causes arteriolar dilatation as well as increased capillary permeability with loss of intravascular volume, and an attendant reduction in venous return and cardiac output, leading to a marked reduction in arterial pressure, and reductions in central venous and pulmonary capillary wedge pressures and hemoconcentration.

TREATMENT   This should be directed toward the rapid restoration of cardiac output and tissue perfusion. The patient should be treated in a properly equipped intensive care unit, where continuous monitoring of intraarterial, pulmonary artery wedge, and central venous pressures is possible. Frequent determinations of arterial blood gases, pH, and serum electrolytes are necessary. However, general supportive measures must be undertaken immediately, even before transfer to the unit. Whether shock results from decreased cardiac output due to a primary reduction in intravascular volume or from a reduction of "effective blood volume" with pooling of blood in the venous bed, the most effective means of restoring adequate circulation is by the rapid infusion of volume-expanding fluids (whole blood, plasma, plasma substitutes, or isotonic electrolyte solutions) to restore systolic arterial pressure to above 100 mmHg in a previously normotensive person, with central venous and pulmonary artery wedge pressures below approximately 15 and 20 mmHg, respectively.

However, when shock is secondary to, or is accompanied by, cardiac failure with increased pulmonary vascular and central venous pressures, the infusion of volume-expanding fluids may result in pulmonary edema. Here attention must be directed toward restoring cardiac function with cardiotonic drugs such as digitalis glycosides and isoproterenol (Chap. 182), and an attempt should be made to support arterial pressure at levels sufficient to maintain the coronary perfusion pressure (Chap. 190). Intraaortic balloon counterpulsation, together with augmentation of contractility with a sympathomimetic amine, and adjustment of preload to an optimal level of left ventricular filling pressure (approximately 20 mmHg) may be used to treat this state. Arrhythmias, which may also contribute to the low cardiac output, should be corrected (Chaps. 183 and 184).

The appearance of the external jugular veins may be helpful in differentiating between shock with high or low central venous pressure. However, catheters inserted into the superior vena cava and, if possible, into the pulmonary artery (a Swan-Ganz balloon-tipped catheter) are the best means for continuously monitoring ventricular filling pressure and of considerable value in guiding therapy. Serial measurements of central venous pressure, urine flow rate, heart rate, and the clinical and mental state of the patient often provide more important indexes of the efficacy of therapy than arterial pressure changes do. In patients with cardiogenic shock, the balloon-tipped catheter "floated" into the pulmonary artery at the bedside without the aid of fluoroscopy is essential in guiding treatment (Chap. 190). Shock secondary to cardiac tamponade may be recognized by the presence of a paradoxical pulse, jugular venous distention, and pericardial fluid detected by echocardiography (Chap. 194). Pericardiocentesis may be life-saving. Adequate ventilation with 100% O_2 must be assured. In patients with infection, appropriate antibiotics and, if necessary, surgical debridement are required.

There is considerable debate concerning the efficacy of vasoconstrictor drugs in shock. In patients with severe peripheral constriction these agents are often ineffective and may actually reduce the already impaired tissue perfusion. However, these drugs may be helpful in patients with inadequate vasoconstrictor responses who are not in heart failure. The use of alpha-adrenergic blocking agents or massive doses of adrenal glucocorticoids in shock secondary to gram-negative septicemia with endotoxin release is also a matter of considerable controversy. The release of the endogenous opiate β-endorphin in many forms of stress has led to trials with the specific opiate antagonist naloxone, with favorable responses having been reported in patients with septic shock.

Following immediate attention to improvement of perfusion in patients with shock, efforts should be directed to treating the underlying etiologic factors, such as gastrointestinal hemorrhage, diabetic acidosis, or septicemia (Table 29-1). Normal pH and serum electrolyte patterns should be restored. After hypovolemia has been corrected, consideration must also be given to the function of other organ systems, particularly the lungs and kidneys, with treatment of ARDS and acute tubular necrosis as outlined elsewhere (Chaps. 216 and 219, respectively). It should be remembered that death secondary to failure of the lungs, kidney, and/or liver occurs not infrequently in patients whose circulation has been restored after they have experienced prolonged shock.

CHRONIC HYPOTENSION

Although many patients have been treated for chronic "low blood pressure," most of them, with systolic pressures in the range of 90 to 110 mmHg, are normal and may actually have a greater life expectancy than those with "normal" pressures. Patients with true chronic hypotension may complain of lethargy, weakness, easy fatigability, and dizziness or faintness, especially if arterial pressure is lowered further when the erect position is assumed. These symptoms are presumably due to a decrease in perfusion of the brain, heart, skeletal muscle, and other organs.

Chronic hypotension occasionally results from severe reductions of the cardiac output. The major endocrine causes of chronic hypotension are associated with deficient gluco- and mineralocorticoid secretion and resultant reductions of the extracellular fluid volume. Hypotension is usually more pronounced in patients with primary adrenocortical insufficiency than in those with hypopituitarism because

secretion of the salt-retaining adrenocortical hormone, aldosterone, is partially preserved in pituitary insufficiency (Chap. 325).

Malnutrition, cachexia, chronic bed rest, and a variety of neurologic disorders may result in chronic hypotension, especially in the standing position. Interference with the neural pathways anywhere between the vasomotor center and the efferent sympathetic nerve endings on the blood vessels or heart may prevent the vasoconstriction and increase in cardiac output which occur as a normal response to a reduction in arterial pressure. Multiple sclerosis, amyotrophic lateral sclerosis, subacute combined sclerosis, syringomyelia, tabes dorsalis, peripheral neuropathies, spinal cord section, diabetic neuropathy, extensive lumbodorsal sympathectomy, and the administration of drugs interfering with nerve transmission in the sympathetic nervous system are all associated with orthostatic hypotension.

IDIOPATHIC ORTHOSTATIC HYPOTENSION (PRIMARY AUTONOMIC INSUFFICIENCY) This is a rare condition occurring mostly in older men in which there is degeneration of central and/or peripheral autonomic nervous structures, which may result in such severe orthostatic hypotension that syncope or seizures occur when the patient arises from recumbency. This condition is progressive and characterized by ascending anhidrosis and loss of hair, decreased basal metabolic rate (BMR), reduced norepinephrine production, deficient secretion of lacrimal and salivary glands, ileus, bladder atony, and absence of tachycardia on standing despite marked reduction of blood pressure. Hypertension may occur in the supine position.

Those patients with orthostatic hypotension and central nervous system disease (*Shy-Drager syndrome*) have degeneration of the extrapyramidal tracts, the basal ganglia, and the dorsal nucleus of the vagus and have normal resting plasma norepinephrine levels, while those with only peripheral autonomic disease have depressed levels at rest. Both groups fail to increase their circulating concentrations of the neurotransmitter normally during standing and exercise. Thus, it appears that patients with orthostatic hypotension and central nervous system disease have an intact peripheral sympathetic nervous system, but are unable to activate it, while those without central disease have true insufficiency of the peripheral autonomic nervous system with depletion of norepinephrine in sympathetic nerve endings.

Specific therapy is not available for most of the neurologic causes of orthostatic hypotension, and treatment with sympathomimetic drugs has not proved effective over prolonged periods. However, the expansion of extracellular volume, which may be achieved with a high-salt diet (10 to 20 g per day), and/or the potent synthetic salt-retaining steroid, 9α-fluorohydrocortisone (0.1 to 0.5 mg per day) may be useful but often results in hypertension when the patient is supine. Tight, full-length elastic supportive hose to reduce orthostatic pooling of blood in the legs may also be helpful in sustaining arterial pressure, and in the most severe cases pressurized aviator suits may be necessary to permit ambulation. Occasionally, favorable results may be achieved with sympathomimetic amines such as dihydroergotamine, hydroxyamphetamine, or L-dopa in combination with a monoamine oxidase inhibitor, such as tranylcypromine, with indomethacin or propranolol.

HYPERTENSION (See also Chap. 196)

DIAGNOSIS Patients with elevations of arterial pressure are usually asymptomatic, and the blood pressure abnormality often arouses attention only incidentally during military, life insurance, or other periodic physical examinations. Because hypertension results in secondary organ damage and a reduced life span, it should be evaluated and, when appropriate, treated.

Often, however, the first question is whether patients with a moderately elevated routine blood pressure recording are truly hypertensive. It is well established that anxiety, discomfort, physical activity, or other stress can acutely and transiently raise arterial pressure. Arterial pressure should be measured with the patient sitting comfortably and having been at rest for at least 5 min. Most persons have a higher pressure when initially examined than after several measurements made in the course of a single visit; in order to establish the diagnosis of hypertension, it is necessary to document in the course of at least two separate examinations in each of which arterial pressure is measured at least twice, that arterial pressure remains elevated. This precaution need not be taken in patients with markedly elevated blood pressure and/or in those in whom significant target organ damage is already manifest. Patients with transient or "labile" hypertension may not require immediate treatment but should be reexamined periodically, since over the course of time they may develop sustained hypertension. A diastolic pressure that is consistently ≥90 mmHg is considered to be abnormal; in the presence of a normal diastolic pressure, a systolic pressure ≥160 mmHg represents isolated systolic hypertension.

MECHANISM Regardless of the primary cause, the hemodynamic abnormality in most patients with fixed hypertension is increased vascular resistance, especially at the level of the smaller muscular arteries and arterioles, though some patients may have an increased cardiac output, particularly in the early stages of the illness.

Peripheral resistance is determined by the intrinsic physical characteristics of the resistance vessels, i.e., the ratio of lumen to wall thickness, as well as the neurohumoral influences that act on vascular smooth muscle; the latter include the neurotransmitters norepinephrine, a vasoconstrictor, and in some vessels, acetylcholine, a vasodilator. Humoral and locally acting substances include angiotensin II and vasopressin (vasoconstrictors) and prostaglandins and kinins (vasodilators). Hypoxia and products of metabolism, such as H^+, lactic acid, and, perhaps most important, adenosine, also exert potent *local* vasodilating influences.

Systolic hypertension is most commonly seen in elderly patients with decreased compliance of the aortic wall and, like diastolic hypertension, is a risk factor for the development of atherosclerosis. When systolic hypertension is due to an elevated stroke volume, as in patients with severe bradycardia, thyrotoxicosis, severe anemia, aortic valvular regurgitation, arteriovenous shunts or fistulas, patent ductus arteriosus, or the hyperkinetic heart syndrome, it is usually accompanied by a reduced diastolic pressure and a normal mean pressure, and under these circumstances it does not appear to be a risk factor for atherosclerosis.

ETIOLOGY A specific cause for the elevated arterial pressure cannot be defined for most patients with hypertension. The percentage of patients with so-called idiopathic, essential, or primary hypertension is high, varying from 80 to 95 percent depending on both the patient population and how extensive the "routine" evaluation is. More specific etiologic relationships have been established for a smaller group of patients with systemic hypertension, i.e., secondary hypertension (Table 196-1). Primary renal vascular and renal parenchymal diseases associated with the development of serious hypertension (as distinguished from renal damage secondary to hypertension) are well recognized, as are a number of endocrine disorders, including Cushing's syndrome, primary hyperaldosteronism (Chap. 325), acromegaly (Chap. 321), and pheochromocytoma (Chap. 326).

EFFECTS OF HYPERTENSION Patients with untreated hypertension die prematurely, most commonly due to heart disease (Chaps. 182 and 196), with strokes (Chap. 343) and renal failure (Chap. 227) also frequently occurring.

APPROACH TO THE PATIENT WITH HYPERTENSION The physician's first task is to determine whether or not a patient with a given level of arterial pressure has hypertension. Then, determinations of the extent of pretreatment evaluation, whether or not to treat, how to treat, and how frequently to reevaluate are necessary. In general, it is preferable to measure arterial pressure on several occasions prior to starting therapy. Initial history, physical examination, and laboratory evaluation should be directed at uncovering correctable secondary forms of hypertension (Table 196-1).

An assessment of the following areas in the medical history is particularly important: family or personal history of hypertension; drugs or dietary factors which may aggravate the hypertension, e.g., high salt intake, oral contraceptives, and hormones; cardiovascular risk factors including diabetes mellitus, smoking, lipid abnormalities, or strokes; cardiac or renal disease; and symptoms suggestive of secondary forms of hypertension, e.g., muscle cramps and weakness associated with primary aldosteronism (Chap. 325) or episodic headaches, palpitations, and sweating associated with pheochromocytoma (Chap. 326).

The *physical examination* should include a standing blood pressure, height, weight, funduscopic examination, assessment of thyroid size, bruits in neck or abdomen, peripheral pulses including determination of synchrony between upper and lower extremities, examination of the heart for size, rate, murmurs, gallops, auscultation of the lungs, examination of the abdomen for masses, and particularly kidney size, and a neurologic examination to assess the presence of deficits associated with a stroke.

The basic *laboratory evaluation* should consist of hematocrit, urinalysis, blood urea nitrogen or creatinine, serum potassium, ECG, and chest x-ray. Often blood glucose, uric acid, and cholesterol determinations and a blood count are also useful, particularly since they may be part of a battery of automated blood tests that as a group are about the same price as the individual tests listed above. Other studies to identify secondary forms of hypertension may be indicated on the basis of the response to initial therapy or physical examination.

If the diastolic pressure is consistently higher than 90 mmHg, therapy is almost always indicated unless contraindications exist.

Therapy should be directed at reducing the arterial pressure to or near normal levels, since studies have documented that morbidity and mortality are reduced. Ideally, this will be accomplished with agents directed at correcting the underlying mechanism(s) responsible for the elevated blood pressure in the individual patient. When the underlying mechanism(s) is(are) unknown or no specific therapy is available, then a "stepcare approach" has been advocated to achieve this goal. The principle involves initiating therapy with a small dose of a single drug, either a thiazide diuretic or a beta-adrenergic blocker, if necessary increasing the dose of that drug, and then adding the other drug and, if necessary, other agents one at a time (Chap. 196). The therapeutic regimen should be revised as dictated by the arterial pressure measured at periodic intervals. The frequency of reevaluation should be as often as weekly while blood pressure is being lowered in patients with initial diastolic pressures greater than 115 mmHg, and approximately every 4 months in symptom-free patients on stable treatment programs.

The specific drugs are discussed elsewhere (Chap. 196). However, it is important to emphasize here that control of arterial pressure is a lifelong endeavor, the success of which is often dependent on the physician's ability to motivate the patient to adhere to the therapeutic program and to recognize the pharmacologic interactions and adverse reactions of antihypertensive agents.

REFERENCES

ABBOUD FM: Pathophysiology of hypotension and shock, in Hurst JW (ed): *The Heart*, 6th ed. New York, McGraw-Hill, 1986, p 370

ABBRUZZESE JL et al: Postural hypotension. Johns Hopkins Med J 148:127, 1981

BERNTON EW et al: Opioids and neuropeptides: Mechanisms in circulatory shock. Fed Proc 44:290, 1985

GENEST J (ed): *Hypertension: Physiopathology and Treatment*, 2d ed. New York, McGraw-Hill, 1983

GUYTON AC: Circulatory shock and physiology of its treatment, in *Textbook of Medical Physiology*, 7th ed. Philadelphia, Saunders, 1986, p 326

———: Arterial pressure regulation, in *Textbook of Medical Physiology*, 7th ed. Philadelphia, Saunders, 1986, p 244

HOLCROFT JW, BLAISDELL FW: Shock: Causes and management of circulatory collapse, in *Davis-Christopher Textbook of Surgery*, 13th ed, DC Sabiston Jr (ed). Philadelphia, Saunders, 1986, p 38

THE JOINT NATIONAL COMMITTEE ON DETECTION, EVALUATION AND TREATMENT OF HIGH BLOOD PRESSURE: The 1984 Report of the Joint National Committee on Detection, Evaluation, and Treatment of High Blood Pressure. Arch Intern Med 144:1045, 1984

KAPLAN NM: Systemic hypertension: Therapy, in *Heart Disease*, 2d ed, E Braunwald (ed). Philadelphia, Saunders, 1984, p 902

KIRKENDALL WM et al: AHA Committee Report: Recommendations for human blood pressure determination by sphygmomanometers. Circulation 62:1146A, 1980

LEDINGHAM IM et al: Prognosis in severe shock. Brit Heart J 284:443, 1982

MANNING DM et al: Miscuffing: Inappropriate blood pressure cuff application. Circulation 68:763, 1983

ROCK P et al: Efficacy and safety of naloxone in septic shock. Crit Care Med 13:28, 1985

SOBEL BE: Cardiac and noncardiac forms of acute circulation failure (shock), in *Heart Disease,* 2d ed, E Braunwald (ed). Philadelphia, Saunders, 1984, p 578

———, ROBERTS R: Hypotension and syncope, in *Heart Disease,* 2d ed, E Braunwald (ed). Philadelphia, Saunders, 1984, p 928

ZIEGLER MG et al: The sympathetic nervous system defect in primary orthostatic hypotension. N Engl J Med 296:293, 1977

30   SUDDEN CARDIOVASCULAR COLLAPSE AND DEATH

BURTON E. SOBEL / EUGENE BRAUNWALD

Sudden cardiac death claims approximately 400,000 lives annually in the United States alone, a frequency on the order of one death per minute. Definitions vary, but most include death occurring unexpectedly and instantaneously or within 1 h of the onset of symptoms in a subject with or without known preexisting heart disease. Usually only several minutes elapse between sudden cardiovascular collapse (without effective cardiac output) and irreversible ischemic changes in the central nervous system. Nevertheless, prolonged survival without functional impairment may result from prompt treatment of certain forms of cardiovascular collapse.

CAUSES

MECHANISMS   Sudden cardiovascular collapse may be due to (1) arrhythmia (Chaps. 183 and 184)—(a) most commonly, ventricular fibrillation or tachycardia, sometimes occurring following a bradyarrhythmia, or (b) severe bradycardia or ventricular asystole, factors generally presaging failure of resuscitative efforts; (2) a marked, abrupt reduction in cardiac output, such as occurs with mechanical blockade of the circulation; massive pulmonary thromboembolism (Chap. 211) and cardiac tamponade are two examples of this form; (3) sudden ventricular (pump) failure, which may occur in the presence of acute myocardial infarction ("nonarrhythmic cardiac death") with or without ventricular rupture (Chap. 190) or critical aortic stenosis (Chap. 187); (4) activation of vasodepressor reflexes, which may contribute to sudden reductions in arterial pressure and heart rate, and which are activated in diverse conditions, including pulmonary thromboembolism, the hypersensitive carotid sinus syndrome (Chap. 12), and primary pulmonary hypertension (Chap. 210). Among the primary electrophysiologic disturbances, the relative incidences of ventricular fibrillation, ventricular tachycardia, and severe bradyarrhythmia or asystole are approximately 75, 10, and 25 percent.

SUDDEN DEATH AND CORONARY ATHEROSCLEROSIS   Sudden death is primarily a complication of severe, multivessel coronary atherosclerosis. Fresh coronary thrombi have been found in a variable percentage of patients, ranging from 25 to 75 percent, studied at postmortem. Plaque fissures causing obstruction have been found in some patients without thrombosis; thus, it appears likely that an acute obstructive event triggers sudden death in the majority of patients with coronary artery disease. In other patients, sudden death may result from functional electrophysiologic instability, detectable with provocative, invasive electrophysiologic testing and persisting for prolonged intervals or indefinitely after myocardial infarction. In victims of sudden death less than 45 years of age, platelet thrombi in the coronary microcirculation are often seen. Approximately 60 percent of patients who die of acute myocardial infarction succumb before they reach the hospital. In fact, in 25 percent of patients with coronary artery disease, death is the first indication of the presence of the disorder (Chap. 190). By extrapolation from experience in coronary care units, in which control of electrical activity of the heart has affected the mortality rate favorably, it would appear that the incidence of sudden death in the community might be reduced substantially by prophylactic therapy in populations at particularly high risk, if such therapy could be demonstrated to be effective, of low toxicity, and convenient to the patient. However, sudden death may be but one mode of expression of coronary artery disease, and effective prevention of sudden death will almost certainly require reduction in the incidence and severity of atherosclerosis. The risk of sudden death, when it is a manifestation of remote, prior infarction, is increased in patients with severe left ventricular dysfunction, complex ventricular ectopic activity, and particularly both.

FACTORS ASSOCIATED WITH INCREASED RISK OF SUDDEN DEATH IN NONHOSPITALIZED PERSONS   When electrocardiograms are recorded for 24 h during the course of normal activities, supraventricular premature contractions are found to occur in most American men over 50 years of age, and ventricular premature contractions occur in almost two-thirds. Simple ventricular premature beats in patients with otherwise normal hearts are not associated with increased risk of sudden death, but conduction abnormalities and couplets or high-grade ventricular ectopic beats (repetitive forms, or R-on-T complexes) are associated with an increased risk, particularly among patients who suffered a myocardial infarction during the preceding year. Among patients with acute myocardial infarction, ventricular ectopic beats occurring late in the cardiac cycle are particularly prone to be associated with malignant ventricular arrhythmia. High-frequency, low-amplitude potentials occurring during the inscription of the terminal portion of the QRS complex and ST segment, detectable by frequency analysis of signal-averaged electrocardiogram (ECG) recordings, may also identify patients at increased risk.

Ventricular premature beats may trigger ventricular fibrillation, particularly in the presence of myocardial ischemia. On the other hand, they may be manifestations of common fundamental electrophysiologic disturbances which predispose to both ventricular premature beats and ventricular fibrillation, or they may be totally independent phenomena associated with electrophysiologic mechanisms different from those responsible for fibrillation. Their role may differ in different persons. Ambulatory electrocardiographic monitoring has revealed that a several hour period of increasingly frequent or complex ventricular arrhythmias often precedes ventricular fibrillation.

In general, ventricular arrhythmias are of greater significance and more ominous in the presence of acute ischemia and of severe left ventricular dysfunction secondary to ischemic heart disease or cardiomyopathy than in their absence.

Severe coronary artery disease, not necessarily accompanied by morphologic evidence of an acute infarction, hypertension, or diabetes mellitus, is present in more than 75 percent of persons dying suddenly, and perhaps more significantly, the incidence of sudden death in persons with at least one of the three abnormalities is substantially increased. More than 75 percent of men without known prior coronary artery disease who die suddenly exhibit at least two of the following four risk factors for the development of atherosclerosis: hypercholesterolemia, hypertension, hyperglycemia, and cigarette smoking. Obesity and electrocardiographic criteria of left ventricular hypertrophy are also associated with an increased incidence. The incidence of sudden death is higher in cigarette smokers than in nonsmokers, perhaps because of the elevation of circulating catecholamines and fatty acids and the production of increased circulating carboxyhemoglobin with consequently diminished oxygen-carrying capacity by the blood. The proclivity of cigarette smoking to cause sudden death is not cumulative and appears to be reversible when smoking is discontinued.

Cardiovascular collapse on exertion occurs only rarely in patients with ischemic heart disease undergoing exercise testing, and with appropriate personnel and facilities these episodes respond promptly to electrical defibrillation. Rarely, acute emotional stress may precipitate acute myocardial infarction and sudden death, a finding which is in keeping with recent clinical observations of an association of these events with type A personality and experimental observations of increased susceptibility to ventricular tachycardia and ventricular fibrillation after coronary occlusion in emotionally stressed animals or those with augmented sympathetic activity, and protection of experimental animals with selected central nervous system neurotransmitter precursors.

Two major clinical syndromes may be recognized in patients who die suddenly and unexpectedly; both are generally associated with ischemic heart disease. In the larger group, the arrhythmia occurs totally unexpectedly and without preceding symptoms or prodromata. This form is *not* associated with acute myocardial infarction although most patients afflicted exhibit criteria of remote myocardial infarction or other types of organic heart disease. After resuscitation, there is a propensity for early recurrence, probably reflecting the myocardial electrical instability responsible for the intitial episode, and a relatively high 2-year mortality rate (approximately 50 percent). Clearly, these patients can be salvaged only by a rapidly responsive system and aggressive evaluation and management with drugs, surgery, implantable defibrillators, or programmable pacing devices. Pharmacologic prophylaxis probably enhances survival. The second, smaller group consists of patients who, following resuscitation, exhibit evidence of acute myocardial infarction. These patients often exhibit prodromal symptoms—chest pain, dyspnea, and syncope—and show a much lower recurrence and 2-year mortality rate (15 percent). Survival in this subgroup is similar to that following resuscitation from ventricular fibrillation complicating acute myocardial infarction in the coronary care unit. The propensity for developing ventricular fibrillation at the time of acute infarction is of short duration, in contrast to the prolonged interval of high risk among patients in whom fibrillation occurs without acute infarction. However, the risk of sudden death remains particularly high among some survivors of infarction. Risk factors include extensive infarction; severe impairment of ventricular function; persistent, complex ventricular ectopic activity; QT prolongation after the acute episode; loss of the normal hypertensive response to exercise after convalescence; and persistently positive myocardial infarct scintigrams.

OTHER CAUSES OF SUDDEN DEATH Sudden cardiovascular collapse may result from a number of disorders other than coronary atherosclerosis (Table 30-1). Severe aortic stenosis (congenital or acquired) with sudden arrhythmias or pump failure, hypertrophic cardiomyopathy, and myocarditis or cardiomyopathy associated with arrhythmia may be responsible. Massive pulmonary embolism leads to circulatory collapse and death within minutes in approximately 10 percent of patients; some of the remainder succumb gradually with progressive right ventricular failure and hypoxia. Acute circulatory collapse may be presaged by smaller emboli occurring at variable intervals before the lethal attack. Accordingly, implementation of therapy during the premonitory sublethal phase, including anticoagulant administration, may be lifesaving (Chap. 211). Cardiovascular collapse and sudden death are rare but always potential complications of infective endocarditis (Chap. 188).

A number of less common causes of sudden death have been recognized increasingly in recent years. Sudden cardiac death has been associated with liquid-protein, modified-fast diet programs. Distinguishing features include QT prolongation as well as the less specific morphologic cardiac lesions typical of cachexia seen in autopsied cases. Primary degeneration of the atrioventricular conduction system, with or without deposition of calcium or cartilage, may lead to sudden death in the absence of severe coronary atherosclerosis. Trifascicular atrioventricular (AV) block is often seen in these conditions, which account for more than two-thirds of the cases of chronic AV block in adults (Chap. 183). However, the risk of

sudden death is substantially greater with impaired conduction associated with ischemic heart disease than that due to primary conduction system disease itself. Electrocardiographic QT-interval prolongation, nerve deafness, and autosomal recessive inheritance (the Jervell and Lange-Nielsen syndrome) are associated with a high proportion of cases of ventricular fibrillation. The same electrocardiographic abnormality and electrophysiologic instability without nerve deafness (the Romano-Ward syndrome) appears to be inherited in an autosomal dominant mode. Electrocardiographic changes in these disorders may be manifest only after exercise. The overall risk of sudden death in afflicted subjects is approximately 1 percent per year. Congenital deafness, history of syncope, female gender, and documented torsades de pointes (see below) or ventricular fibrillation are independent risk factors for sudden cardiac death. Although left stellate ganglionectomy exerts transitory prophylactic benefit, long-term salutary effects have not been substantiated.

Other conditions with QT prolongation and increased temporal dispersion of repolarization, such as hypothermia and a number of drugs (including quinidine, disopyramide, procainamide, the phenothiazines and tricyclic antidepressants), hypokalemia, hypomagnesemia, and acute myocarditis, have been associated with sudden death, particularly when preceded by episodes of torsades de pointes, a form of rapid ventricular tachycardia with distinctive electrocardiographic and pathophysiologic features (Chap. 184). Sinoatrial arrest or block with depression of lower pacemakers or the sick sinus syndrome, usually accompanied by conduction system dysfunction as well, may also lead to asystole. Rarely, fibromas or inflammatory processes in the region of the sinus or AV nodes and conduction system elements (ganglionitis and neuritis) may precipitate sudden death in subjects without prior manifestations of heart disease. Sudden rupture of a papillary muscle, the ventricular septum, or free wall, usually occurring within the first few days following acute myocardial infarction, occasionally causes sudden death (Chap. 190). Sudden cardiovascular collapse is also a major, and frequently the terminal, event in patients with major cerebrovascular accidents, particularly subarachnoid hemorrhage, sudden alterations of intracranial pressure, or lesions affecting the brainstem. It may also occur with asphyxia. Digitalis toxicity may result in life-threatening arrhythmias, leading to sudden cardiovascular collapse and, if treatment is not immediate, to death (Chap. 182). Paradoxically, antiarrhythmic drugs may exacerbate arrhythmia or predispose to ventricular fibrillation in as many as 15 percent of patients.

TABLE 30-1 Conditions associated with cardiovascular collapse and sudden death in adults

Ischemic heart disease secondary to coronary atherosclerosis (including acute myocardial infarction)
Prinzmetal's variant angina; coronary artery spasm
Congenital coronary artery disease (including anomalous origins, coronary arteriovenous fistula)
Coronary embolism
Acquired, nonatherosclerotic coronary disease (including aneurysms occurring with Kawasaki's disease)
Myocardial bridges that demonstrably impair perfusion
Wolff-Parkinson-White syndrome
Hereditary or acquired QT-interval prolongation (with or without congenital deafness)
Sinoatrial node disease
Atrioventricular block (Stokes-Adams syndrome)
Secondary disease of the conduction system (e.g., amyloid, sarcoid, hemochromatosis, thrombotic thrombocytopenic purpura, myotonia dystrophica)
Drug toxicity or idiosyncrasy (e.g., digitalis, quinidine)
Electrolyte derangements (with myocardial magnesium and potassium deficiencies having been implicated)
Valvular heart disease, especially aortic stenosis
Infective endocarditis
Myocarditis
Cardiomyopathies, particularly idiopathic hypertrophic subaortic stenosis
Liquid-protein, modified-fast diet programs
Pericardial tamponade
Mitral valve prolapse (extremely uncommon cause of sudden death)
Cardiac tumor
Ruptured or dissecting aortic aneurysm
Pulmonary thromboembolism
Cerebrovascular accident, particularly hemorrhage

ELECTROPHYSIOLOGIC MECHANISMS Potentially lethal ventricular arrhythmias in patients with acute myocardial infarction may result from reentry, derangements of automaticity, or both. It would appear that reentry plays a dominant role in early arrhythmia, for example, within the first hour, and that derangements of automaticity are an important contributing factor later.

Several factors appear to set the stage for ventricular fibrillation and other rhythms dependent upon reentry early after the onset of ischemia (see also Chap. 184). Local accumulation of hydrogen ions, an increased ratio of extra- to intracellular potassium, and regional adrenergic stimulation tend to shift diastolic transmembrane potentials toward zero and elicit anomalous depolarizations possibly mediated by calcium currents or indicative of depressed, fast sodium-mediated depolarizations. This type of depolarization appears to contribute to slowed conduction required for the development of reentry early after the onset of ischemia.

Another mechanism implicated in reentry early after ischemia is focal reexcitation. Anoxia results in abbreviation of the duration of the action potential. Accordingly, during electrical systole, cells within an ischemic zone may be repolarized before cells in adjacent nonischemic tissue. The consequent disparity between prevailing transmembrane potentials may give rise to an uneven depolarization of adjacent cells and hence contribute to arrhythmia dependent upon reentry. Concomitant pharmacologic or metabolic factors may predispose toward reentry. For example, quinidine may depress conduction velocity disproportionately to its prolongation of refractoriness, thereby facilitating arrhythmias dependent upon reentry early after the onset of ischemia.

The so-called vulnerable period, corresponding to the ascending limb of the T wave, represents that portion of the cardiac cycle when temporal dispersion of ventricular refractoriness is maximum and, accordingly, when reentrant rhythms leading to sustained, repetitive activity can be initiated most readily. In patients with severe myocardial ischemia, the vulnerable period is prolonged and the intensity of stimulus required to evoke repetitive tachycardia or ventricular fibrillation is reduced. Temporal dispersion of refractoriness may be increased in nonischemic tissue in the presence of a slow heart rate. Accordingly, profound bradycardia due to decreased automaticity of the sinus node or AV block may also be particularly dangerous in patients with acute myocardial infarction since it may potentiate reentry.

Ventricular tachycardia occurring more than 8 to 12 h after the onset of ischemia appear to be dependent in part on derangements of automaticity or triggered activity of Purkinje fibers and possibly of myocardial cells as well. This rhythm resembles the slow ventricular tachycardia often occurring between a few hours and a day after coronary ligation in experimental animals. It does not generally degenerate into ventricular fibrillation or other malignant arrhythmia. Reduction of diastolic transmembrane potential in response to regional biochemical alterations induced by ischemia may contribute to the derangements of automaticity by facilitating repetitive depolarizations of Purkinje fibers triggered by a single depolarization. Since catecholamines facilitate propagation of such slow-current responses, enhanced regional adrenergic stimulation may be an important contributing factor. The apparent efficacy of beta-adrenergic blockade in suppressing some ventricular arrhythmias and the relative inefficacy of conventional antiarrhythmic agents such as lidocaine in patients with sympathetic hyperactivity may be reflections of the importance of regional adrenergic stimulation to enhanced automaticity.

Asystole and/or profound bradycardia are less common electrophysiologic mechanisms underlying sudden death caused by coronary atherosclerosis. They may be manifestations of complete right coronary artery occlusion and usually presage failure of resuscitative efforts. They often result from failure of impulse formation in the sinus node, AV block, and failure of subsidiary pacemakers to function effectively. Sudden death associated with these manifestations is usually a consequence of diffuse myocardial disease in most patients rather than the AV block per se.

TREATMENT AND PREVENTION

IDENTIFICATION OF HIGH-RISK SUBJECTS The difficulties entailed in ambulatory electrocardiographic monitoring or other procedures for mass screening to detect candidates at risk for sudden death are formidable, since the population at risk comprises more than one-third of all men 35 to 74 years of age, and since ventricular ectopic activity occurs so commonly and is so variable from day to day in the same subject. At greatest risk are the following: (1) patients who have previously experienced primary ventricular fibrillation without associated acute myocardial infarction; (2) patients with ischemic heart disease who exhibit bouts of rapid ventricular tachycardia; (3) patients seen within 6 months after recovery from acute myocardial infarction with frequent, early, or multifocal ventricular premature contractions at rest, during physical activity, or during psychological stress, particularly those who also have severe left ventricular dysfunction with ejection fraction <40 percent or overt heart failure; (4) patients with prolonged QT intervals and frequent premature contractions, particularly those who present with a history of syncope. Although identification of patients at high risk is particularly important, selection of an effective prophylactic regimen remains difficult, and none has clearly demonstrated effectiveness in reducing the risk. For survivors of sustained ventricular tachycardia or fibrillation induction of the arrhythmia by ventricular stimulation techniques with catheter electrodes and selection of a pharmacologic regimen based on abolition of subsequent induction of the arrhythmia appear to be predictive of the efficacy of specific pharmacologic regimens for preventing or interrupting recurrent malignant arrhythmia, particularly ventricular tachycardia. In addition, it identifies patients refractory to conventional management and facilitates selection of candidates for aggressive measures such as administration of investigational drugs, implantation of automatic defibrillators, or cardiac surgery (Chap. 184).

PHARMACOLOGIC THERAPY Treatment with antiarrhythmic drugs in doses sufficient to maintain "therapeutic" drug levels has been claimed to be effective in reducing recurrent ventricular tachycardia and/or fibrillation in survivors of sudden death, if during acute drug testing advanced grades of ventricular premature contraction (early or repetitive forms) can be eliminated or reduced. For those survivors of sudden cardiac death who exhibit frequent and complex ventricular ectopic activity occurring between episodes of ventricular tachycardia and/or fibrillation (approximately 30 percent), prophylactic treatment should be employed on an individual basis, with pharmacologic efficacy defined by suppression of the intercedent arrhythmia. Conventional doses of long-acting procainamide (30 to 50 mg/kg per day by mouth in divided doses every 6 h), quinidine gluconate (15 mg/kg per day by mouth in divided doses every 6 h), or disopyramide (6 to 10 mg/kg per day by mouth in divided doses every 6 h) may be effective in suppressing these arrhythmias. Dosage of quinidine may be increased up to 3 g per day if found necessary, unless gastrointestinal disturbances or electrocardiographic evidence of toxicity occurs. Amiodarone (an investigational drug in the United States, 5 mg/kg intravenously over 5 to 15 min or 300 to 800 mg per day by mouth with or without a loading dose of 1200 to 2000 mg per day in divided doses for 1 to 4 weeks) has striking antifibrillatory actions but a very slow rate of onset with peak effects seen only after several days or weeks of administration. Toxicity may occur both acutely and with chronic administration (Chap. 184). Although amiodarone is an unequivocally effective antifibrillatory drug, its use should be reserved for conditions refractory to less toxic agents or alternative approaches.

For most survivors of sudden cardiac death, frequent or complex ventricular ectopic activity is manifest only rarely or not at all between episodes of ventricular tachycardia and/or fibrillation. For such patients, selection of an appropriate prophylactic regimen should be based upon favorable responses to specific regimens reflected by results of provocative, invasive electrophysiologic testing, as described in Chap. 184. Ambulatory electrocardiographic monitoring with or without exercise stress may be particularly helpful in documenting the efficacy of treatment, since the incomplete knowledge regarding the pathogenesis of sudden death makes rational prophylactic drug selection and dosage difficult and a stereotyped regimen for all patients impractical. However, because of the marked variability of spontaneous arrhythmias on Holter recordings, which should be characterized for each subject, profound reduction of ectopic activity (at least 80 percent over a 24-h period) must be documented before attributing pharmacologic efficacy to a specific regimen. Even when such efficacy is demonstrable, it does not necessarily imply comparable protection against ventricular fibrillation. Some patients require concomitant administration of multiple drugs. Since the fundamental electrophysiologic derangements underlying ventricular fibrillation and premature beats may not be the same, even documented suppression of premature beats, while desirable, provides no reassurance of prevention of sudden death.

Decreased incidence of sudden death in a random selection of patients surviving acute myocardial infarction has been documented in several prospective double-blind studies utilizing beta-adrenergic blocking agents, although the effect of treatment on arrhythmia was not quantified and the mechanism of apparent protection has not yet been identified. The incidence of sudden cardiac death was significantly decreased, in proportion to an overall decrease in mortality, during follow-up intervals of several years among survivors of myocardial infarction by treatment with beta blockers initiated several days after the infarct.

Delays by the patient, physician, and transportation system and in the emergency room after the occurrence of acute myocardial infarction are significant impediments to prevention of sudden death. The median elapsed time between onset of symptoms of acute infarction and hospitalization averages 3 to 5 h in most areas of the United States. Denial by the patient of the seriousness of the condition and indecision by both the patient and physician contribute most to total delay.

SURGICAL APPROACHES In carefully selected survivors of sudden cardiac death with recurrent malignant arrhythmia, described in Chap. 184, surgical approaches may be indicated. In some patients prophylaxis with an automatic implantable defibrillator may enhance survival, although the unpleasant nature of the discharges of the device and the possibility of physiologically inappropriate discharges are serious disadvantages.

COMMUNITY EFFORTS Experience gained in Seattle, Washington, has shown that in order to deal effectively on a communitywide basis with the problem of sudden cardiovascular collapse and death, it is necessary to develop a system that provides rapid and effective response for these emergencies. Important elements of the system include a citywide emergency call number through which the system can be activated, a well-trained group of paramedical personnel such as fire fighters to respond, a short average time of response (under 4 min), and a large number of lay people trained in techniques of resuscitation. Clearly, the success in immediate resuscitation and for long-term survival is directly related to how soon following collapse resuscitation efforts are initiated. The availability of special ambulances (mobile coronary care units) equipped and staffed to handle acute cardiac emergencies appears to reduce delay by increasing community and physician awareness of the urgency of prompt medical attention. Such a system can be effective in resuscitating more than 40 percent of patients who have undergone cardiovascular collapse. Involvement of well-trained citizens in a communitywide program of "bystander cardiopulmonary resuscitation" appears to increase the likelihood that resuscitation will lead to a favorable outcome, reflected by an increased fraction of successful hospital discharges among patients sustaining prehospital cardiac arrest (30 to 35 percent compared with 10 to 15 percent in the absence of such a program). Long-term survival may be increased also from a 50 percent 2-year rate to 70 percent or more. Advocates of bystander resuscitation are

presently exploring the use of portable home defibrillators designed for safe use by lay persons with only a modicum of training required.

PATIENT EDUCATION Providing instructions to susceptible persons on how to seek medical care on an emergency basis upon the development of symptoms of myocardial infarction is of great importance in the prevention of sudden cardiac death. This strategy includes instructing the patient that prompt entry into an effective emergency care system is not only urgent but also what the physician expects of the patient, regardless of whether symptoms suggestive of myocardial infarction occur during the day or night (Chap. 190); this concept also means instructing the patient to bypass the physician and to contact the emergency care system directly. Unsupervised physical stress, such as jogging, should be discouraged in patients with known ischemic heart disease and prohibited in those at high risk of sudden death, as defined above.

APPROACH TO THE PATIENT WITH SUDDEN CARDIOVASCULAR COLLAPSE

Sudden death can often be averted even when cardiovascular collapse has occurred. When a patient under close medical observation develops sudden collapse from arrhythmia, the immediate goal must be restoration of effective cardiac rhythm. Circulatory collapse must be recognized and confirmed immediately. Its cardinal features are (1) loss of consciousness and seizures; (2) absent peripheral arterial pulses; and (3) absent heart sounds. Since external cardiac massage provides only limited cardiac output, presently no more than 30 percent of the lower limit of normal, definitive restoration of effective rhythm should be the immediate goal, and in the absence of evidence to the contrary, abrupt circulatory collapse should be assumed to be due to ventricular fibrillation. If the physician sees the patient within 1 min of the collapse, time should not be wasted by attempting to achieve oxygenation. An immediate blow to the precordium ("thump version") may be attempted, since this is occasionally effective and takes only seconds. Rarely, when circulatory collapse is due to ventricular tachycardia and the patient is still conscious when first seen, a vigorous cough may terminate the arrhythmia. In the absence of immediate restoration of the circulation, electrical defibrillation (Chap. 184) should be attempted immediately thereafter, without necessarily even pausing first to record an electrocardiogram on separate equipment, although use of portable defibrillators capable of electrocardiographic recording directly from the defibrillating electrodes may be helpful. Maximum electrical output of conventionally available equipment (320 W·s) is generally adequate, even for obese patients, and should be used. Efficacy is potentiated by application of the electrode paddles with firm pressure, and delivery of the electrical discharge promptly and before the energy requirements for defibrillation increase with the duration of ventricular fibrillation. Devices with automated impedance adjustment are promising because they can minimize the hazards of unnecessarily high energy discharges while avoiding ineffectively low discharges for patients with higher-than-anticipated impedance. If these immediate attempts are unsuccessful, external cardiac massage and complete cardiopulmonary resuscitation with prompt establishment and maintenance of a good airway should be implemented.

If collapse is due to unequivocal asystole, transthoracic or transvenous electrical pacing should be implemented immediately. Intracardiac epinephrine, 5 to 10 mL of 1:10,000 solution, may facilitate the heart's response to artificial pacing or be helpful when a slow ventricular focus is present but ineffective. If these initial definitive measures fail despite adequate technical performance, prompt restitution of a favorable metabolic milieu and monitoring are necessary. This is best accomplished by these three procedures:

1 External cardiac massage.
2 Correction of acid-base balance, often requiring intravenous sodium bicarbonate administration in an initial dose of 1 meq/kg. One-

half the dose should be repeated every 10 to 12 min as needed based on frequent determinations of arterial pH.

3 Assessment and correction of electrolyte imbalance. Definitive efforts to restore an effective cardiac rhythm should be attempted again as soon as possible, certainly within minutes. When effective cardiac rhythm is restored but rapidly degenerates again into ventricular tachycardia or fibrillation, lidocaine should be administered as a bolus, 1 mg/kg intravenously, •then continued by intravenous infusion at a rate up to 1 to 5 (mg/kg)/h, and countershock repeated.

CARDIAC MASSAGE (Fig. 30-1) External cardiac massage was designed by Kouwenhoven and coworkers to establish perfusion of vital organs by sequential, manual compression of the chest. Adherence to several aspects of technique is essential. (1) If efforts to rouse the patient by shaking the shoulders and calling fail, the patient should be placed supine on a firm surface (a wooden board serves well). (2) An open airway should be established by a maneuver such as chin lift, performed by tilting the patient's head backward with firm pressure applied to the forehead while bringing the mandible anteriorly with the fingers of the other hand under the chin. (3) If a carotid pulse is not palpable during a 5-s observation interval,

FIGURE 30-1 *Cardiopulmonary resuscitation (CPR) and external chest compression. A diagrammatic representation of the steps required for resuscitation by a single rescuer. [Modified from Standards and guidelines for cardiopulmonary resuscitation (CPR) and emergency cardiac care (ECC). JAMA 244:453, 1980.]*

compression of the chest should be performed with the heel of one hand at the midsternal region with the inferior portion two finger-breadths cephalad to the xiphoid process (to avoid lacerations of the liver) and the other hand applied with the fingers locked on top of the first. (4) Chest compression of 3 to 5 cm should be delivered at a frequency of one per second to permit adequate time for ventricular filling. (5) The resuscitator's waist must be higher than the patient's chest to permit application of the approximately 50-kg force required, and the elbows should be straight. (6) Depression and release of the chest wall should each occupy 50 percent of the cycle. Sudden compression may elicit a pressure wave palpable at the femoral or carotid artery but one able to eject little blood. (7) Massage should not be interrupted, even for a moment, because cardiac output increases cumulatively during the first 8 to 10 compressions, and even brief interruptions are detrimental. (8) Effective ventilation must be maintained throughout at a rate of approximately 12 breaths per minute and monitored by arterial blood gas analyses. If the latter are clearly abnormal, endotracheal intubation should be carried out expeditiously with no more than a 20-s pause in the external chest compression sequence.

Each external cardiac compression unavoidably limits venous return, to some extent. Thus, the optimal anticipated cardiac index during external massage approximates only 40 percent of the lower limit of normal, well below that seen in most patients after spontaneous ventricular contractions have returned. Therefore, prompt restoration of effective cardiac rhythm is essential.

It is likely that some modifications of the classical technique of cardiopulmonary resuscitation (CPR) will become established in the near future aimed at (1) augmenting intrathoracic pressure during compression (positive airway pressure, simultaneous ventilation and compression, abdominal binding, initiating compression at end-inspiration), (2) reducing intrathoracic pressure during relaxation (negative airway pressure during this phase), and (3) reducing intrathoracic aortic and systemic arterial collapse during compression (augmentation of vascular volume and antishock inflatable trousers). One application of these concepts that has already been employed is "cough CPR," a technique with which a still-conscious patient can maintain cardiac output despite ventricular fibrillation, at least for brief intervals, by repetitive, rhythmic coughing which phasically augments intrathoracic pressure, simulating the changes induced by conventional chest compression. Because of effects of CPR on blood flow, needed drugs should be given intravenously via upper extremity or central (not femoral) lines and generally by bolus injection rather than by continuous infusion. Isotonic agents can be given after dilution in saline by injection into the endotracheal tube because absorption occurs through the bronchial circulation.

Rarely, organized electrocardiographic activity unaccompanied by effective cardiac contraction (electromechanical dissociation) may occur. Intracardiac epinephrine (5 to 10 mL of 1:10,000 solution) or calcium gluconate (1 g) may be helpful in restoring mechanical function. Alternatively, calcium chloride (10%) can be given intravenously in a dose of 5 to 7 mg/kg. Refractory or repetitively recurrent ventricular fibrillation may respond to lidocaine, 1 mg/kg followed by 0.5 mg/kg at 10- to 12-min intervals to a maximum of 225 mg; procainamide, 20 mg every 5 min to a maximum of 1000 mg followed by an infusion of 2 to 6 mg/min; or bretylium tosylate, 5 to 12 mg/kg given over several minutes followed by infusion of 1 to 2 mg/kg per minute. Cardiac massage should be terminated as soon as effective cardiac contractions serve to produce a detectable pulse and systemic arterial blood pressure.

The therapeutic approach outlined above is based on several considerations: (1) irreversible brain damage often occurs after a few (approximately 4) minutes of circulatory collapse; (2) the likelihood of restoring effective cardiac rhythm and successfully resuscitating the patient diminishes rapidly with time; (3) 80 to 90 percent survival can be anticipated in patients developing primary ventricular fibrillation, as when undergoing cardiac catheterization or exercise testing, in whom definitive treatment is prompt; (4) survival rates in the general hospital setting are much lower, approximately 20 percent, depending in part on the coexisting or underlying disease process; (5) survival rates in the community approach zero, unless special emergency care systems have been perfected, probably because of unavoidable delays in initiating definitive therapy and limitations of equipment and available personnel; and (6) external cardiac massage can provide only a limited cardiac output. When ventricular fibrillation occurs, the earliest application of electrical countershock is the one most likely to succeed. Thus, when circulatory collapse is a primary event, therapy must be directed toward prompt restoration of effective cardiac rhythm.

COMPLICATIONS External cardiac massage is not free from significant complications, including rib fracture, hemopericardium and tamponade, hemothorax, pneumothorax, liver laceration, fat embolus, and ruptured spleen with late, occult blood loss. However, these complications can be minimized by proper technique and, if appropriately considered, can be readily recognized and often managed effectively. The decision to terminate unsuccessful cardiopulmonary resuscitation is always difficult. In general, if effective cardiac rhythm has not been restored and if the patient's pupils are fixed and dilated despite 30 min or more of cardiac massage, a successful resuscitation cannot be expected.

REFERENCES

BETA-BLOCKER HEART ATTACK TRIAL RESEARCH GROUP: A randomized trial of propranolol in patients with acute myocardial infarction. I. Mortality results. JAMA 247:1707, 1982

BIGGER JT JR et al: THE MULTICENTER POST-INFARCTION RESEARCH GROUP: The relationships among ventricular arrhythmias, left ventricular dysfunction, and mortality in the 2 years after myocardial infarction. Circulation 62:250, 1984

CHANDRA N et al: Simultaneous chest compression and ventilation at high airway pressure during cardiopulmonary resuscitation. Lancet 1:175, 1980

COBB LA et al: Sudden cardiac death. A decade's experience with out-of-hospital resuscitation. Mod Concepts Cardiovasc Dis 49:31, 1980

DAVIES MJ, THOMAS AC: Thrombosis and acute coronary-artery lesions in sudden cardiac ischemic death. N Engl J Med 310:1137, 1984

————, ————: Plaque fissuring: The cause of acute myocardial infarction, sudden ischaemic death, and crescendo angina. Br Heart J 53:363, 1985

ECHT DA et al: Clinical experience, complications, and survival in 70 patients with the automatic implantable cardioverter/defibrillator. Circulation 71:289, 1985

HALPERIN HR et al: The determinants of vital organ flow during cardiac arrest in dogs. Circulation, vol. 73, March, 1986

JAMES TN (ed): *15th Bethesda Conference Report: Sudden Cardiac Death.* J Am Coll Cardiol 5(Suppl):1B, 1985

LEVER HM et al: Sudden death in hypertrophic cardiomyopathy. Clev Clin Quart 51:65, 1984

LEWIS BH et al: Detailed analysis of 24 hour ambulatory electrocardiographic recordings during ventricular fibrillation of torsade de pointes. J Am Coll Cardiol 2:426, 1983

LEWIS RP et al: Reduction of mortality from prehospital myocardial infarction by prudent patient activation of mobile coronary care system. Am Heart J 103:123, 1982

McINTYRE KM, LEWIS AJ (eds): *Textbook of Advanced Cardiac Life Support.* Dallas, American Heart Association, 1981

MILLER JM et al: Subendocardial resection for ventricular tachycardia: Predictors of surgical success. Circulation 70:624, 1984

ROTH R et al: Out-of-hospital cardiac arrest: Factors associated with survival. Ann Emerg Med 13:237, 1984

SMITH WM, GALLAGHER JJ: "Les Torsades de Pointes": An unusual ventricular arrhythmia. Ann Intern Med 93:578, 1980

TRESCH DD et al: Long-term survival after prehospital sudden cardiac death. Am Heart J 108:1, 1984

VINCENT R et al: A community training scheme in cardiopulmonary resuscitation. Brit Med J 288:617, 1984

WEAVER WD et al: Improved neurologic recovery and survival after early defibrillation. Circulation 69:943, 1984

section 5 Alterations in gastrointestinal function

31 ORAL MANIFESTATIONS OF DISEASE

PAUL GOLDHABER

DISTURBANCES OF THE TEETH AND DENTAL TISSUES

DENTAL CARIES, PULPAL AND PERIAPICAL INFECTION, AND SEQUELAE Dental caries, the principal cause of tooth loss up to the fourth decade of life, is characterized by a bacteria-induced progressive destruction of the mineral and organic components of the outer enamel and underlying dentin. Numerous long-term studies have clearly shown that the artificial fluoridation of drinking water supplies to a level of 1 part per million leads to a 50 to 75 percent reduction in the occurrence of dental caries in permanent teeth of children, presumably because of an alteration of the developing enamel crystals during tooth formation which makes them more resistant to acid dissolution.

If the carious lesion progresses unchecked, there is eventual infection of the dental pulp, giving rise to an *acute pulpitis.* During the early stages of pulpitis moderately severe pain may result from thermal changes, particularly with cold drinks. As more of the pulp becomes involved because of advanced caries, heat or reclining may stimulate the onset of even more severe and continuous pain. At this stage, damage to the pulp is irreversible, and treatment consists of either extraction or thorough removal of the remaining contents of the pulp chamber and root canals followed by sterilization and filling with an inert material (root canal therapy).

If the pulpitis is not treated, infection may spread beyond the apex of the tooth into the periodontal ligament, giving rise to pain on chewing or percussion. The most common manifestation of periapical disease is the *periapical granuloma,* a localized mass of chronic granulation tissue which slowly expands at the expense of the surrounding alveolar bone. The *chronic periapical granuloma* may present the above symptoms or may be asymptomatic. If allowed to persist untreated, the periapical granuloma may give rise to a *periapical cyst* or a *periapical abscess*—all three lesions appearing as radiolucent areas on roentgenograms. The acute periapical abscess may extend into the surrounding bone marrow, resulting in an *osteomyelitis.* More frequently, the abscess perforates the cortical plate and, following the path of least resistance, spreads through various tissue spaces, giving rise to cellulitis and bacteremia, or discharges into the oral cavity, into the maxillary sinus, or through the skin.

The symptoms produced by cellulitis depend on which tissue space is affected. For example, *Ludwig's angina* originates from an infected mandibular molar, involves the submaxillary space, and subsequently extends into the sublingual and submental spaces. Clinically, this is manifested by swelling of the floor of the mouth, elevation of the tongue, and difficulty in swallowing and breathing. With continued swelling, there may be edema of the glottis, necessitating an emergency tracheotomy. Spread of the infection to the parapharyngeal spaces may lead to cavernous sinus thrombosis.

EFFECT OF SYSTEMIC FACTORS ON TEETH   Systemic factors, occurring in utero or in infancy during the stages of crown formation, may influence the development and structure of the teeth. *Enamel hypoplasia* of the primary and/or permanent teeth, manifested by alterations ranging from white spots to gross defects in the surface structure of the crowns, may be caused by disturbances of calcium and phosphate metabolism such as are found in vitamin D-refractory rickets, hypoparathyroidism, gastroenteritis, and celiac disease. Premature birth or high fevers may also give rise to enamel hypoplasia. Tetracycline, given during the last half of pregnancy, infancy, and childhood up to 8 years of age, causes both a permanent discoloration of the teeth and enamel hypoplasia. Daily ingestion of more than 1.5 mg fluoride can result in enamel discoloration (mottling). Prenatal factors appear to influence crown size. Larger teeth are associated with maternal diabetes, maternal hypothyroidism, and large birth size. Tooth size is reduced in *Down's syndrome*. Premature loss of the deciduous dentition is frequently the first symptom in *juvenile hypophosphatasia*. Systemic disease may give rise to pain that simulates pulpal disease. *Maxillary sinusitis* is frequently manifested by pain in the maxillary teeth, including sensitivity to thermal changes and percussion. *Cardiac disease* with *angina pectoris* may result in referred pain to the lower jaw.

PERIODONTAL DISEASE

After the third decade chronic destructive periodontal disease *(periodontitis)* is responsible for the loss of more teeth than dental caries. It begins as a marginal inflammation of the gingivae (gingivitis), which slowly spreads to involve the underlying alveolar bone and periodontal ligament. As the disease progresses, the alveolar bone is resorbed, resulting in loss of periodontal ligament fiber attachment from the tooth to the bone. The separation of the soft tissue from the tooth surface results in "pocket" formation, the inner aspect of which bleeds readily on probing or spontaneously during chewing. Frank pus sometimes exudes from under the gingival margin, accounting for the use of the now outmoded term *pyorrhea*. With continued loss of alveolar bone the involved teeth become mobile. As the periodontal pockets deepen, the pocket orifice may become occluded, leading to the formation of a *periodontal abscess*. The prognosis for teeth with advanced bone loss, extreme mobility, and recurrent abscess formation is usually poor or hopeless, and the usual treatment is extraction.

The most important local etiologic factors associated with this disease are thought to be *poor oral hygiene,* resulting in the accumulation of grossly visible adherent masses of bacteria *(bacterial plaque),* calculus (mineralized bacterial plaque), and food impaction. The margins of overextended fillings also play a role as local irritating factors. Occlusal trauma, particularly trauma due to grinding and clenching habits, may be involved. Therapy is aimed at elimination of these factors and the development of a local environment which can be maintained in health by good oral hygiene. It appears that specific groups of organisms found subgingivally correlate with the different types and severity of periodontal disease. In advanced periodontitis, the flora is dominated by motile rods and spirochetes.

Systemic factors are thought to modify the response of the host to the local factors, but their nature is more obscure. Reduced neutrophil functions, such as chemotaxis and phagocytosis, appear to predispose to *juvenile periodontitis,* a form of periodontitis characterized by early and severe alveolar bone loss and a familial pattern of occurrence. Of possible etiologic importance is the finding that a sonic extract of *Actinobacillus actinomycetemcomitans,* a microorganism consistently isolated from patients with juvenile periodontitis, contains a leukotoxin which specifically kills human polymorphonuclear leukocytes and monocytes. *Capnocytophaga,* another organism implicated in periodontal disease, has also been reported to be associated with morphologic and functional abnormalities of neutrophils. On the other hand, patients with IgA deficiency and agammaglobulinemia have less periodontal disease and dental

caries than matched immunocompetent controls. Individuals with *Down's syndrome* seem to be particularly susceptible to periodontal disease and may demonstrate advanced alveolar bone loss around the permanent mandibular incisors and maxillary first molars. Severe chronic periodontal disease may be present in uncontrolled *diabetes mellitus*. In some instances, however, there are characteristic alterations in the gingiva in response to a number of specific systemic conditions. For example, during *pregnancy* the gingiva may become edematous and friable, with a raspberry-like appearance of the interdental papillae. Occasionally, a tumorlike mass may develop in an interdental area; this usually regresses following parturition. Oral contraceptives may lead to an increase in gingival inflammation. The use of the anticonvulsant drug *phenytoin* (Dilantin) frequently results in fibrous hyperplasia of the gingiva, which may actually cover the teeth, interfere with mastication, and cause a serious aesthetic problem. A similar clinical picture, although usually more generalized and extensive, occurs in *idiopathic familial fibromatosis*. The latter condition appears to be hereditary.

A relatively common gingival disease, found predominantly in young adults, is *acute necrotizing ulcerative gingivitis* (Vincent's infection, trench mouth). This disease is characterized by tender or painful gingivae, bleeding on pressure, and the pathognomonic sign of papillary or marginal gingival necrosis and ulceration. Clinical evidence suggests that the cause of this disease has a psychosomatic component. Vincent's infection differs from *acute herpetic gingivostomatitis,* with which it is most frequently confused, because fever or malaise rarely develops, and patients respond rapidly to penicillin or broad-spectrum antibiotics.

It should be noted that both infected periapical lesions and periodontal disease provide potential sources of infection which may spread to other sites. Transient bacteremias have been demonstrated after simple massage of inflamed gingivae or use of an oral irrigative device, as well as during tooth extraction. The frequent association of tooth extraction with the subsequent occurrence of subacute bacterial endocarditis has led to the prophylactic use of antibiotics in dental patients with a history of rheumatic fever or other evidence of valvular disease. Similar precautions should be taken with dental patients having heart valve or joint prostheses. Prophylactic extraction of healthy teeth in leukemic patients is not justified.

DISEASES OF THE ORAL MUCOSA AND TONGUE

HEMATOLOGIC DISTURBANCES   Oral manifestations are common in both the acute and chronic forms of all types of leukemia, particularly *monocytic leukemia*. They consist of local gingival bleeding, enlargement, and necrosis. Petechiae and ulceration of the oral mucosa may also be evident. Extensive ulcerations of the gingivae, buccal mucosa, lips, soft palate, pharynx, and tonsils may also occur in *agranulocytosis*. In thrombocytopenic states multiple petechiae, ecchymoses, and bleeding gingivae may be observed. The mucous membranes of the oral cavity, including the papillae of the tongue, are atrophic in the *Plummer-Vinson syndrome* (see Chaps. 32 and 234). As a result, the tongue is red, smooth, and sore, and there is difficulty in swallowing. Of interest is the finding that the atrophic mucous membranes have a predisposition toward the development of oral carcinoma. The oral symptoms in *pernicious anemia* are similar (see Chap. 285). Ulceration, mucositis, xerostomia, and infection (bacterial or fungal) are relatively common oral complications among patients receiving chemotherapy and/or radiotherapy for malignancies not involving the head or neck.

VITAMIN DEFICIENCIES   *The oral effects of deficiency of the B group of vitamins* involve the soft tissues primarily, giving rise to reddening and ulceration of the oral mucosa and tongue, swelling and burning of the tongue, and fissuring at the corners of the lips *(angular cheilosis)*. Severe vitamin C deficiency *(scurvy)* is manifested by petechiae in the oral mucosa; swollen, ulcerated, bleeding gingivae; and loosening of teeth.

PIGMENTATIONS (See Table 31-1) The spread of irregular spots or blotches or brown pigment throughout the oral mucosa, primarily the buccal mucosa, may be the first sign of *Addison's disease*. The pigmentation associated with the *Peutz-Jeghers syndrome* is readily differentiated because of its characteristic distribution around the lips, eyes, and nostrils, as well as its intraoral distribution. Both *lead poisoning* and *bismuth poisoning* may be manifested by a dark line along the gingival margin, particularly in individuals who have poor oral hygiene. Bismuth poisoning may also demonstrate pigmented patches elsewhere in the oral mucosa.

INFECTIONS See Tables 31-2 and 31-3.

DERMATOLOGIC DISEASES See Tables 31-2 and 31-3 and Chaps. 47 to 52.

TONGUE ALTERATIONS See Table 31-4.

MALODOROUS BREATH A distinctly unpleasant odor of the breath (halitosis) may emanate from any patient with *infections of the upper part of the respiratory tract*, especially in bronchiectasis and lung abscess. Halitosis may occur with oral sepsis as in *stomatitis*, *gingivitis*, or extensive *caries*. Some persons who smoke excessively may have halitosis. Occasionally otherwise normal persons will have halitosis without obvious cause. The primary oral sources of bad breath are inflamed periodontal pockets and the coating on the dorsoposterior surface of the tongue. A *fishy odor* of the breath is found in patients with hepatic failure (fetor hepaticus), an *ammoniacal* or *urinary odor* is found in azotemia, and a *sweet, fruity odor* is typical of diabetic ketoacidosis.

DISEASES OF THE SALIVARY GLANDS

Conditions affecting the salivary glands include mumps parotitis (Chap. 141), Mikulicz's disease, Sjögren's syndrome (Chap. 266), and sarcoidosis. Inflammation of the salivary glands (*sialadenitis*) is usually associated with the presence of a salivary stone (*sialolithiasis*) in the duct of one of the major salivary glands. The classic history of pain and swelling of the gland at mealtimes is due to the partial blockage of salivary flow by the stone. Localization of the stone may be accomplished by palpation or by roentgenograms with or without the use of an intraductal injection of radiopaque material (*sialography*). Acute or recurrent parotitis, with or without a defined microorganism, may occur in children and is marked by sudden onset of swelling of the whole gland or side of the face, accompanied by suppuration from Stensen's duct.

Xerostomia, or dryness of the mouth, is due to salivary gland dysfunction and may be temporary or permanent. Among the factors which cause temporary dryness are emotional factors (such as fear), infection of the glands, and administration of drugs such as atropine, antihistamines, or tricyclic antidepressants and phenothiazines. Radiation of the area may produce a more permanent xerostomia because of atrophy of the glands. A similar dryness may occur in Sjögren's syndrome. The dry mouth may give rise to rampant caries, particularly if sugar-containing candies are sucked in an attempt to stimulate salivary flow. Other symptoms may include disturbances in taste, difficulty in speech or swallowing, and inflammation of the oral mucosa. Altered taste (dysgeusia) may also be due to central nervous system diseases or trauma. Extensive dental caries, especially around the gum margins of the teeth, may be seen in drug addicts and alcoholics, presumably due to xerostomia and lack of oral hygiene and dental care. Xerostomia-induced caries may be prevented or arrested by the daily topical application of a 1% sodium fluoride gel. The soft tissue complications may be relieved by the utilization of an artificial saliva or by oral administration of pilocarpine.

Benign or malignant tumors may arise in the major or minor salivary glands. The benign *mixed tumor* accounts for the vast majority of all salivary gland tumors and has a relatively high recurrence rate. Malignant tumors of the parotid gland may affect the facial nerve.

ORAL CANCER

Oral cancer constitutes more than 5 percent of all human cancers. *Squamous cell carcinoma* is the most common malignant oral tumor, accounting for approximately 90 to 95 percent of all oral malignant tumors. Most of these tumors occur on the lips, primarily the lower lip, rather than intraorally. About half the intraoral tumors involve the tongue, primarily the posterior two-thirds and the lateral borders. The major etiologic factor in lip cancer appears to be exposure to intense sunlight. Predisposing factors for intraoral carcinoma include tobacco (usually in the form of cigar or pipe smoking, or snuff placed in the mucobuccal fold), excessive consumption of alcohol, syphilitic glossitis, and the atrophic mucosa of the Plummer-Vinson syndrome. Although numerous instances of carcinoma of the tongue adjacent to a sharp tooth or dental appliance have been reported, animal studies with chronic irritation per se, as well as epidemiologic studies, cast doubt on this apparent relationship. The most common *precancerous lesion* in the oral cavity is *leukoplakia*, a whitish patch on the mucosa that histologically shows hyperkeratosis, acanthosis, and dyskeratosis.

TABLE 31-1 Pigmented lesions of the oral mucosa

Condition	Usual location	Clinical features	Course
Black, hairy tongue	Dorsum of tongue	Elongation of filiform papillae of tongue, which take on a brown to black coloration	Long-lasting but may disappear spontaneously
Heavy metal pigmentation (bismuth, mercury, lead)	Gingival margin	Thin blue-black pigmented line along gingival margin due to prior treatment for syphilis with bismuth or mercury or from accidental absorption of lead	Long-lasting
Drug ingestion (tranquilizers, oral contraceptives, antimalarials)	Any area in mouth	Brown, black, or gray areas of pigmentation	Disappears following cessation of drug
Amalgam tattoo	Gingiva and mucobuccal fold	Small blue-black pigmented areas associated with embedded amalgam particles in soft tissues; these will show up on radiographs as radiopaque particles	Remains indefinitely
Fordyce's disease	Buccal and labial mucosa	Aggregation of numerous, small yellowish spots just beneath mucosal surface; no subjective symptoms	Remains without apparent change indefinitely
Addison's disease	Any area in mouth but mostly on buccal mucosa	Blotches or spots of bluish-black to dark-brown pigmentation occurring early in the disease, accompanied by diffuse pigmentation of skin; other symptoms of adrenal insufficiency	Condition controlled by steroid therapy
Peutz-Jeghers syndrome	Any area in mouth	Dark brown spots on lips, buccal mucosa, and palate with characteristic distribution of pigment around lips, nose, eyes, and on hands; concomitant intestinal polyposis	Lesions remaining indefinitely
Malignant melanoma	Any area in mouth	May appear as a raised, painless, brown-black lesion or may be amelanotic; may be ulcerated and infected	Early metastasis leading to death

TABLE 31-2 Vesicular, bullous, or ulcerative lesions of the oral mucosa

Condition	Usual location	Clinical features	Course
VIRAL DISEASES			
Acute herpetic gingivostomatitis (herpes simplex, type 1)	Lip and oral mucosa	Labial vesicles which rupture and crust, and intraoral vesicles which quickly ulcerate; extremely painful to pressure; acute gingivitis, fever, malaise, foul odor, and cervical lymphadenopathy; occurs primarily in infants and children	Heals spontaneously in 10–14 days unless secondarily infected
Recurrent herpes labialis	Mucocutaneous junction of lip	Eruption of groups of vesicles which may coalesce, then rupture and crust; painful to pressure or spicy foods	Lasts about 1 week, but condition may be prolonged if secondary infection occurs
Primary herpes, type 2	Mouth, oral pharynx, and genitalia	Large, painful, discrete vesicles on zone of erythema; anterior cervical glands enlarged	Lasts several weeks; may recur
Herpangina (coxsackievirus A; also possibly coxsackievirus B and echovirus)	Oral mucosa, pharynx, tongue	Sudden onset of fever, sore throat, and oropharyngeal vesicles usually in children under 4 years, during summer months; diffuse pharyngeal injection and vesicles (1–2 mm), grayish white surrounded by red areola; vesicles enlarge and ulcerate	Incubation period 2–9 days; fever for 1–4 days; recovery uneventful
Hand, foot, and mouth disease (type A coxsackieviruses)	Oral mucosa, pharynx, palms, and soles	Fever, malaise, headache with oropharyngeal vesicles which become painful, shallow ulcers	Incubation period 2–18 days; lesions heal spontaneously in 2–4 weeks
Chickenpox	Gingiva and oral mucosa	Skin lesions may be accompanied by small vesicles on oral mucosa that rupture to form shallow ulcers; may coalesce to form large bullous lesions that ulcerate; mucosa may have generalized erythema	Lesions heal spontaneously within 2 weeks
Herpes zoster	Cheek, tongue, gingiva, or palate	Unilateral vesicular eruption and ulceration in linear pattern following sensory distribution of trigeminal nerve	Gradual healing without scarring
Infectious mononucleosis	Oral mucosa	Fatigue, sore throat, malaise, low-grade fever, and enlarged cervical lymph nodes; numerous small ulcers usually appear several days before lymphadenopathy; gingival bleeding and multiple petechiae at junction of hard and soft palates	Oral lesions disappear during convalescence
Warts	Any place on skin and oral mucosa, primarily lips and vestibule	Single or multiple papillary lesions, with thick, white, keratinized surfaces containing many pointed projections	Lesions grow rapidly and spread
BACTERIAL OR FUNGAL DISEASES			
Acute necrotizing ulcerative gingivitis ("trench mouth," Vincent's infection)	Gingiva	Painful, bleeding gingiva characterized by necrosis and ulceration of gingival papillae and margins plus lymphadenopathy and foul odor	Continued destruction of tissue followed by remission, but may recur
Prenatal (congenital) syphilis	Palate, jaws, tongue, and teeth	Gummatous involvement of palate, jaws, and facial bones; Hutchinson's incisors, mulberry molars, glossitis, mucous patches, and fissures of corners of mouth	Tooth deformities in permanent dentition irreversible
Primary syphilis (chancre)	Lesion appears where organism enters body; may occur on lips, tongue, or tonsillar area	Small papule developing rapidly into a large, painless ulcer with indurated border; unilateral lymphadenopathy; chancre and lymph nodes containing spirochetes; serologic tests positive by third to fourth weeks	Healing of chancre in 1–2 months, followed by secondary syphilis in 6–8 weeks
Secondary syphilis	Oral mucosa frequently involved with mucous patches, primarily on palate but also at commissures of mouth	Maculopapular lesions of oral mucosa, about 5–10 mm in diameter with central ulceration covered by grayish membrane; eruptions occurring on various mucosal surfaces and skin accompanied by fever, malaise, and sore throat	Lesions may persist from several weeks to a year
Tertiary syphilis	Palate and tongue	Gummatous infiltration of palate or tongue followed by ulceration and fibrosis; atrophy of tongue papillae may produce characteristic bald tongue and glossitis	Gumma may destroy palate, causing complete perforation
Gonorrhea	Lesions may occur in mouth at site of inoculation or secondarily by hematogenous spread from a primary focus elsewhere	Earliest symptoms are burning or itching sensation, dryness, or heat in mouth followed by acute pain on eating or speaking; tonsils and oropharynx most frequently involved; oral tissues may be diffusely inflamed or ulcerated; saliva develops increased viscosity and fetid odor; submaxillary lymphadenopathy with fever in severe cases	Lesions resolve with appropriate antibiotic therapy
Tuberculosis	Tongue, tonsillar area, soft palate	A solitary, irregular ulcer covered by a persistent exudate; ulcer has an undermined, indurated border	Lesion may persist
Cervicofacial actinomycosis	Swellings in region of face, neck, and floor of mouth	Infection may be associated with an extraction, jaw fracture, or eruption of molar tooth; in acute form resembles an acute pyogenic abscess, but contains yellow "sulfur granules" (gram-positive mycelia and their hyphae)	Acute form may last a few weeks; chronic form lasts months or years; prognosis excellent; actinomycetes respond to antibiotics (tetracyclines or penicillin) but not to antifungal drugs
Histoplasmosis	Any area in mouth, particularly tongue, gingiva, or palate	Numerous small nodules which may ulcerate; hoarseness and dysphagia may occur because of lesions in larynx, usually associated with fever and malaise	May be fatal

TABLE 31-2 Vesicular, bullous, or ulcerative lesions of the oral mucosa (*Continued*)

Condition	Usual location	Clinical features	Course
DERMATOLOGIC DISEASES			
Mucous membrane pemphigoid	Primarily mucous membranes of the oral cavity, but may also involve the eyes, urethra, vagina, and rectum	Painful, grayish white collapsed vesicles or bullae with peripheral erythematous zone; gingival lesions desquamate, leaving ulcerated area	Protracted course with remissions and exacerbations; involvement of different sites occurs slowly; corticosteroids may control severe cases
Erythema multiforme (Stevens-Johnson syndrome)	Primarily the oral mucosa and skin of hands and feet	Intraoral ruptured bullae surrounded by an inflammatory area; lips may show hemorrhagic crusts; the "iris," or "target" lesion, on the skin is pathognomonic; patient may have severe signs of toxicity	Onset very rapid; condition may last 1–2 weeks; may be fatal
Pemphigus vulgaris	Oral mucosa and skin	Ruptured bullae and ulcerated oral areas; mostly in older adults	With repeated recurrence of bullae, toxicity may lead to cachexia, infection, and death within 2 years
NEOPLASTIC DISEASES			
Squamous cell carcinoma	Any area in mouth, most commonly on lower lip, tongue, and floor of mouth	Ulcer with elevated, indurated border; failure to heal, pain not prominent; lesions tend to arise in areas of leukoplakia or in smooth or atrophic tongue	Invades and destroys underlying tissues or may metastasize to regional lymph nodes
Acute leukemia	Gingiva	Gingival swelling and superficial ulcerations followed by hyperplasia of gingiva with extensive necrosis and hemorrhage; deep ulcers may occur elsewhere on the mucosa complicated by secondary infection	Fatal
Lymphoma	Gingiva, palate, tongue, and tonsillar area	Elevated, ulcerated area which may proliferate rapidly, giving the appearance of a traumatic inflammatory lesion; swelling of regional lymph nodes	Fatal
Metastatic tumors	Deep in jaw bone, usually in premolar-molar area of mandible	May arise from carcinoma of distant organ, such as breast, lung, or kidney; advanced lesion may expand and destroy bone, loosen and spread teeth, involve inferior alveolar nerve, cause pain and numbness of lower lip	Fatal
OTHER CONDITIONS			
Recurrent aphthous stomatitis	Any place on oral mucosa	Single or clusters of painful ulcers with surrounding erythematous border, found anywhere on mucosa; lesions may be 1–15 mm in diameter	Lesions heal in 1–2 weeks but may recur monthly or several times a year. Topical corticosteroid ointments give symptomatic relief in mild cases. Systemic corticosteroids are used in severe cases. A tetracycline oral suspension may decrease ulcer severity.
Behçet's syndrome	Oral mucosa, eyes, and genitalia	Multiple aphthouslike ulcers in mouth; inflammatory ocular changes and ulcerative lesions on genitalia	Ulcers may persist for several weeks and heal without scarring
Traumatic ulcers	Any place on oral mucosa; dentures frequently responsible for ulcers in vestibule	Localized, discrete ulcerated lesion with red border; produced by accidental biting of mucosa, penetration by a foreign object, or chronic irritation by a denture	Lesion usually heals in 7–10 days when irritant is removed, unless secondarily infected

TABLE 31-3 White lesions of oral mucosa

Condition	Usual location	Clinical features	Course
Pachyderma oralis	Any area in mouth	Elevated white lesion due to hyperkeratosis and thickening of the oral epithelium secondary to chronic irritation	Removal of irritant leads to healing in 2–3 weeks
Leukoplakia	Any area in mouth	White patch or raised plaque with sharply defined borders; in more severe cases the lesion is indurated and rough, and may be fissured and eroded; pain not present in early lesions	Carcinoma frequently arises in the more severe type of lesion
Lichen planus	Any area in mouth but most often on buccal mucosa	Varied appearance of lesion due to arrangement of grayish-white papules which coalesce to make up the pattern; a reticular network is most common; oral lesions may precede skin lesions; lichenoid lesions may be drug-induced	May disappear spontaneously
Candidiasis (moniliasis, thrush)	Any area in mouth	Creamy white curdlike patches which reveal a raw, bleeding surface when scraped; found in sick infants, debilitated elderly patients, patients receiving high doses of corticosteroids or broad-spectrum antibiotics, or in patients with acquired immunodeficiency syndrome (AIDS)	Responds favorably to antifungal therapy after correction of predisposing causes
Chemical burns	Any area in mouth	White slough due to necrosis of epithelium and underlying connective tissue caused by contact with agents (e.g., aspirin) applied locally or the use of undiluted sodium perborate or hydrogen peroxide as a mouthwash; removal of slough leaves a raw, painful surface	Lesion heals in several weeks if not secondarily infected

Nodular leukoplakias have a much higher potential for malignant transformation than homogeneous leukoplakias. Recent evidence suggests that the asymptomatic, red velvety (erythroplastic) lesion of the floor of the mouth, ventrolateral aspect of the tongue, or soft palate–anterior pillar complex is more likely to be carcinoma in situ or invasive carcinoma than is the white lesion. *All chronic ulcerative lesions which fail to heal within 1 to 2 weeks should be considered potentially malignant* and must be biopsied in order to make the definitive diagnosis. It is noteworthy that in their early stages intraoral epidermoid carcinomas are rarely painful, in contrast to similar-appearing inflammatory lesions.

The prognosis for patients with carcinoma of the lip is usually good, since these malignant tumors are noted sooner and apparently metastasize later. Patients with carcinoma of the tongue have a poorer prognosis, particularly as the tumor occurs more posteriorly on the tongue. Intraoral carcinomas may spread by direct invasion to the underlying bone. Depending on the site of origin of the intraoral carcinoma, metastases usually spread to the submaxillary or cervical lymph nodes. Death may result from recurrent or uncontrollable disease above the clavicles; metastatic disease beyond the neck; treatment complications; or a second primary cancer, usually in the oral cavity or the upper parts of the gastrointestinal or respiratory tract. Metastatic tumors to the jaw may occur from carcinomas of the lung, breast, kidney, or gastrointestinal tract.

NEUROLOGIC DISTURBANCES

A number of neurologic disturbances have a direct effect on oral and paraoral structures. *Trigeminal neuralgia* (tic douloureux) is an example of a syndrome involving the trigeminal nerve. It is characterized by extremely severe, unilateral, lancinating pain of the face occurring spontaneously or set off by pressure on a "trigger zone" on the face (see Chap. 352). In some cases of idiopathic trigeminal neuralgia, dental and oral pathoses, primarily in the form of jawbone

cavities at sites of previous extractions, may be major etiologic factors. Facial palsy is a unilateral disturbance of the motor branch of the facial nerve due to either trauma, surgical sectioning, or tumor involvement. When it is of acute onset and unknown cause, possibly a localized infection in the nerve, it is called *Bell's palsy*. It may be due to cranial herpes zoster in some instances. The condition is manifested by drooping of the corner of the mouth, inability to close the eye on the same side, and difficulty in speech and eating. In mild cases the symptoms may disappear spontaneously within a month. Alteration in taste sensation in the anterior two-thirds of the tongue due to disturbance of the sensory component of the facial nerve occurs in some cases and indicates a more central location of the lesion in the nerve (see Chap. 352). Taste acuity declines with age for salty and bitter, but not for sour and sweet. This change may be associated in part with the number of missing teeth and the size of any artificial prosthesis used, thereby influencing food preferences, palatability, intake, and nutritional status of the elderly.

The pain associated with the *glossopharyngeal neuralgia syndrome* is similar in type and intensity to that found in trigeminal neuralgia, being set off by a trigger zone in the pharynx and affecting the posterior region of the tongue, pharynx, soft palate, and ear. Disturbance of the hypoglossal nerve leads to dysfunction of the tongue musculature and atrophy. Bilateral nerve involvement prevents protrusion of the tongue; unilateral involvement leads to deviation of the protruded tongue toward the affected side.

DISTURBANCES OF THE TEMPOROMANDIBULAR JOINT

Pain in the area of the temporomandibular joint frequently causes the patient to seek therapy. It may be due to posterior displacement of the condyle in the fossa leading to displacement of the meniscus and chronic trauma. *Dislocation of the condyle anteriorly* beyond the articular eminence due to sudden stretching or tearing of the capsular ligament may result in a locking of the mandible in an open position. In *osteoarthritis* the clinical signs and symptoms may be minimal despite extensive changes in the condyle. Temporomandibular joint involvement occurs less frequently in *rheumatoid arthritis*. When affected, the joints are swollen and painful, leading to limitation of movement, particularly on arising in the morning. In children the disease may lead to malocclusion. *Ankylosis* of the joint may occur eventually, necessitating a condylectomy (see Chap. 263).

The myofascial pain syndrome, the most common disorder of the temporomandibular joint, is characterized by facial pain and mandibular dysfunction in the absence of clinical or radiologic evidence of organic disease. The pain is often localized in the ear or jaw and may extend to the neck and shoulder. The mandibular dysfunction is manifested by limitation of movement, particularly an inability to open the jaw to the fullest extent. It is thought that such patients have increased musculature tension and hyperexcitable reflexes related to emotional tension. The precipitating factor appears to be the stretching of an abnormal focus of pain which initiates a self-sustaining pain-spasm-pain cycle. Treatment of the pain-dysfunction syndrome involves emotional support, stress reduction, and the use of drugs to relieve the pain, lessen cortical excitability, and relax the muscles. Local heat therapy, elimination of gross occlusal discrepancies, and jaw-opening exercises are also used. Local anesthetics are used intramuscularly in the region of the trigger zone or as superficial sprays in an attempt to break the pain-spasm-pain cycle.

TABLE 31-4   Alterations of the tongue

Type of change	Clinical features
SIZE OR MORPHOLOGY CHANGES	
Macroglossia	Enlarged tongue which may be part of a syndrome found in developmental conditions such as Down's syndrome; may be due to tumor (hemangioma or lymphangioma), metabolic disease (such as primary amyloidosis), or endocrine disturbance (such as acromegaly or cretinism)
Fissured ("scrotal") tongue	Dorsal surface and sides of tongue covered by painless shallow or deep fissures which may collect debris and become irritated
Median rhomboid glossitis	Congenital abnormality of tongue with ovoid, denuded area in the median posterior portion of the tongue
COLOR CHANGES	
"Geographic" tongue ("wandering rash")	Asymptomatic inflammatory condition of the tongue, with rapid loss and regrowth of filiform papillae, leading to appearance of denuded red patches "wandering" across the surface of the tongue
Hairy tongue	Elongation of filiform papillae of the medial dorsal surface area due to failure of keratin layer of the papillae to desquamate normally; brownish-black coloration may be due to staining by tobacco, food, or chromogenic organisms
"Strawberry" and "raspberry" tongue	Appearance of tongue during scarlet fever due to the hypertrophy of fungiform papillae plus changes in the filiform papillae
"Bald" tongue	Complete atrophy of papillae which may occur in pernicious anemia, severe iron-deficiency anemia, pellagra, or syphilis; may be accompanied by painful, burning sensations

REFERENCES

BEITMAN RG: Oral manifestations of gastrointestinal disease. Dig Dis Sci 26:741, 1981

GOLDMAN HS, MARDER MZ: *Physician's Guide to Disease of the Oral Cavity*. Oradell, NJ, Medical Economics, 1982

LYNCH MA et al: *Burket's Oral Medicine, Diagnosis, and Treatment*, 8th ed. Philadelphia, Lippincott, 1984

ROSE LF, KAYE D: *Internal Medicine for Dentistry*. St. Louis, Mosby, 1983

SHAFER WG et al: *A Textbook of Oral Pathology,* 4th ed. Philadelphia, Saunders, 1983
SHKLAR G: *Oral Cancer: The Diagnosis, Therapy, Management, and Rehabilitation of the Oral Cancer Patient.* Philadelphia, Saunders, 1984
SONIS ST et al: *Principles and Practice of Oral Medicine.* Philadelphia, Saunders, 1984
WOOD NK, GOAZ PW: *Differential Diagnosis of Oral Lesions.* St. Louis, Mosby, 1980

32 DYSPHAGIA

RAJ K. GOYAL

Dysphagia is defined as a sensation of "sticking" or obstruction of the passage of food through the mouth, pharynx, or the esophagus.

Dysphagia should be distinguished from other symptoms related to swallowing. *Aphagia* signifies complete esophageal obstruction which is usually due to bolus impaction and represents a medical emergency. *Difficulty in initiating a swallow* occurs in disorders of the voluntary phase of swallowing. Once initiated, however, swallowing is completed normally. *Odynophagia* means painful swallowing. Frequently, odynophagia and dysphagia occur together. *Globus hystericus* is the sensation of a lump lodged in the throat. No difficulty, however, is encountered when actual swallowing is performed. *Phagophobia,* meaning fear of swallowing, and *refusal to swallow* may occur in hysteria, rabies, tetanus, and pharyngeal paralysis due to fear of aspiration. Painful inflammatory lesions that cause odynophagia may also cause refusal to swallow. Some patients may feel the food as it goes down the esophagus. This esophageal sensitivity is not associated with sticking of the food or obstruction, however. Similarly, the *feeling of fullness in the epigastrium* that occurs after a meal or after swallowing air should not be confused with dysphagia.

PHYSIOLOGY OF SWALLOWING The process of swallowing begins with a voluntary (oral) phase during which a bolus of food is pushed backward into the pharynx. The bolus activates oropharyngeal sensory receptors which initiate the involuntary (pharyngeal and esophageal) phase, or deglutition reflex. The deglutition reflex is a complex series of events which serves both to propel food through the pharynx and the esophagus and to prevent its entry into the airway. At the same time as the bolus is propelled backward by the tongue, the larynx moves forward and the upper esophageal sphincter opens. As the bolus moves into the pharynx, contraction of the superior pharyngeal constrictor against the contracted soft palate initiates a peristaltic contraction that proceeds rapidly downward to move the bolus through the pharynx and the esophagus. The lower esophageal sphincter opens as the food enters the esophagus and remains open until the peristaltic contraction has swept the bolus into the stomach. Peristaltic contraction in response to a swallow involves the entire swallowing passages and is called *primary peristalsis.* Local distention of the esophagus due to food activates intramural reflexes in the smooth muscle which result in *secondary peristalsis,* limited to the lower esophagus. *Tertiary contractions* are nonperistaltic as they occur simultaneously over a long segment of the esophagus. Tertiary contractions may occur in response to a swallow or esophageal distention, or they may occur spontaneously.

PATHOPHYSIOLOGY OF DYSPHAGIA The normal transport of an ingested bolus through the swallowing passage depends on (1) the size of the ingested bolus, (2) the luminal diameter of the swallowing passage, (3) the peristaltic contraction, and (4) deglutitive inhibition, which includes normal relaxation of upper and lower esophageal sphincters during swallowing and inhibition of persisting contractions in the esophageal body, for example, due to an immediately preceding swallow. Dysphagia caused by a large bolus or luminal narrowing is called *mechanical dysphagia,* while dysphagia due to incoordination or weakness of peristaltic contractions or to impaired deglutitive inhibition is called *motor dysphagia.*

Mechanical dysphagia Mechanical dysphagia could be caused by luminal factors, intrinsic narrowing or extrinsic compression of the lumen. In an adult, the esophageal lumen can distend to a diameter of well over 4 cm because of the elasticity of the esophageal wall. When the esophagus cannot dilate to more than 2.5 cm in diameter, dysphagia can occur, but it is always present when it cannot distend beyond 1.3 cm. Circumferential lesions produce dysphagia more consistently than eccentric lesions. Eccentric benign tumors and lesions causing extrinsic compression cause dysphagia infrequently. The causes of mechanical dysphagia are listed in Table 32-1. Common causes are carcinoma, peptic and other benign strictures, and lower esophageal ring.

Motor dysphagia Motor dysphagia may result from difficulty in initiating a swallow or abnormalities in peristalsis and deglutitive inhibition due to diseases of the esophageal skeletal or smooth muscle.

Diseases of the skeletal muscle involve the pharynx, upper esophageal sphincter, and the upper part of the esophagus. The striated muscle is innervated by a somatic component of the vagus with cell bodies of the lower motor neurons located in the nucleus ambiguus. These neurons are cholinergic and excitatory and are the sole determinant of the muscle activity. Peristalsis in the skeletal muscle segment is due to sequential central activation of neurons innervating muscles at different levels. Motor dysphagia of the pharynx results from neuromuscular disorders causing muscle paralysis, simultaneous nonperistaltic contraction, or loss of opening of

TABLE 32-1 Causes of mechanical dysphagia

I Luminal
  A Large bolus
  B Foreign body
II Intrinsic narrowing
  A Inflammatory condition causing edema and swelling
    1 Stomatitis
    2 Pharyngitis, epiglottitis
    3 Esophagitis (e.g., viral, monilial)
  B Webs
    1 Pharyngeal (Plummer-Vinson syndrome)
    2 Esophageal
  C Lower esophageal ring
    1 Mucosal ring (Schatzki ring)
  D Benign strictures
    1 Peptic
    2 Caustic and drug-induced
    3 Inflammatory (Crohn's disease, moniliasis, epidermolysis bullosa)
    4 Ischemic
    5 Postoperative, postirradiation
    6 Congenital
  E Malignant tumors
    1 Primary carcinoma
      a Squamous cell carcinoma
      b Adenocarcinoma
      c Carcinosarcoma
      d Pseudosarcoma
      e Lymphoma
      f Melanoma
    2 Metastatic carcinoma
  F Benign tumors
    1 Leiomyoma
    2 Lipoma
    3 Angioma
    4 Inflammatory fibroid polyp
    5 Epithelial papilloma
III Extrinsic compression
  A Cervical spondylitis
  B Vertebral osteophytes
  C Retropharyngeal abscess and masses
  D Enlarged thyroid gland
  E Zenker's diverticulum
  F Vascular compression
    1 Aberrant right subclavian artery
    2 Right-sided aorta
    3 Left atrial enlargement
    4 Aortic aneurysm
  G Posterior mediastinal masses
  H Pancreatic tumor, pancreatitis
  I Postvagotomy hematoma and fibrosis

NOTE: *Some lesions can occur anywhere along the swallowing passages while others occur in a specific location.*

the upper esophageal sphincter. Loss of opening of the upper sphincter is caused by paralysis of geniohyoid and other suprahyoid muscles or loss of deglutitive inhibition of the cricopharyngeus muscle. Because each side of the pharynx is innervated by ipsilateral nerves, a lesion of motor neurons occurring only on one side leads to unilateral pharyngeal paralysis. Although lesions of skeletal muscle also involve the upper part of the esophagus, the clinical manifestations of pharyngeal dysfunction usually overshadow the manifestations due to esophageal involvement.

Diseases of the smooth muscle segment involve the lower part of the esophagus and the lower esophageal sphincter. This smooth muscle is innervated by the parasympathetic component of the vagal preganglionic fibers and postganglionic noncholinergic neurons in the myenteric ganglia. These nerves exert a predominantly inhibitory influence on the lower esophageal sphincter and cause inhibition followed by contraction in the esophageal body. Peristalsis in this segment is due to neuromuscular mechanisms in the wall of the esophagus itself. Dysphagia results when the peristaltic contractions are weak or nonperistaltic or when the lower sphincter fails to open normally. Loss of contractile power occurs due to muscle weakness, as in scleroderma, or to loss of myenteric neurons, as in achalasia. The cause of simultaneous onset of contractions, typically seen in diffuse esophageal spasm, is not understood. Impairment of deglutitive inhibition of the lower esophageal sphincter is associated with a

TABLE 32-2 Causes of motor (neuromuscular) dysphagia

I Difficulty in initiating swallowing reflex
  A Oral lesions and paralysis of tongue
  B Oropharyngeal anesthesia
  C Lack of saliva
  D Lesions of sensory components of vagus and glossopharyngeal nerves
  E Lesions of swallowing center
II Disorders of pharyngeal and esophageal skeletal muscle
  A Muscle weakness
    1 Lower motor neuron lesion (bulbar paralysis)
      a Cerebrovascular accident
      b Motor neuron disease
      c Poliomyelitis
      d Polyneuritis
      e Amyotrophic lateral sclerosis
      f Familial dysautonomia
    2 Neuromuscular
      a Myasthenia gravis
    3 Muscle disorders
      a Polymyositis
      b Dermatomyositis
      c Myopathies (myotonic dystrophy, oculopharyngeal myopathy)
  B Simultaneous onset contractions or impaired deglutitive inhibition
    1 Pharynx and upper esophagus
      a Rabies
      b Stiff-man syndrome
      c Extrapyramidal tract disease
      d Upper motor neuron lesions (pseudobulbar paralysis)
    2 Upper esophageal sphincter (UES)
      a Paralysis of suprahyoid muscles (causes same as paralysis of pharyngeal musculature)
      b Cricopharyngeal achalasia
III Disorders of esophageal smooth muscle
  A Paralysis of esophageal body causing weak contractions
    1 Scleroderma and related collagen vascular diseases
    2 Myotonic dystrophy
    3 Metabolic neuromyopathy (amyloid, alcohol?, diabetes?)
    4 Achalasia (classical)
  B Simultaneous-onset contractions or impaired deglutitive inhibition
    1 Esophageal body
      a Diffuse esophageal spasm
      b Achalasia (vigorous)
      c Variants of diffuse esophageal spasm
    2 Lower esophageal sphincter (LES)
      a Achalasia
        (1) Primary
        (2) Secondary
          (a) Chagas' disease
          (b) Carcinoma
          (c) Lymphoma
          (d) Intestinal pseudoobstruction syndrome
          (e) Toxins and drugs
          (f) Irradiation
      b Lower esophageal muscular (contractile) ring

defect in inhibitory nerves to the sphincter and is the major cause of dysphagia in achalasia.

The causes of motor dysphagia are listed in Table 32-2. The important causes are achalasia, diffuse esophageal spasm and related motor disorders, pharyngeal paralysis, cricopharyngeal achalasia, and scleroderma of the esophagus.

APPROACH TO THE PATIENT WITH DYSPHAGIA History The history can provide a correct presumptive diagnosis in over 80 percent of patients. The type of food causing dysphagia provides useful information. Difficulty only with solids implies mechanical dysphagia with a lumen that is not severely narrowed. The impacted bolus may be forced through the narrowed area by drinking liquids. In advanced obstruction dysphagia occurs with liquids as well as solids. In contrast, motor dysphagia due to achalasia and diffuse esophageal spasm is equally affected by solids and liquids from the very onset. Patients with scleroderma have dysphagia to solids that is unrelated to posture and to liquids in the recumbent but not in the upright posture. When peptic stricture develops in these patients dysphagia becomes more persistent.

The duration and course of dysphagia are helpful in diagnosis. Transient dysphagia of short duration may be due to an inflammatory process. Progressive dysphagia of a few weeks' to a few months' duration is suggestive of carcinoma of the esophagus. Episodic dysphagia to solids of several years' duration indicates a benign disease and is characteristic of a lower esophageal ring.

The localization of dysphagia is helpful when it is described in the chest, where the site of dysphagia generally correlates with the site of esophageal obstruction. However, localization of dysphagia to the neck is of no diagnostic value because lesions of the pharynx, cervical esophagus, and even lower esophagus may cause dysphagia to be perceived in the neck.

Associated symptoms provide important diagnostic clues. Nasal regurgitation and tracheobronchial aspiration with swallowing are hallmarks of pharyngeal paralysis or a tracheoesophageal fistula. Tracheobronchial aspiration unrelated to swallowing may be secondary to achalasia, a Zenker's diverticulum, or gastroesophageal reflux. Severe weight loss out of proportion to the degree of dysphagia is highly suggestive of carcinoma. When hoarseness precedes dysphagia, the primary lesion is usually in the larynx. Hoarseness following dysphagia may suggest involvement of the recurrent laryngeal nerve by extension of esophageal carcinoma beyond the walls of the esophagus. Sometimes hoarseness may be due to laryngitis secondary to gastroesophageal reflux. Association of laryngeal symptoms and dysphagia also occurs in various neuromuscular disorders. Hiccups suggest a lesion in the distal portion of the esophagus. Unilateral wheezing with dysphagia indicates a mediastinal mass involving the esophagus and a large bronchus. Chest pain with dysphagia occurs in diffuse esophageal spasm and in related motor disorders. Chest pain resembling diffuse esophageal spasms also may occur in acute aphagia due to a large bolus. A prolonged history of heartburn and reflux preceding dysphagia indicates peptic stricture. Similarly, a history of prolonged nasogastric intubation, ingestion of caustic agents, previous radiation therapy, or associated mucocutaneous diseases may provide the cause of esophageal stricture. If odynophagia is present, monilial or herpes esophagitis should be suspected, particularly in debilitated patients with carcinoma or those receiving immunosuppressive therapy.

Physical examination Physical examination is important in motor dysphagia due to skeletal muscle, neurologic, and oropharyngeal diseases. Signs of bulbar or pseudobulbar palsy, including dysarthria, dysphonia, ptosis, tongue atrophy, and hyperactive jaw jerk, in addition to evidence of generalized neuromuscular disease, should be carefully searched for. The neck should be examined for thyromegaly or a spinal abnormality. A careful inspection of the mouth and pharynx should disclose lesions that may cause interference with passage of food from the mouth or esophagus because of pain or obstruction. Changes in the skin and extremities may suggest a diagnosis of scleroderma and other collagen vascular diseases, or mucocutaneous diseases such as pemphigoid or epidermolysis bullosa which may involve the esophagus. Metastatic diseases to lymph nodes and liver may be evident. Pulmonary complications of acute aspiration pneumonia or chronic aspiration may be present.

Diagnostic procedures Dysphagia is one of the major symptoms of esophageal disease, and a cause for this symptom can invariably be determined. Therefore, all patients with dysphagia must be thoroughly investigated until a specific cause is determined. This is particularly important because the treatment depends upon the underlying cause of dysphagia. Barium swallow with cineradiography, esophagogastroscopy with biopsy and exfoliative cytology, and esophageal motility study are the main diagnostic procedures (see Chap. 234).

REFERENCES

CASTELL DO, JOHNSON LF (eds): *Esophageal Function in Health and Disease.* New York, Elsevier Biomedical, 1983
ENTERLINE H, THOMPSON, J: *Pathology of the Esophagus.* New York, Springer-Verlag, 1984
GIDDA JS, GOYAL RK: Regional gradient of initial inhibition and refractoriness in esophageal smooth muscle. Gastroenterology 89:843, 1985
GOYAL RK, COBB BW: Motility of pharynx, esophagus and esophageal sphincter, in *Physiology of the Gastrointestinal Tract,* LR Johnson (ed). New York, Raven Press, 1981, pp 359–391
SCHULZE-DELNIEU K, CHRISTENSEN J: The esophagus, in *The Gastroenterology Annual,* F Kern, A Blum (eds). New York, Elsevier Science, 1984, pp 1–28

33 INDIGESTION

LAWRENCE S. FRIEDMAN / KURT J. ISSELBACHER

Indigestion, or *dyspepsia,* is a term frequently used by patients to describe a variety of symptoms generally appreciated as distress associated with the intake of food. The term is nonspecific and may not have the same meaning for the patient and physician. Thus, in approaching the patient with indigestion, it is important for the physician first to elicit a precise description of this complaint. To some patients indigestion refers to actual abdominal pain, pressure, or heartburn. Others may use the term to describe a sense of abdominal fullness or a vague feeling that digestion has not proceeded naturally. Still others may use it to describe belching, a feeling of excessive gas, or flatulence. These complaints are considered in this chapter. Discussed elsewhere are the closely related symptoms of dysphagia, anorexia, and nausea and vomiting (Chaps. 32 and 34).

After having ascertained the patient's definition of indigestion, it is important to determine (1) the location and duration of the discomfort, (2) the temporal relation of the symptoms to the ingestion of food, and (3) the possible relation of the symptoms to the ingestion of specific types of food (e.g., milk, fatty foods) or drugs.

Indigestion may occur in association with diseases of the gastrointestinal tract or pathologic states in other organ systems. As a result of a systematic clinical and laboratory investigation, a definable pathophysiologic process often can be shown to be responsible for the symptoms in a given case of indigestion. Frequently, however, a clear etiologic explanation for the patient's complaint of indigestion is not established. Such cases are often designated as "functional indigestion," with a strong implication that psychosomatic factors underlie the complaint. Although it is clear that psychological factors may lead to symptoms of indigestion, the designation of "functional indigestion" is rarely a satisfactory explanation, serving only to rephrase the patient's description of the symptoms. Moreover, on the basis of electrophysiologic studies of the intestine it appears likely that some cases of functional indigestion result from subtle distur-

bances of gastrointestinal motility. Indeed, some patients with functional indigestion also have other features of the irritable bowel syndrome, suggesting a diffuse motility disturbance of the gastrointestinal tract (see Chap. 239).

SYNDROMES COMMONLY DESCRIBED AS INDIGESTION

PAIN Pain patterns A careful elucidation of the pattern of pain may provide important diagnostic information. True visceral abdominal pain is mediated by visceral afferent nerves which accompany the abdominal sympathetic pathways (see Chap. 5). Visceral pain is generally described as dull and aching in nature, with a diffuse midline localization, or as fullness or pressure. The location of the discomfort corresponds generally to the segmental level of neural innervation of the affected organ. Abdominal visceral pain can be produced experimentally by artificially increasing pressure in a hollow viscus. Usually this pain is the result of distention or exaggerated muscular contraction of a viscus. Inflammation generally lowers the threshold for pain from such stimuli.

The visceral pain of indigestion should be distinguished from the sharp, localized pain patterns of many acute abdominal processes involving the peritoneum. In contrast to true visceral pain, this pain is mediated by cerebrospinal afferent nerves.

In view of the diffuse nature of true visceral abdominal pain, the main clue to the cause comes from the *location of the pain* and the corresponding segmental level of neural innervation; however, in any given segmental region there is no way of determining which of several viscera is the source of the pain (Table 33-1). The following rules, already described in Chap. 5, are useful: *Substernal pain* of gastrointestinal origin usually arises from disorders of the esophagus or cardia of the stomach. Because pain in this area frequently emanates from the heart, cardiac disease must be carefully considered and excluded. *Epigastric pain* is generally of gastric, duodenal, biliary, or pancreatic origin. (The epigastrium is also a frequent location for "functional" pain.) As pathologic processes in the biliary tract or pancreas become more intense, pain may lateralize and localize, e.g., biliary pain to the right upper quadrant and tip of the scapula and pancreatic pain to the left upper quadrant and back. *Periumbilical pain* is generally associated with disease involving the small intestine. *Pain below the umbilicus* is often of appendiceal, colonic, or pelvic origin.

Temporal relationships The unraveling of the *temporal relationships* of the patient's symptoms often provides additional diagnostic

TABLE 33-1 Distribution of visceral pain and examples of disorders frequently involving the specific organ

Organ	Location of pain	Examples of disorders
Esophagus	Substernum, epigastrium	Peptic esophagitis, stricture, esophageal spasm, carcinoma
Stomach	Epigastrium	Gastritis, gastric ulcer, carcinoma
Duodenum (first and second portions)	Epigastrium	Duodenal ulcer
Small intestine (excluding first and second portions of duodenum)	Periumbilical	Infectious gastroenteritis, regional enteritis, lymphoma, intestinal obstruction
Gallbladder	Epigastrium, right upper quadrant, right upper back	Cholelithiasis, cholecystitis
Pancreas	Epigastrium, left upper quadrant, left side of back	Pancreatitis, pancreatic carcinoma
Liver	Right upper quadrant	Hepatitis, cirrhosis, passive congestion
Colon	Below umbilicus	Infectious colitis, ulcerative colitis, carcinoma, partial obstruction

clues. It is important to ascertain whether the symptoms are *constant* (continually present over extended periods of time), as may occur, for example, with an infiltrating gastric carcinoma, or *intermittent,* as in acute gastritis or biliary colic. The symptoms may have a *diurnal* pattern as in the case of reflux esophagitis in which pain often occurs nocturnally and with recumbency. Pain that awakens the patient from a sound sleep occurs most often with duodenal ulcer. Occasionally symptoms are *seasonal,* as in peptic ulcer disease, in which some patients experience more discomfort in the spring and autumn than at other times.

Another helpful diagnostic feature is the relation of pain to the *ingestion of food. Early postprandial symptoms* may reflect esophageal disease, acute gastritis, or gastric carcinoma. *Late postprandial indigestion,* i.e., that occurring several hours after eating, may reflect failure of the stomach to empty adequately, as in gastric outlet obstruction or atony, or duodenal ulcer, in which case pain results from exposure of ulcerated mucosa to acid secreted by the stomach and unbuffered by food. Conversely, the relief of pain following ingestion of food or antacids is characteristic of duodenal ulcer and is presumably due to the neutralization of the acid. Late postprandial indigestion also may result from impaired digestive and absorptive processes, as in pancreatic insufficiency.

It is important to recognize that the pain patterns and relationships to the intake of food described above are generalizations, and many cases do not conform to classic "textbook" descriptions. For example, although pain limited to the right upper quadrant is often caused by gallbladder disease, about half of patients with this condition experience only epigastric pain. Similarly, there are some patients with peptic ulcer whose pain is not relieved by antacids, while there are other patients with functional indigestion and even gastric carcinoma whose pain improves with antacids.

HEARTBURN   Heartburn, or pyrosis, is a sensation of warmth or burning located substernally or high in the epigastrium with radiation into the neck and occasionally to the arms. Occasional heartburn is common in normal persons, but frequent and severe heartburn is generally a manifestation of esophageal dysfunction. Heartburn may result from abnormal motor activity or distention of the esophagus, reflux of acid or bile into the esophagus, or direct esophageal mucosal irritation (esophagitis).

Heartburn is most often associated with gastroesophageal reflux (see Chap. 234). In this setting, heartburn occurs after a large meal, with stooping or bending, or when the patient is supine. It may be accompanied by the spontaneous appearance in the mouth of fluid which may be salty ("water brash"), sour (gastric contents), or bitter and green or yellow (bile). Heartburn may arise following the ingestion of certain foods (e.g., citrus fruit juices) or drugs (e.g., alcohol and aspirin). Characteristically heartburn is alleviated promptly, even if only temporarily, by antacids.

Heartburn may also occur in the absence of a demonstrable or motor pathologic condition. In this setting, it is frequently accompanied by aerophagia, which may represent an attempt by the patient to relieve discomfort, and is often attributed to psychological factors for lack of other explanation.

FOOD INTOLERANCE   In some persons specific foods or types of foods appear to be related to indigestion. Careful documentation of this relationship is sometimes of great help in arriving at an etiologic diagnosis.

Some foods may be poorly tolerated because of their consistency. Patients with esophageal stricture or carcinoma may tolerate liquids well but may experience discomfort, especially substernal distress, after ingesting solids (see Chap. 234). Certain foods may be tolerated poorly because of impaired intestinal digestion or absorption. This condition may occur following the ingestion of fatty foods in patients with pancreatic or biliary tract disease. Citrus fruits, with their relatively low pH, often provoke symptoms in patients with peptic ulcer disease or peptic esophagitis.

Persons may have a congenital or acquired *lack or deficiency of a specific enzyme* required for intestinal absorption of a certain nutrient. One example is the deficiency of lactase, the intestinal mucosal enzyme which catalyzes the hydrolysis of lactose. In persons who are lactase-deficient, the ingestion of milk (which contains lactose) results in abdominal cramps, distention, diarrhea, and flatulence (Chap. 237). Also, certain substances may lead to profound systemic effects because of *biochemical defects* in the patient which render the substances particularly hazardous. An example of the latter is galactose intolerance in persons with galactosemia (see Chap. 314).

There are a number of other conditions in which specific foods are tolerated poorly. For example, some foods may initiate *allergic reactions,* which should be suspected when symptoms occur immediately after ingestion of the food, recur on challenge testing, and are associated with other features of an allergic reaction, such as lip swelling, urticaria, angioedema, asthma, or rarely anaphylactic shock. Other foods may exert *toxic effects* on the intestinal tracts of susceptible persons (e.g., gluten in patients with celiac sprue).

The mechanisms described above do not explain the majority of clinical situations in which indigestion is associated with the ingestion of specific foods. For example, a history of fatty food intolerance or an inability to eat spicy foods is commonly obtained from patients with indigestion. However, the mechanisms underlying the production of symptoms in these circumstances are still unclear.

AEROPHAGIA, GASEOUSNESS, FLATULENCE   A number of common clinical syndromes which may be described by the patient as indigestion appear to be related to increased quantities of or sensitivity to gas in the intestinal tract.

Aerophagia   Patients with a complaint of *chronic, repetitive eructation* (belching) can be observed to precede each belch with a swallow of air, most of which passes only partway down the esophagus and is then regurgitated. Thus, excessive eructation results from *aerophagia,* or air swallowing, not from excessive gas production in the stomach or the intestine. A degree of aerophagia occurs in normal persons, but some individuals gulp air excessively because of chronic anxiety, rapid eating, drinking carbonated beverages, gum chewing, postnasal drip, or poorly fitting dentures. Because eructation which follows aerophagia may provide a temporary sense of relief to the patient, a vicious cycle of aerophagia and eructation may ensue.

About 20 to 60 percent of intestinal gas represents swallowed air. Because N_2 (nitrogen) and O_2 (oxygen) are the only gases present in the atmosphere in appreciable concentrations and because they are not produced in the gastrointestinal tract, the detection of these gases on gas chromatographic analysis of intestinal gas indicates that swallowed air must be the source. Swallowed air that is not eructated passes on to the stomach and intestinal tract. Accumulation of swallowed air in the stomach may lead to postprandial fullness and pressure and the finding on an abdominal radiograph of a large amount of air in the gastric fundus. This symptom complex, referred to as the *magenblase* (i.e., gastric bubble) *syndrome,* may occur when a patient lies supine after a large meal so that the gastric air is "trapped" below the gastroesophageal junction by overlying fluid and cannot be eructated. Acute gastric distention by swallowed air can occasionally produce sharp pains which may mimic angina pectoris. Swallowed air which successfully passes the stomach may either produce diffuse abdominal distention or become trapped in the splenic flexure of the colon. The latter condition, known as the *splenic flexure syndrome,* is characterized by a sensation of left upper quadrant fullness and pressure with radiation to the left side of the chest. Relief of pain often follows defecation or the expulsion of flatus. The diagnosis is suggested by the finding of increased tympany in the extreme left lateral portion of the upper abdomen on physical examination or of large amounts of air in the splenic flexure of the colon on a plain abdominal radiograph.

Gaseousness, bloating, and flatulence   Despite the widely held belief that feelings of *diffuse abdominal pain and bloating* are often caused by excessive quantities of intestinal gas, studies employing an intestinal gas wash-out technique suggest that patients complaining of excessive gas have normal volumes of intestinal gas. The primary abnormality causing functional bloating and pain in such persons appears to be a motility disturbance that causes the patient to perceive pain with an intestinal gas volume that is well tolerated by normal subjects. Alternatively, intestinal motility may be normal in such persons, but they may be excessively responsive to normal impulses arising from the intestinal tract.

A major source of intestinal gas is the fermentative action of intestinal bacteria on carbohydrates and proteins within the lumen. Normally such bacteria are limited to the colon, and the principal gases produced are CO_2 (carbon dioxide) and H_2 (hydrogen) (in addition to minute quantities of odoriferous gases which give flatus its characteristic odor). In the upper small bowel CO_2 is also produced when hydrochloric acid from the stomach or ingested fatty acids are neutralized by bicarbonate. (This may explain, in part, indigestion associated with fatty foods.) In addition, about one-third of the adult population produces appreciable quantities of CH_4 (methane) in the colon, a characteristic which appears to be a familial trait and unrelated to food ingestion. An increase in intraluminal gas production with resulting *abdominal distention, bloating,* and *flatulence* occurs following the ingestion of certain foods, such as legumes and some grains, which contain significant quantities of nonabsorbable carbohydrates that pass into the colon where they supply gas-forming substrate for the colonic bacteria. The best studied example of this is the case of beans, which contain the oligosaccharides stachyose and raffinose that cannot be split by the mucosal enzymes of the small intestine. As stated above, increased intraluminal gas production may also occur in patients with carbohydrate malabsorption states, such as lactose malabsorption due to intestinal lactase deficiency. Abnormal bacterial colonization of the small intestine (bacterial overgrowth syndrome) or infection with *Giardia lamblia* may also lead to an increase in intraluminal gas production, resulting in distention, pain, diarrhea, and flatulence.

INDIGESTION DUE TO DISEASE OUTSIDE THE INTESTINAL TRACT

A number of extraintestinal diseases may result in indigestion by mechanisms which are poorly understood, For example, indigestion may be the presenting complaint in congestive heart failure, pulmonary tuberculosis, neoplastic disease, and uremia. Also, a variety of drugs such as aspirin, nonsteroidal anti-inflammatory agents, and corticosteroids may cause symptoms of indigestion because of their ulcerogenic properties.

DIAGNOSTIC APPROACH TO THE PATIENT WITH INDIGESTION

Indigestion represents a challenging and difficult diagnostic problem because of the nonspecific nature of its manifestations. The cornerstone of the evaluation of indigestion is obtaining a clear and detailed description of the specific symptoms, particularly the patient's definition of the term *indigestion*. The nature of the distress, its frequency and time of occurrence, its relationship to meals, and the special circumstances which lead to its exacerbation or relief should be elicited. Associated intestinal symptoms such as nausea and vomiting, abnormal bowel habits, diarrhea, steatorrhea, and melena should be sought, and an assessment of nutritional status, appetite, and changes in weight should be made. A careful history should also include an assessment of the patient's general health, including the possible presence of extraintestinal disorders which may produce indigestion. A careful evaluation of psychological factors is crucial, because they often play an etiologic or contributory role to the patient's problems. Of particular importance are anxiety, depressive symptoms, and hysteria (see Chap. 11).

Physical examination rarely establishes the specific diagnosis, but it may be useful in detecting diseases in other organ systems which

can affect intestinal function (e.g., congestive heart failure). Stools should be examined for appearance and occult blood.

Whether further diagnostic studies are indicated depends on the specific nature of the patient's complaints and the patient's age (concern about the possibility of gastrointestinal malignancy being greater in older patients). Abdominal pain may be evaluated with radiologic studies of the esophagus, stomach, small intestine, colon, pancreas, and biliary tract. Esophagogastroscopy, endoscopic cholangiopancreatography, sigmoidoscopy, or colonoscopy may also be helpful or necessary. On the other hand, in patients under age 30 with epigastric pain typical of acid-peptic disease, routine diagnostic studies are unlikely to disclose serious diseases (such as gastric carcinoma) and are often negative; thus, an empiric trial of antacids or possibly H_2-blocking drugs may be appropriate before proceeding with further diagnostic tests. In individuals complaining of excessive eructation, a simple demonstration that aerophagia reproduces the symptoms may suffice to confirm the diagnosis and break the patient of the habit. Patients complaining of excessive gas, bloating, distention, and flatulence must be questioned carefully about dietary preferences and the relation of symptoms to specific foods. In some cases elimination of certain foods (e.g., milk) from the diet followed by rechallenge may confirm the role of that food in producing the patient's symptoms. In other cases a more detailed evaluation, including stool examination for fat and muscle fibers and for parasites such as *Giardia lamblia,* breath tests to detect carbohydrate malabsorption, and intestinal motility studies, may be helpful.

Even after completion of careful diagnostic studies, many cases of indigestion will turn out to have no clear explanation. Some of these are psychogenic and may respond to appropriate psychiatric measures. Others represent subtle physiologic derangements which are undetectable by currently available diagnostic methods. In some such instances, an empiric trial of dopamine antagonists, such as metoclopramide, which augment gastrointestinal motility may be beneficial. Still other cases represent early stages of actual disease processes which may only be diagnosable by conventional methods at a later date. The ultimate evaluation of indigestion requires, therefore, the utmost in sensitivity, diligence, and concern on the part of the examining physician.

REFERENCES

BOND JH, LEVITT MD: Gaseousness and intestinal gas. Med Clin North Am 62:155, 1978

HEALTH AND PUBLIC POLICY COMMITTEE, American College of Physicians: Endoscopy in the evaluation of dyspepsia. Ann Intern Med 102:266, 1985

HORROCKS JC, DEDOMBAL FT: Clinical presentation of patients with "dyspepsia." Gut 19:19, 1978

LASSER RB et al: The role of intestinal gas in functional abdominal pain. N Engl J Med 293:524, 1975

LEVITT MD: Intestinal gas production—recent advances in flatology. N Engl J Med 302:1474, 1980

MEAD GM et al: Use of barium meal examination in dyspeptic patients under 50. Br Med J 1:1460, 1977

34 ANOREXIA, NAUSEA, AND VOMITING

KURT J. ISSELBACHER

ANOREXIA Anorexia, or loss of the desire to eat, is a prominent symptom in a wide variety of intestinal and extraintestinal disorders. It must be clearly differentiated from satiety and from specific food intolerance. Anorexia occurs in many disorders and as a result *by itself is of little specific diagnostic value*. The mechanisms whereby hunger and appetite are modified in various disease states are poorly understood. Normally food intake is regulated by two hypothalamic centers—a lateral "feeding center" and a ventromedial "satiety center.'' The latter inhibits the feeding center following a meal, leading to the sensation of satiety. There is some evidence to suggest that the brain-gut peptide cholecystokinin (CCK) has a satiety effect and is involved in the regulation of feeding behavior.

Anorexia is commonly seen in diseases of the gastrointestinal tract and liver. For example, it may precede the appearance of jaundice in hepatitis, or it may be a prominent symptom in gastric carcinoma. In the setting of intestinal disease, anorexia should be clearly differentiated from *sitophobia,* or fear of eating because of subsequent or associated discomfort. In such circumstances, appetite may persist, but the ingestion of food is curtailed nonetheless. Sitophobia may be seen, for example, in regional enteritis (especially with partial obstruction) or in patients with gastric ulcer following partial or total gastrectomy.

Anorexia may also be a prominent feature of severe extraintestinal diseases. For example, anorexia may be profound in severe congestive heart failure and is often associated with cardiac glycoside intoxication. It may be a major symptom in patients with uremia, pulmonary failure, and various endocrinopathies (e.g., hyperparathyroidism, Addison's disease, and panhypopituitarism). Anorexia also often accompanies psychogenic disturbances, such as anxiety or depression. For a discussion of anorexia nervosa, see Chap. 73.

NAUSEA AND VOMITING   Nausea and vomiting may occur independently of each other, but generally they are so closely allied that they may conveniently be considered together. *Nausea* denotes the feeling of the imminent desire to vomit, usually referred to the throat or epigastrium. *Vomiting* refers to the forceful oral expulsion of gastric contents; *retching* denotes the labored rhythmic respiratory activity that frequently precedes emesis. Extremely forceful *projectile vomiting* is a special form of vomiting which has significance because it may connote the presence of increased intracranial pressure.

Nausea often precedes or accompanies vomiting. It is usually associated with diminished functional activity of the stomach and alterations of the motility of the duodenum and small intestine. Accompanying severe nausea there is often evidence of altered autonomic (especially parasympathetic) activity: pallor of the skin, increased perspiration, hypersalivation, and the occasional association of hypotension and bradycardia (vasovagal syndrome). Anorexia is also often present.

Following a period of nausea and a brief interval of retching, a sequence of involuntary visceral and somatic motor events occurs, resulting in emesis. The stomach plays a relatively passive role in the vomiting process, the major ejection force being provided by the abdominal musculature. With relaxation of the gastric fundus and gastroesophageal sphincter, a sharp increase in intraabdominal pressure is brought about by forceful contraction of the diaphragm and abdominal wall. This, together with concomitant annular contraction of the gastric pylorus, results in the expulsion of gastric contents into the esophagus. Increased intrathoracic pressure results in the further movement of esophageal contents into the mouth. Reversal of the normal direction of esophageal peristalsis may play a role in this process. Reflex elevation of the soft palate during the vomiting act prevents the entry of the material into the nasopharynx, whereas reflex closure of the glottis and inhibition of respiration help to prevent pulmonary aspiration.

Repeated emesis may have deleterious effects in a number of different ways. The process of vomiting, if forceful, may lead to pressure rupture of the esophagus (Boerhaave's syndrome) or linear mucosal tears in the region of the cardioesophageal junction, resulting in massive hematemesis (Mallory-Weiss syndrome). Prolonged vomiting may lead to dehydration and the loss of gastric secretions (especially hydrochloric acid), resulting in metabolic alkalosis with hypokalemia. Finally, in states of central nervous system depression (coma, etc.), gastric contents may be aspirated into the lungs, with a resulting aspiration pneumonitis.

Vomiting mechanism   The act of vomiting is under the control of two functionally distinct medullary centers: the *vomiting center* and the *chemoreceptor trigger zone*. They lie close to each other near other brainstem centers regulating vasomotor and autonomic functions. The vomiting center controls and integrates the actual act of emesis. It receives afferent stimuli from the intestinal tract and other parts of the body, from higher cortical centers, especially the labyrinthine apparatus, and from the chemoreceptor trigger zone. The important efferent pathways in vomiting are the phrenic nerves (to the diaphragm), the spinal nerves (to the abdominal musculature), and visceral efferent nerves (to the stomach and esophagus).

The chemoreceptor trigger zone is also located in the medulla but by itself is incapable of mediating the act of vomiting. Activation of this zone results in efferent impulses to the medullary vomiting center, which in turn initiates the act of emesis. Dopamine receptors in the chemoreceptor trigger zone can be activated by many stimuli, including drugs such as apomorphine and levodopa, after decarboxylation to dopamine.

Phenothiazine derivatives such as prochlorperazine and metoclopramide inhibit cerebral dopamine receptors and can be effective against both nausea and vomiting. Metoclopramide is the prototype of selective dopamine antagonists called *substituted benzamides.* In contrast to the phenothiazines, which have anticholinergic effects, metoclopramide has powerful cholinergic effects. These effects, together with its dopamine antagonism, have made metoclopramide a useful agent equal or superior to drugs such as prochlorperazine in the treatment of nausea and vomiting. The usual oral dosage is 10 mg four times daily. Metoclopramide is also effective in hastening esophageal clearance, accelerating gastric emptying, and shortening small-bowel transit. It may be used intravenously in doses up to 1 to 3 mg/kg as prophylaxis prior to potent chemotherapy agents (e.g., cisplatin).

Clinical classification   Nausea and vomiting are common manifestations of organic and functional disorders. The precise mechanisms triggering vomiting in the various clinical states are poorly understood, making classification of mechanisms difficult. The categories mentioned below serve to illustrate some of the many disorders which may be accompanied by nausea and vomiting.

Many *acute abdominal emergencies* which lead to the "surgical abdomen" are associated with nausea and vomiting. Notably, vomiting may be seen with inflammation of a viscus as in acute appendicitis or acute cholecystitis, obstruction of the intestine, or acute peritonitis (see Chap. 5).

In many of the disorders involving *chronic indigestion* (see Chap. 33) nausea and vomiting may be prominent. Emesis may be either spontaneous or self-induced and may lead to relief of symptoms, as, for example, in uncomplicated peptic ulcer. Nausea and vomiting may accompany the distention and pain seen in the aerophagic syndromes. Often in patients with chronic indigestion, nausea and vomiting may be provoked by specific foods (e.g., fatty foods), for reasons that are poorly understood.

Acute systemic infections with fever, especially in young children, are frequently accompanied by vomiting and often by severe diarrhea. The mechanism whereby infections remote from the gastrointestinal tract produce these manifestations is unclear. Viral, bacterial, and parasitic infections of the intestinal tract may be associated with severe nausea and vomiting, often with diarrhea. Severe nausea and vomiting may be prominent in viral hepatitis, even before the appearance of jaundice.

Central nervous system disorders which lead to increased intracranial pressure may be accompanied by vomiting, often projectile. Brain swelling due to inflammation, anoxemia, acute hydrocephalus, neoplasms, etc., may thus be complicated by vomiting. Disorders of the labyrinthine apparatus and its central connections which underlie vertigo may be accompanied by vomiting with nausea and retching. Acute labyrinthitis and Ménière's disease are examples of such disturbances. Migraine headaches, tabetic crises, and acute meningitis are additional examples of disorders of the nervous system which may lead to vomiting. In the reactive phase of hypotension with syncope, there may also be nausea and vomiting.

Severe nausea and vomiting may be present in *acute myocardial infarction,* especially of the posterior wall of the heart. Nausea and vomiting may also be seen in *congestive heart failure,* perhaps in relation to congestion of the liver. The possibility that these symptoms may be due to drugs (e.g., opiates or digitalis) should always be borne in mind in patients with cardiac disease.

Nausea and vomiting commonly accompany several *endocrinologic disorders,* including diabetic acidosis and adrenal insufficiency, especially adrenal crisis. The morning sickness of early pregnancy is another instance of nausea and vomiting possibly related to hormonal changes.

The *side effects of many drugs and chemicals* include nausea and vomiting. In some instances this is because of gastric irritation which stimulates the medullary vomiting center. The ingestion of a *toxin* (e.g., food poisoning) may also cause acute vomiting.

Psychogenic vomiting means vomiting which may occur as part of any emotional upset on a transitory basis or more persistently as part of a psychic disturbance. Close observation will usually disclose the condition to be one of regurgitation rather than of vomiting, and weight loss may not correspond at all to the patient's description of the frequency and severity of vomiting. As discussed in Chap. 73, anorexia nervosa is an emotional disturbance which may be associated not only with anorexia but also with vomiting. Often patients with emotional disorders and vomiting maintain a relatively normal state of nutrition because a relatively small amount of the ingested food is vomited.

Differential diagnosis Vomiting should be distinguished from *regurgitation,* which refers to the expulsion of food in the absence of nausea and without abdominal diaphragmatic muscular contraction which is part of vomiting. Regurgitation of esophageal contents may occur with esophageal stricture or diverticula. Regurgitation of gastric contents is generally seen with gastroesophageal sphincter incompetence, especially with hiatus hernia or in association with peptic ulcer, usually when pylorospasm supervenes.

The temporal relationships of vomiting to eating may be of help diagnostically. Vomiting which occurs predominantly in the morning is often seen early in pregnancy and uremia. Alcoholic gastritis is commonly accompanied by early-morning emesis, the so-called dry heaves. Vomiting which occurs shortly after eating may suggest pylorospasm or gastritis. On the other hand, vomiting which occurs 4 to 6 h or longer after eating and involves the elimination of large quantities of undigested food often indicates gastric retention (e.g., diabetic gastric atony or pyloric obstruction). However, with gastric retention vomiting may also occur early (e.g., 30 to 90 min) after a meal.

The character of the vomitus offers clues to the diagnosis. If the vomitus contains free hydrochloric acid, the obstruction may be due to an ulcer; absence of free hydrochloric acid is more compatible with gastric malignancy. A feculent or putrid odor reflects the results of bacterial action on the intestinal contents. Such vomiting may be seen with low-intestinal obstruction, peritonitis, or gastrocolic fistula. Bile is commonly present in gastric contents whenever vomiting is prolonged. It has no significance unless constantly present in large quantities, when it may signify an obstructive lesion below the ampulla of Vater. The presence of blood in the gastric contents usually denotes bleeding from the esophagus, stomach, or duodenum.

REFERENCES

FELDMAN M: Nausea and vomiting, in *Gastrointestinal Disease,* 3d ed, MH Sleisenger, JS Fordtran (eds). Philadelphia, Saunders, 1983, pp 160–177

HERZOG DB, COPELAND PM: Eating disorders. N Engl J Med 313:295, 1985

SMITH GP: Satiety effect of gastrointestinal hormones, in *Polypeptide Hormones,* RF Beers, EG Bassett (eds). New York, Raven Press, 1980, pp 413–420

WESER E: Anorexia and obesity in *Gastrointestinal Disease,* 3d ed, MH Sleisenger, JS Fordtran (eds). Philadelphia, Saunders, 1983, pp 135–144

35 GAIN AND LOSS IN WEIGHT

DANIEL W. FOSTER

GENERAL PRINCIPLES In normal persons weight is stable because caloric intake is matched to caloric expenditure by the coordinated activity of "feeding" and "satiety" centers presumably located in the hypothalamus. The signals that regulate the interactions of these centers are not known; regulation is probably multifactorial, and both short- and long-term controls are thought to be operative. Whatever the mechanisms the system is normally efficient over periods of months to years.

Gain or loss in tissue mass is determined by the net balance between caloric intake and caloric expenditure. Caloric intake is determined by availability and attractiveness of food and by emotional and physical factors. The bulk of energy expenditure is due to basal metabolism and physical activity. The former is defined as the total caloric requirement when the body is in the supine position, motionless except for quiet respiration, e.g., the energy required to maintain structural and functional integrity of the organism in the absence of physical activity. About half the total daily caloric intake is normally consumed by basal processes. Active persons spend about 40 percent of calories in physical activity; athletes may utilize 50 percent or more of ingested energy in exercise. Persons sedentary because of habit, illness, or obesity may expend far less in activity. In nonobese, nonsedentary subjects 10 percent of ingested calories is released as heat associated with the absorption of food, a process called dietary thermogenesis. This fraction, previously designated specific dynamic action, is usually considered a separate component of energy costs. Heat generated during and after exercise and that released for maintenance of body temperature (regulatory thermogenesis) are included in the energy costs of physical activity and basal metabolism, respectively.

Change in body weight as a consequence of voluntary alteration in diet or exercise is never worrisome; change in weight that is not deliberately sought, on the other hand, is a frequent reason for consultation with the physician and often indicates the presence of disease. Changes in weight may reflect alteration in either tissue mass or body fluid content. Rapid swings usually indicate the latter. Even when tissue mass is changing, fluid loss or gain plays a major role in the measured change in weight, particularly over the short run. This point is illustrated in Table 35-1, where the composition of weight loss was estimated during a 24-day period of semistarvation in 13 normal men (daily intake, 1010 kcal). During the first 3 days 70 percent of the decrease in weight was due to water loss, while in subsequent stages a diminution of protein and fat accounted for essentially all the weight loss. This varying contribution of fluid explains why a fixed formula cannot be used for predicting weight loss or gain. It is frequently stated that a net change of 7700 kcal will be accompanied by a 1-kg change in body mass (3500 kcal/lb). While this estimate is reasonable for long-term changes in caloric intake, the apparent caloric cost per kilogram of weight lost or gained varies with the accompanying fluid shifts. In the experiment summarized in Table 35-1, for example, a negative balance of only 2596

TABLE 35-1 Percentage composition of mean daily weight loss in 13 young men during caloric restriction for 24 days

Days	Mean weight loss, kg/day	Water, %	Fat, %	Protein, %	Calorie equivalents of weight loss, kcal/kg
1–3	0.80	70	25	5	2596
11–13	0.23	19	69	12	7043
22–24	0.17	0	85	15	8700

SOURCE: *After Brožek et al.*

kcal resulted in the loss of a kilogram of weight between days 1 and 3, while between days 22 and 24, loss of a kilogram required a deficit of 8700 kcal. In general if weight loss or gain has occurred over a period of weeks or months, it is safe to assume that change in tissue mass has occurred; weight loss or gain limited to a several-day period may be due to fluid shifts alone. Occasionally true loss of tissue mass is obscured by fluid retention as in the case of the cirrhotic patient who develops ascites or the patient with anorexia nervosa who has significant edema.

WEIGHT GAIN

While obesity is a major public health concern (see Chap. 317), its diagnosis is usually uncomplicated. Obese subjects often deny over-eating, but the true situation can be assessed either by tabulating actual food intake and determining its caloric content from standard tables or by interviewing the patient's family and friends.

Regardless of history, excess caloric intake is the cause of obesity in the majority of cases. Pathologic causes are rare. In the adult, Cushing's syndrome can result in acquired obesity in a previously nonobese patient, but usually the diagnosis is suggested by the pattern of fat distribution and the clinical picture. Other endocrine diseases such as hypothyroidism, hypogonadism, and insulin-secreting tumors are frequently listed in the differential diagnosis of obesity but do not represent significant diagnostic problems. Congenital diseases that cause obesity such as the Prader-Willi, Laurence-Moon-Biedl, and Alström syndromes are readily recognizable and appear early in life. Rarely, a disease involving the hypothalamus, particularly craniopharyngioma, may cause acquired obesity. Extensive workup of the central nervous system in obesity is not indicated, however, in the absence of suspicious symptoms (headache, visual difficulties, vomiting, or endocrine changes).

WEIGHT LOSS

Weight loss in the absence of deliberate dieting is a more serious problem than weight gain because there is a high chance that organic disease is present. Mechanisms include decreased appetite, accelerated metabolism, and loss of calories in urine or stool, acting singly or in combination. No attempt will be made to list all diseases capable of causing weight loss, but in one prospective study 26 percent of patients had no identifiable physical or psychiatric illness to which the weight loss could be attributed. If uncontrolled and symptomatic, any serious illness can cause weight loss; the usual mechanism is anorexia due either to direct pathophysiologic consequences (e.g., congestion of the liver and gastrointestinal tract in right-sided heart failure) or malaise and depression. The following categories are singled out for special comment because the primary illness may be masked at the time of initial presentation.

DIABETES MELLITUS Initial weight loss with the onset of diabetes is largely fluid and is due to the osmotic diuresis induced by hyperglycemia. Subsequently, loss of tissue mass occurs in the insulin-dependent form of the disease as a result of caloric wastage (the consequence of glycosuria) and of the hormonal abnormalities that characterize the illness. Insulin deficiency and glucagon excess result in impaired synthesis of protein and fat and simultaneously cause accelerated proteolysis and lipolysis such that the net energy state is catabolic. Weight loss in diabetes is frequently associated with increased food intake.

ENDOCRINE DISEASE While weight loss is not inevitable (indeed, thyrotoxicosis may rarely be found in a patient who has gained weight), it is common in hyperthyroidism. Increased appetite and food intake are the rule, and patients often consume a high-carbohydrate diet. Caloric expenditure is enormous, primarily because of an increased metabolic rate, but increased motor activity also plays

a role. The molecular mechanism whereby thyrotoxicosis causes weight loss is not settled, but thyroid hormone is thought to increase sodium-potassium adenosine triphosphatase (ATPase) activity in many tissues, suggesting that the diminished efficiency of ingested calories is due to futile cycle of adenosine triphosphate (ATP) synthesis and breakdown with energy lost as heat. In "apathetic" hyperthyroidism weight loss and weakness may predominate with little evidence of nervousness or other symptoms. Another cause of weight loss due to hypermetabolism is pheochromocytoma, the inducing agent being catecholamine release. Panhypopituitarism and adrenal insufficiency may also be associated with weight loss, largely as a consequence of diminished appetite secondary to cortisol deficiency.

GASTROINTESTINAL DISEASE Overt or occult steatorrhea due to sprue, chronic pancreatitis, or cystic fibrosis may produce wasting despite major increases in food intake. Chronic diarrhea due to inflammatory bowel disease (with or without fistulas) or parasites, esophageal disease with reflux or vomiting, and even ordinary peptic ulcer have to be considered in the differential diagnosis. The mechanism of weight loss in alimentary tract disease is generally either decreased food intake or malabsorption, though inflammation per se probably plays a role in the weight loss of ulcerative colitis and regional enteritis.

INFECTION Hidden infection must always be sought in patients with unexplained weight loss. Tuberculosis, fungal disease, amebic abscess, and subacute bacterial endocarditis should be high on the list of suspects. The mechanism probably involves both anorexia and inflammation-induced acceleration of cellular metabolic demands. Glucagon may play a role in the negative nitrogen balance and tissue wastage of inflammation, but the catabolic state probably also requires changes in other hormones.

MALIGNANCY Occult malignancy is probably the most common cause of weight loss in the absence of major signs and symptoms. In the search for malignancy particular emphasis must be placed on the gastrointestinal tract, pancreas, and liver. Lymphoma and leukemia should also be considered. While silent (except for weight loss) malignancy can occur in any organ, the gastrointestinal tract is the most common site. Mechanisms of weight loss in cancer vary, and more than one factor often plays a role. For example, although anorexia is almost invariably present in carcinoma of the pancreas, malabsorption appears to play the predominant role, with weight gain frequently occurring when pancreatic enzymes are provided. In other tumors, particularly lymphomas and leukemias, the mechanism appears to be increased metabolism with caloric wastage.

PSYCHIATRIC DISEASE The classic psychiatric illness associated with profound weight loss is anorexia nervosa (Chap. 73). Conversion disorders, schizophrenia, and depression may also cause weight loss due to decreased food intake. While organic disease causing both anorexia and depression has to be ruled out, ordinarily the psychiatric nature of the problem will be clear.

RENAL DISEASE One of the earliest manifestations of uremia is anorexia. As a consequence all patients with unexplained weight loss should be given screening renal function tests.

SUMMARY

Weight loss is more often a diagnostic problem than weight gain and more often a sign of serious organic illness. If the weight loss is associated with increased food intake, the diagnosis is likely diabetes, thyrotoxicosis, or malabsorption; less frequently, leukemias, lymphomas, or pheochromocytoma cause weight loss in the presence of increased food intake. If food intake is normal or decreased, malignancy, infection, renal disease, psychiatric syndromes, or endocrine deficiency is more common.

REFERENCES

BROŽEK J et al: Changes in body weight and body dimensions in men performing work on a low calorie carbohydrate diet. J Appl Physiol 10:412, 1957

FOSTER DW: Eating disorders: Obesity and anorexia nervosa, in *Williams Textbook of Endocrinology,* 7th ed, JD Wilson, DW Foster (eds). Philadelphia, Saunders, 1985, p 1081

GARFINKEL PE et al: Differential diagnosis of emotional disorders that cause weight loss. Can Med Assoc J 129:939, 1983

KHOURY P et al: Weight change since age 18 years in 30- to 55-year-old whites and blacks. Associations with lipid values, lipoprotein levels, and blood pressure. JAMA 250:3179, 1983

KONISHI F: Food energy equivalents of various activities. J Am Diet Assoc 46:186, 1965

MARTON KI et al: Involuntary weight loss: Diagnostic and prognostic significance. Ann Intern Med 95:568, 1981

PEREZ MM et al: Assessment of weight loss, food intake, fat metabolism, malabsorption, and treatment of pancreatic insufficiency in pancreatic cancer. Cancer 52:346, 1983

RUNCIE J, HILDITCH TE: Energy provision, tissue utilization and weight loss in prolonged starvation. Br Med J 2:352, 1974

YANG M-U, VAN ITALLIE TB: Composition of weight loss during short-term weight reduction. Metabolic responses of obese subjects to starvation and low calorie ketogenic and non-ketogenic diets. J Clin Invest 58:722, 1976

36 CONSTIPATION, DIARRHEA, AND DISTURBANCES OF ANORECTAL FUNCTION

STEPHEN E. GOLDFINGER

NORMAL COLONIC FUNCTION Each day approximately 9 liters of fluid enters the digestive tract; 2 liters represents ingested fluids and the remainder comes from salivary, gastric, biliary, pancreatic, and intestinal secretions that are needed to provide an appropriate milieu for food digestion. Most of this fluid is absorbed in the upper bowel. Approximately 1 liter containing undigested dietary residue and cellular debris passes across the ileocecal valve to the colon. Little of nutritional value remains following the extensive digestive processing and absorption that occurs in the small intestine. The colon's principal function is to convert this liquid ileal effluent to solid feces before it is advanced to the rectum and evacuated. Several important physiologic processes underlie normal colonic function; among these are *absorption* of fluid and electrolytes; *peristaltic contractions* that facilitate mixing, dessication, and passage of feces to the rectum; and, finally, *defecation.*

Absorption of fluid and electrolytes (see also Chap. 237) In western societies where dietary fiber content is relatively low, the average daily stool weight is less than 200 g, of which 60 to 80 percent is water. Thus, the colon normally absorbs approximately 80 to 90 percent of the fluid it receives, and this occurs well within its absorptive capacity of 6 liters water and 800 meq sodium per day. Fluid and electrolyte absorption occurs primarily in the ascending and transverse colon. Water absorption occurs passively, osmotically following the active transport of sodium and chloride ions. In addition, bicarbonate is secreted in exchange for chloride. The secreted bicarbonate is converted, in part, to carbon dioxide by reacting with acids produced by colonic bacteria.

The term *diarrhea* generally connotes *frequent* or *loose* stools. Based on physiologic events described above, diarrhea may be defined more quantitatively as a fecal output exceeding 200 g per day when dietary fiber content is low. Diarrhea can be further classified on the basis of underlying mechanisms (see Table 36-1). In *secretory diarrhea,* fecal fluid rich in sodium and potassium is lost as a consequence of impaired absorption and/or excessive secretion of electrolytes by the bowel. In *osmotic diarrhea,* absorption of water is decreased by the osmotic effect of nonabsorbable, intraluminal molecules. *Exudative diarrhea* is caused by an outpouring of necrotic mucosa, colloid, fluid, and electrolytes from an inflamed colon which,

in addition, is less able to carry out its normal absorptive function. Increased amounts of arachidonic acid metabolites present in inflamed mucosa may also promote increased ion secretion. *Anatomic derangements* of the bowel and *motility disorders* cause diarrhea by reducing the surface area or the contact time necessary for adequate absorption to occur.

Colonic innervation and motility The colon and rectum are innervated by fibers that release norepinephrine, acetylcholine, and a variety of other neurotransmitters, which may include bioactive amines, peptides, and nucleotides. Signals transmitted by autonomic nervous system fibers originating centrally, local reflex arcs confined to the autonomous "enteric nervous system," and intrinsic contractile responses of smooth muscle all play a part in the coordination of colonic motility. Parasympathetic nerves, which stimulate peristaltic contraction as well as electrolyte secretion, dominate the neurogenic regulation of colonic motor activity; adrenergic tone inhibits cholinergic stimulation and also increases electrolyte absorption. The precise integration of all neural and nonneural mediators of colonic motility and ion transport remains poorly understood.

The basal motor activity of the colon corresponds to the function of its various segments. In the ascending colon, where most fluid absorption occurs, rhythmic, retrograde contractions occur to prolong fecal contact time. In the midcolon, segmental contractions continue the process of absorption while feces are gradually advanced to the left colon. The most distal portion of the colon, which is under the greatest neurogenic control, propels feces caudally in preparation for defecation. In addition, massive peristalsis occurs several times per day.

Since colonic motility plays an important role in both absorption and movement of contents to the rectum, alterations of bowel tone occurring as a result of disease, stress, or various drugs tend to have an important influence on bowel movements. In view of the number of pharmacologic agents that may influence smooth muscle contractility, it is essential to take a careful drug history when evaluating patients with constipation or diarrhea of recent onset.

Defecation The defecatory reflex is initiated by acute distention of the rectum. When it is allowed to progress by supraspinal centers, sigmoidal and rectal contractions heighten the pressure within the rectum and also obliterate the rectosigmoidal angle. Concomitant relaxation of the internal and external anal sphincters then permits the evacuation of feces. This can be augmented by an increase in intraabdominal pressure created by the Valsalva maneuver. Conversely, defecation may be consciously prevented by the voluntary contraction of the striated muscles of the pelvic diaphragm and

TABLE 36-1 Classification of diarrhea

Type	Mechanism	Stool characteristics	Examples
Secretory	↑ Secretion of electrolytes ↓ Absorption of electrolytes	Clear $Na^+ + K^+$ $\simeq 2 \times$ osmolality No polymorphs	Cholera Diarrheogenic islet cell tumors Bile salt enteropathy
Exudative	Impaired colonic absorption; outpouring of cells and colloid	Purulent Polymorphs present Gross or occult blood	Ulcerative colitis Shigellosis Amebiasis
Decreased absorption			
Osmotic	Nonabsorbable intraluminal molecules	Clear $Na^+ + K^+$ $\simeq 2 \times$ osmolality No polymorphs	Lactase deficiency Mg^{2+}-containing cathartics
Anatomic derangement	Decreased absorption surface	Variable	Subtotal colectomy Gastrocolic fistula
Motility disorder	Decreased contact time	Variable	Hyperthyroidism Irritable bowel syndrome

external anal sphincter. The functional value of voluntary control of defecation requires little elaboration, but the opportunity for individuals to resist the defecatory urge, when abused, may lead to chronic rectal distention, reduced afferent signals, lax tone, and chronic constipation.

DIARRHEA AND CONSTIPATION The bowel habits of apparently healthy persons vary widely. For this reason, the complaint of *diarrhea* and *constipation* should be evaluated in terms of the degree of change from an individual's customary pattern. Reasonably detailed information is important in either abnormality. When patients complain of diarrhea, it is important to obtain an estimate of the volume as well as frequency of fecal output and, whenever possible, to examine directly a stool sample for consistency, blood, oiliness, and malodor. For example, the repeated elimination of small quantities of solid material admixed with gas, so typical in the irritable bowel syndrome, has a far different connotation than the same number of movements of liquid, blood-tinged feces. It is also useful to learn if fecal incontinence is present. Involuntary loss of feces may be an embarrassing complaint for a patient to verbalize, but such information may point to a potentially correctable anal sphincter abnormality. The term *constipation* may be used by the patient to refer to a variety of changes including reduction in frequency of defecation, a constant sensation of rectal fullness with incomplete evacuation of feces, and sometimes painful defecation due to hard stools or perianal pathology. Excessively hard stools are usually due to increased absorption of fluid as a result of prolonged contact of the luminal contents with the colonic mucosa consequent to delayed transit. In an assessment of complaints of diarrhea or constipation, it is important to consider the patient's emotional state since in many instances the recent onset of psychological stress is the major reason for altered bowel habits. However, it can be hazardous to assume this to be the case, even when the relationship seems convincing. For this reason, the judicious use of laboratory, proctoscopic, and radiologic procedures is recommended to make certain that organic disease will not be overlooked.

Acute diarrhea Diarrhea of abrupt onset occurring in otherwise healthy persons is usually due to an infectious cause. A variety of accompanying symptoms are often observed, including fever, headache, anorexia, vomiting, malaise, and myalgia, but they cannot be used to distinguish with certainty among viral, bacterial, and protozoal causes. Because bacterial and protozoal pathogens are usually not recovered from the feces, so-called nonspecific diarrhea is often considered to be of viral etiology. However, the demonstration of enterotoxins produced by strains of *Escherichia coli*, which are not distinguishable from "normal flora" on routine culture, suggests that these bacteria may account for a number of cases that are usually ascribed to viral infection.

Acute diarrhea presumed to be of viral etiology typically persists for a period of 1 to 3 days; death is extremely rare except in previously debilitated individuals who become severely dehydrated. When human volunteers have been infected with the Norwalk virus, which is believed to account for approximately one-third of epidemics of acute viral diarrhea in American adults, transient malabsorption of fat and xylose has been described. Changes in the small intestine include abnormalities of intestinal cell morphology such as villous shortening, an increase in the number of crypt cells, and increased cellularity of the lamina propria. The colonic mucosa is unaffected in viral diarrhea; this is consistent with the absence of polymorphonuclear leukocytes when fresh stool is examined microscopically after preparation with Loeffler's methylene blue.

Bacterial diarrhea may be suspected if there is a history of a similar and simultaneous illness in individuals who have shared contaminated food with the patient. Diarrhea developing within 12 h of the meal is most likely due to ingestion of a preformed toxin (e.g., staphylococcal exotoxin). A lag period of up to 3 days after consumption of contaminated food can occur with salmonellosis. The pathogenesis of bacterial diarrhea is due to two principal mechanisms, *mucosal invasion* and *enterotoxin-induced hypersecretion*. Bacterial

invasion of the colonic wall leads to mucosal hyperemia, edema, leukocytic infiltration, and frank ulceration. Lower abdominal cramps and tenderness are prominent, as are tenesmus and rectal urgency. In severe cases the stool is grossly bloody. At other times, microscopic examination of the stool will reveal erythrocytes along with pus cells. In *shigellosis*, diarrhea is mainly due to mucosal destruction by the invading microorganisms, but small intestinal hypersecretion may also occur in the early stage of enteritis caused by some enterotoxin-producing strains of *Shigella*. The prototype of hypersecretory bacterial diarrhea is *cholera*, in which the organism *Vibrio cholerae* adheres to, but does not invade, the surface epithelial cells and releases an enterotoxin which stimulates massive secretion of fluid and electrolytes by the small intestine. This may be produced experimentally in animals by placing the enterotoxin, free of the organism itself, into isolated intestinal loops. Hypersecretion reaches a peak at 4 to 6 h and is mediated by the stimulation of mucosal adenylate cyclase by the toxin. It should be emphasized that in cholera, mucosal morphology is essentially normal and intestinal absorptive capacity is preserved. This provides the basis for oral rehydration therapy with solutions containing simple sugars and sodium chloride, the former stimulating absorption of the latter. Because other species of bacteria, such as *E. coli, Clostridium,* and *Salmonella,* have been shown to produce enterotoxins, the finding of an exudate-free stool does not preclude bacterial infection as the cause of diarrhea.

Protozoal infections may also be responsible for acute diarrhea. *Entamoeba histolytica,* prevalent in some areas of the United States and in the homosexual male population, produces an inflammatory colitis which can closely mimic idiopathic ulcerative colitis. Giardiasis is a cause of prolonged, watery diarrhea that often afflicts travelers returning from endemic areas where the water supply has been contaminated. *Cryptosporidial* infection, initially described as occurring in immunocompromised patients, has also been linked to diarrheal illness in otherwise normal persons. Careful microscopic examination of fresh stools by experienced personnel is required for the diagnosis of protozoal infection. Duodenal samples in the form of aspirate and biopsy touch preparations may be necessary to make the diagnosis of giardiasis and cryptosporidiosis (see Chaps. 160, 161).

Travelers' diarrhea may result from any one or several of the pathogens described above. When no specific agent is identified, the etiology is usually assumed to be due to enterotoxin-producing coliform organisms or viruses; both Norwalk virus and rotavirus have been implicated. Not infrequently prolonged bowel irregularity will occur following the acute illness.

Ulcerative colitis and *Crohn's disease* may begin as acute diarrhea (Chap. 238). Bloody stools, abdominal cramping, tenderness, and fever are often observed. When Crohn's disease is limited to the small bowel (regional enteritis), the diarrhea tends to be milder, is often nonbloody, and is associated with right lower quadrant pain and tenderness. Diarrhea may be caused by a variety of *drugs,* including cholinergic agents, magnesium-containing antacids, antimetabolites used in cancer chemotherapy, and many antibiotics. A necrolytic toxin produced by *Clostridium difficile* is the cause of pseudomembranous colitis occurring during or after antibiotic use. Diarrhea due to *diverticulitis* is usually accompanied by fever, tenesmus, and rectal urgency, together with cramps and tenderness in the left lower quadrant (Chap. 239). When there is no evidence of acute inflammation, diarrhea in the presence of colonic diverticula is probably due to a spastic (irritable) colon, a disorder which may set the stage for the development of diverticula. In elderly and debilitated individuals with *fecal impaction,* the presenting symptom may be the frequent expulsion of small amounts of liquid stool overflowing from colonic distention behind the impaction. This is sometimes termed *paradoxical diarrhea.* Fecal incontinence due to anal sphincter impairment is a problem that may be encountered in certain neurologic disorders or following local surgical procedures (e.g., hemorrhoidectomy, episiotomy). Acute *psychological stress* can cause diarrhea at any age.

DIAGNOSTIC APPROACH   The appropriate tempo and approach in the evaluation of acute diarrhea depend so heavily on the clinical setting in which it occurs that only very general guidelines can be offered. It is entirely reasonable to withhold studies in mild, self-limited cases such as are seen as part of an epidemic viral illness. When dealing with sporadic severe diarrhea or when a suggestive epidemiologic history is obtained, bacterial cultures and microscopic examination of the stool for parasites and inflammatory cells are appropriate. Proctoscopy is generally reserved for patients with bloody diarrhea, or those who do not show improvement within 10 days. Likewise, radiologic studies should usually be deferred until the initial course of the illness has been observed. In cases of massive fluid loss, measurement of serum electrolytes is useful to aid in determining replacement therapy.

TREATMENT   General and nonspecific treatment of acute diarrhea includes rest, encouragement of fluid intake, and prescription of opiate-containing agents by mouth. Intravenous fluid and electrolyte replacement may be desirable and necessary in infants and the elderly. As a result of success achieved with cholera patients, the use of oral sugar-electrolyte solutions is being extended to the treatment of patients with acute diarrhea considered to be due to other enterotoxin-producing bacteria. Biofeedback therapy has proved helpful for some patients who suffer from fecal incontinence due to anal sphincter impairment.

Chronic diarrhea   Diarrhea persisting for weeks or months, whether constant or intermittent, may be a functional symptom or a manifestation of serious illness. For this reason, it is incumbent upon the physician to search carefully for evidence of organic disease, such as fever, weight loss, malnutrition, or anemia. Abdominal tenderness and fever suggest the presence of inflammation. When there is involvement of the large bowel, the major diseases to be considered include ulcerative colitis, Crohn's disease of the colon, amebiasis, and diverticulitis. Crohn's disease of the small intestine may involve one or more of its segments. The ileum is most frequently affected. Other diarrheal conditions which may resemble Crohn's disease radiographically include tuberculous and fungal enteritis, lymphoma, amyloidosis, and argentaffin (carcinoid) tumors of the small bowel.

Prolonged diarrhea without evidence of inflammation may reflect impairments of absorption, secretion, or digestion. Selective derangements, such as those due to *bile salt enteropathy* and *lactase deficiency*, are usually not accompanied by weight loss or malnutrition. *Mucosal disorders*, best exemplified by sprue, are frequently associated with weight loss, malodorous stools, abdominal distention, and anemia, and, when more severe, with osteomalacia, bleeding due to hypoprothrombinemia, avitaminotic neuropathies, and tetany. *Pancreatic insufficiency* resulting from chronic pancreatitis, carcinoma, resection, or cystic fibrosis produces steatorrhea and weight loss of varying severity. A number of mechanisms may be responsible for *postgastrectomy diarrhea* (see Chap. 235). These include the dumping syndrome, postvagotomy motility derangements, inadequate stimulation of pancreatic digestive enzymes, and incomplete mixing of these enzymes with food. On rare occasions severe postgastrectomy diarrhea and malnutrition are due to the inadvertent creation by the surgeon of a gastroileostomy instead of a gastrojejunostomy. *Bacterial overgrowth* in the small intestine, as may occur with extensive diverticulosis and prolonged bowel stasis secondary to disorders of peristalsis (e.g., scleroderma, diabetic visceral neuropathy), can also lead to chronic diarrhea and weight loss. This has been attributed to bacterial deconjugation of bile salts and hydroxylation of long-chain fatty acids, to consumption of nutrients by the organisms, and to mucosal abnormalities believed to be caused by bacteria or their metabolites (see Chap. 237). At times, diarrhea may accompany stasis in the absence of bacterial overgrowth.

Endocrine disorders that may be accompanied by chronic diarrhea include thyrotoxicosis, diabetes mellitus, adrenal insufficiency, and hypoparathyroidism. The release of potent secretagogues from neoplastic tissue in the Zollinger-Ellison syndrome (gastrin), medullary carcinoma of the thyroid (calcitonin, prostaglandins), and pancreatic cholera syndrome (vasoactive intestinal peptide) makes diarrhea a prominent feature of these disorders. *Rectal villous adenomas* may secrete large quantities of fluid and electrolytes, which are promptly evacuated as a clear, odorless liquid. When marked fluid loss occurs, hypokalemia and dehydration may result.

Habitual *cathartic abuse* must be suspected when the cause of prolonged diarrhea remains perplexing. Even if this is denied by the patient, a stool sample should be alkalinized with sodium hydroxide; this will produce a lavender color if phenolphthalein-containing laxatives have been surreptitiously ingested. The observation of melanosis coli by sigmoidoscopy indicates chronic usage of anthraquinone laxatives.

Constipation   Constipation is a common complaint often resulting from the inordinate expectation of ''regularity'' in bowel-conscious individuals. Stools are described as infrequent, incomplete, or unduly hard; unusual straining may be required to achieve defecation. A review of the patient's habits often reveals contributory and correctable causes, such as insufficient dietary roughage, lack of exercise, suppression of defecatory urges arising at inconvenient moments, inadequate allotment of time for full defecation, and prolonged travel. Appropriate adjustments of these patterns and reassurance are preferable to the prescription of laxatives and may be all that is required for improvement. When the patient also has symptoms such as fatigue, malaise, headaches, or anorexia, the possibility should be considered that such symptoms reflect an underlying depression of which constipation is but one component. Decreased colonic motility is responsible for the constipation associated with the use of parasympatholytic drugs, spinal cord injury, scleroderma, and Hirschsprung's disease.

Hemorrhoids, anal fissures, perineal abscesses, and rectal strictures often prevent easy and adequate stool evacuation. When constipation and tenesmus of recent onset are reported, the possibility of carcinoma of the rectum or sigmoid colon must be seriously considered. In such instances sigmoidoscopic and barium enema examinations should be obtained early and are virtually obligatory if fecal blood has been observed or if occult blood is detected on any of three successive stool specimens. Stools of abnormally thin caliber occur in patients with rectal or sigmoid colon carcinoma but are even more commonly due to a spastic colon. Other mechanical causes of constipation include volvulus of the sigmoid colon, diverticulitis, intussusception, and hernias. A variety of metabolic abnormalities, such as hypothyroidism, hypercalcemia, hypokalemia, porphyria, lead poisoning, and dehydration are often associated with constipation. Prolonged fecal retention, leading to impaction, may occur in certain neurologic disorders (e.g., spinal cord injury, multiple sclerosis, cerebral palsy, senility), and in these instances, when autonomic regulation of evacuation is unachievable, vigorous and sustained enema programs are often necessary.

IRRITABLE BOWEL   The irritable bowel syndrome (also referred to as *spastic colon* and *mucous colitis*) is one of the most frequent gastrointestinal disorders (see Chap. 239). This condition is characterized by periodic or chronic bowel symptoms which include diarrhea, constipation, and abdominal pain. These symptoms are often secondary to mental distress, but the anxiety produced by the bowel disturbance is sometimes regarded by the patient as the fundamental cause of the emotional upset. During periods of discomfort, stools are apt to become thin, fragmented, or pelletlike, and accompanied by excessive mucus and gas. Efforts to ameliorate symptoms with mild cathartics or antispasmodic drugs may yield adverse and exaggerated responses. A variety of therapeutic approaches, including the avoidance of foods which tend to upset the patient, addition of bulk-forming agents, judicious use of antispasmodics and tranquilizers, and psychotherapy may provide some degree of relief. If the patient's life goals can be shifted away from the quixotic search for the perfect stool, much can be accomplished. At the same time, it must be remembered that such individuals are not exempt from developing bowel cancer, and any worrisome deviation from their general pattern of derangement must be seriously evaluated.

FLATULENCE   A significant amount of flatus is passed each day by normal persons, and the complaint of flatulence often reflects a heightened and embarrassing awareness of this natural occurrence. Excessive quantities of flatus may be caused by aerophagia or the formation of increased amounts of gas by intestinal bacteria. The latter process can be associated with malabsorption syndromes but is more frequently a consequence of eating foods such as beans, broccoli, and cabbage which have a high content of nondigestible polysaccharides. The oligosaccharides stachyose and raffinose, isolated from beans, are particularly effective substrates for fermentation to carbon dioxide, hydrogen, and methane by colonic flora. Chromatographic analysis of a sample of flatus will show these gases to predominate, in contrast to the high nitrogen levels that occur when excessive flatus is caused by aerophagia. The treatment of flatulence is generally undertaken to reduce embarrassment and consists of measures to decrease aerophagia along with avoidance of foods that cause excessive gas.

REFERENCES

BLACKLOW NR, CUKOR GC: Viral gastroenteritis. N Engl J Med 304:397, 1981

CHRISTENSEN J: Motility of the colon, in *Physiology of the Gastrointestinal Tract*, LR Johnson et al (eds). New York, Raven Press, 1981, vol 1, chap 14

DROSSMAN DA et al: The irritable bowel syndrome. Gastroenterology 73:811, 1977

FIELD M et al (eds): *Secretory Diarrhea*, Clinical Physiology Series. Bethesda, Md, American Physiological Society, 1980

GERSHON MD, ERDE SM: The nervous system of the gut. Gastroenterology 80:1571, 1981

LIEBERMAN DA: Common anorectal disorders. Ann Intern Med 101:837, 1984

PLOTKIN GR et al: Gastroenteritis: Etiology, pathophysiology and clinical manifestations. Medicine 58:95, 1979

READ NW et al: Chronic diarrhea of unknown origin. Gastroenterology 78:2644, 1980

SCHULTZ SG: Ion transport by mammalian large intestine, in *Physiology of the Gastrointestinal Tract*, LR Johnson et al (eds). New York, Raven Press, 1981, vol 2, chap 38

SNOOKS SJ et al: Damage to the innervation of the pelvic floor musculature in chronic constipation. Gastroenterology 89:977, 1985

WOLFSON JS et al: Cryptosporidiosis in immunocompetent patients. N Engl J Med 312:1278, 1985

37   HEMATEMESIS, MELENA, AND HEMATOCHEZIA

KURT J. ISSELBACHER / JAMES M. RICHTER

Hematemesis is defined as the vomiting of blood, and *melena* as the passage of stools rendered black and tarry by the presence of altered blood. These symptoms of gastrointestinal hemorrhage should bring the patient to medical attention and, within certain limits, suggest the anatomic site of bleeding. Exsanguinating gastrointestinal hemorrhage will rarely occur without the appearance of altered or gross blood passed by mouth or rectum. The color of vomited blood will vary depending on the concentration of hydrochloric acid in the stomach and its admixture with the blood. Thus, if vomiting occurs shortly after the onset of bleeding, the vomitus appears red; if there is a delay in vomiting, the appearance will be dark red, brown, or black. Precipitated blood clots in the vomitus will produce a characteristic "coffee grounds" appearance. Hematemesis usually indicates bleeding proximal to the ligament of Treitz, since blood entering the gastrointestinal tract below the duodenum rarely enters the stomach.

While bleeding sufficient to produce hematemesis usually results in melena, less than half of patients with melena have hematemesis. *Melena* usually denotes bleeding from the esophagus, stomach, or duodenum, but lesions in the jejunum, ileum, and even ascending

colon may cause melena provided the gastrointestinal transit time is sufficiently prolonged. Approximately 60 mL of blood is required to produce a single black stool; acute blood loss greater than this may produce melena for up to 3 days. After the stool color returns to normal, tests for occult blood may remain positive for up to a week or longer.

The black color of stools secondary to intestinal bleeding results from contact of the blood with hydrochloric acid to produce hematin. Characteristically, such stools are tarry ("sticky"). This tarry consistency is in contrast to black or dark stools occurring after the ingestion of iron, bismuth, or licorice. Similarly, red stools may result from the ingestion of beets or intravenous administration of sulfobromophthalein. Gastrointestinal bleeding, even if detected only by positive tests for occult blood, indicates potentially serious disease and must be further investigated.

Hematochezia, the passage of bright-red blood per rectum, generally signifies bleeding from a source distal to the ligament of Treitz. However, since blood must remain in the gut for approximately 8 h to produce melena, rapid hemorrhage into the esophagus, stomach, or duodenum may also result in hematochezia.

The clinical manifestations of gastrointestinal bleeding depend upon the extent and rate of hemorrhage, and the presence of coincidental diseases. Blood loss of less than 500 mL is rarely associated with systemic signs; exceptions include bleeding in the elderly or in the anemic patient in whom smaller amounts of blood loss may produce hemodynamic alterations. Rapid hemorrhage of greater volume results in decreased venous return to the heart, decreased cardiac output, and increased peripheral resistance due to reflex vasoconstriction. Orthostatic hypotension greater than 10 mmHg usually indicates a 20 percent or greater reduction in blood volume. Concomitant symptoms include syncope, lightheadedness, nausea, sweating, and thirst. When blood loss approaches 40 percent of blood volume, shock frequently ensues with pronounced tachycardia and hypotension. Pallor is prominent, and the skin is cool.

It is important to recognize that the hematocrit, when determined immediately after the onset of bleeding, may not accurately reflect blood loss, since equilibration with extravascular fluid and hemodilution require several hours. Common laboratory findings include mild leukocytosis and thrombocytosis which develop within 6 h after the onset of bleeding. The blood urea nitrogen may be mildly elevated, particularly in upper gastrointestinal bleeding, due to breakdown of blood proteins to urea by intestinal bacteria as well as from a mild reduction in the glomerular filtration rate.

ETIOLOGY OF UPPER GASTROINTESTINAL BLEEDING   A careful history and physical examination of the oropharynx and nasal cavity should serve to exclude swallowed blood as a source of hematemesis or melena.

The four most common causes of upper gastrointestinal hemorrhage are (1) peptic ulceration, (2) erosive gastritis, (3) variceal bleeding, and (4) Mallory-Weiss syndrome. These entities account for up to 90 percent of all cases of upper gastrointestinal hemorrhage in which a definite lesion can be found.

Peptic ulcer   Peptic ulcer is probably the most common cause of upper gastrointestinal bleeding; the majority of such ulcers are found in the duodenum. Approximately 20 to 30 percent of patients with documented ulcers will have significant bleeding sometime during the course of their disease. Because hemorrhage may be the initial manifestation of a peptic ulcer, this lesion should be seriously considered even when a history characteristic of ulcer disease is not obtained.

Gastritis   Gastritis may be associated with recent alcohol ingestion or with the use of anti-inflammatory drugs, such as aspirin or indomethacin. Gastric erosions also frequently develop in patients with major trauma, surgery, and severe systemic disease, particularly burn victims and patients with increased intracranial pressure. Because there are no characteristic physical findings, the diagnosis of gastritis must be suspected when the appropriate clinical setting is encountered.

When a specific diagnosis is required, gastroscopy is usually needed to confirm the diagnosis since radiologic examination generally lacks the sensitivity required to detect gastritis.

Variceal bleeding Variceal bleeding is characteristically abrupt and massive; chronic gastrointestinal blood loss is unusual. Bleeding from esophageal or gastric varices is usually the result of portal hypertension, secondary to cirrhosis. Although alcoholic cirrhosis is the most prevalent cause of esophageal varices in the United States, any condition producing portal hypertension, even in the absence of hepatic disease (i.e., portal vein thrombosis or idiopathic portal hypertension), may result in variceal bleeding. Further, while the presence of varices usually connotes long-standing portal hypertension, acute hepatitis or severe fatty infiltration of the liver may occasionally produce varices which disappear once the hepatic abnormality resolves. It should be emphasized that although upper gastrointestinal bleeding in a patient with cirrhosis suggests a variceal source, approximately half those patients will be bleeding from other lesions (e.g., gastritis, ulcers). Consequently, it is essential to exclude nonvariceal causes of bleeding so that the appropriate treatment can be instituted.

MALLORY-WEISS SYNDROME With the advent of esophagogastroduodenoscopy, the Mallory-Weiss syndrome has been demonstrated with increasing frequency as a cause of acute upper gastrointestinal hemorrhage (see also Chap. 34). This syndrome refers to a mucosal laceration in the region of the esophagogastric junction which is often characterized historically by retching or nonbloody vomiting followed by hematemesis.

OTHER LESIONS Less common bleeding esophageal lesions include esophagitis and carcinoma; these generally cause chronic blood loss and rarely produce massive bleeding.

Gastric carcinoma may result in chronic gastrointestinal bleeding. Lymphoma, polyps, and other tumors of the stomach and small bowel are uncommon and, consequently, are infrequent causes of hemorrhage. Leiomyoma and leiomyosarcoma are likewise rare, but they can lead to massive hemorrhage. Bleeding from duodenal and jejunal diverticula is relatively unusual. Vascular insufficiency of the mesenteric vessels, including occlusive and nonocclusive disease, may lead to bloody diarrhea.

Arteriosclerotic aortic aneurysms may rupture into the small intestine; such an event is almost always fatal. Rupture may also occur following arterial reconstructive surgery with fistula formation between synthetic graft and bowel lumen. A small or herald bleed may precede a sudden massive hemorrhage from an aortoenteric fistula. Sudden bleeding may also occur after trauma resulting in hepatic laceration; this may result in blood loss into the bile ducts (i.e., hemobilia).

Primary blood dyscrasias, including leukemia, thrombocytopenic states, the hemophilias, and disseminated intravascular coagulation may result in significant gastrointestinal bleeding. Polycythemia vera may be associated with an increased incidence of peptic ulceration, and may also result in gastrointestinal bleeding due to mesenteric or portal vein thrombosis. Periarteritis nodosa, Henoch-Schönlein purpura, and other forms of vasculitis may lead to gastrointestinal blood loss. Gastrointestinal bleeding may be seen with amyloidosis, Osler-Weber-Rendu disease, other arteriovenous malformations, pseudoxanthoma elasticum, Turner's syndrome, intestinal hemangiomas, neurofibromatosis, Kaposi's sarcoma, and Peutz-Jeghers syndrome. Uremia may produce gastrointestinal blood loss; the most common presentation is chronic, occult bleeding from diffuse involvement of the mucosa of the stomach and small bowel.

ETIOLOGY OF LOWER GASTROINTESTINAL BLEEDING Anal and rectal lesions Small amounts of bright red-blood on the surface of the stool and toilet tissue are often caused by hemorrhoids; such bleeding is generally precipitated by the strained passage of a hard stool. Anal fissures and fistulas may present in a similar fashion. Proctitis is another source of rectal bleeding; it is frequently seen in young adults, especially in male homosexuals. In the latter situation, proctitis may be due to gonorrheal or mycoplasma infections or may be idiopathic. Rectal trauma is a cause of hematochezia, and the placement of foreign objects in the rectal vault may precipitate perforation as well as acute rectal hemorrhage. It must be emphasized that anal pathology does not preclude other sources of blood loss, and these must be sought and excluded.

Colonic lesions Carcinoma of the colon, as well as colonic polyps, may produce chronic blood loss. Angiodysplastic lesions, usually involving the ascending colon, are a major source of acute or chronic bleeding in elderly patients; such vascular lesions can be identified by angiography or colonoscopy. Frankly bloody diarrhea is common and may be the presenting symptom in patients with ulcerative colitis; it is less frequent in granulomatous colitis, but occult blood may be present in the stool. Bleeding may also accompany diarrhea due to infections such as shigellosis, amebiasis, campylobacterosis, and rarely, salmonellosis. In the elderly patient, ischemic colitis may be a cause of bloody diarrhea; this lesion may also be seen in younger women who use oral contraceptive agents.

Diverticula Colonic diverticula are most often located in the sigmoid colon; however, diverticular bleeding may originate anywhere in the colon. Bleeding from colonic diverticula is a cause of massive lower gastrointestinal hemorrhage. The usual presentation of a diverticular hemorrhage is that of painless passage of a maroon-colored stool. Meckel's diverticulum, a congenital anomaly of the distal ileum, is present in about 2 percent of the population and may cause bleeding. Although only about 15 percent of these diverticula contain gastric mucosa, half of the lesions which cause acute bleeding contain gastric mucosa. This anomaly is an important cause of acute hemorrhage in children and young adults.

APPROACH TO THE PATIENT WITH GASTROINTESTINAL BLEEDING The approach to the bleeding patient depends upon the site, extent, and rate of bleeding. Patients with hematemesis have usually bled greater amounts (often greater than 1000 mL) than those who have melena alone (usually 500 mL or less), and mortality with the former is about twice that of the latter. When first seen, the patient may be in shock. Prior to taking a history and performing a thorough physical examination, vital signs should be noted, blood sent for typing and cross-matching, and a large-bore intravenous line placed for infusion of saline or other plasma expanders. The physician initiating the evaluation of the bleeding patient must be aware that the primary consideration is the necessity of maintaining adequate intravascular volume and hemodynamic stability during the diagnostic workup.

History A history or symptoms suggestive of prior ulcer disease may provide a useful clue. Similarly, recent abuse of alcohol or ingestion of anti-inflammatory drugs should make erosive gastritis more suspect. If alcohol abuse has been long-standing, esophageal varices may be a more likely source of hemorrhage. Aspirin use may also cause gastroduodenitis, peptic ulceration, and bleeding. Prior history of gastrointestinal bleeding may be helpful, as may a family history of intestinal disease or hemorrhagic diathesis. Recent retching followed by hematemesis should suggest the possibility of the Mallory-Weiss syndrome. The acute onset of bloody diarrhea may indicate the presence of inflammatory bowel disease or an infectious colitis. It is also important to exclude associated systemic illnesses or recent trauma, since bleeding from erosive gastritis is frequently seen under such conditions.

Physical examination Following evaluation for orthostatic changes in pulse and blood pressure and institution of volume repletion, the patient should be examined for clues to the underlying illness. A nonintestinal bleeding source should be excluded by careful examination of the oral cavity and nasopharynx. Dermatologic examination may disclose the characteristic telangiectasia of Osler-Weber-Rendu disease (although these will not be visible if severe anemia is present), the perioral pigmentation of Peutz-Jeghers syndrome, the dermal fibromas of neurofibromatosis, the sebaceous cysts and bony tumors of Gardner's syndrome, the palpable purpura frequently seen with vasculitis, or the diffuse pigmentation seen in hemochromatosis. Stigmata of chronic liver disease such as spider angiomata, gynecomastia, testicular atrophy, jaundice, ascites, and hepatosplenomegaly should suggest portal hypertension resulting in bleeding from esophageal or gastric varices. Significant lymph node enlargement or abdominal masses may reflect underlying intraabdominal malignancy. Careful rectal examination is important to exclude local pathology as well as to observe the color of the stool.

Laboratory studies   Initial studies should include the hematocrit, hemoglobin, careful assessment of red blood cell morphologic features (hypochromic, microcytic red blood cells suggest that blood loss is chronic), white blood cell count, differential, and platelet count. Prothrombin time, partial thromboplastin time, and other coagulation studies may be in order to exclude primary or secondary clotting defects. A radiograph of the abdomen is rarely helpful in establishing a diagnosis unless a perforated viscus is suspected. Though the initial studies are valuable and essential, repeated evaluation of the laboratory data is important as one follows the clinical course of the bleeding.

Diagnostic and therapeutic approach   The diagnostic approach to the patient with gastrointestinal hemorrhage must be individualized. The initial management of gastrointestinal bleeding may be under the direction of the internist, but it is prudent to consult a surgeon in the event that surgery is required.

When there is a history of melena or hematemesis or the suspicion of bleeding from the upper part of the gastrointestinal tract, the patient should have a nasogastric tube passed to empty the stomach and to determine whether the bleeding is in the upper part of the gastrointestinal tract. If the initial nasogastric aspirate is clear, the tube should be left in place for several hours, since active duodenal bleeding may occur with an initially clear nasogastric aspirate. If the aspirate is negative for blood during a period of active bleeding, it is reasonable to conclude that active bleeding is not occurring in the gastroduodenal region, and the nasogastric tube can be removed. However, if there is no evidence of active bleeding at the time the nasogastric tube is placed, one cannot assume bleeding did not come from the stomach or duodenum and endoscopy may be required.

If red blood or "coffee grounds" material is aspirated from the nasogastric tube, saline irrigation of the stomach should be initiated. Irrigation serves two purposes: it provides the clinician with an assessment of the rapidity of the bleeding, and clears the stomach of old blood prior to possible endoscopy. Subsequent diagnostic maneuvers will depend on whether bleeding continues; this can be assessed by vital signs, transfusion requirements, and the number and consistency of stools. Most medical centers now have available experienced endoscopists as well as radiologists with facilities for selective arteriography so that it is possible to have emergency endoscopic or angiographic studies performed within hours of the patient's admission to the hospital. It must be emphasized that demonstration of a lesion in a patient with gastrointestinal bleeding should also be accompanied by evidence that this lesion is the site of bleeding (Fig. 37-1).

If the bleeding has stopped, and the patient is stable, one may proceed with either esophagogastroduodenoscopy or upper gastrointestinal barium studies. Although *endoscopy* provides a higher diagnostic yield, it has not been proved conclusively that survival is increased by early endoscopy. *Barium examination* may identify a potential source of hemorrhage, but there are important limitations to such x-rays. First, lesions such as erosive gastritis and Mallory-Weiss lacerations are not visualized by x-ray. Second, if the patient rebleeds following a barium exam, the retained contrast material will make endoscopy difficult and angiography impossible. Clearly the approach in this setting must be individualized. The decision to employ esophagogastroduodenoscopy or barium studies will depend on several variables, including the availability of an experienced endoscopist and the condition of the patient. Although studies have shown that emergency endoscopy and a vigorous diagnostic approach do not generally decrease patient morbidity or mortality, emergency endoscopy may be important in planning therapy in certain patients with cirrhosis or previous gastric surgery. By identifying other patients with visible vessels and thus a high risk for recurrent bleeding, possible complications can be anticipated. Newer techniques for coagulation of bleeding ulcers or sclerosis of varices via the endoscope may broaden the indications for and utility of early endoscopy in the future.

Persistent upper gastrointestinal hemorrhage must be viewed differently, and most clinicians would proceed immediately to esophagogastroduodenoscopy. Determination of the site and cause of bleeding is essential to plan for appropriate therapy, particularly if varices are suspected. Thus, anticipation of surgery, angiography, or the suspicion of bleeding varices are strong indications for esophagogastroduodenoscopy in the evaluation of the patient with persistent upper gastrointestinal bleeding. In contrast, esophagogastroduodenoscopy is more difficult in the evaluation of *massive* hemorrhage, since large amounts of blood obscure visualization of mucosal pathology, and angiography may be required in addition to endoscopy.

Should bleeding continue and endoscopy fail to reveal the bleeding source, the site of hemorrhage may be beyond the ligament of Treitz. In this situation angiography is frequently valuable in establishing a diagnosis. Angiographic demonstration of the bleeding site requires blood loss at a rate of at least 0.5 mL/min. Clinical correlates reflecting this degree of blood loss include postural hypotension and the necessity for blood transfusion to maintain stable vital signs. Emergency angiography may localize the site of bleeding; however, the cause of the bleeding may not be determined unless varices, vascular malformations, or aneurysms are present.

FIGURE   37-1 *Endoscopic photographs from a patient with hematemesis. A. A gastric ulcer along the lesser curvature of the stomach is identified (arrows). B. The same ulcer is bleeding actively from a spurting artery (arrows).*

Therapeutic angiography is a helpful approach to the control of persistent hemorrhage. Continuous intraarterial infusion of vasoconstrictor agents, such as vasopressin, is often successful in controlling hemorrhage due to gastric ulcer or Mallory-Weiss tear. Additionally, embolic material may be injected directly into the artery perfusing the bleeding site. However, intravenous infusions of vasopressin and endoscopic sclerosis for control of variceal bleeding are more valuable than angiographic techniques.

If bleeding esophageal varices are identified on upper endoscopy, peripheral infusions of vasopressin may control the bleeding. The response to such therapy depends upon the general condition of the patient as assessed by clinical and laboratory parameters. It has been shown that intraarterial vasopressin is no more effective than intravenous administration in the control of variceal bleeding. Varices may also be controlled by balloon tamponade with a Sengstaken-Blakemore tube. Unlike vasopressin, this technique is generally used as a preoperative stabilizing measure which should be followed by definitive therapy within 48 h whenever possible. Endoscopic sclerosis of varices has emerged as an effective therapy for bleeding esophageal varices and when available should be attempted prior to surgery.

In the evaluation of *lower gastrointestinal bleeding* the most important procedures are the digital examination, anoscopy, and sigmoidoscopy. The last of these may identify a bleeding site or document bleeding coming from above the range of the instrument. Colonoscopy is a valuable technique for the evaluation of patients with small to moderate lower gastrointestinal bleeds. Preparation of the colon with saline lavage solutions permits a colonoscopic evaluation of the bowel within hours. Most colonic abnormalities, including angiodysplasia, can be detected and treated with polypectomy or electrocoagulation. If brisk bleeding continues, arteriography may serve to localize the bleeding site and allow local infusion of vasoconstrictor agents to control bleeding. Because arteriography detects actively bleeding lesions only when blood loss exceeds 0.5 mL/min and gastrointestinal bleeding tends to be intermittent, arteriography is often nondiagnostic. Radiolabeled erythrocyte scanning is more sensitive than arteriography in detecting blood loss of 0.1 mL/min and may be used to investigate less severe bleeding. However, bleeding scans are less specific than arteriography, generally localizing the lesion and seldom making a discrete diagnosis. Bleeding scans are most helpful in detecting active, low-grade, or intermittent bleeding in order to better time arteriography and obtain the maximal diagnostic yield. Finally, a barium enema has a limited role in the evaluation of acute rectal bleeding. Although it may localize potential bleeding sources, it will not define the bleeding site. Furthermore, if brisk bleeding recurs, subsequent colonoscopy or angiography will be difficult to interpret due to retained contrast material. Therefore, it is advisable to withhold barium studies of both the upper and lower bowel for at least 48 h after the cessation of active bleeding.

REFERENCES

ATHANASOULIS CA: Angiography. Its contribution to the emergency management of gastrointestinal hemorrhage. Radiol Clin North Am 14:265, 1976

CELLO JP et al: Endoscopic sclerotherapy versus portocaval shunt in patients with severe cirrhosis and variceal hemorrhage. N Engl J Med 311:1589, 1984

CHOJKIER M et al: A controlled comparison of continuous intra-arterial and intravenous infusions of vasopressin in hemorrhage from esophageal varices. Gastroenterology 77:540, 1979

FLEISCHER D: Endoscopic therapy of upper gastrointestinal bleeding. Gastroenterology 90:217, 1986

LICHTENSTEIN JL: Accuracy and reliability of endoscopy and x-ray in upper gastrointestinal bleeding. Dig Dis Sc 26:70s, 1981

LUK GD et al: Gastric aspiration in localization of gastrointestinal hemorrhage. JAMA 241:576, 1979

PETERSON WL et al: Routine early endoscopy in upper gastrointestinal tract bleeding: A randomized, controlled trial. N Engl J Med 304:925, 1981

PRIEBE HJ et al: Antacid versus cimetidine in preventing acute gastrointestinal bleeding. A randomized trial in 75 critically ill patients. N Engl J Med 302:426, 1980

RICHTER JM et al: Angiodysplasia: Clinical presentation and colonoscopic diagnosis. Dig Dis Sci 29:481, 1984

STEER ML, SILEN W: Diagnostic procedures in gastrointestinal hemorrhage. N Engl J Med 309:646, 1983

38 JAUNDICE AND HEPATOMEGALY

KURT J. ISSELBACHER

JAUNDICE

Jaundice, or *icterus,* refers to the yellow pigmentation of the skin or scleras by bilirubin. This in turn is a result of elevated levels of bilirubin in the bloodstream. Jaundice may be brought to clinical attention by a darkening of the urine or a yellow discoloration of the skin or sclera; the latter often is the site where clinical icterus may first be detected. Scleral pigmentation is attributed to richness of this tissue in elastin, which has a special affinity for bilirubin. Jaundice must be distinguished from other causes of yellow pigmentation such as carotenemia (see Chaps. 51 and 76), which is due to carotenoid pigments in the bloodstream and is associated with a yellowish discoloration of the skin but not of the sclera.

Normal serum bilirubin concentrations range from 0.3 to 1.0 mg/dL (or 5.1 to 17 μmol per liter), and normally most of this is unconjugated (see Fig. 38-1). The precise level at which jaundice becomes clinically evident varies, but it can usually be recognized when the total serum bilirubin exceeds 2 to 2.5 mg/dL. With pronounced jaundice the skin may take on a greenish hue because of

FIGURE 38-1 *The sources and precursors of bilirubin and steps in its subsequent metabolism and excretion.*

the conversion of bilirubin to biliverdin, an oxidation product of bilirubin. Oxidation occurs more readily with conjugated bilirubin, and hence a greenish hue is seen more frequently in conditions with pronounced conjugated hyperbilirubinemia. When bilirubin is exposed to visible blue light (430 to 470 nm), metastable isomers of bilirubin are produced. These photoisomers are polar (because they permit no intramolecular hydrogen bonding) and can be excreted by the liver into bile without having to be conjugated (see below and Fig. 38-2).

PRODUCTION AND METABOLISM OF BILIRUBIN Normal sources of bilirubin (Fig. 38-2)

Most bilirubin is derived from the catabolism of hemoglobin present in senescent red blood cells. This normally accounts for about 80 to 85 percent of the daily bilirubin production. When a circulating red blood cell reaches the end of its normal life span of approximately 120 days, it is destroyed in the reticuloendothelial system. In the catabolism of hemoglobin, globin is first dissociated from heme, after which the heme moiety (ferroprotoporphyrin IX) is oxidatively cleaved and converted to biliverdin by a microsomal heme oxygenase. This enzyme system requires oxygen and a cofactor, reduced nicotinamide adenine dinucleotide phosphate (NADPH). Bilirubin (in the chemical form of bilirubin IXα) is then formed from biliverdin by biliverdin reductase.

About 15 to 20 percent of the bilirubin is derived from sources other than senescent erythrocytes. One source is the *destruction of maturing erythroid cells in the bone marrow,* or so-called ineffective erythropoiesis (see Chap. 287). The other is *nonerythroid components,* especially in the liver, and involves the turnover of heme and heme proteins (such as cytochrome, myoglobin, and heme-containing enzymes). These two sources of bilirubin are collectively referred to as the *early labeled fraction,* a term derived from experiments with labeled glycine and Δ-aminolevulinic acid (ALA). Thus when labeled glycine is administered to a normal subject, approximately 15 percent of the label appears in stool urobilinogens in the first 3 to 5 days; 85 percent of the label appears over a broad range with the peak at about 120 days and reflects bilirubin produced from the normal destruction of senescent red blood cells.

Transport of bilirubin Following liberation of unconjugated bilirubin into the plasma, virtually all the pigment is tightly *bound to albumin.* The maximum binding capacity is 2 mol bilirubin per mole of albumin in a reversible, noncovalent manner. Certain organic anions, such as sulfonamides and salicylates, compete with bilirubin for common binding sites on albumin and may displace bilirubin from albumin, permitting it to enter tissues such as the central nervous system. Most of the evidence for albumin binding has been obtained from studies using unconjugated bilirubin. Conjugated bilirubin is also bound to albumin, but in both a reversible and an irreversible manner. The reversible binding is similar to the noncovalent binding of unconjugated bilirubin, but the binding is much weaker. The second type involves a very tight, irreversible albumin-bilirubin complex that appears in the serum when hepatic excretion of bilirubin is impaired (i.e., with cholestasis). Due to the nature of the binding, the complex does *not* appear in urine. Also this bilirubin-albumin conjugate may remain detectable in the serum for several weeks after the relief of the obstruction or during recovery from hepatocellular jaundice.

Bilirubin is found in body fluids (cerebrospinal fluid, joint effusions, cysts, etc.) in proportion to the albumin content of the fluids and is absent from true secretions such as tears, saliva, and pancreatic juice. The appearance of jaundice is also influenced by blood flow and edema. Paralyzed extremities and edematous areas tend to remain uncolored, and "unilateral" jaundice in patients with hemiplegia and edema may be seen if jaundice develops.

Hepatic metabolism of bilirubin (Fig. 38-3) The liver occupies a central role in the metabolism of the bile pigments. Three distinct phases are recognized: (1) *hepatic uptake,* (2) *conjugation,* and (3) *excretion* into bile. Of these three steps, excretion appears to be the

FIGURE 38-2 *Scheme showing the conversion of bilirubin IXα to water-soluble derivatives by photoisomerization or conjugation. In A the normal, unconjugated pigment Z-Z isomer is shown; the dashed line shows the upright position of the hydrogen at the methene bridges linking the pyrrole molecules. B shows the effect of light leading to the formation of the water-soluble E-E isomer; the dashed-line box serves to emphasize the inversion of the hydrogens at the methene bridges between the pyrrole molecules. C shows the formation of water-soluble bilirubin diglucuronide formation; the dashed-line box encloses one of the two glucuronic acid moieties.*

BILIRUBIN IX α
(Z–Z isomer)

Light

Conjugation

BILIRUBIN IX α
(E–E isomer, water soluble)

BILIRUBIN IX α—DIGLUCURONIDE
(water soluble)

rate-limiting step and the one most susceptible to impairment when the liver cell is damaged.

UPTAKE Unconjugated bilirubin bound to albumin is presented to the liver cell, and upon entry the pigment and albumin become dissociated. The uptake phase and subsequent hepatocyte storage of bilirubin involves binding of bilirubin to certain cytoplasmic anionic binding proteins, especially ligandin. This binding may prevent efflux of bilirubin back into the plasma.

CONJUGATION Unconjugated bilirubin is water-insoluble and must be converted to a *water-soluble derivative* in order to be excreted by the liver cell into bile. This is accomplished by conjugation whereby bilirubin is predominantly converted to bilirubin glucuronide. The reaction occurs in the endoplasmic reticulum of the hepatocytes by action of bilirubin glucuronyl transferase. As shown in Fig. 38-3, this appears to be a two-step reaction, resulting first in the formation of the monoglucuronide followed by the production of the diglucuronide. Normally, bile contains 85 percent of bilirubin diconjugates and 15 percent monoconjugates. Unconjugated bilirubin usually is *not* excreted by the liver into the bile (except following photooxidation, see below).

EXCRETION OR SECRETION INTO BILE Normally, for bilirubin to be excreted into bile, *the pigment must be in the conjugated form.* Although the overall process is not well understood, the excretion of conjugated bilirubin into bile appears to be an energy-dependent and *rate-limiting* step in the hepatic metabolism of bilirubin. When this step is compromised, two consequences occur: (1) decreased excretion of bilirubin into the bile, and (2) "regurgitation," or reentry of conjugated bilirubin from the liver cells into the bloodstream.

As indicated above, bilirubin IXα can exist as four geometric isomers. The naturally occurring isomer is the Z-Z form (see Fig. 38-2), which permits intramolecular hydrogen bonding, making the molecule hydrophobic. The other isomers (Z-E, E-Z, and E-E, depending on the position of the hydrogens at the two bridge double bonds) can be formed upon exposure to blue light and are unstable. They are *water-soluble* because their geometric configuration prevents intramolecular hydrogen bonding. Thus, these isomers (photoisomers) can be *excreted* into bile *without having to be conjugated*. The natural Z-Z isomer is also rendered water-soluble by conjugation with glucuronic acid. Bilirubin glucuronide formation prevents intramolecular hydrogen bonding, makes the molecule polar, and permits excretion of the pigment into bile (Fig. 38-2).

Intestinal phase of bilirubin metabolism After its appearance in the intestinal lumen, bilirubin glucuronide may be excreted in the stool or metabolized to urobilinogen and related products. Because of its polarity, *conjugated bilirubin is not reabsorbed* by the intestinal mucosa, a mechanism which may serve to rid the body of this pigment. The formation of urobilinogen from conjugated bilirubin

requires the action of bacteria and occurs in the lower part of the small intestine and colon.

In contrast to conjugated bilirubin, *urobilinogen is reabsorbed* from the small intestine into the portal blood and is thus subject to the enterohepatic circulation. Some urobilinogen is reexcreted by the liver into the bile; the rest is excreted in the urine in an amount usually not exceeding 4 mg daily. When the hepatic excretory mechanism is impaired (e.g., in hepatocellular disease) or the production of bilirubin is greatly increased (e.g., in hemolytic anemia), the urinary urobilinogen may increase significantly.

The normal output of fecal urobilinogen ranges from 50 to 280 mg per day. Under conditions of decreased excretion of conjugated bilirubin into the intestine (e.g., liver disease, bile duct obstruction) or suppression of intestinal flora by antibiotics, fecal output will be diminished. In hemolytic anemia, urinary and fecal urobilinogen excretion is greatly increased.

In a normal person with a blood volume of 5 liters and a hemoglobin concentration of 15 g/dL, the total circulating hemoglobin is 750 g. Because approximately 0.8 percent of the red blood cells are destroyed daily, 6.3 g hemoglobin is released for catabolism.

Renal excretion of bilirubin Normally the urine contains no bilirubin that can be detected by the methods usually employed, although traces may be detectable by sensitive spectrophotometric procedures. Unconjugated bilirubin, being tightly bound to albumin, is not filtered by the renal glomeruli, and because there is no tubular secretory process for bilirubin, *unconjugated bilirubin (as the IXα, Z-Z isomer) is not excreted in urine.* On the other hand, conjugated bilirubin is less tightly bound to albumin, and a small fraction (about 5 percent) is unbound. The unbound fraction is dialyzable and is filtered by the renal glomeruli. Thus, in contrast to the unconjugated pigment, a fraction of plasma *conjugated bilirubin appears in the urine.* Bile salts enhance the dialyzability of conjugated bilirubin, and in obstructive jaundice, the elevated level of plasma bile acids may account for an increased renal excretion of conjugated bilirubin. This may also explain why in biliary tract obstruction, serum conjugated bilirubin levels tend to plateau and not to exceed 30 to 40 mg/dL, while with severe hepatocellular injury bilirubin levels higher than this may occur.

CHEMICAL TESTS FOR BILE PIGMENTS The most widely employed chemical test for the bile pigments in serum is the van den Bergh reaction. In this reaction the bilirubin pigments are diazotized with sulfanilic acid, and the chromogenic products are measured colorimetrically. The van den Bergh reaction can be used to distinguish between unconjugated and conjugated bilirubin because of the different solubility properties of the pigments. When the reaction is carried out in an *aqueous* medium, the water-soluble conjugated bilirubin reacts to give the so-called direct van den Bergh reaction. When the reaction is carried out in *methanol*, the intramolecular hydrogen bonds

FIGURE 38-3 *Scheme of bilirubin uptake, conjugation, and excretion by the liver cell. Although the conversion of BMG to BDG appears to be catalyzed by glucuronyl transferase, some have also postulated its formation by a plasma membrane transglucuronidase. B = bilirubin; BMG = bilirubin monoglucuronide; BDG = bilirubin diglucuronide; UDP = uridine diphosphate.*

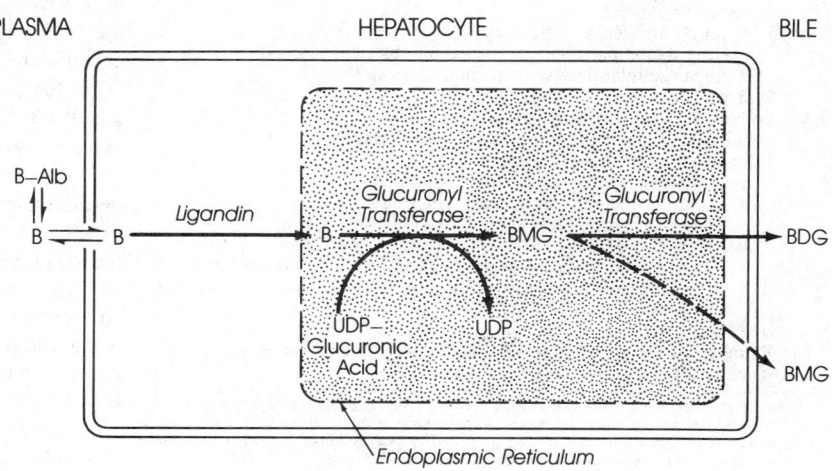

of unconjugated bilirubin are broken; thus both conjugated and unconjugated pigments react, giving a measure of the *total* bilirubin level. The total minus the direct-reacting bilirubin give the *indirect* value, which is a measure of the unconjugated bilirubin level.

In the direct van den Bergh reaction, the most accurate measurements are those carried out at 1 min. If the reaction is allowed to proceed longer, a small amount of the unconjugated pigment may begin to react in the aqueous medium. As a result, if the reaction is carried out at 30 min in a patient with unconjugated hyperbilirubinemia, falsely low values for the indirect-reacting bilirubin may be obtained. This serves to emphasize that the direct and indirect van den Bergh reactions represent *approximations* (not absolute measurements) of the conjugated and unconjugated pigments.

The most accurate method for measuring bilirubin in biologic fluids involves the formation of bilirubin methyl esters (by alkaline methanolysis) and measuring the products by high-performance liquid chromatography (HPLC). Studies with this procedure show that *normal serum contains mostly unconjugated bilirubin* with less than 4 percent of the total bilirubin being conjugated. This confirms the long-held suspicion that the small amount of "direct-reacting" bilirubin measured by the van den Bergh method (0.1 to 0.3 mg/dL) is not correct and is an overestimate of the amount of conjugated

bilirubin actually present in normal serum. The HPLC method also shows that in patients with liver disease and conjugated hyperbilirubinemia, the serum contains significant amounts of *monoconjugates as well as diconjugates*. A summary of the key differences in the properties and reactions of the bilirubin pigments is presented in Table 38-1.

The qualitative measurement of bilirubin in the urine may be carried out with Ictotest tablets or the dipstick method. The foam test is also a simple and qualitatively valid procedure. When normal urine is vigorously shaken in a test tube, the foam is absolutely white. In urine containing bilirubin, the foam will be yellow. This difference may be subtle and may become evident only by comparing a normal urine specimen and one containing bilirubin side by side.

Except for concentrated urine, the most common cause of a deep-yellow-brown or dark urine is bilirubinuria. However, other mechanisms and diseases associated with a dark urine need to be considered. These include yellow urine due to drugs (e.g., sulfasalazine); red urine due to porphyria, hemoglobinuria, myoglobinuria, or drugs (e.g., pyridium); and dark-brown or black urine due to homogentisic acid (in ochronosis) or melanin (with melanoma).

APPROACH TO THE PATIENT WITH JAUNDICE　Once jaundice is recognized clinically or chemically, it is important to determine whether it is predominantly due to unconjugated or conjugated hyperbilirubinemia. *A simple clue in this regard is to determine whether bilirubin is present in the urine.* Its absence in the urine suggests unconjugated hyperbilirubinemia (since this pigment is not filtered by the glomerulus); its presence indicates conjugated hyperbilirubinemia. One can then proceed to the chemical measurement of the bilirubin pigments in the serum. In predominantly unconjugated hyperbilirubinemia, 80 to 85 percent of the total serum bilirubin is measured as unconjugated by the van den Bergh reaction, but more than 96 percent by the more accurate HPLC method. The patient is considered to have predominantly conjugated hyperbilirubinemia when more than 50 percent of the serum bilirubin is of the conjugated type. The serum of such patients will contain both mono- and diglucuronide conjugates.

An approach to the classification of jaundice based on this important distinction is presented in Table 38-2. Derangements of bilirubin metabolism may occur through any of four mechanisms: (1) overproduction, (2) decreased hepatic uptake, (3) decreased hepatic conjugation, and (4) decreased excretion of bilirubin into bile (due to both intrahepatic and extrahepatic factors). Jaundice may also be described on the basis of the pathogenetic mechanisms or disease processes leading to increased bilirubin levels. Thus, the terms *hemolytic jaundice, hepatocellular jaundice,* and *obstructive* (or *cholestatic) jaundice* are often used. Though these classifications and terms are helpful, in any one patient more than a single derangement or more than one "type" of jaundice may be present. For example, a patient with cirrhosis may have not only impaired liver cell function (and hence hepatocellular jaundice) but also hemolysis. Furthermore, obstructive jaundice may be due to either *mechanical* obstruction of the biliary radicles or *functional* factors causing impaired hepatic excretion of bilirubin into bile.

In the present chapter a brief description of the major types of jaundice is given. A more detailed discussion of the individual disease entities is found in Chap. 246.

TABLE 38-1　Comparison of the major differences between conjugated and unconjugated bilirubin

Properties and reactions	Unconjugated*	Conjugated
Water solubility	0	+
Affinity for lipids	+	0
Renal excretion	0	+
van den Bergh reaction	Indirect (total minus direct)	Direct
Binding to serum albumin (reversible)	+ + +	+
Formation of bilirubin-albumin complex (irreversible)	0	+ †

* *These properties apply to the naturally occurring bilirubin IXα. Other geometric and photoisomers behave like conjugated bilirubin. See text for details.*
† *Detectable in plasma under conditions of cholestasis (see text).*

TABLE 38-2　Classification of jaundice based on underlying derangement of bilirubin metabolism

I Predominantly *unconjugated* hyperbilirubinemia
　A Overproduction
　　1 Hemolysis (intra- and extravascular)
　　2 Ineffective erythropoiesis
　B Decreased hepatic uptake
　　1 Drugs (e.g., flavaspidic acid)
　　2 Prolonged fasting (< 300 cal per day)
　　3 Sepsis
　C Decreased bilirubin conjugation (decreased glucuronyl transferase activity)
　　1 Gilbert's syndrome (*mild* decrease in transferase)
　　2 Crigler-Najjar type II (*moderate* decrease in transferase)
　　3 Crigler-Najjar type I (*absent* transferase)
　　4 Neonatal jaundice
　　5 Acquired transferase deficiency
　　　a Drug inhibition (e.g., pregnanediol, chloramphenicol)
　　　b Hepatocellular disease (hepatitis, cirrhosis)*
　　6 Sepsis
II Predominantly *conjugated* hyperbilirubinemia
　A Impaired hepatic excretion (intrahepatic defects)
　　1 Familial or hereditary disorders
　　　a Dubin-Johnson syndrome; Rotor syndrome
　　　b Recurrent (benign) intrahepatic cholestasis
　　　c Cholestatic jaundice of pregnancy
　　2 Acquired disorders
　　　a Hepatocellular disease* (e.g., viral or drug-induced hepatitis)
　　　b Drug-induced cholestasis (e.g., oral contraceptives, methyltestosterone)
　　　c Sepsis
　B Extrahepatic biliary obstruction (mechanical obstruction, e.g., stones, stricture, tumor of bile duct)

* *In hepatocellular disease (hepatitis and cirrhosis) there is usually interference in the three major steps of bilirubin metabolism—uptake, conjugation, and excretion. However, excretion is the rate-limiting step and is usually impaired to the greatest extent. As a result, conjugated hyperbilirubinemia predominates.*

Jaundice with predominantly unconjugated bilirubin in the serum
OVERPRODUCTION OF BILIRUBIN　When an increased amount of hemoglobin is released from red blood cells into either the bloodstream or tissues, increased bilirubin production occurs. This is reflected by an increase in unconjugated bilirubin levels in the serum, but with levels rarely exceeding 3 to 4 mg/dL. There may also be a slight increase in conjugated bilirubin, but on a percentage basis the amount is comparable to what is found in normal serum, i.e., 4 percent or less of total bilirubin. For a detailed description of the causes of increased bilirubin production, see Chap. 246.

IMPAIRED HEPATIC UPTAKE OF BILIRUBIN   As indicated previously, the uptake of bilirubin by the liver cell involves dissociation of the pigment from albumin, and then binding to ligandin. In some cases of drug-induced jaundice (e.g., due to flavaspidic acid) and possibly in some patients with Gilbert's syndrome, there may be a derangement in this phase of bilirubin metabolism (see Chap. 246).

IMPAIRED GLUCURONIDE CONJUGATION   Both acquired and genetic derangements in hepatic glucuronyl transferase occur. In the fetus and at birth, glucuronyl transferase activity is low and appears to account in part for the *neonatal jaundice* normally found between the second and the fifth days of life. *Mild* decreases in glucuronyl transferases occur in Gilbert's syndrome, *moderate* decreases are found in Crigler-Najjar syndrome type II, and the enzyme is totally *absent* in the rare Crigler-Najjar syndrome type I (see Chap. 246).

Acquired defects in bilirubin glucuronyl transferase activity may be produced by drugs (i.e., enzyme inhibition) or intrinsic liver disease. However, with liver cell damage, the excretory capacity of the liver is impaired to a greater extent than is the conjugating capacity. Therefore in most hepatocellular diseases, the hyperbilirubinemia is predominantly of the conjugated type (see Chap. 246).

Jaundice with predominantly conjugated bilirubin in the serum

IMPAIRED EXCRETION OF BILIRUBIN BY THE LIVER   The impaired excretion of bilirubin into the biliary canaliculi, whether due to functional or mechanical factors, results in predominantly conjugated hyperbilirubinemia and bilirubinuria. The presence of *bilirubin in the urine is evidence of conjugated hyperbilirubinemia* and is a most important point in the differential diagnosis of jaundice. Such findings are identical to those occurring in complete obstruction of the bile duct, emphasizing that *jaundice due to hepatocellular disease can seldom be differentiated from that due to extrahepatic obstruction solely on the basis of changes in bile pigment metabolism.* Indeed there are often instances when the two conditions are not distinguishable by any biochemical criteria, and liver biopsy or other diagnostic procedures (e.g., ultrasound) are needed for the definitive diagnosis.

When there is interference in the excretion of conjugated bilirubin into bile, by what mechanism does this pigment enter the systemic circulation? Several postulates have been proposed for this "reentry": (1) rupture of the bile canaliculi secondary to the necrosis of the hepatic cells that constitute their walls; (2) occlusion of the canaliculi by inspissated bile or their compression by swollen hepatic cells; (3) obstruction of the terminal intrahepatic bile ducts (cholangioles) by inflammatory cells; (4) altered hepatic cell permeability; and (5) impaired excretion, resulting in accumulation of conjugated bilirubin in the hepatocytes, and secondary diffusion into the plasma. Although some of these postulates are speculative, it is likely that several of these mechanisms occur. For example, occasionally in histologic sections, escape of bile through rents in the walls of canaliculi in areas of necrosis is apparent. Also, microscopic studies of the liver of rats injected with fluorescent dyes have shown reflux of bile from canaliculi into sinusoids. However, no anatomic damage needs to be invoked, because when unconjugated bilirubin is infused into normal subjects at high rates, conjugated hyperbilirubinemia occurs; this is explained most logically by passive diffusion.

EXTRAHEPATIC BILIARY OBSTRUCTION   Complete obstruction of the extrahepatic bile ducts leads to jaundice with predominantly conjugated hyperbilirubinemia, bilirubinuria, and clay-colored stools. Failure of bile to reach the intestine results in virtual disappearance of urobilinogen from the stool and urine. The concentration of bilirubin rises progressively but then usually plateaus at a level of 30 to 40 mg/dL. To some extent this plateau may be explained by a balance between renal excretion and diversion of bilirubin to other metabolites. In hepatocellular jaundice, such a plateau tends not to occur, and bilirubin levels in excess of 50 mg/dL may be found, in part due to concomitant hemolysis and renal insufficiency.

Partial obstruction of the extrahepatic bile ducts can also give rise to jaundice but only if the intrabiliary pressure is increased, because the excretion of bilirubin does not diminish until the intraductile pressure approaches the maximal secretory pressure of approximately 250 mmHg bile. Jaundice may occur at much lower pressures if the obstruction is complicated by infection of the ducts or hepatocellular injury. Therefore, jaundice, bilirubinuria, and clay-colored stools are inconstant findings in partial biliary obstruction, and the amount of urobilinogen in urine and stool varies with the degree of occlusion.

The functional reserve of the liver is so great that *occlusion of the intrahepatic bile ducts* does not give rise to jaundice unless the drainage of bile from a large segment of the parenchyma is interrupted. Either of the two major hepatic ducts or a large number of secondary radicles may be occluded without production of jaundice. In experimental animals the ducts draining at least 75 percent of the parenchyma must be occluded before jaundice appears.

Additional points of terminology   In clinical practice, a patient may be described as having *obstructive,* or *cholestatic,* jaundice. By this is meant that clinically, and especially biochemically, there is little to suggest hepatocellular damage and that the main features point to interference with, or obstruction in, the flow of bile. Typically one would expect such a patient to show (1) predominantly conjugated hyperbilirubinemia, (2) minimal biochemical changes of parenchymal liver damage, and (3) a moderate to a marked increase in the serum alkaline phosphatase level [usually three or four times normal (or greater than 250 IU per liter)]. As emphasized in Chaps. 244 and 245, an *elevated alkaline phosphatase level* in a patient with jaundice or liver disease, in the absence of other disorders such as bone disease, is most suggestive of interference with bile secretion or an infiltrative process in the liver. However, *laboratory tests alone may not permit differentiation of intrahepatic from extrahepatic cholestasis.*

Some clinicians reserve the term obstructive jaundice for those cases in which anatomic obstruction can be demonstrated and use the term cholestatic jaundice for cases of parenchymal liver disease in which the obstructive phase is on a functional basis. Nevertheless, because these two entities frequently are indistinguishable by clinical and biochemical criteria, the terms obstructive jaundice and cholestatic jaundice are often used interchangeably.

Hepatocellular disorders in which jaundice associated with an obstructive, or cholestatic, phase occurs include (1) occasional cases of viral hepatitis, (2) drug reactions, especially those due to chlorpromazine and methyltestosterone, (3) some cases of alcoholic hepatitis or alcohol-induced fatty liver, (4) jaundice in the last trimester of pregnancy, (5) most cases of Dubin-Johnson or Rotor syndrome, (6) benign recurrent intrahepatic cholestasis, and (7) certain types of postoperative jaundice. These and other conditions are discussed in Chaps. 246 and 247.

In summary, all forms of conjugated hyperbilirubinemia have by definition an impairment in the excretion of bilirubin into bile. In most cases of parenchymal liver disease, a broad derangement is shown by the biochemical tests of liver function. However, when the major detectable alterations of liver function tests include (1) conjugated hyperbilirubinemia and (2) moderate to marked elevation of the serum alkaline phosphatase level, the terms obstructive or cholestatic jaundice may be appropriate. Additional procedures, including operation, are often needed to determine the cause of the cholestasis (see Chaps. 243 and 245).

HEPATOMEGALY

In the supine position, the major part of the liver lies beneath the right rib cage. In some normal persons the liver edge may be palpable 1 to 2 cm below the right costal margin, and a palpable liver edge by itself does not necessarily indicate hepatomegaly. In evaluating liver size by physical examination, two factors other than ability to palpate the liver edge need to be considered, namely, (1) the location of the upper border of liver dullness by percussion, and (2) the body habitus.

Normally, the upper edge of liver dullness on the right side in the midclavicular line is at the level of the fifth rib, but in asthenic habitus it may be lower. The liver edge normally descends 1 to 3 cm with deep inspiration. In hypersthenic subjects, the liver may extend over to the left side of the abdominal wall, with the lower edge high and not palpable; in hyposthenic subjects with a very acute costal angle, the liver may lie in the right half of the abdomen, the edge being palpable by as much as 6 to 8 cm below the right costal margin lateral to the right rectus abdominis muscle. Thus, palpability does not necessarily imply hepatomegaly.

In determining liver enlargement by palpation, one should be certain that the liver is being palpated rather than other right upper quadrant masses such as gallbladder, colonic neoplasm, or fecal material in the colon. Liver enlargement is often confirmed by radiologic studies, including hepatic scintiscans, computerized tomography, and ulrasonography.

In many cases of generalized liver enlargement, the left lobe will be felt in the epigastrium between the xiphoid and umbilicus. The liver should be carefully palpated during deep inspiration to determine whether the edge is tender, regular or irregular, firm or soft, rounded and thickened, or sharp. The edge is tender and often rounded with hepatic inflammation, as in hepatitis, or when the liver is acutely congested, as in cardiac decompensation. Pulsation of the liver may be found with tricuspid valvular incompetence. A carcinomatous liver may be rocklike in hardness; the cirrhotic liver is very firm in consistency. The largest livers are often found with carcinoma (primary or metastatic), marked fatty infiltration, congestive cardiac decompensation, Hodgkin's disease, and amyloidosis. Rapid decrease in liver size may occur with improvement of congestive failure, mobilization of fat from the liver, or massive hepatic necrosis.

In a patient with hepatomegaly, auscultation is sometimes helpful. A friction rub may be audible (and palpable) in the right upper quadrant; it is usually due to a recent biopsy, tumor, or perihepatitis. In portal hypertension a venous hum may be audible between the umbilicus and the xiphoid. An arterial murmur or bruit over the liver may indicate tumor, usually hepatocellular carcinoma.

Some of the causes of a palpable liver and hepatomegaly are given in Table 38-3.

TABLE 38-3   Causes of a palpable liver and hepatomegaly

I Palpable liver without hepatomegaly
  A Right diaphragm displaced downward (e.g., emphysema, asthma)
  B Subdiaphragmatic lesion (e.g., abscess)
  C Aberrant lobe of liver (Riedel's lobe)
  D Extremely thin or relaxed abdominal muscles
  E Occasionally present in normal persons
II Hepatomegaly
  A Vascular congestion (e.g., congestive heart failure, hepatic vein thrombosis)
  B Bile duct obstruction (e.g., lesion in common duct leading to hepatomegaly and subsequently to biliary cirrhosis)
  C Infiltrative disorders
    1 Bone marrow and reticuloendothelial cells
      a Extramedullary hematopoiesis
      b Leukemia
      c Lymphoma
    2 Fat
      a Fatty liver (e.g., secondary to alcohol, diabetes, or toxins)
      b Gaucher's disease and some other lipidoses
    3 Glycogen (e.g., diabetes, especially after insulin excess)
    4 Amyloid
    5 Iron (hemochromatosis and hemosiderosis)
    6 Granuloma (tuberculosis, sarcoid)
  D Inflammatory disorders
    1 Hepatitis—due to drugs or infectious agents
    2 Cirrhosis—except in late stages when prolonged scarring may lead to a *small*, shrunken liver
  E Tumors—primary or metastatic
  F Cysts—polycystic disease, congenital hepatic fibrosis

REFERENCES

BERLIN N, BERK P: Quantitative aspects of bilirubin metabolism for hematologists. Blood 57:983, 1981

BLANKAERT N, SCHMID R: Physiology and pathophysiology of bilirubin metabolism, in *Hepatology: A Textbook of Liver Disease*, D Zakim, T Boyer (eds). Saunders, Philadelphia, 1982, pp 246–296

MCDONAGH AF et al: Blue light and bilirubin excretion, Science 208:145, 1980

VAN HOOTEGEM P et al: Serum bilirubins in hepatobiliary disease: Comparison with other liver function tests. Hepatology 5:112, 1985

WEISS JS et al: The clinical importance of a protein-bound fraction of serum bilirubin in patients with hyperbilirubinemia. N Engl J Med 309:147, 1983

WOLKOFF AW et al: Hereditary jaundice and disorders of bilirubin metabolism, in *The Metabolic Basis of Inherited Disease*, 5th ed, JB Stanbury et al (eds). New York, McGraw-Hill, 1983, pp 1385–1420

39   ABDOMINAL SWELLING AND ASCITES

ROBERT M. GLICKMAN / KURT J. ISSELBACHER

ABDOMINAL SWELLING   Abdominal swelling or distention is a common problem in clinical medicine and may be the initial manifestation of a systemic disease or of otherwise unsuspected abdominal disease. *Subjective* abdominal enlargement, often described as a sensation of fullness or bloating, is usually transient and is often related to a functional gastrointestinal disorder when it is not accompanied by objective physical findings of increased abdominal girth or local swelling. *Obesity* and lumbar lordosis, which may be associated with prominence of the abdomen, may usually be distinguished from true increases in the volume of the peritoneal cavity by history and careful physical examination.

Clinical history   Abdominal swelling may first be noticed by the patient because of a progressive increase in belt or clothing size, the appearance of abdominal or inguinal hernias, or the development of a localized swelling. Often, considerable abdominal enlargement has gone unnoticed for weeks or months, either because of coexistent obesity or because the ascites formation has been insidious, without pain or localizing symptoms. Progressive abdominal distention may be associated with a sensation of "pulling" or "stretching" of the flanks or groins and vague low back pain. Localized *pain* usually results from involvement of an abdominal organ (e.g., a passively congested liver, large spleen, or colonic tumor). Pain is uncommon in cirrhosis with ascites and when it is present, pancreatitis, hepatoma, or peritonitis should be considered. Tense ascites or abdominal tumors may produce increased intraabdominal pressure, resulting in *indigestion* and *heartburn* due to gastroesophageal reflux or *dyspnea*, *orthopnea*, and *tachypnea* from elevation of the diaphragm. A coexistent pleural effusion, more commonly on the right, presumably due to leakage of ascitic fluid through lymphatic channels in the diaphragm, may also contribute to respiratory embarrassment. The patient with diffuse abdominal swelling should be questioned about increased alcoholic intake, a prior episode of jaundice or hematuria, a change in bowel habits, or a past history of rheumatic heart disease. Such historical information may provide the clues that will lead one to suspect an occult cirrhosis, a colonic tumor with peritoneal seeding, congestive heart failure, or nephrosis.

Physical examination   A carefully executed *general physical examination* can yield valuable clues concerning the etiology of abdominal swelling. Thus palmar erythema and spider angiomas suggest an underlying cirrhosis, while supraclavicular adenopathy (Virchow's node) should raise the question of an underlying gastrointestinal malignancy. *Inspection* of the abdomen is an important but often cursorily performed aspect of the abdominal examination. By noting the abdominal contour, one may be able to distinguish localized from generalized swelling. The tensely distended abdomen with tightly stretched skin, bulging flanks, and everted umbilicus is characteristic of ascites. A prominent abdominal venous pattern with the direction of flow away from the umbilicus often is a reflection of portal hypertension; venous collaterals with flow from the lower part of the abdomen toward the umbilicus suggest obstruction of the inferior vena cava; flow downward toward the umbilicus suggests superior vena cava obstruction. "Doming" of the abdomen with visible ridges from underlying intestinal loops is usually due to intestinal obstruction or distention. An epigastric mass, with evident peristalsis proceeding from left to right, usually indicates underlying pyloric obstruction. A liver with metastatic deposits may be visible as a nodular right upper quadrant mass moving with respiration.

Auscultation may reveal the high-pitched, rushing sounds of early intestinal obstruction or a succussion sound due to increased fluid and gas in a dilated hollow viscus. Careful auscultation over an enlarged liver occasionally reveals the harsh bruit of a vascular tumor, especially a hepatoma, or the leathery friction rub of a surface nodule. A venous hum at the umbilicus may signify portal hypertension and an increased collateral blood flow around the liver. A fluid wave and flank dullness which shifts with change in position of the patient are important signs that indicate the presence of peritoneal fluid. In obese patients, small amounts of fluid may be difficult to demonstrate; on occasion the fluid may be detected by abdominal percussion with patients on their hands and knees. Doubt about the presence of peritoneal fluid may be resolved by careful paracentesis with a small-gauge (no. 19 or 20) needle. Careful percussion should serve to distinguish generalized abdominal enlargement from localized swelling due to an enlarged uterus, ovarian cyst, or distended bladder. Percussion can also outline an abnormally small or large liver. Loss of normal liver dullness may result from massive hepatic necrosis; it may also be a clue to free gas in the peritoneal cavity, as from perforation of a hollow viscus.

Palpation is often difficult with massive ascites, and ballottement of overlying fluid may be the only method of palpating the liver or spleen. A slightly enlarged spleen in association with ascites may be the only evidence of an occult cirrhosis. When there is evidence of portal hypertension, a soft liver suggests that obstruction to portal flow is extrahepatic; a firm liver suggests cirrhosis as the likely cause of the portal hypertension. A very hard or nodular liver is a clue that the liver is infiltrated with tumor, and when accompanied by ascites, it suggests that the latter is due to peritoneal seeding. The presence of a hard periumbilical lymph node (Sister Marie Joseph's nodule) suggests metastatic disease from a pelvic or gastrointestinal primary tumor. A pulsatile liver and ascites may be found in tricuspid insufficiency.

An attempt should be made to determine whether a mass is solid or cystic, smooth or irregular, and whether it moves with respiration. The liver, spleen, and gallbladder should descend with respiration unless they are fixed by adhesions or extension of tumor beyond the organ. A fixed mass not descending with respiration may indicate that it is retroperitoneal. Tenderness, especially if localized, may indicate an inflammatory process such as an abscess; it may also be due to stretching of the visceral peritoneum or tumor necrosis. Rectal and pelvic examinations are mandatory; they may reveal otherwise undetected masses due to tumor or infection.

Radiographic and laboratory examinations are essential for confirming or extending the impressions gained on physical examination. Upright and recumbent films of the abdomen may demonstrate the dilated loops of intestine with fluid levels characteristic of intestinal obstruction or the diffuse abdominal haziness and loss of psoas margins suggestive of ascites. Ultrasonography is often of value in detecting ascites, determining the presence of a mass, or evaluating the size of the liver and spleen. Computerized axial tomography (CT scanning) provides similar information. A plain film of the abdomen may reveal the distended colon of otherwise unsuspected ulcerative colitis and give valuable information as to the size of the liver and spleen. An irregular and elevated right side of the diaphragm may be a clue to a liver abscess or hepatoma. Studies of the gastrointestinal tract with barium or other contrast media are usually necessary in the search for a primary tumor.

ASCITES The evaluation of a patient with ascites requires that the *cause* of the ascites be established. In most cases ascites will appear as a part of a well-recognized illness, i.e., cirrhosis, congestive heart failure, nephrosis, or disseminated carcinomatosis. In these situations, the physician should determine that the development of ascites is indeed a consequence of the basic underlying disease and not due to the presence of a separate or related disease process. This distinction is necessary even when the cause of ascites seems obvious. For example, when the patient with compensated cirrhosis and minimal ascites develops progressive ascites that is increasingly difficult to control with sodium restriction or diuretics, the obvious temptation is to attribute the worsening of the clinical picture to progressive liver disease. However, an occult hepatoma, portal vein thrombosis, spontaneous bacterial peritonitis, or even tuberculosis may be responsible for the decompensation. The disappointingly low success in diagnosing tuberculous peritonitis or hepatoma in the patient with cirrhosis and ascites reflects the too-low index of suspicion for the development of such superimposed conditions. Similarly, the patient with congestive heart failure may develop ascites from a disseminated carcinoma with peritoneal seeding. The thorough evaluation of each patient with ascites, even in the presence of an "obvious" cause, will help avoid these errors.

Diagnostic paracentesis (50 to 100 mL) should be part of the routine evaluation of the patient with ascites. The fluid should be examined for its gross appearance, protein content, cell count, and differential cell count, as well as Gram's and acid-fast stains and culture. Cytologic and cell-block examination may disclose an otherwise unsuspected carcinoma. Table 39-1 presents some of the features of ascitic fluid typically found in various disease states. In some disorders, such as cirrhosis, the fluid has the characteristics of a transudate (less than 2.5 g protein per deciliter and a specific gravity less than 1.016); in others, such as peritonitis, the features are those of an exudate. Although there is variability of the ascitic fluid in any given disease state, some features are sufficiently characteristic to suggest certain diagnostic possibilities. For example, blood-stained fluid with more than 2.5 g protein per deciliter is unusual in uncomplicated cirrhosis but is consistent with tuberculous peritonitis or neoplasm. Cloudy fluid with a predominance of polymorphonuclear cells and a positive Gram stain are characteristic of bacterial peritonitis; if most cells are lymphocytes, tuberculosis should be suspected. The complete examination of each fluid is most important, for occasionally only *one* finding may be abnormal. For example, if the fluid is a typical transudate but contains more than 250 white blood cells per cubic millimeter, the finding should be recognized as atypical for cirrhosis, nephrosis, or congestive heart failure and should warrant a search for tumor or infection. This is especially true in the evaluation of cirrhotic ascites where occult peritoneal infection may be present with only minor elevations in the white blood cell count of the peritoneal fluid (300 to 500 cells per cubic millimeter). Since Gram's stain of the fluid may be negative in a high proportion of such cases, careful culture of the peritoneal fluid is mandatory. Direct visualization of the peritoneum (laparoscopy) may disclose peritoneal deposits of tumor, tuberculosis, or metastatic disease of the liver. Biopsies are taken under direct vision often adding to the diagnostic accuracy of the procedure.

Chylous ascites refers to a turbid, milky, or creamy peritoneal fluid due to the presence of thoracic or intestinal lymph. Such a fluid shows Sudan-staining fat globules microscopically and an increased triglyceride content by chemical examination. A turbid fluid due to leukocytes or tumor cells may be confused with chylous fluid (pseudochylous), and it is often helpful to carry out alkalinization and ether extraction of the specimen. Alkali will tend to dissolve cellular proteins and thereby reduce turbidity; ether extraction will lead to clearing if the turbidity of the fluid is due to lipid. Chylous ascites is most often the result of lymphatic obstruction from trauma, tumor, tuberculosis, filariasis (see Chap. 163), or congenital abnormalities. It may also be seen in the nephrotic syndrome.

Rarely, ascitic fluid may be *mucinous* in character, suggesting either pseudomyxoma peritonei (Chap. 242) or rarely a colloid carcinoma of the stomach or colon with peritoneal implants.

TABLE 39-1 Ascitic fluid characteristics in various disease states

Condition	Gross appearance	Specific gravity	Protein, g/dL	Cell count — Red blood cells, >10,000/mm³	Cell count — White blood cells, per mm³	Other tests
Cirrhosis	Straw-colored or bile-stained	<1.016 (95%)*	<2.5 (95%)	1%	<250 (90%);* predominantly endothelial	
Neoplasm	Straw-colored, hemorrhagic, mucinous, or chylous	Variable, >1.016 (45%)	>2.5 (75%)	20%	>1000 (50%); variable cell types	Cytology, cell block, peritoneal biopsy
Tuberculous peritonitis	Clear, turbid, hemorrhagic, chylous	Variable, >1.016 (50%)	>2.5 (50%)	7%	>1000 (70%); usually >70% lymphocytes	Peritoneal biopsy, stain and culture for acid-fast bacilli
Pyogenic peritonitis	Turbid or purulent	If purulent, >1.016	If purulent, >2.5	Unusual	Predominantly polymorphonuclear leukocytes	+Gram's stain, culture
Congestive heart failure	Straw-colored	Variable, <1.016 (60%)	Variable, 1.5–5.3	10%	<1000 (90%); usually mesothelial, mononuclear	
Nephrosis	Straw-colored or chylous	<1.016	<2.5 (100%)	Unusual	<250; mesothelial, mononuclear	If chylous, ether extraction, Sudan staining
Pancreatic ascites (pancreatitis, pseudocyst)	Turbid, hemorrhagic, or chylous	Variable, often >1.016	Variable, often >2.5	Variable, may be blood-stained	Variable	Increased amylase in ascitic fluid and serum

* Since the conditions of examining fluid and selecting patients were not identical in each series, the percentage figures (in the parentheses) should be taken as an indication of the order of magnitude rather than as the precise incidence of any abnormal finding.

On occasion, ascites may develop as a seemingly isolated finding in the absence of a clinically evident underlying disease. It is then that a careful analysis of ascitic fluid may indicate the direction the evaluation should take. A useful framework for the workup starts with an analysis of whether the fluid is an exudate or transudate. *Transudative ascites* of unclear etiology is most often due to occult cirrhosis, right-sided venous hypertension raising hepatic sinusoidal pressure, or hypoalbuminemic states such as nephrosis or protein-losing enteropathy. Cirrhosis with well-preserved liver function (normal albumin) resulting in ascites invariably is associated with significant portal hypertension (see Chap. 249). Evaluation should include liver function tests, liver spleen scan or other hepatic imaging procedure (i.e., CT or ultrasound) to detect nodular changes in the liver, or a colloid shift of isotope to suggest portal hypertension. On occasion a wedged hepatic venous pressure can be useful to document portal hypertension. Finally, if clinically indicated, a liver biopsy will confirm the diagnosis of cirrhosis and perhaps suggest its etiology. Other etiologies may result in hepatic venous congestion and resultant ascites. Right-sided cardiac valvular disease and particularly constrictive pericarditis should raise a high index of suspicion and may require cardiac imaging and cardiac catheterization for definitive diagnosis. Hepatic vein thrombosis is evaluated by visualizing the hepatic veins using imaging techniques (angiography, CT scans, magnetic resonance imaging) to demonstrate obliteration, thrombosis, or obstruction by tumor. Uncommonly, transudative ascites may be associated with benign tumors of the ovary, particularly fibroma (Meigs's syndrome) with ascites and hydrothorax.

Exudative ascites should initiate an evaluation for primary peritoneal processes, most importantly infection and tumor. Routine bacteriologic culture of ascitic fluid often will yield a specific organism causing infectious peritonitis. Tuberculous peritonitis (Table 39-1) is best diagnosed by peritoneal biopsy, either percutaneously or via laparoscopy. Histologic examination invariably shows granulomata which may contain acid-fast bacilli. Since cultures of peritoneal fluid and biopsies for tuberculosis may require 6 weeks, characteristic histology with appropriate stains allows antituberculosis therapy to be started promptly. Similarly the diagnosis of peritoneal seeding by tumor can be made by cytologic analysis of peritoneal fluid or by peritoneal biopsy. Appropriate diagnostic studies can then be undertaken to determine the nature and site of the primary tumor. Pancreatic ascites (Table 39-1) is invariably associated with an extravasation of pancreatic fluid from the pancreatic ductal system, most commonly from a leaking pseudocyst. Ultrasound or CT examination of the pancreas followed by visualization of the pancreatic duct by direct cannulation (viz. endoscopic retrograde cholangiopancreatography, ERCP) will usually disclose the site of leakage and permit resective surgery to be carried out.

An analysis of the physiologic and metabolic factors involved in the production of ascites (see Chap. 249 for details), coupled with a complete evaluation of the nature of the ascitic fluid, will invariably disclose the etiology of the ascites and permit appropriate therapy to be instituted.

REFERENCES

BAR-MEIR S: Analysis of ascitic fluid in cirrhosis. Dig Dis Sc 24:136, 1979

CATTAN EL JR et al: The accuracy of the physical examination in the diagnosis of suspected ascites. JAMA 247:1146, 1982

CONN HO: Spontaneous bacterial peritonitis: Multiple revisitations. Gastroenterology 70:455, 1976

GARCIA-TSAO G et al: The diagnosis of bacterial peritonitis. Hepatology 5:91, 1985

GRAKE TMS et al: Peritoneoscopy in the diagnosis of tuberculous peritonitis. Gastrointest Endosc 27:66, 1981

RECTOR WG JR, REYNOLDS TB: Superiority of the serum: Ascites albumin difference over the ascites total protein concentration in separation of "transudative" and "exudative" ascites. Am J Med 77:83, 1984

40 ALTERATIONS IN URINARY FUNCTION

FREDRIC L. COE

AZOTEMIA, OLIGURIA, AND ANURIA

AZOTEMIA Measurements of urea and creatinine concentrations in serum are often obtained to assess the glomerular filtration rate (GFR). Both substances are produced at a reasonably constant rate, by the liver and muscles, respectively. As discussed in Chap. 218, they undergo complete glomerular filtration and are not reabsorbed extensively by the renal tubules; hence their clearances tend to reflect the GFR. An increase in their serum concentrations, termed *azotemia* (*azo*, "containing nitrogen"), occurs as the GFR falls. Creatinine is a more reliable index of GFR than urea because of the latter's lower back diffusion from tubule lumen to peritubular blood. The GFR may be reduced by a fall in the filtration rates of individual functioning nephrons or by a reduction in the total number of functioning nephrons. (See Table 40-1.)

Reduced single-nephron glomerular filtration rate TUBULAR FUNCTION NORMAL An important response of the normal kidney to a severe sodium-conserving stimulus, such as extracellular fluid volume depletion, is reduction of the single-nephron glomerular filtration rate (SNGFR) and subsequent reabsorption of an increased fraction of the reduced amounts of NaCl and water that enter the tubules. The

resulting azotemia is called *prerenal azotemia*, in which urinary Na concentration falls below 20 (often below 1) meq per liter (see Table 40-1). The fractional excretion of Na can be calculated (see Chap. 219) and used as an additional index of prerenal azotemia. Secretion of vasopressin is stimulated by depletion of extracellular fluid volume, and as a consequence, the distal tubules and collecting ducts become fully permeable to water. The concentrating mechanisms in the inner medulla (Chap. 218) are very efficient when flow rates through the loops of Henle and the collecting ducts are low. As a result, the filtrate that escapes reabsorption in the proximal tubule undergoes maximal osmotic concentration, the urine volume becomes small, and it has a high osmolality, above 500 mosmol per kilogram of water. Most of the filtered creatinine escapes tubular reabsorption, and consequently the ratio of the urine-to-plasma (U/P) creatinine concentrations is very high, 40 or more. Because urea can back-diffuse more completely than creatinine, the blood urea nitrogen (BUN) level rises more than the serum creatinine concentration. Normally, the ratio of BUN to serum creatinine concentration is 10:1; with depletion of the extracellular fluid volume this ratio rises. An elevated ratio can also be produced by unrelated factors such as tetracycline administration, adrenocortical steroid therapy, the presence of blood in the gastrointestinal tract, and increased protein turnover due to trauma or burn.

Prerenal azotemia can occur in any edema-forming condition during the phase in which NaCl and water accumulate. Typical examples include the nephrotic syndrome and hepatic cirrhosis with ascites (Chaps. 28 and 223). When a diuretic is being administered to inhibit the tubular reabsorption of NaCl, urine volume and Na concentration may be normal or elevated, even though SNGFR falls

TABLE 40-1 Pathophysiologic mechanisms of azotemia

Mechanism of reduced GFR	Clinical examples	Laboratory findings					
		Oliguria	Urine osm, mosmol/kg	Urine [Na⁺], meq/L	$\left(\dfrac{U}{P}\right)_{creat}$	$\left(\dfrac{U}{P}\right)_{urea}$	$\dfrac{BUN}{Serum\ creat}$
REDUCED SNGFR							
Tubules normal (prerenal azotemia)	Severe dehydration, edema-forming states, diuretic agents, systemic hypotension, acute glomerular disease,* acute urinary obstruction, incomplete renal vascular obstruction	Nearly always present	>500	<20	>40	>8	>10
Tubules damaged (acute renal failure)	Acute tubular necrosis, nephrotoxic agents, glomerulonephritis with tubule injury	Common	<350	>40	<20	>2	10
REDUCED NEPHRON NUMBER							
Elevated SNGFR	Chronic tubulointerstitial-renal disease / Surgical loss of renal tissue	Rare†	[290	>40	3–10	3–10]	10
Normal SNGFR	Diffuse chronic glomerulonephritis / Diabetic nephropathy	Rare†	[100–350‡	10–100‡	>10	>3]	>10
Reduced SNGFR	Any of the factors that can reduce SNGFR (listed above) may lower SNGFR in a patient who has a reduced number of functioning nephrons	Common	290	>20	>10	<3	>10

* *Acute obstruction causing reduced SNGFR is called postrenal azotemia.*
† *Occurs only when total GFR is below 5% normal; urine chemistry values are helpful only when oliguria is present and are therefore enclosed in brackets.*
‡ *Varies with diet and with the level of GFR. When GFR is below 20% normal, osmotic concentration of the urine is usually impossible.*
NOTE: = *osm = osmolality; creat = creatinine concentration; U = urine; P = plasma.*

in response to the combination of the underlying edema-forming stimulus and further extracellular fluid volume depletion from the drug. Oliguria may appear upon withdrawal of the drug as the renal tubules resume intense reabsorption of NaCl and water. Prerenal azotemia may also be seen when renal blood flow is reduced by systemic hypotension, incomplete renal arterial or venous occlusion, or other cause (Chap. 127). Acute incomplete obstruction of the ureter and acute glomerular injury may also reduce SNGFR and leave tubule function relatively intact; postrenal azotemia is a term often applied when acute obstruction lowers SNGFR and causes azotemia. Whenever chronic obstruction of any portion of the urinary tract or glomerulonephritis damages nephrons extensively, the high urinary osmolality, U/P ratios for creatinine or urea, and low urinary Na concentrations disappear, and the kidneys behave as they do when nephron number is reduced.

TUBULE FUNCTION IMPAIRED   Certain acute renal diseases which produce azotemia lower SNGFR and at the same time damage the tubules sufficiently to reduce or even abolish their reabsorptive function, producing *acute renal failure.* Acute tubular necrosis, exposure to nephrotoxic agents, and all forms of acute tubulointerstitial disease are excellent examples. Azotemia and oliguria appear, but the urinary Na concentration exceeds 20 meq and usually 40 meq per liter; the U/P ratios for urea and creatinine are below 2 and 20, respectively; and urine osmolality is below 350 mosmol per kilogram of water. The ratio of BUN to serum creatinine is not elevated (see Chap. 219).

Reduced nephron number   INCREASED SNGFR   If one kidney is removed, the other grows larger, its nephrons enlarge, and the SNGFR increases until the total GFR becomes nearly normal for two kidneys. The tubules are overperfused with filtrate, but they appear to cope well with their increased reabsorptive burdens, perhaps in part because they are longer and wider and possess more cells. If more kidney tissue is removed, the remnant nephrons enlarge further, and their SNGFR rises. Extreme overperfusion of the tubules interferes with Na conservation. At the same time, total GFR comes to depend more and more upon expansion of the extracellular fluid volume largely because the increase in SNGFR is due not only to anatomic growth of the glomeruli but also to a relatively high rate of blood flow per glomerulus. Nephron adaptations to reduced nephron number are detailed in Chap. 218.

Azotemia occurs because the total GFR, i.e., the product of the elevated SNGFR and the markedly reduced nephron number, is low. Tubular conservation of filtered H_2O and Na conservation are poor, so fluid and salt intake must be liberal. Clinical states that produce this picture include surgical loss of renal substance secondary to trauma, neoplasm, stone, and destruction of kidneys by bacterial infection or tuberculosis, polycystic and medullary cystic renal diseases, and all the chronic tubulointerstitial nephropathies (Chaps. 226 and 228). In each of these disorders, the nephrons that remain viable are either fully intact or behave as though the SNGFR is better preserved than tubule function.

SNGFR NORMAL   The SNGFR does not appear to increase despite a reduction of nephron number in diseases such as glomerulonephritis and diabetic glomerulosclerosis, where the glomerulus is the primary site of damage. In these diseases total GFR falls directly with nephron number and is not supported by elevated SNGFR. Since the tubules are not confronted with an excessive reabsorptive burden, sodium conservation is adequate. In these disorders, superimposed conditions that lower SNGFR, such as depletion of extracellular fluid volume, can cause oliguria with low urine sodium concentration and U/P ratios for creatinine and urea above 20 and 3, respectively. The serum urea to creatinine ratio will rise distinctly.

SNGFR REDUCED   In patients with chronic renal disease in whom total GFR has been sufficient to support life only because of a very high SNGFR, inadvertent dehydration or any other factor (Table 40-1 and Chaps. 218 and 219) that lowers the SNGFR can provoke oliguria and severe azotemia. Under these circumstances, urine Na concentration falls, but not below 20 meq per liter, as in the normal person, because SNGFR, though reduced from a previously elevated level, may still be above normal. The U/P ratios for creatinine and urea will be low, usually below 10 and 3, respectively, despite oliguria, and urine osmolality will not rise above the plasma level. The serum urea to creatinine ratio may rise, but not above 20. In less extreme situations, reduction of SNGFR will worsen azotemia and alter urine chemistry in the same directions but to a lesser extent.

OLIGURIA AND ANURIA   *Oliguria* refers to a urine volume insufficient to sustain life, usually less than 400 mL per 24 h in an adult of average size. Daily urine volume is difficult to measure when flow rate is low, because small absolute errors of volume measurement, in the range of 50 to 100 mL of urine each day, or of timing of collection, may represent large percentage errors.

Anuria, which is the absence of urine flow, is caused mainly by urinary obstruction, which must be excluded as a first step (Chap. 230). Total renal arterial and venous occlusion is another important cause. Severe renal diseases such as cortical necrosis and rapidly progressive glomerulonephritis produce anuria in the adult, but so rarely that anuria should never be ascribed to a primary renal disease until patency of the urinary tract and major renal blood vessels has been established.

Approach to the patient with azotemia or oliguria   A critical issue is whether azotemia has been stable and long-standing (chronic renal failure, Chap. 217) or is recent and increasing (acute renal failure, Chap. 219; pre- and postrenal azotemia). If azotemia is recent, and oliguria present, the most discriminating additional measurements include serum urea and creatinine concentrations, and the Na, urea, and creatinine concentrations and osmolality of a concurrent urine sample. Reduction of SNGFR with well-preserved tubule function is usually present when urine osmolality exceeds 500 mosmol per kilogram of water, Na < 20 meq per liter, the U/P ratios for urea and creatinine > 8 and 40, respectively, the urinalysis is normal, and the BUN is more than 10 times the serum creatinine concentration. The prognosis for recovery of adequate GFR is good, if the cause of reduced SNGFR can be reversed. When urine osmolality is below 350 mosmol per kilogram of water, Na > 40 meq, the U/P values for urea and creatinine < 2 and 20, respectively, and the BUN exceeds the serum creatinine by only tenfold, tubule function has been lost, and some form of acute or chronic renal failure usually is present.

ABNORMAL URINARY CONSTITUENTS

PROTEINURIA   Normal adults may excrete up to 150 mg protein daily. Of this, only 10 to 15 mg is albumin; the rest is composed of over 30 different plasma proteins and of glycoproteins that derive from the renal cells. Tamm-Horsfall mucoprotein, the most prevalent of the urine proteins that do not arise from plasma, is produced by the cells of the ascending limb of the loop of Henle and is excreted at the rate of 25 mg per day. Daily excretion of more than 150 mg protein is properly termed *pathologic proteinuria,* but in common usage the word *proteinuria* suffices. Protein excretion above 3.5 g per 24 h is termed *massive* proteinuria and usually occurs when glomeruli have been damaged enough to allow plasma proteins, especially albumin, to enter the urine. Urinary albumin loss lowers serum albumin concentration, and the consequent fall in intracapillary oncotic pressure fosters the accumulation of tissue edema (Chap. 28); serum lipids rise, for reasons detailed in Chap. 223. The combination of *massive proteinuria, hypoalbuminemia, edema,* and *hyperlipidemia* is often called the *nephrotic syndrome;* but this term is becoming synonymous with massive urinary protein loss alone. Hypoalbuminemia, elevated blood lipids, and edema are pathophysiologic consequences of massive proteinuria and occur only when hepatic albumin synthesis, though normal or even increased, fails to compensate for urine albumin losses; these features are not a direct result of renal disease.

Detection of proteinuria Proteinuria is usually detected by urine "dipsticks" that register a trace result in response to as little as 50 mg protein per liter, and a distinct color change of the 1+ level at about 300 mg protein per liter. Since proteinuria can be missed if the urine is very dilute, fasting morning samples that tend to be concentrated are usually studied. Dipsticks respond best to albumin, so that a negative result can occur when large amounts of other protein, or protein fragments such as light chains, are being excreted. Dipstick proteinuria requires additional evaluation by the measurement of 24-h excretion rate. If total protein excretion is abnormal, it is helpful to characterize the proportions of albumin and globulins in the urine by cellulose acetate electrophoresis or other methods. Immunoelectrophoresis is required to identify immunoglobulin fragments, kappa or lambda light chains, when their presence is suggested by a monoclonal peak on routine urine electrophoresis.

Mechanisms of proteinuria TUBULAR PROTEINURIA Normal low-molecular-weight (<40,000) serum proteins, such as beta$_2$ microglobulin (11,600 mol wt), lysozyme (14,000 mol wt), or light chains (22,000 mol wt) are readily filtered by the glomeruli but are reabsorbed so efficiently that only trace amounts enter the urine. Diseases that selectively damage the tubules more than glomeruli (Chap. 226) cause excessive excretion of these small proteins with little or no increase in albumin excretion. The resulting proteinuria is usually between 1 and 3 g per 24 h, and edema and lipid disorders do not occur because albumin losses are small. Bence Jones protein, which is probably a dimer of two light chains, light chains themselves, and myoglobin are examples of proteins whose plasma concentrations may increase as a consequence of disease. If their filtered load rises enough to exceed tubular reabsorptive capacity, "overflow" proteinuria may occur.

GLOMERULAR PROTEINURIA Normal glomeruli filter very little albumin or globulin. Glomerular capillary endothelial cells form a barrier penetrated by pores of about 1000 Å diameter that holds back cells and other particles but offers no impediment to most proteins. The glomerular basement membrane traps molecules about 50 Å in effective radius, above 100,000 daltons molecular mass. The *foot processes (podocytes)* of the visceral epithelial cells (Fig. 40-1) cover the urinary aspect of the glomerular basement membrane and produce a series of narrow channels through which molecules that traverse the basement membrane must pass. Anionic molecules, like albumin, are filtered less freely than are neutral or positively charged molecules of the same size, so little albumin enters the filtrate. This charge selectively appears to be due to anionic glycoproteins that cover the surfaces of the foot processes and contribute to the matrix structure of the basement membrane (Chap. 218). The glycoproteins are anionic because they contain the dicarboxylic amino acids, glutamic and aspartic acid, and sialic acid. At the pH of blood (7.4) or urine (4.5 to 7.5) carboxylic and sialic acid residues are dissociated and, therefore, have a negative charge; albumin also carries an overall negative charge. The negatively charged portions of the glycoproteins repel those of albumin and retard filtration.

Glomerular disease can disrupt any of these filtration barriers. Injury limited to the polyanion glycoproteins would tend to produce selective losses of anionic proteins, such as albumin, that would be filtered more completely by the normal glomerulus but for their charge. Extensive injury that involves the entire basement membrane, not only its polyanion components, may increase losses of very large proteins as well as albumin.

The selectivity of proteinuria varies with the extent of glomerular injury. However, the clinical value of measuring selectivity has not been fully defined. The basis of such measurements is to express the excretion rate of a protein as a fraction of its theoretical maximal filtered load, which is the product of its serum concentration and the GFR. This fraction must reflect the relative filtration efficiency of the protein to that of a completely filtered GFR marker, usually inulin

or creatinine, provided that tubular reabsorption and renal production or catabolism are negligible. The slope of a plot of such a clearance ratio against the molecular weight for a variety of serum proteins is one index of filtration selectivity. A more practical version of this test is based upon the ratio of the clearance fractions of two proteins of different molecular weight, such as IgG and transferrin (Chap. 223).

Approach to the patient with proteinuria Given dipstick proteinuria of the 1+ level or more, 24-h urine protein excretion should be measured. If it is above 150 mg, electrophoresis should be carried out to determine the proportions of albumin and other proteins. Excretion mainly of albumin signifies a glomerular lesion. When the total daily protein excretion exceeds 3.5 g, by definition the nephrotic syndrome is considered to be present; milder albuminuria is called an *asymptomatic urinary abnormality*. The initial steps in evaluating proteinuria are outlined in Chap. 217. Subsequent details of differential diagnosis are in Chaps. 223 and 224. Tubular proteinuria usually reflects a hereditary or acquired tubular disorder (Chap. 228) or tubulointerstitial nephropathy (Chap. 226). The presence of large amounts of Bence Jones protein suggests that multiple myeloma may be present (Chap. 258).

HEMATURIA AND CASTS Isolated hematuria Bleeding in the urinary tract from the urethra to the renal pelvis produces isolated hematuria, without significant proteinuria, cells, or urinary casts. Total hematuria, which occurs evenly throughout voiding, means that blood has had the opportunity to mix fully with the bladder urine. When bleeding occurs mainly at the beginning or end of micturition, a prostatic or urethral origin is more likely.

FIGURE 40-1 *Top. Diagram showing normal structures separating the capillary lumen and urinary space in the glomerulus. In the process of glomerular filtration, an ultrafiltrate of plasma traverses the glomerular capillary wall through endothelial fenestrae, basement membrane, and slit diaphragms. Macromolecules in the plasma are believed to be restricted from entry into glomerular urine by each of these wall structures. In addition, circulating polyanions (e.g., albumin) are thought to be retarded by negatively charged glycosialoproteins, which, as shown by the shaded area in the upper panel, are distributed throughout the glomerular wall. Bottom. A corresponding electron micrograph of the same structures. (Drawing by NL Gahan from BM Brenner, R Beeuwkes, Hosp Prac, vol 13, no 7, 1978. Reproduced with permission.)*

Common causes of *isolated* hematuria are urinary tract stones, benign and malignant neoplasms of the urinary tract, tuberculosis, trauma, and prostatitis; few primary renal diseases cause it. As discussed in Chaps. 217 and 223, *focal glomerulitis,* in the syndrome of benign recurrent hematuria or in Berger's disease, i.e., IgA nephropathy, is usually associated with red blood cell casts. Analgesic nephropathy and sickling states cause isolated hematuria, but modest proteinuria; papillary necrosis or azotemia often is present and suggests a renal origin. Hemoglobin electrophoresis is appropriate whenever a sickling disorder is suspected.

Examination of the prostate and external urethra is the basic first step in the evaluation of isolated hematuria. Intravenous pyelography and renal ultrasonography are the next. If no lesion is found and no obvious cause of bleeding such as renal stone passage is present, cystoscopy and retrograde pyelography may become necessary. At cystoscopy, blood may be found to issue from only one ureter, a helpful clue which indicates a localized lesion rather than a primary renal disease. Disorders of coagulation, and thrombocytopenia, as well as urinary infection, must be excluded. Because infection with tuberculosis and fungi may be difficult to detect, multiple urine samples must be cultured and examined by microscopy. Computerized tomography of the kidney and sometimes renal arteriography may be needed to disclose anatomic lesions such as cysts or tumors.

Hematuria associated with urinary tract infection   Bacterial infection of the lower urinary tract or of the kidneys frequently causes hematuria. The presence of associated pyuria suggests the diagnosis of infection, and the demonstration of pathogenic bacteria in concentrations above 10^5 colonies per milliliter of urine establishes it. Acute cystitis or urethritis in women is an especially common cause of gross hematuria; in such symptomatic patients infection is documented by colony counts above 10^2 colonies per milliliter. Urinary tuberculosis can produce isolated hematuria, but pyuria often is present as well.

Hematuria with evidence of renal disease   NEPHRONAL HEMATURIA   Blood that enters the tubular fluid anywhere along the nephron can be trapped in a cylindrical mold of gelled Tamm-Horsfall protein to produce red blood cell casts. Tamm-Horsfall protein gels when concentrated at a low pH, as occurs during dehydration, or when exposed to myoglobin, hemoglobin, albumin, Bence Jones protein, and pyelographic contrast media. Degenerated red blood cells and clumps of hemoglobin can produce deeply pigmented casts that have the same significance—nephronal hematuria—as red blood cell casts.

Nephronal hematuria always connotes significant renal disease such as glomerulonephritis, tubulointerstitial injury, or a vasculitis that has damaged the circulation of the nephron. Glomerular or tubular proteinuria often accompanies renal bleeding, as a consequence of nephron injury. In general, nephronal hematuria of proteinuria alone arises from primary renal diseases that have a better prognosis than those in which proteinuria and hematuria occur in combination (Chap. 217).

Hematuria with proteinuria or casts   Frequently, hematuria is accompanied by proteinuria, but red blood cell and deeply pigmented granular casts are absent. The presumption then is that bleeding is of nephronal origin, but a coincident independent lesion of the urinary tract must always be considered, because common renal diseases, such as diabetic glomerulosclerosis and arteriolar nephrosclerosis associated with hypertension, produce mainly proteinuria.

TYPES OF CASTS   Heavy albuminuria or dehydration can cause showers of transparent, refractile "hyaline" casts. During heavy proteinuria, tubule cells fill with cholesterol-rich lipid droplets that display a Maltese-cross appearance in polarized light. Casts that incorporate these cells are called *fatty casts* because the lipid droplets are prominent. The same lipid-rich cells free in urine are called *oval fat bodies.*

White blood cell and epithelial cell casts can occur in any inflammatory state that involves the nephrons. White blood cell casts are particularly common in pyelonephritis, in nephritis associated with systemic lupus erythematosus, and during transplant rejection. When white blood or epithelial cells degenerate, they form granular nonpigmented casts that contain cellular debris and aggregated proteins. So-called *waxy* casts, with few granules and very distinct margins, arise when cell debris has broken down to a fine dispersion so that granules are no longer visible and are most common in chronic and progressive renal diseases.

Broad casts, of unusual width, are thought to arise in the dilated tubules of enlarged nephrons that have undergone compensatory hypertrophy in response to a reduction of functioning renal mass. A urine sample that contains a combination of broad and waxy casts as well as cellular or granular casts or red blood cells indicates a chronic smoldering process and has been termed a *telescoped* urine. This abnormality, first described in polyarteritis nodosa and systemic lupus erythematosus, can also be found in many chronic forms of glomerulonephritis with active glomerulitis.

Approach to the patient with hematuria   Many urinalyses should be performed to determine whether the hematuria is isolated or associated with other features of primary renal disease, i.e., cells, casts, or proteinuria. The magnitude and type of associated proteinuria should be determined. As a general rule intravenous pyelography should be performed, if it can be done safely, even when the hematuria is of definite nephronal origin. Not only lesions of the urinary tract, but renal tumors or cysts, discrete areas of papillary necrosis, or signs of renal venous obstruction may be present. The source of isolated hematuria must always be ascertained, and this means a detailed examination of the urinary tract by cystoscopy, retrograde pyelography, and arteriography to disclose tumor, stone, cysts, or other cause. Renal ultrasonography and computer-assisted tomography are particularly helpful in detecting and evaluating renal cysts and tumors and should precede cystoscopy and arteriography. If all the studies disclose normal structures, a nephronal origin of hematuria is likely even if no red blood cell casts are present. The role of renal biopsy in such cases is detailed in Chaps. 223, 224, and 226. Hematuria with infection or overt renal disease usually requires no steps beyond intravenous pyelography. Evaluation of hematuria is detailed further in Chap. 217.

POLYURIA AND NOCTURIA

POLYURIA   A reasonable definition of polyuria is a urine volume above 3 liters per day, but this should be qualified to exclude normal individuals who desire a large fluid intake and therefore form large volumes of urine. Patients cannot always distinguish polyuria from urinary frequency, the frequent voiding of small volumes. Since voiding volumes may not be clear from the history, polyuria must be substantiated by 24-h urine collection before one begins an investigation of causes.

Causes   Polyuria can arise from inadequate secretion of vasopressin, failure of the renal tubules to respond to vasopressin, solute diuresis, or natriuresis (Table 40-2). It may also occur as a physiologic adaptation to deliberate excessive water drinking. The normal physiology of urine formation and mechanisms responsible for renal water conservation are discussed in Chap. 218.

DIABETES INSIPIDUS (see also Chap. 323)   The term *diabetes insipidus* is applied to situations in which inadequate renal water conservation causes polyuria and secondary thirst. Either vasopressin insufficiency (central diabetes insipidus) or renal unresponsiveness to vasopressin (nephrogenic diabetes insipidus) may be responsible. In both, water reabsorption is reduced all along the distal nephron, because passive water movement from tubules into the hypertonic outer and inner medullary interstitium is slow. But even though the rate of water movement out of the collecting ducts is low for a given osmotic difference between the tubule lumen and interstitial fluid, the fluid that enters the collecting ducts is so abnormally dilute and copious in volume that more water enters the inner medulla than under normal circumstances and medullary solutes are washed out into the vasa recta. Wash-out is incomplete and vasopressin administration can lead to formation of an osmotically concentrated urine, but the maximal urine osmolality that can be attained is below normal.

Vasopressin-sensitive (central) diabetes insipidus may be idiopathic or secondary to hypophysectomy or trauma or to neoplastic, inflammatory, vascular, or infectious causes (Table 40-2). Idiopathic diabetes insipidus can be inherited as an autosomal dominant trait; but more commonly it is sporadic and appears in childhood. In both forms there is selective destruction of the neurons that produce vasopressin in the supraoptic nucleus.

Rarely, nephrogenic diabetes insipidus is familial and congenital; but usually it is acquired from renal disease (Table 40-2). Hypercalcemia and hypokalemic nephropathy are important reversible causes of nephrogenic diabetes insipidus. Lithium carbonate, methoxyflurane (1,1-difluoro-2,2-dichloroethyl methyl ether) anesthetic, and demeclocycline, a tetracycline derivative, can also produce nephrogenic diabetes insipidus.

SOLUTE DIURESIS Excessive filtration of a poorly resorbed solute such as glucose, mannitol, or urea can depress reabsorption of NaCl and water in the proximal tubule and cause their loss in the urine, producing polyuria. Urine Na concentration is below that of blood, so that more water than salt is lost from the body and serum hypertonicity can be produced. Glucosuria in diabetes mellitus is a common cause of solute diuresis. Iatrogenic solute diuresis may arise from mannitol infusion, angiographic contrast media, and high-protein gavage feedings, which produce an excessive excretion of urea. Any degree of solute diuresis can cause polyuria, so further evaluation of renal concentrating ability should be postponed until the solute diuresis is corrected.

NATRIURETIC SYNDROMES Excessive chronic Na loss may occur during the course of tubulointerstitial or cystic renal diseases. Polyuria and polydipsia are accompanied by an unusually large daily Na requirement. Examples of this phenomenon include medullary cystic disease, Bartter's syndrome, and the diuretic phase of acute tabular necrosis, in which Na and water losses are very large.

PRIMARY POLYDIPSIA Whether because of habit, predilection, psychiatric disorder, a specific lesion in the brain, or medication (Table 40-2), some people drink enough water every day to produce polyuria. The body and the kidneys rarely if ever are injured by chronic polydipsia, but the condition can be confused with diabetes insipidus, which it resembles closely. During deliberate polydipsia, extracellular fluid volume is normal or high, and vasopressin secretion is reduced to a basal level because serum osmolality tends to be near the lower limits of normal. Reabsorption of water from the end distal convoluted tubule and collecting ducts is reduced so that all the surplus water can be excreted into the urine. The inner medulla loses its urea and NaCl gradients because of wash-out, as in diabetes insipidus. Wash-out may be more severe than in diabetes insipidus because primary polydipsia tends to cause expansion of the extracellular fluid volume, whereas primary renal water loss does the opposite. Volume expansion raises total delivery of NaCl and water to the thick ascending limb of Henle's loop and therefore to the inner medulla, all things being equal. It also raises renal blood flow, and increased flow through the vasa recta reduces their ability to trap solutes in the medulla.

Approach to the patient with polyuria Solute diuresis and natriuretic syndromes usually are apparent from the history, physical examination, urinalysis (glucosuria), clinical setting, blood count, blood glucose, and serum creatinine or the BUN. Diagnostic problems occur mainly when stable, chronic polyuria and polydipsia of uncertain origin are present. Here, one must try to distinguish between vasopressin-sensitive diabetes insipidus, nephrogenic diabetes insipidus, and primary polydipsia; the best-established way to do this is by measuring the response of urine osmolality to water deprivation and the administration of vasopressin.

The patient should have free access to water and receive a normal diet that provides approximately 100 mmol NaCl per day for 3 days; then a total fast is instituted. During the fast, pulse and blood pressure should be measured every 30 min and body weight every hour, using an accurate balance. When 3 percent of the initial body weight has been lost or 14 h have elapsed, urine and serum osmolality are measured. A normal subject will lower urine volume below 0.5 mL/min and raise urine osmolality to above 700 mosmol per kilogram of water. In complete diabetes insipidus, nephrogenic or vasopressin-sensitive, the urine osmolality will remain below 200 mosmol/kg and urine flow will remain above 0.5 mL/min, but some rise in osmolality and fall in flow will occur given incomplete diabetes insipidus. If urine osmolality is below 700 mosmol/kg, by the end of the fasting period, 5 mU/min of aqueous vasopressin is administered by intravenous drip. Patients with complete or partial vasopressin-sensitive diabetes insipidus will raise their urine osmolality above the level achieved by fasting alone by more than 9 percent (see Chap. 323). No increase will occur given complete nephrogenic diabetes insipidus, although incomplete forms of nephrogenic diabetes insipidus will permit some response to vasopressin. Infusion of hypertonic saline (Chap. 323) is useful in defining defects of osmoregulator function.

The response of patients with primary polydipsia is quite different. During fluid restriction the secretion of vasopressin increases, and at the completion of the test the flow rate and osmolality of the urine will reflect a physiologic level of vasopressin acting upon normal tubules that traverse a medullary interstitium whose urea and NaCl concentrations have been reduced by chronic wash-out. In other words, the wash-out will set the upper limit on urine osmolality, and patients with primary polydipsia thus demonstrate a submaximal concentrating ability in spite of intact vasopressin secretion. Exogenous vasopressin can increase urine osmolality very little, <9 percent, because medullary wash-out, not vasopressin insufficiency or insensitivity, is the main limiting factor. Usually the urine osmolality will be above 400 mosmol/kg by the end of the fluid deprivation test, in contrast to the lower values of approximately 200 mosmol/kg encountered in patients with diabetes insipidus; but it may be impossible to distinguish incomplete diabetes insipidus from primary polydipsia, in some cases, by using the fluid deprivation test alone. However, measurement of serum antidiuretic hormone levels by radioimmunoassay may increase diagnostic accuracy.

NOCTURIA Whether an individual sleeps through the night without urinating depends upon a diurnal rhythm in which the volume of urine formed during sleep does not exceed bladder capacity, because of reduced renal osmotic concentration, high sodium excretion, solute diuresis, or low bladder capacity.

All the polyuric states may cause nocturia. Urinary concentrating

---

TABLE 40-2 Causes of polyuria

I Inadequate renal water conservation
  A Diabetes insipidus
    1 Vasopressin-sensitive (posthypophysectomy; posttrauma; postpituitary ablation; idiopathic, supra- or intrasellar tumors or cysts; histiocystosis or granuloma; encroachment by aneurysm; Sheehan's syndrome, meningoencephalitis; Guillain-Barré's syndrome; fat embolus; empty sella)
    2 Nephrogenic
      a Acquired tubulointerstitial renal disease (pyelonephritis, analgesic nephropathy, multiple myeloma, amyloidosis, obstructive uropathy, sarcoidosis, hypercalcemic or hypokalemic nephropathy, Sjögren's syndrome, sickle cell anemia, renal transplantation)
      b Drugs or toxins (lithium, demeclocycline, methyoxyflurane, ethanol, diphenylhydantoin, propoxyphene, amphotericin)
      c Congenital (hereditary nephrogenic diabetes insipidus, polycystic or medullary cystic disease)
  B Solute diuresis (glucosuria, high-protein tube feedings, urea or mannitol infusion, radiographic contrast media, chronic renal failure)
  C Natriuretic syndromes (salt-losing nephritis, diuretic phase of acute tubular necrosis, diuretic agents)
II Primary polydipsia
  A Psychogenic
  B Hypothalamic disease
  C Drugs (thioridazine, chlorpromazine, anticholinergic agents)

ability falls in most renal diseases (Chap. 218), often at an early stage. Even though overt polyuria may be absent, overnight urine volume frequently exceeds bladder capacity. Nocturia also occurs in edema-forming states. In congestive heart failure, nephrotic syndrome, and hepatic cirrhosis with ascites, fluid accumulates preferentially in dependent portions of the body during the day. At night, with recumbency, tissue capillary forces change and some edema fluid is mobilized, producing the effect of an intravenous saline infusion. Venous insufficiency may produce dependent edema of the legs that is often also mobilized at night, causing nocturia.

Reduced bladder capacity also causes nocturia. Infection, tumor, or stone can cause inflammation and increased irritability. Chronic partial bladder-outflow obstruction, from prostatic hypertrophy, urethral stricture, or benign or malignant neoplasm or stone, causes a frequent stimulus to void and also a thickening of the muscular wall that reduces its compliance. Frequent small voidings may be a clue to this lower urinary tract cause of nocturia, but in its earlier phases chronic obstruction may lead to only one nocturnal voiding of reasonable volume.

DYSURIA, FREQUENCY AND URGENCY, INCONTINENCE, AND ENURESIS

DYSURIA, FREQUENCY, AND URGENCY *Dysuria* refers to pain or burning during urination. *Urinary frequency* means voiding at abnormally brief intervals, due to a sense of bladder fullness that is due not to a full bladder but to a bladder that is irritable and feels full even when it is not. *Urgency* is an exaggerated sense of needing to urinate, due to an irritable or inflamed bladder.

Mechanisms of dysuria REDUCED BLADDER COMPLIANCE When the bladder has a decreased ability to expand, frequency, nocturia, and urgency usually result. When decreased expansion is due to inflammation of the mucosa (cystitis) from infection, radiation, chemicals, or foreign bodies (catheters, stones), burning usually is more prominent than when it is due to infiltration of the muscle by tumors of the bladder or from adjacent organs (prostate, rectum, uterus).

INFECTION Acute bacterial cystitis, which occurs more frequently in women, usually causes great frequency day and night, burning on urination, and, not infrequently, gross hematuria. Prostatitis or prostatocystitis in men can cause a picture similar to acute cystitis in women. When only the prostate is involved, milder symptoms such as vague pain or discomfort in the lower abdomen, groin, perineum, rectum, testes, or penis occur. The symptoms may be associated with urination but more frequently are noticed at times other than during micturition or ejaculation.

PSYCHOSOMATIC CYSTITIS The functional bladder syndrome and chronic glandular urethrotrigonitis are synonyms for a very common but poorly understood affliction of middle-aged and older women, in which pain is usually vague, aching in nature, and in the lower abdomen or vagina. There is daytime frequency without nocturia; pyuria is absent. A complete urologic evaluation usually becomes necessary because symptoms are chronic and hard to eradicate. The functional bladder syndrome must be distinguished from the effects of a cystocele, which can be repaired surgically. (See also Chap. 225.)

Approach to the patient with dysuria The medical history should focus on past as well as present urinary problems. A pelvic examination in women and prostatic examination in men are necessary components of the physical examination. Microscopic examination of a two-glass urinary sediment in all patients and of the prostatic fluid in men, obtained by prostatic massage, is also necessary. The first 20 mL of a voiding, if collected separately, may contain a higher concentration of leukocytes and bacteria than the remainder of the voided urine, when the urethra is the principal site of inflammation or infection.

Normal prostatic fluid, not subjected to centrifugation, contains less than 10 leukocytes per high-power field; excessive leukocytes in the prostatic fluid are an important clue to prostatitis and may, when prostatis is chronic, be the only detectable abnormality. Further diagnostic studies will depend upon such positive findings as a history of chronic or recurrent episodes or associated fever, which are rare in lower urinary tract infections except in acute prostatitis, or an abnormality on physical examination such as a pelvic or rectal mass or tenderness, hematuria or pyuria, or excessive leukocytes and macrophages in the prostatic fluid. Serum acid phosphatase may be elevated when carcinoma of the prostate has extended beyond the boundary of the prostatic capsule.

Additional evaluation of dysuria, when the cause is not evident from clinical examination, may include cultures of urine and prostatic fluid for aerobic and anaerobic bacteria, tubercle bacilli, and mycoplasma; excretory urography; and voiding cystourethrography. If these examinations do not reveal the diagnosis, but symptoms are troublesome, urologic evaluations, including cystoscopy and urethroscopy with endoscopic biopsies of visualized abnormalities, and dynamic urinary tract studies may be useful.

INCONTINENCE *Incontinence* refers to the inability to retain urine in the bladder. It results from neurologic or mechanical disorders of the complicated system that controls normal micturition.

Normal bladder function The detrusor muscle, which provides the propulsive force for emptying the bladder, consists of interlacing fibers of smooth muscle that are under parasympathetic autonomic control through the pelvic nerves from sacral spinal cord segments S2, S3, and S4. The smooth muscle of the trigonal portion of the bladder, between the ureteral orifices and the posterior area of the bladder outlet, is innervated by motor fibers from thoracolumbar segments (T11 to L2) of the sympathetic nervous system, in which alpha receptor sites predominate. This layer of muscle extends into the posterior urethra and acts as an involuntary internal sphincter that helps maintain urinary continence even in the absence of voluntary control. The external urethral sphincter and perineal muscles are under voluntary control via the pudendal nerves.

Sensory tracts of pain, temperature, and distention pass from the bladder via the pelvic nerves to sacral spinal levels S2, S3, and S4, creating a simple spinal voiding reflex between the bladder and the sacral spinal cord. The sensory tracts from the bladder further ascend through sacrobulbar pathways to the medulla of the brain and ultimately to cortical centers, from which impulses arise, pass back down the lateral and ventral reticulospinal tracts, and normally suppress the sacral spinal reflex arc controlling bladder emptying.

The normal adult bladder can accommodate as much as approximately 400 mL fluid without a significant increase in intravesical pressure (<20 cmH$_2$O). Above this point, sensations of fullness are transmitted to the sacral cord. If not suppressed by cortical control, the sacral cord reflexly discharges motor impulses that cause powerful sustained detrusor contraction. Urination can be prevented by cortical suppression of the reflex arc or by voluntary contraction of the external sphincter and perineal muscles. Infants, and adults with spinal cord damage above S2, urinate spontaneously when the bladder fills sufficiently.

Normal micturition is initiated by voluntary suppression of cortical inhibition of the reflex arc and by relaxation of the muscles of the pelvic floor and the external sphincter. The base of the bladder falls; then the trigone contracts, an action that occludes the ureters as they pass through the bladder wall and helps to prevent vesicoureteral reflux of urine during voiding. Finally, the detrusor contracts and voiding occurs.

Causes of incontinence DETRUSOR INSTABILITY In this condition, the bladder becomes prone to uncontrollable contractions—that cause incontinence—because inhibitory neural pathways are damaged. Among the elderly, detrusor instability causes as much as 70 percent of urinary incontinence, and arises from diseases of the central nervous system such as cerebrovascular accidents, Alzheimer's dementia, neoplasm, and, possibly, normal pressure hydrocephalus. Any lesion that disrupts the lateral and vertical reticulospinal tracts can reduce or abolish descending inhibiting impulses to the sacral spinal reflex and can result in detrusor instability. If the descending tracts are completely destroyed, the bladder will empty automatically. Bladder or pelvic infection or tumor, fecal impaction, uterine prolapse, and prostatic hypertrophy are other causes. Whatever the cause, the usual clinical picture is of unpredictable, involuntary voiding, usually >160 mL each time. Imipramine, 25 mg at bedtime, or calcium channel blockers (such as nifedipine) reduce detrusor contractions, and improve continence. Local infection, tumors, or fecal impaction are treated conventionally.

STRESS INCONTINENCE   This condition is common in postmenopausal parous women. The structures of the female urethra atrophy when deprived of estrogen, and many become unable to resist the passage of urine under the stress of increased intraabdominal pressure during coughing, sneezing, climbing stairs, and other physical activity, so small amounts of urine escape. Parturition may damage the pelvic support of the bladder so that the bladder and urethra can slip downward from their normal position above the pelvic diaphragm. As they do, the urethra shortens, and the normal urethrovesical angle, important in closing the urethral sphincter, is lost. In men, stress incontinence usually is secondary to prostatic surgery for benign prostatic hypertrophy or prostatic carcinoma. If the external sphincter has also been damaged during operation, total incontinence may result. Surgical elevation of the urethrovesicle angle is helpful in women. Estrogen replacement therapy may prevent atrophy of the urethral mucosa.

MECHANICAL INCONTINENCE   Some congenital anomalies, extrophy of the bladder, patent urachus, and ectopic ureteral openings distal to the vesical neck cause mechanical incontinence. They are all correctable only by surgery. Acquired mechanical incontinence can follow transurethral resection of the prostate in which damage has occurred to both the internal and external sphincter mechanisms. Pelvic surgery or irradiation of the uterus or rectum may cause incontinence because of vesicovaginal, ureterovaginal, vesicoperineal, or ureteroperineal fistulas.

OVERFLOW OR PARADOXICAL INCONTINENCE   This form of incontinence arises from large residual volumes of urine secondary to obstruction at the bladder neck or along the urethra (urethral stricture) or from neurologic damage. Benign prostatic hypertrophy afflicts upward of 75 percent of older men. It is manifested by nocturia, reduced size and force of the urinary stream, straining to urinate, and terminal dribbling, all due to outflow obstruction. Functional outflow obstruction can occur because of spinal cord disease; the detrusor and external sphincter contract dyssynergistically, i.e., at the same time. Hypotonic neurogenic bladders may occur in diseases which produce autonomic peripheral neuropathy, such as diabetes mellitus, uremia, hypothyroidism, chronic alcoholism, Guillain-Barré syndrome, collagen vascular diseases, and toxic neuropathies associated with some carcinomas (especially lung and kidney). It also may occur because of prolonged overdistention of the bladder. Hydronephrosis and impaired renal function can occur in patients with chronic overflow incontinence. All causes produce a dilated, palpable bladder. Especially in diabetes, patients can control micturition but lose their sensory awareness of bladder filling. Their incontinence can be avoided by scheduled reminders. Outlet obstruction is treated surgically. If the bladder has become adynamic because of prolonged overfilling, bethanechol chloride, 50 to 100 mg per day, may improve emptying.

PSYCHOGENIC AND FUNCTIONAL INCONTINENCE   Children, and even some young adults, draw attention to themselves by feigning incontinence and thereby derive some secondary emotional satisfaction. A complete diagnostic evaluation usually is necessary to rule out organic disease even when psychogenic incontinence is strongly suspected. In elderly people, especially those who have a limited ability to walk

or who are confused because of central nervous system disease or drugs, incontinence may be *functional*, i.e., due simply to an inability to reach a toilet in time. Treatment depends upon correcting the individual problem in each case.

ENURESIS   *Enuresis* refers to the involuntary passage of urine at night or during sleep—hence, the synonym bed-wetting. Some clinicians reserve the term enuresis for those bed wetters who have no gross urologic abnormalities, but it should be used for bed-wetting in general.

The sacral spinal reflex arc alone controls urination in the infant; therefore, enuretic incontinence is normal under the age of 2 years. As the nervous system matures, cortical control over the spinal reflex arc results in the voluntary control over urination and defecation by the age of $2\frac{1}{2}$ years. Even so, enuresis beyond the age of 3 years occurs to some degree in approximately 10 percent of all otherwise normal children and probably is due to a delay in maturation of bladder control, which may be familial.

Although the majority of bed wetters will be dry by the age of puberty, organic diseases, especially infections of the urinary tract, obstructive lesions with overflow incontinence, neurovesical dysfunction, and polyuric conditions that overload the bladder must be suspected in any child who is enuretic beyond the age of 3 years. Patients with organic disease usually, but not always, are incontinent during the day as well as at night. For the majority, who have no overt lesions, imipramine (75 mg at bedtime) may be useful.

REFERENCES

Azotemia, oliguria, and anuria

ABUELO JG: Proteinuria: Diagnostic principles and procedures. Ann Intern Med 98:186, 1983

BRENNER BM et al: Molecular basis of proteinuria of glomerular origin. N Engl J Med 298:826, 1978

BRIDGES CR et al: Glomerular charge alterations in human minimal charge nephropathy. Kidney Int 22:677, 1982

GLASSOCK RJ et al: Primary glomerular diseases, in *The Kidney*, 3d ed, BM Brenner, FC Rector Jr (eds). Philadelphia, Saunders, 1986, p 929

KURTZMAN NA (ed): *Seminars in Nephrology: Acute Renal Failure*, JP Knochel (guest ed). New York, Grune & Stratton, 1981

——— (ed): *Seminars in Nephrology: Chronic Renal Failure*, G Eknoyan (guest ed). New York, Grune & Stratton, 1981

OKEN DE: On the differential diagnosis of acute renal failure. Am J Med 71:916, 1981

PARDO V et al: Benign primary hematuria: Clinicopathologic study of 65 patients. Am J Med 67:817, 1979

Polyuria and nocturia

BERL T (ed): Disorders of water metabolism, in *Seminars in Nephrology*, vol 4. New York, Grune & Stratton, 1984, p 285

ROBERTSON GL, BERL W: Pathophysiology of water metabolism, in *The Kidney*, 3d ed, BM Brenner, FC Rector Jr (eds). Philadelphia, Saunders, 1986, p 385

SCHRIER RW, BICHET DG: Osmotic and nonosmotic control of vasopressin release and the pathogenesis of impaired water excretion in adrenal, thyroid, and edematous disorders. J Lab Clin Med 98:1, 1981

ZERBE RL, ROBERTSON GL: A comparison of plasma vasopressin measurements with a standard indirect test in the differential diagnosis of polyuria. N Engl J Med 305:1539, 1981

Dysuria, frequency and urgency, incontinence, and enuresis

BRADLEY WE: Diagnosis of urinary bladder dysfunction in diabetes mellitus. Ann Intern Med 92:323, 1980

BRADLEY WE, SCOTT FB: Physiology of the urinary bladder, in *Urology*, 4th ed, JH Harrison et al (eds). Philadelphia, Saunders, 1978, vol 1, p 87

DEGROAT WC, BOOTH AM: Physiology of the urinary bladder and urethra. Ann Intern Med 92:312, 1980

HINDMARSH HR, BYRNE PO: Adult enuresis: A symptomatic and urodynamic assessment. Br J Urol 52:88, 1980

MEARES EM JR: Prostatitis syndromes: New perspectives about old woes. J Urol 123:141, 1980

MIKKELSEN EJ, RAPOPORT JL: Enuresis: Psychopathology, sleep stage, and drug response. Urol Clin North Am 7:361, 1980

PLATT R: Quantitative definition of bacteriuria. Infectious Diseases Symposium, July 28, 1983, p 44, Supplement to Am J Med

TURNER-WARWICK R, WHITESIDE CG (eds): *Symposium on Clinical Urodynamics: The Urologic Clinics of North America*, vol 6. Philadelphia, Saunders, 1979

WILLIAMS ME, PANNELL FC: Urinary incontinence in the elderly. Ann Intern Med 97:895, 1982

41   FLUIDS AND ELECTROLYTES

NORMAN G. LEVINSKY

SODIUM AND WATER

PHYSIOLOGIC CONSIDERATIONS (See also Chap. 218) Both physiologically and clinically, sodium and water metabolism are closely interrelated. The sodium content of the body depends on the balance between dietary intake and renal excretion of sodium. In health, extrarenal losses of sodium are negligible. Renal sodium excretion is closely regulated to match dietary content. Within 2 to 4 days after sodium intake stops, urinary excretion decreases to 5 meq per day or less. If dietary sodium is abruptly increased, sodium excretion promptly rises and equals intake within a few days. Thus, in normal persons the sodium content of the body remains quite constant despite wide variations in sodium intake; over the range of 0 to 400 meq per day, total body sodium varies only by about 10 percent.

Renal sodium excretion is regulated by the interplay of multiple control mechanisms. Sodium loads or deficits tend to produce corresponding changes in the central blood volume. Receptors, apparently located in the atria and central arteries, respond to changes in local pressure or flow which signal the volume/capacity relation of the central circulation (*effective blood volume*). If the effective volume is depleted, salt retention is induced, while expansion triggers multiple factors that favor natriuresis. With volume (salt) depletion, renal blood flow falls, due to decreased cardiac output, increased renal sympathetic nerve activity, and activation of the renin-angiotensin system. Glomerular filtration also tends to fall, which reduces filtered sodium. Tubular reabsorption of sodium is enhanced. Proximal reabsorption is stimulated by changes in Starling forces (e.g., increased plasma protein concentration) in the peritubular circulation and by sympathetic nerves which innervate proximal segments directly. Distal tubular reabsorption is enhanced by aldosterone, which is secreted at an increased rate in response to stimulation of the adrenal gland by angiotensin. Volume expansion leads to the opposite changes in renal hemodynamics and in these various regulators of tubular transport. Moreover, one or more natriuretic hormones are secreted in response to increased extracellular volume. Their nature and role are less well defined than that of aldosterone. Peptides in the cardiac atria can increase sodium excretion acutely by hemodynamic or tubular mechanisms. There is some evidence for another natriuretic hormone which decreases tubular salt transport by inhibiting Na-K adenosine triphosphatase (ATPase). Prostaglandins reduce sodium reabsorption in distal nephron segments.

Undoubtedly, other regulatory mechanisms remain to be defined. The multiplicity of control mechanisms prevents abnormalities of any single mechanism from grossly distorting the regulation of sodium excretion. For example, increased aldosterone secretion leads only to limited and transient sodium retention, because the initial accumulation of sodium stimulates opposing natriuretic factors such as increased glomerular filtration and decreased proximal tubular sodium reabsorption.

All but 2 to 5 percent of the sodium in the body is located in the extracellular fluids. (Approximately 40 percent of total body sodium is located in bone, but this fraction does not participate significantly in most physiologic processes and will not be considered further.) Except for minor differences in concentration due to the Gibbs-Donnan effect of plasma proteins, the electrolyte compositions of plasma and interstitial fluid are essentially equal. Consequently, plasma composition can be considered representative of the entire extracellular compartment. Total extracellular volume approximates 20 percent of body weight. Of this, 5 percent represents plasma volume and 15 percent the volume of interstitial fluids. Thus, in a 70-kg individual with plasma sodium concentration of 140 meq per liter, extracellular sodium content will approximate 2000 meq. The volume of intracellular fluid is approximately twice as great as that of extracellular fluid, i.e., about 40 percent of body weight. However, since intracellular sodium concentration is less than 5 meq per liter, total intracellular sodium content is only about 100 to 150 meq. The asymmetric distribution of sodium across cell membranes is maintained by expenditure of a large fraction of the energy derived from cell metabolism, which is required constantly to pump sodium out of cells against its electrochemical gradient. All the principal electrolytes are asymmetrically distributed across cell membranes. The principal electrolytes of the extracellular fluids are sodium, chloride, and bicarbonate. The major electrolytes of the intracellular fluids are potassium, magnesium, calcium, and organic anions, including proteins.

Since sodium salts account for more than 90 percent of the total osmolality of the extracellular fluid, variations in plasma sodium concentration are almost always reflected in equivalent changes in plasma osmolality. Exceptions due to accumulation of other solutes in plasma are discussed later. Although the electrolyte compositions of intracellular and extracellular fluids differ markedly, they are always in osmotic equilibrium, since water moves rapidly across cellular membranes to dissipate osmotic gradients. Therefore, although sodium is largely confined to extracellular fluids, plasma sodium concentration is an index of not only the relative proportions of sodium and water in those fluids but also the relation between total body solute and total body water. An example is the effect of shift of sodium from extracellular to intracellular fluid without a change in total body solute. Movement of sodium into cells would not cause hyponatremia, since water would shift into cells with the sodium. On the other hand, a primary decrease in the concentration of osmotically active solute within cells would decrease total body solute; although there would be no change in total body sodium or water, hyponatremia would result from the shift of intracellular water into the extracellular compartment.

A very effective mechanism involving the *hypothalamus,* the *neurohypophysis,* and the kidney regulates plasma osmolality. Changes of 2 percent or less in plasma osmolality can be detected by osmoreceptors in the hypothalamus. Small increases in osmolality stimulate the secretion of antidiuretic hormone (ADH) from the neurohypophysis, while small decreases suppress secretion of the hormone. Normal plasma osmolality is approximately 280 to 300 mosmol per kilogram of water; the exact level is determined by the "set" of the hypothalamic osmoreceptors in a given individual. When ADH secretion is maximal, urine volume will be about 500 mL per day, and urine osmolality will be 800 to 1400 mosmol/kg. In the absence of ADH, minimal urine osmolality is 40 to 80 mosmol/kg, and maximum water diuresis can reach 15 to 20 liters per day or more. The capacity of this receptor-effector system is sufficient to maintain plasma osmolality within narrow limits despite large variations in the volume and concentration of dietary fluids. ADH secretion is also regulated by changes in extracellular volume. A reduction of 10 percent or more may trigger ADH release even in the absence of changes in plasma osmolality. If volume contraction is sufficiently severe, volume-mediated stimulation of ADH may override osmotic signals and cause water retention despite progressive dilution of body fluids. Conversely, extracellular volume expansion tends to suppress ADH release even if the body fluids are hypertonic.

The total sodium *content* of the body is determined by the renal sodium regulatory mechanisms described earlier. However, the principal determinant of plasma sodium *concentration* is water metabolism rather than total body sodium content. If excess sodium were to be ingested and retained, hypernatremia would be only transient. Water intake would increase because of thirst, and the fluid ingested would be retained because hypernatremia (hyperosmolality) would stimulate ADH secretion. Expanded extracellular volume, not hypernatremia, would be the end result. Conversely, if the osmoregulatory system is functioning normally, loss of moderate amounts of sodium without water would not result in permanent reduction of plasma sodium concentration. The initial reduction would shut off secretion of ADH, and a water diuresis would ensue. The final outcome would be contraction of extracellular volume, while plasma sodium concentration would be restored to normal. It follows that changes in total sodium content tend to cause changes in extracellular volume. In this sense, the sodium content of the extracellular fluid determines extracellular volume. On the other hand, changes in plasma sodium concentration reflect altered regulation of water excretion, not changes in total body sodium content alone. Clinically, plasma sodium concentration per se gives no information about the amount of sodium present in the body. Total body sodium content is determined by the volume of extracellular fluids as well as by the concentration of sodium in these fluids. Extracellular volume is usually the dominant factor since changes in volume tend to be proportionately greater than changes in sodium concentration. Plasma sodium concentration reflects the relative proportions of sodium and water (or, more exactly, of total body solute and water), not the absolute amount of sodium in the body. Either hyponatremia or hypernatremia may occur when total body sodium content is decreased, normal, or increased.

CLINICAL DISORDERS Deficits and excesses of sodium and water occur in a great variety of clinical circumstances. The manifestations of the underlying illness may overshadow the clinical features of the fluid and electrolyte disorder. Theoretically, disturbances of sodium and water metabolism can be classified into four categories, reflecting a primary excess or deficit of water or sodium. Practically, such isolated disturbances are uncommon. A primary excess of sodium leads to edema; it is not ordinarily considered as an electrolyte disorder but as a feature of underlying disease, such as congestive heart failure, hepatic cirrhosis, or nephrotic syndrome. Primary sodium deficits are nearly always accompanied by water depletion, leading to the clinical syndrome of extracellular volume depletion. Pure or disproportionate water excess leads to hyponatremia, relative or absolute water depletion to hypernatremia. A practical clinical classification of disorders of sodium and water metabolism is given in Table 41-1.

VOLUME DEPLETION Combined sodium and water deficits are far more frequent than isolated deficits of either constituent. Although the term *dehydration* is often used for combined deficits, this usage is confusing. Dehydration should be used to describe relatively pure water depletion leading to hypernatremia; *volume depletion* or some similar term should be used for combined deficits.

Pathogenesis As noted earlier, elimination of sodium from the diet will not by itself lead to sodium depletion in the presence of normal renal function, since urinary sodium excretion will quickly fall to very low levels. Therefore, sodium depletion is always due either to extrarenal losses or to abnormal renal losses.

GASTROINTESTINAL The most common cause of volume depletion is loss of a significant fraction of the 8 to 10 liters of gastrointestinal fluids normally secreted daily. Since the principal secretions contain potassium and hydrogen ion or bicarbonate in large amounts, volume depletion due to gastrointestinal losses is often combined with potassium depletion and acidosis or alkalosis.

Significant volume depletion may be caused by sequestration of secretions within an obstructed gastrointestinal tract or within the peritoneal cavity in peritonitis. Rapid reaccumulation of ascites after paracentesis may cause contraction of the effective circulating blood volume.

SKIN The sodium concentration of sweat varies from 5 to 50 meq per liter; sodium concentration increases with higher rates of sweating and in adrenal insufficiency. Because sweat is always a hypotonic solution, sweating leads to water deficits out of proportion to sodium losses. In burns, capillary damage may lead to sequestration of large amounts of sodium and water in the injured skin.

RENAL Abnormal losses of sodium and water in the urine may occur in both acute and chronic renal diseases. Early in the recovery (diuretic) phase of *acute renal failure,* urinary sodium concentration tends to be high (50 to 100 meq per liter), and substantial deficits of both sodium and water may ensue. With rare exceptions, severe sodium and water wasting does not persist beyond the first few days. It is important to discriminate between increased excretion, which represents elimination of excess retained during the oliguric period, and true tubular sodium and water wasting, which depletes normal extracellular volume. Only the latter requires replacement. Acute salt and water wasting due to tubular damage may also occur immediately after relief of prolonged *obstruction* of the urinary tract. Although such a postobstructive diuresis may be severe, it rarely persists for more than several days as a clinically important phenomenon.

Patients with *chronic renal failure* have limited ability to decrease sodium and water excretion in response to decreased intake. They will become progressively volume-depleted if their intake is restricted by the anorexia, nausea, and vomiting characteristic of uremia or because of their physician's instructions. Large deficits may develop insidiously over many days or weeks. A "self-perpetuating cycle" may result, in that volume depletion will tend further to compromise renal function. Severe sodium-wasting renal disease, i.e., negative sodium balance when dietary sodium is normal, is rare. It occurs in occasional patients with tubulointerstitial diseases of the kidney, especially medullary cystic disease.

Renal sodium wasting in the presence of normal intrinsic renal function occurs in three clinical circumstances. Perhaps the most common is sodium depletion due to continued administration of potent *diuretics* to patients after edema has been relieved or to patients whose edema is sequestered and cannot be mobilized. For example, attempted treatment of cirrhotics with ascites may result in depletion of overall extracellular volume rather than mobilization of ascitic

---

TABLE 41-1   Disorders of sodium and water metabolism

I Combined sodium and water depletion (volume depletion)
  A Extrarenal losses
    1 Gastrointestinal (vomiting, diarrhea, gastrointestinal suction, fistulas)
    2 Abdominal sequestration (peritonitis, rapid reaccumulation of ascites)
    3 Skin (sweating, burns)
  B Renal losses
    1 Renal disease (chronic renal failure, salt-wasting tubular disease, diuretic phase of acute renal failure, postobstructive diuresis)
    2 Diuretic excess
    3 Osmotic diuresis (diabetic glycosuria)
    4 Mineralocorticoid deficiency (Addison's disease, hypoaldosteronism)
II Hyponatremia
  A Associated with extracellular volume depletion (see list of causes above)
  B Associated with extracellular volume excess and edema
  C Associated with normal or modestly expanded extracellular volume (no edema)
    1 Acute and chronic renal failure
    2 Temporary impairment of water diuresis (pain, drugs, emotion)
    3 Syndrome of inappropriate secretion of antidiuretic hormone (SIADH)
    4 Severe polydipsia
    5 Endocrine (glucocorticoid deficiency, hypothyroidism)
    6 Essential ("sick cell syndrome")
  D Without plasma hypoosmolality
    1 Osmotic (hyperglycemia, mannitol)
    2 Artifactual (hyperlipemia, hyperproteinemia, laboratory error)
III Hypernatremia
  A Due solely to water loss
    1 Extrarenal
      a Skin (insensible losses)
      b Lungs
    2 Renal
      a Diabetes insipidus (central, nephrogenic)
    3 Hypothalamic dysfunction
  B Due to water loss associated with sodium loss
    1 Extrarenal
      a Sweat
    2 Renal
      a Osmotic diuresis (glycosuria, urea)
  C Due to sodium gain
    a Excessive sodium administration
    b Adrenal hyperfunction (hyperaldosteronism, Cushing's syndrome)

fluid. An obligatory *osmotic diuresis* may also cause renal sodium and water wasting despite normal renal function. Marked glycosuria in uncontrolled diabetes mellitus is the most frequent clinical example. Administration of osmotic diuretics such as mannitol is a common iatrogenic cause. Volume depletion in patients receiving high-protein enteral or parenteral alimentation may be due to an osmotic diuresis of urea formed by protein metabolism. Finally, renal sodium wasting despite normal intrinsic function occurs in Addison's disease and hypoaldosteronism due to a *deficiency* of *mineralocorticoids*.

Clinical features and diagnosis   The cause of volume depletion can usually be suspected from a history of inadequate salt and water intake together with vomiting, diarrhea, or excessive sweating; the symptoms of poorly controlled diabetes mellitus or of renal or adrenal disease may be elicited. The key findings on physical examination are those of plasma and extracellular volume depletion. Decreased skin turgor is usually present in patients with significant volume contraction but may be difficult to evaluate in the elderly. It can be estimated clinically by noting the slow rate of return of skin to its original position when it is raised between the examiner's fingers. An area of skin normally free of wrinkles and not subject to wide variations in the thickness of subcutaneous tissue, such as that over the sternum, should be selected for this maneuver. Oral mucous membranes may be dry and axillary sweating decreased; these are less reliable diagnostic features than decreased skin turgor. With moderate volume depletion, blood pressure is usually normal when the patient is recumbent, although resting tachycardia may be present. Postural hypotension, i.e., a drop of at least 5 to 10 mmHg in the sitting or standing position, is often present. With greater degrees of volume depletion, even recumbent blood pressure is reduced, and frank shock may occur. The patient with moderate or severe degrees of volume contraction is often lethargic, weak, confused, or obtunded. Such patients are usually oliguric, even when recumbent blood pressure is normal. However, an osmotic diuresis, as occurs in hyperglycemia, tends to prevent oliguria despite volume contraction.

LABORATORY FINDINGS   The hematocrit and plasma protein concentration are increased, but values within the normal range are interpretable only if prior values are known. Plasma sodium concentration may be decreased, normal, or increased, depending upon the proportion between deficits of sodium and of water. Plasma creatinine and urea nitrogen are usually increased, since the glomerular filtration rate is decreased ("prerenal azotemia"). Urinary sodium concentration may be of value in differentiating extrarenal and renal sources of sodium loss if the probable cause is not clear from the history. With extrarenal losses, urinary sodium concentration will be less than 10 meq per liter; the concentration will usually exceed 20 meq per liter if renal or adrenal disorders are at fault. However, urinary sodium may ultimately fall below this level even in patients with renal salt wasting if sodium depletion becomes severe.

Treatment   The principal clinical manifestations of extracellular volume depletion are due to reduction of plasma and interstitial fluid volume. Since there is no convenient clinical method for assessing these volumes, the effect of treatment must be determined by following the clinical changes in parameters such as blood pressure, urine output, and skin turgor. Modest deficits of sodium and water can often be corrected by increased oral intake in patients not suffering from gastrointestinal disorders. Severe depletion requires therapy with intravenous solutions. Isotonic saline (0.85%) is the infusion of choice in patients whose serum sodium concentration is approximately normal. The amount to be infused can be estimated from the history of prior losses and from the severity of the physical findings of extracellular volume contraction. Patients with moderate volume contraction usually require replacement with 2 to 3 liters of saline, while patients with severe depletion may require much larger volumes. The need for correction of other concurrent electrolyte abnormalities may alter the composition of the required infusion; e.g., some of the sodium may be given as bicarbonate to patients with volume contraction and metabolic acidosis, or potassium may be added in patients with concurrent potassium depletion. In estimating the total amount to be infused, allowance for ongoing losses must be included. Since the amount to be infused cannot be calculated precisely, patients should be monitored carefully to avoid fluid overload and congestive failure.

HYPONATREMIA Pathophysiology   Hyponatremia indicates that the body fluids are diluted by an excess of water relative to total solute. Hyponatremia is not equivalent to sodium depletion, which is only one of the clinical states in which it may occur (see Table 41-1). Most types of hyponatremia result from defective urinary dilution. The normal response to dilution of body fluids is a water diuresis, which corrects the hypoosmotic state. Normal water diuresis requires three factors: (1) Secretion of ADH must be suppressed. (2) Sufficient sodium and water must reach the diluting sites of the nephron, in the ascending limb of Henle's loop and the distal convoluted tubule. (3) These nephron segments must function normally, reabsorbing sodium while remaining impermeable to water.

Correspondingly, three types of mechanisms may cause defective water diuresis in patients with hyponatremia. (1) Secretion of ADH may continue "inappropriately" despite hypotonicity of extracellular fluid, which normally shuts off secretion of the hormone. This may be due to unregulated release of ADH by neoplasms or to nonosmotic stimuli to ADH secretion. The latter include volume depletion and neural factors such as pain and emotion. (2) Insufficient sodium may reach the diluting segments to permit the formation of an adequate amount of dilute urine. Inadequate delivery of tubular fluid to distal sites may be due to reduced glomerular filtration and/or enhanced proximal tubular reabsorption. Even in the absence of ADH, distal tubular segments are not absolutely impermeable to water; small amounts of water continue to leak from the hypotonic tubular fluid into the isotonic cortical and slightly hypertonic medullary interstitial fluid. The amount of water leaking back in this manner becomes an increasingly larger fraction of the volume of dilute urine formed, as the diluting process is progressively limited by decreasing delivery. Hence, urine osmolality rises progressively. In some instances, this mechanism may even result in excretion of a urine hypertonic to plasma, despite the absence of ADH. (3) Sodium transport in the diluting segments may be defective, or water permeability may be excessive at these sites even in the absence of ADH. One of these three factors can account for most types of hyponatremia, as described below.

Types of hyponatremia (Table 41-1)   In patients with extracellular *volume depletion,* delivery of sodium and water to the diluting segments of the nephron is reduced because of decreased glomerular filtration, increased proximal tubular reabsorption, or both. ADH secretion is stimulated by the volume contraction. These changes in renal function and hormone secretion limit water diuresis during extracelluar volume depletion. Hyponatremia per se is usually of little clinical significance in sodium (volume) depletion. The major features are those of extracellular volume contraction, described above. Reduction of plasma sodium concentration by more than 10 to 15 meq per liter is rare in the absence of obvious decreases in skin turgor, postural or recumbent hypotension, and some degree of azotemia. Treatment is directed to correction of the volume deficits. In the occasional symptomatic patient with sodium depletion whose plasma sodium concentration is less than 125 meq per liter, some of the intravenous sodium replacement fluids should be administered as hypertonic saline.

In *edematous states* such as congestive heart failure, cirrhosis, and the nephrotic syndrome, hyponatremia paradoxically appears to result from mechanisms similar to those that cause hyponatremia in patients with volume depletion. Although plasma or extracellular volume is normal or increased in most edematous patients, it is believed that the "effective" volume is reduced by decreased cardiac output or sequestration of fluid outside the central circulation. The decrease in "effective" volume results in diminished delivery of sodium and water to nephron diluting segments, because of reduced glomerular filtration, increased proximal tubular reabsorption, or both. Volume-mediated secretion of ADH is also triggered in these conditions. In some edematous patients essential hyponatremia may be an additional mechanism (see below). In edematous states, the severity and frequency of hyponatremia correlate to some extent with the magnitude of the edema and the seriousness of the underlying condition. Hyponatremia is usually present in patients with advanced disease unless water intake is restricted. The hyponatremia itself is often of little clinical significance. The principal features are those of the underlying disease. However, symptomatic hyponatremia may occur, most often in connection with vigorous diuretic therapy or excessive oral or parenteral intake of dilute fluids.

Hyponatremia associated with edema responds to effective treatment of the underlying disease. Moderate nonprogressive hyponatremia in edematous patients usually does not cause symptoms. Attempts to correct such hyponatremia by restriction of fluid intake induce thirst and discomfort without improving the clinical picture or longevity. Patients with severe or progressive hyponatremia may require some restriction of water intake, especially during vigorous treatment with diuretics. However, moderate limitation to the range of 1000 to 1500 mL per day will often suffice to avoid symptoms of progressive hyponatremia. More severe restriction should be instituted only if specific clinical or laboratory observations warrant. Since edematous subjects have excess total extracellular sodium, hypertonic saline should not be administered except in rare instances in which clinical manifestations of extreme hyponatremia, such as coma or convulsions, justify emergency measures. Furosemide should be given concurrently in such cases to avoid further expansion of the extracellular space. Dialysis can also be used to correct severe hyponatremia without increasing volume in edematous patients.

Multiple factors contribute to hyponatremia caused by *diuretics*. Salt loss may cause volume depletion, which limits water diuresis by mechanisms already described. Furosemide, ethacrynic acid, and thiazides inhibit salt reabsorption in the diluting segments of the nephron and thereby directly limit water diuresis. Thiazides appear to be the diuretics most commonly associated with hyponatremia, probably because they interfere with elaboration of a hypotonic urine by inhibiting sodium reabsorption in the distal convoluted tubule but, unlike loop diuretics, do not limit urine concentration and water retention by interfering with salt transport in the loop of Henle. In addition, potassium depletion caused by many diuretics contributes to hyponatremia through uncertain mechanisms. Hyponatremia due to diuretic therapy is frequent but usually minor in severity. However, moderate or severe hyponatremia may occur in patients who receive diuretics and who drink large quantities of water or other hypotonic fluids. Progressive hyponatremia is an important complication of diuretic therapy in edematous patients, in whom the underlying disease tends to cause hyponatremia (see above) and to whom large doses of diuretics may be given. The treatment of hyponatremia due to diuretics is water restriction and repletion of potassium deficits.

Hyponatremia may result from *impaired water excretion* not associated with a substantial deficit or excess of salt. In this case, extracellular volume is only modestly expanded. Since excess water is distributed throughout both intracellular and extracellular fluids in proportion to their volumes, only one-third of a water excess will be retained in the extracellular compartment. *Oliguric* patients develop dilutional hyponatremia if the volume of oral and intravenous fluids is not restricted appropriately. The ability to excrete a normal volume of dilute urine is progressively limited in advancing *chronic renal failure*. Regulation of water intake by thirst usually prevents dilutional hyponatremia. However, hyponatremia may be precipitated by increased fluid intake (for example, if the patient is instructed to force fluids). Since the ability to regulate salt excretion is also limited in chronic renal failure, in many patients hyponatremia is associated with edema or salt depletion. In patients with normal renal function, water diuresis may be limited temporarily by ADH secretion induced by various neural stimuli such as pain and narcotics. In the postoperative state, these factors, together with administration of large

volumes of hypotonic fluids, may cause hyponatremia. The etiology of hyponatremia is usually evident from the clinical setting and a careful review of fluid intake and output. This type of hyponatremia is treated by water restriction. Only if severe symptoms occur is hypertonic saline infusion required.

Hyponatremia in patients with the *syndrome* of chronic *inappropriate* secretion of *antidiuretic hormone* (SIADH) is principally due to water retention, but continued urinary losses of sodium also contribute to a mild negative sodium balance. Renal sodium wasting is related to modest volume expansion, since it can be eliminated by restricting fluid intake. The mechanisms by which extracellular expansion increases sodium excretion have been discussed above. Clinically, SIADH is defined by a unique group of features: (1) Urine osmolality is not maximally dilute even when marked hyponatremia is induced by water loading. In most cases, urine osmolality exceeds plasma osmolality. (2) Plasma creatinine and urea are normal or low, indicating that the glomerular filtration rate is normal or increased. (The elaboration of hypertonic urine is presumptive evidence of ADH secretion if the glomerular filtration rate is normal.) (3) During fluid loading (even if the fluid is saline), hyponatremia increases due to water retention and urinary sodium wasting. It should be noted that sodium wasting during volume expansion may be minimal or even absent in patients with extreme degrees of hyponatremia. (4) During restriction of fluid intake, hyponatremia and urinary sodium wasting are corrected. This response is helpful in occasional patients in whom it may be difficult to distinguish SIADH from mild volume depletion as the cause of hyponatremia. The plasma uric acid also may be of value in making this distinction. Since uric acid excretion tends to vary with "effective" extracellular volume, hyperuricemia is common in volume depletion while hypouricemia is usual in SIADH.

SIADH has been found frequently in patients with oat cell carcinoma of the lung but has also been described in patients with a variety of other *neoplasms*. In some of these patients the tumor secretes ADH or a substance with analogous biologic activity (see also Chap. 323). The syndrome has also been reported in patients with various disorders of the *central nervous system*, including meningitis, encephalitis, tumors, trauma, stroke, and porphyria. It is assumed that ADH in these patients is secreted in response to direct stimulation of the hypothalamic osmoreceptors. *Pulmonary* diseases associated with SIADH, in addition to tumors, include a wide variety of infections.

Pharmacologic agents that induce SIADH include (1) the oral hypoglycemic agents chlorpropamide and tolbutamide; (2) the antineoplastic and immunosuppressive agents vincristine and cyclophosphamide; (3) psychoactive drugs such as haloperidol, thioridazine, carbamazepine, and amitriptyline; and (4) clofibrate. These agents exert their antidiuretic effect either by potentiating the tubular action of small amounts of ADH or by stimulating inappropriate secretion of ADH.

Hyponatremia due to SIADH responds to limitation of fluid intake; restriction to the range of 1000 to 1200 mL per day is ordinarily adequate. Occasional patients who are symptomatic despite water restriction may be treated by enhancing water excretion. This can be accomplished either by increasing solute excretion (by taking a high-salt, high-protein diet or ingesting urea) or by antagonizing ADH with demeclocycline or lithium. Initial therapy with hypertonic saline infusions may be required in a few patients with marked hyponatremia. Concurrent administration of furosemide may facilitate correction of hyponatremia in those patients who do not respond promptly to hypertonic saline alone.

Hyponatremia may occur in certain endocrine disorders, notably adrenal insufficiency and hypothyroidism. Multiple factors appear to play a role in limiting water diuresis in patients with *adrenal insufficiency*. Deficient secretion of mineralocorticoid hormones may lead to sodium depletion, with consequent reduction of glomerular filtration and enhancement of proximal tubular sodium reabsorption. Moreover, glucocorticoid deficiency directly reduces filtration. Therefore, adrenal insufficiency will tend to decrease delivery of sodium to diluting sites. In addition, glucocorticoid deficiency prevents the maintenance of normal water impermeability in distal diluting segments of the nephron. This appears to be due to inappropriate secretion of ADH, although glucocorticoid deficiency may have a direct effect on water permeability of distal tubular epithelium. Since patients with adrenal insufficiency may have the combination of defective dilution of the urine and sodium wasting, hyponatremia due to Addison's disease can occasionally be confused with SIADH. Usually, other clinical features of adrenal insufficiency such as hyperkalemia, pigmentation, and hypoglycemia suggest the correct diagnosis. However, specific tests of adrenal function are indicated whenever the diagnosis is in doubt. Hyponatremia due to adrenal insufficiency is corrected by appropriate hormonal therapy.

Hyponatremia may develop in moderate or severe *hypothyroidism.* Decreased delivery of tubular fluid to diluting segments and persistent release of ADH both limit water excretion in this condition. The diagnosis of this type of hyponatremia is made by recognizing the clinical features of hypothyroidism and from the response to treatment with thyroid hormone.

The normal kidney can excrete 15 to 20 liters of dilute urine per day. Normal water intake, regulated by thirst and habit, is a small fraction of this maximum excretory capacity. Rarely, *psychogenic polydypsia* may be so severe that the rapid ingestion of huge quantities of fluids may overwhelm normal excretory capacity and produce symptomatic dilutional hyponatremia despite normal renal diluting mechanisms. Hyponatremia of this type is diagnosed from the history of massive fluid intake, most often in patients with other evidence of psychiatric illness. Since water excretory capacity is normal, the urine is maximally dilute in this condition. Hyponatremia due to psychogenic polydypsia responds to water restriction. Rare patients who are symptomatic due to extreme degrees of hyponatremia may require intravenous infusion of hypertonic saline.

Some patients may be hyponatremic in the absence of a defect in water diuresis. The terms *essential hyponatremia* and *sick cell syndrome* have been applied to this category. Osmoreceptor cells in the hypothalamus are thought to be "reset" to maintain a decreased level of body fluid osmolality as though it were normal. Urine becomes dilute or concentrated, respectively, if plasma sodium falls or increases slightly from the new "normal" level for the particular patient. The genesis of such a syndrome is speculative. Changes in cellular metabolism may lead to a primary reduction in cellular osmolality. Another possibility is that essential hyponatremia is a variant of SIADH in which there is a nonosmotic stimulus to ADH secretion. When plasma osmolality is reduced sufficiently, osmotic suppression of ADH secretion overcomes the nonosmotic stimulus.

Essential hyponatremia may occur in a variety of chronic illnesses, such as pulmonary tuberculosis, congestive heart failure, and hepatic cirrhosis. This type of hyponatremia is asymptomatic; skin turgor, blood pressure, and renal function are normal, unless altered by the primary disease. Definitive diagnosis of essential hyponatremia requries the demonstration of normal urinary dilution in response to water loading, normal urinary concentration during dehydration, and normal renal sodium excretory responses to sodium loading and restriction. This type of hyponatremia does not require treatment.

Hyponatremia due to *accumulation* of *osmotically active solutes* in the plasma is the sole exception to the rule that hyponatremia means decreased plasma osmolality. In this type of hyponatremia, plasma osmolality is increased. Plasma sodium is diluted by movement of water out of cells along the osmotic gradient created by the addition of a solute such as glucose or mannitol. (High plasma urea levels in patients with renal failure do not cause hyponatremia because urea concentration is equal across cell membranes.) The diagnosis of hyponatremia due to increased plasma concentrations of osmotically active solutes is usually apparent from the history and clinical features of uncontrolled diabetes. Plasma sodium concentration will decrease by about 1.6 meq per liter with every elevation of 100 mg/dL in plasma glucose above normal. This type of hyponatremia should also be considered whenever there is a history of recent administration of mannitol, especially to oliguric patients unable to excrete it promptly. Since plasma osmolality is increased, clinical manifestations of hypotonicity are absent in this type of hyponatremia.

In patients with severe hyperlipemia or, very rarely, with extreme hyperproteinemia, *artifactual* hyponatremia may be reported by the laboratory. In severe hyperlipemia part of any unit volume of plasma

FIGURE 41-1 *Flow chart for differential diagnosis of causes of hyponatremia. Categories (A, B, C, D) and types (C1–6) are keyed to Table 41-1. Abbreviations: Nl = normal; ECF = extracellular fluid; creat = creatinine;* *CHF = congestive heart failure; BP = blood pressure; Uosm = urinary osmolality; U_{Na} = urinary Na, meq per liter; ↓ = decreased, ↑ = increased.*

taken for analysis will be lipid, which is sodium-free. This type of hyponatremia rarely occurs unless the plasma is grossly milky. In patients with extreme hyperproteinemia, proteins occupy more than the normal 7 percent of plasma volume, thereby reducing the proportion of aqueous sodium-containing fluid per unit of plasma taken for analysis. In both cases, hyponatremia will be reported by the laboratory because the sodium concentration will be low in milliequivalents per liter of plasma. However, sodium concentration per liter of plasma water and plasma osmolality are normal; hence, this type of hyponatremia has no clinical significance.

Differential diagnosis Although the type of hyponatremia can be defined easily in most patients, precise diagnosis may be difficult in some. More than one type of hyponatremia may occur in a specific disease entity. For example, hyponatremia in patients with hepatic cirrhosis is usually associated with edema or is due to excessive administration of diuretics, but essential hyponatremia may also occur in this condition. Moreover, current categories may prove artificial or inaccurate when the pathophysiology of hyponatremia is more completely understood and specific diagnostic tests such as a radioimmunoassay for ADH are readily available. Despite these limitations, the classification outlined above is a useful framework for diagnosis and treatment.

Figure 41-1 is a flow chart that outlines the major steps in determining the cause of hyponatremia. First, assess extracellular fluid (ECF) volume. The history and physical examination are usually sufficient to determine whether the hyponatremia is associated with a decreased, increased, or normal extracellular volume. In occasional patients, moderate volume depletion may not readily be separable from normovolemia by clinical examination. In that event, measurement of blood urea nitrogen (BUN) and plasma creatinine may be helpful. The plasma creatinine, and especially the BUN, tend to be increased when hyponatremia is associated with volume depletion and normal or decreased when it is associated with a normal or expanded extracellular volume, as in SIADH. The various types of normovolemic hyponatremia can frequently be recognized by a careful review of specific features of the history, such as associated diseases, drug therapy, and fluid intake. However, laboratory tests, such as measurement of serum cortisol, may be needed to confirm a diagnosis.

Measurements of urinary sodium concentration and osmolality are common in the workup. *Urinary sodium concentration* is low (under 10 meq per liter) if hyponatremia is associated with edema or with volume depletion due to extrarenal causes. Urine sodium concentration usually exceeds 20 meq per liter if hyponatremia is due to renal salt losses or to renal failure with water retention. In SIADH, urine sodium concentration usually exceeds 20 meq per liter unless fluid intake has been restricted. Since impaired water diuresis is the mechanism of most types of hyponatremia, measurement of *urinary osmolality* is not usually of value. A maximally dilute urine would be expected only in hyponatremia due to extreme polydipsia or at times in essential hyponatremia. With other causes, urinary osmolality exceeds 150 mosmol per kilogram of water; usually the urine is hypertonic to plasma.

Clinical manifestations Neurologic dysfunction is the principal clinical manifestation of hyponatremia. It is due to intracellular movement of water, leading to swelling of brain cells. The severity of symptoms is related both to the degree of hyponatremia and to the rapidity with which it develops. In chronic hyponatremia, the degree of brain swelling caused by any given reduction in body fluid osmolality is reduced because solute, largely potassium chloride, is lost from the cells. Patients may be lethargic, confused, stuporous, or comatose. If hyponatremia develops rapidly, signs of hyperexcitability such as muscular twitches, irritability, and convulsions may occur. Hyponatremia rarely causes clinical symptoms when plasma sodium is above 125 meq per liter, although occasionally symptoms may occur at higher levels if the decrease in concentration has been rapid.

Treatment Appropriate therapy for the various types of hyponatremia has been outlined. Hyponatremia itself is often of little significance and requires no specific treatment. If severe, symptomatic hyponatremia requires intravenous treatment; the amount of sodium given should be calculated by multiplying the deficit in plasma sodium concentration (milliequivalents per liter) by the total body water (approximately 50 to 60 percent of body weight). Although the administered sodium will remain in the extracellular compartment, the osmotic effect of hypertonic saline will cause water to shift out of cells. The amount needed to raise plasma sodium concentration to the range of 125 to 130 meq per liter should be calculated and infused over several hours. The patient's symptoms and clinical status, especially with respect to circulatory congestion, should be carefully assessed throughout the infusion. Furosemide may be given if fluid overload is present initially or develops during the infusion. Complete correction of hyponatremia, if indicated, is usually best carried out more slowly by water restriction or oral sodium supplementation if possible. Some studies, although controversial, have raised the possibility that rapid, complete correction of hyponatremia may cause neurological damage (central pontine myelinolysis).

HYPERNATREMIA Pathophysiology Hypernatremia is due to a deficit of body water relative to total body solute or sodium content. Without exception, hypernatremia indicates that the body fluids are hypertonic. Normally, minimal increases in tonicity stimulate both thirst and release of ADH. Although renal water retention induced by ADH helps to correct hypernatremia, thirst appears to be the principal defense mechanism. Hypernatremia is usually modest in patients with diabetes insipidus, who lack ADH and may excrete 15 liters or more of urine per day. Thirst stimulates water intake enough to balance even such large water losses. Severe persistent hypernatremia occurs only in patients who cannot respond to thirst by voluntary ingestion of fluid, e.g., infants or mentally obtunded patients. In such individuals, loss of dilute body fluids progressively elevates body fluid osmolality. Initial losses of water are from the extracellular compartment, but water deficits are rapidly equilibrated throughout total body water. The rise in extracellular fluid tonicity causes intracellular water to shift into the extracellular compartment. In effect, approximately two-thirds of pure water deficits are derived from intracellular fluid. Hence, extracellular volume depletion occurs in patients with relatively pure deficits of water only when such deficits are large. The principal clinical features are attributable to decreased intracellular volume, especially dehydration of cells in the central nervous system. Brain cells appear to adapt to chronic hyperosmolality by accumulating increased intracellular solute. When hyperosmolality is rapidly corrected, the increase in total intracellular solute may promote brain swelling even at normal or slightly elevated plasma osmolality. These mechanisms may account for the fact that rapid correction of hypertonicity sometimes causes deterioration of central nervous function. The identity of the excess brain solute is uncertain; electrolyte accumulation accounts for only part of the excess.

Pathogenesis (Table 41-1) For clinical purposes it is useful to classify hypernatremia as due to water loss alone; to water deficits associated with, but proportionately in excess of, sodium deficits; or to retention of sodium. Pure water deficits may be due to extrarenal or renal water losses that are not replaced. Insensible losses of water from the skin or lungs may reach several liters per day, especially in patients with fever, increased respirations, or extensive burns. Renal losses may lead to hypernatremia in diabetes insipidus. Alert patients with diabetes insipidus ordinarily maintain normal or only slightly hypertonic body fluids despite massive renal water wasting by increasing fluid intake appropriately. However, diabetes insipidus may develop acutely after cerebral trauma or neurosurgical procedures. In such patients, careful attention to replacement of urinary losses is mandatory to avoid severe hypernatremia. Defective thirst and ADH regulation occurs in rare patients with hypothalamic disorders, which may be idiopathic ("essential hypernatremia") or due to specific causes such as tumors, granulomas, and cerebrovascular accidents.

Water losses leading to hypernatremia are often associated with sodium deficits. In such cases, the clinical features of extracellular volume depletion and hypernatremia may both be present, and either may predominate. Extrarenal losses of salt and water due to profuse sweating and renal losses due to osmotic diuresis are the major causes of hypernatremia in this category. Since sweat is hypotonic, hypernatremia will develop if profusely sweating patients cannot drink. In an osmotic diuresis, urinary sodium concentration is less than plasma concentration; therefore, hypernatremia tends to occur. Hypernatremia due to a urea diuresis may develop when patients unable to complain of thirst are placed on high-protein feeding. Examples include patients with severe cerebrovascular accidents who are unable to swallow and postoperative neurosurgical patients. In the syndrome of hyperosmolar nonketotic diabetic coma, severe hyperosmolality of the body fluids is due to a combination of hyperglycemia and relative or absolute hypernatremia. The hypernatremia is a consequence of an intense glucose osmotic diuresis in patients who are unable to ingest fluids. Since hyperglycemia itself causes hyponatremia by inducing a shift of water from cells, the presence of hypernatremia in the face of extreme hyperglycemia indicates that total body water is severely depleted.

Infrequently, hypernatremia may result from an absolute excess of sodium rather than from water depletion. Examples are hypernatremia caused by accidental substitution of salt for sugar in infant feeding formulas and administration of excessive amounts of hypertonic sodium chloride or bicarbonate infusions to comatose adults unable to drink. The cause of the common mild hypernatremia in patients with adrenal hyperfunction is uncertain. Presumably, stimulation of renal tubular sodium reabsorption by adrenal steroids initiates the hypernatremia, and the hypervolemia that results resets upward the threshold for ADH release. It is not known why the thirst mechanism fails to maintain normal body fluid osmolality.

Clinical features and diagnosis The principal manifestations of hypernatremia are observed in the central nervous system. Confusion and other evidence of altered mental state; increased neuromuscular irritability, such as twitching and seizures; and obtundation, stupor, or coma may all occur. The magnitude of symptoms depends on the severity of the hyperosmolality. The symptoms are similar whether hyperosmolality is due to hypernatremia or extreme hyperglycemia. The neurologic symptoms appear to be due to dehydration of brain cells. The clinical manifestations of acute hypernatremia are more marked than those of slowly developing hypernatremia. Severe hyperosmolality may cause irreversible neurologic sequelae, apparently due to vascular consequences such as venous sinus thrombosis and hemorrhage from vessels that rupture when the brain shrinks. High mortality rates are associated with extreme hyperosmolality, especially in children and in the elderly.

In patients with pure water deficits, manifestations of extracellular volume depletion are minimal because only one-third of the deficit is derived from extracellular fluid. As noted, combined deficits are common, especially in patients who sweat or experience an osmotic diuresis; in such individuals, the signs and symptoms of volume depletion may overshadow those of hypernatremia.

The cause of hypernatremia can usually be inferred from the history when it is due to extrarenal water loss, an osmotic diuresis, or sodium excess. In these cases, the urine is hypertonic to plasma. The differential diagnosis of pituitary and nephrogenic diabetes insipidus, in which urine concentrating ability is impaired, is discussed in Chap. 323.

Treatment Hypernatremia itself is corrected with water by mouth or by intravenous infusion of 5% dextrose in water. Calculation of water requirements must be based on total body water, since water deficits are drawn from both intracellular and extracellular fluid and both must be repleted. For example, suppose a 70-kg man has a plasma sodium of 160 meq per liter which is to be lowered to 140.

Total body water is estimated as 60 percent of 70 kg, which is 42 liters. To reduce plasma sodium, this volume must be increased to $(160/140) \times 42$ liters, which equals 48 liters. Thus, a positive water balance of 6 liters $(48 - 42)$ is required. Hypernatremia should be corrected slowly; no more than half the water deficit should be replaced in the first 12 to 24 h. As stated above, rapid correction of hypertonicity may cause central nervous function to deteriorate.

In patients with associated sodium deficits, saline solutions should be infused. If the predominant clinical feature is extracellular volume depletion with circulatory insufficiency, treatment should begin with 0.9% saline to replete extracellular volume promptly. If the neurologic effects of hypertonicity predominate, therapy can start with 0.45% saline. In patients with hyperosmolar diabetic coma, sodium deficits are usually large, due to prior glucose osmotic diuresis. Plasma hypertonicity is due to both hyperglycemia and hypernatremia. Treatment consists of isotonic saline (0.9%) to replete extracellular volume and insulin to lower plasma glucose and thereby partly correct hypertonicity. Later, hypotonic saline (0.45%) can replace the remaining water and salt deficits and return plasma sodium to normal.

POTASSIUM

PHYSIOLOGIC CONSIDERATIONS Potassium is the principal intracellular cation. Active transport mediated by Na^+-K^+-stimulated ATPase in cell membranes maintains a cellular concentration of approximately 160 meq per liter, 40 times that in extracellular fluid. All but 2 percent of the 2500 to 3000 meq potassium in the body is within cells. Since potassium is a large fraction of total cellular solute, it is a major determinant of the volume of the cell and the osmolality of the body fluids. Moreover, potassium is an important cofactor in a number of metabolic processes. Extracellular potassium, while a small fraction of the total, greatly influences neuromuscular function. The ratio of intracellular to extracellular potassium concentration is the principal determinant of membrane potential in excitable tissues. Since extracellular potassium concentration is low, small deviations in concentration produce large variations in this ratio; conversely, only large changes in intracellular potassium influence the ratio significantly. These relationships have practical consequences. For example, toxic effects of hyperkalemia can be mitigated by inducing movement of potassium from extracellular fluid into cells.

The relation between plasma and cellular potassium is complex and is influenced by a number of factors, including acid-base balance. Acidosis tends to shift potassium out of cells, and alkalosis favors movement from extracellular fluid into cells. The relation between blood pH and plasma potassium is complex and is influenced by several factors, including the type of acidosis, the duration of the altered acid-base state, and the change in plasma bicarbonate per se. In general, plasma potassium changes less with respiratory acidosis than with metabolic acidosis and less with alkalosis than with acidosis. While the magnitude of the change in plasma potassium cannot be predicted from changes in blood pH alone, a patient with normal total body potassium tends to be hyperkalemic if acidotic and hypokalemic if alkalotic. Hormones also influence the distribution of potassium between extracellular fluid and cells. Insulin, beta-adrenergic catecholamines, and possibly aldosterone promote movement of potassium into cells. These hormones appear to be important parts of the mechanism for moving potassium loads out of plasma. Conversely, alpha-adrenergic agonists impair potassium uptake into cells.

During potassium depletion, plasma potassium initially decreases about 1 meq per liter for each 100 to 200 meq lost. However, plasma potassium falls more slowly after it reaches 2 meq per liter. Thus, a plasma potassium in the range of 2 to 3.5 meq per liter is a reasonably accurate guide to the magnitude of depletion, but plasma potassium concentrations less than 2 meq per liter may reflect a wide range of deficits, from moderate to severe. Plasma concentration increases about 1 meq per liter after acute administration of 100 to 200 meq potassium. Assuming an extracellular volume of 15 liters, 150 meq would be expected to raise plasma potassium by about 10 meq per liter. Thus, the largest fraction of administered potassium rapidly enters cells. Renal excretion also increases promptly. Chronic exposure to high-potassium diets enhances both tissue uptake and renal excretion of the ion; the mechanism of these adaptations is uncertain. Sustained hyperkalemia rarely is caused by excess intake, because these mechanisms normally function so efficiently. Impaired renal excretion and cellular transfer are the usual causes of hyperkalemia.

Of the usual potassium intake of 50 to 150 meq per day, most is excreted in the urine. Normally, stool and sweat contain only about 5 meq per day. As noted, the kidneys respond to acute and chronic changes in potassium intake by corresponding changes in excretion. Excess potassium is excreted promptly; about half of an acute load appears in the urine within 12 h. The renal response to potassium depletion is more sluggish. Excretion does not fall to minimal levels for 7 to 14 days. During this period, a deficit of 200 meq or more may develop in an individual on a potassium-deficient diet. Renal excretory mechanisms for potassium are complex. Potassium in the urine is secreted in the distal convoluted tubule and collecting duct; filtered potassium is nearly quantitatively reabsorbed in more proximal segments. Potassium secretion appears to be determined by the potassium concentration of tubular cells and by an electrochemical gradient favoring diffusion of the ion into tubular fluid. Net excretion is the resultant of secretion and concurrent reabsorption in the distal segments. Among the key influences on this complex system are aldosterone, distal tubular fluid flow rate, acid-base balance, and factors that alter distal tubular electronegativity. Aldosterone stimulates potassium secretion. Thus, hyperkalemia increases potassium excretion by two mechanisms: it stimulates adrenal secretion of aldosterone, and it directly enhances renal secretion, presumably via increased tubular cell potassium. Potassium secretion in the distal tubule is flow-dependent; increased distal delivery of tubular fluid favors potassium excretion. For example, loop diuretics, which enhance distal volume delivery, increase potassium excretion, especially in patients with edema and secondary aldosteronism. Alkalosis enhances and acidosis depresses renal potassium secretion, probably by inducing corresponding changes in tubular cell potassium. If delivery to distal segments of sodium salts of unreabsorbable anions such as excess bicarbonate or carbenicillin is augmented, tubular electronegative potential will increase as sodium is reabsorbed. The enhanced electrical gradient will promote potassium excretion.

POTASSIUM DEPLETION AND HYPOKALEMIA Pathogenesis The

principal causes of potassium depletion are listed in Table 41-2. As noted, renal excretion of potassium falls slowly in persons on potassium-deficient diets. During the 10 to 14 days before balance is achieved, significant deficits may occur. Thus, in contrast to sodium, moderate potassium depletion may result from *poor intake* alone. Potassium deficiency is frequent in *gastrointestinal disorders* in which vomiting, diarrhea, or loss of gastrointestinal secretions is prominent. Diarrhea may cause large potassium deficits, since the potassium concentration of liquid stool is 40 to 60 meq per liter. *Loss of gastric secretions* through vomiting or vasogastric suction is also a common cause of potassium depletion. The potassium concentration of gastric fluid is 5 to 10 meq per liter; direct losses contribute only modestly to negative potassium balance. The potassium deficit is primarily due to increased renal excretion. Potassium excretion appears to be stimulated by three mechanisms. Loss of gastric acid leads to *metabolic alkalosis,* which increases tubular cell potassium concentration. The elevated plasma bicarbonate concentration also increases delivery of bicarbonate and fluid to the distal nephron. Finally, secondary hyperaldosteronism due to associated extracellular volume contraction may play a role in maintaining potassium excretion at high levels despite potassium depletion.

All *diuretics* in common use except spironolactone, triamterene, and amiloride promote potassium excretion. In edematous patients with secondary aldosteronism, these agents often cause hypokalemia

and potassium depletion. Although hypokalemia also occurs in patients receiving diuretics for treatment of hypertension, potassium depletion is modest if dietary potassium is normal and there are no other factors that stimulate potassium excretion. Potassium excretion is increased during an *osmotic diuresis*. This mechanism leads to potassium depletion in patients with diabetic ketoacidosis, in whom the osmotic diuresis is due to glycosuria and to increased excretion of keto acid anions. However, potassium depletion may be masked by the shift of potassium out of tissues caused by the diabetic acidosis. Failure to recognize potassium depletion may lead to serious cardiotoxicity from sudden hypokalemia when the acidosis is corrected with insulin or alkali. A normal plasma potassium concentration in an acidotic patient strongly suggests potassium depletion.

Urinary potassium loss is often due to *excessive mineralocorticoid activity*. Hypokalemia is characteristic of *primary aldosteronism* but may be minimal in patients with restricted sodium intake. *Secondary aldosteronism* causes renal potassium wasting and hypokalemia in patients with malignant hypertension, Bartter's syndrome, and renin-secreting renal tumors. *Licorice* contains a compound with mineralocorticoid activity; patients who consume huge amounts may become hypokalemic. Excessive levels of *glucocorticoids* stimulate secretion of renal potassium (and hydrogen), leading to hypokalemia and alkalosis in patients with *Cushing's syndrome* and those receiving *therapeutic steroids*.

Renal tubular potassium wasting is a feature of *renal tubular acidosis* (Chap. 228). Some patients with monocytic or myelomono-cytic *leukemia* develop hypokalemia. The mechanism is uncertain. Renal potassium wasting in some patients appears to correlate with lysozymuria, and the enzyme may interfere with tubular function. In *Liddle's syndrome,* a rare familial disorder (Chap. 228), renal potassium wasting is an intrinsic tubular abnormality. Certain *antibiotics* may cause hypokalemia by increasing potassium excretion. Carbenicillin in large amounts promotes distal tubular secretion by acting as an unreabsorbed anion; amphotericin B alters distal tubular permeability. Gentamicin has also been reported to cause hypokalemia by unknown mechanisms.

Magnesium depletion can cause potassium depletion, apparently due to increased renal and possibly gastrointestinal losses. Increased aldosterone secretion may play a role in stimulating potassium excretion. Hypokalemia in this condition is associated with hypocalcemia.

Clinical features and diagnosis The most prominent features of hypokalemia and potassium depletion are neuromuscular. Moderate degrees of depletion may be asymptomatic, especially if they develop slowly. Some patients, however, complain of muscle weakness, especially in the lower extremities. With more severe or acute degrees

TABLE 41-2 Causes of potassium depletion and hypokalemia

I Gastrointestinal
   A Deficient dietary intake
   B Gastrointestinal disorders (vomiting, diarrhea, villous adenoma, fistulas, ureterosigmoidostomy)
II Renal
   A Metabolic alkalosis
   B Diuretics, osmotic diuresis
   C Excessive mineralocorticoid effects
      1 Primary aldosteronism
      2 Secondary aldosteronism (including malignant hypertension, Bartter's syndrome, juxtaglomerular cell tumor)
      3 Licorice ingestion
      4 Glucocorticoid excess (Cushing's syndrome, exogenous steroids, ectopic ACTH production)
   D Renal tubular diseases
      1 Renal tubular acidosis
      2 Leukemia
      3 Liddle's syndrome
      4 Antibiotics
   E Magnesium depletion
III Hypokalemia due to shift into cells (no depletion)
   A Hypokalemic periodic paralysis
   B Insulin effect
   C Alkalosis

of hypokalemia and potassium deficiency, marked and generalized weakness of skeletal muscles is prominent. Very severe or abrupt development of hypokalemia may lead to virtually total paralysis, including the respiratory muscles. Rhabdomyolysis may occur. On physical examination, in addition to decreased motor power, the patient may demonstrate decreased or absent tendon reflexes. The smooth muscle of the gastrointestinal tract may be affected, resulting in paralytic ileus.

Abnormalities in the electrocardiogram are common (Chap. 178). The characteristic changes include flattening and inversion of the T wave, increased prominence of the U wave, and sagging of the ST segment. These alterations are not well correlated with the severity of the disturbance in potassium metabolism and cannot be relied on as indexes of the clinical significance of a potassium deficit. Although moderate potassium depletion rarely affects cardiac action, severe or rapid reduction in serum potassium may cause cardiac arrest. Potassium deficiency enhances the cardiac toxicity of digitalis preparations. A variety of atrial and ventricular arrhythmias may occur in hypokalemia, especially in patients receiving digitalis.

Renal tubular function is markedly impaired by potassium depletion (Chap. 226). The most prominent abnormality is decreased concentrating ability, which may cause polyuria and polydipsia. Glomerular filtration rate is normal or slightly reduced; moderate reductions may occur with chronic potassium depletion nephropathy. Renal regulation of potassium excretion remains normal. The urinalysis is benign: protein excretion is normal or minimally increased, and the urinary sediment is normal or demonstrates only a slight increase in hyaline or granular casts.

DIAGNOSIS   The cause of hypokalemia and potassium depletion is usually evident from the history. However, patients whose potassium deficiency is caused by chronic abuse of laxatives; psychogenic, self-induced vomiting; or surreptitious use of diuretics rarely volunteer an accurate history. Patients with villous adenomas of the rectum sometimes report that their feces are formed; careful questioning will reveal the elimination of the characteristic mucous secretion of the tumor.

When the history is obscure, *evaluation of urinary potassium excretion* may be helpful in determining the origin of the potassium deficit (Fig. 41-2). If gastrointestinal losses have occurred, urinary excretion is usually less than 20 to 25 meq per liter or per day. Although renal conservation of potassium is slow, excretion falls to these levels by the time that clinically significant deficits of potassium have accumulated. On the other hand, when renal potassium wasting is the cause, urinary concentration usually exceeds 20 meq per liter and excretion is more than 25 meq per day. However, lower concentrations and lower excretion rates may be found in severe depletion, in those patients with excessive mineralocorticoid activity while on low sodium intake, and in patients whose diuretics have been stopped at the time of examination. *Measurement of blood pH* also may help in differential diagnosis. A normal pH or alkalosis is present in most patients who are potassium-depleted. Hypokalemia is associated with acidosis in renal tubular acidosis, diarrhea, and diabetic ketoacidosis, and in patients treated with carbonic anhydrase inhibitors. A third clue to diagnosis is the presence of *hypertension,* which suggests hyperaldosteronism (except Bartter's syndrome) or glucocorticoid excess. Blood pressure is normal in patients whose potassium depletion is due to the other causes listed in Table 41-2. Figure 41-2 is a flow chart which outlines the steps in differential diagnosis of hypokalemia when the cause is not evident from the history.

Treatment   When possible, potassium depletion should be corrected by increased dietary intake or supplementation with potassium salts. Potassium chloride is the salt of choice, especially in alkalotic patients. It may be given in the form of an elixir or in tablets in which potassium chloride crystals are imbedded in a wax. Enteric-coated potassium chloride tablets have been responsible for ulceration of the small bowel, due to release of high concentrations of potassium salts. Organic salts such as gluconate or citrate are adequate in patients who are not severely alkalotic and often are used to treat hypokalemia due to renal tubular acidosis. In edematous patients treated with diuretics that cause hypokalemia, potassium deficits should be prevented or treated by increased dietary potassium intake, supplementation with potassium chloride, or addition of "potassium-sparing" diuretics such as spironolactone. More controversial is the need for routine dietary supplements in patients receiving diuretics for treatment of hypertension. Patients with adequate dietary potassium intake usually do not develop significant hypokalemia and probably do not require routine supplements to prevent potassium depletion. However, those who do develop hypokalemia despite adequate diets should probably receive potassium salts, since hypokalemia may be associated with an increased frequency of arrhythmias.

Intravenous treatment is required for patients with gastrointestinal

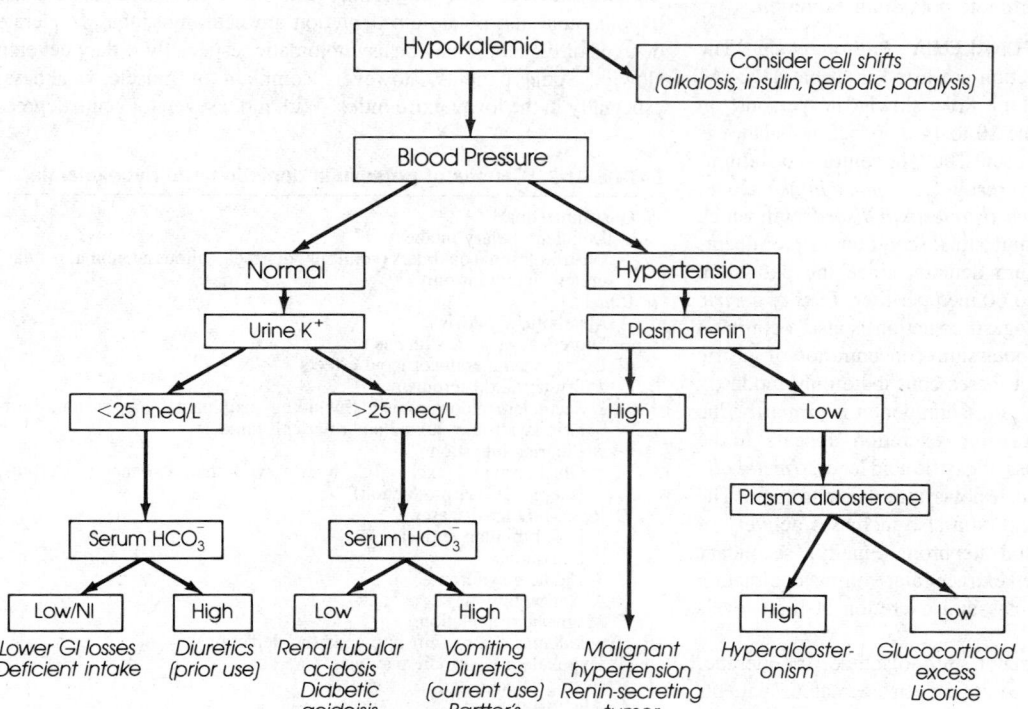

FIGURE 41-2 *Flow chart for differential diagnosis of principal causes of hypokalemia.*

disorders or when the potassium deficiency is severe. It must be emphasized that the potassium *concentration* in commonly available intravenous solutions of potassium chloride is 2000 meq per liter. Concentrations in intravenous infusions should not exceed 40 or at the most 60 meq per liter. The rate of infusion should not exceed 20 meq/h or approximately 200 to 250 meq per day, unless the need for more rapid infusion has been demonstrated in the individual patient by evidence of continuing losses large enough to justify more intensive therapy. The results of treatment are best monitored by repeated determinations of plasma potassium and evaluation of clinical symptoms such as muscular weakness or paralysis. Disappearance of electrocardiographic abnormalities correlates only roughly with improvement in total body potassium content. However, during rapid intravenous administration of potassium, the electrocardiogram should be monitored to avoid cardiac toxicity from inadvertent hyperkalemia.

Hypokalemia and hypocalcemia may occur together, for example, in patients with malabsorption syndrome. The neuromuscular effect of each electrolyte abnormality is masked by the other. Treatment of either disorder alone may precipitate symptoms. Thus, treatment of hypokalemia alone may precipitate tetany, and conversely, treatment of hypocalcemia without correcting the hypokalemia may exacerbate the manifestations of potassium deficiency.

HYPERKALEMIA Pathogenesis The causes of hyperkalemia are shown in Table 41-3. *Inadequate renal excretion* is the most frequent cause (see also Chaps. 220 and 221). When oliguria or anuria is present, as in acute renal failure, progressive hyperkalemia is the rule. Plasma potassium rises by about 0.5 meq per liter per day if there are no abnormal loads. Chronic renal failure does not cause severe or progressive hyperkalemia unless oliguria supervenes. Adaptive changes of unknown etiology increase potassium excretion per residual nephron as chronic renal failure progresses. However, patients with chronic renal failure function at the limits of their excretory capacity. Hence, hyperkalemia may develop rapidly if the potassium load is increased or excretory capacity is limited, e.g., by administration of spironolactone. Selective renal *tubular potassium secretory defects* have been described with renal disease caused by lupus erythematosus, sickle cell disease, rejection of a transplanted kidney, or obstructive uropathy.

Hyperkalemia is a cardinal feature of adrenal insufficiency (Addison's disease) and of selective *hypoaldosteronism.* The common form of the latter disorder in adults is *hyporeninemic hypoaldosteronism* (Chap. 325). Inhibition of the activity of the renin-angiotensin-aldosterone system by beta-adrenergic blockers, nonsteroidal antiinflammatory drugs, or converting enzyme inhibitors also may induce hyperkalemia.

A kilogram of tissue such as muscle or erythrocytes contains about 80 meq potassium, and damaged cells release potassium into the plasma. Hence hyperkalemia may be seen when there is *muscle-crushing injury, hemolysis,* or *internal hemorrhage.* Acidosis drives potassium out of cells and leads to hyperkalemia. Severe progressive hyperkalemia is not ordinarily a consequence of increased release of potassium from damaged or acidotic tissues alone. However, acidosis and tissue damage often occur together with acute renal insufficiency; under these circumstances, severe hyperkalemia may develop quickly. In contrast to the increase of 0.5 meq per liter per day typical of uncomplicated anuria, plasma potassium in anuric patients with tissue damage may increase 2 to 4 meq per liter per day. Such rapidly progressive hyperkalemia may be an important cause of death in military casualties. In patients with trauma, burns, or neuromuscular diseases such as paraplegia and multiple sclerosis, the muscle relaxant succinylcholine may cause dangerous hyperkalemia. This agent apparently releases potassium from muscle by depolarizing cell membranes. *Arginine hydrochloride,* used to treat metabolic alkalosis, drives potassium out of cells. If potassium excretion is impaired, clinically significant hyperkalemia may occur during arginine infusions. Extreme digitalis poisoning may cause severe hyperkalemia; potassium leaks out of cells because Na^+-K^+-ATPase is inhibited by the drug. *Beta-adrenergic blockers* may induce hyperkalemia by interfering with the action of endogenous beta-catecholamines to enhance movement of potassium into tissues. *Metabolic acidosis* causes hyperkalemia by shifting potassium out of cells. Respiratory acidosis has less striking effects. *Hyperosmolality* also enhances potassium movement from cells. *Insulin deficiency* is conducive to hyperkalemia because the action of insulin to promote potassium movement into cells is diminished. Hyperosmolality or metabolic acidosis may be additional mechanisms of hyperkalemia in insulin-deficient patients. In *hyperkalemic periodic paralysis,* the hyperkalemia is associated with repeated attacks of muscular paralysis. The mechanism of this syndrome is not understood. Ingestion of increased amounts of potassium may precipitate attacks.

The severity of hyperkalemia caused by large oral or intravenous potassium loads is influenced by factors that modulate tissue uptake and renal excretion of potassium. For example, insulin deficiency and treatment with beta-adrenergic blockers tend to augment hyperkalemia by limiting tissue uptake. Volume depletion enhances hyperkalemia by limiting the rate at which the kidney excretes such loads.

Patients with extreme thrombocytosis or, more rarely, extreme leukocytosis in leukemia may demonstrate the phenomenon of pseudohyperkalemia. Platelets or white blood cells release potassium during blood clotting in vitro. While serum potassium may be grossly abnormal, plasma potassium is not increased. Artifactual elevation of plasma potassium may occur if blood is drawn after repeated fist clenching to make veins more prominent during application of a tourniquet. Artifactual hyperkalemia may be suspected when electrocardiographic abnormalities are absent despite apparently marked elevation of serum potassium.

Clinical features and diagnosis The most important toxic effects of hyperkalemia are cardiac arrhythmias. The characteristic sequence of electrocardiographic changes is shown in Fig. 178-15. The earliest manifestation is the development of high-peaked T waves, especially prominent in precordial leads. Hyperkalemia does not prolong the QT interval, unlike other disorders which induce peaking of the T waves. Later changes include prolongation of the PR interval, complete heart block, and atrial asystole. As plasma potassium rises further, ventricular complexes may deteriorate. The QRS complex becomes progressively prolonged and finally tends to merge with the T wave in a sine wave configuration. Terminally, ventricular fibrillation and standstill may occur.

Occasionally moderate or severe hyperkalemia has striking effects on peripheral muscles. Ascending muscular weakness can occur, progressing to flaccid quadriplegia and respiratory paralysis. Cerebral and cranial nerve function are normal, as is sensation.

TABLE 41-3 Causes of hyperkalemia

I Inadequate excretion
  A Renal failure
    1 Acute renal failure
    2 Severe chronic renal failure
    3 Tubular disorders
  B Adrenal insufficiency
    1 Hypoaldosteronism
    2 Addison's disease
  C Diuretics which inhibit potassium secretion (spironolactone, triamterene, amiloride)
II Shift of potassium from tissues
  A Tissue damage (muscle crush, hemolysis, internal bleeding)
  B Drugs: succinylcholine, arginine, digitalis poisoning, beta-adrenergic antagonists
  C Acidosis
  D Hyperosmolality
  E Insulin deficiency
  F Hyperkalemic periodic paralysis
III Excessive intake
IV Pseudohyperkalemia
  A Thrombocytosis
  B Leukocytosis
  C Poor venipuncture technique
  D In vitro hemolysis

Treatment   In considering therapy, it is helpful to classify hyperkalemia according to degree of severity. The seriousness of hyperkalemia is best estimated by considering both the plasma potassium and the electrocardiogram. When the plasma potassium is less than 6.5 meq per liter and electrocardiographic changes are limited to peaking of T waves, hyperkalemia is mild. When the plasma potassium is 6.5 to 8 meq per liter and T-wave peaking is the only electrocardiographic abnormality, hyperkalemia is moderate. Severe hyperkalemia is present if the plasma potassium exceeds 8 meq per liter or if electrocardiographic abnormalities include absent P waves, widened QRS complexes, or ventricular arrhythmias. Minimal hyperkalemia can usually be treated by elimination of a cause, such as potassium-sparing diuretics, or by treatment of accompanying acidosis. More severe or progressive hyperkalemia requires vigorous therapy. Severe cardiac toxicity responds most rapidly to infusion of calcium; 10 to 30 mL of 10% calcium gluconate may be infused intravenously within a period of 1 to 5 min under constant electrocardiographic monitoring. While calcium infusions do not alter plasma potassium, they counteract the adverse effects of potassium on neuromuscular membranes. The effect of calcium infusions, while almost immediate, is transient if the hyperkalemia is not treated directly.

In moderately severe hyperkalemia, infusion of hypertonic glucose solutions decreases toxicity by shifting potassium into cells. In the first 30 min, 200 to 500 mL of 10% glucose may be given. An additional 500 to 1000 mL may be infused over the next several hours. Ten units of regular insulin may be given subcutaneously, although this is probably necessary only in insulin-deficient diabetic patients. This treatment may reduce serum potassium by 1 to 2 meq per liter, and effects persist for a number of hours. The infusion of sodium bicarbonate also helps lower serum potassium rapidly by causing potassium to shift into cells; 50 to 150 meq alkali (two to three ampuls) may be added to a liter of glucose. Although this agent is most valuable in acidotic patients, it also is effective in individuals with normal acid-base status. The effect occurs within 1 h and persists for a number of hours. The infusion of hypertonic sodium solutions may also be effective in reversing cardiac toxicity, especially in hyponatremic or volume-depleted patients. In part, the effect depends simply on dilution of plasma potassium, but there may be a direct effect of elevated plasma sodium to antagonize hyperkalemic neuromuscular toxicity as well. Glucose, bicarbonate, and sodium may be combined in a "therapeutic cocktail," formulated by adding an ampul or two of sodium bicarbonate to a liter of 5% dextrose in 0.9% saline.

None of the measures just described removes potassium from the body. Cation exchange resins such as sodium polystyrene sulfonate may be given by retention enema in the treatment of moderate or severe hyperkalemia. Enough potassium may be removed by a single enema to reduce potassium by 0.5 to 2 meq per liter within an hour, and repeated enemas can be given. These resins can also be given repeatedly by mouth to maintain low plasma potassium concentration. Twenty grams is given three or four times a day together with 20 mL of a 70% sorbitol solution, as required to ensure the passage of several loose stools daily. In patients with renal failure, hemodialysis and peritoneal dialysis effectively control hyperkalemia. However, they are relatively slow techniques, and patients with severe hyperkalemia should be treated first with one of the methods previously discussed.

REFERENCES

Sodium and water

BARTTER FC: The syndrome of inappropriate secretion of antidiuretic hormone (SIADH). Dis Month Nov, 1973

BERL T et al: Clinical disorders of water metabolism. Kidney Int 10:117, 1976

MILLER M, MOSES AM: Drug-induced states of impaired water excretion. Kidney Int 10:96, 1976

NARINS RG et al: Diagnostic strategies in disorders of fluid, electrolyte and acid-base homeostasis. Am J Med 72:496, 1982

ROBERTSON GL: Thirst and vasopressin function in normal and disordered states of water balance. J Lab Clin Med 101:351, 1983

———, BERL T: Pathophysiology of water metabolism, in The Kidney, 3d ed, BM Brenner, FC Rector Jr (eds). Philadelphia, Saunders, 1986, p 385

WEINER M, EPSTEIN FH: Signs and symptoms of electrolyte disorders. Yale J Biol Med 43:76, 1970

ZERBE R et al: Vasopressin function in the syndrome of inappropriate diuresis. Ann Rev Med 31:315, 1980

Potassium

BIA MJ, DeFRONZO RA: Extrarenal potassium homeostasis. Am J Physiol 240:F257, 1981

HOLLENBERG NK, BROWN RS (eds): Electrolytes and cardiovascular disease. Am J Med 77(5A):1, 1984

KNOCHEL JP: The syndrome of hyporeninemic hypoaldosteronism. Ann Rev Med 30:145, 1979

———: Neuromuscular manifestations of electrolyte disorders. Am J Med 72:521, 1982

RICHARDSON RMA, KUNAU RT JR: Renal regulation of potassium: Abnormal, in The Kidney: Physiology and Pathophysiology, 2d ed, DW Seldin, G Giebisch (eds). New York, Raven Press, 1985, p 1251

STERNS RH et al: Internal potassium balance and the control of the plasma potassium concentration. Medicine 60:339, 1981

WRIGHT FS: Sites and mechanisms of potassium transport along the renal tubule. Kidney Int 11:415, 1977

---

42   ACIDOSIS AND ALKALOSIS

NORMAN G. LEVINSKY

PHYSIOLOGIC CONSIDERATIONS   Acids are produced continuously during normal metabolism. Despite the addition of some 20,000 mmol of carbonic acid and 80 mmol of nonvolatile acids to body fluids daily, the free hydrogen ion concentration of these fluids is fixed within a narrow range. The pH of extracellular fluid is normally between 7.35 and 7.45 (hydrogen ion, 45 to 35 nmol per liter). The pH of intracellular fluids cannot be determined with precision, but most methods suggest a mean intracellular pH in the range of 6.9. Intracellular hydrogen ion concentration is not uniform; it varies among intracellular organelles within individual cells. Although the free hydrogen ion concentration of body fluids is low, protons are so reactive that even minute changes in concentration influence enzymatic reactions and physiologic processes. Immediate defense against untoward changes in pH is provided by buffers that can take up or release protons instantaneously in response to changes in acidity of body fluids. Regulation of pH ultimately depends on the lungs and the kidneys.

The principal acid product of metabolism is carbon dioxide, equivalent to potential carbonic acid. The normal concentration of carbon dioxide in body fluids is fixed at 1.2 mmol per liter (P_{CO_2} = 40 mmHg) by the lungs; at this concentration, pulmonary excretion equals metabolic production. Although carbon dioxide reacts with water and body buffers during transport from cells to pulmonary alveoli, no net change in body fluid composition results, since the CO_2 excreted by the lungs is equal to the CO_2 produced by cells. When a nonvolatile acid is produced by metabolism, the protons are removed instantaneously from body fluids by reaction with buffers. In extracellular fluid, bicarbonate is converted to water and carbon dioxide, which is excreted by the lungs. Although this mechanism minimizes changes in acidity, it destroys bicarbonate and uses up cell buffer capacity. The total buffer capacity of the body fluids is about 15 meq per kilogram of body weight. Thus, the normal rate of production of nonvolatile acids would be sufficient to deplete the body buffers completely in 10 to 20 days, were it not for the ability of the kidney to eliminate protons from the body by secretion into the urine, thereby regenerating bicarbonate and cell buffer capacity.

The principal source of nonvolatile acid is metabolism of methionine and cystine in dietary proteins, which produces sulfuric acid. Additional sources include the incomplete combustion of carbohydrates and fats, which produces organic acids; the metabolism of nucleoproteins, which produces uric acid; and the metabolism of organic phosphorus compounds, which releases protons and inorganic phosphates. The diet does not normally contain significant amounts of preformed acid or alkali, but significant amounts of potential acid (e.g., an excess of cationic acids, such as lysine) or alkali (e.g., citrate) may be present.

The principal functions of the kidney in acid-base metabolism can be viewed as retention of existing bicarbonate and generation of new bicarbonate to replace that used to buffer nonvolatile acids. Bicarbonate is reabsorbed in both proximal and distal segments by secretion of protons into tubular fluid. New bicarbonate is generated by secretion of protons onto urinary buffers. Normally, one-third is titrated onto phosphate, converting HPO_4^{2-} to $H_2PO_4^-$, and the remainder onto ammonia. The amount of free acid which can be excreted in the urine is negligible, even at the minimum urine pH of 4.8. However, acidification of the urine is essential for titration of acid onto phosphate and ammonia. Changes in the pH of body fluids lead to regulatory responses by the kidney. Acidosis stimulates renal hydrogen ion secretion. Ammonia production increases, and more protons can be excreted as ammonium. In extreme acidosis, ammonia production may increase tenfold or more above the normal rate of 40 to 50 meq per day. The bicarbonate concentration of extracellular fluid is, in effect, set by the renal rate of proton secretion (bicarbonate reabsorption and generation). If plasma bicarbonate rises without an increase in renal reabsorptive capacity, bicarbonate is excreted rapidly and normal plasma bicarbonate is restored promptly. For example, chronic ingestion of even large amounts of sodium bicarbonate normally produces only minimal sustained elevation of plasma bicarbonate. The rate of proton secretion is influenced by a number of factors, important among them carbon dioxide tension of body fluids, extracellular volume, aldosterone, and body potassium stores. Bicarbonate reabsorption is directly related to carbon dioxide concentration; hypercapnia tends to stimulate, and hypocapnia tends to inhibit, renal bicarbonate retention. Contraction of extracellular volume enhances tubular bicarbonate reabsorption, while volume expansion has the opposite effect. Aldosterone stimulates renal proton secretion; by this effect, hyperaldosteronism promotes metabolic alkalosis, while hypoaldosteronism causes acidosis. In experimental animals, renal bicarbonate reabsorption is inversely related to body potassium stores. In humans, the relation is less clear, but severe potassium depletion has been associated with increased bicarbonate reabsorption and metabolic alkalosis.

The respiratory response to changes in blood pH is almost instantaneous. Acidosis stimulates and alkalosis depresses ventilation. The respiratory center in the medulla appears to respond to a pH intermediate between those of blood and cerebrospinal fluid.

EVALUATION OF ACID-BASE BALANCE In practice, classification of acid-base disorders is based on measurements of changes in the bicarbonate–carbonic acid system, the principal buffer of extracellular fluid. Because intracellular and extracellular buffers are functionally linked, measurement of the plasma bicarbonate system provides useful information about total body buffers. The relationship among the elements of the bicarbonate system is usually described in terms of the Henderson-Hasselbalch equation:

$$pH = pK + \log \frac{[HCO_3^-]}{[H_2CO_3]}$$

(The pK of carbonic acid is 6.1. $[H_2CO_3]$ is calculated as αP_{CO_2}; α, the solubility factor for carbon dioxide in body fluids, is 0.031 mmol per liter per mmHg P_{CO_2}. For a normal P_{CO_2} of 40 mmHg, $[H_2CO_3]$ is calculated to be 40 x 0.031 = 1.2 mmol per liter.)

Acidosis is defined as a disturbance which tends to add acid or remove alkali from body fluids, while *alkalosis* is any disturbance which tends to remove acid or add base. Since compensatory processes may minimize or prevent a change in the hydrogen ion concentration of the plasma, some authors prefer to use the terms *acidemia* and *alkalemia* to indicate those situations in which the pH of the plasma is measurably altered. *Respiratory* disorders are those in which the primary change is in the concentration of carbon dioxide (carbonic acid). As can be seen from the Henderson-Hasselbalch equation, a fall in carbon dioxide concentration causes alkalemia, while an increase in carbon dioxide concentration causes acidemia. *Metabolic* disorders are those in which the primary disturbance is in the concentration of bicarbonate. Since bicarbonate appears in the numerator of the buffer salt/acid ratio in the Henderson-Hasselbalch equation, increased bicarbonate concentration causes alkalemia while a decrease in bicarbonate causes acidemia.

A major problem in the assessment of acid-base disorders results from the compensatory responses of the lungs and the kidney. A primary change in carbon dioxide concentration induces a compensatory renal response which alters plasma bicarbonate in the same direction. Conversely, a primary alteration of plasma bicarbonate induces compensatory changes in plasma carbon dioxide. Consider a patient with chronic respiratory insufficiency who has the following set of acid-base parameters: P_{CO_2} = 70 mmHg, $[HCO_3^-]$ = 31 mmol per liter, pH = 7.25. The clinician needs to know whether the elevation of plasma bicarbonate is merely the appropriate renal response to the primary hypercapnia or a metabolic acid-base disorder is superimposed. No calculations or a priori reasoning will provide the answer to this key question. Such information can be derived only from in vivo observations in which the usual compensatory response to a given degree of chronic hypercapnia is determined.

Clinical and experimental observations in humans (and animals) have been made in all common primary acid-base disturbances. They are most readily visualized and used for analysis of clinical acid-base disorders by the ''confidence band'' technique, as shown in Fig. 42-1. Each band represents the mean ± 2 SD, that is, 95 percent of observations, for the compensatory response to each primary disturbance. In the example under discussion, inspection of the confidence band marked *chronic respiratory acidosis* indicates that 95 percent of individuals with chronic elevation of P_{CO_2} to 70 mmHg would have $[HCO_3^-]$ between 34 and 44 meq per liter, due to renal compensation. Thus, the $[HCO_3^-]$ of 31 meq per liter in the example cannot be interpreted as the sole result of an appropriate compensatory response to chronic hypercapnia. A second acid-base disorder, presumably metabolic acidosis, must be superimposed. Obviously, the use of this figure is no panacea, nor does it obviate the need for commonsense clinical evaluation of alternative possibilities. For example, if the patient under discussion had only recently developed

FIGURE 42-1 *Nomogram, showing bands for uncomplicated respiratory or metabolic acid-base disturbances in intact subjects. Each ''confidence'' band represents the mean ±2 SD for the compensatory response of normal subjects or patients to a given primary disorder. Ac = acute; chr = chronic, resp = respiratory; met = metabolic; acid = acidosis; alk = alkalosis. (Modified from Arbus.)*

hypercapnia, the [HCO_3^-] of 31 meq per liter would be too high for a purely compensatory response to acute respiratory acidosis and would be interpreted as superimposed metabolic alkalosis. The difference between these two interpretations depends entirely on the clinical recognition of the chronicity of the primary respiratory disorder. The use of Fig. 42-1 in each type of acid-base disturbance is described in the appropriate section of this chapter.[1]

METABOLIC ACIDOSIS

PATHOPHYSIOLOGY Metabolic acidosis is caused by one of three mechanisms (see Table 42-1): (1) increased production of nonvolatile acids, (2) decreased acid excretion by the kidney, (3) loss of alkali. In intracellular fluid excess protons replace potassium, which shifts out of cells, tending to elevate plasma levels. Extracellular bicarbonate is reduced by reaction with hydrogen ions or, in patients wasting alkali, by loss of bicarbonate in urine or stool. The decrease in pH stimulates respiration, and P_{CO_2} is lowered. Inspection of the confidence band for metabolic acidosis (Fig. 42-1) indicates that a decrease in P_{CO_2} of about 1.2 mmHg can be expected for each decrement of 1 mmol per liter in plasma bicarbonate. Complete respiratory compensation for primary metabolic acidosis does not occur. Respiratory compensation for acute acidosis tends to be somewhat greater than for chronic metabolic acidosis. The minimum level of P_{CO_2} which can be attained is approximately 10 mmHg; levels below 15 to 20 mmHg are rarely maintained in chronic metabolic acidosis. When kidney function is normal, net acid excretion increases promptly in response to metabolic acidosis. Most of the initial rise is due to increased titration of urinary phosphate as urine pH falls below 5.2. Over several days, ammonia production by the kidney increases and becomes the most important mechanism for excreting excess protons. Net acid excretion may increase 5 to 10 times above normal, reaching a maximum of several hundred milliequivalents per day.

The most common cause of *acute* metabolic acidosis is increased production of nonvolatile acids. In *diabetic ketoacidosis,* acetoacetic and β-hydroxybutyric acids are produced more rapidly than they can be metabolized (Chap. 327). Severe ketoacidosis may occur in *association* with *acute* and *chronic alcoholism.* Typically patients give a history of prolonged abstention from food, protracted vomiting, and appreciable alcohol intake just before development of the ketoacidosis. β-Hydroxybutyrate, acetoacetate, and lactate accumulate in the plasma. The ketosis may be overlooked because the ratio

---

[1] *Although the confidence band method does not permit automatic identification of simple or complicated acid-base disorders, it is preferable to techniques such as "buffer base" or "base excess-deficit" for reasons discussed in detail by Schwartz and Relman, N Engl J Med 268:1382, 1963. These terms are not used in this chapter.*

TABLE 42-1 Causes of metabolic acidosis

Increased anion gap
I Increased acid production
  A Ketoacidosis
    1 Diabetic
    2 Alcoholic
    3 Starvation
  B Lactic acidosis
    1 Secondary to circulatory or respiratory failure
    2 Associated with various disorders (see text)
    3 Drugs and toxins
    4 Enzyme defects
  C Poisoning (salicylates, ethylene glycol, methanol)
II Renal failure

Normal anion gap (hyperchloremic)
III Renal tubular dysfunction
  A Renal tubular acidosis
  B Hypoaldosteronism
  C "Potassium-sparing" diuretics
IV Loss of alkali
  A Diarrhea
  B Ureterosigmoidostomy
  C Carbonic anhydrase inhibitors
V Ammonium chloride, cationic amino acids (excess intake)

of β-hydroxybutyrate to acetoacetate tends to be high; the nitroprusside test used for clinical detection of plasma ketones responds only to the latter. Blood sugar is usually normal or mildly elevated in these patients. The mechanism of the syndrome is uncertain. *Starvation* may cause mild ketoacidosis because of increased fat metabolism.

Several types of *lactic acidosis* have been recognized (Chap. 328). The most common is *secondary* to severe acute circulatory or respiratory failure, with poor tissue perfusion or arterial oxygen desaturation. The clinical features of shock are usually present. In these patients, lactic acidosis probably is due both to increased production of lactate by hypoxic tissues and to decreased utilization by the liver. Lactic acidosis may also be *associated* with acute hepatic necrosis, leukemia, solid tumors, and uncontrolled diabetes mellitus. The biguanide oral hypoglycemic agents, such as phenformin, were the drugs most often responsible for *drug-induced* lactic acidosis; they are no longer in general use. Certain sugars used for parenteral alimentation, such as fructose, may cause lactic acidosis. Increased lactic acid production contributes to acidosis in *poisoning* by methanol and salicylates. In infants and children, congenital defects in enzymes of carbohydrate metabolism have been identified as causes of lactic acidosis. Primary lactic acidosis in patients without an underlying disease has been reported, but the existence of such a spontaneous disorder is uncertain.

Poisoning and drug toxicity are causes of acute metabolic acidosis. Among the more common agents are salicylates, ethylene glycol, and methyl alcohol (Chap. 171). Salicylates create a metabolic block, which leads to production of a mixture of endogenous organic acids. Methanol and ethylene glycol are converted to acid metabolites, methanol to formic acid and ethylene glycol to glyoxylic and oxalic acids. In addition, these intoxicants create metabolic blocks, which may lead to increased production of endogenous organic acids. Salicylates have the additional effect of stimulating the respiratory center directly. Respiratory alkalosis is the earliest derangement in salicylate intoxication and may be the only acid-base disorder in some patients.

Renal disease is the most common cause of chronic metabolic acidosis. In *chronic renal failure* (Chap. 220), the principal defect is decreased ability to excrete ammonium, but some patients also waste bicarbonate, especially at plasma levels of 18 mmol per liter or above. Acidification of the urine and formation of titratable acidity are usually normal. Plasma bicarbonate tends to fall progressively as renal insufficiency becomes increasingly severe, but plasma bicarbonate usually stabilizes at levels of 12 to 18 mmol per liter; it rarely falls below 10 mmol per liter, even in advanced uremia. The mechanisms of stabilization are thought to be (1) stimulation of acid excretion by advancing acidosis, which occurs to some extent even in the diseased kidney; and (2) buffering of the daily metabolic acid load by carbonate and phosphate in bone. In *acute renal failure* (Chap. 219), plasma bicarbonate decreases by only 1 to 2 mmol per liter per day if reduced renal acid excretion is the only cause of metabolic acidosis. Greater rates of fall suggest the presence, in addition, of some cause of increased acid production.

Chronic metabolic acidosis is the hallmark of *renal tubular acidosis* (Chap. 228), which may be an isolated disorder of tubular acid excretion; part of a Fanconi syndrome, in which other tubular functions are also abnormal; or associated with nonrenal primary disorders (Chap. 307). The acidosis is due to defective renal tubular acidification mechanisms, which limit renal conservation and regeneration of bicarbonate.

Aldosterone stimulates distal tubular acid and potassium secretion. In *hypoaldosteronism,* loss of this effect leads to metabolic acidosis and hyperkalemia. The acidosis is due not only to loss of the direct effect of aldosterone on acid excretion but also to the hyperkalemia, which decreases renal ammonia production. The same factors account for metabolic acidosis caused by the diuretic spironolactone, which blocks the action of aldosterone, and other "potassium-sparing" diuretics such as triamterene and amiloride, which directly inhibit distal tubular secretion of acid and potassium.

Loss of alkali may cause acute or chronic metabolic acidosis. Severe *diarrhea* or intestinal malabsorption usually causes mild to moderate acidosis due to the loss of bicarbonate in liquid stool, in which concentrations of 40 to 60 mmol per liter may be present. Ureterosigmoidostomy, i.e., transplantation of the ureters into the sigmoid colon, leads to metabolic acidosis both because of exchange of chloride for bicarbonate by intestinal epithelium and because renal disease (obstructive uropathy and pyelonephritis) often develops. However, acidosis is not a problem with the more modern technique for urinary diversion, in which a bladder is formed from a small isolated loop of ileum. Carbonic anhydrase inhibitors, such as acetazolamide, cause mild to moderate acidosis by increasing bicarbonate loss in the urine.

Acidosis can be caused by administration of ammonium chloride and lysine or arginine hydrochloride, which form HCl during metabolism. This type of acidosis also may occur during parenteral alimentation with amino acid infusates that contain an excess of the cationic amino acids arginine, lysine, and histidine.

CLINICAL FEATURES AND DIAGNOSIS

There are few specific symptoms or signs of metabolic acidosis; diagnosis depends on recognition of the clinical setting and appropriate laboratory studies. In acute metabolic acidosis, hyperventilation is usual and may be intense (Kussmaul respiration). However, it is ordinarily impossible to detect increased respiration by physical examination in patients with chronic metabolic acidosis, despite substantial reduction of P_{CO_2}. Acute, severe acidosis produces a variety of nonspecific symptoms ranging from fatigue through confusion, stupor, and coma. Cardiovascular effects include decreased cardiac contractility and vasodilatation, which may lead to heart failure or hypotension. Chronic metabolic acidosis may produce no symptoms or may be associated with fatigue and anorexia, although it is usually difficult to determine whether these symptoms reflect the acidosis per se or are related to the underlying disease.

The characteristic laboratory features are reduction of plasma bicarbonate and blood pH, together with a compensatory reduction in P_{CO_2} (see Fig. 42-1). Hyperkalemia is often present, due to shift of potassium out of cells. This phenomenon may mask significant potassium depletion (see Chap. 41). Hypokalemia is a clue to conditions in which concomitant potassium depletion is severe, for example, diarrhea or diabetic ketoacidosis, or in which renal potassium-regulating mechanisms are affected, such as renal tubular acidosis or administration of carbonic anhydrase inhibitors.

When the cause of metabolic acidosis is not evident from the history or clinical setting, calculation of unmeasured anions (anion gap) may help in differential diagnosis. Unmeasured anions are calculated by subtracting the sum of plasma bicarbonate and chloride from plasma sodium concentration; the normal value is 8 to 16 mmol per liter. The negative charges on plasma proteins, principally albumin, make up most of the anion gap. Phosphate, sulfate, and organic acid anions normally contribute to unmeasured anions to a lesser degree. When metabolic acidosis is due to increased acid production or renal insufficiency (categories I and II, Table 42-1), the anion gap is usually increased. In acidosis resulting from increased acid production, the increased anion gap is due to accumulation in plasma of the anions of the various acids such as acetoacetate or lactate, which are produced faster than they can be metabolized or excreted. In renal failure, the anion gap increases because sulfate, phosphate, and organic acid anions are not excreted efficiently. In all other types of metabolic acidosis (categories III, IV, V, Table 42-1), the anion gap is normal since there is neither increased production nor decreased excretion of organic acids, sulfate, and phosphate. Plasma chloride concentration is increased approximately as much as plasma bicarbonate is decreased (hyperchloremic acidosis).

In diabetic ketoacidosis a variety of plasma acid-base patterns may develop, depending on the balance between production and renal excretion of ketoacid anions. In most patients there is renal dysfunction, and the anions are retained, leading to an anion-gap acidosis in which the elevation in plasma unmeasured anion is about equal to the reduction in bicarbonate concentration. Patients whose renal function is not impaired may present with a component of hyperchloremic acidosis due to renal excretion of ketone anions and retention of chloride. After therapy that repairs volume depletion and hence renal dysfunction, most patients develop some degree of hyperchloremia, due to the same mechanisms.

TREATMENT

The treatment of metabolic acidosis depends on its cause and severity. In *chronic renal failure,* mild or moderate metabolic acidosis does not require treatment. When plasma bicarbonate falls below 15 mmol per liter, it is reasonable to treat patients with oral alkali, such as sodium bicarbonate or sodium citrate. The dose is gradually increased until plasma bicarbonate concentration rises to about 18 to 20 mmol per liter. Some patients appear to benefit symptomatically from elevation of bicarbonate to this level, and fatigue, anorexia, and malaise tend to be alleviated. Caution must be exerted to avoid excessively rapid alkalination of the plasma, which may precipitate tetany; excess sodium given with alkali may aggravate hypertension or edema. Acidosis should be corrected as completely as possible in patients with type 1 (distal) *renal tubular acidosis;* this will avoid hypercalciuria, osteomalacia, nephrocalcinosis, and lithiasis. In type 2 (proximal) renal tubular acidosis, therapy is usually not required (see Chap. 228). Patients with *acute renal failure* also do not ordinarily require specific therapy for acidosis. Dialysis instituted for management of the renal failure should maintain an adequate plasma bicarbonate.

Diabetic *ketoacidosis* responds to insulin, and most patients do not require treatment with alkali (see Chap. 327). However, when acidosis is extreme (pH less than 7.1 or [HCO_3^-] less than 6 to 8 meq per liter), intravenous bicarbonate therapy is justified. The ketoacidosis associated with alcoholism responds rapidly to infusions of glucose and saline. Insulin is not required, nor should alkali be given unless acidosis is extreme. The ketoacidosis of starvation is mild and requires no specific treatment.

Lactic acidosis secondary to acute circulatory or respiratory failure is corrected if treatment of the underlying disorder is successful (see Chap. 328). Since this type of lactic acidosis is usually associated with severe acute circulatory or respiratory failure, the mortality rate is high. Lactic acidosis occurring in other disorders is usually resistant to treatment. Rapid administration of several hundred milliequivalents of alkali may raise plasma bicarbonate in some patients, but in others net production of lactic acid is so rapid that correction of acidosis is difficult. Since vigorous administration of alkali may lead to circulatory overloading, dialysis may be useful. Despite rapid administration of alkali, the mortality rate in these patients is high.

The acidosis due to *diarrhea* or loss of alkaline upper intestinal secretions is usually associated with other volume depletion and potassium deficiency. Treatment of such electrolyte disorders with intravenous infusions appropriate for the patient's specific abnormalities may be required.

Some general points about therapy with alkali are worth emphasis. Oral treatment with sodium bicarbonate should usually begin with 1 g three times daily and be increased to maintain the desired plasma bicarbonate level. Some patients find that sodium bicarbonate leads to upper gastrointestinal discomfort; a 10% sodium citrate solution may be more palatable. In the intravenous treatment of acute metabolic acidosis, sodium bicarbonate is the agent of choice. The amount of bicarbonate to be given depends upon the severity of the acidosis and any associated disorders of serum sodium concentration. Typically, concentrations of bicarbonate between 50 and 150 meq per liter are achieved by adding one to three vials of sodium bicarbonate to a liter of dextrose in water. The concentration of bicarbonate in these vials is 1000 meq per liter (50 meq in 50 mL); these bicarbonate solutions should never be given undiluted in the treatment of acidosis, since rapid infusion may induce serious or even fatal cardiac arrhythmias, especially if given as a bolus through a central venous catheter. The total amount of alkali needed to raise plasma bicarbonate can be estimated from the effects of administration of acid loads. Approximately equal amounts of acid appear to be buffered by extracellular bicarbonate and by intracellular buffers. (In severe acidosis, a greater fraction of the acid load may be buffered within cells.) Therefore, it is appropriate to calculate the amount of alkali needed by assuming that approximately half will accept protons from intracellular buffers and be destroyed; the other half will elevate plasma bicarbonate concentration. Thus, the calculation would be: millimoles of bicarbonate required equals desired increment in plasma concentration (millimoles per liter) times 40 percent of body weight. The 40 percent figure represents twice the extracellular volume. It is rarely desirable to infuse enough alkali to elevate plasma bicarbonate to normal. Possible untoward effects include hypokalemic cardiac toxicity in patients who are substantially potassium-depleted, tetany in patients with renal failure or hypocalcemia, and congestive failure due to excess sodium. Moreover, alkalosis may supervene. Cerebrospinal fluid bicarbonate does not equilibrate rapidly with plasma. Hence the respiratory center, which responds to acidity both of blood and cerebrospinal fluid, maintains some degree of hyperventilation as plasma bicarbonate is increasing. This type of respiratory alkalosis may sometimes persist for several days after correction of metabolic acidosis. In acute acidosis due to overproduction of metabolic acids, successful treatment of the primary disorder will cause rapid metabolic conversion of lactate and ketone bodies to bicarbonate. Thus, excessive administration of bicarbonate early in therapy also may lead to metabolic alkalosis at a later stage of treatment, when endogenous bicarbonate has been reconstituted by improvement in metabolism.

METABOLIC ALKALOSIS

PATHOPHYSIOLOGY Metabolic alkalosis is usually initiated by increased loss of acid from the stomach or the kidney. However, excretion of bicarbonate at high plasma concentrations is normally so rapid that alkalosis will not be sustained unless bicarbonate reabsorption is enhanced or alkali is continuously generated at a great rate. Clinically, maintenance of metabolic alkalosis is most often due to stimulation of bicarbonate reabsorption by a volume (chloride) deficit. During volume depletion, renal conservation of sodium takes precedence over other homeostatic mechanisms, such as correction of alkalosis. Since in alkalosis a large fraction of plasma sodium is paired with bicarbonate, complete reabsorption of filtered sodium requires reabsorption of bicarbonate as well. Alkalosis is sustained until volume depletion is corrected by administration of sodium chloride. This diminishes tubular avidity for sodium and provides chloride as an alternative anion for reabsorption with sodium; excess bicarbonate can then be excreted with sodium.

The other major mechanism which can maintain metabolic alkalosis is hypermineralocorticoidism. Mineralocorticoids stimulate renal hydrogen ion secretion. In patients with excess mineralocorticoid activity, elevation of plasma bicarbonate is initiated by increased urinary loss of protons as ammonium and titratable acidity. Stimulation of tubular acid secretion also enhances bicarbonate reabsorption, thereby sustaining the metabolic alkalosis. Patients with excess mineralocorticoid activity are not volume- or chloride-deficient. Hence, this type of metabolic alkalosis does not respond to sodium chloride administration.

TABLE 42-2   Causes of metabolic alkalosis

I Associated with volume (chloride) depletion
  A Vomiting or gastric drainage
  B Diuretic therapy
  C Posthypercapnic alkalosis
II Associated with hyperadrenocorticism
  A Cushing's syndrome
  B Primary aldosteronism
  C Bartter's syndrome
III Severe potassium depletion
IV Excessive alkali intake
  A Acute
  B Milk-alkali syndrome

The relation between metabolic alkalosis and potassium is incompletely understood. Alkalosis and hypokalemia often occur together. Alkalosis may cause hypokalemia and potassium depletion through mechanisms discussed in Chap. 41. Conversely, potassium depletion may help to sustain metabolic alkalosis because tubular acid secretion, and hence bicarbonate reabsorption, is stimulated. Whether potassium depletion alone can generate metabolic alkalosis is uncertain; if so, severe potassium depletion is required.

Respiratory compensation for metabolic alkalosis is limited. Alveolar ventilation decreases, and P_{CO_2} is elevated. However, since this response is limited by hypoxia, P_{CO_2} rarely rises above 50 to 55 mmHg.

PATHOGENESIS The principal causes of metabolic alkalosis are outlined in Table 42-2. *Vomiting* and *gastric drainage* usually induce only minimal or moderate alkalosis, but occasional patients, especially those with increased gastric acid secretion, e.g., with acid-peptic disease or the Zollinger-Ellison syndrome, may develop very severe alkalosis. Loss of hydrochloric acid in the gastric fluid initiates the alkalosis. Water and sodium chloride are lost in the vomitus or gastric aspirate. Initially, sodium is lost in the urine as well, coupled to increased bicarbonate excretion (which results from elevation of plasma bicarbonate above the tubular reabsorptive threshold). These losses cause a volume (chloride) deficit, which stimulates tubular reabsorption of bicarbonate and thus maintains the elevated plasma bicarbonate generated by gastric losses of hydrochloric acid.

Alkalosis may be present in patients treated with any *diuretic* except those that specifically inhibit bicarbonate reabsorption, such as acetazolamide, or inhibit distal cation secretion, such as spironolactone and triamterene. The diuretics cause extracellular volume contraction. They inhibit chloride reabsorption in the loop of Henle or distal convoluted tubule, which increases delivery of tubular fluid to more distal nephron segments. The volume deficit and consequent hyperaldosteronism stimulate proton secretion in these segments, generating and maintaining the alkalosis. Alkalosis due to oral treatment with diuretics is usually mild. Acute administration of potent intravenous diuretics such as ethacrynic acid to patients on low-sodium diets may induce more severe alkalosis due to rapid loss of sodium chloride in the urine. Sudden contraction of extracellular volume elevates plasma bicarbonate; renal excretion of excess bicarbonate is prevented by the mechanism discussed above.

Patients with chronic hypercapnia due to respiratory insufficiency maintain high plasma bicarbonate concentrations (see "Respiratory Acidosis," below). If respiration improves, P_{CO_2} falls promptly. However, urinary excretion of excess bicarbonate previously generated by renal compensatory mechanisms takes a number of days. In patients on low-salt diets or diuretics who have a volume (chloride) deficiency, *posthypercapnic* alkalosis of this type may persist indefinitely unless sodium or potassium chloride is added to the diet. The mechanism in this condition is the same as that which causes persistent alkalosis in vomiting, described earlier.

Alkalosis is variable in patients with excess mineralocorticoid activity. Minimal or moderate alkalosis is usually present in patients with *Cushing's syndrome* or *primary aldosteronism*. More marked alkalosis may be seen in patients with extreme adrenal hyperfunction associated with ACTH-secreting tumors, such as bronchogenic carcinoma. Moderate alkalosis is typical of patients with *Bartter's syndrome*.

Although alkalosis and *potassium depletion* are often associated, mild or moderate potassium depletion does not cause sustained metabolic alkalosis. However, extreme degrees of potassium depletion (serum potassium usually 2 meq per liter or less) may cause metabolic alkalosis. This type of alkalosis is not corrected by administration of sodium chloride but does respond to administration of potassium.

For reasons noted earlier, alkalosis due to administration of alkali cannot be sustained unless large amounts are given. When renal function is compromised, alkalosis may be sustained by small exogenous loads. This is apparently the mechanism of alkalosis in the milk-alkali syndrome, in which hypercalcemic nephropathy and alkalosis develop in response to excessive intake of absorbable alkali. The nephropathy limits bicarbonate excretion, thus maintaining the alkalosis.

CLINICAL FEATURES AND DIAGNOSIS There are no specific clinical signs or symptoms. Severe alkalosis may cause apathy, confusion, and stupor. If serum calcium is borderline or low, rapid development of alkalosis may lead to tetany. The diagnosis of metabolic alkalosis depends on recognition of the clinical setting and appropriate laboratory studies. Plasma bicarbonate is increased. P_{CO_2} increases by about 0.6 mmHg for each milliequivalent per liter. Elevation of P_{CO_2} is insufficient to prevent alkalemia (see Fig. 42-1). Plasma potassium concentration is often reduced, and the electrocardiogram may reveal changes in T and U waves typical of hypokalemia (Chap. 178). These changes may be due to alkalosis itself or to associated alterations in potassium metabolism. Despite elevation of plasma bicarbonate, the urine pH is usually less than 7 in patients with sustained metabolic alkalosis. This "paradoxical aciduria" reflects the fact that bicarbonate reabsorption must be increased if metabolic alkalosis is to be sustained.

Differential diagnosis is usually made from clinical features, such as a history of vomiting or the manifestations of Cushing's syndrome. The urinary chloride concentration may be a helpful clue if the diagnosis is not evident. When the alkalosis is associated with volume contraction (category I, Table 42-2), urinary chloride is low, usually less than 10 meq per liter. When the alkalosis is caused by hyperadrenocorticism or severe potassium depletion (categories II and III), urinary chloride is higher, usually 20 meq per liter or more.

TREATMENT Mild or moderate metabolic alkalosis rarely requires specific treatment. In patients with gastric alkalosis, infusion of saline solutions is usually sufficient to enhance renal bicarbonate excretion and to correct alkalosis by mechanisms discussed above. Administration of potassium chloride is also helpful in treating or preventing alkalosis in these patients and those with diuretic-induced alkalosis. In patients with adrenal hyperfunction, alkalosis is corrected by specific treatment of the underlying disease. In Bartter's syndrome hypokalemia, potassium wasting, and alkalosis may be partly corrected by treatment with prostaglandin synthetase inhibitors such as indomethacin. Whenever alkalosis and potassium depletion occur together, potassium depletion should be treated with potassium chloride, not with an organic salt of potassium.

Rarely, with prolonged gastric metabolic alkalosis losses may be severe enough to require intravenous therapy with acidifying agents. Dilute hydrochloric acid or acidifying salts such as ammonium chloride or arginine hydrochloride may be given slowly under such circumstances. In most patients the use of acidifying agents can be avoided by appropriate treatment with saline and potassium chloride. In patients who are volume-expanded or in whom volume loading is inadvisable, therapy with acetazolamide, which enhances renal bicarbonate excretion, may be helpful.

RESPIRATORY ACIDOSIS

PATHOPHYSIOLOGY Failure of ventilation promptly increases P_{CO_2} (carbonic acid) because metabolic production of carbon dioxide is so rapid. Acute respiratory acidosis is modulated to a limited degree by tissue buffers. As can be seen from the curve labeled *acute respiratory acidosis* in Fig. 42-1, immediate tissue buffering elevates plasma bicarbonate only slightly, by about 1 meq per liter for each increase of 10 mmHg in P_{CO_2}. If hypercapnia is sustained, renal acid excretion is enhanced, and bicarbonate reabsorption is stimulated. Over a period of several days, plasma bicarbonate rises approximately 3 meq per liter for each increase of 10 mmHg in P_{CO_2}, thereby minimizing the degree of acidemia. The increment in plasma bicarbonate attributable to renal activity is represented by the difference between the curves marked *chronic respiratory acidosis* and *acute respiratory acidosis*.

PATHOGENESIS (See also Table 215-1) *Acute* respiratory acidosis occurs whenever there is a sudden failure of ventilation. Common causes include depression of the respiratory center by cerebral disease or drugs, neuromuscular disorders, and cardiopulmonary arrest. *Chronic* respiratory acidosis occurs in pulmonary diseases such as chronic emphysema and bronchitis, in which ventilation and perfusion are mismatched and effective alveolar ventilation is decreased. Chronic hypercapnia may also result from primary alveolar hypoventilation or from alveolar hypoventilation related to extreme obesity (Pickwickian syndrome). Acute and chronic diseases characterized principally by interference with alveolar gas exchange, such as chronic pulmonary fibrosis, pneumonia, and pulmonary edema, usually cause hypocapnia rather than hypercapnia. In these conditions, hypoxia stimulates increased ventilation; since carbon dioxide is much more diffusible than oxygen, excretion of carbon dioxide is enhanced despite the barrier to gas exchange. Hypercapnia occurs only with respiratory fatigue or extremely severe disease.

CLINICAL FEATURES AND DIAGNOSIS It is often difficult to separate the manifestations of respiratory acidosis from those of associated hypoxia. Moderate hypercapnia, especially if it develops slowly, probably has no specific clinical features. When P_{CO_2} exceeds 70 mmHg, patients become progressively confused and obtunded. Asterixis may be present. Papilledema may occur, apparently because intracranial pressure is increased by the cerebral vasodilation characteristic of hypercapnia. Dilatation of conjunctival and superficial facial blood vessels may be noted.

The diagnosis of acute respiratory acidosis is usually evident from the clinical situation, especially if respiration is obviously depressed. Proof requires laboratory confirmation that P_{CO_2} is elevated. Acidemia is always present in patients with *acute* hypercapnia. Acidosis in acute cardiopulmonary arrest is usually a combination of a metabolic lactic acidosis and acute respiratory acidosis. Patients with chronic hypercapnia are usually acidemic. However, some individuals with minimal or moderate chronic hypercapnia may have normal or even slightly elevated plasma pH, as may be seen from Fig. 42-1. The mechanism of full compensation or of "overcompensation" in such instances is unknown. However, significant elevation of pH in patients with chronic hypercapnia is almost always due to complicating metabolic alkalosis. Diuretics, low-sodium diets, and posthypercapnic alkalosis are frequent causes of this type of superimposed acid-base disorder.

Because of the differences between plasma bicarbonate in acute hypercapnia and in chronic hypercapnia, proper interpretation of acid-base parameters in respiratory acidosis depends on clinical information.

TREATMENT The only worthwhile approach to treatment of respiratory acidosis is correction of the underlying disorder. Rapid infusion of alkali is justified in cardiopulmonary arrest. In other circumstances, infusions of alkali have no role in practical management of respiratory acidosis.

RESPIRATORY ALKALOSIS

PATHOPHYSIOLOGY Acute reduction in carbon dioxide concentration releases hydrogen ion from tissue buffers, which minimize alkalemia by reducing plasma bicarbonate. Acute alkalosis also enhances glycolysis; increased production of lactic and pyruvic acids lowers serum bicarbonate and raises plasma concentrations of the corresponding anions by a millimole or two. In chronic hypocapnia, plasma bicarbonate is further reduced because the decreased P_{CO_2} inhibits tubular reabsorption and generation of bicarbonate. As in respiratory acidosis, compensation for the chronic state is much more complete than for the acute (Figure 42-1). In acute hypocapnia, plasma bicarbonate falls only about 2 meq per liter for each 10-mm reduction in P_{CO_2}. In chronic hypocapnia, plasma bicarbonate is reduced by 4 to 5 meq per liter for each 10-mm decrease in P_{CO_2}.

The decrement in plasma bicarbonate attributable to renal compensatory activity is shown by the difference between the curves labeled acute and chronic respiratory alkalosis in Fig. 42-1.

PATHOGENESIS   Respiratory alkalosis is due to acute or chronic hyperventilation, which lowers P_{CO_2}. The causes of respiratory alkalosis are shown in Table 42-3.

CLINICAL FEATURES AND DIAGNOSIS   Depending on its severity and acuteness, hyperventilation may or may not be clinically apparent. In acute respiratory alkalosis, the clinical picture is rather characteristic: patients complain of paresthesias, numbness, and tingling; of light-headedness; and, if alkalosis is sufficiently severe, of manifestations of tetany. Alkalosis directly enhances neuromuscular excitability; this effect, rather than the modest decrease in ionized plasma calcium induced by alkalosis, is probably the major cause of tetany.

TABLE 42-3   Causes of respiratory alkalosis

I Hypoxia
  A Acute (e.g., pneumonia, asthma, pulmonary edema)
  B Chronic (e.g., pulmonary fibrosis, cyanotic heart disease, high altitudes)
II Respiratory center stimulation
  A Anxiety
  B Fever
  C Salicylate intoxication
  D Cerebral disease (tumor, encephalitis, etc.)
III Exercise
IV Gram-negative sepsis
V Hepatic cirrhosis
VI Pregnancy
VII Excessive mechanical ventilation

Severe respiratory alkalosis may cause confusion or loss of consciousness, perhaps due to cerebral vasospasm induced by hypocapnia.

The diagnosis may be suspected from the clinical setting but must be confirmed by analysis of the plasma bicarbonate system. Hypocapnia together with a variable degree of alkalemia is found; plasma bicarbonate is decreased but is rarely below 15 mmol per liter.

TREATMENT   The only successful treatment for respiratory alkalosis is elimination of the underlying disorder. In the acute hyperventilation syndrome, sedation, reassurance, and if symptoms are sufficiently severe, rebreathing into a bag will usually terminate the attack.

REFERENCES

ARBUS GS: An in vivo acid-base nomogram for clinical use. Can Med Assoc J 109:291, 1973

BATTLE DC, KURTZMAN NA: Renal regulation of acid-base homeostasis: Integrated response, in *The Kidney: Physiology and Pathophysiology,* 2d ed, DW Seldin, G Giebisch (eds). New York, Raven Press, 1986, p 1539

——— et al: Clinical and pathophysiologic spectrum of acquired distal renal tubular acidosis. Kidney In 20:398, 1981

COGAN MG, RECTOR FC JR: Acid-base disorders, in *The Kidney,* 3d ed, BM Brenner, FC Rector Jr (eds). Philadelphia, Saunders, 1986, p 457

EMMETT M, NARINS RG: Clinical use of the anion gap. Medicine 56:38, 1977

KASSIRER JP, MADIAS NE: Respiratory acid-base disorders. Hosp Practice 15:57, 1980

LEVY LH et al: Ketoacidosis associated with alcoholism in non-diabetic subjects. Ann Intern Med 78:213, 1973

NARINS RG, EMMETT M: Simple and mixed acid-base disorders: A practical approach. Medicine 59:161, 1980

SCHWARTZ WB, RELMAN AS: A critique of the parameters used in the evaluation of acid-base disorders. N Engl J Med 268:1382, 1963

STINEBAUGH BJ et al: Pathogenesis of distal renal tubular acidosis. Kidney Int 19:1, 1981

TANNEN RL: Control of acid excretion by the kidney. Ann Rev Med 31:35, 1980

section 7   Alterations in reproductive and sexual function

43   DISTURBANCES OF MENSTRUATION AND SEXUAL FUNCTION IN WOMEN

BRUCE R. CARR / JEAN D. WILSON

Complaints related to the female reproductive tract can usually be categorized either as disturbances of menstruation, pelvic pain, disturbances in sexual function, or infertility. However, a single disorder, for example leiomyoma of the uterus, can present with symptoms referable to any one or more of these categories. Furthermore, sexual dysfunction can interdigitate with other complaints in several ways. On the one hand, in women who present with complaints related to other reproductive tract functions, the underlying problem may actually be severe sexual dysfunction or marital conflict. Alternatively, women who have severe organic diseases of the pelvis, for example pelvic inflammatory disease, may present with a problem of sexual function such as dyspareunia, which in fact is only a minor manifestation of the underlying disease.

Since normal reproductive function depends on the integrated action of the central nervous system, the endocrine glands, and the reproductive organs, menstrual cycle abnormalities, sexual dysfunction, and infertility may be the result of a variety of systemic and psychological disorders as well as of primary defects in the endocrine and reproductive organs. The endocrine and physiologic changes—normal and abnormal—associated with puberty, reproductive life, and menopause are discussed in Chap. 331. The focus of this chapter is on the initial evaluation of women with disturbances of the reproductive tract.

DISTURBANCES IN MENSTRUATION   Disorders of menstruation can be divided into abnormal uterine bleeding and amenorrhea.

Abnormal uterine bleeding   The menstrual cycle is defined as the interval between the onset of one bleeding episode and the onset of the next. In normal women of reproductive age the cycle averages 28 ± 3 days, the mean duration of menstrual flow is 4 ± 2 days, and the average blood loss is 40 to 100 mL. Between the menarche and the menopause almost every woman experiences one or more episodes of abnormal uterine bleeding, here defined as any bleeding pattern outside the parameters of frequency, duration, and/or amount of blood loss described above. The decision to evaluate a patient with an abnormal bleeding pattern is based on the severity and frequency of the abnormal bleeding episodes.

When uterine bleeding is suspected, it is essential to establish first that the blood observed by the patient is derived from the uterine endometrium. Rectal, bladder, cervical, or vaginal sources of bleeding must be excluded. Once the bleeding is documented to be uterine in origin, a pregnancy-related disorder (such as threatened or incomplete abortion or ectopic pregnancy) must be excluded by physical examination and appropriate laboratory tests. Abnormal uterine bleeding may also be the initial or principal manifestation of a generalized bleeding diathesis. The remaining causes of abnormal uterine bleeding fall into two general categories: those associated with ovulatory cycles and those associated with anovulatory cycles.

OVULATORY CYCLES Menstrual bleeding with ovulatory cycles is spontaneous, regular in onset, predictable in duration and amount of flow, and frequently associated with discomfort. Uterine bleeding with ovulatory cycles is due to progesterone withdrawal at the end of the luteal phase and requires prior estrogen priming of the endometrium during the follicular phase of the cycle. When deviations from an established pattern of menstrual flow occur but the cycles are still regular, the usual cause is organic disease of the outflow tract. For example, regular, prolonged, excessive bleeding episodes unassociated with a bleeding diathesis are commonly due to abnormalities of the uterus such as submucous leiomyomas, adenomyosis, or endometrial polyps. On the other hand, cyclic, predictable menstruation characterized by spotting or light bleeding is often due to obstruction of the outflow tract as with uterine synechiae or scarring of the cervix. Intermittent bleeding between cyclic ovulatory menses is often due to cervical or endometrial lesions.

ANOVULATORY CYCLES Uterine bleeding that is irregular in occurrence and unpredictable as to amount and duration of flow is called dysfunctional uterine bleeding. Such bleeding is usually painless. Dysfunctional uterine bleeding is the result of a failure of normal follicular maturation with consequent anovulation and may be either transient or chronic. Transient disruption of the synchronous hypothalamic-pituitary-ovarian hormonal patterns necessary for ovulatory cycles occurs most often in the early menarcheal years, during the perimenopausal period, or as the secondary consequence of a variety of stresses and intercurrent illnesses. Persistent dysfunctional uterine bleeding during the reproductive years can occur in several organic diseases that affect ovarian function and is most often due to estrogen breakthrough bleeding. Estrogen breakthrough bleeding occurs when prolonged continuous estrogen stimulation of the endometrium is not interrupted by cyclic progesterone withdrawal. For example, chronic acyclic estrogen production not associated with ovulation can occur in polycystic ovarian disease.

Amenorrhea Amenorrhea is defined as failure of menarche by age 16, regardless of the presence or absence of secondary sexual characteristics, or the absence of menstruation for 6 months in a woman with previous periodic menses. Amenorrhea in a woman who has never menstruated is termed primary; cessation of menses is termed secondary amenorrhea. Because some disorders can cause both primary and secondary amenorrhea, we prefer a functional classification based upon the nature of the underlying defect, namely anatomic defects of the outflow tract (uterus, cervix, or vagina), ovarian failure, and chronic anovulation.

Anatomic defects of the outflow tract include congenital defects of the vagina, imperforate hymen, transverse vaginal septa, cervical stenosis, intrauterine adhesions (synechiae), absence of the vagina or uterus, and uterine maldevelopment. The diagnosis of an anatomic defect is usually made by physical examination and confirmed by demonstrating failure of bleeding following administration of estrogen plus a progestogen for 21 days.

Causes of *ovarian failure* include gonadal dysgenesis, deficiency of 17α-hydroxylase or 17,20-desmolase, resistant ovary syndrome, and premature ovarian failure. Ovarian failure encompasses those disorders in which the ovary is deficient in germ cells and those in which the germ cells are resistant to FSH (follicle-stimulating hormone). The diagnosis of ovarian failure as the cause of amenorrhea is confirmed by a plasma FSH greater than 40 mIU/mL.

Women with *chronic anovulation* fail to ovulate spontaneously but have the capability of ovulating with appropriate therapy. In some patients with chronic anovulation estrogen production is adequate, but estrogen is not secreted in a cyclic fashion. In others estrogen production is deficient.

Women who have adequate estrogen production and demonstrate withdrawal bleeding after progesterone challenge usually have polycystic ovarian disease (see Fig. 331-7). Unusual causes include hormone-secreting ovarian and adrenal tumors. Women with deficient or absent estrogen production, and therefore with absence of withdrawal bleeding after progesterone treatment, usually have hypogonadotropic hypogonadism due either to organic or functional disorders of the pituitary or central nervous system such as brain tumors, pituitary tumors (especially prolactin-secreting adenomas), primary hypopituitarism, or Sheehan's syndrome.

PELVIC PAIN Pelvic pain may originate in the pelvis or be referred from some other region of the body. A pelvic source for such pain is often suggested by the history (for example, dysmenorrhea and dyspareunia) and physical findings, but a high index of suspicion must be entertained for extrapelvic disorders that refer to the pelvis, such as appendicitis, cholecystitis, intestinal obstruction, and urinary tract infections (see Chap. 5).

"Physiologic" pelvic pain PAIN ASSOCIATED WITH OVULATION ("MITTELSCHMERZ") Many women experience low abdominal discomfort with ovulation, typically a dull aching pain at midcycle in one lower quadrant lasting from a few minutes to hours. It is rarely severe or incapacitating. The relationship of the pain to the mechanisms of ovulation is unknown. It may result from peritoneal irritation by follicular fluid released into the peritoneal cavity at the time of ovulation. The onset at midcycle and a short duration of pain are often diagnostic.

PREMENSTRUAL OR MENSTRUAL PAIN In normal ovulatory women somatic symptoms during the few days prior to menses may be insignificant or disabling. Such symptoms include edema, breast engorgement, and abdominal bloating or discomfort. A symptom complex of cyclic irritability, depression, and lethargy is known as the *premenstrual syndrome*. The cause is unknown but may be prostaglandin-mediated.

Severe or incapacitating cramping in women with ovulatory menses but no demonstrable disorders of the pelvis is termed *primary dysmenorrhea*.

Pelvic pain due to organic causes Severe dysmenorrhea associated with disease of the pelvis is termed *secondary dysmenorrhea*. Organic causes of pelvic pain can be classified as (1) uterine, (2) adnexal, (3) vulvar or vaginal, and (4) pregnancy-associated.

UTERINE PAIN Pain of uterine etiology is often chronic and continuous and increases in intensity during menstruation and intercourse. Causes include leiomyomas of the uterus (particularly submucous and degenerating leiomyomas), adenomyosis, and cervical stenosis. Infections of the uterus associated with intrauterine manipulation following dilatation and curettage or with intrauterine devices can also cause significant pelvic pain (see Chap. 331). Pelvic pain due to endometrial or cervical cancer is usually a late manifestation of disseminated disease (see Chap. 331).

ADNEXAL PAIN The most common cause of pain in the adnexae (fallopian tubes and ovaries) is infection (see Chap. 104). Acute salpingo-oophoritis presents as low abdominal pain, fever, and chills, beginning a few days after a menstrual period, and is most often a consequence of chlamydia or of gonococcal disease with or without a superimposed pyogenic infection. Chronic pelvic inflammatory disease results from either a single episode or multiple episodes of infection and may present as infertility associated with chronic pelvic pain that increases in intensity with menses and intercourse. On physical examination the adnexa are tender, and adnexal thickening with or without masses may be present. Pelvic inflammatory disease may become a surgical emergency if peritonitis results from rupture of a tuboovarian abscess. Ovarian cysts or neoplasms may cause pelvic pain that becomes more severe with torsion or rupture of the mass, and ectopic pregnancy must also be considered in the differential diagnosis (see below). Endometriosis involving fallopian tubes, ovaries, or peritoneum may cause both chronic low abdominal pain and infertility; the magnitude of tissue involvement does not always correlate with the severity of symptoms. Endometriosis pain typically increases with menstruation and, if the posterior ligaments of the uterus are involved, with intercourse.

VULVAR OR VAGINAL PAIN   Pain in these areas is most often due to infectious vaginitis caused by organisms such as *Monilia, Trichomonas,* or *Gardnerella* and is characteristically associated with vaginal discharge and pruritus. Herpetic vulvitis, condyloma acuminata, and cysts or abscesses of Bartholin's glands may also cause vulvar pain.

PREGNANCY-ASSOCIATED DISORDERS   Pregnancy must be considered in the differential diagnosis of pelvic pain in women during the reproductive years. Threatened abortion or incomplete abortion often presents with uterine cramping, bleeding, or passage of tissue following a period of amenorrhea. Ectopic pregnancy may be insidious in presentation and result in severe intraperitoneal hemorrhage and maternal death.

The evaluation of pelvic pain includes a careful history and pelvic examination. This often leads to the correct diagnosis and institution of appropriate treatment. If the pain is severe and the diagnosis is unclear, the workup should follow that outlined for the acute abdomen (Chap. 5). A culdocentesis is indicated if a ruptured ectopic pregnancy is suspected. If there is a question of an adnexal mass such as a tubal pregnancy or if the patient is so obese as to preclude a thorough pelvic examination, sonography may be helpful in the evaluation. Serial human chorionic gonadotropin (hCG) measurements may be helpful in establishing a diagnosis of tubal pregnancy. Finally, diagnostic laparoscopy and laparotomy may be indicated with severe or prolonged pain of undetermined etiology.

SEXUAL DYSFUNCTION   Some women with sexual dysfunction describe minor complaints related to the reproductive tract as a means of bringing sexual problems to the attention of the physician. Alternatively, sexual dysfunction may be thought to be the cause of low abdominal discomfort or dyspareunia when the actual etiology is an organic lesion. However, more and more women seek medical advice because of sexual problems that interface in provenance between medicine and sociology.

The normal sexual response begins with sexual arousal which causes genital vasocongestion that results in vaginal lubrication in preparation for intromission. The lubrication is due to the formation of a transudate in the vagina and in conjunction with genital congestion produces the so-called orgasmic platform prior to orgasm. Sexual stimuli (visual, tactile, auditory, and olfactory) as well as healthy vaginal tissue are prerequisites for genital vasocongestion and vaginal lubrication. During the second stage of the sexual response a series of involuntary contractions of the muscles of the pelvis under control of the autonomic nervous system results in a pleasurable cortical sensory phenomenon known as orgasm. Direct or indirect stimulation of the clitoris is important in the production of the female orgasm. In simple terms, sexual dysfunction can be due to interference with the arousal or orgasmic phases of the sexual response. Either disorder can be due to organic or functional cause or both.

Illnesses that impair neurologic function such as diabetes mellitus or multiple sclerosis may prevent normal sexual arousal. Local pelvic diseases such as vaginitis, endometriosis, and salpingo-oophoritis may preclude normal sexual response because of resulting dyspareunia. Debilitating systemic diseases such as cancer and cardiovascular diseases may impair normal sexual response indirectly.

More commonly, failure of a normal sexual response is due to psychological problems that impair sexual arousal. Such problems include misinformation, for example, the perception of sexual satisfaction as bad, or feelings of guilt about previous psychologically traumatic events such as incest, rape, or unwanted pregnancy. In addition, women who have had previous hysterectomy or mastectomy may perceive themselves as "incomplete." Stresses such as anxiety, depression, fatigue, and marital or interpersonal conflicts may lead to failure of the vasocongestive response and prevent normal vaginal lubrication. Women with such experiences may be unable to achieve normal sexual response unless they receive professional counseling by a family physician, psychologist, psychiatrist, or sex therapist. Such problems are approached by attempting to identify and reduce the causative stresses.

Failure to achieve orgasm is a specific form of sexual dysfunction. Many women enjoy sexual encounters to variable degrees without experiencing orgasm because of the pleasure derived from closeness in a cherished relationship particularly with a loving partner. However, for other women sexual relations with rare or absent orgasms are frustrating and unsatisfying. In many instances, failure of orgasm is due to insufficient clitoral stimulation and may be rectified by appropriate counseling and patient education.

A specific entity, "vaginismus," painful, involuntary contractions of the musculature surrounding the entrance to the vagina, is a rare cause of dyspareunia. It is a conditioned response to a previous real or imagined frightening or traumatic sexual experience. Treatment is directed to elimination of the conditioned response by progressive vaginal dilation by the patient in conjunction with marital therapy.

REPRODUCTION   Problems of infertility are discussed in detail in Chap. 331. The approach to infertile couples always involves evaluation of both the man and woman. The initial evaluation includes a thorough history and physical examination. The history should elicit information as to the frequency of intercourse, the sexual responses of both, the use of contraceptives or lubricants, previous or past medical illnesses, and all medications taken.

Male-associated factors account for a third of infertility problems. Therefore, one of the first procedures in the workup of infertile couples should be a semen analysis (see Chap. 330). The initial evaluation of the female includes documentation of normal ovulatory cycles. A history of regular, cyclic, predictable, spontaneous menses usually indicates ovulatory cycles, which may be confirmed by basal body temperature graphs, properly timed endometrial biopsies, or plasma progesterone measurements during the luteal phase of the cycle. Also, the diagnosis of luteal-phase dysfunction can be established by these methods. If the woman is anovulatory, attempts to induce ovulation can be undertaken by a variety of methods including clomiphene citrate, human menopausal gonadotropins, bromocryptine mesylate, luteinizing hormone releasing hormone (LHRH) agonists, or wedge resection of the ovaries (Chap. 331).

The most common cause of infertility in women is tubal disease, usually due to infection (pelvic inflammatory disease) or endometriosis. Tubal disease can be evaluated by obtaining a hysterosalpingogram or by diagnostic laparoscopy. The treatment of tubal causes of infertility is primarily surgical.

A cervical factor as a cause of infertility is evaluated by a properly timed postcoital examination. During this examination the sperm motility in cervical mucus is observed. Also, immunologic etiologies for infertility may be present and can be tested for by a variety of laboratory tests. We are unable to account for a cause of infertility in 10 percent of couples.

The desire for fertility control or contraception is also a frequent cause for women to seek medical treatment or evaluation. The most widely used methods for fertility control include (1) rhythm and withdrawal techniques, (2) barrier methods, (3) intrauterine devices, (4) oral steroid contraceptives, (5) sterilization, and (6) abortion. A discussion of these methods and the possible complications of each is found in Chap. 331.

REFERENCES

FORDNEY DS: Dyspareunia and vaginismus. Clin Obstet Gynecol 21:205, 1978
HATCHER RA et al: *Contraceptive Technology 1984–1985.* New York, Irvington, 1984
KASE NG et al: *Principles and Practice of Clinical Gynecology.* New York, Wiley, 1983
MASTERS W, JOHNSON V: *Human Sexual Response.* Boston, Little, Brown, 1966
———, ———: *Human Sexual Inadequacy.* Boston, Little, Brown, 1970
PRITCHARD JH et al: *Williams Obstetrics,* 17th ed. Norwalk Ct., Appleton-Century-Crofts, 1985
SPEROFF L et al: *Clinical Gynecologic Endocrinology and Infertility,* 3d ed. Baltimore, Williams & Wilkins, 1983

44 IMPOTENCE AND INFERTILITY IN MEN

PATRICK C. WALSH / JEAN D. WILSON

A coordinated sequence of physiologic events (psychic, endocrine, vascular, and neurologic) controls normal sexual and reproductive function in men. In this chapter, the discussion is focused on the clinical presentation of sexual disorders in men. (Also see Chaps. 45, ''Medical Aspects of Sexuality,'' and 330, ''Disorders of the Testis.'')

SEXUAL FUNCTION

NORMAL SEXUAL FUNCTION   Simply stated, normal male sexual function can be divided into five events, each of which is under diverse regulation: libido, erection, ejaculation, orgasm, and detumescence.

The first, sexual desire or libido, is regulated by psychic factors and by testicular androgens. Castration produces a decline in libido that can be restored by treatment with testosterone.

The second phase, erection, is primarily a neurologic event that results in modification of the vascular supply to the penis, causing it to become engorged with blood. The neurologic aspect of erection is controlled by both reflex and psychic stimuli. The sensory portion begins with fibers that originate in pacinian corpuscles of the penis and pass via the pudendal nerve to the S2–S4 dorsal root ganglia. The efferent limb begins with parasympathetic preganglionic fibers from S2–S4 which synapse in the perivesicular, prostatic, and cavernous plexuses. From there, postganglionic fibers pass to blood vessels of the corpora cavernosa. Efferent fibers from S3–S4 also travel in the pudendal nerve to the ischiocavernosus and bulbocavernosus muscles. Sympathetic innervation of the male genitalia originates in fibers from the lateral columns of T12 and L1, the so-called thoracolumbar erection center, that synapse in the pelvic and perivesicular plexuses. Postganglionic fibers innervate the smooth muscle of the vas deferens, seminal vesicle, and internal sphincter of the bladder. Sympathetic innervation can act synergistically with the sacral parasympathetics to mediate erection initiated by psychic stimuli but is not mandatory for erection, because most men have normal potency after bilateral complete sympathectomy. The central nervous system modulates erectile response via pathways thought to descend in the lateral columns of the spinal cord. The effect of the central nervous system on erection can either be stimulatory or inhibitory, thus the importance of psychic factors for erection.

While erection is controlled by the parasympathetic nervous system, the transformation of the penis from a flaccid to an erect state is a vascular phenomenon. Blood reaches the penis via terminal branches of the right and left internal pudendal arteries. The erectile tissue of the penis consists of two corpora cavernosa lying side by side on the dorsal aspect of the penis and the corpus spongiosum that surrounds the urethra. This erectile tissue consists of an irregular spongelike system of vascular spaces interspersed between arteries and veins.

Erection is initiated by a decrease in arterial resistance resulting in increased arterial blood flow with a subsequent decrease in venous outflow. The neurotransmitter responsible for these events has not been identified, but vascular or cavernosal smooth muscle relaxation may result from mediation by beta-adrenergic, cholinergic, or vasoactive intestinal polypeptide (VIP) mechanisms. Furthermore, alpha-adrenergic antagonists can cause increased blood flow to the corpus and hence erection.

The third phase, ejaculation, is under control of the sympathetic nervous system and consists of two processes, seminal emission and true ejaculation. Emission results from the contraction of the vas deferens, prostate, and seminal vesicles which causes seminal fluid to enter the urethra. True ejaculation results from contraction of the muscles of the pelvic floor including the bulbocavernosus and ischiocavernosus muscles. Retrograde ejaculation into the bladder is prevented by partial bladder neck closure mediated by the sympathetic nerves.

The fourth phase, orgasm, is a cortical sensory phenomenon in which the rhythmic contraction of the bulbocavernosus and ischio-cavernosus muscles is perceived as pleasurable. It is purely psychic. The fact that orgasm can occur without either erection, ejaculation, or bladder neck closure explains why some drugs that prevent erection or ejaculation do not interfere with orgasm.

Detumescence after orgasm and ejaculation may be the result of vasoconstriction of the arterioles supplying blood to the erectile tissue, thus allowing venous drainage to empty the sinuses and the penis to become flaccid. Following orgasm, there is a refractory period that varies with age, physical condition, and psychic factors during which erection and ejaculation are inhibited.

IMPOTENCE   Male sexual dysfunction, often termed *impotence,* may be manifested in various ways: loss of desire, inability to obtain or maintain an erection, premature ejaculation, absence of emission, inability to achieve orgasm. Many subjects complain of more than one abnormality simultaneously. These complaints can be secondary to other chronic or debilitating diseases, the consequence of specific disorders of the urogenital or endocrine systems, or the result of psychiatric disturbance. It is mandatory in all instances to exclude organic (and in some instances potentially correctable or treatable) causes.

Loss of desire   Because androgens have a major influence on sexual desire in men, a decrease in libido may indicate androgen deficiency arising from either pituitary or testicular disease. This possibility can be tested by the measurement of plasma testosterone and gonadotropins. However, since the level of testosterone required to maintain libido is usually less than the amount necessary for full stimulation of the prostate and seminal vesicles, absence of emission also occurs when the loss of libido is due to hypogonadism. Conversely, if the semen volume is normal, it is unlikely that endocrine factors are responsible for their sexual dysfunction.

Failure of erection   The organic causes of erectile impotence can be grouped into endocrine, drug, local, neurologic, and vascular causes (Table 44-1).

Endocrine causes of testicular failure that result in impotence usually cause such profound changes that the disorders are not difficult to recognize (Chap. 330). However, hyperprolactinemia may cause impotence in some patients with pituitary tumors and may not be obvious on physical examination (see Chaps. 321 and 332); hyperprolactinemia suppresses LHRH (luteinizing hormone–releasing hormone) production, resulting in plasma gonadotropins and testosterone values in the low normal range. Bromocriptine mesylate, a dopamine agonist, may lower prolactin levels and reverse impotence in such patients.

Many drugs cause impotence including antihistamines, antihypertensives, anticholinergics, psychogenic agents, and drugs of habituation or addiction. The usual explanation is neurologic blockade, and this may well be the case for those drugs with peripheral parasympatholytic actions such as the tricyclic antidepressants. Others may act by enhancing prolactin secretion. It is not clear whether impotence caused by drugs of addiction such as alcohol, methadone, and heroin is due to reduced testosterone levels or the general condition of the patient.

Penile diseases that cause impotence can almost always be diagnosed by history and physical examination and include previous priapism, penile trauma, and Peyronie's disease.

Many types of neurologic disorders can cause impotence including lesions in the anterior temporal lobe, spinal cord disorders, insufficiency of sensory input such as can occur in diabetic neuropathy and tabes dorsalis, or damage to parasympathetic nerves, for example, following surgical procedures such as total prostatectomy. Transurethral prostatectomy, in contrast, does not cause organic impotence. Furthermore, the nerve supply to the penis (the nervi erigentes) runs through the lateral pedicle of the prostate, and if the nerves are preserved during radical prostate surgery, potency can be preserved in most men. If spinal cord injury is above the thoracolumbar region, reflex erections may occur. Diffuse injury of the spinal cord results in total impotence. Diabetes mellitus deserves special comment. As many as half of diabetic men develop impotence within 6 years of the onset of diabetes, and impotence may be the first clinical manifestation of diabetic neuropathy. However, when a careful neurologic examination is performed including measurement of the cystometrogram, other evidences of neurologic disturbance are usually uncovered. Many of the other polyneuropathies described in Chap. 354 have similar effects.

Vascular insufficiency causes impotence because blood flow into the vascular network of the penis is insufficient to obtain (or maintain) the erect state. The prototype of impaired penile blood supply is the Leriche syndrome. Here impedance to the blood flow into the penis occurs as the result of obstruction of the distal aorta. This usually presents as claudication and impotence; either can occur separately. Likewise, occlusion in smaller vessels supplying the penis can also lead to impotence. Together with neuropathy, vascular insufficiency contributes to the impotence in many men with diabetes mellitus. Decreased blood flow to the penis may be detected using the Doppler technique. By dividing the penile systolic blood pressure by the simultaneously determined supine brachial systolic pressure, the penile/brachial index is obtained. An index of over 0.75 is normal, and one of less than 0.6 is suggestive of vasculogenic impotence. An index of 0.6 to 0.75 is indeterminate. Due to overlap of such abnormal results with those in older potent men it is not possible to be certain that arterial insufficiency is the cause of impotence in a given individual. Normal values exclude arterial insufficiency; abnormal values require confirmatory arteriography.

Premature ejaculation   This disorder seldom has an organic cause. It is usually related to anxiety in the sexual situation, unreasonable expectations about performance, or emotional disorder. A variety of successful therapeutic modalities have been described by Levine.

Absence of emission   This symptom may be produced by (1) retrograde ejaculation, (2) sympathetic denervation, (3) androgen deficiency, or (4) drugs. Retrograde ejaculation may occur following surgery on the bladder neck or may develop spontaneously in diabetic men. Demonstration of sperm in a postcoital urine specimen will establish the diagnosis. Following sympathectomy or occasionally after extensive retroperitoneal surgery, the autonomic innervation of the prostate and seminal vesicles is lost, resulting in absence of smooth-muscle contraction at the time of ejaculation. Androgen deficiency results in a decrease in secretions of the prostate and seminal vesicles and in a diminution of the volume of ejaculate. Finally, drugs such as guanethidine, phenoxybenzamine, and phentolamine primarily impair ejaculation rather than erection or libido.

Absence of orgasm   If libido and erectile function are normal, the absence of orgasm is almost always due to a psychiatric disorder.

Failure of detumescence   Priapism is a persistent painful erection, often unrelated to sexual activity. Priapism is usually idiopathic but can be associated with sickle cell anemia, chronic granulocytic leukemia, or spinal cord injury. The disorder is thought to be secondary to clotting within the penile vascular network. The persistent erection disrupts the network and can lead to fibrosis and subsequent erectile impotence. Early surgical relief of priapism by shunting procedures may prevent subsequent impotence.

Evaluation of impotence   The commonest cause of prolonged impotence is an anxiety or depression state. These closely related conditions can be diagnosed by the criteria enunciated in Chap. 11. Other psychological factors such as disinterest in the sexual partner, fear of sexual incompetence, marital discord, deviant sexual attitudes, worry, fatigue, and ill health often operate in various combinations to reduce sexual impulse. The central issue in the evaluation of impotence is to separate those instances due to psychological factors from those due to organic causes (Table 44-1). Usually, the separation can be made on the basis of history. From early childhood through the eighth decade, erections occur during normal sleep. This phenomenon, termed *nocturnal penile tumescence* (NPT), occurs during rapid eye movement sleep, and the total time of NPT averages 100 min per night. Consequently, if the impotent man gives a history of turgid erections under any circumstances (often when awakening in the early morning), the psychic, efferent neurologic, and circulatory systems that mediate erection are intact, and dysfunction is probably due to a psychiatric disorder. In these patients the physical and laboratory examinations should be limited. (Occasional patients with sensory neuropathy may have nocturnal erections.)

If the history of nocturnal erections is questionable, measurements of NPT can be made with the use of a strain gauge attached to a recorder. Alternatively, the penis can be wrapped with gummed, perforated paper; failure to break the perforations on three successive nights suggests absence of nocturnal erections. Although false-negative and false-positive results are possible, these procedures help to differentiate psychogenic and organic impotence. Interestingly, psychogenically impotent men may experience longer and more frequent nocturnal erections than do normal men. Other factors in favor of organic impotence include a similar degree of erectile dysfunction under all circumstances, onset not associated with any

TABLE 44-1   Some organic causes of erectile impotence in men

I Endocrine causes
   A Testicular failure (primary or secondary)
   B Hyperprolactinemia
II Drugs
   A Antihistamines
      1 Cimetidine
      2 Diphenhydramine
      3 Hydroxyzine
   B Antihypertensives
      1 Clonidine
      2 Methyldopa
      3 Propranolol
      4 Reserpine
      5 Spironolactone
      6 Thiazides
   C Anticholinergics
   D Antidepressants
      1 Amitriptyline
      2 Doxepin
      3 Isocarboxazid
   E Antipsychotics
      1 Chlorpromazine
      2 Haloperidol
      3 Thioridazine
   F Tranquilizers
      1 Diazepam
      2 Barbiturates
      3 Chlordiazepoxide
   G Drugs of habituation or addiction
      1 Alcohol
      2 Methadone
      3 Heroin
III Penile diseases
   A Previous priapism
   B Penile trauma
   C Peyronie's disease
IV Neurologic diseases
   A Anterior temporal lobe lesions
   B Diseases of the spinal cord
   C Loss of sensory input
      1 Diabetes mellitus and various polyneuropathies
      2 Tabes dorsalis
      3 Disease of dorsal root ganglia
   D Disease of nervi erigentes
      1 Complete prostatectomy
      2 Rectosigmoid operations
      3 Aortic bypass surgery
V Vascular disease
   A Leriche syndrome

particular psychiatric symptomatology, a previous uninterrupted period of normal erectile function, and persistent sexual desire.

Having deduced an organic cause, the fundamental problem is the differential diagnosis of the etiology (Table 44-1). The history should be probed for symptoms of diabetes mellitus, symptoms of peripheral neuropathy or bladder dysfunction, symptoms referable to the vascular system such as intermittent claudication, and symptoms of local disease such as a history of priapism. A thorough drug history should be obtained, and inquiry concerning past operations that may have produced neurologic damage should be made.

Physical examination should include a thorough genital examination to identify abnormalities of the penis. The testes should be palpated for size and abnormal masses; if the length is less than 3.5 cm, hypogonadism should be considered. Evidence of feminization such as gynecomastia and abnormal body hair distribution should be sought. All pulses should be palpated, including the penile pulse, which can be felt by pressing both corpora between the thumb and forefinger and palpating to either side of the midline. However, because only a portion of the superficial dorsal arteries reach the corpus cavernosum, normal dorsal pulse pressures do not exclude the presence of deep cavernous arterial occlusion. If there is an indication from either history or physical examination of a vascular etiology, a Doppler procedure or arteriography may be indicated.

The neurologic exam should measure anal sphincter tone, perineal sensation, and the bulbocavernosus reflex. This reflex is elicited by squeezing the glans penis and noting the degree of anal sphincter constriction. An examination for peripheral neuropathy, including distal muscle weakness, loss of tendon reflexes in the legs, and tests for impairment of vibratory, position, tactile, and pain sensation should also be performed (see Chap. 354). In the absence of a concomitant neurogenic bladder, electromyographic sacral signal tracing of the bulbocavernosus reflex may be a useful ancillary procedure for detection of localized peripheral neuropathy; the methodology involves measurement of bulbocavernosus response latencies following electrical stimulation of the glans. Although this procedure has not been studied exhaustively, improvement by revascularization surgery is unlikely if the test is abnormal.

Laboratory evaluation is probably of minimal value. Measurement of serum testosterone in the absence of evidence of feminization or hypogonadism is seldom helpful.

Treatment of impotence Medical therapy with androgens offers little more than placebo benefit except in hypogonadal men. If a prolactin-secreting pituitary tumor is present, however, either surgical removal or treatment with bromocriptine usually results in return of potency. Surgical therapy may be useful in the treatment of decreased potency related to aortic obstruction; however, potency can be lost rather than improved after aortic operation if the autonomic nerve supply to the penis is damaged. This complication is minimized if an endarterectomy is done or, in a grafting procedure, if the reconstruction of the distal end is performed above the origin of the external iliac arteries.

A useful surgical technique for improvement of potency in refractory patients such as individuals with diabetic neuropathy is the implantation of a penile prosthesis, namely the insertion within the corpora of a small, blunt Silastic rod. The patient must be made aware that full erection is not produced and that the device only prevents buckling during intercourse. Furthermore, the complication rate is high in some series. Alternatively, an inflatable prosthetic device has been devised for implantation on either side of the corpora. A connecting reservoir of material is placed in the perivesicular space and pumps are located in the scrotum. By means of these pumps the penis can be made to become nearly fully erect at the appropriate time and to relax after intercourse. Intracavernous injections of papaverine and/or phentolamine in patients with nonvascular causes for impotence can cause transitory penile tumescence sufficient for coitus. Whether self-injection of these agents will be successful for the management of sexual dysfunction is not clear.

In the larger group of anxiety states and depressive illnesses,

measures directed at their alleviation may restore sexual potency, and sexual counseling, education, and psychotherapy are beneficial in alleviating psychogenic factors.

REPRODUCTION

Approximately a tenth of marriages in the United States are barren, and another tenth result in fewer children than desired. The husband is the cause of the infertility in about a third of these marriages.

Infertility can be due to either disorders of the hypothalamic-pituitary system, disorders of the testes, or abnormalities of the ejaculatory system (Table 330-1). When obtaining a history, the physician should collect information about the duration of infertility, fertility in prior marriages of both the husband and wife, the presence of acquired or congenital disease that may lead to infertility, technique and frequency of intercourse, and family history of infertility. To exclude gross abnormalities of the endocrine system, the physical examination should evaluate the distribution of body hair, the presence of gynecomastia, the development of the scrotum and penis, the location of the urethral meatus, and the presence of normal vasa deferentia and epididymides. The size of each testis should be estimated. Because the seminiferous tubules account for more than 75 percent of the testicular mass, a reduction in testicular size (less than 3.5 cm in length) indicates a deficiency in the spermatogenic function of the testis. Finally, with the patient in the upright position, the Valsalva maneuver should be utilized to test for the presence of a varicocele.

The semen analysis provides a semiquantitative estimation of the severity of the dysfunction. The findings are usually considered normal if the semen coagulates and then liquefies, the volume is 2 to 5 mL, the sperm count is greater than 20 million per milliliter, more than 60 percent of the sperm are actively motile, and more than 60 percent have normal morphology. If no sperm are present, the term *azoospermia* is used; if sperm are present but the count is less than 20 million per milliliter, the patient is considered to have *oligospermia*. In the azoospermic man with normal-sized testes, the differential diagnosis includes hyalinization of the seminiferous tubules, Sertoli cell–only syndrome, gonadotropin deficiency, ductal obstruction, and maturation arrest. Plasma testosterone, LH (luteinizing hormone), and FSH (follicle-stimulating hormone) measurements are helpful in separating these conditions. With hyalinization of the seminiferous tubules LH and FSH are elevated, and plasma testosterone is low or borderline normal. Men with Sertoli cell–only syndrome usually have normal LH and testosterone, but elevated FSH levels. In gonadotropin deficiency LH, FSH, and testosterone are low, and in ductal obstruction or maturation arrest all endocrine studies are normal. To differentiate between the last two disorders, a testicular biopsy is necessary. In oligospermic patients, if the history and physical examination are normal, it is unlikely that any further laboratory investigation will be useful in defining the etiology. These patients are usually classified in the large group termed *idiopathic oligospermia*.

REFERENCES

Impotence

BENSON GS: Mechanisms of penile erection. Invest Urol 19:65, 1981
BUVAT J et al: Comparative investigations in 26 impotent and 26 nonimpotent diabetic patients. J Urol 133:34, 1985
COLE NJ: Drugs that influence sexual expression. Consultant 20:3281, 1980
DAVIDSON JM et al: Effects of androgen on sexual behavior in hypogonadal men. J Clin Endocrinol 48:955, 1979
ERCOLE JJ et al: Changing surgical concepts in the treatment of priapism. J Urol 125:210, 1981
FISHMAN JF et al: Experience with inflatable penile prosthesis. Urology 23:86, 1984
FURLOW WL (ed): Male sexual dysfunction. Urol Clin North Am 8:1, 1981
LEVINE SB: Marital sexual dysfunction: Ejaculation disturbances. Ann Intern Med 84:575, 1976
LUE TF et al: Hemodynamics of erection in the monkey. J Urol 130:1237, 1983

MARSHALL PG et al: Nocturnal penile tumescence with stamps: A comparative study under sleep laboratory conditions. J Urol 130:88, 1983

MEYER J: Disorders of sexual function, in *Williams Textbook of Endocrinology*, JD Wilson, DM Foster (eds). Philadelphia, Saunders, 1985, vol 7, pp 476–491

NATH RL et al: The multidisciplinary approach to vasculogenic impotence. Surgery 89:124, 1981

NEWMAN HF et al: Mechanism of human penile erection: An overview. Urology 17:399, 1981

SPARK RF et al: Impotence is not always psychogenic. JAMA 243:750, 1980

VAN ARSDALEN KN et al: Erectile physiology, dysfunction and evaluation: I. Physiology of erection. Monogr Urol 1983, 4:137–156

——— et al: Erectile physiology, dysfunction and evaluation: II. Etiology and evaluation of erectile dysfunction. Monogr Urol 1983, 4:165–185

WALSH PC et al: Impotence following radical prostatectomy: Insight into etiology and prevention. J Urol 128:492, 1982

WINTER CC: Priapism. Urol Surv 28:163, 1978

ZORGNIOTTI AW: Auto-injection of the corpus cavernosum with a vasoactive drug combination for vasculogenic impotence. J Urol 133:39, 1985

Infertility

AMELAR RD et al: *Male Infertility*. Philadelphia, Saunders, 1977, p 153

GREENBERG SH et al: Experience with 425 subfertile male patients. J Urol 119:507, 1970

SHERINS RJ et al: Male infertility, in *Campbell's Urology*, 5th ed, PC Walsh et al (eds). Philadelphia, Saunders, 1985, vol 1, chap 12

---

45   MEDICAL ASPECTS OF SEXUALITY

PETER REICH

Sexual problems are common in the general population. In one study of healthy, married, middle-aged couples, 40 percent of the men and 63 percent of the women had sexual dysfunctions, primarily impotence and premature ejaculation in men and inability to achieve orgasm in women. In another study 53 percent of outpatients in a general medical group practice described sexual problems when the issue was brought up by the physician during a medical evaluation.

These surveys also showed that patients tend to be reticent about sexual concerns unless they are asked about sexual function by their physicians. Only a fraction of those who were impotent had complained spontaneously of the problem in previous medical contacts. Even those patients who develop erectile dysfunction after taking medications frequently fail to report the problem. Married couples with sexual dysfunctions tend to modify their behavior to compensate for the problem rather than seek medical help.

The reason that many patients find it difficult to discuss sexuality

TABLE 45-1   An outline of the sexual history recommended for the initial data base

Introductory question
1 Have you noticed any problems in your ability to have and enjoy sexual relations (sex)?
  If positive response, have patient elaborate, then continue with questions.
  If negative response, continue with questions.
Men
2 Do you have any problems having or maintaining an erection? If so, in what situations?
3 Do you have any problems having an orgasm (ejaculating) (coming) (too soon, or not soon enough)? If so, in what situations?
Women
2 Do you have any pain during penetration?
3 Do you have any difficulty coming to orgasm? If so, in what situations?
Men and women
4 Are you sexually active?
5 Has your present illness affected your sexual functioning?
6 Do you have any questions or concerns about your sexual functioning?
Clarification of problems
1 How much of a problem is this?
2 How long has this been a problem? When was it better or worse?
3 Do you have any ideas about what causes this problem?
4 Have you ever sought help for this or any other sexual concerns?
5 How do you feel about getting some help now?

SOURCE: *Ende et al.*

with physicians has not been studied systematically. Some may be inhibited by shyness, embarrassment, guilt, shame, anxiety, or feelings of inadequacy. Old attitudes tend to persist in spite of the current openness about sexuality in general. A common finding in surveys of sexual dysfunction is that patients are often grateful when they are asked about their sexual function and generally perceive the physician as being more competent, thorough, and caring after such questions are asked.

The physician in turn may inadvertently discourage the patient from bringing up sexual concerns by subtle indications of discomfort, disapproval, or embarrassment or by failing to ask appropriate and timely questions. Physicians may avoid the subject because of fears of starting an emotionally charged discussion with insufficient time to resolve it. In truth, most physicians can make an initial assessment of sexual symptoms, and a brief inquiry seldom leads to the need for a lengthy discussion.

An objective approach to sexual issues reduces tensions and enables both patient and physician to deal with sensitive material. Often patients harbor fears and misconceptions that may be relieved by open discussion. Sexual symptoms may be the first manifestation of organic disorders, and a change in sexual function at any time of life is an indication for a thorough medical evaluation. Thus, it is the responsibility of the physician to establish an accurate and complete diagnosis including both physiologic and psychological factors and to evaluate the significances of sexual problems in the context of the patient's background and lifestyle. The yield from this aspect of a general medical evaluation can be high in terms of relieving suffering, understanding the patient's medical status, and achieving a good doctor-patient relationship.

THE GENERAL APPROACH TO THE PATIENT   More often than in other areas of medicine, the physician needs to take an active role in initiating the discussion of sexual matters. The inclusion of routine screening questions in the review of systems is one way to ensure that the area is not overlooked. Sexuality can be brought up comfortably after questions about menstrual function in women or questions about urinary function in men. Some clinicians prefer linking questions about sexual function to inquiries about relationships and personal satisfactions. To be effective, screening questions should be nonspecific, should not assume that the patient is heterosexual, and should project a nonjudgmental attitude.

Table 45-1 gives an outline of the brief sexual history recommended by Ende et al. for screening purposes. Similar guides can be found in standard texts of psychiatry and of obstetrics and gynecology. It is useful to have such a framework in mind when obtaining a sexual history. A detailed guide to the assessment of sexual function has been published by the Group for Advancement of Psychiatry.

Screening questions vary with the age and the circumstances of the patient. Such questions should be routine or the physician may overlook problems, may return to the subject as an afterthought, or may experience tension or show embarrassment when trying to think of a screening question during the history.

When a sexual complaint is elicited or volunteered, a detailed history of the manifestations and associated symptoms should be obtained. The assessment of a sexual problem is similar to the assessment of a problem involving any other system. The history of a sexual complaint necessarily includes information about relationships with partners; tensions, anxieties, preconceptions, attitudes, and interpersonal factors must be taken into account. A complete history that includes careful attention to multiple determinants, a thorough evaluation of the patient as a person, and a consideration of the context of the symptoms usually yields a working diagnosis that enables the physician either to treat the patient or to make an appropriate referral.

The physician has the special responsibility of initiating a discussion of sexuality when coexisting medical problems are likely to affect sexual function. Patients may fear sexual activity after myocardial infarction or episodes of cardiac arrhythmia or may anticipate loss of sexual function after transurethral prostatectomy, hysterectomy, or other procedures or conditions involving the urogenital tract. Other disorders affect sexuality directly or indirectly through loss of libido or changes in body image (Chaps. 43 and 44). By anticipating sexual problems the physician can help the patient make adjustments and can sometimes prevent disorders that are secondary to fears or misconceptions.

Reassurances about confidentiality may be necessary during the discussion of sexual matters even though such confidentiality is ordinarily assumed in the doctor-patient relationship. The assurance of confidentiality is especially important when the physician also treats other members of the family or when the patient needs to discuss extramarital, deviant, or extralegal behavior.

The dignity of the patient should be kept in mind as the history is taken by observing such simple practices as using scientific words for sexual parts and sexual activities. Vernacular or slang expressions, which are sometimes used in a mistaken effort to put the patient at ease, and jokes or other informal remarks should be avoided even with a patient who uses them. Comments that may seem casual to the physician tend to live on in the patient's mind.

Anticipation of discomfort may lead physicians to choose an evasive route of inquiry while patients might appreciate a direct question. Alternatively, some patients allude to sexual problems indirectly with idiomatic phrases, such as "changing nature" or "problems in relationships"; unless the physician is sensitive to feelings and language the reference may be missed, and the patient may assume that the physician is not interested in further information. Sometimes sexual problems appear indirectly through other complaints relating to the urogenital system.

Two types of patients—the elderly and the homosexual—present special problems in regard to the evaluation of sexual function. The sexuality of elderly patients is often not well understood by physicians. With reasonable health, men retain sexual interest and potency into old age. Impotence at any age is pathologic. Women also retain their sexual response but are more likely to suffer loss of their partner. Physicians may refrain from asking questions because they incorrectly assume that sexual satisfactions can no longer be achieved because of the aging process. Alternatively, patients silently accept a loss of sexual function because of similar misconceptions about the effects of illness or of aging. Depression may be a factor in such instances. Here the questions of the physician, coupled with some reassuring statements about the tendencies of many persons to assume mistakenly they will never be able to enjoy sexual relations again, bring the issue into the open and awaken new hopes in the patient.

Homosexual patients with disorders of sexual function often do not receive sympathetic medical care from heterosexual physicians. In one study of gynecologic care for lesbians a major hindrance in communication was the assumption by physicians that all patients are heterosexual. Homosexual men have similar problems in relating to heterosexual physicians. Some homosexual patients prefer going to homosexual physicians or to clinics run by homophile organizations. Many physicians share with the public at large serious misconceptions about homosexual behavior.

Kinsey and his coworkers showed how common homosexuality is in western societies. In his survey of more than 16,000 American men and women, Kinsey reported that approximately 4 percent of the men and 2 percent of the women are exclusively homosexual throughout their lives, and another 13 percent of the men are predominantly homosexual for at least 3 years of their lives. Occasional or intermittent homosexual contact was common in men and women. Approximately one-third of the men surveyed had had one or more homosexual contacts after puberty. In studies of homosexual men and women no association has been found between homosexuality and family structure, childhood experiences, or parental influences. Early gender nonconformity was the only predictor of homosexual development. Homosexuality was not a conscious choice of the individual but appeared to arise in a predetermined pattern. Homosexuality is also not associated with psychopathology or personality disorder and is compatible with normal productivity in society. In spite of increased acceptance of homosexuality in our culture, gay men and lesbian women often encounter personal rejection and job discrimination. Expectations of rejection may lead patients to conceal homosexuality from their physicians.

With the current epidemic of the acquired immunodeficiency syndrome (AIDS) in homosexual males, it is especially important for the physician to know the sexual orientation of male patients. This information may also provide insight into other disorders to which homosexual men are predisposed, such as hepatitis and proctitis. Homosexual women may also receive better medical care when their sexual orientation is understood. As in other areas of sexuality, a simple direct approach to the issue is generally welcomed by the patient. One experienced clinician advocates asking all patients whether they are homosexual or heterosexual; others simply ask all patients to identify their sexual preference. Whether or not AIDS is a clinical concern, male homosexual patients may be suffering from hidden fears of the disease and would be relieved by an explicit discussion. Even married patients may have covert homosexual activities that have important clinical implications. The parents of homosexual individuals often appeal to physicians for help. They need the reassurance that it is not their fault and that their children can lead satisfying, productive lives while accepting their homosexual orientation. It is important to emphasize that homosexuality is not a disorder and is not associated with psychopathology. It is not a choice taken by the individual and is not amenable to change.

EVALUATION Once a sexual complaint has been elicited, a detailed history of specific behavior should be obtained. Terms for sexual disorders may be misused, exaggerated, or misunderstood by patients. Other sexual complaints reflect misconceptions, ignorance, or fears, and the problems prove to be nonexistent when the behavior is explored in detail. Patients may overestimate or underestimate the extent of a problem, depending upon their psychological orientation. For example, one woman believed herself to be frigid because her sexual partner, for neurotic reasons of his own, compared her in a disparaging way to his previous partners. Much can be learned from the first instance of a sexual problem, from the pattern of behavior after the onset of symptoms, and from inquiring whether the problem is present consistently or varies with the circumstances or nature of the sexual practice.

In every disorder there is a complex interaction between the physical and the emotional, and every sexual symptom needs to be evaluated in the context of the relationships between the patient and the sexual partners and in the context of the sexual practices and attitudes of the patient. A past history, including early experiences, attitudes of parents, and attitudes toward childhood sexuality, development, marriage, and pregnancy may be relevant. Establishing the relationship of sexual function to general health is of fundamental importance, and it is essential to take a complete drug history on every patient, both in regard to drug abuse and to use of prescribed drugs. An understanding of the daily habits of a patient may provide important clues to diagnosis. Fatigue, anxiety, and stress, as well as the timing of the use of alcohol, drugs, and medications, can provide insight into the underlying cause.

A general physical examination with special attention to an examination of the genitalia is essential. At times patients conceal or are unaware of abnormalities of the genitalia. On the other hand, otherwise sophisticated patients may harbor irrational misconceptions or feelings of shame about their bodies and may require concrete reassurance about the adequacy of the genital apparatus. Even if the diagnosis is that of a psychogenic basis for the sexual dysfunction, the patient may disregard assurances that there is no organic basis unless the workup for possible medical causes of the complaint has been thorough.

Appropriate laboratory tests to screen for systemic illnesses together with the specific test for various endocrinopathies, neurologic conditions, and other systemic disorders that may present with sexual problems may be indicated (see Chaps. 43 and 44). Attention to the mental status, including assessment of mood, affect, thought content, judgment, and reality testing, enables the physician to determine whether the sexual symptom is an aspect of a mental disorder. Rarely, sexual problems, especially loss of libido, may be the presenting sign of a disorder of the central nervous system; an examination of mental status can reveal early signs of dementia or of other organic brain conditions.

DIAGNOSTIC CONSIDERATIONS   Specific disorders of sexual function are discussed in Chaps. 43 and 44. All of them can vary in severity, from complete loss of function under all circumstances to relatively minor disturbances in specific circumstances or with specific partners. Patients also may vary in their reactions to sexual symptoms, some ignoring or concealing severe disability, others reacting with panic about minor disturbances.

When significant organic factors are present, a useful distinction can be made between sexual symptoms that arise *directly* from organic disorders, such as structural disorders of the urogenital system, neurologic disorders affecting the innervation of the sexual organs, and endocrinopathies that influence sexual physiology, and those that are *secondary* to changes in general health, such as sexual disturbances associated with rheumatoid arthritis, malignancies, renal failure, and other chronic diseases, or those that occur with acute debilitating conditions, such as myocardial infarction, major surgery, and hepatitis. Patients with primary organic disorders may need counseling to help them adjust to permanent losses of sexual function if medical measures cannot reverse the process. Although libido may be affected adversely by a general loss of vitality and by toxic and metabolic factors, the sexual disturbances associated with physical illnesses can also be the expression of hopelessness, depression, or anxiety and may be perpetuated by psychological factors long after the organic problems have disappeared. Persistent sexual dysfunction after a heart attack may reflect fear of sudden death during sexual excitement.

The apparent absence of an organic etiology does not necessarily mean a sexual dysfunction is psychogenic. Subtle vascular or neurologic changes not found on routine evaluations of impotence may underlie some instances of erectile dysfunction. The diagnosis of psychogenic impotence should be reserved for cases in which positive evidence of emotional disturbance can be found. Psychological factors that can interfere with the sexual response include fears and conflicts about sex, emotional disturbances that are antithetical to sexual excitement, and anger or dissatisfaction with a partner. Once a sexual failure has occurred for any reason, performance anxiety can develop and lead to further impairment by worry about subsequent encounters. In one study of impotence only 14 percent of cases were diagnosed as psychogenic. In many instances of sexual dysfunction, psychological factors interact with an organic vulnerability to produce overt symptoms.

Primary psychogenic disturbances, those that have been present since puberty, can be distinguished from *secondary* disturbances, those that represent decompensations from previous adequate levels of function. The former often reflect chronic and deep-seated sexual conflicts. When a patient seeks help for a chronic disturbance, the key diagnostic issue may be why help has been sought at this particular time. A secondary decompensation may be the presenting symptom of a psychological defeat or a disturbance in a relationship. Some sexual problems occur in connection with life stresses or transitions, such as retirement, pregnancy, work crises, or bereavement.

Other sexual disorders are manifestations of major mental disorders and respond only to treatment directed at the mental disorders themselves. Diminished sexual responsiveness, impotence, or ejaculatory disturbances may be indications of depression. Bizarre sexual complaints with increased or diminished sexual activity can indicate incipient psychosis. The strange qualities of the symptoms or the intensity of the associated feelings may be the best diagnostic clue to the presence of a psychosis. Hypersexuality can also occur with the onset of mania or as a manifestation of depression, especially in postmenopausal women.

Alcohol may play a significant role in impairment of potency. Often the first episode of secondary impotence is associated with the use of alcohol, and the midlife depressive syndrome that is often related to secondary impotence may be further complicated by alcohol abuse. Barbiturates and opiates also can cause reduced libido and impotence. Antihypertensive agents, tranquilizers, hypnotics, analgesics, and sedatives may also impair sexual function, particularly in the male.

Sexual disturbances may develop after traumatic incidents. For example, impotence can develop after cystoscopic examination or after vasectomy, even though neither procedure has any direct physiologic effect upon sexual function. An automobile accident, assault, pregnancy, contraceptive difficulties, disturbing sexual encounters, and a host of other emotionally significant episodes may cause sudden changes in sexual functioning. In women, either sexual assault or childhood sexual abuse can lead to long-standing sexual inhibition and dysfunctions. Many women are reluctant to share the history of a rape or of an incestuous experience; others may have little memory of traumatic events, especially when they occurred in childhood, although these events may exert a profound effect on adult sexuality.

The diligent physician may inadvertently overdiagnose sexual disturbances. Most patients have self-doubts and sexual dissatisfactions even though they are functioning adequately. It is well to have in mind the concept of a threshold of disturbance to separate the normal vicissitudes from problems that require treatment.

TREATMENT   Some sexual problems resolve spontaneously during the evaluation process, especially during an extensive workup. With those problems that persist, the physician must decide whether to treat the patients or to refer them elsewhere. The management of sexual dysfunction due to organic causes is described in Chaps. 43, 44, 330, and 331; sexual problems related to such physical illnesses are appropriately handled by the same physician who treats the physical disorder. Generally, the secondary or reactive psychogenic disorders are most amenable to brief counseling, especially when they occur in response to stress. Patients with more deep-seated problems may best be handled by psychiatrists.

The technique for counseling by the family physician cannot be mapped in a formal way. Sufficient time, a relaxed atmosphere, and genuine interest shown by the physician are necessary. The patient should be encouraged to tell the full story with careful attention to the circumstances surrounding the onset of symptoms, to the attitudes of the patient and partner, to the nature of the patient's relationships, and to factors that might lead to anxiety or depression. Although it may be necessary to review the physical details of the sexual practices, resolution of symptoms may occur with only indirect reference to sexual techniques. Sexual inadequacies often produce anxiety, which in turn leads to further defeats and to inhibition of libido. Without reduction of anxiety and lifting of depression, the process cannot be reversed.

Some physicians choose not to attempt sexual counseling, while others find it a satisfying aspect of practice. In either case, physicians should be familiar with the resources in their communities and understand the capabilities and limitations of various treatments. Physicians who do not undertake sexual counseling themselves usually have referral relationships with gynecologists, urologists, and psychiatrists. In addition, many communities have family services and counseling services. Referral should be tailored to the problems and to the lifestyle and personality of the patient. Some patients prefer to discuss the intimate details of a sexual problem only with a gynecologist or urologist. Others should be directed to a reputable clinic where behavioral approaches to the treatment of sexual dysfunctions are available.

Referral is often a difficult transition for a patient because it implies turning to a stranger after having confided in a physician who has understood the problem. A previously eager patient may lose motivation when referred elsewhere. Some physicians have counselors associated with them in their offices. This system has the advantage of maintaining the personal relationship between counselors and physicians but has the disadvantage of encouraging physicians to rely on counselors for the evaluation of emotional problems rather than carrying through the diagnostic phase themselves. If physicians keep in touch with patients through the process of therapy, it enables them to evaluate the efficacy of the treatment program and to provide support and reassurance.

A few examples will illustrate some of the principles involved in the treatment of patients with sexual disorders.

A.R., a 56-year-old attorney who had recently suffered a myocardial infarct, complained to his physician of loss of libido. He was an energetic, competitive, aggressive self-made man, who enjoyed athletics and was "top man" in his firm. The physician asked him about the details of his daily life and found that the loss of libido was only one of many inhibitions. He avoided arguments, stopped playing handball, reduced his work load, lost weight, and developed insomnia and anorexia. Further questioning revealed fears of sudden death and the fatalistic belief that his days were numbered. He assumed that strict reduction of activity was mandatory. His wife shared his fears and urged him to avoid stress. Together they had decided not to have sexual relations during the period immediately after his heart attack, and he had no desire to resume. In the course of several sessions of counseling the physician reassured him that his fears were exaggerated and that many patients with heart trouble experienced similar feelings, clarified the extent of his disability, and helped him and his wife to plan realistic resumption of many of his previous activities, including sexual relations.

L.D., a 26-year-old woman, consulted a physician because of frigidity. She had left her husband after 6 years of an unfulfilling marriage and had sought satisfaction in a series of brief affairs. The interview revealed a restless, competitive, chronically dissatisfied person who was unhappy in her career and experienced disappointment in close relationships. After careful evaluation of the physical aspects of her sexual difficulties and experiences, the physician decided that her problem reflected long-standing psychological conflicts and referred her to a psychiatrist.

M.B., a 34-year-old salesman, complained to his physician of impotence. He was a nervous, insecure, ineffectual man who worked for his older brother. His wife, an active real estate broker, had become withdrawn and bitter, and his two adolescent children were involved in minor delinquency. The impotence was confined to his relationship with his wife; in a recent extramarital affair he had performed adequately. He said he was unable to satisfy his wife in any way; she was either withdrawn or overly demanding. The physician determined that the impotency had no organic basis and referred the patient to a service agency where the family could be worked with as a unit. Here the wife was found to be depressed and received psychiatric treatment. Later the patient reported that when her depression improved, his potency returned.

C.W., a woman with breast cancer, was asked about her marriage. She reported that her husband had stopped having sexual relations with her when it was discovered that she had metastatic disease. The physician then saw the husband, who confessed to an extramarital affair and the wish to leave his wife. He also described irrational anger directed to his wife and feelings of shame and worthlessness. It emerged that the marriage had been an unusually close one and that he could not bear the anticipation of his wife's death. Sexual contact with her reminded him of his impending loss. His anger and the extramarital affair were responses to grief. The physician met with him for several sessions. By avoiding a moralistic position and by indicating that many spouses of patients with serious diseases have similar feelings and may even find solace in extramarital relationships, the physician helped him to overcome his shame and to share his grief. The process brought dramatic relief, and with occasional contact with the physician he was able to remain with his wife and be helpful to her throughout her terminal illness.

MARITAL COUNSELING BY THE PHYSICIAN The evaluation of sexual problems almost invariably requires some attention to marital or other sexual relationships. Counseling that focuses primarily on these relationships has been designated *marital counseling*. Instead of the usual medical relationship, which emphasizes the individual patient, marital counseling involves both partners, although each may be seen separately at times.

The specific nature of the counseling depends upon the complaints or upon the time of life of the couple. The main requisite is a willingness for physicians to set aside time for this kind of undertaking and to develop an interest in the functional health of patients beyond the specific issues raised by disease. The stresses and transitions in the early years of a marriage should be appreciated as well as the pressures exerted by children. In later years, job problems and conflicts over roles may emerge, followed by development of the "empty nest" syndrome, menopausal and midlife issues, and the male-depressive syndrome as horizons close in and the realities of aging appear.

Most marital problems are not due to sexual difficulties, although sexual problems may be the leading edge, especially in the climate where sexual adjustment is so widely publicized. Sexual satisfaction is dependent on the broader aspects of the relationship between partners and on mental and physical health. The alert physician should probe to these deeper levels during marriage counseling. In this sense, counseling about sexual problems is dependent upon the successful outcome of marriage counseling. Early in the approach the motivation of both partners should be assessed. If one partner is determined to break up the marriage, the counseling may consist of communicating this information to the other partner and perhaps advising legal assistance. On the other hand, apparent determination to seek divorce by either partner needs to be evaluated because it may mask depression, a paranoid reaction, or a hidden problem that is being avoided by flight, such as shame over an affair, fear, illness, or personal failure.

In marital counseling, as with other medical counseling, it is well to avoid giving direct advice about interpersonal relationships. By defining the problem, the physician may enable the patient to arrive at a decision on a course of action. By taking sides in family conflicts or by espousing an ethical position, physicians can inadvertently introduce their own biases or allow themselves to be manipulated by one of the marital partners.

REFERENCES

BELL AP et al: *Sexual Preference: Its Development in Men and Women.* Bloomington, Indiana University Press, 1981

ENDE J et al: The sexual history in general medicine practice. Arch Intern Med 144:558, 1984

FRANK E et al: Frequency of sexual dysfunction in "normal" couples. N Engl J Med 299:111, 1978

GROUP FOR THE ADVANCEMENT OF PSYCHIATRY, COMMITTEE ON MEDICAL EDUCATION: *Assessment of Sexual Function.* New York, Jason Aronson, 1974

KOLODNY RC et al: *Textbook of Sexual Medicine.* Boston, Little, Brown, 1979

LIEF HI et al: *Sexual Problems in Medical Practice.* American Medical Association, 1981

LUDEMAN K: The sexuality of the older person: Review of the literature. Gerontologist 21:203, 1981

MAGGEE MC: Psychogenic impotence: A critical review. Urology 15:435, 1980

MEYER J: Disorders of sexual function, in *Williams' Textbook of Endocrinology,* 7th ed, JD Wilson, DW Foster (eds). Philadelphia, Saunders, 1985, p 312

MUNJACK DJ, OZIER LJ: *Sexual Medicine and Counseling in Office Practice: A Comprehensive Treatment Guide.* Boston, Little, Brown, 1980

SLAGG MF et al: Impotence in medical clinic outpatients. JAMA 249:1736, 1983

---

46 HIRSUTISM AND VIRILIZATION

WILLIAM J. KOVACS / JEAN D. WILSON

Hirsutism, the growth of hair in women in a pattern characteristic of men, is a common and perplexing problem. The distribution and growth of hair in normal persons is under complex genetic and endocrine control so that there is considerable variability in hair growth in normal men and women. As a consequence, abnormal hair growth is sometimes difficult to define: Some patients may seek medical attention because of what the physician may consider an insignificant cosmetic defect. Others, because of personal or cultural differences, may be undisturbed by surprising degrees of hirsutism. The central issue in dealing with such patients is the separation of those infrequent instances in which hirsutism is a manifestation of an underlying virilizing or defeminizing syndrome from the vast majority of hirsute women in whom excess hair is fundamentally a cosmetic problem.

CONTROL OF NORMAL HAIR GROWTH AND DISTRIBUTION Endocrine control Androgens are the major determinants of hair distribution in both sexes. There are three principal circulating androgens in women—dehydroepiandrosterone, derived from the adrenal; androstenedione, which is derived equally from adrenal and ovary; and testosterone, which is both secreted by the ovary and adrenal and formed in peripheral tissue from circulating dehydroepiandrosterone and androstenedione. The production of adrenal androgen is regulated primarily by ACTH, while ovarian androgen secretion is regulated by luteinizing hormone (LH). These various androgens must be converted to testosterone (or dihydrotestosterone) before they can bind to the androgen receptor of target cells and induce an androgenic response. Thus, adrenal androgens virilize only in so far as they serve as precursors for testosterone and dihydrotestosterone.

Several types of relationships can be defined between hair growth and androgens in normal individuals. Eyebrows, eyelashes, and lanugo (fine, downy hair) are not dependent on androgens, while axillary and lower pubic hair are sensitive to the small amounts of androgen secreted by the adrenal. Hair in these regions therefore grows approximately equally in men and women. Hair growth in areas typical of males appears to require the greater androgen levels normally produced by the testes; such areas include the face, upper pubic triangle, chest, and ears. Finally, scalp hair exhibits androgen-mediated regression. The reason different body regions respond differently to the same or similar androgen is unknown. Theoretically, the metabolism of androgens might differ in the various sites, or hormone receptors might vary. The hair follicle, like some other androgen-responsive cells, requires conversion of testosterone to dihydrotestosterone for expression of androgen action, and hair follicles from all regions of the body perform this conversion equally well. Moreover, the same receptor that is essential for androgen action in other cells (Chap. 330) is necessary for the action of dihydrotestosterone in the hair follicle. Genetic disorders with normal testosterone production but absent androgen receptor have deficient or absent axillary, pubic, facial, truncal, and limb hair (Chap. 333). Regional differences in androgen responsiveness of hair in normal individuals may be the consequence of regional differences in the amount of androgen receptor in hair follicles.

Genetic factors Despite similar hormone levels, there is considerable diversity in the distribution of hair between individuals and among different racial groups in regard to facial, truncal, and pubic hair. Dark-haired, darkly pigmented whites of either sex tend to be more hirsute than blond or fair-skinned persons. Orientals, American Indians, and blacks on average are less hirsute than whites. Orientals rarely have facial or body hair except in the pubic and axillary regions, and American Indians, in addition, rarely develop baldness in either sex. Heterogeneity of hair patterns also exists within families.

The inheritance of hair patterns is complex and probably polygenic in nature.

Other factors Aging is a prerequisite for the expression of some types of hair development. For example, in men hair on the trunk and extremities frequently increases for several years after maximal levels of plasma androgens have been reached. Conversely, loss of androgen may not result in diminution of normal hair growth in men or reverse hirsutism completely in women. The appearance of pubic hair is frequently the heralding event of puberty in females. Women in the first trimester of pregnancy commonly observe increased hairiness of the face, extremities, and breasts. Menopause is often associated with the loss of hair in the pubic area, axillae, and extremities, whereas growth of hair on the face increases in postmenopausal women. The physiologic basis for these changes is unclear and cannot be explained entirely by changes in androgen levels.

PATHOLOGIC HAIR GROWTH AND DISTRIBUTION In evaluating women for hirsutism the most important feature is whether virilization or defeminization is also present (Table 46-1). In patients with overproduction of androgen defeminizing signs, such as disturbances of menstruation, are more consistent than are the signs of virilization. Virilization should be interpreted with caution for at least two reasons. First, signs of virilization (clitoromegaly, balding, coarsening of the hair, hirsutism) indicate androgen excess at some time in the patient's life but do not necessarily mean that active disease is present at the time of evaluation. It is necessary to measure plasma androgen levels and/or production rates to determine if androgen excess is ongoing. Second, severe overandrogenization may exist in the absence of marked virilization; i.e., at the same level of androgen production clitoromegaly may be present in one patient and not another.

Diagnostic considerations DRUGS Excessive hair growth can be caused by drugs that do not produce other defeminizing or virilizing signs. Such drugs include phenytoin, minoxidil, diazoxide, and hexachlorobenzene. Androgens produce hirsutism as well as virilization. Some synthetic progestogens have androgenic activity.

TUMORS The rapid onset of hair growth with or without accompanying signs of frank virilization suggests a neoplastic source of androgen. Such tumors include androgen-secreting adenomas and carcinomas of the adrenal and ovarian tumors such as arrhenoblastoma, which secrete androgens directly, and Krukenberg tumors of the ovary, which stimulate the surrounding ovarian stromal tissue to produce excess androgen.

POLYCYSTIC OVARIAN DISEASE The most common cause of ovarian hyperandrogenism is polycystic ovarian disease. This disorder has a broad clinical spectrum that ranges from mild hirsutism to complete amenorrhea and virilization. The salient feature for the diagnosis is the pubertal onset of chronic anovulation and hirsutism; enlarged cystic ovaries, obesity, and amenorrhea (i.e., the Stein-Leventhal syndrome) are present in only half or fewer of women with this disorder and need not be present for the diagnosis (see Chap. 331). The fundamental abnormality in polycystic ovarian disease is not fully understood. Elevation of plasma LH concentration causes enhanced androgen secretion by stromal and thecal cells of the ovary.

ATTENUATED FORMS OF ADRENAL HYPERPLASIA The adrenal can also be the source of excess androgen in the absence of tumor. Heritable defects in adrenal steroidogenesis (congenital adrenal hyperplasia) such as 21-hydroxylase deficiency, 11β-hydroxylase deficiency, and 3β-hydroxysteroid dehydrogenase deficiency can produce virilization, and each of these enzyme deficiencies can occur in a "late-onset" form in which hirsutism or virilization and menstrual irregularities appear at the time of expected puberty or in adulthood (see Chap. 333). The clinical presentation in these cases may be indistinguishable from polycystic ovarian disease. Late-onset 21-hydroxylase deficiency is most common and has been most extensively studied; its incidence in the general population of hirsute, oligomen-

TABLE 46-1 Clinical signs of defeminization and virilization

Signs of defeminization	Signs of virilization
Amenorrhea	Frontal balding
Decrease in breast size	Increase in size of shoulder girdle muscles
Loss of female body contours	Clitoromegaly
	Coarsening of the voice
	Acne

SOURCE: *After Karp L, Herrmann WL: Diagnosis and treatment of hirsutism in women. Obstet Gynecol 41:283, 1973* orrheic women is probably on the order of a few percent. The presence of elevated plasma levels of adrenal androgens (such as dehydroepiandrosterone sulfate) or of dexamethasone-suppressible hyperandrogenism does not necessarily imply that the overandrogenization is due to a specific adrenal steroidogenic defect, but these findings may be useful as a guide to therapy.

IDIOPATHIC HIRSUTISM In many women with hirsutism a specific diagnosis cannot be made. The term idiopathic hirsutism applies to those women with evidence of androgen excess but with normal menses, normal-sized ovaries, no evidence of tumors of the adrenal or ovary, and normal adrenal function. Slight elevations of plasma androstenedione and testosterone are commonly present in such women, and testosterone production rates are increased above normal, although to a lesser degree than in patients with polycystic ovarian disease.

Experience with the antiandrogen cyproterone acetate (not available in the United States) indicates that this form of hirsutism is androgen-mediated, since therapy results in improvement. Women with idiopathic hirsutism could constitute the extreme end of a normal continuum of androgen production or represent a true pathologic subset. Some women with the tentative diagnosis of idiopathic hirsutism actually have mild or early polycystic ovarian disease, but in most, hirsutism is not accompanied by or followed by signs of ovarian dysfunction. If such women are merely extremes of the normal range of androgen production, then their hirsutism is fundamentally a cosmetic defect.

DIAGNOSTIC EVALUATION The decision as to when to undertake a complex diagnostic evaluation depends on several factors. Such evaluation is appropriate in all women with hirsutism and virilization; whether it should be performed in women with isolated hirsutism depends upon the severity, distribution, and rate of hair growth. An approach to the diagnostic evaluation of hirsute patients is shown in Fig. 46-1. The clinical history is taken with particular attention to drug ingestion and to the details of pubertal development and menstrual history and their relation to the onset of excessive hair growth. The physical examination is directed to the assessment of sites of growth of androgen-dependent hair (pubic, axillary, facial, truncal, and extremity) and evaluation for signs of virilization, which correlate with higher levels of androgen overproduction and raise the concern of androgen-producing neoplasms. Such signs include laryngeal enlargement (deepening of the voice), temporal balding, clitoromegaly, and increased muscle mass in the limb girdles. Signs of cortisol excess (plethora, centripetal obesity, striae, and cervical and supraclavicular fat pads) should also be sought. Pelvic examination should include a search for palpable ovarian masses. Appropriate laboratory tests include measurement of serum androgens and, when appropriate, radiologic imaging of ovaries and adrenal glands. Basal measurements of dehydroepiandrosterone sulfate greater than 800 ng/dL or of serum testosterone over 200 ng/dL suggest neoplastic sources of androgen excess; plasma testosterone levels in the normal range are more difficult to interpret because total levels in women do not necessarily reflect the free or unbound levels of hormone under conditions when testosterone-binding globulin levels are either increased or decreased. Suspected Cushing's syndrome should be evaluated with standard dexamethasone supression testing if a screening test (such as urinary free cortisol excretion or overnight dexamethasone suppression test) is abnormal. The diagnosis of polycystic ovarian disease is made from the history and clinical features in a woman with chronic anovulation. Women with severe hirsutism associated with cystic acne may be screened for delayed-onset adrenal hyperplasia by the short cosyntropin stimulation test and measurement of plasma 17-hydroxyprogesterone (see Chap. 325).

MANAGEMENT In the case of drug-induced hirsutism and neoplastic disease of the ovary or adrenals treatment is straightforward; administration of the drugs should be stopped, or the tumor should be removed. Adrenal steroidogenic defects are treated with glucocorticoids to suppress excess ACTH and hence inhibit adrenal androgen secretion. In most instances (polycystic ovarian disease as well as idiopathic hirsutism) both cosmetic treatment and suppression of androgen production or antagonism of its action at the receptor level need to be employed.

Cosmetic therapy is directed at the concealment or removal of hair from exposed skin areas. Small amounts of hair can be bleached with hydrogen peroxide. Methods for removal of hair are classified as depilatory (removal of hair from the surface of the skin) or epilatory (removal of the intact hair with the root). Depilatory techniques include shaving and chemical methods. Shaving does not have an adverse effect on hair growth rate or coarseness (although the blunt ends may feel coarse), but shaving of areas other than axillae or legs is unacceptable to most women. Chemical depilatories are effective for limited areas of hair removal and are generally safe if used properly. Most available depilatories are substituted mercaptans, such as thioglycollic acid, which reduce the disulfide bonds in the peptide chains of keratin. The hair fiber swells and softens to a consistency that can be washed from the skin. Care must be taken to avoid skin irritation because of the alkalinity of these preparations. Temporary epilation can be achieved by plucking (useful only for isolated hairs) or wax treatment. The waxes are melted and applied to the skin.

FIGURE 46-1 *Diagnostic approach to the hirsute patient. T = testosterone; DHEA-S = dehydroepiandrosterone sulfate.*

When the wax cools and sets, it is stripped off, removing hair with it. The procedure is uncomfortable, and best results can be obtained by salon treatments. Permanent epilation can be achieved only by electrolysis. The treatments are expensive and time-consuming, and success depends on the skill of the electrologist.

While cosmetic treatment is undertaken, attempts to suppress androgen overproduction may also be appropriate. Treatment with combination oral contraceptives suppresses ovarian androgen secretion when restoration of fertility is not an objective. To minimize side effects the lowest effective dosage of estrogen should be used. Women over 35 years of age, smokers, and those with hypertension, a history of thromboembolic disease, impaired liver function, or suspected estrogen-dependent neoplasm should not be treated with oral contraceptives. Suppression of adrenal androgen overproduction can be achieved with small doses of dexamethasone and is useful in the treatment of women with late-onset 21-hydroxylase deficiency.

Antagonism of the effects of androgens at the hair follicle is the basis for the other main treatment modality, the antiandrogens. Cyproterone acetate has been used with success but is unavailable in the United States. Spironolactone has a dual action of blocking the androgen receptor and of inhibiting androgen production and is a useful alternative therapy. Cimetidine also binds to the androgen receptor and acts as an androgen antagonist, but it is not of general benefit in the treatment of hirsutism.

If pharmacologic therapy is undertaken, the patient should be prepared to make a commitment of 6 months for an adequate trial of efficacy. Even when treatment is long-term, dramatic reversal of established hair growth is unlikely to be achieved by interference with androgen synthesis or action. Such hormonal manipulations can arrest or slow the rate of hair growth, but established hair must be dealt with by use of cosmetic treatment.

REFERENCES

CUMMING DC et al: Treatment of hirsutism with spironolactone. J Am Med Assoc 247:1295, 1982

GIVENS JR: Normal and abnormal androgen metabolism. Clin Obstet Gynecol 21:115, 1978

KIRSCHNER MA et al: Idiopathic hirsutism—an ovarian abnormality. N Engl J Med 294:637, 1976

KUTTENN F et al: Late-onset adrenal hyperplasia in hirsutism. N Engl J Med 313:224, 1985

LUCKY AW et al: Plasma androgens in women with acne vulgaris. J Invest Dermatol 81:70, 1983

RAJ SG et al: Normalization of testosterone levels using a low estrogen-containing oral contraceptive in women with polycystic ovary syndrome. Obstet Gynecol 60:15, 1982

RUBENS R: Androgen levels during cyproterone acetate and ethinyl oestradiol treatment of hirsutism. Clin Endocrinol 20:313, 1984

WILLIAMS GH: Hirsutism, in Office Practice of Medicine, WT Branch (ed). Philadelphia, Saunders, 1986, in press

section 8 Alterations in the skin

47 INTERPRETATION OF ALTERATIONS IN THE SKIN

THOMAS B. FITZPATRICK / HARLEY A. HAYNES

CLINICAL EXAMINATION OF THE SKIN

The identification of skin lesions, or alterations, is a problem similar to the recognition of cells in a blood smear: the minute details are of the greatest importance. Lesions may be the presenting complaint of the patient or may be incidental findings during the routine physical examination; or they may be incidental to some major presenting complaint such as fever, cough, arthralgia, and the like. The recognition of the important and nonimportant skin lesions commonly encountered during the routine physical examination of the skin is a requisite part of the physician's task.

Inasmuch as the identification of skin lesions is the *sine qua non* of dermatologic diagnosis, the examiner's eye is undoubtedly the most valuable instrument at his or her disposal. Adequate illumination, preferably with natural light, is necessary. The observation of the total skin surface should begin with an overall, "low-power" general assessment of the completely disrobed patient. The systematic approach to the examination of skin should be as follows: first the fingernails and then the anterior and posterior aspects of the arm; then, in sequence, the scalp, the face, the trunk, the lower extremities and the skin between the toes; and then the mucous membranes, including the mouth and anogenital areas. The examiner of dermatologic lesions should consider (1) the specific *type* of lesion, (2) the *shape* of the lesion, (3) the *arrangement* of the groups of lesions, such as linear, arciform, annular, polycyclic, herpetiform, zosteriform, and serpiginous, and (4) *distribution* of the lesions.

Types of skin lesions can be classified by determining the topographic level of the lesions in relation to the normal skin (Table 47-1). For example, it is possible to distinguish lesions that are in or that protrude from or are superimposed above or below the level of the normal skin. The lesions that are encompassed within the scope of dermatology are listed in Fig. 47-1 and Table 47-1, and the histologic aspects are illustrated in Figs. 47-2 through 47-13.

The *shape* of the individual lesion and the *arrangement* of two or more lesions in relation to each other sometimes constitute important diagnostic clues. A *linear* arrangement of lesions often is indicative of an exogenous cause; also, linear lesions may occur because the pathologic process involves a vein, a lymphatic component, or an arteriole. Linearity can often be seen in various types of cutaneous hamartomas involving epidermal cells or melanocytes or even dermal connective tissue. In contrast, *annular* and *arciform* lesions and annular and arciform arrangements are relatively common and therefore only rarely lead to a specific diagnosis. The *iris* lesion (also called "target" lesion), however, a special and important type of annular lesion, is an erythematous annular or concentric macule or papule with either a purplish papule or vesicle in the center. Iris lesions are characteristic of the erythema multiforme syndrome. Annular macules may be observed in drug eruptions, secondary syphilis, and lupus erythematosus. Annular lesions with scale often suggest dermatophytosis or pityriasis rosea or psoriasis. The wheals that occur in creeping eruptions as well as the nodules in late syphilis are arranged in a *serpiginous* (snake-like) pattern.

Lesions that are contiguous are described as *grouped* and are of relatively little diagnostic value except in the special pattern, *herpetiform,* which is virtually pathognomonic for herpes simplex or herpes zoster. Similarly, the special arrangement, *zosteriform,* follows a dermatome in a bandlike pattern and is characteristically seen in herpes zoster; a zosteriform arrangement of skin nodules is occasionally seen in metastatic carcinoma of the breast. A *reticular* (netlike) arrangement often results from vascular dilatation and is observed in cutis marmorata and livedo reticularis.

The *distribution* of sites of localization of skin eruptions has been greatly overemphasized in dermatologic diagnosis; of far more importance are the type, shape, and arrangement of the lesions. The distribution of eruptions can be classified as *isolated, regional,* or *generalized;* the term *total* (universal) denotes an involvement of all the skin, including the hair and the nails. When the eruption occurs in a bilateral and symmetric distribution, the pathologic stimulus is usually endogenous, i.e., hematogenously disseminated. Bilateral symmetry is characteristic of hypersensitivity and is a common response to a drug. In photosensitivity eruptions, lesions are localized to the parts of the body that are exposed to sunlight. The exposed areas of the face that are usually spared include the fold of skin in the upper eyelids, the skin of the hair-covered scalp, the region below the chin, and the area behind the ears.

LABORATORY AND OTHER AIDS IN EXAMINATION OF THE SKIN

There are certain technical, clinical, and laboratory aids and procedures that are indispensable in the clinical examination and interpretation of skin conditions.

VISUAL AIDS   Magnification   Certain diagnostic signs can be revealed only by magnification of the skin lesions, e.g., the follicular plugging indicative of lupus erythematosus, the fine telangiectasia and translucent raised border indicative of basal cell carcinoma, and, if present, the bluish color indicative of early primary malignant melanoma. A pocket magnifier (7×) is necessary for proper identification.

Transillumination   Oblique lighting of skin lesions which is done in a darkened room is often required to detect slight degrees of elevation or depression, and is also sometimes useful in estimating the extent of the eruption.

Diascopy   Diascopy is an essential technique for the examination of skin because it permits the differentiation of purpura from erythematous macules. Diascopy consists of firmly pressing a micro-

TABLE 47-1   Types of skin lesion

Flat lesions (in plane of skin)	Elevated lesions (above plane of skin)	Depressed lesions (below plane of skin)
Macule	Vesicle and bulla	Atrophy*
Infarct†	Pustule	Sclerosis†‡
Sclerosis†‡	Abscess§	Erosion
Telangiectasia‡	Cyst‡	Excoriation
	Papule	Scar‡
	Wheal	Ulcer
	Plaque	Sinus§
	Nodule§	Gangrene*
	Vegetation	
	Keratosis	
	Desquamation (scales)	
	Exudate† (crusts)	
	Lichenification	

* *May also be in the plane of the skin.*
† *May also be below the plane of the skin.*
‡ *May also be above the plane of the skin.*
§ *May also be in or below the plane of the skin.*
SOURCE: *TB Fitzpatrick, in Dermatology in General Medicine, 3d ed, TB Fitzpatrick et al (eds), New York, McGraw-Hill, 1987.*

scope slide or a piece of clear plastic over the skin lesion; if the lesion is erythematous, the pressure will reveal compressible capillary dilatation rather than an extravasation of blood, which cannot be blanched. Sarcoidosis, lymphoma, and tuberculosis of the skin are suggested if diascopy of the nodules exhibits either a characteristic hyaline, yellowish-brown, or an "apple-jelly" appearance.

Long-wave ultraviolet light, or Wood's lamp   Long-wave ultraviolet light (360 nm), or Wood's lamp, is a necessary source of illumination for complete examination of the skin. Wood's lamp consists of a high-pressure mercury arc lamp with a specially compounded glass filter made of nickel oxide and silica (Wood's filter). This filter permits the passage of a band of radiation of 360 nm, which will reveal fluorescence when light passed through the filter impinges upon certain structures.

FIGURE 47-1   *Common lesions, shown on anterior and posterior views of the patient, encountered during the physical examination of the skin. (From Fitzpatrick et al.)*

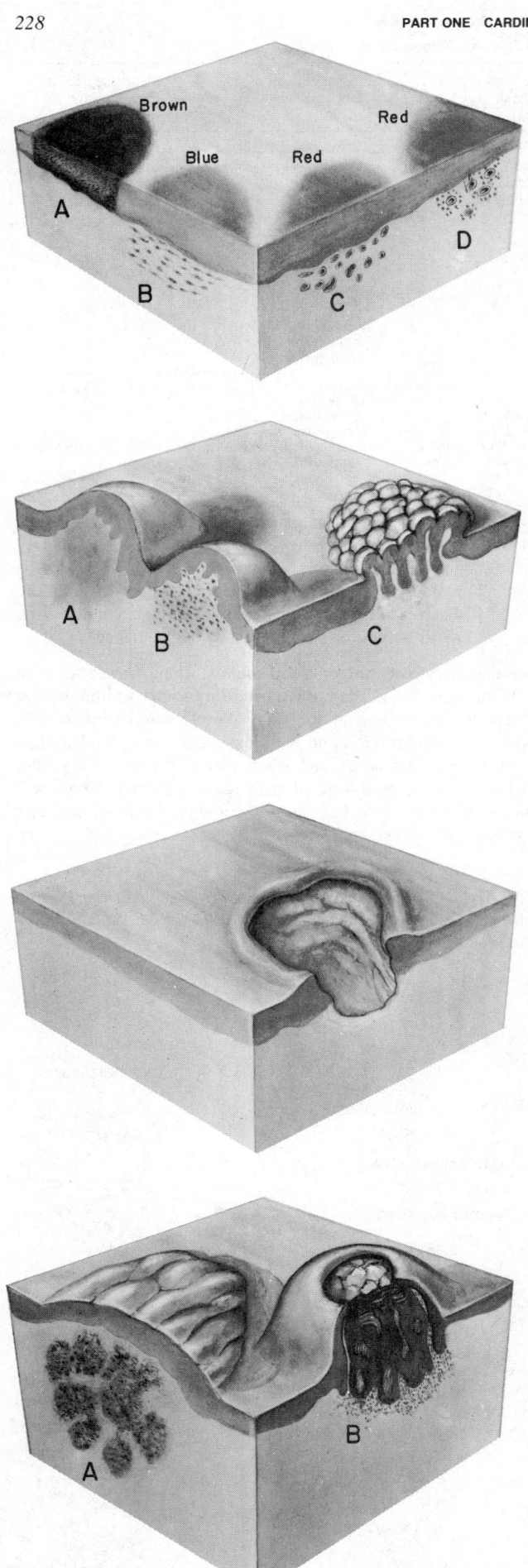

MACULE

FIGURE 47-2 *A* macule *is a circumscribed area of change in normal skin color without elevation or depression of the surface relative to the surrounding skin. The macules may be of any size and are the result of hypopigmentation (e.g., vitiligo) or hyperpigmentation—melanin (A) or hemosiderin (D)—such as café au lait spots and Mongolian spots (B), or permanent vascular abnormalities of the skin, as in a capillary hemangioma or transient capillary dilation (erythema) (C). Pressure of a glass slide (diascopy) on the border of a red lesion is a simple and reliable method for detecting the extravasation of red blood cells. If the redness remains under the pressure of the slide, the lesion may be purpuric (D); if the redness disappears, the lesion is erythematous and is due to vascular dilation (C).*

PAPULE

FIGURE 47-3 *A* papule *is a solid lesion, generally considered as less than 1 cm in diameter. Most of it is elevated above, rather than deep within, the plane of the surrounding skin. The elevation is caused by metabolic deposits (A) in the dermis or by localized infiltrates (B) in the dermis or by localized hyperplasia of cellular elements (C) in the dermis or epidermis. Superficial papules with distinct borders are seen when the lesion is the result of an increase in the number of epidermal cells (C) or melanocytes. Deeper dermal papules resulting from cellular infiltrates have indistinct borders. The topography of a papule or plaque may consist of multiple, small, closely packed, projected elevations that are known as a vegetation (C).*

ULCERS

FIGURE 47-4 *An* ulcer *is a lesion in which there has been destruction of the epidermis and the upper papillary layer of the dermis. Certain features that are helpful in determining the cause of ulcers include location, borders, base, discharge, and any associated topographic features of the lesions, such as nodules, excoriations, varicosities, hair distribution, presence or absence of sweating, and adjacent pulses.*

NODULE

FIGURE 47-5 *A* nodule *is a palpable solid, round, or ellipsoidal lesion deeper than a papule and is in the dermis or subcutaneous tissue (A) or in the epidermis (B). The depth of involvement rather than the diameter primarily differentiates a nodule from a papule. Nodules result from infiltrates (A), neoplasms (B), or metabolic deposits in the dermis or subcutaneous tissue and often indicate systemic disease. Late syphilis, tuberculosis, the deep mycoses, lymphoma, and metastatic neoplasms, for example, can present as cutaneous nodules. Therefore, biopsy should be performed on unidentified persistent nodules, and a portion of excised tissue should be ground in a sterile mortar and cultured for fungi. Nodules can develop as a result of a benign or malignant proliferation of keratinocytes, as in keratoacanthoma (B), verruca vulgaris, and squamous cell and basal cell carcinoma.*

WHEAL

FIGURE 47-6 *A wheal is a rounded or flat-topped, pale-red elevation in the skin that is characteristically evanescent, disappearing within hours. Observation of the borders of wheals that have been traced with a skin-marking pencil reveals that the wheals shift relatively rapidly from the involved to the uninvolved adjacent areas. Wheals are the result of edema in the upper layer of the dermis.*

VESICLE

FIGURE 47-7 *A vesicle (less than 0.5 cm) or a bulla (more than 0.5 cm) is a circumscribed elevated lesion containing fluid. Often the walls are so thin that they are translucent, and the serum, lymph fluid, blood, or extracellular fluid can be seen. Vesicles and bullae arise from a cleavage at various levels of the skin; the cleavage may be within the epidermis (i.e., intraepidermal vesication), or at the epidermal-dermal interface (i.e., subepidermal).*

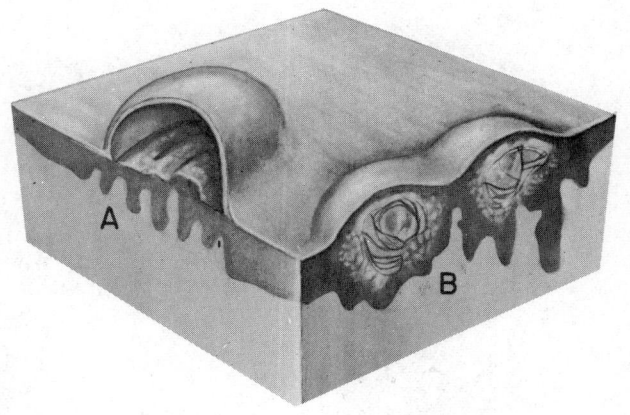

BULLA (A, subcorneal; B, spongiotic)

FIGURE 47-8 *When the cleavage is just beneath the stratum corneum, a subcorneal vesicle or bulla results (A), as seen in impetigo and subcorneal pustular dermatosis. Intraepidermal vesication may result from intercellular edema, or spongiosis (B), as characteristically seen in delayed hypersensitivity reactions of the epidermis (e.g., in contact eczematous dermatitis), and in dyshidrotic eczema (B). Spongiotic vesicles may or may not be seen clinically as vesicles.*

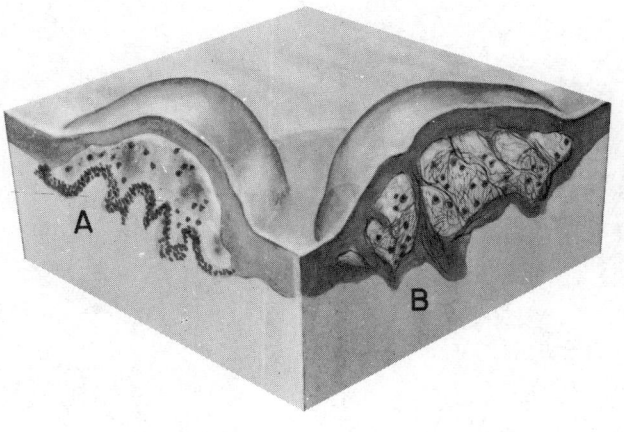

VESICLE (A, acantholytic; B, viral)

FIGURE 47-9 *Loss of intercellular bridges, or desmosomes, is known as acantholysis (A), and this type of intraepidermal vesication is seen in the vesicles or bullae of pemphigus vulgaris; the cleavage is usually just above the basal layer, as in pemphigus vulgaris, but may occur just below the subcorneal layer, as in pemphigus foliaceous. Viruses cause a curious "ballooning degeneration" of epidermal cells (B), as in herpes zoster, herpes simplex, variola, and varicella. Viral bullae often have a depressed ("umbilicated") center.*

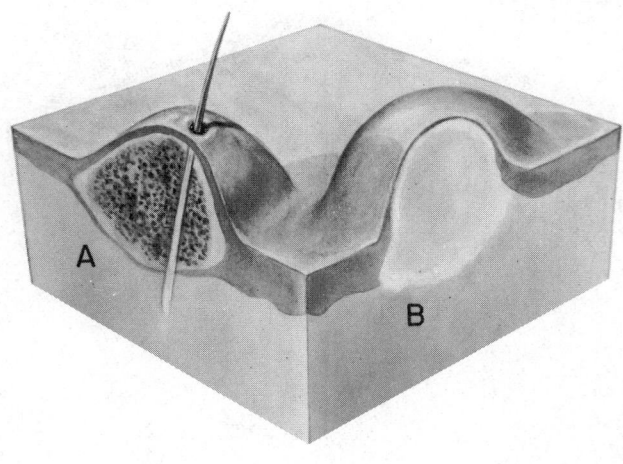

PUSTULE

FIGURE 47-10 *A* pustule *is a circumscribed elevation of the skin that contains a purulent exudate that may be white, yellow, or greenish yellow. This process may arise in a hair follicle (A) or independently (B). Pustules may vary in size and shape; follicular pustules, however, are always conical and usually contain a hair in the center. The vesicular lesions of the viral diseases (varicella, variola, vaccinia, herpes simplex, and herpes zoster) may secondarily become pustular. A Gram's stain and culture should be done on all pustules for identification of intracellular gram positive cocci.*

PLAQUE

FIGURE 47-11 *A* plaque *is an elevation above the skin surface that occupies a relatively large suface area in comparison with its height above the skin. Frequently, it is formed by a confluence of papules, as in psoriasis and mycosis fungoides. Lichenification is a proliferation of keratinocytes and stratum corneum forming a plaquelike structure. The skin appears thickened, and the skin markings are accentuated. The process results from repeated rubbing, and frequently develops in persons with atopy. Lichenification occurs in eczematous dermatitis.*

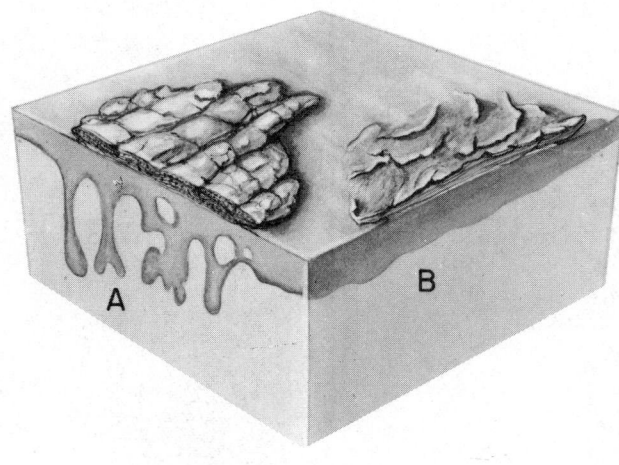

SCALES

FIGURE 47-12 *Epidermal cells are completely replaced every 27 days. The end product of this holocrine process is the stratum corneum. This outermost layer of skin, the stratum corneum, normally does not contain nuclei and is imperceptibly lost. With an increased rate of proliferation of epidermal cells, as in psoriasis, the stratum corneum is not formed normally, and the outermost layers of the skin retain the nuclei. These desquamating layers of skin are seen clinically as scales. Densely adherent scales that have a gritty feel (like sandpaper) result from a localized increase in the stratum corneum and are typically seen in solar keratosis (B).*

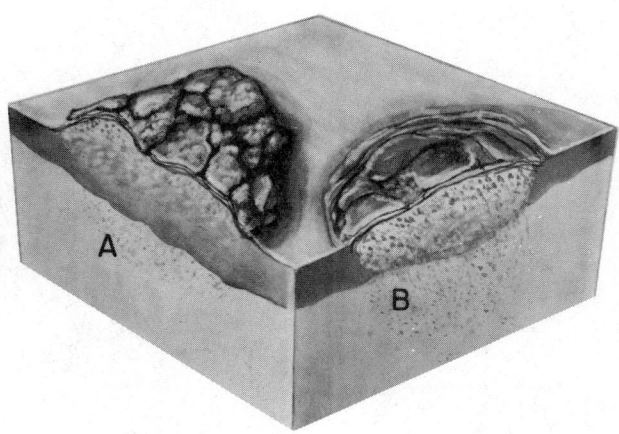

CRUSTS

FIGURE 47-13 Crusts, *resulting when serum, blood, or purulent exudate dries on the skin surface, are the hallmark of pyogenic infection. Crusts may be thin, delicate, and friable (A) or thick and adherent (B). Crusts are yellow when formed from dried serum, green or yellow-green when formed from purulent exudate, or brown or dark red when formed from blood. Superficial crusts occur as honey-colored, delicate, glistening particulates on the surface (A) and are typically seen in impetigo. When the exudate involves the entire epidermis, the crusts may be thick and adherent, and this condition is known as ecthyma (B).*

Wood's lamp is important for the detection of the pinkish-red fluorescence of the urine of patients with porphyria cutanea tarda; the addition of 5% hydrochloric acid greatly intensifies the fluorescence, owing to the oxidation of porphyrin precursors to porphyrins.

Wood's lamp is also a great help in estimating variation in the pigmentation of the skin; it reveals both increased and decreased pigmentation. Inasmuch as melanin is a universal absorber of ultraviolet light, areas of increased melanin will show an increased intensity under Wood's lamp; conversely, areas of decreased melanin will show a decrease in intensity (or an increased reflection) because the ultraviolet light is not absorbed. In this respect, Wood's lamp may be the only means of recognizing the sometimes indistinguishable hypomelanotic macules in tuberous sclerosis, a dominantly inherited trait associated with mental retardation and seizures. The white spots are present at birth and remain throughout life, and therefore represent important markers of this serious genetic disorder. Wood's lamp can be used in mass screening for detection of the fluorescence of dermatophytosis present *in the hair shaft* in ringworm of the scalp.

CLINICAL TESTS **Patch testing** Patch testing is primarily used by dermatologists to detect contact sensitivity. Some contactants are listed in Fisher's monograph on the subject.

Darier's sign One useful clinical response of the skin, Darier's sign, is used as a test for urticaria pigmentosa, and is evoked by the vigorous rubbing of a pigmented macule with the blunt end of a pen. In urticaria pigmentosa (mastocytosis), a palpable red wheal occurs within a few minutes after the physical trauma, owing to the release of histamine by the mast cells in the skin.

LABORATORY PROCEDURES **Examination for bacteria in crusts and biopsy specimens** Gram's stains and bacterial cultures of exudates should be performed on all lesions consisting of crusts and purulent exudates. Ulcers and nodules should be biopsied by removal of a wedge of tissue that extends from the surface down to the subcutaneous fat. The biopsy specimen should be minced in a sterile mortar and cultured for bacteria (including typical and atypical mycobacteria) and fungi.

Examination for mycelia The presence of mycelia may be ascertained by the application of 10% potassium hydroxide to a single tiny portion of scale, which is then gently heated. For fungi and yeasts, scales and hair should be cultured on Sabouraud's medium.

Tzanck test The Tzanck test, or the microscopic examination of cells from the base of vesicles, determines the presence of giant epithelial cells and multinucleated giant cells that occur in herpes simplex, herpes zoster, and varicella. Material taken from the base of a vesicle by gentle curettage with a scalpel is spread gently on a glass slide and prepared with Giemsa's or Wright's stain for the examination.

Dark-field examination of serum for *Treponema pallidum* Dark-field examination of serum from ulcers and erosions on the male and female genitalia is essential for the detection of *Treponema pallidum*. Dark-field examination of material obtained from the oral cavity is not diagnostic because of the presence of nonpathogenic treponemas that are indistinguishable from *T. pallidum*.

BIOPSY Microscopic examination of tissue is particularly applicable in dermatology because biopsies of the lesions can be easily obtained. Although the classic method is an elliptical incision followed by suturing, a satisfactory method for diagnostic purposes is "punch" biopsy. Biopsy of the skin enables correlation of gross and microscopic pathology. For punch biopsy, a small, 3.0- to 4.0-nm, disposable tubular blade is rotated between the thumb and index finger to cut through the entire thickness of the abnormal skin; the resulting cylinder of skin is then lifted out with forceps, and the skin is cut off at its base with a pointed scissors. This simple operation is done under local anesthesia, and the bleeding can be stopped by the use of pressure or absorbable foam; suturing is not usually necessary.

TABLE 47-2 Approach to dermatologic diagnosis

I History
  A Duration of lesions: days, weeks, months, years
  B Relationship of skin lesions to season, heat, cold, previous treatment, drug ingestion
  C Skin symptoms: pruritus, pain, paresthesia
  D Constitutional symptoms
    1 "Acute illness" syndrome: headache, chills, feverishness, weakness
    2 "Chronic illness" syndrome: fatigue, weakness, anorexia, weight loss, malaise
  E System review
II Physical examination
  A Appearance of patient: uncomfortable, "toxic," well
  B Changes in body temperature: elevated
  C Normal skin color: white, brown, black
  D Skin—four major skin signs: (1) type, (2) shape, (3) arrangement, (4) distribution of lesions
    1 Type of lesion

Basic lesions	Sequential lesions
Macule	Scale
Papule-plaque	Exudation: dry (crust)
Wheal	wet (weeping)
Nodule	Erosion
Cyst	Scar
Vesicle-bulla	Lichenification
Pustule	
Ulcer (also sequential)	
Hyperkeratosis (also sequential)	
Sclerosis	
Atrophy (also sequential)	
Telangiectasia	
Infarct	
Purpura	

    Color of lesions or of skin (if diffuse involvement): "skin color," white, leukoderma, hypomelanosis; red, erythema, pink, violaceous; brown, hypermelanosis, black, blue, gray, orange, yellow. Red purpuric lesions do not blanch with pressure (diascopy).

    Palpation
    Consistency (soft, firm, hard, fluctuant, boardlike)
    Deviation in temperature (hot, cold)
    Mobility of lesion or of skin
    Presence of tenderness
    Estimate of the depth of lesion (i.e., dermal or subcutaneous)

    2 *Shape* of individual lesions: round, oval, polygonal, polycyclic, annular (ring-shaped), iris, serpiginous (snake-like), umbilicated
    3 *Arrangement* of multiple lesions
      Grouped: herpetiform, zosteriform, arciform, annular, reticulated (netlike), linear, serpiginous (snake-like)
      Disseminated: scattered discrete lesions or diffuse involvement, i.e., without identifiable borders
    4 *Distribution* of lesions
      Extent: isolated (single lesion), localized, regional generalized, universal
      Pattern: symmetric, exposed areas, sites of pressure, intertriginous areas, follicular localization, random
      Characteristic patterns: scabies, secondary syphilis, psoriasis, seborrheic dermatitis, lichen planus, pityriasis rosea, dermatitis herpetiformis, atopic dermatitis, vitiligo, acne, erythema multiforme, candidiasis, contact dermatitis, lupus erythematosus, erythrasma, ichthyosis, pemphigus, pemphigoid, porphyria cutanea tarda, xanthoma, necrotizing angiitis (vasculitis)
  E Hair and nails
  F Mucous membranes
  G Miscellaneous physical findings: lymphadenopathy, hepatosplenomegaly, cardiac findings, neurologic findings, ophthalmologic findings
III Laboratory and special examinations
  A Dermatopathology
    1 Light microscopy: site, process, cell types
    2 Immunofluorescence
    3 Special techniques: stains, electron microscopy, etc.
  B Microbiologic examination of skin material: scales, crusts, or exudate
    1 Direct microscopic examination of skin
      For yeast and fungus: 10% potassium hydroxide preparation
      For bacteria: Gram stain
      For virus: Tzanck smear
      For spirochetes: Dark-field examination
      For parasites: Scabies mite from a burrow
    2 Culture
      Bacterial: for granulomas, culture
      Mycologic: minced tissue
  C General laboratory examinations: blood
    Bacteriologic: culture
    Serologic: ANA, STS

TABLE 47-2 Approach to dermatologic diagnosis (continued)

Hematologic: hematocrit or hemoglobin, cells, differential smear, erythrocyte sedimentation rate
Chemistry: Fasting blood sugar, blood urea nitrogen, creatinine

D Wood's light examination

Urine: pink-orange fluorescence in porphyria cutanea tarda (add 5.0% hydrochloric acid)
Hair (in vivo): green fluorescence in tinea capitis (hair shaft)
Skin (in vivo):

	Erythrasma	Coral-red fluorescence
Compared to visible light examination	Hypomelanosis	Decrease in intensity
	Brown hypermelanosis	Increase in intensity
	Blue hypermelanosis	No change in intensity

E Radiographic studies

TABLE 47-3 Clinical classification of skin lesions and syndromes according to the component of the skin primarily involved

I Epidermis (keratinocytes and melanocytes)
 A Keratinocytes
  1 Scaling macules, papules, or plaques
  2 Vesicles and bullae
  3 Pustules
  4 Exudative (impetiginized) lesions
  5 Eczematous dermatitis
  6 Erythroderma syndrome (exfoliative dermatitis)*
  7 Atrophy, diffuse* or circumscribed
 B Melanocytes
  1 Hypomelanotic macules
  2 Diffuse hypomelanosis*
  3 Hypermelanotic (brown) macules
  4 Diffuse brown hypermelanosis*
II Dermis (connective tissue and blood vessels)
 A Connective tissue component
  1 Papules and nodules (with and without inflammation)
  2 Ulcers
  3 Sclerosis, diffuse* or circumscribed
  4 Edema*
  5 Atrophy, diffuse* or circumscribed
 B Blood vessels
  1 Morbilliform and scarlatiniform eruptions
  2 Urticarial syndromes
  3 Erythema multiforme syndrome
  4 Purpura (with and without inflammation)
  5 Infarcts
  6 Telangiectasia
III Panniculus adiposus (connective tissue and blood vessels)
 A Connective tissue component
  1 Nodules, noninflammatory, usually nontender
  2 Atrophy
 B Blood vessels
  1 Nodules, inflammatory, usually tender and red
   a Erythema nodosum syndrome

* *Pathologic changes affect large areas of skin, and there are no discrete, circumscribed lesions.*
SOURCE: *TB Fitzpatrick, in Dermatology in General Medicine, 3d ed, TB Fitzpatrick et al (eds), New York, McGraw-Hill, 1987.*

This technique is as harmless and simple as a venipuncture, and supplies enough tissue to permit a definitive histologic diagnosis in most cases.

APPROACH TO DIAGNOSIS In Tables 47-2 and 47-3 an orderly sequence is suggested as a method of establishing a diagnosis in a patient presenting with skin lesions.

REFERENCES

FISHER AA: *Contact Dermatitis*, 2d ed. Philadelphia, Lea & Febiger, 1973
FITZPATRICK TB et al (eds): *Dermatology in General Medicine*, 3d ed. New York, McGraw-Hill, 1987
LAZARUS GS, GOLDSMITH LA: *Diagnosis of Skin Disease*. Philadelphia, Davis, 1980, p 506
ROOK A, WILKINSON DS: The principles of diagnosis, in *Textbook of Dermatology*, A Rook et al (eds). Oxford, Blackwell Scientific, 1979, p 37

---

48 SKIN LESIONS OF GENERAL MEDICAL SIGNIFICANCE

THOMAS B. FITZPATRICK / JEFFREY D. BERNHARD

The skin is one of the best indicators of serious disease; even an untrained eye can recognize cyanosis, jaundice, or the ashen pallor of shock. The competent physician must be able to detect the subtle skin signs of life-threatening diseases and cutaneous clues to diseases in other organs. Skin lesions are frequently critical in the final resolution of puzzling diagnostic medical problems. Thus, certain cutaneous "marker syndromes," such as erythema nodosum, can be indications of multisystem disease and therefore demand thorough medical evaluation.

The skin (Fig. 48-1) is composed of three layers: (1) the *epidermis,* the outermost part, which consists of two main cell types, keratinocytes and melanocytes; (2) the *dermis,* upon which the epidermis rests, which is composed of a mélange of connective tissue elements, nerves, blood and lymph vessels, glands, appendages, and a few cells (mast cells, fibroblasts, histiocytes); and (3) the *panniculus adiposus* (subcutaneous tissue), which acts as a cushion between the outer layers and the underlying bone. Keratinocytes produce and retain in their cytoplasm the intermediate filament keratin. They constantly turn over, about 27 days are required to complete differentiation and maturation. During maturation the keratinocyte loses its nucleus and retains only the cytoplasm. The latter becomes a highly ordered, two-phase system of keratin filaments embedded in an amorphous matrix, much like the cellulose-lignin system of wood fiber, which is known to be well adapted to withstand shearing and compression forces. The anucleate outermost portion of the epidermis is the *stratum corneum,* which acts as a tough, keratinous membrane. The stratum corneum functions structurally as a "waterproof" wall between the internal fluid milieu and the environment. It is the major barrier of the skin and protects the body against loss of fluids and entrance of toxic agents. It also serves as a passive membrane—some substances move across the skin by passive diffusion in the direction of the concentration gradient.

The skin has a relatively limited number of pathologic responses. If the individual skin lesions are taken to represent the letters of the alphabet, then groups of lesions can be said to form recognizable words or phrases. To the trained eye, these may lead to recognition of a clinically meaningful reaction pattern or diagnosis. The lesions in the majority of patients seen by the general physician can be classified in one of the groups of clinical reaction patterns (see Table 47-3) or types of skin lesion listed in Table 47-1. These skin lesions or clinical reactions may consist of one type of lesion, such as a vesicle or a nodule, or aggregates of various types of lesions, such as papules or vesicles. One or more solitary lesions or one or more groups of lesions may be distributed any place on the body. In some pathologic processes the borders of the lesions may not be defined; this type of diffuse involvement occurs in systemic sclerosis and in pigmentation disorders.

Cutaneous signs of systemic disease not discussed in this chapter include generalized pruritis (Chap. 50), photosensitivity (Chap. 52), and the cutaneous manifestations of internal malignancy (Chap. 300). Cutaneous markers for diseases of other organ systems, such as hyperpigmentation in Addison's disease (Chap. 51) and café au lait macules in neurofibromatosis, are also discussed elsewhere in the text.

In the physician's attempts to identify the specific types of lesions, it is essential to try to estimate the component of the skin that is *primarily* affected, i.e., the epidermis, the dermis, the blood vessels, or the panniculus adiposus. Inasmuch as there are a finite number of disorders that produce pathologic changes in the various individual components, this method of approach will improve the physician's diagnostic acumen. For example, even though erythema multiforme involves the dermis and the epidermis, the *primary component* affected is the blood vessel, and it is this involvement that explains the erythematous macules; the inflammatory process leads subsequently to the development of the cellular infiltrates seen clinically as papules and to destruction of the basement membrane and the development of bullae.

CLASSIFICATION OF LESIONS ACCORDING TO THE COMPONENT OF THE SKIN PRIMARILY AFFECTED

EPIDERMIS   Scaling macules, papules, or plaques   Generalized scaling macules, papules, or plaques are frequent and important diagnostic problems and are usually a presenting complaint of the patient (see Figs. 47-2, 47-3, and 47-11).

The sudden onset of symmetric, scaling, erythematous macules or papules is often indicative of drug-induced hypersensitivity reactions. Scaling erythematous papules on the scalp and extensor aspects of the arms and legs are suggestive of *psoriasis;* psoriatic lesions often are accentuated on the sites of repeated trauma, such as the elbows and knees. The papules or plaques of psoriasis are often surmounted by a silvery white micaceous scale that is relatively easily removed in layers. In psoriasis, there is a severalfold increase in the normal number of the basal cells of the epidermis. This increase in the basal cell population reduces the turnover time of the epidermis from the normal 27 days to 3 to 4 days. With the consequent shortened interval of epidermal cell migration from the basal layer to the skin surface, the normal events of cell maturation and keratinization do not occur (see A in Fig. 47-12); this failure of maturation is reflected by an array of abnormal morphologic and biochemical changes. In association with the basal cell hyperplasia, there is enhanced metabolism and accelerated synthesis and degradation of nucleoproteins, resulting in an elevated urinary excretion of nucleic acid metabolites such as uric acid. In addition, the subepidermal vasculature proliferates to support the increased rate of cell division. These numerous cytologic, histologic, histochemical, and biochemical alterations are now known to be the result, rather than the cause, of the disease process. The only main fact known at this time about the fundamental cause of psoriasis is that the predisposition to its development is genetically transmitted. An erosive joint disease, *psoriatic arthritis,* is discussed in Chap. 276.

The treatment of psoriasis still remains within the province of the dermatologist. The most effective treatment in the control of *localized psoriasis,* for most patients, is the use of topical corticosteroids, topical coal-tar preparations, and ultraviolet light or sunlight exposures. Corticosteroids can also be injected directly into small, resistant plaques. Systemic corticosteroids are not only ineffective in psoriasis but may cause generalization of the process and are absolutely contraindicated. With certain patients who have generalized psoriasis, it has been necessary to use a variety of systemic chemotherapeutic agents, especially methotrexate; the latter has the capacity to inhibit cell replication without a proportionate inhibition of cell function, i.e., keratinization.

In 1974, a new form of photochemotherapy was introduced which uses oral methoxsalen and a high-intensity, long-wave ultraviolet light source. This approach may replace many of the other forms of therapy. In this so-called PUVA treatment, psoralen (P) is administered by mouth 2 h before total-body irradiation with a special light system that emits predominantly long-wave (320- to 400-nm) ultraviolet light (UV-A). The light alone is ineffective in producing erythema or remission of psoriatic lesions; however, in the presence of one of the psoralens (methoxsalen) the UV-A becomes a potent photoactive agent and produces a remission of psoriatic lesions after multiple exposures. The mechanism of action is probably related in part to the binding of psoralen to DNA by the action of UV-A. Multicenter clinical trials in the United States and Europe involving over 5000 patients have shown that oral methoxsalen photochemotherapy is highly effective in the control of severe psoriasis; in over 80 percent of such patients the psoriasis completely cleared in 3 to 4 weeks of treatment using two or four exposures per week. After clearing, the patients may be given maintenance exposures once per week or less frequently. While methoxsalen photochemotherapy is effective, it requires specialized knowledge and equipment in order to deliver precisely measured amounts of UV-A. PUVA treatment is recommended only for patients with disabling psoriasis because long-term sequelae include premature aging of the skin, skin cancers in certain susceptible patients (i.e., with history of previous exposure to arsenic or ionizing radiation), and cataracts. In extremely disabling and recalcitrant cases, it may be necessary to combine PUVA or UV-B (middle-wave ultraviolet) with other modalities, such as systemic methotrexate, either sequentially or in combination.

The general physician does not always appreciate the impact of psoriasis as a major cause of disability and of disfigurement. Psoriasis affects between 2 and 8 million persons in the United States; about 100,000 are severely affected.

Psoriasiform lesions occurring on the face, lower abdomen, buttocks, groin, perineum, and legs occur in the *glucagonoma syndrome.* The lesions may be almost indistinguishable from subacute psoriasis, but they often have superficial necrosis in the center of the plaques; stomatitis, anemia, and marked weight loss are also present. Hyperglycemia may or may not be present. The eruption disappears rapidly on removal of the glucagon-secreting tumor of the pancreas. Psoriasiform lesions are also seen in Reiter's syndrome (keratoderma blennorrhagicum), mycosis fungoides (cutaneous T-cell lymphoma), nummular eczematous dermatitis, parapsoriasis, certain drug reactions, and dermatophytosis.

Symmetric scaling macules or papules localized on the palms and soles are often seen as the presenting signs of *secondary syphilis;* very frequently generalized lymphadenopathy and oral erosions are present as well.

A relatively common and often baffling generalized scaling eruption is seen in *pityriasis rosea.* In this condition, the scale at the periphery of the lesion is very thin and forms a collarette; the center of the lesion may or may not be scaly. Pityriasis rosea typically has a "fir-tree" type of distribution, especially evident on the back. Very

FIGURE 48-1   *Anatomy of the skin. (Copyright 1967 CIBA Pharmaceutical Company, division of CIBA-Geigy Corporation. Reproduced, with permission from the Clinical Symposia, illustrated by Frank H Netter, MD. All rights reserved.)*

often, but not always, a preceding, single, isolated scaling lesion—the herald patch—is present for several days before generalization of the lesions.

Scaling macules and papules are seen in *dermatophytosis* and *candidiasis,* and it is therefore necessary that some of the scales be examined for the presence of mycelia whenever scaling is present (see "Laboratory Procedures," in Chap. 47).

The various types of *dermatophytosis* (so-called ringworm infections) are confined to the epidermis, hair, toenails, and fingernails, and all (except tinea versicolor) respond to oral griseofulvin. Dermatophytosis is due to three types of fungus: *Microsporum, Epidermophyton,* and *Trichophyton. Microsporum audouini,* a parasite of humans, is the principal pathogen causing epidemic urban fungous infection of the scalp. *Microsporum canis,* which affects the scalp and also the face, where it causes boggy nodules, is a parasite of animals and originates largely from young (usually) farm animals and pets (kittens, puppies, and calves). *Trichophyton rubrum, T. mentagrophytes,* and *E. floccosum,* which also are parasites of humans, are the agents that usually cause dermatophytosis of the feet, the most common site of mycotic infection.

Susceptibility to superficial dermatophyte infection is variable, and appears to depend, at least in part, on individual host responses. The response of dermatophyte infections to oral griseofulvin varies, especially with regard to site of infection. Griseofulvin is effective, even in short courses, in fungous infection of the scalp, trunk, and groin, but even prolonged therapy rarely controls infection of the hands, fingernails, or toenails. Topical treatment with any of the imidazole antifungals is quite effective in infection of the feet, trunk, and groin, but is ineffective for infections of the fingernails or toenails.

The other major category of mycotic infections is represented by candidiasis (monilial infections). These infections do not respond at all to oral griseofulvin and are caused chiefly by *Candida albicans,* and occasionally by *C. tropicalis, C. krusei,* and *C. stellatoidea. C. albicans* can exist as a harmless saprophyte in the gastrointestinal tract and in the vagina. It is more common in females, and is most often present in those who are pregnant or who are taking oral contraceptives or broad-spectrum antibiotics. The association with diabetes mellitus, however, is so common that all patients (regardless of sex) with candidiasis should be screened for this disease.

Despite the fact that *C. albicans* is a normal saprophytic fungus in the vagina and gastrointestinal tract, it is rarely isolated from the exposed surface of the normal skin. *C. albicans* can invade the epidermis when the skin is exposed to high humidity and when the skin becomes macerated; therefore, candidiasis commonly occurs in the intertriginous areas (under the breasts and in the umbilicus, groin, and axillae) and in the oral, as well as the vaginal, mucous membranes. Chronic paronychia is usually caused by *C. albicans.* Candidiasis also may involve the lungs, urinary tract, and heart (see Chap. 147).

The treatment of candidiasis of the skin and mucous membranes depends on the site of the infection and the type of lesion. Maceration of the skin should be treated by air-drying of the area. Lotions and dusting powders containing nystatin are also very useful for intertriginous areas. Oral administration of nystatin is not of value in cutaneous moniliasis. Unless the sexual partner is treated when candidiasis is present, there will be constant retransfer of the infection. For monilial paronychia, 2% alcohol solutions of gentian violet are still the best treatment. Systemic administration of ketoconazole is indicated in certain situations, such as chronic mucocutaneous candidiasis.

Differentiation between dermatophytosis caused by any of the three types of fungus already mentioned and candidiasis may be difficult, if not impossible, without cultures of the fungus. Direct examination of the scales from a scaling eruption in the intertriginous area is not diagnostic because it may reveal mycelia in both dermatophytosis and candidiasis; spores, however, are seen only in candidiasis. Too often, the general physician starts treatment with topical antifungal agents or with griseofulvin without establishing whether the eruption is a type of dermatophytosis or candidiasis. Inasmuch as candidiasis does not respond to systemic griseofulvin and dermatophytes do not respond to nystatin, prescribing these agents for an undiagnosed eruption may result in prolonged disability for the patient. Newer agents such as haloprogin and miconazole are effective against both dermatophytosis and candidiasis.

In the past few years, fungous diseases have assumed a new significance in medicine because of the increased number of patients under treatment with chemotherapeutic agents for leukemia and other neoplasms. Almost all of the saprophytic fungi can invade the tissues of patients who are being treated with chemotherapeutic agents or who have had kidney transplants.

Vesicles and bullae   Some diseases may occasionally be associated with vesicles or bullae, such as erythema multiforme or porphyria cutanea tarda, but blisters (vesicles and bullae) are the major feature of a number of disorders: certain bacterial and viral infections; allergic contact dermatitis (such as poison ivy); trauma from mechanical, thermal, or chemical agents; and most important, the bullous diseases of unknown cause (such as pemphigus and pemphigoid).

Grouped vesicles occur in herpes zoster and herpes simplex, whereas scattered, discrete vesicles occur in varicella. A helpful sign in determining the nature of the vesicles is the Tzanck test (see "Laboratory Procedures," in Chap. 47). Epithelial giant cells are present in herpes simplex, herpes zoster, and varicella but are absent in vaccinia and variola. Skin biopsy will also establish the nature of the vesicle or bulla; that is, whether it is intraepidermal (as in virus infections and pemphigus) or subepidermal (as in bullous pemphigoid) (see Figs. 47-7 to 47-9).

Vesicles arranged in linear streaks are characteristic of poison ivy dermatitis. The most reliable clue to the diagnosis of both allergic and primary-irritant contact dermatitis is the localization of vesicles to the skin areas likely to have been exposed to the agent in question. Isolated vesicles and bullae on the dorsal pressure areas of the dorsa of the hands and the face may be the only sign of porphyria cutanea tarda and the variegate porphyria; the diagnosis of the former is immediately confirmed by examination of the urine, using Wood's lamp. These patients do not present with photosensitivity, though the distribution of lesions suggests that sunlight plays a role in their localization.

Scattered, isolated bullae in adults represent a special and serious problem in diagnosis and treatment. *Bullous pemphigoid* and *pemphigus* are chronic and occur primarily in adults; one of them, pemphigus, has serious consequences for the patient. These two disorders need to be distinguished by biopsy of the skin and by immunofluorescence techniques. It is impossible on the basis of clinical diagnosis alone to distinguish between bullous pemphigoid, which is usually a chronic and relatively benign disorder, of limited duration, and *pemphigus vulgaris,* which is a serious disease leading in a relentless course to death, unless treatment with immunosuppressive agents is instituted. Four separate types of pemphigus occur, but pemphigus vulgaris is the most important for the general physician to recognize. Pemphigus vulgaris may begin in the nasal or oral mucous membrane, and the patient may consult the dentist or otolaryngologist first for persistent erosions of the larynx (hoarseness), the mouth, or a bloody nasal discharge. The lesions tend to involve other parts of the body in an unpredictable fashion, but localize chiefly on the umbilicus, scalp, and trunk, although there is no specific distribution pattern. Pemphigus vulgaris affects primarily the middle-aged, particularly between the ages of 40 and 60. It rarely occurs before the age of 17 or after the age of 75. The clinical lesions appear as flaccid bullae from the beginning; they break easily and rarely become very large. The denuded areas (erosions) that form at the site of the ruptured bullae increase in size as the epidermis detaches itself. Occasionally, almost the entire surface may be involved by large, denuded areas; this represents a serious problem in the management of secondary infection and in maintenance of fluid balance—more or less the same problems that occur in a severely burned patient. Oral or nasal mucosal lesions occur in nearly all patients, and more than half have lesions in the mucous membrane of the mouth as the first manifestation of the disease. The disease often starts with only a few lesions in the mouth and may remain limited in extent for several weeks; it then gradually spreads to other parts of the body.

The diagnosis of pemphigus is made on the basis of the light-microscopic examination of the biopsy of an early vesicle and direct immunofluorescence. The earliest change in pemphigus vulgaris consists of intercellular edema followed by disappearance of intercellular bridges in the lower epidermis (see A in Fig. 47-9). This results in loss of cohesion between the epidermal cells (acantholysis) and leads to the formation of clefts and then bullae that are predominantly in suprabasal locations; in other words, the basal cells, although separated from one another, remain attached to the dermis much like a "row of tombstones."

Immunofluorescence allows detection of IgG antibodies specific for an intercellular substance of the skin and mucosa in the serum of patients with pemphigus, and makes possible a differentiation of pemphigus and pemphigoid by the localization of the antibody. The fluorescence is localized precisely to the site of acantholysis in pemphigus; IgG is confined to the intracellular glycocalyx of epidermal cells. In bullous pemphigoid, however, the antibodies react with an antigen in the basement membrane region, and the fluorescence is localized there.

Treatment of pemphigus with systemic corticosteroids, sometimes in combination with azathioprine, is quite successful. Azathioprine alone can control the disease in some patients.

Pustules This skin reaction (see Fig. 47-10) may result from infections or from sterile inflammation. Pustules may arise from preexisting vesicles of any etiology. Infection by pyogenic bacteria, especially staphylococci, as well as by certain fungi and mycobacteria, can produce pustules without a preceding vesicular stage. Noninfectious causes of pustules include acne, pustular psoriasis, and hypersensitivity to drugs, particularly sulfonamides, iodides, or bromides. Purpuric pustules in an acral distribution are characteristic of disseminated gonococcemia, but may also be seen in other forms of bacterial sepsis.

Exudative (impetiginized) lesions Acute infection with gram-positive cocci can occur as a primary process or may be superimposed on eczematous dermatitis or occasionally on any of the vesiculobullous diseases, and is characterized by the presence of crusts (see Fig. 47-13). Such infection on the skin has the same implications as a streptococcal pharyngitis, inasmuch as acute glomerular nephritis develops in a significant percentage of patients with impetiginized dermatitis. Patients with impetiginized dermatitis must be treated with full courses of systemic antibiotics.

Eczematous dermatitis Eczematous dermatitis is not a specific disease entity but a characteristic inflammatory response of the skin due to both endogenous and exogenous agents. Eczematous dermatitis therefore requires a qualifying etiologic term, e.g., *atopic eczematous dermatitis*. Eczematous dermatitis is sufficiently serious to account for the highest incidence of skin disease. Approximately one-third of all patients in the United States seen by dermatologists have eczema. It is responsible for incalculable losses of time and productivity in industry. In Tables 48-1 and 48-2 some of the types of eczematous dermatitis are summarized (see also B in Fig. 47-8 and Fig. 47-11). For the general physician, atopic eczematous dermatitis is the most important disease of this group of disorders. Over 30 percent of atopic patients develop respiratory allergic manifestations (asthma and hay fever). Furthermore, the disease may persist for 15 to 20 years. Cataracts develop in 15 percent of young patients. Finally, patients with atopic eczematous dermatitis are particularly susceptible to infections with herpes simplex and vaccinia. The majority of patients with severe atopic eczematous dermatitis have elevated serum levels of IgE. Control of the intractable pruritus in this disease is difficult, and best results are obtained by judicious use of topical corticosteroids, tar gels, oil baths, lubrication with emollients, and limitation of emotional stress.

Erythroderma syndrome (exfoliative dermatitis) The erythroderma syndrome is an important disorder that may occur as a drug reaction, as a generalized extension of a preexisting dermatitis, such as psoriasis or atopic dermatitis; or in association with lymphoma and leukemia. This syndrome consists of a generalized, erythematous, scaling eruption involving all of the skin surface, and has important implications in general medicine because of the systemic effects occasioned by the massive and continuous exfoliation of the skin. The severity of the metabolic response to exfoliation depends on the duration and

TABLE 48-1 Various types of eczematous dermatitis* of uncertain etiology

Clinical type	Suspected pathogenesis	Diagnostic considerations
Atopic eczematous dermatitis	Hereditary predisposition plus precipitating factors	Eczematous dermatitis, especially localized to the antecubital and popliteal fossae and to the face
Lichen simplex chronicus	Hereditary predisposition plus repeated local trauma	One or more lichenified plaques (see Fig. 47-11), especially on neck
Prurigo nodularis	Repeated local trauma	One or more nodules, especially on extremities
"Neurodermatitis"	Hereditary predisposition plus repeated scratching	Generalized or localized eczematous eruption at sites of repeated trauma
Stasis dermatitis	Chronic venous insufficiency	Signs of venous insufficiency
Nummular eczematous dermatitis	Various precipitating factors (contact irritants, xerosis, emotional stress, etc.)	Discrete coin-shaped patches, usually on extremities and trunk
"Dyshidrotic" eczematous dermatitis	Emotional stress plus other factors‡	Vesicles and bullae on palms and soles
Seborrheic dermatitis	Constitutional diathesis	Greasy scaling patches on scalp, eyebrows, and nasolabial area
Various patterns of eczematous dermatitis	Association with gastrointestinal malabsorption	Eczematous eruption in patient with steatorrhea and abnormal biopsy specimens of the jejunal mucosa
"Eczematous-like eruptions"† with systemic disease: Wiskott-Aldrich syndrome X-linked agammaglobulinemia Phenylketonuria Ahistidinemia Hurler's syndrome Hartnup disease Acrodermatitis enteropathica	Metabolic and immunologic disorders	Related features of clinical syndrome plus immunologic deficiency or biochemical abnormality

* This term is used by many clinicians for at least four types of eczematous dermatitis that may be exclusively localized to the hands (atopic eczematous dermatitis, allergic contact eczematous dermatitis, nummular eczematous dermatitis, and "dyshidrotic" eczematous dermatitis). Possibly, contact irritants to which the hands are frequently exposed may precipitate or aggravate one of the above-mentioned basic types of eczematous dermatitis.

† These eruptions are reported in the literature as eczematous dermatitis, but clear, careful clinical descriptions with cutaneous biopsy specimens are frequently lacking.

‡ Such as constitutional diathesis and contact dermatitis.

TABLE 48-2 Various types of eczematous dermatitis of known etiology

Clinical type	Pathogenesis	Diagnostic considerations
Allergic contact eczematous dermatitis	Chemical allergens (plants, medicaments, cosmetics, metals, fabrics, etc.)	Site and configuration are clues to causal agent; patch tests may confirm diagnosis; avoidance of cause cures eruption
Photoallergic contact eczematous dermatitis	Ultraviolet radiation plus topical chemicals (in soaps, perfumes, citrus fruits, etc.), which then become allergens	Occurs on exposed skin; photopatch tests confirm diagnosis
Polymorphous light-induced eruption—eczematous type	Ultraviolet radiation; sometimes visible light	Occurs on exposed skin; diagnosis implies that all known causes of light-induced eruptions have been eliminated
"Infectious eczematoid dermatitis"	Bacterial products from draining focus (e.g., ear infection)	Occurs near site of infection; responds to treatment of primary infection
Eczematous dermatophytosis	Fungus	Fungi demonstrated in scales or exudate

severity of the process itself. Serious metabolic effects of chronic exfoliative dermatitis occur when the rate of scaling reaches 17 g/m² per 24 h. Patients with extensive exfoliative dermatitis may have negative nitrogen balance, edema, hypoalbuminemia, and loss of muscle mass. Another salient feature in these patients is the large extrarenal water loss, due to markedly increased transepidermal water loss across the defective cutaneous barrier. The etiology of exfoliative dermatitis determines its course: the disease eventually clears in patients with psoriasis or atopic dermatitis, whereas the prognosis is relatively poor in patients with lymphoma and leukemia. Approximately 60 percent of patients with exfoliative dermatitis recover within 8 to 10 months, 30 percent die, and 10 percent have a persistent problem unresponsive to therapy.

Atrophy, diffuse or circumscribed Epidermal atrophy is manifested by an almost transparent epidermis and is associated with a decrease in the number of epidermal cells. Atrophic epidermis may or may not retain normal skin markings and is often associated with some alteration in the dermis. Circumscribed epidermal atrophy occurs in discoid lupus erythematosus, in necrobiosis lipoidica diabeticorum, and in striae cutis distensae; diffuse epidermal atrophy occurs with aging and in scleroderma.

The most important atrophic-type disorder is *necrobiosis lipoidica diabeticorum* (NLD) (Plate 5-1). These lesions, which are usually asymptomatic, occur more frequently in women and *on areas subject to trauma* such as the anterior and lateral surfaces of the lower legs. Lesions may also occur on the arms and even on the face. The lesion begins as a small, reddish, elevated nodule with a sharply circumscribed border, gradually enlarges, and becomes flattened and depressed as the skin becomes atrophic. The brownish-yellow–to–orange color is prominent, and blood vessels are readily seen because the atrophic epidermis is smooth, thin, and translucent. The lesions of NLD are often indolent, but shallow ulcerations that are very slow to heal may develop. NLD may apparently occur when diabetes mellitus cannot be detected, but full tests of glucose tolerance, such as the cortisone-glucose tolerance test, have not been done in large numbers of patients who fall into this catgory. NLD is characterized by focal changes in the dermis that present as acellular and intense eosinophilic areas of necrosis bordered by inflammation. Granulomatous inflammation with epithelioid cells, histiocytes, and multinucleated giant cells is a central feature. The blood vessels are always involved, with endothelial proliferation and sometimes even occlusion of arterioles and arteries deep within the dermis; capillary walls are thickened with focal deposits of PAS-positive material. NLD can be controlled with careful intralesional injections of suspensions of triamcinolone acetonide in some patients.

Hypomelanotic macules See Chap. 51.

Diffuse hypomelanosis See Chap. 51.

Hypermelanotic macules See Chap. 51.

Diffuse brown hypermelanosis syndrome See Chap. 51.

DERMIS Papules and nodules (with or without inflammation) Papules and nodules without epidermal change (i.e., scaling) may be either skin color, erythematous, or even slightly pigmented (yellow or brown). Dermal papules and all nodules require a biopsy for definitive diagnosis because they often represent processes that have general medical significance, such as sarcoidosis, or histiocytosis X, tuberculosis, lymphoma, or metastatic carcinoma. Inasmuch as dermal nodules may be present in deep mycotic infections such as coccidioidomycosis, it is necessary to obtain a biopsy not only to rule out malignancy but to culture a portion of the excised tissue for fungi. Cultures of nodules must be made from tissue ground by mortar and pestle. The histologic specimen should be carefully studied for the presence of acid-fast bacilli, since nodules are the presenting feature of leprosy and tuberculosis. Nodules removed from common areas of localization for leishmaniasis (face and arms) should be carefully examined for the presence of parasites.

Papules and nodules with and without inflammation can occur in disorders of the sebaceous glands. Sebaceous glands are distributed largely on the face and scalp, although they can also occur in the labia minora and on the scrotal skin, trunk, nipples, and eyelids. The sebaceous gland is a holocrine gland in which the entire cell is cast off into the excretory stream. Sebum is a complex lipid mixture of squalene (a major product of the steroid pathway), triglycerides, and wax esters. Sebaceous glands are controlled by direct hormonal stimulation by androgens, derived largely from the gonads in both sexes; in the female, but not in the male, adrenal androgens may be important factors in maintaining sebum production. The major disease of the sebaceous gland in humans is *acne vulgaris* which occurs predominantly on the face and, to a lesser degree, on the back, chest, and shoulders. It is characterized by a variety of clinical lesions. These lesions may be either noninflammatory or inflammatory papules and nodules. The noninflammatory papules are called comedones, and these may be either open (blackheads) or closed (whiteheads). Closed comedones are the precursors of papules, pustules, and large inflammatory nodules. In addition, cysts and scars of various sizes may occur; the typical acne scar is a sharply punched-out pit. Pustular and cystic lesions, despite a large amount of purulent exudate that may be recovered following incision, are usually sterile but may contain *Propionibacterium acnes*.

The initial stimulus to the formation of comedones (both the closed and open types) is not precisely known at this time, but the initial histologic event in comedone formation is excessive keratinization within the follicular canal. It is currently believed that lypolysis of triglycerides by *Propionibacterium acnes* releases fatty acids; it is thought that these fatty acids are capable of eliciting an inflammatory process in the follicle wall, which may then rupture. Discharge of the follicular content leads to perifollicular inflammation. The inflammatory infiltrate is lymphocytic, but later, as a result of the presence of keratinous material, gram-positive diphtheroids, and sebum, the infiltrate consists essentially of a foreign-body giant cell reaction.

There should be a careful search of the histologic material, with acid-fast stains, for tubercle and lepra bacilli, for tissue parasites (in leishmaniasis, echinococcus, cysticercosis, schistosomiasis, onchocerciasis, and myiasis), and for fungi (of actinomycosis, blastomycosis, sporotrichosis, coccidioidomycosis, and dermatophytosis). It is necessary to examine tissue sections with the polarizing microscope to detect zirconium and silicon and uric acid crystals. Acne vulgaris is a serious problem, especially common during adolescence, and its therapy is complex and prolonged. Moderate to severe acne vulgaris is best treated by dermatologists who are trained in a number of modalities: topical agents, incision and drainage of cystic lesions, ultraviolet light therapy, and judicious use of systemic antibiotics; x-ray therapy has no place in the treatment of acne vulgaris.

How antibiotics such as tetracycline improve acne is not completely understood, but these drugs are known to suppress the number of propionibacteria and to cause a reduction of free fatty acids on the skin. Because the organisms have been shown to have lipolytic activity in vitro, it is presumed that the antibiotic causes this reduction of free fatty acids. Benzoyl peroxide lotions and gels probably act as antibacterial agents and decrease the bacterial population; these agents are very effective and are widely used by dermatologists.

Estrogens combined with progestins (oral contraceptives) were initially considered to be effective in controlling acne; however, they have been of only limited value in the treatment of acne in females and cannot be given to males. There is no convincing evidence to suggest that particular foods have any effect on the course or severity of acne vulgaris. Acne vulgaris may begin as early as the eighth year or may not appear until the twentieth. It lasts for several years and then subsides spontaneously, usually in the early twenties. In some patients, however, acne vulgaris may continue into the third and fourth decades. Topical antibiotic solutions such as clindamycin or erythromycin are effective new agents for treatment of acne vulgaris. The most dramatically effective new treatment for severe cystic acne is orally administered 13-*cis*-retinoic acid. This drug acts rapidly and is very effective, but it is teratogenic and cannot be used in women of child-bearing age unless effective contraception is guaranteed. Other side effects, such as xerosis and hypertriglyceridemia, and bony spur formation mandate that it be used only in severe cases in which conventional modalities have failed.

Pretibial myxedema (PM) also may cause nodules on the legs and dorsa of the feet. The lesions are usually bilateral and consist of elevated, firm dermal nodules and plaques that are not easily movable. They may be skin color, pink, or, rarely, brown, and, when diascoped, appear yellow and waxy. The epidermis over the nodules may appear normal or may have a marked verrucous (warty) surface. The pathogenesis of pretibial myxedema is not clear. Pretibial myxedema may occur with or without hyperthyroidism (Graves' disease) or before or after treatment of hyperthyroidism, and its development does not parallel the ocular changes (if present). The nodules in pretibial myxedema are accumulations of mucopolysaccharides, which can be demonstrated by special staining of the histopathologic material. LATS (long-acting thyroid stimulator), which is associated in the plasma with immunoglobulin G (7 S gamma globulin), has been implicated in the pathogenesis of pretibial myxedema, exophthalmos, and acropachy; the role of LATS in the pathogenesis of pretibial myxedema has not been established.

Ulcers Ulcers occur as a result of destruction of the epidermis and, at least, the papillary layer of the dermis (see Fig. 47-4). All ulcers of the skin that do not heal within a period of a month must be assumed to be carcinoma until proved otherwise, and it is essential that a biopsy be obtained to rule out malignancy. Ulcers can be divided into two categories: lesions that occur on the legs and feet, and lesions that occur elsewhere on the body. Ulcers not occurring on the legs are rather rare except in primary cancer of the skin or in malignant metastases to the skin. Ulcers arising in nodules with inflammation should be approached in the manner suggested previously for nodules—that is, a biopsy should be obtained, and the tissue examined for bacterial, mycotic, and parasitic diseases. Chancre-like ulcerations and noduloulcerative lesions with regional lymphadenopathy may occur in primary syphilis, primary tuberculosis, and in tularemia, anthrax, glanders, and bubonic plague. Isolated noduloulcerative lesions may be seen in sporotrichosis, coccidioidomycosis, leishmaniasis, cryptococcosis, and tertiary syphilis. Serologic studies are necessary in the diagnosis of syphilis.

The most important etiologic factors in ulceration on the legs and feet are disturbances of circulation. Chronic venous insufficiency leads to ulceration, especially on the medial aspect of the ankle or lower leg, and the ulcers develop in areas of skin with brownish hemosiderin pigmentation and occasionally where there is edema or sclerosis of the area. Hypertensive or ischemic ulcerations tend to start on the lateral aspect of the ankle. Ulceration can also occur as a result of tissue infarction in areas supplied by either large or small blood vessels (arteries, arterioles); infarction may occur as the result of occlusion or constriction due to a variety of etiologic factors, in addition to those already mentioned: emboli, thrombosis, cryoagglutinins, macroglobulinemia, cryoglobulinemia, thrombotic thrombocytopenic purpura, polycythemia, systemic lupus erythematosus, Raynaud's phenomenon, arteriosclerosis obliterans, and thromboangiitis obliterans. Ulceration of the lower extremities also occurs in hemolytic anemia, including sickle cell anemia, thalassemia, and hereditary spherocytosis.

Some ulcers show extensive necrosis of the edges, such as those in *pyoderma gangrenosum,* an indolent ulcer usually on the lower extremities and often associated with ulcerative colitis or regional ileitis. The ulcers in pyoderma gangrenosum have ragged bluish-red overhanging edges and a necrotic base. These lesions often start as pustules or tender red nodules at the site of trauma, and then gradually increase in size until liquefaction necrosis occurs and an irregular ulcer develops. The ulcers are often multiple and may cover large areas of the leg. The histopathologic findings are not specific. The healing of the ulcers usually parallels the activity of the ulcerative colitis, and, inasmuch as the ulceration extends into and involves the reticular layer of the dermis and the subcutis, scarring occurs. Pyoderma gangrenosum and variants of it also occur in association with a number of other conditions such as myeloproliferative disorders and rheumatoid arthritis.

The term *"tropical" ulcer,* in addition to cutaneous leishmaniasis, now also includes ulceration due to cutaneous diphtheria, treponemal disorders (syphilis, yaws, and bejel), and phagedenic ulcer, a chronic ulcer of the feet and legs caused by mixed bacteria that occurs in persons suffering from starvation and neglect.

Ulcers can be associated with peripheral neuropathy ("neuropathic" ulcer, or malum perforans) seen in diabetes mellitus, tabes dorsalis, polyneuritis, leprosy, congenital anesthesia, or hereditary sensory radicular neuropathy.

Anal and perianal ulcers are seen in histiocytosis X and in amebiasis. A hanging-drop preparation is necessary to detect *Entamoeba histolytica.*

Ulcers with artificial and bizarre shapes must be suspected of being self-induced by means of destructive agents such as acid and lighted cigarettes. Factitial ulcers are overstudied and, unfortunately, underdiagnosed by most physicians.

Stony-hard, noduloulcerative lesions, particularly around joints (elbows, knees, and fingers) are suggestive of calcinosis cutis or gout; roentgenographic examination enables the detection of calcinosis cutis but shows no opaque bodies in gout.

Sclerosis, diffuse or circumscribed Diffuse sclerosis of the skin is most often seen on the upper extremities, chest, and face in systemic scleroderma (sometimes called progressive systemic sclerosis). Initially, the skin appears yellowish and shows slight nonpitting edema; later, however, it becomes indurated, bound down, and may be markedly hyperpigmented. Calcinosis cutis and Raynaud's phenomenon commonly occur.

Circumscribed sclerosis occurs in *morphea,* which consists of one or more round or oval, firm, reddish plaques up to several centimeters in diameter that become white or yellow centrally, often with a lilac-colored, telangiectatic border. This disorder is not associated with any other organ involvement and is a localized cutaneous form of scleroderma. Another type of localized scleroderma is *linear scleroderma,* in which the morphologic change is the same as that seen in morphea except that the process occurs in bands extending parallel to the long axis of the extremity or along the paramedian line of the forehead and scalp. This form of scleroderma has no relationship to progressive systemic sclerosis.

Edema In addition to the various causes of localized edema and generalized edema, there is a type of edema of the lower extremities that is not often recognized by the physician. This is a bilateral pedal edema which is common in patients with subacute or chronic dermatitis of the lower extremities. This type of edema is most often seen with chronic eczematous dermatitis and psoriasis, but is unrelated to cardiac failure or lymphatic obstruction. It is most probably due to an increased permeability as a result of local capillary damage, which is part of the inflammatory process in the skin. The increased capillary permeability leads to an increased transfer of fluid from the intravascular to the extravascular component of the extracellular fluid space. This type of pitting edema disappears completely when the dermatitis has resolved.

Atrophy, diffuse or circumscribed Dermal atrophy results from a decrease of the papillary or reticular connective tissue and is manifested in the skin as a depression. Circumscribed dermal atrophy may follow trauma, or may occur in association with epidermal atrophy, as in the striae of pregnancy or Cushing's disease.

PANNICULUS ADIPOSUS (SUBCUTIS) Nodules (inflammatory, usually tender, red) Nodules in the subcutis may be recognized by the fact that the skin is usually movable over the nodule; occasionally, however, in inflammatory processes, the nodule may involve both the dermis and panniculus adiposus, and the skin will then not be movable over the nodule. Acute, tender, red nodules on the leg are characteristically found in two disorders: *erythema nodosum syndrome* and *nodular subcutaneous fat necrosis* associated with pancreatitis.

The erythema nodosum syndrome refers to the occurrence of multiple bilateral tender nodules appearing principally on the anterior aspect of the lower extremities and occasionally on the upper extremities and face. The erythema nodosum syndrome is associated with a number of disorders that are unrelated to each other, except for their ability to elicit this distinctive hypersensitivity reaction.

The nodules in erythema nodosum are only slightly elevated, edematous, and sometimes exquisitely tender. Bruising is a characteristic feature of the disease and is due to hemorrhage, leading to the formation of contusions. The lesions never ulcerate or become indurated and very seldom leave any scarring or atrophy. Erythema nodosum is associated with primary tuberculosis and primary coccidioidomycosis, histoplasmosis, *Yersinia* infection, beta-hemolytic streptococcal infections, lymphogranuloma venereum, leprosy, sarcoidosis, ulcerative colitis, Crohn's disease, regional enteritis, drugs (penicillin, sulfonamides, bromides, iodides), and oral contraceptives containing ethynylestradiol and norethynodrel.

Tender, red subcutaneous nodules may also appear on the legs in association with acute pancreatitis and with pancreatic neoplasms and are often erroneously called erythema nodosum. This disorder has been termed *nodular liquefying panniculitis* (NLP). These lesions are distinctive. Their morphologic features are different from those of classic erythema nodosum. The lesions in NLP vary in size from a few millimeters to several centimeters, and, in contrast to the lesions of erythema nodosum, are movable. The lesions of NLP involute in 2 to 3 weeks and may leave a hyperpigmented scar that is slightly depressed. The nodules are often associated with abdominal pain and may also be accompanied by fever and arthralgia. Rarely, lesions may be present on other parts of the body besides the legs. Some of the larger nodules may undergo an abscess-like change, become fluctuant, rupture, and exude a whitish, creamy, or oily viscous material; abscess formation with drainage rarely, if ever, occurs in erythema nodosum. The most common pancreatic neoplasm associated with NLP is an acinous adenocarcinoma of the pancreas. In *Weber-Christian panniculitis,* the subcutaneous nodules, which at first are slightly mobile, become adherent to the overlying skin; then, as the edema subsides in the area of induration, a central depression occurs.

In addition to the above-mentioned entities, various types of vasculitis may also produce tender subcutaneous nodules. Therefore,

diagnosis of these lesions often requires an excisional or incisional biopsy.

Nodules (noninflammatory, usually nontender, nonerythematous) Movable, painless, noninflammatory-appearing nodules occur around joints in rheumatic fever, rheumatoid arthritis, and in certain metabolic diseases such as xanthoma, gout, and calcinosis. Metastatic carcinoma or metastatic malignant melanoma may appear as movable, nontender subcutaneous nodules. Sarcoidosis may be manifested in the skin solely as subcutaneous nodules on the lower extremities. Subcutaneous nodules also occur in onchocerciasis and loiasis. *Lipomas*, relatively common causes of subcutaneous nodules, are benign tumors composed of adipose tissue and may be single or multiple and are frequently lobulated; they are often rubbery or compressible and occur most often on the trunk and back of the neck and forearms. Occasionally, subcutaneous lipoma may be painful and associated with marked obesity; this condition, known as *Dercum's disease,* is most common in middle-aged females.

Atrophy, diffuse or circumscribed Atrophy of the panniculus adiposus produces depressions in the skin; these depressions are seen in progressive lipodystrophy, in liquefying panniculitis, and in the localized fat atrophy that occurs at the site of injections of insulin. About 25 percent of diabetics who receive insulin (most often females under the age of 20) have this type of atrophy. The depressed areas of localized fat atrophy show a complete absence of the panniculus, and there is no inflammation. In lipodystrophy, diffuse atrophy of the skin may involve large portions of the body.

BLOOD VESSELS Morbilliform and scarlatiniform eruptions Morbilliform (measles-like) and scarlatiniform eruptions are macular and papular exanthems and can be due to drug hypersensitivities, measles, German measles, erythema infectiosum, other viral exanthems, rickettsial diseases including endemic murine typhus and Rocky Mountain spotted fever, scarlet fever, and secondary syphilis. Many of the diseases manifested by macules or papules and occurring in acutely ill patients with a fever are listed in Table 48-3.

Urticaria Urticaria is characterized by wheals, of which the outstanding feature is their persistence for only a few hours (see Fig. 47-6). This short duration differentiates urticarial wheals from the otherwise almost identical papules of erythema multiforme, which persist for more than 1 or 2 days rather than for a few hours. An acute onset of urticaria is usually related to ingestion of drugs or certain types of foods (shellfish, fresh berries).

Chronic recurrent urticaria is a special problem, and its causes are not easily established. Most patients with this disorder require a careful examination for cryptic diseases such as lymphoma, systemic lupus erythematosus, primary or metastatic carcinoma, intestinal parasites, acute hepatitis, systemic vasculitis, or dermatomyositis. It is especially important, even in chronic urticarias, to carry out a painstaking interrogation of the patient in search of a history of drugs. Aspirin is one of the most common causes of chronic urticaria and can often be missed even in a careful drug history because many patients do not consider aspirin a drug. It is probably true that some patients with chronic urticaria can relate their problem to emotional stress, but this should be considered only after excluding all possible organic causes.

Erythema multiforme syndrome Erythema multiforme syndrome is a characteristic response of the skin and mucous membranes that is related to a number of possible etiologies, including infectious agents (herpesvirus hominis, *Mycoplasma pneumoniae*) and drugs (especially penicillin, antipyretics, barbiturates, hydantoins, and sulfonamides). In 50 percent of patients no etiology is ascertained. The major pathologic change is an acute lymphohistiocytic inflammatory infiltrate around blood vessels and at the dermal-epidermal interface. Degenerative changes in the endothelial cells of the capillaries, marked papillary dermal edema, and keratinocyte necrosis are also seen. There is some evidence for an immune-complex etiology with hypocomplementemic vasculitis.

The lesions occur in a characteristic symmetric distribution and favor the extensor areas of the distal parts of the limbs, the backs of the hands, and the dorsa of the feet; the palms and soles are often involved, even to the exclusion of the dorsal surfaces. Oral lesions, first as blisters and then erosions, occur on the buccal mucous membrane, gums, and tongue, and there is often swelling and crusting of the lips. The syndrome may also include severe toxemia and prostration, high fever, cough, and "patchy" inflammation of the lungs. The skin lesions are often characterized by a vivid redness that gradually becomes duller, and they become more indurated, with the development of centers that are pale or may have bullae; these "target" or "iris" lesions, which are characteristic of erythema multiforme but do not invariably occur, are identified by the clear red area at the periphery that surrounds a pale pink zone and a central livid area, which may contain a bulla. The efficacy of systemic corticosteroids has not been proved, but this therapy is commonly used.

Purpura (with and without inflammation) A purpuric eruption demands immediate exploration for its etiology. Purpura arises in the skin of the vascularized dermis and is almost always confined to the dermis. Purpuric macules gradually disappear after days or weeks, depending on their size. Punctate or tiny purpuric spots are termed *petechiae,* larger (>2.0 cm) macules are spoken of as *suggillations,* and extensive purpuric macules are called *ecchymoses* (see D in Fig. 47-2).

Purpura with inflammation is usually "palpable," i.e., papular, and is seen in systemic vasculitis and in bacteremias such as staphylococcemia, gonococcemia, and meningococcemia. In these bacteremias and in vasculitis, the examination of biopsied skin may establish a diagnosis within 8 h (the time required for processing the tissue). Gentle scraping of the purpuric lesions will produce enough material for a Gram's stain; intracellular gram-negative diplococci are occasionally found in the lesions in acute, but not in chronic, meningococcemia, and are rarely found in acute gonococcemia. The differential diagnosis of palpable purpuric lesions and infarcts occurring in *systemic vasculitis* (necrotizing vasculitis) as compared with those in chronic meningococcemia is not easy. The skin lesions in systemic vasculitis are usually bilateral, and almost symmetric, in their distribution. They tend to be concentrated on the lower extremities, especially on the lower portion and around the ankles and the dorsa of the feet. The lesions in chronic meningococcemia are more randomly distributed, with occurrence on the trunk, lower and upper extremities, and face. Nevertheless, in meningococcemia, lesions can occur in a bilateral distribution, which makes the distinction between chronic meningococcemia and systemic vasculitis difficult, if not impossible, at times. The individual lesions in both chronic meningococcemia and systemic vasculitis may be identical, consisting of a mixture of palpable purpura and urticarial-type papules without purpura. Unfortunately, the histologic findings in biopsy specimens of the lesions in both diseases do not permit a distinction. Therefore, a patient with bilaterally distributed palpable purpuric lesions and fever is best treated with antibiotics before the results of blood cultures are available.

Purpura without inflammation is completely macular, and examination of a blood smear can quickly establish the presence of platelets; if platelets are seen in the smear, thrombocytopenic purpura can be safely ruled out as a possibility.

On the lower legs of older people, a great variety of inflammatory skin diseases, including various types of contact dermatitis, may be associated with purpura; under these circumstances, the purpura does not have the same importance as it does when present on the trunk or upper extremities. Perifollicular purpura, however, on the lower extremities (usually accompanied by follicular hyperkeratosis) is almost pathognomonic of scurvy.

Purpura frequently develops in amyloidosis when the lesions (waxy macules and papules) are pinched. This "pinch" purpura, however, may also occur in the normal skin of patients with thrombocytopenic purpura or in the skin of apparently normal elderly persons. (For a full discussion of the classification and differential diagnosis of purpura, see Chaps. 54 and 279.)

Infarcts Infarcts in the skin are usually not pale like those that occur in the kidney but have a variegated dusky red, grayish hue. They are irregularly shaped macules, sometimes slightly depressed below the plane of the skin, and often surrounded by a pink zone of hyperemia. Infarcts are usually slightly tender.

Cutaneous infarctions are important and often diagnostic signs of serious multisystem disease, including both acute and chronic meningococcemia, streptococcal and staphylococcal septicemia, gonococcemia, pseudomonas septicemia, systemic vasculitis, purpura fulminans, systemic lupus erythematosus, and, rarely, dermatomyositis. Degos' disease (malignant atrophic papulosis), in which porcelain-white macules are surrounded by a narrow telangiectatic and erythematous rim, is often associated with similar infarctions in the gastrointestinal and central nervous system.

Telangiectasia Redness of the skin is most frequently caused by transient dilatation of blood vessels (erythema). In contrast to the color produced by fixed blood pigments, as in purpura, the erythema will disappear under the pressure of a glass or plastic slide (see "Diascopy," in Chap. 47). Telangiectasia is the condition in which redness of the skin results from a permanent enlargement in the caliber of small blood vessels (which will be revealed by examination with a hand lens) and an increase in the number of the vessels. Telangiectasia may be composed of fine linear branches of blood vessels appearing distinctly red (i.e., not blue), which are often seen on the nose and face, or of confluent macular areas that appear as a permanent erythema. Erythema in discoid and systemic lupus ery-

TABLE 48-3 Rash and fever in the acutely ill patient: Diagnosis according to type of lesion

DISEASES MANIFESTED BY MACULES OR PAPULES

Drug hypersensitivities	Rocky Mountain spotted fever
Scarlet fever	(early lesions)*
Erythema infectiosum (fifth	Pityriasis rosea
disease)	Erythema multiforme
Measles (rubeola)	Erythema marginatum
German measles (rubella)*	Systemic lupus erythematosus*
Enterovirus (echo- and cox-	Dermatomyositis
sackievirus) infections	"Serum sickness"* (manifested
Adenovirus infections	only as wheals)
Typhoid fever	Urticaria, acute (viral hepatitis)
Secondary syphilis	Urticaria, persistent (necrotizing an-
Typhus, murine (endemic)	giitis)
	Lyme disease

DISEASES MANIFESTED BY VESICLES, BULLAE, OR PUSTULES

Drug hypersensitivities	Variola†
Dermatitis from plants	Enterovirus (echo- and cox-
Rickettsialpox	sackievirus) infections, including
Varicella (chickenpox)†	hand-foot-mouth disease
Generalized herpes zoster†	Toxic epidermal necrolysis
Disseminated herpes simplex†	Staphylococcal scaled-skin syn-
Eczema herpeticum†	drome
Disseminated vaccinia†	Erythema multiforme bullosum
Eczema vaccinatum†	

DISEASES MANIFESTED BY PURPURIC MACULES, PURPURIC PAPULES, OR PURPURIC VESICLES

Drug hypersensitivities	Enterovirus (echo- and coxsackievi-
Bacteremia:‡	rus) infections
Meningococcemia (acute or	Rickettsial diseases:
chronic)*	Rocky Mountain spotted fever*
Gonococcemia*	Typhus, louse-borne (epidemic)
Staphylococcemia	"Allergic" vasculitis*‡
Pseudomonas bacteremia	Purpura fulminans‡
Subacute bacterial endocarditis	Acquired immunodeficiency syn-
	drome

* May have arthralgia or musculoskeletal pain.
† One characteristic lesion of these exanthems is an umbilicated papule or vesicle.
‡ Often present as infarcts.
SOURCE: *TB Fitzpatrick, RA Johnson, in Dermatology in General Medicine, 3d ed, TB Fitzpatrick et al (eds), New York, McGraw-Hill, 1987.*

thematosus, dermatomyositis, and psoriasis is caused largely by the presence of telangiectasia.

Telangiectasia may also occur in a scattered, discrete fashion on the upper trunk or on the extremities and is seen characteristically in progressive systemic sclerosis (systemic scleroderma). Telangiectasia occurring around the nail beds, i.e., periungual telangiectasia, is an important diagnostic sign in lupus erythematosus (both discoid and systemic) and in dermatomyositis; these lesions are seen rarely, if at all, in systemic scleroderma or rheumatoid arthritis.

Sharply outlined, red macules or papules 1 to 2 mm in diameter, with an area of radiating telangiectasia, are seen in *hereditary hemorrhagic telangiectasia* (Chap. 281). These occur on the lips, tongue, nasal mucosa, face, and hands.

Generalized telangiectasia occurring in the form of red macules over most of the body surface may be the presenting sign of mastocytosis or urticaria pigmentosa.

Telangiectasia is a prominent and diagnostic feature of *ataxia-telangiectasia,* or Louis-Bar syndrome. Telangiectasia may be present as early as the second year of life but usually develops by the fifth year; it appears first on the bulbar conjunctiva and subsequently involves the ears, the eyelids, the butterfly area of the face, the upper aspect of the chest, and the extremities.

Telangiectasia may occur in a characteristic form known as the *arterial spider,* or spider nevus, spider angioma, or naevus araneus. The main vessel of the spider is an arteriole, and it is usually faintly pulsating, which will show under the diascope. A less common skin lesion usually found with vascular spiders in liver disorders is the telangiectatic *mat* or net, a small red patch composed of intermeshed fine vessels that blanch on pressure. Spider angiomas, usually three or fewer, occur not infrequently in normal children and adults. Numerous spider angiomas often develop during pregnancy or after the ingestion of progestational agents or in rheumatoid arthritis or thyrotoxicosis. Most patients with numerous and prominent vascular spiders, however, have some form of underlying diffuse liver disease, e.g., alcoholic cirrhosis. The progression of subacute hepatitis is often paralleled by the appearance of crops of spiders, and in alcoholic and postnecrotic cirrhosis, almost half the patients have multiple vascular spiders. The mechanism responsible for the development of spider angiomas in liver disease is not known, nor has it been firmly established that the lesions result from disordered metabolism of estrogens by the liver.

REFERENCES

Braverman I: *Skin Signs of Systemic Disease.* Philadelphia, Saunders, 1981

Farber EM, Cox AJ (eds): *Psoriasis: Proceedings of the Third International Symposium.* New York, Yorke Medical, 1981

Fitzpatrick TB, Bernhard JD: The structure of skin lesions and fundamentals of diagnosis, in *Dermatology in General Medicine,* 3d ed., TB Fitzpatrick et al (eds). New York, McGraw-Hill, 1987

Henseler T et al: Oral 8-methoxypsoralen photochemotherapy of psoriasis. Lancet 1:853, 1981

Honigsmann H et al: Oral photochemotherapy with psoralens and UVA (PUVA): Principles and practice, in *Dermatology in General Medicine,* 3d ed, TB Fitzpatrick et al (eds). New York, McGraw-Hill, 1987

Leyden JJ, Kligman AM: The role of bacteria in acne vulgaris, in *Progress in Diseases of the Skin,* R Fleischmajer (ed). Orlando, Grune & Stratton, 1984, pp 21, 29

Parrish JA et al: Photochemotherapy of psoriasis with oral methoxsalen and longwave ultraviolet light. N Engl J Med 291:1207, 1974

Peck GL et al: Prolonged remissions of cystic acne with 13-*cis*-retinoic acid. N Engl J Med 300:329, 1979

49   RASH AND FEVER

LAWRENCE COREY / PHILIP KIRBY

Because many infectious and noninfectious diseases produce cutaneous lesions, specific diagnosis of an acutely ill febrile patient with a rash is a clinical skill with important therapeutic implications. Some exanthems are unique to a particular pathogen; others are common to numerous etiologic agents. Classification of exanthematous illness into (1) maculopapular, (2) vesicular, or (3) petechial eruptions is useful in determining the etiology and in understanding the pathogenesis of an exanthem.

PATHOGENESIS Exanthems are cutaneous eruptions due to systemic or contiguous spread of an organism. The pathogenesis of an exanthem may be caused by (1) multiplication of the pathogen in the skin, (2) carriage of the agent in plasma or in infected hematopoietic cells (leukocytes and/or lymphocytes) into integumentary blood vessels, or (3) antigen-antibody or delayed hypersensitivity reactions to antigens derived from the infecting microorganism.

Maculopapular exanthems may be caused by either direct viral or bacterial invasion of the skin or local or systemic immune responses to the microorganism. For example, rubella virus can be recovered from rubella maculopapules as well as from areas of the body not involved by the exanthem. Administration of pooled immune serum globulin after exposure to rubella may not eliminate rubella viremia but does prevent rash. The exanthem of rubeola may be a manifestation of an Arthus reaction produced by the deposition of viral antigen in the endothelium of dermal capillaries. The complex interplay between the host and the pathogen may influence the duration and pattern of a rash. In many viral illnesses, such as enterovirus infections, initial viral replication occurs in the infected mucosal surface and regional lymphatic tissue. A primary viremia then ensues, and "seeding" of the virus into target organs, such as liver, muscle, central nervous system, or heart, may occur. Continued viral replication and a secondary viremia with hematogenous spread of the virus to the skin may then follow. The regional multiplication of the virus, primary viremia, and visceral dissemination of virus prior to the development of the exanthem help explain why the initial clinical manifestations of many illnesses occur prior to the development of the rash. Humoral and cellular immune responses which prevent or ameliorate secondary viremia may prevent the development of rash and may explain why exanthems associated with enteroviruses occur more frequently in younger children than in adolescents or adults; young children do not possess cross-reacting antibodies or cannot mount an anamnestic immune response to the infecting agent.

As with maculopapular eruptions, vesicular exanthems can be caused either by direct invasion into the skin by organisms such as herpes simplex virus, varicella-zoster virus, or the coxsackieviruses causing hand-foot-and-mouth disease; by elaboration of a toxin such as in staphylococcal scalded skin syndrome, or by host immune responses such as bullous erythema multiforme or pemphigus.

Petechial eruptions may arise from direct invasion of the cutaneous vasculature by a microorganism, as occurs with septic emboli, or may result from immunologic injury to the vascular endothelium. In Rocky Mountain spotted fever, for example, *Rickettsia rickettsiae* can be demonstrated in the smooth muscle wall of arterioles. Vascular damage, microinfarction, and extravasation of red blood cells produce the characteristic petechial exanthem. Occasionally, a petechial eruption may complicate previous maculopapular or vesicular exanthems, usually coinciding with the development of diffuse intravascular coagulation. In some petechial eruptions, direct evidence of viral or bacterial invasion can be obtained by direct aspiration and culture of the lesion, by demonstration of the agent with Gram's stain, or by immunofluorescent stain to detect microbial agents.

CLINICAL DIAGNOSIS OF MACULOPAPULAR ERUPTIONS Table 49-1 lists the numerous viral, bacterial, rickettsial, and noninfectious agents that may be associated with maculopapular exanthems. One helpful approach to the physical examination of viral maculopapular (not vesicular) rashes is that these eruptions relatively spare the palms and soles in contrast to eruptions associated with drug reactions, bacteria, mycoplasma, and rickettsial and/or immunologic diseases. In the last two entities, a prominent palmar or plantar distribution is often present.

While some exanthematous diseases produce characteristic cutaneous patterns, e.g., measles or erythema infectiosum, overlap in the cutaneous manifestations of viral induced maculopapular exanthems is the rule. Therefore, the presence of associated signs or symptoms as well as the epidemiologic characteristics of the disease, such as the season of the year, the patient's age, and history of exposure and previous immunization, are useful in formulating a diagnostic impression. Because viral maculopapular exanthems are manifestations of the agent's systemic spread, evidence of mucosal viral replication in the form of an enanthem is often a valuable aid in determining the etiology of a viral rash. Koplik's spots in rubeola, ulcerative lesions of the hard and soft palate with herpangina due to coxsackievirus A, and palatal petechiae in early infectious mononucleosis are all helpful clinical signs. Associated clinical findings such as coryza, conjunctivitis, and cough with rubeola; mild fever and posterior auricular lymphadenopathy in rubella; or localized mastitis or furunculosis in staphylococcal scalded skin syndrome should be looked for. Concomitant arthritis, renal disease, and/or heart disease generally suggest entities such as acute rheumatic fever, subacute bacterial endocarditis, serum sickness, or collagen vascular disease.

The distribution of the rash provides important information. Erythema infectiosum presents with a diffuse erythema of the cheeks ("slapped cheeks"). In addition, central clearing of the eruption on the extremities results in a lacelike appearance of the exanthem. Erythema marginatum occurs in 10 percent of patients with acute rheumatic fever and is characterized by a ringed eruption which rapidly spreads to the trunk and extremities. Scarlet fever due to erythrogenic toxin elaborated by a group A streptococcus produces a rash that starts on the neck and spreads to the trunk and extremities within 36 h. The rash consists of numerous punctate papular lesions at the site of hair follicles and feels like rough sandpaper. Circumoral pallor, large red fungiform papillae (strawberry tongue), extension of the rash into body folds including the antecubital fossae, concomitant tonsillitis and cervical lymphadenopathy, and the subsequent desquamation of the rash, especially on the palms and soles, confirm the clinical diagnosis. Erysipelas due to group A (uncommonly group G) streptococci and staphylococci is characterized by an edematous indurated superficial cellulitis. Characteristically, the rash is shiny with a sharply demarcated edge. Occasionally streptococci can be demonstrated on Gram's stain and culture of material aspirated from the advancing edge of the lesion.

Some strains of *Staphylococcus aureus* (phage group 2) can elaborate a toxin which produces a diffuse erythema of the skin (staphylococcal scalded skin syndrome). The development of bullae resulting from the easy separation of the epidermis (Nikolsky's sign) may occur but is not specific for this entity.

Staphylococcal toxic shock syndrome is characterized by the acute onset of fever, hypotension, vomiting, diarrhea, vaginal discharge, and the development of a diffuse scarlatiniform rash with subsequent desquamation (see Chap. 94). This syndrome was reported with increasing frequency in the United States between 1978 and 1980 especially in young menstruating women using tampons. *Staphylococcus aureus,* often in pure culture, was isolated from nearly all of these patients not receiving antimicrobials. Relapses of disease, which are usually milder, are occasionally seen. The staphylococcal strains isolated from these patients appear to elaborate newly described toxin(s).

The course of the eruption is also helpful in differentiating the etiology of viral exanthems. Rubeola usually starts in the hairline area and spreads downward until the involved areas coalesce into a diffuse morbilliform eruption. In contrast, the eruption of

TABLE 49-1 Differential diagnosis of patients with rash and fever

Macules or papules	Vesicles & pustules	Petechiae-purpura
VIRAL		
Rubeola	Herpes simplex	Enteroviruses (echovirus)
Rubella	Varicella-zoster	
Enteroviruses	Vaccinia	Viral hemorrhagic fevers
Cytomegalovirus	Enteroviruses (herpangina)	
Hepatitis B		Dengue
Erythema infectiosum	Hand-foot-and-mouth disease (A16)	Adenoviruses
Exanthem subitum		Yellow fever
Adenoviruses	Orf	Atypical measles
Arboviruses	Molluscum contagiosum	
Rhabdovirus group		
Reoviruses	Vesicular stomatitis virus	
Live virus vaccines (measles, rubella)		
BACTERIAL		
Group A streptococci:	Staphylococcal scalded-skin syndrome	Severe sepsis with diffuse intravascular coagulation
Scarlet fever		
Erysipelas	Bullous impetigo	Meningococcemia
Erythema marginatum		Gonococcemia
Staphylococcal scalded-skin syndrome		*Haemophilus influenzae* (type B)
Staphylococcal toxic shock syndrome		*Pseudomonas* sepsis
Subacute bacterial endocarditis		Subacute bacterial endocarditis
Secondary syphilis		*Listeria monocytogenes*
Typhoid fever		
Erysipelothrix		
Myobacterium leprae		
Rat bite fever		
Leptospirosis		
Chronic meningococcemia		
Pseudomonas sepsis		
Erythema chronicum migrans (Lyme disease)		
RICKETTSIAL		
Rocky Mountain spotted fever (early)	Rickettsialpox	Rocky Mountain spotted fever
Murine typhus		Epidemic (louse-borne) typhus
FUNGAL		
Candidiasis		
Sporotrichosis		
Cryptococcosis		
Tinea versicolor		
Pityriasis rosea		
Tinea corporis		
CHLAMYDIAL		
Psittacosis		
PROTOZOAL		
Toxoplasmosis		Trichinosis
Trichinosis		Plasmodia (blackwater fever)
Scabies		
IMMUNOLOGIC		
Erythema multiforme	Erythema multiforme	Immune thrombocytopenic purpura
Systemic lupus erythematosis	Pustular psoriasis	
Dermatomyositis	Reiter's syndrome	Thrombotic thrombocytopenic purpura
Relapsing polychondritis	Sweet's syndrome	Henoch-Schönlein purpura
	Behçet's syndrome	
Rheumatoid arthritis	Bowel bypass syndrome	Polyarteritis nodosa
Erythema nodosum	Acne fulminans	Wegener's granulomatosis
Urticarial vasculitis		
Leukemic infiltrate		Cholesterol embolization
UNKNOWN		
Mucocutaneous lymph node syndrome		
DRUGS		
Drug eruptions	Drug eruptions	Drug eruptions

rubella tends to disappear from its original sites of involvement as it spreads.

The rash of Rocky Mountain spotted fever usually starts on the extremities and spreads centripetally to the trunk. In contrast, the rash of roseola subitum starts on the trunk and spreads centrifugally to the arms and legs. Pityriasis rosea is characterized by the development of papular lesions along the lines of cleavage of the trunk ("fir tree" effect). The development of the earlier appearing "herald patch" and the lack of fever characterize this exanthem.

While papular lesions may be a manifestation of viral disease, systemic bacterial and/or fungal disease may also produce these lesions. Chronic meningococcemia may be associated with pale-rose-colored maculopapular lesions that may be mistaken for erythema nodosum when located on the lower extremities. The cutaneous lesions tend to wax and wane with fever. Organisms usually are not demonstrated in Gram's stain or cultures of these lesions. However, blood cultures taken during febrile periods may be positive. The development of discrete papules on the trunk in a patient with a previous history of diarrhea should suggest the possibility of typhoid fever. These "rose spots" are 1- to 3-mm papules which disappear in 3 to 4 days. In the untreated patient new lesions will emerge over the next 2 to 3 weeks. *Pseudomonas* bacteremia can also produce small painless papules on the trunk. The papulosquamous lesions of secondary syphilis often involve the trunk, palms, soles, and mucous membranes and may be present for days to several weeks. The serology (VDRL) is invariably positive in secondary syphilis. Erythema chronicum migrans is an exanthem characteristically seen in Lyme disease, an illness caused by the spirochete *Borrelia burgdorferi*. The lesion starts as a small red papule or macule which may gradually expand over a period of days to weeks. Multiple annular or secondary lesions are common. A history of tick bite and associated neurologic, cardiac, and rheumatologic findings are important factors in considering Lyme disease.

Papulonodular lesions can be identified in 10 to 15 percent of patients with disseminated candidiasis. The appearance of these lesions in febrile immunosuppressed patients who fail to respond to antimicrobials should suggest the possibility. Biopsy and culture of the lesions should demonstrate the blastospores and pseudohyphae of *Candida* species.

Noninfectious causes of maculopapular eruptions and fever Drug eruptions are probably the most common noninfectious causes of maculopapular rash and fever. Drug eruptions may be urticarial, bullous, exfoliative, and lichenoid, but the typical drug eruption resembles the exanthem of measles and is often called morbilliform. Drug eruptions begin centrally and extend centrifugally to the extremities, often affecting the palms and soles. They usually begin within one to several weeks after starting a drug, but may be delayed. While most drugs occasionally produce rashes, those most commonly associated with fever and rash include sulfonamides, phenytoin, barbiturates, sulfones, iodides, and bromides. Past and current exposure to the drug is a most important part of the diagnosis.

Several collagen vascular diseases produce distinctive papular rashes and fever. Systemic lupus erythematosus is best known for malar erythema in a "butterfly" distribution, but may also include scaly "discoid" plaques or bullae. Dermatomyositis is less commonly associated with fever, but has a heliotrope erythema of the periorbital skin and flat violaceous papules over the knuckles (Gottron's papules). Relapsing polychondritis causes episodes of fever and erythema over cartilaginous structures, particularly the superior portion of the ear. Rheumatoid arthritis may present with fever and transient erythematous macules prior to the onset of joint complaints. The diagnosis of collagen vascular diseases usually rests on evidence of specific organ involvement and serologic studies, but recognition and biopsy of skin lesions may be helpful.

Erythema nodosum is a form of panniculitis occurring most commonly in young women. Patients have fever, arthralgias, and exquisitely tender erythematous nodules over the pretibial region bilaterally. Erythema nodosum is often idiopathic, but can be associated with inflammatory bowel disease, streptococcal infection, oral contraceptives, sarcoidosis (Lofgren's syndrome), and many other diseases. Biopsy may be needed for diagnosis and to exclude other forms of panniculitis, such as Weber-Christian syndrome. Erythema multiforme may occur as a papular eruption, but is discussed with vesicular disease. Leukemic or lymphomatous infiltration of the skin may present with fever and adenopathy. Acute monocytic leukemia, myelomonocytic leukemia, chronic lymphocytic leukemia, and non-Hodgkin's lymphoma may all produce nontender plum-colored papules which usually involve the upper body. Biopsy is diagnostic.

CLINICAL DIAGNOSIS OF VESICULAR AND PUSTULAR ERUPTIONS The distribution of the eruption is often helpful in determining a clinical and etiologic diagnosis of a vesicular exanthem. Varicella begins on the trunk, spreads centrifugally, and demonstrates lesions in all stages of healing, i.e., vesicles, ulcers, and crusts. Variola usually begins on the extremities, spreads centripetally, and is characterized by lesions in similar stages of development. The vesicular ulcerative pharyngeal lesions of herpangina are present only on the palate, whereas primary herpes simplex gingivostomatitis also involves the anterior gingival area and/or the lips. Hand-foot-and-mouth disease due to coxsackievirus A16 presents as multiple linear vesicles or pustules on the palms and soles; this is an unusual distribution for either herpes simplex or varicella-zoster virus.

First-episode primary herpes simplex virus (HSV) infection is often accompanied by constitutional symptoms such as fever, malaise, and myalgias; numerous bilaterally distributed lesions; and tender regional lymphadenopathy. In contrast, patients with recurrent HSV are usually afebrile and have only a few clustered unilateral lesions which last from 5 to 12 days. Patients will often complain of a "prodrome," a tingling sensation near or at the eventual site of lesion, from 2 to 48 h prior to the appearance of vesicles. Occasionally, HSV infection will present in a dermatomal distribution that is usually characteristic of herpes zoster. Because cytologic techniques do not differentiate between these two agents, viral cultures or use of specific techniques such as immunofluorescence must be employed in order to differentiate these two viruses.

The appearance of vesicles may be helpful. Herpes simplex and varicella lesions have a surrounding zone of erythema and a thin vesicular roof, and they are tender when irritated. The lesions of molluscum contagiosum are umbilicated, contain an expressible white core, and are usually not tender when scraped gently.

NONINFECTIOUS CAUSES OF VESICULAR AND PUSTULAR ERUPTION Erythema multiforme is a hypersensitivity reaction affecting skin and mucous membranes. The spectrum of erythema multiforme ranges from mild papular reactions to life-threatening bullous diseases referred to as Stevens-Johnson syndrome and toxic epidermal necrolysis. Erythema multiforme has been associated with an extensive list of conditions and often occurs idiopathically, but the most common causes are drugs and infections. Infectious causes include herpes simplex and mycoplasma. Common drug etiologies are phenytoin, sulfonamides, phenobarbital, and penicillins. Recurrent erythema multiforme is usually due to herpes simplex. The classic lesion of erythema multiforme is the target, or iris, lesion with a central dusky papule or vesicle surrounded by concentric rings of erythema and pallor. Lesions are most frequent on the extremities and face, but may be generalized.

Pustular eruptions can be particularly difficult to distinguish from bacterial and viral infections. Culture and biopsy are usually needed to define an etiology. Pustular psoriasis is a rare condition affecting persons both with and without a prior history of psoriasis. The onset is abrupt with disseminated erythematous papules and plaques with superficial pustules and lakes of pus. Annular lesions are common and the oral mucosa is often involved. Progression to erythroderma and death rarely occurs with modern treatment modalities. Reiter's syndrome may produce similar lesions which begin as pustules and become crusted papules called keratoderma blennorrhagicum. The triad of urethritis, arthritis, and conjunctivitis is usually present.

Sweet's syndrome, acute febrile neutrophilic dermatosis, is characterized by fever, leukocytosis, arthralgia, and single or multiple painful erythematous, pustular plaques of the face and upper body. Sweet's syndrome is most frequent in women, may be recurrent, and has been associated with prior upper respiratory infection and myeloproliferative disease. Cultures are negative and biopsy is diagnostic.

Behçet's syndrome is characterized by oral and genital ulceration, uveitis, arthritis, thrombophlebitis, and pustular skin lesions. A characteristic of Behçet's syndrome is formation of pustules at sites of minor trauma such as needle puncture.

Bowel bypass syndrome is believed to be an immune-complex disease due to antigens associated with bacterial overgrowth in an intestinal blind loop. Patients have episodes of fever and sterile pustules of the skin.

Acne fulminans is a rare disease of adolescent males, frequently with no prior history of acne. The onset is sudden, with fever, leukocytosis, arthralgias, and extensive inflammatory cysts of the chest, back, and face. Less common findings include lytic bone lesions and a positive blood culture for *Propionibacterium acnes.*

PETECHIAL ERUPTIONS Infectious causes Many hematologic and immunologic entities produce thrombocytopenia as a result of defects in the production, maturation, sequestration, or destruction of platelets. A consequence is the development of petechiae. The physician who is presented with an acutely ill patient with a petechial exanthem must be concerned with systemic, bacterial, or rickettsial disease. The common microorganisms associated with petechial exanthems are listed in Table 49-1. However, any microorganism that is capable of initiating the cascade of hematologic events termed disseminated intravascular coagulation may produce a petechial exanthem.

Petechiae due to septic embolization are characteristic of subacute bacterial endocarditis. Lesions may occur anywhere on the skin and/or mucous membranes but are most common over the upper anterior trunk. Splinter hemorrhages under the nails are difficult to differentiate from traumatic lesions and may be seen in hematologic, malignant, and other infective disorders.

Petechial lesions associated with meningococcemia are small, irregularly shaped, slightly raised, pale-grayish lesions with a vesiculopustular center. The lesions are usually asymmetric and are seen most often on the trunk and extremities, although the conjunctivas and mucous membranes may also be affected. Fulminant meningococcal infection may produce coalescence of the petechiae into grossly ecchymotic areas (purpura fulminans).

Gonococcal infections usually produce lesions on the distal extremities, often over joints. The presence of these pustular, hemorrhagic skin lesions in patients with asymmetric tenosynovitis or polyarthritis, involving the wrists, fingers, knees, or ankles, should suggest the gonococcal arthritis-dermatitis syndrome. The majority of patients with disseminated gonococcal infection do not have symptoms of urogenital, anorectal, or pharyngeal gonococcal disease.

The metastatic lesions of staphylococcal bacteremia include pustules, subcutaneous abscesses, and purulent petechiae. Aspiration of material from the purulent center of the lesion will often reveal gram-positive cocci in clumps. *Pseudomonas* septicemia may produce ecthyma gangrenosum, a round, indurated, painless, necrotic eschar usually located in the anogenital or axillary area. In addition, hemorrhagic lesions with surrounding erythema resembling erythema multiforme may be associated with *Pseudomonas* sepsis.

Rickettsial disease may produce an arteriolar vasculitis that results in a petechial exanthem. The rash of Rocky Mountain spotted fever generally starts as a blanching maculopapular exanthem on the extremities, and after 2 to 4 days petechiae appear in the involved areas. The lesions no longer fade, and increased capillary fragility, manifested by a positive Rumpel-Leede test, is often present. These cutaneous findings in a patient with abrupt onset of fever, chills, headache, myalgias, and arthralgias should suggest this diagnosis. If the patient comes from an endemic area, and a tick bite or tick exposure is present, appropriate therapy should be instituted.

Summer febrile illness due to enteroviruses, especially the echovirus group, may occasionally produce a petechial eruption. While involvement of the face is common, the distribution of the exanthem is usually not distinctive, and because fever, headache, and meningismus may also be present, the clinical differentiation between *Neisseria meningitidis* infection and viral aseptic meningitis may be difficult.

Atypical measles is another viral exanthem that produces a petechial eruption. It begins on the arms and legs and spreads to the trunk and face. The rash differs from typical measles because it has features of raised papules, blisters, and pinpoint hemorrhages into the skin. Koplik's spots are not present, while high fever, cough, bilateral interstitial pulmonary infiltrates, and eosinophils usually are. Patients with this syndrome have a history of previous immunization with inactivated (killed) measles vaccine or of receiving live measles vaccine within 3 months after killed vaccine. The history of previous antigenic exposure to measles virus plus eosinophilia suggests a "hypersensitivity" reaction. A fourfold rise in measles complement fixation antibody titer between acute and convalescent specimens may be demonstrated.

Petechial eruptions and profuse mucosal bleeding are often major manifestations of the viral hemorrhagic fevers. This syndrome is associated with a number of the arenaviruses (Lassa, Junin), arthropod-borne viruses (dengue), and rhabdoviruses (Ebola, Marburg). A history of recent travel to endemic or epidemic areas, involvement of the liver, spleen, heart, kidneys, and lungs, and evidence of diffuse intravascular coagulation are usually present.

Noninfectious causes of petechiae An important differential point in evaluating a patient with a purpuric eruption is between palpable and nonpalpable purpura. Nonpalpable purpura suggests hemorrhage from thrombocytopenia or coagulopathy, but palpable purpura suggests vasculitis. Diseases associated with fever and nonpalpable purpura include immune thrombocytopenic purpura and thrombotic thrombocytopenic purpura. Palpable purpura is usually an indication for skin biopsy for histology and immunofluorescence to confirm and characterize the vasculitis. It is often difficult to distinguish the various types of vasculitis from just the physical examination. Small vessel vasculitis, such as Henoch-Schönlein purpura, serum sickness, and cryoglobulinemia, usually produces symmetric round and oval lesions, located in dependent areas. Larger vessel vasculitis, such as polyarteritis nodosa and Wegener's granulomatosis, produces asymmetric, irregularly shaped lesions which may ulcerate.

Allergic vasculitis (Henoch-Schönlein purpura) is found most frequently in children less than 16 years of age. The presence of symmetric purpuric papules, commonly on the lower extremities, accompanied by abdominal pain, gastrointestinal bleeding, renal involvement (edema, hypoproteinemia, hematuria), and arthralgias characterizes this entity. Cholesterol embolization can mimic polyarteritis nodosa and occurs most commonly as a complication of angiography. Biopsy shows intravascular clefts from cholesterol crystals.

LABORATORY DIAGNOSIS The laboratory studies most useful in determining the etiology of an exanthem in an acutely febrile patient are directed at demonstrating the microorganism at the cutaneous site. Gram's stain and culture of the lesions, dark-field microscopy of spirochetal lesions, and the use of immunofluorescent microscopy of skin scrapings or skin biopsy specimens for the detection of microbial antigens should be employed. Because exanthems are generally manifestations of a systemic illness, blood cultures should be taken prior to antimicrobial therapy. Isolation of the agent from other sites may also be useful, e.g., demonstration of gonococci in throat or urethral smears. Histologic identification of organisms from skin biopsies of lesions may be of great help, especially with slowly growing agents such as fungi or mycobacteria.

Because local viral invasion is characteristic of vesicular exanthems, isolation of the agent from these lesions provides the diagnosis. The development of rapid viral diagnostic testing has been especially useful in the differential diagnosis of vesicular lesions. Biopsies or scrapings of exfoliated cells from vesicular lesions of herpes group viruses (varicella-zoster, herpes simplex virus) contain multinucleated giant cells and/or intranuclear inclusions. However, because the Tzanck smear is only 40 to 70 percent as sensitive as viral isolation, the absence of giant cells does not rule out herpes infection. Herpes simplex and zoster can be differentiated by viral isolation as well as by antigen detection techniques such as fluorescent microscopy or enzyme-linked immunoabsorbent assays (ELISA). Immunofluorescence may also be useful in confirming the diagnosis of immunologically related diseases such as pemphigus vulgaris and vasculitis.

Electron microscopy may be useful for distinguishing the distinct morphology of poxviruses, vaccinia, variola, and molluscum from herpes viruses. In addition, molluscum bodies can be demonstrated by light microscopy with use of a 10% KOH preparation.

In viral exanthems, demonstration of local viral replication in throat secretions or rectal swabs provides presumptive evidence of the etiology of the exanthem; an example is the demonstration of coxsackievirus A16 in throat secretions of patients with hand-foot-and-mouth syndrome. In Behçet's syndrome or in collagen vascular disease, the absence of viruses in an early vesicular or active ulcerative lesion is useful in relating these mucosal lesions to the underlying multisystem illness.

Serologic determinations of acute phase serums are helpful in the diagnosis of syphilis, leptospirosis, streptococcal disease, Epstein-Barr virus infection, hepatitis B, toxoplasmosis, typhoid fever, and occasionally rickettsial disease. Evidence of autoantibody fixation may be useful in diagnosing some collagen vascular diseases. Demonstration of a fourfold or greater rise in antibody titer between acute and convalescent serums will confirm the diagnosis in rubella, rubeola, cytomegalovirus, or rickettsial or chlamydial infection.

MUCOCUTANEOUS LYMPH NODE SYNDROME (KAWASAKI'S DISEASE)
Mucocutaneous lymph node syndrome is a multisystem disease of children.

This entity was first described in Japan in the 1960s, but is now frequently recognized in the United States. It affects children from 2 months to 9 years of age, with 50 percent of cases occurring in children under 2 years of age. Occasional cases in young adults have been documented. Characteristically, the patient presents with a fever between 38.3 and 40°C of 1 to 2 weeks' duration which is unresponsive to antimicrobials. Bilateral conjunctivitis; dryness, redness, and fissuring of the lips; diffuse erythema of the oral and pharyngeal mucosa; "strawberry tongue"; and cervical adenopathy may be present. On the third to fifth day of illness, a macular erythematous eruption, usually starting on the extremities, appears. Pronounced reddening of the palms and soles is present, and the child's hands and feet may swell due to an indurative edema. Characteristically during the second week of illness desquamation of the rash starts at the junction of the nails and skin of the fingers and toes. Myocardial involvement is common, with abnormal electrocardiogram findings in over 50 percent of patients. Coronary angiography may reveal aneurysms and pathologic changes in the vessels similar to infantile periarteritis nodosa in 7 to 40 percent of cases. In severe cases, myocardial infarction due to coronary thrombosis may occur. Laboratory abnormalities include an elevated sedimentation rate, normal antistreptolysin O (ASO) titers, elevated C-reactive protein, peripheral leukocytosis, thrombocytosis, high levels of circulating immune complexes, and hypergammaglobulinemia. In the United States, cases have been clustered geographically and temporally. Children of Asian ancestry appear to be at higher risk than white children. The etiology of this entity is unknown. Investigations of outbreaks have revealed no evidence of person-to-person transmission or a common source of exposure. Aspirin in doses (100 mg/kg per day) to produce serum salicylate levels of 15 to 25 mg/dL is used during the acute stage of illness. When fever is controlled, the aspirin may be lowered and given in antithrombotic dosages (10 mg/kg per day). Trials evaluating

the use of high-dose intravenous gamma globulin (400 mg/kg) are also underway.

REFERENCES

CENTERS FOR DISEASE CONTROL: Multiple outbreaks of Kawasaki syndrome—United States. Morb Mort Week Rep 34:33, 1985

COOPER PH et al: Acute febrile neutrophilic dermatosis (Sweet's syndrome) and myeloproliferative disorders. Cancer 51:1518, 1983

FURUSHO K et al: High dose intravenous gammaglobulin for Kawasaki disease. Lancet 2:1055, 1984

GILCHEST B, BARDEN HP: Photodistribution of viral exanthems. Pediatrics 54:136, 1974

HEGGIN AD: Pathogenesis of rubella exanthems. J Infect Dis 137:74, 1978

KIMURA A et al: Measles rash, light and electron microscopic study of measles skin eruptions. Arch Virol 47:295, 1975

KOREN MD et al: Probable efficacy of high dose salicylates in reducing coronary involvement in Kawasaki disease. JAMA 254:767, 1985

MELISH ME: Kawasaki syndrome: A new infectious disease? J Infect Dis 143:317, 1981

SHANDS KN: Toxic shock syndrome in menstruating women: Its association with tampon use and Staphylococcus aureus and the clinical features of 52 cases. N Engl J Med 303:1436, 1980

STEERE AC: The early clinical manifestations of Lyme disease. Ann Intern Med 99:76, 1983

TODD J et al: Toxic shock syndrome associated with phage-group-1 staphylococci. Lancet 2:1116, 1978

TONNESON MG, SOTER NA: Erythema multiforme. J Am Acad Dermatol 1:357, 1979

VANARSDEL PP: Allergy and adverse drug reactions. J Am Acad Dermatol 6:833, 1982

50 GENERALIZED PRURITUS

THOMAS B. FITZPATRICK / JEFFREY D. BERNHARD

Generalized pruritus is a frequent and important problem in differential diagnosis for the general physician. Since it may be due to factors as trivial as dryness or as serious as an underlying lymphoma or endocrine abnormality, the evaluation of the patient presenting with pruritus of undetermined origin requires as much clinical judgment as it does knowledge and expertise in examining the skin. For the most part, no particular qualities of pruritus due to an underlying systemic illness permit a specific diagnosis; for example, obstructive biliary disease versus hyperthyroidism or lymphoma. The clinician must rely on the history, physical examination, and laboratory studies to establish the diagnosis.

Itch and pain share common neuroanatomic pathways but are distinct sensory modalities. Free-nerve endings that act as receptors for itch stimuli reside in the papillary layer of the dermis near the dermoepidermal junction, but there are no specific end organs for itching. A variety of diffusable mediators are apparently involved in both peripheral and central aspects of itching. Histamine, trypsin, proteases, and bile salts all cause pruritus when introduced intracutaneously. Prostaglandin E lowers the threshold to itching evoked by both histamine and papain. Prostaglandins are increased in inflamed skin, and may thereby potentiate pruritus in inflammatory dermatoses. Central nervous system opiate peptides and receptors seem to be involved in the perception of itch. The opiate naloxone hydrochloride leads to diminution of itching in several experimental and clinical settings. This may provide a clue as to how opiates relieve pain but exacerbate pruritus.

Patients with pruritus associated with obvious skin lesions, such as vesicles and papules, usually have a primary dermatologic disease. Some of the dermatologic disorders in which pruritus is a common symptom are listed in Table 50-1. Specialized dermatologic approaches, particularly biopsy of the skin, are often required in order to establish the diagnosis.

The itching patient without an apparent skin eruption and with or without the sequelae of chronic scratching (excoriations) and rubbing (lichenification, polished nails) poses a diagnostic challenge. Initially, a search should be undertaken for the primary lesions and subtle evidence of a primarily cutaneous disorder (Table 50-1).

Thorough evaluation of the patient with generalized pruritus in an attempt to discover an underlying systemic disease should include,

TABLE 50-1 Conditions in which pruritus occurs with diagnostic skin lesions

Infestation
  Scabies
  Pediculosis
  Insect bites (especially flea and bedbug)
Inflammatory
  Dermatitis herpetiformis
  Bullous pemphigoid
  Atopic dermatitis
  Lichen planus (inconstant)
  Miliaria
  Urticaria (inconstant)
  Dermographism
  Aquagenic pruritus
  Drug hypersensitivity
  Polymorphic light eruption
Infectious
  Varicella
  Dermatophytosis
  Folliculitis
Neoplastic
  Mycosis fungoides
Miscellaneous or idiopathic
  Xerosis
  Anogenital pruritus
  Mastocytosis
  Sunburn
  Exfoliative dermatitis
  Lichen sclerosis et atrophicus

SOURCE: *Bernhard.*

in addition to the history and physical examination, the following basic laboratory screening tests: complete blood count; sedimentation rate, urinalysis; blood glucose, liver, thyroid, and renal function tests; chest x-ray; Papanicolaou smear; and stool exam for ova, parasites, and occult blood. Additional tests such as serum protein electrophoresis and radiologic surveys should be performed when indicated. A psychological assessment is helpful. Attributing generalized pruritus of uncertain etiology to a psychological disturbance is unwise until other possibilities have been adequately considered.

Psychogenic pruritus as a reaction to stress occurs but must be considered a diagnosis of exclusion, especially given that the torment of severe itching is stressful in itself. This type of pruritus often affects the skin of the scalp, and may be associated with other sensory complaints such as a bitter taste in the mouth or burning of the tongue. Some patients with psychogenic pruritus are convinced that the itching is caused by some sort of parasite in their skin that cannot be seen by themselves or the physician. Such patients may scratch their skin to the point of ulceration and then assert that the itching has disappeared, owing, they believe, to removal of a parasite or "germ."

Pruritus due to dry skin is a common occurrence in the elderly. On occasion, elderly persons who do not have obviously dry skin experience generalized pruritus that cannot be attributed to emotional stress or to an underlying systemic or cutaneous illness. Such so-called senile pruritus is usually most severe when the patients disrobe to go to bed. It usually begins in one area, particularly the back, and

spreads to involve the entire body. Neither psychogenic nor senile pruritus leads to a loss of sleep.

A subtle and important cause of pruritus without a visible rash may be a reaction to drugs, such as aspirin, opiates and their derivatives, and quinidine. Some drugs, such as chlorpromazine, may cause pruritus by inducing cholestasis.

The itching associated with pediculosis corporis may be so intense that it will interfere with sleep. Long linear excoriations along the back are characteristic. The insect can be found in the clothing, particularly along the seams. In scabies, itching is most pronounced at bedtime. The web spaces of the fingers, groin, axillae, and buttocks are most often involved.

For a list of conditions in which generalized pruritus occurs without any evidence of primary skin disease, see Table 50-2.

Generalized pruritus may frequently be the first sign of biliary cirrhosis and may occur many months before the onset of jaundice. It may be the first sign also of lymphoma, and, rarely, of carcinoma. The pruritus may be of sudden onset and may be very severe. It often begins in the palms of the hand and soles of the feet. It is often improved by oral cholestyramine (see Chap. 249).

The treatment of generalized pruritus is unsatisfactory if the primary cause cannot be corrected or eliminated. Exceptions are the excellent response of uremic pruritus to ultraviolet radiation therapy (UV-B) and the response of patients with various forms of cholestasis to oral cholestyramine or activated charcoal. Not one of the systemic medications has been shown to be effective in generalized pruritus. A topical preparation containing 0.5% menthol and 1% phenol in an emollient such as Nivea oil is somewhat helpful in relieving pruritus temporarily. Topical anesthetics containing benzocaine should be avoided because of the high risk of allergic sensitization. When the patient with pruritus also has insomnia, a hypnotic or a sedative should be prescribed. Antihistamines are of little value except in pruritus due to urticaria, but may be of some help in itching due to other causes. It is a general clinical impression that aspirin is helpful in pruritus of any origin, but this has not been proven. The development of drugs that control pruritus remains one of the great challenges of medical research. It is paradoxical that severe pain can be immediately controlled with a variety of agents but there is not yet a single agent so effective for generalized pruritus.

REFERENCES

BERNHARD JD: Clinical aspects of pruritus, in *Dermatology in General Medicine,* 3d ed, TB Fitzpatrick et al (eds). New York, McGraw-Hill, 1987

BERNSTEIN JE: Neuropeptides and the skin, in *Biochemistry and Physiology of the Skin,* LA Goldsmith (ed). New York, Oxford University, 1983, pp 1217–1233

CUNLIFFE WJ: The skin and the nervous system, in *Textbook of Dermatology,* 3d ed, A Rook et al (eds). Oxford, Blackwell, 1979

GILCHREST BA et al: Ultraviolet phototherapy of uremic pruritus. Ann Intern Med 91:17, 1979

GREAVES M: Pathophysiology of pruritus, in *Dermatology in General Medicine,* 3d ed, TB Fitzpatrick et al (eds). New York, McGraw-Hill, 1987

HERNDON, JH, JR: Itching: The pathophysiology of pruritus. Int J Dermatol 14:465, 1975

TABLE 50-2 Conditions in which generalized pruritus may occur without diagnostic skin lesions

Metabolic and endocrine conditions	Malignant neoplasms	Drug ingestion	Infestations	Renal disease	Hematologic disease	Hepatic disease	Psychogenic states	Miscellaneous conditions
Hyperthyroidism Diabetes mellitus Carcinoid syndrome	Lymphoma and leukemia Abdominal cancer CNS tumors Multiple myeloma Mycosis fungoides	Opium derivatives Subclinical drug sensitivities	Pediculosis corporis Scabies* Hookworm (ancylostomiasis) Onchocerciasis Ascariasis Trichinosis Certain zoonoses	Chronic renal failure	Polycythemia vera Paraproteinemia Iron deficiency	Cholestasis (intra- or extrahepatic) Pregnancy (intrahepatic cholestasis)	Transitory: periods of emotional stress Persistent: delusions of parasitosis Psychogenic pruritus Neurotic excoriation	Dry skin (xerosis) "Senile" pruritus† Mastocytosis Pregnancy

* *Diagnostic lesions may be present.*
† *Unexplained intense pruritus in patients over 65 years without obvious "dry skin" and with no apparent emotional stress.*
SOURCE: *Bernhard.*

51   PIGMENTATION OF THE SKIN AND DISORDERS OF MELANIN METABOLISM

THOMAS B. FITZPATRICK / DAVID B. MOSHER

THE MELANOCYTE SYSTEM

DEFINITION OF MELANIN The relative quantities of melanin, oxyhemoglobin, reduced hemoglobin, and carotene account for the wide variations of normal human skin color; melanin is, however, the principal pigment responsible for the color of human skin, hair, and eyes. Melanin is also a density filter that decreases the harmful effects of ultraviolet light on the skin and thereby provides protection against acute sunburn reaction and chronic actinic damage, including skin cancer.

Derived from the Greek word *melas,* "black," melanin is a protein-bound polymer formed by the oxidation of tyrosine by tyrosinase to dihydroxyphenylalanine (dopa) within melanocytes, which are specialized epidermal dendritic cells of neural crest origin. The structure of melanin is unknown because eumelanin is so insoluble that all attempts to degrade it into identifiable fragments have failed. However, all animal melanins are known to contain indoles and are composed basically of indole 5,6-quinone units, in contrast to plant melanins which contain catechols. Pheomelanins are yellow-brown sulfur-containing pigments that, unlike eumelanin, are readily soluble in dilute alkali. Pheomelanins are only present in hair and are the pigments in human red hair.

Skin color is derived from the presence of melanin within the keratinocytes, which are receptor cells for melanocyte-formed mel-

FIGURE 51-2 *Epidermal melanin unit. Four biologic processes in melanin pigmentation underscore the differences in melanosome formation and packaging between blacks and whites: (1) Formation of melanosomes in melanocytes; (2) melanization of melanosomes in melanocytes; (3) secretion of melanocytes by keratinocytes; and (4) transport of melanocytes by keratinocytes, either with degradation of melanosomes within lysosome-like organelles (in whites) or without apparent degradation of melanosomes (in blacks). Note the difference in size between the melanosomes in the black and white epidermal keratinocytes. In the black keratinocytes, the melanosomes are nonaggregated. In the white keratinocytes, groups of several melanosomes are aggregated within membrane-limited lysosome-like organelles, and the melanosomes often appear fragmented (G, Golgi apparatus; N, nucleus; I to IV, the four stages in the development of the melanosome). The epidermal melanin unit is shown at the top. The melanocyte supplies melanosomes to a group of keratinocytes.*

FIGURE 51-1 *Diagram showing the embryonic origin, dispersal, and developmental fate of melanocytes in humans. [By permission from JB Stanbury et al (eds), The Metabolic Basis of Inherited Disease, 5th ed, New York, McGraw-Hill, 1983.]*

anin-containing organelles called *melanosomes.* Normal skin color is genetic or "constitutive"—that of habitually unexposed skin, as on the buttocks—and "facultative"—that resulting from the sun-induced tanning reaction or from increased pigmentation by pituitary melanocyte-stimulating hormones (MSH).

BIOSYNTHESIS OF MELANIN The melanocyte system is composed of melanocytes found at the dermoepidermal interface, in the hair bulb, uveal tract, retinal pigment epithelium, inner ear, and leptomeninges (Fig. 51-1). The melanocyte system is analogous to, but not known to be related to, the chromaffin system, the cells of which

COOH

Tyrosine

(O)

Dopa

(O)

Melanin

5,6,-Dihydroxyindole

FIGURE 51-3 *Biosynthesis of melanin from tyrosine.*

are also derived from the neural crest and which possess biochemical mechanisms for the hydroxylation of tyrosine to dopa. However, in the latter system the enzyme is not tyrosinase, but tyrosine hydroxylase, and dopa is converted to adrenochrome and not to tyrosine melanin.

Melanocytes within the epidermis at the dermoepidermal interface are dendritic cells that are functionally linked to a number of keratinocytes; each melanocyte and its corresponding associated 36 keratinocytes compose an *epidermal melanin unit* (Fig. 51-2). This functional unit permits organized transfer of specialized tyrosinase-containing, melanin-producing organelles, or melanosomes, to associated keratinocytes. Melanosomes are ellipsoidal organelles which are thought to arise in the area of the endoplasmic reticulum and Golgi apparatus; they are formed as unmelanized spherical structures that darken and become more dense and oval in shape with increasing melanization.

Tyrosinase, the principal enzyme in the pathway of melanin production, is one of a large group of copper-containing aerobic oxidases that catalyze the oxidation of both monohydroxy and *o*-dihydroxy phenols to orthoquinones. In humans and other mammals, this oxidase catalyzes the hydroxylation of the melanin precursor, tyrosine, to dopa and dopa quinone (Fig. 51-3). Tyrosinase is required only for the first step in the biosynthesis of tyrosine melanin, i.e., the orthohydroxylation of tyrosine. It is noteworthy that zinc ions catalyze the conversion of dopachrome to 5,6-dihydroxyindole and that melanosomes have been shown to contain high concentrations of zinc. Recently some new factors have been shown to augment or block the synthesis of melanin *after* the action of tyrosinase.

BIOLOGY OF MELANIN PIGMENTATION Melanin pigmentation (Fig. 51-4), from the clinical point of view, results from the melanin present in the keratinocytes. Inasmuch as the ratio of keratinocytes to melanocytes in the epidermis is 36:1, it is apparent that the amount of melanin present in the keratinocytes must be the predominant factor in the determination of skin color. The relationship of skin color to the location of melanin in the epidermis was studied with the light microscope in American blacks of various hues of brown coloration. In lightly pigmented skin, there was a great variation in

both the number and location of melanin particles within the epidermis; only scanty melanin deposits were in the malpighian layer, and no deposits were in the stratum corneum. In fact, in the most lightly pigmented skin, the only melanin particles were in the keratinocytes of the basal layer. In the most heavily pigmented skin, there were melanin particles in the keratinocytes of the basal layer, throughout the malpighian cells, and in the stratum corneum. Based on studies of various skin colors in American blacks and their progeny, it has been estimated that between three to six gene pairs may account for the black-white color gradient. The genetic control of *facultative* color change is not known; it is broadly related to levels of constitutive skin color.

It is apparent from studies of normal skin and of pigmentary disorders, that the intensity of pigmentation, as viewed clinically, depends not only on the rate of melanosome production but also on the number of melanosomes that are transferred to the keratinocytes (Fig. 51-2). Another factor that determines normal and abnormal melanin pigmentation is the degree of melanization of the individual melanosomes. Until recently, three factors—melanosome formation, melanosome melanization, and melanosome secretion—were considered to be the major variables in normal and abnormal melanin pigmentation. In the past few years, however, a fourth variable has been implicated in melanin pigmentation, i.e., the phenomenon of aggregation and degradation of melanosomes that occurs during their transport in the keratinocytes.

Melanosomes are present in melanocytes mainly as nonaggregated (single), membrane-delimited, discrete organelles. In keratinocytes, however, melanosomes occur either as single, or nonaggregated, particles or as aggregates of three or more within a membrane-delimited organelle. These melanosome-containing organelles resemble the melanosome-containing organelles within macrophages that have been identified as lysosomes. In the epidermal keratinocyte, melanosomes appear to undergo a gradual degradation. In heavily pigmented skin, however, intact melanosomes are present in the stratum corneum, indicating that some melanosomes are apparently not degraded with the lysosomes in the epidermis. The regulation of

FIGURE 51-4 *Melanogenesis in human skin, as seen in the light and the electron microscopes and at the molecular level.*

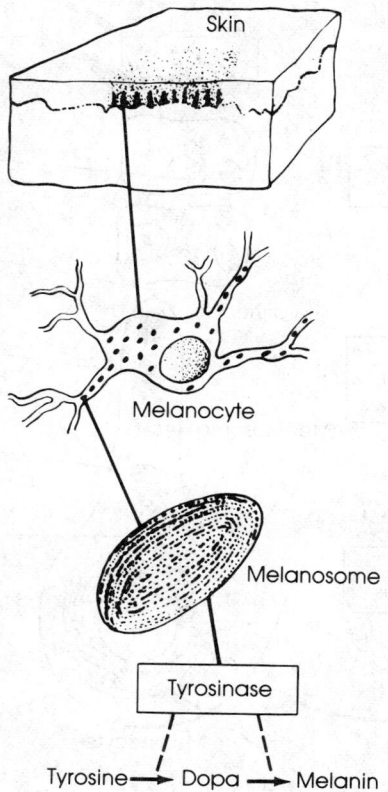

Skin

Melanocyte

Melanosome

Tyrosinase

Tyrosine → Dopa → Melanin

melanogenesis and melanin pigmentation is controlled by three major determinants: genes, hormones, and ultraviolet radiation. These three factors may act independently or in combination. In addition, specific chalones and glycopeptides may markedly affect melanogenesis and melanin pigmentation by exerting negative feedback control and regulating the mitotic activity of melanocytes and keratinocytes. The rate of transfer of melanosomes to keratinocytes may, in fact, regulate the amount of melanosome synthesis. Chalones may also regulate adenylate cyclase activity as well as melanocyte and keratinocyte division. Hormones (MSH) appear to act by a direct effect on adenylate cyclase, which results in increased cyclic AMP leading to increased tyrosinase and melanosome synthesis.

Melanin pigmentation of the skin is related to 10 biologic processes as shown in Fig. 51-5. Aggregation and dispersion of melanosomes probably play little part in the pigmentary anomalies of humans. Such movement has thus far been observed only in specialized effector cells, *melanophores*, present only in vertebrates below mammals in the phylogenetic scale; this movement of melanosomes is under neural and hormonal control in these animals.

In humans, melanocytes by means of their production and transfer of melanin, provide defense against the biologic damage caused by visible and ultraviolet radiation (UVR). Melanin in the uveal tract and in the retinal pigment epithelium protects the eye from visible and longer wavelength (UV-A) radiant energy while UV-B is largely filtered by the cornea. Melanized human epidermis shields the epidermis and dermis by effectively reducing the transmission of UV-B and UV-A radiant energy.

In humans, furthermore, this defense against UVR is highly developed in that exposure of skin to this portion of the electromagnetic spectrum causes the activation of an integrated mechanism (tanning) for the formation of dense organelles containing chromoprotein (melanosomes) and the delivery of these to epidermal cells. Within the epidermal cells, melanosomes scatter and adsorb ultraviolet radiation and remove the damaging free radicals that are generated in the skin after exposure to UVR.

In a heavily pigmented skin, the epidermal cells and the stratum corneum are filled with myriads of melanosomes. Melanosomes contain about 30 percent melanin and, because of their density and universal absorption of UVR, can protect against solar damage. The perinuclear localization of melanosomes in epidermal cells may serve to protect the vulnerable DNA-containing nuclei by reducing the direct impact of the photons.

The role of melanin in protecting against the damaging effects of UVR is quite generally accepted. Negroes and dark-skinned Caucasians are far less susceptible to acute and chronic actinic damage than fair-skinned Caucasians. Sun-induced skin cancer on the exposed areas of the face and upper extremities is very rare in black people living in geographic regions with high UV-B flux; on the other hand, black albinos living in these areas are very susceptible to skin cancer and develop solar keratoses and skin cancer in childhood. Finally, since many of these deleterious biologic processes are involved in skin aging, melanin provides protection against environmentally induced premature aging.

DISORDERS OF THE MELANOCYTE SYSTEM: HYPOMELANOSES AND HYPERMELANOSES

Disorders of melanin pigmentation have been increasingly found to be markers for diseases of other organ systems (Tables 51-1 and 51-2) and may be classified as hypomelanoses (decreased or absent epidermal melanin, leukoderma) or hypermelanoses (increased epidermal or dermal melanin). Hypomelanoses, in general, result from a defect of one or more of over 10 steps in the melanian pathway, such as absence of melanocytes, failure of formation of normal melanosomes, or failure of transfer of melanosomes to keratinocytes. The hypermelanoses are further classified as *epidermal* pigment disorders which present as brown, or as *dermal* pigment disorders which are blue, blue-gray, or gray. Brown hypermelanoses (melanoderma) arise from increased melanin in the epidermis, resulting from increased melanocyte activity, increased numbers of secretory melanocytes, increased numbers of melanosomes, or increased size of melanosomes. The blue-gray hypermelanoses (ceruloderma) represent a virtual "melanin tattoo"—the presence of melanin in the dermis

FIGURE 51-5 *Morphologic and metabolic pathway of epidermal melanin pigmentation.*

TABLE 51-1 Pigmentary Changes as Diagnostic Signs in General Medicine

Chief complaint or presenting problem	Pigmentary change	Diseases	Systemic changes
ADDISONIAN BROWN HYPERPIGMENTATION			
"Getting dark"	Generalized diffuse brown hypermelanosis	Addison's disease	Adrenal insufficiency
		Hemochromatosis	Cirrhosis of liver, diabetes
		ACTH-producing tumors	Pituitary tumor, primary; metastatic cancer
		Systemic scleroderma (early)	Dysphagia; pulmonary insufficiency
		Porphyria cutanea tarda	Liver: increased iron stores
			Diabetes mellitus (25%)
CIRCUMSCRIBED BROWN MACULES			
"Abdominal pain, brown spots on lips, fingers"	Circumscribed, mostly small dark-brown macules (many)	Peutz-Jegher syndrome	Polyposis of small intestine
"Brown spots all over"	Circumscribed small dark-brown macules	"LEOPARD" syndrome	Abnormal ECG Pulmonary stenosis
"Birth mark"; hypertension; precocious puberty	Circumscribed, uniformly brown macules, small or large (café au lait) (few or many)	Von Recklinghausen's neurofibromatosis	Neurofibromatosis of skin and peripheral nervous system; pheochromocytoma; Eye: pigmented hamartoma (Lisch nodules)
		Albright's syndrome	Polyostotic fibrous dysplasia Precocious puberty
		Watson's syndrome	Pulmonary stenosis
"Many dark moles"	Circumscribed dark-brown macules or slightly raised papules with irregular borders and variegation of color (few or many)	Dysplastic nevus syndrome	
CIRCUMSCRIBED WHITE MACULES			
"White spots"	Circumscribed, mostly large white macules (few or many)	Vitiligo Hypothyroidism Thyrotoxicosis Pernicious anemia Adrenal insufficiency Diabetes mellitus	
		Sarcoidosis	Pulmonary findings Uveitis
		Leprosy	Skin (anesthetic white macules) Peripheral neuropathies Hepatosplenomegaly
"Convulsions"; mental retardation	Congenital circumscribed small (1–3 cm) white macules (more than 3)	Tuberous sclerosis	Mental retardation, abnormal EEG Abnormal CT scan Rhabdomyoma of heart
"Eye trouble"; deafness	Circumscribed white macules, poliosis	Vogt-Koyanagi-Harada disease	Uveitis, dysacousia
"Deafness"	White forelock, congenital circumscribed large white macules	Waardenburg's syndrome	Nerve deafness, heterochromia
UNIVERSAL HYPOMELANOSIS			
"Sun sensitivity"; decreased vision	Universal hypomelanosis of skin, hair, and uveal tract	Oculocutaneous albinism, recessive	Decreased visual acuity, iris translucency, nystagmus
"Sun sensitivity"; "Poor tanner"	Type I or type II skin	Oculocutaneous albinoidism, dominant	Iris translucency, normal vision, nystagmus (rare)

in ectopic dermal melanocytes or in dermal macrophages which, because of the Tyndall effect, imparts a characteristic gray, slate, or blue color to the skin. Blue or slate-gray coloration of the skin may also arise from nonmelanin sources—ochronosis, tattoos, pharmacologic agents (chlorpromazine, amiodarone, minocycline), and deposition of other foreign materials in the dermis.

Clinical recognition of circumscribed hypomelanosis ("white spots") and of gray or slate or blue hypermelanosis is usually not difficult. When the degree of hypomelanosis is very slight, when the patient's normal skin color is very light, or when the patient's skin is untanned, the hypomelanotic lesions may be inapparent, and the diagnosis may be facilitated by the use of black light (Wood's lamp; see Chap. 47), which will heighten the contrast between abnormal epidermal pigmentation and normal skin but will not increase the contrast between increased dermal pigmentation and normal skin. Differentiation between abnormal diffuse brown hyperpigmentation (e.g., Addison's disease) normal pigmentation or between diffuse hypomelanosis (e.g., albinism) and normal pigmentation frequently

poses a problem because there is such a wide range of skin coloration in normal individuals. Diffuse color changes may be insidious; often patients themselves have been unaware of an unusual or unexplained progressive or gradual deepening of their skin color, such as a summer tan that did not fade. The degree of hypermelanosis that develops is related to the basic skin color of the patient involved. With the onset of Addison's disease, a patient of Mediterranean descent (such as Italian, French, or Spanish) may become intensely pigmented, whereas a light-skinned individual may have only a minimal degree of hypermelanosis. The appearance of pigmentation in mucous membranes and in certain specific areas, such as the axillae and the palmar creases, is usually easier to identify as abnormal than generalized brown hyperpigmentation.

GENETIC MELANIN DISORDERS Patients with pigmentary changes may present with complaints such as "I'm getting dark," "I have many dark moles," "white spots," or "birth spots" (see Table 51-1). Others present with disorders such as deafness, iritis, and seizures,

TABLE 51-2 Disturbances of human melanin pigmentation

Hypomelanosis[a] (Leukoderma) White	Hypermelanosis[a] (Melanoderma) Brown, gray, slate, or blue[b]	Hypomelanosis[a] (Leukoderma) White	Hypermelanosis[a] (Melanoderma) Brown, gray, slate, or blue[b]
GENETIC FACTORS		CHEMICAL AND PHARMACOLOGIC AGENTS	
Piebaldism[c]	Café au lait and freckle-like macules in neurofibromatosis[c]	Hydroquinone, monobenzylether[c]	Arsenical intoxication[f]
Waardenburg's syndrome[b]	Melanotic macules in polyostotic fibrous dysplasia (Albright's syndrome)[c]	Hydroquinone[c,e]	Busulfan administration[f]
Vitiligo[c,d]		Miscellaneous catechol and phenol compounds[f]	Photochemical agents (topical or systemic drugs)[c]
Hypomelanotic macules in tuberous sclerosis[c,e]	Ephelides (freckles)[c]	Chloroquine and hydroxychloroquine[h]	5-Fluorouracil, systemic[f]
Albinism, oculocutaneous:[f,g]	Lentigines[c]	Arsenical ingestion[c]	Cyclophosphamide[f]
Tyrosinase-negative	Lentigines with cardiac arrhythmias[c]	Corticosteroids, topical and intradermal[c,e]	Nitrogen mustard, topical[c]
Tyrosinase-positive	Becker's nevus[c]		Bleomycin[c]
Yellow mutant	Neurocutaneous melanosis[c]		Fixed (drug) eruption[b,c]
Brown Rufous	Xeroderma pigmentosum[c]		Adriamycin
Hermansky-Pudlak syndrome	Acanthosis nigricans[.]		BCNU
Chédiak-Higashi syndrome	Fanconi's syndrome[c]		
Cross-McKusick-Green syndrome	Dermal melanocytosis (Mongolian spot)[b,c]	PHYSICAL AGENTS	
Albinism, ocular[c,g,h]	Incontinentia pigmenti[b,c]	Burns: Thermal, ultraviolet, ionizing radiation[c,d]	Ultraviolet light (suntanning)[c]
Albinoidism, oculocutaneous[f,g,h]		Trauma[c,d]	Thermal radiation[c]
Pigmentary dilution with immunodeficiency			Alpha, beta, and gamma ionizing radiation[c]
Phenylketonuria[f,g,h]			Trauma (e.g., chronic pruritus)[c]
Fanconi's syndrome[h]			
Homocystinuria[f,h]		INFLAMMATION AND INFECTION	
Histidinemia[f]		Sarcoidosis[c,e]	Postinflammation melanoses (exanthems, drug eruptions)[c]
Menkes' kinky hair syndrome[h]		Pinta[c]	Lichen planus[c]
Canities, premature[h]		Yaws[c]	Lupus erythematosus, discoid[c]
		Leprosy[c,e]	Lichen simplex chronicus[c]
METABOLIC FACTORS		Tinea versicolor[c,e]	Atopic dermatitis[i]
	Hemochromatosis[f]	Post–kala azar[c]	Psoriasis[c]
	Hepatolenticular disease (Wilson's disease)[f]	Eczematous dermatitis[c,e]	Tinea versicolor[c]
	Porphyria (congenital erythropoietic, variegata and cutanea tarda)[f]	Psoriasis[c]	Pinta in exposed areas[b,c]
		Discoid lupus erythematosus[c]	
	Gaucher's disease[i]	Vagabond's leukoderma[c]	
	Niemann-Pick disease[i]	Miscellaneous postinflammatory hypomelanoses[c,e]	
	Biliary cirrhosis[i]		
	Chronic renal failure	NEOPLASMS	
		Leukoderma acquisitum centrifugum (including halo nevus)[c]	Malignant melanoma[c,m]
ENDOCRINE FACTORS		Vitiligo-like hypomelanosis[c,e] associated with melanoma	Mastocytosis (urticaria pigmentosa)[c]
Hypopituitarism[f]	ACTH-producing and MSH-producing pituitary and other tumors[f]		Acanthosis nigricans, with adenocarcinoma and lymphoma[c]
Addison's disease[c]			Slate-gray dermal pigmentation with metastatic melanoma and melanogenuria[f]
Hyperthyroidism[c]	ACTH therapy[f]		
	Pregnancy[i]		
	Addison's disease[f]	MISCELLANEOUS FACTORS	
	Melasma[c,j]	Vogt-Koyanagi-Harada syndrome[c]	Scleroderma, systemic[f]
		Scleroderma, circumscribed or systemic[c]	Chronic hepatic insufficiency[f]
NUTRITIONAL FACTORS		Canities[h]	Whipple's syndrome[f]
Chronic protein deficiency or loss:[h,k]	Pellagra[i]	Alopecia areata[n]	Lentigo, senile ("liver spots")[c]
Kwashiorkor	Sprue[i]	Horner's syndrome, congenital and acquired[g]	Cronkhite-Canada syndrome[c]
Nephrosis	Vitamin B_{12} deficiency[i]	Idiopathic, guttate hypomelanosis[c]	POEMS syndrome
Ulcerative colitis	Chronic nutritional insufficiency[c]		
Malabsorption			
Vitamin B_{12} deficiency[h]			

[a] Listing includes the pigmentation disorder itself or the condition with which it is associated.
[b] Gray, slate, or blue color results from the presence of dermal melanocytes or phagocytized melanin in the dermis.
[c] Pigment change is circumscribed.
[d] Total loss of pigment in the skin and hair may occur.
[e] Loss of pigmentation is usually partial (hypomelanosis); viewed with Wood's lamp, the lesions are not completely devoid of pigment (amelanosis), as in vitiligo.
[f] Pigment change is diffuse, not circumscribed, and there are no identifiable borders.
[g] Pigment is decreased in the iris.
[h] Pigment is decreased in the hair.
[i] Pigment change may be diffuse or circumscribed.
[j] Idiopathic or due to progestational agents.
[k] Hair is gray or reddish.
[l] There is a loss of melanocytes.
[m] Areas of brown may be admixed with the slate-gray and blue discoloration.
[n] Regrown hair is white.
SOURCE: Modified from: DB Mosher et al, in Dermatology in General Medicine, 2d ed, TB Fitzpatrick et al (eds), New York, McGraw-Hill, 1979.

and the pigmentary change is incidental. The following presentation is, however, arranged by etiology rather than by symptoms.

Oculocutaneous albinism is an autosomal recessive trait characterized by congenital, decreased, uniform hypomelanosis of skin and hair; albinism involving the skin alone has not been reported, but ocular albinism with minimal or no cutaneous involvement has been observed. The classic constellation of findings in oculocutaneous albinism includes marked hypomelanosis or amelanosis of skin, white or faintly blondish hair, photophobia, nystagmus, hypopigmented fundus oculi, and translucent irides. Oculocutaneous albinism may be classified according to the presence or absence of tyrosinase in plucked hair follicles of the scalp (the hair bulb incubation test). In normal individuals hair bulbs darken when incubated with tyrosine; in some persons with oculocutaneous albinism the hair follicles darken when incubated in tyrosine, i.e., *tyrosinase-positive,* while in others no such darkening occurs, i.e., *tyrosinase-negative.* These two types of albinism are known to have separate gene loci. In oculocutaneous albinism melanocytes are present, but formation of melanosomes is interrupted in the early stages so that few mature melanosomes are present in albino skin or hair. Whatever tyrosinase is present must be functionally defective and unable to convert enzymatically tyrosine to dopa. Other variants of oculocutaneous albinism include yellow mutant, Hermansky-Pudlak syndrome (hemorrhagic diathesis secondary to storage pool platelet defect), and Chédiak-Higashi syndrome (recurrent infections, hematologic and neurologic abnormalities, and early death from lymphoma). The deficiency of melanin in oculocutaneous albinism has two disturbing consequences for humans: decreased visual acuity and an abnormal degree of intolerance to sunlight. The sensitivity of human albinos to ultraviolet light often leads to the development of carcinoma in exposed areas of the skin. Nearly all albinos in the tropics have actinic keratoses or skin cancers by the third decade. Daily use of effective topical sunscreens and avoidance of unnecessary sun exposure are indicated for all albinos (see Chap. 52).

A syndrome of congenital diffuse pigmentary dilution with immunodeficiency has been described. It is associated with hepatosplenomegaly, neutropenia, thrombocytopenia, and defective helper-T-cell function.

Phenylketonuria is an autosomal recessive disorder of phenylalanine metabolism in which there is a single metabolic block in the conversion of phenylalanine to tyrosine. There is pigmentary dilution of the skin, hair, and irides. The lightening of hair, which is characteristically light blond to dark brown, may be appraised only by comparison with uninvolved siblings. The melanocytes are normal but lack a full complement of melanosomes. Decreased melanin formation results from the fact that excess phenylalanine and its metabolites, present in serum and extracellular fluid, act as competitive inhibitors of tyrosinase and block melanin synthesis.

Vitiligo is an idiopathic, acquired, circumscribed hypomelanosis which is familial in about 30 percent of cases and is characterized by progressively enlarging amelanotic macules (Table 51-3). Vitiligo may be localized, segmental (one or more dermatomes), or generalized. On occasion, vitiligo may become so extensive that all or nearly all the skin becomes white. Characteristic distribution patterns of vitiligo involve extensor surfaces and bony prominences (elbows, knees), the small joints in the hands, and the area around the eyes and mouth. The low back, axillae, and flexor wrists may also be involved. Genitalia, palms and soles, and mucous membranes are often affected. Typically, the vitiligo macules gradually enlarge centrifugally, and new macules appear. In up to 30 percent of cases some minimal and inconsequential spontaneous repigmentation occurs, particularly in sun-exposed areas of skin. White hairs are common in macules of vitiligo, but may also be normally pigmented. Most vitiligo patients are generally healthy, although thyroid disease, diabetes mellitus, Addison's disease, and pernicious anemia occur with increased frequency. Thyroid disease—hyperthyroidism, thyroiditis, hypothyroidism, and nontoxic goiter—may, in fact, be a common coexisting disorder with vitiligo in patients over the age of 50, especially hypothyroidism. Syndromes with multiple endocrinopathies and with hyperthyroidism, hypoparathyroidism, Addison's disease, chronic mucocutaneous candidiasis, and alopecia areata have been described. Iritis may occur in over 10 percent of patients. The pathogenesis of vitiligo is unresolved, but classic hypotheses include destruction of melanocytes by toxic melanin precursors or lymphocytes. Antibodies to normal melanocytes have also been reported.

Electron microscope studies show a total absence of melanocytes in the white vitiligo macules and decreased numbers of melanocytes in "trichrome" areas (macules or margins of vitiligo patches in which a color intermediate between the normal skin color and the vitiligo white is present). Abnormal keratinocytes (with vacuolation) have been observed with transmission electron microscopy in clinically "normal" skin of patients with idiopathic vitiligo. Vitiligo is thus

both a marker for multisystem disease and also a tragic social problem for brown and black peoples. The internist should never regard the problem as simply a cosmetic disorder; having ruled out subclinical thyroid disease, Addison's disease, pernicious anemia, and polyglandular endocrinopathy, the brown or black patient should be referred to a dermatologist capable of offering the options for control of the disease. Fair-skinned persons often can learn to "live with their disease" and will not accept treatment.

Options for treatment of vitiligo include sunscreens, cosmetic cover-up, repigmentation, or depigmentation. In over half the patients treated with PUVA photochemotherapy, psoralens, and ultraviolet A [UV-A (sunlight or an artificial UV-A light system; see Chap. 52)] significant repigmentation occurs, particularly on the face and neck, and usually on the trunk, upper arms, and legs. Up to 200 or more treatments may be required, however. In some older patients with extensive areas of depigmentation, irreversible depigmentation of the remaining pigmented skin with topical monobenzylether of hydroquinone cream (Benoquin) is a more practical and feasible approach. These persons look essentially normal but must use sun-protective lotions daily.

Piebaldism is a congenital, autosomal dominant, stable, circumscribed hypomelanosis which resembles vitiligo except that it has a characteristic distribution pattern different from vitiligo and does not usually progress or resolve over time. The hypomelanosis in piebaldism occurs in circumscribed areas on the extremities and anterior surface of the thorax. A white forelock is typical. The eyes are normal, and the patients are otherwise healthy.

Tuberous sclerosis is an autosomal dominant disease which manifests itself by the presence of congenital, circumscribed, white macules in up to 98 percent of cases, and classically by the development (by the fourth year) of seizures, mental retardation, and adenoma sebaceum. The white macules are characteristically located on the trunk or buttocks, are hypomelanotic, number from 3 to 100,

TABLE 51-3   Disorders associated with circumscribed vitiligo-type hypomelanosis

Associated disorder
GENETIC
Vitiligo, with or without: Hyper/hypothyroidism Diabetes mellitus Addison's disease Pernicious anemia Hypoparathyroidism Addison's disease Chronic mucocutaneous candidiasis syndrome Piebaldism Waardenburg's syndrome Tuberous sclerosis Ataxia-telangiectasia
CHEMICAL EXPOSURE
Phenolic germicides (O-Syl, Phebocide, etc.) Hydroquinone, monobenzylether of Hydroquinone, monomethylether of
NEOPLASTIC
Malignant melanoma (in sites of regression) Melanocytic nevi (halo nevi)
INFECTIOUS
Leprosy Pinta Tinea versicolor
IDIOPATHIC
Vogt-Koyanagi-Harada syndrome Postinflammation: atopic dermatitis, psoriasis Sarcoidosis Scleroderma

and are of typical shape—oval, lance-ovate, or polygonal, like a "thumbprint." The most characteristic, though not the most frequent, is the lance-ovate or American mountain "ash-leaf" macule, which is usually less than 3 cm in its longest dimension and off-white, not pure white, in color. The macules are oriented transversely on the trunk and axially on the extremities. The size and color of these lesions do not change over time. Histologically, these macules contain melanocytes which have decreased numbers of small melanosomes. The presence of three or more circumscribed macules in a patient is strongly suggestive of tuberous sclerosis. Examination with Wood's lamp is often necessary to visualize the lesions.

All persons with unexplained seizures or mental retardation should be screened with a Wood's lamp examination for the presence of white spots to exclude tuberous sclerosis. In addition, examination of parents and siblings with CT scans or magnetic resonance imaging (MRI) is necessary to detect the location, size, and shape of calcifications and intraventricular nodules. MRI may facilitate diagnosis of solid tumors.

Neurofibromatosis (von Recklinghausen's disease) is an autosomal dominant trait characterized by the appearance, usually by the age of 3 and primarily on the trunk and the extremities, of numerous pale yellow-brown macules, or café au lait spots, that vary in diameter from less than 1 cm to more than 15 cm. Spotty generalized pigmentation and axillary freckling may also be present. Often, a few or many soft, rounded, cone-shaped, or pendulous cutaneous tumors covered by normal skin appear by the first or second decade.

The presence in an adult of six or more café au lait spots—which are uniformly hypermelanotic, circumscribed, oval macules with a diameter greater than 1.5 cm (over five greater than 0.5 cm in a child)—is characteristic of neurofibromatosis even in the absence of a positive family history. Lisch nodules (pigmented hamartomas of the iris detected by slit lamp examination) in patients above 6 years are diagnostic of von Recklinghausen's neurofibromatosis; they are not present in Albright's syndrome or in bilateral acoustic neurofibromatosis. In *Albright's syndrome* (polyostotic fibrous dysplasia), however, there are rarely more than three or four such macules, which are usually unilaterally distributed on the buttocks or cervical areas. A single, large, isolated café au lait spot of neurofibromatosis is indistinguishable from the macule of Albright's syndrome. It is possible, however, using light microscopy, to detect melanin macroglobulins in whole amounts of epidermis prepared from café au lait macules of neurofibromatosis; these melanin macroglobulins are usually not found in the pigmented macules present in Albright's disease or in the café au lait macules observed in 10 percent of the normal population.

Moynahan's syndrome, or "LEOPARD" syndrome, is an autosomal dominant trait in which generalized lentigines (multiple, diffuse, small, dark-brown, circumscribed hypermelanotic macules) have been associated with ECG abnormalities and, in its fully expressed form, with other findings (lentigines, ECG abnormalities, ocular hypertelorism, pulmonary stenosis, abnormal genitalia, retardation of growth, and deafness).

Peutz-Jeghers syndrome is an autosomal dominant disorder in which hyperpigmented, brown to blue macules on the lips and buccal mucosa are associated with similar cutaneous lesions and gastrointestinal polyps. The cutaneous macules, but not the buccal pigmented lesions may fade, by adulthood. This disease is discussed in Chap. 239.

METABOLIC FACTORS   Generalized brown hypermelanosis of the skin is a characteristic manifestation of *hemochromatosis, porphyria cutanea tarda,* and *variegate porphyria.* The hyperpigmentation observed in hemochromatosis may be grayish brown or brown and indistinguishable from that of Addison's disease. The diagnosis of hemochromatosis may be established from a skin biopsy which shows hemosiderin deposition in the sweat glands. Melanin deposition is also apparent. Porphyria cutanea tarda may be diagnosed by the clinical presence of vesicles, bullae, atrophic macules, sclerodermoid changes, and milia on the skin of the dorsal hands and face, and in

the laboratory by red fluorescence of acidified urine, or the presence of increased urinary uroporphyrin (uroporphyrin to coproporphyrin ratio usually is greater than 3:1). Similar changes may be seen in patients with *variegate porphyria,* which has a distinctive porphyrin profile, especially a high fecal protoporphyrin. The lesions in variegate porphyria are identical to porphyria cutanea tarda and the diseases must be differentiated as they have different responses to treatment and very different associated medical problems (see Chaps. 52 and 312). Primary biliary cirrhosis may be associated with hyperpigmentation in normally sun-exposed areas. Chronic renal failure may also be associated with diffuse hyperpigmentation.

NUTRITIONAL FACTORS   In *chronic nutritional deficiency,* in general, macules of dirty-brown hyperpigmentation appear, especially on the trunk. In selective deficiencies, such as protein deficiency in *kwashiorkor,* or when there is protein loss as in *chronic nephrosis, ulcerative colitis,* and *malabsorption syndrome,* there is sometimes dilution of hair color so that the hair becomes a reddish-brown and eventually gray. In other selective deficiencies, such as sprue, there may be a brown hypermelanosis over any area of the body. In *pellagra,* however, the pigmentation is limited to areas of skin exposed to light or to trauma. In *vitamin B$_{12}$ deficiency,* there is premature graying of hair and a hypermelanosis most apparent overlying the small joints of the hands.

ENDOCRINE FACTORS   Diffuse brown hypermelanosis is a striking feature of primary adrenocortical insufficiency (Addison's disease). There is a marked hyperpigmentation over certain areas, namely, the pressure points (vertebrae, knuckles, elbows, and knees), and in body folds, palmar creases, and gingival mucous membrane. An identifiable type of diffuse hyperpigmentation has also been reported to follow adrenalectomy in patients with Cushing disease. In these patients, there usually are signs and symptoms of pituitary tumors; all tumors recorded have been chromophobe adenomas. A third example of the Addisonian type of melanosis has also been observed in patients with pancreatic and lung tumors. The generalized brown hypermelanosis found in all these conditions results from overproduction of melanocyte-stimulating hormone (MSH) and adrenocorticotropic hormone (ACTH), which share common amino acid sequences. It appears that an excess of α-MSH plays a dominant role in the abnormal pigmentation that occurs in Addison's disease. Both MSH and ACTH are increased in adrenal insufficiency as a result of decreased output of cortisol by the adrenals. Hypermelanosis of the Addisonian type can be produced in adrenalectomized human subjects by the administration of large amounts of homogeneous ACTH and α-MSH. α-MSH is a single-polypeptide chain of 13 amino acid residues and is identical in sequence to the terminal portion of ACTH except for the acetylation of the terminal serine residue. Recent evidence has shown that the polypeptide hormones themselves are produced by cleavage of the larger polypeptides. In mammals, MSH causes a significant darkening of skin as early as 24 h after administration. Mammalian melanocytes have been shown to be uniquely sensitive to α-MSH. Melanocytes appear to possess a unique membrane-bound receptor molecule that is present in the G$_2$ phase of the cell cycle. Following interaction of this receptor with α-MSH, an enzyme also found within the membrane, adenylate cyclase, is stimulated, leading to an increase in the formation and level of intracellular cyclic AMP. Eight hours following treatment with MSH, tyrosinase activity begins to increase. This effect is followed at 16 h by an increase in melanin formation. Current information suggests that cyclic AMP is the mediator of the MSH effect; this evidence includes the fact that cyclic AMP levels rise soon after exposure to MSH.

Melasma, or the "mask of pregnancy," is found in pregnant women, women on oral contraceptives, and in some otherwise normal women and men. This is a circumscribed brown hypermelanosis of the epidermis, (with a dermal or blue-gray component in some), usually of the forehead, cheeks, upper lip, and chin. MSH levels are normal in these patients. Melasma-like hyperpigmentation has also been observed in patients taking phenytoin or mesantoin. Treatment with topical depigmenting agents in conjunction with opaque covering is effective in about 50 percent of the patients.

CHEMICAL FACTORS Exposure to or use of various chemicals, particularly para-substituted phenol derivatives may cause depigmentation. Topical use of hydroquinone induces a temporary lightening which may be useful in some patients with melasma; monobenzylether of hydroquinone, however, causes a permanent vitiligo-like leukoderma, even remote from the site of application, and is used only to depigment completely the uninvolved pigmented normal skin in patients with extensive vitiligo. Addisonian-like hypermelanosis of the skin follows busulfan therapy, and hypermelanosis may also be seen after use of cyclophosphamide and nitrogen mustard. Inorganic trivalent arsenicals may also produce generalized Addisonian-like hypermelanosis as well as scattered macular hypomelanosis and punctate keratosis of the palms and soles. Blue-gray nonmelanin pigmentation has been observed due to prolonged high doses of chlorpromazine, minocycline, and amiodarone.

PHYSICAL FACTORS Mechanical trauma, as well as burns caused by heat, ultraviolet light, or alpha, beta, and gamma radiation, can lead to hypomelanosis or hypermelanosis. The effects of these physical agents on pigmentation are determined by the intensity and duration of exposure and are limited to the site of injury. Hypomelanosis results from destruction of melanocytes.

INFLAMMATORY AND INFECTIOUS FACTORS Many epidermal proliferative processes resolve and leave aberrations of pigmentation at the sites of involvement; both postinflammatory hypermelanosis (blue-gray, brown, or both) and hypomelanosis may occur following resolution of lupus erythematosus, eczema, psoriasis, lichen planus, drug reactions, pemphigus, viral exanthems, etc. Usually the epidermal hypermelanoses disappear spontaneously within several months, but dermal hypermelanoses are much slower to resolve. White halos surrounding psoriatic plaques are a result of abnormal prostaglandin synthesis and are not an abnormality of melanin biology.

Tinea versicolor, a hypomelanotic, not amelanotic, scaling, circumscribed eruption of the upper anterior and posterior chest in young people, results from the presence in the skin of *Pityrosporum orbiculare* which contains an enzyme that forms azelaic acid, a melanocyte toxin, and results in decreased melanin pigmentation. Sun exposure will result in repigmentation only after appropriate topical antifungal therapy.

Tuberculoid and *lepromatous leprosy* have hypomelanotic macules and papules that are anesthetic. The color, unlike vitiligo, is not pure white, rather, off-white, and the margins of these macules are characteristically indiscrete.

NEOPLASTIC FACTORS Disorders of melanin pigmentation are uncommon features of skin neoplasms. Hypomelanosis has been found around benign nevi (halo nevi) in healthy patients but may also be found in or around malignant melanoma (the primary or metastatic lesion); vitiligo-like hypomelanotic macules remote from the melanoma may also occur. *Leukoderma acquisitum centrifugum* (LAC) refers to the presence of a macule of hypomelanosis surrounding a central pigmented lesion. LAC is most common around nevocellular nevi. Such halo nevi occur in healthy individuals but may also be found in or around melanoma (primary or metastases). The halo is usually eccentrically placed around malignant lesions but concentric around benign ones. *Mycosis fungoides,* which is a cutaneous T-cell lymphoma, may present with vitiligo-like macules. Plaque and systemic lymphoma stages invariably follow after several to many years.

A Vogt-Koyanagi-Harada syndrome has been reported following bacillus Calmette-Guérin (BCG) therapy of melanoma. During terminal stages of malignant melanoma, striking development of blue hypermelanosis may be observed, associated with large amounts of a conjugated derivative of 5,6-dihydroxyindole excreted in the urine (melanogenuria). This intermediate in the metabolic pathway from tyrosine to melanin (Fig. 51-3) can be oxidized to melanin in the absence of tyrosinase; therefore, melanin can be synthesized at almost any site in which oxidation can take place. Diffuse black pigmentation is seen in the peritoneum, liver, heart, muscle, and dermis of patients during the late stages of malignant melanoma. The brown melanin in the dermal phagocytes appears clinically as blue in the skin because of the Tyndall light-scattering phenomenon.

Acanthosis nigricans is characterized by velvety textured hypermelanotic (brown) macules which may be found in the axillae and other areas in patients with various carcinomas, particularly adenocarcinomas of the gastrointestinal tract. Acanthosis nigricans may also be congenital or benign and associated with diabetes mellitus, Cushing's disease, Addison's disease, pituitary adenoma, and other disorders.

Urticaria pigmentosa is characterized by multiple, irregular, round or oval, yellowish brown to reddish brown macules and papules related to the presence of melanin in the epidermis overlying clusters of mast cells. Vigorous rubbing of such lesions results in the development of urticarial wheals (Darier's sign). In children, the skin lesions usually appear in infancy and often spontaneously disappear in several years. The usual course is quite benign, but symptoms of flushing, itching, and urticaria occur in about 30 percent of patients; less than 15 percent experience vomiting, syncope, or shock. The symptoms are presumed to be due to histamine release from mast cells and often coincide with increased urinary excretion of free histamines and metabolites. Urinary levels of 5-hydroxyindoleacetic acid are normal. Antihistamines are of little value. Systemic mastocytosis, in which mast cells infiltrate diffusely into the liver, spleen, gastrointestinal system, and bones, is a rare condition. Mast cell leukemia occasionally develops.

UNKNOWN CAUSES Generalized brown hypermelanosis of the type seen in Addison's disease may be associated with *systemic scleroderma* early in the course of the disorder. Generalized hyperpigmentation occasionally develops in patients with *chronic hepatic insufficiency,* especially that due to portal cirrhosis. The pathogenesis of the pigmentation in both conditions is unknown; MSH levels are not elevated. *Cronkhite-Canada syndrome* is the association of acquired lentigo-like brown macules with gastrointestinal polyposis from the stomach to the rectum. Diarrhea, weight loss, and abdominal pain usually precede the pigmentary changes by several months. Hypopigmented macules with perifollicular hyperpigmented macules are seen in *scleroderma;* such depigmented macules are devoid of melanocytes. Hypomelanotic macules may also be found in a small percentage of patients with *sarcoidosis.* These macules are characteristically not pure white and are circumscribed with indiscrete margins. They may overlie dermal nodules, particularly on the extremities but also at times on the trunk.

REFERENCES

FITZPATRICK TB et al: *Biology and Diseases of Dermal Pigmentation.* Tokyo, University of Tokyo, 1981

KORNER AM, PAWLEK J: Dopachrome conversion, a possible control point in melanin biosynthesis. J Invest Derm 75:192, 1980

MOSHER DB et al: Abnormalities of pigmentation, in *Dermatology in General Medicine,* 3d ed, TB Fitzpatrick et al (eds). New York, McGraw-Hill, 1987

―――― et al: Vitiligo: Etiology, pathogenesis, diagnosis and treatment, in *Update: Dermatology in General Medicine,* TB Fitzpatrick (ed). New York, McGraw Hill, 1983

ORTONNE JP et al: *Vitiligo and Other Hypomelanoses of Hair and Skin.* New York, Plenum, 1983

QUEVEDO WC et al: Biology of melanocytes, in *Dermatology in General Medicine,* 3d ed, TB Fitzpatrick et al (eds). New York, McGraw-Hill, 1987

WICK MJ et al: Biochemistry of melanization, in *Dermatology in General Medicine,* 3d ed, TB Fitzpatrick et al (eds). New York, McGraw-Hill, 1987

WITKOP CV et al: Albinism, in *The Metabolic Basis of Inherited Diseases,* 5th ed, JB Stanbury et al (eds). New York, McGraw-Hill, 1983

52 PHOTOSENSITIVITY AND OTHER REACTIONS TO LIGHT

MADHUKAR A. PATHAK / THOMAS B. FITZPATRICK / JOHN A. PARRISH

Humans have evolved in sunlight and depend upon it for much more than an indirect source of food and maintenance of the earth's temperature. Natural light has always been recognized for, and endowed with, health-giving powers. Our skin, eyes, blood vessels, and certain endocrine gland functions respond to radiation from the electromagnetic spectrum of the sun. The formation of vitamin D from sterol precursors in the skin by solar ultraviolet radiation (UVR) exposure has long been recognized in the management of rickets. Certain of our daily biorhythms are dependent upon the cycles of sunlight. Yet, sunlight can be harmful and damage or kill living cells. Sunlight causes sunburn, damage to deoxyribonucleic acid (DNA), skin cancer, wrinkling and aging changes in the skin, eye inflammation, and possibly cataracts. During the past decade, interest in the reaction of human skin to light has been renewed as a result of

1 The public's obsession with sunbathing, resulting in premature "aging" of the skin (solar elastosis).
2 Demographic data indicating that exposure to sunlight is an important cause of basal cell and squamous cell carcinoma and even melanoma of the sun-exposed parts of the body.
3 The widespread use of certain drugs such as phenothiazines, thiazides and related sulfonamide diuretics, and antibiotics (demethylchlortetracycline), which alter the cutaneous responses to sunlight and cause undesirable photosensitivity reactions.
4 Increased awareness that sunlight is a major cause of discomfort and photosensitivity reactions in patients with certain types of porphyria, especially for those with erythropoietic protoporphyria.
5 The emergence of a new science of photomedicine and photochemotherapy based on the recent advances in molecular photobiology and the availability of high-intensity ultraviolet irradiation

TABLE 52-1   Diseases induced or exacerbated by light

I By light alone
  A Genetic: ephelides (freckles)
  B Idiopathic
    1 Acute solar skin damage (sunburn)
    2 Connective tissue degeneration (wrinkling)
    3 Telangiectasia
    4 Solar keratoses and solar lentigo
    5 Basal cell carcinoma
    6 Squamous cell carcinoma
    7 Malignant melanoma
    8 Polymorphous photodermatosis
    9 Solar urticaria
    10 Actinic reticuloid
II By light plus exogenous agents
  A Chemical or drug
    1 Phototoxic reactions
    2 Phytophotodermatitis
    3 Lupus erythematosus (with hydralazine, procainamide)
  B Chemical and immunologic: photoallergic reactions
III By light plus metabolite(s)
  A Porphyrias
  B Porphyria cutanea tarda associated with hexachlorobenzene, estrogens, alcohol
IV By light plus preexisting disease
  A Genetic
    1 Xeroderma pigmentosum
    2 Oculocutaneous albinism
    3 Vitiligo
    4 Hartnup's syndrome
  B Nutritional or metabolic
    1 Pellagra
    2 Malignant carcinoid
  C Viral: herpes simplex
  D Unknown: lupus erythematosus (cutaneous, systemic)

systems; this has enabled both researchers and practicing physicians to use UVR and visible radiation with or without the systemic administration of the drug to achieve a striking, therapeutic response in diseases such as psoriasis, polymorphic photodermatitis, mycosis fungoides, lichen planus, vitiligo, uremic pruritus, etc. Visible radiation also has been successfully used in newborn infants in the treatment of neonatal jaundice to prevent bilirubin encephalopathy. Light emitted by certain types of lasers is being increasingly used in the treatment of port-wine stains, telangiectasia, and other vascular lesions.

6 The increased recognition that the exposure of UVR can alter the function and viability of cellular components of the immune system; normal and abnormal immune responses can be altered and can result in local alterations of immune function at the site of exposure or some specific systemic alterations at distant nonexposed sites.

There are more than 25 human disorders that are either caused by or aggravated by exposure of the skin to sunlight. These range from degenerative and neoplastic changes to disability and discomfort associated with chemically induced photosensitivity reactions. These abnormal reactions to light in humans are briefly presented in Table 52-1.

This chapter will be concerned with (1) common conditions such as sunburn, the degenerative and neoplastic conditions associated with solar radiation (basal cell carcinoma, squamous cell carcinoma, malignant melanoma, solar keratoses), and chronic sun-induced degeneration; (2) photosensitivity related to drugs and to increased production of photosensitizing porphyrins in patients with all types of porphyrias (except acute intermittent porphyria); (3) certain idiopathic forms of commonly occurring photodermatoses; (4) photochemotherapy; and (5) photoprotection.

The unit of wavelength most commonly used to measure and express nonionizing UVR or visible light is the nanometer (1 nm = 10^{-9} m = 10 Å).

Electromagnetic emanations from the sun comprise a wide range of radiation and include electric waves, radio waves, infrared rays, visible light, UVR, roentgen rays (x-rays), gamma rays, and cosmic rays. The shortest wavelengths that reach the surface of the earth through the atmosphere are about 286 to 290 nm. Wavelengths shorter than 286 nm are principally absorbed by ozone in the stratosphere. In terrestrial sunlight, the UVR region extends from 290 to 400 nm, the visible spectrum from 400 to 760 nm, and the near-infrared and infrared spectrum from wavelengths longer than 760 nm.

The solar spectrum that can affect human skin includes wavelengths of 290 to 760 nm; however, infrared radiation (1.5 to 1000 μm) can produce thermal effects (including burn) and potentiate the photochemical and biologic reactions initiated by UVR or visible radiation. For practical reasons, UVR is often arbitrarily subdivided into three bands designated as (1) UV-A (320 to 400 nm, or long-wave ultraviolet), (2) UV-B (290 to 320 nm, or sunburn spectrum), and (3) UV-C (shorter than 290 nm, or germicidal radiation).

The amount and type of solar radiation, especially UVR, that may reach a given part of the earth at any given time are determined by a great variety of factors, including latitude, time of day, season, altitude, local atmospheric conditions (smog, cloudiness, haze, smoke, dust, fog, humidity, aerosol particles), variations in the thickness of the ozone layer, and height of the sun above the horizon.

Approximately 50 percent of the sun's radiant energy is in the visible portion of the spectrum (400 to 760 nm), about 44 percent in the infrared region, and about 6 percent in the UV region. The damage to skin (sunburn, skin cancer) is evoked by 3 percent of the ultraviolet radiation wavelengths, namely, from 290 to 360 nm.

The transmission of radiant energy varies with wavelength and different areas of the human skin; it may range from 0 to 70 percent. Shorter wavelengths (<285 nm) are mostly absorbed by the dead-cell layer of the stratum corneum; wavelengths that produce sunburn (290 to 315 nm) are also mostly absorbed in the epidermis. About 5 to 15 percent of the impinging UV-B radiation penetrates to the papillary dermis, and the depth of UV-B penetration depends upon the degree of melanin pigmentation of the skin. Longer wavelengths (320 to 760 nm) penetrate more deeply into the dermis. Transmission of different wavelengths depends upon (1) the regional thickness of the epidermis, (2) the degree of hydration, (3) the concentration of UV and visible light-absorbing components such as melanin, proteins (keratin, elastin, collagen), nucleic acid, urocanic acid, carotenoids, and hemoglobin, and (4) the number and spatial arrangement of melanosomes and of blood vessels. In fair-skinned individuals, about 85 to 90 percent of 290- to 315-nm radiation is absorbed by the epidermis and only about 5 to 15 percent can penetrate through the epidermis to reach the dermis. In dark-skinned individuals, nearly 90 to 95 percent of 290- to 315-nm radiation is absorbed by the epidermis. The transmission through the epidermis of long-wave UV radiation (320 to 400 nm) and visible radiation (400 to 760 nm) may range from 20 to 70 percent. The optical properties of hypopigmented epidermis of fair-skinned individuals are such that approximately 2 to 5 percent of 250-nm (germicidal) radiation, about 12 to 15 percent of 300-nm radiation, and about 50 percent of 360-nm radiation can be transmitted to the dermis. Since cutaneous blood flow is about 500 mL/min, the equivalent entire blood volume of an adult person at rest can circulate through the skin every 11 min. Thus, UVR penetrating through the epidermis and impinging on the network of capillaries and small vessels can affect lymphocytes circulating through the skin, and prolonged exposure (over 90 min) may damage a significant portion of the circulating cells. It is now known that UVR induces loss of mononuclear cell viability; they are most sensitive to UV-C (<290 nm) and less sensitive to UV-B and UV-A radiation (sensitivity ratios of 10^4:10:1). UV-induced alterations in immune function appear to be involved in the pathogenesis of experimental photocarcinogenesis in mice. The significance of the alteration of lymphocyte function following exposure to UVR is not well understood, but it is possible that such alterations may play a role in the pathogenesis of UV-induced skin cancer, lupus erythematosus, and some photosensitivity disorders. The alteration of lymphocyte function and immune responses may explain the beneficial effects of phototherapy and photochemotherapy in certain skin diseases.

The most detrimental effect of UVR is cell death. Other effects include mutagenesis, carcinogenesis, interference or inhibition in the synthesis of DNA, RNA, and protein, and also in immune functions. The mutagenic and carcinogenic effects appear to be mediated largely through the action of UV-B radiation on DNA. The most common reactions, such as sunburn, tanning or melanin pigmentation, synthesis of vitamin D, keratosis, and skin aging are also caused by UV-B radiation. Although the longer wavelengths (UV-A, or 320 to 400 nm or 400 to 760 nm) penetrate more deeply and in greater amount into the skin than UV-B, they are much less effective at causing these types of photobiologic phenomena. UV-A radiation is about 800 to 1000 times less effective than UV-B in evoking erythema and other degenerative changes. However, in the presence of certain chemical agents (e.g., drugs that are given orally or endogenous porphyrins in certain porphyrias), these wavelengths become highly damaging and can cause severe skin photosensitization at quite low doses.

Protection against this damage to the "normal" skin has been the subject of much investigation, and many commercially available sunscreens can be recommended in the prevention of sunburn, skin cancer, aging of skin, and in various types of photosensitivity disorders.

SUNBURN AND TANNING

CLINICAL CHANGES Erythema, or sunburn reaction Erythema is caused principally by 290- to 320-nm radiation, maximum solar effectiveness being 300 to 307 nm. UVR emitted by artificial light sources produces erythema maximally at 297 and 254 nm. Radiation greater than 320 nm (320 to 760 nm) is generally considered to be

nonerythemogenic, although prolonged exposure to 320- to 400-nm radiation (1.5 to 2 h of midday summer sun in northern latitudes) can produce mild sunburn in normal subjects. The minimal erythema dose (MED) is defined as the lowest UVR dose which produces perceptible redness up to 24 h following exposure to a defined spectral band (either UV-B or UV-A). In fair-skinned individuals, the MED of UV-B is approximately 20 to 50 mJ/cm² (equivalent to approximately 12 to 25 min in northern latitudes during June and July). UV-B doses larger than 3, 6, or 9 times the MED have a short latent period, and the subsequent erythema reaction is more severe; marked erythema, edema, and even bullae may occur. If the total dose is large, pain and systemic symptoms such as fever may occur. The MED of 320 to 400 nm (UV-A) is approximately 25 to 100 J/cm² or about 800 to 1000 times greater than that of UV-B.

Sunburn, suntan, and peeling are experiences familiar to almost the entire fair-skinned population. Individuals vary in their susceptibility to sunburn and suntan. Personal history of sunburning (e.g., easy, moderate, severe, or difficult), peeling, and the ability to acquire tan (minimal, moderate, profuse, etc.) is very helpful to classify people of different ethnic backgrounds into six sun-reactive types as described in Table 52-2.

The sunburn reaction is a complex inflammatory process. The observed histologic changes include the appearance of dyskeratotic cells (containing pyknotic nuclei), spongiosis, vacuolation of keratinocytes, and edema. The dermal changes include an inflammatory infiltrate (mostly lymphocytes), endothelial swelling, and capillary leakage manifested by extravasation of red blood cells. The severity of these changes and the rate at which they evolve depend on the exposure dose, the incident wavelength, and degree of skin pigmentation. Hypopigmented, fair-skinned individuals (e.g., red-haired, freckled individuals such as the Irish or Scottish) are more susceptible to sunburn than pigmented individuals who tan well. The nature of the chromophore that absorbs the light energy which initiates the primary photochemical responses is not well established, although the bulk of evidence suggests that nucleic acids (DNA) are primary targets for the absorption of the 290- to 320-nm radiation. Vasodilatation which accompanies the sunburn reaction appears to result from the activation and release of one or more chemical mediators (e.g., prostaglandins, kinins, serotonin, histamine).

There has been considerable focus on the role of prostaglandins (PG) and related derivatives of arachidonic acid as mediators of the delayed erythema reaction induced by UV-B. Prostaglandins of the PGE and PGF series are low-molecular-weight, oxygenated fatty acid structures synthesized by microsomal enzymes (PG synthase, lipoxygenase, and cyclooxygenase) present in all mammalian cells, including epidermal cells. Increased levels of prostaglandins (PGE series) have been observed in widely different types of cutaneous inflammation reaction, including the UV-induced sunburn reaction. Indomethacin, a nonsteroidal anti-inflammatory agent, when applied topically or given intradermally, can decrease a delayed sunburn response of human skin produced by UV-B radiation. Since indomethacin is known to inhibit prostaglandin synthesis, these findings support the possible role of prostaglandins as mediators of the delayed erythemal response to UV-B radiation. It is of interest to note that prostaglandin levels are increased in skin exposed to an erythemogenic dose of UV-C (germicidal) radiation. However, a PUVA (psoralen + UV-A)–induced phototoxic reaction does not seem to generate elevated levels of prostaglandins, and indomethacin, applied topically

TABLE 52-2 Classification of sun-reactive skin types*

Skin type	History of sunburning and tanning
I	Always burn, never tan, often peel
II	Always burn, tan slightly
III	Always burn, tan moderately (average whites)
IV	Sometimes burn (minimally), always tan (olive skin)
V	Rarely burn, tan easily and substantially (brown skin)
VI	Never burn, tan profusely (blacks)

* After first exposure to approximately 45 min (3 MED) of summer sun.

or given intradermally, has no effect in decreasing the intensity of the erythema reaction, suggesting that the mechanism of photosensitization reaction evoked by PUVA is not mediated by PGs. Other mediators including histamine are also believed to be involved in UV-B–induced immediate as well as delayed erythema reaction. Ultraviolet radiation may also have a direct effect on the blood vessels of the upper layer of the dermis (capillaries, venules, and arterioles). The formation of reactive oxygen species such as singlet oxygen, peroxides, superoxide anions, or free radicals appears to play an important role in the damage to cell membranes and lysosomal membranes associated with lipid oxidation. In fair skin, 290- to 320-nm spectrum is known to produce damaging free radicals (molecules with unpaired electrons).

Melanin pigmentation, or tanning   Tanning (increase in melanin pigment) that follows exposure of the skin to solar radiation involves two distinct photobiologic processes. The first, *immediate pigment darkening* (IPD), or darkening of preformed pigment in the epidermis, is elicited by wavelengths of 320 to 720 nm. The second, *melanogenesis*, or delayed tanning reaction, is an intricate process that consists of the *erythema response (sunburn)* followed usually in 3 to 4 days by formation of new pigment. Immediate pigment darkening reaction is oxygen-dependent and results from oxidation of melanin through the production of semiquinone-like free radicals in the melanin polymer; transfer of melanosomes from melanocytes and redistribution of already existing melanosomes within the keratinocytes also may occur.

Melanogenesis involves (1) an increase in the number of functional melanocytes, resulting from increased proliferation of melanocytes, and activation of dormant melanocytes; (2) increased arborization of melanocytic dendrites; (3) an increase in the number of melanosomes in proliferating melanocytes; (4) an increase in tyrosinase activity; and (5) an increase in the transfer of melanosomes from melanocytes to keratinocytes. The degree of melanin pigmentation, however, that can be achieved in an individual by exposure to solar radiation is genetically predetermined. People with fair skin who burn easily but do not tan or tan poorly (skin types I and II) cannot with repeated sun exposures achieve that degree of tanning which can be easily achieved by someone genetically able to tan profusely with minimal exposure. Delayed tanning reaction appears to have a protective effect on the skin against subsequent exposures.

CELLULAR AND MOLECULAR CHANGES Hyperplasia   Within 72 h after exposure, there is an increase in the number of epidermal cells with a high rate of mitotic activity. The rate of cell proliferation decreases after 7 to 10 days, and the thickness of the epidermis gradually returns to normal within the next 30 to 60 days. In UV-induced hyperplasia the activities of polyamine biosynthetic enzymes, ornithine-decarboxylase (ODC) and S-adenosyl-methionine decarboxylase are increased in UV-B irradiated skin, resulting in the elevation of putrescine and spermidine. PUVA and UV-C also induce increased epidermal ODC activity, reflecting the potential role of polyamines in cell growth and hyperplasia.

DNA and RNA changes   Damage to DNA by sunburn-producing UV light (290 to 320 nm) may result in mutation or cell death. The principal epidermal DNA photoproducts are pyrimidine dimers (e.g., thymine dimers); these are of the cyclobutane type and are formed between adjacent pyrimidine bases. Cell membranes, DNA, RNA, protein, and other molecules may be altered, and the synthesis of DNA, RNA, and protein may be temporarily inhibited immediately after irradiation. New synthesis is evident by 24 h and is maximal by 60 to 70 h.

Mitosis   Inhibition of epidermal mitosis and retardation of basal cell turnover occur within 1 h after irradiation. The epidermal cell cycle is interrupted at the S phase of DNA synthesis. Inhibition of mitosis can persist for 7 to 24 h; it is followed by an acceleration of mitotic rate and basal cell turnover that reaches a peak by 48 to 72 h and is associated with epidermal hyperplasia. The mitotic cycle appears to be interrupted in the G_2 stage, in the prophase stage, or in both. The increased mitotic activity and the associated hyperplasia may last for 30 to 60 days. This hyperplasia appears to be due to a combination of the removal of the epidermal mitotic inhibitors (chalones) and stimulation of growth by the action of cyclic adenosine monophosphate (AMP) and guanosine 5′-monophosphate (GMP).

Formation of vitamin D   The skin has long been recognized as the site for sun-induced photosynthesis of vitamin D. The action spectrum (290–320 nm) and the photochemical mechanisms involved in the synthesis of vitamin D_3 have been recently elucidated and are described in Chap. 274.

SUN-INDUCED SKIN CANCER

The malignancies and premalignancies unequivocally associated with sun exposure (primarily UV-B radiation) include solar or actinic keratoses, basal cell epitheliomas, squamous cell carcinomas, and keratoacanthomas. Some studies have established that carcinoma of the skin occurs more frequently on the parts of the body habitually exposed to sunlight; thus, the lesions of the head and hands are concentrated on the nose, central portions of the cheeks, eyelids, and dorsum of the hands. In fair-skinned whites who sunburn easily, these cancers are limited almost exclusively to the exposed portions of the face, head, neck, arms, and hands. Black skin, on the other hand, is remarkably resistant to the development of skin cancer on the exposed surfaces, and a similar resistance is seen among the pigmented whites (e.g., East Indians), American Indians, and Asiatics.

Carcinoma of the exposed skin is more prevalent among persons who are outdoors a great deal and is the common cause of cancer in whites in Australia, South Africa, and the southern parts of the United States. The action spectrum for photocarcinogenesis is similar to that of sunburn reaction.

Several studies based on the distribution of local populations in the United States, Australia, and Ireland have emphasized that skin cancer develops earlier and more frequently in people who have light skin and freckles, who burn easily and do not tan on exposure to the sun, and who are of mostly Celtic ancestry (people with skin types I and II). *Australia, with the highest reported incidence of skin cancer in the world*, has a population largely descended from British stock, with about 25 percent claiming Celtic (i.e., Irish, Scottish, and Welsh) extraction. In all three countries surveyed, persons of Celtic ancestry were found to have a disproportionately high incidence of skin cancer. Dark-pigmented races and people who tan well (skin types IV to VI) are least susceptible to skin cancer. Chronically exposed areas of many fair-skinned individuals may develop small hyperkeratotic lesions commonly referred to as *solar keratoses*. These may progress to squamous cell or basal cell carcinomas and may be seen as early as the third decade. Susceptible individuals may exhibit more than one lesion. These can be readily recognized by the use of topical 5-fluorouracil.

All varieties of skin cancer develop in patients with *xeroderma pigmentosum*, an autosomal recessive disorder. This rare defect represents, in the extreme, the basic problem of solar radiation and skin cancer. Patients with this disease have a greatly increased susceptibility to malignant tumors of the skin in the light-exposed areas. The characteristic skin manifestations are atrophy, telangiectasia, hyperpigmented macules, keratoses, and ulcerations, all occurring in sun-exposed areas. Within the first few years of life, basal cell or squamous cell carcinomas or sarcomas or malignant melanomas develop. An inherited enzyme defect may be responsible, at least in part, for the cancer-forming potential in patients with xeroderma pigmentosum. Cultured fibroblasts from patients with xeroderma pigmentosum are incapable of releasing thymine dimers from DNA and, in consequence, are deficient in their ability to repair their UV-damaged DNA. Xeroderma pigmentosum is the most notable human disease in which there is a defect in the excision repair process involving the removal of UV-induced dimers followed by the synthesis and re-forming of new segments of DNA. This enzymatic deficiency may result in a high somatic mutation rate of skin cells after sun exposure and, eventually, in cancer formation. The fact that mutagenesis is largely the result of errors made during the repair of photodamaged DNA and that UVR is known to be mutagenic suggests that the first step toward UV-induced carcinogenesis may be the result of an error made during the repair and replication of the damaged DNA (see Chap. 51 for discussion of sun and melanoma).

SUN-INDUCED DEGENERATIVE CHANGES OF THE SKIN (DERMATOHELIOSIS)

Degenerative skin changes (wrinkling, telangiectasia, keratoses) are more frequent in white-skinned people living in areas where the intensity of UVR is great (e.g., southwestern United States, Australia, South Africa). The term *solar degeneration* or *dermatoheliosis* implies a group of changes in the exposed areas of the skin, including wrinkling, atrophy, hypermelanotic and hypomelanotic macules, telangiectasia, yellow papules and plaques, and keratoses. The furrowed and leathery condition of the skin is seen particularly in persons who have fair skin and poor tanning ability and are constantly exposed to the sun. The most conspicuous and characteristic change may result from biochemical and structural alterations of connective tissue (elastin as well as collagen). The degenerative changes are primarily caused by sunburn-producing (290- to 320-nm) wavelengths and to a limited extent by UV-A (320- to 400-nm) radiation that can penetrate deeply into the dermis. Heat (infrared radiation) may accelerate actinic degeneration.

Chronically light-damaged human epidermis shows shortening or flattening of the rete ridges, thinning of the epidermis (decrease in malpighian cells), and many abnormal cells in disorderly arrangement. There is a progressive degeneration in the papillary and subpapillary zones of the dermis. Other changes include (1) the development of vascular ectasia, (2) accumulation of acid mucopolysaccharides, (3) appearance of abnormal fibrocytes, (4) loss of collagen, (5) degeneration of elastic tissue ("actinic elastosis") and disorganization of the connective tissue into amorphous masses. In actinically damaged skin the concentration of elastin may be increased and collagen decreased. These changes are mostly irreversible but can be minimized by daily topical application of effective sunscreens.

PHOTOTOXICITY AND PHOTOALLERGY

Sensitivity to sunlight is a common clinical problem. Continuous daily exposure to sun alone may be the major factor responsible for irreversible skin changes (e.g., freckles, telangiectasia, wrinkling, keratoses, atrophy, hypermelanotic and hypomelanotic macules, and carcinomas in the sun-exposed regions). Apart from these chronic changes, human skin can also become hypersensitive to UVR and visible light. The interface between humans and their environment is the skin, and the physical (light) and chemical agents acting directly on it are important etiologic or precipitating factors in photosensitivity disorders.

EFFECT OF DRUGS AND OTHER CHEMICALS IN ASSOCIATION WITH LIGHT EXPOSURE   Some chemicals and drugs by themselves may not act as contact irritants and are generally innocuous to skin in the absence of light exposure. However, when the skin is challenged with proper concentrations of the agent and the appropriate light wavelengths, these agents can induce undesirable skin reactions.

Cutaneous photosensitivity is a general term used to refer to the abnormal reaction of the human skin to the stimulus of light. Chemical or drug photosensitivity reactions may be defined clinically as adverse skin responses resulting from the combination of exposure to certain therapeutic or chemical agents and UVR. In most of the drug or chemical photosensitivity reactions, the wavelengths that evoke abnormal reactions are usually but not always in the 320- to 400-nm

region. Adverse cutaneous reactions can occur in some individuals who either have ingested certain drugs or have been in contact with certain chemicals (Tables 52-3 and 52-4). These reactions may include an acute, abnormal sunburn response, namely, edema, papules, macules, vesicles, bullae, or acute eczematous or urticarial reactions. There may be desquamation and hyperpigmentation or hypopigmentation. These adverse photosensitivity reactions are classified into two broad categories: (1) phototoxic reactions and (2) photoallergic reactions.

Phototoxic reactions are those reactions exaggerated by UVR in which there is no evidence of participation of the immune system; these reactions usually can be elicited in almost everyone with enough light energy of the appropriate wavelengths and when appropriate concentrations of the agent are either applied topically or given orally. Light plus the offending agent leads to an exaggerated sunburn reaction, with or without painful edema. The reaction can occur within 5 to 18 h after exposure to the sun and is usually maximum at 36 to 72 h. Hyperpigmentation and desquamation can also occur. The reaction is usually confined to the site of exposure. If the applied concentration of the implicated agent is high, bullae or small vesicles may develop. The most common chemicals that induce phototoxicity reactions in humans are (1) anthraquinone dyes; (2) chlorothiazides; (3) chlorpromazines and phenothiazines; (4) coal tars containing anthracene, acridine, phenanthrene, etc.; (5) nalidixic acid; (6) protriptyline; (7) psoralens (8-methoxypsoralen and 4,5',8-trimethylpsoralen); (8) sulfonamides; and (9) tetracycline (demethylchlortetracycline, etc.) (see Table 52-4).

Certain *phototoxic reactions* require the presence of molecular oxygen (e.g., hematoporphyrin, several dyes). The oxygen-dependent reactions are referred to as *photodynamic reactions*. On the other hand, many phototoxic reactions can occur in the absence of oxygen (e.g., psoralen photosensitization). Most reactions have been reported to require UV-A (320- to 400-nm) radiation; however, certain phototoxic reactions can be initiated by the UV-B (290- to 320-nm) as well as by the visible (400- to 700-nm) spectra. The phototoxic reactions in general should be regarded as the undesirable sequelae of augmentation of the primary photochemical reactions that underlie the inflammatory response of skin evoked by UVR. It is believed that a deleterious amount of radiant energy is absorbed by the skin and the photosensitizing agents. This absorbed energy can directly cause cell damage by creating a covalent linking of the sensitizing molecule to the pyrimidines (e.g., thymine) in the cellular DNA. This linkage (the formation of cyclobutane photoadducts of the sensitizer and the pyrimidines) can be lethal to the cell. Photosensitizers like the psoralens selectively intercalate between two base pairs and produce single-strand photoadducts with pyrimidine bases in DNA or interstrand cross-links with epidermal DNA. In addition, the photosensitizing molecule can transfer the absorbed energy and promote formation of free radicals (molecules with unpaired electrons that are highly reactive) and cause damage to the cell membranes and lysosomes. In the presence of certain porphyrins (e.g., hematoporphyrin, protoporphyrin), a reactive singlet form of oxygen can be generated by these photosensitizing molecules. Drug-induced phototoxic reactions may thus involve damage to the DNA, RNA, lysosomes, cell membranes, and other organelles. Certain drugs (chlorpromazine, benoxaprofen) may operate by both photodynamic and photoallergic mechanisms.

Photoallergy to drugs is an acquired and altered capacity of the skin to respond to light in the presence of a photosensitizer, and involves the immune system. Rather than an exaggerated sunburn, the clinical reaction may consist of an eczematous eruption or discrete eruption or discrete papules and plaques. The absorbed light energy may promote a photochemical reaction between the drug and the skin proteins. The drug may act to form a haptenic group and either combines directly with the protein to form a photoantigen or is altered by the absorbed energy; this altered haptenic group then reacts with the proteins to form an antigen. The photoantigen is then processed by macrophages and is believed to come in contact with T cells to

TABLE 52-3 Contact photosensitizers: Chemicals that induce photosensitivity reactions in humans

Name	Use	Reported clinical observations
Halogenated salicylanilides; 3,3′,4′,5-tetrachlorosalicylanilide; 3,4′,5- and 3,3′,5-trichlorosalicylanilide; 3,4′,5- and 3,3′,5-tribromosalicylanilide; 3,5- and 4,5′-dibromosalicylanilide	Deodorant, bacteriostatic agents in soaps	Phototoxic and eczematous photoallergic reactions, burning, itching, cross-photosensitivity reactions
Hexachlorophene	Antimicrobial, antiseptic	Phototoxic reactions
Bithionol or bis(2-hydroxy-3,5-dichlorophenyl) sulfide	Antimicrobial, antiseptic	Photoallergic reactions
Fentichlor (2,2′-dihydroxy-5,5′-dichlorodiphenyl sulfide); multifungin (bromochlorosalicylanilide); Jadit (4-chloro-2-hydroxybenzoic acid N-n-butylamide)	Antifungal	Phototoxic and photoallergic reactions
5-Flurouracil	Antineoplastic	Acceleration of inflammatory process
p-Aminobenzoic acid (PABA) and esters of PABA	Sunscreen	Photoallergic reactions
4,4′-Bis(3-phenylureido)-2,2′-stilbenedisulfonic acid or blankophor	Fluorescent brightening agent for cellulose, nylon, or wool fibers	Phototoxic and photoallergic reactions
Cadmium sulfide	In tattoos	Erythema
Furocoumarins: psoralen, 8-methoxypsoralen, 5-methoxypsoralen, 4,5′,8-trimethylpsoralen	In vitiligo for increased pigment formation and sun tolerance	Marked erythema, vesicles, bullae, hyperpigmentation
Essential oils: oil of bergamot, oil of lime, oil of cedar, oil of lavender, oil of citron, oil of sandalwood	Cosmetics and beauty aids	Phototoxic reactions and postinflammatory hyperpigmentation
Plants: Umbelliferae, Rutaceae	Used in perfumes or flavorings or as spices	Phytophotodermatitis, hyperpigmentation, vesicles, bullae
6-Methylcoumarin	Used in cosmetics	Photoallergic reactions
Musk ambrette	Used in cosmetics	Photoallergic reactions
Dyes: acriflavine, fluorescein, rose bengal, eosin, erythrocine, trypaflavin, orange red, paraphenylenediamine, methylene blue, toluidine blue, trypan blue, anthraquinone	Cosmetics and dye industry	Erythema, edema, vesicles, pigmentation, phototoxic reaction
Coal tar and coal tar derivatives containing anthracene, phenanthrene, naphthalene, thiophene, and many phenolic agents; pitch, acridine	In therapy for psoriasis and chronic eczema; in hair shampoos	Smarting, exaggerated sunburn, urticarial wheals, tar melanosis

SOURCE: *TB Fitzpatrick et al, in Sunlight and Man: Normal and Abnormal Photobiologic Responses, MA Pathak et al (eds), Tokyo, University of Tokyo Press, 1974.*

manifest any ordinary type of delayed hypersensitivity immunologic response. The complete photoantigen is recognized on subsequent exposure to sensitized T cells in the form of a papulovesicular or an eczematous response.

The clinical manifestations in drug-induced photoallergic reactions may range from acute urticarial lesions, developing within a few minutes after exposure, to eczematous or papular lesions appearing within 24 h or later. The eruption may extend beyond the exposed areas. In recurrent cases, flare-ups of distant, previously uninvolved sites may also occur. Some edema and vasodilatation are common in most of these eruptions. The action spectrum is generally in the long-wave range (320 to 400 nm), and less energy is required than is necessary for the production of phototoxic reactions. In general, photoallergy is much less common than phototoxic reaction, and the light-microscopic examination of a lesional biopsy reveals a characteristic, though not diagnostic, dense perivascular round cell infiltrate.

The various systemic therapeutic agents and their effects on the skin in the presence of light (whether phototoxic or photoallergic reactions) are listed in Table 52-4. The biologic action spectra that induce either the phototoxic or photoallergic reactions are also given.

EFFECT OF PLANTS PLUS LIGHT *Phytophotodermatitis* (phototoxic reactions) can develop as the result of contact with many plants (belonging principally to the families Rutaceae and Umbelliferae, e.g., certain limes, parsley, celery, bishop's weed, figs) and subsequent exposure of the skin to sunlight. The photodermatitis involves a mild-to-severe erythematous reaction with or without vesicles or bullae. Dense postinflammatory hyperpigmentation is visible within 3 to 5 days. Perfumes and colognes containing oil of bergamot are also known to induce hyperpigmentation with or without erythema. The pigmentation in berloque dermatitis occurs in configurations that seem bizarre but actually represent the areas to which the scent was applied; sometimes the hyperpigmentation may be droplike or pendant-like, and has therefore been named accordingly (*berloque* or *berlock,*

meaning trinket or pendant). This phytophotodermatitis, as well as that which follows contact with various other plants, is thought to be caused by furocoumarins (e.g., 5-methoxypsoralen, 8-methoxypsoralen, and other psoralens) characteristically present in these plants. The combination of exposure to long-wave UVR (320 to 400 nm) and furocoumarins greatly enhances the erythema and the pigmentation response.

Treatment Therapy of acute phototoxic reactions induced by topical or systemic agents is best achieved by removal of the offending agent and avoidance of exposure to the sun, or both. If necessary, the usual dermatologic procedures for minimizing the discomforts of the inflammatory response should be undertaken. However, in instances in which continued systemic use of the drug is vital, cutaneous photoreactions may be prevented by instructing the patient to remain indoors or by avoiding exposure to sunlight between 10 A.M. and 4 P.M. Generally the problem subsides within a week after discontinuation of the stress (sun and the drug). Sunscreens listed in Table 52-5 also should be prescribed.

EFFECT OF LIGHT PLUS ENDOGENOUS PHOTOSENSITIZERS
This category includes several photosensitivity reactions in patients with various types of porphyria (see Chap. 312). The photosensitivity reactions are related to the overproduction in vivo of either proto-, uro-, or coproporphyrins and their precursors. In the porphyrias, endogenously synthesized porphyrin molecules, when exposed to light, cause burning, itching, urticaria, edema, crusting and scarring, vesiculation, atrophy, and many other disabling cutaneous changes. The light-absorbing molecules involved in evoking the cutaneous reactions are a complex of oxidized porphyrins present in abnormal amounts in red blood cells, plasma, skin, liver, stool, and urine. The photodermatitis is optimally produced by a narrow band of light in the region of 400 to 410 nm, which corresponds to one of the absorption peaks of porphyrins. Patients, however, are sensitive to

wavelengths from 380 to 600 nm. The most disabling types of photosensitivity reactions are encountered in erythropoietic (congenital) porphyria (Gunther's disease) and in erythropoietic protoporphyria (Chap. 312). Symptoms and signs of sensitivity to sunlight occur in early childhood.

The adverse cutaneous responses to sunlight in patients with erythropoietic protoporphyria (EPP) have been found to be ameliorated by oral ingestion of β-carotene (Chap. 312). Patients who take β-carotene are able to withstand prolonged exposures to sunlight and experience relief from their usual photosensitivity reactions. A recommended treatment is the daily oral ingestion of β-carotene (Solatene) sufficient to maintain blood levels of 600 to 800 µg/dL (usually adults receive a dose of 120 to 180 mg per day; children under 12 years receive 30 to 90 mg per day). Photoprotective effect of β-carotene is observed after 4 to 6 weeks, and the therapy is generally continued throughout the year. In vitro, β-carotene has been found to be an effective quencher for the ''singlet'' oxygen-generated photoactivated porphyrins. During porphyrin-mediated photosensitivity reactions, peroxide radicals (HO_2^0) are also generated which damage the lipid membranes. It is presumed that β-carotene is preferentially oxidized and that by quenching the ''singlet'' oxygen, it inhibits lipid peroxide formation.

POLYMORPHOUS LIGHT ERUPTIONS

Polymorphous light eruption (PMLE) is an idiopathic, acquired syndrome characterized by a delayed abnormal response to light and varied morphology. The clinical patterns are pleomorphic or polymorphic in nature. The most common pattern consists of multiple small papules, or papules and vesicles that may become confluent and present at times an eczematous clinical picture. Lichenification due to scratching of the pruritic lesions is not common but certainly occurs. Less frequently, the primary lesion is a large papule that may present an erythema multiforme–like pattern or become confluent to form plaques. This variety is usually, but not exclusively, confined to the face and neck. The only consistent histologic feature in all cases is a dense perivascular infiltrate in the upper and middle dermis. The infiltrate is predominantly lymphocytic and the infiltrating mononuclear cells are mostly T cells. Typically the lesions appear in early spring and after each exposure. The latent period between exposure and the appearance of rash may range from a few hours to 2 days, with the most common interval being 24 to 36 h. Itching is frequent and may occur during sun exposure and even preceding the eruption. Irritating papules may coalesce into plaques, and frequently excoriate and subside within 2 to 5 days if sun exposure is avoided. In the majority of patients, the PMLE condition is seasonal, occurring in the early spring and summer months. Patients tend to improve as the summer progresses. The familial or hereditary form of polymorphous light eruptions has been reported in North American and Latin American Indians.

The sunburn-producing spectrum (UV-B, or 290 to 320 nm) is the most effective waveband for eliciting abnormal PMLE responses. However, in many instances, the action spectrum may extend into the UV-A (320- to 400-nm) region; in some instances it may extend into the visible region. Even alpha particles, x-rays, and germicidal

TABLE 52-4 Systemic photosensitizers: Chemicals that induce photosensitivity reactions in humans

Name	Uses	Clinical observations	Action spectrum, nm
SULFONAMIDES			
Sulfanilamide, sulfathiazole, sulfapyridine, sulfamethazine, sulfaguanidine, sulfisoxazole, monochlorphenamide	Chemotherapy, antibacterial agents	Phototoxic and photoallergic reactions	290–320
SULFONYLUREA			
Carbutamide, tolbutamide (Orinase), chlorpropamide (Diabinese)	Hypoglycemic or antidiabetic drugs	Phototoxic reactions	290–360
CHLORTHIAZIDES			
6-Chloro-7-sulfamyl-3,4-dihydro-1,2,4-thiodiazine 1,1-dioxide (HydroDiuril)	Diuretics, antihypertensive	Papular and edematous eruption, plaques	290–320
Quinethazone (Diuril)	Antihypertensive	Phototoxic and photoallergic reactions	320–400
PHENOTHIAZINES			
Chlorpromazine (Thorazine), promethazine (Phenergan), mepazine, Stelazine, trimeprazine, Compazine, promazine (Sparine)	Tranquilizer, nematode infestation agent, urinary antiseptic, antihistamine	Exaggerated sunburn, maculopapular and urticarial eruptions, gray-blue hyperpigmentation	290–400
ANTIBIOTICS			
Demethylchlortetracycline (Declomycin), chlortetracycline, oxytetracycline, doxycycline	Broad-spectrum antibiotic	Exaggerated sunburn, phototoxic reaction	320–400
Griseofulvin	Antimycotic	Exaggerated sunburn, phototoxic and photoallergic reactions	320–400
Nalidixic acid (NegGram)	Antibacterial	Erythema, bullae	320–400
FUROCOUMARINS: PSORALENS			
4,5′,8-Trimethylpsoralen (trioxsalen), 8-methoxypsoralen (methoxsalen), psoralen	In photochemotherapy of psoriasis and vitiligo; for sun tolerance and increased pigment formation	Erythema, bullae, hyperpigmentation	320–400
ESTROGENS AND PROGESTERONES			
Mestranol and norethynodrel, diethylstilbestrol	Oral contraceptives	Melasma, phototoxic reactions	?290–320
Chlordiazepoxide (Librium)	Tranquilizer, psychotropic	Eczematous eruption	290–360
Triacetyldiphenolisatin	Laxative	Eczematous photoallergic reaction	290–320
Cyclamates, calcium cyclamate, sodium cyclohexylsulfamate	Artificial sweeteners	Phototoxic and photoallergic reactions	290–360

SOURCE: *TB Fitzpatrick et al, in Sunlight and Man: Normal and Abnormal Photobiologic Responses, MA Pathak et al (eds), Tokyo, University of Tokyo Press, 1974.*

TABLE 52-5 Sun protection factors of some brand name sunscreens under indoor or outdoor conditions

Trade name	Ingredients	Type of sunscreen	Sun protection factor (SPF) Indoor solar simulator	Outdoor sunlight	Resistance to Sweating	Water immersion
PABA sunscreens:						
PreSun-15		Clear lotion	15–18	10–12	Excellent	Poor
Pabanol	5% PABA in 50–70% ethyl alcohol	Clear lotion	15–18	6–8	Fair	Poor
Sunbrella		Clear lotion	15	6	Fair	Poor
PreSun-15		Gel	15	10–12	Good	Fair
PABA ester sunscreens:						
Block out	3.3% isoamyl-*p*-N,N-dimethyl aminobenzoate (padimate A)	Lotion/gel	6–8	6	Good	Fair
PABAFILM	3.3% isoamyl-*p*-N,N-dimethyl aminobenzoate (padimate A)	Lotion/gel	6–8	4–6	Good	Fair
Sundown	3.3% isoamyl-*p*-N,N-dimethyl aminobenzoate (padimate A)	Lotion	8–10	4–6	Good	Fair
Original Eclipse	3.5% padimate A + 3.0% octyldimethyl PABA	Lotion	8–10	4–6	Fair	Fair
Aztec	5.0% homomenthyl salicylate + 2.5% amyl-*p*-dimethyl aminobenzoate	Lotion	6–8	4	Fair	Poor
Sea & Ski	3.3% octyldimethyl PABA	Cream	7–8	4	Fair	Poor
Marbert Sun Creme	Benzyliden-camphor + phenyl-benzimidazole-5-sulfonic acid + isopropyl dibenzoyl methane	Cream	15	13–14	Good	Poor
PABA-ester combination sunscreens:						
Coppertone Super Shade-15	7% octyldimethyl PABA + 3% oxybenzone	Milky lotion	15–18	10–12	Excellent	Excellent
Total Eclipse-15*	2.5% glyceryl PABA + 2.5% octyldimethyl PABA + 2.5% oxybenzone	Milky lotion	15–18	10–14	Excellent	Good
MMM-What-A-Tan!	3.0% octyldimethyl PABA + 2.5% benzophenone-3	Milky lotion	15–20	10–12	Excellent	Good
PreSun-15 (water-resistant)	8% padimate O + 3% oxybenzone	Milky lotion	15–20	8–10	Excellent	Good
Clinique-19	Phenyl-benzimidazole-5-sulfonic acid + 2.5% octyldimethyl PABA	Milky lotion	15–19	7–8	Good	Fair
Sundown-15* (sunblock)	7% padimate O + 5% octylsalicylate + 4% oxybenzone	Milky lotion	15–20	10–11	Excellent	Good
Bain de Soleil	7.0% padimate O + 2.5% oxybenzone + 0.5% dioxybenzone	White cream	15–18	9	Excellent	Fair
Elizabeth Arden Suncare Creme-15	Padimate O + oxybenzone	White cream	15–20	14	Good	Excellent
Estee Lauder-15	Phenyl-benzimidazole-5-sulfonic acid + dimethyl PABA	White cream	15–20	9	Good	Fair
Rubenstein Gold Beauty-15	Ethyl-hexyl-*p*-methoxycinnamate + octyldimethyl PABA	Yellow gel	10–12	9	Fair	Poor
Block Out-15	7% octyldimethyl PABA + 3% oxybenzone	Creamy lotion	15	5–8	Good	Good
Shiseido-15	6.5% titanium dioxide + 2.5% octyldimethyl PABA + 0.3% benzophenone-3	Lotion	15–20	8–10	Good	Good
Non-PABA sunscreens:						
Piz Buin-8†	5% ethyl-hexyl-*p*-methoxycinnamate + 3% 2-hydroxy-4-methoxybenzophenone + 4% 2-phenyl-benzimidazole sulfonic acid	Cream	15–20	10–12	Excellent	Good
Piz Bun-8†	5% ethyl-hexyl-*p*-methoxycinnamate + 3% 2-hydroxy-4-methoxybenzophenone	Milky lotion	20–22	10–12	Excellent	Good
TIScreen-15		Milky lotion	16–20	10–12	Excellent	Good
Piz Buin-4*	4.5% ethyl-hexyl-*p*-methoxycinnamate	Milky lotion	10–12	4–6	Fair	Poor
UVAL	10% 2-hydroxy-4-methoxy-benzophenone-5-sulfonic acid	Milky lotion	10–12	4	Poor	Poor
Coppertone	8% homomenthylsalicylate	Lotion	3.5–4	2	Poor	Poor
Ultra Vera-20 (Cheesebrough-Pond's)	Octylmethoxycinnamate + 2-hydroxy-4-methoxy-benzophenone	Milky lotion	12–15	6	Fair	Fair
Piz Buin Gletsher Creme-15	Cinnamide + dibenzoylmethane	Yellow lotion	15	12–13	Excellent	Excellent
Piz Buin-12	4.5% octyl-methoxycinnamate + 4.5% zinc oxide + 4.5% talc + 2.2% benzophenone-3	Milky lotion	15–20	12–14	Excellent	Excellent
Physical sunscreens:						
A-Fil		Cream	6–8	4–6	Good	Fair
RV Paque		Cream	10–12	4–6	Good	Fair
Shadow	Titanium dioxide + zinc oxide + talc, kaolin, iron oxide, or red veterinary petrolatum	Cream	4–6	6–8	Good	Fair
Reflecta		Cream	10–12	2–4	Good	Good
Covermark		Cream	10–12	6–8	Good	Fair
Clinique		Cream	10–12	4–6	Good	Fair

KEY: *Excellent = SPF value retained is over 90 to 100% after stress of 45-min swimming; good = SPF value retained is over 75 to 90% after stress of 45-min swimming; fair = SPF value retained is over 50 to 75% after stress of 45-min swimming; poor = SPF value retained is less than 50% after stress of 45-min swimming.*
* *Ingredients may include octyldimethyl PABA + oxybenzone.*
† *Not available in the United States.*
NOTE: *Eyes should always be protected with ultraviolet-opaque goggles or sunglasses while sunbathing or skiing.*
SOURCE: *Pathak et al, in Dermatology in General Medicine, 2d ed, TB Fitzpatrick et al (eds), New York, McGraw-Hill, 1979.*

radiation (290 nm) may produce PMLE. Although the mechanisms underlying these reactions are not known, the evidence suggests a delayed hypersensitivity reaction to an antigen induced by radiation.

TREATMENT Photoprotection with the use of highly effective sunscreens (Table 52-5) or through the avoidance of outdoor activities between 9 A.M. and 5 P.M. during summer months and appropriate long-sleeved clothes may significantly reduce the severity of the clinical response. The synthetic antimalarials are effective in PMLE, but they must be used with great caution to prevent retinopathy and optic nerve atrophy. One of the effective treatments for PMLE is to induce tolerance or hardening of the skin by oral methoxsalen (0.6 mg/kg) photochemotherapy. This tolerance or desensitization by repeated graduated exposures to sunlight or to artificial radiation (UV-A) in combination with psoralens (methoxsalen) is attributed to thickening of epidermis and increased pigmentation and appears to account for the rarity of PMLE in Australia, where the fair-skinned population is exposed to the sun year round. Oral administration of β-carotene (Solatene) has been found to be of limited value.

Several other idiopathic forms of photodermatoses are seen that constitute a rare but large group of light-induced abnormal reactions. *Solar urticaria* following brief exposure to sunlight or artificial radiation is a rare but distinctive condition. The exposed skin reddens, scattered wheals appear and coalesce, and an erythematous flare develops around the wheals with or without urticaria; the cause is unknown. In some patients exposure to UV-B, UV-A, or visible radiation has been followed by the elevation of histamine, degranulation of mast cells, and elevated levels of eosinophil and neutrophil chemotactic factors into the circulation, suggesting that mast cells may play a role. Although antihistamines may benefit some patients, topical broad-spectrum sunscreens and gradual induction of tolerance to natural or artificial radiation by repeated and graded exposures to radiation of appropriate wavelengths have been found to diminish the urticarial reaction.

Actinic reticuloid is another form of chronic, persistent photodermatitis occurring mainly in males who are middle-aged or elderly. It is a most distressing form of persistent photosensitivity characterized by erythematous papular and eczematous eruption; pruritus is generally severe. Lymphomatoid infiltrate is observed histologically with microscopic features implied by the term reticuloid. The patients are severely sensitive to UV-B, UV-A, and even visible radiation. There is a frequent history of eczema present for many years; in some, photosensitivity starts with photocontact dermatitis to a chemical agent. Oral psoralen photochemotherapy appears to help the clearance of photodermatoses.

PHOTOTHERAPY AND PHOTOCHEMOTHERAPY

Phototherapy refers to the therapeutic effectiveness of UVR (usually 290 to 320 nm) or visible radiation without the systemic use of a drug. Photochemotherapy, on the other hand, involves the combination of nonionizing electromagnetic radiation and a systemically administered, photochemically reactive agent. Generally in the doses used, neither the drug alone nor the radiation alone has any therapeutic response; only the combination of the photoactive drug and the radiation, administered at the appropriate time, is therapeutic. Indications for phototherapy include various dermatoses, uremic pruritus, and neonatal hyperbilirubinemia. Phototherapy with blue visible light (430 to 500 nm) causes the photoisomerization of bilirubin, and the resulting water-soluble bilirubin photoproducts are readily excreted in bile and urine. Psoriasis, eczema, and pityriasis rosea may improve with controlled sun exposures. UV-B radiation (290 to 320 nm) is, therefore, a part of the therapeutic regimen for these dermatoses.

The treatment of psoriasis and other proliferative diseases of the skin has involved attempts to inhibit cellular proliferation and DNA synthesis.

The topical application of crude coal-tar products followed by subsequent UV exposure has been a standard treatment for severe generalized psoriasis and was first described by W. H. Goeckerman, M.D., of the Mayo Clinic more than 50 years ago. Although tar-induced phototoxicity affecting DNA synthesis is believed to be responsible for therapeutic effects, it is not yet clear whether the beneficial effects are due to the chemical ingredients of tar alone or the photosensitizing action of UV-A (320 to 400 nm) or UV-B.

ORAL PSORALEN PHOTOCHEMOTHERAPY Psoralens are naturally occurring furocoumarins that are tricyclic compounds, many of which are photochemically reactive [e.g., 8-methoxypsoralen (methoxsalen) and 4,5′,8-trimethylpsoralen (trioxsalen)]. It has been shown that in the presence of psoralens irradiation with UV-A (320 to 400 nm) can result in covalent binding of psoralens to pyrimidine bases in DNA. This photoconjugation may lead to interstrand cross-linking of psoralen between base paired strands of DNA, inhibition of DNA synthesis, and cell death. Psoralens in combination with UV-A (PUVA) are now widely used in treating psoriasis, vitiligo, and mycosis fungoides. Two hours after ingestion of methoxsalen (0.6 mg/kg), patients are exposed to a measured dose of UV-A radiation. The initial dose depends on the patient's skin reactivity to UVR (skin type) and degree of melanin pigmentation of skin. Repeated oral psoralen plus UV-A treatments cause disappearance of psoriatic lesions; a total of 20 treatments given two or three times weekly will usually result in clearance of psoriasis. Maintenance treatments are recommended, once weekly for two months. The scalp and areas to which UV-A does not penetrate do not respond to therapy. Data verifying the efficacy of PUVA have come from several carefully designed, prospective clinical trials involving over 5000 patients at university medical centers throughout the United States and western Europe.

In vitiligo, a disease characterized by amelanotic macules of varying sizes and absence of melanocytes, PUVA treatment can be used in restoring the normal skin color to pigmentless areas of vitiligo macules. Over 70 percent of repigmentation in vitiliginous areas can be achieved. Over 100 to 200 treatments are needed, and this long duration of treatment can often be frustrating, especially when the pigment response is slow, unpredictable, and subject to the presence of functional melanocytes and their proliferation.

The potential long-term concerns of photochemotherapy include premature aging (irreversible changes in connective tissue, blood vessels, and keratinocytes), cataracts, and skin cancer. Oral methoxsalen photochemotherapy using long-wave UVR sources is a new approach. Although over 200,000 patients with psoriasis and thousands of patients with vitiligo have been treated, well-documented examples of actinic keratoses or early squamous cell carcinoma have been infrequently observed in fair skinned patients (skin type I–III) receiving over 80 treatments. Prior history of skin cancer, exposure to ionizing radiation, and arsenic ingestion appear to be predisposing factors for increased incidence of squamous cell carcinoma. However, there is no evidence of cataractogenesis in vitiligo patients treated with psoralens and sunlight over the past 33 years, and adequate eye protection with appropriate UV-A–opaque lenses would largely obviate this risk. Photochemotherapy is an effective treatment which, when compared with other available treatments for generalized psoriasis or vitiligo, appears to have the most acceptable risk/benefit ratio.

Another type of photochemotherapy that appears to be promising is the treatment of tumors with a photosensitizer and visible light. A hematoporphyrin derivative in combination with visible radiation is now being increasingly used for the local treatment of a wide variety of malignant lesions (e.g., metastatic breast carcinoma), including those involving skin. The therapy is based upon the ability of hematoporphyrin to localize in the tumor mass, and its photodynamic efficiency in killing of malignant cells by the photoactivated hepatoporphyrins through the generation of reactive singlet oxygen and subsequent damage to the DNA and other cellular components.

TOPICAL SUNSCREENS IN HEALTH AND DISEASES

Since exposure of skin to UVR is the major cause of skin cancer and actinic aging, the risk can be significantly reduced by decreasing the quantity of harmful radiation reaching the skin with topical application of effective sunscreens. Sunscreens protect viable cells of the skin by absorbing and reflecting the radiation impinging on the skin (see Table 52-5). The majority of sunscreens are designed to protect the user against UV-B (290 to 320 nm). Sunscreens that contain two or more UVR-absorbing chemicals [e.g., benzophenones + cinnamic acid derivatives or benzophenones + PABA ester (padimate O)] appear to filter out both UV-B and UV-A radiation, and at times are referred to as broad-spectrum sunscreens. The effectiveness of a sunscreen is rated on the basis of the sun protection factor (SPF), a term that designates a ratio of MED of the sunscreen-protected skin to the MED of the nonprotected skin; the higher the SPF, the better the skin protection. In counseling people in the prevention of sunburn, skin cancer, aging of the skin, actinic elastosis, and various forms of sun sensitivity, the choice and recommendations of sunscreen depend upon several factors. The most important consideration should be the individual's reactivity to sunlight. People with fair skin, blue eyes, with or without freckles, who burn easily and tan poorly (skin types I and II, Table 52-2) should be given those sunscreens that have an SPF of 10 or greater (Table 52-5). Individuals with skin types III and IV, who burn moderately or minimally but tan well, may be recommended sunscreens with an SPF of 6 to 8. Habitually exposed areas, e.g., face, ears, neck, arms, and hands, should be protected by daily application of a nonoily lotion.

For the greatest protection patients should apply sunscreens with SPF of 10 or more 1 h before exposure. Although many new sunscreens are water-resistant (see Table 52-5), the patient should reapply the sunscreen after swimming or during prolonged sunbathing. In many instances patients may be exquisitely sensitive, irrespective of skin type, and they may require combination therapy with two or more sunscreens (preferably an opaque sunscreen). The drug-induced photosensitization reactions can be minimized or prevented by prescribing topical sunscreens containing benzophenones (Table 52-5). Sunscreens containing PABA or its derivatives should *not* be prescribed for individuals who are photosensitive to certain drugs and manifest phototoxic or cell-mediated delayed hypersensitivity reactions. In patients receiving antihypertensive thiazide diuretics or sulfonamides there may be a cross-reaction with PABA leading to eczematous dermatitis. These patients should be prescribed sunscreens containing benzophenones (see Table 52-5) or opaque sunscreens containing zinc oxide, titanium oxide, and other light-scattering agents such as kaolin.

Individuals with acute sunburn reaction manifesting severe erythema, edema, and painful blistering reaction may be treated with systemic corticosteroids. Oral prednisone, beginning with 40 to 60 mg and tapering over 4 to 8 days, will help to control the severe sunburn reaction.

REFERENCES

HARBER LC, BICKERS DR: *Photosensitivity Diseases: Principles of Diagnosis and Treatment.* Philadelphia, Saunders, 1981

MAGNUS IA: *Dermatological Photobiology.* Oxford, Blackwell, 1976

PARRISH JA: Phototherapy and photochemotherapy of skin diseases. J Invest Dermatol 77:167, 1981

———— et al: Photomedicine, in *Dermatology in General Medicine*, 3d ed, TB Fitzpatrick et al (eds). New York, McGraw-Hill, 1987

PATHAK MA, DUNNICK JK: *Photobiologic, Toxicologic, and Pharmacologic Aspects of Psoralens*, National Cancer Institute Monograph 66, US Department of Health and Human Services, National Cancer Institute, Bethesda, MD, 1984

———— et al: Evaluation of topical agents that prevent sunburn. N Engl J Med 280:1459, 1969

———— et al (eds): *Sunlight and Man: Normal and Abnormal Photobiologic Responses.* Tokyo, University of Tokyo Press, 1974

———— et al: Sunscreens: Topical and systemic approaches for protection of human skin against harmful effects of solar radiation. J Am Acad Dermatol 7:285, 1982

section 9   Hematologic alterations

53   ANEMIA

H. FRANKLIN BUNN

By definition patients with anemia have a significant reduction in red cell mass and a corresponding decrease in the oxygen-carrying capacity of the blood. Normally, blood volume is maintained at a nearly constant level. Therefore, anemia entails a decrease in the concentration of red cells or hemoglobin in peripheral blood.

Under unusual circumstances, the blood values do not accurately reflect alterations in the red cell mass. For example, hemoglobin level and hematocrit are falsely elevated in patients who have sustained an acute reduction in plasma volume owing to hemorrhage, extensive burns, vigorous diuresis, or other types of severe dehydration. In contrast, the blood values may be falsely low in patients who have an expanded blood volume, as in pregnancy or congestive heart failure.

Normal blood values for individuals of various ages are shown in the Appendix. In women in the childbearing age group the blood values are 10 percent lower than in men. At high altitudes, higher values are found, roughly in proportion to the elevation above sea level. Anemia may be defined as a reduction of more than 10 percent below the mean values for the sex. However, since the variations in normal hemoglobin values approach this limit, the documentation of mild anemia may be uncertain.

SIGNS AND SYMPTOMS OF ANEMIA   The clinical presentation of the anemic patient depends on the underlying disease as well as on the severity and chronicity of the anemia. The manifestations of anemia per se can be explained by the pathophysiologic principles outlined in this chapter and in Chap. 283. Most of these signs and symptoms represent cardiovascular and ventilatory adjustments which compensate for the decrease in red blood cell mass.

The degree to which symptoms occur in an anemic patient depends on several contributing factors. If the anemia has developed rapidly, there may not be adequate time for compensatory adjustments to take place, and the patient may have more marked symptoms than if an anemia of equivalent severity had developed insidiously. Furthermore, the patient's complaints may depend on the presence of local vascular disease. For example, angina pectoris, intermittent claudication, or transient cerebral ischemia may be unmasked by the development of anemia.

Individuals with mild anemia are often asymptomatic. They may complain of fatigue as well as dyspnea and palpitation, particularly following exercise. Severely anemic patients will often be symptomatic at rest and unable to tolerate significant exertion. When the hemoglobin concentration falls below 7.5 g/dL, resting cardiac output rises significantly with an increase in both heart rate and stroke volume. The patient may be aware of this hyperdynamic state and complain of palpitation or a pounding pulse. Symptoms of cardiac failure may develop if the patient's myocardial reserve is reduced.

The symptoms of severe anemia extend to other organ systems. Patients often complain of dizziness and headache and may experience syncope, tinnitus, or vertigo. Many patients are irritable and have difficulty sleeping or concentrating. Because of decreased blood flow to the skin, patients may become hypersensitive to cold. Gastrointestinal symptoms such as anorexia, indigestion, and even nausea or bowel irregularity are attributable to shunting of blood away from the splanchnic bed. Females commonly develop abnormal menstruation, both amenorrhea and increased bleeding. Males may complain of impotence or loss of libido.

Physical findings *Pallor* is the physical finding most commonly associated with anemia. However, the usefulness of this sign is limited by other factors that affect the color of the skin. The thickness and texture of the skin vary widely among individuals. Furthermore, the blood flow to the skin can undergo wide fluctuations. Normal individuals will appear sallow when blood is shunted away from the skin, whereas anemic patients may appear flushed when overheated or during periods of excitement. The concentration of melanin in the epidermis is another important determinant of skin color. Individuals with a fair complexion may look pale even though they are not anemic. Conversely, pallor is difficult to detect in deeply pigmented individuals. Furthermore, acquired disorders of melanin pigmentation (e.g., Addison's disease, hemochromatosis) or jaundice may interfere with detection of pallor. Nevertheless, even in blacks, the presence of anemia may be suspected by the color of the palms or of noncutaneous tissues such as oral mucous membranes, nail beds, and palpebral conjunctivas. The color of the creases of the palm is a useful sign. When they are as pale as the surrounding skin, the patient usually has a hemoglobin of less than 7 g/dL.

Two factors contribute to the development of pallor in patients with anemia. There is, of course, a decrease in the hemoglobin concentration of blood perfusing the skin and mucous membranes. Also, blood is shunted away from the skin and other peripheral tissues, permitting enhanced blood flow to vital organs. Redistribution of blood flow is an important mode of compensation in anemia.

Other physical findings associated with anemia include tachycardia, wide pulse pressure, and a hyperdynamic precordium. A systolic ejection murmur is often heard over the precordium, particularly at the pulmonic area. In addition, a venous hum may be detected over the neck vessels. These cardiac findings disappear when the anemia is corrected. Patients with hemolytic anemia often have icterus and splenomegaly and occasionally develop superficial skin ulceration over the ankle bones.

APPROACH TO THE PATIENT WITH ANEMIA In evaluating the anemic patient, the physician should proceed in an orderly fashion so that the correct diagnosis can be established with a minimum of laboratory tests and procedures. As in other clinical disciplines, a comprehensive history and meticulous physical examination are of paramount importance in the initial workup of the anemic patient. For example, a family history which reveals a dominant inheritance pattern provides strong support for the diagnosis of hereditary spherocytosis. The discovery of a heart murmur and splenomegaly raises the possibility that the anemic patient may have subacute bacterial endocarditis.

The evaluation of the anemic patient should be based on a firm understanding of the pathophysiologic principles outlined in Chap. 283. As shown in Table 53-1, the clinician must first ask whether the anemia is due to a decreased production of red cells or to enhanced destruction. Moreover, the possibility of blood loss either as the sole etiology or as a contributing factor must always be considered. The

examination of the stool for occult blood is an indispensable part of the evaluation of all anemic patients. At this crossroad, laboratory information can be gathered which will establish whether the patient is failing to produce an adequate number of circulating red cells or is undergoing hemolysis.

The *reticulocyte count* is the most useful laboratory test for answering this question. When an appropriate supravital stain is applied to a sample of peripheral blood, the 1- to 2-day-old red cells exhibit a network of purple strands which are aggregates of ribosomes. Reticulocytosis is a reflection of the release of an increased number of young cells from the bone marrow. The degree of increased erythropoiesis can be assessed more quantitatively by determining the reticulocyte index, which uses the hematocrit or packed cell volume (PCV) and is calculated as follows:

$$\text{Reticulocyte index} = \text{reticulocyte \%} \times \frac{\text{patient's PCV}}{\text{normal PCV}}$$

This measure fails to consider the distribution of reticulocytes between the bone marrow and the peripheral blood. When the marrow is greatly stimulated, marrow reticulocytes enter the circulation prematurely. Since the circulation of these "shift reticulocytes" in the peripheral blood is prolonged, the reticulocyte index should be divided by about 2. This factor varies from 1.5 to 3 depending upon the severity of the anemia and the degree of erythropoietin stimulation. This correction should always be made if normoblasts are encountered in the peripheral blood since this finding indicates the premature release of red cell precursors into the circulation. On a routinely prepared smear, "shift reticulocytes" appear larger than average and have a lavender hue, so-called polychromatophilia.

A failure to produce red cells is reflected in an inappropriately low reticulocyte count. In contrast, a significant elevation of reticulocytes is suggestive of hemolysis. Exceptions include (1) the brisk reticulocyte response that is seen in a patient with hemorrhage, (2) reticulocytosis encountered in patients recovering from impaired erythropoiesis (e.g., an individual with pernicious anemia who received an injection of vitamin B_{12} 1 week earlier), and (3) mild to moderate elevations in reticulocytes (3 to 7 percent) encountered in myelophthisic anemia in which the orderly release of cells is affected by alterations of the marrow stroma owing to tumor, fibrosis, or granulomata. These exceptions are often readily appreciated in the initial evaluation of the patient. Furthermore, a number of ancillary laboratory tests described below are useful in determining to what extent hemolysis is occurring. The measurement of unconjugated bilirubin in the serum is a particularly useful guide to the presence of accelerated red blood cell breakdown. Once this information is obtained, the workup can be directed toward the establishment of a specific etiology.

Three additional baseline studies are of critical importance in the initial workup of the patient with anemia: *measurement of red cell indexes, examination of the peripheral blood smear,* and, in many patients, *bone marrow examination.*

Red cell indexes Red cell indexes can be calculated from determinants of hematocrit, hemoglobin concentration, and red blood cell

TABLE 53-1 Initial evaluation of anemia

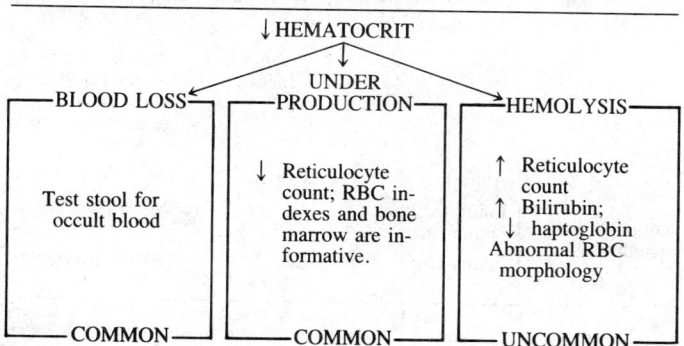

	↓ HEMATOCRIT	
BLOOD LOSS	UNDER PRODUCTION	HEMOLYSIS
Test stool for occult blood	↓ Reticulocyte count; RBC indexes and bone marrow are informative.	↑ Reticulocyte count ↑ Bilirubin; ↓ haptoglobin Abnormal RBC morphology
COMMON	COMMON	UNCOMMON

count. Measuring the hematocrit or PCV is the simplest and one of the most precise ways to ascertain the concentration of red cells in the blood. Generally, a small sample of anticoagulated blood is drawn into a capillary tube which is sealed at one end and centrifuged. The PCV is the ratio of the volume of packed red cells to the total volume. Alternatively, the concentration of hemoglobin can be determined spectrophotometrically from the absorbance of the cyanmethemoglobin form at a specific wavelength. With the advent of automated red blood cell counting technology, very precise measurements of red blood cell indexes are now readily available in nearly all hospitals and clinical laboratories. The electronic counter makes a direct measurement of the red cell count (RBC/μL) and the mean red cell volume (MCV):

$$\text{MCV (fl)} = \frac{\text{PCV (liters/liters)}}{(\text{RBC}/\mu\text{L}) \times 10^{-9}}$$

This instrument calculates the PCV from the direct measurement of MCV and RBC/μL. In addition, hemoglobin concentration is measured directly on a separate channel. The mean corpuscular hemoglobin concentration (MCHC) is then computed as follows:

$$\text{MCHC (g/dL)} = \frac{\text{Hb (g/dL)}}{\text{PCV (liters/liters)}}$$

A third red blood cell index, the mean corpuscular hemoglobin (MCH), is determined as follows:

$$\text{MCH (pg)} = \frac{\text{Hb (g/dL)}}{(\text{RBC}/\mu\text{L}) \times 10^{-7}}$$

When calculated by an electronic counter, the MCHC is not reliable and is of little use to the clinician. Generally, an automated system provides a printout which includes hemoglobin concentration, red cell count, packed cell volume, and the three red cell indexes (MCV, MCHC, and MCH).

As Table 53-2 shows, the MCV is particularly useful in classifying the anemias due to decreased red cell production. Microcytic anemias have low values for MCV. On microscopic examination, the red cells appear small and often pale. In contrast, in the macrocytic anemias the MCV is elevated and large oval cells (macroovalocytes) are seen on microscopic examination. Unlike the anemias of underproduction, nearly all the hemolytic anemias are normocytic or slightly macrocytic owing to the preponderance of young red cells. Exceptions include

TABLE 53-2   Anemias due to decreased red cell production

RBC Indexes	Marrow	Additional lab tests	Diagnosis
Hypochromic, microcytic ($\downarrow$ MCV)	0 Iron	$\downarrow$ Fe, $\uparrow$ TIBC	Iron deficiency
	+ Iron	$\uparrow$ Hb A$_2$, $\uparrow$ Hb F $\downarrow$ Hb A$_2$	β Thalassemia
	Ring sideroblasts		Sideroblastic anemia
Macrocytic ($\uparrow$ MCV)	Megaloblastic	$\downarrow$ Serum B$_{12}$, achlorhydria	Vitamin B$_{12}$ deficiency, pernicious anemia
		$\downarrow$ Serum folate	Folic acid deficiency
Normochromic, normocytic	Normal	$\downarrow$ Fe, $\downarrow$ TIBC	Anemia of chronic inflammation
		$\uparrow$ Creatinine	Anemia of uremia
		Abn LFT	Anemia of liver disease
		$\downarrow$ T$_4$	Anemia of myxedema
	Aplastic	Pancytopenia	Aplastic anemia
Normoblasts, teardrops	Infiltrated: tumor, lymphoma, etc.		Myelophthisic
	Fibrosis	$\uparrow$ LAP	Myeloid metaplasia

NOTE: *Fe, iron; TIBC, total iron-binding capacity; Hb, hemoglobin; LAP, leukocyte alkaline phosphatase; LFT, liver function tests; Abn, abnormal; MCV, mean corpuscular volume.*

the severe forms of thalassemia in which microcytic red cells are accompanied by brisk hemolysis.

Examination of the blood smear   In the evaluation of patients with anemia, the physician should take the time to examine a well-stained peripheral blood film. Figures A5-1 to A5-12 show examples of abnormalities in red cell morphology encountered in various types of anemia. Many subtleties escape the attention of the technologist whose primary purpose in examining the slide is to obtain a white cell differential count. Furthermore, the clinician can approach the specimen with a prepared mind and can scrutinize it for specific abnormalities. As suggested above, the examination can confirm the size and color of red cells as estimated by RBC indexes. Furthermore, while these indexes provide mean statistical values, the microscopic examination can reveal variation in red cell size (anisocytosis) or shape (poikilocytosis), changes which are helpful in the diagnosis of specific anemias. Examination of the blood smear is particularly important in evaluating a patient with hemolysis. Most hemolytic anemias have characteristic morphologic abnormalities. Finally, this practice may yield unexpected dividends. The finding of rouleaux suggests the presence of dysproteinemia as occurs in multiple myeloma. The examination may provide the initial clue that the patient has significant thrombocytopenia.

Bone marrow examination   A microscopic examination of the bone marrow is generally indicated in the workup of any *unexplained* anemia. Study of the bone marrow is particularly informative in the anemias of underproduction. The more severe the anemia, the more likely that the procedure will be informative. An assessment of the quantity and quality of red cell precursors may determine whether there is a primary defect in cell production. A marrow biopsy is particularly useful in estimating overall cellularity. The normal differential of nucleated cells in the marrow is shown in the Appendix. The ratio of myeloid (M) to erythroid (E) precursors is normally about 2:1 but may be artifactually increased by the inclusion of circulating leukocytes. The ratio is increased in patients with infection, a leukemoid reaction, or neoplastic proliferation of myeloid cells. Rarely, a high M/E ratio is due to selective aplasia of the red cell precursors. A decreased M/E ratio indicates erythroid hyperplasia (seen in hemolysis or hemorrhage) or ineffective erythropoiesis (e.g., megaloblastic and sideroblastic anemias). The morphology of the precursors may reveal a maturation deficit such as megaloblastic anemia. The bone marrow examination is also important in demonstrating the presence of cellular infiltrates such as those found in leukemia, lymphoma, or multiple myeloma. The demonstration of tumor, fibrosis, or granulomata usually requires a biopsy. A portion of the marrow specimen should be stained with Prussian blue. In addition to providing an assessment of iron stores, the iron stain is required for the identification of sideroblasts.

ANEMIA DUE TO BLOOD LOSS   This form of anemia varies considerably in its clinical presentation depending upon the site, severity, and rapidity of the hemorrhage. At opposite extremes are acute fulminant bleeding producing hypovolemic shock and chronic occult blood loss leading to iron-deficiency anemia.

Patients who have sustained an acute hemorrhage generally present with signs and symptoms secondary to hypoxia and hypovolemia. Depending on the severity of the process, the patient will have weakness, fatigue, light-headedness, stupor, or coma and will often appear pale, diaphoretic, and irritable. Vital signs are a reflection of cardiovascular compensation for the acute blood loss (Chap. 29). The patient will have hypotension and tachycardia in proportion to the degree of hemorrhage. Elicitation of postural signs is useful in the initial evaluation of patients with acute blood loss. If the pulse rises 25 percent or more, or the systolic blood pressure falls 20 mmHg or more upon going from a supine to sitting position, the patient is likely to have significant hypovolemia (blood loss >1000 mL) and requires prompt replacement. Acute blood loss in excess of 1500 mL usually leads to cardiovascular collapse.

If the blood loss has been acute and recent, the peripheral blood may not reveal a significant decrease in packed cell volume or hemoglobin, since the red cell mass and plasma volume are contracted in parallel. There often is a moderate leukocytosis and a "shift to the left" in the white cell differential count. Thrombocytosis may be encountered in both acute and chronic blood loss, particularly when the patient is iron-deficient. During the first few days following an acute hemorrhage there is usually an increase in reticulocytes. Occasionally nucleated red cells may appear in the peripheral blood. Since young red cells are larger than old ones, the patient may develop slightly macrocytic red cell indexes (MCV = 95 to 105 fl). As mentioned above, sustained reticulocytosis will be seen if significant blood loss continues, or until iron stores have been exhausted. Internal bleeding may be accompanied by an increase in unconjugated bilirubin. This abnormality is a reflection of an increase in catabolism of heme from extravasated red cells. Patients with acute gastrointestinal blood loss will often have an elevation of blood urea nitrogen owing to impaired renal blood flow and perhaps to the absorption of digested blood protein.

It is of critical importance to assess these patients promptly and institute treatment without delay. A large-bore intravenous line should be placed. While blood is being typed and cross matched, saline, Ringer's lactate, or, preferably, a colloid such as 5% albumin should be infused to correct hypovolemia. Whole blood is then administered as soon as it is available. Monitoring of vital signs and central venous pressure is useful in determining the appropriate amount of volume replacement. During and following these emergency measures, diagnostic studies may reveal the site or sites of bleeding. If the bleeding is unexplained an emergency coagulation profile should be obtained. Demonstration of bleeding from the gastrointestinal tract may require the insertion of a nasogastric tube. Appropriate radiologic studies may be indicated to determine sites of internal bleeding such as retroperitoneal hemorrhage.

Chronic blood loss is usually due to lesions in the gastrointestinal tract or the uterus. The testing of stool specimens for occult blood is an essential, though frequently overlooked, part of the evaluation of anemia. It may be necessary to examine serial specimens over a prolonged period of time since gastrointestinal bleeding is often intermittent. The hematologic manifestations of chronic blood loss are those of iron-deficiency anemia, discussed in detail in Chap. 284.

ANEMIAS DUE TO DECREASED RBC PRODUCTION

As shown in Table 53-2, red cell indexes are useful in classifying the anemias due to underproduction of red cells. They can be conveniently grouped into three major categories: microcytic, macrocytic, and normocytic.

The *microcytic* anemias include iron-deficiency anemia (Chap. 284), sideroblastic anemias (Chap. 284), and the thalassemias (Chap. 288). Collectively, they represent a decrease in the availability or synthesis of one of the three major constituents of the hemoglobin molecule: iron, porphyrin, and globin. Since hemoglobin makes up over 90 percent of the protein within the erythrocyte, it is not surprising that these defects in hemoglobin synthesis result in the formation of small, pale red cells. These disorders involve a variable degree of ineffective erythropoiesis (Chap. 283). In addition, the anemias of chronic inflammation and malignancy may be slightly microcytic (Chap. 286). This phenomenon is due to a defect in the availability of iron. However, these disorders are more often normocytic and have been so classified in Table 53-2. Measurement of serum iron and iron-binding capacity and evaluation of marrow iron stores are particularly useful in distinguishing between these anemias.

The *macrocytic* anemias generally are associated with megaloblastic morphology in the bone marrow. In most cases, a deficiency of either vitamin B_{12} or folic acid results in an impairment of the replication of DNA, particularly in cells having a high turnover rate. Because nuclear maturation lags behind cytoplasmic development, large red cells tend to be produced in the bone marrow. Megaloblastic anemias are discussed in detail in Chap. 285. Like the microcytic anemias, these disorders are maturation defects associated with ineffective erythropoiesis. Macrocytosis, generally of a lesser degree, may also be encountered in patients with liver disease, hypothyroid-

ism, acute blood loss, hemolytic anemia, aplastic anemia, and alcoholism. However, in these conditions, the red cell precursors in the bone marrow do not appear megaloblastic. The macrocytes in liver disease and hypothyroidism may be related to an increased deposition of lipid in the red cell membrane.

The *normocytic* anemias of underproduction comprise a diverse group of disorders. As shown in Table 53-2, this group can be conveniently subdivided into two categories: those secondary to some other underlying disease and those due to intrinsic pathology within the bone marrow.

The primary disorders of the bone marrow are best approached by microscopic examination of a marrow aspirate and biopsy. This group of anemias is often accompanied by leukopenia and thrombocytopenia. Pancytopenia, usually to a lesser degree, can also be seen in hypersplenism and in the megaloblastic anemias. Aplastic anemia and the myelophthisic anemias are discussed in Chap. 290.

The diagnosis of anemia secondary to some underlying disease is usually quite straightforward. Conversely, the presence of an unexplained normocytic anemia should prompt the search for an underlying disorder such as chronic renal failure, infection, or myxedema. If the presence of such an illness is established, the physician is obliged to investigate whether other factors such as blood loss or a nutritional deficiency contribute to the patient's anemia. Generally, the anemias due to liver disease, chronic inflammation, or an endocrinopathy are of only moderate severity. Unlike the other "secondary" anemias, that due to chronic renal failure can be severe. All these anemias are discussed in more detail in Chap. 286.

HEMOLYTIC ANEMIAS Hemolytic anemias (Table 53-3) are encountered much less frequently than the anemias due to decreased red cell production. Although they are a diverse group, the hemolytic anemias have a number of clinical features in common. Signs and symptoms of patients with hemolysis are briefly mentioned above.

A number of laboratory tests are available to establish the presence of accelerated breakdown of red cells. The reticulocyte count is the single most useful test. Patients with hemolysis nearly always have an elevated reticulocyte count. A variety of serum and urine tests are useful in confirming the presence of hemolysis and assessing its magnitude. Serum haptoglobin and unconjugated bilirubin are particularly useful (Table 53-1). Others are described in detail in Chap. 287 and are summarized in Table 287-2.

Classification of hemolytic anemias Once the presence of hemolysis is established, a large battery of laboratory tests is available for determining the specific diagnosis. Some of these tests are listed in Table 53-3. No other area of internal medicine is better suited to detailed and fruitful diagnostic probing. In the interest of time and

TABLE 53-3 Hemolytic anemias

Blood smear	Additional lab tests	Diagnosis
Schistocytes, helmet cells		Traumatic hemolytic anemia
Spherocytes	+ Coombs' test	Immunohemolytic anemia
	↑ Osmotic fragility	Hereditary spherocytosis
Spur cells	Abnormal LFT	Spur cell anemia
	+ Sucrose lysis	Paroxysmal nocturnal hemoglobinuria
Sickle cells	+ Sickle prep	Sickle cell syndromes
Target cells	Abn Hb electrophoresis	Hb C, D, etc.
Heinz bodies	Abn Hb electrophoresis	Congenital Heinz body hemolytic anemia
	↓ G6Pd	G6PD deficiency

NOTE: *Hb, hemoglobin; G6PD, glucose 6-phosphate dehydrogenase; LFT, liver function tests; Abn, abnormal.*

money, the clinician should use the available tests in an orderly fashion. This complex group of disorders is easier to approach diagnostically if a concise and workable classification is used. The hemolytic anemias can be grouped in several ways: congenital versus acquired, intracorpuscular versus extracorpuscular, or by anatomic site of the erythrocyte defect. The various kinds of hemolytic anemia are discussed in Chap. 287.

THERAPEUTIC CONSIDERATIONS The effective treatment of anemia, like other disorders, is predicated upon a thorough diagnostic evaluation. There is no reason to administer hematinics such as iron, vitamin B$_{12}$, or folic acid unless a specific deficiency of these substances has been demonstrated or is anticipated. Although the indiscriminate administration of vitamin B$_{12}$ is not deleterious per se, it lulls both the patient and the physician into false security. In contrast, the inappropriate use of iron preparations over a prolonged period of time can be directly harmful, leading to a state of iron overload. Pyridoxine is indicated only in the treatment of sideroblastic anemias.

Many kinds of anemias can be corrected if a precipitating cause can be uncovered and reversed. If a drug or toxin can be incriminated, its withdrawal may allow full recovery. The outcome of the "secondary" anemias is dependent on whether the underlying condition can be corrected. Anemias due to an endocrinopathy or infection should respond favorably to appropriate treatment. Occasionally, the anemia of malignancy is corrected by the removal of the primary tumor. One of the most dramatic sequelae of a successful renal transplant is the prompt correction of the "anemia of uremia." In chronic disorders such as hepatic cirrhosis or rheumatoid arthritis, the anemia is likely to persist, along with the underlying disease.

Primary disorders of the bone marrow such as aplastic anemia or myelophthisic anemia are often irreversible and are treated with supportive measures. *Androgens* are sometimes employed in this group of anemias, but their efficacy is marginal. Many of these patients require transfusions of red cells and platelets. Because prognosis is so bleak in these disorders, a radical approach to treatment seems justified. As described in Chaps. 290 and 291, bone marrow transplantation and immunosuppressive therapy are now reasonable therapeutic alternatives in selected cases of severe aplastic anemia and acute leukemia.

Several factors should be weighed in determining whether an anemic patient should be transfused. The risks and complications of the administration of blood products are discussed in Chap. 282. Patients with chronic or long-standing anemias are able to compensate in several ways, discussed earlier in this chapter. A considerable reduction in red cell mass can be surprisingly well tolerated, especially if the patient is young or sedentary. Transfusion is seldom indicated in a patient with a chronic anemia whose hemoglobin is 9 g/dL or greater. Those who are expected to respond to the administration of a specific agent such as iron, folic acid, or vitamin B$_{12}$ can usually be spared transfusions. If the anemia has precipitated an episode of congestive heart failure or myocardial ischemia, prompt but cautious administration of packed red cells is indicated. In general, whole blood should be given only if the patient is hypovolemic.

Corticosteroids have only a limited role in the treatment of anemia. These agents are not effective in stimulating erythropoiesis. High doses of a glucocorticoid are indicated in the treatment of immunohemolytic anemia, thrombotic thrombocytopenic purpura, and pure red cell anemia. Otherwise, steroids should be prescribed sparingly unless some coexisting condition dictates their use.

Splenectomy is indicated in the treatment of certain hemolytic anemias. The efficacy of splenectomy correlates with the degree to which the abnormal or defective red cells are sequestered. Splenectomy is virtually curative in hereditary spherocytosis. The operation may be beneficial in selected patients with immunohemolytic anemia, congestive splenomegaly, spur cell anemia, and certain hemoglobinopathies and enzymopathies. Splenectomy has also been recommended early in the treatment of thrombotic thrombocytopenic purpura. The operative morbidity and mortality from elective sple-

nectomy are very low. Occasional patients develop a left subphrenic abscess. Following splenectomy, young children are at risk of developing overwhelming septicemia. This complication is much rarer in adults. Thrombocytosis generally develops promptly following splenectomy. However, in most cases, it is transient. In patients with continued hemolysis or a myeloproliferative disorder (Chap. 289), the thrombocytosis usually persists and may occasionally be associated with thromboembolic phenomena.

REFERENCES

BABIOR BM, STOSSEL TP: *Hematology, A Pathophysiological Approach*. New York, Churchill Livingston, 1984
BECK WS (ed): *Hematology*. Boston, MIT Press, 1985
CROSBY WH: Red cell mass: Its precursors and perturbations. Hosp Prac 15:2, 71, 1980
ERSLEV AJ, GABUZDA TG: *Pathophysiology of Blood*. Philadelphia, Saunders, 1985
HILLMAN RS, FINCH CA: *Red Cell Manual*. Philadelphia, Davis, 1974
WILLIAMS WJ et al (ed): *Hematology*, 2d ed. New York, McGraw-Hill, 1983
WINTROBE MM (ed): *Blood, Pure and Eloquent*. New York, McGraw-Hill, 1980

54 BLEEDING AND THROMBOSIS

ROBERT I. HANDIN

Hemorrhage, intravascular thrombosis, and embolism are common clinical manifestations of many diseases. The hemostatic system usually limits blood loss by precisely regulated interactions between components of the vessel wall, circulating blood platelets, and plasma proteins. However, when disease or trauma damage large arteries and veins, excessive bleeding may occur, despite a normal hemostatic stystem. Less frequently, hemorrhage is caused by an inherited or acquired disorder of the hemostatic machinery itself. A large number of such bleeding disorders have now been identified.

In addition, unregulated activation of the hemostatic system may cause thrombosis and embolism, which can reduce blood flow to critical organs like the brain and myocardium. Although we understand less about the pathophysiology of thrombosis than of hemostatic failure, certain patient groups have been identified that are particularly prone to thrombosis and embolism. These include patients (1) immobilized after surgery, (2) with chronic congestive heart failure, (3) with atherosclerotic vascular disease, (4) with malignancy, or (5) who are pregnant. Most of these "thrombosis-prone" patients have no identifiable hemostatic disorder. However, there are certain patient groups who have inherited or acquired a "hypercoagulable" or "prethrombotic" state which predisposes them to recurrent thrombosis.

The cardinal manifestations of disordered hemostasis which cause bleeding or thrombosis are discussed below, along with the clinical approach to diagnosis and evaluation of these patients. Certain information in the patient's history, such as the mode of onset and sites of bleeding, a family bleeding tendency, and a record of drug ingestion help establish the correct diagnosis. Physical examination can identify bleeding in the skin or joint deformities due to previous hemarthroses. Ultimately, however, bleeding disorders are diagnosed by laboratory tests. General screening tests are utilized first, to document a systemic disorder, and are supplemented by specific tests of coagulation protein or platelet function to arrive at an accurate diagnosis.

The hypercoagulable or prethrombotic patient can also be identified by a careful history. There are three important clues to this diagnosis: (1) repeated episodes of thromboembolism without an obvious predisposing condition; (2) a family history of thrombosis; and (3) well-documented thromboembolism in adolescents and young adults. There are, as yet, no clinically useful screening tests for the prethrombotic state. However, several of the prethrombotic disorders can be diagnosed with specific immunologic and functional assays.

NORMAL HEMOSTASIS

Accurate diagnosis and treatment of patients with either bleeding or thrombosis requires some knowledge of the pathophysiology of hemostasis. The process can be divided into primary and secondary components and is initiated when trauma, surgery, or disease disrupt the vascular endothelial lining and blood is exposed to subendothelial connective tissue. *Primary hemostasis* involves the rapid formation of platelet plugs at sites of injury. This occurs within minutes of injury and is of prime importance in stopping blood loss from capillaries, small arterioles, and venules (see Fig. 54-1). *Secondary hemostasis,* or fibrin formation, results from reactions of the plasma coagulation system and may require a longer time for completion. In this reaction, fibrin strands strengthen the primary hemostatic plug. This is particularly important in larger vessels and prevents secondary bleeding hours or days after the initial injury. Although presented here as separate events, primary and secondary hemostasis are closely linked. For example, activated platelets, accelerated coagulation reactions, products of coagulation, such as thrombin, stimulate platelet aggregation.

Effective primary hemostasis requires three critical events— platelet adhesion, granule release, and platelet aggregation. Within a few seconds of injury, platelets adhere to collagen fibrils in vascular subendothelium. As shown in Fig. 54-2, this interaction is facilitated by the von Willebrand's factor, an adhesive glycoprotein which allows platelets to remain attached to the vessel wall despite the high shear forces generated within the vascular lumen. Von Willebrand's factor accomplishes this task by forming a link between platelet receptor sites and subendothelial collagen fibrils. The adherent platelets then generate and secrete mediators like those depicted in Fig. 54-1.

As in other cells, platelet activation and secretion are regulated by changes in the level of cyclic nucleotides, the influx of calcium, hydrolysis of membrane phospholipids, and phosphorylation of critical intracellular proteins. The relevant pathways are depicted in Figs. 54-3 and 54-4. The binding of agonists such as epinephrine, collagen, or thrombin to platelet surface receptors activates two membrane enzymes—phospholipase C and phospholipase A_2. These enzymes catalyze the release of arachidonic acid from two of the major membrane phospholipids, phosphatidylinositol and phosphatidylcholine. Initially, a small quantity of the released arachidonic acid is converted to thromboxane A_2 (TXA_2), which, in turn, can activate phospholipase C. The formation of TXA_2 from arachidonic acid is mediated by the enzyme cyclooxygenase (see Fig. 54-3). This enzyme is inhibited by aspirin and nonsteroidal anti-inflammatory drugs. Inhibition of TXA_2 synthesis is a common cause of bleeding, as well as the basis for the action of some antithrombotic drugs.

Hydrolysis of the membrane phospholipid, phosphatidylinositol 4,5-biphosphate (PIP_2), produces diacylglycerol (DAG) and inositol triphosphate (IP_3), which play a critical role in platelet metabolism. IP_3 mediates the movement of calcium into the platelet cytosol and stimulates the phosphorylation of myosin light chains. The latter interact with actin to facilitate granule movement and platelet shape change. DAG activates protein kinase C which, in turn, phosphorylates a 47,000-dalton protein that controls platelet granule secretion.

There is a finely balanced mechanism which controls the rate and extent of platelet activation which is illustrated in Fig. 54-3. TXA_2, a platelet product of arachidonic acid, increases phospholipase C activity, which stimulates platelet activation and secretion. In contrast, prostacyclin (PGI_2), an endothelial cell product of arachidonic acid, inhibits phospholipase C activity by raising the intraplatelet cyclic AMP levels which in turn inhibits platelet activation. Similar pathways to regulate activation and secretion occur in other cells.

Following activation, platelets secrete their granule contents into plasma. Endoglycosidases and a heparin cleaving enzyme are released from lysosomes; calcium, serotonin, and adenosine diphosphate (ADP) from the dense granules; and several proteins including von Willebrand's factor, fibronectin, thrombospondin, and a heparin-neutralizing protein (platelet factor 4) from alpha granules. Released ADP modifies the platelet surface so that fibrinogen can attach to a complex formed between membrane glycoproteins IIb and IIIa and link adjacent platelets into a hemostatic plug (Fig. 54-2). Platelet-derived growth factor (PDGF), another alpha granule protein, stimulates the growth and migration of fibroblasts and smooth muscle cells within the vessel wall, which is an important part of the repair process.

As the primary hemostatic plug is being formed, plasma coagulation proteins are activated to initiate secondary hemostasis. An

FIGURE 54-1 *Schematic presentation of the major events in primary hemostasis. The first event is platelet adhesion, the interaction of platelets with a nonplatelet surface such as vascular subendothelium. This is followed by platelet activation and secretion. Some of the products secreted by platelets are depicted. Abbreviations—ADP, adenosine diphosphate; PDGF, platelet-derived growth factor, vWF, von Willebrand's factor. The final event is the binding of activated platelets to the adherent monolayer in the process of platelet aggregation.*

Activation / Secretion

ADP

Factor Ⅴa

Thrombospondin

Thromboxane A_2

PDGF

Heparinase

vWF

Fibrinogen

Fibronectin

Adhesion

Aggregation

FIGURE 54-2 *The molecular basis of platelet adhesion and aggregation. Adhesion of platelets to vascular subendothelium is facilitated by the von Willebrand's factor which forms a bridge between collagen fibrils in the vessel wall and receptors on platelet glycoprotein Ib (GpIb). In a similar manner, platelet aggregation is mediated by fibrinogen which links adjacent platelets via receptors on the platelet glycoprotein IIb and IIIa complex (GpIIb–IIIa).*

overall picture of the coagulation scheme, including the role of various inhibitors, is shown in Fig. 54-5. The coagulation pathway can be broken down into a series of reactions (outlined in Fig. 54-6) which culminate in the production of sufficient thrombin to convert a small portion of plasma fibrinogen to fibrin. Each of the reactions requires the formation of a surface bound complex, the conversion of inactive precursor proteins into active proteases by limited proteolysis, and is regulated by plasma and cellular cofactors and calcium.

In *reaction 1*, the intrinsic or contact phase of coagulation, three plasma proteins, Hageman factor (factor XII), high-molecular-weight kininogen (HMWK), and prekallikrein (PK), form a complex with vascular subendothelial collagen. After binding to HMWK, factor

FIGURE 54-3 *Generation of thromboxane A_2 in platelets and prostacyclin (PGI$_2$) in endothelial cells.*

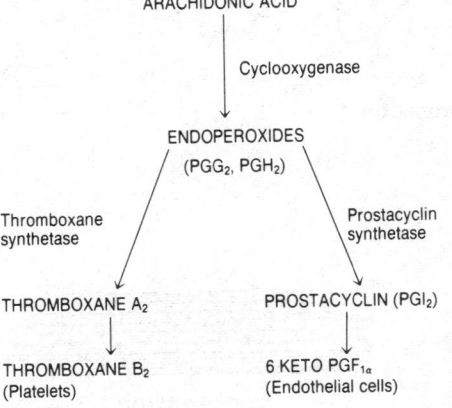

XII is slowly converted to an active protease (XIIa), which converts both PK to kallikrein and factor XI to its active form (XIa). Kallikrein accelerates XII conversion to XIIa, while XIa participates in subsequent coagulation reactions.

Reaction 2 provides a second pathway to initiate coagulation by converting factor VII to an active protease. In this extrinsic or tissue-factor-dependent pathway, a complex is formed between factor VII, calcium, and tissue factor, a ubiquitous lipoprotein present in cellular membranes which is exposed following cellular injury. Factor VII and three other coagulation proteins—factors II (prothrombin), IX, and X—require calcium and vitamin K for biologic activity. These proteins are synthesized in the liver, where a vitamin K–dependent carboxylase catalyzes a unique posttranslational modification by adding a second carboxyl group to certain glutamic acid residues. Pairs of these di-γ-carboxyglutamic acid (Gla) residues bind calcium, which anchors these proteins to negatively charged phospholipid surfaces. The inhibition of this posttranslational modification by vitamin K antagonists (e.g., warfarin) is the basis of one of the most common forms of anticoagulant therapy.

In *reaction 3*, factor X is activated by the proteases generated in the two previous reactions. In one reaction, a calcium- and lipid-dependent complex is formed between factors VIII, IX, and X. Within this complex, factor IX is first converted to IXa by factor XIa that was generated within the intrinsic pathway (reaction 1). Factor X is then activated by factor IXa in concert with factor VIII. Alternatively, factor X can be activated more directly by factor VIIa generated via the extrinsic pathway (reaction 2). Factor X activation provides an important link between the intrinsic and extrinsic coagulation pathways (see Fig. 54-5).

Reaction 4, the final step, converts prothrombin to thrombin in the presence of factor V, calcium, and phospholipid. Although prothrombin conversion can take place on various natural and artificial phospholipid-rich surfaces, it accelerates several thousand-fold on the surface of activated platelets. Thrombin, the product of this reaction, has multiple functions in hemostasis. Although its principal role in hemostasis is the conversion of fibrinogen to fibrin, it also activates factors V, VIII, and XIII and stimulates platelet aggregation and secretion. Following the release of fibrinopeptides A and B from the alpha and beta chains of fibrinogen, the modified molecule, now called fibrin monomer, polymerizes into an insoluble gel. The fibrin polymer is then stabilized by the cross-linking of individual chains by factor XIIIa, a plasma transglutaminase.

Vessel repair begins immediately after the formation of the definitive hemostatic plug. Tissue plasminogen activator (TPA) diffuses from endothelial cells and converts plasminogen adsorbed to the fibrin clot into plasmin (see Fig. 54-7). Plasmin then degrades fibrin polymer into small fragments which are cleared by the monocyte-macrophage scavenger system. Although plasmin can also degrade fibrinogen, the reaction remains localized because (1) TPA activates plasminogen more effectively when it is adsorbed to fibrin clots, and (2) any plasmin that enters the circulation is rapidly bound and neutralized by the alpha$_2$ plasmin inhibitor. The importance of this inhibitor is underscored by the fact that patients who lack it have unchecked fibrinolysis and bleed.

As noted above, the plasma coagulation system is tightly regulated so that only a small quantity of each coagulation enzyme is converted to its active form and the hemostatic plug does not propagate beyond the site of injury. Regulation is important since there is enough clotting potential in a single milliliter of blood to clot all the fibrinogen in the body in 10 to 15 s. Blood fluidity is maintained by the flow of blood itself, which reduces the concentration of reactants, the adsorption of coagulation factors to surfaces, and the presence of multiple inhibitors in plasma. Antithrombin and proteins C and S are the most important inhibitors which help regulate coagulation reactions.

These inhibitors have distinct modes of action. Antithrombin forms complexes with all the serine protease coagulation factors except factor VII (see Fig. 54-5). Rates of complex formation are accelerated by heparin and heparin-like molecules on the surface of the endothelial cells. This ability of heparin to accelerate the activity of antithrombin is the basis for heparin's action as a potent anticoagulant. Protein C is converted to an active protease by thrombin after it is bound to an endothelial cell protein called thrombomodulin. Activated protein C then inactivates the two plasma cofactors V and VIII to slow down two critical coagulation reactions. Protein C may also stimulate the release of tissue plasminogen activator from endothelial cells. The inhibitory function of protein C is enhanced by protein S. As one might predict, reduced levels of antithrombin, or proteins C and S or dysfunctional forms of the molecule, result in a hypercoagulable or prethrombotic state.

This biochemical description of blood coagulation implies that the process is uniform throughout the body. In fact, the nature of the blood clot varies with the site of injury. In addition, there is little difference between hemostatic plugs, which are a physiologic response to injury, and pathologic thrombi. To underscore the similarity, thrombosis is often described as coagulation occurring in the wrong place or at the wrong time. Hemostatic plugs or thrombi that form in veins where blood flow is slow are richly endowed with fibrin and trapped red blood cells and contain relatively few platelets. They are often called red thrombi due to their appearance in surgical and pathologic specimens. The friable ends of these red thrombi, which often form in leg veins, can break off and embolize to the pulmonary circulation. Conversely, clots that form in arteries under conditions of high flow are predominantly composed of platelets and have little fibrin. These white thrombi may readily dislodge from the arterial

wall and embolize to distant sites to cause temporary or permanent ischemia. This is particularly common in the cerebral and retinal circulation and may lead to transient neurologic dysfunction (transient ischemic attacks) including temporary monocular blindness (amaurosis fugax) or strokes. In addition, there is increasing evidence that many episodes of myocardial infarction are due to thrombi which form within atherosclerotic coronary arteries.

CLINICAL EVALUATION

HISTORY Certain elements of the history are particularly useful in determining whether bleeding is due to an underlying hemostatic disorder rather than to a local anatomic defect. One clue is a history of repeated bleeding episodes with common hemostatic stresses such as dental extraction, childbirth, or minor surgery. Bleeding that is sufficiently severe to require a blood transfusion merits special attention. A family history of bleeding and bleeding from multiple sites that cannot be linked to trauma or surgery also suggest a systemic disorder. Since bleeding can be mild, lack of a family history of bleeding does not exclude an inherited hemostatic disorder.

It may be possible to localize the defect to the platelet or plasma coagulation system (Table 54-1). Bleeding from a platelet disorder is usually localized to superficial sites such as the skin and mucous membranes, comes on immediately after trauma or surgery, and is readily controlled by local measures. In contrast, bleeding from

FIGURE 54-4 *The biochemical basis of platelet activation and secretion. Binding of agonists such as thrombin, epinephrine, or collagen sets in motion a chain of events which hydrolyzes membrane phospholipids, inhibits adenylate cyclase, mobilizes intracellular calcium, and phosphorylates critical intracellular proteins. The net result is shape change, movement of granules to the canalicular system, generation of mediators like thromboxane A$_2$, and* granule secretion. Abbreviations—A.C., adenylate cyclase; G, guanine nucleotide binding protein; PIP$_2$, phosphatidylinositol 4,5-biphosphate; PLC, phospholipase C; DAG, diacylglycerol; PLA$_2$, phospholipase A$_2$; PC, phosphatidylcholine; AA, arachidonic acid; CO, cyclooxygenase; AA, arachidonic acid; O$_2$, oxygen; IP$_3$, inositol triphosphate; cAMP, cyclic AMP; Ca-CM, calcium calmodulin complex; MLCK, myosin light chain kinase.

FIGURE 54-5 *A schematic diagram of some of the clinically important coagulation reactions. The unactivated or precursor proteins are indicated by roman numerals, and the active form by the addition of a lower case "a"—a standard convention. Other abbreviations are HMWK, high-molecular-weight kininogen; PK, prekallikrein; PL, phospholipid; TM, thrombomodulin; Ca^{2+}, calcium. There are two independent activation pathways, the* contact system and the tissue factor–mediated or extrinsic system. They both merge at the point of factor X activation and lead to the generation of thrombin, which converts fibrinogen into fibrin. These reactions are regulated by antithrombin, which forms complexes with all of the coagulation protein serine proteases except factor VII, and the protein C–protein S system which inactivates factors V and VIII.

FIGURE 54-6 *The major coagulation reactions are subdivided and depicted in schematic form to emphasize their similarity. They all rely on the formation of surface bound enzyme, cofactor complexes. Abbreviations are PK, prekallikrein; K, kallikrein; HMWK, high-molecular-weight kininogen; TF, tissue factor; Ca^{2+}, calcium; PT, prothrombin; Thr, thrombin. By convention other* coagulation factors are indicated by roman numerals, with a lower case "a" appended to indicate their active form. The ∧∧∧ is used to indicate the Gla (di-γ-carboxyglutamic acid) containing domains of factors VII, IX, X, Xa, and PT which bind calcium and phospholipid. Hatching is used to indicate proteins that adhere to surfaces by hydrophobic interaction.

secondary hemostatic or plasma coagulation defects occurs hours or days after injury and is unaffected by local therapy. Such bleeding most often occurs in deep subcutaneous tissues, muscles, joints, or body cavities.

PHYSICAL EXAMINATION In conjunction with a careful history, physical examination can also be of help in evaluating patients with hemostatic disorders. The most common site to observe bleeding is in the skin and mucous membranes. Collections of blood in the skin are called *purpura* and may be subdivided on the basis of the site of bleeding in the skin. Small pinpoint hemorrhages into the dermis due to the leakage of red cells through capillaries are called *petechiae* and are characteristic of platelet disorders—in particular, severe thrombocytopenia. Larger subcutaneous collections of blood due to leakage of blood from small arterioles and venules are *ecchymoses* (common bruises) or, if somewhat deeper and palpable, *hematomas.* They are also common in patients with platelet defects and result from minor trauma. There are other skin and mucous membrane lesions like dilated capillaries or *telangiectasia* that may cause bleeding without any hemostatic defect. In addition, the loss of connective tissue support for capillaries and small veins that accompanies aging increases the fragility of superficial vessels, such as those on the dorsum of the hand, leading to extravasation of blood into subcutaneous tissue—*senile purpura.* Menorrhagia is a serious problem in women with severe thrombocytopenia or platelet dysfunction. In addition, some patients with primary hemostatic defects, especially von Willebrand's disease, may have recurrent gastrointestinal hemorrhage.

As mentioned previously, bleeding into body cavities, retroperitoneum, and joints is a common manifestation of plasma coagulation defects. Repeated joint bleeding may cause synovial thickening, chronic inflammation, and fluid collections and may erode articular cartilage and lead to chronic joint deformity and limited mobility. Such deformities are particularly common in factor VIII and IX deficiency, the two sex-linked coagulation disorders referred to as the hemophilias. For unclear reasons, hemarthroses are much less common in other plasma coagulation defects. Blood collections in various body cavities or soft tissues can cause secondary necrosis of tissues or nerve compression. Retroperitoneal hematomas can cause femoral nerve compression, and large collections of poorly coagulated blood in soft tissues may occasionally mimic malignant growths— the pseudotumor syndrome. Two of the most life-threatening sites of bleeding are in the oropharynx, where bleeding can compromise the airway, and in the central nervous system. Intracerebral hemorrhage is one of the leading causes of death in patients with severe coagulation disorders.

LABORATORY TESTS The most important screening tests of the primary hemostatic system are (1) a *bleeding time* (a sensitive measure of platelet function) and (2) a *platelet count.* The latter is particularly useful as it is readily available and correlates well with the propensity to bleed. The normal platelet count is 150,000 to 450,000 platelets per cubic millimeter of blood. As long as the count

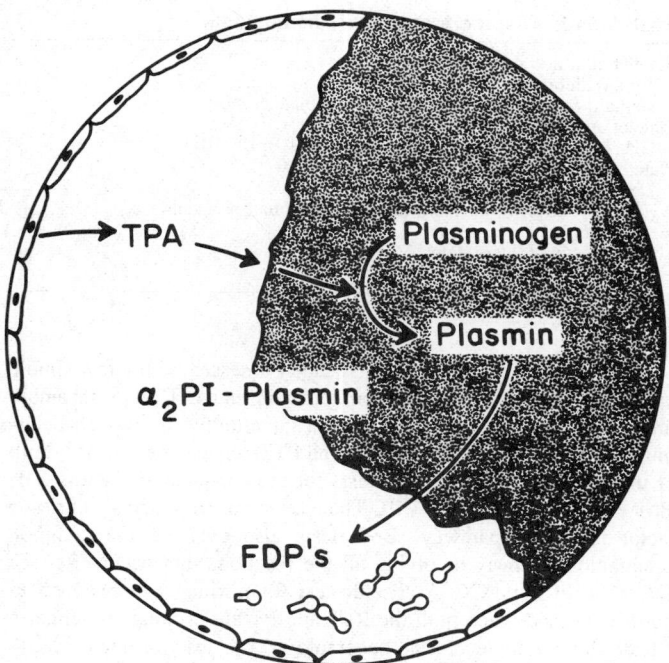

FIGURE 54-7 *A schematic diagram of the fibrinolytic pathway. TPA (tissue plasminogen activator) is released from endothelial cells, enters the fibrin clot, and activates plasminogen to plasmin. Any free plasmin is complexed with a_2 PI (alpha$_2$ plasmin inhibitor). Fibrin is degraded to low-molecular-weight fragments, abbreviated as FDPs, fibrin degradation products.*

is above 100,000 per cubic millimeter, patients are not symptomatic and the bleeding time remains normal. Platelet counts of 50,000 to 100,000 per cubic millimeter cause mild prolongation of the bleeding time so that bleeding occurs only with severe trauma or other stress. Patients with platelet counts less than 50,000 per cubic millimeter have easy bruising, which is manifested by skin purpura with minor trauma and bleeding after mucous membrane surgery. Patients with a platelet count below 20,000 per cubic millimeter have an appreciable incidence of spontaneous bleeding, usually have petechiae, and may have intracranial or other spontaneous internal bleeding. The major causes of thrombocytopenia are outlined in Table 54-2.

Patients with qualitative platelet abnormalities have a normal platelet count and a prolonged bleeding time (Table 54-3). Although any patient with a bleeding time over 10 min has a slightly increased risk of bleeding, the risk does not become great until the bleeding time exceeds 15 or 20 min. When a defect in primary hemostasis is uncovered, specialized testing is needed to determine the cause of the platelet dysfunction (Table 54-3). A precise diagnosis is important since patients with bleeding due to a primary hemostatic disorder may need therapy with platelets, corticosteroids, or plasma fractions, depending on the nature of the disorder.

TABLE 54-1 Differential diagnosis of primary and secondary hemostatic disorders

	Primary hemostasis (platelet defect)	Second hemostasis (plasma proteins)
Onset of bleeding after trauma	Immediate	Delayed—hours or days
Sites of bleeding	Superficial—skin; mucous membranes; nose; gastrointestinal, genetourinary tracts	Deep—joints, muscle, retroperitoneum
Physical findings	Petechiae, ecchymoses	Hematomas, hemarthroses
Family history	Autosomal dominant	Autosomal or X-linked recessive
Response to therapy	Immediate; local measures effective	Requires sustained systemic therapy

TABLE 54-2 Causes of thrombocytopenia

I Decreased marrow production of megakaryocytes
  A Marrow infiltration with tumor, fibrosis
  B Marrow failure—aplastic, hypoplastic anemias
II Splenic sequestration of circulating platelets
  A Splenic hypertrophy—tumor, portal hypertension
III Increased destruction of circulating platelets
  A Nonimmune destruction
    1 Vascular prostheses, cardiac valves
    2 Disseminated intravascular coagulation
    3 Sepsis
    4 Vasculitis
  B Immune destruction
    1 Autoantibodies to platelet antigens
    2 Drug-associated antibodies
    3 Circulating immune complexes—systemic lupus erythematosus, viral agents, bacterial sepsis

TABLE 54-3   Disorders of primary hemostasis

Platelet adhesion defects:
  Von Willebrand's disease
  Bernard-Soulier syndrome (absence of platelet GpIb)*
Platelet aggregation defects:
  Glanzmann's thromboasthenia (absence of BpIIb–IIIa)
Platelet release defects:
  Decreased cyclooxygenase activity
    Drugs—aspirin, nonsteroidal anti-inflammatory agents
    Congenital
  Granule storage pool defects
  Uremia

* Gp = glycoprotein.

Plasma coagulation function is readily assessed with a few simple laboratory tests—the partial thromboplastin time (PTT), prothrombin time (PT), thrombin time (TT), or a quantitative fibrinogen determination (Fig. 54-5, Table 54-4). The PTT screens the intrinsic limb of the coagulation system and tests for the adequacy of factors XII, HMWK, PK, XI, IX, and VIII. The PT screens the extrinsic or tissue factor-dependent pathway. Both tests also evaluate the common coagulation pathway involving all the reactions that occur after the activation of factor X. A specific test for fibrinogen conversion to fibrin is needed when both the PTT and PT are prolonged—either a TT or fibrinogen level can be employed. A test for factor XIII–dependent fibrin cross-linking, such as clot solubility in 5-M urea, should be ordered when the PT and PTT are both normal but there is a strong history of bleeding. The fibrinolytic system can be assessed by measuring the rate of clot lysis with the euglobulin lysis or whole blood clot lysis tests and by measuring the level of alpha₂ plasmin inhibitor. When abnormalities are noted in any of the screening tests, more specific coagulation factor assays can be ordered to determine the nature of the defect.

There are no clinical tests to screen patients suspected of having hypercoagulable or prethrombotic disorders, although tests are being developed in research laboratories which measure small peptides or enzyme-inhibitor complexes generated during coagulation. For example, radioimmunoassays have been developed for fibrinopeptides A and B, for the thrombin-antithrombin complex, and for prothrombin cleavage fragments. Elevated levels of these products have been reported in patients with prethrombotic disorders and in patients with thromboembolism. At present, patients suspected of having a hypercoagulable state, on the basis of clinical information, should have specific assays to screen for the small number of known defects. Currently available tests can identify 10 to 20 percent of the cases of familial thrombosis and represent only a small fraction of the many patients who present to physicians with thromboembolism.

Inhibitor syndromes or circulating anticoagulants are usually due to antibodies which impair coagulation factor activity. They are an infrequent cause of bleeding which require specialized diagnostic testing. Inhibitors are likely when screening test abnormalities cannot be reversed by adding normal plasma to patient plasma. Antibodies against specific coagulation factors may develop in (1) postpartum females; (2) patients with autoimmune disorders such as systemic lupus erythematosus; (3) patients taking drugs like penicillin and streptomycin; and (4) otherwise healthy elderly individuals. In addition, between 10 and 20 percent of patients with severe hemophilia who have received multiple plasma infusions develop inhibitor antibodies. Some patients, especially those with systemic lupus erythematosus may also have a nonspecific form of anticoagulant antibody which interferes with phospholipid binding of coagulation factors and prolongs the PT and PTT but does not cause clinical bleeding. Occasionally, patients develop inhibitors that are not antibodies. For example, several patients with circulating mucopolysaccharides that have heparin-like activity have had clinical bleeding.

REFERENCES

BLOOM AL, THOMAS DP (eds): *Haemostasis and Thrombosis.* London, Churchill-Livingstone, 1981

COLMAN RW et al (eds): *Hemostasis and Thrombosis: Basic Principles and Clinical Practice.* Philadelphia, Lippincott, 1982

HANDIN RI: Hemorrhagic Disorders II. Platelets and purpura, in *Hematology,* 4th ed, W Beck (ed). Cambridge, MIT Press, 1985, pp 433–456

ROSENBERG RD: Hemorrhagic disorders I. Protein interactions in the clotting mechanism, in *Hematology,* 4th ed, W Beck (ed). Cambridge, MIT Press, 1985, pp 401–431

TABLE 54-4   Relationship between secondary hemostatic disorders and coagulation test abnormalities

Prolonged partial thromboplastin time (PTT):
  No clinical bleeding—factors XII, HMWK, PK
  Mild or rare bleeding—factor XI
  Frequent, severe bleeding—factors VIII and IX
Prolonged prothrombin time (PT):
  Factor VII deficiency
  Vitamin K deficiency—early
  Warfarin anticoagulant ingestion
Prolonged PTT and PT:
  Factor II, V, or X deficiency
  Vitamin K deficiency—late
  Warfarin anticoagulant ingestion
Prolonged thrombin time (TT):
  Mild or rare bleeding—afibrinogenemia
  Frequent, severe bleeding—dysfibrinogenemia
  Heparin-like inhibitors or heparin administration
Clot solubility in 5-M urea:
  Factor XIII deficiency
  Inhibitors or defective cross-linking
Rapid clot lysis
  Alpha₂ plasmin inhibitor

NOTE: *HMWK = high-molecular-weight kininogen; PK = prekallikrein.*

---

55   ENLARGEMENT OF LYMPH NODES AND SPLEEN

BARTON F. HAYNES

Lymph nodes and spleen constitute a major portion of the peripheral immune system, and become enlarged in a wide spectrum of infectious, malignant, autoimmune, and metabolic diseases. Enlargement of lymph nodes (lymphadenopathy) and spleen (splenomegaly) are common clinical findings that can lead to a wide range of diagnostic and therapeutic procedures. The goal of this chapter is to serve as an introduction to these two components of the immune system and to highlight clinical features and diagnostic evaluation of some of the diseases in which lymphadenopathy and splenomegaly occur.

LYMPH NODE STRUCTURE AND FUNCTION   Lymph nodes are peripheral lymphoid organs that are connected to the circulation by afferent and efferent lymphatic vessels (Fig. 55-1) and by postcapillary high-endothelial venules. A number of cell types make up the lymph node supportive framework and stroma. Fibroblasts are the predominant cell type in the lymph node capsule and trabeculae. Fibroblast-derived reticular cells are supporting cells found frequently in bone marrow–derived (B) cell areas (follicles and germinal centers) of lymph nodes. Tissue macrophages derived from circulating monocytes are present throughout the normal node. Within cortical areas are interdigitating reticular cells (also called dendritic cells) and Langerhans cells both of which are specialized nonphagocytic, Ia-bearing cells of bone marrow origin that along with macrophages participate in antigen presentation to thymus-derived (T) and B cells (Chap. 62). The outer lymph node cortex contains lymphoid follicles with germinal centers that are the B-cell areas of lymph node (Fig. 55-1). Primary lymphoid follicles are aggregates of IgM- and IgD-bearing B cells and T4⁺ helper (inducer) T cells prior to antigenic challenge. Secondary lymphoid follicles are the result of antigen stimulation, and contain an outer or mantle layer of IgM- and IgD-bearing B cells and an inner zone (germinal center) of activated B cells, macrophages, reticular cells, and scattered T4⁺ helper T cells. Between primary and secondary follicle areas (interfollicular zones) and inner lymph node medullary regions are T-cell (paracortical) areas. The majority of T cells in lymph nodes are T4+ helper T cells (approximately 80 percent) while the minority are T8+ suppressor/cytotoxic T cells (approximately 20 percent).

The two most important factors contributing to the composition and distribution of lymphoid cells within lymph node are (1) generation of memory B and T cells de novo from proliferation of antigen-stimulated percursors within lymph nodes, and (2) selective recirculation to and homing of specific types of lymphoid cells to lymph nodes from the circulation. Traffic through lymph nodes is via two general routes (Fig. 55-1). Afferent lymph, containing lymphocytes, macrophages, and antigens, enters the lymph node via the subcapsular space, and drains through paracortical and medullary areas into medullary sinuses that converge to form efferent lymphatic vessels through which lymph exits. B cells from bone marrow and T cells from the thymus enter lymph nodes from the circulation by binding to specific receptors on cells of postcapillary high-endothelial venules. After activation by antigen and clonal expansion, sensitized T and B cells and antibody-secreting plasma cells leave the node in efferent lymph and rejoin the peripheral blood circulation via the thoracic duct.

Lymph nodes function as sites of macrophage, T-cell and B-cell contact with antigen, with a specialized structure that gives rise to optimal T cell, B cell, and macrophage interactions that result under normal conditions in efficient recognition of antigen, activation of the cellular and humoral arms of the immune response, and ultimate elimination of antigen (see Chap. 62).

Lymph node enlargement can be due to (1) an increase in the number of benign lymphocytes and macrophages during response to antigens, (2) infiltration by inflammatory cells in infections involving lymph nodes (lymphadenitis), (3) in situ proliferation of malignant lymphocytes or macrophages, (4) infiltration of nodes by metastatic malignant cells, or (5) by infiltration of lymph nodes by metabolite-laden macrophages in lipid storage diseases.

In normal immune responses, antigen stimulation of macrophages and lymphocytes in lymph nodes exerts profound influences on lymphocyte traffic. One of the earliest effects of antigen is to increase blood flow through the affected node, which during antigen stimulation may reach 10 to 25 times normal levels. Lymphocytes accumulate in antigen-stimulated nodes by increase in traffic through the node, decreased egress of lymphocytes from antigen-stimulated nodes, and by proliferation of responding T and B cells. A lymph node may thus reach 15 times its normal size 5 to 10 days after antigenic stimulation.

DISEASES ASSOCIATED WITH LYMPHADENOPATHY Under normal conditions in adults, the inguinal lymph nodes may be palpable, and are generally 0.5 cm up to 2 cm in size. Elsewhere in the body, smaller lymph nodes due to past infections may be present normally. Enlargement of lymph nodes requires investigation when there are one or more new nodes present equal to or greater than 1 cm in diameter, and not known to arise from a previously recognized cause. However, this is not a rigid criterion and under certain circumstances new multiple or single smaller lymph nodes may warrant investigation as well. Important factors in assessing the significance of enlarged lymph nodes are (1) the patient's age, (2) the physical characteristics of the lymph node, (3) node locations, and (4) the clinical setting associated with lymphadenopathy. Lymphadenopathy reflects significant disease more often in adults than in children because children are more likely to respond to minor stimuli with lymphoid hyperplasia. Lymphadenopathy in patients under 30 years of age is due to benign causes in approximately 80 percent of cases whereas in patients greater than 50 years of age lymphadenopathy is due to benign causes in only 40 percent of cases.

The physical characteristics of peripheral nodes are important. Nodes of lymphomas tend to be rubbery, firm, matted together, and nontender. Nodes involved with metastatic carcinomas are usually hard and fixed to underlying tissue. In acute infections, nodes are tender, asymmetrically enlarged, matted together, and the overlying skin may be erythematous.

The clinical setting is important in assessing lymphadenopathy. In a young college student with fever and recent onset of lymph node enlargement, infectious mononucleosis syndromes are important to consider. In homosexuals, hemophiliacs, and intravenous drug users with systemic lymphadenopathy, the acquired immunodeficiency syndrome (AIDS) or an AIDS-related complex syndrome should be considered (see Chap. 257).

The location of enlarged lymph nodes may suggest important clues to the diagnosis. Enlarged posterior cervical nodes are frequently present in scalp infections, toxoplasmosis, and rubella, whereas anterior auricular nodes suggest infections of the eyelids and conjunctiva. Lymphomas commonly involve cervical lymph nodes and can occasionally involve posterior auricular and occipital nodes as well. Enlarged suppurative cervical nodes are seen in mycobacterial lymphadenitis (scrofula). Unilateral jugular or mandibular lymph node enlargement suggests lymphoma or nonlymphoid head-and-neck malignancy. Supraclavicular and scalene lymph node enlargement is always significant, and frequently results from metastasis from intrathoracic or gastrointestinal malignancies or from lymphomas. Virchow's node is an enlarged left supraclavicular lymph node infiltrated with metastatic tumor usually from the gastrointestinal tract. Unilateral epitrochlear node enlargement is usually due to hand infections; bilateral epitrochlear node enlargement is seen in sarcoidosis, tularemia, and secondary syphilis.

Unilateral axillary adenopathy can be seen with breast carcinoma, lymphomas, infections of the upper extremities, cat-scratch disease, and brucellosis.

Bilateral inguinal adenopathy can be seen in a variety of venereal infections; however, lymphogranuloma venereum and syphilis are associated with unilateral inguinal adenopathy. Progressive inguinal lymph node enlargement without obvious infection suggests malignant disease. Femoral node involvement has been reported to occur in *Pasteurella pestis* infections and lymphomas.

Symptoms that should raise the suspicion of hilar or mediastinal node enlargement are cough or wheezing due to airway compression, recurrent laryngeal nerve compression with hoarseness, paralysis of the diaphragm, dysphagia with esophageal compression, and swelling of the neck, face, or arms due to superior vena cava or subclavian vein compression. Bilateral mediastinal adenopathy is frequently seen in lymphomas, especially the nodular sclerosing type of Hodgkin's disease. Unilateral hilar adenopathy indicates a high likelihood of metastatic carcinoma (usually lung), while bilateral hilar adenopathy is more often benign and is seen in sarcoidosis, tuberculosis, and systemic fungal infections. Bilateral hilar adenopathy in asymptomatic patients or in association with erythema nodosum or uveitis is almost always due to sarcoidosis (Chap. 270). The association of bilateral

FIGURE 55-1 *Schematic lymph node structure. Lymph flows into nodes via afferent lymphatics (A) and leaves nodes via efferent lymphatics (E). B-cell areas are primary and secondary follicles in lymph node cortex while T cells are concentrated in paracortical areas.*

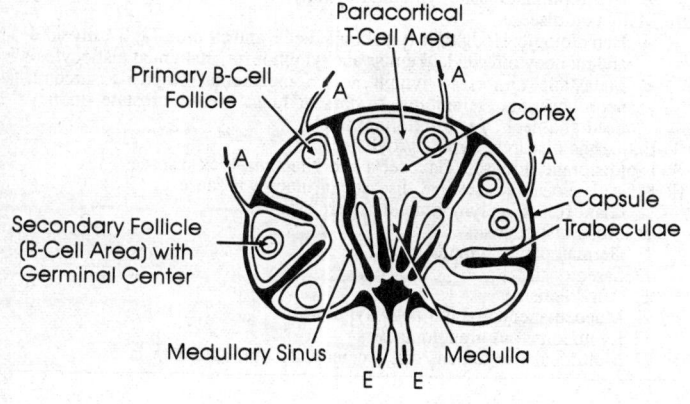

hilar adenopathy with an anterior mediastinal mass, pleural effusion, or pulmonary mass suggests neoplastic disease.

Enlarged retroperitoneal and intraabdominal nodes are not usually inflammatory in origin, but are frequently due to lymphomas or other neoplastic diseases. Tuberculosis can cause mesenteric lymphadenitis with large matted and sometimes calcified nodes.

Some of the diseases associated with lymph node enlargement are listed in Table 55-1 and fall into six general categories: infectious diseases, immunologic diseases, malignant diseases, endocrine diseases, lipid storage diseases, and miscellaneous.

The manifestations of infectious diseases are protean and are best considered according to the type of infectious agent. The most common viral infection associated with systemic lymphadenopathy is Epstein-Barr (EB) virus–associated infectious mononucleosis (see Chap. 138). A variety of other viral diseases including viral hepatitis, cytomegalovirus, rubella, and influenza can cause clinical syndromes similar to those induced by the EB virus. AIDS has recently been shown to be caused by a human retrovirus, human T-cell lymphotropic virus type III (HTLV III), also called lymphadenopathy-associated virus (LAV). In the HTLV III/LAV–associated lymphadenopathy syndrome, cervical, axillary, and occipital nodes are the most commonly involved (see Chap. 257).

Chronic bacterial infections as well as fungal infections may produce considerable lymph node enlargement without signs of local inflammation. Cat-scratch disease is a regional lymphadenitis occurring approximately 2 weeks following a cat scratch or bite. The nodes involved relate to lymph drainage of the wound site with upper extremity adenopathy being the most common, occurring in 50 percent of cases. Fungi associated with primary pulmonary infections (coccidioidomycosis, histoplasmosis) can cause hilar adenopathy. Acute and chronic mycobacterial, parasitic, and spirochetal diseases against which there is a profound cellular and humoral immune response all can result in either systemic or regional enlarged lymph nodes depending on the clinical syndrome in question. Virtually any disease characterized by immune cell activation (systemic lupus erythematosus, rheumatoid arthritis, serum sickness, reactions due to

drugs such as diphenylhydantoin, angioimmunoblastic lymphadenopathy) can be associated with regional or systemic adenopathy. Lymph node enlargement associated with malignant disease may be due to direct node involvement by tumor, lymphoid hyperplasia in response to tumor, or both. Generalized lymphoid hyperplasia may occur with hyperthroidism. Patients with lipid storage diseases such as Gaucher's and Niemann-Pick disease can have enlarged lymph nodes, particularly in the abdomen, due to accumulation of lipid-laden macrophages.

A number of diseases of unknown cause are associated with lymphadenopathy and in many of the diseases in this group, lymphadenopathy is a major manifestation of the disease. Sarcoidosis frequently presents with generalized lymph node enlargement, especially in cervical, inguinal, and epitrochlear areas (Chap. 270). Although giant follicular lymph node hyperplasia can occur in extrathoracic lymph nodes, mediastinal or hilar nodes are involved in 70 percent of cases. In sinus histiocytosis, massive cervical lymph node enlargement often associated with generalized lymphadenopathy occurs and is associated with fever and leukocytosis. Patients with exfoliative dermatitis or other dermatologic syndromes can develop enlarged superficial lymph nodes (called dermatopathic lymphadenitis) which usually regress with resolution of the dermatitis. Lymph node involvement occurs in approximately 30 percent of cases of primary and secondary amyloidosis; only rarely is amyloid lymphadenopathy the major or the only organ involvement. The mechanism of node enlargement in amyloidosis is the accumulation of extracellular masses of amyloid fibrils that compress and eventually obliterate normal lymph node architecture (Chap. 259).

Mucocutaneous lymph node syndrome (Kawasaki's disease) is a systemic lymphadenopathy syndrome, the hallmarks of which are fever, conjunctivitis, erythema of the tongue with protrusion of papillae (strawberry tongue), a truncal exanthem with desquamation of palms and soles, and acute nonsupportive enlargement of cervical lymph nodes (see Chaps. 49 and 269).

Lymphomatoid granulomatosis is a disease characterized by infiltration of various organs (lungs, skin, central nervous system) with an angiocentric and angioinvasive polymorphic cellular infiltrate consisting of atypical lymphocytes and macrophages. The disease has characteristics of both an inflammatory granulomatous process and a lymphoproliferative disease, with progression to frank lymphoma in up to 50 percent of cases. Lymphadenopathy in the prelymphoma state of lymphomatoid granulomatosis occurs in 40 percent of cases affecting primarily intrathoracic nodes while peripheral adenopathy occurs only rarely (10 percent) (see Chap. 269).

Angioimmunoblastic lymphadenopathy is a disease characterized by fever, generalized lymphadenopathy, hepatosplenomegaly, polyclonal hypergammaglobulinemia, and Coombs-positive hemolytic anemia. Although it is not thought to be a malignant disease, it evolves into B-cell lymphoma in 35 percent of patients, (see Chap. 294).

Diseases characterized by benign and malignant proliferation of tissue macrophages (histiocytes) or of specialized bone marrow–derived cells called Langerhans cells have been termed *histiocytoses* or *histiocytosis X*. In the past, these terms encompassed a number of diseases including unifocal and multifocal eosinophilic granuloma, Hand-Schüller-Christian syndrome, Letterer-Siwe disease, and frank neoplasms of undifferentiated histiocytes. Recently, the identification of the Langerhans cell as the predominant cell in forms of eosinophilic granuloma has prompted reevaluation of these syndromes.

One term currently in use for eosinophilic granuloma syndromes is *Langerhans cell (eosinophilic) granulomatosis,* and this term will be used here. The term histiocytosis X is an outmoded term that refers to a spectrum of diseases encompassing both the benign disorder of Langerhans cell (eosinophilic) granulomatosis and malignant lymphomatous disease.

The classic triad of the *Hand-Schüller-Christian syndrome* (exophthalmus, diabetes insipidus, and destructive bone lesions) occurs with 25 percent of cases of multifocal eosinophilic granuloma but also may occur in malignant lymphoma and carcinoma. *Letterer-Siwe*

TABLE 55-1   Diseases associated with lymph node enlargement

I Infectious diseases
  A Viral infections: infectious hepatitis, infectious mononucleosis syndromes (cytomegalovirus, EB virus), AIDS, rubella, varicella–herpes zoster, vaccinia
  B Bacterial infections: streptococci, staphylococci, salmonella, brucella, Francisella tularensis, *Listeria monocytogenes, Pasteurella pestis, Hemophilus ducreyi,* cat-scratch disease
  C Fungal infections: coccidioidomycosis, histoplasmosis
  D Chlamydial infections: Lymphogranuloma venereum, trachoma
  E Mycobacterial infections: tuberculosis, leprosy
  F Parasitic infections: trypanosomiasis, microfilariasis, toxoplasmosis
  G Spirochetal diseases: syphilis, yaws, endemic syphilis (bejel), leptospirosis
II Immunologic diseases
  A Rheumatoid arthritis
  B Systemic lupus erythematosus
  C Dermatomyositis
  D Serum sickness
  E Drug reactions—diphenylhydantoin, hydralazine, allopurinol
  F Angioimmunoblastic lymphadenopathy
III Malignant diseases
  A Hematologic: Hodgkin's lymphoma, acute and chronic T-, B-, myeloid, and monocytoid cell leukemias and lymphomas, malignant histiocytosis
  B Metastatic tumors to lymph nodes: melanoma, Kaposi's sarcoma, neuroblastoma, seminoma, tumors of lung, breast, prostate, kidney, head and neck, gastrointestinal tract
IV Endocrine diseases: hyperthyroidism
V Lipid storage diseases: Gaucher's and Niemann-Pick diseases
VI Miscellaneous diseases and diseases of unknown cause
  A Giant follicular lymph node hyperplasia
  B Sinus histiocytosis
  C Dermatopathic lymphadenitis
  D Sarcoidosis
  E Amyloidosis
  F Mucocutaneous lymph node syndrome
  G Lymphomatoid granulomatosis
  H Multifocal Langerhans cell (eosinophilic) granulomatosis

disease is an acute clinical syndrome of unknown etiology in infants that consists of hepatosplenomegaly, lymphadenopathy, hemorrhagic diathesis, anemia, no familial occurrence, and generalized hyperplasia of tissue macrophages in a variety of organs. It is currently felt that Letterer-Siwe disease represents an unusual form of malignant lymphoma, and is distinct from forms of eosinophilic granuloma.

Histologically, Langerhans cell granulomatosis consists of aggregates of mature eosinophils and Langerhans cells. Langerhans cells are bone marrow–derived cells normally found among epidermal cells of skin and rarely in B-cell areas of lymph node and the medulla of thymus. Langerhans cells contain distinct cytoplasmic granules (Birbeck granules) and contain adenosine triphosphatase and alpha naphthyl acetate esterase. Surface markers of Langerhans cells include class II major histocompatibility complex antigens (Ia-like) and the T6 antigen that is also expressed by the cortical (immature) thymocytes (see Chap. 62).

Unifocal Langerhans cell (eosinophilic) granulomatosis is a benign disease of children and young adults, predominantly in males. Occasionally, it occurs as late as 60 to 70 years of age, and presents as a solitary osteolytic lesion in the femur, skull, vertebrae, ribs, or occasionally the pelvis. Since there are no consistent accompanying laboratory abnormalities, the diagnosis of unifocal Langerhans cell granulomatosis requires biopsy of the lytic bone lesion. Treatment of choice of this condition is excision or curettage of the lesion. Rarely, lesions in inaccessible sites such as cervical vertebrae require moderate doses of irradiation (300 to 600 rads). After initial bone scan and radiographic survey to assess extent of disease, follow-up studies should be performed at 6-month intervals for 3 years. If no additional lesions are present 12 months after diagnosis, development of subsequent lesions is unlikely.

Multifocal Langerhans cell (eosinophilic) granulomatosis also usually presents in childhood, and is characterized by the development of multiple bony lesions at virtually any site—though less commonly in the feet and hands.

Transient or permanent diabetes insipidus due to granulomatous involvement of the hypothalamus occurs in one-third of patients; 20 percent develop hepatomegaly, 30 percent splenomegaly, and one-half of the patients have focal or generalized lymph node involvement. Lesions may also involve the skin, vulva, gingiva, lung, and thymus. Laboratory studies are rarely helpful in the diagnosis of multifocal Langerhans cell granulomatosis, necessitating biopsy of lesions. While generally a benign disease, multifocal Langerhans cell granulomatosis is best treated with low to moderate doses of methotrexate, prednisone, or vinblastine, usually with regression of lesions.

EVALUATION OF THE PATIENT WITH LYMPHADENOPATHY
Good physical examination techniques for palpation and assessment of lymph nodes are essential for providing useful information on which diagnostic and therapeutic decisions can be based. For serial evaluation of nodes, the documentation of each node with regard to size, location, consistency, and mobility at each examination is critical. For cervical nodes the examiner may stand behind or in front of the seated patient to palpate the neck and to examine in sequence the sites of various groups of nodes. Submental nodes are under the chin in the midline and on either side; submandibular nodes are under the jaw near its angle; jugular nodes are along the anterior border of the sternocleidomastoid muscle; supraclavicular nodes are found behind the mid portion of the clavicle. Suboccipital nodes are found in the apex of the posterior cervical triangle, and pre- and postauricular nodes are found in front of and behind the ear pinnae, respectively. Central axillary nodes occur near the middle of the thoracic wall of the axilla; lateral axillary nodes are located near the upper part of the humerus along the axillary vein and are best felt by having the patient's arm elevated. Subscapular nodes can be felt under the anterior edge of the latissimus dorsi muscle, and pectoral nodes are beneath the lateral edge of the pectoralis major muscle. Infraclavicular nodes can be felt under the distal end of the clavicle. Epitrochlear nodes are located approximately 3 cm proximal to the medial humeral epicondyle. Palpation of epitrochlear nodes is best accomplished by palpation across the epitrochlear node area in an anterior to posterior direction. Enlarged abdominal lymph nodes can be difficult to palpate and may only be felt if the patient has a shallow abdominal cavity. Pelvic nodes are best evaluated with deep palpation of the lower abdomen by rolling the extended fingers over the pelvic brim.

The investigation of lymphadenopathy can be organized according to where nodes occur and the type of clinical symptoms present. Enlarged supraclavicular nodes most often result from lymphoma, gastrointestinal, or intrathoracic tumors and should be biopsied. Acute onset of cervical adenopathy in young adults in the absence of head-and-neck infections suggests the diagnosis of infectious mononucleosis syndromes. If localized cervical node enlargement persists and serologic evaluation for EB virus, cytomegalovirus, and toxoplasmosis infections as well as chest x-ray and intermediate-strength PPD skin test are negative, then lymph node biopsy is indicated to seek lymphoma, sarcoidosis, carcinoma, and other diseases listed in Table 55-1.

Unilateral cervical adenopathy warrants a careful ear, nose, and throat examination for malignancy. In the asymptomatic patient with persistent new axillary and/or inguinal adenopathy, a biopsy specimen should be obtained. If fever and constitutional symptoms are present, the cause of infectious mononucleosis–like syndromes should be sought prior to node biopsy.

Generalized lymph node enlargement can be caused by systemic infections, drug reactions, malignancy, or one of the systemic lymphadenopathy syndromes (Table 55-1). History and physical examination can yield clues regarding the possibility of these diagnoses and direct further evaluation (e.g., complete blood count, blood cultures, chest x-ray, serologies, skin tests). If systemic adenopathy persists without an obvious cause being identified, lymph node biopsy is warranted. Once the decision to perform lymph node biopsy has been made, tissue should be processed for culture of appropriate organisms, frozen in liquid nitrogen for lymphocyte typing or other special diagnostic studies for malignant cell types, and processed for routine pathologic evaluation. One can expect information that will lead to a diagnosis in 50 to 60 percent of lymph node biopsies. About 25 percent of patients with nondiagnostic lymph node biopsies will subsequently develop within a year a disease (usually a lymphoma) related to the indication for biopsy. Therefore there should be little hesitation to repeat a nondiagnostic biopsy, especially if enlarged lymph nodes and symptoms persist.

The term *atypical hyperplasia of lymph nodes* refers to neither a clinical nor a pathologic entity, but designates cases in which the pathologist expresses concern about neoplasia and is unable to unequivocally diagnose lymphoma. Since 30 percent of patients whose lymph node biopsies are read as atypical hyperplasia subsequently develop lymphoma, a repeat biopsy is recommended at a later date if node enlargement persists. Needle aspiration biopsy is a safe technique for initial evaluation of superficial adenopathy. While lymph node aspiration can aid in the diagnosis of metastatic tumor and infections, it is rarely helpful in the diagnosis of lymphomas and other hematologic malignancies.

SPLEEN STRUCTURE AND FUNCTION The spleen is a lymphoreticular organ that serves at least four major physiologic functions. First, it is an organ of the immune system and a major site of clearance of microorganisms and particulate antigens from the bloodstream and of generation of humoral or cellular responses to foreign antigens. Second, the spleen is instrumental in sequestration and removal of normal and abnormal blood cells. Third, the vasculature of the spleen plays a role in regulation of portal blood flow. Fourth, while hematopoiesis in the normal adult takes place primarily in the bone marrow, under pathologic conditions when the marrow is replaced or overstimulated to respond, the spleen may become a major site of extramedullary hematopoiesis.

The spleen is arranged into units of areas called red and white pulp (Fig. 55-2). Red pulp contains blood-filled sinuses and pulp

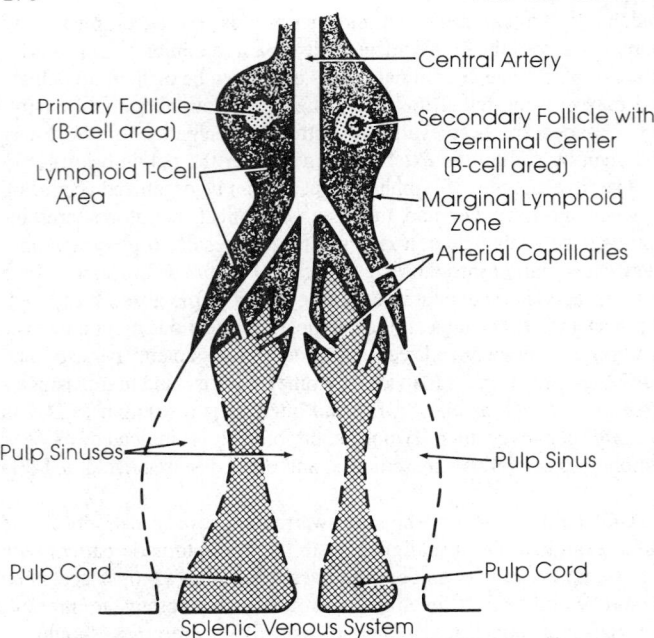

FIGURE 55-2 *Schematic spleen structure. The spleen is made up of multiple units of red and white pulp centered around small branches of the splenic artery called central arteries. White pulp areas of spleen are lymphoid areas while red pulp areas include pulp sinuses and pulp cords. In white pulp, B-cell areas are primary and secondary follicles and the marginal lymphoid zone, while T-cell areas are lymphoid cells around follicles and arterial capillaries. Redrawn with permission from Videbaek et al.*

cords lined by reticuloendothelial cells. White pulp contains centrally located arterioles, surrounded by densely packed small lymphocytes, which are primarily $T4^+$ helper T lymphocytes. Adjacent to the T-cell periarteriolar lymphocyte sheath is the follicular zone of B lymphocytes which also contains germinal centers made up of B cells and macrophages. The outermost portion of white pulp is another B-cell layer called the marginal zone which blends into red pulp areas.

The blood supply and the route of blood flow is unique in the spleen, and splenic anatomy can best be defined in terms of route of blood flow (Fig. 55-2). Blood enters the spleen by the splenic artery. The splenic artery divides into branches which penetrate into the spleen via connective tissue projections called trabeculae and from the trabeculae branch into smaller arteries called central arteries. From central arteries the bloodstream reaches the arterial capillaries. The periarteriolar lymphoid sheaths of T cells surrounding B-cell follicles persist around the arterial vessels until they become small arterioles. Blood in central arterioles empties partly through arterial capillaries directly into splenic venules and then into splenic veins. The central arterioles also empty into macrophage-lined sinuses of red pulp and into the fibrous network of reticuloendothelial cells and tissue macrophages called pulp cords. Blood in red pulp sinuses and pulp cords empties directly into the splenic venous system. During red blood cell passage from central arteries to pulp cords, and finally to spleen sinuses, red cells are concentrated in the macrophage-rich pulp cords. Normally circulating red cells accumulate in pulp cords with subsequent passage through critical small openings of sinus endothelium into red pulp sinuses and on to the splenic venous system. Packing of red cells in pulp cords with subsequent passage through small slits into sinuses is termed *erythrocyte conditioning*. Upon senescence, red cells become less deformable and are unable to pass into sinuses; they are retained in pulp cords and phagocytosed by macrophages—a process termed *culling*. Erythrocyte particulate matter such as nuclear material (Howell-Jolly bodies), denatured hemoglobulin (Heinz bodies), or malaria parasites can be pinched off during passage of red cells from pulp cords into sinuses and retained in the spleen while the rest of the red cell passes back into the circulation—a process termed *pitting*.

Many of the mechanisms of spleen enlargement are exaggerated forms of normal spleen function. While there is a wide variety of diseases associated with enlargement of the spleen, there are six basic pathophysiologic mechanisms of splenic enlargement. (1) Splenic enlargement occurs from reticuloendothelial or immune system hyperplasia in infectious diseases such as bacterial endocarditis or in immune diseases such as Felty's syndrome. Reticuloendothelial hyperplasia also occurs in diseases associated with destruction of abnormal red blood cells such as hereditary spherocytosis, thalassemia, or early in the course of sickle cell disease. (2) Splenic enlargement occurs due to altered splenic blood flow in hepatic cirrhosis or splenic, hepatic, or portal vein thrombosis. (3) Malignant neoplasms can involve the spleen either primarily as with lymphomas or angiosarcomas, or secondarily with leukemias or metastatic solid tumors. (4) Splenic enlargement can occur in situations leading to extramedullary hematopoiesis in the spleen such as in myeloid metaplasia or other myelophthisic syndromes. (5) Infiltration of the spleen with abnormal material in amyloidosis and Gaucher's disease can result in splenomegaly. (6) Splenomegaly can also result from space-occupying lesions such as hemangiomas and cysts.

DISEASES ASSOCIATED WITH SPLENIC ENLARGEMENT A wide variety of diseases lead to an increase in cellularity and vascularity of the spleen (Table 55-2). Increase in cellularity in infections is due to lymphocyte and macrophage proliferation in both red and white pulp areas. Splenomegaly is often present in acute systemic bacterial infections. Infectious granulomas due to mycobacterial and fungal infections occur in both red and white pulp. In diseases associated with disordered immunoregulation such as rheumatoid arthritis and

TABLE 55-2 Diseases associated with enlargement of the spleen

I Infections
  A Infectious mononucleosis
  B Bacterial septicemias
  C Bacterial endocarditis
  D Tuberculosis
  E Malaria
  F Leishmaniasis
  G Trypanosomiasis
  H Acquired immunodeficiency syndrome
  I Viral hepatitis
  J Congenital syphilis
  K Splenic abscess
  L Disseminated histoplasmosis
II Diseases of disordered immunoregulation
  A Rheumatoid arthritis (Felty's syndrome)
  B Systemic lupus erythematosus
  C Immune hemolytic anemias
  D Angioimmunoblastic lymphadenopathy
  E Drug reactions with serum sickness syndromes
  F Immune thrombocytopenias and neutropenias
III Diseases of disordered splenic blood flow
  A Laennec's and postnecrotic cirrhosis
  B Hepatic vein obstruction
  C Hepatic schistosomiasis
  D Portal vein obstruction or cavernous sinus transformation
  E Splenic vein obstruction
  F Chronic congestive heart failure
  G Splenic artery aneurysm
IV Diseases associated with abnormal erythrocytes
  A Spherocytosis
  B Sickle cell disease
  C Ovalocytosis
  D Thalassemia
V Infiltrative diseases of the spleen
  A *Benign*—amyloidosis, Gaucher's disease, Niemann-Pick disease, Hurler's syndrome, Tangier disease, multifocal Langerhans cell (eosinophilic) granulomatosis, extramedullary hematopoiesis, hamartomas, fibromas, hemangiomas, lymphangiomas, splenic cysts
  B *Malignant*—leukemias, lymphomas, Hodgkin's lymphoma, primary splenic tumors, angiosarcomas, metastatic tumors, myeloproliferative syndromes
VI Miscellaneous diseases or diseases of unknown cause
  A Idiopathic splenomegaly
  B Thyrotoxicosis
  C Iron-deficiency anemia
  D Sarcoidosis
  E Berylliosis

systemic lupus erythematosus, splenic enlargement is often due to lymphoid hyperplasia with enlarged lymphoid follicles present in white pulp areas and increased number of plasma cells and macrophages around red pulp arterioles and pulp cords. Splenic enlargement associated with abnormal splenic blood flow is most commonly due to chronic passive congestion from increased portal vein pressure, or from portal vein obstruction. *Banti's syndrome is congestive splenomegaly* with hypersplenism associated with cirrhosis and portal hypertension and is manifested histologically by red pulp congestion with accumulation and concentration of erythrocytes in widened pulp cords and sinuses. In congestive splenomegaly, reticuloendothelial hyperplasia occurs with proliferation of cells lining red pulp cords and sinuses. In splenic enlargement in conditions associated with abnormal erythrocytes such as hereditary spherocytosis, there is pooling of abnormal red cells in sinuses and pulp cords because of increased red cell rigidity and therefore decreased ability to traverse the red pulp sinusoidal endothelium.

Myelosclerosis with myeloid metaplasia is characterized by splenic intrasinusoidal extramedullary hematopoiesis involving all three myeloid cell lines associated with dilated and distended pulp sinuses. In cases of secondary extramedullary hematopoiesis such as in myelophthisic syndromes, extramedullary hematopoiesis may only involve one or two cell lineages, particularly red cells. Infiltrative malignant disease can cause focal or generalized increases in white pulp lymphoid cells as in the case of Hodgkin's disease and lymphocytic lymphoma, or infiltration of red pulp areas with malignant cells as in chronic granulocytic leukemia, acute leukemia syndromes, systemic mast cell disease, and metastatic carcinoma. Infiltrative diseases of the spleen such as Gaucher's and Niemann-Pick disease produce splenic enlargement by increase in number of splenic red pulp histocytes. Thyrotoxicosis can be associated with splenomegaly and is due to thyroid hormone–induced lymphoid hyperplasia. Sarcoidosis causes splenic enlargement by the development of areas of granulomatous inflammation in white pulp lymphoid tissue. A splenic artery aneurysm may cause unexplained splenomegaly, cramping, and left upper abdominal pain; a calcified ring in the splenic area may be seen on x-ray.

The degree of splenomegaly varies with the disease entity. Slight or mild enlargement occurs in chronic passive congestion of the liver due to congestive heart failure, acute malaria, typhoid fever, bacterial endocarditis, systemic lupus erythematosus, rheumatoid arthritis, and thalassemia minor. Moderate splenic enlargement occurs in hepatitis, cirrhosis, lymphomas, infectious mononucleosis, hemolytic anemias, splenic abscesses and infarcts, and amyloidosis. Massive enlargement of the spleen occurs in chronic myelocytic leukemia, agnogenic myeloid metaplasia with myelofibrosis, hairy cell leukemia, Gaucher's and Niemann-Pick diseases, sarcoidosis, thalassemia major, chronic malaria, congenital syphilis, leishmaniasis, and in some cases of portal vein obstruction.

DIAGNOSTIC EVALUATION OF THE PATIENT WITH SPLENIC ENLARGEMENT When normal in size and position, the spleen is generally inaccessible to abdominal palpation. A normal-sized spleen is about 12 cm long and 7 cm wide. Because of the oblique orientation of the spleen to the abdominal cavity, its long axis lies behind and parallel to the tenth rib in the midaxillary line, with splenic width located between the ninth and eleventh ribs. Therefore, to percuss for splenic dullness the patient is placed on the right side and the ninth intercostal space is located by finding the tip of the scapula lying in the seventh intercostal space and counting down to the ninth intercostal space. Dullness outside the ninth and eleventh intercostal spaces suggests splenomegaly, although fluid in the stomach and feces in the colon can cause splenic area dullness as well. Palpation of the left upper quadrant is performed with the patient supine or on the right side by the examiner's right hand; the examiner's left hand is placed under the lower thorax grasping the lower ribs posteriorly. Palpation for spleen enlargement is performed with the patient taking deep breaths to permit the examiner to feel the inferior tip of an enlarged spleen. To avoid missing a massively enlarged spleen, palpation of the left upper quadrant should begin in the lower abdominal cavity with gradual movement up to the left upper quadrant.

Demonstration of mild to moderate splenic enlargement by physical examination may be difficult, particularly in obese patients. Other techniques for assessment of spleen size include ^{99}Tc-colloid liver-spleen scan, computerized axial tomography, and ultrasound scanning of the left upper quadrant. These three techniques can be useful in defining splenic defects such as cysts, infarct, or tumors, or in defining accessory splenic tissue that may be due to congenital accessory spleens or residual foci of splenic tissue following splenic rupture (splenosis).

In the evaluation of the patient with splenomegaly, it is helpful to consider splenomegaly with acute or subacute illnesses separately from splenomegaly with chronic illness. Acute left upper quadrant pain with an enlarged tender spleen suggests subcapsular hematoma, splenic rupture, or splenic infarcts. Rupture of the spleen with splenic hematoma most often follows direct or remote trauma but can occur as well in the setting of infectious diseases such as malaria, typhoid fever, and EB virus–induced infectious mononucleosis. Splenic infarcts due either to in situ red cell sickling (in sickle cell disease) or to emboli (from mural thrombus, atrial myxoma, or cardiac valve vegetation) can usually be detected by spleen scan or arteriogram. More unusual disorders presenting acutely are diffuse splenic metastatic disease and hemorrhage into a splenic cyst.

An acute febrile illness associated with splenomegaly may be due to bacterial endocarditis, infectious mononucleosis syndromes, tuberculosis, and histoplasmosis. Fever, peripheral adenopathy, and splenomegaly, with or without a rash or arthralgias should suggest, in addition to infection mononucleosis, sarcoidosis, Hodgkin's lymphoma, a collagen vascular disease such as systemic lupus erythematosus, or a serum sickness syndrome.

An acute illness with splenomegaly associated with the signs and symptoms of anemia, with or without bleeding, suggests autoimmune hemolytic anemia, myeloproliferative syndromes, or acute leukemia.

Splenomegaly with signs and symptoms of chronic illness suggests a wide range of disorders, many of which are listed in Table 55-2. Liver disease with portal hypertension is a common etiology of splenomegaly in this setting. Patients with congestive splenomegaly from liver disease or portal or splenic vein thrombosis are often asymptomatic. With clinical features of rheumatoid arthritis and leukopenia, Felty's syndrome should be considered. The presence of lymphadenopathy should suggest chronic lymphocytic leukemia or lymphoma. Plethora and an elevated hematocrit suggest polycythemia vera or chronic lung disease, with right heart failure and congestive splenomegaly. Weight loss or other signs of chronic illness suggest leukemia or other myeloproliferative syndromes as well as a variety of hemoglobinopathies. Bone marrow aspiration and biopsy can aid in the diagnosis of leukemia and lymphoma, lipid storage diseases, disseminated fungal or mycobacterial diseases, metastatic malignant diseases, and amyloidosis.

Occasionally laparotomy and splenectomy are indicated in the evaluation of splenomegaly. The decision to perform diagnostic laparotomy in a patient with unexplained splenomegaly is difficult and must take into account the patient's age and clinical signs, symptoms, and laboratory abnormalities present. One study has documented palpable spleens in 3 percent of entering college freshman and no increased risk of any disease during the ensuing 6 years. In another study of older subjects (average age 49) who had undergone splenectomy for undiagnosed splenomegaly and had signs and symptoms of chronic illness, a diagnosis of an underlying disorder was obtained in the majority of patients by splenectomy.

HYPERSPLENISM The term hypersplenism applies to any clinical situation in which the spleen removes excessive quantities of erythrocytes, granulocytes, or platelets from the circulation. General mechanisms of removal of formed blood elements include increased sequestration of cells due to hemodynamic abnormalities of splenic blood flow, or by production of anti-red cell, granulocyte, or platelet antibodies, making the cells vulnerable to clearance by splenic macrophages. Situations in which passive congestion of the spleen occurs produce abnormal sludging of blood in sinuses and red pulp cords. Under these conditions there is plasma pooling, producing marked intrasplenic hemoconcentration and hypoxia, making blood cells more vulnerable to the phagocytic action of pulp cord macrophages. Criteria for diagnosis of hypersplenism include (1) splenomegaly, (2) splenic destruction of one or more cell lines in the peripheral blood, (3) normal or hyperplastic cellularity of bone marrow with normal representation of the cell line deficient in the circulation, and (4) variably, evidence of increased cell turnover in the cell lines affected, i.e., reticulocytosis, increased band forms of neutrophils, or circulating immature platelet forms.

Therapy for hypersplenism relates in large part to the underlying disease or the underlying pathophysiologic process. If the underlying disorder responsible for hypersplenism cannot be corrected, splenectomy is an option for cases in which a severe deficit is present (see below for indications for splenectomy).

HYPOSPLENISM The terms hyposplenia or asplenia are used to indicate diminished or absent splenic function. The usual causes of hyposplenism are splenectomy, congenital absence of the spleen, sickle cell anemia in patients older than 5 years (with autosplenectomy due to repeated infarcts), and splenic irradiation. In sickle cell anemia, persistence of a palpable spleen after age 5 suggests coexisting alpha thalassemia. Findings in the peripheral blood that indicate diminished splenic function include the presence of nucleated red cells, erythrocyte Howell-Jolly bodies, erythrocyte Heinz bodies, as well as target and burr forms of red cells.

Splenectomized patients or patients with functional asplenia (such as in sickle cell disease) are prone to bacterial infections, which are frequently overwhelming and life-threatening, particularly with encapsulated organisms such as *Streptococcus pneumoniae, Neisseria meningitidis, Escherichia coli*, and *Haemophilus influenzae*. This is due to a reduction or absence of the filtration function of the spleen for clearance of antibody-coated bacteria as well as to decreased production of IgG and IgM antibodies (opsonins) needed to bind bacteria. Immunization with pneumococcal vaccine is recommended in patients older than 2 years with hyposplenism and prior to elective splenectomy. The presence of peripheral blood manifestations of hyposplenism (Howell-Jolly bodies) in the presence of a normal-sized or enlarged spleen suggests the presence of splenic infiltrative disease such as a primary splenic angiosarcoma.

INDICATIONS FOR SPLENECTOMY Splenic trauma, whether accidental blunt trauma or intraoperative iatrogenic injury, is the most common indication for splenectomy. En bloc removal of the spleen may be indicated either because of tumor involvement or for a splenorectal shunt. Staging laparotomy with splenectomy remains a major diagnostic procedure for many early stage Hodgkin's disease patients being considered for radiation therapy alone. Splenectomy for selected patients with idiopathic splenomegaly is often necessary when other investigations fail to produce a diagnosis; however, the spleen should not be removed simply because it is palpable. Hypersplenism in lymphomas can cause persistent cytopenias and in select cases responds to splenectomy. B-cell hairy cell leukemia frequently presents with hypersplenism, and splenectomy is often beneficial, producing remission in the majority of cases with a 5-year survival of 50 percent.

Felty's syndrome (rheumatoid arthritis and hypersplenism) and Gaucher's disease both require splenectomy when splenomegaly leads to symptomatic neutropenia or other complications of hypersplenism. Immune thrombocytopenic purpura which persists after trials of medical therapy may benefit from splenectomy (see Chap. 279). Of the hemolytic anemias, hereditary spherocytosis, hereditary elliptocytosis, immune hemolytic anemia with warm-reacting IgG antibody, and pyruvate-kinase deficiency have been improved by splenectomy. Splenectomy is usually necessary late in the course of thalassemia major when neutropenia or thrombocytopenia develops, or when transfusion requirements double. Chronic lymphocytic leukemia (CLL),

chronic granulocytic leukemia, and agnogenic myeloid metaplasia may be complicated by symptomatic hypersplenism or, in the case of CLL, immune hemolytic anemia and thrombocytopenia, often necessitating splenectomy. (Chaps. 289 and 292.)

REFERENCES

Lymph node enlargement

BUTCHER E, WEISSMAN I: Lymphoid tissues and organs in *Fundamental Immunology*, WE Paul (ed). New York, Raven, 1984, pp 109–127

GREENFIELD S, JORDAN MC: The clinical investigation of lymphadenopathy, in primary care practice. JAMA 240:1388, 1978

IOACHIM HL: *Lymph Node Biopsy*. Philadelphia, Lippincott, 1982

LENNERT K, STEIN H: The germinal center, in *Morphology, Histochemistry, and Immunohistology in Lymphoproliferative Diseases of Skin*, M Goos, E Christopher (eds). Berlin, Heidelberg, New York, Springer-Verlag, 1982

LIEBERMAN PH et al: A reappraisal of eosinophilic granuloma of bone, Hand-Schüller-Christian syndrome, and Letterer-Siwe syndrome. Medicine 48:375, 1969

NATHWANI BN et al: Malignant lymphoma arising in angioimmunoblastic lymphadenopathy. Cancer 41:578, 1978

POPPEMA S et al: Distribution of T cell subsets in human lymph nodes. J Exp Med 153:30, 1981

SCHROER KR, FRANSSILA KO: Atypical hyperplasia of lymph nodes: A follow-up study. Cancer 44:1155, 1979

SINCLAIR S et al: Biopsy of enlarged, superficial lymph nodes. JAMA 228:602, 1974

THOMAS JA et al: Combined immunological and histochemical analysis of skin and lymph node lesions in histiocytosis X. J Clin Pathol 35:327, 1982

WINTERBAUER RH et al: A clinical interpretation of bilateral hilar adenopathy. Ann Intern Med 78:65, 1973

YEN-TSU N et al: Lymph node biopsy for diagnosis: A statistical study. J Surg Oncol 14:53, 1980

Splenic enlargement

BUTLER JJ: Pathology of the spleen in benign and malignant conditions. Histopathology 7:453, 1983

EICHNER ER, WHITFIELD CL: Splenomegaly: An algorithmic approach to diagnosis. JAMA 246:2858, 1981

ENRIQUEZ E, NEIMAN RS (eds): *The Pathology of the Spleen: A Functional Approach*. Chicago, American Society of Clinical Pathologists, 1976

HERMANN RE et al: Splenectomy for the diagnosis of splenomegaly. Ann Surg 168:896, 1964

LEWIS SM (ed): *Clinics in Haematology*, vol 12: *The Spleen*. London, Saunders, 1983, pp 361–608

McINTYRE OR, EBAUGH FG: Palpable spleens in college freshmen. Ann Intern Med 66:301, 1967

STEINBERG MH et al: Evidence of hyposplenism in the presence of splenomegaly. Scand J Haematol 31:437, 1983

VIDEBAEK A et al: *The Spleen in Health and Disease*. Chicago, Yearbook, 1982

---

56 DISORDERS OF PHAGOCYTIC CELLS

JOHN I. GALLIN

Leukocytes are the major cellular components of inflammatory and immune responses and include neutrophils, lymphocytes, monocytes, eosinophils, and basophils. The blood is the most readily obtainable source of leukocytes and serves as the vehicle for their delivery to the various tissues from the bone marrow, where they are produced. Normal blood leukocyte counts in adults range from 4.5 to 11 × 10⁶ cells per cubic millimeter; a table of normal values for different ages can be found in the Appendix. The most prevalent cells are neutrophils (54 to 62 percent), followed by lymphocytes (25 to 33 percent), monocytes (3 to 7 percent), eosinophils (1 to 3 percent), and basophils (0 to 0.75 percent). The various leukocytes are thought to derive from a common stem cell in the bone marrow. Three-fourths of the nucleated cells of bone marrow are committed to the production of leukocytes. Leukocyte maturation in the marrow is generally thought to be under the regulatory control of a number of different factors which are incompletely defined. Because an alteration in the number and type of leukocytes is a frequent association with disease processes, a total white blood count (WBC) (cells per cubic millimeter) and differential counts are obtained frequently. The lymphocytes and basophils are discussed elsewhere. This chapter focuses on the neutrophils, monocytes, and eosinophils.

NEUTROPHILS

MATURATION Important events in the neutrophil life are summarized in Fig. 56-1. In normal humans neutrophils are only produced in the bone marrow. Best estimates indicate that the appropriate number of stem cells necessary to support hematopoiesis is between 400 and 500. There is convincing evidence that human blood monocytes and tissue macrophages produce colony-stimulating factors, hormone(s) required for the growth of monocytes and neutrophils in the bone marrow. The hematopoietic system not only produces enough neutrophils (approximately 1.3×10^{11} cells per 80-kg person per day) to carry out physiologic functions but also has a large reserve stored in the marrow which can be mobilized in response to inflammation or infection. An increase in the number of blood neutrophils is called *neutrophilia*, and the presence of immature cells is termed a "shift to the left." A diminution in the number of blood neutrophils is referred to as *neutropenia*.

Neutrophils evolve from pluripotent stem cells. The final stages of hematopoiesis are characterized by the appearance of cells with distinct morphologic features. The myeloblast is the first recognizable precursor cell and is followed by the *promyelocyte*. The promyelocyte evolves when the classic lysosomal granules, called the *primary* or *azurophil granules*, are produced. The primary granules contain hydrolases, elastase, myeloperoxidase, and cationic proteins. The promyelocyte divides to produce the *myelocyte*, a cell responsible for the synthesis of the *specific* or *secondary granules* which contain unique (specific) constituents such as lactoferrin, vitamin B_{12}–binding proteins, and probably cytochrome b, histaminase, and receptors for certain chemoattractants and adherence promoting factors. The secondary granules do not contain acid hydrolases and therefore are not classic lysosomes. They are readily released extracellularly, and their mobilization is probably important in modulating inflammation. During the final stages of maturation there is no cell division and the cell passes through the *metamyelocyte* stage and then to the *band* neutrophil with a sausage-shaped nucleus. As the band cell matures the nucleus assumes a lobulated configuration.

In settings of severe acute bacterial infection, prominent neutrophil cytoplasmic granules called *toxic granulations* are occasionally seen. Toxic granulations are thought to be immature or abnormally staining azurophil granules. Cytoplasmic inclusions (*Doehle bodies*) can also be seen during infection and probably represent fragments of endoplasmic reticulum. Large neutrophil vacuoles are often present in acute bacterial infection and probably represent pinocytosed (internalized) membrane.

Neutrophils have long been thought to be a homogeneous population of cells. However, studies of neutrophil function have suggested they are heterogeneous. Recently monoclonal antibodies have been developed that recognize only a subset of mature neutrophils. The meaning of neutrophil heterogeneity is not known.

MARROW RELEASE AND CIRCULATING COMPARTMENTS Specific signals, including interleukin 1 (endogenous pyrogen) or the complement fragment C3e, mobilize leukocytes from the bone marrow and deliver them to the blood in an unstimulated state. Under normal conditions about 90 percent of the neutrophil pool is in the bone marrow, 2 to 3 percent in the circulation, and the remainder in the tissues. The blood pool exists as two compartments: the marginated pool adherent to endothelial cells and the freely flowing circulating pool. In response to chemotactic stimuli from tissues (e.g., the complement product C5a, the arachidonic acid derivative leukotriene B_4, or the bacterial product N-formylmethionylleucylphenylalanine), neutrophil adhesiveness increases and the circulating cells aggregate to each other and adhere to the endothelium. An increased expression of a glycoprotein receptor for C3bi (also called CR3) appears to be intimately involved with the increased adhesion. Receptors for chemoattractants and opsonins are probably also mobilized; the cells orient toward the chemoattractant source in the extravascular space, increase their motile activity (chemokinesis), and migrate with direction (chemotaxis) into tissues. The process of migration into tissues is called *diapedesis* and involves the crawling of neutrophils between postcapillary endothelial cells which open junctions between adjacent cells to permit leukocyte passage. The endothelial responses (increased blood flow secondary to increased vasodilation and permeability) are mediated by anaphylatoxins (e.g., complement products C3a and C5a) as well as vasodilators such as bradykinin and prostaglandins E and I. In the healthy adult most neutrophils leave the body by migration through the mucous membrane of the gastrointestinal tract. Normally neutrophils spend a relatively short time in the circulation with a half-life of 6 to 7 h. Once in the tissues neutrophils release enzymes such as collagenase and elastase, which may help establish abscess cavities. Neutrophils ingest (phagocytose) pathogenic materials that have been properly altered (opsonized) by substances such as immunoglobulin G (IgG) and the complement product C3b. Fibronectin and the tetrapeptide tuftsin facilitate the phagocytic process.

Concomitant with phagocytosis there is a burst of oxygen consumption and activation of the hexosemonophosphate shunt. Nicotinamide-adenine dinucleotide phosphate (NADPH) oxidase is activated, and through a complex enzyme system containing flavoproteins and cytochrome b, toxic oxygen products (e.g., hydrogen peroxide and hydroxyl radical) are generated. Hydrogen peroxide + chloride + neutrophil myeloperoxidase provide a particularly toxic system that generates hypochlorous acid, hypoclorite, and chlorine. These products oxidize and halogenate microorganisms and tumor cells and when uncontrolled, can damage host tissue. Strongly cationic proteins also participate in microbial killing, and other enzymes, such as lysozyme and acid proteases, help digest microbial debris. After 1 to 4 days in tissues neutrophils die. The second wave of inflammation,

FIGURE 56-1 *Schematic diagram of the life cycle of the neutrophil.*

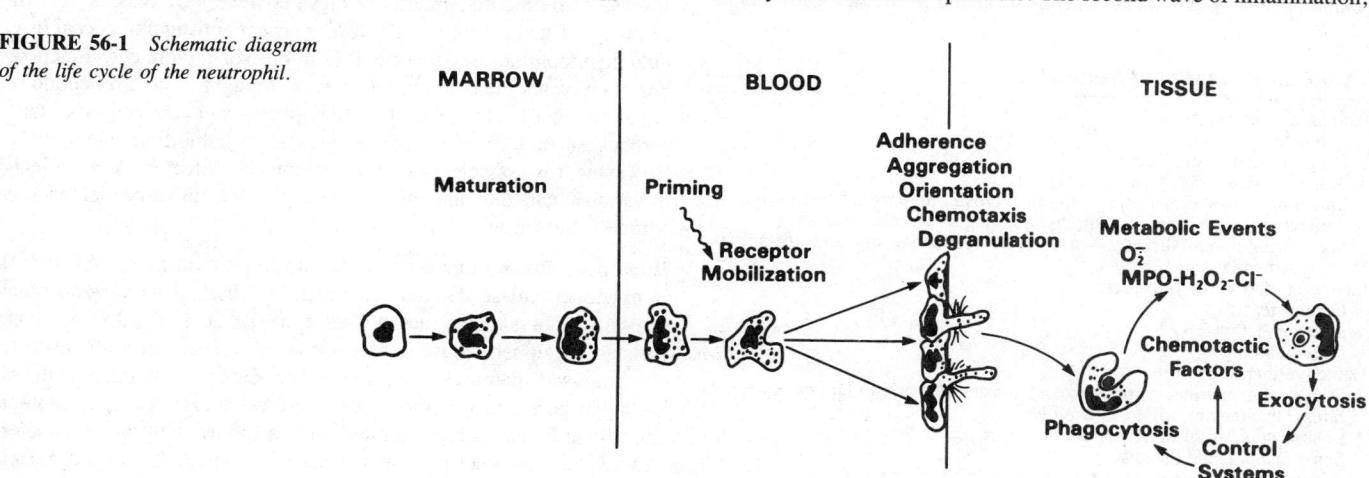

TABLE 56-1 Causes of neutropenia

Decreased production:
Hematologic diseases—idiopathic, cyclic neutropenia, Chédiak-Higashi syndrome, aplastic anemia, infantile genetic disorders
Drug-induced—alkylating agents (nitrogen mustard, busulfan, chlorambucil, cyclophosphamide); antimetabolites (methotrexate, 6-mercaptopurine, 5-flurocytosine); noncytotoxic agents [antibiotics (chloramphenicol, penicillins, sulfonamides), phenothiazines, tranquilizers (meprobamate), certain diuretics, anti-inflammatory agents, antithyroid drugs, many others]
Tumor invasion, myelofibrosis
Nutritional deficiency—vitamin B_{12}, folate (especially alcoholics)
Infection—tuberculosis, typhoid fever, brucellosis, tularemia, measles, infectious mononucleosis, malaria, viral hepatitis, leishmaniasis
Peripheral destruction:
Antineutrophil antibodies and/or splenic trapping:
Autoimmune disorders—Felty's syndrome
Drugs—aminopyrine, α-methyldopa, phenylbutazone, mecurial diuretics, some phenothiazines
Peripheral pooling:
Overwhelming bacterial infection
Hemodialysis
Cardiopulmonary bypass

monocyte accumulation, occurs within 6 to 12 h of initiation of inflammation. Neutrophils, monocytes, microorganisms in various states of digestion, and altered local tissue cells make up pus, which derives its characteristic green color from myeloperoxidase. Myeloperoxidase and other factors may be important in turning off the inflammatory process by inactivating chemoattractants and immobilizing phagocytic cells.

NEUTROPHIL DYSFUNCTION A defect anywhere in the neutrophil life cycle summarized in Fig. 56-1 can lead to dysfunction and compromised host defenses. The clinical result is often recurrent and severe bacterial and fungal infections creating novel and often difficult management problems.

Neutropenia The consequences of absent neutrophils represent a dramatic demonstration of their importance in host defense. When the neutrophil count is below 1000 per cubic millimeter, there is an increased risk for infection (Chap. 84); when there are fewer than 200 cells per cubic millimeter, the inflammatory process is absent. The causes of neutropenia are multiple and are related to depressed production, peripheral destruction, and peripheral pooling (Table 56-1).

In the newborn severe neutropenia may be seen in the setting of acute bacterial or viral infection and is due to the infant's poor bone marrow reserve. Congenital forms of neutropenia exist and include Kostmann's syndrome (less than 100 neutrophils per cubic millimeter), which is often fatal; more benign chronic idiopathic neutropenia (300 to 1500 neutrophils per cubic millimeter); the hair-cartilage-hypoplasia syndrome; Shwachman syndrome associated with pancreatic insufficiency; and neutropenias associated with other immune defects (X-linked agammaglobulinemia, ataxia-telangiectasia, IgA deficiency). Cyclic neutropenia, an autosomal dominant trait, may occur in infancy. Maternal factors associated with neutropenia in the newborn include

TABLE 56-2 Causes of neutrophilia

Increased production:
Idiopathic
Drug-induced—corticosteroids
Infection—bacterial, fungal, rarely viral
Inflammation—thermal injury, tissue necrosis, myocardial and pulmonary infarction, hypersensitivity diseases, collagen vascular diseases
Myeloproliferative diseases—myelocytic leukemia, myeloid metaplasia, polycythemia vera
Increased marrow mobilization:
Corticosteroids
Acute infection
Inflammation
Defective margination:
Drugs—epinephrine, corticosteroids, nonsteroidal anti-inflammatory agents
Stress, excitement, vigorous exercise
Leukocyte C3bi receptor deficiency
Some chemotactic defects

transplacental transfer of IgG directed against antigens on fetal neutrophils and drugs (e.g., thiazide) ingested during pregnancy.

The presence of immunoglobulin (IgG) directed toward neutrophils is seen in Felty's syndrome (triad of rheumatoid arthritis, splenomegaly, and neutropenia) (Chap. 263). Patients with Felty's syndrome who respond to splenectomy with an increase in their neutrophil count lower their postoperative serum granulocyte-binding IgG, suggesting that one beneficial effect of splenectomy is reduction in antineutrophil antibody. Drugs that produce neutropenia by increased destruction or sequestration appear to act by serum antibody interaction with drug (antigen) absorbed to the neutrophil. The drugs that cause neutropenia by this mechanism have varying latent periods for their toxicity, although following drug rechallenge neutropenia occurs within hours.

Neutrophilia Neutrophilia results from increased production, marrow release, or defective margination (Table 56-2). Increased production is associated with chronic inflammation or infection and certain myeloproliferative diseases. Increased marrow release is induced by corticosteroids. Release of epinephrine, as with vigorous exercise, excitement, or stress, will demarginate neutrophils and double the neutrophil count. Leukocytosis to 10,000 to 25,000 cells per cubic millimeter occurs in response to infection or other forms of acute inflammation and results from both release of the marginated pool and mobilization of marrow reserves. Persistent neutrophilia of 30,000 to 50,000 cells per cubic millimeter or greater is called a *leukemoid reaction*, a term often used to distinguish this degree of neutrophilia from leukemia. In a leukemoid reaction the circulating neutrophils are usually mature.

ABNORMAL NEUTROPHIL FUNCTION Congenital deficiencies and acquired abnormalities of phagocyte function are described in Table 56-3. The resulting diseases are best considered in terms of the functional defects of adherence, chemotaxis, and microbicidal activity. The distinguishing features of the important congenital lesions are shown in Table 56-4, several of which are discussed below.

C3bi (CR3) receptor deficiency Patients with congenitally (autosomal recessive) abnormal phagocyte adherence lack the plasma membrane receptor for the fragment of the third complement component called C3bi (CR3 by other terminology). Clinically most patients with this syndrome have recurrent bacterial and fungal infections, severe periodontal disease, persistent leukocytosis (15,000 to 20,000 neutrophils per cubic millimeter), and usually a history of delayed separation of the umbilical stump. Neutrophils (and monocytes) from these patients have defective adherence, spreading, aggregation, and chemotaxis.

Hyperimmunoglobulin E–recurrent infection (Job's) syndrome Abnormal neutrophil and monocyte chemotaxis occurs in the hyperimmunoglobulin E–recurrent infection (Job's) syndrome. These patients have recurrent infections with *Staphylococcus aureus* (Chap. 84), and often have characteristically coarse facies, "cold" cutaneous abscesses, dermatitis, markedly elevated levels of plasma IgE including antistaphylococcal IgE, low or absent antistaphylococcal IgA, mild eosinophilia, and abnormal T-suppressor lymphocyte function. For many years the cold abscesses were thought to be a reflection of impaired chemotaxis with too few phagocytes arriving too late, perhaps secondary to a lymphocyte factor inhibiting chemotaxis. However, it is now clear that the chemotactic defect in these patients is variable and the fundamental basis for the impaired defenses is complex and inadequately delineated.

Myeloperoxidase deficiency The most common neutrophil defect is myeloperoxidase deficiency, which is inherited as an autosomal recessive trait and has an incidence of about 1 in 2000 persons. Isolated myeloperoxidase deficiency is not associated with severely compromised defenses, because other defense systems such as hydrogen peroxide generation are accelerated. However, if another underlying defect in host defense, such as poorly controlled diabetes mellitus, accompanies myeloperoxidase deficiency, then host defenses

TABLE 56-3 Types of neutrophil dysfunction

Function	Drug-induced	Acquired disease	Congenital disorder
Adherence-aggregation	Aspirin; colchicine; alcohol; corticosteriods; ibuprofen; piroxicam	Neonates, hemodialysis	C3bi receptor deficiency
Deformability		Leukemia, neonates, diabetes mellitus, immature neutrophils	
Chemokinesis-chemotaxis	Corticosteroids (high-dose); auranofin; colchicine (weak effect); phenylbutazone, naproxen; indomethacin	Thermal injury; malignancy; malnutrition; periodontal disease; neonates; systemic lupus erythematosus; rheumatoid arthritis; diabetes mellitus; sepsis; influenza virus infection; herpes simplex virus infection; acrodermatitis enteropathica; Down's syndrome; α-Mannosidase deficiency; severe combined immunodeficiency; Wiskott-Aldrich syndrome	Hyper IgE–recurrent infection (Job's) syndrome; Chédiak-Higashi syndrome; specific granule deficiency
Microbicidal activity	Colchicine; cyclophosphamide; corticosteroids (high-dose)	Leukemia; aplastic anemia; certain neutropenias; tuftsin deficiency; thermal injury; sepsis; neonates; diabetes mellitus; malnutrition	Chédiak-Higashi syndrome; specific granule deficiency; chronic granulomatous diseases

are likely to be significantly compromised. An acquired form of myeloperoxidase deficiency occurs in myelomonocytic leukemia and acute myeloblastic leukemia. In acute myelogenous leukemia, pink-staining, apparently aberrant large primary granules, called Auer bodies, are seen.

Chédiak-Higashi syndrome (CHS) CHS is a rare disease with autosomal recessive inheritance characterized clinically by recurrent pyogenic infections (Chap. 84), periodontal disease, partial oculo-cutaneous albinism, nystagmus, and progressive peripheral neuropathy. About 50 percent of the patients develop a lymphomatous (accelerated) phase of the disease at adolescence. Neutrophils and all cells containing lysosomes from patients with CHS characteristically have large granules. CHS neutrophils and monocytes have impaired chemotaxis and abnormal rates of microbial killing due to slow rates of fusion of the lysosomal granules with phagosomes.

Chronic granulomatous diseases Chronic granulomatous disease (CGD) represents a group of patients with disorders of neutrophil and monocyte oxidative metabolism. Although CGD is rare, occurring in about one in 1 million individuals, it is an important model of defective neutrophil oxidative metabolism. Most often CGD is inherited as an X-linked recessive pattern, although in 15 percent of patients the disease is inherited with an autosomal recessive pattern

and an autosomal dominant pattern has been reported in one family. Leukocytes from patients with CGD have severely diminished hydrogen peroxide production. Defects anywhere in the leukocyte's hexose-monophosphate shunt or the NADPH oxidase enzyme system can lead to clinical disease. Patients with CGD characteristically have increased infection with catalase-positive microorganisms (organisms which destroy their own hydrogen peroxide). These patients have an increased propensity to infection with such microorganisms as *Staphylococcus aureus*, *Escherichia coli*, *Serratia marcescens*, *Chromobacterium violaceum*, *Nocardia*, and certain fungi (*Aspergillus* and *Candida albicans*) (Chap. 84). They do not have an increased incidence of infection with catalase-negative microorganisms such as *Streptococcus pneumoniae*. When patients with CGD become infected, they often have extensive inflammatory reactions and lymph node suppuration is common despite the administration of appropriate antibiotics. Aphthous ulcers, gingivitis, and chronic inflammation of the nares are usually present. Granulomas are frequent and can obstruct the gastrointestinal or genitourinary tracts. The excessive inflammatory reactions probably reflect abnormal turnoff of inflammation by failure to degrade chemoattractants and antigens which cause persistent neutrophil accumulation. Impaired killing of intracellular microorganisms by macrophages may lead to persistent cell-mediated immunity and granuloma formation. Surgery is required for thorough drainage of abscesses in the lung, liver, and bones.

TABLE 56-4 Distinguishing features of congenital phagocyte dysfunction syndromes

Disease	Defect	Clinical manifestations
C3bi receptor deficiency	Adherence, aggregation, spreading, chemotaxis, leukemoid reaction	Delayed separation of umbilical stump, depressed inflammation, bacterial infections, gingivitis, periodontal disease
Hyperimmunoglobulin E–recurrent infection (Job's) syndrome	Variable chemotactic defects, very high IgE with anti-*S. aureus* IgE; low anti-*S. aureus* IgA	"Coarse" facies in most patients, "cold" cutaneous abscesses; recurrent pulmonary, bone, upper airway infections with *S. aureus* or *Haemophilus influenza;* mild eosinophilia; mucocutaneous candidiasis
Myeloperoxidase deficiency	Absent myeloperoxidase	Minimal unless another defect, then *Candida albicans* or other fungal infections
Chédiak-Higashi syndrome	Giant lysosomal granules; neutropenia, chemotaxis, degranulation, microbicidal activity, excess O_2 consumption and H_2O_2 production	Recurrent pyogenic infections, especially with *S. aureus;* many patients get lymphomatous-like illness during adolescence; periodontal disease; partial oculocutaneous albinism, nystagmus, progressive peripheral neuropathy
Specific granule deficiency	Absent specific granules; chemotaxis, O_2^- production, bactericidal activity decreased	Recurrent cutaneous, ear, and pulmonary bacterial infections; diminished inflammation
Chronic granulomatous disease	H_2O_2 production absent in neutrophils and monocytes; defective "turn-off" of inflammation	Severe infections of skin, ears, lungs, liver, bone with catalase (+) microorganisms such as *S. aureus, Pseudomonas cepacia, Aspergillus* sp, *Chromobacterium violaceum;* often hard to culture organism; excessive inflammation with granulomas; frequent lymph node suppuration; granulomas can obstruct gastrointestinal or genitourinary tracts; gingivitis, aphthous ulcers

MONONUCLEAR PHAGOCYTES

The mononuclear phagocyte system is defined as a continuum linking monoblasts, promonocytes, and monocytes with the structurally diverse tissue macrophages which make up what was previously referred to as the reticuloendothelial system. Macrophages are long-lived phagocytic cells capable of many of the functions of neutrophils. They are important secretory cells that, through their receptors and secretory products, participate in many complex immunologic and inflammatory processes not attributed to neutrophils. Monocytes leave the circulation by diapedesis more slowly than neutrophils and have a half-life in the blood of 12 to 24 h.

After blood monocytes arrive in the tissues, they differentiate into macrophages with specialized functions suited for specific anatomic locations. Alveolar macrophages, liver Kupffer cells, splenic macrophages, peritoneal macrophages, bone marrow macrophages, lymphatic macrophages, brain microglial cells, and dendritic macrophages all have specialized functions. Macrophage secreted products include lysozyme, neutral proteases, acid hydrolases, arginase, numerous complement components, enzyme inhibitors (plasmin, α_2-macroglobulin), binding proteins (transferrin, fibronectin, transcobalamin II), nucleosides, and interleukin 1 (pyrogen). Interleukin 1 (see Chap. 9) has many important functions including stimulating the hypothalamus to initiate fever, mobilizing leukocytes from the bone marrow, as well as activating lymphocytes and neutrophils. Other macrophage secreted products include reactive oxygen metabolites, bioactive lipids (arachidonate metabolites and platelet activating factors), a neutrophil chemoattractant, factors regulating synthesis of proteins by other cells, bone marrow colony-stimulating factors, factors stimulating fibroblast and microvasculature proliferation as well as factors inhibiting replication of lymphocytes, tumors, viruses, and certain bacteria (Listeria monocytogenes). Macrophages are key effector cells in the elimination of intracellular microorganisms. Their ability to fuse to form giant cells which coalesce into granulomas in response to some inflammatory stimuli is important in the elimination of intracellular microbes and may be under the control of γ-interferon.

Macrophages play an important role in the immune response (see Chap. 62). They process antigen for presentation to lymphocytes, their secreted products modulate lymphocyte function, and macrophages participate in autoimmune phenomena by removing immune complexes and other immunologically active substances from the circulation. Furthermore, they play a role in wound healing, in the disposal of senescent cells, and in the development of atheromas.

DISORDERS OF THE MONONUCLEAR PHAGOCYTE SYSTEM
Many disorders of neutrophils extend to mononuclear phagocytes. Thus drugs which suppress neutrophil production in the bone marrow usually lead to monocytopenia. Transient monocytopenia can also be seen after stress or corticosteroid administration. Monocytosis is associated with certain infections such as tuberculosis, brucellosis, subacute bacterial endocarditis, Rocky Mountain spotted fever, and malaria. Monocytosis is also seen in kala azar, malignancies, leukemias, myeloproliferative syndromes, hemolytic anemias, chronic idiopathic neutropenias, granulomatous diseases such as sarcoidosis, regional enteritis, and some collagen vascular diseases. Patients with neutrophil C3bi receptor deficiency, the hyperimmunoglobulin E–recurrent infection (Job's) syndrome, Chédiak-Higashi syndrome, and chronic granulomatous diseases all have defects in the mononuclear phagocyte system.

Certain viral infections impair mononuclear phagocyte function. For example, influenza virus infection is associated with abnormal monocyte chemotaxis. Abnormal monocyte chemotaxis and clearance of IgG-coated erythrocytes (discussed below) is also seen in the acquired immunodeficiency syndrome (AIDS), which is caused by a human retrovirus (see Chap. 257). It is likely that the defects of the monocyte-macrophage system in AIDS contribute to the increased susceptibility to opportunistic infection due to intracellular microorganisms such as Pneumocystic carinii and Mycobacterium avium-intracellulare. T lymphocytes produce a factor, possibly deficient in

AIDS, that induces Fc-receptor expression and phagocytosis by mononuclear phagocytes. In other diseases, such as T-cell lymphomas, excessive release of such a T-cell factor is thought to cause erythrophagocytosis by splenic macrophages.

Specific defects of the mononuclear phagocytes have been described in certain autoimmune diseases. Removal of IgG-coated radiolabeled autologous erythrocytes, presumably via the Fc receptor of splenic macrophages, is profoundly abnormal in patients with active systemic lupus erythematosus. Patients with other autoimmune diseases characterized by tissue deposition of immune complexes, as seen in Sjögren's syndrome, mixed cryoglobulinemia, dermatitis herpetiformis, and chronic progressive multiple sclerosis, also have defects in Fc-receptor function as judged by clearance of IgG-coated erythrocytes (see Chap. 261). Clinically, normal subjects with genetic haplotypes commonly associated with autoimmune disease (i.e., HLA-B8/DRw3) also have an increased incidence of defective Fc receptor–specific functional activity, suggesting that this defect may predispose individuals with this genetic profile to immune complex disease.

EOSINOPHILS

Eosinophils and neutrophils share similar morphology, many lysosomal constituents, most chemotactic responses, phagocytic capacity, and oxidative metabolism. However, there are major differences between the two cell types, and little is known about the natural function of eosinophils. Eosinophils are much longer lived than neutrophils and, unlike neutrophils, tissue eosinophils can recirculate. During most infections eosinophils do not appear to have any important function. However, in invasive parasite infections, such as hookworm, schistosomiasis, strongyloidiasis, toxocariasis, trichinosis, filariasis, echinococcosis, and cysticercosis, the eosinophil likely plays a central role in host defense. Eosinophils are also associated with bronchial asthma, cutaneous allergic reactions, and other hypersensitivity states.

The characteristic red-staining eosinophil granules (Wright's stain) contain a number of unique constituents. The distinctive feature of the eosinophil granule is its crystalline core consisting of an arginine-rich protein (major basic protein) with histaminase activity, which is probably important in host defense against parasites. Eosinophil granules also contain a unique eosinophil peroxidase which catalyzes the oxidation of many substances by hydrogen perioxide and may facilitate killing of microorganisms. Eosinophil peroxidase, in the presence of hydrogen perioxide and halide, initiates mast cell secretion in vitro and thereby may contribute to inflammation. Other substances found in eosinophils include cationic proteins, some of which bind to heparin and reduce its anticoagulant activity. Eosinophil cytoplasm contains Charcot-Leyden crystal protein, a hexagonal bipyramidal crystal first described in leukemia and then in sputum from asthma patients, which is a lysophospholipase and may function to restrict the toxicity of certain lysophospholipids. Eosinophils also contain a powerful neurotoxin. Because patients with hypereosinophilic syndrome and cerebral spinal fluid eosinophilia exhibit varied neurologic abnormalities, eosinophil-derived neurotoxin may play an important role in central nervous system disease.

Several factors enhance the eosinophil's function in host defense. For example, T-cell-derived eosinophil stimulation promoter enhances the ability of eosinophils to kill parasites. Mast-cell-derived eosinophil chemotactic factor of anaphylaxis (ECFa) increases the number of eosinophil complement receptors and enhances eosinophil killing of parasites. In addition, eosinophil colony-stimulating factors produced by macrophages may not only increase eosinophil production in the bone marrow but also activate eosinophils to kill parasites.

EOSINOPHILIA More than 500 eosinophils per cubic millimeter of blood is common in many settings besides parasite infection. The most common cause of eosinophilia is probably allergic reactions to drugs such as iodides, aspirin, and sulfonamides. Allergies such as hay fever, asthma, and eczema commonly are associated with eosinophilia. Eosinophilia is also seen in collagen vascular diseases (e.g., rheumatoid arthritis, eosinophilic fasciitis, allergic angiitis, and granulomatosis) and malignancies (e.g., Hodgkin's disease, mycosis fungoides) as well as the hyperimmunoglobulin E–recurrent infection (Job's) syndrome and the chronic granulomatous diseases; the mechanism for the eosinophilia in these diseases is not known. The most dramatic increases in eosinophils occur in hypereosinophilic syndromes incuding Loeffler's syndrome, eosinophilic leukemia, as well as idiopathic hypereosinophilic syndrome (with counts as high as 50,000 to 100,000 eosinophils per cubic millimeter).

The idiopathic hypereosinophilic syndrome represents a heterogeneous group of disorders with the common feature being prolonged eosinophilia of unknown cause and associated organ system dysfunction, including the heart, central nervous system, kidneys, lungs, gastrointestinal tract, and skin. The bone marrow is involved in all subjects, but the most severe complications involve the heart and central nervous system. Eosinophils are found in the involved tissues and are thought to cause tissue damage by local deposition of toxic eosinophil proteins such as eosinophil cationic protein and eosinophil major basic protein. In the heart the pathological changes lead to thrombosis which may result in endocardial fibrosis and restrictive endomyocardiopathy. Similar pathological changes are thought to contribute to the damage of tissues in other organ systems. Although the mechanism for the hypereosinophilia is not known, it has been shown that chemotherapy with corticosteroids usually induces remission. In patients unresponsive to corticosteroids, a cytotoxic agent, such as hydroxyurea, has been used successfully to lower the peripheral blood eosinophil counts and to improve markedly prognosis. Aggressive medical and surgical approaches are also employed when managing patients with cardiovascular complications.

EOSINOPENIA This occurs with stress, such as acute bacterial infection, and following administration of corticosteroids. The mechanism of eosinopenia of acute bacterial infection is unknown but is independent of endogenous corticosteroids since it occurs in animals following total adrenalectomy. There is no known adverse effect of eosinopenia.

DIAGNOSIS AND MANAGEMENT OF PHAGOCYTE DYSFUNCTION

Diagnosis of phagocytic cell disorders is suggested from clinical evaluation. Neutropenia or impaired neutrophil function is frequently associated with depressed inflammation. Aphthous ulcers of the mucous membranes (gray ulcers without pus) are not uncommon. Gingivitis is common and periodontal disease is frequent in some patients. Characteristically, patients with phagocyte defects have recurrent and often severe bacterial or fungal infections which often present as difficult management problems. Patients with congenital defects can have infections within the first few days of life. In some disorders the frequency of infection is variable and patients can go months or even years without major infection. Adults over 30 years of age with congenital defects are unusual, suggesting that patients with such defects die at an early age. However, in recent years, with aggressive management, adults with these diseases are being seen with increasing frequency. Skin, ear, upper and lower respiratory tract and bone infections are common. Sepsis and meningitis are rare.

Initial studies of white blood count and differential and often bone marrow exam are followed by assessment of bone marrow reserves (steroid challenge test), marginated circulating pool of cells (epinephrine challenge test), and marginating ability (endotoxin challenge test). In vivo assessment of inflammation is possible with a Rebuck skin window test, in which the ability of leukocytes to accumulate at a superficial abrasion and adhere to a glass coverslip is tested. In

vivo clearance of IgG-coated erythrocytes provides a useful way to monitor the mononuclear-phagocyte (reticuloendothelial) system. In vitro tests of phagocyte aggregation, adherence, chemotaxis, phagocytosis, degranulation, and microbicidal activity (for *Staphylococcus aureus*) help pinpoint cellular or humoral lesions which can then be further characterized at the molecular level. Deficiencies of oxidative metabolism are screened with the nitroblue tetrazolium dye (NBT) test, which is based on the ability of products of oxidative metabolism to reduce yellow, soluble NBT to blue-black formazan, an insoluble material which precipitates intracellularly and can be seen microscopically. Further aspects of neutrophil oxidative metabolism are defined by studies of superoxide and hydrogen perioxide production.

The most important aspect of patient management is to appreciate that patients often have delayed inflammatory responses. Therefore, clinical manifestations may be minimal despite overwhelming infection, and unusual infections must always be suspected in some patients. Early signs of infection demand prompt, aggressive use of antibiotics and surgical drainage of abscesses. Prolonged antibiotics are often required, and in life-threatening infections daily white blood cell transfusions (enriched for neutrophils) are probably beneficial, although their use is still controversial. In patients with the chronic granulomatous diseases, prophylactic antibiotics (trimethoprim-sulfamethoxazole) probably diminish the frequency of life-threatening infections. Rigorous oral hygiene reduces but does not eliminate the discomfort of gingivitis, periodontal disease, and aphthous ulcers; tooth brushing with a hydrogen peroxide–sodium bicarbonate paste helps some patients. Ketoconazole has caused dramatic improvement of mucocutaneous candidiasis in patients with the hyperimmunoglobulin E–recurrent infection (Job's) syndrome. Treatment to restore myelopoiesis in patients with neutropenia due to impaired production has included use of androgens, glucocorticoids, lithium, and immunosuppressive therapy. Cure of some congenital phagocyte defects is theoretically possible by bone marrow transplantation (see Chap. 291). However, complications of bone marrow transplantation are still great, and with rigorous medical care many patients with phagocytic disorders can go for years without a life-threatening infection.

REFERENCES

ADAMS DO: Macrophage activation and secretion. Fed Proc 41:2193, 1982

ANDERSON DC et al: The severe and moderate phenotypes of heritable Mac1, LFA-1 deficiency: Their quantitative definition and relation to leukocyte dysfunction and clinical features. J Infect Dis 152:668, 1985

BABIOR BM: The respiratory burst of phagocytes. J Clin Invest 73:599, 1984

BUESCHER ES et al: Use of an X-linked human neutrophil marker to estimate timing of Lyonization and size of the dividing stem cell pool. J Clin Invest 76:1581, 1985

DALE DC et al: Chronic neutropenia. Medicine 38:128, 1979

DINARELLO, CA: Interleukin 1. Rev Infect Dis 6:51, 1984

DONABEDIAN H, GALLIN JI: The hyperimmunoglobulin E–recurrent infection (Job's) syndrome. A review of the NIH experience and the literature. Medicine 62:195, 1983

DRESKIN SC et al: Immunoglobulins in the hyperimmunoglobulin E and recurrent infection (Job's) syndrome. Deficiency of anti-*Staphylococcus aureus* immunoglobulin A. J Clin Invest 75:26, 1985

FAUCI AS et al: The idiopathic hypereosinophilic syndrome: Clinical, pathophysiologic, and therapeutic considerations. Ann Intern Med 97:78, 1982

GALLIN JI: Abnormal phagocyte chemotaxis: Pathophysiology, clinical manifestations, and management of patients. Rev Infect Dis 3:1196, 1981

———: Neutrophil heterogeneity exists, but is it meaningful? Blood 63:977, 1984

———: Neutrophil specific granule deficiency. Ann Rev Med 36:263, 1985

———, FAUCI AS (eds): *Advances in Host Defense Mechanisms*, vol. 1: *Phagocytic Cells*. New York, Raven, 1982

——— et al: Recent advances in chronic granulomatous disease. Ann Intern Med 99:657, 1983

GLEICH GJ, LOEGEUNG DA: Immunobiology of eosinophils. Ann Rev Immunol 2:429, 1984

SMITH PD, et al: Monocyte function in the acquired immune deficiency syndrome. Defective chemotaxis. J Clin Invest 74:2121, 1984

TAUBER AI et al: Chronic granulomatous disease: A syndrome of phagocyte oxidase deficiences. Medicine 62:286, 1983

section 1 Genetics and human disease

57 GENETIC ASPECTS OF DISEASE

JOSEPH L. GOLDSTEIN / MICHAEL S. BROWN

GENETIC PRINCIPLES

More than one-fifth of the proteins (and hence genes) in each human being exist in a form that differs from the one present in the majority of the population. This remarkable genetic variability, or polymorphism, among "normal" people accounts for much of the normal variation in body traits such as height, intelligence, and blood pressure. These genetic differences also determine the ability of each individual to meet environmental challenges, including those that produce disease. All human diseases can be considered to result from an interaction between an individual's unique genetic makeup and the environment. In certain diseases, the genetic component is so overwhelming that it expresses itself in a predictable manner without a requirement for extraordinary environmental challenges. Such diseases are termed *genetic disorders*.

MOLECULAR BASIS OF GENE EXPRESSION All hereditary information is transmitted from parent to offspring through the inheritance of deoxyribonucleic acid (DNA). DNA is a linear polymer composed of purine and pyrimidine bases whose sequence ultimately determines the sequence of amino acids in every protein made by the body. The four types of bases in DNA are arranged in groups of three, each triplet forming a code word, or codon, that signifies a particular amino acid. A *gene* represents the total sequence of bases in DNA that specifies the amino acid sequence of a single polypeptide chain of a protein molecule.

Genetic information encoded in the DNA of the chromosomes is first transcribed into a *ribonucleic acid* (RNA) copy. During transcription the ribose nucleotides align themselves along the DNA according to base-pairing rules. Thus, adenine of DNA pairs with uridine of RNA, cytosine pairs with guanine, thymine pairs with adenine, and guanine pairs with cytosine. The ribose bases are joined together by RNA polymerase. The resulting *RNA transcript* forms the template for translation into the amino acid sequence of a protein. Figure 57-1 shows the DNA and mRNA code words for each of the amino acids in protein.

Figure 57-2 illustrates a schematic diagram of the genetic control of protein synthesis in higher organisms, including humans. The DNA of most genes is fragmented into discrete coding regions (exons) separated by noncoding regions (introns or intervening sequences). The *coding regions* contain the bases that specify the sequence of amino acids in the polypeptide chain. The *intervening sequences* are

FIGURE 57-1 *The genetic code.*

Second nucleotide

		A or U			G or C			T or A			C or G			
A or U	AAA AAG AAT AAC	UUU UUC UUA UUG	Phe / Leu	AGA AGG AGT AGC	UCU UCC UCA UCG	Ser	ATA ATG ATT ATC	UAU UAC UAA UAG	Tyr / Stop	ACA ACG ACT ACC	UGU UGC UGA UGG	Cys / Stop / Trp	A or U G or C T or A C or G
G or C	GAA GAG GAT GAC	CUU CUC CUA CUG	Leu	GGA GGG GGT GGC	CCU CCC CCA CCG	Pro	GTA GTG GTT GTC	CAU CAC CAA CAG	His / Gln	GCA GCG GCT GCC	CGU CGC CGA CGG	Arg	A or U G or C T or A C or G
T or A	TAA TAG TAT TAC	AUU AUC AUA AUG	Ile / Met	TGA TGG TGT TGC	ACU ACC ACA ACG	Thr	TTA TTG TTT TTC	AAU AAC AAA AAG	Asn / Lys	TCA TCG TCT TCC	AGU AGC AGA AGG	Ser / Arg	A or U G or C T or A C or G
C or G	CAA CAG CAT CAC	GUU GUC GUA GUG	Val	CGA CGG CGT CGC	GCU GCC GCA GCG	Ala	CTA CTG CTT CTC	GAU GAC GAA GAG	Asp / Glu	CCA CCG CCT CCC	GGU GGC GGA GGG	Gly	A or U G or C T or A C or G

First nucleotide (left margin) / Third nucleotide (right margin)

Note: The DNA codons appear in boldface type; the complementary RNA codons are in italics. A = adenine, C = cytosine, G = guanine, T = thymine, U = uridine (replaces thymine in RNA). In RNA, adenine is complementary to thymine of DNA; uridine is complementary to adenine of DNA; cytosine is complementary to guanine, and vice versa. "Stop" = termination. The amino acids are abbreviated as follows:

Ala = alanine	*Cys = cysteine*	*His = histidine*	*Met = methionine*	*Thr = threonine*
Arg = arginine	*Gln = glutamine*	*Ile = isoleucine*	*Phe = phenylalanine*	*Trp = tryptophan*
Asn = asparagine	*Glu = glutamic acid*	*Leu = leucine*	*Pro = proline*	*Tyr = tyrosine*
Asp = aspartic acid	*Gly = glycine*	*Lys = lysine*	*Ser = serine*	*Val = valine*

composed of bases that act as spacers between the coding regions; they are not translated into protein. The transcription of DNA produces a faithful copy of the entire gene sequence; thus, the RNA transcript contains altering coding and intervening sequences. The RNA transcript is edited in the nucleus before it passes into the cytoplasm. In the editing process, the intervening sequences are excised, and the coding regions are spliced together to form one continuous gene (Fig. 57-2).

After processing, the edited RNA, which is called *messenger RNA* (mRNA) leaves the nucleus and enters the cytoplasm where it becomes associated with *ribosomes* and thereby serves as a template for the ribosomal synthesis of proteins. Each of the 20 amino acids is attached in the cell cytoplasm to a specific molecule called *transfer RNA* (tRNA). Each tRNA contains a triplet sequence of purine and pyrimidine bases that is "complementary" to a specific codon in the mRNA. These tRNA molecules with their attached amino acids line up along the mRNA molecule in the precise order dictated by the genetic code. Under the action of cytoplasmic enzymes (initiation factors, elongation factors, and termination factors), peptide bonds are formed between the various amino acids, and the completed protein is released from the ribosome. For a more detailed account of the molecular basis of gene expression, see Chap. 58.

MAINTENANCE OF GENETIC DIVERSITY THROUGH TRANSMISSION AND SEGREGATION OF GENES   The amount of DNA in the nucleus of each human cell is sufficient to code for more than 50,000 genes and hence to specify more than 50,000 polypeptide chains. The genes are arranged in a linear sequence of DNA that together with certain histone proteins form rod-shaped bodies called *chromosomes*. Each somatic cell contains 46 chromosomes, arranged in 23 pairs, one of each pair derived from each parent. Thus, each individual inherits two copies of each chromosome and hence two copies of each gene. The chromosomal location of the two copies of each gene is termed the *genetic locus*. When a gene occupying a genetic locus exists in two or more different forms, these alternate forms of the gene are referred to as *alleles*.

In humans, a given gene always resides at a specified genetic locus on one particular chromosome. For example, the genetic locus for the Rh blood group is on the short arm of chromosome 1; at this site there are two Rh genes, one on chromosome 1 derived from the mother and the other on chromosome 1 derived from the father. When two genes at the same genetic locus are identical, the individual is a *homozygote*. When the two genes differ (i.e., two different alleles are present at the locus), the individual is a *heterozygote*. Each normal human is heterozygous at approximately 20 percent of

genetic loci and homozygous at 80 percent. Figure 57-3 shows a map of human chromosome 1, illustrating the location of a representative sample of genes that have been assigned loci on this chromosome.

The genetic information carried on chromosomes is transmitted to daughter cells under two different sets of circumstances. One of these occurs whenever a somatic cell (i.e., a nongerm cell) divides. This process, called *mitosis,* transmits identical copies of each gene to each daughter cell, thus maintaining a uniform genetic makeup in all cells of a single individual. The other set of circumstances prevails when genetic information must be transmitted from one individual to an offspring. This process, called *meiosis,* produces germ cells (i.e., ova or spermatozoa) that possess only one copy of each parental chromosome, thus allowing for new combinations of chromosomes to occur when ovum and sperm cell fuse during fertilization.

During meiosis, the 46 chromosomes of an immature germ cell arrange themselves in 23 pairs at the center of the nucleus, each pair being composed of one chromosome derived from the mother and its homologous chromosome derived from the father. At a specified point in the meiotic process, the two partner chromosomes separate, only one of each pair going into each daughter cell, or gamete. Thus, meiosis produces gametes with a reduction in the number of chromosomes from 46 to 23, each gamete having received one chromosome from each of the 23 pairs. The assortment of the chromosomes within each pair is random so that each germ cell receives a different combination of maternal and paternal chromosomes. During the process of fertilization, the fusion of ovum and sperm cell, each of which has 23 chromosomes, produces an individual with 46 chromosomes.

The independent assortment of chromosomes into gametes during meiosis produces an enormous diversity among the possible genotypes of the progeny. For each 23 pairs of chromosomes, there are 2^{23} different combinations of chromosomes that could occur in a gamete, and the likelihood that one set of parents will produce two offspring with the identical complement of chromosomes is one in 2^{23} or one in 8.4 million (assuming no monozygotic or identical twins).

RECOMBINATION   Adding to the genetic diversity in humans is the phenomenon of *genetic recombination*. During meiosis, when homologous chromosomes are paired, bridges frequently form between corresponding regions of the chromosome pair. These bridges, or *chiasmata,* are regions in which the two chromosomes break at identical points along their length and subsequently rejoin, the distal segments having been switched from one homologous chromosome to another. This process is designated *crossing over*. Although no net change in the amount of genetic material occurs during crossing

FIGURE 57-2 *A schematic diagram of the genetic control of protein synthesis, illustrating the flow of genetic information from the base sequence of DNA to the RNA transcript (transcription) to mRNA (processing) to the polypeptide chain of a protein molecule (translation). Although DNA exists in a double-stranded form, only one of the two strands is used as a template for transcribing the RNA transcript. Solid sections represent coding regions in DNA, RNA transcript, mRNA, and amino acid sequence in polypeptide chain; dotted sections represent intervening sequences in DNA and RNA transcript.*

over, a recombination of genes does occur. For example, consider a chromosome with two loci, A and B, located at opposite ends of the same chromosome. On this particular chromosome, the A locus has a rare allele x, and the B locus also has a rare allele y. Without the phenomenon of recombination every offspring that inherited the x allele at the A locus would also inherit the y allele at the B locus. However, if recombination occurs, the A locus with the x allele would then be on the opposite chromosome from the B locus with the y allele. In this case any offspring that inherited the x allele at the A locus could not inherit the y allele at the B locus.

Crossing over occurs with great frequency in every meiosis in humans, and the resultant recombination of genes may occur at any point on a chromosome. The farther apart two genes are on the same chromosome, the greater is the likelihood that a crossing over will occur in the space between them. When two genes are on the opposite ends of a long chromosome, the probability of recombination is so great that their respective alleles are transmitted to offspring almost independently of one another, just as if the two gene loci were on different chromosomes. On the other hand, gene loci that are close together on the same chromosome are said to be *linked* so that there is a great likelihood that offspring will inherit the same combination of alleles that are present on the parental chromosome.

Several examples of *gene linkage* can be seen from the map of human chromosome 1 (Fig. 57-3). For example, the locus for the gene specifying the Rh blood group factor and the locus for the gene producing one form of the dominant trait hereditary elliptocytosis occur in close proximity on this chromosome. Thus, if a subject with hereditary elliptocytosis transmits the disease to an offspring, the offspring will usually inherit the allele that is present at the Rh locus on this chromosome. If the Rh allele happens to be a rare one in the population (such as r'), one can assume that whichever offspring inherits the r' allele at the Rh locus will also inherit the abnormal allele at the elliptocytosis locus. On the other hand, if an offspring does not exhibit the r' allele, he or she will not usually have elliptocytosis. The concept of linkage does not imply an association between any particular set of Rh alleles and the disease state elliptocytosis, rather between the two genetic loci. Thus, in different families the abnormal elliptocytosis allele may be linked to the R^1, R^0, r_2, or any other allele at the Rh locus, depending on the allele that happened to be at that locus when the elliptocytosis mutation occurred. Stated another way, the elliptocytosis locus is linked to the Rh locus in every family, but the particular Rh allele with which it is associated differs from family to family.

MUTATION Broadly defined, a *mutation* is a stable, heritable alteration in DNA. Although the causes of mutation in humans are largely unknown, a variety of environmental agents, such as radiation, viruses, and chemicals, are among the factors that are implicated.

Mutations can involve a visible alteration in the structure of a chromosome, such as a deletion or translocation of a portion of a chromosome, or they can involve a minute change in one of the purine or pyrimidine bases of a single gene. Most commonly, such "point" mutations consist of the substitution of one base for another, changing the meaning of the codon containing that base, hence their designation as *missense mutations*. For example, in the gene coding for the β chain of hemoglobin, the sixth position normally contains the nucleotide triplet CTC, which codes for the amino acid glutamic acid (Fig. 57-1). The mutation that gives rise to hemoglobin C produces a change of the first base of this triplet from cytosine to thymine, changing the triplet to TTC, which codes for lysine. On the other hand, the mutation that gives rise to hemoglobin S produces a change in the second base of the same triplet (from thymine to adenine), producing CAC, which codes for valine. Thus, in the sixth position of the β chain of hemoglobin, the normally occurring glutamic acid may be replaced with either lysine (producing hemoglobin C) or valine (producing hemoglobin S). More than 90 such single-base mutations in the hemoglobin β chain have been identified, and many of these mutations produce distinct clinical syndromes. Of

all the mutations so far elucidated in humans, most involve such single-base changes.

Besides producing an amino acid substitution, a single-base substitution can also cause another abnormality in protein synthesis—premature chain termination. Three mRNA code words (UAA, UAG, and UGA) normally do not specify an amino acid but constitute the signal that the message has ended and that the protein chain should be released from the ribosome (Fig. 57-1). If a change occurs in DNA that produces one of these mRNA code words [for example, a switch in an mRNA triplet from UAU (tyrosine) to UAA (termination)], the polypeptide chain would be terminated prematurely when translation had reached that point. Such mutations, called *non-sense mutations*, produce short fragments of proteins that have reduced function.

CELLULAR MECHANISM BY WHICH MUTANT GENES PRODUCE DISEASES Critical to the understanding of heredity is the concept that the only information transmitted from generation to generation is the sequence of bases in DNA and that these sequences in turn specify only the primary structure of RNA and protein molecules. All other chemical reactions—such as the synthesis of complex lipids and carbohydrates, the formation of membranes and other cellular organelles, and the accumulation and partitioning of inorganic ions—occur as a secondary consequence of the action of specific proteins. Many of these proteins are enzymes that catalyze the biochemical conversion of one molecule into another. Others are structural proteins such as collagen and elastin, and still others are regulatory proteins that dictate how much of each enzyme and each structural protein is made.

Since proteins are the cellular molecules whose structures are encoded by genes, mutations in genes exert their deleterious effects by altering the structure of enzymes, structural proteins, or regulatory

FIGURE 57-3 *Gene map of human chromosome 1, illustrating a representative sample of the genes that have been localized to this chromosome. The black bands represent those genetic regions of the chromosome that stain brightly by a fluorescent dye such as quinacrine; the white bands are the negatively staining regions; the hatched area is a variable region that stains differently (i.e., either brightly or negatively) in the chromosomes of different individuals. Each gene is listed opposite its genetic locus on the right. (Data provided by VA McKusick.)*

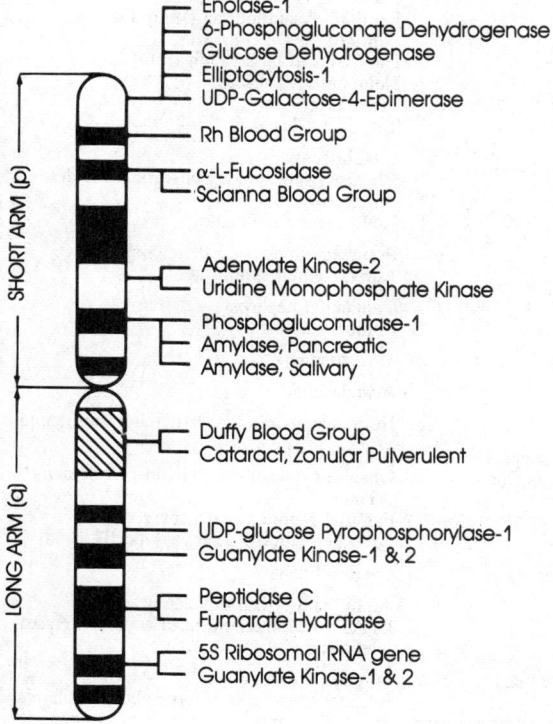

SHORT ARM (p)

- Enolase-1
- 6-Phosphogluconate Dehydrogenase
- Glucose Dehydrogenase
- Elliptocytosis-1
- UDP-Galactose-4-Epimerase
- Rh Blood Group
- α-L-Fucosidase
- Scianna Blood Group
- Adenylate Kinase-2
- Uridine Monophosphate Kinase
- Phosphoglucomutase-1
- Amylase, Pancreatic
- Amylase, Salivary

LONG ARM (q)

- Duffy Blood Group
- Cataract, Zonular Pulverulent
- UDP-glucose Pyrophosphorylase-1
- Guanylate Kinase-1 & 2
- Peptidase C
- Fumarate Hydratase
- 5S Ribosomal RNA gene
- Guanylate Kinase-1 & 2

proteins. For example, in a disease such as glycogen storage disease, type I (von Gierke's disease), massive accumulation of glycogen in the liver is due not to a primary structural abnormality in the polysaccharide glycogen but to a structural abnormality in a protein, glucose 6-phosphatase, an enzyme that is required to liberate glucose so as to permit glycogen breakdown. Other examples of the biochemical mechanisms by which mutant genes alter cellular metabolism are discussed below under "Simply Inherited Disorders."

GENETIC HETEROGENEITY   When two or more mutations can produce a similar clinical syndrome, genetic heterogeneity is said to exist. Hemophilia is one example of a genetically heterogeneous syndrome. A clinically similar bleeding disorder can be caused by mutations at either of two loci on the X chromosome, one leading to a deficiency of factor VIII (classic hemophilia) and the other causing a deficiency of factor IX (Christmas disease). Most, if not all, hereditary diseases, when carefully analyzed, will probably prove to be genetically heterogeneous.

Genetic heterogeneity may result from the existence of a series of different mutations at a single genetic locus (allelic mutations) or from mutations at different genetic loci (nonallelic mutations). For example, drug-induced hemolysis of red blood cells can occur in patients with several different types of allelic mutations at the glucose 6-phosphate dehydrogenase locus. On the other hand, hemophilia is an example of a syndrome in which nonallelic mutations can produce a similar clinical picture (see above).

In some cases of heterogeneity, both the genetic locus and the mode of inheritance differ. Diseases such as spastic paraplegia, Charcot-Marie-Tooth peroneal muscular atrophy, and retinitis pigmentosa are inherited as autosomal dominant traits in some families,

TABLE 57-1   Examples of simply inherited disorders that occur with increased frequency in specific ethnic groups

Ethnic group	Simply inherited disorder
African blacks	Hemoglobinopathies, especially Hb S, Hb C, persistent Hb F, α and β thalassemias Glucose 6-phosphate dehydrogenase deficiency
Armenians	Familial Mediterranean fever
Ashkenazi Jews	Abetalipoproteinemia Bloom's syndrome Dystonia musculorum deformans (recessive form) Factor XI (PTA) deficiency Familial dysautonomia (Riley-Day syndrome) Gaucher's disease (adult form) Neimann-Pick disease Pentosuria Tay-Sachs disease
Chinese	α thalassemia Glucose 6-phosphate dehydrogenase deficiency Adult lactase deficiency
Eskimos	Pseudocholinesterase deficiency Adrenogenital syndrome
Finns	Congenital nephrosis Mulibrey nanism
French Canadians	Tyrosinemia
Japanese	Acatalasemia
Lebanese	Homozygous familial hypercholesterolemia
Mediterranean peoples (Italians, Greeks, Sephardic Jews)	β thalassemia Glucose 6-phosphate dehydrogenase deficiency Familial Mediterranean fever Glycogen storage disease, type III
Northern Europeans	Cystic fibrosis
Scandinavians	Alpha₁-antitrypsin deficiency LCAT (lecithin:cholesterol acyltransferase) deficiency
South African whites	Porphyria variegata Homozygous familial hypercholesterolemia

as autosomal recessives in others, and as X-linked recessives in still others. The identification of such genetic heterogeneity in these disorders is of obvious importance for correct genetic counseling.

TAKING THE FAMILY HISTORY

The investigation of a patient with a possible genetic disorder begins with the *family history*. The first step is to obtain certain information on the *proband* or *index case* (i.e., the clinically affected person who has brought the family to attention) and on each of the *first-degree relatives* (i.e., the parents, siblings, and offspring of the proband). This information includes the given name, surname, maiden name, birth date or current age, age at death, cause of death, and name or description of any disease or defect.

The second step is to ask questions designed to survey the family for the presence of disease or defect. (1) Has any relative an identical or similar trait? (2) Has any relative a trait that is absent in the proband but is known to occur in some patients with the same disease? This question requires that the physician have some knowledge about the manifestations of the disease in question. For example, when obtaining the family history from a proband with dissecting aneurysm caused possibly by Marfan's syndrome, one should ask about the occurrence of eye abnormalities, cardiac abnormalities, and skeletal abnormalities in the relatives. (3) Has any relative a trait that is recognized to be genetically determined? The purpose of this question is to ascertain the occurrence of hereditary disease in the family even though the particular patient may not be involved. (4) Has any relative an unusual disease, or has any relative died of a rare condition? The purpose of this question is to identify a condition that might be genetically determined though not recognized as such by the informant. In addition, this question may help to identify conditions in relatives that might be etiologically related to the patient's problem. For example, a patient with pheochromocytoma should be suspected of having von Recklinghausen's disease if he or she has a brother with scoliosis and mental retardation, both of which can be manifestations of the neurofibromatosis (von Recklinghausen's) gene. (5) Is there any consanguinity in the family? This inquiry should be made directly. In addition, one should ask whether common last names appear in the families of husband-wife pairs. Consanguineous marriage may be the source of a rare autosomal recessive syndrome, and sometimes its presence in the family may not be known by the proband. (6) What is the ethnic origin of the family? Persons of various ethnic origins, such as blacks, Jews, and Greeks, have increased chances of specific genetic diseases. Table 57-1 lists examples of simply inherited disorders that are found with increased frequency in various ethnic groups.

CATEGORIES OF GENETIC DISORDERS

Genetic diseases generally fall into one of three categories: (1) *Chromosomal disorders* involve the lack, excess, or abnormal arrangement of one or more chromosomes, producing excessive or deficient genetic material. (2) *Mendelian or simply inherited disorders* are determined primarily by a single mutant gene. These disorders display inheritance patterns which can be classified into autosomal dominant, autosomal recessive, or X-linked types. (3) *Mulifactorial disorders* are caused by an interaction of multiple genes and multiple exogenous or environmental factors. Although many of these multifactorial disorders, such as essential hypertension and cleft lip and palate, are said to run in families, the inheritance pattern is complex and the risk to relatives is less than in the single-gene (mendelian) disorders. Each of these categories presents different problems with respect to causation, prevention, diagnosis, genetic counseling, and treatment.

CHROMOSOMAL DISORDERS   The karyotype of an individual (i.e., the number and structure of the chromosomes) can be ascertained from readily accessible body tissues, such as peripheral blood lymphocytes or skin, by growing them in tissue culture until active cell proliferation occurs and then preparing single cells for examination of chromosomes by microscopy. Each individual chromosome can be identified by special staining of DNA sequences, for example, by the affinity of fluorescent dyes (such as quinacrine hydrochloride) for certain chromosomal segments that can be visualized by fluorescence microscopy or by treatment with special dyes (Giemsa) and proteolytic enzymes (trypsin). These techniques produce characteristic *banding patterns* for each chromosome (Fig. 57-4).

The number of chromosomes in normal individuals is 46, of which 44 are the 22 pairs of *autosomes* and the other two are the *sex chromosomes*. Women have two X chromosomes (XX), and men have one X chromosome and one Y chromosome (XY). Each of the 22 pairs of autosomes and the two sex chromosomes can be distinguished on the basis of size, location of the centromere (which divides the chromosome into arms of equal or unequal length), and the unique banding pattern (Fig. 57-4). The relative length of the arms and the position of the centromere are used as further criteria to divide the human chromosomes into seven groups (designated A to G) (Fig. 57-4).

For a complete discussion of the etiology and clinical features of chromosomal abnormalities affecting humans, the reader is referred to Chap. 60.

SIMPLY INHERITED DISORDERS Disorders caused by the transmission of a single mutant gene show one of three simple (or mendelian) patterns of inheritance: (1) autosomal dominant, (2) autosomal recessive, or (3) X-linked. The distinction between "dominant" and "recessive" is one of convenience in pedigree analysis and does not imply a fundamental difference in genetic mechanism. The term *dominant* implies that a mutation is clinically manifest when an individual has a single dose of this mutation (or is *heterozygous* for it), while *recessive* implies that a double dose (or *homozygosity*) is required for clinical detection. Genes are never dominant or recessive; their effects, however, produce clinical patterns that are classified as dominant or recessive. Despite their overall clinical "normality," individuals who are heterozygous for "recessive" genes often have biochemical abnormalities that are demonstrable in the laboratory; on the other hand, those who are homozygous for "dominant" genes are usually more severely affected than are the heterozygotes.

With few exceptions, each of the approximately 1200 mendelian diseases is rare. However, as a group these disorders constitute an important cause of morbidity and death, accounting directly for more than 5 percent of all hospital admissions.

The genes for more than 100 simply inherited diseases have been assigned to specific chromosomes. Disease-producing genes assigned to the X chromosome outnumber those so far assigned to any single autosome. This is because assignment to the X chromosome requires only pedigree studies showing X-linked inheritance (see below). Assignment to an autosome is more complicated, requiring sophisticated techniques of somatic cell hybridization or pedigree studies showing linkage between a disease-producing gene and a "marker" gene that is known to be on a certain chromosome. Table 57-2 shows a partial list of those human genetic diseases that have been mapped to specific chromosomes.

The demonstration that a particular disease or syndrome shows one of the three mendelian patterns of inheritance implies that its pathogenesis, no matter how complex, is due to an abnormality in a single protein molecule. For example, in sickle cell anemia, the entire clinical syndrome, including such seemingly unrelated disturbances as anemia, pain crises, nephropathy, and predisposition to pneumococcal infections, are all the physiologic consequences of having thymine instead of adenine at a specific site in the gene that codes for the β chain of hemoglobin, producing a substitution of a valine for a glutamic acid in the sixth amino acid position in the protein sequence.

In many mendelian disorders, especially in those with dominant

inheritance, it is not possible to demonstrate directly the protein that is primarily altered by the mutation. In such cases (e.g., adult polycystic kidney disease and tuberous sclerosis) only the distal physiologic effects of the mutation are recognizable. Nevertheless, it is safe to assume that a single primary defect exists whenever a disease is transmitted by a single gene mechanism and that the various manifestations of the disease all can be related to the mutational event by a more or less complicated "pedigree of causes." Table 57-3 lists the most commonly encountered mendelian disorders affecting adults.

Autosomal dominant disorders Dominant diseases are those manifest in the heterozygous state, that is, when only one abnormal gene (*mutant allele*) is present and the corresponding partner allele on the homologous chromosome is normal. The gene responsible for an autosomal dominant disorder is located on one of the 22 autosomes, and both males and females can be affected. Since alleles segregate independently at meiosis, there is a 1 in 2 chance that the offspring of an affected heterozygote will inherit the mutant allele and, similarly, a 1 in 2 chance of the offspring inheriting the normal allele.

Figure 57-5 shows a typical pedigree involving an autosomal dominant trait. The following features are characteristic: (1) Each affected individual has an affected parent (unless the condition arose by a new mutation or is mildly expressed in the affected parent); (2) an affected individual will bear, on the average, both normal and affected offspring in equal proportions; (3) normal children of an affected individual will have only normal offspring; (4) males and females are affected in equal proportions; (5) each sex is equally likely to transmit the condition to male and female offspring, with male-to-male transmission occurring; and (6) vertical transmission of the condition through successive generations occurs, especially when the trait does not impair reproductive capacity.

While half of the offspring of an individual with an autosomal dominant condition will inherit the disease, it is not necessarily true that each affected person must have an affected parent. In every autosomal dominant disease a certain proportion of affected persons owe their disorder to a new mutation rather than to an inherited mutation. Since the estimated frequency of mutation is 5×10^{-6} mutations per gene per generation and since a dominant trait, by definition, requires a mutation in only one of a pair of alleles, one would expect that about 1 in 100,000 newborn persons would possess a new mutation at any given genetic locus. Many of these mutations

FIGURE 57-4 *The karyotype of a normal male showing the chromosomes of a single somatic cell in the metaphase stage of cell division. The photographic images of the chromosomes have been cut out and arranged according to descending length and varying arm ratio. The chromosomes have been stained by the Giemsa technique, which allows each chromosome pair to be identified by its unique banding pattern. Chromosomes 1 to 22 are the autosomes. The sex chromosomes in this normal male are an X and a Y. The normal female has an identical karyotype except for the absence of the Y chromosome and the presence instead of a second X chromosome. (Courtesy of K Hirschhorn.)*

either do not impair the function of the gene product or involve a recessive function so that the mutation is clinically silent. Others, however, cause a defective gene product that gives rise to a dominant trait. The parent in whose germ cells the mutation arose is clinically normal. Likewise, the siblings of the affected individual are normal since the mutation affects only a single germ cell. However, the affected individual transmits the disease to half of his or her children.

The proportion of patients with dominant disorders who represent

TABLE 57-2   Partial list of human genetic diseases that have been mapped to specific chromosomes

Chromosome	Disease
1	Elliptocytosis
	RH erythroblastosis
	Gaucher's disease (severe form)
2	Carbamoylphosphate synthetase deficiency
3	Generalized gangliosidosis
	Orotic aciduria
4	Huntington's chorea
	Analbuminemia
5	Sandhoff's disease
	Maroteaux-Lamy's syndrome (mucopolysaccharidosis VI)
6	Complement C2 deficiency
	Complement C4 deficiency
	Hemochromatosis
	Congenital adrenal hyperplasia (21-hydroxylase deficiency)
7	Argininosuccinic aciduria
	Ehlers-Danlos syndrome (one form)
	Osteogenesis imperfecta (one form)
9	Citrullinemia
	Galactosemia
	Nail-patella syndrome
10	Hexokinase deficiency (hemolytic anemia)
	Cholesteryl ester storage disease, Wolman's syndrome
11	Acatalasemia
	Syndrome of Wilms's tumor, aniridia, gonadoblastoma, retardation
	β thalassemia; sickle cell anemia
	Acute intermittent porphyria
12	Phenylketonuria
	Triosephosphate isomerase deficiency (hemolytic anemia)
13	Retinoblastoma
14	Nucleoside phosphorylase deficiency (immunodeficiency)
	Alpha$_1$-antitrypsin deficiency
15	Prader-Willi syndrome
	Tay-Sachs disease
16	α thalassemia
	Gout due to adenine phosphoribosyltransferase deficiency
	LCAT deficiency
17	Growth hormone deficiency (type 1A)
	Glycogen storage disease II (acid maltase deficiency)
19	Familial hypercholesterolemia
	Familial type 3 hyperlipoproteinemia
	Myotonic dystrophy
	Complement C3 deficiency
20	Adenosine deaminase deficiency (immunodeficiency)
22	Metachromatic leukodystrophy
	Hurler's syndrome (mucopolysaccharidosis I)
	Scheie's syndrome (mucopolysaccharidosis V)
X	X-linked ichthyosis due to placental steroid sulfatase deficiency
	Ocular albinism
	Chronic granulomatous disease
	Duchenne muscular dystrophy
	Testicular feminization syndrome
	Phosphoglycerate kinase deficiency (hemolytic anemia)
	Fabry's disease
	Lesch-Nyhan syndrome
	Fragile site associated with X-linked mental retardation
	Color blindness
	Hemophilia A
	Glucose 6-phosphate dehydrogenase (G6PD) deficiency

SOURCE: *McKusick.*

TABLE 57-3   Some relatively frequent mendelian disorders affecting adults

AUTOSOMAL DOMINANT DISORDERS

Familial hypercholesterolemia
Hereditary hemorrhagic telangiectasia
Marfan's syndrome
Hereditary spherocytosis
Adult polycystic kidney disease
Huntington's chorea
Acute intermittent porphyria
Osteogenesis imperfecta tarda
von Willebrand's disease
Myotonic dystrophy
Idiopathic hypertrophic subaortic stenosis (IHSS)
Noonan's syndrome
Neurofibromatosis
Tuberous sclerosis

AUTOSOMAL RECESSIVE DISORDERS

Deafness
Albinism
Wilson's disease
Hemochromatosis
Sickle cell anemia
β thalassemia
Cystic fibrosis
Hereditary emphysema (alpha$_1$-antitrypsin deficiency)
Homocystinuria
Familial Mediterranean fever
Friedreich's ataxia
Phenylketonuria

X-LINKED DISORDERS

Hemophilia A
Glucose 6-phosphate dehydrogenase deficiency
Fabry's disease
Ocular albinism
Testicular feminization
Chronic granulomatous disease
Hypophosphatemic rickets
Color blindness

new mutations is inversely proportional to the effect of the disease in question on biologic fitness. The term *biologic fitness* refers to the ability of an affected individual to produce children who survive to adult life and reproduce. In the extreme case, if a dominant mutation produced absolute infertility, then all observed cases would of necessity represent new mutations, and it would be impossible to prove the genetic transmission of the trait. In less severe disorders, as in tuberous sclerosis, the severe mental retardation reduces biologic fitness to about 20 percent of normal, and the proportion of cases due to new mutations is about 80 percent. Other examples of the relation between biologic fitness and the proportion of new mutations in dominant disorders are shown in Table 57-4.

Many new mutations appear to occur in the germ cells of fathers who are of relatively advanced age. Such a "paternal age effect" is seen, for example, in Marfan's syndrome in which the average age of fathers of sporadic or "new mutation" cases (37 years) is in excess of the mean age of fathers generally (30 years) and also in excess of the age of fathers who transmit Marfan's disease due to an inherited mutation (30 years).

Before one concludes that a dominant disorder in a given patient with unaffected parents is the result of a new mutation, it is important to consider two other possibilities: (1) that the gene may be carried by one parent in whom the disease is of low expressivity (discussed below), and (2) that extramarital paternity may have occurred. The latter is found in about 3 to 5 percent of randomly studied children in the United States.

Most autosomal dominant disorders show two characteristic features that are not usually seen in recessive syndromes: (1) *delayed age of onset* and (2) *variability in clinical expression.* Delayed age of onset is seen in disorders such as Huntington's chorea and adult polycystic kidney disease. These disorders do not manifest clinically

FIGURE 57-5 *Pedigree pattern of an autosomal dominant trait. Note the vertical pattern of inheritance.*

1 Islet Cell Adenomas
Parathyroid Adenomas
Lipomas
2 Lipomas, Kidney Stones
3 Islet Cell Adenomas
Parathyroid Adenomas
Pituitary Adenoma
Lipomas

4 Peptic Ulcer
Disease
5 Pituitary
Adenoma

FIGURE 57-6 *Pedigree of a family affected with the multiple endocrine adenoma–peptic ulcer syndrome, a disorder inherited as an autosomal dominant trait. Circles denote females; squares, males. Open circles and squares denote unaffected relatives; closed circles and squares denote affected relatives. Deceased relatives are indicated by the oblique line. The age of each relative is indicated below his or her symbol. Note the marked variation in clinical expression among living affected heterozygotes.*

until adult life, even though the mutant gene is present from the time of conception. Variability in clinical expression is illustrated dramatically by the multiple endocrine adenoma–peptic ulcer syndrome. Patients in the same family inheriting the same abnormal gene may have hyperplasia or neoplasia of one or more endocrine glands (including the pancreas, parathyroid glands, and pituitary gland), as well as of adipose tissue. The resulting clinical manifestations are diverse; different members of the same family may develop peptic ulcers, hypoglycemia, kidney stones, multiple lipomas of the skin, or bitemporal hemianopsia. The recognition that each family member suffers from the same genetic abnormality can be difficult, as illustrated by the family pedigree in Fig. 57-6.

Dominant mutations involve a type of gene product that produces clinical symptoms when only 50 percent of the gene product is defective. The defective genes usually do not encode enzymes, since a 50 percent deficiency of most enzymes produces no symptoms (see "Recessive Disorders" below). Rather, dominant diseases are likely to involve abnormalities in two classes of proteins: (1) those that regulate complex metabolic pathways, such as membrane receptors and rate-limiting enzymes in pathways under feedback control, and (2) key structural proteins, such as hemoglobin or collagen.

The basic biochemical defects have been identified in only a handful of the approximately 600 autosomal dominant disorders. These include familial hypercholesterolemia (abnormal cell surface receptor that binds plasma low-density lipoprotein and thereby regulates cholesterol metabolism); hereditary methemoglobinemia and several hemolytic anemias due to unstable forms of hemoglobin (abnormal hemoglobin molecule); hereditary angioneurotic edema (abnormal protein inhibitor of an enzyme involved in the serum complement system); acute intermittent porphyria (abnormal enzyme that catalyzes a rate-limiting step in the heme biosynthetic pathway); and pseudohypoparathyroidism, type 1 (abnormal guanine nucleotide-binding regulatory component or *G*-protein of the adenylate cyclase system).

Autosomal recessive disorders Autosomal recessive conditions are clinically apparent only in the homozygous state, that is, when both alleles at a particular genetic locus are mutant. By definition, the gene responsible for an autosomal recessive disorder must be on one of the 22 autosomes; thus, both males and females can be affected.

Figure 57-7 shows a pedigree in which an autosomal recessive trait is present in the family. The following features are characteristic: (1) the parents are clinically normal; (2) only siblings are affected, and vertical transmission does not occur; and (3) males and females are affected in equal proportions.

The relative infrequency of recessive genes in the population and the requirement for two abnormal genes for clinical expression combine to create special conditions for autosomal recessive inheritance: (1) the more infrequent the mutant gene in the population, the stronger the likelihood that affected individuals are the product of consanguineous matings (see below); (2) if a husband and a wife are both carriers for the same autosomal recessive gene, 25 percent of the children will be normal, 50 percent will be heterozygous carriers, and 25 percent will be homozygous and affected with the disease; (3) if an affected individual marries a heterozygote (as may occur with consanguineous marriage), half the children will be affected, and a pedigree simulating dominant inheritance will result; and (4) if two individuals with the same recessive disease marry, all their children will be affected.

The clinical picture in autosomal recessive disorders tends to be more uniform than that of dominant diseases, and the age of onset is often early in life. As a general rule, recessive disorders are more commonly diagnosed in children, while dominant diseases are more frequently encountered in adults.

Since with recessive inheritance only one of four children in a sibship is expected to be affected, multiple cases in a family may

TABLE 57-4 Approximate proportion of patients affected by new mutations in some autosomal dominant disorders

Disorder	Percentage
Achondroplasia	80
Tuberous sclerosis	80
Neurofibromatosis	40
Marfan's syndrome	30
Myotonic dystrophy	25
Huntington's chorea	4
Adult polycystic kidney disease	1
Familial hypercholesterolemia	Very low

FIGURE 57-7 *Pedigree pattern of an autosomal recessive trait. Note the horizontal pattern of inheritance.*

not occur. This is especially true in a society in which small families are common. Consider, for example, 16 families in which both parents are heterozygous for the same recessive disorder. If each family has two children, 9 of the families will have no affected children, 6 will have one affected and one normal child, and only 1 of the 16 families will have two affected children. In the United States physicians usually see sporadic or isolated cases of a recessive disorder without an affected sibling to alert them to the possibility of a genetic disorder. Fortunately, because of the relatively uniform clinical picture of recessive disorders and because most can be diagnosed directly by biochemical tests, the correct diagnosis can usually be made even when no other members of a family are clinically affected.

The basic biochemical lesions underlying many autosomal recessive disorders have been identified. Of the three types of proteins in which mutations could occur (i.e., enzymes, structural proteins, and regulatory proteins), the enzymes have been the easiest to study. A mutation that destroys the catalytic activity of an enzyme generally does not impair the health of a heterozygote (i.e., an individual who has one mutant allele specifying a functionless enzyme and one normal allele on the partner chromosome specifying a normal enzyme). In this situation each cell in the body usually produces about 50 percent of the normal number of active enzyme molecules. However, normal regulatory mechanisms function to avert any clinical consequences of this 50 percent deficiency, and so heterozygotes usually are clinically normal. On the other hand, when an individual inherits functionless alleles at both loci specifying an enzyme, the reduction in enzyme activity is too great for a compensatory mechanism to overcome, and a disease results. For example, heterozygotes for phenylketonuria have half the normal activity of phenylalanine hydroxylase, but they are clinically asymptomatic because the body compensates for the half-normal level of the enzyme by raising the substrate concentration approximately twofold. Under these conditions a normal amount of phenylalanine can be metabolized with no symptoms. On the other hand, the homozygote for phenylketonuria has such a severe reduction in phenylalanine hydroxylase activity that enormous levels of phenylalanine and its derivatives accumulate, causing detrimental brain development. As in the case of phenylketonuria, the majority of enzyme deficiency states produce *simultaneously* both a simple accumulation of one or more metabolites preceding the enzymatic block and a deficient production of other metabolites distal to the block in the metabolic pathway.

Most of the genetic enzyme deficiencies that have been elucidated are not only inherited as recessive traits but also tend to involve enzymes that participate in catabolic pathways. Frequently these enzymes degrade organic molecules that are ingested in the diet, such as galactose (galactosemia), phenylalanine (phenylketonuria), and phytanic acid (Refsum's syndrome). A special class of such catabolic diseases is that in which the deficiency affects an acid hydrolase that occurs within lysosomes. In these *lysosomal storage disorders* the substrate, usually a complex lipid or polysaccharide, accumulates within swollen lysosomes in specific organs, giving the cells a foamy appearance. Examples of such lysosomal diseases include the mucopolysaccharidoses such as Hurler's syndrome (α-iduronidase deficiency) and the lipid storage diseases such as Gaucher's disease (glucocerebrosidase deficiency).

In general, recessive diseases are rare because the reduced biologic fitness of homozygotes acts to remove the mutant gene from the population. However, a few recessive disorders, such as cystic fibrosis and sickle cell anemia, are common. To explain this paradox, it has been postulated that the biologic fitness of heterozygotes is greater than that of noncarriers for these genes. In such a case the frequency of the gene in the population depends on the balance between the increased fitness of the relatively numerous heterozygotes and the reduced fitness of the less common homozygotes. A small selective advantage of the heterozygote over the normal results in a high gene frequency and hence a high birth frequency of homozygotes even when the disease is lethal. Thus, about 1 in 22 Caucasians is a heterozygous carrier for the genetically lethal disease cystic fibrosis, and the disease occurs in about 1 in 2000 Caucasian births. To maintain such a high gene frequency, heterozygotes for cystic fibrosis must have a definite reproductive advantage over noncarriers, but the nature of this advantage is unknown. In sickle cell anemia, another recessive disorder with high frequency among certain populations, heterozygotes appear to have increased resistance to malaria.

Inasmuch as recessive diseases require the inheritance of a mutation at the same genetic locus from each parent, when the genes are rare, the likelihood of any two parents being carriers for the same defect becomes small. However, if the parents have a common ancestor and if that ancestor was a carrier for the recessive gene, then the likelihood that two of the descendants have inherited the gene becomes relatively great. The rarer the recessive gene, the stronger the likelihood that an affected individual will have resulted from such a consanguineous mating. On the other hand, certain recessive genes are so common in the population that the likelihood of two random parents being carriers is great enough to eliminate the need for consanguinity. For common traits such as sickle cell anemia, phenylketonuria, cystic fibrosis, and Tay-Sachs disease, all of which have a high carrier frequency in certain populations, consanguinity in the parents is unusual.

In general, consanguinity is infrequent in families with recessive diseases in the United States. This is because the rate of consanguinity in the general population is low. In most of the United States (as opposed to areas with relative geographic isolation such as northern Norway and Switzerland), a disorder must indeed be rare before it is associated with an important frequency of consanguinity. For example, consanguinity is expected in a large proportion of families having children with very rare disorders such as the Laurence-Moon-Biedl syndrome and abetalipoproteinemia.

Genetic compounds represent a special type of recessively inherited disorder in which the affected individual's two mutant genes, although located at the same genetic locus, are not identical. The mutations in the paternal and maternal alleles presumably involve different alterations in the DNA of the same gene. SC hemoglobinopathy is an example of such a *heteroallelic* compound state in which individuals have a gene for sickle cell hemoglobin on one chromosome and a gene for hemoglobin C on the homologous chromosome.

X-linked disorders   The genes responsible for X-linked disorders are located on the X chromosome; therefore, the clinical risk and severity of the disease are different for the two sexes. Since a female has two X chromosomes, she may be either heterozygous or homozygous for a mutant gene, and the trait may therefore demonstrate either recessive or dominant expression. Males, on the other hand, have only one X chromosome, so they can be expected to display the full syndrome whenever they inherit the gene regardless of whether the gene behaves as a recessive or as a dominant trait in the female. Thus, the terms *X-linked dominant* or *X-linked recessive* refer only to the expression of the gene in women.

An important feature of all X-linked inheritance is the absence of male-to-male (i.e., father-to-son) transmission of the trait. This follows because a male must always contribute his Y chromosome to his sons; hence, he can never contribute his X chromosome. On the other hand, a male contributes his one X chromosome to all his daughters.

The pedigree in Fig. 57-8 illustrates the characteristic features of X-linked recessive inheritance. (1) In contrast to the vertical transmission in dominant traits (parents and children affected) and the horizontal transmission in autosomal recessive traits (siblings affected), the pedigree pattern in X-linked recessive traits tends to be oblique because of the occurrence of the trait in the sons of normal carrier sisters of affected males (uncles and nephews affected) (Fig. 57-8A); (2) male offspring of carrier women have a 50 percent chance of being affected; (3) all female offspring of affected males are carriers, and affected males do not transmit the disease to their sons (Fig. 57-8C); (4) unaffected males do not transmit the trait to any

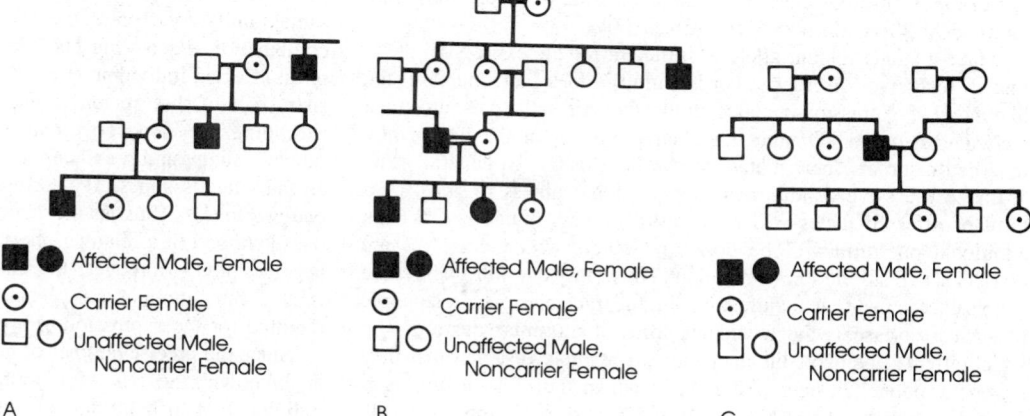

FIGURE 57-8 *Pedigree patterns of an X-linked recessive trait. A. Note the oblique pattern of inheritance. B. An affected female can result from the mating of an affected male and a carrier female, as in the consanguineous marriage shown here. C. An affected male mating with a normal noncarrier female has all normal sons and all carrier daughters.*

offspring; and (5) affected homozygous females occur only when an affected male fathers the child of a carrier female (Fig. 57-8*B*).

Examples of X-linked recessive disorders in humans include hemophilia A, nephrogenic diabetes insipidus, the Lesch-Nyhan syndrome, Duchenne form of muscular dystrophy, glucose 6-phosphate dehydrogenase deficiency, testicular feminization, and Fabry's disease. Color blindness is also inherited as an X-linked recessive trait, but it is sufficiently frequent (occurring in about 8 percent of white males) that the occurrence of homozygous color-blind females is no rarity.

X-linked dominant inheritance is illustrated by the pedigree in Fig. 57-9. Its characteristic features are as follows: (1) Females are affected about twice as often as males; (2) an affected female transmits the disorder to half of her sons and half of her daughters; (3) an affected male transmits the disorder to all his daughters and to none of his sons; and (4) the syndrome is more variable and less severe in heterozygous affected females than in hemizygous affected males. One common trait, the Xg(a+) blood group, is inherited as an X-linked dominant trait, as is vitamin D–resistant rickets (hypophosphatemic rickets).

Some rare conditions may be inherited as X-linked dominant traits in which there is lethality in the hemizygous male. The characteristics of this form of inheritance are illustrated by the pedigree in Fig. 57-10: (1) The disorder occurs only in females who are heterozygous for the mutant gene, (2) an affected mother transmits the trait to half of her daughters, (3) an increased frequency of abortions occurs in affected women, the abortions representing affected male fetuses. Conditions that appear to be transmitted by this mode of inheritance include incontinentia pigmenti, focal dermal hypoplasia, orofaciodigital syndrome, and hyperammonemia due to ornithine transcarbamylase deficiency.

Expression of X-linked traits in females tends to be variable because of the phenomenon of X-chromosome inactivation. Early in embryonic development one of the two X chromosomes in each somatic cell of a female is inactivated. The inactivation process is random, so that for each cell there is an equal probability that the paternally or maternally derived X chromosome will be inactivated. The inactivated X chromosome is rendered permanently nonfunctional, so that all progeny of the initial cell inherit the same active and inactive X chromosomes. Thus, each female is a mosaic; on the average, half of her cells express the X chromosome of the father, and half express the X chromosome of the mother. If a mutation in a gene is carried on one of her X chromosomes, about one-half of the cells in each tissue will be normal and the other half will manifest the mutant phenotype. However, chance or selection of one or the other set of clones of cells may disturb these proportions in any given individual. Depending on the proportions of mutant and normal X chromosomes in each tissue, a genetically heterozygous female may either be clinically normal or have mild or severe manifestations of the disease. To illustrate, mothers of boys with the X-linked recessive

Duchenne form of muscular dystrophy may occasionally show mild manifestations of the disease, such as limb girdle weakness or hypertrophied calves.

In each female cell the nonfunctional X chromosome can be visualized by several techniques. By ordinary staining, the inactivated X chromosome in metaphase appears heteropyknotic (condensed in appearance), and it replicates late in the mitotic cycle ("late-labeling" with tritiated thymidine). In nondividing cells the inactivated X chromosome can be observed as a clump of chromatin at the periphery of the nucleus—the so-called X chromatin or Barr body. In abnormal states with more than two X chromosomes such as 47, XXX, all but

FIGURE 57-9 *Pedigree pattern of an X-linked dominant trait.*

FIGURE 57-10 *Pedigree pattern of an X-linked dominant trait lethal in the hemizygous male.*

one of the X chromosomes are inactivated, so female cells may have multiple X chromatin bodies (see Chap. 60).

Since a single mutant allele is sufficient for the expression of X-linked recessive disorders, consanguinity does not increase the likelihood of expression in males, unlike the case in the rare autosomal recessive disorders. On the other hand, just as in the dominantly inherited disorders, new mutations can be a factor. In general, if an X-linked recessive condition reduces biologic fitness to zero, one-third of affected males will be a result of new mutations, and an additional one-third will be born to mothers who themselves are carriers as a result of a new mutation. Thus, only one-third will come from a classic pedigree manifesting oblique transmission. An example of such a disease is the Duchenne form of muscular dystrophy in which affected hemizygous males are so severely disabled that they never reproduce. In hemophilia A, in which the biologic fitness is greater than zero, about 20 percent of affected males represent new mutations.

In families in which only one male is affected with an X-linked recessive disease and there is no other family history of the trait, it is essential for proper genetic counseling that the mother undergo biochemical tests or other relevant studies to determine whether she is a carrier. If she is a carrier, half of her daughters will be carriers and half of her sons will be affected. On the other hand, if her affected son represents a new mutation, only his daughters will inherit the gene. At present, biochemical tests can identify female carriers for several X-linked diseases including the Lesch-Nyhan syndrome, Fabry's disease, Hunter's syndrome, hemophilia, and the Duchenne form of muscular dystrophy.

The distinction between X-linked inheritance and *sex-influenced autosomal dominant inheritance* is important. Baldness is probably inherited as an autosomal dominant trait, yet it is manifested mainly in men and rarely in women. Heterozygous females express the baldness gene only when a source of testosterone becomes available as occurs with a masculinizing tumor of the ovary.

MULTIFACTORIAL GENETIC DISEASES   The common chronic diseases of adults (such as essential hypertension, coronary heart disease, diabetes mellitus, peptic ulcer disease, and schizophrenia) as well as the common birth defects (such as cleft lip and palate, spina bifida, and congenital heart disease) have been long known to "run in families." They fit best into the category of *multifactorial genetic diseases*. The genetic element in these disorders rarely manifests itself in an all-or-none fashion as it does in the simply inherited (mendelian) disorders and in chromosomal aberrations. Instead, it is the interaction of multiple genes with multiple environmental factors that produces the familial aggregation.

In the multifactorial genetic diseases, there is a *polygenic component* consisting of a series of genes that interact in a cumulative fashion. An individual who inherits the right combination of these genes passes beyond a "threshold of risk," at which point an *environmental component* determines whether and to what extent that

person is clinically affected. In order for another individual in the same family to express the same syndrome, the same or similar combination of genes must be inherited. Since the first-degree relatives of an affected individual (i.e., parents, siblings, and offspring) each share half of that person's genes, they are all at increased risk of exhibiting the same polygenic syndrome. Second-degree relatives (uncles, aunts, and grandparents) share on the average one-fourth of an individual's genes $(\frac{1}{2})^2$, and third-degree relatives (cousins) share one-eighth $(\frac{1}{2})^3$. Thus, as the degree of relation becomes more distant, the likelihood of a relative inheriting the same combination of genes becomes less. Moreover, the chances of any relative inheriting the right combination of risk genes decrease as the number of genes required for the expression of a given trait increases.

Since the precise number of genes responsible for polygenic traits is unknown, the risk of inheritance for a relative of an affected individual is difficult to calculate, and the standard is based on empiric risk figures (i.e., a direct tally of the proportion of affected relatives in previously reported families). In contrast to the simply inherited disorders in which 25 or 50 percent of the first-degree relatives of an affected proband are at genetic risk, multifactorial genetic disorders are generally observed empirically to affect no more than 5 to 10 percent of first-degree relatives. Moreover, in contrast to mendelian traits, the recurrence risk of multifactorial conditions varies from family to family, and its estimation is significantly influenced by two factors: (1) the number of affected persons already present in the family, and (2) the severity of the disorder in the index case. The greater the number of affected relatives and the more severe their disease, the higher the risk to other relatives. For example, the risk of cleft lip in the siblings of a child with unilateral cleft lip is about 2.5 percent, but if the lesion in the index case is bilateral, the risk in the siblings rises to 6 percent. Table 57-5 lists the empiric risk figures for the familial recurrence of a number of multifactorial genetic diseases.

The hypothesis of a polygenic component in the inheritance of multifactorial diseases has been given a sound basis in recent years by the demonstration that at least one-third of all gene loci harbor polymorphic alleles that vary among individuals. Such a large degree of variation in normal genes undoubtedly provides the substrate for variations in genetic predisposition with which environmental factors can interact. So far, the genetic loci most strikingly associated with predisposition to specific diseases are those that constitute the HLA system (also called the *major histocompatibility gene complex*) (see Chap. 63). The HLA gene complex is located on the short arm of chromosome 6. It consists of four closely linked but distinct loci (A, B, C, and D). The products of these genes are proteins that are found on the surface of body cells and that enable an individual's immune system to distinguish its own cells from those of someone else. Each HLA locus in the population consists of multiple alleles, each of which produces an immunologically distinct protein. For example, an individual may inherit any 2 of 20 alleles at the HLA-B locus.

An important observation of recent years has been the finding that certain alleles at the HLA loci predispose individuals to certain specific diseases. For example, if the B27 allele at the HLA-B locus is inherited by an individual, that person has a 121-fold greater chance of developing ankylosing spondylitis than an individual who lacks this allele (Table 57-6). Ankylosing spondylitis remains a multifactorial disease, however, because its development clearly requires one or more other factors in addition to the B27 allele. Thus, less than 15 percent of people who inherit this allele develop this disease. Table 57-6 lists some of the diseases associated with alleles at the HLA loci. Several of them are suspected to be of viral etiology, suggesting that the HLA loci may dictate the mode of expression of certain viral diseases. A more detailed discussion of the HLA system is presented in Chap. 63.

Multifactorial disorders are heterogeneous in the sense that the relative contribution of the polygenic factors ("risk genes") and environmental factors to the etiology vary greatly from patient to patient. However, it is important to remember that among common

TABLE 57-5   Empiric risks for some common multifactorial genetic diseases affecting adults

Disorder in index case	Estimated absolute risk for first-degree relatives, %
Cleft lip and/or palate	3
Congenital heart disease	4
Coronary heart disease	8 for male relatives
	3 for female relatives
Diabetes mellitus	5–10
Epilepsy	5–10
Hypertension	10
Manic-depressive psychosis	10–15
Psoriasis	10–15
Schizophrenia	15
Thyroid disease (autoimmune disorders including hyperthyroidism, thyroiditis, primary myxedema, simple goiter)	10

phenotypes which are largely multifactorial, often a small proportion will be created by major mutant genes. For example, although coronary heart disease is usually of multifactorial etiology, about 5 percent of subjects with premature myocardial infarctions are heterozygotes for familial hypercholesterolemia, a single-gene disorder that produces atherosclerosis in the absence of any other predisposing factor. Similarly, in a small proportion of patients with other common diseases such as peptic ulcer disease or "essential" hypertension, the condition is not multifactorial but determined by a single gene, as in the multiple endocrine adenoma–peptic ulcer syndrome or the medullary thyroid carcinoma–pheochromocytoma syndrome, respectively.

INTERACTION BETWEEN SINGLE GENETIC AND ENVIRONMENTAL FACTORS

Many diseases result from an interaction between a specific genotype and a specific environmental factor. In particular, inherited single-gene mutations may produce clinically significant and often life-threatening idiosyncratic responses to certain drugs.

Table 57-7 lists the most important of these *pharmacogenetic disorders,* which encompass all the mendelian modes of inheritance. Perhaps the most common is glucose 6-phosphate dehydrogenase deficiency, an X-linked recessive trait in which a variety of drugs may precipitate a hemolytic anemia. Plasma pseudocholinesterase deficiency and hepatic transacetylase deficiency are examples of autosomal recessive traits which alter drug catabolism so that when the muscle relaxant suxamethonium or the antituberculous drug isoniazid is administered, apnea or peripheral neuropathy, respectively, may ensue. Malignant hyperthermia is an autosomal dominant trait in which acute hyperpyrexia, muscle rigidity, and hyperkalemic cardiac arrest may be induced by administration of any one of several anesthetic agents. Acute intermittent porphyria is another example of a genetic disorder that is exacerbated by drugs, such as barbiturates.

TABLE 57-6 Alleles at the HLA loci associated with multifactorial genetic diseases

Disease	HLA locus	Specific allele	Relative risk*
Ankylosing spondylitis	B	B27	121
Reiter's syndrome	B	B27	40
Psoriasis with arthritis	B	B27	5
Celiac disease	B	B8	10
Chronic active hepatitis	B	B8	4
Myasthenia gravis	B	B8	4
Diabetes mellitus (insulin-dependent)	DR	DR3/DR4	33
Hyperthyroidism	DR	DR3	4
Addison's disease	B	B8	7
	DR	DR4	10
Multiple sclerosis	DR	DR2	7

* Relative risk *is the probability of the disease developing in an individual with the specific allele, divided by the probability of its development in an individual who does not possess this specific allele.*

Misinterpretation of adverse drug reactions may result in serious harm to patients. In general, all unusual idiosyncratic reactions should be considered to be genetically determined until proved otherwise. Fortunately, the pharmacogenetic disorders are a group of diseases for which therapy is straightforward: avoidance of the noxious drug by patient and relatives.

In addition to drugs, other factors in the environment may aggravate specific genetic traits. Cigarette smoke may have deleterious effects on persons homozygous and possibly heterozygous for alpha$_1$-antitrypsin deficiency, who are predisposed to the development of emphysema. Patients with xeroderma pigmentosa and anhydrotic ectodermal dysplasia are unusually sensitive to sunlight and high temperatures, respectively. Avoidance of milk at an early age prevents many of the complications ordinarily seen in persons with galactosemia.

Genetic-environmental interactions are particularly important in pregnancy. Women who are affected with phenylketonuria may

TABLE 57-7 Examples of inherited disorders involving an abnormal response to drugs

Disorder	Molecular abnormality	Mode of inheritance	Frequency	Clinical effect	Drugs producing abnormal response
Slow inactivation of isoniazid	Isoniazid acetylase in liver	Autosomal recessive	~50% of U.S. population	Polyneuritis	Isoniazid, sulfamethazine, sulfamaprine, phenelzine, dapsone, hydralazine
Suxamethonium sensitivity	Pseudocholinesterase in plasma	Autosomal recessive	Several mutant alleles; most common affects 1 in 2500	Apnea	Suxamethonium, succinylcholine
Warfarin insensitivity	? Altered receptor or enzyme in liver with increased affinity for vitamin K	Autosomal dominant	Rare	Inability to achieve anticoagulation with usual doses of drug	Warfarin
Glaucoma	Unknown	? Autosomal dominant	Common	Increased intraocular pressure	Corticosteroids
Malignant hyperthermia	Unknown	Autosomal dominant	~1 in 20,000 anesthetized patients	Severe hyperpyrexia, muscle rigidity, death	Such anesthetics as halothane, succinylcholine, methoxyfluorane, ether, cyclopropane
Unstable hemoglobins: Hemoglobin Zurich	Arginine substitution for histidine at sixty-third position of β chain of hemoglobin	Autosomal dominant	Rare	Hemolysis	Sulfonamides
Hemoglobin H	Hemoglobin composed of four β chains	Autosomal dominant	Rare	Hemolysis	Sulfisoxazole
Glucose 6-phosphate dehydrogenase deficiency	Glucose 6-phosphate dehydrogenase in erythrocytes	X-linked recessive	~ 1×10^8 affected persons in world; common in persons of African, Mediterranean, Asiatic origin; multiple mutant alleles	Hemolysis	Analgesics, sulfonamides, antimalarials, nitrofurantoin, other drugs

SOURCE: *ES Vesell, N Engl J Med 287:904, 1972.*

develop high plasma phenylalanine levels during pregnancy, and thus their offspring may suffer from a variety of phenylalanine-induced birth defects even though the offspring may not themselves have phenylketonuria. Other examples of diseases resulting from an adverse genetic relation between the mother and fetus include erythroblastosis caused by Rh incompatibility and diabetic embryopathy, a term that refers to a series of major birth defects occurring in about 5 percent of the offspring of women who are clinically diabetic during pregnancy.

REFERENCES

HARRIS H: *The Principles of Human Biochemical Genetics*, 3d ed. New York, American Elsevier, 1980

LEWIN B: *Genes*, 2d ed. New York, Wiley, 1985

MCKUSICK VA: *Mendelian Inheritance in Man: Catalogs of Autosomal Dominant, Autosomal Recessive and X-Linked Phenotypes*, 6th ed. Baltimore, Johns Hopkins, 1983

——: The human gene map. *Clin Genet* 27:207, 1985

STANBURY JB et al: *The Metabolic Basis of Inherited Disease*, 5th ed. New York, McGraw-Hill, 1983

VOGEL F, MOTULSKY AG: *Human Genetics: Problems and Approaches*, 2d ed. Berlin, Springer-Verlag, 1986

58   MOLECULAR GENETICS AND MEDICINE

ARTHUR L. BEAUDET

The human genome contains about 3×10^9 (3 billion) base pairs of DNA and encodes 30,000 to 100,000 gene products. The length of DNA frequently is quantitated in thousands of bases (kilobases, kb), e.g., the human genome is 3 million kb in length. Each individual inherits two copies of this genome, and the DNA is packaged as 23 pairs of chromosomes. Each chromosome contains a single linear duplex DNA molecule. Most of the DNA sequences that encode proteins occur as unique (single copy) sequences in the genome. Many gene products show similarities in amino acid sequence and can be viewed as members of large gene families, e.g., the globin gene family. A large amount of DNA in the genome appears not to be functional. Hundreds or thousands of repetitive DNA sequences of uncertain function are present in the genome; some are dispersed, and some are clustered.

If one were to print *one copy* of *one strand* of the human genome, it would fill a text 170 times the size of *Harrison's*. The analogy of the human genome to a large book can be carried further. The book can be envisioned as being bound into 46 separate volumes, each the equivalent of one chromosome. Individuals would inherit one paternal set of 23 volumes and one maternal set of 23 volumes. Sickle cell anemia would be the equivalent of changing a single letter on one page of one volume from each of the sets, while deletion of the alpha-globin gene cluster in alpha thalassemia might represent the equivalent of the loss of one or two pages of text in each set. Digestion of genomic DNA with restriction enzymes, which recognize specific short DNA sequences and cut DNA at these sites, would be the equivalent of cutting the line of text each time a specific word occurred.

The human genome is polymorphic in two ways. One way is by differences in primary DNA sequence, and the second involves the biologic significance of such variations. Beginning at the single nucleotide level, the DNA sequence for the human genome can be variable or relatively constant at a given position. As an example, a DNA base would be highly variable if 50 percent of genes in the population had an A (adenine) nucleotide at the position, 40 percent of genes had a G (guanine) nucleotide there, and 10 percent of genes had a C (cytosine) nucleotide. Nucleotide positions where more than 1 percent of genes show a nonmajority sequence are designated *polymorphic sites*. Only 1 in 200 to 1 in 500 nucleotide positions qualify as polymorphic. Most nucleotide positions are relatively invariant, the vast majority having the same sequence. The remaining positions have intermediate frequencies of variation. Nucleotide sequence variation is greater in nonfunctional parts of the genome, less in regions of the genome that encode protein sequence or have other important functions. The consequence is that each copy of the human genome varies from every other copy in millions of sequence-specific ways. The nucleotide variations might be envisioned as a multimillion digit serial number embedded within each copy of the human genome. The variability in primary sequence goes beyond single-base changes to include presence or absence of whole segments of DNA. Indeed, considerable length variations occur in the human genome. Inversions of DNA sequence also occur, and translocations between chromosomes also cause DNA variation.

The second type of genetic variation involves phenotypic effect. The alteration of a single nucleotide or single gene may have a dramatic effect. Indeed, certain DNA sequence alterations may be lethal at the stage of the gamete, fertilized egg, or preimplantation embryo. These instances in which a single alteration has a large effect on the phenotype are single-gene disorders; such disorders have been the focus of most efforts to understand human genetic disease up to the present. However, most of the nucleotide differences between human genomes do not cause any significant phenotypic effect. A continuum exists whereby variations in DNA sequence have phenotypic effects ranging from none to minuscule, to small, to moderate, to large, or to overwhelming. In many instances, multiple genetic loci may interact with each other and/or with environmental factors to produce a phenotypic effect. For example, genetic variations in lipoprotein genes, lipoprotein receptor genes, genes that influence intermediary metabolism, and other genes probably interact with diet, smoking, and additional environmental factors to determine susceptibility to atherosclerosis. Together, variations in DNA sequence and in the biologic effect caused by these differences create individuality. Individuals are probably as heterogeneous in susceptibility to hypertension, atherosclerosis, cancer, psychiatric symptoms, and obesity as in their facial appearance and fingerprint patterns.

ANALYSIS OF THE HUMAN GENOME

POWER OF THE RECOMBINANT DNA TECHNIQUES   The size, the complexity, and the variability of the human genome constitute barriers to the analysis of individual traits and genes. The feasibility for such analysis was greatly enhanced by the development of recombinant DNA technology. This technology allows for the analysis of one DNA fragment at a time and has provided an index for the human genome and made it possible to locate and isolate individual genes, segments of genes, or nucleotide sequences from the vast DNA library. One of the most powerful of these techniques, so-called cloning of DNA, makes it possible to isolate individual genes or portions of genes, to make an unlimited number of copies of such DNA fragments, and to transcribe and translate the genes so isolated. The various genes and gene products can then be utilized for diverse studies of gene structure and function in normal and disease states. Other recombinant DNA techniques make it possible to analyze genetic variation in individuals directly using clinical samples. Using DNA-hybridization techniques and restriction fragment length polymorphisms (RFLP), to be described below, disease traits can be analyzed both directly and by genetic linkage of polymorphic sites.

The cloning of DNA involves isolation of DNA fragments and insertion of a sequence into the nucleic acid from another biologic source (vector) for manipulation and propagation. The most widely used vectors for this purpose are bacterial plasmids, which have a genome of small, circular, double-stranded DNA. Among other properties, these plasmids can encode resistance to multiple antibiotics, and hence bacteria containing the plasmids can be isolated by virtue of their antibiotic resistance. The plasmids contain a site of origin for DNA replication, and they exist in the bacterial cell as extrachromosomal DNA. Many copies of the plasmid genome can be present in a single bacterium, allowing both high levels of expression of the cloned genes and easy isolation of plasmid DNA.

Another group of vectors are derived from modifications of bacteriophage λ. These bacteriophages can accommodate up to about 15,000 base pairs of inserted DNA and are suitable for preparation of DNA libraries. Cosmid vectors are constructed from fragments of bacteriophages and plasmids; such cosmids can accommodate even larger segments of inserted DNA and combine some technical advantages of λ vectors and of plasmid vectors. Recombinant DNA molecules are grown and manipulated in a host organism such as *Escherichia coli*. Frequently, host strains with impaired genes for recombination are utilized to reduce rearrangements in the cloned foreign DNA.

The development of techniques for the cloning of genes and of other applications of recombinant DNA technology was dependent on the specificity of nucleic acid hybridization and the use of enzymes that cleave DNA at specific sites (restriction endonucleases).

Nucleic acid hybridization Many of the steps in recombinant DNA analysis take advantage of the fact that the complementary nature of nucleic acid interaction is the result of base pairing during the synthesis of DNA and RNA (see Chap. 57). Linear pieces of double-stranded (native) DNA can be treated with heat or alkali to dissociate the two strands to yield single-stranded (denatured) DNA. The denatured DNA can be incubated under conditions that allow for nucleic acid hybridization, i.e., the recognition of two complementary strands and re-formation of double-stranded molecules by base pairing. Nucleic acid hybridization is so sensitive that a single-stranded DNA molecule can be hybridized specifically to a complementary strand of RNA or DNA present at about 1 part in 10,000. Many recombinant DNA studies involve the preparation of one radioactive strand of nucleic acid which is then used as a "probe" in the analysis. It is possible to identify and distinguish both fully homologous sequences and partially homologous sequences. The specificity of nucleic acid hybridization, sometimes in combination with other techniques, allows detection of a single gene among tens of thousands or of a viral sequence in the midst of other nucleic acid sequences.

Restriction endonucleases The discovery in microorganisms of restriction endonucleases, commonly known as restriction enzymes, facilitated recombinant DNA manipulations. The enzymes recognize a specific oligonucleotide sequence in double-stranded DNA and cleave the DNA at this site. Many of these enzymes recognize different DNA sequences (Fig. 58-1). Some enzymes recognize sequences only four nucleotides in length. For example, the enzyme *Hae* III cleaves the sequence 5′-GGCC-3′. Other enzymes recognize sequences six nucleotides in length. The enzyme *Hin*d III cleaves the sequence 5′-AAGCTT-3′ (T = thymine). Other enzymes, such as *Mst* II, recognize a seven-base-pair sequence but tolerate any nucleotide pair in the middle position. The sequence specificity of restriction enzymes is a powerful tool in dissection of large genomes. When human DNA is digested with a particular restriction enzyme, hundreds of thousands of DNA fragments are generated with remarkable reproducibility. Such fragments can vary from a few nucleotides to several thousand nucleotides in length, depending on the enzyme used. Restriction enzymes that recognize a sequence only four base pairs long cleave the DNA into smaller fragments than enzymes that recognize a six-base-pair sequence. With the use of multiple restriction enzymes to analyze a particular segment of DNA, it is possible to define a detailed map of restriction endonuclease cleavage sites for the region. Such a map can span a region of from several hundred to tens of thousands of base pairs of DNA. As described below, variations in the sequences of those cleavage sites can be utilized to analyze variations in the human genome. In addition, the sequence specificity of restriction endonucleases has been used

$$Hae\ III \qquad \begin{array}{l} 5'-G-G\ |\ C-C-3' \\ 3'-C-C\ \downarrow\ G-G-5' \end{array}$$

$$Hind\ III \qquad \begin{array}{l} 5'-A\ |\ A-G-C-T-T-3' \\ 3'-T-T-C-G-A\ |\ A-5' \end{array}$$

$$Mst\ II \qquad \begin{array}{l} 5'-C-C\ |\ T-N-A-G-G-3' \\ 3'-G-G-A-N-T\ |\ C-C-5' \end{array}$$

FIGURE 58-1 *DNA sequence specificity and nuclease activity for three restriction endonucleases. Hae III leaves a blunt end while the other enzymes leave single-stranded ends.*

to analyze for differences in the sequence of a particular site in the human genome as will be demonstrated below.

Southern blotting Many analyses of the human genome involve a specific application of DNA-DNA hybridization, the blotting procedure developed by E.M. Southern. For clinical analysis, *Southern blotting* (Fig. 58-2) begins with the isolation of genomic DNA from cells such as peripheral leukocytes or amniotic fluid cells. The high-molecular-weight genomic DNA is digested with a restriction enzyme

FIGURE 58-2 *Southern blotting analysis of genomic DNA.*

GENOMIC DNA

RESTRICTION ENZYME DIGESTION

RFLP

DELETION

AGAROSE GEL ELECTROPHORESIS

MEMBRANE

GEL

HYBRIDIZATION WITH RADIOACTIVE PROBE

AUTORADIOGRAM

to yield a series of reproducible fragments. These DNA fragments are separated by electrophoresis in agarose gels. After electrophoresis, the DNA is transferred from the gel to a membrane that binds the DNA. The membrane is treated to denature the DNA and is soaked in a solution containing a radioactive single-stranded nucleic acid probe. The probe will form a double-stranded nucleic acid complex at sites on the membrane where homologous DNA is present. The membrane is washed to remove unbound radioactivity, and regions on the membrane where homologous DNA sequences were bound are detected using x-ray film. The sensitivity of Southern blotting is achieved by splitting the DNA into small segments, fractionating the fragments, and applying a sensitive detection method to pick out specific fragments (nucleic acid hybridization). Overall, this method can detect genomic DNA fragments that represent a single gene or about 1 part in 1 million in the genome. The clinical power of Southern blotting resides in the ability it gives to analyze a tiny portion of the primary structure of human genomic DNA taken from an individual.

An analogous procedure starting with RNA for analysis has been termed *northern* (in contrast to Southern) *blotting*. In this procedure, the presence or absence of a particular mRNA as well as its approximate size can be determined. The term *western blotting* describes a derivative procedure designed to analyze protein antigens. Proteins are separated by electrophoresis and transferred to a solid membrane through a blotting procedure. The membrane is analyzed by incubation with antibodies followed by a second step for enzymatic or radioactive detection of bound antibody. Thus, Southern blotting, northern blotting, and western blotting each combines a fractionation and a detection method to provide a sensitive technique for the analysis of DNA, RNA, and protein, respectively (Table 58-1).

Illustrative strategy for DNA cloning   Technical aspects of DNA cloning will be described briefly; for details see Watson. Many of the early successful efforts to clone eukaryotic genes involved purification of mRNA from tissues where a gene product, such as globin, immunoglobulin, and albumin, was found in abundance. Reverse transcriptase was used to copy a first strand of DNA complementary to the mRNA (cDNA). *E. coli* DNA polymerase was used to copy a second strand of DNA from the first strand. Insert DNA and vector DNA were hybridized and introduced into *E. coli* where the mosaic molecules were repaired and ligated to yield recombinant DNA plasmids containing foreign cDNA inserts. Growth and multiplication of the *E. coli* then resulted in production of unlimited amounts of the DNA sequence in question. This general strategy for cloning cDNA sequences is still useful.

Current strategies for cloning genes or DNA sequences use some combination of the following approaches: availability of antibodies to a gene product; availability of amino acid sequence data for a gene product; nucleic acid hybridization specificity; knowledge of the biology of a differentiated system; or analysis for a biologic function of the cloned gene product.

Immunoprecipitation of polysomes with antibodies to a protein allows for partial purification of the specific mRNA, which can be cloned as described above. Another strategy involves preparation of cDNA libraries from mRNA isolated from specific sources such as liver, brain, or cultured human fibroblasts. Each mRNA will be represented approximately according to its abundance in each tissue. After the cloning process, these libraries can be screened to identify sequences expressed in the appropriate tissue.

Occasionally, functional properties of a gene can facilitate cloning of DNA sequences. Enzymes produced may complement bacterial deficiencies, or products of eukaryotic genes produced by bacteria may have biologic properties that are assayable or can be identified with specific antibodies. If amino acid sequence data are available for a protein, the specificity of the genetic code allows for reverse translation of this sequence into a nucleic acid sequence with limited ambiguity. Single-stranded oligonucleotide probes then can be synthesized and used to screen cloned DNA libraries by hybridization techniques to identify sequences that could encode the protein (see Chap. 57). Using various strategies, more than 300 mammalian genes have been cloned. Isolation of a cloned gene in other mammalian species usually is sufficient to isolate the human equivalent by using the nonhuman clone as a probe to screen human cDNA and genomic DNA libraries using nucleic acid hybridization techniques.

Construction of recombinant DNA libraries is an essential part of strategies for recombinant DNA analysis of human biology, and cDNA libraries are available from most human tissues. Construction of genomic DNA libraries is designed to achieve a series of clones that will include all human sequences without regard to expression. These libraries usually are constructed by restriction enzyme digestion of total human genomic DNA followed by insertion into appropriate recombinant DNA vectors. Genomic DNA libraries have also been prepared from individual human chromosomes that are separated by fluorescence-activated sorting prior to cloning.

For more detailed analysis of genes or DNA, cloned DNA fragments can be sequenced to determine their nucleotide structure. Using these methods, the normal sequence and the mutant sequence for many human genes have been determined.

RFLP MAP OF THE GENOME   In 1978, Kan and Dozy demonstrated genetic variation in the size of fragments generated after digestion of normal human DNA with restriction endonucleases. These differences are caused by the DNA sequence polymorphisms discussed above. Restriction enzyme digestion and Southern blotting analysis make it possible to identify these polymorphisms and utilize them as markers for specific sites within the genome. If one of the base pairs in the recognition sequence for a restriction enzyme is variable between individual copies of the genome, or if there is a length variation in the DNA, there will be variation in the size of DNA fragments generated by the restriction enzyme digestion. When the probe for Southern blotting analysis identifies a unique DNA sequence, the pattern of resulting fragments is simple. These restriction fragment length polymorphisms (RFLP) reflect the polymorphisms in normal DNA and are inherited according to mendelian principles. Typical RFLPs are demonstrated in Fig. 58-3. Highly polymorphic sites occur when a sequence is tandemly repeated a variable number of times to give extensive length variation at the site. Although each restriction enzyme detects only a portion of nucleotide variation, the large number of different restriction enzymes available and the extent of genetic heterogeneity allow for detection of almost unlimited numbers of RFLPs.

The ability to analyze primary DNA structure in clinical samples and the availability of gene markers in the form of RFLPs have made it possible to generate a detailed human gene map. Multiple RFLPs detectable in a small region can be linked together to form a series, or haplotype, of tightly clustered DNA markers to enhance the informativeness of such analyses (see "Disorders of globin genes" below). Such haplotypes are equivalent to determination of tiny bits of the unique "serial number" in each copy of the genome. It is also possible to demonstrate linkage of RFLPs to genes for human disease. In the cases of Huntington's disease, cystic fibrosis, and adult polycystic kidney disease the availability of RFLPs made it possible to obtain cloned DNA markers near the disease genes before the identity of the mutant gene or its normal allele was known. "Chromosome walking" (cloning immediate flanking DNA fragments) over short distances is possible, and strategies have been suggested for hopping longer distances to adjacent DNA. It will eventually be possible to clone the gene responsible for any mendelian disorder. A

TABLE 58-1   Analytical blotting procedures

Blot method	Material analyzed	Fractionation	Detection
Southern	DNA	Electrophoresis	Nucleic acid hybridization
Northern	RNA	Electrophoresis	Nucleic acid hybridization
Western	Protein	Electrophoresis	Immunologic

FIGURE 58-3 *Examples of restriction fragment length polymorphisms in human DNA. The solid blocks indicate segments of DNA used as probe. Parents are homozygous and children are heterozygous for the left panel,* while the parents are heterozygous and children are homozygous for the right panel. Symbols above the arrows indicating cutting (+) or noncutting (−) by the restriction endonuclease. Numbers indicate DNA length in kilobases.

detailed human gene map would also make it possible to analyze the role of individual loci in diseases with polygenic or multifactorial etiologies. RFLPs should not be confused with mutant genes. Mutations that cause disease are almost always too rare to be classified as polymorphisms, and only occasionally can they be detected directly with restriction enzymes.

Genetic linkage and linkage disequilibrium
The general concepts of genetic recombination and linkage are discussed in Chap. 57. For autosomal genes, each new individual inherits one copy of each chromosome from each parent. Each chromosome is a unique mosaic of polymorphic DNA sequences derived by crossing-over between grandparental chromosomes through the process of meiotic recombination (Fig. 58-4). Genes on different chromosomes are inherited independently, but genes close together on the same chromosome are inherited together unless a meiotic crossover occurs between the two genes. Genes far apart on the same chromosome are inherited as if they were on different chromosomes because of the high likelihood of meiotic crossovers between two distant loci. Genetic distance is expressed in centimorgans (cM) and is a measure of the likelihood of crossover between two loci. The usual clinical concern is whether the disease gene or the normal gene was transmitted from an individual to the next generation. This is true for prenatal diagnosis, presymptomatic diagnosis, and heterozygote detection. If the mutant gene in question can be detected directly by DNA analysis, genetic linkage need not be considered. However, diagnostic analysis frequently relies on a genetic variation near the disease locus for clinical diagnosis. In current terms, this usually means utilization of an RFLP as the nearby genetic marker. If the cloned disease gene is available

as a probe, there is negligible likelihood of a crossover between the disease gene and a nearby RFLP (RFLP #1, Fig. 58-4). If the cloned disease gene is not available, it may be possible to use another cloned DNA fragment near the disease gene. In this instance, there will be occasional crossover between the disease locus and the RFLP (RFLP #2, Fig. 58-4). Other RFLPs may be so far from the disease locus that no functional linkage is demonstrable (RFLP #3, Fig. 58-4). There are on average 30 to 35 crossovers during meiosis in males and perhaps twice as many during meiosis in females. The frequency of meiotic crossing-over is not uniform along the length of chromosomes.

For clinical linkage analysis, it is essential that some genetic marker near the disease gene be informative. This means that the individual who is heterozygous for the disease locus must also be heterozygous for a nearby genetic marker. Most analyses can be made informative, since RFLPs are frequent and since it is usually possible to identify useful polymorphisms at important sites. A second requirement is the need to know the *phase* between the two loci for genetic analysis. If an RFLP yields a 10-kb DNA fragment and a 5-kb DNA fragment, it is necessary to know whether the disease gene is linked with the 10-kb fragment and the normal gene with the 5-kb fragment or vice versa. With this knowledge of phase, analysis of which fragment size was transmitted will indicate whether the disease gene or the normal gene was transmitted. The accuracy of such predictions depends upon the proximity of the two genetic loci and the possibility for crossover. Determination of phase usually rests upon previous occurrence of disease within a family or the use of biologic tests to determine the phenotype or genotype. Examples of RFLP analysis in clinical situations will be presented below.

FIGURE 58-4 *Depiction of two chromosomes (one in solid lines and one in dotted lines) from an individual before (above) and after (below) meiotic crossing over. The individual is heterozygous for a disease locus with a normal allele (filled square) and a disease allele (open square) and for three RFLPs with alleles A/B, M/N, and Y/Z. See discussion in text.*

Linkage disequilibrium refers to the fact that certain genes occur together in homogeneous populations more frequently than can be explained by chance. Any new mutation at a specific site must occur on a chromosome of a particular genotype and near preexisting polymorphic sites. If no crossovers occur, after a few generations, all of the daughter chromosomes that contain the mutant gene also will contain the same immediate neighboring DNA sequences. If a few crossovers occur, the extent of this association between close neighbors will be partially disrupted. Linkage disequilibrium describes the fact that two closely linked traits tend to be found together more often than their overall frequency in the gene population would predict if they were each distributed randomly (i.e., in equilibrium). The association patterns reflect the history of crossover events between very close genetic loci. Therefore, a particular RFLP haplotype frequently may be inherited together with a disease gene.

Linkage disequilibrium was demonstrated with the first RFLP described by Kan and colleagues near the beta-globin locus. The enzyme *Hpa* I gives rise to a 13-kb, 7.6-kb, or 7-kb fragment of the beta-globin gene based on a polymorphism in the 3′ flanking region of the gene. The sickle cell mutation is found preferentially with the 13-kb variant in some west African and Mediterranean populations. Linkage disequilibrium affects clinical analyses in two principal ways. First, when developing a haplotype for adjacent RFLPs, extensive linkage disequilibrium is common, so that only a portion of all possible haplotypes (RFLP combinations) are observed. Second, occasional strong linkage disequilibrium between an RFLP haplotype and a disease allele may be of diagnostic value as discussed for alpha$_1$-antitrypsin deficiency below.

Finding a DNA marker near a disease gene Development of a detailed human gene map based on DNA markers made it possible to search for genetic linkages for all common important mendelian disorders. Figure 58-5 depicts analysis for linkage to an autosomal disorder using two randomly selected DNA markers, one of which has A and B alleles and resides near the disease gene on the same chromosome, and one of which has Y and Z alleles and is on a different chromosome. Inspection of the family data suggests linkage of the marker with A and B alleles to the disease locus, and analysis of sufficient pedigree data can provide conclusive evidence that a DNA polymorphic marker is near a disease gene. The frequency of crossovers can be used to estimate the genetic distance between the two markers. Any DNA clone can be mapped to a chromosome. This strategy was used to identify an anonymous (random) DNA segment linked to the Huntington's chorea locus at a distance of 3 to 5 cM on the short arm of chromosome 4. Likewise, a highly polymorphic DNA region near the alpha-globin cluster is linked to the adult polycystic kidney disease locus on chromosome 16. Analogous efforts can be applied to autosomal recessive diseases; for example, the cystic fibrosis gene was mapped to chromosome 7 using this strategy.

CURRENT VIEW OF A TYPICAL GENE A typical gene produces an mRNA that is translated into a protein (Fig. 58-6) (also see Chap. 57). The end of the gene where transcription (RNA synthesis) originates is referred to as the 5′ end, relative to the orientation of the mRNA. The site where transcription begins is referred to as the Cap site. At least some of the DNA sequences required for initiation

AUTOSOMAL DOMINANT MEDICAL DISORDER

D   DISEASE ALLELE
N   NORMAL ALLELE
■,● DISEASE PHENOTYPE
□,○ NORMAL PHENOTYPE

FIGURE 58-5 *Example of a search for linkage of DNA markers to an autosomal dominant disease. A and B are DNA marker alleles at one site, and Y and Z are alleles at another site. Two pairs of chromosomes are depicted for each parent. The B haplotype and the disease allele are inherited together from the father except for the last-born child in whom a crossover occurred, and the A haplotype was inherited with the disease allele.*

FIGURE 58-6 *A typical gene encoding a protein product. Sequences included in mature mRNA (exons) are represented by open blocks with narrower regions for untranslated sequences. Introns (intervening sequences) are shown as hatched blocks.*

FIGURE 58-7 *A splicing mutation in the beta-globin gene. Exons are numbered and introns are hatched. A mutation in the first nucleotide in the second intron causes the formation of two abnormal mRNA products (right).*

and regulation of transcription are located upstream from this region (opposite from the direction of transcription, to the left in Fig. 58-6). Many upstream regions contain sequences referred to as TATA boxes and CAAT boxes, which are involved in the initiation and control of transcription. Important sequences for gene regulation may also occur even further upstream and downstream from the Cap site. The segments of DNA sequence that are retained in mature processed mRNA are called exons. These exons are separated by segments called intervening sequences (IVS) or introns, which initially are copied into RNA but which are spliced out in the formation of mature mRNA; i.e., the initial transcript contains an RNA copy of both introns and exons, whereas mature mRNA contains copies only of exons. Untranslated RNA sequences are present in mature mRNA and occur upstream from the protein initiator (AUG) codon and downstream from the terminator (UAA, UAG, or UGA) codon. Transcription proceeds beyond the site where mature mRNA will end. The initial RNA transcript is processed by nuclease cleavage at a poly-A recognition site and subsequent addition of A (adenine) nucleotides to the 3′ end of the mRNA.

Many types of mutation are known. The gene can be entirely deleted. The gene can be rearranged by partial deletion, insertion, or inversion of significant segments. Single-base changes in the coding region generate missense or nonsense codons that cause amino acid substitution or premature chain termination. Mutations in the initiator or terminator codon also can cause disease. In addition, mutations can cause abnormalities of mRNA splicing, usually by changing conserved sequences near intron-exon boundaries. These abnormalities of splicing usually generate mRNAs that do not produce a functional product (Fig. 58-7). Mutations also can occur in control regions and in the polyadenylation signal. In addition, disease mutations may occur in parts of the genome that do not encode proteins, although there are few examples of such instances. The diversity of mutations means that detection of mutant genes at a DNA level can be quite complex.

CLINICAL APPLICATIONS OF MOLECULAR DIAGNOSIS

DISORDERS OF GLOBIN GENES The most extensive experience in the molecular analysis of disease involves globin chain abnormalities, and insights applicable to other genes have come from the study of these mutations. For large deletions of major portions of a globin chain cluster, Southern blotting analysis can be used to demonstrate the presence of a homozygous defect (Fig. 58-8). Gene deletion is a common cause for alpha thalassemia, and prenatal diagnosis of these defects is straightforward using either cDNA or genomic DNA probes. Identification of heterozygous deletions requires either careful quantitation or demonstration of abnormal junction fragments from the

deleted site. Large deletions are a less frequent cause of mutations in the beta-globin cluster, but such deletions can be demonstrated in hereditary persistence of fetal hemoglobin (Fig. 58-8) and in some forms of delta-beta thalassemia.

By comparison, most single nucleotide changes in the genome are not demonstrated readily by Southern blotting analysis. The first method for molecular diagnosis of sickle cell anemia involved the

FIGURE 58-8 *Depiction of Southern blot analysis of human globin genes. Above, DNA was isolated from a normal individual and from patients with homozygous hereditary persistence of fetal hemoglobin (HPFH) or homozygous alpha thalassemia. DNA was digested with the enzyme Eco RI. A mixed DNA probe was prepared by reverse transcription of reticulocyte globin mRNA. Below, arrows indicate Eco RI cut sites in the alpha- and beta-globin regions, and numbers indicate DNA fragment sizes in kilobases. (Adapted from YW Kan, AM Dozy, Proc Natl Acad Sci, USA 75:5631, 1978.)*

use of the previously mentioned RFLP flanking the 3' end of the beta-globin gene. This type of analysis was useful only in some families, and the phase could not always be deduced with certainty (see above and "Autosomal Recessive Disorders" below). One of the alternative procedures developed for the direct demonstration of the sickle mutation utilizes a variation of the Southern blotting technique in which the hybridization probe is a synthetic 19-base oligonucleotide that represents a perfect match for either the β^S sequence or the β^A sequence (Fig. 58-9). The oligonucleotide method may be useful in other instances where a particular mutation accounts for a large proportion of disease in the population but has two drawbacks: first, most genetic diseases are heterogeneous at the molecular level, and specific oligonucleotides are required for each mutation; second, the method is so demanding technically as to limit widespread application.

Another method for direct detection of the sickle cell mutation circumvents these technical difficulties. A portion of the nucleotide sequence in the β^A gene is 5'-CCTGAGG-3', and the corresponding sequence in the sickle gene is 5'CCTG*T*GG-3'. The GAG to GTG change causes the glutamic acid to valine substitution. The restriction enzyme *Mst* II cuts the sequence 5'CCTNAGG-3' and hence will cut the β^A but not the β^S sequence at this site (Fig. 58-10A). Digestion of genomic DNA with the enzyme *Mst* II yields a 1.15-kb fragment for the normal gene and a 1.35-kb fragment for the β^S gene. Southern blotting analysis using *Mst* II and the appropriate beta-globin fragment as a DNA probe allows identification of the AS, AA, and SS genotypes (Fig. 58-10B). This is the method of choice for prenatal diagnosis of sickle cell anemia but is not applicable to most other

diseases. Indeed, it is unusual for a mutation to both cause disease and be common enough to cause RFLP.

The molecular heterogeneity in beta thalassemia illustrates the magnitude of the task involved in application of DNA analysis for genetic diagnosis. Small DNA alterations, primarily single-nucleotide changes, that cause premature chain termination and splicing aberrations are common among beta-thalassemia alleles. Mutations involving 5' upstream regulatory regions or the polyadenylation signal also cause thalassemia. Indeed, 17 different splicing mutations, 10 different frameshift or nonsense mutations, and 6 different transcriptional mutations are known for the beta-globin gene (Fig. 58-11). One approach for genetic diagnosis of beta thalassemia involves analysis of RFLPs in the beta-globin cluster. Such variations can be assembled into a haplotype for each chromosome (Fig. 58-12). Assuming that haplotype analysis is informative, prenatal diagnosis can be accomplished in instances where a previous affected child has occurred. In general, each new mutation is associated with a particular haplotype and occurs with limited geographic distribution. In isolated populations, hematologic analysis for heterozygote detection and haplotype analysis can identify carriers and establish a presumed genetic phase for heterozygote screening and prevention of thalassemia. Such analysis becomes much more complicated with admixture of various thalassemia mutations as a consequence of population movements. For example, in Greek or Italian populations in North America, it can be difficult to perform prenatal diagnosis using haplotype analysis if a couple has not had a previous affected child to establish the phase. Direct demonstration of mutant genes using oligonucleotide probes, diagnostic restriction enzyme digestions, or some other method has advantages since requirements for informative markers and determination of phase are eliminated. However, because of the heterogeneity of molecular defects, each family represents a substantial diagnostic project. Comparison of sickle cell anemia, where a single mutation accounts for all of a particular disease phenotype, with beta thalassemia, where extreme molecular heterogeneity is involved in the generation of a particular phenotype, provides important lessons for the study of other loci.

OTHER SINGLE-GENE DISORDERS   The term autosomal dominant describes a condition in which heterozygous individuals have a significant disease phenotype. For autosomal recessive disorders, heterozygous individuals are healthy, and only homozygous or compound heterozygous individuals have a disease phenotype (see Chap. 57). These distinctions remain important when considering molecular diagnosis of single-gene disorders.

Autosomal recessive disorders   DNA analysis of fetal cells sometimes provides an opportunity for prenatal diagnosis of autosomal recessive disorders such as alpha$_1$-antitrypsin deficiency, phenylketonuria (PKU), and cystic fibrosis. Although these disorders represent a range of disease burden and although few couples at risk may or may not choose prenatal diagnosis, the diseases illustrate the principles involved for autosomal recessive disorders. A hypothetical series of PKU families is illustrated in Fig. 58-13. Phenylalanine hydroxylase is the defective enzyme in PKU, and at least eight RFLPs are detectable using the cloned cDNA for the gene. Each family depicted has a previous child with PKU. For family 1, the analysis is informative, and the phase can be deduced; both parents are heterozygous for an RFLP, and the first affected child indicates that the 5-kb fragment is with the disease gene in both parents. For family 2, the analysis is informative only for the father. For family 3, both parents are heterozygous for the RFLP, but the phase cannot be determined adequately, and the analysis is only partially informative. For family 4, the analysis is uninformative since both parents are homozygous at the RFLP site. For family 5, complete information can be obtained using two RFLPs, since the father is informative for one analysis and the mother is informative for the other analysis. Because more than one RFLP is potentially informative, most families are fully informative, and prenatal diagnosis can be provided to the majority of families with a previously affected child. DNA analysis

FIGURE 58-9   *Southern blot analysis using oligonucleotide probes to diagnose sickle cell anemia. The 19 base probes were Hβ19A' for the normal sequence and Hβ19S for the sickle gene. The genotype for individuals is indicated above each lane, and DNA was digested with a restriction enzyme. HβG1 represents cloned normal globin gene DNA. The smear in the upper region is nonspecific hybridization. (From BJ Conner et al, Proc Natl Acad Sci, USA 80:278, 1983, with permission.)*

FIGURE 58-10 *Southern blot analysis to diagnose the sickle globin mutation directly. Arrows indicate* Mst II *sites, including the one corresponding to amino acid positions 5, 6, and 7. The* Mst II *fragment of 1.15 kb is the probe; see text. (From JC Chang, YW Kan, N Engl J Med 307:30, 1982; reprinted with permission.)*

may also detect heterozygous relatives such as aunts, uncles, and siblings in families with an affected child.

In the case of alpha₁-antitrypsin deficiency, precise genotypic diagnosis and heterozygote detection can be achieved postnatally using protein electrophoresis. A few mutations, primarily the Z allele (a single-nucleotide change causing an amino acid substitution), account for most instances of the disease. Prenatal diagnosis can be carried out using oligonucleotide probes to distinguish the transmission of the Z allele or the normal allele from each parent to the fetus. In addition, linkage disequilibrium involving an RFLP occurs in the 5′ flanking region of the alpha₁-antitrypsin gene, and the presence of a particular RFLP haplotype in this region is virtually diagnostic of the presence of the Z allele. This degree of linkage disequilibrium is unusual. Because of the feasibility of population-based identification of specific alleles for alpha₁-antitrypsin, it would be possible to offer prenatal diagnosis to couples both of whom have the MZ genotype, even if they have not had a previous affected child.

Diagnosis using linked DNA probes is not in widespread use for autosomal recessive disorders, but the identification of DNA markers near the cystic fibrosis gene should alter this situation. The *met* oncogene and a random DNA marker are closely linked (about 1 cM) to the cystic fibrosis gene on chromosome 7. These DNA markers provide the opportunity for prenatal diagnosis and heterozygote detection in cystic fibrosis families. The principles are similar to those discussed for PKU (Fig. 58-13) except that crossovers between the DNA marker and the cystic fibrosis gene will occur. In attempts to carry out prenatal diagnosis in a family with one previously affected child, there are four opportunities for crossing over, two in the first affected child who is used to determine the phase in the parents and two for the fetus. If a linked DNA marker were 1 cM from the disease gene, there would be a risk of erroneous diagnosis of almost 4 percent. Thus, linkage diagnosis of this type requires RFLP markers that are close to the mutant gene. Such DNA markers allow for

heterozygote detection within affected families but not within the general population.

One rare autosomal recessive form of growth hormone deficiency is due to homozygous deletion of the growth hormone gene. This disorder exemplifies the usefulness of molecular analysis. First, DNA analysis can establish the etiology of severe growth failure in such an infant. Second, the analysis has prognostic significance, since such children are more likely to produce antibodies to exogenous growth hormone and may be resistant to growth hormone replacement therapy. Third, the analysis identifies this as a recessive defect with a high risk of recurrence. Fourth, DNA analysis can make prenatal diagnosis possible for such families. DNA analysis also is useful for prenatal diagnosis of recessive disorders, such as carbamyl phosphate synthetase deficiency, in which enzyme activity is not expressed in cultured amniotic cells.

DNA analysis has less to offer when a deficient enzyme can be measured in amniotic cells and the techniques for prenatal diagnosis are well established. Biologic tests such as enzyme assay make it possible to detect defective function without regard to heterogeneity of the molecular defect. For example, prenatal diagnosis and heterozygote detection for lysosomal storage disorders such as Tay-Sachs disease are likely to be uninfluenced by cloning of the mutant genes.

Autosomal dominant disorders   Some genes involved in autosomal dominant disorders have been cloned, the low-density lipoprotein (LDL) receptor and antithrombin III being two examples. For the LDL receptor genetic heterogeneity is common; most cases of familial hypercholesterolemia are due to inherited mutant alleles rather than new mutation. At least one RFLP has been identified using gene

FIGURE 58-11   *Location of 30 mutations causing beta thalassemia. Symbols are (△), frameshift and nonsense mutations; (◇), RNA splicing mutants; (●), transcriptional mutants; (○), RNA cleavage mutant. (From SE Antonarakis et al, Hum Genet 69:1, 1985.)*

β - Globin Gene

Haplotypes

	Hinc II	Hd III	Hd III	Hinc II		Ava II	Bam HI
I	+	−	−	−	−	+	+
II	−	+	+	−	+	+	+
III	−	+	−	+	+	+	−

FIGURE 58-12 *Examples of RFLP haplotypes at the beta-globin cluster. Restriction fragment length RFLPs are indicated by arrows. Only three of the many possible haplotypes are presented; (+) indicates cleavage by the restriction enzyme and (−) indicates no cleavage. (Adapted from SH Orkin et al, Nature 296:627, 1982.)*

probes for the LDL receptor so that presymptomatic diagnosis should be possible in some instances.

Linked DNA markers have been identified for Huntington's disease and for adult polycystic kidney disease. As of 1985, the nearest DNA markers are at distances between 2 and 6 cM from the disease loci. Although these markers are major research tools, the occurrence of crossovers complicates their clinical application. Identification of closer DNA markers or the disease genes themselves is needed. For Huntington's disease, presymptomatic diagnosis is not usually warranted because it may lead to an unacceptable psychological burden for affected individuals, but it is possible to make both presymptomatic and prenatal diagnosis of the disorder. Hypothetical examples of Huntington's disease families and haplotype analyses based on RFLPs are presented in Fig. 58-14. For this illustration, it is assumed that the DNA marker is 3 cM away from the disease gene and that the chance of a crossover for meiosis in males or females would be 3 percent. For family 1, the analysis is informative, and the Huntington's disease allele is in phase with the B haplotype. It can be predicted with approximately 97 percent certainty that the pregnant mother has inherited Huntington's disease, and prenatal diagnosis can be offered with about 94 percent accuracy. In family 2 numerous individuals are dead, and presymptomatic diagnosis cannot be offered to the pregnant woman, although one form of prenatal diagnosis can be offered. If the fetus inherits the B (grandpaternal) haplotype from the mother, there is a high risk of Huntington's disease, while there is

low risk of Huntington's disease if the fetus inherits the A (grand-maternal) haplotype from the mother. If all pregnancies for this couple with fetal haplotypes BB or BC were terminated, and those with AB or AC were continued, half of all pregnancies would be terminated, but the risk of transmission of Huntington disease would be reduced without clarifying the mother's risk. Using this approach, the terminated pregnancies would likely be affected with Huntington's disease in about half of these families where the parent is affected but would be unaffected in the half of families where the parent is unaffected. Because of the early death of affected individuals, the circumstances in family 2 may be common. The circumstances for adult polycystic kidney disease are similar but differ in that presymptomatic diagnosis using renal ultrasound is generally accurate. A highly polymorphic marker, the result of length variation in tandem repetitive sequences, is closely linked to the adult polycystic kidney disease locus (Fig. 58-15). Availability of linked probes offers the opportunity for prenatal diagnosis of adult polycystic disease, but the acceptability of prenatal testing within affected families is not established.

Certain general features can be recognized for autosomal dominant disorders. In instances such as defects of the LDL receptor where molecular heterogeneity is common, haplotype analysis using RFLPs should be useful. In instances such as Huntington's disease where the great majority of the disease may occur in descendents from one or a few mutations (e.g., molecular heterogeneity would be limited or absent), it would be important to clone the disease gene and identify the molecular defect. Direct identification of the mutation would make presymptomatic and prenatal diagnosis possible in all cases. DNA analysis would be expected to be of limited usefulness in disorders such as achondroplastic dwarfism, where the majority of disease is due to new mutations. There is no opportunity to anticipate the occurrence of new mutations, and molecular prenatal diagnosis is impractical for the new mutation cases since a test must detect all molecular defects and would have to be used in all pregnancies. Thus, cloning the gene for achondroplasia would not provide a

FIGURE 58-13 *Hypothetical families with a child affected with phenylketonuria. Simplified but realistic examples of Southern blot analyses using the phenylalanine hydroxylase cDNA as a probe are depicted. Families are numbered above, and restriction fragment sizes are indicated in kilobases; see text.*

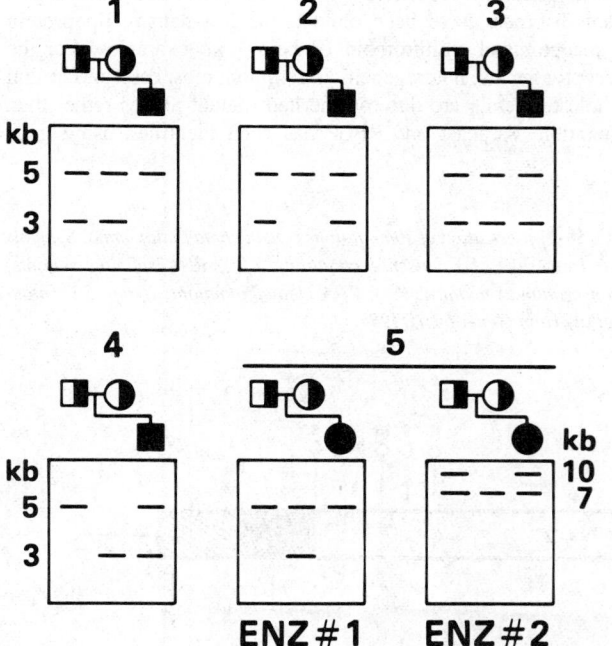

FIGURE 58-14 *Hypothetical families with Huntington's disease. A, B, and C indicate haplotypes for RFLPs detectable with a linked DNA probe. Solid symbols are symptomatic individuals, and P indicates a pregnancy; see text.*

FIGURE 58-15 *Southern blotting analysis of a family affected with adult polycystic kidney disease. Alleles C, D, G, J, and H are detected with a linked, highly polymorphic probe. Designations above each lane refer to pedigree positions, and every person with the C allele also has polycystic disease. (From ST Reeders et al, Nature 317:542, 1985; reprinted with permission.)*

FIGURE 58-16 *Families with hemophilia A. The A and B haplotypes are based on RFLPs detected using the factor VIII gene as a probe. Solid squares indicate affected males, a dot in a circle indicates an obligate carrier female, P = pregnancy; see text.*

practical option for prenatal detection of most cases. Furthermore, diagnosis by DNA analysis is likely to be handicapped by extensive molecular heterogeneity for disorders such as Marfan's syndrome, tuberous sclerosis, and others, where there are usually few affected individuals in each family. Molecular diagnosis is particularly complicated in disorders involving collagen genes because of the size and complexity of the genes and the degree of molecular heterogeneity (see Chap. 319). Some mutations in a collagen gene cause autosomal dominant disorders, while different mutations in the same gene cause autosomal recessive phenotypes.

X-Linked disorders The same principles apply with modifications for X-linked disorders for which the cloned gene is available, as for factor VIII deficiency (hemophilia A) or factor IX deficiency (hemophilia B). Deletion, gross rearrangement of the gene, or fortuitous mutation within a restriction enzyme site allows for direct detection of the mutation in occasional cases. Alternatively, it may be necessary to rely on linkage analysis using RFLPs detected with the cloned gene as a probe. Analysis of males establishes the phase of linkage between the RFLP and the disease gene, even when the males do not transmit the disease, because males have a single X chromosome. Hypothetical families with hemophilia A are presented in Fig. 58-16, where the cloned factor VIII gene has been used as the DNA probe. In family 1, the analysis is informative, and the phase (hemophilia gene with the B haplotype) can be deduced from analysis of the affected grandson or the unaffected grandfather. Family 2 illustrates the advantages of direct detection of mutations, as compared to RFLP analysis, when it is unclear if the propositus is the result of inherited or new mutation. It is possible to determine if the pregnant woman is a heterozygote only if the mutation can be detected directly and not by RFLP analysis. If the mutation cannot be detected directly, heterozygote testing for this woman depends on analysis of factor VIII activity and antigen. It is possible to offer prenatal diagnosis to family 2 by establishing that if the mother is a carrier, only male fetuses with the B haplotype are at increased risk and that if the mother is a noncarrier, male fetuses are not at risk. In family 3, two brothers, one affected and one normal, inherited the same haplotype. Since the chance of a crossover within the factor VIII gene is low, it is probable that the affected child is the result of new mutation, the mother is not a carrier, and the pregnancy is not at significant risk for a second new mutation. Because random X-inactivation complicates heterozygote detection for X-linked diseases using enzyme

assays, DNA analysis when possible is preferable for heterozygote detection.

Some of the complications in the use of linkage analysis for determination of linkage phase are illustrated for a hypothetical X-linked disorder in Fig. 58-17. In each instance the pregnant woman is an obligate carrier, and the DNA marker is 10 cM from the disease locus. In family 1, the probability that the A haplotype is with the disease gene in the mother is .90, based on the findings in the grandson, and prenatal diagnosis in males would be about 81 percent accurate because of the combined uncertainty regarding phase and chance of crossover for the fetus. Family 2 is identical to family 1 except that haplotype information is available for the grandfather, indicating that the disease gene is in phase with the B haplotype in the mother. The affected boy in family 2 must be the result of a crossover, and prenatal diagnosis of males would be about 90 percent accurate. Note that fetuses of haplotype A are predicted to be affected for family 1 and normal for family 2. For family 3, the probability that the phase links the B haplotype with the disease allele is .99, because two affected sons exhibit the same phase (note difference from family 1 with only one affected). The accuracy of prenatal diagnosis in males would be about 90 percent. Similar principles apply in determining phase with autosomal markers.

The advantages of two flanking linked markers are depicted in Fig. 58-18, again using X-linked inheritance as an example. Assuming each marker is 10 cM from the disease locus, prenatal diagnosis can be carried out with 90 percent accuracy if only one marker is informative. If both markers are informative, there will be a 20 percent chance of crossover between the two DNA markers and about a 1 percent chance of a double crossover. Thus, for about one-fifth of families, the analysis will be inconclusive, but such analysis would be 99 percent accurate if the linkage phase were preserved between the two flanking markers.

CLINICAL GUIDELINES Some of the diseases where DNA analysis is helpful are listed in Table 58-2. Molecular studies should be offered to families affected with these diseases as part of prereproductive

FIGURE 58-17 *Issues involved in the determination of phase of linkage using an X-linked example. A and B represent haplotypes based on RFLPs detected using a DNA marker 10 cM from the disease locus; P = pregnancy; see text.*

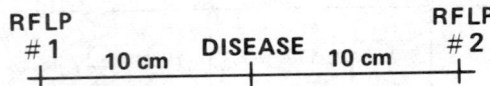

ONE MARKER INFORMATIVE

– 100% OF FAMILIES, 90% ACCURATE

TWO MARKERS INFORMATIVE

– 81% OF FAMILIES, 99% ACCURATE

– 19% OF FAMILIES, NO DIAGNOSIS

FIGURE 58-18 *Demonstration of the effect of flanking linked genetic markers for an X-linked disease; see text.*

evaluation and counseling. Blood for DNA should be stored from patients affected with Huntington's disease, Duchenne's muscular dystrophy, cystic fibrosis, and polycystic kidney disease. Lack of DNA from affected individuals or from older family members may prevent genetic diagnostic testing for younger family members.

In summary, RFLP analysis with a linked marker is useful, and

TABLE 58-2 Role of molecular analysis for diagnosis of genetic disease

Disease	Detection of mutation*	RFLPs with gene probe	RFLPs with linked marker	Comments
Sickle cell anemia	+ + + +			*Mst* II analysis
Beta thalassemia	+ +	+ +		Very heterogeneous
Alpha thalassemia	+ + +	+		Many deletions
Hemophilia A	+	+ +	+	
Hemophilia B	+	+ +	+	
Phenylketonuria		+ + + +		
Alpha₁ antitrypsin ZZ	+ +	+ +		
Antithrombin III deficiency	+	+ +		Biologic tests valuable
Familial hypercholesterolemia	+	+ +		Biologic tests valuable
Growth hormone deficiency	+			Rare form
Lesch-Nyhan syndrome	+ +	+ +		Heterozygote detection
Retinoblastoma			+ + +	Inherited form
Huntington's disease			+ + +	Delay over ethical concerns
Myototonic dystrophy			+ +	
Adult polycystic kidney disease			+ + +	
Ornithine transcarbamylase deficiency	+	+ + +		Prenatal and heterozygote
Carbamyl phosphate synthetase deficiency		+ + +		
X-linked retinitis pigmentosa			+ + +	
Fragile X syndrome			+ + +	
Cystic fibrosis			+ + +	

* Plus symbols indicate relative importance of an approach as of the end of 1985. Additional diseases and new clones and techniques should expand and change this tabulation rapidly.

RFLP analysis with the disease gene as the probe is better; direct detection of the mutation is optimal but more difficult because it requires both isolating the gene itself and a method to identify each mutation. The examples also emphasize the complexity of identifying new mutations, determining heterozygote status, establishing linkage phase, and ascertaining if a linkage analysis will be informative.

MOLECULAR CYTOGENETICS Recombinant DNA techniques provide a bridge between single-gene disorders and cytogenetics (see Chap. 60). Genetic alterations range from single-base changes to gain or loss of an entire chromosome. As an example, some patients with Duchenne's muscular dystrophy have gross cytogenetic abnormalities, other patients have large deletions of DNA with apparently normal cytogenetic analysis, and presumably others will prove to have single-base changes.

Cytogenetic abnormalities can be studied using either Southern blotting analysis or in situ hybridization. Southern blotting can be used to perform a dosage analysis regarding any unique DNA segment as exemplified in Fig. 58-19. For any chromosomal deletion, duplication, or translocation, it is possible to determine if a particular DNA probe falls within the abnormal region. Indeed, DNA analysis detects heterozygous deletions that are too small to document by conventional cytogenetics. For example, about half of the patients with the Prader-Willi syndrome have deletions or other abnormalities of the proximal portion of the long arm of chromosome 15. Molecular studies of those patients with normal cytogenetic findings might identify deletions too small to detect microscopically. For research purposes, Southern blotting can be applied to the analysis of somatic cell hybrids that contain translocated or rearranged chromosomes separated from their normal homologues. With these techniques, it is possible to determine the location of any DNA marker relative to any cytogenetic breakpoint.

The technique of in situ hybridization involves the use of radioactive DNA probes for direct reannealing to chromosomal DNA in fixed tissue preparations. Such annealing can be detected by autoradiographic techniques over chromosomal regions that contain unique complementary DNA sequences. Clinically, the technique can be used to determine the presence or absence of a DNA segment within an abnormal chromosome and hence to determine whether a segment is deleted or to demonstrate the position of a DNA segment relative to a balanced translocation breakpoint. DNA analysis has also been used to detect Y chromosome–specific sequences in 46 XX males and 46 XX true hermaphrodites (see Chap. 333).

MOLECULAR ONCOLOGY At least three types of molecular changes, all of which alter the expression of the oncogenes, are known to be associated with human tumors (see Chap. 59). These include single-base changes in the coding region of the normal oncogenes, amplification of the copy number, and chromosomal translocations with breakpoints in or adjacent to oncogenes. Each of these alterations can be recognized with Southern blotting. Analysis of tumor DNA for changes in oncogene sequence, for oncogene amplification, and for relevant translocations may ultimately provide diagnostic and therapeutic information for individual patients.

Other tumors are associated with the loss of function of both alleles at specific sites in the genome, for example, at regions of the genome that normally function to suppress tumor formation. If one normal allele for such a gene is inactivated by a first event, loss or alteration of a segment of the other chromosome in this region would cause loss of suppressor function. This was first demonstrated for an association of retinoblastoma with a region of chromosome 13q and subsequently was demonstrated for chromosome 11p in Wilm's tumor. Loss of the second functional gene frequently involves a mechanism that affects adjacent DNA (e.g., cytogenetic deletion). It is possible to compare tumor DNA and uninvolved DNA from the same individual and deduce whether loss of heterozygosity has occurred near the "suppressor" locus. In the case of dominantly inherited retinoblastoma, linkage analysis using DNA markers is useful for genetic counseling, and the heterozygosity analysis of a tumor can be used

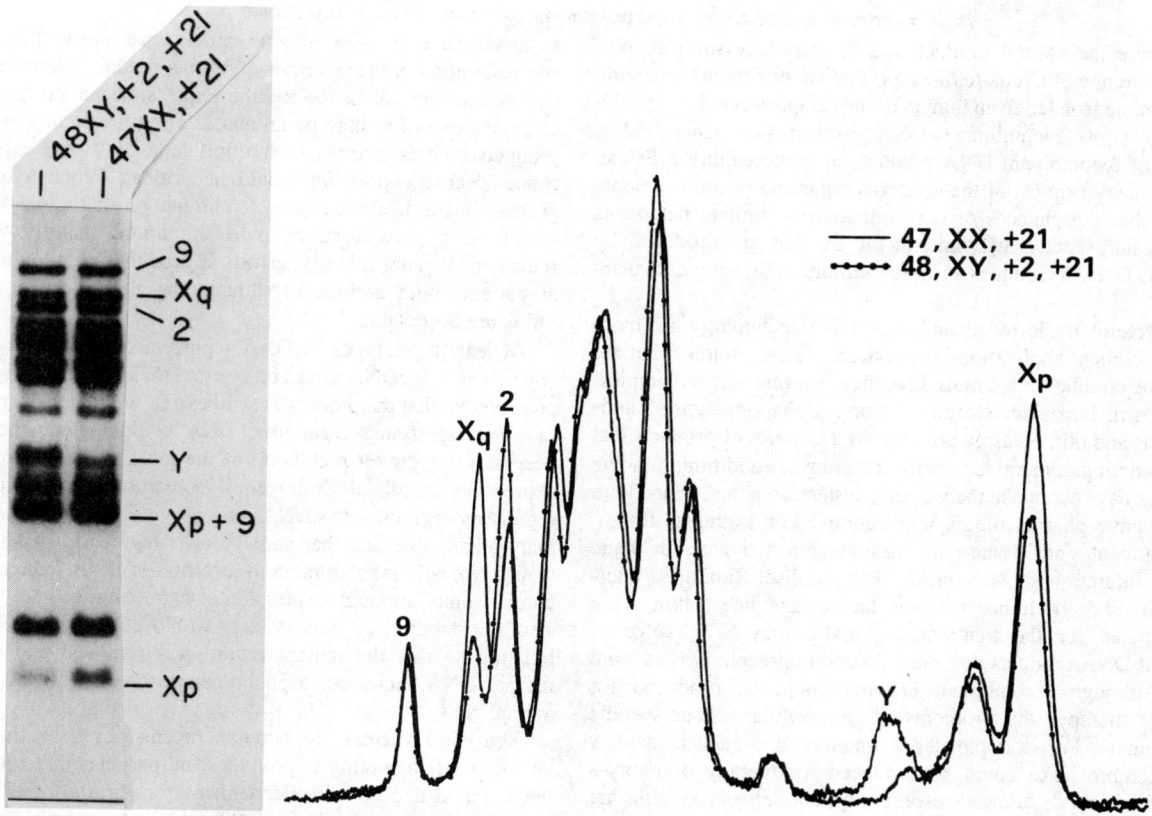

FIGURE 58-19 *Example of dosage analysis using cytogenetically abnormal cell lines. Southern blotting was performed using a cDNA probe which cross-reacts with genomic DNA sequences on 11 different chromosomes including X and Y. Chromosome composition is indicated above the lanes in panel A.*

Densitometric tracings are presented in panel B with dosage differences for DNA sites on chromosomes 2, Xp, Xq, and Y, but similar dosage for a site on chromosome 9. (From TS Su et al, Am J Hum Genet 36:954, 1984.)

to determine the phase of linkage, with the retained allele marking the defective chromosome and the lost allele marking the normal constitutional chromosome.

DIAGNOSTIC VIROLOGY AND MICROBIOLOGY

Virtually all microorganisms have DNA or RNA genomes that can be detected by nucleic acid hybridization techniques. As discussed above, such hybridization techniques are sensitive and specific, and in human specimens, such as stool, urine, blood, and tissue biopsies, they can be used to detect nucleic acid sequences from microorganisms. These techniques may prove especially suitable for diagnosing cytomegalovirus, rotovirus, Epstein-Barr virus, and other viruses.

MISCELLANEOUS APPLICATIONS

DNA fragments that hybridize with multiple, repeated, highly polymorphic sequences in the genome can be used to define polymorphic differences between individuals in a single analysis, even when each variant fragment cannot be readily assigned to a particular chromosomal site. This type of analysis is very useful for quickly detecting nonidentity between individuals. For example, a single Southern blot analysis can distinguish between nonidentical twins and between host cells and donor cells after bone marrow transplantation. These probes offer considerable advantages over conventional genetic markers and may be useful for paternity testing and as a forensic tool to link individuals to semen, blood, and hair root samples. Tissue typing at the HLA loci is also feasible using RFLPs, and such DNA studies may complement or supplant immunologic methods.

CLINICAL PRODUCTS FROM RECOMBINANT DNA

Cloned DNA sequences can be used for the synthesis of proteins and peptides. The major advantages of this strategy are the ability to produce an unlimited amount of a purified product and the avoidance of contamination by pathogens. Production can be carried out in bacteria or in yeast.

Bacteria do not splice eukaryotic messenger RNA properly so that the coding region is usually provided as cDNA clones or as synthetic DNA sequences. The coding region must be linked to bacterial DNA segments that control transcription and initiation of translation. The major difficulties involve the lack of eukaryotic mechanisms for posttranslational processing. Almost all bacterial and eukaryotic proteins undergo proteolytic cleavage at the amino terminus to remove the initiator methionine, and multiple proteolytic cleavages may be involved, as in the production of various hormones from the pro-opiomelanocortin gene. Other forms of posttranslational modification include carbohydrate addition, phosphorylation, acylation, formation of disulfide bridges, and vitamin K–dependent carboxylation. Improperly or incompletely processed proteins may not function normally and may be antigenic.

These obstacles have been overcome for the synthesis of human insulin. Ordinarily, production of mature insulin involves the formation of three disulfide bridges in a single polypeptide chain followed by proteolytic cleavage to remove the C peptide and leave the α and β chains linked. One strategy was to produce the α and β chains separately from synthetic DNA sequences. Because the mature insulin chains do not contain the amino acids methionine and tryptophan (an unusual and fortuitous circumstance), it was possible to remove the initiator methionine chemically. The chains were then combined, and the proper disulfide bridges formed in vitro.

For the production of growth hormone, bacterial peptidase does not remove the amino terminal methionine from the protein. This results in the production of a growth hormone with an extra methionine residue at the amino terminus. Although the methionyl growth hormone is active in humans, concern regarding immunologic effects delayed release for general use. Growth hormone represents an instance where the natural product was in extremely short supply, and the occurrence of Creutzfeldt-Jakob disease in patients receiving growth hormone isolated from human tissues emphasizes the potential advantages of the recombinant DNA product (see Chap. 322). Production of recombinant DNA products in tissue culture cells can circumvent many or most of the concerns regarding posttranslational processing, but the chances of contamination by human pathogens may be greater. Factor VIII and factor IX that are produced by recombinant DNA techniques in tissue culture cells have coagulant activity.

Some proteins made by recombinant DNA technology are more suitable for clinical applications than others. Those proteins that are present in the circulation are most amenable to replacement therapies. Insulin, growth hormone, clotting factors, alpha$_1$-antitrypsin, antithrombin III, and other plasma proteins are examples of products that could be used for parenteral replacement therapy. In addition, biologic products that have actions in the vascular system or in the extracellular space may have pharmacologic applications. For example, thrombolytic treatment with tissue-type plasminogen activator for acute myocardial infarction shows considerable promise. Similarly, interferon (α, β, and γ), tumor necrosis factor, and interleukin 2 are being evaluated for the treatment of malignancy. The value of recombinant DNA products that must function intracellularly is more tenuous. Although recombinant enzyme could be produced for replacement therapy, the problems of intracellular, tissue-specific targeting remain. For example, large amounts of α-galactosidase A and glucocerebrosidase could be produced for therapy of Fabry's disease and Gaucher's disease, respectively, but delivery systems are unproven. Proteins for which there is no mechanism for endocytosis and proteins required in the central nervous system are unlikely candidates for such replacement therapy. While the majority of recombinant DNA products undergoing trials at present are not completely modified to the mature, posttranslational state, most are biologically active.

Recombinant DNA technology also is useful for the preparation of diagnostic reagents and vaccines. Routine methods for vaccine production involving inactivation of viral particles or development of attenuated live-virus strains carry risks. Occasionally, inactivation of virus is incomplete, or other viruses may contaminate vaccines. Furthermore, preparations of hepatitis B vaccine from human plasma may be contaminated by proteins that cause reactions in allergic individuals. Live attenuated viral strains are subject to change and may cause disease in immunologically compromised recipients. Production of viral proteins by recombinant techniques may provide an acceptable antigen for vaccination. A vaccine for the virus that causes foot-and-mouth disease in cattle is available, and a hepatitis B antigen made in yeast is being tested in humans. An alternative approach to production of new vaccines involves the insertion of one or more DNA sequences encoding antigens into the vaccinia virus genome to produce a polyvalent vaccine. For example, a DNA sequence from influenza virus was recombined with vaccinia to yield a vaccine to protect against vaccinia and influenza.

Diagnostic reagents also can be prepared with recombinant DNA techniques. For example, viral antigens for acquired immune deficiency syndrome (AIDS) and for hepatitis B can be produced for use in radioimmunoassays for viral diagnosis. Various enzymes for diagnostic tests and many of the restriction endonucleases and nucleic acid polymerases used in recombinant DNA diagnosis are produced using the cloned genes for these enzymes.

RESEARCH POTENTIAL

THE PROSPECTS OF GENE REPLACEMENT THERAPY   For human genetic disorders in which the mutant gene is identified and the cloned normal gene is available, a number of strategies can be considered for gene replacement therapy (Table 58-3). Gene replacement therapy has a major theoretical advantage over enzyme or factor replacement, since a single treatment could provide permanent correction. If the disease is caused by simple deficiency of the product,

as in the case of most enzyme deficiencies and clotting disorders, any restoration of the synthesis of normal product might be beneficial, and neither normal tisuse-specific expression nor precise regulation of gene expression may be an absolute requirement. For other gene products such as globins, an appropriate level of gene expression and tissue-specific expression would be critical. When a mutant gene product has a deleterious effect, elimination of the deleterious gene might be as necessary or more important than provision of a replacement gene. Initially, efforts at gene therapy should be directed at patients with serious life-threatening illness where risk-benefit ratios are acceptable.

At least three types of DNA replacement can be envisioned. In one instance, a cDNA might be inserted under the control of a foreign promoter so that the product is synthesized without proper regulation. In a second strategy, genomic DNA could include the sequences necessary for proper regulation of the level and tissue specificity of expression. Artificial "minigene" constructions that link genomic regulatory regions with cDNA may provide constructions that are of manageable size and that show proper regulation. These strategies would typically involve random insertion of DNA sequences into the chromosome, although expression of extrachromosomal sequences is also a possibility. A third strategy would utilize site-specific recombination so that the mutant region was removed and replaced by normal DNA sequence, a phenomenon that is difficult to effect in animal cells.

Retroviral vectors are potential agents for gene therapy. Such vectors have the ability to produce viral particles that encode foreign nucleic acid and contain mechanisms for chromosomal integration. One current strategy (Fig. 58-20) involves insertion of cDNA or minigene DNA constructions between two viral long terminal repeats (LTRs) in a plasmid vector. These constructions can be introduced into cultured cell lines that provide the viral proteins necessary to package pseudovirus particles that include the gene sequence of interest. For example, bone marrow cells could be removed from a patient with a specific defect, bone marrow stem cells could be infected with these viral particles, and the patient's bone marrow could be repopulated with the altered cells. Delivery to tissues such as liver would be more complex, but can be envisioned.

Alternative strategies might include packaging of DNA in liposomes, development of other viral vectors, and use of vectors that remain in an extrachromosomal state. The risk-benefit ratio for somatic gene replacement therapy must be estimated on an individual basis. Random insertion of DNA sequences into the genome is likely to have some risk for carcinogenesis. However, based on the experience with retroviruses that do not contain oncogenes, this risk might be relatively low if viral progeny are not produced in the recipient. Such risks may be acceptable in patients with life-threatening illness where no reasonable alternative therapy is available. Adenosine deaminase deficiency is a possible candidate disorder for early attempts. Other enzyme deficiencies and clotting factor deficiencies may also be candidate disorders. If proper regulation of globin genes could be achieved, disorders such as sickle cell anemia and thalassemia would constitute important opportunities because of the accessibility of bone marrow for in vitro treatment, because of the frequency of the diseases, and because of their serious nature. Disorders that require careful regulation of gene expression or tissue-specific expression, such as in the central nervous system, are more challenging.

BASIC RESEARCH   Over 300 genes have been cloned from human and other mammalian sources. Many of these genes are part of complex functional systems that are only partially understood. A group of genes that control segment differentiation in *Drosophila* have been cloned, and homologous sequences are present in humans and could have functional similarities. Efforts to characterize and clone the genes for Huntington's disease, polycystic kidney disease, cystic fibrosis, and Duchenne's muscular dystrophy should allow for the understanding of the biology of the normal alleles for these genes and could lead to the development of new therapies for some of these disorders.

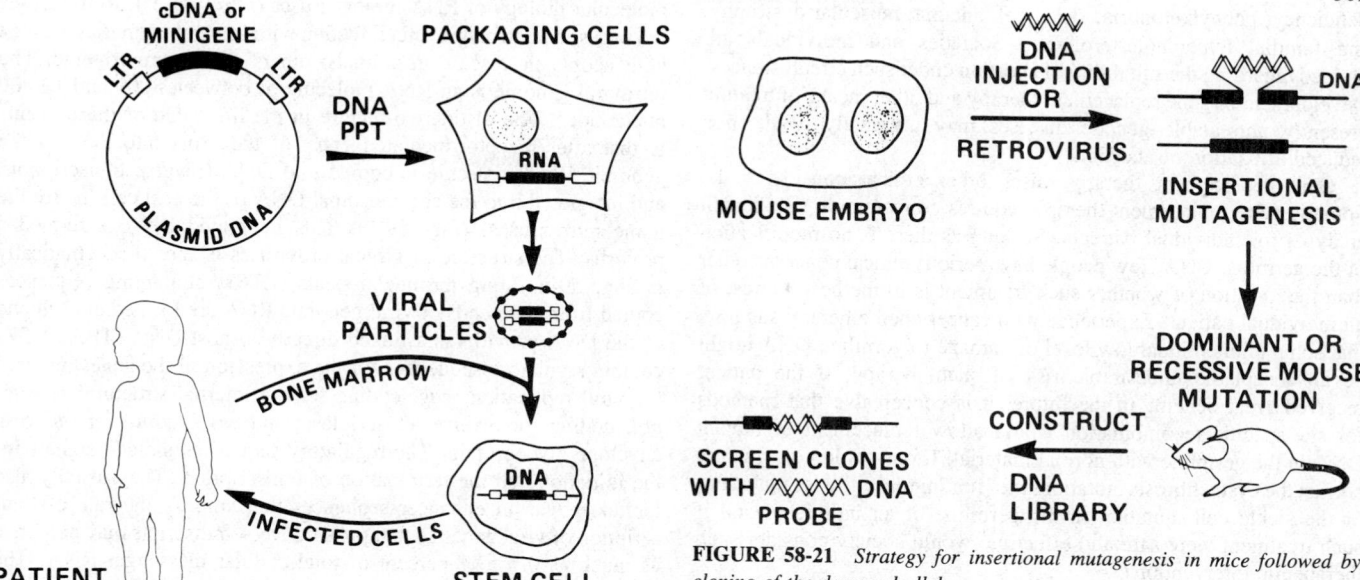

FIGURE 58-20 *One strategy for attempting gene replacement therapy.*

FIGURE 58-21 *Strategy for insertional mutagenesis in mice followed by cloning of the damaged allele.*

Recombinant DNA techniques are likely to be powerful tools for studies of neurobiology and developmental biology. Libraries of cDNA clones can be generated from specific parts of the central nervous system and at specific times in embryogenesis. Another strategy involves the generation of new mutations in mice through insertional mutagenesis (Fig. 58-21). Foreign DNA can be inserted randomly into the genome of early mouse embryos using direct DNA injection or retroviral infection. A functional region of DNA may be interrupted, giving a recessive or dominant phenotype. Phenotypes of biologic interest can be selected such as those causing developmental abnormalities or neurologic dysfunction. The inserted foreign DNA can be used as a probe to clone the damaged region of DNA. Thus, one can generate an informative mutant phenotype and immediately clone the relevant gene. The cloned sequences can be used to search for mRNA sequences to determine the site of tissue-specific expression and the timing of gene expression. If the region encodes a protein, the nucleic acid sequence can be used to deduce the structure of peptides that can then be synthesized and used to generate antibodies. Such antibodies can be used to determine the tissue-specific and cell-specific location of a protein. For example, this insertional mutagenesis strategy was used to identify an embryonic lethal mutation in a type I collagen gene in mice. These tools make it possible to induce informative phenotypes, to explore the molecular basis of the phenotype, and to deduce the related normal biology and physiology.

The availability of a detailed human gene map greatly increases the feasibility of searching for genetic variations associated with predisposition to disease. The fact that there are many known disease associations for the HLA region may be due to a preferential localization of disease susceptibility genes in this region or may reflect the greater opportunity to gather data for highly polymorphic markers. As other parts of the genome become well charted with RFLPs, additional associations may be established between diseases and genetic markers. Such associations may allow identification of genes whose variability predisposes to polygenic or multifactorial diseases.

ETHICAL CONSIDERATIONS Prenatal diagnosis is now possible for diseases with a wide range of burden, such as alpha₁-antitrypsin

TABLE 58-3 Human diseases as candidates for gene replacement therapy

Disorders	Burden of disease	Alternative treatment	Disease frequency	Requirement for tissue specificity	Regulation	Relative feasibility*
Hemoglobinopathies	Great	Transfusion, fair to poor	1 in 600 in ethnic groups	Erythroid	Required	+ +
Lesch-Nyhan	Great	Poor	Rare	Brain, ?other	?Not essential	+ +
Adenosine deaminase and nucleoside phosphorylase	Great	Transplant, fair to poor	Very rare	Bone marrow	?Not essential	+ + + +
Phenylketonuria	Small to moderate	Diet, good	1 in 11,000	Liver, ?other	?Not essential	+ +
Urea cycle disorders	Moderate to great	Diet, drug, good to poor	1 in 30,000 for all types	Liver, ?other	?Not essential	+ + +
Alpha₁ antitrypsin	Moderate	Poor	1 in 3500	Liver, ?other	?Not essential	+ + +
Hemophilia A & B	Moderate to great	Replacement, fair (AIDS)	1 in 10,000 males	?Any organ, factor VIII	?Not essential	+ + + +
Lysosomal storage diseases	Great	Poor	1 in 1500 for all types	Brain for many	?Not essential	+
Familial hypercholesterolemia	Great	Diet, drug, fair	1 in 500 heterozygotes	Liver, ?other	Some importance	+ +
Cystic fibrosis	Great	Supportive, fair to poor	1 in 2000 whites	?	?	No clone
Duchenne's muscular dystrophy	Great	Poor	1 in 10,000 males	?Muscle	?	No clone
Huntington's disease	Great	Poor	1 in 20,000	?Brain	?	No clone

* *Relative feasibility attempts to take into account requirements for regulation, accessibility of target organ, alternative treatment, and risk-benefit considerations.*

deficiency, phenylketonuria, sickle cell anemia, muscular dystrophy, and familial hypercholesterolemia. Societies and individuals are divided regarding the suitability of abortion under such circumstances. Development of gene replacement therapy and other means of treating presently untreatable genetic diseases may ultimately result in a reduced utilization of abortion.

Gene replacement therapy raises other ethical considerations. Somatic gene replacement therapy requires conventional risk-benefit analyses for individual patients. So long as there is no modification of the germline DNA, few people have serious ethical concerns other than the question of whether such treatment is in the best interest of an individual patient. Experience with cancer chemotherapy suggests that some unintentional low level of damage to germline DNA might be an acceptable undesirable risk of such therapy, if the patient received great benefit. In the future, it is conceivable that methods for site-specific recombination would allow replacement of mutant DNA in the germline with normal material. If one could permanently correct the cystic fibrosis mutation, the Huntington's disease mutation, or the sickle cell mutation in the germline of an individual and if such treatment were safe and effective, would society consider such therapeutic intervention?

REFERENCES

ANTONARAKIS SE et al: DNA polymorphism and molecular pathology of the human globin gene clusters. Hum Genet 69:1, 1985

BEAUDET AL: Bibliography of cloned human and other selected DNAs. Am J Hum Genet 37:386, 1985

BOTSTEIN D et al: Construction of a genetic linkage map in man using restriction fragment length polymorphisms. Am J Hum Genet 32:314, 1980

GILL P et al: Forensic application of DNA ''fingerprints.'' Nature 318:577, 1985

GUSELLA JF et al: DNA markers for nervous system diseases. Science 225:1320, 1984

LAWN RM et al: The molecular genetics of hemophilia: Blood clotting factors VIII and IX. Cell 42:405, 1985

MONACO AP et al: Detection of deletions spanning the Duchenne muscular dystrophy locus using a tightly linked DNA segment. Nature 316:842, 1985

NEWMARK P: Testing for cystic fibrosis. Nature 318:309, 1985

REEDERS ST et al: A highly polymorphic DNA marker linked to adult polycystic kidney disease on chromosome 16. Nature 317:542, 1985

WATSON JD et al: Recombinant DNA, A Short Course. Scientific American Books. Distributed by WA Freeman Co. New York, 1983

WILLIAMS DA et al: Introduction of new genetic material into pluripotent haematopoietic stem cells of the mouse. Nature 310:476, 1984

59 ONCOGENES AND NEOPLASTIC DISEASE

PAUL NEIMAN

Upon dividing, cancer cells transmit the neoplastic phenotype to daughter cells. For that reason, it has been generally assumed that the inheritance of the neoplastic phenotype is determined by specific genes. This assumption explains the great appeal of oncogenic viruses for cancer researchers. In spite of their relative genetic simplicity, these agents are capable of inducing all the pathologic and clinical changes associated with neoplastic disease, and in some cases a virus introduces into a normal cell a single gene (oncogene) whose product can initiate and maintain the neoplastic state. These oncogenes represent altered forms of cellular proto-oncogenes, which have important cellular functions in the normal state. Human homologues of some of these oncogenes may play a role in human cancer. This situation prompts a number of questions about the nature of oncogenes, the control of their expression, the biochemical nature of their gene products, and the mechanism of interaction with the metabolism of the host cell.

RETROVIRAL ONCOGENES **Interaction of retroviruses with host cells** The discovery of oncogenes was a result of the study of the molecular biology of RNA tumor viruses (retroviruses). Retroviruses are widespread in nature, and infection with some of them is associated with neoplastic disease in animals; others are nontumorigenic. The retroviral genome is an RNA molecule of between 8000 and 10,000 nucleotides. The distinctive feature in the life cycle of these agents is that after receptor-mediated entry of the virus into the cell the genomic RNA molecule is copied into DNA (reverse transcription) and integrated into the chromosomal DNA of the host cell (hence the name retroviruses) (Fig. 59-1). This integrated DNA is termed a provirus. The structure of typical proviruses is shown schematically in Fig. 59-2. Long terminal repeats (LTRs) containing sequences copied from both ends of viral genomic RNA are located at each end of the DNA provirus and linked directly to host DNA. These LTRs contain regulatory sequences for the expression of the genes required for viral replication: *gag*, coding for the internal structural protein; *pol*, coding for reverse transcriptase; and *env*, coding for the viral envelope glycoprotein. The regulatory sequences include signals for the initiation and the termination of transcription. They usually also include powerful enhancer sequences that amplify the rate of transcription of viral genes so that proviral RNA transcripts may comprise as much as 0.1 to 1 percent of total cellular messenger RNA. The transcriptional promoter-enhancer sequences usually function only when introduced into particular cell types, accounting for tissue-specific expression of viral genes. In other cases the activity of these enhancer sequences is regulated by steroid hormones. In contrast to many other viruses, retroviruses usually do not kill the host cell when the replicative process is completed; instead their life cycle results in the introduction and expression of exogenous genes and thus in alteration of the phenotype of the host cells.

Acute transforming retroviruses and their oncogenes Infection of animals with retroviruses encoding only the *gag, pol,* and *env* genes results in neoplastic disease after a long latent period. In contrast, acute transforming retroviruses can induce neoplastic disease in vivo in days to weeks and can transform cultured cells in vitro. The prototype of this class of viruses is the Rous sarcoma virus.

The structure of proviruses from these two classes of oncogenic agents is illustrated in Fig. 59-2. Almost all known acute transforming retroviruses are defective, that is, they have lost part of the genes required for replication and hence require co-infection with a standard helper retrovirus for propagation. Such defects result from the replacement of replicative genes of the virus by an oncogene that mediates the direct transforming properties of the virus. (An exception to this general pattern is represented by some strains of Rous sarcoma virus that have both the replicative genes and the viral oncogene.) Although there is variability as to which segment of the viral genome is replaced by the oncogene, the common configuration for acute transforming retroviruses is as depicted in Fig. 59-2. In this case, the oncogene is fused to a 5' portion of the viral *gag* gene, resulting in the synthesis of a transforming protein that contains *gag* peptides at its amino terminus.

Table 59-1 lists some viral oncogenes (designated by their acronyms), the natural host species, and the types of tumors they induce. In the case of the Rous sarcoma virus, the role of the *src* gene in neoplastic transformation was established by genetic and biochemical means. Mutations that cause reversible inactivation of the *src* gene product at elevated temperature (so-called temperature-sensitive mutations) bring about a reversal of the transformed phenotype to the normal state when infected cells are exposed to elevated temperatures. When the temperature is lowered, the cells again revert to the transformed state. Likewise, deletions of the *src* gene destroy the ability of this virus to induce acute neoplasms. Similar but less complete data exist for other viruses listed in Table 59-1.

Almost all the acute transforming viruses can be detected in vitro by their ability to induce transformation of cultured cells. The standard assay is the formation by infected fibroblasts (or fibroblast-like cell lines) of morphologically altered cells. Some of the leukemia-inducing viruses can transform macrophages and/or hematopoietic cells in vitro.

FIGURE 59-1 *Replication of retroviruses. (1) Envelope glycoprotein on the surface of viral particles (virions) recognizes receptors which mediate entry into the cell and release of viral genomic RNA. (2) There are two viral RNA molecules per virion which are copied by reverse transcriptase into circular, supercoiled viral DNA molecules. (3) Some of the circular DNA molecules integrate into host chromosomal DNA at a precise point on the viral DNA molecule and a random, or near random, site on host chromosomes. (4) The integrated viral DNA copy, or provirus, is transcribed into both messenger RNA, which is translated into viral proteins on cellular polysomes (5), and full-length genomic viral RNA, which contains specific sequences serving as packaging signals for virus assembly. (6) Viral RNA and proteins are assembled into particles which bud from the cell surface. The whole process can occur without cytopathic effects on host cells.*

PROTO-ONCOGENES   The oncogenes of retroviruses are closely related to normal cellular genes. This relationship was deduced from the discovery of nucleotide sequence homology between the transforming oncogene of Rous sarcoma virus, v-*src* (viral-*src*), and a normal chicken gene, c-*src* (cellular-*src*). Apparently, Rous sarcoma virus originated from a recombination event between c-*src* and an ancestral standard avian retrovirus. This mechanism, recombination between a viral gene and a gene of host origin, is the apparent explanation for the formation of the transforming viruses listed in Table 59-1. The function of the normal genes and their role in nonviral tumor formation is, therefore, a subject of intense interest and investigation.

The normal forms of the oncogenes are highly conserved in nature. There are human homologues of each, and homologues of some are present in all eukaryotic organisms, including invertebrate species and yeasts. This conservation implies that these genes have vital functions in normal cells and suggests that the oncogenic potential of the genes is acquired only after functionally significant alteration (such as occurs from recombination with a retrovirus). Such genes are referred to as *proto-oncogenes* (c-*onc*).

The nucleotide sequences of the protein coding regions of viral oncogenes differ from those of the proto-oncogenes. There are also major differences in the regulation of expression of the viral and cellular genes. For example, the normal cellular form of an oncogene can be expressed without transforming the cell, although usually at a lower level and/or more strictly regulated than with viral oncogenes expressed from proviruses. The relative contributions of overexpression, altered regulation, and structural mutation to the transforming activity of viral oncogenes is not fully resolved. All of these elements may be important to degrees that vary with the individual oncogene and target cell type.

Infection with retroviruses that lack oncogenes can induce neoplastic disease in some animals after a long latent period. A common mechanism for this oncogenic activity is the activation of cellular proto-oncogenes, as illustrated by the induction of lymphomas in the bursa of Fabricius of chickens by avian leukosis virus (ALV). In these neoplasms, a proto-oncogene called c-*myc* is expressed at high levels as a result of the integration fo the promoter-enhancer of the ALV genome near c-*myc*. The fact that these tumors are clonal and that c-*myc* activation occurs only in the tumor cells, coupled with the known oncogenic potential of v-*myc*, supports the idea that c-*myc* plays an important role in these tumors. Table 59-2 lists cellular proto-oncogenes that are known to be activated in retrovirus-induced

neoplasms of long latency. Some (*myc* and *erbB*) are homologues of known viral oncogenes. Others (*Int*-1, *Int*-2, *Pim*-1, *Mlvi*-1, and *Mlvi*-2) have not been identified as part of the genomes of acute-transforming viruses. Their oncogenic potential is inferred by analogy.

Human retroviruses   Human T-cell leukemia viruses (HTLV) are retroviruses that appear to replicate preferentially in human lymphocytes. Infection with HTLV type I is associated with the development of a specific type of adult T-cell leukemia that occurs with increased frequency in southern Japan and the Caribbean basin. In vitro infection on human T cells by HTLV-I in culture confers a capacity for growth that is independent of exogenous T-cell growth factors (immortali-

FIGURE 59-2 *Comparative structure of the proviruses of standard replication competent and acute transforming retroviruses. In both cases the provirus is bounded by direct long terminal repeat sequences (LTRs) which contain essential regulatory elements including transcriptional promoters and enhancers, signals for the termination of viral RNA transcripts (polyA addition signals), and for integration into the host DNA. Inside the LTRs of standard retroviruses are three genes: gag (internal structural proteins), pol (reverse transcriptase), and env (envelope glycoprotein), which are required for infection and replication. In the acute transforming viruses, all or part of the replicative genes have been replaced by a transforming oncogene which mediates the oncogenic properties of the virus. The most common structure is a fusion of the 5' portion of the gag gene with the oncogene. The standard provirus is transcribed into full-length genomic viral RNA and spliced messenger RNAs for viral proteins. The acute transforming provirus often expresses only one size RNA transcript. It is replication defective and requires co-infection with a standard retroviral "helper" in order to replicate. The Δgag symbol indicates that part of the gag sequence is missing because it has been deleted.*

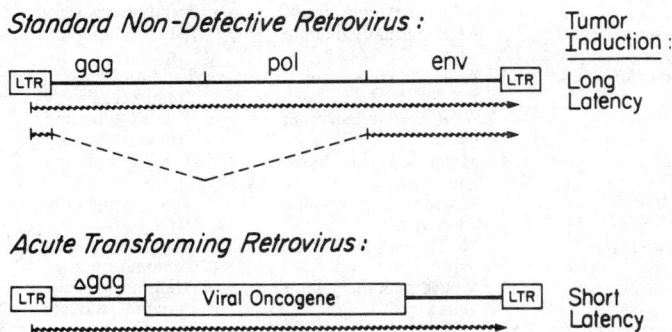

TABLE 59-1   Viral oncogenes that cause acute transformation

Name	Virus	Tumors in vivo
CHICKEN		
src	Rous sarcoma virus (RSV)	Sarcomas
yes	Y73 sarcoma virus	Sarcomas
fps/fes	Fujinami sarcoma virus	Sarcomas
ros	UR11 avian sarcoma virus	Sarcomas
erbB	Avian erythroblastosis virus (AEV)	Erythroid leukemia
myb	Avian myeloblastosis virus (AMV)	Myeloid leukemia
myc	Avian myelocytomatosis virus (MC-29)	Leukemia, endothelioma
ski	Avian SKV770 virus	Unknown
TURKEY		
rel	Reticuloendotheliosis virus (REV)	Lymphomas
MOUSE		
abl	Abelson leukemia virus	B lymphomas
mos	Moloney murine sarcoma virus (MoMSV)	Sarcomas
fos	FBJ osteosarcoma virus	Osteosarcoma
raf	3611 murine sarcoma virus	Sarcomas
RAT		
Ha-ras1	Harvey murine sarcoma virus (HaMSV)	Sarcomas, erythroid leukemia
Ki-ras2	Kirsten murine sarcoma virus (KiMSV)	Sarcomas, erythroid leukemia
CAT		
fes/fps	Snyder Thielen feline sarcoma virus (ST-FeSV)	Sarcomas
fms	McDonough feline sarcoma virus (SM-FeSV)	Sarcomas
fgr	Gardner-Rasheed feline sarcoma virus (GR-FeSV)	Sarcomas
MONKEY		
sis	Simian sarcoma virus (SSV)	Sarcomas

zation). Infection with a different virus called HTLV-III or lymph-adenopathy associated virus (LAV) is associated with the acquired immunodeficiency syndrome. The HTLVs do not appear to contain a host cell–related oncogene. Instead, unique transacting viral regulatory proteins may alter host cell behavior.

Normal human DNA contains structures that appear to be proviruses and that are genetically transmitted in the germline. Their significance is unknown.

TABLE 59-2   Proto-oncogenes and putative proto-oncogenes activated in tumors by nearby integration of retroviral proviruses

Target gene or locus	Virus	Tumor
c-myc	Avian leukosis virus	B-cell lymphomas (chicken)
c-myc	Feline leukemia virus	Lymphomas (cat)
c-myc	AKR-murine leukemia virus	T-cell lymphoma (mouse)
c-erbB	Avian leukosis virus	Erythroid leukemia (chicken)
Pim-1	AKR-murine leukemia virus	T-cell lymphoma (mouse)
Mlvi-1	Moloney murine leukemia virus	T-cell lymphoma (rat)
Mlvi-2	Moloney murine leukemia virus	T-cell lymphoma (rat)
Int-1	Mouse mammary tumor virus	Mammary adenocarcinoma (mouse)
Int-2	Mouse mammary tumor virus	Mammary adenocarcinoma (mouse)

ACTIVATED CELLULAR ONCOGENES DETECTED BY TRANSFECTION **The transfection assay for oncogenes**   Certain established cell lines have the property of incorporating exogenous DNA into chromosomal DNA with an efficiency that makes experimental gene transfer practical in tissue culture. The transfection technique commonly involves precipitating the DNA onto the surface of the target cells with calcium phosphate followed by the uptake of the DNA into cells by pinocytosis. Some of the ingested DNA molecules are transported to the cell nucleus where they are integrated into the chromosomal DNA. If the transfected DNA contains a gene that can be expressed as a dominant, selectable marker in the recipient cells, transfected cells expressing this trait can be recovered with efficiencies of up to about one in 10^5 possible transfection events. Many of the viral oncogenes in Table 59-1 can induce transformation in this type of assay. Such transformation can be achieved either with pure oncogene DNA or with total chromosomal DNA from cells transformed by retroviruses.

Activated cellular oncogenes can also be detected by this technique in the DNA of tumors not known to be induced by viruses. For example, DNA from chemically transformed animal cells and DNA from a variety of naturally occurring animal and human tumor cells contain transforming genes. Normal high-molecular-weight human DNA does not transform cells, but transforming genes can be activated by fragmentation of normal cellular DNA. These findings support the concept that proto-oncogenes in the normal genome are activated during tumor formation but do not distinguish whether the activation of transforming genes is a cause or an effect of the neoplastic phenotype. Although only a fraction of human tumor DNAs will transform in transfection assays, these observations opened the way for analysis of the molecular genetics of human neoplasia.

The ras family of cellular oncogenes   Some of the transforming genes detected by transfection of cells with DNA from human tumor cells have been identified (Table 59-3). The most common oncogenes belong to a family of genes called ras. The first to be identified was the human homologue of the oncogene of Harvey murine sarcoma virus (Table 59-1) called c-ras^H, which codes for a protein of 21,000 mol wt called p21 and is activated in a human cell line derived from bladder carcinoma. In cells transformed by Harvey sarcoma virus, p21 is expressed at high levels, and high-level expression of c-ras^H by experimental linkage of the cellular gene to viral regulatory elements is sufficient to induce cellular transformation. Nevertheless, c-ras^H is not expressed at high levels in those human tumor cell lines in which it is detectable. Instead, the ability to transform cells appears to be conferred by point mutations that cause amino acid changes either at amino acid position 12 or 61 of the p21 protein. Thus, either altered regulation or mutations of protein structure can activate this proto-oncogene.

A second member of the ras family is more frequently activated in human tumors, e.g., the human homologue of the transforming gene of the Kirsten murine sarcoma virus called c-ras^K. Between 10 and 20 percent of human tumor DNA from diverse neoplasms contains a c-ras^K gene that transforms cells in transfection assay (Table 59-3). A protein encoded by c-ras^K is also a p21 molecule, and the transforming activity is due to a structural mutation of this protein similar to that seen for c-ras^H. This mutation is not present in DNA derived from normal tissues of individuals with carcinomas containing an activated c-ras^K gene, suggesting that activation is a somatic event which occurs during tumor formation. Finally, in transfection experiments with DNA from some tumors a third member of this family called ras^N induces transformation. Activation of ras^N occurs in 10 to 20 percent of human acute myeloid leukemias.

Activation of ras is a regular event in some chemically induced epithelial carcinomas in rodents, implying that these genes are activated by chemical carcinogens. However, activated ras genes are found only in a fraction of tumors in humans. As yet unidentified alterations of ras may occur in human tumors, or alteration of other genes might act in place of altered ras genes during tumor development. Neither of these possibilities may be detectable in the standard transfection assays. Alternatively, activation of all oncogenes could be a result of the neoplastic state, rather than an underlying cause. Formal proof for a causative role of activated *ras* genes in the human tumors in which they are found is lacking.

Possible lineage-specific oncogenes In contrast to the *ras* family, which appears to be involved in many types of neoplasms, activation of other oncogenes may be specific to neoplasms of particular cell lineages. The first of these to be identified is called *ChBlym*-1. DNA from chicken lymphomas induced by avian leukosis virus transforms cells in transfection assays, while DNA from normal tissues of the same birds does not have this property. A gene believed to be responsible for this activity, *ChBlym*-1, was obtained from cells transformed by DNA from a bursal lymphoma cell line. It appears to be unrelated to *ras* or the other viral oncogenes described in Table 59-1. As with other oncogenes, nucleotide sequences related to *ChBlym*-1 are conserved in evolution and are present in human DNA.

Human Burkitt's lymphoma resembles the virus-induced lymphomas of chickens in that it is composed of similar B cells at about the same stage of differentiation. The DNA from most Burkitt's lymphoma cell lines can transform cells in transfection assays. This property appears to be due to a gene called *HuBlym*-1, which has about 50 percent homology at the DNA sequence level to *ChBlym*-1. Thus, *Blym* oncogenes are activated in B-cell lymphomas in both chickens and humans but have not been found in other types of tumors. The normal homologues of these transforming genes have not been characterized, so that the cause for activation of the *Blym* oncogenes is not known.

Other B-cell and T-cell neoplasms and adenocarcinomas of the breast contain transforming genes that appear to be distinct for each tumor type. For example, a transforming gene in neoplasms with an intermediate stage of T-cell differentiation, called *Tlym*-1, is distinct from other known oncogenes.

ONCOGENES IMPLICATED IN TUMOR FORMATION BY CHROMOSOMAL TRANSLOCATIONS AND OTHER REARRANGEMENTS A third line of evidence for the activation of oncogenes during tumor formation is derived from the analysis of cytogenetic changes in human neoplasms. Most human tumors are clonal or oligoclonal, that is, composed of cell populations dominated by the progeny of single cells. The dominant cell clones of certain neoplasms are marked by consistent chromosomal abnormalities, such as reciprocal translocations between chromosome 9 and chromosome 22 in chronic myelogenous leukemia (producing the Philadelphia chromosome, Ph′) or between chromosomes 8 and 14 in Burkitt's lymphoma. Indeed, characteristic nonrandom chromosomal changes have been identified in many neoplasms. Genes at or near the site of the DNA rearrangements underlying these cytogenic changes might play a role in the development of the tumors. Advances in in situ hybridization and other techniques of somatic cell genetics have also made it possible to locate the approximate positions of a number of proto-oncogenes on human chromosomes (Table 59-4). Some of these genes are located near the breakpoints of chromosomes that are translocated in particular tumors.

Rearrangement of the c-myc locus in Burkitt's lymphoma As noted in Table 59-4, the human c-*myc* gene is located on chromosome 8. This chromosome is invariably involved in a translocation in Burkitt's lymphoma. At the DNA level the translocation involves recombination between the c-*myc* locus on chromosome 8 and an immunoglobulin gene locus, usually near a heavy chain gene on chromosome 14, less often near a light chain gene on chromosomes 2 or 22. This translocation does not appear to affect the structure of the protein coding portion of the c-*myc* locus but instead affects the regulation of its expression. Similar translocations resulting in recombination between c-*myc* and immunoglobulin genes occur in mouse plasmacytomas.

Alteration of c-abl expression as a result of chromosomal translocation in chronic myelogenous leukemia The Ph′ chromosome

TABLE 59-3 Oncogenes detected in human tumors by transfection of NIH/3T3 cells

Oncogene	Tumors or tumor-derived cell lines
c-*ras*^H	Cell lines derived from EJ/T24 bladder carcinoma, lung carcinoma, and mammary carcinosarcoma
c-*ras*^K	Lung, colon, bladder, pancreatic, and ovarian carcinomas; rhabdomyosarcoma
ras^N	Neuroblastoma, fibrosarcoma, promyelocytic and acute myelogenous leukemia, Burkitt's lymphoma, and colon carcinoma
HuBlym-1	Burkitt's lymphoma cell lines (several)
Tlym-1	T-cell lymphoma–derived cell lines*

* The cloned Tlym-1 gene is of mouse origin. A similar transforming gene appears to be activated in human T-cell lymphoma lines as judged by patterns of inactivation by restriction endonucleases.

is present both in leukemic cells and in normal marrow cell lineages from most patients with chronic myelogenous leukemia (CML). In this disease, the marrow and peripheral blood are thought to be populated by the progeny of a hematopoietic stem cell that retains its ability to differentiate into red cells, megakaryocytes, and granulocytes. The proliferation of granulocytes, however, is abnormal and excessive, producing the clinical manifestations of CML. Genes whose expression is altered as a consequence of the formation of the Ph′ chromosome are candidates for involvement in the development of CML. The human homologue of the proto-oncogene c-*abl* (Table 59-1) is located near the breakpoint on chromosome 9 for the 9-22 translocation and is transferred to chromosome 22 in the exchange. In the Ph′ chromosome the expression of c-*abl* appears to be both quantitatively and qualitatively altered. The levels of c-*abl* RNA are increased, and both the predominant RNA transcript of the gene and the c-*abl* protein are larger than the c-*abl* RNA and protein molecules in normal cells. The RNA and protein gene products of the c-*abl* focus in CML cells are thought to include a fusion production of the c-*abl* gene and a gene called *bcr* (breakpoint cluster region) at the breakpoint on the recombinant Ph′ chromosome. If this alteration in c-*abl* plays a role in CML, it must be at an early stage of the disease.

Amplified proto-oncogenes in human tumors An increase in gene copy number per cell (gene amplification) can sometimes be manifested at the cytogenetic level by the formation of small chromosome-like structures called double minute chromosomes or by the appearance of homogeneous staining regions (HSRs) on regular chromosomes. HSRs are the result of amplification of segments of DNA within the chromosome to the extent that they are identifiable cytogenetically. As a consequence, the structure contains multiple copies of the gene(s) encoded by the DNA segment. Gene amplification in nontransformed cells can sometimes be induced by growing the cells

TABLE 59-4 Localization of some proto-oncogenes on human chromosomes.

Gene	Chromosome	Chromosomal sublocalization, or band*
c-*myc*	8	q24
c-*abl*	9	q34
c-*mos*	8	q22
c-*fes*	15	q24–q25
c-*myb*	6	q22–q24
c-*mil* (raf)	3	p25
N-*ras*	1	cen→p21
c-*ras*^H	11	p14.1
c-*ras*^K	12	p12.05→ter
c-*ets*	11	q23–q24
c-*erbB*	7	pter→q22
c-*erbA*	17	q21–q22
HuBlym-1	1	p32
c-*fms*	5	q34
c-*fos*	14	q21→q31
c-*ski*	1	NA
c-*sis*	22	q11→ter
c-*src*-1	20	p34–p36
c-*src*-2	1	q12→ter

* q = long arm, p = short arm, cen = centromere, ter = terminal, NA = not available

under special conditions. For example, cells containing an amplification of the dihydrofolate reductase gene, which is required for DNA replication, can be selected when cells are grown in the presence of low levels of methotrexate, an inhibitor of dihydrofolate reductase. This increase in gene copy number enhances the amount of enzyme in the cell and overcomes the effects of the inhibitor. Double minute chromosomes and HSRs are present in a variety of tumor cells, suggesting that genes critical to the growth of neoplastic cells may amplify during tumor formation.

The first amplified oncogene recognized in a human tumor cell was the c-*myc* gene which was expressed at a high level in one case of promyelocytic leukemia, both in fresh tumor cells and in a derived cell line. Amplification of c-*myc* appears to be a rare event in this neoplasm and has not been observed in other promyelocytic leukemias. However, double minute chromosomes, amplification of c-*myc* genes, and elevated levels of c-*myc* RNA have been reported in some gastric cancers and small cell carcinomas of the lung, and amplification of the c-*myc* proto-oncogene has been reported in two cell lines derived from human colon carcinoma. Human neuroblastomas are characterized by a high frequency of double minute chromosomes and HSRs. A gene called N-*myc*, which is related to the c-*myc* gene, is amplified and/or expressed at a high level in most neuroblastomas, in cell lines derived from neuroblastomas, and in other neuroendocrine tumors. Considerable heterogeneity occurs within the tumor cell population with respect to the degree of amplification and/or expression of N-*myc*.

FUNCTIONS OF ONCOGENES Studies of the proteins encoded by the viral oncogenes and their normal cellular homologues have provided insight into the functions of these genes. The protein product of the v-*src* gene of Rous sarcoma virus acts as a tyrosine protein kinase, and the oncogenic properties of v-*src* depend upon this enzymatic activity. Five additional viral oncogene proteins (those encoded by *fes/fps*, *yes*, *ros*, *abl*, and *fgr*) are also tyrosine protein kinases. The problem has been to identify the cellular proteins that are modified by these kinases and that are critical for transformation. For example, in cells transformed by Rous sarcoma virus, a number of cellular proteins are modified by the addition of phosphate groups to tyrosine residues, but a role for such changes in oncogenesis has not been established.

Growth factors and receptors An important conceptual advance has come from separate lines of research on oncogene function and growth factor function (Fig. 59-3). The proliferation and differentiation of normal cells are regulated by signals derived from the binding of growth factors to receptors on the cell surface. Two of the better characterized growth factors are platelet-derived growth factor (PDGF), which promotes the growth of connective tissue and smooth muscle cells, and epidermal growth factor (EGF), which is required for

optimal growth of epithelial cells in vitro. The receptors for PDGF and EGF possess a tyrosine protein kinase which is activated by binding of PDGF or EGF. Whether the growth factor receptor and oncogene tyrosine protein kinases modify some of the same target proteins inside the cells is not known.

A protein encoded by the viral oncogene of Simian sarcoma virus, *sis*, is closely related to PDGF. The *erbB* oncogene of avian erythroblastosis virus appears to be a truncated form of the receptor molecule for EGF. The *fms* oncogene of a strain of feline sarcoma virus may be related to the receptor of a macrophage growth factor called CSF-1. These observations have led to the postulate that the unregulated growth signal involved in neoplastic transformation might result from changes in growth factors, their receptors, or other elements in the pathway.

***Ras* oncogene proteins** The proteins encoded by *ras* oncogenes are associated with the inner surface of the cell membrane. They share a functional activity, the binding of guanosine triphosphate (GTP), with a family of GTP-binding or G proteins. G proteins are found in association with the adenylate cyclase complex on the inner surface of the cell membrane, and they participate in the transmission of signals from the cell surface that result in changes in intracellular cyclic nucleotide levels (see Chap. 67). In yeast, *ras* genes act through the adenylate cyclase–protein kinase pathway. Thus, transforming *ras* proteins may be a class of altered G proteins that transmit a constitutive growth signal.

Oncogene proteins in the cell nucleus The proteins encoded by three of the oncogenes in Table 59-1, *myb*, *myc*, and *fos*, are located in the cell nucleus. The normal homologue of *myb* is expressed predominantly in the G1 phase of the cell cycle in some but not all cells. The other two genes appear to be closely tied to the growth factor pathway. When growth-arrested fibroblasts are exposed to PDGF, a specific set of genes (estimated to be between 10 and 30) is expressed, including the proto-oncogenes c-*fos* and c-*myc*, and cellular messenger RNA levels for these genes increase. Expression of c-*myc* is also enhanced in resting B and T lymphocytes after exposure to appropriate mitogens. Once cells enter the growth cycle the expression of c-*myc* remains fairly constant. When cells lose the ability to divide, for example, in postmitotic, differentiated cells, c-*myc* expression ceases. These proto-oncogenes, therefore, may function normally as regulators of cell "activation," growth, and differentiation and may be nuclear targets for growth-factor-derived signals. When altered or deregulated, they may provide a constitutive drive for the uncontrolled cell growth and abnormal differentiation that characterize the neoplastic state. Both the *myc* and *myb* proteins have DNA binding activity, but the mechanism of action of nuclear proteins is not known.

EXTRA-CELLULAR	plasma membrane	CYTOPLASM	NUCLEUS		EFFECTS
Growth Factors (Sis)	Receptors (Erb B)	Adenylate Cyclase → Protein Kinases G-Proteins : (Ras) Tyrosine Protein Kinases (Src, Yes, Fes/Fps, Fgr, Abl, Ros)	Myc → Myb Fos		Activation Growth Differentiation

FIGURE 59-3 *Possible relationship of the molecular biology of growth factors to the function of oncogenes. Growth factors are small molecules that signal cell activation, replication, and differentiation by binding to specific receptors on the surface of target cells. As shown, a number of the proteins made by oncogenes fit into the general pathway for growth factor activity. Oncogenes may transform cells by transmitting a constitutive, unregulated signal for cell growth from their particular position in the pathway. For details see text.*

EXPERIMENTAL INTRODUCTION OF ACTIVE ONCOGENES INTO GERM CELLS AND SOMATIC TISSUE STEM CELLS

One approach to demonstrating the oncogenic potential of tumor-associated oncogenes is to transfer activated oncogenes into normal cells in vivo and to observe the effects of these genes on development. Several different genes, such as those specifying immunoglobulin and growth hormone, have been introduced by microinjection into fertilized mouse eggs. The injected "trans-genes" become integrated into the genome of progeny mice and, in some cases, are expressed in appropriate cell types (for example, immunoglobulin trans-genes are expressed predominately in B lymphocytes).

The introduction by this technique of a T antigen gene from the DNA tumor virus SV40 into the germline of mice resulted in the formation of choroid plexus papillomas. Likewise, the introduction of altered c-*myc* trans-genes with promoter-enhancer sequences derived from mouse mammary tumor virus into the germline of mice caused the development of mammary tumors in some of the mice. The introduced oncogene appeared to act as a predisposing factor for the accelerated development of mammary carcinomas, but additional events may be required for the full development of mammary tumors in these animals.

Introduction of oncogenes into transplantable stem cells of bone marrow and lymphoid organs is done by infecting stem cells ex vivo with viral vectors containing the genes and then transplanting the cells into appropriately prepared hosts. The introduction of the v-*myc* gene by this technique into the stem cells of the chicken bursa induced pre-neoplastic proliferative lesions that precede the development of B-cell lymphomas. This occurred in the absence of activation of transforming genes like *Blym*-1 that are found in more advanced neoplasms of this type. Consequently, activated *myc* oncogenes may be responsible for the early pre-neoplastic stages of lymphoma formation in this system, while additional events, such as activation of *Blym*-1, may be required for neoplastic progression.

ONCOGENES AND MULTISTAGED TUMORIGENESIS

Human cancer and chemically induced neoplasia in animals usually develop as a multistep process in which an abnormal pre-neoplastic cell type evolves into a cell population successively dominated by clones with increasingly malignant characteristics. This evolution of tumor development is thought to be preceded by a latent period, and the whole process may take a significant fraction of the life span of the affected individual. In contrast, acute transforming viruses carrying activated forms of oncogenes that are implicated in nonviral cancer appear to induce neoplasms within days or weeks, i.e., with kinetics that suggest a single-step process. This difference may be due to several factors. First, many of the viral oncogenes encode kinases with multiple cellular targets and may induce abrupt changes that would require several different mutations in more slowly evolving neoplasms. Second, expression of the viral oncogenes is driven by powerful regulatory elements (promoters and enhancers in the proviral LTRs). The transforming potential of the cellular homologues of these same genes can be activated by mechanisms that do not involve such high-level expression, for example, the point mutations at amino acids 12 or 61 of the proteins encoded by the human *ras* tumor-associated oncogenes. In these situations the concerted activity of several genes may be required to induce the same transformed phenotype that can be induced by very high level, unregulated expression of just one of the genes (as occurs with acute transforming retroviruses).

This point is illustrated by transfection experiments suggesting cooperation between oncogenes in inducing transformation of cultured fibroblasts. The activated *ras* genes from human tumor cells can transform immortalized cell lines but cannot induce full morphologic transformation of primary cell cultures. The combination of activated *myc* and *ras* gene clones, however, produces the fully transformed phenotype in primary cell cultures. Thus, in this system *myc* (and other oncogenes that do not alter these cells by themselves) can complement the transforming activating of human *ras* oncogenes. However, when powerful transcriptional enhancer sequences are engineered into the activated *ras* oncogene, this gene can itself transform primary fibroblast cultures, presumably because of a higher level of expression of the oncogene. The requirement for multiple genes in transformation may be conditioned, in part, by the level of oncogene expression, and more than one cellular oncogene may be activated in neoplasms in vivo.

IMPLICATIONS OF ONCOGENE RESEARCH FOR CLINICAL ONCOLOGY

The clinical impact of the identification and analysis of human oncogenes and their products may be extensive, indeed revolutionary. For example, efforts to identify and control environmental and nutritional factors that may cause or prevent cancer depend heavily on epidemiologic techniques, animal studies, and clinical trials where disease incidence and mortality are endpoints for measurement. Knowledge of the specific proto-oncogenes that are the targets of environmental carcinogens and of the nature of the changes induced may provide better methods for assessing the actual role of candidate carcinogens and for devising preventive approaches. Delineation of the molecular anatomy of neoplastic change in specific cell lineages should also add new dimensions to diagnosis. An example would be the use of rapid techniques for detecting alteration of the c-*abl* RNA and/or protein for analysis of chronic myelogenous leukemia cells. Knowledge of the molecular mechanisms employed by oncogenes to transform cells may also provide more precise and more specific means for targeting pharmacologic intervention.

REFERENCES

BISHOP JM, VARMUS H: Functions and origins of retroviral transforming genes, in *Molecular Biology of Tumor Viruses; RNA Tumor Viruses,* 2d ed, R Weiss et al (eds). New York, Cold Spring Harbor Laboratory, 1982, pp 999–1108
COHEN S: The epidermal growth factor (EGF). Cancer 51:1787, 1983
COOPER GM, LANE MA: Cellular transforming genes and oncogenes. Biochim Biophys Acta 738:9, 1984
FIALKOW PJ: Clonal origin of human tumors. Ann Rev Med 30:135, 1979
HUNTER T: The proteins of oncogenes. Sci Am 251:70, 1984
LAND H et al: Cellular oncogenes and multistep carcinogens. Science 222:771, 1983
LEDER P et al: Translocations among antibody genes in cancer. Science 222:765, 1983
STILES CD: The molecular biology of platelet-derived growth factor. Cell 33:653, 1983
WEINSTEIN IB: Multistage carcinogenesis involves multiple genes and multiple mechanisms, in *Cancer Cells,* AJ Levine et al (eds). New York, Cold Spring Harbor Laboratory, 1984, pp 229–237
YUNIS JJ: The chromosomal basis of human neoplasia. Science 221:227, 1983

60 CYTOGENETIC ASPECTS OF HUMAN DISEASE

JAMES L. GERMAN III

The chromosome complement of humans, like that of other species, is guarded carefully against change; most chromosome mutations, either structural or numerical, are deleterious. Only rarely is a balanced structural rearrangement (one that results in neither deficiency nor duplication of significant chromosome segments) introduced into the population and transmitted from generation to generation. (Figure 60-1 shows the normal human chromosome complement. In the legend of the figure several terms used in human cytogenetics are defined.) As a rule an abnormal number of autosomes results in early death, except for trisomy of the shortest chromosome. In contrast, an abnormal number of sex chromosomes is often tolerated reasonably well, although infertility or subfertility usually is present. Nevertheless, among human embryos abnormalities in chromosome structure and number are common and are, in fact, the major known cause of embryonic and early fetal wastage. However, not every fetus with an abnormal chromosome complement is aborted, and those that survive constitute the material of medical cytogenetics.

Clinical disorders resulting from chromosome imbalance present varying features including abnormal anatomic development, mental

FIGURE 60-1 *Normal human lymphocyte chromosomes arrested in metaphase and stained for G bands (G standing for Giemsa). The inset shows the arrangement of chromosomes in an intact cell, and the remainder of the figure shows their ordered arrangement into a karyotype. By the time mitosis begins, each chromosome consists of two identical parts called sister chromatids and is identified by the relative length, the location of the centromere, and a distinctive sequence of bands of varying lengths and depth of staining. The number of bands visible microscopically varies from cell to cell, depending on the degree of chromosome condensation. The 300 to 400 bands seen in this particular cell can be increased to several times that number if cells with longer chromosomes are chosen for analysis, i.e., many of the bands seen here will resolve into subbands. Normally, the G-band patterns of the two chromosomes of a pair are alike, with the exception of certain polymorphic regions, examples of which are shown in Fig. 60-4.*

The centromere of a chromosome divides it into a short arm (p) and a long arm (q). Numbers 13 to 15, 21, 22, and Y are called acrocentric because *of the nearly terminal positions of their centromeres; the minute p of each acrocentric autosome bears a nucleolus-organizing region which often causes a secondary constriction in the metaphase chromosome (the constriction at the centromere being the primary constriction).*

By standard nomenclature, this karyotype is described as 46,XY, indicating that its chromosome number is 46, its sex chromosomes are an X and a Y, and the autosomes (those besides the X and Y) number 44. The following examples show the general use of this nomenclature: A normal female karyotype is described as 46,XX. A female cell with an extra chromosome 18 (trisomic for 18) would be described as 47,XX, + 18. A cell with only one sex chromosome, an X, and with deletion in the short arm of chromosome 5 would be described as 45,X,5p − . A male cell with a translocation between the long arm of chromosome 2 and the short arm of chromosome 3 would be described as 46,XY,t(2q;3p); exact breakpoints could be indicated by additional characters and symbols.

deficiency, behavioral disorders, and disturbances in growth and sexual development. Sometimes infertility, repeated abortion, or the birth of malformed children is the presenting complaint of persons with abnormal chromosome complements whose own general development is normal.

The disorders just referred to are due to chromosome imbalance that affects tissues throughout the body. In addition, change can occur in the chromosome complement in a single cell of some somatic tissue. Such a mutant cell may have a proliferative advantage over normal cells, in which case a clone bearing the abnormal chromosome complement can develop among otherwise normal cells. Although such mutant clones are in many cases clinically insignificant, much

evidence suggests that they are also important in the etiology of cancer.

This chapter is addressed to those aspects of normal chromosome structure and function that constitute the basis for an understanding of the chromosome alterations in human disease. In addition, the chromosome alterations important in adult medicine and their consequences are summarized.

CHROMOSOME STRUCTURE AND FUNCTION The human autosomes are numbered 1 through 22, and the sex chromosomes are denoted X and Y (Fig. 60-1). Each is recognizable microscopically by morphologic features such as relative length and position of the centromere and by staining characteristics (banding pattern). A mammalian chromosome is believed to be composed of one double-stranded chain of deoxyribonucleic acid (DNA) that extends from one end through the centromere to the other end.

Cell-division cycle Chromosomes must duplicate before cell division can occur. This duplication occurs over a period of several hours prior to the onset of mitosis or meiosis in a phase of the cell cycle termed S, for synthesis of DNA (Fig. 60-2). Thus, from the completion of S to the completion of metaphase, each chromosome contains two identical double-stranded helices of DNA, and the nucleus contains four times as much DNA as a spermatozoon or ovum. During mitosis chromosomes are condensed, and the two sister chromatids can be visualized by late prophase or early metaphase (Fig. 60-1). (Metaphase is the stage in the cell-division cycle ordinarily employed for cytogenetic analysis.)

At the onset of anaphase the centromeric regions of each chromosome separate, and the two chromatids move quickly to opposite poles of the mitotic spindle. As soon as each pole receives one full complement of chromatids (now called chromosomes), a nuclear membrane—it had been disassembled late in prophase—is assembled about each cluster to complete formation of the nuclei of the two sister cells that emerge at telophase. The sister cells emerge in what usually is called the G_1 phase of the cell cycle, in which they remain unreplicated unless another division is to be prepared for, whereupon they enter the S phase. Cells engaged in some differentiated function ordinarily remain unreplicated.

Most normal cells in the human body are diploid; i.e., they have twice the haploid number of chromosomes, the number in a gamete (haploid = 23, diploid = 46). In the germ line, which is devoted to gamete formation, cells destined eventually to differentiate into spermatozoa or ova undergo mitotic cell cycles until they enter the two specialized divisions termed *meiosis*. In meiosis, pairing of homologous chromosomes occurs (the paternally derived chromosome 1 with the maternally derived chromosome 1, and so on), and genetic recombination takes place (see Chap. 57). At the first meiotic division homologous chromosomes are segregated, and the diploid chromosome number is reduced to the haploid; i.e., each cell then contains one of each of the 22 (duplicated) autosomes plus one (duplicated) sex chromosome. No S phase takes place between the first and second meiotic divisions (depicted in Fig. 60-2, right), so that at the second division, in which sister chromatids separate, emerging cells maintain the haploid number of chromosomes but are reduced in their content of DNA to half the amount of diploid G_1 cells of somatic tissues. With fertilization of an ovum by a spermatozoon, both the chromosome constitution and the DNA content of the zygote are restored to that of a G_1 somatic cell. An S period in the zygote then permits reinstitution of regular cell-division cycles characteristic of the somatic cells.

Chromosome differentiation A chromosome is differentiated along its length, and some aspects of this differentiation are resolvable in the light microscope. The DNA is complexed with a number of proteins in a highly specific way. The DNA-protein complex together with some associated ribonucleic acid (RNA) is referred to as *chromatin*. The fine structure and the manner in which the DNA is compacted and interacted with proteins are thought to pertain to the control of RNA production and DNA replication, and perhaps to cellular differentiation as well.

The sequences of nucleotide bases in DNA that constitute the genes and that can be transcribed into messenger RNA are distributed throughout the length of the various chromosomes. (These sequences are too short to be resolved microscopically.) Over 400 genes have been mapped to specific chromosomes, in many cases to specific regions of a chromosome. The locations of a few of the many genes of interest in clinical medicine and that have been mapped are shown in Fig. 60-3.

Certain segments of at least 12 chromosomes vary in length among individuals. These segments can be delineated by their staining characteristics (Fig. 60-4). The variable segments consist of nontranscribed, highly repetitive nucleotide sequences of DNA and are transmitted from parent to child in a straightforward mendelian fashion. Techniques of molecular genetics, which are useful as an extension of the microscopic observation of human chromosomes, permit the identification and molecular definition of an even greater number of variable segments of DNA, ones that are submicroscopic. These sometimes are referred to as *restriction fragment-length polymorphisms* (RFLPs). Variations in both the microscopically visible and invisible segments are unassociated with detectable phenotypic effect. However, they can serve as useful cell markers in prenatal diagnosis when they have been shown to lie very close to disease-associated loci (e.g., Duchenne's muscular dystrophy) and in determination of zygosity of twins, paternity, and survival of transplants.

Other microscopically recognizable segments in the short arms of the acrocentric autosomes are devoted to the production of ribosomal RNA and nucleoli. As mitosis progresses, these nucleolus-organizer regions tend to remain relatively uncondensed later than other regions. Consequently, at metaphase they appear understained and thereby demarcate condensed segments of chromatin distal to them on the chromosome arms—*satellites*. (Satellites are examples of the polymorphic segments just mentioned.) Several other regions that remain relatively uncondensed at metaphase and that are seen more often than the remainder of the chromatin to undergo outright disruption ("breakage") are recognizable in a low percentage of cells from some normal individuals and sometimes are called *fragile sites*. In a few cases studied the tendency for such fragile sites to be visible at metaphase is a dominantly transmitted trait. The only such region known to be of significance in relation to a human trait is one located near the distal end (the end away from the centromere) of the long arm of the X chromosome; it segregates in certain families as an X-linked trait in association with a syndrome that features mental defectiveness, a characteristic facies, and macroorchia—the "fragile-X syndrome." (This locus is one of the mapped loci indicated in Fig. 60-3.) Other examples of segmental specialization along the chromosome include *telomeres* and *centromeres*. Telomeres, the distal termini of each arm, have some relationship to the nuclear membrane and probably are important in the maintenance of order in the interphase nucleus; centromeric regions are sites of microtubule attachment at metaphase.

FIGURE 60-2 *Schematic representation of the mitotic and meiotic cell-division cycles, as described in the text. G_1 and G_2 = time gaps before and after S, the period in which DNA replicates. Each of these intervals is several hours in duration; together they constitute interphase. M = mitosis; I and II = the two divisions of meiosis. The DNA content of the cycling cells is indicated on the vertical axis: 1c = the content in a gamete; 2c = that in either an egg immediately postfertilization or a somatic cell emerging from mitosis; 4c = the amount in a cell which has completed chromosome duplication and is ready to enter mitosis or meiosis.*

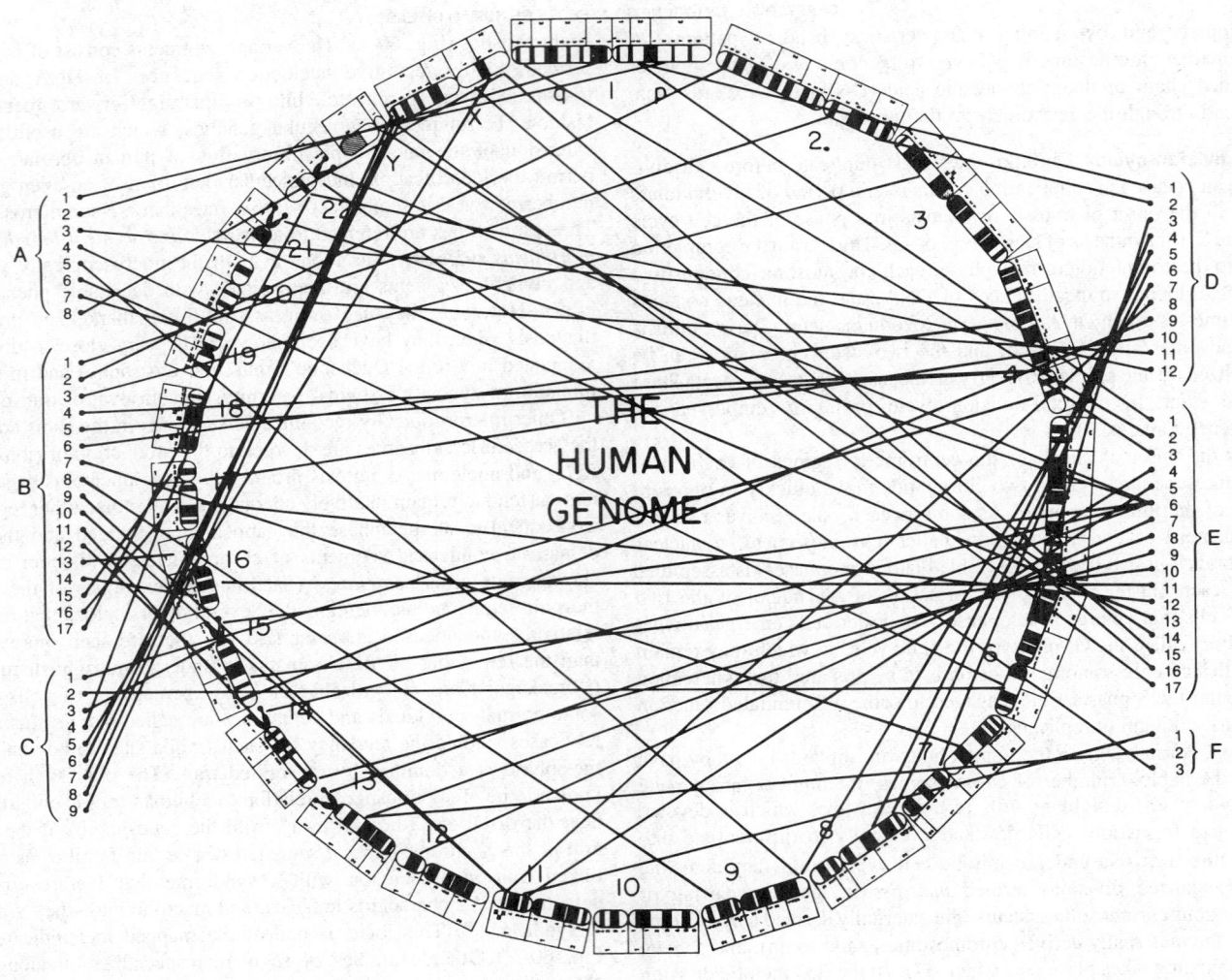

A: CELL SURFACE ANTIGENS
1 = Rhesus
2 = Duffy
3 = MNSs
4 = MHC
5 = ABO
6 = Lewis
7 = Lutheran
8 = Xg

B: DIFFERENTIATED CELL PRODUCTS
1 = Immunoglobulin kappa-light chain
2 = Glucagon
3 = Transferrin
4 = Albumin
5 = Alpha-fetoprotein
6 = Fibrinogen
7 = Collagen I
8 = Interferon (leukocyte)
9 = Insulin
10 = Hemoglobin-beta
11 = Immunoglobulin heavy chain
12 = Beta-2-microglobulin
13 = Hemoglobin-alpha
14 = Haptoglobin
15 = Myosin heavy chain
16 = Growth hormone
17 = Immunoglobulin lambda-light chain

C: GENES FOR DISEASE
1 = Huntington's chorea
2 = Congenital adrenal hyperplasia
3 = Prader-Willi syndrome
4 = Familial hypercholesterolemia
    (LDL receptor)
5 = Duchenne's muscular dystrophy
6 = Hunter's syndrome
7 = Hemophilia B
8 = Hemophilia A
9 = X-linked mental deficiency

D: CELLULAR ONCOGENES
1 = N-ras
2 = N-myc
3 = myb
4 = erb B
5 = mos
6 = myc
7 = abl
8 = H-ras
9 = fes
10 = erb A
11 = src
12 = sis

E: MISCELLANEOUS
1 = Phosphoglucomutase
2 = 55 ribosomal RNA
3 = Phosphoglucomutase-2
4 = Dihydrofolate reductase
5 = Lactate dehydrogenase A
6 = Ribosomal RNA
7 = Lactate dehydrogenase B
8 = Esterase D
9 = DNA segment D14S1
10 = Hexosaminidase-A
11 = Metallothionein
12 = Thymidine kinase
13 = Superoxide dismutase-1
14 = Testis-determining factor
15 = Steroid sulfatase
16 = DNA segment DXS7
17 = G-6-PD

F: "CANCER GENES"
1 = Wilms's tumor
2 = Retinoblastoma
3 = Meningioma

FIGURE 60-3 *The 24 human chromosomes arrayed in a circle. The distinctive bands demonstrable by several cytogenetic techniques are shown, with the numerical designations that were agreed upon by a series of international conferences. From the several hundred genes that have been mapped to specific chromosome regions, a few of interest in medicine have been selected and their locations indicated. (For a current listing of all known human gene localizations, see McKusick.)*

A further example of chromosome differentiation is the established sequence by which various segments replicate during S; certain segments replicate early, others late. In general, late replication of a chromosome segment correlates with genetic inertness. This correlation is exemplified by one of the two X chromosomes in female cells; the chromosome inactivated by the Lyon effect is almost entirely late-replicating (see Chap. 57 for an explanation of X-chromosome inactivation).

A little-understood type of chromatin is that which long has been referred to as *heterochromatin*. It is tightly condensed, not just at metaphase but throughout interphase. Such condensation of chromatin correlates positively with genetic inactivity and also with late replication. Some regions are condensed and inactive in all cells (constitutive heterochromatin), while others, for example, the X chromosome, may be either condensed and inactive or decondensed and active (facultative heterochromatin). Many chromosome imbalances that permit viability beyond intrauterine life involve chromosome segments that are rich in this apparently inactive, or inactivatable, type of chromatin, e.g., chromosomes that can be trisomic in liveborn individuals or, in the case of X, monosomic. The activity of genes can sometimes be affected, even inactivated, if they are positioned near regions of heterochromatin, as can occur as a result of chromosome breakage and rearrangement.

Therefore, in chromosomal imbalance both the specific genetic loci and the particular types of chromatin deleted or duplicated are important. Also, the significance of a structural rearrangement probably depends on the new and abnormal positioning of structural and regulatory genes in relation to each other and to heterochromatin.

Fortunately for the cytologist, several differentiated features of the chromosome correlate with cytological artifacts that can be produced and visualized in the laboratory. A number of techniques are now in use to display a pattern of bands of various lengths and staining characteristics (Figs. 60-1 and 60-4). These patterns are identical in each chromosome 1, each chromosome 2, etc., varying only in the inert polymorphic regions mentioned above, so that they can be used in clinical cytogenetics to identify chromosomes and to detect and define structural rearrangements.

Sources of error Every aspect of the cell-division cycle is complicated. Doubtless a large number of genetic loci must be active to produce the numerous enzymes and structural proteins required to initiate and complete a cycle. Remarkable precision and accuracy are demanded over and over in matters such as the passage of a cell from G_1 into S, orderly progression of replication, assembly of the mitotic spindle, and spindle function in segregating chromatids during mitosis. An additional battery of loci is activated to permit a cell of the germ line to pass successfully through the complicated stages of meiotic prophase, including pairing of homologous chromosomes, genetic recombination, and then disjoining of chromosomes. Probably all these mechanisms and processes are subject to errors, some spontaneous, others promoted by some unfavorable environmental influence (e.g., Fig. 60-5) or by the presence of deleterious mutations involving one of the many steps just mentioned. Furthermore, the genetic material itself is subject to damage, and certain types of unrepaired or erroneously repaired lesions in DNA theoretically may predispose to chromosome rearrangement. Errors at many of these steps lie behind chromosome imbalance. Errors that occur in germ cells, during fertilization, and in early postfertilization divisions are important in relation to embryonic maldevelopment and infertility; errors in somatic cells are important in relation to neoplasia.

CHROMOSOME ABNORMALITIES Mutations of a single base in a gene and deletions and duplications of chromosome segments involving even hundreds of base pairs are not visible to the cytogeneticist. In fact, for the normal chromosome banding pattern to be detectably disturbed, a lengthy segment of DNA must be deleted, duplicated, or transposed. This means that a chromosome mutation that is microscopically detectable must involve relatively huge amounts of DNA. It is noteworthy, however, that the same environmental

FIGURE 60-4 *Metaphase chromosomes stained for C bands (C standing for centromeric or constitutive heterochromatin), showing inherited variation in lengths of C bands in chromosome 1 (arrows).*

agents known to produce point mutations (mutagens in the usual sense) are in general also chromosome-breaking agents, and vice versa. Thus, it seems safe to assume the existence of a spectrum extending from mutations visible to the cytogeneticist all the way down to those that must be defined by nucleotide sequencing. Mutations visible to the cytogeneticist ordinarily exert a more widespread effect on development than do point mutations; ordinary genes—often many of them—as well as other specialized types of chromatin whose function usually is unknown, are involved in cytologically visible mutations.

If an entire chromosome is affected in an imbalance, the genome is said to be either trisomic or monosomic for the chromosome (thus, trisomy 13, monosomy X). Genes and chromatin carried on the affected chromosome then are present in triple or single dose, respectively, rather than the normal double dose. Abnormal dosage affecting less than an entire chromosome, the result of chromosome

FIGURE 60-5 *Breaks and rearrangements (arrows) in metaphase chromosomes of a blood lymphocyte that received ionizing irradiation before being stimulated by phytohemagglutinin to enter S and divide.*

breakage and rearrangement, is often termed *partial trisomy* or *partial monosomy*, to indicate that segments rather than entire chromosomes are involved (thus, partial trisomy 13q, partial monosomy 4p). The commoner chromosome imbalances, both numerical and structural, are listed in Table 60-1.

Incidence The frequency with which chromosomal imbalance is detectable depends on the population investigated. It is estimated that a minimum of 1 in 10 recognized human conceptions has a chromosome abnormality. In human embryos and fetuses aborted spontaneously, the incidence of chromosome imbalance is higher the earlier in pregnancy the sampling is made. The contribution of imbalance to late abortion and stillbirth, though not well studied, probably also is significant. In the more than 65,000 consecutive or random live-born babies that now have been examined in different laboratories, approximately 1 in 200 has a significant chromosome abnormality, either numerical or structural. In such studies, at least 1 in 700 newborns is trisomic for one of the autosomes 21, 18, or 13; about 1 in 350 newborn males has the complement 47,XXY or 47,XYY. One in every several thousand newborns has monosomy X. One in five hundred has some structural rearrangement, most of which are genetically balanced. Samplings of the general adult population reveal an occasional inherited balanced structural rearrangement as well as the expected number of XXY, XYY, and XXX complements; the inherited, apparently innocuous segmental polymorphisms (e.g., Fig. 60-4) and minor structural rearrangements demonstrable by banding techniques are found in abundance.

In populations of individuals with mental deficiency, 10 to 15 percent have a chromosome abnormality, the proportion being greater if the individuals also have anatomic malformations. In some groups of male criminals and in infertile men an increased incidence of individuals with an extra sex chromosome, an X or a Y, is found. Infertile women also include many individuals with extra or missing sex chromosomes and an appreciable number with structural chromosome rearrangement; approximately one-fourth of women with primary amenorrhea have some abnormality of the X chromosome. Among infertile men and women, individuals with genes that interfere with meiosis, so-called meiotic mutants, are also found occasionally.

Numerical abnormalities Trisomy (47 chromosomes) is the most common chromosome imbalance in early spontaneous abortuses, followed by monosomy (45 chromosomes) and triploidy (69 chromosomes). The extra or missing chromosomes can be either paternal or maternal in origin, and the error in segregation of chromosomes

TABLE 60-1　The commoner chromosome imbalances that recur in the human population and that can result in clinically recognizable syndromes*

Imbalance	Chromosomes affected	Karyotypes†	Clinical features‡
Monosomy	Sex chromosome: X	45,X	Turner's syndrome
Segmental deficiency—"partial monosomy"	X	46,XXp-; 46,XXq-; 46,X,r(X); 46,X,iso(Xp); 46,X,iso(Xq);	Turner's syndrome or some features of it
	Y	46,XYp-; 46,XYq-; 46,X,r(Y); 46,X,iso(Yp); 46,X,iso(Yq)	Turner's syndrome, or some features of it; "mixed gonadal dysgenesis" syndrome may result when a 45,X cell line coexists; risk of testicular neoplasia
	Autosome: 4	46,XY,4p-	Gr, Cf, Mi, Ey, Sk, Ge, Ht, Co, Me
	5	46,XY,5p-	Cri-du-chat syndrome: Cr, Mi, Cf, Me
	11	46,XY,11p-	WT, Ge, Me
	13	46,XY,13q-	RB, Cf, Me
	15	46,XY,15q-	Prader-Willi syndrome
	18	46,XY,18p-	Gr, Cf, Ea, Te, Po, Sk, Ht, Me
	18	46,XY,18q-	Cf, Hy, Sk, Ey
	21	46,XY,r(21)	Cf, Hp, Ea, Me
Trisomy	Sex chromosome: X	47,XXX	Se, Me (mild), Ps
	X	47,XXY	Klinefelter's syndrome
	Y	47,XYY	Ta, Ac, Su, B; but often normal
	Autosome: 8	46,XY/47,XY,8+	Cf, Sk, Me (moderate)
	13	47,XY,13+	Trisomy 13 syndrome: Cp, Ey, Pd, Po, Ht, D, V, Sc, F, Ar, Me
	18	47,XY,18+	Trisomy 18 syndrome: Cf, Ea, V, F, Gr, D, He, Me
	21	47,XY,21+	Trisomy 21 syndrome (Down's syndrome)
Segmental duplication—"partial trisomy"	Sex chromosome: Y	46,X,t(X;Y)§	True hermaphroditism or XX male
	Autosome: 9	+9p†	Cf
	22	+22q¶	Gr, Cf, Ea, Cp, He, Hy, Co
Chimerism	Entire complement	46,XY/46,XX	Pseudo- or true hermaphroditism; dimorphism of blood-cell-surface antigens

* *For complete listing, consult DeGrouchy and Turleau.*
† *The sex chromosome constitution might be either XY or XX, but in the example karyotypes given, XY arbitrarily is used.*
‡ *The clinical features given include only some of the more constant ones. Deficiency of one segment often is accompanied by duplication of another, and the phenotypic effect is the consequence of the combined imbalance.*
§ *Translocation onto an X of the minute segment of the Y responsible for testicular differentiation. Random inactivation of either the normal X or the one bearing Y material determines the gonadal phenotype(s)—testis or ovary, respectively.*
¶ *Brought about through any of several rearrangements.*
NOTE: *Abbreviations: Ac, acne; Ar, arrhinencephaly; B, behavior disorder; Cr, characteristically abnormal cry; Cf, characteristic craniofacial dysmorphism; Co, convulsions; Cp, cleft lip–palate; D, early death; Ea, characteristically abnormal ears; Ey, eye anomaly; F, characteristically flared, overlapping fingers; Ge, abnormality of external genitalia; Gr, severe growth deficiency; Hp, hypertonia; Ht, cardiac malformation; Hy, infantile hypotonia; Me, intellectual deficit; Mi, microcephaly; Po, characteristically abnormal posture; Pd, polydactyly; Ps, psychotic predisposition; RB, retinoblastoma; Sc, scalp defect; Se, secondary amenorrhea; Sk, skeletal anomalies; Su, subfertility; Ta, tallness; Te, characteristically abnormal teeth; V, visceral anomalies; WT, Wilms's tumor with aniridia.*

can occur in the germ line, fertilized egg (zygote), or early embryo. Trisomy of every chromosome except the no. 1 has been observed in spontaneous abortions, trisomy 16 most frequently.

Sex chromosomal trisomy (XXY, XYY, and XXX) is compatible with intrauterine survival; in contrast, autosomal trisomy rarely permits survival to term. However, a small proportion of autosomal trisomics is live-born. For practical purposes these are only trisomy 21, 18, and 13, in decreasing frequency. Trisomies 18 and 13 cause death during infancy. Therefore trisomies of significance in adults are trisomy 21, XXY, XXX, and XYY. A few other autosomal trisomies, such as trisomy 8, have occasionally been reported, usually in mosaicism with a normal cellular component. (Mosaicism is the coexistence of multiple, genetically different populations of cells, all derived originally, however, from a single zygote.)

Autosomal monosomy is rare even among abortion material. In contrast, monosomy X (45,X) occurs in approximately 1.5 percent of recognized conceptions. It is common among spontaneously aborted human embryos (approximately 10 percent) and is present in one in every several thousand live-born babies. The reason for the death of 45,X embryos and fetuses is unknown, although developmental abnormalities doubtless contribute; cardiovascular and renal anomalies are common in the few that survive. In monosomy X, the missing sex chromosome can be either a Y or an X and is either paternal or maternal in origin. Often the second sex chromosome is not completely absent but is replaced by a structurally rearranged Y or X. Mosaicism is common in live-borns with monosomy X; here, tissues are populated not only by cells with a 45,X complement but by other cells, perhaps with a normal complement, either 46,XY or 46,XX, or with a complement in which the second sex chromosome is rearranged in some way.

Triploidy is rare in live-born babies and usually leads to early death, even when in a mosaicism with normal cells: 46,XY/69,XXY. The phenotypic effects of the autosomal trisomies, of 47,XXY, and of monosomy X (45,X) are characteristic and well defined so that their diagnosis usually is not difficult (see Chap. 333). The effects of the 47,XYY and 47,XXX constitutions are less striking, and therefore these complements are underdiagnosed. Mosaicism with coexistence of abnormal and normal populations of cells can cause an abnormal phenotype to approach the normal.

The mechanisms responsible for the numerical abnormalities are undefined and may be multiple. A striking but unexplained maternal age effect exists in trisomies 21, 18, 13, XXY, and XXX. In the case of trisomy 21 (at least), the maternal age effect is present regardless of whether the sperm or the egg contributes the extra chromosome at fertilization. Over one-third of babies with trisomy 21 are born to women over 35, whereas only one-tenth of all births occur in this group. The frequency of trisomy 21 rises from 0.5 to 0.7 per 1000 live births between ages 21 and 23 to 3.1 per 1000 at age 35, 10.5 per 1000 at age 40, and 33.6 per 1000 at age 45. (A paternal age effect may also exist in trisomy 21.) Maternal x-ray irradiation in low dosage is also associated with an increased incidence of trisomy 21. After a child with trisomy 21 is born, the risk to the parents of recurrence in future pregnancies is increased to approximately 1 percent. As to the etiology of monosomy X, the frequent association of the 45,X complement in mosaicism with normal complements and with structural rearrangements of the X and Y suggests that the zygote or the preimplantation embryo may often be the target of a chromosome-breaking event.

Structural abnormalities Some structural chromosome rearrangements are inherited, and others represent new mutations. The etiology of the new rearrangements is unknown, although they are assumed to be partly spontaneous and partly the effect of environmental agents such as mutagenic chemicals or ionizing radiation acting on the germ line, zygote, or early embryo (Fig. 60-5). The majority of de novo rearrangements are paternal in origin.

Many of the known chromosome rearrangements have been detected only once or a few times. Others are detected repeatedly, the same one occurring in unrelated individuals and families. For example, the commonest translocation, one that can occur either as a result of de novo mutation or by inheritance, affects one chromosome 13 and one 14 at or near their centromeres. In this translocation, only inert chromatin is lost from the tiny short arms. Also common is a similar translocation affecting chromosomes 14 and 21.

Chromosome complements bearing rearrangements can be genetically balanced or effectively so, thus imparting no unfavorable phenotypic effect to their bearers; about two-thirds of rearrangements detected during surveys of consecutive live-born babies are balanced. Or, the complement can be unbalanced and affect development adversely, the usual case when rearrangements are detected during surveys of spontaneous abortuses or of individuals with multiple anomalies and mental deficiency.

Some balanced rearrangements are transmitted from generation to generation without producing clinical effects. In other cases, however, they are profoundly important to members of the kindred transmitting them, by being responsible for the conception of embryos with unbalanced genomes. For example, bearers of some 13;14 translocations (mentioned above) are at risk of having children with the trisomy 13 syndrome, and inherited translocations involving chromosome 21 predispose to the trisomy 21 syndrome. Approximately 5 percent of live-borns with the trisomy 21 syndrome have a translocation, and in about a fifth of those it is detectable in one of the parents. Because most babies with the trisomy 21 syndrome due to translocation are born to women under 30, a search for a translocation is important when a child with this clinical syndrome is born to young parents.

Different translocations bestow on their carriers different risks of having offspring with unbalanced rearrangements. These risks cannot be predicted on the theoretical basis of the way the translocation might be expected to behave during meiosis. Useful empiric risk figures have been accumulated for common translocations; e.g., the 14;21 translocation bestows a 2 percent risk on a balanced male carrier and more than a 10 percent risk on a female carrier of having a child with the trisomy 21 syndrome. In contrast, the balanced carrier of a 21;21 translocation can expect only unbalanced offspring. Information of this type is indispensable to those undertaking genetic counseling in relation to chromosome disorders.

DISEASE ASSOCIATIONS Various combinations of abnormalities in malformed and defective individuals have been correlated with variations in the chromosome complement. In this way, clinical syndromes due to specific chromosome imbalances have been defined. (Many of the pediatric conditions are of little significance in adult medicine because of their lethality in infancy or early childhood.)

Autosome imbalance Of the three autosomal trisomies found in live-born babies, only trisomy 21 is compatible with survival past infancy. The phenotype produced by the presence of an extra chromosome 21, formerly known as *mongolism* but now termed the *Down syndrome* or *trisomy 21 syndrome,* is characteristic and easily diagnosed from birth: mental deficiency, short stature, muscular hypotonia, brachycephaly, short neck, typical facies (oblique orbital fissures, flat nasal bridge, small simple or folded ears, nystagmus, mouth hanging open), narrow palate, short broad hands with incurving fifth fingers, gaps between the first and second toes, and characteristic dermatoglyphics. Additional findings may include congenital heart disease, blepharitis, and conjunctivitis, Brushfield's spots of the iris, straight pubic hair, abnormal teeth, a protruding furrowed tongue, a high-arched palate, loose skin of the neck, transverse palmar creases, and hyperflexibility of the joints. Cardiac malformations lead to death in infancy in a third of individuals with trisomy 21, and other malformations and infections may also cause early death. However, subjects who survive infancy often reach adulthood, and some even old age. The proneness to develop leukemia in affected infants is not maintained in later life. Females occasionally become pregnant, and, as expected, approximately half their children have trisomy 21.

Mosaicism of trisomy 21 with normal cells (46/47,+21) may occur in individuals with modified features of the trisomy 21 syndrome, and it is probable that many individuals with this mosaicism go undiagnosed. The risk of such persons having trisomic children is increased, but unfortunately their mosaicism is usually detected only after they have had an affected child. Partial trisomy, partial monosomy, or a combination of the two explains many of the instances in both children and adults of multiple developmental defects combined with mental deficiency. Sometimes a balanced autosomal translocation is detected in normally developed adults who have repeated spontaneous abortion or subnormal fertility, with or without abnormal liveborn children.

Although the phenotypic effects of many of the different segmental chromosome imbalances which can occur are varied and nonspecific, the resulting anomalies sometimes compose recognizable clinical syndromes. Two examples are the following: (1) If a rearrangement causes partial trisomy of just the distal band of the long arm of 21, the clinical features composing the full syndrome associated with an extra chromosome 21 develop. (A triple dose of other segments of the long arm of chromosome 21 also produces adverse effects but not the trisomy 21 syndrome.) (2) Partial monosomy of a short segment within the short arm of chromosome 5 causes mental deficiency, a characteristic facies, and a characteristic cry during infancy. This group of signs is known as the *5p −* (five-p-minus) or *cri-du-chat syndrome.*

Because of the large number of karyotype-phenotype correlations made in recent years, additional specific syndromes produced by imbalance of many different segments now are known (Table 60-1), e.g., the 4p −,9p partial trisomy, 13q −, and 18q − syndromes, to name a few. Rearrangements not previously described and their corresponding clinical syndromes are still being recognized. Any of these syndromes may appear as a result either of de novo chromosome rearrangement or through formation of a genetically unbalanced gamete in a person carrying in balanced state a rearrangement affecting the segment involved.

In most individuals with chromosome imbalance, regardless of which segments are affected, a degree of phenotypic similarity is present. These recurring and nonspecific features include mental deficiency, growth deficiency, dysmorphic ears, nose, and mouth, cardiac malformations of standard types, abnormalities of dermal ridges and creases, and dysmorphic digits. (As a rule, autosomal imbalance need not be considered in the etiology of anatomic defects unaccompanied by mental deficiency.) Why similar abnormalities occur with so many different segmental imbalances is unknown, but when several such features are observed in a single individual, they can be a valuable clinical indication for cytogenetic analysis. Imbalance affecting certain segments also causes specific phenotypic changes; an example is the anomalous cry in the 5p − syndrome mentioned above. Other examples of specificity are retinoblastoma, which may develop when one particular band of chromosome 13 is present in single dose, and the Prader-Willi syndrome, which is often associated with a disturbance of a band near the centromere of chromosome 15. Whereas the nonspecific changes serve to call the clinician's attention to the possibility of some chromosome imbalance, the specific features can suggest the exact segment of the genome affected.

Sex chromosome imbalance (see also Chap. 333) In contrast to autosome imbalance, sex chromosome imbalance has relatively mild phenotypic effects. This is because X chromosomes beyond one in the complement of somatic cells are usually almost totally inactivated and because the Y chromosome bears few genes other than the testis determinants. X-linked loci (in contrast to autosomal loci) function normally in single dose: the male is hemizygous for X-linked genes, having only one X chromosome (with the possible exception of a few loci on the Y that may be homologous to a segment on the X); the female is functionally hemizygous through the Lyon effect. The addition of an extra sex chromosome to the normal male or female complement has a phenotypic effect but insufficient to interfere with intrauterine survival. Since major anatomic defects are usually absent,

individuals with the complements 47,XXY and 47,XYY, both of whom are males, and 47,XXX, who are females, ordinarily go unrecognized till adolescence or later, often never to be diagnosed at all.

The *Klinefelter syndrome* (Chap. 333), which in classic form consists of small testes, infertility, gynecomastia, and variable degrees of underandrogenization, sometimes with mild mental deficiency, antisocial behavior, or both, is the consequence of the addition of an extra X to the male complement: 47,XXY. The extra X interferes in some way with the survival of germ cells, and atrophy of the spermatogenic tubules and azoospermia are the consequence. Sometimes the phenotypic effects are surprisingly mild, the testicular atrophy being the only noteworthy feature in otherwise healthy and socially well-adjusted men. The mosaicism 46,XY/47,XXY sometimes occurs and may ameliorate the phenotypic effect of the extra X. More extreme phenotypic effects and mental deficiency result when more than one extra sex chromosome is added to the normal male complement: 48,XXXY or 49,XXXXY.

The phenotypic effect of 47,XYY is less well defined; although increased height, behavioral difficulties, and infertility are common, the extra Y is sometimes found in otherwise normal men. The rare complement 48,XXYY results in infertility, probably because of the extra X, as in the 47,XXY Klinefelter's syndrome. The phenotype associated with 47,XXX is also poorly defined, but women with mild mental deficiency, psychosis, and menstrual abnormalities are increased in frequency; this complement is sometimes detected in normal, healthy women. Further clarification is needed concerning the effects on personality and behavior of all three of the complements 47,XXY, 47,XYY, and 47,XXX.

Loss of the Y or of the second X has drastic effects on development. If it does not cause abortion, it may or may not be recognizable at birth. Loose nuchal skin folds and edema of the hands and feet in a newborn girl, with or without renal or cardiovascular anomalies, may point to the diagnosis of the 45,X complement. The *Turner syndrome* (gonadal dysgenesis) is the manifestation in subsequent life (Chap. 333): short stature resistant to all treatment, infantilism of otherwise normal female external and internal genitalia, germ-cell-free gonads referred to as gonadal streaks, and variable renal, cardiovascular, skeletal, and ectodermal anomalies. Without estrogen administration breast development remains infantile and menstruation does not occur. Although mental deficiency is not a feature, a poorly defined emotional immaturity is common.

The Turner syndrome may be the developmental consequence of several chromosome constitutions besides 45,X. Mosaicism as well as structural abnormalities of a second sex chromosome, either a Y or an X, cause a spectrum of disorders at both the clinical and cytogenetic levels. A normal male or normal female cellular component may be present along with the 45,X cellular component, or one component may bear a structurally abnormal chromosome. Common abnormalities of the Y and X are isochromosome formation (one arm deleted and the other duplicated) or deletion of part or all of one arm. In some affected individuals, all cells have 46 chromosomes, with one normal X plus an abnormal Y or X, for example, 46,XXp −, deletion of a segment of the short arm of one of the X chromosomes. In others, a second or third cellular component may be present as well, for example, 45,X/46,XX/46,XXp −. Clinically pure Turner syndrome may be found in association with various combinations of these karyotypes if one of them is either monosomic or partially monosomic for X. However, when Y-bearing cells coexist with the 45,X cells, for example, 45,X/46,XY, genital ambiguity often develops, and gonads may vary from streaks to functional testes (the syndrome of *mixed gonadal dysgenesis*); here the risk of malignant gonadal neoplasia is significant. When 46,XX cells coexist with 45,X, varying degrees of ovarian function may be maintained, including ovulation. Although the phenotype may approach a normal male or female pattern when normal and abnormal cells coexist, the effects of mosaicism are unpredictable. Thus, the clinical syndrome associated with monosomy X and structurally abnormal Ys or Xs ranges from a predominantly male phenotype through Turner syndrome to an almost normal female phenotype.

Two other rare conditions deserve mention—*true hermaphroditism* and the *46,XX male* (see also Chap. 333): true hermaphroditism is present when both testicular and ova- and follicle-containing ovarian tissue exist in the same individual. In most cases 46,XX is the chromosome complement, and it appears normal by banding. Exceptionally, true hermaphrodites have the complement 46,XY; rarely is the chimerism 46,XY/46,XX found, each of the two cellular components having been derived from a different zygote. Second, males occasionally have the complement 46,XX. As in 47,XXY men, the second X interferes with meiosis, and azoospermia results. In both the 46,XX true hermaphrodite and the 46,XX male, the rule that a Y is required for testicular differentiation appears to break down. However, the two conditions may have the same etiologic basis; the most plausible explanation is occult translocation of the testis-determining segment of the Y to another chromosome.

X-linked mental deficiency In the general population more males than females are mentally deficient, and mental deficiency when familial affects males preferentially. In some such kindreds, severe mental deficiency segregates as an X-linked trait.

Although chromosome imbalance is not responsible, one cause, as mentioned above, can be diagnosed by cytogenetic techniques. In a significant proportion of families in which mental deficiency is segregating, the X in the affected males and that same X in their mothers is, or can be made, recognizable cytogenetically by technical manipulations. Near the end of its long arm (Xq) this phenotypically unusual X chromosome, in a variable but usually small proportion of metaphases from affected persons, exhibits an attenuated, and therefore faintly staining, segment. Because this segment usually can be seen to have broken in some of the metaphases, it is sometimes referred to as a fragile site, and the condition the *fragile-X syndrome*. (The "fragile X" is not demonstrable in all families with X-linked mental deficiency.)

Chromosome change in cancer The theory that an alteration in the chromosomal complement may be the cause of cancer was advanced almost seven decades ago, but the matter is still unsettled. Chromosome changes are plentiful in cancer, but this very fact—too many changes—has been a major reason many have rejected them as of etiologic significance. However, support for the idea that chromosome alteration is significant in the etiology of human cancer has come from two observations: (1) the known environmental "causes" of human cancer (carcinogenic chemicals and ionizing radiation) are also chromosome-breaking agents (Fig. 60-5); and (2) three recessively inherited disorders result in increased chromosome breakage and rearrangement in cells in culture, and in each the risk of cancer is increased—Bloom's syndrome, Fanconi's anemia, and ataxia-telangiectasia. Thus, the known environmental and the known genetic causes of increased chromosome mutation all predispose to cancer.

Most human cancers have altered chromosome complements. Table 60-2 lists some of those found with regularity. In the leukemias, lymphomas, and certain myeloproliferative disorders, the alterations are less extensive than in solid tumors and, therefore, easier to define. In certain lymphomas, chromosome 14 is often found to have undergone structural rearrangement, with the breakpoint at one specific segment. In over 95 percent of chronic granulocytic leukemias, a translocation affecting chromosome 22 (usually chromosome 9 is the other chromosome affected) is detected, the so-called Ph¹ chromosome and a no. 22 lacking much of its long arm can be demonstrated in most cases; if the disease progresses into a "blastic" phase, the karyotype often evolves, certain additional chromosome changes being added stepwise in a nonrandom sequence. In this and certain other leukemias, the various chromosome changes have diagnostic value, as well as a limited value in prognosis and choice of therapy.

Solid tumors, which generally are studied later in their course than conditions affecting the bone marrow, show extensive karyotypic changes, both structural and numerical. Different cells from a single tumor have similar numerical changes and structural rearrangements, but in the same type tumor from another person the changes usually seen are different. This apparent lack of specificity is partly due to the complexity of the changes, however, and a few examples of chromosome alterations specific for a solid tumor are known; for example, meningiomas are associated with a deletion of chromosome 22 in almost every case. The cytogenetic findings in both solid tumors and leukemias demonstrate the clonal nature of human cancer.

TECHNICAL CONSIDERATIONS Human metaphase chromosomes can be examined in any tissue in which sufficient cells are cycling. Preparations can therefore be made directly from almost any embryonic tissue and from adult bone marrow, lymphoid tissue, and selected malignant tissues. In searches for mosaicism, the study of multiple tissues is often required. Some tissues unlikely to yield cells in metaphase can be placed in culture, and chromosome preparations can be made from cells that reach mitosis in vitro. Blood T lymphocytes stimulated to enter cell-division cycles by phytohemagglutinin are the standard material for diagnosing constitutional chromosome imbalance. In some myeloproliferative disorders and leukemias, unstimulated circulating blood cells divide spontaneously after a few hours in culture. Long-term cultures of fibroblasts can be derived from minute skin biopsies or from fragments of many other types of tissue, although more elaborate laboratory facilities and a longer period of time are required before cytogenetic preparations can be made. Amniotic fluid is among the sources of cells suitable for culture, and the cells, which are fetal in origin, are widely used in the prenatal diagnosis of chromosome imbalance, particularly in pregnancy in women of advanced age or who already have borne a child with a chromosome imbalance. Metaphase preparations also can be made from chorionic villi biopsied in the first trimester of pregnancy.

Nucleated cells in interphase can be used for the study of sex chromatin. Cells from buccal mucosa and hair follicles are perhaps the most readily obtained, but surgical and autopsy specimens or cells in culture are at times useful also. X chromatin (formerly called the Barr body), a condensed body apposed to the nuclear membrane

TABLE 60-2 Some of the recurring chromosome abnormalities encountered in human neoplasms

Neoplasm	Aberration	Chromosome regions affected
Leukemia:		
Chronic granulocytic	Translocation	9q34 and 22q11
Acute nonlymphocytic:		
M1	Translocation	9q34 and 22q11
M2	Translocation	8q22 and 21q22
Me	Translocation	15q22 and 17q11
Chronic lymphocytic	Trisomy	12
Acute lymphocytic		
L1–L2	Translocation	9q34 and 12q11
L2	Translocation	4q21 and 11q23
L3	Translocation	8q24 and 14q32
Lymphoma:		
Burkitt's	Translocation	8q24 and 14q32
Follicular	Translocation	14q32 and 18q21
Solid tumors:		
Benign:		
Meningioma	Deletion or monosomy	22
Parotid, mixed	Translocation	3p25 and 8q21
Malignant:		
Lung, small cell	Deletion	Bands 3p14 to 3p23
Neuroblastoma	Deletion	Bands 1p31 to 3p36
Ovary, cystadenocarcinoma	Translocation	6q21 and 14q24
Retinoblastoma	Deletion	Band 13q14
Wilms's tumor	Deletion	Band 11p13

NOTE: *The FAB (French-American-British) classification of leukemias is employed above. The chromosome breakpoint and band nomenclature is that of the Paris Conference* (Birth Defects: Original Articles Series VIII (7):1–46, 1971). *The chromosome and chromosome-arm designation (e.g., 9q means the long arm of chromosome no. 9) appears first and is followed by the chromosome region and band on that arm (e.g., 9q34 means the fourth band in the third region of the long arm of chromosome no. 9).*

and present in normal female cells, is composed of the chromatin of one X chromosome. The X responsible for X chromatin in any particular cell is the one genetically inactivated and late-replicating. Therefore, the number of X-chromatin masses is an indication of the number of X chromosomes in excess of 1. Y chromatin, a predominantly genetically inactive segment of the Y chromosome demonstrated by quinacrine staining and fluorescence microscopy, is present in interphase nuclei of Y-bearing cells (for example, 48,XXYY cells contain one X-chromatin and two Y-chromatin masses).

Meiotic chromosome preparations from testicular biopsies are sometimes useful in obscure cases of infertility. Here translocations and genetically determined disturbances in meiotic pairing may be identified.

Recombinant DNA technology has been employed in conjunction with conventional cytogenetic techniques to define chromosome abnormalities in finer detail. As probes for specific loci or chromosome segments have become available, it has been possible to identify segments of chromosomes involved in rearrangements in which banding techniques had lacked the required resolution. In prenatal diagnosis, probes for RFLPs (mentioned earlier) sometimes are used to identify which chromosome has been inherited by the fetus. This can be useful in pregnancies at risk of X-linked disease, determining in male fetuses whether the single X chromosome is the one that bears a particular undesirable locus that one of the parents is known to carry, such as that for Duchenne's muscular dystrophy or hemophilia. Recombinant technology also can be useful in conditions that follow a dominant pattern of inheritance, such as Huntington's chorea, determining whether the undesired mutant gene is present in the complement of the fetus by determining whether an RFLP closely linked to the mutant gene is or is not present. In a few instances, probes for undesirable mutant genes themselves are available. Probes specific for the Y chromosome can define the sex of an embryo or fetus if a few cells can be obtained, for example by chorionic villus biopsy or amniocentesis. They also can be of diagnostic value in obscure cases of intersex in which a Y chromosome, or a segment of the Y, is being sought.

Sometimes, metaphase chromosomes are analyzed to determine whether damage to the genetic material has been induced by some environmental agent (radiation, chemical, virus). Cells that have proliferated in vivo may be used in search of evidence of damage to the genetic material of a given person or of a population. Alternatively, cultured cells can be treated with the agent in question to determine whether the agent is clastogenic (capable of breaking chromosomes) or whether it promotes chromatid exchange and rearrangement. A test system less laborious than metaphase-chromosome analysis, but one capable of showing that chromosome breakage has occurred either in vivo or in vitro, is the determination of the proportion of nondividing cells having micronuclei. A micronucleus is produced when a chromosome fragment lacking a centromere lags at anaphase (as it will be obliged to do) and is encompassed in a separate nuclear at telophase. The micronucleus assay is useful in the survey of populations for clastogen exposure, which is equivalent to mutagen and carcinogen exposure.

REFERENCES

Berg K et al (eds): *Cytogenetics and Cell Genetics*, vol 32: *Human Gene Mapping 6 (1981). Sixth International Workshop.* Basel, Karger, 1982

De Grouchy J, Turleau C: *Clinical Atlas of Human Chromosomes*, 2d ed. New York, Wiley, 1984

German JL: Studying human chromosomes today. Am Sci 58:182, 1970

McKusick VA: The human gene map. Clin Genet 27:207, 1985

Schwarzacher HG: *Methods in Human Cytogenetics.* New York, Springer-Verlag, 1974

Simpson JL: *Disorders of Sexual Differentiation.* New York, Academic, 1976

61   PREVENTION AND TREATMENT OF GENETIC DISORDERS

JOSEPH L. GOLDSTEIN / MICHAEL S. BROWN

APPROACHES TO PREVENTION

The trend for couples to have smaller families has heightened the concern that children should be healthy and free of genetic diseases. Thus, primary-care physicians are called upon to play a more active role in the prevention and treatment of hereditary diseases. In most situations, genetic advice can be given by the primary physician once the relatively simple principles of medical genetics (Chap. 57) and genetic counseling (discussed below) have been mastered.

RETROSPECTIVE GENETIC COUNSELING The prevention of genetic diseases requires the identification of matings that are capable of producing defective genotypes. These may involve matings in which one of the two individuals carries a dominant or X-linked gene mutation or a balanced translocation, or matings in which both individuals are carriers of a deleterious recessive gene at the same locus. Such individuals are usually identified through an affected child or near relative, in which case retrospective genetic counseling can be provided.

When advising family members about the risk of transmitting a disorder that has already affected someone in the family, the counselor's first step is to be certain of the *correct diagnosis*—in particular, to make certain that the problem in question is really of genetic origin. This is especially important in disorders that may have either a genetic or a nongenetic etiology, such as deafness or mental retardation. Second, if the disease has a hereditary element, the possibility of *genetic heterogeneity*, i.e., a situation in which clinically similar genetic disorders show varying patterns of inheritance, must be considered. For example, there are two types of hereditary methemoglobinemia that resemble each other quite closely, but one shows autosomal recessive and the other autosomal dominant inheritance.

To estimate the *recurrence risk*, one must initially determine what is known of the genetic mechanisms controlling the relevant disorder. When more than one genetic mechanism exists, or when environmental factors can cause clinically indistinguishable traits, the *relative probabilities* of the different mechanisms operating in the particular family are computed. For conditions determined by simple mendelian inheritance, there is no difficulty in predicting the probability of an offspring being affected, provided that the genotypes of the parents can be recognized. Identification of the parental genotype is easiest for autosomal recessive and X-linked disorders since the basic lesions in these two forms of mendelian inheritance frequently involve simple enzyme deficiencies for which biochemical tests are now available.

For autosomal dominant disorders, identification of the parental genotype is more difficult since the basic defect is known for only a few of these disorders, and the diagnosis of the heterozygote for a dominant disorder depends almost exclusively on the clinical evaluation and a careful pedigree analysis. In counseling a family in which one relative is affected with a dominant disorder, it is important that appropriate clinical examination of all first-degree relatives and selected distant relatives be carried out. If relatives appear unaffected, the clinical symptoms may be masked by *delayed age of onset* and *variability in expression*, or the possibility of a new dominant mutation must be entertained. Table 61-1 lists the most commonly encountered dominant disorders affecting adults and the methods available for detection of the heterozygote.

When advising families about multifactorial genetic diseases, such as diabetes mellitus, in which the inheritance pattern is not clear-cut, the physician must resort to empiric risk estimates that have been derived from retrospectively assembled data (Table 57-5).

TABLE 61-1 Methods for detection of asymptomatic heterozygotes in frequently encountered dominantly inherited disorders

Disorder	Method of heterozygote detection		Therapeutic advantage of early diagnosis
	Physical findings	Laboratory tests	
GASTROINTESTINAL, LIVER, AND PANCREAS			
Gilbert's disease		Serum bilirubin	Avoid confusion with more serious forms of liver disease
Peutz-Jeghers syndrome	Melanin spots on lips, buccal mucosa, and digits	X-ray of small intestine	Clarify cause of gastrointestinal bleeding
Familial polyposis		X-ray of colon; colonoscopy	Prevent colon carcinoma
Gardner's syndrome	Multiple sebaceous cysts; lipomas; fibromas; osteomas; dental abnormalities; desmoid tumors	X-ray of colon and small intestine; colonoscopy	Prevent colon carcinoma
METABOLIC AND ENDOCRINE			
Medullary thyroid carcinoma-pheochromocytoma syndrome		Serum calcitonin; measurement of blood pressure	Prevent thyroid carcinoma and complications of hypertension
Multiple endocrine adenomatosis	Multiple lipomas	Serum calcium, gastrin, blood sugar; x-rays of sella turcica, stomach, and small intestine	Prevent complication of hyperparathyroidism, hypoglycemia, peptic ulcer, metastatic cancer
Familial hyperparathyroidism		Serum calcium, parathyroid hormone	Prevent renal damage and other complications of hypercalcemia
Familial hypercholesterolemia	Tendon xanthomas, xanthelasma, arcus corneae	Serum cholesterol; low-density lipoprotein receptor activity of cultured fibroblasts	Prevent premature coronary heart disease
HEART AND VASCULAR			
Holt-Oram syndrome	Abnormality of thumb and carpals; murmur of atrial septal defect	X-ray of hands; cardiac evaluation	Prevent complications of atrial septal defect
Noonan's syndrome	Hypertelorism; small chin; low-set ears; ptosis; pectus deformity; cryptorchidism; murmur of pulmonic stenosis	Cardiac evaluation; x-ray of skeleton; intravenous pyelogram (renal anomalies)	Prevent heart failure
Idiopathic hypertropic subaortic stenosis (asymmetric septal hypertrophy)	Presystolic gallop; characteristic carotid arterial pulse	ECG; echocardiogram	Prevent sudden death, syncope, angina, heart failure
Dominantly inherited form of atrial septal defect	Heart murmur	ECG showing first-degree heart block, right bundle branch block, right axis deviation	Prevent complications of atrial septal defect
HEMATOLOGIC			
Hereditary spherocytosis	Splenomegaly; jaundice	Blood smear; reticulocyte count; hemoglobin; osmotic fragility test	Prevent anemia, cholelithiasis
Hereditary hemorrhagic telangiectasia	Telangiectasia of tongue, lips, conjunctiva, ears, fingers; pulmonary AV fistula	X-ray of lungs	Clarify cause of nosebleeds and gastrointestinal bleeding
Von Willebrand's disease		Immunologic and functional assays of plasma antihemophilic globulin levels; bleeding time	Prevent gastrointestinal and urinary bleeding
CONNECTIVE TISSUE AND BONE			
Ehler-Danlos syndromes (types I, II, III)	Loose-jointedness; fragile, stretchable, bruisable skin; subcutaneous calcified spherules		
Marfan's syndrome	Ectopic lens; mitral and aortic murmurs; excessive length of extremities	Slit-lamp examination; metacarpal index by x-ray	Reduce risk of aortic dissection; prevent blindness
Osteogenesis imperfecta	Multiple fractures; loose-jointedness; blue scleras; deafness; aortic regurgitation	X-ray of bones	
RENAL			
Alport's syndrome	Nerve deafness; cataracts, lenticonus, spherophakia	Urinalysis, slit-lamp examination	Prevent uremia
Nail-patella syndrome	Dysplastic nails; absent patellas	X-ray of pelvis (iliac horns); urinalysis	Clarify cause of hematuria and azotemia
Polycystic kidney disease		Urinalysis; intravenous pyelogram; renal arteriogram; measurement of blood pressure	Prevent uremia and complications of hypertension
Renal tubular acidosis		X-ray of kidneys (nephrocalcinosis); urine pH, calcium; serum electrolytes, calcium	Prevent acidosis, osteoporosis, kidney stones

Disorder	Method of heterozygote detection		Therapeutic advantage of early diagnosis
	Physical findings	Laboratory tests	
RESPIRATORY			
Hereditary angioneurotic edema		Serum level of Cl esterase inhibitor of complement	Reduce risk of sudden death caused by laryngeal edema and clarify cause of acute abdominal pain
DERMATOLOGIC			
Neurofibromatosis	Café au lait spots; neurofibromas; scoliosis		Prevent malignant degeneration of neurofibromas
Waardenburg syndrome	Wide bridge of nose; frontal white blaze of hair; heterochromia iridis; white eyelashes; deafness		Clarify cause of deafness
Basal-cell nevus syndrome	Multiple basal-cell carcinomas; jaw cysts; pits on palms and soles; skeletal defects (ribs, spina bifida, scoliosis)	X-rays of skull (calcification of falx cerebri) and skeleton	Removal of cutaneous cancers; provide cosmetic surgery
NEUROLOGIC			
Charcot-Marie-Tooth disease	Pes cavus; atrophy of anterior tibial and calf muscles ("stork legs"); absence of deep tendon reflexes	Biopsy of muscle and of sural cutaneous nerve	Improve walking by corrective shoes and orthopedic measures
Myotonic dystrophy	Myotonia; muscle wasting of temporal and sternocleidomastoid muscles; cataracts; frontal baldness; signs of hypogonadism	Slit-lamp examination; electromyography; measurement of serum immunoglobulins; electrocardiogram	Anticipate complete heart block
Acute intermittent porphyria		Measurement of uroporphyrinogen synthetase activity in red blood cells	Reduce risk of neuropathic attacks by avoidance of aggravating drugs such as barbiturates
Tuberous sclerosis	Adenoma sebaceium; cutaneous white macules; shagreen patch; periungual fibromas		Prevent seizures
Huntington's chorea	Paranoia, other personality changes; choreic movements; dementia		
Periodic paralysis syndromes (hypo-, hyper-, and normokalemic types)	Cold-induced myotonia	Electromyogram; serum potassium	Reduce frequency of attacks by avoidance of aggravating agents such as high-carbohydrate diet and exposure to cold
PHARMACOGENETIC			
Malignant hyperthermia		Serum creatine phosphokinase	Prevent fatal episode of hyperthermia induced by general anesthesia

Once the parental genotypes are determined, the genetic prognosis is usually presented in terms of probability that a given couple will produce an affected offspring. The physician must make certain that the couple understands not only the meaning of such risk figures, but also the severity of the disease and the variability in clinical expression. In other words, in dealing with a disorder such as neurofibromatosis, it is important for the parents to realize not only that they have a 50 percent risk of producing a child with this disorder but also that a certain proportion of patients with the disorder have severe disease, a certain proportion have mild disease, etc. They should also have an understanding of the potential impact of the disease on their family; a disease that is lethal at birth might be classified as more "severe" than one that is lethal at age 16, but the latter is likely to have a more profound impact on the family.

Although different families react in different ways to the same risk, most couples who seek genetic advice take a responsible course of action that is based on the information quoted. Generally, the physician should avoid giving direct advice as to whether a couple "should" or "should not" have children. For serious genetic disease, with a recurrence risk equal to or greater than 1 in 10, most parents are deterred from planning further children. When the risk is less than 1 in 10, most parents continue with additional pregnancies.

PROSPECTIVE GENETIC COUNSELING In contrast to retrospective genetic counseling in which advice is given after the birth of at least one affected family member, in prospective genetic counseling advice is provided to possible carriers of recessive genes before an affected individual is born. As a first step, this requires the identification of heterozygous individuals by a population-screening procedure. Second, unmarried heterozygotes are instructed about the risk of their having affected children if they marry another heterozygote for the same gene. Finally, if two heterozygotes are already married, there is the possibility of interrupting the birth of affected infants if the disease can be diagnosed in utero by amniocentesis.

Population screening for heterozygote detection is possible for several autosomal recessive disorders (such as sickle cell anemia, thalassemia major, and Tay-Sachs disease) that occur in certain populations with high frequency. For example, 8 percent of the American black population carries the sickling gene, and 4 percent of Ashkenazi Jews are carriers of the Tay-Sachs gene.

Screening programs raise many ethical and social problems. Informing a healthy person that he or she is carrying a specific mutant gene that may cause disease in the children if a certain type of mate is chosen differs from counseling parents who have already had an affected child. Little is known about the social and psychologic effects as well as occupational discrimination that may result from discovering that a person carries a "bad" gene.

PRENATAL DIAGNOSIS The use of transabdominal amniocentesis permits diagnosis of certain genetic diseases at a stage early enough

TABLE 61-2 Inborn errors of metabolism for which prenatal diagnosis is feasible (partial list)

DISORDERS OF CARBOHYDRATE METABOLISM

Glycogen storage diseases—Types II, III, and IV
Galactosemia
Galactokinase deficiency
Pyruvate decarboxylase deficiency

DISORDERS OF AMINO ACID METABOLISM

Argininosuccinicaciduria
Citrullinemia
Homocystinuria
Maple syrup urine disease
Methylmalonic aciduria
Isovaleric acidemia
Ketotic hyperglycinemia

DISORDERS OF LIPOPROTEIN AND LIPID METABOLISM

Homozygous familial hypercholesterolemia (receptor-negative type)
Refsum's syndrome

DISORDERS OF LYSOSOMAL ENZYMES

Mucopolysaccharidosis, type I (Hurler's syndrome)
Mucopolysaccharidosis, type II (Hunter's syndrome)
Mucopolysaccharidosis, type III (Sanfillipo's syndrome, types A and B)
Mucopolysaccharidosis, type VI (Maroteaux-Lamy syndrome)
Mucopolysaccharidosis, type VII (β-glucuronidase deficiency)
I-cell disease
Lysosomal acid phosphatase deficiency
Wolman's syndrome and cholesteryl ester storage disease
Fabry's disease
Gaucher's disease
Krabbe's disease (globoid cell leukodystrophy)
Metachromatic leukodystrophy
Niemann-Pick disease
Tay-Sachs disease
Sandhoff's disease
Generalized gangliosidosis
Juvenile gangliosidosis
Fucosidosis
Mannosidosis
Farber's disease (lipogranulomatosis)

DISORDERS OF STEROID METABOLISM

21-Hydroxylase deficiency—congenital adrenal hyperplasia
Steroid sulfatase deficiency (X-linked ichthyosis)

DISORDERS OF PURINE AND PYRIMIDINE METABOLISM

Lesch-Nyhan syndrome
Hereditary orotic aciduria
Xeroderma pigmentosum
Adenosine deaminase deficiency (combined immunodeficiency)

DISORDERS OF METAL METABOLISM

Menkes' syndrome

DISORDERS OF PORPHYRIN AND HEME METABOLISM

Acute intermittent poryphyria

DISORDERS INVOLVING CONNECTIVE TISSUE, MUSCLE, AND BONE

Hypophosphatasia (some types)

DISORDERS OF THE BLOOD AND BLOOD-FORMING TISSUES

Sickle cell anemia
α Thalassemias
β Thalassemias
Glucose 6-phosphate dehydrogenase deficiency

DISORDERS OF TRANSPORT

Cystinosis

centesis consists of the transabdominal aspiration of amniotic fluid from the uterus. The procedure is preferably performed between the fourteenth and sixteenth weeks of pregnancy. When performed by a trained gynecologist, the technique is safe for both mother and fetus.

Direct examination of the amniotic fluid itself may be diagnostic. For example, an elevated level of α-fetoprotein is a relatively good indicator of the presence of spina bifida or another neural tube abnormality. More frequently, prenatal diagnosis requires culture of the fetal cells in vitro, a process which usually takes 3 weeks. By this means the karyotype of the fetus can be determined to ascertain fetal sex and to detect chromosomal aberrations. Moreover, many inborn errors of metabolism can be detected by assays of specific enzyme activities or restriction length DNA polymorphisms (Chap. 58) in the cultured fetal cells. Table 61-2 lists those inborn errors for which prenatal diagnosis is currently feasible. More disorders are constantly being added to this list.

A promising new approach to prenatal diagnosis, called chorionic villus sampling, allows the identification of genetic abnormalities between the ninth and twelfth week of gestation. The technique involves passing a catheter through the cervix into the placenta and obtaining a sample of developing chorionic villi, which consists of trophoblastic and mesenchymal cells. A single aspiration typically yields 10 to 25 mg of wet tissue, which is sufficient for studies of chromosomes, enzyme activities, and DNA polymorphisms. Ongoing clinical trials suggest that this is a relatively safe procedure with a miscarriage rate of about 4 percent, a figure that does not exceed the rate in the general population.

Prenatal diagnosis is currently indicated in the following high-risk situations: (1) couples having a previous child with spina bifida or anencephaly, (2) couples having a previous child with a chromosomal aberration such as the trisomy 21 form of Down's syndrome, (3) couples in whom either the husband or wife carries a balanced translocation chromosome for Down's syndrome, (4) couples at high risk for having a child with a detectable inborn error of metabolism, and (5) pregnant women 35 years of age and older. Table 61-3 lists the major indications for prenatal diagnosis, the risks involved, and methods by which the abnormal fetus can be detected.

APPROACHES TO TREATMENT

The goal of treatment for genetic diseases is to modify the natural history of the genetic trait so that an affected person may live a

TABLE 61-3 Major indications for prenatal diagnosis

Clinical situation	Estimated risk to fetus, %	Method of detection of abnormal fetus
Couples having a previous child with spina bifida or anencephaly	5	Measurement of α-fetoprotein in amniotic fluid
Couples having a previous child with a chromosomal disorder such as the trisomy 21 form of Down's syndrome	2	Chromosomal analysis of cultured amniotic fluid cells
Couples in whom either the husband or wife carries a balanced translocation for Down's syndrome	5–20	Chromosomal analysis of cultured amniotic cells
Pregnant women 35 years of age and older whose risk of having a child with Down's syndrome is increased	1–2	Chromosomal analysis of cultured amniotic fluid cells
Couples at risk for having a child with a detectable inborn error of metabolism (see Table 61-2)	25 or 50	Biochemical analysis of cultured amniotic fluid cells

to terminate a pregnancy and to prevent the birth of a defective child. This procedure gives high-risk couples the opportunity to have unaffected children provided they are willing for the pregnancy to be terminated in the event that an abnormal fetus is detected. Amnio-

TABLE 61-4 Some treatable hereditary disorders affecting adults

Method of treatment	Disorder	Method of treatment	Disorder
DIETARY RESTRICTION OF SUBSTRATE		**AMPLIFICATION OF ENZYME ACTIVITY**	
Lactose	Lactase deficiency	Pyridoxine (vitamin B_6)	Homocystinuria
Galactose	Galactosemia and galactokinase deficiency	Vitamin B_{12}	Methylmalonic aciduria
Fructose	Fructose intolerance	Phenobarbital	Crigler-Najjar variant and other forms of unconjugated hyper-bilirubinemia
Neutral fats	Familial lipoprotein lipase deficiency		
Phytanic acid	Refsum's syndrome	**REPLACEMENT OF MUTANT PROTEIN**	
Phenylalanine	Phenylketonuria	Gamma globulin	Agammaglobulinemia
REPLACEMENT OF DEFICIENT END PRODUCT		Factor VIII (AHG)	Hemophilia
		Infusion of irradiated erythro-cytes containing adenosine de-aminase	Severe combined immunodeficiency disease
Vitamin D and phosphate	Hypophosphatemic rickets		
Cortisol	Adrenogenital syndromes	**ORGAN TRANSPLANTATION**	
Thyroxine	Familial goiters		
Uridine	Orotic aciduria	Kidney	Fabry's disease, cystinosis, Alport's syndrome, polycystic kidney disease (adult form)
DEPLETION OF STORAGE SUBSTANCE		Allogeneic bone marrow	Lymphopenic hypogamma-globulinemia (Swiss type), Wiscott-Aldrich syndrome, severe combined immunodeficiency disease
Sterol removal by bile-acid binding resins heterozygotes	Familial hypercholesterolemia and inhibitors of cholesterol synthesis		
Cystine removal by D-penicilla-mine	Cystinuria	Liver	Familial hypercholesterolemia (homozygotes)
Copper removal by D-penicilla-mine	Wilson's disease	**SURGERY**	
Iron removal by phlebotomy	Hemochromatosis	Splenectomy	Hereditary spherocytosis
Uric acid removal by uricosuric agents	Gout	Portacaval shunt	Glycogen storage disease (type I) and homozygous familial hypercholesterolemia
		Colectomy	Familial polyposis of the colon
		Thyroidectomy	Medullary thyroid carcinoma syndrome

comfortable and healthy life despite a mutant genotype. Such treatment can be achieved for a number of inherited diseases using a variety of approaches, including (1) the exclusion or restriction of toxic foods, (2) metabolic supplementation, (3) removal of toxic products, (4) surgery, and (5) organ transplantation. Table 61-4 lists examples of hereditary diseases affecting adults that can be successfully treated at the present time.

REFERENCES

EMERY AEH, RIMOIN DL: *Principles and Practice of Medical Genetics,* vols 1 and 2. Edinburgh, Churchill Livingstone, 1983

EPSTEIN CJ et al: Recent developments in the prenatal diagnosis of genetic diseases and birth defects. Ann Rev Genet 17:49, 1983

JACKSON, LG: First-trimester diagnosis of fetal genetic disorders. Hosp Pract 20(3):39, 1985

STANBURY JB et al: *The Metabolic Basis of Inherited Disease,* 5th ed. New York, McGraw-Hill, 1983

section 2 Clinical immunology

62 INTRODUCTION TO CLINICAL IMMUNOLOGY

BARTON F. HAYNES / ANTHONY S. FAUCI

Basic research in immunology has resulted in advances in many clinical areas, ranging from allergy and rheumatology to neurology and cardiology. Monoclonal antibody technology has revolutionized the study of cell surface antigens of effector and regulatory immune cells and provided monospecific reagents to essentially any target molecules. The isolation, cloning, and sequencing of genes for antigen receptors on B cells (immunoglobulins) and T cells (α and β chains of T-cell antigen receptor) and of products of the major histocompatibility locus (HLA antigens) have yielded the probes necessary to begin to understand immune effector function. These include diversification of the T- and B-cell antigen repertoire, induction of self-tolerance (self-antigen nonreactivity), and regulation of immune cell growth and differentiation. Molecular biology techniques have likewise provided genetic probes for study and production of large quantities of secreted molecules (products from lymphocytes, *lymphokines;* from monocytes, *monokines*) that regulate immune cell function. Finally, the discovery of the human T-cell lymphotropic virus (HTLV) family of retroviruses (see Chap. 293) that causes forms of leukemia (HTLV type I, adult T-cell leukemia) and immunodeficiency [HTLV III/LAV (lymphadenopathy-associated virus), acquired immunodeficiency syndrome (AIDS)] and analysis of the genetic mechanisms of HTLV alteration of normal T-cell growth has led to understanding of some aspects of normal and abnormal immune cell growth. This knowledge regarding control of immune cell growth and differentiation will lead to new and specific modes of therapy for diseases of disordered immunoregulation such as autoimmune diseases, immunodeficiency diseases, and malignant diseases of the immune system. The aim of this chapter is to provide the essentials of immunology with particular emphasis on those principles relevant to understanding at a basic level the protean clinical and laboratory manifestations of disordered immunity.

PHENOTYPE AND FUNCTION OF IMMUNE CELLS

The dual limbs of the immune system are the thymus-derived (T) lymphocyte and the bone marrow–derived or bursa-equivalent (B) lymphocyte, both of which derive from a common stem cell. Other cell types such as the monocyte-macrophage play major roles in the inductive, regulatory, and effector phases of the immune response. The principal effector and regulatory cells of the immune system are T, B, and large granular lymphocytes and monocyte-macrophages. Nonlymphoid cells such as neutrophils, eosinophils, and basophils play roles in the inflammatory response that results from certain immune-mediated reactions and as such must be considered in the scheme of immune cell function (Table 62-1). The proportion and distribution of immunocompetent cells in various tissues reflect cell traffic, homing patterns, and functional capabilities. Bone marrow contains pluripotent stem cells capable of giving rise to all hematopoietic cell types and is the major site of maturation of B cells, monocyte-macrophages, and granulocytes. T-cell precursors also arise from bone marrow stem cells but leave bone marrow while immature and home to thymus for completion of maturation. Mature T lymphocytes, B lymphocytes, and monocytes enter the circulation and home to peripheral lymphoid organs (lymph nodes, spleen) and the gut-associated lymphoid tissue (tonsil, Peyer's patches, and appendix) and await activation via interaction with foreign antigens. Mature myeloid effector cells (neutrophils, eosinophils, basophils) leave the bone marrow and circulate in peripheral blood as well as home to tissues to perform effector functions associated with the response to foreign antigens (Fig. 62-1).

T CELLS

T lymphocytes arise from bone marrow precursor cells that migrate to the thymus during fetal and early postnatal life. T lymphocytes differ from other immune effector cell types in that the pool of effector T cells is established in the thymus early in life and is maintained throughout life by antigen-driven expansion of long-lived T cells that reside primarily in peripheral lymph organs and recirculate in blood and lymph. Mature T lymphocytes contribute 70 to 80 percent of normal peripheral blood lymphocytes, 90 percent of thoracic duct lymphocytes, 30 to 40 percent of lymph node cells, and 20 to 30 percent of spleen lymphoid cells. In lymph nodes T cells occupy deep paracortical areas around B-cell germinal centers and in spleen are in periarteriolar areas of white pulp (see Chap. 55). T cells are the primary effectors of cell-mediated immunity with subsets of T cells maturing into cytotoxic cells capable of lysis of viral infected or foreign cells. T cells are also the primary regulator cells of T- and B-lymphocyte and monocyte function via the production of lymphokines and direct contact; in addition, T cells regulate erythroid cell maturation in bone marrow.

Human T cells express cell surface proteins that are markers of discrete stages of intrathymic T-cell maturation; many of these molecules mediate or augment specific T-cell functions (Table 62-1). The earliest identifiable cells of T lineage are prothymocytes located in the subcapsular cortical region of thymus (Fig. 62-2), many of which express the sheep-erythrocyte-binding protein, T11, and the pan-T-cell specific protein, 3A1-p40 (stage I). With further maturation, prothymocytes enter the inner thymic cortex, acquire the cortical thymocyte protein T6, and coexpress T-lineage molecules T4 and T8 (stage II). More than 90 percent of stage II thymocytes that arise in the inner cortex die intrathymically, with only a minority of thymocytes achieving phenotypic and functional maturity. Mature T cells located in small foci within the inner cortex and throughout the thymic medulla express the T-cell antigen receptor-associated T3 molecules (20,000 to 25,000 mol wt), p80 molecules thought to be

important in T-cell homing to peripheral lymphoid tissues, and high-density cell surface HLA-A, -B, and -C antigens (stage III). With maturity, T-cell expression of the T6 antigen ceases, and T-cell subset antigens T4 and T8 are reciprocally expressed. Mature T4⁺ cells induce B-cell differentiation, induce T8⁺ cytotoxic T-cell proliferation, produce various lymphokines, and regulate certain stages of erythropoiesis. A subset of T4⁺ cells may also function as cytotoxic effector cells, and recognize foreign antigen in the context of major histocompatibility complex (MHC) class II (Ia) antigens. T8⁺ cells function as suppressor T cells of B-cell antibody synthesis and as cytotoxic effector T cells that recognize foreign antigen associated with class I antigens (see Chap. 63).

TABLE 62-1 Characteristics of human immune and inflammatory effector cells

Cell type	Functional surface molecules	Cellular function mediated via surface molecules
T lymphocyte	T3/T-cell antigen receptor complex	Antigen recognition, T-cell activation.
	Sheep erythrocyte receptor (T11 antigen)	T-cell activation.
	T4 antigen	Marker of inducer-helper T cells, and a subset of cytotoxic T cells. T4 molecule facilitates antigen recognition by T4⁺ cells, and is a surface recognition molecule via which HTLV III/LAV (AIDS) virus infects this subset.
	T8 antigen	Marker of suppressor and cytotoxic T cells. T8 molecule facilitates T8⁺ cell recognition of antigen via class I MHC molecules.
	Interleukin 2 (IL-2) receptor	Present on activated T cells, binds IL-2.
B lymphocyte	Surface immunoglobulins (sIg)	Antigen recognition, cell activation.
	IgG Fc receptors	Bind immune complexes.
	C3 receptors	Bind immune complexes.
Large granular lymphocyte (LGL)	IgG Fc receptors	Bind immune complexes.
Monocyte-macrophage	IgG Fc receptors	Bind and phagocytose immune complexes.
	C3 receptors	Bind and phagocytose immune complexes.
	MHC class II (Ia) antigens	Antigen presentation to T and B cells.
	Chemotactic receptors	Cellular polarization and chemotaxis.
Neutrophil	IgG Fc receptors	Bind and phagocytose immune complexes.
	Chemotactic receptors	Cell polarization and chemotaxis.
	C3 receptors	Bind and phagocytose immune complexes.
Eosinophil	IgG Fc receptors	Bind immune complexes.
	C3 receptors	Bind immune complexes.
Basophil–mast cell	IgE Fc receptors C3 receptors	Release of granules containing mediators of immediate hypersensitivity after cross-linking of Fc-bound IgE with allergen (antigen).

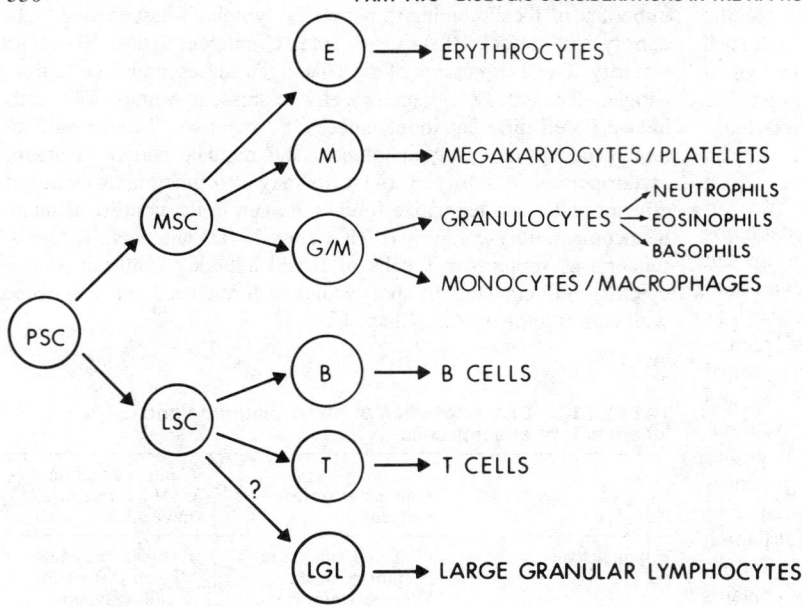

FIGURE 62-1 *Model of hematopoietic stem cell differentiation. Multipotential hematopoietic stem cells (HSC) may give rise to more restricted progenitor cells with self-renewal capacity. Thus, lymphocyte-committed stem cells (LSC) give rise to T and B cells. Another group of hematopoietic cells, for which the immediate progenitor is a more differentiated myeloid stem cell (MSC), includes erythrocytes, megakaryocytes, and platelets as well as the granulocyte, monocyte-macrophage series; the origin of large granular lymphocytes in this schema is hypothetical. (Adapted from MD Cooper et al, with permission.)*

T-cell maturation stages I, II, and III are clinically relevant in that T-cell malignancies can be grouped generally as being derived from one of these stages. T-cell acute lymphoblastic leukemia and lymphomas share phenotypic similarities with stages I or II T cells and thus are malignancies of immature T cells. Forms of cutaneous T-cell lymphoma (mycosis fungoides, Sézary syndrome) and the syndrome of adult T-cell leukemia (associated with HTLV I infection) share the phenotype of stage III T cells and therefore are malignancies of mature T cells.

The structural basis for the association of T-cell functional competence and surface expression of the T3 antigen results from the fact that two of the T3 proteins are bound to the T-cell antigen

FIGURE 62-2 *Model of human intrathymic T-cell maturation. Immature T cells in subcapsular cortex (stage I) and inner cortex (stage II) give rise to mature T cells in small foci in thymic inner cortex and medulla (stage III). Stage III thymocytes migrate to the periphery (peripheral blood, lymph nodes, spleen) and after challenge with antigen, expand into memory-T-effector-cell populations.*

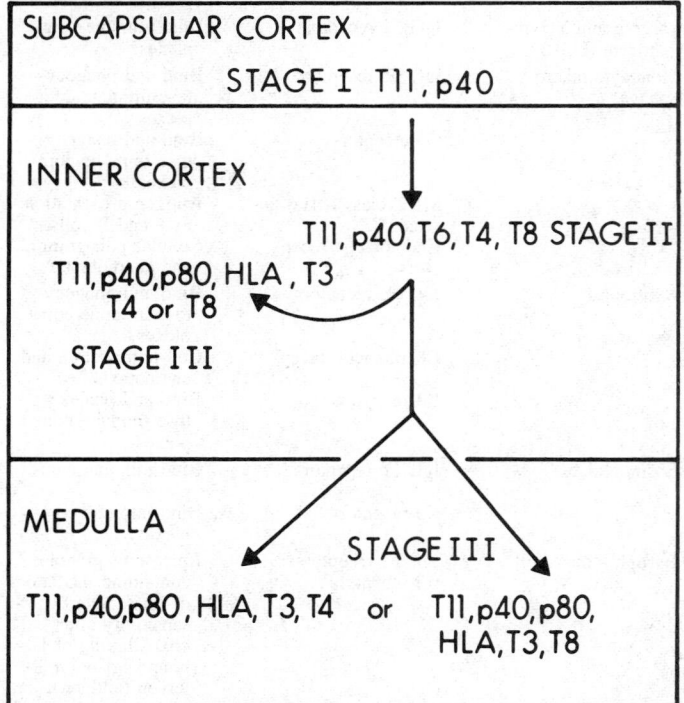

receptor. The T-cell antigen receptor, called Ti, is a 90,000-mol wt heterodimer composed of one 50,000-mol wt and one 43,000-mol wt B chain. The α and β T-cell antigen receptor molecules possess amino acid sequence homology and structural similarities to immunoglobulin heavy and light chains. The Ti β chain contains four separately encoded regions, namely the V (variable), D (diversity), J (joining), and C (constant) regions, and the Ti α chain consists of at least V, J, and C regions. Thus, the T-cell antigen receptor has constant and variable regions, and the gene for the α and β chains of the T-cell antigen receptor undergo gene rearrangement during T-cell maturation culminating in synthesis of the completed Ti molecule.

The epithelial component of the thymus is arranged in zones that correspond to those seen in Fig. 62-2 for thymocyte subsets. Thymic epithelial cells containing the thymic hormones thymopoietin, thymulin, and thymosin α_1 are located primarily in the subcapsular cortical and medullary thymic zones. Thymic hormones are thought to play important roles in supporting early stages of T-cell maturation. The specificity of mature T cells is largely determined within the thymus. For example, elimination of T cells capable of reacting against autologous (self) antigens may occur intrathymically, thus preventing autoimmune reactivity. Positive selection likely occurs intrathymically as well. T cells recognize foreign antigens in association with cell surface molecules encoded for by the major histocompatibility complex (MHC) on antigen-presenting cells. Specifically, cytotoxic T8$^+$ T cells recognize antigens in association with class I (HLA-A, -B, and -C) MHC molecules, and T4$^+$ helper and T4$^+$ cytotoxic T cells recognize and respond to foreign antigens in the context of class II (Ia-like) MHC molecules. The association between surface phenotype of T cells and the class of MHC molecules recognized suggests that the T4 and T8 antigens themselves are required to facilitate recognition of, or binding of, T cells to foreign antigens. This ability to corecognize foreign antigen with autologous class I and II MHC antigens on monocyte-macrophages is referred to as *MHC restriction* of immune cell interactions.

B CELLS Mature B cells comprise 10 to 15 percent of human peripheral blood lymphocytes, 50 percent of splenic lymphocytes, and approximately 10 percent of bone marrow lymphocytes and express on their surface intramembrane immunoglobulin molecules that function as B-cell antigen receptors. B cells also express surface receptors for the Fc region of IgG molecules as well as receptors for activated complement components (C3d, C3b). The primary function of B cells is to produce antibodies. Mature B cells are derived from bone marrow precursor cells that arise continuously throughout life (Figs. 62-1 and 62-3). Like myeloid and erythroid cells, B cells are constantly replaced every few days through cell division from marrow precursor cells. However, the maturation of B lymphocytes differs from myeloid and erythroid cell lineages in that B lymphocytes have antigen-dependent and antigen-independent phases of maturation (Fig. 62-3). Pre-B cells arise from precursor cells in bone marrow and are identified by the presence of cytoplasmic immunoglobulin M (cIgM) (initially IgM heavy chain followed by cytoplasmic light chain synthesis). Pre-B cells mature to immature B cells that no longer express cIgM but rather express surface IgM molecules (sIgM). Immature B cells migrate to the periphery and continue antigen-independent maturation, expressing surface IgD, diversifying the B-cell antigen repertoire, and switching the B-cell surface immunoglobulin isotype such that either surface IgM, IgG, IgA, or IgE is expressed along with IgD. Only one Ig heavy and light chain variable region and thus only one antigen specificity is expressed by each B cell. In lymph organs, B cells are the principal cells in lymph node cortical germinal centers and medullary cords and in primary and secondary germinal centers in the white pulp of spleen (see Chap. 55). On contact with antigen, mature B cells in peripheral lymph nodes and spleen either terminally differentiate into antibody-secreting plasma cells or proliferate to form populations of long-lived memory B cells that are capable of interaction with antigen when rechallenged with the same antigen (Fig. 62-3).

LARGE GRANULAR LYMPHOCYTES   Large granular lymphocytes (LGL) (previously called "null cells") constitute approximately 5 to 10 percent of peripheral blood lymphocytes, and are nonadherent, nonphagocytic cells with large azurophilic cytoplasmic granules. LGL express surface receptors for the Fc portion of IgG (see Table 62-1), and many LGL express T lineage markers and proliferate in response to interleukin 2 (T-cell growth factor). Functionally LGL share features with both monocyte-macrophages and neutrophils in that subsets of LGL mediate antibody-dependent cellular cytotoxicity (ADCC) and natural killer cell activity. ADCC is the binding of an opsonized (antibody-coated) target cell to an Fc receptor–bearing effector cell via the Fc region of antibody resulting in lysis of the target by the effector cell. Natural killer (NK) cell activity is the nonimmune (i.e., effector cell never having had previous contact with the target), non-antibody-mediated killing of target cells, usually malignant cell types. Thus, LGL that mediate natural killer activity may play an important role in immune surveillance and destruction of cells that spontaneously undergo malignant transformation in vivo.

MONOCYTE-MACROPHAGES   Monocytes arise from precursor cells within bone marrow (Fig. 62-1) and circulate with a half-life ranging from 1 to 3 days. Monocytes leave the peripheral circulation by marginating in capillaries and then migrating into a vast extravascular pool. Tissue macrophages arise by migration of monocytes from the circulation and by proliferation of macrophage precursors in tissue. Common locations of tissue macrophages (and some of their specialized names) are lymph node, spleen, bone marrow, perivascular connective tissue, serous cavities such as peritoneum, pleura, synovium, skin connective tissue, lung (alveolar macrophage), liver (Kupffer cell), bone (osteoclast), and central nervous system (microglia).

The monocyte-macrophage system plays a major role in the expression of immune reactivity by mediation of functions such as the presentation of antigen to lymphocytes and the secretion of factors such as interleukin 1 (IL-1) that are central to activation of T lymphocytes. Under certain circumstances monocytes can also mediate immunoregulatory functions such as suppressor cell activity. In addition, monocyte-macrophages mediate effector functions such as destruction of antibody-coated bacteria, tumor cells, or even normal hematopoietic cells in certain types of autoimmune cytopenias. Activated macrophages can also mediate NK-like activity and eliminate cell types such as tumor cells in the absence of antibody. Monocyte-macrophages express surface receptors for a number of molecules, including the Fc region of IgG, activated complement components, and various lymphokines (macrophage inhibitory and activating factors) (Table 62-1). In addition, monocyte-macrophages express cell surface MHC class II (Ia-like) antigens and specific cell surface differentiation antigens. Finally, macrophage secretory products are more diverse than those known for any other cell of the immune system. These secretory products allow the macrophage to exert both pro- and anti-inflammatory effects and to regulate other cell types. Among monocyte-macrophage–secreted products are hydrolytic enzymes, products of oxidative metabolism, and IL-1, also called leukocytic pyrogen and lymphocyte-activating factor, which affects lymphocytes, hepatocytes, fibroblasts, synoviocytes, and cells within the hypothalamus.

NEUTROPHILS, EOSINOPHILS, AND BASOPHILS   Granulocytes are a feature of nearly all forms of inflammation and represent a nonspecific amplification and effector component to a specific response. Unchecked accumulation and activation of granulocytes can lead to host tissue damage as seen in neutrophil- and eosinophil-mediated necrotizing vasculitis. Granulocytes are derived from stem cells in bone marrow (Fig. 62-1). Each type of granulocyte (neutrophil, eosinophil, basophil) is derived from a different subclass of progenitor cell which is stimulated to proliferate by proteins tropic for each cell type. During terminal maturation stages of granulocytes, class-specific nuclear morphology, and cytoplasmic granules appear that allow for histologic identification of granulocyte type. Neutrophils express Fc receptors for IgG and activated complement components (C3b, C3d)

FIGURE 62-3   *Model of B-cell differentiation. B cells undergo antigen-independent and antigen-dependent maturation stages that culminate in terminal differentiation into either antibody-secreting plasma cells or memory B cells.*

TABLE 62-2   Mediators released from human mast cells and basophils

Mediator	Actions
Histamine	Smooth muscle contraction, increased vascular permeability
Slow reacting substance of anaphylaxis (SRSA) (leukotriene D4)	Smooth muscle contraction
Eosinophil chemotactic factor of anaphylaxis (ECF-A)	Chemotactic attraction of eosinophils
Platelet-activation factor	Activation of platelets to secrete serotonin and other mediators
Neutrophil chemotactic factor (NCF)	Chemotactic attraction of neutrophils
Leukotactic activity (leukotriene B4)	Chemotactic attraction of neutrophils
Heparin	Anticoagulant
Basophil kallikrein of anaphylaxis (BK-A)	Cleavage of kininogen to form bradykinin

(Table 62-1). Upon neutrophil interaction by immune complexes, azurophilic granules (containing myeloperoxidase, lysozyme, elastase, and other enzymes) and specific granules (containing lactoferrin, lysozyme, collagenase, and other enzymes) are released, and microbicidal superoxide radicals (O_2^-) are generated at the neutrophil surface. The generation of superoxide is thought to lead to inflammation by direct injury to tissue and cells and by alteration of macromolecules such as collagen and DNA.

Eosinophils express Fc receptors for IgG and are potent cytotoxic effector cells for various parasitic targets. Intracytoplasmic contents of eosinophils, such as major basic protein, eosinophil cationic protein, and eosinophil-derived neurotoxin, are capable of directly damaging tissues and may be responsible in part for the organ system dysfunction in the hypereosinophilic syndromes (see Chap. 56). Since the eosinophil granule contains anti-inflammatory types of enzymes (histaminase, arylsulfatase, phospholipase D), eosinophils may downregulate or terminate ongoing inflammatory responses in normal homeostasis.

The normal functions of basophils are not known; the capacity of basophil mediators to increase local delivery of antibodies and complement by increasing vascular permeability is hypothetical. Thus, the basophil is identified principally with allergic reactions and some delayed cutaneous hypersensitivity states. Certainly the promotion of increased vascular permeability by basophils is important in the genesis of inflammatory lesions in some vasculitis syndromes (see Chap. 269). Basophils express surface receptors for IgE, and upon cross-linking of basophil-bound IgE by antigen, basophils release their granules containing histamine, eosinophil chemotactic factor of anaphylaxis, heparin, platelet-activating factor, and slow reacting substance of anaphylaxis—all mediators of components of immediate

(anaphylaxis) hypersensitivity responses (Table 62-2). In addition basophils express surface receptors for activated complement components (C3a, C5a).

HUMORAL MEDIATORS OF IMMUNITY: IMMUNOGLOBULINS   Immunoglobulins are the products of differentiated B cells and mediate the humoral arm of the immune response. Their primary functions are to bind to antigen and bring about the inactivation or removal of the offending toxin, microbe, parasite, or other foreign substance from the body. The structural basis of immunoglobulin molecule function and immunoglobulin gene organization has provided insight into the role of antibody in normal protective immunity and in the mediation of unwanted immune-mediated damage by immune complexes, and autoantibody formation against host determinants.

All immunoglobulins have the basic structure of two heavy and two light chains (Fig. 62-4). Immunoglobulin isotype is determined by the type of heavy and light chain present. IgG and IgA can further be divided into subclasses (IgG1, IgG2, IgG3, IgG4, and IgA1, and IgA2) based on specific antigenic determinants on heavy chains. The characteristics of human immunoglobulins are outlined in Table 62-3. The four chains are covalently linked by disulfide bonds. Each chain is made up of a variable (V) region and constant (C) regions (also called domains) made up of homologous units of 110 amino acids. Light chains have one variable (VL) and one constant (CL) region; heavy chains have one variable region (VH) and three or four constant (CH) regions, depending on isotype. As the name suggests, constant regions are made up of homologous sequences and share the same primary structure as all other chains of the same isotype and subclass. Constant regions are involved in biologic functions of immunoglobulin molecules. The CH_2 domain of IgG and the CH_4 domain of IgM are involved with binding complement components. The CH region at the carboxy terminus end of the IgG molecule, the Fc region (Fig. 62-4), binds to surface Fc receptors of macrophages, LGL, B cells, neutrophils, and eosinophils.

Variable regions (VL and VH) constitute the antibody-binding (Fab) region of the molecule. Within the VL and VH regions are hypervariable regions of extreme sequence variability that constitute the antigen-binding site unique to each immunoglobulin molecule. The idiotype is the specific region of the Fab portion of the immunoglobulin molecule to which antigen binds. Antibodies against the idiotype portion of an antibody molecule are called *anti-idiotype* antibodies. The formation of anti-idiotype antibodies in vivo during a normal B-cell antibody response may generate a negative (or "off") signal to B cells to terminate antibody production (see "Autoimmunity").

IgG makes up approximately 75 percent of the total serum immunoglobulin. The four IgG subclasses are numbered in order of their level in serum, IgG1 is found in greatest amounts and IgG4 the least. IgG subclasses have clinical relevance in their variability in binding macrophage and neutrophil Fc receptors and in their variability to activate complement (Table 62-3). IgG antibodies are frequently the antibodies made after rechallenge of the host with antigen (secondary antibody response). Of the immunoglobulin isotypes only IgG crosses the placenta. IgM antibodies normally circulate as a 950,000-mol wt pentamer with 160,000 monomers joined by a molecule called the J chain, a 15,000-mol wt nonimmunoglobulin molecule that also effects polymerization of IgA molecules. IgM is the first immunoglobulin to appear in the immune response (primary antibody response) and is the initial type of antibody made by neonates. Membrane IgM in the monomeric form also functions as a major antigen receptor on the surface of the mature B cell. IgM is an important component of immune complexes in autoimmune diseases. For instance, IgM antibodies against IgG molecules (*rheumatoid factors*) are present in high titers in rheumatoid arthritis, other collagen diseases, and some infectious diseases (subacute bacterial endocarditis). IgM antibody binds the C1 component of complement via the CH_4 domain and thus is a potent activator of complement. IgA makes up only 10 to 15 percent of total serum immunoglobulin but is the predominant class of immunoglobulin in secretions. IgA

FIGURE 62-4   *Schematic structure of the immunoglobulin G (IgG) molecule.*

TABLE 62-3 Characteristics of human immunoglobulins

Isotype	Molecular weight	Heavy chain	Light chain	Adult average serum level (mg/dL)	Half-life (days)	Complement activation		Binding to cells via Fc	Other biologic properties
						Classical pathway	Alternative pathway		
IgG	150,000	$\gamma_1, \gamma_2, \gamma_3, \gamma_4$	κ or γ	1250 ± 300	23.0	IgG1, IgG2, IgG3, yes; IgG4 no	IgG1, IgG2, IgG3, no; IgG4 yes	Macrophages, neutrophils, eosinophils large granular lymphocytes	Placental transfer
IgM	190,000 (950,000)*	μ	κ or λ	125 ± 50	5.1	Yes	No	Lymphocytes	Primary antibody response, rheumatoid factor
IgA	160,000 (385,000)†	α_1, α_2	κ or λ	210 ± 50	5.8	No	Yes	Lymphocytes	Antibody in mucous secretions
IgD	175,000	δ	κ or λ	4	2.8	No	Yes	None	Primary lymphocyte surface molecule
IgE	190,000	ϵ	κ or λ	0.03	2.5	No	Yes	Mast cells, basophils	Mediates anaphylaxis, allergy

* IgM circulates as a pentameric molecule.
† Secretary IgA is a dimer.
SOURCE: *Adapted with permission from DJ Jeske, JD Capra, Immunoglobulin: Structure and Function, in Fundamental Immunology, WE Paul et al (eds), New York, Raven, 1984.*

in secretions (tears, saliva, nasal secretions, gastrointestinal tract fluid, and human milk) is in the form of secretory IgA (sIgA), a polymer consisting of two IgA monomers, a joining molecule called J chain, and a glycoprotein called the secretory piece.

Of the two IgA subclasses (IgA1 and IgA2), IgA1 is primarily found in serum, whereas IgA2 is more prevalent in secretions. IgA fixes complement via the alternative pathway and has potent antiviral activity in human beings by prevention of virus binding to respiratory and gastrointestinal epithelial cells. IgD is found in minute quantities in serum (Table 62-3) and along with IgM is a major receptor for antigen on the B-cell surface. Present in serum in very low concentrations (Table 62-3), IgE is the major class of immunoglobulin involved in arming mast cells and basophils by binding to these cells via the IgE Fc region. Antigen cross-linking of IgE molecules on basophil and mast cell surfaces results in release of mediators of immediate hypersensitivity responses (Table 62-2).

Similar to the genes for the T-cell antigen receptor, the heavy and light chains of immunoglobulin are each encoded by multiple genetic elements physically separated in germline DNA but brought together to create a single active gene in B cells.

The variable regions of light chains (e.g., κ light chains) are constructed from two genes called VK and JK. These genes, though on the same chromosome, are far apart in the germline but during B-lymphocyte maturation are brought close together with excision of intervening DNA sequences (gene rearrangement). There are approximately 300 VK genes and 5 JK genes resulting in the pairing of VK and JK genes to create 1500 different light chain combinations. The number of distinct κ light chains that can be generated is increased by somatic mutational events within the VK and JK genes, which thus create a large number of specificities from a limited amount of germline genetic information.

Heavy chain immunoglobulin gene rearrangement is more complex than for light chains. The VH domain is created by the joining of three types of germline genes called VH, DH, and JH, thus allowing for even greater diversity in the variable region of heavy chains than in that of light chains.

CELLULAR INTERACTIONS INVOLVED IN REGULATION OF THE NORMAL IMMUNE RESPONSE

The net result of activation of the humoral (B-cell) and cellular (T-cell) arms of the immune system by foreign antigen is the elimination of antigen directly by effector cells or in concert with the production of specific antibody. In addition, a series of regulatory cells are activated which modulate T-effector-cell activation and B-cell antibody production. Figure 62-5 is a simplified schematic diagram of the immune system outlining some of these cellular interactions.

MONOCYTE–T CELL INTERACTIONS Many of the activation and regulatory effects of lymphocytes and monocytes occur via soluble mediators. Monocyte-macrophages are required for optimal activation of T cells by antigens or by mitogens (nonspecific activators of lymphocytes). A soluble macrophage product, IL-1, can substitute in some cases for intact macrophages. Upon contact with antigens or mitogens, macrophages secrete IL-1, two effects of which are (1) the induction of receptors for T-cell growth factor or interleukin 2 (IL-2) on T cells and (2) the induction of IL-2 secretion. IL-2 in turn effects activation of T cells resulting in expansion of effector and regulatory T cells that have also been induced to express IL-2 receptors. Effector T cells mediate a variety of functions including the killing of virally infected cells, graft rejection, graft-versus-host reaction, delayed type of hypersensitivity, and the release of lymphokines (Table 62-4).

T CELL–T CELL AND T CELL–B CELL INTERACTIONS The expression of immune cell function is the result of a complex series of phases. Both T and B lymphocytes mediate immune functions, and each of these cell types when given appropriate signals passes through stages, from activation and induction to proliferation, differentiation, and ultimately effector functions. The effector function expressed may be at the end point of a response, such as secretion of antibody by a differentiated plasma cell, or it might serve a regulatory function that modulates other functions such as is seen with inducer or suppressor T lymphocytes which modulate both differentiation of B cells and activation of cytotoxic T cells. As shown schematically in Fig. 62-5, upon activation via IL-1 and IL-2, regulatory T-cell subsets are generated that exert positive and negative forces on effector cells. Thus, for B cells and cytotoxic (T4+ or T8+) T cells, there are T4+ inducer and T8+ suppressor cells that either facilitate or downregulate effector cell function. For B cells, trophic effects are mediated by a variety of cytokines, particularly T cell–derived B-cell growth factor (BCGF) and B-cell differentiating factor (BCDF) which act at sequential stages of B-cell maturation resulting in the induction and propagation of B-cell proliferation, differentiation, and ultimately antibody secretion. For T cells, trophic factors include inducer-T-

FIGURE 62-5 *Schematic representation of cellular interactions involved in the generation of cell-mediated and humoral immunity. [Adapted with permission from AS Fauci, in WN Kelly et al (eds).]*

cell secretion of IL-2. These complex cellular and humoral interactions involve a delicate balance among positive and negative influences and ultimately result in expression of an appropriate immune response. The slightest imbalance in these immunoregulatory circuits may result in aberrant immune function leading to clinically apparent immune-mediated disease.

THE COMPLEMENT SYSTEM The complement system is a cascading series of enzymes, regulatory proteins, and proteins capable of cell lysis. There are two arms of the complement system (Fig. 62-6). Activation of the classical complement pathway via C1, C4, C2, and activation of the alternative complement pathway via factor D, C3, and factor B lead to cleavage and activation of C3. C3 is a protein whose products are critical for opsonization (antibody and complement coating in preparation for phagocytosis) of bacteria and other foreign antigens. A protein fragment (C3b) results from the activation of C3 and is necessary for activation of the terminal complement components. These components (C5 to C9) when acti-

vated form a molecule called the membrane attack complex which inserts into cell membranes resulting in osmotic lysis of the cell. C3b also joins with a cleavage product of factor B (called Bb) to form C3bBb, also known as the alternative pathway C3 convertase. Activation of the classical complement pathway results in cleavage of C4 and C2 with a resulting complex of fragments called C4b2a, also called the classical pathway C3 convertase. Both the classical C3 convertase (C4b2a) and the alternative pathway C3 convertase (C3bBb) function to cleave C3 to form active C3b, thus driving activation of terminal complement components and the C5 to C9 membrane attack complex. The fact that C3b can combine with Bb to form the alternative C3 convertase gives rise to a potent positive feedback loop for production of C3b and thus continued activation of terminal complement components. Activation of the classical complement pathway is by interaction of antigen and antibody-forming immune complexes that bind C1q, a subunit of C1. Immunoglobulin isotypes that bind C1q and activate the classical pathway are IgM, IgG1, IgG2, and IgG3. In contrast, IgA1, IgA2, and IgD activate complement via the alternative pathway. In addition, nephritic factors (IgG autoantibodies against C3bBb, the alternative pathway C3 convertase) are present in serum of some patients with membranoproliferative glomerulonephritis, and binding of nephritic factors to C3bBb results in stabilization of C3bBb enzyme activity and favors positive feedback into the C3b alternative pathway amplification loop. Activation of the complement cascade via the classical pathway by IgG- or IgM-containing immune complexes is rapid, efficient, and leads to activation of terminal complement components. In contrast, activation of the alternative pathway via IgA-containing immune complexes or by bacterial endotoxin is slower and less efficient in terminal component activation. Thus, the immunoglobulin isotype composition of immune complexes is a critical factor in determining complement activation, and therefore in determining efficiency of clearance of immune complexes by Fc receptor–bearing cells within the immune system (see Chap. 261).

In addition to the role of complement in opsonization and cell lysis, several complement component fragments are potent mediators of cell activation. C3a and C5a bind to receptors on mast cells and basophils resulting in release of histamine and other mediators of anaphylaxis. C5a is also a potent chemoattractant for neutrophils and monocyte-macrophages (Table 62-5).

TABLE 62-4 Soluble mediators of the immune response and the targets of their action

Target cells	Factors
Monocyte-macrophage	Migration-inhibitory factor (MIF) Leukotrienes Prostaglandins
Lymphocytes	Lymphocytotoxin (LT) T-cell growth factor, interleukin 2 (IL-2) Gamma interferon B-cell growth factor (BCGF) B-cell differentiation factor (BCDF)
Neutrophils	Leukocyte-inhibitory factor (LIF) Chemotactic factors
Other cell types	Eosinophil chemotactic factor (ECF) Basophil chemotactic factor (BCF) Interferons (IF) Colony-stimulating factor (CSF) Osteoclast-activating factor (OAF)

CLASSICAL PATHWAY OF ACTIVATION

Recognition of Antigen-Antibody Complexes

Rapid and Efficient

C1qrs
C4
C2

ALTERNATIVE PATHWAY OF ACTIVATION

Recognition of Bacteria and Other Activating Surfaces

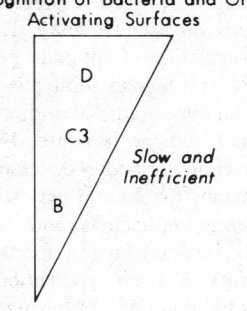

D
C3
B

Slow and Inefficient

C3→C3a + C3b
Mast Cell Degranulation
Opsonization
Recruitment of the Alternative Pathway
Initiation of the Membrane Attack Complex

C5
C6
C7   Membrane Attack
C8   Complex
C9

LYSIS

FIGURE 62-6 *Components of the complement system. [Adapted with permission from WE Paul, in WE Paul (ed).]*

TABLE 62-5 Biologic activities of some complement components

Component	Activity
C4, C2 kinin	Increases vascular permeability.
C3a	Anaphylatoxin; evokes histamine release from basophils, serotonin from platelets.
C5a	Anaphylatoxin; evokes histamine release from basophils; potent chemoattractant for monocytes and neutrophils.
C3b	Enhancement of phagocytosis by neutrophils and monocytes. Promotes immune-complex binding to cells within the monocyte-macrophage system, as well as neutrophils. With Bb forms alternative pathway C3 convertase and amplifies alternative pathway. Promotes solubilization of immune complexes.
C5–C9	Membrane attack complex; forms transmembrane channels leading to cell destruction.

SOURCE: *Adapted with permission from S Ruddy, in WN Kelly et al (eds).*

MECHANISMS OF IMMUNE DAMAGE Several scenarios of host defense in response to foreign antigen culminate in the rapid and efficient elimination of nonself substances (Table 62-6). These scenarios interface those classic arms of the immune system (T cells, B cells, macrophages) with cells and soluble products that are mediators of inflammatory responses (neutrophils, eosinophils, basophils, kinin and coagulation systems, and complement cascade). Three general phases of host defense involve (1) specific and nonspecific recognition of foreign antigens mediated by T and B lymphocytes, macrophages, and the alternative complement pathway, (2) amplification of the inflammatory response with recruitment of specific and nonspecific effector cells by complement components, lymphokines and monokines, kinins, arachidonic acid metabolites, and mast cell–basophil products, and (3) macrophage, neutrophil, and lymphocyte participation in the phase of antigen destruction and ultimate removal of antigen by phagocytosis of antigen particles (macrophage, neutrophil) or by direct cytotoxic mechanisms (macrophage, neutrophil, lymphocyte). Under normal circumstances, orderly progression of host defenses through these phases results in a well-controlled immune and inflammatory response that protects the host from the offending antigen. However, regulatory dysfunction of any of the systems involved in host defense can damage host tissue and produce clinically apparent disease.

IMMUNE-COMPLEX FORMATION (TYPE III REACTION) Clearance of antigen by immune-complex formation between antigen and antibody is a highly effective mechanism of host defense. However, depending on the level of immune complexes formed and their physicochemical properties, immune complexes may or may not result in host and foreign cell damage. After antigen exposure, certain types of soluble antigen-antibody complexes freely circulate and, if not cleared by the reticuloendothelial system, can be deposited in blood vessel walls and in other tissues such as renal glomeruli. The precise mechanisms whereby immune complexes damage tissues, particularly blood vessels, are discussed in detail in Chaps. 261 and 269.

IGE-MEDIATED ALLERGIC REACTIONS AND ANAPHYLAXIS (TYPE I) Mast cells and basophils have receptors for the Fc portion of IgE, and cell-bound IgE effectively "arms" basophils. Basophil mediator release is triggered by antigen interaction with Fc receptor–bound IgE; the mediators released are responsible for the pathophysiologic changes of allergic disease (Table 62-2). The mediators released from mast cells can be divided into three broad categories of actions:

1 Those that increase vascular permeability and contract smooth muscle (histamine, SRS-A, BK-A)
2 Those that are chemotactic for or activate other inflammatory cells (ECF-A, NCF, leukotriene B4)
3 Those that modulate the release of other mediators (BK-A, platelet-activating factor)

CYTOTOXIC REACTIONS OF ANTIBODY (TYPE II) In this type of immunologic injury, complement-fixing (C1 binding) antibodies against normal or foreign cells or tissues (IgM, IgG1, IgG2, IgG3) bind complement via the classical pathway and initiate a sequence of events similar to those initiated by immune-complex deposition resulting in cell lysis or tissue injury. Examples of type II antibody-mediated cytotoxic reactions include red cell lysis in transfusion reactions, Goodpasture's syndrome with anti-glomerular basement membrane antibody formation, and possibly juvenile-onset diabetes mellitus with anti-islet cell antibody production.

TABLE 62-6 Mechanisms of immunologically mediated inflammation

Mechanism type	Characteristics of inflammatory response	Clinical disease type
I Allergic (IgE-mediated)	Basophil and mast cell products leading to immediate flare-and-wheal.	Atopy, anaphylaxis
II Cytotoxic or tissue-specific antibody (IgM- or IgG-mediated)	Acute inflammation via phagocytic cells and deposition of complement in tissues, lysis or phagocytosis of target cells.	Goodpasture's syndrome, anti-red cell antibodies in transfusion reactions
III Immune complex (IgG-, IgM-, IgA-mediated)	Accumulation of neutrophils, macrophages, complement components.	Systemic necrotizing vasculitis, systemic lupus erythematosus, serum sickness syndromes
IV Delayed hypersensitivity	T cell–induced mononuclear cell accumulation of regulatory and effector T cells and macrophages. Lymphokines and monokines released. Often granuloma formation.	Tuberculosis, sarcoidosis, rheumatoid arthritis, Wegener's granulomatosis

CLASSIC DELAYED HYPERSENSITIVITY REACTIONS (TYPE IV)

Inflammatory reactions initiated by mononuclear leukocytes and not by antibody alone have been termed delayed hypersensitivity reactions. The term *delayed* has been used to contrast the secondary cellular response which appears 48 to 72 h after antigen exposure to an "immediate" hypersensitivity response generally seen within 12 h of antigen challenge initiated by basophil mediator release or preformed antibody. For example, in an individual previously infected with *Mycobacterium tuberculosis* (TB) organisms, intradermal placement of TB protein purified derivative (PPD) as a skin test challenge results in an indurated area of skin at 48 to 72 h, indicating previous exposure to TB. The cellular events that result in classic delayed hypersensitivity responses are centered around T cells, their soluble products, and macrophages. In the general schema outlined in Fig. 62-5, antigen is processed by macrophages and presented to T cells expressing a cell surface receptor specific for the antigen. Macrophage-secreted IL-1 amplifies antigen-induced T-cell triggering; antigen-specific T cells clonally expand; and lymphokines are secreted to recruit other T cells and macrophages nonspecifically to participate in the inflammatory response. Once recruited, macrophages frequently undergo epithelioid cell transformation and form giant cells. This type of mononuclear cell infiltrate is termed *granulomatous inflammation*. Examples of diseases in which delayed-type hypersensitivity plays a major role are fungal infections (*histoplasmosis*), mycobacterial infections, chlamydial infections (*lymphogranuloma venereum*), helminth infections (*schistosomiasis*), reactions to toxins (*berylliosis*), and hypersensitivity reactions to organic dusts (*hypersensitivity pneumonitis*). In addition, delayed-type hypersensitivity responses may play a role in *rheumatoid arthritis* and Wegener's granulomatosis.

AUTOIMMUNE DISEASE Autoimmune diseases are characterized by production of either antibodies that react with host tissue or immune effector T cells that are autoreactive. Since B-cell responses in human beings generally require inducer T cells, a B-cell autoantibody response directly implies disordered T-cell immunoregulatory control. Examples of clinically relevant autoantibodies are antithyroid antibodies in thyroiditis, and anti-DNA, antierythrocyte, and anti-platelet antibodies in systemic lupus erythematosus.

The clonal selection theory was put forth by Burnet in 1949 to explain autoimmunity. Burnet proposed that the contact of antibody-forming cells with their respective antigens during fetal or early postnatal life lead to their elimination. Thus, in this theory self-reactive clones are avoided unless they arise in later life by somatic mutation of lymphocytes. The progeny of such mutant cells would give rise to self-reacting antibodies. As the study of autoimmunity has progressed, it has become clear that the genesis of autoimmune B and T cells is far more complex than originally thought. Certain drugs (procainamide, phenytoin) and infectious agents (Epstein-Barr virus, *Mycoplasma pneumoniae*) can elicit the production of auto-antibodies to a wide array of host antigens in otherwise normal persons. Moreover, normal mice produce autoantibodies when given injections of nonspecific activators of lymphocytes (mitogens). In all of these circumstances, the autoantibodies combine with ubiquitous antigens: DNA, IgG (as the target of an IgM rheumatoid factor), phospholipids (cardiolipins), erythrocytes, lymphocytes, or cytoskeletal components (vimentin, keratins). Thus, production of autoantibodies is an inherent property of the normal immune system. The immune system controls the tendency to produce autoantibodies by a network of feedback controls exerted by T and B cells. It is generally thought that B cells normally are inhibited from terminal differentiation by suppressor T cells, a lack of inducer T cells, or both. In autoimmunity an imbalance between the two types of T cells can perturb the immunoregulatory network; this may be associated with activation of autoreactive B cells. In some instances, autoantibodies may arise by a normal T- and B-cell response activated by foreign organisms or substances that contain antigens, particularly polysaccharides, that cross-react with similar polysaccharides in body tissues.

As mentioned above in the description of immunoglobins, the unique portion of the variable region of the immunoglobulin molecule where antigen binds is called the *idiotype*, and an antibody reactive specifically with the idiotypic region of an antibody molecule is called an *anti-idiotypic* antibody. The specificity of antibody molecules and the regulation of antibody production have been probed by making rabbit anti-human idiotypic antibodies. There are also autologous anti-idiotypes (auto-anti-idiotypes) that arise during the course of the normal immune response. For example, auto-anti-idiotypes against antitetanus antibodies develop during normal immunization of humans to tetanus toxoid and may serve to deliver "off" signals to B cells secreting antitetanus antibodies. Idiotypes and auto-anti-idiotype antibodies may be an important component of the immunoregulatory network. Anti-idiotype antibodies may also be relevant to two types of autoimmunity: (1) dysfunction of the idiotype–anti-idiotype antibody system could lead to B-cell hyperreactivity by lack of generation of "off" signals for B-cell differentiation, and (2) some anti-receptor antibodies produced in autoimmune diseases (anti-acetylcholine receptor antibodies in myasthenia gravis, anti-insulin receptor antibodies in forms of type I diabetes mellitus, and anti-thyrotropin receptor antibodies in thyrotoxicosis) may be anti-idiotype antibodies made against the antibody combining site (idiotype) of an autoantibody.

Finally, genetic factors likely play a role in the genesis of autoimmune disease, either by selecting for inherent B-cell hyperreactivity and tendency toward autoantibody formation or via other unknown factors. Linkage of autoimmune diseases with known genetic loci such as the major histocompatibility complex has provoked great interest. Myasthenia gravis, thyrotoxicosis, and pernicious anemia are all associated with HLA-B8 (class I) and -DR3 (class II) alloantigen expression (Chap. 63) and are also associated with certain immunoglobulin heavy chain allotypic markers. Genetic marker systems such as HLA types and immunoglobulin heavy chain allotypic antigens may be associated with autoimmunity by making the host susceptible in some way to antiself immune cell activation. Thus, multiple genes and/or events are operative in the ultimate generation of the clinical autoimmune state.

CLINICAL EVALUATION OF IMMUNE FUNCTION Clinical assessment of immunity requires investigation of the four major components of the immune system that participate in host defense and in pathogenesis of autoimmune diseases: humoral immunity (B cells), cell-mediated immunity (T cells, monocytes), phagocytic cells of the reticuloendothelial system (polymorphonuclear cells, macrophages), and complement. Clinical problems that require an evaluation of immunity include chronic infections, recurrent infections, unusual infecting agents, and certain autoimmune syndromes. The type of clinical syndrome under evaluation can provide information regarding possible immune defects. Defects in cellular immunity generally result in viral, mycobacterial, and fungal infections. An extreme example of deficiency in cellular immunity is the acquired immunodeficiency syndrome (see Chap. 257). Antibody deficiencies result in recurrent bacterial infections, frequently with organisms such as *Streptococcus pneumoniae* and *Haemophilus influenzae* (Chap. 256). Disorders of phagocyte function frequently are manifest by recurrent skin infections, often due to *Staphylococcus aureus* (Chap. 56). Finally, deficiencies of early complement components are associated with autoimmune phenomena, and deficiencies of late complement components are associated with recurrent *Neisseria* infections (Table 62-7). Table 62-8 summarizes useful initial screening tests of immune function. For evaluation of antibody-mediated immunity, measurement of total serum immunoglobulin levels, measurement of specific antibody titers to commonly administered antigens (such as tetanus toxoid), and determination of isohemagglutinin titers yield information necessary for institution of appropriate therapy. In certain cases of hypogammaglobulinemia, quantitation of B-cell markers and in vitro B-cell functional assays are of use.

For assessment of cell-mediated immunity, the total lymphocyte count coupled with an appropriately placed battery of intradermal

TABLE 62-7 Clinical syndromes associated with complement deficiencies

Deficient protein	Clinical syndrome*
C1q	Glomerulonephritis and poikiloderma congenitale
C1r	Glomerulonephritis, SLE
C1s	SLE-like syndrome
C1 1NH	Hereditary angioedema, SLE
C4	SLE, Sjögren's syndrome
C2	SLE, discoid lupus, polymyositis, common variable hypogammaglobulinemia, Hodgkin's disease, glomerulonephritis
C3	Glomerulonephritis, SLE, *Neisseria* infections
C5	*Neisseria* infections
C6	*Neisseria* infections
C7	SLE, RA, Raynaud's phenomenon, vasculitis, *Neisseria* infections
C8	SLE, *Neisseria* infections
C9	*Neisseria* infections

* *SLE = systemic lupus erythematosus, RA = rheumatoid arthritis.*
SOURCE: *Adapted with permission from S Ruddy, in WN Kelly et al (eds).*

skin tests provides a useful index of T-cell and macrophage response to antigens in vivo.

Anergy is the absence of an appropriate delayed hypersensitivity reaction and can be general anergy with lack of T-cell responses to many types of antigens or specific anergy with lack of T-cell responses to one antigen type. Anergy is determined by absence of reactivity in delayed hypersensitivity skin testing to antigens against which the patient is sensitized. For example, a battery of skin tests including *Candida*, histoplasmin, trichophytin, and *Mycobacterium tuberculosis* are placed intradermally. Most normal adult subjects should react to one of these four antigens. If there is no response on two separate occasions, the subject is said to be *anergic*. The causes for anergy vary in different diseases. Generalized anergy occurs in chronic fungal and TB infections and in sarcoidosis. An example of specific anergy is lack of T-cell responses to *Candida* antigen in mucocutaneous candidiasis.

Quantitation of total T cells and T4 and T8 T-cell subsets can be clinically useful. However, changes in the T4/T8 ratio occur in many clinical conditions and are not specific. In certain situations such as evaluation of a transplant recipient for response to donor antigens, the measurement of lymphocyte activation by determination of the amount of tritiated thymidine incorporated into lymphocyte DNA in response to donor antigens and mitogens is of use.

The evaluation of patients with recurrent cutaneous skin infections such as Job's syndrome and chronic granulomatous disease requires quantitation of neutrophil numbers and tests of neutrophil function. Functional neutrophil tests include nitroblue tetrazolium test, superoxide generation, chemotaxis, and quantitation of the ability of neutrophils to kill bacteria (Chap. 56).

TABLE 62-8 Initial screening tests of immune function

Humoral immunity
 Quantitative immunoglobulin levels, IgG, IgM, IgA, IgE
 Tests of specific antibody formation (antitetanus toxoid)
 Isohemagglutinin titer (anti-A, anti-B): measures IgM response
Cell-mediated immunity
 White blood cell count with differential: measures total lymphocytes
 Delayed hypersensitivity skin tests: measures specific T-cell and macrophage response to antigens
Phagocytosis
 White blood cell count with differential: measures total neutrophils
 Nitroblue tetrazolium test (NBT), superoxide production: measures metabolic function
 Chemotaxis: measures cell motility
 Quantitative measurement of intracellular bacterial killing
Complement
 Total hemolytic complement (CH_{50}): quantitates complement activity
 Assay of individual complement components: defines complement component deficiencies

SOURCE: *Adapted with permission from AJ Ammann, Immunodeficiency diseases, in Basic and Clinical Immunology 5th ed, DP Stites et al (eds), Los Altos, Lange Medical, 1984.*

The total hemolytic complement (CH_{50}) determination measures the ability of a test sample of serum to lyse 50 percent of a standard suspension of sheep erythrocytes coated with rabbit anti-sheep erythrocyte antibody. This reaction requires the entire classical complement reaction sequence. For the classical activation pathway (C1, C4, C2) or the terminal sequence (C5 to C9) the CH_{50} determination is a reliable screen for homozygous deficiencies. A normal CH_{50}, however, does not exclude heterozygous partial deficiencies of classical complement components. When the CH_{50} level is subnormal, individual component measurements (usually by radioassay) are required to determine specific component deficiency states.

REFERENCES

ACUTO O, REINHERZ EL: The human T cell receptor: Structure and function. N Engl J Med 311:1019, 1984

BUTCHER E, WEISSMAN IL: Lymphoid tissues and organs, in *Fundamental Immunology,* WE Paul (ed). New York, Raven, 1984, pp 109–127

COOPER MD et al: Lymphocytes, in *Fundamental Immunology,* WE Paul (ed). New York, Raven, 1984

FAUCI AS et al: Activation and regulation of human immune responses: Implications in normal and disease states. Ann Intern Med 99:61, 1983

HAYNES BF: The human thymic microenvironment. Adv Immunol 36:87, 1984

KEHRL JH et al: Human B cell activation, proliferation and differentiation. Immunol Rev 78:75, 1984

KELLY WN et al (eds): *Textbook of Rheumatology,* 2d ed. Philadelphia, Saunders, 1985, chaps 2,7,9, and 10

PAUL WE: Introduction to the immune system, in *Fundamental Immunology,* WE Paul (ed). New York, Raven, 1984

PLAUT M, LICHTENSTEIN LM: Cellular and chemical basis of the allergic inflammatory response, in *Allergy: Principles and Practice,* E Middleton et al (eds). St. Louis, Mosby, 1978, pp 115–138

ROMAIN PL, SCHLOSSMAN SF: Human T cell subsets: Functional heterogeneity and surface recognition structures. J Clin Invest 74:1559, 1984

SHOENFELD Y, SCHWARTZ RS: Immunologic and genetic factors in autoimmune disease. N Engl J Med 312:100, 1985

STITES DP et al (eds): *Basic and Clinical Immunology,* 5th ed. Los Gatos, Lange Medical, 1984

63 THE MAJOR HISTOCOMPATIBILITY GENE COMPLEX

CHARLES B. CARPENTER

Antigenic differences between members of a species are called *alloantigens,* and when these play a determining role in the rejection of allogeneic tissue grafts they are called *histocompatibility antigens.* Evolution has conserved a single closely linked region of histocompatibility genes, the products of which are prominently displayed on cell surfaces and provide a strong barrier to allotransplantation. The terms *major histocompatibility antigens* and *major histocompatibility gene complex* (MHC) refer to the gene products and genes of this chromosomal region. Many minor histocompatibility antigens, in contrast, are encoded throughout the genome. They represent weaker allotypic differences on molecules that serve a variety of functions. Structures bearing MHC antigens play a major role in immunity and in self-recognition in the differentiation of cells and tissues. Much of the evidence for MHC control of the immune response comes from work in animal models in which immune-response genes have been mapped within the mouse (H-2), rat (RT1), and guinea pig (GPLA) MHC. In humans the MHC is called *HLA.* The individual letters of HLA have various meanings, and by international agreement HLA is the logo for the human MHC.

Several generalizations can be made about the MHCs. *First,* three classes of gene products are encoded within the small [<2 cM (centimorgans)] region of the MHC. Class I molecules, expressed on virtually all cell surfaces, consist of one heavy and one light polypeptide chain and are the products of three reduplicated loci: HLA-A, HLA-B, and HLA-C. Class II molecules, restricted in expression to B lymphocytes, some monocytes, and activated T lymphocytes, consist of two polypeptide chains (α and β) of unequal length and are the products of several closely linked genes, collectively termed the HLA-D region. Class III molecules are the C4, C2, and Bf components of complement. *Second*, class I and class II molecules either form complexes with nominal antigens or the histocompatibility antigens and nominal antigens are conjointly recognized by T lymphocytes having appropriate antigen receptors. Self versus nonself discrimination in the initiation and effector phase of the immune response is thereby intimately directed by class I and II molecules. *Third*, restricted cell-to-cell interactions involving suppressor T lymphocytes are not clearly defined in humans, but HLA genes are important for some suppressor activities. *Fourth*, genes for enzyme systems having no apparent relationship to immunity are located in the region of the MHC, as are genes of importance in skeletal growth and development. The known loci of the HLA region on the short arm of chromosome 6 are shown in Fig. 63-1.

LOCI OF THE HLA SYSTEM   Class I antigens

HLA antigens of the class I type are defined serologically by human sera, principally from multiparous females, and to a limited extent by monoclonal antibodies. They are present in varying densities in most body tissues, including B cells, T cells, and platelets but not in mature red blood cells. The number of serologically defined specificities is large, and the HLA system is the most polymorphic genetic system known in humans. Three clearly defined loci are recognized within the HLA complex for class I, serologically defined (SD), HLA antigens. Each class I antigen consists of an 11,500-dalton beta$_2$ microglobulin subunit and a 44,000-dalton heavy chain that carries the antigenic specificities (Fig. 63-2). There are 70 clearly defined A and B specificities, and eight C-locus specificities are known. Antigens of the major complex are prefixed by HLA, but this may be omitted when the context is clear. Antigens tentatively accepted by the World Health Organization have a *w* after the locus designation. The number following the locus designation is the name of the antigen. The HLA antigens of African, Asian, and Oceanic peoples are not well defined

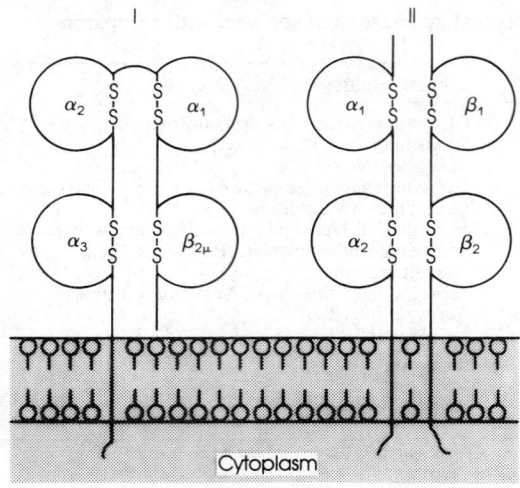

FIGURE 63-2 *Schematic representation of classes I and II molecules on the cell surface. Class I molecules are composed of two polypeptide chains. The 44,000-dalton heavy chain passes through the plasma membrane. Its external portion consists of three domains (α_1, α_2, α_3) formed by disulfide bonding. The beta$_2$-microglobulin ($\beta_{2\mu}$) light chain (11,500 daltons) encoded by chromosome 15 is noncovalently bound to the heavy chain. Amino acid sequence homologies among class I molecules is 80 to 85 percent, falling to 50 percent or less in portions of α_1 and α_2 which most likely represent the sites of alloantigenic polymorphism. Class II molecules consist of two noncovalently associated polypeptide chains, a 34,000-dalton α and a 29,000-dalton β. Each chain has two domains formed by disulfide bridging. [From CB Carpenter and EL Milford, Renal Transplantation: Immunobiology in The Kidney, B Brenner, F Rector (eds), Saunders, New York, 1985, with permission.]*

at present, although they include some of the antigens commonly found in people of West European ancestry. The distribution of HLA antigens is distinctive for certain racial groups and can serve as anthropologic markers in the study of migration patterns and diseases.

Since chromosomes are paired, each individual has six serologically defined HLA-A, HLA-B, and HLA-C antigens, three from each parent. Each of these chromosomal sets is termed a *haplotype*, and by simple mendelian inheritance one-fourth of siblings have identical haplotypes, half share a haplotype, and the remaining one-fourth are completely incompatible (Fig. 63-3). Evidence that this gene complex plays the major role in the transplantation response comes from the fact that haplotype-matched sibling donor-recipient combinations show excellent results in kidney transplantation, in the vicinity of 85 to 90 percent long-term survival (see Chap. 221).

Class II antigens   The HLA-D region is adjacent to the class I loci on the short arm of chromosome 6 (Fig. 63-1). This region encodes a series of class II molecules, each consisting of a 29,000-dalton α chain and a 34,000-dalton β chain (Fig. 63-2). Incompatibility for this region, particularly concerning the DR antigens, determines the in vitro proliferative response of lymphocytes to mismatched haplotypes. This mixed lymphocyte response (MLR) is assessed by the degree of proliferation of a *mixed lymphocyte culture* (MLC) and is positive even when HLA-A, HLA-B, and HLA-C antigens are identical (Fig. 63-3). HLA-D antigens are defined by reference-stimulating lymphocytes that are homozygous for HLA-D and are inactivated by x-irradiation or mitomycin C to make the reaction unidirectional. There are 19 such antigens (HLA-Dwl-19) recognized by homozygous typing cells.

Attempts to define HLA-D by serology first established a series of D-related (DR) antigens expressed on class II molecules of B lymphocytes, monocytes, and activated T lymphocytes. Other closely related antigen systems were soon discovered and given various local names (MB, MT, DC, SB). The separate identity of sets of class II

FIGURE 63-1 *Schematic representation of human chromosome 6, showing the location of the HLA region in the 21 region of the short arm. The HLA-A, HLA-B, HLA-C loci encode class I heavy chains (44,000 daltons), while the beta$_2$ microglobulin light chain (11,500 daltons) of the class I molecule is encoded by genes of chromosome 15. HLA-D region (class II) is centromeric to the A, B, C loci, with genes for closely linked complement components C4A, C4B, Bf, and C2 in the B-D region. The order of the complement genes is uncertain. Each D region class II molecule is made up of an α and a β chain. They appear on the cell surface in distinct sets, DP, DQ, and DR. The numbers preceding α or β indicate that there are different genes for the chains of a given set; e.g., for DR, there are three β-chain genes, so that the expressed molecule may be $1\beta\alpha$, $2\beta\alpha$, or $3\beta\alpha$. The antigens DRw52 (MT2) and DRw53 (MT3) are on the 2β chain, while DR is on 1β. DRα is not polymorphic, while molecules bearing the DQ antigens have polymorphism in both α and β chains ($2\alpha2\beta$). The other DQ set ($1\alpha1\beta$) has limited polymorphism. Polymorphism in DP is confined to the β chains. The overall length of the HLA region is about 3 cM.*

Haplotypes:

a = A1, Cw3, B8, Dw3
b = A29, Cw4, Bw35, Dw1
a$_r$ = A1, Cw3, B8, Dw1
b$_r$ = A29, Cw4, Bw35, Dw3

Inheritance:

ab x cd

ac   ad   bc   bd

FIGURE 63-3 *HLA region, chromosome 6: inheritance of HLA haplotypes. Each chromosomal segment of linked genes is termed a haplotype, and each individual inherits one haplotype from each parent. The A, B, C, and D antigens of haplotypes a and b are shown for this hypothetical individual in chromosomal order on the diagram, and also below as they would be written in text. If individual ab were to marry cd, their offspring would be of four types only, as far as HLA is concerned. Occasionally (dotted cross) recombination occurs in the germ line (meiosis) of a parent, resulting in an altered haplotype. The frequency of recombinant children is a measure of the map distance (1 percent recombination frequency = 1 cM; see Fig. 63-1). (From CB Carpenter, Kidney International, 14:283, 1978.)*

molecules is now established, and the genes for their respective α and β chains have been isolated and sequenced. The class II gene map shown in Fig. 63-1 describes a minimal number of genes and molecular sets. Although a class II molecule may be composed of a DRα from one parental haplotype and a DRβ from the other parent (transcomplementation), α and β combinatorial possibilities outside of each DP, DQ, DR set rarely, if ever, occur. DR, and to some extent DQ, molecules provide the stimuli for the primary MLR. The secondary MLR is called the *primed lymphocyte test* (PLT) and occurs rapidly over 24 to 36 h instead of 6 to 7 days. DP alloantigens were discovered from their ability to provide PLT stimulation, although they do not produce a primary MLR. While B lymphocytes and activated T lymphocytes express all three sets of class II molecules, DQ antigens are not expressed on 60 to 90 percent of monocytes, which are virtually all DP- and DR-positive.

Molecular genetics Each polypeptide chain of class I and class II molecules bears several polymorphic sites in addition to the "private" antigen defined by alloantisera. In the *cell-mediated lympholysis* (CML) test the specificity of killer T cells (T$_c$), which arise during the proliferative events in MLR, is determined by testing upon target cells from donors other than those providing the MLR stimulus. Antigen systems defined by this method show a close but imperfect correlation with class I private antigens. Cloning of cytotoxic cells has revealed the presence of a variety of polymorphic target determinants on HLA molecules, some of which are identifiable by alloantisera or monoclonal antibodies derived from immunization of mice with human cells. Some of these reagents can be used to identify private determinants of HLA, while others are directed to more "public" (sometimes called supertypic) determinants. One such system of public HLA-B antigens has two alleles, Bw4 and Bw6. Most HLA-B private antigens are associated with either Bw4 or Bw6. Other systems are restricted to subsets of HLA antigen groups. For example, HLA-B-bearing heavy chains carry additional sites that are common to B7, B27, Bw22, and B40 or to B5, B15, B18, and Bw35. Other types of shared antigenic determinants exist, as exemplified by a monoclonal antibody which reacts with a site shared between HLA-A and HLA-B heavy chains.

The amino acid sequence and peptide maps of several HLA molecules show that the class I hypervariable regions are clustered in outer α$_1$ domain (Fig. 63-2) and the adjacent portion of α$_2$. Variability in the sequences of class II molecules differs from locus to locus. Remarkably, the class I α$_3$ domain, the class II α$_2$ and β$_2$ domains, and the portions of the T8 (Leu 2) cell surface molecule which function in T-cell interactions (see Chap. 62) all show significant

amino acid sequence homologies with immunoglobulin constant regions. These findings suggest evolutionary elaboration within a family of gene products which have immune recognition functions. When genomic DNA for HLA is examined, typical exon-intron sequences of DNA have been found for class I and class II, exons having been identified for signal peptides (5'), each of the domains, a transmembrane hydrophobic segment, and a cytoplasmic segment (3'). cDNA probes are available for most of the HLA chains, and enzymatic digests have been used to study patterns of *restriction fragment length polymorphisms* (RFLP), many of which correlate with class II serologic and MLR patterns. There are 20 to 30 class I genes, however, making assessment of polymorphism by RFLP difficult. Many of these genes are not expressed (pseudogenes), while some could represent additional class I loci that are expressed only on activated T cells, and are of uncertain function. Development of HLA-A or HLA-B locus specific probes will help to resolve this complexity.

Complement (class III) Structural genes for three complement components, C4, C2, and Bf, are present in the HLA-B-D region (Fig. 63-1). There are two loci for C4, coding for C4A and C4B, formerly recognized as the Rodgers and Chido red blood cell antigens, respectively. These antigens are, in fact, absorbed plasma C4 molecules. Other complement components are not closely linked to HLA. No crossovers have been found between the C2, Bf, and C4 loci. They are all encoded within a 100-kilobase segment between HLA-B and HLA-DR. There are two alleles of C2, four of Bf, seven of C4A, and three of C4B, plus blanks for each locus (QO). The extensive polymorphism of complement types (complotypes) makes them useful for genetic studies. The four most common extended haplotypes found in people of western European ancestry are shown in Table 63-1. MLRs between unrelated individuals who are matched for these extended haplotypes are nonreactive, whereas reactivity is common if unrelated individuals are matched for only HLA-DR and -DQ. Such identical extended haplotypes may be conserved from a common ancestor.

Other sixth-chromosome genes Deficiency of steroid 21-hydroxylase, an autosomal recessive trait, results in the syndrome of congenital adrenal hyperplasia (Chaps. 325 and 333). The gene for the enzyme is localized in the HLA-B-D region. The 21-hydroxylase gene adjacent to C4A is deleted in affected individuals along with C4A (C4AQO), and the HLA-B locus gene may have been altered to convert B13 to the rare Bw47 found only in affected haplotypes. A late-onset variant of 21-hydroxylase deficiency is also linked to HLA, although congenital adrenal hyperplasia due to 11β-hydroxylase deficiency is not HLA-linked. Idiopathic hemochromatosis, an autosomal recessive disorder, is linked to HLA, as has been shown in several family studies (see Chap. 310). Although the pathogenesis of this disease is unknown, the gene that modulates gastrointestinal iron absorption is near HLA-A (Table 63-2).

Immune response genes HLA-D is analogous to the mouse H-2I region as established by studies of in vitro responses to synthetic polypeptide antigens, keyhole limpet hemocyanin, collagen, and tetanus toxoid. Presentation of antigenic fragments on the surfaces of macrophages or other cells bearing class II molecules requires conjoint recognition of a class II + antigen complex by T lymphocytes bearing the appropriate receptor(s) (see Chap. 62). The crux of this "self + X" or "altered self" hypothesis is that in the T-dependent immune response, help from the T helper/inducer cell (T$_H$) occurs

TABLE 63-1 Common extended HLA haplotypes

HLA-B	HLA-DR	BF	C2	C4A	C4B
8	3	S	C	QO	1
7	2	S	C	3	1
57	7	S	C	6	1
44	7	F	C	3	1

TABLE 63-2 Linkage of genetic defects to HLA

	Gene location	Common haplotype found
C2 deficiency	HLA-B-D	Aw25, B18, BfS, DR2
21-OH deficiency	HLA-B-D	A3, Bw47, BfF, DR7
21-OH deficiency (late onset)	HLA-B-D,	B14, BfS, DR1
Idiopathic hemochromatosis	HLA-A	A3, B14
Paget's disease	HLA-A-D	
Spinocerebellar ataxia	HLA-A-D	
Hodgkins' disease	HLA-A-D	

only if the appropriate class II determinant can be synthesized. The genes for the latter are Ir genes. Since allogeneic class II determinants are perceived as already altered, the allogeneic MLR response represents a model for the immune system in which additional nominal antigen does not need to be added (Fig. 63-4). Effector phases of immunity require recognition of nominal antigen together with a self structure. The latter in humans, as in mice, is the molecule bearing class I histocompatibility antigens. Human cell lines infected with influenza virus are lysed by immune cytotoxic T lymphocytes (T_c) only if an HLA-A- or HLA-B-locus antigen is shared between the attacking and target cells. Again, the allogeneic MLR provides a model for development of class I restricted cytotoxic T lymphocytes (Fig. 63-4). When primed cells are propagated and cloned, an array of restrictions to different class I and II molecules and epitopes can be discerned. At the level of the antigen presenting cell, for example, a given T_H clone recognizes an antigenic fragment conjointly with a specific site on a class II molecule via its receptor (T_i). The restriction elements for some microbial antigens are DR or Dw alleles. Suppression of immune responses (i.e., low responder status) to cedar pollen, streptococcal antigen, and schistosomal antigen is linked to HLA as a dominant trait, suggesting the existence of immune suppressor (Is) genes. Specific allele associations with immune response (e.g., ragweed Ra5 antigen with DR2 and collagen with DR4) have also been demonstrated.

DISEASE ASSOCIATIONS   If the major histocompatibility complex serves a critical natural biologic function, what might that be? One hypothesis is that it plays a role in immune surveillance against neoplastic cells that develop in the course of an individual's lifetime. The system could also play an important role in pregnancy because of the histoincompatibility that always exists between the mother and the fetus. The high degree of polymorphism may also ensure survival

of the species in relation to the large numbers of microbiologic agents present in the environment. Self-tolerance which happens to cross-react with microbiologic agents would produce a high degree of susceptibility, resulting in lethal infection, whereas the polymorphism in the HLA system ensures that segments of the population recognize offending agents as foreign and initiate the appropriate response. All these hypotheses relate to the survival value of the system under selective evolutionary pressures, and there is some evidence for each of them.

Circumstantial evidence for the role of the HLA complex in immunobiology comes from the finding that a number of disease processes are positively associated with certain HLA antigens within the population. The search for such associations has been stimulated by the discovery of immune response genes linked to the H-2 complex in the mouse. Table 63-3 summarizes the most significant HLA and disease associations.

Most striking is the increased frequency of HLA-B27 in certain rheumatic diseases, particularly ankylosing spondylitis, a condition with a strong familial tendency. B27 is present in about 7 percent of people of West European ancestry, while it appears in 80 to 90 percent of patients with ankylosing spondylitis. Expressed as a relative risk, the antigen B27 confers a susceptibility to the development of ankylosing spondylitis that is 87 times that in the general population. Similarly, acute anterior uveitis, Reiter's syndrome, and reactive arthritis to at least three bacterial infections (yersinia, salmonella, and gonococcus) show a high degree of association with B27. Although the ordinary form of juvenile rheumatoid arthritis (JRA) also shows a similar association with B27, the pauciarticular form of JRA with iritis is DR5-associated. The increased incidence of B27 in psoriatic arthritis is also significant for the central type of the disorder, while Bw38 is associated with both the central and peripheral types. Psoriasis is associated with Cw6. Patients with degenerative arthritis or gout show no alteration in antigen frequencies.

Most other disease associations are with HLA-D region antigens. For example, gluten-sensitive enteropathy (celiac disease, nontropical sprue) in children and adults is associated with DR3 (relative risk = 21). The actual percentage of such patients having this antigen ranges from 63 to 96 percent compared to 22 to 27 percent of controls. The same antigen is also present in increased frequency in patients with chronic active hepatitis and in patients with dermatitis herpetiformis who also have gluten-sensitive enteropathy. Juvenile-onset insulin-dependent diabetes mellitus (type I) is associated with DR4 and DR3 and is negatively associated with DR2. Maturity-onset diabetes is not HLA-associated. A rare allele of Bf (F1) is also found in 17 to 25

ALLOGRAFT RESPONSE

FIGURE 63-4 *Schema of the relative roles of HLA-A, HLA-B, HLA-C, and HLA-D antigens in initiation of the alloimmune response and in the development of effector cells and antibodies. Two main classes of T lymphocytes recognize antigens: T_c, the precursors to the cytotoxic "killer" cells, and T_H, the helper cells for amplification of the cytotoxic response. T_H also provide help to B lymphocytes for production of a fully mature IgG response. Note that T_c generally recognize class I antigens, while the T_H signal is provided principally by HLA-D, which has class II antigens closely associated. (From CB Carpenter, Kidney International, 14:283, 1978.)*

percent of cases of type I diabetes. Hyperthyroidism in the United States is associated with B8, Dw3, while in Japanese populations the association is with Bw35. More extensive studies of healthy and diseased members of various races will help in clarification of which HLA markers are universal. For example, B27 is rare in healthy Japanese but is common in subjects with ankylosing spondylitis. Also, DR4 seems to be the common marker for type I diabetes in all races. Sometimes an HLA marker is clearly associated only with a subgroup within a syndrome. For example, myasthenia gravis without thymoma is more strongly B8, DR3-associated, and the association of DR2 with multiple sclerosis is strong in patients with rapidly progressive deterioration. Goodpasture's syndrome due to autoimmunity to glomerular basement membrane, idiopathic membranous glomerulonephritis, which may be an autoimmune process involving antibodies to an antigen of the glomerulus, and gold-induced membranous nephritis are strongly HLA-DR-associated.

LINKAGE DISEQUILIBRIUM Although the distribution of HLA alleles varies in racial and ethnic populations, the most salient feature of population genetics of HLA antigens is the presence of linkage disequilibria among certain antigens of the A and B, B and C, and B, D, and complement loci. Linkage disequilibrium means that antigens of closely linked loci appear together more frequently than predicted by random association. The classic example is the linkage disequilibrium present between the A-locus antigen, HLA-A1, and B-locus antigen, HLA-B8, in people of western European ancestry. The coincidence of A1 and B8 should be the product of their individual gene frequencies, or 0.17 times 0.11 equals approximately 0.02. The observed frequency of A1 and B8 is 0.08, four times that expected, an increase of 0.06. The latter value is termed Δ (delta), and is a measure of the disequilibria. Other A- and B-locus haplotype disequilibria have been recognized and include (A3, B7), (A2, B12), (A29, B12), and (A11, Bw35). Furthermore, some D-region determinants are in linkage disequilibrium with B-locus antigens (for example, DR3 and B8), as are some B-locus and C-locus antigens. Serologically defined HLA antigens can serve as markers for the genes of an entire haplotype within a family and as markers for specific genes within a population but only where a linkage disequilibrium exists.

Linkage disequilibrium is of importance because such gene associations may have some bearing on their function. For example, selective pressures during the course of evolution may have been the major factor in the survival of certain gene combinations in a haplotype. Such a theory would suggest, for example, that A1 and B8, along with certain D-region and other determinants, conferred a selective advantage in the face of epidemics such as the plague or smallpox. It would also follow that the descendants of the survivors may display susceptibility to certain diseases because their unique gene complex happens to confer an abnormal response to other environmental agents. The major difficulty with this hypothesis is the assumption that selection must work on several genes simultaneously to account for the observed Δ's; however, the need for complex interactions among the products of the several loci of the major histocompatibility complex is only beginning to be appreciated, and selection might force multiple linkage disequilibria. The conservation of certain extended haplotypes, mentioned above, supports this view.

On the other hand, the selection hypothesis is not necessary to explain linkage disequilibrium. When a population lacking certain antigens is crossed with one in which a high frequency of antigens is in equilibrium, a Δ can develop within a few generations. For example, the increasing Δ value for A1, B8 found in populations from east to west, from India to western Europe, can be explained on the basis of migration and fusion. In smaller groups, consanguinity, founder effects, and gene drift may account for disequilibria. Finally, certain linkage disequilibria could occur as a result of nonrandom crossing over during gametic meiosis, because of chromosomal segments which are either more or less likely to break. Unless there are selective pressures or restrictions in crossing over, linkage

TABLE 63-3 HLA antigens and disease, showing the most highly associated antigens

Disease	Antigen	Relative risk*
RHEUMATIC		
Ankylosing spondylitis	B27	87.0
Reiter's syndrome	B27	37.0
Acute anterior uveitis	B27	10.3
Reactive arthritis (yersinia, salmonella, gonococcus)	B27	18.0
Psoriatic arthritis, central	B27	10.7
	Bw38	9.1
Psoriatic arthritis, peripheral	B27	2.0
	Bw38	6.5
Juvenile rheumatoid arthritis	B27	4.5
	DRw8	3.6
Juvenile arthritis, pauciarticular	DR5	5.2
Rheumatoid arthritis	Dw4/DR4	6.0
Sjögren's syndrome	Dw3	9.7
Systemic lupus erythematosus	DR3	5.8
Systemic lupus erythematosus (hydralazine)	DR4	5.6
GASTROINTESTINAL		
Gluten-sensitive enteropathy	DR3	21.0
Chronic active hepatitis	DR3	6.8
Ulcerative colitis	B5	3.8
HEMATOLOGIC		
Idiopathic hemochromatosis	A3	8.2
	B14	26.7
	A3, B14	90.0
Pernicious anemia	DR5	5.4
SKIN		
Dermatitis herpetiformis	Dw3	15.4
Psoriasis vulgaris	Cw6	4.8
Psoriasis vulgaris (Japanese)	Cw6	10.7
Pemphigus vulgaris (Jews)	DR4	14.4
	A10	5.9
Behçet's disease	B5	6.3
ENDOCRINE		
Type 1 diabetes mellitus	DR4	6.4
	DR3	3.3
	DR2	0.2
	BfF1	15.0
Hyperthyroidism	B8	3.6
	Dw3	3.7
Hyperthyroidism (Japanese)	Bw35	3.9
Adrenal insufficiency	Dw3	10.5
Subacute thyroiditis (de Quervain)	Bw35	13.7
Hashimoto's thyroiditis	DR5	3.2
NEUROLOGIC		
Myasthenia gravis	B8	2.7
	DR3	2.5
Multiple sclerosis	DR2	3.9
Manic-depressive disorder	Bw16	2.3
Schizophrenia	A28	2.3
RENAL		
Idiopathic membranous glomerulonephritis	DR3	12.0
Goodpasture's syndrome (anti-GBM)	DR2	15.9
Minimal change disease (steroid response)	B12	3.5
Polycystic kidney disease	B5	2.6
IgA nephropathy	DR4	4.0
Gold nephropathy	DR3	14.0
INFECTIOUS		
Tuberculoid leprosy (Asians)	B8	6.8
Paralytic polio	Bw16	4.3
Low vs. high response to vaccinia virus	Cw3	12.7
IMMUNODEFICIENCY		
IgA deficiency (blood donors)	DR3	13.0

$$* \ Relative \ risk = \frac{(\% \ antigen\text{-}positive \ patients)(\% \ antigen\text{-}negative \ controls)}{(\% \ antigen\text{-}negative \ patients)(\% \ antigen\text{-}positive \ controls)}.$$

disequilibria disappear over a period of several generations. A large number of nonrandom associations occur throughout the HLA gene complex, and elucidation of the reasons for their existence may provide insight into the mechanism underlying certain disease susceptibilities.

LINKAGE AND ASSOCIATION   The diseases listed in Table 63-2 are examples of HLA linkage wherein the inherited conditions are marked within families by the relevant HLA haplotypes. For C2 deficiency, 21-hydroxylase deficiency, and idiopathic hemochromatosis the mode of inheritance is recessive, with heterozygotes showing partial deficiencies. These genetic defects are also HLA-associated, with an excess of certain HLA alleles in affected unrelated individuals. Also, C2 deficiency is commonly linked to the HLA-Aw25, B18, BS5, D/DR2 haplotype, and idiopathic hemochromatosis exhibits both linkage and strong association with HLA-A3 and B14. The high degree of linkage disequilibria in these HLA-linked diseases may result from mutations in a single founder, and a sufficient period of time may not have passed to bring the gene pool back into equilibrium. In this view, the HLA antigens are simple markers for the linked gene. Alternatively, expression of the defect may require interaction with specific HLA alleles. This latter hypothesis would require a higher mutation rate, with defective gene expression occurring only when linked with certain HLA genes.

Paget's disease and spinocerebellar ataxia are HLA-linked autosomal dominant traits in families having multiple affected members, and Hodgkins disease shows an HLA-linked recessive pattern of inheritance. No HLA associations have been discerned for these disorders, suggesting that there were multiple founders with mutations in linkage with different HLA alleles.

HLA linkage is readily recognized when recessive or dominant inheritance patterns are clear-cut, i.e., when expressivity is high and the process is mostly, if not entirely, determined by a single gene defect. In most of the associations HLA markers represent risk factors involving the operation and modulation of the immune response under the influence of multiple genes. An example of a polygenic immunologic disease is atopic allergy, in which the association to HLA may be evident only in individuals whose genetically controlled (non-HLA) levels of IgE production are low. Another is IgA deficiency (Table 63-3), which is HLA-DR3-associated.

CLINICAL APPLICATIONS   The clinical value of HLA typing for diagnosis of disease is limited to B27 and ankylosing spondylitis, where nevertheless there are 10 percent false-positive and false-negative rates. HLA studies are also of value in genetic counseling and early recognition of disease in families with idiopathic hemochromatosis or congenital adrenal hyperplasia due to steroid 21-hydroxylase deficiency, particularly as HLA typing can be performed upon cells obtained by amniocentesis. The high degree of polymorphism of the HLA system also makes it a powerful tool for paternity testing and other medicolegal applications. The implications for diseases such as type I diabetes mellitus and the other diseases showing HLA associations require further study of the components of the HLA system and their role in the pathogenesis of disease.

REFERENCES

ALBERT E, MAYR W (eds): *Histocompatibility Testing, 1984*. Berlin, Springer-Verlag, 1984

ANDERSSON M et al: Genomic hybridization with class II transplantation antigen cDNA probes as a complementary technique in tissue typing. Hum Immunol 11:57, 1984

BODMER J, BODMER W: Histocompatibility, 1984. Immunol Tod 5:251, 1984

COHEN D et al: Clusters of HLA class IIβ restriction fragments describe allelic series. Proc Natl Acad Sci USA 81:7870, 1984

DEGOS L, DAUSSET J: Human migrations and linkage disequilibrium of HLA system. Immunogenetics 3:195, 1974

KAUFMAN JF et al: The class II molecules of the human and murine major histocompatibility complex. Cell 36:1, 1984

LARKHAMMAR D et al: Complete amino acid sequence of an HLA-DR antigen–like beta chain as predicted from the nucleotide sequence: Similarities with immunoglobulins and HLA-A, -B, and -C antigens. Proc Natl Acad Sci USA 79:3687, 1982

MARSH DG et al: Epidemiology and genetics of atopic allergy. N Eng J Med 305:1551, 1981

MÖLLER G (ed): Structure and function of HLA-DR. Immunol Rev 66:1982 (entire volume)

——— (ed): HLA and disease susceptibility. Immunol Rev 70:1983 (entire volume)

NISHIMURA Y, SASAZUKI T: Suppressor T cells control the HLA-linked low responsiveness to streptococcal antigen in man. Nature 302:67, 1983

QVIGSTAD E et al: Antigen-specific T cell clones restricted by DR, DRw53 (MT), or DP (SB) class II HLA molecules. Inhibition studies with monoclonal HLA-specific antibodies. Hum Immunol 11:207, 1984

RYDER LP et al (eds): *HLA and Disease Registry: Third Report*. Copenhagen, Munksgaard, 1979

WHITE PC et al: HLA-linked congenital adrenal hyperplasia results from a defective gene encoding a cytochrome P-450 specific for steroid 21-hydroxylation. Proc Natl Acad Sci USA 81:7505, 1984

section 3 Clinical pharmacology

64   PRINCIPLES OF DRUG THERAPY

JOHN A. OATES / GRANT R. WILKINSON

QUANTITATIVE DETERMINANTS OF DRUG ACTION

Safe and effective therapy with drugs requires their delivery to target tissues in concentrations within the narrow range that yields efficacy without toxicity. Optimal precision in achieving concentrations of drug within this therapeutic "window" can be achieved with regimens that are based on the kinetics of the drug's availability to target sites. This chapter deals with the principles of drug elimination and distribution that form the basis for loading and maintenance regimens for the average patient and considers instances in which elimination of the drug is impaired (e.g., renal failure). The kinetic basis for optimal utilization of plasma level data is also discussed.

PLASMA LEVELS AFTER A SINGLE DOSE   The levels of lidocaine in plasma following intravenous administration decline in two phases as illustrated in Fig. 64-1; such a biphasic decline is typical for many drugs. Immediately following rapid injection, essentially all of the drug is in the plasma compartment, and the high initial plasma level reflects its confinement to this small volume. Subsequently, the drug is transferred into the extravascular compartment, and the period of time during which this occurs is referred to as the *distribution phase*. For lidocaine the distribution phase is virtually complete within 30 min; then a slower rate of fall ensues, referred to as the *equilibrium phase* or *elimination phase*. During this latter phase, the drug levels in plasma and those in the tissues are in pseudoequilibrium.

Distribution phase   Pharmacologic events during the distribution phase depend on whether the level of drug at the receptor site is similar to that in the plasma. If this is the case, the pharmacologic effects, whether favorable or adverse, may be inordinately great during this period. For example, following a small bolus dose (50 mg) of lidocaine, antiarrhythmic effects may be evident during the

FIGURE 64-1 *Concentrations of lidocaine in plasma following the administration of 50 mg intravenously. The half-life of 108 min is computed as the time required for levels to fall from any given value during the equilibrium phase (Cp$_{initial}$) to one-half that level. Cp$_0$ is the hypothetical concentration of lidocaine in plasma at time zero if equilibrium had been achieved instantly.*

early distribution phase but disappear as levels fall below those that are minimally effective and even before equilibrium between plasma and tissue is reached. Thus, larger single doses or multiple small doses must be administered to achieve an effect that is sustained into the equilibrium phase. The toxicity of high levels of some drugs during the distribution phase precludes administration of a single intravenous loading dose that will achieve therapeutic levels during the equilibrium phase. For example, the administration of a loading dose of phenytoin as a single intravenous bolus can cause cardiovascular collapse due to the high levels during the distribution phase. If a loading dose of phenytoin is administered intravenously, it must be given in fractions at intervals sufficient to permit substantial distribution of the prior dose before the next is given (for example, 100 mg every 3 to 5 min). For similar reasons, the loading dose of many potent drugs that rapidly equilibrate with their receptors is divided into fractional doses for intravenous administration.

After an oral dose that delivers an equivalent amount of drug into the systemic circulation, plasma levels during the distribution phase do not rise as steeply as after an intravenous bolus dose. Because the drug is not absorbed instantly after oral administration and is delivered into the systemic circulation more slowly, much of the drug is distributed by the time absorption is complete. Thus, procainamide, which is almost totally absorbed after oral administration, can be given as a single 750-mg loading dose with little risk of hypotension; in contrast, loading of the drug by the intravenous route is more safely accomplished by giving the dose in fractions of about 100 mg at 5-min intervals to avoid the hypotension that might ensue during the distribution phase if the entire loading dose were given as a single bolus.

In contrast, other drugs are distributed slowly to their sites of action during the distribution phase. For example, levels of digoxin at the receptor site (and its pharmacologic effect) do not reflect plasma levels during the distribution phase. Digoxin is transported (or bound) to its cardiac receptors more slowly by a process that proceeds throughout distribution. Thus, plasma levels fall during a distribution phase of several hours, while levels at the site of action and pharmacologic effect increase. Only at the end of the distribution phase, when the drug has reached equilibrium with the receptor, does the concentration of digoxin in plasma reflect pharmacologic effect. For this reason, there should be a 6- to 8-h wait after the distribution phase before plasma levels of digoxin are obtained for a guide to therapy.

Equilibrium phase   After distribution has proceeded to the point where the concentration of drug in plasma is in equilibrium with that in the tissues outside the vascular compartment, the levels in plasma and tissues fall in parallel as the drug is eliminated from the body.

Thus, the *equilibrium phase* is sometimes also referred to as the *elimination phase.*

Most drugs are eliminated as a first-order process. During the equilibrium phase, a characteristic of the first-order process is that the time required for the level of drug in plasma to fall to one-half the original value (the half-life, $t_{1/2}$) is the same regardless of which point on the plasma level curve is chosen as a starting point for the measurement. Another characteristic of the first-order process is that a semilogarithmic plot of the concentrations in plasma versus time during the equilibrium phase is linear. From such a plot (Fig. 64-1) it can be seen that the half-life of lidocaine is 108 min.

One can calculate what amount of the administered dose remains in the body at any multiple of the half-life interval following administration:

Number of half-lives	Amount of dose remaining in the body, %
1	50
2	25
3	12.5
4	6.25
5	3.125

In theory, the elimination process never reaches completion. From a clinical standpoint, however, elimination is essentially complete when it has reached 90 percent. Therefore, for practical purposes, *a first-order elimination process reaches completion after 3 to 4 half-lives.*

DRUG ACCUMULATION—LOADING AND MAINTENANCE DOSES

With repeated administration of a drug, the amount in the body accumulates if the elimination of the first dose is incomplete when the second dose is given, and both the amount of drug in the body and its pharmacologic effect increase with continuing administration until they reach a plateau. The accumulation of digoxin administered in repeated maintenance doses (without a loading dose) is illustrated in Fig. 64-2. As digoxin's half-life is about 1.6 days in a patient with normal renal function, 65 percent of digoxin remains in the body at the end of 1 day. Thus, the second dose will raise the amount of digoxin in the body (and average plasma level) to 165 percent of that following the first dose. Each subsequent dose will result in greater amounts in the body until a plateau is attained. At the plateau, or *steady state,* drug intake per unit of time is the same as the rate of drug elimination. For *all* drugs with first-order kinetics, the time required to achieve steady-state levels can be predicted from the half-life because accumulation also is a first-order process with a half-life identical to that for elimination. Hence, accumulation reaches 90

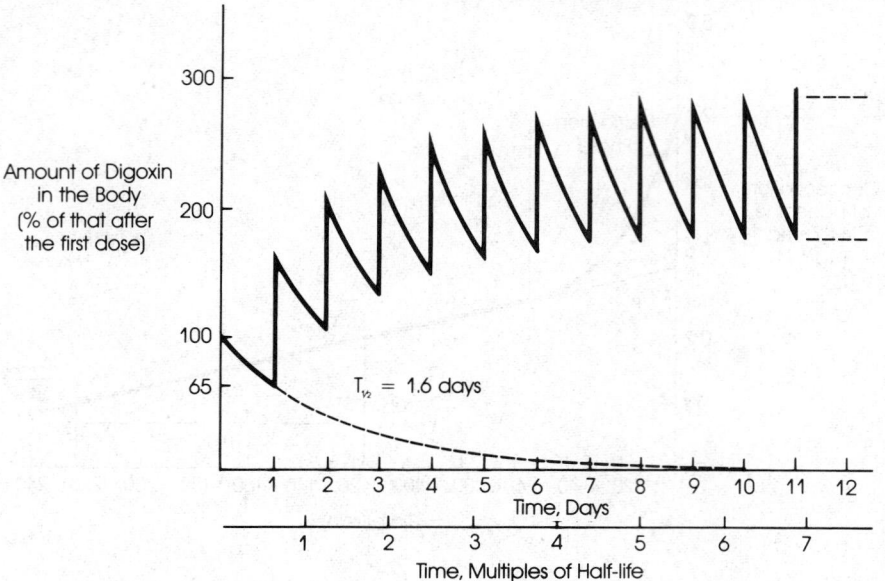

FIGURE 64-2 *The time course of digoxin accumulation when a single daily maintenance dose is given without a loading dose. Note that accumulation is more than 90 percent complete by the end of 4 half-lives.*

percent of steady-state levels at the end of 3 to 4 half-lives. For digoxin, with a half-life of 1.6 days (with normal renal function), accumulation will be practically complete in 5 days. Continuing infusion of a drug at a constant rate also will result in progressive accumulation to a steady state with a time course predictable from the elimination curve for that drug (Fig. 64-3).

When the time required to reach steady-state levels is longer than one wishes to wait, plasma levels may be achieved more rapidly by the administration of a *loading dose*. Loading entails the administration of an amount that will bring the concentration in plasma (at equilibrium) to the level present during steady state. This may be accomplished by the administration of the loading amount as a single dose, or in the case of drugs with low therapeutic indexes (the therapeutic index is the ratio of the toxic dose to the therapeutic dose) the loading amount is administered in a series of fractions of the total loading amount. As the accumulation of procainamide to 90 percent of steady state by infusion would require approximately 10 h (the $t_{1/2}$ is 3 h), a loading regimen is almost always desirable. The load required to suppress an arrhythmia, however, varies among individuals from 300 to 1000 mg, and rapid intravenous administration of the *average loading dose* causes hypotension during the distribution phase in some patients. Therefore, the intravenous loading dose of procainamide is given in fractions (e.g., 100 mg every 5 min) until the arrhythmia is controlled or adverse effects such as hypotension indicate that no further drug should be given. Dividing the loading dose into fractions is appropriate for most drugs that have a low

therapeutic index. This permits better individualization of the loading amount and minimizes adverse effects.

The size of loading dose required to achieve the plasma levels at steady state can be determined from the fraction of drug eliminated during the dosage interval and the maintenance dose (in the case of intermittent drug administration). For example, if the fraction of digoxin eliminated daily is 35 percent and the planned maintenance dose is to be 0.25 mg daily, then the loading dose to achieve steady-state levels should be 100/35 times the maintenance dose, or approximately 0.75 mg. Thus,

$$\frac{\text{Loading}}{\text{dose}} = \frac{100}{\substack{\% \text{ of drug eliminated} \\ \text{per dosage interval}}} \times \text{maintenance dose}$$

The fraction of drug eliminated during any dosage interval can be determined from a semilogarithmic graph, in which the total amount in the body at time zero is set at 100 percent and the fraction remaining at the end of 1 half-life is 50 percent.[1] Conversely, if the loading dose is known, the maintenance dose can be similarly calculated.

---

[1] *Alternatively, the fraction of drug lost from the body during a dosage interval can be determined nongraphically from this equation:*

$$\text{Fraction of drug lost from body} = 1 - e^{-kt}$$

Values for e^{-kt} can be obtained from a table of natural exponential functions or by a calculator, where k ($= 0.693/t_{1/2}$) is the fractional elimination constant (described in the next section) and t is the time interval after drug administration.

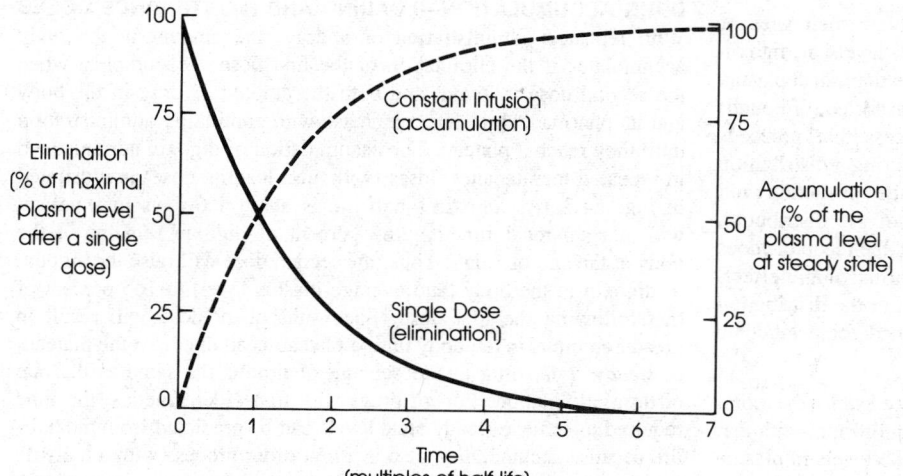

FIGURE 64-3 *The time course of plasma levels of a drug following a single intravenous dose (———) compared with those during a constant intravenous infusion (----). This relationship applies to all drugs that rapidly achieve equilibrium between plasma and tissues.*

Regardless of the size of the loading dose, *after maintenance therapy has been given for 3 to 4 half-lives, the amount of drug in the body is determined by the maintenance dose.* The independence of the plasma levels at steady state from the load is illustrated in Fig. 64-3, which indicates that the elimination of any drug would be practically complete after 3 to 4 half-lives.

DETERMINANTS OF PLASMA LEVELS DURING THE EQUILIBRIUM PHASE

An important determinant of the level of drug in plasma during the equilibrium phase after a single dose is the extent to which the drug is distributed outside the plasma compartment. For example, if the distribution of a 3-mg dose of a large macromolecule is confined to a plasma volume of 3 liters, then the concentration in plasma will be 1 mg per liter. However, if a different drug is distributed so that 90 percent of it leaves the plasma compartment, then only 0.3 mg will remain in the 3-liter plasma volume, and the concentration in plasma will be only 0.1 mg per liter. The extent of extravascular distribution at equilibrium can be expressed by the *apparent volume of distribution*, or V_d. V_d expresses the relationship between the amount of drug in the body and the plasma concentration at equilibrium:

$$V_d = \frac{\text{amount of drug in body}}{\text{plasma concentration}}$$

The amount of drug in the body is expressed as mass (e.g., milligrams), and the plasma concentration is expressed as mass per volume (e.g., milligrams per liter). Thus V_d is a hypothetical volume into which a quantity of drug would distribute if its concentration in the entire volume were the same as that in plasma. Although it is not a real volume, it is an important concept because it determines the fraction of total drug in the plasma and therefore the fraction available to the organs of elimination. An approximation of V_d in the equilibrium phase can be obtained by estimating the concentration of drug in plasma at time zero (Cp_0) by back-extrapolation of the equilibrium phase plot to zero time as illustrated in Fig. 64-1. Then, after intravenous administration when the amount in the body at time zero is the dose, we have

$$V_d = \frac{\text{dose}}{Cp_0}$$

For the administration of the large macromolecule mentioned above, the measured Cp_0 of 1 mg per liter after a 3-mg dose indicates a V_d that is a real volume, the plasma volume. This is the exception, however, for the V_d of most drugs is larger than plasma volume; many drugs are so extensively taken up by cells that cellular levels exceed those in plasma. For such drugs, the hypothetical V_d is large, even greater than the volume of body water. For example, Fig. 64-1 indicates that the Cp_0 obtained by extrapolation after administration of 50 mg lidocaine is 0.42 mg per liter, yielding a V_d of 119 liters.

As elimination is performed largely by the kidney and liver, it is useful to consider the elimination of drugs according to the *clearance* concept. For example, in the kidney, regardless of the extent to which removal of drug is determined by filtration, secretion, or reabsorption, the net result is a reduction of the concentration of drug in plasma as it passes through the organ. The extent to which the concentration is reduced is expressed as the *extraction ratio*, or E, which is constant as long as first-order elimination occurs.

$$E = \frac{C_a - C_v}{C_a}$$

where C_a = arterial plasma concentration
C_v = venous plasma concentration

If the extraction is complete, $E = 1$. If the total plasma flow to the kidneys is Q (mL/min), the total volume of plasma from which drug is completely removed in a unit time (clearance from the body, Cl) is determined as

$$Cl_{renal} = QE$$

If the renal extraction ratio of penicillin is 0.5 and renal plasma flow is 680 mL/min, then penicillin's renal clearance is 340 mL/min. If the extraction ratio is high, as is the case for renal extraction of aminohippurate or hepatic extraction of propranolol, then clearance is a function of organ blood flow.[2]

Clearance from the body is the sum of clearance from all organs of elimination and is the best measure of the efficiency of the elimination processes. If a drug is removed by both the kidney and liver, then

$$Cl = Cl_{renal} + Cl_{hepatic}$$

Thus, if penicillin is eliminated by both renal clearance (340 mL/min) and hepatic clearance (36 mL/min) in a normal individual, total clearance is 376 mL/min. If renal clearance is reduced to half, total clearance is 170 + 36 or 206 mL/min. In anuria, total clearance equals hepatic clearance.

Only the drug in the vascular compartment can be cleared during each passage through an organ. To ascertain the effect of a given plasma clearance by one or more organs on the rate of removal of drug from the body, the clearance must be related to the volume of "plasma equivalents" to be cleared, that is, the volume of distribution. If the volume of distribution is 10,000 mL and clearance is 1000 mL/min, then one-tenth of the drug in the body is eliminated per minute. This fraction, Cl/V_d, is known as a *fractional elimination constant* and is designated as k:

$$k = \frac{Cl}{V_d}$$

If the fraction k is multiplied by the total amount of drug in the body, the actual rate of elimination at any given time can be determined:

$$\text{Rate of elimination} = k \times \text{amount in body} = ClCp$$

This is the general equation for all first-order processes and expresses the fact that rate is proportional to the declining quantity in a first-order process.

As half-life is a temporal expression of the exponential first-order process, half-life ($t_{1/2}$) can be related to k as follows:

$$t_{1/2} = \frac{0.693}{k}$$

Because $k = \dfrac{Cl}{V_d}$

then $t_{1/2} = \dfrac{0.693V_d}{Cl}$

As shown in the section on drug dosage in renal failure, the linear relationship of k to creatinine clearance makes k a useful parameter upon which to estimate changes in drug elimination with reduction in creatinine clearance in renal insufficiency. Half-life is not linearly related to clearance.

The important relationship

$$t_{1/2} = \frac{0.693V_d}{Cl}$$

expresses clearly the influence of both clearance and volume of distribution on half-life. Thus, half-life is shortened when phenobarbital induces the enzymes responsible for hepatic clearance of a drug, and half-life is lengthened when a drug's renal clearance is attenuated in renal failure. Also, the half-life of some drugs is shortened when their volume of distribution is reduced. If, as in the case of cardiac failure, the volume of distribution is reduced at the same time that clearance is reduced, there may be little change in drug half-life to reflect the impaired clearance, but plasma levels will be increased,

---

[2] *When drug is present in the formed elements of blood, then calculation of extraction and clearance from blood is more physiologically meaningful than from the plasma.*

as is the case with lidocaine. In treating patients after an overdose, the effects of hemodialysis on a drug's elimination are dependent on its volume of distribution. When the volume of distribution is large, as with tricyclic antidepressants (V_d of desipramine equals more than 2000 liters), the removal of drug, even with a high-clearance dialyzer, proceeds slowly.

The extent to which a drug is bound to plasma protein also determines the fraction extracted by the organ(s) of elimination. Altered binding changes the extraction ratio significantly, however, only when elimination is limited to the unbound (free) drug in plasma. The extent to which binding influences elimination depends on the relative affinity of the plasma binding versus the affinity of the drug for the extraction process. The high affinity of the renal tubular anion transport system for many drugs leads to extraction of bound and unbound drug, and the efficient process by which the liver removes propranolol extracts most of this highly bound drug from blood.

STEADY STATE With a constant infusion of drug, the infusion rate equals elimination rate at steady state. Therefore,

$$\underset{\text{(amt/unit time)}}{\text{Infusion rate}} = \underset{\text{(amt/vol)}}{Cp} \times \underset{\text{(vol/unit time)}}{\text{Cl}}$$

when the units for amount, volume, and time are consistent.

Thus, if clearance (Cl) is known, the infusion rate to achieve a given plasma level can be calculated. Estimation of drug clearance is discussed in the section on renal disease.

When the dose is given intermittently instead of by infusion, the above relationship between plasma concentration and the dose administered at each dosage interval can be expressed as

$$\text{Dose} = Cp_{av} \times \text{Cl} \times \text{dosage interval}$$

The average plasma concentration (Cp_{av}) implies, as seen in Fig. 64-2, that levels can be higher and lower than the average during the dosage interval.

When a drug is given orally, only a fraction (F) of the administered dose may reach the systemic circulation. This *bioavailability* may reflect a poorly formulated dosage form that fails to disintegrate or dissolve in the gastrointestinal fluids. Regulatory standards have reduced the extent of this problem. Drug interactions also can impair absorption after oral dosing. Bioavailability may also be reduced due to drug metabolism in the gastrointestinal tract and/or the liver during the absorption process, the *first-pass effect*. This is a particular problem for drugs that are extensively extracted by these organs, and considerable interpatient variability often exists in bioavailability. Lidocaine for the control of arrhythmias is not administered orally because of the first-pass effect. Drugs that are injected intramuscularly may also have low bioavailability, e.g., phenytoin. An unexpected drug response should lead to consideration of bioavailability as a possible factor. Calculation of a dosage regimen should be corrected for bioavailability:

$$\underset{\text{dose}}{\text{Oral}} = \frac{Cp_{av} \times \text{Cl} \times \text{dosage interval}}{F}$$

DRUG ELIMINATION THAT IS NOT FIRST-ORDER The elimination of some drugs such as phenytoin, salicylate, and theophylline does not follow first-order kinetics when amounts of drug in the body are in the therapeutic range. For these drugs, the clearance changes as levels in the body fall during elimination or after alterations in dose. This pattern of elimination is said to be *dose-dependent*. Accordingly, the time for the concentration to fall to one-half becomes less as plasma levels fall; this halving time is not truly a half-life, because the term *half-life* applies to first-order kinetics and is a constant. The elimination of phenytoin is dose-dependent, and when very high levels are present (in the toxic range), the halving time may be longer than 72 h, whereas, as the concentration in plasma declines, the clearance increases and the concentration in plasma will halve in 20 to 30 h. When a drug is eliminated by first-order kinetics, the plasma level at steady state is directly related to the amount of the maintenance

dose, and a doubling of the dose should lead to doubling of the steady-state plasma level. However, for drugs with dose-dependent kinetics, increases in the dose may be accompanied by disproportionate increases in plasma level. Thus, if the daily dose of phenytoin is increased from 300 to 400 mg, plasma levels rise by more than 33 percent. The extent of increase is not predictable because of the interpatient variability in the extent to which clearance deviates from first order. Salicylates are also eliminated by dose-dependent kinetics at high plasma levels, and in children particular caution must be taken with the administration of high doses. Ethanol metabolism also is dose-dependent, with obvious implications. The mechanisms involved in dose-dependent kinetics may include the saturation of the rate-limiting step in metabolism or a feedback inhibition of the rate-limiting enzyme by a product of the reaction.

INDIVIDUALIZATION OF DRUG THERAPY

Recognition of factors modifying drug action is essential for therapy that provides optimal benefit and minimal risk to each patient.

ALTERATION OF DRUG DOSAGE IN RENAL DISEASE Where urinary excretion is an important route of elimination, renal failure results in decreased drug clearance and therefore slower removal of the drug from the body, so that administration of the usual dosage leads to greater accumulation and an increased likelihood of toxicity. The goal in such cases is to modify the dosage schedule so that the average drug concentration in the plasma of the patient with renal insufficiency is the same and so that the steady state is reached after a similar time interval as in the patient with normal renal function. This is particularly appropriate for drugs with long half-lives and narrow therapeutic indexes (e.g., digoxin).

One approach is to calculate the *fraction of the normal dose* that is to be given at the usual dosage interval. This fraction can be determined from either drug clearance (Cl) or the fractional rate constant (k), based on the fact that both renal clearance and k are proportional to creatinine clearance (Cl_{cr}). Creatinine clearance is best determined directly. However, serum creatinine (C_{cr}) may be used to estimate the value by the following equation which is applicable to men:

$$Cl_{cr} = \frac{(140 - \text{age}) \times \text{weight (kg)}}{72 \times C_{cr} \text{ (mg/dL)}} \text{ (mL/min)}$$

For women, the value should be reduced to 85 percent of that estimated by this equation. This approach to estimation of Cl_{cr} is invalid in severe renal insufficiency ($C_{cr} > 5$ mg/dL) or with rapidly changing renal function.

The clearance approach Calculation of drug dosage is most accurately based on the clearance of a drug. From data on the clearance of a drug, the dose in renal insufficiency ($Dose_{ri}$) may be calculated as follows:

$$Dose_{ri} = Dose \times \frac{Cl_{ri}}{Cl}$$

where ri = renal insufficiency
   Cl = clearance from the whole body with normal renal function
   Cl_{ri} = clearance from the whole body with renal insufficiency
   Dose = maintenance dose with normal renal function ($Cl_{cr} \sim$ 100 mL/min)

The normal clearance and that in renal impairment can be obtained by employing the data in Table 64-1 in the following equations:

$$Cl = Cl_{renal} + Cl_{nonrenal}$$

$$Cl_{ri} = Cl_{renal} \times \frac{\text{measured } Cl_{cr}}{100 \text{ mL/min}} + Cl_{nonrenal}$$

The Cl_{renal} values in Table 64-1 are those found with $Cl_{cr} = 100$ mL/min, and the renal clearance of drug in renal insufficiency is obtained by multiplying Cl_{renal} by the ratio of measured Cl_{cr} (in milliliters per minute) to 100 mL/min.

For gentamicin, with a normal Cl_{renal} of 78 mL/min and $Cl_{nonrenal}$ of 3 mL/min, Cl = 81 mL/min. Therefore, with a Cl_{cr} of 12 mL/min, Cl_{ri} = 78 × (12/100) + 3 = 12.4 mL/min. If the dose of gentamicin for a given infection should be 1.5 mg/kg per 8 h in the presence of normal renal function, then

$$Dose_{ri} = \frac{1.5 \text{ mg/kg}}{8 \text{ h}} \times \frac{12.4 \text{ mL/min}}{81 \text{ mL/min}} = \frac{0.23 \text{ mg/kg}}{8 \text{ h}}$$

In the patient with renal insufficiency, this computation provides an average plasma level during a dosage interval that is the same as the average plasma level during the dosage interval with normal renal function; the fluctuations between peaks and troughs, however, will be less pronounced.

In some instances it may be desirable to calculate a dose that will yield a certain plasma level at steady state. This approach is most appropriate for constant intravenous infusions where 100 percent of the dose is delivered to the systemic circulation. When clearance of a drug in a patient with renal insufficiency is calculated as above, then

$$\underset{\text{(amt/unit time)}}{Dose_{ri}} = \underset{\text{(vol/unit time)}}{Cl_{ri}} \times \underset{\text{(amt/vol)}}{Cp}$$

where the time, amount, and volume terms are uniform.

If a plasma concentration of carbenicillin of 100 μg/mL is the therapeutic objective in a patient with a creatinine clearance of 25 mL/min, the infusion rate is calculated as follows. Carbenicillin clearance is

$$Cl_{ri} = 68 \times \frac{25}{100} + 10 = 27 \text{ mL/min}$$

Therefore, carbenicillin should be infused at a rate of 2700 μg/min.

Should the method of calculating dose based on the desired plasma level be applied to intermittent-dose therapy, particular attention should be given to the fact that the calculation is based on an *average* plasma level and that peak plasma levels will be higher. In addition, if an oral drug is not completely absorbed, the computed dose must be divided by the fraction (F) that reaches the systemic circulation (see "Steady State" above).

The fractional rate constant (k) approach   For many drugs, clearance data in renal failure are not available. In these cases, the fraction of the normal dose that is required in a patient with renal failure can be approximated from the ratio of the fractional rate constant for elimination from the body in renal failure (k_{ri}) to that with normal renal function (k). This approach requires the assumption that the distribution of the drug (V_d) is not affected by renal disease. The approach is the same as that employed with clearance data:

$$Dose_{ri} = Dose \times \frac{k_{ri}}{k}$$

As the ratio k_{ri}/k is the fraction of the usual dose employed in a given degree of renal insufficiency, it is termed the *dose fraction* and may be estimated from the information in Table 64-2 and the nomogram (Fig. 64-4). Table 64-2 gives the fraction of the usual dose of a drug required at a creatinine clearance of zero (dose fraction$_0$). The nomogram presents the dose fraction as a linear function of creatinine clearance.

To calculate the dose fraction$_{ri}$, the dose fraction$_0$ is obtained from Table 64-2, plotted on the left ordinate of the nomogram, and connected by a straight line to the upper right-hand corner of the nomogram. This line describes the dose fraction over a range of creatinine clearances from 0 to 100 mL/min. The point of intersection between the measured creatinine clearance (on the lower abscissa) and this dose fraction line is a coordinate with the dose fraction (on the left ordinate) corresponding with that particular creatinine clearance. For example, if a patient with a creatinine clearance of 20 mL/min requires penicillin G for an infection that would be treated with

TABLE 64-1   Clearance of drugs

Drug	Renal clearance,* mL/min	Nonrenal clearance, mL/min
Ampicillin†	340	12
Carbenicillin	68	10
Digoxin†	110	36
Gentamicin	78	3
Kanamycin	60	0
Penicillin G‡	340	36

* The "normal" renal clearances are those associated with a clearance of creatinine of 100 mL/min.
† The fraction of digoxin absorbed after an oral dose (F) is approximately 0.75 and F for ampicillin is 0.5.
‡ One microgram of penicillin G = 1.6 units.

10 million units daily in patients with normal renal function, then an appropriate dose would be 2.8 million units daily. This dose is estimated by plotting the dose fraction$_0$ for penicillin G (0.1) on the left-hand ordinate and connecting it to the top right-hand corner of the nomogram (Fig. 64-4). On this dose fraction line for penicillin G, the coordinate for a creatinine clearance of 20 mL/min corresponds on the left ordinate with a dose fraction of 0.28. Hence, the dose is 0.28 × 10 million units daily.

TABLE 64-2   Estimated fraction of usual dose of drug required for a patient with a creatinine clearance of zero (dose fraction$_0$) and average overall fractional elimination rate constant for a patient with normal renal function (k)

Drug	Dose fraction$_0$	k, per hour
ANTIBIOTICS		
Amikacin	0.01	0.4
Amoxicillin	0.15	0.7
Ampicillin	0.1	0.6
Carbenicillin	0.1	0.6
Cephalexin	0.04	0.7
Cephaloridine	0.08	0.4
Cephalothin	0.02	1.4
Cephazolin	0.06	0.35
Chloramphenicol	0.8	0.3
Clindamycin	0.8	0.2
Cloxacillin	0.25	1.2
Colistimethate	0.3	0.2
Dicloxacillin	0.5	1.2
Doxycycline	0.8	0.03
Erythromycin	0.7	0.5
Gentamicin	0.02	0.3
Isoniazid:		
Fast inactivators	0.8	0.5
Slow inactivators	0.5	0.25
Kanamycin	0.03	0.35
Lincomycin	0.4	0.15
Methicillin	0.12	1.4
Minocycline	0.9	0.06
Nafcillin	0.4	1.2
Oxacillin	0.25	1.4
Oxytetracycline	0.2	0.08
Penicillin G	0.1	1.4
Polymyxin B	0.12	0.15
Rifampin	1.0	0.25
Streptomycin	0.04	0.25
Sulfadiazine	0.45	0.7
Sulfamethoxazole	0.85	0.07
Tetracycline	0.12	0.08
Tobramycin	0.02	0.35
Tricarcillin	0.1	0.6
Trimethoprim	0.45	0.06
Vancomycin	0.03	0.12
MISCELLANEOUS DRUGS		
Chlorpropamide	0.4	0.02
Lidocaine	0.9	0.4
Sulfinpyrazone	0.55	0.3
CARDIAC GLYCOSIDES		k, per day
Digitoxin	0.7	0.1
Digoxin	0.3	0.45

The loading dose In addition to adjusting the maintenance dose in renal failure, consideration must also be given to the loading dose. Since this dose is designed to bring the plasma concentration, or more particularly the amount of drug in the body, rapidly to the level at steady state, there is no need to modify the usual loading dose, if one is normally used. The elimination of many drugs is sufficiently rapid that the time required to reach steady state is not significant, and no loading dose is usually used. On the other hand, in renal failure where the half-life may be significantly prolonged, this accumulation period may become unacceptably long. In such a case, a loading dose may be calculated as described in "Drug Accumulation" above for a drug given intermittently. For an infusion, the loading dose may be approximated (when all units are consistent):

$$\text{Loading dose}_{ri} = \frac{\text{infusion rate}_{ri}}{k_{ri}}$$

General considerations for determining dosage in renal insufficiency Because of the differences in volumes of distribution and rates of metabolism, calculations of drug dose in renal failure must be viewed as valuable approximations which prevent the use of doses that are grossly excessive or inadequate for most patients. However, *maintenance dosages are most accurate when plasma level data are employed to enable adjustment of the dose where necessary.*

In all the above calculations, it is assumed that the nonrenal clearance and nonrenal k are constant in renal failure. In fact, when cardiac failure accompanies renal failure, metabolic clearance for many drugs is reduced. Accordingly, when a drug with a narrow therapeutic index, such as digoxin, is used in cardiac failure, an appropriate precaution would be to reduce the value for nonrenal clearance (or k) to about one-half.

Active or toxic metabolites of drugs also may accumulate in renal failure. Meperidine, for example, is cleared largely by metabolism, and its concentration in plasma is little altered by renal insufficiency. However, the plasma concentration of one of its metabolites, normeperidine, is increased when its renal elimination is impaired. As normeperidine has more convulsant activity than meperidine, its accumulation in patients with renal failure probably accounts for the signs of central nervous system excitation such as irritability, twitching, and seizures that result from the administration of multiple doses of meperidine to patients in renal insufficiency.

The metabolite of procainamide, N-acetylprocainamide, has similar cardiac effects to those of the parent drug. As N-acetylprocainamide

is eliminated almost entirely by the kidney, its concentration in plasma is increased by renal failure. Thus, the potential of procainamide to produce toxicity in renal insufficiency cannot be assessed by measuring the plasma concentration of procainamide alone.

LIVER DISEASE In contrast to the predictable decline in renal clearance of drugs when glomerular filtration is reduced, it is not possible to make a general prediction of the effect of liver disease on hepatic biotransformation of drugs (Chap. 243). Rather, in hepatitis and cirrhosis changes may range from impaired to increased drug clearance. Even in advanced hepatocellular disease, the magnitude of impairment in drug clearance usually is only about two- to fivefold. The extent of such changes, however, cannot be predicted by the common tests of liver function. Consequently, even when it is suspected that drug elimination is altered in liver disease, there is no quantitative base upon which to adjust the dosage regimen other than assessment of clinical response and concentration of drug in plasma.

Portacaval shunting creates a special situation because the effective hepatic blood flow is reduced. This situation has its greatest effect on drugs that normally have a high hepatic extraction ratio so that their clearance is largely a function of blood flow; thus the clearance of such drugs (e.g., propranolol and lidocaine) is remarkably reduced by portacaval shunting. In addition, the fraction of an administered oral dose reaching the systemic circulation is increased, because drug that is shunted around the liver during the absorption process escapes the first-pass metabolism by this organ (e.g., meperidine, pentazocine).

CIRCULATORY INSUFFICIENCY—CARDIAC FAILURE AND SHOCK Under conditions of decreased tissue perfusion, redistribution of the cardiac output occurs to preserve blood flow to the heart and brain at the expense of other tissues (Chap. 29). As a result, the drug is distributed into a smaller volume of distribution, higher drug concentrations are present in the plasma, and the tissues are exposed to these higher concentrations. If either the brain or heart is sensitive to the drug, an alteration in response will occur.

Furthermore, the decreased perfusion of the kidney and liver may impair drug clearance by these organs directly or indirectly. Thus, in severe congestive heart failure, in hemorrhagic shock, and in cardiogenic shock, the response to the usual dose of drug may be excessive, and dosage modification may be necessary. For example, the clearance of lidocaine is reduced by about 50 percent in cardiac failure, and therapeutic plasma levels are achieved at infusion rates of only about half of those usually required. In cardiac failure there also is a significant reduction in lidocaine's volume of distribution which results in the requirement of a smaller loading dose. Similar situations are thought to exist for procainamide, theophylline, and possibly quinidine. Unfortunately, predictors of these types of pharmacokinetic alterations are unavailable. Therefore, loading doses should be conservative, and continued therapy should be monitored closely, following clinical indicators of toxicity and plasma levels.

DISEASE-INDUCED CHANGES IN PLASMA BINDING Many drugs circulate in the plasma partly bound to the plasma proteins. Since only the unbound or free drug can distribute to the site of pharmacologic action, the therapeutic response should be related to the free rather than the total circulating plasma drug concentration. In most cases the degree of binding is fairly constant across the therapeutic concentration range so that significant error is not caused by individualizing therapy on the basis of total drug levels in plasma. However, states such as hypoalbuminemia, liver disease, and renal disease can decrease the extent of drug binding, particularly of acidic and neutral drugs, so that at any total plasma level there is a greater concentration of free drug and a risk of increased response and toxicity. Other conditions, e.g., myocardial infarction, surgery, neoplastic disease, rheumatoid arthritis, and burns, that lead to an increased plasma concentration of the acute-phase reactant alpha$_1$-acid glycoprotein have the opposite effect from basic drugs that are bound to this macromolecule. The drugs for which such changes are important are those that are normally highly bound in the plasma (>90 percent)

FIGURE 64-4 *Nomogram for estimation of the dose fraction (k_{ri}/k) in patients with renal insufficiency. The application of the nomogram is described in the text.*

because a small alteration in the extent of binding produces a large change in the amount of drug in the unbound form.

The consequences of these binding changes, particularly with respect to total drug levels, depend on whether the clearance and distribution are dependent on the unbound or total drug. For many drugs, elimination and distribution are largely restricted to the unbound fraction, and therefore a decrease in binding leads to an increase in the clearance and distribution of the drug. The relative magnitudes of these changes are such that the net effect is to shorten the half-life. The appropriate modification of the dosage regimen in conditions with reduced drug binding is simply to administer the usual daily dose of the drug but in divided doses at more frequent intervals. Individualization of therapy can then be based on either the clinical response or the plasma concentration of unbound drug. It is critical that the patient not be titrated into the usual therapeutic range for concentration of *total* drug in plasma since this will lead to excessive response and toxicity.

In the case of drugs bound to alpha$_1$-acid glycoprotein, the disease-induced increase in binding has the opposite effects of reducing the clearance and distribution of drug. Accordingly, constant rate infusion of lidocaine to control arrhythmias after myocardial infarction leads to an accumulation of drug. However, the clearance of unbound and pharmacologically active drug remains essentially unchanged. Again, it is critical that the patient not be dosed on the basis of total drug concentrations in the plasma since this will be associated with subtherapeutic levels of unbound drug.

INTERACTIONS BETWEEN DRUGS

The effect of some drugs can be altered markedly by the administration of other agents. Such interactions can sabotage therapeutic intent by producing excessive drug action (with adverse effects) or decreasing the action of a drug, rendering it ineffective. Drug interactions must be considered in the differential diagnosis of unexpected responses to drugs, recognizing that patients often come to the physician with a legacy of drugs acquired during previous medical experiences. A meticulous drug history will minimize the unknown elements in the therapeutic milieu; it should include examination of the patient's medications and calls to the pharmacist to identify prescriptions, if necessary.

There are two principal types of interactions between drugs. *Pharmacokinetic interactions* result from alteration in the delivery of drugs to their sites of action. *Pharmacodynamic interactions* are those in which the responsiveness of the target organ or system is modified by other agents.

An index of the drug interactions discussed in this chapter is provided in Table 64-3. Included are interactions which have verified significance in patients and a few of such potential danger that cognizance should be taken of experimental data or case reports suggesting their likely occurrence.

I PHARMACOKINETIC INTERACTIONS CAUSING DIMINISHED DRUG DELIVERY

A **Impaired gastrointestinal absorption** Cholestyramine, an ionic exchange resin, binds thyroxine, triiodothyronine, and the cardiac glycosides with sufficiently high affinity to impair their absorption from the gastrointestinal tract. This resin probably also interferes with the absorption of other drugs, and it is safest not to give it within 2 h of their administration. Aluminum ions, present in antacids, form insoluble chelates with the tetracyclines, thereby preventing absorption of these drugs. Ferrous ions similarly block tetracycline absorption. Kaolin-pectin suspensions bind digoxin, and when the drugs are administered together, digoxin absorption is reduced by about one-half. However, when kaolin-pectin is administered 2 h after digoxin, there is no effect on absorption of digoxin.

Ketoconazole is a weak base that dissolves well only at acidic

pH. Thus, histamine-2 antagonists such as cimetidine, by neutralizing gastric pH, impair the dissolution and subsequent absorption of ketoconazole. Oral administration of aminosalicylate interferes with the absorption of rifampin by an unknown mechanism.

Impaired absorption results in reduction in the total amount of drug absorption, with reduced area under the plasma level curve, reduced peak plasma levels, and lower steady-state concentrations of the drug involved.

B **Induction of hepatic drug-metabolizing enzymes** When the elimination of the drug is largely by metabolism, an increase in the rate of metabolism reduces its availability to sites of action. The metabolism of most drugs occurs largely in the liver, because of its mass, high blood flow, and concentration of enzymes that metabolize drugs. The initial step in metabolism of many drugs is executed by a group of mixed-function oxidase isoenzymes in the endoplasmic

TABLE 64-3 Drug interaction index

Drug	Section of chapter describing interaction
Acetohexamide	IIB
Allopurinol	IIA
p-Aminosalicylate	IA
Amiodarone	IIC
Amphetamine	IC
Antidepressants, tricyclic (desipramine, nortriptyline, imipramine, doxepin, protriptyline, amitriptyline)	IC
Aspirin	IIB, III
Azathioprine	IIA
Barbiturates (class)	IB
Bethanidine	IC
Carbamazepine	IB
Chloramphenicol	IIA
Chlorpromazine	IC
Cholestyramine	IA
Cimetidine	IA, IIA, IIB
Clofibrate	IIA
Clonidine	IC
Cyclosporine	IB
Dexamethasone	IB
Dicumarol	IIA, IIB
Digitoxin	IA, IB, IIC
Digoxin	IA, IIC
Disulfiram	IIA
Ephedrine	IC
Ethanol	IIA
Guanethidine	IC
Indomethacin	III
Isoniazid	IIA
Kaolin-pectin	IA
Ketoconazole	IA
Lidocaine	IIA
6-Mercaptopurine	IIA
Methadone	IB
Methotrexate	IIB
Metronidazole	IB, IIA
Metyrapone	IB
Nifedipine	IIA
Nonsteroidal anti-inflammatory drugs	III
Oral contraceptive steroids	IB
Phenobarbital	IB
Phenylbutazone	IIA, IIB
Phenytoin (diphenylhydantoin)	IB, IIA
Piroxicam	III
Potassium	III
Prednisone	IB
Probenicid	IIB
Procainamide	IIB
Propranolol	III
Quinidine	IB, IIA, IIC
Ranitidine	IA, IIA
Rifampin	IA, IB
Salicylate	IIB
Spironolactone	III
Tetracycline	IA
Thiazide diuretics	III
Tolbutamide	IIA
Triamterene	III
Verapamil	IIC
Warfarin	IB, IIA, III

reticulum. These enzyme systems containing cytochrome P_{450} oxidize the molecule by a variety of reactions including aromatic hydroxylations, N-demethylations, O-demethylations, and sulfoxidations. The products of these reactions are usually more polar (and more readily excreted by the kidney).

The biosynthesis of some of the mixed-function oxidase isoenzymes is under regulatory control at the transcriptional level, and their content in the liver can be induced by a number of drugs. Phenobarbital is the prototype of these inducers, and all barbiturates in clinical use increase mixed-function oxidase isoenzymes. Induction with phenobarbital can occur with doses of as little as 60 mg daily. Mixed-function oxidases also are induced by rifampin, carbamazepine, phenytoin, and glutethimide, by occupational exposure to chlorinated insecticides such as DDT, and by chronic alcohol ingestion.

Phenobarbital and other inducers lower plasma levels of many drugs, including warfarin, digitoxin, quinidine, cyclosporine, dexamethasone, prednisolone (the active metabolite of prednisone), oral contraceptive steroids, methadone, metronidazole, and metyrapone. These interactions all have obvious clinical significance. With the coumarin anticoagulants, the patient is placed at major risk when an appropriate level of anticoagulation is achieved while the coumarin drug is coadministered with an inducing agent. Should the inducer then be discontinued, e.g., following discharge from the hospital, plasma levels of the coumarin anticoagulant will rise as the induction effect wears off, leading to excessive anticoagulation. Barbiturates have been shown to lower the plasma levels of phenytoin in some patients, but the clinical effect of reduced phenytoin levels is probably counterbalanced by the anticonvulsant effects of phenobarbital.

There is considerable variation among individuals in the extent to which drug metabolism can be induced. In some patients phenobarbital leads to marked acceleration in the rate of drug metabolism, whereas little induction is seen in others.

In addition to inducing certain of the mixed-function oxidase isoenzymes, phenobarbital has other effects on hepatic function. It increases liver blood flow, bile flow, and the hepatocellular transport of organic anions. The conjugation of drugs and bilirubin may also be enhanced by inducing agents.

C Inhibition of cellular uptake or binding The guanidinium antihypertensives, guanethidine and bethanidine, are transported to their site of action in adrenergic neurons by an energy-requiring membrane transport system for biogenic monoamines. Although the physiologic function of the transport system is reuptake of the adrenergic neurotransmitter, it also transports a variety of ring-substituted bases, including guanethidine and bethanidine, into the adrenergic neuron against a concentration gradient. Inhibitors of norepinephrine uptake prevent the uptake of the guanidinium antihypertensives into adrenergic neurons and thereby block their pharmacologic effects. The tricyclic antidepressants are potent inhibitors of norepinephrine uptake. Consequently, concomitant administration of clinical doses of tricyclic antidepressants including desipramine, protriptyline, nortriptyline, and amitriptyline almost totally abolishes the antihypertensive effects of guanethidine and bethanidine. Although they are less potent inhibitors of norepinephrine uptake, doxepin and chlorpromazine, when given in doses of greater than 100 mg daily, produce dose-related antagonism of the action of the guanidinium antihypertensives. In patients with severe hypertension, the loss of control of blood pressure from these drug interactions can lead to stroke and malignant hypertension.

Amphetamine also antagonizes the antihypertensive effect of guanethidine by displacing it from its site of action within the adrenergic neuron (Chap. 196). Ephedrine, a component of many drug combinations used in asthma, also antagonizes the effect of guanethidine, probably by both inhibition of uptake and displacement from the neuron.

The antihypertensive effect of clonidine is partially antagonized by tricyclic antidepressants. Clonidine lowers arterial pressure by reducing sympathetic outflow from the blood-pressure-regulating centers in the hindbrain (Chap. 196). This central hypotensive action is antagonized by the tricyclic antidepressants.

II PHARMACOKINETIC INTERACTIONS CAUSING INCREASED DRUG DELIVERY

A Inhibition of drug metabolism If the active form of a drug is cleared largely by biotransformation, inhibition of its metabolism leads to a reduced clearance, prolonged half-life, and accumulation of the drug during maintenance therapy. Excessive accumulation due to inhibited metabolism can lead to significant adverse effects.

Cimetidine is a potent inhibitor of the oxidative metabolism of warfarin, quinidine, nifedipine, lidocaine, theophylline, phenytoin, and propranolol. Adverse reactions, many of them severe, have resulted from the administration of these drugs in conjunction with cimetidine. Cimetidine is a more potent inhibitor of mixed-function oxidases than ranitidine, whereas ranitidine is more potent as a histamine-2 antagonist. Thus, ranitidine, when administered in doses of 150 mg twice daily, does not inhibit the oxidative metabolism of most drugs; where reduced drug elimination has been observed, the effects of ranitidine have been less than those of cimetidine and devoid of appreciable pharmacodynamic consequence. Doses of ranitidine higher than 150 mg, however, may produce greater inhibition of drug oxidation.

The metabolism of phenytoin is also inhibited by a number of other drugs. Clofibrate, phenylbutazone, chloramphenicol, dicumarol, and isoniazid can raise the steady-state plasma levels of phenytoin by more than twofold. Impaired metabolism of tolbutamide with severe hypoglycemia has resulted from coadministration of clofibrate, phenylbutazone, and chloramphenicol. Excessive anticoagulation by warfarin may result from inhibition of its metabolism by disulfiram, metronidazole, or phenylbutazone, or by ingestion of ethanol. Warfarin is administered as a racemic mixture, and its $S(-)$ isomer has five times the anticoagulant potency of the $R(+)$ isomer. Phenylbutazone selectively inhibits the metabolism of the $S(-)$ isomer, and only when this isomer is examined specifically can the substantial reduction in its metabolism produced by phenylbutazone be unmasked.

Azathioprine is readily converted in the body to an active metabolite, 6-mercaptopurine, which in turn is oxidized by xanthine oxidase to 6-thiouric acid. When allopurinol, a potent inhibitor of xanthine oxidase, is administered concurrently with standard doses of azathioprine or 6-mercaptopurine, life-threatening toxicity (bone marrow suppression) can result.

B Inhibition of renal elimination A number of drugs are secreted by the renal tubular transport systems for organic anions. Inhibition of this tubular transport system can cause excessive accumulation of a drug. Phenylbutazone, probenecid, salicylates, and dicumarol competitively inhibit this transport system. Salicylate, for example, reduces the renal clearance of methotrexate, an interaction that may lead to methotrexate toxicity. Renal tubular secretion contributes substantially to the elimination of penicillin, which can be inhibited by probenecid.

Inhibition of the tubular cation transport system by cimetidine impedes the renal clearance of procainamide and its active metabolite N-acetylprocainamide.

C Inhibition of clearance by multiple mechanisms The concentrations of digoxin and digitoxin in plasma are elevated by quinidine, due largely to inhibition of renal elimination and in part from inhibition of nonrenal clearance as well. An increase in cardiac arrhythmia may occur when quinidine is given in conjunction with a cardiac glycoside.

Amiodarone and verapamil also increase the concentration of digoxin in plasma.

III PHARMACODYNAMIC AND OTHER INTERACTIONS BETWEEN DRUGS Therapeutically useful interactions occur in which the combined effect of two drugs is greater than that of either drug alone.

These favorable drug combinations are described in specific therapeutic sections in this text, and the following is directed toward those interactions that create unwanted effects. Two drugs may act on separate components of a common process and yield effects greater than either alone. For example, small doses of aspirin (less than 1 g daily) do not alter the prothrombin time appreciably in patients who are on warfarin therapy. However, the addition of aspirin to patients anticoagulated with warfarin increases the risk of bleeding because aspirin inhibits platelet aggregation. Thus the combination of impaired functions of platelets and the clotting system increases the potential for hemorrhagic complications in patients receiving warfarin therapy.

Indomethacin, piroxicam, and probably other nonsteroidal anti-inflammatory drugs antagonize the antihypertensive effects of beta-adrenergic receptor blockers, diuretics, converting enzyme inhibitors, and other drugs. The resultant elevation in blood pressure ranges from trivial to severe. Aspirin and sulindac, however, do not elevate the blood pressure in treated hypertensive patients.

The administration of supplemental potassium leads to more frequent and more severe hyperkalemia when potassium elimination is reduced by concurrent treatment with spironolactone or triamterene.

VARIABLE ACTIONS OF DRUGS CAUSED BY GENETIC DIFFERENCES IN THEIR METABOLISM

ACETYLATION Isoniazid, hydralazine, procainamide, and a number of other drugs are metabolized by acetylation of a hydrazino or amino group. This reaction is catalyzed by *N*-acetyl transferase, an enzyme in the liver cytosol that transfers an acetyl group from acetyl coenzyme A to the drug. Individuals differ markedly in the rate at which drugs are acetylated, and there is a bimodal distribution of the population into "rapid acetylators" and "slow acetylators." The rate of acetylation is under genetic control; rapid acetylation is an autosomal dominant trait.

Responses to hydralazine therapy are dependent upon the acetylation phenotype. The hypotensive effect of hydralazine is greater in patients who acetylate the drug slowly, and the lupus erythematosus-like syndrome produced by hydralazine occurs almost exclusively in those with slow acetylation. Thus it may be of value to know the acetylation phenotype as a predictor of which patients with hypertension might benefit from an increase in the dose of hydralazine above the 200 mg daily that can be safely employed in the population at large.

Acetylation phenotype can be determined by measuring the ratio of acetylated to nonacetylated dapsone or sulfamethazine in plasma or urine following administration of a test dose of these acetylation substrates. The ratio of monoacetyldapsone to dapsone in plasma at 6 h after dapsone administration is less than 0.35 for slow acetylators and greater than 0.35 for rapid acetylators. At 6 h following the administration of sulfamethazine, less than 25 percent of the drug in the plasma is in the acetylated form in slow acetylators (rapid acetylators, more than 25 percent); in the urine collected in the 5- to 6-h interval after administration, less than 70 percent of the drug is in the acetylated form in slow acetylators (rapid acetylators, more than 70 percent).

METABOLISM BY MIXED-FUNCTION OXIDASES In healthy individuals taking no other medications, the major determinant of the rate of metabolism of drugs by the hepatic mixed-function oxidases is genetic. Hepatic endoplasmic reticulum contains a family of cytochrome P_{450} isoenzymes with different substrate specificities. Many drugs undergo oxidative metabolism by more than one isoenzyme, and the steady-state concentrations of such drugs in the plasma is a function of the sum of the activities of these and other metabolizing enzymes. When a drug is metabolized by multiple pathways, the catalytic activities of the participating enzymes are regulated by a number of genes so that the frequency of clearance rates and steady-state concentrations of the drug tend to distribute unimodally within the population. The range of activity may differ markedly (tenfold or more) between different individuals, as is the case for chlorpromazine, and there is no way to make a prior prediction of the rate.

For certain metabolic pathways bimodally distributed activity suggests control by a single gene, and several polymorphisms have been identified. As a result, two phenotypic populations are usually present analogous to the situation with *N*-acetylation (see above). A majority of the population are extensive metabolizers (EM), and a smaller group of individuals of the poor metabolizer phenotype (PM) have an impaired, if not an absent, ability to metabolize the drug. For example, about 8 to 10 percent of whites are unable to form the 4-hydroxy metabolite of the test drug debrisoquin, and this trait is inherited in an autosomal recessive fashion. Importantly, the putatively involved cytochrome P_{450} isoenzyme is also involved in the biotransformation of other drugs whose metabolic fate, therefore, cosegregates with the debrisoquin trait. A similar situation occurs with other oxidative polymorphisms that characterize the metabolism of tolbutamide, mephenytoin, and nifedipine. The situation is further complicated by interethnic differences in the frequency of the polymorphisms. For example, impaired hydroxylation of mephenytoin is present in only 3 to 5 percent of whites, but the incidence is about 20 percent in individuals of Japanese descent; likewise, the frequency of the PM phenotype for debrisoquin hydroxylation appears to decrease as one moves from Western (8 to 10 percent) to Eastern (0 to 1 percent) population groups.

Polymorphisms in drug metabolizing ability may be associated with large differences in the disposition of the drug among individuals, especially when the involved pathway is a major contribution to the overall elimination of the drug. For example, the oral clearance of mephenytoin differs 100- to 200-fold between individuals of the EM and PM phenotypes. As a result, peak plasma concentrations and bioavailability after oral administration may be profoundly increased and the rate of drug elimination decreased in PM individuals. This in turn results in drug accumulation and exaggerated pharmacologic responses, including toxicity, when usual drug dosages are administered to patients with the PM phenotype. Effective individualization of drug therapy is even more critical when using drugs exhibiting polymorphic drug metabolism.

CONCENTRATION OF DRUGS IN PLASMA AS A GUIDE TO THERAPY

Optimal individualization of therapy is assisted by measuring the concentration of certain drugs in plasma. Genetic variation in elimination rates, interactions with other drugs, disease-induced alterations in elimination and distribution, and other factors combine to yield a wide range of plasma levels in patients given the same dose. Furthermore, the problem of noncompliance with prescribed regimens during continuing therapy is an endemic and elusive cause of therapeutic failure (see below). Clinical indicators assist the titration of some drugs into the desired range, and no chemical determination is a substitute for careful observations of the response to treatment. However, the therapeutic and adverse effects are not precisely quantifiable for all drugs, and in complex clinical situations estimates of the action of a drug may be misleading. For example, previously existing neurologic disease may obscure the neurologic consequences of intoxication with phenytoin. Because clearance, half-life, accumulation, and steady-state plasma levels are difficult to predict, the measurement of plasma levels is often useful as a guide to the optimal dose. This is particularly so when there is a narrow range between the plasma levels yielding therapeutic and adverse effects. For drugs having such characteristics, e.g., digoxin, theophylline, lidocaine, aminoglycosides, and anticonvulsants, numerous dosing methods have been developed in an attempt to improve the relationship between dosing, plasma drug concentration, and response. Some of these

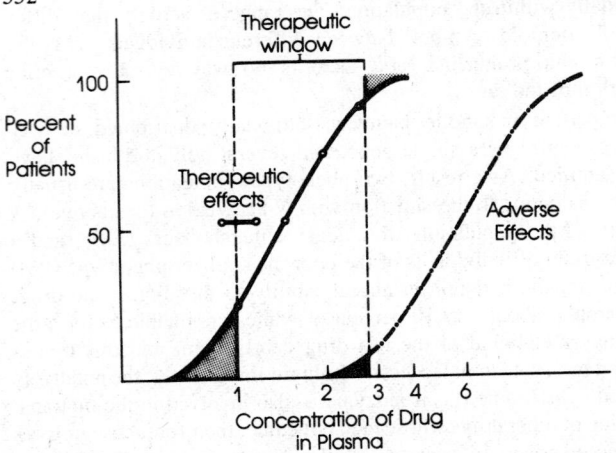

FIGURE 64-5 *The cumulative percentage of patients responding to increasing levels of drug in plasma with both therapeutic and adverse effects. The therapeutic "window" defines the range of concentrations of drug that will achieve therapeutic effects in most patients with adverse effects in only a small percentage.*

methods are accurate and useful, for example, the Bayesian feedback approach, but others are not accurate or have not been sufficiently validated. Further examination of their cost effectiveness is necessary to establish their place in routine patient care.

The variability among individual responses to given plasma levels must be recognized. This is illustrated by a hypothetical population dose-response curve (Fig. 64-5) and its relationship to the therapeutic range or therapeutic "window" of desired plasma levels. The defined therapeutic window should include the levels at which the majority of patients achieve the intended pharmacologic effect. However, a few people are sensitive to the therapeutic effects of most drugs, responding to lower levels, whereas others are sufficiently refractory as to require levels that impose the likelihood of adverse effects as a price for therapeutic benefit. For example, a few patients with strong seizure foci require plasma levels of phenytoin exceeding 20 µg/mL to control seizures. Dosages to achieve this effect may be appropriate.

As also illustrated in Fig. 64-5, some patients are prone to adverse effects at levels that are tolerated by most of the population, and therefore elevation of levels to those with a high probability of therapeutic effect may bring on unwanted actions in the exceptional patient. Table 64-4 presents the concentrations of a number of drugs

TABLE 64-4   Concentrations of drugs in plasma: Relation to efficacy and adverse effects

Drug	Efficacy*	Adverse effects†
Amikacin	20 µg/mL	40 µg/mL
Carbenicillin	100 µg/mL ‡	300 µg/mL
Carbamazepine	3 µg/mL	10 µg/mL
Digitoxin	12 ng/mL	25–30 ng/mL
Digoxin	0.8 ng/mL	2.0 ng/mL
Ethosuximide	40 µg/mL	100 µg/mL
Gentamicin	4 µg/mL §	12 µg/mL
Lidocaine	1.5 µg/mL	5 µg/mL
Lithium	0.5 meq/liter	1.3 meq/liter
Penicillin G	1–25 µg/mL¶	
Phenytoin (diphenylhydantoin)	10 µg/mL	20 µg/mL
Procainamide	4 µg/mL	8 µg/mL
Quinidine	2.5 µg/mL	6 µg/mL
Theophylline	8 µg/mL	20 µg/mL

* *The therapeutic effect is infrequent or slight at levels below these.*
† *The frequency of adverse effects increases sharply when these levels are exceeded.*
‡ *Minimal inhibitory concentration (MIC) for most strains of Pseudomonas aeruginosa. MIC for other, more sensitive, organisms is less.*
§ *Dependent on the MIC. Higher levels (up to 8 µg/mL) may be desired when host defenses are impaired.*
¶ *There is a wide range of MIC of penicillin for various organisms, and the MIC of all those for which penicillin is used is < 20. "Massive" penicillin therapy with 20 million units daily achieves levels of 20 to 25 µg/mL in patients with clearance of creatinine of 100 mL/min.*

in plasma that are associated with adverse and therapeutic effects in most patients. Its use within the guidelines discussed should permit more effective and safer therapy for those patients who are not "average."

EFFECTIVE PARTICIPATION OF THE PATIENT IN THERAPEUTIC PROGRAMS   Measurement of the concentration of a drug in plasma is the most effective approach to determining when patients have failed to take the drug. Such "noncompliance" is a frequent problem in the long-term treatment of diseases such as hypertension and epilepsy, occurring in 25 percent or more of patients in therapeutic environments that lack special efforts to involve patients in the responsibility for their own health. Occasionally, noncompliance can be uncovered by sympathetic, nonincriminating questioning, but more often it is recognized only after determining that the concentration of drug in plasma is nil or is recurrently low. Because other factors can cause plasma levels to be lower than expected, comparison with levels obtained during in-patient treatment may be required to confirm that noncompliance did, in fact, occur. Once the physician is certain of noncompliance, a nonaccusatory discussion of the problem with the patient may elucidate a reason for the noncompliance and serve as a basis for more effective participation of the patient in the care subsequently. Many approaches have been tried to enhance the patients' exercise of responsibility for their own treatment, most based on improved communication regarding the nature of the disease and the expectations of treatment success and treatment failure. This communication includes an opportunity for the patient to relate problems associated with treatment, and it may be improved by involving nurses and other paramedical personnel in the process. Minimizing the complexity of the regimen is helpful, both in terms of the number of drugs and the frequency of administration. Educating patients to assume the principal role in their own health care requires a blend of the art and science of medicine.

REFERENCES

BENET LZ, SHEINER LB: Design and optimization of dosage regimens: Pharmacokinetic data, in *Goodman and Gilman's The Pharmacological Basis of Therapeutics*, 7th ed. AG Gilman et al (eds). New York, Macmillan, 1985, p 1663, Appendix II.

BURTON ME et al: Comparison of drug dosing methods. Clin Pharmacokinet 10:1, 1985

CHENNAVASIN P, BRATER DC: Nomograms for drug use in renal disease. Clin Pharmacokinet 6:193, 1981

DETTLI L: Elimination kinetics and dosage adjustment of drugs in patients with kidney disease. Prog Pharmacol, vol 1, no 4, 1977

SHAND DG et al: Pharmacokinetic drug interactions, in *Handbook of Experimental Pharmacology*, vol 28: *Concepts in Biochemical Pharmacology*, JR Gillette, JR Mitchell (eds). New York, Springer-Verlag, 1975, p 272

SHEINER LB, TOZER TN: Clinical pharmacokinetics: The use of plasma concentrations of drugs, in *Clinical Pharmacology: Basic Principles in Therapeutics*, 2d ed, KL Melmon, HF Morrelli (eds). New York, Macmillan, 1978, p 71

WILKINSON GR, SHAND DG: A physiological approach to hepatic drug clearance. Clin Pharmacol Ther 18:377, 1975

65   ADVERSE REACTIONS TO DRUGS

ALASTAIR J. J. WOOD / JOHN A. OATES

The beneficial effects of drugs are coupled with the inescapable risk that they may also cause untoward effects. The morbidity and mortality that result from these untoward effects often present diagnostic problems, for these drugs can involve every organ and system of the body.

Major advances in the investigation, development, and regulation of drugs ensure in most instances their uniformity, effectiveness, and relative safety, as well as identify their recognized hazards. However, the extremely large number and variety of drugs and drug products available over the counter (OTC) or by prescription from a physician make it impossible for patient or physician to obtain or retain the knowledge necessary to use all these drugs well. It is understandable, therefore, that many OTC drugs are used unwisely by the public and that restricted drugs may be prescribed incorrectly by physicians.

Most physicians use no more than 50 drug products in their practice, gaining familiarity with their effectiveness and safety. Most patients probably use only a limited number of OTC drugs. Nevertheless, many patients receive care and drug prescriptions from more than one physician, and surveys have shown that in any 30-day period patients may consume more than three different OTC drug products containing nine or more different chemical agents.

Twenty-five to fifty percent of patients may make errors in self-administration of prescribed medicines, and this can be responsible for adverse drug effects. Elderly patients are most likely to commit such errors. One-third or more of patients also may not take their prescribed medications. It also seems likely that many patients commit similar errors in taking OTC drugs by not reading or following the directions for use of the medicines provided on the containers. Physicians must recognize that providing directions with prescriptions does not always guarantee their patients' compliance.

Every drug can produce untoward consequences, even when used according to standard or recommended methods of administration. When used incorrectly, the drug's effectiveness may be reduced, or adverse reactions can be expected to occur more frequently. The administration of several drugs during the same period of time also may result in adverse interactions between drugs (see Chap. 64).

In the hospital all the drugs a patient is given should be under the control of a physician, and patient compliance is, in general, ensured. Errors may occur nevertheless, in that the wrong drug or dose may be given, or the drug may be given to the wrong patient, although systems improving drug distribution and administration in hospitals have reduced this problem. On the other hand, there are no means for controlling how ambulatory patients take prescription or OTC drugs.

EPIDEMIOLOGY Epidemiologic studies of adverse drug reactions have been helpful in evaluating the magnitude of the overall problem, in calculating the rate of reactions to individual drugs, and in characterizing some of the determinants of adverse drug effects.

Patients receive on the average 10 different drugs while hospitalized. The sicker the patient, the more drugs are given, and as expected, there is a corresponding increase in the likelihood of adverse drug reactions. When fewer than 6 different drugs are given to hospitalized patients, the probability of an adverse reaction is about 5 percent, but if more than 15 drugs are given, the probability is over 40 percent. Retrospective analysis of ambulatory patients has revealed a history of some adverse drug effects in 20 percent of them.

Thus, the magnitude of the problem posed by drug-induced disease has become exceedingly large. Two to five percent of patients are admitted to the medical and pediatric services of general hospitals because of illnesses attributed to drugs. The case/fatality ratio from drug-induced disease in hospitalized patients varies from 2 to 12 percent. A proportion of fetal or neonatal abnormalities may be due to medicines taken by the mother during pregnancy or parturition.

Women experience twice as many gastrointestinal manifestations of adverse drug effects as do men.

A small group of widely used drugs account for a disproportionate number of reactions. A number of studies have shown that aspirin, digoxin, anticoagulants, diuretics, antimicrobials, steroids, and hypoglycemic agents account for as many as 90 percent of all reactions.

ETIOLOGY Most adverse reactions to drugs may be classified into one of two groups. The most frequent are those that result from the exaggerated but predicted pharmacologic action of the drug. Other adverse reactions ensue from toxic effects on cells that result from mechanisms unrelated to the intended pharmacologic actions. These therefore are often unpredictable, are frequently severe, and result from a number of recognized as well as undiscovered mechanisms. Some of the mechanisms of extrapharmacologic toxicity include direct

cytotoxicity, the initiation of abnormal immune responses, and the perturbation of metabolic processes in individuals rendered susceptible by genetic enzymatic defects.

EXAGGERATION OF THE INTENDED PHARMACOLOGIC EFFECT By prior consideration of the known factors that modify drug action, these adverse reactions often are preventable.

Abnormally high drug concentration at the receptor site (site of action) due to the pharmacokinetic variability discussed in Chap. 64 is the usual cause. For example, reduction in the volume of distribution, in the rate of metabolism, or in the rate of excretion will all result in higher than expected concentration of the drug at the receptor site with consequent increase in pharmacologic effect.

Alteration in the dose-response curve due to increased receptor sensitivity will result in an increase in drug effect at the same concentration. An example of this is seen in the excessive response to the anticoagulant warfarin at normal and lower than normal blood levels in the elderly.

The shape of the dose-response curve itself also determines the likelihood of the development of adverse drug reactions. These drugs with a steep dose-response curve are more likely to be associated with dose-related toxicity because of the small increase in dose required to produce a large change in pharmacologic effect. An increase in the dose of drugs which exhibit nonlinear kinetics, such as phenytoin (see previous chapter), may produce a proportionately greater increase in the blood level, resulting in toxicity.

Concomitant drug therapy may affect the pharmacokinetics or pharmacodynamics of other drugs. Pharmacokinetics may be affected by alterations in bioavailability, protein binding, or the rate of metabolism or excretion. Pharmacodynamics may be altered by competition for receptor sites, by prevention of the drug's reaching its site of action, or by antagonism or enhancement of the drug's pharmacologic effect. These subjects are discussed in detail in the previous chapter.

TOXICITY UNRELATED TO A DRUG'S PRIMARY PHARMACOLOGIC ACTIVITY Cytotoxic reactions Our understanding of these so-called idiosyncratic reactions has greatly improved recently as it has become clear that many of these reactions are due to irreversible binding of drug or metabolites to tissue macromolecules by shared electron (covalent) bonds. Some chemical carcinogens such as the alkylating agents combine directly with DNA. However, it is more commonly only after metabolic activation to chemically reactive metabolites that covalent binding occurs. This metabolic activation usually occurs in the microsomal mixed-function oxidase system, the hepatic enzyme system which is responsible for the metabolism of many drugs (Chap. 64). During the course of drug metabolism by these pathways, reactive metabolites of some drugs may be produced which covalently bind to tissue macromolecules, causing tissue damage. Because of the highly reactive nature of these metabolites, covalent binding often occurs close to the site of production, such as the liver, but the mixed-function oxidase system is found in other tissues as well.

An example of this type of adverse drug reaction is the hepatotoxicity associated with isoniazid, which is metabolized principally by acetylation (Fig. 65-1) to acetylisoniazid, which is then hydrolyzed to acetylhydralazine. The further metabolism of acetylhydralazine by the mixed-function oxidase system liberates reactive metabolites which covalently bind to hepatic macromolecules, causing hepatic necrosis. The administration of drugs known to increase the activity of the mixed-function oxidase system, such as phenobarbital or rifampin, together with isoniazid, is associated with the production of increased amounts of reactive metabolites, increased covalent binding, and hepatic damage.

The hepatic necrosis produced by overdosage of acetaminophen is caused by the covalent binding of reactive electrophilic metabolites to hepatic macromolecules. Normally these reactive metabolites are detoxified by combining with hepatic glutathione. When glutathione becomes exhausted, the metabolites bind instead to hepatic macromolecules with resultant hepatocyte damage. The hepatic necrosis produced by the ingestion of large quantities of acetaminophen can be prevented, or at least attenuated, by the administration of substances such as N-acetylcysteine, which reduce the binding of electrophilic metabolites to hepatic proteins with resultant hepatic necrosis. The risks of hepatic necrosis are increased in patients also receiving drugs such as phenobarbital which increase the rate of drug metabolism and rate of production of toxic metabolite(s).

It is likely, though as yet unproved, that other idiosyncratic reactions are caused by the covalent binding of reactive metabolites to tissue macromolecules, with either direct cytotoxicity or via the initiation of an immunologic response.

Immunologic mechanisms Most pharmacologic agents are poor immunogens since they consist of small molecules with molecular weights less than 2000. Stimulation of antibody synthesis or sensitization of lymphocytes by a drug or one of its metabolites usually requires in vivo activation and covalent linkage to protein, carbohydrate, or nucleic acid.

Drug stimulation of antibody production may mediate tissue injury by one of several mechanisms. The antibody may attack the drug affixed to a cell by covalent linkage and thereby destroy the cell, as occurs in penicillin-induced hemolytic anemia. Complexes of antibody-drug-antigen may be passively adsorbed by a bystander cell which is destroyed by activation of complement; this occurs in quinine- and quinidine-induced thrombocytopenia. Drugs or their reactive metabolites may alter host tissue, rendering it antigenic, and stimulate autoantibodies; for example, hydralazine and procainamide can chemically alter nuclear material, stimulate formation of antinuclear antibodies, and occasionally cause lupus erythematosus. Autoantibodies may be stimulated by drugs which neither interact with the host antigen nor have any chemical similarity to the host tissue; for example, alpha methyldopa frequently stimulates formation of antibodies to host erythrocytes, yet the drug does not itself attach to the erythrocyte or share any chemical similarities with the antigenic determinants on the erythrocyte.

Serum sickness (Chap. 260) results from deposition of circulating drug-antibody complexes on endothelial surfaces. Complement activation occurs, chemotactic factors are generated locally, and an inflammatory response appears at the site of complex entrapment. Arthralgias, lymphadenopathy, glomerulonephritis, or cerebritis may result. Penicillin is the most common cause of serum sickness today. Many drugs, particularly the antimicrobial agents, induce production of IgE, which affixes to mast cell membranes. Contact with a drug antigen initiates a series of biochemical events within the mast cell and results in the release of mediators which may produce urticaria,

wheezing, rhinorrhea, and occasionally hypotension characteristic of anaphylaxis.

Drugs may also excite cell-mediated immune responses. Topically administered substances may interact with sulfhydryl or amino groups in the skin and react with sensitized lymphocytes to produce the rash characteristic of contact dermatitis. Other types of rashes may also appear from the interaction of serum factors, drugs, and sensitized lymphocytes. The role of drug-activated lymphocytes in the immune mechanisms governing destruction of visceral tissue is unknown.

Toxicity associated with genetically determined enzymatic defects In the porphyrias, drugs which increase the activity of enzymes proximal to the deficient enzyme in the biosynthetic pathway of porphyrins can increase the quantity of porphyrin precursors that accumulate proximal to the deficient enzyme (Chap. 312). These drugs are listed in Table 65-1.

Patients with a deficiency of glucose 6-phosphate dehydrogenase (G6PD) will develop hemolytic anemia on primaquine and a number of other drugs (Table 65-1) which do not cause hemolysis in patients who have adequate quantities of this enzyme (Chap. 287).

Diagnosis The manifestations of drug-induced diseases frequently resemble those associated with other diseases and may be produced by different and dissimilar drugs. Recognition of the role of a drug or drugs responsible for illness is dependent upon appreciation of the possible implication of adverse reactions to drugs in any disease, identification of a temporal relationship between drug administration and development of illness, and familiarity with the manifestations most often caused by particular drugs. Although specific reactions have been described as resulting from the use of particular drugs, there is always a "first," and any drug should be suspected of causing an adverse effect if the clinical setting is appropriate.

Illness related to a drug's pharmacologic action may be more easily recognized than illness attributable to immunologic or other mechanisms. For example, side effects such as cardiac arrhythmias in patients receiving digitalis, hypoglycemia in patients given insulin, and bleeding in patients receiving anticoagulants are more easily related to the prescribed drug than are symptoms like fever or rash, which may be caused by many drugs or by other factors.

Once an adverse reaction is suspected, discontinuance of the suspected drug followed by disappearance of the reaction is presumptive evidence of a drug-induced illness. Reappearance of the reaction upon cautious readministration of the drug may provide confirmatory evidence of the relationship if such confirmation adds useful information to the future management of the patient without entailing undue risk. With concentration-dependent adverse reactions, lowering the dosage may also be followed by disappearance of the reaction, and increasing the dose may cause it to reappear. When the reaction is thought to be allergic, however, readministration of the drug may be hazardous, since anaphylactic shock may develop. Readministration is unwise under these conditions unless alternate drugs are not available and treatment is mandatory.

If the patient is receiving many different drugs when an adverse reaction is suspected, the drugs most likely to be incriminated can usually be identified. All drugs may be discontinued at once, or if this is not practical, then drugs should be discontinued one at a time, starting with the drug under greatest suspicion, and the patient observed for signs of improvement. It must be remembered that the time taken for the disappearance of a concentration-dependent adverse effect will depend on the time taken for the concentration to fall below the range associated with the adverse effect, and this in turn will depend on the initial blood level and on the rate of elimination or metabolism of the drug. Adverse effects of drugs such as phenobarbital which have long half-lives will take a considerable time to disappear.

To assist in the identification of adverse reactions, a table of the drugs recognized as producing a number of reactions appears in this chapter (Table 65-1). This table is not intended to be exhaustive but rather includes well-documented reactions and some less well-

FIGURE 65-1 *Biotransformation of isoniazid to a hepatotoxic metabolite.*

TABLE 65-1 Clinical manifestations of adverse reactions to drugs

I Multisystem
  A Fever
    Penicillins
    Novobiocin
    p-Aminosalicylic acid
    Amphotericin B
    Antihistamines
    Cephalosporins
    Barbiturates
    Phenytoin
    Quinidine
    Sulfonamides
    Iodides
    Thiouracil
    Phenolphthalein
    Methyldopa
    Asparaginase
    Bleomycin
    Procainamide
  B Drug-induced lupus erythematosus
    Acebutolol
    Hydralazine
    Procainamide
    Isoniazid
  C Serum sickness
    Aspirin
    Penicillins
    Streptomycin
    Sulfonamides
    Propylthiouracil
  D Anaphylaxis
    Bromsulfophthalein
    Penicillins
    Cephalosporins
    Streptomycin
    Dextran
    Iron dextran
    Procaine
    Insulin
    Demeclocycline
    Iodinated drugs or contrast media
    Lidocaine
II Endocrine
  A Disorders of thyroid function tests
    Oral contraceptives
    Bromsulfophthalein
    Phenindione
    Iodides
    Tolbutamide
    Chlorpropamide
    Lithium
    Acetazolamide
    Gold salts
    Dimercaprol
    Clofibrate
    Phenothiazines (long-term)
    Phenylbutazone
    Sulfonamides
    Phenytoin
  B Addisonian-like syndrome
    Busulfan
  C Gynecomastia
    Estrogens
    Testosterone
    Spironolactone
    Digitalis
    Reserpine
    Methyldopa
    Isoniazid
    Ethionamide
    Griseofulvin
  D Galactorrhea (may also cause amenorrhea)
    Methyldopa
    Phenothiazines
    Reserpine
    Tricyclic antidepressants
    Dexamphetamine
  E Sexual dysfunction
    1 Impaired ejaculation
      Guanethidine
      Debrisoquin
      Bethanidine
      Thioridazine
    2 Decreased libido and impotence
      Oral contraceptives
      Sedatives
      Major tranquilizers
      Lithium

      Methyldopa
      Clonidine
III Metabolic
  A Hyponatremia
    1 Dilutional
      Vincristine
      Cyclophosphamide
      Chlorpropamide
      Diuretics
    2 Salt wasting
      Diuretics
      Corticosteroid (withdrawal)
      Enemas
      Mannitol
  B Hyperkalemia
    Spironolactone
    Triamterene
    Amiloride
    Cytotoxics
    Corticosteroid (withdrawal)
    Succinylcholine
    Digitalis overdose
    Potassium salts of drugs
    Potassium preparations including salt substitute
    Lithium
  C Hypokalemia
    Diuretics
    Laxative abuse
    Corticosteroids
    Amphotericin B
    Alkali-induced alkalosis
    Insulin
    Osmotic diuretics
    Carbenoxolone
    Gentamicin
    Degraded tetracycline
    Vitamin B_{12}
  D Metabolic acidosis
    Paraldehyde (degraded)
    Phenformin
    Acetazolamide
    Spironolactone
    Salicylates
  E Hypercalcemia
    Antacids with absorbable alkali
    Vitamin D
    Thiazides
  F Hyperuricemia
    Thiazides
    Chlorthalidone
    Ethacrynic acid
    Furosemide
    Aspirin
    Cytotoxics
    Hyperalimentation
    Fructose (IV)
  G Hyperglycemia
    Corticosteroids
    Oral contraceptives
    Chlorthalidone
    Ethacrynic acid
    Thiazides
    Furosemide
    Diazoxide
    Growth hormone
  H Porphyria exacerbation
    Barbiturates
    Chlordiazepoxide
    Meprobamate
    Sulfonamides
    Estrogens
    Oral contraceptives
    Chlorpropamide
    Phenytoin
    Glutethimide
    Griseofulvin
    Rifampin
  I Hyperbilirubinemia
    Rifampin
    Novobiocin
IV Dermatologic
  A Exfoliative dermatitis
    Penicillins
    Sulfonamides
    Barbiturates
    Phenytoin
    Phenylbutazone
    Gold salts

    Quinidine
  B Toxic epidermal necrolysis (bullous)
    Barbiturates
    Phenylbutazone
    Phenytoin
    Sulfonamides
    Phenolphthalein
    Penicillins
    Allopurinol
    Iodides
    Bromides
    Nalidixic acid
  C Erythema multiforme or Steven-Johnson syndrome
    Sulfonamides
    Barbiturates
    Phenylbutazone
    Chlorpropamide
    Thiazides
    Sulfones
    Phenytoin
    Ethosuximide
    Salicylates
    Tetracyclines
    Codeine
    Penicillins
  D Erythema nodosum
    Penicillins
    Sulfonamides
    Oral contraceptives
  E Fixed drug eruptions
    Phenolphthalein
    Barbiturates
    Sulfonamides
    Salicylates
    Phenylbutazone
    Quinine
    Captopril
  F Photodermatitis
    Tetracyclines, particularly demeclocycline
    Griseofulvin
    Sulfonamides
    Sulfonylureas
    Thiazides
    Furosemide
    Phenothiazines
    Nalidixic acid
    Oral contraceptives
    Chlordiazepoxide
  G Urticaria
    Aspirin
    Penicillins
    Sulfonamides
    Barbiturates
  H Nonspecific rashes
    Ampicillin
    Barbiturates
    Allopurinol
    Phenytoin
    Methyldopa
  I Pigment changes (hyperpigmentation)
    ACTH
    Busulfan
    Phenothiazines
    Hypervitaminosis A
    Oral contraceptives
    Gold salts
    Chloroquine and other antimalarials
    Cyclophosphamide
    Bleomycin
  J Alopecia
    Cytotoxics
    Ethionamide
    Heparin
    Oral contraceptives (withdrawal)
  K Purpura (see also thrombocytopenia)
    Corticosteroids
    Aspirin
  L Lichenoid eruptions
    Chlorpropamide
    Gold salts
    Antimalarials
    PAS
    Methyldopa
    Phenothiazines
  M Eczema (contact dermatitis)
    Topical antimicrobials
    Topical local anesthetics
    Topical antihistamines

Cream and lotion preservatives
Lanolin
N Acne
Anabolic and androgenic steroids
Corticosteroids
Bromides
Iodides
Oral contraceptives
Isoniazid
Troxidone

V *Hematologic*
A Pancytopenia (aplastic anemia)
Chloramphenicol
Phenytoin
Mephenytoin
Trimethadione
Phenylbutazone
Oxyphenbutazone
Gold salts
Mepacrine
Quinacrine
Potassium perchlorate
Sulfonamides
Cytotoxics
B Agranulocytosis (see also pancytopenia)
Chloramphenicol
Sulfonamides
Phenylbutazone
Oxyphenbutazone
Gold salts
Indomethacin
Propylthiouracil
Methimazole
Carbimazole
Phenothiazines
Cytotoxics
Tolbutamide
Cotrimoxazole
Tricyclic antidepressants
Captopril
C Thrombocytopenia platelet dysfunction
(see also pancytopenia)
Quinidine
Quinine
Furosemide
Chlorthalidone
Thiazides
Gold salts
Cotrimoxazole
Aspirin
Indomethacin
Phenylbutazone
Oxyphenbutazone
Chlorpropamide
Acetazolamine
Phenytoin and other hydantoins
Methyldopa
Carbamazepine
Digitoxin
Novobiocin
Carbenacillin
D Megaloblastic anemia
Folate antagonists
Cotrimoxazole
Phenytoin
Primidone
Phenobarbital
Triamterene
Trimethoprim
Oral contraceptives
E Hemolytic anemia
Methyldopa
Levodopa
Mefenamic acid
Melphalan
Isoniazid
Rifampin
Sulfonamides
Penicillins
Cephalosporins
Insulin
Quinidine
Chlorpromazine
Phenacetin
p-Aminosalicylic acid
Dapsone
Procainamide
F Hemolytic anemia (in G6PD deficiency)
Antimalarials, e.g., primaquine

Chloramphenicol
Dapsone
Nalidixic acid
Nitrofurantoin
Sulfonamides
Aspirin
Phenacetin
p-Aminosalicylic acid
Quinidine
Vitamin C
Vitamin K
Cotrimoxazole
Probenecid
Procainamide
G Lymphadenopathy
Phenytoin
Primidone
H Leukocytosis
Lithium
Corticosteroids
I Eosinophilia
Erythromycin estolate
Sulfonamides
Chlorpropamide
p-Aminosalicylic acid
Imipramine
Nitrofurantoin
Procarbazine
Methotrexate

VI *Cardiovascular*
A Exacerbation of angina
Vasopressin
Oxytocin
Ergotamine
Methysergide
Propranolol withdrawal
Excessive thyroxin
Alpha blockers
Hydralazine
B Cardiomyopathy
Emetine
Sympathomimetics
Phenothiazines
Lithium
Sulfonamides
Daunorubicin
Adriamycin
C Pericarditis
Procainamide
Hydralazine
Methysergide
Emetine
D Fluid retention or congestive heart failure
Estrogens
Steroids
Carbenoxolone
Phenylbutazone
Indomethacin
Propranolol
Mannitol
Diazoxide
Minoxidil
Verapamil
E Arrhythmias
Sympathomimetics
Thyroid hormone
Digitalis
Quinidine
Procainamide
Verapamil
Atropine
Propranolol
Guanethidine
Emetine
Propellants in aerosols
Tricyclic antidepressants
Phenothiazines, particularly thioridazine
Lithium
Anticholinesterases
Papaverine
Daunomycin
Adriamycin
Lincomycin (intravenous)
F Hypotension (see also arrythmias)
Nitroglycerin
Phenothiazines
Morphine
Diuretics
Citrated blood

Levodopa
Nifedipine
Verapamil
G Hypertension
Oral contraceptives
Sympathomimetics
Clonidine withdrawal
Monoamine oxidase inhibitors with sympathomimetics
Tricyclic antidepressants with sympathomimetics
Corticosteroids
ACTH
Phenylbutazone
H Thromboembolism
Oral contraceptives

VII *Respiratory*
A Nasal congestion
Reserpine
Guanethidine
Isoproterenol
Oral contraceptives
Decongestant abuse
B Respiratory depression
Aminoglycosides
Polymixins
Trimethaphan
Opiates
Sedatives
Hypnotics
C Airway obstruction (bronchospasm, asthma;
see also anaphylaxis)
Beta blockers
Nonsteroidal anti-inflammatory drugs,
e.g., aspirin, indomethacin
Cholinergic drugs
Tartrazine (drugs with yellow dye)
Penicillins
Cephalosporins
Streptomycin
Pentazocine
D Pulmonary infiltrates
Amiodarone
Nitrofurantoin
Methysergide
Bleomycin
Chlorambucil
BCNU
Procarbazine
Busulfan
Melphalan
Cyclophosphamide
Azothioprine
Methotrexate
Mitomycin C
Sulfonamides
E Pulmonary edema
Heroin
Methadone
Hydrochlorthiazide
Propoxyphene
Contrast media

VIII *Gastrointestinal*
A Dental discoloration
Tetracycline
B Gingival hyperplasia
Phenytoin
C Oral ulceration
Aspirin
Isoproterenol (sublingual)
Cytotoxics
Pancreatin
Gentian violet
D Taste disturbances
Penicillamine
Biguanides
Griseofulvin
Metronidazole
Lithium
Rifampin
Captopril
E Dry mouth
Anticholinergics
Levodopa
Tricyclic antidepressants
Clonidine
Methyldopa
F Swelling of salivary gland
Phenylbutazone

Guanethidine
Bethanidine
Bretylium
Clonidine
Iodides
G Peptic ulceration or hemorrhage
  Aspirin
  Phenylbutazone
  Indomethacin
  Ethacrynic acid
  Reserpine (large doses)
H Intestinal ulceration
  Enteric-coated potassium chloride
I Nausea or vomiting
  Digitalis
  Opiates
  Estrogens
  Levodopa
  Potassium chloride
  Ferrous sulfate
  Aminophylline
  Tetracyclines
J Diarrhea or colitis
  Lincomycin
  Clindamycin
  Broad-spectrum antibiotics
  Magnesium in antacids
  Guanethidine
  Debrisoquin
  Methyldopa
  Reserpine
  Digitalis
  Colchicine
  Purgatives
  Lactose excipients
K Constipation or ileus
  Ganglionic blockers
  Tricyclic antidepressants
  Phenothiazines
  Opiates
  Aluminum hydroxide
  Calcium carbonate
  Barium sulfate
  Ion exchange resins
  Ferrous sulfate
L Malabsorption
  Broad-spectrum antibiotics
  Neomycin
  Cholestyramine
  Colchicine
  p-Aminosalicylic acid
  Biguanides
  Phenytoin
  Primidone
  Phenobarbital
  Cytotoxics
M Pancreatitis
  Corticosteroids
  Thiazides
  Azathioprine
  Oral contraceptives
  Sulfonamides
  Opiates
  Furosemide
  Ethacrynic acid
N Diffuse hepatocellular damage
  Halothane
  Methoxyflurane
  Methyldopa
  Isoniazid
  Rifampin
  Aminosalicylic acid
  Ethionamide
  Phenytoin and other hydantoins
  Acetaminophen (paracetamol)
  Salicylates
  Allopurinol
  Sulfonamides
  Tetracyclines
  Erythromycin estolate
  Ketoconazole
  Propylthiouracil
  Methimazole
  Oxyphenisatin
  Methotrexate
  Pyridium
  Propoxyphene
  Monoamine oxidase inhibitors
  Sodium valproate

Nitrofurantoin
Aprindine
O Cholestatic jaundice
  Phenothiazines
  Androgens
  Anabolic steroids
  Oral contraceptives
  Erythromycin estolate
  Chlorpropamide
  Gold salts
  Methimazole
  Acetohexamide
  Nitrofurantoin
IX Renal
A Nephrotic syndrome
  Penicillamine
  Gold salts
  Phenindione
  Probenecid
  Captopril
B Tubular necrosis
  Amphotericin B
  Aminoglycosides
  Polymixins
  Cephaloridine
  Tetracyclines
  Colistin
  Sulfonamides
  Radioiodinated contrast medium
  Methoxyflurane
  Cyclosporin
C Interstitial nephritis
  Penicillins, particularly methicillin
  Sulfonamides
  Phenindione
  Furosemide
  Thiazides
  Allopurinol
D Nephropathies
  Due to analgesics (e.g., phenacetin)
E Concentrating defect with polyuria (or
  nephrogenic diabetes insipidus)
  Vitamin D
  Lithium
  Demeclocycline
  Methoxyflurane
F Renal tubular acidosis
  Degraded tetracycline
  Amphotericin B
  Acetazolamide
G Calculi
  Acetazolamide
  Vitamin D
H Obstructive uropathy
  Intrarenal: cytotoxics
  Extrarenal: methysergide
I Hemorrhagic cystitis
  Cyclophosphamide
J Bladder dysfunction
  Anticholinergics
  Monoamine oxidase inhibitors
  Tricyclic antidepressants
  Disopyramide
X Genital (see also endocrine)
A Vaginal carcinoma
  Diethylstilbestrol (administered to mother)
B Impairment of spermatogenesis or oogenesis
  Cytotoxics
XI Neurologic
A Peripheral neuropathy
  Isoniazid
  Hydralazine
  Nitrofurantoin
  Vincristine
  Mustine
  Streptomycin
  Polymyxin, colistan
  Clioquinol
  Phenelzine
  Tricyclic antidepressants
  Chloramphenicol
  Procarbazine
  Ethambutol
  Ethionamide
  Glutethimide
  Demeclocycline
  Nalidixic acid
  Tolbutamide
  Chlorpropamide

Methysergide
Phenytoin
Metronidazole
Clofibrate
Chloroquine
Perhexiline
Disopyramide
B Exacerbation of myasthenia
  Aminoglycosides
  Polymixins
C Extrapyramidal effects
  Butyrophenones, e.g., haloperidol
  Phenothiazines
  Tricyclic antidepressants
  Methyldopa
  Levodopa
  Reserpine
  Metoclopramide
  Oral contraceptives
D Seizures
  Amphetamines
  Analeptics
  Phenothiazines
  Isoniazid
  Lidocaine
  Theophylline
  Penicillins
  Nalidixic acid
  Physostigmine
  Tricyclic antidepressants
  Vincristine
  Lithium
E Stroke
  Oral contraceptives
F Pseudotumor cerebri (or intracranial
  hypertension)
  Corticosteroids
  Oral contraceptives
  Tetracyclines
  Hypervitaminosis A
G Headache
  Hydralazine
  Bromides
  Glyceryl trinitrate
  Ergotamine (withdrawal)
  Indomethacin
XII Ocular
A Corneal opacities
  Vitamin D
  Mepacrine
  Chloroquine
  Indomethacin
B Corneal edema
  Oral contraceptives
C Cataracts
  Phenothiazines
  Corticosteroids
  Busulfan
  Chlorambucil
D Glaucoma
  Mydriatics
  Sympathomimetics
E Retinopathy
  Chloroquine
  Phenothiazines
F Optic neuritis
  Clioquinol
  Chloramphenicol
  Streptomycin
  Isoniazid
  Ethambutol
  Quinine
  Phenothiazines
  Penicillamine
  PAS
  Phenylbutazone
G Alteration in color vision
  Troxidone
  Sulfonamides
  Streptomycin
  Methaqualone
  Barbiturates
  Digitalis
  Thiazides
XIII Ear
A Vestibular disorders
  Aminoglycosides
  Quinine
  Mustine

B Deafness	Amphetamines	E Delirious or confusional states
Aminoglycosides	Lysergic acid	Digitalis
Ethacrynic acid	Levodopa	Anticholinergics
Furosemide	Tricyclic antidepressants	Bromides
Quinine	Monoamine oxidase inhibitors	Sedatives and hypnotics
Bleomycin	Bromides	Phenothiazines
Chloroquine	Corticosteroids	Antidepressants
Mustine	B Depression	Corticosteroids
Aspirin	Centrally acting antihypertensives	Isoniazid
Nortriptyline	(reserpine, methyldopa, clonidine)	Levodopa
XIV Musculoskeletal	Propranolol	Amantadine
A Myopathy or myalgia	Corticosteroids	Penicillins
Corticosteroids	Amphetamine withdrawal	Aminophylline
Chloroquine	Levodopa	Methyldopa
Clofibrate	C Hypomania, mania, or excited reactions	F Sleep disturbances
Oral contraceptives	Levodopa	Anorexiants
Amphotericin B	Sympathomimetics	Levodopa
Carbenoxolone	Corticosteroids	Monoamine oxidase inhibitors
B Bone disorders	MAO inhibitors	Sympathomimetics
1 Osteoporosis	Tricyclic antidepressants	G Drowsiness
Corticosteroids	D Hallucinatory states	Anxiolytic drugs
Heparin	Amantadine	Major tranquilizers
2 Osteomalacia	Narcotics	Tricyclic antidepressants
Anticonvulsants	Pentazocine	Antihistamines
Glutethimide	Propranolol	Methyldopa
Aluminum hydroxide	Levodopa	Clonidine
XV Psychiatric disorders	Tricyclic antidepressants	Reserpine
A Schizophrenic-like or paranoid reactions	Meperidine	

documented reactions which are sufficiently devastating as to require their consideration. It should be used to suggest the likely causative drug, but the absence of a drug from the table should not be interpreted to mean that it is not responsible for the reaction.

Serum antibody has been demonstrated in some persons with drug allergy involving cellular blood elements, as in agranulocytosis, hemolytic anemia, and thrombocytopenia. For example, both quinine and quinidine can produce platelet agglutination in vitro in the presence of complement and the serum from a patient who has developed thrombocytopenia following this drug.

Eliciting a drug history from patients is important for diagnosis. Attention must be directed to nonprescription, or OTC, as well as to prescription drugs. Each type can be responsible for adverse drug effects, and frequently adverse interactions occur between drugs purchased by patients over the counter and those prescribed by physicians. In addition, it is common for patients to be cared for by several physicians; and duplicative, additive, counteractive, or synergistic drugs may therefore be taken if the physicians are not aware of the patients' drug histories. Every physician should determine what drugs a patient has been taking, at least during the preceding 30 days, before prescribing any medications. A history of previous adverse drug effects in patients is common. Since these patients have a predisposition to other drug-induced illnesses, familiarity with such a history should dictate added caution in prescribing drugs.

Patients with biochemical abnormalities such as erythrocyte G6PD deficiency can be identified; patients with the defect are usually blacks or of Mediterranean descent. Drug-induced hemolytic crisis can be avoided by testing for the enzyme defect before administering these drugs. Similarly, persons with an abnormal serum pseudocholinesterase may have abnormally prolonged apnea when given succinylcholine.

General comments No drug is completely without side effects, and it is important to remember that a side effect in one patient may be the desired pharmacologic effect in another. Recent improvements in drug regulation allow physicians to prescribe drugs with considerable confidence in their purity, bioavailability, and effectiveness. However, while regulatory bodies try to ensure that drugs with serious toxic potential are not marketed, they have to constantly weigh the potential toxicity against the possible benefits. Thus toxicity which would be acceptable for an effective antineoplastic agent would not be permitted in, for example, an oral contraceptive. In addition, because of the necessarily small number of patients treated in premarketing studies, rare adverse reactions cannot be identified, so that the first responsibility for identifying and reporting these effects

must rest with the practicing clinician through the use of the various national adverse reaction reporting systems, such as those operated by the Food and Drug Administration in the United States and the Committee on Safety of Medicines in Great Britain. The publication of a newly recognized adverse reaction can in a short time stimulate a very large number of similar such reports which previously had gone unrecognized.

The prevention of adverse drug reactions must first involve a high index of suspicion that the development of a new symptom or sign may be drug-related. Reduction of the dose or discontinuation of the suspected agent will usually clarify the position in concentration-dependent toxic reactions. Physicians should be familiar with the common adverse effects of the drugs they use and, if they are in doubt, should consult the literature.

REFERENCES

DAVIES DM: *Textbook of Adverse Drug Reactions,* 2d ed. New York, Oxford University Press, 1981

GOLDSTEIN RA: Drug allergy: Prevention, diagnosis, and treatment. Ann Intern Med 100:302, 1984

ROSSI AC, KNATT D: Discovery of new adverse drug reactions. JAMA 252:1030, 1984

STEEL K et al: Iatrogenic illness on a general medical service at a university hospital. N Engl J Med 304:398, 1981

TIMBRELL JA: Drug hepatotoxicity. Br J Clin Pharmacol 15:3, 1983

66 PHYSIOLOGY AND PHARMACOLOGY OF THE AUTONOMIC NERVOUS SYSTEM

LEWIS LANDSBERG / JAMES B. YOUNG

FUNCTIONAL ORGANIZATION OF THE AUTONOMIC NERVOUS SYSTEM

The autonomic nervous system innervates vascular and visceral smooth muscle, exocrine and endocrine glands, and parenchymal cells throughout the various organ systems. Functioning below the conscious level, the autonomic nervous system responds rapidly and continuously to perturbations that threaten the constancy of the internal environment. The many functions governed by this system include the distribution of blood flow and the maintenance of tissue perfusion, the regulation of blood pressure, the regulation of the volume and composition of the extracellular fluid, the expenditure of metabolic energy and supply of substrate, and the control of visceral smooth muscle and glands.

Autonomic responses, like those of the somatic nervous system, are induced promptly and dissipated quickly, in contrast to the slower, more prolonged effects of circulating hormones. The autonomic nervous system, like the endocrine system, regulates the rate of processes that have intrinsic activities of their own, while the somatic nervous system initiates responses de novo. Although certain autonomic responses are discriminating, many are generalized and influence a variety of effectors in different organs. The interface between the autonomic nervous system and the endocrine system is exemplified by the adrenal medulla. This gland, homologous in many respects with the postganglionic sympathetic neuron, secretes a hormone (epinephrine) into the circulation to interact with adrenergic receptors throughout the body.

ANATOMIC ORGANIZATION The autonomic neurons, located in ganglia outside the central nervous system, give rise to the postganglionic autonomic nerves that innervate organs and tissues throughout the body. The activity of autonomic nerves is regulated by central neurons responsive to diverse afferent inputs. After central integration of afferent information, autonomic outflow is adjusted to permit the functioning of the major organ systems in accordance with the needs of the organism as a whole. Connections between the cerebral cortex and the autonomic centers in the brainstem coordinate autonomic outflow with higher mental functions.

The sympathetic and parasympathetic divisions The preganglionic neurons of the parasympathetic nervous system leave the central nervous system in the third, seventh, ninth, and tenth cranial nerves and in the second and third sacral nerves, while the preganglionic neurons of the sympathetic nervous system exit the spinal cord between the first thoracic and the second lumbar segments. Responses to sympathetic and parasympathetic stimulation are frequently antagonistic, as exemplified by their opposing effects on heart rate and gut motility. This antagonism reflects highly coordinated interactions within the central nervous system; the resultant changes in parasympathetic and sympathetic activity, often reciprocal, provide more precise control of autonomic responses than could be achieved by the modulation of a single system.

Neurotransmitters *Acetylcholine* (ACh) is the preganglionic neurotransmitter for both divisions of the autonomic nervous system, as well as the postganglionic neurotransmitter of the parasympathetic neurons. Nerves that release ACh are said to be cholinergic. *Norepinephrine* (NE) is the neurotransmitter of the postganglionic sympathetic neurons; these nerves are said to be adrenergic. Within the sympathetic outflow postganglionic neurons innervating the eccrine sweat glands (and perhaps some blood vessels supplying skeletal muscle) are of the cholinergic type.

THE SYMPATHETIC NERVOUS SYSTEM AND THE ADRENAL MEDULLA

CATECHOLAMINES All three of the naturally occurring catecholamines, NE, *epinephrine* (E), and *dopamine,* function as neurotransmitters within the central nervous system. NE, the neurotransmitter of postganglionic sympathetic nerve endings, exerts its effects locally, in the immediate vicinity of its release. E, the circulating hormone of the adrenal medulla, influences processes throughout the body. A peripheral dopaminergic system also exists but has not been characterized in detail.

Biosynthesis (Fig. 66-1) Catecholamines are synthesized from the amino acid tyrosine, which is sequentially hydroxylated to form dihydroxyphenylalanine (dopa), decarboxylated to form dopamine,

and hydroxylated on the beta position of the side chain to form NE. The initial step, the hydroxylation of tyrosine, is rate-limiting and is regulated so that synthesis of dopa is coupled to norepinephrine release. This regulation is achieved by alterations in both the activity and the amount of tyrosine hydroxylase. In the adrenal medulla and in those central neurons utilizing E as neurotransmitter, NE is *N*-methylated to E by the enzyme phenylethanolamine-*N*-methyltransferase (PNMT). A major portion of the blood perfusing the adrenal medulla is enriched with corticosteroids from the adrenal cortex, and since adrenal PNMT is inducible by glucocorticoids, the capacity of the adrenal medulla to form E may be related to its strategic location within the adrenal cortex.

Catecholamine metabolism (Fig. 66-1) The major metabolic transformations of catecholamines involve *O*-methylation at the meta-hydroxyl group and oxidative deamination. *O*-methylation is catalyzed by the enzyme catechol-*O*-methyltransferase (COMT), and oxidative deamination is promoted by monoamine oxidase (MAO). COMT in liver and kidney is important in the metabolism of circulating catecholamines. MAO, a mitochondrial enzyme present in most tissues including nerve endings has a lesser role in the metabolism of circulating catecholamines but is important in regulating the catecholamine stores within the peripheral sympathetic nerve endings. The metanephrines and 4-hydroxy-3-methoxymandelic acid (VMA) are the major end products of N and NE metabolism. Homovanillic acid (HVA) is the end product of dopamine metabolism.

STORAGE AND RELEASE OF CATECHOLAMINES Both in the adrenal medulla and sympathetic nerve endings catecholamines are stored in subcellular granules and released by exocytosis. The large stores of catecholamines in these tissues provide an important physiologic reserve that maintains an adequate supply of catecholamines in the face of intense stimulation.

Adrenal medulla The adrenal medullary chromaffin tissue in a pair of normal human adrenal glands weighs about 1 g and contains approximately 6 mg of catecholamines, 85 percent of which is E. Catecholamines are maintained in high concentration within the storage (chromaffin) granule by an active uptake process involving the granule membrane and by an intragranular storage complex that appears to involve ATP, calcium, and a specific granule protein (chromagranin A). Catecholamine secretion, stimulated by ACh from the preganglionic sympathetic nerves, occurs after calcium influx triggers fusion of the chromaffin granule membrane and cell membrane; obliteration of the cell membrane at the point of fusion and extrusion of the entire soluble contents of the granule into the extracellular space complete the process of exocytosis (Fig. 66-1). Approximately 2 to 10 percent of the total adrenal medullary catecholamine store is turned over each day.

Peripheral sympathetic nerve endings The peripheral sympathetic nerve endings form a reticulum or ground plexus that brings the terminal fibers into close contact with effector cells. All the NE in peripheral tissues is in the sympathetic nerve endings, and heavily innervated tissues contain as much as 1 to 2 μg per gram of tissue. NE stored in the nerve endings is in discrete subcellular particles analogous to the adrenal medullary chromaffin granules. MAO in the mitochondria of the nerve endings plays an important role in regulating the local concentration of NE (Fig. 66-1). Amines in storage vesicles are protected from oxidative deamination; amines within the cytoplasm, however, are deaminated to inactive metabolites. Release from the nerve ending occurs in response to action potentials propagated in terminal sympathetic fibers (Fig. 66-1).

THE PERIPHERAL ADRENERGIC NEUROEFFECTOR JUNCTION
Neuronal uptake The peripheral sympathetic nerve endings possess an amine transport system that actively takes up amines from the extracellular fluid. A variety of synthetic and naturally occurring amines are substrates for this process. Neuronal uptake or recapture of locally released NE terminates the action of the transmitter and contributes to the constancy of the NE stores (Fig. 66-1).

FIGURE 66-1   *Catecholamine biosynthesis, release, and metabolism. Schematic representation of a peripheral sympathetic nerve ending is shown at the top; the bulbous areas on the terminal fiber represent varicosities identified by histochemical fluorescence techniques as areas of high neurotransmitter concentration. The processes of biosynthesis, release, modulation, and reuptake are shown sequentially for demonstration purposes only; in vivo they proceed concurrently. Adrenal medullary chromaffin cells are shown at the bottom of the diagram. (TH = tyrosine hydroxylase, AAD = aromatic-L-amino acid decarboxylase, DA = dopamine, DBH = dopamine-β-hydroxylase, NE = norepinephrine, PNMT = phenylethanolamine-N-methyltransferase, E = epinephrine, COMT = catechol-O-methyltransferase, NMN = normetanephrine, MAO = monoamine oxidase, DHMA = 3,4-dihydroxymandelic acid, VMA = 3-methoxy-4-hydroxymandelic acid.)*

Prejunctional modulation   A variety of factors alter the relationship between neuronal impulse traffic and NE release. Diminished temperature and acidosis, for example, both decrease the amount of NE released in response to sympathetic impulses. Several chemical mediators operate at the peripheral sympathetic nerve ending (referred to as prejunctional or presynaptic sites) to modify sympathetic neurotransmission by influencing the amount of NE released in response to nerve impulses. Prejunctional modulation may be either inhibitory or facilitatory. Certain modulators, such as catecholamines and ACh, may either inhibit or facilitate NE release, antagonistic effects that are mediated by different adrenergic or cholinergic receptors, respectively. Those compounds exerting an *inhibitory* effect on NE release at the prejunctional nerve ending include the following: catecholamines (alpha₂ receptor), ACh (muscarinic receptor), dopamine (D-2 receptor), histamine (H-2 receptor), serotonin, adenosine, enkephalins, and prostaglandins. *Facilitatory* prejunctional modulators include catecholamines (beta₂ receptor), ACh (nicotinic receptor), and angiotensin II. The overall significance of prejunctional modulation, as well as the relative importance of the various mediators, has yet to be established.

PREJUNCTIONAL ADRENERGIC RECEPTORS   Catecholamines reduce NE release via prejunctional alpha receptors in a classical negative feedback system. Feedback regulation is complicated by the fact that beta-receptor activation facilitates NE release. Two hypotheses have been advanced to explain how the antagonistic alpha and beta effects on NE release may be integrated physiologically. One hypothesis is that beta-mediated effects occur at lower agonist concentrations than those mediated by the alpha receptor, whereas alpha-mediated responses predominate at higher concentrations of agonist. During low levels of sympathetic stimulation, therefore, when NE concentrations in the synaptic cleft are low, beta-mediated positive feedback may predominate with facilitation of NE release. Conversely, at higher levels of sympathetic stimulation with increased NE concentration in the synaptic cleft, alpha-mediated negative feedback predominates and NE release is inhibited. The other hypothesis is that prejunctional beta receptors are more sensitive to E than NE; circulating levels of E, therefore, might stimulate the prejunctional beta receptors, thereby augmenting NE release and enhancing sympathetic neurotransmission.

PREJUNCTIONAL CHOLINERGIC RECEPTORS   Though both inhibitory and facilitatory effects of ACh on NE release have been described, the inhibitory effect of ACh, mediated by the muscarinic cholinergic receptor, occurs at lower ACh concentrations and is probably of greater physiologic significance. This peripheral inhibitory effect of ACh on adrenergic neurotransmission may reinforce the reciprocal changes in central parasympathetic and sympathetic outflow that occur in the regulation of numerous physiologic responses.

CENTRAL REGULATION OF SYMPATHOADRENAL OUTFLOW
Brainstem sympathetic centers   Sympathetic outflow is initiated from the reticular formation of the medulla oblongata and pons and from centers in the hypothalamus. Descending fibers originating from these centers synapse in the intermediolateral cell column of the spinal cord with the preganglionic sympathetic neurons. The brainstem sympathetic centers, which have an intrinsic activity of their own, are regulated by many stimuli, including impulses from more rostral areas of the central nervous system (cortex, limbic lobe, hypothalamus); neural afferents that interact at the level of the brainstem centers and at the higher centers; and changes in the physical and chemical properties of the extracellular fluid, including the circulating levels of hormones and substrates. The higher centers, which have connections with the brainstem, coordinate sympathetic outflow with higher mental functions, emotional reactions, and the homeostatic needs of the internal environment. Although the hallmark of intense sympathoadrenal stimulation is a global response (the fight-or-flight reaction

of Cannon), discrete changes in sympathetic outflow to different organ systems influence many autonomic functions.

RELATIONSHIP BETWEEN THE SYMPATHETIC NERVOUS SYSTEM AND THE ADRENAL MEDULLA   Sympathetic nervous system activity and adrenal medullary secretion are coordinated but not always congruent. During periods of intense sympathetic stimulation, such as cold exposure and exhaustive exercise, the adrenal medulla is progressively recruited, and circulating E reinforces the physiologic effects of sympathetic stimulation. In other situations the sympathetic nervous system and the adrenal medulla are stimulated independently. The response to upright posture, for example, involves predominantly the sympathetic nervous system while hypoglycemia stimulates only the adrenal medulla.

Sympathetic regulation of the cardiovascular system   The sympathetic nervous system plays a major role in the regulation of the circulation. Stretch receptors in the systemic and pulmonary arteries and veins continuously monitor intravascular pressures; the resulting afferent impulses, after relay and integration in the brainstem, alter sympathetic activity in defense of blood pressure and blood flow to critical areas (Fig. 66-2).

ARTERIAL BARORECEPTORS   An increase in blood pressure stimulates receptors in the carotid sinus and aortic arch. The ensuing afferent impulses, after relay within the nucleus of the solitary tract (NTS) in the brainstem, suppress the brainstem sympathetic centers (Fig. 66-2). This baroreceptor reflex arc forms a negative feedback loop in which a rise in arterial pressure results in the inhibition of central sympathetic outflow. A brainstem noradrenergic pathway interacts with the NTS to participate in suppression of sympathetic outflow. This noradrenergic inhibitory pathway is stimulated by centrally acting alpha-adrenergic agonists and may be involved in the action of certain antihypertensive drugs, such as clonidine, that potentiate the baroreceptor-mediated vasodepressor response (Chap. 196). In the opposite manner, when the blood pressure falls, decreased afferent impulses diminish central inhibition, resulting in an increase in sympathetic outflow and a rise in arterial pressure.

CENTRAL VENOUS PRESSURE   Receptors in the walls of the great veins and within the atria are also involved in the regulation of sympathetic outflow. Stimulation of these receptors by high venous pressure suppresses the brainstem sympathetic centers; when central venous pressure is low, sympathetic outflow increases. The central connections are poorly understood, but the afferent impulses are carried in the vagus (Fig. 66-2).

ASSESSMENT OF SYMPATHOADRENAL ACTIVITY   The clinical assessment of sympathoadrenal activity involves the measurement of catecholamines in plasma and of catecholamines and catecholamine metabolites in urine. Quantitation of urinary catecholamines and metabolites is useful in the diagnosis of pheochromocytoma (Chap. 326).

Plasma catecholamines   Catecholamines in human plasma may be measured by radioenzymatic isotope derivative techniques or by high performance liquid chromotography in conjunction with electrochemical detection. Plasma catecholamine measurements provide an index of sympathetic nervous system and adrenal medullary activity and have been widely used to assess sympathoadrenal activity in clinical investigation in human subjects. The usefulness of plasma catecholamine measurements is, however, compromised by factors that alter the relationship between the plasma concentration of catecholamines and the functional state of the sympathoadrenal system. The clinical usefulness of plasma catecholamine levels is limited to the evaluation of patients with autonomic insufficiency (Chap. 29) and, on occasion, patients with suspected pheochromocytoma (Chap. 326).

Basal plasma NE concentrations are in the range of 150 to 350 pg/mL; basal E levels are about 25 to 50 pg/mL. The half-time of disappearance of NE from the circulation is approximately 2 min. The plasma NE level is markedly affected by a variety of factors,

including posture; accordingly, the conditions under which blood is obtained for assay must be controlled. By convention, basal plasma NE levels are those obtained through an indwelling intravenous line after the patient has rested supine in a relaxed environment for 30 min.

PLASMA NE RESPONSE TO UPRIGHT POSTURE   The predictable increase in circulating NE concentration during upright posture provides a convenient test of sympathetic nervous system function. Five minutes of quiet standing results in a two- to threefold increase in plasma NE level. A normal response requires an intact afferent system, appropriate central nervous system relays, and an intact peripheral sympathetic nervous system; a defect of any of these components reduces the increment in circulating NE.

Plasma E levels are also dependent on the physical and mental state of the subject. Change in plasma E with upright posture is usually small. Hypoglycemia and various types of mental stress, however, can cause large increments in the plasma E level.

PERIPHERAL DOPAMINERGIC SYSTEM

In addition to its role as neurotransmitter in the central nervous system, dopamine functions as an inhibitory transmitter in the carotid body and the sympathetic ganglia. A distinct peripheral dopaminergic system is also believed to exist. Dopamine elicits a variety of responses not attributable to stimulation of classic adrenergic receptors; it relaxes the lower esophageal sphincter, delays gastric emptying, causes vasodilation in the renal and mesenteric arterial circulation, suppresses aldosterone secretion, and stimulates renal sodium excretion. The mediation of these dopaminergic effects in vivo is poorly understood. Dopamine does not appear to be a circulating hormone. Unequivocal evidence of peripheral autonomic dopaminergic nerves has not been produced, although such nerves may be present in the kidney. The kidney, furthermore, produces much of the dopamine in the urine since the amount excreted each day (approximately 200 μg per 24 h) cannot be accounted for by clearance of plasma dopamine. Decarboxylation of circulating dopa, which is present in high concentration in the plasma (1500 pg/mL) may contribute to urinary dopamine production. Dopamine generated from the decarboxylation

FIGURE 66-2   *Sympathetic regulation of the circulation. Receptors in the venous and arterial circulations are stimulated by stretch, caused by an increase in pressure; afferent impulses from these receptors are carried to the central nervous system by the ninth and tenth cranial nerves. The net result of these afferent impulses, after relay in the brainstem, is to inhibit central sympathetic outflow. The arterial baroreceptor reflex involves a relay in the nucleus of the tractus solitarius (NTS). (+ = stimulation; − = inhibition.)*

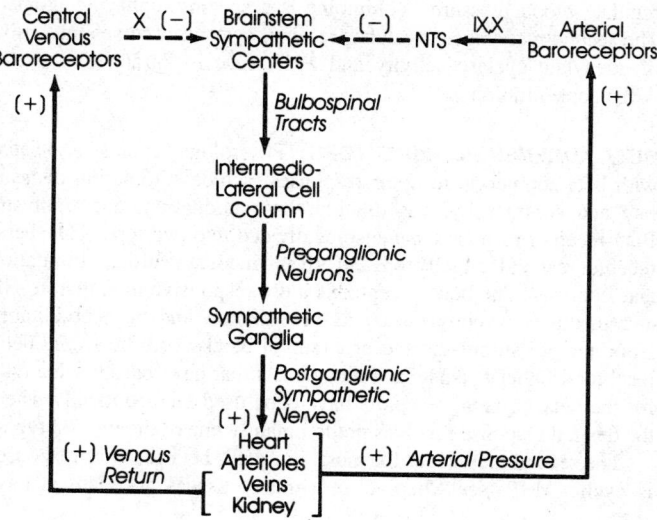

of circulating dopa might also be involved in the mediation of dopaminergic effects in the kidney and other sites. Thus, the nature of the peripheral dopaminergic system is obscure, but the existence of a dopaminergic system in those tissues that respond uniquely to dopamine seems likely.

ADRENERGIC RECEPTORS

Catecholamines influence effector cells by interacting with specific *receptors* on the cell surface. When stimulated by catecholamines, the adrenergic receptor initiates a series of membrane changes followed by a cascade of intracellular events that culminates in a measurable response. Compounds that elicit the response are referred to as *agonists;* those that block the interaction of the agonist with the receptor are referred to as adrenergic *receptor blocking agents* or *antagonists.*

Two major categories of response to catecholamines reflect the activation of two populations of adrenergic receptors, designated *alpha* and *beta.* Selective agonists and antagonists are available, enabling pharmacologic stimulation or blockade of the physiologic effects mediated by one receptor without influencing those mediated by the other. Both alpha and beta receptors have been further divided into subtypes that serve different functions and are susceptible to differential stimulation and blockade.

ALPHA-ADRENERGIC RECEPTORS The alpha-adrenergic receptor mediates vasoconstriction, intestinal relaxation, and pupillary dilatation. E and NE are approximately equipotent as alpha-receptor agonists. Distinct $alpha_1$- and $alpha_2$-receptor subtypes are also recognized. Originally the postsynaptic or postjunctional alpha-adrenergic receptors on effector cells were designated $alpha_1$, while the prejunctional alpha-adrenergic receptors on the sympathetic nerve endings were designated $alpha_2$. Several additional nonneuronal (postsynaptic) processes appear to be mediated by the $alpha_2$ receptor. The $alpha_1$ receptor mediates the classic alpha effects including vasoconstriction; phenylephrine and methoxamine are selective $alpha_1$ agonists, and prazosin is a selective $alpha_1$ antagonist. The second messenger for $alpha_1$-mediated processes has not been identified with certainty but may involve changes in intracellular calcium concentration or in membrane phosphatidylinositol turnover. The $alpha_2$ receptor mediates presynaptic inhibition of NE release from adrenergic nerves and other responses including inhibition of ACh release from cholinergic nerves, inhibition of lipolysis in adipocytes, inhibition of insulin secretion, stimulation of platelet aggregation and, perhaps, initiation of vasoconstriction. Specific $alpha_2$ agonists include clonidine and α-methylnorepinephrine; these agents, the latter derived from α-methyldopa in vivo, exert an antihypertensive effect by interacting with $alpha_2$ receptors within the brainstem sympathetic centers that regulate blood pressure. Yohimbine is a specific $alpha_2$ antagonist. The second messenger for $alpha_2$-receptor systems involves inhibition of adenylate cyclase activity and a decrease in intracellular cyclic AMP concentration.

BETA-ADRENERGIC RECEPTORS Physiologic events associated with beta-adrenergic receptor responses include stimulation of heart rate and contractility, vasodilation, bronchodilation, and lipolysis. Beta-receptor responses can also be divided into two types. The $beta_1$ receptor responds equally to E and NE and mediates cardiac stimulation and lipolysis. The $beta_2$ receptor is more responsive to E than to NE and mediates responses such as vasodilation and bronchodilation. Isoproterenol stimulates and propranolol blocks both $beta_1$ and $beta_2$ receptors. Other agonists and antagonists that have partial selectivity for the $beta_1$ or $beta_2$ receptors have been used therapeutically where the desired response involves predominantly one of the two subtypes.

The second messenger for most, if not all, beta-receptor responses is cyclic AMP (see Chap. 67). In many tissues correlations have been shown between beta-receptor occupancy and stimulation of adenylate cyclase, on the one hand, and between intracellular cyclic AMP accumulation and physiologic response, on the other. While in some systems sequential enzymatic activations involving cyclic AMP–mediated protein phosphorylation couple beta-receptor stimulation and physiologic response, in many tissues the molecular events that mediate beta-adrenergic responses are unknown.

DOPAMINERGIC RECEPTORS Specific dopaminergic receptors, distinct from the classic alpha- and beta-adrenergic receptors, are present in the central and peripheral nervous system and in several nonneural tissues. Two types of dopaminergic receptor serve different functions and have different second messengers. Dopamine is a potent agonist of both types of receptor; the action of dopamine is antagonized by phenothiazines and thioxanthenes. The dopamine-1 receptor mediates vasodilation in the renal, mesenteric, coronary, and cerebral vascular beds. The effects are mediated by a stimulatory effect on adenylate cyclase and an increase in intracellular cyclic AMP. Fenoldopam is an investigational agonist selective for the dopamine-1 receptor. The dopamine-2 receptor inhibits transmission in the sympathetic ganglia, inhibits NE release from sympathetic nerve endings by an effect on the presynaptic membrane (Fig. 66-1), inhibits prolactin release from the pituitary, and causes vomiting. The second messenger for some dopamine-2–mediated processes involves the inhibition of adenylate cyclase. Selective agonists of the dopamine-2 receptor include bromocriptine, lergotrile, and apomorphine, while butyrophenones such as halolperidol (active within the central nervous system) and domperidone (does not cross blood-brain barrier readily) and the benzamide, sulpiride, are relatively selective dopamine-2 antagonists.

REGULATION OF ADRENERGIC RECEPTORS Radiolabeled adrenergic-receptor agonists and antagonists have been utilized as ligands to study adrenergic receptors. In combination with studies of peripheral tissue sensitivity these studies demonstrated that changes in adrenergic receptors occur under a variety of physiologic conditions. Prolonged exposure to alpha- or beta-adrenergic agonists decreases the number of corresponding adrenergic receptors on effector cells. Although the biochemical mechanisms involved are obscure, internalization of the beta-adrenergic receptor within the cell occurs during agonist exposure in some systems, suggesting that internal translocation causes the decrease in receptor number. Alteration in agonist concentration may also affect the affinity of the receptor for the agonist. Adrenergic receptors that utilize adenylate cyclase for the second messenger (beta receptors, $alpha_2$ receptors) exist in high and low affinity states; exposure to agonist diminishes the proportion of receptors in the high affinity state. Such alterations in adrenergic receptors induced by adrenergic agonists are termed homologous regulation. Agonist-induced alterations in adrenergic-receptor density and affinity are believed to contribute to the diminished physiologic response that occurs after prolonged exposure of an effector tissue to adrenergic agonist, a phenomenon known as *tachyphylaxis* or *desensitization.*

Adrenergic receptors are also influenced by factors other than adrenergic agonists, so-called heterologous regulation. Enhanced alpha-adrenergic-receptor affinity, for example, may underlie the potentiation of alpha-adrenergic responses that occur in response to lowered environmental temperatures. Thyroid hormones potentiate beta-receptor responses by alterations in beta-receptor number and in the efficiency of coupling receptor occupancy with physiologic response. Estrogen and progesterone alter the sensitivity of the myometrium to catecholamines by effects on alpha-adrenergic receptors. Glucocorticoids may influence adrenergic function by antagonizing agonist-induced decreases in adrenergic receptors, thereby counteracting tachyphylaxis in response to intense adrenergic stimulation.

Alterations in sensitivity to catecholamines also occur as a consequence of postreceptor changes.

PHYSIOLOGY OF THE SYMPATHOADRENAL SYSTEM

Catecholamines influence all the major organ systems. The effects take place in seconds as compared with the minutes, hours, or days that characterize the actions of the endocrine system and most other control systems that regulate bodily processes. The sympathoadrenal system, moreover, may respond in anticipation of physiologic requirement. An increase in sympathoadrenal activity prior to strenuous exercise, for example, lessens the impact of exercise on the internal environment.

DIRECT EFFECTS OF CATECHOLAMINES Cardiovascular system
Catecholamines stimulate vasoconstriction in the subcutaneous, mucosal, splanchnic, and renal vascular beds by an alpha-receptor-mediated mechanism. Since vasoconstriction in the coronary and cerebral circulations is minimal, flow to these areas is maintained. The adaptive significance of this priority given the heart and brain is clear; in both of these organs the metabolic requirements relative to blood flow are high, and continuous perfusion is essential for life. Skeletal muscle vasculature contains beta receptors sensitive to low circulating levels of E so that skeletal muscle blood flow is augmented during adrenal medullary activation.

The effects of catecholamines on the heart are mediated by beta$_1$ receptors and include increase in heart rate, enhancement of cardiac contractility, and increase in conduction velocity. The increase in myocardial contractility is illustrated by a leftward and upward shift of the ventricular function curve (Fig. 181-5) that relates cardiac work to ventricular diastolic fiber length; at any initial fiber length catecholamines increase cardiac work. Catecholamines also enhance cardiac output by stimulating venoconstriction, enhancing venous return, and by increasing the force of atrial contraction, thereby augmenting diastolic volume and hence fiber length. The acceleration of conduction in the junctional tissues results in a more synchronous, and hence more effective, ventricular contraction. Cardiac stimulation increases myocardial oxygen consumption, a major factor in the pathogenesis and treatment of myocardial ischemia.

Metabolism Catecholamines increase metabolic rate. The biochemical processes involved and the sites of the increased heat production are not known in humans; in small mammals mitochondrial respiration in brown adipose tissue is uncoupled.

SUBSTRATE MOBILIZATION In a variety of tissues catecholamines stimulate the breakdown of stored fuel with the production of substrate for local consumption; glycogenolysis in the heart, for example, provides substrate for immediate metabolism by the myocardium. Catecholamines also accelerate fuel mobilization in liver, adipose tissue, and skeletal muscle, liberating substrates (glucose, free fatty acids, lactate) into the circulation for use throughout the body. Activation of enzymes involved in fuel breakdown occurs by a beta-receptor (beta$_1$) mechanism for adipose tissue lipolysis and by alpha- and beta-receptor (beta$_2$) mechanisms for hepatic glycogenolysis and gluconeogenesis. In skeletal muscle catecholamines stimulate glycogenolysis (beta receptor) thereby increasing lactate efflux.

Fluids and electrolytes Catecholamines contribute to the regulation of the volume and composition of extracellular fluid. By a direct action on the renal tubule, NE stimulates sodium reabsorption, thereby defending extracellular fluid volume. Dopamine, in contrast, promotes sodium excretion. NE and E also promote cellular uptake of potassium, thereby defending against the development of hyperkalemia. Effects of catecholamines on calcium, magnesium, and phosphate metabolism are complex and depend on a variety of factors.

Viscera Catecholamines affect visceral function by actions on smooth muscle and glandular epithelium. Urinary bladder and intestinal smooth muscle are relaxed while the corresponding sphincters are stimulated. Gallbladder emptying also involves sympathetic mechanisms. Catecholamine-mediated smooth-muscle contraction in the female aids ovulation and ovum transport along the fallopian tubes, and in the male provides propulsive force for the seminal fluid during ejaculation. Inhibitory alpha$_2$ receptors on cholinergic neurons within the gut contribute to intestinal relaxation. Catecholamines induce bronchodilation by a beta$_2$ receptor mechanism.

INDIRECT EFFECTS OF CATECHOLAMINES The ultimate physiologic response induced by catecholamines involves changes in hormone secretion and in blood flow distribution, both of which support and amplify the direct effects of catecholamines.

Endocrine system Catecholamines influence the secretion of renin, insulin, glucagon, calcitonin, parathormone, thyroxine, gastrin, erythropoietin, progesterone, and, possibly, testosterone. Secretion of each of these hormones is governed by complex feedback loops. With the exception of thyroxine and the gonadal steroids, each is a polypeptide not under the direct control of the pituitary gland. Sympathoadrenal input into the secretion of these hormones provides a mechanism for regulation by the central nervous system and ensures a coordinated hormonal response in accord with the homeostatic needs of the organism.

RENIN The juxtaglomerular apparatus of the kidney is heavily innervated. Sympathetic stimulation increases renin release by a direct beta-receptor effect independent of vascular changes within the kidney. The renin response to volume depletion is sympathetically mediated and is initiated by a fall in central venous pressure. Since renin secretion activates the angiotensin-aldosterone system, angiotensin-induced vasoconstriction supports the direct effects of catecholamines on blood vessels, while aldosterone-mediated sodium reabsorption complements the direct increase in sodium reabsorption induced by sympathetic stimulation. Beta-receptor blocking agents suppress renin secretion.

INSULIN AND GLUCAGON The pancreatic islets also receive an extensive sympathetic innervation. Stimulation of pancreatic sympathetic nerves or an elevation in circulating catecholamines suppresses insulin and increases glucagon release. Inhibition of insulin secretion is mediated by the alpha$_2$ receptor, and stimulation of glucagon is mediated by the beta receptor. This combination of effects supports substrate mobilization, reinforcing the direct effects of catecholamines on hepatic glucose output and lipolysis. Although alpha-receptor-mediated suppression of insulin release usually predominates, a beta-receptor mechanism may augment insulin secretion under some circumstances.

SYMPATHOADRENAL FUNCTION IN SELECTED PHYSIOLOGIC AND PATHOPHYSIOLOGIC STATES Support of the circulation
The sympathetic nervous system functions to maintain an adequate circulation. During upright posture and volume depletion, reduction of afferent venous and arterial baroreceptor impulse traffic diminishes an inhibitory input to the vasomotor center, thereby increasing sympathetic activity (Fig. 66-2) and reducing efferent vagal tone. As a result, heart rate is increased, and cardiac output is diverted from the skin, subcutaneous tissues, mucosa, and viscera. Sympathetic stimulation of the kidney increases sodium reabsorption, and sympathetically mediated venoconstriction enhances venous return. With pronounced hypotension, the adrenal medulla is recruited and E reinforces the effects of the sympathetic nervous system. A similar pattern of sympathetic activation occurs in the postprandial state when blood and extracellular fluid are sequestered in the splanchnic circulation and in the lumen of the gut, respectively.

CONGESTIVE HEART FAILURE The sympathetic nervous system also provides circulatory support during congestive heart failure (Chap. 182). Venoconstriction and sympathetic stimulation of the heart increase cardiac output while peripheral vasoconstriction directs blood flow to the heart and brain. The afferent signals are less clear than in simple volume depletion since the venous pressure is usually elevated. In severe heart failure depletion of cardiac NE may impair the effectiveness of sympathetic circulatory support.

TRAUMA AND SHOCK   In acute traumatic injury or shock, adrenal catecholamines support the circulation and mobilize substrates. It is presumed, but unproved, that the sympathetic nervous system is activated as well. In the chronic, reparative phase following injury catecholamines contribute to substrate mobilization and to the elevation in metabolic rate.

EXERCISE   Sympathetic activation during exercise increases cardiac output, maintains blood flow, and ensures sufficient substrate to meet the increased needs. Central neural factors, such as anticipation, and circulatory factors, such as fall in venous pressure, trigger the sympathetic response. Mild degrees of exercise stimulate the sympathetic nervous system alone; during more severe exertion the adrenal medulla is activated as well. Conditioning is associated with a decrease in sympathetic nervous system activity both at rest and during exercise.

Hypoglycemia   Hypoglycemia causes a marked increase in adrenal medullary E secretion. When glucose concentrations fall below overnight fasting levels, regulatory glucose-sensitive neurons in the central nervous system initiate a prompt increase in adrenal medullary secretion. The increase is especially intense when plasma glucose levels drop below 50 mg/dL when plasma E levels increase 25 to 50 times above baseline, thereby increasing hepatic glucose output, providing alternative substrate in the form of free fatty acids, suppressing endogenous insulin release, and inhibiting insulin-mediated glucose utilization in muscle. Many clinical manifestations of hypoglycemia, such as tachycardia, palpitations, nervousness, tremor, and widened pulse pressure, are secondary to increased E secretion.

Cold exposure   The sympathetic nervous system plays a critical role in the maintenance of normal body temperature during exposure to a cold environment. Receptors in the skin and central nervous system respond to a fall in temperature by activating hypothalamic and brainstem centers that increase sympathetic activity. Sympathetic stimulation leads to vasoconstriction in the superficial vascular beds, thereby diminishing heat loss. Heat production is simultaneously increased by shivering, generation of metabolic heat, and substrate mobilization. Acclimatization during chronic cold exposure increases the capacity for metabolic heat production in response to sympathetic stimulation.

Dietary intake   Fasting suppresses and overfeeding stimulates the sympathetic nervous system. The reduction in sympathetic activity during fasting or starvation may contribute to the decrease in metabolic rate, bradycardia, and hypotension in these states. Enhanced sympathetic activity during periods of increased caloric intake may

contribute to the elevation in metabolic rate associated with a chronic increase in dietary intake.

Hypoxia   Chronic hypoxia is associated with stimulation of the sympathoadrenal system, and some of the cardiovascular changes in hypoxia may be dependent upon catecholamines.

PARTICIPATION OF THE SYMPATHETIC NERVOUS SYSTEM IN THE PATHOGENESIS OF SELECTED DISEASE STATES

HYPERTENSION (See also Chaps. 29 and 196)   As shown in Fig. 66-3, regulation of arterial pressure by the sympathetic nervous system involves blood vessels, the heart, and the kidneys. The sympathetic nervous system increases peripheral resistance by direct stimulation of the resistance vessels and by activation of the renin-angiotensin system. Increased cardiac output is the result of enhanced cardiac contractility and augmented venous return, the latter a result of venoconstriction and increased renal sodium reabsorption. Stimulation of sodium retention diminishes the capacity of the kidney to compensate for the increase in blood pressure. Antiadrenergic agents lower blood pressure by interacting at many of the sites shown in Fig. 66-3.

The sympathetic nervous system plays at least a permissive role in the maintenance of hypertension (Chap. 29). Despite the elevated blood pressure, sympathetic nervous system activity is not suppressed in hypertensive patients, and reflex control of the circulation is retained, due in part to upward resetting of the baroreceptors. In addition, peripheral sensitivity of the vasculature to NE is either normal or enhanced. The maintenance of sympathetic nervous system activity in patients with hypertension accounts for the hypotensive effects of antiadrenergic agents.

During antihypertensive treatment with vasodilators or diuretics the sympathetic nervous system may be activated in response to decreased pressure in either the venous or arterial circulation (Fig. 66-2). The heightened sympathetic activity that results, in addition to causing tachycardia, may oppose the antihypertensive therapy by activating the various effector systems shown in Fig. 66-3. Antiadrenergic agents, therefore, have a fundamental role in the therapy of most hypertensive patients.

ANGINA PECTORIS (Chap. 189)   Sympathetic stimulation of the cardiovascular system increases myocardial oxygen consumption as a consequence of elevated heart rate, enhanced myocardial contractility, and increased myocardial wall tension. Attacks of angina, therefore, are often precipitated by situations associated with sympathetic activation such as exercise, eating, and cold exposure. Beta blockade is beneficial in the treatment of angina (Chap. 29) because

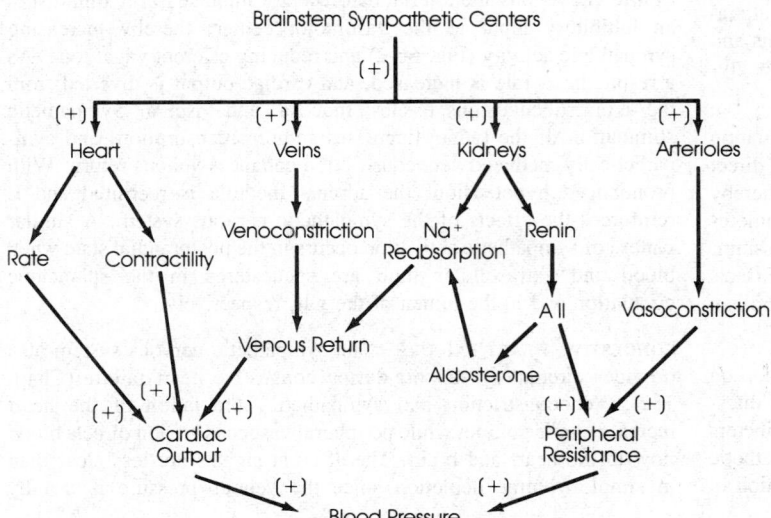

FIGURE 66-3   *Sympathetic nervous system effects on blood pressure. Sympathetic stimulation (+) increases blood pressure by effects on the heart, the veins, the kidneys, and the arterioles. The net result of sympathetic stimulation is an increase in both cardiac output and peripheral resistance. (From JB Young, L Landsberg, in P Sleight et al (eds). Scientific Foundations of Cardiology, London, Heinemann, 1981.)*

of reduction in sympathetic stimulation of the heart. Alpha-adrenergically mediated coronary vasoconstriction may also contribute to coronary spasm.

HYPERTHYROIDISM (Chap. 324)   Many of the peripheral manifestations of hyperthyroidism suggest a hyperadrenergic state. Enhancement of beta-receptor responses in hyperthyroidism is due in part to effects on the beta receptor. Thyroid hormone, in some tissues and in some species, increases receptor number; in other tissues, even when beta-receptor number is not increased, coupling of receptor occupancy to the adenylate cyclase cyclic-AMP system is augmented to amplify catecholamine-induced responses. Since thyroid hormone excess does not suppress sympathetic nervous system activity (plasma NE levels are normal in thyrotoxic patients), a "normal" level of sympathetic activity may evoke an exaggerated physiologic response. Many of the adrenergic manifestations of hyperthyroidism are diminished by treatment with beta-receptor blocking agents.

ORTHOSTATIC HYPOTENSION (Chap. 29)   The maintenance of arterial pressure during upright posture depends upon an adequate blood volume, an unimpaired venous return, and an intact sympathetic nervous system. Significant postural hypotension, therefore, often reflects extracellular fluid volume depletion or dysfunction of the circulatory reflexes. Diseases of the nervous system, such as tabes dorsalis, syringomyelia, or diabetes mellitus, may disrupt these sympathetic reflexes with resultant orthostatic hypotension. Although any antiadrenergic agent may impair the postural sympathetic response, orthostatic hypotension is most prominent with drugs that block neurotransmission within the ganglia or adrenergic neurons.

The term *idiopathic orthostatic hypotension* refers to a group of degenerative diseases involving either the pre- or postganglionic sympathetic neurons. Involvement of the peripheral sympathetic nervous system is characterized by low basal NE levels, while involvement at the level of the central nervous system or preganglionic sympathetic neurons is associated with normal basal plasma NE levels. In both cases the plasma NE response to upright posture is deficient. Orthostatic hypotension caused by disruption of the preganglionic autonomic neurons within the intermediolateral cell column of the spinal cord often occurs in association with degenerative changes of basal ganglia and other portions of the central nervous system. In the latter situation, known as *multiple systems atrophy*, or the *Shy-Drager* syndrome, orthostatic hypotension occurs along with a variety of neurologic disturbances including Parkinson's disease.

Treatment of orthostatic hypotension is usually unsatisfactory except in the mildest cases. There is no way of reestablishing the normal relationship between fall in venous return and sympathetic neuronal activation. Volume expansion with fludrocortisone and a liberal salt diet in conjunction with fitted stockings to the waist, and elevation of the head of the bed to avoid recumbency, will maintain plasma volume and venous return and frequently provide symptomatic improvement. Rarely a beneficial response may be obtained from treatment with sympathomimetic amines (including clonidine).

PHARMACOLOGY OF THE SYMPATHOADRENAL SYSTEM

A variety of therapeutic agents affect sympathetic nervous system function or interact with adrenergic receptors, making it possible to stimulate or suppress effects mediated by catecholamines with some degree of specificity (Table 66-1).

SYMPATHOMIMETIC AMINES   Sympathomimetic amines may directly activate adrenergic receptors (direct acting) or release NE from the sympathetic nerve endings (indirect acting). Many agents have both direct and indirect effects.

Epinephrine and norepinephrine   The naturally occurring catecholamines act predominantly by the direct stimulation of adrenergic receptors. NE is employed to support the circulation and elevate the blood pressure in hypotensive states (Chap. 29). Peripheral vasoconstriction is the major effect although cardiac stimulation occurs as well. E, also employed as a pressor, has special usefulness in the treatment of allergic reactions, especially those associated with anaphylaxis. E antagonizes the effects of histamine and other mediators on vascular and visceral smooth muscle and is useful in the treatment of bronchospasm.

Dopamine   *Dopamine* is used in treating hypotension, shock (Chap. 29), and certain forms of heart failure (Chap. 182). At low infusion rates it exerts a positive inotropic effect both by a direct action on the cardiac beta$_1$ receptors and by the indirect release of NE from sympathetic nerve endings in the heart. At low doses direct stimulation of dopaminergic receptors in the renal and mesenteric vasculature also results in vasodilation in the gut and kidney and facilitates sodium excretion. At higher infusion rates interaction with alpha-adrenergic receptors results in vasoconstriction, an increase in peripheral resistance, and an elevation of blood pressure.

Beta-receptor agonists   *Isoproterenol*, a direct-acting beta-receptor agonist, stimulates the heart, decreases peripheral resistance, and relaxes bronchial smooth muscle. It raises the cardiac output and accelerates atrioventricular conduction while increasing the automaticity of ventricular pacemakers. Isoproterenol is used in the treatment of heart block and bronchoconstriction. *Dobutamine*, a congener of dopamine with relative selectivity for the beta$_1$ receptor and with a greater effect on myocardial contractility than on heart rate, is also used in the treatment of congestive heart failure, often in combination with vasodilators (Chap. 182).

SELECTIVE BETA$_2$-RECEPTOR AGONISTS   The cardiac stimulation caused by nonselective beta agonists, such as isoproterenol or epinephrine, is occasionally dangerous when these agents are used in the treatment of bronchoconstriction. Selective beta$_2$ agonists (*metaproterenol*, *albuterol*, *terbutaline*, and *isoetharine*) improve the therapeutic ratio by achieving bronchial dilatation with less activation of the cardiovascular system (Chaps. 202 and 208); selectivity is relative, and some cardiac stimulation occurs with these agents, particularly at the higher dose levels. *Ritodrine*, another selective beta$_2$ agonist, is used as a tocolytic agent (as is *terbutaline*) to relax the uterus and antagonize premature labor.

Alpha-adrenergic agonists   *Phenylephrine* and *methoxamine* are direct-acting alpha agonists that elevate blood pressure by increasing peripheral vasoconstriction. They are used primarily in the treatment of hypotension and paroxysmal supraventricular tachycardia (Chap. 184), in the latter case by increasing cardiac vagal tone through reflex baroreceptor stimulation. Phenylephrine and a related proprietary compound, *phenylpropanolamine*, are common constituents of decongestant medications (often combined with antihistamines) for the treatment of allergic rhinitis and upper respiratory infections.

Miscellaneous sympathomimetic amines with mixed actions   *Ephedrine* has both direct beta-receptor agonist properties and an indirect effect on sympathetic nerve endings, from which it releases NE, and is used primarily as a bronchodilator. *Sudephedrine*, a congener of ephedrine, is less potent at dilating bronchi and serves as a nasal decongestant. *Metaraminol* has both direct and indirect effects on sympathetic nerve endings and is employed in the treatment of hypotensive states.

Dopaminergic agonists   The dopamine-2-receptor agonist *bromocriptine* is used to suppress prolactin secretion (Chap. 321). *Apomorphine*, another dopamine-2-receptor agonist, is used to induce emesis.

ANTIADRENERGIC OR SYMPATHOLYTIC AGENTS (See also Chap. 196)   **Agents inhibiting central sympathetic outflow**   The antihypertensive agents *methyldopa*, *clonidine*, and *guanabenz* diminish central sympathetic outflow by stimulating a central alpha-adrenergic pathway (alpha$_2$ receptor) that diminishes vasomotor outflow. Central limited use in the treatment of intestinal and bladder smooth-muscle dysfunction such as occurs in paralytic ileus and atonic urinary bladder. Cholinesterase inhibitors induce a vagotonic response in the heart and may be useful in terminating attacks of paroxysmal supraventricular tachycardia (Chap. 184).

Cholinergic-receptor blocking agents   *Atropine* blocks muscarinic cholinergic receptors, with little effect on cholinergic transmission at the autonomic ganglia and the neuromuscular junctions. Many of the central nervous system actions of atropine and atropine-like drugs are attributable to blockade of central muscarinic synapses. The related alkaloid, *scopolamine,* is similar to atropine but causes drowsiness, euphoria, and amnesia, effects that make it suitable as a preanesthetic medication.

Atropine increases heart rate and enhances atrioventricular conduction, actions that may be useful in combating the bradycardia or heart block associated with heightened vagal tone. In addition, atropine reverses cholinergically mediated bronchoconstriction and diminishes respiratory tract secretions. These effects contribute to its utility as a preanesthetic medication.

Atropine also decreases gastrointestinal tract motility and secretion. Although various derivatives and congeners of atropine (such as *propantheline, isopropamide,* and *glycopyrrolate*) have been advocated in patients with peptic ulcer or with diarrheal syndromes, the chronic use of such agents is limited by other manifestations of parasympathetic inhibition such as dry mouth and urinary retention. The investigational selective M-1 inhibitor pirenzepine inhibits gastric secretion at doses that have minimal anticholinergic effects at other sites; this agent may be useful in the treatment of peptic ulcer. Atropine and its congener *ipratropium,* when given by inhalation, cause bronchodilation and have been used experimentally in the treatment of asthma.

REFERENCES

FRISHMAN WH: Beta-adrenoceptor antagonists: New drugs and new indications. N Engl J Med 305:500, 1981

———: Pindolol: A new B-adrenoceptor antagonist with partial agonist activity. N Engl J Med 308:940, 1983

INSEL PA: Identification and regulation of adrenergic receptors in target cells. Am J Physiol 247:E53, 1984

LANDSBERG L, YOUNG JB: Catecholamines and the adrenal medulla, in *Williams Textbook of Endocrinology,* 7th ed, JD Wilson, DW Foster (eds). Philadelphia, Saunders, 1985, p 891

———, ———: The influence of diet on the sympathetic nervous system, in *Neuroendocrine Perspective,* vol 4, EE Muller et al (eds). Amsterdam, Elsevier, 1985, p 191

LIMBIRD LE: GTP and Na+ modulate receptor-adenyl cyclase coupling and receptor-mediated function. Am J Physiol 247:E59, 1984

MOSES JW, BORER JS: Beta-adrenergic antagonists in the treatment of patients with heart disease. DM 27:1, 1981

WEINER N, TAYLOR P: Neurohumoral transmission: The autonomic and somatic motor nervous systems, in *The Pharmacologic Basis of Therapeutics,* 7th ed, AG Gilman et al (eds). New York, Macmillan, 1985, p 66

67   THE ADENYLATE CYCLASE SYSTEM

HENRY R. BOURNE

Cyclic 3′,5′-monophosphate (cyclic AMP) acts as an intracellular "second messenger" for a diverse array of peptide hormones and biogenic amines, drugs, and toxins. Consequently, an understanding of the adenylate cyclase system is essential for understanding the pathophysiology and management of many diseases. Investigation of the second messenger role of cyclic AMP advanced our understanding of endocrine, neural, and cardiovascular regulation. Conversely, research aimed at unraveling the biochemical basis of certain diseases has contributed to understanding the molecular mechanisms by which the synthesis of cyclic AMP is regulated.

BIOCHEMISTRY   The enzymatic steps involved in the actions of hormones (first messengers) that work via cyclic AMP are depicted in Fig. 67-1, and the hormones that work via this mechanism are listed in Table 67-1. The actions of these hormones are initiated by binding to specific receptors on the external surface of the plasma membrane. The hormone-receptor complex activates the membrane-bound enzyme, adenylate cyclase, which synthesizes cyclic AMP from intracellular ATP. Within the cell cyclic AMP relays the hormonal message by combining with and activating its own receptor, cyclic AMP–dependent protein kinase. The activated protein kinase transfers the terminal phosphate of ATP to specific protein substrates (usually enzymes). Phosphorylation of these enzymes enhances (or in some cases, inhibits) their catalytic activities. Altered activities of these enzymes produce the characteristic effects of the hormone on its target cell.

A second class of hormones acts by binding to membrane receptors that inhibit adenylate cyclase. The action of these hormones, denoted H_i to distinguish them from stimulatory hormones (H_S), is described in more detail below. Figure 67-1 also shows an additional set of biochemical mechanisms that limit the action of cyclic AMP. These mechanisms may also be regulated by hormones. Such regulation allows fine tuning of cell function by additional neural and endocrine pathways.

Biologic role of cyclic AMP   Each of the protein molecules involved in the intricate push-pull mechanisms of Fig. 67-1 represents a potential site for regulation of hormonal responsiveness, for therapeutic and toxic actions of drugs, and for pathologic alterations in disease. Specific instances of such interactions are discussed in later sections of this chapter. To set these in context, the general biologic functions of cyclic AMP as a second messenger should be considered. These functions are conveniently illustrated by reference to the regulation of the release of glucose from hepatic glycogen stores (the biochemical system in which cyclic AMP was discovered) by glucagon and other hormones.

TRANSDUCTION OF HORMONAL SIGNALS ACROSS THE PLASMA MEMBRANE   The biologic stability and structural complexity of peptide hormones like glucagon make them useful carriers of diverse hormonal messages between cells but impair their ability to penetrate cell membranes. Hormone-sensitive adenylate cyclase allows the information content of the hormonal signal to cross the membrane, although the hormone itself may not.

AMPLIFICATION   By binding to a few specific receptors (probably less than 1000 per cell), glucagon stimulates synthesis of a much larger number of cyclic AMP molecules. These cyclic AMP molecules stimulate cyclic AMP–dependent protein kinase, which causes activation of thousands of molecules of hepatic phosphorylase (the enzyme that limits glycogen breakdown) and the subsequent release of millions of glucose molecules from a single cell.

METABOLIC COORDINATION AT THE LEVEL OF A SINGLE CELL   In addition to stimulating phosphorylase and causing degradation of glycogen to glucose, cyclic AMP–dependent protein phosphorylation simultaneously deactivates the enzyme that synthesizes glycogen (glycogen synthase) and stimulates enzymes responsible for hepatic gluconeogenesis. Thus, a single chemical signal, glucagon, mobilizes energy reserves via more than one metabolic pathway.

TRANSDUCTION OF DIVERSE MESSAGES INTO A SINGLE METABOLIC PROGRAM   Because hepatic adenylate cyclase can be stimulated by epinephrine (acting through beta-adrenergic receptors) as well as glucagon, cyclic AMP allows regulation of hepatic carbohydrate metabolism by two chemically distinct hormones. If the second messenger did not exist, each of the regulatory enzymes involved in hepatic mobilization of carbohydrates would have to be able to recognize both glucagon and epinephrine.

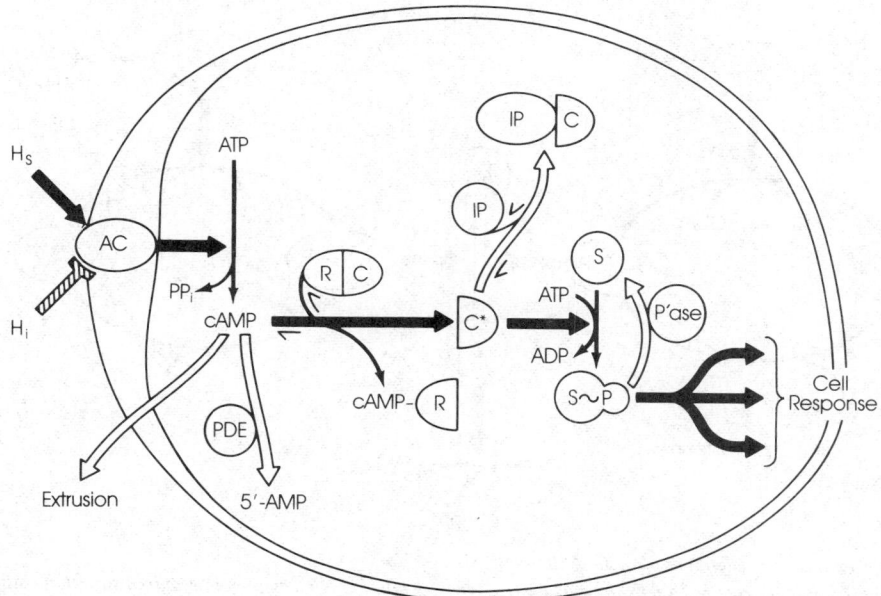

FIGURE 67-1 *Cyclic AMP as an intracellular second messenger for hormones. The diagram depicts an idealized cell containing the protein molecules (enzymes) involved in mediating actions of hormones that work via cyclic AMP. Filled arrows indicate the flow of information from stimulatory hormone (H_s) to cellular response, while open arrows indicate opposing processes that act to modulate or inhibit the flow of information. Extracellular hormones stimulate (H_s) or inhibit (H_i) the membrane enzyme, adenylate cyclase (AC), as described in the text and in Fig. 67-2. AC converts ATP into cyclic AMP (cAMP) and pyrophosphate (PP_i). The intracellular concentration of cyclic AMP depends upon a balance between its rate of synthesis and two processes that remove it from the cell: degradation by cyclic nucleotide phosphodiesterases (PDE), which convert cyclic AMP to 5'-AMP, and extrusion from the cell by an energy-dependent transport system. The intracellular actions of cyclic AMP are mediated or regulated by at least five additional classes of proteins. The first of these, the cyclic AMP–dependent protein kinases (RC), are composed of regulatory (R) and catalytic (C) subunits. In the RC holoenzyme the C subunit is catalytically inactive (inhibited by R). Cyclic AMP acts by binding to the R subunits, freeing C from the cyclic AMP-R complex. Free catalytic subunits (C^*) catalyze transfer of the terminal phosphate of ATP to specific protein substrates (S), e.g., phosphorylase kinase. In the phosphorylated state ($S{\sim}P$) these substrate proteins (usually enzymes) initiate the characteristic actions of cyclic AMP within the cell (e.g., activation of glycogen phosphorylase, inhibition of glycogen synthetase). The proportion of the kinase substrate proteins in the phosphorylated ($S{\sim}P$) state is regulated by two additional classes of proteins: Kinase inhibitor protein (IP) binds reversibly to C^*, rendering it catalytically inactive (IP-C). Phosphatases (P'ase) recycle $S{\sim}P$ back to S by removing covalently bound phosphate.*

COORDINATED REGULATION OF DIFFERENT CELLS AND TISSUES BY A FIRST MESSENGER   In the classic "fight-or-flight" response to stress, catecholamines bind to beta-adrenergic receptors in heart, adipose tissue, blood vessels, and many other tissues including liver. If cyclic AMP were not available to mediate most of the responses to beta-adrenergic catecholamines (e.g., increased heart rate and contractility, dilatation of vessels supplying skeletal muscle, mobilization of energy from carbohydrate and lipid stores), a huge panoply of distinct enzymes in these tissues would have to possess specific binding sites for regulation by catecholamines.

Similar examples of the biologic functions of cyclic AMP could be adduced from the other first messengers listed in Table 67-1. Cyclic AMP acts as an intracellular mediator for each of these hormones, signifying their presence on the cell surface. Like all good mediators, cyclic AMP provides a simple, economical, and highly specific way of communicating diverse and complex messages.

HORMONE-SENSITIVE ADENYLATE CYCLASE   The pivotal enzyme that mediates this system is hormone-sensitive adenylate cyclase. This enzyme is composed of at least five classes of separable proteins, each embedded in the lipid bilayer of the plasma membrane (Fig. 67-2).

Two classes of hormone receptors, R_s and R_i, are exposed on the outer surface of the cell membrane. They contain specific recognition sites for binding hormones that stimulate (H_s) or inhibit (H_i) adenylate cyclase.

The catalytic unit of adenylate cyclase (AC), exposed on the cytoplasmic face of the plasma membrane, converts intracellular ATP to cyclic AMP and pyrophosphate. Two classes of guanine nucleotide–binding regulatory proteins also face the cytoplasm. These proteins, G_s and G_i, mediate the stimulatory and inhibitory effects of R_s and R_i, respectively.

Both the stimulatory and inhibitory coupling functions of the G proteins depend upon their capacity to bind guanosine triphosphate (GTP) (Fig. 67-2). Only the GTP-bound forms of the G proteins

TABLE 67-1   Hormones that utilize cyclic AMP as a second messenger

Hormone	Target organ/tissue	Characteristic effect
Adrenocorticotropic hormone	Adrenal cortex	Cortisol production
Calcitonin	Bone	↓ Serum calcium
Catecholamines (beta-adrenergic)	Heart	↑ Rate, contractility
Chorionic gonadotropin	Ovary, testis	↑ Production of sex steroids
Follicle-stimulating hormone	Ovary, testis	↑ Gametogenesis
Glucagon	Liver	Glycogenolysis, release of glucose
Luteinizing hormone	Ovary, testis	↑ Production of sex steroids
Luteinizing hormone–releasing hormone	Pituitary	↑ Release of luteinizing hormone
Melanocyte-stimulating hormone	Skin (melanocytes)	↑ Pigmentation
Parathyroid hormone	Bone, kidney	↑ Serum calcium, ↓ serum phosphate
Prostacyclin, prostaglandin E_1	Platelets	↓ Platelet aggregation
Thyrotropin	Thyroid	↑ Production and release of T_3, T_4
Thyrotropin-releasing hormone	Pituitary	↑ Release of thyrotropin
Vasopressin	Kidney	↑ Concentration of urine

NOTE: *Only the best-documented cyclic AMP–mediated effects are listed here, although many of these hormones produce multiple effects in several target organs.*

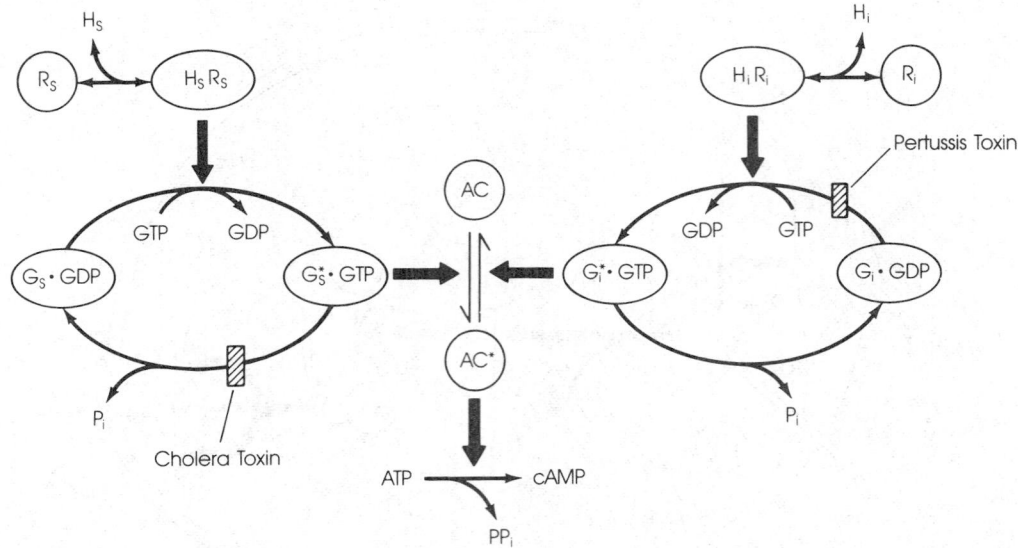

FIGURE 67-2 *Molecular mechanism of regulation of cyclic AMP synthesis by hormones, hormone receptors, and G proteins. Adenylate cyclase (AC) in its active form (AC*) converts ATP to cyclic AMP (cAMP) and pyrophosphate (PP_i). Activation and inhibition of AC are mediated by formally identical systems, shown on the left and right of the diagram. In each system the G protein oscillates between an inactive state, bound to GDP (G-GDP) and an active GTP-bound state (G*-GTP); only the active state of each protein can stimulate (G_s) or inhibit (G_i) AC activity. Each G-GTP complex possesses an intrinsic GTPase activity which converts it to the inactive G-GDP complex. In order to return the G protein to its active state, stimulatory or inhibitory hormone receptor complexes (H_sR_s and H_iR_i, respectively) promote replacement of GDP by GTP at the G protein's guanine nucleotide–binding site. Note that* while the HR complex is required to initiate stimulation or inhibition of AC by G_s or G_i, hormone can dissociate from receptor independently of regulation of AC, which instead depends upon the duration of the GTP-bound state of the appropriate G protein, regulated by its intrinsic GTPase. Two bacterial toxins regulate adenylate cyclase activity by catalyzing ADP-ribosylation of the G proteins (see text). ADP-ribosylation of G_s by cholera toxin inhibits its GTPase activity, stabilizing G_s in its active state and thereby increasing cyclic AMP synthesis. In contrast, ADP-ribosylation of G_i by pertussis toxin prevents it from interacting with the H_iR_i complex and stabilizes G_i in the inactive GDP-bound state; as a result, pertussis toxin prevents hormonal inhibition of AC.*

regulate cyclic AMP synthesis. Neither stimulation nor inhibition of AC is permanent; instead, the terminal phosphate of GTP in each G-GTP complex is eventually hydrolyzed, and G_s-GDP or G_i-GDP cannot regulate AC. For this reason, sustained stimulation or inhibition of adenylate cyclase requires continued recycling of G-GDP to G-GTP. In both pathways, hormone-receptor complexes (H_sR_s or H_iR_i) promote the exchange of GDP for GTP. This recycling mechanism temporally and spatially separates the binding of hormones to receptors from the regulation of cyclic AMP synthesis, using the energy stored in the terminal phosphate bond of GTP to amplify the effects of hormone-receptor complexes.

This scheme explains how several different hormones can stimulate or inhibit cyclic AMP synthesis within a single cell. Because receptors are physically distinct from adenylate cyclase, the array of receptors expressed on a cell surface determines the cell's specific pattern of responsiveness to external chemical signals. An individual cell may express three or more different inhibitory receptors and six or more distinct stimulatory receptors. In contrast, all cells appear to contain similar (perhaps identical) G and AC components.

The molecular components of hormone-sensitive adenylate cyclase provide control points for changing the sensitivity of a given tissue to hormonal stimulation. Both R and G components are critical in physiologic regulation of hormonal sensitivity, and alterations of the G proteins are implicated as the primary lesion of four diseases discussed below.

Regulation of sensitivity to hormones (see also Chap. 66) Repeated administration of a hormone or drug often causes gradually increasing resistance to its effects. This phenomenon is variously termed desensitization, refractoriness, tachyphylaxis, or tolerance.

Hormones or neurotransmitters may induce desensitization that is receptor-specific or "homologous." For example, administration of beta-adrenergic catecholamines induces specific refractoriness of heart muscle to readministration of the same amines but not to drugs that do not act via beta-adrenergic receptors. Receptor-specific desensitization involves at least two separate mechanisms. The first, which

develops rapidly (within minutes) and is rapidly reversed upon removal of the hormone, functionally "uncouples" receptors from G_s protein and therefore reduces their ability to stimulate adenylate cyclase. The second process involves actual reduction in the number of receptors on the cell membrane, a process termed *receptor down-regulation*. The down-regulation process may require hours to occur and is not readily reversible.

These desensitization processes are part of normal regulation. Removal of normal physiologic stimuli may result in increased sensitivity of a target tissue to pharmacologic stimulation, as in denervation supersensitivity. A potentially important clinical correlate of this increase in receptor number may occur in patients in whom therapy with propranolol, a beta-adrenergic blocking agent, is abruptly withdrawn. Such patients often have transient signs of elevated sympathetic tone (tachycardia, elevation of blood pressure, headaches, tremor, etc.) and may develop symptoms of coronary insufficiency. Peripheral blood leukocytes of subjects receiving propranolol exhibit elevated numbers of beta-adrenergic receptors, and receptor number returns slowly to normal when propranolol is withdrawn. Although the more numerous receptors in leukocytes do not mediate the cardiovascular symptoms and signs of propranolol withdrawal, receptors in myocardium and other tissues likely undergo similar changes.

Sensitivity of cells and tissues to hormones may also be regulated in a "heterologous" fashion—i.e., the sensitivity to one hormone is regulated by a second hormone, acting through a different set of receptors. Regulation of cardiovascular sensitivity to beta-adrenergic amines by thyroid hormones is the most prominent clinical example of heterologous regulation. Thyroid hormones cause an accumulation of an increased number of beta-adrenergic receptors in heart muscle. This increase in receptors partially accounts for the increased cardiac sensitivity of hyperthyroid patients to catecholamines. However, the fact that in experimental animals the increase in number of beta-adrenergic receptors produced by administration of thyroid hormones is not sufficient to account for the increased cardiac sensitivity to catecholamines suggests that thyroid hormones also affect components of the hormone response distal to receptors, possibly including, but not limited to, G_s. Other examples of heterologous regulation include control by estrogen and progesterone of uterine sensitivity to relaxation by beta-adrenergic agonists and the increased responsiveness of many tissues to epinephrine that is produced by glucocorticoids.

A second type of heterologous regulation involves inhibition of hormonal stimulation of adenylate cyclase by agents that act via R_i and G_i, as noted above. Acetylcholine, opiates, and alpha-adrenergic catecholamines act through distinct classes of inhibitory receptors (muscarinic, opioid, and alpha-adrenergic) to decrease the sensitivity of adenylate cyclase in certain tissues to stimulation by other hormones. Although the clinical importance of this type of heterologous regulation is not established, inhibition of cyclic AMP synthesis by morphine and other opiates could account for some aspects of tolerance to opiates. Similarly, relief of such inhibition may be involved in producing the syndrome that follows withdrawal of opiates.

Pseudohypoparathyroidism (see also Chap. 336)   A genetic defect involving the G_s component of adenylate cyclase is the molecular basis of pseudohypoparathyroidism type I (PHP-I). This rare inherited disease is characterized by hypocalcemia and hyperphosphatemia, elevated serum parathyroid hormone (PTH), and resistance to the metabolic effects of exogenously administered PTH.

PTH regulates calcium homeostasis at least in part by stimulating adenylate cyclase in kidney and bone. Administration of PTH to normal subjects (and to patients with idiopathic or surgical hypoparathyroidism) causes greatly increased excretion of cyclic AMP in urine. In contrast, PTH causes little or no increase in the urinary cyclic AMP of PHP-I patients. This finding initially raised the possibility that PHP-I is caused by a defect in the PTH receptor, rendering it less capable of stimulating cyclic AMP synthesis.

A defect confined to the PTH receptor, however, could not account for the fact that many PHP-I patients are also partially resistant to other hormones, including thyrotropin (TSH), antidiuretic hormone, glucagon, and gonadotropins. Indeed, some PHP-I patients require replacement therapy for symptomatic hypothyroidism, because of thyroid resistance to TSH. Resistance to the action of the other hormones is for the most part clinically silent and can be detected only with specialized tests.

The fact that these hormones utilize cyclic AMP as a second messenger suggests that PHP-I is caused by a defect distal to hormone receptors, affecting some component common to all cyclic AMP–mediated responses. For many PHP-I patients that component is the G_s protein. Activity of G_s is reduced by about 50 percent in erythrocytes, platelets, and skin fibroblasts of most PHP-I patients. G_s activity was found to be reduced in the kidney of one PHP-I patient and is probably reduced in other endocrine target cells as well, including bone, thyroid, liver, etc.

If G_s deficiency is generalized in PHP-I, why are most of its important clinical consequences related to resistance to a single hormone, PTH? While this question cannot be answered with certainty, it is likely that most hormone responses mediated by cyclic AMP are maintained—in spite of partial G_s deficiency—by a variety of compensatory mechanisms, including elevation of circulating concentrations of the stimulating hormone. Elevated circulating PTH does not suffice to maintain normal calcium homeostasis in PHP-I, however, presumably because the actions of PTH are more critically dependent upon normal activity of G_s. Fortunately, the defect in PTH responsiveness can be bypassed by treatment with vitamin D, which restores serum calcium and phosphate to normal.

Cholera (see also Chap. 115)   Elevated cyclic AMP in intestinal mucosal cells causes the massive secretion of water and electrolytes that results in the diarrhea of cholera. Pathogenic *Vibrio cholerae* produce a protein exotoxin that can stimulate cyclic AMP synthesis in virtually all animal cells. The clinical disease is limited to intestinal mucosa because the toxin is not absorbed from the gastrointestinal tract, and other tissues are thus not accessible to the toxin produced by bacteria growing in the intestinal lumen.

Unlike stimulation of adenylate cyclase by hormones, the effect of cholera toxin is slow in onset and does not disappear immediately when the toxin is removed. The reason for this difference is that cholera toxin does not act by reversible binding to a stimulatory receptor but instead acts as an enzyme, producing a stable covalent modification of the G_s protein component of adenylate cyclase. Following binding of the toxin to cells, one of its peptide subunits penetrates the cell membrane, where it catalyzes ADP-ribosylation of G_s, using intracellular nicotinamide adenine dinucleotide (NAD^+) as a substrate:

$$G_s + NAD^+ \xrightarrow{\text{toxin}} G_s\text{-ADP-ribose} + \text{nicotinamide} + H^+$$

ADP-ribosylation of G_s increases cyclic AMP synthesis, apparently by decreasing the rate of hydrolysis of GTP in the G_s-GTP-C complex that synthesizes cyclic AMP (Fig. 67-2).

This biochemical mechanism may explain why the diarrhea of cholera can be produced by a relatively small number of pathogenic organisms and why the diarrhea can persist after the organisms have been eradicated. The first phenomenon stems from the fact that the toxin is an enzyme, so that small numbers of toxin molecules suffice to ADP-ribosylate a substantial fraction of the G_s molecules in a cell. Persistently elevated cyclic AMP synthesis after removal of the toxin, at least in experimental studies, correlates with stability of G_s-ADP-ribose. Most cells apparently lack enzymes capable of removing ADP-ribose from G_s, so that the effect of the toxin disappears only when the G_s-ADP-ribose molecules are replaced by newly synthesized G_s molecules. Recovery from the clinical disease may even require replacement of the mucosal cells themselves. Elucidation of the molecular basis for the action of cholera toxin served as a valuable tool in the discovery and characterization of G_s and advanced our understanding of the biochemical basis of hormone action.

Pertussis (see also Chap. 109)   The molecular pathogenesis of pertussis in bronchi closely parallels that of cholera in the gut. Neither organism invades tissues; instead, both cause disease by producing exotoxins that alter cyclic AMP synthesis in host cells. *Bordetella pertussis* secretes two pathogenic exotoxins: The molecular target of one, termed pertussis toxin, is the inhibitory guanine nucleotide–binding protein of adenylate cyclase, G_i. The other toxin is itself an adenylate cyclase molecule.

Like cholera toxin, pertussis toxin catalyzes transfer of ADP-ribose from NAD^+ to a membrane protein; in this case, the protein is G_i. The ADP-ribosylated form of G_i is unable to interact with R_i (Fig. 67-2); as a result, pertussis toxin prevents inhibition of adenylate cyclase by inhibitory ligands such as muscarinic, alpha-adrenergic, and opiate agonists.

The key bronchial target cells for pertussis toxin and the molecular pathways that link ADP-ribosylation of G_i to signs and symptoms of the disease are largely unknown. The ADP-ribosylation reaction does, however, provide an explanation for one puzzle: Antibiotic treatment of pertussis infection does little to limit intensity and duration of disease; indeed, symptoms can persist for 3 weeks or more after organisms have disappeared from the tracheobronchial tree. ADP-ribosylation of G_i (like that of G_s, as described above) is not readily reversible by cellular enzymes. Probably, the disease persists, even in the absence of additional toxin, until the modified G_i proteins or the cells that contain them have been replaced.

The second pathogenic product of *B. pertussis*, adenylate cyclase toxin, remains enzymatically inert until it enters host cells. There it is activated by binding to calmodulin, with a resulting profound elevation of cellular cyclic AMP. Unlike the effect of pertussis toxin, that of the adenylate cyclase toxin rapidly disappears when the source of the toxin is removed; cellular enzymes degrade the bacterial enzyme, and cellular cyclic AMP rapidly returns to normal.

While most of the links between molecular actions of these toxins and the resulting disease are poorly understood, in vitro experiments show that both toxins can interfere with function of human neutrophils—cells that play a crucial role in defense against infection. Cyclic AMP accumulation caused by the adenylate cyclase toxin impairs the neutrophil's ability to kill ingested microorganisms. Pertussis toxin, by ADP-ribosylating G_i or G_i-like molecule, blocks neutrophil responses (chemotaxis, release of lysosomal hydrolases, etc.) to complement and other chemotactic factors. Either or both of these effects could contribute to increased susceptibility to pulmonary infection by other organisms, a frequent complication of pertussis infection.

Aside from their role as tools for exploring transduction of hormonal signals, knowledge of these toxins can produce real clinical dividends. Although the present practice of immunizing with extracts of whole pertussis organisms effectively prevents infection, the immunization itself produces considerable morbidity. Pertussis organisms specifically incapable of producing either of the two toxins are rendered harmless to animal hosts. Accordingly, immunization with purified toxin preparations should prevent disease and may reduce the morbidity of immunization. Results of preliminary clinical trials support both predictions.

Anthrax (see also Chap. 98) Cutaneous infection by *Bacillus anthracis* produces a characteristic lesion, with central necrosis surrounded by prominent subcutaneous edema. While the necrotic lesion appears not to involve the cyclic AMP system, the organism's "edema factor" is in fact adenylate cyclase. Like the adenylate cyclase toxin of pertussis, edema factor gains access to host cells, is activated by cellular calmodulin, and increases intracellular cyclic AMP. Interestingly, there are rare instances of patients who ingest anthrax organisms and develop a watery diarrhea indistinguishable from cholera. Diarrhea in such instances probably results from penetration of edema factor into cells of the intestinal mucosa, with resulting cyclic AMP elevation and secretion of salt and water.

CYCLIC AMP IN CLINICAL MEDICINE A large number of hormones and neurotransmitters act by stimulating adenylate cyclase, and several pharmacologic antagonists act by blocking their binding to specific receptors—e.g., propranolol at beta-adrenergic receptors and cimetidine at H_2-histamine receptors. The therapeutic actions of these agents depend upon elevations or decreases in cyclic AMP content of target cells and tissues in patients. In addition, the methylxanthines (caffeine and theophylline) block cyclic nucleotide phosphodiesterases and may produce some of their therapeutic effects (e.g., bronchodilatation) by elevating cellular cyclic AMP.

In clinical practice, measurements of cyclic AMP in the urine are useful in diagnosing disorders that involve PTH and calcium homeostasis. A substantial fraction of urinary cyclic AMP is made in proximal tubular cells responding to circulating PTH. Thus, urinary cyclic AMP provides a convenient "window" for assessing effects of PTH on the kidney and can reflect elevated PTH (in hyperparathyroidism), decreased PTH (in hypoparathyroidism), or end-organ resistance to PTH (in PHP-I) (see Chap. 336).

At present, however, the real importance of cyclic AMP for medicine is as a tool in understanding normal and pathologic regulation and in developing new drugs. Adenylate cyclase assays are now routinely used to screen new compounds for their ability to stimulate or block adrenergic, histaminergic, and many peptide receptors. Hormone receptors are not the only critical and specific control points in regulation mediated by cyclic AMP; it seems likely that the other proteins depicted in Fig. 67-1 will serve as targets of future therapeutic agents.

OTHER SECOND MESSENGERS Although cyclic AMP is the most thoroughly studied hormonal second messenger, some hormones act by increasing intracellular concentrations of other chemical signals, including calcium ion and cyclic guanosine 3',5'-monophosphate (cyclic GMP). Certain effects of alpha-adrenergic and cholinergic (muscarinic) agents, for example, appear to be mediated by elevated cytoplasmic concentrations of calcium. Many cell types contain guanylate cyclase, cyclic GMP phosphodiesterases, and protein kinases that are specifically stimulated by cyclic GMP. Nonetheless, the role of this second cyclic nucleotide in normal and pathologic regulation is not well defined.

REFERENCES

FARFEL Z et al: Pseudohypoparathyroidism: Inheritance of deficient receptor-cyclase coupling activity. Proc Natl Acad Sci USA 78:3098, 1981

GILMAN AG: Guanine nucleotide–binding regulatory proteins and dual control of adenylate cyclase. J Clin Invest 73:1, 1984

LEPPLA SH et al: Anthrax toxin edema factor: A bacterial adenylate cyclase that increases cyclic AMP concentrations in eukaryotic cells. Proc Natl Acad Sci USA 79:3162, 1982

WEISS AA et al: Pertussis toxin and extra-cytoplasmic adenylate cyclase as virulence factors of *Bordetella pertussis*. J Infect Dis 150:219, 1984

68 ARACHIDONIC ACID METABOLITES RELEVANT TO MEDICINE

R. PAUL ROBERTSON

This chapter focuses on the formation and mechanism of action of the physiologically active metabolites of arachidonic acid and on the biologic phenomena in which these compounds may be involved.

FORMATION OF THE EICOSANOIDS Prostaglandins, the first arachidonic acid metabolites to be recognized, were so named because they were originally identified in seminal fluid and thought to be secreted by the prostate. As other active metabolites were characterized, two major pathways—the cyclooxygenase and the lipoxygenase pathways—became apparent. These synthetic pathways are summarized schematically in Fig. 68-1, and structures of representative metabolites are shown in Fig. 68-2. All products of both the cyclooxygenase and the lipoxygenase pathways are called *eicosanoids*. The products of the cyclooxygenase pathway—the prostaglandins and the thromboxanes—are termed *prostanoids*.

The initial synthetic step for both pathways involves the cleavage of arachidonic acid from phospholipid in the plasma membrane of cells. Free arachidonic acid can then be oxygenated by the cyclooxygenase or lipoxygenase pathway. The first product of the cyclooxygenase pathway is the cyclic endoperoxide prostaglandin G_2 (PGG_2), which is converted to prostaglandin H_2 (PGH_2). PGG_2 and PGH_2 are the key intermediates in the formation of physiologically active prostaglandins (PGD_2, PGE_2, $PGF_{2\alpha}$, and PGI_2) and thromboxane A_2 (TXA_2). The first product of the 5-lipoxygenase pathway is 5-hydroperoxyeicosatetraenoic acid (5-HPETE) which is an intermediate in the formation of 5-hydroxyeicosatetraenoic acid (5-HETE) and the leukotrienes (LTA_4, LTB_4, LTC_4, LTD_4, and LTE_4). Two fatty acids other than arachidonic acid [3,11,14-eicosatrienoic acid (dihomo-γ-linolenic acid) and 5,8,11,14,17-eicosapentaenoic acid] can be converted to metabolites closely related to these eicosanoids. Prostanoid products of the former substrate carry the subscript 1; the leukotriene subscript is 3. Prostanoid products of the latter substrate have the subscript 3 while leukotrienes have the subscript 5. Arachidonic acid forms prostaglandin products with subscripts 2 and leukotrienes with the subscript 4. (The subscripts designate the number of double bonds between carbon atoms in the side chains.)

Virtually all cells have the necessary substrates and enzymes to form some of the metabolites of arachidonic acid, but tissues differ in the enzymes they possess and consequently in the products they form. Eicosanoids are synthesized according to immediate need and are not stored in significant amounts for later release.

The cyclooxygenase products Prostaglandins D_2, E_2, $F_{2\alpha}$, and I_2 are formed from the cyclic endoperoxides PGG_2 and PGH_2. Of these, PGE_2 and PGI_2 exert the broadest physiologic effects. PGE_2 has notable effects in, and is synthesized by, many tissues. PGI_2 (also called prostacyclin) is a dominant product of arachidonic acid in the endothelial and smooth muscle cells of vessel walls and in some nonvascular tissues. PGI_2 is a vasodilator and an inhibitor of platelet

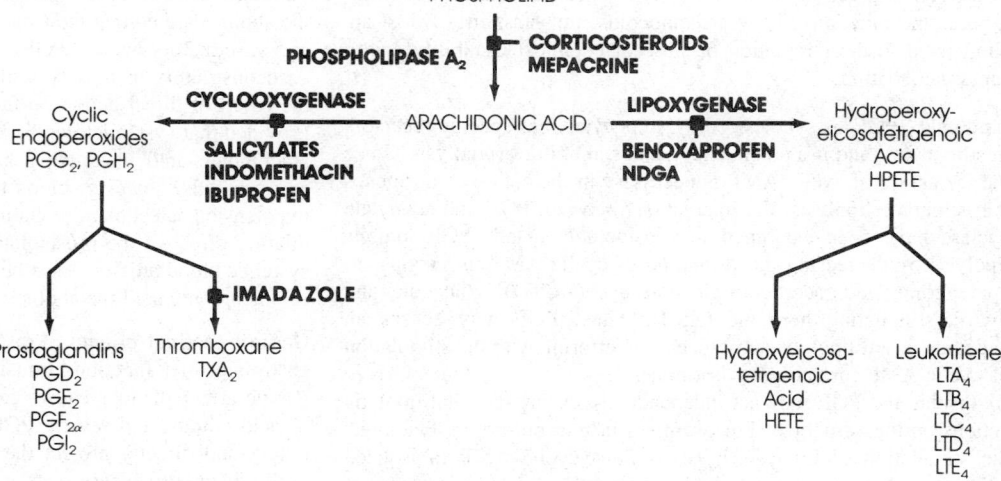

FIGURE 68-1 *The overall scheme of arachidonic acid metabolism. The various drugs act at the various enzymatic steps to inhibit the reactions. The major pathways are the cyclooxygenase and the lipoxygenase pathways. Phospholipase A_2 is inhibited by corticosteroids and mepacrine; cyclooxygenase is inhibited by certain salicylates, indomethacin, and ibuprofen; and lipoxygenase is inhibited by benoxaprofen and nordihydroguaiaretic acid (NDGA). Imidazole prevents TXA_2 synthesis.*

aggregation. PGD_2 is also believed to play a role in platelet aggregation and brain function. $PGF_{2\alpha}$ plays a role in uterine and ovarian function.

Thromboxane synthetase catalyzes the incorporation of an oxygen atom into the ring of the endoperoxide PGH_2 to form the thromboxanes. TXA_2 is synthesized by platelets and enhances platelet aggregation.

The lipoxygenase products The leukotrienes and HETE are the end products of the lipoxygenase pathway. The leukotrienes have histamine-like actions, including induction of increased vascular permeability and of bronchospasm, and appear to have mediator activities for leukocytes. LTC_4, LTD_4, and LTE_4 together have been identified as slow-reacting substance of anaphylaxis (SRS-A). (The pathophysiology of the leukotrienes is discussed in detail in Chap. 202.)

EFFECTS OF DRUGS ON THE SYNTHESIS OF EICOSANOIDS

Many drugs block the synthesis of eicosanoids by inhibiting one or more enzymes in their biosynthetic pathways. Glucocorticoids and antimalarial drugs such as mepacrine interfere with the cleavage of arachidonic acid from phospholipids (Fig. 68-1). Cyclooxygenase is directly inhibited by nonsteroidal anti-inflammatory drugs including salicylates, indomethacin, and ibuprofen. Benoxaprofen, another nonsteroidal anti-inflammatory drug, inhibits the lipoxygenase-mediated conversion of arachidonic acid to HPETE. Tranylcypromine, an antidepressant drug, inhibits the conversion of cyclic endoperoxides to PGI_2, and imidazole inhibits thromboxane synthesis. The fact that a drug inhibits the synthesis of a certain eicosanoid does not mean that a given drug effect is the direct result of a deficiency of that eicosanoid. Most of these drugs inhibit early reactions in the synthetic pathways and therefore block the formation of more than one product. Additionally, some of these drugs have other effects. For example, indomethacin not only inhibits formation of cyclic endoperoxides by cyclooxygenase but may also disrupt calcium flux across membranes, inhibit cyclic adenosine monophosphate (cyclic AMP)–dependent protein kinase and phosphodiesterase, and inhibit one of the enzymes responsible for degradation of PGE_2.

No truly specific synthesis inhibitors nor specific receptor antagonists for individual arachidonic acid metabolites are suitable for human use. The lack of such drugs is a major barrier to elucidating the role of these metabolites in physiologic and pathophysiologic processes.

METABOLISM AND ASSAY OF EICOSANOIDS

Arachidonic acid metabolites are catabolized rapidly in vivo. Prostaglandins of the E and F series, although chemically stable, are almost completely degraded during a single passage through the liver or the lung. Thus, essentially all nonmetabolized PGE_2 measurable in urine is derived from renal and seminal vesicle secretion, whereas PGE_2 metabolites in urine represent total-body PGE_2 synthesis. PGI_2 and TXA_2 are both chemically unstable and also rapidly catabolized. Because PGE_2,

PGI_2, and TXA_2 are short-lived in vivo, measurement of their inactive metabolites is commonly used as an index of the rates of their formation. PGE_2 is converted to 15-keto-13,14,-dihydro-PGE_2, PGI_2 is converted to 6-keto-$PGF_{1\alpha}$, and TXA_2 is converted to TXB_2. Five methods are available to measure arachidonic acid metabolites in physiologic fluids: bioassay, radioimmunoassay, chromatography, receptor assay, and mass spectrometry. With each method certain precautions must be taken in handling samples because prostaglandin synthesis may be enhanced during the collection of biologic samples. For example, if blood is allowed to clot or if platelets are not carefully separated from plasma, the generation of large amounts of PGE_2 and TXA_2 during processing can lead to erroneous results. Use of an inhibitor of prostaglandin synthesis in the collection tube minimizes this problem.

PHYSIOLOGY Prostaglandins and leukotrienes have specific receptor sites on the plasma membranes of cells such as liver, corpus luteum, adrenal gland, adipocytes, thymocytes, uterus, pancreatic islets, platelets, and red blood cells. Most of the binding sites exhibit specificity for eicosanoids of a given type. For example, the liver plasma membrane PGE receptor binds PGE_1 and PGE_2 with high affinity but not prostaglandins of the A, F, and I configurations. The postreceptor mechanisms by which the binding of the prostaglandins alters cell function are poorly understood. The normal physiologic actions of eicosanoids are not mediated via the plasma. Instead, eicosanoids act as local, intercellular, and/or intracellular modulators

FIGURE 68-2 *Structures of representative biologically active eicosanoids.*

Prostaglandin	5-HETE
PGE_2	5-HETE
Prostacyclin	Leukotriene
PGI_2	LTD (SRS-A)
Thromboxane	
TXA_2	

of biochemical activity in the tissues in which they are formed (e.g., a paracrine function). They are autocoids, not hormones. Most are short-lived in the circulation because of chemical instability and/or rapid degradation.

Lipolysis PGE_2 is synthesized by adipocytes, has specific receptors in adipocytes, and is a potent endogenous inhibitor of lipolysis. Since the formation of cyclic AMP is necessary in the action of hormones that stimulate lipolysis, the interactions between PGE and adenylate cyclase have been examined in considerable detail. PGE inhibits lipolysis by decreasing the formation of cyclic AMP in response to epinephrine, adrenocorticotropic hormone (ACTH), glucagon, and thyroid-stimulating hormone (TSH). Thus, PGE may act as an endogenous antilipolytic substance by interfering with the stimulation of cyclic AMP formation by hormones.

Insulin and PGE may act independently during their antilipolytic actions on the adipocyte. For example, insulin but not PGE inhibits the stimulation of lipolysis by exogenous cyclic AMP in isolated adipocytes, but both agents inhibit hormone-stimulated generation of cyclic AMP. This suggests a site of action of insulin distal to the stimulation of adenylate cyclase. In some animals PGE inhibits glucagon-induced lipolysis whereas insulin does not.

Sodium and water balance The renin-angiotensin-aldosterone system is a major regulator of sodium homeostasis, and vasopressin exerts the principal control over water balance. Arachidonic acid metabolites influence both systems. PGE_2 and PGI_2 stimulate renin secretion, and inhibitors of prostaglandin synthesis have the opposite effect. PGI_2 and PGE_2 decrease renal vascular resistance and increase blood flow; this results in redistribution of blood flow from the outer renal cortex to the juxtamedullary region of the kidney. Conversely, inhibitors of prostaglandin synthesis, such as indomethacin and meclofenamate, decrease total renal blood flow and shunt the remaining flow to the outer cortex, which can lead to acute renal venoconstriction and acute renal failure in circumstances such as volume depletion and edematous states. PGE_2 is natriuretic whereas cyclooxygenase inhibitors cause sodium and water retention.

Indomethacin also increases sensitivity to exogenous vasopressin in dogs. Conversely, PGE_2 decreases vasopressin-stimulated water transport. Since this effect of PGE_2 is circumvented by the administration of dibutyryl–cyclic AMP, PGE_2 most likely interferes with the stimulation of adenylate cyclase by vasopressin.

Platelet aggregation Platelets synthesize PGE_2, PGD_2, and TXA_2. Although a physiologic role has not been established for PGE_2 and PGD_2 in platelet function, TXA_2 is a potent stimulator of platelet aggregation; in contrast PGI_2, formed by the endothelial cells of blood vessel walls, is a potent antagonist of platelet aggregation. TXA_2 and PGI_2 may exert their opposing effects by decreasing and increasing, respectively, platelet generation of cyclic AMP.

Inhibitors of endogenous prostaglandin synthesis interfere with platelet aggregation. For example, a single dose of aspirin can suppress normal platelet aggregation for 48 h and longer, presumably by suppressing cyclooxygenase-mediated TXA_2 synthesis. Cyclooxygenase inhibition by a single dose of aspirin is of longer duration in platelets than in other tissues, because the platelet, in contrast to nucleated cells that can synthesize new proteins, does not have the machinery to form new enzyme. Consequently, the effect of aspirin persists until newly formed platelets have been released. Endothelial cells, on the other hand, rapidly recover cyclooxygenase activity following discontinuation of treatment with aspirin, and PGI_2 production is thus restored. This is one reason that patients taking aspirin are not predisposed to excessive formation of platelet thrombi. In addition, the platelet is more sensitive than the endothelial cell to aspirin.

Endothelial damage may lead to platelet aggregation along the blood vessel wall by causing a local decrease in PGI_2 synthesis, thereby allowing unbridled platelet aggregation at the site of vessel wall damage.

Vascular effects The vasoactive properties of arachidonic acid metabolites are among their most impressive actions. PGE_2 and PGI_2 are vasodilators where $PGF_{2\alpha}$, TXA_2, and LTC_4-LTD_4-LTE_4 are vasoconstrictors in most vascular beds. These effects appear to be the result of direct action on the smooth muscle of the vessel wall. Provided that systemic blood pressure is maintained, the vasodilatory arachidonic acid metabolites act to increase blood flow. If blood pressure falls, however, blood flow decreases because with systemic hypotension catecholamine-induced vasoconstriction offsets the vasodilatory effect of the prostaglandins. Thus, significant alterations in systemic blood pressure must be excluded when evaluating the effects of arachidonic acid metabolites on organ blood flow.

Gastrointestinal effects Prostaglandins of the E series influence gastrointestinal function. Infusion of either PGI_2 or PGE_2 into the gastric artery of dogs causes increases in blood flow and inhibition of acid output, and several PGE analogues both inhibit gastric acid output and directly protect the gastrointestinal mucosa when taken orally. In in vitro experiments prostaglandins stimulate gastrointestinal smooth muscle and thereby increase motility, but it is not clear whether these actions are physiologically important.

Neurotransmission PGE inhibits egress of norepinephrine from sympathetic nerve terminals. The effect of PGE on norepinephrine secretion appears to be prejunctional, i.e., at a site on the nerve terminal proximal to the synaptic cleft, and can be reversed by increases in calcium concentration in the perfusing medium. Therefore, PGE_2 may inhibit norepinephrine release by blocking calcium influx. Inhibitors of PGE_2 synthesis can augment norepinephrine release in response to stimulation of adrenergic nerves.

Catecholamines can release PGE_2 from a variety of tissues, probably by an alpha-adrenergic–mediated mechanism. For example, in innervated tissues such as the spleen, nerve stimulation or injection of norepinephrine causes release of PGE_2. This release is blocked after denervation or administration of alpha-adrenergic blockers. Thus, a stimulus that activates the nerve causes release of norepinephrine, which in turn stimulates synthesis and release of PGE_2; PGE_2 then feeds back at the prejunctional level of the nerve terminal to decrease the amount of norepinephrine released.

Pancreatic endocrine function PGE_2 has both stimulatory and inhibitory effects on insulin secretion by the pancreatic beta cell in vitro. In vivo, insulin responses to intravenous glucose in humans are inhibited by PGE_2. This inhibitory effect appears to be specific for glucose because the insulin responses to other secretagogues are not influenced by PGE_2. Studies with inhibitors of prostaglandin synthesis support the concept that endogenous PGE_2 acts in vivo to inhibit insulin secretion. In general, such drugs augment insulin secretion and improve carbohydrate tolerance. An exception is indomethacin, which inhibits glucose-induced insulin secretion and can cause hyperglycemia. The discordant results with indomethacin are likely due to some action other than inhibition of cyclooxygenase. The lipoxygenase pathway appears to play a role in potentiating insulin secretion by participating in stimulus-secretion coupling. In this case a likely active arachidonic acid product may be 12-HPETE.

Luteolysis In the sheep hysterectomy during the luteal phase of the ovarian cycle results in maintenance of the corpus luteum, suggesting that the uterus normally produces a luteolytic substance. A candidate for this substance is $PGE_{2\alpha}$ since it can cause luteal regression.

PATHOPHYSIOLOGY Most postulated roles for arachidonic acid metabolites in disease involve excessive production, but a few disorders may be the result of decreased production. The latter could result from dietary deficiency of arachidonic acid (an essential fatty acid), from damage to a tissue required for prostaglandin synthesis, or from therapy with drugs that inhibit enzymes in the synthetic pathway.

Bone resorption: Hypercalcemia of malignancy (also see Chaps. 303 and 336) Hypercalcemia occurs in association with nonparathyroid malignancies of many different types. Parathyroid hormone excess, as the result either of autonomous production by parathyroid tissue or ectopic formation by the tumor itself, causes a portion of these cases. However, most patients with hypercalcemia of malignancy do not have elevated plasma levels of parathyroid hormone, and the etiology of the hypercalcemia has been the subject of considerable interest.

Prostaglandin E_2 is a potent inducer of bone resorption and of calcium release from bone, and PGE_2 production is elevated in certain hypercalcemic animals with transplantable tumors. Treatment of these animals with inhibitors of PGE_2 synthesis causes reduction of PGE_2 levels and a concomitant decrease in hypercalcemia. Likewise, some patients with hypercalcemia and malignancy have excessive amounts of PGE_2 metabolites in urine, whereas equally elevated levels do not occur in normocalcemic patients with otherwise similar malignancies. Drugs that inhibit prostaglandin synthesis decrease circulating calcium levels in some patients with hypercalcemia of malignancy. Thus, a subset of approximately 5 to 10 percent of patients with hypercalcemia and malignancy have elevated PGE production and can be treated with drugs that inhibit prostaglandin synthesis.

The source of the excess PGE_2 in these patients has not been identified. Increased liver and lung degradation of PGE would be expected to compensate if large amounts of PGE were present in the circulation. It is possible, of course, that such large amounts of PGE_2 are released by a tumor into the circulation that liver and lung degradation cannot handle the load. Alternatively, if lung metastases are present, the venous drainage from the tumors could be delivered into the systemic circulation without passing through lung tissue. A third possible mechanism involves metastatic seeding of bone. Tumor cells synthesize PGE in culture, and metastatic tumor cells in bone could synthesize PGE that acts locally to cause bone resorption. Hypercalcemia of malignancy can occur in the absence of demonstrable bone metastases, but the clinical tools for excluding such metastases, such as radioisotope scans, may not be sensitive enough to detect many small lesions.

Bone resorption: Rheumatoid arthritis and dental cysts (see Chap. 263)

Overproduction of PGE_2 has been postulated as a cause of the juxtaarticular osteoporosis and bony erosions in some patients with rheumatoid arthritis. Rheumatoid synovia synthesize PGE_2 in tissue culture, and media from these cultures promote bone resorption; moreover, the inclusion of indomethacin in the culture medium blocks this resorptive capacity. Since indomethacin does not prevent bone resorption due to preformed PGE_2, the PGE_2 produced by the synovia is presumed to be responsible for the resorptive activity.

Cells from benign dental cysts also cause bone resorption and synthesize PGE_2 in tissue culture. Again, bone resorption caused by the culture medium from such cells is decreased if indomethacin is added prior to the incubation. A related problem is that of alveolar bone resorption in patients with periodontal disease, a common inflammatory disease of the gums. PGE_2 levels in inflamed gingiva are greater than in healthy gingival tissue. Thus, it is possible that alveolar resorption might be due, in part at least, to local overproduction of these metabolites.

Bartter's syndrome (see Chap. 228)

Bartter's syndrome is characterized by elevated levels of plasma renin, aldosterone, and bradykinin; resistance to the pressor effect of angiotensin; hypokalemic alkalosis; and renal potassium wasting in the presence of normal blood pressure. The basis for the postulated role of prostaglandins in the disorder is that PGE_2 and PGI_2 stimulate the release of renin and that the pressor response to infused angiotensin is blunted by the vasodilator effects of PGE_2 and PGI_2. The increase in renin release leads to increased aldosterone secretion, which in turn can increase urinary kallikrein activity.

In keeping with this postulate, elevated levels of PGE_2 and 6-keto-$PGF_{1\alpha}$ are present in urine of patients with the syndrome. Hyperplasia of renal medullary interstitial cells (which synthesize PGE in culture) has also been demonstrated. These findings led to

therapeutic trials of inhibitors of prostaglandin synthesis in the disorder. Indomethacin (and other inhibitors) reverse virtually all the abnormalities except hypokalemia. Thus, a prostaglandin, probably PGE_2 and/or PGI_2, probably mediates some of the manifestations of Bartter's syndrome.

Diabetes mellitus (see Chap. 327)

Intravenous administration of large amounts of glucose to normal individuals causes a sudden (first-phase) increase in secretion of insulin into plasma followed by a slower, more prolonged response termed second-phase insulin secretion. Patients with type II (non-insulin-dependent, adult-onset) diabetes mellitus have absent first-phase insulin release in response to glucose and a variable decrease in second-phase insulin secretion. Insulin response to other secretagogues, such as arginine, isoproterenol, glucagon, and secretin, is preserved. Thus, diabetics appear to have a specific defect that interferes with normal perception of glucose signals. Since PGE inhibits glucose-induced insulin secretion in normal individuals, inhibitors of endogenous prostaglandin synthesis have been given to patients with type II diabetes mellitus to ascertain whether insulin secretion can be improved. Both sodium salicylate and aspirin elevate basal plasma insulin levels, partially restore the first-phase insulin response, increase second-phase insulin secretion, and improve glucose tolerance.

Patent ductus arteriosus (see Chap. 185)

The ductus arteriosus in sheep is sensitive to the vasodilatory properties of PGE_2, and PGE-like material is present in the ductal wall. Thus, enhanced endogenous PGE_2 might maintain prenatal patency of the ductus. Since inhibitors of prostaglandin synthesis cause constriction of the ductus of fetal lambs, trials with indomethacin were undertaken in premature human infants with isolated patent ductus arteriosus. Such treatment for several days is followed by closure of the vessel in the majority, although some require a second course of therapy, and a minority require surgical ligation. Infants under 35 weeks of gestational age are most likely to respond.

Patients with certain types of congenital heart disease require a patent ductus arteriosus to survive. Ductus-dependent pulmonary blood flow is essential under circumstances in which the ductus is the major channel by which nonoxygenated blood reaches the lungs from the aortic arch, for example, in pulmonary atresia and tricuspid atresia. Since PGE relaxes the smooth muscle in the lamb ductus arteriosus, clinical trials of intravenous PGE were undertaken to attempt to maintain patency of the ductus in such patients as an alternative to emergency surgery. Such PGE infusions for a short time cause a temporary increase in blood flow to the lungs and improve arterial oxygen saturation until the necessary corrective heart surgery can be performed. The large right-to-left shunt in these cardiac malformations allows the intravenously infused PGE_2 to escape pulmonary degradation before arriving at the ductus. In this instance, the disease process itself facilitates delivery of the therapeutic agent.

Peptic ulcer disease (see Chap. 235)

Excessive gastric acid secretion in patients with peptic ulcer disease is involved in damaging the mucosa. Various analogues of PGE_2 inhibit gastric acid secretion and are also inherently cytoprotective. These agents are more effective than placebo in relieving pain and decreasing gastric acid secretion in patients with ulcer disease. Moreover, acceleration of the healing of ulcer craters as assessed by endoscopic criteria has been reported in patients receiving PGE analogues as compared with placebo-treated groups.

Dysmenorrhea (see Chap. 331)

Dysmenorrhea is usually associated with increased uterine contractions. The fact that some analgesics used to treat this disorder also inhibit prostaglandin synthesis suggests that arachidonic acid metabolites may play a role in the pathogenesis of dysmenorrhea. Prostaglandins of the E and F series are present in human endometrium. Intravenous infusion of either produces uterine contractions, and PGF and PGE levels in menstrual blood are decreased by administration of prostaglandin synthesis inhibitors. Controlled trials comparing prostaglandin synthesis inhibitors with placebo in women with dysmenorrhea suggest that symptomatic improvement is greater following drug therapy.

Asthma (see Chap. 202)

Inflammatory response and immune response (see Chaps. 62 and 260)   Drugs such as aspirin have antipyretic, anti-inflammatory, and analgesic effects. Several arguments support a relation between inflammation and the arachidonic acid metabolites: (1) Inflammatory stimuli such as histamine and bradykinin release endogenous prostaglandins in parallel. (2) Leukotriene C_4-D_4-E_4 is more potent than histamine in causing bronchoconstriction. (3) Several arachidonic acid metabolites cause vasodilatation and hyperalgesia. (4) PGE_2 and LTB_4 are present in areas of inflammation. Polymorphonuclear cells release these products during phagocytosis, and they are chemotactic for leukocytes. (5) Some prostaglandins cause increased vascular permeability, a feature of the inflammatory response that gives rise to local edema. (6) Vasodilation induced by PGE is not abolished by atropine, propranolol, methysergide, or antihistamines, known antagonists of other possible mediators of the inflammatory response. Thus, PGE may have a direct inflmmatory effect, and some mediators of inflammation may act by influencing PGE release. (7) Some arachidonic acid metabolites can cause pain in animal models and hyperalgesia or an increased sensitivity to pain in humans. (8) PGE can cause fever after injection into the cerebral ventricles or into the hypothalamus of animals. (9) Pyrogens cause increased concentrations of prostaglandins in cerebrospinal fluid, whereas prostaglandin synthesis inhibitors decrease fever and decrease release of prostaglandins into cerebrospinal fluid.

Arachidonic acid metabolites may also play a role in the immune response. Small amounts of PGE_2 can suppress stimulation of human lymphocytes by mitogens such as phytohemagglutinin, and the inflammatory response is associated with the local release of arachidonic acid metabolites; thus, these substances may act as negative modulators of lymphocyte function. The release of PGE by mitogen-stimulated lymphocytes may constitute a portion of a negative feedback control mechanism by which lymphocyte activity is regulated. Sensitivity of lymphocytes to the inhibiting effects of PGE_2 increases with age, and indomethacin augments lymphocyte responsiveness to mitogens to a greater degree in the elderly. Lymphocytes cultured from patients with Hodgkin's disease release more PGE_2 after the addition of phytohemagglutinin, and lymphocyte responsiveness is enhanced by indomethacin. When suppressor T cells are removed from the cultures, the amount of PGE_2 synthesized is diminished, and the responsiveness of the lymphocytes from the Hodgkin's patients and controls is no longer different. Depressed cellular immunity in patients with Hodgkin's disease may be the result of PGE inhibition of lymphocyte function.

REFERENCES

ROBERTSON RP (ed): Symposium on prostaglandins in health and disease. Med Clin North Am 65:711, 1981

METZ SA et al: Prostaglandins as mediators of paraneoplastic syndromes: Review and update. *Metabolism* 30:299, 1981

GOETZL EJ, SCOTT WA (eds): Regulation of cellular activities by leukotrienes and other lipoxygenase products of arachidonic acid. *J Allergy Clin Immunol* 74:309, 1984

69   THE ENDOGENOUS OPIATE PEPTIDES

MICHAEL ROSENBLATT

The endogenous opiate peptides, the enkephalins and endorphins, are present in the hypothalamus and brain, endocrine glands (pituitary, adrenals, ovaries, and testes), and gastrointestinal tract (including pancreas). These peptides constitute a class of approximately 10 to 15 substances that range in length from 5 to 31 amino acids. Some of them share common biosynthetic and secretory pathways with hormones such as adrenocorticotropin (ACTH), α-melanocyte-stimulating hormone (α-MSH), β-melanocyte-stimulating hormone (β-MSH), and β-lipotropin (β-LPH). They have (1) morphine-like analgesic properties; (2) behavioral effects; and (3) neurotransmitter and neuromodulator functions. Indeed, these peptides may play a role in many functions such as memory, learning, response to stress, reproduction, pain transmission, and regulation of appetite, temperature, and respiration (Table 69-1). In addition, the placebo response, acupuncture-mediated analgesia, stress-induced amenorrhea, and the pathogenesis of shock may be mechanistically linked to the enkephalins and the endorphins. Tranquilization, irritability, agitation, violent behavior, catalepsy, narcolepsy, and catatonia may also be related to the endorphins. Other behavioral phenomena, such as the smoking habit; alcoholism, and drug addiction, may reflect biochemical abnormalities of the system.

The discovery of the enkephalins and endorphins began with opiate receptors, which were identified and characterized before the first endogenous opiate peptides were isolated. The presence of receptors that bind opiate alkaloids such as morphine in the central nervous system and other tissues raised the teleologic issue of the reason for their existence. It seemed unlikely that the receptors were present to interact with exogenously administered drugs; endogenous substances with morphine-like properties were postulated to exist, and efforts were made to identify them.

In 1975, Hughes, Kosterlitz, and colleagues published a report of their discovery of two small (five-amino acid) brain peptides that bind to opiate receptors and are more potent than morphine. They named these substances *enkephalins* (meaning ''in the head''). Within months, three more opiate peptides, larger in size than the enkephalins, were isolated from hypothalamic-pituitary extracts and named endorphins (a contraction for ''endogenous morphine''). Later dynorphin, α-neoendorphin, and other structures were added to the list. The term *endorphin* is used by some as a general term for all opiate peptides.

STRUCTURE AND BIOSYNTHESIS   The structure of several endogenous opiates is provided in Fig. 69-1. Although these substances are chemically unrelated to morphine, molecular modeling studies indicate that the morphine molecule can mimic a predicted conformation of the enkephalins and endorphins that may occur at the instant of interaction with receptor.

Structurally, these substances are identical in the four amino acids at their amino terminus, which constitutes their ''active core,'' although each has different biologic effects. The endorphins as a class bind better to opiate receptors than does morphine itself and are 20 to 700 times more potent than the morphine alkaloids in a variety of in vitro and in vivo bioassays. Rapid lability may cause underestimation of potency in some assays and is the result of enzymatic degradation of the smallest of these substances, the enkephalins.

Although the opiate peptides have common chemical features, they arise via different biosynthetic pathways. In the pituitary β-endorphin, the most abundant endorphin, is synthesized as part of a larger precursor molecule (pro-opiomelanocortin or POMC) that also contains the full sequence of ACTH, α-MSH, β-MSH, and β-LPH (Fig. 69-2). This precursor molecule also has the potential to generate

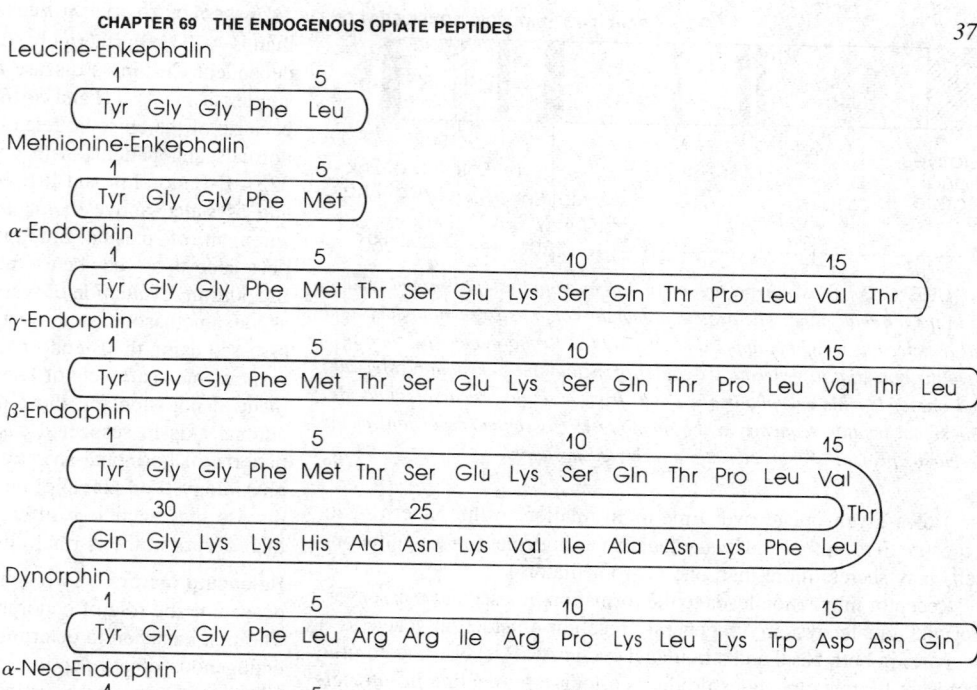

FIGURE 69-1 *Structure of several endogenous opiate peptides. The amino-terminal (leftmost) four amino acids are identical in each peptide. At position 5, a methionine or leucine is found.*

other forms of endorphin, fragments termed α-endorphin and γ-endorphin. "Prohormone-type" cleavage sites exist within POMC and allow the generation of each of the above-mentioned peptides in some anatomic sites. Hence, β-lipotropin is likely a prohormone for β-endorphin. Although β-lipotropin has its own spectrum of biologic properties, its physiologic significance in humans has not been determined. Most importantly, this biosynthetic pathway represents the only means by which the pituitary gland produces ACTH. Therefore, the biosyntheses of ACTH and β-endorphin are inextricably linked in the pituitary by derivation from a single gene that encodes both hormones. Whenever the pituitary secretes ACTH, it also secretes β-endorphin.

Differential processing of POMC occurs within different tissues. Such processing may include metabolic inactivation of peptides generated from the precursor at certain anatomic sites. For instance, although the pituitary gland does not metabolize ACTH to smaller fragments, the hypothalamus converts the precursor molecule to α-MSH. β-MSH is generated in the intermediate lobe of lower species. Humans lack an intermediate lobe as a distinct anatomic entity and hence only produce β-MSH in scattered cells within the pituitary. The cells of the pituitary gland secrete β-endorphin, β-lipotropin, and ACTH. In other cells, the final secretory products are determined by the pattern of cleavage of the large peptide precursor by the enzymatic machinery within that cell. Although several cell types may synthesize the same primary gene product, the final profile of hormone secretion can differ completely.

The enkephalins are derived from different precursors. For example, the adrenal glands biosynthesize enkephalins as part of a large (50,000-mol wt) protein, proenkephalin A, that contains six repeats of the Met-enkephalin sequence and one Leu-enkephalin structure (Fig. 69-3). Again, typical "prohormone-type" cleavage sites delineate the enkephalin structures. Dynorphins and neoendorphins are derived from a third distinct precursor molecule, proenkephalin B.

Additional ("cryptic") peptides are encoded within the structures of these precursor proteins and have the potential to be released by "prohormone-type" cleavages. It is not known whether these cryptic peptides are secreted in vivo, but some have been chemically synthesized and found to have biologic effects.

MECHANISM OF ACTION Like other peptide hormones, the initial step in expression of biologic activity for the opiate peptides is binding to specific receptors on the plasma membrane of target cells.

TABLE 69-1 Biologic effects and possible physiologic roles of endogenous opiates

Analgesia
Catatonic-like state
Seizures
Temperature regulation
Appetite control
Reproductive function (endocrine)
Sexual behavior
Blood pressure decline
Stress response
Release of hypothalamic/pituitary hormones
Memory alteration
Regulation of respiration
Modulation of immune response

At least five functional types of opiate receptors have been characterized: taken together with the multiple forms of endogenous opiate peptides, the complexity of the system is great. The complexity is further increased by variation in response (desensitization, tolerance,

FIGURE 69-2 *Biosynthetic pathway for β-endorphin in the pituitary gland. A single precursor protein, pro-opiomelanocortin (POMC) (molecular weight of approximately 31,000), is initially synthesized from translation of a gene that encodes the structure of adrenocorticotropin (ACTH), β-lipotropin (β-LPH), and β-endorphin. Prohormone-type cleavages can generate other hormones from the same precursor, although this occurs in tissues other than the pituitary. Abbreviations: MSH = melanocyte-stimulating hormone; LPH = lipotropin; CLIP = corticotropin-like intermediate peptide; ACTH = adrenocorticotropin.*

FIGURE 69-3 *Biosynthetic precursor for enkephalins (pre-proenkephalin A) in the adrenal gland. The protein precursor contains 260 amino acids and has a molecular weight of approximately 50,000. Prohormone-type cleavages have the potential to generate six copies of methionine-enkephalin (Met-enk) and one of leucine-enkephalin (Leu-enk) from a single precursor molecule. The signal peptide sequence at the amino terminus (leftmost portion) of the precursor protein is characteristic of secreted proteins.*

etc.) to a given opiate over time or in relation to the pattern of its exposure to receptors and by the fact that a single neuron (or endocrine cell) may secrete more than one neuromediator.

Receptor interaction leads to the formation of a second messenger. For the opiate system in general, receptor interaction leads to a decrease in both basal and stimulated cyclic AMP levels, and chronic exposure to opiate peptides produces a long-term decline in intracellular cyclic AMP levels. As a compensatory response, however, the number of adenylate cyclase units gradually increases with time. This biochemical change may be the physiologic correlate of tolerance and tachyphylaxis, requiring higher doses of opiate to suppress cyclic AMP levels. Sudden withdrawal of opiates at a time when the cell is enriched in adenylate cyclase releases these units from inhibition, resulting in "overshoot" of cyclic AMP levels, and perhaps contributing to development of the opiate withdrawal syndrome.

ENDOCRINOLOGY OF ENDOGENOUS OPIOID PEPTIDES   Endocrine physiology

ACTH, β-endorphin, and β-lipotropin biosynthesis and secretion by the pituitary gland are linked both in normal and in abnormal states. Under normal conditions, β-lipotropin circulates in higher molar concentrations than does β-endorphin, but the radioimmunoassays used clinically recognize both entities. Hence, levels of immunoreactive β-endorphin reflect the combined levels of β-endorphin and β-lipotropin. Such radioimmunoassays provide clinical evidence of the biosynthetic link between ACTH and β-endorphin. For instance, in Addison's disease the plasma levels of both ACTH and immunoreactive β-endorphin are elevated; likewise, glucocorticoid replacement decreases both ACTH and β-endorphin levels. Administration of corticotropin-releasing factor (CRF) stimulates release of both ACTH and immunoreactive β-endorphin in a parallel manner. In Nelson's syndrome (development of a pituitary tumor after bilateral adrenalectomy for Cushing's disease), both plasma ACTH and immunoreactive β-endorphin levels are elevated. Ectopic production of ACTH by tumors is also accompanied by immunoreactive β-endorphin excess. In the latter case, measurement of immunoreactive β-endorphin can be useful as a tumor marker and in some cases serves to monitor treatment.

Cushing's disease   Immunoreactive β-endorphin is easily detected and less prone to destruction during sample storage and handling

TABLE 69-2   Endocrine effects of endogenous opiate peptides and opiate antagonists

Hormone	Opioid peptide	Naloxone
Luteinizing hormone (LH)	↓	↑
Follicle-stimulating hormone (FSH)	↓	↑
Growth hormone (GH)	↑	↔
Prolactin (Prl)	↑	↔ or ↓
Antidiuretic hormone (ADH)	↑	↑
Adrenocorticotropin (ACTH)	↓	↑
Cortisol	↓	↑
Insulin	↑	↔
Glucagon	↑	↔
Somatostatin	↓	↔

than is ACTH. Furthermore, differentiation of patients with pituitary-dependent Cushing's disease from normal subjects on the basis of a single plasma ACTH and cortisol determination is generally unreliable because of the episodic release and rapid clearance of ACTH in both normals and patients with Cushing's disease (see Chaps. 321 and 325). β-Endorphin and β-lipotropin have a longer half-life in blood and as stated above cross react in most radioimmunoassays. Measurement of plasma immunoreactive β-endorphin, together with plasma cortisol, may be useful for the diagnosis of Cushing's disease. In addition, evaluation of response of the pituitary to maneuvers such as dexamethasone suppression or metyrapone stimulation can be assessed using the β-endorphin radioimmunoassay. Hence, measurement of plasma levels of β-endorphin and β-lipotropin may supplement, if not supplant, those of ACTH in evaluation of the pituitary-adrenal axis in suspected cases of Cushing's disease. Furthermore, patterns of hormonal secretion may be altered in states of abnormal physiology. For example, pituitary tumors responsible for Cushing's disease may secrete a different ratio of β-lipotropin to β-endorphin than occurs in the normal pituitary.

Releasing factors   Two general approaches have been employed to determine the role of endorphins in normal physiology (Table 69-2). The first has been to determine the effects of direct administration of endogenous opiate peptides to animals or humans via the systemic circulation or the cerebrospinal fluid. For example, the pharmacologic administration of β-endorphin produces an increase in the secretion of growth hormone (GH), prolactin (Prl), and arginine vasopressin (AVP) and a decrease in the secretion of ACTH, cortisol, luteinizing hormone (LH), and follicle-stimulating hormone (FSH). The effects of β-endorphin on the pituitary gland are not thought to result from direct action on the pituitary but by modulating release of hypothalamic hormones. Hence, they are not direct hypothalamic releasing factors.

An alternate approach to determining the role of the endogenous opiate peptides is to assess the effects of selective antagonists of the opiates, such as naloxone. Such agents block the effects of endogenously secreted opiates, revealing the tonic or physiologic role of opiate peptides. Naloxone administration causes elevations in LH, FSH, and ACTH levels and prevents the stress-mediated rise in prolactin levels. However, naloxone does not cause sustained lowering of GH levels in patients with acromegaly or Prl levels in patients with prolactinomas.

Reproductive endocrinology   Administration of opiate antagonists alters the secretory patterns of gonadotropins, suggesting a role for the endorphins in normal reproduction. The effects depend on the sex, age, species, and levels of sex steroids at the time of study. Administration of opiate antagonists causes an increase in the frequency and amplitude of pulsatile secretion of LH, suggesting that gonadotropins are tonically inhibited by endogenous opiate peptides. β-Endorphins are present in hypothalamic portal blood of primates: they are high during the midfollicular and luteal phases of the menstrual cycle but virtually undetectable at the time of menses. Similarly, β-endorphin levels in the hypothalamic portal circulation are low or undetectable in oophorectomized animals, suggesting that ovarian steroids may modulate or play a permissive role in hypothalamic endorphin secretion and that β-endorphin may play a regulatory role in the normal menstrual cycle.

In addition, endorphins may play a role in puberty. Steady increases in plasma β-endorphin levels occur during human puberty, and a decline in the sensitivity of the hypothalamic-pituitary axis to opiate-mediated inhibition of LH secretion occurs in animals as they mature. Thus, "escape" from tonic inhibition may signal the onset of puberty.

Abnormal reproductive function in some women may be linked to alterations in endogenous opiate peptide levels. Extreme stress often produces a delay in the onset of puberty in girls. Similarly, women may develop irregular or absent menses during times of stress, possibly reflecting the effects of stress-increased central endorphin levels and subsequent suppression of pituitary gonadotropin secretion. Female narcotic addicts rarely have normal menses (even prior to marked weight loss), again suggesting a link between opiate receptor activation and inhibition of endocrine reproductive function. Finally, peripheral levels of immunoreactive β-endorphin (reflecting pituitary secretion) increase several-fold with intensive and regular exercise, and the development of oligomenorrhea or amenorrhea in women athletes may reflect the effects of exercise-induced β-endorphin on gonadotropin secretion. Hence, under several conditions of "stress," endogenous opiate peptides may serve to suppress ovulation. Finally, in adddition to brain and pituitary, the pro-ACTH/endorphin precursor system is present in the ovaries, testes, and placenta, further suggesting a role for endogenous opiates in reproduction.

Diabetes mellitus Endorphin-containing cells are in close proximity to insulin-containing cells in the endocrine pancreas. β-Endorphin stimulates insulin and glucagon release and inhibits somatostatin secretion, effects that can be reversed by naloxone. Patients with non-insulin-dependent diabetes who receive chlorpropamide develop facial flushing after taking alcohol. This flushing response is blocked by naloxone and reproduced by opiate peptides and is thought to be related to increased sensitivity to endogenous opiates in diabetics. However, a significant role for endorphins in carbohydrate metabolism or a contribution of β-endorphin to the pathophysiology of diabetes has not been established.

NEUROPHYSIOLOGY OF ENDOGENOUS OPIATE PEPTIDES **Anatomic location** β-Endorphin is present in the pituitary gland and in the brain. In the human pituitary, ACTH and endorphin-containing cells are found in the anteromedial region of the anterior lobe, at the posterior boundary of the anterior lobe, and in nerve fibers of the posterior lobe. By histochemical criteria, the pituitary is the richest site of endorphin in the body.

The hypothalamus contains neurons that biosynthesize endorphin. These neurons have long projections to other regions of the brain. For example, regions of the brain associated with the limbic system contain substantial quantities of immunoreactive β-endorphin, suggesting a role in memory, learning, and emotions.

Neurons containing the enkephalins are distributed even more widely in the central nervous system. Concentrations are particularly high in the dorsal columns of the spinal cord, a region that contains opiate receptors and that is involved in the transmission of pain (see Chap. 3). Enkephalins are also present in the gastrointestinal tract. Concentrations in the myenteric plexus of the longitudinal muscles of the gut are higher than in the brain. Enkephalins are synthesized in the chromaffin cells of the adrenal medulla and packaged together with the catecholamines in the same secretory granules. Enkephalin is released as part of the sympathetic response to stress together with epinephrine and norepinephrine (Fig. 69-4). Similarly, enkephalin levels in blood are high in pheochromocytoma.

Pain transmission and amelioration The endogenous opiate peptides play a role in regulating pain transmission. In the dorsal horn of the spinal column, enkephalins are released by interneurons that impinge on afferent pain-sensing fibers from the periphery. These pain-transmitting fibers form synapses in the gray matter of the dorsal horn with a second set of neurons, which cross and ascend through the spinal cord as the lateral spinothalamic tract. The release of enkephalins (which may be influenced by descending neuronal input from higher centers) inhibits release of substance P, a neurotransmitter that mediates pain, from afferent fibers entering the dorsal horn (see Chap. 3).

Microinjections of β-endorphin into the central nervous system produce analgesia in animals. Electrical stimulation of regions of the brain involved in pain transmission, such as the periventricular gray area, produces analgesia accompanied by an increase in cerebrospinal fluid levels of endorphins or enkephalins. In the decerebrate cat, localized administration of enkephalin selectively blocks spontaneous firing of neurons involved in pain transmission.

In humans, increased β-endorphin levels have been found in the cerebrospinal fluid of patients with chronic pain from malignancy or causalgia. As in animals, electrical stimulation of periventricular sites produces analgesia accompanied by increased immunoreactive β-endorphin levels, and direct administration of β-endorphin into the cerebrospinal fluid of subjects with terminal malignancies has produced long-lasting analgesia without systemic morphine-like side effects.

Acupuncture and placebo effects The induction of analgesia by acupuncture may be mediated by endogenous opiate peptides. In some studies, the induction of analgesia by acupuncture is accompanied by increased cerebrospinal fluid levels of endorphins whereas coadministration of naloxone (the opiate antagonist) blocks acupuncture-mediated analgesia. Likewise, the effects of placebos may reflect the capacity of an individual to recruit the endogenous opiate peptide system. In studies in which tooth extraction was the pain stimulus, placebo analgesia can be reversed by the administration of naloxone. Similarly, the phenomena of placebo tolerance and dependence are consistent with known properties of the endogenous opioid system.

Behavioral effects Administration of opiate peptides to animals at doses below those required to produce analgesia generates specific and striking behavioral responses. Rats who receive intracerebral β-endorphin display a "catonic-like" behavior, as a consequence of massive hippocampal seizures. Certain stereotyped forms of behavior are also seen, such as the production of "wet-dog shakes." In cats, a rage response is elicited.

Furthermore, it has been suggested that abnormal levels of endogenous opioids or their receptors may play a causal or contributory role in major psychiatric disorders. In one study of schizophrenia, the frequency of auditory hallucinations decreased in patients receiving naloxone. However, other attempts to correlate levels of β-endorphin with states of depression, mania, or other psychiatric disorders have been unsuccessful.

Addictive behavior in humans has also been postulated to be linked to altered levels of endogenous opiate peptides. The susceptibility to chronic abuse of narcotics might be a genetically predetermined disorder of the endogenous opiate system. In addition, certain types of habitual behavior have been described as "addictive." Marathon running and other forms of intensive exercise dramatically increase β-endorphin levels, leading to the hypothesis that such activity creates an internal (central) "self-reward." However, supporting data regarding central nervous system levels of endogenous opiates (perhaps at highly localized anatomic sites) have not been obtained.

OTHER PHYSIOLOGIC AND PATHOPHYSIOLOGIC RESPONSES
Thermogenesis The opiate peptides may play a role in the adaptive response to heat. Chronic exposure of animals to high temperature

FIGURE 69-4 *Hormonal response to stress indicating release of endogenous opiate peptides and other hormones into the systemic circulation and cerebrospinal fluid. Abbreviations: CRF = corticotropin-releasing hormone; EPI = epinephrine; NE = norepinephrine; CNS = central nervous system; ACTH = adrenocorticotropin.*

followed by administration of naloxone produces a rapid increase in body temperature. Peptides encoded in the precursor molecule and related to endorphin, such as γ-melanocyte-stimulating hormone (γ-MSH), produce rapid decreases in body temperature.

Stress   Increased secretion of β-endorphin and β-lipotropin accompanies the increased ACTH and cortisol levels during stress. Similarly, serum prolactin levels increase in stress. The increase in serum prolactin is blocked by administration of naloxone, suggesting that stress-mediated prolactin release is in part stimulated by endogenous opiates. In certain species, stress-induced eating is blocked by naloxone. The endocrinologic and central role of corticotropin-releasing factor (CRF) as a "stress hormone" links pituitary β-endorphin and β-lipotropin secretion to ACTH and cortisol as part of the stress response, although the target organ(s) for β-endorphin and β-lipotropin action are not known (Fig. 69-4).

Appetite control   Endorphins may play a role in normal regulation of appetite and in eating disorders. Genetically obese mice and rats have marked increases in the pituitary content of β-endorphin, β-lipotropin, and ACTH. Injection of β-endorphin into the brain of such animals or injection of morphine subcutaneously produces further increase in food intake. This increase in feeding in genetically obese animals but not in their normal counterparts is blocked by naloxone. Decreased food intake has also been observed in humans given opiate antagonists. The site of action of endorphin in feeding behavior appears to be the hypothalamic paraventricular nucleus. In addition to potential central nervous system sites of endorphin action, opiate receptors are present in the gastrointestinal tract. Furthermore, β-endorphin is synthesized in the pancreas, where it acts (in a paracrine fashion) to stimulate insulin release, perhaps leading to increased food intake and altered glucose utilization.

Blood pressure and shock   Severe hypotension or shock stimulates the pituitary release of ACTH, β-lipotropin, and β-endorphin and a subsequent increase in blood cortisol levels. However, a large component of the stress response may not be to the advantage of the organism. In sepsis, immunoreactive β-endorphin levels in blood rise prior to the development of hypotension. Administration of naloxone partially or completely restores blood pressure in experimental hemorrhagic, "neurogenic" or spinal, and septic shock, resulting in decreased mortality in the latter condition. The amount of β-endorphin that is released under these circumstances appears to be regulated (at least in some species); administration of naloxone during endotoxin-mediated shock produces even greater increases in β-endorphin levels, suggesting that β-endorphin secretion is under feedback control. The putative short feedback-inhibitory loop from the pituitary to the hypothalamus could occur via the general circulation since the median eminence of the hypothalamus is one region of the brain which lies outside the blood-brain barrier. Alternatively, one study suggests that pituitary endorphins may ascend to the hypothalamus via the hypothalamic-pituitary portal circulation in what is conventionally regarded as a retrograde direction. It is important to note that several biochemical mediators may contribute to the development of septic shock. For example, platelet-activating factor, arachidonic acid metabolites, kinins, immunoregulatory peptides, and other substances (in addition the endogenous opiates) may participate in septic shock. The relative contribution of these factors to hypotension appears to vary from species to species. Hence, the role of endorphins and enkephalins in the pathophysiology of septic shock in humans requires further study.

Regulation of respiration   Opiate receptors are present in regions of the brainstem responsible for regulation of respiration, but a role for these agents in regulation of respiration is not established. In one study treatment of patients with chronic obstructive pulmonary disease with naloxone increased the magnitude of the ventilatory response to airway resistance and caused an increase in dyspnea. However, in another study naloxone did not increase responsiveness to carbon dioxide rebreathing. Furthermore, the ventilatory response to short-term hypoxia is not altered by naloxone in normal adults. Hence, it is unlikely that endorphins serve a major regulatory role in respiration.

Rather, they may participate in the fine-tuning of ventilation and may be responsible for variations in respiratory drive among individuals. Alternatively, their effects may be amplified when normal regulatory mechanisms are disturbed.

Immune system interactions   The endogenous opiates may provide a biochemical link between the brain, the neuroendocrine system, and the immune system and might provide an explanation for the concept that emotional stress may be associated with compromised immune response, perhaps leading to increased infection and unmasking of malignancy when immune surveillance is nonoptimal.

Opiate receptors are present on human granulocytes, lymphocytes, and monocytes, and there is some evidence that lymphocytes produce a β-endorphin–like substance. Unfortunately, attempts to define a potential regulatory role for opiate peptides in the immune response suggest both suppressive and stimulatory effects, depending on the assay system employed. Opiate peptides stimulate human macrophage chemotaxis, inhibit or increase lymphocyte proliferation, and variably affect natural killer cell activity. The integrated effects of the opiates on immune system responsiveness in vivo remain to be clarified.

CLINICAL IMPLICATIONS   Insights gathered from the study of the endogenous opiate peptides hold therapeutic promise in several disorders, particularly in the areas of reproduction, appetite control, and obesity. Elucidation of the pathways and means of transmission of pain has important implications for treatment of pain. Further understanding of the mechanism of action and the cellular responses to the opiate peptides may provide insight into the pathophysiology of addiction, tolerance, and withdrawal from narcotics and into the management of these disorders. Information regarding psychiatric health and disease may also be afforded by study of the endogenous opiates, and naloxone is under investigation as part of the therapeutic regimen for septic shock.

Knowledge of the structure of the endogenous opiates has permitted chemical synthesis of these substances and the design of analogues. Analogues containing any of the following properties might be clinically useful: long duration of action, oral bioavailability, increased potency, selectivity within the spectrum of action of opiates, decreased side effects, and nonaddictive properties.

Many important principles have emerged from the study of the endogenous opiate peptides. The biologic properties of a naturally occurring peptide depend not only on its structure but also on its location and the type of cell with which it interacts. For example, the same chemical substance may act both as a neuromodulator for analgesia and as a hormone that influences gonadotropin secretion.

In addition, study of the opiate peptide system has demonstrated a fundamental pharmacologic principle. Receptors that bind drugs normally interact with endogenous ligands. Such endogenous substances may belong to a chemical class different from the drug (i.e., morphine is an alkaloid, and endorphin is a peptide). Furthermore, the endogenous substances may be more potent and possess fewer side-effects than the currently utilized pharmacologic agent. Exploitation of this principle might uncover endogenous compounds with digoxin-like, tricyclic antidepressant–like, or benzodiazepine-like effects. Isolation of these substances and determination of their structure should provide new biologically active agents.

REFERENCES

CARR DB, ROSENBLATT MR: Endorphins in the normal and abnormal pituitary. Proceedings of the International Symposium on Pituitary Tumors, June 1983, in PM Black et al (eds), *Secretory Tumors of the Pituitary Gland (Progress in Endocrine Research and Therapy).* New York, Raven, 1984, pp 245–261

HUGHES J et al: Identification of two related pentapeptides from the brain with potent opiate agonist activity. Nature 258:577, 1975

MARTIN WR: Pharmacology of opioids. Pharmacol Rev 35:283, 1984

MORLEY JE: The endocrinology of the opiates and opioid peptides. Metabolism 30:195, 1981

PERT CB et al: Neuropeptides and their receptors: A psychosomatic network. J Immunol 135:820s, 1985

PFEIFFER A, HERZ A: Endocrine actions of opioids. Horm Metabol Res 16:386, 1984

WATKINS LR, MAYER DJ: Organization of endogenous opiate and nonopiate pain control systems. Science 216:1185, 1982

70 NUTRITIONAL REQUIREMENTS

DANIEL RUDMAN

ESSENTIAL AND NONESSENTIAL NUTRIENTS AND THEIR THRESHOLDS (REQUIREMENTS, ALLOWANCES, AND TOLERANCES) Over the past few decades diverse factors, including increased personal income, expanded public assistance programs, and vitamin and mineral enrichment of food, have reduced the prevalence of the classic nutritional deficiency diseases. Nevertheless, malnutrition, both overt and subclinical, remains a major problem, especially among the poor, the elderly, alcoholics, the chronically ill, and hospital populations. All too often the patient's nutritional status is ignored during the clinical evaluation, and complete nutritional needs are not met during hospitalization. To approach nutritional care rationally, the physician, understanding how disease affects the two types of nutrient thresholds (requirement and tolerance), must assess the patient's preexisting nutritional status, calculate the needs for maintenance and repletion, and institute the appropriate diet therapy.

The body contains many thousands of species of organic molecules but requires for health the intake of only 24 organic compounds in addition to a source of energy and water: 9 essential amino acids, 2 fatty acids, and 13 vitamins. The vast majority of organic molecules in food, although metabolized or assimilated by the body, are "nonessential" in the sense that their deletion from the diet does not cause illness. The simplicity of the nutritional requirements, compared with the complexity of body composition, is the result of the remarkable capacity for endogenous biosynthesis.

Of the inorganic compounds in food, 15 are believed to be nutritionally essential: calcium, phosphorus, iodine, iron, magnesium, zinc, copper, potassium, sodium, chloride, cobalt, chromium, manganese, molybdenum, and selenium. (It is possible that arsenic, vanadium, and tin may also be essential trace elements.)

The requirement of an essential nutrient is defined as the smallest quantity that maintains normal mass, chemical composition, morphology, and physiologic functions of the body and prevents any clinical or biochemical sign of the corresponding deficiency state. In children, an additional criterion is a normal rate of growth. When the intake of an essential nutrient is limited, the body may conserve that nutrient by increasing absorption (e.g., calcium, iron); by slowing catabolism (e.g., amino acids, calories); by minimizing excretion (e.g., sodium, potassium, magnesium, chloride, phosphate, water); and by mobilizing body reserves (e.g., vitamin A, vitamin B_{12}, essential fatty acids). Only when these homeostatic reactions are inadequate does the nutritional deficiency state appear. The time that elapses, after the intake of an essential nutrient is interrupted (for example, during total parenteral nutrition with an incomplete formula), before a deficiency state develops is proportional to the ratio of body stores divided by daily requirement.

Because requirements vary among individuals due to numerous genetic and environmental circumstances, the recommended dietary allowances (RDA) provide a margin of safety sufficient to meet the needs of 90 to 95 percent of the healthy population (Tables 70-1 and 70-2). RDA is determined as follows:

1 In healthy adults the requirements of protein (or its constituent amino acids) and macrominerals (requirements greater than 100 mg per day) can be assessed by balance techniques. The daily balance of each element equals intake minus output (urinary plus fecal). The requirement of each amino acid or macromineral is the smallest intake that maintains zero balance for nitrogen or for the mineral under study. A negative balance of any essential element, if it persists long enough, leads to illness and death.

2 In the infant or growing child the requirement of energy and essential nutrients is the smallest amount of each that maintains an optimal rate of growth while all others are fed in adequate amounts.

3 For micronutrients (requirement less than 100 mg per day) the requirement is the smallest daily intake that prevents eventual appearance of the nutrient-specific deficiency state.

Table 70-3 lists the amino acids required by infants and adults to illustrate the effect of age on nutrient requirements. Table 70-4 describes the main features of the illness which ensues when each essential nutrient is deficient.

Another nutritional threshold is the maximal tolerance of a nutrient. Just as intake of any essential nutrient below a specific level causes disease, intake above a certain level for many nutrients (either essential or nonessential) disturbs body structure or function. Intakes exceeding tolerance can lead to acute reversible symptoms, acute permanent damage, or progressive systemic impairments (Table 70-5). A physiologic diet provides intakes of each nutrient between the two thresholds of minimal requirement and maximal tolerance. The recognition that tolerance for a nutrient can be exceeded is particularly important during parenteral nutrition, when the gastrointestinal mechanisms (anorexia, emesis, incomplete absorption, diarrhea) that ordinarily help protect the individual from the effects of excessive nutrient intake are bypassed. Although allowance values have been established for the essential nutrients, the actual maximal tolerance levels in many cases are uncertain.

FACTORS ALTERING NUTRITIONAL THRESHOLDS The recommended allowance and the maximal tolerance of each essential nutrient are influenced by many factors: rate of growth, age, exercise, pregnancy and lactation, chemical composition of the diet, diseases, drugs. In addition, the route, rate, and timing of alimentation influence requirements and tolerances. As the "window" between requirement and tolerance narrows, nutritional management becomes more difficult (e.g., protein intake of a cachectic, encephalopathic, cirrhotic patient).

Physiologic factors Growth, exercise, pregnancy, and lactation (Table 70-1) increase the daily requirements per unit of body weight for energy and for most essential nutrients. In the aged person, basal energy requirements per kilogram of lean body mass are the same as those of a younger person; nevertheless, energy requirements decline with age due to the reduced lean body mass and reduced activity. Amino acid and calcium requirements may be higher in old age; optimal nutrient intakes for the elderly are, in general, still uncertain.

Composition of the diet Given diets with identical contents of nitrogen, digestible carbohydrates, fat, vitamins, and minerals, the metabolic availability of the nutrients may vary widely. Thus, all proteins are not equally effective in meeting the daily requirement because of differences in digestibility or in content of essential amino acids (Table 70-6). Gastrointestinal absorption of some minerals is influenced by the presence in the diet of other reactive components; the utilization of vitamins may be influenced by level of intake of organic macronutrients. Examples are given in Table 70-7.

Route, rate, and time (see Chap. 74) The allowances listed in Tables 70-1 to 70-3 apply to enteral nutrition. For some nutrients, different amounts are required for parenteral nutrition. Net gastrointestinal absorption of ingested amino acids, carbohydrates, fats, sodium, chloride, and potassium normally is greater than 90 percent (Table 70-8), and these nutrients have the same RDAs for the intravenous as for the enteral route. For others of the essential minerals, however, net absorption is only 50 percent or less (Table

TABLE 70-1 Recommended daily dietary allowances[a]

Age, years	Weight, kg	Height, cm	Energy, kcal	Protein, g	Fat-soluble vitamins Vitamin A RE[b], μg	Vitamin D, μg[c]	Vitamin E, mg αTE[d]
INFANTS							
0.0–05	6	60	kg × 115	kg × 2.2	420	10	3
0.5–1.0	9	71	kg × 105	kg × 2.0	400	10	4
CHILDREN							
1–3	13	90	1300	23	400	10	5
4–6	20	112	1700	30	500	10	6
7–10	28	132	2400	34	700	10	7
MALES							
11–14	45	157	2700	45	1000	10	8
15–18	66	176	2800	56	1000	10	10
19–22	70	177	2900	56	1000	7.5	10
23–50	70	178	2700	56	1000	5	10
51+	70	178	2400	56	1000	5	10
FEMALES							
11–14	46	157	2200	46	800	10	8
15–18	55	163	2100	46	800	10	8
19–22	55	163	2100	44	800	7.5	8
23–50	55	163	2000	44	800	5	8
51+	55	163	1800	44	800	5	8
PREGNANCY							
			+300	+30	+200	+5	+2
LACTATION							
			+500	+20	+400	+5	+3

[a] The allowances are intended to provide for individual variations among most normal persons as they live in the United States under usual environmental stresses. Diets should be based on a variety of common foods in order to provide other nutrients for which human requirements have been less well defined.
[b] Retinol equivalents; 1 retinol equivalent = 1 μg retinol or 6 μg β-carotene.
[c] As cholecalciferol; 10 μg cholecalciferol = 400 IU vitamin D.
[c] α-Tocopherol equivalents; 1 mg d-α-tocopherol = 1 αTE.
[e] Niacin equivalents; 1 NE = 1 mg niacin or 60 mg dietary tryptophan.

70-8); consequently the intravenous requirement is only a fraction of the oral one. It is also likely that the requirements of amino acids are not identical by enteral and parenteral routes. After ingestion and absorption into the portal venous system, a portion of the absorbed amino acids is catabolized or transformed during the "first pass" through the liver, where many of the enzymes of amino acid degradation and intermediary metabolism are located. Intravenously infused amino acids, in contrast, partially bypass these catabolic and biosynthetic pathways and reach sites of protein synthesis in muscle and other extrahepatic tissues.

Timing can be important. For example, all of the essential amino acids must be supplied simultaneously to support protein synthesis. If one such essential amino acid, e.g., tryptophan, is administered at a different time than the other amino acids, assimilation of all into protein is curtailed. Similarly, when amino acids, glucose, lipids, and minerals are infused at separate times during the day or week,

as often happens in parenteral feeding, assimilation may be impaired. For example, omission of phosphorus or potassium from hyperalimentation solutions impairs retention of the nitrogen furnished by the same fluid.

For these various reasons, the daily requirements of essential nutrients delivered by the parenteral route still remain uncertain.

Disease Nutritional requirements and tolerances may be altered by disease through at least seven mechanisms (see also Table 70-9):

1 *Increased utilization of nutrients.* Fever, infection, and trauma increase resting metabolic rate and, as a consequence, daily caloric requirements. Folate is utilized more rapidly in patients with hemolysis and increased cell turnover (hemolytic anemia, psoriasis, cancer). Many nutritional requirements are greater during repletion from cachexia than during maintenance of normal nutriture. In this respect, the repletion process in adults resembles growth in children.

TABLE 70-2 Estimated safe and adequate daily dietary intakes of additional selected vitamins and minerals[*][†]

	Vitamins Age, yr	Vitamin K, μg	Biotin, μg	Pantothenic acid, mg	Trace elements Copper, mg	Manganese, mg	Fluoride, mg	Chromium, mg	Selenium, mg
Infants	0–0.5	12	35	2	0.5–0.7	0.5–0.7	0.1–0.5	0.01–0.04	0.01–0.04
	0.5–1.0	10–20	50	3	0.7–1.0	0.7–1.0	0.2–1.0	0.02–0.06	0.02–0.06
Children and adolescents	1–3	15–30	65	3	1.0–1.5	1.0–1.5	0.5–1.5	0.02–0.08	0.02–0.08
	4–6	20–40	85	3–4	1.5–2.0	1.5–2.0	1.0–2.5	0.03–0.12	0.03–0.12
	7–10	30–60	120	4–5	2.0–2.5	2.0–3.0	1.5–2.5	0.05–0.20	0.05–0.20
	11+	50–100	100–200	4–7	2.0–3.0	2.5–5.0	1.5–2.5	0.05–0.20	0.05–0.20
Adults		70–140	100–200	4–7	2.0–3.0	2.5–5.0	1.5–4.0	0.05–0.20	0.05–0.20

* Because there is less information on which to base an allowance, these are not given in the main table of dietary allowances but are provided here in the form of ranges of recommended intakes.
† Because the toxic levels for many trace elements may be only several times usual intakes, the upper levels for the trace elements given in this table should not be habitually exceeded.

Water-soluble vitamins							Minerals					
Ascorbic Acid, mg	Thiamin, mg	Riboflavin, mg	Niacin, mg NE^d	Vitamin B$_6$, mg	Folacin, µg^f	Vitamin B$_{12}$, µg	Calcium, mg	Phosphorus, mg	Magnesium, mg	Iron, mg	Zinc, mg	Iodine, µg
35	0.3	0.4	6	0.3	30	0.5	360	240	50	10	3	40
35	0.5	0.6	8	0.6	45	1.5^g	540	360	70	15	5	50
45	0.7	0.8	9	0.9	100	2.0	800	800	150	15	10	70
45	0.9	1.0	11	1.3	200	2.5	800	800	200	10	10	90
45	1.2	1.4	16	1.6	300	3.0	800	800	250	10	10	120
50	1.4	1.6	18	1.8	400	3.0	1200	1200	350	18	15	150
60	1.4	1.7	18	2.0	400	3.0	1200	1200	400	18	15	150
60	1.5	1.7	19	2.2	400	3.0	800	800	350	10	15	150
60	1.4	1.6	18	2.2	400	3.0	800	800	350	10	15	150
60	1.2	1.4	16	2.2	400	3.0	800	800	350	10	15	150
60	1.1	1.3	15	1.8	400	3.0	1200	1200	300	18	15	150
60	1.1	1.3	14	2.0	400	3.0	1200	1200	300	18	15	150
60	1.1	1.3	14	2.0	400	3.0	800	800	300	18	15	150
60	1.0	1.2	13	2.0	400	3.0	800	800	300	18	15	150
60	1.0	1.2	13	2.0	400	3.0	800	800	300	10	15	150
+20	+0.4	+0.3	+2	+0.6	+400	+1.0	+400	+400	+150	^{h}	+5	125
+40	+0.5	+0.5	+5	+0.5	+100	+1.0	+400	+400	+150	^{h}	+10	250

^{f} The folacin allowances refer to dietary sources as determined by Lactobacillus casei *assay after treatment with enzymes ("conjugases") to make polyglutamyl forms of the vitamin available to the test organism.*

^{g} The RDA for vitamin B$_{12}$ in infants is based on average concentration of the vitamin in human milk. The allowances after weaning are based on energy intake (as recommended by the American Academy of Pediatrics) and consideration of other factors such as intestinal absorption.

^{h} The increased requirement during pregnancy cannot be met by the iron content of habitual U.S. diets nor by the existing iron stores of many women; therefore, the use of 30 to 60 mg of supplemental iron is recommended. Iron needs during lactation are not substantially different from those of nonpregnant women, but continued supplementation of the mother for 2 to 3 months after parturition is advisable in order to replenish stores depleted by pregnancy.

2 *Malabsorption.* For each nutrient absorbed less efficiently than normal in malabsorption states, the daily requirement is increased correspondingly.

3 *Impaired ability to activate or utilize a nutrient.* The requirement for vitamin D is increased by renal disease that impairs hydroxylation of the vitamin; requirements for folate, thiamin, and pyridoxine in subjects with cirrhosis of the liver may be greater than normal because of impaired hepatic capacity to transform these vitamins into their active forms. Injured or infected patients may utilize glucose and triglyceride less efficiently than healthy individuals.

4 *Abnormally large losses of nutrients.* Impaired conservation of electrolytes or amino acids because of renal disease, burns, blood loss, nasogastric suction, diarrhea, or hemodialysis leads to loss of nutrients. One criterion of normal nutriture for nitrogen and minerals in the adult is zero elemental balance, i.e., enteral or parenteral intake equal to urinary plus fecal output. If output of nitrogen or mineral is increased by abnormal renal or extrarenal loss, then intake must be correspondingly higher to maintain zero balance.

5 *Impaired catabolic or excretory pathways.* Metabolic defects can reduce both requirement and tolerance, because the rate of degradation or excretion of a nutrient is slowed. In children with phenylketonuria or maple syrup urine disease, the requirements for phenylalanine or branched-chain amino acids, respectively, are less than normal. Patients with uremia have a reduced dietary requirement for nonessential amino acids.

6 *Hyperabsorption.* Increased absorption can result in a decrease in both requirement and tolerance. Examples are calcium in hyperabsorptive hypercalciuria, iron in hemochromatosis, and copper in Wilson's disease.

7 *Drugs.* Pharmacologic agents can alter nutritional requirements by

Molybdenum, mg	Electrolytes		
	Sodium, mg	Potassium, mg	Chloride, mg
0.03–0.06	115–350	350–925	275–700
0.04–0.08	250–750	425–1275	400–1200
0.05–0.10	325–975	550–1650	500–1500
0.06–0.15	450–1350	775–2350	700–2100
0.10–0.30	600–1800	1000–3000	925–2775
0.15–0.50	900–2700	1525–4575	1400–4200
0.15–0.50	1100–3300	1875–5625	1700–5100

TABLE 70-3 Recommended daily allowances of the essential amino acids per kilogram of body weight for infants, children, and adult male subjects

Amino acid	Infants*	Children	Adults
L-Threonine	68	28	8
L-Valine	92	25	14
L-Isoleucine	83	28	12
L-Leucine	135	42	16
L-Lysine	99	44	12
L-Tryptophan	21	4	3
L-Methionine-cystine	49	22	10
L-Phenylalanine-tyrosine	141	22	16
L-Histidine	33	?†	?†

* The preterm infant has additional requirements for arginine, tyrosine, cystine, and taurine.

† Essentiality has been established by long-term nitrogen balance and plasma amino acids; however, recommended levels of intake have not been established.

TABLE 70-4 Symptoms and manifestations of nutrient deficiency

Nutrient	Disorders and symptoms of deficiency	Laboratory tests
Water	Thirst, poor tissue turgor, dry mucous membranes, vascular collapse, altered mental status	Serum electrolytes ↑, serum osmolarity ↑, total body water ↓
Calories (energy)	Weakness and physical inactivity, loss of subcutaneous fat, muscle wasting, bradycardia	Weight loss, MAFA ↓, MAMA ↓, creatinine/height ↓, BMR ↓
Protein	Psychomotor change, dyspigmented, sparse, and easily plucked hair, "flaky-paint" dermatitis, edema, muscle wasting, hepatomegaly, ↓ growth	MAMA ↓, serum albumin, transferrin, retinol binding protein ↓, anemia, creatinine/height ↓, serum nonessential/essential amino acids ↑, urine urea/creatinine ↓
Linoleic acid	Xerosis, desquamation, thickening of skin, hair loss, fatty liver, delayed wound healing	Serum ratio of triene to tetraene fatty acids ↑
Linolenic acid	Visual defect	↓ Serum ω3 fatty acids, thrombocytopenia, abnormal liver function tests
Vitamin A	Xerosis of eye and skin, xerophthalmia, Bitot's spot, follicular hyperkeratosis, hypogeusia, hyposmia	Plasma vitamin A ↓, dark adaptation time ↑
Vitamin D	Rickets and growth failure in children, osteomalacia in adults	Serum alkaline phosphatase concentration ↑, plasma 25-hydroxycholecalciferol ↓, serum Ca^{2+} and P ↓
Vitamin E	Anemia	Plasma α-tocopherol ↓, hemolysis of RBC in dilute H_2O_2
Vitamin K	Bleeding diathesis	Prothrombin time ↑
Vitamin C (ascorbic acid)	Scurvy, petechiae, ecchymoses, perifollicular hemorrhage, spongy and bleeding gums (if not edentulous)	Ascorbic acid concentration in plasma, platelets, whole blood, and white blood cells ↓; urinary ascorbic acid ↓
Thiamin (vitamin B_1)	Beriberi, muscle tenderness and weakness, hyporeflexia, hypesthesia, tachycardia, cardiomegaly, congestive heart failure, encephalopathy	Erythrocyte thiamine pyrophosphate and transketolase activity ↓ and in vitro effect thereon of thiamin pyrophosphate ↑, urinary thiamin ↓, blood pyruvate and α-ketoglutarate levels ↑, lactic acidosis
Riboflavin (vitamin B_2)	Angular stomatitis (or angular scars), cheilosis, magenta tongue, atrophic lingual papillae, corneal vascularization, angular blepharitis, dyssebacia, scrotal (vulvar) dermatosis	EGR activity ↓, and in vitro effect on EGR activity of flavin adenine dinucleotide ↑, pyridoxal phosphate oxidase activity ↓ and in vitro effect thereon of riboflavin ↑, ↓ urinary riboflavin
Niacin	Pellagra, scarlet and raw tongue, atrophic lingual papillae, tongue fissuring, pellagrous dermatosis, diarrhea, dementia	Urinary N^1-methylnicotinamide ↓, urinary 2-pyridone/N^1-methylnicotinamide ratio ↓
Pyridoxine (vitamin B_6)	Nasolabial seborrhea, glossitis, kidney stones, peripheral neuropathy, muscular twitching, convulsions, microcytic anemia	EGOT activity ↓ and in vitro effect of pyridoxal phosphate on EGOT activity ↑, tryptophan load test ↓ (urinary excretion of xanthurenic and quinolinic acids), urinary vitamin B_6 excretion ↓
Folacin	Pallor, glossitis, stomatitis, diarrhea, anemia	Erythrocyte and serum folate concentration ↓, urine formiminoglutamic acid excretion ↑ after histidine load, macrocytic anemia, polymorphonuclear leukocytes hypersegmented, megaloblastic bone marrow
Vitamin B_{12}	Pallor, mild icterus, anorexia, diarrhea, paresthesia, ataxia, optic neuritis, mental changes	Serum vitamin B_{12} ↓, peripheral blood and bone marrow morphology
Biotin	Fatigue, depression, nausea, dermatitis, muscular pains	Urinary biotin ↓, whole blood biotin ↓
Pantothenic acid	Fatigue, sleep disturbances, impaired coordination, nausea	Urinary pantothenic acid ↓
Calcium	Stunted growth, rickets, osteomalacia, convulsions	Osteopenia by x-ray, serum Ca^{2+} ↓
Phosphorus	Weakness, osteomalacia, ↓ phagocytosis, hemolysis, ↓ cardiac function, neurological syndromes, respiratory failure	Osteopenia by x-ray, serum P ↓
Magnesium	Growth failure, behavioral disturbances, weakness, tremor, tetany, seizures, cardiac arrhythmias	Serum, urine, and RBC Mg ↓
Iron	Pallor, weakness, reduced resistance to infection, angular stomatitis, atrophic lingual papillae, koilonychia	Plasma and marrow iron ↓, serum ferritin ↓, microcytic hypochromic anemia
Zinc	Psoriasiform rash, eczematous scaling, growth restriction, hypogonadism, delayed puberty, slow wound healing, hypogeusia, photophobia, anergy	Plasma and 24-h urine zinc ↓
Iodine	Goiter, symptoms of hypothyroidism	TSH ↑, T_4 and T_3 ↓, 24-h urine iodine ↓, RAI uptake ↑
Copper	Pallor	Neutropenia, hypochromic microcytic anemia, hypoferremia, osteopenia, plasma and urine copper ↓, ceruloplasmin ↓
Fluorine	Higher frequency of tooth decay	
Chromium	Glucose intolerance	Serum chromium ↓, urinary chromium ↓
Selenium	Cardiomyopathy, muscle pain	Plasma, RBC selenium ↓, glutathione peroxidose activity ↓
Sodium	Muscle weakness and cramps, confusion, apathy, anorexia, hypotension, oliguria	Serum Na^+ ↓, BUN/creatinine ↑
Potassium	Lassitude, polyuria, ileus, muscular weakness	Serum and urine K^+ ↓, body ^{40}K ↓, abnormal ECG
Chloride	Muscle cramps, apathy, anorexia, alkalosis	Serum Cl^- ↓

NOTES: *BMR* = basal metabolism rate; *BUN* = blood-urea nitrogen; *creatinine/height* = 24-h urine creatinine/height ratio; *ECG* = electrocardiogram; *EGOT* = erythrocyte glutamic-oxaloacetic transaminase; *EGR* = erythrocyte glutathione reductase; *MAFA* = midarm fat area; *MAMA* = midarm muscle area; *RAI* = radioactive iodine; *RBC* = red blood cell; T_3 = triiodothyroxine; T_4 = thyroxine; *TSH* = thyroid-stimulating hormone.

causing malabsorption or renal loss of a nutrient, by preventing its metabolic utilization, or by accelerating its degradation.

INDIVIDUAL ESSENTIAL NUTRIENTS Water

A reasonable allowance is 1 mL/kcal for adults and 150 mL/kg body weight for infants. The minimum requirement, considerably less than the customary allowance, depends on the preformed and potential solutes ingested (largely protein, sodium, chloride, and potassium), the concentrating ability of the kidney, and extrarenal losses. Normally 50 to 100 mL per day is excreted in the feces, 500 to 1000 mL is lost by exhalation and evaporation (insensible loss), and the remainder is excreted in the urine. Water intake must equal these losses to avoid under- or overhydration. Water supply is often inadequate in quantity or quality for impoverished populations in developing nations.

TABLE 70-5 Syndromes that can result from excessive intake or absorption of nutrients by oral route or from excessive infusion by parenteral route

Nutrient	Manifestation of overnutrition
Water	Edema, headache, nausea, hypertension
Calories	Obesity
Proteins	Exacerbation of inborn errors in amino acid catabolism or "nitrogen accumulation diseases, renal damage"
Fat	In predisposed individuals, hyperlipemia
Vitamin A	Headache, vomiting, peeling of skin, anorexia, swelling of long bones, cirrhosis
Vitamin D	Hypercalcemia, nephrolithiasis, impaired renal function
Vitamin K	At high doses may cause jaundice
Ascorbic acid (vitamin C)	Hyperoxaluria
Calcium	Hypercalcemia, mental and renal dysfunction
Magnesium	Diarrhea
Iron	Siderosis, hemochromatosis
Zinc	Fever, nausea, vomiting, diarrhea
Iodine	Depression of thyroid activity, goiter, occasional hyperthyroidism
Copper	Wilson's disease, vomiting
Manganese	Generalized disease of nervous system
Fluorine	Mottling of teeth, increased bone density, neurological disturbances
Sodium chloride	Hypertension, edema, heart failure
Potassium	Muscular weakness, arrhythmia, death

TABLE 70-7 Some essential nutrients for which the daily dietary requirement is influenced by other dietary components

Nutrient	Influence by other dietary component
Protein	Requirement inversely related to calories when the latter are deficient
Essential amino acids	Utilization curtailed if any essential amino acid is deficient
Phenylalanine	Requirement inversely related to tyrosine intake
Methionine	Requirement inversely related to cystine intake
Valine, leucine, isoleucine	Requirement of each is increased by excess of the other branched-chain amino acid(s)
Vitamin E	Requirement proportional to intake of polyunsaturated fat
Thiamin	Requirement proportional to calories
Niacin	Requirement inversely related to tryptophan intake
Vitamin B$_6$	Requirement increased by protein
Folacin	Requirement increased by alcohol intake
Calcium	Urinary excretion increased by high protein intake
Calcium, magnesium, nonheme iron, zinc	Absorption decreased by phytates
Nonheme iron	Absorption improved by vitamin C or sulfur-containing amino acids
Copper	Absorption decreased by calcium, requirement increased by excess dietary zinc

Maximal tolerance normally is more than 5 liters daily because of the kidney's large capacity for free water clearance. Water requirement and tolerance are increased by factors that cause increased losses in urine, feces, or sweat. The obligatory urinary loss is proportional to the excretion of solutes and the kidney's concentrating capacity; it is increased in proportion to the intake of protein, sodium, potassium, and chloride. Water requirements are increased by deficiency of antidiuretic hormone and decreased when the hormone is secreted inappropriately. Fecal loss of water may increase to over 5 liters per day in severe diarrhea. Nasogastric suction, ileostomy, gastrointestinal fistulas, and burns similarly increase daily water requirements. Water loss is excessive during fever, heavy exercise, or exposure to high environmental temperature. Each degree Celsius of fever causes an obligatory loss of about 200 mL water per day.

Energy To maintain stable weight, energy intake must equal energy output. The output can be divided into basal and activity components. Basal metabolic rate (BMR) is usually measured in the fasting, resting subject immediately after waking (Table 70-10). Values during sleep are about 10 percent less. After each meal, the metabolic rate increases by as much as 30 percent; this thermic effect of food (dietary thermogenesis or specific dynamic action) accounts for about 6 percent of the basal energy expenditure. BMR falls by 20 percent between 30 and 90 years of age; however, this decline disappears when BMR is expressed per kilogram of lean body mass.

Mild, moderate, or severe exercise increases energy expenditure by roughly 30, 50, or 100 (or more) percent, respectively. Energy expenditures in specific types of activity are described in Chap. 317.

The daily energy requirement equals the sum of expenditures incurred by basal metabolism, specific dynamic action, and physical activity. The requirement can be estimated by assessing basal energy expenditure per day from the subject's surface area (Table 70-10), using ideal body weight in this calculation. Subtract 10 percent from basal during the sleeping hours. Add 6 percent to the 24-h basal estimate to cover dietary thermogenesis. From an activity-energy chart, such as is given in Chap. 317, calculate the energy expenditure of the subject's physical activities during a typical day. The daily energy expenditure can be estimated as the sum of basal requirements (minus correction for sleep) plus dietary thermogenesis plus energy requirement for physical activity. Since, on average, 93 percent of energy intake is utilized and 7 percent is lost in feces and urine, the estimated energy requirement for zero balance equals 107 percent of the calculated energy expenditure.

In actual practice, a simpler formula can be used. The Harris-Benedict equations account for sex, weight, height, and age in estimating basal energy expenditure (Table 70-11). To this basal expenditure, 30, 50, or 100 percent is added for sedentary, moderate, or strenuous activity, respectively. Nonstressed hospitalized patients usually require 120 percent of basal energy expenditure, whereas catabolic patients usually require 150 to 200 percent of basal energy expenditure to minimize tissue breakdown or to allow anabolism. Weight is monitored weekly, and if weight increases or decreases in the absence of edema, calories are adjusted accordingly. Short-term changes in weight, however, primarily reflect fluid balance.

Energy expenditure is increased by fever (about 13 percent over basal per degree Celsius), burns (40 to 100 percent), trauma (40 to

TABLE 70-6 Biologic value of food proteins*

Protein source	Biologic value
Milk	93
Egg	93
Beef	76
Peanut meal	74
Potato	69
Oat	65
Rice	65
Corn	50
Soy flour	41
Wheat gluten	40

* As determined from nitrogen balance studies conducted in the rat, generally at a dietary protein concentration of 5 percent. Tests in the rat at other concentrations, or in other species, give generally similar but not identical biologic values.

TABLE 70-8 Net absorption of nutrients in normal adults on diets containing mixtures of plant and animal foods

Element	Percent	Element	Percent
Carbohydrate	>90	Manganese	<5
Protein	>90	Fluorine	80–90
Fat	>95	Chromium	1–3
Calcium	5–40	Selenium	>50
Phosphorus	50–60	Molybdenum	40–50
Magnesium	25–50	Cobalt	>50
Iron	5–15	Sodium	>95
Zinc	33	Potassium	80–90
Iodine	>50	Chlorine	>95
Copper	25		

TABLE 70-9   Disorders that alter nutrient requirements by the oral route

Nutrient	Increases dietary requirement	Reduces dietary requirement
Calories	Fever, hyperthyroidism, trauma, malabsorption	Coma, hypothyroidism
Protein	Fever, hyperthyroidism, trauma, azotorrhea	Nitrogen accumulation diseases, inborn errors of urea synthesis
Phenylalanine		Phenylketonuria
Branched-chain amino acids		Maple syrup urine disease
Linoleic acid and fat-soluble vitamins	Malabsorption syndromes	
Folacin	Increased cell turnover	
Calcium	Malabsorption syndromes	Hyperabsorptive hypercalciuria
Phosphorus	Malabsorption syndromes	Renal insufficiency
Magnesium	Malabsorption syndromes	
Iron	Malabsorption syndromes	Hemochromatosis
Zinc	Acrodermatitis enteropathica	
Copper	Malabsorption syndromes	Wilson's disease
Carnitine*	Advanced cirrhosis	

* *No requirement normally.*

100 percent), elective surgery (10 to 20 percent), sepsis (40 to 80 percent), and hyperthyroidism (10 to 100 percent). Hypometabolism, whether due to hypothyroidism, starvation, or other cause, lowers the energy expenditure and, therefore, the energy requirement.

Patients with severe malabsorption may absorb as little as 25 percent of their ingested fat calories and as little as 50 percent of carbohydrate and protein calories, compared with the normal value of over 95 percent. In this situation the oral energy requirement is higher than normal and may prove impossible to achieve if diarrhea is aggravated by increased nutrient intake. In such patients only parenteral nutrition can prevent progressive starvation.

Protein   Dietary protein provides a mixture of amino acids for endogenous protein synthesis and is also a metabolic fuel for energy. Healthy adults require nine essential amino acids in amounts varying from 250 to 1100 mg per day. About 7 g of nitrogen as nonessential amino acids is also required for protein synthesis. The requirement and allowance of dietary protein depend on the biologic value of the proteins ingested. Biologic value is defined as the proportion of absorbed protein retained by the body under standard test conditions and is a function of the content of essential amino acids. Nearly optimal ratios of the 9 essential and 11 nonessential amino acids are present in egg and milk proteins, which consequently have the highest biologic values, viz., 90 to 95 (Table 70-6). The biologic value of proteins follows the general order: animal products > legumes > cereals (rice, wheat, corn) > roots. The adult RDA for protein given in Table 70-1, about 50 g per day, assumes a biologic value of about

TABLE 70-10   Basal energy requirements of normal subjects

Age, years	Males, (kcal/m²)/h	Females, (kcal/m²)/h
14–16	46.0	43.0
16–18	43.0	40.0
18–20	41.0	38.0
20–30	39.5	37.0
30–40	39.5	36.5
40–50	38.5	36.0
50–60	37.5	35.0
60–70	36.5	34.0
70–80	35.5	33.0

SOURCE: *EF DuBois, Basal Metabolism in Health and Disease, 3d ed. Philadelphia, Lea & Febiger, 1936, p 151*

TABLE 70-11   Calculation of basal energy expenditure (BEE) by Harris-Benedict equations

WOMEN

$$BEE = 655 + (9.6 \times W) + (1.8 \times H) - (4.7 \times A)$$

MEN

$$BEE = 66 + (13.7 \times W) + (5 \times H) - (6.8 \times A)$$

NOTE: *W = ideal body weight in kilograms, H = height in centimeters, A = age in years*

80, a characteristic value for animal products. The lower the biologic value, the higher the daily protein requirement.

Plant proteins have low biologic value because one or more essential amino acids are usually deficient. Thus for corn (maize), lysine and tryptophan are limiting; for soybeans and green peas, methionine; for rice, lysine and threonine; for wheat, lysine. Therefore, mixtures of vegetable proteins deficient in different essential amino acids have a higher biologic value than either protein separately.

While the usual reason for low biologic value of a particular protein or mixtures of proteins is the limiting content of one or more essential amino acids, a change in the proportion of amino acids or an excess of amino acids can impair the value. For example, when a mixture of amino acids lacking histidine is added to a marginally adequate protein source containing histidine, rats become anorexic and cease growing. This amino acid imbalance is corrected by adding the most limiting amino acid, histidine. An excess of certain amino acids, e.g., methionine and tyrosine, can cause toxic reactions. Requirements for other amino acids can be enhanced by an excess of a structurally similar amino acid, e.g., the branched-chain amino acids, leucine, isoleucine, and valine. These are important considerations in planning the composition of synthetic amino acids for parenteral or enteral feeding, particularly because the anorectic reaction which normally protects against an imbalanced diet is being bypassed.

In other cases essential amino acids may be "spared" by chemically related amino acids. For example cystine and tyrosine, which are synthesized from methionine and phenylalanine, respectively, exert a "sparing" effect in that 80 percent of the methionine requirement and 70 percent of the phenylalanine requirement could be met by giving cystine and tyrosine, respectively.

The daily requirement of a protein, or its constituent amino acids, is influenced by energy intake; the values for protein allowances given in Table 70-1 assume adequate energy intake. When the energy requirement is met by nonprotein calories, a substantial portion of ingested amino acids is utilized for protein synthesis. In contrast, if caloric intake is deficient, some amino acids are diverted from protein synthesis into oxidative metabolism and gluconeogenesis. Under these circumstances, the daily protein requirement is inversely proportional to the energy intake ("protein-sparing effect of nonprotein calories"). Thus, energy undernutrition makes a person more vulnerable to protein starvation, an interaction which accounts for the high prevalence of the combined deficiency state protein-energy undernutrition (see Chap. 72).

The protein-sparing effect of nonprotein calories depends on the source. Carbohydrate spares protein, but in the absence of carbohydrate, fat does not have this action. Protein sparing is maximal when the nonprotein calories include 100 to 150 g carbohydrate per day; the remainder may then be given as fat, carbohydrate, or a mixture of the two.

The daily protein requirement per unit body weight is increased by growth, pregnancy, lactation, fever, infection, trauma, and malabsorption. More protein is required during repletion from cachexia. Protein requirements may be increased in some of the elderly.

To understand how the "nitrogen accumulation diseases," hepatic and renal insufficiency, alter the requirement and tolerance of dietary protein, consider the scheme of amino acid metabolism shown in Fig. 70-1. The daily adult allowance of about 50 g protein serves to maintain protein synthesis (reaction 2) at a rate equal to protein breakdown (reaction 3). Tolerance for protein is normally greater than 250 g per day because of the high capacity of the degradative pathway (reactions 4, 6, 7, and 9). Note that 25 to 40 percent of urea formed in the liver is hydrolyzed by bacteria within the colon and recyles at least once as ammonia (reaction 8). When step 10 is blocked (uremia), the requirement for nonessential nitrogen may be reduced because a small proportion of the ammonia released by urea breakdown is utilized for the synthesis of nonessential amino acids; the carbon skeletons of these acids are readily produced by the intermediary metabolism of glucose. This pathway for endogenous synthesis of nonessential amino acids is the theoretic basis for treating uremics with a diet furnishing a limited amount of protein rich in essential amino acids ("Giovanetti diet"). If to such a diet are added the carbon skeletons (α-keto derivatives) of the essential amino acids, the requirement for the latter nutrients (except for threonine and lysine) is further reduced in part because of the reversibility of transamination (reaction 5 in Fig. 70-1), and in part because the branched-chain keto acids retard the breakdown of proteins in skeletal muscles. Similar considerations apply in the dietary management of cirrhosis of the liver and of hereditary disorders of urea synthesis.

Not only is the daily requirement for protein in some uremics and cirrhotics lower than normal, but the maximal tolerance is curtailed as well. As little as 20 g of protein a day can precipitate or aggravate symptoms of hepatocerebral disease in susceptible patients with liver disease. Intakes of protein customary for healthy subjects in the United States (80 to 100 g per day) can also intensify the uremic syndrome.

One theory to explain the clouded sensorium in liver failure is based on the imbalance of the plasma amino acid profile, namely increased aromatic and decreased branched-chain amino acids. This abnormal ratio, which probably reflects impaired metabolic clearance of aromatic amino acids, might lead to increased synthesis of false neurotransmitters in the brain and subsequent disturbances of neurotransmission. According to this theory, patients with liver failure require a higher ratio of branched-chain to aromatic amino acids in the diet than do individuals with normal liver function.

Reactions 2 and 3 in Fig. 70-1 represent whole-body protein turnover, estimated at about 200 g per day in the 70-kg adult. The major source of amino acids presented for metabolism is from endogenous protein breakdown (reaction 2). Metabolic stress (fever, trauma, infection) increases turnover and reduces efficiency of amino acid reutilization (reaction 3). To achieve nitrogen balance, the protein requirement is increased in the stressed patient by as much as 50 percent.

Fat While the average adult in the United States consumes 40 percent of calories as fat (around 90 g), the dietary requirement is only about 5 percent of total calories as polyunsaturated fatty acids. To minimize the risk of atherosclerosis, the National Institutes of Health have recommended that all Americans (except children under 2 years of age) should reduce total dietary fat intake from the current average level to 30 percent of total calories, reduce saturated fat intake to less than 10 percent of total calories, increase polyunsaturated fat intake but to no more than 10 percent, and reduce daily cholesterol intake to less than 300 mg.

Both the quality and the quantity of the dietary polyunsaturated fatty acids are significant for health. The body contains four classes of unsaturated fatty acids, designated according to the location of the double bond closest to the methyl-terminal, or ω, carbon. Thus, oleic, palmitoleic, linoleic, and linolenic acids, respectively, are 18:1ω9, 16:1ω7, 18:2ω6, and 18:3ω3. Each of these four fatty acids is a precursor for a series of polyunsaturated fatty acids of the same ω class. Only the ω9 and ω7 series can be synthesized by mammals; the ω6 and ω3 compounds are obtained from vegetable and fish or marine animal dietary sources, respectively.

Animals fed a fat-free diet develop a generalized nutritional deficiency syndrome consisting of growth failure, dermatitis, fatty liver, and neurologic and visual abnormalities. Most of these defects are corrected or prevented by the ω6 precursor linoleic acid, but the

FIGURE 70-1 *Overview of amino acid metabolism.*

neurologic-visual changes reflect depletion of the ω3 class and require linolenic acid for correction. It is now recommended that the human diet contain about 4 percent of calories as linoleic acid and 1 percent as linolenic acid.

Furthermore, the series of 20-carbon-chain eicosanoids (prostaglandins, thromboxanes, prostacyclins, and leukotrienes) derived from each class of polyunsaturated fatty acids has a different profile of bioactivities (see Chap. 68). The ω3 eicosanoids have the unique ability to reduce platelet adhesiveness and lower serum triglycerides. These properties may lower the prevalence of coronary heart disease in populations with a high intake of marine oils.

Naturally occurring animal, fish, and vegetable triglyceride fatty acids are largely 16 or 18 carbons in length. Medium-chain triglycerides (12 to 14 carbons) are clinically useful because they are absorbed through the portal vein, not the splanchnic lymphatics, they are cleared from the circulation more rapidly than long-chain triglycerides, and their fatty acids can be oxidized by carnitine-independent mechanisms in the mitochondria.

Minerals and vitamins The daily allowances and the influence of various conditions on these thresholds are listed in Tables 70-1, 70-2, 70-7, and 70-9. The deficiency syndromes corresponding to each nutrient are listed in Table 70-4, and some clinical effects of exceeding the daily tolerance are given in Table 70-5 (see also Chap. 76). It is important to realize that the mineral and vitamin requirements of the elderly have not been established and that the present recommendations are based on studies of young subjects. Thus, the optimal daily intake of calcium in postmenopausal women is now considered to be 50 percent higher than in youth.

NONESSENTIAL SUBSTANCES Fiber Dietary fiber is a mixture of cellulose, hemicellulose, pectins, algae, polysaccharides, and lignin and contributes 15 to 25 g to the average U.S. diet. The soluble components of these undigestible polymers bind ions, sterols, and bile salts, and the insoluble components add bulk to and accelerate the transit time of the intraluminal contents. Claims have been made for the beneficial effects of dietary fiber on diverticulosis, colon cancer, gallstones, diabetes, and coronary artery disease. Much work is still needed in this area.

Choline, carnitine, inositol These organic compounds have biologic activity, but they have not been considered essential vitamins because several animal species including humans can synthesize them. However, a limited capacity for biosynthesis may be present in immature animals and in certain genetic and acquired disorders; therefore, under these circumstances an exogenous source should be considered.

REFERENCES

FOOD AND NUTRITION BOARD: *Recommended Dietary Allowances.* Washington, D.C. National Academy of Sciences, 1979

GLOMSET JA: Fish, fatty acids and human health. N Engl J Med 312:1253, 1985

MUNRO HN: Nutritional requirements in health. Crit Care Med 8:2, 1980

———: Nutrition-related problems of middle age. Proc Nutr Soc 43:281, 1984

NUTRITIVE VALUE OF AMERICAN FOODS: Agriculture Handbook #456. Agricultural Research Service, USDA, 1975

PHILLIPSON BE et al: Reduction of plasma lipids, lipoproteins, and apoproteins by dietary fish oils in patients with hypertriglyceridemia. N Engl J Med 312:1210, 1985

RECOMMENDED DIETARY ALLOWANCES: National Research Council, Washington, D.C., National Academy of Sciences, 1980

REEDS PJ, GARLICK J: Nutrition and protein turnover in man. Adv Nutr Res 6:93, 1984

RUDMAN D, WILLIAMS PJ: Pathophysiologic principles of nutrition, in *Pathophysiology: The biological principles of disease*, 2d ed, LH Smith Jr, SO Thier (eds). Philadelphia, Saunders, 1985

SANDSTEAD HH: Trace metals in human nutrition. Curr Concepts Nutr 13:37, 1984

71   ASSESSMENT OF NUTRITIONAL STATUS

DANIEL RUDMAN

Undernutrition is a common contributor to morbidity and mortality. As a peculiar discrepancy, however, undernutrition rarely appears in the list of diagnoses or in the progress notes. Consequently, quantitative tests of nutritional status are infrequent in the initial clinical workup, and the progress of the nutritional state is rarely monitored regularly during the course of illness. As a result, undernutrition tends to be recognized late, when it is severe and difficult to treat. This chapter defines feasible methods for identifying and quantifying the deficiency syndromes, for investigating their cause, and for monitoring their course.

MASS AND COMPOSITION OF THE BODY COMPARTMENTS

Consideration must first be given to the normal mass and chemical composition of the major body compartments, which are altered by nutritional deficiencies in characteristic ways. The body can be viewed as consisting of four compartments: extracellular fluid, protoplasm (intracellular compartment), bone, and adipose tissue. The first three make up the lean body mass.

The body compartments of a healthy "reference man," 70 kg in weight, 172 cm tall, 35 years old, are summarized in Table 71-1. Typical masses of extracellular fluid, protoplasm, bone, and adipose tissue are 17, 35, 5, and 13 kg, respectively. Chloride is localized almost exclusively in the extracellular fluid, where its average concentration is 96 meq per liter; nitrogen and potassium are largely located in protoplasm, with normal concentrations of 27 g and 150 meq per kilogram of wet weight, respectively; calcium is found primarily in bone, where its concentration averages 260 g per kilogram

TABLE 71-1   Approximate mass and major elemental composition of body compartments in a 70-kg healthy "reference man"

	Protoplasm	Extracellular fluid	Bone	Adipose tissue
Mass	35 kg	17 kg	5 kg	13 kg
Body weight	50%	24%	7%	19%
Elemental composition, kg wet wt	27 g N 97 mmol P 150 meq K	140 meq Na 96 meq Cl	260 g Ca 115 g P	

TABLE 71-2   Reifenstein equations for determining change in mass of body compartments

ΔProtoplasm, g	$= 27 \times \Delta N$, g
ΔECF, *g	$= 9.6 \times \Delta Cl$, meq
ΔBone, g	$= 0.1 \times \Delta Ca$, meq
ΔAdipose tissue, g	$= \Delta BW,\dagger$ g $- [\Delta$ protoplasm, g $+ \Delta ECF$, g $+ \Delta$ bone, g]

* *Extracellular fluid.*
† *Body weight.*

of wet weight. The adipose tissue contains insignificant levels of these elements.

DIRECT AND INDIRECT METHODS FOR MEASURING MASS OF BODY COMPARTMENTS

If one assumes that the concentrations of chloride, nitrogen, potassium, phosphorus, and calcium remain normal in extracellular fluid, protoplasm, and bone during a period of observation involving expansion or contraction of these compartments, and if one knows the balance (i.e., intake and output) of each element (termed Δ nitrogen, Δ phosphorus, etc.) during this period, then from the equations in Table 71-2 one can calculate the change (Δ) in the mass of each compartment during the period under consideration. The equations are based on the fact that each kilogram of extracellular fluid, protoplasm, or bone gained or lost by the body contains a characteristic amount of chloride, nitrogen, or calcium, respectively.

The urinary excretion of urea nitrogen is accelerated in the patient with trauma, infection or inflammation. A bedside estimate of daily nitrogen balance in grams can be made as follows:

$$\frac{\text{Daily protein intake (g)}}{6.25} - [\text{24-h urine urea nitrogen (g)} + 2.5\text{g}^1]$$

For clinically stable patients, protein intake can be estimated in grams as [24-h urine urea nitrogen (in grams) + 2.5] × 6.25. This approximation is useful in monitoring compliance of patients on low protein diets and in evaluating protein intake of subjects at risk for malnutrition.

Metabolic balance techniques of this type allow estimation of the change in mass of each compartment during the period of observation but provide no information about the absolute mass of the compartment at the beginning and end. Such absolute measurements can be made by several methods: whole-body analysis of potassium (total-body protoplasm), measurement of total-body nitrogen by neutron activation analysis, measurement of extracellular fluid by isotope dilution, measurement of total-body nitrogen by neutron activation analysis, measurement of extracellular fluid by isotope dilution, measurement of total-body water by isotope dilution, calculation of intracellular water (closely related to protoplasmic mass) as total-body water minus extracellular water, measurement of adipose mass by determining whole-body density. These methods are largely restricted to research units. Fortunately, several indirect methods for estimating the mass of body compartments are available to the clinician:

1 In the nonedematous patient, body weight as percent of ideal is a useful indicator of adipose tissue plus lean body mass. Ideal body weight can be estimated from the height/weight tables of the Metropolitan Life Insurance Company or from the following simple formula: in women, 45 kg for the first 152 cm and 0.9 kg for each centimeter over 152; in men, 48 kg for the first 152 cm and 1.1 kg for each centimeter over 152. Reduction of the body weight/ ideal body weight ratio to 80 percent in nonedematous patients usually means mild protein-energy undernutrition; a reduction to 70 to 80 percent indicates moderate protein-energy undernutrition; a decline to 70 percent or less indicates severe protein-energy undernutrition.

2 Anthropometric analysis of the midarm requires only a tape measure and caliper. The principle is illustrated in Fig. 71-1; the arm consists of a cylinder of muscle within a sheath of adipose tissue. From the external circumference of the nondominant midarm and the width of the adipose layer (equal to one-half the triceps skin fold), midarm muscle area and midarm fat area can be calculated. The midarm muscle and fat areas are indicators of the body's masses of skeletal muscle and adipose tissue, respectively. Normal average values for adult men and women, respectively, are midarm muscle area, 50.91 and 42.81 cm², and midarm fat area, 17.04 and 21.28 cm². By taking skinfold measurements at the biceps, subscapular, and suprailiac sites, in addition to the triceps, one

---

¹ *Two-and-one-half grams is the approximate sum of urinary nonurea nitrogen plus fecal and integumental losses of nitrogen.*

Normal Values (adults)	Male	Female
Triceps skinfold, mm	12.5	16.5
Midarm muscle circumference, cm	25.3	23.2
Midarm fat area, cm²	17.0	21.3
Midarm muscle area, cm²	50.9	42.8

Calculation of Mid Upper Arm Muscle Circumference

C_1 = mid upper arm circumference in centimeters

S = triceps skinfold in centimeters

d_1 = arm diameter

d_2 = muscle diameter

Skinfold $(S) = 2 \times$ subcutaneous fat $= d_1 - d_2$

Circumference $(C_1) = \pi d_1$

Muscle circumference $= C_1 - \pi S$

Midarm muscle area $= \dfrac{(C_1 - \pi S)^2}{4\pi}$

Midarm fat area $= \dfrac{(S)(C_1)}{2} - \dfrac{\pi(S^2)}{4}$

FIGURE 71-1 *Anthropometric measurement of muscle and adipose compartments of the mid-upper arm. Midarm circumference is measured with a tape measure and triceps skinfold with a caliper. (After C Butterworth and C Blackburn, Nutr Today 10:8, 1974.)*

can calculate total adipose mass by the method of Durnin and Womersley. Lean body mass is derived from the difference between fat mass in kilograms and body weight.

3 Urine creatinine is related to lean body mass by the equation:

$$\text{Lean body mass (kg)} = 7.138 + 0.02908 \times (\text{mg creatinine/24 h})$$

The ratio of 24-h creatinine excretion (in grams) to height (in centimeters) is considered a measure of muscle mass and can be used as an index to determine protein depletion. Three qualifying conditions should be considered: (a) diets containing meat influence the quantity of creatinine excreted; (b) impaired renal function results in falsely low creatinine excretion; and (c) creatinine excretion declines with age as a result of smaller muscle mass. In normal men and women the creatinine/height ratio averages 10.5 and 5.8 mg/cm, respectively. In men, ratios in the ranges 8.4 to 9.5, 7.4 to 8.4, and less than 7.4 mg/cm signify mild, moderate, and severe degrees of protein depletion, respectively.

4 Sagittal or horizontal radiograms or computerized tomography (CT) scans of an extremity also provide quantitative information about the mass of representative skeletal muscles but are more expensive.

Skeletal muscle makes up about 30 percent of the lean body mass and atrophies progressively in protein-energy starvation, the most common deficiency state in U.S. hospitals (see Chap. 72). By monitoring the creatinine/height ratio and midarm muscle area, the clinician can identify protein-energy starvation easily and monitor its course.

The visceral compartment, which maintains tissue function, blood protein synthesis, and the immune response, comprises 20 percent of the lean body mass. Under conditions of nutritional inadequacy, protein synthesis declines, metabolic pathways are altered, and the immune system is impaired. Certain blood proteins are sensitive indicators of these events and are used to detect malnutrition and monitor nutritional repletion (Table 71-3). Prealbumin and retinol binding protein have the shortest half-lives (1 to 2 days) and thus

TABLE 71-3 Laboratory tests for the evaluation of nutritional status (adults)

Nutrient evaluation	Test	Deficient (often with clinical manifestations)	Low (usually without clinical manifestations)	Acceptable
Protein	Serum albumin, g/dL	<3.0	3.0–3.5	>3.5
Protein	Serum transferrin, mg/dL	<180–260		180–260
Protein	Serum prealbumin, mg/dL	<20–50		20–50
Protein	Serum retinol binding protein, μg/mL	<30–45		30–45
Protein	Creatinine/height ratio	<90% of Standard	90–95%	>95%
Protein	Nitrogen balance, g	>(−)3	(−)1–3	0–3
Protein, Fe, folacin, vitamin B_{12}	Hemoglobin, g/dL	<12	12–14	>14
Iron	Serum iron, μg/dL	<60		>60
Vitamin A	Plasma retinol, μg/dL	<10	10–20	>20
Vitamin D	Serum Ca × P product, mg/dL	<40		>40
Vitamin D	Alkaline phosphatase, King-Armstrong units/dL	>40	15–40	8–14
Vitamin C	Serum ascorbic acid, mg/dL	<0.20	0.20–0.30	>0.30
Thiamin	Erythrocyte transketolase (% thiamin disphosphate stimulation)	>20	15–20	<15
Riboflavin	Erythrocyte glutathione reductase activity coefficient	>1.40	1.20–1.40	<1.20
Niacin	N-Methylnicotinamide excretion, mg/g creatinine	<0.5	0.5–1.59	>1.6
Vitamin B_6	Erythrocyte aminotransferase activity coefficients:			
	Erythrocyte ALT	>1.25		<1.25
	Erythrocyte AST	>1.5		<1.5
Vitamin B_6	Tryptophan load test (xanthurenic acid), mg/day	>50	25–50	<25
Folacin	Serum folate, ng/mL	<3	3.0–6.0	>6.0
Folacin	Erythrocyte folate, ng/mL	<140	140–160	>160
Vitamin B_{12}	Serum vitamin B_{12}, pb/mL	<150	150–200	>200
Ca	24-h urine Ca^{2+}, mg	<50	50–100	>100
P	24-h urine P, mg	<100	100–300	>300
Mg	24-h urine Mg^{2+}, meq	<4	4–8	>8
Na	24-h urine Na^+, meq	<20	20–40	>40
K	24-h urine K^+, meq	<20	20–40	>40

can be used to monitor patients at high risk of developing protein-energy malnutrition and to evaluate the initial repletion. Presently, these immunoassays are expensive. Transferrin, with a half-life of 8 days, is also useful in monitoring repletion, although concurrent iron-deficiency anemia makes interpretation difficult. Albumin (half-life, 14 days) is the most useful prognostic indicator of protein-energy malnutrition. Albumin synethesis may be impaired in liver disease; nevertheless, in undernourished cirrhotics the albumin level usually rises with nutritional repletion.

SYNDROMES OF UNDERNUTRITION   When any of the 39 essential nutrient requirements (Chap. 70) are not met, undernutrition syndromes result. Undernutrition of such micronutrients as nitrogen, sodium, chloride, potassium, calcium, and phosphorus reduces the mass of one or more body compartments, often with associated abnormalities in compartmental chemistry, structure, and function. For example, deficiencies of nitrogen (protein), sodium, and calcium erode protoplasm, extracellular fluid, and bone, respectively. Undernutrition of a micronutrient tends to cause a specific morphologic or functional abnormality in certain tissues without alteration in compartmental mass or elemental composition. While in theory 39 different types of human malnutrition could occur, undernutrition syndromes usually occur in groups rather than in ''pure'' form.

Deficiency of each essential nutrient can be characterized in terms of symptoms, signs, and chemical and radiographic abnormalities, but deficiency syndromes have several principles in common:

1 Undernutrition can be either primary or secondary in origin. The primary form is due to an inadequate supply of food containing the essential nutrients. In secondary undernutrition an adequate diet is available, but because of illness or medical treatment, nutrients cannot be ingested, absorbed, or metabolized adequately, or the rate of utilization of external losses is excessive. Primary and secondary mechanisms frequently reinforce each other; for example, the hypermetabolism and anorexia of infection precipitate nutritional deficiencies more rapidly in patients who previously subsisted on marginal diets than in well-nourished individuals. To determine whether undernutrition in a particular patient is primary or secondary, the physician must obtain a dietary history, assess personal habits and living conditions, and examine the patient for organic disease.
2 Nutritional deficiency syndromes tend to evolve through three stages. Many essential nutrients are stored in the tissues of the well-nourished subject; for example, iron and vitamins B_{12}, A, and

D in liver; essential fatty acids in adipose tissue; nitrogen in a labile reserve in muscle and liver. When intake falls below the daily requirement, these reserves temporarily maintain normal blood levels and forestall manifestation of deficiency (stage 1). In stage 2, blood levels of the nutrient or nutrient-dependent metabolic products decline, but the patient is asymptomatic. In stage 3, clinical signs and symptoms develop. Methods for assessing the nutritional status should ideally be capable of detecting all stages of deficiency. Available techniques, however, usually reveal only stages 2 and 3.
3 Because anorexia is a major mechanism in protein-energy undernutrition in the United States, the intake of nutrients must be measured in one of three ways: by recall, by diary (outpatient), or by observation (inpatient).
4 Change in weight may be ambiguous. In the absence of edema various proportions of weight loss are due to depletion of adipose tissue and lean body mass. In the presence of edema body weight changes are even more difficult to intrepret. Gain in weight can reflect an accumulation of edema, masking erosion of protoplasm; conversely, loss of weight can reflect diuresis with simultaneous expansion of the protoplasmic compartment. An initially obese patient can lose 15 kg because of chronic wasting illness and present with a normal body weight, the still substantial adipose organ masking a shrinkage in the lean body mass. In such instances, direct or indirect estimation of the size of the protoplasmic compartment is essential as described above.
5 The undernourished patient is usually deficient in several nutrients. Common patterns are deficiency of two or more water-soluble vitamins (usually including folate, vitamin C, and/or thiamine) and deficiency of both calcium and magnesium in patients with malabsorption.

The various physical, chemical, and radiographic characteristics of each type of undernutrition are summarized in Table 70-4. The most commonly used chemical indexes of nutrient deficiency are listed in Table 71-3, which gives three average concentration ranges for each test: normal, subnormal without clinical manifestations, and subnormal with clinical signs or symptoms of deficiency. Although these tests are of value in population surveys and in following the response of patients to therapies, coexisting conditions, such as the effect of renal disease on 24-h urinary creatinine, must be taken into consideration.

The clinician must select a reasonable number of historical, physical, and laboratory items to use as a ''nutritional data base'' for screening for undernutrition. Table 71-4 presents a selection of historical and physical items that reveal most deficiency states in hospital patients. Mullen has shown that a nutritional index based on triceps skin fold, skin reactivity to recall antigens, and serum levels of albumin and transferrin, is a valuable predictor of complications and death after surgery.

Most of the quantitative indexes of nutritional status so far considered are ''static'' measurements of body composition or of concentrations of nutrients or nutrient-dependent products in body fluids. ''Functional'' indexes sensitive to nutritional deficiencies include work capacity, dark adaptation, taste acuity, phagocytic activity of leukocytes, cognitive ability, capillary fragility, and reproductive performance. The measurement of such nutrient-dependent physiologic functions is especially important in identifying marginal deficiency syndromes and in documenting the impact of nutritional supplements on the health of populations.

MONITORING THE COURSE OF MALNUTRITION   Besides defining the type, severity, and mechanism for the development of undernutrition, it is important to ascertain the rate of progression. This is accomplished by periodic monitoring of body weight, albumin, hematocrit, creatinine excretion, midarm muscle area, midarm fat area, and appropriate blood or urine concentrations of nutrition-dependent variables. An example of the course of progressive protein-energy malnutrition is shown in Fig. 71-2.

TABLE 71-4   Nutritional data base

HISTORY

Previous weight curve
Dietary intake by retrospective recall and prospective diary
Alcohol intake
Socioeconomic and family status, including income
Anorexia, vomiting, diarrhea
Blood loss
Pregnancy, lactation, menses
Vitamin and mineral supplements
Use of drugs that might affect nutrition

PHYSICAL EXAMINATION

General: weight as percent of ideal body weight; triceps skinfold; midarm muscle circumference
Skin: xerosis, follicular hyperkeratosis, pellagrous dermatitis, petechiae, ecchymoses, perifollicular hemorrhages, flaky paint dermatitis, pallor
Hair: dyspigmentation, easy pluckability, thinning, straightening
Head: temporal wasting, parotid enlargement
Eyes: Bitot spots, conjunctival and scleral xerosis, keratomalacia, corneal vascularization, angular palpebritis
Mouth: cheilosis, angular stomatitis, magenta tongue, atrophic lingual papillae, tongue fissuring, glossitis, spongy gums, state of dentition
Heart: cardiomegaly, findings of congestive heart failure
Abdomen: hepatomegaly
Extremities: edema, koilonychia
Neurologic: irritability, weakness, calf tenderness, loss of deep tendon reflexes

FIGURE 71-2   *The course of a patient with protein-calorie depletion during repletion by nasogastric hyper-alimentation.*

REFERENCES

BISTRIAN BR: A simple technique to estimate severity of stress. Surg Gynecol Obstet 148:675, 1979

BLACKBURN GL, THORNON PA: Nutritional assessment of the hospitalized patient. Med Clin North Am 63:1103, 1979

DURNIN J, WOMERSLEY J: Body fat assessed from total body density and its estimation from skinfold thickness: Measurement on 481 men and women from 16 to 72 years. Br J Nutr 32:77, 1974

FORBES GB: Urinary creatinine excretion and lean body mass. Am J Clin Nutr 29:1361, 1976

HERBERT V: The five possible causes of all nutrient deficiency: Illustrated by deficiencies of vitamin B_{12} and folic acid. Am J Clin Nutr 26:77, 1973

MAGHAN KJ et al: The relative proportions of fat, muscle and bone in the normal human forearm as determined by computed tomography. Clin Sci 66:683, 1984

MULLEN JL et al: Implications of malnutrition in surgical patients. Arch Surg 114:121, 1979

PHILLIPS LS, UNTERMAN T: Somatomedin activity in disorders of nutrition and metabolism. Clin Endocrinol Metab 13:145, 1984

REIFENSTEIN EC et al: The accumulation, interpretation, and presentation of data pertaining to metabolic balances, notably those of calcium, phosphorus, and nitrogen. J Clin Endocrinol Metab 5:367, 1945

RUSSELL DM, JEEJEEBHOY KN: The assessment of the functional consequences of malnutrition. Curr Concepts Nutr 13:113, 1984

SAUBERLICH HE: Implications of nutritional status on human biochemistry, physiology, and health. Clin Biochem 17:132, 1984

SOLOMONS NW, ALLEN LH: The functional assessment of nutritional status: Principles, practice and potential. Nutr Rev 41:33, 1983

SUTPHEN JL: Growth as a measure of nutritional status. J Pediatr Gastroenterol Nutr 4:169, 1985

VASWANI AN et al: Effects of caloric restriction on body composition and total body nitrogen as measured by neutron activation. Metabolism 32:185, 1983

VITERI FE, ALVARADO J: The creatinine height index: Its use in the estimation of the degree of protein depletion and repletion in protein calorie malnourished children. Pediatrics 46:696, 1970

72   PROTEIN AND ENERGY UNDERNUTRITION

DANIEL RUDMAN

RELEVANCE TO CONTEMPORARY MEDICINE   Protein-energy undernutrition was described in developing nations in the 1930s. The syndrome affects the structure and function of every organ in the body. The causes, manifestations, and treatment have been intensively studied in African and Asian children, in whom the prevalence of the primary form of the disorder is high. The secondary varieties of protein-energy deficiency are common within hospital populations in developed nations. Subacutely or chronically ill patients living longer under the protection of modern therapeutics but handicapped by anorexia, hypermetabolism, or malabsorption may rapidly develop protein-energy malnutrition. A third cause of protein-energy undernutrition in the western world is the syndrome of anorexia nervosa in young women.

DEFINITION AND ETIOLOGY   The progressive loss of both lean body mass and adipose tissue results from insufficient consumption of protein and energy, although one or the other may play the dominant role in a given individual. The inadequate intake may be primary or secondary, as discussed in Chap. 71. Synergism between the two mechanisms is common. Patients with scanty reserves of protein and energy develop clinical protein-energy starvation more rapidly than well-nourished subjects when challenged by the hypermetabolism, catabolism, and anorexia of infection or other illnesses.

On a global basis the primary mechanism predominates. Socioeconomic factors that limit the quantity and quality of the diet are paramount. Particularly important is the poor biologic value of many vegetable proteins. The problem is accentuated if energy is inadequate because a large proportion of the dietary amino acids must then be oxidized as fuel instead of used to synthesize tissue and plasma protein. In developed countries, protein-energy malnutrition is often the result of inadequate nutrient intake due to drug or alcohol abuse; to depression and isolation in the aged; or to anorexia, malabsorption, or hypermetabolism in the hospitalized patient.

EPIDEMIOLOGY   The prevalence of protein-energy undernutrition can be assessed by measuring percent reduction in midarm fat area, midarm muscle area, 24-h urinary creatinine/height ratio, and serum albumin (see Chap. 71). The rate of growth of the children is a sensitive index of the nutritional state of a population: subnormal height for age ("stunting") usually indicates chronic protein-energy deficiency, and subnormal weight for height ("wasting") manifests recent energy deficit.

Estimates of prevalence of protein-energy depletion in various population groups are given in Table 72-1. In the United States, subclinical protein deficiency is more common in the south than in the north, in blacks and Latin Americans than in whites, and in the poor and the elderly than in the general population. In contrast to developing nations, protein-energy depletion in the general population in the United States tends to be mild and subclinical. In hospitals, on the other hand, severe as well as mild deficiencies are frequent and are usually associated with other types of malnutrition and with underlying organic disease. The widespread prescription of low protein diets to treat hepatic encephalopathy, chronic progressive renal disease, and uremia has created new groups at risk for protein deficiency.

PATHOPHYSIOLOGY   Energy and protein deficiencies have been studied most extensively in children of developing nations in whom inadequate or marginal diets, the augmented nutritional requirements of growth, and frequent episodes of infectious disease combine to cause florid manifestations of deficiency. Two syndromes have been distinguished: (1) marasmus, manifested by stunted growth, loss of adipose tissue, and generalized wasting of lean body mass without edema; and (2) kwashiorkor, manifested by growth failure (in children), hypoalbuminemia, edema, fatty liver, and preservation of adipose tissue. Mixed forms (kwashiorkor-marasmus) are common.

In adult secondary protein-energy undernutrition, Bistrian has defined weight loss >10 percent or body weight <80 percent of ideal, without hypoalbuminemia, as "adult marasmus." Hypoalbuminemia alone is termed "adult kwashiorkor." The distinction seems to be useful because in hospital practice the latter group experiences greater morbidity and mortality than the former.

METABOLIC AND ENDOCRINE ASPECTS   **Energy deficiency**   The events during calorie undernutrition can be viewed as adaptations serving to conserve the lean body mass. The first level of adaptation involves reduction of physical activity and energy expenditure. In early life, if the food intake of balanced diets is reduced to 60 percent of the ad lib intake, growth rate is slowed, puberty is delayed, and adult size is reduced. In rats, mice, and dogs, a moderate degree of underfeeding with a balanced diet (to about 60 percent of ad lib) leads to small, healthy adults. Interestingly, the life span of dogs is increased by a factor of 1.2 to 1.8 compared with ad lib–fed animals; the improved longevity reflects less cancer, better immunity, and preservation of renal function in later life.

Further reduction in caloric intake, or semistarvation, exceeds these adaptations and now leads to adverse effects throughout the body, with increased morbidity, shortened life span, and diminished work capacity. The body responds to semistarvation with an orderly physiologic adaptation, engineered in large part by a reduced secretion of insulin, augmented plasma levels of glucagon and cortisol, curtailed hepatic production of triiodothyronine (T_3) from thyroxine (T_4), and diminished hepatic secretion of somatomedin C despite augmented growth hormone release. The fall in plasma insulin permits free fatty acids and amino acids to be mobilized from adipose tissue and muscle to provide carbon for the continuing oxidative metabolism of the

body, while glucose tends to be spared for the central nervous system. The impaired glucose tolerance of starvation sometimes reflects a component of insulin resistance; excessive production of growth hormone, cortisol, catecholamines, free fatty acids, and interleukins may all contribute, especially in the stressed patient. When energy balance is negative, oxidative metabolism claims first priority in the utilization of dietary protein. During starvation, the carbon chains of amino acids also provide substrate for gluconeogenesis, since a continuing supply of glucose is required by the central nervous system. The augmented secretion of ACTH and cortisol contributes to the acceleration of gluconeogenesis. As amino acids are diverted from protein synthesis into oxidative metabolism and gluconeogenesis, protein synthesis is curtailed, particularly in muscle. The low somatomedin level in the underfed child is a probable cause for the slowing of the growth rate. The metabolic rate gradually declines, because of diminished extrathyroidal conversion of T_4 to T_3, decreased synthesis of the T_3 receptor, curtailed production and turnover of catecholamines, and a decrease in dietary thermogenesis. During partial or total deprivation of calories, both lean body mass and adipose tissue contract, but the latter does so more rapidly. In prolonged starvation, the adipose organ may be totally consumed when lean body mass has contracted by only 30 or 40 percent.

During the first week of total starvation, the average patient loses 4 to 5 kg of body weight which consists of about 25 percent adipose tissue, 35 percent extracellular fluid, and 40 percent protoplasm. Losses of nitrogen, potassium, sodium, and chloride represent 3 to 8 percent of the total body content of each element. Negative balances of magnesium, phosphorus, and calcium are also considerable. During ensuing weeks, as further adaptive endocrine and enzymatic adjustments occur, losses of nitrogen and other elements continue but at a slower rate. Ketone bodies now tend to replace glucose as substrate for oxidation in the brain, thereby sparing gluconeogenesis and protein catabolism.

The intracellular compartment does not contract at the same rate in all tissues. The central nervous system does not lose weight. Skeletal muscle atrophies more rapidly than cardiac muscle, and the gastrointestinal tract and liver lose mass more rapidly than kidneys. Mobilization of amino acids from muscle to liver permits the latter to continue to synthesize some albumin and lipoproteins; as a consequence, hypoalbuminemia and fatty liver are not conspicuous. When the loss of muscle mass in protein-energy undernutrition reaches 50 percent, survival is limited; thus, it is unusual to find midarm muscle circumference less than 50 percent of standard in chronically ill adults.

Protein deficiency   Frequently the intake of protein is more limited than that of calories. This occurs because dietary protein is more expensive than carbohydrate or fat; because protein of high biologic value (chiefly animal) is more expensive than protein of low biologic value (chiefly vegetable); because high-calorie, low-protein foods (many snack foods, ethanol, starchy root-based vegetables) are in common use in the United States and abroad; and because physicians may administer glucose as the sole organic nutrient in the intravenous feeding of the patient who cannot eat. The deficiency state under these conditions is analogous to kwashiorkor in children. The reduction of insulin secretion, which is a central mechanism in the adaptation to energy starvation, is circumvented. Insulin secreted in response to the dietary or intravenous carbohydrate promotes lipogenesis and retards lipolysis; adipose tissue is preserved, and free fatty acids are not available for oxidation in place of amino acids. The high plasma insulin also impairs mobilization and redistribution of amino acids from skeletal muscle to liver. Plasma amino acids fall, and the total body rate of protein synthesis declines. The synthesis of albumin and transport proteins by the liver is curtailed. Fatty infiltration of the liver is common. Two biochemical mechanisms are probably involved in the steatosis: (1) lack of methionine limits phospholipid synthesis, secondarily impairing lipoprotein formation, and (2) hepatic synthesis of triglycerides from glucose continues. Decreased concentrations of plasma albumin, plasma transferrin, and hemoglobin reflect severe

TABLE 72-1   Prevalence of protein-energy malnutrition in selected groups

Group	Criterion of deficiency	Prevalence of deficiency, %
Children <5 years, 28 developing countries*	Body weight <80% (kwashiorkor) or <60% of standard (marasmus)	25
Pediatric patients, Children's Hospital Medical Center, Boston†	Weight/height <90% of standard; midarm muscle area <15th percentile	37
Cancer patients, Emory University Hospital‡	Creatinine/height <60% std., triceps skin fold <80% std.	50
General surgical patients, Boston City Hospital¶	Midarm muscle circumference, triceps skin fold, serum albumin more than two standard deviations below normal mean	48

* *J Bengou, J Trop Pediatr 13:169, 1967.*
† *R Merritt, Am J Clin Nutr 32:1320, 1979.*
‡ *D Nixon, Am J Med 68:683, 1980.*
¶ *BR Bistrian et al, JAMA 230:858, 1974.*

protein starvation. Edema is characteristic of this stage and results in part from the hypoalbuminemia.

The account above describes the sequence of events in primary protein deficiency. However, variable degrees of energy and protein starvation commonly occur together. A further complication in secondary undernutrition is that the metabolic stress of trauma, infection, fever, or inflammation can cause the release of interleukins that inhibit albumin synthesis. In such patients, the rate of albumin catabolism and its movement from intravascular to extravascular sites are accelerated. Hypoalbuminemia correlates with morbidity and mortality in secondary protein-energy undernutrition, but its pathogenesis is complex.

Mineral metabolism   Protein-energy undernutrition is generally associated with a depletion of body minerals. In part this reflects the contraction of protoplasmic and extracellular fluid compartments with their constituent elements (nitrogen, phosphorus, potassium, and magnesium within cells; sodium and chloride in extracellular fluid) being excreted into the urine in the same proportions as in the lean body mass. However, mineral losses are often out of proportion to the contraction of lean body mass. One reason is a shift of potassium and magnesium from muscle to plasma in exchange for sodium. In addition, potassium, magnesium, phosphorus, and calcium intakes may be even less adequate than those of protein and energy (e.g., during prolonged intravenous nutrition with magnesium- or phosphorus-free solutions). Finally, renal and extrarenal losses of these elements may be significant (diuresis, diarrhea, fistulas, etc.).

STRESSED VERSUS NONSTRESSED PROTEIN-ENERGY MALNUTRITION   Simple starvation in an otherwise healthy individual, as described above, involves maintenance of glucose production at the expense of muscle tissue. Unchecked protein catabolism would quickly lead to death, but a gradual metabolic adaptation mitigates the effects: the need for gluconeogenesis from amino acids is reduced as the central nervous system adapts to ketone bodies as a fuel source, and basal energy expenditure is reduced.

Protein-energy undernutrition in a patient stressed by trauma, burn, infection, or inflammation proceeds more rapidly. Muscle especially is catabolized at an accelerated rate. The loss of 1.5 to 2 kg of protoplasm in the first week of simple starvation should be compared to the loss of 1.0 to 2.5 kg of protoplasm per day under conditions of severe metabolic stress.

The accelerated pace of protein-energy undernutrition in "stressed semistarvation" has several causes: (1) augmented consumption of glucose because of hypermetabolism and because of the glucose requirement of inflammatory tissues; (2) extra utilization of protein for immune function and wound repair; (3) the exaggerated catecholamine and cortisol responses contributing to hypermetabolism (up to +100 percent), gluconeogenesis, and insulin resistance; (4) production of interleukins. Activated phagocytic cells release one or more metabolically active peptides, variously termed leukocyte pyrogen, leukocyte endogenous mediator, or interleukin 1, which causes prostaglandin E_2 to accumulate in brain, liver, muscle, and adipose tissue, with resultant fever, protein breakdown in muscle, synthesis of acute phase proteins in liver, fat mobilization, insulin resistance, and movement of iron and zinc from the circulation into storage sites in the liver. These features are all prominent in stressed semistarvation.

Studies with heavy isotopes have shed some light on the catabolic response to injury. The rate of turnover of whole-body protein in the normal adult is of the order of 200 g per day. Eighty to ninety percent of the amino acids released by this process are normally reutilized; the remaining 10 to 20 percent are supplied by the diet. The efficiency of the reutilization process depends upon an adequate supply of energy. In unstressed starvation, the rate of protein breakdown remains unchanged, while the rate of protein synthesis declines, with a resultant loss of body protein. In stressed starvation, both protein breakdown and protein synthesis are accelerated, but the former to a greater extent, thereby increasing the loss of body protein. The efficiency of reutilization of the amino acids released by catabolism

is reduced in the febrile or injured patient. Branched-chain amino acids may become limiting in the reutilization process, and an increased intake of these building blocks improves muscle protein synthesis in some catabolic patients.

CARDIOVASCULAR-RESPIRATORY AND RENAL RESPONSES
The heart and kidneys lose mass progressively during the course of protein-energy starvation. These losses are generally proportional to the erosion of lean body mass, so that ratios of heart mass/lean body mass and kidney mass/lean body mass remain normal. Consequently, a functional insufficiency of these two shrunken organs is not a usual feature of protein-energy depletion. Cardiac output declines in parallel with the falling metabolic rate. Blood pressure is reduced by the fall in cardiac output. The ventilatory response to hypoxia is blunted. Glomerular filtration rate and renal blood flow are lowered. The ability of the kidney to excrete an acid load or to respond to antidiuretic hormone may be impaired. Although these changes in cardiac and renal structure and function are in part appropriate to the reduced lean body mass and hypometabolic state, they may become important handicaps during vigorous nutritional repletion, acute infection, or other circumstances that require rapid increases in cardiac output, metabolic rate, and urinary excretion of solutes. Heart failure and death may occur during the rapid repletion of subjects with severe protein-energy undernutrition.

BLOOD   Reduced blood volume, hematocrit, albumin, transferrin, retinol-bending protein, and total lymphocyte count are characteristic in the wasted patient. The anemia of "pure" protein-energy depletion is normocytic and normochromic and usually results from a decreased production of red blood cells, perhaps reflecting the protein requirement for globin synthesis.

In most patients with protein-calorie undernutrition, there are complicating factors such as multiple micronutrient deficiencies; concurrent bacterial, viral, or parasitic infestation; or major underlying disease. In the primary undernutrition in developing nations, iron deficiency is apparent in about 25 percent of patients on admission and becomes evident in 90 percent during recovery. Folate is deficient on admission in 10 to 20 percent. Serum erythropoietin is high. Feeding an adequate diet quickly causes reticulocytosis.

STRUCTURE AND FUNCTION OF GASTROINTESTINAL TRACT
AND PANCREAS   The gastrointestinal tract and pancreas atrophy. In the small intestine, villous height, mitotic index, and content of disaccharidases and dipeptidases all decline. Exocrine elements of the pancreas atrophy as well, and the production of digestive enzymes is reduced. Bacterial overgrowth may occur in the small intestine. Hypoalbuminemia may lead to edema of the small bowel. These factors combine to produce malabsorption and lactose intolerance. The structural and functional regression of the small intestine results, in part, from decreased oral feeding rather than systemic malnutrition, since patients fully repleted by the parenteral route still exhibit the same lesion.

IMMUNE SYSTEM   Lymphatic tissues atrophy. Impaired cell-mediated immunity is evident by all standard tests (blastogenic response of lymphocytes to mitogens, total lymphocyte count, and skin testing with recall antigens). Bactericidal activity of polymorphonuclear leukocytes is decreased. Diminished thymic hormone activity retards the maturation of T cells, and the proportion of circulating T cells of the null variety is increased. Deficiencies of zinc and water-soluble vitamins contribute to the T-cell defects. Plasma B-cell functions (plasma immunoglobin concentrations and humoral responses to antigens) are preserved. Protein-energy-starved patients experience increased morbidity and mortality during common infections and are subject to infection by opportunistic organisms (gram-negative bacteria, *Candida*, herpes simplex). Impaired respiratory function, leading to atelectasis and pneumonia, is a common cause of death. The extent of cutaneous anergy correlates both with the severity of nutritional deficiency and with morbidity and mortality rates.

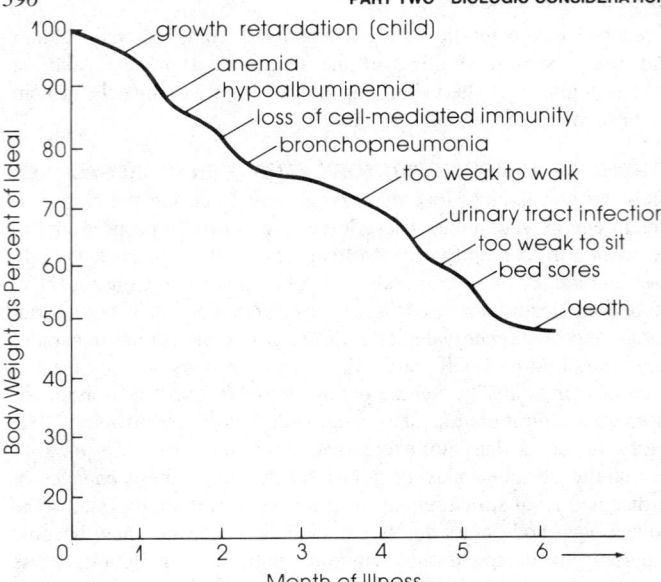

FIGURE 72-1 *Course of a typical case of progressive protein-energy starvation.*

WOUND HEALING The response of fibroblasts to surgical wounds is impaired. Consequently, incisions and enteric anastomoses heal more slowly in undernourished patients; wound dehiscence is common.

TEMPERATURE REGULATION In the absence of fever, basal metabolic rate is reduced. Hypothermia is common. The underlying mechanisms are reduced heat production due to low plasma T_3, possible decreased adrenergic function, loss of thermal insulation when subcutaneous adipose tissue is gone, and resetting of the thermostat in the preoptic nuclei of the hypothalamus. Hypoglycemia may occur (see Chap. 329).

REPRODUCTION Nearly every phase of the reproductive process is impaired in women of child-bearing age. Diminished secretion of luteinizing hormone–releasing hormone (LHRH) by the hypothalamus may cause amenorrhea. Fertility is reduced: if implantation occurs, the risk of early fetal resorption is high. If gestation is completed, the progeny are substandard in weight and length. Lactation is impaired so that postnatal undernutrition is common. Even if postnatal nutrition is adequate, stunted growth in the malnourished infant is in part irreversible, and impairment in learning capacity may be life-long.

In wasted men, plasma total and free testosterone tend to be low due to various combinations of primary gonadal defect and diminished hypothalamic LHRH production.

CLINICAL MANIFESTATIONS   History A primary component in the etiology can be uncovered only by reviewing protein and caloric intake and the biologic quality of the dietary protein during the

TABLE 72-2 Undesirable practices affecting the nutritional health of hospital patients

1 Failure to record height and weight on admission
2 Lack of a weight curve in the hospital chart
3 Prolonged use of glucose and saline intravenous feedings
4 Failure to measure patient's food intake
5 Withholding meals because of diagnostic tests
6 Use of tube feedings of inadequate amount and uncertain composition
7 Ignorance of the composition of nutritional products
8 Failure to recognize increased nutritional needs due to injury or illness
9 Delay of nutrition support until the patient is in an advanced state of depletion
10 Limited availability of laboratory tests to assess nutritional status; failure to use those that are available
11 Failure to correct inadequate dentition or the edentulous state

SOURCE: *After Butterworth.*

preceding months. Factors that predispose to a secondary etiology include the presence of a known chronic medical problem, prolonged fever, anorexia or other gastrointestinal symptoms, and lack of teeth.

In children failure to gain height and weight is an early sign. In adults weight loss is usual, but a body weight equal to or greater than ideal does not exclude the presence of deficiency of caloric intake, protein, or both. Thus, progressive loss of protoplasm and adipose tissue may be masked by edema; or the patient may have been previously obese, and a substantial loss of lean body mass during the current illness may be masked by a residue of obesity. Listlessness, easy fatigability, sensation of coldness, swollen ankles, and dry, cracked skin are frequent in patients with protein-energy malnutrition.

Physical signs The facies is drawn, temporal regions are concave and fleshless, intercostal spaces are excavated, and the skin hangs in folds on the wasted extremities. "Flaky paint" dermatitis and dyspigmentation of skin and hair are common. The patient is pale and may be edematous. Signs of vitamin deficiency may be present. Decubiti and skin ulcers are common in advanced stages.

Vital signs The blood pressure is decreased. The pulse is slow, and the extremities are cool; central temperature may be decreased.

Anthropometrics The midarm fat area and midarm muscle area are reduced in varying ratios dependent on previous nutritional state and relative severity of the energy and protein deficiencies.

Laboratory and x-ray findings The ratio of 24-h urinary creatinine/height is decreased. In the absence of renal disease, this is the most sensitive and practical clinical indicator of protein starvation and should be monitored at monthly intervals in the chronically ill hospital patient. These analyses are valid only in the afebrile state, since urinary excretion of creatinine is increased by fever. Other signs of protein-energy malnutrition include a decrease in serum albumin, serum transferrin, and hematocrit, but these changes are less specific. Nevertheless, protein depletion may be the most common cause of hypoalbuminemia in hospitalized patients, even in patients with hepatic disease. Plasma levels of essential and nonessential amino acid concentrations, and urine urea and creatinine levels are reduced. T-lymphocyte cell function is decreased, as revealed by cutaneous anergy and peripheral lymphopenia (absolute lymphocyte count <1200 cells per cubic millimeter). Glucose tolerance is impaired. Plasma cortisol is often increased (in part because of retarded metabolic clearance), T_3 is decreased, reverse T_3 (rT_3) may be increased, and basal metabolic rate is low. Plasma somatomedin C is low. Heart size is small on chest film. Echocardiography shows a small heart with decreased cardiac output. Sagittal or cross-section x-rays of the arm show a diminished muscle mass.

Course A typical case is illustrated in Fig. 72-1. In children, an early manifestation is slowing of growth. As the protein-energy depletion becomes more severe, pallor, fatigue, and amenorrhea appear. Loss of cell-mediated immunity predisposes to infections. The hypermetabolism and anorexia of intercurrent infection accelerate the progress of cachexia. In advanced undernutrition (midarm fat area <2 cm², creatinine/height ratio <60 percent of standard), decubiti, hypothermia, and terminal infection are the rule.

Relation to other deficiency states Usually other nutrients are also depleted. Folic acid, thiamine, riboflavin, nicotinic acid, pyridoxine, ascorbic acid, and vitamin A deficiencies are relatively common in hospital populations in the United States (see Table 72-2). Body content of most minerals is also reduced, but a distinction must be made between absolute and relative decreases. As protoplasmic protein is consumed to supply metabolic fuel and substrate for gluconeogenesis in the underfed patient, the intracellular minerals potassium, phosphorus, and magnesium and some of the microminerals are excreted in parellel with the nitrogen. Such loss is absolute but not relative, since the intracellular and extracellular concentrations of potassium, phosphorus, and magnesium usually remain normal. If the diet is also deficient in potassium, phosphorus, or magnesium, a further deficiency occurs, and the intracellular, extracellular, and urinary concentrations may become subnormal. Similar considerations apply to the body content of essential fatty acids. Whether the depletion of potassium, phosphorus, magnesium, or essential fatty acids is absolute or relative, repletion with a feeding solution deficient in that nutrient may lead to chemical and clinical manifestations of the corresponding deficiency state within a few days. Life-threatening hypokalemia, hypophosphatemia, or hypomagnesemia can occur. By similar mechanisms, plasma levels of trace minerals decline during hyperalimentation if adequate rations of these nutrients are not provided.

REFERENCES

ALLEYNE GAO et al: Protein-energy malnutrition. London, Butler & Tanner, 1977

BARACOS V et al: Stimulation of degradation of muscle proteins during fever. A mechanism for the increased degradation of muscle proteins during fever. N Engl J Med 308:553, 1983

BECKER DJ: The endocrine responses to protein calorie malnutrition. Ann Rev Nutr 3:187, 1983

BEISEL WR: Magnitude of the host nutritional responses to infection. Am J Clin Nutr 30:1236, 1977

————: Metabolic effects of infection. Prog Food Nutr Sci 8:43, 1984

BISTRIAN BR et al: Prevalence of malnutrition in general medical patients. JAMA 235:1567, 1976

———— et al: Protein status of general surgical patients. JAMA 230:858, 1974

BUTTERWORTH CE: The skeleton in the hospital closet. Nutr Today 9:4, 1974

CAHILL GF: Starvation in man. N Engl J Med 282:668, 1970

CHANDRA RK: Numerical and functional deficiency in T helper cells in protein energy malnutrition. Clin Exp Immunol 51:126, 1983

CORMAN LC: The relationship between nutrition, infection and immunity. Med Clin North Am 69:519, 1985

CUTHBERTSON DP: Post-traumatic metabolism: A multidisciplinary challenge. Surg Clin North Am 58:1045, 1978

DAVIES L: Nutrition and the elderly: Identifying those at risk. Proc Nutr Soc 43:295, 1984

DINARELLO CA: Interleukin 1. Rev Infect Dis 6:51, 1984

DOWD PS, HEATLEY RV: The influence of undernutrition on immunity. Clin Sci 66:241, 1984

FERNANDES G: Nutritional factors: Modulating effects on immune function and aging. Pharmacol Rev 36:123S, 1984

GRAHAM GG: Poverty, hunger, malnutrition, prematurity, and infant mortality in the United States. Pediatrics 75:117, 1985

GRANTHAM-MCGREGOR S: Chronic undernutrition and cognitive abilities. Hum Nutr Clin Nutr 38:83, 1984

KEUSCH GT: Nutrition as a determinant of host response to infection and the metabolic sequellae of infectious diseases. Seminars in Infectious Disease 2:265, 1979

LEEVY CM et al: Incidence and significance of hypovitaminemia in a randomly selected municipal hospital population. Am J Clin Nutr 17:259, 1965

LONG CM: Energy balance and carbohydrate metabolism in infection and sepsis. Am J Clin Nutr 30:1301, 1977

LUNDHOLM KG: Nutritional problems in trauma. Acta Chir Scand (suppl) 522:183, 1985

MASORO EJ: Nutrition as a modulator of the aging process. Physiologist 27:98, 1984

MOLDAWER LL et al: Muscle proteolysis in sepsis and trauma. N Engl J Med 309:494, 1983

PURI S, CHANDRA RK: Nutritional regulation of host resistance and predictive value of immunologic tests in assessment of outcome. Pediatr Clin North Am 32:499, 1985

ROE DA: *Drug-Induced Nutritional Deficiencies*. Westport, Conn, AVI, 1976

STEFFEE W: Malnutrition in hospitalized patients. JAMA 244:2630, 1980

TEN-STATE NUTRITION SURVEY. 1968–1970. US Department of Health, Education and Welfare Publication (HSM) 72, 1972

---

73 ANOREXIA NERVOSA AND BULIMIA

DANIEL W. FOSTER

Anorexia nervosa and bulimia are eating disorders in young, previously healthy women who develop a paralyzing fear of becoming fat. The population at risk consists largely of white women from middle- and upper-class backgrounds. The disorders rarely occur in black or oriental women, are unusual in the poor, and are almost never seen in men. The driving force is the pursuit of thinness, all other aspects of life being secondary. In the anorexia nervosa syndrome this aim is achieved primarily by radical restriction of caloric intake, the end result being emaciation. In bulimia massive binge eating is followed by vomiting and excessive use of laxatives. Weight loss in bulimic subjects is not great despite the obsession with food. Some authors consider anorexia nervosa and bulimia to be distinct illnesses, while others classify bulimia as a variant of anorexia nervosa. Clearly, overlap syndromes exist since emaciated patients fulfilling the criteria of true anorexia nervosa may exhibit bulimic behavior, while subjects with bulimia often pass through a phase of anorexia. In this chapter it will be assumed that the two disorders represent different clinical expressions of a primary psychologic disturbance focused on an obsession with body weight.

PREVALENCE Estimates of prevalence for anorexia nervosa range from 0.4 to 1.5 per 100,000 population. In adolescent white girls from middle- or upper-class families rates as high as 1 per 100 have been reported. Prevalence is believed to be increasing. Subclinical variants may be present in up to 5 percent of the socioeconomic group at highest risk. The incidence of bulimia is less certain. Vomiting after eating may occur in as many as 18 percent of women college students. The figure for self-induced vomiting in the general population is probably 1 to 2 percent, but the full-blown bulimic syndrome is less frequent.

DIAGNOSIS The diagnosis of both anorexia nervosa and bulimia is made on clinical grounds. No specific diagnostic tests exist. For many years the criteria of Feighner et al. (Table 73-1) were the basis for diagnosis in research studies. Less strict requirements were formulated for the Diagnostic and Statistical Manual of Mental Disorders III (DSM-III) of the American Psychiatric Association:

1 Intense fear of becoming obese, which does not diminish as weight loss progresses

2 Disturbance of body image; e.g., claiming to "feel fat" even when emaciated

3 Weight loss of at least 25 percent of original body weight, or if under 18 years of age, weight loss from original body weight plus weight gain expected from growth charts may be combined to make 25 percent

4 Refusal to maintain body weight over minimal normal weight for age and height

The uniqueness of the disturbance in body image in patients with eating disorders has been questioned, and some authorities have recommended its omission on the grounds that many normal young women demonstrate the same perceptual distortion. Similarly, the 25 percent figure for weight loss may be too restrictive, particularly in children. A presumptive diagnosis of anorexia nervosa is justified if the following elements are elicited: (1) a history of major weight loss; (2) absence of organic disease sufficient to account for weight loss; (3) absence of severe primary psychiatric illness which might account for failure to eat; (4) extreme restriction of food intake with or without intermittent induction of vomiting; (4) ritualized exercise; and (5) denial of hunger, fatigue, or emaciation.

The criteria for the diagnosis of bulimia in DSM-III appear to be less useful. The picture is that of a normal or near normal weight subject whose life is dominated by gorging and regurgitation in the

TABLE 73-1 Criteria for the diagnosis of anorexia nervosa

1 Onset prior to age 25
2 Anorexia with weight loss of at least 25 percent of original body weight
3 Distorted attitude toward eating, food, or weight that overrides hunger, admonitions, reassurances, and threats
4 No known medical illness that could account for the weight loss
5 No other known psychiatric disorder
6 At least two of the following manifestations:
  a Amenorrhea
  b Lanugo hair
  c Bradycardia (persistent resting pulse of 60 beats per minute or less)
  d Periods of overactivity
  e Episodes of bulimia
  f Vomiting (may be self-induced)

SOURCE: *After Feighner et al.*

absence of the physical changes or symptoms of profound weight loss.

ETIOLOGY   The cause of anorexia nervosa and bulimia is unknown. Although primary dysfunction of the hypothalamus has been postulated, the associated hypothalamic abnormalities revert to normal with weight gain and thus are secondary rather than causal.

Most investigators favor a psychiatric etiology, but there is disagreement about its nature. One view holds that the disorders begin in response to inadequate or destructive interpersonal relationships in upper middle class families that are goal-oriented and highly achieving. Despite an outward appearance of normality, interpersonal communication among family members tends to be inadequate, frequently following a pattern in which the father seeks success in his work while the mother turns to her children for fulfillment and in the process becomes overdirective. It is often stated that the families are "enmeshed," meaning that generational boundaries are blurred and that parents and children are constantly involved in each other's problems. Psychoanalytic interpretation tends to focus on anorexia as a mechanism whereby the patient reestablishes control of her own life in a way that cannot be controlled by parental direction. It is not clear how this sequence might result in the intense fear of being fat that is the central feature of both classic anorexia and bulimia.

Although the absence of psychiatric disease is one criterion for diagnosis (Table 73-1), it is now widely held that depression plays a significant role in the eating disorders. Abnormalities of neurotransmitter concentrations have been reported in cerebrospinal fluid, but it is not known whether they are primary or secondary. One report claims an increased prevalence of the HLA-Bw16 haplotype in anorexia nervosa, but this antigen may correlate better with depression than with eating disorders per se.

Cultural issues are likely also important in the prevalence of anorexia nervosa. The quest for health and slimness is a powerful force in modern western society and may reinforce the fear of fatness in patients with established anorexia or tip the borderline case into full-blown disease. Occupation may play a role since dancers have a prevalence of anorexia nervosa 10 times that of the general population. Likewise athletes, particularly runners, often seek to decrease body fat to very low levels (5 to 7 percent).

Whatever the mechanism(s) involved, the behavioral response is obsessive and is difficult to treat.

CLINICAL PICTURE   While anorexia nervosa and bulimia may coexist in the same patient, the clinical pictures are ordinarily distinct (Table 73-2).

TABLE 73-2   The eating disorders

	Anorexia nervosa	Bulimia
Predominant sex	Female	Female
Method of weight control	Restriction of intake	Vomiting
Binge eating	Uncommon	Invariant
Weight at diagnosis	Markedly decreased	Near normal
Ritualized exercise	Usual	Rare
Amenorrhea	~100%	~50%
Antisocial behavior	Rare	Frequent
Cardiovascular changes (bradycardia, hypotension)	Common	Uncommon
Skin changes (hirsutism, dryness, carotenemia)	Usual	Rare
Hypothermia	Usual	Rare
Edema	+/-	+/-
Medical complications	Hypokalemia, cardiac arrhythmias	Hypokalemia, cardiac arrhythmias, aspiration of gastric contents, esophageal or gastric rupture

NOTE: *These features are characteristic of pure anorexia nervosa and pure bulimia. Overlap syndromes occur, and anorexia may evolve to bulimia (the bulimia → anorexia transformation is rare).*

Anorexia nervosa   The anorexia nervosa syndrome usually begins before or shortly after puberty but may appear later (rarely later than the middle twenties). Many patients have been overweight in childhood. Emaciation is equivalent to that seen in the concentration camp victims of World War II. Despite profound weight loss the patients deny hunger, thinness, or fatigue. They are often physically active, and ritualized exercise programs are common. Frenzied calisthenics or running may follow food intake. There is a preoccupation with food, and elaborate meals may be prepared for others. If social circumstances require them to eat more than usual, vomiting is induced as soon as possible, often in a public restroom. As noted, episodic binge eating may occur and is also followed by emesis. Amenorrhea is nearly always present. It usually accompanies or follows weight loss but in a sixth of patients may appear prior to any physical change. Constipation and cold intolerance are common. The latter are presumably due to a defect in regulatory thermogenesis secondary to hypothalamic dysfunction.

In advanced cases bradycardia, hypothermia, and hypotension are present. Body fat is undetectable, and the bones protrude through the skin. Interestingly, breast tissue is often preserved. The skin may be dry and scaly and is often yellow due to carotenemia, (particularly visible in the palms). Body hair is often increased; it is usually of fine, lanugo quality, but frank hirsutism may occur. Parotid glands may be enlarged as in other forms of starvation. Edema in the absence of hypoalbuminemia is thought to be due to failure of extracellular fluid volume to diminish proportionately with body mass during weight loss. Because of edema in the legs and parotid enlargement, which gives a fullness to the face, the true state of emaciation may be masked when the patient is fully dressed.

Laboratory abnormalities include anemia and leukopenia (with hypocellularity of the bone marrow), hypokalemia, and hypoalbuminemia. Serum β-carotene levels tend to be elevated. Prerenal azotemia may occur if vomiting or laxative use are prominent. The blood urea nitrogen may be as high as 60 to 70 mg/dL. Renal concentrating ability is impaired, possibly due to blunted responsiveness to antidiuretic hormone. Release of vasopressin in response to an osmotic stimulus is also abnormal. Plasma cholesterol is occasionally high, but triglyceride levels are not increased despite low activities of hepatic and lipoprotein lipases. Glucose tolerance is abnormal as in other forms of starvation.

Miscellaneous abnormalities include low levels of IgG, IgM, and a variety of proteins in the complement pathways. Despite these findings immune function is generally preserved, and serious infections are rare. Plasma iron and ceruloplasmin are normal, but iron binding capacity is decreased. Serum zinc and copper are decreased, but concentrations of these metals are normal in hair. Serum amylase may be increased in the absence of signs or symptoms of pancreatitis.

A variety of endocrine abnormalities are seen. Basal levels of luteinizing hormone (LH) and follicle-stimulating hormone (FSH) are low when weight loss is severe, and the LH response to luteinizing hormone–releasing hormone (LHRH) is impaired. FSH response to LHRH is normal, although time to peak increase may be delayed. Studies of the 24-h circadian pattern of LH secretion show regression of the maturational stage to the pattern characteristic of prepubertal or early pubertal girls; i.e., episodic LH release is missing or occurs only during sleep. These findings presumably account, at least in part, for the amenorrhea. Menses return with weight gain, although the weight required for reinitiation of menstruation may be somewhat higher (~ 10 percent) than that needed for the original induction of menarche. Ovulatory menses may be induced in subjects with anorexia nervosa by prolonged treatment with LHRH, suggesting that pituitary gonadotropin release is impaired because of hypothalamic dysfunction. Prolactin levels are normal. Plasma estradiol levels are low, and plasma testosterone is in the normal female range. Testosterone concentrations are low in men with anorexia nervosa.

Growth hormone (GH) in the basal state may be normal or elevated. A rise in GH occurs after injection of thyrotropin-releasing hormone (TRH), as in other states with elevated basal levels of GH such as acromegaly, uremia, and protein-calorie malnutrition. Insulin-like growth factor I (somatomedin C) concentrations are low. Plasma cortisol levels are high despite normal production rates; this is due to decreased metabolism of cortisol and prolongation of the plasma half-life. Dexamethasone suppression tests may be abnormal. Norepinephrine concentrations in plasma are depressed.

Thyroxine (T_4) levels tend to be slightly low but free T_4 is normal. Triiodothyronine (T_3) concentrations are reduced while reverse T_3 (rT_3) levels are increased. Basal levels of thyroid-stimulating hormone (TSH) are usually normal, and TSH response to TRH is intact. The primary defect in thyroid hormone metabolism is decreased activity of the 5'-deiodinase that converts T_4 to T_3 and rT_3 to diiodothyronine in nonthyroidal tissues. These changes are characteristic of starvation and wasting diseases and are not specific for anorexia nervosa.

Bone density is decreased in women with anorexia nervosa. The mechanism is thought to be estrogen deficiency rather than an abnormality in vitamin D metabolism.

Bulimia Bulimia, which means "ox-hunger," refers to the episodic ingestion of large amounts of food in a compulsive fashion, coupled with awareness that the eating pattern is abnormal, a fear that eating cannot be stopped voluntarily, and feelings of depression at completion of the act. Bulimics have a morbid fear of becoming fat. While binge eating may occur in several types of emotional disorders, a high percentage of patients give a history of overt or cryptic anorexia nervosa, suggesting that bulimia is commonly a variant of anorexia nervosa. Episodes of binge eating are followed by induced vomiting, with or without the subsequent ingestion of large quantities of laxatives. Initially vomiting is induced by placing a toothbrush or fingers in the throat, but eventually most patients learn to vomit reflexly.

Binge eating generally occurs daily in the active phase; in a series of 40 patients the mean number of episodes per week was 12, ranging from 1 to 46. The duration of the eating period averaged 1.2 h but could last as long as 8 h. The amount of food ingested can be enormous, up to 50,000 calories a day, although the mean number of calories consumed in a single episode is around 3500. High-carbohydrate foods are favored, and more than one food is usually eaten. The order of frequency in one report was: ice cream→bread→candy→donuts→soft drinks. The term "dietary chaos" describes the eating pattern. Because of the high sugar content of the diet, dental caries are frequent.

Other behavioral abnormalities are common. Secrecy about the eating-vomiting sequence is characteristic so that family and friends are often unaware. Stealing is common, and food is the item most often taken. There is a high rate of alcohol and drug abuse. Depression tends to be more severe than in anorexia nervosa, making suicide a definite risk. Hysterical behavior may occur. Families of patients with bulimia have a higher incidence of affective disorders, alcoholism, and illicit drug use than is seen in families of patients with classic anorexia nervosa.

Despite the close relationship with true anorexia nervosa, a number of differences are noted. While many patients with bulimia are thin, weight loss to the point of emaciation is not seen; generally weight is within 15 percent of the normal range as defined by life insurance tables of ideal weight. Fluctuating weight is common, with cyclical gains and losses. Some patients are modestly overweight. In contrast to anorexia nervosa, about half of the patients continue to menstruate, and a number have become pregnant. Persistent menstruation probably reflects the absence of extreme weight loss. Sexual activity is greater in bulimic subjects than in those with anorexia.

The physical findings associated with bulimia are usually minimal, although subjects with more extensive weight loss may manifest some of the changes seen with anorexia nervosa.

The most common laboratory abnormality is hypokalemia with metabolic alkalosis secondary to vomiting and laxative use. Evaluation of the endocrine system has not been systematically carried out.

PROGNOSIS The course of anorexia nervosa is variable. In long-term follow-up about 50 percent of patients achieve normal weight, 20 percent improve but remain underweight, 20 percent continue anorexic, 5 percent become obese, and 6 percent die. Even when weight gain occurs, signs of persistent illness remain since intermittent dieting, binge eating, vomiting, and laxative use persist in up to two-thirds of patients. Death is usually due to starvation (cardiac arrhythmias primarily) or suicide. Poor prognostic signs include older age of onset, longer duration of illness, history of bulimia or vomiting, extreme weight loss, and presence of significant depression.

The prognosis in bulimia is worse than that of anorexia nervosa, probably because the accompanying psychiatric disturbances are more severe. Suicide occurs twice as frequently. Aspiration pneumonia, acute gastric dilatation, gastric or esophageal rupture, and pancreatitis contribute to higher mortality rates.

TREATMENT There is no specific treatment for anorexia nervosa or bulimia. The intense fear of becoming fat coupled with a perceptual disturbance that causes overestimation of body size results in powerful resistance to therapy. The benefits of psychiatric intervention are marginal. The same can be said of behavior modification techniques and for group and family therapy. Supportive care by an understanding physician may accomplish as much as formal psychotherapy. The patient should be seen regularly for a review of weight change, diet, and exercise patterns. It is often useful to establish a mutually agreeable explicit contract; e.g., if the patient weighs 65 pounds and ideal body weight determined from life insurance tables is 115 pounds, a goal of 90 pounds might be set as a first stage. At every visit the patient should be reassured by the physician that "we will not let you get fat." A calm but realistic review of the dangers of starvation, including sudden death, should be given, coupled with statements like "my job is to help you deal with this illness so that you can have a normal life expectancy with reasonable happiness." The physician must be perceived not as an enemy or a parental surrogate but an advisor and partner in the struggle.

A similar approach should also be used with bulimic patients. Even if the gorging-regurgitation cycle cannot be stopped, the lesser goal of limiting the load of food ingested (to minimize the chance of aspiration or gastric rupture) and decreasing the frequency of events may be achieved. Because depression and antisocial behavior are more common in bulimia, psychiatric therapy is usually required.

Drugs such as phenytoin and cyproheptadine are ineffective in the eating disorders. It is now common to use antidepressants in both anorexia nervosa and bulimia. Imipramine and phenelzine may be the best choices. Potassium supplementation may be required for vomiters.

Hospitalization may be a life-saving measure with severe anorexia nervosa. Sudden death may occur at weights more than 35 percent below ideal, particularly if weight loss has been rapid. Hypokalemia, hypotension, and prerenal azotemia due to volume depletion are other indications for hospitalization. If the patient refuses to eat, a nasogastric tube will be required, but it is better to persuade the patient to eat. Supervision of every meal is initially required, ideally by the same person. During the hospitalization the patient should never be allowed to eat alone. Total parenteral nutrition is rarely indicated. Training in nutrition, occupational therapy, group work with the family, and individual psychotherapy should be included in the treatment plan. The "safety" of eating and assurances that obesity will not result should be emphasized repetitively. Some specialists feel that all seriously affected anorexia patients benefit from initial hospitalization, but this is not a universal view. Hospitalization for bulimic subjects is normally only required for medical complications (e.g., aspiration).

Treatment of patients with the anorexia-bulimia syndrome is a long-term proposition, rife with failure, and requires perseverance by the afflicted subject, the family, and the physician.

REFERENCES

FEIGHNER JP et al: Diagnostic criteria for use in psychiatric research. Arch Gen Psychiatry 26:57, 1972

FOSTER DW: Eating disorders: Obesity and anorexia nervosa, in *Williams Textbook of Endocrinology*, 7th ed, JD Wilson, DW Foster (eds). Philadelphia, Saunders, 1985, pp 1081–1107

HARRIS RT: Bulimarexia and related serious eating disorders with medical complications. Ann Intern Med 99:800, 1983

HERZOG DB, COPELAND PM: Eating disorders. N Engl J Med 313:295, 1985

MITCHELL JE et al: Frequency and duration of binge-eating episodes in patients with bulimia. Am J Psychiatry 138:835, 1981

PYLE RL et al: Bulimia: A report of 34 cases. J Clin Psychiatry 42:60, 1981

SCHWABE AD et al: Anorexia nervosa. Ann Intern Med 94:371, 1981

74   DIET THERAPY

DANIEL RUDMAN

Dietary modifications are indicated in many clinical situations. (1) The pathogenesis of certain chronic diseases is influenced by the long-term intake of dietary factors: sodium in hypertension, calcium in osteomalacia, and calories in obesity are examples of such situations. (2) The symptomatic stage of other disorders can be ameliorated or worsened by dietary components, for example, sodium in congestive heart failure, protein in uremia, and gluten in celiac disease. (3) Protein-energy undernutrition, the consequence of numerous subacute or chronic diseases, can often be prevented or corrected with newer techniques of nutritional support. (4) Drug therapy can modify the requirement for certain nutrients; for example, hydantoin anticonvulsants decrease serum levels of folic acid. Conversely, some foods may influence the effectiveness of drugs; for example, calcium-containing foods chelate oral tetracycline and prevent its absorption.

For these reasons, a controlled diet may be a critical aspect of a therapeutic program. The appropriate period of regulation may be temporary or permanent. In some circumstances, the physical composition and even the route of alimentation may need to be changed, with little or no alteration desired in the content of essential or nonessential nutrients. In other circumstances, a specific nutrient may need to be controlled. The physician who wishes to regulate a specific nutrient without causing a deficiency or excess of other nutrients and without the loss of palatability needs to understand the nutrient composition of the common foods.

DISTRIBUTION OF NUTRIENTS AMONG FOOD GROUPS   Because nutrients are not evenly distributed, a variety of foods must be eaten to achieve adequate nutrition. The average diet contains nearly 200 different food items. Isocaloric servings of meat and fruit, for example, have totally dissimilar nutrient contents.

Because of this complexity, foods have been arranged into groups of similar nutrient content. Milk-dairy products, meats-legumes, fruits-vegetables, and breads-cereals are the four groups commonly used (Table 74-1). The recommended number of servings from these groups meets the requirements for approximately three-fourths of the essential nutrients. Additional food selections should be made to fulfill the requirements for energy and certain vitamins and minerals.

It is often desirable to control (either increase or reduce) the intake

TABLE 74-1   The nutrient content of the four food groups compared to the recommended dietary allowances (RDAs)*

Food	Recommended servings	Energy, kcal	Protein, g	Fat, g	Carbohydrate, g	Vitamin A, mg RE	Vitamin E, mg	Ascorbic acid, mg	Thiamine, mg	Riboflavin, mg	Niacin, mg	Vitamin B$_6$, mg	Vitamin B$_{12}$, µg	Folacin, µg
MILK GROUP														
2% low fat	2 cups	288	20	10	29	117	0.19	5	0.2	1.0	0.5	0.19	1.9	5
MEAT GROUP														
Egg	1	70	6	5	0	156	0.23	0	0.1	0.1	0.1	0.05	1.0	3
Meat, fish, poultry	4 oz	285	31	18	0	26	0.26	0	0.3	0.2	7.3	0.59	1.6	9
VEGETABLE-FRUIT GROUP														
Leafy green and deep yellow	¼–⅓ cup	12	1	0	2	254	0.47	20	0	0.1	0.3	0.08	0	22
Other vegetables	¼–⅓ cup	19	1	0	4	35	0.16	7	0	0	0.4	0.05	0	14
Potato	1 medium	113	3	0	26	0	0.05	24	0.1	0	2.0	0.21	0	9
Citrus fruit	1 serving	44	1	0	10	12	0.04	44	0.1	0	0.3	0.03	0	3
Other fruit	1 serving	92	1	0	22	50	0.22	5	0	0	0.4	0.10	0	5
BREAD-CELL GROUP														
Cereal, enriched or whole grain	¾ cup	135	4	1	29	0	0.22	0	0.1	0	1.3	0.04	0	15
Bread, enriched or whole grain	3 slices	205	7	2	39	0	0.21	0	0.2	0.1	2.0	0.08	0	17
Fortified margarine	4 tsp	144	0	16	0	66	10.0	0	0	0	0	0	0	0
Totals		1300	75	62	161	716	12.0	105	1.9	1.5	14.6	1.42	4.5	102
RECOMMENDED DIETARY ALLOWANCES†														
Women (23–50 yr)		2000	44			800	12	60	1.0	1.2	13	2.0	3.0	400
Men (23–50 yr)		2700	56			1000	15	60	1.4	1.6	18	2.2	3.0	400

* Values represent the average nutrient content of a food group
† Taken from Recommended Dietary Allowances.
‡ Because there is less information on which to base an allowance, ranges of recommended intakes are given.

of a specific food component or nutrient, such as sodium, potassium, lactose, or oxalate. For this purpose, lists have been compiled of foods that are the richest sources of the relevant substances (Table 74-2). In addition, for use in diabetes mellitus, an exchange food-grouping system (Table 74-3) has been adapted for the basic four food groups. This system makes it easy to exchange one food for another within a food group and allows flexibility and variety in planning a diet.

To meet therapeutic goals, food groups or specific foods can be restricted or augmented. However, such a modification may lead to deficiency or excess of other nutrients present in high concentrations in those foods that were removed from, or added to, the diet.

DIET MODIFICATION Consistency The consistency of the diet can be altered from solid to pureed to liquid. *Soft* denotes a general diet altered by method of food preparation to allow easier chewing. Meats, for example, can be ground. *Pureed* signifies a nutritionally adequate, general diet that has been homogenized for edentulous patients or those who have difficulty swallowing solid foods. *Full liquid* diets contain only liquids or foods that liquefy at room temperature and are often used as a step in the reintroduction of foods to patients in whom oral intake has been withheld and in those recovering from oral or facial surgery. However, it is not suitable for prolonged use because it may contain large amounts of lactose and cholesterol and can be inadequate in iron, folic acid, and vitamin B_6. *Clear liquid* means liquids or frozen foods that are clear. Because there is no fiber residue, this diet is used to prepare the bowel for diagnostic workups or surgery and to serve as the initial step in progressing from nothing by mouth to solid foods. A clear liquid diet provides water, sodium, potassium, and small amounts of carbohy-

TABLE 74-2 Foods containing large amounts of certain nutrients*

SODIUM

Salt, catsup, mustard	Cheese, buttermilk
Soy sauce, steak-barbeque sauce	Salted nuts, peanut butter
Worcestershire sauce	Self-rising flour, biscuit mixes
Bouillon cubes	Salted crackers, chips, popcorn
Commercially prepared or cured meats, fish	Pickles, olives
	Commercial salad dressings
Canned foods (except fruit)	Instant cooked cereals

POTASSIUM

Milk	Vegetables: Artichoke, bamboo
Meat, fish, poultry	shoots, beet greens, chard, dried
Fruit: Apricots, avocado, banana,	beans, mushrooms, potato, spin-
cantaloupe, dates, honeydew,	ach, sweet potato, tomatoes, win-
orange, prunes, raisins	ter squash

OXALATE

Spinach	Almonds, cashew nuts
Rhubarb	Chocolate, cocoa
Dandelion greens	Tea

LACTOSE

Milk, milk products	Milk chocolate, chewing gum
Cheese	Some sugar substitutes
Commercial bread and dessert mixes	Foods with these ingredients: Milk, milk solids, dry milk, curd,
Commercial creamed and breaded meats	whey, whey solids, demineralized whey, lactose
Creamed and dehydrated soups	
Creamed, breaded, buttered vegetables	

* *Adapted from Handbook of Chemical Dietetics and Rudman et al.*

drate; therefore, it is usually used for short periods. When clear liquids are desired for a longer period of time, low-residue enteral feedings should be included in the diet. *Liquid formulas* are nutritionally complete and provide adequate nutrition on a prolonged basis either as a supplement to solid food or as complete nutritional support via enteral tube feeding.

Residue or fiber content The residue or fiber content of a diet can be supplemented or restricted. *Dietary fiber* refers to plant material that is not digested. *Residue* signifies the fecal solids, which are made up of undigested and unabsorbed food and metabolic and bacterial products. In the normal bowel, dietary fiber is the main source of fecal residue.

Low-fiber, low-residue diet contains foods with a minimum of fiber and connective tissue. It is used to limit fecal output and prevent the formation of an obstructing bolus in patients with a narrowed intestinal lumen or with an ileostomy. Patients in an acute phase of diverticulitis, ulcerative colitis, or infectious enterocolitis may also benefit from a low-fiber diet. Low-fiber, high-residue foods (milk, prune juice) may also need to be limited.

High fiber signifies a diet with increased amounts of fiber from fruits, vegetables, and grains. Fiber is a natural laxative. It is useful to (1) increase the volume of residue reaching the colon, (2) increase gastrointestinal motility, (3) decrease intraluminal colonic pressure,

Pantothenic acid, mg	Calcium, mg	Phosphorus, mg	Magnesium, mg	Iron, mg	Zinc, mg	Sodium, mg	Potassium, mg	Dietary fiber, g
1.6	698	547	62	0.5	1.9	298	854	0
0.8	24	90	6	1.1	0.5	54	57	0
0.8	14	274	33	3.1	5.4	88	430	0
0.1	34	22	13	0.6	0.3	12	127	2.0
0.1	19	22	13	0.5	0.2	30	105	1.4
0.3	11	79	14	0.8	0.3	5	614	3.5
0.2	19	17	11	0.3	0.1	1	174	0.4
0.2	10	16	13	0.6	0.2	2	176	1.5
0.2	13	75	21	1.1	0.5	303	73	3.8 / 6.4
0.4	68	126	38	1.9	0.8	414 / 200	143	0 / 19
0	4	12	0	0	0	1407	4	
4.7	914	1280	224	10.5	10.2		2758	
4–7‡	800	800	300	18	15	1100–	1875–	
4–7‡	800	800	350	10	15	3300‡	5625‡	

TABLE 74-3 Diabetic exchange list

	Serving size	Carbohydrate, g	Protein, g	Fat, g
Milk, skim	8 oz	12	8	0
Meat:	1 oz			
Lean		0	7	3
Medium fat		0	7	5
High fat		0	7	8
Bread-cereal	1 slice or ½ cup	15	2	0
Vegetables	½ cup	5	2	0
Fruit	Per list	10	0	0
Fat	1 tsp	0	0	5

and (4) reduce insulin requirements in some diabetics by delaying absorption of simple sugars. Patients with chronic diverticulitis or irritable bowel syndrome may benefit from a gradual increase in dietary fiber. Increasing fiber by a mixed diet is preferred to the exclusive use of bran, which interferes with the absorption of calcium, zinc, and iron. It has been suggested that people who habitually consume high-fiber diets may receive some protection from colorectal cancer because of more rapid fecal excretion or reduced production of carcinogens formed from bile acids by colonic bacteria.

Omission of foods Certain foods can be omitted because they irritate the patient or interfere with certain diagnostic tests.

Bland diet previously referred to the extensive use of milk and omission of roughage; highly seasoned foods, condiments, and spices; and caffeine. The rationale for avoiding chemical or mechanical irritation has not been supported by medical research. Therefore, the bland diet has been redefined to exclude only those items documented to cause (1) gastric irritation—red and black pepper, chili powder, caffeine, decaffeinated coffee, tea, cocoa, cold beverages, and alcohol; or (2) decreased lower esophageal sphincter pressue—tomatoes, citrus juices, chocolate, caffeine, decaffeinated coffee, peppermint, and excessively fatty foods. Individuals with gastric or duodenal ulcers or esophageal reflux may benefit from this diet and an eating pattern of frequent, small meals.

Elimination diets are useful in identifying food excitants that cause allergies. Milk, eggs, seafood, nuts, seeds, chocolate, oranges, and tomatoes, the most common excitants, are removed from the diet for a few weeks. If symptoms abate, foods are added back singly and at intervals until the offending foods are determined. Diets to control food allergies should be reviewed for nutritional adequacy.

A *serotonin- and 5-hydroxyindoleacetic acid-restricted diet* eliminates foods that lead to a false-positive diagnosis of malignant carcinoid tumors (see Chap. 299). Bananas, plantains, tomatoes, plums, avocados, pineapples, and walnuts should be omitted for 24 h prior to urine collection for such a workup.

Restriction or supplementation of foods PROTEIN MODIFICATION Protein-modified diets comprise low- and high-protein, altered-amino-acid, low-purine, tyramine-free, and gluten-free diets.

Low-protein diets reduce the intake from an average of 80 to 100 g to 0 to 60 g per day by reducing high-protein items such as meat, eggs, milk, and legumes. Symptoms of nitrogen accumulation (as in hepatic encephalopathy, renal insufficiency, and genetic defects in urea synthesis) respond favorably to such restriction. Selection of proteins with high biologic value minimizes the negative nitrogen balance, but prolonged use of a severely restricted diet can lead to protein malnutrition and other nutrient deficiencies.

The original purpose of treating uremic patients with low-protein diets was to minimize azotemia and metabolic acidosis. It was then reported that, in patients so treated, the loss of residual renal function was slower than in their counterparts eating ad lib. Brenner proposed that chronic consumption of excess dietary protein causes sustained increases in renal blood flow and glomerular filtration rate, with resulting intrarenal hypertension and progressive glomerular sclerosis. Clinical trials are now underway testing the theory that reduction of protein intake to the minimum compatible with nitrogen balance will retard the progress of chronic renal disease.

Patients with chronic hepatic or renal disease or with an inborn error of nitrogen metabolism, who are treated with low-protein diets, must be monitored for manifestations of protein deficiency as described in Chap. 72. Compliance with these diets can be determined from the 24-h urine urea content.

High-protein diets, 100 to 120 g, may be prescribed for emaciated or hypermetabolic patients. Generally, high-protein diets also have increased amounts of other nutrients and a higher energy content. When energy intake is adequate, the nitrogen balance in healthy individuals is not enhanced by increasing protein intake above the recommended dietary allowance (RDA). There are, however, two common situations in which a high protein to calorie ratio improves

nitrogen balance: the "stressed" patient (infection, trauma, inflammation, or fever) and the protein-starved patient. In addition, high-protein diets also stimulate ventilatory drive, an effect which can be used to expedite weaning of ventilator-dependent patients.

Altered-amino-acid diets are sometimes useful in the treatment of nitrogen accumulation disorders. Synthetic mixtures of amino acids reduce the accumulation of excess plasma amino acids and tend to return the plasma amino acid profile toward normal, sometimes with clinical improvement. However, protein adequacy must be monitored periodically. Examples of such diets include essential-amino-acid mixtures in uremia, altered ratios of branched-chain to aromatic amino acids in hepatic encephalopathy and the catabolic response to injury, and various altered-amino-acid mixtures in genetic errors of nitrogen metabolism.

Low-purine diets contain reduced amounts of uric acid precursors, as an adjunct in the treatment of gout and uric acid calculi. Sweetbreads, anchovies, sardines, shrimp, mackerel, liver, kidney, meat extracts, and dried legumes are excluded from the diet.

A *tyramine-, dopamine-free diet* eliminates foods containing tyramine or dopamine and fermented or aged foods containing bacteria capable of forming amines. Aged cheese and meats, yeast-containing products, alcoholic beverages, and bananas are omitted. This diet prevents amine-mediated hypertensive crises in patients taking monoamine oxidase inhibitors and is useful in preventing false elevations of urinary catecholamine excretion in the workup of suspected pheochromocytomas.

A *gluten-free diet* eliminates wheat, rye, oat, barley, and their derivatives which contain glutens. This diet provides symptomatic control of gluten-induced enteropathy.

CARBOHYDRATE MODIFICATION   Carbohydrate-modified diets restrict total carbohydrates, disaccharides, or monosaccharides.

Low total carbohydrate diets reduce carbohydrates from the customary 50 percent to 20 to 30 percent of total calories. A carbohydrate intake of less than 70 g per day is ketogenic and is helpful in certain forms of childhood epilepsy. Postgastrectomy "dumping" may also be responsive to a diet that limits the intake of osmotically active substances. Therefore, a diet containing 140 g or less of carbohydrate with restricted mono- and disaccharides and administered in small, frequent feedings is recommended.

High carbohydrate diets increase CO_2 production, an effect which can cause respiratory distress or failure in patients with compromised pulmonary function, or impede weaning from the ventilator. A diet high in fat and low in calories is used to decrease CO_2 production.

Lactose- or sucrose-restricted diets reduce the lactose content of the diet from 25 to 30 g to 0 to 10 g per day, depending on the severity of the lactose deficiency (Table 74-2); sucrose is reduced to 5 to 15 g per day in subjects with a sucrase-isomaltase deficiency. Lactose restriction requires the omission of milk and dairy products, the primary sources of calcium in the diet, and therefore calcium supplements should be given when the diet is needed on a long-term basis.

A *galactose-free diet* eliminates all sources of galactose (and thereby lactose) for the treatment of individuals with galactosemia (see Chap. 314).

The *300-g carbohydrate diet* has been advocated by some for 3 days prior to a glucose tolerance test. However, a balanced diet providing at least 150 g of carbohydrate results in a valid test. Individuals on hypocaloric or low-carbohydrate diets should receive a balanced or high-carbohydrate diet for 3 days before the test.

FAT MODIFICATION   Fat-modified diets may be restricted in total fat (largely triglycerides), in cholesterol, or both, and may be supplemented with medium-chain triglycerides. These diets are used to treat various types of hyperlipemia (see Chap. 315) or malabsorption.

A typical *low-fat, low-cholesterol diet* for hyperlipemic states furnishes 30 to 35 percent of calories as fat, the composition of which is altered to provide more polyunsaturated and less saturated fat and less than 300 mg cholesterol per day. Some types of hyperlipemia also require restrictions of carbohydrate and calories. Increasing the polyunsaturated/saturated fatty acid ratio requires decreasing the intake of beef, pork, lamb, cheese, and egg yolks and increasing the use of chicken, turkey, veal, and fish. Skim milk is used rather than whole milk, and margarines made with polyunsaturated vegetable oils are substituted for butter. Reducing cholesterol to 300 mg per day or less involves restricting egg yolks to three per week as well as limiting fat from animal sources. Such a change in eating habits requires long-term reinforcement.

For the patient with fat malabsorption, severe chylomicronemia, or chylous ascites, long-chain triglycerides should be restricted to 20 to 50 g per day (10 to 25 percent of total calories). When fat intake is severely restricted, medium-chain triglycerides, which are absorbed independently of long-chain fatty acids, should be added to provide sufficient energy. To document fat malabsorption, a diet containing 100 g fat is eaten during a 3-day stool collection. Actual fat intake must be estimated to determine the extent of malabsorption.

ENERGY MODIFICATION   Energy-modified diets are designed for weight reduction, weight gain, or weight maintenance. Conditions that benefit from energy-modified diets include obesity, hypertension, diabetes mellitus, hyperlipemia, cachexia, and hypermetabolic states due to trauma, infection, and burns.

Low-kilocalorie diets usually furnish 800 to 1200 kcal for women and 1000 to 1500 kcal for men. Although a weight-reduction diet is designed to include selections from the four food groups, it may be inadequate to meet all of the recommended daily allowances if the caloric content is severely restricted; therefore, vitamin and mineral supplements may be needed.

High-kilocalorie diets (2800 to 4000 kcal per day) usually are designed to provide the estimated basal energy expenditure of the individual plus an additional 100 to 200 percent for repletion or hypermetabolism. If the patient is not able to consume the required caloric intake as solid food, liquid supplements can be used between meals.

Appropriate *diabetic diets* are fundamental to the treatment of diabetes mellitus with the major goals being restrictions of the intake of sucrose and free glucose and achievement of ideal body weight (see Chaps. 317 and 327). Energy requirements are based on the basal energy expenditure (see Chap. 70) plus an additional allowance of 25, 50, or 75 percent for sedentary, moderate, or strenuous activity levels, respectively. The recommended distribution of caloric intake is 50 to 60 percent from carbohydrate, 12 to 20 percent from protein, and 30 to 35 percent from fat. Three meals per day are usually planned for the obese, non-insulin-dependent diabetic. The type of insulin prescribed and the timing of insulin administration determine the meal patterns in the insulin-dependent diabetic. Usually, each of three meals and an evening snack provide three-tenths and one-tenth, respectively, of the allowed carbohydrate and caloric content. Patients receiving intermediate acting insulins such as NPH insulin may require a midafternoon snack to avoid hypoglycemia during the peak activity of the insulin.

ELECTROLYTE AND MINERAL MODIFICATION   Electrolyte-mineral–modified diets consist of low-sodium, low- or high-potassium, low- or high-calcium, and low-phosphorus intakes.

Low-sodium diets reduce sodium consumption from an average daily intake of 4 g (176 meq, 10 g NaCl) to 0.5 to 2 g (22 to 88 meq, 1.3 to 5 g NaCl). Patient compliance is often poor if daily intake is restricted to less than 2 g sodium. The 2-g sodium diet eliminates the foods listed in Table 74-2 and controls the use of milk, salted breads and cereals, and salted margarines but does not require the use of salt-free milk, breads, and margarines, which are expensive and have a low palatability. Patients with persistent edema or ascites may require restriction of sodium of 1 g or even 0.5 g a day.

Low-potassium diets reduce intake from an average of 6 g (153 meq) to 2 g (51 meq) for the patient with hyperkalemia. *High-potassium diets* provide an intake greater than 5.8 g (150 meq) and may be indicated when potassium-wasting diuretics are used (Table

74-2). *Low-calcium diets* reduce the calcium intake from an average of 800 mg to 200 to 400 mg and are used to treat hypercalcemia and some types of nephrolithiasis. The long-term consequences of a low-calcium diet on bone are unknown. A *high-calcium diet* indicates a 1000-mg calcium diet, which is used in the evaluation of hypercalciuria, and a 1500-mg calcium diet for women with postmenopausal osteoporosis. A *low-phosphorus diet,* 700 to 800 mg per day, is used to prevent hyperphosphatemia and secondary enhancement of parathyroid hormone secretion in renal disease. A *low-oxalate diet* is designed to eliminate exogenous sources of chronic oxalate and is useful in hyperoxaluria and in calcium oxalate nephrolithiasis.

Alteration of the feeding route   The route of delivery can be changed from oral to enteral tube feeding. Technological improvements in nasoenteral tubes, formulas, and infusion pumps have improved the efficacy and safety of tube feedings. The enteral route has three advantages over intravenous feeding. (1) It maintains the integrity of the intestinal mucosa, and nutrients are handled in a more physiologic manner, (2) it causes fewer metabolic and technical complications, and (3) it can be less expensive than intravenous alimentation. Consequently, clinicians should consider enteral tube feeding before resorting to parenteral nutrition (see Chap. 75).

PATIENT SELECTION   Oral intake can be inadequate because of anorexia or mechanical obstruction, increased nutrient losses, or hypermetabolism. Wasting disorders in which enteral feedings may be useful include cerebral vascular accidents, head and neck cancer, anorexia nervosa, trauma, and burns. Contraindications to tube feeding include intractable vomiting, upper gastrointestinal bleeding, and intestinal obstruction. Steatorrhea is a handicap but may be surmounted by the use of chemically defined "elemental" formulas or with antidiarrheal drugs.

TUBE PLACEMENT   Several enteral tube placements are used: nasogastric, nasoduodenal, nasojejunal, gastrostomy, jejunostomy, or placement of a gastrostomy feeding tube by percutaneous endoscopy. Because the latter three require surgery or endoscopy, the nasogastric or nasoduodenal route is most frequently chosen. Small-bore Silastic or polyurethane tubing minimizes the complications of nasopharyngitis, rhinitis, otitis media, parotitis, and subsequent stricture. Insertion and maintenance of proper placement are facilitated by a removable wire stylet and a mercury-weight tip. A properly irrigated tube may remain in place for months.

Patients who require permanent tube feedings benefit from gastrostomy: the cosmetic problems of the nasogastric tube are avoided, and there is no need to rely on expensive formulas since the large-bore tube allows the use of blended foods.

Jejunal feedings may be desirable when an obstruction or fistula is proximal to the jejunum. An advantage of the jejunostomy is the reduced risk of aspiration from gastric reflux.

SELECTION OF INFUSION METHOD   One of the early disadvantages of enteral tube feedings was the lack of control of the infusion rate, and as a consequence patients sensitive to large volumes or hyperosmolar solutions often developed osmotic diarrhea and cramping. Enteral infusion pumps are now available to ensure a constant drip rate. When large volumes (3000 mL) of a hyperosmolar solution (>500 mosmol per liter) are necessary for repletion, either of two approaches can be tried. A full-strength formula can be begun at 50 mL/h for 24 h, and the rate of infusion daily can be increased as tolerated until the desired volume is achieved. Alternately, the formula can be made isotonic by dilution and infused from the start at a rate of 125 mL/h for 24 h; the concentration of the formula can then be gradually increased each day until full strength is reached. Infusion periods of less than 24 h may be preferable when aspiration is a potential problem.

FORMULA SELECTION   Over 80 enteral formulas are available in the United States alone to meet nutritional requirements. Choosing from this array is made easier by the knowledge that the products fall into four categories: elemental (''monomeric''), polymeric, modular, and altered amino acids.

Elemental formulas are composed of di- and tripeptides and/or crystalline amino acids, glucose oligosaccharides, and vegetable oil or medium-chain triglycerides. Residue is minimal, and little digestive action is required. An elemental formula may be of use in patients with the short-bowel syndrome, partial bowel obstruction, pancreatic insufficiency, inflammatory bowel disease, radiation enteritis, or bowel fistulas.

Polymeric formulas are composed of complex nutrients, e.g., protein as casein, lactalbumin, or soy protein; carbohydrate as corn syrup solids or maltodextrins; and fat as vegetable oils or milk fat. There is heterogeneity with regard to lactose content, sodium content, caloric density, content of medium-chain triglycerides, and palatability. Most patients with a functional gastrointestinal tract and few specialized nutrient requirements can utilize a formula from the polymeric group. Unless malabsorption is present, polymeric products are preferable to monomeric ones because the hyperosmolarity of the latter may cause gastrointestinal reactions.

Single nutrient modules, available for protein, carbohydrate, and fat, can be combined or added to a monomeric or polymeric formula to create a formula that meets specialized nutrient requirements. The simplest modular formula involves adding a carbohydrate source to a formula to increase caloric value. For example, a cachectic cirrhotic patient with ascites and encephalopathy may benefit from a high-caloric, low-protein, low-sodium formula.

Altered-amino-acid formulas are indicated in patients with genetic errors of nitrogen metabolism: phenylketonuria, maple syrup urine disease, homocystinuria, tyrosinemia, methylmalonic acidemia, and propionic acidemia. In the acquired disorders of nitrogen accumulation (chronic renal failure and cirrhosis), synthetic formulas are designed to either limit or increase the intake of certain amino acids and thereby provide symptomatic improvement. Patients who are catabolic because of injury or infection may show improved nitrogen balance when the branched-chain amino acid content of their nutritional formula is increased.

PATIENT MONITORING   Successful enteral tube feeding requires continual, careful monitoring for possible mechanical, gastrointestinal, fluid, and electrolyte complications. Common examples are as follows. Mechanical: clogging of tube by formula, pulmonary aspiration, esophageal erosion, tube dislodgement; gastrointestinal: vomiting, diarrhea; metabolic: hyperglycemia, hyperosmolar coma, edema, hypernatremia, hypercalcemia; cardiovascular: congestive heart failure.

The guidelines given in Chap. 71 for nutritional assessment should be used to evaluate the effectiveness of the nutrition support.

INDICATIONS FOR DIET THERAPY   The majority of diseases would probably be benefited by a dietary modification, either in terms of prevention or palliation. Consequently, the clinical indications for dietary modification are too numerous to be listed here. Some examples are given in Table 74-4. For a comprehensive treatment of this subject, see texts on clinical dietetics.

DRUG-NUTRIENT INTERACTIONS   Certain foods or meal patterns can alter drug effectiveness, and certain drugs can alter nutrient requirements. Many drugs influence appetite and food intake. Examples of hypophagic drugs are chemotherapeutic agents, narcotics, digitalis, amphetamines, and phenylbiguanides. Some hyperphagic drugs are tranquilizers, insulin, glucocorticoids, metoclopramide, and antihistamines.

The absorption of a drug is generally slower when it is taken with food, an effect that may be important when rapid onset of drug action is desired. Complete inhibition of drug absorption occurs when calcium-containing foods or iron salts chelate tetracycline, making it insoluble. Enhanced drug absorption results when lipid-soluble drugs are given with fat-containing meals or when alcohol is taken with a timed-release medicine that is alcohol-soluble. Gastric irritation by a drug is lessened if it is taken with meals. The optimal timing of each

drug with regard to meals should be specified when it is prescribed; pharmacology texts can be consulted for details.

Drugs frequently alter either the gastrointestinal absorption, the utilization, or the urinary excretion of nutrients, with a resulting increase of nutrient requirements. For example, anticonvulsants cause a deficiency of 1,25-dihydroxycholecalciferol, aluminum hydroxide prevents absorption of dietary phosphate and iron, and glucocorticoids reduce absorption of calcium; broad-spectrum antibiotics suppress synthesis of vitamins by the intestinal flora and can cause a deficiency of vitamin K or biotin; isoniazide impairs the utilization of vitamin B_6; and oral contraceptives interfere with the utilization of folic acid; thiazides, furosemide, and penicillamine cause urinary hyperexcretion of potassium, magnesium, zinc, or copper, or several of these. This subject is treated comprehensively in Roe's monograph. In brief, the patient treated with one or more drugs for extended periods is often a risk for a nutritional deficiency. Conversely, the desired action of a drug can be blocked by a nutrient, such as pyridoxine versus levodopa, or vitamin K versus warfarin.

THE PRINCIPLES OF DIET PRESCRIPTION   Several considerations are involved in formulating effective diet therapy. The *dietary modifications* appropriate for a given clinical situation must be selected (change in food consistency, removal of specific foods, reduction or increase of specific nutrients, or change in route of nutrient delivery). The appropriate *degree of restriction* or supplementation should be determined, recognizing that the extreme ranges of dietary modifications may cause noncompliance. Does a cardiac patient need a 2- or 0.5-g sodium diet; does a dysphagic patient require a soft or pureed diet; does a patient with wasting febrile illness require a 2000 − or 3000-kcal diet? When more than one dietary modification is appropriate, a decision must be made as to which is the most important. Some combinations are virtually incompatible, such as a low-kilocalorie, high potassium diet; a high-calcium, lactose-free diet; or a high-protein, low-fat diet. The *duration* of the diet prescription must be estimated. Diets with severely limited nutrients should be used for as short a time as possible.

By using the type of information shown in Tables 74-1 to 74-3 and in the American Dietetic Association's *Handbook of Clinical Dietetics,* the dietitian implements the prescribed diet and reports how closely the implemented diet conforms to the desired modifications and whether undesired dietary imbalances may have been created by the prescription. Severely altered diets may be deficient or augmented in nutrients not considered in the original diet prescription; for example, a lactose-free diet is also low in calcium and riboflavin. Therefore, further manipulations may be necessary to prevent secondary deficiencies or excesses inherent in the original diet order. Three examples of prescribed diets and their implementations are given below.

Example 1

I Diagnosis: Obesity and hypertension.
II Physician's order: 1200 kcal, 2 g Na, high-potassium diet.
III Dietitian's response: High potassium (>5.8 g, 150 meq) is difficult to achieve when a kilocalorie restriction is ordered. Potassium supplements may be necessary.

	Energy, kcal*	Na, mg*	K, mg*
2 cups milk, skim	180	240	710
6 oz meat, lean	330	150	780
4 servings bread	280	800	180
4 servings vegetables	100	40	1440
3 servings fruit	120	0	1140
4 servings margarine, oil	180	200	40
	1190	1430 (62 meq)	4290 (110 meq)

* *Values represent the average nutrient content of a food group.*

Nutritional analysis: No deficiencies or excesses of essential nutrients.

TABLE 74-4 Examples of clinical disorders that benefit from appropriate diet therapy

Clinical disorder	Recommended diet therapy	Comments	Clinical disorder	Recommended diet therapy	Comments
GASTROINTESTINAL DISORDERS			**PULMONARY DISORDERS**		
Dysphagia	Pureed, liquid supplements		Sarcoidosis	Low-calcium	If patient is hypercalcemic
Reflux esophagitis	Bland, frequent small meals		**ENDOCRINE-METABOLIC DISORDERS**		
Gastric ulcers	Frequent small meals		Diabetes mellitus	Kilocalorie-carbohydrate, fat-controlled	Achieve and maintain ideal body weight
Posgastrectomy dumping	Low-carbohydrate, frequent small meals		Reactive hypoglycemia	High-protein, low-carbohydrate, frequent small meals	
Fat malabsorption	Low-fat—MCT supplemented	Mg and vitamin A, D, E, and K supplements	Obesity	Low-kilocalorie	
			Osteoporosis	High-calcium	Vitamin D supplement
Celiac disease	Gluten-free				
Lactose intolerance	Lactose-free	Ca supplement	Gout, uric acid stones	Low-purine	
HEPATIC DISORDERS			Nephrogenic diabetes insipidus	Low-sodium, protein-controlled	
Alcoholic liver disease:			Hypoparathyroidism	High-calcium	1,25-$(OH)_2D_3$ supplement
Alcoholic hepatitis	High-kilocalorie, high-protein	Multivitamin and folate supplements	Hyperparathyroidism	Low-calcium	
Cirrhosis	High-kilocalorie, high-protein	Multivitamin and folate supplements	Steroid therapy	Low-sodium, high-protein	
Encephalopathy	Low-protein, low-ammonia		**GENETIC DISORDERS**		
Ascites	Low-sodium, high-kilocalorie, high-protein		Galactosemia	Galactose-free	
			Sucrose-maltose deficiency	Low-sucrose	
RENAL DISORDERS			Phenylketonuria	Low-phenylalanine, tyrosine supplemented	
Acute, chronic renal failure	Protein, phosphorus, sodium, potassium reduced	1,25-$(OH)_2D_3$, Ca supplements	Maple syrup urine disease	Low-leucine, -isoleucine, -valine	Thiamine, when responsive
Nephrotic syndrome	Low-sodium		Homocystinuria	Low-methionine, cystine	Pyridoxine, when responsive
Renal osteodystrophy	Low-phosphorus	1,25-$(OH)_2D_3$, Ca supplements	Adrenogenital syndrome	High-sodium	
Potassium wasting	High-potassium		Propionic acidemia	Low-protein	Biotin, when responsive
Hypercalciuric nephrolithiasis	Low-calcium, oxalate-free		Methylmalonic acidemia	Low-protein	Vitamin B_{12}, when responsive
CARDIOVASCULAR DISORDERS			Hypophosphatemic rickets		P, 1,25-$(OH)_2D_3$ supplements
Hyperlipemia:			Urea cycle disorders	Low-protein	
Type I	Low-fat	No alcohol			
Type IIa	Low-cholesterol, low-saturated-fat, increased-polyunsaturated-fat				
Type IIb, III	Carbohydrate-controlled, low-cholesterol, low-saturated-fat	Achieve and maintain ideal body weight			
Type IV	Carbohydrate-controlled, low-cholesterol, low-saturated fat	Achieve and maintain ideal body weight			
Type V	Low-fat, low-cholesterol	No alcohol, achieve and maintain ideal body weight			
Hypertension	Low-sodium	Achieve and maintain ideal body weight			
Congestive heart failure	Low-sodium				

NOTE: *Note: 1,25(OH)_2D_3 = 1,25-dihydroxycholecalciferol.*

Example 2

I Diagnosis
  A Cirrhosis of the liver
    1 Encephalopathy
    2 Ascites
  B Chronic pancreatitis
  C Malnutrition

II Physician's order: 40 g protein, low ammonia, 1 g Na, low-fat diet with increased calories.

III Dietitian's response: Increased caloric intake (>2500 kcal) is difficult to achieve when protein and long-chain fatty acids can contribute only 610 kcal. Medium-chain triglycerides (MCT) and foods containing largely sucrose will be needed to increase kilocalories.

	Protein, g*	Na, mg*	Fat, g*	Energy, kcal*
½ cup milk, whole	4	60	4	75
3 oz meat or eggs	21	75	15	220
4 servings bread or cereal	8	800	0	280
4 servings vegetables	8	40	0	100
10 servings fruit	0	0	0	400
5 servings low-protein desserts	0	0	10	460
4 servings salt-free margarine	0	0	20	180
18 servings MCT mayonnaise	0	0	90	810
	41	975 (42 meq)	139	2525

* *Values represent the average nutrient content of a food group.*

Nutritional analysis: This diet is deficient in calcium, thiamine, riboflavin, and niacin and needs to be supplemented.

Example 3

I Diagnosis: Same patient as in Example 2, with a fourth problem, anorexia.

II Physician's order: 40 g protein, 1 g Na, low fat, enteral tube feeding.

III Dietitian's response: Modular formula.

	Protein, g	Na, mg	Fat, g	Energy, kcal
750 mL Isocal	25	390	33	790
18 g Casec	15	27	0	60
360 mL Polycose	0	220	0	720
105 mL MCT oil	0	0	105	945
250 mL water				
1500 mL	40	637	138	2515

Nutritional analysis: This diet needs to be supplemented with vitamins A, D, and B$_6$, and folic acid, iodine, iron, and zinc.

ASSESSMENT OF DIETARY COMPLIANCE Assessment of compliance and evaluation of effectiveness are the final steps in successful diet therapy. When a ''calorie count'' is ordered for a hospitalized patient, the dietitian can estimate the daily intake of protein, carbohydrate, fat, and kilocalories. Some nutrients can be monitored by blood or urine analysis; for example, compliance with a low-sodium diet can be determined by urinary sodium analysis. An outpatient food intake diary is useful in assessing the home compliance. Improvements in symptoms and signs of the disorder also serve as indicators of effective dietary modification.

REFERENCES

AMERICAN DIETETICS ASSOCIATION: *Handbook of Clinical Dietetics*. New Haven, Yale, 1981

BRENNER BM et al: Dietary intake and the progressive nature of kidney disease. N Engl J Med 307:652, 1982

CRAPO PA: Simple versus complex carbohydrate: Use in the diabetic diet. Ann Rev Nutr 5:95, 1985

GOODHART RS, SHILS ME (eds): *Modern Nutrition in Health and Disease*, 6th ed. Philadelphia, Lea & Febiger, 1980

HATHCOCK JG: Metabolic mechanisms of drug-nutrient interactions. Fed Proc 44:124, 1985

KRAUSE MV, MOHER KL: *Food, Nutrition and Diet Therapy: Textbook of Nutritional Care*, 7th ed. Philadelphia, Saunders, 1984

KROMHOUT D et al: The inverse relation between fish consumption and 20-year mortality from coronary heart disease. N Engl J Med 312:1205, 1985

MIZOCK BA: Branched-chain amino acids in sepsis and hepatic failure. Arch Intern Med, 145:1284, 1985

RANDALL HT: Enteral nutrition: Tube feeding in acute and chronic illness. J Parenter Nutr 8:113, 1984

ROBINSON CH, LAWLES MR: *Normal and Therapeutic Nutrition*, 16th ed. New York, Milwaukee Publishing Co, 1982

ROE DA: Nutrient and drug interactions. Nutr Rev 42:141, 1984

SCHNEIDER HA et al: *Nutritional Support of Medical Practice*. Hagerstown, MD, Harper & Row, 1983

WALSER M: Therapeutic aspects of branched-chain amino and keto acids. Clin Sci 66:1, 1984

75 PARENTERAL NUTRITION

KHURSHEED N. JEEJEEBHOY / JEFFREY P. BAKER

Nutritional support is indicated when a normal oral diet cannot be ingested, absorbed, or tolerated for a significant period of time. When possible the route of support should be enteral (see Chap. 74). However, in patients who cannot eat, do not absorb an oral diet efficiently, or deteriorate on oral feeding, partial or complete nourishment by the parenteral route is indicated until they can be fed and can absorb nutrients orally.

INDICATIONS FOR TOTAL PARENTERAL NUTRITION Total parenteral nutrition (TPN) is indicated in the following situations:

1 In patients who are unable to eat or absorb normally. The rate of development of malnutrition is based on a number of factors, including previous dietary history and the coexisting illness. The diagnosis of malnutrition is based upon evidence of muscle wasting, hypoalbuminemia, edema, reduced skin fold thickness, and reduced body weight (see Chap. 71). Weight loss alone is not sufficient evidence of malnutrition because edema or previous obesity may mask the degree of nitrogen depletion actually present.

2 In well-nourished who are temporarily unable to eat. An estimate has to be made as to the length of time that oral nutrition will not be available. If the period is likely to exceed 7 to 10 days, then total parenteral nutrition should be administered to avoid undue wasting and malnutrition. This is especially important if sepsis or trauma complicate the clinical picture by accelerating catabolism and tissue wasting.

3 In patients with Crohn's disease, intestinal fistulas, and pancreatitis. In such patients food ingestion may exacerbate symptoms and high caloric wastage through fistulas, thus preventing healing. When such patients are given nothing by mouth and receive TPN, they may improve by healing fistulas and reducing the size of inflammatory masses while maintaining good nutritional status.

4 In subjects with prolonged coma when tube feeding is not possible.

5 For nutritional support in patients with marked hypercatabolism or protein loss, as in those with severe trauma and burns, even if some oral intake is possible.

6 For nutritional support during therapy for malignant disease, especially when malnutrition has been caused by diminished food intake rather than by uncontrolled tumor growth. Chemotherapy and complications of radiation therapy are particularly prone to cause anorexia and mucosal inflammation that may limit oral intake. TPN given prior to and with chemotherapy results in an improved nutritional status in these patients.

7 Occasionally, in malnourished patients, as in patients likely to undergo surgery.

NUTRIENT REQUIREMENTS DURING TPN Energy and fluid requirements The Harris-Benedict equation is an excellent guide to total energy requirements.

For men:

$$\text{Energy (kcal/24h)} = 66.473 + 13.7516 \times \text{wt(kg)} + 5.0033 \times \text{ht(cm)} - 6.7550 \times \text{age (years)}$$

For women:

$$\text{Energy (kcal/24h)} = 655.0955 + 9.5634 \times \text{wt(kg)} + 1.8496 \times \text{ht(cm)} - 4.6756 \times \text{age (years)}$$

In general, the needs for weight maintenance in afebrile patients are those predicted by these equations. For weight increase, an additional 30 percent of calories is required. Similarly, in septic patients basal energy needs should be increased by 30 percent. As a general rule, 32 kcal/kg per day is sufficient for weight maintenance, and 40 kcal/kg per day is adequate for maintenance in septic patients or for weight gain. In burn patients, when the area of burn exceeds 40 percent of the surface area, caloric requirements may increase by as much as 100 percent.

Basal fluid infusion should be about 1 to 1.2 mL/kcal. To this should be added a volume equivalent to losses from diarrhea, stomal output, nasogastric suction, and fistula drainage. In oliguric patients a basal intake of 750 to 1000 mL should be given, plus a volume equal to that of urine and other losses. In patients with cardiac failure, about 40 mL/kg can be infused provided that the sodium intake is restricted to between 20 and 40 meq per day.

Amino acid requirements The efficient functioning of the body requires maintenance of the integrity of the musculoskeletal system and viscera, together with normal levels of enzymes, hormones, and plasma proteins. All are dependent on new protein synthesis to meet the demands of normal turnover; protein synthesis in turn requires that amino acids be available. A major objective of parenteral nutrition is to provide an adequate supply of amino acids for protein synthesis. Although the amount required is influenced by several factors, nitrogen balance and protein synthesis (including albumin formation) are proportional to the amount of amino acid infused within the range of zero to 2 g amino acids per kilogram of body weight per day. In addition, as mentioned above, severe injury, sepsis, and burns increase nitrogen losses, making it necessary to infuse larger amounts of amino acids. The pattern of amino acids infused is important, since unbalanced mixtures do not support protein synthesis. Enrichment of amino acid mixtures with branched chain amino acids and/or branched chain keto acids may aid protein synthesis in septic patients. Requirements are larger if amino acids are the sole energy source than if some caloric demands are met by fat or carbohydrate.

In ordinary starvation the infusion of 100 g of glucose per day reduces urinary nitrogen loss but does not produce positive nitrogen balance. Infusion of amino acids alone also reduces net nitrogen deficits, and in large amounts (~2 g per kilogram of body weight per day) it can induce a slight positive nitrogen balance. However, amino acids are more efficiently utilized when they are infused along with nonprotein energy sufficient to meet calorie requirements. Positive nitrogen balance is achieved in most malnourished patients (who are not suffering abnormal losses) by infusing 0.5 to 1.0 g of amino acids per kilogram of ideal body weight per day, together with optimal nonprotein calories. Unusual losses, as in protein-rich exudates from burns or in upper gastrointestinal tract contents rich in pancreatic secretions, increase requirements to between 1.5 and 2.0 g/kg per day. As the input of nonprotein energy is increased, nitrogen retention is augmented at all levels of amino acid intake. The protein-sparing effect of carbohydrate and fat is most obvious as intake increases from none to an amount approximating the metabolic rate but is also observed to a lesser degree until the intake approximates 55 to 60 kcal per kilogram of ideal body weight. Beyond this point, additional calories in adults do not significantly improve nitrogen retention.

Relation of nitrogen retention to the source of nonprotein energy

Both carbohydrates and lipids can be infused with amino acids to provide sufficient nonprotein energy to meet the metabolic requirements. The two types of substrates are equal in efficacy in malnourished and septic patients after an initial 3- to 4-day period for adaptation to the source of the energy. Hence the source of nonprotein energy chosen depends on factors other than its effect on nitrogen retention.

The first factor of importance in choosing the source of nonprotein energy is osmotic pressure. Concentrated glucose solutions are hyperosmolar and cause thrombosis when administered by peripheral vein. TPN regimens using glucose as the primary energy source thus require placement of a catheter in the superior vena cava where rapid blood flow quickly dilutes the hypertonic infusion. A second factor is the metabolic state of the patient. Glucose requires insulin for utilization, and hypertonic glucose solutions are not ideal for diabetic subjects. In such individuals, lipid infusions avoid or diminish the need for additional insulin and for frequent monitoring of blood glucose. Conversely, triglyceride emulsions may be contraindicated in hyperlipiproteinemic states. A third consideration is that infusing glucose as the sole source of calories causes an increase in the metabolic rate and carbon dioxide production and thus may accentuate ventilatory demands. In such patients, giving half the nonprotein calories as fat reduces carbon dioxide excretion.

Glucose infusion mixtures consist of 25 percent dextrose, 2 percent amino acids, vitamins, and minerals. Lipid emulsions are mixtures of triglyceride, phospholipid (as an emulsifying agent), and glycerol (added to maintain isotonicity). Lipid can be infused concurrently with amino acid–dextrose mixtures using a Y connector and can provide 50 to 80 percent of nonprotein calories. Combinations of these nutrients are sometimes supplied in a single bag and are stable under refrigeration for up to 4 days. These concentrations can be given by peripheral vein without fear of thrombosis. Insulin is not required for metabolism of the fat; indeed, plasma insulin levels are low and free fatty acids and ketones are high when lipid is the major source of nonprotein calories. Lipid infusions can also be discontinued abruptly without danger of hypoglycemia because insulin levels are not elevated. This aspect is important in critically ill patients who may require repeated and unpredictable alterations in therapy, especially when surgery may be performed on short notice. Finally, lipid infusions meet essential fatty acid requirements; linoleic acid is present in sufficient quantities if as little as 500 mL of commercially available triglyceride emulsion (Intralipid) is given daily. While essential fatty acid deficiency is ordinarily rare in adults, lipid deficiency may develop in as little as 1 week with TPN and cause abnormal liver function and skin rash.

It is also possible to administer TPN with a ratio of 1:1 (calorie:calorie) of glucose and lipid calories. Substrate and hormone profiles in the blood following infusion of such a mixture are similar to those in the postprandial state.

Recommendations regarding source (type) of nonprotein energy

Lipid-free systems are required only in patients with hyperchylomicronemia. Other patients should receive lipid as a part of the regimen for total parenteral nutrition. The 80 percent lipid system can be given by peripheral vein, minimizing the threat of catheter sepsis and other catheter-related complications. However, the authors recommend a 1:1 (calorie:calorie) lipid-glucose solution, given through a central venous line. This regimen simulates the normal diet and causes neither hyperinsulinemia nor hyperglycemia, thus almost eliminating the need for exogenous insulin.

TABLE 75-1 Vitamin input and blood or plasma vitamin levels in six patients on long-term TPN

Vitamin	Input* provided by: MVI, per 5 mL	Soluzyme + vitamin C, per 10 mL	Consequent average daily input	Daily (oral) recommended requirement	Plasma/blood vitamin level Average level observed in six patients	Normal range
A	5000 IU		2500 IU	5000 IU	41.6	25–70 μg/dL
D	500 IU		250 IU	400 IU	34.4	28–42 ng/mL
E	5 mg		27.5 mg†	30 mg	0.65	0.8–1.2 ng/dL
B₁	22 mg	10 mg	16.0 mg	1.5 mg	226	10–64 ng/mL
B₂	5 mg	10 mg	7.5 mg	2.0 mg		
Niacinamide	50 mg	250 mg	150 mg	20.0 mg	16	3–6 μg/mL
Pantothenate	12 mg	45 mg	28 mg	10.0 mg	689	150–400 ng/mL
Pyridoxine	6 mg	5 mg	5.5 mg	2.5 mg	40	30–80 ng/mL
Ascorbic acid	500 mg	500 mg	500 mg	75 mg	2.0	0.4–1 mg/dL
Folic acid		5 mg	2.5 mg	0.15 mg	48	4–20 ng/mL
B₁₂		25 μg	12.5 μg	1.0 μg	872	100–900 pg/mL
Biotin				300 μg	63	200–500 pg/mL

* *Given on alternate days.*
† *Of the average of 27.5 mg vitamin E per day 25 mg is provided by infusing 500 mL Intralipid per day.*
SOURCE: *After KN Jeejeebhoy, Ann Coll Physicians Surg Can 9:287, 1976.*

TABLE 75-2 Recommended electrolyte intake per day (mmol)

	Na	K	Ca	Mg	P
Basal*	100–120	80–100	7.5–10	10–12	12–16
Cardiac failure	20–50	80–100	10–15	10–12	12–16
Renal failure	20	†		†	

* To this basal intake, amounts of Na, K, Cl, and HCO₃ are added to meet losses from fistulas, nasogastric tube drainage, diarrhea, and stomal output.
† These ions are added as needed, on the basis of initial and continuing measurements of their circulating level and the clinical state of the patient.

Other requirements VITAMINS Vitamin requirements are given in Table 75-1. Amounts of vitamins sufficient to meet these needs must be added to the basic solution for parenteral feeding. Excessive amounts of fat-soluble vitamins, in particular vitamins A and D, should not be given because of the danger of hypercalcemia and other toxic effects. (See Chap. 76.) A combination of 5 mL Multivitamin Infusion (MVI) with 10 mL Soluzyme plus vitamin C on alternate days meets the requirements for vitamins A and D and for most water-soluble vitamins. These solutions should be supplemented with vitamin K (5 mg) and vitamin B₁₂ (200 μg) initially and at intervals of 3 weeks. Folate (5 mg) is given weekly. Biotin deficiency may occur in infants on TPN, as manifested by acidosis, rash, and alopecia.

ELECTROLYTES Electrolytes are an essential component of total parenteral nutrition. Potassium, magnesium, and phosphorus are necessary for optimal nitrogen retention and tissue formation; sodium and chloride are required to maintain osmolality and acid-base balance. Calcium is required to prevent demineralization of bone. Recommended ranges of intake are given in Table 75-2.

TRACE ELEMENTS Trace elements, in particular zinc, copper, and chromium, are needed when parenteral nutrition exceeds 1 to 2 weeks.

Zinc is essential for wound healing, for defense against infection, and as a cofactor for many enzymes. In its absence ageusia, loss of hair, night blindness, and a skin rash occur. The skin rash is often associated with superficial infection due to staphylococci and yeast and responds only to zinc supplementation. Zinc deficiency also interferes with delayed hypersensitivity. In the absence of excessive gastrointestinal losses, 3 mg zinc per day is sufficient to meet needs. For each liter of intestinal fluids lost through fistulas, stomal output, suction, or diarrhea in patients with extensive resection of the small bowel, an additional 12 mg should be added. If the small bowel is intact, zinc losses are greater, and about 17 mg zinc is required per liter of intestinal fluids lost per day.

Copper deficiency causes anemia and neutropenia. The daily requirement is estimated to be between 0.3 and 0.5 mg, with the larger intake to be given in patients with major losses of gastrointestinal fluid. Copper should not be given to patients with obstructive jaundice. *Manganese* requirement is about 0.8 mg per day. This element also should not be given if obstructive jaundice is present. *Chromium* deficiency is associated with glucose intolerance and neuropathy. The chromium requirement is about 20 μg daily. *Selenium* deficiency has been associated with congestive cardiomyopathy and possibly with muscle disease. Selenium requirements are probably somewhat greater than 10 μg per day.

ROUTES OF ADMINISTRATION Central venous catheterization This route allows infusion of fluids irrespective of osmolality and minimizes the need for repeated venipuncture. However, there is a risk of septicemia and thrombosis if the catheter is not properly inserted and cared for during therapy.

Basic principles of catheter insertion and care are as follows:

1 Catheters should be placed and handled using aseptic technique. Face mask and sterile gloves are required.
2 It should be documented radiologically that the catheter is in the superior vena cava prior to commencement of TPN with hypertonic fluids. If the tip is in another central vein (e.g., the internal jugular), thrombosis may occur.
3 Catheters should be introduced via puncture of a large central vein and not via a peripheral vein.
4 The catheter should not be used to withdraw blood or to measure central venous pressure.
5 The skin puncture site should be cleansed weekly with a detergent, painted with a povidone-iodine solution, and occluded with a dressing. An occlusive, transparent plastic dressing is recommended because the insertion site can then be easily inspected for infection, drainage, and bleeding.
6 Barium-impregnated silicone rubber catheters (e.g., Silastic, Extracorporeal Medical Specialities, Inc.) do not traumatize the central veins and are less likely to be surrounded with a fibrin clot.

Peripheral venous infusion This route is safe and not a likely source of sepsis or thrombotic complications. However, the infused fluids must be isotonic or only mildly hypertonic. To achieve these conditions, nonprotein energy must be given mainly as lipid.

REPRESENTATIVE PROTOCOLS FOR ADMINISTRATION OF TOTAL PARENTERAL NUTRITION The sample protocols in Table 75-3 are designed for a 60-kg individual, are intended to be administered over 24 h, and provide 1 g amino acids and 40 nonprotein calories per kilogram of body weight. Proportionate modifications can be made for larger or smaller persons. Nonprotein energy is provided either as (1) glucose, (2) 50 percent glucose and 50 percent lipid, or (3) 85 percent lipid and 15 percent glucose. The latter is suitable for peripheral venous administration. The infusion materials must be

TABLE 75-3 Representative daily protocols for total parenteral nutrition

Component solutions	100% dextrose regimen[a]	50% dextrose–50% lipid regimen[a]	15% dextrose–85% lipid regimen[a]
Amino acid 2.1%, dextrose 25%, mL	3000	—	—
Amino acid 4.2%, dextrose 25%, mL	—	1500	—
Amino acid 5%, dextrose 12.5%,[b] mL	—	—	1500
Lipid 10%,[c,d] mL	—	1000	1500
Electrolyte mix,[e] mL	60	60	60
Trace element mix,[f] mL	5	5	5
Vitamins,[g] mL	10	10	10
Total volume, mL	3075	2575	3075
Total electrolytes[h]			
Na⁺, meq	125	125	132.5
K⁺, meq	81	80	87
Ca²⁺, meq	10	10	10
Mg²⁺, meq	22	22	16
Cl⁻, meq	193	192	148
Ac⁻, meq	96	95	112.5
P, mg	582	582	693
Total protein, g	60	60	75
Total nonprotein calories, kcal	2550	2375	2286

[a] All values represent total 24-h amount. Percentage of total calories derived from dextrose and lipid as noted.
[b] Obtained by mixing equal volumes of commercially available 10% amino acid and 25% dextrose.
[c] The triglyceride and dextrose–amino acid mixture are infused concurrently through a central venous line using a connector for continuous mixing.
[d] Intralipid 10% (Cutter Laboratories) or Liposyn 10% (Abbott Laboratories).
[e] Electrolyte mix contains 80 meq Na⁺, 10 meq Ca²⁺, 16 meq Mg²⁺, 42 meq K⁺, and 148 meq Cl⁻ per 60 mL.
[f] Trace-element mix contains 1 mL each of (1) 0.5 mg/mL elemental Cu as cupric chloride (CuCl₂·2H₂O), 20 μg/mL elemental Cr as chromic nitrate [Cr(NO₃)₃], and 120 μg/mL of elemental Se as selenious acid (H₂SeO₃); (2) 120 μg/mL elemental I as potassium iodide (KI); (3) 3 mg/mL elemental Zn as zinc sulfate (ZnSO₄·7H₂O); and (4) 0.7 mg/mL elemental Mn as manganous chloride (MnCl₃·4H₂O).
[g] Vitamins include MVI injection (USV Pharmaceutical Corporation) once weekly and Soluzyme (Upjohn) six times weekly. Vitamin K is given as Synkayvite (Roche) 10 mg weekly.
[h] Total electrolytes are calculated on the assumption that the amino acid mixture used contains electrolytes. The total input of electrolytes in this table has been found to be capable of maintaining balance in patients without abnormal losses of gastrointestinal secretions.

prepared with care. In most centers such preparation is done exclusively by specially trained pharmacists.

HOME PARENTERAL NUTRITION (HPN)

Home parenteral nutrition has revolutionized the lives of persons who otherwise would require prolonged hospitalization for long-term nutritional support. A permanent silicone rubber catheter is placed in the superior vena cava via a subclavian or jugular vein and brought to the outside through a subcutaneous tunnel. These catheters may be left in place for years without need for replacement. The patient receives periodic supplies of prepackaged nutrients ready for infusion. The nutrients are infused during sleep. A simple pneumatic cuff placed around the plastic bags containing the prepackaged infusion fluids is safe, inexpensive, and less cumbersome than electromechanical delivery systems. The system is disconnected after the overnight infusion, and the catheter is capped and filled with a heparin solution. The patient is then free to carry out normal activities during the day.

PARTIAL PARENTERAL NUTRITION

It is debatable whether amino acids should replace glucose and electrolyte solutions in the management of patients unable to eat for short periods (up to 1 week) following surgery, strokes, or other acute illnesses. In 7 days a patient has (on average) a net negative nitrogen balance of 100 to 110 g when receiving only glucose replacement. If amino acids are given at a level of 1 g per kilogram of body weight per day, the nitrogen loss is cut to 35 to 45 g. This difference is equal to about 3 percent of the total nitrogen content of a 60-kg man. Since such a small deficit probably does not make any difference in clinical outcome (the nitrogen content is quickly replenished when food intake is restored) and since amino acid solutions are expensive, amino acid infusion is not recommended for fasts of up to 1 week. Beyond 1 week, full TPN should probably be given.

In some patients oral intake is possible, but the amounts ingested are inadequate for full nutrition. In such cases an estimate is made of the amount taken orally, and the deficiency is made up by parenteral means. When there is a question about how much of the ingested diet is absorbed (e.g., after bowel resection or with intestinal fistulas), the amount of nutrition given parenterally must be determined by trial and error, using weight gain and other signs of clinical improvement as a guide.

COMPLICATIONS

Technical complications Most technical complications are due to improper central venous catheter placement. These can be minimized by restricting the placement to designated, trained persons. Complications during insertion include injury to lung and pleura causing pneumothorax and hemothorax, embolism due to shearing off the catheter during placement, and brachial plexus injury. The needle used to locate the subclavian vein should be kept anterior, just behind the clavicle. Catheter embolism is caused by attempting to withdraw the catheter while keeping the needle stationary, thus severing the catheter. The needle and catheter should be withdrawn as a unit. Attention to these two simple principles can minimize serious problems.

Technical complications resulting from inappropriate catheter placement include infusion of nutrients into pleura and mediastinum due to a misplaced catheter and thrombosis of jugular and central veins. These can be avoided by infusing only normal saline solution until it has been established radiographically that the catheter is in the lower superior vena cava. High placement or misplacement may result in venous thrombosis if hypertonic solutions are not diluted by a rapid flow of blood; such dilution occurs in the superior vena cava. Late problems can arise from air embolism or catheter clotting. Air embolism can be avoided by using Luer-Lok connections. If catheter thrombosis occurs it can be unblocked by injecting urokinase; it is rarely necessary to remove a blocked catheter.

Septic complications Septic complications may occur because the cutaneous puncture site and catheter tract form a direct route for access of bacteria and fungi to the central veins. The presence in this tract of a foreign body, such as the catheter, aids the process. Hence,

catheter sepsis can be avoided by inserting it under strict aseptic conditions after proper skin preparation and by regular cleansing and dressing of the catheter site using strict aseptic technique. Catheter placement and care by specially trained teams can reduce sepsis to below 2 to 3 percent. It should be recognized that fever in a patient with a catheter is often *not* due to catheter sepsis. Hence where fever develops despite good catheter care, it is recommended that the TPN be stopped and electrolyte solutions infused while the cause of fever is investigated. Careful physical examination and history review are performed to identify other causes of fever. Blood cultures are taken from peripheral and central venous catheters, and cultures of sputum, wound, and urine are obtained. If no other cause for sepsis is found and blood cultures are positive, the catheter is removed and the patient is carefully watched. With pure catheter sepsis prompt defervescence should ensue. A new catheter can be inserted 48 hours after the fever has subsided. The common error is to assume that the fever is caused by catheter sepsis and thus to deny TPN to a patient who then becomes more malnourished and even more prone to sepsis.

Metabolic complications In patients with sepsis hyperglycemia may occur owing to insulin resistance and high levels of counterregulatory hormones such as catecholamines and cortisol. The treatment is to replace glucose calories with lipid calories and/or to add insulin. During TPN the blood glucose levels should not be allowed to go below 150 mg/dL because of the danger of hypoglycemia. The unexpected appearance of hyperglycemia may herald a febrile episode caused by sepsis. In contrast, hypoglycemia may occur either owing to the sudden stopping of the hypertonic glucose infusion or rarely in a patient receiving TPN and insulin whose sepsis has been cured.

Hyperammonemia and a picture resembling hepatic encephalopathy may occur in patients who have been infused with a mixture of essential amino acids containing little or no arginine. In such patients, care should be taken to give only minimal nitrogen infusions.

Hypertriglyceridemia may occur with overfeeding. The treatment is to reduce total calorie intake and to discontinue lipid infusions.

Electrolyte disturbances Anabolism is associated with the cellular uptake of potassium, magnesium, and phosphorus. This can result in hypokalemia, hypomagnesemia and hypophosphatemia. The latter can cause disorientation, convulsions, and coma because hypophosphatemia results in low red cell levels of 2,3-diphosphoglycerate (2,3-DPG) and thus reduced oxygen transfer to tissues. These abnormalities should not occur with the use of the mixtures given in Table 75-2 and with proper monitoring.

Acid-base balance The metabolism of the basic amino acids in their chloride forms results in the production of protons and chloride, which, if unbuffered, can accumulate and cause hyperchloremic acidosis. For this reason all current amino acid mixtures contain sodium acetate. The conversion of acetate to bicarbonate serves to buffer the protons produced by the metabolism of basic amino acids. Hence, disturbances of acid-base balance do not occur unless there is loss of bicarbonate from other sources, such as diarrhea, or unless lactic acid acidosis develops.

Liver disease Minimal elevations of serum alkaline phosphatase and aminotransferase are common (70 to 90 percent) during TPN and are usually not associated with jaundice. These abnormalities are as frequent in patients given glucose-electrolyte solutions or those fed by mouth as in those given TPN, which suggest that TPN is only one factor in their development. In occasional patients (1.5 to 2 percent) jaundice and cholestasis develop with minimal hepatocyte injury; hyperbilirubinemia is common in septic patients. Minor abnormalities of liver function are of no consequence, but sepsis should be treated appropriately.

During TPN, "sludge" accumulates in the gall bladder and may lead to obstructive changes in the biliary tract. In some patients cholecystectomy for gall bladder disease has been followed by relief of jaundice despite continuing TPN.

An enlarged, tender, fatty liver may develop if excess calories are given as carbohydrate. The treatment is to reduce caloric intake and replace 50 percent of it with lipid. The pathogenesis appears to be conversion of a portion of the infused carbohydrate to fat. The fat accumulates in the liver as triglyceride. Decreasing or replacing infused carbohydrate reduces the fatty liver.

Hypercalcemia and pancreatitis Pancreatitis associated with hypercalcemia can occur during TPN. This may be relieved by eliminating vitamin D from the infusion.

Metabolic bone disease In some patients receiving home TPN, osteomalacia and osteoporosis have occurred, leading to bone pain and fractures. The mechanism for these changes is not clear.

REFERENCES

ANDERSON GH et al: Design and evaluation by nitrogen balance and blood aminograms of an amino acid mixture for total parenteral nutrition of adults with gastrointestinal disease. J Clin Invest 53:904, 1974

———— et al: Dose-response relationships between amino acid intake and blood levels in newborn infants. Am J Clin Nutr 30:1110, 1977

BAKER JP et al: A randomized trial of total parenteral nutrition in critically ill patients. Gastroenterology 87:53, 1984

BATSTONE GF et al: Metabolic studies in subjects following thermal injury. Intermediary metabolites, hormones and tissue oxygenation. Burns 2:207, 1976

BLACKBURN GL et al: Protein sparing therapy during periods of starvation with sepsis or trauma. Ann Surg 177:588, 1973

CAHILL GF JR et al: Starvation in man. N Engl J Med 282:668, 1970

CRAIG RP et al: Intravenous glucose, amino acids and fat in the postoperative period. Lancet 2:8, 1977

GREENBERG GR et al: Protein-sparing therapy in postoperative patients. Effects of added hypocaloric glucose or lipid. N Engl J Med 294:1411, 1976

IZSAK EH et al: Pancreatitis in association with hypercalcemia in patients receiving total parenteral nutrition. Gastroenterology 79:555, 1980

JEEJEEBHOY KN et al: Metabolic studies in total parenteral nutrition with lipid in man: Comparison with glucose. J Clin Invest 57:125, 1976

———— et al: Total parenteral nutrition at home: Studies in patients surviving 4 months to 5 years. Gastroenterology 71:943, 1976

————: Protein sparing effect of amino acids, in *Clinical Nutrition Update: Amino Acids*, HL Green et al (eds). Chicago, American Medical Association, 1977

————: Role of measuring albumin synthesis as a way of measuring protein body repletion, in ibid.

KORETZ RL, MEYER JH: Elemental diets—Facts and fantasies. Gastroenterology 78:393, 1980

MENG HC, WILMORE DW (eds): *Fat Emulsions in Parenteral Nutrition*. Chicago, American Medical Association, 1976

MESSING B: Does total parenteral nutrition induce gallbladder sludge formation and lithiasis? Gastroenterology 84:1012, 1983

ROULET M et al: A controlled trial of the effect of parenteral nutrition support on patients with respiration failure and sepsis. Clin Nutr 2:97, 1983

RUDMAN D et al: Elemental balances during intravenous hyperalimentation of underweight adult subjects. J Clin Invest 55:94, 1975

SHIKE M et al: A possible role for Vitamin D in the genesis of parenteral-nutrition-induced metabolic bone disease. Ann Int Med 95:560, 1981

76 VITAMIN DEFICIENCY AND EXCESS[1]

JEAN D. WILSON

The role of vitamins in disease has changed within the past few decades. Deficiencies of single vitamins are now rarely endemic, even in developing nations, and instead occur either as a portion of states of malnutrition, as a result of food faddism, as a complication of more widespread disease such as malabsorption, as a complication of complex therapy such as hemodialysis or total parenteral nutrition, or as the result of an inborn error of metabolism. Indeed, disorders of vitamin excess may now be more common than vitamin deficiency.

In considering the pathophysiology of vitamins several points are worth emphasis. (1) The fact that organic compounds cannot be synthesized within the body and are required constituents of the diet is the result of mutations, and the provision of vitamins in the diet is a form of therapy for an inborn error of metabolism. In some instances, such as the limited ability to synthesize thiamine, the requirement is common to many if not all animals, and the mutation must have occurred early in evolution; in others, such as the single-gene defect that prevents ascorbic acid synthesis, humans share the defect with only a few other species, such as the guinea pig. (2) The feature that separates vitamins from other necessary organic constituents in the diet is that small amounts of them are required, in contrast to the relatively large amounts of essential amino acids and essential fatty acids. This is a consequence of the fact that vitamins function not as building blocks of tissue mass or as substrates for energy production but rather as prosthetic groups for quantitatively minor tissue constituents or as catalytic cofactors for biologic reactions; like most catalysts they are required only in small amounts. (3) Deficiency of some vitamins has never been described in humans (e.g., pantothenic acid) implying that these vitamins are either so ubiquitous in food sources or are conserved so efficiently by the body that deficiency can become manifest, if at all, only in the context of a mixed nutritional and vitamin deficiency. (4) Alcoholism is the background upon which many vitamin deficiencies develop in the United States. This is the consequence of several interlocking factors including diminished intake, impairment of absorption and storage of vitamins, and in some cases predisposing genetic factors. In those instances in which alcoholism is not associated with an increased frequency of disease (e.g., pellagra), the etiology of the disorder is more complicated than a simple deficiency state. (5) Biochemical means of proving vitamin deficiency, once suspected, are limited, and the role of vitamin deficiency in disease states is frequently not recognized because nonspecific vitamin therapy is a common part of standard supportive care. As a consequence, understanding the manifestations of vitamin deficiency and a high index of suspicion in the appropriate clinical setting are essential for considering the diagnosis, and demonstration of a response to replacement therapy may be the most accurate way to confirm a diagnosis. (6) The widespread consumption of excessive amounts of vitamins can occur either as the indirect consequence of dietary practice or, more commonly, as the result of deliberate ingestion. The toxicity of the fat-soluble vitamins A and D has long been established, whereas the toxicity syndromes produced by the water-soluble vitamins are inconsistent and less well characterized.

DEFICIENCY STATES

NIACIN (PELLAGRA) **Biochemistry** *Niacin* is the generic term for nicotinic acid (3-pyridinecarboxylic acid) and derivatives that exhibit the nutritional activity of nicotinic acid (Fig. 76-1). In one sense niacin is not a vitamin since it can be formed from the essential amino acid tryptophan. In the human an average of about 1 mg of niacin is formed from 60 mg of dietary tryptophan. Accordingly, estimates of the adequacy of dietary intake must take into account the tryptophan content of the diet as well as the content of niacin. Many foodstuffs, especially cereals, contain bound forms of niacin from which the vitamin is not nutritionally available.

The absorption, tissue distribution, and metabolism of the vitamin are poorly understood. Approximately one-fifth of the vitamin is decarboxylated, and the remainder is excreted in the urine as methylated products, largely *N*-methylnicotinamide and its derivatives.

Mechanism of action Niacin is an essential component of nicotinamide adenine dinucleotide (NAD) and nicotinamide adenine dinucleotide phosphate (NADP), coenzymes for many oxidation-reduction reactions.

Requirements The requirements and recommended daily allowances for niacin and tryptophan are listed in Tables 70-1 and 70-2. In contrast to most vitamins, the requirement for niacin does not appear to be increased during pregnancy. Requirement is primarily determined by the amino acid composition of the diet.

[1] For vitamin D, see Chap. 337 and for the hematologic vitamins, see Chap. 285.

Experimental depletion After the institution of a diet deficient in niacin and tryptophan, the urinary excretion of niacin metabolites reaches minimal values (<1.5 mg per day) after 1 to 2 months and remains constant thereafter. Clinical deficiency develops shortly after excretion becomes stable at a low level and consists of dermatitis, glossitis, stomatitis, diarrhea, proctitis, mental depression, abdominal pain, vaginitis, dysphagia, and amenorrhea, findings similar to those in pellagra.

Clinical deficiency Pellagra was previously an endemic disease in the American south and in many other parts of the world. The endemic disease is usually associated with a high intake of maize (American corn) and can be cured by the administration of niacin; nevertheless, the fact that large populations of people exist on a diet in which maize is the major source of protein but nevertheless are free of endemic pellagra implies that the relation between maize intake and the development of the disease is not straightforward. As a consequence, the concept of the pathogenesis of pellagra has evolved from that of a pure vitamin deficiency or a mixed deficiency of tryptophan and available niacin in the diet to a more complicated etiology. The disorder may be due to an imbalance in dietary amino acids; the niacin equivalent (available niacin and tryptophan) of

maize, although low, is no lower than that of some cereals that are unassociated with endemic pellagra. Furthermore, the leucine content of common varieties of maize is high, whereas a hybrid strain of maize, opaque 2, has lower leucine but similar tryptophan and niacin contents. Dogs fed a diet rich in conventional maize or a diet rich in opaque 2 maize supplemented with leucine develop experimental pellagra, whereas dogs fed the opaque 2 maize alone do not. This finding presumably explains why pellagra can result from a diet rich in millet (sorghum, jowar), which has a leucine content similar to that of maize but a niacin and tryptophan content (and availability) equivalent to that of rice. Leucine is believed to inhibit the synthesis of nicotinic acid mononucleotide and consequently the synthesis of NAD and NADP. Thus, development of symptomatic niacin "deficiency" may depend on the amino acid content of the rest of the diet as well as upon the intake of the vitamin and its precursors. The second possibility is that the milling of maize influences the bioavailability of the niacin in the cereal. On the one hand, treatment of maize with alkali in the preparation of foods in Latin America may serve to hydrolyze bound nicotinic acid and to inactivate toxins that may accumulate in stored grain contaminated with molds. On the other hand, degermination of the cereal during the usual milling process in the United States may inhibit the liberation of bound

FIGURE 76-1 *The structure and principal functions of some of the vitamins associated with human disorders.*

Vitamin	Active Derivative or Cofactor Form	Principal Function
Niacin	Nicotinamide Adenine Dinucleotide Phosphate (NADP) and Nicotine Adenine Dinucleotide (NAD)	Coenzymes for Oxidations and Reductions
Thiamine	Thiamine Diphosphate	Coenzyme for Cleavage of Carbon-Carbon Bonds
Pyridoxine	Pyridoxal Phosphate	Cofactor for Enzymes of Amino Acid Metabolism
Riboflavin	Flavin Mononucleotide (FMN) and Flavin Adenine Dinucleotide (FAD)	Cofactor for Oxidation-Reduction Reactions and Covalently Attached Prosthetic Groups for Some Enzymes
Ascorbic Acid	Ascorbic Acid and Dehydroascorbic Acid	Participation as a Redox Ion in Many Biological Oxidation Reactions
Vitamin A	Retinol, Retinal, and Retinoic Acid	Formation of Carotenoid Proteins (Vision) and Glycoproteins (Epithelial Cell Function)
Vitamin E	Tocopherol	Antioxidant
Vitamin K	Menaquinone	Cofactor for Post-Translational Carboxylation of Many Proteins Including Essential Clotting Factors

niacin. The effect of these treatments, respectively, would be to prevent or to predispose to the development of pellagra when maize is a major element of the diet.

Whatever the cause, endemic pellagra disappeared coincident with the improvement of nutritional education and with the widespread supplementation of grain cereals with niacin. At present, pellagra is an occasional secondary manifestation of two disorders that profoundly affect tryptophan metabolism, the carcinoid syndrome, in which up to 60 percent of tryptophan is catabolized by what is ordinarily a minor pathway of metabolism (see Chap. 303), and Hartnup disease (see Chap. 307), an inherited disorder in which several amino acids including tryptophan are absorbed poorly from the diet. In both disorders pellagra is due to diminished availability of effective niacin equivalents and can be cured by the administration of large amounts of the vitamin.

Pellagra is a chronic wasting disease typically associated with dermatitis, dementia, and diarrhea. The dermatitis is bilateral, symmetric, and present in sites exposed to sunlight, and is due to photosensitivity. The mental changes are less discrete; fatigue, insomnia, and apathy may precede the development of an encephalopathy characterized by confusion, disorientation, hallucination, loss of memory, and eventually, frank organic psychosis. Paresthesias and polyneuritis may be the result of coexisting deficiencies of other vitamins. Diarrhea, when it occurs, results from widespread inflammation of the mucous surfaces; other mucosal abnormalities include achlorhydria, glossitis, stomatitis, and vaginitis. The course is progressive over a several-year period, and death is usually due to secondary complications.

The relation between the known coenzyme function of NAD and NADP and these various symptoms has not been defined. Levels of NAD and NADP in erythrocytes are lower in patients with pellagra than in normal individuals, but the coenzymes are essential to so many reactions in intermediary metabolism that profound deficiency of the coenzymes is incompatible with life. The mental changes in pellagra may be associated with diminished conversion of tryptophan to serotonin.

No biochemical test is of diagnostic value, and diagnosis must be based upon suspicion and response to replacement therapy. As predicted, excretion in the urine of the metabolites of nicotinic acid and tryptophan is lower than average but not lower than in patients with generalized malnutrition (Table 71-4). Plasma tryptophan and erythrocyte NAD and NADP levels are also low. The skin lesions are characterized by hyperkeratosis, hyperpigmentation, and desquamation.

The administration of small amounts of niacin (10 mg per day) in the face of limiting amounts of dietary tryptophan is sufficient to cure endemic pellagra. Large amounts (40 to 200 mg per day) may be required in Hartnup disease and in the carcinoid syndrome.

THIAMINE (BERIBERI)   Biochemistry   Thiamine contains pyrimidine and thiazole moieties linked by a methylene bridge (Fig. 76-1). The vitamin is synthesized by a variety of plants and microorganisms but not ordinarily by animals. However, rats and pigeons fed a thiamine-free diet can be protected from deficiency by large quantities of the pyrimidine and thiazole moieties, suggesting a small capacity to couple the subunits together. Limited amounts of the vitamin may be synthesized by microorganisms in the gastrointestinal tract. Thiamine is absorbed both by an active-transport process and by passive diffusion. The capacity to absorb the vitamin in the human intestine is limited to about 5 mg per day. Approximately 25 to 30 mg are stored in the body, 80 percent as thiamine diphosphate (pyrophosphate), 10 percent as thiamine triphosphate, and the remainder as free thiamine monophosphate. Large amounts are present in skeletal muscles (about one-half of body stores), heart, liver, kidneys, and brain. A number of thiaminase enzymes inactivate thiamine by splitting the vitamin into its two component parts. Several metabolites are excreted in the urine, principally thiamine itself (which is secreted by the renal tubules), an acetylated derivative, and end products of thiamine catabolism, mainly derivatives of thiazole acetate and pyrimidine carboxylate.

Mechanism of action   Thiamine diphosphate acts as a coenzyme for several reactions that cleave carbon-carbon bonds—the oxidative decarboxylation of α-keto acids (pyruvate and α-ketoglutarate) and keto analogues of leucine, isoleucine, and valine, and the transketolase reaction in the pentose phosphate pathway. Many features of thiamine deficiency are the result of inhibition of these enzymatic reactions and/or the accumulation of the proximal metabolites. Thiamine may also have a specific role in neurons independent of its coenzymatic function in general metabolism; thiamine and its esters are present in axonal membranes, and electrical stimulation of nerves effects the hydrolysis and release of thiamine diphosphate and triphosphate.

Requirements   The recommended daily allowances for thiamine are given in Tables 70-1 and 70-2. The vitamin has a widespread distribution in food and is absent only from oils, fats, cassava, and refined sugar. In vegetable products the vitamin is largely in the form of thiamine. The outer layers of cereal grains are especially rich in the vitamin; hence, machine-milled rice is a poor source. In animal tissues thiamine is present largely in the form of phosphate esters. The esters are dephosphorylated by phosphatases in the intestine, and only the free vitamin is absorbed. A substantial loss of the vitamin takes place during cooking above 100°C.

Several factors influence the absorption and metabolism of the vitamin (and hence alter daily requirements). One is the presence of thiaminases in foods including fresh fish, clams, shrimp, mussels, and some raw animal tissues, and in microorganisms in the colon. Two, daily needs decrease when fat forms a large part of the diet and increase as carbohydrate intake increases. Requirements are increased in pregnancy, during lactation, in thyrotoxicosis, and by fever. Accelerated loss of thiamine from the body may occur with diuretic therapy, hemodialysis, peritoneal dialysis, and diarrhea. Defective intestinal absorption can occur in malabsorption states, alcoholism, chronic malnutrition, and folate deficiency.

Experimental depletion   Following the institution of a thiamine-free diet in control subjects, thiamine excretion in the urine decreases to 5 percent of the control value after a week and becomes undetectable after 2 weeks. However, the excretion of the pyrimidine and thiazole catabolites of thiamine remains unchanged for as long as a month, indicating that the body pool is slowly utilized during a period of deficient intake.

Within a week after the institution of a deficient diet, subjects develop a resting tachycardia, followed by the onset of weakness, decreased deep tendon reflexes, and (in some) a sensory neuropathy. Subjective symptoms include generalized malaise, headache, nausea, and aching of the muscles. Appearance of these symptoms is paralleled by a fall in red blood cell transketolase activity. Within a week of thiamine repletion (2 mg per day) all abnormal physical findings disappear, and the subjective symptoms clear after 2 weeks. (Experimental depletion in humans has never been carried to the point of development of severe cerebral or cardiovascular symptoms.)

Clinical deficiency   In developed nations thiamine deficiency occurs in alcoholics or food faddists or in the context of special clinical situations, such as chronic peritoneal dialysis, hemodialysis, refeeding after starvation, or after the administration of glucose to asymptomatic but thiamine-depleted patients. In developing countries the disorder is commonly due to the consumption of milled rice or foods containing thiaminases or (possibly) other antithiamine factors.

Development of thiamine deficiency in chronic alcoholics is due to low thiamine intake, impaired thiamine absorption and storage, accelerated destruction of thiamine diphosphate, and varying degrees of energy expenditure. However, clinical manifestations develop in only a fraction of alcoholics and other chronically malnourished persons. Genetic factors may be involved in susceptibility. For example, in fibroblasts cultured from patients with the Wernicke-Korsakoff syndrome the thiamine-requiring transketolase binds thiamine diphosphate only one-tenth as avidly as in those of controls. This finding implies that an underlying genetic polymorphism is clinically silent when the diet is adequate but becomes overt if thiamine intake is low or marginal.

The two major manifestations of thiamine deficiency involve the cardiovascular (wet beriberi) and nervous systems (dry beriberi and the Wernicke-Korsakoff syndrome). The typical patient has mixed symptoms involving both the cardiovascular and nervous systems, but pure cardiovascular, pure polyneuritic, and pure cerebral forms also occur. The factors that determine the relative preponderance of these manifestations are related in part to the duration and severity of the deficiency, the degree of physical exertion, and the caloric intake. Severe physical exertion, high carbohydrate intake, and a moderate degree of chronic deficiency favor wet beriberi with little or no peripheral neuritis, whereas an equal deficiency with caloric restriction and relative inactivity favors the development of dry beriberi.

Beriberi heart disease comprises three major physiologic derangements: (1) peripheral vasodilation leading to a high-output state, (2) biventricular myocardial failure, and (3) retention of sodium and water leading to edema. In the chronic form peripheral vasodilatation leads to increased arteriovenous shunting of blood, rapid circulation time, tachycardia, increased cardiac output, and a venous congestive state characterized by elevated peripheral venous pressure, elevated right ventricular end-diastolic pressure, decreased arteriovenous extraction of oxygen, sodium retention, and edema. Disordered blood flow (decreased cerebral and renal blood flow and increased flow to muscles) is common. Cardiac output increases so that notwithstanding the lowered peripheral vascular resistance ventricular work, arterial blood pressure, and pulmonary wedge pressure tend to be elevated. Temporary appearance or worsening of hypertension may occur during thiamine repletion, presumably due to closing of arteriovenous shunts and temporary volume overload.

In acute fulminant cardiovascular (shoshin) beriberi, the myocardial lesion is the central feature of a course in which severe dyspnea, restlessness, and anxiety eventuate in acute cardiovascular collapse and death within hours to days. Physical findings include stocking-glove cyanosis, extreme tachycardia, marked cardiomegaly, hepatomegaly, arterial bruits, and neck vein distention. The venous pressure is high, and the circulation time is rapid. Because of the fulminant course edema may be minimal or absent. Administration of thiamine rapidly restores peripheral vascular resistance, but improvement in the myocardial abnormality may be delayed so that low-output failure supervenes during treatment.

Three types of nervous system involvement occur: peripheral neuropathy, Wernicke's encephalopathy (cerebral beriberi), and the Korsakoff syndrome. The neuropathy may or may not be painful and is characterized by a symmetric impairment of sensory, motor, and reflex function that affects the distal segments of limbs more severely than the proximal ones. The histologic lesion is a noninflammatory degeneration of myelin sheaths. No meaningful distinction can be made between this disorder and so-called alcoholic neuropathy on the basis of either clinical or neurologic criteria.

Wernicke's encephalopathy ordinarily develops in an orderly sequence and consists of vomiting, nystagmus (horizontal more commonly than vertical), palsies of the rectus muscles leading to unilateral or bilateral ophthalmoplegia (and decrease in the nystagmus), fever, ataxia, and progressive mental deterioration that eventuates in a global confusional state and may progress to coma and death. Improvement occurs after thiamine replacement, although Korsakoff's syndrome may supervene. Thus, the eye palsies are corrected, the nystagmus improves in one-half, the ataxia improves or disappears in two-thirds, and the global confusional state disappears to be replaced by Korsakoff's syndrome. The latter consists of retrograde amnesia, impaired ability to learn, and (usually) confabulation. The patient is usually alert and responsive and exhibits no serious defect in behavior. Recovery (complete or partial) from Korsakoff's syndrome can be expected only in one-half.

In summary, Wernicke's encephalopathy and the amnesic psychosis of Korsakoff's syndrome are not separate clinical events; instead, the changing ocular and ataxic signs, the transformation of the global confusional state into the amnesic-confabulatory syndrome, and the development of a nonconfabulatory amnesic state are successive stages in the recovery from a single process. The clinical features, differential diagnosis, course, and pathology of cerebral beriberi are discussed in detail in Chap. 349.

Various biochemical tests to detect thiamine deficiency include the measurement of blood thiamine, pyruvate, α-ketoglutarate, lactate, and glyoxylate; measurement of the urinary excretion of thiamine and thiamine metabolites; a thiamine-loading test; and measurement of urinary methylglyoxal. The most reliable is the measurement of whole-blood or erythrocyte transketolase activity. Any enhancement in enzymatic activity resulting from added thiamine diphosphate (TPP) is referred to as the TPP effect (expressed in percent). If the activity of the enzyme is increased more than 15 percent by the added thiamine diphosphate, then a deficiency state is probably present (Table 71-4). Due to variability in activity, measurement of isolated transketolase levels is not useful, but demonstration of an increase in activity after treatment coupled with a significant stimulation in vitro by added thiamine diphosphate prior to treatment suggests the presence of thiamine deficiency.

Another criterion for the diagnosis is the assessment of clinical response to thiamine administration. Clinical improvement may be dramatic in cardiovascular beriberi, and an increase in blood pressure and decrease in heart rate may be seen within 12 h after start of therapy. Diuresis and reduction in heart size may be apparent within 1 to 2 days.

Prompt administration of thiamine is indicated when beriberi is diagnosed or suspected. Fifty milligrams per day should be given intramuscularly for several days after which 2.5 to 5 mg per day can be administered by mouth. Larger amounts are usually not absorbed. All patients should also receive other water-soluble vitamins in therapeutic quantities.

Thiamine-responsive inborn errors of metabolism   A number of thiamine-responsive inborn errors of metabolism have been described in which patients respond to pharmacologic doses of thiamine. These include thiamine-responsive megaloblastic anemia, for which the mechanism is unknown; thiamine-responsive lactic acidosis, which is due to low activity of pyruvate carboxylase in liver; thiamine-responsive branched-chain ketoaciduria, which is due to low activity of a ketoacid dehydrogenase; and intermittent cerebellar ataxia which may result from an abnormal pyruvate dehydrogenase. In addition, the autosomal recessive disorder subacute necrotizing encephalomyelopathy (Leigh's disease) may be related to a diminished amount of thiamine triphosphate in neural tissue; a factor has been isolated from the urine of such patients that inhibits the enzyme that synthesizes thiamine triphosphate. The clinical response of patients with Leigh's disease to pharmacologic doses of the vitamin appears to be minor, however.

PYRIDOXINE (VITAMIN B$_6$)   Biochemistry   The biologic activity of the vitamin B$_6$ group is displayed by pyridoxine, pyridoxal, and pyridoxamine and their 5-phosphate esters (Fig. 76-1). The coenzyme form is pyridoxal 5-phosphate, and the other compounds owe their activity to conversion to pyridoxal 5-phosphate. The vitamin is widely and uniformly distributed in all foods; muscle meats, liver, vegetables, and whole-grain cereals are among the best sources.

Mechanism of action   Pyridoxal phosphate acts as a cofactor for many enzymes involved in amino acid metabolism, including transaminases, synthetases, and hydroxylases. In humans the vitamin is of particular importance in the metabolism of tryptophan, glycine, serine, glutamate, and the sulfur-containing amino acids. Pyridoxal phosphate is also required for the synthesis of the heme precursor δ-aminolevulinic acid. A large portion of body stores of pyridoxine is in muscle phosphorylase, where it functions to stabilize the enzyme rather than as a catalyst. It also plays a poorly understood role in neuronal excitability, possibly as a result of its function in transsulfuration reactions or in γ-aminobutyric acid metabolism

Requirements   The recommended daily allowances are described in Tables 70-1 and 70-2. Even more than for most vitamins, the requirement is increased in pregnancy and by the ingestion of estrogens. In both conditions abnormal tryptophan metabolites are excreted in urine, and this can be prevented by supplementation with pyridoxine. Estrogens appear to inhibit the role of pyridoxal phosphate in tryptophan metabolism. Pyridoxine requirement may also be increased by high protein intake. The ingestion of ethanol interferes with the metabolism of pyridoxal phosphate, the ethanol metabolite acetaldehyde displacing the coenzyme from proteins and thus enhancing its degradation.

Experimental depletion   The feeding of pyridoxine-deficient diets leads to chemical evidence of deficiency (increased xanthurenic acid and decreased pyridoxine in urine) within a week. Electroencephalographic abnormalities are demonstrable within 3 weeks, and some subjects have grand mal seizures. Deficiency induced with the pyridoxine antagonist deoxypyridoxine causes, in addition, seborrheic dermatitis, cheilosis, glossitis, nausea, vomiting, weakness, and dizziness.

Clinical deficiency   The widespread occurrence of the vitamin in food is probably the reason that the naturally occurring pure pyridoxine deficiency does not occur except when the pyridoxine content of food is either destroyed or converted to less available protein-bound forms during processing, as has happened in some infant formulas. It is a paradox, therefore, that pyridoxine deficiency is now frequent due to the fact that many commonly used drugs act as pyridoxine antagonists. Hydrazines such as *isoniazid* induce peripheral neuritis that can be prevented by pyridoxine supplementation; these drugs combine with pyridoxal and pyridoxal phosphate to form hydrazones. The hydrazones inhibit enzymes such as pyridoxal kinase, induce convulsions directly, and accelerate pyridoxine loss in the urine and thus induce a vitamin deficiency. *Cycloserine* also causes an increase in the excretion of the vitamin in the urine and produces profound neurologic effects, presumably by forming a complex with pyridoxal phosphate that competes with the cofactor for apoenzymes. *Penicillamine* acts as an antagonist by forming a thiazolidine derivative with pyridoxal phosphate. In each of these instances abnormal tryptophan metabolism and convulsions can be prevented by supplementation with the vitamin.

Estimates of vitamin deficiency have been based upon the correction of clinical signs of deficiency following administration of the vitamin, measurement of the excretion of tryptophan metabolites after tryptophan-loading tests, measurement of various amino acid transferase activities in blood, and measurement of the excretion of pyridoxine or its metabolites or of oxalate in urine (Table 71-4). The most commonly used index is the measurement of urinary tryptophan metabolites, particularly xanthurenic acid, following tryptophan loading. Alternatively, cystathionine can be assayed after administration of a methionine load. In vitro measurement of red blood cell glutamic pyruvic transaminase in the presence and absence of pyridoxal phosphate may be a better indicator of pyridoxine status than either loading test.

The appropriate management is prevention of deficiency. Supplementation of the diet with 30 mg of pyridoxine returns tryptophan metabolism to normal in pregnancy, in users of oral contraceptives, and in patients taking isoniazid. Doses as high as 100 mg per day may be required in subjects taking penicillamine.

Pyridoxine-responsive diseases   Several genetic disorders cause abnormalities in vitamin B_6 metabolism. In one group, infants develop convulsions and brain damage and die if not provided with large daily supplements of pyridoxine; these children have an apoenzyme for glutamic acid decarboxylase that has a decreased binding affinity for pyridoxal phosphate. Consequently they do not form normal amounts of γ-aminobutyric acid, a physiologic inhibitor of neuro-

transmission. Another group of patients has pyridoxine-responsive chronic anemia; pyridoxine supplementation results in prompt hematologic improvement but does not correct the morphologic abnormality in the erythrocytes.

The synthesis of cystathionine from homocystine and serine and its cleavage to cysteine and homoserine are catalyzed by two pyridoxal phosphate enzymes. The changes that occur in deficiency of these two enzymes and in xanthurenic aciduria due to kynureninase deficiency have been reviewed by Mudd. Some patients with vitamin B_6–responsive xanthurenic aciduria or cystathioninuria have a mutant apoenzyme that interacts abnormally with pyridoxal phosphate, a defect that can be largely corrected by elevated concentrations of the cofactor. In contrast, the vitamin B_6 response in patients with homocystinuria due to cystathionine synthetase deficiency is due to an enhancement of the activity of the residual amount of normal enzyme present rather than a restoration of the affected enzyme levels to normal.

RIBOFLAVIN   Riboflavin in the form of the coenzymes flavin mononucleotide (FMN) and flavin adenine dinucleotide (FAD) participates in a variety of oxidation-reduction reactions (Fig. 76-1). In addition, covalently attached flavins are essential to the structure of such enzymes as succinate dehydrogenase and monoamine oxidase. The vitamin is absorbed from the gastrointestinal tract either as free riboflavin or the 5′-phosphate by a specific transport process. The requirements and recommended daily allowances are listed in Tables 70-1 and 70-2. Covalently linked vitamin accounts for less than one-tenth of the tissue pool. The vitamin is excreted in urine predominantly in the free form although a small fraction of the daily turnover is the result of catabolism by microorganisms in the gastrointestinal tract.

Riboflavin deficiency can be induced in humans by feeding a riboflavin-deficient diet or by the administration of riboflavin antagonists such as galactoflavin. The deficiency syndrome is characterized by sore throat, hyperemia and edema of the pharyngeal and oral mucous membranes, cheilosis, angular stomatitis, glossitis, seborrheic dermatitis, and normochromic, normocytic anemia due to red cell hypoplasia of the bone marrow. These features can be rapidly and completely reversed by riboflavin administration. Thyroid hormones and adrenal steroids enhance FMN and FAD synthesis; certain psychotropic agents (phenothiazines and tricyclic antidepressants) competitively inhibit flavin coenzyme biosynthesis, but these agents alone do not induce deficiency. Instead, riboflavin deficiency almost invariably occurs in combination with other vitamin deficiencies.

VITAMIN C (SCURVY)   Biochemistry   In most animals ascorbic acid (vitamin C) can be synthesized from glucose. However, humans, other primates, and the guinea pig are unable to synthesize L-ascorbic acid and require vitamin C in the diet. These species can perform the various reactions required for the biosynthesis of the vitamin from D-glucose except for one step, the conversion of L-gluconogammalactone to L-abscorbic acid. The enzyme that catalyzes this reaction (L-gluconolactone oxidase) is missing because of a mutation; thus the need for vitamin C in the diet is the result of an inborn error in carbohydrate metabolism.

Mechanism of action   L-Ascorbic acid readily undergoes reversible oxidation and reduction as follows:

$$\text{L-ascorbic acid} \rightleftharpoons \text{dehydro-L-ascorbic acid} + 2H^+ + 2e$$

This property of the vitamin is the key to understanding its role as a redox agent for biologic oxidation. However, ascorbic acid does not act as a conventional cofactor since its requirement can usually be replaced by other compounds with similar redox properties. The best understood function is in the synthesis of collagen; absence of the vitamin leads to impairment of peptidyl hydroxylation of procollagen and a reduction in collagen formation and secretion by connective tissue. Nonhydroxylated collagen is unstable and cannot form the triple helix required for normal tissue structure. Many features of scurvy result from this defect in collagen synthesis, including the capillary fragility that underlies the hemorrhagic features, the poor healing of wounds, and (in part) the bony abnormalities of children. Collagens that normally have the highest content of hydroxyproline are most severely affected, accounting for the early disruption of the adventitia, media, and basal laminae of blood vessels. Ascorbic acid also functions to prevent oxidation of tetrahydrofolate and thus protect the active folic acid pool and to regulate iron distribution and storage, probably by influencing the valence of stored iron and maintaining a normal ratio of ferritin to hemosiderin. Scorbutic patients excrete incompletely oxidized products of tyrosine metabolism, but the significance is not clear.

Requirements The recommended daily allowances for vitamin C are described in Tables 70-1 and 70-2. The vitamin is present in milk and some meats (kidney, liver, fish) and is widely distributed in fruits and vegetables. A portion is lost after prolonged storage of unprocessed fruits and vegetables (for example, potatoes), but it is partially preserved (half or greater) by most means of food processing (boiling, steaming, pressure cooking, preserving jams and jellies, freezing, dehydration, and canning). As a consequence the recommended daily allowances can be met with even a modest intake of fruits and vegetables. The utilization of the vitamin is increased during pregnancy and lactation and in thyrotoxicosis, and absorption is decreased in diarrheal states and in achlorhydria.

Experimental depletion The total-body pool of vitamin C varies from 1.5 to 3 g. When a deficient diet is instituted, the pool is depleted at a constant rate that may be as high as 4 percent per day. In monkeys the major catabolic pathway involves oxidation of the alcohol at carbon 6 to an aldehyde and then to an acid. Because of differences in initial pool size and rates of turnover, differences in the completeness of deficiency in various experimental diets, and variation among normal subjects at the cellular or enzymatic level, the time required for development of symptoms ranges from 1 to 3 months in different studies. Manifestations of deficiency correlate better with the total pool size than with plasma or blood levels. The first symptoms (petechial hemorrhages and ecchymoses) develop when the pool size is less than 0.5 g; with further depletion (pool size 0.1 to 0.5 g) abnormalities include gum involvement, hyperkeratosis, congested hair follicles, arthralgias, Sjögren's syndrome, coiled hairs, and joint effusions. When depletion is extreme (pool size <0.1 g), dyspnea, edema, oliguria, and neuropathy supervene. Progress of the disease may then be rapid.

Symptoms do not improve until the normal pool is repleted, and the larger the therapeutic dose, the more rapid the repletion. However, with doses as small as 6.5 mg per day the body pool eventually returns to normal, and amelioration of symptoms follows.

Clinical deficiency Clinical scurvy now occurs for the most part in areas of urban poverty. An increased incidence occurs at 6 to 12 months of age in infants whose processed milk formulas are unsupplemented with citrus fruit or vegetables as a result of maternal error or neglect. Another peak occurs in middle and old age; edentulous men who live alone and cook for themselves are particularly prone to develop scurvy. Clinical scurvy is more severe than the experimental disease, doubtlessly because affected individuals usually have deficiencies of other dietary constituents as well and because the groups at risk (infants and the elderly) are especially vulnerable. The disorder has different clinical features in adults and children.

In adults the features include perifollicular hyperkeratotic papules in which hairs become fragmented and buried; perifollicular hemorrhages; purpura beginning on the backs of the lower extremities coalescing to become ecchymoses (Fig. 76-2); hemorrhage into the muscles of the arms and legs with secondary phlebothromboses; hemorrhages into joints; splinter hemorrhages in the nail beds; gum involvement (only in people with teeth) that includes swelling, friability, bleeding, secondary infection, and loosening of the teeth; poor healing of wounds and breakdown of recently healed wounds; petechial hemorrhages in the viscera; and emotional changes. Symptoms resembling those of Sjögren's syndrome may occur. Terminally,

icterus, edema, and fever are common, and convulsions, shock, and death may occur abruptly.

In infancy and childhood hemorrhage into the periosteum of long bones causes painful swellings and may result in epiphyseal separation. The sternum may sink inward, leaving a sharp elevation at the rib margins (scorbutic rosary). Purpura and ecchymoses may develop in the skin, and gum lesions occur if the teeth have erupted. Retrobulbar, subarachnoid, and intracerebral hemorrhages rapidly culminate in death if treatment is delayed.

Severe to moderate anemia is common both in children and in adults, is usually normochromic and normocytic, and is due to bleeding into tissues. The anemia may be macrocytic and/or megaloblastic (one-fifth of patients in one series). Many foods that contain vitamin C also contain folate, and diets that cause scurvy may also cause folate deficiency. However, ascorbic acid deficiency also results in an increased oxidation of formyl tetrahydrofolic acid to inactive folate metabolites and may cause a decrease in the active folate pool. Whether changes in iron distribution and storage are involved in the pathogenesis of the anemia is unclear. Whatever the mechanism, the anemia is corrected with refeeding and replenishment of vitamin C and the institution of a balanced diet.

In some hospitals platelet ascorbic acid levels are useful in diagnosing scurvy and are usually less than one-fourth of the normal value (52 ± 22 μg per 10^{10} platelets). Plasma levels of the vitamin correlate less well with the clinical state (Table 71-4). In infants x-ray changes of the bones may be diagnostic. Indirect bilirubin is frequently elevated. Capillary fragility is abnormal. The remainder of the laboratory tests are nondiagnostic.

Scurvy is potentially fatal; if the diagnosis is suspected, blood should be obtained, and ascorbic acid therapy should be instituted

FIGURE 76-2 *Hemorrhages and ecchymoses in a patient with scurvy. (Photograph, courtesy of Dr. Leonard L. Madison.)*

promptly. The usual dose in adults is 100 mg three to five times a day by mouth until 4 g has been administered, then 100 mg per day. In infants and children administration of 10 to 25 mg three times a day is adequate. A diet rich in vitamin C should be initiated simultaneously. Spontaneous bleeding usually ceases within 24 h, muscle and bone pains subside quickly, and the gums begin to heal within 2 to 3 days. Even large ecchymoses and hematomas resolve in 10 to 12 days, although pigmentary changes in areas of extensive hemorrhage may persist for months. Serum bilirubin becomes normal within 3 to 5 days, and the anemia is ordinarily corrected within 2 to 4 weeks.

VITAMIN A　Biochemistry　Vitamin A (retinol) can either be ingested or synthesized within the body from plant carotenoids (Fig. 76-1). Preformed vitamin A is present in animal tissues, and the best sources are liver, milk, and kidney, where it occurs largely in the form of fatty acid esters. The esters are hydrolyzed during digestion, absorbed in the free form, reesterified with fatty acids within the intestinal mucosa, and enter the circulation in association with lymph chylomicrons. The carotenoid substrates for synthesis of vitamin A, mainly β-carotenes, are widely distributed in plants. β-Carotene can either be absorbed intact or cleaved at the central double bond in the intestinal mucosa (or lumen) to form two molecules or retinaldehyde. Retinaldehyde is subsequently reduced by an aldehyde reductase to retinol. Retinol from whatever source is stored as retinyl esters in the parenchymal cells of the liver. The normal body retinol pool varies from 300 to 900 mg.

Prior to release from the liver retinyl esters are hydrolyzed, and the free alcohol is mobilized bound to a specific transport protein, retinol-binding protein (RBP), for transport to peripheral tissues. In vitamin A deficiency the release of RBP from the liver is inhibited, and the protein accumulates in liver; with repletion RBP is rapidly released from preformed stores. The pathway by which retinol is catabolized and excreted has not been defined; approximately equal amounts are excreted in the bile and urine.

Mechanism of action　The best-defined function of vitamin A is its role in vision; in the retina vitamin A constitutes the prosthetic group of a series of carotenoid proteins that provide the molecular basis for visual excitation. In addition, vitamin A is required for growth, reproduction, and the maintenance of life. Retinol-phosphate-mannose glycolipid is present in a variety of cell membranes, and the vitamin plays a primary role in sugar transfer reactions involved in the synthesis of glycoproteins. The importance of glycoprotein to every cell implies that this is an equally important function of the vitamin.

Requirements　The recommended daily allowances for vitamin A are listed in Tables 70-1 and 70-2. The assumed utilization efficiency for the conversion of β-carotene to vitamin A in the human is one-sixth (0.167). Other carotenoids with provitamin A activity have, on the average, one-half the activity of β-carotene. Pregnancy and disease states in which there is impaired absorption or storage, excessive utilization, or increased excretion of vitamin A may lead to increased requirements.

Experimental depletion　When experimental subjects are fed a diet deficient in both retinol and carotene, plasma levels fall to less than 10 μg/dL, and the body pool shrinks to less than one-half the control value. Deficiency is manifested by follicular hyperkeratosis, impaired dark adaptation, and abnormalities of the electroretinogram. These changes are corrected after supplementation with 150 μg of retinol or 300 μg of β-carotene per day.

Clinical deficiency　Endemic results from inadequate amounts of the vitamin and of the carotene provitamins in the diet and probably always occurs in conjunction with deficiency of other nutrients or complicating diseases. In some developing countries vitamin A deficiency is a major cause of blindness in the young as a consequence of failure to incorporate green leafy vegetables or other sources of the provitamin or vitamin into the diet. Vitamin A deficiency may also accompany protein-calorie malnutrition, and here the deficiency

is due in part to a defective release mechanism from the liver secondary to inadequate retinol-binding protein. In developed nations vitamin A deficiency is usually due either to intestinal malabsorption (as in sprue or after intestinal bypass surgery), abnormal storage (liver disease), or enhanced destruction or excretion of the vitamin (proteinuria). Vitamin A deficiency has also occurred in patients receiving total parenteral nutrition because of loss of vitamin A after prolonged storage of intravenous fluid.

Night blindness is the earliest symptom of deficiency, followed by degenerative changes in the retina. The bulbar conjunctiva becomes dry (xerosis), and small gray plaques with foamy surfaces develop (Bitôt's spots). These early lesions are reversible with vitamin A. The more serious effects of vitamin A deficiency are ulceration and necrosis of the cornea (keratomalacia), leading to perforation, endophthalmitis, and blindness. Patients may also have dryness and hyperkeratosis of the skin.

Vitamin A levels in plasma are not reliable for the assessment of stores in individual cases. Measurements of dark adaptation, rod scotometry, and electroretinography are reliable indicators of vitamin A stores but require trained personnel and expensive equipment; consequently, the diagnosis is usually based upon a high index of suspicion in malnourished children or in patients with known predisposing factors for its development.

Night blindness and the milder conjunctival changes respond well to 30,000 IU of vitamin A daily for a week. Corneal damage constitutes a therapeutic emergency, and the usual treatment is 20,000 IU per kilogram of body weight per day for 5 days.

VITAMIN E　Biochemistry　Eight naturally occurring tocopherols possess vitamin E activity. The structure of alphatocopherol, the most widely distributed and most active of the tocopherols, is shown in Fig. 76-1. The vitamin is absorbed from the gastrointestinal tract by a mechanism similar to that for other fat-soluble vitamins and enters the bloodstream via the lymph, associated first with chylomicrons and then with plasma betalipoproteins. Indeed, plasma levels correlate closely with plasma lipid levels. The vitamin is stored in all tissues, and the tissue stores can protect against vitamin deficiency for long periods. Approximately three-fourths of the vitamin is excreted in bile, and the balance is excreted as glucuronides in urine. Metabolites with quinone structures (including one similar to ubiquinone) are present in tissues.

Mechanism of action　The vitamin probably acts as an antioxidant rather than as a specific cofactor. In so acting it presumably inhibits oxidation of essential cellular constituents and prevents the formation of toxic oxidation products. Other antioxidants such as selenium, sulfur-containing amino acids, and the ubiquinone group can reverse the symptoms of vitamin E deficiency in animals.

Requirements　The estimated daily requirement is 10 to 30 mg per day (Tables 70-1 and 70-2). Diets containing large amounts of polyunsaturated fatty acids increase and diets containing antioxidants decrease the requirement. The vitamin is widely distributed in food, so that a primary deficiency state has never been recognized in otherwise healthy children or adults. Newborn infants have plasma concentrations about one-fifth that of maternal levels, implying poor placental transfer, but human milk (in contrast to cow's milk) has sufficient levels to meet the requirements in infants.

Experimental depletion　In long-term studies of vitamin E depletion vitamin E concentrations in plasma declined significantly only after months on a deficient diet. No manifestations of the depletion were detected in normal volunteers, making it difficult to establish that tocopherol is a human vitamin.

Clinical deficiency　In the appropriate clinical setting vitamin E deficiency is associated with a discrete syndrome. Intestinal malabsorption can cause deficiency of all fat-soluble vitamins including vitamin E, and children with chronic cholestatic liver disease appear to be particularly susceptible, due to a combination of malabsorption of vitamin E and trapping of the vitamin in plasma by the associated hyperlipemia, so that tissue stores may be depleted despite a normal tocopherol level in serum. Indeed, the ratio of serum vitamin E to total serum lipid is the preferred index for assessing vitamin E status. The manifestations of deficiency include areflexia, gait disturbance, decreased proprioceptive and vibratory sensation, and paresis of gaze and are associated with degeneration of the posterior columns of the spinal cord, selective loss of large-caliber, myelinated axons in peripheral nerves, and appearance of spheroids in the gracile and cuneate nuclei of the brain. Treatment (50 to 100 IU per day by mouth) is most effective when initiated early in the course of the disease.

VITAMIN K Vitamin K consists of a quinone ring attached to a side chain (labeled *R* in Fig. 76-1) that varies depending on the source of the vitamin. Vitamin K_1 (phylloquinone) is present in most edible vegetables, particularly in green leaves, and vitamin K_2 is produced by intestinal bacteria. The many compounds with vitamin K activity are structurally related to the simpler compound, 2-methyl-1,4-naphthoquinone (menadione). Menadione is formed in the gut by the removal of the side chain from the vitamin by intestinal bacteria. After absorption, menadione is converted in the body to the active menaquinone. The vitamin is a component of a specialized microsomal enzyme system that effects the posttranslational γ carboxylation of glutamic acid in proteins of the plasma, bone, kidney, and urine, including the precursor proteins for the clotting factors VII, IX, X, and possibly V. Death from hemorrhage in deficiency states ensues before deficiency of the other carboxylated proteins becomes manifest.

Under ordinary circumstances about 80 percent of vitamin K is absorbed from the small bowel into the intestinal lymph. Because the naturally occurring forms of vitamin K are fat-soluble and are poorly stored in the body, deficiency can occur in association with diseases that interfere with fat absorption. In addition, long-term treatment with antimicrobial drugs may temporarily eliminate intestinal bacterial as a source for vitamin K. The warfarin anticoagulant drugs induce hypoprothrombinemia by inhibiting the γ carboxylation of the precursor protein.

Newborn infants tend to be deficient in vitamin K and have low plasma levels of several coagulation factors in the prothrombin complex. Such deficiencies result from minimal stores of vitamin K at birth, lack of an established intestinal flora, and a limited dietary intake of the vitamin.

Routine determination of prothrombin should be performed prior to surgical procedures or delivery. Subjects with levels below 70 percent of normal should receive therapy with vitamin K. Vitamin K deficiency can be separated from hypoprothrombinemia of liver disease by measurement of the noncarboxylated prothrombin precursor that accumulates in plasma in the vitamin deficiency.

VITAMIN EXCESS

Fat-soluble vitamins are stored to a variable extent in the body and hence are more likely to cause adverse effects when taken in excess; excess states for vitamins D (see Chap. 337) and A are particularly well characterized. Water-soluble vitamins are readily excreted in the urine and stored only to a limited extent. Consequently, toxicity states for these vitamins only occur when large amounts are taken for prolonged periods.

VITAMIN A AND CAROTENES Carotenemia Carotenemia results from excessive intake of vitamin A precursors in foods, principally carrots. Excess carotene is not injurious apart from the cosmetic effect; the fact that carotenemia does not cause hypervitaminosis A indicates that the conversion of carotene to vitamin A must be regulated. Carotenemia is manifested by yellowing of the skin with greatest intensity on the palms and soles and by a corresponding yellowness of serum. The yellowing of the skin can be distinguished from jaundice in that the scleras remain white. Hypothyroid patients are particularly susceptible. The omission of carrots from the diet leads to the rapid disappearance of the pigmentation. Discoloration of the skin can also result from the consumption of excessive amounts of other colored fruits and vegetables.

Vitamin A toxicity Hypervitaminosis A can result from accidental overingestion by hunters or explorers (polar bear liver), as the result of food faddism (usually caused by overly solicitous parents), or as a side effect of inappropriate therapy. Acute toxicity from a single massive dose consists of abdominal pain, nausea, vomiting, headache, dizziness, sluggishness, papilledema, and in infants a bulging fontanel followed within a few days by generalized desquamation of the skin and recovery. Chronic toxicity occurs following ingestion of 40,000 units or more daily for protracted periods and is characterized by bone and joint pain, hyperostoses, hair loss, dryness and fissures of the lips, anorexia, benign intracranial hypertension, low-grade fever, weight loss, and hepatosplenomegaly. The only diagnostic laboratory finding is elevation of the vitamin in serum, chiefly in the form of retinyl esters. The concentration of retinol-binding protein is normal, and the excess vitamin A circulates in association with lipoprotein. Relief is prompt on withdrawal of the vitamin from the diet.

VITAMIN E Relatively large doses of vitamin E have been taken by some for extended periods without causing apparent harm. In others, a variety of nonspecific complaints have been reported including malaise, gastrointestinal complaint, headaches, and possibly hypertension. However, true toxicity appears to occur in two situations—in subjects receiving oral anticoagulants and in premature infants. In large amounts, vitamin E can apparently antagonize vitamin K and inhibit prothrombin time; this phenomenon results in a marked potentiation of oral anticoagulants. Premature infants given parenteral vitamin E are reported to have developed ascites associated with hepatosplenomegaly, cholestatic jaundice, azotemia, and thrombocytopenia.

VITAMIN K Dietary supplements high in vitamin K can block the effects of oral anticoagulants and when given to pregnant women can cause jaundice in the newborn.

PYRIDOXINE Most adults can consume up to 10 times the recommended daily allowance of 2 mg pyridoxine per day without adverse effects. However, severe peripheral neuropathies have developed after ingestion of several grams per day for prolonged periods; symptoms include ataxia, perioral numbness, and clumsiness of the hands and feet, and the findings include loss of position and vibration sense without impairment of reflexes or sensory function. Recovery is slow after ingestion ceases. Lower doses (25 mg per day) can antagonize the effects of levodopa in Parkinson's disease and decrease the anticonvulsant effects of phenytoin.

VITAMIN C Vitamin C is widely used in megavitamin therapy because of the claim that large doses of the vitamin (a gram or greater per day) are effective in preventing or minimizing the symptoms of the common cold. However, in controlled studies, no significant differences in occurrence, severity, or duration have been demonstrated in subjects treated with a placebo compared with the vitamin. Use of the vitamin in this way is unwarranted and probably unwise. The long-term use of ascorbic acid in these doses can interfere with the absorption of vitamin B_{12}, cause uricosuria, and predispose to formation of oxalate kidney stones. In addition, large doses enhance the development of metabolizing enzymes in the fetus and may cause rebound scurvy in the offspring of mothers who have ingested large amounts of the vitamin during pregnancy. However, pharmacologic doses (200 mg daily) may correct leukocyte abnormalities in patients with the Chédiak-Higashi syndrome (see Chap. 56).

NIACIN Large doses of niacin have been used for treatment of hypercholesterolemia and occasionally for other purposes. The vitamin causes release of histamine, which in turn can cause severe flushing, pruritis, and gastrointestinal disturbances and may aggravate asthma. Acanthosis nigricans may occur. In doses of 3 g per day niacin has been reported to cause elevation of serum uric acid and of fasting glucose.

REFERENCES

Niacin deficiency

BOLLET AJ: The conquest of pellagra. Resid Staff Physician 28:31, May 1982

CASTIELLO RJ, LYNCH PJ: Pellagra and the carcinoid syndrome. Arch Dermatol 105:574, 1972

DARBY WJ et al: Niacin. Nutr Rev 33:289, 1977

DE LANGE DJ, JOUBERT CP: Assessment of nicotinic acid status of population groups. Am J Clin Nutr 15:169, 1964

GOLDSMITH GA: Experimental niacin deficiency. J Am Dietetic Assoc 32:312, 1956

GOPALAN C, RAO KSJ: Pellagra and amino acid imbalance, in Vitamins and Hormones, PL Munson et al (eds). New York, Academic, 1975, vol 33, p 505

JEPSON JB: Hartnup disease, in The Metabolic Basis of Inherited Disease, 4th ed, JB Stanbury et al (eds). New York, McGraw-Hill, 1978, p 1563

SCHOENTAL R: Mouldy grain and aetiology of pellagra: The role of toxic metabolites of Fusarium, Biochem Soc Trans 8:147, 1980

Thiamine deficiency

BLASS JP, GIBSON GE: Abnormality of a thiamine-requiring enzyme in patients with Wernicke-Korsakoff syndrome. N Engl J Med 297:1367, 1977

BROWN GM: Biogenesis and metabolism of thiamine, in Metabolic Pathways, 3d ed, DM Greenberg (ed), Academic, New York, 1970, p 369

HOYUMPA AM: Mechanisms of thiamine deficiency in chronic alcoholism. Am J Clin Nutr 33:2750, 1980

KAWAI C et al: Reappearance of beriberi heart disease in Japan. Am J Med 69:383, 1980

KOZAM RL et al: Cardiovascular beriberi. Am J Cardiology 30:418, 1972

KURIYAMA M et al: Blood vitamin B_1, transketolase, and thiamine pyrophosphate (TPP) effect in beriberi patients. Clin Chim Acta 108:159, 1980

PINCUS JH et al: Thiamine derivatives in subacute necrotizing encephalomyelopathy. Pediatrics 51:716, 1973

SCRIVER CR: Vitamin-responsive inborn errors of metabolism. Metabolism 22:1319, 1973

VICTOR M et al: The Wernicke-Korsakoff Syndrome, Philadelphia, Davis, 1971

ZIPORIN ZZ et al: Excretion of thiamine and its metabolites in the urine of young adult males receiving restricted intakes of the vitamin. J Nutr 85:287, 1965

Pyridoxine deficiency

FRIMPTER GW et al: Vitamin B_6-dependency syndromes: New horizons in nutrition. Am J Clin Nutr 22:794, 1969

GERSHOFF SN: Vitamin B_6, in Nutrition Reviews' Present Knowledge in Nutrition, 4th ed, DM Hegsted et al (eds). Washington, DC, The Nutrition Foundation, 1976, p 149

HARRIS JW, HORRIGAN DL: Pyridoxine-responsive anemia-prototype and variations on the theme, in Vitamins and Hormones, RS Harris et al (eds). New York, Academic, 1964, vol 22, p 721

JAFFE IA: The antivitamin B_6 effect of penicillamine: Clinical and immunological implications, in Advances in Biochemical Psychopharmacology, MS Ebodi et al (eds). New York, Raven, 1972, vol 4

LUHBY AL et al: Vitamin B_6 metabolism in users of oral contraceptive agents: I. Abnormal urinary xanthurenic acid excretion and its correction by pyridoxine. Am J Clin Nutr 24:684, 1971

MUDD SH: Pyridoxine-responsive genetic disease. Fed Proc 30:970, 1971

SAUBERLICH HE et al: Biochemical assessment of the nutritional status of vitamin B_6 in the human. Am J Clin Nutr 25:629, 1972

Riboflavin deficiency

MERRILL AH JR et al: Formation and mode of action of flavoproteins. Ann Rev Nutr 1:281, 1981

PINTO J et al: Inhibition of riboflavin metabolism in rat tissue by chlorpromazine, imipramine, and amitriptyline. J Clin Invest 67:1500, 1981

RIVLIN RS: Hormones, drugs, and riboflavin. Nutr Rev 37:241, 1979

Ascorbic acid deficiency

BAKER EM et al: Ascorbic acid metabolism in man. Am J Clin Nutr 19:371, 1966

BARNES MJ, KODICEK E: Biological hydroxylations and ascorbic acid, in Vitamins and Hormones, P Munson et al (eds). New York, Academic, 1972, vol 30, p 1

BARNESS LA: Nutritional aspects of vegetarianism, health foods and fad diets. Nutr Rev 59:153, 1977

BOXER LA et al: Correction of leucocyte function in Chédiak-Higashi syndrome by ascrobate. N Engl J Med 295:1041, 1976

HODGES RE: Clinical manifestations of ascorbic acid deficiency in man. Am J Clin Nutr 24:432, 1971

SATO P, UDENFRIEND S: Studies on ascorbic acid related to the genetic basis of scurvy, in Vitamins and Hormones, P Munson et al (eds). New York, Academic, 1978, vol 36, p 33

TOLBERT BM et al: New information on synthesis and metabolism of ascorbic acid. Nutr Rev 35:22, 1977

VILTER RW: Effects of ascorbic acid deficiency in man, in The Vitamins, WH Sebrell Jr et al (eds). New York, Academic, 1967, vol 1, p 457

WALLERSTEIN RO, WALLERSTEIN RO JR: Scurvy. Sem Hematol 13:211, 1976

Vitamin A deficiency

DELUCA LM: The direct involvement of vitamin A in glycosyl transfer reactions of mammalian membranes, in Vitamins and Hormones, PL Munson et al (eds). New York, Academic, 1977, vol 35, p 1

HOWARD L et al: Vitamin A deficiency from long term parenteral nutrition. Ann Intern Med 93:576, 1980

SAUBERLICH HE et al: Vitamin A metabolism and requirements in the human studied with the use of labeled retinol, in Vitamins and Hormones, RS Harris et al (eds). New York, Academic, 1974, vol 32

SMITH FR, GOODMAN DS: Vitamin A transport in human vitamin A toxicity. N Engl J Med 294:805, 1976

————, ————: Vitamin A metabolism and transport, in Present Knowledge in Nutrition, 4th ed, DM Hegsted et al (eds). Washington, DC, The Nutrition Foundation, 1976

SOMER A et al: Clinical characteristics of vitamin A responsive and nonresponsive Bitot's spots. Am J Ophthalmol 90:160, 1980

SRIKANTIA SG: Human vitamin A deficiency, in World Review of Nutrition and Dietetics, GH Bounre (ed). Basel, S Karger, 1975, vol 20, p 185

WALD G: Molecular basis of visual excitation. Science 162:230, 1968

Vitamin E deficiency

GUGGENHEIM MA et al: Progressive neuromuscular disease in children with chronic cholestasis and vitamin E deficiency: Diagnosis and treatment with alpha tocopherol. J Pediatr 100:51, 1982

HORWITT MK: Interrelations between vitamin E and polyunsaturated fatty acids in adult men, in Vitamins and Hormones, GF Marrian and KV Thimann (eds). New York, Academic, 1962, vol 20, p 541

ROSENBLUM JL et al: A progressive neurologic syndrome in children with chronic liver disease. N Engl J Med 304:503, 1981

SOKOL RJ et al: Vitamin E deficiency with normal serum vitamin E concentrations in children with chronic cholestasis. N Engl J Med 310:1209, 1984

———— et al Mechanism causing vitamin E deficiency during chronic childhood cholestasis. Gastroenterology 85:1172, 1983

Vitamin K deficiency

BERTINA RM et al: New method for the rapid detection of vitamin K deficiency. Clin Chim Acta 105:93, 1980

DOISY EA JR, MATSCHINER JT: Biochemistry of vitamin K, in Fat-Soluble Vitamins, RA Morton (ed). Elmsford, NY, Pergamon, 1970, vol 9, p 293

OLSON RE, SUTTIE JW: Vitamin K and α-carboxyglutamate biosynthesis, in Vitamins and Hormones, PL Munson et al (eds). New York, Academic, 1977, vol 35, p 59

SHEARER MJ et al: Studies on the absorption and metabolism of phylloquinone (vitamin K) in man, in Vitamins and Hormones, RS Harris et al (eds). New York, Academic, 1974, vol 32, p 513

SUTTIE JW: Vitamin K Metabolism and Vitamin K-Dependent Proteins. Baltimore, University Park Press, 1980

Vitamin excess

ALHADEFF L: Toxic effects of water-soluble vitamins. Nutr Rev 42:33, 1984

CHALMERS TC: Effects of ascorbic acid on the common cold. Am J Med 58:532, 1975

CORRIGAN JJ JR: The effect of vitamin E on warfarin-induced vitamin K deficiency. Ann NY Acad Sci 82:361, 1982

HERBERT V: The vitamin craze: Arch Intern Med 140:173, 1980

LORCH V et al: Unusual syndrome with fatalities among premature infants: Association with a new intravenous vitamin E product. Morb Mort Week Rep 33:198, 1984

LOMBAERT A, CARTON H: Benign intracranial hypertension due to A-hypervitaminosis in adults and adolescents. Eur Neurol 14:340, 1976

ROBERTS HJ: Perspective on vitamin E therapy. JAMA 246:129, 1981

SCHAUMBURG H et al: Sensory neuropathy from pyridoxine abuse: A new megavitamin syndrome. N Engl J Med 309:445, 1983

STEIN HB et al: Ascorbic acid–induced uricosuria: A consequence of megavitamin therapy. Ann Intern Med 84:385, 1976

77   DISTURBANCES IN TRACE ELEMENT METABOLISM

KENNETH H. FALCHUK

CLASSIFICATION AND FUNCTIONS   The "trace elements" comprise metals in biologic fluids at concentrations below one microgram per gram of wet weight. Most are essential nutrients for human beings (Table 77-1). Others (As, Ni, Sn, V, Si) are essential for some plants and/or vertebrates including mammals and may be required by humans. The functions of trace elements and of other, more abundant metals (Na, K, Ca, Mg) are determined, in part, by their charges, mobilities, and binding constants to biologic ligands. Elements in one group (Na, K) bind weakly to negatively charged ligands and can cross cellular membranes without major impediment. They are used by living systems as charge carriers to conduct electric impulses along nerves, etc. Those in a second group (Mg, Ca) form moderately stable but not tight complexes with enzymes, nucleic

TABLE 77-1 Requirements and functions of trace elements in humans

Element	Requirements, mg/day*	Amount† Total, g per 70 kg body weight	Blood μg/dL	Serum μg/dL	Selected biochemical functions	Enzymes Class	Example
Fe	10–20	4.0	45000	100	Oxygen transport	Oxidoreductases	Cytochrome oxidase
Zn	15–20	3.0	800	100	Nucleic acid and protein synthesis and degradation, alcohol metabolism	Transferases, hydrolases, lyases, isomerases, ligases, oxidoreductases	Carboxypeptidases, alcohol dehydrogenases, alkaline phosphatases
Cu	2–6	0.25	100	100	Hemoglobin synthesis, connective tissue metabolism, bone development	Oxidoreductases	Superoxide dismutase, ferroxidase (ceruloplasmin)
Co	0.0001	1.1	0.02	0.0007	Methionine metabolism	Transferases	Homocysteine methyltransferase
Mn	2–5	0.02	0.09	0.06	Oxidative phosphorylation; fatty acid, mucopolysaccharide, and cholesterol metabolism	Oxidoreductases, hydrolases, ligases	Diamine oxidase, pyruvate carboxylase
Mo	0.15–0.5	0.07	1.5	0.07	Xanthine metabolism	Oxidoreductases	Xanthine oxidase
Se	0.05–0.2	(−)	20	13	Antioxidant	Oxidoreductases, transferases	Glutathione peroxidase
Ni	(−)	(−)	2.5	0.1	?Stabilizing RNA structure	Oxidoreductases, hydrolases	Urease
Cr	0.005–0.2	0.0006	(−)	0.02	?Binding of insulin to cells, glucose metabolism		

* Requirements may differ for different age groups and physiologic states, e.g., pregnancy.
† Reported normal values vary owing to differences in sample preparation, analytical instruments, and small quantities present in biologic materials.
(−), reported values variable or not available.

acids, and other ligands. They act as biochemical "triggers," altering and/or controlling the functions of these molecules, e.g., Ca affects muscle contraction and relaxation (Chap. 357). Those in a third group (Fe, Zn, Cu, and others) form strong, static complexes with and become integral functional components of enzymes (Table 77-1).

METAL DEFICIENCY OR TOXICITY All metals can cause disease through deficiency, imbalance, or toxicity. Deficiency usually results when dietary intake is inadequate or when intake is adequate but other conditioning factors come into play. Deficiencies can be caused by metal malabsorption in chronic diarrheal diseases, surgical resection of the small intestine, or formation of metal complexes with dietary components that are not readily absorbed, e.g., between phytates and Zn. Deficiency states can also result from increased losses through urine, pancreatic juice, or other exocrine secretions or from metabolic imbalances produced by antagonistic or synergistic interactions between metals. Large amounts of Ca, for example, decrease the absorption of and induce deficiency of Zn. Similarly, Mo and Cu compete with each other; excessive Mo in cattle leads to Cu deficiency characterized by diarrhea and wasting. Proven manifestations of trace element deficiencies in humans, except for iron, were previously rare but have been recognized more frequently with the use of total parenteral nutrition (TPN) (Chap. 75). Clinical criteria for the recognition of deficiency states include decreases in metal content of whole blood, serum, hair and/or other accessible fluids and tissues, changes in the activities of metalloenzymes, and characteristic signs and symptoms (Table 77-2).

Toxic effects are dependent on the chemical form, the amount ingested, the route of entry into the body, the biologic ligands associated with the metal, the tissue distribution, the concentration achieved, and the excretion rate. Mechanisms of toxicity include inhibition of enzyme activity by binding to essential amino acid residues, alterations in nucleic acid function and structure, alteration in protein synthesis, effects on membrane permeability, and inhibition of phosphorylation, among others. Metal toxicity in patients undergoing chronic renal dialysis is important because of the frequency and severity of the resulting problems and because of the number of metals involved, e.g., Al, Zn, Cu, Ni, and Sn (Chap. 221). For example, even when it is present only in trace amounts in dialysis fluids, Al is readily absorbed into blood and accumulates in brain,

bone, and erythroid tissues, causing disabling neurologic, skeletal, and hematologic disorders. These include malaise, memory loss, asterixis, dementia, twitches, and other manifestations of metabolic encephalopathy including seizures and death. Osteomalacia unresponsive to vitamin D, fractures, muscular pain, weakness, and anemia may occur. Documentation of increase in plasma Al concentration following deferoxamine administration is diagnostic.

DISORDERS OF METABOLISM OF SPECIFIC METALS Zinc Zn absorption in the small intestine is decreased by fibers, phytate, phosphate, Ca, and Cu. In contrast, amino acids, peptides, iodoquinol and other chelating agents increase Zn absorption. Excretion of Zn occurs principally through secretions of the pancreas and intestine. Nearly 99 percent of total-body Zn is inside cells, the remainder is in plasma and extracellular fluids. Serum Zn, approximately 70 percent of which is loosely bound to albumin and other proteins, is the source of metal for cellular needs. Serum Zn content does not normally vary, but it decreases when intake or absorption is reduced (e.g., in regional enteritis) or when urinary losses are increased (e.g., in nephrotic syndrome; in cirrhosis of the liver or other hypoalbuminemic states; during the administration of penicillamine or other chelating agents; in high catabolic states as after trauma, burns, or surgery; and in hemolytic anemias and sickle cell disease). Plasma Zn also decreases in the acute phase of myocardial infarction, infections, malignancies, and hepatitis and other diseases. The decreases may be due to redistribution from plasma to tissues and are probably mediated by ACTH, cortisol, and/or a leukocyte protein (leukocyte endogenous mediator). Clinical deficiency may follow these decreases in serum content. The Zn requirement of the developing fetus, pregnant woman, and growing child or adolescent is higher than that of adult men or nonpregnant women. Therefore, the former groups are more susceptible to Zn depletion. Zn deficiency in pregnant animals can lead to fetal Zn deficiency, which results in high mortality rates or congenital malformations of nearly all organ systems. Zinc deficiency has not been described in pregnant women, but has been reported in adolescents who eat dirt, in patients who receive TPN without supplemental Zn (see Chap. 75), and in patients with the autosomal recessive defect acrodermatitis enteropathica. In the latter disease, deficiency in plasma Zn may be the consequence of a defect in Zn absorption. The onset of symptoms often occurs when an affected infant is weaned from human to cow's milk. Zn may also play a role in the maintenance of normal taste and in wound healing.

Tissues with a high cellular turnover, including skin, gastrointestinal mucosa, chondrocytes, spermatogonia, and thymocytes are characteristically affected (Table 77-2). The dermatologic abnormalities (hyperkeratosis, parakeratosis, acrodermatitis, and alopecia) call attention to the possibility of Zn deficiency. The usual distribution of the keratotic lesions is in areas that are readily traumatized (elbows, knees), but the lesions can develop in other areas as well. The keratotic lesions can become pustular or crusting, red, scaly plaques. Superinfections are common with either fungi or bacteria.

Toxicity follows inhalation of Zn fumes (by welders), oral ingestion, or intravenous administration. Inhalation of high concentrations of zinc oxide fumes leads to an acute illness called *metal-fume fever* or *brass chills*, manifested by fever, chills, excessive salivation, headaches, cough, and leukocytosis. Dialysis fluids can be contaminated with Zn from the adhesive plaster used on the dialysis coils or from galvanized pipes. The toxic syndrome associated with hemodialysis is characterized by anemia, fever, and central nervous system disturbances (Table 77-2). Toxic amounts of Zn decrease chemotaxis, phagocytosis, pinocytosis, and platelet aggregation.

Copper   The liver, kidney, heart, and brain contain the highest amounts of Cu. Over 90 percent of plasma Cu is associated with ceruloplasmin, while 60 percent of that in red blood cells is bound to superoxide dismutase. The major excretory pathway is through the bile. The serum Cu concentration is normally constant. Increases occur in patients with acute myocardial infarction, leukemia, solid tumors, infections, portal and biliary cirrhosis, hemochromatosis, thyrotoxicosis, and connective tissue disorders. The consequences of the increases are unknown. Conversely, decreases occur in the nephrotic syndrome, kwashiorkor, the hepatolenticular degeneration of Wilson's disease (see Chap. 311), severe diarrheal diseases with malabsorption, and other conditions associated with increased excretion or decreased synthesis of ceruloplasmin. Premature infants who are fed diets deficient in Cu develop decreased serum ceruloplasmin and Cu levels, anemia, osteopenia, skin and hair depigmentation, and psychomotor retardation. Cu deficiency in subjects receiving TPN causes anemia and neutropenia.

A more complex disorder of Cu metabolism occurs in Menkes' disease, an X-linked recessive disorder. Intestinal Cu uptake is normal, and tissue Cu content varies; that of intestinal, kidney, and skin (fibroblast) cells is normal or high, while that of serum, liver, brain, and (likely) vascular cells is low. Ceruloplasmin content and the activities of some Cu enzymes (e.g., connective tissue amine oxidases) also are decreased. The clinical picture is similar to that of nutritional Cu deficiency in animals except that anemia does not occur (Table 77-2). The patients have kinky hair, and decreased amounts of mature collagen and elastin cause dissecting aneurysms, sudden cardiac rupture, emphysema, and osteoporosis. Death usually occurs in the first 5 years of life.

Excessive oral intake of Cu or hemodialysis with water contaminated with Cu is toxic. The acute symptoms include hemolytic anemia, nausea, vomiting, and diarrhea. The renal and hepatic failure and the central nervous system disorders that eventually develop (Table 77-2) are typical of the Cu toxicity syndrome in hepatolenticular degeneration (Wilson's disease). (See Chap. 311.)

Cobalt   Co is a component of vitamin B_{12}, and deficiency syndromes are those associated with deficiency of the vitamin (see Chap. 286). Pharmacologic doses of Co induce erythropoiesis. Chronic administration blocks iodine uptake by the thyroid, resulting in development of goiter.

Cardiomyopathy, congestive heart failure with pericardial effusions, polycythemia, thyroid enlargement, and neurologic abnormalities have been reported as manifestations to Co toxicity in drinkers of beer to which the metal had been added as a foam stabilizer. Co accumulates in the heart, forms a complex with lipoic acid, and interferes with decarboxylation reactions critical to both pyruvate and fatty acid metabolism.

Manganese   Mn acts both as an activator of enzymes and as a component of metalloenzymes (Table 77-1). Defects of the skeletal, central nervous, and gonadal systems occur in Mn deficiency in animals. Humans obtain sufficient Mn throughout normal dietary intake so that a deficiency syndrome is rare. In one reported instance an increase in prothrombin time, unresponsive to Vitamin K, was noted. In serum, Mn is bound to transmanganin. Mn is excreted primarily in bile and pancreatic secretions.

Serum Mn increases following myocardial infarction and decreases for unknown reasons in children with convulsive disorders. Miners who inhale large quantities of Mn dust over long periods of time develop asthenia, anorexia, apathy, headache, impotence, leg cramps, speech disturbances, and occasionally even more severe toxic symptoms (Table 77-2).

TABLE 77-2   Disorders of metal metabolism in humans

Element	Deficiency	Toxicity*
Fe	Anemia	Hepatic failure, diabetes, testicular atrophy, arthritis, cardiomyopathy, peripheral neuropathy, hyperpigmentation
Zn	Growth retardation, alopecia, dermatitis, diarrhea, immunologic dysfunction, failure to thrive, psychological disturbances, gonadal atrophy, impaired spermatogenesis, congenital malformations.	Gastric ulcer, pancreatitis lethargy, anemia, fever, nausea, vomiting. respiratory distress, pulmonary fibrosis
Cu	Anemia, growth retardation, defective keratinization and pigmentation of hair, hypothermia, degenerative changes in aortic elastin, mental deterioration, scurvy-like changes in skeleton	Hepatitis, cirrhosis, tremor, mental deterioration, Kayser-Fleischer rings, hemolytic anemia, renal dysfunction (Fanconi-like syndrome)
Mn	Bleeding disorder (increased prothrombin time)	Encephalitis-like syndrome, Parkinson-like syndrome, psychosis, pneumoconiosis
Co	Anemia (B_{12} deficiency)	Cardiomyopathy, goiter
Mo	? Esophageal cancer	? Hyperuricemia
Cr	? Impairment of glucose tolerance	Renal failure, dermatitis (occupational), pulmonary cancer
Se	Cardiomyopathy, congestive heart failure, striated muscle degeneration	Alopecia, abnormal nails, emotional lability, lassitude, garlic odor to breath
Ni	?	Dermatitis (occupational), lung and nasal carcinomas, liver necrosis, pulmonary inflammation
Si	? Impaired early bone development	Pulmonary inflammation, granuloma, fibrosis
F	? Impaired bone and dental structure	Motted dental enamel, nausea, abdominal pain, vomiting, diarrhea, tetany, cardiovascular collapse

* Symptoms are dependent on route of entry and tissue distribution (see text).

Selenium Se is a component of glutathione peroxidase and plays a critical role in the control of oxygen metabolism, particularly in catalyzing the breakdown of H_2O_2. The metal is required for the growth of human fibroblasts and other cells in tissue culture. Furthermore, Se cures or prevents Keshan disease, a syndrome that is endemic to Keshan Province in China where the soil may be deficient in the metal. Keshan disease is characterized by multifocal myocardial necrosis and reduced blood and serum Se content. The clinical severity varies from severe arrhythmias and cardiogenic shock to a mild form with cardiac enlargement as the only significant finding. Peripheral myopathies may develop as a consequence of muscle degeneration (Table 77-2). Children and women of child-bearing age are particularly susceptible. Se protects animals from a number of carcinogenic chemicals and viral agents; a role in human cancer prevention is not established. Se binds Cd, Hg, and other metals and mitigates their toxic effects, even though the measurable levels of the metals remain elevated.

Se toxicity occurs in animals, but humans who have consumed vegetables grown in soil containing high selenium content have not become ill. Se poisoning has been reported due to ingestion of water containing large amounts of the metal.

Other trace elements *Silicon* is present in bone and skin and may play a role in the cross-linkage of collagen. Deficiency in animals results in decreased growth, abnormal early bone development, and decreased hexosamine content of epiphyses and epiphyseal plates. No instance of deficiency in humans has been described. Inhalation of fine particles of SiO_2 causes granuloma formation and chronic fibrosis (silicosis) of the lungs (see Chap. 204).

Fluoride is a constituent of teeth and bone. It prevents dental caries, and its use in patients with osteoporosis has resulted in increased mineralized bone (see Chap. 339). Complications of long-term ingestion by such patients include calcification of bony ligaments and tendons. Chronic intake of fluorides also causes fluorosis, a syndrome characterized by weakness, weight loss, anemia, brittle bones, and mottling of teeth (if taken during stages of enamel formation). Acute ingestion of toxic amounts, as found in some insect poisons, causes severe abdominal pain, nausea, vomiting, diarrhea, and hypocalcemia. Eventually, tetany and cardiorespiratory arrest occur.

A deficiency of any one of *arsenic, nickel, tin,* and *vanadium* causes pathologic manifestations in plants and some vertebrates. Their roles in human health are undefined.

REFERENCES

FALCHUK KH: Effect of acute disease and ACTH on serum zinc proteins. N Engl J Med 296:1129, 1977

KARCIOULU ZA, SARPER RM: *Zinc and Copper in Medicine,* Springfield, Ill., Charles C Thomas, 1980

Metabolic and physiological consequences of trace element deficiency in animals and man. Philos Trans R Soc Lond [Biol] 294:1, 1981

MILLINER DS et al: Use of the deferoxamine infusion test in the diagnosis of aluminum-related osteodystrophy. Ann Intern Med 101:775, 1984

PRASAD AS: *Trace Elements in Human Health and Disease.* New York, Academic, 1976, vol II

REINHOLD JG: Trace elements—A selective survey. Clin Chem 21:476, 1975

TING-KAI L, VALLEE BL: The biochemical and nutritional roles of other trace elements, in *Modern Nutrition in Health and Disease,* 6th ed, RS Goodhart and ME Shils (eds). Philadelphia, Lea and Febiger, 1980

UNDERWOOD EJ: *Trace Elements in Human and Animal Nutrition,* 3d ed. New York, Academic, 1971

WILLIAMS RJP: The Tilden lecture. Q Rev Chem Soc (Lond) 24:331, 1970

section 5 Neoplastic diseases

78 PRINCIPLES OF NEOPLASIA

JOHN MENDELSOHN

INTRODUCTION The last few years have witnessed remarkable progress in understanding the biologic and biochemical bases for cancer. This is not to imply that the problem of neoplastic disease is solved. Gains in the treatment of cancer in adults have been gradual and have focused upon those malignancies characterized by unusual sensitivity to radiation and chemotherapy. These include primarily acute myelocytic leukemia, the lymphoproliferative malignancies, testicular cancer, and breast cancer. New treatment modalities involving immunotherapy and agents that promote normal cell maturation remain experimental and are under intensive investigation. Meanwhile, the search has begun for compounds which can interact with oncogene products, gene regulators, and growth factors and their receptors. Research employing modern technology in molecular genetics and immunology promises to provide a new array of anticancer agents which could move rapidly into clinical trials. This is possible because understanding cancer as a pathologic process is buttressed by new knowledge of cancer as an acquired genetic derangement.

This chapter provides an overview of the biology, etiology, and clinical sequelae of the neoplastic process, followed by a description of the general methods for diagnosing cancer and determining its stage, or extent of spread. Cancer treatment is presented in the following chapter, and the details of managing patients with specific types of malignant disease will be found in the chapters devoted to disorders of various specific organs.

Definition The terms cancer, neoplasia, and malignancy are usually used interchangeably in both the technical and popular literature. The disease called cancer is best defined by four characteristics which describe how cancer cells act differently from their normal counterparts.

1 *Clonality:* In most cases, cancer originates from a single stem cell which proliferates to form a clone of malignant cells.
2 *Autonomy:* Growth is not properly regulated by the normal biochemical and physical influences in the environment.
3 *Anaplasia:* There is a lack of normal, coordinated cell differentiation.
4 *Metastasis:* Cancer cells develop the capacity for discontinuous growth and dissemination to other parts of the body.

Properties similar to each of these characteristics *can* be expressed by normal, nonmalignant cells at certain appropriate times—for example, during embryogenesis and wound repair—but in cancer cells the characteristic is inappropriate or excessive. The process by which a normal cell is converted into one which exhibits these characteristic traits is termed *malignant transformation.*

THE CLINICAL PROBLEM One-third of all individuals in the United States will develop cancer. The 5-year relative survival rate for these

TABLE 78-1 Estimated new cases and deaths for major sites of cancer—1984

Site or type	Number of cases	Deaths
Lung	139,000	121,000
Colon-rectum	130,000	59,000
Breast	116,000	38,000
Prostate	76,000	25,000
Uterus	55,000*	10,000
Urinary tract	57,000	19,000
Mouth	27,000	9,000
Pancreas	25,000	23,000
Leukemia	24,000	17,000
Ovary	18,000	12,000
Melanoma	18,000†	7,000

* *Includes cervix. If carcinoma in situ is included, cases total over 99,000.*
† *Estimated new cases of skin cancer (nonmelanoma) = about 400,000.*
NOTE: *Estimates are based on rates from the N.C.I. SEER program 1973–1979.*

patients (the probability of escaping death from cancer for 5 years following diagnosis) has risen to nearly 50 percent as a result of progress in the early diagnosis and the therapy of this disease. However, cancer remains second only to cardiac disease as a cause of death in this country. Twenty percent of Americans die from cancer; this amounted to 450,000 deaths in 1984. Half of the deaths were due to the three most common types of cancer: lung, breast, and colon-rectum. Lung cancer is more prevalent in males, while breast cancer is the commonest form of malignancy in females. Cancer of the colon and rectum is equally common in males and females.

Information is provided yearly by the American Cancer Society, summarizing the incidence and mortality rates for the common types of cancer. Table 78-1 and Fig. 78-1 present just a small portion of the extensive data available. Of particular importance is the clear documentation in Fig. 78-1 that deaths from lung cancer are increasing in the face of stable or falling rates for a number of other types of malignant disease.

Cancer typically presents to the physician as an abnormal growth, or tumor, which causes illness by production of biochemically active molecules, by local expansion, or by invasion into adjacent or distant tissue sites. The symptoms of the illness depend upon the specific molecular products and the location(s) of the tumor. Each type of cancer has a relatively distinctive natural history that describes the likely clinical course of the particular neoplastic process. Designing a proper treatment plan for an individual patient with malignant disease depends upon determining the extent of disease spread, together with a knowledge of the natural history and the available therapeutic alternatives for the particular type of cancer.

TUMOR CELL BIOLOGY AND BIOCHEMISTRY Since all cells in an organism originate from a single fertilized egg (zygote), all carry the identical genetic information. The proliferation and differentiation of this cell into an embryo, and eventually into a mature organism, involve selective and coordinated expression of the genomic repertoire. Control of gene expression is accomplished through incompletely understood molecular interactions which can be modulated, in part, by chemical influences in the environment. The genomic repertoire includes information which permits cells to expand clonally, to function with varying degrees of autonomy, to differentiate and dedifferentiate, and to move from one part of the organism to another in a coordinated way. In the adult, the process of wound healing activates expression of these cellular characteristics in a more "embryo-like" fashion, but under well-coordinated control. In the case of malignancy, the normal control process is subverted or bypassed due to the anomalous activities of a select group of genes (oncogenes) which have central importance to the regulation of cellular activities. A detailed discussion of oncogenes is provided in Chap. 59.

Clonality Careful cytogenetic analysis of metaphase chromosome preparations from cancer cells has yielded a wealth of information about the neoplastic process. It has become clear that virtually all solid tumors and a majority of hematopoietic malignancies display abnormalities in the karyotype which are inherited by the population of tumor cells. These may involve translocations of chromosomal fragments into new locations, as well as additions or deletions of parts of chromosomes or whole chromosomes. A particular karyotypic alteration often occurs in a substantial fraction of all patients with a form of cancer. The first and most well known example of this is the Philadelphia chromosome (Ph¹) observed in 85 percent of patients with chronic myelogenous leukemia (CML), in which the long arm of chromosome 22 is translocated onto the long arm of chromosome 9. This alteration is so characteristic of CML that when analysis of some cases of acute lymphocytic leukemia demonstrated the identical translocation, it was inferred that the disease represented an unusual conversion from CML (which usually progresses to acute myelocytic leukemia). Characteristic chromosomal rearrangements have been described in a number of other human cancers.

The observation of uniform karyotypic abnormalities in all cells within a tumor provides strong evidence for the clonal origin of the

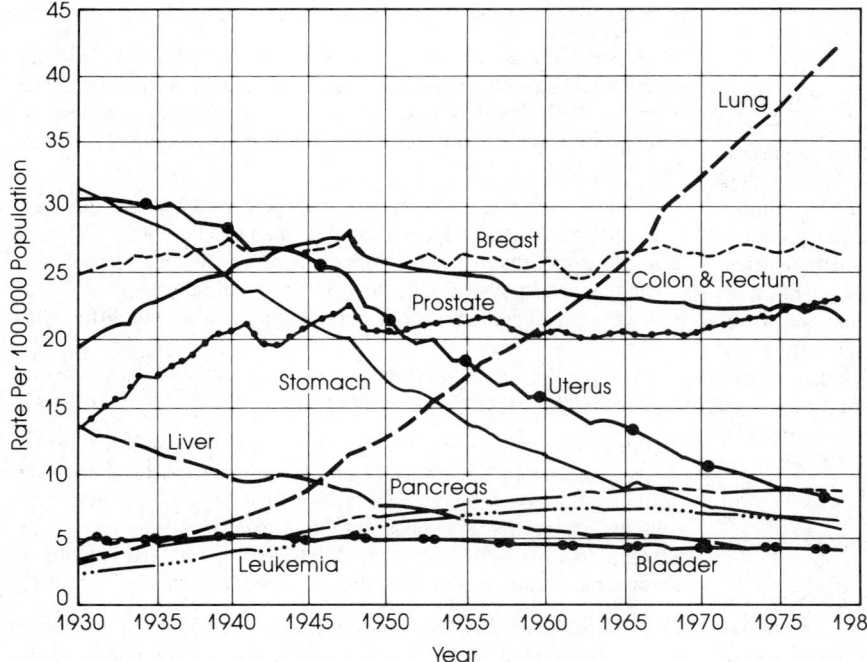

FIGURE 78-1 *Cancer death rates by site in the United States, 1930 to 1979. (Prepared by the American Cancer Society from data provided by the National Center for Health Statistics and the Bureau of the Census.)*

FIGURE 78-2 *A schematic model of clonal progression. The N cell is normal. Five hypothetical genetic changes are noted. The first does not result in malignancy but the second does. The third adds invasiveness, the fourth confers the capacity to disseminate and produce metastases, and the fifth provides resistance to chemotherapy. Each may be accompanied by incremental alterations in the karyotype, with an increasing tendency to aneuploidy during further clonal evolution.*

tumor. In turn, the chromosomal abnormalities serve as markers of the presence of a common malignant state in the individual cells.

A remarkable concordance between the chromosome locations of a number of human cellular oncogenes and the break points involved in chromosome translocations in human malignancies has been demonstrated. Furthermore, in many cases, these locations correlate with "fragile" sites in the chromosome. Treatment of cultured cells with agents that inhibit the DNA repair process induces chromosomal breaks far more frequently at many of these loci. A reasonable hypothesis, currently under investigation, links these phenomena and suggests that chromosomal rearrangements may result in activation of cellular oncogenes. For example, in Burkitt's lymphoma, the typical translocation between chromosomes 8 and 14 places the cellular *myc* gene adjacent to the immunoglobulin heavy chain locus, a site of gene activation in the normal lymphocyte.

Studies of the selective expression of the X-linked isoenzymes of glucose 6-phosphate dehydrogenase in heterozygotic patients have provided further evidence for the clonal origin of most cancers from single progenitor cells. Examination of both glucose 6-phosphate dehydrogenase isoenzymes and karyotypes in CML patients has demonstrated clonal abnormalities in erythroid, myeloid, and megakaryocytic cells, as well as B lymphocytes, suggesting that this malignancy originates in a precursor cell common to all of these cell lineages.

While there is convincing evidence for the origin of cancer from genetic alterations in a single cell, further heritable alterations commonly occur, resulting in the presence of a heterogeneous mixture of subclones in a mature tumor cell population which has proliferated enough to be clinically detectable. This heterogeneity can be demonstrated by assaying a variety of characteristics in the subpopulations within a tumor; for example, further abnormalities in the karyotype, varied drug sensitivites and metastatic capacities, differences in growth rates, and the presence or absence of hormone receptors or particular cell surface glycoproteins. With time, therefore, the progressive accumulation of heritable abnormalities in tumor subpopulations typically results in highly significant phenotypic changes which have their clinical counterpart in development of resistance to previously effective therapy or in increased metastatic spread. The appearance of new chromosomal abnormalities in patients with PH[1]-positive CML heralds the onset of a rapidly progressive, fatal phase of the disease. A schematic model of this process of clonal progression is shown in Fig. 78-2. It remains to be determined when in the life history of a typical malignancy the process of clonal progression occurs: the sequence of genetic alterations may occur early, with later expansion of selected subpopulations from a heterogeneous mixture of cells as circumstances change; alternatively the genetic alterations may occur close to the time when they are detected by changes in the behavior of the tumor cells.

Following the discovery of cellular oncogenes, evidence rapidly accumulated to show that successive activation of two or more of these genes may be the molecular genetic explanation for clonal progression in tumor cell subpopulations. Activation of cellular oncogenes may be due to a variety of genetic mechanisms in addition to translocation. These mechanisms include gene amplification, or insertion of promoters of transcription adjacent to (*cis*) or in a *trans* relationship to a cellular oncogene, with or without accompanying mutations of specific nucleotides in the oncogene DNA sequence. Many of these changes are undetectable in the karyotype, but can be identified by restriction digest analysis of cellular DNA or by DNA sequencing.

Autonomy Environmental influences which regulate the proliferation of normal cells are circumvented when the process of malignant transformation occurs. This is demonstrable by a variety of experimental assays which document, in different ways, the capacity of the malignant cells to continue to proliferate under normally nonconducive conditions. These assays are listed in Table 78-2.

At least initially, the autonomy of human malignancies is relative rather than absolute. The well-known experiments of Huggins and associates in the 1950s led to a new form of cancer therapy which took advantage of the initial dependence of certain tumors upon the normal influences of sex hormones. The conversion of many prostatic and breast cancers from sensitivity to resistance to hormone therapy vividly demonstrates the further development of autonomy through clonal progression.

Many tumor cell lines can proliferate in culture medium without the usual requirement for serum, provided that a "cocktail" containing three to five essential growth factors and other growth-promoting agents is added. Examples of such factors are epidermal growth

TABLE 78-2 Experimental detection of malignant transformation

Assay	Normal cell	Transformed cell
Capacity of single cells to form colonies in agar suspension	Unsuccessful	Successful
Density-dependent inhibition of cell proliferation in liquid culture	Yes	No
Generations obtained by continuous division in liquid culture	Limited to about 50	Unlimited
Requirements for serum or growth factors	Invariable	Reduced or absent
Capacity to grow as xenografts	Absent	Present

factor, platelet-derived growth factor, the carrier protein transferrin, and the hormone insulin. Malignant cells may obviate the requirements for even these essential factors. One mechanism, demonstrated experimentally and possibly of clinical significance, involves production of a growth factor (or its analogue) by the tumor cells themselves, a process called *autocrine secretion*. In this situation a glycoprotein secreted by the tumor cells may have the capacity to bind to a receptor on the surface of the tumor cells, resulting in autostimulation (Fig. 78-3). The first autocrine tumor growth factor to be described was transforming growth factor alpha, an analogue of epidermal growth factor. In other situations, the tumor cell may activate an internal biochemical process ordinarily dependent upon binding of a specific growth factor to a cell surface receptor, thereby completely bypassing the need for the growth-promoting agent.

Anaplasia Lack of normal differentiation is a most useful characteristic in the pathologic diagnosis of malignancy. While cancer cells usually bear some of the morphologic characteristics of their normal mature counterparts, they display cellular and histologic abnormalities readily detectable with the light microscope. The cells tend to have large nuclei, with more apparent chromatin and prominent nucleoli. There are increased mitoses, as well as abnormal mitoses and giant cells containing multiple nuclei, reflecting aneuploidy and/or a failure of karyokinesis. The degree of morphologic derangement typically correlates with the extent of disease spread or the metastatic potential of the tumor. The histologic appearance of malignancy is one of disarray, with partial or complete loss of normal tissue architecture. Partial formation of structures such as glands or villi may be suggested, even in poorly differentiated malignancies.

Although the term is not used this way, the process of anaplasia may be expressed at a biochemical level as production of hormones or hormone-related peptides, which are either improperly regulated by normal feedback mechanisms (e.g., excessive corticosteroid production by an adrenal carcinoma), or are not appropriate for the particular cell type if it were normally differentiated (e.g., ACTH production by a carcinoma of the lung). In such cases, the genomic repertoire of the malignant cell is expressed inappropriately. Another example is the unregulated production of immunoglobulin (partial or complete chains) by neoplastic derivatives of B lymphocytes.

Histologic features which are abnormal but do not meet the criteria of anaplasia (loss of differentiation) are designated *dysplastic*. Such changes may be seen in "premalignant" situations, for example, in the epithelial lining of the bronchi of cigarette smokers. These abnormalities are often reversible. Cessation of smoking can lead to normalization of the lung epithelium over a period of 5 years.

Metastasis This term encompasses a number of phenotypic traits which together result in the clinical problem which most often leads to death from cancer. The cells lose their adherence and restrained

position within an organized tissue, move into adjacent sites, develop the capacity both to invade and to egress from blood vessels, and become capable of proliferating in unnatural locations or environments. These changes in growth patterns are accompanied by biochemical alterations which have the capacity to promote the metastatic process. Invasive tumors may secrete a variety of tissue-degrading enzymes including collagenases and lysosomal hydrolases. Plasminogen activators which lead to promotion of fibrinolysis are also produced. Conversely, procoagulant compounds may be released into the environment of the tumor cells at stages when focal aggregation of cells might be of survival value. In experimental situations where tumor cells show a propensity to select a particular organ as a preferred site of metastasis, surface molecules on the metastatic cells appear to have a high affinity for endothelial cells in the vasculature of the specific target organ. A large number of biochemical steps are involved in the progression of a tumor from a homogeneous proliferating clone to a group of heterogeneous subpopulations of cells, some of which have progressively accumulated the entire array of enzymes and surface molecules required for metastasis. It may be for this reason that the rate of metastasis is low during early tumor growth, in spite of the well-documented fact that malignant cells are often released from a tumor into the circulation continuously and in large numbers. Agents which could block critical steps in the metastatic process would be of great value in the armamentarium of antineoplastic agents.

It appears that clonal progression of a tumor generates biochemical or physiologic alterations which confer greater autonomy, greater degrees of anaplasia, and a greater capacity to metastasize. Because there is progressive selection for cells with increased tumorogenic capacity, the process has been called clonal evolution and has been compared to Darwinian evolution, in this case at a cellular level.

ETIOLOGY Patterns of cancer incidence vary with sex, race, and geographic location. In addition, the types of tumors observed vary with age. Hereditary traits and variations in the internal environments around cells explain some of the differences in cancer incidence. It is clear from epidemiologic investigations that variations in diet and exposure to chemical and physical agents in the external environment contribute to the development of neoplasia. The environmental agents which have been linked to the incidence of cancer fall into three broad categories: radiation, a variety of chemicals, and viruses.

Genetic factors For many of the common malignancies, the incidence of cancer is higher among patients with positive family histories than among unselected patients, usually in the range of up to threefold. However, the risk can rise to as high as twenty-five- to thirtyfold in certain groups of patients with a familial history of breast cancer or bowel cancer. In addition, there are a number of uncommon inherited disorders involving either (1) a high risk for the occurrence of a particular neoplasm, or (2) the presence of multiple preneoplastic lesions that can progress to frank malignancy.

The hereditary neoplasms (Table 78-3) may occur as the only manifestation of a gene defect, or as part of a generalized syndrome involving multiple developmental abnormalities. The inheritance patterns in these disorders are generally autosomal dominant, with varying penetrance. Half of the children of patients with these disorders will inherit the gene defect.

The preneoplastic states are grouped into four major categories by Fraumeni (Table 78-3). The hamartomatous syndromes show autosomal dominant inheritance patterns. The most common is neurofibromatosis, occurring in 1 of 3000 live births. The neurofibromas undergo sarcomatous changes in about 10 percent of patients, with development of gliomas in the brain or optic nerve, meningiomas, acoustic neuromas, or pheochromocytomas. The genodermatoses are rare autosomal recessive genetic disorders which conspicuously involve the skin. Chromosome breakage disorders are characterized by the recessive inheritance of chromosomal instability and rearrangements of karyotypes; patients have an increased incidence of acute leukemia. The immune deficiency ataxic telangiectasia is also char-

FIGURE 78-3 *A diagrammatic representation of autocrine, paracrine, and endocrine secretion. Peptide growth factors are shown in latent form within the cell. The thickened, semicircular regions of the cell membrane represent receptor sites. (From MB Sporn, GJ Todaro, N Engl J Med 303:878, 1980.)*

Endocrine   Paracrine   Autocrine

acterized by chromosomal fragility. Patients with hereditary or acquired immunodeficiency states have an increased incidence of neoplasia, most commonly the lymphoproliferative malignancies.

Race is a genetic factor in the incidence of cancer, but interpretation of epidemiologic data is made difficult by the concurrent effects of environmental and socioeconomic influences. Both the incidence and the death rate from cancer is higher in American blacks than in American whites, with all of the difference being accounted for by the higher cancer rate in black males. It is believed that later detection and less adequate treatment may account for part, but not all, of the difference in survival. The important effect of environmental factors is made clear by documented differences in cancer incidence for Asians living in Hawaii and in California.

Radiation

It is estimated that less than 3 percent of cancers result from exposure to radiation. Radiation that can remove electrons from atoms is called ionizing radiation. It includes electromagnetic waves such as x-rays and gamma rays, as well as charged particles such as protons. The unit of radiation dose measures the energy absorbed in matter as a result of exposure to radiation: 1 rad = 100 erg/g; 1 gray = 1 joule/kg = 100 rad.

Information on the capacity of radiation in relatively large doses to induce cancer in humans comes from studies on survivors of atomic bomb blasts, on individuals accidentally exposed to irradiation or radiative fallout, and on patients exposed to radiation for diagnostic purposes or for therapy. It has been learned that nearly all tissues are susceptible to tumor induction by radiation, but with variable sensitivity. The most sensitive tissues are the bone marrow, breast, and thyroid. The latent period is only 2 to 5 years for acute leukemia, and 5 to 10 years for most solid tumors. There is a higher incidence of leukemia in patients who have received radiation therapy for neoplastic diseases and for ankylosing spondylitis, and of thyroid cancer in children irradiated for thymic enlargement.

Solar radiation, resulting from exposure to electromagnetic radiation from the sun, is the primary risk factor in skin cancer. The evidence for this linkage comes from a variety of epidemiologic and experimental observations. Skin cancer is rare in blacks and the deeply pigmented racial groups, whereas it is especially common in fair-complexioned individuals. It occurs primarily on the parts of the body exposed to sunlight and has a higher incidence in outdoor workers. Patients with genetic diseases such as xeroderma pigmentosa and albinism, which are exacerbated by sunlight, have very high risks for the development of skin cancer.

The carcinogenic effect of solar irradiation is greatest in the spectral range of 290 to 320 nm (UV-B radiation), which produces delayed erythema in human skin (sunburn). This range of wavelengths correlates with the action spectrum for UV-induced damage to DNA.

Exposure to solar ultraviolet irradiation is also a risk factor in melanoma. As with skin cancer, there is a higher incidence of melanoma among populations living at a latitude nearer the equator, where exposure to UV irradiation is greatest.

Tobacco

Numerous epidemiologic studies have demonstrated that the principal carcinogenic agent in our environment is inhaled tobacco smoke. The incidence of lung cancer is more than tenfold higher in male smokers than in nonsmokers. Furthermore, tobacco smoking is associated with increased rates of cancer of the oral cavity, esophagus, kidney, bladder, and pancreas. Particulate matter in tobacco smoke, known as "tar," contains a long list of chemicals, primarily polycyclic hydrocarbons, which have been shown experimentally to be contact carcinogens. In addition, the metabolic activation of tobacco components, for example, the cyclic N-nitrosamines, can produce carcinogens with the capacity to act upon the cells of internal organs. Tobacco-related malignancies account for one-third of all cancer deaths among men in the United States and for 5 to 10 percent of all female cancer deaths. Unfortunately, this figure is rising in females. As a result of increased use of tobacco by women in the period since World War II, the incidence of lung cancer in females is expected to pass that of breast cancer by 1990.

TABLE 78-3 Hereditary cancer syndromes

I Hereditary neoplasms
   Retinoblastoma
   Nevoid basal cell carcinoma syndrome
   Multiple endocrine adenomatosis (Werner's syndrome)
   Pheochromocytoma and medullary thyroid carcinoma (Sipple's syndrome)
   Chemodectomas
   Polyposis coli
   Gardner's syndrome
   Tylosis with esophageal carcinoma

II Preneoplastic states
   A Hamartomatous syndromes
      Neurofibromatosis
      Tuberous sclerosis
      von Hippel–Lindau syndrome
      Multiple exostoses
      Peutz-Jeghers syndrome
      Cowden's multiple hamartoma syndrome
   B Genodermatoses
      Xeroderma pigmentosum
      Albinism
      Werner's syndrome
      Epidermodysplasia verruciformis
      Polydysplastic epidermolysis bullosa
      Dyskeratosis congenita
   C Chromosome breakage disorders
      Bloom's syndrome
      Fanconi's syndrome
   D Immune deficiency syndromes
      Ataxia-telangiectasia
      Wiskott-Aldrich syndrome
      Late-onset immunologic deficiency
      X-linked agammaglobulinemia

SOURCE: *From JF Fraumeni, Jr, in JF Holland, E Frei.*

Clearly the single most effective action which could be taken against cancer at the present time involves not an application of molecular genetic research, but cessation of smoking. Fortunately, it appears that smoking cessation results in a gradual decrease in risk, so that after 10 to 15 years, exsmokers have nearly the same risk of lung cancer as nonsmokers. Because the habit of smoking is difficult to break, the physician's role in cessation of smoking is of critical importance. Doctors should deliver a *firm* antismoking message.

Occupational exposure

The first report of cancer related to occupational hazards was Percival Pott's observation of an unusually high frequency of scrotal cancer among London chimney sweeps in 1775. It is now known that skin cancer (including scrotal) can be induced by a variety of coal tar products, such as the materials contacted in the London chimneys. Epidemiologic studies also have related lung cancer to exposure to coal by-products. Table 78-4 provides a partial listing of industrial agents which are known to cause cancer.

Air pollution

It is clear that lung cancer incidence is increased by tobacco smoking and by certain industrial and occupational exposures (primarily related to coal tar and combustion by-products). Once the risks resulting from exposure to these factors are taken into account, the epidemiologic evidence that links ambient air pollution to lung cancer remains inconclusive. Studies correlating the incidence of lung cancer with increased levels of polycyclic hydrocarbons and benzo(a)pyrene in urban air are complicated by the difficulty of eliminating the contribution of exposure to these compounds through tobacco smoking as well as occupational exposure.

TABLE 78-4 Examples of occupational causes of cancer

Etiology	Site of malignancy
Arsenic (inorganic)	Lung, skin, liver
Asbestos	Mesothelium, lung
Benzene	Leukemia
Benzidine	Bladder
Chromium compounds	Lung
Radiation (mining, dial painting)	Numerous locations
Mustard gas	Lung
Polycyclic hydrocarbons (coal by-products)	Lung, skin
Vinyl chloride	Angiosarcoma of liver

Medications   Certain drugs and hormones have been shown to be carcinogenic. The synthetic nonsteroidal estrogen diethylstilbestrol (DES), which was used for a period of time to reduce fetal wastage in pregnant women, caused an increased incidence of vaginal and cervical cancer in daughters who were exposed in utero. Conjugated estrogens have been shown to increase the incidence of endometrial cancer in patients treated for menopausal symptoms. The use of progesterone concomitantly, together with decreased estrogen dose, may obviate this problem.

Alkylating agents have been shown to cause an increased incidence of acute myelocytic leukemia and probably other malignancies. They are used in therapeutic situations in which the poor prognosis of malignancy far outweighs the increased risk of an additional cancer in the future. However, because of this risk, new drug regimens which avoid the use of alkylating agents are being explored in situations where substantial long-term benefits from chemotherapy have been demonstrated, for example, in Hodgkin's disease.

The recipients of organ transplants who are treated with immunosuppressive agents, such as azathioprine and prednisone, have an increased incidence of histiocytic lymphoma as well as a variety of solid tumors. A similar increased incidence is observed in individuals with inherited and acquired immunodeficiency, for example, AIDS. This has been attributed to reduced immune surveillance, but a variety of other explanations are equally likely, such as activation of a latent oncogenic virus or chronic immunostimulation in conjunction with a compromised and malfunctioning immune system.

Diet   The role of diet and nutrition in carcinogenesis has been the subject of intensive investigation and equally intensive controversy. There are numerous nutritional hypotheses of carcinogenesis. Some of these have led to unconventional forms of cancer therapy that are based upon no scientific evidence. Unfortunately, these putative dietary therapies are propagated upon a patient population for which proven treatment modalities are often unsuccessful in achieving cure, and at a time when there is a popular emphasis on healthful nutrition.

Epidemiologic analyses of international variations in cancer incidence and comparisons of the types and frequencies of cancer in populations with different dietary habits have yielded a great deal of evidence that cancers of most major sites are influenced by diet. These studies were reviewed in an authoritative publication, *Diet, Nutrition, and Cancer*. Interim dietary guidelines are suggested which are both consistent with good nutritional practices and likely to reduce the risk of cancer: (1) Reduce the intake of fat, saturated and unsaturated, from its present average level (40 percent) to 30 percent of total calories in the diet. (2) Include fruits (especially citrus), vegetables (especially carotene-rich and cruciferous), and whole cereal grain (fiber) in the daily diet; these provide amounts of vitamins A and C as well as fiber adequate to obviate the need for dietary supplements. (3) Minimize consumption of salt-cured or smoked food. (4) Use alcoholic beverages in moderation, since they increase the risk of certain cancers, especially when combined with cigarette smoking.

Experimental data lend support to the inferences from epidemiologic studies, but additional research is necessary to understand how dietary factors influence carcinogenesis. For example, epidemiologic evidence strongly correlates the intake of fat with the occurrence of cancer at several sites, especially the breast and colon. Possible explanations for this observation include increased adiposity, leading to greater conversion of androstenedione to estrone, which could influence carcinogenesis in the breast; and stimulation of increased bile salt excretion which could alter gut flora and thereby augment the production of carcinogenic substances by the bacteria in the colon. Vitamin C may act to prevent cancer by blocking endogenous formation of *N*-nitroso compounds in the gastrointestinal tract, but there are no data showing that taking vitamin C will prevent cancer in human beings. Dietary fiber enhances the rapid transit of potential carcinogens through the colon, which could explain the low incidence of bowel cancer and rectal cancer in tropical Africa.

It is important to stress that the accumulated scientific evidence does not support the anticarcinogenic value of particular vitamins, minerals, or nutritional supplements in amounts greater than provided by a prudent diet. Certainly their use in high doses in the therapy of established malignant disease is not indicated. The physician must be alert to the scientifically unproven dietary treatments which patients with cancer may be urged to undertake. Of course the greatest tragedy occurs when patients whose malignancy could be cured by proven therapeutic modalities are misled into depending upon such dietary manipulations.

Viruses   Although there has been extensive research on viral oncogenesis with experimental murine tumors, viruses have been implicated as the cause of only one human cancer, an uncommon malignancy of T lymphocytes. There are a number of situations in which viruses are linked to the occurrence of specific cancers with a high incidence in particular geographic locations, although a causative role has not been established. The Epstein-Barr virus is closely associated with African Burkitt's lymphoma as well as nasopharyngeal carcinoma in Asia. Cofactors in the development of these malignancies might be holoendemic malaria in African Burkitt's lymphoma, and a particular configuration of histocompatibility antigens in the case of nasopharyngeal carcinoma among Chinese. While the Epstein-Barr virus can infect human B lymphocytes (infectious mononucleosis) and transform them in cell culture, evidence is lacking that such a transformation is the cause of clinical malignancy.

Hepatitis B infection is correlated with the incidence of hepatocellular carcinoma, but again there is no evidence for a causal relationship. Chronic hepatocyte infection by the virus might predispose to carcinogenesis in these cells. There may be a variety of contributing factors, including malaria, malnutrition, and exposure to aflatoxin. There also is a statistical correlation between herpes simplex 2 viral infection, which is sexually transmitted, and the incidence of cervical cancer.

Risk of cancer   Knowledge of genetic and environmental factors that may contribute to cancer incidence can be utilized by the conscientious physician to identify patients who have an increased risk of malignancy. The presence of certain hereditary diseases in a patient's family may suggest procedures that can lead to early detection and prevention, for example, early surveillance by colonoscopy and prevention by prophylactic colectomy in persons who have familial polyposis of the colon. Environmental factors that increase cancer risks should be identified and avoided. It is evident, however, that changing an individual's life-style in order to avoid exposure to a carcinogen can require an extraordinary level of effort on the part of both the patient and the physician.

CLINICAL SEQUELAE   The presence of a malignant lesion may not, in itself, cause symptoms in a patient with cancer. The primary lesion may, for a period of time, be unnoticed and unimportant for the normal maintenance of body functions, in which case its clinical significance is due to its potential for growth and spread. In addition, the presence of metastasis need not result in symptomatic illness. Patients with carcinoma of the bowel, whose disease may have spread beyond the limits of surgical curability, may live for many months or even years with easily detectable metastatic lesions in the lung or abdomen, yet remain free of symptoms until the function of a vital organ is compromised or obstructive problems appear.

Malignancies produce clinical symptoms in three general ways (Table 78-5): by direct effects resulting from invasion or compression of normal tissues; by release of cytokines, hormones, and other biologically active agents into the local and systemic environment; and by secondary psychological effects upon the patient. Each of these factors may contribute profoundly to the degree of illness experienced by the patient. Clinical symptoms resulting from released biologically active agents, as well as systemic problems caused by as yet undetermined mechanisms, are usually grouped under the category of "paraneoplastic syndromes."

TABLE 78-5   Symptoms caused by malignant diseases

I Mass effects
  A Ablation by crowding or by invasion
  B Obstruction of vessels, tubes, and ducts
  C Rupture of blood vessels
II Remote effects (paraneoplastic syndromes)
  A Ectopic hormone production
  B Neuropathies and CNS abnormalities
  C Dermatologic abnormalities
  D Metabolic disorders
    1 Anorexia, weight loss
    2 Fever
    3 Chronic inflammation
  E Hematologic disorders
  F Immunosuppression
  G Collagen vascular disorders
III Psychosocial effects
  A Loss of control
  B Acceptance of personal finitude
  C Fear of pain and mutilation
  D Separation and loneliness

Mass effects of malignancy   In most cases tumors produce clinical problems as a result of local expansion, with obliteration of normal tissues, as the malignant cells proliferate within the confines of the involved organ: marrow replacement by leukemia results in reduced production of the normal cellular elements of the blood; lung cancer compromises oxygen exchange in involved alveoli; primary or metastatic cancer in bone causes weakened trabecular architecture, resulting in pathologic fractures; hepatomas replace normal hepatocytes and interfere with liver function. A second result of local expansion is compression of normal structures, with partial or complete obstruction of tubular organs, blood vessels, and lymphatics: colonic cancer may obstruct the gastrointestinal tract; lung cancer blocks airflow through bronchi and can obstruct pulmonary venous return; hepatic and biliary malignancies produce obstructive jaundice; a variety of intraabdominal neoplasms can encase the ureters, causing renal failure; in the extreme case, penetration of blood vessels can violate the integrity of the vasculature, resulting in hemorrhage. A third result of local expansion is pain, due to pressure on or stretching of nerve fibers. When neoplasia causes increased pressure on nervous tissue within the confines of the skull, the symptoms include headache and vomiting as well as seizure disorders and brain dysfunction.

Paraneoplastic syndromes   The malignant process is felt to develop as a result of the unregulated and/or inappropriate expression of certain genes crucial to cell proliferation and differentiation. The aggressiveness of the malignant process is increased by the subsequent uncovering of additional genetic information. In this evolutionary process, abnormal genetic information may be expressed which results in severe physiologic effects upon the patient. As noted above, there may be excessive synthesis of a gene product which is normally found in the particular cell type, or the malignant cell may produce a molecule which does not ordinarily originate from its normal counterpart.

A common type of molecule produced by malignant tumors falls into the category of polypeptide hormones. The synthesis of antidiuretic hormone or ACTH by small cell carcinoma of the lung or parathormone by some squamous cancers are examples. These can produce clinical illness by mediating normal physiologic functions to an excessive degree. Other active molecules have been detected which are homologous with or identical to known growth factors. The potential for autonomous stimulation of proliferation mediated by production of essential growth-promoting agents has been discussed.

From this brief introduction, it can be seen that biologically active agents produced by malignant cells can be clinically important for a number of reasons:

1 They may serve as markers for the presence of a type of tumor. Detection of such markers early in the course of the disease might increase chances for cure. They also may be used to follow the clinical progress of the disease and anticipate recurrence.

2 They may produce symptoms as a result of their intrinsic biologic activity. In some cases these can become the major clinical problems determining survival (e.g., hypercalcemia).

3 They may serve to promote the growth of the tumor directly. In turn, growth-promoting agents of this type may become the focus of new approaches to anticancer treatment.

The paraneoplastic sequelae of cancer which involve ectopic hormone production are described in Chap. 303, and the neurologic manifestations of neoplasia in Chap. 304. Cutaneous manifestations of internal malignancy are discussed in Chap. 300. The association of malignancy with certain metabolic disorders, hematologic abnormalities, and immunosuppression will be further described here.

Metabolic disorders   One of the major and most characteristic problems seen with cancer is weight loss, usually associated with anorexia. The extensive wasting which results is known as cachexia. The cause for this commonly observed and often life-limiting disturbance remains to be determined in spite of the fact that many contributing factors have been identified. Abnormalities of taste and smell, physiologic malfunction of the gastrointestinal tract, excessive energy demands made by the tumor, and failure to adapt energy expenditure to the levels of nutrient intake have been implicated as causes of cachexia in patients with cancer. Biochemical abnormalities in energy metabolism have been well-characterized in these patients. Fatty acids are oxidized in preference to glucose, and anaerobic glucose metabolism is increased while oxidative phosphorylation is reduced. This results in an inefficient expenditure of ATP, which might lead to an energy deficit. However, none of these observations is felt to account for the magnitude of the problem.

Typically, the anorectic patient simply cannot ingest food, in spite of a clear understanding of the need for increased nourishment. The chief complaint is unpalatability. An aversion to meat has been clearly documented. While nausea may be a component of the syndrome, emesis occurs rarely. This may be because the patient feels so satiated that no food intake is tolerated.

Provision of alimentation through enteral tubes or by the intravenous route has the potential to provide total parenteral nutrition (TPN) to patients with cancer, and the techniques for performing these procedures have been well described by investigators managing nonmalignant disease. At present there is no indication that the provision of nutritional support at this level can, by itself, affect the course of malignant disease. However, clinical trials have suggested a role for nutritional supplementation, including TPN, in preparing nutritionally deprived cancer patients for potentially beneficial surgical procedures or chemotherapy programs which otherwise might not have been tolerated due to the wasted state of the patient.

A polypeptide produced by macrophages has been isolated and named cachectin. This molecule can mimic the syndrome of cachexia in experimental animals. It may ultimately explain the pathogenesis of this puzzling and vexing syndrome.

Fever is another sign associated with malignancy, and it is usually attributable to infection. Because of the debility which often accompanies cancer, and the depression in circulating granulocytes and mononuclear cells resulting from aggressive therapeutic measures, the types of infection seen may be unusual. Infection by endogenous bacteria, fungi, viruses, and protozoa must be considered when evaluating fever of unknown etiology in patients with malignancy (see Chap. 9). There remain unusual instances when fever can not be explained by infection and must be attributed to a cause intrinsic to the neoplasm itself.

Hematologic abnormalities   Anemia is found with increased incidence in advanced stages of malignant disease. The mechanisms accounting for anemia are, in nearly all cases, extrinsic to the tumor, and may be due to several mechanisms. Increased destruction of erythrocytes can result from hypersplenism, microangiopathic hemolysis, and autoantibodies, seen especially in the lymphoproliferative malignancies. Anemia due to occult bleeding is one of the cardinal signs of malignancy in the gastrointestinal tract. Decreased production of erythrocytes may result from iron deficiency related to bleeding, vitamin B_{12} or folate deficiency, erythron depletion due to tumor crowding in the marrow, toxicity secondary to chemotherapy or radiotherapy, and the anemia associated with chronic inflammatory disease.

Granulocytopenia is commonly associated with marrow infiltration by hematologic malignancies, and also results from chemotherapy. The etiologies of thrombocytopenia are comparable to those associated with anemia. Depression in one or all of the circulating hematopoietic elements may result from one of the various forms of marrow failure or aplastic anemia which are known to be preleukemic.

An increase in the formed elements of the blood may also occur. Erythrocytosis resulting from inappropriate production of erythropoietin is observed not only in polycythemia vera, but also in renal cell carcinoma, hepatoma, and cerebellar hemangioma. An elevated granulocyte count may result from marrow infiltration by tumor cells, or an inflammatory response to malignancy, and frank leukemoid reactions may be seen with nonhematopoietic tumors. Thrombocytosis unrelated to primary marrow disease is commonly associated with a systemic malignancy.

A hypercoagulable state is a rare clinical complication of malignancy, although it may be far more prevalent at a subclinical level. Mucin-producing tumors and adenocarcinomas, especially those of the pancreas and stomach, head the list of tumors reported to be associated with clinical disseminated coagulopathy (DIC). This may present as a migratory thrombophlebitis of unknown etiology, which can produce venous thrombosis as well as pulmonary embolism. Hypercoagulation also may be associated with marantic (nonbacterial) endocarditis and resultant thromboembolic episodes, which further complicate the clinical picture. The treatment of the primary malignancy is the only successful therapeutic attack on the problem. Anticoagulation, following the principles for treatment of DIC (Chaps. 54 and 281), may provide short-term benefits in acute situations, but with attendant risks.

Acute promyelocytic leukemia is often associated with abnormalities of hemostasis related to a hypercoagulable state. The malignant immature granulocytes can release procoagulant materials which initiate DIC. In this case, the addition of anticoagulation to the initial phase of antileukemia therapy results in an improved chance for a successful outcome.

Immunosuppression   Advanced cancer is accompanied by abnormalities in immune function which can be demonstrated by skin testing against common antigens and by examination of lymphocyte responses to mitogenic stimulation in vitro. Moreover, in general, the extent of malignant disease correlates well with the degree of immune dysfunction. In spite of a vast experimental literature on this subject, the two significant questions concerning immunosuppression in cancer patients continue to be unanswered: (1) What is the mechanism(s) of inhibition? (2) Is the immunosuppression merely secondary to the malignant state, or could it play an etiologic role (failure of "immune surveillance")?

Experimental data have implicated defects in both T- and B-cell function, as well as abnormalities of macrophages, in the etiology of the reduced immune competence in cancer patients. Primary malignancies of lymphocytes are accompanied by abnormalities in the functioning of the particular cell type involved. Some of the lymphoproliferative malignancies are characterized by an increase in autoimmune reactions, most notably in 25 percent of patients with chronic lymphocytic leukemia. In addition, both chemotherapy and radiotherapy can produce long-standing suppression of immune function.

One approach to cancer treatment involves attempts to stimulate an effective immune response with the hope that immune antitumor activity can act alone or in concert with the standard therapeutic modalities to eliminate the malignant cell population. Monoclonal antibodies against antigens present in relatively increased quantities on tumor cells may provide ways to reconstitute or hyperconstitute immune responses to malignancy. Treatment with cytokines such as the interferons has produced some interesting preliminary results, and therapy with high concentrations of interleukin 2 is under active investigation.

Psychosocial effects   The diagnosis of cancer immediately raises in the mind of the patient and his or her family a host of questions and fears which require the undivided attention of an empathetic, considerate, and skilled physician. This is especially true when the particular form of cancer has a poor chance for cure, or when malignancy has recurred.

Of the variety of psychosocial problems experienced by patients, two which are particularly difficult to deal with are helplessness and loss of control. These involve both economic control and personal control of one's activity and one's future. Closely tied to these problems and adding to the feeling of helplessness is the difficulty of accepting personal finitude. A third major source of mental anguish is the fear of pain and mutilation. Finally, separation from loved ones, both anticipated and real, creates a void of loneliness and a fear of abandonment.

The reactions to the mental stresses which are produced by these problems can only be dealt with effectively by a professional who has become familiar with the patient's personality and his or her social and intellectual environment. Although one or another emotion may dominate at a particular time, the responses commonly observed include anger, denial, withdrawal, and depression. Added to these problems is the complexity resulting from the response of the patient's family to the illness and to the patient's own response to the illness. In spite of these stresses, some patients with incurable malignancies are able to adapt and reorient their lives in a creative and meaningful way. The intellectual and emotional challenge to the physician is obvious, and careful attention must be given to managing the patient's (and the family's) responses to malignancy in addition to providing specific treatment for the disease.

Does the patient's psychological attitude have a role in the cause or treatment of malignant disease? The question is a complex and controversial one. There is evidence, which is contested, that life stresses can predispose to systemic illness by producing anxiety or depression. One theory postulates that stress leads to a reduction in immunologic function, resulting in inadequate immune surveillance, but this explanation for the pathogenesis of cancer is not adequately supported by available clinical data. There are also claims that correction of emotional difficulties and development of positive attitudes can serve as effective anticancer therapy. In favor of psychological support and counseling is the clear benefit to the quality of life which can be achieved by helping patients with malignancy to develop positive attitudes and to gain some measure of control over *how* they are living. However, scientific evidence does not demonstrate that the patient's psyche can achieve regression or cure of the malignant process. Some of the strongest and most responsible advocates of counseling and attitudinal approaches to cancer patient management also stress the need for concurrent treatment with standard anticancer therapies.

DIAGNOSIS AND STAGING   There are four general goals in evaluating a patient for the presence of malignancy. First, information must be gathered leading to biopsy of a candidate lesion, which alone can establish the pathologic diagnosis of neoplasia. The second goal is to determine as precisely as possible the extent of tumor spread, both at the site of origin and as metastases. The process of obtaining this information is known as *staging*. The third goal is to determine the growth rate and time course of the neoplasm in the particular patient undergoing diagnostic evaluation. The dictum that "every person is different" holds for cancers as well. Each malignancy is different, although there is a natural history which broadly characterizes each type of neoplasm. The rate of tumor growth can be determined by sequential assessment, using physical examinations or radiologic techniques, occasionally aided by the measurement of serum markers of tumor activity. The physician's ingenuity and persistence often come into play; an example is determining the existence of past radiologic studies, locating them, and obtaining them for review. The fourth goal in the evaluation is to determine the effects of the malignancy upon the health and performance of the patient. The importance of this in the design of a management plan is obvious, since control of symptoms and proper modification of acitivity levels will improve the well-being of the patient. In addition, it has become increasingly evident that the patient's performance status provides important data in predicting prognosis as well as response to anticancer therapy.

There are two widely used clinical scales of performance status, the Karnofsky scale and a modification developed by the Eastern Cooperative Oncology Group. The influence of performance status upon prognosis is demonstrated by a report correlating performance and median survival in patients with inoperable lung cancer (Table 78-6).

Pathologic diagnosis The diagnosis of cancer is made by pathologic examination. While there are definite limitations to histologic and cytologic examination of tumor specimens, this procedure is essential in order to exclude inflammatory processes as well as hyperplasia or benign tumors. In addition, the tissue of origin of a malignancy must be known in order to select the appropriate therapy. Specimens for pathologic examination are usually obtained by biopsy of a suspicious lesion. The procedure may involve a surgical operation under general anesthesia, but in many cases tissue specimens can be obtained through local incision (e.g., breast cancer) or by removal of a piece of tissue under direct visualization (bronchoscopy, colonoscopy). When direct visualization is not possible because of the internal location of a suspected lesion, it is often possible to obtain tissue fragments or clumps of cells by fine-needle biopsy aspiration, guided by computerized axial tomography or fluoroscopy. In addition, suitable cytologic preparations can be obtained by washing or scraping surface lesions, as is commonly done to evaluate lesions on the cervix or in bronchi. Finally, in the case of malignancy involving the hematopoietic system or growing in body cavities (e.g., ascites), needle aspiration of tumor cells in suspension can be performed.

To make the diagnosis of cancer the pathologist looks for histologic and cytologic features characteristic of the disease. These include pleomorphism of cellular and nuclear structure, a high rate of mitosis and the presence of large or multiple nuclei, disordered tissue architecture, destruction or invasion of normal tissue boundaries, and the presence of cells in inappropriate locations (metastases). Special stains are useful for identifying chemical components characteristic of particular cell types and tissues. Additional evidence can be brought to bear upon the pathologic diagnosis, using the results of immuno-histochemical studies, flow cytometry data on cellular DNA content, karyotype analysis, and electron microscopy. However, in the over-whelming majority of cases, the diagnosis is made with the light microscope, on the basis of morphologic evaluation of the cells individually and as organized into tissue structures.

After the pathologic diagnosis of malignancy is established, the description usually includes three characteristics which classify the neoplasia:

1 The tissue of origin (e.g., adenocarcinoma, epidermoid carcinoma, sarcoma, leukemia)
2 Anatomic origin (e.g., colon, lung, breast)
3 Degree of differentiation (e.g., well-differentiated or poorly differentiated)

Each of these characteristics gives the therapist information relevant to the selection of treatment and to the prognosis. Although this terminology for classification is followed in general, there are many examples of exceptions based upon customary nomenclature involving particular tissues of origin or on the use of eponyms (e.g., Hodgkin's disease, glioblastoma multiforme).

Staging of cancer The staging of a cancer patient involves the detection of the anatomic extent of the tumor, both in its primary

TABLE 78-6 Influence of pretreatment performance status on patients with inoperable lung cancer*

Performance status scale†			Median survival (weeks)	Patients in group (percent)
ECOG	Karnofsky	Definitions		
0	100	Asymptomatic, normal activity	34	2
1	80–90	Symptomatic, but ambulatory	24–27	32
2	60–70	Symptomatic, in bed less than 50% of day, needs minimal assistance	14–21	40
3	40–50	Symptomatic, in bed more than 50% of day, requires considerable assistance	7–9	22
4	20–30	100% bedridden, severely disabled	3–5	5

* $N = 5022$ males with inoperable lung cancer of all histologic types entered onto VA Lung Group protocols from 1968–1978.
† Eastern Cooperative Oncology Group (ECOG) performance status scale, and DA Karnofsky et al, Cancer 1:634, 1948.
SOURCE: Adapted from JD Minna et al, in VT DeVita, Jr et al.

location and in metastatic sites. This process is of critical importance in the clinical management for a number of reasons:

1 The optimal treatment plan for an individual patient is selected on the basis of the stage of disease.
2 By determining the presence of early metastatic disease, treatment can often be designed which can increase the chance for cure, or delay the development of symptoms even if cure is not achievable.
3 Staging provides information from which the physician can better evaluate the prognosis.
4 Because half of the cases of cancer cannot be cured by the therapies available today and because rapid advances in the development of anticancer treatment are occurring, management of an individual patient often involves new drugs or experimental procedures which are in the process of being evaluated for toxicity and efficacy. Staging to determine the extent of disease accurately is essential for evaluating factors influencing the results of such new treatments.

The anatomic extent of disease is best described and communicated to other professionals by a standardized nomenclature known as the TNM system. The three elements characterized in this system are the primary *t*umor, the regional lymph *n*odes, and *m*etastases (Table 78-7). The details of classification were decided upon by the International Union against Cancer (UICC) and the American Joint Committee for Cancer Staging (AJCCS). There is a scale of subcategories with designations ranging from 0 to 4 for each of the three tumor characteristics listed in the table. These scales were chosen because they can provide useful predictions of the clinical course. The primary tumor is classified by its size and the extent of local involvement. The involvement of lymph nodes is typically stratified by the spread to locations at a varying distance from the primary lesion and by the number of involved nodes. The most relevant information regarding metastases is their presence or absence. The details of stratification within the TNM system vary for each type of malignancy and are highly individualized. They depend on the characteristic growth patterns and lymphatic drainage patterns of neoplasms of the various

TABLE 78-7 TNM system of anatomic staging

T: Primary tumor
  T0   No evidence of primary tumor
  T1–4 Ascending degrees of increase in tumor size and involvement
N: Regional lymph nodes
  N0   No evidence of disease in lymph nodes
  N1–4 Ascending degrees of nodal involvement
M: Distant metastasis
  M0   No evidence of metastasis
  M1–4 Ascending degrees of metastatic involvement

TABLE 78-8 Tumor (T), node (N), metastasis (M) classification and stage grouping lung cancer*

Occult cancer	TX	N0	M0
Stage Ia	T1,T2	N0	M0
Stage Ib	T1	N1	M0
Stage II	T2	N1	M0
Stage III	T3	N0,N1	M0
	Any T	N2	M0
Stage IV	Any T	Any N	M1

* TX, positive cytology; T1, less than or equal to 3 cm, no invasion; T2, more than 3 cm, extension to hilar region must be at least 2 cm distal to carina; T3, gross extension, effusion, atelectasis of an entire lung; N1, hilar nodes; N2, mediastinal nodes; M1, distant metastasis.
SOURCE: *P. Rubin; modified from American Joint Committee.*

organs. There is not always agreement about the definitions of the TNM characteristics, which can create confusion.

The stage of the tumor is typically divided into three or four categories (e.g., I to IV). For each type of malignancy, the various T, N, and M designations are assigned to one of four stages, in order to develop separation into groupings which correlate with data on prognosis and clinical responses to therapy. This is best described by mentioning a specific example. For the neoplasm with the highest mortality rate, non-small cell carcinoma of the lung, the therapy which has the best chance for curing the patient is surgery. The staging system for lung cancer (Table 78-8) is designed in a way which stratifies patients into groups, for which different treatment protocols are indicated. For the stages I and II patients, surgery is the treatment of choice. The extent of the surgical procedure depends on the extent of disease designated by the T and N classification within these two stages. Total excision of all tumor is the therapeutic goal, with 5-year postresection survival rates of 50 percent for stage I and 15 percent for stage II. Only occasional patients with stage III come to surgery, because of the usual nonresectability of the disease at this stage and the lack of survival benefit from removal of the primary tumor in the presence of unresectable metastases.

Clinical evaluation How does the clinician proceed to evaluate a patient for the presence of malignant disease? Early detection depends primarily on awareness of the hereditary and environmental factors contributing to the incidence of cancer, combined with thorough exploration for symptoms and signs which could lead to further diagnostic workup. The seven warning signals widely publicized by the American Cancer Society are useful to remember (Table 78-9) and are usually covered in a review of systems. A careful physical examination is especially useful in detecting early breast cancer, cancer of the colon, skin cancer, and head-and-neck cancers. Three diagnostic screening tests have proved of value in early detection: (1) the exfoliative cytology ("Pap smear") screen for cervical cancer, (2) fecal occult blood testing, accompanied by periodic sigmoidoscopy, and (3) mammograms.

The prudent guidelines for early cancer detection provided by the American Cancer Society can be summarized as follows. A cancer-related checkup is recommended every 3 years for those 20 to 40 years of age. For breast cancer screening, an examination of patients in this age group by a physician is recommended every 3 years, a self-examination every month, and one baseline breast x-ray between the ages of 35 and 40. For detection of cervical and uterine cancer, a pelvic examination is recommended every 3 years and a Pap test at least every 3 years after two initial negative tests 1 year apart.

In the age group of 40 and over, a yearly cancer checkup is recommended by the American Cancer Society. Women over 40 are

TABLE 78-9 Cancer's seven warning signals

Change in bowel or bladder habits
A sore that does not heal
Unusual bleeding or discharge
Thickening or lump in breast or elsewhere
Indigestion or difficulty in swallowing
Obvious change in wart or mole
Nagging cough or hoarseness

SOURCE: *American Cancer Society.*

advised to have a professional breast examination every year, a self-examination every month, and a breast x-ray every 1 to 2 years for those 40 to 49 years of age, and every year for those 50 and over. For screening of cervical and uterine cancer in this age group, a pelvic examination is recommended every year, a Pap test at least every 3 years after two negative tests a year apart, and an endometrial tissue sample at menopause if the patient has high-risk factors. For colon and rectal cancer, a digital rectal examination is suggested every year after 40, and a stool occult blood test every year after 50 as well as a sigmoidoscopic examination every 3 to 5 years after two initial negative tests 1 year apart.

The three most common malignancies involve bowel, lung, and breast, and it is significant that screening tests are suggested for only two of these. Unfortunately, trials of mass screening for lung cancer with chest x-rays and sputum cytology have not resulted in reduced mortality, even when subjects believed to be at high risk were followed. However, the physician who is evaluating a patient in order to attempt to detect cancer early must learn whether or not the patient smokes cigarettes and should attempt to intervene.

The approach to a patient who presents to the physician with a history of symptoms or with abnormal physical findings which could be attributed to cancer involves selection of appropriate diagnostic procedures from a wide variety of available radiologic tests and laboratory studies (Table 78-10). The choice of diagnostic procedures used in the staging of cancer patients is guided by the natural history of the various types of malignancy. For example, knowledge that distant spread of breast cancer most frequently occurs to the lung, liver, bone, brain, and contralateral breast leads to consideration of studies of each of these organs as part of the staging workup. In addition, the diagnostician must know the probability of spread to these various metastatic sites in the presence or absence of abnormal findings in the history, physical examination, and standard blood studies. For the asymptomatic patient with breast cancer who has no abnormal physical findings outside of a small palpable breast lesion, and normal hematologic and blood chemistry values, a chest x-ray and a mammogram are the tests typically performed to stage the patient prior to a decision for definitive therapy. Evaluation of the other organs to which breast cancer commonly metastasizes has not been proven to be worthwhile in this situation. Similar considerations go into planning the diagnostic workup for patients with each of the various forms of malignancy. It is for this reason that a thorough familiarity with the natural history of malignancies of the various organs, as well as the efficacy of a wide variety of diagnostic procedures in detecting these cancers, is essential.

Tumor markers A tumor marker is an abnormality which is specific for a particular type of malignancy. For example, the Ph^1 chromosome abnormality in the karyotype is a marker for chronic myelogenous leukemia, and the exclusive presence of either κ or λ chains on the surface of a population of lymphocytes is a marker of the lympho-proliferative malignancies. Often, the term *marker* is used in a more restrictive sense, referring to molecules which are produced in abnormal amounts or under abnormal circumstances and are released into the circulation. Assays of such markers may be of great help to the clinician in a number of ways: (1) screening of high-risk individuals for the presence of malignancy, (2) diagnosis of malignancy, (3) monitoring of the effectiveness of therapy, (4) early detection of recurrence, and (5) immunodetection of metastatic sites, using radioactive-labeled antibodies against the markers.

The utility of tumor markers depends upon the sensitivity of assays for their presence, and the specificity of the markers for a particular malignant cell type. Data collected from a large number of studies have demonstrated that absolutely specific tumor markers do not exist, except for idiotypic immunoglobulin chains produced by malignant lymphocytes. However, the anaplasia and autonomy of the tumor cells permit production of molecules in greater than normal amounts or at inappropriate times in the life of the organism, and in this sense the abnormalities may become specific.

The tumor marker of greatest use to the clinician is human

chorionic gonadotropin (HCG), which has specificity because of its nearly exclusive production by the trophoblastic epithelium of the placenta under normal circumstances. HCG levels rise during pregnancy. The hormone also may be secreted into the blood by trophoblastic tumors, as well as germ cell neoplasms of the testes and ovaries. Other neoplasms have been reported to be associated with elevated HCG levels, but the serum concentration rarely exceeds 10 ng/mL, whereas trophoblastic tumors can produce concentrations over 100,000 ng/mL. The usefulness of the assay for HCG is markedly enhanced by clinical data which show that changes in the serum HCG concentration in patients with secreting trophoblastic malignancies accurately reflect changes in the tumor burden. Therefore, decisions on the appropriate time to discontinue therapy can be based on the time course of serum levels, and decisions to reinstate therapy for recurrent disease are made on the basis of reappearance of HCG in the serum. The clinical test for HCG utilizes a radioimmunoassay for the beta subunit, to avoid cross reactivity with luteinizing hormone.

Two clinically useful tumor markers are products of genes which are expressed during the normal differentiation of fetal tissue but are partially or completely suppressed in the adult. These markers have been termed oncofetal antigens. Carcinoembryonic antigen (CEA) was originally thought to be specific for bowel cancer, but further studies have shown it to be a nonspecific tumor-associated antigen which also may be elevated in a variety of benign conditions. In the gastrointestinal tract, the molecule, a glycoprotein with a molecular weight of 180,000, is concentrated in the glycocalyx of epithelial cells, from which it is released into the lumen of the bowel. In the presence of malignancy, CEA concentrations may be elevated in the blood and other body fluids. Serum levels of CEA above the normal concentration of 2.5 ng/mL are found in greater than 50 percent of neoplasms involving the colon, pancreas, stomach, lung, and breast. A variety of common nonmalignant conditions are associated with elevation of CEA, but typically not over 10 ng/mL. These include cigarette smoking, chronic pulmonary disease, alcoholic cirrhosis, hepatitis, and inflammatory bowel disease. CEA is not selective for cancer, and measurements of its levels should not be used in screening for the presence of malignant disease. However, serial measurements of CEA levels in patients with secreting malignancies can provide valuable information on the efficacy of treatment and the recurrence of disease. The possibility that early elevation of serum CEA can predict recurrence of bowel cancer soon enough to allow further surgical resection for cure is under study.

The second clinically useful oncofetal antigen is alpha fetoprotein (AFP), which is produced by the liver and gastrointestinal tract epithelium during gestation and which falls to levels less than 20 ng/mL after birth. Serum levels are elevated in 70 percent of patients with hepatocellular cancer, the majority of patients with nonseminomatous testicular cancer, and occasional patients with neoplasms of the gastrointestinal tract. As with CEA, the serum concentration of AFP may be elevated in benign conditions, especially in inflammatory disease of the liver. Its utility is in monitoring tumor activity, especially in the case of testicular tumors.

Elevation of either AFP or HCG is found in 80 to 90 percent of all nonseminomatous germ cell tumors of the testes. However, absence

TABLE 78-10 Methods for clinical evaluation

I History
II Physical examination, including examination of oropharynx, Pap test, and proctoscopy
III Radiologic studies
  A Roentgenogram
  B Ultrasound
  C Computerized axial tomography
  D Angiography and lymphangiography
  E Nuclear medicine
  F Magnetic resonance imaging
IV Laboratory studies
  A Hematologic evaluation
  B Chemical tests of internal organ function
  C Tumor markers
V Pathologic examination of tissue

or normal levels of these biochemical markers of malignancy cannot be interpreted as proof that there is no tumor. Some tumors do not produce these marker molecules. Furthermore, because of tumor heterogeneity, it is possible for marker concentrations to fall in the presence of tumor, if a nonproducing subclone begins to grow preferentially. For this reason, recurrence of disease need not be accompanied by recurrence of elevated marker levels.

Other biochemical markers with clinical utility include calcitonin, with which familial medullary carcinoma of the thyroid can be detected in individuals who appear to be normal. Prostatic acid phosphatase levels are useful in determining the extent (stage) of prostatic cancer, and in monitoring the response to therapy.

There are many tumors which, because of increased cellular mass or loss of normal regulation, produce excessive quantities of polypeptides normally secreted into the circulation by the tissue of origin. Examples include the immunoglobulin molecules produced in multiple myeloma, and insulin or gastrin hypersecretion by islet cell tumors. In addition, tumors may secrete molecules which ordinarily are not produced in the tissue from which they are derived. This phenomenon has already been discussed in the description of the paraneoplastic syndromes, because in many cases these marker molecules have biologic activities which can produce clinical illness in the patient. In some cases of malignant disease, cultures of tumor cells have been found to secrete a variety of polypeptide hormones atypical of the tissue of origin. In addition, molecules related to normal hormones or to their precursor forms may be present in the patient's serum, in the absence of any demonstrable clinical effects. These observations provide evidence for the broad scope of genetic deregulation which may accompany the process of oncogene expression and carcinogenesis.

REFERENCES

CALABRESI P et al: *Medical Oncology: Basic Principles and Clinical Management of Cancer.* New York, Macmillan, 1985

DEVITA VT JR et al: *Cancer: Principles and Practices of Oncology.* Philadelphia, Lippincott, 1985

GROBSTEIN C et al: *Diet, Nutrition and Cancer.* Washington DC, National Academy Press, 1982

HOLLAND JF, FREI E: *Cancer Medicine.* Philadelphia, Lea & Febiger, 1982

RUBIN P: *Clinical Oncology for Medical Students and Physicians.* New York, American Cancer Society, 1983

SCHOTTENFELD D, FRAUMENI JF JR: *Cancer Epidemiology and Prevention.* Philadelphia, Saunders, 1982

79 PRINCIPLES OF CANCER THERAPY

VINCENT T. DeVITA, JR.

BIOLOGY OF TUMOR GROWTH

The principles of cancer therapy are based on our knowledge of the biology of tumor growth. The realization, two decades ago, that even small primary cancers shed viable tumor cells into the circulatory system as they grow in their primary site fundamentally altered the thinking about the likelihood of eradicating cancers using methods of local control alone and led to the development of systemic methods of treatment such as chemotherapy and biologic therapy. The cancer phenotype appears to be created by alterations in genetic mechanisms important in developmental biology. A family of highly conserved genes exists in the normal genome as proto-oncogenes, and alteration in their structure, or rearrangement of their location within the genome, appears to be responsible for deregulation of growth by production of abnormal proteins or abnormal quantities of proteins vital to cell growth. Although originally identified in defective oncogenic retroviruses, the existence of proto-oncogenes in normal tissue and oncogenes in many human cancers has been proved by DNA transfection experiments (see Chap. 59). Increased or abnormal expression has been shown in small cell lung cancer, colon and breast cancers, and lymphomas. The malignant phenotype is most likely the end result of the expression of the cascade of these genes. That the products of these genes are important in cell growth is underscored by their partial homology with some growth factors and receptors of growth factors. Experiments in transgenic mice (mice given single copies of oncogenes by insertion into the fertilized eggs) are providing powerful tools for identifying the cascade of genes activated for each histologic type of cancer and approaches for controlling the expression of these genes as a future means of preventing, diagnosing, or treating human cancer. For example, methylphosphonate derivatives of nucleosides complementary to the DNA of known oncogenes that can penetrate cell membranes have been shown to be capable of blocking the translation of messenger RNA and interfering with the function of these genes in vitro.

If proto-oncogenes are important regulatory elements in embryonic growth, it should not be surprising that deregulation could lead to abnormally sustained growth. In addition to uncontrolled growth, cancer cells migrate and kill largely by metastasizing and crowding out other vital organs. Several groups have cloned the genes that appear to regulate the capacity of cells to metastasize suggesting that like regulation of growth, the capacity to metastasize represents the deregulation of genetic mechanisms once responsible for normal cell migration. The capacity to metastasize appears to be related to the ability of a malignant cell to express receptors for the basement membrane protein laminen and of enzymes such as collagenases that are necessary to fix the cell to the basement membrane and to disrupt it, to allow the cell to escape from its primary site. In human studies, breast cancer cells have been shown to express large numbers of laminen receptors with a direct correlation between expression of laminen receptors and involvement of axillary lymph nodes. Developing the capacity to metastasize may be a relatively late step in the genetic cascade leading to clinically relevant cancers, a fact that would account for late metastases associated with some large tumors of certain histologic subtypes. Interfering with the ability of cancer cells to migrate has therapeutic implications. Blocking laminen receptors with laminen fragments in vitro has been shown to interfere with metastatic potential in vivo.

Once cells become malignant, the kinetics of their growth can be easily determined and are similar to the growth of normal tissues. There are three general classes of normal tissue with regard to growth characteristics: renewing (marrow and germ cells), expanding (liver, kidney, and endocrine glands), and static (neurons and striated muscle). For static tissues such as neurons, the cells live for the duration of the life of the host and are normally not replaced if lost. For expanding tissue, mitotic potential becomes apparent in cells only when cell loss takes place (trauma, surgical resection), and then the tissue is replenished. Adult cells of renewing populations have a finite, usually short, life span, and continued replacement from a stem cell pool normally takes place. As long as cell birth does not exceed cell loss, a neoplastic process is not evident even though, in a strict sense, cells of renewing tissue like bone marrow "metastasize." Regardless of the tissue of origin, the kinetics of growing populations of tumor cells resemble those of renewing populations of normal tissue. Growth characteristics of expanding tumor masses are best described as a Gompertzian function. As the mass increases, the growth is matched by exponential retardation of growth. The tumor doubling time (the time required for a given mass to double its volume) is a complex value influenced by the cell cycle time, the fraction of cells in the population undergoing cell division, and the rate of cell loss from the mass. The phases of a cell cycle are illustrated in Fig. 79-1. Cells not in cycle but viable and capable of entering cell division under proper circumstances are said to be in a resting phase (G_0). The fraction of cells in cycle in a given population (proliferative pool, growth fraction) determined by incorporation of tritiated thymidine into DNA (labeling index) markedly influences the growth of the tumor. Although cell cycle times are relatively constant in tumors of a given histologic type, considerable species differences exist in cycle times of normal and tumor tissue. For a given cycle time, a tumor with a high growth fraction will double faster than a tumor with a low growth fraction if cell loss (death, metastasis, shedding) is constant. High rates of cell loss account for long doubling times in tumors known to have high growth fractions. Cell loss begins early in the growth of a tumor. Even small (1 to 2 mm), apparently localized tumors can be assumed to shed cells into surrounding tissue (e.g., shedding from the surface of a colon cancer into the lumen of the bowel) or into lymphatics and/or the bloodstream. Cell loss may be due to departure of cells with active metastatic potential or to shedding of cells unable to produce viable colonies. The fact that some cancers can be cured by local treatment reaffirms the fact that many shed cells are unable to establish metastatic colonies for a variety of reasons, one of which may be that deregulation of the genes controlling migration may not yet have taken place.

CLONAL EVOLUTION OF CANCER The concept that cancer originates from a single transformed cell, or clone, is supported by cytogenetic studies of human neoplasms. The classic example is multiple myeloma, a malignant proliferation of antibody-secreting plasma cells, which is characterized by elevated levels of a single immunoglobulin molecule in blood or urine. In addition, tumor-specific abnormalities in chromosome structure have been demonstrated in more than 95 percent of all tumors. The first example described was the Philadelphia chromosome, which occurs in approximately 95 percent of patients with chronic myelogenous leukemia (CML) (Chap. 289). The abnormal chromosome 22 has been identified in hematopoietic precursor cells, in some cases, several years prior to the onset of overt leukemia. The clonal evolution of this disease is further supported by studies of X-inactivation mosaicism. Each cell of the female determines at the early stage in embryogenesis whether the paternal- or maternal-derived X chromosome will remain

FIGURE 79-1 *The cell cycle. The gap terminology divides the cell cycle into phases M, G_1, S, and G_2. M is the period of cell division. G_1 is the period of normal cell metabolism but without replicative DNA synthesis; cells that stay in G_1 for long periods are often referred to as being in the G_0 phase. The S, or DNA synthetic, phase is the period of doubling of the DNA content; it is followed by the G_2, or tetraploid, phase, which precedes cell division. Normal and cancer cells have similar cycle times, in general: M, 0.5 to 1 h; G_1, 2 h to infinity; S, 6 to 24 h; G_2, 2 to 8 h.*

Cell Cycle   Mitosis

Prophase

Metaphase

Anaphase

Telophase

active or suppressed. The X-linked enzyme glucose 6-phosphate dehydrogenase (G6PD) has proved a useful marker for such studies of clonal origin because it is polymorphic in the black population. Women who are heterozygous at the G6PD locus for the common gene Gd^B and the variant Gd^A normally have two distinct cell populations reflected in their enzyme electrophoretic pattern. While the nonleukemic G6PD heterozygotes have both the A and B enzyme type in white blood cells, patients with chronic myelogenous leukemia demonstrate only one enzyme type in their leukemic granulocytic series, suggesting that the disorder originated from a single cell. Oncogenes have been located at some translocation sites including loci on chromosome 9 (c-*abl*) and 22 (c-*sis*) in CML and on chromosome 14 (c-*myc*) in Burkitt's lymphoma. In this instance, the c-*myc* gene product appears normal but is constitutively expressed because it has been brought under control of the promoter sequences of the heavy chain immunoglobulin gene on chromosome 14. Cytogenetic abnormalities in malignancies such as acute myelogenous leukemia appear to be predictors of response to treatment and to be characteristic of specific cell types. In patients who relapse after complete remission attained by chemotherapy, the original cytogenetic abnormality usually reappears but may be associated with additional translocations. In follicular lymphomas, biclonal tumors have been identified by examining the rearrangement of their immunoglobulin genes. Two other hereditary tumors, neurofibroma and trichoepithelioma, have demonstrated a double enzyme phenotype, indicating multicellular origin. These exceptions suggest that the somatic mutation theories of oncogenesis may not be valid for all neoplasms.

CHEMOTHERAPEUTIC AGENTS USED FOR THE SYSTEMIC TREATMENT OF CANCER

CYTOTOXIC DRUGS Radiotherapy and surgery offer ways of reducing the tumor mass in specific regions of the body amenable to surgical excision or high doses of radiotherapy. Neither is applicable to the destruction of the widely disseminated or circulating tumor cells characteristically present in most patients with cancer. The stimulus for the development of systemic treatment of cancer can be traced to the success in identifying and using antibiotics for bacterial infections and antiprotozoan drugs for malaria. Drug development for cancer began with the accidental identification of the lympholytic activity of mustard gases used in World Wars I and II. Nitrogen mustard, an antitumor drug, is a derivative of mustard gas and was used to treat lymphomas in the 1940s. Because all of the successfully treated patients subsequently relapsed, the initial success in the treatment of Hodgkin's disease and lymphocytic lymphomas with this drug was followed by an overwhelming disappointment and skepticism that cancer could be successfully treated by drugs. Further excitement was created with the identification of the effectiveness of the antimetabolite methotrexate, first used successfully against acute childhood leukemia and then in the treatment of choriocarcinoma. In that instance, remissions produced by the drug appeared permanent. The need for a standardized approach to the development of anticancer drugs was recognized in the 1950s. Since then, many synthetic drugs, fermentation, and plant products have been identified as possessing antitumor activity against rodent tumors. These compounds have been selected both by rational synthesis and random screening. Six major classes of antitumor agents: alkylating agents, antimetabolites, plant alkaloids, antitumor antibiotics, endocrine agents, and biologicals as well as some miscellaneous drugs are now available either commercially or in investigational clinical studies. These are shown with their acute and delayed toxicity in Tables 79-1 and 79-2. Detailed discussions of the mechanism of action and pharmacology of these agents are found in the references.

THE DEVELOPMENT OF DRUG RESISTANCE Limitations of cancer surgery are related to the tolerable removal of normal tissue. Resistance to radiotherapy is relative to the dose of radiation tolerated by the adjacent normal tissue. While toxicity to normal tissue limits the use

of cancer drugs at very large doses, permanent resistance to a cancer drug is an inherent property of the cancer cell itself. Drug resistance can be viewed as either temporary or permanent. Temporary resistance refers to the inability of drugs to kill cancer cells because the cells are in the wrong phase of the cell cycle, are in pharmacologic sanctuaries such as the central nervous system or testis, where drugs may not penetrate in sufficient doses, or are in the center of a poorly vascularized tumor, unreachable by the active moiety of a drug. Permanent resistance refers to ways by which the organism alters a fundamental mechanism of activating, deactivating, or transporting a drug or of repairing damage caused by the agent. Methods of overcoming temporary drug resistance have been quite successful and include treating tumors when the number of cells is small and growing actively, introducing drugs into pharmacologic sanctuaries (such as intrathecal use of methotrexate in leukemia), and reducing tumor mass by surgery or radiotherapy to facilitate drug exposure of individual cells by reducing residual mass size, such as in ovarian cancer, where omentectomy and removal of all resectable tumor masses appears to influence subsequent capacity to respond to chemotherapy. Explanations based on cell kinetics are inadequate to explain the invariably inverse relationship between curability and cell number because in rodent tumors, resistance has been shown to develop over an increase in tumor cell number from 10^3 to 10^8. At these population sizes, cell cycle kinetics have been shown to remain constant. Also, in human adjuvant studies, the use of chemotherapy in the early stages of cancer has only been slightly more effective in curing patients than use of the same drugs in patients with advanced disease in spite of the favorable kinetics in micrometastases.

In 1979, Goldie and Coldman proposed that development of permanent resistance to cancer drugs occurred in a fashion similar to the development of resistance in bacteria to bacteriophage and was a spontaneous genetic effect. They proposed a model by which mutation to drug resistance was related to both the mutation rate and the cell number. There are several important implications of this model. First, because of the sharp relationship to cell number at any given mutation rate, the likelihood of curability decreases rapidly over small increases in tumor mass encompassing as few as six tumor doublings or a 2 log increase in cell number. If the mutation rate is 10^{-6} or greater, the likelihood of a singly or a doubly drug-resistant line appearing in a population of cells of less than 10^9, the usual level of clinically detectable tumor, is almost a certainty. These data suggest that the failure of drugs to cure many patients with advanced cancer is due to the presence of multiple permanently drug-resistant cell lines. If the mutation rate is in the range of 10^{-6}, the *absolute number* of resistant cell lines in a mass should be low enough, however, not to negatively influence the initial response to treatment. Complete remissions should be possible, but cell lines resistant to treatment would regrow and account for relapse in the phase of continued exposure to the effect of chemotherapy (Fig. 79-2). This is consistent with the clinical observations that initially responsive tumors will regrow during continued exposure to drug therapy in some cases. Also, the mutation rate is a stochastic phenomenon in bacteria and probably in the genetically unstable cancer cell. It may be different in tumors of the same type and stage, accounting for the variable responses and cure rates of uniformly staged and treated patients of the same histologic type.

The most persistent chemotherapeutic puzzle has been the unresponsiveness of tumors of visceral origin to chemotherapy when compared to childhood cancers and those of the hematologic system; in many cases, responses to chemotherapy are not observed in some visceral cancers at all. While at first this seemed inconsistent with the Goldie-Coldman hypothesis, there are several ways to account for this observation. First, these tumors may be inherently resistant to drugs as a result of the constant exposure of their normal tissue counterpart to the environment. They may possess detoxification mechanisms developed to protect them from exposure to natural toxins from which many anticancer drugs have been developed. Second, the mutation rate in tumors developed from these tissues

TABLE 79-1   Some commercially available anticancer drugs and hormones (dose-limiting effects are italicized)

Drug	Acute toxicity	Delayed toxicity*
Aminoglutethimide (Cytadren—Ciba)	Drowsiness; nausea; dizziness	Hypothyroidism (rare); bone marrow depression; fever; hypotension; masculinization
Asparaginase (Elspar–Merck)	*Nausea and vomiting; fever;* chills; headache; hypersensitivity, anaphylaxis; abdominal pain; hyperglycemia leading to coma	CNS depression or hyperexcitability; acute hemorrhagic pancreatitis; coagulation defects; thrombosis; renal damage; hepatic damage
Bleomycin (Blenoxane—Bristol)	*Nausea and vomiting; fever;* anaphylaxis and other allergic reactions	*Pneumonitis and pulmonary fibrosis; rash;* stomatitis; alopecia; Raynaud's phenomenon
Busulfan (Myeleran—Burroughs Wellcome)	*Nausea and vomiting;* rare diarrhea	*Bone marrow depression;* pulmonary infiltrates and fibrosis; hyperpigmentation; alopecia; gynecomastia; ovarian failure; azospermia; leukemia; chromosome aberrations; cataracts; Addisonian syndrome
Carmustine (BCNU; BiCNU—Bristol)	*Nausea and vomiting;* local phlebitis	*Delayed leukopenia and thrombocytopenia* (may be prolonged); pulmonary fibrosis (may be irreversible); delayed renal damage; gynecomastia; reversible liver damage
Chlorambucil (Leukeran—Burroughs Wellcome)	Minimal nausea at low doses	*Bone marrow depression;* pulmonary infiltrates and fibrosis; leukemia; hepatic toxicity; hallucinations
Cisplatin (cis-diamine-dichloroplatinum; cis-DDP; Platinol—Bristol)	*Nausea and vomiting;* anaphylactic reactions; fever; hemolytic-uremic syndrome; Raynaud's syndrome	*Renal damage;* bone marrow depression; ototoxicity; hemolysis; hypomagnesemia; peripheral neuropathy; hypocalcemia; hypokalemia; dementia
Cyclophosphamide (Cytoxan—Bristol; Neosar—Adria)	*Nausea and vomiting;* type 1 (anaphylactoid) hypersensitivity; facial burning with IV administration	*Bone marrow depression;* alopecia; hemorrhagic cystitis; sterility (may be temporary); pulmonary infiltrates and fibrosis; hyponatremia; leukemia; bladder cancer
Cytarabine HCl (cytosine arabinoside; Cytosar-U—Upjohn)	*Nausea and vomiting;* diarrhea; anaphylaxis	*Bone marrow depression;* conjunctivitis; megaloblastosis; oral ulceration; hepatic damage; fever; pulmonary edema and encephalopathy with high doses
Dacarbazine (DTIC; DIC; DTIC—Dome-Miles)	*Nausea and vomiting;* diarrhea; anaphylaxis; pain on administration; flulike syndrome	*Bone marrow depression;* alopecia; renal impairment; hepatic necrosis; facial flushing, paresthesia; photosensitivity
Dactinomycin (actinomycin D; Cosmegen—Merck)	*Nausea and vomiting;* diarrhea; local reaction and phlebitis; anaphylactoid reaction	*Stomatitis; oral ulceration; bone marrow depression;* alopecia; folliculitis; dermatitis in previously irradiated areas
Daunorubicin (daunomycin; Cerubidine—Ives)	*Nausea and vomiting;* diarrhea; red urine (not hematuria); severe local tissue damage and necrosis on extravasation; transient (EKG changes); anaphylactoid reaction	*Bone marrow depression; cardiotoxicity* (may be irreversible); alopecia; stomatitis; anorexia; diarrhea; fever and chills
Doxorubicin (Adriamycin—Adria)	*Nausea and vomiting;* red urine (not hematuria); severe local tissue damage and necrosis on extravasation; diarrhea; transient ECG changes; ventricular arrhythmia; anaphylactoid reaction	*Bone marrow depression; cardiotoxicity* (may be irreversible, but may be decreased by weekly schedule); alopecia; stomatitis; anorexia; diarrhea, fever; chills; conjunctivitis
Estramustine phosphate sodium (estracyt; Emcyt—Roche)	*Nausea and vomiting;* diarrhea	Mild gynecomastia; increased frequency of vascular accidents; myelosuppression (uncommon); edema dyspnea; pulmonary infiltrates and fibrosis; leukemia
Etoposide (VP16-213; Vepesid—Bristol)	*Nausea and vomiting;* diarrhea; fever	*Bone marrow depression;* alopecia; peripheral neuropathy; allergic reactions; hepatic damage
Floxuridine (FUDR—Roche)	*Nausea and vomiting;* diarrhea	*Oral and gastrointestinal ulceration; bone marrow depression;* alopecia; dermatitis
Fluorouracil (5-FU; Fluorouracil—Roche; Adrucil—Adria)	*Nausea and vomiting;* diarrhea; hypersensitivity reaction	*Oral and gastrointestinal ulcers; bone marrow depression;* neurologic defects, usually cerebellar; alopecia
Hydroxyurea (Hydrea—Squibb)	*Nausea and vomiting;* allergic reactions to tartrazine dye	*Bone marrow depression;* stomatitis; dysuria; alopecia; rare neurologic disturbances
Lomustine (CCNU; Cee-NU—Bristol)	*Nausea and vomiting*	*Delayed (4 to 6 weeks) leukopenia and thrombocytopenia* (may be prolonged); transient elevation of transaminase activity; neurologic reactions; pulmonary fibrosis
Mechlorethamine (nitrogen mustard; HN2; Mustargen— Merck)	*Nausea and vomiting;* local reaction phlebitis	*Bone marrow depression;* alopecia; diarrhea; oral ulcers; pulmonary infiltrates and fibrosis; leukemia
Melphalan (Allkeran—Burroughs Wellcome)	Mild nausea; hypersensitivity reactions	*Bone marrow depression* (especially platelets); pulmonary infiltrates and fibrosis; leukemia
Mercaptopurine (6-MP; Purinethol—Burroughs Wellcome)	*Nausea and vomiting;* diarrhea	*Bone marrow depression; cholestasis and rarely hepatic necrosis; oral and intestinal ulcers;* pancreatitis; allopurinol may increase overall toxicity
Methotrexate (MTX; Methotrexate—Lederle; Mexate—Bristol; Folex—Adria)	*Nausea and vomiting;* diarrhea; fever; anaphylaxis	*Oral and gastrointestinal ulceration* (perforation may occur); *bone marrow depression;* hepatic toxicity including cirrhosis and acute hepatic necrosis; renal toxicity; pulmonary infiltrates and fibrosis; osteoporosis; chills, fever; alopecia; depigmentation; infertility; menstrual dysfunction; encephalopathy and anaphylactoid reactions with high doses

TABLE 79-1 Some commercially available anticancer drugs and hormones (dose-limiting effects are italicized) *(continued)*

Drug	Acute toxicity	Delayed toxicity*
Mitomycin (Mutamycin—Bristol)	*Nausea and vomiting;* local reaction if extravasation; fever; hemolytic-uremic syndrome	*Bone marrow depression* (cumulative); stomatitis; alopecia; pulmonary fibrosis; hepatotoxicity; renal toxicity
Mitotane (o, p′-DDD; Lysodren—Bristol)	*Nausea and vomiting;* diarrhea	*CNS depression;* rash; visual disturbances; adrenal insufficiency; brain damage with long-term high dosage; hematuria; hemorrhagic cystitis; albuminuria; hypertension; orthostatic hypotension; cataracts
Plicamycin (Mithracin—Miles)	*Nausea and vomiting;* diarrhea; fever	*Hemorrhagic diathesis; bone marrow depression* (thrombocytopenia); coagulation abnormalities; hepatic damage; hypocalcemia and hypokalemia; stomatitis; renal damage
Procarbazine HCl (Matulane—Roche)	*Nausea and vomiting;* CNS depression; Antabuse-like effect with alcohol	*Bone marrow depression;* stomatitis; peripheral neuropathy; pneumonitis; leukemia
Streptozocin (streptozotocin; Zanosar—Upjohn)	*Nausea and vomiting;* local pain; chills and fever	*Renal damage;* hypoglycemia; hyperglycemia; liver damage; diarrhea; bone marrow depression (uncommon); fever; eosinophilia
Tamoxifen citrate (Nolvadex—Stuart)	*Nausea and vomiting;* hot flashes; transient increased bone or tumor pain	Vaginal bleeding and discharge; rash; hypercalcemia; thrombocytopenia; peripheral edema; depression; dizziness; headache; decreased visual acuity; corneal changes; retinopathy
Thioguanine (6-TG; Tabloid Brand Thioguanine—Burroughs Wellcome)	*Occasional nausea and vomiting*	*Bone marrow depression;* hepatic damage; stomatitis
Thiotepa (triethylene-thiophosphoramide; Thiotepa—Lederle)	*Nausea and vomiting;* local pain	*Bone marrow depression;* menstrual dysfunction; interference with spermatogenesis; pulmonary infiltrates and fibrosis; leukemia
Vinblastine sulfate (Velban—Lilly)	*Nausea and vomiting;* local reaction and phlebitis with extravasation	*Bone marrow depression;* alopecia; stomatitis; loss of deep tendon reflexes; jaw pain; muscle pain; paralytic ileus; inappropriate antidiuretic hormone (ADH) secretion
Vincristine sulfate (Oncovin—Lilly)	Local reaction with extravasation	*Peripheral neuropathy;* alopecia; mild bone marrow depression; constipation; paralytic ileus; inappropriate ADH secretion; hepatic damage; jaw pain

* *Cutaneous reactions (sometimes severe), hyperpigmentation, and ocular toxicity have been reported with virtually all nonhormonal anticancer drugs.*
SOURCE: *Adopted from* The Medical Letter *(Feb. 15, 1985), with permission.*

may also be higher due to the exposure to potential carcinogens such as those in cigarette smoke and other chemicals. Third, the impression that tumors of 1 cm in size have gone through 30 doublings to reach 10^9 cells as shown below in Fig. 79-3 is based on the assumption of exponential growth, a rare event in both animal and human tumors. Cell loss approaches 90 percent in some well-studied human visceral malignancies effectively requiring as many as 1200 doublings to reach 10^9 cells. If the likelihood of a mutation to resistance is related to the number of generation cycles, then such tumors could be largely composed of resistant cell lines at the time of diagnosis, at which time they are also unresponsive to multiple chemotherapeutic agents. This is consistent with the clinical data on the doubling times of some highly drug-resistant human cancers, such as colon cancer, which have been reported to be about 2 years.

The clinical implications of the Goldie-Coldman hypothesis are profound. First, it is the only reasonable explanation for the effectiveness of combination chemotherapy and the invariably inverse relationship between cell number and curability. Second, it underscores the need to treat with drugs early in the natural history of the disease. Third, it strongly suggests that delays in treatment as short as a few weeks to a month may markedly alter tumor curability by drugs. Such an effect has been suggested in one human breast cancer adjuvant drug trial where a delay of chemotherapy by 1 month negatively influenced the outcome of the study. It also provides an explanation for the failure of adjuvant chemotherapy to be more effective than initially expected since in most circumstances, the sum total of multiple deposits of micrometastases very likely exceeds 10^9 cells.

FIGURE 79-2 *Various compartments and flow between compartments in a hypothetical tumor mass.*

Tumor Stem Cell Compartments

*Resistant phenotypes also may go into and out of resting phase, but they remain T/R cells.

TABLE 79-2 Investigational drugs

Drug	Acute toxicity	Delayed toxicity	Drug	Acute toxicity	Delayed toxicity
Amsacrine (AMSA—Bristol, Parke-Davis)	Nausea and vomiting; diarrhea; pain or phlebitis on infusion	Bone marrow depression; hepatic injury; convulsions; stomatitis; ventricular fibrillation; alopecia	Interferon (Roferon-A—Roche; Intron-A—Schering; Wellferon—Burroughs Wellcome)	Fever; chills, myalgias; fatigue; hypotension	Bone marrow depression; anorexia; renal damage; hepatic damage
Azacitidine (Mylosar—Upjohn)	Nausea and vomiting; diarrhea; fever	Leukopenia (may be prolonged); thrombocytopenia; hepatic damage; muscle pain and weakness; bone marrow depression; possibly cardiotoxicity	*Leuprolide (LH-releasing hormone analogue—Lupron-Abbott)	Transient increase in bone pain; hot flashes	Impotence; gynecomastia
Bisantrene (ADC, ADAH—Lederle)	Nausea and vomiting; hypotension; flulike illness; fever; phlebitis	Leukopenia; thrombocytopenia	Mitobronitol (Myelobromol—Sinclair, UK)	Gastrointestinal disturbances	Bone marrow depression; alopecia
Deoxycoformycin (DCF)		Nephrotoxicity	Mitolactol	Mild nausea	Bone marrow depression
Flutamide (Eulexin—Schering)	Nausea	Gynecomastia; impotence	*Mitoxantrone HCL (DHAD; Novantrone—Lederle)	Green pigment in urine, green sclera; nausea	Bone marrow depression; cardiotoxicity; alopecia, white hair
*Hexamethylmelamine (HMM)	Nausea and vomiting	Bone marrow depression; CNS depression; peripheral neuritis; visual hallucinations	Tegafur (ftorafur—Mead Johnson)	Nausea and vomiting; CNS symptoms including dizziness and lethargy	Stomatitis; bone marrow depression; alopecia; dermatitis
Ifosfamide (Ifex—Mead Johnson)	Nausea and vomiting	Bone marrow depression; hemorrhagic cystitis; alopecia; sterility (may be temporary)	*Teniposide (VM-26—Bristol)	Nausea and vomiting; diarrhea; phlebitis; anaphylactoid symptoms	Bone marrow depression; alopecia; peripheral neuropathy
			*Vindesine sulfate (Eldisine—Lilly)	Local reaction if extravasation; fever; nausea and vomiting; diarrhea	Bone marrow depression; alopecia; peripheral neuropathy; jaw pain

* *Commercially available in Canada.*
SOURCE: *Adopted from* The Medical Letter *(Feb. 15, 1985), with permission.*

Many mechanisms of specific permanent resistance to available chemotherapeutic agents have been identified, and most occur on a genetic basis demonstrated by gene transfer experiments. These are listed in Table 79-3. Two require special mention. Pleiotropic resistance, development of resistance to multiple different classes of antitumor agents without prior exposure, has been described in rodent and human cancers. In a single step, pleiotropic resistance produces cross-resistance to most of the best and most available anticancer agents, the large complex plant- and microbial-derived products. It is often associated with the appearance of a surface glycoprotein, 170,000 daltons in size, the quantity of which is related to the degree of resistance. The presence of this protein may prove to be a useful way of identifying such lines before therapy is initiated. Pleiotropic resistance appears to be associated with defective drug accumulation due to increased drug efflux. A wide variety of drugs, including many which themselves do not possess any antitumor activity, have been demonstrated in various experimental systems to potentiate cytotoxic effects of certain chemotherapeutic drugs (Table 79-4). The calcium antagonists, calmodulin inhibitors, polyene antibiotics, triparonal analogues, and antiarrhythmic agents all appear to exert their effect, at least in part, by increasing the net accumulation of antineoplastic drugs in resistant tumor cells. Since pleiotropic drug

FIGURE 79-3 *A schematic representation of the life cycle of a human tumor. Number of cells present in the body is shown on the ordinate with number of population doublings on the abscissa. Clinical phenomena are related to expected size of tumor mass on plotted line. Most tumors have completed at least two-thirds of their growth (32 doublings) at the time of diagnosis of a 1-cm mass.*

TABLE 79-3 Mechanisms of resistance to cytotoxic drugs

General mechanism	Drug	Specific alteration
Defective transport	Methotrexate Melphalan Mechlorethamine	Decreased carrier-mediated uptake
	Cytarabine	Decreased membrane nucleoside binding sites
Defective metabolism to active species	Cytarabine	Decreased deoxycytidine kinase activity
	5-Azacitidine	Decreased uridine-cytidine kinase activity
	5-Fluorouracil	Decreased uridine kinase activity, decreased orotic acid phosphoribosyltransferase, decreased uridine phosphorylase
	6-Mercaptopurine 6-Thioguanine	Decreased HGPRT activity
	Methotrexate	Defection polyglutamation
	Doxorubicin	Decreased P_{450} or flavin reductase
Increased drug inactivation	6-Mercaptopurine 6-Thioguanine	Increased membrane alkaline phosphatase
	Cytarabine	Increased cytidine deaminase activity
	Alkylators	Increased intracellular glutathione or metallothioneine
Altered DNA repair	Alkylators Cisplatin Doxorubicin	Increased efficiency of excision of damaged bases and/or ligation of excised segment
Gene amplification with increased target protein	Cadmium	Increase in metallothioneine gene copy number
	N-Phosphonacetyl-L-aspartic acid	Increase in aspartate transcarbamylase gene copy number
	Methotrexate	Increase in DHFR gene copy number
	5-Fluorouracil	? Increase in thymidylate synthetase gene copy number
	Pentostatin	? Increase in adenosine deaminase gene copy number
Altered targets	Methotrexate	Altered DHFR
	Vincristine	Altered tubulin
	5-Fluorouracil	Altered thymidylate synthetase
	Hydroxyurea	Altered ribonucleotide reductase
	Steroids	Altered steroid receptor Altered steroid receptor complex binding to DNA
Altered nucleotide pools	Cytarabine 5-Fluorouracil	Increased intracellular CTP and dCTP pools
Salvage pathways	Methotrexate	Increased purine salvage
	5-Fluorouracil	Increased thymidine kinase activity
Pleiotropic drug resistance	Doxorubicin Vinca alkaloids	Defective drug accumulation due to increased energy-dependent efflux
	Dactinomycin Other natural products	? Specific membrane glycoprotein markers

resistance is associated with a decreased accumulation of antineoplastic drugs, the agents which increase cellular drug levels are attractive candidates for clinical trials aimed at reversing primary acquired resistance as well as the broad cross-resistance frequently observed in cancer patients who have relapsed.

Finally, gene amplification has been shown to be associated with drug resistance. This plasticity of the human genome appears to occur as a result of the reduplication of transcription if it is halted or slowed down and can be induced by agents that slow DNA synthesis such as low doses of alkylating agents and x-irradiation. Thus, marginally effective chemotherapeutic agents and/or exposure to radiation therapy may induce resistance to drugs like methotrexate without prior exposure to the drug, a factor which is influencing the design sequence of these cancer treatments. The realization that permanent specific drug resistance is a spontaneous event that can be studied and possibly circumvented is the working hypothesis for a new generation of clinical investigations in cancer therapy which emphasize early chemotherapy, in some cases *prior to* surgery (head and neck, and breast cancers), to determine if the tumor is inherently sensitive, and shorter and more intensive adjuvant chemotherapy courses to maximize the therapeutic effect while minimizing the exposure of surviving cancer cells to chemotherapeutic agents that might increase their mutation rate.

DIFFERENTIATING AGENTS There is increasing evidence that in some cases, cancers such as the leukemias represent an arrest in development. Drugs such as the polar planar compound hexamethylbisacetamide, retinoid derivatives, and biologicals such as interferon have been shown to cause leukemia cells to differentiate in vitro, and in a few reports, the retinoid 13-*cis*-retinoic acid has been shown to cause some differentiation in human acute myelogenous leukemia. Two drugs, dimethylformamide and hexamethylbisacetamide, developed only because of their ability to differentiate cells rather than their cytotoxicity, have reached clinical trials.

ENDOCRINE THERAPY Tumors such as those originating in the prostate and uterine endometrium or lymphoid tissue may respond to hormonal manipulation. The mechanism of interaction of hormones and receptors has been carefully studied. Hormones bind to receptors in the cytoplasm and nucleus and sterically alter the shape of the receptor protein itself, which interacts with DNA and is responsible for initiating specific messenger RNA and protein synthesis. Following this interaction, cytoplasmic receptor concentration is restored and the cycle can be repeated. The adrenal corticosteroids are unique among the steroid hormones because they exert some antitumor effect in tissues not normally considered to be endocrine organs, such as the malignant cells in acute lymphatic leukemia. Receptors for corticosteroids have been identified in the cytosol of leukemic cells which, along with other nonspecific effects of the corticosteroids, probably explains their antitumor action. Receptors also exist for progesterones and androgens.

TABLE 79-4 Modulation of drug resistance

Drugs	Antineoplastic* drugs affected	Proposed mechanism of increased cytotoxicity

Calcium antagonists
  Verapamil
  Nifedipine
  Nitrendipine
  Caroverine
	VCR, DNR,
	ADR
		Increased accumulation by blocking efflux

Calmodulin inhibitors
  Prenylamine
  Trifluoperazine
  Clomipramine
	VCR, DNR
	ADR
		Same as above

Amphotericin	ADR, ACT-D, BCNU	Alterations in lipid composition of plasma membrane leading to increased accumulation
Tween 80	ADR	
Perhexiline maleate	ADR	
Triparanol analogues Tamoxifen	ADR	Increased drug accumulation
Antiarrhythmic drugs Quinidine	ADR, VCR	Increased drug accumulation
Antihypertensive Reserpine	ADR	Increased drug accumulation
Thiol depleter Buthionine sulfoximine	L-PAM, PLAT, ADR	Drug inactivation, free radical metabolism, protection/repair of DNA

* Abbreviations: VCR, vincristine; DNR, daunorubicin; ADR, adriamycin; L-PAM, melphalan; PLAT, cisplatin. BCNU, 1,3 bis(2 chloroethyl)1-nitrosourea; ACT-D, actinomycin-D.

Although prostate and uterine fundal cancers have been shown to possess binding proteins for their respective hormones, the correlation between the frequency and quantity of binding proteins and the response to hormonal therapy has been most carefully studied in breast cancer. While hormones are effective alone, they are being used increasingly with other modalities of therapy either to synchronize tumor cells and increase their vulnerability to cytotoxic drugs (in breast cancer) or as noncytotoxic components of combination drug programs (in leukemias, lymphomas, breast and prostate cancers). Agonists of hypothalamic neuropeptides have been used to down-regulate receptors on hormone-responsive tissues as a new approach to hormone blockade, sometimes in combination with hormone antagonists. In prostate cancer, this has produced impressive early clinical results without the cardiovascular toxicity associated with estrogen use.

BIOLOGICALS AND CANCER THERAPY Since the host's immunologic system may be involved in the control of malignant processes, immunologic approaches to cancer treatment have been under investigation for over two decades. Manipulation of the exquisite information available on the complex network of the immune system holds considerable promise for the development and use of very specific biologicals as an integral part of the systemic approach for the treatment of cancer. Since the development of the hybridoma technique in 1975, large quantities of monoclonal antibodies have become available that react to tumor-associated antigens on tumors such as colon, lung, pancreas, and melanoma, and leukemias and lymphomas. Clinical studies are in progress to evaluate their role used alone when they are complementing fixing antibodies; coupled with toxins, such as a chain of the chemical toxin ricin or *Pseudomonas* toxin; or coupled with radioisotopes, especially alpha particle emitters. Early clinical studies have shown that monoclonal antibodies can produce temporary regressions in leukemias and lymphomas. Recombinant DNA techniques have also led to the cloning of genes for potent lymphokines, and large quantities of purified biologicals once only available in minute amounts for laboratory studies are now available for clinical trials. These include T-cell growth factor (interleukin 2), tumor necrosis factor, and interferon. In experimental systems, biologicals work best when the tumor burden is small, and thus their use after surgery or radiotherapy or after chemotherapy-induced remissions is an important investigational area. Antitumor agents are immunosuppressive, but as patients recover from their effects, their immunologic reactivity may be enhanced temporarily, and this could be the optimal time for biologic therapy.

Purified interleukin 2 (IL 2) has been used to amplify and activate a population of lymphocytes referred to as LAK cells (lymphokine-activated killer cells) which differ from natural killer cells by virtue of their ability to kill fresh autologous tumor cells from both rodents and humans regardless of their immunogenicity. Combinations of IL 2 and LAK cells have produced cures in well-controlled rodent experiments in animals with metastatic tumors. Investigational trials in humans using large doses of recombinant IL 2 and LAK cells concomitantly have produced complete and partial remissions in patients with advanced metastatic melanoma, colon cancer, and renal and lung cancers, and this holds promise as a new form of biologic therapy in adjuvant studies for earlier stages of these diseases.

Local nonspecific immunotherapy is sometimes useful and utilizes delayed hypersensitivity reactions at the site of skin tumors. Bacillus Calmette-Guérin (BCG) injections into skin nodules of patients with recurrent breast cancer or melanoma can be an effective way of controlling local disease although not often used. Delayed hypersensitivity has been produced in patients by cutaneous application of dinitrochlorobenzene. Subsequent application of this substance in superficial epidermoid and basal cell carcinomas has a cure rate equal to topical chemotherapy with 5-fluorouracil. The macrophage plays an important role as a sensor cell in the modulation of the immunologic response to antigenic tumors in rodents. Studies aimed at stimulating macrophages are in progress with levamisole, an antiprotozoan drug that improves depressed lymphocyte function by stimulating macro-phages. Coupled with 5-fluorouracil, levamisole has significantly reduced the relapse rate and improved survival in one adjuvant program in colon cancer.

INFLUENCE OF TUMOR MASS ON CURABILITY AND DOSE-RESPONSE RELATIONSHIPS

The growth and size of a tumor are generally measured in order of magnitude or logs. A human tumor, when first diagnosed as, for example, a 1.0-cm mass, contains approximately 1 billion cancer cells, whereas 10^{12} cells has been estimated to represent a lethal body burden for some malignancies. Tumor mass is an important variable for all modalities of treatment.

SURGERY The mass of the primary tumor is directly correlated with the degree of local invasion, and, in turn, the degree of local invasion is a constant predictor of the likelihood of metastases in most malignancies especially in colon and breast cancer and malignant melanoma. Within a given histologic subset of each cancer, tumor mass exerts a profound effect on curability by surgery alone.

DOSE RESPONSE AND RADIATION THERAPY For clinical purposes, a dose-response curve for radiotherapy can be constructed for specific tumors in which local tumor control is plotted as a function of dose. For a specific type of cancer, the larger the mass, the less the likelihood of destroying the tumor without severe damage to normal surrounding tissues. The radiation dose-response curve is illustrated in Fig. 79-4. The fraction of surviving cells is plotted on a log scale against radiation dose. The slope of the exponential portion of the curve, usually referred to as D_0 (mean lethal dose) is a standard reference point. D_0 is the dose required to place one inactivating event in each pertinent biologic entity. The more radiosensitive the cell, the steeper the curve. Owing to the random nature of these energy deposits, some energy will be deposited in a cell which has already been destroyed, while some will escape altogether. According to the Poisson distribution, instead of destroying all the cells, the D_0 destroys only 63 percent of them. Therefore, the dose required to reduce the number of cells in a population to 37 percent of the original number is the D_{37}, which is an index of radiosensitivity. For most cells, this value lies between 0.80 and 2 Gy (80 and 200 rad). The surviving fraction after two mean lethal doses is 37×37 percent or 13.7 percent, and after three mean lethal doses, it is 5.1 percent, etc. In practice, the logarithmic curve is not exactly a straight line. There is a small shoulder to overcome before the curve is exponential. With a strictly exponential curve, $D_0 = D_{37}$. The shoulder on the curve reflects doses below which the cell can repair radiation-induced damage. The dose at which the curve becomes exponential (D_q) is the threshold dose. Repair of radiation-induced damage can take place within 2 h. The identification of D_q, D_0, D_{37} repair time, and mechanisms of repair has important implications in clinical dose fractionation, particularly in studies combining drugs with radiation therapy.

DOSE RESPONSE AND CHEMOTHERAPY When chemotherapy was first developed, it was reserved in the main for advanced cases, after surgery and radiation therapy had failed. Most chemotherapy is able to reduce cell numbers by one to 3 logs; this is capable of producing only minimal palliation in a patient with 10^{12} tumor cells due in part to the relatively large number of cancer cells out of cell cycle less vulnerable to drugs that kill by virtue of interfering with cell growth or division. Total eradication of tumor cells is therefore not possible in advanced metastatic cancer in all but the most drug-sensitive malignancies. The cytotoxic action of anticancer agents is defined by first-order kinetics; they kill a constant fraction of cells rather than a constant number. A course of therapy with a capacity to kill 10^3 tumor cells will reduce a tumor with 10^{10} cells to 10^7, or a neoplasm of 10^5 to 10^2 cells. The majority of single drugs have a limited cell kill potential.

The implication of the fractional killing effect is that to effectively eradicate a drug-sensitive tumor population, it is necessary either to increase the dose of drug(s) within limits tolerable to the host or to begin treatment when the number of cells is sufficiently small to allow tumor destruction at reasonably tolerated doses. The killing effect of cancer chemotherapeutic agents has a definite selectivity for cancer cells over normal cells. The clinical counterpart of animal experiments showing a markedly increased sensitivity to drugs of tumor cells over normal cells can be inferred from the dramatic antitumor effects noted in some patients with drug-sensitive tumors without permanent damage to the patients' bone marrow or gastrointestinal tract.

Conceptually, tumor cells can be divided into three distinct kinetic compartments, each with its particular significance in relation to the effectiveness of chemotherapy (Fig. 79-2). First, there is the fraction of tumor cells sensitive to chemotherapy and actively growing that is most vulnerable to drug treatment. Second, there is a population of cells which are temporarily nondividing but, nevertheless, have the capability of returning to a replicative stage. In terms of cell cycle kinetics, these cells are in an extended G_1 or G_0 phase and are considerably less sensitive to antitumor agents, particularly the cell cycle phase–specific antimetabolites, even though this type of resistance may be temporary. Then there is a compartment of cells that have permanently lost proliferative capacity but which still contribute to the estimated mass of the tumor at the bedside until they die and are absorbed. The dose-response curves for both toxicity and therapeutic effect for cancer drugs are steep. In some rodent experiments, a 20 percent reduction in dose leads to a 50 percent reduction in cure rate. The observation has been extended to doses of single drugs within effective drug combinations. Loss of the curative effect of a combination of drugs is seen with modification of the most effective agent in the combination to accommodate the toxicity of other drugs used with it. Dose rate refers to the administration of a given amount of a drug over a finite time. Since most chemotherapeutic agents are toxic to dividing cells, intervals between treatment cycles are dictated by the recovery of normal renewing tissue pools, most often the bone marrow, which takes approximately 18 to 28 days in humans. Prolonged intervals between cycles of treatment, even if drugs are given at full doses, reduces the dose rate and may allow for both regrowth of tumors and development of permanent resistance. This has been clearly demonstrated in animal models and in the clinic in the treatment of acute myelogenous leukemia, Hodgkin's disease, and small cell lung cancer. Since the effect of most drug treatment programs is reported on the basis of a fixed dose rate, ad hoc alterations of the use of specific treatment regimens in the clinic for purposes of convenience, an all too common event, very likely reduce the reported good effects of the treatment program.

TREATMENT OF LOCALIZED OR REGIONAL TUMOR

SURGICAL THERAPY Surgery is still considered the primary treatment for most early cancers. However, many tumors are operable but not fully resectable, and some that appear resectable (control of the tumor and lymph node compartments) have micrometastatic disease outside the tumor field. This point can best be illustrated using colon and breast carcinoma as examples. Lymph nodes involved in breast cancer (stage II) and colon cancer (Duke's C) serve as indicators of metastatic potential and are associated with low 5-year survivals without further treatment. Increasingly radical surgery in both these cancers has not been demonstrated to provide additional benefit, but minimal surgical procedures, such as lumpectomy with radiotherapy to the breast, give results as good as those attained with radical or modified radical mastectomy. As surgery has become less radical, the complexity of the procedures has sometimes increased, such as in limb-sparing surgery for extremity sarcomas.

LASER SURGERY Laser surgery is another way of excising benign or malignant lesions. The biologic effects of laser surgery in general and the commonly used CO_2 laser surgery in particular are unique. The wavelength of the CO_2 laser is readily absorbed by all biologic structures with very little scatter. When focused appropriately, the incision may be quite fine with minimal damage to adjacent tissue. Combined with an operating microscope, laser surgery is a precise technique. Biologic material is vaporized rather than cauterized. Blood vessels and lymphatics up to 0.5 mm are sealed during treatment. These features minimize trauma, facilitate healing, and shorten hospital stays. The chief drawbacks to laser surgery are the inability to cauterize larger vessels and destroy larger regions of tissue. Carbon dioxide laser surgery is used in cancers of the head and neck region and in the tracheobronchial tube, where its controlled depth of penetration is useful in avoiding perforation. It is under evaluation in the treatment of brain tumors. No claims have been made for improved survival, but significant palliation can be achieved in obstructing tracheobronchial and esophageal lesions treated through a rigid endoscope. It may also be more advantageous than cold knife surgery in patients with blood dyscrasias and in seriously ill patients. Complications are serious heat damage to patients and operating personnel and eye damage from reflected light, both of which can be easily avoided.

Surgeons also perform nontherapeutic procedures in newly diagnosed patients for staging purposes only, such as laparotomy in Hodgkin's disease and other lymphomas (see Chap. 294) and second-look procedures in ovarian and colon cancer. Indications for use of these procedures vary with treatment options, and they should never be performed by the surgeon in vacuo, without prior consultation with the physician, or team of physicians, who will eventually be called upon to provide the definitive treatment.

Indications for more mutilating radical surgical procedures such as hemicorporectomy, pelvic exenteration, and radical head and neck surgery have diminished as methods of combining treatments have proved successful. They are offered to patients with locally advanced primary tumors or locally recurrent tumors for which no other means of controlling the regional tumor or systemic treatment is available. If the patient understands fully the degree of mutilation involved, a careful search reveals no metastases, the risk of recurrent disease is not unreasonably great, and the operation is technically feasible, then the risks of mortality must be weighed against the chance for controlling the tumor. These are very individual decisions shared by the patient, the family, and the physician. Significant advances in reconstructive surgery of the head, neck, and pelvic regions have been made and the greater availability of more acceptable prostheses may make these radical procedures more acceptable.

FIGURE 79-4 *Radiation dose-response curve (see text).*

RADIATION THERAPY Radiation therapy is another regional form of treatment used for the control of localized cancers. The ideal in radiation therapy of malignant disease is achieved when the tumor is completely eradicated and the surrounding normal tissues in the treated volume show little or no evidence of structural or functional injury. The important factor in successful treatment is the difference in radiosensitivity of neoplastic and normal cells. The difference depends on the capacity for intracellular repair of normal and neoplastic cells and the ability of normal organs to continue to function well if they are only segmentally damaged. If surrounding tissue can tolerate twice the radiation dose of a given tumor, then the tumor is radiosensitive. On the other hand, tumor which extensively involves both lungs and may be cured by a dose of 30 Gy (3000 rad) cannot be treated effectively with radiation therapy because of the greater radiosensitivity of the surrounding lung tissue. As with normal tissue, however, different tumors have a different range of radiosensitivity, some being responsive to as little as a few hundred rad, and others being incurable with as much as 100 Gy (10,000 rad). This range of sensitivity can exist even within a specific tumor type.

TYPES OF RADIOTHERAPY EQUIPMENT The term *x-ray* or *roentgen ray* is applied to electromagnetic, nonparticulate, ionizing radiations produced by man-made machines, whereas gamma rays emanate from naturally occurring or artificially produced radioactive elements such as radium or cobalt 60. These radiations of very short wavelengths have extremely high penetrating power in materials of low atomic number such as water and tissue, but are stopped effectively in materials of high atomic number such as lead. The ionizing events following irradiation lead to the production of free radicals in the water molecules of the cell microenvironment. Such free radicals and oxidizing agents interact with DNA molecules and produce a large number and variety of DNA breaks and damage. The exact lesion of x-ray irradiation remains undefined, but once alterations in nucleotide sequences occur, a change in transcription, or defective repair, results in cell death. At one time, the best-available apparatus for "deep therapy" operated at 200 to 250 kV, referred to as the *kilovoltage range*. The *supervoltage energy range* is generally taken to be 2 to 10 MeV, and *megavoltage energies* are those above 10 MeV. Radium emits gamma rays from about 1 MeV, while the artificially produced isotope cobalt 60 (^{60}Co) emits gamma rays of about 1.4 MeV. The mere presence in a unit of a quantity of ^{60}Co does not make it a true supervoltage instrument. The great tissue penetration which characterizes the supervoltage range is obtained only when the radiation source is far removed (preferably 70 cm to 1 m) from the surface of the patient. Since the output of the source decreases inversely as the square of its distance from the patient, units containing very large amounts of ^{60}Co (7.4×10^{13} to 11.1×10^{13} Bq, or 2000 to 3000 Ci) are required to produce adequate intensities and reasonably short treatment times at treatment distances of 1 m or greater. The units which contain smaller amounts of ^{60}Co and are operated at a distance of 50 cm or less should not be thought of as supervoltage devices since the physical distribution of gamma ray beams from these sources is comparable with kilovoltage rays. Linear (electron) accelerators are able to generate high-energy radiations without employing high voltages, and those operating in the range of 4 to 10 MeV are commercially available. A similar device, the betatron, accelerates electrons magnetically in a circular path within a vacuum tube. Commercial units presently available produce electrons and x-rays at a peak energy of 18 to 30 MeV.

Megavoltage radiation equipment has almost completely replaced kilovoltage sources in cancer therapy. Because of reduced skin doses and lesser internal scatter with megavoltage irradiation, higher doses of irradiation can be delivered to tumors at any depth in the body. Linear accelerators in the 4- to 35-MeV range and cobalt sources are the photon generators most widely employed. Linear accelerators deliver radiation with sharper beam margins than do cobalt machines. Linear accelerators can also provide electrons, which are particulate and penetrate approximately 0.25 to 0.5 cm per megaelectronvolt of energy with a relatively abrupt falloff in tissues, so that deeper normal tissues are spared from irradiation. The low penetrance of electron beams is proving useful in intraoperative radiotherapy, which seeks to avoid radiation to normal tissues distal to the target organ and those moved aside at surgery.

Other forms of particulate irradiation which are more penetrating than the electron and which have very favorable physical and biologic characteristics for the treatment of cancer are being developed. These include fast neutrons, charged particles such as protons or helium ions, and negative pi mesons. These particles cause a more intense deposition of energy per unit path in the tissue [high linear energy transfer (LET)] than does ordinary photon radiation. They also have the theoretical advantage of greater relative biologic effectiveness (RBE), in part because of lower oxygen-enhancement ratios (OER), which should treat hypoxic fractions of tumors more effectively. Fast neutrons are now being tested in clinical trials using medically dedicated neutron generators. Preliminary results suggest some advantage in patients with head and neck cancers and striking improvements in patients with salivary gland cancers. Attempts to avoid toxicity to normal tissues and improve fractionation techniques include the use of intraoperative radiotherapy for abdominal primaries where normal bowel can be moved outside of the radiation field. Clinical studies in the United States and Japan have shown that dose fractions much larger than conventional fractions can be delivered at the time of surgery and may improve local control in gastric and pancreas cancers; effects on survival have not yet been demonstrated.

Doses of radiation are expressed in units called grays (Gy). One gray equals 100 rad or 1 rad equals 0.01 Gy. These units indicate the amount of absorbed energy per unit volume of tissue. The biologic effects of irradiation are dependent on the time over which the radiation is delivered and the dose per fraction. Usual dose fractionation is about 10 Gy (1000 rad) per week, delivered in 1.5- to 2.5-Gy (150 to 250 rad) fractions. Delivering tumoricidal doses with kilovoltage sources required prolonged periods of time and utilization of many fractions when skin tolerance was the major limiting factor. With megavoltage irradiation this is no longer the case, and shorter and more intense irradiation dose fractionation is being developed and studied.

RADIOSENSITIZERS; CHEMICALS Tumor masses have been shown to contain significant fractions of hypoxic cells due to the inadequacy of the blood supply (as the mass increases) in large tumors. Since the free radical state of molecular oxygen interacts with ionization products created by radiation beams, radiation therapy to such tumors is less effective than to fully oxygenated tumors. In experimental tumor systems, the size of the hypoxic fraction has been shown to be directly proportional to the failure rate of local treatment.

Attempts to improve the cell kill of hypoxic cells have involved the use of hypoxic cell sensitizer drugs. Of the compounds tested as hypoxic cell sensitizers, the 2-nitroimidazoles appear to have the greatest potential because of pharmacologic properties that promote distribution of drug to the central portion of tumors in spite of poor blood supply. Among these, metronidazole and another experimental derivative, misonidazole have been active in animal model systems. These compounds act by mimicking oxygen in fixing DNA damage caused by radiation. They improve radiosensitivity of hypoxic cells as tested both in vitro and in vivo. They do not sensitize normal oxic cells to radiation and therefore exert a selective effect between tumors and normal tissues. The use of hypoxic radiosensitizers has been limited in clinical trials due to neurotoxicity. Newer studies are examining different dosing and fractionation to avoid this side effect, and newer, less lipophilic compounds are in early clinical trials.

There are other compounds that are not hypoxic cell sensitizers that enhance the effect of radiotherapy. One group is the thiol-depleting agents. All cells contain thiols, some of which are nonprotein sulfhydryls that act to protect DNA from radiation damage. Compounds such as *N*-ethylmaleimide or a synthesis blocker like buthionine sulfoximine can render cells radiosensitive. Some chemicals are radioprotectors and theoretically can protect normal tissue from the effects of radiotherapy. So far, only one radioprotector, a sulfhydryl compound—ethiofos— has been developed. In animal studies, it protects normal and tumor tissue equally.

Cytotoxic drugs also act as radiosensitizers to both normal and tumor tissue. Pyrimidine analogues, particularly bromodeoxyuridine and idoxuridine, constitute such a class of radiosensitizers when used in noncytotoxic doses. Radiosensitization occurs when a halogenated pyrimidine is substituted for thymidine in cellular DNA. Sensitization requires prolonged infusion since these compounds are incorporated into the cell only during DNA synthesis. Clinical studies in brain tumors using prolonged intravenous infusions are yielding promising results. In some cases, the use of cancer drugs in cytotoxic doses concurrently with radiotherapy (small cell lung cancer; stage II breast cancer) has improved local control and survival. The toxic effects of drugs like doxorubicin, dactinomycin, and bleomycin are enhanced on normal tissues such as the skin, heart, and lungs when used with radiotherapy.

HYPERTHERMIA Cell sensitivity to heat in the range of 43 to 45°C is increased in the presence of low pH, hypoxia, poor perfusion, and low nutrient supply, conditions found in the interior of many tumors, and tumor cells have been found to be more sensitive to heat than normal cells. Heat tends to kill cells in S phase, the most radioresistant phase of the cell cycle. In animal studies, closely spaced or concurrent use of heating and radiation therapy produces more effective tumor control than either modality alone, and in some cases, allows lower doses of radiation therapy to be used. Experimental data suggest that the antitumor effect of hyperthermia also includes inhibition of radiation damage repair. There are major technical problems, however, with the three chief ways of delivering hyperthermia in the clinics (microwaves, ultrasound, and radio frequency currents) largely related to heat distribution in tumors of varying size and depth and to thermometry techniques to measure heat distribution. Hyperthermia's potential in the treatment of cancer is clear; microwave hyperthermia has received Federal Drug Administration (FDA) approval for use with photon radiotherapy, and several important clinical studies are in progress. Hyperthermia also sensitizes cells to chemotherapy, and clinical trials using whole-body hyperthermia are in progress to evaluate the combination of drugs, heat, and radiotherapy to overcome the limitations of hyperthermia used as a regional treatment.

PHOTODYNAMIC THERAPY A new approach to treatment of cancers limited to geographic regions, photodynamic therapy (PDT), combines exposure to radiated light in the visible range and non-cytotoxic drug therapy. Light-absorbing chemicals such as hemato-porphyrin derivatives are selectively retained by cancer cells. The cancer cells are killed when exposed to certain wavelengths of light. Dramatic responses have been reported in rodents and humans with superficial lesions such as skin tumors or in intrabronchial tumors when hematoporphyrin-exposed cells are exposed to laser beams of the appropriate wavelengths through an endoscope. Experiments in rodents with ascites tumors show that complete resolution of ascites is possible since the entire abdominal cavity can be exposed to light. PDT is relatively nontoxic, but its limitations are similar to radiation therapy in that all tumor cells must be exposed to light. Such a circumstance is difficult to achieve with cells in circulation.

CHOICE OF LOCAL MODALITY Treatment with radiotherapy instead of surgery, using more sophisticated equipment, has the advantage of being less mutilating and, where it provides equivalent results, is the preferred approach. This choice will depend in some cases on the expertise in a given institution. For example, in the treatment of stage I carcinoma of the cervix, either modality provides equal survival rates. In localized carcinoma of the vocal cords because radiotherapy has a high cure rate and spares the vocal cords, it is preferred to surgery. In carcinoma of the prostate, with stage A and B, radiotherapy is the preferred approach because it produces survival figures equivalent to those with surgery with far lower risk of impotence. In women with breast tumors less than 4 cm in size, radiotherapy to the breast and axillary nodes is the primary treatment after lumpectomy if the institutional radiotherapist has the necessary

technical skills. In carcinoma of the rectum below the peritoneal reflection, radiotherapy alone in small, nonulcerated, and superficial lesions is quite effective in controlling the tumors; radiotherapy can improve survival figures when used in conjunction with surgery and chemotherapy in patients with rectal cancer which is more extensive. In epidermoid cancers of the anal canal, radiotherapy with chemotherapy has replaced abdominoperineal resection and colostomy while producing equivalent survival rates.

In some cases, however, the routine use of radiotherapy as an adjunct to surgery should be avoided. In carcinoma of the breast, routine postmastectomy radiotherapy of the *chest wall* and lymph node areas adds nothing to the results of surgery, does not improve survival, but does cause significant morbidity. Local recurrences are rare in the absence of systemic metastases, and local recurrences can be controlled by radiotherapy or drug treatment when they occur.

In stage IIB carcinoma of the ovary (limited to the pelvis), radiotherapy alone should be discouraged since further drug therapy is usually required. Its use as the primary treatment of stage III ovarian cancer (widespread intraabdominal disease) is also contraindicated. Except in rare instances, routine radiotherapy in lung cancer has been ineffective, although it improves local control and survival when used concurrently with effective drug treatment of small cell carcinoma. In testicular cancer, the routine use of retroperitoneal radiotherapy following lymphadenectomy is no longer used in patients with nonseminomatous tumors. Routine preoperative or postoperative therapy of stage I uterine fundal cancer may not offer additional benefit to surgery.

TREATMENT OF ADVANCED CANCER

CHEMOTHERAPY The most important aspect of cancer chemotherapy trials conducted in the 1960s and realized in the 1970s was the demonstration that drugs could cure patients with some types of advanced cancer. The most important initial goal of the more intensive drug treatment programs is similar to the goal of surgery and radiation therapy for localized tumor—that is, to erase all clinical evidence of disease (complete remission). The length of time the patient remains free of disease after all therapy is discontinued is used as an indication of the magnitude of the reduction of tumor cell number. These indicators of successful treatment have been valid, and survival has improved commensurate with an increase in the rates and duration of complete remission for metastatic cancers when drug combinations have been compared with single agents.

Cancers can generally be grouped into categories according to the effectiveness of systemic treatment. Table 79-5 lists types of cancers for which current chemotherapeutic programs have major activity and are clinically quite useful. In some cases, patients are curable even though the body burden of tumor cells is very high. In most cases maximum benefit is achievable only by drug combinations. In Hodgkin's disease, acute childhood leukemia, diffuse large cell lymphomas, and testicular tumors, disease-free survival after cessation of treatment extends to over 15 years. Considering the tumor volume in most of these patients at the time of treatment ($\pm$ 10^{11} cells), these results are quite remarkable. The break in the survival curve varies for each disease. A 2-year disease-free interval from the end of treatment is sufficient to consider patients cured with such virulent, rapidly growing tumors as choriocarcinoma, Burkitt's lymphoma, and diffuse large cell lymphomas, while 4 or more years are required to evaluate the results of treatment in Hodgkin's disease, acute childhood leukemia, breast cancer, and testicular cancer. Widespread use of these treatment programs has resulted in marked improvement in relative survival rates concomitant with a sharp decrease in national mortality in patients with Hodgkin's disease and other lymphomas, testes cancer, acute leukemia of childhood, other pediatric neoplasms, ovarian carcinoma, and premenopausal women with breast cancer. Chemotherapy has moderate and useful activity in the cancers listed in Table 79-6, although cure is not generally possible once the diseases have metastasized. Adjuvant studies have proved positive in

TABLE 79-5 Diseases in which chemotherapy has major activity

Cancer type	Drugs currently preferred	Alternative drugs	Cancer type	Drugs currently preferred	Alternative drugs
Acute lympho-cytic leukemia (ALL)	Induction: vincristine + prednisone ± asparagi-nase ± doxorubicin	Daunorubicin, cyclo-phosphamide, cytara-bine, thioguanine, vin-desine,* teniposide,* mitoxantrone,* etopo-side	Diffuse large cell lym-phoma	Prednisone + metho-trexate-leucovorin dox-orubicin + cyclophos-phamide + etoposide—mechlorethamine + vincristine + procarba-zine + prednisone (ProMACE-MOPP)	Bleomycin, chlorambu-cil, lomustine, carmus-tine, cytarabine, etopo-side, teniposide,* amsacrine,* asparagi-nase, methotrexate, high-dose cytarabine, ifosfamide*
	CNS prophylaxis: in-trathecal methotrexate ± radiotherapy	CNS prophylaxis: high-dose IV methotrexate		Methotrexate, doxorubi-cin, cyclophosphamide, vincristine, prednisone, bleomycin (MACOP-B)	
	Maintenance: combina-tion chemotherapy with methotrexate + mer-captopurine or other combinations	Maintenance: doxorubi-cin and/or asparaginase in addition to metho-trexate and mercaptopu-rine		Bleomycin + doxorubi-cin + cyclophospha-mide + vincristine + dexamethasone + methotrexate with leu-covorin rescue (M-BACOD)	
Acute myelocytic leukemia (AML)	Daunorubicin + cytara-bine ± thioguanine	Amsacrine,* azaciti-dine,* high-dose cytara-bine, teniposide,* eto-poside, mitoxantrone*		Bleomycin + doxorubi-cin + cyclophospha-mide + vincristine + prednisone + procarba-zine (COP-BLAM)	
Anal cancer	Fluorouracil + mitomy-cin†			Cyclophosphamide + vincristine + metho-trexate-leucovorin + cytarabine (COMLA)	
Brain					
Adult gliomas†	High-dose methotrexate with citrovorum factor rescue; carmustine or lomustine	Procarbazine, doxorubi-cin, vincristine	Follicular lym-phoma	Investigational protocols similar to those used in diffuse large cell lym-phomas or observation for low-grade follicular lymphomas; combina-tion chemotherapy for intermediate or high-grade	Cyclophosphamide or chlorambucil or vincris-tine or prednisone or etoposide (combinations not demonstrably supe-rior to single agents); cytarabine, asparagi-nase, methotrexate, in-terferon,* anti-idiotype monoclonal antibody*
Medulloblas-toma†	Vincristine + carmustine ± mechlorethamine ± methotrexate				
	Mechlorethamine + vin-cristine + procarbazine + prednisone (MOPP)				
Breast cancer†	Tamoxifen, progestins; cyclophosphamide + methotrexate + fluo-rouracil ± prednisone (CMF or CMFP); cy-clophosphamide + doxorubicin ± fluo-rouracil (AC or CAF)	Vincristine, vinblastine, mitomycin, mitolactol,* mitoxantrone,* tenipo-side,* estrogens, andro-gens, prednisone, ami-noglutethimide	Mycosis fun-goides	Mechlorethamine (topical in ointment base); com-bination chemotherapy as in Hodgkin's disease or non-Hodgkin's lym-phoma	Vinblastine, methotrex-ate, psoralen + ultravi-olet light (PUVA), interferon,* deoxyco-formycin*
Choriocarcinoma	Methotrexate ± dactino-mycin	Vinblastine, chlorambu-cil, bleomycin, etopo-side, cisplatin, 6-mer-captopurine			
Embryonal rhab-domyosarcoma†	Vincristine + dactino-mycin + cyclophos-phamide (VAC) ± doxorubicin	Methotrexate, thiotepa	Ovary	Melphalan (or cyclo-phosphamide) ± cis-platin ± doxorubicin (CP, CAP); cyclophos-phamide + hexame-thylmelamine* + dox-orubicin + cisplatin (CHAP); high-dose cis-platin plus cyclophos-phamide	Hexamethylmelamines,* fluorouracil, chlorambu-cil, thiotepa, vincris-tine, ifosfamide,* megestrol acetate
Ewing's sarcoma†	Cyclophosphamide + doxorubicin + vincris-tine (CAV)	Dactinomycin			Intraperitoneal: fluorour-acil, methotrexate, mel-phalan, or doxorubicin
Hairy cell leuke-mia	Interferon,* deoxycoformycin*	Chlorambucil			
Hodgkin's disease	Mechlorethamine + vin-cristine + procarbazine + prednisone (MOPP) Doxorubicin + bleomy-cin + vinblastine + dacarbazine (ABVD) MOPP alternated with ABVD	Lomustine, carmustine, etoposide, teniposide,* streptozotocin	Osteogenic sar-coma†	Doxorubicin and/or high-dose methotrexate + leucovorin rescue ± bleomycin ± cyclo-phosphamide ± dacti-nomycin anal	Melphalan, mitomycin, cisplatin
Lung			Sarcomas† (soft tissue, adults)	Doxorubicin + cyclo-phosphamide	Vincristine, methotrex-ate, ifosfamide,* dacar-bazine
Small cell (oat cell)	Cyclophosphamide + doxorubicin + vincris-tine (CAV); cyclophos-phamide, methotrexate, lomustine (CMC)	Cyclophosphamide + doxorubicin + vincris-tine + etoposide (CAVE)	Testicular	Cisplatin + vinblastine + bleomycin (PVB); ± etoposide for bulky tumor	Vinblastine + dactino-mycin + bleomycin + cyclophosphamide + cisplatin (VAB-6)
	Etoposide + cisplatin	Procarbazine, mechlor-ethamine		Bleomycin + etoposide + cisplatin (BEP)	Etoposide, cyclophos-phamide, methotrexate, plicamycin, dactinomy-cin, melphalan, chlor-ambucil
Lymphocytic lym-phoma					
Burkitt's lym-phoma	Cyclophosphamide	Carmustine, methotrex-ate, ifosfamide*	Wilms's tumor	Dactinomycin + vincris-tine for favorable his-tology; ± doxorubicin for unfavorable prog-nostic factors	Doxorubicin, cyclophos-phamide
	Cyclophosphamide + vincristine + metho-trexate				

* Available only for investigational use.
† Drugs have major activity when combined with surgical resection, radiotherapy, or both (primary multimodal therapy).
SOURCE: Modified from The Medical Letter (Feb. 15, 1985).

TABLE 79-6 Diseases in which chemotherapy has moderate activity

Cancer type	Drugs currently preferred	Alternative drugs	Cancer type	Drugs currently preferred	Alternative drugs
Adrenocortical carcinoma	Mitotane	Doxorubicin, aminoglutethimide, cyclophosphamide, cisplatin	Islet cell carcinoma	Streptozocin ± fluorouracil	Cyclophosphamide, doxorubicin, dacarbazine
Bladder	Cisplatin and/or doxorubin ± methotrexate ± vinblastine; thiotepa or doxorubicin instillation	Mitomycin, fluorouracil, vinblastine, methotrexate, instillation of mitomycin or BCG*	Kaposi's sarcoma (epidemic)	Etoposide or interferon*	
			Lung cancer		
			Non-small cell	Cyclophosphamide + doxorubicin + cisplatin†	Methotrexate, etoposide, lomustine, fluorouracil, ifosfamide,* mitomycin, mitomycin + vinblastine
Cervix	Cisplatin + bleomycin ± methotrexate	Cyclophosphamide, vincristine, methotrexate, mitomycin, fluorouracil, doxorubicin, vinblastine		Vindesine* + cisplatin	
	Bleomycin + mitomycin + vincristine ± cisplatin			Vinblastine + cisplatin	Mitomycin + vinblastine + cisplatin
					Fluorouracil + doxorubicin + mitomycin (FAM)
Chronic lymphocytic leukemia	Chlorambucil ± prednisone	Cyclophosphamide, vincristine			
Chronic myelocytic leukemia (CML)			Myeloma	Melphalan (or cyclophosphamide) + prednisone	Carmustine, vincristine, lomustine, doxorubicin, interferon*
Stable phase	Busulfan; hydroxyurea	Mitobronitol,* mercaptopurine, thioguanine, melphalan			
Acute phase	Daunorubicin + cytarabine + vincristine + prednisone ± thioguanine	Amsacrine,* azacitidine,* vincristine		Melphalan + carmustine + cyclophosphamide + prednisone	
				Dexamethasone + doxorubicin + vincristine	
	Vincristine + prednisone for lymphoid variant		Neuroblastoma	Doxorubicin + cyclophosphamide + cisplatin + teniposide*	Mechlorethamine, daunorubicin, dacarbazine, vinblastine, prednisone, cisplatin, teniposide,* etoposide
Endometrial	Megestrol acetate or hydroxyprogesterone caproate or medroxyprogesterone	Fluorouracil, tamoxifen, melphalan			
	Doxorubicin ± cyclophosphamide		Prostate	Leuprolide* ± flutamide*	Diethylstilbesterol, estramustine, megestrol acetate, fluorouracil, cyproterone,* flutamide ± (antiandrogen), methotrexate; cisplatin ± cyclophosphamide ± doxorubicin
Gastric	Fluorouracil + doxorubicin + mitomycin (FAM)	Cisplatin			
	Fluorouracil + doxorubicin + semustine*				
Head and neck, squamous cell	Bleomycin + cisplatin ± methotrexate; cisplatin + fluorouracil	Vinblastine, cyclophosphamide, mitomycin, doxorubicin	Retinoblastoma	Doxorubicin + cyclophosphamide	

* Available only for investigational use.
† Drugs have major activity only when combined with surgical resection, radiotherapy, or both (adjuvant chemotherapy).
SOURCE: Modified from The Medical Letter (Feb. 15, 1985).

non-small cell lung cancer and head and neck cancers that, if confirmed, could change the outlook of these diseases in a major way.

Tumors listed in Table 79-7 are frequently thought of as resistant to treatment, but on occasion significant palliation can be provided for patients by the careful use by an experienced physician of existing chemotherapeutic agents. However, studies using adjuvant 5-fluorouracil plus levamisole have shown a statistically significant improvement in relapse-free and overall survival at 4 years in Duke's B_2 and C colon cancer, and the combination of 5-fluorouracil and radiation therapy has been shown to improve survival in patients with locally unresectable pancreatic cancer. These studies are being reconfirmed in larger-scale clinical trials. Biological therapy with interleukin 2 and activated lymphocytes has produced significant regression of metastases in patients with colon, renal, lung cancer, and malignant melanoma; and preliminary results with specific monoclonal antibodies have shown useful responses in a few patients with colorectal and pancreas cancer and malignant melanoma.

CONTINUOUS INFUSION CHEMOTHERAPY Two advances in technology have reawakened an interest in the methods of delivery of chemotherapy to sites of specific tumor involvement: the availability of improved infusion devices, and sensitive methods for measuring the active moiety of both drugs and their cellular targets within the biologically active range. Organ-directed chemotherapy holds considerable promise as a component of multimodal therapy to deliver drugs at higher concentrations for prolonged periods. This approach

can ovecome pharmacokinetic problems in drugs with short half-lives and cell kinetic problems by exposing tumor cells to effective concentrations for periods well in excess of their cell cycle times. In liver perfusions, advantage can be taken of drugs that are metabolically inactivated by the normal liver to avoid systemic toxicity. At the

TABLE 79-7 Diseases in which chemotherapy has minor activity

Cancer type	Drugs currently preferred	Alternative drugs
Colorectal	Fluorouracil;† intraarterial floxuridine	Methotrexate
Esophagus	Cisplatin + vinblastine + bleomycin	5-Fluorouracil, doxorubicin
Liver	Doxorubicin; fluorouracil ± methotrexate	Fluorouracil, floxuridine, amsacrine,* intraarterial floxuridine, vinblastine
Melanoma	Dacarbazine	Dactinomycin, carmustine, procarbazine, vinblastine, interferon*
Pancreatic	Fluorouracil + doxorubicin + mitomycin (FAM); fluorouracil + radiation†	Streptozocin + mitomycin + fluorouracil (SMF); mitomycin, doxorubicin, streptozocin, semustine,* ifosfamide*
Renal	No good choice	Vinblastine, lomustine, interferon*

* Available only for investigational use.
† Clinically useful only in patients with locally unresectable diseases.
SOURCE: Modified from The Medical Letter (Feb. 15, 1985).

present time, however, continuous intravenous infusions of anticancer drugs have not shown a clear benefit over pulse or short-term infusions with the possible exception of the continuous intravenous infusion of bromodeoxyuridine or iododeoxyuridine coupled with radiotherapy in the treatment of gliomas. Intraarterial infusion therapy is presently being restudied in patients with metastases from colon cancer limited to the liver. While the results suggest some improvement in terms of increased response rates, most studies are not well enough controlled to recommend the therapy over systemic treatment except under investigational conditions, and because survival has not been improved. The combined use of 5-fluorodeoxyuridine infusions coupled with external radiation therapy to the liver appears to offer some advantage in survival. Attempts are being made to redirect the blood supply away from normal liver to liver metastases by using vasoconstrictors or by trapping drugs in the tumor vasculature temporarily by administration with starch granules which are subsequently dissolved by amylase. Studies are needed to couple infusion therapy with resection of hepatic metastases to focus on minimal residual disease. Intraperitoneal therapy of ovarian cancer using dialysis techniques appears promising and takes advantage of the rapid systemic clearance of many anticancer drugs and the slow diffusion out of the peritoneal cavity of large, non-lipid-soluble molecules. Its use in early-stage disease is still experimental.

Implantable elastomer access ports with self-sealing silicone diaphragms are being used to administer continuous infusions and have reduced the risk of infection associated with tunneled central venous catheters. Extravasation during infusions into the ports remains a problem with drugs such as adriamycin. Several new portable infusion pumps are available as delivery devices. The totally implantable Infusaid pump driven by an internal fluorocarbon energy source is an effective tool in evaluating organ-directed therapy. Implantable access ports and infusion devices are already allowing greater flexibility of scheduling in experimental protocols, with greater comfort to the patient.

THE USE OF SURGERY AND RADIOTHERAPY AS AN ADJUNCT IN PATIENTS WITH ADVANCED CANCER   Surgery and radiotherapy, although considered treatment of localized primary cancers, have an increasingly important role in the treatment of patients with advanced metastatic cancer either in an attempt to cure or to palliate. Seemingly solitary brain metastases should be removed surgically, particularly in young people, if at all possible, since the likelihood of rapid demise without such treatment is high, and occasional long-term control is possible. Pulmonary metastases of a variety of sarcomas can be resected even when multiple nodules are present and long-term survival is possible. This has been true particularly in patients whose tumors can be shown to have long doubling times prior to surgery. Removal of metastases to the lungs is important in patients with testicular tumors because of the histologic heterogeneity of this tumor and the likelihood that a metastasis has resulted from growth of a clone of a histologic type resistant to the drugs employed. The resection of apparently localized hepatic metastases of colorectal cancer has resulted in long-term disease-free survival in as many as 25 percent of such patients. These results coupled with the recent information on the biochemistry of metastases have altered the previous universally pessimistic attitude toward patients who develop recurrent tumors. Reducing tumor bulk by resecting major masses of tumor in patients with widespread disease to reduce the body burden of tumor prior to chemotherapy has, however, not proved as useful as anticipated except in ovarian cancer. In one controlled clinical trial, in locally advanced testis tumor, debulking surgery did not improve the ultimate results of chemotherapy.

Surgeons are often asked to provide palliation for patients whose conditions are incurable by any modality. The operative risks are often high and the therapeutic yield, from the surgical point of view, low, but considerations of comfort and ability to return home during the terminal months of illness often make such procedures worthwhile. Palliation should be considered, for example, in intestinal obstruction due to ovarian and pancreatic cancer, in gastrointestinal bleeding, and for urinary diversions; and to relieve pain with neurosurgical procedures. The primary physician often is in the best position to make the judgment regarding the feasibility of such palliative procedures.

In highly radiosensitive tumors, radiotherapy may be used to reduce the areas of prior tumor involvement in patients with advanced metastatic cancers to enhance the cure rate with drugs, as in patients with some types of lymphomas. In diseases that are systemic at diagnosis, such as leukemia and small cell lung cancer, prophylactic use of radiotherapy to treat the brain and meninges before disease is evident has been successful as an ancillary method to drug treatment and has resulted in prolonged disease-free survival. Palliative radiotherapy has many applications in patients with metastatic cancer. In emergency situations, it can be used in conjunction with drugs to provide rapid relief of superior mediastinal obstruction, or to relieve ureteral obstruction in patients with lymphomas or testicular tumors which are drug-resistant. It can provide frequent and useful relief of bone pain and may prevent fractures, if used prophylactically to treat lesions of weight-bearing bones. In these cases, the primary treatment is usually with drugs and the radiation field should be only as large as required to control the lesion in question. For lytic lesions of weight-bearing bones, greater than 2.5 cm in diameter, especially those involving the cortex, prophylactic internal fixation followed by radiation therapy is the treatment of choice. Radiation of the brain and spinal cord are important examples of palliation which, when used early and effectively, can prevent catastrophic neurologic incapacitation in the final months of illness.

MULTIMODAL PRIMARY (ADJUVANT) TREATMENT

A major reduction in national mortality rates from the common visceral cancers appears likely to occur only if current and future systemic treatment programs are applied more effectively in the perioperative period to the treatment of those large numbers of patients who develop recurrences if treated with surgery or radiotherapy alone. Multimodal therapy began by combining the standard surgical and/or radiotherapeutic approaches with newly developed systemic treatment, without alterations, for their use in combination. This approach, while effective in many cases, was often quite toxic. Multimodal primary therapy has now evolved to a process of tailoring each component of the treatment program to maximize the strength of the modality while minimizing the toxicity. This approach has not only improved survival but has markedly altered the methods and morbidity of local control in a significant number of cancers. In cancers in which systemic treatment can cure patients with visible metastases, the effect has been most dramatic. In choriocarcinoma, chemotherapy has replaced hysterectomy; in Hodgkin's disease, chemotherapy alone has become the treatment of choice in stage III, or in combination with radiotherapy, in some patients with stage II disease; in pediatric tumors, in the 60 percent of patients with Wilms's tumor who have favorable histology, surgery and a two-drug combination has replaced the use of surgery, radiotherapy, and a three-drug combination (which included doxorubicin), sparing the patient the growth-retarding effects of radiotherapy and the cardiotoxicity of doxorubicin; in diffuse large cell lymphoma, chemotherapy has proved effective enough in advanced disease that it has replaced radiotherapy as the treatment of choice in stage II disease and in some cases of stage I disease; in nonseminomatous testicular cancer, chemotherapy with the use of sensitive biologic markers has become the primary treatment once orchiectomy is performed; in small cell lung cancer, better local control and improved survival has been achieved if radiotherapy is used concurrently with chemotherapy. In tumors where cure of visible metastatic disease is not yet possible with combination chemotherapy but a major clinical effect is achievable against micrometastases, there has also been an influence on methods of local control which has in some cases resulted in improvement in survival as well. In breast cancer, equivalent local control is achieved with lumpectomy and radiotherapy for women with tumors less than 4 cm; improved survival and decreased mortality is possible when chemotherapy is added in patients with lymph node tumor metastases; in extremity sarcomas a marked improvement in survival is observed with limb-sparing surgery and radiotherapy coupled with combination chemotherapy; and in anorectal cancers equivalent local control and survival without the need for colostomy is attainable with concurrent use of radiotherapy and chemotherapy.

The four most important considerations in the development of drug programs for post- and perioperative use are the following: (1) the identification of populations of patients who, even after optimal surgery or radiotherapy for their primary disease, have a high risk of recurrence and death from their cancer (e.g., stage II breast cancer, Duke's C colon cancer); (2) the availability of a proven systemic form of treatment; (3) the weighing of the potential benefits of treatment against short- and long-term risks of added drug treatment, keeping in mind that a fraction of patients exposed to adjuvant drug treatment would not have developed recurrent tumor; and (4) proper study design. Since measuring the reduction of tumor masses is not a possible end point during adjuvant studies, few can be accepted unless comparisons of treated groups and untreated controls are made, or the risk of recurrence is known to be very high and is spread over so narrow a time frame as to obviate the need for concurrent controls. In the latter case, historical controls may suffice. An example of a tumor requiring controls in adjuvant studies is stage II (T_1,N_1,M_0) melanoma. Sex, site, level of invasion of the primary, and degree of nodal involvement all affect not only the risk but the time of recurrence, which may be spread over periods from a few months to several years.

The most difficult question is the level of effectiveness required of systemic therapy in patients with advanced metastatic tumor before it is feasible to use it in an adjuvant program. Clinical studies have shown that changes in measurements of tumor masses in patients with metastatic disease are sufficiently variable to render partial response rates of 10 percent or less in drug-treated patients the equivalent of "biologic noise." Presently, only single agents, drugs and biologicals, or combinations of both with response rates of 20 percent or higher are considered acceptable for postoperative treatment programs. The attractiveness of a candidate program is enhanced considerably if some fraction of treated patients attain complete rather than partial responses. There is uncertainty as to whether drugs which are apparently inactive against advanced cancer are potentially useful against a small number of cancer cells present in the postoperative period when fewer resistant cell lines are likely to be present and vulnerability to drugs may be different.

The sequencing of chemotherapy and radiation therapy has varied from site to site with the use of radiotherapy before, during, and after chemotherapy. The standard method of using radiotherapy with chemotherapy in the past has been to give radiotherapy first followed by chemotherapy. Numerous clinical trials are now in progress testing the alternative approaches described above. The limit of tolerance for radiotherapy on normal tissue has been the operative guide to therapy rather than the ability to control the tumor and to determine whether combinations of radiation and drugs are additive, synergistic, or inhibitory. There is increasing evidence that the concurrent use of chemotherapy and radiotherapy produces superior results as in brain tumors, breast cancer, extremity sarcomas, anal cancers, and pediatric tumors and lymphomas. These observations are consistent with the Goldie-Coldman hypothesis, which predicts that either concurrent or alternating cycles of chemotherapy and radiotherapy could maximize reduction of resistant cell lines in major tumor masses. Although the concurrent use of radiation therapy and chemotherapy tends to be more toxic, alterations in dosing and fractionation may be possible with less toxicity.

COMPLICATIONS OF THERAPY

Each side effect of treatment must be weighed against the potential benefit to be derived. Patients must be apprised of all the risks involved, both in undergoing therapy and in refusing it. In a disease highly treatable with chemotherapy, it is rare that nausea, vomiting, and temporary hair loss should be of sufficient significance to withhold or reduce treatment. Many treatments are carcinogenic to some degree. The opportunity to identify this risk has come about only following the advent of successful treatment of patients with metastatic cancer, since long disease-free survival provides the follow-up time necessary to bring this to light. Radiation therapy is known to be carcinogenic, but the risk, when it is used alone, is relatively low in a given treatment field. Combinations of drugs and x-rays, however, are associated with a higher risk of second malignancies such as acute myelocytic leukemia and tumors in the irradiated field. This has been noted in long-term survivors of Hodgkin's disease who had received both combination chemotherapy (MOPP) and radiation therapy. In several studies, it is estimated that patients treated with both extensive radiation therapy and MOPP chemotherapy have an incidence of acute myelocytic leukemia between 5 and 10 percent within 10 years. Patients who are long-term survivors of Wilms's tumors treated with both radiation and drug therapy have also had a high incidence of secondary malignancies in the radiation treatment field. In addition, there is some evidence that long-term exposure to alkylating agents in patients with otherwise normal bone marrow may be associated with late marrow dysplasia which may eventuate in acute myelocytic leukemia. These potential risks are particularly germane to the use of these drugs in adjuvant treatment programs although in several large series of studies, the risk of leukemia in drug-treated breast cancer patients was less than 0.5 percent and the benefit far outweighed the risks.

The physician should be familiar with normal tissue tolerance for radiation and its acute and late effects. Acute radiation effects are largely on cell-renewal tissue—skin, oropharyngeal mucosa, small intestine, rectum, bladder mucosa, and vaginal mucosa. Acute radiation effects such as skin reactions, weight loss, nausea and vomiting, mucositis, and blood count depression may appear during or near the end of treatment and are usually reversible. Others, such as pneumonitis, may not appear until several weeks or months following treatment and then resolve. Since the effect on rapid-cell-renewal tissues will be dependent on the balance between cell birth and cell death, it will be crucially affected by the time allowed for repopulation. It will also be dependent upon the cell kill per fraction. Therefore, fraction size will be important. The radiotherapist frequently observing the oral mucosa and seeing an excessive reaction knows that a small decrease in fraction size or a small treatment break may allow rapid resolution of the problem since these changes will permit reconstitution of normal tissue. Late consequences of radiation therapy are its dose-limiting effect, which often progresses with time and is usually irreversible. They include necrosis, fibrosis, fistula formation, nonhealing ulceration, and damage to specific organs such as spinal cord transection or blindness. Normal tissues and organs differ in radiosensitivity. The risk of complications increases with dose and, if delivery is by megavoltage sources in the usual fractions, occurs when the dose exceeds the following: both lungs 15 Gy (1500 rad); both kidneys 24 Gy (2400 rad); liver 30 Gy (3000 rad); heart 35 Gy (3500 rad); spinal cord 40 Gy (4000 rad); intestine 55 Gy (5500 rad); brain 60 Gy (6000 rad); bone 75 Gy (7500 rad). While the mechanisms of late toxicity are not clear, they do not appear to depend primarily on the rapid proliferation of a cell-renewal tissue. Clinically, late effects appear to be much more dependent on the total dose of radiation and the size of the radiation fraction. Only if the same fractionation scheme is used with the same normal tissue end point, the same volume irradiated, and the same treatment technique can acute and late effects be correlated. If any of the treatment parameters is varied, the acute reactions to radiation may be dissociated from eventual late effects. Rather than serve as a guide, these acute reactions will then be misleading. There are a number of examples in radiation therapy in which the total dose has been increased, the fraction size increased or maintained constant, but the time has been extended to minimize acute effects. Such maneuvers have resulted in unacceptable late complications.

There are two hypotheses for the mechanism of late radiation effects. One theory holds that all late effects are due to damage to vascular-connective tissue stroma. A variation on this hypothesis is that damage to the endothelial cells determines late effects. An alternative hypothesis suggests that both the acute and late effects of radiation and cytotoxic chemotherapy are due to depletion of the major target cell-renewal tissues. Acute effects depend on the balance between cell killing and compensatory cellular replication of both the stem and proliferative compartments. The development of late effects requires that stem cells have only a limited proliferative capacity. Compensation for extensive or repeated cell killing may exhaust this capacity, resulting in eventual tissue failure.

Chemical and radiation therapy produce sterilization in both sexes which may be reversible but often is not. If at all reversible, the time necessary for reversal may be several years. Anticancer drugs and radiotherapy are teratogenic. It should never be assumed that chemotherapy and radiotherapy themselves are sufficient methods of contraception. All patients in the childbearing age who are treated with radiation and/or drugs should be fully informed of the risks and be advised of contraceptive measures. When pregnancy occurs during chemotherapy or exposure to radiotherapy, abortion should be considered because of the high risk of teratogenesis if the pregnancy is discovered in the first trimester, even though there are abundant case reports of normal children born to women treated with drugs in the first trimester. Treatment of women who develop tumors while pregnant is best withheld until delivery, which may need to be hastened. Chemotherapy can be used safely in the third trimester, but because of the uncertain long-term effects on the fetus, should not be employed unless the situation is critical.

NUTRITION AND CANCER

A profound state of malnutrition, the cachexia of malignancy, is frequently the most debilitating feature of this disease process. In many instances, it can be attributed to anorexia with an associated distortion of taste sensation or acquired aversion to specific foods, particularly meat. There are, however, patients in whom the extent of weight loss far exceeds the deficit in quantity and quality of calories consumed. In addition to the loss of adipose tissue and protein stores, these patients have a marked degree of insulin resistance with abnormal glucose tolerance. It has been demonstrated that malignancies can cause an augmentation of hepatic and renal gluconeogenesis secondary to enhanced Cori cycle activity, as well as an excessive utilization of fatty acids as metabolic fuel, which can theoretically contribute to a net energy loss by normal tissue. Hyperalimentation with total parenteral nutrition (TPN) with solutions based on 50 percent glucose and mixtures of essential amino acids and vitamins, containing about 3000 calories per day, is used to restore nutritionally depleted patients who have a chance for tumor control by surgery, chemotherapy, and/or radiotherapy. TPN through a catheter placed in the superior vena cava is also indicated in patients with pain on deglutition, fistulas, or intestinal obstruction. When possible, oral hyperalimentation is preferred and effective. TPN in patients who have lost 10 lb or more body weight is associated with an average weight gain of 6 lb in a mean of 24 days, even when chemotheray and radiotherapy are given simultaneously. There is no evidence that TPN preferentially enhances tumor growth. Catheter-related sepsis occurs in about 2 percent of patients. Hyperosmolar, nonketotic coma can be avoided with gradual increases in the concentration of glucose.

HYPERURICEMIA AND OTHER CONSEQUENCES OF RAPID CELL LYSIS

Hyperuricemia is most common in patients with acute leukemia but occasionally occurs in other malignancies. The high serum uric acid levels are due to the increased formation and destruction of tumor cells and accompanying breakdown of nucleoproteins. Chemotherapy and radiotherapy may cause further elevations in serum uric acid and urinary urate excretion. Uric acid is actively secreted by the kidney, and its solubility is highest in alkaline urine. When the concentration exceeds the solubility, uric acid precipitates in the tubules causing obstruction, decreased glomerular filtration, and eventually anuria. Allopurinol prevents the formation of uric acid from xanthine and hypoxanthine. Prophylactic use of this drug in patients with a large volume of tumor prior to treatment, in anticipation of high urate load, should obviate the need to treat uric acid nephropathy. Urate nephropathy can also be prevented by ensuring a water diuresis. Administration of sodium bicarbonate to maintain the urinary pH above 7.0 is helpful. Secondary gout is uncommon except in patients with polycythemia vera. The excessive production of lactate by suboxygenated masses of tumor causes lactic acidosis in patients with leukemia and Burkitt's lymphoma. The lactic acidosis can be reversed by cytotoxic chemotherapy directed against the tumor. The elaboration of large quantities of lactic dehydrogenase (LDH) has been observed in these settings. Cytotoxic therapy in highly drug-sensitive tumors can cause rapid tumor lysis with release of intracellular phosphates and potassium leading to serious hyperkalemia, hypocalcemia, and potentially fatal cardiotoxicity.

REFERENCES

AARONSON SA, TRONICK SR: The role of oncogenes in human neoplasia, in *Important Advances in Oncology*, VT DeVita et al (eds). Philadelphia, Lippincott, 1985, pp 3–15

CHABNER BA (ed): *Pharmacologic Principles of Cancer Treatment*. Philadelphia, Saunders, 1982

———, MYERS CE: Clinical pharmacology of cancer chemotherapy, in *Cancer: Principles and Practice of Oncology*, 2d ed, VT DeVita et al (eds). Philadelphia, Lippincott, 1985, pp 290–328

DEVITA VT et al: The effect of combined modality therapy on local control and survival. Int J Radiat Oncol Biol Phys (in press)

GOLDIE GH, COLDMAN AJ: The genetic origin of drug resistance in neoplasms: Implications for systemic therapy. Cancer Res 44:3643, 1984

LIOTTA LA: The mechanisms of cancer invasion and metastasis, in *Important Advances in Oncology*, VT DeVita et al (eds). Philadelphia, Lippincott, 1985, pp 28–41

section 6 Geriatric medicine

80 THE BIOLOGY OF AGING

WILLIAM R. HAZZARD

The phenomenon of aging has always fascinated mankind. This interest probably derives from the fact that until comparatively recently only a small fraction of people actually lived into old age. The concept of retirement, for example, did not exist until the latter portion of the nineteenth century. However, several forces have brought aging and its consequences into the social and scientific limelight. These forces can best be appreciated by contrasting representative longevity curves of the populations of developing and developed nations (Fig. 80-1). The curves reflect the high birthrates and high infant and childhood mortality rates that are characteristic of developing nations and the correspondingly low rates observed in developed countries. Socioeconomic development results in improved nutrition, housing, education, personal and public hygiene, and eventually in a reduced birthrate. These factors are also responsible for increases in the median age of the population and in expected longevity at birth. However, once maturity has been achieved, extension of longevity is less pronounced. This upper limit of longevity is depicted in Fig. 80-1. Note the similar ages at which the upper ends of longevity curves from populations with disparate degrees of socioeconomic development intersect the abscissa. Survival beyond 120 years of age has not been documented beyond question.

Hence, the change in the modern era is not an increase in the upper limit of the human life span but is an increase in the proportion and number who survive to approach that limit. This trend is the result of a narrowing of the gap between *primary aging,* which is genetically determined and immutable, and *secondary aging,* which is attributable to personal, social, and environmental factors that may be subject to change. When large numbers of individuals age in concert, society itself reflects the aging process. The United States is now experiencing such a redistribution of population toward an older median age. A steady state, with about a fourth of the total population in the ages 1 to 19 years and another fourth in the age group over 55 years, will be reached in another half century (Fig. 81-1). Unless more efficient and effective means are devised for meeting the needs of an aging population, health and social services for the elderly will be overwhelmed.

AGING AT THE CELLULAR LEVEL Clinical and epidemiologic research on aging has lagged behind studies of aging at the cellular

level. This has occurred in large part because of the difficulty in separating the primary effects of aging from the secondary effects of the diseases that accompany aging. Only when reduced to the simplest unit of organization, the cell, can aging be studied independently of age-related disease. Even at this level knowledge about aging is primitive, and several theories of aging remain extant. Research in this area was given its major impetus when human skin fibroblasts were found to have a limited potential for replication, about 50 population doublings under the most favorable conditions (the Hayflick phenomenon). This limit is an inherent property of the fibroblasts themselves and not of their environment. A finite and relatively fixed number of doublings is also characteristic of the proliferative potential of certain other cells, such as arterial smooth-muscle cells. Consistent with the suggestion that these cell culture studies may reflect aging in vivo, the actual number of potential doublings of a given fibroblast in vitro is inversely related to the age of its donor. Furthermore, fibroblasts from donors with Werner's syndrome, a single gene defect that causes dramatic acceleration of aging, undergo fewer doublings than cells from age-matched controls.

As a consequence of these findings in cultured cells, several theories have been advanced to attempt to explain senescence on the basis of alteration at the genomic level. One theory, Szilard's mutation hypothesis, holds that as DNA mutations accumulate in somatic cells, chromosomal inactivation and cell death ensue. Related theories suggest that senescence occurs via cumulative errors in formation of RNA or through progressive errors in protein synthesis, resulting in an "error catastrophe" (a theory that has receded from favor, as formal tests have failed to document such cumulative errors in aging cells). Such mutations have also been invoked to explain the age-related increase in autoimmunity. However, the effects of mutation need not be permanent. Indeed, the capacity for DNA repair in fibroblasts and the amount of reserve or redundant DNA sequences may correlate with longevity of various species. Finally, it has been proposed that the accumulation of free radicals that occurs with aging (the result of decreased activity of superoxide dismutase) may cause reduced resistance to intra- and extracellular injury.

These theories of "intrinsic" aging have been challenged because they are based on in vitro phenomena and hence are far removed from processes occurring in the aging whole organism. In addition, such theories do not explain the marked differences in replicative potential observed among various cell types. For instance, while fibroblasts exhibit senescence in vitro, cells of gastrointestinal and hematopoietic origin appear capable of replication throughout their life span, and kidney and liver cells replicate at all ages in response to unilateral nephrectomy or partial hepatectomy. Still other cells,

FIGURE 80-1 *Survival curves in different countries varying in degree of socioeconomic development. Diagonal arrow indicates change accompanying such development. (Reprinted by permission from L Hayflick, N Engl J Med 295:1302, 1976.)*

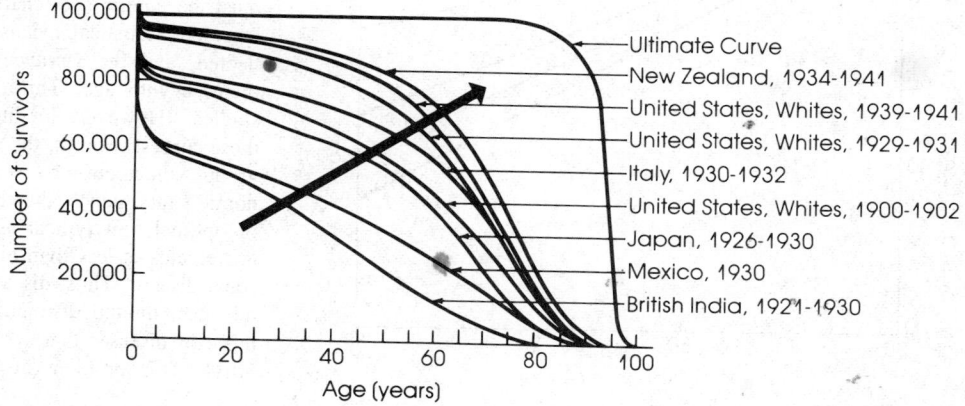

- Ultimate Curve
- New Zealand, 1934-1941
- United States, Whites, 1939-1941
- United States, Whites, 1929-1931
- Italy, 1930-1932
- United States, Whites, 1900-1902
- Japan, 1926-1930
- Mexico, 1930
- British India, 1921-1930

such as those of the central nervous system and striated muscle, do not replicate during adult life. However, regardless of replicative potential, no nonmalignant cell—and this includes all of the hematopoietic cells—survives indefinitely (in contrast to cancer cells). Thus, while considerable variation occurs in generation time and replicative potential of different cell types within a given species and of the same cell type among species, senescence at the cellular level appears to be a universal feature of normal cells.

But do these in vitro phenomena relate to aging in vivo? Even the strongest proponents of the intrinsic school of cellular aging acknowledge that the probability is small that organisms age solely because one or more cell populations lose proliferative capacity. Perhaps, in aging cells, decrements in functional capacities other than proliferative capacity render the organism vulnerable to death. This possibility has been supported in other studies by Hayflick and his colleagues, who have reported that fibroblasts lose the capacity to synthesize and lyse collagen prior to the loss of replicative capacity. Therefore, attention has been focused upon the regulatory processes that control the functions of tissues and whole organisms, specifically the nervous, endocrine, and immune systems.

One school has focused upon the role of central nervous system monoamines, notably dopamine, norepinephrine, and serotonin. These neurotransmitters are altered in certain age-related neurologic diseases. Parkinson's disease, for instance, is associated with major deficiencies of monoamines (e.g., striatal dopamine) and can be partially treated by L-dopa replacement. Furthermore, changes in catecholamine metabolism occur in the normal aging brain, and the elderly are more susceptible to development of parkinsonian symptoms following treatment with phenothiazines. Hence, age-related changes in dopamine uptake and catecholamine metabolism may lower the threshold for induction of parkinsonian symptoms by drugs that deplete or antagonize catecholamines. Such changes may also account for the late onset of postencephalitic Parkinson's disease, in which aging unmasks an earlier viral insult. Other age-related changes, perhaps attributable to alterations in central nervous system monoamines, include changes in circadian rhythms, sleep patterns, libido, and thermoregulation. Alternatively, cholinergic changes in the central nervous system may account for certain alterations in behavior and mental function. The fact that patients with senile dementia of the Alzheimer type demonstrate selective loss of cholinergic neurons of the nucleus basalis of Meynert has led to trials of agents that enhance central nervous system levels of acetylcholine [e.g., phosphatidylcholine (lecithin) and the cholinesterase inhibitor physostigmine].

Changes in endocrine function with aging may be related to these neurotransmitter alterations. For example, normal aging is accompanied by a decline in glucose tolerance, and the incidence of diabetes mellitus is increased in the aged. The higher prevalence of nonketotic hyperosmolar coma in the elderly diabetic may be due to the impaired osmoregulation and diminished thirst perception that are common even among the healthy elderly. Clinical and subclinical thyroid deficiency is also more common. Thyroid insufficiency and perhaps the increased incidence of diabetes mellitus may be secondary to age-related increases in autoimmunity. Another age-related change in endocrine function relates to events associated with the menopause in women. It is not established whether the cessation of ovulation is due solely to depletion of primordial follicles within the ovary or whether changes in the neuroendocrine regulation of the ovary that accompany aging are also in part responsible. Whatever the etiology, menopausal endocrine changes, including diminished estradiol secretion, diminished negative feedback control of gonadotropin production at the level of the hypothalamus, compensatory increases in follicle-stimulating hormone (FSH) and luteinizing hormone (LH) secretion, and abnormal thermoregulation, have profound consequences at both psychological and physiologic levels. The endocrine changes in the aging male—though less dramatic—may be of equal import. These include both a decrease in mean plasma testosterone (most evident at the morning peak of the circadian cycle) and an increase in mean plasma estrogens, so that increasing feminization in aging men parallels diminished estrogen production in women.

The immune system may function as the pacemaker of the aging process. The thymus normally reaches maximal size in childhood and begins involution after puberty. Other lymphoid tissues generally reach maximal size soon after puberty and undergo gradual atrophy thereafter. Such atrophy is characterized by a reduction in lymphoid cells and their replacement by connective tissue. In addition there is a reduction in T-cell function that is even greater than the reduction in T-cell number. Other age-related changes in immune function include a decrease in the primary immune response of B cells, especially in those responses requiring T-cell interaction. Specific changes in lymphocyte function include (1) decreases in the proliferative responses to mitogens such as phytohemagglutinin and concanavalin A, (2) decreased suppression of B lymphocytes by T cells, and (3) decreased cytotoxic activity of T cells. These changes may have relevance to certain diseases of the elderly. For example, compared to young adults, the elderly have four to five times the case rate for cancer and tuberculosis and six to seven times the fatality rate from pneumonia.

The changes with age in neurotransmitters, endocrine function, and the immune system may be interlinked. For instance, production of thymic hormones may decrease with age, and this in turn may be under neuroendocrine regulation. Other endocrine changes, such as altered responses to glucocorticoids or changes in glucocorticoid secretion, may also affect the immune response.

While these regulatory systems may be of importance in the aging of the whole organism, age-related decrements occur in nearly all physiologic systems (Fig. 80-2). Such decrements at the organ system level reflect functional decrements at the cellular level. These data must be interpreted cautiously, for several reasons. First, they represent statistical means. Second, individual variation is not reflected, and the variance in physiologic performance appears to increase with age. Third, they were derived from cross-sectional studies. (However, longitudinal follow-up has largely reproduced these curves.) Fourth, the study subjects were all men and of an elite group, volunteers who were highly educated and in upper socioeconomic strata; hence, the changes depicted are perhaps representative of optimal, not typical aging. Nevertheless, the magnitude of the decrements is less than that associated with functional disability or frank disease. Thus, disease, not aging, is a threat to homeostasis at all ages, though distinguishing the primary effects of aging from those of diseases that occur with aging remains a challenge (Table 80-1). This problem of distinguishing between the primary and

FIGURE 80-2 *Physiologic functions in normal men aged 30 to 80 years, expressed as percent of average values for 30-year-olds. a. Fasting blood glucose. b. Nerve conduction velocity, cellular enzymes. c. Cardiac index (resting). d. Vital capacity, renal blood flow. e. Maximum breathing capacity. f. Maximum work rate, maximum oxygen uptake. (From NW Shock.)*

TABLE 80-1 Primary vs. secondary aging. Examples of primary age-related changes and age-related disease effects

Organ system	Clinical manifestation	Primary age-related change	Secondary aging factors (disease and time-related factors including drug effects)
Skin	Wrinkling Purpura with minor trauma Susceptibility to pressure sores and slower healing Dry skin/pruritis Hair loss; hair graying	Atrophy (especially subcutaneous), decreased elasticity, increased vascular fragility, decreased sweating and sebaceous gland secretions, decreased hair and hair pigment, diminished cell replication	Sun exposure Chemical exposure
Eyes	Presbyopia, decreased dark adaptation Cataract Glaucoma Macular degeneration	Altered lens elasticity Altered biochemistry and physiology of vitreous and retina	Diabetes ? Cataract ? Glaucoma ? Macular degeneration Drug effects (miosis)
Ears	Decreased hearing, esp. high frequency; decreased sound discrimination Diminished position sense—"dizziness," falls	Diminished function of hair cells in the vestibular apparatus Diminished vestibular function	Traumatic hearing loss Ménière's disease Drug toxicities "Benign positional vertigo"
Nose and mouth	Decreased taste and food enjoyment Dry mouth	Diminished olfaction Diminished number of taste buds; diminished taste levels and salivation	Zinc deficiency Periodontal disease Drug-induced dry mouth, decreased salivation Diminished social eating cues
Gastrointestinal tract	Dysphagia, gastroesophageal reflux Hypochlorhydria with bacterial overgrowth Constipation Altered drug metabolism	Diminished esophageal motility and sphincter function Diminished acid, pepsin, and trypsin secretion Decreased intestinal motility Altered hepatic enzymes	Hiatal hernia Pernicious anemia Constipation secondary to low-residue diet, laxative abuse Chemical abuse altering drug metabolism (smoking, alcohol)
Respiratory system	Decreased vital capacity, FEV_1, maximum breathing capacity	Diminished lung elasticity Diminished respiratory musculature	Chronic obstructive pulmonary disease secondary to smoking, pollution Diminished respiratory muscle power secondary to lack of exercise
Cardiovascular system	Diminished cardiac reserve, increased pulse pressure, increased vulnerability to hypotension and syncope	Diminished myocardial cell number, increased left ventricular and arterial resistance, diminished chronotropic response, diminished vascular baroreceptor (adrenergic) sensitivity	Atherosclerosis-related ischemia, ventricular dysfunction, arrhythmias, hypertensive heart disease, congestive heart failure
Renal-urinary system	Decreased glomerular filtration rate, tubular reabsorption Obstructive uropathy and overflow incontinence Stress incontinence	Diminished number of nephrons, changes in tubular function Decreased bladder tone, decreased bladder capacity, diminished sphincter tone, prostatic hyperplasia (men), diminished tone of pelvic musculature (women)	Hypertension-related nephrosclerosis Drug-induced renal disease (aminoglycosides, nonsteroidal anti-inflammatory agents) Urinary tract infections
Endocrine-metabolic system	Menopause (vasomotor symptoms, vaginal atrophy) Diminished male libido, potency, sexual drive Relative glucose intolerance Diminished thyroid reserve	Hypogonadism Relatively abrupt (women) Relatively slow (men) Diminished insulin response to glucose load, decreased insulin sensitivity (increased adiposity) Diminished thyroid response	Surgical hypogonadism (oophorectomy), hypogonadism secondary to alcohol abuse Increasing incidence of diabetes mellitus Autoimmune thyroiditis and hypothyroidism; hyperthyroidism (often apathetic)
Musculoskeletal system	Decreased strength Increased vulnerability to fracture Joint stiffness and inflammation	Decreased muscle fiber number and diameter Diminished bone mineral content Diminished bone formation Increased stiffness of tendons, connective tissue Diminished joint cartilage	Disuse atrophy (sedentary lifestyle) Gonadal steroid deficiency; diet-, alcohol-, tobacco-, and drug-related osteoporosis Osteomalacia secondary to Vitamin D deficiency (deficient diet and lack of sun exposure) Drug-induced osteoarthritis (fluoride) Traumatic osteoarthritis (occupational, recreational)
Central nervous system	Hypothermia Hyperthermia Dehydration Postural hypotension, "dizziness," syncope, falls Slowness of movement Retarded rate of learning Retarded positional correction, falls Altered sleep patterns	Diminished tolerance to temperature variation Diminished thirst and drinking Diminished postural reflexes and autonomic regulation Neuronal loss in the nucleus basalis, decreased cholinergic neurotransmitters and choline acetyltransferase activity Diminished basal ganglia function Diminished dorsal column function	Hypothermia from hypothyroidism Hyperosmolar, nonketotic coma in diabetes mellitus Drug-induced dehydration Autonomic insensitivity Drug-induced cognitive dysfunction Delirium Drug-induced parkinsonism Alzheimer's disease Parkinson's disease Drug-induced ataxia, alcoholic cerebellar degeneration
Immune system	Increased susceptibility to infections and malignancy Impaired response to immunization Increased autoantibodies	Diminished cellular immunity (decreased helper cells) Diminished primary antibody response Increased abnormal immunoglobulins and autoimmunity	Nutritional deficiency Autoimmune diseases (thyrotoxicosis, thyroiditis, pernicious anemia)

secondary effects of aging will become more difficult as average longevity increases (death rates are declining most rapidly among the elderly and notably among those over 85), particularly since age-related decrements in functional capacity can pose a threat to the independence of the individual even in the absence of clear-cut disease. Thus age-related decrements may produce morbid symptoms in the elderly, especially under conditions of stress and acute illness. The simultaneous impairment of multiple systems in the elderly patient may explain the cascade of complications that can be initiated by a seemingly trival perturbation as well as the exponential rise in death rate among the very old (e.g., above age 93). The longevity curve of individuals above age 93 suggests that death may occur almost as a random phenomenon.

SUMMARY AND PROJECTION Aging occurs in all cells except those that undergo malignant transformation. While age-related phenomena may be most readily detected in assays of cellular replication in vitro, changes in cell function of a more subtle nature may be more relevant to aging of the whole organism. Such changes are likely to be amplified in systems that regulate metabolism and function of the whole organism, such as the nervous, endocrine, and immune systems. The aging phenomenon in its entirety must represent a mixture of cellular and systemic physiologic changes intrinsic to the species and of environmental insults that interact with the intrinsic processes.

Enhanced survival into old age is predominantly the result of changes in the environment that accompany socioeconomic development. During the twentieth century such changes have resulted in an increased average longevity in developed nations. However, there is little evidence that the upper limit of the human life span, ca. 120 years, has been altered, nor is there a realistic prospect for such a change. Hence, biologic aging in the human, though poorly understood, proceeds inexorably, resulting in a maximal life span that appears to be relatively fixed.

Many physiologic functions decline in an age-related manner, and attempts have been made to estimate physiologic (as contrasted to chronologic) age by application of a battery of tests to presumably healthy individuals of different ages. Although such profiles of performance may permit a gross estimate of biologic age that is useful in predicting a specific outcome in groups of subjects, these tests have no clinical utility in dealing with individuals. Hence, while general awareness of the limited reserve in many systems is of importance in geriatric practice, a careful search for disease-specific causes of decline is imperative in the elevation of patients of all ages.

REFERENCES

ADLER WH et al: Aging and immune function, in *The Biology of Aging*, JA Behnke et al (eds). New York, Plenum, 1978, p 221

GOLDBERG AP et al: Diabetes mellitus in the elderly, in *Principles of Geriatric Medicine*, R Andres et al (eds). New York, McGraw-Hill, 1985, p 750

FINCH CE: The regulation of physiological changes during mammalian aging. Quart Rev Biol 51:49, 1976

FRIES J: Aging, natural death, and the compression of morbidity. N Engl J Med 130:135, 1980

GOLDSTEIN S: The biology of aging. N Engl J Med 285:1120, 1971

HAYFLICK L: Theories of biological aging, in *Principles of Geriatric Medicine*, R Andres et al (eds). New York, McGraw-Hill, 1985, p 9

MARTIN GM et al: Replicative lifespan of cultivated human cells: Effects of donor's age, tissue, and genotype. Lab Invest 23:86, 1970

SHOCK NW: Physiological and chronological age, in *Aging—Its Chemistry*, AA Dietz (ed). Washington, D.C., American Association for Clinical Chemistry, 1980, p 3

81   HEALTH PROBLEMS OF THE ELDERLY

WILLIAM R. HAZZARD / JOHN R. BURTON

Increased concern for the health problems of the elderly is a result of the changing distribution of the population by age that occurs as nations develop socioeconomically (Fig. 81-1), a redistribution that is producing a rise in the proportion of the oldest segments of the American population (Fig. 81-2). This special concern reflects several phenomena: the close association between the aging process and the disease accumulated by the elderly (Table 80-1), the multiple disabilities, both apparent and potential, among those who survive into old age, the chronic and progressive nature of many of these disabilities, the disproportionate per capita consumption of health care resources by the elderly because of their vulnerable health status, and concern about the magnitude of health care expenditures as a proportion of gross national product. The challenge to the system for health and social care is to match the resources of the system to the needs of an aging population so as to improve both efficiency and effectiveness.

The principles of geriatric medicine overlap the principles of internal medicine. Information relevant to the medical care of the elderly is dispersed throughout this text, and a companion volume, *The Principles of Geriatric Medicine*, is available. Accordingly, this chapter is addressed to integrative aspects of geriatric medicine, including comprehensive assessment, preventive medicine, nutrition, and pharmacology of the elderly.

COMPREHENSIVE GERIATRIC ASSESSMENT Comprehensive geriatric assessment is indicated in various circumstances, all having in common a change in social, physical, or health care status. The profile of a typical patient would be one 75 years of age or older (a common threshold to define the younger end of the geriatric age spectrum) (1) whose physician has died or retired, (2) whose physician desires consultation or is not prepared to undertake long-term management of such a problem, (3) whose family perceives a change in health status that may require intervention, (4) whose locale has changed perhaps in response to a deteriorating health status, or (5) who has experienced a new medical problem or social crisis (or any combination of the five). Commonly this assessment is part of the decision-making process about the advisability of admission to a long-term care facility. The purpose of assessment is to review the physical, mental, and social situation with the view toward detecting and treating reversible causes of disease and disability, stabilizing those that may be progressing unnecessarily, introducing rehabilitative strategies to restore function, or adjusting the social or physical environment to provide independence and/or support in a deteriorating situation. The search for a cure for a given disease or even the establishment of a specific diagnosis is less often a primary goal than the formulation of a strategy, often practical in nature, to preserve independence, dignity, and function in a multiply disabled and frail individual. Since hospitalization is itself a risk to the precarious homeostasis of the elderly, this assessment should be carried out in the ambulatory setting wherever possible, the hospital being reserved for the treatment of acute disease.

Dimensions of assessment A comprehensive geriatric assessment includes five dimensions: physical health, mental health, social/economic status, environmental circumstances, and, most important, functional status.

Sometimes patients have undergone multiple previous assessments by generalists or specialists. The physician performing a geriatric assessment therefore may begin with a detailed review of available records so as to avoid redundancy in laboratory or radiologic testing. This aims both at avoiding the risk and cost of unnecessary testing and at identifying any points of uncertainty that remain after previous

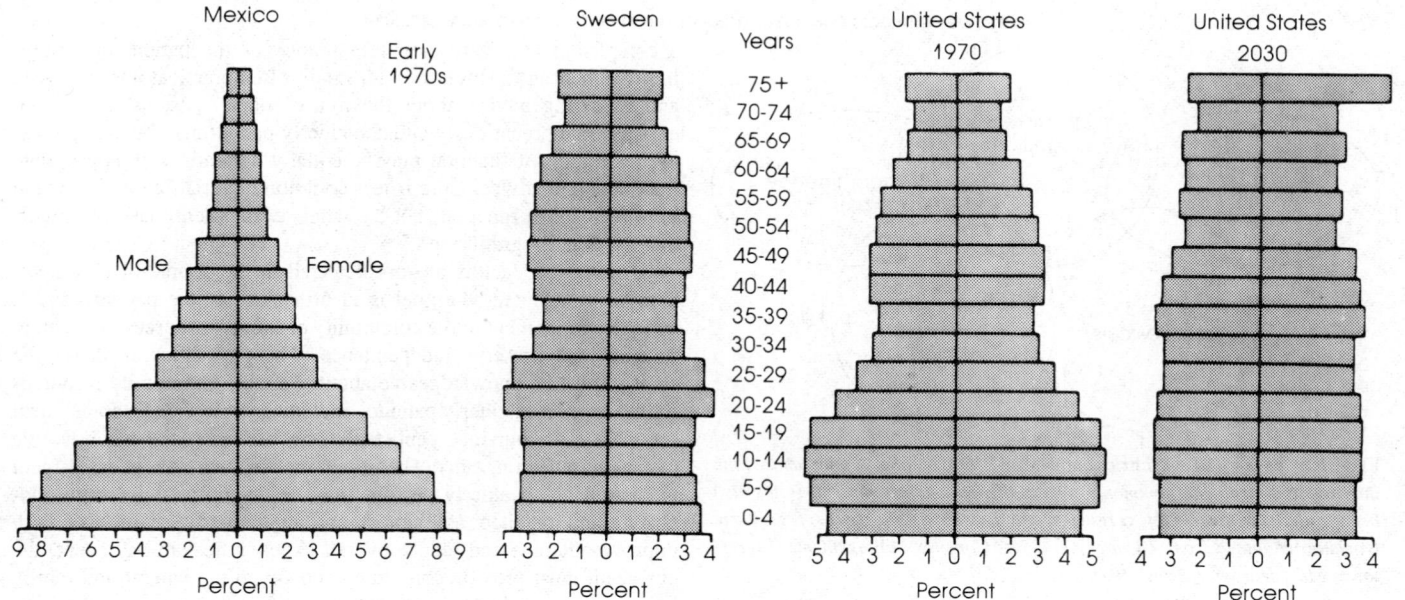

FIGURE 81-1 *Comparative profiles of population age and sex distributions among three nations in the present era and in the United States in 2030 (when a steady state will be approached). From AR Somers, The high cost of health care for the elderly: Diagnosis, prognosis, and some suggestions for therapy, J Health Politics, Policy, and Law 3(2):163, 1978.*

assessments. When geriatric assessment is performed as a consultation, few if any additional laboratory or radiologic examinations may be required. To assist in the systematic collection of requisite clinical and sociologic data, one of the several instruments developed for such assessment may be used, such as the Older American's Resources and Service Group (OARS) assessment form (Duke University Center for the Study of Aging and Human Development, Durham, NC 27710), which takes approximately 1 h to administer. A useful and somewhat shortened version of the OARS instrument, taking approximately half the time to administer, is the Functional Assessment Inventory (FAI) (Suncoast Gerontology Center, University of South Florida Medical Center, Tampa, FL 33612). A general limitation of all such assessment forms is that they have been developed for research use in groups of subjects rather than for the management of an individual patient. They are also less useful in circumstances of rapidly changing physical and mental status (such as in the hospital setting) than in a more stable circumstance over the long term. Therefore, physicians often develop individual approaches to geriatric assessment, commonly relying upon selected portions of the OARS or FAI for the cataloguing of social and economic resources and upon their own assessments of physical and mental health. All mechanisms of assessment, however, should include a systematic analysis of several dimensions.

PHYSICAL HEALTH   Physical health should be assessed through the traditional medical history and physical examination, though the evaluation may have to be tailored to the limited physical and mental reserves of the elderly patient; e.g., perhaps conducted over a series of short office visits. Special care must also be taken to compensate for impediments to communication with the elderly patient. For example, the patient may have a problem with mobility, may not understand or be confused by questions, may have difficulty in vision or with hearing, and may become fatigued. Aids for the hearing impaired may be helpful, and the light should be facing the examiner to allow an element of lip-reading by the patient. The physician must be especially careful to evaluate those systems more often the focus of the interest of subspecialists outside the realm of internal medicine: the eyes, the ears, the teeth and mouth, the skin, and the nervous system. Problems such as immobility and incontinence may bridge more than one discipline (Fig. 81-3).

MENTAL HEALTH   Depressive illness, delirium, dementia, and other mental disorders are especially debilitating in the elderly: hence, special focus upon cognitive function and mood is required. Systematic evaluation may be enhanced by use of simple scales or standards such as those for measuring depression or mental assessment.

SOCIAL AND ECONOMIC RESOURCES   Social circumstances often heavily influence the physical and mental status and represent constraints to problem-solving. Critical areas for social/economic assessment include identification of those who will provide care for the patient in time of need. These "supporters" are critical for the maintenance of the elderly patient in the community and commonly include the spouse, adult children, or perhaps neighbors or landlords. Especially important is identification of those who will provide support of unlimited duration (usually confined to family members). Sources of intermittent or indirect support include church, community, and relevant social agencies. A cardinal rule of geriatric medicine is to "support the supporters," and supporter fatigue may precipitate a geriatric assessment, hospitalization, or long-term institutionalization. Not uncommonly, sickness or death of a prime supporter may be catastrophic for an elderly patient previously living independently in the community. The review of social resources also includes the taking of a financial inventory and establishing the degree to which public or private resources may need to be marshalled in support of the patient.

ENVIRONMENTAL CIRCUMSTANCES   The physician should understand the physical environment in which the patient lives: Are there stairs to be climbed? Is the bathroom accessible to the precariously mobile individual? Are there hazards to ambulation in the dwelling (loose

FIGURE 81-2 *Percentage change from 1970 to 1980 in the population of United States residents by age groups. (Adapted from Bureau of Census: General population characteristics, 1980 Census of Population, Washington, DC, US Department of Commerce.)*

Age	
85+	48.3
80-84	28.5
75-79	25.0
70-74	24.9
65-69	25.6
60-64	17.1

FIGURE 81-3 *The geriatric quintet or "O complex" emphasizes the interaction of problems commonly seen in the frail elderly patient. It has also been called the five Is of geriatrics and represents the core of geriatric teaching. (Adapted from R Cape, Aging: Its Complex Management, Hagerstown, Md., Harper & Row, 1978.)*

cords or rugs, clutter, sharp-edged furniture, etc.)? Are there fire hazards, especially for the cognitively impaired patient (e.g., open-flame stoves)?

FUNCTIONAL STATUS Care provided to the frail elderly patient must conform to the patient's functional ability. Scales of the activities of daily living (ADL) and "instrumental" activities of daily living (IADL) have been developed. Perhaps the most well-known and widely used is the Katz Functional Assessment Scale (Table 81-1). Six basic functions are assessed: bathing, dressing, toileting, transferring, continence, and feeding. More complex activities necessary for independent living include meal preparation, shopping, financial management, housekeeping, transportation, medication taking, and laundering. A strong association between specific diseases and functional capacity is often lacking, and the latter appears to predict outcome better than the former. Functional disability is the final common pathway of many chronic disorders that are prevalent among the elderly, and serial assessment of functional status may provide the most meaningful means of monitoring patient status with time.

Value of assessment A major goal of geriatric medicine is the preservation of function and independence in the elderly. At the time of assessment the patient is commonly in a state of flux: one or more chronic conditions may be in exacerbation, the social circumstances may be changing for the worse, or mental deterioration and depression may have supervened. The comprehensive geriatric assessment will dissect the components of such change and instability, the primary

TABLE 81-1 Areas and levels of assessment in the Katz Index of Independence in Activities of Daily Living*

Bathing	_____ Receives no assistance
	_____ Receives assistance in bathing only one part
	_____ Receives assistance in bathing more than one part
Dressing	_____ Gets clothes and dresses without assistance
	_____ Needs assistance in tying shoes only
	_____ Needs assistance greater than above or stays undressed
Toileting	_____ Needs no assistance
	_____ Needs assistance only in getting to toilet room or in cleaning self
	_____ Does not go to toilet room
Transferring	_____ Needs no assistance from another person
	_____ Needs assistance with transferring
	_____ Does not get out of bed
Continence	_____ Continent
	_____ Occasional accident
	_____ Needs supervision, uses catheter, or is incontinent
Feeding	_____ Needs no assistance
	_____ Needs assistance in cutting meat or buttering bread
	_____ Needs more assistance or is tube- or intravenously fed

* From S Katz et al, Studies of illness in the aged: The Index of ADL, JAMA 185:94, 1963.

accomplishment often being reassurance of the patient or family, improvement in function through small, often practical interventions, and rendering advice about the future course. Just as the rate of collapse in a precariously situated elderly patient may be precipitous, the restitution of function may be equally dramatic with appropriate treatment and advice. Cure is less common in geriatric medicine than improvement in function, but the latter, even when relatively minor, may be equally gratifying.

If reversible factors are not detected in the course of a comprehensive assessment, the goal is identification of the patient's needs and the arrangement of the community or family resources to maintain function and preserve independence. The physician caring for the elderly must be knowledgeable about available community resources for the support of elderly patients, including professional, nonmedical services (e.g., nursing, dentistry, social services, the rehabilitative therapies, nutrition, etc.). The importance of such careful assessment is clear. Half of elderly persons may be inappropriately institutionalized, and detailed assessment and rehabilitative care may both improve outcome and reduce overall expenditures. In any event, the physician must provide continuing support to the patient and family because few problems are short-term and because needs may change abruptly. Home visits for assessment and intermittent care allow evaluation of the environmental conditions and also allow assessment of interactions of the patient with family and other supporters. Such home visits are especially important for the physician who does not have access to a multidisciplinary assessment team (e.g., social worker, rehabilitation therapists).

PREVENTIVE MEDICINE IN THE ELDERLY Effective intervention to retard or prevent many of the time-related chronic disease processes that pass the clinical threshold in old age must begin long before age 75: hypertension must be treated, dyslipoproteinemia must be diagnosed and managed, bone demineralization must be prevented or retarded, pulmonary function must be preserved by cessation of cigarette smoking, etc. "Preventive gerontology" involves intervention throughout the lifespan. Among the elderly, preventive medicine should focus upon short-term problems and solutions, balancing the risks and costs as well as the potential benefits of intervention (including their estimated duration). Particular attention should focus on the prevention of phenomena that may trigger catastrophic collapse such as immunizations (notably one-time polyvalent pneumococcal vaccination, maintenance of adequate tetanus protection, and annual influenza vaccination), elimination of environmental hazards (classically the scatter rug), and preservation of adequate physical activity, nutrition, and social interactions. Furthermore, even in the frail elderly, systematic exercise programs may improve the sense of well being. This type of preventive medicine is an important part of the periodic health evaluation of the elderly patient with its emphasis upon social, psychological, and functional issues in addition to the usual physical and mental evaluation.

Nutrition and aging A frequent final common pathway of functional decline in the elderly is malnutrition, notably when acute illness is superimposed on chronic disease and disability. Few data have been gathered relative to the prevalence, incidence, and severity of such malnutrition. For example, micro- and macronutrient requirements have not yet been defined for the elderly. By ordinary criteria, significant malnutrition among free-living elderly is common only among the poor and sick. On the other hand, barriers to adequate nutrition are imposed both by primary aging and by the common disease concomitants of the aging process: decline in smell and taste perception causes diminished enjoyment of food; salivation decreases, and mastication is commonly impaired through dental losses and disease; swallowing may be difficult, choking is common, and esophageal motility is diminished; gastric acid and pepsin secretion are diminished, and gastric motility may be reduced (as may that of the small and large intestine, constipation being common); biliary secretion is commonly impaired, and gall bladder disease is common;

perhaps most important, since physical activity is diminished, appetite is also suppressed, and the intake of both macro- and micronutrients may be decreased to the point of marginal deficiency. Social and psychological cues to eating frequently are lacking, and depression is common; for example, death of a spouse may jeopardize intake not only because of the anorexia of the depression associated with bereavement but also by removing the incentive to prepare a tasteful and nutritious meal. The impact of accompanying weight loss and malnutrition is immediately apparent. Weight loss, a cardinal manifestation of disease at all ages, should signal an exhaustive search for its cause in the elderly, for whom it represents a proximate and ominous sign of decline. The cause may be obvious, e.g., malignancy, or cryptic; e.g., tuberculosis or endogenous depression. Just as often the cause cannot be determined, and long-term assessment may be required before the cause of the weight loss can be ascertained. As with geriatric medicine in general, the search for iatrogenic or social causality is of prime importance: e.g., digitalis intoxication; lack of enjoyment through an enforced diet (for example, one that is severely fat- or carbohydrate-restricted); or depression following translocation of a patient from a supportive social environment to one of isolation, as in a retirement community providing no interaction. In any event the prognostic significance of weight loss is nowhere more evident than among the elderly, since malnutrition may represent a serious barrier to recovery from illness and is correlated with the development of pressure sores, infections, muscle wasting, and weakness that prevent ambulation and self care.

Nutritional assessment in the elderly is not unlike that in the nonelderly. Laboratory tests such as serum albumin, lymphocyte count, or transferrin levels appear to add little to the clinical assessment of weight/height (commonly expressed as the Quetelet or body mass index [BMI], weight/height^2), or more valuable, documentation of a change in weight. Measurement of skinfold thickness also adds an objective dimension to evaluation (see Chap. 71), though it is subject to imprecision because of increased skin flaccidity and the lack of adequate standards for the elderly. Calorie counts or reviews of dietary intake may be useful, particularly if food avoidance is suspected. If inadequate intake is documented in the hospitalized patient, intervention is indicated with oral, enteral, or parenteral supplements. Other laboratory measurements are of derivative use only; e.g., folate and/or B_{12} levels if the patient demonstrates a macrocytic anemia.

Nutritional therapy is frequently attempted in the elderly, though success may be elusive and difficult to document. Oral multivitamin and mineral supplements are taken commonly with or without physician advice. The rationale for such supplementation is apparent, however, given the low risk of "one-a-day" vitamin supplementation and the relatively high risk of micronutrient deficiency in the elderly patient whose nutritional status is marginal. Increased calcium intake (1000 to 1500 mg per day) is also recommended in middle-aged and elderly women to prevent or retard osteoporosis. The addition of liquid, calorie-rich supplements in the malnourished patient may be helpful and at times essential (e.g., in the patient with oral pathology or dysphagia for solid foods). However, in the anorectic patient these seldom suffice to overcome antecedent weight loss and may create a false sense of security. Where functional impediments exist (e.g., a swallowing disorder following a stroke), a specific nutritional regimen may be critical in promoting recovery, for example, enteral or parenteral feeding with early consideration of gastrostomy in those requiring chronic enteral alimentation. While many formulations with varying degrees of osmolality, caloric density, and caloric distribution have been introduced for such feeding (see Chap. 74), caloric restitution is of primary importance given adequate protein and micronutrient replacement. Whereas the determinants of disease usually play the dominant role and nutritional supplements only a permissive role in recovery, malnutrition per se can be the cause of depression and even anorexia itself; correction by hyperalimentation may increase activity, positive mood, and eating and permit wound healing and recovery from infection.

Pharmacology in the elderly Iatrogenic disease is one of the major problems of geriatric medicine (Fig. 81-3) and is of primary concern to the physician caring for the elderly. Pharmacologic misadventures are prominent in this concern. Since the elderly commonly have multiple disorders, treatment with multiple medications ("polypharmacy"), both appropriate and inappropriate, is common. While special characteristics of the elderly place them at risk from side effects of drugs, no principle is as important as that multiple drugs enhance the hazard of complications from those drugs.

Approximately 90 percent of the elderly take at least one medication, and the majority take two or more. The most commonly prescribed drugs are those for the treatment of cardiovascular disease, antihypertensives, analgesics, and anti-inflammatory agents. Over-the-counter medications account on average for some 40 percent of the drugs consumed by the elderly; inventory of these agents is important in the search for pharmacologic causes of disease and disability. Patients confined to long-term care facilities commonly take even more medications, psychotropic agents surpassing all others in such institutions (in up to 75 percent of institutionalized as opposed to 25 percent of ambulatory patients). As a consequence of this high prevalence of drug ingestion, adverse drug reactions occur in 6 to 40 percent of those over 60 years of age in various series, are a common cause of hospitalization, and may be difficult to detect. The risk factors for such reactions, in addition to multiple drug usage, include being a woman (perhaps attributable to small body size and failure to adjust dosage accordingly), hepatic or renal insufficiency (leading to drug accumulation), and previous drug reactions. Whether age is a factor independent of its association with disease is not established; what is clear, however, is that the elderly are at particularly high risk to drug misadventures.

Other aspects of drug therapy in the elderly are also relevant. Compliance is of particular concern. In some studies 25 to 50 percent of outpatients fail to take their medications, underscoring the impor-

TABLE 81-2 Summary of factors affecting drug disposition in the geriatric patient

Pharmacokinetic parameter	Age-related physiologic changes	Pathologic conditions	Environmental factors
Absorption	Increased gastric pH Decreased absorptive surface Decreased splanchnic blood flow Decreased gastrointestinal motility	Achlorhydria Diarrhea Gastrectomy Malabsorption syndromes Pancreatitis	Antacids Anticholinergics Cholestyramine Drug interaction Food or meals
Distribution	Decreased total-body water Decreased lean body mass Increased body fat	Dehydration Hepatic failure Malnutrition Renal failure	Protein-binding displacement
Metabolism	Decreased hepatic mass Decreased enzyme activity Decreased hepatic blood flow	Congestive heart failure Fever Hepatic insufficiency Malignancy Malnutrition Thyroid disease Viral infection or immunization	Dietary composition Drug interaction Acceleration of metabolism Inhibition of metabolism Insecticides Tobacco (smoking)
Excretion	Decreased renal blood flow Decreased glomerular filtration rate Decreased tubular secretion	Hypovolemia Renal insufficiency	Drug interactions

SOURCE: *Vestal*

TABLE 81-3   Examples of drugs usually given in reduced dosage in the elderly*

Drug (or drug class)	Possible consequences of standard dosage regimen
Aminoglycosides	Ototoxicity and nephrotoxicity
Benzodiazepines	Unwanted CNS depression—more common with larger doses
Carbamazepine	Drowsiness or ataxia may develop
Chlormethiazole	Confusion possible with larger doses
Digoxin	Digitalis toxicity
Haloperidol	Extrapyramidal reactions
Levodopa	Hypotension common
Meperidine	Respiratory depression
Metoclopramide	Confusion common
Thioridazine	Confusion common
Thyroxine	Myocardial infarction
Vitamin D	Renal toxicity

* *The drugs listed are examples only; this is not intended to be an exhaustive listing*
SOURCE: *From World Health Organization, Health care in the elderly: Report of the technical group on use of medicaments by the elderly, Drugs 22:279, 1981.*

tance of careful review of drug-taking practices at the initial and subsequent assessments in the outpatient setting. In one study 59 percent of ambulatory patients above age 60 made one or more medication errors (26 percent potentially serious ones), and multiple errors are common (especially in patients above 75 years of age). The causes of errors in drug taking include problems in communication and understanding on the part of the patient or supporter, the use of multiple drugs, and the employment of complicated and changing regimens.

Age-related differences also exist in pharmacokinetics (summarized in Table 81-2). In the elderly body water and lean body mass are diminished relative to adipose mass. Hence water-soluble drugs are distributed in a smaller space (i.e., at a higher concentration per dose administered). Alcohol is one such agent that not only has a higher concentration after a given oral dose in the elderly because of a diminished space of distribution but also appears to have an increased effect (producing gait disturbances with smaller amounts ingested, for example). Since renal clearance may decline progressively with age, drugs cleared by the kidney (such as digoxin) must be given in reduced doses. However, some drugs (such as beta-adrenergic blocking agents) are actually of diminished potency in the elderly. Overall, prudence in drug prescription should be exercised both as to the quantity of each agent made available and the number of such agents prescribed (see Table 81-3). The principles for prescribing drugs in the elderly are summarized in Table 81-4.

TABLE 81-4   Principles of drug prescription for geriatric patients

1 Evaluate the need for drug therapy.
  a Not all diseases afflicting the elderly require drug treatment.
  b Avoid drugs if possible, but do not withhold on account of age drugs that might enhance the quality of life.
  c Strive for a diagnosis prior to treatment.
2 Take a careful history of habits and drug use.
  a Patients often seek advice and receive prescriptions from several physicians.
  b Knowledge of existing therapy, both prescribed and nonprescribed, helps anticipate potential drug interactions.
  c Smoking, alcohol, and caffeine may affect drug response.
3 In general, use smaller doses in the elderly.
  a Often the standard dose is too large for the elderly patient.
  b While the effect of age on drug metabolism by the liver is less predictable, renal excretion of drugs and their active metabolites tends to decline.
  c The elderly are particularly sensitive to drugs affecting central nervous system function.
4 Titrate drug dosage with patient response.
  a Establish reasonable therapeutic endpoints.
  b Adjust dosage until endpoints are reached or unwanted side effects prevent further increases.
  c Use an adequate dose, particularly in the treatment of pain associated with malignancy.
  d Sometimes combination therapy is appropriate and effective.
5 Simplify the therapeutic regimen and encourage compliance.
  a Try to avoid intermittent schedules. Once- or twice-daily dosage is ideal.
  b Select a dosage form appropriate for the patient.
  c Label drug containers clearly. When appropriate, specify standard containers.
  d Give careful instructions to both patient and a relative or friend. Explain why the drug(s) is (are) being prescribed.
  e Suggest the use of a medication calendar or diary.
  f Encourage the return or destruction of outdated medications.

SOURCE: *Vestal*

REFERENCES

ANDRES R et al: *Principles of Geriatric Medicine.* New York, McGraw-Hill, 1984

BRESLOW L, SOMERS AR: The lifetime health monitoring program: A practical approach to preventive medicine. N Engl J Med 296:601, 1977

HAZZARD WR: Preventive gerontology: Strategies for healthy aging. Post-Graduate Medicine 27(1):22, 1983

KANE RA, KANE RL: *Assessing The Elderly: A Practical Guide to Measurement,* Lexington, MA, Lexington Books, 1981

RUBENSTEIN LZ et al: Effectiveness of a geriatric evaluation unit. N Engl J Med. 31:1664, 1984

VESTAL RE: Clinical pharmacology, in *Principles of Geriatric Medicine,* R Andres et al (eds). New York, McGraw-Hill, 1984

WILLIAM TF et al: Appropriate placement of the chronically ill and aged: A successful approach by evaluation. JAMA 226:1332, 1973

PART THREE DISORDERS CAUSED BY BIOLOGIC AND ENVIRONMENTAL AGENTS

section 1 Important considerations in infectious diseases

82 AN APPROACH TO INFECTIOUS DISEASES

ROBERT G. PETERSDORF / RICHARD K. ROOT

THE SCOPE OF INFECTIOUS DISEASES The vast majority of human and animal diseases of known etiology are produced by biologic agents: viruses, rickettsias, bacteria, mycoplasma, *Chlamydia,* fungi, protozoa, or nematodes. No small part of the past and present importance of infectious diseases in medical practice is attributable to their enormous frequency and the public health implications of their contagiousness. However, developments in sanitary engineering, vector control, immunization, and specific chemotherapy have modified the situation favorably. Although important exceptions remain, infectious diseases as a class are more easily prevented and more easily cured than any other major group of disorders. Despite the elimination of some infectious diseases such as smallpox and the profound reduction in the morbidity and mortality rates of many, humans are by no means free of infection. In fact, the total human load of disease produced by microbial parasites has decreased only modestly, primarily through smallpox and malaria control and better health care in developing countries. As certain specific microbial infections have been controlled, others have emerged as troublesome therapeutic and epidemiologic problems. With the introduction of cytotoxic drugs, massive irradiation in the treatment of malignant diseases, and immunosuppressive agents to control the rejection of transplanted organs, the insertion of prosthetic devices into the bloodstream, and the progressive longevity of people with chronic degenerative diseases, infections due to organisms previously considered saprophytic or commensal have increased. These infections have also been termed *opportunistic.* Worldwide concern has been aroused by the occurrence of infection of T lymphocytes by retroviruses causing either their malignant transformation or cytolysis. The profound immunosuppression characteristic of human lymphotrophic virus III lymphadenopathy-associated virus (HTLV III/LAV) infection and lysis of T helper cells is known as the *acquired immunodeficiency syndrome* (AIDS) (see Chap. 257). Multiple opportunistic infections cause death in the majority of patients with AIDS.

Because of better environmental sanitation and other measures that now prevent contact with many microbial agents, and the development of acquired immunity early in childhood, certain infections have been seen more frequently in adults. For example, as contact with poliomyelitis virus in childhood declined in many countries, paralytic poliomyelitis became more common in young adults. *Haemophilus influenzae* meningitis and pneumonia is being reported more frequently in adults than heretofore, and decreasing infection with the tubercle bacillus raises questions about the status of antituberculous immunity in adults. For reasons that are not clear, hepatitis A is predominantly a disease of young adults, while non-A, non-B hepatitis tends to occur in individuals over 35 years of age.

As antimicrobial agents reduce the mortality associated with certain common infections, other microbes emerge as important causes of human disease. If an infection occurs during or immediately following a course of chemotherapy, it is often caused by a microorganism that is resistant to the drug that was given; such an infection is termed a *superinfection.* While it is relatively unusual nowadays for patients to die of uncomplicated pneumococcal pneumonia, a disease readily handled with available antimicrobials, it is common to see serious disease produced by microorganisms which are much more resistant even though they are often part of the normal microbial flora in humans. These include staphylococci, gram-negative enteric bacilli, and a variety of anaerobes and fungi. One important mechanism by which resistance is conferred on gram-negative enteric bacteria is the action of R factors (see Chap. 85).

Agents not previously known as causes of human disease are being identified rapidly. *Legionella pneumophila* (see Chap. 117) was first described in 1976 and in the ensuing 6 years much of the epidemiology, microbiology, pathogenesis, clinical course, prognosis, and treatment have been worked out. Since the original description of *L. pneumophila* less virulent but related microorganisms that cause pneumonia have been described (see Chap. 117). However, in contrast to *L. pneumophila,* these organisms turned out not to be new pathogens. Rather, they had been described in the past and given different names and the discovery of *L. pneumophila* placed them into the proper taxonomic and clinical framework. A different manifestation of an old organism is the relationship between *Staphylococcus aureus* and the toxic shock syndrome (see Chap. 94). In this situation a well-known organism appears to be elaborating a toxin that causes a severe systemic illness. The precise mechanism whereby this toxin produces disease is not known. Yet another relatively new entity that was presumed to be of infectious etiology, Lyme arthritis (see Chap. 277), has been found to be caused by a spirochete. These brief descriptions of new diseases are cited to illustrate the ever-changing array of infectious diseases.

Particularly striking is the spectrum of infections that are seen in AIDS patients in addition to malignancies such as Kaposi's sarcoma and lymphomas (see Chap. 257). AIDS patients who present with opportunistic infections caused by viruses [cytomegalovirus (CMV), herpes simplex], bacteria (*Mycobacterium avium-intracellulare, M. tuberculosis*), parasites (*Pneumocystis carinii, Toxoplasma gondii, Cryptosporidium*), and fungi (*Cryptococcus neoformans, Histoplasma capsulatum,* and *Candida albicans*) invariably die despite transiently effective antimicrobial therapy, and current attempts at immune reconstitution. This tragic outcome emphasizes the vital role of the cellular immune defenses in protection against these organisms and in surveillance against certain malignancies. No wonder one-quarter of people that seek medical attention, even in developed countries, do so for infections, and the number is much higher in the developing world. It should also come as no surprise that, in the United States, 25 percent of prescriptions that are written are for antibiotics.

In this and the subsequent chapters, principles of host-parasite interaction, the usefulness of diagnostic procedures, important epidemiologic issues, principles of chemotherapy, major infectious syndromes not associated with specific organ systems (which are found under diseases of these organ systems), and approaches to preventing infections are stressed. In subsequent chapters of this section, diseases caused by specific etiologic agents are described. Together, the syndromic as well as etiologic approach provides a thorough compendium to the study of infectious diseases.

THE PARASITE AND THE HOST   The interaction between microorganism and humans that results in infection and disease is complex. Much has been learned about the way in which microbes enter the body, the ways in which they produce tissue injury, the influence of specific immunity and "nonspecific" resistance of the host in contributing to the manifestations of both infection and protection, and the mechanisms of recovery. It is not yet possible to transfer in any specific way much of the information that has been acquired to the individual patient with an infection. However, considerable progress is being made. Examples are the sexual transmission of hepatitis A virus; the major role that *Chlamydia* are found to play in the causation of pelvic inflammatory disease (see Chap. 91); the role of Norwalk and rotaviruses in infectious diarrheas (see Chap. 89); and advances in antimicrobial therapy in containing heretofore difficult-to-treat bacteria (see Chap. 88).

INFECTION AND CLINICAL DISEASE   Microorganisms of different species or different strains of the same species vary widely in their capacity to produce disease, and human beings are not equally susceptible to the disease caused by a given bacterium or virus. Furthermore, while a specific infectious disease will not occur in the absence of the causative organism, the mere presence of the organism in the body does not lead invariably to clinical illness. Indeed, the production of symptoms in humans by many parasites is the exception rather than the rule, and the *subclinical infection* or the "carrier state" is the usual host-parasite relationship. *Disease* in a clinical sense is not synonymous with the presence of the organism or *infection* in a microbiologic sense. In fact, for most organisms the number of subclinical infections far exceeds that of clinical disease.

MECHANISMS OF INJURY   It is customary to refer to bacteria or other microorganisms that are capable of producing disease as *pathogenic. Virulence,* the *degree* of pathogenicity, should be distinguished from *invasiveness,* the ability to spread and disseminate in the body. For example, *Clostridium tetani* is pathogenic and, by virtue of its exotoxin, highly virulent, but it is almost completely lacking in invasiveness. Moreover, in certain circumstances and in certain anatomic locations, mildly "pathogenic" organisms can produce fatal disease, or highly "pathogenic" species can multiply without producing any harmful effect.

A few microorganisms produce *toxins* that account for the tissue damage and physiologic alterations of infection. *Hypersensitivity* to components of the organism is demonstrable in several infections to account for the manifestations of disease. For many pathogenic agents, an explanation of their damaging effects upon the host is incomplete or wholly lacking. Generally, therefore, the aim of therapy is to stop multiplication or to kill the microorganisms with appropriate drugs; in diseases caused by toxin-producing organisms, the use of antitoxin (as in tetanus or diphtheria) is the definitive procedure, and chemotherapy is of secondary importance. A relatively new example of a toxin-mediated infection is the toxic shock syndrome, in which the toxin is elaborated by *S. aureus.* In this situation, this ordinarily invasive organism does not usually invade local tissues.

The tendency of certain pathogenic organisms to *localize in certain cells or organs* and to produce disease in a specific anatomic site or evoke a combination of symptoms referable to certain organs often suggests the identity of the causative organism. For example, the pneumococcus usually causes infection in the lung but almost never in the kidney, and *H. influenzae* infections are confined almost solely to the respiratory tract and meninges. Similarly, in the presence of disease known to be caused by a given agent, involvement of other tissues can be anticipated or predicted. Examples include the multiple lung abscesses which are so characteristic of hematogenously disseminated staphylococcal disease and the metastatic skin lesions which complicate *Pseudomonas* bacteremia.

Frequently, the proper management of infectious disease involves the use of techniques completely unrelated to microbiology or chemotherapy, in an effort to support the function of damaged organs. Survival in varicella pneumonia usually depends upon treatment of respiratory failure; in the management of endocarditis, valve replacement is often more difficult than the eradication of the causative organism; in cholera the repletion of the volume deficit and in Weil's disease the treatment of acute renal failure with peritoneal or hemodialysis are the important therapeutic objectives.

RESISTANCE AND SUSCEPTIBILITY   Many so-called host factors are known to influence the likelihood that disease will occur if organisms enter the tissues, or to play a determining role in the outcome once the infection has become established. These include the integrity of mucocutaneous barriers, the action of local macrophages, the adequacy of polymorphonuclear leukocyte responses, the function of the complement systems, and the presence or absence of specific antibodies or specific cellular immunity. In the earliest stages of infection, the balance between nonspecific defenses and virulence factors of organisms determines whether or not infection progresses to become clinically apparent.

In experimental animals, sex, microbial strain, age, route of infection, the presence of specific antibody, associated diseases, nutritional state, and the use of such procedures as exposure to ionizing radiation or high environmental temperature, administration of antimetabolites, adrenal steroids, epinephrine, and metabolic analogues can be shown to exert a profound effect on infection by bacteria, viruses, fungi, and other agents.

In humans, these factors are no less important, although controlled studies are lacking for many. Alcoholism; diabetes; deficiency or absence of immunoglobulins (see Chap. 256); defects in cellular immunity (see Chap. 260); malnutrition; chronic administration of steroid hormones; chronic lymphedema; ischemia; the presence of foreign bodies such as bullets, calculi, or bone fragments; obstruction of a bronchus, the urethra, or any hollow tube; agranulocytosis or congenital defects in bactericidal or virucidal activity; various blood dyscrasias, and many other circumstances influence susceptibility to systemic or local infection. Furthermore, in those instances where the extenuating condition is remediable, the probability of recovery is enhanced. An interesting example is provided by the high incidence of tuberculous and fungal infections in patients undergoing jejunoileal bypass for morbid obesity. In some of these patients, the infection could not be reversed until the bypass was reconstructed.

Racial differences in susceptibility, such as the poor resistance of dark-skinned people to tuberculosis and their predilection for developing disseminated coccidioidomycosis, are well established. Resistance to infection may be determined genetically. The relation of sickle cell trait to malaria is one example. The increased frequency and severity of some infections in children, of others in pregnant women, and still others in the aged are familiar. In the elderly, it is important to distinguish between infections complicating age-related diseases (e.g., urinary tract infection in prostatic hypertrophy) versus age-related alterations in specific immunity (e.g., tuberculosis reactivation from suppressed cellular immunity).

Prior contact with an organism or its products, whether by active infection or by artificial immunization, increases resistance to some infections, such as measles, diphtheria, and pertussis, by stimulating antibody production, but seems to have little influence on resistance to others, such as gonorrhea.

Knowledge of all the factors involved in human resistance and susceptibility to infection is incomplete. While various disorders can be shown to alter nonspecific or specific immune mechanisms, the precise contributions of such alterations to clinical manifestations often remain incompletely defined. Given the multiplicity of defenses against microorganisms, profound depression of one or more is usually required to cause repeated or unusually severe infections. For example, unless granulocyte counts fall below 1000 per cubic millimeter (normal >1800 per cubic millimeter), or a major bactericidal mechanism is deleted from all polymorphonuclear leukocytes (e.g., oxygen-forming capacity), as in chronic granulomatous disease (see Chap. 272), life-threatening bacterial or visceral fungal infections are not increased in incidence. Many individuals (~1 in 500) may lack serum or secretory IgA, yet relatively few suffer infectious complications. Similarly, many patients with deficiencies of serum complement components may have no infectious complications or long infection-free intervals. While coexistent infection with CMV, Epstein-Barr virus (EBV), hepatitis, or other sexually transmitted pathogens may serve as promotors for HTLV III/LAV infection in exposed patients, life-threatening opportunistic infections do not occur, as a rule, until the T-helper population is markedly depleted. Not all patients who become colonized with *Haemophilus influenzae* B or *Neisseria meningitidis* develop clinically apparent or severe infection in the absence of specific antibodies. These observations highlight the complex nature of the interactions between microorganisms and the human host which determine the outcome of encounters with infectious agents.

PATHOGENESIS OF INFECTION   With relatively minor variations, the development of an infectious disease follows a consistent pattern. The parasites enter the body through the skin, nasopharynx, lung, intestine, urethra, or other portal. A number of microorganisms adhere to their site of primary attack through fimbriae, pili, and surface antigens; the adherence of *Bordetella pertussis* to respiratory epithelium, the gonococcus to urethral epithelium, and possibly some gram-negative urinary pathogens known as "adhesins" to the epithelium of the renal pelvis are some examples. These surface factors couple to specific cellular receptors, the availability, distribution, and turnover of which play a major role in regulating the character of the local microbial flora. Once established in the host, the organisms can multiply and, in so doing, establish a local or primary lesion. From this site, there may be local spread along fascial planes or tubular structures, such as a bronchus or ureter. The next step may be systemic spread of the microorganisms via the circulating blood. Bacteria can enter the bloodstream by direct invasion of vessels, a relatively unusual occurrence, or more commonly by traversing peripheral lymph nodes to enter the thoracic duct lymph and thence the venous system. In the bloodstream, they spread to other tissues and can produce distant or secondary lesions. In infections such as tetanus and diphtheria, distant lesions are produced by toxins elaborated at the primary site without systemic spread of the bacteria. The infectious process may terminate in recovery or death at any stage: the local lesion, systemic spread, or distant lesion.

The apparent inconsistency of this pattern in clinical medicine is attributable to the fact that the infection is recognized as a clinical entity only at the stage when symptoms are most likely to appear. For example, pneumococcal pneumonia is a local lesion, and the distant lesion, pneumococcal meningitis, is referred to clinically as a complication. In meningococcal infections, the local lesion, nasopharyngitis, is rarely symptomatic and has no status as a clinical entity, but the stage of spread, meningococcemia, and the commonest distant lesion, meningitis, are clinical entities. A rarer distant lesion, arthritis, is called a complication. In a patient who has osteomyelitis, a clinical entity, a recent furuncle may be referred to as a predisposing factor. In another patient with extensive furunculosis who develops osteomyelitis, the infection in bone may be regarded as a complication of the superficial infection. The stages mentioned are in no way limited to bacterial diseases; the primary lesion of poliomyelitis is intestinal and is usually asymptomatic, viremia may occur without

neurologic involvement, or a distant lesion manifested by symptomatic involvement of the central nervous system may be established.

Because clinical usage and terminology are based upon the symptomatic illness that leads patients to seek medical aid, the consistency of this general sequence in the pathogenesis of infection is often not recognized. However, the concept is useful and offers some basis for systematizing what may otherwise seem to be a miscellaneous collection of unrelated clinical signs and symptoms.

CLINICAL MANIFESTATIONS OF INFECTIONS   So varied are the disorders attributable to infection or infestation of humans by lower organisms that generalizations about them are difficult. The clinical manifestations of infection can duplicate those of diseases of any other etiology. However, certain clinical features are highly suggestive of infection, including abrupt onset, fever, chills, myalgia, photophobia, pharyngitis, acute lymphadenopathy and splenomegaly, gastrointestinal upset, and leukocytosis or leukopenia. It is obvious that the presence of one, several, or all of these features does not constitute proof of the microbial origin of illness in a given patient. Conversely, serious, even fatal, infectious disease may exist in the absence of fever or other signs and symptoms.

Although there is no infallible clinical criterion of infection, it is possible to recognize accurately many specific infectious diseases from information obtained by *history, physical examination, blood count, and urinalysis.* The importance of interrogation about past illness, predisposing factors such as alcoholism, familial disease, exposure to ill persons, contact with animals or insects, ingestion of contaminated food, type and order of onset of symptoms, and recent or remote residence in endemic areas is discussed in the subsequent chapters that deal with specific diseases and etiologic agents. Cardinal physical signs are also described for each entity.

The mechanisms that produce most of the signs and symptoms of human infection are incompletely known. The endogenous production of a family of polypeptides known collectively as interleukin 1 (IL-1) appears instrumental in producing many of the clinical manifestations of infection including chills and fever, leukocytosis, myalgias, lassitude, and a negative nitrogen balance (see Chap. 8). The physiologic alterations underlying "malaise," "postinfectious asthenia," "toxicity," and other common complaints are completely mysterious. The factors responsible for leukocytosis or leukopenia are only partially understood (see Chap. 56). Why the rash of typhus begins on the trunk while that of another rickettsiosis, Rocky Mountain spotted fever, begins on the extremities is unanswered. Failure to understand these manifestations does not impair their clinical usefulness, although it is probable that understanding them might lead to more accurate diagnosis and better management.

DIAGNOSTIC PROCEDURES   The specific procedures for the diagnosis of infectious disease have become sufficiently complex to warrant separate discussion. This is provided in Chap. 83.

Importance of specific diagnosis in infectious diseases   The diagnostic procedures employed for infectious diseases are no more absolute than those in other diseases; they cannot be blindly equated with the science of microbiology. The responsibility for interpreting the facts supplied by the bacteriologist, immunologist, and virologist in the total context of a patient's illness remains that of the physician. A positive tuberculin skin test certainly does not indicate that a patient has active tuberculosis. The finding of *Candida albicans* in a stool culture does not necessarily mean that a patient's diarrhea is caused by intestinal candidiasis. The presence of staphylococci in nasal cultures from a patient with headaches does not establish a diagnosis of staphylococcal sinusitis. A throat culture containing group A beta-hemolytic streptococci does not rule out diphtheria, nor does such a culture establish that a febrile illness in a patient with mitral stenosis is a recurrence of acute rheumatic fever rather than bacterial endocarditis. A positive serologic test for syphilis may indicate a treponematosis other than syphilis, syphilis that is active or inactive, or an unrelated disease such as systemic lupus erythematosus.

The etiologic agent   From a practical point of view, two important steps are vital to the correct diagnosis of infection: (1) the organ(s) or organ systems involved must be found, and (2) the etiologic agents causing the infections must be identified precisely. Chapter 83 deals with the diagnostic approaches that are available. Most of the remaining chapters in this part take up the specific bacteria, spirochetes, fungi, rickettsias, viruses, *Mycoplasma,* and protozoa which cause infections. The common syndromes caused by these agents are described either in chapters dealing with specific organisms or in chapters dealing with infections in individual organ systems such as pneumonia (see Chap. 205), bacterial endocarditis (see Chap. 188), urinary tract infections (see Chap. 230), osteomyelitis (see Chap. 340), meningitis (see Chap. 346), and infectious arthritis (see Chap. 277).

When confronted with specific organ involvement, it is important to know the most common pathogens which cause disease in the involved organ. Table 82-1 provides a listing of those pathogens. The disease syndrome may be modified by previous conditions or therapy, thus emphasizing the need for specific diagnostic studies. Used in conjunction with the individual chapters dealing with specific agents and the summary of chemotherapy (see Chap. 88), the table should provide a rational guide to treatment which often must be instituted before the results of cultures and antimicrobial sensitivity tests are available.

ANTIMICROBIAL THERAPY   The impact of chemotherapy upon mortality and morbidity from infection and upon epidemic disease is a matter of record. These therapeutic agents, however, have in no way lessened the importance of specific diagnosis; indeed, their availability has increased the need for obtaining exact etiologic information. It requires but a moment's reflection to realize that the substitution of a prescription for a broad-spectrum antibiotic or a quick injection of penicillin for the systematic collection of facts and thoughtful consideration of diagnostic possibilities is a fallacious, unwise, and dangerous practice. Numerous antibiotics with overlapping spectra are now available, dosages for different infections vary widely, the drugs themselves are potentially dangerous, and their administration entails considerable expense. They should never be prescribed as placebos, antipyretics, or substitutes for diagnosis. In the vast majority of instances in which this is done, patients recover just as they would if no "therapy" had been given, and the drugs are wasted. More importantly, an inadequate dosage of a drug or the wrong agent may suppress symptoms temporarily without achieving cure and may make isolation of the etiologic agent difficult, delay recognition of the true nature of an illness, and postpone the institution of curative treatment. Furthermore, antibiotics may select out resistant variants or facilitate the transfer of R factors between pathogenic and commensal enterobacteria. Resistant variants can then replace sensitive strains and pose the additional hazard of spread to others. Finally, to expose a patient to the risk of a drug reaction without proper indication is inexcusable, whether the drug is an antibiotic, a sedative, a laxative, or a narcotic.

EPIDEMIOLOGIC CONSIDERATIONS   Just as the decision to administer antibiotics to a patient with a febrile illness of presumed infectious etiology must be made on an individual basis, the selection of cases in which extensive cultural and serologic testing is required is a matter of judgment. The majority of common grippe-like illnesses subside spontaneously, and symptomatic treatment is sufficient. However, because of this tendency toward spontaneous recovery and also because the results of serologic tests may not be available until after recovery has taken place, the effort to determine the specific

TABLE 82-1   The syndromic approach to treatable infections

Type of infection	Etiologic agents		
	Common	Relatively common	Unusual but important
Skin and subcutaneous tissue	*Staphylococcus aureus*	*Streptococcus pyogenes, Candida,* superficial fungi	Gram-negative bacilli (burns, wounds)
Sinusitis	*Streptococcus pneumoniae, Haemophilus influenzae*	*S. pyogenes, H. influenzae, S. aureus*	Mucorales
Pharyngitis	Respiratory viruses, *S. pyogenes*	Gonococcus	*Corynebacterium diphtheriae*
Epiglottitis	*H. influenzae*		
Otitis, mastoiditis	*S. pneumoniae, H. influenzae* (children)	*S. aureus, S. pyogenes*	*Pseudomonas, Proteus*
Pneumonitis	*S. pneumoniae, Mycoplasma pneumoniae, Mycobacterium tuberculosis*	*S. aureus, Klebsiella-Enterobacter,* respiratory viruses, *Legionella pneumophilia*	*S. pyogenes,* gram-negative enteric bacilli, psittacosis, systemic fungi, *Pneumocystis, H. influenzae, Pasteurella multocida*
Empyema and lung abscess	*S. aureus,* anaerobic streptococcus, *Bacteroides, Fusobacterium*	*Klebsiella* (abscess)	
Bacterial endocarditis	*Streptococcus viridans, S. aureus,* enterococcus	*S. pneumoniae,* anaerobic streptococci	*Pseudomonas, Candida, Staphylococcus epidermidis, Listeria monocytogenes*
Gastroenteritis	*Salmonella, Shigella,* enteric viruses, *Campylobacter jejuni, Escherichia coli* (enterotoxic)	*S. aureus,* clostridia, *Giardia*	*Yersinia enterocolitica, Entamoeba histolytica, Vibrio cholerae, V. parahemolyticus*
Peritonitis, cholangitis, intraabdominal abscess	*E. coli,* enterococcus, *Bacteroides,* anaerobic streptococcus, *Fusobacterium*	*Klebsiella-Enterobacter, Proteus* spp.	Clostridia, *S. aureus*
Urinary infection (cystitis, pyelonephritis)	*E. coli, Klebsiella-Enterobacter,* paracolon, *Proteus,* enterococcus	*Pseudomonas*	*S. aureus, S. saprophyticus*
Urethritis	Gonococcus, *Chlamydia trachomatis*	*Treponema pallidum, Mycoplasma*	
Pelvic inflammatory disease	Gonococcus, *E. coli, Bacteroides,* anaerobic streptococci, *Chlamydia trachomatis*	*Klebsiella-Enterobacter,* enterococcus, *Fusobacterium*	Clostridia, *S. aureus*
Bones (osteomyelitis)	*S. aureus*	*Salmonella*	*S. pyogenes*
Joints	*S. aureus,* gonococcus, *S. pneumoniae, H. influenzae*	*S. pyogenes, Neisseria meningitidis*	
Meninges	*S. pneumoniae, H. influenzae, N. meningitidis*	*E. coli, Klebsiella-Enterobacter, Proteus, Pseudomonas*	*S. pyogenes, M. tuberculosis, Cryptococcus, S. aureus, Listeria monocytogenes*

etiology of illness is often considered an impractical, "academic" procedure. If pursued universally such an attitude fails to recognize that in addition to the individual patient, the welfare of the community must be considered. For example, a clinical diagnosis of "virus pneumonia" may turn out, following serologic tests, to be psittacosis. Although the "index" patient may have recovered completely, others in the community may be at risk until the pet parakeet which was the source of the illness has been eliminated. Even more pertinent is the tracing of sexual contacts of patients with sexually transmitted infections. There is no way to eradicate the present-day epidemic of sexually transmitted diseases without this essential "shoe-leather epidemiology." Equally important is the tracing of tuberculosis, particularly in the refugees from southeast Asia who are populating many communities in the United States, and in whom the prevalence of the disease is very high. The physician must be alert to the possibilities of disease transmission or recognize important clustering of cases in caring for patients with infectious diseases.

Pursuing the diagnosis of obscure, often self-limited, illnesses may be academic, but this approach has led to clarification of some important etiologic relations. For example, the syndrome of infectious mononucleosis has been linked with development of antibody to a herpes-like virus, the EB virus (see Chap. 138), which also has a causal relationship to Burkitt's lymphoma and carcinoma of the posterior nasopharynx. Some congenital anomalies have been related to prenatal viral infections; this relationship is well known for rubella (see Chap. 133), but a number of other viruses (CMV, varicella, herpes simplex) have been implicated, although with less certainty. The finding of bacteria-like bodies in the intestinal mucosa of patients with Whipple's disease and the improvement of these patients with tetracycline therapy provides another example of an entity of unknown etiology entering the realm of infectious diseases. The virus etiology of a number of severe fatal demyelinating diseases of the central nervous system has been well established (see Chap. 347). A variety of DNA and retroviruses have now been implicated in the pathogenesis of specific neoplasms in human beings, and their relationship to endogenous "oncogenes" defined.

The recent past has witnessed several striking examples of how careful epidemiologic observations can be wedded to excellent microbiologic and serologic techniques to define the causes of previously mysterious or new diseases. These include the establishment of *Legionella* species in aqueous reservoirs as a cause of epidemic pneumonia or grippe-like illness in normal and immunosuppressed hosts, the documentation of a tick-borne *Borrelia* species as the cause of Lyme disease (see Chap. 127), and the isolation of a newly occurring retrovirus infecting T lymphocytes as the agent responsible for AIDS. Not only has the etiology of newly recognized diseases been defined by these approaches, but linkage to other disorders for which the pathogenesis remains obscure has been suggested. For example, host responses to infection with *Borrelia burgdorferii* provide clues to mechanisms involved in chronic arthritis. The infectious and neoplastic complications of AIDS demonstrate the manner in which cellular immunity may both regulate responses to chronic intracellular infections and participate in surveillance against neoplasia. It seems likely that the continued pursuit of the potential role of infectious agents in other disorders of unknown etiology will disclose new pathogenetic relationships.

REFERENCES

GALLIN JI, FAUCI AS (eds): *Advances in Defense Host Mechanisms*, vol 5, *Acquired Immunodeficiency Syndrome (AIDS)*. New York, Raven, 1985

International Conference on Acquired Immunodeficiency Syndrome. Ann Intern Med 103:653, 1985

MANDELL GL et al (eds): *Principles and Practice of Infectious Diseases*, 2d ed. New York, Wiley, 1985

ROOT RK: Infectious diseases: Pathogenetic mechanisms and host responses, in *Pathophysiology—The Biological Principles of Diseases*, 2d ed, LH Smith Jr, SO Thier (eds). Philadelphia, Saunders, 1985

83 THE DIAGNOSIS OF INFECTIOUS DISEASES

JAMES J. PLORDE

The diagnosis of an infectious disease requires the direct or indirect demonstration of a pathogenic microbe on or within the tissues of the afflicted host. The major ways in which this is accomplished are described in this chapter.

DIRECT MICROSCOPIC EXAMINATION The direct microscopic examination of body fluids, exudates, and tissues is both the simplest and one of the most helpful laboratory procedures available for the diagnosis of infectious diseases. In many situations the examination allows an accurate, highly specific identification of the causative agent. Examples include the recognition of *Borrelia* or *Plasmodium* species in blood smears taken from patients with relapsing fever or malaria. More commonly, only a tentative identification can be made on the basis of microbial morphology. Nevertheless, this is often sufficiently precise to allow the selection of an appropriate chemotherapeutic agent pending the results of more definitive investigations. A variety of techniques are used in direct microscopy. If the agent being sought is sufficiently large or characteristic, the specimen can be prepared as an unstained wet mount and examined by light-field, dark-field, or phase contrast microscopy. More commonly, a dried smear is made; this allows the application of a variety of stains which assists the visualization and identification of the microbe in question.

Wet mounts Dark-field examination of fluid from genital lesions for the spirochete of syphilis is a well-known, but neglected, procedure. More often, wet mounts are used for the diagnosis of fungal and parasitic infections. The examination of hair fragments, skin scrapings, or nail clippings in a drop of 10% KOH is useful in establishing the presence of superficial mycoses. At times, as for tinea versicolor infections, the fungous elements will be sufficiently characteristic to allow the specific identification of the causative agent. Occasionally a presumptive diagnosis of a systemic fungus infection can also be established with this procedure. Two examples are cryptococcal meningitis diagnosed by demonstrating the encapsulated organism in an india ink preparation of cerebrospinal fluid, and coccidioidomycosis identified by finding characteristic spherules in expectorated sputum.

Examination of wet mounts of stool or duodenal drainage is also the initial step in establishing the diagnosis of intestinal protozoal infections such as amebiasis, giardiasis, and cryptosporidiosis. Moreover, it is the definitive procedure diagnosing intestinal helminthic infections including ascariasis, trichuriasis, strongyloidiasis, and hookworm. Finally, filariasis and sleeping sickness can be recognized by demonstrating the characteristic motility of microfilariae and trypanosomes in blood or other body fluids.

Stain-enhanced microscopy Despite many recent technical advances in the field of microbiology, Gram's stain remains, after 90 years of use, the best single technique available for the rapid diagnosis of bacterial infections. It can be applied to virtually all clinical specimens and is of particular value in the examination of exudates, aspirates, and body fluids, including cerebrospinal fluid and urine. Gram's stains are examined first under the lower-power objective to demonstrate the presence of pink-staining inflammatory cells. The paucity of such cells in the presence of many squamous epithelial cells suggests that the specimen was contaminated during the process of collection and may not be representative of the inflammatory process. The smear is then examined for the presence of bacteria using the oil immersion lens; bacteria appear either as dark-blue (gram-positive) or pink (gram-negative) bodies. Their color and morphologic appearance often make possible a presumptive identification of the genus and occasionally the species of the organism. The demonstration of pneumococci in the sputum, Enterobacteriaceae in the urine, staphylococci in localized abscesses, gonococci in urethral exudates, clostridia in foul-smelling discharge, and pneumococci, meningococci, or *Haemophilus influenzae* in stained smears of the cerebrospinal fluid permits the initiation of specific chemotherapy with the assurance that the regimen is the proper one. In some immunosuppressed patients *Candida* blastoconidia and pseudohyphae can be found in blood smears several days before candidemia is demonstrable by culture.

A variety of other stains are available for the demonstration of specific microbes. Mycobacteria have the unique capacity to resist the decolorization by strong mineral acid alcohol solutions once they have been stained with basic carbol-fuchsin or one of the fluorochromes. This allows their immediate recognition in body tissues and fluids. The presence of a large number of acid-fast bacilli in the expectorated sputum establishes the presumptive diagnosis of respiratory tuberculosis and is sufficient evidence for initiating isolation procedures and antituberculosis therapy once additional specimens are collected for culture. Subsequent examination of the sputum with acid-fast stains is an important element in monitoring the success of therapy. The traditional Ziehl-Neelsen and Kinyoun stains are being supplanted by the fluorochromes which allow a much more rapid scanning of smears using relatively low magnification.

Acid-fast smears can also be used to identify *Cryptosporidium* in the stool of patients with diarrhea. If mineral acid rather than acid-alcohol is used for decolorization, pathogenic strains of *Nocardia* may be visualized in body fluids or exudates. When an even weaker decolorizing agent such as organic acid is used, organisms such as *Actinomyces* may also be seen.

Both Giemsa's and iodine stains may be used to diagnose chlamydial infections involving the eye, urethra, or cervix. When epithelial cells obtained by scraping these areas are stained with Giemsa's stain, a typical semilunar dense inclusion body composed of many blue- or purplish-staining particles is seen adjoining the nucleus of the cell. Iodine stains reveal a similar reddish-brown mass in scrapings from the eye but are not useful in cervical specimens.

A number of stains are available for the definitive identification of parasites. *Pneumocystis carinii* can be recognized in transbronchial brush biopsies using a modified Wright's stain, toluidine blue, or methenamine silver. The latter produces a very distinctive black-stained cyst. Blood and tissue protozoa such as plasmodia and *Leishmania* can be demonstrated best with Romanowsky-type mixtures containing methylene blue and eosin. These render the nuclei red to violet and the cytoplasm blue. The identification of intestinal protozoa, on the other hand, requires the use of stains such as iron hematoxylin or trichome to demonstrate the taxonomically important nuclear detail.

Immune microscopy   This method combines the specificity of immunologic procedures with the speed of direct microscopy. In the immunofluorescent technique, smears thought to contain viral, bacterial, fungal, or parasitic organisms are stained with specific antibody preparations labeled with fluorescent compounds and examined with a fluorescent microscope. The most useful application of this technique is the examination of brain tissue for herpes simplex or rabies virus; lung tissue, pleural fluid, and sputum for *Legionella* spp.; and cervical, urethral, and conjunctival scrapings for trachoma-inclusion conjunctivitis agent. Direct fluorescent antibody staining of nasal epithelial cells may also be used for the rapid diagnosis of influenza, parainfluenza, and respiratory syncytial virus infections. The direct immunofluorescence technique for detecting antibody-coated bacteria in the urinary sediment has been useful in distinguishing kidney from bladder infection in females.

The accuracy and reliability of immunofluorescent techniques continues to improve as older polyclonal antiserums are replaced with more specific monoclonal reagents. The need for expensive fluorescent microscopes, the poor quality of many of the commercially available conjugated antiserums, and the need for well-trained technologists restrict the routine use of these procedures to reference laboratories.

Enzyme-linked immunosorbent assay (ELISA) tests are similar to the immunofluorescence test except that the antiserum is reacted with an enzyme-labeled antispecies conjugate. After treatment with an appropriate substrate, a color change can be visualized with the ordinary light microscope, obviating the need for expensive equipment.

Electron microscopy   The electron microscopic examination has been useful in the identification of certain viruses which do not produce cytopathic effects in cell cultures. It has been particularly valuable in the detection of rotaviruses in the stool specimens of infants and small children suffering from gastroenteritis. The large number and characteristic appearance of these virus particles allow specific identification to be made on morphologic grounds alone. Electron microscopy has also been used in the diagnosis of the so-called winter vomiting disease caused by the Norwalk and Hawaii agents. These agents are morphologically similar to those of the picornavirus group, and specific identification requires aggregation of the virus particles with immune serum. This technique of immune electron microscopy may have wide application in virology and has been used to identify virus-like particles associated with non-A, non-B hepatitis in experimental animals.

DETECTION OF MICROBIAL ANTIGENS, BY-PRODUCTS, AND GENOMES   The relative nonspecificity of many direct microscopic methods and the delay inherent in culture procedures have resulted in the introduction of a variety of techniques aimed at the rapid detection of microbial antigens, by-products, or genomes.

Counterimmunoelectrophoresis   The most widely used of the antigen detection techniques is counterimmunoelectrophoresis (CIE). In this variation of the agar gel diffusion test, the specimen being tested for antigen is placed in an agar well and specific antiserum in a second apposed well. An electric current is then passed through the agar resulting in rapid confluence of antigen and antibody with the formation of a precipitant within a matter of minutes. CIE has proved most useful for the rapid diagnosis of bacterial meningitis in childhood where the cerebrospinal fluid is checked for the presence of pneumococcal, meningococcal, group B streptococcal, or *H. influenzae* antigens. The technique has approximately the same order of sensitivity as Gram's stain but has the advantage of heightened specificity. CIE has also been used for the detection of the above-mentioned bacterial antigens in serum, pneumococcal capsular antigens in sputum, and the detection of rotavirus and enterovirus in stool.

Particle agglutination   These tests have been utilized in many of the same situations as CIE and require less technical skill for their performance. Although greater sensitivity has been claimed for particle agglutination, both latex and coagglutination tests have been plagued by false-positive reactions from heat-labile serum components and rheumatoid factor. Perhaps their greatest usefulness has been in the detection of bacterial antigens in the urine and spinal fluid of children with acute meningitis and cryptococcal antigen in the blood and spinal fluid of patients with chronic meningoencephalitis. Particle agglutination tests have been introduced for the detection of pneumococci in the sputum, group A streptococci in throat swabs, *Candida* antigen in serum, and rotavirus, as well as the enterotoxin of *C. difficile* in stool. The place of these newer tests remains to be determined.

Radioimmunoassay (RIA)   The most spectacular application of this technique is in the detection of hepatitis B surface antigen–associated (HBsAg-associated) infection and in the prevention of such infections by the screening of blood and blood products for the presence of the antigen. This procedure is highly sensitive, and results can be obtained within a few hours with commercially available test kits. In this method HBsAg-labeled ^{125}I competes with antigen in a test serum for a specific antibody in the test mixture. Free and bound antigens are separated by washing. The reactivity of the antigen-antibody complex is then analyzed with a gamma counter. Experimental RIA procedures have also been developed for the detection of circulating antigens in disseminated fungal infections.

Enzyme-linked immunosorbent assays The method, as described above under "Direct Microscopic Examination," can be adapted for the visual or spectrophotometric detection of microbial antigens. Increasingly, it is coming to replace radioimmunoassay techniques in the diagnosis of hepatitis A and B infections and is extensively utilized to ascertain the presence of rotavirus in the diarrheal stool of infants. It has been successfully used to detect circulating antigens in candidiasis, aspergillosis, and toxoplasmosis. Enzyme immunoassays may soon play an important role in the diagnosis of *C. trachomatis* and gonococcal cervicitis and urethritis.

Urine screening tests A number of nonmicroscopic bacteriuria screening tests are commercially available. Each is designed to decrease the time and cost involved in the diagnosis of urinary tract infections. Bioluminescence, filtration-colorimetry, or chemical procedures are employed to determine the presence or absence of bacterial and/or leukocytic enzymes in the urine specimen. The tests can be performed reliably by individuals with minimal technical training and require only minutes to complete. Generally, specimens demonstrating a positive screening test are cultured; a negative result is reported as such, and the specimen discarded. The sensitivity, specificity, and reproducibility of these tests do not differ significantly from those obtained with a microscopic examination of a stained urine smear conducted by a competent microbiologist; all reliably detect specimens containing 10^5 or more colony-forming units (CFU) per milliliter of urine, but are insufficiently sensitive at lower colony counts. The considerably higher cost of the screening tests vis-à-vis microscopic examination is partially offset by their technical simplicity. The ultimate role of these screening tests in the detection of bacteriuria remains uncertain.

DNA probes The utilization of recombinant DNA techniques has made it possible to isolate, reproduce, and label single-stranded nucleotide sequences from the genome of specific microorganisms that are unique to that particular strain, species, genus, or group. These labeled DNA fragments, or probes, can be added to body fluids, exudates, or tissues thought to contain the pathogen in question, and the mixture treated with heat or chemicals to separate the microbial DNA into single strands. Following treatment, the DNA strands reanneal. This reassociation, or hybridization, is highly specific occurring only between strands bearing complementary nucleotide sequences. If the specimen contains nucleotide sequences complementary to those of the probe, they will be hybridized and labeled.

The potential advantages of such probes are in their unique specificity, their capacity to detect a single pathogen among a plethora of others, and the capacity to identify microorganisms that are either difficult or impossible to recover by cultural methods. Their most immediate impact will be on the diagnosis of viral, chlamydial, mycobacterial, enteric bacterial, and parasitic infections. Probes have already been developed for a wide variety of agents, including herpes simplex virus I and II, cytomegalovirus, enteroviruses, Epstein-Barr virus, hepatitis B virus, adenovirus, varicella-zoster virus, rotavirus, human T-cell leukemia virus, enterotoxigenic *E. coli, Yersinia enterocolitica, Salmonella* spp., *Shigella* spp., *Campylobacter* spp., *Mycobacteria* spp., *Leishmania mexicana, L. braziliensis,* and *Plasmodium falciparum*. To date, only the *E. coli* probes have undergone large-scale clinical trials.

Ultimately, the utility of DNA probes in clinical medicine will rest on the simplification and commercialization of the hybridization procedure and the development of practical, highly sensitive labels. To date, most probes have utilized radioisotopic markers (usually ^{32}P). These demonstrate a high level of sensitivity but require prolonged processing for autoradiographic detection, have an extremely limited shelf life, and require the storage and disposal of radioactive materials, making them impractical for the clinical laboratory. Colorimetrically detected enzymatic labels have been developed which circumvent these drawbacks; to date, however, all appear to be somewhat less sensitive than the radiometric labels and decidedly less sensitive than most cultural procedures. With the anticipated development of more satisfactory, nonradiometric labels, the DNA probe may well alter the diagnosis and management of infectious diseases in a dramatic and fundamental way. They are unlikely, however, to displace cultural methods for infections in which the recovery, characterization, and susceptibility testing of the pathogenic agent is critical to the management of the sick patient.

Gas chromatography This method involves the direct examination of clinical specimens by gas-liquid chromatography for the detection of characteristic microbial by-products. It has been thought helpful in differentiating aerobic from anaerobic organisms in pus and blood. It has also been used to differentiate staphylococcal, streptococcal, and gonococcal from traumatic arthritis and to detect *Candida* in the blood of patients with fungemia. Although the role of gas chromatography in the identification of anaerobic bacteria is established, its usefulness in the direct analysis of clinical specimens remains to be determined.

CULTURE Despite the time and complexity, the isolation of the etiologic agent by cultivation in artificial media, tissue cultures, or animals is generally the most definitive procedure available.

The diagnostic value of a culture specimen, however, depends to a large extent on the likelihood that it has been collected free of contamination with the resident microbial flora and transported to the laboratory in a fashion that ensures survival of fastidious organisms.

Specimen collection When specimens from deep closed lesions are collected, the site of percutaneous needle aspiration should be cleansed first by using 70% isopropyl or ethyl alcohol and then disinfected with a 2% tincture of iodine or an appropriate iodophor. The iodine is applied in a concentric fashion beginning at the site of aspiration and allowed to act for 1 to 2 min before the aspiration is performed. The area should not be probed or manipulated unless sterile gloves are worn or the involved fingers have also been disinfected. If the initial attempt at collection fails, subsequent efforts should be carried out with a new needle through a freshly disinfected site. At the completion of the procedure the iodine should be removed with alcohol to avoid the danger of sensitization. If the specimen for culture is drawn through an indwelling cannula, the site of withdrawal must be disinfected in the same fashion.

When specimens are to be collected from the uterus or a draining wound or sinus tract, the orifice must be thoroughly cleansed and disinfected as described above, a sterile intravenous catheter or multilumen tube is introduced as deeply as possible through the orifice, and the specimen aspirated into a sterile syringe. Culture from an open lesion may be collected by biopsy, aspiration from the margin, or by swabbing the surface. In the first two situations the wound is prepared as for a deep closed lesion. For swab cultures, the wound surface is cleansed only with sterile saline to remove debris and saprophytic flora.

Transportation All specimens submitted for microbial culture should be transported to the laboratory as rapidly as possible, preferably within 1 h. Delay beyond this time may result in death of fastidious organisms, overgrowth of contaminants, and/or change in the number of bacteria unless special procedures are employed to overcome these problems. Rapid transportation is particularly important when dealing with blood, body fluids, and exudates which may harbor pathogenic *Neisseria* or anaerobes. The container should be clean, sterile (stool specimens excepted), and appropriately labeled. Respiratory secretions, urine, large pieces of tissue, and large volumes of fluid can be safely transmitted in plastic containers with leakproof lids. Aspirates are conveniently and safely transported in the same syringe used in the collection procedure, providing all air is expressed from the syringe and the needle is capped with a sterile holder. Alternatively, such fluid may be injected into a sealed gassed-out vial suitable for transport of anaerobic specimens. If such vials are used, it is important that the indicator in the vial be checked to ascertain whether it is still colorless. A pink or blue color indicates the presence of oxygen and suggests that the vial is no longer adequate for the transport of specimens for anaerobic culture. Small pieces of tissue (less than 1 cm²) are transported best in sterile rubber-stoppered gassed-out tubes. After the anaerobic indicator is checked, the tube is held upright to minimize the loss of the heavy inert gas, the stopper removed, specimen inserted, and the tube recapped.

Swabs submitted for the culture of group A beta-hemolytic streptococci can be transported in dry sterile test tubes. All other swabs should be submitted in one of several commercially available transport media. These prevent both the desiccation of organisms implanted on the swab and the overgrowth of hardy organisms at the expense of more fastidious ones. Although special anaerobic transport materials are available, use of swab cultures for the recovery of such organisms is not encouraged.

Culture of specific specimens UPPER RESPIRATORY TRACT   Because the throat and nasopharynx are normally heavily colonized by both saprophytic and potentially pathogenic bacteria, culture of this area is seldom useful except when a particular bacterial pathogen is being sought, e.g., *Streptococcus pyogenes*, *Bordetella pertussis*, *Corynebacterium diphtheriae*, meningococci, or gonococci.

Throat cultures. When throat cultures are submitted to the laboratory without specifying the pathogen being sought, the laboratory will generally report only the presence or absence of *S. pyogenes*. Since a single properly obtained throat swab will detect at least 90 percent of patients with streptococcal pharyngitis, a negative culture is very helpful in excluding the possibility of this disease. Similarly, a heavy or predominant growth of group A beta-hemolytic streptococci in patients presenting with the signs and symptoms of streptococcal pharyngitis is highly predictive of an antibody response to streptococcal antigens and, therefore, presumably disease. It is far more difficult to interpret cultures with a light or nonpredominant growth of *S. pyogenes*. A large proportion of these patients do not mount an appreciable immunologic response, suggesting that bacterial growth represents a carrier state.

Throat cultures may not be indicated in adults presenting with sore throat if they lack fever, cervical lymphadenopathy, or recent exposure to another patient with streptococcal pharyngitis since fewer than 5 percent of this population have positive cultures. Conversely, adults with temperatures of 38°C or higher, tender cervical lymphadenopathy, or pharyngeal exudate are so frequently culture positive that immediate antibiotic therapy is more cost-effective than waiting for the result of culture.

Mouth cultures. Usually massively mixed flora of aerobic and anaerobic bacteria is present in mouth cultures, and they are not clinically useful except when a careful attempt to avoid contamination with indigenous flora has been made. This is particularly true for the isolation of *Actinomyces israelii*. This organism is part of the normal oropharyngeal flora, and the time and effort required for its isolation is not justified unless an uncontaminated specimen can be provided.

LOWER RESPIRATORY TRACT   Although culture of expectorated sputum is the most frequently employed technique for the diagnosis of lower respiratory tract infections, both its sensitivity and specificity are open to question. Studies of patients with bacteremic pneumococcal pneumonia have shown the etiologic agent to be present in the sputum in only 50 to 94 percent of cases. Moreover, expectorated sputum is almost always contaminated with oropharyngeal flora including, in many cases, bacterial species commonly associated with pulmonary infections. Even when a potential pathogen is recovered, its role in the causation of a lower respiratory tract infection is uncertain. Attempts to remove saliva and nasal secretions from the sputum by repeated washing or to differentiate upper and lower tract organisms on the basis of quantitative sputum culture have been ineffective or unacceptably tedious. Some confusion can be avoided if the specimen is collected appropriately and screened carefully for both gross and microscopic characteristics prior to inoculation of the culture. Ideally, sputum specimens should be collected early in the morning under direct supervision of a physician or respiratory therapist. If the patient is unable to produce sputum, coughing may be stimulated by lowering

the head of the patient's bed for a few minutes or exposing the patient to an aerosol of warm hypertonic saline.

Because sputum is rarely homogeneous, it should be examined carefully for bits of pus and blood. These should then be used to prepare a Gram's stain smear which is examined for the presence of squamous epithelial cells (SEC) and leukocytes under the low-power objective (10×) of the microscope. If there are fewer than 10 SEC and greater than 25 leukocytes per field, the results of the culture are more likely to represent lower tract flora. This is particularly true if a single or clearly predominant bacterial type grows, or, in the case of chronic obstructive pulmonary disease, if both pneumococci and *H. influenzae* are isolated. If squamous epithelial cells number more than 10 per low-power field, the specimen can be considered heavily contaminated with oropharyngeal flora and should be discarded. In most cases a second carefully collected expectorated sputum will yield a satisfactory specimen.

Direct endotracheal or endobronchial aspiration may be employed when a satisfactory expectorated sputum cannot be produced. However, such specimens are subject to contamination by oropharyngeal flora which is introduced during the passage of the aspiration instrument. Fiberoptic bronchoscopy, which allows the direct visualization and aspiration of bronchial secretions, is a relatively inocuous procedure and may result in a somewhat better specimen. When it is accompanied by a brush biopsy performed through an occluded double-lumen tube, the material obtained is unlikely to be diluted with saliva or topical anesthetics and may be utilized for anaerobic cultures. Alternatively, the specimen may be collected by a technique that totally bypasses the oropharynx. The most widely used is transtracheal aspiration. This method entails a definite risk of hemoptysis, subcutaneous and mediastinal emphysema, vagal discharge, or respiratory embarrassment and is contraindicated in the presence of a bleeding diathesis. It should be used only when results from expectorated sputum are unsatisfactory and the infection is severe enough to merit the attendant risks. The technique produces a more reliable sputum specimen than expectoration and is probably the only other satisfactory method for collecting specimens for anaerobic culture. However, some 20 percent of specimens from patients without clinical evidence of pneumonia yield potential respiratory pathogens. These "false-positive" specimens are primarily from patients who have chronic pulmonary disease, who have recently suffered minor bouts of aspiration, or in whom the tip of the catheter was coughed into the hypopharynx during the collection procedure.

Needle aspiration of a pulmonary infiltrate under fluoroscopic control also produces specimens of excellent quality. The percutaneous method gives both a high yield and accurate results but has at least a 5 percent chance of complications, particularly pneumothorax. The morbidity risk is greater than with transtracheal aspiration biopsy, but the diagnostic yield may be superior.

Whatever technique is used to sample the lower respiratory tract, a concomitant blood culture should always be obtained. If a pleural effusion is present, it should also be aspirated and cultured.

In addition to bacterial pathogens, pneumonia can be caused by viruses, *Rickettsia*, *Chlamydia*, *Mycoplasma pneumoniae*, and *Legionella* and related agents. Techniques for the recovery of these agents from the sputum are generally not available in a routine clinical microbiology laboratory, and the diagnosis is most frequently made by clinical and/or serologic methods. *L. pneumophila* can be cultured from expectorated sputum, lung tissue, or empyema fluid. In addition, it can be demonstrated by direct fluorescent antibody staining in these specimen types and in transtracheal aspirates. This allows early diagnosis and rapid institution of appropriate therapy. For discussion of the techniques used for the recovery of mycobacteria and fungi from the lower respiratory tract, the chapters devoted to these organisms should be consulted.

URINE CULTURES   Voided urine, like expectorated sputum, is usually contaminated with the normal microbial flora, in this case from the urethra and external genitalia. Urine cultures, however, are more reliable than those of expectorated sputum, because the periurethral area can be disinfected and the urethra itself flushed with the first portion of the urine stream before a sample is taken. In addition, quantitation of the bacterial growth is helpful in separating contaminated specimens from true infection. In general, bacterial counts exceeding 100,000 organisms per milliliter of urine indicate true bacteriuria while those less than 1000 organisms per milliliter reflect contamination with perineal or urethral flora. Before a high bacterial count can be accepted as evidence of infection, however, the following factors need to be considered: (1) the adequacy of the disinfection procedures, (2) the sex of the patient, (3) the interval between specimen collection and plating, and (4) the number of bacterial species isolated. Patients must be carefully instructed in the techniques of collecting clean voided specimens or the collection supervised by a trained attendant. In females, the labia must be separated and the periurethral area repeatedly cleansed with an appropriate disinfectant and then rinsed with warm sterile water. Cleansing procedures appear to be unnecessary in males. During the void, the first 20 to 25 mL is discarded, and the specimen is caught directly in a sterile container without interrupting the stream. The cup should be held in a way to avoid contact with the legs or perineal area. When this procedure is followed conscientiously, a single specimen from a male which yields a colony count in excess of 100,000 organisms per milliliter is highly indicative of bacteriuria. In women, the colony count must exceed 100,000 organisms per milliliter in two consecutive urine specimens before infection can be considered to be present. Because urine is a good culture medium, contaminating organisms will multiply to large numbers if the urine is allowed to stand at room temperature for prolonged periods of time. For this reason, specimens which cannot be dispatched to the laboratory within an hour should be refrigerated. They can be held at 4°C for 4 to 6 h without an appreciable change in the bacterial colony count. In most instances, urinary tract infections are caused by a single bacterial species. The isolation of three or more species in a urine culture usually reflects contamination even when the colony count is high. True polymicrobial bacteriuria does occur but is generally restricted to patients with chronic indwelling urethral catheters. In contrast, colony counts of less than 100,000 organisms per milliliter may represent true bacteriuria. For example, $\geq 10^2$ CFU per milliliter in symptomatic dysuric women and $\geq 10^3$ in symptomatic men are significant counts. In fact, up to one-third of urinary tract infections are associated with counts less than 100,000 organisms per milliliter. Patients receiving antimicrobial therapy and specimens obtained by ureteral or urethral catheterization and by suprapubic aspiration also are likely to contain a low number of organisms.

When an adequate clean-voided urine specimen cannot be obtained, or when anaerobic cultures are desired, suprapubic aspiration may be employed. Specimens obtained in this manner are unlikely to be contaminated, and even slight growth may be significant. When an indwelling catheter is in place, a specimen should be collected directly from the catheter by means of a sterile needle and syringe after careful disinfection of the exterior surface or sampling port. Urine should not be taken from the drainage tube or bag, because these are frequently contaminated. Occasionally Foley catheter tips are submitted to the laboratory for culture when a catheterized patient shows signs or symptoms of urinary tract infection. Statistical analysis has shown this practice to be both futile and potentially misleading.

Examination of a Gram's stain smear of uncentrifuged urine is often helpful in the rapid diagnosis of urinary tract infection. The presence of many squamous epithelial cells and mixed bacterial flora indicates contamination and the need for another specimen. In the absence of the epithelial cells, the presence of one or more bacterial cells per 20 oil immersion fields usually indicates true bacteriuria especially when accompanied by one or more leukocytes.

BLOOD CULTURES Cultures should be obtained from all febrile patients who have rigors, are seriously ill, are thought to have endocarditis or intravascular infection, or are immunosuppressed. If viremia, fungemia, brucellosis, tularemia, leptospirosis, or an infection with cell wall–deficient bacteria is suspected, the laboratory should be contacted for special instructions. The sensitivity of most culture techniques is volume-dependent, with yields increasing approximately 2 percent for each milliliter of blood drawn over 5 mL. In general, three blood cultures of 10 to 30 mL taken at intervals of no less than 60 min are adequate to document the presence of bacteremia in an adult. In emergent situations, two cultures taken simultaneously from different anatomic sites will usually suffice. In patients who have received antimicrobial agents within the previous 2 weeks or in whom endocarditis is suspected, a total of six cultures taken over a 2-day period may be useful. If the patient is receiving antimicrobial agents, the cultures should be taken immediately prior to the next dose, and the laboratory should be notified to allow the addition of penicillinase, use of an antibiotic removal device, or extensive dilution of the blood specimen. The collection of specimens over and above the number listed above is seldom helpful in detecting occult bacteremia unless the culture procedures, media, or conditions of incubation are altered to allow detection of fastidious organisms.

Specimens are best collected by percutaneous venipuncture. If possible, aspirations from the femoral vein should be avoided since disinfecting the skin of the groin is often difficult and the concentration of organisms in the venous drainage of the lower extremity is generally less than that found in the venous blood of the arms. The increasingly common practice of drawing blood for culture through an indwelling intravascular cannula often results in a higher level of contamination without substantially improving the detection of bacteremia. Similarly there is no evidence that arterial blood cultures possess any advantage over venous cultures. Bone marrow cultures may reveal the etiologic agent when it cannot be obtained by other means in occasional patients with disseminated salmonellosis, tuberculosis, and deep mycoses.

To minimize the chance of contamination with skin flora, the site of aspiration should be carefully disinfected as described above. Following aspiration, the blood should be inoculated into both aerobic and anaerobic broths immediately. The dilution ratio of blood to broth should be at least 1:5 to minimize the normal bactericidal activity of serum and the activity of any antimicrobial agents that may be present. If direct inoculation into broth is not feasible, the blood may be drawn into a sterile Vacutainer tube containing sodium polyethanol sulfanate (SPS). This anticoagulant is anticomplementary and inactivates leukocytes and certain aminoglycoside and polypeptide antibiotics. Nevertheless, it will not delay bacterial death indefinitely, and Vacutainer specimens should be sent to the laboratory for dilution in broth within 30 min of the time the blood is drawn. If fungemia is suspected, the laboratory should be notified since some of the standard techniques described above are less satisfactory for the isolation of fungi.

Gram's stain examination of buffy coat smears is seldom indicated. Although a number of microorganisms, particularly meningococci and staphylococci, can be detected within granulocytes in approximately 4 percent of submitted blood culture specimens, the procedure is time-consuming and seldom of therapeutic value. It may be justified if fungemia is suspected. The toxicity of amphotericin B therapy precludes initiation of treatment without strong evidence of systemic fungal infection. Because these organisms may require 2 to 5 days to grow, a positive buffy coat smear would be of obvious therapeutic importance.

Approximately two-thirds of blood cultures from bacteremic patients are found to be positive within 24 h and 90 percent within 3 days. Despite strict adherence to disinfectant procedures on the ward and sterile technique in the laboratory, contamination occasionally occurs. The following are characteristics of "false-positive" blood cultures: (1) repeat cultures are seldom positive for the same organism, (2) bacterial growth in broth generally occurs after 2 days of incubation, and (3) the organisms are often identified as diphtheroids, Bacillus, or Staphylococcus epidermidis. However, any of these species can occasionally be responsible for true bacteremia, particularly in immunosuppressed patients.

CEREBROSPINAL FLUID   Examination of the cerebrospinal fluid (CSF) from patients suspected of having meningitis represents one of the major emergency procedures faced by the clinical microbiology laboratory. Bacterial meningitis can be rapidly fatal if treatment is delayed or inadequate, and appropriate therapy often requires specific identification of the etiologic agent. Because of the clinical urgency, CSF specimens should be collected as soon as the diagnosis is considered, and the specimen promptly transported to the laboratory. The laboratory should be notified if the specimen has been collected from an abscess within the central nervous system to ensure that it is cultured both aerobically and anaerobically. If possible, at least 2 mL CSF should be obtained and the specimen sent for glucose, quantitative protein level, and cell count in addition to microbiologic studies. A simultaneous blood sugar also should be drawn for correlation with the CSF glucose level. Fastidious organisms, particularly *Neisseria meningitidis*, may not survive prolonged storage at temperatures below that of the body. If a delay in CSF examination cannot be avoided, specimens should be held at 37°C.

After receipt, the specimen is concentrated by centrifugation or filtration, Gram stained, and cultured. The inflammatory response in the CSF is helpful in distinguishing acute bacterial meningitis from nonbacterial forms of the disease. In bacterial meningitis, polymorphonuclear leukocytes predominate, while in tuberculous, fungal, or protozoal meningitis, the inflammatory cells usually consist of lymphocytes, and the response is less intense. Although polymorphonuclear leukocytes may dominate early in the course of aseptic meningitis, there is usually a clear shift to mononuclear cells within 8 h. Cytologic changes in the CSF may also be seen in patients with brain abscess. However, smears and cultures are generally negative in these cases unless the abscess ruptures into the subarachnoid space or into the ventricles. The Gram's stain smear of the CSF should be examined carefully for stainable organisms, particularly meningococci, pneumococci, *Enterobacteriaceae*, *Listeria*, and staphylococci in patients with atrioventricular shunts. Stainable, but nonviable, organisms occasionally contaminate sterile plastic containers and may result in a ''false-positive'' Gram's stain. In addition, in cases of partially treated bacterial meningitis there is a tendency for gram-positive organisms to stain gram-negative.

When a large number of organisms are present and specific antiserums are available, the etiologic agent can often be rapidly identified by the quellung reaction or a precipitin test. Counterimmunoelectrophoresis and particle agglutination tests are even more sensitive and may be positive when the Gram's stain is not. Moreover, detection of microbial antigens in the CSF is often the only method of identification of an infectious agent from a patient with partially treated meningitis. In the presence of a significant number of mononuclear cells without stainable bacteria, encapsulated cryptococci or cryptococcal antigen can be identified with the India ink preparation or latex agglutination tests, respectively.

Regardless of the results of these studies, the CSF must be cultured and any resulting growth identified to the species level. Mycobacterial and fungal cultures should be set up on patients who present with chronic meningitis and a mononuclear inflammatory response in the CSF.

Naegleria fowleri, the cause of amoebic meningoencephalitis, can often be recognized by its amoeboid movements in wet-mount preparations of cerebrospinal fluid. This organism should be looked for in patients who develop hemorrhagic meningoencephalitis during the summer months (see Chap. 153).

GASTROINTESTINAL TRACT   Cultures of the mouth, periodontal lesions, or saliva usually yield a mixed flora of aerobic and anaerobic organisms including *A. israelii* and *Candida* spp. The isolation of these organisms is without significance unless the specimen was collected in a way which avoided contamination with indigenous flora. If actinomycosis is suspected, the laboratory should be contacted for special instructions. The diagnosis of oral thrush and Vincent's infection can be made with stained smears from scrapings of the suspected lesion.

Cultures of ileostomy or colostomy stomas, gastrointestinal fistulas, and rectal fissures invariably grow both aerobic and anaerobic intestinal flora. They are seldom helpful, therefore, unless a search is made for specific intestinal pathogens.

Fecal cultures are helpful in determining the etiology of diarrhea and in detecting carrier states. Such specimens are routinely cultured for species of *Salmonella*, *Shigella*, and *Arizona*. Many laboratories are now also looking for *Vibrio parahemolyticus*, *Yersinia enterocolitica*, *Campylobacter jejuni*, and *Clostridium difficile*, the agent of antibiotic-associated pseudomembranous enterocolitis. Cell culture and particle agglutination techniques can be used for the direct detection of *C. difficile* toxin in the stool of diarrheal patients. There is at present no convenient and reliable cultural method of identifying enterotoxogenic strains of *E. coli*, the Norwalk-like viruses, or rotaviruses in the clinical laboratory. The laboratory should be alerted as to whether any of these, or any other unusual infection such as candidiasis, clostridial food poisoning, or cholera, are suspected.

Although rectal swabs are adequate for the diagnosis of bacterial diarrhea, they are less satisfactory for the detection of carrier states. If swabs are used, they should show obvious soiling and be sent to the laboratory in appropriate transport media. Whole stool should be collected free of urine, placed in clean waxed cardboard cartons, and promptly dispatched to the laboratory. If delivery cannot be made within 1 h, the stool should be preserved in phosphate-buffered glycerol to prevent death of fastidious organisms such as *Shigella* spp. It is seldom necessary to submit more than three consecutive daily specimens.

GENITAL TRACT   Genital specimens are submitted primarily for the diagnosis of venereal disease including gonorrhea, syphilis, herpes, chancroid, trichomoniasis, and chlamydial infections. Instructions for the collection of specimens should be sought in the sections of the text dealing with these specific diseases. In addition to the venereal pathogens, a number of organisms may infect the endometrium, tuboovarian tissues, and vagina. Endometrial cultures must be collected through a double- or triple-lumen tube inserted through a decontaminated cervical os if contamination with vaginal and cervical flora is to be avoided. The specimens should be delivered to the laboratory in either a gassed-out vial or a sealed syringe to ensure recovery of anaerobic organisms. When a patient presents with vaginitis, a specimen is collected by swabbing the vaginal fornix under direct visualization. If trichomoniasis is suspected, the swab should be placed in a small amount of sterile saline and sent to the laboratory immediately. If the concentration of organisms is large, and if the swab is received within 10 to 15 min, the organism can be identified without difficulty by its characteristic motility in a wet-mount preparation. The use of special culture techniques improves the likelihood of detecting light infections. Cultural examination usually focuses on the recovery of agents thought capable of causing vaginitis such as *Gardnerella vaginalis*, group B beta-hemolytic streptococci, *Mobiluncus* spp., and *Candida albicans*.

EXUDATES AND BODY FLUIDS   Pus from undrained abscesses as well as pericardial, pleural, peritoneal, and synovial fluids is best collected by syringe and needle aspiration through disinfected skin. Prior rinsing of the syringe with a sterile anticoagulant such as heparin or SPS will help prevent formation of clots. Because anaerobic organisms are commonly involved in infection of these areas, the syringe should be sealed and sent immediately to the microbiology laboratory. Alternatively, the aspirate may be injected into a gassed-out anaerobic transport vial. The use of swabs is not encouraged since the sample size is small and fastidious organisms including anaerobes are unusually susceptible to desiccation and oxidation. Deep suppurative lesions which communicate with the surface of the body through fistulas or sinus tracts present a difficult problem in specimen collection. The communicating pathway is generally colonized by a wide variety of bacterial flora which contaminate drainage being ejected through the fistula opening. The degree of contamination can be lessened in many instances by carefully disinfecting the orifice and aspirating material via a sterile plastic catheter inserted deep into the sinus. Even when these precautions are taken, however, sinus tract cultures often fail to correlate well with pathogens isolated from operative specimens. For this reason, a bacteriologic diagnosis of draining suppurative lesions should be based on a culture of currettings or biopsy rather than sinus drainage. If actinomycosis is suspected, the draining sinus tract may be covered with gauze which is left in place until it is thoroughly saturated. The gauze is then submitted to the laboratory where it is carefully examined for the presence of granules which can be picked out and then identified.

SKIN, SOFT TISSUE, AND SUPERFICIAL WOUNDS Specimens collected from these areas are usually heavily contaminated with the normal flora of their respective sites. Swab cultures should be obtained only if gross pus is present or if there is need to confirm the presence or absence of only a single bacterial pathogen, such as *C. diphtheriae;* in this case, the wound should first be cleansed mechanically with saline to remove as much exudate as possible. Material from bullae and areas of cellulitis is best obtained with a syringe. Successful aspiration of an area of cellulitis may require several thrusts and withdrawals, care being taken to maintain the tip of the needle beneath the surface of the skin and a significant vacuum in the barrel of the syringe. If sterile saline is injected prior to aspiration, this solution should not contain a preservative which may affect the viability of some bacteria. Alternatively, a punch biopsy may be obtained of the area after appropriate disinfection. Similarly, cultures from open lesions may be obtained by biopsy or by aspirating from the margins of these lesions using a syringe and needle. Semiquantitative cultures of burn eschars are useful in identifying patients at risk of bacteremia.

Intravenous and intraarterial catheter segments are best collected by disinfecting the area of the skin penetrated by the catheter, carefully withdrawing the catheter, and aseptically cutting off the 5-cm section that had been located just under the skin into a sterile container. This is then delivered to the microbiology laboratory where semiquantitative cultures are done. In general, catheters which are contaminated during removal will have only a few colonies on agar plates, while infected catheters will show heavy growth.

SKIN TESTS Exposure to antigens of certain types, by various routes, and under circumstances not completely understood often results in the development of immediate (anaphylactic, atopic) hypersensitivity or delayed (bacterial, tuberculin) hypersensitivity.

Active infection with some, but not all, bacteria and viruses results in delayed hypersensitivity to the infecting agent in some, but not all, individuals. Clinically, this allergic state is detected by intradermal injection of the organism or one of its components; in a sensitive individual, induration and erythema will appear at the local site within 24 to 48 h. If an individual is highly "sensitive" or if the amount of antigen injected is excessive, there may be extensive local inflammation with necrosis, vesicle formation, edema, regional lymphadenopathy, and even malaise and fever. Antigens prepared in concentrations unlikely to provoke severe reactions are generally available for intradermal testing for tuberculosis, leprosy, mumps, lymphogranuloma venereum, cat-scratch disease, chancroid, brucellosis, tularemia, glanders, toxoplasmosis, blastomycosis, histoplasmosis, coccidioidomycosis, and many other infections. The immune reaction to vaccination is also an example of delayed dermal hypersensitivity.

The reliability, specificity, and usefulness of the individual tests differ and are discussed in the chapters on specific infection.

Intradermal injection of antigens derived from sources other than microorganisms usually produces an immediate *wheal-and-erythema* reaction which subsides promptly. The greatest clinical usefulness of this type of reaction is in the detection of allergy to foreign serums, pollens, and animal dander (see Chap. 260). The skin tests for demonstrating infestation with helminths (trichinosis, filariasis) produce reactions of the immediate type in allergic individuals, but many

of the antigens employed are so nonspecific that they are of little use in diagnosis.

IMMUNOLOGIC METHODS These diagnostic methods are intended to supply evidence of past or present infection by demonstrating antibodies in serum or other body fluids, or indicating changed reactivity of the host (hypersensitivity, allergy) to products of the organism.

Serologic tests The finding on a single occasion that a patient's serum contains antibody which reacts with a certain antigen merely indicates that the patient has had previous contact with the antigen or a closely related substance. For this reason, with rare exceptions, the clinical interpretation of serologic tests depends on serial determinations. If the antibody titer is found to *rise or fall significantly,* the response likely is a result of recent contact with the antigen. In subsequent chapters, the need for serologic testing of acute phase and convalescent serum is emphasized repeatedly. *In any patient with a puzzling illness, a sterile specimen of serum should be preserved in a frozen state so that it can, if necessary, be studied and compared with serum collected at a later date.*

Prior contact with an antigen may be the result of past immunization with vaccines; interpretation of serum agglutinin titers for typhoid bacilli is often made difficult by prior immunization. The so-called anamnestic reaction, a nonspecific stimulation of antibody formation by an acute illness (e.g., a rise in *Brucella* agglutinins in a patient with acute tularemia), occurs only when the two organisms are antigenically related, and rarely presents a serious problem.

Some mention of "nonspecific" serologic changes may serve to emphasize again that clinical laboratory tests have come into use *only because they have been found to correlate reasonably well with clinical findings.* In several diseases it has been found, often accidentally, that serum antibody develops which will react with antigens derived from sources other than the etiologic agent (which may actually be unknown). Common examples are heterophil agglutinins in infectious mononucleosis, cold agglutinins in mycoplasma pneumonia, and the agglutination of certain strains of *Proteus* bacilli by serum of patients with rickettsial diseases. The VDRL test for syphilis and related flocculation tests are performed with antigens derived from sources completely unrelated to *Treponema pallidum.*

The results of serologic tests must be interpreted in the light of other information about the patient, including such factors as previous immunizations and illnesses, the possibility of exposure to chemically but etiologically unrelated antigens, and the importance of a changing titer in serial tests as opposed to a single isolated observation.

VIROLOGIC SPECIMENS The selection of specimens for the diagnosis of viral illness depends on both the stage of the disease and its clinical presentation. If the patient is seen early in the course of illness, frequently it is possible to demonstrate viral antigen in body tissue or fluids and/or to recover the virus by appropriate culture techniques. If the patient is seen later, during the recovery or convalescent stages, the diagnosis is often best established by serologic means. The type of specimen submitted for culture and the method of specimen transport depend to some extent on the nature of the illness. Throat swabs are helpful in the diagnosis of most viral infections. Because respiratory viruses are extremely labile, the swabs are placed in a buffered, high-protein transport medium containing antibiotic agents. If the specimen is to be transported to another institution, the specimen should be stored at $-60°C$ and shipped on dry ice.

Cerebrospinal fluid from patients presenting with meningitis or encephalitis can also be submitted for culture. As with throat swabs, these specimens should be stored at low temperatures and shipped on dry ice. Stool should be collected in patients with respiratory illnesses, meningitis, or encephalitis, if either adenoviruses or enteroviruses are thought to be involved. Since these organisms are hardy, the feces can be collected in any sterile screw-top bottle and dispatched without refrigeration. Urine cultures are seldom helpful except in the diagnosis of cytomegalovirus and rubella infections. Vesicular fluid is a rich source of virus and viral antigen in patients presenting with exanthems. Pericardial fluid may be of help in patients with myocarditis or pericarditis. Viral blood cultures are seldom useful except in the diagnosis of arboviral infections. Isolation techniques for these viruses are highly specialized and are not available in most virus laboratories. Buffy coat cultures for cytomegalovirus and herpesvirus may be of help in immunosuppressed patients. Brain biopsy is the best single method for diagnosing herpes simplex encephalitis (see Chap. 136). The biopsy specimen should be placed in a sterile screw-top bottle and stored and dispatched in the frozen state.

REFERENCES

EISENBERG HD et al: Collection, handling and processing of specimens, in *Manual of Clinical Microbiology*, 4th ed, EH Lennette et al (eds). Washington, DC, American Society for Microbiology, 1985

ENGLEBERG NC, EISENSTEIN BI: The impact of new cloning techniques on the diagnosis and treatment of infectious diseases. N Engl J Med 311:892, 1984

PLORDE JJ: Newer methods in microbial diagnosis, in *Contemporary Issues in Infectious Diseases*, vol 4: *Septic Shock*, RK Root, MA Sande (eds). New York, Churchill Livingstone, 1985

TODD JK: Nonculture techniques using blood specimens for the diagnosis of infectious disease, in *Proceedings of a Symposium: Body Fluids and Infectious Diseases*, Am J Med, July 28, 1983, vol 75, pp 37–43

WASHINGTON JA II: Bacteria, fungi and parasites, the clinician and microbiology laboratory, in *Principles and Practice of Infectious Diseases*, 2d ed, GL Mandell et al (eds). New York, Wiley, 1985

84 INFECTIONS IN THE COMPROMISED HOST

HENRY MASUR / ANTHONY S. FAUCI

DEFINITION Patients who lack resistance to infection because of a deficiency in any of their multifaceted host defenses are referred to as compromised hosts. Other terminologies such as "abnormal host," "immunosuppressed host," or "immunocompromised patient" are often used, but these terms have different connotations. The latter two terms refer specifically to a subpopulation of compromised hosts whose major deficiency in antimicrobial activity is related to their defective immune response.

An expanding spectrum of diseases can now be controlled or cured by complex and aggressive surgery, implantation of foreign bodies, or powerful cytotoxic or anti-inflammatory drugs. As noninfectious complications such as hemorrhage or uremia or graft rejection are being managed with increasing success, infection is becoming the major threat to the quality and duration of survival in many different patient populations.

HOST DEFENSE MECHANISMS

Antimicrobal defense mechanisms (Table 84-1) consist of complex, interacting systems that protect the host from endogenous and exogenous microbes. The degree to which a patient becomes abnormally susceptible to infection by this microbial environment depends on which mechanisms are compromised, how severe the derangements are, and how these derangements interact. For instance, as isolated abnormalities, total absence of serum IgA or complement component C9 would probably have minor, if any, impact on host susceptibility to infection. Isolated abnormalities such as total absence of circulating neutrophils, serum IgG, or complement component C3 would, in contrast, lead to recurrent and life-threatening infections. Similarly, partial deficiencies in host defense mechanisms can have variable impact on susceptibility to infection depending on the specific mechanism, the degree of deficiency, and the presence of concomitant

abnormalities. A modest decrease in circulating neutrophil count to 25 percent of the lower limit of normal or a decrease in serum IgG concentration to 50 percent of the lower limit of normal would probably be managed with only moderate difficulty if either was an isolated and transient abnormality. If such a neutrophil count were present concurrently with a major defect in the skin or mucous membrane for a prolonged period of time, patient survival would far more likely be threatened.

Recognition of which specific and nonspecific host defenses are compromised is important in order to develop effective clinical strategies for predicting the probable onset of infection and the most likely causative organisms; for formulating the appropriate diagnostic approach; and for developing the optimal therapeutic and preventive plan. However, based on an understanding of the mechanisms of host defenses, such an approach must be supplemented by clinical experience with specific patient populations. Because there are complexities of various host defense mechanisms that are not fully understood, it cannot be assumed that all patient populations with the same measured deficiency in antimicrobial defense (as assessed by current laboratory techniques) will behave identically. For example, patients with cytomegalovirus infection (Chap. 137) have immunologic profiles that are similar in certain respects to the profile of patients in the early phases of the acquired immunodeficiency syndrome (AIDS) (Chap. 257). However, the susceptibility of these two populations to life-threatening opportunistic infection is vastly different, with AIDS patients being far more susceptible.

PHYSICAL AND CHEMICAL BARRIERS Physical and chemical barriers (Table 84-1) are part of a complex and interacting system of nonspecific host defense mechanisms that are essential for preventing the introduction and spread of microbial pathogens. These barriers utilize a wide variety of properties to protect the host, including the physical presence of structural barriers (e.g., morphologic integrity of skin or mucous membranes, epiglottis, sphincters); chemical processes (e.g., gastric acidity, pancreatic enzymes, cutaneous fatty acids or lysozyme); physical removal of organisms (e.g., peristalsis, sloughing of squamae, urine flow); and competition from less virulent flora. Interference with any of these mechanisms can increase the host's susceptibility to infection.

INFLAMMATORY RESPONSES Circulating phagocytes (neutrophils, monocytes, eosinophils, and basophils) arise from the bone marrow and upon appropriate signals enter the peripheral circulation and are distributed to local tissues, where they form the cornerstone of the inflammatory response. Recruitment of phagocytes from the bloodstream is a complicated process which involves the phagocytes' aggregation, adherence to the vascular endothelium, passage through endothelial spaces, and migration to local tissue sites (Chap. 56). An effective inflammatory response depends on the ability of the phagocyte to adhere, deform, have random locomotion, and respond to a chemical signal with directed movement. Humoral mediators influence local structures in ways that affect the phagocyte's ability

TABLE 84-1 Mechanisms of host defense

Physical and chemical barriers
  Morphologic integrity of skin, mucous membranes
  Sphincters
  Epiglottis
  Normal secretory and excretory flow
  Endogenous microbial flora
  Gastric acidity
Inflammatory response
  Circulating phagocytes
  Complement
  Other humoral mediators (bradykinins, fibrinolytic systems, arachidonic acid cascade)
Reticuloendothelial system
  Tissue phagocytes
Immune response
  T lymphocytes and their soluble products
  B lymphocytes and immunoglobulins

to reach various loci: an example is the influence the complement cascade (especially C3a and C5a) has on the potential spaces between endothelial cells. Humoral mediators including the complement system, the arachidonic acid cascade, kinin-generating systems, and products of cellular elements (fibroblasts, neutrophils, macrophages, lymphocytes, and microorganisms) also guide directly the locomotion of the phagocytes. Once the phagocyte arrives at a focus of infection, it can adhere to the microorganism, ingest it, and digest it, particularly if the organism has been opsonized by antibodies or complement products. A wide variety of gram-positive and gram-negative bacteria as well as fungi are killed by neutrophils in this manner.

RETICULOENDOTHELIAL SYSTEM Circulating microorganisms are cleared from the bloodstream by tissue phagocytes that are derived from circulating monocytes. These phagocytes include macrophages in the liver (Kupffer cells), spleen, lymph nodes, lung (alveolar macrophages), and brain (microglial nodules). The antimicrobial activities of these monocytes and macrophages are strongly influenced by opsonins such as IgG or C3b which enhance the rate of particle ingestion, and by a large variety of soluble mediators produced primarily by mononuclear leukocytes. The efficacy of the reticulo-endothelial system is also influenced by characteristics of specific organisms which often possess adaptive properties allowing the microbes to resist specific steps necessary for microbial activity such as phagocytosis (cryptococci), lysosome-phagosome fusion (toxo-plasma), or lysosomal degradation (leishmania).

Immune response The major cellular components of the immune response are T lymphocytes and B lymphocytes (Chap. 62). These cells are distributed throughout the body in the bloodstream and at tissue sites. They interact in a highly complex fashion among themselves and with monocytes, macrophages, immunoglobulins, and the complement cascade. T lymphocytes are the major cellular component of the cell-mediated immune system. They secrete a multitude of soluble products which influence the functional status of other T lymphocytes, B lymphocytes, monocytes, and macro-phages. B lymphocytes and plasma cells secrete specific antibodies which have important roles in eradicating certain infections. As noted above, the ability of the monocytes and macrophages to ingest and kill a wide variety of bacteria, fungi, and protozoa is dependent on the ability of the T lymphocyte to activate these cells. Any process which requires opsonization with antibody, such as the process which occurs between neutrophils and many bacteria, can also be profoundly influenced by the regulatory effect of T lymphocytes on B lymphocytes (Chap. 62).

ETIOLOGY AND PATHOGENESIS OF INFECTION

In compromised hosts the occurrence of infectious diseases reflects the impaired interaction of immunologic and nonimmunologic host defense mechanisms with the host's endogenous and exogenous microbial environment. Potentially pathogenic microorganisms may arise from the host's endogenous flora, and factors which change this microbial flora have an important impact on the organisms that are likely to cause disease. Such factors include antimicrobial therapy, nonsterile invasive procedures or trauma, ingestion or inhalation of infected material, and hospitalization itself. Infectious diseases in compromised patients are more often related directly to alterations in host defense mechanisms than to changes in the microbial flora, although both factors are undoubtedly important. Numerous processes can predispose to serious infection by compromising the anatomic and physical barriers of host defense. For example, the skin and mucous membranes can be breached by conditions such as tumor invasion, tumor necrosis, or vascular insufficiency induced by arteritis or atherosclerosis; by injury such as burns, pressure, or trauma; by therapy such as radiation or cytotoxic chemotherapy; by a drug-induced cutaneous slough; and by procedures such as venipuncture or surgery. The respiratory tract can become the site of infection

when its anatomic barriers are disrupted: the epiglottis may fail to protect the lower tract when the patient's consciousness is impaired or during intubation or bronchoscopy. The patient's ability to expel organisms may be adversely affected if infection, tumor, or drugs that alter the state of consciousness or prevent coughing; if mucociliary transport is disrupted by a congenital disorder of ciliary subunits (such as Kartagener's syndrome) or by smoke or other inhaled toxins, anesthetic agents, or cytotoxic therapy; or if an airway is obstructed by tumor, a foreign body, or lymph node enlargement. The gastroin-testinal tract can become a less effective barrier against entry of organisms if gastric acidity is abolished by a surgical procedure or antacid therapy (infections with *Salmonella* and *Mycobacterium* are particularly important in this regard); or if its mucosa is eroded by tumor or cytotoxic therapy, especially in neutropenic patients. Ob-struction of the intestinal or biliary tract by tumor, a stricture, or a stone also allows endogenous or introduced flora to gain access to capillary and lymphatic systems. The genitourinary tract can become a portal of entry for infections if its mucosa is eroded by tumor, irradiation, or cytotoxic therapy. Obstruction of urine flow by tumor, strictures, stones, or prostatic hypertrophy also allows organisms to multiply and gain access to the capillaries and lymphatic systems. Renal failure associated with oliguria or anuria deprives the geni-tourinary system of the ability to flush out microorganisms and obviates the antimicrobial effects of urine itself. The insertion of foreign bodies into the urethra during catheterization or cystoscopy is an iatrogenic cause for exogenous organisms to be introduced into this system. Any locus in the body can become the site of infection if devitalized tissue or foreign bodies are seeded by bacteria or become infected by direct penetration. Spontaneous or traumatic hematomas, necrotic tissue, infarcts, calcified heart valves, and prosthetic devices (joints, heart valves, or central nervous system appliances) are particularly prone to infection.

Defects in inflammatory and immune function may permit infec-tions that would normally be promptly eradicated to progress and cause clinically important disease. These quantitative or qualitative defects may be related to a congenital disorder, an underlying acquired disease, or drug therapy. Several specific types of defects are associated with particularly frequent or severe infectious complica-tions.

LEUKOCYTE DISORDERS The clinical consequences of leukocyte disorders depend on which subpopulations of leukocytes are numer-ically or functionally affected, and how prolonged the dysfunction is (Table 84-2) (Chap. 56). Neutropenia (less than 3000 neutrophils per cubic millimeter) is the most commonly encountered defect in inflammatory host defense mechanisms (Chap. 56). As the neutrophil count falls below 1000 cells per cubic millimeter, there is a progressive increase in susceptibility to bacterial and fungal infections and a progressive decrease in the clinical signs and symptoms of inflam-mation which ordinarily provide clinical clues to the location of the infection. Susceptibility to infection increases dramatically when the peripheral neutrophil count falls below 500 cells per cubic millimeter and increases even more markedly when the count falls below 100 cells per cubic millimeter. The rate of decline and the duration of neutropenia are also important indexes which influence the clinical consequences. Neutropenia can occur because of bone marrow failure, peripheral destruction of cells, or pooling or sequestration of cells. The most common causes of neutropenia are antineoplastic or cytotoxic chemotherapy, neoplastic invasion of the bone marrow, aplastic anemia, and idiosyncratic drug reactions.

Neutrophil dysfunction can also result in a substantial predispo-sition to serious infection. Dysfunction may be a manifestation of a congenital disorder such as chronic granulomatous disease or Chédiak-Higashi syndrome (Chap. 56). Neutrophil dysfunction can also be a consequence of drug therapy, e.g., corticosteroids. In this regard, certain multiple drug chemotherapeutic regimens may alter both the number and the function of circulating neutrophils.

Lymphopenia in adults is defined as less than 1000 lymphocytes per cubic millimeter. The clinical consequences of lymphopenia

TABLE 84-2 Infections associated with common defects in inflammatory or immunologic response

Host defect	Examples of diseases or therapies associated with defects	Common etiologic agents of infections	Host defect	Examples of diseases or therapies associated with defects	Common etiologic agents of infections
INFLAMMATORY RESPONSE				Acquired immunodeficiency syndrome	*Pneumocystis carinii*
Neutropenia	Hematologic malignancies	Gram-negative bacilli			Cytomegalovirus
	Cytotoxic chemotherapy	*Staphylococcus aureus*			*Herpes simplex*
	Aplastic anemia	*Candida* species			*Mycobacterium avium-intracellulare*
		Aspergillus species			*Cryptococcus neoformans*
Chemotaxis	Chédiak-Higashi syndrome	*Staphylococcus aureus*			*Candida* species
		Streptococcus pyogenes	T lymphocyte	Mucocutaneous candidiasis	*Candida* species
	Job's syndrome	*Staphylococcus aureus*		Purine nucleoside phosphorylase deficiency	Fungi
		Haemophilus influenzae			Viruses
	Protein-calorie malnutrition	Gram-negative bacilli	B-cell deficiency/dysfunction	Bruton's X-linked agammaglobulinemia	*Streptococcus pneumoniae*
Phagocytosis (cellular)	Systemic lupus erythematosus	*Streptococcus pneumoniae*			Other streptococci
	Chronic myelogenous leukemia	*Haemophilus influenzae*		Agammaglobulinemia	*Haemophilus influenzae*
	Megaloblastic anemia			Chronic lymphocytic leukemia	*Neisseria meningitidis*
Microbicidal defect	Chronic granulomatous disease	Catalase-positive bacteria and fungi:			*Staphylococcus aureus*
		Staphylococci		Multiple myeloma	*Streptococcus pneumoniae*
		Escherichia coli			*Staphylococcus aureus*
		Klebsiella species			*Klebsiella pneumoniae*
		Pseudomonas aeruginosa			*Escherichia coli*
		Candida species			*Giardia lamblia*
		Aspergillus species		Dysglobulinemia	*Pneumocystis carinii*
		Nocardia species			Enteroviruses
	Chédiak-Higashi syndrome	*Staphylococcus aureus*		Selective IgM deficiency	*Streptococcus pneumoniae*
		Streptococcus pyogenes			*Haemophilus influenzae*
COMPLEMENT SYSTEM					*Escherichia coli*
C3	Congenital	*Staphylococcus aureus*		Selective IgA deficiency	*Giardia lamblia*
	Liver disease	*Streptococcus pneumoniae*			Viral hepatitis
	Systemic lupus erythematosus	*Pseudomonas* species			*Streptococcus pneumoniae*
		Proteus species			*Haemophilus influenzae*
C5	Congenital	*Neisseria* species	Mixed T- and B-cell deficiency/dysfunction	Common variable hypogammaglobulinemia	*Pneumocystis carinii*
		Gram-negative rods			Cytomegalovirus
C6, C-7, C-8	Congenital	*Neisseria meningitidis*			*Streptococcus pneumoniae*
	Systemic lupus erythematosus	*Neisseria gonorrhoeae*			*Haemophilus influenzae*
Alternate pathway	Sickle cell disease	*Streptococcus pneumoniae*			Various other bacteria
	Splenectomy	Salmonella species		Ataxia-telangiectasia	*Streptococcus pneumoniae*
IMMUNE RESPONSE					*Haemophilus influenzae*
T-lymphocyte deficiency	Thymic aplasia	*Listeria monocytogenes*			*Staphylococcus aureus*
	Thymic hypoplasia	*Mycobacterium* species			Rubella
	Hodgkin's disease	*Candida* species			*Giardia lamblia*
	Sarcoid	*Aspergillus* species	Severe combined immunodeficiency	*Candida albicans*
	Lepromatous leprosy	*Cryptococcus neoformans*			*Pneumocystis carinii*
		Herpes simplex			Varicella
		Herpes zoster			Rubella
					Cytomegalovirus
				Wiskott-Aldrich	Infections seen in T- and B-cell abnormalities

depend on which subset(s) is affected; regardless of the total lymphocyte count, severe infections of various types may occur if profound deficiencies of either B lymphocytes or T lymphocytes are present. Substantial reductions in helper T lymphocytes have particularly important consequences in terms of susceptibility to infection. The most common causes of lymphopenia are hematologic malignancies, corticosteroid therapy, antilymphocyte globulins, cytotoxic drugs, and infection with certain viruses such as cytomegalovirus (Chap. 137) and HTLV III (Chap. 257). Congenital lymphopenias can also have severe consequences.

Lymphocyte dysfunction can predispose to life-threatening infection even if lymphocyte number is normal. Lymphocyte dysfunction is most often a consequence of corticosteroids or of cytotoxic antineoplastic or anti-inflammatory therapy.

IMMUNOGLOBULIN DISORDERS Profound decrease in the ability to synthesize functional immunoglobulin, particularly IgG, can cause a marked increase in susceptibility to microbial disease (Chap. 62). Patients with significant reductions in IgG (usually less than 200 to 300 mg/dL) characteristically have recurrent infections due to encapsulated bacteria, particularly *Streptococcus pneumoniae*, *Hemophilus influenzae*, and *Neisseria meningitidis*, and to certain protozoa (*Pneumocystis carinii* and *Giardia lamblia*). Selective IgA deficiency, when severe, can be associated with similar infections, particularly due to *Giardia lamblia*, as well as severe viral hepatitis. The few documented cases of significant selective IgM deficiency have also been associated with severe infections, particularly those associated with gram-negative organisms such as *Neisseria meningitidis*. Causes of clinically important immunoglobulin deficiency or dysfunction include both congenital and acquired disorders, malignancies (multiple myeloma, chronic lymphocytic leukemia), sickle cell disease, and childhood splenectomy (Table 84-2) (Chap. 256).

COMPLEMENT DISORDERS The consequences of total absence of functional complement proteins depend on which of the specific components are deficient (Table 84-2) (Chap. 62). Deficiencies of the early components (C1, C4, C2) have been associated with pneumococcal infections while deficiencies of C3, C5, C6, C7, or C8 may lead to relapsing *Neisseria meningitidis* or *Neisseria gonorrhoeae* infections. The majority of severe deficiencies are reported with inherited disorders, although there are reports relating significant deficiencies to systemic lupus erythematosus, cirrhosis, and splenectomy.

SPLENECTOMY The spleen is a major site for T cell–independent immune responses, and a large number of B lymphocytes reside there as do monocytes and macrophages. The spleen has an important role in the phagocytosis of circulating opsonized organisms. Following splenectomy young children are at high risk for fulminant infections due to *Streptococcus pneumoniae*, *Haemophilus influenzae*, and *Neisseria meningitidis*. In contrast, when otherwise healthy adults undergo splenectomy, they probably are at only modestly increased risk for these infections, especially during the first 3 years after surgery. However, they may be at risk for developing fulminant infection with intraerythrocytic protozoa such as *Plasmodium malariae* and *Babesia*.

DIAGNOSIS

The diagnosis of infections in compromised patients requires special attention because the clinical manifestations of infection may be atypical. Unusual causative organisms may require special considerations for optimal specimen acquisition and processing, and microbial diseases may become life-threatening with remarkable rapidity. It is important to recognize patients who are at high risk of infection in advance of the onset of their microbial disease so that subtle symptoms and signs can be sought prospectively, especially at those times and in those sites where a particular patient population has been shown to be most susceptible. For instance, fever during the second or third postoperative week following insertion of a prosthetic heart valve or removal of a large traumatic abdominal hematoma should alert the clinician to look for the source even if the temperature elevation is not impressive, as infected prosthetic heart valves or abdominal clots may be fatal rapidly if not treated aggressively. Because of surgical trauma and instrumentations, kidney transplant recipients are known to be at very high risk for bacterial wound and urinary tract infections during the first postoperative month, while opportunistic viral, fungal, or protozoan diseases occur characteristically during the second through sixth months. A patient with a hematologic malignancy needs particular scrutiny when the neutrophil count falls precipitously to 100 cells per cubic millimeter (a time that is usually predictable from the pharmacokinetics of the chemotherapeutic regimen). Similar scrutiny would be appropriate for an adult with recently diagnosed multiple myeloma, an infant who had recently undergone splenectomy, or an AIDS patient whose total helper-T-lymphocyte population had fallen close to zero. Knowledge of these patterns should not substitute for a comprehensive clinical evaluation in any individual patient, but such information does allow the clinician to focus on times, sites, and microorganisms that are highly likely to be causing or soon to be causing clinical disease.

THERAPY

In compromised patients the therapy of infectious complications ideally should include reconstitution of deficient antimicrobial defenses, drainage of localized collections of infected material, and specific antimicrobial therapy. In actively infected patients some antimicrobial defense mechanisms can be augmented and improved. Examples include the infusion of fresh frozen plasma to augment complement components, the administration of immune serum globulin to restore IgG levels, and the tapering of immunosuppresive drugs (such as corticosteroids or cytotoxic agents) to restore cell-mediated immune mechanisms or neutrophil production. Neutropenia is the most common host defense mechanism which predisposes to recurrent life-threatening infections. Augmentation or replacement of neutrophils can be achieved temporarily by white blood cell transfusions or permanently by bone marrow transplantation. However, both of these procedures are expensive, technically difficult, and not always effective.

The administration of antimicrobial chemotherapy to various populations of compromised patients is associated with many critical but unresolved controversies. Should empiric therapy be initiated or should the institution of antimicrobial therapy be postponed until the etiologic agent is identified? Which antimicrobial drugs and which combinations provide optimal empiric or specific therapy? What duration of therapy is optimal considering the etiologic agent and the deficient host defense system?

Empiric therapy is clearly appropriate for some patient populations. Profoundly neutropenic patients who have a spiking fever benefit as a group from prompt empiric therapy using a broad-spectrum regimen directed against the major gram-positive and gram-negative pathogens. In contrast, patients who are compromised because of achlorhydria, a recently resected colon carcinoma, or a bronchoscopic examination usually do not benefit from empiric therapy initiated solely because of a temperature elevation.

INFECTION PREVENTION

In compromised patients certain types of infections can be prevented by avoiding damage to physical barriers, bolstering host defenses, reducing acquisition of new potential pathogens, and suppressing colonizing flora. Damage to physical barriers can be minimized by avoiding invasive procedures such as venipuncture, indwelling vessel catheters, urinary catheterization, or surgery. Bolstering host defenses can be accomplished directly in some patient groups. For example, immune serum globulin can be given prophylactically to hypogammaglobulinemic patients; hyperimmune varicella-zoster immunoglobulin can prevent or reduce the severity of varicella-zoster virus disease after acute exposure; immunization with vaccines against pneumococcal, haemophilus, meningococcal, or other likely pathogens may be helpful for groups with specific susceptibilities such as splenectomized individuals; bolstering nutritional status may also be of benefit in certain patients. Unfortunately, most methods to enhance depressed cell-mediated immunity or to mobilize or supplement low neutrophil counts have been clinically ineffective. Reducing the acquisition of potential pathogens can be faciliated by simple techniques such as having hospital personnel wash their hands before patient contact and by appropriate isolation from specific potentially contagious organisms such as *Herpes zoster*, *Mycobacterium tuberculosis*, or multiply antibiotic-resistant gram-negative bacilli. More stringent measures such as laminar flow isolation or control of the sterility of food and water have not proved to be useful or cost-effective when the survival of most patient populations is assessed, although these measures will decrease the rate of infection for patients with prolonged and profound granulocytopenia. Suppression of endogenous organisms is an important concept since more than 80 percent of organisms causing disease in neutropenic cancer patients can be found in the endogenous flora of the host. From a practical point of view, gut sterilization or prophylactic systemic antibiotics have not been effective consistently in recent studies. However, antimicrobial prophylaxis of certain specific infections that have exceedingly high attack rates in certain defined populations can be quite effective. The impressive protection which trimethoprimsulfamethoxazole provides against *Pneumocystis carinii* pneumonia in children with acute lymphocytic leukemia is a striking example.

REFERENCES

Brown AE, Armstrong DA: Symposium on infectious complications of neoplastic disease. Am J Med 76:413, 631, 1984

Eraklis AJ et al: Hazard of overwhelming infection after splenectomy in childhood. N Engl J Med 276:1255, 1967

Gallin JI, Fauci AS: *Advances in Host Defense Mechanisms*, vol 1: *Phagocytic Cells.* New York, Raven, 1982

———: *Advances in Host Defense Mechanisms*, vol. 2: *Lymphoid Cells.* New York, Raven, 1983

———: *Advances in Host Defense Mechanisms*, vol 3: *Chronic Granulomatous Disease.* New York, Raven, 1983

Kapadia SB: Multiple myeloma: A clinicopathologic study of 62 corresponding autopsy cases. Medicine 5:380, 1980

Lau WK et al: Comparative efficacy and toxicity of amikacin/carbenicillin versus gentamicin/carbenicillin in leukopenic patients. Am J Med 62:959, 1977

Notter DT et al: Infections in patients with Hodgin's disease: A clinicial study of 300 consecutive adult patients. Rev Infect Dis 2:761, 1980

Pizzo PA et al: Empiric antibiotic and antifungal therapy for cancer patients with prolonged fever and granulocytopenia. Am J Med 72:101, 1982

——— et al: Fever in the pediatric and young adult patient with cancer: A prospective study of 1001 episodes. Medicine 61:153, 1982

———, Schimpff SC: Strategies for the prevention of infection in the myelosuppressed or immunosuppressed cancer patient. Cancer Treat Rep 67:223, 1983

Ross SC, Densen P: Complement deficiency states and infection. Epidemiology, pathogenesis and consequences of neisserial and other infections in an immune deficiency. Medicine 63:243, 1984

Rubin RH, Young LS: *The Clinical Approach to Infection in the Immunocompromised Host.* New York, Plenum, 1981

Tramont, EC: General or non-specific host defense mechanisms, in *Principles and Practice of Infectious Diseases*, 2d ed, GL Mandell et al (eds). New York, Wiley, 1985, pp 25–31

85   HOSPITAL-ACQUIRED INFECTIONS

PIERCE GARDNER / PAUL M. ARNOW

DEFINITIONS   Hospital-acquired infections (also called nosocomial infections) are significant causes of human morbidity and mortality. They are defined as infections occurring in patients after admission to the hospital that were neither present nor in incubation at the time of admission. Infections acquired in the hospital but not manifest until after the patient is discharged are also included. Although many of these infections can be prevented, some cannot, and the term *hospital-acquired infection* should not be equated with *iatrogenic infection,* which indicates an infection caused by a diagnostic or therapeutic intervention such as the insertion of a urethral or intravenous catheter. *Opportunistic infections* occur in patients with impaired host defenses and are commonly caused by infectious agents that do not ordinarily produce disease in healthy individuals. Many

opportunistic infections are caused by organisms in the patient's own flora (*autochthonous infections*) and are often unavoidable because they are related to defects in mucosal barriers or other host defenses rather than preventable environmental risks.

ETIOLOGY AND EPIDEMIOLOGY   Incidence and cost   Hospital-acquired infections occur in from 2 to 10 percent (average, 5 percent) of patients admitted to general hospitals. The highest infection rates are reported from municipal hospitals and tertiary-care centers, while the prevalence of these infections is much lower in community hospitals. These differences in rates appear to be due to the greater severity of underlying disease of patients in municipal and tertiary-care hospitals and may also reflect greater utilization of invasive procedures and diagnostic tests in the management of these patients. On the average, hospital-acquired infections have a mortality rate of 1 percent and contribute to the death of at least an additional 3 percent of cases. Therefore the estimated 2 million hospital-acquired infections which occur annually in the United States result in approximately 20,000 deaths and contribute to the mortality of an additional 60,000 patients. Nosocomial infections add over 7.5 million hospital days and over 1 billion dollars to the national health care costs.

Causative pathogens   Gram-negative bacilli lead the list of nosocomial pathogens (Table 85-1). Their statistical importance is due in large part to their role in urinary tract infections, but gram-negative bacilli also are important pathogens at other sites. Many of these organisms, especially pseudomonads and *Klebsiella,* require minimal nutrients and are able to establish reservoirs in the inanimate hospital environment, as well as in patients. In addition, gram-negative bacilli develop resistance to antibiotics more readily than gram-positive cocci. In large part, resistance among gram-negative bacilli is due to the acquisition of plasmids called *resistance factors* (R factors). R-factor plasmids consist of extrachromosomal circular DNA, which mediates antibiotic resistance by coding for enzymes that inactivate the drug or by modifying systems involved in antibiotic uptake. Several properties of plasmids are of major public health concern: (1) Resistance to several antibiotics is often linked on the same R factor; (2) R-factor transfer can occur across species and even genera of gram-negative bacilli; (3) small gene fragments encoding for a single antibiotic-inactivating enzyme have been incorporated into diverse plasmids which are spread among many genera of gram-negative bacilli. Certain gram-negative bacilli (most often *Enterobacter, Pseudomonas,* and *Serratia*) have developed an additional chromosomal mechanism of resistance to penicillin and cephalosporin drugs, i.e., the induction of β-lactamase enzymes. Because production of these enzymes is enhanced by exposure to β-lactam antibiotics (especially the newer cephalosporins), widespread use of these antibiotics in hospitals exerts selective pressure for the emergence of these difficult-to-treat gram-negative bacilli.

Among gram-positive cocci, *Staphylococcus aureus,* the scourge of the 1950s and early 1960s, remains the most important pathogen.

TABLE 85-1   The percentage distribution of the most frequently isolated nosocomial pathogens by site of infection, 1983

Pathogen	Urinary tract	Surgical wound	Lower respiratory tract	Blood-stream	Skin	Other	Total isolates	%
E. coli	31.7	11.4	7.1	9.5	7.7	7.3	5779	18.6
S. aureus	1.6	19.0	12.8	12.8	33.3	16.4	3356	10.8
Enterococci	14.9	11.4	1.6	7.3	9.5	7.3	3308	10.7
P. aeruginosa	12.5	8.1	15.1	6.1	7.2	6.2	2288	7.4
Klebsiella spp.	7.6	4.8	12.8	9.1	4.4	4.0	2288	7.4
Coagulase-negative staphylococci	3.7	8.4	1.1	14.2	9.5	11.1	1892	6.1
Enterobacter spp.	4.4	6.9	10.0	6.9	4.1	4.1	1811	5.8
Proteus spp.	7.3	5.0	4.4	1.7	3.5	3.2	1667	5.4
Candida spp.	5.1	1.4	4.2	5.6	4.5	13.4	1570	5.1
Serratia spp.	1.2	2.0	5.6	2.8	1.8	1.8	691	2.2
All others	10.0	21.6	25.3	24.0	14.5	25.2	5364	17.1
Number of isolates	13,165	6163	4490	2292	1798	3104	31,012	100.0

SOURCE: *Centers for Disease Control, National Nosocomial Infections Study, 1983, Morb Mort Week Rep (Suppl)* 33:2SS, 1984.

Multiply antibiotic-resistant strains of *S. aureus* have appeared in many hospitals in Europe and North America in recent years and have been responsible for epidemics of infections, primarily in critical care units. These strains are generally resistant to all β-lactam agents and often to erythromycin, clindamycin, and the aminoglycosides as well. For serious infections caused by these strains, vancomycin is the drug of choice. There is epidemiologic and laboratory evidence to suggest that resistant *S. epidermidis* strains are an important reservoir of genes mediating multiple resistance and can transfer these genes to *S. aureus*. Bacterial tolerance (organisms are inhibited but not killed by bactericidal drugs) is common among currently isolated strains of *S. aureus*, but the clinical significance of this in vitro observation has not been clearly defined in human infections. The enterococcus (group D streptococcus), long recognized as an important pathogen in nosocomial urinary tract infections, is emerging as a significant wound pathogen particularly in patients who have received broad-spectrum cephalosporins (to which enterococci are uniformly resistant).

The spectrum of microorganisms recognized to be important nosocomial pathogens has expanded considerably. Opportunistic infections caused by low-virulence bacteria (*Staphylococcus epidermidis*, JK diphtheroid) and fungi (*Aspergillus, Candida,* and agents causing mucormycosis) have become commonplace. Respiratory viruses, especially respiratory syncytial virus and influenza, have gained increased recognition as causes of significant morbidity when acquired during hospitalization. Other viruses transmissible in blood (hepatitis viruses, HTLV III) are of concern to hospital personnel as well as patients.

Transmission of nosocomial pathogens Contact with hospital personnel remains the principal means of transmission of nosocomial pathogens and hand-washing by hospital personnel remains the principal control measure. Other less important modes of transmission include the airborne route, by which infections such as chickenpox and tuberculosis are spread, and contact with environmental sources. The inanimate hospital environment usually is not the source of infecting pathogens, and improved understanding of the epidemiology of nosocomial infections has generally focused attention on other aspects of infection control. However, environmental reservoirs have proved to be of primary importance in clusters of cases of aspergillosis caused by inhalation of spores from dust or fireproofing material, and in epidemics of Legionnaires' disease linked to contaminated cooling towers or hot tap water in hospitals.

Host factors The age and underlying disease of patients, the integrity of their mucosal and integumentary surfaces, and the status of their immunologic defenses are among the major determinants of both the incidence and outcome of hospital-acquired infections (see Chap. 84).

COMMON HOSPITAL-ACQUIRED INFECTIONS Urinary tract infections These infections account for approximately 40 percent of hospital-acquired infections and are usually a consequence of instrumentation of the urethra, bladder, or kidneys. The most common predisposing factor is the insertion of an indwelling urethral catheter which bypasses the normal anatomic barriers to ascending infection. Hospital surveys show that 10 to 15 percent of all adult patients have indwelling urinary catheters, many of which are unnecessary. Because the urinary tract is the most common site of infection resulting in gram-negative bacteremia, steps to prevent catheter-related infections merit special emphasis and include the following:

1 Restrict the use of indwelling catheters except when required for management of bladder outlet obstruction or for close monitoring of fluid and electrolyte balance in severely ill patients.

2 Rigorously adhere to sterile technique during insertion of the catheter.

3 Maintain a system of closed drainage. Good technique can usually keep the urine sterile for 5 to 7 days. After that, the risk of infection increases with time, 5 to 10 percent for each day of catheterization.

4 Keep the collecting tubing and bag unobstructed and in a dependent position.

5 When urine specimens are required, aspirate the specimen from the sampling port in the collecting tubing by use of a sterile needle and syringe rather than by breaking the closed drainage system.

6 Consider intermittent straight catheterization for patients with anticipated short-term needs for bladder drainage in order to avoid using an indwelling catheter altogether.

Wound infections Most surgical wound infections are caused by organisms introduced directly into the tissues at the time of operative procedures. Most infecting organisms originate from the resident flora of the patient, although personnel in the operating theater may occasionally be the source of infection, especially with group A streptococci or *S. aureus*. The major factors affecting the incidence of wound infection include the type of operation, its duration, the skill of the surgeon, and the basic health of the patient. Operations involving contaminated sites, such as the bowel or vagina, are more likely to be complicated by infection than operations on sites which are sterile prior to surgery. Operations of long duration, or ones in which devitalized tissue, foreign bodies, or hematomas are left behind, are associated with increased rates of wound infection. Other factors predisposing to wound infection include advanced age, poor nutritional status, the presence of distant foci of infection, diabetes mellitus, renal failure, and corticosteroid therapy.

Most wound infections become apparent from 3 to 7 days following surgery. Early postoperative wound infections (those occurring within 24 to 48 h of surgery) are commonly caused by group A *Streptococcus* or *Clostridium* spp. Staphylococcal wound infections characteristically become evident 4 to 6 days after surgery, and those caused by gram-negative bacilli and anaerobic bacteria may not appear for a week or more. If perioperative antibiotics are used, the manifestations of infection may be delayed. Gram-stained smears of wound exudate, together with culture, often provide valuable early clues to the bacterial cause of wound infections.

In addition to emphasis on maintaining sterility in the operating room and insistence on operative techniques that minimize tissue trauma and blood loss, increasing attention is being given to preventing postoperative wound infections with short prophylactic courses of systemic antibiotics during the perioperative period. The principles that should govern the use of antibiotics in this situation include (1) beginning the drug during the immediate preoperative period but not earlier, (2) ensuring adequate tissue levels throughout the surgery, giving intraoperative doses of antibiotics if necessary, and (3) discontinuing antibiotic prophylaxis within 24 to 48 h following surgery. These brief courses of antibiotics do not appear to alter the patient's flora or promote colonization with resistant strains. Prolonged pre- and postoperative courses are unnecessary, expensive, and potentially harmful because of the increased risk of drug toxicity and superinfection. Antibiotic prophylaxis administered according to these principles has reduced infectious morbidity in a wide variety of operative procedures that are traditionally associated with major risk of infection including colon surgery and vaginal hysterectomy.

Nonsurgical wounds that are common sites of nosocomial infection include burns, decubitus ulcers, and cutaneous ulcers resulting from venous or arterial occlusive disease. In general, the offending pathogens are similar to those found in surgical wound infections, except that burn wound infections are frequently caused by *Pseudomonas aeruginosa*, and ulcers of the pelvis and lower extremities usually contain fecal flora. Bacteremic *Pseudomonas* infections may result in bacterial vasculitis and cutaneous infarction manifested by hemorrhagic bullae (ecthyma gangrenosum, see Chap. 105).

Pneumonia Lower respiratory tract infections are the leading cause of mortality among hospital-acquired infections, although they rank third in incidence behind urinary tract infections and wound infections. The major pathogens are the gram-negative bacilli and *S. aureus*, all of which characteristically cause a necrotizing bronchopneumonia. These organisms usually reach the lower respiratory tract by aspiration from the pharynx rather than by hematogenous spread. This is consistent with the observation that the pharyngeal flora of seriously ill patients contains an increased number of gram-negative bacilli. The three settings in which nosocomial pneumonias occur most commonly are in (1) obtunded patients whose gag reflex and cough are ineffective, (2) patients with underlying pulmonary disease or congestive heart failure whose pulmonary clearance mechanisms are impaired, and (3) patients who require respiratory tract instrumentation or ventilatory assistance.

Because antibiotic treatment of nosocomial pneumonia is often ineffective, preventive measures assume special importance. Positioning the patient in a swimmer's or Gatch position is the cornerstone of prevention of aspiration in obtunded patients. Treatment of congestive heart failure will improve the effectiveness of the lung's defenses and will reduce lung edema fluid that serves as an excellent culture medium. Emphasis should be placed on sterile technique when performing tracheal toilet, and the breathing circuits on ventilatory assistance equipment must be properly maintained. The routine use of positive pressure breathing machines in perioperative care is unnecessary and subjects patients to the risk of infection inherent in exposure to ventilatory equipment.

Although patients with pulmonary tuberculosis are now diagnosed and managed in general hospitals, nosocomial spread of the tubercle bacillus is uncommon. Recognition of active cases of pulmonary tuberculosis and prompt institution of respiratory isolation and appropriate chemotherapy are the principal means by which in-hospital spread of the disease can be limited. General hospitals located in communities with an appreciable incidence of tuberculosis should maintain an active surveillance program for their employees.

Hospital transmission of viral respiratory pathogens is common, especially on pediatric services but except for influenza and respiratory syncytial virus, rarely results in severe disease. It is now recognized that hospital personnel often become infected by patients' respiratory viruses and that direct and indirect contact spread of viruses on the hands of personnel is a more important route of transmission than airborne spread. When influenza A is widespread in the community, amantadine prophylaxis, as well as immunization, should be considered for unimmunized hospital patients identified as being at high risk for complications of influenza. Increasing the immunization levels among hospital personnel is likely to reduce the risk of nosocomial transmission of influenza viruses.

Bacteremia   Although invasion of the bloodstream can occur in any nosocomial infection, the infected vascular cannula is the most common and also most preventable cause of hospital-acquired primary bacteremia and fungemia. Annually in the United States more than 10 million persons (more than one in four hospitalized patients) receive intravenous therapy, and therefore even a low rate of infection assumes major clinical significance. Infections related to intravenous therapy account for about 5 percent of all nosocomial infections and 10 percent of all positive blood cultures. The most common causative organisms are S. epidermidis, S. aureus, gram-negative bacilli, and enterococci; when hyperalimentation fluid is administered through the catheter, Candida also is an important pathogen. Although microorganisms can enter a fluid delivery system at any point, contamination most commonly occurs at the site of entry into the

skin during cannula insertion or subsequent manipulation and may be followed by migration of organisms along the cannula into the bloodstream. Occasionally hematogenous seeding of the cannula may occur. Intravenous fluids may become contaminated as a result of adding medications, or, rarely, in the process of manufacture. A clue to the possible presence of infusate contamination is unexpected bacteremia caused by one of the few pathogens (Enterobacter, Klebsiella, Serratia, Pseudomonas cepacia, or Citrobacter freundii) capable of sustained growth in intravenous solutions containing 5% dextrose.

The type of cannula, the choice of insertion site, the adequacy of skin preparation, and the duration of cannula use determine the risk of cannula-related septic complication. Stainless steel needles, especially scalp vein needles, are preferable to plastic cannulas, which carry greater risks of local phlebitis, contamination, and sepsis. Suppurative phlebitis, one of the most feared complications of cannula-related infections, is virtually unknown with steel needles. Arms are better insertion sites than legs owing to lower rates of phlebitis and sepsis. When cannula infection is suspected, semiquantitative microbiologic evaluation of the removed cannula tip by culture or by direct examination of a Gram-stained catheter segment is very useful in identifying patients with heavily colonized cannulas who are at high risk of developing bacteremia or fungemia. Preventive measures designed to reduce the incidence of intravenous-associated infections are listed in Table 85-2. With meticulous care, central venous catheters used for parenteral hyperalimentation can be maintained free of infection for prolonged periods. However, infectious complications, particularly Candida sepsis, are not uncommon in this setting. Intravascular catheters used for pressure monitoring pose many of the same risks as those used for infusion therapy; in addition, the presence of an indwelling pulmonary artery catheter during a period of bacteremia may increase the risk of developing endocarditis.

Transient bacteremia following diagnostic or therapeutic manipulations of the mouth or respiratory, gastrointestinal, or genitourinary tract are usually well-tolerated by the normal host. However, the patient with valvular or congenital heart disease or a prosthetic valve may be at risk of developing endocarditis during such episodes and should receive antibiotic prophylaxis when undergoing procedures associated with significant risk of bacteremia. These procedures include dental manipulations, urinary tract instrumentation, abdominal surgery, and other surgery involving infected tissue. For patients with prosthetic heart valves, these recommendations have been extended. Detailed programs of prophylaxis are given in the chapter on infective endocarditis (see Chap. 188).

NOSOCOMIAL INFECTIONS OF SPECIAL INTEREST   **Hepatitis B**
The risk of hospital-acquired hepatitis B is significant not only for patients but also for hospital personnel who work with infected patients or handle their blood specimens. Patients at special risk of hepatitis B virus infection include those who receive blood products or undergo hemodialysis. The widespread practice of screening blood products for the presence of hepatitis B surface antigen (HBsAg) has markedly reduced the incidence of posttransfusion hepatitis B, and most posttransfusion hepatitis is now caused by other hepatitis viruses (non-A, non-B hepatitis). However, transmission of hepatitis B virus remains an endemic problem on many hemodialysis units and oncology services. For poorly understood reasons, hepatitis B virus infections are often more severe in previously healthy personnel than in patients.

Measures to prevent nosocomial hepatitis B infections should include (1) meticulous attention to precautions designed to limit spread of pathogens by needle accidents or direct contact; (2) labeling and careful handling of all blood and tissue specimens from infected patients; (3) encouragement of hepatitis B immunization for hospital personnel whose work places them at high risk of infection, (4) prompt passive-active immunization with hepatitis B immune globulin and hepatitis B vaccine for susceptible personnel or patients who have had a specific hepatitis B risk (i.e., needle-stick from an infectious patient).

Considerable concern has been generated about the infectivity of

TABLE 85-2   Guidelines to reduce the risk of infusion-associated infections

1   Limit use of vascular cannulas to specific clinical circumstances when other routes of administration of fluids or drugs are not feasible.
2   Avoid high-risk infection sites, such as the legs.
3   Use stainless steel needles in preferences to plastic catheters when possible.
4   Adequately disinfect skin over the insertion site.
5   Use sterile technique in insertion of cannulas.
6   Securely anchor the cannula to limit to-and-fro motion.
7   Apply sterile dressing over the insertion site (antibiotic ointment optional).
8   Inspect insertion site daily and remove the cannula if inflammation, phlebitis, or cannula malfunction is present.
9   Change peripheral cannulas at frequent (48–72 h) intervals.

the approximately 1 percent of physicians and dentists who are asymptomatic carriers of HBsAg. Although several instances of transmission of infection from health care workers to patients have been identified, the great majority of HBsAg-positive health care personnel do not appear to present a hazard to their patients. They should be encouraged to pay particular attention to personal hygiene and hand-washing and should wear gloves during invasive procedures or contact with mucous membranes. If these precautions are observed, their patient-related activities need not be restricted.

Acquired immunodeficiency syndrome (AIDS) Epidemiologic and laboratory evidence indicates that human T-cell lymphotrophic virus III is spread primarily by the same routes (blood and intimate sexual contact) as hepatitis B but is less transmissible. Blood and secretion precautions appear adequate to protect other patients and hospital personnel participating in the care of patients with AIDS. The risk of transmission of opportunistic pathogens from patients with AIDS to other patients also appears to be very low, although in patients with active *Pneumocystis* pneumonia the potential for cross-infection may warrant respiratory precautions.

Legionnaires' disease Nosocomial Legionnaires' disease has been widely reported in the United States and Europe, usually affecting immunocompromised patients. Although contamination of hospital cooling tower water accounts for some cases, sustained epidemic or hyperendemic problems have almost always been traced to heavy contamination of hot tap water by *Legionella* species. Infectious aerosols of tap water can be produced presumably by showers and during operation of some humidifiers and respiratory devices filled with tap water. A causative role of contaminated hospital tap water has been substantiated by the efficacy of hyperchlorination or super-heating of hospital tap water in curtailing epidemics.

Clostridium difficile, colitis Bacterial superinfection with *C. difficile* is a consequence of alteration of bowel flora by antimicrobial therapy. Patients with *C. difficile* colitis excrete large numbers of organisms and represent a risk to other patients. Therefore, enteric precautions and thorough cleaning of bathroom areas of patients with *C. difficile* disease should be implemented.

CONTROL MEASURES Infection control team The goals of those concerned with infection control are (1) to reduce the risk of patients acquiring infections in the hospital, (2) to provide adequate care for patients with a potentially communicable infection, and (3) to minimize the infectious risks of employees, visitors, and community contacts. The functions of the infection control team include (1) development of enforceable policies necessary for appropriate management of patients with communicable infections; (2) development of a surveillance system which identifies patients with communicable infections, quantitates the incidence and prevalence of hospital-acquired infection, and investigates problems that are likely to be remediable; (3) feedback to physicians and other staff regarding identified problem areas and surveillance finds, including surgical wound infection rates; (4) liaison with personnel from nursing, central supply, housekeeping, maintenance, pharmacy, and other hospital services to ensure that an appropriate infection control environment is maintained; (5) education of employees in appropriate techniques to prevent the spread of infectious agents within the hospital; (6) communication with employee health services to ensure adequate immunization of hospital employees and to provide care when personnel are exposed to a potentially communicable disease; and (7) monitoring of antibiotic utilization and susceptibility patterns of common nosocomial pathogens. Generally an effective infection control program can reduce nosocomial infection rates by one-third. Most large hospitals employ full-time personnel, nurses and/or physicians, to lead the multidisciplinary team effort that is necessary to carry out these functions.

Prevention The basic principles of hand-washing between patient contacts, appropriate isolation of patients harboring communicable microorganisms, and application of epidemiologic methods to identify and correct potential sources of infection remain the cornerstones of prevention of nosocomial infections.

EMPLOYEE HEALTH SERVICE Preventive medicine applies not only to patients but also to hospital personnel. The employee health service should maintain an employee surveillance program for communicable diseases such as tuberculosis and routinely immunize personnel who are susceptible to measles, mumps, poliomyelitis, diphtheria, or tetanus. In addition, personnel of both sexes who are likely to come into contact with pregnant women should be tested for rubella antibodies, and, if susceptible, immunized before being allowed to work in areas where contact with pregnant women is likely. Personnel whose work will involve frequent handling of blood or direct contact with patients at high risk of having hepatitis B should receive hepatitis B vaccine. Annual influenza immunization should be encouraged both to reduce the risk of nosocomial influenza transmission to patients and to minimize winter absenteeism.

Hospital personnel who develop significant infectious diseases should be removed from patient contact during the period of communicability. The dangers of paronychias and other pustular lesions due to *S. aureus* or group A streptococci are often underestimated by the staff, and it is commonly forgotten that susceptible contacts may develop chickenpox following exposure to persons with herpes zoster.

ADMISSION SCREENING A patient scheduled for elective admission who has, or is thought to be incubating, a communicable disease should not be admitted until the period of communicability has passed. Screening on admission for communicable infections is particularly important for pediatric patients and for patients being admitted to oncology and transplant services where there may be a concentration of immunocompromised patients. Infections usually considered to be of minor importance, such as chickenpox or measles, can be devastating in such patients.

CONTAINMENT Each pathogen has its characteristic mode(s) of spread, and, on the basis of this knowledge, isolation precautions can be tailored to fit the situation. Isolation procedures are time-consuming and expensive and can hinder essential patient care activities if applied too rigidly. They should be used only when necessary and for the shortest period consistent with good medical practice. The following types of isolation and precautions are in common use:

1 Strict isolation, where both airborne and contact transmission of an organism are possible, e.g., varicella pneumonia
2 Respiratory isolation, where the infectious agent is contained in airborne droplet nuclei of respirable size, e.g., tuberculosis
3 Wound skin precautions, where direct or indirect contact with infected skin lesions or dressings may transmit the organism, e.g., a staphylococcal wound infection
4 Enteric precautions, where transmission usually occurs via the fecal-oral route and where contact with articles contaminated by feces is to be avoided, e.g., hepatitis A
5 Protective (reverse) isolation, where the precautions are designed to protect an unusually susceptible patient with impaired host defenses from organisms in the environment, e.g., patients with burns
6 Blood precautions, where transmission is by accidental percutaneous or mucous membrane inoculation with blood or serum, e.g., hepatitis B
7 Resistant-organism precautions, where precautions are designed to reduce the spread of multiply resistant bacteria to other patients and the hospital environment

If preventive measures fail and a communicable infection develops in an inpatient, the following principles of containment should be observed:

1 Prevent further transmission of disease by the index case by either isolating the patient or, if the patient's condition allows, arranging for discharge from the hospital.

2 Identify all contacts of the index case and determine their susceptibility and degree of exposure.

3 If prophylactic measures are available, administer them appropriately to exposed susceptible individuals.

4 Design a plan to prevent the spread of the infectious agent from the exposed susceptibles to other patients and personnel. This plan must recognize the epidemiology of the communicable disease in question, the effectiveness and feasibility of various control measures, and the potential consequences of further disease transmission.

Methods commonly employed to limit the tertiary spread of communicable diseases by exposed susceptibles are (1) early discharge of patients when feasible, (2) arranging assignments of exposed personnel to avoid patient contact during the period of communicability, and (3) cohorting exposed susceptible patients and personnel together and treating them as an epidemiologic unit. Although cohorting is cumbersome, it remains a major measure for control of hospital outbreaks of chickenpox and epidemic diarrhea.

PROGNOSIS Most nosocomial infections are diseases of medical progress, and the ever-increasing orientation of modern medicine to technologically sophisticated procedures, both diagnostic and therapeutic, makes it likely that the risk of patients acquiring infections in the hospital will continue to increase. On the other hand, many of the factors that promote infections in the hospital have been identified, and measures for their control have been developed. Influencing hospital personnel to carry out these control measures, such as handwashing, catheter care, and restraint in the use of antibiotics, remains a major challenge.

REFERENCES

BENNETT JV, BRACHMAN PS (eds): *Nosocomial Infections.* Boston, Little, Brown, 1979

COMMITTEE ON IMMUNIZATIONS: *Guide for Adult Immunization.* Philadelphia, American College of Physicians, 1985

CONTE JE JR et al: Infection control guidelines for patients with the acquired immunodeficiency syndrome (AIDS). N Engl J Med 309:740, 1983

COOPER GL, HOPKINS CC: Rapid diagnosis of intravascular catheter–associated infection by direct gram staining of catheter segments. N Engl J Med 312:1142, 1985

DIXON RE (ed): Symposium on nosocomial infections. Am J Med 70:379, 478, 631, 744, 899, 986, 1981

GARNER JS, SIMMONS BP: CDC guidelines for isolation precautions in hospitals. Infect Contr 4:249, 1983

HALEY RW et al: The efficacy of infection surveillance and control programs in preventing nosocomial infections in US hospitals. Am J Epidemiol 121:182, 1985

KIM K-H et al: Isolation of *Clostridium difficile* from the environment and contacts of patients with antibiotic-associated colitis. J Infect Dis 143:42, 1981

MEYER RD: *Legionella* infections: A review of five years of research. Rev Infect Dis 5:258, 1983

86 SEPTIC SHOCK

DAVID C. DALE / ROBERT G. PETERSDORF

DEFINITION Septic shock is characterized by inadequate tissue perfusion, following bacteremia most frequently with gram-negative enteric bacilli. Hypotension, oliguria, tachycardia, tachypnea, and fever are observed in most patients. The circulatory insufficiency is due to diffuse cell and tissue injury and the pooling of blood in the microcirculation.

ETIOLOGY Septic shock may be associated with gram-positive infections, notably those due to staphylococci, pneumococci, and streptococci, although it is more common following gram-negative bacteremia. The most frequently causative organisms are *Escherichia coli, Klebsiella-Enterobacter, Proteus, Pseudomonas,* and *Serratia. Neisseria meningitidis* bacteremia and gram-negative anaerobic bacteremia with *Bacteroides* spp are also important causes of septic shock. In gram-negative bacteremia, the shock syndrome is not due to bloodstream invasion with bacteria per se but is related to toxins from the organisms. Endotoxin, the lipopolysaccharide moiety of the microbial cell wall, is the best-studied of these toxins.

EPIDEMIOLOGY Gram-negative bacteremia and septic shock occur primarily in hospitalized patients who usually have underlying diseases which render them susceptible to bloodstream invasion. Predisposing factors include diabetes mellitus; cirrhosis; leukemia, lymphoma, or disseminated carcinoma; cancer chemotherapy and immunosuppressive drugs; and a variety of surgical procedures and antecedent infections in the urinary, biliary, or gastrointestinal tracts. Particularly at risk are neonates, childbearing women, and elderly men with prostatic obstruction. The incidence of gram-negative bacteremic sepsis is increasing, and it is now as high as 12 cases per 1000 admissions in some large urban hospitals. In addition to the predisposing factors mentioned above, the widespread use of antibiotics, adrenal steroids, intravenous catheters, humidifiers and other hospital equipment, and the increasing longevity of patients with chronic diseases contribute to this serious problem (see Chaps. 84 and 85).

PATHOGENESIS AND PATHOLOGY Most of the bacteria causing gram-negative sepsis are normal commensals in the gastrointestinal tract. From there they may spread to contiguous structures, as in peritonitis after appendiceal perforation, or they may migrate from the perineum into the urethra or bladder. Gram-negative bacteremia follows infection in a primary focus, usually the genitourinary tract; biliary tree; gastrointestinal tract or lungs; and, less commonly, the skin, bones, and joints. In burn patients and in patients with leukemia, the skin or the lungs are often portals of entry. In many instances, notably in patients with debilitating diseases, cirrhosis, and cancer, no primary focus is apparent. When bacteremia is followed by metastatic lesions in distant sites, classic abscess formation occurs. More often, however, the autopsy findings in gram-negative sepsis reflect primarily the infection at the primary locus and show involvement of target organs: pulmonary edema, hemorrhage, and hyaline membrane formation in the lungs; tubular or cortical necrosis in the kidney; patchy necrosis in the myocardium; superficial ulceration in the gastrointestinal tract; and thrombi in the capillaries in many tissues.

PATHOPHYSIOLOGY Basic mechanisms Septic shock occurs because bacterial products react with cell membranes and components of the coagulation and complement systems to activate coagulation, injure cells, and alter blood flow, particularly through the microcirculation. Experimental studies conducted by injection of bacteria and endotoxin suggest that many of these responses are stimulated simultaneously; much of the present understanding of the pathophysiology of septic shock depends on studies of the effects of bacterial endotoxin and its toxic component, lipid A.

Endotoxin and other bacterial products activate cell membrane phospholipases to liberate arachidonic acid and initiate synthesis and release of leukotrienes, prostaglandins, and thromboxanes. In cells containing phospholipase A_2 (e.g., neutrophils, monocytes, platelets), platelet activating factor (PAF) is also generated. These inflammatory mediators have major influences on vasomotor tone, microvascular permeability and the aggregation of leukocytes and platelets. For instance, thromboxane A_2 and prostaglandin $F_{2\alpha}$ produce marked pulmonary vasoconstriction, leukotrienes C_4 and D_4 induce microvascular leakage, and leukotriene B_4 and PAF promote neutrophil aggregation and activation. Although the opposing actions and interactions of these substances are complex, their net effect in initiating the shock state appears to be very significant (see Chap. 68, "Prostanoids and Eicosanoids").

Microorganisms activate the classic complement pathway, and endotoxin activates the alternate pathway; both result in generation of C3a and C5a with effects on leukocyte and platelet aggregation and vascular tone. Complement activation, leukotriene generation, and the direct effects of endotoxin on neutrophils lead to accumulation of these inflammatory cells in the lungs, release of their enzymes, and production of toxic oxygen radicals which damage the pulmonary endothelium and initiate the acute respiratory distress syndrome (ARDS). Activation of the coagulation system results in thrombin generation and platelet thrombi formation in the microcirculation in many tissues.

Infusion of gram-negative bacteria or endotoxin stimulates release of catecholamines and glucocorticosteroids by the adrenals, histamine from mast cells, and serotonin from platelets. Opioid secretion in the central nervous system, bradykinin generation from kininogen, and the production of the vasoactive arachidonate derive from many cells simultaneously. Tachycardia, hypotension, and eventual circulatory collapse are attributed to the combined effects of these vasoactive substances. Inhibitors and antagonists of these substances are used experimentally and clinically to alter the course of septic shock. It has been recognized for some time that glucocorticosteroid infusion before administration of endotoxin in experimental animals is protective, an effect attributed to the prevention of arachidonic acid release from cell membranes. If the endotoxin is given first, the effect of glucocorticoids is far less impressive. Opioid secretion, i.e., β-endorphins and enkephalins, may be critical in the development of the shock state. Naloxone, an opiate antagonist, significantly improves cardiovascular function in several experimental situations.

Septic shock results in cell injury and death from the direct effects of endotoxin and other bacterial products, from the indirect effects of endogenous mediators, and from tissue anoxia. The vascular endothelium is particularly exposed; experimental studies demonstrate diffuse injury to and vacuolization and desquamation of these cells. Anoxia and the release of hormones (e.g., catecholamines, glucagon, insulin, glucocorticoids) dramatically shift tissue metabolism from aerobic to anaerobic and cause abnormal lipid metabolism, protein catabolism, hypoglycemia, and lactic acidosis. Many clinical consequences of septic shock are a result of these metabolic changes.

Hemodynamic alterations Early in the development of shock, blood pools in the capillary bed and plasma proteins leak into the interstitial fluid. This, in turn, results in a sharp decrease in effective circulating blood volume, lowered cardiac output, and systemic arterial hypotension. Further sympathetic activity, vasoconstriction, and selective reduction of blood flow to visceral organs and skin follow. If ineffective perfusion of vital organs is permitted to continue, metabolic acidosis and severe parenchymal damage ensue, and shock is then irreversible. In humans, the kidneys and lungs are the organs particularly susceptible to endotoxin; oliguria as well as tachypnea and, in some instances, pulmonary edema develop early. In general, the heart and brain are spared early in shock, and myocardial failure and coma are late and often terminal manifestations of the shock syndrome. There is also experimental evidence that, after the administration of live gram-negative bacteria, significant arteriovenous shunting occurs around the capillary beds of susceptible organs. This intensifies tissue anoxia. In some instances the injured cells seem unable to utilize available oxygen. The net result of defective tissue perfusion is a sharp decrease in arteriovenous (AV) oxygen difference and lactic acidemia.

Early in septic shock, the picture is usually one primarily of vasodilatation with an increase in cardiac output, a decrease in systemic vascular resistance, a decrease in central venous pressure, and an increase in stroke volume. In contrast, later in septic shock, the predominant picture is one of vasoconstriction with an increase in systemic vascular resistance, a decrease in cardiac output, a decrease in central venous pressure, and a decrease in stroke volume. The study of large groups of patients with septic shock has revealed certain patterns of clinical and laboratory abnormalities:

1 Shock characterized by a normal cardiac output, normal blood volume, normal circulation time, normal or high central venous pressure, normal or high pH, and *reduced* peripheral resistance. These patients have warm, dry skin. While hypotension, oliguria, and lactic acidemia are present, the prognosis is generally good. Shock in this group has been attributed to shunting of blood through AV communications, making it unavailable for perfusion of vital organs.

2 Patients with low blood volume, low central venous pressure, high hematocrit, increased peripheral resistance, low cardiac output, hypotension, oliguria, but only a moderate elevation of blood lactate and normal or slightly high pH. These patients may be hypovolemic before bacteremia, and their prognosis is reasonably good, provided intravascular volume is restored, bacteremia is treated with appropriate antibiotics, septic foci are removed or drained, and vasoactive drugs are given.

3 Shock characterized by normal blood volume, high central venous pressure, normal or high cardiac output, reduced peripheral resistance but *marked metabolic acidosis,* oliguria, and very high blood lactate, indicating ineffective tissue perfusion or impaired oxygen utilization. Despite the presence of warm, dry extremities in these patients, the prognosis is unfavorable.

4 Shock characterized by low blood volume, low central venous pressure, low cardiac output, marked decompensated metabolic acidosis, and severe lactic acidemia. In these patients the extremities are cool and cyanotic. The prognosis is extremely poor.

These observations suggest that there are various stages of septic shock, from hyperventilation, respiratory alkalosis, vasodilatation, and high or normal cardiac output in early shock, to perfusion failure characterized by high-grade lactic acidemia, metabolic acidosis, low cardiac output, and small AV oxygen difference in irreversible, late shock. Moreover, in some patients there is little correlation between the outcome and the hemodynamic abnormalities.

COMPLICATIONS Coagulation defects In most patients with septic shock there is a deficiency in several clotting factors, due to consumption of these factors, a syndrome termed *disseminated intravascular coagulation* (DIC). The pathogenesis of this syndrome involves the activation of the intrinsic clotting system by factor XII (Hageman factor) followed by deposition of fibrin-platelet aggregates on the capillary thrombi that have formed as a result of the generalized Shwartzman reaction. The fibrin-platelet aggregates are typical of DIC, which is characterized by a decrease in factors II, V, and VIII, fibrinogen, and platelets. There may be some degree of fibrinolysis, with appearance of split products. These clotting abnormalities are present to some degree in most patients with septic shock, but usually there is no clinical bleeding, although hemorrhagic phenomena due to thrombocytopenia or deficiency in clotting factors occur occasionally. A more important effect of further disseminated intravascular coagulation is development of capillary thrombi, particularly in the lung. Unless there is bleeding, the coagulopathy requires no therapy and disappears spontaneously as shock is treated.

Respiratory failure Respiratory failure is the most important cause of death in patients with shock, particularly after the hemodynamic aberrations have been corrected. This important cause for the acute respiratory distress syndrome (ARDS) is characterized by pulmonary edema, hemorrhage, atelectasis, hyaline membrane formation, and formation of capillary thrombi. The severe pulmonary edema may be a consequence of a marked increase in capillary permeability. It may occur in the absence of heart failure. Respiratory failure may develop and progress even as other abnormalities return to normal. Pulmonary surfactant decreases, and pulmonary compliance becomes progressively compromised.

Renal failure Oliguria occurs early in shock and is probably due to low intravascular volume and inadequate renal perfusion. If renal perfusion remains inadequate, acute tubular necrosis develops. In an occasional patient, renal cortical necrosis, as occurs in the generalized Shwartzman reaction, is seen.

Cardiac failure Many patients with septic shock develop myocardial failure even though they were free of heart disease before development of shock. On the basis of experimental data, heart failure has been attributed to a product of lysosomal enzyme activity in the ischemic splanchnic region. This product has been termed myocardial depressant factor (MDF). Functionally, there is left ventricular failure as indicated by an increase in left ventricular end-diastolic pressure.

Other organs Superficial ulcerations of the gastrointestinal tract manifested by hemorrhage are common, as are abnormalities in liver function, characterized by hypoprothrombinemia, hypoalbuminemia, and mild jaundice.

CLINICAL MANIFESTATIONS Usually gram-negative bacteremia begins abruptly with chills, fever, nausea, vomiting, diarrhea, and prostration. When septic shock develops, there are, in addition, tachycardia; tachypnea; hypotension; cool, pale extremities, often with peripheral cyanosis; mental obtundation; and oliguria. When present in its full-blown form, gram-negative shock is detected readily, but occasionally the findings are quite subtle, particularly in old, debilitated patients or in infants. Unexplained hypotension, increasing confusion, and disorientation or hyperventilation may be the only clues to septic shock. Some patients are hypothermic, and in the absence of fever the diagnosis is often missed. Jaundice occurs occasionally and signifies infection in the biliary tree, intravascular hemolysis, or "toxic" hepatitis. As shock progresses, oliguria persists, and heart failure, respiratory insufficiency, and coma supervene. Death usually occurs from pulmonary edema, generalized anoxemia secondary to respiratory insufficiency, cardiac arrhythmias, disseminated intravascular coagulation with bleeding, cerebral anoxia, or a combination of these factors.

LABORATORY FINDINGS The laboratory data in septic shock vary greatly and depend in many instances on the cause of the shock syndrome and on the stage of shock. The hematocrit is often elevated and falls to below normal as the volume deficit is repaired. There usually is *leukocytosis* with a white blood cell count between 15,000 and 30,000 per cubic millimeter with a shift to the left. However, the white blood cell count may be normal, and some patients have leukopenia. The *platelet count* is usually decreased, and the prothrombin time and partial thromboplastin times may be abnormal, reflecting a consumption of *clotting factors*.

The *urinalysis* shows no specific abnormalities. Initially, the specific gravity is high; as oliguria persists, isosthenuria develops. The *blood urea nitrogen* (BUN) and *creatinine* are elevated, and creatinine clearance is reduced.

Simultaneous measurements of urine and plasma osmolalities are a useful clue to impending renal failure. If the urinary osmolality is greater than 400 mosmol and the ratio of urine to plasma osmolality is greater than 1.5, renal function is preserved and oliguria is probably due to volume depletion. On the other hand, a urine osmolality of less than 400 mosmol and a urine/plasma ratio less than 1.5 signify renal failure. Other useful clues to suggest prerenal azotemia are urine sodium less than 20 meq per liter, a urine creatinine/serum creatinine ratio greater than 40, or a BUN/serum creatinine ratio greater than 20. Electrolyte patterns vary considerably, but there is a tendency to *hyponatremia* and hypochloremia. The serum potassium may be high, low, or normal. The *bicarbonate concentration* is usually low and *blood lactate* is elevated. A low blood pH and high level of blood lactate are the most reliable clues to poor tissue perfusion.

Early in endotoxin shock there is *respiratory alkalosis* manifested by a low P_{CO_2} and high arterial pH, probably because of progressive anoxemia and an attempt to blow off CO_2 to compensate for developing lactic acidemia. As shock progresses, *metabolic acidosis* develops. There often is striking *anoxemia*, and P_{O_2} values below 70 mmHg are common. The *electrocardiogram* generally shows depression of the ST segment, inversion of the T waves, and a variety of arrhythmias, and may mistakenly suggest the diagnosis of myocardial infarction.

In untreated septic shock, the blood cultures should reveal the causative pathogens, but bacteremia may be intermittent and the blood cultures may be negative. Furthermore, many patients will have received antimicrobial agents when they are first seen, masking the bacteriologic diagnosis. *A negative blood culture does not exclude the diagnosis of septic shock.* Culture of the primary septic focus may aid in the diagnosis, but the bacteriology may have been altered by prior chemotherapy. The ability of endotoxin to coagulate the blood of the horseshoe crab *Limulus* is the basis of a test for endotoxemia, but this test is not widely available and is of limited clinical usefulness.

DIAGNOSIS The diagnosis of septic shock is not difficult in the presence of chills, fever, and an overt focus of infection. However, none of the obvious clues may be present. Elderly, debilitated patients, in particular, may have severe infections in the absence of fever. Unexplained confusion and disorientation and hyperventilation without abnormal chest x-rays should call the diagnosis to mind. Pulmonary embolism, myocardial infarction, cardiac tamponade, aortic dissection, and silent hemorrhage are entities often confused with septic shock.

COURSE The rational treatment of septic shock depends upon careful monitoring of patients. A flow sheet for recording clinical data is very helpful. Specifically four basic indexes need to be followed at the bedside:

1 The status of the *pulmonary circulation* and, to a lesser extent, of left ventricular function should be monitored by insertion of a Swan-Ganz catheter. A pulmonary wedge pressure in excess of 15 to 18 cmH2O signifies fluid overload. When a Swan-Ganz catheter is not available, the *central venous pressure* (CVP) should be measured. Insertion of a catheter into the great veins or right atrium provides an accurate index of the relation between right ventricular competence and effective blood volume and should be used as a guide to fluid replacement therapy. When the CVP exceeds 12 to 14 cmH2O, there is some danger of overloading the circulation and precipitating pulmonary edema. It is important to be sure that the flow through the catheter is free and that the catheter is not in the right ventricle. Either a Swan-Ganz catheter or a CVP line should be placed in every patient with septic shock.
2 The *pulse pressure* serves as an estimate of stroke volume.
3 *Cutaneous vasoconstriction* provides a clue to peripheral resistance, although it does not reflect accurately blood flow to kidney, brain, or gut.
4 Hourly *urine output* should be used to monitor splanchnic blood flow and visceral perfusion. Usually this requires placement of an indwelling urethral catheter.

By means of these four measurements the patient with shock can be followed carefully and managed intelligently. Indirect arterial blood pressure does not provide an accurate picture of the hemodynamic situation, and perfusion of vital organs may be adequate in patients with hypotension; conversely, some patients with normal blood pressures may have marked pooling and inadequate visceral blood flow. Direct measurement of arterial pressure is helpful but not necessary. Where possible, these patients should be treated in intensive care units in hospitals that have laboratories available for measurement of arterial pH, blood gases, blood lactate, renal function, and electrolytes.

TREATMENT   Support of respiration In many patients with septic shock arterial P_{O_2} is markedly depressed. It is essential to establish an airway at the outset and to administer oxygen nasally, or by mask or by endotracheal intubation. Ventilatory support with a respirator should be employed early to avoid acidosis and hypoxia.

Volume replacement With the CVP or pulmonary wedge pressure as a guide, blood volume should be replaced with blood (if anemia is present), plasma, or other colloids, especially human serum albumin, and appropriate electrolyte solutions, primarily dextrose-saline and bicarbonate (which is preferable to lactate for treating the acidosis). Bicarbonate should be given to increase the blood pH to about 7.2 to 7.3 but not higher under most circumstances. The quantity of fluid required may be considerably in excess of "normal" blood volume and may amount to 8 to 12 liters in only a few hours. Large quantities may be required even when the cardiac index is normal. *Oliguria in the presence of hypotension is not a contraindication to continued vigorous fluid therapy.* In order to guard against pulmonary edema, diuresis with furosemide should be attempted when the CVP reaches a level of approximately 10 to 12 cmH₂O and the pulmonary artery pressure 16 to 18 cmH₂O.

Antibiotics Blood cultures and cultures of relevant body fluids or exudates should be taken before instituting antimicrobial therapy. Drugs should be given intravenously, and bactericidal agents used when possible. When the results of blood cultures and sensitivities are known, one of the appropriate drugs recommended in the chapters dealing with the specific infections and discussed in Chap. 88 should be given. Without specific knowledge of the infecting organism, the first principle of initial therapy is that it should be comprehensive, covering all of the pathogens likely to be involved. Clinical clues often guide the initial antimicrobial choices. For example, a young woman with dysuria, chills, and flank pain and septic shock is likely to have *Escherichia coli* bacteremia. Gram-negative sepsis in a burn patient is probably caused by *Pseudomonas*. During an epidemic of influenza, treatment should include coverage for *Staphylococcus aureus* because this is a frequent and serious cause of bacterial superinfection and pneumonia in this setting.

When the cause of septic shock is unknown, therapy should be initiated with both gentamicin (or tobramycin) and a cephalosporin or a penicillinase-resistant penicillin; many physicians add carbenicillin to this regimen. Because of their toxic effect on the vestibular portion of the eighth nerve, gentamicin, tobramycin, and other aminoglycosides must be given cautiously to oliguric patients. If *Bacteroides* is suspected, chloramphenicol, 7-chlorlincomycin (clindamycin), or carbenicillin can be added. As soon as culture results become available, therapy can be adjusted appropriately.

Surgical intervention Many patients with septic shock have an abscess, infarcted or necrotic bowel, inflamed gallbladder, infected uterus, pyonephrosis, or other local situations which lend themselves to surgical drainage or excision. As a rule, successful treatment of shock requires surgical intervention even if the patient is desperately ill. Operations should not be postponed "to get the patient in shape" because these patients' condition will continue to deteriorate unless the septic focus is removed or drained.

Vasoactive drugs Usually, septic shock is accompanied by maximal stimulation of alpha-adrenergic receptors, and pressor agents which act by stimulating these receptors, such as norepinephrine, levarterenol, and metaraminol, are generally not indicated. The two groups of drugs which have been of value in septic shock are beta-receptor stimulants (notably isoproterenol and dopamine) and alpha-receptor blocking agents (phenoxybenzamine and phentolamine).

Dopamine hydrochloride is used widely for treatment of shock. Unlike other vasoactive agents, this drug increases renal blood flow and with it glomerular filtration, sodium excretion, and urine flow. This effect is seen at low doses [1 to 2 (μg/kg)/min]. At a dose of 2 to 10 (μg/kg)/min, the beta receptors in the heart are stimulated with a resulting increase in cardiac output but without increase in heart rate or blood pressure. Between 10 and 20 (μg/kg)/min there is some effect on the alpha receptors with a rise in blood pressure. Above 20 (μg/kg)/min, alpha stimulation predominates, and vasoconstriction may reverse the dopaminergic effects on the renal and splanchnic circulations. Treatment should be started at 2 to 5 (μg/kg)/min and the dose increased until urine flow and blood pressure respond. Most patients respond to doses of 20 (μg/kg)/min or less. Side effects include ectopic rhythms, nausea and vomiting, and occasionally tachyarrhythmias. They usually disappear with reduction in dosage.

Isoproterenol counteracts arteriolar and venous constriction in the microcirculation by its direct vasodilating effect. In addition, the drug exerts a direct inotropic effect on the heart. Cardiac output is increased by stimulation of the myocardium and by reduction of cardiac work as peripheral resistance decreases. The dose of isoproterenol is 2 to 8 μg/min for the average adult. Ventricular arrhythmias

may result from this drug, and shock may be made worse if fluid administration does not keep pace with relieved vasoconstriction.

Phenoxybenzamine, an adrenolytic agent, effects a central phlebotomy by reducing resistance and increasing intravascular capacity. Hence there is a redistribution of blood. Blood leaves the lungs, relieving pulmonary edema and enhancing gas exchange. Central venous pressure and left ventricular end-diastolic pressure fall, cardiac output rises, and peripheral venous constriction regresses. The recommended dose is 0.2 to 2.0 mg/kg intravenously. Small doses can be injected instantaneously and large doses over a period of 40 to 60 min. Fluids must be given simultaneously to compensate for the increment in venous capacitance; failure to do so aggravates shock. Phenoxybenzamine[1] is not available for general use, and experience with phentolamine has not been great enough to recommend it.

Diuretics and digitalis It is important to maintain urine flow to try to prevent the development of renal tubular necrosis. Once the volume status of the patient is repaired, a diuretic, preferably furosemide, should be given to keep the hourly urine output up to greater than 30 to 40 mL/h. In patients who remain hypotensive despite an elevated CVP or pulmonary wedge pressure, digoxin may be beneficial but should be given cautiously because of the frequent occurrence of acid-base abnormalities, hyperkalemia, and impaired renal function in shock patients.

Glucocorticosteroids Numerous experimental studies provide a rationale for the use of corticosteroid therapy to ameliorate the effects of endotoxemia and septic shock. Steroids appear to protect cell membranes from endotoxin-mediated injury, to prevent transformation of arachidonic acid to its vasoactive derivatives, to decrease platelet aggregation, and to reduce the extracellular release of leukocyte enzymes. Some studies suggest that steroids also may have a direct effect on reducing peripheral vascular resistance. Because of the complexity of the clinical circumstances surrounding the patient with endotoxic shock, it has been difficult to prove that steroid therapy is clearly helpful. Some controlled studies have demonstrated a benefit for treating patients with methylprednisolone (30 mg/kg) or dexamethasone (3 mg/kg) as soon as shock was recognized. Therapy was repeated in 4 h in the most severely ill patients. These studies and experience in many shock centers support the early use of steroids in high doses for relatively brief periods (24 to 48 h). Late in septic shock, steroids are probably of no benefit. Prolonged steroid therapy substantially increases the problems of hyperglycemia, gastrointestinal bleeding, and other steroid side effects and should be avoided.

Other measures Hemorrhage must be controlled with whole blood, fresh frozen plasma, cryoprecipitate, or platelet transfusion, depending on the clotting abnormality. The use of naloxone, prostaglandin synthesis inhibitors, and prostacyclin is still experimental. Treatment of disseminated intravascular coagulation with heparin remains a controversial and hazardous procedure. Hyperbaric oxygen has been tried in gram-negative bacteremia with indifferent results.

PROGNOSIS The measures described above usually will resuscitate most patients, at least temporarily. Indicators of a favorable response are

1 Improved sensorium and general appearance
2 Decreased peripheral cyanosis
3 Warming of the skin over the extremities
4 Urine output of 40 to 50 mL/h
5 Increased pulse pressure
6 Return of CVP and pulmonary artery pressure to normal
7 Increased blood pressure

The ultimate outcome, however, is dependent upon several other factors:

1 Ability to eliminate the source of infection with surgery or

---

[1] *This drug has not been approved for this purpose by the Food and Drug Administration at the time of publication.*

antibiotics. The prognosis of urinary tract infections, septic abortions, abdominal abscesses, gastrointestinal or biliary fistulas, and subcutaneous or anorectal abscesses is better than that of primary foci in the skin or lungs. However, extensive abdominal surgery, even if necessary, is associated with a poor prognosis.

2 Previous contact with the organism. Patients with chronic urinary tract infections who develop bacteremia rarely have severe gram-negative shock, perhaps because they have become tolerant to the endotoxin.

3 Underlying disease. Patients with lymphoma or leukemia who develop septic shock while their hematologic disease is out of control rarely recover; conversely, if hematologic remission is achieved, the shock is more likely to respond to therapy. Patients with antecedent heart disease and with diabetes mellitus also have a poor prognosis.

4 Metabolic status. The development of severe metabolic acidosis and lactic acidemia—irrespective of cardiac output—is associated with a poor prognosis.

5 Development of pulmonary insufficiency even after the hemodynamic abnormalities have been corrected is associated with an unfavorable outcome.

The overall mortality rate of septic shock remains 50 percent; however, with better monitoring and more physiologic treatment, the outcome should improve.

PREVENTION   The poor results in the treatment of septic shock are not due to lack of potent antibiotics or vasoactive agents. Rather, failure to institute therapy sufficiently early is a major roadblock to success. Septic shock usually is recognized too late, all too often after irreversible changes have taken place. Because 70 percent of patients who are likely to develop septic shock are in the hospital *before* signs and symptoms of shock appear, it is essential to watch patients who are candidates for development of shock assiduously, to treat their infections vigorously and early, and to perform appropriate surgery before catastrophic complications occur. It is particularly important to watch for infected venous and urinary catheters which may act as portals of entry for the organisms that cause gram-negative sepsis and to remove them from all patients as soon as feasible. There is some preliminary evidence that early therapy of septic shock improves the ultimate outcome. Finally, the protective effect of antiserum in experimental animals may, at some time in the future, be applicable to humans.

REFERENCES

BERNTON EW et al: Opioids & neuropeptides: Mechanisms in circulatory shock. Fed Proc 44:290, 1985

BRYAN CS et al: Analysis of 1,186 episodes of gram-negative bacteremia in non-university hospitals: The effects of antimicrobial therapy. Rev Infect Dis 5:629, 1983

HOUSTON MC et al: Shock diagnosis and management. Arch Intern Med 144:1433, 1984

HOUTCHENS BA, WESTENSKOW DR: Oxygen consumption in septic shock: Collective review. Circ Shock 13:361, 1984

KREGER BE et al: Gram-negative bacteremia: III. Reassessment of etiology, epidemiology and ecology in 612 patients. Am J Med 68:332, 1980

————: Gram-negative bacteremia: IV. Re-evaluation of clinical features and treatment in 612 patients. Am J Med 68:344, 1980

McCABE WR et al: Pathophysiology of bacteremia. Am J Med 75:225, 1983

MIZOCK B: Septic shock—a metabolic perspective. Arch Intern Med 144:579, 1984

PARKER MM, PARRILLO JE: Septic shock: Hemodynamics and pathogenesis. JAMA 250:3324, 1983

ROOT RK, SANDE MM: *Septic Shock.* New York, Churchill Livingstone, 1985

SCHUMER W: Steroids in the treatment of clinical septic shock. Ann Surg 184:333, 1976

SPRUNG CL et al: The effects of high-dose corticosteroids in patients with septic shock. N Engl J Med 311:1137, 1984

87   LOCALIZED INFECTIONS AND ABSCESSES

JAN V. HIRSCHMANN

GENERAL CONSIDERATIONS

While many bacterial diseases are conveniently described by their specific etiologic pathogens, in some their location primarily determines the clinical picture. Examples of such infections include abscesses, soft tissue infections, bacterial endocarditis (see Chap. 188), pyogenic infections of the central nervous system (see Chap. 346), urinary tract infections (see Chap. 225), lung abscess (see Chap. 205), mediastinitis (see Chap. 214), appendicitis and appendiceal abscess (see Chap. 241), diverticulitis (see Chap. 239), osteomyelitis (see Chap. 340), and infections of the pericardium (see Chap. 194). Many pathogens can cause infections in these sites; although their bacteriologic identification may be time-consuming, knowledge of the usual flora causing infection in certain anatomic loci should permit appropriate therapy before the results of cultures are available.

ETIOLOGY   Localized pyogenic infection can develop in any region or organ of the body, and may be initiated by *trauma* and secondary bacterial contamination, by some *alteration in local conditions* that renders a tissue susceptible to infection with organisms already present as part of the "normal flora" to which it is ordinarily resistant, by *contiguous spread* from a nearby lesion, or by *metastatic implantation* of microorganisms carried in blood or lymph.

Under appropriate conditions of lowered local host defenses, almost any common bacteria can initiate an infectious process. Cultures from open lesions such as those of the skin or from intraabdominal foci arising from perforations of the gastrointestinal tract frequently contain several bacterial species; as expected, the organisms found most frequently are the "normal flora" of these regions.

Infection in some areas is more likely to be caused by certain organisms, such as staphylococci in the skin and coliform bacteria in the urinary tract, and special features of the tissue reaction produced by some bacterial species make it possible to recognize infection by them with considerable accuracy. The *staphylococci* produce rapid necrosis and early suppuration with large amounts of creamy yellow pus (see Chap. 94). Group A beta-hemolytic streptococcal infections (see Chap. 95) tend to spread rapidly through tissues, causing intense edema and erythema but relatively little necrosis and thin, serumlike exudate; anaerobic bacteria (see Chap. 102) produce necrosis and profuse, brownish, foul-smelling pus.

The identification of infecting organisms is important in the choice of antimicrobial chemotherapy. However, when infection occurs in certain areas, as in paranasal sinuses or cutaneous ulcers, or shows up in sputum, it is unlikely that treatment will render cultured specimens sterile. In these locations, serial cultures during antimicrobial administration are typically unhelpful, and therapy should be guided largely by the clinical response.

PATHOGENESIS   Factors predisposing to the initiation and persistence of infection in a tissue include trauma, obstruction of normal drainage (sweat glands, biliary tract, bronchial tree, urinary tract), ischemia (infarction, gangrene), chemical irritation (by gastric contents, bile, or intramuscularly injected drugs), hematoma formation, accumulation of fluid (lymphatic obstruction, cardiac edema), foreign bodies (bullets, splinters, sutures), and others such as the occurrence of stasis or turbulence in the vascular system.

Infection in soft tissue usually begins as a *cellulitis,* a diffuse acute inflammation with hyperemia, edema, and leukocytic infiltration but little or no necrosis and suppuration. With some organisms, this is followed by necrosis, liquefaction, accumulation of leukocytes and debris, suppuration, loculation of the pus, and formation of one or more *abscesses*. Abscess formation is particularly likely to follow infection in a preexisting space or cavity, such as the fallopian tubes or lung cysts.

The local spread of infection generally follows the path of least resistance along fascial planes; proper surgical treatment requires a knowledge of these routes, which will be described for specific infections later in this chapter. Lymphatic spread may lead to lymphangitis, lymphadenitis, or, if the regional nodes suppurate, to the formation of a *bubo*. Involvement of local venules or large veins may cause infective thrombophlebitis with resulting bacteremia, septic embolization, and systemic dissemination of infection. Staphylococci, streptococci, and *Bacteroides* are notorious for frequently producing vascular lesions of this type.

Depending upon the infecting organism and the anatomy of the affected region, a small abscess may subside completely; there may be gradual encapsulation of the accumulated pus and persistence of the focus in a quiescent state; or the lesion may "point" and rupture into adjacent tissues or to the outside surface of the body, as usually happens with furuncles. Spontaneous drainage ordinarily leads to resolution of a superficially situated suppurative focus. However, if the abscess is deeply situated and well encapsulated, persistence of a fistulous tract and the formation of a chronic, draining sinus often occur. *The development of persistent sinuses over an area of suppuration produced by ordinary pyogenic bacteria should always suggest involvement of underlying bone or the presence of a foreign body.* Fistulas that open onto the skin are, of course, soon colonized by microorganisms from the external environment. Ordinary bacterial cultures of drainage fluid almost invariably show a mixed flora and are unreliable for the etiologic diagnosis of the underlying disease. This is particularly important in disorders that characteristically lead to persistent sinus formation, such as tuberculosis and actinomycosis. In these situations, superficial organisms about the opening of the sinus tract may mask the true nature of the lesion by obscuring the real pathogen.

MANIFESTATIONS Secondary infection of wounds and cutaneous ulcers is usually recognizable by inspection. Infections of the skin and subcutaneous tissues almost invariably produce the classic manifestations: *redness, tenderness, heat,* and *swelling*. Reddish streaks extending proximally and associated with tender enlargement of regional lymph nodes indicate lymphangitis. Systemic symptoms may be absent or mild, or there may be fever, malaise, prostration, and leukocytosis.

Infection and suppuration in deeper tissues or in body cavities often cause local pain and tenderness, but locating and determining the exact nature of the lesion may be difficult. Palpating a tender mass is helpful, but muscle spasm and intervening structures often interfere. Abdominal or pelvic examination under anesthesia is sometimes useful in these circumstances.

Auscultation may reveal a friction rub over an abdominal viscus, the pleura, or the pericardium. The rapid development of an effusion in the pericardium, pleura, abdomen, or a joint should suggest infection. Similarly, fluid detected by transillumination of paranasal sinuses or inspection of the tympanic membrane may be the first sign of infection.

Depending on the location of an abscess, symptoms and signs referable to encroachment upon adjacent structures may dominate the picture. Respiratory obstruction may be the first sign of mediastinal abscess; dysphagia often first calls attention to peritonsillar or retropharyngeal abscesses; and tamponade is sometimes the initial clue to pericardial infection. Localizing signs of dysfunction are especially striking and important with brain and spinal cord abscesses, although brain abscesses may be clinically silent (see Chap. 346). In some patients local pain and tenderness or signs of dysfunction are mild or equivocal, and fever, prostration, and weight loss dominate the picture. The fever may be low-grade but is often hectic, with repeated rigors and drenching night sweats. Fatigue and anemia are frequent, and weight loss may be so rapid that emaciation occurs within a few weeks. A patient with these symptoms and signs may have chronic subphrenic, perinephric, or other abscess in the complete absence of any detectable physical sign pointing to the location of a large accumulation of pus. Because of prior antimicrobial therapy, some deep-seated abscesses present the picture of a chronic illness manifested by no more than malaise, easy fatigability, low-grade fever, mild anemia, and an elevated sedimentation rate.

Fluctuation of a mass on palpation is a reliable sign that it contains fluid, perhaps pus, but failure to detect this sign when examining deeper structures does not exclude suppuration as a cause, indicate that the mass is noninfectious, or prove that drainage is unnecessary.

LABORATORY FINDINGS Peripheral polymorphonuclear leukocytosis is frequent with abscesses, and significant unexplained elevation of the white blood cell count in any patient should lead to a search for localized suppuration. Depending on the severity and duration of infection, there may be a chronic normocytic, normochromic anemia. The sedimentation rate is almost always rapid. Mild albuminuria, occasionally noted in febrile patients, has no diagnostic import.

Pus or fluid obtained by needle aspiration or incision of a suspected lesion should *always* be stained and examined directly in addition to being cultured aerobically and anaerobically. Pus is a poor metabolic substrate, and bacteria may fail to grow in cultures from an abscess of long standing. In such instances, the findings on microscopic examination may be the only guide in choosing proper chemotherapy. *Failure to examine exudates with Gram's stain is the single greatest deterrent to appropriate antimicrobial therapy;* the internist as well as the surgeon should be sure that this procedure is performed.

Blood cultures are often positive in intravascular infections such as septic thrombophlebitis and endocarditis and in pyogenic infections in which localized abscesses are metastatic, as in staphylococcal, streptococcal, and *Salmonella* bacteremias. Moreover, manipulation, including surgical incision, of any localized infection may cause transient bacteremia.

Noninvasive techniques are often helpful in the diagnosis of abscess. X-ray examinations may indicate localized collections of pus when they show atypical collections of gas, displacement of organs, and tissue densities in abnormal locations. Radionuclide scans may demonstrate abscesses in brain, liver, spleen, and thyroid. The isotope [^{67}Ga] gallium citrate is selectively concentrated in areas of suppuration, but in noninfectious inflammation and neoplasms as well, and many have found gallium scans of limited value in locating abscesses. Scans using ^{111}In-labeled leukocytes may be more accurate. The technique of diagnostic ultrasound is not only useful in localizing abscess but also may provide clues to the size of the abscess and to the presence of multiple abscesses or loculation. Computerized tomography (CT scan) is very helpful in demonstrating abscesses, especially in the brain and abdominal cavity, including the retroperitoneum.

THERAPEUTIC CONSIDERATIONS Recognition of the striking symptomatic improvement that follows spontaneous evacuation of a suppurative focus led long ago to the adoption of *surgical incision* for the treatment of abscesses. The exact reasons that local and constitutional manifestations improve with adequate drainage of pus are unknown, but clinically the benefits are unequivocal.

Incision of infected tissue before the stage of liquefaction and accumulation of pus is often deleterious, fails to relieve discomfort, and may even at times facilitate spread of infection. For this reason, it is sometimes necessary to wait until an abscess "ripens," i.e., localizes and "comes to a head." The *application of heat* to an area of superficial inflammation will relieve pain and often speed the subsidence of cellulitis without suppuration. If necrosis of tissue is already under way, hot applications appear to facilitate localization of the process and accumulation of pus, making incision and drainage feasible at an earlier time. Another procedure that helps reduce swelling and relieve pain is *elevation of the affected part*.

The availability of specific chemotherapeutic drugs has modified the need for heat, elevation, and incision surprisingly little. The early administration of chemotherapeutics has reduced the incidence of suppurative complications in many disorders, but once suppuration has appeared, antimicrobial drugs become remarkably incapable of eradicating the infecting organisms, although they may mask the classic clinical features of abscess formation.

Some antimicrobials, notably the penicillins, appear to retain their antibacterial activity in the presence of pus, while others, exemplified by the aminoglycosides, are at least partially inactivated. However, inability of the drug to penetrate into an area of suppuration is rarely the reason for therapeutic failure. Although this possibility exists in some infections, such as osteomyelitis, it is usually overcome by increasing dosage. Because direct instillation of the antibiotic into an infected area is not, by itself, a curative procedure, other factors are probably more important than faulty diffusion of the agent into the purulent focus.

An established inflammatory exudate is a relatively poor environment for bacterial multiplication. Because the penicillins and cephalosporins are bactericidal only against multiplying organisms, failure of these antibiotics to eradicate bacteria in an abscess may be related to the organisms' inactive metabolic state. Although the mechanism of their antibacterial action differs from that of the penicillins, bacteriostatic agents such as tetracycline or chloramphenicol also are incapable of eradicating bacteria in the static phase of growth. By definition, these drugs only inhibit multiplication of bacteria and usually exert no direct lethal action; the death of organisms in any infection treated with bacteriostatic agents depends on other mechanisms. For most pyogenic bacteria, phagocytosis is one of the most important of these (although there must be others not so carefully studied), and, in the absence of phagocytes or in circumstances which inhibit their activity, bacteriostatic drugs are relatively ineffective. In fluid-filled cavities, particularly in the metabolically unfavorable milieu of an abscess, phagocytosis is greatly reduced. Consequently, despite inhibition of bacterial multiplication, organisms can remain dormant and survive for long periods of time. It is probably a combination of these two circumstances, decreased multiplication of bacteria and decreased phagocytosis, that makes infection in the heart valves, for example, so relatively resistant to antimicrobial therapy. Large doses of bactericidal drugs for long periods are needed to achieve cure.

Antimicrobial drugs may obviate suppuration if given early or prevent spread of an existing abscess, but usually are no substitute for surgical drainage. Indeed, their use in the face of a lesion requiring evacuation of pus is one of the most common serious errors in treating pyogenic infections.

In empyema, suppurative pericarditis, or pyarthrosis, excellent therapeutic results are sometimes achieved by aspiration of pus and systemic antimicrobial therapy. Success, however, depends as fully on the adequacy of drainage as it does upon the administration of the antibiotic, and if loculation occurs or the exudate becomes too viscid to remove, surgical incision and drainage become mandatory.

In infective thrombophlebitis, surgical interruption of the veins by ligation or, in some cases, by total excision of an infected segment is sometimes indicated to prevent seeding of other organs by infected emboli.

CLINICAL FEATURES OF INFECTIONS IN VARIOUS REGIONS

SUPERFICIAL ABSCESSES   Skin and subcutaneous tissues   *Impetigo* is a superficial infection caused by group A hemolytic streptococci, sometimes combined with *Staphylococcus aureus*. It is primarily a disease of children, common in warm weather, characterized by multiple erythematous lesions which vesiculate and are intensely pruritic. In adults impetigo is most commonly an infectious complication of a chronic dermatitis. Local spread occurs through scratching and release of infected vesicle fluid. Serious complications

are metastatic abscesses and acute glomerulonephritis. Treatment consists of local and general cleansing of the skin, appropriate systemic antibiotics, and therapy of any underlying dermatologic condition present.

Deeper infections of the skin are almost invariably staphylococcal in origin and are described in Chap. 94. Erysipelas, a characteristic dermal lesion produced by group A streptococci, is described in Chap. 95.

Lymphadenitis with or without suppuration may complicate any pyogenic skin lesion and is often striking with superficial streptococcal infections. Specific diseases characterized by suppurative regional lymphadenitis include lymphogranuloma venereum (see Chap. 150), cat-scratch disease (see Chap. 118), tularemia (see Chap. 113), and bubonic plague (see Chap. 114).

Infections of the hand   These are almost invariably secondary to trauma. Because of the rapidity with which infection can spread through the complex fascial spaces of the hand, wrist, and forearm, and produce irreparable functional damage, *any deep infection in this area should receive expert surgical attention immediately.* The availability of antibiotics has in no way lessened the importance of such care.

The ordinary *paronychia,* or ''run-around,'' is a superficial infection of the epithelium lateral to a nail, usually a result of tearing a hangnail and most frequently caused by staphylococcus. Hot applications will lead to subsidence of paronychial cellulitis, but often a superficial blister of pus appears. A small incision or simply separation of the nail fold from the nail will promote adequate drainage. If the infection burrows beneath the nail to form a painful *subungual abscess,* incision and drainage with partial or complete removal of the nail are necessary. Recurrence is common, especially in nail biters, and this seemingly trivial infection can cause painful disability. Chronic paronychial inflammation, usually from *Candida,* occurs in those with prolonged or frequent immersion of hands in water.

What appears to be a small furuncle of the webs of the fingers sometimes produces a *collar-button abscess,* consisting of a superficial and deep compartment connected by a narrow tract. Evacuation of the shallow pocket without emptying the deeper abscess can lead to puzzling persistence of infection. Sometimes a foreign-body granuloma forms in the skin of the digital webs. This is most common in barbers, in whom a hair is the core of the foreign-body granuloma, the ''barber's interdigital pilonidal sinus.''

Infection of the distal phalanx of a finger, usually acquired by pinprick, thorn prick, etc., may lead to the formation of a *felon,* or *whitlow.* This is a suppurative infection in the tightly enclosed fibrous compartments of the finger pulp, the ''anterior closed space,'' which can compromise the distal blood supply by compression of the digital arteries, with consequent necrosis of bone and the development of osteomyelitis. The manifestations are swelling, extreme pain, and tenderness of the palmar surface of the fingertip. The treatment is immediate incision directly over the lesion, sometimes by the use of a trephine, and cutting all the fibrous septa that radiate from the periosteum to the subcutaneous fascia.

Suppurative tenosynovitis, usually a complication of a puncture wound, is an even more serious infection of the hand; early diagnosis and treatment are mandatory to prevent permanent disability from destruction of the tendon or its sheath. The three cardinal manifestations of tenosynovitis are (1) exquisite tenderness limited to the course of the sheath, (2) flexion of the fingers, and (3) excruciating pain, most marked at the base of the digit, on extension of the involved finger. *Immediate incision* of the sheath is indicated, not only to prevent damage to the tendon itself but also to avoid proximal extension of the process into the major fascial spaces of the hand or forearm. Vigorous antibiotic treatment should accompany surgery. The definitive treatment of any serious infection of the hand is a matter for a skilled surgeon, but the early recognition of the need for surgery often falls to other physicians.

Human bites lead to very important hand infections which, if neglected, almost invariably produce a highly destructive, necrotizing lesion contaminated by a mixture of aerobic and anaerobic organisms. A deliberately inflicted bite on the hand or elsewhere is usually recognized as dangerously contaminated, but wounds on the knuckles produced by striking an opponent's teeth with the fists may not be recognized as potentially dangerous. In general, bite wounds should be cleaned thoroughly and not sutured. Patients should be given prophylaxis for tetanus and antibiotics, preferably both a penicillinase-resistant penicillin and ampicillin.

Chronic cutaneous ulcers

A partial list of the causes of chronic ulcers of the skin includes circulatory disturbances, such as varicose veins and obliterative arterial disease, extensive injury from frostbite or burns, trophic changes accompanying many neurologic disorders, bedsores or decubiti, systemic diseases such as sickle cell disease, neoplasms, and various infections. No matter what the underlying disease, secondary infection is very likely to occur and to interfere with healing, complicate grafting or other restorative procedures, or produce extension of the process.

The management of secondary bacterial infection in skin ulcers associated with obliterative arterial disease, a common problem in diabetics, is especially important, because infection frequently precipitates spreading gangrene and makes amputation necessary.

The microflora of chronic cutaneous ulcers almost invariably comprises bacteria of many species, including staphylococci, aerobic and anaerobic streptococci, coliform bacilli, and members of the *Proteus* and *Pseudomonas* groups. Depending on the patient's environment and on systemically or locally administered antimicrobial drugs, the predominating bacterial species show great variation in serial cultures. Resistant strains or species commonly replace sensitive organisms during the course of chemotherapy.

Treatment of chronic dermal ulcers should be directed toward the underlying disorder but should also include *local debridement* and *chemotherapy.* Debridement by surgical excision is often needed, but the local application of wet-to-dry dressings or other forms of "medical debridement" frequently suffice. Intensive systemic administration of antibiotics should be carried out only in conjunction with definitive surgical procedures or when infection can be controlled in no other way. The prevention of infection by "prophylactic" administration of antimicrobial drugs is futile because it results in the development of a flora resistant to the drugs being used. The *local application of antibacterial agents* is sometimes highly effective, and in managing chronic mixed infections of this type several potent but toxic antibiotics have great value. An ointment or solution containing neomycin, bacitracin, and polymyxin exerts a bactericidal effect against a wide variety of organisms and will sometimes temporarily sterilize a chronic lesion. Other useful topical medications are furacin and 3% acetic acid, which is especially helpful in *Pseudomonas* infections.

Diphtheritic ulcer of the skin is discussed in Chap. 96.

INFECTIONS OF THE HEAD AND NECK

Pustules of the nose and upper lip may be particularly dangerous, because they can extend intracranially through the angular vein to the cavernous sinus. These lesions should be treated conservatively, manipulation or incision should be avoided if possible, and systemic antibiotics should be used if local swelling or redness appears.

Suppurative parotitis

Typically, suppurative parotitis occurs in elderly and chronically ill patients who have a dry mouth from decreased oral intake, following general anesthesia and surgery, or from medications with atropine-like effects, such as antihistamines or phenothiazines. In most patients, it is an ascending infection due to *S. aureus,* which normally colonizes the opening to Stensen's duct. Occasionally, there is an obstructing calculus. Its onset, usually sudden, is heralded by unilateral local pain and swelling, frequently with fever and chills. Frank pus can often be expressed from the duct and may show gram-positive cocci in clumps. The gland itself is firm and tender, often with redness and edema of the overlying skin.

Treatment consists of systemic antimicrobial therapy with a penicillinase-resistant penicillin or some other agent effective against *S. aureus,* unless another organism is isolated, combined with improved hydration and oral hygiene. Massage of the gland and sialagogues, like lemon drops, help promote drainage through the duct. Surgery is usually unnecessary and should be reserved for patients failing to improve after 4 to 5 days of medical management.

Miscellaneous infections

Antibiotics have reduced the incidence of many formerly common suppurative complications of streptococcal pharyngitis. However, as a result of streptococcal sore throat, *Bacteroides* infections of the pharynx, or introduction of infection by trauma to the floor of the mouth or the pharyngeal wall, abscesses of the deep cervical structures still occur. *Suppurative cervical adenitis,* once an all-too-common sequel to streptococcal pharyngitis in children, is now rare. *Peritonsillar abscess (quinsy)* is manifested by fever, sore throat, cervical lymphadenopathy, unilateral pain radiating to the ear on swallowing, and enlargement of the tonsil with redness and swelling of the adjacent soft palate. Treatment with penicillin and irrigations of warm saline solution sometimes suffices, but if digital palpation reveals fluctuation, needle aspiration or surgical drainage is indicated. Some recommend tonsillectomy immediately or several weeks later; others reserve it for patients with recurrent tonsillar infections. Organisms associated with peritonsillar abscess include *Streptococcus pyogenes* and oral anaerobic bacteria.

The course of *deep cervical infections* depends upon the anatomic arrangement of fascial planes. Infection in this area is serious and is attended by fever, prostration, and leukocytosis. A tender mass may be palpated, but *surgical evacuation of such an infection should not be delayed because of failure to detect fluctuation,* which is usually absent because of the dense fascial layers.

Infection of the *sublingual* and submandibular spaces, so-called Ludwig's angina, causes brawny induration of the submaxillary region, edema of the floor of the mouth, and elevation of the tongue. It usually originates from apical abscesses of the second and third mandibular molars. There are severe pain, dysphagia, and, within hours, dyspnea from respiratory obstruction. The causative organisms of this and other neck abscesses are mainly streptococci and oral anaerobes. Mortality was formerly about 50 percent. *Treatment* consists of large doses of penicillin and careful observation. With significant airway obstruction, tracheostomy is necessary. Since the infection is largely a cellulitis, incision and drainage are reserved for evidence of fluctuation.

The retropharyngeal space lies between the muscles anterior to the cervical vertebrae and the pharyngeal mucosa. *Retropharyngeal abscess,* formerly common in children, is manifested by dysphagia, progressive stridor, pain, and fever. The bulging mass is easily seen and can completely occlude the airway within hours. Incision and drainage are mandatory; spontaneous rupture may lead to death by aspiration. Esophageal perforation during endoscopy may result in abscess as a late complication. Tuberculous abscess, secondary to spinal disease, occasionally appears in the retropharyngeal space; it is painless, and relief of obstruction follows surgical incision.

Submastoid abscess, or suppuration in the submastoid space, known as *Bezold's abscess,* is usually secondary to otitis and produces nuchal rigidity, which may lead to a mistaken diagnosis of otogenous meningitis. Infection can extend down the carotid sheath to the mediastinum. A suppurative thrombophlebitis of the jugular vein usually accompanies this infection, and the vessel is easily felt as a tender cord. Bacteremia and systemic spread of infection are common, and the involved venous segment may require excision. Spontaneous rupture of the carotid artery with rapid death from exsanguination is a rare complication.

Therapy of head and neck abscesses includes surgical incision and drainage, open treatment of infected wounds, and systemic antibiotics, which should include agents active against anaerobic organisms, particularly if there is foul-smelling pus. Penicillin is usually the drug of choice.

INTRAABDOMINAL ABSCESSES

A useful classification divides intraabdominal abscesses, according to location, into three major types, each with several subdivisions: (1) intraperitoneal, (2) retroperitoneal, and (3) visceral (Table 87-1). The clinical features vary but usually include fever, with no characteristic pattern (ranging from mild to hectic), leukocytosis, and an elevated erythrocyte sedimentation rate. Common, but not universal, are pain near the abscess, anorexia, weight loss, nausea, vomiting, and altered bowel habits. A tender mass may be palpable. Plain abdominal films may suggest an abscess by showing a soft tissue density, displacement of adjacent organs, or extraintestinal gas from a perforated viscus or produced by the infecting organisms within the abscess cavity.

The most useful noninvasive diagnostic techniques are ultrasound and CT examinations. Ultrasound has a diagnostic accuracy of about 80 to 90 percent and is most effective in detecting abscesses in the right upper quadrant, retroperitoneum, and pelvis. It shows a sonolucent mass that may have internal echoes when debris and septations are present. The appearance is usually indistinguishable from other fluid-filled masses, but clinical features and, if necessary, needle aspiration of the mass should discriminate among the possible causes. Since gas blocks the beam, ultrasound is not useful when large amounts of gas are present, as occurs in the stomach and splenic flexure, which makes the left upper quadrant a difficult area to examine. Similarly, loops of gas-filled bowel impair evaluation of the midabdomen. Since the transducer must have good skin contact, wounds, fistulas, stomata, and surgical dressings may make ultrasound examination impossible.

These factors do not affect CT scans, which are therefore especially useful in the postoperative patient, when there are no focal signs or symptoms, or when the area of concern is the left upper quadrant, pancreas, or midabdomen. CT scans are positive in over 90 percent of patients with abscesses, characteristically demonstrating fluid collections with well-defined walls that enhance following intravenous administration of contrast material. Unless gas lies within the mass, however, these findings do not distinguish abscesses from simple cysts, old hematomas, or mucinous metastases. Clinical features or needle aspiration should determine the correct diagnosis.

Effective treatment must include antimicrobial agents active against the responsible organisms. While the infecting flora varies, it commonly comprises bowel organisms, a complex mixture of aerobic and anaerobic bacteria, including *Bacteroides fragilis*. An appropriate therapeutic choice is a combination of an aminoglycoside, such as gentamicin, and an antianaerobic agent such as clindamycin, chloramphenicol, or metronidazole. Cefoxitin alone is an effective alternative, but an aminoglycoside should be added if the infection is hospital-acquired or the patient has received previous antimicrobial therapy.

Antimicrobial therapy alone is often sufficient for some abscesses—appendiceal, renal, and some hepatic—but cure usually also requires drainage of pus, either by surgery or percutaneous catheters, inserted with ultrasonic or CT guidance. Criteria for percutaneous drainage include (1) pus thin enough to be evacuated through the catheter; (2) no more than two abscess cavities or loculations; (3) the absence of a continuing source of contamination, such as a perforated viscus; (4) a drainage route that does not traverse bowel, uncontaminated organs, or sterile pleural or peritoneal spaces. The third criterion excludes appendiceal and diverticular abscesses and the fourth excludes most pelvic and interloop abscesses. Overall, percutaneous drainage is appropriate for less than 50 percent of intraabdominal abscesses. It is also not very successful in pancreatic abscesses. When used appropriately, however, its success rate is about 85 percent, with the catheters typically remaining in place for about 10 to 20 days.

INTRAPERITONEAL ABSCESS　These infections usually arise from a generalized peritonitis caused by perforated abdominal viscera, penetrating trauma, or postoperative infections. Some derive from localized peritonitis when infection extends from a contiguous site. With generalized peritonitis, the effects of gravity, intraabdominal pressure, and respiratory movements favor localization to the subphrenic spaces, the pelvis, and paracolic gutters lateral to the ascending and descending colon.

Subphrenic abscess　These abscesses occur in the subphrenic space, arbitrarily defined as lying between the diaphragm and the transverse colon and possessing four subdivisions. The *suprahepatic* and *subhepatic* spaces are located on the right side; on the left there is a single *subphrenic* space plus the *lesser sac,* a space posterior to the stomach and anterior to the pancreas. About 55 percent of subphrenic abscesses are right-sided, 25 percent left-sided, and 20 percent multiple. Over 90 percent are complications of abdominal surgery, especially on the biliary tract, stomach, and duodenum. The contamination causing infection can occur during surgery or afterward, especially from anastomotic leaks. Symptoms typically begin 3 to 6 weeks after surgery, but occasionally develop only months later. Fever, nearly universal, is often mild, rather than dramatic. Abdominal pain is usual, but localized tenderness less common, and a palpable mass rare. By causing diaphragmatic irritation, inflammation that spreads to the pleural cavity, and abdominal distention, subphrenic abscesses often produce thoracic symptoms such as cough, dyspnea, and chest pain. Shoulder discomfort, referred pain from an irritated diaphragm, and hiccups sometimes occur. On chest examination there may be dullness to percussion, diminished breath sounds, basilar crackles, and rarely, a pleural friction rub. Chest roentgenograms, usually abnormal, may demonstrate ipsilateral atelectasis, pleural effusion, elevated hemidiaphragm, and basilar pneumonia.

Midabdominal abscess　These abscesses include those in the right and left lower quadrants and between loops of bowel (interloop abscesses). *Right lower quadrant abscesses* usually arise as a complication of acute appendicitis, but occasionally from colonic diverticulitis, Crohn's disease, or upper alimentary tract perforations that drain down into the right paracolic gutter. Most commonly, fever, right lower quadrant pain, and a palpable mass occur following symptoms suggesting acute appendicitis. Occasionally, the abscess causes partial or complete small bowel obstruction. Appendiceal abscesses are usually treatable with antibiotics alone. *Left lower quadrant abscesses* complicate left colonic perforations, usually from diverticulitis, carcinoma, or Crohn's disease, and cause fever, left lower quadrant pain, and a palpable mass. *Interloop abscesses* are collections of pus between the folded surfaces of the small and large intestines and their mesenteries, generally arising from anastomotic disruptions, bowel perforations, or Crohn's disease. The clinical features, which are often very subtle, include mild fever, with or without vague abdominal discomfort. Abdominal tenderness, mechanical bowel obstruction, or a palpable mass occasionally occurs. Plain abdominal roentgenograms may show bowel wall edema,

TABLE 87-1　Intraabdominal abscesses

Intraperitoneal:
　Subphrenic:
　　Right suprahepatic
　　Right subhepatic
　　Left subphrenic
　　Lesser sac
　Midabdominal:
　　Right lower quadrant
　　Left lower quadrant
　　Interloop
　Pelvic
Retroperitoneal:
　Anterior retroperitoneal
　Perinephric
Visceral:
　Hepatic
　Splenic
　Pancreatic
　Renal

separation of bowel loops, localized ileus, and air-fluid levels on upright films.

Pelvic abscess These are complications of acute appendicitis, colonic diverticulitis, or acute salpingitis. The major symptoms are fever and lower abdominal discomfort. Those adjacent to the colon may cause diarrhea; those next to the bladder may cause urinary frequency and urgency. On abdominal examination tenderness is common, but peritoneal signs, guarding, or a palpable mass are unusual. Rectal or vaginal examination may reveal a mass anterior to the rectum or in the cul-de-sac. Pelvic abscesses usually require surgical drainage, but those arising from acute salpingitis typically resolve with antibiotic therapy alone.

RETROPERITONEAL ABSCESS The retroperitoneum is the space between the posterior peritoneum and the transversalis fascia lining the posterior portion of the abdominal cavity. The *anterior retroperitoneal* space, lying between the posterior peritoneum and the anterior renal fascia, contains the extraperitoneal portion of the alimentary tract: the ascending and descending colon, the duodenal loop, and the pancreas. Abscesses in this space usually develop from pancreatitis or perforations in these extraperitoneal parts of the intestines. The major clinical features are fever, abdominal or flank pain and tenderness, and a palpable mass.

The *perinephric* space, situated between the anterior and posterior layers of the renal (Gerota's) fascia on each side of the body, contains the kidney, adrenal, and ureter. Perinephric abscesses almost always occur from rupture of a renal parenchymal abscess through the renal capsule. Such an abscess may be staphylococcal following hematogenous dissemination from another site, usually the skin, but more commonly it arises from pyelonephritis, especially associated with renal calculus disease. The causative organisms, therefore, are usually *Escherichia coli, Proteus* sp., and *Klebsiella-Enterobacter.* The major symptoms are fever, chills, and unilateral flank pain. Dysuria is frequent, and most patients have unilateral flank or abdominal tenderness, often with a palpable mass. Leukocytosis, pyuria, and a positive urine culture are typical. Blood cultures are positive in 20 to 40 percent of patients. Perinephric abscess usually differs clinically from uncomplicated acute pyelonephritis by the longer duration of symptoms before hospitalization (usually more then 5 days) and the failure of patients to become afebrile within 5 days after receiving antimicrobial therapy. Chest roentgenograms often show ipsilateral pneumonia, atelectasis, pleural effusion, or elevated hemidiaphragm. Findings on excretory urogram include a nonvisualizing or poorly visualizing kidney, distorted calyces, anterior renal displacement, and unilateral fixation of the kidney, best demonstrated by fluoroscopy or inspiration-expiration films. Ultrasound and CT are very effective in detecting these abscesses. Treatment includes appropriate systemic antibiotics, surgical drainage, and relief of any urinary obstruction; occasionally, nephrectomy is necessary.

VISCERAL ABSCESS   Hepatic abscess These abscesses are usually amebic (see Chap. 153) or bacterial (pyogenic). Bacterial liver abscesses usually develop by one of five mechanisms: (1) portal vein bacteremia arising from an infected intraabdominal site, such as appendicitis, diverticulitis, or perforated bowel; (2) systemic bacteremia originating from a distant site, in which bacteria reach the liver via the hepatic artery; (3) ascending cholangitis in a biliary tract completely or partially obstructed by stone, malignancy, or stricture; (4) direct extension from a contiguous focus of infection outside the biliary tract, such as a subphrenic abscess; or (5) trauma, either penetrating, with direct introduction of organisms into the liver, or blunt, causing a hematoma that becomes secondarily infected. In most cases the cause is apparent, but in some the pathogenesis of the abscess is unexplained (''cryptogenic''). Most abscesses are single; multiple abscesses are typically microscopic and are associated with systemic bacteremia or complete biliary tract obstruction. In these cases, the onset is acute, and the clinical features of the predisposing disease predominate.

Most other cases of hepatic abscess have a subacute onset, and an illness lasting several weeks is the rule. Fever is nearly always present and is accompanied by such nonspecific symptoms as chills, nausea, vomiting, anorexia, weight loss, and weakness. Right upper quadrant abdominal pain or tenderness is present in about one-half of patients, as is hepatomegaly. Some complain of right pleuritic chest pain. Jaundice is usually evident only when there is biliary tract obstruction.

Laboratory findings in most patients include one or more of the following: anemia, leukocytosis, increased erythrocyte sedimentation rate, increased alkaline phosphatase, decreased serum albumin, and usually mildly increased serum bilirubin. The chest roentgenogram is abnormal in about one-half of patients and shows right-sided basilar atelectasis, pneumonia, pleural effusion, or an elevated hemidiaphragm.

The radionuclide liver scan demonstrates filling defects for most abscesses greater than 2 cm in diameter. Ultrasound scans are usually positive and can distinguish fluid-filled from solid masses, helping to discriminate between infectious and neoplastic lesions. Computerized tomography is the most accurate method of demonstrating multiple abscesses.

The bacteriology of liver abscesses depends upon the cause. With systemic bacteremia staphylococci or streptococci are common. Abscesses originating from an intraabdominal infection, however, usually contain aerobic gram-negative rods, especially *E. coli* and *Klebsiella-Enterobacter;* anaerobic bacteria, especially anaerobic gram-positive cocci, *Fusobacterium nucleatum,* and *B. fragilis;* or a mixture of aerobes and anaerobes. Blood cultures are positive in about half of patients but may not grow all the organisms present in the abscess.

Treatment consists of surgical or percutaneous catheter drainage supplemented by appropriate antibiotic therapy. When the bacteriology is unknown, chloramphenicol or a combination of clindamycin and an aminoglycoside should be effective. Antibiotics are usually continued for several weeks following drainage. In uncomplicated pyogenic abscesses, antimicrobial therapy alone may be curative following diagnostic needle aspiration to determine the pathogens.

In correctly diagnosed and treated patients the mortality rate is about 20 to 40 percent, and is higher in those with multiple rather than single abscesses.

In patients with a clinical picture suggesting a liver abscess and an abnormal hepatic radionuclide, CT, or ultrasound scan, it is important to distinguish between a bacterial and an amebic abscess, since the latter rarely requires drainage. Features suggesting an amebic etiology are age under 50; single rather than multiple abscesses; a history of diarrhea, especially if bloody; the presence of *Entamoeba histolytica* in the stool; and the absence of a condition predisposing to bacterial liver abscess. The most helpful differential point is that nearly all patients with amebic liver abscesses have a positive serology for *E. histolytica.*

Splenic abscess Most splenic abscesses are multiple, small, and clinically silent lesions found incidentally at autopsy and occurring as a terminal manifestation of uncontrolled infection elsewhere. Clinically important splenic abscesses are generally solitary and arise from (1) systemic bacteremia originating in another site, such as endocarditis or salmonellosis; (2) infection, probably by the hematogenous route, of a spleen damaged by bland infarction (as occurs in hemoglobinopathies, especially sickle cell trait or sickle cell disease), trauma, penetrating or blunt (with superinfection of a subcapsular hematoma), or other diseases (malaria, hydatid cysts); or (3) extension from a contiguous focus of infection, such as a subphrenic abscess. The most common organisms are staphylococci, streptococci, anaerobes, and aerobic gram-negative rods, including *Salmonella.*

The onset is typically subacute, and the major features are fever and left-sided pain which is often pleuritic and located in the upper abdomen, lower chest, or flank. The pain may radiate to the left shoulder. Left upper quadrant abdominal tenderness and splenomegaly are common, but an audible splenic friction rub is rare. Leukocytosis is usually present.

Radiographic findings may include (1) a left upper quadrant soft tissue abdominal mass, (2) extraintestinal gas from gas-forming organisms in the abscess, (3) displacement of other organs, including the colon, kidney, and stomach, (4) elevation of the left hemidiaphragm, and (5) left pleural effusion. A liver-spleen radionuclide scan is valuable in detecting abscesses larger than 2 or 3 cm, and an ultrasound scan may be positive for macroscopic splenic abscesses, but CT scan is the most reliable diagnostic test.

Treatment consists of appropriate systemic antibiotics and splenectomy. Splenic abscesses should be considered a possible, although rare, cause of continued bacteremia in acute endocarditis despite appropriate chemotherapy, and splenectomy may be necessary to achieve final eradication of the infection.

Pancreatic abscess   These abscesses usually occur in a site of pancreatic necrosis following acute pancreatitis. Typically, the patient improves after the attack of pancreatitis, but about 10 to 21 days later fever, abdominal pain and tenderness, nausea, vomiting, and sometimes persistent ileus occur. Less commonly, the abscess develops shortly after the attack begins. In those cases, persistent fever, leukocytosis, and abdominal findings beyond 7 to 10 days should suggest an abscess. A mass is palpable in about half of the cases. The serum amylase is irregularly elevated, but leukocytosis is usually present. The serum alkaline phosphatase may be increased and the albumin decreased.

Chest roentgenograms often show a left pleural effusion, basilar atelectasis or pneumonia, or a raised hemidiaphragm. Ultrasound is very useful in revealing fluid-filled pancreatic masses but may be unable to distinguish infected from uninfected fluid. CT is the most accurate test for abscesses and may show pancreatic gas, peripancreatic fluid collections, or masses, but only pancreatic gas is diagnostic of infection.

Treatment is surgical drainage and appropriate antibiotic therapy. Since the usual organisms are coliforms, staphylococci, streptococci, and anaerobes in varying combinations, chloramphenicol or clindamycin and an aminoglycoside are reasonable choices until culture results return. Even with surgical drainage the mortality rate is about 40 percent, and recurrent abscesses requiring reoperation are common.

Renal abscess   Single or multiple abscesses of the renal *cortex* may be the result of metastatic implantation of staphylococci from another focus. There is no relationship to previous renal disease; the infection occurs in younger individuals, is usually unilateral, and occurs on the right side oftener than on the left. Many patients give a history of recent skin infection such as furuncle. Although acute pyelonephritis is a diffuse disease with foci of cellular infiltrates in the interstitium of the renal medulla, these inflammatory foci may coalesce to form single or multiple distinct abscess cavities in the medulla. This situation probably ensues more frequently than is generally appreciated.

The onset of renal abscess is abrupt, with chills and fever, followed by costovertebral pain and tenderness. If the abscess is cortical, the urine contains *no white blood cells;* medullary abscesses are usually accompanied by pyuria. The stained urinary sediment may show myriads of gram-positive cocci in cortical abscesses and gram-negative organisms in medullary abscesses. Transient gross or microscopic hematuria may occur at the onset. The white blood cell count is usually elevated and may exceed 30,000 cells per cubic millimeter. Physical signs are usually localized to the region of the kidney, but abdominal spasm may lead to confusion with appendicitis, cholecystitis, or pancreatitis. Early in the disease, ureteral calculus or acute hydronephrosis may be considered as possible diagnoses. Sudden onset of *fever, leukocytosis, and renal pain in the absence of pyuria* should suggest the diagnosis of a renal cortical abscess, especially in a patient with infection elsewhere. Obstruction of the ureter by pus or cellular debris may also yield a urine sediment sparse in white blood cells and bacteria. Excretory urograms typically reveal an intrarenal mass, and ultrasound and CT scans usually demonstrate the abscess as a fluid-filled defect. *Treatment* consists of appropriate antibiotics, adequate fluids, and relief of pain. An abscess may suddenly discharge into the renal pelvis, with relief of pain and the passage of cloudy urine containing enormous numbers of leukocytes and bacteria. Recovery is ordinarily prompt, and chronic sequelae are rare. Failure to achieve prompt defervescence following treatment suggests an incorrect diagnosis or the necessity of drainage, either by needle aspiration or by surgery.

MISCELLANEOUS ABSCESSES

RETROFASCIAL ABSCESS   The retrofascial space, lying between the transversalis and psoas fascias, contains the psoas and quadratus lumborum muscles. Abscesses in this area usually derive from infections in the vertebrae, ilium, and sacroiliac joints. Less frequently, they represent extensions from abscesses in the anterior retroperitoneal space. Sometimes no adjacent source of infection is apparent; these "primary" infections are usually staphylococcal and almost surely have a hematogenous origin. The symptoms of retrofascial abscesses are abdominal pain in the iliac or inguinal region and, particularly with psoas muscle involvement, hip pain and posterior thigh pain and paresthesias. Careful palpation of the lower abdomen or groin often reveals a mass, and rectal or vaginal examination may disclose fullness and tenderness. Pain on hip motion is common, the hip is flexed, and extension or internal rotation of the hip is very painful. Plain abdominal films may demonstrate a mass or loss of the psoas shadow; excretory urograms may show displacement of the kidney or ureter and scoliosis with concavity on the side of infection. Ultrasound usually reveals a soft tissue mass, but CT scans typically provide more precise information, including evaluation of the adjacent bones. Treatment consists of drainage and appropriate antimicrobial therapy.

PROSTATIC ABSCESS   These abscesses, typically occurring in middle age, are complications of acute prostatitis, cystitis, urethritis, or epididymitis. Most patients are *afebrile* and have urinary frequency, retention, or dysuria. Less common features are hematuria, perineal pain, and a purulent urethral discharge. Some patients have persistent or recurrent urinary infections despite apparently adequate antimicrobial therapy. Rectal examination may reveal prostatic tenderness or fluctuance, but sometimes there is only prostatic enlargement or even no abnormality at all. Pyuria and positive urine cultures are usual, but not invariably so. Many of these abscesses are unexpected discoveries at prostatic surgery or endoscopy performed for apparent benign prostatic hypertrophy. Treatment is appropriate antibiotics and surgical drainage by transurethral or perineal incision. The usual pathogens are aerobic gram-negative rods and, less frequently, *Staphylococcus aureus.*

RECTAL ABSCESS   Most of these infections are superficial and involve the perirectal region, and many are associated with fistulas. Infection in the apocrine glands (hidradenitis) or folliculitis in the perianal region, extension of cryptitis or obstructions in the "anal glands" which open into the crypts of Morgagni, and contamination of submucosal hematomas, sclerosed hemorrhoids, or anal fissures may lead to abscess formation. In most patients, the cause of infection is not apparent. These are usually painful, easily palpable, often visible on inspection. Treatment is incision and drainage. Antibiotics are rarely necessary unless there is extensive perineal cellulitis.

Difficulties in diagnosis are likely to arise with infections higher in the rectum. Most are in the ischiorectal area, but those above the pelvic diaphragm, the so-called supralevator abscess, are particularly elusive. Patients with this type of infection often have fever, malaise, and leukocytosis for several days or even weeks before any symptoms referable to the rectum develop. There is vague pelvic discomfort, relieved by defecation, and constipation punctuated by short episodes of diarrhea is common. In males, the inflammation often involves the base of the bladder, and urinary urgency or retention may occur, falsely centering attention on the urinary tract as the source of fever and malaise. Eventually, the abscess produces severe pain, chills, and fever; palpation and instrumentation will reveal the swelling in the rectal ampulla. Such an abscess may surround the rectum and produce narrowing that is differentiated from neoplasm by the fact that the mucosa remains intact. A useful sign of deep rectal abscess is severe pain with pressure in the region between the anus and the coccyx. The supralevator space is continuous with the ischiorectal space, with both the gluteal and obturator regions, and with the retroperitoneal space. In neglected cases, the abscess may drain through the skin of the perineum, the groin, or the buttock or may extend as high as the perirenal areas. Rectal abscesses are not uncommon in patients with preexisting anorectal disease, diabetes, alcoholism, and neurologic disease; infections in this area are also peculiarly frequent in patients with acute leukemia, especially when neutropenia is present. Because the clinical picture may be that of "fever of unknown origin" for a long period, it is important that thorough digital and endoscopic examination of the rectum be carried out in patients with unexplained fever. Patients with diabetic ketoacidosis should receive a careful rectal examination because a rectal abscess may be the infection responsible for precipitating the ketoacidosis.

A rectal abscess may be a forerunner of both ulcerative colitis and regional enteritis, and may occur months and even years before other overt manifestations of these diseases. For this reason, proctosigmoidoscopy, colonoscopy, barium enema, and, often, upper gastrointestinal roentgenograms are indicated in nonhealing or recurrent rectal lesions.

Treatment of high rectal abscesses consists of incision and drainage, analgesics, and antibiotics directed at *E. coli, Klebsiella-Enterobacter, Bacteroides,* and a variety of streptococci, which constitute the polymicrobial flora of these lesions.

REFERENCES

BARTLETT JG et al: Anaerobic infections of the head and neck. Otolaryngol Clin North Am 9:655, 1976

CHOW AW et al: Orofacial odontogenic infections. Ann Intern Med 88:392, 1978

FEDERLE MP et al: Computed tomography of pancreatic abscesses. Am J Roentgenol 136:879, 1981

GOLIGHER JC: *Surgery of the Anus, Rectum, and Colon,* 5th ed. New York, Macmillan, 1984

HAU T et al: Pathophysiology, diagnosis, and treatment of abdominal abscesses. Curr Probl Surg 21:8, 1984

HOVERMAN IV et al: Intrarenal abscess: Report of 14 cases. Arch Intern Med 140:914, 1980

LINSCHEID RL et al: Common and uncommon infections of the hand. Orthop Clin North Am 6:1063, 1975

MCDONALD MI et al: Single and multiple pyogenic liver abscesses. Medicine 63:291, 1984

SART MG, ZUIDEMA GD: Splenic abscess—Presentation, diagnosis and treatment. Surgery 92:480, 1982

SIMONS GW et al: Retroperitoneal and retrofascial abscesses. J Bone Joint Surg 65-A:1041, 1983

88 CHEMOTHERAPY OF INFECTIONS

HAROLD C. NEU

INTRODUCTION There are many reasons for the plethora of new antimicrobial agents. The most important are changes in the host, the appearance of new pathogens, and the resistance of new and old pathogens to previously available antimicrobial agents. Changes in the host include prolonged survival of critically ill patients due to use of cancer chemotherapy, transplantation, and prosthetic devices. The problem of resistance has been particularly severe due to the worldwide dissemination of plasmids which have the ability to convey

resistance to multiple antimicrobial agents simultaneously. Most antimicrobial agents in general use act by inhibiting the growth of the infecting microorganism rather than by enhancing host defense mechanisms. In the past, physicians often were faced with few choices of antimicrobial agents with which to treat an infection. Today that situation has been changed due to the discovery of new agents or the molecular modification of existing compounds. In addition to considerations of efficacy and toxicity which have the major impact on the selection of antimicrobial agents, cost is becoming increasingly important. This chapter deals with some general observations on antimicrobial therapy, and a description of most antibacterial agents. Recommendations for therapy of infections are made in the chapters dealing with individual diseases. Tables 88-1 and 88-2 summarize important information concerning the drugs discussed in this chapter.

FACTORS INFLUENCING SELECTION OF ANTIMICROBIAL AGENTS AND OUTCOME OF THERAPY Several factors bear directly on the selection of an antimicrobial agent. First there must be a knowledge of the infecting microorganism. In many situations this is not the case at the time therapy is initiated. As a consequence, antimicrobial therapy is started empirically in many situations. Even empiric selection of an antimicrobial agent, however, should be based on a knowledge of the likely pathogens and their antimicrobial susceptibility. For example, it is recognized that the most common cause of urinary tract infections is gram-negative bacilli and that *Escherichia coli* is the most common source of outpatient urinary tract infections. Hence, in most instances, therapy should be selected to inhibit this microorganism. However, therapy for treatment of a nosocomial urinary tract infection might be quite different. Bacteria other than *E. coli* are likely to produce this infection, particularly in the presence of an indwelling urethral catheter, and nosocomial pathogens are likely to be resistant to many antibiotics.

The host plays an extremely important role in the selection of an antimicrobial agent, as the antibiotics chosen to treat a febrile, neutropenic patient will be different than those for a healthy individual with a minor infection. Host factors also have an important impact on the route of administration of antimicrobial agents and upon the duration of therapy.

IDENTIFICATION OF THE INFECTING ORGANISMS There are a number of techniques for the rapid identification of the infecting microorganism. A Gram stain is a simple, inexpensive, and rapid method to identify many bacteria and fungi. This technique should be applied to all available body fluids such as urine, wound exudate, synovial fluid, pleural fluid, peritoneal fluid, and cerebrospinal fluid (CSF). Gram stains of sputum, if properly collected, are useful in the diagnosis of the causative organisms involved in bacterial pneumonia. *Campylobacter* can be identified in stains of stool. Another technique which may be useful is antigen detection in body fluids such as CSF (see Chap. 83).

In situations in which material for diagnosis is not available, knowledge of the most likely pathogens will be beneficial in directing the selection of an antimicrobial agent. For example, following an animal bite an organism such as *Pasteurella multocida* should be suspected. Cellulitis in the foot of a diabetic patient should suggest hemolytic streptococci of groups A, B, or G and *Staphylococcus aureus,* as well as mixed infections including anaerobes.

ANTIMICROBIAL SUSCEPTIBILITY OF INFECTING MICROORGANISMS There are a number of different methods for determining the susceptibility of bacteria to antimicrobial agents. Susceptibility of viruses and fungi is in a less well developed state, and very few laboratories have the ability to determine susceptibility of parasites to antiparasitic drugs.

A commonly used method to determine bacterial susceptibility to antibiotics is a disk diffusion method, which is simple, inexpensive, and provides data within 24 h. It is only semiquantitative and is not useful for many slow-growing or fastidious organisms, and has not been adequately standardized for anaerobic bacteria. With the disk

TABLE 88-1 Serum and body fluid levels after oral administration of various antibiotics

Drug	Unit dose* (oral)	Average peak level, μg/mL Blood†	Urine‡	Bile§	CSF¶	Half-life, h C_{cl} >80mL	C_{cl} <10mL	Dose adjustment renal failure
Amoxicillin	0.5 g	10	1000	10	NA	1	6	Minor
Ampicillin	0.25 g	1.5	50	5	NA	1	6	Minor
Cephalexin	0.25 g	8	500	3	NA	1	8–20	Major
Cephradine	0.25 g	8	500	85	NA	1	8	Major
Chloramphenicol	1 g	13	100	3	6	2	5	Minor
Ciprofloxacin	0.75 g	4	100–300	8	1	3	5–10	Major
Clindamycin	0.15 g	2	30	20	NA	2	6–10	Minor
Cloxacillin	0.5 g	8	200	—	NA	1	4	Minor
Dicloxacillin	0.5 g	15	200	—	NA	1	2–4	Minor
Doxycycline	100 mg	2.5	100	15	NA	15–20	15–20	No
Erythromycin estolate	0.25 g	1.4	200	800	NA	1.5–2	4–6	No
Indanyl carbenicillin	1 g	15	600	NA	NA	1–2	15	Major
Metronidazole	0.25 g	5	50	5	2	8	8	Minor
Minocycline	100 mg	2.5	100	15	NA	15	15–25	Minor
Norfloxacin	500 mg	4	200	—	NA	3–8	8–20	Major
Oxfloxacin	400 mg	6	100–500	5–15	NA	5–10	10–20	Major
Penicillin V	0.25 g	2	300	4	NA	1	2	No
Rifampin	8 mg/kg	10	50	100	0.5	1.5–5	1.5–5	No
Sulfadiazine	1.0 g	25	100	25	15	10	12–25	Major
Tetracycline	0.25 g	2.2	100	15	NA	6–8	30–50	Major
TMP/SMX	0.16 g TMP + 0.8 g SMX	1 + 30	10 + 100	3 + 30	0.5 + 15	10	25	Major

* *Doses listed are the lowest doses that would normally be employed for adults or children over 32 kg with normal renal function in the treatment of systemic infections.*
† *Blood levels are at 1–2 h after IM or at the end of 20–30 min IV infusion. In most instances considerably higher serum levels are attainable with higher dosages. For example, 2g of ampicillin would yield a peak blood level of 70–90 μg/mL, 2g of cefoxitin a peak blood level of 120–140 μg/mL.*
‡ *Drug concentrations may be significantly lower if the patient is producing a very dilute urine or if creatinine clearance is below 10 mL/min. Concentration based on mean levels for the first 4 h after drug is administered.*
§ *Assuming normal liver function.*
¶ *Meningeal inflammation; in meningitis higher doses than those listed would normally be employed resulting in higher CSF levels.*
NOTE: *NA = not appropriate therapy for meningitis; — = data not available; TMP/SMX = trimethoprim/sulfamethoxazole*

TABLE 88-2 Serum and body fluid levels after parenteral administration of various antibiotics

Drug	Unit dose[a] (parenteral)	Average peak level, μg/mL Blood[b]	Urine[c]	Bile[d]	CSF[e]	Half-life, h C_{cl} >80mL	C_{cl} <10mL	Dose adjustment renal failure	Effect of hemodialysis
Amdinocillin	1 g	70	>1000	5–30	1–5[f]	1	4	Minor	Yes
Amikacin	5 mg/kg IM or IV	25	200	5	5	2	30	Major	Yes
Ampicillin	1.0 g IV	35	500	10	3[f]	1	4	Minor	Yes
Azlocillin	3.0 g IV	190	>2000	100	—	1	4	Minor	Yes
Aztreonam	1 g	160	>1000	5–10	1–5[f]	1.5–2	6	Minor	Yes
Carbenicillin	4.0 g IV	250	>1000	50	20	1	15	Major	Yes
Cefamandole	1.0 g IV	70	1000	100	NA	0.7	8	Minor	Yes
Cefazolin	1.0 g IV	110	>1000	50	NA	2	25	Major	Yes
Ceftizoxime	1.0 g IV	80	>1000	30	1–10[f]	1.6	19	Major	Yes
Cefoperazone	2.0 g IV	250	>1000	>100	NA	2	2–4	No	No
Cefotaxime	1.0 g IV	80	>1000	15	10[f]	1	4	Minor	Yes
Cefoxitin	1.0 g IV	70	1000	100	1–5	0.8	10	Major	Yes
Cefuroxime	0.75 g	40	>1000	10–30	1–30[f]	1.5	20	Major	Yes
Ceftazidime	1 g	80	>1000	5–10	1–30[f]	1.8	1.5	Major	Yes
Ceftriaxone	1 g	150	>1000	200	1–30[f]	8	16	No	Yes
Cephalothin	1.0 g IV	70	500	10	0.7	0.5	8	Minor	Yes
Cephapirin	1.0 g IV	70	500	10	NA	0.5	8	Minor	Yes
Chloramphenicol	1.0 g IV	15	100	3	10	1–2	3–5	No	Yes
Ciprofloxacin	200 mg	4	100	5	?	3–4	5–10	Yes	Yes
Clindamycin	0.6 g IV	15	30	40	NA	2	6–10	No	No
Erythromycin	1 g IV	10	20	80	1	1–2	4–6	No	No
Gentamicin	1.5 mg/kg IM or IV	6	50	2	1	1–2	4–6	Major	Yes
Imipenem	0.5 g IV	30	100	10	1	1	6	Major	Yes
Kanamycin	5.0 mg/kg IM or IV	20	200	5	NA	2	35	Major	Yes
Methicillin	2.0 g IV	80	1000	30	5	0.5	4	Minor	Yes
Metronidazole	8.0 mg/kg IM	25	100	20	10	8	8	Minor	Yes
Mezlocillin	3.0 g IV	190	>2000	100	—	1	4	Minor	Yes
Moxalactam	1.0 g IV	100	>1000	60	1–30[f]	2	19	Major	Yes
Nafcillin	1.0 g IV	70	150	40	2	1	2	Minor	No
Oxacillin	1.0 g IV	70	500	2.5	1	1	2	Minor	No
Penicillin G	3 million units IV	115	300	15	6	1	4	Minor	Yes
Piperacillin	3.0 g IV	190	>2000	50	20	1	4	Minor	Yes
Ticarcillin	3.0 g IV	190	>2000	50	20	1	15	Major	Yes
Tobramycin	1.5 mg/kg IM or IV	6	50	2	1	2	35	Major	Yes
Vancomycin	0.5 g IV	30	100	3	3	6	120	Major	No

[a] *Doses listed are the lowest doses that would normally be employed for adults or children over 32 kg with normal renal function in the treatment of systemic infections.*
[b] *Blood levels are at 1–2 h after IM or at the end of 20–30 min IV infusion. In most instances considerably higher serum levels are attainable with higher dosages. For example, 2g of ampicillin would yield a peak blood level of 70–90 μg/mL, 2g of cefoxitin a peak blood level of 120–140 μg/mL.*
[c] *Drug concentrations may be significantly lower if the patient is producing a very dilute urine or if creatinine clearance is below 10 mL/min. Concentration based on mean levels for the first 4 h after drug is administered.*
[d] *Assuming no biliary obstruction.*
[e] *Meningeal inflammation; in meningitis higher doses than those listed would normally be employed resulting in higher CSF levels.*
[f] *Value at higher dose*
NOTE: *NA = not appropriate therapy for meningitis; — = data not available*

method, results are usually given as susceptible, resistant, and intermediate. A *susceptible* zone of inhibition correlates with serum and urine levels that are readily achievable with standard doses of the agent being tested. A *resistant* reading indicates that the zone of inhibition, using regression analysis, is less than that which would correspond to a concentration that could be achieved in blood or serum under normal circumstances. *Intermediate* susceptibility means that the organism falls into a category that is necessary because of the splay in data correlating zone size with minimum inhibitory concentrations (MIC). This is particularly true if the infecting organism is found in a urine specimen in which the concentration of antimicrobial agent would be much higher than in blood or tissues.

Quantitative data on the susceptibility of particular organisms can be determined by micro or macro broth-dilution techniques. These methods detect the lowest concentration of antimicrobial agent that prevents visible growth after an 18- to 24-h incubation period. This is referred to as the minimal inhibitory concentration (MIC). To understand MIC values it is essential to understand the pharmacokinetics of an antimicrobial agent. In general, an organism is considered susceptible when the MIC is no more than one-fourth of the readily obtainable peak serum level of the antimicrobial agent. Using the microdilution method, it is also possible to determine the minimal bactericidal concentration (MBC) or minimal lethal concentration (MLC). This is defined as the concentration of drug that reduces the original inoculum by 99.9 percent as judged by subculture on antibiotic-free medium. MBC determinations are necessary in only a few situations that will be discussed below.

The large number of antimicrobial agents has made it difficult for laboratories to test routinely all antimicrobial agents against an isolate. Many laboratories will use a particular compound as the class representative for a group of compounds. For example, among the first-generation cephalosporins, cephalothin is the representative drug that, either in a disk or in a broth-dilution system, is used to represent susceptibility to cephapirin, cefazolin, cephalexin, and cephradine.

Occasionally, susceptibility tests provide incorrect information. For example, methicillin-resistant *S. aureus* appear susceptible to cephalosporin antibiotics, but are not. Most susceptibility tests do not readily identify a resistant subpopulation.

Some microorganisms have remained susceptible to the same drugs since antibiotics were discovered, and in them development of resistance is exceedingly rare. Examples are group A streptococci which are susceptible to penicillins and cephalosporins. Hence most laboratories do not report susceptibilities of group A streptococci. However, group A streptococci may be resistant to erythromycin, and if the use of this drug is contemplated, susceptibility tests may be necessary. Most strains of *Streptococcus pneumoniae* remain susceptible to penicillin. However, some isolates have intermediate susceptibility; that is, the MICs are between 0.1 and 1.0 mL. Although such penicillin concentrations can readily be achieved in the blood and lung, it may be difficult to achieve cerebrospinal fluid concentrations that are tenfold this level. For this reason, pneumococci isolated from the CSF should be tested for penicillin susceptibility, particularly in patients who do not respond promptly to the drug.

CLINICAL PHARMACOLOGY Knowledge of the clinical pharmacology of antimicrobial agents has become increasingly important in selecting therapeutic programs that are both effective and safe. Antimicrobial agents can be administered by the oral, intramuscular, intravenous, intraperitoneal, or topical routes. After absorption they dissolve in the plasma and are variably bound to plasma proteins. From the plasma they are distributed to various extracellular tissues and fluids in which they may be free or bound. As an antibiotic is distributed into extravascular compartments, there is an initial fall in plasma concentration. Peak concentrations of antimicrobial agents after intravenous infusion occur at the end of the infusion. In contrast, after intramuscular injection, and after oral ingestion, there is an initial slow distribution phase, that is, a combination of absorption and simultaneous excretion or metabolism. Peak serum levels following oral ingestion of antimicrobial agents usually occur at 1 to 2 h.

Continued decrease in serum levels of antimicrobial agents is related to renal and biliary excretion and to the hepatic metabolism of some drugs. The amount of drug that reaches the extravascular tissues in which the infection is present depends not only on the concentration gradient from serum to tissue, but also on protein binding in serum and in tissues and the diffusibility of the agent. The diffusibility of antimicrobial agents is a function of their molecular size, dissociation constant, and lipid solubility.

There are several pharmacokinetic indexes that are useful in adjusting dosage of antimicrobial agents. The half-life of a drug is the time required for the plasma concentration to fall by one-half as it is being eliminated from the body. Half-life refers to the drug elimination phase after the absorption of the drug has been completed and the drug has been distributed throughout its entire volume of distribution. The assumption is that the fall in plasma concentration parallels the fall in the total amount of drug in the body. However, direct extrapolation of the frequency of dosing from half-life considerations is not completely appropriate. The MIC of the infecting organism, site of infection, and host defense mechanisms must be considered in determining dose frequency.

Another pharmacokinetic index that may be useful for guiding therapy is the volume of distribution (V_d). This is the volume in which the total amount of drug in the body would have to be uniformly distributed in order to give the observed plasma concentration. Simplistically it is calculated by the formula $V_d = A/C_p$, where A is amount of drug administered and C_p is plasma concentration. The volume of distribution does not correspond to an actual anatomic or physiologic space. It is useful for determining initial or loading doses and in calculating subsequent or maintenance doses to achieve safe, therapeutic plasma concentrations. When a drug dose is given repetitively at regular intervals, the peak concentration and the minimal concentration eventually reach a constant state if there is no change in the rate of drug elimination. With most antimicrobial agents it is not necessary to use an initial loading dose. However, when agents such as the aminoglycosides are used to treat serious infections such as suspected bacteremia or pneumonia, a loading dose which will provide an initial plasma and tissue concentration well above the MIC of the suspected infecting microorganisms is usual.

The half-life distribution data of many antibiotics have been determined in healthy young males. Prolongation of a drug half-life often may result from renal or hepatic dysfunction. Half-life may also be influenced by age and may be shortened in certain disease states. Other drugs administered concomitantly can also either prolong or shorten a drug's half-life.

HOST FACTORS THAT AFFECT ANTIMICROBIAL CHEMOTHERAPY A number of different host factors have a significant influence on the efficacy and toxicity of antimicrobial agents.

Allergic history It is critical to obtain a history of previous adverse reactions to antimicrobial agents since similar reactions may occur to drugs within the same class.

Age Certain antimicrobial agents should not be given to individuals in some age groups. For example, sulfonamides should not be administered to pregnant females or to newborns because sulfonamides bind to serum albumin, displacing bilirubin, which may result in kernicterus. Premature and newborn babies produce an inadequate amount of glucuronyltransferase, the enzyme that inactivates chloramphenicol, and some newborns treated with this drug may develop the "gray baby syndrome," which is characterized by progressive pallor, cyanosis, vasomotor collapse, and death. Tetracyclines should not be administered to pregnant females, newborn infants, or to children below 8 years of age because the drugs bind to developing bone and tooth structure, which may cause brownish discoloration of the teeth.

Renal function The majority of antimicrobial agents are removed from the body by renal excretion. There are several periods in life when renal function has not achieved complete development or has begun to deteriorate. Glomerular and some tubular functions do not develop to adult levels until at least 2 months of age, and drugs administered to premature or newborn infants must be given at different dosage schedules than those used for older children or adults. With advancing age, renal function decreases, and approximately 1 percent of glomerular clearance is lost per year over the age of 30. Antimicrobial agents removed from the body purely by glomerular filtration will accumulate as glomerular filtration declines, resulting in toxicity to other organs or to the kidney itself. Even compounds removed from the body by tubular secretion will accumulate as renal function falls below creatinine clearance of 20 mL/min. Toxic levels of certain penicillins, aminoglycosides, tetracyclines, and quinolones may develop in the presence of markedly reduced renal function. Serum creatinine or blood urea nitrogen may not reflect the true state of renal function in an elderly individual with a small body mass. Hence in calculating the dose of antimicrobial agent it is necessary to consider age, sex, and body weight.

Hepatic function   Some antimicrobial agents are metabolized and removed from the body primarily by hepatic mechanisms. These include some of the macrolides, rifamycins, imidazoles, chloramphenicol, and linconoid drugs. Reductions in dose may be necessary to avoid toxic concentrations of these agents. Chloramphenicol is likely to accumulate in patients with impaired hepatic function, while clindamycin and tetracyclines accumulate in patients with severe liver disease. The half-lives of both rifampin and isoniazid are prolonged in patients with extensive hepatic disease. Some drugs which are excreted by biliary mechanisms are excreted by the kidney in the presence of marked elevations of bilirubin. Conversely, some compounds that are normally excreted by the kidney are excreted in the bile in the presence of renal failure. In the presence of combined biliary and hepatic disease, toxic levels may be reached. Examples would be a cephalosporin such as cefoperazone, which is primarily excreted by biliary mechanisms, or carbenicillin and ticarcillin, which are primarily renally excreted; in the presence of combined hepatic and renal failure these drugs accumulate in tissues to a greater extent.

Pregnancy   Antimicrobial agents cross the placenta to varying degrees. Most penicillins, cephalosporins, and erythromycins are not teratogenic and are safe in pregnant women. Tetracyclines should not be used in pregnancy not only because of their effect upon fetal dentition but also because they have a propensity to cause fatty necrosis of the liver, pancreatitis, and possible renal damage in pregnant females. If streptomycin is used to treat tuberculosis in pregnancy, it can cause abnormalities of vestibular function and hearing in the child.

Genetic factors   A number of different antimicrobial agents will produce hemolysis in patients with glucose 6-phosphate dehydrogenase deficiency. These include sulfonamides, nitrofurantoin, furazoline, chloramphenicol, pyrimethamine, and various sulfones.

The rate at which isoniazid is inactivated by acetylation in the liver is genetically determined. In the United States and North European populations, 50 to 60 percent of individuals are slow inactivators of this drug. Polyneuritis is seen more frequently as a complication of isoniazid therapy in individuals who are slow acetylators.

Site of infection.   The site of infection is one of the most important factors in determining the choice of an antimicrobial agent and the dose and route by which the antimicrobial agent is administered. For antimicrobial therapy to be effective, adequate concentrations of a drug must be delivered to the site of the infection. In many situations, if the local concentration of an antimicrobial equals or exceeds the minimum inhibitory concentration of the infecting microorganism, cure will result. This statement is true only for those areas of the body in which there are adequate host defenses such as polymorphonuclear cells, complement, and antibody. In those areas of the body in which these factors are inadequate or absent, such as in the spinal fluid or on the heart valves, concentrations at least fourfold and preferably five- to tenfold above the MIC, or even MBC, are needed

to achieve a cure. In some situations, even though concentrations above the MICs of the infecting organisms may not be achieved, there will be a significant effect on the microorganisms that will aid the host's defenses against the infection. Subinhibitory concentrations of antimicrobial agents alter the adherence properties of microorganisms; treated bacteria then do not accumulate to a number adequate to achieve further invasion. Subinhibitory concentrations also alter surface structures, reducing opsonic requirements and enhancing phagocytosis. Subinhibitory concentrations of antibiotics, by binding to the surface of microorganisms, enhance the intracellular killing of bacteria ingested by phagocytic cells. These factors may explain the unusual circumstances in which antimicrobial agents in seemingly inadequate doses result in clinical cure. Nonetheless, the major goal of therapy should be to achieve concentrations above the MIC in all tissues.

In general, antimicrobial agents are widely distributed and achieve adequate concentrations in many infected sites. These include the pleural, pericardial, and infected joint fluids, and infections in muscles or skin structures associated with cutaneous infection. Important exceptions to this statement include vegetations on the heart valves in endocarditis. Although the heart valve is exposed to the circulation, the bacteria often are trapped deep within the fibrin vegetation. The organisms are growing less rapidly making them less susceptible to many antibiotics and there is inadequate phagocytic function in the focal infection on the heart valve. Because of these factors, therapy of bacterial endocarditis requires agents that are bactericidal, that are administered for long periods of time, and that achieve such high concentration in the blood so that diffusion of the antibiotic into the vegetation is facilitated (see Chap. 188).

Meningitis is another disease in which the concentration of antimicrobial agent in the infected space is critical. Many antimicrobial agents cross the blood-brain barrier poorly and do not produce adequate cerebrospinal fluid levels. For example, aminoglycoside antibiotics do not produce effective cerebrospinal fluid levels when given parenterally. Lipid-soluble agents can cross the spinal fluid barrier easily, accounting for the utility of chloramphenicol. This agent has proved highly effective in the therapy of meningitis due to *Streptococcus pneumoniae, Haemophilus influenzae,* and *Neisseria meningitidis* because of the achievable bacteriostatic and bactericidal concentrations it produces in the cerebrospinal fluid. Chloramphenicol is not useful in treating meningitis due to *E. coli* or *Klebsiella penumoniae,* even if the organisms are susceptible in vitro, because the drug is not bactericidal for these organisms, and concentrations eightfold above the MIC cannot be achieved within the cerebrospinal fluid. Fortunately a number of new bactericidal antimicrobials such as cefotaxime, ceftizoxime, ceftriaxone, ceftazidime, and moxalactam all enter the cerebrospinal fluid in concentrations adequate to treat both the common causes of meningitis and the less frequently encountered gram-negative organisms. However, experience with any of these agents is relatively sparse, and it is not clear whether reasonable drug levels are achieved in brain abscesses.

Another infectious site that may be particularly refractory to treatment involves bones in areas of devitalized tissue, as occurs in diabetics and other patients with inadequate blood supply due to vascular insufficiency. Here the penetration of the antimicrobial agents to the site of the infection may be only borderline or inadequate. For this reason antimicrobial agents must be administered in high concentrations for prolonged periods of time to yield adequate concentration within bone. Even with extended periods of therapy, many cases of chronic osteomyelitis are never completely cured since some of the bacteria are in a resting state and do not come into contact with the antimicrobial agent.

Abscesses present a particular problem, and in many instances the surgeon's knife is the only mechanism by which an abscess can be cured. Certain exceptions to this dictum exist, however. For example, lung abscess can be treated without surgical intervention in most situations since the abscess can drain via the bronchi, and the antimicrobial agents kill bacteria in the surrounding inflammatory tissue. However, lung abscesses 8 to 10 cm in diameter frequently do not respond to antimicrobial therapy alone since there is inadequate diffusion of the antimicrobial agent into the cavity and organisms persist. Hence the size of the abscess may influence the ultimate outcome. Other abscesses which respond to antimicrobial therapy alone are those of the ovary, brain, and liver. Ultrasound, computer tomography scanning (CT), and magnetic resonance imaging (MRI) have demonstrated detectable decreases in abscess size. The question that remains unanswered is whether these "imaged abscesses" are equivalent to the abscesses that were in the past diagnosed clinically, and that were remanded to surgery. In general, abscesses in other parts of the abdomen require external drainage, since antimicrobial agents by themselves fail to sterilize the majority of them. Exceptions to this rule have been noted with some anaerobic microorganisms; compounds such as metronidazole diffuse into the abscess and destroy the anaerobic organisms.

Local factors within an abscess can have an important impact upon the activity of certain antimicrobial agents. For example, in the case of a mixed aerobic and anaerobic abscess, the anaerobic organisms may produce β-lactamases that will destroy the β-lactam compound which is being used to inhibit the aerobic gram-negative bacilli. Aminoglycoside antibiotics are significantly less active in an anaerobic abscess since they require an aerobic environment for antimicrobial activity. This class of drugs is also dependent on oxidative phosphorylation to achieve transport across the cell membrane.

Other local circumstances may have a marked impact upon the effectiveness of antimicrobial agents. Aminoglycoside antibiotics are less effective at an acid pH than they are at pH 7.4. Gentamicin or tobramycin might inhibit a *Klebsiella* at 0.1 μg/mL in a Mueller-Hinton broth of pH 7.4, but this condition is not present in the infected lung, where the pH in infected areas is 6.4 to 6.5. Aminoglycosides are ten- to thirtyfold less active at this pH than they are at pH 7.4. Cellular debris from decaying white cells will complex with aminoglycosides and reduce their activity. In a hyperosmolar environment some β-lactam antimicrobial agents may be less effective because they will not produce death of the microorganism but merely change its cell shape. Agents such as methenamine, nitrofurantoin, and chlortetracycline are more active at an acid pH; the activities of erythromycin, clindamycin, and aminoglycosides are greater in an alkaline milieu.

Foreign bodies have an extremely important effect on the response to antimicrobial agents. For example, infections of prosthetic heart valves or joint implants usually are not cured by antimicrobial agents even though the organisms infecting the foreign body are highly susceptible to bactericidal β-lactam or aminoglycoside antibiotics. The reasons for this are complex, but probably involve the development of a glycocalyx which adheres to the foreign material and provides a cover for the microorganisms. A number of studies have revealed that organisms such as *Staphylococcus epidermidis* send projections into small defects in the polypropylene material which is used in catheters and other foreign devices. The methylacrylate used in artificial joints provides a large number of interstices in which microorganisms hide, covered by fibrinous material, and are not exposed to antimicrobial agents. Indwelling urethral catheters are another example of a foreign body which makes it virtually impossible to eradicate infecting microorganisms. Even silicone catheters have a deposit of gelatinous material on the inner aspect of the catheter. Microorganisms persist within this material, and unless the catheter is removed, the organisms will not be eradicated. Other examples of foreign material are suture materials. Even though wire sutures are much less likely to cause infection than braided fiber sutures, sternal wound infections following cardiac surgery usually cannot be completely eradicated as long as the wire sutures remain in place and the infection remains undrained. Calculi, whether in the urinary or biliary tracts, provide a haven for microorganisms. The microorganisms are incorporated into the calculus and will periodically be released as the calculi undergo remodeling. Thorough knowledge of the mechanical, metabolic, and physiologic factors involved in infection is essential

in planning therapy to bring about optimal results in infections located in different parts of the body, and different strategies must be applied to infections within the urinary, pulmonary, and central nervous systems.

ANTIMICROBIAL COMBINATIONS   Although the majority of infections can be treated with a single antimicrobial agent, there are definite situations in which the combination of antimicrobial agents is necessary. Combination antimicrobial therapy is used much more frequently than necessary. It provides a false sense of security, suggesting that all possible causes have been dealt with and a successful outcome will be more likely. In certain situations inappropriate use of combinations of antimicrobial agents may actually have deleterious results.

The combination of two or three antimicrobial agents may result in one of three different effects. Drugs are said to be *additive* when the activity of the drugs in combination equals the sum of their separate, independent activities. *Synergistic* activity implies that the activity of two or three antimicrobials is greater than the sum of their independent activities. Drugs are considered *antagonistic* when the activity of the combination is less than the sum of the independent effects.

A number of reasons have been advanced for the use of antimicrobial combinations. Preventing the emergence of resistant organisms is one of the most common indications for combination therapy, but this is true only for tuberculosis. The mycobacteria causing tuberculosis consist of a population of organisms of varying susceptibility to antituberculous drugs. In any focus of infection containing a large number of bacilli, particularly in a tuberculous lung cavity, there will be a small percentage of organisms that are intrinsically resistant to the antituberculous agent. In this setting the organisms reach such large numbers that they include a number of drug-resistant mutants which occur naturally and spontaneously at a rate of 1 in 10^{-6} organisms. For this reason, two or three drugs are utilized in the treatment of this disease. The concept of the use of multiple drugs in the treatment of tuberculosis is particularly important when isoniazid-resistant organisms are found in specific patient populations such as those from the far east or the Caribbean.

Another example of preventing the emergence of resistance has been to use rifampin to treat infections other than those caused by mycobacteria. Use of rifampin as a single agent to treat staphylococcal infections rapidly results in the emergence of strains resistant to the antibiotic. However, the combination of a β-lactam antibiotic with rifampin reduces the chance for the emergence of such resistant strains. It has been suggested that the combination of an aminoglycoside with aminothiazolyl cephalosporins (see below) or monobactams (aztreonam) will prevent the emergence of resistance in *Enterobacter* or *Citrobacter* species. Although it is possible to demonstrate this phenomenon in the test tube, there are no clinical studies demonstrating that such a combination is less likely to result in the emergence of resistant organisms. This is particularly true when resistance to gram-negative bacteria is mediated by R factors. These plasmids often code for several enzymes leading to the development of resistance to multiple drugs simultaneously.

A second major reason for combination therapy is to treat polymicrobial infections. Intraperitoneal and pelvic infections are usually due to an aerobic and anaerobic flora. Although some antimicrobial agents inhibit both aerobic and anaerobic species, it may not always be feasible to use these drugs clinically. Combination therapy might include an agent effective against the anaerobic organism and an agent effective against the aerobic gram-negative rod. Another example of this might be the use of an agent such as clindamycin and a third-generation cephalosporin to treat hospital-acquired aspiration pneumonia caused by an anaerobic oral flora, which would be inhibited by the clindamycin and organisms acquired in the hospital such as *Klebsiella* which would be inhibited by the cephalosporin. Brain abscesses are frequently caused by *Bacteroides* and anaerobic or microaerophilic streptococci. Metronidazole penetrates extremely well into the abscess and has excellent activity against the *Bacteroides* species. However, it is not active against streptococcal species. Penicillin will penetrate the brain adequately to kill the streptococcal species but could not be used singly since it would be destroyed in the brain abscess by the β-lactamases frequently elaborated by the *Bacteroides* strains.

A theoretical reason for the use of drug combinations is to lower concentrations of compounds that have toxic potential. Although this is an interesting concept, there is little clinical evidence to substantiate the use of two drugs at lower concentrations than that at which they would normally be utilized. For example, using amphotericin B and 5-fluorocytosine to treat cryptococcal meningitis with lower doses of amphotericin has not decreased nephrotoxicity from the amphotericin. This illustrates that in practice it is difficult to reduce toxicity while continuing therapy with toxic drugs.

One of the major indications for combined antimicrobial therapy is to provide a broad spectrum of coverage for the patient who is neutropenic and has significantly compromised host defenses. It has been the practice to use a broad-spectrum antipseudomonas penicillin combined with an aminoglycoside as an initial therapy for the febrile neutropenic patient. Studies of new highly active β-lactam compounds such as ceftazidime which inhibit the major pathogens causing bacteremia in these patients open this concept to question. Nevertheless, combination therapy will probably continue to be used in such patients since gram-negative organisms continue to be a major cause of infection in neutropenic patients, and it is necessary to provide antimicrobial activity against aerobic gram-negative species, staphylococci, and *Corynebacterium* species until the true pathogen becomes apparent.

Although synergism can be demonstrated in the laboratory with many antimicrobial combinations, in only a few clinical settings has combination therapy proved more effective than single agents. The most widely accepted combination therapy is penicillin G or ampicillin with an aminoglycoside, streptomycin or gentamicin, for the treatment of enterococcal endocarditis. There is clear clinical evidence that this combination is more effective treatment for this infection than a single drug. The penicillin enhances the uptake of the aminoglycosides by the enterococci, which are killed as a result. Similar synergism can be demonstrated between semisynthetic penicillinase-resistant penicillins, such as nafcillin or oxacillin, and gentamicin against *S. aureus*. However, clinical data do not show that this combination has advantages over use of a single drug. Combinations of antipseudomonas penicillins such as carbenicillin, ticarcillin, azlocillin, or piperacillin with gentamicin, tobramycin, or amikacin are synergistic against many strains of *Pseudomonas aeruginosa*. Both animal experiments and clinical trials have demonstrated the superiority of these combinations in neutropenic hosts. However, there are no convincing data that treatment of neutropenic patients infected with organisms such as *E. coli*, *Klebsiella*, *Serratia*, or other members of the *Enterobacteriaceae* with two agents will result in a more favorable outcome, despite the demonstration of synergism in vitro.

There are several other examples of synergism in vitro that have clinical application. One of these is the combination of trimethoprim with sulfamethoxazole. These two agents act by inhibiting two critical points in the folic acid cycle which is part of the production pathway of DNA nucleotides. In vitro and animal experiments readily demonstrate that on a milligram basis, the two drugs are more effective than either drug singly. However, the major situation in which such a combination is absolutely necessary is in treatment of *Pneumocystis carinii* infection. In urinary tract infections trimethoprim alone is as effective as the combination of the two agents. Trimethoprim has not been compared to the combination in the treatment of serious infections outside the urinary tract.

Combination of a β-lactam drug with a β-lactamase inhibitor is another example of the synergistic combination of two drugs. Augmentin is a combination of amoxicillin and clavulanate and timentin a combination of ticarcillin and clavulanate. This combination of a β-lactamase-susceptible β-lactam with a β-lactamase inhibitor enhances the antibacterial spectrum of the drug that would normally be destroyed by β-lactamase. Augmentin inhibits *Haemophilus*, *Branhamella*, *E. coli*, *Salmonella*, and *S. aureus* strains which are resistant to amoxicillin. In the case of timentin, the ticarcillin is effective against *Bacteroides* species, *Klebsiella*, and staphylococci which would normally destroy the agent. Sulbactam is another β-lactamase inhibitor which has been combined with ampicillin or cefoperazone to prevent their destruction by β-lactamases.

Another form of synergy has been to use compounds which interfere with cell wall synthesis but inhibit different enzymes. The amdino, amdinocillin, which binds to a specific penicillin-binding protein different from the penicillin-binding proteins to which other penicillins and cephalosporins bind, when combined with various β-lactams has been shown to be synergistic both in vitro and in animal models. Clinical studies have also demonstrated that such synergy is possible. However, it is not clear that this approach is more effective than utilizing a single drug which has activity superior to the two-combination compounds. Combinations of fosfomycin, a cell wall inhibitor, and β-lactams are synergistic in experimental situations, but clinical studies showing the superiority of such combinations are not available.

Disadvantages of antimicrobial combinations   There are a number of examples of antagonism of antimicrobial agents. The most impressive historical example was the demonstration that penicillin alone was more effective than a combination of penicillin and chlortetracycline for the treatment of pneumococcal meningitis. There have been other reports that the treatment of meningitis with a combination of ampicillin and chloramphenicol has been associated with a higher mortality than the use of ampicillin alone. One of the most common uses of combination therapy has been in the treatment of meningitis due to β-lactamase-producing *Haemophilus influenzae* or to relatively resistant *Streptococcus pneumoniae*. The effectiveness of cephalosporins such as cefuroxime, cefotaxime, and ceftriaxone for treatment of childhood meningitis make it unnecessary to use combination therapy, although experience with the newer drugs is limited, and to date they are more costly.

There are in vitro examples of antagonism between β-lactams. For example, cefoxitin will induce β-lactamase production in *P. aeruginosa* and *Enterobacter cloacae*. The combination of cefoxitin and an antipseudomonas penicillin can be shown to be antagonistic in vitro. Certain animal experiments have also shown that this combination is antagonistic. Nonetheless, many patients have been treated with the combination of cefoxitin and azlocillin or other antipseudomonas penicillins without evidence of reduced efficacy. In general, however, it seems wise to avoid combined use of a β-lactam that is a good β-lactamase inducer and other β-lactams that might be inactivated by high levels of the enzyme. This is particularly likely to occur during treatment of *Pseudomonas*, *Enterobacter*, *Serratia*, and *Citrobacter* infections.

Combination therapy may on occasion result in superinfection with other organisms, particularly fungi, since the combination obliterates the normal protective flora of the oropharynx and the intestine. This problem can be avoided by discontinuing unnecessary empiric combination therapy once the diagnosis has been established.

Another adverse effect of combination therapy may be increased drug reactions or other metabolic side effects. Examples of such toxicity are the combination of cephalothin and gentamicin, resulting in increased nephrotoxicity. There is a slightly increased risk of hepatic toxicity in patients receiving both isoniazid and rifampin, but this is outweighed by the more rapid eradication of tubercle bacilli and the more rapid clinical improvement seen with this combination.

ROUTE OF ADMINISTRATION OF ANTIMICROBIAL AGENTS   Having determined the most appropriate agent to treat a given infection, the most appropriate route of administration should be determined. The choice usually lies between the oral and the parenteral route. Oral administration of antimicrobial agents has generally been for infections that are mild and are treated on an outpatient basis. As hospital costs have risen, reevaluation of this concept is necessary. Some serious infections initially may be treated parenterally; then therapy can be completed with an oral antibiotic. Examples would be osteomyelitis, or severe skin infections that have begun to respond to parenteral therapy. When drugs are administered by the oral route, it is important to be certain that the patient takes the drug in a manner that will result in the best serum and tissue levels. The absorption of many antimicrobial agents is markedly decreased by food. Some compounds such as the tetracyclines form a soluble chelate with magnesium, calcium, aluminum, or iron. In a number of infections it may be possible to administer an oral antimicrobial agent twice a day rather than four times a day. This may be an important way to achieve patient compliance.

The parenteral route is generally used for agents that are not absorbed from the gastrointestinal tract, and for serious infections in which a high concentration of the antimicrobial agent is needed immediately. Examples are suspected bacteremia, meningitis, and gram-negative pneumonia. Intravenous administration of most drugs is preferred since it provides for high serum concentration. There are no definitive data that show whether bolus, 3- to 5-min injection, infusion over 15 to 30 min, or continuous administration of a drug by the intravenous route is more effective in curing bacterial infection. Serum concentrations adequate to treat many infections will be achieved after intramuscular administration. With some agents with extremely long half-lives it may be possible to complete therapy of serious infections by administration of the drug intramuscularly once a day. It is rarely necessary to instill antimicrobial agents into infected cavities. There are certain exceptions to this, however. Peritonitis in patients receiving peritoneal dialysis may respond better to administration of the antimicrobial agent in the dialysis solution. Certain forms of meningitis will require intraventricular or intrathecal therapy. This is true for meningitis due to *Coccidioides immitis* and some gram-negative species.

MONITORING PATIENT RESPONSE TO ANTIMICROBIAL THERAPY With some antimicrobial agents it is essential that serum levels of the agent be monitored. This is true for the aminoglycoside antibiotics, for which peak levels should be obtained to determine that effective concentrations are being achieved and trough levels should be measured to determine that the drugs are not accumulating and producing nephrotoxicity or ototoxicity. In most situations, it is not necessary to monitor serum concentrations of β-lactam antibiotics. The one exception to this would be in renal failure, where the drugs may accumulate to toxic levels.

Serum bactericidal titers, defined as the dilution of serum which will kill the infecting pathogen in vitro, have been used extensively to monitor therapy of bacterial endocarditis. There has been wide variation in the performance of serum bactericidal titers, but guidelines for their use have been developed. If a standardized inoculum of organisms is used and standard media and techniques employed, the tests are useful in certain clinical situations. For example, a peak serum bactericidal titer >1:64 correlates with a 98 percent bacteriologic cure of endocarditis. However, clinical cure cannot be predicted since damage to the valve as a result of the endocarditis may result in valvular insufficiency requiring surgery. Most experts feel that a peak serum bactericidal titer greater than 1:8 correlates with a successful outcome in osteomyelitis, bacteremia, septic arthritis, and empyema.

SPECIFIC ANTIMICROBIAL AGENTS

PENICILLINS Penicillins can be conveniently divided into several classes on the basis of antibacterial activity. There are overlaps among the groups, but differences within the groups usually are pharmacologic rather than clinical.

Natural penicillins Penicillin G and penicillin V are the two natural penicillins. Penicillin G is available as an orally, intramuscularly, and intravenously administered compound. Penicillin G is combined with procaine as a 1:1 molar salt which extends the half-life of the drug, and it is combined with benzathine to produce a long-acting repository form of penicillin. Penicillin V is available only for oral use. The antibacterial activity of penicillin G and penicillin V includes *S. pneumoniae*, beta-hemolytic streptococci, viridans group streptococci, and microaerophilic and anaerobic streptococci. Most *S. aureus* and *S. epidermidis* produce β-lactamases which destroy both penicillin G and V. *Neisseria meningitidis* are susceptible to penicillin G as are many *N. gonorrhoeae*. However, in certain parts of the world penicillinase-producing *N. gonorrhoeae* are a significant problem. Penicillin G has excellent activity against clostridial species and also inhibits many of the oral *Bacteroides* species and *Fusobacterium* species. Penicillin V does not have good activity against species such as *Haemophilus* or *Branhamella*, which may be important pathogens causing sinusitis, otitis, and other upper respiratory infections. Infrequently encountered organisms for which penicillin G remains an excellent drug are *Erysipelothrix, Listeria monocytogenes, Pasteurella multocida, Streptobacillus, Spirillum, Fusospirochetes, Treponema pallidum*, and *Actinomyces israelii*, as well as the *Borrelia* which causes Lyme disease.

Penicillin G is not stable in gastric acid and should not be used as an oral preparation. In contrast, penicillin V is 60 percent absorbed when given orally, and food causes only a minor decrease in absorption. Penicillin V is an effective agent in treatment of streptococcal infections and less serious forms of pneumococcal pneumonia. It should not be used, however, to treat syphilis, gonorrhea, or *Haemophilus* infections. Procaine penicillin G remains a useful drug administered twice daily for the therapy of pneumococcal pneumonia, but oral penicillins probably are equally useful. Although procaine penicillin is still used in the treatment of gonorrhea, oral ampicillin or amoxicillin can be used, combined with tetracycline, since the treatment of urethritis usually is directed against both gonorrhea and *Chlamydia* (see Chap. 90). Penicillin G remains the treatment of choice for viridans group streptococcal endocarditis and for pneumococcal and meningococcal meningitis. Since penicillin G has a short half-life due to rapid tubular secretion, it must be administered on a 4- or 6-hourly basis. Only minor dosage adjustments are necessary until the creatinine clearance falls below 30 mL/min. Even in the presence of renal failure, doses of 4,000,000 to 6,000,000 units per day can be administered safely. Benzathine penicillin, which has a half-life of a week, can be used in the treatment of streptococcal pharyngitis, in the therapy of primary and early syphilis, and in the prevention of recurrences of rheumatic fever when administered once monthly.

Aminopenicillins Aminopenicillins are so-called because of the presence of an amino group on the β-acyl side chain of the penicillin nucleus. A number of different compounds are available. They differ microbiologically to a minor degree. Ampicillin was the first aminopenicillin. Subsequently, amoxicillin was produced, and other agents such as bacampicillin, cyclacillin, epicillin, hetacillin, and pivampicillin have been synthesized. Aminopenicillins retain the in vitro activity of penicillin G. In addition, they inhibit *H. influenzae* and are more active against *Streptococcus faecalis*, and *S. faecium* than is penicillin G. Many *E. coli* are inhibited by aminopenicillins, as are *Proteus mirabilis*. In the United States, many *Salmonella* species and *Shigella* species are inhibited by ampicillin, but in developing countries most strains are resistant to aminopenicillins. Aminopenicillins inhibit most mouth organisms, but do not inhibit *Pseudomonas* species, *Klebsiella, Enterobacter,* and the majority of *Bacteroides fragilis* species. In some parts of the United States, 25 percent of *H. influenzae* contain a β-lactamase, making them resistant to the aminopenicillins.

Amoxicillin and bacampicillin are absorbed approximately twice as well as ampicillin. Bacampicillin is an ester of ampicillin that is converted in the intestinal mucosa and in serum to free ampicillin. Administered parenterally, ampicillin is well distributed to body compartments and achieves therapeutic concentrations in the cerebrospinal, pleural, joint, and peritoneal fluids in the presence of inflammation. Urinary levels are high, even in the presence of markedly reduced renal function. Although ampicillin can be administered intramuscularly, orally administered amoxicillin will produce serum levels comparable to those achieved by intramuscular injection of similar amounts of ampicillin. Ampicillin currently is used in the treatment of outpatient urinary tract infections, upper respiratory infections, otitis media, sinusitis, bacterial exacerbations of bronchitis, and community-acquired pneumonia. It is effective therapy for pneumococcal and meningococcal meningitis, and is used in the therapy of enterococcal endocarditis, always in combination with an aminoglycoside. In the oral form, amoxicillin should replace ampicillin due to its better absorption. The one clinical setting in which amoxicillin is inferior to ampicillin is in the treatment of shigellosis. This is probably related to better absorption of the drug so that less of the active compound is present within the intestine. Amoxicillin and bacampicillin can be administered in most situations three times a day, and still achieve adequate blood, tissue, and urinary levels for treatment of susceptible organisms.

Although allergic reactions of the hypersensitivity type to the aminopenicillins occur with the same frequency as with penicillin G or V, there is an increased risk of skin rash with oral ampicillin. It is estimated that 8 to 10 percent of patients receiving oral ampicillin develop a skin rash. As many as 90 percent of patients with infectious mononucleosis receiving ampicillin develop a maculopapular rash beginning approximately 4 days after therapy is instituted. This rash does not represent true penicillin allergy and does not mean that the patient can never receive a penicillin again.

Penicillinase-resistant penicillins   A number of different penicillinase-resistant penicillins were developed for the treatment of staphylococcal infections. These agents inhibit *S. aureus* and *S. epidermidis*, as well as *S. pyogenes* and *S. pneumoniae*. None of them has activity against *S. faecalis* (enterococcus) or against aerobic or anaerobic gram-negative bacilli. Methicillin was the first antistaphylococcal β-lactamase-stable penicillin.

S. aureus resistant to all β-lactams are referred to as methicillin-resistant. These isolates have an altered penicillin-binding protein as the basis of their resistance, and hence these *S. aureus* and similar strains of *S. epidermidis* are resistant to all penicillins and to cephalosporins as well. In vitro tests of methicillin-resistant staphylococci against cephalosporins tend to be unreliable, and may show these organisms to be sensitive when, in fact, they are resistant. Methicillin-resistant staphylococci may be inhibited by carbapenems, such as imipenem, or by other penem antibiotics. However, the drug of choice for methicillin-resistant staphylococci is vancomycin.

Methicillin can only be used parenterally since it is not acid-stable, and it has a short half-life, necessitating intravenous administration every 4 h. Since interstitial nephritis is a relatively common side effect, methicillin is rarely used today.

Nafcillin has more intrinsic activity than methicillin against both staphylococci and streptococci. It is excreted primarily by the liver, and to a lesser extent by the kidney. Nafcillin should not be used orally since absorption by this route is erratic, whether the drug is taken fasting or with food. The usual dosage of nafcillin is 4 to 12 g per day, depending upon the severity of the infection, and 100 to 200 mg/kg per day for children. Intravenous nafcillin may result in more severe phlebitis than other antistaphylococcal penicillins, and in high doses may result in more suppression of white cells.

The isoxazolyl penicillins consist of oxacillin, which should be used only parenterally due to poor oral absorption, and the oral preparations cloxacillin and dicloxacillin. In many countries, flucloxacillin is also available as an oral drug and in some countries cloxacillin is available for parenteral use. Although dicloxacillin produces higher blood levels than cloxacillin, it is slightly more protein-bound, 96 vs. 94 percent, than cloxacillin. The active antibiotic

levels of the two drugs are actually quite similar. In general, cloxacillin or dicloxacillin are administered in doses of 0.5 or 0.25 g four times a day, respectively.

Although the primary indication for the use of antistaphylococcal penicillins is infection due to penicillinase-producing staphylococci, they are often administered before the etiologic agent is known. Blood levels with the penicillinase-resistant penicillins are adequate to inhibit *S. pneumoniae* and most hemolytic streptococci; therefore, it is not necessary to give both a penicillinase-resistant penicillin and penicillin G simultaneously. However, infections caused by *S. faecalis* (enterococcus) and *Neisseria* do not respond to penicillinase-resistant penicillins, and ampicillin should also be used if these organisms are suspected.

Carboxy penicillins   Carbenicillin was the first penicillin with activity against *P. aeruginosa* and certain indole-positive *Proteus* species. Ticarcillin is also a carboxy penicillin, but it is fourfold more active than carbenicillin. Both of these compounds are destroyed by β-lactamases of gram-positive and some gram-negative organisms, but they are less readily destroyed by the β-lactamases of species such as *Pseudomonas, Enterobacter, Morganella,* and *Proteus-Providencia.* Carbenicillin and ticarcillin are less active than ampicillin against *S. pyogenes, S. pneumoniae,* and *Streptococcus faecalis* (enterococcus). However, they have excellent activity against non-β-lactamase-producing *Haemophilus, N. meningitidis,* and *N. gonorrhoeae.* In general, the antibacterial activity of the carboxy penicillins against *E. coli, Proteus, Salmonella,* and *Shigella* species is similar to ampicillin. They are inactive against *Klebsiella* since they are destroyed by the β-lactamase of these organisms.

Ticarcillin and carbenicillin have activity against oral and intestinal *Bacteroides* species, although higher concentrations are required than are needed to inhibit the Enterobacteriaceae. Both carbenicillin and ticarcillin act synergistically with aminoglycosides to inhibit *P. aeruginosa.* The pharmacokinetics of ticarcillin and carbenicillin are virtually identical. Because of the greater in vitro activity of ticarcillin, it has replaced carbenicillin. The drugs are rarely used intramuscularly since peak serum levels are only 20 μg/mL after a 1-g dose. These levels are inadequate for tissue *Pseudomonas* infections, but provide adequate concentrations in the urine. Both agents are administered in dosages of 200 to 300 mg/kg per day, divided into 4- or 6-hourly doses for 24 h. Both carbenicillin and ticarcillin are excreted by the renal tubules and accumulate in the presence of renal dysfunction. Since each drug contains 4.7 meq of sodium, full doses of 12 to 30 g per day may precipitate congestive heart failure. Hypokalemia may also result since the nonreabsorbable portion of the anion is delivered to the distal tubule where it triggers a hydrogen ion exchange, resulting in potassium loss. Carbenicillin and other penicillins bind to ADP receptor sites on platelets, and prevent normal platelet aggregation. Bleeding times are prolonged and clinical bleeding may occur in the presence of high serum levels. Carbenicillin or ticarcillin cannot be administered in the same solution as aminoglycosides since they complex with the aminoglycoside, rendering the aminoglycoside inactive. This does not normally occur in the body, except in the presence of renal failure, when very high concentrations of the antipseudomonas penicillins result in complexing with aminoglycosides. Ticarcillin has proved useful in the therapy of aspiration pneumonia in the hospital setting, in the therapy of the febrile neutropenic patient, in treatment of intraabdominal infection, and in treatment of gynecologic infections.

In the United States, there is only one oral antipseudomonas penicillin, indanyl carbenicillin. This is an alpha-carboxy ester of carbenicillin that has no intrinsic activity of its own, but is acid-stable and moderately well absorbed in the gastrointestinal tract, where it is hydrolyzed to yield free carbenicillin. Indanyl carbenicillin does not provide adequate serum or tissue levels for systemic infection and is useful only for the treatment of urinary tract infections or prostatitis. In the presence of decreased renal function, urine levels may be lower and may be inadequate to treat *Pseudomonas* urinary tract infections.

Ureido penicillins Ureido penicillins, azlocillin, mezlocillin, piperacillin, and apalcillin,[1] in contrast to the carboxy penicillins, are derivatives of ampicillin in which the presence of a side chain linked to the amino group on the alpha carbon provides increased binding to penicillin-binding proteins and more rapid passage through porin channels of gram-negative bacteria. Ureido penicillins are destroyed by β-lactamases of *S. aureus, E. coli, Klebsiella,* and *Bacteroides.* Azlocillin is 8 to 16 times more active than carbenicillin against *P. aeruginosa* and is less active against indole-positive *Proteus* species. It has the same activity as ampicillin against streptococcal species. It is not absorbed orally and must be given by the intravenous route to provide adequate serum levels to treat *Pseudomonas* infections. Since ureido penicillins show nonlinear pharmacokinetics, these drugs should be used in a larger dose administered at intervals of 6 h, rather than the 4-h interval used for carbenicillin. Azlocillin also does not accumulate in the blood in renal failure to the same degree as do carbenicillin and ticarcillin. Its half-life increases to a maximum of only 4 h, even when renal insufficiency is present, necessitating less adjustment in dosage. Azlocillin has been shown to enter the cerebrospinal fluid in the presence of meningeal inflammation, but levels are only 10 percent of serum levels. The drug is used primarily to treat *Pseudomonas* infections; the usual dose is 12 to 18 g per day.

Mezlocillin is a ureido penicillin that differs from carbenicillin and ticarcillin by being more active against streptococci, particularly enterococci. Its activity against streptococci is similar to ampicillin's. It also inhibits approximately 60 percent of *Klebsiella* in a concentration of 16 μg/mL; virtually no *Klebsiella* are inhibited by carbenicillin or ticarcillin. It is also more active against *B. fragilis* and *H. influenzae.* Mezlocillin has activity against *P. aeruginosa* similar to that of ticarcillin. Mezlocillin can be given at 6-hourly intervals, and the dose needs to be reduced only moderately as renal function declines. Mezlocillin is the least likely of the broad-spectrum penicillins to alter bleeding times, but the clinical significance of this is unknown. The drug has been effective in the treatment of respiratory, urinary, gynecologic, and surgical infections. Usual doses are 12 to 18 g per day for adults.

Piperacillin has excellent activity against streptococcal species, *Neisseria, Haemophilus,* and it is the most active penicillin, and probably the drug of choice against *P. aeruginosa.* It also inhibits many *P. cepacia* which are increasingly important organisms in hospital infections. Like the other acyl ureido penicillins, it is destroyed by β-lactamases. It inhibits many community-acquired *Klebsiella* and *Bacteroides* species but will not inhibit Enterobacteriaceae which contain the plasmid β-lactamase. The human pharmacology of piperacillin is similar to the other ureido penicillins. It should be administered in a dose of 12 to 18 g per day, at 6-hourly intervals.

Other penicillins Amdinocillin is penicillin active only against gram-negative species since it does not bind to the penicillin-binding proteins of gram-positive organisms. It has poor activity against *Haemophilus* and *Neisseria,* but is extremely active against *E. coli,* many *Klebsiella, Enterobacter,* and *Citrobacter* species. It has variable activity against *Proteus* species and does not inhibit *Pseudomonas* or *Bacteroides fragilis.* Amdinocillin acts synergistically with other penicillins and has been used in this way. Amdinocillin is not acid-stable and cannot be used orally except as the pivolyl ester which is well absorbed and immediately hydrolyzed, yielding the free compound in serum.

Temocillin[1] is a 6-alpha-methoxy derivative of ticarcillin. This penicillin is not destroyed by plasmid- or chromosomally mediated β-lactamases, but it has markedly reduced activity against gram-positive species and *Pseudomonas.* Temocillin inhibits the majority of *E. coli, Klebsiella, Enterobacter, Proteus, Serratia,* and *Citrobacter* at readily achievable concentrations. *Bacteroides* are resistant. Temocillin has a half-life in humans of 4 to 6 h. It can be administered

twice or three times daily. It accumulates in the presence of renal failure and is only partially removed by hemodialysis. Temocillin is not available in the United States, but is currently used in Europe to treat urinary infections and soft tissue infections due to gram-negative bacilli.

Untoward reactions to penicillins The major adverse effects of penicillin are hypersensitivity reactions which range from minor rashes to immediate anaphylaxis. Anaphylactic reactions and accelerated urticarial reactions are due to IgE antibody. Patients who have had such reactions should not receive penicillins. Drug fever is common with all penicillins. Intestinal side effects produced by penicillins are diarrhea or bouts of enterocolitis, some of which are due to overgrowth of *Clostridium difficile.* Neutropenia, platelet dysfunction, and hemolytic anemia have followed the use of all the penicillins. Minor elevations in serum glutamic oxaloacetic transaminase (SGOT) occur most often with oxacillin, nafcillin, or carbenicillin. Neurologic adverse effects in the form of seizures will occur if penicillin G is administered in high doses to patients with decreased renal function. Renal toxicity has varied from allergic angiitis to interstitial nephritis most commonly with methicillin, but this complication can occur with all penicillins.

CEPHALOSPORINS Cephalosporins differ from penicillins by the presence of a dihydrothiazine ring rather than the five-membered thiazolidine ring fused to the four-membered β-lactam ring. Because of their structural configuration, cephalosporins have been modified chemically to produce compounds with different microbiologic and pharmacologic properties. In order to understand their antimicrobial activity, it is useful to divide cephalosporins into so-called generations. In a particular group of cephalosporins, there may be marked differences in microbiologic activity and pharmacologic properties. Like the penicillins, cephalosporins inhibit cell wall biosynthesis and are bactericidal. First-generation cephalosporins include some compounds that can be used only parenterally and some that can be used orally. The parenteral agents are cephalothin, cephapirin, cephaloridine, cefazolin, and cephradine. Oral compounds are cephalexin, cephradine, cefadroxil, and cefaclor.

First-generation cephalosporins First-generation cephalosporins inhibit group A, B, C, and G streptococci and most viridans group streptococci. They are active against *S. pneumoniae, S. aureus,* and *S. epidermidis.* Among the Enterobacteriaceae, *E. coli, P. mirabilis,* and *Klebsiella* species are inhibited. None of these first-generation drugs inhibit *Serratia, Enterobacter,* indole-positive *Proteus, P. aeruginosa,* or *B. fragilis* species. Although a number of the drugs inhibit *H. influenzae,* only cefaclor can be considered therapeutically useful against *Haemophilus.* None of these agents is therapeutic for *Neisseria* species, although all of them have some inhibitory activity against these organisms in vitro.

In some hospitals, 20 to 30 percent of *E. coli* and *Klebsiella* are resistant to first-generation cephalosporins. Nonetheless, one of these agents, cefazolin, has continued to be both useful and heavily used. Cefazolin has a half-life of approximately 2 h and can be administered either by the intramuscular or intravenous routes. It accumulates in the body in the presence of decreased renal function, and dosage adjustments must be made in the presence of renal failure. It is normally administered in doses of 0.5 to 1 g every 6 to 8 h. Cefazolin has proved useful as therapy of respiratory, skin, and urinary tract infections, and as therapy of endocarditis due to viridans streptococci in penicillin-allergic patients. It is also appropriate therapy for osteomyelitis due to staphylococcal species. Cefazolin is useful as a prophylactic antimicrobial agent at the time of orthopedic surgery, prosthetic valve surgery, and upper gastrointestinal operations. Cephalothin and cephapirin have extremely short half-lives, 4 h, and are converted in the body to less active desacetyl derivatives. These drugs should be administered every 4 h, and for this reason they are used much less frequently today.

Both cephalexin and cephradine are well absorbed after oral ingestion, yielding peak blood levels in the range of 15 to 20 μg/mL

---

[1] *Not available in the United States.*

after a 0.5-g dose. Although these cephalosporins are less active against *S. aureus* than the parenteral first-generation cephalosporins, serum and tissue concentrations are adequate to treat many minor staphylococcal infections in penicillin-allergic patients. Both drugs have a half-life of approximately 1 h and are usually administered three or four times daily. The drugs are totally excreted in the urine, yielding high concentrations inhibitory to common urinary pathogens.

Cefadroxil is a parahydroxy derivative of cephalexin which has a longer half-life, allowing it to be administered twice daily. Otherwise, its antimicrobial activity is identical to that of cephalexin.

Cefaclor has found utility primarily as a therapeutic agent for respiratory infections in children caused by *H. influenzae* or other susceptible organisms. It is poorly β-lactamase stable but the concentrations in ear fluid are adequate to eradicate β-lactamase-producing *H. influenzae*. It should not be used for serious infections caused by β-lactamase-producing strains and is ineffective in urinary tract infections due to β-lactamase-producing *E. coli* and *Klebsiella*.

Second-generation cephalosporins   Second-generation cephalosporins probably should not be grouped as a class since the compounds within this class have markedly different antibacterial and pharmacologic properties. All of these agents are administered parenterally and can be used either intramuscularly or intravenously, although they are most frequently used by the intravenous route. Cefamandole has excellent activity against streptococcal and staphylococcal species with the exception of *S. faecalis* (enterococcus). It is more active than first-generation cephalosporins against *E. coli* and *Klebsiella* and has increased activity against *H. influenzae*. It is destroyed by β-lactamases of some gram-negative species, and is not active against *Bacteroides* or *Pseudomonas* species. Although a number of *Enterobacter* and *Citrobacter* strains are inhibited by cefamandole in vitro, clinically it is not useful to treat infections due to these organisms because resistance develops rapidly. Cefamandole has a relatively short half-life, 0.7 h, and it is administered every 4 to 6 h in doses of 1 to 2 g. The drug does not produce adequate concentrations in the cerebrospinal fluid, and it should not be used in patients in whom meningitis is suspected.

Cefuroxime is a β-lactamase-stable cephalosporin that inhibits most streptococcal and staphylococcal species, *H. influenzae*, penicillinase-producing *N. gonorrhoeae*, and β-lactamase-producing Enterobacteriaceae. It is not active against *S. faecalis* (enterococcus), *Bacteroides fragilis*, or *P. aeruginosa*. Cefuroxime has a half-life of approximately 1.5 h, permitting administration at 8-hourly intervals. It enters the cerebrospinal fluid in concentrations adequate to treat meningitis due to *H. influenzae*, *S. pneumoniae*, and *N. meningitidis*. CSF concentrations are inadequate to treat meningitis due to *E. coli* or *Klebsiella* species. Cefuroxime has been used in the therapy of respiratory infections, biliary tract infections, soft tissue infections, osteomyelitis, and urinary tract infections. It can also be used for therapy of meningitis in children and young adults.

Cefonicid is a cephalosporin structurally related to cefamandole. However, substitution of a different moiety at position 3 of the dihydrothiazine ring has provided the compound with a long half-life of approximately 4 to 5 h. Cefonicid activity is similar to that of cefamandole and cefuroxime, with the exception of lower activity against *S. aureus* that may not be clinically important. Cefonicid has been used in a single daily dose administered either intravenously or intramuscularly to treat respiratory, skin, and urinary tract infections due to susceptible organisms. It should not be used to treat meningeal infections.

Ceforanide is similar in structure and antimicrobial activity to cefamandole, but is somewhat less active against *H. influenzae*. Higher serum levels are achieved following intramuscular injection since the drug is highly protein-bound. It has a half-life of approximately 3½ h, and has been used in a single or twice-daily dose to treat susceptible infections.

Cefotiam[1] is a second-generation cephalosporin with activity against streptococci, staphylococci, and most Enterobacteriaceae. It is not β-lactamase-stable and possesses high activity because of its affinity for penicillin-binding proteins. Cefotiam has a short half-life of 0.5 h, similar to many of the first-generation cephalosporins. Therefore, it must be administered every 4 h. Cefotiam is not available in the United States, but is used in Europe and Japan.

Cefoxitin is a cephalosporin which possesses a methoxy group affixed to the β-lactam ring. This provides excellent β-lactamase resistance, but decreases activity against gram-positive organisms such as staphylococci. Cefoxitin inhibits most staphylococci at concentrations of 2 to 4 μg/mL, and *S. pneumoniae* are inhibited at similar concentrations. It possesses no activity against *S. faecalis* (enterococcus). Cefoxitin inhibits *E. coli* and *Klebsiella* species resistant to first-generation and other second-generation cephalosporins. It lacks activity against *Enterobacter* and *Citrobacter* species, and does not inhibit *Pseudomonas*. Cefoxitin has excellent activity against *B. fragilis*, inhibiting the majority of clinical isolates at a concentration between 16 to 32 μg/mL, which is readily achieved in humans. Cefoxitin has a half-life of approximately 0.8 h. It is widely distributed to body sites, but does not yield adequate concentrations within the CSF. The drug accumulates in the presence of decreased renal function, and dose adjustments must be made when renal failure is present. Cefoxitin has been widely used as therapy of mixed aerobic and anaerobic intraabdominal infections and in the treatment of gynecologic infections. In some centers, cefoxitin combined with doxycycline is the therapy of choice for pelvic inflammatory disease. Cefoxitin has also been used as a parenteral prophylactic agent administered at the time of intraabdominal surgery on the colon, particularly in patients in whom oral prophylactic programs are not feasible. Cefoxitin has also proved useful in the therapy of anaerobic pleuropulmonary disease where it is an alternative to penicillin or clindamycin therapy. It is effective for treatment of gonorrhea due to penicillinase-producing *Neisseria*.

Third-generation cephalosporins   Third-generation cephalosporins can be grouped into several convenient classes. The first of these are the aminothiazolyl iminomethoxy cephalosporins which consist of cefotaxime, ceftizoxime, cefmenoxime, and ceftriaxone. These agents possess excellent activity against hemolytic streptococci and *S. pneumoniae*, inhibiting these species at concentrations <0.1 μg/mL. They do not inhibit *S. faecalis* (enterococci). The compounds are highly active against *H. influenzae*, *N. meningitidis*, and *N. gonorrhoeae*, including β-lactamase-producing strains. Because of their high affinity for penicillin-binding proteins, these compounds inhibit the majority of the Enterobacteriaceae at concentrations below 4.0 μg/mL, although some *Enterobacter* and *Citrobacter* are resistant. These four agents do not have much activity against *P. aeruginosa* and *Acinetobacter*, and they are much less active than cefoxitin against *B. fragilis*.

Cefotaxime has a half-life of approximately 1 h, and it is converted to a desacetyl derivative which has a half-life of approximately 1.6 h. Although the desacetyl derivative is less active than the parent compound, it is more active than most second-generation cephalosporins and acts synergistically with the parent compound to inhibit some microorganisms. Cefotaxime produces concentrations in the CSF ranging from 1 to 30 μg/mL, depending upon the degree of inflammation and the dose used. It has proved effective as therapy of meningitis due to group B streptococci, *E. coli*, *H. influenzae*, *N. meningitidis*, *S. pneumoniae*, *Klebsiella*, and some infections due to *Enterobacter* and *Serratia*, although failures have occurred with these organisms. Agents that have been employed more frequently (penicillin, ampicillin) should be used unless the patient is allergic to them or the organism is resistant. Although cefotaxime has a relatively short half-life, its high activity and the presence of an active metabolite indicate that it can be administered 8-hourly in most infections, except in febrile neutropenic patients.

Ceftizoxime has a slightly longer half-life than cefotaxime at 1.6 h. It also has proved useful in the therapy of gram-negative meningitis and can be administered every 8 to 12 h in the majority of infections.

Cefmenoxime[1] has a half-life of 1 h. It is normally administered

LINCOMYCIN AND CLINDAMYCIN Lincosamide antibiotics inhibit many of the same organisms as do the erythromycins. Lincomycin is rarely used today and clindamycin is the primary agent in this class. Clindamycin inhibits *S. pneumoniae*, *S. pyogenes*, and viridans group streptococci. It does not have activity against *S. faecalis* (enterococcus). Many strains of *S. aureus* and *S. epidermidis* are inhibited by clindamycin, and it has excellent activity against most anaerobic species, including *Clostridium* and *Bacteroides*. It also inhibits *Chlamydia*.

Clindamycin is well-absorbed following oral ingestion and can also be administered intramuscularly or intravenously. The serum half-life is approximately 2.5 h, and the drug is metabolized primarily in the liver. Dosage adjustments are minor except in the presence of hepatic failure. Clindamycin produces high concentrations in bone, and has been found to enter white blood cells. Its most significant toxic effect is diarrhea, which has often been associated with pseudomembranous colitis caused by *C. difficile*. If diarrhea develops during clindamycin therapy, the drug should be discontinued. If diarrhea persists, proctoscopy or assay for *C. difficile* toxin should be performed and therapy with oral vancomycin or metronidazole instituted.

The major therapeutic use of clindamycin is for anaerobic infections or as a combination with an aminoglycoside. Clindamycin provides coverage against streptococcal, staphylococcal, and anaerobic species while the aerobic gram-negative organism is attacked by the aminoglycoside. Clindamycin has also been successfully combined with the monobactam aztreonam replacing the aminoglycoside. Clindamycin has proved to be an excellent agent for the therapy of anaerobic pulmonary disease, particularly in patients who have failed to respond to penicillin. Topical solutions of clindamycin are useful in the treatment of severe acne.

RIFAMPIN Rifampin is a macrocyclic antibiotic produced by a *Streptomyces*. Rifampin is available in the United States only for oral use. The drug has been used primarily in the treatment of tuberculosis. However, rifampin has a broad range of activity, inhibiting many microorganisms. It is extremely active against both coagulase-positive and -negative staphylococci. It also inhibits *N. meningitidis*, *N. gonorrhoeae*, and *H. influenzae*. It is the most active agent known against *L. pneumophila* and is also effective against *L. micdadei*. It inhibits *C. difficile* at concentrations less than 1 μg/mL and inhibits the majority of streptococci and *S. pneumoniae* at concentrations of less than 0.1 μg/mL. Although rifampin inhibits many of the Enterobacteriaceae and some strains of *Pseudomonas*, resistance develops rapidly. The drug inhibits *Chlamydia*, but *Ureaplasma urealyticum* and *Treponema pallidum* usually are resistant.

Rifampin is well-absorbed from the gastrointestinal tract and, following ingestion of 600 mg in an adult or 10 mg/kg in children, peak serum concentrations of approximately 7 μg/mL are reached. Concentrations increase over the first several days that the drug is taken. With repeated doses, drug levels decrease because the drug stimulates the hepatic enzymes responsible for its metabolism. The drug is approximately 75 percent protein-bound. Rifampin is both metabolized and excreted by the liver. The desacetyl derivative is not reabsorbed and is excreted via the stool; only 5 to 30 percent of the dose is excreted in the urine. In general, dosage adjustment is unnecessary in renal failure, but a lower dose should be used in patients with severe hepatic dysfunction. Food will interfere with the absorption of rifampin, lowering and delaying peak blood levels. Rifampin penetrates into all body tissues and enters white cells. High concentrations are found in lacrimal and salivary secretions; the drug penetrates well into bone. Cerebrospinal fluid levels as high as 1.3 μg/mL have been observed during treatment of meningitis.

The adverse effects of rifampin are few. On occasion, it will produce a flulike syndrome in individuals who take the drug intermittently. There have also been reports of interstitial nephritis, thrombocytopenia, and hemolytic anemia. Rifampin alters the metabolism of a number of drugs; it decreases the effect of exogenous steroids and interferes with birth control pills. It artificially lowers the serum concentration of thyroxin; tri-iodothyronine remains normal. Patients should be warned that rifampin will cause red discoloration of urine and can cause permanent staining of soft contact lenses. Rifampin crosses the placenta and has produced teratogenic effects in rodents, but such effects have not been observed in humans. However, the drug should only be used during pregnancy for severe tuberculosis. The major use of rifampin is in short-term (6 to 9 months) treatment of tuberculosis, combined with isoniazid (see Chap. 119). It is also used as prophylaxis for contacts of patients with meningococcal meningitis in a dose of 600 mg for 2 days in adults and 20 mg/kg for 2 days in children. It has also been recommended for prophylaxis of children under 4 years of age who have had close contact with a child with *H. influenzae* type B meningitis. Rifampin, combined with cloxacillin, has proved quite effective in eradicating nasal carriage in individuals with recurrent furunculosis. It may also be used to eradicate methicillin-resistant staphylococci when used in combination with vancomycin or trimethoprim-sulfamethoxazole. Rifampin has been used in the therapy of endocarditis due to tolerant *S. aureus* and for treatment of *Corynebacterium* species endocarditis. It is useful in patients who have failed to respond to erythromycin in Legionnaire's disease. Rifampin also may be useful combined with nafcillin or vancomycin in the treatment of chronic staphylococcal osteomyelitis.

METRONIDAZOLE Metronidazole is a nitroimidazole which is a potent bactericidal agent. It kills organisms within a twofold dilution of the inhibitory concentration: 99 percent of *B. fragilis* are inhibited by 8 μg/mL and 100 percent of *Fusobacterium* by 4 μg/mL. Most clostridial species are inhibited by 4 μg/mL. However, anaerobic gram-positive cocci may be less susceptible, as are *Actinomyces* and *Arachnida*. It is highly active against *C. difficile*. *Proprionibacterium acnes* are resistant, but *Gardnerella vaginalis*, *Campylobacter fetus*, oral *Spirochaeta*, and *Treponema* are inhibited by metronidazole.

Metronidazole is rapidly and almost completely absorbed when given orally. It can also be absorbed by rectal instillation and is available as an intravenous solution. There is minimal protein binding; the drug has a long half-life of 8 h. Absorption of metronidazole is not affected by food although peak levels are markedly delayed. Metronidazole is metabolized in the liver to a variety of hydroxy and glucuronide derivatives. Both metronidazole and its metabolites are eliminated in the urine and in the feces. Metronidazole dosage does not need to be adjusted in renal failure, but the drug is rapidly removed by hemodialysis. Therefore, additional doses should be given after dialysis. Although metronidazole is usually administered every 6 h, with its prolonged half-life, this frequent dosing is probably unnecessary. The standard dose is 500 mg every 6 h, but 500 mg every 8 h is adequate.

There are a number of adverse effects related to metronidazole. Rare but important reactions are seizures and encephalopathy, peripheral neuropathy, disulfiram-like reaction with alcohol, potentiation of the effects of warfarin, and, extremely rarely, pseudomembranous colitis. Minor problems that are associated with the drug are development of gastrointestinal disturbance, metallic taste, maculopapular rashes, or vaginal burning. Metronidazole is tumorigenic in rats. There is no evidence that this occurs in humans. Nevertheless, the drug should probably not be used in pregnancy.

Metronidazole is effective in treatment of serious anaerobic infections, with some exceptions. It is not useful in actinomycosis, and it has not been very effective in aspiration pneumonia, probably because of the large number of streptococci found in this infection. It is particularly useful in intraabdominal infections since it is able to penetrate abscesses and kill *Bacteroides* within the abscess. It has also been used in other anaerobic infections including bacteremia, osteomyelitis, and head-and-neck infections. Metronidazole can be used in the management of pseudomembranous colitis due to *C. difficile;* it is extremely inexpensive when administered orally. It is the drug of choice if oral vancomycin is not available. Metronidazole is a useful drug in the treatment of *Trichomonas* vaginitis and has also proved useful in the therapy of amebic liver abscess and intestinal amebiasis. It may be useful in *Blastocystis hominis* infections. Metronidazole has been used as prophylaxis for elective colonic surgery and gynecologic surgery or at the time of emergency appendectomy. However, the drug has no activity against gram-positive or gram-negative aerobic organisms.

POLYMYXINS Polymyxins are cyclic basic polypeptides. There are two compounds available, polymyxin B sulfate and polymyxin E, or colistin. Polymyxins are active only against aerobic gram-negative bacteria such as *Pseudomonas* and members of the Enterobacteriaceae. The compounds are not absorbed when given orally and must be administered parenterally. They are rapidly sequestered within the kidney and liver, reducing their clinical value. Both drugs produce very serious neuro- and nephrotoxicity. In view of the large number of other compounds available, there is no reason to use them.

SULFONAMIDES AND TRIMETHOPRIM Sulfonamides are bacteriostatic and act by interfering with folic acid metabolism in bacteria. They are generally classified as short-, medium-, or long-acting sulfonamides, sulfonamides limited to the gastrointestinal tract, and topical sulfonamides. Sulfonamides inhibit a variety of gram-positive bacteria and members of the Enterobacteriaceae, including *E. coli*, *Klebsiella*, and *Proteus*. They are also active against *Haemophilus*, but do not have activity against *P. aeruginosa*. The major problem with sulfonamides is that bacteria rapidly become resistant on the basis of plasmid-mediated production of altered enzymes. Most sulfonamides are administered orally, although sulfamethoxazole is available for intravenous use. Sulfonamides are absorbed rapidly from the small intestine and stomach. The compounds are distributed throughout the body and enter the CSF, synovial, pleural, and peritoneal fluids in concentrations that approximate 80 percent of serum levels. Sulfonamides are metabolized in the liver by acetylation and glucuronidation. They are excreted via glomerular filtration with partial reabsorption and tubular secretion. Sulfonamides differ widely in their protein binding, plasma half-life, metabolism, and solubility.

One of the major reasons that sulfonamide use has fallen off is that these agents produce a large number of serious side effects. These include a rash that appears in 3 to 5 percent of individuals, fever, jaundice, serum sickness–like syndrome, and acute hemolysis in the G6PD-deficient patient. They also may cause agranulocytosis, thrombocytopenia, and leukopenia. Sulfonamides cannot be administered during the last month of pregnancy since they cross the placenta and displace bilirubin from albumin and increase the risk of kernicterus. Long-acting sulfonamides have been associated with fatal hypersensitivity reactions; this has been noted with the longer-acting sulfonamides used in malarial preparations. By binding to albumin sites, sulfonamides may displace drugs such as warfarin, methotrexate, and hypoglycemic agents such as chlorpropamide. Sulfonamide concentrations are increased by indomethacin, salicylates, and probenecid. Tubular necrosis due to deposition of sulfa crystals within the kidney rarely occurs today.

Sulfadiazine is the most active sulfonamide attaining the highest blood and cerebrospinal fluid levels. However, it tends more often to produce crystalluria; hence sulfisoxazole and sulfamethoxazole are used more frequently. Mixtures of three sulfonamides are also available and can be used in the treatment of toxoplasmosis. Long-acting sulfonamides should be avoided because of the risk of severe erythema multiforme. Topical sulfonamide preparations such as silver-sulfadiazine or mafenide are extremely useful to reduce the number of bacteria in burn eschars.

Trimethoprim is a 2,4-diaminopyrimidine that is a dihydrofolate reductase inhibitor. Trimethoprim is active against most gram-positive cocci and gram-negative rods with the exception of *P. aeruginosa* and *Bacteroides*. It also has relatively poor activity against *Neisseria* species, and against *Chlamydia* and *Nocardia*. Resistance to trimethoprim has been fairly slow to develop. However, in the far east, strains of *Salmonella* and *Shigella* have become resistant, and toxigenic *E. coli* have been isolated in Central America which are resistant to trimethoprim and the combination of trimethoprim and sulfamethoxazole.

Trimethoprim is available as a single agent or a combined agent in a fixed combination of one part trimethoprim to five parts sulfamethoxazole. It is also available as an intravenous combination which contains one part trimethoprim and five parts sulfamethoxazole. Like the sulfonamides, trimethoprim is well-absorbed from the gastrointestinal tract. Most of the drug is excreted in the urine via tubular secretion; it has a serum half-life of 9 to 11 h in normal individuals. Trimethoprim-sulfamethoxazole can usually be given to patients with creatinine clearances greater than 30 mL/min in the usual doses and given in half doses to patients whose creatinine clearances are in the range of 15 to 30 mL/min. Trimethoprim itself may cause fever and rash and depression of white cells and platelets. This problem often can be avoided by the simultaneous administration of folinic acid. Pseudomembranous enterocolitis also can occur following use of trimethoprim-sulfamethoxazole.

Trimethoprim-sulfamethoxazole has been useful in the treatment of urinary tract infections, acute bacterial exacerbations of chronic bronchitis, and gastrointestinal infections due to *Salmonella*, *Shigella*, and toxigenic *E. coli*. Trimethoprim also is useful in the treatment of gonorrhea. Trimethoprim-sulfamethoxazole is used in high-dose oral or intravenous therapy of *Pneumocystis carinii* infections. Trimethoprim-sulfamethoxazole has also proved useful as prophylaxis in neutropenic children and in chronic granulomatous disease of childhood. The combination has been of particular value in the prevention of recurrent bacteriuria in women with recurrent urinary tract infections.

QUINOLONES Quinolones are synthesized chemically. They include nalidixic acid which inhibits gram-negative bacteria and, to a lesser extent, gram-positive organisms. It has been used primarily for the treatment of urinary tract infections. Nalidixic acid is a naphthyridine derivative while the new quinolones, which are some thousandfold more active than nalidixic acid, are true quinolone compounds. All of these agents bind to an enzyme, DNA gyrase, which is involved in the production of new DNA molecules.

The compounds can be considered in groups; nalidixic acid, oxolinic acid, and cinoxacin are one group. They inhibit the majority of strains of *E. coli*, *P. mirabilis*, *Klebsiella*, and *Enterobacter* at concentrations that readily can be achieved in urine. *Pseudomonas* species are resistant as are most gram-positive organisms, *S. aureus*, *S. pneumoniae*, and *S. faecalis*. Cross-resistance occurs between all three of the compounds. These agents are given by the oral route and are almost completely absorbed from the gastrointestinal tract. They are metabolized in the liver to biologically active and inactive compounds that are excreted by the kidney. The major difficulty with these agents has been the rapid development of resistance to them; hence they have not proved very effective in the treatment of urinary tract infections.

The new carboxyfluoroquinolones such as norfloxacin, enoxacin, pefloxacin, ofloxacin, and ciprofloxacin differ from the previously mentioned drugs because they have an extended antibacterial spectrum. All of these agents inhibit virtually all of the Enterobacteriaceae at concentrations below 1 μg/mL. In addition, they show varying activity against *Pseudomonas*, depending upon the particular compound. For example, ciprofloxacin is extremely active against *P. aeruginosa* and other *Pseudomonas* species, inhibiting isolates resistant to β-lactam and aminoglycoside antibiotics. The agents also inhibit *Haemophilus*, *Branhamella*, and methicillin-resistant staphylococci. They tend to have less activity against *S. pneumoniae* and generally do not inhibit *Bacteroides* and many clostridial species except at high concentrations.

These agents differ in their oral absorption. Oxfloxacin and enoxacin are more readily absorbed than are norfloxacin and ciprofloxacin. Absorption is markedly reduced in the presence of antacids, but not by H-2-blocking agents. The compounds are widely distributed in the body and are metabolized to both active and inactive products within the liver. The majority of these excretion products leave the body via the urinary tract, and they tend to accumulate in the presence of decreased renal function. The quinolones have been known to enter the CSF at therapeutic concentrations against *H. influenzae,* *N. meningitidis,* and Enterobacteriaceae, but they do not yield adequate concentrations for treatment of *S. pneumoniae* infections. High concentrations are achieved in bone, and studies of experimental osteomyelitis have demonstrated that the agents are superior to aminoglycosides. Several of these agents are available in Europe and Japan, but at present none are available for use in the United States. The compounds have been used in the treatment of urinary tract infections, respiratory tract infections, gastrointestinal disease due to *Salmonella* and *Shigella,* and pathogenic *E. coli* and *Campylobacter.* They have been successfully used in the treatment of osteomyelitis and skin infections. Ciprofloxacin has been extremely effective in therapy of *Pseudomonas* infections, including those occurring in cystic fibrosis patients.

Toxic and adverse reactions to these agents have been fairly rare. Gastrointestinal side effects have included nausea, vomiting, and occasionally diarrhea. Nonspecific rashes and urticaria have occurred. Ophthalmologic side effects have consisted of decreased visual and color perception, both of which have returned to normal with cessation of therapy. Central nervous system symptoms noted with nalidixic acid include headache, vertigo, seizures, and psychosis, but such reactions have not been reported with the 4-quinolones. It is too early to determine the precise role of these compounds in the chemotherapy of infection. However, they appear to be new and exciting agents to treat multiresistant microorganisms.

ANTITUBERCULOSIS DRUGS (See Chap. 119) Isoniazid remains one of the most important drugs for the treatment of tuberculosis. It should be included in any regimen for the treatment of patients with tuberculosis at any site. Isoniazid is well absorbed orally and can also be administered intramuscularly in patients unable to take oral medication. It enters the cerebrospinal fluid in concentrations adequate to treat tuberculous meningitis. The major concern with the use of isoniazid involves its hepatotoxicity. Approximately 15 percent of individuals who receive isoniazid develop elevations in SGOT. Individuals under 20 years of age rarely if ever have significant liver toxicity, but the frequency of hepatotoxicity in adults over 50 approximates 2 to 3 percent. The mechanism of toxicity remains unknown. Peripheral neuropathy may be seen in individuals who receive large doses and is more likely to be seen in individuals with alcoholism, diabetes, or uremia, and in particular those who are slow acetylators of the drug. Pyridoxine will not alter isoniazid's action, but will ameliorate the neuropathy. Isoniazid may also produce fever, skin eruption, and sideroblastic anemia. The most important aspect of monitoring isoniazid use is to follow liver function tests in older individuals.

Ethambutol is a tuberculostatic agent that is administered orally. It is well-absorbed from the gastrointestinal tract and is widely distributed throughout the body, including the cerebrospinal fluid. Resistance to the drug develops readily and hence it must always be used as a second drug to a primary compound such as isoniazid or rifampin. Retrobulbar neuritis occurs if the drug is used in large doses. For this reason, the dose should be kept under 15 mg/kg per day. Although complete blindness has occurred, visual acuity usually returns when the drug is stopped, and eventually patients' visual acuity will gradually return to normal.

Pyrazinamide is an analogue of nicotinamide that is used in short-course therapy for tuberculosis because of its bactericidal action against the tubercle bacillus. It may prove to be an extremely useful agent since it is active at an acid pH which is present in tuberculous cavities. Moreover, the compound appears to enter cells where the pH may be acid. Pyrazinamide is well absorbed orally and distributed throughout the body, including the CSF. It is metabolized in the liver, and its metabolic products are excreted in the urine. It should not be administered to individuals with renal failure. At doses of 20 to 35 mg/kg per day, the drug appears to cause a minimal amount of hepatotoxicity. Liver function tests should be monitored in individuals receiving pyrazinamide, particularly if they are receiving rifampin and isoniazid at the same time. The drug has been reported

to cause gout. In certain settings, pyrazinamide can be administered once a week, and it is well tolerated in a twice-weekly program of 50 mg/kg when used in short courses.

There are a number of studies of the use of investigational antituberculous drugs to treat *M. avium-intracellulare* infections, which are a major problem in AIDS patients. One of these, ansamycin, is a rifampin derivative. Another agent is clofazimine, a drug that is ordinarily used in the treatment of leprosy. Results to date are not too encouraging. In vitro, ciprofloxacin, a new quinolone, has proved quite effective against atypical mycobacteria.

ANTIFUNGAL AGENTS See Chap. 146.

ANTIVIRAL AGENTS See Chap. 129.

ANTIPARASITIC AGENTS See Chap. 151 for a general discussion and Chaps. 153 to 168 for treatment of specific diseases.

REASONS FOR FAILURE OF CHEMOTHERAPY

This chapter, as well as the chapters which deal with specific disease entities, has documented that there are few microorganisms with the exception of fungi and viruses that are not susceptible to some antimicrobial agents. Nonetheless, a large number of patients who develop infections continue to die. In these patients, antimicrobial agents have failed. The failure of chemotherapy often is more apparent than real, and may be attributed to a number of different causes.

First, the infection being treated may not be due to a treatable microorganism but to a viral infection that will not respond to the chemotherapeutic agents that are being used. Antibiotics do not prevent bacterial complications of many viral infections.

A second common reason for failure of antimicrobial therapy is that purulent material has not been drained, or that a focus of obstruction or a foreign body has not been removed. Antimicrobial agents do not work well in these situations.

Third, fever may continue, not due to the infection, but as the result of development of hypersensitivity to one of the agents being used to treat the patient. Drug fever is particularly common with many of the antimicrobial agents of the β-lactam and sulfonamide class.

Occasionally, chemotherapy fails because the incorrect drug has been chosen or the culture results have been misinterpreted. This may be particularly true in respiratory infections. One of the most common errors when such a patient is not responding is to add more antimicrobial agents indiscriminately, when the correct course would be to discontinue therapy and observe the patient.

With many of the new antimicrobial agents, failure to provide an adequate dose of antibiotic is less frequently a problem than it was formerly. However, this still may be true in certain infections in which penetration of the antimicrobial agent to the particular area of the body is inadequate unless large doses are utilized.

Perhaps most importantly, the type of patient requiring antimicrobial therapy has shown a marked change in the past decade. More and more, today's patients lack host defenses, and include premature infants, elderly patients with degenerative and debilitating diseases, or patients who have received multiple antimicrobial agents, antineoplastic or immunosuppressive drugs, or who have undergone major surgical procedures. These individuals will tend to have much more difficulty in responding to antimicrobial therapy than normal uncompromised hosts, most of whom remain free of life-threatening infections.

REFERENCES

BARZA M: Imipenem: First of a new class of beta-lactam antibiotics. Ann Intern Med 103:552, 1985

GERDING DN (ed): Role of aminoglycosides as first-line therapy in multiple clinical settings. Am J Med 79(1A):1, 1985

NEU HC (ed): Advances in cephalosporin therapy: Beyond the third generation. Am J Med 79(2A):1, 1985

———— (ed): β-Lactamase inhibition: Therapeutic advances. Am J Med 79(5B):1, 1985

REMINGTON JS (ed): Carbapenems: A new class of antibiotics. Am J Med 78(6A):1, 1985

SCULLY BE, NEU HC: Use of aztreonam in the treatment of serious infections due to multiresistant gram-negative organisms, including *Pseudomonas aeruginosa*. Am J Med 78:251, 1985

SNAVELY SR, HODGES GR: The neurotoxicity of antibacterial agents. Ann Intern Med 101:92, 1984

WINSTON DJ et al: Moxalactam plus piperacillin versus moxalactam plus amikacin in febrile granulocytopenic patients. Am J Med 77:442, 1984

89   ACUTE INFECTIOUS DIARRHEAL DISEASES AND BACTERIAL FOOD POISONING

CHARLES C. J. CARPENTER

Acute diarrheal illnesses caused by bacterial, viral, or protozoal pathogens vary from slightly annoying bowel dysfunction to fulminant, life-threatening diseases. Largely because of the recognition of enterotoxigenic *Escherichia coli* as a major cause of acute diarrheal disease in adults and the identification of rotavirus as a frequent cause in young children, specific etiologic agents have been isolated from 80 to 85 percent of patients with acute diarrheal illnesses. Those illnesses caused by bacterial pathogens are more often life-threatening, at least among adults, and for that reason they will be addressed first. This chapter is aimed at presenting an overview of these diseases; in most instances, the entities are discussed in more detail in the chapters dealing with the specific etiologic agent.

In considering the bacterial diarrheas, it is useful to divide them into two groups, those caused by invasive and those caused by noninvasive microorganisms. The invasive pathogens, of which *Shigella* (see Chap. 108) may be considered the prototype, generally cause abdominal pain, fever, and other systemic symptoms, often including headache and myalgia. Illness caused by the noninvasive pathogens, of which cholera (see Chap. 115) is the prototype, is generally characterized by the absence of fever and few systemic symptoms (except those directly related to intestinal fluid loss). The invasive pathogens characteristically destroy gut mucosal cells, typically involving the terminal ileum and colon, and both leukocytes and erythrocytes are present, to a variable degree, in the stool. Inflammatory cells are generally absent from the stool in acute diarrheal disease caused by noninvasive bacterial pathogens.

NONINVASIVE BACTERIAL PATHOGENS

ENTEROTOXIGENIC *ESCHERICHIA COLI*   Etiology and epidemiology   Enterotoxin-producing *E. coli* (ETEC), which have the dual capacity to adhere to small-bowel epithelial cells and to produce one or more diarrheagenic toxins, are recognized as a major cause of acute diarrheal disease throughout most of the world and are the most common cause of "traveler's diarrhea." Largely because current techniques for demonstrating toxigenicity remain cumbersome, the epidemiology of ETEC diarrhea is poorly understood. ETEC are responsible for the majority of cases of traveler's diarrhea in visitors to the developing nations in South America, Africa, and Asia. ETEC are also one of the two (with rotavirus) leading causes of acute diarrheal illnesses in children throughout the developing world. ETEC have been implicated as a major cause of fulminant, cholera-like diarrheal disease in adult patients in south and southeast Asia but generally cause milder, self-limited diarrhea in adults in other parts of the developing world. There is no satisfactory explanation for the difference in severity in diarrhea caused by ETEC in different geographic areas. ETEC are rarely incriminated in episodic diarrheal illness in children and adults in the United States.

Pathogenesis   The ability to cause diarrheal disease is not restricted to any one *E. coli* serotype but appears to be dependent upon the presence of both a plasmid-mediated colonization factor, which allows the *E. coli* to adhere to small-bowel mucosal cells, and one or more plasmids which code for the production of one or both of the two diarrheagenic toxins which may be produced by *E. coli*. The kinetics and mode of action of one of the toxins, which is heat labile (LT) and of relatively high molecular mass (~83,000 daltons), are similar to those of cholera enterotoxin (see Chap. 115); the diarrheagenic effect results from stimulation of adenylate cyclase in the gut epithelial cells. The other toxin, which is heat stable (ST) and of a lower molecular mass (<2000 daltons), has a more rapid onset of action and probably exerts its effect through stimulation of guanylate cyclase in the gut mucosal cells. Either or both toxins may be produced by ETEC. Most isolates from patients with severe diarrheal disease in Bangladesh produce both LT and ST, whereas isolates from patients in other developing nations have shown widely varying capacities for the production of LT, ST, or both. The wide clinical spectrum may be, in part, related to the predominant production of either LT or ST by the culpable microorganisms. The nutritional status of the host may also be a factor in determining the clinical response to ETEC.

Manifestations   Both clinical observations and volunteer studies indicate that the incubation period is generally between 24 and 72 h. The illness which follows is quite variable, ranging from the fulminant, cholera-like disease often seen on the Indian subcontinent to the much milder Mexican "turista," in which the symptoms of mild, watery diarrhea, abdominal cramps, and occasional low-grade fever are more troublesome than life-threatening. Vomiting occurs in fewer than half the adults with *E. coli* diarrhea and is seldom responsible for major fluid losses.

In fulminant cases, the severe diarrhea seldom lasts longer than 24 to 36 h, and the response to either oral or intravenous electrolyte repletion is predictable and dramatic. With milder disease, the symptoms subside more gradually, occasionally persisting for a week or longer.

Laboratory findings   As with cholera, no erythrocytes and few, if any, polymorphonuclear leukocytes are seen in a stool preparation stained with Loeffler's methylene blue. Because *E. coli* occurs normally among stool flora, and because its ability to produce enterotoxin is not restricted to any specific serotype, there is no rapid and simple means to make the laboratory diagnosis of enterotoxigenic *E. coli*. Bioassays for LT, based on the ability of *E. coli* isolates to produce fluid in isolated intestinal loops of experimental animals or to stimulate adenylate cyclase in cells in tissue culture, as well as the suckling mouse bioassay for ST, are reliable but of little value in patient management. Newer technology, utilizing DNA probes for rapid identification of the genes responsible for ST and LT production, appears promising and may be adapted for widespread use for epidemiologic purposes in the future.

Treatment   The intestinal fluid losses are qualitatively identical to those in cholera. Therefore, in those patients who develop clinically significant saline depletion, the principles of fluid administration are identical to those described for cholera (see Chap. 115). Oral solutions containing electrolytes plus glucose or sucrose are consistently effective in correcting the saline depletion. Antibiotics (tetracycline, 30 mg/kg per day, given orally at 6-h intervals for 48 h; trimethoprim, 200 mg twice daily for 5 days; or trimethoprim, 160 mg, with sulfamethoxazole, 800 mg, twice daily for 5 days) are effective in decreasing the duration of illness but are not essential. Bismuth subsalicylate, 60 mL hourly for four doses, provides symptomatic relief (less frequent stools, less severe abdominal cramps). Both diphenoxylate and loperamide may provide rapid relief of abdominal cramps, but neither drug has been shown to alter the volume of intestinal fluid loss.

Prognosis   With even the more fulminant cases of disease caused by ETEC with adequate fluid replacement, the prognosis is excellent.

Prevention   Careful hygienic practices, with special attention to ingestion of clean water and adequately cooked foods, provide the most certain protection against enterotoxigenic *E. coli.* Doxycycline, 100 mg per day, is 60 to 90 percent effective as a prophylactic agent, the effectiveness varying with the tetracycline sensitivity of the ETEC in the geographic area. Trimethoprim, 160 mg, with sulfamethoxazole, 800 mg, taken once daily, is also effective in prophylaxis against traveler's diarrhea caused by ETEC.

CHOLERA   See Chap. 115.

OTHER ENTEROTOXIGENIC ENTEROBACTERIACEAE   Noninvasive strains of *Klebsiella* and *Enterobacter* occasionally have been implicated in acute diarrheal disease in developing areas of the world. The clinical illness produced is indistinguishable from the milder cases of diarrhea caused by enterotoxigenic *E. coli,* and treatment is the same.

CLOSTRIDIUM PERFRINGENS (See Chap. 101)   This organism remains a significant cause of diarrheal disease and is implicated in many cases of acute food poisoning in the United States. Both the epidemiologic background and the clinical picture of *C. perfringens* diarrhea differ strikingly from those of *E. coli. Clostridium perfringens* diarrhea tends to occur in a microepidemic pattern following ingestion of contaminated meat, poultry products, or legumes. The relatively short incubation period of 6 to 12 h is an important diagnostic clue. Typically, two or more patients who have ingested the same meat dish become ill at roughly the same time. The production of a specific enterotoxin by the actively sporulating microorganisms in the intestinal tract appears to be responsible for all the symptoms. The clinical picture of diarrhea caused by *C. perfringens* is different from that caused by enterotoxigenic *E. coli* in one important respect, because moderately severe cramping abdominal pain, which is usually less prominent with *E. coli,* is a major presenting symptom. Treatment consists of symptomatic therapy with codeine to alleviate the cramping abdominal pain and intravenous fluid therapy in the small proportion of patients in whom there is clinical evidence of saline depletion. The illness is self-limited and rarely lasts for more than 24 h. Because of the relatively short natural course of the illness, antimicrobial therapy is of no value. Because *C. perfringens* normally inhabits mammalian and avian intestinal tracts, prevention is dependent upon adequate cooking and handling of meat and poultry products. The practice of allowing cooked meat products to cool slowly toward room temperature over 12 to 24 h permits germination of contaminating clostridial spores; this practice must be avoided.

STAPHYLOCOCCUS AUREUS (See Chap. 94)   Acute staphylococcal diarrhea, classic "food poisoning," is due entirely to ingestion of preformed enterotoxin, and the causative organisms are often absent from the stool during the acute illness. This form of diarrhea often occurs in institutional outbreaks and is characterized by a short incubation period (2 to 6 h), relatively short duration (usually less than 10 h), and very high attack rates (often greater than 75 percent of the population at risk). In addition to its distinctive epidemiologic features, acute staphylococcal diarrhea differs from other noninvasive bacterial diarrheas by the prominence of vomiting, which is an almost constant feature and is apparently mediated by a direct effect of the absorbed toxin on the central nervous system. Treatment is directed toward correction of the saline depletion (intravenous fluids are required in 10 to 20 percent of patients) and, when necessary, toward symptomatic relief of vomiting. Because staphylococcal food poisoning is caused by preformed enterotoxin and is not perpetuated by viable microorganisms, antimicrobials are of no value.

A good example of the explosive nature of staphylococcal food poisoning was provided by an outbreak on a jet liner flying from Anchorage to Copenhagen. In this episode, 57 percent of 343 passengers developed an acute illness characterized by vomiting, diarrhea, and cramping abdominal pain. Of the 200 affected individuals, 30 required intravenous fluids, but none had serious sequelae. The food, contaminated by a pustule on the hand of a food handler,

had not been adequately refrigerated aboard the plane, allowing abundant growth of the staphylococcus, with production of enterotoxin. Since staphylococci are ubiquitous, the prevention of massive contamination is dependent largely on control of growth conditions, primarily temperature. *Staphylococcus aureus* can multiply at temperatures from 4 to 46°C, and if contaminated food is allowed to remain at ambient temperatures after cooking, these organisms have ample opportunity to multiply, especially in such items as cream pastries, potato salad, and mayonnaise.

BACILLUS CEREUS   *Bacillus cereus* is a cause of acute diarrheal disease which, although uncommon, has been identified with increasing frequency in Europe. The illness results from gross contamination of food with this gram-positive rod, which is capable of producing at least two discrete enterotoxins, one having characteristics similar to those of the labile enterotoxin of *E. coli* and the other having effects similar to that of staphylococcal enterotoxin. *Bacillus cereus* may, therefore, cause two distinct clinical syndromes, a diarrheal form resulting from the *E. coli* LT type of enterotoxin and an emetic form caused by the staphylococcal type of enterotoxin. The diarrheal syndrome caused by *B. cereus* is generally similar to that caused by enterotoxin-producing *E. coli,* with the exceptions that abdominal cramps are more common (75 percent of cases) and both the incubation period (6 to 14 h) and median duration of illness (20 h) are shorter. The emetic syndrome is clinically indistinguishable from that caused by staphylococcal enterotoxin, with a short incubation period (median 2 h), short duration (median 9 h), and prominent vomiting (100 percent compared with less than 25 percent in the diarrheal syndrome). Because both syndromes are self-limited and generally mild, no specific therapy is indicated. When *B. cereus* food poisoning is suspected clinically, the diagnosis can be confirmed by demonstration of 10^5 or more *B. cereus* organisms per gram in epidemiologically incriminated food. *Bacillus cereus* grows readily on simple laboratory media, including blood agar, but will not generally be identified as a pathogen unless such identification is specifically requested. Isolation of *B. cereus* from stool alone does not establish it as the etiologic agent because the organism is frequently found in the fecal flora of normal individuals. Since *B. cereus* is ubiquitous in soil, as well as in many raw, dried, and processed foods, proper food handling is the only practical means of preventing this form of food poisoning. The emetic form of *B. cereus* food poisoning almost invariably has been associated with ingestion of contaminated fried rice. *Bacillus cereus* is commonly present in uncooked rice, and its spores survive boiling and germinate, with production of the enterotoxin, when boiled rice is left unrefrigerated. Brief rewarming before serving is not adequate to destroy the relatively heat-stable toxin. Prompt refrigeration of boiled rice will prevent transmission of the disease.

INVASIVE AND/OR DESTRUCTIVE ENTERIC PATHOGENS

INTRODUCTION   Shigellae characteristically invade the colon and terminal ileum, destroy segments of intestinal mucosa, cause extensive inflammatory changes in the lamina propria, and are the prototype of the invasive enteric bacterial pathogens. Other important invasive bacterial enteric pathogens include *Salmonella, Yersinia enterocolitica, Campylobacter jejuni, Vibrio parahemolyticus,* and invasive *E. coli,* which may have the capacity both to damage intestinal mucosa and to produce an enterotoxin. As opposed to the noninvasive pathogens, the invasive enteric organisms frequently cause systemic symptoms, including headache, myalgias, chills, and fever. As a general rule, antiperistaltic agents such as opiates, diphenoxylate, loperamide, and atropine are contraindicated in diarrheal disease caused by invasive enteric pathogens because they clearly worsen the clinical course in human shigellosis, as well as in salmonellosis and shigellosis in animal models.

The major therapeutic challenge in invasive bacterial diarrheas is that of distinguishing between (1) shigellosis and yersiniosis, in which antimicrobial therapy decreases the duration and severity of illness and shortens the period of fecal shedding of the pathogen, and (2) infections caused by *Salmonella*, which are characterized primarily by watery diarrhea and few systemic symptoms and in which antimicrobial therapy does not alter the duration of illness and may cause prolonged excretion of the pathogen.

SHIGELLOSIS   See Chap. 108.

SALMONELLOSIS   See Chap. 107.

YERSINIA ENTEROCOLITICA   See Chap. 114.

CAMPYLOBACTER JEJUNI
Etiology and epidemiology *Campylobacter jejuni* was first implicated in acute diarrheal disease in humans in 1972; by 1979 *C. jejuni* was second only to *Giardia lamblia* among recognized causes of waterborne diarrheal disease outbreaks in the United States. Attack rates have been highest in adolescents and young adults. *C. jejuni* occurs in the intestinal flora of many wild and domestic animals and poultry, and can be transmitted to humans by milk and water polluted by such animal carriers. The distribution of *C. jejuni* is worldwide, and *C. jejuni* appears to cause from 5 to 10 percent of acute diarrheal illnesses in both the industrialized and the developing areas of the world. Ingestion of raw milk and of water from contaminated mountain streams has been implicated in *Campylobacter enteritis* in North Ameria; in outbreaks associated with ingestion of raw milk, attack rates have reached 60 percent.

Pathogenesis *C. jejuni* causes patchy destruction of mucosa of both the small intestine, especially the distal ileum, and the colon; the stools, therefore, regularly contain pus cells and are occasionally grossly bloody. *C. jejuni* rarely produces transient bacteremia; when it does, it is likely to occur in an immunocompromised host.

Manifestations An incubation period of 2 to 6 days, longer than that of most bacterial enteric pathogens, is followed by fever, cramping abdominal pain, and diarrhea that is initially watery but later contains blood and mucus. The diarrhea, generally mild but occasionally voluminous, usually ceases within 2 to 5 days without specific antimicrobial therapy; on rare occasions the diarrhea may persist for 3 to 4 weeks. In some cases, the abdominal pain may be more prominent than the diarrhea, and the clinical picture may simulate acute appendicitis or, rarely, pancreatitis. (This may also be true in *Yersinia* enterocolitis; see Chap. 114.) In such cases, laparotomy has revealed acutely inflamed mesenteric lymph nodes as well as patchy inflammation of the small bowel. Acute reactive arthritis, similar to that associated with other invasive bacterial diarrheas (*Shigella, Salmonella, Yersinia*) may follow *C. jejuni* enteritis and is often associated wtih the HLA-B27 antigen.

Laboratory findings Diagnosis depends upon isolating *C. jejuni* from stool. Since this curved, motile bacillus does not compete well with other enteric flora on standard enteric media, it will rarely be isolated from stool unless special techniques are utilized. These include incubation at 42°C in a microaerobic atmosphere on blood agar to which a number of antimicrobials have been added. Serologic diagnosis is rarely helpful, as there are many serotypes of *C. jejuni*, and agglutination tests require use of the homologous organism.

Treatment Since *C. jejuni* usually produces a short, self-limited illness, antimicrobial therapy is not essential to management. Erythromycin, 30 mg/kg per day, does, however, significantly decrease the duration of fecal shedding of *C. jejuni* and may shorten the mean duration of illness. In the occasional patient who develops clinical signs of saline depletion, oral and/or intravenous fluids of the same sort used in cholera are uniformly effective (see Chap. 115).

OTHER *CAMPYLOBACTER* INFECTIONS
The observation of small, curved, gram-negative rods with characteristic corkscrew-like motility in many stool specimens from which *C. jejuni* cannot be isolated has led to the identification of several additional species of *Campylobacter*

which are associated with human disease. All such species, like *C. jejuni*, appear to be epizootic, but precisely which animals are the most common vectors for specific *Campylobacter* species is not known. This discussion will be limited to three species of *Campylobacter*, which represent the spectrum of illness caused by these microorganisms.

Campylobacter coli, although slightly different in biochemical characteristics, is identical to *C. jejuni* in morphology, growth characteristics and epidemiology, as well as in the illness which it produces.

Campylobacter fetus is similar to *C. jejuni* in morphology and growth characteristics but has a marked predilection for patients with chronic renal, hepatic, and neoplastic disease, alcoholism, and compromised immune function. Although the intestinal tract of the compromised host is the presumed site of entry, the intestinal infection may be mild or subclinical, and overshadowed by a bacteremic illness, associated with high fever, which often follows a prolonged or relapsing course and may be complicated by endocarditis, infection of preexisting aortic aneurysms, and/or septic phlebitis. Persistent bacteremia may be enhanced by the relative resistance of *C. fetus* to the bactericidal activity of normal serum.

Although occasional patients have had self-limited *C. fetus* sepsis, *C. fetus* bacteremia is usually fatal unless treated with antimicrobials. Gentamicin is thought to be the drug of choice, although no controlled observations are available. At least 4 weeks of antimicrobial treatment is recommended because of the tropism of *C. fetus* for intravascular sites.

Campylobacter cinaedi sp. n. has been the most frequently isolated of four *Campylobacter*-like organisms (CLOs) which have been associated with proctitis, proctocolitis, and enteritis in homosexual males. Although morphologically similar to *C. jejuni*, the CLOs grow poorly at 42° (and are therefore missed by the standard technique used to isolate *C. jejuni* and *C. fetus*), and prototype CLO strains show little (< 2 percent) DNA homology with *C. jejuni* and *C. fetus*. The CLO organisms grow slowly in a microaerophilic environment on modified brucella agar supplemented with 10% sheep blood.

Despite the differing growth characteristics, the CLOs produce changes which are indistinguishable from those caused by *C. jejuni* on sigmoidoscopic and histologic examination. Although the CLOs are sensitive to erythromycin, no controlled studies of antimicrobial therapy are available.

VIBRIO PARAHEMOLYTICUS
Etiology and epidemiology *Vibrio parahemolyticus* is a curved, aerobic, nonmotile, gram-negative bacillus. Although present in coastal waters throughout the temperate zone, it has most commonly been associated with acute diarrheal illness in Japan, presumably because of the frequency of ingestion of raw seafood. It is regarded as the prototype of the halophilic vibrios because it grows more rapidly in 6% NaCl solutions than in the isotonic or hypotonic media used to culture most bacterial pathogens. *V. parahemolyticus* is responsible for a relatively small (< 10 percent) proportion of acute diarrheal illnesses in both adults and children in rural Bangladesh, where an association with seafood is less clearly established. It has been implicated in several outbreaks of acute diarrheal disease in the coastal United States, always as a common-source outbreak related to ingestion of inadequately cooked seafood, usually shrimp. Secondary cases caused by person-to-person transmission occur rarely. Several epidemics of *V. parahemolyticus* infections on cruise ships have been reported.

Pathogenesis Although *V. parahemolyticus* produces a toxin capable of causing intestinal fluid accumulation in experimental animals, the role of this toxin in human disease is not certain. *V. parahemolyticus* causes patchy mucosal damage in both distal ileum and colon; stools usually contain numerous polymorphonuclear leukocytes and are occasionally grossly bloody. The volume of fluid lost with *V. parahemolyticus* infection is relatively small, and intravenous fluids are seldom required. The illness is self-limited, with a median duration of just under 24 h.

Manifestations Within 6 to 48 h after ingestion of raw or inadequately cooked seafood, the patient develops an acute diarrheal illness. The volume of fluid lost is not great, moderately severe abdominal cramps may be a prominent feature, and chills and fever are observed in roughly half the cases. Vomiting is generally not prominent and occurs in no more than one-third of patients. The illness is self-limited, and no deaths have been reported in outbreaks involving over a thousand patients in the United States.

Laboratory findings When a common-source outbreak of acute diarrheal disease occurs in a group exposed to fresh or frozen seafood, the index of suspicion should be high and the diagnosis should be confirmed by plating a rectal swab on thiosulfate–citrate–bile salt–sucrose (TCBS) agar, on which typical colonies of *V. parahemolyticus* appear in 24 h. (This organism grows poorly and is therefore easily overlooked on deoxycholate culture plates.) The stool generally has numerous polymorphonuclear leukocytes and a smaller number of erythrocytes, but these findings are less prominent than in shigellosis.

Treatment No therapy is required by the large majority of patients. Antimicrobial therapy shortens neither the course nor the duration of pathogen excretion. Antiperistaltic agents are not of clear-cut benefit. An occasional patient may lose sufficient quantities of intestinal fluid to require oral or intravenous fluid therapy.

Prognosis The outcome is almost always good. Fatal cases, occasionally reported from Japan, have occurred in rare instances in patients with serious underlying disease.

VIBRIO MIMICUS *Vibrio mimicus* has been identified as a pathogen in sporadic outbreaks of acute diarrheal disease, occurring in previously healthy individuals of all age groups who have ingested raw seafood (especially oysters) along the Gulf Coast. The epidemiology of *V. mimicus* infections differs from that caused by *V. parahemolyticus* in that, with the exception of one small outbreak, all isolates have represented single, sporadic cases. Although *V. mimicus*, like *V. cholerae*, is not a halophilic vibrio (it grows more rapidly in 1% NaCl than in higher salt solutions), it does not produce cholera enterotoxin, and it causes an illness in which the presenting features are clinically indistinguishable from those caused by *V. parahemolyticus*.

Fever occurs in at least 40 percent of cases and bloody diarrhea in roughly 15 percent. Since the illness is self-limited, treatment is symptomatic. Antibiotic therapy is of no value.

INVASIVE *ESCHERICHIA COLI* Invasive *E. coli*, which are far less common pathogens than enterotoxigenic *E. coli*, may cause a clinical syndrome quite similar to shigellosis with the exceptions that vomiting seldom occurs with the invasive *E. coli* and the illness is of shorter duration. Diarrhea caused by invasive *E. coli* is rare in the United States but has been a significant cause of short-term disability in eastern Europe and southeast Asia. Since the illness caused by invasive *E. coli* is relatively short-lived, antimicrobial therapy has not been shown to be helpful.

CYTOTOXIC *ESCHERICHIA COLI* A single *E. coli* strain, 0157:H7, has been implicated in widely distributed sporadic cases of hemorrhagic colitis in the United States. Undercooked meat, especially hamburger, has been the most frequently identified mode of transmission. All age groups have been affected, and the clinical illness has been indistinguishable from shigellosis. Colonoscopy has demonstrated inflammation, edema, and/or hemorrhage, primarily in the ascending and proximal transverse colon. The mean duration of illness has been 8 days.

All *E. coli* 0157:H7 isolates tested have been noninvasive (Sereny test negative) but have produced Vero cytotoxin which is immunologically indistinguishable from the Shiga toxin produced by *Shigella dysenteriae* type I. Available data indicate that the hemolytic-uremic syndrome is as frequent following *E. coli* 0157:H7 colitis, as it is following shigellosis caused by *S. dysenteriae* type I.

With the exception of the few individuals who developed the hemolytic-uremic syndrome, the illnesses have been self-limited. Treatment with appropriate antimicrobials has not been shown to alter the duration or severity of the illness, but the sporadic occurrence of cases has prevented controlled studies of antibiotic therapy.

ACUTE VIRAL DIARRHEAS

Acute viral gastroenteritis is discussed in detail in Chap. 139. These illnesses are both more common and more life-threatening in small children than adults. In the United States, rotaviruses account for a large proportion of diarrheal illnesses during the first 2 years of life and usually occur during the winter. They have seldom been implicated in adult illness. In rural Bangladesh, infection with rotavirus accounts for roughly 60 percent of episodes of diarrhea in children from 6 to 24 months of age and for about 5 percent in the 2- to 5-year-old age group; it seldom occurs in adolescents and adults. The illness usually presents with vomiting followed by watery diarrhea and low-grade fever, with little or no associated abdominal pain. Vomiting is a prominent and almost constant early manifestation of rotavirus enteritis but rarely persists beyond the first 24 h. Diarrhea often persists for 4 to 8 days. Although the illness is generally not life-threatening, many patients require fluid and electrolyte repletion. Since the vomiting is usually short-lived, fluid repletion can generally be achieved by the oral route, using the same fluids that are effective in the treatment of cholera (see Chap. 115).

The diagnosis can be confirmed by a variety of tests including demonstration of the virus in stool by electron microscopy, a rise in complement-fixing antibody titers, and radioimmunoassay. The most useful and reliable test for rapid diagnosis under field conditions consists of direct demonstration of the antigen in stool by the enzyme-linked immunosorbent assay (ELISA).

Norwalk and Norwalk-like viruses, now implicated in roughly a third of episodes of epidemic gastroenteritis involving adults in the United States, usually cause relatively mild, short (< 36 h), and self-limited disease, for which neither fluid nor drug therapy is necessary (see Chap. 139).

ACUTE PROTOZOAL DIARRHEAS

Giardia lamblia has emerged as a major cause of acute diarrheal disease (see Chap. 160). Although formerly thought to be a pathogen only in children and later considered to be a significant cause of diarrheal disease only in developing nations, this organism is the pathogen most commonly incriminated in outbreaks of waterborne diarrheal disease in the United States where it occurs most commonly in the Rocky Mountain states and more frequently causes disease in visitors than in the indigenous population. The illness characteristically presents with the sudden onset of watery diarrhea and malabsorption, accompanied by mild to moderate abdominal discomfort, bloating, and flatulence. Symptoms may occasionally persist for weeks unless appropriate antimicrobials are administered. Prolonged disease with malabsorption occurs from time to time in previously normal individuals but is particularly common in patients with IgA deficiency, who tend to have the most severe form of giardiasis.

The attack rate may be quite high (> 50 percent) in individuals exposed to contaminated water sources. In certain groups of North American travelers returning from Leningrad, where the water supply appears to be heavily contaminated with *Giardia* cysts, up to 60 percent of individuals have developed clinical giardiasis. The usual incubation period is 10 to 20 days. The illness, therefore, frequently develops after a traveler returns home, and the travel history is a critical element in suspecting the diagnosis. Occasionally the disease occurs endemically in individuals who have not traveled. The diagnosis can be confirmed in approximately half the cases by examining the stool for cysts; if the stool examination is negative in a patient with characteristic clinical features, duodenal aspirates or biopsies will usually yield the characteristic trophozoites. Treatment with quina-crine, 100 mg tid for 5 to 7 days, is generally curative; metronidazole, 250 mg tid for 7 days, is an equally effective alternative regimen.

TRAVELER'S DIARRHEA

Diarrhea is by far the most common health problem of travelers to developing countries. Of more than 16 million travelers annually from industrialized nations to developing countries, approximately one-third will develop diarrhea. The incidence of traveler's diarrhea (TD) varies markedly by destination.

ETIOLOGY AND EPIDEMIOLOGY Virtually all cases of TD are caused by infectious agents, acquired through ingestion of fecally contaminated food and/or water. Especially risky foods include raw vegetables, raw meats, and raw seafood. Foods sold by street vendors are a common source of enteropathogens. Bacterial pathogens account for the great majority of episodes. Overall, the most common etiologic agents in TD are enterotoxigenic *E. coli* (ETEC), which are responsible for 50 to 75 percent of episodes. The culpable ETEC may produce LT, ST, or both enterotoxins, with considerable geographic variation. Other recognized enteropathogens can be isolated from most of the remainder of cases, but with great regional differences in prevalence. For example, *Shigella* causes up to 10 percent of TD in Mexico but is an unusual etiologic agent in North Africa. *Vibrio parahemolyticus* is a relatively common cause of TD in Japanese travelers in Asia but has not been associated with TD in South America. Viruses (rotavirus, Norwalk-like virus) and protozoa (amoebas, *Giardia*) are collectively responsible for fewer than 10 percent of cases of TD.

PATHOGENESIS The pathogenesis varies with the culpable etiologic organism, but most cases of TD, even when caused by *Shigella*, are self-limited illnesses and have not been associated with serious sequelae in previously healthy individuals.

MANIFESTATIONS Episodes of TD usually begin abruptly, with urgent diarrhea, abdominal cramps, nausea, and often low-grade fever. In the great majority of cases, the fluid loss is not voluminous, and symptoms subside within 3 to 5 days.

TREATMENT For the great majority of patients, fluid losses do not demand specific replacement fluids. Patients want relief from the two specific problems of abdominal cramps and diarrhea. Bismuth sub-salicylate, taken as Pepto-Bismol liquid, in a dose of 60 mL qid, can decrease the severity of symptoms. Diphenoxylate and loperamide both provide symptomatic relief, but should not be used in the rare patient with high fever or blood in the stool; the antimotility agents should be discontinued if symptoms persist beyond 48 h. Patients with more severe symptoms (e.g., more than three loose stools within 8 h) may benefit from antimicrobial treatment. Trimethoprim, 160 mg, with sulfamethoxazole, 800 mg, twice daily, or trimethoprim alone, 200 mg twice daily for 3 days, has proved effective in shortening the mean duration of symptoms from 4 to 1.5 days. It is not certain that these antimicrobials will prove equally effective in all parts of the developing world.

PREVENTION The only sure prevention is to avoid ingestion of contaminated water and food, a goal that is not practical for most travelers. Carefully controlled studies have demonstrated that two antimicrobials, doxycycline and trimethoprim-sulfamethoxazole, when taken prophylactically, are consistently effective in reducing the incidence of TD by 50 to 86 percent in various parts of the developing world. Because of the calculable risks of administration of prophylactic antimicrobials to several million travelers annually, balanced against the generally self-limited course of TD, prophylactic antimicrobials are not routinely recommended for prevention of TD. Travelers are advised, however, to obtain therapeutic doses of effective antimicro-bial agents (vide supra) prior to travel to high-risk areas, so that the more severe episodes of TD can be treated early, without recourse to potentially dangerous over-the-counter drugs.

REFERENCES

BARKER WH JR et al: *Vibrio parahemolyticus* outbreak in Covington, Louisiana, in August, 1972. Am J Epidemiol 100:316, 1974

BLACKLOW NR, CUKOR G: Viral gastroenteritis. N Engl J Med 304:397, 1981

BLASER MJ et al: *Campylobacter* enteritis in the United States: A multicenter study. Ann Intern Med 98:360, 1983

———, RELLER BL: *Campylobacter* enteritis. N Engl J Med 305:1444, 1981

CARPENTER CCJ, SACK RB: Infectious diarrheal syndromes, in *Update I: Harrison's Principles of Internal Medicine*, KJ Isselbacher et al (eds). New York, McGraw-Hill, 1981, pp 209–229

CONSENSUS CONFERENCE: Traveler's diarrhea. J Am Med Assoc 253:2700, 1985

DUPONT HL et al: Pathogenesis of *Escherichia coli* diarrhea. N Engl J Med 285:1, 1971

——— et al: Symptomatic treatment of diarrhea with bismuth subsalicylate among students attending a Mexican university. Gastroenterology 73:715, 1977

——— et al: Treatment of traveler's diarrhea with trimethoprim/sulfamethoxazole and with trimethoprim alone. N Engl J Med 307:841, 1982

GORBACH SL et al: Traveller's diarrhea and toxigenic *Escherichia coli*. N Engl J Med 292:933, 1975

GRIFFIN MR et al: Foodborne Norwalk virus. Am J Epidemiol 115:178, 1982

GUERRANT RL et al: Role of toxigenic and invasive bacteria in acute diarrhea of childhood. N Engl J Med 293:576, 1974

——— et al: Campylobacteriosis in man: Pathogenic mechanisms and review of 91 bloodstream infections. Am J Med 65:584, 1978

KAPLAN JE et al: Epidemiology of Norwalk gastroenteritis and the role of Norwalk virus in acute nonbacterial gastroenteritis. Ann Intern Med 96:756, 1982

MERSON MH et al: Traveler's diarrhea in Mexico. A prospective study of physicians and family members attending a Congress. N Engl J Med 294:1299, 1976

QUINN TC et al: Infections with *Campylobacter jejuni* and *Campylobacter*-like organisms in homosexual men. Ann Intern Med 101:187, 1984

REMIS RS et al: Sporadic cases of hemorrhagic colitis associated with *Escherichia coli* 0157:H7. Ann Intern Med 101:624, 1984

SACK DA et al: Oral rehydration in rotavirus diarrhea: A double blind comparison of sucrose with glucose electrolyte solution. Lancet 2:280, 1978

——— et al: Prophylactic doxycycline for traveller's diarrhea. N Engl J Med 298:758, 1978

SACK RB et al: Enterotoxigenic *Escherichia coli* isolated from patients with severe cholera-like disease. J Infect Dis 123:378, 1971

——— et al: Human diarrheal disease caused by enterotoxigenic *Escherichia coli*. Annu Rev Microbiol 29:333, 1975

TAYLOR DN et al: *Campylobacter* enteritis from untreated water in the Rocky Mountains. Ann Intern Med 99:38, 1983

TERRANOVA W et al: Current concepts: *Bacillus cereus* food poisoning. N Engl J Med 298:143, 1978

ZEN-YOJI H et al: Epidemiology, enteropathogenicity and classification of *Vibrio parahemolyticus*. J Infect Dis 115:436, 1965

---

90   SEXUALLY TRANSMITTED DISEASES

KING K. HOLMES / H. HUNTER HANDSFIELD

Venereology encompasses not only the five "venerable" venereal diseases (syphilis, gonorrhea, chancroid, lymphogranuloma vene-reum, and granuloma inguinale) but also a growing number of other diseases which might be considered the "new generation" of sexually transmitted diseases (STDs). The most recently recognized STD is the acquired immunodeficiency syndrome, caused by the AIDS retrovirus (see Chaps. 257 and 293). Like gonorrhea, many of these newer STDs became epidemic in nearly all countries of the world during the past quarter-century. With increasing interest in these diseases and improved methods for diagnosis has come awareness of the growing consequences of STD on health and society, which extend beyond the traditional sphere of venereology; for example, major impact of the newer STDs has been noted on maternal and infant morbidity and on human infertility and reproduction.

CLASSIFICATION OF SEXUALLY TRANSMITTED DISEASES These diseases can be classified on the basis either of their etiologies or their clinical manifestations. Table 90-1 gives an etiologic clas-sification of STD. Sexual transmission has been implicated as an important factor in the propagation of each of the pathogens listed in this table. There have been sporadic case reports of sexual transmission of many other pathogenic agents, but the diseases caused by these other agents are not generally considered, since sexual transmission seems to be a minor factor in their propagation. For each of the agents listed in Table 90-1, there are one or more diseases or syndromes known to be caused by the agent, and others (indicated by a question mark) for which a causal association is suspected but not proven.

APPROACH TO SEXUALLY TRANSMITTED DISEASE

The STDs are viewed throughout the world as a related set of infections for several reasons: knowledge of infectious diseases and dermatology are important for diagnosis and management; skills in the genitourinary examination are required; they are sexually transmitted; and coinfections are common. However, the principal reason for dealing with STDs as a unique set of infections is that no single STD can be regarded as an isolated problem. STDs are not endogenous or transmitted by fomites, food, flies, or casual contact. *An infected partner always exists.* The sexual history and management of sexual partners are therefore of paramount importance. Failure to identify and examine or refer at least one partner represents a failure in management, both at the community level (since sources of spread of infection are not identified) and at the patient level (since reinfection is not prevented). Most persons with genital discharges, lesions, or pain cease sexual activity and seek medical care. Accordingly, those who transmit infection usually are among the minority who are infected but asymptomatic, or who do not understand the implications of their symptoms. Therefore, they do not seek medical attention spontaneously, and physicians must see that they are examined and treated, or referred. In the United States, local health departments will usually identify and treat contacts of some diseases (e.g., syphilis, gonococcal pelvic inflammatory disease), but for most STDs this responsibility is shared by the patient and the physician. With the increasing importance of potentially incurable viral STDs (AIDS retrovirus infection, genital herpes, genital papillomaviruses, hepatitis B virus carriage), the role of counseling to reduce transmission is growing. It is necessary for the clinician to consider the approach to STD syndromes before an etiologic diagnosis is established. Table 90-2 lists some of the most common clinical syndromes and their complications associated with sexually transmitted pathogens. Strategies for the management of some of the common syndromes are outlined below.

MALE URETHRITIS

Urethritis in the male is classified as gonococcal or nongonococcal. The incidence of gonococcal urethritis has stabilized in many western countries, while that of nongonococcal urethritis (NGU) continues to rise, suggesting that current measures for control of NGU are relatively ineffective. In general, gonorrhea and NGU are equally common among men seen in STD clinics in the United States, whereas NGU is approximately three times as common as gonorrhea among men seen by physicians in private practice and 10 times as common as gonorrhea among college students.

About 40 percent of NGU is caused by *Chlamydia trachomatis.* Herpes simplex virus and *Trichomonas vaginalis* each cause a small additional proportion of NGU cases in the United States, but about 50 percent of cases cannot be attributed to any of these three pathogens. *Ureaplasma urealyticum* has been implicated in case-control studies as a probable cause of many of the *Chlamydia*-negative cases. A newly described organism, *Mycoplasma genitalium,* is also under investigation as a possible cause of this syndrome. Since facilities for detection of *U. urealyticum* and *M. genitalium* are not widely available, and the role of these agents is not certain, the diagnosis of male urethritis usually does not include cultures for either organism. However, diagnostic testing for *C. trachomatis* is increasingly available, using isolation of the agent in tissue cell culture, or direct immunofluorescent staining of urethral exudate or enzyme-linked immunosorbent assay for detection of chlamydial antigen. The following steps should be taken in evaluating sexually active men with symptoms of urethral discharge and/or dysuria:

1 *Establish the presence of urethritis.* Commonly in NGU, and less often in gonorrhea, discharge can be demonstrated only by milking the urethra after the patient has not voided for several hours, preferably overnight. If no overt discharge is demonstrable, urethral inflammation can be documented by inserting a small urethrogenital

TABLE 90-1 Twenty-four sexually transmitted pathogens and the diseases they cause

Agent	Disease or syndrome
BACTERIA	
Neisseria gonorrhoeae	Urethritis, epididymitis, proctitis, cervicitis, endometritis, salpingitis, perihepatitis, bartholinitis, pharyngitis, conjunctivitis, prepubertal vaginitis, ?prostatitis, accessory gland infection, amniotic infection syndrome, disseminated gonococcal infection, chorioamnionitis, premature rupture of membranes, and premature delivery
Chlamydia trachomatis	Urethritis, epididymitis, proctitis, cervicitis, endometritis, salpingitis, perihepatitis, bartholinitis, prepubertal vaginitis, otitis media in infants, ?chorioamnionitis, ?premature rupture of membranes, ?premature delivery, inclusion conjunctivitis, infant pneumonia, trachoma, and lymphogranuloma venereum
Mycoplasma hominis	Postpartum fever, ?salpingitis
Ureaplasma urealyticum	?Nongonococcal urethritis, ?chorioamnionitis, ?premature delivery
Treponema pallidum	Syphilis
Gardnerella vaginalis and other vaginal bacteria	Bacterial vaginosis
Haemophilus ducreyi	Chancroid
Calymmatobacterium granulomatis	Donovanosis (granuloma inguinale)
Shigella spp.	Shigellosis in homosexual men
Campylobacter spp.	Enteritis, proctocolitis in homosexual men
Group B streptococcus	Neonatal sepsis, neonatal meningitis
VIRUSES	
AIDS retrovirus (HTLV III/LAV)	Acute mononucleosis-like syndrome, AIDS-related complex (including persistent generalized lymphadenopathy), acquired immunodeficiency syndromes, ?subacute encephalitis and other neurologic syndromes
Herpes simplex virus	Initial and recurrent genital herpes, aseptic meningitis, neonatal herpes, cervical dysplasia and carcinoma, ?carcinoma in situ of the vulva
Hepatitis B virus	Acute hepatitis B, chronic active hepatitis, persistent (unresolved) hepatitis, polyarteritis nodosa, chronic membranous glomerulonephritis, ?mixed cryoglobulinemia, ?polymyalgia rheumatica, hepatocellular carcinoma
Hepatitis A virus	Acute hepatitis A
Cytomegalovirus	Heterophil-negative infectious mononucleosis, congenital infection, gross birth defects and infant mortality, cognitive impairment (e.g., mental retardation, sensorineural deafness), varied manifestations in the immunosuppressed host
Human papilloma virus types 6, 11, 16, 18, 31	Condyloma acuminatum, laryngeal papilloma, cervical dysplasia, Bowen's papulosis, ?squamous cell carcinoma of the cervix, vulva, penis, and anus
Molluscum contagiosum virus	Genital molluscum contagiosum
PROTOZOA	
Trichomonas vaginalis	Trichomonal vaginitis
Entamoeba histolytica	Amebiasis in homosexual men
Giardia lamblia	Giardiasis in homosexual men
FUNGI	
Candida albicans	Vulvovaginitis, balanitis
ECTOPARASITES	
Phthirius pubis	Pubic lice infestation
Sarcoptes scabiei	Scabies

TABLE 90-2 Selected syndromes and complications with corresponding sexually transmitted etiologic agents*

Syndrome	Agent
MEN	
Urethritis	N. gonorrhoeae, C. trachomatis, herpes simplex virus, T. vaginalis U. urealyticum
Epididymitis	C. trachomatis, N. gonorrhoeae
Intestinal infections:	
Proctitis	N. gonorrhoeae, herpes simplex virus, C. trachomatis
Proctocolitis or enterocolitis	Campylobacter spp., Shigella spp., E. histolytica
Enteritis	G. lamblia
Hepatitis	Hepatitis A and B viruses, cytomegalovirus, T. pallidum
Acquired immunodeficiency and related syndromes	AIDS retrovirus (HTLV III/LAV)
WOMEN	
Lower genitourinary tract infection:	
Vulvitis	C. albicans, herpes simplex virus
Vaginitis	T. vaginalis, C. albicans, ?G. vaginalis
Cervicitis	N. gonorrhoeae, C. trachomatis, herpes simplex virus
Urethritis	N. gonorrhoeae, C. trachomatis, herpes simplex virus
Pelvic inflammatory disease	N. gonorrhoeae, C. trachomatis, ?Mycoplasma hominis
Infertility:	
Postsalpingitis, postobstetric, postabortion	N. gonorrhoeae, C. trachomatis, ?M. hominis
Pregnancy morbidity: Chorioamnionitis, amniotic fluid infection, prematurity, premature rupture of membranes, postpartum endometritis, ectopic pregnancy	Several STD agents have been implicated in one or more of these conditions
MEN AND WOMEN	
Neoplasia	
Squamous cell epithelial dysplasia and cancer (cervix, vulva, penis, anus)	?Human papillomavirus, ?herpes simplex virus
Hepatocellular carcinoma	Hepatitis B
Kaposi's sarcoma Non-Hodgkin's lymphomas	AIDS retrovirus (?cofactors)
Genital ulceration with or without regional lymphadenopathy	Herpes simplex virus, T. pallidum, H. ducreyi, Cal. granulomatis, C. trachomatis (LGV strains)
Acute arthritis with urogenital or intestinal infection	N. gonorrhoeae, C. trachomatis, Shigella spp., Campylobacter spp.
Genital warts, molluscum contagiosum	Human papilloma virus, molluscum contagiosum virus
Ectoparasite infestations	Sarcoptes scabiei, Phthirius pubis
Heterophil-negative mononucleosis	Cytomegalovirus, ?Epstein-Barr virus
NEONATES AND INFANTS	
TORCHES syndrome†	Cytomegalovirus, herpes simplex virus, T. pallidum
Conjunctivitis	C. trachomatis, N. gonorrhoeae
Pneumonia	C. trachomatis, ?U. urealyticum
Otitis media	C. trachomatis
Sepsis, meningitis	Group B streptococcus
Cognitive impairment, deafness	Cytomegalovirus, herpes simplex virus, T. pallidum
AIDS and AIDS-related diseases	AIDS retrovirus

For each syndrome, some cases cannot yet be ascribed to any cause and must currently be considered idiopathic.

† TORCHES is an acronym for toxoplasmosis, rubella, cytomegalovirus, herpes, and syphilis. The syndrome consists of various combinations of encephalitis, hepatitis, dermatitis, and disseminated intravascular coagulation.

swab 2 to 3 cm into the urethra and examining the Gram-stained direct smear prepared from this swab for leukocytes. Five or more leukocytes per 1000× field in areas containing cells suggests urethritis. Patients with symptoms who lack objective confirmatory evidence of urethritis on two occasions 1 week apart may have functional problems and generally do not benefit from repeated courses of antibiotics.

2 *Exclude complications or alternative diagnoses.* Epididymitis and systemic complications, such as the gonococcal arthritis-dermatitis syndrome and Reiter's syndrome, should be excluded by brief history and examination. Bacterial prostatitis and cystitis should be excluded by appropriate tests in men with dysuria who lack signs of urethritis. However, digital examination of the prostate gland is seldom informative in patients with urethritis, unless concomitant symptoms such as perineal, suprapubic, or rectal discomfort are present.

3 *Evaluate for gonococcal and chlamydial infection.* The diagnosis of gonorrhea is confirmed by demonstrating typical gram-negative diplococci within neutrophils. The diagnosis of NGU is warranted if gram-negative diplococci are not found. Smears containing only extracellular or atypical gram-negative diplococci are equivocal. In most settings, an attempt should be made to isolate *N. gonorrhoeae* by culture in order to document antimicrobial susceptibility, and also because the predictive value of Gram-stained urethral smears is dependent on the experience of the laboratory. Diagnostic testing for *C. trachomatis* (culture or detection of antigen by immunodiagnosis) should also be performed if resources are available, regardless of the presence or absence of gonorrhea, since coinfection with *N. gonorrhoeae* and *C. trachomatis* is common in men with urethritis. Treatment recommended for gonorrhea includes antimicrobials also effective against *C. trachomatis*, but detection of *Chlamydia* in the male will facilitate management of sexual partners. An approach to the diagnosis of urethritis is illustrated in Fig. 90-1. The treatment of gonorrhea and chlamydial infections is discussed in Chaps. 104 and 150, respectively.

EPIDIDYMITIS Acute epididymitis is almost always unilateral and must be differentiated from testicular torsion, tumor, and trauma. Torsion, a surgical emergency, usually occurs in adolescents and young adults and is suggested by sudden onset of pain, elevation of the testicle within the scrotal sac, and absence of blood flow on Doppler examination or ^{99}Tc scan. In sexually active men under age 35, acute epididymitis is usually caused by *C. trachomatis*, or less commonly by *Neisseria gonorrhoeae*, and is usually associated with overt or subclinical urethritis. Antimicrobial agents are the mainstay of therapy; optimal treatment for epididymitis due to *C. trachomatis* is doxycycline 100 mg twice daily for 10 days. For gonococcal epididymitis, this regimen should be preceded by a single dose of an antibiotic active against both penicillin-sensitive and penicillin-resistant *N. gonorrhoeae*, such as ceftriaxone 125 to 250 mg intramuscularly. Bed rest and scrotal elevation may hasten symptomatic relief.

Acute epididymitis in older men or following urinary tract instrumentation is usually caused by urinary pathogens such as coliform bacteria or *Pseudomonas aeruginosa*. Urethritis is usually absent, but bacteriuria is present. Treatment should be initiated with a broad-spectrum, parenteral antibiotic (e.g., tobramycin) and continued with the appropriate antibiotics as determined by sensitivity tests. An algorithm for diagnosis and management of acute epididymitis in sexually active men is presented in Fig. 90-2.

LOWER GENITOURINARY TRACT INFECTION IN WOMEN Infections of the female urinary tract, cervix, vulva, and vagina produce dysuria, vulvar irritation, dyspareunia, and altered quality or increased quantity of vaginal discharge. Diagnostic confusion may be attributable not only to the symptomatology, which is nonspecific, but also to the lack of consistent application of available laboratory tests, and to the difficulty in differentiating true inflammatory conditions from functional genitourinary complaints. Two steps are required in the evaluation of lower genitourinary symptoms in women: (1) differentiation among cystitis, urethritis, vaginitis, cervicitis, and cervical ectopy, and (2) exclusion of associated upper tract disease (e.g., pyelonephritis, salpingitis).

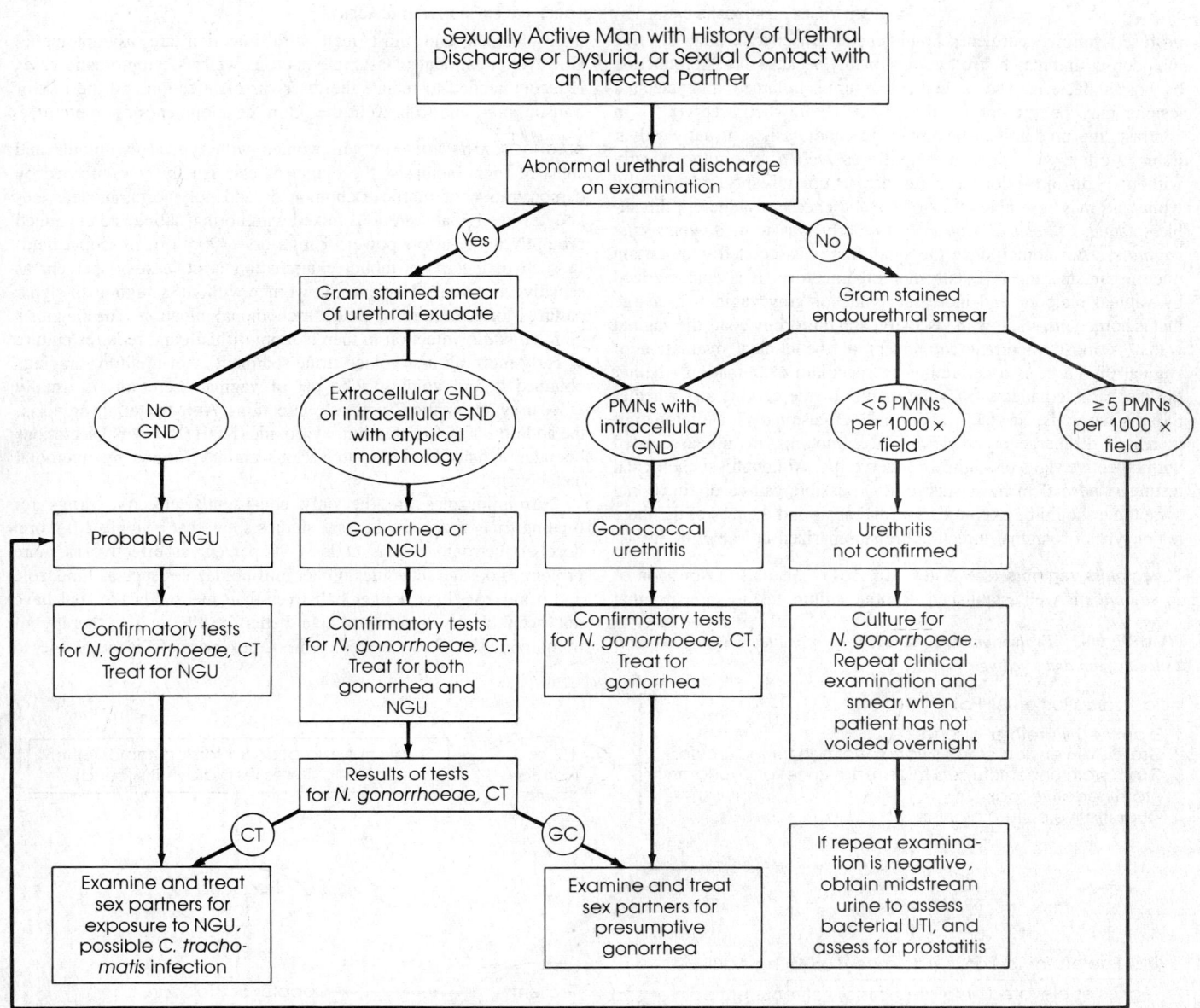

FIGURE 90-1 *Evaluation of sexually active men with suspected urethritis. PMN = polymorphonuclear leukocyte; GND = gram-negative diplococci; NGU = nongonococcal urethritis; UTI = urinary tract infection.*

Cystitis and urethritis Although dysuria is more common in bacterial urinary tract infection (UTI) than in vaginitis, dysuria is often attributable to vaginitis in young women because vaginitis is substantially more common than UTI. Localization of dysuria as "internal" is suggestive of UTI or "urethritis," while "external" dysuria (caused by painful contact of urine with the labia) is associated with vulvovaginitis. In a study of female college students with dysuria, urgency, or frequency without vaginal infection, about half had bacterial cystitis with 10^5 bacteria or more per milliliter of urine, and one-quarter had bacterial cystitis with less than 10^5 bacteria per milliliter (usually between 10^2 and 10^5 per milliliter). About one-quarter had urethral symptoms without bacteriuria—often termed the *urethral syndrome* or *dysuria-frequency syndrome*. In the latter group, about half had pyuria, and most of these were infected with *C. trachomatis*, while most of those without pyuria had no demonstrable infection and improved with placebo therapy. In populations whose risk of gonorrhea is higher than that of college students, *N. gonorrhoeae* is also a common cause of the urethral syndrome.

DIAGNOSIS AND THERAPY   As outlined in Fig. 90-3, the first step in the evaluation of dysuria and frequency in sexually active women is the differentiation of cystitis or urethritis from vaginitis by history and examination. Among women without vaginitis, bacterial UTI must then be differentiated from the urethral syndrome. The finding of a single conventional urinary pathogen, such as *Escherichia coli* or *Staphylococcus saprophyticus*, in a concentration of $\geq 10^2$ per milliliter in a properly collected midstream urine specimen from a symptomatic woman with pyuria indicates probable bacterial UTI, whereas pyuria with fewer than 10^2 conventional uropathogens per milliliter of urine ("sterile pyuria") suggests the diagnosis of acute urethral syndrome due to *C. trachomatis* or *N. gonorrhoeae*. Gonorrhea should be excluded by culture of the cervix and urethra. Chlamydial infection should be excluded by culture or specific immunologic tests for chlamydial antigen in urethral and cervical specimens. Treatment with tetracycline (e.g., tetracycline HCl, 500 mg four times daily for 7 days) has been shown to alleviate symptoms in women with "sterile" pyuria and dysuria, but not in women without pyuria or isolation of a pathogen. The sexual partners of such patients should also be examined and considered for treatment.

VAGINITIS   In self-referred women attending STD clinics, vaginitis is the most common diagnosis. In most patients, bacterial vaginosis is the most common cause of vulvovaginal symptoms, followed by candidiasis, with trichomoniasis least common.

Vaginal infection, without UTI, is characterized by one or more of the following: increased volume of discharge; abnormal yellow color of discharge caused by increased concentration of polymorphonuclear leukocytes; vulvar itching, irritation, or burning; dyspareunia; and malodor. *Trichomonas vaginalis* characteristically produces a profuse, yellow, purulent, homogeneous discharge that is often malodorous and may be frothy, presumably because of gas production by vaginal bacteria. The vaginal epithelium is inflamed, and petechial lesions may be present on the cervix (''strawberry cervix''). In contrast, the predominant symptom in candidiasis is usually vulvar itching, often with signs of vulvitis as well as vaginitis, usually without a distinct odor. The discharge, often scanty, is typically white and may resemble curds of cottage cheese or adherent thrush-like plaques. *Bacterial vaginosis* formerly was termed *nonspecific vaginitis,* a misnomer since the syndrome is associated with certain microorganisms and is usually noninflammatory. It is characterized by vaginal malodor and increased white or gray vaginal discharge that is homogeneous, low in viscosity, and uniformly coats the vaginal walls. A most important component of the clinical evaluation of vaginal discharge is ascertaining by speculum examination whether the discharge emanates from the vagina or the cervix, and whether the discharge is, in fact, abnormal. Occasionally, symptoms of increased discharge or other vaginal symptoms are not associated with objective signs of vaginitis or cervicitis. Although psychological testing is normal in most such cases, possible causes of functional symptoms should be explored. The diagnosis and therapy of the three major types of vaginal infection are summarized in Table 90-3.

T. vaginalis vaginitis (see also Chap. 161)   Sexual transmission of *T. vaginalis* is well established. Routine culture testing indicates that

many women and most men with infection are asymptomatic. However, treatment of asymptomatic as well as symptomatic cases is recommended to reduce the reservoir of infection and the risk of transmission, and to prevent the future development of symptoms.

DIAGNOSIS AND THERAPY   In women with typical symptoms and signs of trichomoniasis, the diagnosis can usually be confirmed by demonstration of motile trichomonads and polymorphonuclear leukocytes in vaginal secretions mixed with normal saline and examined promptly under a low-power or high dry (400×) microscopic field. In such patients, wet-mount examination is at least 80 percent as sensitive as culture. However, in women without symptoms or signs, culture is often required to detect trichomonal infection. The diagnosis of *T. vaginalis* infection in men is more difficult and requires culture of early morning first-voided urine sediment or of urethral scrapings obtained before voiding. The pH of vaginal secretions is usually ≥5.0 in symptomatic *T. vaginalis* infections. As in bacterial vaginosis, the addition of 10% potassium hydroxide (KOH) to vaginal secretions liberates a fishy odor due to various amines formed by microbial metabolism.

Nitroimidazoles are the only consistently effective drugs for treating trichomoniasis. Several studies show that a single 2.0-g oral dose of metronidazole is at least 90 percent as effective as more prolonged dosage schedules. Other nitroimidazoles such as tinidazole and ornidazole have longer half-lives than metronidazole, but have not been clearly shown to give better results in the therapy of trichomoniasis. Routine treatment of sex partners is advisable to

FIGURE 90-2 *Evaluation and management of patients with unilateral testicular pain and swelling.*

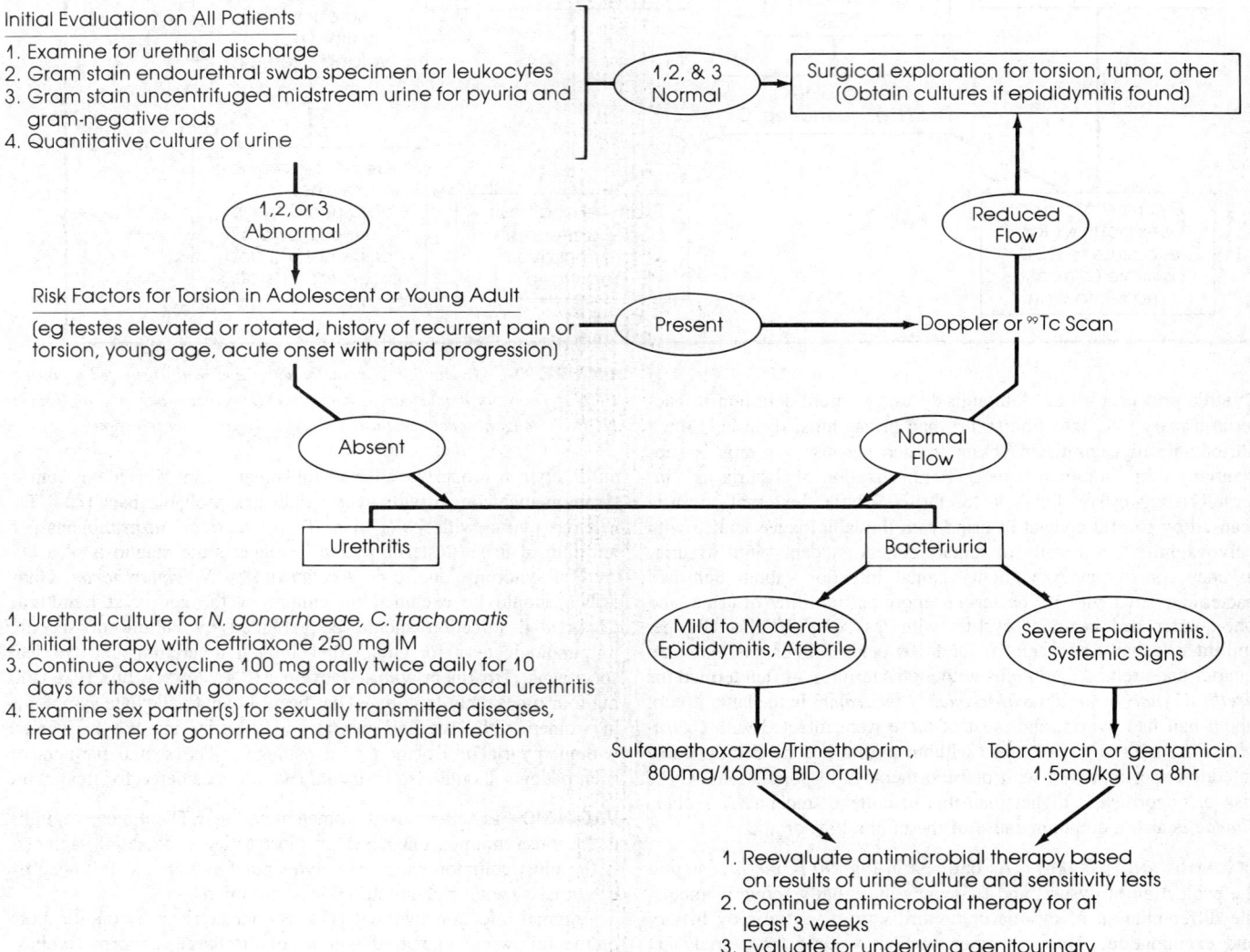

Bed rest and scrotal elevation are recommended for all patients with acute epididymitis.

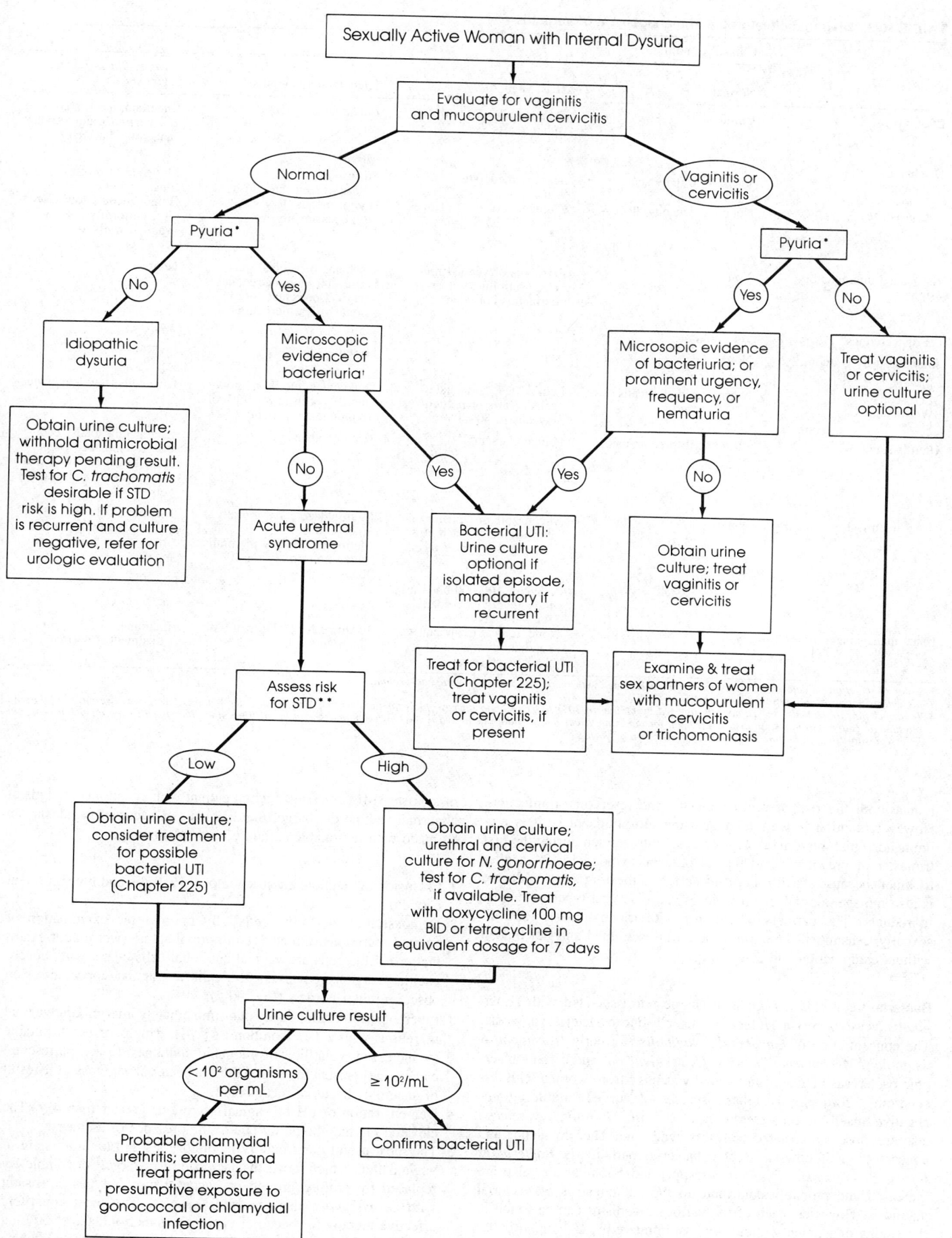

FIGURE 90-3 *Evaluation of sexually active women with "internal" dysuria.*
*Pyuria is defined as ≥ 20 WBC per 400× microscopic field of a centrifuged midstream urine specimen, or ≥ 1 WBC per 400× field of uncentrifuged urine.

†Microscopic evidence of bacteriuria is the presence of ≥ 1 bacillus per 400× field of an uncentrifuged midstream specimen of urine.
**Evaluation of STD risk is based on number and nature of sexual partner(s), recent change in partner, marital status, past history of STD, etc.

TABLE 90-3 Diagnostic features and management of vaginitis

	Clinical Condition			
	Normal	Yeast vaginitis	Trichomonal vaginitis	*Gardnerella*-associated vaginosis
Etiology	Uninfected	*Candida albicans* and other yeasts	*Trichomonas vaginalis*	Uncertain; associated with *G. vaginalis* and various anaerobic bacteria
Discharge: Amount Color* Consistency	Variable; usually scant Clear or white Nonhomogeneous, flocculant	Scant to moderate White Clumped; adherent plaques	Profuse Yellow, green, brownish Homogeneous, low viscosity; occasionally frothy	Moderate to profuse Clear or white Homogeneous, low viscosity, uniformly coating vaginal walls; occasionally frothy
Associated inflammatory signs	None	Erythema of vaginal mucosa, introitus; vulvar dermatitis common	Erythema of vaginal mucosa, introitus; occasional cervical petechiae; occasional vulvar dermatitis	None
pH of secretions†	≤4.5	≤4.5	≥5.0	>4.5
Amine (''fishy'') odor with 10% KOH‡	None	None	Present	Present
Microscopy Wet mount	Normal epithelial cells	Leukocytes, epithelial cells; yeasts or pseudomycelia in 50–80%	Leukocytes; motile trichomonads seen in 80–90% of symptomatic patients	Clue cells; few leukocytes
Gram's stain	Lactobacilli predominate	Fungal elements	Trichomonads	Lactobacilli totally or largely replaced by profuse flora consistent with *G. vaginalis* and anaerobes
Usual treatment	None	Miconazole or clotrimazole intravaginally, each 50–100 mg daily for 7 days Nystatin, 100,000 units intravaginally twice daily for 7–14 days	Metronidazole 2.0 g orally (single dose) Metronidazole 250 mg orally three times daily for 10 days	Metronidazole 500 mg orally twice daily for 7 days
Usual management of sex partners	None	None; topical treatment if candidal dermatitis of penis is present	Examine for STD; treat with metronidazole	Examine for STD; no treatment if normal

* Color of secretions is determined by examining a swab coated with secretions against a white background.
† pH determination is not useful if blood is present.
‡ To detect fungal elements, secretions are digested by boiling in 10% KOH prior to microscopic examination; to examine for other features, secretions are mixed (1:1) with physiologic saline. Gram's stain also is excellent for detecting yeasts and pseudomycelia and is the only technique useful for distinguishing lactobacilli from other bacteria, but is less sensitive than the saline preparation for detection of T. vaginalis.

reduce both the risk of reinfection and the reservoir of infection. However, caution is warranted in using nitroimidazoles. It is recommended that metronidazole not be given to women during the first trimester of pregnancy and that alcohol be avoided for 24 h after treatment because of a disulfiram-like effect of the drug. Metronidazole is also mutagenic, and massive doses cause several types of tumors in rodents. The partners of patients with trichomoniasis (and all sexually transmitted infections) should be examined and not treated without examination and counseling.

Bacterial vaginosis Vaginal discharge not associated with *T. vaginalis,* yeast, or cervical infection is usually due to bacterial vaginosis. The concentration of *Gardnerella vaginalis* (formerly *Haemophilus vaginalis*), *Mycoplasma hominis, U. urealyticum,* and certain anaerobic bacteria is increased in vaginal washings from women with this syndrome. Two closely related species of curved, motile, gram-negative anaerobic rods (*Mobiluncus curtisii, Mobiluncus mulieris*) also are closely associated with this syndrome. The prevalence and concentration of other anaerobic bacteria, particularly *Bacteroides bivius, B. capillosis, Peptococcus* spp., and *Eubacterium,* also are increased and probably contribute to the pathogenesis of bacterial vaginosis. However, each of the various organisms can be found in the vagina of women without this syndrome; e.g., *G. vaginalis* has been isolated from the vagina of up to 50 percent of normal women. Metronidazole treatment of the male sex partners of women with bacterial vaginosis does not prevent recurrence of the syndrome in the female.

DIAGNOSIS AND TREATMENT In a patient with symptoms or signs of abnormal vaginal discharge, the diagnosis of bacterial vaginosis can be made with reasonable certainty by the following:

1 Exclusion of candidal and trichomonal vaginitis and mucopurulent cervicitis.
2 Demonstration of ''clue cells'' by microscopic examination of vaginal secretions diluted 1:1 in normal saline (wet-mount examination). Clue cells are vaginal epithelial cells coated with coccobacillary organisms, giving the cells a granular appearance and obscuring their borders (Fig. 90-4).
3 Liberation of a distinct fishy odor immediately after mixing vaginal secretions with a 10% solution of KOH. This odor is attributable to increased volatility of biogenic diamines (e.g., putrescine, cadaverine) present in vaginal fluid in bacterial vaginosis, the result of anaerobic bacterial metabolism.
4 Demonstration of pH of vaginal secretions greater than 4.5. The elevated pH may be partly due to the presence of amines.
5 The most useful confirmatory laboratory test is the Gram stain of vaginal fluid, which shows that lactobacilli are largely or completely replaced by profuse growth of bacterial morphotypes consistent with *G. vaginalis* plus anaerobic species. The most consistent effective therapy for bacterial vaginosis is metronidazole, 500 mg twice daily for 7 days, perhaps because of the role of the anaerobes, which are highly susceptible to metronidazole in this infection. Ampicillin, 500 mg four times daily for 7 days, has been effective in about 40 to 50 percent of cases of bacterial vaginosis, and is

the primary alternative to metronidazole. Sulfonamide-containing vaginal creams are usually ineffective, probably because sulfonamides are inactive against both *G. vaginalis* and many vaginal anaerobes. Tetracycline therapy also is usually ineffective. Treatment of male partners of women with this syndrome does not affect recurrence rates and is not indicated.

Vulvovaginal candidiasis *Candida albicans* accounts for about 80 percent of yeasts isolated from the vagina, while *Torulopsis glabrata* and other less commonly encountered *Candida* species are found in the remainder. Overt vulvovaginitis is more common among women colonized by *C. albicans* than among those colonized with *T. glabrata* or other species. Most cases of vulvovaginal candidiasis probably result from increased growth of yeasts that previously colonized the vagina, or by spread of organisms from the anus. Some cases of recurrent vulvovaginal candidiasis may be due to sexual transmission from a colonized male.

DIAGNOSIS AND THERAPY   The diagnosis of yeast vaginitis involves demonstration of fungal elements by microscopic examination of vaginal secretions in saline or 10% KOH, or by Gram's stain. Demonstration of pseudohyphae strengthens the diagnosis of vaginitis due to *C. albicans*. Microscopic examination is less sensitive than culture, but culture has the disadvantage of detecting asymptomatic carriage in women who may not require therapy. The pH of vaginal secretions is usually less than 4.5, and the vaginal odor is normal. Vulvitis often accompanies vaginitis and may result in superficial erosions that must be differentiated from genital herpes. In most circumstances, therapy for candidal vaginal infection is indicated only if the patient is symptomatic. The usual treatment is intravaginal miconazole or clotrimazole, 100 mg once daily for 7 days; intravaginal nystatin is less effective. Simultaneous therapy with oral nystatin, with the intent of eradicating colonic colonization with *Candida*, does not reduce the risk of recurrent yeast vaginitis. Treatment of the sex partner is not routinely indicated, although this has not been studied rigorously.

MUCOPURULENT CERVICITIS   Mucopurulent cervicitis refers to inflammation of the columnar epithelium and subepithelial lesions of the endocervix, and of any contiguous columnar epithelium that lies exposed in an ectopic position on the exocervix. Mucopurulent cervicitis in the female can be regarded as the "silent" partner of urethritis in the male, being equally common and caused by the same agents but more difficult to recognize. It is the most common major STD syndrome in women and can lead to pelvic inflammatory disease, and in pregnant women may lead to obstetrical complications. Improved recognition and treatment of this syndrome would greatly improve the control of STD. Mucopurulent cervicitis usually is caused by *C. trachomatis*, sometimes by *N. gonorrhoeae*. About one-third of cases are associated with neither of these organisms; these have been correlated with *U. urealyticum* infections, but this requires confirmation. The syndrome can usually be differentiated clinically from cervicitis caused by primary or recurrent herpes simplex virus infection, which produces lesions on the stratified squamous epithelium of the exocervix, as well as on the columnar epithelium; and from vaginitis caused by *C. albicans* or *T. vaginalis*.

DIAGNOSIS AND THERAPY   The diagnosis is made by demonstrating mucopurulent discharge from the cervical os (analogous to demonstrating abnormal exudate in the male urethra) or by demonstrating increased numbers of polymorphonuclear leukocytes in Gram-stained or Papanicolaou smears of endocervical discharge from women without visible mucus (analogous to criteria now widely used to diagnose urethritis in men without overt urethral discharge). Cervical ectopy (see below) that is edematous and bleeds readily when swabbed is also a common sign of mucopurulent cervicitis due to *C. trachomatis*. Cervical biopsy in such cases shows infiltration of the stroma and epithelium predominantly by lymphocytes, plasma cells, and histiocytes characteristically with lymphoid germinal centers (follicular cervicitis).

A simple way to demonstrate mucopurulent discharge from the cervix, which augments the visual documentation of abnormal exudate, is to observe the color of cervical mucus on a white swab removed from the endocervix; a yellow color indicates the presence of mucopus. After the results of this "swab test" are noted, the cervical mucus should be rolled *thinly* on a slide for Gram staining. An area of the slide should be identified which contains strands of cervical mucus which are not contaminated by vaginal squamous epithelial cells or bacteria. The presence of ≥10 polymorphonuclear cells per 1000× microscopic field within strands of cervical mucus suggests cervicitis. In studies in STD clinics and student gynecology clinics, the prevalence of *C. trachomatis* infection has been approximately 50 percent among women with mucopurulent cervicitis by the above criteria and 10 percent among women without it. The presence of a characteristic pattern of inflammatory cells on Papanicolaou smears of endocervical cells is also increasingly being used by cytopathologists to suggest the possibility of chlamydial infection and the need for specific confirmatory testing.

Mucopurulent cervicitis requires antimicrobial therapy. An etiologic diagnosis should always be established to guide management of sexual partners, but therapy should usually be initiated against the most likely causes of this syndrome, while results of diagnostic tests are pending. The diagnosis of gonococcal cervicitis is made by Gram's stain and culture of an endocervical specimen. If a specimen is properly collected from within the endocervix after first wiping the cervix clean to remove vaginal material, then the sensitivity of the Gram's stain showing intracellular gram-negative diplococci (in comparison with culture) is about 50 percent. However, the specificity approaches 100 percent, and observation of intracellular gram-negative diplococci by an experienced microscopist indicates gonococcal

FIGURE 90-4 *A. Vaginal epithelial "clue cells." Note granular appearance due to adherent G. vaginalis and indistinct cell margins. 400×. B. Normal vaginal epithelial cells. The cell margins are distinct and lack granularity.*

A

B

infection, even if the culture is negative. The sensitivity of a single endocervical culture for *N. gonorrhoeae* is 80 to 90 percent.

Chlamydial infection of the cervix can be confirmed by culture or antigen detection. The sensitivity of a single endocervical culture for *C. trachomatis* is estimated to be 80 percent or more. The sensitivity of antigen detection approaches that of isolation of the organism in cell culture. Antigen detection by direct immunofluorescence is specific in experienced hands, but detection by enzyme immunoassay may be less specific. While diagnostic test results are pending, therapy can be initiated with a single-dose regimen effective for gonorrhea, plus tetracycline hydrochloride, 500 mg four times per day, or doxycycline, 100 mg twice daily, orally for 1 week. For pregnant women, erythromycin base or stearate, in a dose of 500 mg four times daily for 7 to 14 days, can be substituted for the tetracycline-doxycycline treatment. The male sex partners of women with non-gonococcal mucopurulent cervicitis should be examined for urethritis and other STD, and treated for exposure to any infection found in the female. If cultures for *C. trachomatis* are not available, the male partners should be treated for presumptive chlamydial infection, regardless of whether urethritis is documented.

Cervical ectopy Cervicitis must be differentiated from cervical ectopy, which is often mislabeled "cervical erosion." Ectopy represents the presence of the 1-cell-thick columnar endocervical epithelium in an exposed visible "ectopic" position on the cervix, where it appears redder than the 20-cell-thick stratified squamous vaginal epithelium. When ectopy is present, the cervical os may contain clear or slightly cloudy mucus, but not mucopus. Colposcopy shows that the epithelium is intact and not ulcerated. Ectopy is normally present during early adolescence and gradually recedes as squamous metaplasia replaces the ectopic columnar epithelium. Oral contraceptive usage or pregnancy favors persistence or reappearance of ectopy. The use of cauterizing procedures to eliminate ectopy is controversial. The presence of ectopy may make the cervix more susceptible to infection with *N. gonorrhoeae* or *C. trachomatis* by exposing a larger surface area of susceptible columnar epithelium. When mucopurulent cervicitis supervenes, the area of ectopy may become edematous and fragile, with bleeding induced by gentle swabbing. In addition, edema of the cervix may result in eversion of the os, enlarging the apparent area of ectopy.

ULCERATIVE LESIONS OF THE GENITALIA Genital skin lesions can be classified as ulcerative or nonulcerative. Nonulcerative genital lesions include several sexually transmitted infections such as scabies, genital warts, *Candida* balanitis or vulvitis, or genital molluscum contagiosum, as well as a broad spectrum of nonsexually transmitted dermatologic conditions.

The incidence and etiology of ulcerative lesions of the genitalia vary greatly in different areas of the world (Table 90-4). In Asia and Africa, genital ulcers are seen as frequently as gonorrhea in some STD clinics, and chancroid is the commonest cause, while genital herpes is relatively uncommon. In the industrialized western countries, genital ulcers are considerably less common than urethritis or vaginitis, and genital herpes is the commonest form, with chancroid being relatively uncommon. Syphilis has been the second commonest form

of genital ulcer in all areas of the world and must always be excluded. Lymphogranuloma venereum (LGV) and donovanosis (granuloma inguinale) are rare causes of genital ulceration.

DIAGNOSIS AND THERAPY In industrialized countries, the differential diagnosis of genital ulceration, when trauma and excoriated lesions are excluded, usually rests among genital herpes simplex virus (HSV) infection, syphilis, and, rarely, chancroid. Epidemiologic factors that increase the likelihood of chancroid, LGV, or donovanosis include acquisition of infection in a developing country and sexual contact with a prostitute, a homosexual, or an individual of low socioeconomic status. The clinical findings are occasionally definitive (e.g., presence of herpetic vesicles), and clinical findings plus epidemiologic considerations usually help to guide initial therapy pending further studies. Nevertheless, most genital ulcerations cannot be diagnosed confidently on clinical grounds. It is axiomatic to exclude syphilis by appropriate serology in all cases. Dark-field examination should also be performed, by experienced technicians when possible, on lesions suggesting primary or secondary syphilis. Direct immunofluorescence using monoclonal antibodies to *T. pallidum* is at least as sensitive and specific as dark-field microscopy for detection of *T. pallidum* in lesion exudate, and can be performed on specimens sent to a central laboratory. This procedure should become available in the future. Chancroid should not be used as "wastebasket" diagnosis for all ulcerative lesions not attributable to syphilis or genital herpes since few such lesions are confirmed as chancroid, except in developing nations, or in certain local outbreaks (e.g., Manitoba, California, New York City, or Florida in recent years). Selective enrichment media are available for isolation of *Haemophilus ducreyi* from such cases.

The following general guidelines are recommended for management of ulcerative genital lesions (Fig. 90-5):

1 *If typical painful herpetic vesicles or pustules are present:* In this case the clinical diagnosis of herpes is warranted, although a serologic test for syphilis should be performed. If desired, the diagnosis can be confirmed by isolation of HSV in 90 percent and by cytology (Papanicolaou smear) in about two-thirds of patients with intact vesicles or pustules. Immunochemical detection with specific monoclonal antibody is also a promising technique.

2 *If painful nonvesicular ulcer(s) raise the suspicion of herpes or chancroid:* If the lesions(s) or inguinal node(s) is painful or has other features suggestive of herpes or chancroid, attempts to demonstrate HSV or *H. ducreyi* are indicated. All methods of HSV detection are somewhat less sensitive in the ulcerative stage than in the vesicular stage. Syphilis should be excluded by dark-field examination and serologic testing, both of which should be repeated 1 to 2 weeks later if negative initially and if other diagnoses cannot be confirmed.

3 *If painless ulcerative lesions suggest the diagnosis of syphilis:* If lesions are at all suggestive of syphilis, or there are epidemiologic reasons to suspect syphilis, such as recent exposure, then dark-field examination and a rapid serologic test for syphilis should be performed for prompt diagnosis. If these are negative, two more dark-field examinations on successive days are recommended, and

TABLE 90-4 Etiology of genital ulcers in six studies, showing marked difference in populations*

	Percent of patients†					
	Detroit (N = 100)	Seattle (N = 82)	Nairobi (N = 97)	Swaziland (N = 155)	Johannesburg/ Soweto (N = 102)	Papua (New Guinea) (N = 101)
Chancroid	2	1	62	44	61	0
Genital herpes	40	55	5	12	17	0
Syphilis	17	12	11	19	9	50
Lymphogranuloma venereum	0	0	0	12	1	23
Donovanosis	0	0	0	1	1	46
Other	12	12	5	0	4	
Unknown	37	21	24	15	15	15

* Only men were studied in Detroit, and only women in Papua; the other series included both sexes.
† A variable proportion of patients in each series had multiple etiologies; therefore, percentages total >100.

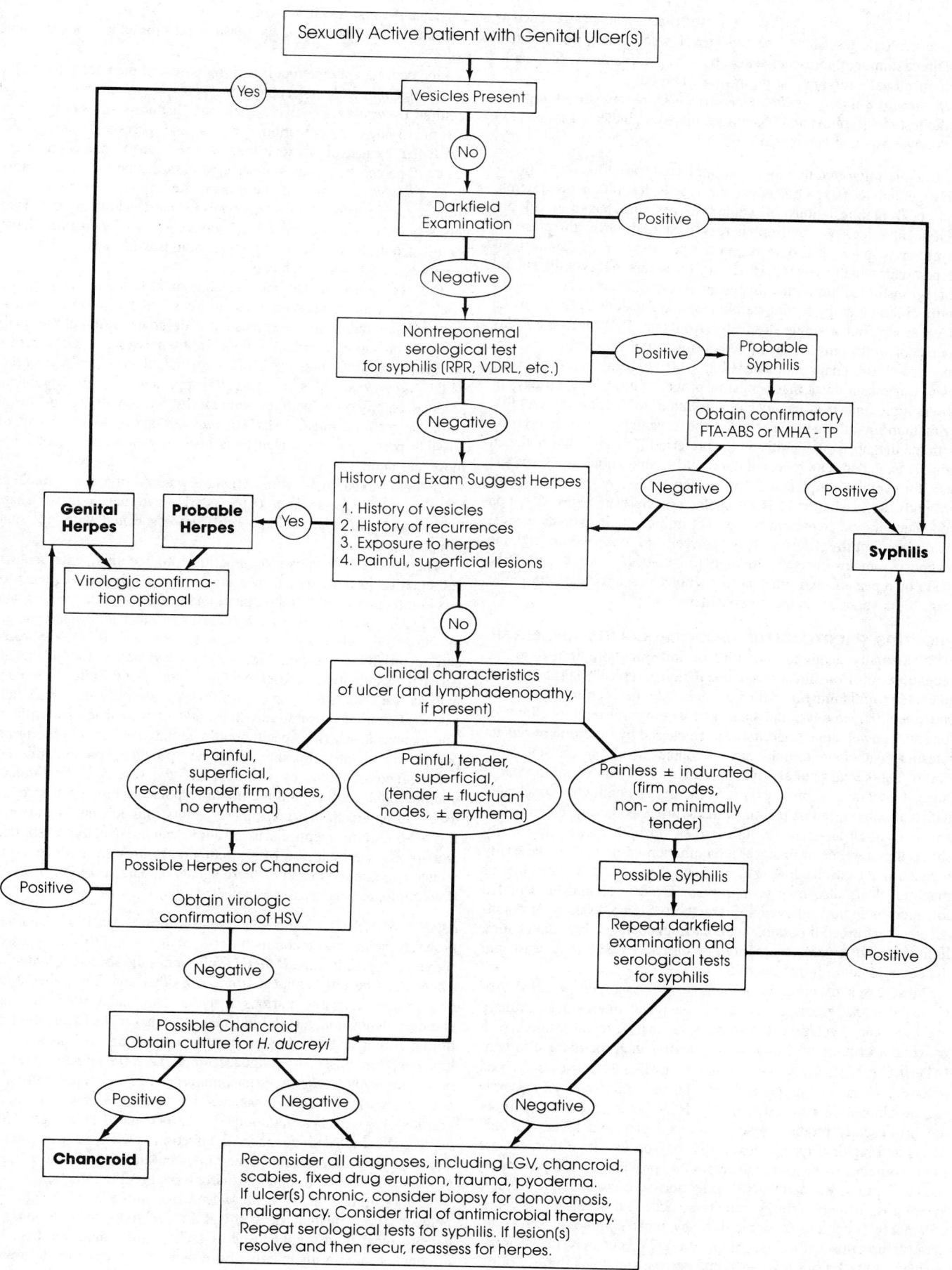

FIGURE 90-5 *Evaluation of sexually active persons with genital ulcer–inguinal lymphadenopathy syndromes.*

the serologic test should be repeated 1 week and 6 weeks later. Direct immunofluorescent detection of *T. pallidum* with specific monoclonal antibody is a promising technique.

4 *If chronic painless genital ulceration progresses:* In addition to the tests for syphilis and chancroid, biopsy is indicated to exclude donovanosis and carcinoma.

Oral antimicrobial therapy is not indicated for undiagnosed ulcerative genital lesions. Oral acyclovir speeds resolution of systemic and local manifestations of genital herpes and has a small but significant effect on recurrent herpes if started early; therefore, if acyclovir is given, it should be started promptly if the diagnosis of herpes seems likely (see Chap. 136). Treatment for syphilis should not be instituted until the diagnosis is established. The value of antimicrobial therapy for idiopathic ulcerative lesions of the genitalia is uncertain, but a single dose of ceftriaxone, 250 mg, or a 7-day course of erythromycin or trimethoprim-sulfamethoxazole, as recommended for chancroid (see Chap. 110), seems reasonable for lesions of recent onset that persist or progress during several days of observation and that cannot be attributed to herpes or syphilis. Trimethoprim-sulfamethoxazole has the advantage of not interfering with the diagnosis of syphilis and is preferred if syphilis has not been reliably excluded, and repeated dark-field examinations and serologic tests for syphilis are planned. Antimicrobial therapy should be given promptly when chancroid is probable, especially if regional lymph node suppuration is present or appears imminent. If patients worsen or do not improve during 1 or 2 weeks of observation and the diagnosis remains obscure, attempts to isolate *H. ducreyi* should be made or repeated, and other noninfectious and infectious etiologies (e.g., donovanosis) should be considered.

PROCTITIS, PROCTOCOLITIS OR ENTEROCOLITIS, AND ENTERITIS   Sexually acquired proctitis, or inflammation limited to the rectum, results from direct rectal inoculation of typical STD pathogens. In contrast, inflammation which extends from the rectum to the colon (proctocolitis), involves the small and large bowel (enterocolitis), or the small bowel alone (enteritis) can be caused by ingestion of typical intestinal pathogens through sexual contact involving oral-fecal exposure. Anorectal pain and mucopurulent or bloody rectal discharge suggest proctitis or proctocolitis. Proctitis is commonly associated with tenesmus and constipation, whereas proctocolitis and enterocolitis are more often associated with diarrhea. In both, anoscopy usually shows the presence of mucosal inflammation with exudate and easily induced mucosal bleeding (i.e., positive "wipe test"). Petechial or mucosal ulcers also may be observed. Exudate should be sampled for microbiologic studies and Gram stain. Sigmoidoscopy or colonoscopy, performed if possible without an enema, shows inflammation limited to the rectum in proctitis, or disease extending at least into the sigmoid colon in proctocolitis.

Most cases of proctitis are due to *N. gonorrhoeae,* HSV, or *C. trachomatis;* these are acquired via rectal intercourse. Primary and secondary syphilis can also produce anal or rectal lesions, with or without symptoms. Gonococcal proctitis and proctitis due to non-LGV strains of *C. trachomatis* typically involve the most distal rectal mucosa and the anal crypts and are clinically mild, without systemic manifestations. In contrast, primary HSV proctitis and LGV proctocolitis usually produce severe anorectal pain and fever. Perianal ulcers and inguinal lymphadenopathy may occur with either, but are more common with anorectal herpes. Approximately 50 percent of men with primary anorectal HSV infection have associated neurologic symptoms, usually urinary retention, S5-S5 dysesthesias or, less commonly, impotence. Sigmoidoscopy most commonly shows ulcerative proctitis with either herpes or LGV, but may reveal intact vesicopustular lesions with anorectal herpes. In herpes, biopsy of the rectal mucosa shows microulcerations and may show intranuclear inclusions or perivascular lymphocytic cuffing. In LGV, biopsy typically shows crypt abscesses, granulomas, and giant cells, findings indistinguishable from those of Crohn's disease or idiopathic ulcerative proctocolitis. Syphilis can also produce rectal granulomas, usually

associated with infiltration by plasma cells or other mononuclear cells.

Proctocolitis and enterocolitis in homosexual men are most often caused by *Campylobacter* spp. or *Shigella* spp., which are primarily acquired by oral-anal contact. These are diagnosed by stool culture and microscopic examination for ova and parasites. *Entamoeba histolytica,* a cause of proctocolitis, has also been extremely prevalent (up to 25 percent) in studies of selected homosexual men, but strains of *E. histolytica* found in these men are reported to be of low virulence and of uncertain relationship to intestinal symptoms. Two new species of *Campylobacter* (*C. cinaedi* and *C. fennellae*) have been isolated almost exclusively from homosexual men, and appear to be associated with proctocolitis.

The occurrence of diarrhea and abdominal bloating or cramping pain, without anorectal symptoms, in association with normal anoscopy and sigmoidoscopy, is consistent with inflammation of the small intestine or more proximal colon. In homosexual men, enteritis limited to the small intestine is often attributable to *Giardia lamblia,* while *Campylobacter* spp., *Shigella* spp. and *E. histolytica* can produce enterocolitis with or without lesions involving the distal colon or rectum. *Blastocystis hominis,* an intestinal protozoan of possible pathogenic significance, is also very prevalent among homosexual men.

In homosexual men with AIDS, a variety of other pathogens [including *Cryptosporidium* (Chap. 161), cytomegalovirus (Chap. 137), and *C. albicans* (Chap. 146)] are associated with intestinal symptoms.

The etiologic diagnosis of proctitis, proctocolitis, enterocolitis, and enteritis in homosexual men is confounded by the frequency of mixed infection. For example, nearly half of those with proctitis who have rectal gonorrhea also have at least one other intestinal or rectal infection. For this reason, the diagnostic evaluation is complicated and potentially expensive. The minimum evaluation should include perianal examination, anoscopy, Gram stain, and culture of rectal mucosa (or exudate, if present) for *N. gonorrhoeae,* dark-field examination of any ulcerative lesions, and a serologic test for syphilis. The manner in which a specific etiologic diagnosis should be further pursued is dictated by the syndrome (proctitis, proctocolitis, or enteritis/enterocolitis), by the expense, the results of preliminary microbiologic studies, and the initial response to empiric therapy, if used. An approach that takes these factors into account is shown in Fig. 90-6. All the agents discussed above can be sexually transmitted, and appropriate treatment of sex partners, to prevent reinfection and reduce community spread of these agents, can be accomplished only if an etiologic diagnosis is established.

ACUTE ARTHRITIS   The gonococcal arthritis-dermatitis syndrome probably is the most common form of acute arthritis in sexually active young adults, and Reiter's syndrome is the second commonest. These must be differentiated from each other and from other forms of infective arthritis, various diseases associated with immune-complex deposition, crystal-induced arthritis, acute rheumatoid arthritis, and other less common rheumatic disorders such as systemic lupus erythematosus. Meningococcemia, *Yersinia* infection, sarcoidosis, and syphilis are other uncommon causes of acute arthritis. In one series of consecutive patients hospitalized because of acute arthritis of 2 weeks' or less duration, 52 percent of those aged 15 to 30 had disseminated gonococcal infection (DGI), 13 percent had Reiter's syndrome, and in another 5 percent the arthritis was directly or indirectly related to other sexually transmissible infections.

Demonstration of *N. gonorrhoeae* by culture or a specific immunochemical method in synovial fluid, blood, skin lesions, or cerebrospinal fluid is diagnostic of DGI. Failing this, the diagnosis of gonococcal arthritis is virtually certain if all three of the following criteria are met: (1) *N. gonorrhoeae* is recovered from a mucosal site of infection or from the patient's sex partner; (2) typical pustular or hemorrhagic skin lesions are distributed primarily on the extremities; and (3) a therapeutic antibiotic trial produces prompt defervesence and improvement of the arthritis. If only two of the above three

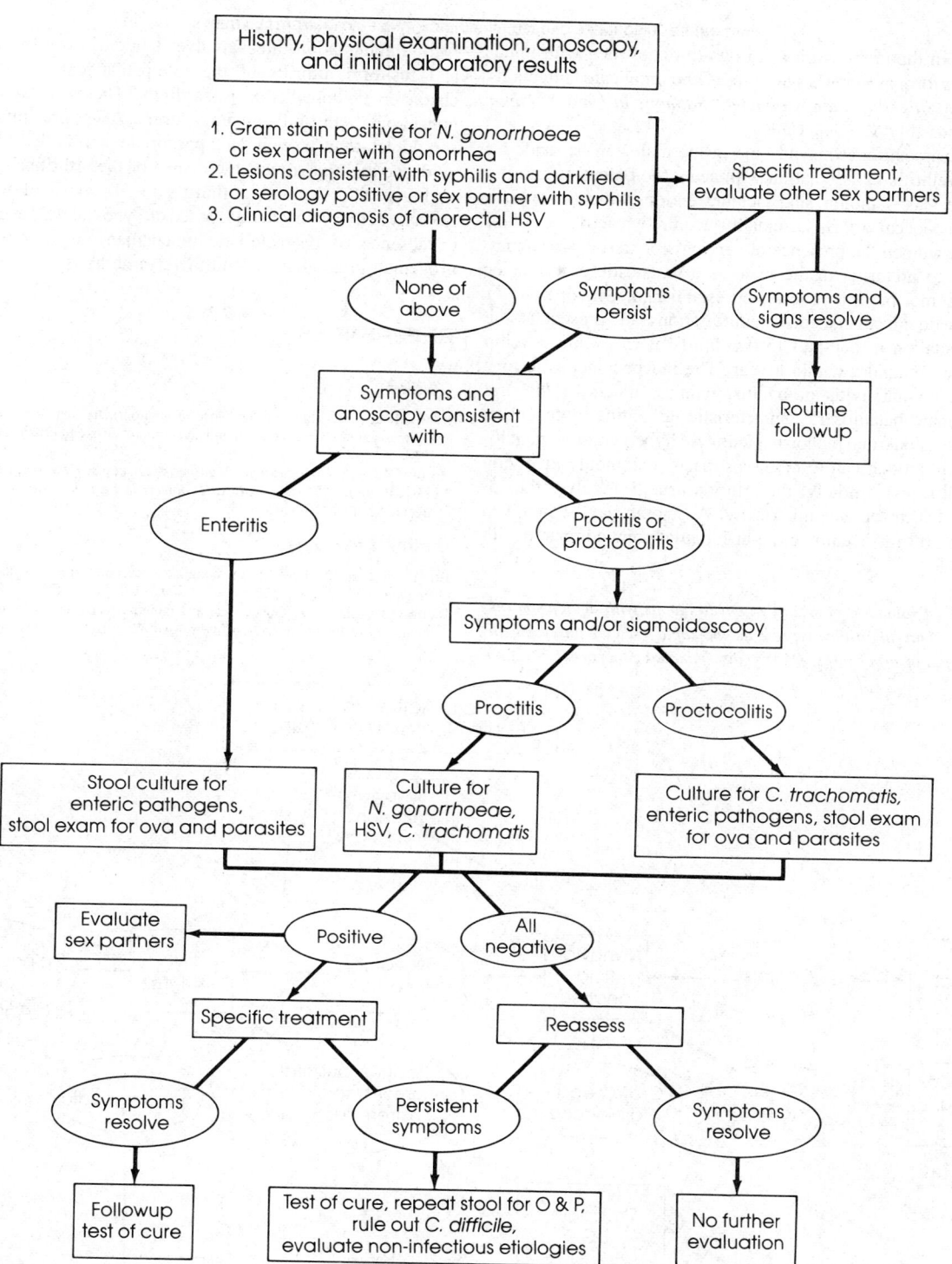

FIGURE 90-6 *Algorithm for management of anorectal and/or intestinal symptoms in homosexually active men. Anoscopy, cultures for* N. gonorrhoeae, *and a serologic test for syphilis should be performed in all cases. Empirical therapy for enteritis or proctitis could be given pending results of microbiologic studies. HSV = herpes simplex virus; O + P = ova and parasites.*

criteria are met, the diagnosis of gonococcal arthritis remains highly probable, especially if the other diagnoses listed above are excluded.

DGI due to penicillinase-negative strains of *N. gonorrhoeae* is best treated with intravenous crystalline penicillin G, 10 million units per day until clear-cut clinical improvement occurs, followed by oral ampicillin 500 mg four times daily to complete 7 to 10 days of antibiotic therapy. Patients who are allergic to penicillin may be given 7- to 10-day courses of cefoxitin or cefotaxime 4 to 6 g daily intravenously, or ceftriaxone 1 to 2 g daily intravenously; mildly ill patients may be given tetracycline 500 mg four times daily for 7 to 10 days. Cefoxitin, cefotaxime, or ceftriaxone should be used for DGI due to penicillinase-producing gonococci. Patients with gonococcal arthritis with highly purulent synovial effusions occasionally have persistent fever and arthritis despite adequate antimicrobial therapy, and they may require repeated closed-joint irrigations with saline before improvement occurs.

Reiter's syndrome occurs in a sporadic (apparently sexually transmitted) form and a postdysenteric form, which sometimes occurs in discrete epidemics. Reiter's syndrome is most commonly diagnosed in men, although some series include many women. Approximately 80 percent of patients have the HLA-B27 haplotype, compared with fewer than 10 percent of the general population. The pathogenesis of Reiter's syndrome is not understood, but it is believed that any of several mucosal infections in a predisposed (e.g., HLA-B27–positive) host triggers an immune response that causes the arthritis and mucocutaneous lesions. *C. trachomatis* is believed to be the most common precipitating infectious agent in the sporadic form and can be isolated from the urethras of up to two-thirds of men with initial episodes of this form of Reiter's syndrome. Other implicated infectious agents include *Shigella, Campylobacter, Salmonella,* and *Yersinia* species, and possibly *N. gonorrhoeae.*

The diagnosis of Reiter's syndrome in the male can be made on the basis of urethritis in association with acute, noninfective arthritis that persists at least 1 month, and includes entities which have been called postgonococcal arthritis, sexually acquired reactive arthritis, and others. In women the presence of cervicitis or sterile pyuria may be equivalent to urethritis in the male as a diagnostic criterion for Reiter's syndrome, but this is less well established. One or more of the characteristic mucocutaneous manifestations are present at the time of presentation in one-half to two-thirds of cases and develop in most of the remainder within a year. The mucocutaneous lesions include acute conjunctivitis or uveitis, painless ulcers of the oral mucosa, circinate balanitis (a characteristic dermatitis of the glans penis), and keratoderma blenorrhagicum (a hyperkeratotic papulo-squamous eruption that can resemble psoriasis, commonly involving the palms and soles). Initially, the arthritis usually involves four or fewer joints, distributed asymmetrically. Any joint may be involved and sacroiliac arthritis is common, a differential point compared with

DGI. Inflammation often involves tendon insertions (enthesopathy), and fusiform arthritis of the interphalangeal joints produces the characteristic so-called sausage digits. The mainstay of treatment is nonsteroidal anti-inflammatory drugs. The precipitating infection should be treated with an appropriate antibiotic, but there is no evidence that this affects the course of the arthritis.

Figure 90-7 is an algorithm for the diagnosis of acute arthritis in sexually active young adults, based on synovial fluid analysis, presence or absence of characteristic mucocutaneous lesions, evidence of urogenital inflammation, and therapeutic trials with antibiotics.

REFERENCES

General

BERG AO et al: Establishing the cause of genitourinary symptoms in a family practice: Comparison of clinical examination and comprehensive microbiology. JAMA 251:620, 1984

HOLMES KK et al (eds): *Sexually Transmitted Diseases.* New York, McGraw-Hill, 1984

TAYLOR-ROBINSON D (ed): *Clinical Problems in Sexually Transmitted Diseases.* Dordrecht, Martinus Nijhoff, 1985

Urethritis in males

BOWIE WR et al: Etiology of nongonococcal urethritis: Evidence for *Chlamydia trachomatis* and *Ureaplasma urealyticum.* J Clin Invest 59:735, 1977

JACOBS NF, KRAUS SF: Gonococcal and nongonococcal urethritis in men: Clinical and laboratory differentiation. Ann Intern Med 82:7, 1975

FIGURE 90-7 *Evaluation of sexually active patients with acute, nontraumatic arthritis. This algorithm represents the logic used in analyzing the results of the tests or procedures. DGI = disseminated gonococcal infection.*

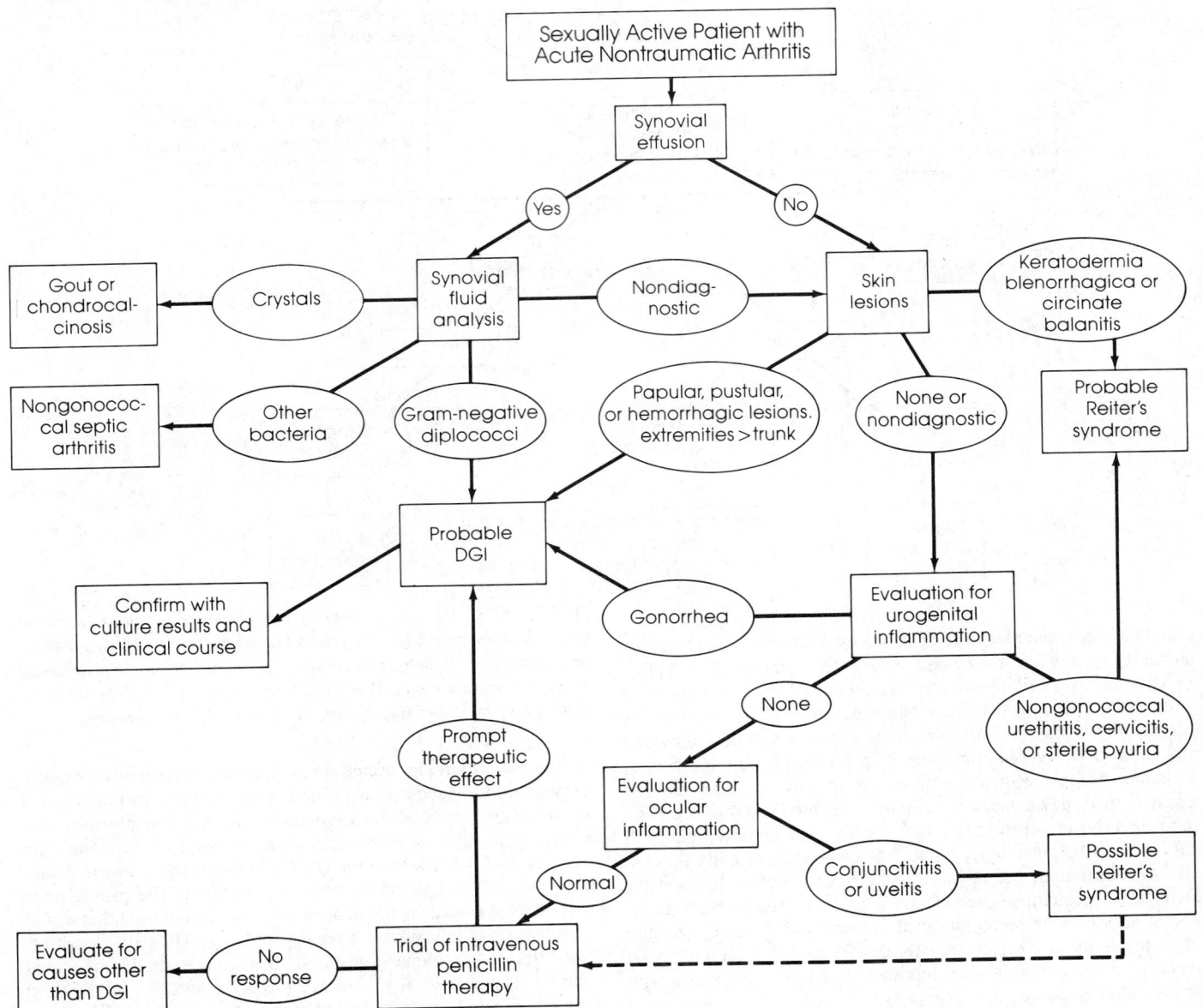

Epididymitis

BERGER RE et al: Etiology, manifestations, and therapy of acute epididymitis: Prospective study of 50 cases. J Urol 121:750, 1979

Urethral syndrome

STAMM WE et al: Causes of the acute urethral syndrome in women. N Engl J Med 303:409, 1980

Vaginitis

HOLMES KK: Lower genital tract infections in women, in Sexually Transmitted Diseases, KK Holmes et al (eds). New York, McGraw-Hill, 1984, pp 557–589
KRAUS SF: Trichomonas vaginalis: Reevaluation of its clinical presentation and laboratory diagnosis. J Infect Dis 141:137, 1980
MÅRDH PA, TAYLOR-ROBINSON D (eds): Bacterial Vaginosis. Stockholm, Almqvist & Wiksell, 1984
ORIEL JD et al: Genital yeast infections. Br Med J 4:761, 1972
SPIEGEL CA et al: Anaerobic bacteria in nonspecific vaginitis. N Engl J Med 303:601, 1980

Cervicitis

BRUNHAM RC et al: Mucopurulent cervicitis—the ignored counterpart in women of urethritis in men. N Engl J Med 311:1, 1984
KIVIAT NB et al: Cytologic manifestations of cervical and vaginal infections: I. Epithelial and inflammatory cellular changes. JAMA 253:989, 1985

Genital ulcers

CHAPEL TA et al: The microbiological flora of penile ulceration. J Infect Dis 137:50, 1978
KRAUS SJ: Genital ulcer adenopathy syndrome, in Sexually Transmitted Diseases, KK Holmes et al (eds). New York, McGraw-Hill, 1984, pp 706–714
NSANZE H et al: Genital ulcers in Kenya: Clinical and laboratory study. Br J Vener Dis 57(6):378, 1981

Proctitis, proctocolitis, enterocolitis, enteritis

QUINN TC et al: The polymicrobial etiology of intestinal infections in homosexual men. N Engl J Med 309:576, 1983

Arthritis

HOLMES KK et al: Disseminated gonococcal infection. Ann Intern Med 74:979, 1971
POLLOCK PS, HANDSFIELD HH: Arthritis, in Sexually Transmitted Diseases, KK Holmes et al (eds). New York, McGraw-Hill, 1984, pp 745–760

91 PELVIC INFLAMMATORY DISEASE

KING K. HOLMES

DEFINITION The term *pelvic inflammatory disease (PID)* usually refers to ascending infection of the uterus, fallopian tubes, and broad ligaments. Intrauterine infection can be primary (spontaneously occurring and usually sexually transmitted) or secondary to invasive intrauterine surgical procedures (e.g., dilatation and curettage, termination of pregnancy, insertion of an intrauterine device, or hysterosalpingography), or to parturition. Endometritis or endomyometritis is particularly common following delivery by cesarean section.

PID is uncommon during pregnancy itself. The uterotubal junction is closed as early as the seventh week of pregnancy, and the choriamnion becomes approximated to the endocervical os, sealing off the intrauterine cavity, at the twelfth to fifteenth week of gestation. As a consequence, ascending intrauterine infection prior to the twelfth week of gestation may be associated (either as cause or effect) with endometritis and spontaneous abortion, while ascending infection after the twelfth week may be associated with chorioamnionitis. Rarely, infection may extend secondarily to the pelvic organs from adjacent foci of inflammation, such as appendicitis, regional ileitis, or diverticulitis; as a result of hematogenous dissemination, such as tuberculosis; or as a rare complication of certain tropical diseases, such as schistosomiasis. However, the great majority of cases of PID arise spontaneously, without predisposing surgical trauma, obstetrical events, other systemic infection, or adjacent intraabdominal disease.

Spontaneously occurring PID can be divided into chronic and acute types. Chronic PID due to tuberculosis has become uncommon in developing countries; other forms of chronic PID, due to chronic infection with *Chlamydia trachomatis* or secondary to IUD usage, have been described but have not been adequately studied.

The term *PID* is most often used today to refer to cases of acute spontaneously occurring infection ascending from the cervix or vagina. The clinical diagnosis of PID is imprecise. About 10 percent of women with suspected acute PID are found at laparoscopy to have other problems, such as acute appendicitis, endometriosis, ectopic pregnancy, fallopian tube torsion, or corpus luteum bleeding, while another quarter have no laparoscopic evidence of acute disease, and only about 65 percent have laparoscopic evidence of acute salpingitis. Use of endometrial biopsy together with laparoscopy provides evidence of a continuum, progressing from cervicitis alone to endometritis, to salpingitis, to pelvic peritonitis, to generalized peritonitis, to perihepatitis, or to pelvic abscess. In this chapter, the term *PID* is used to refer to the clinical syndrome which includes each of these conditions, and the term *salpingitis* is restricted to patients with visually or histopathologically confirmed inflammation of the fallopian tubes. The distinction between endometritis and salpingitis may be important, because long-term sequelae are common after salpingitis. These sequelae include infertility due to bilateral tubal occlusion, peritubal adhesions, ectopic pregnancy due to tubal damage without occlusion, chronic pelvic pain, and recurrent PID.

ETIOLOGY The etiology of PID has seemed to vary greatly in several studies for reasons related to patient selection as well as methodology. As is summarized in Table 91-1, the agents most often implicated in acute PID include those which are primary causes of cervicitis (*Neisseria gonorrhoeae* and *C. trachomatis*) and those which can be regarded as abnormal components of the vaginal flora.

In the United States, gonococci were isolated from 44 percent of women with acute PID in a multicity cooperative study during the 1970s. From 1980 through 1985 in Seattle, *N. gonorrhoeae* and *C. trachomatis* have each been found in about half of all patients with proven PID: about one-fourth had gonorrhea alone, one-fourth had chlamydial infection alone, and one-fourth had both infections. However, in Scandinavian countries, where gonococcal infection is under better control, endocervical gonococcal infection has been found in less than one-fourth of women with PID during the past decade, while chlamydial infection has been roughly twice as common as gonococcal infection in this group. In general, PID is most often associated with gonorrhea in populations having a high incidence of gonorrhea in developing countries and in indigent, central city urban populations in developed countries. In several studies of women with PID, up to two-thirds with positive endocervical cultures for *N. gonorrhoeae* have had positive endometrial, peritoneal, or tubal cultures for this organism. Similarly, studies of women with proven PID have shown that *C. trachomatis* can be demonstrated by

TABLE 91-1 Cervical and vaginal organisms most often implicated in acute PID

Cervical pathogens	Vaginal flora		Mycoplasma
	Anaerobic bacteria	Facultative bacteria	
N. gonorrhoeae	Bacteroides spp.	Enterobacteriaceae	M. hominis
C. trachomatis	Peptococci	H. influenzae	U. urealyticum
	Peptostreptococci	G. vaginalis	
	Mobiluncus spp.	Streptococcus, groups B, D	
	Actinomyces spp.		

culture or immunofluorescent staining in the endometrium or tubes of the majority of those who have endocervical chlamydial infection.

Anaerobic and facultative anaerobic organisms (especially *Bacteroides* species, anaerobic gram-positive cocci, *Escherichia coli*, and group B and group D streptococci) and genital mycoplasmas have been isolated from specimens obtained at laparoscopy from the peritoneal fluid or fallopian tubes in a varying proportion—typically one-fourth to one-third—of women with PID studied in the United States. These vaginal organisms can be found in association with chlamydial or gonococcal infection, as well as in women without them, and have been implicated particularly often in women wearing intrauterine contraceptive devices. The importance of vaginal organisms in salpingitis has probably been overestimated in studies based on culture obtained by culdocentesis or endometrial aspiration, procedures in which contamination of the aspirated specimen by vaginal flora could occur. However, as noted above, specimens obtained by laparoscopy have also contained anaerobic and facultative species in some patients with PID.

It should be apparent that it is extremely difficult to determine the exact microbial etiology in the individual patient with PID because of the frequency of mixed infection, the difficulty in sampling the fallopian tube itself, and the complexity of microbiologic techniques required to detect the various fastidious pathogens which most often cause this disorder.

In general, first episodes of acute PID are particularly likely to be caused by *N. gonorrhoeae* and/or *C. trachomatis*. These sexually transmitted pathogens are somewhat less often implicated in recurrent bouts of acute PID, episodes occurring in IUD users, and episodes precipitated by invasive intrauterine diagnostic or therapeutic procedures, which are often associated with ascending infection caused by the more virulent components of the endogenous vaginal flora.

EPIDEMIOLOGY   It has been estimated that the annual incidence of PID in the United States during the mid-1970s was about 850,000 cases per year, and the direct and indirect costs of PID and its complications (excluding the cost of fetal death due to ectopic pregnancies) totaled an estimated $1.25 billion per year. These cost estimates do not include the growing costs of tubal microsurgery and in vitro fertilization for women rendered infertile because of salpingitis. PID is not a reportable disease in the United States; survey data from the National Drug and Therapeutic Index and the National Ambulatory Medical Care Survey suggest that the incidence of PID increased from the mid-1960s through the mid-1970s and may have decreased since then. The incidence of one of the major sequelae of salpingitis, ectopic pregnancy, progressively rose each year from 13,200 cases in 1967 to 67,000 cases in 1981. Similar trends in ectopic pregnancies have been seen in Canada and England. There is some evidence that the percentage of involuntary infertility has also increased in the United States during the same period.

Acute PID is almost exclusively a disease of sexually active women. The risk appears to be several times greater in sexually active teenagers who are 15 to 16 years old than among women 20 to 24 years of age. Important risk factors other than young age include a previous history of gonorrhea or of salpingitis, and use of an intrauterine device, particularly the Dalkon shield. In most studies, the relative risk of PID among IUD users was higher in nulliparous women than in parous women. On the other hand, women using oral contraceptives appear to be at decreased risk of PID, particularly gonococcal PID, and for this reason some experts advocate use of oral contraceptives by women at high risk for PID. Barrier methods of contraception prevent PID by reducing the risk of chlamydial and gonococcal infection. Tubal sterilization reduces (but does not completely eliminate) the risk of salpingitis by preventing intraluminal spread of infection into the tubes.

PATHOGENESIS   Factors cited as possibly contributing to intracanalicular upward spread of gonococci and *Chlamydia* from the endocervix to the endometrium and endosalpinx include estrogen-dominated (thin) cervical mucus, attachment to sperm which migrate upward into the tubes, use of an intrauterine device, and menstruation. The onset of symptoms of gonorrhea-associated PID and of *Chlamydia*-associated PID often occurs during or just after the menstrual period. In fallopian tube organ cultures in vitro, gonococci attach to the surface of the secretory columnar cells (but not the ciliated cells) of the endosalpinx. Gonococcal pili and perhaps other surface proteins are important in this attachment. Gonococci then are taken into the secretory cells by endocytosis. They pass through the cells, and perhaps between cells, and are extruded through the base of the cell into the submucosal connective tissue. Ciliary motion ceases, and then ciliated cells, although not directly invaded by gonococci, are sloughed from the mucosa during this process—a factor which may render the tubes more susceptible to superinfection by other organisms. It is uncertain whether this loss of ciliated cells is irreversible in vivo. Gonococcal endotoxin and peptidoglycan are at least partly responsible for these cytotoxic effects.

Gonococci associated with PID are significantly more resistant to penicillin and less likely to belong to the Arg-Hyx-Ura- auxotype than are strains causing uncomplicated gonorrhea. Also, gonococci isolated from the fallopian tubes reportedly form transparent colonies, whereas paired isolates from the cervix more often form opaque colonies, reflecting phenotypic changes in the protein composition of the gonococcal outer membrane which may be important in the pathogenesis of PID.

C. trachomatis also infects the columnar cells of the fallopian tube, but produces little damage in tubal organ cultures, perhaps because the host response is more important in the pathogenesis of chlamydial salpingitis. Chlamydial endometritis and salpingitis have been better studied than gonococcal endometritis or salpingitis in vivo, partly because animal models have been developed for chlamydial salpingitis, but not for gonococcal salpingitis. In chlamydial mucopurulent cervicitis (MPC), cervical biopsies show inclusions containing *Chlamydia* within columnar cells, and submucosal and stromal infiltration by mononuclear cells, polymorphonuclear leukocytes, and lymphoid aggregates containing transformed lymphocytes. Routine endometrial biopsies from consecutive women with chlamydial MPC show endometritis in approximately one-half. Although endometritis detected in this way is correlated with uterine tenderness, abnormal menstrual bleeding, and leukocytosis, symptoms of abdominal pain and fever are usually lacking, underscoring the subclinical nature of many cases of upper genital tract chlamydial infection. It is not known what proportion of those with endometritis also have salpingitis, since laparoscopy has not been performed in the absence of more suggestive symptoms and signs of salpingitis. However, among women with chlamydial MPC who do have symptoms and signs suggestive of salpingitis, the great majority who undergo endometrial biopsy and laparoscopy have both endometritis and salpingitis. Chlamydial inclusions are demonstrable by direct immunofluorescence in columnar epithelial cells of the endometrium and endosalpinx. The endometrial biopsies show plasma cells in the superficial endometrial stroma—a finding also seen to a lesser extent in gonococcal endometritis, but never in the uninfected endometrium. In addition, there is dense infiltration of the surface epithelium by acute and chronic inflammatory cells, lymphoid aggregates containing transformed lymphocytes in the stroma, and acute and chronic inflammatory cells in the lumens of the endometrial glands. Experimental inoculation of the fallopian tubes of lower primates produces mild acute salpingitis and ciliary sloughing, which is completely reversible. However, if experimental tubal inoculation is preceded by repeated inoculation of the cervix, a more intense salpingitis results and progresses to peritubular scarring. This suggests that in the female genital tract, as in the eye, it is repeated exposure to *C. trachomatis* which leads to the greatest degree of tissue inflammation and damage.

The pathogenesis of PID attributable to mycoplasmas or other vaginal anaerobic or facultative organisms is less well studied. It is possible that other vaginal organisms implicated in PID cause tubal infection in women whose tubes have already been damaged by a primary sexually transmitted pathogen (i.e., *N. gonorrhoeae* or *C. trachomatis*). Since the anaerobic organisms and mycoplasmas implicated in PID are found in the vagina most often and in greatest concentration in bacterial vaginosis (nonspecific vaginitis), it is possible that bacterial vaginosis itself is a predisposing risk factor for PID (in the same manner that poor oral hygiene is a risk factor in aspiration pneumonia).

Certain other iatrogenic factors, such as dilatation and curettage or cesarean section, are known to pose a greater risk of causing PID in women with endocervical gonococcal or chlamydial infection. It remains to be determined whether such procedures are also a greater risk in women with bacterial vaginosis.

CLINICAL MANIFESTATIONS Tuberculous salpingitis
Unlike nontuberculous salpingitis, genital tuberculosis often occurs in older women, and about half are postmenopausal. In a large review of cases in Sweden, 38 percent had had previously diagnosed tuberculosis. The commonest presenting symptoms were abnormal vaginal bleeding (41 percent), pain including dysmenorrhea (25 percent), and infertility (13 percent). Most had normal bimanual pelvic examinations, though about one-quarter had adnexal masses. The most common method of diagnosis was endometrial biopsy, showing tuberculous granulomas, associated with a positive culture in many cases.

Nontuberculous salpingitis The evolution of symptoms classically proceeds from a mucopurulent vaginal discharge caused by cervicitis—possibly associated with dysuria and frequency due to urethritis, or with anorectal pain, tenesmus, rectal discharge, and bleeding due to proctitis—to midline abdominal pain and abnormal vaginal bleeding caused by endometritis, to bilateral lower abdominal and pelvic pain caused by salpingitis, to nausea and vomiting and increased abdominal tenderness caused by peritonitis. Some patients have generalized abdominal pain caused by generalized peritonitis, or pleuritic right upper quadrant pain caused by perihepatitis. The pattern in which symptoms evolve varies from patient to patient and is also related to the etiology of the PID.

The onset of IUD-associated PID is typically gradual, and may be preceded by typical malodorous vaginal discharge characteristic of bacterial vaginosis. The onset of gonococcal PID is typically more acute than that of chlamydial PID, although both are often associated with menses.

The abdominal pain is usually described as dull or aching. In some cases, pain is lacking or is atypical, and active inflammatory changes can be found in the course of an unrelated evaluation or procedure such as a tubal ligation or laparoscopic evaluation for infertility. Metrorrhagia precedes or coincides with the onset of pain in about 40 percent of women with PID, symptoms of urethritis occur in 20 percent, and symptoms of proctitis in 7 percent of patients.

Speculum examination shows evidence of mucopurulent cervicitis in the majority of women with gonococcal or chlamydial PID. Cervical motion tenderness is produced by stretching of the adnexal attachments on the side toward which the cervix is pushed. Bimanual examination reveals uterine fundal tenderness due to endometritis, and abnormal adnexal tenderness due to salpingitis which is usually, but not necessarily, bilateral. Adnexal swelling is palpable in about one-half of women with acute salpingitis, but evaluation of the adnexae in a patient with marked tenderness is not completely reliable, even by an experienced examiner. An initial temperature >38°C is found in only about one-third of patients with acute salpingitis, and fever is not required for the diagnosis.

Laboratory findings include elevation of the erythrocyte sedimentation rate (ESR) in 75 percent and elevation of the peripheral white blood cell count in about 60 percent of patients with salpingitis. C-reactive protein is elevated in most women with acute PID. Microscopic examination of a saline wet-mount preparation of vaginal fluid has revealed more than one polymorphonuclear leukocyte per vaginal epithelial cell in nearly all patients with laparoscopically confirmed salpingitis in Swedish studies, and some experts consider the absence of white blood cells in vaginal fluid or cervical mucus as incompatible with the diagnosis of acute PID.

Certain clinical manifestations of acute PID have been correlated with etiologic findings. For example, the onset of salpingitis is related to menses in women with gonorrhea or chlamydial infection. Women with gonorrhea or chlamydia-associated salpingitis are significantly younger than women with other forms of salpingitis. As is summarized in Table 91-2, women with chlamydia-associated salpingitis tend to have an indolent disease with mild symptoms of significantly longer duration and with less fever when compared to women who have gonorrhea-associated salpingitis, but paradoxically, those with chlamydia-associated salpingitis have had significantly higher erythrocyte sedimentation rates and more severe inflammatory reactions seen in laparoscopy. It is suspected that for all recognized cases of symptomatic *Chlamydia* salpingitis, there is an equal number of unrecognized cases of indolent subclinical *Chlamydia* salpingitis, and that subclinical chronic or recurrent *Chlamydia* salpingitis may be a major cause of infertility in women.

IUD-associated PID also tends to be indolent and is less often associated with fever, but more often with adnexal masses, than is PID not associated with IUD use.

Perihepatitis and periappendicitis Symptoms of perihepatitis, including pleuritic upper abdominal pain and tenderness, usually localized to the right upper quadrant, occur in 5 to 10 percent of women with acute PID. The onset of symptoms of perihepatitis occurs during or after onset of symptoms of PID and may overshadow the lower abdominal symptoms, leading to a mistaken diagnosis of cholecystitis. In up to a quarter of all cases of acute salpingitis in some studies, laparoscopy performed early reveals inflammation ranging from edema and erythema of the liver capsule to exudate with fibrinous adhesions between the visceral and parietal peritoneum. When treatment is delayed, and laparoscopy is performed late, dense "violin-string" adhesions are seen over the liver; these cause chronic exertional or positional right upper quadrant pain when traction is placed on the adhesions. Although perihepatitis, also known as the Fitz-Hugh–Curtis syndrome, was for many years attributed to gonococcal PID, it has been recognized that most cases of perihepatitis have been associated with chlamydial salpingitis. In patients with chlamydial salpingitis, serum microimmunofluorescent antibody titers against *C. trachomatis* are typically much higher when perihepatitis is present than when it is absent, and it has been suggested that repeated chlamydial infections are responsible for perihepatitis.

Physical findings include right upper quadrant tenderness and usually show evidence of adnexal tenderness and cervicitis, even in patients whose symptoms are not suggestive of salpingitis.

Liver function tests are nearly always normal, since inflammation is largely limited to the liver capsule, usually sparing the parenchyma.

TABLE 91-2 Characteristics of laparoscopically verified salpingitis associated with *C. trachomatis* alone, *N. gonorrhoeae* alone, or neither agent (from Svensson et al, 1980)

	Chlamydia-associated, % (N = 68*)	Gonococcus-associated, % (N = 19†)	Not gonococcus- or chlamydia-associated, % (N = 64)
Temperature >38°C	27	74	30
Duration pelvic pain >3 days	85	68	62
ESR >30	65	32	28
Laparoscopic appearance of tubes, moderately severe or severe	78	74	47

* *C. trachomatis isolated from cervix, urethra, rectum, or tubes; or serologic evidence of acute chlamydial infection.*
† *N. gonorrhoeae isolated from cervix, urethra, or tubes; no cultural or serologic evidence of C. trachomatis infection.*
SOURCE: *Svensson et al.*

Oral cholecystogram may show nonfunction of the gallbladder, but ultrasonography of the right upper quadrant is normal. The presence of mucopurulent cervicitis and pelvic tenderness in a young woman with subacute pleuritic right upper quadrant pain with normal ultrasonography of the gallbladder points to a diagnosis of perihepatitis.

Periappendicitis (appendiceal serositis which does not involve the intestinal mucosa) has been found in approximately 5 percent of patients undergoing appendectomy for suspected appendicitis, and can occur as a complication of gonococcal or chlamydial salpingitis.

DIAGNOSIS Early diagnosis and initiation of therapy are essential to minimize tubal scarring. Appropriate treatment must not be withheld from patients who have an equivocal diagnosis. Since delay in therapy may lead to progression of tubal scarring, it is better to err on the side of overdiagnosis and overtreatment. On the other hand, it is essential to differentiate between salpingitis and other pelvic pathology, particularly surgical emergencies such as appendicitis and ectopic pregnancy.

No clinical or laboratory finding short of laparoscopy is pathognomonic for salpingitis, and there is reluctance to perform laparoscopy in all cases of suspected salpingitis. The following minimum criteria for the clinical diagnosis of salpingitis are advocated: (1) lower abdominal pain of <3 weeks' duration; (2) pelvic tenderness on bimanual pelvic examination; and (3) evidence of lower genital tract infection (e.g., white blood cells outnumber all other cells in the vaginal fluid). Approximately 60 percent of such patients have salpingitis at laparoscopy.

The presence of additional findings such as a rectal temperature >38°C, a palpable adnexal mass, and elevation of the ESR >15 mm/h also raise the probability of salpingitis, which was found at laparoscopy in 68 percent of patients with one of these additional findings, 90 percent of patients with two or more, and 96 percent of patients with three or more additional findings. However, only 17 percent of all patients with laparoscopy-confirmed salpingitis had three additional findings. The serum C-reactive protein is usually elevated in women with confirmed PID.

Mucopurulent cervicitis is probably responsible for the presence of leukocytes in vaginal fluid in PID, and it is likely that mucopurulent cervicitis would be a useful discriminatory sign in differentiating PID from other causes of lower abdominal pain.

Several clinical features other than the presence of cervicitis favor a diagnosis of salpingitis. These include onset with menses, history of recent abnormal menstrual bleeding, presence of an IUD, history of previous salpingitis, and exposure to a male with urethritis. Detection of polymorphonuclear leukocytes in fluid aspirated by culdocentesis supports a diagnosis of suspected salpingitis. Urethritis or proctitis may occur in chlamydial or gonococcal infection but may also represent a urinary tract infection or an intestinal source for the patient's symptoms. Early onset of nausea and vomiting would favor appendicitis or other disorders of the gut. A missed menstrual period dictates evaluation for ectopic pregnancy. The more sensitive assays

for human chorionic gonadotropin which are now available are usually, but not always, positive.

Ultrasonography is sometimes useful to differentiate pelvic abscess from an inflammatory mass involving tubes, ovary, bowel, and omentum, but is not sufficiently sensitive to detect salpingitis.

Laparoscopy is the most specific method for diagnosis of acute salpingitis. Although it may be normal if inflammation is limited to the endosalpinx or endometrium, patients with suspected PID who have normal laparoscopy have a better prognosis, with few if any sequelae, when compared with patients who have abnormal laparoscopic findings. The primary and uncontested value of laparoscopy in women with lower abdominal pain is exclusion of other surgical problems. Table 91-3 clearly shows that the most common and serious problems that may be confused with salpingitis are usually unilateral. Unilateral pain or pelvic mass, though not incompatible with PID, is a strong indication for laparoscopy unless the clinical picture warrants laparotomy instead. Atypical clinical findings such as the absence of lower genital tract infection, a missed menstrual period, or failure to respond to appropriate therapy are other frequent indications for laparoscopy.

Laparoscopic criteria used for the diagnosis of salpingitis include (1) erythema of the fallopian tube; (2) edema of the fallopian tube; and (3) seropurulent exudate or fresh, easily lysed adhesions at the fimbriated end or on the serosal surface of a fallopian tube. Laparoscopic findings are further scored as mild, where the above manifestations are mild and the tubes are freely movable and patent; moderate, when the above manifestations are more marked, tubes are not freely movable, and patency is uncertain; and severe, when findings consist of an inflammatory mass.

Endometrial biopsy showing plasma cell endometritis is relatively sensitive and highly specific for the diagnosis of PID, being found in at least two-thirds or more of women with laparoscopically confirmed salpingitis, and absent in women without PID.

The etiologic diagnosis of PID can be further studied by cultures or specimens obtained by endocervical swab, endometrial aspiration, or culdocentesis, or by laparoscopy or laparotomy. Endocervical swab specimens should be examined by Gram stain for granulocytes and gram-negative diplococci and by culture for *N. gonorrhoeae*. The sensitivity of Gram stain is about 60 percent and specificity >95 percent, compared with culture. The endocervical swab specimen should also be tested for *C. trachomatis* whenever possible. Although isolation of either *N. gonorrhoeae* or *C. trachomatis* from the cervix does not prove that either agent is also present in the upper genital tract, this should strongly support the diagnosis of PID. A 1985 study showed that the clinical diagnosis of PID made by expert gynecologists was confirmed by laparoscopy or endometrial biopsy in only 60 percent of all consecutive patients, but in 90 percent of those who also had positive cultures for *N. gonorrhoeae* or *C. trachomatis*. There is no evidence that isolation of anaerobes or facultative anaerobes from the cervix or vagina correlates with the presence of these organisms in the upper genital tract in acute PID, but this has not been well studied. The value of culture of culdocentesis and endometrial aspirate specimens is disputed because of the risk of contamination of the specimen with vaginal flora. When laparoscopy is performed, material can be obtained directly from the cul-de-sac or the fimbriated opening of the tube, or by tubal aspiration if pyosalpinx is present. Such specimens should be cultured for anaerobic and facultative pathogens, as well as for *N. gonorrhoeae* and *C. trachomatis*.

TREATMENT Hospitalization should be considered in all women with PID. Hospitalization is strongly recommended when (1) the diagnosis is uncertain, (2) surgical emergencies such as appendicitis and ectopic pregnancy must be excluded, (3) a pelvic abscess is suspected, (4) severe illness precludes outpatient management, (5) the patient is pregnant, (6) the patient is assessed as unable to follow or tolerate an outpatient regimen, (7) the patient has failed to respond to outpatient therapy, or (8) clinical follow-up after 48 to 72 h of instituting antibiotic treatment cannot be arranged. The treatment of

TABLE 91-3 Laparoscopic findings in patients with false-positive or false-negative clinical diagnoses of acute PID

False-positive clinical diagnosis		False-negative clinical diagnosis, unexpected PID at laparoscopy	
Laparoscopic diagnosis	Percent	Clinical diagnosis	Percent
Acute appendicitis	24	Ovarian tumor	20
Endometriosis	16	Acute appendicitis	18
Corpus luteum bleeding	12	Ectopic pregnancy	16
Ectopic pregnancy	11	Chronic salpingitis	6
Pelvic adhesions only	7	Acute peritonitis	6
Benign ovarian tumor	7	Endometriosis	5
Chronic salpingitis	6	Uterine myoma	5
Miscellaneous	15	Atypical pelvic pain	6
		Miscellaneous	6

SOURCE: *Jacobsen and Weström.*

choice is not established. No single agent is active against the entire spectrum of pathogens (Table 91-4). Several antimicrobial combinations do provide a broad spectrum of activity against the major pathogens in vitro, but many have not been adequately evaluated for clinical efficacy in PID.

Examples of combination regimens with broad activity against major pathogens in PID

1 Doxycycline 100 mg, twice a day, IV, plus cefoxitin 2.0 g, four times a day, IV. These drugs should be continued IV for at least 4 days and at least 48 h after the patient defervesces. Doxycycline should be continued in a dose of 100 mg by mouth, twice a day, after discharge from the hospital to complete 14 days of therapy. This regimen provides excellent coverage for N. gonorrhoeae, including penicillinase-producing N. gonorrhoeae (PPNG), and C. trachomatis.

2 Clindamycin 600 mg, four times a day, IV, plus gentamicin 2.0 mg/kg, IV, followed by 1.5 mg/kg, three times a day, IV, in patients with normal renal function. These drugs should be continued for at least 4 days and at least 48 h after the patient defervesces. Clindamycin should be continued in a dose of 450 mg, by mouth, four times a day, after discharge from the hospital to complete 14 days of therapy. This regimen provides optimal activity against anaerobes and facultative gram-negative rods, and limited data suggest that it is active against C. trachomatis and N. gonorrhoeae when recommended doses are used.

Patients who are not hospitalized should also receive a combined regimen with broad activity, such as cefoxitin 2.0 g, IM, followed by doxycycline 100 mg, by mouth, twice a day for 14 days. Although a single loading dose of amoxicillin, ampicillin, or procaine penicillin with probenecid, as recommended for uncomplicated gonorrhea (see Chap. 104), could be used in place of cefoxitin, these regimens are not effective against PPNG and have less activity against anaerobes and facultative gram-negative rods. Tetracycline could also be used in a dose of 500 mg, four times a day, in place of doxycycline, but it is less active against certain anaerobes, and requires more frequent dosing; both represent major drawbacks in the treatment of PID.

Management of sexual partners
All persons who are sexual partners of patients with PID should be examined for STD and promptly treated with a regimen effective against uncomplicated gonococcal and chlamydial infection.

Follow-up
All patients who are treated as outpatients should be clinically reevaluated in 48 to 72 h. Those not responding favorably should be hospitalized. A culture to test whether cure has been achieved should be performed as needed.

Removal of an intrauterine device
Although the exact effect of IUD removal on the response of acute salpingitis to antimicrobial therapy and on the risk of recurrent salpingitis is unknown, removal of the IUD is recommended soon after antimicrobial therapy has been initiated. When an IUD is removed, contraceptive counseling is necessary.

Surgery
Surgery is necessary only rarely for treatment of salpingitis, except in the face of life-threatening infection such as rupture or threatened rupture of a tuboovarian abscess, or for drainage of an abscess. Ultrasonography is useful for diagnosing and following pelvic abscesses. When surgery is performed, conservative procedures are usually sufficient. Pelvic abscesses can often be drained by posterior colpotomy, and peritoneal lavage can be used if there is generalized peritonitis.

PROGNOSIS Of women treated for PID on an ambulatory basis with IM penicillin followed by a 10-day course of ampicillin, or with a 10-day course of tetracycline alone, in a cooperative trial in the United States, nearly 20 percent treated with either drug were judged to be clinical failures. Among 900 women who underwent long-term follow-up for a mean period of 8 years after successful treatment of the acute episode with various regimens in Sweden, late sequelae included infertility due to bilateral tubal occlusion, ectopic pregnancy due to tubal scarring without occlusion, chronic pelvic pain, and recurrent salpingitis. Chronic pain lasting longer than 6 months was seen in 18 percent of patients and infertility due to tubal occlusion in 17 percent; 4 percent of pregnancies that did occur were ectopic, representing approximately a sixfold increase over the expected rate of ectopic pregnancies.

The rate of infertility after salpingitis was found to be related to age of the patient, etiology of salpingitis, duration of symptoms when treatment was started, severity of salpingitis by laparoscopy at the time of diagnosis, and number of episodes of salpingitis. The rate of infertility due to tubal occlusion among women exposed to a chance of pregnancy was 14 percent for women 15 to 24 years of age and 26 percent for women 25 to 34 years of age; the risk for women of all ages combined was 11 percent after one episode of salpingitis, 23 percent after two episodes, and 54 percent after three or more episodes. The risk was 6 percent after one episode of N. gonorrhoeae–associated salpingitis and 21 percent after one episode of nongonococcal salpingitis. Infertility was demonstrated in about 20 percent of women after one episode of C. trachomatis–associated salpingitis.

Although the rate of infertility after C. trachomatis–associated salpingitis has not been determined in a similar prospective study, a preliminary analysis of such cases suggests about a 10 percent rate of tubal occlusion after therapy. A striking relationship has also been shown in several countries between infertility due to tubal occlusion and the prevalence and titer of antibody to C. trachomatis.

Recurrent salpingitis has been seen in approximately 15 to 25 percent of women treated for salpingitis in various studies.

PREVENTION Prevention of PID depends first on the effective use of current methods for control of gonococcal and chlamydial infection. These methods include providing ready access to modern methods of diagnosis and effective treatment, and treatment of sex partners to control further spread. The decline in popularity of the intrauterine device, particularly in nulliparous women, has undoubtedly helped to reduce the incidence of PID. It is possible, but not proven, that increased use of oral contraceptives might reduce the risk of PID,

TABLE 91-4 Approximate activity of the antimicrobial agents most commonly used to treat PID against the pathogens most commonly implicated in PID

	N. gonorrhoeae	C. trachomatis	Vaginal anaerobes		Facultative GNR	M. hominis
			GPC*	GNR†		
Ampicillin/penicillin G	4+	1+	4+	2+	2+	0
Tetracycline HCl	3+	4+	4+	2+	2+	0
Doxycycline	3+	4+	4+	3+	2+	2+
Cefoxitin	4+	0	4+	3+	2+	2+
Gentamicin/tobramycin	3+	0	1+	0	4+	0
Clindamycin	0	2+	4+	4+	4+	2+?
Metronidazole	0	0	4+	4+	0	3+

* GPC = Gram-positive cocci (peptococci, peptostreptococci).
† GNR = Gram-negative rods (anaerobic GNR include Bacteroides; facultative GNR include Enterobacteriaceae, H. influenzae).
NOTE: No single antimicrobial agent offers optimal activity against all of these pathogens, but certain combinations (e.g., cefoxitin plus doxycycline, gentamicin plus clindamycin) have complimentary activity against these pathogens.

particularly the risk of recurrent PID among women who have already experienced one episode of PID.

The complications of salpingitis can be minimized by early diagnosis and prompt treatment. It seems logical, but is unproven, that broad-spectrum therapy effective against all of the common causes of PID would offer the best outcome. Similarly, hospitalization to ensure rest and adequate compliance may improve the rather dismal long-term prognosis for tubal function. One placebo-controlled study showed that concurrent anti-inflammatory therapy with prednisolone hastened the reduction of acute inflammatory changes but did not improve the end results as measured by fertility, hysterosalpingographic findings, or chronic pain. However, since the dose of prednisolone used was relatively low, and since the antibiotics used concurrently would not be very effective against chlamydial or anaerobic infection, the potential value of anti-inflammatory therapy has not been adequately evaluated.

REFERENCES

Acute Pelvic Inflammatory Disease (PID): 1985 STD Treatment Guidelines. Morb Mort Week Rep 34(4S):92S, 1985

ESCHENBACH DA et al: Polymicrobial etiology of acute pelvic inflammatory disease. N Engl J Med 293:166, 1975

FALK V: Treatment of acute nontuberculous salpingitis with antibiotics alone and in combination with glucocorticoids. Acta Obstet Gynecol Scand 44(Suppl):1, 1965

—— et al: Genital tuberculosis in women. Am J Obstet Gynecol 138:974, 1980

GJØNAESS H et al: Pelvic inflammatory disease: Etiologic studies with emphasis on chlamydial infection. Obstet Gynecol 59:550, 1982

HENRY-SUCHET J et al: *Chlamydia trachomatis* associated with chronic inflammation in abdominal specimens from women selected for tuboplasty. Am J Obstet Gynecol 138:1022, 1980

JACOBSEN L, WESTRÖM L: Objectivized diagnosis of acute pelvic inflammatory disease. Am J Obstet Gynecol 105:1088, 1969

MÅRDH PA et al: *Chlamydia trachomatis* infection in patients with acute salpingitis. N Engl J Med 296:1377, 1977

MØLLER BR et al: Pelvic infection after elective abortion associated with *Chlamydia trachomatis*. Obstet Gynecol 59:210, 1982

OSSER S, PERSSON K: Epidemiologic and serodiagnostic aspects of chlamydial salpingitis. Obstet Gynecol 59:206, 1982

PAAVONEN J et al: Comparison of endometrial biopsy and peritoneal fluid cytologic testing with laparoscopy in the diagnosis of acute pelvic inflammatory disease. Am J Obstet Gynecol 151:645, 1985

ST JOHN RK, BROWN ST (eds): International symposium on pelvic inflammatory disease. Am J Obstet Gynecol 138:845, 1980

SVENSSON L et al: Differences in some clinical and laboratory parameters in acute salpingitis related to culture and serologic findings. Am J Obstet Gynecol 138:1017, 1980

—— et al: Infertility after acute salpingitis—with special reference to *Chlamydia trachomatis*–associated infections. Fertil Steril 40:322, 1983

THOMPSON SE et al: High failure rates in outpatient treatment of salpingitis with either tetracycline alone or penicillin/ampicillin combination. Am J Obstet Gynecol 152:635, 1985

WASSERHEIT JN et al: Microbial causes of proven pelvic inflammatory disease and efficacy of clindamycin with tobramycin. Ann Intern Med (in press)

WØLNER-HANSSEN P et al: Endometrial infection in women with chlamydial salpingitis. Sex Transm Dis 9:84, 1982

92 PREVENTION OF INFECTION: IMMUNIZATION AND ANTIMICROBIAL PROPHYLAXIS

LAWRENCE COREY / ROBERT G. PETERSDORF

There are three major ways to prevent infections: (1) by reducing exposure, (2) by acquiring or inducing immunity, and (3) by using antimicrobial agents to prevent colonization and infection. Exposure can be reduced by diminishing the prevalence of the infecting agent, by community-wide vaccination programs, and by isolating infected patients in cohorts. On an individual basis, however, the most reliable way to prevent infectious disease is to provide effective immunization or chemoprophylaxis against the causative agent. This chapter sum-

marizes current immunization practices and principles of antimicrobial prophylaxis. Additional details are provided in the chapters dealing with individual diseases.

IMMUNIZATION

Immunity may be defined as the ability of the individual to resist or overcome infection; it may be innate or acquired. For many infectious diseases, immunity is acquired during recovery from an infection or induced by the administration of vaccines prepared from inactivated or live microorganisms of modified disease-producing potential, or from specific antigen(s) derived from these organisms. The purpose of immunization, therefore, is to provoke a specific immunologic response to a selected microbial agent or its antigens with the expectation that this will result in humoral, and/or secretory, and/or cell-mediated immunity. While this protection may diminish over time, future exposures to the same stimulus will result in a rapid return of the immune response because of heightened reactivity of antibody-forming, phagocytic, and other cells that mediate immune mechanisms (see Chap. 62).

Certain infectious diseases present special situations that impede the development of vaccines. For example, *Salmonella* organisms and rhinoviruses consist of several hundred antigenically unique strains, making production of a vaccine difficult. Second, the portal of entry of an organism and the role of local immunity are important in determining whether a vaccine given parenterally will offer protection from either infection or disease. Third, even when effective immunizing agents are available, difficulties in delivering them to the susceptible population may preclude their use.

GENERAL PRINCIPLES OF IMMUNIZATION   Infections can be prevented or controlled by active and/or passive immunization. Active immunization with live attenuated vaccines generally results in subclinical or mild clinical illness which duplicates, to a limited extent, the disease that is marked for prevention; generally, it provides both local and durable humoral immunity. "Killed" or inactivated vaccines, such as influenza, rabies, typhoid, and cholera vaccines, maintain immunogenicity, without infectivity, but have several disadvantages including the large amount of antigen that must be administered by the parenteral route and the greater time period between administration of the antigen and the appearance of a protective effect. Table 92-1 summarizes active immunizing agents.

The use of any biological substance requires balancing its benefits and risks, and each vaccine must be evaluated accordingly. While some immunizations, such as diphtheria, tetanus, and poliomyelitis, are recommended for all individuals, others should be used only in those who have an increased risk of either acquiring the disease or developing complications. Pneumococcal polysaccharide vaccine, influenza vaccine, hepatitis B vaccine, bacillus Calmette-Guérin (BCG) vaccine, and meningococcal vaccine are some examples.

Inactivated vaccines can be administered simultaneously at separate sites, although vaccines known to be associated with severe side effects should generally be given on separate occasions. Some vaccines contain trace amounts of preservatives or antibiotics to which patients may be sensitive, and, although reactions to them are unusual, reviewing the manufacturers' package insert prior to use of these agents may be helpful. Live virus vaccines prepared by growing viruses in cell culture are usually devoid of potential allergic substances. Many live virus vaccinations can be given simultaneously; measles, mumps, and rubella are some examples. However, when more than one dose of live viral vaccine is required, repeated administration should be separated by at least 1 month. After administration of an immunobiologic, the patient should be given a written record of its receipt and information about the necessity and timing of subsequent doses.

Contraindications to vaccination   Virus replication following administration of live attenuated virus vaccines can be accentuated in immune-deficiency diseases and in patients whose immune responses have been suppressed as in leukemia, lymphoma, or generalized malignancy or following therapy with corticosteroids, alkylating drugs, antimetabolites, and radiation. Such patients should not be given live attenuated virus vaccines. Vaccination of persons with severe febrile disease should be deferred to avoid superimposing the adverse effects of the vaccine on the underlying illness. Because of a theoretical risk to the developing fetus, live attenuated virus vaccines generally should not be given to pregnant women. For some vaccines, particularly live attenuated rubella vaccine, pregnancy is an absolute contraindication to vaccination. Passively acquired antibody can interfere with the response to live attenuated virus vaccines; therefore, administration of live vaccine should be postponed until approximately 3 months after passive immunization.

IMMUNIZATION IN ADULTS Most immunization policies have been directed at vaccinating infants and children. A substantial portion of the morbidity and mortality from vaccine-preventable diseases occurs in adolescents and adults. Foreign students, immigrants, and refugees are often at increased risk of vaccine-preventable illnesses. A systematic approach to immunization is needed by all adult health care providers to ensure that their patients are protected against those diseases that can be averted or mitigated by vaccination.

Diphtheria Because of the widespread use of diphtheria toxoid, the incidence of diphtheria in the United States has declined drastically, and only 11 cases were reported between 1980 and 1982. However, 62 percent of adults aged 18 to 39, and over 50 percent of those over 60 lack protective levels of circulating antitoxin to diphtheria. The myocardial and peripheral nervous system involvement associated with *Corynebacterium diphtheriae* is due to elaboration of an exotoxin (see Chap. 96). Diphtheria toxoid is a cell-free preparation of diphtheria toxin treated with formaldehyde. The quantity of toxoid varies among products, and the concentration of diphtheria toxoid in adult preparations is lower than in the pediatric formulation. Adverse reactions are thought to be related to dose and age. Diphtheria immunization is at least 95 percent effective in reducing both the risk of diphtheria and the severity of clinical illness. Diphtheria toxoid provides protection against only the toxin and not the somatic components of *C. diphtheriae*, and local infection, either in the respiratory tract or skin, may occur in immune individuals. Nontoxigenic strains also may cause mild, focal infections.

All children under 7 years should receive routine immunization against diphtheria in the form of absorbed diphtheria and tetanus toxoids and pertussis vaccine (DPT). Absorbed toxoids are produced by the addition of aluminum compounds to the formaldehyde-inactivated toxoid and are more antigenic than the fluid (plain) preparation. Children should receive a primary series of three doses of DPT vaccine before they are a year old, a booster at 18 months, and another when they enter school. A preparation without pertussis vaccine is available for primary immunization of children who are unable to tolerate the pertussis vaccine (DT). Because pertussis is less common and less severe in older children and adults, the preparation recommended for use in adults is a combination of tetanus and diphtheria toxoid in which the diphtheria toxoid is reduced to a maximum of two flocculating units per dose to avoid the febrile reactions that may accompany repeated exposure to diphtheria toxoid. This vaccine (Td) is recommended for primary immunization of adults and children older than 6 years of age and is also routinely used for booster immunization, both for the prevention of tetanus at the time of injury and for diphtheria prophylaxis. For primary immunization in adults, three intramuscular doses of Td should be given, the second dose 1 to 2 months after the first, and the third 6 to 12 months later. Thereafter, boosters at 10-year intervals should be given.

Tetanus (see Chap. 99) The incidence of tetanus has decreased dramatically with the routine use of tetanus toxoid, a formaldehyde-detoxified bacteria-free filtrate of *Clostridium tetanus*. The 75 cases of tetanus that are reported yearly in the United States almost exclusively occur in adults who are unimmunized or inadequately immunized. Two doses of the absorbed toxoid or three doses of fluid toxoid usually result in a protective level of antibody, 0.01 unit per milliliter tetanus antitoxin. Immune pregnant women confer temporary protection to their infant through placental transfer of maternal antibodies. Tetanus toxoid may be used singly or in combination with diphtheria toxoid (DT or Td), or with both diphtheria toxoid and pertussis vaccine (DPT). When used singly, primary immunization with the fluid toxoid is given in three doses at least 1 month apart with a booster 8 to 12 months later. The absorbed form should be given in two doses, 1 month apart. Primary immunization with tetanus toxoid is highly recommended for all children and adults. Clinical tetanus does not necessarily provide immunity against subsequent tetanus. Boosters after wound infection are recommended at 5-year intervals. Routine boosters at 10-year intervals (at mid-decade ages (25, 35, 45) are recommended. Systemic reactions after toxoid (Td) are uncommon. Arthus-like hypersensitivity reactions beginning 2 to 8 h after injection may be seen in persons who have received multiple boosters of tetanus toxoid. A history of a severe hypersensitivity or neurologic reaction from a previous booster constitutes a contraindication to further booster shots. Local side effects do not preclude a booster at 10-year intervals.

Pertussis Endemic pertussis infection is prevalent throughout the world. Complications and mortality of infection are greatest in children, especially those under 6 months. While controversy about the use of pertussis vaccine has occurred, routine use of the vaccine reduces the morbidity and mortality associated with pertussis infection in the neonate. Pertussis infection in adults and older children is usually mild, while systemic and local side effects from vaccination are increased in older children and adults. Pertussis vaccination is routinely recommended for children 1 year of age. Vaccination is *not* recommended for use in adults or children over 6 years of age. In exceptional cases such as persons with chronic pulmonary disease exposed to children with pertussis, or health care personnel exposed during outbreaks of pertussis, a booster dose of adsorbed pertussis vaccine (0.20 to 0.25 mL) may be useful.

Poliomyelitis (see Chap. 139) Routine polio vaccination of adults residing in the United States is not necessary because most are immune and the risk of exposure is small. However, susceptible adults at increased risk by virtue of travel or exposure to wild or vaccine poliovirus should receive primary immunization with either inactivated or wild attenuated polio vaccines. Both a live attenuated oral polio vaccine (OPV) and an inactivated polio vaccine (IPV) are licensed in the United States. A primary vaccination series with either OPV or IPV produces immunity to all three types of poliovirus in over 95 percent of recipients. OPV has been favored over IPV because it is easier to administer, orally versus injection; some studies indicate that it confers more resistance in the alimentary tract to reinfection; and it interferes with simultaneous infection by wild polioviruses. These properties are of special value during epidemics of poliomyelitis. Vaccination with OPV results in shedding of virus contained in the vaccine, and spread of virus to unvaccinated persons occurs. Rarely, recipients of oral vaccine or people in contact with them have contracted paralytic polio. The risk of vaccine-associated polio has been estimated to be one case per 9 million doses distributed to vaccinees and one case per 7 million doses distributed in household contacts. The relative risk of paralytic disease is slightly higher in susceptible adults than in children. Oral trivalent polio vaccine is the principal vaccine used in the United States. IPV is recommended in selective circumstances such as primary immunization of susceptible adults and in persons with immunodeficiencies and their household contacts. Primary immunization with IPV consists of four doses: three at 1- to 2-month intervals and a booster 6 to 12 months after the third. Booster doses at 2- to 3-year intervals either with IPV or with one dose of OPV after primary immunization with IPV will sustain long-lasting immunity.

For infants and children, the primary series of vaccination with

TABLE 92-1 Active immunization in adults (continued)

	Type of vaccine	Administration and frequency*	Comments
ALL ADULTS			
Tetanus and diphtheria	Adsorbed toxoid	IM at least every 10 years	Usually administered together as Td vaccine
Poliomyelitis	Live attenuated	Oral polio vaccine (OPV)	Preferred for routine use and during epidemics
	Formalin-inactivated	Inactivated polio vaccine (IPV)	Selective use in unimmunized adults
Measles, mumps, rubella	Live attenuated	SC once	All adults born after 1957 should have measles—see text for specific recommendations re: mumps and rubella vaccine
WOMEN OF CHILDBEARING AGE			
Rubella vaccine	Live attenuated	SC once	Postpartum vaccination of antibody negative persons
POSTPUBERTAL MALES			
Mumps	Live attenuated	SC once	Prevention of orchitis in susceptible seronegative males
PERSONS AT HIGH RISK OF ACQUIRING DISEASE OR DEVELOPING COMPLICATIONS OF DISEASE			
Influenza vaccine	Inactivated	SC yearly	Directed at reducing morbidity and mortality in those at risk of complications of influenza, e.g., chronic heart and lung disease and those over 65 years
Pneumococcal polysaccharide vaccine	Purified polysaccharide vaccine	SC once	Same population as influenza vaccine, functional or surgical asplenia, agammaglobulinemia, cirrhosis, multiple myeloma, and nephrotic syndrome
Hepatitis B vaccine	Inactivated subunit vaccine	3 doses IM at 0, 1, and 6 months	High-risk groups for acquisition of hepatitis B, including household contacts of hepatitis B patients, patients requiring a large volume of clotting factors, illicit drug users, homosexual men, and selected medical and dental personnel
Haemophilus influenzae type B	Purified capsular polysaccharide	SC once	Routine use in children more than 24 months of age; selected populations (day care of children 18–24 months and adults at high risk of getting invasive *H. influenzae* disease, e.g., asplenia, hypogammaglobulinemia)
POPULATIONS EXPOSED TO LOCALIZED OUTBREAKS			
Meningococcal vaccine	Purified capsular polysaccharide	SC once	Control of localized epidemics and adjunct to chemoprophylaxis in household contacts
Measles vaccine	Live attenuated	SC once	Control of outbreaks usually among adolescents or young adults
BCG vaccine	Live attenuated	SC or intradermally, once	Used in groups with excessive risk of new infection with tuberculosis or individuals persistently exposed to sputum-positive tuberculosis
Adenovirus vaccine	Live attenuated bivalent (types 4 and 7)	PO once	Used only for military recruits
Typhoid vaccine	Inactivated bacilli	SC in two doses	Household contact of documented *Salmonella typhi* carrier
Rubella vaccine	Live attenuated	SC once	Control of outbreaks among adolescents and young adults
TRAVELERS TO FOREIGN COUNTRIES			
Smallpox	Live vaccinia virus	Intradermally, every 3–5 years	No indications for smallpox vaccine in civilians
Yellow fever	Live attenuated	SC once per 10 years	Administered at yellow fever vaccination centers
Cholera	Phenol-inactivated suspension of *Vibrio cholerae*	SC approximately every 6 months	Only 50% effective and not effective in decreasing transmission of disease
Typhoid	Inactivated bacilli	SC in half doses 4 weeks apart	70–90% efficacy in ''normal'' exposure

TABLE 92-1 Active immunization in adults *(continued)*

	Type of vaccine	Administration and frequency*	Comments
Plague	Formaldehyde-inactivated *Yersinia pestis*	Primary series = three IM doses. First dose 1 mL; second dose 4 weeks later, 0.2 mL; third dose 5 months later, 0.2 mL	Agricultural workers who reside in plague-endemic areas
Poliomyelitis	Oral or inactivated polio vaccine	See text	Unimmunized adults should receive a complete primary series or at least 2 doses of IPV 1 month apart; if not, then a single dose of OPV is recommended; for high-risk travel in immunized adults, a single dose of OPV or IPV is recommended
Japanese encephalitis	Inactivated, purified mouse-brain vaccine	2 doses IM, 7–10 days apart	Not licensed in U.S.
Hepatitis A	Immune serum globulin	IM every 3 months	See ''Passive Immunization'' in this chapter

* *PO, orally; SC, subcutaneously; IM, intramuscularly.*

OPV consists of three doses. The first two should be given not less than 6 and preferably 8 weeks apart. The third dose should follow 8 to 12 months after the second dose. A booster dose of trivalent OPV should be given when the child enters kindergarten or first grade. Additional preadolescent immunization (at age 11 to 12) has been recommended to provide additional protection during adulthood. Live attenuated oral polio vaccine is acceptable for adults who have been vaccinated previously or whose circumstances do not allow adequate time for administration of IVP and who are not in a category in which oral vaccine is contraindicated.

Measles (see Chap. 132) While measles vaccine has markedly reduced the incidence of measles in the United States, localized outbreaks, particularly among teenagers and young adults, continue to occur. Measles mortality and encephalitis are greatest in adults, and efforts to eliminate measles in both the child and adult populations is currently underway. Measles vaccine is an attenuated live virus (Schwarz) vaccine derived from passage of the Edmonston strain of measles virus grown in a culture of chick embryo cells. The current vaccine differs from the older live attenuated Edmonston strain vaccine which was administered with human immune globulin.

Vaccination with the Schwarz strain produces life-long immunity in more than 95 percent of recipients. Revaccination of previously immune persons is not associated with significant adverse effects. Measles vaccine is recommended for all persons born after 1957 who lack documentation of prior vaccination on or after their first birthdays or who lack a firm diagnosis of measles. Persons born before 1957 can generally be considered immune. During measles outbreaks, it is recommended that all susceptible children, as well as adolescents and adults at risk, be immunized. Individuals who received measles vaccine before 12 months of age or who received killed measles vaccine followed within 3 months by live vaccine or a measles vaccine of unknown type between 1963 and 1967 should be revaccinated; travelers should be immune to measles before leaving the United States. Repeat vaccination with live measles vaccine poses no increased risk for individuals who have previously had natural measles or who have been vaccinated.

Up to 15 percent of vaccinated children will have fever lasting up to 5 days between the fifth and twelfth days after vaccination. Local induration and edema at the injection site may occur in persons who previously received killed measles vaccine.

IMMUNIZATION IN WOMEN OF CHILDBEARING AGE Rubella (see Chap. 133) The purpose of rubella vaccination is to prevent rubella embryopathy in the fetus. The direct approach to this goal would be to immunize all women before they become pregnant. However, the difficulty is being sure that a woman is not pregnant at the time of vaccination, and the increased risk of joint symptoms associated with vaccination in women has rendered this approach impractical. Because children are a major source of spread of rubella to pregnant females, rubella vaccination has been routinely recommended for all children older than 12 months. When given in combination with measles antigen, rubella vaccine should be administered when a child is about 15 months of age to achieve the maximum rate of measles seroconversion.

Since 1969 when rubella vaccine was first licensed, the incidence of rubella has declined steadily. However, 954 cases of the congenital rubella syndrome have been reported in the United States since the vaccine was introduced. An estimated 10 to 15 percent of young adults are susceptible to rubella, and outbreaks continue to occur at universities and places of employment that entail a higher risk, such as hospitals. Routine premarital rubella antibody determinations would help identify susceptible females before their first pregnancy. Testing for rubella antibody during the perinatal or antepartum period and vaccination of susceptible women in the immediate postpartum period is recommended. Rubella immunization of both male and female medical personnel having frequent contact with pregnant women is also recommended.

Rubella vaccine is prepared in cell cultures and is administered by subcutaneous injection. A single dose induces antibodies in approximately 95 percent of susceptible persons. There is no risk to susceptible contacts of vaccinees. Rubella vaccine virus has been demonstrated to cross the placenta and infect the fetus. Through 1983, 214 susceptible pregnant women who inadvertently received rubella vaccine within 3 months before or after conception and who continued their pregnancies to term have been evaluated. None of these infants had recognizable malformations attributable to rubella. However, fetal infection with vaccine-like rubella virus may produce pathologic changes in developing organs. The risk of teratogenicity is felt to be much lower from the vaccine virus than from the wild virus. If a pregnant woman is inadvertently vaccinated or if she becomes pregnant within 3 months of vaccination, she should be advised of the low (3 percent) risk of congenital infection to the fetus, and the theoretical risk of congenital rubella syndrome.

VACCINATION DURING PREGNANCY When a vaccine or toxoid is to be given during pregnancy, waiting until the second or third trimester to minimize concern about teratogenicity is advisable. Pregnant women not previously vaccinated against tetanus or diphtheria should receive two doses of Td. For those with an incomplete primary series, the completion of the series should be achieved. Booster doses of Td may be given during pregnancy. While live virus vaccines are not usually administered to pregnant women, if immediate protection against poliomyelitis or yellow fever is required, these vaccines may be administered. If yellow fever protection is necessary only for travel, then a waiver letter may be obtained. Indications for the administration of human immune globulin and inactivated vaccine such as hepatitis B, influenza, and rabies are not altered by pregnancy.

VACCINATION OF SUSCEPTIBLE POSTPUBERTAL MALES

Mumps (see Chap. 141)   Mumps is primarily a disease of school-aged children; only about 15 percent of the cases occur in adolescents and adults. Most mumps infections are subclinical or self-limited. Meningoencephalitis occurs in up to 15 percent of cases and is usually uncomplicated and benign, although nerve deafness may be seen in 1 in 15,000 cases. Orchitis, usually unilateral, may occur in 20 percent of postpubertal males. The incidence of subsequent sterility is low. Live attenuated mumps vaccine (Jeryl-Lynn strain) grown in chick embryo cell cultures has been available since 1967. Mumps vaccination is recommended for all children older than 1 year and especially in children approaching puberty, adolescents, and adults, particularly males, who have not had mumps or who have no serologic evidence of mumps immunity. Skin testing is not a reliable indication of past infection. Persons with prior mumps or who have received vaccine are not at risk from live mumps vaccine. A single dose is given subcutaneously; continuing protection against infection and protective antibodies have both been shown to persist for at least 12 years after vaccination. Parotitis after vaccination is very rare. Patients with severe febrile illness or hypersensitivity to egg products, with malignancy who are receiving immunosuppressive therapy, or who are pregnant should not be vaccinated. Mumps vaccine virus has been shown to infect the placenta, but virus has not been isolated from fetal tissue.

VACCINATION OF PERSONS WITH CHRONIC HEART, PULMONARY, AND METABOLIC DISEASE Influenza (see Chap. 130)

Influenza occurs every year in the United States but with variation in incidence and geographic distribution. Epidemics occur periodically; more are caused by influenza A viruses than by influenza B. More importantly, influenza A epidemics are notable for causing mortality in excess of what is usually expected. In the 1957 to 1958 Asian influenza epidemic, nearly 70,000 excess deaths were reported in the United States during the 12-week epidemic period. Most nationwide influenza epidemics have resulted in 10,000 to 20,000 excess deaths. Hospitalization rates in high-risk groups will increase two- to fivefold. During influenza epidemics, deaths occur primarily among persons with chronic cardiovascular, pulmonary, renal, metabolic, or immunologic diseases. Surveys indicate that almost 50 percent of elderly persons have high-risk conditions, but only 25 percent of these get vaccinated. Vaccination of high risk populations has been shown to reduce mortality and complications associated with influenza. Vaccination of the entire population has not been considered a reasonable public health policy because protection is of limited duration owing to both the antigenic drift of the virus, as well as the short-lived antibody response to the inactivated vaccine, and the low incidence of serious infections in healthy persons.

Influenza vaccines are inactivated products of the prevalent circulating types of influenza virus. The vaccine usually contains influenza A and influenza B prototype antigens. Two types of vaccines are available, whole virus vaccines and "split-product" or subunit vaccines. Generally, whole virus vaccines are more immunogenic but have a slightly higher reaction rate than split-product vaccines. Studies with both preparations indicate a 60 to 95 percent protection rate, depending upon the population group studied and the relationship between the "epidemic" strain and the vaccine strain. In adults either form of vaccine can be used, but because of the high frequency of febrile reactions, children under 12 should receive two doses of split-product vaccine at approximately 3- to 6-week intervals. Vaccine is generally administered during the fall of the year and is given subcutaneously. While intradermal vaccination may elicit a good humoral antibody response, the clinical efficacy of this route of administration has not been well documented. Because even the zonally centrifuged inactivated influenza vaccines contain trace amounts of egg protein, patients who are allergic to egg or egg protein should not receive this vaccine. Severe adverse reactions to influenza vaccine are uncommon. Among recipients of A/New Jersey/76 swine influenza vaccine, an excess risk of Landry-Guillain-Barré syndrome occurred (10 cases for every million vaccinated), an incidence five to six times higher than in unvaccinated persons, but more recent (nonswine) influenza vaccines have not been associated with an increased risk of the Landry-Guillain-Barré syndrome.

Influenza vaccine is the preferred form of prophylaxis, because of its low cost, efficacy, and slight toxicity. Amantadine hydrochloride has been effective in preventing influenza infection especially during interepidemic intervals. Patients at risk of developing the complications of influenza who failed to receive their annual influenza vaccination should be placed on 100 mg amantadine hydrochloride twice daily during the period in which influenza A virus is identified in the community or until adequate protection after receipt of influenza vaccine has occurred.

Pneumococcal vaccine (see Chap. 93)   Despite antibiotic therapy, the morbidity and mortality of pneumococcal disease remains a problem. Bacteremic pneumococcal disease appears to be more common in persons with sickle cell anemia, anatomic or functional asplenia, agammaglobulinemia, multiple myeloma, nephrotic syndrome, cirrhosis, alcoholism, diabetes mellitus, chronic cardiorespiratory disease, and after organ transplantation; in these situations vaccination is generally indicated. Other situations in which pneumococcal vaccine may be of benefit include closed populations in which systemic pneumococcal disease has been identified as an epidemic or endemic problem, or where an antibiotic-resistant strain of pneumococcus has emerged.

The pneumococcal polysaccharide vaccine licensed for use in the United States contains purified capsular material extracted separately from 23 types of *Streptococcus pneumoniae* (Danish types 1, 2, 3, 4, 5, 6F, 7F, 8, 9N, 9V, 10A, 11A, 12F, 14, 15B, 17F, 18C, 19A, 19F, 20, 22F, 23F, and 33F). These 23 types are responsible for about 87 percent of bacteremic pneumococcal disease in the United States. One dose of vaccine contains 25 μg of each polysaccharide. The majority of adults and most children over 2 years of age respond with development of measurable humoral antibody 2 to 3 weeks after vaccination. Immunity exists only against the pneumococcal types contained in the vaccine, although theoretically there may be some degree of cross-protection among immunologically similar types. The duration of protection is unknown, but elevated antibody levels appear to persist 3 to 5 years after immunizations. Booster doses are not recommended because of accentuated local adverse reactions. Persons who received the previous tetradecavalent (14-type) vaccine should not get the newer 23 valent vaccine. Vaccination reduces the likelihood of acquiring the pneumococcal types in the vaccine in the nasopharynx. There has been no evidence of a relative increase in disease caused by other microbial pathogens among vaccine recipients. Vaccination appears to reduce the incidence of pneumococcal pneumonia and bacteremia due to types in the vaccine by about 70 percent. Efficacy may be slightly lower in persons with cirrhosis or renal failure. Two-thirds of persons with serious pneumococcal disease have been hospitalized in the prior 5 years. This suggests that vaccination of high-risk patients who come to hospitals should be performed. Local erythema and pain at the injection site occur in approximately half the patients. Fever and myalgias are reported in fewer than 1 percent of recipients. Serious adverse reactions are rare, about 5 per 1 million doses.

Hepatitis B vaccine   Hepatitis B vaccine (HBV) is a subunit, inactivated preparation containing the hepatitis B surface antigen (HBsAg). It is manufactured by concentration purification and inactivation of the hepatitis B virus from human donors with high titers of hepatitis B surface antigen in their plasma. Hepatitis B vaccine contains 20 μg/mL of HBsAg protein. Three 1-mL doses of vaccine given 1 and 6 months apart are recommended; O.5-mL (10 μg) doses are recommended for infants and children from 3 months to 9 years of age. For immunosuppressed patients and patients undergoing hemodialysis three 40-μg doses are recommended. Anti-HBs can be detected in the serum of both adults and children in over 90 percent of recipients after a complete vaccination series. Vaccine should be administered in the deltoid; lower seroconversion rates are seen with buttock injections. The protective efficacy of hepatitis B vaccine for the prevention of clinical hepatitis B has been approximately 95 percent in homosexual men, 90 percent in medical staff of hemodialysis units with endemic hepatitis B, and 75 percent in patients with renal insufficiency undergoing chronic hemodialysis in units with endemic hepatitis B. The duration of vaccine-induced protection and the need for boosters are not known.

Because of the cost and limited availability of vaccine, vaccination strategy is based on selective immunization of high-risk groups. These include susceptible household and sexual contacts of patients with acute and/or chronic hepatitis B, illicit users of injectable drugs, homosexual men, patients requiring blood clotting factor concentrations and large-volume transfusions, residents and staff of institutions and hemodialysis units, infants born to HBsAg-positive women, and closed communities where hepatitis B is endemic. Selective vaccination of health care personnel, including laboratory personnel who handle blood and blood products, nursing staff, and medical and dental personnel having frequent contact with groups with hepatitis B or blood products, is also recommended. These persons should be vaccinated as soon as possible after they begin work in a high-risk environment. The vaccine appears to have no effect on patients who are carriers of hepatitis B surface antigen and has not been associated with either resolution or worsening of chronic hepatitis B infection.

Postexposure immunization with a combination of hepatitis B immune globulin (HBIG) plus hepatitis B vaccine is useful in some clinical situations, such as immunoprophylaxis of infants born to mothers with acute or chronic hepatitis B, sexual contacts of patients with acute or chronic hepatitis B, or needle stick exposure from a known HBsAg carrier. When administered at a different site, HBIG does not appear to alter the subsequent development of anti-HBs after hepatitis B vaccine, and the combination of HBV and HBIG obviates the need for a second dose of HBIG.

Haemophilus influenzae vaccine (see Chap. 109) *H. influenzae* type B infection is largely a disease of children, with peak attack rates between 6 months and 1 year of age. After 5 years of age, *H. influenzae* disease is not usually a significant problem. A polysaccharide vaccine has been newly licensed in the United States for routine use in all children at age 24 months. The vaccine could be used at age 18 months in high-risk groups, such as children attending day-care centers. Insufficient data are available on the efficacy and immunogenicity of vaccine in older children and adults. The vaccine should be used in children with chronic conditions associated with a high risk of type B disease such as hypogammaglobulinemia, asplenia, and Hodgkin's disease.

VACCINES USEFUL IN LOCALIZED OUTBREAKS Meningococcal

vaccine (see Chap. 103) Meningococcal disease is endemic throughout the world. Occasionally, epidemics occur. In civilians in the United States meningococcal infections occur primarily in single isolated cases; serogroup B cause most of the illnesses, with serogroups C and W-135 accounting for the remainder. Secondary cases occur more frequently in household contacts than in the general population, and appropriate antibiotic prophylaxis has been the principal method of reducing the risk for immediate contacts. Vaccines have been used to curtail outbreaks of groups A and C meningococcal disease, and when epidemic meningococcal disease due to groups A or C occurs, the population at risk should be identified and vaccinated. Vaccination also should be considered as an adjunct to antibiotic prophylaxis for household contacts of cases of meningococcal disease caused by serogroups A, C, Y, or W-135. Because half of the secondary cases in families occur more than 5 days after the primary case, this is enough time to allow potential benefit from vaccination if antibiotic chemoprophylaxis has not been successful.

Two meningococcal polysaccharide vaccines, bivalent A-C, and quadrivalent A, C, Y, and W-135, are licensed for selective use in the United States. These vaccines are chemically defined antigens consisting of purified capsular polysaccharides and induce specific immunity to the serologic groups. The vaccine is administered

parenterally as a single dose. Adverse reactions consist principally of localized erythema lasting 1 to 2 days. The vaccine appears effective in all age groups beyond the first year of life, and there is suggestive evidence of efficacy in children as young as 3 months of age. The duration of immunity and the need for booster doses has not been established.

BCG vaccine Efforts to control tuberculosis in the United States are directed toward the early identification and treatment of active cases and preventive therapy with isoniazid. Use of BCG vaccine should be considered for uninfected persons (skin test negative to 5 tuberculin units) who are exposed repeatedly to untreated or inadequately treated individuals or to individuals harboring resistant organisms, or health care workers and others with an annual infection rate of greater than 1 percent despite control measures. The protection from BCG vaccine is relative, and neither permanent nor predictable. BCG recipients should have repeat skin tests 2 to 3 months later; if they are negative, vaccination should be repeated. The World Health Organization (WHO) recommends that BCG vaccine be administered by the intradermal route, but vaccine for percutaneous administration is also available. Severe ulceration at the vaccination site occurs in about 1 percent of vaccinees. BCG should not be given to persons with impaired immune responses, and although no harmful effects of BCG on the fetus have been observed, it is best to avoid vaccination during pregnancy.

Adenovirus vaccine The epidemiologic syndrome of epidemic acute respiratory disease due to adenovirus 4 or 7 is almost exclusively a problem of military recruits. While an effective oral attenuated adenovirus vaccine has been manufactured, clinical illness caused by these adenoviruses has not been associated with significant morbidity or mortality in the civilian population, and hence use of this vaccine outside the military is not recommended.

Typhoid vaccine Routine typhoid vaccination is not recommended in the United States. Selective immunization is indicated for persons who are household contacts of a documented typhoid carrier or travelers to areas where typhoid is endemic. Typhoid vaccine is generally not necessary for persons affected by flooding or other natural disasters or for those in rural summer camps. Typhoid vaccine consists of whole typhoid bacilli that have been killed, concentrated, and preserved by various methods. The vaccine should be given in two doses of 0.5 mL subcutaneously or 0.1 mL intradermally, according to the manufacturers' recommendations. Booster doses at intervals of 3 years or more are recommended. Local reactions such as erythema, induration, and moderate fever for about 24 h may occur. Controlled trials indicate a 70 to 90 percent protection rate from clinical typhoid. Immunity may be overcome by exposure to high inocula of *Salmonella,* and localized gastrointestinal infection accompanied by diarrhea may still occur. A newly developed *oral* typhoid vaccine affords protection and is much easier to administer, particularly in endemic areas.

VACCINATION OF TRAVELERS TO FOREIGN COUNTRIES There

are two objectives for immunization of foreign travelers: (1) to satisfy a country's requirements, as modified by international regulations, regarding prevention of the introduction and spread of disease (e.g., yellow fever, cholera, and smallpox), and (2) to protect the traveler.

Smallpox vaccination (see Chap. 134) In May 1980, the WHO declared the world free of smallpox. A smallpox vaccination certificate is not required by any country as a condition of entry for international travel. In May 1983, the distribution of smallpox vaccine for civilian use in the United States was discontinued. In the United States, smallpox vaccination is recommended only for persons who work in high-security laboratories with variola virus. Smallpox vaccine should *not* be used for the treatment of warts or prevention of recurrent herpes simplex virus infections.

Yellow fever vaccine Many countries require a current international certificate of vaccination against yellow fever from persons older than 6 months who have been in the countries reporting yellow fever (South America and the African subcontinent) in the preceding 6 days. Because these requirements change and often vary with the length of stay in the country, all travelers to areas where yellow fever is endemic should seek current information from health departments or international airlines before departing. Yellow fever vaccine must be administered at a designated yellow fever center. Vaccination certificates are valid for a period of 10 years, beginning 10 days after vaccination. The only yellow fever vaccine licensed in the United States is a live attenuated vaccine produced in chick embryos which must be administered subcutaneously in 0.5-mL amounts. Fever and malaise occur in 10 percent of recipients, but major reactions such as encephalitis are very rare. While pregnant females should generally not be vaccinated with live attenuated virus, the risk to the fetus is small, and pregnant women who must travel to areas where the risk of yellow fever is high should be vaccinated. Yellow fever virus vaccine should not be given to patients with severe underlying diseases such as leukemia or those receiving immunosuppressive therapy.

Cholera (see Chap. 115)   Travelers to the Middle East, Asia, and Africa may require evidence of cholera vaccination. Ideally, travelers to these countries should be vaccinated 1 month prior to their departure. A single primary series or booster dose of vaccine is generally sufficient. The risk of cholera for travelers who use ordinary tourist accommodations is very slight, and currently available cholera vaccines are only about 50 percent effective in reducing the incidence of clinical illness for a period of only 3 to 6 months. They do not prevent transmission of disease.

Typhoid   Travelers going to regions where food and water sanitation is poor may wish to receive typhoid vaccine. However, care in selecting food and water is the best protection.

Japanese encephalitis (see Chap. 143)   Cases of Japanese encephalitis have occurred in travelers. An effective inactivated mouse-brain vaccine is available from Japan. While currently not licensed in the United States, the vaccine may be obtained under an investigational permit from the Centers of Disease Control. Candidates for the vaccine are persons who plan a visit of 3 or more weeks during the time of peak encephalitis activity to those areas in which Japanese encephalitis occurs and whose itinerary includes extensive travel to rural areas and intensive exposure to mosquito vectors. Short visits to urban areas are not an indication for vaccination.

Plague (see Chap. 114)   Immunization against *Yersinia pestis* is recommended only for laboratory workers and for individuals such as Peace Corps volunteers or agricultural advisors who reside in plague-enzootic or plague-epidemic rural areas where avoidance of rodents and fleas is difficult. Travelers to countries or areas reporting endemic plague do not need to receive vaccine.

UNUSUAL OCCUPATIONAL EXPOSURES   In general, vaccination of personnel such as laboratory or field workers whose vocation or avocation puts them at particular risk of developing an immunizable disease should receive preexposure immunization. For example, laboratory workers involved with rabies, *Y. pestis*, smallpox, *Rickettsia prowazekii*, *R. rickettsii*, yellow fever virus, or Venezuelan or Eastern equine encephalitis viruses, anthrax bacillus, or tularemia should be vaccinated against the appropriate agent. Occupational exposure requiring vaccination includes preexposure immunization against rabies for veterinarians, spelunkers, and other animal handlers exposed to potentially rabid dogs, cats, skunks, foxes, and bats; *Yersinia* vaccination for field workers in endemic areas; and anthrax vaccination for industrial workers who process hides, hair, bone meal, and wool of potentially infected animals.

PASSIVE IMMUNIZATION (Table 92-2)   Prophylaxis or therapy of infection can also be accomplished by passive immunization which involves the administration of preformed antibody obtained from humans or other animals who have been actively immunized. Because animal antiserum can induce a hypersensitivity response in the recipient, antiserums from humans are preferable. The duration of immunity provided by passive immunization is brief. Intracellular virus generally is not affected by antibody, and once infection has been initiated, the role of antibody is limited to resisting the spread of the virus.

Hepatitis A (see Chap. 247)   Immune serum globulin (ISG) administered before exposure and during the incubation period of hepatitis A is 80 to 90 percent effective in preventing or modifying the disease. The prophylactic effect of ISG is greatest when given early in the incubation period, and the use of ISG more than 2 weeks after exposure or after onset of clinical illness is not indicated. Immune serum globulin is recommended for household contacts of patients with hepatitis A but not for contacts at school, hospital, or work. In institutional settings where periodic epidemics of hepatitis A are common, the administration of ISG to residents and staff may limit the spread of the disease. The dose of ISG for postexposure prophylaxis is 0.02 mL per kilogram of body weight.

The risk of hepatitis A for residents of the United States traveling abroad is small. Travelers to tropical areas or to developing countries who bypass the usual tourist routes should probably be given ISG. For travelers at risk for 2 to 3 months, a single intramuscular dose of 0.02 mL/kg is recommended. Travelers staying in developing countries or in tropical areas longer than 3 months should receive a single injection of ISG, 0.06 mL per kilogram of body weight, every 5 months. Immune globulin modified for intravenous administration may be given as prophylaxis to those for whom intramuscular preparations are contraindicated because of thrombocytopenic or hemorrhagic disorders. The manufacturer's recommendations should be closely followed concerning dose and route of administration.

Hepatitis B (see Chaps. 85 and 247)   Hepatitis B immune globulin (HBIG) alone or in combination with hepatitis B vaccine is used for postexposure prophylaxis of hepatitis B. Some controversy exists about the relative efficacy and/or cost benefit of ISG-containing antibody to hepatitis B surface antigen (anti-HBs) or hyperimmune globulin containing a high titer of anti-HBs [hepatitis B immunoglobulin (HBIG)]. HBIG is recommended for susceptible health care personnel who are anti-HBs-negative and who have a percutaneous or mucous membrane exposure to blood from documented HBsAg-positive donors. Ideally, a single dose of HBIG (0.06 mL/kg or 5 mL for adults) should be administered within 48 h of exposure. Because of its lower cost and more likely potential for preventing non-A, non-B hepatitis, ISG may be used in susceptible persons with needle exposures from unknown sources. A series of 3 doses of hepatitis B vaccine should also be initiated within 1 week of exposure. Vaccine and HBIG may be given simultaneously, but in different sites. For those who do not choose to take hepatitis B vaccine, a second dose of HBIG should be given 1 month later. HBIG and hepatitis B vaccine are 90 percent effective in preventing chronic hepatitis B infection in neonates born to mothers with acute or chronic hepatitis B. HBIG should be given to the infant within 24 h of birth (preferably in the delivery room), and hepatitis vaccination should be initiated within the first week of life. For homosexual exposure to an HBsAg-positive male, a single dose of HBIG should be given to susceptible contacts within 14 days of sexual exposure. Hepatitis B vaccine should then be initiated. For heterosexual exposure to persons with acute hepatitis B, a single dose of HBIG is also recommended. If the index case remains HBsAg-positive for 3 months and exposure is continuous, a second dose of HBIG and vaccination should be considered.

Varicella-zoster serum immune globulin (VZIG)   If administered within 72 h after exposure, VZIG may prevent or ameliorate varicella-zoster among immunosuppressed susceptible patients. Indications for the use of VZIG are listed in Chap. 135. VZIG is not indicated in established varicella-zoster or in adults with a past history of varicella.

Diphtheria antitoxin (see Chap. 96)   Diphtheria antitoxin may be useful in the prophylaxis of asymptomatic unimmunized household

TABLE 92-2 Passive immunization

Disease	Preparation	Route	Comments
Hepatitis A	ISG, human	IM (0. mL/kg) IV (10	Household contacts
Hepatitis B	Human hepatitis B immuno-globulin	IM (0.; two doses 4 wee	HBIG is preferred prophylaxis for direct paren-teral exposure (needle stick) or mucous-membrane contact in susceptibles; if unavail-able, ISG should be given. HBIG should be administered to neonates born to mothers with hepatitis B.
	ISG, human	IM (0.t; two doses 4 wee	
Vaccinia immuno-globulin	Human VIG	IM (0.:	Use in eczema vaccinatum, disseminated vacci-nia, vaccinia in pregnancy
Herpes zoster	Human varicella-ZIG	IM (12er 10 kg, up to 625	Prevention and amelioration of varicella in sus-ceptible immunosuppressed patients
Diphtheria	Diphtheria antitoxin, horse	IM or D0–100,000 units)	Dose dependent on extent of membrane and degree of toxicity; may also be used in unim-munized household contacts
Tetanus	Human tetanus immuno-globulin (TIG)	IM (25(	When given with tetanus toxoid, use separate syringes and sites
Rabies	Human rabies immuno-globulin	One-hal and one-half IM/kg)	Used for postexposure prophylaxis with rabies vaccine
	Equine antirabies globulin	One-hal and one-half IM/kg)	Same as above
Pertussis	Pertussis immunoglobulin, human	IM (1.5peat in 5–7 days)	No studies suggest efficacy in susceptible infants
Measles	ISG, human	IM (0.2 or 20–30 mL)	Susceptible household contacts less than 1 year old, exposed susceptible pregnant females, or immunodeficient persons
Rubella	ISG, human	IM (20–	Exposed susceptible pregnant females who will not consider termination
Botulism (Chap. 100)	Horse serum, trivalent AB	One-halfd one-half IV (8–32 r	Use only therapeutically: greatest efficacy in type E
Snake bite (Chap. 170)	Polyvalent crotaline anti-venom (pit vipers)	IV (dosen of severity of bite)	See Chap. 170
Spider bite (Chap. 170)	Equine	IM (2.5	*Latrodectus* (black widow spider) poisoning

* IM, intramuscularly; IV, intravenously.

contacts along with (1) chemoprophylaxis with either oral erythro-mycin or intramuscular benzathine penicillin or (2) immunization with diphtheria toxoid. The risk of diphtheria among household contacts, which was approximately 20 percent before the antibiotic era but is negligible now, must be weighed against that of serum sickness from equine antiserum before this product is used.

Tetanus immune globulin (TIG) (see Chap. 99) The product of choice when contaminated wounds are present in persons whose history of previous tetanus immunization is uncertain or inadequate is TIG. The current recommended prophylactic dose of TIG is 250 to 1000 units given intramuscularly. TIG does not interfere with the primary immune response to tetanus toxoid given at the same time but at a different site.

Rabies (see Chap. 142) Postexposure prophylaxis for rabies consists of both passive and active immunization. Human rabies immune globulin is the preferred immunizing agent. The dose is 20 IU per kilogram of body weight given half intramuscularly and half intra-venously.

Pertussis (see Chap. 109) Hyperimmune pertussis globulin does not appear effective in preventing disease among unvaccinated susceptible neonates.

Measles (see Chap. 132) Immune serum globulin should not be used to control measles outbreaks. Live measles vaccination can usually prevent development of disease if administered within 2 days of exposure. Immune serum globulin should be reserved for susceptible household contacts of measles patients, particularly for those under 1 year of age, exposed pregnant females, or persons in whom measles vaccine is contraindicated, such as immune deficient hosts. The usual dose is 10 to 20 mL intramuscularly.

Rubella (see Chap. 133) After exposure to rubella, ISG will not prevent infection or viremia with rubella virus but may modify or

press symptoms. The routine use of ISG for postexposure pro-laxis of rubella in early pregnancy is not recommended, and nts with congenital rubella have been born to women who were n ISG shortly after exposure.

EMOPROPHYLAXIS OF INFECTION

E OF A SINGLE DRUG Antibiotics have been used prophylac-lly to (1) prevent the acquisition of an exogenous organism, (2) vent a resident organism from infecting a normally sterile site, (3) prevent a dormant pathogenic organism from causing disease. neral, antimicrobial prophylaxis with a single drug, administered r a moderate period of time and directed at a single pathogen, been successful. Examples of this type of prophylaxis employing doses of "narrow-spectrum" antimicrobials include the preven-of recurrent episodes of rheumatic fever secondary to group A ptococcal disease with benzathine penicillin, of malaria with roquine, and of influenza A with amantadine. Table 92-3 lists e clinical situations where prolonged chemoprophylaxis either to vent exposure to an exogenous organism or reactivation of a mant organism in a uniquely susceptible host has been useful. There are also situations in which the short-term use of antibiotics y prevent bacteremia, as in prophylaxis of bacterial endocarditis ndividuals with acquired or congenital heart disease, or may abort alized mucosal infections. Here the use of antibiotics is based on rationale that brief exposure to an antimicrobial, early in the ase before bacterial multiplication has led to established infection, y prevent full-blown disease. Some examples of short-term pro-laxis are given in Table 92-4.

TIBIOTICS PROPHYLAXIS IN SURGERY Controlled evaluations short courses of prophylactic antimicrobials have indicated that selective use of antibiotics, particularly in operative procedures

TABLE 92-3 Drugs that may be administered prophylactically for prolonged exposure or for extended periods of time

Disease or organism	Drug
Group A streptococcus (rheumatic fever) (Chap. 186)	Penicillin G, sulfonamide
Influenza A infection* (Chap. 130)	Amantadine
Malaria (Chap. 154)	Chloroquine and/or pyrimethamine, sulfadoxine
Tuberculosis contacts (Chap. 119)	Isoniazid
Recurrent urinary tract infection in females (Chap. 225)	Trimethoprim-sulfamethoxazole, nitrofurantoin
Recurrent otitis media (Chap. 212)	Sulfisoxazole, ampicillin, trimethoprim-sulfamethoxazole

IMMUNOSUPPRESSED PATIENTS

Pneumocystis carinii in cancer patients receiving cytotoxic agents* (Chap. 158)	Trimethoprim-sulfamethoxazole
Bacterial infections in granulocytopenic patients (Chap. 84)	Trimethoprim-sulfamethoxazole, liquid nonabsorbable antibiotics (vancomycin, gentamycin, nystatin)
Bacterial infection in persons with defective antibody synthesis	Immune serum globulin for intravenous use
Herpes simplex virus infections in patients receiving cytotoxic agents (Chap. 136)	Acyclovir†
Cytomegalovirus infection in renal transplant patients (Chap. 137)	Leukocyte interferon†

* *May require only short courses.*
† *Not licensed by the Food and Drug Administration.*

involving potentially contaminated surgical sites, will lower the rate of postoperative infections. The following principles should be applied in using antimicrobial prophylaxis in surgery (Table 92-5): (1) there must be a high prevalence of postoperative infections that are potentially severe before employing antimicrobial drugs; (2) the prophylactic antimicrobial must be effective against the most frequent postoperative pathogens; (3) the drug should be administered from immediately before and during the operation, and for only a short period thereafter; and (4) where possible, prophylaxis should be carried out with a single drug. In studies of cardiac, colorectal

TABLE 92-4 Short-term antimicrobial prophylaxis

Disease	Antibiotic
USUALLY EFFECTIVE	
Subacute bacterial endocarditis:	
Streptococcus viridans	Penicillin V or procaine penicillin G plus streptomycin
Enterococcus	Ampicillin or penicillin G or vancomycin plus gentamicin or streptomycin
Neisseria gonorrheae (ophthalmia)	Silver nitrate, penicillin, tetracycline
Neisseria gonorrheae (genital infection)	Tetracycline
Nongonococcal urethritis	Tetracycline
Congenital or incubating syphilis	Penicillin
Toxigenic *Escherichia coli* ("tourista")	Tetracycline, trimethoprim-sulfamethoxazole, bismuth subsalicylate
Enteropathogenic *E. coli* diarrhea	Neomycin or kanamycin
Neisseria meningitidis	Sulfonamides (sensitive strains only), rifampin, minocycline
Corynebacterium diphtheriae	Erythromycin, clindamycin, penicillin, benzathine penicillin
SOMETIMES EFFECTIVE	
Shigellosis	Ampicillin, neomycin
Chronic bronchitis*	Ampicillin, tetracycline
Short-term urethral catheterization (<24 h)	Ampicillin, tetracycline, nitrofurantoin, trimethoprim-sulfamethoxazole

* *Prophylaxis may require prolonged administration.*

al, and biliary tract surgery, single-dose antibiotic prophylaxis [has] been as effective as multiple postoperative administration of [antibi]otics. Antibiotic prophylaxis is recommended in clean surgical [proc]edures that involve insertion of prostheses where the development [of in]fections can be severe or fatal. Other operations such as those [invo]lving clean-contaminated, contaminated, or "dirty" wounds, [whe]re the infection rates vary from 10 to 40 percent, also warrant [prop]hylactic antibiotics. This topic is also discussed in Chap. 85. [For] choice of the appropriate agent, Chap. 88 should be consulted.

[ANTI]BIOTICS IN SUSCEPTIBLE HOSTS In contrast to short-term [anti]microbial prophylaxis with a single drug, which is unlikely to be [dele]terious, attempts to prevent infection with multiple drugs administered in high doses for relatively prolonged periods are much more [like]ly to be harmful. Adverse effects of "prolonged" antimicrobial [prop]hylaxis include (1) superinfection (defined as an infection with [a re]sistant organism that has developed during antibiotic therapy), [(2)] increased incidence of toxic or allergic reactions to drugs, (3) [incr]eased cost, and last but not least, (4) a sense of false security on [the] part of attending physicians or surgeons, resulting in less stringent [obs]ervation of the patient. However, many of the patients who are [giv]en antibiotics prophylactically are precisely the ones who are [su]sceptible to complicating infections, and particular care must be [ta]ken to watch assiduously for the development of infection and to [tre]at it promptly when it occurs. Such policy is often superior to the [us]e of antimicrobial prophylaxis.

Prophylactic antibiotics have not been useful in preventing bacterial [co]mplications of antecedent viral respiratory illness such as influenza

[TA]BLE 92-5 Systemic antimicrobial prophylaxis in surgery

	Antibiotic
[PR]OPHYLAXIS INDICATED	
[O]bstetric-gynecologic surgery:	
Vaginal and abdominal hysterectomy	A cephalosporin (cefazolin), metronidazole
Caesarean section after prolonged rupture of membranes	A cephalosporin
[C]olorectal surgery	Neomycin and erythromycin base, doxycycline, cefoxitin, metronidazole, gentamicin plus clindamycin, cefamycin
Appendectomy	Doxycycline, cefoxitin, ampicillin
Cardiac surgery (including coronary artery bypass)	A cephalosporin
Valvular, noncardiac thoracic surgery	A cephalosporin
Orthopedic surgery (joint replacement, prosthesis, compound fractures)	A cephalosporin or penicillinase-resistant penicillin
Peripheral artery surgery with graft replacement	A cephalosporin
Contaminated surgical wounds	A cephalosporin
Prostatectomy with preoperative bacteriuria	Treat according to bacterial sensitivity tests
PROPHYLAXIS OF VALUE IN SELECTED PATIENTS	
Gastroduodenal surgery (obstructing duodenal ulcer, achlorhydria, chronic cimetidine therapy, gastric ulcer, malignancy, bypass for obesity)	A cephalosporin
Biliary tract surgery (elderly, obstructed)	A cephalosporin
Microsurgical craniotomy	A cephalosporin
Extensive ear, nose, or throat surgery	A cephalosporin
PROPHYLAXIS UNLIKELY TO BE OF VALUE	
Clean abdominal surgery	
Gynecologic surgery (other than mentioned above)	
Genitourinary surgery in persons with sterile urine	
Simple lacerations	

CHAPTER 93 PNEUMOCOCCAL INFECTIONS

TABLE 92-6 Antibiotic prophylaxis in susceptible hosts in whom its use is not indicated

OUTPATIENT USE

Viral respiratory disease
Viral exanthems
Preventing acute exacerbations of asthma

HOSPITALIZED PATIENTS

Preventing pneumonia in comatose patients
Preventing tracheal colonization with pathogenic organisms
Preventing infections in patients with congestive heart failure
Prolonged urethral catheterization (>24 h)
Prolonged intravenous catheterization (>48 h)
High-dose steroid therapy
Prematurity
Shock

or in preventing colonization of pathogenic organisms in intensive care units. Indeed, in these and many other clinical situations the risk of superinfection with resistant, difficult-to-treat organisms outweighs the unlikely effectiveness of prophylactic antibiotics (Table 92-6). However, in some populations, such as victims of severe burns or patients with severe granulocytopenia, antibiotic prophylaxis may be useful. Infections in granulocytopenic patients are often life-threatening. Most infections develop in persons with prolonged (>14 days) and profound (<100 granulocytes per milliliter) granulocytopenia. Mucosal damage by tumor therapy allows invasion of organisms colonizing the alimentary and respiratory tracts and the oral cavity, resulting in pneumonitis, esophagitis, colitis, and perianal infections. Many infections are due to the patient's indigenous flora, and others are due to organisms acquired from the hospital environment. In selected patients, reduction of indigenous flora and prevention of colonization by microbial suppression using oral nonabsorbable antibiotics such as gentamicin, vancomycin, and nystatin (GVN) with or without laminar airflow rooms or selective suppression of alimentary canal microbial flora with trimethoprim-sulfamethoxazole with or without antifungal agents such as ketoconazole have been effective.

The necessity of maintaining continuous GVN therapy, the difficulty of patient compliance, the emergence of trimethoprim-sulfamethoxazole–resistant organisms, and the existence of localized outbreaks of unusual organisms indicate that continued evaluation of these prophylactic antibiotic regimens is needed. Among organ transplant patients, the use of systemic acyclovir to prevent endogenous reactivation of herpes simplex virus infections has been demonstrated. Immunobiogens, such as the interferons or immunoglobulins, have been effective in prevention of cytomegalovirus infections in selected instances, and their further evaluation is indicated.

REFERENCES

Adult immunization: Recommendations of the immunization practices advisory committee. Morb Mort Week Rep 33, no. 15, 1984

BROOME CV: Pneumococcal disease after pneumococcal vaccination. N Engl J Med 303:549, 1980

Centers for Disease Control: 1985 STD treatment guidelines. Morb Mort Week Rep 34(4S), 1985.

COMMITTEE ON IMMUNIZATION, COUNCIL OF MEDICAL SOCIETIES: Guide to adult immunization. Am Coll Phys 1985

DUPONT HL: Chemotherapy and chemoprophylaxis of traveler's diarrhea. Ann Intern Med 102:258, 1985

GOLDMAN PG, PETERSDORF RG: Prophylactic antibiotics: Controversies give way to guidelines. Drug Ther June 1979, pp 57–77

HIRSCHMANN JV, INUI TS: Antimicrobial prophylaxis: A critique of recent trials. Rev Infect Dis 2:1, 1980

IMMUNIZATION PRACTICES ADVISORY COMMITTEE, CDC: Poliomyelitis prevention. Ann Intern Med 96:630, 1982

KRUGMAN S: Effect of human immune serum globulin on infectivity of hepatitis A virus. J Infect Dis 34:70, 1975

LEVIN S: Selected overview of nongynecologic surgical intraabdominal infections: Prophylaxis and therapy. Am J Med 79(suppl 5B):146, 1985

RUBEN FL: Antitoxin responses in the elderly to tetanus-diphtheria (Td) immunization. Am J Epidemiol 108:145, 1978

SCHIMPFF SE: Infection prevention during profound granulocytopenia. Ann Intern Med 93:358, 1980

SHAPIRO ED: Controlled evaluation of the protective efficacy of pneumococcal vaccine for patients at high risk of serious pneumococcal infection. Ann Intern Med 301:325, 1984

WEISS BP: Tetanus and diphtheria immunity in an elderly population in Los Angeles County. Am J Public Health 73:802, 1983

section 2 Diseases caused by gram-positive organisms

93 PNEUMOCOCCAL INFECTIONS

ROBERT AUSTRIAN

ETIOLOGY The pneumococcus *(Streptococcus pneumoniae)* is a gram-positive encapsulated coccus that usually grows in pairs or short chains. In the diplococcal form, the adjacent margins are rounded and the opposite ends slightly pointed, giving the organisms a lancet shape. In stained preparations of exudate, gram-negative forms are sometimes present. Pneumococcal colonies are surrounded by greenish discoloration on or in blood agar and are confused at times with other alpha-hemolytic streptococci to which they are closely related. Their isolation from respiratory secretions may be facilitated by inclusion of 5 μg gentamicin per milliliter in the medium. Pneumococci can be distinguished by their bile solubility and mouse virulence or by serologic typing. Another method with approximately 90 percent specificity, utilizing inhibition of pneumococci by Optochin-impregnated paper disks, is less cumbersome.

The capsular substances are complex polysaccharides and are the basis for dividing pneumococci into serotypes. Organisms exposed to type-specific antiserum show a positive capsular precipitin reaction, the *Neufeld quellung reaction;* by this means, 84 serotypes have been identified. All are pathogenic for human beings, but types or groups 1, 3, 4, 7, 8, 9, and 12 are encountered most frequently in clinical practice. Types or groups 6, 14, 19, and 23 often cause pneumonia and otitis media in children but are less common in adults.

Specific typing of pneumococci remains of great clinical importance if pneumococcus is to be identified with regularity, and recognition of pneumococcus has decreased significantly since the abandonment of capsular typing by most clinical laboratories. The detection of pneumococcal capsular polysaccharides in sputum and in other body fluids by immunologic methods such as counterimmunoelectrophoresis (CIE) or latex agglutination provides an alternative to bacteriologic techniques for the presumptive diagnosis of pneumococcal infection. Because of cross reactions between the polysaccharides of pneumococci and of other bacterial species, immunologic diagnosis is less specific than bacteriologic diagnosis.

PATHOGENESIS The mechanism by which pneumococci damage the mammalian host is obscure, and no toxin elaborated by the organism has been shown to play a major pathogenic role in pneumococcal infection, although components of the cell wall may cause inflammation. The capsular polysaccharides, though nontoxic, are known to be necessary factors in virulence and to protect the organism to a certain extent from phagocytosis.

Although "pneumococcal pharyngitis" is a doubtful entity, invasion of the tissue of the nasopharynx may occur in the infant and occasionally in the nonimmune adult and be followed by spread to the circulation via the cervical lymphatics. At times, secondary infection of serous cavities in the absence of demonstrable focal infection of the upper or lower respiratory tract may occur. The organisms multiply readily in vivo and may produce acute inflammation of the lungs, serous cavities, and endocardium.

The normal human respiratory tract is provided with a variety of mechanisms which guard the lungs from infection. The lower respiratory tract is protected by the glottis and larynx, and material passing these barriers stimulates the expulsive cough reflex. Removal of small particles impinging on the walls of the trachea and bronchi is facilitated by their mucociliary lining; and growth of bacteria reaching normal alveoli is inhibited by their relative dryness and by the phagocytic activity of alveolar macrophages. Any anatomic or physiologic derangement of these coordinated defenses tends to augment the susceptibility of the lungs to infection. Anesthesia, alcoholic intoxication, convulsions, and disturbed innervation of the larynx depress the cough reflex and may permit aspiration of infected material. Alterations in the tracheobronchial tree leading to anatomic changes in the epithelial lining or to localized obstruction increase the vulnerability of the lungs to infection. Pulmonary edema, local or generalized, resulting from viral infection, inhalation of irritant gases, cardiac failure, or contusion of the chest wall, provides a fluid menstruum in the alveoli for the growth of bacteria and their spread to adjacent areas of the lung. Viral infection of the respiratory epithelium with concomitant disruption of its component cells interferes significantly with the clearance of bacteria from the lungs, an observation in accord with the high incidence of pneumococcal pneumonia during epidemics of viral influenza and its frequent clinical association with sporadic viral respiratory infections.

Pneumonia begins usually in the right lower, right middle, or left lower lobe, those areas to which gravity is most likely to carry upper respiratory secretions aspirated during sleep. Bronchial embolization with infected mucinous secretions during the course of an upper respiratory infection appears to be the initiating factor in many cases of pneumococcal pneumonia. Protected initially from phagocytosis by mucinous material, the bacteria multiply and, in infected alveoli, evoke the outpouring of proteinaceous fluid which serves both as a nutrient and as a vehicle for spread to adjacent alveoli. Soon thereafter, polymorphonuclear leukocytes migrate from the pulmonary capillaries to phagocytize a part of the pneumococcal population before the appearance of detectable antibody. Delay in the polymorphonuclear leukocytic response occurs during alcoholic intoxication and certain forms of anesthesia, permitting spread of infection. Glucocorticosteroids may also interfere with leukocyte migration. Later, as the pneumonic lesion evolves, macrophages appear in the exudate and remove the debris of fibrin and cells. It is probable that antibody to the capsular polysaccharide of the invading pneumococcus makes its appearance locally in the lung before being detectable in the circulation. Such antibody increases the efficiency of phagocytosis approximately twofold and causes agglutination of the organisms and their adherence to alveolar walls, thereby slowing their dissemination in the lung. The outcome of infection depends, therefore, on the rate at which bacteria can multiply in the edema fluid and spread, and on the host's ability to immobilize and destroy them by phagocytosis. Individuals with hypogammaglobulinemia and patients with multiple myeloma (see Chap. 258) incapable of producing anticapsular antibody are prone to recurrent attacks of pneumococcal pneumonia. Repeated infection with the same pneumococcal type should always prompt a search for dysgammaglobulinemia.

Failure of local defense mechanisms in the lung results in lymphatic spread of pneumococci to the hilar lymph nodes. In the sinusoids of these organs, a sequence of events not unlike that in the lung ensues. If infection is not checked in this secondary line of defense, organisms find their way into the thoracic duct and then into the circulation. Although transient bacteremia may occur at the onset of many cases of pneumococcal pneumonia, it is detectable in only 20 to 30 percent of cases. Bacteremia, which reflects the body's inability to localize the pulmonary infection, is a poor prognostic sign and carries with it the danger of metastatic infection. The mortality of treated or untreated bacteremic pneumococcal pneumonia is four times that resulting from comparably managed nonbacteremic infections. Metastatic infection secondary to bacteremia may occur in the meninges, joints, or peritoneum or on the endocardium. Direct spread from the infected lung may give rise to empyema or to pericarditis.

Natural recovery from pneumococcal infection coincides usually, but not invariably, with the appearance of detectable type-specific antibody in the circulation and is often accompanied by a dramatic and abrupt fall in temperature, the so-called crisis. Antibody aids recovery by increasing the efficiency of phagocytosis and by limiting dissemination of the organisms. Bacteriostatic drugs, such as sulfonamides, facilitate control of the infection by limiting the size of the pneumococcal population, but the host's defense mechanisms are still required for the elimination of the bacteria. Bactericidal agents, such as penicillin, cause the death of pneumococci in the lung and are effective when some of the host's defense mechanisms are compromised. With the arrest of infection, the alveolar exudate undergoes liquefaction, the inflammatory debris is removed by expectoration and via the lymphatic channels, and the lung is restored to its normal state. Necrosis of pulmonary tissue as a result of pneumococcal infection is distinctly uncommon. Primary pneumococcal lung abscess is a rare clinical entity, although the diagnosis is mistakenly made at times when pneumococcal infection complicates lung abscess of other origins.

In addition to causing pneumonia and its metastatic sequelae, pneumococcus can extend from the nasopharynx to its adjacent structures, giving rise to otitis media, mastoiditis, paranasal sinusitis, or conjunctivitis. Soft tissue abscesses are rare but may occur.

PNEUMOCOCCAL PNEUMONIA

Pneumococcal pneumonia is a disease of considerable uniformity, in contrast to other infections such as typhoid fever and tuberculosis. The diseases produced by different pneumococcal serotypes show little variation in severity or in clinical manifestations. The prognosis in type 3 pneumococcal pneumonia is usually regarded as poor, probably because type 3 infections occur frequently in the aged and in patients with other debilitating diseases, such as diabetes and congestive heart failure. The usual lesion in adults is segmental or lobar in distribution, but in children and the aged, bronchopneumonia, characterized by patchy involvement, is frequent.

MANIFESTATIONS Pneumonia is often preceded for a few days by coryza or some other form of common respiratory disease. The onset is frequently so abrupt that the patient can state the exact hour that illness began. There is a sudden *shaking chill* in more than 80 percent of the cases and a rapid rise in temperature, with corresponding tachycardia and an increase in respiratory rate (tachypnea). Most patients with pneumococcal pneumonia have a single rigor unless antipyretic drugs are administered, and repeated chills should suggest another etiologic agent.

About 75 percent of patients develop severe *pleuritic pain* and *cough,* productive of pinkish or "rusty" mucoid sputum within a few hours. The chest pain is agonizing, and respirations become rapid, shallow, and grunting as the patient tries to splint the affected side. Many patients are mildly cyanotic as a result of hypoxia caused by $\dot{V}/\dot{Q}$ (ventilation perfusion ratio) abnormality or shunt, which accompanies altered respiration, and show dilatation of the alae nasi when first seen. Patients appear acutely ill; but nausea, headache, and malaise are not prominent, and most individuals are alert. Pleuritic pain and dyspnea are the dominant complaints.

In the untreated disease, there are sustained fever of 102.5 to 105°F (39.2 to 40.5°C), continued pleuritic pain, cough, and expectoration; and *abdominal distention* is frequent. *Herpes labialis* is a common complication. After 7 to 10 days, there are diaphoresis, abrupt defervescence, and dramatic improvement in well-being, the "crisis."

In cases which terminate fatally, there is usually extensive pulmonary involvement, and dyspnea, cyanosis, and tachycardia are prominent. Circulatory collapse or a picture resembling adult respiratory distress syndrome has been observed. Death in a few patients is associated with empyema or some other suppurative complication such as meningitis or endocarditis.

Physical examination reveals restricted motion of the affected hemithorax. Tactile fremitus may be decreased during the initial day of illness but is usually increased when consolidation is fully established. Deviation of the trachea away from the affected lung suggests pleural effusion or empyema. The percussion note is dull, and if the lesion is in an upper lobe, impaired motion of the diaphragm can be detected on the affected side. Very early in the course of infection, breath sounds are diminished, but as the lesion evolves, they become tubular or bronchial in quality, and bronchophony and whispered pectoriloquy can be elicited. These findings are accompanied by fine crepitant rales.

EFFECT OF SPECIFIC CHEMOTHERAPY Pneumococcal pneumonia usually improves promptly when an appropriate antimicrobial drug is given. Within 12 to 36 h after initiation of treatment with penicillin, temperature, pulse, and respiration begin to fall and may reach normal values, pleuritic pain subsides, and the spread of the inflammatory process is halted. The temperature of approximately half the patients, however, requires 4 days or longer to become normal, and failure of the patient's temperature to reach normal in 24 to 48 h should not prompt a change in antibacterial therapy in the absence of other indications.

COMPLICATIONS The typical course of pneumococcal pneumonia can be modified by the development of one or more local or distant complications:

In the lung ATELECTASIS Atelectasis of all or part of a lobe may occur during the active stage of pneumonia or after treatment has been instituted. The patient may complain of sudden recurrence of pleuritic pain and show rapid respirations. Small areas of atelectasis are often detected by x-ray in the absence of symptoms. These areas usually clear with coughing and deep breathing, but bronchoscopic aspiration is occasionally necessary. If atelectasis is allowed to persist, the affected area becomes fibrotic and functionless.

DELAYED RESOLUTION Return to normal of physical findings in the lung after pneumococcal pneumonia is usually complete within 2 to 4 weeks. X-ray evidence of residual pulmonary consolidation, however, may persist as long as 8 weeks, and other radiologic manifestations of the infection (volume loss, stranding, and pleural disease) may persist for up to 18 weeks. The process of resolution may require a longer time in those over 50 years of age and in those with chronic obstructive airway disease or alcoholism.

ABSCESS Lung abscess is a rare sequel to pneumococcal infection, although pneumococcal pneumonia is a not uncommon complication of lung abscess of other origins. It is manifested by continued fever and profuse expectoration of purulent sputum. X-ray shows one or more cavities. This complication is exceedingly rare in patients who receive penicillin therapy and is most likely to follow infection with pneumococcus type 3.

In adjacent structures PLEURAL EFFUSION Pleural effusion detectable in lateral decubitus x-rays of the chest occurs in approximately half of patients with pneumococcal pneumonia and is associated with delay in the initiation of therapy and with bacteremia. Usually the effusion is sterile and is absorbed spontaneously within a week or two. At times, however, the effusion is large and requires aspiration or drainage.

EMPYEMA Before the introduction of effective chemotherapy, empyema occurred in 5 to 8 percent of patients with pneumococcal pneumonia; it is now observed in less than 1 percent of treated cases. It is manifested by persistent fever or pleuritic pain, together with signs of pleural effusion. In the early stages, the gross appearance of infected fluid may not differ from that of a sterile pleural effusion; later, there is a profuse outpouring of polymorphonuclear leukocytes and fibrin, resulting in an exudate of thick greenish pus containing large clots of fibrin. The quantity of exudate may become large enough to displace mediastinal structures. In neglected cases, this process leads to extensive pleural scarring, with limitation of thoracic movement. Rupture and drainage through the chest wall *(empyema necessitatis)* occurs, but is rare. Metastatic *brain abscess* is an occasional complication of chronic empyema.

PERICARDITIS A particularly serious complication is spread of infection to the pericardial sac. This lesion is characterized by pain in the precordial region, a friction rub synchronous with the heartbeat, and distention of cervical veins, although one or all of these findings may be absent. The possibility of coexisting purulent pericarditis should be considered whenever a very ill patient with pneumonia develops empyema.

Metastatic infections *Arthritis* occurs more often in children than in adults. The affected joint is swollen, red, and painful, with a purulent effusion. It usually subsides promptly with systemic administration of penicillin, although aspiration and intraarticular injection of penicillin may be necessary in adults.

Acute bacterial endocarditis complicates pneumococcal pneumonia in fewer than 0.5 percent of cases. Its manifestations and treatment are discussed below. *Meningitis,* another complication of pneumococcal pneumonia, is also discussed subsequently.

Paralytic ileus Gaseous abdominal distention is commonly present and in severely ill patients may assume such serious proportions that the term *paralytic ileus* is justified. This complication further impairs respiratory movement by elevation of the diaphragm and constitutes a difficult problem in management. A rarer and more serious gastrointestinal complication is acute gastric dilatation.

Impaired liver function Alterations in hepatic function are common during the course of pneumococcal pneumonia, and mild jaundice is not at all rare. The pathogenesis of the jaundice is not entirely clear, although in some patients it appears to be related to glucose 6-phosphate dehydrogenase deficiency.

LABORATORY FINDINGS *Sputum* should be obtained in the physician's presence before the administration of antimicrobial drugs to ensure its quality. Although resort to transtracheal aspiration or lung puncture may be necessary on occasion to establish the cause of pneumonia, routine use of these invasive techniques is not recommended because of their attendant, albeit infrequent, complications. When stained by Gram's method, the sputum shows polymorphonuclear leukocytes and variable numbers of gram-positive cocci, singly and in pairs. These can be typed directly by the Neufeld quellung technique, and this procedure should be used to facilitate diagnosis whenever possible. The *blood culture* is positive for pneumococci during the first days of untreated illness in 20 to 30 percent of cases. The white blood count usually shows a polymorphonuclear *leukocytosis* ranging from 12,000 to 25,000 cells per cubic millimeter. A normal white count or leukopenia is sometimes observed in patients with overwhelming infection and bacteremia. Occasionally, pneumococci may be seen directly in granulocytes of patients with bacteremia by examining the buffy coat after staining with Wright's stain. These patients often have asplenia. *X-ray of the chest* usually reveals a homogenous density in the affected area of the lung. In well-established cases, the density may occupy one or more entire lobes. Atypical patterns of consolidation may be seen in patients with underlying chronic pulmonary disease.

EXTRAPULMONARY PNEUMOCOCCAL INFECTION

PNEUMOCOCCAL MENINGITIS The pneumococcus is second only to the meningococcus as a cause of purulent meningitis in adults; in children, meningitis caused by *Haemophilus influenzae* is also more frequent than pneumococcal infection.

Pneumococcal meningitis can develop as a "primary" disease without preceding signs of infection elsewhere; as a complication of pneumococcal pneumonia; by extension from otitis, mastoiditis, or sinusitis; or following a skull fracture which creates an opening between the subarachnoid space and the nasal cavity or paranasal sinuses. Patients with pneumococcal endocarditis frequently develop meningeal infection. Patients with multiple myeloma and with sickle cell disease seem to be prone to pneumococcal infection of the meninges, just as they are to pneumonia.

The *manifestations* are of those of any acute pyogenic meningitis (see Chap. 346) and include chills, fever, headache, nuchal rigidity, Kernig's and Brudzinski's signs, delirium, and cranial nerve palsies. Evidence of otitis, sinusitis, or pneumonia should be carefully sought by physical and roentgenographic examination in all patients.

The *spinal fluid* is under increased pressure, appears cloudy, often with a greenish tint, and shows a high protein and low glucose content. Stained smears usually reveal gram-positive diplococci and polymorphonuclear leukocytes; in some patients, the number of cells in the spinal fluid is surprisingly small, and much of the cloudiness is produced by the bacterial content. The diagnosis can be established rapidly by identification of pneumococci in the spinal fluid by Gram's stain. Immunologic tests (CIE or latex agglutination) are positive in approximately 80 percent of culture-positive cases and may provide a presumptive bacterial cause of infection in some patients from whose spinal fluid no organism is recovered.

With appropriate chemotherapy, recovery can be expected in 70 percent of cases; the prognosis is better in children than in infants or in adults. Relapse may occur but is unusual if adequate treatment is carried out. Subarachnoid block, the result of accumulation of large amounts of thick exudate in the meningeal space and at the base of the brain, is an unusual complication.

PNEUMOCOCCAL ENDOCARDITIS Endocarditis is usually a complication of pneumonia or meningitis. The clinical picture is that of acute bacterial endocarditis (see Chap. 188), with remittent fever, splenomegaly, and metastatic infection of the lungs, meninges, joints, eye, and other tissues. Petechiae are uncommon. The infection can attack normal valves and is particularly likely to occur on the aortic valve. The valvular infection is destructive, and loud murmurs and heart failure develop rapidly. Rupture or perforation of cusps or even rupture of the aorta may occur. The blood culture is consistently positive for the pneumococcus in the absence of treatment with antimicrobial drugs; yet at the same time antibodies to the infecting organism may be demonstrable in the blood, a combination of findings seldom observed except in endocarditis or brucellosis. Although the infection is relatively easy to cure with penicillin, damage to valve leaflets, especially to the cusps of the aortic valve, may be followed by rapidly progressive heart failure. Surgical repair or replacement of damaged valvular structures should be carried out early, before heart failure becomes intractable.

PNEUMOCOCCAL PERITONITIS Pneumococcal peritonitis is a rare disease and is probably the sequel to transient pneumococcal bacteremia, although, because of its somewhat greater frequency in young girls, it has been hypothesized that the organism may gain entry to the peritoneum via the vagina and fallopian tubes. Peritonitis was formerly a common complication of the nephrotic syndrome, particularly in children, but it occurs now with a frequency of less than 2 percent. In adults, the disease is seen in association with cirrhosis or with carcinoma of the liver. The diagnosis is made by examination of the ascitic fluid; blood cultures are often positive, and a polymorphonuclear leukocytosis is the rule.

TREATMENT

SPECIFIC ANTIMICROBIAL THERAPY Although resistance of pneumococci to antimicrobial drugs has not been regarded as a significant problem in the past, some strains have been found to be resistant to one or all of the following agents: penicillins, cephalosporins, tetracyclines, chloramphenicol, erythromycin, clindamycin, co-trimoxazole, and aminoglycosides. For this reason sensitivity of the infecting organism to the drug(s) to be used should be determined, particularly in treating extrapulmonary infection. In the absence of resistance or of hypersensitivity to it, penicillin G (benzylpenicillin) is the drug of choice for all manifestations of pneumococcal infection. Strains of pneumococcus manifesting increased resistance to penicillin have been recovered infrequently from humans; and although the level of such resistance does not often preclude treatment with this antibiotic, awareness of the phenomenon is necessary. Although the minimum curative dose for *pneumonia* caused by strains of usual sensitivity to penicillin is less than 60,000 units daily and a dose of 600,000 units daily provides a good margin of safety in treating adults with bacteremic or nonbacteremic infection with such strains in the absence of an extrapulmonary focus, the occurrence of pneumococci showing increased resistance to penicillin makes the initiation of therapy with larger amounts desirable today. Treatment may be started with doses of 600,000 units of aqueous crystalline penicillin G or procaine penicillin administered at 12-h intervals to be continued until the patient has been afebrile for 48 to 72 h. Pneumococcal pneumonia can be treated with an oral penicillin, preferably one resistant to gastric acid (see Chap. 92), in dosage equivalent to 2.4 to 4.8 million units of penicillin G. *Peritonitis* caused by sensitive strains responds usually within 36 to 48 h to 2 to 4 million units of penicillin daily.

Pneumococcal meningitis in adults should be treated with 18 to 24 million units of penicillin G daily intravenously. In some clinics, even larger amounts are used, though care must be taken to avoid neurotoxicity from excessive dosage. Intrathecal administration of penicillin is unnecessary, and supplementation of penicillin with broad-spectrum bacteriostatic drugs such as tetracyclines may exert a deleterious effect. All pneumococcal isolates from cerebrospinal fluid should be tested promptly for their sensitivity to antibacterial drugs. Vancomycin appears currently to be the drug of choice for treatment of meningitis caused by pneumococci resistant to multiple antimicrobial agents.

Moderate doses of penicillin G are used to treat pneumococcal endocarditis—8 to 12 million units daily by intravenous infusion. Rapidly developing heart failure as a result of valvular injury and a tendency to form myocardial abscess, however, often lead to a fatal outcome despite the use of antibiotics. Prompt surgical repair or replacement of damaged heart valves should be considered when cardiac failure develops.

Cephalosporins in parenteral doses of 1 to 2 g daily are effective in pneumococcal pneumonia but must be administered with caution to those hypersensitive to penicillin. Many members of this class of β-lactam drugs cannot be used to treat meningitis because of their poor ability to penetrate the blood–cerebrospinal fluid barrier. Several of the newer cephalosporins, including cefotaxime and ceftriaxone, show promise of efficacy in treating pneumococcal meningitis although experience with each is limited. The tetracyclines in doses of 1 to 2 g daily, erythromycin in doses of 1.6 g daily, or clindamycin in doses of 1.2 g daily are effective treatment for pneumococcal pneumonia if it is caused by a sensitive strain, but they are recommended only for patients who have had untoward reactions to penicillins or cephalosporins. Despite its efficacy, chloramphenicol should not be used to treat pneumococcal infections other than meningitis in patients hypersensitive to penicillin who are infected with a drug-sensitive strain. For patients with illness caused by multiply drug-resistant pneumococci, vancomycin in doses of 2 g daily is the drug of choice. Sulfonamides have little place in the present-day treatment of pneumococcal pneumonia and are useless in endocarditis and meningitis. Aminoglycosides, such as gentamicin, tobramycin, and amikacin, should not be employed to treat pneumococcal infection.

Pneumococcal arthritis responds to systemic penicillin, but aspiration and intraarticular instillation of the drug may be necessary.

Empyema should be detected and treated as early as possible. When an effusion is found, fluid should be removed and examined for bacteria, leukocytes, glucose concentration, and pH. The presence of bacteria, pus, a pH below 7.0, and/or a pleural fluid glucose below 40 mg/dL are indications for institution of closed-chest tube drainage. Failure of early cure of empyema may be followed by pleural fibrosis and necessitate subsequent surgical decortication of the lung to restore pulmonary function.

OTHER MEASURES Oxygen administered through a face mask should be used to treat significant cyanosis, cardiac failure, and delirium. In the presence of adult respiratory distress syndrome, positive end-expiratory pressure may be indicated. Codeine, 32 to 64 mg every 4 h, will usually control pleuritic pain. When pain is severe, it may require intercostal nerve block with 1 to 2% procaine for relief.

PROGNOSIS AND PREVENTION

Although the mortality from pneumococcal pneumonia has diminished significantly since the advent of antimicrobial drugs, available evidence indicates that the incidence of the disease has changed little, if at all. The fatality rate in patients over the age of 12 years with bacteremic pneumococcal pneumonia treated with an antibiotic is 18 percent, and in patients over the age of 50 and in those with underlying systemic illness, it is significantly higher.

Signs of poor prognosis in pneumonia include leukopenia, bacteremia, multilobar involvement, any extrapulmonary focus of pneumococcal infection, presence of preexisting systemic disease, circulatory collapse, and occurrence of the infection in the first year of life or after the age of 55. Infection with pneumococcus type 3 has a higher mortality rate than that caused by other pneumococcal types. Death is most likely to occur in individuals sustaining irreversible physiologic damage early in the course which is unaltered by antimicrobial therapy. Until the nature of the injury produced by pneumococcus is understood and ways are devised to repair it, vaccination will remain the principal means of protecting those at high risk of a fatal outcome.

A 23-valent vaccine containing the capsular polysaccharides of pneumococcal types 1, 2, 3, 4, 5, 6B, 7F, 8, 9N, 9V, 10A, 11A, 12F, 14, 15B, 17F, 18C, 19F, 19A, 20, 22F, 23F, and 33F, which include the serotypes or groups responsible for 90 percent of bacteremic infections in the United States, is recommended for prevention of pneumococcal infection caused by these serotypes in individuals at high risk of a fatal outcome. Those at higher-than-average risk are individuals over the age of 55 and patients with a variety of chronic systemic illnesses including heart disease, chronic bronchopulmonary disease, hepatic disease, renal insufficiency, diabetes, and a variety of malignancies. Persons of all ages with sickle cell disease have an increased risk of developing pneumococcal infection, and the vaccine is recommended for those with this disorder over the age of 2 years. Since anatomic or functional asplenia is associated with fulminant overwhelming pneumococcal septicemia with disseminated intravascular coagulation, giving rise to a clinical picture resembling the Waterhouse-Friderichsen syndrome, such individuals should also be immunized. However, the vaccine does not contain the antigens of all pneumococcal types, and infection caused by antigens not included may occur occasionally in immunized subjects. Reactions to the vaccine are usually absent or mild, although in the occasional individual they may resemble those following immunization with typhoid vaccine: local pain, erythema, and elevation of temperature. The most severe local and systemic reactions to the vaccine appear to be associated with preexisting high levels of antibody to one or more of the antigens in the vaccine. Because of the persistence of pneumococcal antibodies after a single injection of vaccine, reimmunization in less than 5 years after the initial injection is not recommended. The vaccine is 80 to 90 percent effective in immunocompetent adults but may afford little, if any, protection to those with agamma- or dysgammaglobulinemia or to patients who have been subjected recently to intensive antitumor chemotherapy and radiation. In children under 6 years, immunologic responsiveness to different capsular antigens develops at different times as a result of maturational characteristics of the human immune system, and protection may be of shorter duration than in the adults. Further data are needed to define the utility of the vaccine in childhood. If necessary, pneumococcal vaccine may be administered concomitantly with influenza viral vaccine, provided each vaccine is injected from a separate syringe at a separate site.

REFERENCES

AUSTRIAN R, GOLD J: Pneumococcal bacteremia with especial reference to bacteremic pneumococcal pneumonia. Ann Intern Med 60:759, 1964

—— et al: Prevention of pneumococcal pneumonia by vaccination. Trans Assoc Am Phys 89:184, 1976

FRUCHTMAN SM et al: Adult respiratory distress syndrome as a cause of death in pneumococcal pneumonia. Chest 83:598, 1983

GOPAL V, BISNO AL: Fulminant pneumococcal infections in "normal" asplenic hosts. Arch Intern Med 137:1526, 1977

HEFFRON R: *Pneumonia with Special Reference to Pneumococcus Lobar Pneumonia.* Cambridge, Harvard, 1979

KAPLAN SL: Antigen detection in cerebrospinal fluid—pros and cons. Am J Med 75:109, 1983

LIGHT RW et al: Parapneumonic effusions. Am J Med 69:507, 1980

MARINO PL et al: Bacteremic pneumococcal pneumonia and myoglobinuric renal failure. Am J Med 80:521, 1986

ROBBINS JB et al: Considerations for formulating the second-generation pneumococcal capsular polysaccharide vaccine with emphasis on the cross-reactive types within groups. J Infect Dis 148:1136, 1983

SHAPIRO ED, CLEMENS JD: A controlled evaluation of the protective efficacy of pneumococcal vaccine for patients at high risk of serious pneumococcal infections. Ann Intern Med 101:325, 1984

STEPHEN JJ et al: The radiographic resolution of *Streptococcus pneumoniae* pneumonia. N Engl J Med 293:798, 1975

TUOMANEN E et al: The induction of meningeal inflammation by components of the pneumococcal cell wall. J Infect Dis 151:859, 1985

WARD J: Antibiotic-resistant *Streptococcus pneumoniae*: Clinical and epidemiologic aspects. Rev Infect Dis 3:254, 1981

94 STAPHYLOCOCCAL INFECTIONS

RICHARD M. LOCKSLEY

The staphylococci, of which *S. aureus* is the most important human pathogen, are hardy gram-positive bacteria that colonize the skin of most human beings. If the skin or mucous membranes are disrupted by surgery or trauma, staphylococci may gain access to and proliferate in the underlying tissues, giving rise to a typically localized, superficial abscess. Although these cutaneous infections are most commonly harmless and self-limited, the multiplying organisms may invade the lymphatics and the blood, leading to the potentially serious complications of staphylococcal bacteremia. These complications include septic shock, which may be indistinguishable from that caused by gram-negative bacteria, and serious metastatic complications, including endocarditis (see Chap. 188), arthritis (see Chap. 277), osteomyelitis (see Chap. 340), pneumonia (see Chap. 205), and abscesses (see Chap. 87) in virtually any organ in the body. Certain strains of *S. aureus* produce toxins that can cause skin rashes or that mediate multisystem dysfunction, as in toxic shock syndrome. Coagulase-negative staphylococci, particularly *S. epidermidis*, are important nosocomial pathogens, with a particular predilection for infecting vascular catheters and prosthetic devices. *S. saprophyticus* is a common cause of urinary tract infection.

ETIOLOGY AND MICROBIOLOGY   Staphylococci are gram-positive, nonmotile, aerobic or facultatively anaerobic, catalase-positive cocci within the family Micrococcaceae. The name derives from the typical clustering of organisms (the Greek *staphyle*, ''bunch of grapes'') observed microscopically in stained specimens taken from colonies grown on solid media. Pathogenic staphylococci are distinguished from nonpathogenic micrococci by the ability of staphylococci to ferment glucose anaerobically and by their sensitivity to lysostaphin endopeptidase. *S. aureus*, the most important human pathogen in the genus, is named for the golden color of colonies grown aerobically on solid media, the color results from the production of carotenoids. All staphylococcal strains producing coagulase are designated *S. aureus*. In contrast to coagulase-negative staphylococci, *S. aureus* ferments mannitol, produces DNase, and displays greater susceptibility to lysostaphin. *S. aureus* is generally hemolytic when cultured on blood agar. Commercially available kits using specific antibodies linked to latex particles or beads can distinguish *S. aureus* from coagulase-negative staphylococci by particle agglutination. *S. aureus* strains typically exhibit greater expression of biochemical activity (production of coagulase, toxins, hemolysins) than coagulase-negative staphylococci.

There are currently 12 recognized and 2 proposed species of coagulase-negative staphylococci, of which *S. epidermidis* and *S. saprophyticus* are the most important clinically. *S. saprophyticus* can be identified by its resistance to novobiocin and nalidixic acid, although this is reliable only for urinary isolates.

Differentiation among strains of *S. aureus* or *S. epidermidis* has been used to identify a common source during epidemics or intrahospital outbreaks of staphylococcal disease. Strains of *S. aureus* may be distinguished by antimicrobial susceptibility profiles, by patterns of lysis by staphylococcal bacteriophages (phage typing), and by analysis of plasmids within the organism. Of these three tests, antibiotic susceptibility testing has the least and plasmid analysis the most discriminatory ability. Attempts to differentiate strains of *S. epidermidis* using biotyping, antimicrobial susceptibility, or serotyping alone have been generally unsatisfactory. Only 20 to 40 percent of hospital isolates of *S. epidermidis* can be typed by standard phage typing. Plasmid analysis is the most reliable method distinguishing among strains.

EPIDEMIOLOGY   The coagulase-negative staphylococci are part of the normal flora of the skin, mucous membranes, and lower bowel; *S. epidermidis* is the commonest species isolated. *S. aureus* transiently colonizes the anterior nares in 70 to 90 percent of persons and may be recovered for relatively prolonged periods of time in 20 to 30 percent of them. Nasal carriage is often accompanied by secondary colonization of the skin. Independent colonization of the perineal area occurs in 5 to 20 percent of persons, and vaginal carriage has been demonstrated in 10 percent of menstruating females. Higher carriage rates of *S. aureus* have been documented in hospital employees (including physicians and nurses), hospitalized patients, and patients whose care requires frequent puncture of the skin, e.g., insulin-dependent diabetic patients, dialysis-dependent renal failure patients, and patients receiving frequent desensitization injections for allergies. Drug abusers who use needles also have enhanced *S. aureus*

carriage rates. Presumably, disturbances in the local cutaneous barrier allow *S. aureus* to establish and maintain colonization successfully.

S. saprophyticus demonstrates enhanced adherence to urothelial cells compared to *S. epidermidis*. Approximately 5 percent of healthy males and females have low colony counts of *S. saprophyticus* in the urethral or periurethral areas.

Although staphylococci can survive in the environment for prolonged periods of time, and airborne spread of organisms can be demonstrated, person-to-person transfer via contaminated hands is the most important mechanism for transmission of staphylococci. Hospitalized patients with active staphylococcal infection or those who become heavily colonized, particularly at cutaneous sites (surgical wounds, burns, decubitus ulcers), constitute the greatest reservoir for nosocomially acquired infection. Such patients shed an enormous number of organisms, and the hands of hospital personnel caring for these patients become readily colonized. Failure to use aseptic technique and neglect of hand washing allows transmission of the organisms to the skin of other patients. Strains of both *S. aureus* and *S. epidermidis* may become endemic in areas of the hospital housing patients with large integumental defects, particularly when widespread antimicrobial use favors the acquisition of multiply resistant strains (burn units, intensive care units, bone marrow transplant units). Less frequently, otherwise healthy hospital employees who are nasal carriers have been implicated in nosocomial outbreaks. Upon careful examination, most of these carriers will have active dermatologic infections during the time that effective transmission of staphylococci is documented.

If infections arising from the urinary tract are excluded, *S. aureus* and *S. epidermidis* together have become the most common cause of nosocomial infection in United States hospitals. They are the most frequently isolated pathogens in both primary and secondary bacteremias, and in cutaneous and surgical wound infections.

PATHOGENESIS   Infection by staphylococci usually results from a combination of bacterial virulence factors and diminution in host defense. Important microbial factors include the ability of the staphylococcus to survive under harsh conditions, its cell wall constituents, the production of enzymes and toxins that promote tissue invasion, its capacity to persist intracellularly in certain phagocytes, and its potential to acquire resistance to antimicrobials. Important host factors include an intact mucocutaneous barrier, an adequate number of functional neutrophils, and removal of foreign bodies or devitalized tissues.

Microbial factors   Cell wall components of *S. aureus* include a large peptidoglycan complex that confers rigidity to the organism and enables it to survive under unfavorable osmotic conditions, a unique teichoic acid linked to peptidoglycan, and protein A, found both attached to peptidoglycan over the outermost parts of the cell and released in soluble form. Both peptidoglycan and teichoic acid are capable of activating the complement cascade via the alternative pathway. Although important for opsonization of organisms for ingestion by phagocytes, complement activation may also play a role in the pathogenesis of shock and disseminated intravascular coagulation. Protein A binds to the Fc portion of certain classes of IgG as well as to the Fc receptor on phagocytes and may serve as a blocking factor preventing neutrophil ingestion of the organisms. Specific receptors for laminin, the major glycoprotein of the vascular basement membrane, may mediate the widespread metastatic potential of *S. aureus*. Some strains of *S. aureus* may be coated by an antiphagocytic capsule that requires specific antibodies for ingestion. The cell wall of certain strains of *S. epidermidis* is also capable of activating complement; shock and disseminated intravascular coagulation during infections by these organisms have been described, although less frequently than with *S. aureus*. The capacity of *S. epidermidis* to adhere to intravascular cannulas and prosthetic devices may explain the propensity of these organisms to cause foreign body infections; the nature of the adherence ligands is unknown.

Certain enzymes produced by *S. aureus* may play a role in virulence. Catalase degrades hydrogen peroxide and may protect the organism during phagocytosis when it must withstand the phagocyte's respiratory burst. This may be important in intracellular persistence of some ingested staphylococci. Coagulase is present in both soluble and cell-bound forms, and causes plasma to clot by formation of thrombinlike material. The high correlation between coagulase production and virulence suggests that this substance is important in the pathogenesis of staphylococcal infections, but its precise role as a determinant of pathogenicity has not been determined. Many strains also produce hyaluronidase, an enzyme that degrades hyaluronic acid in the connective tissue matrix and that may promote spreading of infection. *S. saprophyticus* produces urease, an enzyme capable of breaking down urea to ammonium, alkalinizing the urine, and favoring the formation of struvite stones.

S. aureus may produce numerous extracellular toxins. Toxins may be encoded by chromosomal or plasmid DNA. At least one toxin, enterotoxin A, is encoded by bacteriophage DNA integrated into the bacterial chromosome. Four different red cell hemolysins—designated alpha, beta, gamma, and delta toxins—have been identified. Alpha toxin is also dermonecrotic when injected subcutaneously into animals. Delta toxin inhibits water absorption by elevating cAMP in guinea pig ileum and may play a role in the acute watery diarrhea seen in some cases of staphylococcal infection. Leukocidin lyses granulocyte and macrophage membranes by producing membrane pores permeable to cations.

While the role of the above factors in virulence is incompletely understood, the staphylococcal enterotoxins, exfoliatin toxins A and B, and the toxic shock syndrome toxin—TSST-1—each have been implicated in disease. Five serologically distinct enterotoxins (A through E) have been implicated in food poisoning due to *S. aureus*. The toxins enhance intestinal peristalsis and seem to induce vomiting via a direct effect on the central nervous system. The exfoliatin toxins mediate the dermatologic manifestations of the staphylococcal scalded skin syndrome. The toxins cause intraepidermal cleavage of the skin at the stratum granulosum, leading to bullae formation and denudation. Antibodies to the toxins are protective in both humans and animals. Toxins have been suggested to mediate toxic shock syndrome (TSS) because of the multisystem dysfunction present in the absence of positive blood cultures. TSST-1, so designated because of evidence for additional toxins, is produced by over 90 percent of *S. aureus* recovered from women with menstrual TSS and over 60 percent of nonmenstrual cases. The toxin causes hypotension, conjunctival and cutaneous hyperemia, and fever when injected into rabbits; death may result from multisystem failure and mimics human TSS. TSST-1 induces human monocytes to release interleukin 1 (endogenous pyrogen), which may mediate some of the symptoms of TSS. Interleukin 1 produces fever, neutrophilia, acute phase protein synthesis, and, through its influence on cellular arachidonic acid metabolism, muscle proteolysis, and, potentially, diarrhea and hypotension. Low magnesium ion concentrations enhance the production of TSST-1. The gene encoding TSST-1 has been cloned and seems to be missing or rearranged in toxin-negative strains of *S. aureus*.

Antimicrobial resistance by staphylococci favors their persistence in the hospital environment. Over 90 percent of both hospital and community strains of *S. aureus* causing infection are resistant to penicillin. Resistance is due to the production of β-lactamases, usually by plasmids. Introduction of the penicillinase-resistant antimicrobials was followed shortly by the isolation, initially in Europe and Scandinavia, of the so-called methicillin-resistant *S. aureus* (MRSA). These organisms are resistant to all the β-lactam antimicrobics, as well as to the cephalosporins, despite the fact that standard disk susceptibility testing may indicate sensitivity to cephalosporin drugs. Resistance of MRSA is chromosomally mediated and is not due to enzymatic alteration of the drug. It probably involves alterations of staphylococcal penicillin-binding proteins. Not uncommonly, MRSA has acquired R plasmids mediating some combination of resistance to erythromycin, tetracycline, chloramphenicol, clindamycin, and

aminoglycosides. MRSA has become increasingly common worldwide, particularly in tertiary care referral hospitals. In the United States, approximately 5 percent of hospital isolates of *S. aureus* are MRSA; one-third of hospitals surveyed have experienced bacteremias due to MRSA. Despite the theoretic survival advantage of MRSA, the isolation of these organisms has remained relatively constant since 1980. Outbreaks continue to occur periodically in the form of intrahospital epidemics. The community carriage rate of MRSA is low, although selected patient populations, like parenteral drug abusers, may have MRSA at the time of admission to the hospital. These isolates remain susceptible to vancomycin.

Tolerance to β-lactams is an in vitro phenomenon characterized by resistance of the organism to the lethal action of normally cidal antimicrobials. It is characterized by a marked discrepancy between the minimal inhibitory and the minimal bactericidal concentrations of the drug. The mechanism may relate to a defect in the normal activation of autolytic enzymes of the bacteria by cell wall–active antimicrobials. Demonstration of the trait is influenced markedly by physicochemical conditions, and the nature and significance of tolerance remains controversial. Although tolerance has been reported to influence the outcome of severe staphylococcal infection adversely, it has been difficult to incriminate tolerance to β-lactams as a significant cause of antibiotic failure in animal models of infection. This may reflect the in vitro observation that continued treatment with β-lactams will kill tolerant *S. aureus*, although killing proceeds more slowly.

Most instances of *S. epidermidis* infection are nosocomially acquired and typically express greater variability and degrees of antimicrobial resistance than those of *S. aureus*. Virtually all isolates contain R plasmids that produce β-lactamase and are resistant to penicillin. Approximately one-third are resistant to aminoglycosides and two-thirds are resistant to tetracycline, erythromycin, clindamycin, and chloramphenicol. Hospital isolates of *S. epidermidis* containing multiple antimicrobial-resistant plasmids can serve as important reservoirs for the acquisition of resistance by *S. aureus*; transfer of R plasmids from *S. epidermidis* to *S. aureus* via conjugation has been demonstrated both in vitro and on the skin.

Methicillin resistance is common among *S. epidermidis* strains; over 80 percent of isolates from cases with prosthetic valve endocarditis in one study were methicillin-resistant. Methicillin resistance is heterotypic among *S. epidermidis*—only one in 10^4 cells may express resistance under nonselective conditions. Conditions of temperature, pH, osmolality, and the presence of chelating agents and heavy metals all may influence the demonstration of resistance. Methicillin-resistant isolates may appear susceptible by routine susceptibility testing. The most reliable identification of these organisms is by their growth from a large inoculum (10^7 cells) spread on agar containing 20 µg/mL methicillin. Cross-resistance to the other β-lactam antimicrobials and to the cephalosporins is always present, although as with MRSA, these bacteria may appear susceptible to cephalosporins using conventional disk testing. As with *S. aureus*, *S. epidermidis* strains remain susceptible to vancomycin and usually to rifampin, although resistance to the latter may occur rapidly when the drug is used alone.

Host factors The importance of host factors in resisting staphylococcal infections is demonstrated by the observation that enormous numbers of bacteria are required to establish experimental infections in humans and animals. Areas where skin or mucosal continuity is broken provide portals of entry for staphylococci. More than 50 percent of serious staphylococcal infections of deep tissues arise from cutaneous foci; a smaller number originates from the respiratory, gastrointestinal, or less frequently, genitourinary tract. Direct inoculation of organisms into the blood is an important route of infection in hospitalized patients with intravenous catheters and in drug abusers.

Staphylococci often invade the integument via plugged hair follicles and sebaceous glands, or areas involved by burns, wounds, abrasions, insect bites, or dermatitis. Colonization and invasion of the lungs may occur when the normal mucociliary clearance mechanisms are either bypassed, as occurs with endotracheal intubation, or depressed, as occurs following viral infections of the lung (influenza) or in patients with cystic fibrosis. Mucosal damage to the gastrointestinal tract following cytotoxic chemotherapy or radiotherapy predisposes to invasion from that site.

Once the integument has been breached, local bacterial multiplication is accompanied by inflammation and tissue necrosis at the site of infection. Neutrophils rapidly enter the area and ingest large numbers of staphylococci. Thrombosis of surrounding capillaries occurs; fibrin is deposited about the periphery; later, fibroblasts create a relatively avascular wall about the area. The fully developed staphylococcal abscess consists of a central core of dead and dying leukocytes and bacteria which gradually liquefies to form characteristic thick, creamy pus, surrounded by a fibroblastic wall. When host mechanisms fail to contain the cutaneous or submucosal infection, staphylococci may enter the lymphatics and the bloodstream. Common sites of metastatic seeding include the diaphyseal ends of long bones in children, and the lungs, kidneys, cardiac valves, myocardium, liver, spleen, and brain.

Polymorphonuclear leukocytes capable of normal chemotaxis, ingestion, and killing appear to be the major protective mechanisms against staphylococcal disease. Persons with inherited or acquired defects in any of these leukocyte functions, or with neutropenia itself, are particularly susceptible to staphylococcal infections. A low number of staphylococci is capable of surviving within phagocytes, which may account for the relatively slow response of staphylococcal infections to antimicrobials and the potential for relapse.

Although infections may occur in all age groups, serious staphylococcal infections most commonly afflict the young and the old—particularly those with underlying debilitating diseases. Primary staphylococcal pneumonia is common in infants but rare in adults. Acute staphylococcal osteomyelitis is almost exclusively a disease of children. Superficial staphylococcal pyoderma is more frequent in infants, whereas actual abscess formation occurs more often in adults. While these examples suggest some role for immunity in resistance against staphylococci, there has been no satisfactory demonstration that human staphylococcal disease is followed by effective immunity or that infection can be modified significantly by vaccination. Virtually 100 percent of adults possess antistaphylococcal antibodies in their serum. Except for the neutralizing antibodies to the exfoliatin toxin and the suggestion of a protective effect of antibodies against TSST-1, the role of humoral immunity in modifying or protecting against staphylococcal infection is unclear.

The presence of a foreign body such as a suture or a prosthetic device markedly decreases the inoculum of staphylococci required to produce experimental infection. Once established, such infections are very difficult to cure without removal of the foreign body. Strains of *S. epidermidis* are capable of adhering firmly to and invading plastic catheters, and of secreting a protective glycocalyx covering the adherent colonies. Neutrophil function is also altered in the presence of a foreign body; phagocytosis and killing of *S. aureus* are diminished.

DIAGNOSIS   The diagnosis of all staphylococcal infections is made by Gram's stain and culture of purulent material, either aspirated pus or involved tissue, or by culture of normally sterile body fluids. Typical clustering of organisms may not be seen in clinical specimens; individual cocci and even short chains of three or four organisms may be present. Bacteria in the static phase or within leukocytes may appear gram-negative. Abundant neutrophils, many containing intracellular organisms, are usually present, except in severely neutropenic patients.

SPECIFIC DISEASES   Superficial infections   Infection of hair follicles manifested by a minute erythematous nodule without involvement of the surrounding skin or deeper tissues is termed folliculitis. A more extensive and invasive follicular or sebaceous gland infection with some involvement of subcutaneous tissues is termed a furuncle, or boil. Itching and mild pain are followed by progressive local swelling and erythema, and the overlying skin becomes exquisitely painful on pressure or motion. Relief of pain occurs promptly after spontaneous or surgical drainage.

Furuncles occur most commonly in areas subjected to maceration or friction, poor personal hygiene, or involved by acne or dermatitis. The face, neck, axillae, buttocks, and thighs are common sites. Staphylococcal infection may involve the apocrine sweat glands in the axilla or groin (hidradenitis suppurativa). These infections may be deep-seated, slow to localize and drain, and are prone to recurrence and scarring.

Staphylococcal infections within the thick, fibrous, inelastic skin of the back of the neck and upper part of the back lead to formation of a carbuncle. The relative thickness and impermeability of the overlying skin lead to lateral extension and loculation, and a large, indurated, painful lesion with multiple ineffective drainage sites results. Carbuncles produce fever, leukocytosis, extreme pain, and prostration. Bacteremia is common.

Staphylococci frequently colonize impetiginous lesions, but most impetigo is due to group A streptococci. However, staphylococcal impetigo does occur, and while it cannot be clearly differentiated on the basis of its clinical features from streptococcal impetigo, it tends to produce multiple superficial, localized lesions, at different stages of development, has a grayish rather than golden yellow crust, and less often produces high fever.

Treatment of most superficial infections does not require the use of antibiotics. Local moist heat, attention to personal hygiene, and washing with germicidal soaps that leave an inhibitory residue on the skin (hexachlorophene, chlorhexidine, triclosan) are usually sufficient. For more severe or recurrent disease, oral antibiotic therapy with dicloxacillin or cloxacillin (2 g per day in four divided doses) for 7 to 10 days may be effective. Incision and drainage should be utilized selectively. Disease presenting with prominent constitutional symptoms or facial or periorbital infection, should be treated with intravenous doses of appropriate antimicrobials as outlined in the section on bacteremic disease.

Toxin-mediated staphylococcal diseases   STAPHYLOCOCCAL SCALDED SKIN SYNDROME (SSSS)   SSSS is a generalized exfoliative dermatitis complicating infection by toxin (exfoliatin)-producing strains of *S. aureus*. The disease typically occurs in newborns (Ritter's disease) and in children under the age of 5; it is rare in adults. Strains of *S. aureus* causing SSSS in the United States are frequently phage group II, type 71. The disease begins with a localized cutaneous infection often accompanied by a nonspecific viral-like prodrome. Fever and leukocytosis are mild. A scarlatiniform rash begins in the perioral area, becomes generalized over the trunk and extremities, and finally desquamates. The disease may consist of rash alone (staphylococcal scarlet fever), or large, flaccid bullae develop that may be localized (more common in adults) or generalized. The bullae burst, resulting in red, denuded skin resembling a burn. Friction applied to healthy areas of skin cause the epidermis to wrinkle and separate (Nikolsky's sign). *S. aureus* can usually be recovered from the skin and nasopharynx. Therapy includes antistaphylococcal antibiotics and local skin care. Recovery usually occurs.

In adults, SSSS has been grouped with other severe scalding syndromes such as toxic epidermal necrolysis (Lyell's disease). Drug reactions are the most frequent cause of toxic epidermal necrolysis in adults, and the syndrome may be differentiated from SSSS by skin biopsy. Cleavage of the skin in drug-induced toxic epidermal necrolysis occurs at the basal cell layer resulting in full-thickness denudation, with a greater potential for superinfection and significant fluid and electrolyte loss. In SSSS, cleavage occurs within the epidermis. Kawasaki's disease and toxic shock syndrome should also be considered in the differential diagnosis of SSSS.

TOXIC SHOCK SYNDROME   Toxic shock syndrome (TSS) was described in 1978 as a multisystem disease presenting with high fever, a "sunburn" rash that went on to desquamate, and hypotension in children who had group I *S. aureus* isolated from mucosal or sequestered sites. In 1980 TSS became epidemic among young, primarily white, women, with onset during menstruation. A strong correlation was found between TSS and recovery of *S. aureus* from vaginal or cervical cultures of affected patients. The occurrence of a rash, the infrequency of bacteremia, and the association with *S. aureus* suggested a toxin-associated illness. Subsequently a marker toxin, TSST-1, which is produced by most TSS staphylococcal isolates and is believed to mediate the syndrome, was identified. Other undiscovered toxins may mediate TSS among TSST-1–negative isolates. Most *S. aureus* isolates belong to group I.

Epidemiologically, TSS was associated with the introduction of certain brands of hyperabsorbent tampons. Their prolonged intravaginal use, together with the capacity of the materials used in these tampons to bind magnesium, has been associated with increased growth of intravaginal *S. aureus* and enhanced TSST-1 production. Public education and removal of hyperabsorbent tampons from the market have resulted in a marked decrease in the number of reported cases of TSS. Although the majority of cases continue to occur among menstruating females, nonmenstrual TSS now accounts for 25 to 30 percent of TSS cases in the United States.

The diagnosis of TSS is based on clinical criteria that include high fever, a diffuse "sunburn" rash that desquamates on the palms and soles over the subsequent 1 to 2 weeks, hypotension that may be orthostatic, plus evidence of involvement in three or more organ systems. These commonly include gastrointestinal dysfunction (vomiting or diarrhea), renal or hepatic insufficiency, mucous membrane hyperemia, thrombocytopenia, myalgias with elevated creatinine phosphokinase (CK) levels, and disorientation with a normal cerebrospinal fluid examination. Milder forms of the syndrome have been reported.

The onset is acute and typically occurs around the start of menses in a young woman using tampons. The vaginal mucosa is hyperemic, and *S. aureus* can be cultured from the vaginal discharge. Blood cultures are usually negative. Clinical findings are the same in nonmenstrual-associated TSS. Cutaneous infections, postpartum vaginal and cesarean-section wound infections, surgical wound infections, focal tissue infections (abscesses, empyema, osteomyelitis), and rarely primary staphylococcal bacteremia have been associated with TSS. Signs of infection may be minimal among patients with postoperative wound infections where the onset typically occurs on the second day after surgery. The mortality rate of TSS is 3 percent and is most often due to refractory hypotension and the development of the adult respiratory distress syndrome (ARDS) with or without disseminated intravascular coagulation.

Treatment is directed at correcting shock and treating renal failure, pulmonary insufficiency, and disseminated intravascular coagulation when present. Antistaphylococcal antibiotics should be administered parenterally. Focal collections of *S. aureus* must be drained. Up to 30 percent of menstruating women with TSS may have recurrences with subsequent menses, although these are generally milder. The use of antistaphylococcal antibiotics to treat TSS and discontinuation of tampon use significantly decrease the likelihood of recurrences.

The differential diagnosis of TSS includes Rocky Mountain spotted fever, meningococcemia, streptococcal scarlet fever, toxic epidermal necrolysis, and Kawasaki's syndrome.

Staphylococcal food poisoning   See Chap. 89.

Invasive staphylococcal infections   BACTEREMIA AND ENDOCARDITIS   Bacteremia due to *S. aureus* may arise from any local infection, either at extravascular (cutaneous infections, burns, cellulitis, osteomyelitis, arthritis) or intravascular foci (intravenous catheters, dialysis access sites, intravenous drug abuse). Up to one-third of patients do not have an identifiable focus.

Rarely, patients with bacteremia die within 12 to 24 h with high fever, tachycardia, cyanosis, and vascular collapse. Nonencapsulated strains may trigger disseminated intravascular coagulation, producing a disease mimicking meningococcemia. Commonly, the disease progresses more slowly, with hectic fever and metastatic abscess

formation in the bones, kidneys, lungs, myocardium, spleen, brain, or other tissues.

A major complication of *S. aureus* bacteremia is endocarditis (see Chap. 188). *S. aureus* is the second most common cause of endocarditis, and the commonest cause among drug addicts. Among nonaddicts, normal valves are involved in 30 to 60 percent of cases, and older, frequently hospitalized, patients with underlying medical disease are most often infected. The mitral, aortic, or both valves may be involved. The disease typically pursues an acute course with high fever, progressive anemia, and frequent embolic and extracardiac septic complications. Progressive valvular insufficiency leads to significant murmurs in 90 percent of patients. Valve ring and myocardial abscesses are common. The mortality rate is 20 to 30 percent. Infection of the aortic valve, the development of uncontrolled congestive heart failure, or evidence of central nervous system involvement are poor prognostic signs; these patients frequently require surgical intervention.

Among addicts, *S. aureus* most frequently involves the tricuspid valve. Evidence for septic pulmonary emboli (chest pain, hemoptysis, nodular infiltrates) is common. Audible murmurs and peripheral stigmata of endocarditis are less common than in nonaddicts. Myalgias and back pain may be the major presenting symptoms and obfuscate the diagnosis. The mortality rate is 2 to 10 percent.

Differentiation of isolated bacteremia from endocarditis may be difficult. Patients with normal heart valves with an identifiable, easily managed or removable primary focus of infection, who receive and respond promptly to appropriate antibiotic therapy, and who do not develop evidence of metastatic complications during the subsequent 2 weeks on therapy, usually can be treated for bacteremia alone. Patients with underlying valvular disorders, with murmurs of valvular regurgitation, with community-acquired disease and no obvious focus, with infection secondary to drug abuse, with evidence for embolic events, or with echocardiographic evidence for vegetations should be treated for endocarditis. The presence of antibodies to the teichoic acid cell-wall component of *S. aureus* after 2 weeks of illness has been used to discriminate between endocarditis or bacteremia with metastatic foci, and uncomplicated bacteremia. Although a negative test supports the diagnosis of simple bacteremia, a positive titer is less specific for complicated disease.

Three carefully collected blood cultures are adequate for the diagnosis in most instances; usually all are positive for *S. aureus*. More cultures may be required if the patient has previously received antibiotics. Purulent skin lesions and urine should also be cultured before starting antibiotic therapy. The urine may be positive in up to a third of cases of staphylococcal bacteremia (with colony counts typically lower than 10^5 per millimeter), and staphylococcal bacteriuria in this setting does not indicate metastatic renal infection.

Intravenous therapy should be initiated with a penicillinase-resistant agent. Nafcillin (1.5 g every 4 h) and oxacillin (2.0 g every 4 h) are preferred to methicillin because of the high incidence of interstitial nephritis with methicillin. Gentamicin (1 mg/kg every 8 h, adjusted for renal function) is frequently added for the first 48 to 72 h because of evidence for synergy with β-lactam antimicrobials against *S. aureus* and the tendency for patients treated with both drugs to defervesce more rapidly and to achieve earlier sterilization of the bloodstream. Rare isolates that do not produce β-lactamase should be treated with intravenous penicillin G (4×10^6 units every 4 h). First-generation cephalosporins (cephalothin, cefazolin) have also been used successfully in infections with both penicillinase-positive and -negative strains of *S. aureus*. Patients with serious penicillin allergy or with infections due to methicillin-resistant *S. aureus* should be treated with vancomycin (0.5 g every 6 h, adjusted by monitoring blood levels).

Cases of uncomplicated *S. aureus* bacteremia can be treated for 2 weeks. These patients should be followed carefully; relapses should be treated as endocarditis. Right-sided endocarditis in drug addicts has been successfully treated with 2 weeks of intravenous therapy followed by 4 weeks of oral dicloxacillin (1 to 1.5 g every 6 h). All other cases of endocarditis should receive 4 to 6 weeks of parenteral antimicrobials. Prosthetic valve endocarditis should be treated with an appropriate penicillin or vancomycin, plus gentamicin, with or without rifampin, for 6 weeks. Most cases will require surgery as well.

The response to antimicrobials in staphylococcal endocarditis may be slow. The fever may not disappear until the second week of therapy. Persistent fever or signs of sepsis should prompt a search for metastatic abscesses that require drainage.

S. epidermidis is the most common isolate in primary nosocomial bacteremias and the most frequent organism infecting intravenous access devices. It has been recognized as a major cause of bacteremia among neutropenic cancer patients, arising either from long-term, indwelling central catheters or from the gastrointestinal tract. Continued fever, progressive sepsis, multiple pulmonary abscesses, and death may result if this complication is left untreated.

Although an uncommon cause of native valve endocarditis, *S. epidermidis* is the commonest cause of prosthetic valve endocarditis (40 percent of cases). Most cases are due to inoculation of organisms at the time of surgery but may not become clinically apparent until 1 year later. Infections frequently involve the valve ring and require surgical intervention. Over 50 percent of patients die.

Because coagulase-negative staphylococci are frequent blood culture contaminants, distinguishing infection from contamination can be difficult. Positive blood cultures demand careful inspection of catheter sites and repeat blood cultures, even in the absence of symptoms, in patients with indwelling catheters, or with prosthetic heart valves or vascular grafts. Speciation of multiple isolates may be useful if isolates can be demonstrated to be the same; plasmid analysis may be required. Catheters should be removed and cultured, although antibiotic therapy alone has been successful for treatment of bacteremic catheter-related infections.

Hospital-acquired *S. epidermidis* infections are usually multiply antibiotic resistant. Methicillin resistance is heterotypic and difficult to exclude. For these reasons, all serious *S. epidermidis* infections should be treated with vancomycin in doses used for *S. aureus.* Prosthetic valve endocarditis should be treated for 6 weeks with vancomycin plus gentamicin, with or without rifampin.

OSTEOMYELITIS   *S. aureus* is responsible for the majority of cases of acute osteomyelitis (see Chap. 340). This infection occurs most commonly in children under the age of 12, but adults are also susceptible to acute osteomyelitis, especially of the spine. Approximately 50 percent of patients give a history of a furuncle or superficial staphylococcal infection preceding osteomyelitis. In children, the frequent localization in the diaphyseal end of the long bones is thought to be due to the endarterial circulation of the diaphysis. Many patients give a history of preceding trauma to the involved area. Clavicular osteomyelitis has complicated septic thrombosis of a catheterized subclavian vein.

Once established, infection spreads through the newly formed juxtaepiphyseal bone to the periosteum or along the marrow cavity. If the infection reaches the subperiosteal space, the periosteum is lifted, a subperiosteal abscess forms, and rupture with infection of the subcutaneous tissues may occur. Rarely, the joint capsule is penetrated, producing pyogenic arthritis. There is death of bone, producing a sequestrum, followed by new bone formation, the involucrum. Occasionally indolent staphylococcal infections of bone may persist for years within dense granulation tissue about a central necrotic cavity, a so-called Brodie's abscess.

Osteomyelitis in children may present as an acute process beginning abruptly with chills, high fever, nausea, vomiting, and progressive pain at the site of bony involvement. Muscle spasm about the affected bone is a common early sign, and the child may refuse to move the affected limb. Leukocytosis is common. Blood cultures are positive for *S. aureus* in 50 to 60 percent of cases early in disease. The tissues overlying the involved bone become edematous and warm, and the skin becomes erythematous. Anemia develops during the course of untreated disease.

Staphylococcal vertebral osteomyelitis in the adult differs considerably from acute osteomyelitis in the child. The onset is less abrupt, and there is a greater tendency for bony fusion with obliteration of the disk space. The lumbar spine is most frequently affected.

Osteomyelitis should be suspected in any child with fever, limb pain, and leukocytosis. Similarly, back or neck pain in an adult, when accompanied by fever, should raise the possibility of vertebral osteomyelitis. A history of a preceding cutaneous infection, local tenderness over the bone, and culture of *S. aureus* from the blood are confirmatory. Roentgenograms are usually normal during the first week, but radionuclide scans may be abnormal. Bony rarefaction, local periosteal elevation, and new bone formation can frequently be seen during the second week. Needle aspiration or bone biopsy should be performed if necessary to obtain a specific etiologic diagnosis prior to institution of chemotherapy. In chronic osteomyelitis, sinus tracts are often present, but cultures of the sinus tracts are not reliable in the diagnosis.

Therapy should be initiated parenterally using a penicillinase-resistant semisynthetic penicillin as outlined for bacteremia and endocarditis, and continued for 4 to 6 weeks. Cephalosporins and clindamycin have also been used. Uncomplicated osteomyelitis in children has been managed with 2 weeks of intravenous therapy followed by 2 to 4 weeks of oral therapy. Vancomycin can be used in penicillin-allergic patients and in infections due to methicillin-resistant organisms. Surgery may be required to remove devitalized bone and to drain soft tissue and periosteal abscesses. Neurologic findings due to epidural abscess and cord compression complicating vertebral osteomyelitis demand early surgical intervention. Aggressive treatment of acute osteomyelitis has decreased the incidence of chronic osteomyelitis, with its penchant for recurrent flare-ups and fistula formation. The cure rate for acute staphylococcal osteomyelitis is approximately 90 percent, and death is rare.

PNEUMONIA (See Chap. 205)   *S. aureus* causes approximately 1 percent of community-acquired bacterial pneumonias. This disease occurs sporadically except during influenza outbreaks, when staphylococcal pneumonia is relatively more common, although still less frequent than pneumococcal pneumonia.

Primary staphylococcal pneumonia in infants and children frequently presents with high fever and cough. Multiple thin-walled abscesses, or pneumatoceles, are present on the chest roentgenogram. Empyema formation is common. Cough may be nonproductive, and blood cultures are usually negative, frequently necessitating empiric antistaphylococcal therapy. In older children and healthy adults staphylococcal pneumonia is generally preceded by an influenza-like respiratory infection (influenza, measles, or other viruses). Onset of staphylococcal involvement is abrupt, with chills, high fever, progressive dyspnea, cyanosis, cough, and pleural pain. The sputum may be bloody or frankly purulent.

Staphylococci frequently colonize the bronchiectatic airways in children with cystic fibrosis and may cause recurrent episodes of bronchopneumonia. Nosocomial staphylococcal pneumonia typically occurs in intubated patients in intensive care units and in debilitated patients who are prone to aspiration. Residents of nursing homes may have an increased incidence of staphylococcal pneumonia. Infections distal to an obstructing bronchogenic carcinoma may also be caused by *S. aureus.* These infections can begin insidiously, with increasing fever, tachycardia, and tachypnea the only indications of infection. The disease may also be less abrupt when pulmonary involvement occurs during the course of staphylococcal bacteremia, as in patients with right-sided endocarditis. Cavitation, pleural involvement, and empyema are common.

The course of staphylococcal pneumonia may be stormy despite adequate antimicrobial therapy. Gradual defervescence starting 48 to 72 h after the initiation of therapy is typical.

Staphylococcal pneumonia must be differentiated from other pneumonias. The preceding influenza-like illness, rapid onset of pleural pain, cyanosis, and prostration out of proportion to physical findings should suggest primary staphylococcal pneumonia. Sputum

Gram's stain showing masses of neutrophils and gram-positive intraleukocytic cocci provides supportive evidence. Leukocytosis is generally present. When pneumonia develops suddenly or insidiously in debilitated hospitalized patients, staphylococci should be considered in the differential diagnosis.

Parenteral therapy should be initiated with antistaphylococcal antimicrobials as outlined for serious bacteremia and endocarditis. Two weeks of intravenous therapy is usually adequate if complications do not develop. The presence of an empyema usually necessitates chest tube drainage and may be complicated by the formation of loculations or bronchopleural fistulas. Ultrasound or computerized tomography scan may be required to identify loculated collections of pus for drainage.

URINARY TRACT INFECTION *S. saprophyticus* is, after *Escherichia coli*, the most common cause of primary, nonobstructive urinary tract infection in sexually active young women. It is responsible for 10 to 20 percent of infections in healthy outpatients. Symptoms of urgency, frequency, and burning are indistinguishable from urinary infections due to other agents. Fever is absent or low-grade. Although lower tract infection is most common, pyelonephritis has been reported.

The diagnosis is established by examination of the urinary sediment, which characteristically reveals pyuria, microscopic hematuria, and cocci in clumps. The organism may be identified by its resistance to novobiocin and nalidixic acid. *S. saprophyticus* grows readily on blood agar, but less well on MacConkey agar and may be missed by currently available rapid diagnostic methods that depend on nitrate reduction or glucose utilization. The criterion for greater than 10^5 bacteria per milliliter developed for gram-negative urinary tract infection is unreliable.

The organism is susceptible to most antimicrobials used for urinary tract infection, including ampicillin, trimethoprim, sulfonamides, and nitrofurantoin. Relapses after appropriate therapy should raise the consideration of infected renal calculi, which may be formed because of the organism's capacity to produce urease.

Isolation of *S. aureus* from a well-collected urine specimen should prompt consideration of staphylococcal bacteremia, which may have been complicated by renal, perinephric, or prostatic abscesses.

Miscellaneous infections *S. epidermidis* and *S. aureus* rank first and second among pathogens infecting prosthetic devices and intravascular grafts. *S. epidermidis* infections tend to be more insidious and frequently pursue a prolonged course with high morbidity due in part to the temptation to regard positive cultures as contaminants. Subtle clinical findings are common—prosthetic hip infections may present with pain and loosening of the prosthesis, and cerebrospinal fluid shunt infections may present as hypocomplementemic glomerulonephritis due to circulating immune complexes.

S. aureus is a frequent cause of mastitis in nursing mothers; the infant is usually colonized. Although *Clostridium difficile* is the most common cause of postantibiotic colitis, overgrowth of *S. aureus* in the ileum and cecum may be responsible occasionally. *S. epidermidis* is a common cause of endophthalmitis complicating ocular surgery.

CONTROL OF INTRAHOSPITAL OUTBREAKS OF STAPHYLOCOC-CAL DISEASE (See Chap. 85) Hospital outbreaks of staphylococcal disease may develop rapidly in burn units, intensive care units, or neonatal care units—areas housing debilitated patients under continuous antibiotic pressure. The index case is frequently a patient recently discharged or transferred from another hospital where the organism is endemic. The implicated strains of *S. aureus* are frequently methicillin-resistant (MRSA).

Control demands the rapid identification of the patient reservoir in the affected care units by cultures of wounds, nares, and perineum; urine cultures should be obtained from patients with indwelling urinary catheters. Isolation of culture-positive patients together with reinforcement of the need for proper aseptic technique and hand washing by hospital personnel decreases transmission. Housekeeping antisepsis using phenolic cleaning agents should be carried out in the rooms of colonized patients. Early discharge of colonized patients

should be encouraged. Charts should be labeled and patients returned to strict isolation upon readmission to the hospital until shown to be culture-negative.

Although nasal carriers among hospital personnel may transmit the organism, efficient dissemination occurs by persons with cutaneous diseases (eczema, atopic dermatitis) that have become colonized with *S. aureus*. Such personnel should be removed from clinical duties until they become culture-negative either spontaneously or following therapy.

Decolonization of the skin and nares in patients and personnel has been accomplished by whole-body washing with antiseptic soaps that leave an inhibitory residue on the skin—hexachlorophene, chlorhexidine, or triclosan. Topical antibiotics are ineffective. Oral antibiotics may be required to abolish the carrier state. Rifampin (600 mg every day for 5 days) has been used successfully alone or, depending on the sensitivity of the staphylococcal isolate, combined with trimethoprim-sulfamethoxazole, doxycycline, or dicloxacillin to prevent the emergence of rifampin resistance.

REFERENCES

ARCHER GL: *Staphylococcus epidermidis* and other coagulase-negative staphylococci, in *Principles and Practice of Infectious Diseases*, GC Mandell et al (eds). New York, Wiley Medical, 1985, pp 1117–1123

CHAMBERS HF et al: *Staphylococcus aureus* endocarditis: Clinical manifestations in addicts and nonaddicts. Medicine 62:170, 1983

GARBE PL et al: *Staphylococcus aureus* isolates from patients with nonmenstrual toxic shock syndrome. Evidence for additional toxins. JAMA 253:2538, 1985

HOVELIUS B, MARDH P-A: *Staphylococcus saprophyticus* as a common cause of urinary tract infections. Rev Infect Dis 6:328, 1984

LOWY FD, HAMMER SM: *Staphylococcus epidermidis* infections. Ann Intern Med 99:834, 1983

SHEAGREN JN: *Staphylococcus aureus*. The persistent pathogen. New Engl J Med 310:1368, 1437, 1984

WALDVOGEL FA: *Staphylococcus aureus* (including toxic shock syndrome) in *Principles and Practice of Infectious Diseases*, GC Mandell et al (eds). New York, Wiley Medical, 1985, pp 1097–1117

95 STREPTOCOCCAL INFECTIONS

ALAN B. BISNO

Streptococci are among the commonest bacterial pathogens of humans. They are responsible for a diverse spectrum of diseases including pharyngitis and tonsillitis, scarlet fever, erysipelas, impetigo, lymphangitis, and perinatal infections of mother and child. Certain representatives of this genus are prominent causes of endocarditis and urinary tract infections. In addition to their role in causing acute pyogenic infections, strains of *Streptococcus pyogenes* are capable of giving rise to the delayed nonsuppurative sequels of acute rheumatic fever and acute glomerulonephritis.

ETIOLOGY AND CLASSIFICATION Streptococci are spherical or ovoid bacterial cells which grow in pairs or chains of varying lengths. Most are facultative anaerobes, although some taxonomists include certain strict anaerobes in the genus. The organisms are gram-positive, usually nonmotile, non-spore-forming, and catalase-negative. No single system of classification suffices to differentiate this heterogeneous group of organisms. Instead, classification depends upon a combination of features, including patterns of hemolysis observed on blood agar plates, antigenic composition, growth characteristics, and biochemical reactions.

When cultivated on blood agar plates, streptococci may produce one of three different patterns of hemolysis. Alpha-hemolytic colonies are surrounded by a zone of partial hemolysis; in addition, such organisms usually produce a greenish discoloration in the medium due to the presence of an unidentified reductant of hemoglobin. This greening reaction gives rise to the designation "viridans" streptococcus, which is often applied to alpha-hemolytic strains. Strains of *S. pneumoniae* are alpha-hemolytic, as are many other streptococci which normally inhabit the upper respiratory and gastrointestinal tracts. Beta-hemolytic colonies are surrounded by clear colorless zones within which the red blood cells in the medium have been completely lysed. This pattern of complete hemolysis is shown by *S. pyogenes* and many of the other streptococci pathogenic for humans. Gamma streptococci fail to produce hemolysis upon blood agar plates.

Although classification of streptococci on the basis of hemolytic reactions is quite useful in certain clinical situations, more precise identification of streptococci is accomplished by differentiation into serogroups, as originally described by Lancefield, on the basis of antigenic differences in cell wall carbohydrates or teichoic acids. These antigens are readily extracted from streptococcal cell walls and identified by precipitin reactions using specific antiserums. The majority of beta-hemolytic streptococci isolated from human infections belong to groups A to D and G. Certain alpha-hemolytic and nonhemolytic strains also contain group-specific antigens. The most important of these are the group D streptococci, including the so-called enterococci, among which many strains fail to show beta hemolysis. There are 21 recognized species of streptococci. Species designation is based upon growth characteristics under varying conditions of temperature, pH, and media composition. Five species do not possess group antigens, and, conversely, a number of serogroups do not encompass any of the recognized species.

Anaerobic streptococci include members of the family Peptococceae, genus *Peptostreptococcus*; five species are recognized. Hemolytic reactions of these organisms are variable, and no satisfactory method of classifying them has been devised.

GROUP A STREPTOCOCCAL INFECTIONS

Streptococci of Lancefield's group A (*S. pyogenes*) are uniquely important because of the frequency with which they cause human infections and their role as precursors of rheumatic fever and glomerulonephritis.

ETIOLOGY The *group-specific carbohydrate* of group A streptococci is a polymer of rhamnose and *N*-acetylglucosamine. There are approximately 80 recognized and provisional group A serotypes. The typing system is based upon antigenic differences in a cell wall constituent known as *M protein*, which is the principal virulence factor of group A organisms. Strains rich in M protein are highly resistant to phagocytosis by polymorphonuclear leukocytes in vitro and are capable of initiating disease in humans and experimental animals. Strains lacking M protein are avirulent. The antiphagocytic effect of M protein is due, at least in part, to its ability to prevent opsonization of the organism by the complement system. Acquired human immunity to streptococcal infection is based upon development of opsonic antibodies directed against the antiphagocytic moiety of M protein. This immunity is type-specific and lasts for many years, perhaps indefinitely. M proteins of certain types share antigenic determinants with human heart tissue.

T protein serves as the basis of a subsidiary typing system which has been useful in classifying strains not typeable by the M systems; unlike M protein, the T antigen plays no role in virulence. *Lipoteichoic acid*, a substance which has a marked affinity for biological membranes, has been found to play a crucial role in colonization by binding group A streptococci to fibronectin and to specific receptor sites on human epithelial cells. The streptococcal *cell membrane* contains a number of antigenic structures, certain of which have been reported to share determinants with constituents of human heart and with basement membrane of the renal glomerulus. During the early logarithmic phase of replication, streptococci are enveloped in a slimy *hyaluronic acid capsule* which serves to retard phagocytosis and, therefore, represents an accessory virulence factor. Streptococcal

hyaluronate is nonantigenic in humans, presumably because it is identical to that found in human connective tissue.

As streptococci grow in vitro or in vivo, they elaborate a number of extracellular products. *Erythrogenic toxin (pyrogenic exotoxin)*, which is induced by lysogeny with a temperate bacteriophage, is responsible for the rash of scarlet fever. There are four serologically distinct toxins, the effects of which may be neutralized by antibody. Two distinct hemolysins are elaborated. *Streptolysin O* is reversibly inhibited by oxygen (hence exerting its effect primarily on subsurface colonies) and irreversibly inhibited by cholesterol. It is produced by almost all group A strains as well as by many group C and G organisms. Titration of antistreptolysin O (ASO) antibodies in human serums is the most widely used serologic procedure to detect group A streptococcal infection in clinical practice. Hemolysis on the surface of blood agar plates is due primarily to the action of *streptolysin S*. Although streptolysin S differs from streptolysin O in being oxygen-stable and nonantigenic, both hemolysins possess the capacity to damage membranes of polymorphonuclear leukocytes, platelets, and subcellular organelles. A number of other extracellular products exert effects which might serve to facilitate the organisms' survival in vivo by liquefying pus [streptokinase and deoxyribonucleases (DNases) A to D] or by allowing spread through tissue planes (*hyaluronidase and proteinase*). The role of these substances in streptococcal virulence remains unproved.

The two most frequent types of group A streptococcal infection are pharyngitis and pyoderma. They differ markedly in their epidemiologic, clinical, and bacteriologic characteristics.

STREPTOCOCCAL PHARYNGITIS　Epidemiology The incidence of this ubiquitous infection is highest in children aged 5 to 15 years; males and females are affected equally. The great majority of such infections are due to group A streptococci, but strains of other serogroups, particularly group C or G, are involved occasionally. The organism is ordinarily transmitted directly from person to person, most likely by droplet spread, and crowding markedly facilitates interpersonal transmission. This may account for the increased incidence of streptococcal pharyngitis in northern latitudes during the colder months of the year, as well as for the explosive outbreaks which occur in military recruit camps and other crowded institutional settings. Common-source epidemics of streptococcal sore throat with high attack rates occasionally occur following contamination of a food item with beta-hemolytic streptococci.

Patients with acute streptococcal pharyngitis harbor large numbers of organisms in the anterior nares and throat. If antibiotics are not administered, the organisms may persist in the upper respiratory tract for weeks to months after symptoms have subsided. However, as the length of the carrier state increases, the organisms decrease in number, disappear from the anterior nasal secretions, and lose detectable M protein. Therefore, convalescent carriers are less likely than acutely ill patients to transmit group A streptococci to exposed individuals. Group A pharyngeal carriage rates vary with geographic location, season of the year, and age group. Among school-age children, rates of 15 to 20 percent have been reported; the carriage rate among adults is considerably lower.

Symptoms The usual incubation period of streptococcal pharyngitis is between 2 and 4 days. The classic syndrome, as observed in older children and adults, is ushered in by the rather abrupt onset of sore throat, particularly by pain on swallowing. Associated symptoms include headache, malaise, feverishness, and anorexia. Chilliness is a frequent symptom, but true rigors are rare. Nausea, vomiting, and abdominal pain are common in children.

Physical signs The patient appears moderately ill with tachycardia and fever which frequently exceeds 38.3°C (101°F). There is diffuse erythema, edema, and lymphoid hyperplasia of the posterior pharynx. The uvula is edematous. The tonsils, if present, are enlarged, reddened, and covered by a punctate or coalescent exudate which may be yellow, gray, or white. Discrete areas of pinhead-size exudate may be present on the hypertrophied lymphoid follicles of the posterior pharynx. On the soft palate, small, red, raised follicular lesions with yellowish centers (''doughnut lesions'') are occasionally seen. The anterior cervical lymph nodes at the angles of the jaw are enlarged and tender. Cough and hoarseness, if present, are mild and, in the absence of the signs and symptoms indicated above, do not suggest the diagnosis of streptococcal pharyngitis. Laryngeal involvement with loss of voice is not a feature of streptococcal infection.

The full-blown clinical syndrome of acute exudative tonsillopharyngitis is seen frequently during explosive epidemics of streptococcal disease, particularly those occurring in institutional settings such as military recruit camps. In endemically occurring infections among civilian populations, however, the illness is frequently much milder. Indeed, in such circumstances, only about half the children with sore throats and positive cultures for group A streptococci will have tonsillar exudate, and a third or less may have fever greater than 38.3°C (101°F) or marked leukocytosis. Patients who have undergone tonsillectomy tend to experience a milder clinical syndrome. In infants, streptococcal upper respiratory infections tend to be less sharply localized to the lymphoid tissue of the faucial and posterior pharyngeal areas. Infections at this age are characterized by rhinorrhea with excoriation of the nares, low-grade fever, anorexia, and a protracted clinical course. Exudative pharyngitis in children under 3 is rarely streptococcal in etiology.

Course The course of streptococcal pharyngitis is usually brief and self-limited. Fever abates within a week, usually within 3 to 5 days. Constitutional symptoms and sore throat disappear with defervescence or shortly thereafter. Several weeks may be required, however, for the tonsils and lymph nodes to return to normal size.

SCARLET FEVER When streptococcal pharyngitis is due to a lysogenic strain producing erythrogenic toxin, and when the host does not possess neutralizing antibody to the toxin, scarlet fever ensues. The situation may be more complex than was previously thought, because a preexisting state of hypersensitivity to streptococcal products may predispose to the development of scarlet fever.

The rash usually appears within 2 days after onset of sore throat, involves first the neck, upper chest, and back, then spreads over the remainder of the trunk and the extremities, and spares the palms and soles. The rash may be difficult to appreciate in black patients. It consists of a diffuse erythema, which blanches on pressure, with numerous 1- to 2-mm punctate elevations that impart a ''sandpaper'' texture to the skin. Discrete lesions are absent from the face, but there is a generalized facial flush which contrasts with the prominent circumoral pallor. The rash is more intense along skin folds, such as those of the antecubital fossae and axillary folds, and in these locations often produces linear striations of confluent petechiae known as *Pastia's lines*, which are due to increased capillary fragility.

The exanthem of scarlet fever is accompanied by an enanthem, consisting of punctate erythema and petechiae on the soft palate. Early in the disease, the tongue is covered with a white coat through which hypertrophied papillae protrude as islands of red (white strawberry tongue). By the fourth or fifth day the coating is gone and the entire tongue appears beefy red (red strawberry or raspberry tongue). In rare cases, scarlet fever may be complicated by jaundice, pleural effusion, and arthralgia.

The rash usually lasts 4 to 5 days and is followed by extensive desquamation which begins as early as a few days or as late as 3 to 4 weeks after onset of the disease and is often a striking feature of the convalescent phase of scarlet fever.

Although scarlet fever usually follows upper respiratory infection due to group A streptococci, rarely erythrogenic toxins are produced by streptococci of other groups and by certain strains of staphylococci. Moreover, scarlet fever may follow streptococcal impetigo or secondary streptococcal infection of superficial wounds or surgical incisions. The disease must be differentiated from various of the childhood exanthems (e.g., rubeola, rubella, exanthem subitum), toxic shock syndrome, Kawasaki disease, infectious mononucleosis when the latter is associated with rash, miliaria, and drug eruptions.

The management of scarlet fever consists of adequate treatment of the causative infection.

Complications Streptococcal pharyngitis may give rise to suppurative complications, among which acute otitis media and acute sinusitis are the most frequent. Suppurative cervical lymphadenitis may also occur. Inflammation of the faucial area induced by streptococcal infection may give rise to peritonsillar cellulitis, peritonsillar abscess, or retropharyngeal abscess. The abscesses themselves, however, usually contain a variety of oropharyngeal flora, including anaerobic bacteria, with or without group A streptococci. A variety of other complications, common in the past, are almost never seen in the antibiotic era: (1) extension up the cribriform plate of the ethmoid or via the mastoid, giving rise to meningitis, brain abscess, or thrombosis of cerebral venous sinuses; and (2) bacteremia with metastatic foci of infection such as suppurative arthritis, endocarditis, osteomyelitis, or liver abscess. Streptococcal pharyngitis is associated with two delayed nonsuppurative sequels: acute rheumatic fever (ARF) and acute glomerulonephritis (AGN). These are discussed in Chaps. 186 and 223, respectively.

Diagnosis Sore throat due to group A streptococci must be differentiated from that caused by a number of other agents. *Diphtheria* is rare in immunized populations. It is characterized by the presence of an extensive diphtheritic membrane, and in severe cases by respiratory embarrassment due to laryngeal involvement, as well as by myocarditis and cranial nerve palsies. Cultures on Loeffler's medium will be positive for *Corynebacterium diphtheriae*. Gonococcal tonsillopharyngitis should be suggested by a history of homosexuality or fellatio and confirmed by appropriate cultures. *Vincent's angina* is characterized by sore throat and tonsillopharyngeal exudate. Unlike streptococcal sore throat, however, there is an insidious onset without constitutional symptoms, pharyngeal ulcerations are frequent, and the disease is usually unilateral.

The major differential diagnostic confusion is with viral upper respiratory infections, which occur more frequently than streptococcal infections. In many cases, the viral etiology may be suspected because of the more prominent catarrhal, ''common cold–like'' quality of these viral infections. *Adenoviruses* may cause an exudative pharyngitis which is indistinguishable clinically from that due to group A streptococci. *Infectious mononucleosis* also produces severe exudative pharyngitis with fever and toxicity and at times is accompanied by a rash which may be confused with scarlet fever. The generalized lymphadenopathy, splenomegaly, prolonged fever, and presence of abnormal lymphocytes and heterophile antibodies in the peripheral blood serve to differentiate this entity. Pharyngitis due to group A coxsackieviruses (*herpangina*) or to primary infection with *herpes simplex* is characterized by formation of vesicles, which rupture and leave shallow ulcers. *Influenza* virus infections frequently occur in epidemics; they are accompanied by severe myalgias, bronchitis is a frequent clinical feature, and all age groups are affected. *Mycoplasma pneumoniae* infections may cause pharyngitis that at times may be exudative. Bullous myringitis, if present, should suggest this diagnosis.

Although use of algorithms incorporating combinations of epidemiologic data, symptoms, and signs may enhance diagnostic accuracy, in many instances it is impossible to differentiate streptococcal from nonstreptococcal sore throat on clinical grounds alone. For this reason, precise diagnosis requires identification of the infecting organism in the pharynx. This is achieved most reliably by a throat culture. In obtaining the culture, it is important to rub the cotton swab over both tonsils or tonsillar fossae, the oropharynx, and the nasopharynx posterior to the uvula. The swab should be inoculated onto a sheep blood agar plate to allow evaluation of patterns of hemolysis after overnight incubation. If beta-hemolytic streptococci are isolated, they may be identified presumptively as group A if growth is inhibited around a low-potency (0.04-unit) bacitracin disk. Definitive identification may be accomplished by fluorescent antibody, agglutination, or precipitin techniques. A number of the positive cultures obtained, particularly those with relatively few organisms on the culture plate, will represent streptococcal carriers rather than cases of acute infection. It is not possible to differentiate cases from carriers confidently on the basis of culture results, but culture does serve to exclude from antimicrobial therapy the bulk of patients with sore throat (approximately 70 percent) who have negative cultures for beta-hemolytic streptococci. A number of commercial kits are available which allow detection of group A antigen directly from throat swabs by immunologic means. These kits provide results within less than an hour, some within a few minutes. The direct antigen tests are highly specific, and the physician may proceed confidently on the basis of a positive result. Although the immunologic tests are in general quite sensitive, they fail to identify reliably patients with very weakly positive cultures. Many such patients are, however, asymptomatic carriers. The precise role of group A antigen tests, which provide rapid results at the expense of somewhat reduced sensitivity compared to throat culture, has not been established.

In selecting patients for throat culture or antigen testing, it should be borne in mind that group A streptococcal pharyngitis and acute rheumatic fever are extremely rare in children under 3 in the United States. Likewise, first attacks of rheumatic fever are rare in older adults. Routine use of streptococcal diagnostic procedures is less cost-effective in these groups.

Assays of serum antibodies to streptococcal extracellular products (e.g., ASO) provide confirmatory evidence of recent streptococcal infection in patients suspected of having ARF or AGN, but such tests are of no value in the diagnosis of acute streptococcal infection.

Treatment   Therapy of streptococcal pharyngitis is directed primarily toward prevention of ARF and of suppurative sequelae. It is unclear whether treatment of the antecedent streptococcal infection will prevent development of AGN. Prevention of ARF depends upon eradication of the infecting organism from the pharynx, and attainment of this objective requires prolonged antibiotic treatment. Penicillin is the drug of choice. It is inexpensive and nontoxic and all group A streptococci have remained exquisitely sensitive to it. A single intramuscular injection of benzathine penicillin G, 600,000 units for children weighing 27 kg (60 lb) or less and 1.2 million units for all others, ensures a prolonged penicillinemia and is the most effective form of therapy. Given the current low risk of ARF in most areas of the United States, many physicians now choose oral therapy for compliant patients. This is an attractive alternative because the risk of severe allergic reactions is presumed to be less with oral than with intramuscular penicillin. A full 10 days of therapy is required, however, and this is often difficult to achieve, because patients are usually asymptomatic well before the 10 days have elapsed. If oral therapy is elected, penicillin V, 125 to 250 mg, three to four times daily, is the treatment of choice.

Penicillin-allergic individuals may be treated with oral erythromycin. Prescribing information for the various formulations should be consulted for the precise dosage. For most preparations, the dose is 40 mg per kilogram of body weight per day, to be administered in two to four equally divided portions. The total daily dose should not exceed 1 g.

Nearly all group A streptococci in the United States have remained susceptible to erythromycin, but extensive resistance has been reported in certain areas of the world such as Japan. On the other hand, tetracycline-resistant strains are encountered with some frequency in the United States, and this drug is not recommended. Sulfonamides are ineffective in eradication of established streptococcal infection, although they are useful prophylactically in preventing new pharyngeal acquisitions of group A streptococci and in preventing recurrences of ARF (see Chap. 186).

Because of the very low incidence of ARF and because a high proportion of "treatment failures" occur in streptococcal carriers rather than in acutely infected patients, routine follow-up cultures are not needed in asymptomatic individuals. Exceptions should be made, however, if there is a history of ARF in the patient or family contacts.

Appropriate antibiotic therapy is effective in preventing ARF,

even when initiated as long as 9 days after the onset of acute pharyngitis. Therefore, in the patient seen early in the course of illness, the delay in initiating therapy occasioned by processing a throat culture is not ordinarily a matter of concern. Although treatment also speeds resolution of fever, sore throat, and systemic symptoms associated with streptococcal pharyngitis, the effect of antibiotics is in most cases not dramatic. Indeed, given the self-limited course of the illness, it is difficult to demonstrate clinical improvement in antibiotic-treated vs. placebo-treated patients if therapy is initiated more than 24 h after onset of symptoms. Unless patients have high fever, severe systemic toxicity, or evidence of suppurative complications, initiation of antimicrobial therapy can await the results of throat culture.

In patients judged to be more severely ill, therapy may be initiated at the time of the initial visit after a throat culture has been obtained. If oral antibiotic therapy is elected, the throat culture serves as a guide to the necessity of completing a full 10-day course or, alternatively, of recalling the patient for definitive therapy with an injection of benzathine penicillin G.

Patients with more severe suppurative complications, such as mastoiditis or ethmoiditis, require larger doses of penicillin than those used for treatment of uncomplicated sore throat. When streptococcal upper respiratory infection is complicated by the development of abscesses associated with suppurative cervical adenitis or in the peritonsillar or retropharyngeal soft tissues, incision and drainage are usually required.

The role of tonsillectomy, if any, in the management of patients with frequent recurrences of acute pharyngitis or in the prevention of ARF remains undefined. Clinical episodes of pharyngitis occur less frequently and tend to be milder following tonsillectomy, but this may possibly make detection and appropriate treatment of immunologically significant streptococcal infections more difficult.

Family contacts of patients with streptococcal sore throat frequently develop symptomatic infections or become asymptomatic pharyngeal carriers. Symptomatic secondary cases in families should be treated appropriately. Asymptomatic family contacts should also be cultured in high-risk circumstances. These include the presence of a rheumatic subject in the family or of known cases of ARF occurring in the general area. In situations where the risk is lower, cultures of asymptomatic family contacts need not be performed routinely.

STREPTOCOCCAL SKIN INFECTIONS Erysipelas   Also known as Saint Anthony's fire, erysipelas is an acute infection of the skin, with marked involvement of cutaneous lymphatic vessels, caused by group A streptococci. Other streptococci and *Staphylococcus aureus* have been implicated on rare occasions. The disease most frequently affects infants, young children, and elderly individuals. The commonest site of involvement is the face, where cutaneous infection originates from an upper respiratory source, presumably by way of small or inapparent breaks in the skin. Erysipelas may also result from streptococcal infection of wounds, surgical incisions, or even areas of dermatophytosis, in which case any portion of the body may be involved.

The onset is usually abrupt; initial symptoms include malaise, chilliness, feverishness, headache, and vomiting. The skin lesion may begin with itching and mild discomfort at the site of infection and is followed shortly thereafter by a small area of erythema which enlarges during the ensuing hours. The lesion spreads rapidly, reaching its maximum extent in 3 to 6 days. It is warm, pink to deep red in color, and has an advancing elevated margin which protrudes irregularly into the surrounding areas of normal skin. Vesicles and bullae may appear; these rupture leaving crusts on the surface. While the advancing margin remains inflamed, central clearing may be evident with a return of the skin to normal appearance or with residual pigmentation. The eruption may be less well demarcated in areas where the skin is loose, but edema and erythema are constant features. Facial erysipelas commonly involves the bridge of the nose and one or more cheeks in a "butterfly" distribution (Fig. 95-1).

The disease process may be accompanied by high fever and bacteremia. Recovery is usually apparent by the end of a week, but

FIGURE 95-1 *This patient with facial erysipelas exhibits the characteristic "butterfly" distribution of the lesion. The picture was obtained after 48 h of penicillin therapy when the acute inflammation and systemic toxicity had abated slightly.*

this varies with the severity of the infection. The substantial mortality attending bacteremic cases of erysipelas in the preantibiotic era has been markedly reduced by penicillin. Fatalities still occur among children within the first few months of life and elderly, debilitated, immunosuppressed individuals. The disease is noted for its propensity to recur, especially in areas of chronic lymphatic obstruction.

The diagnosis of erysipelas is primarily clinical. Group A streptococci may at times be isolated from the respiratory tract or the bloodstream. Culture of edema fluid or of saline injected intracutaneously and then withdrawn from the advancing margin may yield streptococci, but this maneuver is rarely successful.

Pyoderma This term is used collectively to denote localized purulent streptococcal skin infections. Some pyoderma lesions represent obvious secondary infections of wounds or burns. For the most part, however, the term is used synonymously with streptococcal impetigo or impetigo contagiosa and refers to discrete purulent lesions which appear to be primary infections of the skin. Streptococcal impetigo differs from streptococcal pharyngitis in a number of particulars (Table 95-1). Epidemiologically, impetigo is more prevalent among underprivileged children residing in warm, humid climates such as the southeastern United States or the tropics. However, the disease may also occur during the summer in northern settings, such as the American Indian reservations of Minnesota. The peak incidence is in young children (2 to 6 years), and there is no definite sex or racial predisposition.

The mode of spread of streptococcal pyoderma is unknown, but personal contact and insect vectors such as *Hippelates* flies are probably both important. "Skin strains" of group A streptococci (i.e., strains of M and T types usually associated with pyoderma) are capable of contaminating unbroken skin, from where they may be inoculated intradermally by local scratches, abrasions, or insect bites. Nasal and pharyngeal carriage of skin strains is frequent in children with impetigo, but such carriage does not ordinarily occur until after establishment of cutaneous carriage or overt infection.

The pattern of immunologic responses to streptococcal impetigo differs from that associated with upper respiratory infection. In particular, the ASO response to impetigo is weak, perhaps because streptolysin O is inactivated by lipids present in the skin. Brisk antibody responses to anti-DNAse B and anti-hyaluronidase, as well as to the Streptozyme slide hemagglutination reagent, are observed, however. Type-specific anti-M responses are variable, depending in

part upon the antigenicity of the infecting strain, but in general such responses are weaker than in pharyngeal infections. The role of type-specific antibodies in protection against reinfection in pyoderma has not been adequately studied.

Streptococcal impetigo occurs on exposed areas of the body, most frequently on the lower extremities. The lesions remain well-localized but are frequently multiple. They begin as papules but rapidly evolve into vesicles surrounded by an area of erythema. The vesicular lesions are rarely recognized clinically; they give rise to pustules which gradually enlarge, then break down over 4 to 6 days to form characteristic thick crusts. The lesions heal slowly, leaving depigmented areas. A deeply ulcerated form of impetigo is known as *ecthyma*. Although regional lymphadenitis often occurs, systemic symptoms are not ordinarily present.

In addition to the indolent, impetiginous skin infections of young children, a more severe and extensive form of pyoderma has been observed in combat troops serving in hot, wet environments such as the jungles of southeast Asia. During the Vietnam conflict, such "jungle sores" became a major medical problem among infantry personnel. In their most common form, they consist of multiple ecthymatous ulcers located on the ankle or dorsum of the foot. The ulcers are usually circular, punched-out lesions 0.5 to 3.0 cm in diameter, have borders, and are surrounded by a zone of erythema. They are filled with purulent material and covered with grayish-yellow adherent crusts. Secondary cellulitis or lymphadenitis may be present.

The diagnosis of streptococcal pyoderma is made by culture. Adequate cultures require removal of the surface crusts in order to obtain specimens from the base of the lesions. Although both *S. pyogenes* and *Staphylococcus aureus* may be isolated from the lesions, the former is the major pathogen. Morphologically characteristic lesions respond well to penicillin therapy, even when penicillinase-resistant staphylococci are recovered. These lesions contrast with bullous impetigo, which is ordinarily due to *S. aureus* and not to streptococci. Antibiotic regimens are the same as those for pharyngitis, and benzathine penicillin G, oral penicillin V, or oral erythromycin all result in cure rates in excess of 95 percent. Topical antiseptics and antibiotics are of little or no value. Prevention of pyoderma depends primarily upon adherence to good personal hygiene, with special attention to frequent scrubbing with soap and water.

Streptococcal pyoderma does not give rise to ARF. This observation remains unexplained, but may indicate a requirement for infection at the pharyngeal site, with its rich endowment of lymphoid tissue, in order to initiate the immunologic events leading to ARF. On the other hand, studies of populations in which ARF and AGN occur simultaneously indicate that the streptococcal strains responsible for each sequela are distinct and suggest that "pyoderma strains" of

TABLE 95-1 Comparative features of pharyngitis and pyoderma due to group A streptococci

	Pharyngitis	Pyoderma
Predominant geographic distribution	Ubiquitous	Subtropic-tropic
Season (temperate zone)	Winter-spring	Summer-fall
Peak age group	5–15 years	2–5 years
Mode of spread	Direct contact (droplet)	Unknown (?insects)
Clinical illness	Acute	Indolent
Streptococcal types	Generally lower-numbered M types	Generally higher-numbered M types
ASO responses	Good	Weak
Type-specific antibody responses	Generally good	Variable, often poor
Nonsuppurative sequelae	Acute rheumatic fever, acute glomerulonephritis	Acute glomerulonephritis

SOURCE: *Modified from Wannamaker LW, N Engl J Med 282:23, 1970* group A streptococci may be nonrheumatogenic. When pyoderma is due to a nephritogenic strain of group A streptococcus, AGN may ensue. Indeed, pyoderma is by far the commonest antecedent of poststreptococcal glomerulonephritis in subtropical and tropical regions of the world. Strains of a number of M types (49, 55, 57, and others) have been associated with both sporadic cases and large epidemics of pyoderma-associated nephritis in diverse geographic areas. There are no conclusive data to indicate that treatment of an individual case of pyoderma will prevent the subsequent occurrence of AGN in that patient. Such treatment is important, however, in eradicating nephritogenic streptococci from the environment in epidemiologic settings in which these strains are prevalent.

Cellulitis Streptococcal cellulitis may occur in areas of tissue damage due to trauma, operative wounds, or stasis ulceration. Although such infections are frequently due to group A organisms, beta hemolytic streptococci of groups G, B, or C may be responsible. Cellulitis is an acute inflammation of the skin and subcutaneous tissues marked by pain, tenderness, erythema, fever, and often regional lymphadenopathy. In contrast to erysipelas, the margins of the lesions are neither elevated nor sharply demarcated from the surrounding uninvolved tissue. Rarely such lesions may progress to frank gangrene. Certain patients who have undergone saphenous venectomy for coronary bypass surgery experience recurrent bouts of acute streptococcal cellulitis in the months to years after surgery. The cellulitis always involves the saphenous donor extremity. Frequently the patients suffer from tinea pedis, and uncontrolled observations suggest that eradication of the superficial fungal infection, which may serve as a nidus for streptococcal colonization, may result in abolition of the recurrent attacks.

Cellulitis of the perianal area may be manifested by painful defecation or by pruritus; asymptomatic anal colonization has been the source of several outbreaks of hospital-acquired streptococcal infection. Vaginal colonization by group A streptococci has a number of features in common with perianal involvement. In both instances there is a close epidemiologic association with streptococcal upper respiratory infection. Anal and vaginal streptococcal infection may be either symptomatic or asymptomatic. At least one outbreak of nosocomial streptococcal infection has been attributed to an asymptomatic vaginal carrier.

LYMPHANGITIS AND PUERPERAL SEPSIS Local trauma, whether or not complicated by frank cellulitis, may give rise to *acute lymphangitis*. This entity is characterized by the appearance of red linear streaks extending from the portal of entry to the draining regional lymph nodes, which are enlarged and tender. Systemic symptoms, including chills, fever, malaise, and headache, are prominent, and the process may be accompanied by demonstrable bacteremia.

Streptococcal bacteremia, from whatever cause, may give rise to metastatic foci of infection, such as suppurative arthritis, osteomyelitis, peritonitis, endocarditis, meningitis, or visceral abscesses. Streptococcal bacteremia may complicate parenteral drug abuse; such infections are often associated with local abscesses at the injection site and/or infective endocarditis (see Chap. 94). The clinical course of streptococcal bacteremia may be fulminant and lead rapidly to prostration, shock, purpura fulminans, disseminated intravascular coagulation, and death.

Puerperal sepsis follows abortion or childbirth when streptococci invade the endometrium and surrounding structures and then the lymphatics and bloodstream. The process may be further complicated by pelvic cellulitis, septic pelvic thrombophlebitis, peritonitis, or pelvic abscess. The causative organism may be transmitted to the pregnant woman directly by medical personnel or attendants, as was demonstrated by Semmelweiss in the mid-nineteenth century. Group B streptococci have supplanted other organisms as the most frequent cause of perinatal streptococcal infections of mother and child (see below). Anaerobic streptococci, along with other anaerobic organisms, have also been implicated.

PNEUMONIA AND EMPYEMA Pneumonia due to group A streptococci is uncommon and usually occurs following influenza, measles, pertussis, or varicella. The illness occurs in epidemic form in military recruit camps and is characterized by abrupt onset of fever, chills, myalgia, dyspnea, cough, pleuritic chest pain, and hemoptysis. Patients are severely ill and often cyanotic. Pathologically and radiologically, this is usually a bronchopneumonia, and lobar consolidation is uncommon. A characteristic feature of streptococcal pneumonia is the early and rapid accumulation of copious amounts of thin, serosanguinous empyema fluid. Bacteremia occurs in 10 to 15 percent of cases. Extension of the pneumonic process to the pericardium may give rise to a purulent pericarditis. Other potential complications include mediastinitis, pneumothorax, and bronchiectasis. Therapy consists of at least 4 to 6 million units of parenteral penicillin daily in the form of aqueous procaine penicillin G, given every 6 to 12 h intramuscularly, or intravenous aqueous crystalline penicillin G, and adequate drainage of empyema fluid, which usually requires insertion of a chest tube.

GROUP B STREPTOCOCCAL INFECTIONS

Streptococci belonging to serogroup B have been of interest to veterinarians because of their association with bovine mastitis, an association which led to their species designation as *S. agalactiae*. The organisms are beta-hemolytic and usually, but not uniformly, resistant to bacitracin. In addition to the presence of group B carbohydrate in their cell walls, *S. agalactiae* may be identified by biochemical means, including their production of hippuricase and so-called CAMP factor and their failure to hydrolyze bile esculin agar. Group B streptococci may be subdivided by means of surface polysaccharides and protein antigens into five serotypes: Ia, Ib, Ic, II, and III.

Human strains of group B streptococci, which appear to be biologically distinct from bovine strains, frequently colonize the female genital tract as well as the throat and rectum. Asymptomatic vaginal carriage rates in postpubertal women generally have ranged between 6 and 25 percent, depending on the bacteriologic methods employed and on the socioeconomic status and geographic residence of the women sampled. The majority of serious group B infections occur as perinatal events. Maternal infections include chorioamnionitis, septic abortion, and puerperal sepsis. *Streptococcus agalactiae* now ranks with *Escherichia coli* as one of the two most frequent causes of neonatal sepsis and meningitis. Neonatal disease takes one of two forms. Early-onset disease, occurring within the first 10 days of life, is usually due to organisms acquired from the maternal genital tract. It involves primarily the lungs, probably as a result of aspiration of infected amniotic fluid, but the organism can be cultured from the blood, nasopharynx, skin, and myocardium. Early-onset group B streptococcal infection occurs in approximately two of every thousand live births (the incidence is higher following prolonged or complicated delivery) and is attended by a high mortality rate. Late-onset disease occurs in infants over 10 days old, may be due to nosocomial transmission of group B streptococci, is manifested primarily by meningitis and bacteremia, and has a lower mortality rate than early-onset disease. Although the serotypes involved in early-onset illness are variable, type III organisms predominate as the cause of late-onset meningeal infection. Transplacentally acquired antibodies to type III organisms may protect against late-onset disease: they are reported to be present in serums of most women delivering healthy babies but are usually lacking in serums of mothers whose offspring develop late-onset meningitis due to type III group B streptococci.

Group B streptococci also cause a group of adult infections not associated with the puerperium. These include urinary tract infections in both sexes; the infections in men often occur in elderly individuals, perhaps due to associated prostatism. A second syndrome occurs in patients with adult-onset insulin-dependent diabetes mellitus, peripheral vascular insufficiency, and suppurative gangrenous lesions, infected with *S. agalactiae*. Bacteremia may accompany this syndrome. Other adult infections due to group B organisms include endocarditis, pyogenic arthritis, pneumonia, empyema, meningitis, peritonitis, and terminal bacteremia in patients with malignancy. Although recovered from a small proportion of throat cultures, group B streptococci are rarely, if ever, the cause of clinically significant pharyngitis. All strains are susceptible to penicillin, which is the drug of choice, although group B organisms have higher minimal inhibitory concentrations for penicillin than do group A strains. Life-threatening group B infections in neonates are often treated initially with aminoglycosides in addition to high doses of penicillin, because this combination is synergistic in vitro and because of occasional reports of penicillin tolerance in group B strains. Only occasional strains are resistant to erythromycin. Tetracyclines should not be used without prior susceptibility testing because resistance to them is quite common.

OTHER STREPTOCOCCAL INFECTIONS

Although streptococci of groups C and G are human commensals, both are capable of causing pharyngitis, and epidemics of upper respiratory disease due to these organisms have been reported, particularly following ingestion of contaminated foods. Strains of both serogroups produce streptolysin O, and pharyngeal infections with groups C and G elicit rises in ASO titer. Streptococci of groups C and G are highly susceptible to penicillin.

Most human infections with group C are due to *S. equisimilis*. There have, however, been several reports of outbreaks of human disease due to *S. zooepidemicus*, in which the vehicle was unpasteurized or inadequately pasteurized milk or cheese. Clinical manifestations have included pharyngitis, cervical adenitis, and disseminated deep tissue infections. In two outbreaks, cases of poststreptococcal glomerulonephritis ensued.

Group G streptococcal bacteremia often arises from cutaneous foci such as localized cellulitis or decubitus ulcers, and chronic lymphatic obstruction and venous insufficiency are important predisposing factors. The patients involved frequently have underlying conditions such as malignancy, alcoholism, or parenteral drug abuse. Bacteremia may lead to severe or even life-threatening complications such as endocarditis, meningitis, or septic arthritis.

Lancefield's group D streptococci consist of enterococcal species (*S. faecalis*, *S. faecium*, *S. durans*) and nonenterococci (*S. bovis*, *S. equinus*). Group D streptococci are frequent causes of urinary tract infection in patients with structural abnormalities of the urinary tract and are responsible for 10 percent or more of cases of bacterial endocarditis. They are isolated from infected decubitis ulcers and intraabdominal abscesses, usually in combination with other bacteria. These microorganisms are ordinarily alpha-hemolytic or nonhemolytic but may be beta-hemolytic. The treatment of severe enterococcal infections, particularly bacterial endocarditis, is complicated by the fact that the organisms are resistant to many antibiotics and are relatively resistant to the penicillins. In the therapy of enterococcal endocarditis, a combination of intravenous penicillin G or ampicillin in high doses plus an aminoglycoside antibiotic should be used, because this combination exerts a synergistic effect in the killing of enterococci (see Chap. 188). Formerly, streptomycin was the aminoglycoside of choice, but high-level resistance ($>$2000 µg/mL) to streptomycin and kanamycin has been found in a significant number of enterococcal isolates and synergy is not observed in the presence of such high-level resistance. Gentamicin is the drug of choice along with penicillin or ampicillin in treatment of serious enterococcal infections due to organisms which are highly resistant to streptomycin. The combination of penicillin and tobramycin is not lethal in vitro for strains of *S. faecium*.

Certain enterococcal strains have developed resistance by a variety of mechanisms to many of the aminoglycoside antibiotics. Fortunately, gentamicin remains an effective synergistic agent for treatment of most deep tissue enterococcal infections encountered in the United

States. In treatment of individual cases, however, it is advisable to rule out the presence of high-level gentamicin resistance by in vitro testing. Treatment of life-threatening enterococcal infections in patients who cannot tolerate penicillin is difficult. Cephalothin and clindamycin are of no value, but vancomycin, in combintion with gentamicin, is likely to be effective.

Nonenterococcal group D streptococci, of which *S. bovis* is the major pathogen, remain extremely sensitive to penicillin and are amenable to therapy with this agent alone. Bacteremia or endocarditis due to *S. bovis* has been associated with carcinoma of the colon. Laboratory differentiation of *S. bovis* from enterococci is sometimes difficult. Likewise, *S. mutans*, a penicillin-sensitive viridans streptococcus which is normally found in the mouth and occasionally causes endocarditis, may be confused with group D streptococci. A series of precise biochemical tests is required to identify the various species correctly. In particular, enterococci grow in 6.5% sodium chloride, while *S. bovis* and *S. mutans* do not.

Streptococci of most groups have been isolated at least occasionally from infected heart valves, soft tissues, or visceral abscesses. Such infections may occur as "opportunists" following surgical manipulation or in patients with malignant disease. Danish and Dutch investigators have reported a number of instances of meningitis and bacteremia in humans due to streptococci of serogroup R, a group of organisms well-known as pathogens of swine. In nearly all human cases there had been a history of contact with pigs.

Viridans streptococci are normal inhabitants of the oropharynx and gastrointestinal tract. They remain the most frequent causative agents of subacute bacterial endocarditis (see Chap. 186). The taxonomy of these organisms is confused, but one classification scheme recognizes five species (in addition to *S. pneumoniae*): *salivarius*, *mitior*, *milleri*, *sanguis*, and *mutans*. Although viridans streptococci are not usually considered to be highly invasive, *S. milleri* is capable of causing serious pyogenic infections such as liver and brain abscesses, peritonitis, and empyema. Cases of endocarditis due to *S. milleri* are more likely to be complicated by abscess formation in peripheral tissues than are similar infections due to other species of viridans streptococci. *Streptococcus milleri* is usually considered "microaerophilic," and its clinical behavior is similar to that of the anaerobic streptococci. All the viridans species, including *S. milleri*, are susceptible to penicillin. Modest increases in the minimal inhibitory concentrations of oral streptococci to penicillin occur following prolonged oral therapy or high-dose intravenous therapy with this antibiotic.

Anaerobic streptococci (see Chap. 102) abound in the mouth, intestinal tract, and vagina. They may be found, often in combination with other anaerobic and aerobic microorganisms, in abscess cavities throughout the body. In the head and neck, anaerobic streptococci may be found in infected paranasal sinuses, brain abscess, dental abscess, infections of the retropharyngeal or lateral pharyngeal spaces, and in cases of Ludwig's angina. In the chest, these organisms occur in lung abscesses and empyema fluids. Abscesses of the liver and other intraabdominal viscera, as well as perirectal abscesses and pelvic abscesses in women, may be due in part to peptostreptococci. These organisms may also thrive in dead or devitalized muscle, skin, or subcutaneous tissue. *Streptococcal myositis* is characterized by marked edema, crepitant myositis, pain, and the presence of chains of gram-positive cocci in a seropurulent exudate. *Hemolytic streptococcal gangrene* may occur after trauma or surgery or without an obvious portal of entry. It is characterized by necrosis of subcutaneous and dermal tissues with spread along fascial planes. *Progressive synergistic gangrene* usually develops about a surgical incision and consists of an ulcerated lesion surrounded by gangrenous skin. The infection is associated particularly with the use of through-and-through sutures after abdominal surgery, and is thought most often to be due to the synergistic action of *S. aureus* and microaerophilic streptococci. *Chronic burrowing ulcer* is a deep soft tissue infection caused by microaerophilic streptococci which erodes through subcutaneous tissue to emerge as an ulcer at a distant site. Management of anaerobic streptococcal infections consists of drainage of abscesses, debridement of devitalized tissues, and high-dose intravenous penicillin therapy.

REFERENCES

AMERICAN HEART ASSOCIATION, COMMITTEE ON RHEUMATIC FEVER AND BACTERIAL ENDOCARDITIS: Prevention of rheumatic fever. Circulation 70:1118A, 1984

AUCKENTHALER R et al: Group G streptococcal bacteremia: Clinical study and review of the literaure. Rev Infect Dis 5:196, 1983

BADDOUR LM, BISNO AL: Recurrent cellulitis after coronary bypass surgery: Association with superficial fungal infection in saphenous venectomy limbs. JAMA 251:1049, 1984

————: Non-group A beta-hemolytic streptococcal cellulitis. Am J Med 79:155, 1985

BREESE BB, HALL CB: Beta Hemolytic Streptococcal Diseases. Boston, Houghton Mifflin, 1978

BRENNAN RO, DURACK DT: The viridans streptococci in perspective, in Current Clinical Topics in Infectious Diseases, JS Remington, MN Swartz (eds). New York, McGraw-Hill, 1984

EDWARDS MS, BAKER CJ: Streptococcus agalactiae (group B streptococcus), in Principles and Practice of Infectious Diseases, 2d ed, GL Mandell et al (eds). New York, Wiley, 1985

GALLAGHER PG, WATANAKUNAKORN C: Group B streptococcal bacteremia in a community teaching hospital. Am J Med 78:795, 1985

LAM K, BAYER AS: Serious infections due to group G streptococci. Am J Med 75:561, 1983

SCHWARTZ RH et al: Penicillin V for group A streptococcal pharyngotonsillitis: A randomized trial of seven vs ten days' therapy. JAMA 246:1790, 1981

SHULMAN ST: Pharyngitis: Management in an Era of Declining Rheumatic Fever. New York, Praeger, 1984

STOLLERMAN GH: Rheumatic Fever and Streptococcal Infection. New York, Grune & Stratton, 1975

96 DIPHTHERIA

JAMES P. HARNISCH

DEFINITION Diphtheria is an acute infectious disease produced by *Corynebacterium diphtheriae*. It is characterized by a local inflammatory lesion, usually in the upper part of the respiratory tract, and a toxic reaction involving primarily the heart and peripheral nerves.

ETIOLOGY *Corynebacterium diphtheriae* is a gram-positive, nonsporulating, nonmotile rod. There is a characteristic swelling at one end of the bacillus, which gives it a club shape. A Chinese-letter configuration is usually seen in stained smears owing to the alignment of the bacilli at sharp angles with each other. Diphtheria bacilli have been classified into *mitis, gravis,* and *intermedius* groups on the basis of colonial morphology, appearance on tellurite medium, fermentation reactions, and ability to produce hemolysis. European workers have suggested that there is a significant difference in the clinical manifestations and in the severity of disease related to the strain; gravis and intermedius infections are thought to be accompanied by more severe toxic manifestations and a higher death rate. In the United States, the gravis strain is comparatively uncommon, and less significance is attached to the relationship of the type of organism and the clinical form of the disease.

Corynebacterium diphtheriae produces a protein exotoxin which is responsible for many of the clinical manifestations; as little as 0.0001 mg is lethal for guinea pigs. Strains of diphtheria bacilli which elaborate exotoxin are lysogenic with the temperate β-converting phage. Absence of lysogeny generally is associated with lack of toxin formation and virulence. However, symptomatic diphtheria may also follow invasion by strains of *C. diphtheriae* that cannot be shown to produce toxin.

EPIDEMIOLOGY Diphtheria occurs primarily in the temperate zone and is still very common in some parts of the world. Since 1966, there has been an irregular increase in the number of cases of diphtheria in the United States. Two outbreaks in Texas early in the 1970s accounted for most of the cases. However, since 1973, more than 75 percent of the cases were reported from the Pacific northwest and the southwest. The western provinces of Canada experienced a similar increase in diphtheria. Until this geographic trend was recognized, the highest frequency had been in children between 1 and 9 years of age. The attack rate for unimmunized children was 70 times higher than the rate for children who had received primary immunization. Within the United States since 1980, few cases have been reported annually, and 70 percent have occurred in adults. In the Pacific northwest, isolates have been obtained predominantly from indigent adults with symptomatic skin lesions. A high incidence is observed among native Americans both in urban centers and on tribal lands. Another striking change has been a decrease in the incidence of laryngeal involvement. In general, diphtheria is acquired by droplet transmission from active cases or carriers, but fomites may play a role in the spread of cutaneous infection. Each diphtheria infection must be classifed as either a case or a carrier. A *case* is an individual who is colonized in the respiratory tract with *C. diphtheriae* and is symptomatic. The concomitant presence of other organisms, such as beta-hemolytic streptococci, does not change the definition or prognosis of a diphtheria case. A *carrier* is colonized with *C. diphtheriae* but lacks symptoms. No attempt should be made to classify an instance of cutaneous diphtheria as a case or a carrier.

PATHOGENESIS AND PATHOLOGY The commonest portal of entry for the diphtheria bacillus is the upper respiratory tract. The skin, genitalia, eye, and middle ear may also be sites of invasion. Growth of the organism is superficial in most cases, and there is little tendency to invade the lymphatics or bloodstream except in the terminal stages. The exotoxin elaborated in the local lesion is absorbed and carried by the blood to all parts of the body. The intensity of the toxic effects is greatest when the primary lesion is in the pharynx, less when it is in the larynx, and least when it is on the nasal mucosa or skin. Simultaneous involvement of the pharynx, larynx, trachea, and bronchial tree is associated with most severe intoxication.

The *membrane,* the primary lesion of diphtheria, is thick, leathery, and blue-white and is composed of bacteria, necrotic epithelium, phagocytes, and fibrin. It is surrounded by a narrow zone of inflammation and is firmly adherent to the underlying tissues; bleeding follows its forcible removal. Ulceration is not a regular feature. Regional lymphadenitis is frequent.

The *toxic manifestations* involve primarily the heart, kidneys, and peripheral nerves. The brain is rarely affected. Cardiac enlargement is frequent; this appears to be related to myocarditis rather than hypertrophy. The kidneys may be enlarged and reveal cloudy swelling and interstitial changes. Bronchopneumonia due to *C. diphtheriae* or to secondary invading organisms occurs in some patients, especially those with laryngeal involvement. Membrane is present throughout the bronchial tree when the diphtheria bacillus is responsible for the pulmonary infection. The peripheral nerves may reveal fatty degeneration, disintegration of the medullary sheaths, and involvement of the axis cylinder. Both motor and sensory fibers are affected, but the main impact is on the motor innervation. The anterior horn cells and the posterior columns of the spinal cord may be damaged. Other central nervous system involvement includes cerebral hemorrhage, meningitis, and encephalitis. Petechial and purpuric lesions are occasionally present in the kidneys, skin, or adrenals. Endocarditis due to *C. diphtheriae* is rare.

Death results from respiratory obstruction by membrane or edema, or from the effects of toxin on the heart, nervous system, or other organs.

IMMUNITY Susceptibility to the complications of diphtheria is related to the presence or absence of circulating antibody to exotoxin. The Schick test yields a rough estimate of the quantity of antitoxin in the circulation. This test is carried out in the following manner: 0.1 mL purified diphtheria toxin (one-fiftieth the minimum lethal dose) dissolved in buffered human serum albumin is injected intradermally on the volar surface of the forearm; 0.1 mL purified diphtheria toxoid is injected into the other arm as a control. These areas are examined at 24 and 48 h and between the fourth and seventh days and interpreted in the following way:

1 *Positive reaction.* The site of injection of toxin begins to redden in 24 h; the reddening increases and reaches a maximum in about a week, at which time the lesion may be as large as 3 cm in diameter and moderately swollen and tender. There is usually a small (1 to 1.5 cm) dark-red central zone which gradually turns brown, desquamates, and leaves a pigmented area. The area of toxoid injection shows no reaction. A positive test indicates little or no circulating antitoxin and no immunity.

2 *Negative reaction.* There is no reaction at the site of injection of either toxoid or toxin. This is consistent with a blood antitoxin level of 1/30 to 1/100 unit and immunity to ordinary exposure.

3 *Pseudoreaction.* Inflammation at both sites of injection within 12 to 14 h, which reaches a maximum in 48 to 72 h and then fades. This usually indicates immunity plus hypersensitivity to the toxin or other materials in the solution.

4 *Combined reaction.* This begins like the pseudoreaction, but the inflammatory response at the toxin site persists after that in the area of toxoid injection has faded. It indicates delayed sensitivity to toxin or other proteins and either low levels or no antitoxin. The incidence of combined reactions increases with age and is highest in unimmunized groups living in areas where diphtheria is prevalent.

Individuals with negative Schick tests occasionally contract diphtheria, and some persons with positive Schick reactions do not develop the disease after exposure. In some parts of the United States fewer than 50 percent of adults have "protective" levels of circulating antitoxin. The Schick test is not used routinely in the United States, and the lack of ability to perform it should not delay the treatment of asymptomatic contacts of diphtheria.

Second attacks of respiratory diphtheria are rare despite the fact that about 10 percent of patients who have had the disease remain Schick-positive. This suggests that factors other than antitoxin may play a role in protection against infection. Recidivism with cutaneous diphtheria has been observed during large outbreaks. Underlying chronic dermatoses constitute a common feature of this phenomenon. In general, immunized patients have a milder illness than unimmunized ones when the initial clinical picture and level of circulating antitoxin are the same. Early therapy of diphtheria with antibiotics may lead to recurrence of the disease if exposure to fresh infections occurs shortly after discontinuation of treatment, suggesting that the development of antitoxic immunity is suppressed in these cases. Full immunization with diphtheria toxoid does not prevent nasopharyngeal carriage of the organism but significantly reduces the case fatality ratio. It also ameliorates the symptoms of active disease.

CLINICAL MANIFESTATIONS

The incubation period of diphtheria is 1 to 7 days. The local symptoms vary with the site of the primary lesion. A membrane is not always present. The constitutional reaction usually is of only minor to moderate severity in uncomplicated disease. Fever is usually low [37.8 to 38.3°C (100 to 101°F)], unless infection with another organism (often group A *Streptococcus pyogenes*) supervenes. When toxic manifestations are absent, patients feel well except for varying degrees of discomfort at the site of the local lesion. Pallor, listlessness, tachycardia, and weakness are common in more severe cases. Nausea or vomiting is more frequent in young children. Peripheral vascular collapse often develops in the terminal stages of the disease.

Nasal diphtheria Diphtheria is occasionally restricted to the nasal mucosa. It is usually localized to the septum or turbinates in the anterior portion of one side of the nose, does not extend, and may persist for a long time. A foreign body is frequently present. A unilateral serosanguineous discharge is characteristic. When the disease is located in the posterior nasal areas, it commonly extends to the pharynx, from which toxin is absorbed.

Pharyngeal diphtheria The early diphtheritic membrane in the pharynx consists of small areas of soft exudate which wipe off easily and leave no bleeding points. As the disease progresses, the discrete exudate coalesces to form an easily removable thin sheet which spreads to cover tonsils or pharynx, or both. Later, it becomes thicker, bluish white, gray, or black, depending on the degree of hemorrhage, and is so firmly attached to the underlying tissues that attempts to remove it result in bleeding. If infection with group A *Streptococcus pyogenes* is superimposed, the pharynx is diffusely red and edematous. Sore throat is the most common complaint. Pain on swallowing may occur in over 25 percent of the cases and in some patients may be severe. There is a moderate leukocytosis with 15,000 or fewer white blood cells per cubic millimeter.

Local spread of the pharyngeal membrane may occur, and the throat, tonsils, and soft and hard palates become completely covered. Patients with severe disease may develop so-called malignant diphtheria, characterized by marked edema of the submandibular areas and the anterior neck, giving the characteristic "bullneck" appearance. Respiration is noisy, the tongue protrudes, the breath is foul, and the speech thick. The pharyngeal tissues are red and edematous, and the cervical lymph nodes are enlarged. The skin is pale and cool. The patient complains of overwhelming weakness. Purpuric eruptions of the skin, particularly on the neck and anterior chest wall, may appear occasionally. Drowsiness and delirium are common.

Laryngeal diphtheria Involvement of the larynx is usually the result of extension of the diphtheritic membrane from the pharynx. The infection may rarely be limited to the larynx or trachea. This possibility must be considered in the differential diagnosis of all cases of "croup"; it can be ruled out only by direct examination of the airway. The clinical features of this type of disease are described below.

Cutaneous diphtheria Until recently, diphtheria of the skin was a problem primarily in tropical areas where it is responsible for some cases of "jungle sore." However, since 1972, there has been a significant increase in skin diphtheria in the Pacific northwest and the southwest. A high attack rate has occurred in native Americans and in indigent males living in "skid row" areas where crowding and poor personal and community hygiene abound. *Corynebacterium diphtheriae,* being unable to penetrate unbroken skin, invades wounds, burns, or abrasions. Coagulase-positive *Staphylococcus aureus* and/ or beta-hemolytic streptococci frequently are recovered concomitantly. Although the lesions develop most often on the extremities, they may appear at any site including the perianal area. In tropical zones, the typical lesion appears as a round, deep, "punched-out" ulcer, 0.5 cm to several centimeters in diameter. In the early stages, it is covered by a gray-yellow or gray-brown membrane which strips off easily to reveal a clean hemorrhagic base that dries quickly and becomes covered by a thin, leathery, dark-brown or black, adherent membrane. In the untreated case, this separates spontaneously 1 to 3 weeks after infection. The margin of the fully developed ulcer is usually slightly undermined, purple, rolled, and sharply defined. When lesions are infected with a toxigenic strain, anesthesia over the lesion develops within a few weeks. In temperate climates, the lesions are not sufficiently specific to permit visual diagnosis. Cutaneous diphtheria should be suspected in any adult with skin lesions, particularly in the proper epidemiologic setting. Antibiotic therapy will change the character of the skin lesions. Twenty percent of patients with cutaneous diphtheria also have infections in the nasopharynx with the same biotype. Myocarditis or neuropathy occurs in about 3 percent of patients with cutaneous diphtheria. The Landry-Guillain-Barré syndrome develops occasionally.

Diphtheritic lesions in other areas Diphtheria may involve the uterine cervix, vagina, vulva, bladder, urethra, or penis (after circumcision). Toxic manifestations are common. The tongue, buccal mucous membrane, gums, and esophagus may also be affected. Infection of the conjunctiva occurs rarely. Otitis media may occur as an isolated syndrome or secondary to diphtheria in the upper part of the respiratory tract; the aural infection may become chronic; virulent organisms may be isolated from the discharge for many months.

COMPLICATIONS OF DIPHTHERIA   The complications of diphtheria are of two types: (1) those that result from spread of the membrane in the respiratory tract, and (2) those due to the effects of the toxin.

Extension and spread of membrane   The membrane of diphtheria may spread from the fauces over the posterior pharyngeal wall into the larynx, trachea, and, uncommonly, the bronchial tree, leading to severe illness and a high incidence of toxic manifestations. Occlusion of the airway is manifested by tachypnea and, as obstruction increases, restlessness, use of accessory muscles of respiration, cyanosis, and finally death. In some cases, the membrane extends diffusely into the bronchial tree and produces clinical manifestations of pneumonia. Hoarseness and a crouplike cough are seen with laryngeal involvement. Bronchopulmonary diphtheria is very serious, not only because of obstruction but also because of the large surface from which toxin can be absorbed; the death rate is very high. When the pulmonary lesion regresses, pieces of membrane may break off and produce sudden occlusion of the airway; a cast of the bronchial tree may be coughed up. Occasionally, pharyngeal membrane has extended into the esophagus and cardia of the stomach.

Toxic complications of diphtheria   Diphtheria toxin is produced only by isolates of *C. diphtheriae* lysogenic for corynephages that carry the tox structural gene. Nontoxigenic strains can be converted to toxin-producing organisms through transference of this phage. The bacterial host regulates expression of the tox structural gene. The toxin is a single polypeptide chain composed of two fragments. Fragment B recognizes specific surface receptors on sensitive cell membranes, and fragment A crosses the plasma membrane. In the cytoplasm, protein synthesis is inhibited by fragment A through the inactivation of the eukaryotic translocating enzyme, elongation factor 2. A cofactor, nicotinamide adenine dinucleotide, is required for activity of the toxin. The effects of the toxin on the myocardium are thought to result from its ability to decrease the rate of oxidation of long-chain fatty acids by interfering with the metabolism of carnitine. Because of this action, triglycerides accumulate in the myocardium and cause fatty degeneration of muscle.

Myocarditis develops in about two-thirds of patients with diphtheria. However, it is clinically evident in only about 10 percent of cases; alterations in the intensity of the heart sounds, systolic murmurs, bundle branch block, incomplete or complete heart block, atrial fibrillation, and ventricular premature beats or tachycardia, or both, are common. Ventricular fibrillation is a constant threat and is frequently responsible for sudden death. Ninety percent of patients with atrial fibrillation, ventricular tachycardia, or complete heart block die. Overt congestive cardiac failure is uncommon. Evidence of decompensation of the right side of the heart usually develops first; the most common symptom is pain in the right upper quadrant of the abdomen due to rapid engorgement of the liver. Failure of the left side of the heart may appear later. Diphtheritic heart disease is not necessarily "benign" in survivors of the disease; permanent cardiac damage may occur. Fibrosis of the myocardium has been observed in patients who have expired several weeks after "mild" myocarditis was detected electrocardiographically. The degree and extent of fibrotic change have often been greater than could have been predicted on the basis of the type of abnormality present in the ECG.

Peripheral neuritis may occur in the course of diphtheria. Paralysis of the soft palate and posterior pharyngeal wall occasionally appears very early in the disease (2 to 3 days). A more common neuritis (10 percent of cases) usually develops 2 to 6 weeks after onset of the disease. It is characterized by cranial nerve dysfunction; the IIId, VIth, VIIth, IXth, and Xth cranial nerves are most commonly involved. Loss of accommodation, nasal voice, and difficulty in swallowing are the most frequent manifestations. However, any of the peripheral nerves may be affected, with resulting paralysis of the extremities, diaphragm, or intercostal muscles; death may occur from failure of respiration. The peripheral neuritides which appear in the second to the sixth weeks of the disease are characterized primarily by motor loss; sensory changes are uncommon and, when present, are minor. Demyelination is the usual pathologic change. Nerve conduction studies show a marked dissociation between the time course of clinical features and electrophysiologic abnormalities: peripheral nerve conduction velocities are minimally affected early in the disease despite profound weakness. During clinical recovery the electrophysiologic abnormalities are most apparent. Peripheral neuritis may not appear until 2 to 3 months after the onset of diphtheria. In these cases, the clinical picture and course resemble infectious polyneuritis. The outstanding findings are loss of sensation in the "glove-and-stocking" distribution and albuminocytologic dissociation in the cerebrospinal fluid identical with that observed in the Landry-Guillain-Barré syndrome. Motor weakness and areflexia may develop with progression of involvement. Facial diplegia may accompany the other neurologic manifestations. A fatal, rapidly ascending paralysis of the Landry type may develop rarely. Complete recovery is the rule in this late peripheral neuritis, although it may require as long as a year. Encephalitis is a rare toxic complication of diphtheria.

Shock, which develops suddenly and without warning, is an occasional cause of sudden death in this disease. In some instances, this may be a consequence of myocarditis; in others, no cause can be discovered.

Other complications   Cerebral infarction with hemiplegia occurs rarely; it is probably due to embolization from atrial thrombi in patients with myocarditis and cardiac dilatation. Superinfection of the lungs is a risk in all patients with diphtheria who are given antimicrobial agents. Purpuric skin eruptions may be seen in severe, malignant cases; thrombocytopenia occurs rarely. A mild morbilliform rash may be present during the early stage of diphtheria. Secondary invasion of the pharynx by group A *S. pyogenes* may take place in patients who have not received an antibiotic. Serum sickness occasionally follows the use of antitoxin. Relapses of diphtheria may occur when patients given antimicrobial agents are exposed to fresh cases soon after therapy has been discontinued. Bacteremia, endocarditis, and meningitis are rare complications.

COURSE AND PROGNOSIS   The diphtheritic membrane may be present for only 3 to 4 days in mild cases, even when no antitoxin is given; it usually lasts for about a week in cases of moderate severity. Commonly, the pharyngeal lesion increases in extent and thickness during the first 24 h after the administration of antitoxin. As the disease begins to recede, the exudate softens, wipes off easily, leaving no bleeding areas, becomes patchy so that it resembles the picture of "follicular" tonsillitis, and finally disappears, leaving normal underlying mucous membrane.

The fatality rate of diphtheria prior to the use of specific antitoxin was about 35 percent in average cases and 90 percent in those with laryngeal involvement. Since specific serotherapy has been employed, this rate has been reduced to a range of 3.5 to 22 percent, but it is still highest when the larynx is affected. The overall death rate in the United States is about 10 percent. Death is most frequent in the very young and the old. Immunization is a factor of great importance in prognosis. The fatality rate in immunized individuals is one-tenth that in the unimmunized population. Paralysis is 5 times and "malignant" disease 15 times less common in immune than in nonimmune individuals. As a rule, the longer the delay in the administration of antitoxin, the greater the incidence of complications and death. However, antitoxin is ineffective in reducing risks of complications and death if it is given much later than 48 h after diphtheria begins.

A white blood cell count higher than 25,000 per cubic millimeter is associated with a higher risk of complications and death.

DIAGNOSIS   The clinical features of the fully developed diphtheritic membrane, especially in the pharynx, are sufficiently characteristic to suggest the possibility of the disease in most instances. However, the appearance of the pharyngeal exudate alone does not clinch the diagnosis. There are a number of other infections in which pseudo-membranes resembling those of diphtheria are present; among those are infectious mononucleosis, streptococcal pharyngitis, viral exudative pharyngitis, fusospirochetal infection, and acute pharyngeal candidiasis.

The specific diagnosis of diphtheria depends completely on demonstration of the organism in stained smears and their recovery by culture. Methylene blue–stained preparations are positive, in experienced hands, in 75 to 85 percent of cases. Diphtheria bacilli can be recovered by culture on Loeffler's medium in 8 to 12 h if patients have not been receiving antimicrobial agents. *Corynebacterium diphtheriae* also multiplies, but more slowly, on ordinary blood agar. If an antibiotic, especially penicillin or erythromycin, has been administered prior to obtaining cultures, the organisms may not grow for as long as 5 days or may fail to grow at all.

Staining of suspected material with fluorescein-labeled diphtheria antitoxin may allow rapid diagnosis. Toxigenicity of *C. diphtheriae* isolates should be determined by passive agar diffusion (Elek plate method), guinea pig inoculation, or counterimmunoelectrophoresis. Biotype determination will help characterize the epidemiology of an outbreak. Restriction endonuclease digests of *C. diphtheriae* DNA may prove useful in the study of isolates recovered during an occurrence of diphtheria. Comparison of electrophoretic gel patterns of restriction enzyme digests can help identify newly introduced strains from the preexistent resident organisms. Phage typing is too difficult to be of immediate epidemiologic assistance during an outbreak.

TREATMENT Patients with diphtheria should be isolated and kept at strict bed rest; physical effort should be reduced during the early convalescent stages. Local therapy of the diphtheritic pharyngeal lesion is useless. The only specific treatment for diphtheria is antitoxin. Antiserum must never be given until the patient's sensitivity to horse serum, using the eye and skin tests, has been determined. There are several regimens for the administration of antitoxin, and the amount given is often based on an empiric decision. In general, the more severe the disease or the more extensive the membrane formation, the greater the amount of antitoxin required. Mildly symptomatic cases may be treated with 10,000 to 20,000 units. Moderately severe cases, such as those with a pharyngeal membrane, should be given 20,000 to 40,000 units. Severe diphtheria, as with laryngeal involvement, requires 50,000 to 100,000 units. The total dose should be given at one time rather than in split doses over a long period. For doses less than 20,000 units, the intramuscular route is convenient. When this method is used, only one-half the dose should be given intramuscularly and the remainder intravenously in order to expedite delivery of the antitoxin. Alternatively, after appropriate testing for sensitivity, the entire amount of antitoxin may be given intravenously in 100 to 200 mL isotonic saline over a 30-min period. Desensitization should be attempted if the initial skin or eye test is positive. A rare patient may be sensitive to such a high degree that the antiserum cannot be administered without the risk of death.

Antitoxin should be given as early in the course of diphtheria as possible. It is capable of binding or inactivating only the toxin present in blood or extracellular fluid. Once the toxin has entered the cell, the effect cannot be reversed or prevented. Antitoxin must be given when diphtheria is suspected clinically; laboratory confirmation prior to administration of the antitoxin is not necessary. Since mortality increases directly with delay in use of antitoxin, it is better to treat clinically suspect but culture-negative cases than to withhold specific therapy.

A history of military service is not reliable proof of adequate immunization. From World War II until 1956, immunization for diphtheria in the United States military was inconsistent. Since 1957, all branches of the armed forces have routinely immunized their pesonnel. When the immunization history is not clear, it is best to provide antitoxin promptly. Antimicrobial agents do not alter the course, incidence of complications, or outcome of diphtheria.

Patients with laryngeal obstruction should be watched very carefully. In mild cases, inhalation of warm or cool steam may be beneficial. If advancing signs of airway obstruction develop, intubation or tracheostomy is indicated. These procedures must never be delayed until cyanosis appears, because, at this point, stimulation of the pharynx or trachea may produce cardiac standstill and death. Sedative or hypnotic agents should never be given because they may obscure increasing respiratory difficulty.

The pulse and blood pressure should be measured frequently. Little can be done to alter the course of the myocarditis. Quinidine has been tried to prevent and treat arrhythmias but appears to be of no value; there is some suspicion that it may produce deleterious effect. The use of procainamide when ventricular premature beats or tachycardia supervene has been suggested, but no documented observations of its effect have been recorded. The administration of digitalis for cardiac failure in diphtheria is controversial. Some consider this drug to be completely contraindicated; others feel, however, that, used carefully, digitalis may be given safely and with beneficial effects. Shock should be treated according to its etiology (see Chaps. 29 and 139). There is no evidence that corticosteroids and corticotropin are of any value in the treatment of diphtheria or any of its complications. Antibiotics should be used to treat symptomatic cases only after antitoxin is administered. Circulating exotoxin is not affected by antibiotics, and their prompt use may give a sense of false assurance. Patients with diphtheria should be quarantined until two successive cultures of the nose, throat, or other infected areas, taken at 24-h intervals, are negative. If antibiotics have been given, cultures should not be taken until at least 24 h after cessation of therapy.

Treatment of carriers *Corynebacterium diphtheriae* usually disappears from the upper part of the respiratory tract after 2 to 4 weeks in patients who do not receive antimicrobial drugs; in a small number of individuals the organism may persist for a long time or even permanently. The most effective treatment of the acute and chronic carrier state is erythromycin. A dose of 2 g per day orally in divided doses for 7 days appears to be adequate. The enteric-coated base, estolate, and ethyl succinate forms of erythromycin are preferred to ensure adequate serum concentrations without regard to food intake. Alternative antimicrobials include procaine penicillin G, 600,000 units intramuscularly every 12 h for 10 days; clindamycin, 150 mg four times a day orally for 7 days; and rifampin, 600 mg as a single oral dose for 7 days. Tetracyclines, semisynthetic penicillins, aminoglycosides, and oral cephalosporins are inadequate for the eradication of *C. diphtheriae*. Parenteral cephalosporins such as cephalothin or cefamandole are effective. In two areas of North America endemic for cutaneous diphtheria, resistance of *C. diphtheriae* to erythromycin has been recognized. The origin of the plasmid in erythromycin-resistant strains is not clear; fortunately such isolates are uncommon. Initial observations indicate that plasmids are not usually detectable in respiratory isolates of *C. diphtheriae* and are rare in skin isolates. Re-treatment is indicated for carriers whose organisms do not disappear on the first trial. This is preferable to tonsillectomy, which may be considered a last resort should the carrier state persist despite repeated courses of antibiotic. Persistence of the organism after appropriate antimicrobial therapy may represent a lack of compliance rather than drug resistance.

PREVENTION Diphtheria is, for the most part, a preventable disease. Immunization at the age of 3 months should be routine. Diphtheria toxoid is best given together with tetanus toxoid and pertussis vaccine (DPT), because antibody titers are higher with combined immunization than with either agent alone. Booster doses should be administered at the age of 1 year and again just before a child goes to school. Although it has been suggested that Schick testing is not necessary in those who have been immunized, some physicians still carry this out to determine the status of antitoxic immunity. A Schick test acts as a booster. A negative reaction does not indicate absolute protection. The development of highly purified toxoid has made it possible to protect adults with little or no risk of untoward sequelae. In this situation, a combination of adult tetanus-diphtheria (Td) toxoid containing 1 to 2 flocculation (Lf) units per milliliter should be used. With this preparation, severe reactions can be avoided. The Moloney test need not be carried out. Adults should receive booster doses at least every 10 years. Unfortunately, reimmunized adults are the exception, and many elderly patients have low and nonprotective levels of circulating antitoxin. They constitute a high-risk group during any diphtheria outbreak.

Treatment of unimmunized persons exposed to an active case of diphtheria remains controversial. One approach has been to administer 3000 units of equine antitoxin intramuscularly, after appropriate skin and eye tests. In some countries (not in the United States) human diphtheria antitoxin is available. The concentration achieved with this product is sufficient only for passive protection of the asymptomatic, unimmunized contact but is not high enough for treatment of symptomatic disease. If human diphtheria immunoglobulin is used, active immunization must be delayed for 6 weeks. Alternatively, cultures of *C. diphtheriae* can be taken, and a primary series of immunizations initiated. The exposed individual then can be observed closely for signs of active disease. If symptoms occur, antitoxin can be given immediately. In those who have been previously immunized, a booster dose of toxoid is usually sufficient. Cultures from the nasopharynx or open wounds should be obtained from close contacts or family members of a diphtheria case or carrier.

REFERENCES

BELSEY MA, LeBLANC DR: Skin infections and the epidemiology of diphtheria; acquisition and persistence of *C. diphtheriae* infections. Am J Epidemiol 102:179, 1975

BROOKS GR et al: Diphtheria in the United States 1959–1970. J Infect Dis 129:172, 1974

GOOD I: Myocardial changes in fatal diphtheria: A summary of observations in 221 cases. Am J Med Sci 219:257, 1948

GOOR RS, PAPPENHEIMER AM JR: Studies on the mode of action of diphtheria toxin. J Exp Med 126:899, 913, 923, 1967

HARNISCH JP et al: A decade of diphtheria among urban adults: The epidemiology of diphtheria in modern Americans. Ann Intern Med (in press)

IPSEN J: Circulating antitoxin at the onset of diphtheria in 425 patients. J Immunol 54:325, 1946

———: Immunization of adults against diphtheria and tetanus. N Engl J Med 251:459, 1954

KURDI A, ABDUL-KADER M: Clinical and electrophysiological studies of diphtheritic neuritis in Jordan. J Neurol Sci 42:243, 1979

McCLOSKEY RV et al: The 1970 epidemic of diphtheria in San Antonio. Ann Intern Med 75:495, 1971

NAIDITCH MJ, BOWER AG: Diphtheria: A study of 1,433 cases observed during a ten-year period at the Los Angeles County Hospital. Am J Med 17:229, 1954

PAPPENHEIMER AM JR: Diphtheria toxin. Annu Rev Biochem 46:69, 1977

———, MURPHY JR: Studies on the molecular epidemiology of diphtheria. Lancet 2:923, 1983

SCHEID W: Diphtherial paralysis: An analysis of 2,292 cases of diphtheria in adults which include 174 cases of polyneuritis. J Nerv Ment Dis 116:1095, 1952

SCHILLER J et al: Plasmids in *Corynebacterium diphtheriae* and diphtheroids mediating erythromycin resistance. Antimicrob Agents Chemother 18:814, 1980

THOMPSON NL, ELLNER PD: Rapid determination of *Corynebacterium diphtheriae* toxigenicity by counterimmunoelectrophoresis. J Clin Microbiol 7:493, 1978

WITTELS B, BRESSLER R: Biochemical lesion of diphtheria toxin on the heart. J Clin Invest 43:630, 1964

97   INFECTIONS CAUSED BY *LISTERIA MONOCYTOGENES* AND *ERYSIPELOTHRIX RHUSIOPATHIAE*

PAUL D. HOEPRICH

LISTERIA MONOCYTOGENES INFECTIONS

DEFINITION   Listeriosis, a disease caused by *L. monocytogenes*, consists of many clinical syndromes. Perinatal infection, acquired either transplacentally or during parturition, is the most nearly unique form of listeriosis.

ETIOLOGY   *Listeria monocytogenes* are gram-positive, non-acid-fast, microaerophilic, motile bacilli that form smooth colonies but do not produce either capsules or spores. Several serotypes have been defined on the basis of O and H antigens. The epidemiologically essential aid of typing is available from the Centers for Disease Control in Atlanta, Georgia. Types 4b, 1b, and 1a account for more than 90 percent of the cases worldwide. Weakly hemolytic gram-positive bacilli are presumed to be *L. monocytogenes* if they are motile (when grown at 20 to 25°C), reduce 2,3,5-triphenyltetrazolium chloride, hydrolyze esculin, and display characteristic animal pathogenicity: (1) The Anton test—3 to 5 days after inoculation into the conjunctival sac of a rabbit or a guinea pig, *L. monocytogenes* cause a keratoconjunctivitis; (2) general listeriosis (intravenous or intraperitoneal inoculation) typically provokes a monocytosis in rabbits, and focal hepatic necrosis in mice.

EPIDEMIOLOGY AND PATHOGENESIS   Found on every continent save the Antarctic, *L. monocytogenes* are distinct from the nonhemolytic, nonpathogenic, bacilli (found mainly in soil, decaying matter, and feces) that are designated *L. innocua* or assigned to the new genus *Murraya*. *Listeria ivanovii* and *L. seeligeri* have rarely been associated with disease in humans, whereas *L. welshimeri* has not; all three are differentiable from *L. monocytogenes* by biochemical and augmentation hemolysis (CAMP) tests. Although typical *L. monocytogenes* have been isolated from silage, other vegetative sources, and 1 to 5 percent of specimens of human feces, listeriosis is uncommon and occurs sporadically with a frequency of two to three cases per million population per year. Listeriosis is actually more common in urban than rural dwellers, occurring most frequently in July and August (northern hemisphere). The reservoir from which human beings become infected is frequently occult and the mode of transmission often obscure. However, outbreaks associated with the ingestion of coleslaw made from contaminated cabbage, pasteurized milk, and fresh Mexican-style cheese document the importance of food-borne transmission. Transmission from the infected pregnant female to her offspring is well established as a route of infection.

Transplacental perinatal infection results in disseminated fetal listeriosis. The fetus is usually stillborn or is prematurely ejected, virtually always with lethal listeriosis. Fetal listeriosis acquired during delivery is typically not clinically evident for 1 or 2 weeks postpartum and usually presents as a meningitis.

Listeriosis is preponderantly a disease of persons under 1 year and over 55 years of age.

Persons in apparent good health may develop listeriosis. However, other diseases, particularly those with diminished cell-mediated immunity (listerias are cytophilic), facilitate the occurrence of listeriosis: for example, neoplasms (especially of the lymphoreticular system) and any conditions requiring treatment with pharmacologic doses of glucosteroids, irradiation, or cytotoxic agents; alcoholism; cardiovascular disease; diabetes mellitus; and tuberculosis.

MANIFESTATIONS   *Listeriosis of the newborn,* the most nearly unique clinical form of listeriosis, ranges from meningitis that is clinically apparent within 1 month postpartum to diffuse disseminated disease in aborted, premature, stillborn infants, and neonates, who die within minutes to days after birth. If clinical disease is delayed to 1 to 4 weeks postpartum, it is generally localized to the central nervous system, as is the rule when children 1 month to 6 years of age are afflicted.

Infants born alive with listeriosis may or may not have fever; yet these babies are critically ill, with cardiorespiratory distress, vomiting, and diarrhea. Dark-red skin papules are frequent, particularly on the lower extremities. Hepatosplenomegaly may be present. This form of listeriosis is also known as septic or miliary granulomatosis. The findings at necropsy are characteristic and mimic those seen in listeriosis of rodents: widely disseminated abscesses varying in size from grossly visible to microscopic, involving, in order of decreasing frequency, liver, spleen, adrenal glands, lungs, pharynx, gastrointestinal tract, central nervous system, and skin. Typically, the lesions are abscesses, but classic granulomas may be seen, depending principally on the duration of infection before death. Microscopic examination of a Gram-stained smear of meconium from the normal newborn infant does not disclose bacteria; fetal listeriosis results in meconium laden with gram-positive bacilli. For this reason, examination of meconium by Gram's stain and by culture should be carried out whenever there is gross soiling of the amniotic liquid with meconium, prematurity, or unexplained fever in the mother before or at the onset of labor. This is particularly important because listeriosis in the pregnant woman may be asymptomatic or may cause a nonspecific illness. A week to a month prepartum, there may have been malaise, a chill, diarrhea, pain in the back or flanks, and itching. Even when symptomatic, the disease is benign and self-limited in the mother; however, as symptoms subside, a decrease or cessation of fetal movement may be noted. Infection of the fetus may occur as early as the fifth month of gestation but occurs most often in the third trimester. Following delivery of infants with proved fetal listeriosis, cervical cultures are, or soon become, negative for *L. monocytogenes;* subsequent conception, gestation, and delivery of normal offspring are usual.

Meningitis accounts for about three-fourths of the cases verified by culture and is the predominant clinical form of listeriosis. Meningitis caused by *L. monocytogenes* cannot be distinguished on clinical grounds from meningitis caused by other kinds of bacteria.

Nonmeningeal listeriosis of the central nervous system is associated with fever, nausea and vomiting, headache, and listeremia; the cerebrospinal fluid is normal. Localizing neurologic signs may develop (especially if abscess forms), or the picture may be that of an encephalitis.

Listeremia that has no identifiable source and is associated with high fever, and severe prostrating illness (typhoidal listeriosis) occurs most often in patients with cancers and immunosuppression. However, primary listeremia may also develop in patients with cirrhosis, alcoholism, pregnancy, and no discernible underlying disease.

Listerial endocarditis is generally a chronic process without singular manifestations. About half of the patients have no known predisposing cardiac disease.

Other rare forms of listeriosis include ocular infections, dermatitis, infections of serous cavities, and abscesses in various organs.

LABORATORY FINDINGS Although *L. monocytogenes* grow well on the usual culture media, etiologic diagnosis by isolation and identification may be hampered by failure of differentiation from *Corynebacterium* spp., *Erysipelothrix rhusiopathiae*, and *Streptococcus* spp. Recognition of listerial colonies in a mixed culture, as may result with vaginal or cervical specimens, is difficult and may be aided by using selective media and/or enrichment procedures.

Serodiagnosis by assay for agglutinins has not been useful because of the common finding of so-called natural antibodies. Such nonspecific reactions may reflect the known antigenic relationship between *Staphylococcus aureus* and several listerial serotypes. The humoral antibody response to listeriosis in humans is almost exclusively IgM throughout the disease, whereas staphylococci elicit IgG as well as IgM; i.e., treatment of serums with 2-mercaptoethanol may not eliminate nonspecific reactivity.

Monocytosis is not common in human listeriosis. Leukocytosis with neutrophilia, as in any acute bacterial infection, is seen in listerial meningitis, nonmeningeal infection of the central nervous system, primary listeremia, listerial endocarditis, and abscesses in hosts capable of mounting a granulocytic response. In most patients with listerial meningitis, the findings in the cerebrospinal fluid do not differ from those found in other bacterial meningitides, but occasional patients may have a relative increase in mononuclear cells.

DIFFERENTIAL DIAGNOSIS Abortion, premature delivery, stillbirth, and neonatal death are more often due to causes other than listeriosis: Rh incompatibility, syphilis, or toxoplasmosis.

In patients with leptomeningitis, conjunctivitis, endocarditis, bacteremia, or polyserositis, reports of isolation of "diphtheroids" or "nonpathogens" must always be challenged. A statement that *L. monocytogenes* has been excluded should be required.

TREATMENT *Listeria monocytogenes* are susceptible to several antimicrobials in vitro, including penicillin G, ampicillin, erythromycin, rifampin, streptomycin, gentamicin, co-trimoxazole, tobramycin, and the tetracyclines. Tolerance, i.e., inhibition at low concentrations with much higher concentrations needed for killing, is characteristic with the penicillins, erythromycin, rifampin, co-trimoxazole, and streptomycin. Accordingly, combination therapy is necessary for maximally listericidal therapy, e.g., penicillin G [150 to 200 mg (240,000 to 320,000 units) per kilogram of body weight per day, intravenously, as six equal portions every 4 h] plus tobramycin (5 to 6 mg per kilogram of body weight per day, intravenously, as three equal portions every 8 h). Ampicillin and gentamicin (same dosages) may be substituted but offer no advantage. Such treatment is appropriate for listeriosis of the newborn (2 weeks), listeremia in pregnancy (2 weeks), primary listeremia (4 weeks), listerial endocarditis (4 to 6 weeks), and any form of listeriosis outside the central nervous system in immunosuppressed patients (4 to 6 weeks).

As gentamicin and tobramycin do not enter the central nervous system reliably, high-dosage therapy with penicillin G [200 to 300 mg (320,000 to 480,000 units) per kilogram of body weight per day, intravenously, as six equal portions every 4 h] is the primary treatment. Ampicillin may be substituted in the same dose, but the cephalosporins, including the newer derivatives, should not be used. Optimal treatment of patients who are allergic to the penicillins is uncertain; candidate antimicrobials include erythromycin (40 to 50 mg per kilogram of body weight per day, intravenously, as four equal portions every 6 h); doxycycline (3 mg per kilogram of body weight, intravenously as a loading dose, and 1.5 mg per kilogram of body weight per day, intravenously, as two equal portions every 12 h for maintenance); co-trimoxazole (15 and 75 mg per kilogram of body weight, respectively, per day, intravenously, as 3 equal portions every 8 h). Treatment should be continued in full dosage by intravenous injection for 14 to 21 days after defervescence.

PROGNOSIS Prompt, vigorous antimicrobial treatment of the acute forms of listeriosis, excepting fetal listeriosis, is usually curative. On the basis of agglutinin titers, specific antibody disappears during the months following cure. However, reinfection has not been reported.

ERYSIPELOTHRIX RHUSIOPATHIAE INFECTIONS

DEFINITION Erysipeloid is the commonest and most nearly unique form of infection in humans caused by *Erysipelothrix rhusiopathiae*. Infective endocarditis and arthritis are rare forms of erysipelothricosis in human beings.

ETIOLOGY As gram-positive, microaerophilic bacilli, *E. rhusiopathiae* may be confused with nontoxinogenic *Corynebacterium* spp. and *Listeria monocytogenes*. However, *E. rhusiopathiae* is nonmotile and fails to grow on media selective for *Corynebacterium* spp. Also, unlike *L. monocytogenes*, *E. rhusiopathiae* only rarely causes conjunctivitis, following conjunctival inoculation, or monocytosis, after intravenous inoculation, in the rabbit. Because alpha hemolysis is commonly evident after 48 h of incubation of *E. rhusiopathiae*, confusion with streptococci may also occur. Isolates of *E. rhusiopathiae* appear to be serologically homogeneous. Although serodifferentiation from other gram-positive bacilli is possible, few laboratories are capable of definitive serodiagnosis.

EPIDEMIOLOGY AND PATHOGENESIS Primarily a saprophyte, *E. rhusiopathiae* is worldwide in distribution. Human beings are virtually always infected by traumatic dermal inoculation; erysipeloid is the usual result. The disease is almost wholly restricted to persons who in their occupations handle edible or nonedible dead animal products. If the bacilli are not successfully confined to the skin, bacteremia may result and may lead to infective endocarditis; in about two-thirds of the reported cases, there was no evidence of preexisting valvular heart disease.

The seasonal incidence of erysipeloid parallels that of swine erysipelas, being highest in summer and early fall. Yet persons who tend pigs, even pigs ill with porcine erysipelas, do not commonly develop erysipeloid.

MANIFESTATIONS Erysipeloid begins 2 to 7 days after injury, often after the initial lesion has healed. An itching, burning, painful irritation may precede and always accompanies the appearance of the maculopapular, nonvesiculated, sharply defined, raised, purplish-red zone surrounding the site of entry. There is local swelling, and when, as is usual, a finger or the hand is involved, nearby joints may become stiff and painful. Centrifugal spread from the site of inoculation is apparent in a day or so. Movement is slow, 1 to 2 cm per 24 h maximally, and more rapid proximally than distally; involvement of the terminal phalanx of a finger is rare, while spread to other fingers and the hand distal to the wrist is common. With extension, the original center subsides without desquamation or suppuration. There are usually no systemic signs or symptoms; regional lymphangitis and lymphadenitis are rare. Untreated, the disease heals within 3 weeks in most patients, although relapse has been observed.

The manifestations of erysipelothrical endocarditis may be either acute or chronic, depending on the virulence of the infecting strain and on the state of resistance of the host. Usually, there are no classic erysipeloid skin lesions to suggest the disease at the time that endocarditis is clinically evident. However, a history of recent erysipeloid may be helpful.

Erysipelothrical arthritis is not clinically characteristic but usually can be related to erysipeloid or erysipelothrical bacteremia. Isolation of *E. rhusiopathiae* from synovial fluid has not been reported.

LABORATORY FINDINGS The usual culture media are adequate for the growth of *E. rhusiopathiae*. However, differentiation from diphtheroids, listerias, and streptococci depends primarily on the clinician's alerting the laboratory to the possibility of erysipelothricosis.

In erysipeloid, *E. rhusiopathiae* are best recovered by incubating, in broth containing glucose, a full-thickness biopsy of skin removed from the advancing edge of a lesion. Culture of an aspirate obtained after injection of sterile, bacteriostat-free 0.9% NaCl solution into the periphery of a lesion is less likely to yield *E. rhusiopathiae*.

With endocarditis and arthritis, the findings are in keeping with the respective clinical syndromes and are in no way characteristic for *E. rhusiopathiae*.

DIFFERENTIAL DIAGNOSIS The appearance and location of erysipeloid, its slow and limited spread, the lack of constitutional reaction, the history of occupation and injury, all serve to identify this disease. The afflicted skin in *erysipelas* is very erythematous, and the face and scalp are affected; there are regional lymphangitis and lymphadenitis, leukocytosis, fever, and malaise. Eczematous lesions may itch, but they display vesicles and little abnormal color.

The various erythemas have a different location and do not usually itch or burn; they are more apt to be chronic and nonmigratory.

TREATMENT The penicillins, the cephalosporins, erythromycin, clindamycin, the tetracyclines, and chloramphenicol inhibit *E. rhusiopathiae* in vitro at concentrations practical in therapy. Penicillin G is the agent of choice. Erysipeloid is adequately treated by injection of 1.2 million units of benzathine penicillin G. Erythromycin (15 mg/kg per day in four equal portions taken orally for 5 to 7 days) is an alternative. Cure of erysipelothrical endocarditis has been effected by the daily injection of 2 to 20 million units of penicillin per day for 4 to 6 weeks; the dose should be monitored by determination of the bactericidal activity of serum from the patient against the infecting strain. Intractable cardiac failure may oblige surgical excision of an infected valve and insertion of a prosthesis.

PROGNOSIS Penicillin therapy is highly effective in curing erysipelothrical infections. As with infective endocarditis from any cause, the prognosis is primarily a function of the severity of the valvular damage. Of cases reported since penicillin became available, about 25 percent were fatal; earlier diagnosis, and, perhaps, earlier resort to surgical excision and replacement of infected valves, may improve the outcome.

REFERENCES

BOJSEN-MOLLER J: Human listeriosis. Diagnostic, epidemiological and clinical studies. Acta Pathol Microbiol Scand B 229:13, 1972

FLEMING DW et al: Pasteurized milk as a vehicle of infection in an outbreak of listeriosis. N Engl J Med 312:404, 1985

HALLIDAY HL, HIRATA T: Perinatal listeriosis—a review of twelve patients. Am J Obstet Gynecol 133:405, 1979

HOEPRICH PD: Listeriosis, in *Infectious Diseases*, 3d ed, PD Hoeprich (ed). Philadelphia, Lippincott-Harper, 1982, chap 51

————: Erysipeloid, in *Infectious Diseases*, 3d ed, PD Hoeprich (ed). Philadelphia, Lippincott-Harper, 1982, chap 103

Listeriosis outbreak associated with Mexican-style cheese—California. Morb Mort Week Rep 34:357, 1985

NELSON E: Five hundred cases of erysipeloid. Rocky Mount Med J 52:40, 1955

ROCOURT J, GRIMONT PAD: *Listeria welshimeri* sp. nov. and *Listeria seeligeri* sp. nov. Int J Syst Bacteriol 33:866, 1983

SCHLECH WF III et al: Epidemic listeriosis—evidence for transmission by food. N Engl J Med 308:203, 1983

SEELIGER HPR: *Listeriosis*. Basel, Karger, 1961

98   ANTHRAX

DONALD KAYE / ROBERT G. PETERSDORF

DEFINITION Anthrax is a disease of wild and domesticated animals that is transmitted to humans by contact with infected animals or their products, by insect vectors which act as mechanical carriers of the etiologic organism, or, rarely, in some developing parts of the world by direct contact, such as use of common household articles. The characteristic lesion of human anthrax is a necrotic cutaneous ulcer. Occasionally, inhalation can produce a severe infection with mediastinitis and pulmonary manifestations. Rarely, ingestion can cause gastrointestinal or oropharyngeal infection. Meningitis and other forms of dissemination may result from anthrax bacteremia.

ETIOLOGY *Bacillus anthracis* is a large, encapsulated, gram-positive, nonmotile, aerobic, spore-forming microorganism that grows well in most nutrient media. On agar, it produces grayish-white colonies with comma-shaped projections (''Medusa's head''). The colonies are sticky and tend to stand up in stalagmite fashion when lifted with a loop. Microscopic examination of *B. anthracis* from artificial media or in tissue reveals parallel chains of bacilli which resemble boxcars. The pathogenicity of *B. anthracis* for laboratory animals, including mice and guinea pigs, differentiates it from *B. subtilis* and *B. cereus*, which it closely resembles. The spores are killed by boiling for 10 min but can survive for up to 20 years in soil and animal products, an important factor in the persistence and spread of the disease. Uncultivated soil is more favorable to sporulation, and dry climates also favor the persistence of organisms. The anthrax bacillus possesses a capsule of glutamyl polypeptide, which interferes with phagocytosis of the microorganism. In addition, it contains an anticomplementary substance and elaborates a toxin which is probably of importance in determining virulence.

EPIDEMIOLOGY Anthrax is worldwide; repeated outbreaks have occurred in southern Europe, notably Greece and Turkey, the Middle East (particularly Iran), Africa (Zimbabwe and Gambia), Australia and New Zealand, and on both American continents. From 1975 to 1976, under 2000 cases of anthrax were reported to the World Health Organization. This is very likely an underestimate. In the United States, immunization programs for high-risk occupational groups, better industrial protective measures, and decreased contact with contaminated animal products have markedly reduced the number of reported cases of anthrax. No cases were reported in 1981 to 1983, and one case was reported in 1984.

Cattle, horses, sheep, goats, and swine are most commonly infected. There have been outbreaks of anthrax among animals in the United States, centering mostly in South Dakota, Nebraska, Arkansas, Mississippi, Louisiana, Texas, Washington, and California. The disease tends to occur in animals in late summer and early fall. An outbreak of anthrax, acquired from goatskin bongo drum heads and goatskin rugs, occurred in Haiti and was imported into the United States.

The disease in humans is acquired by butchering, skinning, or dissecting infected carcasses or by handling contaminated hides, wool, hair, or other materials. The majority of cases of human anthrax involve workers handling imported and unprocessed wool, hair, or hides, or bone meal used as fertilizer. Gardeners have been infected accidentally by inhaling bone meal fertilizers, and inhalation anthrax has been reported following exposure to exhausts of a tanning plant. The disease usually follows inoculation of bacilli or spores into the skin, often through a wound or abrasion. Intestinal infection has followed ingestion of contaminated meat. In Africa outbreaks of anthrax have been attributed to flies which carry the organism from infected carcasses or to biting flies which may carry the bacillus in their blood. This may account for the absence of lesions on the fingers and hands. In Gambia, under crowded conditions, human-to-human transmission has been implicated through the use of common palm-brushes (loofahs).

PATHOGENESIS Germination of spores occurs within hours of inoculation. The spores germinate, form capsules, and release toxin that causes brawny edema and necrosis. The malignant pustule which follows cutaneous inoculation of anthrax organisms is characterized by vesiculation, neutrophilic infiltration, gelatinous edema, and necrosis. Suppuration is rare in the absence of secondary pyogenic infection; hence, the term *malignant pustule,* which is often used to describe cutaneous anthrax, is inappropriate. Spread of the bacilli to the regional lymph nodes may be followed by systemic dissemination. Examination of tissues from fatal human cases reveals masses of the bacteria in blood vessels, lymph nodes, and the parenchyma of various organs. There is scanty or no cellular exudation at these foci, but hemorrhage and edema are widespread.

In inhalation anthrax the spores are phagocytosed by alveolar macrophages, and germination occurs in mediastinal lymph nodes. There is necrosis of tissue in the nodes and mediastinum resulting in hemorrhagic mediastinitis with associated bacteremia. Respiratory failure may occur either from a hemorrhagic pneumonia secondary to bacteremia or from a direct effect of *B. anthracis* toxin on pulmonary capillaries.

Meningeal anthrax results from bacteremia following a primary cutaneous lesion or from inhalational infection.

Intestinal anthrax occurs by ingestion of infected, poorly cooked animal meat. Spores enter the submucosa and regional lymph nodes where they germinate and cause hemorrhage and necrosis with associated bacteremia. In oropharyngeal anthrax the bacilli damage cervical or submandibular lymph nodes.

B. anthracis toxin has three components: edema factor, lethal factor, and protective antigen. Toxin is important in the pathogenesis of some of the manifestations of the disease. Its persistence may explain delayed response after onset of antimicrobial therapy. Immunity to subsequent infection seems to follow anthrax.

MANIFESTATIONS In the past in the United States, 95 percent of cases were cutaneous and 5 percent were acquired from inhalation. Meningitis occurred in less than 5 percent of cases. Gastrointestinal and oropharyngeal forms of anthrax were extremely rare.

Cutaneous anthrax Human anthrax usually begins on an exposed body surface (such as the upper extremity or face) as a painless pruritic, erythematous papule which vesiculates and ulcerates to form a black eschar. Tiny satellite vesicles are frequent. The ulcer may be surrounded by extensive edematous swelling which is nontender, nonpitting, and so characteristic of anthrax that it is a valuable diagnostic sign. After about 5 days the ulcer begins to subside, but edema may persist for several weeks. Mild tenderness and enlargement of regional lymph nodes are frequently present. Constitutional symptoms are often absent despite extensive local changes, but there may be mild fever, headache, and malaise. Conditions that may resemble cutaneous anthrax are staphylococcal skin infections, plague, tularemia, and orf.

In 10 to 20 percent of untreated cutaneous anthrax, the infection spreads from the hemorrhagic regional lymph nodes to the bloodstream. There is high fever, prostration, and a rapidly fatal course. These cases usually involve the meninges.

Inhalation anthrax Also termed *woolsorter's disease,* this is a highly fatal disseminated infection characterized by cyanosis, dyspnea, mediastinitis, and hemoptysis and is probably dependent on the entry of spores into the lungs. The illness is biphasic and initially consists of an insidious onset of mild fever, malaise, fatigue, myalgia, nonproductive cough, and a feeling of substernal oppression. This phase lasts several days, and there may be some improvement before the acute onset of a second stage consisting of dyspnea, cyanosis, stridor, and shock. Pleural effusions and mediastinal widening on chest x-ray are characteristic. Most patients die within 24 h despite treatment. It has been postulated that underlying lung disease, such as sarcoid, may predispose to inhalation anthrax.

Meningeal anthrax This is an acute fulminant infection. The cerebrospinal fluid is hemorrhagic, purulent, or both.

Intestinal anthrax There is fever, nausea, vomiting, and abdominal pain. Hematemesis, bloody diarrhea, and ascites may develop. Clinically, it may resemble an acute abdomen. The disease usually has been fatal, although a few patients have been cured by resection of the involved bowel.

Oropharyngeal anthrax Patients have fever and cervical or submandibular lymphadenopathy with edema.

LABORATORY DIAGNOSIS The fluid from the cutaneous lesion frequently contains many bacilli, demonstrable by Gram's stain and culture, but when patients have been given topical or systemic antibiotics, cultures and smears may be unreliable. Blood cultures are usually positive in disseminated anthrax, but only 10 percent of patients with cutaneous ulcers have bacteremia. The blood leukocyte count is normal in mild cases, but there is polymorphonuclear leukocytosis in most patients with disseminated disease. Patients with meningeal involvement show bloody spinal fluid, in which the organisms are easily found by direct examination or culture.

A 24-h culture on blood agar shows characteristic colonies. Inoculation of a suspected colony of *B. anthracis* will kill guinea pigs in 24 h, and the organism can be recovered from the left ventricle.

The indirect microhemagglutination test (IMH test) has detected antibodies in 93 percent of patients, 98 percent of vaccinees, and none of the controls. It is useful in confirming the diagnosis.

TREATMENT For cutaneous anthrax, 600,000 units of aqueous procaine penicillin should be given every 6 h until the local edema subsides. Then oral therapy can be continued for a total of 7 to 10 days. In penicillin-allergic patients, erythromycin or tetracycline may be used in doses of 500 mg every 6 h for 7 to 10 days. The eschar goes through its natural evolution in spite of treatment, and lymph node enlargement may persist for several days. *Bacillus anthracis* cannot be recovered from the skin lesion after 24 to 48 h of penicillin. For inhalation anthrax, 20 million units of penicillin should be given intravenously, but it is doubtful that the drug acts sufficiently rapidly to reverse the process. In meningeal anthrax, similar large doses of penicillin plus 300 to 400 mg hydrocortisone should be given. It is not clear whether the addition of steroids affects the outcome favorably.

PREVENTION The potential for infection of personnel in industrial plants where contaminated animal products are handled exists. An outbreak of inhalation anthrax with a high mortality rate was reported in a goat hair processing mill in the United States in the late 1950s. Sterilization of all raw wool, mohair, etc., would probably remove the hazard but has had only limited use. A vaccine prepared from the ''protective'' antigen of *B. anthracis* is available and is effective in reducing the incidence of infection in an exposed population. Spore vaccines of various types are used with good effect in domestic animals in endemic areas but are not suitable for use in humans. Animals dying with anthrax should be disposed of safely.

PROGNOSIS The cutaneous disease was fatal in 20 percent of cases before antimicrobial drugs were available. The mortality rate of cutaneous anthrax now is less than 1 percent with proper treatment. In the rare cases of inhalational, meningeal, and intestinal anthrax the prognosis is poor despite antibiotic therapy.

REFERENCES

Brachman PS: Inhalation anthrax. Ann NY Acad Sci 353:83, 1980

————: Anthrax, in *Bacterial Infections of Humans: Epidemiology and Control*, A Evans, H Feldman (eds). New York, Ms Hilary Evans Publishing, 1982, pp 63–74

Feeley JC, Patton CM: *Bacillus*, in *Manual of Clinical Microbiology, 3*, EH Lennette et al (eds). Washington, DC, American Society of Microbiology, 1980, p 145

Laforce FM: Woolsorters' disease in England. Bull NY Acad Med 54:956, 1978

Nalin DR et al: Survival of a patient with intestinal anthrax. Am J Med 62:130, 1977

Sirisanthana T et al: Outbreak of oral-oropharyngeal anthrax: An unusual manifestation of human infection with *Bacillus anthracis*. Am J Trop Med Hyg 33:144, 1984

99   TETANUS

HARRY N. BEATY

DEFINITION Tetanus is an acute, often fatal, disease caused by an exotoxin produced in a wound by *Clostridium tetani*. It is characterized by generalized increased rigidity and convulsive spasms of skeletal muscles.

ETIOLOGY *C. tetani* is a strictly anaerobic, gram-positive rod which is motile and readily forms a single, spheric, terminal endospore that swells the end of the organism and produces a characteristic ''clubbed'' appearance.

The organism grows well on blood agar at 37°C under anaerobic conditions. *C. tetani* is relatively inert biochemically, with no proteolytic activity and no fermentation of carbohydrates. Vegetative forms are no more resistant to adverse conditions than other bacteria are, but spores are highly resistant to antiseptics and moderately resistant to heat.

Ten types of *C. tetani* can be distinguished on the basis of flagellar antigens. All these types have one or more common somatic antigens and are capable of producing at least two exotoxins. One, a hemolysin, is relatively unimportant clinically. The other, tetanospasmin, generally referred to as tetanus toxin, is a protein with a molecular weight of approximately 145,000 in its dimer form and is responsible for the clinical manifestations of tetanus. The tetanospasmins produced by the various types of *C. tetani* are nearly identical antigenically. For this reason, one antitoxin is needed to neutralize the tetanus toxins produced by all strains.

EPIDEMIOLOGY The tetanus bacillus is found in the superficial layers of soil and as a saprophyte in the intestinal tract of humans and certain animals. It is most frequently encountered in densely populated regions in hot, damp climates and in soil rich in organic matter. Urbanization, mechanization of agriculture, and socioeconomic factors such as poverty and lack of availability of health services also significantly influence the occurrence of this disease.

Worldwide, there are probably 300,000 to 500,000 cases of tetanus each year, with a mortality rate of roughly 45 percent. There is no racial predilection, but the male-to-female ratio is 2.5:1, even among neonates, in which the exposure is presumably equal. In the United States, there are about 100 reported cases each year, which occur almost exclusively in nonimmunized or only partially immunized individuals. The incidence of disease is high among nonwhites in the southern states, and in the last decade, about two-thirds of patients have been 50 or older. However, spores of *C. tetani* are distributed widely throughout urban and rural areas of the entire country, and are found commonly on clothing and in house dust, placing the nonimmune individual at risk after relatively minor household injuries. Tetanus has been known to follow surgery and innocuous procedures such as skin testing or intramuscular injection of medication. The disease is inordinately common in narcotic addicts, perhaps because heroin is frequently ''cut'' with quinine, which drastically lowers the redox potential at the site of injection and favors the growth of *C. tetani*.

Tetanus neonatorum is a major cause of infant mortality in developing countries and is directly related to poor obstetric conditions and lack of maternal immunization programs.

PATHOGENESIS AND PATHOLOGY *C. tetani* is a noninvasive organism. Therefore, tetanus can occur only after spores or vegetative bacteria gain access to tissues and produce toxin locally. The usual mode of entry is through a puncture wound or laceration on an extremity. However, tetanus may follow elective surgery, burn wounds, chronic skin ulcers, otitis media, dental infection, abortion, and pregnancy. Neonatal tetanus usually follows infection of the umbilical stump. Tetanus not infrequently follows trivial injuries not seen by a physician, and in 10 to 20 percent of cases there is neither a history of injury nor a detectable lesion.

Wounds undoubtedly are contaminated frequently with spores of *C. tetani*, but tetanus develops rarely because germination of spores occurs only when the oxygen tension is much lower than that of normal tissue. Spores may survive in the body for months to years and finally produce disease at some later date after minor trauma that alters local conditions. Toxin production in wounds is favored by necrotic tissue, foreign bodies, calcium salts, and associated infections that establish low oxidation-reduction potentials. Infection caused by the tetanus bacillus remains strictly localized, but the toxin produced is transported to the central nervous system via neural pathways. Toxin entering the circulation persists for days, and probably must enter peripheral nerves to spread centrally and cause disease.

The typical clinical manifestations of tetanus are caused by the effect of tetanospasmin on the central nervous system. The toxin attacks synaptic functions to produce disinhibition of both the alpha and gamma motor systems. Generalized muscle rigidity arises from uninhibited afferent stimuli entering the central nervous system from the periphery. When the stimuli become more vigorous, spasms occur. Emotional and, to a lesser extent, visual stimuli can also cause muscle spasm. Tetanus toxin also has other effects. Peripherally it produces neuromuscular blockade similar to that of botulinum toxin, and it acts directly on muscle to produce contraction which is unaccompanied by an action potential in nerves. Certain clinical manifestations suggest that tetanus toxin also has an effect on the sympathetic nervous system.

All the effects of tetanus toxin appear to be self-limited and completely reversible, because patients who recover from the disease have no residual defect. Although there are no distinguishable pathologic changes that are characteristic of tetanus, brainstem lesions have been reported in patients dying from tetanus, and toxic myocarditis has been recognized.

CLINICAL MANIFESTATIONS The *incubation period* of tetanus, i.e., the time between injury and the appearance of unmistakable symptoms, ranges from 2 to 56 days. However, over 80 percent of patients become symptomatic within 14 days. A short incubation period indicates severe disease.

Nonspecific premonitory symptoms such as restlessness, irritability, and headache are encountered occasionally, but the commonest presenting complaints are pain and stiffness in the jaw, abdomen, or back and difficulty swallowing. As the disease progresses, stiffness gives way to rigidity, and patients often complain of difficulty in opening their mouths. In fact, trismus is the commonest manifestation of tetanus and is responsible for the familiar descriptive name of *lockjaw*. As more muscles are involved, rigidity becomes generalized, and sustained contractions of facial muscles produce a characteristic expression called *risus sardonicus*. The intensity and sequence of muscle involvement is quite variable. In a small proportion of patients, only local signs and symptoms develop in the region of the injury. In the vast majority, however, most muscles are involved to some degree, and the signs and symptoms encountered depend upon the major muscle groups affected.

Reflex spasms usually occur within 24 to 72 h of the first symptoms, an interval referred to as the *onset time*. A short onset time is associated with a poor prognosis. Spasms are caused by sudden intensification of afferent stimuli arising in the periphery and may be both painful and dangerous. As the disease progresses, more intense and longer-lasting spasms occur with increasing frequency. Respiration may be impaired by laryngospasm or tonic contraction of respiratory muscles, which prevents adequate ventilation. Hypoxia then may lead to irreversible central nervous system damage and death.

Patients are almost invariably conscious and mentally alert at the time of admission. Low-grade fever, profuse sweating, and tachycardia are common. Deep tendon reflexes are hyperactive, and there may be labile hypertension. The physical examination should be undertaken with care, because reflex convulsive spasms may be precipitated easily. Physical examination should include evaluation of wounds and determination of the extent of rigidity; the severity of trismus; the presence or absence of dysphagia and respiratory embarrassment; the frequency, intensity, and duration of convulsive spasms; and the presence of complications such as respiratory infection.

Characteristically, the manifestations of tetanus increase in severity for about 3 days and then remain stable for the next 5 to 7 days. After about 10 days, spasms begin to occur less frequently, and by the end of 2 weeks, they disappear altogether. Although residual stiffness may persist for a prolonged period, most survivors recover completely in 4 weeks.

Tetanus neonatorum is a severe form of the disease that usually occurs within 10 days of birth. Early signs include difficulty sucking, irritability, and excessive crying, associated with peculiar grimacing. Intense rigidity characteristically produces opisthotonus, flexion of the arms, clenched fists, extension of the legs, and plantar flexion of the toes. Typical spasms occur with minimal stimuli.

Complications Complications contribute significantly to the morbidity and mortality of tetanus. Some result from overly vigorous therapy and prolonged bed rest, while others are attributed to the action of tetanus toxin. Inadequate ventilation is a constant threat. In addition to hypoxia, atelectasis is a common consequence of impaired respiration. Difficulty in swallowing leads to aspiration of secretions, which may also cause atelectasis and initiate pulmonary infection. Thrombophlebitis is occasionally encountered, but bland venous thrombosis is more common and may lead to pulmonary embolization. Cardiovascular complications thought to be due to hyperactivity of the sympathetic nervous system include vasomotor instability, hypertension, tachycardia, arrhythmias, and severe vasoconstriction. Pulmonary edema and hypotension may occur as a consequence of myocarditis. High fever usually signifies secondary infection. Pneumonia is a common late complication of tetanus; other sites of secondary infections include the original wound, decubitus ulcers, and the urinary tract of patients with indwelling bladder catheters. Fractures of midthoracic vertebrae are probably due to severe spasms and are particularly common among children and adolescents. Gastrointestinal complications include acute peptic ulceration, paralytic ileus, and constipation. Hemolysis is seen in a small proportion of patients.

Pneumonia is a major cause of death. Other autopsy findings include congestion of viscera and, occasionally, intracranial hemorrhage or thrombosis. In about 20 percent of cases, no obvious pathology is identified, and death is attributed to the direct effects of tetanus toxin.

LABORATORY FINDINGS There are no laboratory findings characteristic of tetanus. Granulocytosis is seen in about one-third of patients, but anemia is rare. Blood chemistries are almost always normal initially, but various fluid and electrolyte disturbances may arise in the course of the disease. The electrocardiogram usually shows only sinus tachycardia, but occasionally T-wave inversion is seen. Roentgenograms are not helpful except in the evaluation of complications.

The diagnosis of tetanus is entirely clinical and does not depend upon bacteriologic confirmation. *C. tetani* is recovered from the wound in only 30 percent of cases, and not infrequently it is isolated from patients who do not have tetanus. Laboratory identification depends on cultural and morphologic characteristics and demonstration of toxin production in mice.

DIFFERENTIAL DIAGNOSIS No disease resembles fully developed tetanus. However, strychnine poisoning and dystonic reactions due to phenothiazines and metoclopramide produce a syndrome that has been referred to as pseudotetanus. These rare reactions usually follow brief exposure to drugs and subside 24 to 48 h after their administration is discontinued. Early in the course of true tetanus, exclusion of local causes of jaw pain may be difficult, and the combination of neck stiffness and fever may suggest meningitis. However, this can be excluded by lumbar puncture, because in tetanus the spinal fluid is normal. When there is doubt about the diagnosis, clinical observation usually settles the issue within a matter of hours.

TREATMENT In order to formulate a rational plan of therapy, it is useful to assess the severity of tetanus. Because of the poor prognosis of tetanus in older individuals, the disease should be considered moderate to severe in all patients over 50.

General measures Patients must be hospitalized. After initial evaluation, necrotic tissue and foreign bodies should be removed from the infected wound, and abscesses should be drained. Patients should be placed in a quiet room and observed closely for development of complications or unexpected changes in the course of the disease. While it is a good general principle to disturb patients as little as possible, vital signs must be monitored and aspiration must be averted

TIDYMAN M et al: Adjunctive use of dantrolene in severe tetanus. Anesth Analg 64:538, 1985

the toxins are considerably more heat-labile. The toxins are destroyed by boiling for 10 min, or by temperatures of 80°C for 30 min.

PATHOGENESIS For years, botulism was considered a disease that occurred almost exclusively after ingestion of preformed toxin. With the recognition that infant botulism may follow ingestion of *C. botulinum* spores which germinate, proliferate, and produce toxin in the intestinal tract, this concept has been modified. The Centers by positioning the patient carefully and by aspirating nasopharyngeal secretions frequently. Care must be taken to prevent development of decubitus ulcers or contractures, but many routine nursing procedures should be omitted because they may precipitate uncomfortable or

personnel are available to provide controlled mechanical ventilation for the paralyzed patient. It should be reserved for treatment of severe tetanus that is not adequately controlled by other measures. In centers with a team experienced in handling these patients, this approach, in

for Disease Control now report human cases of botulism in four categories: food-borne botulism, infant botulism, wound botulism, and unclassified. The latter includes a small number of adult cases each year for which no ingestion of contaminated food can be documented.

Botulinus toxins exert their major effect by blocking neuromuscular transmission in cholinergic nerve fibers. They either inhibit the release of acetylcholine or bind with it at or near its site of release within presynaptic clefts. Muscle reactivity to acetylcholine applied directly to the motor end plate is unimpaired. Central nervous system cholinergic pathways do not appear to be affected significantly in humans.

Food-borne botulism Food-borne botulism can occur when the following conditions are met: (1) a food product is contaminated with viable *C. botulinum* bacilli or spores; (2) proper conditions for germination of the spores exist; (3) time and conditions permit production of toxin before eating; (4) the food is not heated or is heated insufficiently to destroy botulinus toxin; and (5) the toxin-containing food is ingested by a susceptible host. Though a relatively anaerobic environment and temperatures above 30°C (86°F) are optimal for toxin production, strict anaerobic conditions are not necessary, and toxin production by some type E strains has been observed at temperatures as low as 3°C (38°F).

Although a variety of home-processed foods have been sources of botulism in the United States, certain foods seem to be safer than others. This may be because low pH (acidity) inhibits germination of spores and, therefore, toxin production. Commercially processed foods and improperly handled fresh foods have been implicated in outbreaks of botulism. Contaminated foods may appear putrefied, but frequently look and taste perfectly normal, regardless of toxin type.

Botulinus toxins are absorbed primarily in the stomach and upper part of the small intestine. They are large protein molecules which are absorbed after they have been reduced in size by proteolytic enzymes that do not destroy their activity. Either absorption is incomplete or toxins are inactivated partially by digestion, because the amount of toxin that appears in the bloodstream is variable, and in animals the lethal dose orally is 1000 times greater than the lethal dose intravenously. Toxin that reaches the lower part of the small intestine and colon may be absorbed slowly, which probably accounts for the delayed onset and the prolonged symptoms in many patients.

Infantile botulism It is not clear why botulism occurs in some babies who ingest *C. botulinum* spores and not in others. Age is an important factor; 90 percent of recognized cases have occurred in children under 6 months, and in certain animal models the syndrome can only be reproduced during a few days of early life. The intestinal tract of infants with botulism is colonized with *C. botulinum*, and it is assumed that the manifestations of the syndrome are slowly progressive because toxin is absorbed as it is produced rather than all at once, as is the case in food-borne botulism. Studies comparing the fecal flora of infants who have botulism with that of controls suggest that colonization of the intestine with *C. botulinum* may occur because of a delay in establishment of the normal fecal flora, the presence of organisms that promote or inhibit *C. botulinum* colonization, or a change in intestinal function that favors germination and growth of ingested spores. Diet is an important factor in the development of infant botulism. Honey has been the source of *C. botulinum* spores in a number of cases, and the current recommendation is that honey not be fed to children under 12 months. Honey has not been shown to contain botulinus toxin, so it is a safe food for older children and adults. Breast-feeding may provide relative protection against infant botulism. Supplementary iron may increase a baby's susceptibility to the fulminant form of the disease. Spores can be ingested from a variety of environmental sources, but for the majority of cases no source of *C. botulinum* is identified.

Wound botulism In contrast to food-borne botulism, wound botulism results from toxin produced by *C. botulinum* infecting a wound

that is typically traumatic and contaminated with soil. The wound often seems clinically insignificant. From 1982 to 1983, six cases of this rare syndrome were reported in chronic drug abusers, five of whom abused drugs intravenously, and four of whom had superficial skin infections.

CLINICAL MANIFESTATIONS Botulism may vary from a mild illness for which patients seek no medical advice to a fulminant disease which ends in death within 24 h. Symptoms usually begin 12 to 36 h after ingestion of toxin, although the extremes of 3 h to 14 days are recorded. In general, the earlier symptoms appear, the more serious the disease.

The commonest symptoms are diplopia, blurred vision, and bulbar weakness manifested by dysphonia, dysarthria, dysphagia, and dry mouth. Symmetric paralysis of the extremities appears and may progress rapidly in a descending or ascending manner. Weakness of the respiratory muscles may occur early, but may be asymptomatic until function is moderately impaired.

Impairment of cholinergic autonomic transmission may result in constipation, urinary retention, and reduced salivation and lacrimation. Nausea and vomiting are early symptoms in half the patients, but the absence of these symptoms does not rule out botulism.

On examination, patients are usually alert, oriented, and afebrile, even with severe disease. Ocular signs include ptosis, weakness of extraocular motion, and in some patients failure of accommodation. The pupils are normal in many patients, but in some cases may react sluggishly or may be dilated and unreactive to light. Widespread neuromuscular block results in symmetric flaccid weakness of the palate, tongue, larynx, respiratory muscles, and extremities. Severe paralytic ileus and bladder distention may be present. Deep-tendon reflexes are intact in milder cases, but if significant paralysis is present they are reduced or absent. No pathologic reflexes are detectable. Findings on sensory examination are always entirely normal. Some patients have apparent gait disturbances and incoordination, but this is due to generalized weakness.

Once symptoms are noted, the disease may progress rapidly over several days, with significant changes in status occurring at hourly intervals. A period of stabilization is then followed by gradual recovery over days to months, depending on the severity of intoxication. The mechanism of recovery is not well understood. In wound botulism the patient may be febrile, but the clinical manifestations are otherwise similar. A 10- to 14-day incubation period is common from the time of infection to the onset of toxic symptoms. The clinical spectrum of infant botulism ranges from asymptomatic carriage of *C. botulinum* to a fatal illness indistinguishable from the sudden infant death syndrome. Constipation, poor feeding, and "failure to thrive," alone or in combination, may be the only signs of the illness, but these manifestations may be followed by progressive weakness of skeletal muscles, cranial nerve palsies, "floppiness" of the head, and impaired respiration.

LABORATORY FINDINGS Routine laboratory studies do not aid in diagnosing botulism. When botulism is suspected, public health authorities should be consulted to assist in special studies to confirm the diagnosis. Specimens of blood, feces, and gastric contents, as well as suspected foods and their containers, should be obtained. Because of the extreme potency of botulinus toxin, careful collection and laboratory precautions should be used. The food, stool, and serum should be studied for the presence of toxin by the mouse bioassay technique and submitted for special anaerobic culture. This battery of tests will result in an overall case recognition rate of about 85 percent. Immunofluorescent techniques are useful for the early recognition of the organisms. If wound botulism is suspected, the exudate should be submitted for culture and toxin analysis.

The spinal fluid is usually normal, although mild elevations in protein concentration may occur. Electrocardiographic abnormalities, including minor disturbances in conduction, nonspecific T-wave and ST-segment changes, and various disorders of rhythm, have been described. Electrodiagnostic studies have been shown to be of value in differentiating botulism from other paralytic diseases. The evoked motor action potential may be of low voltage but will facilitate with tetanic stimulation in a manner similar to the myasthenic syndrome (Eaton-Lambert syndrome). Electromyography may show small, short-duration, overly abundant motor units. In severe cases, denervation can occur, resulting in fibrillation activity after several weeks.

DIFFERENTIAL DIAGNOSIS Botulism must be differentiated from other conditions that produce generalized paralysis. In the Guillain-Barré syndrome, mild sensory abnormalities are nearly always present, and the spinal fluid protein is often elevated. The variant of the Guillain-Barré syndrome with ophthalmoplegia, areflexia, and ataxia (Fisher's syndrome) may prove particularly confusing. The course of myasthenia gravis is seldom so acute, and the deep tendon reflexes and pupils are normal. Some patients with botulism may show mild improvement after injection of edrophonium (Tensilon), but this improvement is not of the magnitude seen in myasthenia gravis. In tick paralysis the weakness is generally of an ascending pattern, patients may have paresthesias, and a tick is found. In diphtheria, palatal weakness is frequently the first symptom, and a history of prior pharyngitis may be obtained. Cutaneous diphtheria can be differentiated from wound botulism by appropriate cultures. In poliomyelitis the spinal fluid is abnormal and the weakness is often asymmetric and spares the ocular muscles. Vascular accidents of the brainstem can be recognized by associated neurologic signs. Belladonna poisoning presents with markedly dilated pupils and delirium. In organophosphate poisoning the pupils are markedly miotic. Shellfish poisoning, aminoglycoside antibiotic paralysis, and familial periodic paralysis might also prove confusing.

Patients with marked dry mouth may develop a picture simulating pharyngitis. Patients with gastrointestinal complaints and ileus may appear to have other forms of food poisoning or intestinal obstruction.

TREATMENT The most immediate threat to the survival of patients with botulism is respiratory failure. Patients with symptoms or known exposure should be hospitalized. Close observation is essential, and vital capacity should be measured frequently. If respiratory insufficiency develops, the patient may require assisted ventilation. Respiratory difficulties may develop rapidly; intubation or tracheostomy should be performed before onset of respiratory failure, and may be needed to manage secretions even if ventilation is otherwise adequate.

If there is no ileus, cathartics and enemas should be given to remove unabsorbed toxin from the intestine, but magnesium citrate and magnesium sulfate should not be given, as the magnesium may potentiate the neuromuscular block produced by botulinus toxin. Nasogastric suction and intravenous hyperalimentation may be needed if ileus is severe. If the bladder is atonic, a catheter will be required. Meticulous nursing care and physical therapy are essential.

As soon as the diagnosis of botulism is suspected, the patient should be tested for hypersensitivity to horse serum and treated with trivalent ABE antitoxin (Connaught), which is available from public health authorities. Type-specific antitoxin has been of benefit in several outbreaks of type E intoxication, but the value in type A and B outbreaks is less certain, particularly when paralysis has already occurred. Nonfatal hypersensitivity reactions occur in 15 to 20 percent of patients receiving the equine antitoxin, and those that react to a test dose must be desensitized prior to further treatment. Antibiotics should be reserved for specific infectious complications. In infant botulism, where multiplication of ingested organisms may be a factor, antibiotics have been ineffective in eradicating the organism, though this eventually may occur spontaneously. The value of antibiotic therapy in wound botulism has not been determined. It is essential that public health officials be notified so that toxin-containing foods can be confiscated and persons with possible exposure can be notified.

A number of reports have described the use of guanidine hydrochloride in the treatment of botulism. About two-thirds of the reported cases have shown some improvement with oral doses of 15 to 50 mg/kg per day, but the drug seems ineffective in patients with severe respiratory impairment, and probably has no effect on mortality rate.

Dose-related side effects include gastrointestinal upset, paresthesias, and fasciculations. Idiosyncratic reactions include cardiac arrhythmias and blood dyscrasias.

PROGNOSIS The current mortality rate of food-borne botulism in the United States is about 10 percent, with type A outbreaks having somewhat higher mortality than types B and E. The case/fatality ratio of hospitalized cases of infant botulism is about 2 percent. Death from botulism is due to complications such as respiratory failure and pneumonia. With rapid diagnosis and aggressive supportive care, even severely involved patients can recover fully. Some patients may have mild residual weakness due to denervation atrophy. Artificial respiratory support may be required for many months, and clinical weakness and autonomic symptoms may be noted for as long as 1 year after the onset of disease.

REFERENCES

Arnon SS: Infant botulism. Annu Rev Med 31:541, 1980
Dowell VR et al: Botulism and tetanus: Selected epidemiologic and microbiologic aspects. Rev Infect Dis 6(suppl 1):S202, 1985
Hughes JM et al: Clinical features of types A and B food-borne botulism. Ann Intern Med 95:442, 1981
Long SS et al: Clinical, laboratory, and environmental features of infant botulism in southeastern Pennsylvania. Pediatrics 75:935, 1985
McDonald KL et al: Botulism and botulism-like illness in chronic drug abusers. Ann Intern Med 102:616, 1985
Sellin LC: Botulism—an update. Milit Med 149:12, 1984
Tacket CO: Equine antitoxin use and other factors that predict outcome in type A food-borne botulism. Am J Med 76:794, 1984

101 OTHER CLOSTRIDIAL INFECTIONS

DENNIS L. KASPER

DEFINITION Bacteria of the genus *Clostridium* are gram-positive, spore-forming, obligate anaerobes which are ubiquitous in nature. There are over 60 recognized species of clostridia, many of which generally are considered saprophytic. Some of these species are pathogenic for humans and animals, particularly under conditions of lowered oxidation-reduction potential. Infections associated with these organisms range from localized wound contamination to overwhelming systemic disease. The three major disease categories for which clostridia are responsible include intestinal disorders, skin and soft tissue infections, and bacteremias. Toxins play a major role in some of these syndromes.

ETIOLOGY In humans, clostridia normally reside in the gastrointestinal tract and in the female genital tract, although they occasionally can be isolated from the skin or the mouth. As with other pathogenic anaerobic bacteria, clostridia are quite aerotolerant. Of the known species of the genus *Clostridium*, at least 30 have been isolated from human infections. Clostridia characteristically produce abundant gas in artificial media and form subterminal endospores. *C. perfringens*, the most important of the species discussed in this chapter, is encapsulated, nonmotile, and rarely sporulates in artificial media; the spores usually can be destroyed by boiling. *C. tetani* and *C. botulinum* are discussed in Chaps. 99 and 100, respectively.

Clostridia are present in the normal intestinal flora in concentrations of 10^9 to 10^{10} per gram. Of the 30 or more species which normally colonize humans, *C. ramosum* is the most common, followed by *C. perfringens*. These organisms universally are present in soil in concentrations of up to 10^4 per gram. Although clostridia morphologically are typical gram-positive organisms, many species appear to be gram-negative in clinical material or in stationary phase cultures. Therefore, Gram stains of cultures or clinical material should be interpreted with great care.

C. perfringens is the most common of the clostridial species isolated from tissue infections and bacteremias, followed in frequency by *C. novyi* and *C. septicum*. In the category of enteric infections, *C. difficile* is an important cause of antibiotic-associated colitis, and *C. perfringens* is associated with food poisoning and enteritis necroticans.

PATHOGENESIS Severe infections due to clostridial species are relatively uncommon despite the fact that clostridia can be cultured from most severe, traumatic wounds. Essential to the development of severe disease appears to be the presence of tissue necrosis and a low oxidation-reduction potential. *C. perfringens* requires about 14 amino acids and 6 or 7 additional growth factors for optimum growth. These nutrients are not found in appreciable concentrations in normal body fluids but are present in necrotic tissue. When *C. perfringens* grows in necrotic tissue, a zone of tissue damage due to the toxins elaborated by the organism allows for progressive growth. In contrast, when only a few bacteria leak into the bloodstream from a small defect in the intestinal wall, the organisms do not have the opportunity to multiply rapidly because blood as medium for growth is relatively deficient in certain amino acids and growth factors.

C. perfringens possesses 17 possible virulence factors, including 12 active tissue toxins and enterotoxins. *C. perfringens* has been divided into five types (A through E) on the basis of four major toxins: alpha, beta, epsilon, and iota. The alpha toxin is a phospholipase C (lecithinase) that splits lecithin into phosphorylcholine and diglyceride. This alpha toxin has been associated with gas gangrene and is known to be hemolytic, destroy platelets, and cause widespread capillary damage. When injected intravenously, it causes massive intravascular hemolysis and damages liver mitochondria. Alpha toxin may be important in the initiation of muscle infections which may progress to gas gangrene. Experimentally, the higher the concentration of alpha toxin present in the culture fluid, the smaller the infecting dose of *C. perfringens* required to produce infection. The protective effect of antiserum is directly proportional to its content of alpha antitoxin. Beta, epsilon, and iota toxins are also known to increase capillary permeability.

C. difficile produces a cytotoxin and an enterotoxin. The cytotoxin is potent in tissue culture assays and is a relatively sensitive and specific marker for *C. difficile*–induced enteric disease. The enterotoxin, designated toxin A, appears to be substantially more potent in biologic assays using animal models. Therefore, this toxin may play an important role in the expression of clinical disease.

CLINICAL MANIFESTATIONS **Intestinal disorders** FOOD POISONING *C. perfringens* is the second or third most common cause of food poisoning in the United States. Outbreaks generally have resulted from problems in the cooling and storage of foods cooked in bulk. The food sources primarily involved are meat, meat products, and poultry. Generally, the implicated meats have been cooked, allowed to cool, and then recooked the following day, often in a stew or hash. Strains of *C. perfringens* that contaminate meat manage to survive initial cooking. During reheating, the organisms sporulate and germinate. The disease is associated with an attack rate often as high as 70 percent. Symptoms of food poisoning from type A strains develop 8 to 24 h after ingestion of foods heavily contaminated with the organism. The primary symptoms include epigastric pain, nausea, and watery diarrhea lasting 12 to 24 h. Fever and vomiting are uncommon. Symptoms usually last less than 24 h. Diarrhea appears to be caused by a heat-labile protein enterotoxin. The enterotoxin inhibits glucose transport, damages the intestinal epithelium, and causes protein loss into the intestinal lumen, with minimal activity in the ileum.

ENTERITIS NECROTICANS Enteritis necroticans (*pigbel*), caused by type C strains of *C. perfringens*, has been the cause of necrotizing enteritis and death, occurring after a feast, in children and adults in New Guinea. A similar disease, *darmbrand*, was epidemic in Germany after World War II. It has been proposed that the highlanders of Papua, New Guinea, are susceptible to enteritis necroticans because

their intestinal lumen contains low levels of digestive proteases, as a result of a low-protein diet, and the presence of a heat-stable trypsin inhibitor in sweet potato, their staple food. The low level of intestinal proteolytic activity is thought inadequate to destroy the lethal beta toxin produced by *C. perfringens* type C. Clinical features include acute abdominal pain, bloody diarrhea, vomiting, shock, and peritonitis; death occurs in 40 percent of patients. Pathologically, there is an acute ulcerative process of the bowel restricted to the small intestine. The mucosa is lifted off the submucosa, forming large denuded areas. Pseudomembranes composed of sloughed epithelium are common, and gas may dissect into the submucosa. The source of the organisms may be the patient's own intestinal flora, because cultures of ingested pig have failed to yield the organism. In clinical trials, antitoxin against the beta toxin of *C. perfringens* has been of considerable benefit in changing the course of established disease. In a large-scale trial, children immunized with *C. perfringens* beta toxoid were protected from disease.

ANTIBIOTIC-ASSOCIATED COLITIS Strains of *C. difficile*, which produce toxins detectable in the stool, have been identified as the major cause of colitis in patients with antibiotic-associated diarrhea.

In order to diagnose this type of colitis, there should be no other identifiable cause of diarrhea and the onset of symptoms must occur either during antimicrobial administration or within 4 weeks after the implicated agent has been discontinued. The drugs implicated most commonly in *C. difficile* enterocolitis are clindamycin, ampicillin, cephalosporins, and the aminoglycosides. With the possible exceptions of vancomycin and streptomycin, nearly all antibiotics have been associated with this syndrome. Antibiotic-associated diarrhea is associated with 6.6 to 26 percent of clindamycin usage, and with 5 to 9 percent of ampicillin usage.

Antimicrobial-associated diarrhea can be divided into four anatomic categories: (1) normal colonic mucosa, (2) mild erythema with some edema, (3) granular, friable, or hemorrhagic mucosa, and (4) pseudomembrane formation.

Most commonly, patients with antibiotic-associated diarrhea have a normal, minimally erythematous colonic mucosa with some edema. Occasionally colitis is more severe and characterized by granular, friable, or hemorrhagic mucosa. Stool examination in these patients may reveal large numbers of red blood cells and some leukocytes. Biopsy shows subepithelial edema with round cell infiltration of the lamina propria and focal extravasation of erythrocytes. *C. difficile* toxin has been found in 15 to 46 percent of stools from patients in these first three categories, suggesting that other factors exist in the pathogenesis of antibiotic-associated diarrhea. The most characteristic form of antibiotic-associated colitis caused by *C. difficile* is pseudomembranous colitis (PMC). More than 95 percent of patients with documented PMC have positive stool toxin assays. Close inspection of pseudomembranes reveals exudative punctate raised plaques with skip areas or edematous hyperemic mucosa. These plaques can enlarge and coalesce over large segments of intestine in the later stages of disease. The clinical spectrum of antibiotic-associated PMC is diverse. Diarrhea is the common feature and is usually watery, voluminous, and without gross blood or mucus. Most patients have abdominal cramps and tenderness, fever, and leukocytosis. However, the symptoms may vary considerably. At one end of the spectrum are patients with annoying diarrhea but no systemic signs or symptoms, while at the other end there is severe systemic toxicity, fever to 104 or 105°F, and peripheral white blood cell counts of up to 50,000 per cubic millimeter. Fecal examination frequently reveals leukocytes. Without specific therapy, the course is highly variable. Some patients have prompt resolution of symptoms with discontinuation of the drug, while others have protracted diarrhea with large stool volumes for up to 8 weeks, with resultant hypoalbuminemia and electrolyte imbalance. Severely ill patients with toxic megacolon and colonic perforation have been reported. In those who are severely ill, mortality rates may be as high as 30 percent, while most patients with minimal symptoms have resolution of disease with discontinuation of antibiotics. In the majority of patients, symptoms begin 4 to 10 days after antibiotic therapy is initiated. However, about 25 percent of patients do not have symptoms until the implicated antimicrobial agent has been discontinued, in some cases as long as 4 weeks afterward. A few cases have been reported within hours after initiation of antibiotic therapy.

Diagnostic evaluation of patients with PMC should include examination of the stool for the presence of *C. difficile* cytotoxin. Although several assays are available, the tissue culture assay is the most practical and sensitive. The assay is performed by incubating stool filtrates with tissue culture cells and monitoring for a cytopathic effect which can be neutralized by antitoxin to either *C. sordellii* (which is cross-reactive with *C. difficile*, but does not cause PMC) or *C. difficile*. Endoscopy, although useful in establishing the presence of PMC, does not establish the etiology and should be reserved for more serious disease manifestations to exclude alternative diagnoses. Isolation of *C. difficile* from stool cultures is difficult.

Skin and soft tissue infections   Originally, three categories of traumatic wound infections due to clostridia were described: simple contamination, anaerobic cellulitis, and anaerobic myonecrosis. With the availability of better anaerobic bacteriologic techniques, it has been necessary to expand this classification to encompass other entities in which clostridia are isolated, usually mixed with other bacteria. These infections are frequently suppurative, and the patients may have systemic symptoms. The classification of clostridial soft tissue disease also includes diffuse spreading cellulitis and fasciitis with systemic toxic manifestations.

SIMPLE CONTAMINATION   Clostridia are cultured most often from wounds in the absence of clinical signs of sepsis. As many as 30 percent of battle wounds can be contaminated by clostridia without signs of suppuration, and 16 percent of penetrating abdominal wounds yield clostridia on culture despite treatment with cephalothin and kanamycin. In cases of trauma clostridia are isolated with equal frequency from suppurative and well-healing wounds. Based on these findings, the diagnosis of clostridial infection should be clinical rather than bacteriologic.

SUPPURATIVE INFECTION IN TISSUE   Clostridia are recovered frequently from various suppurative conditions in conjunction with other anaerobic and aerobic bacteria. These conditions exist with severe local inflammation, but without systemic signs induced by clostridial toxins. These infections include intraabdominal sepsis, empyema, pelvic abscess, subcutaneous abscess, frostbite with gas gangrene, infected stumps in amputees, brain abcess, prostatic abscess, perianal abscess, conjunctivitis, and infected aortic grafts.

Clostridia are isolated in approximately two-thirds of patients with intraabdominal infections resulting from intestinal perforation. *C. ramosum*, *C. perfringens*, and *C. bifermentans* are the most commonly isolated species. The clinical presentation does not differ from that of other patients with similar infections in which clostridia are not cultured (Chap. 102).

An interesting association has been made between malignancy and the isolation of *C. septicum* in the absence of grossly contaminated deep traumatic wounds. A major site for these malignancies is the gastrointestinal tract, particularly the colon. An association with leukemia or other solid tumors also has been noted. Some of these patients present with *C. septicum* bacteremia and have a fulminant clinical course; others develop localized suppurative infection in the abdomen or the abdominal wall without bacteremia. Presumably this infection arises from a silent perforation that leads to intraabdominal abscess formation.

Clostridia have been isolated from suppurative infections of the female genital tract, particularly tuboovarian and pelvic abscess. The major species involved here has been *C. perfringens*. Most of these are mild suppurative infections without evidence of uterine gangrene. Isolation of *C. perfringens* has been reported in as many as 20 percent of diseased gallbladders at surgery. One clinical syndrome, emphysematous cholecystitis, is caused by clostridial species at least 50 percent of the time. In this syndrome there is gas formation in the biliary radicles and the wall of the gallbladder. It is seen most often in diabetic patients. Although the mortality rate in this entity is higher than in more common forms of cholecystitis, there is no evidence of myonecrosis.

Clostridia are among the many organisms found in empyema fluids or isolated by transtracheal aspiration from patients with lung abscesses. There is no clinical clue to the presence of clostridia (as opposed to other organisms) in these infections. *C. perfringens* has been reported as a cause of empyema arising from aspiration pneumonia, pulmonary emboli, and infarction. However, the majority of cases of clostridial empyema are secondary to trauma.

LOCALIZED INFECTION OF THE SKIN AND SOFT TISSUE WITHOUT SYSTEMIC SIGNS   This condition was originally referred to as anaerobic cellulitis. It is a localized infection involving the skin and soft tissue due to clostridia in pure or mixed culture. There are no systemic signs of toxicity, although the infection may invade locally, producing necrosis. These infections tend to be relatively indolent, spreading slowly to contiguous areas. Localized infections tend to be relatively free of pain and edema. Perhaps because of the lack of edema, gas that is limited to the wound and the immediately surrounding tissue may be more evident than in gas gangrene. In these localized infections gas is never found intramuscularly. Cellulitis, perirectal abscesses, and diabetic foot ulcers are typical infections from which clostridial species can be isolated. If inadequately treated, these localized infections advance by extension through subcutaneous tissue and fascial planes into muscle and may produce severe systemic disease, with signs of toxemia.

An interesting localized form of suppurative myositis has been described in heroin addicts. These patients develop local pain and tenderness in discrete areas (particularly the thigh and forearm) with the subsequent appearance of fluctuance and crepitance that require surgical drainage. The unusual aspect of these infections is that they remain localized without systemic signs of toxicity. Moreover these local areas are not necessarily sites of trauma or heroin injection. Pathologically there are subcutaneous abscesses, purulent myositis, and fasciitis, from which clostridia are recovered in pure culture; though, on occasion mixed infections involving aerobes and anaerobes are found.

SPREADING CELLULITIS   This condition is best described as diffuse spreading cellulitis and fasciitis, but myonecrosis is absent, and only mild inflammation is seen in muscle. These patients present with the abrupt onset of a syndrome which progresses rapidly through the fascial planes within hours. Patients demonstrate suppuration and gas in soft tissues as well as overwhelming toxemia. This infection is rapidly fatal. On physical examination there is subcutaneous crepitance, but little localized pain. Surgery is of no proven value because there are no discretely involved tissues amenable to resection, as may be the case in myonecrosis.

However, incision of the affected area should be performed, because in rapidly advancing fasciitis, it is still the cornerstone of therapy. The initial local lesion may be quite inocuous and arises from an area involved by tumor or other infection and not from injury. The systemic toxic effects include hemolysis and injury of capillary membranes. Usually, this infection is uniformly fatal within 48 h, despite intensive therapy involving antitoxin and exchange transfusion. This syndrome is seen most commonly in patients with carcinoma, especially of the sigmoid or the cecum. Presumably, the tumor invades the fascia, and tumoral contents leak into the abdominal wall. These patients present with extreme toxicity and occasionally with total-body crepitance. The syndrome differs from necrotizing fasciitis caused by other organisms in three respects: (1) the extreme rapidity of death with clostridia, (2) the rapidity with which the organism moves through tissue, and (3) the systemic effects of the toxin typified by massive hemolysis.

CLOSTRIDIAL MYONECROSIS (GAS GANGRENE)   Clostridial myonecrosis occurs when bacteria invade healthy muscle from adjacent traumatized muscle or soft tissue. The infection originates in a wound contaminated with clostridia. Despite the fact that more than 30 percent of deep wounds are infected with clostridia, the incidence of clostridial myonecrosis is quite low. These infections occur in military or civilian settings. In wartime situations, an essential factor in the genesis of gas gangrene appears to be trauma, particularly involving deep lacerated wounds of muscle. The entity of clostridial myonecrosis is relatively uncommon after simple, through-and-through bullet wounds without shattering of bone, and relatively common following shrapnel fragmentation wounds, particularly when deep muscle is involved. In civilian cases, gas gangrene can occur after trauma or surgery. The trauma need not be severe; however, the wound must be deep, necrotic, and without communication to the surface, conditions which favor anaerobic infection.

The incubation period of gas gangrene is usually short: almost always less than 3 days, and frequently less than 24 h. Eighty percent of cases are caused by *C. perfringens,* while *C. novyi, C. septicum,* and *C. histolyticum* cause most of the other cases. Typically, gas gangrene begins with the sudden appearance of pain in the region of the wound, a point that helps to differentiate it from spreading cellulitis. Once established, the pain steadily increases in severity, but remains localized to the infected area and only spreads if the infection spreads. Soon after pain develops, local swelling and edema, accompanied by a thin, often hemorrhagic exudate appear. These patients frequently develop marked tachycardia, but elevation in temperature may be only minimal. Gas frequently is not obvious at this early stage and may be absent completely. Frothiness of the wound exudate may be noted. The skin is tense, white, often marbled with blue, and cooler than normal. The symptoms rapidly progress; swelling, edema, and toxemia increase and a profuse serous discharge appears. The discharge can have a peculiar sweetish smell. Gram stain of the wound exudate shows many gram-positive rods with relatively few inflammatory cells.

The diagnosis hinges on surgery to demonstrate and define the extent of muscle involvement. At surgery, the muscle is characteristically pale, edematous, and does not contract when probed with the scalpel. As the surgeon dissects further, the muscle appears beefy red and nonviable and can progress to become black, friable, and gangrenous. It is important to establish a diagnosis early, and frozen section biopsy of muscle has been proposed as a diagnostic modality.

Patients with myonecrosis are reported to have peculiar changes in mental status. Despite hypotension, renal failure, and often body crepitance, they have a heightened awareness of their surroundings. This increased mental acuity persists until just before death, when they lapse into toxic delirium and coma. They have a complete appreciation of the gravity of the circumstances, and a most profound and distressing terror of impending death. In untreated cases, as the local wounds progress, the skin becomes bronzed; bullae appear, become filled with dark red fluid, and are accompanied by dark patches of cutaneous gangrene. Gas appears in later phases but may not be as obvious as in anaerobic cellulitis. Jaundice is rarely seen in wound gas gangrene (in contrast to uterine infections), and when it does appear, is almost invariably associated with hemoglobinuria, hemoglobinemia, and septicemia. There have been reports of cases of clostridial myonecrosis without a history of trauma. These patients have bullous lesions and crepitance of the skin; they present with a rapidly worsening course which includes myonecrosis, especially of the extremities.

CLOSTRIDIAL SEPTICEMIA Clostridial septicemia is an uncommon but almost invariably fatal illness occurring after clostridial infection primarily of the uterus, colon, or biliary tract. This entity must be differentiated from transient clostridial bacteremia which is much more common than septicemia. Bacteremia is not necessarily associated with a poor outcome. *C. perfringens* causes the majority of septicemic infections, as well as the majority of cases of transient bacteremia. *C. septicum,* which is more common in patients with malignant disease, and *C. sordellii* and *C. novyi* account for most of the remainder of cases. Clostridia account for 1 to 2.5 percent of all positive blood cultures in major hospital centers. The majority of

these isolates represent transient bacteremia and only rarely true septicemia. In transient bacteremias clostridia are isolated frequently from the blood with other aerobes or anaerobes. Clinically, primary sites of infection can be identified in fewer than half the cases, with pelvic, biliary, or bowel sources the most common.

The majority of cases of clostridial septicemia originate from the female genital tract following septic abortion. In these cases when a foreign body or solution is introduced into the cervix, clostridia are introduced from the foreign object itself or from the perineum or vagina. In the uterus there may be residual necrotic fetal and placental tissues and traumatized endometrium that allow the growth of clostridia. Only a small fraction of cases of septic abortion are followed by serious septicemic illness. Approximately 1 percent of all women hospitalized after septic abortion have clostridial sepsis.

In these patients, sepsis, fever, and chills begin from 1 to 3 days after the attempted abortion. The initial signs are malaise, headache, severe myalgias, abdominal pain, nausea, vomiting, and occasionally diarrhea. Frequently a bloody or brown vaginal discharge is noted. Patients may rapidly develop oliguria, hypotension, jaundice, and hemoglobinuria. The hemolysis, which is secondary to *C. perfringens* alpha toxin, causes a characteristic bronzing of the skin. As in myonecrosis, the mental status of severely ill patients is characterized by increased alertness and apprehension. Local examination of the pelvis reveals foul cervical discharge, occasionally with gas. Frequently laceration marks around the cervix or perforation of the cervical segment are evident. If the infection involves the myometrium or has spread to the adnexa, extreme tenderness, guarding, and an adnexal mass may be found.

Laboratory studies in septicemic patients reveal an elevated white count and may show pink, hemoglobin-tinged plasma. Anemia is proportional to the degree of hemolysis, and the hematocrit may be extremely low. Platelets may be reduced, and there is often evidence of disseminated intravascular coagulation. Oliguria or anuria, increasingly refractory hypotension, and hemorrhage and bruising may develop.

Clostridia may enter the bloodstream from the gastrointestinal or biliary tract. This occurrence is associated with ulcerative lesions or obstruction of the small or large intestine, necrotic or infiltrating malignancy, bowel surgery, or various abdominal catastrophes. The patient may present with an acute febrile illness with chills and fever, but no other signs of localized infection. Intravascular hemolysis occurs in as many as half the cases. Biliary or gastrointestinal symptoms, if present, may be the only clue to the etiology. Positive blood cultures provide the definitive clue for the diagnosis in these patients.

Patients with malignant disease also can develop rapidly fatal clostridial sepsis, particularly from a gastrointestinal focus. The most common species in this setting is *C. septicum.* Characteristic signs and symptoms include fever, tachycardia, hypotension, abdominal pain or tenderness, nausea, vomiting, and preterminally, coma. The tachycardia may be out of proportion to the fever. Only about 20 to 30 percent of patients will develop hemolysis. A striking feature of this syndrome is the rapidity of death, which frequently occurs in less than 12 h.

The relatively common entity of transient bacteremia due to clostridia can arise in any hospitalized patient but is most common with a predisposing focus in the gastrointestinal tract, biliary tract, or uterus. Fever frequently resolves within 24 to 48 h without therapy. Despite the finding of clostridial bacteremia following septic abortions and the frequent isolation of clostridia from the lochia, most of these patients do not have evidence of septicemia. In one series of 60 patients with clostridial bacteremia, half of the cases could be associated with an infected site, while the other half had a totally unrelated illness, such as tuberculous pneumonia, meningitis, or benign gastroenteritis. Frequently, by the time the blood culture reports return, the patients are completely well and sometimes have been discharged. Therefore, when a blood culture report is positive for clostridia, the patient must be assessed clinically rather than simply treated for the positive blood culture alone.

DIAGNOSIS The diagnosis of clostridial disease must be based primarily on clinical findings. Because of the presence of clostridia in many wounds, their mere isolation from any site including the blood does not necessarily indicate severe disease. Smears of wound exudates, uterine scrapings, or cervical discharge may show abundant large gram-positive rods as well as other organisms. Cultures should be placed in selective media and incubated anaerobically for identification of clostridia.

The urine of patients with severe clostridial sepsis may contain protein and casts, and the patients may develop severe uremia. Profound alterations of circulating erythrocytes are seen in such severely toxemic patients. Patients have a hemolytic anemia, which develops extremely rapidly, along with hemoglobinemia, hemoglobinuria, and elevated levels of serum bilirubin. Spherocytosis, increased osmotic and mechanical red blood cell fragility, erythrophagocytosis, and methemoglobinemia have been described. Disseminated intravascular coagulation may be seen in patients with severe infection. In patients with severe septicemia, a Wright or Gram stain smear of peripheral blood or buffy coat may demonstrate clostridia.

X-ray examination sometimes provides an important clue to the diagnosis by revealing gas in muscles, subcutaneous tissue, or the uterus. However, the finding of gas is not pathognomonic for clostridial infection. Other bacteria, particularly anaerobes, mixed with aerobic organisms may produce gas.

The diagnosis of clostridial myonecrosis can be established by frozen section biopsy of muscle. The diagnosis of *C. difficile*–associated colitis is made by the identification of *C. difficile* toxin in stool.

TREATMENT The treatment of choice for clostridial infection is penicillin G, 20,000,000 units a day. In cases of penicillin sensitivity or allergy, other antibiotics should be considered, but all should be tested for in vitro efficacy because of the occasional isolation of resistant strains. Chloramphenicol, 4 g per day, usually is an effective alternative. Clostridia are generally, but not universally, susceptible in vitro to cefoxitin, carbenicillin, clindamycin, metronidazole, doxycycline, minocycline, tetracycline, and vancomycin. The actual choice of antimicrobial agent should be tailored to the specific conditions.

Simple contamination of a wound with clostridia should not be treated with antibiotics.

Localized skin and soft tissue infection can be managed by debridement rather than with systemic antibiotics. Drugs are required when the process extends into adjacent tissue, or when fever and systemic signs of sepsis are present.

Suppurative infections should be treated with antibiotics. Frequently, broad-spectrum antibiotics must be used because of mixed flora in these infections. Aminoglycosides can be used for the aerobic gram-negative bacteria and mixed infections.

The use of a polyvalent gas gangrene antitoxin is still recommended by some authorities. At present the antitoxin is not produced in the United States, and most centers have discontinued its use in management of patients with suspected gas gangrene or clostridial postabortion sepsis because of questionable efficacy and the substantial risk of hypersensitivity to horse serum.

The use of hyperbaric oxygen in the treatment of gas gangrene is also controversial. Studies in humans are not well designed to answer questions on efficacy, but several knowledgeable authors believe that hyperbaric oxygen therapy has contributed to dramatic clinical improvement. It may, however, be associated with untoward effects due to oxygen toxicity and high atmospheric pressure. Some centers without hyperbaric chambers have reported acceptable mortality rates, indicating that expert surgical and medical management and control of complications are probably the most important factors in treating gas gangrene.

Treatment of *C. difficile* enterocolitis The treatment of *C. difficile*–associated colitis requires discontinuation of the offending antimicrobial agent. In some patients symptoms will resolve over a period of 2 weeks. However, specific therapy has been beneficial. The most widely used agent in the treatment of antibiotic-associated diarrhea ascribed to *C. difficile* is oral vancomycin. Most strains of *C. difficile* are susceptible to achievable concentrations of vancomycin. This antibiotic is poorly absorbed after oral administration and high levels appear in the stool. Dosing should begin with 125 mg orally four times a day for 7 to 10 days, but the dose may be increased to 500 mg orally four times a day. It has been reported that oral metronidazole at a dose of 500 mg three times a day for 7 to 10 days is also effective. A few cases of *C. difficile* colitis have developed after oral metronidazole therapy for other infections. Because response to the two treatment regimens is comparable and metronidazole is less costly, it is reasonable to initiate treatment with metronidazole. However, if diarrhea persists, then therapy should be changed to oral vancomycin. Therapy with oral cholestyramine was initially reported to provide dramatic improvement in patients with pseudomembranous colitis (PMC). Subsequent studies have shown that cholestyramine, as well as other anionic resins, bind the cytotoxin produced by *C. difficile*. However, comparative trials in animals have shown that cholestyramine is distinctly inferior to oral vancomycin. Combination therapy with oral vancomycin and cholestyramine in refractory cases has been successful. Although not adequately tested, bacitracin may be promising in the therapy of PMC. This drug is poorly absorbed when administered orally, resulting in high levels in the colonic lumen. Toxin production in PMC persists in 5 to 10 percent of treated patients. Relapses are reported in up to 20 percent of patients, but patients usually respond to a second course of oral vancomycin.

REFERENCES

BARTLETT JG et al: Antibiotic-associated pseudomembranous colitis due to toxin-producing clostridia. N Engl J Med 298:531, 1978

——, TAYLOR NS: Antibiotic-associated colitis, in *Medical Microbiology*, CSF Easman, J Jeljaszewicz (eds). London, Academic Press, 1982, pp 1–48

BORNSTEIN DL: Clostridial myonecrosis, in *Medical Microbiology and Infectious Diseases*, A Braude (ed). Philadelphia, Saunders, 1981, Chap. 239

DORNBUSCH K et al: Antibiotic susceptibility of *Clostridium* species isolated from human infections. Scand J Infect Dis 7:127, 1975

FINEGOLD SM: *Anaerobic Bacteria in Human Disease*. New York, Academic, 1977

GORBACH SL: Other *Clostridium* species (including gas gangrene), in *Principles and Practice of Infectious Diseases*, GL Mandell et al (eds). New York, Wiley, 1985

——, THADEPALLI H: Isolation of *Clostridium* in human infections: Evaluation of 114 cases. J Infect Dis 131:S81, 1975

JENDRZEJEWSKI JW et al: Nontraumatic clostridial myonecrosis. Am J Med 65:542, 1978

KORANSKY JR et al: *Clostridium septicum* bacteremia. Am J Med 66:63, 1979

LAWRENCE G et al: Prevention of necrotizing enteritis in Papua, New Guinea by active immunization. Lancet 1:227, 1979

PRITCHARD JA, WHALLEY PJ: Abortion complicated by *Clostridium perfringens* infection. Am J Gynecol 111:484, 1971

SMITH LDS: Virulence factors of *Clostridium perfringens*. Rev Infect Dis 1:254, 1979

SUTTER VL, FINEGOLD SM: Susceptibility of anaerobic bacteria to 23 antimicrobial agents. Antimicrob Agents Chemother 10:736, 1976

TEASLEY DG et al: Prospective randomized trial of metronidazole versus vancomycin for *Clostridium difficile*–associated diarrhea and colitis. Lancet 2:1043, 1983

THADEPALLI H et al: Abdominal trauma, anaerobes, and antibiotics. Surg Gynecol Obstet 137:270, 1973

102 INFECTIONS DUE TO MIXED ANAEROBIC ORGANISMS

DENNIS L. KASPER

DEFINITIONS Anaerobic bacteria are organisms that require reduced oxygen tension for growth, failing to grow on the surface of solid media in 10% CO_2 in air. Microaerophilic bacteria can grow in 10% CO_2 in air or under anaerobic or aerobic conditions. Facultative bacteria can grow in the presence or absence of air. This chapter addresses infections caused by nonsporulating anaerobic bacteria. In general, anaerobes associated with human infections are relatively aerotolerant. They can survive for as long as 72 h in the presence of oxygen, although generally they will not multiply in this environment. Less pathogenic anaerobic bacteria, which are also part of the normal flora, die after brief contact with oxygen, even in low concentrations.

The nonsporulating anaerobic bacteria exist as normal flora on the mucosal surfaces of humans and animals. The major reservoirs of these bacteria are the mouth, gastrointestinal tract, skin, and the female genital tract. Of the oral flora, anaerobes are the predominant commensal organisms, ranging in concentrations from 10^9 per milliliter in saliva to 10^{12} in gingival scrapings. In the oral cavity the relative concentration of anaerobic to aerobic bacteria ranges from 1:1 on the surface of the tooth to 100 to 1000:1 in the gingival crevice. Anaerobic bacteria are not found in the normal intestine until the distal ileum. In the colon, the proportion of anaerobes increases significantly, as does the overall bacterial count. For example, in the colon there are 10^{11} to 10^{12} organisms per gram of stool, with a ratio of anaerobes to aerobes of approximately 1000:1. In the female genital tract there are approximately 10^9 organisms per milliliter of secretions, with a ratio of anaerobes to aerobes of approximately 10:1. Hundreds of species of anaerobic bacteria have been identified as part of the normal flora of humans. Identification of as many as 500 different anaerobic species in fecal specimens reflects the diversity of the anaerobic flora. Despite the complex array of bacteria which exist in the normal flora, relatively few species are isolated commonly from human infection.

Anaerobic infections occur when the harmonious relationship between the host and bacteria is disrupted. Any site in the body is susceptible to infection with these indigenous organisms when the mucosal barriers or skin are compromised by surgery, trauma, tumor, or situations, such as ischemia or necrosis, which reduce local tissue redox potentials. Because the sites that are colonized by anaerobic bacteria contain many species of bacteria, disruption of anatomic barriers allows penetration of many organisms, resulting frequently in mixed infections involving multiple species of these anaerobes combined with facultative or microaerophilic organisms. Such mixed infections are seen in the head and neck (chronic sinusitis, chronic otitis media, Ludwig's angina, and periodontal abscesses). Brain abscesses and subdural empyema are the most frequent anaerobic infections of the central nervous system. Anaerobes are responsible for pleuropulmonary diseases such as aspiration pneumonia, necrotizing pneumonia, abscesses, or empyema. Similarly, anaerobes play an important role in various intraabdominal infections such as peritonitis, intraabdominal abscesses, and liver abscesses. They are isolated frequently in female genital tract infections such as salpingitis, pelvic peritonitis, tuboovarian abscess, vulvovaginal abscesses, septic abortions, and endometritis. Anaerobic bacteria also are frequently found in infections of the skin, soft tissue, bones, and as a cause of bacteremia.

ETIOLOGY It is useful to consider the classification of these organisms based on Gram-staining characteristics. The major anaerobic gram-positive cocci producing disease are peptostreptococci. The principal anaerobic gram-negative bacilli are the *Bacteroides* family, which includes the *Bacteroides fragilis* group, fusobacteria, and the pigmented *Bacteroides*. The *B. fragilis* group contains the anaerobic pathogens most frequently isolated from clinical infections. Members of this group are part of the normal bowel flora. Several distinct species comprise the group, including *B. fragilis, B. thetaiotaomicron, B. distasonis, B. vulgaris,* and *B. ovatis*. Of this group *B. fragilis* is the most important clinical isolate. However, in the normal fecal flora, the frequency with which *B. fragilis* is isolated is low compared to other *Bacteroides* species. A second major group of *Bacteroides* are part of the indigenous oral flora. These are primarily pigment-producing bacteria which were previously classified under the species *B. melaninogenicus*. Current terminology of this group has changed so that several distinct species are recognized, including *B. gingivalis, B. asaccharolyticus,* as well as *B. melaninogenicus*. Fusobacteria are also isolated from clinical infections, including necrotizing pneumonia and abscesses.

Infections due to anaerobic bacteria most frequently are mixed infections with more than one organism. Infections may be due to one or several anaerobic species, or a combination of anaerobic organisms and aerobic bacteria acting synergistically. The concept of mixed infections requires a restatement of Koch's postulates since the idea of one organism, one disease, which applies to many infections, does not apply to infections caused by multiple strains of bacteria behaving in a cooperative fashion.

APPROACH TO THE PATIENT WITH ANAEROBIC BACTERIAL INFECTIONS There are seven important features to remember when approaching the patient with presumptive infection due to anaerobic bacteria. (1) Most of these organisms are harmless commensals, and very few cause disease. (2) In order for these organisms to cause infection, they must spread beyond the normal mucosal barriers. (3) Conditions favoring the propagation of these bacteria, particularly a lowered oxidation-reduction potential, are necessary. Therefore, these infections arise in sites of trauma, tissue destruction, compromised vascular supply, or as complications of preexisting infections that produce necrosis. (4) A characteristic of anaerobic infections is the complex array of infecting flora. For example, as many as 12 different types of organisms can be isolated from suppurative sites. (5) Anaerobic organisms tend to be found in abscess cavities or in necrotic tissue. The detection of an abscess in a patient which fails to yield organisms on routine culture should alert the physician that this abscess is likely to contain anaerobic bacteria. However, often smears of this "sterile pus" are teeming with bacteria on Gram stain. The malodorous nature of the pus is also an important clue to anaerobe infections. Although some facultative organisms, such as *Staphylococcus aureus,* also are capable of causing abscesses, abscesses in organs or within deeper body tissues should call to mind anaerobic infection. (6) Treatment need not be directed at all of the organisms in the infectious site. However, some species in particular require specific therapy. The best example of this principle is the need to treat *B. fragilis*. Many of these synergistic infections can be cured with antibiotics directed at some, but not all, of the organisms. The hypothesis is that antibiotic therapy, combined with drainage, disrupts the interdependent relationship among the bacteria and that species which are resistant to the antibiotic do not survive without the co-infective organisms. (7) Manifestations of disseminated intravascular coagulation are unusual in patients with infection due to these bacteria.

EPIDEMIOLOGY Difficulties in obtaining appropriate cultures, contamination of cultures by aerobic bacteria or normal flora, and the lack of readily available reliable culture techniques have made accurate incidence or prevalence data on anaerobic infections unavailable. It can be stated, however, that these infections are encountered frequently in hospitals with active surgical, trauma, and obstetric and gynecologic services. In several centers anaerobic bacteria account for approximately 8 to 10 percent of positive blood cultures. In these situations *B. fragilis* predominates. Also, anaerobes have been isolated in up to 50 percent of clinical cultures from other sites.

PATHOGENESIS Because of the specific growth requirements of these organisms and their presence as commensals on mucosal surfaces, conditions must arise which allow these organisms to penetrate mucosal barriers and enter tissue with a lowered oxidation-reduction potential. Therefore, tissue ischemia, trauma, surgery, perforated viscus, shock, or aspiration provide environments conducive to the proliferation of anaerobes. Highly fastidious anaerobes lack the enzyme superoxide dismutase (SOD) that in other organisms reduces toxic superoxide radicals, thereby lessening the potentially lethal effects of superoxide. A general correlation exists between the intracellular concentration of SOD and the oxygen tolerance of anaerobic bacteria; organisms that contain SOD have a selective advantage after exposure to aerobic environments. For example, in the case of a perforated viscus, hundreds of species of anaerobic bacteria are spilled into the peritoneal cavity, but many of these organisms are unable to survive because the highly vascularized tissue provides an adequate oxygen supply. The entry of oxygen into the environment results in selection of aerotolerant organisms.

Anaerobic bacteria produce a number of exoenzymes which are capable of enhancing their virulence. These enzymes include a heparinase elaborated by *B. fragilis* which may contribute to intravascular clotting and lead to a requirement for increased doses of heparin in patients on heparin therapy. Collagenase, produced by *B. melaninogenicus,* may enhance tissue destruction. Both *B. fragilis* and *B. melaninogenicus* possess lipopolysaccharides (endotoxins) which lack the biologic potency characteristic of endotoxins associated with aerobic gram-negative bacteria. The biologic inactivity of the endotoxin may account for the rarity of shock, disseminated intravascular coagulation, and purpura in *Bacteroides* bacteremia compared to facultative and aerobic gram-negative rod bacteremia.

B. fragilis is unique among the various pathogenic anaerobic species in its ability to form abscesses as a sole pathogen. *B. fragilis* has capsular polysaccharides which are a virulence factor, and these polysaccharides stimulate directly the formation of abscesses in experimental models of intraabdominal sepsis. Other anaerobic species require the presence of synergistic facultative species to induce abscesses.

CLINICAL MANIFESTATIONS Anaerobic infections of the head and neck Infections of the mouth can be divided into those infections that arise from the supragingival or subgingival dental plaque. Supragingival plaque formation begins with the adherence of gram-positive bacteria to the tooth surface. This form of plaque is influenced by salivary and dietary components, oral hygiene, and local host factors. Once established, the acquisition of pathogenic bacteria as well as an increase in the amount of plaque is responsible for the ultimate development of gingivitis. Early bacteriologic changes in the supragingival plaque initiate an inflammatory response in the gingiva. These changes include edema, swelling, and increase in gingival fluid and are responsible for the development of caries and endodontic (pulp) infections. Also, these changes are responsible partially for the subsequent pathogenic alteration in the subgingival plaque which arise from poor or inadequate oral hygiene. Subgingival plaque is associated with periodontal disease and disseminated infection arising from the oral cavity. Bacteria that colonize the subgingival area are primarily anaerobic. The black-pigmented gram-negative anaerobic bacilli belonging to the *Bacteroides* group, principally *B. gingivalis* and *B. melaninogenicus*, are the most important. Infections in this area are frequently mixed and involve both anaerobic and aerobic bacteria. After establishment of local infection either in root canals or in the periodontal area, infection may extend into the mandible, causing osteomyelitis; to the maxillary sinuses; or to local tissues in the submandibular or submental spaces, depending upon which teeth are involved. Periodontitis also may result in spreading infection that can involve adjacent bone or soft tissues. This form of infection may be due either to oral *Bacteroides* or to *Fusobacterium.*

GINGIVITIS Gingivitis may become a necrotizing infection (trench mouth, Vincent's stomatitis). The onset of disease is usually sudden and is associated with tender bleeding gums, foul breath, and a bad taste. The gingival mucosa, especially the papillae between the teeth, become ulcerated and may be covered by a gray exudate which is removable with gentle pressure. These patients may become systemically ill, developing fever, cervical lymphadenopathy, and leukocytosis. Occasionally, ulcerative gingivitis can spread to the buccal mucosa, the teeth, and the mandible or maxilla, resulting in widespread destruction of bone and soft tissue. This infection is termed *acute necrotizing ulcerative mucositis* (cancrum oris, noma). This infection destroys tissue rapidly, causing the teeth to fall out and large areas of bone, even the whole mandible, to be sloughed. A strong putrid odor frequently is present, although the lesions are not painful. The gangrenous lesions eventually heal, leaving large disfiguring defects. This infection is seen most commonly following a debilitating illness, or in severely malnourished children in underdeveloped areas of the world. It has been known to complicate leukemia or to develop in individuals with a genetic deficiency of catalase.

ACUTE NECROTIZING INFECTIONS OF THE PHARYNX These occur in association with ulcerative gingivitis, although they also may occur alone. The major complaints are an extremely sore throat, foul breath, and a bad taste in the mouth, accompanied by a sensation of choking and fever. Examination of the pharynx demonstrates that the tonsillar pillars are swollen, red, and ulcerated and covered with a grayish membrane that peels easily. Lymphadenopathy and leukocytosis are common. The disease may last for only a few days or may persist for weeks if not treated. Lesions begin unilaterally but may spread to the other side of the pharynx or the larynx. Aspiration of the infected material by the patient can result in lung abscesses. Soft tissue infection of the oral-facial area may or may not be odontogenic in origin. *Ludwig's angina,* a periodontal infection usually arising from the third molar, may produce submandibular cellulitis that results in marked local swelling of tissues with pain, trismus, and superior and posterior displacement of the tongue. Submandibular swelling of the neck develops, which can result in the inability to swallow and respiratory obstruction. In some cases tracheostomy may be life-saving. Both mixed anaerobic and aerobic infection originating from the oral flora have been implicated in the etiology of this syndrome.

FASCIAL INFECTIONS These arise from the spread of organisms originating in the upper airways to potential spaces formed by the fascial planes of the head and neck. Although there are few well-documented reports on the microbiology of these syndromes, anaerobes from the oral flora have been implicated in many cases studied with adequate bacteriology. *Staphylococcus aureus* and *Streptococcus pyogenes* have been implicated in space infections related to overlying skin infections, such as boils or impetigo, whereas anaerobes are associated with space infections arising from diseases of the mucous membranes, dental manipulations, or occurring spontaneously.

SINUSITIS AND OTITIS While there are a few reports of the role of anaerobic bacteria in acute sinusitis, it is likely that these reports underestimate the frequency with which anaerobes are involved in these infections because of improper collection of specimens. Material for culture is obtained by aspiration at the inferior nasal meatus without decontamination of the nasal mucous membranes. In contrast, no conflict exists concerning the importance of anaerobes in chronic sinusitis. Anaerobic bacteria were found in 52 percent of specimens collected during external frontoethmoidotomy or radical antrotomy via the canine fossa. These methods avoid nasal mucosal bacterial contamination. Similarly, anaerobic bacteria are much more easily implicated in chronic suppurative otitis media than in acute otitis media. Purulent exudate from chronically draining ears has been found to contain anaerobes in up to 50 percent of patients. A variety of anaerobes have been isolated from these chronic infections, particularly *Bacteroides* species. In contrast to other infections of the head and neck, *B. fragilis* has been isolated from up to 28 percent of patients with chronic otitis media.

COMPLICATIONS OF ANAEROBIC HEAD AND NECK INFECTIONS Contiguous spread of these infections craniad may result in osteomyelitis of the skull or mandible, or in intracranial infections such as brain abscesses or subdural empyema. Caudad spread can produce mediastinitis or pleuropulmonary infections. Hematogenous complications also may result from anaerobic infections of the head and neck. Bacteremia, which can occasionally be polymicrobial, has been reported and can lead to endocarditis or other distant infections. When infections spread to produce suppurative thrombophlebitis of the internal jugular vein, a destructive syndrome with prolonged fever, bacteremia, septic emboli to both the lung and brain, and multiple metastatic foci of suppurative infection may develop. This syndrome has been reported with septicemia from species of *Fusobacterium* following exudative pharyngitis. This entity (Lameer's postanginal septicemia) is uncommon in this era of antimicrobial agents.

Central nervous system infections Of the many infections of the central nervous system, brain abscesses most frequently are associated with anaerobic bacteria. If optimal bacteriologic techniques are employed, as many as 85 percent of brain abscesses yield anaerobic bacteria. The anaerobic bacteria found most often in these infections are anaerobic gram-positive cocci, followed in frequency by fusobacteria and *Bacteroides* species. Frequently, facultative or microaerophilic streptococci and coliforms are involved in brain abscesses as mixed infections. Brain abscesses arise from either direct extension of suppurative infection involving the sinuses, mastoids, or middle ear, or from hematogenous dissemination from infection elsewhere, particularly the lungs. Brain abscess is discussed in greater detail in Chap. 346.

Pleuropulmonary infections   Anaerobic pleuropulmonary infections result from the aspiration of oropharyngeal contents, which is associated commonly with an altered state of consciousness or absent gag reflex. There are four clinical syndromes associated with anaerobic pleuropulmonary infection produced by aspiration: simple aspiration pneumonia, necrotizing pneumonia, lung abscess, and empyema.

ANAEROBIC ASPIRATION PNEUMONITIS   Anaerobic aspiration pneumonitis must be distinguished from two other types of aspiration pneumonitis, neither of which are bacterial diseases. One aspiration syndrome results from aspiration of solids, usually food. Obstruction of major airways with resulting atelectasis is typical. Moderate nonspecific inflammation occurs. Therapy consists of removal of the foreign body.

A second aspiration syndrome is more easily confused with bacterial aspiration. This is the so-called Mendelson's syndrome, resulting from regurgitation of stomach contents and aspiration of chemical material, usually gastric juices. Pulmonary inflammation including destruction of alveolar lining with transudation of fluid into the alveolar space occurs with remarkable rapidity. Typically this syndrome develops within hours often following anesthesia when the gag reflex is depressed. The patient becomes tachypneic, hypoxic, and febrile. The leukocyte count may rise, and the chest x-ray may evolve suddenly from normal to a complete whiteout bilaterally within 8 to 24 h. Minimal sputum production occurs. The pulmonary signs and symptoms can resolve quickly with symptomatic therapy or result in respiratory failure with subsequent development of bacterial superinfection over a period of days. Antibiotic therapy is not indicated unless bacterial infection supervenes. The signs of bacterial infection include sputum, persistent fever, leukocytosis, and clinical evidence of sepsis.

In contrast to these syndromes, bacterial aspiration pneumonia develops more slowly. It is seen in patients who are hospitalized and have a depressed gag reflex, elderly patients, or those with transient impaired consciousness such as can result from seizures or alcoholic blackouts. Patients who enter the hospital with this syndrome typically have been ill for several days, generally complain of low-grade fever, malaise, and sputum production. Usually the history reveals a predisposition for aspiration, such as alcohol overdose or residence in a nursing home. Sputum characteristically is not malodorous unless the process has been present for at least a week. Mixed bacterial flora with many polymorphonuclear leukocytes are present on Gram stain; reliable cultures can be obtained only by avoiding contamination with normal oral flora, i.e., by transtracheal aspiration. Chest x-rays show consolidation in dependent pulmonary segments. These dependent areas are the basilar segments of the lower lobes if the patient aspirated while upright or sitting, as is noted commonly in nursing home patients, or in the posterior segment of the upper lobe, usually on the right side, or the superior segment of the lower lobe if aspiration has occurred in the supine position. Organisms isolated reflect the pharyngeal flora; *B. melaninogenicus, Fusobacterium* species, and anaerobic cocci are the most frequent isolates. The patient who aspirates in a hospital setting also may have mixed infection involving facultative bacteria, including enteric gram-negative rods.

NECROTIZING PNEUMONITIS   This is a form of anaerobic pneumonitis characterized by numerous but small abscesses which spread to involve several pulmonary segments. The process can be indolent or fulminating. This syndrome is observed less commonly than either aspiration pneumonia or lung abscess, and includes features of both types of infection.

ANAEROBIC LUNG ABSCESSES   These result from subacute anaerobic pulmonary infection. The clinical syndrome typically involves a history of constitutional symptoms including malaise, weight loss, fever, chills, and foul-smelling sputum which may occur over a period of weeks. Patients who develop lung abscesses characteristically have dental infection and periodontitis, but there are reports of lung abscesses in patients who are edentulous. Abscess cavities may be single or multiple, and generally occur in dependent pulmonary segments. Anaerobic abscesses must be distinguished from tuberculosis, neoplasia, and other causes of lung abscess, despite the fact that the clinical syndrome is usually typical. Oral anaerobes predominate, although *B. fragilis* is isolated in up to 10 percent of cases. *Staph. aureus* may be found as well. Although in vitro resistance by *B. fragilis* to penicillin is common, this antibiotic generally is successful in treatment when combined with vigorous pulmonary toilet, perhaps because of the synergistic nature of the infection. Bronchoscopy is indicated only to rule out the presence of airway obstruction but should be delayed until the antimicrobial has begun to affect the disease process so that it does not spread the infection. Bronchoscopy has no role in enhancing drainage. Surgery is almost never indicated and can be hazardous because of spillage of abscess contents into the lungs.

Empyema   Empyema is a manifestation of long-standing anaerobic pulmonary infection. The clinical presentation resembles other anaerobic pulmonary infections including the presence of foul-smelling sputum. Patients may complain of pleuritic chest pain and marked chest wall tenderness.

Empyema may be masked by overlying pneumonitis and should be considered especially in cases of persistent fever in a patient receiving therapy. Diligent physical examination and the use of ultrasound to localize a loculated empyema are important diagnostic tools. The presence of a foul-smelling exudate obtained by thoracentesis is typical. Drainage is required. Defervescence, a return to a feeling of well-being, and resolution of the process may require several months of therapy for empyema as well as lung abscesses.

Extension from a subdiaphragmatic infection also may result in an anaerobic empyema. Septic pulmonary emboli may originate from intraabdominal or female genital tract infections and can produce anaerobic pneumonia.

Intraabdominal infections   Because anaerobic bacteria outnumber aerobic bacteria in normal bowel flora by 100 to 1000:1, it is not surprising that disruption of the bowel wall will result in peritonitis with a preponderance of anaerobic bacteria. Colonic perforation releases large numbers of these bacteria and therefore entails a high risk of intraabdominal sepsis. Following peritonitis, abscesses may develop in any part of the peritoneal cavity and retroperitoneal spaces. The peritoneum reacts with a marked inflammatory response and effectively walls off the infection in a very short time. If an intraperitoneal abscess is localized, typical signs and symptoms appear (Chap. 87). For example, *subphrenic abscess* may cause an ipsilateral sympathetic pleural effusion, and the patient may have pleuritic type pain and splinting of the hemidiaphragm on the affected side. Constitutional symptoms include fever, chills, and malaise. There is a history of abdominal surgery, trauma, or other conditions that predispose to disruption of the bowel wall. In contrast, more subtle clinical signs must be sought when an intraabdominal abscess is not readily localized. Peritonitis and abscess formation are closely related processes. Often following surgery to repair a bowel perforation, a patient may be febrile without localizing abdominal signs or general clinical deterioration. Persistent leukocytosis may be related to the operative procedure and/or resolving peritonitis. Attention should be directed to the presence and character of wound drainage which if profuse, cloudy, or foul-smelling suggests the possibility of purulent anaerobic infection. Gram stain revealing a mixed fecal flora is frequently helpful. *B. fragilis* is isolated from approximately 70 percent of surgical wounds after trauma involving perforation of the lower gut, and a similar percentage of isolates follows elective colonic surgery. Antibiotics effective against *B. fragilis,* as well as facultative bacteria, are important in therapy, although they are not a replacement for surgical or percutaneous drainage. Appendicitis with perforation and abscess formation is the most common intraabdominal anaerobic infection. Diverticulitis involves nonsporulating anaerobes and can result in perforation followed by generalized peritonitis, but generally results in small walled-off infections that do not require surgical drainage. Abdominal ultrasound, gallium- or indium-labeled neutrophil scans, computerized tomography (CT) scans, or combined liver-spleen and lung scans may be helpful in localizing intraabdominal abscesses. Surgical exploration, however, may be necessary to establish the site of such an infection.

Among visceral abdominal infections involving nonsporulating anaerobes, the most common is *liver abscess;* nonsporulating anaerobes are isolated from approximately 50 percent of liver abscesses. Liver abscess results from both bacteremic spread (sometimes following blunt trauma with localized infarction of hepatic tissue) and from contiguous infection, especially within the peritoneal cavity. Infection may spread from the biliary tract or from the portal venous system (suppurative pyelophlebitis) which results from direct extension of pelvic or intraabdominal sepsis. Symptoms and signs often suggest infection that can be readily localized, but nonspecific symptoms of fever, chills, weight loss, nausea, and vomiting are also seen in many patients. Only half the patients have hepatomegaly, right upper quadrant abdominal tenderness, and jaundice. The diagnosis can be confirmed by ultrasound, CT scan, or radioisotopic scanning. Occasionally more than one diagnostic procedure may have to be utilized. More than 90 percent of patients with liver abscesses have a leukocytosis and elevation of the serum alkaline phosphatase and aspartyl transaminase. Fifty percent have associated anemia, hypoalbuminemia, and elevated serum bilirubin. A basilar pulmonary infiltrate, pleural effusion, or elevated hemidiaphragm can be seen on chest x-ray. One-third of these patients have bacteremia. Open surgical drainage is indicated when an abscess is associated with other lesions requiring surgical drainage. Otherwise, percutaneous drainage using ultrasonography or CT scan to guide the catheter may be combined with antimicrobial therapy. If a liver abscess arises from contiguous gallbladder infection, cholecystectomy is essential.

Pelvic infections   The vagina of a healthy woman is one of the major reservoirs of both anaerobic and aerobic bacteria. In the normal flora of the female genital tract, anaerobes outnumber aerobes by a ratio of approximately 10:1. These anaerobes include anaerobic gram-positive cocci and *Bacteroides* species. Serious infections of the upper female tract contain organisms found in the normal vaginal flora. Anaerobes are isolated from the majority of such patients. The major pathogens consist of *B. fragilis, B. melaninogenicus,* anaerobic cocci, and clostridial species. Anaerobes frequently are encountered in tuboovarian abscess, septic abortion, pelvic abscess, endometritis, and postoperative wound infection, particularly following hysterectomy. Although these infections are frequently mixed, involving both anaerobes and coliforms, pure anaerobic infections without coliform or other facultative bacterial species occur more often in pelvic infections than intraabdominal infections. These infections are characterized by drainage of foul-smelling pus or blood from the uterus, generalized uterine or local pelvic tenderness, and continued fever and chills. Suppurative thrombophlebitis of the pelvic veins may complicate the infections and lead to repeated episodes of septic pulmonary emboli.

Skin and soft tissue infections   Injury to skin, bone, or soft tissue by trauma, ischemia, or surgery creates a suitable environment for anaerobic infections. These infections are most frequently found when the site is prone to contamination with feces or upper airway secretions. Examples include wounds associated with intestinal surgery, decubitus ulcers, or human bites. Anaerobic bacteria can be isolated in cases of crepitant cellulitis, synergistic cellulitis, or gangrene and necrotizing fasciitis. Furthermore, these organisms have been isolated from cutaneous abscesses, rectal abscesses, and axillary sweat gland infections (hydradenitis suppurativa). Anaerobes frequently have been isolated from foot ulcers in diabetic patients. These types of soft tissue or skin infections usually represent processes with mixed flora. A mean of 4.8 bacterial species can be isolated with a roughly 3:2 ratio of anaerobes to aerobes. The most frequently isolated organisms include *Bacteroides* species, anaerobic streptococci, group D streptococci, clostridial species, and *Proteus* species. The presence of anaerobes in these types of infections is associated with a higher frequency of fever, foul-smelling lesions, or a visible foot ulcer.

Anaerobic bacterial *synergistic gangrene* (Meleney's) typically occurs several days postoperatively. This lesion is characterized by the development of a wound infection which is exquisitely painful, red, and swollen, followed by induration. Erythema surrounds a central zone of necrosis. A granulating ulcer which may heal forms at the original center as necrosis and erythema extends outward. Symptoms are limited to pain. Fever is not typical. These infections most usually involve a combination of anaerobic cocci and *Staph. aureus.* Treatment includes surgical removal of necrotic tissue and antimicrobial therapy.

NECROTIZING FASCIITIS   This is a rapidly spreading destructive disease of the fascia, usually attributed to group A streptococci, but it can be caused by anaerobic bacteria including *Peptostreptococcus* and *Bacteroides* species. Similarly, myonecrosis can be associated with mixed anaerobic infection. Fournier's gangrene is an anaerobic cellulitis involving the scrotum, perineum, and anterior abdominal wall in which mixed anaerobic organisms spread along deep external fascial planes and cause extensive loss of skin.

Bone and joint infections   Although *actinomycosis* (Chap. 147) accounts on a worldwide basis for the majority of anaerobic infections in bone, other organisms are frequently isolated in such infections. In particular, anaerobic or microaerophilic cocci, *Bacteroides* species, *Fusobacterium,* and *Clostridium* species can be found. These infections frequently arise in the setting of soft tissue infections in adjacent soft tissues. Hematogenous seeding of bone is uncommon. Oral *Bacteroides* are seen in infections involving the maxilla and mandible, whereas *Clostridium* species have been reported as common anaerobic pathogens in cases of osteomyelitis of the long bones, following fracture or trauma. Fusobacteria have been isolated in pure culture from osteomyelitis adjacent to the perinasal sinuses, and, in the preantibiotic era caused fatal mastoid infections. Anaerobic and microaerophilic cocci have been reported as significant pathogens in infections involving the skull or mastoid.

In cases of anaerobic septic arthritis, the most common isolates are the *Fusobacterium* species. Most of these patients have uncontrolled peritonsillar infections progressing to septic cervical venous thrombophlebitis and resulting in hematogenous dissemination which shows a predilection for the joints. Most of these infections occurred in the preantibiotic era. Following the introduction of antibiotics, the isolation of *Fusobacterium* species from joints has been less common. Unlike anaerobic osteomyelitis, most cases of pyoarthritis caused by anaerobes are not polymicrobial and may be acquired hematogenously. Anaerobes are important pathogens in infections involving prosthetic joints; in these infections the causative organisms are part of the normal skin flora, such as the anaerobic gram-positive cocci and *P. acnes.*

In patients with osteomyelitis, the most reliable source of culture is a bone biopsy obtained free from normal uninfected skin and subcutaneous tissue. If mixed flora is isolated from a bone biopsy, all isolates should be treated. When an anaerobic isolate is recognized as a major or sole pathogen involving a joint, the treatment regimen should be similar to treatment of arthritis caused by aerobic bacteria. Therapy includes management of underlying disease states, appropriate antimicrobial therapy, temporary joint immobilization, percutaneous drainage of effusions, and usually removal of infected prostheses or internal fixation devices. Surgical drainage and debridement such as sequestrectomy are essential for removal of necrotic tissue that would sustain anaerobic infections.

Bacteremia   Transient bacteremia is a well-known event that occurs in healthy people when the anatomic mucosal barriers are injured (e.g., toothbrushing). These bacteremic episodes, which are often due to anaerobes, have no pathologic consequences. However, anaerobic bacteria compose nearly 10 to 15 percent of bacterial blood isolates from clinically ill patients when proper culture techniques are used. *B. fragilis* is the single most frequent anaerobic isolate. The portal of entry can usually be deduced along with the likely underlying problem that led to seeding of the bloodstream, by identification of the organism and understanding its place of normal residence. For example, mixed anaerobic bacteremia including *B. fragilis* implies colonic pathology with mucosal disruption from neoplasia, diverticulitis, or some other inflammatory lesion. The initial manifestations are determined by the portal of entry and reflect the localized condition. However, when bloodstream invasion occurs, patients can become extremely ill with rigors and hectic fevers ranging up to 105°F. The clinical picture may be quite similar to that seen in sepsis with aerobic gram-negative bacilli. Although other complications of anaerobic bacteremia such as septic thrombophlebitis and septic shock have been reported, the incidence of these complications in association with anaerobic bacteremia is low. Anaerobic bacteremia is potentially fatal and requires rapid diagnosis and appropriate therapy. The source of bacteremia must be identified and managed appropriately. The choice of antimicrobial therapy depends on the identification of the infecting organism.

ENDOCARDITIS (Chap. 188)   Endocarditis due to anaerobes is uncommon. However, anaerobic streptococci, which are often classified incorrectly, are responsible for this disease more frequently than is appreciated, although general incidence data are unavailable. Gram-negative anaerobes are unusual causes of endocarditis.

DIAGNOSIS   Because of the time and difficulty involved in the isolation of anaerobic bacteria, diagnosis of these infections must frequently be made on presumptive evidence. Infections caused by these nonsporulating anaerobic bacteria have unique characteristics that serve as useful clues in aiding diagnosis. Certain clinical settings such as avascular, necrotic tissues with lowered oxidation-reduction potential favor the diagnosis of an anaerobic infection. When infections occur in proximity to mucosal surfaces normally harboring anaerobic flora, such as the gastrointestinal tract, female genital tract, or oropharynx, anaerobes should be considered as potential etiologic agents. A foul odor often is present since anaerobes produce certain organic acids as they proliferate in necrotic tissue. Although the presence of these odors is pathognomonic for anaerobic infection, the absence of odor does not exclude these organisms as potential etiologic agents. Fifty percent of documented anaerobic infections lack a characteristic foul odor. Because anaerobes often coexist with other bacteria to form a mixed or synergistic infection, Gram-stained exudate frequently reveals numerous pleomorphic cocci and bacilli suggestive of anaerobes. Sometimes these organisms will have morphologic characteristics associated with specific species.

The presence of gas in tissues is highly suggestive, but not diagnostic, of anaerobes. Culture reports from obviously infected sites which yield no growth or only streptococci or a single aerobic species such as *E. coli,* when a Gram stain reveals mixed flora, imply that the anaerobic microorganisms failed to grow because of inadequate transport and/or culture techniques. Failure of a patient to respond to antibiotics that are not active against anaerobes, for example, aminoglycosides, and, in some circumstances, penicillin, cephalosporins, or tetracyclines, suggests the possibility of anaerobic infection.

There are three critical steps to diagnose anaerobic infection: (1) proper specimen collection, (2) rapid transportation of these specimens to the microbiologic laboratory, preferably in anaerobic transport

media, and (3) proper handling of these specimens by the laboratory. Collection of specimens must be performed by meticulously sampling infected sites avoiding contamination with normal flora. When there is a likely contamination of a specimen with normal flora, the specimen is unacceptable for processing by the bacteriology laboratory. Examples of unacceptable specimens for anaerobic culture include: (1) sputum collected by expectoration, or nasal tracheal suction, (2) bronchoscopy specimens, (3) direct collections through the vaginal vault, (4) collections of urine by voided specimen, and (5) feces. Specimens which can be cultured for anaerobes include blood, pleural fluid, transtracheal aspirates, pus obtained by direct aspiration from an abscess cavity, fluid obtained by culdocentesis, suprapubic bladder aspirates, cerebrospinal fluid, and lung puncture specimens.

Because even brief exposure to oxygen may kill these organisms and result in failure to isolate them in the laboratory, abscess cavities which are aspirated with a syringe should have the air expelled and the needle capped with a sterile rubber stopper. Specimens can be injected into transport bottles containing a reduced medium or brought immediately in syringes to the laboratory for direct culture on anaerobic media. In general, swabs should not be used. However, if a swab must be used, it should be placed in a reduced semisolid carrying medium before transport to the laboratory. It is important to remember that delays in transportation may lead to failure to isolate anaerobes due to exposure to oxygen, or overgrowth of facultative organisms which may eliminate or obscure the anaerobes that are present. All clinical specimens from suspected anaerobic infections should be Gram-stained and examined for organisms with characteristic morphology. It is not unusual for organisms to be observed on Gram stain but not isolated in culture. If purulent materials are found to be sterile, or organisms are seen on Gram stain, but do not grow in the culture, suspicion should be raised that anaerobes are involved and that improper transportation or handling of the specimen in the laboratory has occurred.

TREATMENT   Successful therapy of anaerobic infections involves a combination of appropriate antibiotics, surgical resection, and drainage. Although the operative approach ultimately may be decisive, surgical intervention alone may be inadequate. Drainage of abscess cavities should be carried out as soon as fluctuation or localization occurs. Perforations must be closed promptly, devitalized tissues or foreign bodies removed, closed spaces drained, tissue compartments decompressed, and adequate blood supply established. Appropriate antibiotics should be employed because anaerobic sepsis can continue postoperatively with intermittent symptoms and insidious extension of the process. Frequently it is necessary to begin antimicrobial therapy of anaerobic infections on a presumptive basis before culture and susceptibility data are available. The selection of initial antibiotic therapy should be based on knowledge of the pathogens likely to be present in a specific clinical setting, in combination with the Gram stain findings which should suggest the likelihood of certain species of organisms. Because many anaerobic infections tend to be mixed with coliforms and other facultative organisms, it is advisable, in general, to use drugs active against both anaerobic and aerobic components. In general, if anaerobes are suspected, the choice of antibiotics can be made reliably since patterns of antimicrobial susceptibility are quite predictable. Because *B. fragilis* is resistant to penicillin, a major decision concerns the likelihood of the presence of this organism. *B. fragilis,* in general, does not play a significant role in infections above the diaphragm, including head and neck infections, pleuropulmonary infections, and central nervous system infections. However, septic processes originating below the diaphragm, including in the pelvic and abdominal cavity, frequently contain *B. fragilis,* and specific antimicrobial therapy directed at these organisms should be employed.

In infections arising from sources above the diaphragm, because *B. fragilis* is isolated rarely or is of dubious pathogenic significance, penicillin G is the most widely used antibiotic for treatment. Depending on the site of infection and the severity, the dose of penicillin G recommended is variable. For the treatment of lung abscesses, a dose of 6 to 12 million units per day for at least 4 weeks is recommended (Chap. 205). Infrequently, infections arising from oral organisms will fail to respond to penicillin. In such cases these patients should be treated with drugs effective against penicillin-resistant anaerobes such as clindamycin, chloramphenicol, or cefoxitin. Reports of increasing resistance of *B. melaninogenicus* to penicillin may account for some of these treatment failures.

Infections arising from a colonic source are likely to contain *B. fragilis* and present a different problem. Many therapeutic failures have been noted in patients with documented *B. fragilis* infection who were treated with penicillin or first-generation cephalosporins. In major studies of intraabdominal sepsis, the use of antibiotics effective against anaerobes has clearly reduced the incidence of postoperative infection and serious infectious complications. Based on such data, it is clear that in suspected *Bacteroides* infection, appropriate antimicrobial therapy must be initiated. Although the number of antimicrobial agents effective against *B. fragilis* is somewhat limited, there currently are several choices which are useful; no single regimen has demonstrated clear superiority over another. In general, greater than 80 percent cure rates can be achieved in patients with *B. fragilis* infection when treated with appropriate antimicrobial therapy.

Of the currently available drugs for the treatment of *B. fragilis* infections, several can be considered as potentially useful primary agents. These include clindamycin, metronidazole, and cefoxitin. Although chloramphenicol has produced some good results in studies of intraabdominal and female pelvic infections, there have been case reports of therapeutic failures, including cases of persistent *B. fragilis* bacteremia in the face of adequate treatment. Cefamandole, cefoperazone, cefotaxime, and moxalactam have all had generally higher minimum inhibitory concentrations (MICs) against this organism than the other antibiotics mentioned above.

Regimens for therapy of specific infections must be tailored to the initial infecting site and the clinical situation. For example, intraabdominal sepsis should be treated with either clindamycin, 600 mg intravenously every 8 h, or metronidazole, 7.5 mg/kg every 8 h. An aminoglycoside such as gentamicin or tobramycin should be included in the regimen to treat facultative gram-negative bacilli. Cefoxitin has compared favorably to the regimen of clindamycin and an aminoglycoside in treating serious mixed infections of the abdomen or skin, which frequently include *B. fragilis* among the causative pathogens. However, an aminoglycoside should be added to cefoxitin in patients who have either received prior antibiotic therapy, or who have acquired their infections in the hospital. Such patients are at high risk for infection involving cefoxitin-resistant organisms such as *Enterobacter*, *Pseudomonas*, or *Serratia*.

Chloramphenicol can be used in patients with intraabdominal or central nervous system infections at a dose of 30 to 60 mg/kg per day, depending on the severity of illness. Chloramphenicol has been used successfully in the treatment of central nervous system infections due to anaerobic bacteria. Penicillin G and metronidazole also cross the blood-brain barrier and are bactericidal for the organisms which cause brain abscess. In patients who have meningitis or endocarditis due to anaerobic bacteria, a bactericidal agent is preferred.

Although other semisynthetic penicillinase-resistant penicillins are not active against anaerobes, carbenicillin, ticarcillin, or piperacillin combine the antimicrobial spectrum of penicillin G with increased activity against *B. fragilis* based on the higher dose of drug administered. This group of antibiotics, although not recommended as first-line therapy of anaerobic infection, has been used successfully in some cases.

Nearly all drugs mentioned above have certain significant, toxic side effects. Chloramphenicol produces fatal aplastic anemia in 1:40,000 to 100,000 patients who receive the drug. Clindamycin, the cephalosporins, the penicillins, and even, rarely, metronidazole have been associated with the development of pseudomembranous colitis due to *Clostridium difficile*. Since diarrhea may precede frank development of pseudomembranes, the administration of these drugs should be discontinued if diarrhea develops during therapy.

Due to widespread resistance, tetracycline and doxycycline are not reliable for the therapy of anaerobic infections. Erythromycin and vancomycin have some activity against gram-positive anaerobes but are not recommended for the therapy of serious infection.

Anaerobic infections which have failed to respond to treatment or relapse after initial response should be recultured. The need for surgical drainage or debridement should be reassessed. Superinfection should be considered, potentially due to resistant gram-negative facultative or aerobic bacteria. Drug resistance also must be entertained, particularly if chloramphenicol was the antibiotic used. Repeated cultures should then yield the initial organism.

Other supportive measures in the management of anaerobic infections include careful attention to fluid and electrolyte balance, since extensive local edema formation may lead to hypovolemia; hemodynamic support for septic shock; immobilization of infected extremities; maintenance of adequate nutrition during chronic infections by enteral or parenteral hyperalimentation if oral intake is inadequate; relief of pain; and anticoagulation with heparin for thrombophlebitis. Hyperbaric oxygen therapy is of no value.

REFERENCES

BALOWS A et al: *Anaerobic Bacteria: Role in Disease.* Springfield, Thomas, 1974

BARTLETT JG, FINEGOLD SM: Anaerobic infections of the lung and pleural space. Am Rev Resp Dis 110:56, 1974

FINEGOLD SM: *Anaerobic Bacteria in Human Disease.* New York, Academic, 1977

GORBACH SC: Anaerobic bacteria, in *Principles and Practices of Infectious Diseases,* GL Mandell et al (eds). New York, Wiley, 1985

———, BARTLETT JG: Anaerobic infections. N Engl J Med 290:1177, 1974

HARDING GKM et al: Prospective randomized comparative study of clindamycin, chloramphenicol and ticarcillin, each in combination with gentamicin in therapy for intraabdominal and female tract sepsis. J Infect Dis 142:384, 1980

KASPER DL et al: Virulence factors of anaerobic bacteria. Rev Infect Dis 1:246, 1979

——— et al: Capsular polysaccharides and lipopolysaccharides from two strains of *Bacteroides fragilis.* Rev Infect Dis 6:525, 1984

LEDGER WJ: *Infection in the Female.* Philadelphia, Lea and Febiger, 1977

MANSHEIM BJ, KASPER DL: Infections produced by non-sporulating anaerobic bacteria, in *Seminars in Infectious Diseases VII,* L Weinstein, BJ Fields (eds). New York, Grune & Stratton, 1979

MATHISEN GE et al: Brain abscess and cerebritis. Rev Infect Dis 6:S101, 1984

NAKATA MN, LEWIS RP: Anaerobic bacteria in bone and joint infections. Rev Infect Dis 6:S165, 1984

NEWMAN MG: Anaerobic oral and dental infections. Rev Infect Dis 6:S107, 1984

ONDERDEN K et al: Use of a model of intraabdominal sepsis for studies of the pathogenicity of *Bacteroides fragilis.* Rev Infect Dis 6:S191, 1984

PERERA MR et al: Presentation, diagnosis and management of liver abscess. Lancet 2:629, 1980

SUTTER VL et al: *Wadsworth Anaerobic Bacteriology Manual,* 3d ed. St Louis, Mosby, 1980

section 3 Diseases caused by gram-negative organisms

103 MENINGOCOCCAL INFECTIONS

HARRY N. BEATY

DEFINITION *Neisseria meningitidis* causes a variety of infections, most notably, meningitis and bacteremia.

ETIOLOGY In stained smears, meningococci are gram-negative single cocci or diplococci with flattened adjacent sides. They grow well on solid or semisolid media containing blood, serum, or ascitic fluid, and thrive best at temperatures between 35 and 37°C in an atmosphere reduced in oxygen and containing 5 to 10 percent CO_2. The organism is recovered readily from biologic fluids when fresh specimens are inoculated on warm chocolate agar plates that are incubated 18 to 24 h in a candle jar or in a more sophisticated apparatus that provides a suitable environment.

The biochemical reactions of the *Neisseria* are relatively limited, but they contain cytochrome oxidase, which is responsible for the positive "oxidase" test; the clinically significant species usually are differentiated by their ability to produce acid in glucose, maltose, or sucrose. Typically, the meningococcus ferments both glucose and maltose, but on occasion maltose-negative strains have been isolated.

Meningococci can be divided into serologic groups on the basis of agglutination reactions with immune serum. The present classification includes groups A through Z. Clinically significant new groups encompass Y and W135. The major groups are remarkably heterogeneous, but subclassification with additional serologic markers has been possible. Noncapsular antigens have provided the basis for dividing strains of groups into distinct types.

EPIDEMIOLOGY The natural habitat of meningococci is the nasopharynx of humans, and no other reservoir or vector has been recognized. Transmission from person to person is through inhalation of droplets of infected nasopharyngeal secretions. It is unlikely that the disease is spread by contact with contaminated fomites. Meningococci cause either epidemic or sporadic disease, and historically, there has been a cyclic variation in the prevalence of meningococcal infection with peaks of increased frequency occurring every 8 to 12 years and lasting 4 to 6 years. The last, quite minor, peak occurred in 1965. Subsequently, the incidence has declined to a fairly constant rate of about 1 case per 100,000 population per year. The prevalence of meningococcal infection is also subject to seasonal influences; the lowest attack rate occurs in midsummer and the highest in winter and early spring.

The attack rate of meningococcal disease is highest for children between 6 months and 1 year. The lowest attack rate occurs in individuals over 20. There is no clear-cut reason for sexual predominance, but males develop meningitis and meningococcemia more frequently than females. The attack rate in household contacts of sporadic cases of meningococcal disease is up to 1000 times the overall endemic rate; in epidemic periods, the attack rate among household contacts may be as much as 15,000 times that of the general population. Experience with group A outbreaks in Alaska and the northwestern part of the United States indicates that alcoholics and Alaska natives are at increased risk of infection, as are patients with deficiency in one or more components of complement. Military recruits also are particularly susceptible to meningococcal disease, although outbreaks among this population have disappeared coincident with the routine use of vaccines during the past 10 years.

In the first half of this century, most epidemics of meningococcal disease in the United States were caused by group A organisms. In the past two decades, first group B then group C meningococci were responsible for outbreaks in both the military and civilian populations. Currently, group B is responsible for 50 to 55 percent of reported cases. The proportion of isolates that are groups C, W135, and Y are 20 to 25, 15, and 10 percent, respectively. Only 1 to 2 percent of isolates are group A, but in Alaska and the Pacific Northwest 30 to 60 percent of patients with meningococcal disease are infected with this serogroup.

Studies of meningococci isolated from patients with meningococcal disease show that a very small proportion of strains in the environment cause disease. Common membrane antigens, closely related restriction endonuclease patterns, and the ability to form pili and release endotoxin have been correlated with "virulence."

Coincident with shifts in the predominant serogroup causing disease, there has been a waxing and waning of the proportion of isolates that are resistant to sulfadiazine. In the early 1960s, the majority of group B meningococci were resistant to sulfadiazine; in 1982 over 90 percent were sensitive. Similarly, when group C emerged as the predominant serogroup, sulfadiazine resistance was the rule. While sulfadiazine resistance has been recognized among isolates of all major serogroups, it is now uncommon in all but group B strains, 30 percent of which are resistant.

The potential for the meningococcus to produce serious outbreaks of disease has been reemphasized by epidemics in Brazil, Finland, and parts of Africa. Massive immunization programs curtailed two of these major epidemics.

Carriers Between epidemics, 2 to 15 percent of the individuals in urban centers harbor meningococci in the nasopharynx. When sporadic cases of meningococcal disease occur, the carrier rate in close contacts may rise to 40 percent, and in closed populations or during epidemics, may approach 100 percent. Although some individuals harbor meningococci for years, nasopharyngeal infection is usually transient, and in 75 percent of carriers the organism disappears within a few weeks to a few months. Case-to-case transmission of infection is documented rarely, and carriers, not patients, are the foci from which disease is spread. Even so, the prevalence of meningococcal disease can be attributed to the prevailing carrier rate only in a general way, and the occurrence of clinical disease is most dependent on the immunologic status of the host, other factors that lead to spread of infection beyond the nasopharynx, and strain virulence.

Immunity The fact that meningococcal meningitis is primarily a disease of childhood has suggested that natural immunity develops in most individuals within the first two decades of life. There is a correlation between susceptibility to meningococcal disease and absence of bactericidal antibody in the serum, and most adults have antibodies to pathogenic strains of meningococci. Natural immunization appears to result from asymptomatic carriage of meningococci in the nasopharynx. Not only does the carrier state produce antibodies to the infecting strain, but cross-reacting antibodies may develop, even after colonization with nongroupable organisms. The immunity conferred by meningococcal meningitis or meningococcemia is usually group-specific, and second episodes of meningococcal disease have been encountered. Deficiency of complement components C6, C7, or C8 is a significant risk factor for repeated episodes of bacteremia with the pathogenic *Neisseria,* and is seen more frequently in patients with initial infections than in the general population.

PATHOGENESIS The primary focus of meningococcal infection is the nasopharynx. In most instances, this infection is subclinical, but occasionally localized inflammation occurs and mild symptoms develop. Dissemination of meningococci from the nasopharynx occurs via the bloodstream, and generally is followed by clinical manifestations of meningococcal disease. *Purulent meningitis* is a form of metastatic infection and is either associated with signs and symptoms of meningococcemia or constitutes the predominant clinical expression of illness. Rarely, more extensive inflammation causes an acute diffuse encephalitis.

Although the mechanisms that produce tissue injury are unknown, in laboratory animals, an endotoxin that is biochemically and biologically similar to endotoxins of enteric bacilli appears to be involved. It may be responsible for hypotension and vascular collapse observed in fulminant meningococcemia and may also play a role in the pathogenesis of the purpura and visceral hemorrhages associated with meningococcal bacteremia. Thrombosis of dermal venules, adrenal sinusoids, and renal glomerular capillaries is most commonly seen in patients who die of fulminant meningococcemia and is strikingly similar to the pathologic changes observed in the experimental Shwartzman reaction induced by endotoxin.

CLINICAL MANIFESTATIONS Ninety to ninety-five percent of patients with meningococcal disease have meningococcemia and/or meningitis.

Meningococcemia Thirty to fifty percent of patients who develop overt disease have meningococcemia without meningitis. The onset of clinical illness may be abrupt, but patients usually have nonspecific prodromal symptoms of cough, headache, and sore throat followed by the sudden development of spiking fever, chills, arthralgia, and muscle pains that may be particularly severe in the lower extremities and back. Patients usually appear acutely ill with an inordinate degree of prostration. In addition to high fever, tachycardia, and tachypnea, mild hypotension may be present. However, clinical shock does not occur unless fulminant meningococcemia supervenes. In the course of meningococcal bacteremia, about three-fourths of the patients develop a characteristic petechial rash. Lesions are frequently sparse, and the axillae, flanks, wrists, and ankles are most commonly involved. Often petechiae are located in the center of lighter-colored macules, and they may become nodular as the disease progresses. The diagnosis of meningococcemia occasionally can be established by demonstrating gram-negative diplococci in scrapings from these nodular lesions. In severe cases, purpuric spots or large ecchymoses develop, and a widespread petechial or purpuric eruption suggests fulminating disease. However, the absence of rash does not necessarily indicate that the illness will be mild.

Fulminant meningococcemia, or the Waterhouse-Friderichsen syndrome, is meningococcemia associated with vasomotor collapse and shock. It occurs in 10 to 20 percent of patients with generalized meningococcal infection, and is associated with a high fatality rate. The onset is abrupt, and profound prostration frequently occurs within a few hours. Petechiae and purpuric lesions enlarge rapidly, and hemorrhage into the skin may be extensive. Early in the preshock stage, there is generalized vasoconstriction; patients are alert and pale, with circumoral cyanosis and cold extremities. Upon entering the shock stage, however, coma develops, the cardiac output decreases, and the blood pressure drops. Unless incipient shock is recognized and appropriate therapy is instituted early, death from cardiac and/or respiratory failure almost invariably occurs. Patients who recover may have extensive sloughing of skin lesions or loss of digits because of gangrene.

Chronic meningococcemia is a rare form of meningococcal infection that lasts for weeks or months and is characterized by fever, rash, and arthritis or arthralgia. Typically, the fever is intermittent, and during afebrile periods, which may last several days, patients appear remarkably well. The usual rash is a maculopapular or polymorphous eruption that waxes and wanes with the fever, but petechial or nodular lesions may be seen. Joint involvement is present in two-thirds of the patients, and splenomegaly is detected in about 20 percent. If the diagnosis is not suspected or treatment is otherwise delayed, complications such as meningitis, carditis, or nephritis may occur.

Meningitis Meningitis is a common form of meningococcal disease that occurs primarily in children from 6 months to 10 years. Fever, vomiting, headache, and confusion or lethargy are the commonest symptoms; in about one-fourth of the patients, symptoms begin abruptly and rapidly increase in severity. The more typical patient, however, has symptoms of an upper respiratory tract infection followed by an illness that progresses over several days. Twenty to forty percent of patients have meningitis without clinical evidence of meningococcemia, and the diagnosis depends upon bacteriologic examination of the cerebrospinal fluid. However, when meningitis occurs in association with a petechial or purpuric rash, a presumptive diagnosis of meningococcal disease is warranted, because this pattern of illness is seen only rarely in other infections.

Rarer manifestations The meningococcus is a rare cause of purulent conjunctivitis or sinusitis. Primary pneumonia previously was considered a rare manifestation of meningococcal infection, but increasing numbers of cases are being reported. In one study of military recruits, 68 cases of clinical pneumonia due to group Y meningococci were reported. Bacterial endocarditis, primary pericarditis, arthritis, and osteomyelitis have also been reported. On rare occasion, meningococci have produced genital infections clinically indistinguishable from gonococcal disease. *N. meningitidis* has been isolated with increasing frequency from the genitourinary tract and anal canal of symptomatic and asymptomatic patients of both sexes.

LABORATORY FINDINGS Aside from bacteriologic data, laboratory studies are of little value in establishing the diagnosis of meningococcal infection. Polymorphonuclear leukocyte counts usually range from 12,000 to 40,000 cells per cubic millimeter, but in meningococcemia, normal or low leukocyte counts may be encountered. Anemia is uncommon, and levels of serum electrolytes and blood urea nitrogen are normal unless shock develops. Patients with prominent hemorrhagic manifestations may have low platelet counts and decreased levels of circulating clotting factors as a result of disseminated intravascular coagulation. In meningitis, the cerebrospinal fluid pressure is increased, and the fluid usually contains from 100 to 40,000 polymorphonuclear leukocytes per cubic millimeter. The protein content is increased, and the concentration of glucose is almost always less than 35 mg/dL and often is between 0 and 10 mg/dL.

Meningococci often can be recovered from cultures of blood or spinal fluid, and, on occasion, material aspirated from skin lesions or joints yields the organism. In addition, gram-negative diplococci may be seen in stains of nodular petechiae or the buffy coat of blood from patients with meningococcemia. In meningococcal meningitis, a smear of the spinal fluid is diagnostic in about half the patients but often shows only a few intracellular bacteria which are located with difficulty.

COMPLICATIONS Herpes labialis occurs in 5 to 20 percent of patients with meningococcal disease. Other complications, which result from neurologic damage or secondary foci of infection, are uncommon following appropriate treatment and are often transient. Seizures or deafness occur in 10 to 20 percent of patients during the acute stages of meningitis, but postmeningitic epilepsy is rare, and the frequency of permanent eighth nerve damage is probably less than 5 percent. Peripheral neuropathy, cranial nerve palsies, and hemiplegia are seen occasionally, but usually clear completely within 2 to 4 months. Hydrocephalus and thrombosis of venous sinuses, once frequent sequelae of meningococcal meningitis, are encountered rarely. A number of patients complain of recurrent headache, emotional lability, insomnia, backache, memory loss, and difficulty in concentrating for months after an episode of meningitis. The organic basis for these symptoms is obscure, but they usually disappear a year or two after the infection.

Arthritis is a common metastatic complication of meningococcemia and occurs in 2 to 10 percent of patients. As a rule, multiple joints are involved, and signs and symptoms may not appear until after treatment of meningitis or meningococcemia has been instituted. Joint fluid usually contains many granulocytes, but meningococci are recovered infrequently. Arthritis may be immunologically mediated in those instances when cultures are sterile. Permanent joint changes are rare.

Other purulent complications have become extremely uncommon since antibiotics have gained widespread use. Pneumonia occurs occasionally, but it is uncertain whether it is caused by the meningococcus or coincidental infection with other bacteria. Bacterial endocarditis is quite rare, but a high proportion of patients who die of meningococcal infection have myocarditis. The etiology of these myocardial changes is uncertain, but cardiac failure may be an important factor in the pathogenesis of the shock syndrome in meningococcemia. A pericardial friction rub or electrocardiographic change of pericarditis is seen in about 5 percent of patients, and rarely purulent pericarditis may develop.

DIAGNOSIS   The diagnosis of meningococcal disease depends upon recovering *N. meningitidis* from cultures of blood, spinal fluid, or petechial scrapings from patients with a typical clinical picture. Detection of antigen in spinal fluid by latex agglutination or counterimmunoelectrophoresis is valuable in diagnosing meningococcal meningitis. These techniques do not detect antigens of group B organisms, however. Recovery of meningococci from the nasopharynx does not, in itself, establish the diagnosis of meningococcal disease.

Few diseases need to be considered seriously in the differential diagnosis of meningococcal disease. If meningococcal meningitis is not accompanied by manifestations of bacteremia, it is indistinguishable from meningitis caused by other common pathogens. Occasionally, the common viral exanthems, mycoplasma infection, Rocky Mountain spotted fever (see Chap. 148), and vascular purpuras may be confused with meningococcemia.

TREATMENT   Antimicrobial therapy of suspected or documented meningococcal disease should be instituted as early as possible. Penicillin G is the drug of choice, and should be administered intravenously. The dosage for treatment of meningitis in adults is 12 to 24 million units per day, and in the pediatric age group, 16 million units/m^2 per day. Meningococcemia alone can be treated with 5 to 10 million units per day, because it is not necessary to achieve high levels of antibiotic in the spinal fluid. If treatment with these doses is continued for a minimum of 7 days, or 4 to 5 days after the patient becomes afebrile, relapse is extremely rare. Meningococci are susceptible to chloramphenicol, but it should not be used unless a patient is allergic to penicillin. Then chloramphenicol hemisuccinate 4.0 to 6.0 g per day in divided doses (in adults) is an acceptable alternative. Some of the "third-generation" cephalosporins (see Chap. 88) have been used to treat small numbers of patients with meningococcal meningitis, but they should not be employed routinely until more extensive clinical research documents their efficacy. *Because a significant proportion of meningococci isolated are resistant to sulfonamides, these drugs should not be used alone in the treatment of meningococcal infections,* and their use in combination with penicillin offers no advantage.

Patients with meningococcal infections require supportive treatment as well as antimicrobial therapy. Maintenance of fluid and electrolyte balance and prevention of respiratory complications in comatose patients are of primary concern. When shock occurs, visceral perfusion must be improved by maintenance of an adequate intravascular volume, treatment of heart failure, and support of the blood pressure. Vasoactive drugs should be employed according to the pathophysiologic derangement in each individual case. These derangements can be determined best by carefully monitoring the blood pressure, pulse, arterial blood gases, cardiac output, peripheral resistance, pulmonary artery wedge pressures, and arteriovenous oxygen differences. When blood pressure must be raised immediately, norepinephrine may be indicated. However, if improved tissue perfusion is the primary goal, an agent such as dopamine is likely to be more effective. When heart failure is present, diuretics and digitalis should be given. When disseminated intravascular coagulation is recognized, treatment with heparin, whole blood, or fibrinogen can be tried, but dramatic results should not be expected. Massive doses of adrenal cortical steroids as used in the treatment of septic shock (see Chap. 86) may be helpful, but lower "replacement" doses are of uncertain value.

PREVENTION   With the widespread emergence of sulfonamide-resistant meningococci, alternate methods of preventing meningococcal disease in closed populations were sought. High-molecular-weight polysaccharide antigens from organisms of serogroups A, C, Y, and W135 have been shown to induce a group-specific bactericidal antibody response after subcutaneous injection. Currently, a quadrivalent vaccine containing these antigens is available for use in control of outbreaks. Routine immunization is recommended only for particular high-risk groups. An effective group B vaccine has not yet been developed.

For intimate contacts of sporadic cases of meningococcal disease, chemoprophylaxis should be administered. If the organism isolated from the patient is sensitive to sulfonamides, 2 days of prophylaxis with one of these drugs is recommended. When sensitivities are not known or the organism is resistant to sulfonamides, rifampin in dosage of 600 mg every 12 h for 2 days for adults and 5 to 10 mg/kg every 12 h for children can be expected to eradicate the carrier state temporarily and minimize spread of meningococci.

With increased availability of an effective vaccine, its use as an adjunct to chemoprophylaxis for household or other intimate contacts of sporadic cases of meningococcal disease has been recommended.

PROGNOSIS   Before the introduction of antibiotics, meningococcal meningitis and meningococcemia were almost invariably fatal. With prompt and appropriate chemotherapy, the mortality rate of meningitis without fulminant meningococcemia has dropped to less than 10 percent in the United States, and neurologic sequelae are rare. The mortality of fulminant infection remains high primarily because patients are often in irreversible shock when treatment is instituted. Most deaths occur within 24 to 48 h of admission, and the capacity of the meningococcus to kill a perfectly healthy individual within a few hours remains one of the most awesome characteristics of this disease.

REFERENCES

BAND JD et al: Trends in meningococcal disease in the United States, 1975–1980. J Infect Dis 148:754, 1983

BLACK JR et al: Neisserial antigen H.8 is immunogenic in patients with disseminated gonococcal and meningococcal infections. J Infect Dis 151:650, 1985

BUCHAN H et al: An outbreak of meningococcal disease: Implications for community medicine. NZ Med J 97:860, 1984

CENTERS FOR DISEASE CONTROL: Meningococcal vaccines. Morb Mort Week Rep 34:255, 1985

ROSS SC et al: Complement deficiency states and infection: Epidemiology, pathogenesis and consequences of neisserial and other infections in an immune deficiency. Medicine 63:243, 1984

104   GONOCOCCAL INFECTIONS

KING K. HOLMES

DEFINITION   Gonorrhea, an infection of columnar and transitional epithelium caused by *Neisseria gonorrhoeae*, is the most common reportable communicable disease in the United States. Anatomic sites which can be infected directly by the gonococcus include the urethra, rectum, conjunctivas, pharynx, and endocervix. Local complications include endometritis, salpingitis, peritonitis, and bartholinitis in the female, and periurethral abscess and epididymitis in the male. Systemic manifestations of gonococcemia include arthritis, dermatitis, endocarditis, and meningitis as well as myopericarditis and hepatitis.

ETIOLOGY *Neisseria gonorrhoeae* is a gram-negative coccus usually found in pairs with flattened adjacent sides. It forms oxidase-positive colonies and is differentiated from other *Neisseria* by its ability to utilize glucose but not maltose, sucrose, or lactose, and by specific immunologic reactions.

Colonies examined within 20 h of inoculation from clinical specimens contain organisms covered by fimbria (pili). As the colonies grow older, their appearance changes, reflecting the loss of pili. Piliated organisms cause infection and urethritis after inoculation into the urethras of male volunteers, whereas nonpiliated organisms do not. Pili mediate attachment to various epithelial cells, and interfere with neutrophil phagocytosis. The process by which piliated gonococci throw off nonpiliated variants, and vice versa, is termed *phase variation,* and is mediated by chromosomal rearrangement. Each pilus is composed of repeating peptide subunits (pilin) which have a molecular weight of about 20,000. The pilin subunits consist of conserved and variable regions. The variable regions are prone to rapid antigenic variation in vitro and in vivo. Antigenic variation of pilin may allow gonococci to adapt rapidly to attachment onto different types of epithelial surfaces, and to evade the host's antibody response to pilin.

The trilaminar outer membrane of the gonococcus contains several classes of proteins, including proteins I, II, and III, and lipopolysaccharide (Fig. 104-1). Like pili, protein II also is thought to function as a ligand, mediating the attachment of gonococci to various types of human cells. As in the case with pili, individual strains of gonococci may or may not choose to express protein II, and several antigenic variants of protein II may be expressed at different times by the same strain. The presence or absence of protein II also influences colony morphology, and protein II may be responsible for the clumping of gonococci which is so evident on Gram-stained smears of urethral exudate.

Opaque colonies contain organisms which express protein II, and predominate in isolates from the male urethra, and in cervical isolates obtained from women in midcycle. Transparent colonies lack protein II, and predominate in isolates from women during menses, and in isolates from blood, synovial fluid, or fallopian tubes.

Protein I (32,000 to 36,000 mol wt) is quantitatively the major outer membrane protein, present as a trimer aggregated with protein III. Protein I molecules act as porins, forming transmembrane channels that permit exchange of hydrophilic molecules through the outer membrane. Protein I molecules have been shown to move rapidly from gonococcal outer membranes to the more fluid cytoplasmic membrane of human cells. This process may initiate endocytosis of the gonococcus, representing the first step in gonococcal invasion of the epithelium.

The lipopolysaccharide of the gonococcus contains lipid A and core oligosaccharide, but no repeating polysaccharide side chain. No capsular polysaccharide has yet been isolated, but high-molecular-weight surface polyphosphates have been demonstrated which may have functions similar to those of capsular polysaccharides in other organisms.

Gonococcal typing Gonococcal strains now can be typed on the basis of nutritional requirements (auxotyping) or surface antigenic variation of protein I. Unlike pili and protein II, the protein I expressed by any single strain of gonococcus is antigenically stable, although there is considerable antigenic heterogeneity of protein I between strains. There are two different kinds of protein I, known as IA and IB, and individual strains contain either protein IA or protein IB, but not both. Monoclonal antibodies against different epitopes of protein IA and protein IB can be used to classify gonococci into a large number of serovariants known as serovars IA1 to IA18, and IB1 to IB28.

EPIDEMIOLOGY The only natural hosts for *N. gonorrhoeae* are humans. In the United States the annual age-specific incidence rates tripled from 1963 to 1978, when over 1 million cases were reported and an equal number probably went unreported. During this period of epidemic gonorrhea, the incidence increased fastest in young white females. After 1978, the incidence of gonorrhea fell steadily every year through 1984, when 879,000 cases were reported. In 1985, the incidence again rose unexpectedly by 5 percent. The current increase has been limited to heterosexuals; gonorrhea (and syphilis) in homosexual men has continued to decline rapidly because of fear of AIDS and a decline in homosexual promiscuity. The resurgence of gonorrhea in heterosexuals is unexplained, but could be related to

FIGURE 104–1 *Diagram of the envelope of* N. gonorrhoeae, *showing structures thought to influence pathogenesis, antimicrobial susceptibility, and antigenicity.*

reallocation of public health efforts from gonorrhea control toward control of other sexually transmitted diseases such as AIDS.

Gonorrhea incidence and prevalence rates are known to be related to age, sex, sex preference, race, socioeconomic status, marital status, urban residence, and level of education—risk factors which influence sexual behavior, illness behavior, and accessibility of health care. Among sexually active individuals, the highest rates occur in teen-agers, in non-whites, in the poor and poorly educated, in large cities, and in unmarried persons—particularly those who live alone. Such individuals comprise a "core group" of "efficient transmitters" who play a disproportionate role in the spread of gonorrhea. The incidence is highest in men, while the prevalence is highest in women. The prevalence rate is so high among women in the United States that routine endocervical cultures have been advocated for gonorrhea case detection in asymptomatic women age 30 or under who are considered to be at high risk because of sexual behavior or demographic factors cited above. However, greater reliance should be placed upon contact tracing, which is far more efficient for control of gonorrhea, than upon routine endocervical culturing, which is expensive and does not focus on those most likely to transmit the infection. The single most important axiom about the epidemiology of this disease is that *gonorrhea is usually spread by carriers who have no symptoms or have ignored symptoms.* Symptomatic patients, male or female, have usually been recently infected by such carriers, who must in turn be traced and treated to prevent reinfection. *Men and women with symptomatic gonorrhea should always be interviewed to identify their recent sex contacts, who should be examined and treated if infected.*

There are interesting regional differences in the antibiotic resistance of *N. gonorrhoeae*. In 1976, penicillinase-producing strains of *N. gonorrhoeae* (PPNG), completely resistant to penicillin and ampicillin, appeared almost simultaneously in two areas of the world: in England, where they had probably been imported from west Africa, and in the United States, where they had been imported from the Philippines. The β-lactamase enzymes produced by these strains are encoded on small plasmids identical to plasmids found in *Haemophilus influenzae*. PPNG first became established and then spread in areas of the world where prostitution is exceptionally common and where access to subcurative antimicrobial therapy is unrestricted. PPNG now comprise 50 percent or more of all gonococci in many areas of Africa and Asia, and have by now become well established in many regions of the United States (e.g., Miami, New York, Los Angeles) and Europe. Of equal importance has been the spread of gonococci with chromosomally mediated resistance to penicillin and tetracycline. These strains are referred to as chromosomally mediated resistant *Neisseria gonorrhoeae* (CMRNG). Auxotyping and monoclonal antibody serotyping have shown that in a midsized metropolitan city, as many as 60 to 100 different gonococcal strains are circulating, and new strains are being continuously introduced. Against this background, local outbreaks of PPNG or CMRNG belonging to a single auxotype-serovar class have been identified, and public health efforts have at times been successfully focused on the control of such strains.

CLINICAL MANIFESTATIONS The clinical spectrum of gonococcal infections depends upon the site of inoculation, the duration of infection, the virulence of the infecting strain, and the presence or absence of local or systemic spread of the organism. The influence of inoculum size, variations in host susceptibility, and of coinfection with *C. trachomatis* or other genital pathogens on clinical manifestations has not been well-defined.

Gonorrhea in the male The usual incubation period of gonococcal urethritis ("clap") in the male is 2 to 7 days following exposure, although longer intervals are not infrequent, and some men never develop symptoms. In one study, one fastidious auxotype, which has distinctive nutritional requirements, was associated with 96 percent of asymptomatic infections and only 40 percent of symptomatic infections. Symptoms of urethritis include a purulent urethral discharge, usually associated with dysuria, frequent urination, and meatal erythema. Although approximately 90 to 95 percent of men who

acquire urethral gonococcal infection develop urethral discharge, most symptomatic men seek treatment and are removed from the infectious pool. The remaining men who never develop symptoms or who ignore their symptoms constitute about two-thirds of the infected men at any point in time, and they serve as the main source of spread of infection to women. Before antibiotic treatment became available, symptoms of urethritis persisted for an average of 8 weeks, and unilateral epididymitis occurred in 5 to 10 percent of untreated men. Epididymitis is now an uncommon complication (see below), and gonococcal prostatitis occurs rarely, if at all. Other local complications of gonococcal urethritis which are now unusual include inguinal lymphadenitis, edema of the penis due to dorsal lymphangitis or thrombophlebitis, submucous inflammatory "soft" infiltration of the urethral wall, periurethral abscess or fistula, unilateral inflammation or abscess of Cowper's gland (which lies between the thumb and forefinger when the forefinger is in the anal canal and the thumb is positioned anteriorly on the perineum), and, rarely, seminal vesiculitis.

In homosexual men, rectal and pharyngeal gonococcal infection are common. Gonococcal isolates from homosexual men tend to be more resistant to antimicrobials than are isolates from heterosexuals. This may be due to the fact that certain highly susceptible types are rapidly killed by bile salts and fatty acids in feces and rarely occur in homosexual men, while gonococci possessing a gene for multidrug resistance (*mtr*) are resistant to bile salts and fatty acids and occur with increased frequency in homosexual men. Rectal infection may be asymptomatic from the outset or may produce anorectal pain, pruritus, tenesmus, and a bloody, mucopurulent rectal discharge. Proctoscopy and appropriate laboratory studies are essential to exclude several other conditions which cause similar symptoms (see Chap. 90). These symptoms may subside without treatment, leaving a chronic asymptomatic carrier state. Pharyngeal gonococcal infection occurs in approximately 20 percent of homosexual men or heterosexual women who engage in fellatio with men who have urethral infection, and in a smaller proportion of heterosexual men. Pharyngeal infection may produce exudative tonsillitis but frequently is asymptomatic; asymptomatic pharyngeal gonococcal infection usually clears spontaneously over several weeks, even without therapy.

Gonorrhea in the female Acute uncomplicated gonorrhea in the female often causes dysuria, frequent urination, increased vaginal discharge due to exudative endocervicitis, abnormal menstrual bleeding, and anorectal discomfort. While dysuria and frequency in young men arouse the suspicion of gonococcal urethritis, the same symptoms in a young woman are often automatically attributed to "cystitis." Actually, some of those without bacteriuria have gonococcal or chlamydial infection of the urethra. Young women with dysuria should have a thorough pelvic examination. Compression of the urethra through the anterior vaginal wall against the symphysis pubis may express urethral exudate which can be examined by Gram's stain and culture. Symptomatic young women with "sterile pyuria" (i.e., ≥ 10 neutrophils per $100\times$ microscopic field in the centrifuged sediment of clean-catch midstream urine; no uropathogens isolated from the urine) should be evaluated for gonococcal and chlamydial infection. Acute symptoms of gonococcal urethritis in the female may subside spontaneously or following subcurative therapy with sulfonamides or urinary antiseptics. The proportion of women with gonorrhea who never develop symptoms is undefined.

Asymptomatic gonococcal infection in the female involves the endocervix, urethra, anal canal, and pharynx, in decreasing order of frequency. Extension of infection from the endocervix to the fallopian tubes occurs in at least 15 percent of women with gonorrhea. This tends to occur soon after acquisition of infection or during menstruation and results in acute endometritis, with abnormal menstrual bleeding and midline low abdominal pain and tenderness, followed by *acute salpingitis,* the major complication of gonorrhea. One study suggested one-half of women who became infected after recent exposure to gonorrhea developed signs of pelvic inflammatory disease (PID). Coexisting *C. trachomatis* infection may increase the rate of PID. Extension of infection to the pelvis may produce signs of pelvic peritonitis, accompanied by nausea and vomiting, and may lead to pelvic abscess. Early antibiotic treatment, before development of adnexal masses, restores normal tubal function and fertility in nearly all cases of gonococcal salpingitis. However, if prominent adnexal swelling has occurred before treatment is begun, bilateral tubal damage occurs in 15 to 25 percent.

Spread of gonococci or chlamydia into the upper abdomen may cause *perihepatitis* (Fitz-Hugh–Curtis syndrome) manifested by right upper quadrant or bilateral upper abdominal pain and tenderness, and occasionally by a hepatic friction rub.

Acute inflammation of Bartholin's gland is usually unilateral and frequently is due to gonococcal infection. The acutely infected duct is surrounded by a red halo and exudes pus at the posterior third of the labium majus. Occlusion of the duct results in formation of a Bartholin's abscess. Chronic Bartholin cysts are rarely caused by active gonococcal infection.

There is suggestive evidence that endocervical gonococcal infection is associated with prematurity and premature rupture of membranes.

Gonorrhea in children During childbirth, the gonococcus may infect the conjunctivas, pharynx, respiratory tract, or anal canal of the newborn. The risk of contamination increases with prolonged rupture of membranes. Prevention of gonococcal ophthalmia by prophylactic use of 1% silver nitrate eyedrops has led to the emergence of inclusion conjunctivitis caused by *Chlamydia* as a more common form of ophthalmia neonatorum. Since neonates and young infants lack bactericidal IgM antibody against *N. gonorrhoeae*, they may be at increased risk for gonococcal bacteremia. During the first year of life, infection of the infant usually results from accidental contamination of the eye or vagina by an adult. Between 1 year of age and puberty, many cases of gonorrhea involve vulvovaginitis in females who have been molested by a relative, and medicolegal considerations necessitate a complete bacteriologic diagnosis and child welfare consultation. Auxotyping and serotyping of isolates from the sexual assault victim and accused assailant have been used as evidence in court.

Disseminated gonococcal infection The incidence of disseminated gonococcal infection (DGI) varies with time and place, in relation to the local incidence of infection with strains of gonococci that have a propensity to produce bacteremia. Approximately two-thirds of patients with DGI are women, and symptoms of bacteremia often begin during menses. The majority of men and women with gonococcemia do not have symptoms of urogenital, anorectal, or pharyngeal gonococcal infection. As noted below, serum complement-mediated bactericidal activity appears essential for protection against gonococcal bacteremia.

Patients typically present either with symptoms and signs of gonococcemia, or with purulent arthritis affecting one or two joints. The onset of gonococcemia is characterized by fever, polyarthralgias, and papular, petechial, pustular, hemorrhagic, or necrotic skin lesions. Approximately 3 to 20 such lesions appear, usually on the distal extremities. Gonococci are demonstrable by immunofluorescent staining in about two-thirds of gonococcal skin lesions. The initial joint involvement is characteristically limited to tenosynovitis involving several joints asymmetrically. The wrists, fingers, knees, and ankles are most often involved. Circulating immune complexes have been demonstrated at this stage of infection in some but not all studies. Serum complement levels are normal (except in those with complement deficiency), and the role of immune complexes, if any, is uncertain. Without treatment, the duration of gonococcemia is variable; the systemic manifestations of bacteremia may subside spontaneously within a week. Alternatively, septic arthritis ensues, often without prior symptoms of fever, polyarthralgias, or skin lesions. Pain and swelling then increase in one or, very occasionally, more joints, with accumulation of purulent synovial fluid, leading to progressive destruction of the joint if treatment is delayed. IgM antibody to gonococcal lipopolysaccharide, present in normal human serum, is bactericidal for most strains of gonococci in the presence of complement. Gonococci isolated from patients with DGI

have stable resistance to normal human serum. These strains usually contain protein IA, and are highly susceptible to penicillin. They often require arginine, hypoxanthine, and uracil for growth, and are referred to as belonging to the AHU auxotype. Patients deficient in complement components C5, C6, C7, and C8 are uniquely susceptible to gonococcemia and meningococcemia because they cannot mount a serum bactericidal response to gonococci or meningococci. Gonococci isolated from patients with tenosynovitis and skin lesions are even more resistant to pooled normal human serum than are isolates from patients with purulent arthritis, suggesting that the two different DGI syndromes may be determined by characteristics of the causative organism.

The probability of positive blood cultures decreases after 48 h of illness, and the probability of recovery of gonococci from synovial fluid increases with increasing duration of illness. Gonococci are infrequently recovered from early effusions containing less than 20,000 leukocytes per cubic millimeter, but are usually recovered from effusions containing more than 80,000 leukocytes per cubic millimeter. In the individual patient, gonococci are seldom recovered from blood and synovial fluid simultaneously.

Other common manifestations of disseminated gonococcal infection include mild myopericarditis and "toxic" hepatitis. Endocarditis and meningitis are infrequent but severe complications. Endocarditis is suggested by pathologic or changing heart murmurs, major embolic phenomena, severe myocarditis, deterioration of renal function, or an unusually large number of skin lesions.

PATHOGENESIS Understanding of the pathogenesis of gonorrhea has developed rapidly. Epidemiologic data suggest that only about one-third of men become infected after a single exposure to gonorrhea, and under experimental conditions an inoculum of 10^3 organisms appears necessary to establish urethral infection in 50 percent of male volunteers. Factors which may confer resistance to infection are undefined. Components of the urethral or vaginal flora, such as *Candida albicans*, *Staphylococcus epidermidis*, and certain types of lactobacilli, can inhibit *N. gonorrhoeae* in vitro and may provide some natural resistance in vivo. Lactoferrin is present at mucosal surfaces, where it presumably competes with gonococci for iron, which is required for growth of the organism. AHU strains of gonococci compete poorly with lactoferrin, which could explain the tendency of such strains to cause asymptomatic mucosal infections. Gonococci infect mucus-secreting epithelial surfaces, and mucus could be a physical barrier or competitive inhibitor between the gonococcus and its target cell receptors.

Attachment of gonococci to mucosal cells is mediated in part by pili and by protein II. Local antibody to pili can partially block attachment. Pili also impede phagocytosis of gonococci by neutrophils, and antibody to pili is opsonic. An enzyme produced by the pathogenic *Neisseria*, IgA1 protease, which inactivates sIgA1, may interfere with IgA-mediated antiadherence activity, resulting in increased attachment.

Following attachment to columnar or transitional epithelium, gonococci penetrate through or between cells to reach the subepithelial connective tissue. Transfer of gonococcal protein I into the host cell may initiate endocytosis by the epithelial cell. Gonococcal lipopolysaccharide (LPS) and peptidoglycan are toxic for fallopian tube organ cultures. Gonococci also produce proteases, phospholipases, and elastases which may play a role in pathogenesis. In subepithelial tissue, and in blood, gonococci presumably interact with serum antibody, including natural IgM antibody directed against LPS antigens, with generation of the chemotactic factor C5a and formation of the bactericidal C5b-C9 attack complex. Insertion of the attack complex into the outer membrane of serum-sensitive gonococci results in gonococcal cell lysis. Although an attack complex is also formed when serum interacts with gonococci characterized by stable serum resistance, the insertion of the complex into the outer membrane of the organism has an abnormal configuration which does not result in rapid cell lysis. Furthermore, human serum also appears to contain IgG antibody directed against protein III which blocks the bactericidal action of IgM antibody for strains of gonococci with stable serum resistance. Following phagocytosis by neutrophils, the susceptibility of gonococci to intracellular killing is controversial. During in vivo growth, gonococci apparently develop phenotypic serum resistance and resistance to neutrophil-mediated killing. The mechanisms responsible for these phenotypic changes are largely undefined.

Spread of gonococci from the cervix to the endometrium and salpinges may be enhanced in women using an intrauterine device and impeded by oral contraceptive usage. Menstruation further increases the risk of intraluminal ascent from the cervix and evidently also predisposes to gonococcal bacteremia. Therefore, susceptibility to gonorrhea, to ascending gonococcal PID, and to gonococcemia depends upon a complex interplay of host factors and virulence properties of the organism.

DIFFERENTIAL DIAGNOSIS Gonococcal infection produces several common clinical syndromes which have multiple etiologies or which mimic other conditions. In particular, the epidemiology and clinical manifestations of *Chlamydia trachomatis* infections closely resemble those of gonococcal infections. The differential diagnosis of urethritis, epididymitis, and proctitis in men, vaginitis and cervicitis in women, and of acute arthritis in young adults is discussed in Chap. 90. The differential diagnosis of pelvic inflammatory disease is discussed in Chap. 91.

LABORATORY DIAGNOSIS The Gram's stain of urethral or endocervical exudate is considered diagnostic of gonorrhea when typical gram-negative diplococci are seen within leukocytes, is equivocal if only extracellular or atypical gram-negative diplococci are seen, and is negative if no gram-negative diplococci are seen. When these criteria are employed by experienced microbiologists, the sensitivity and specificity of Gram's stain of the urethral exudate approach 100 percent. Even so, in areas where resistant gonococci are seen, culture should be performed to allow testing of isolates for antimicrobial resistance. The specificity of Gram's stain of purulent cervical exudate also is high, but the sensitivity is only about 50 percent. Thayer-Martin (TM) medium, which contains antibiotics to inhibit most other organisms selectively, is most useful for recovering the gonococcus from the endocervix, rectum, and pharynx, which are colonized by a mixed bacterial flora. The concentration of vancomycin should not exceed 3 μg/mL, and even this concentration may inhibit a small proportion of gonococci. After inoculation, the medium should be placed in an atmosphere containing 3 to 10 percent carbon dioxide to permit growth of the gonococcus. This can be accomplished in a candle jar, by generation of carbon dioxide chemically within packets which are sealed after inoculation, or within special CO_2 incubators. Inoculated media should be incubated at 36°C for 48 h, and putative gonococcal colonies should be confirmed by oxidase reaction, Gram's stain, and sugar utilization tests or agglutination reactions using antiserums which are specific for *N. gonorrhoeae*. The latter two of these tests are especially important for isolates from the pharynx and rectum and for cultures obtained from populations which have a low prevalence of gonorrhea, such as prenatal patients.

In men with incubating or chronic asymptomatic urethral infection without exudate, or as a test of cure following treatment, a very thin swab should be inserted 2 cm into the anterior urethra and used to inoculate TM medium. Cultures of the pharynx and rectum should be obtained from homosexual men with suspected gonorrhea.

The most efficient test for gonorrhea in women is the endocervical culture, which is positive on a single examination in approximately 80 to 90 percent of those with gonorrhea. This diagnostic yield can be increased by performing a second endocervical culture and by performing cultures of the rectum, urethra, and pharynx.

Standard blood culture broth medium containing 3 to 10 percent carbon dioxide should be used in culturing blood and is also recommended for culturing synovial fluid. In pus from skin lesions, *N. gonorrhoeae* is more often demonstrable by immunofluorescent staining than by culture. Techniques designed to detect gonococcal infection by testing of a single serum have been limited by inability

to differentiate antibody due to past gonorrhea from antibody due to current infection, and by false-positive tests caused by cross-reactive antibody to *N. meningitidis*. For these reasons, serologic tests for gonorrhea have had a very low predictive value, and they are not used in clinical practice.

Another diagnostic approach is the detection of gonococcal antigen in urethral or cervical secretion by enzyme-linked immunosorbent assay (ELISA). In men with urethritis, the Gram stain is just as accurate, quicker, and cheaper. In women, these tests may be an acceptable alternative to culture for diagnosis of endocervical gonococcal infection in settings where culture is not at all feasible. However, the positive predictive value of the currently available test requires further study in populations with a low prevalence of gonorrhea; the medical-legal and psychosocial implications of a false-positive diagnosis of gonorrhea can be troublesome.

TREATMENT The preferred drugs for gonococcal infection for several years have been penicillin G, ampicillin, or amoxicillin, tetracycline hydrochloride, and spectinomycin. Although long-acting forms of penicillin (such as benzathine penicillin G) are effective in syphilotherapy, they have *no place* in the treatment of gonorrhea. Penicillin V and the isoxazolyl penicillins are not recommended for the treatment of gonococcal infection. Similarly, first-generation cephalosporins are not used for gonorrhea. In 1985, the Centers for Disease Control issued new treatment guidelines for gonorrhea because of several new developments. The incidence of infections due to penicillinase-producing *N. gonorrhoeae* has increased, and outbreaks have occurred with CMRNG. A high frequency of coexistent chlamydial infection in heterosexual patients with gonococcal infections has been demonstrated, and the importance of serious complications related to chlamydial infections has been established. Several new and more expensive β-lactam antibiotics which are effective in gonococcal infection (especially ceftriaxone) have come onto the market. Spectinomycin resistance has been noted frequently in England, Korea, and occasionally elsewhere. The following guidelines for gonococcal infections attempt to consider these new developments, but they do not represent a comprehensive list of all possible treatment regimens. These guidelines are adapted from recommendations made by a CDC advisory committee in 1985. As is shown in Table 104-1, a regimen combining a single oral dose of amoxicillin or ampicillin plus probenecid, or IM ceftriaxone without probenecid, together with a 7-day course of tetracycline or doxycycline, is recommended for uncomplicated gonococcal infections in heterosexual adults. These combination regimens can be expected to provide adequate therapy for gonorrhea at any site, including the pharynx, and eliminate coexisting *C. trachomatis* infections. In patients who can not tolerate tetracycline, the single-dose oral ampicillin or amoxicillin/probenecid regimen can be followed by erythromycin base or stearate, 500 mg by mouth four times daily for 7 days, or by erythromycin ethylsuccinate, 800 mg by mouth four times daily for 7 days. All tetracyclines are ineffective as single-dose therapy, and even a 7-day course of tetracycline has been ineffective in a small but growing proportion of patients, especially females, with gonorrhea.

Homosexual men with uncomplicated gonococcal infection should be treated with ceftriaxone, 250 mg IM; or with 4.8 million units of aqueous procaine penicillin G, plus 1.0 g of probenecid. Men allergic to penicillin should receive spectinomycin, 2.0 g, in one intramuscular injection. Any of these regimens provides adequate treatment for urethral and anorectal gonorrhea, but spectinomycin is not effective for pharyngeal gonorrhea. Coexisting chlamydial infection is less common in homosexual men with gonorrhea than in heterosexual men with gonorrhea, and therefore the 7-day course of tetracycline is often omitted in treating homosexual males. With parenteral penicillin G, the risk of anaphylaxis in patients who deny previous penicillin allergy has been about 0.04 percent. The risk of procaine reaction due to transient neurotoxic serum concentrations of procaine is probably between 0.1 and 1 percent with the currently recommended dosage.

All patients with gonorrhea should have a serologic test for syphilis at the time of diagnosis. Patients with incubating seronegative syphilis, without clinical signs of syphilis, are likely to be cured by any of the recommended regimens (except spectinomycin) and need not have later follow-up tests for syphilis. However, patients with gonorrhea who also have syphilis or who are established contacts of someone with syphilis should be given additional treatment appropriate to the stage of syphilis. As a test of cure of gonorrhea, follow-up cervical, rectal, and other appropriate cultures should be obtained from women, and urethral and other appropriate cultures from men, 3 to 7 days after completion of therapy.

The patient in whom gonorrhea persists after treatment with one of the nonspectinomycin regimens above should be treated with 250 mg of ceftriaxone intramuscularly or with 2.0 g of spectinomycin intramuscularly (except in areas where spectinomycin resistance is a problem). Most recurrent gonococcal infections after treatment with the recommended schedules are due to reinfection and indicate a need for improved contact tracing and patient education. Since infection by PPNG is a cause of treatment failure, posttreatment isolates should be tested for pencillinase production.

Patients with proven infection by PPNG or CMRNG, or who are likely to have acquired gonorrhea in areas where such strains are common (Africa, Asia, and currently certain metropolitan areas such as Miami), and their sexual partners should receive ceftriaxone, 250 mg, or spectinomycin, 2.0 g, intramuscularly in a single injection. Tetracycline or doxycycline may be added to treat coexistent chlamydial infection. Other newer β-lactam antibiotics (cefotaxime, cefuroxime), and certain new oxyquinolones are also very effective for resistant gonorrhea, but the long half-life of ceftriaxone, together with its in vitro activity, make it the optimal drug for single-dose therapy of resistant gonorrhea at present. Cefoxitin is also effective for PPNG infection in a dose of 2.0 g intramuscularly, together with 1.0 g of probenecid by mouth. Cefoxitin is widely used for PID (with doxycycline) because of its activity against other organisms often implicated in PID, as well as against *N. gonorrhoeae*.

Postgonococcal urethritis (PGU) usually becomes apparent about 2 to 3 weeks after treatment of gonorrhea with a penicillin or a cephalosporin. PGU often is caused by *C. trachomatis* which may have been acquired at the same time as gonorrhea but did not become clinically apparent until later because of the longer incubation period of chlamydial infection. When PGU occurs, it can be managed, like nongonococcal urethritis, with tetracycline, 0.5 g four times a day for at least 7 days. Similarly, mucopurulent cervicitis in women often persists or appears after treatment of gonorrhea with a penicillin, is often caused by *C. trachomatis*, and can be treated like PGU with tetracycline 0.5 g four times a day for 7 days. Men and women exposed to gonorrhea should be examined, cultured, and treated with one of the recommended treatment schedules.

All pregnant women should have endocervical cultures for gonococci at the time of the first visit as an integral part of the prenatal care. A second culture late in the third trimester should be obtained from women at high risk of gonococcal infection.

Drug regimens of choice in pregnancy are ampicillin or amoxicillin, each with probenecid as described above, or ceftriaxone. Women allergic to penicillin, cephalosporins, or probenecid can be treated with spectinomycin, 2.0 g intramuscularly. Erythromycin in the dosage recommended above for chlamydial infection can be added to treat coexistent chlamydial infection. Tetracycline should not be used in pregnant women because of potential toxic effects for mother and fetus.

The management of pelvic inflammatory disease is discussed in Chap. 91. Hospitalization of women with PID is recommended whenever practical. Adequate treatment of women with acute PID must include examination and appropriate treatment of sex partners because of their high prevalence of nonsymptomatic urethral, gonococcal, or chlamydial infection. Failure to treat sex partners may lead to recurrent salpingitis.

Treatment of gonococcal arthritis can be accomplished satisfactorily with several regimens. Gonococci recovered from patients with gonococcal arthritis have been significantly less resistant to penicillin or tetracycline than isolates from patients with uncomplicated gonorrhea. However, because of the threat of endocarditis, meningitis, and joint sepsis, all patients with disseminated infection should preferably be hospitalized and treated with aqueous crystalline penicillin G intravenously, 10 million units per day for at least 3 days, and until clinical improvement occurs. Treatment can then be completed on an outpatient basis with ampicillin or amoxicillin, 2 g per day orally, to complete a 7- to 10-day course of therapy. Treatment with ampicillin, 3.5 g daily orally with 1 g probenecid, followed by 0.5 g four times a day for 7 days, also probably represents adequate therapy for disseminated gonococcal infection. Failure to improve with one of these regimens strongly suggests a diagnosis other than disseminated gonococcal infection. Repeated joint aspiration or closed irrigation of the joint with sterile saline may be required to reduce inflammation in patients with high synovial fluid leukocyte counts. Open drainage is seldom, if ever, required for gonococcal arthritis, except in infants with hip infection. Temporary immobilization of the joint may reduce discomfort for the patient and may be useful during initial ambulation in patients with persistent effusions of the

TABLE 104-1   Recommended treatment for gonococcal infection

Diagnosis	Treatment of choice
Uncomplicated gonococcal infection in adults	Amoxicillin 3.0 g or ampicillin 3.5 g single oral dose, or ceftriaxone 250 mg intramuscularly. Amoxicillin and ampicillin (but not ceftriaxone) to be accompanied by 1.0 g probenecid by mouth. Complete therapy with tetracycline 0.5 g by mouth four times a day or with doxycycline 100 mg by mouth twice daily for 7 days (if penicillin-allergic, give the 7-day tetracycline or doxycycline regimen alone).
Uncomplicated gonococcal infection in homosexual men	Aqueous procaine penicillin G (APPG), 4.8 million units total dose given intramuscularly at two sites, with 1.0 g probenecid by mouth (if penicillin-allergic, give spectinomycin 2.0 g in one intramuscular injection*).
Treatment failures, penicillinase-producing *N. gonorrhoeae*, or chromosomally mediated resistant *N. gonorrhoeae*	Spectinomycin 2.0 g single intramuscular dose* or ceftriaxone 250 mg single intramuscular dose.
Gonorrhea in pregnancy	Same as for uncomplicated gonococcal infection in adults, except that erythromycin should be substituted for tetracycline for coexisting chlamydial infection (see text) (if penicillin-allergic, give spectinomycin 2.0 g single intramuscular dose).
Disseminated gonococcal infection	Hospitalization is recommended. Aqueous crystalline penicillin G, 10 million units intravenously per day for at least 3 days (longer if meningitis or endocarditis occur), followed by ampicillin or amoxicillin, 0.5 g by mouth four times daily to complete 7 days of antibiotic treatment.
Gonococcal PID	Hospitalization is recommended; see Chap. 91 for suggested antimicrobial therapy.
Gonococcal epididymitis	See Chap. 90 for recommended therapy.
Pediatric gonococcal infection	Children who weigh 100 lb (45 kg) should receive adult regimens; for those who weigh less than 100 lb, see discussion in text.

* *Not effective for pharyngeal gonococcal infection (see text).*

knee or ankle. Antibiotics should not be injected directly into the joint. Once the diagnosis of gonococcal arthritis is proven, then occasional patients may benefit from use of anti-inflammatory agents along with antimicrobial therapy. However, if the diagnosis is suspected, but not proven, then early use of anti-inflammatory drugs will prevent monitoring the response to antimicrobial therapy, which is usually rapid and often of diagnostic importance in gonococcal arthritis.

Meningitis and endocarditis caused by the gonococcus require high-dose intravenous penicillin therapy, typically for 10 to 14 days for meningitis and 1 month for endocarditis. In penicillin-allergic patients with disseminated gonococcal infection, ceftriaxone, 1.0 g IV once daily, or cefotaxime, 500 mg IV four times daily for 14 days may be used. Similar doses are acceptable for arthritis, and higher doses may be effective for meningitis and endocarditis, although experience so far is negligible, and cross-allergenicity with penicillin may occur.

Gonococcal conjunctivitis in the adult or newborn should be managed as a medical emergency by irrigation of the conjunctiva with saline, together with penicillin G or ceftriaxone given intravenously.

Pediatric gonococcal infection   The infant born to a mother with gonorrhea is at high risk of infection and requires treatment with a single intravenous or intramuscular injection of aqueous crystalline penicillin G, 50,000 units to the full-term infant or 20,000 units to the low-birth-weight infant. Topical prophylaxis for neonatal ophthalmia is not adequate treatment for infections at other sites. Clinical illness requires additional treatment.

Neonates with gonococcal ophthalmia should be hospitalized and isolated for 24 h after initiation of treatment. Aqueous crystalline penicillin G, 100,000 units per kilogram per day, in four divided daily doses intravenously should be administered for 7 days. Irrigation of the eyes with saline or buffered ophthalmic solutions should be performed immediately and then repeated as often as necessary to eliminate discharge. Topical antibiotic preparations alone are not sufficient or required when appropriate systemic antibiotic therapy is given. Both of the parents of a newborn with gonococcal ophthalmia must be treated for gonorrhea.

Neonates with arthritis and bacteremia should be hospitalized and treated with aqueous crystalline penicillin G, 100,000 units per kilogram per day, intravenously in four divided doses for 7 days (at least 10 days for meningitis).

Uncomplicated gonococcal vulvovaginitis, urethritis, proctitis, or pharyngitis in older children can be treated at a single visit with amoxicillin, 50 mg/kg, orally with probenecid, 25 mg/kg (maximum 1.0 g), or with ceftriaxone, 125 mg IM. This regimen is recommended for proctitis and pharyngitis. Patients should be evaluated for coinfection by chlamydia.

Topical and/or systemic estrogen therapy is of no benefit in gonococcal vulvovaginitis. All children should have follow-up cultures, and the source of infection should be identified, examined, and treated. Child abuse should be carefully considered and evaluated.

Children who are allergic to penicillins can be treated with spectinomycin, 40 mg/kg, intramuscularly. Children older than 8 years may be treated with tetracycline, 40 mg/kg per day, by mouth, in four divided doses for 5 days. For treatment of complicated disease, the alternative regimens recommended for adults may be used in appropriate pediatric dosages.

PPNG infection in neonates should be treated with ceftriaxone, 125 mg intramuscularly, but experience is limited.

Treatment of gonorrhea in developing countries   Ironically, the proportion of gonococcal infections caused by PPNG or CMRNG is highest in developing countries, which can least afford spectinomycin, ceftriaxone, or other new antimicrobials effective against these strains. Inexpensive alternatives to penicillin G and tetracycline, the traditional mainstays of gonorrhea therapy, have been generally disappointing. For example, a sulfonamide-trimethoprim combination which initially cured over 95 percent of cases of gonorrhea in African countries, fell to less than 75 percent efficacy within 2 years after it became a popular regimen in Kenya. One innovative approach has been the use of 4.8 million units of procaine penicillin G intramuscularly plus 1.0 g probenecid orally (a standard regimen for non-PPNG infections) together with 125 mg of clavulanic acid (in the form of one capsule of amoxicillin-clavulanate) to inhibit gonococcal β-lactamase. This inexpensive regimen has been effective in small trials in Kenya, even against PPNG infections. Gentamicin, in a 280-mg single intramuscular dose, has also been used effectively in this setting. Use of newer cephalosporins in lower than recommended doses, to reduce cost, should be discouraged.

PREVENTION AND CONTROL   There is probably no more striking illustration than gonorrhea of the failure of a specific treatment alone to eradicate a communicable disease. Vaccination is not available. A field trial of a purified gonococcal pili vaccine in U.S. soldiers in Korea showed that the vaccine was not effective. Use of the condom can prevent transmission, and the extensive use of condoms for contraception may be responsible for the low rates of gonorrhea in some countries (e.g., Japan). Spermicidal preparations used with a diaphragm probably offer some protection against gonorrhea and chlamydial infection, though this has not been proved convincingly. Prophylactic antibiotics (e.g., 200 mg minocycline or doxycycline taken soon after sexual exposure) reduce the risk of infection, but are not recommended for general use or for individuals with known exposure to gonorrhea, who should receive one of the regimens recommended for established gonorrhea.

To contain the increasing spread of antimicrobial-resistant gonococci, several measures are important: (1) routine use of diagnosis by cultures and testing of isolates for antimicrobial resistance or β-lactamase production; (2) routine use of spectinomycin or ceftriaxone for gonorrhea treatment failures; (3) rapid epidemiologic tracing of contacts of patients with gonorrhea, particularly treatment failures of those known to be infected with resistant gonococci; and (4) routine use of spectinomycin or ceftriaxone in areas where PPNG exceeds a certain threshold proportion (e.g., >5 percent) of all gonococcal isolates. The most effective public health measure now available for control of gonorrhea is tracing sexual contacts of infected patients. Experienced interviewers are able to identify and bring to treatment an average of one additional case for every patient interviewed.

REFERENCES

BRITIGAN BE, SPARLING PF: Gonococcal infection: A model of molecular pathogenesis. N Engl J Med 312:1683, 1985

CENTERS FOR DISEASE CONTROL: 1985 STD treatment guidelines. Morb Mort Week Rep 34(4S):75S, 1985

CURRAN JW et al: Female gonorrhea. Its relations to abnormal uterine bleeding, urinary tract symptoms and cervicitis. Obstet Gynecol 45:195, 1975

EASMON CSF et al: Emergence of resistance after spectinomycin treatment for gonorrhoea due to beta-lactamase–producing strain of Neisseria gonorrhoeae. Br Med J 284:1604, 1982

HANDSFIELD HH et al: Asymptomatic gonorrhea in men. Diagnosis, natural course, prevalence and significance. N Engl J Med 290:117, 1974

—— et al: Treatment of the gonococcal arthritis-dermatitis syndrome. Ann Intern Med 84:661, 1976

—— et al: Epidemiology of penicillinase-producing Neisseria gonorrhoeae infections: Analysis by auxotyping and serogrouping. N Engl J Med 306:950, 1982

HOLMES KK et al: Disseminated gonococcal infection. Ann Intern Med 74:979, 1971

HOOK EH III, HOLMES KK: Gonococcal infections. Ann Intern Med 102:229, 1985

KNAPP JS et al: Serologic classification of Neisseria gonorrhoeae using monoclonal antibodies directed against outer membrane protein I. J Infect Dis 150:44, 1985

PANIKABUTRA K et al: Randomized comparative study of ceftriaxone and spectinomycin in gonorrhea. Genitourin Med 61:106, 1985

PETERSEN BH et al: Neisseria meningitidis and Neisseria gonorrhoeae bacteremia associated with C6, C7, or C8 deficiency. Ann Intern Med 90:917, 1979

ROBERTS M et al: Molecular characterization of two beta-lactamase specifying plasmids isolated from Neisseria gonorrhoeae. J Bacteriol 131:557, 1977

ROBERTS RB: The Gonococcus. New York, Wiley, 1977

SCHOOLNIK GK et al (eds): The Pathogenic Neisseria. Washington, DC, American Society for Microbiology, 1985

105   DISEASES CAUSED BY GRAM-NEGATIVE ENTERIC BACILLI

DENNIS R. SCHABERG / MARVIN TURCK

INTRODUCTION The Enterobacteriaceae are a group of gram-negative nonsporing rods which are aerobic but can grow under anaerobic conditions, and which are commonly found in the gastrointestinal tract. They are characterized biochemically by their ability to ferment glucose, their ability to reduce nitrates to nitrites, and the fact that they are oxidase-negative. The diverse genera in this family, including *Escherichia, Salmonella, Shigella, Klebsiella, Serratia, Enterobacter, Proteus, Morganella, Yersinia, Providencia,* and other less common genera, are differentiated by serologic tests and computerized analysis of biochemical reactions. It is important to make this differentiation, not only taxonomically but also because of epidemiologic and therapeutic implications.

Other gram-negative bacilli which are not members of the family Enterobacteriaceae may also be causes of infection. Important genera include *Pseudomonas, Acinetobacter,* and *Eikenella.*

ESCHERICHIA COLI INFECTIONS

ETIOLOGY *Escherichia coli,* of the family Enterobacteriaceae, is a commensal in the gastrointestinal tract. It may spread from the tract to infect contiguous structures if normal anatomic barriers are interrupted, as occurs in appendiceal perforation. It is believed that the urinary tract is infected from without via urethral contamination, but direct hematogenous spread may also account for renal infection. Once infection has occurred in a primary focus, further spread to distant organs may occur via the bloodstream. A consequence of bacteremia that occurs potentially with all gram-negative bacilli is endotoxin shock (Chap. 86). In more than 50 percent of *E. coli* infections, the urinary tract is the portal of entry; infections emanating from the hepatobiliary tree, peritoneal cavity, skin, and lung are also common. Some patients with *E. coli* bacteremia have no demonstrable portal of entry; they often have neoplastic and hematologic diseases. There may be other defects in host resistance, including diabetes mellitus, cirrhosis, and sickle cell anemia or recent administration of irradiation, cytotoxic drugs, adrenal steroids, or antibiotics. There is also epidemiologic evidence that *E. coli* and other Enterobacteriaceae tend to colonize the skin and mucous membranes of debilitated patients, possibly accounting for the increased frequency of these infections in patients with advanced illness. There is a common misconception that *E. coli* bacterial infections are characterized by a foul-smelling, feculent exudate. Such an odor is caused by anaerobic streptococci or *Bacteroides* species, which are often associated with coliform bacteria in mixed infections.

EPIDEMIOLOGY Strains of *E. coli* are characterized by their somatic (O), flagellar (H), and capsular (K) antigens, and there are hundreds of different serologic varieties. Any of the strains is capable of causing disease. Clinical and epidemiologic studies have demonstrated that certain specific *E. coli* serotypes are more frequently incriminated in diarrheal disease of the infant and newborn as well as in outbreaks of enteric disease in adults. Strains incriminated in infantile diarrhea probably are disseminated within nurseries by symptomatic or asymptomatic infant carriers, mothers, and staff. Although fecal contamination is the usual mode of spread, airborne contamination and fomite spread may also occur.

Some epidemiologic studies have suggested that *E. coli* 04, 06, and 075 are responsible for most *E. coli* infections other than infantile diarrhea. It is unclear whether these strains actually are more virulent or merely are more prevalent than other somatic types.

Strains of *E. coli* with K1 antigen are recovered from an inordinate number of neonates with meningitis. These K antigens have been implicated in promoting adherence to host cells and in resisting phagocytosis.

MANIFESTATIONS   **Urinary tract infections**   *Escherichia coli* accounts for over 75 percent of urinary tract infections, including cystitis, pyelitis, pyelonephritis, and asymptomatic bacteriuria (see Chap. 225). Strains cultured from patients with acute uncomplicated urinary tract infections are almost invariably *E. coli,* whereas other Enterobacteriaceae and strains of *Pseudomonas* become prevalent among patients with chronic infection.

Peritoneal and biliary infections   *Escherichia coli* can usually be cultured from a perforated or inflamed appendix or from abscesses secondary to perforated diverticula, peptic ulcers, subphrenic or lesser sac abscesses, or mesenteric infarction. Often, other organisms, including anaerobic streptococci, clostridia, and *Bacteroides,* are found along with *E. coli.* Acute cholecystitis with gangrene and perforation is often associated with *E. coli* infection. An air-fluid level associated with stones or a circumferential layer of gas in the wall of the gallbladder may be detectable by x-ray and is characteristic of acute emphysematous cholecystitis. From the gallbladder, infection may ascend via the biliary tree to produce cholangitis and multiple liver abscesses. More rarely, *E. coli* infection in the peritoneal cavity may produce a septic thrombophlebitis of the portal vein (pylephlebitis), which in turn is followed by liver abscesses.

Bacteremia   Invasion of the bloodstream is the most serious manifestation of *E. coli* infection; it is characterized usually by the sudden onset of fever and chills but sometimes only by mental confusion, dyspnea, or unexplained hypotension. It is most common in patients with urinary tract infection and biliary or intraperitoneal sepsis. In some patients no portal of entry is evident. Most cases occur in elderly males, presumably because of the high incidence of urethral instrumentation and catheterization in this group. Hyperventilation may be an early sign. Hypotension may be present from the onset but usually occurs within 12 to 16 h after bacteremia; if it is persistent, it is accompanied by oliguria and often by mental confusion, stupor, and coma, a syndrome known as *gram-negative* or *endotoxin shock* (see Chap. 86). Occasionally, *E. coli* bacteremia develops in patients with cirrhosis without an overt portal of entry. This has been attributed to portosystemic shunts both in and around the liver, impaired reticuloendothelial function, and diminution in humoral and cellular defense mechanisms. Persistence or reappearance of bacteremia with *E. coli* or other members of the Enterobacteriaceae on therapy, so-called breakthrough bacteremia, has a poor prognosis and suggests an intraabdominal focus for infection or undrained pus.

Other manifestations   *Escherichia coli* may produce abscesses anywhere in the body. Subcutaneous infections are found at the site of insulin administration in diabetics, in ischemic extremities, and in surgical wounds. Perirectal phlegmons are not uncommon in patients with leukemia. Subcutaneous abscesses, especially among diabetics, are often characterized by formation of gas in tissue, which may be detected by crepitation or by x-ray and which must be differentiated from clostridial infection. This is most rapidly accomplished by Gram's stain. *Escherichia coli* may cause pneumonia de novo; also, *E. coli* are often cultured from sputum in pulmonary superinfections.

Neonatal infection   Neonates, particularly premature infants, often develop *E. coli* bacteremia associated with meningitis and bloodborne pyelonephritis. Fecal soiling and absence of maternal gamma-globulin (IgM) antibody are two of the factors which render this group particularly susceptible to *E. coli* infections.

Gastroenteritis   Children under 2 years of age develop gastroenteritis typified by nausea, vomiting, and diarrhea. Most outbreaks have occurred in nurseries and have been due to specific strains of enteropathogenic *E. coli* (EPEC). These strains can produce toxins, one of which is heat labile (LT) and similar to the toxin elaborated by *Vibrio cholerae,* while the other is heat stable (ST) (see also Chaps. 89 and 115). Fluorescent antibody techniques have been useful in the rapid identification of organisms with serotypes frequently implicated in this syndrome. Although theoretically any *E. coli* strain might be cultured, since the genetic information coding for toxin production is found on a plasmid and can be transferred between *E. coli* strains, the number of different serotypes involved remains restricted. Although diarrhea is usually mediated through production of enterotoxins, occasionally *E. coli* may be enteroinvasive, involving the mucosa and causing disease akin to *Shigella* dysentery. The rapid dehydration, with its attendant high mortality, demands prompt recognition of this condition, isolation of the infants, and treatment of both patients and contacts. *Escherichia coli* is also recognized as a cause of acute diarrheal disease in adults, especially in travelers abroad.

LABORATORY FINDINGS   There are no characteristic laboratory abnormalities. The white blood cell count is usually elevated, and there is a preponderance of granulocytes. At times, however, the white count is normal or low. When *E. coli* infection occurs in previously healthy individuals, anemia is absent, but more commonly there is anemia which is usually related to underlying disease. *Escherichia coli* grows readily in a variety of bacteriologic media and should be cultured from appropriate secretions and blood. In the presence of bacteremia there can be metabolic derangements, including azotemia, metabolic acidosis, hypokalemia, and hyperkalemia as well as a variety of coagulation defects.

DIAGNOSIS   *Escherichia coli* cannot be differentiated from most other gram-negative bacteria on Gram's stain, and culture followed by appropriate biochemical characterization is necessary to identify the organism precisely. Serologic typing of *E. coli* may be useful in individual patients with recurrent urinary tract infections in order to help differentiate between relapse and reinfection.

TREATMENT   As with other infections, drainage of pus and removal of foreign bodies are essential. If *E. coli* is suspected as the etiologic agent in a particular infection, choice of an appropriate antimicrobial will depend upon the site and type of infection as well as upon its severity; outcome is often related to underlying disease. For example, in acute, uncomplicated urinary tract infection in females, the disease is frequently self-limited even without antimicrobial therapy, and there is no evidence that antibiotics are superior to sulfonamides. Conversely, *E. coli* bacteremia in a patient with leukemia may not respond to antimicrobials unless a hematologic remission is achieved simultaneously.

In most situations, antibiotics should be selected on the basis of in vitro susceptibility tests. Although no drug is uniformly active against all strains of *E. coli,* a number of agents are effective against the majority of clinical isolates. Although resistant strains can be encountered, especially in hospital-acquired *E. coli,* ampicillin remains an effective drug when given in doses of 2 to 4 g per day intravenously, intramuscularly, or orally. For severe infections the dose of ampicillin can be raised to 12 g per day, usually given intravenously. The cephalosporins are also effective against *E. coli;* compounds such as cefazolin and cephapirin provide effective therapy. Newer so-called third generation cephalosporins have lower minimal inhibitory concentrations (MICs) for *E. coli*; this increased activity coupled with slightly enhanced CNS penetration make them useful for the therapy of meningitis due to *E. coli* (see Chap. 346). Gentamicin and tobramycin have been employed effectively in the initial treatment of severe *E. coli* infections in doses of 5 mg/kg per day in divided doses every 8 h. Amikacin is very active against isolates which are resistant to the other aminoglycosides in doses of 15 mg/kg per day, divided to be administered every 8 to 12 h. Tetracyclines and chloramphenicol are still used in the treatment of *E. coli* infection, but better drugs are now available. Although combinations of antimicrobials have been recommended there is little need to employ more than one agent in most situations. Nitrofurantoin (400 mg) and nalidixic acid (2 to 4 g) are reserved for treating patients with *E. coli* bacteriuria, and should not be employed when infection is suspected outside the urinary tract. Trimethoprim/sulfamethoxazole is also useful in urinary tract infections.

PREVENTION   Isolation and antimicrobial therapy of infants and contacts are essential to abort epidemic infantile diarrhea. In adults, many *E. coli* infections are hospital-associated, and their incidence can be reduced by limiting use of indwelling urinary and intravenous catheters, by careful surgical aseptic technique, by appropriate isolation of infection-prone patients, and by judicious use of antibiotics, glucocorticosteroids, and cytotoxic agents.

KLEBSIELLA-ENTEROBACTER-SERRATIA INFECTIONS

ETIOLOGY   Next to *E. coli,* strains of *Klebsiella, Enterobacter,* and *Serratia* are the most important enteric organisms infecting humans. These are also of the family Enterobacteriaceae. In many laboratories *Klebsiella* are more resistant to antibiotics than are *E. coli,* and their isolation from blood, purulent exudates, and urine is of more serious epidemiologic and prognostic significance. The Friedlander bacilli (*K. pneumoniae*) are encapsulated gram-negative bacilli found among the normal flora of the mouth and intestinal tracts. *Klebsiella* are closely related to the genera *Enterobacter* and *Serratia* and may be differentiated only by certain amino acid decarboxylase tests. In addition to differentiation by these biochemical tests, which identify the *Klebsiella, Enterobacter,* and *Serratia* groups, strains of *Klebsiella* usually are nonmotile and form large mucoid colonies on solid media, whereas the other species are typically motile. Strains of *Klebsiella* can be further distinguished on the basis of type-specific capsular antigens; more than 75 known capsular types have been identified. There is little evidence that certain types are more virulent than others, and the main role of capsular typing of *Klebsiella* is an epidemiologic tool in nosocomial outbreaks of infection.

Klebsiella rhinoscleromatis is probably the causative agent of rhinoscleroma, and *K. ozenae* has been isolated occasionally from the noses of patients with ozena, a chronic severe rhinitis associated with turbinate atrophy and progressive anosmia. *Klebsiella oxytoca* is the new designation for indole-positive strains of *K. pneumoniae.*

PATHOGENESIS   *Klebsiella, Enterobacter,* and *Serratia* are all capable of causing disease in diverse anatomic sites. However, results of clinical and epidemiologic studies suggest that differences in pathogenicity may exist among these genera and that precise taxonomic identification is of value. Although infections of the respiratory tract with *K. pneumoniae* have been emphasized most in the past, the urinary tract presently accounts for the majority of clinical isolates. In this site clinical manifestations and pathogenesis are similar to those of infections produced by *E. coli,* but *Klebsiella* is more frequently found in patients with complicated and obstructive urinary tract disease. Infections of the biliary tract, peritoneal cavity, middle ear, mastoids, paranasal sinuses, and meninges also are not uncommon. In these locations, *Klebsiella* is more frequent than either *Enterobacter* or *Serratia* and is more likely to produce an illness of greater severity. The apparent increased frequency of infection by *Serratia* represents an increase primarily due to nosocomial spread of this organism. *Enterobacter* species have been incriminated frequently in outbreaks of in-hospital bacteremia attributed to contaminated intravenous solutions.

MANIFESTATIONS   Symptoms and signs of common infections caused by *Klebsiella*—namely, those involving the urinary tract, biliary tree, and peritoneal cavity—are indistinguishable from those caused by *E. coli.* These infections commonly occur in diabetics and in the form of superinfections in patients who have received antimicrobials to which these organisms are resistant. *Klebsiella* infection is also an important etiologic factor in septic shock. *Serratia* and *Enterobacter* are almost exclusively nosocomial pathogens. These organisms have been implicated as pathogens in a wide variety of infections, most frequently pneumonia, urinary tract infections, and bacteremia.

Pneumonia *Klebsiella* is well recognized as a pulmonary pathogen but probably accounts for less than 1 percent of all cases of bacterial pneumonia. The disease is most common in men over 40 years of age and is most frequently found in alcoholics. Other factors associated with increased susceptibility include diabetes mellitus and chronic bronchopulmonary disease. Aspiration of oropharyngeal secretions containing *Klebsiella* organisms is the likely inciting factor among alcoholic patients. The clinical manifestations are indistinguishable from those of pneumococcal pneumonia (see Chap. 93), with sudden onset of chills, fever, productive cough, and severe pleuritic chest pain. Patients are frequently delirious and prostrated, but this may also occur with pneumococcal infection. The pulmonary lesion is most frequent in the right upper lobe but often rapidly progresses and, if untreated, may spread from lobe to lobe. Cyanosis and dyspnea develop rapidly, and jaundice, vomiting, and diarrhea may be present. Physical findings consist primarily of consolidation, unless pleural effusion or necrotizing pneumonitis with rapid cavitation has intervened. The blood leukocyte count may be elevated but is often low, which probably is a reflection of severe infection in an alcoholic patient with poor bone marrow reserve and folate deficiency. Lung abscess and empyema are much more frequent than they are in pneumococcal pneumonia; they are related to the destructive capabilities of this organism. So-called characteristic radiographic features such as bulging fissures and loss of lung volume occur only occasionally; they also may be found in pneumococcal infection as well as in necrotizing pneumonia caused by other gram-negative species.

Klebsiella, *Serratia*, and *Enterobacter* are frequently seen in nosocomial pneumonia. Older patients become colonized with gram-negative bacilli in the oropharynx, and these organisms can then gain access to the respiratory tract and cause pneumonia or purulent bronchitis. Common-source outbreaks, with contamination of a variety of respiratory therapy devices, have been implicated in infections with these pathogens, especially *Serratia*. As a general rule, the most drug-resistant strains of *Serratia* are nonpigmented and account for the majority of nosocomial isolates. However, pigmented and multiply sensitive *Serratia* isolates are also seen in device-related infections. Rarely, infection with *Klebsiella* may progress, often in indolent fashion, to a chronic necrotizing pneumonitis resembling tuberculosis. The principal symptoms are productive cough, weakness, and anemia.

DIAGNOSIS Diagnosis of community-acquired pneumonia is established by an awareness of the clinical setting in which *Klebsiella* infections occur and by isolation of the organism. A presumptive diagnosis of *Klebsiella* pneumonia should be made on the basis of a Gram's stain of the sputum which shows a predominance of short, plump, gram-negative bacilli, frequently surrounded by a clear space because of the capsule. Often these gram-negative organisms occur together with gram-positive cocci, and because the gram-positives are easier to see, the gram-negative bacteria may be ignored and the diagnosis may be missed. This, in turn, may lead to potentially serious delays in instituting therapy. Additional proof of *Klebsiella* infection in the lung is the isolation of the organisms from blood and pleural exudate. In extrapulmonary infections, the organisms are readily seen in, or cultured from, pus or secretions of involved organs.

The diagnosis of nosocomial respiratory infection with these organisms may be more difficult, mainly because colonization has to be distinguished from infection. Careful evaluation of the clinical course is necessary in establishing a diagnosis. Transtracheal aspiration of sputum for culture and Gram's stain may be useful in difficult cases.

TREATMENT *Klebsiella*, *Enterobacter*, and *Serratia* have variable susceptibility to antimicrobial drugs, and cultures of these organisms need to be tested in vitro. Frequently, antimicrobial therapy needs to be begun before results of antibiotic susceptibility tests are available. In general, most strains of *Klebsiella* are susceptible to the aminoglycosides and the newer third generation cephalosporins. *Klebsiella* isolates do not respond to most penicillin analogues, although many isolates are inhibited by newer ureidopenicillins, e.g., mezlocillin. *Serratia* isolates are frequently resistant to many antimicrobials, and resistance to gentamicin and tobramycin is being encountered with increasing frequency. Amikacin has been used effectively in these drug-resistant infections. The antimicrobial regimen of choice in the treatment of *Klebsiella*, *Enterobacter*, and *Serratia* infection will vary from one institution to another depending on the resistance patterns as well as upon the degree of clinical severity of infection. In severely ill patients, the combination of an aminoglycoside such as tobramycin or gentamicin (3 to 5 mg/kg per day) or amikacin (15 mg/kg per day) with cephalothin, cephapirin, or cefazolin (4 to 12 g per day) is usually preferred. The new cephalosporins and/or cephamycins, i.e., cefoxitin, or third generation compounds also may be active against *Klebsiella*, *Enterobacter*, and *Serratia*. Occasionally, one or all of these compounds may be more active than the older cephalosporins, and in vitro susceptibility tests will be required to select the most appropriate agent. Because of the relatively poor blood and tissue levels obtained with the polymyxins, they should not be employed as first-line agents in the treatment of severe *Klebsiella* infections despite apparent in vitro susceptibility. Regardless of the antimicrobial regimen employed, treatment should be continued for a minimum of 10 to 14 days and prolonged if there is extensive cavitation. Pleural effusions must be drained; antibiotic therapy alone is not sufficient treatment for closed-space infections of the pleural cavity. At times, rib resection with open drainage may be necessary and should be considered if effusions recur.

PROGNOSIS Before the introduction of antimicrobials, the fatality rate from these infections varied from 50 to 80 percent, and death within 48 h was not infrequent. Even with antimicrobial treatment the course of these infections is quite variable and the prognosis must be guarded. For the most part, the prognosis reflects the age group involved and the frequent association of *Klebsiella* infections with alcoholism, malnutrition, and severe underlying disease.

PROTEUS, MORGANELLA, AND PROVIDENCIA INFECTIONS

ETIOLOGY The genus *Proteus* of the family Enterobacteriaceae consists of gram-negative bacilli which do not ferment lactose and are characterized by their active motility and spreading growth on solid media. Organisms once thought to be related and once classified as *Proteus* have recently been renamed based on detailed DNA studies. *Proteus morganii* has been reclassified as *Morganella morganii*, while some biogroups of *Proteus rettgeri* have been reclassified as *Providencia stuartii* and *Providencia rettgeri*. *Proteus mirabilis* and *Proteus vulgaris* retain their nomenclature; *Proteus mirabilis* causes 75 to 90 percent of human infections. It is distinguishable from the other organisms mentioned by its inability to form indole. All four split urea, with production of ammonia. Some strains of *Proteus vulgaris* share a common antigen with certain rickettsia, which accounts for the appearance of antibodies against *Proteus* organisms (Weil-Felix reaction) in typhus, scrub typhus, and Rocky Mountain spotted fever. The *Providencia* group of organisms resembles those of the genus *Proteus* closely except for some differences in biochemical tests.

EPIDEMIOLOGY AND PATHOGENESIS These organisms are normally found in soil, water, and sewage and are part of the normal fecal flora. Occasionally, they have been implicated as a cause of epidemic diarrhea in infants, but the evidence for this is inconclusive. They are frequently cultured from superficial wounds, draining ears, and sputum, particularly in patients who have received antibiotics; they replace the more susceptible flora eradicated by these drugs.

MANIFESTATIONS These organisms are rarely primary invaders but produce disease in locations previously infected by other pathogens. These locations include skin, ears and mastoid, sinuses, eyes, peritoneal cavity, bone, urinary tract, meninges, lung, and bloodstream.

Cutaneous infections   These organisms can be isolated from surgical wounds, particularly after antimicrobial therapy, but they do not interfere with normal wound healing provided that the tissues are viable and foreign bodies are not present. Burns, varicose ulcers, and decubitus ulcers may become contaminated with these organisms, often in company with other gram-negative bacilli or staphylococci.

Infections of the ears and mastoid sinuses   Otitis media and mastoiditis, especially with *Proteus mirabilis*, can result in extensive destruction of the middle ear and mastoid sinuses. Fetid otorrhea, cholesteatoma, and granulation tissue constitute a chronic focus of infection in the middle and inner ears and mastoid, and deafness ensues. Paralysis of the facial nerve is an occasional complication. The great danger of these infections lies in intracranial extension, leading to thrombosis of the lateral sinus, meningitis, brain abscess, and bacteremia.

Ocular infections   These pathogens may cause corneal ulcers, usually following trauma to the eye, which occasionally terminate in panophthalmitis and destruction of the eyeball.

Peritonitis   Because they are part of the normal intestinal flora, these organisms may be isolated from the peritoneal cavity following perforation of viscera or mesenteric infarction.

Urinary tract infections   These organisms are a common cause of urinary tract infections, usually in patients with chronic bacteriuria, many of whom have had obstructive uropathy, a history of bladder instrumentation, and repeated courses of chemotherapy. They are often recovered from bacteriuric patients with renal or bladder calculi. This may be related to the urease activity which renders the urine alkaline and provides a fertile medium for formation of ammonium-magnesium-phosphate stones.

Bacteremia   Bloodstream invasion is the most serious manifestation of infection with this organism. In 75 percent of cases, the urinary tract serves as the portal of entry; in the remainder, the biliary tree, gastrointestinal tract, ears and sinuses, and skin are the primary foci. Bacteremia is frequently preceded by cystoscopy, urethral catheterization, transurethral prostatic resection, or other operative procedures. Clinically, the signs, symptoms, and laboratory findings of sepsis—high fever, chills, shock, metastatic abscess, leukocytosis, and rarely thrombocytopenia—are indistinguishable from those of bloodstream infections with *E. coli*, *Klebsiella*, or other gram-negative bacteria.

DIAGNOSIS   The diagnosis of *Proteus*, *Morganella*, or *Providencia* infection depends on culture of the organism from blood, urine, or exudate and its identification by appropriate biochemical tests. It is especially important to separate *Proteus mirabilis*, the indole-negative species, from organisms that are indole-positive, because only *P. mirabilis* is susceptible to the action of penicillin and many other antibiotics. *Proteus* organisms are often present in mixed infections with other pathogens. Particular care should be exercised in the isolation of other organisms growing in the same medium with *Proteus mirabilis* or *Proteus vulgaris* lest they be masked by spreading growth. The spreading character of these bacteria also may make antibiotic sensitivity tests difficult to interpret.

TREATMENT   Most strains of *Proteus mirabilis* are sensitive to penicillin in high concentration (10 units per milliliter or greater), ampicillin, carbenicillin, gentamicin, tobramycin, or amikacin, and the cephalosporin antibiotics. *Proteus mirabilis* bacteriuria can be readily eradicated with any of these drugs during treatment; ampicillin in dosage of 0.5 gm every 4 to 6 h is highly effective. In severe infection, therapy should be parenteral: 6 to 12 g ampicillin or 20 million units of penicillin G plus tobramycin or gentamicin in divided doses of 5 mg/kg per day, if renal function is adequate. There is some evidence that an aminoglycoside is synergistic with ampicillin and penicillin G in *P. mirabilis* infections. In view of the numerous

more effective agents, there is no reason to use chloramphenicol in *P. mirabilis* infections. In general, all strains of *P. mirabilis* are resistant to tetracycline. Most strains other than *P. mirabilis* are predictably sensitive only to aminoglycosides and the third generation cephalosporins. Carbenicillin, ticarcillin, and the new ureidopenicillins are effective against many isolates. Ideally, therapy should be based on in vitro susceptibility, or lacking this, an awareness of local resistance patterns. As with all other gram-negative infections, appropriate attention must be given to drainage of pus, maintenance of fluid and electrolyte status, and, if endotoxin shock is present, treatment of circulatory collapse.

PSEUDOMONAS INFECTIONS

ETIOLOGY   *Pseudomonas aeruginosa* is a motile gram-negative rod which generally is not encapsulated and forms no spores. It grows readily in all ordinary culture media, and on agar it forms irregular, soft, iridescent colonies which usually have a fluorescent yellow-green color because of diffusion into the medium of two pigments, pyocyanin and fluorescin. *Pseudomonas* produces acid but no gas in glucose, and it is proteolytic. It is oxidase-positive and produces ammonia from arginine. A number of different strains have been identified by immunofluorescent techniques or bacteriophage typing. There is no evidence that these strains vary in their virulence for humans. Other *Pseudomonas* species (*P. maltophilia*, *P. cepacia*, *P. fluorescens*, *P. testosteroni*, and *P. putida*) also may cause infection in human beings. For the most part, these organisms have been associated with common-source nosocomial outbreaks; in addition, they have been incriminated in bacteremia, endocarditis, and osteomyelitis in narcotic addicts.

EPIDEMIOLOGY   *Pseudomonas* organisms are present on the skin of some normal persons, particularly in the axilla and anogenital regions. They are uncommon in the stools of adults not receiving antibiotics. In the majority of instances, *Pseudomonas* organisms are cultured as avirulent secondary contaminants in superficial wounds or from the sputum of patients treated with antibiotics. Ordinarily this is of little consequence because the organisms merely fill the bacteriologic vacuum left by the elimination of more sensitive bacteria. Occasionally, however, infections with *Pseudomonas* organisms occur in the ear, lung, skin, or urinary tract of patients, often after the primary pathogen has been eradicated by antibiotics. Serious infections are almost invariably associated with damage to local tissue or with diminished host resistance. Despite the many potential virulence factors shared by strains of *Pseudomonas*, the organism rarely causes disease in healthy persons. Patients compromised by cystic fibrosis and those with neutropenia appear at particular risk to severe infection with *P. aeruginosa*. Premature infants; children with congenital anomalies and patients with leukemia (who are usually receiving antibiotics, adrenal glucocorticosteroids or antineoplastic drugs); patients with burns; and geriatric patients with debilitating diseases are likely to develop *Pseudomonas* infections. Most often these infections occur in the hospital environment, and they generally are exogenous infections with the organism acquired from sources other than the patient's normal flora. In hospitals, the organisms have been cultured from a variety of sources that share in common an aqueous environment, including such items as sinks, antiseptic solutions, and aqueous medications. The organism is prevalent in urine receptacles and on catheters, and on the hands of hospital staff. In several outbreaks, *Pseudomonas* urinary tract infections appear to have been transmitted from patient to patient by human carriers. Similar epidemics have been reported in nurseries among premature infants, and cross infection on burn wards is common. Although *P. aeruginosa* is found in the gastrointestinal tract of only approximately 5 percent of normal adults, carriage rates increase in hospitalized patients.

PATHOGENESIS   The portal of entry of *Pseudomonas* organisms varies with the patient's age and underlying disease. In infancy and childhood, the skin, umbilical cord, and gastrointestinal tract predominate; in old age, the urinary tract is more often the primary focus. Often the infections remain localized to the skin or subcutaneous tissues. In burns, the region below the eschar may become massively infiltrated with bacteria and inflammatory cells and usually serves as the focus for bacteremia, the single most lethal complication. Hematogenous dissemination is characterized by hemorrhagic nodules in many areas, including the skin, heart, lungs, kidneys, and meninges. The histologic picture is one of necrosis and hemorrhage. Typically the walls of arterioles are heavily infiltrated with bacteria, and the vessels are partially or wholly thrombosed.

Most strains of *P. aeruginosa* produce a layer of slime which is rich in carbohydrate and shares heat stable somatic antigenicity with the cell wall. Antibody against the specific serologic type of slime antigen affords protection to experimental challenge. Most isolates also produce a number of exotoxins. Exotoxin A, which shares many properties with diphtheria toxin, is the most potent toxin produced by *P. aeruginosa*. In life-threatening infection with *P. aeruginosa*, high antibody titers against exotoxin A correlate with increased survival.

MANIFESTATIONS *Pseudomonas* infections occur in many locations, including the skin, subcutaneous tissues, bone and joints, eyes, ears, mastoid and paranasal sinuses, meninges, and heart valves. Bacteremia without a detectable primary focus may also occur and should raise the question of contaminated intravenous medications, intravenous solutions, or antiseptics used for preparing an intravenous site, especially when *Pseudomonas* species other than *P. aeruginosa* are isolated.

Infections of the skin and subcutaneous tissues *Pseudomonas* organisms are frequently cultured from surgical wounds, varicose and decubitus ulcers, and burns, particularly following antibiotic therapy. Draining tuberculous or osteomyelitic sinuses may become secondarily infected. The mere presence of *Pseudomonas* in these sites is of little significance provided that bacterial multiplication deep in subcutaneous tissues does not occur and bacteremia does not ensue. Cutaneous infections usually heal after removal or slough of devitalized tissue. *Pseudomonas* organisms may be responsible for green nails in persons whose hands are excessively exposed to water, soap, and detergents, who have onychomycosis, or whose hands are subject to mechanical trauma. The organism can usually be cultured from the nail plate. *Pseudomonas* has been incriminated in whirlpool-associated dermatitis. The disease is benign and resolves spontaneously.

Osteomyelitis Osteomyelitis is unusual with *Pseudomonas* except as a complication of bacteremia, intravenous drug abuse, or puncture wounds. If a puncture wound, especially a nail puncture of the foot in a child, fails to respond to standard therapy within 3 to 4 days, complicating *Pseudomonas* osteomyelitis must be considered.

Infections of the ear, mastoid, and paranasal sinuses Otitis externa is the most common form of *Pseudomonas* infection which involves the ear. It is particularly troublesome in tropical climates and is characterized by chronic serosanguineous and purulent drainage from the external auditory canal. A rapidly progressive, severe infection due to *Pseudomonas* involving the ear, referred to as malignant otitis externa, can develop, especially in diabetics. In contrast to the usual otitis externa, this infection requires aggressive management including surgical debridement and parenteral antimicrobial therapy. Otitis media or mastoiditis usually occurs as a superinfection following eradication of gram-positive organisms by antimicrobial agents.

Infections of the eye Corneal ulceration is the most severe form of ocular *Pseudomonas* infection. It usually follows a traumatic abrasion and may terminate in panophthalmitis and destruction of the globe. Purulent conjunctivitis occurs as a manifestation of *Pseudomonas* infection in premature infants. Contamination of contact lenses or lens fluid may be an important means of infecting the eyes with *Pseudomonas*.

Urinary tract infections *Pseudomonas* organisms are common pathogens in the urinary tract and are usually found in patients with obstructive uropathy who have been subjected to repeated urethral manipulations or to urologic surgery. *Pseudomonas* bacteriuria is in no way unique and cannot be distinguished from infection with other organisms on clinical grounds.

Gastrointestinal tract *Pseudomonas* organisms have been implicated as a cause of epidemic diarrhea of infancy. In addition, a number of infants dying from neonatal sepsis have the classic necrotic, avascular ulcers of *Pseudomonas* bacteremia in the bowel at autopsy. A "typhoidal" form of *Pseudomonas* infection characterized by fever, myalgia, and diarrhea occurs predominantly in the tropics. This illness, also called 13-day fever or Shanghai fever, is self-limited, and the prognosis is good.

Respiratory tract Primary *Pseudomonas* pneumonia is infrequent and culture of this organism from the sputum usually is indicative of aspiration of oropharyngeal contents with secondary infection following eradication of a more sensitive flora with antibiotics. The normal oropharyngeal flora of hospitalized patients is frequently replaced by gram-negative rods, including *Pseudomonas*, early in hospitalization. A variety of nosocomial events, most notably administration of sedative medications, endotracheal intubation, and intermittent positive pressure breathing treatments, can predispose to respiratory infection with *Pseudomonas*. Pulmonary infection is often associated with microabscesses. The organism is often isolated from the sputum of patients with bronchiectasis, chronic bronchitis, or cystic fibrosis who have lingering infections punctuated by multiple courses of chemotherapy, and it is recovered frequently from the stomata of tracheostomy sites. *Pseudomonas* bronchitis and bronchiolitis may be the terminal event in cystic fibrosis, and sputum isolates from these patients often have a characteristic mucoid colonial morphology when cultured on agar.

Meningitis Spontaneous *Pseudomonas* meningitis is unusual, but the bacilli may be introduced into the subarachnoid space by lumbar puncture, spinal anesthesia, intrathecal medication, or head trauma. Shunts performed for hydrocephalus may become contaminated with *Pseudomonas*, and revision or removal of the shunt offers the best hope of cure.

Bacteremia Bloodstream invasion tends to occur in debilitated patients, premature infants, children with congenital defects, patients with lymphomas, leukemias, or other malignant tumors, and elderly patients who have undergone surgery or instrumentation of the biliary or urinary tract. *Pseudomonas* bacteremia is an important cause of death in patients with severe burns. In adults, *Pseudomonas* bacteremia is indistinguishable from bloodstream infection with other bacterial species except for two findings: (1) ecthyma gangrenosum, the classic skin lesion, often located in the anogenital or axillary region as a round, indurated, purple-black area about 1 cm in diameter with an ulcerated center and a surrounding zone of erythema; and (2) rarely, the passage of green urine, presumably due to the hemoglobin pigment verdoglobin. Organisms usually can be cultured from cutaneous lesions and may provide an early clue to the diagnosis.

Bacterial endocarditis A number of cases of *Pseudomonas* subacute bacterial endocarditis have followed open-heart surgery. Usually the organisms become implanted on a silk suture or a synthetic patch employed for closure of septal defects. Reoperation with removal of the vegetation and foreign bodies offers the best hope of cure. *Pseudomonas* endocarditis has been found on normal heart valves in patients with burns and in drug addicts. Metastatic abscesses in bone, joint, brain, adrenal glands, and lungs are frequent consequences of *Pseudomonas* endocarditis.

TREATMENT Localized *Pseudomonas* infection can be treated by irrigation with 1% acetic acid or topical therapy with colistin or polymyxin B. Debridement and drainage of purulent material is essential when deeper tissues are involved. For deep-seated tissue infections and life-threatening infection, such as pneumonia or bacteremia, parenteral therapy must be employed. The aminoglycoside antibiotics, tobramycin and gentamicin, inhibit most strains of *Pseudomonas*. In patients with normal renal function, 5 mg/kg per day in divided doses will provide inhibitory levels. Amikacin is also active against *Pseudomonas* and is especially useful against strains which have developed enzyme-mediated drug resistance to tobramycin and gentamicin. It should be given in doses of 15 mg/kg per day in divided doses. Ticarcillin and mezlocillin are active against most strains of *Pseudomonas* in doses of 16 to 20 g per day. Piperacillin and azlocillin are active in vitro against some isolates not inhibited by ticarcillin. These isolates are usually nosocomial in origin. The combination of an aminoglycoside active against *Pseudomonas* plus an antipseudomonal penicillin is frequently employed to delay emergence of resistance during therapy and provides enhanced activity, especially in granulocytopenic patients with *Pseudomonas* infection. Asymptomatic bacteriuria, particularly when confined to the bladder, should be treated with the least toxic agent, which at times may be a sulfonamide or tetracycline. The antimicrobial susceptibility of *Pseudomonas*, except for *P. aeruginosa*, is variable, and some of these isolates may be resistant to aminoglycoside antibiotics. Some of the newer cephalosporins like cefoperazone and ceftazidime are also active in vitro against many isolates of *Pseudomonas*.

PROPHYLAXIS *Pseudomonas* cross infections in hospitals can be reduced by careful attention to aseptic techniques and good infection control practices (see Chap. 85). Systemic antibiotic prophylaxis aimed at preventing colonization and infection with *Pseudomonas* organisms has been notoriously unsuccessful and should be interdicted. A polyvalent vaccine for *Pseudomonas* has been developed, as well as hyperimmune gamma globulin, but it has not been used widely.

PROGNOSIS The mortality rate in *Pseudomonas* bacteremia is 75 percent and is highest in patients with shock or severe associated disease such as massive third-degree burns, leukemia, or prematurity. When bacteremia originates in the urinary tract and is not accompanied by shock, the prognosis is considerably better. Localized *Pseudomonas* infections do not present a threat to life unless hematogenous dissemination occurs.

ACINETOBACTER INFECTIONS

DEFINITION Organisms of the genus *Acinetobacter* are pleomorphic, gram-negative bacilli which are easily confused with members of the genus *Neisseria*. Severe infections with these organisms, including meningitis, bacterial endocarditis, pneumonia, and bacteremia, have been described with increasing frequency.

ETIOLOGY *Acinetobacter calcoaceticus* var. *lwoffi* was described by DeBord as *Mima polymorpha* in 1939. It is one of two well-characterized varieties of *Acinetobacter*, the other being *Acinetobacter calcoaceticus* var. *anitratus*, formerly called *Herellea vaginicola*. Organisms described as *Bacterium anitratum* and B5W are synonymous with *Acinetobacter*. These organisms are pleomorphic, gram-negative, encapsulated, and nonmotile. They grow well on ordinary media, forming white, convex, smooth colonies. Diplococcal forms predominate in colonies grown on solid media; rods and filamentous forms are more common in liquid media. The species can be differentiated from the Enterobacteriaceae by their negative nitrate reaction and from members of the genus *Neisseria*, which they may resemble morphologically, by their simple growth requirements, their bacillary form in liquid media, and their usually negative oxidase reaction.

EPIDEMIOLOGY AND PATHOGENESIS *Acinetobacter* organisms are ubiquitous. Twenty-five percent of normal subjects are skin carriers of *Acinetobacter*. The striking association of *Acinetobacter* bacteremia with cutdowns or indwelling intravenous catheters favors the skin as a major portal of entry in human beings. The increasing incidence of *Acinetobacter* pneumonia, both as a primary infection and as a superinfection, also points to the respiratory tract as an important portal of entry. It appears that *Acinetobacter* organisms are normal human commensals of relatively low virulence which produce colonization much more frequently than infection. Infections seem to occur in patients subjected to the same epidemiologic pressures encountered with nosocomial, gram-negative bacilli; serious infections are produced under conditions of decreased host resistance, or in the presence of instrumentation, or with prior broad-spectrum antimicrobial therapy. An unexplained predominance of *Acinetobacter* pulmonary infections occurring in late summer has been noted. The role of these organisms as a cause of conjunctivitis, vaginitis, and urethritis requires further documentation.

MANIFESTATIONS Serious infections caused by *Acinetobacter* include (1) meningitis, (2) subacute and acute bacterial endocarditis, (3) pneumonia, (4) urinary tract infections, and (5) bacteremia. Usually, the signs and symptoms associated with infections in these sites are no different from those produced by other pathogens. Occasionally, *Acinetobacter* may be the cause of a fulminating bacteremia, with high fever, vascular collapse, petechiae, and ecchymoses, which is indistinguishable from fulminant meningococcemia. More often, however, bacteremia is associated with an overt portal of entry, such as infected cutdowns or indwelling intravenous catheters, surgical wounds, or burns; it may follow urethral or other surgical instrumentation. The clinical picture presented by these patients is dominated by endotoxemia, and the prognosis is poor.

DIAGNOSIS The diagnosis of *Acinetobacter* infection can be missed, either because the clinical bacteriology laboratory is unfamiliar with these organisms and reports them incorrectly or because they are considered contaminants. The confusion attending the taxonomic classification of these organisms has not simplified matters. For practical purposes, isolation of *Acinetobacter* from blood, spinal fluid, sputum, urine, or pus should be considered significant unless there is no evidence of infection on clinical grounds. Since *Acinetobacter* isolates are resistant to penicillin and members of the genus *Neisseria* are sensitive, differentiation of these organisms is of obvious importance.

TREATMENT Antibiotic sensitivities of *Acinetobacter* strains vary, but most strains are inhibited by gentamicin, tobramycin, amikacin, and the ureidopenicillins such as piperacillin. Sensitivity to the tetracyclines is unpredictable, and most strains are resistant to penicillin, ampicillin, the cephalosporins, erythromycin, and chloramphenicol. For serious systemic infections, the appropriate antibiotic, generally an aminoglycoside, should be administered, and since these organisms may produce localized abscesses, surgical drainage may be necessary.

EIKENELLA INFECTIONS

ETIOLOGY *Eikenella corrodens* is a facultatively anaerobic or capnophilic gram-negative rod which is oxidase-positive. As colonies develop on blood agar, characteristic "pitting" or "corroding" of the agar is seen with many strains and generally requires 48 to 72 h of growth to develop.

EPIDEMIOLOGY *Eikenella corrodens* is an inhabitant of the mouth, upper respiratory tract, and gastrointestinal tract of humans. Infections frequently involve bowel or oral contamination. A striking association between *Eikenella* infections and methylphenidate abuse has been noted, perhaps related to the low redox potential created by "skin popping" of this agent as well as a tendency for needles to become contaminated with oral secretions through needle licking.

MANIFESTATIONS The most common infection caused by *Eikenella* is that of skin or soft tissue. Endocarditis, pneumonia, osteomyelitis, and meningitis are reported but are rare. *Eikenella* infections frequently mimic infections caused by strict anaerobes such as *Bacteroides* *fragilis* or *Peptostreptococcus*. The infections are indolent and frequently mixed with aerobic gram-positive cocci, and drainage is often foul-smelling. Abscess formation is common.

TREATMENT *Eikenella corrodens* is susceptible to penicillin, ampicillin, carbenicillin, and tetracycline. Adequate drainage of purulent material is essential in the management of these infections. Ampicillin or penicillin coupled with surgical drainage generally provides a good response. Of note is the marked resistance of *Eikenella* to clindamycin, making the differentiation between *Eikenella* infections and those caused by mixed anaerobes even more important.

REFERENCES

Enterobacteriaceae: General

KREGER BE et al: Gram negative bacteremia. Am J Med 68:332, 1980
MAKI DG: Nosocomial bacteremia: An epidemiologic overview. Am J Med 70:719, 1981
MOORE RD et al: Association of aminoglycoside plasma levels with therapeutic outcome in gram-negative pneumonia. Am J Med 77:657, 1984
SCHABERG DR et al: Epidemics of nosocomial urinary tract infection caused by multiply-resistant gram-negative bacilli: Epidemiology and control. J Infect Dis 133:363, 1976
TANCREDE CH, ANDREMONT AO: Bacterial translocation and gram-negative bacteremia in patients with hematological malignancies. J Infect Dis 152:99, 1985

Escherichia coli infections

BERK SL, McCABE WR: Meningitis caused by gram-negative bacilli. Ann Int Med 93:253, 1980
CONN HO, FESSEL JM: Spontaneous bacterial peritonitis in cirrhosis. Medicine 50:161, 1971
GERACI JE et al: Endocarditis due to gram-negative bacteria. Mayo Clin Proc 57:145, 1982

Klebsiella-Enterobacter-Serratia infections

COOPER R, MILLS J: *Serratia* endocarditis. Arch Intern Med 140:199, 1980
MELTZ DJ, GRIECO MH: Characteristics of *Serratia marcescens* pneumonia. Arch Intern Med 132:359, 1973
RENNIE RP, DUNCAN IBR: Emergence of gentamicin resistant *Klebsiella* in a general hospital. Antimicrob Agents Chemother 11:179, 1978

Proteus infections

IANNINI PB et al: Multidrug resistant *P. rettgeri*. Ann Intern Med 55:161, 1976
LEWIS J, FEKETY FR: *Proteus* bacteremia. Johns Hopkins Med J 124:151, 1969
MUSCHER DM et al: Role of urease in pyelonephritis resulting from urinary tract infections with *Proteus*. J Infect Dis 131:177, 1975

Pseudomonas infections

BAGEL J, GROSSMAN ME: Subcutaneous nodules in *Pseudomonas* sepsis. Am J Med 80:528, 1986
BODEY GP et al: Infections caused by *Pseudomonas aeruginosa*. Rev Infect Dis 5:279, 1983
COLLINI FJ et al: Ecthyma gangrenosum in a kidney transplant recipient with *Pseudomonas* septicemia. Am J Med 80:729, 1986
DOGGETT RG (ed): *Pseudomonas aeruginosa: Clinical manifestations of infection and current therapy*. New York, Academic, 1979
FLICK MR, CLUFF LE: *Pseudomonas* bacteremia. Review of 108 cases. Am J Med 60:501, 1976
POLLACK M: The role of exotoxin A in *Pseudomonas* disease and immunity. Rev Infect Dis 5(suppl):S979, 1983

Acinetobacter infections

BUXTON AE et al: Nosocomial respiratory tract infection and colonization with *Acinetobacter calcoaceticus*. Am J Med 65:507, 1978
GLEW RH et al: Infections with *Acinetobacter calcoaceticus*: Clinical and laboratory studies. Medicine 56:79, 1977
RETAILLIAU FH et al: *Acinetobacter calcoaceticus*: A nosocomial pathogen with unusual seasonal pattern. J Infect Dis 139:371, 1979

Eikenella infections

BROOKS GF et al: *Eikenella corrodens*, a recently recognized pathogen. Medicine 53:325, 1974
GOLDSTEIN FJC et al: Isolation of *Eikenella corrodens* from pulmonary infections. Am Rev Resp Dis 119:55, 1979

106 MELIOIDOSIS AND GLANDERS

JAY P. SANFORD

MELIOIDOSIS **Definition** Melioidosis is an infection of humans and animals with a protean clinical spectrum. Melioidosis, which means "a resemblance to distemper of asses," bears a striking resemblance to glanders both clinically and pathologically, but is epidemiologically dissimilar.

Etiology Melioidosis is caused by a gram-negative motile bacillus, *Pseudomonas pseudomallei*, which can be differentiated from *P. mallei* by bacteriologic and serologic means. *P. pseudomallei* (also known as Whitmore's bacillus) is a small, gram-negative, motile, aerobic bacillus. When it is stained with methylene blue, Wayson's, or Wright's stain, marked irregularities with a bipolar "safety pin" pattern are observed. It grows well on standard bacteriologic media, with a characteristic wrinkling of colony surfaces after 48 to 72 h of incubation. Two antigenic types have been distinguished, type I (Asian), found widely, including in Australia, and type II (Australian), found mainly in Australia. Both types are equally pathogenic.

Epidemiology The disease is endemic in Southeast Asia where human and animal cases occur commonly. Disease in humans has been reported from adjacent areas including India, Borneo, the Philippines, Guam, Indonesia, Sri Lanka, New Guinea, and Australia (north Queensland, Northern Territory). Cases in humans or animals have been reported from Madagascar, Chad, Kenya, Central West Africa (Niger, Upper Volta), Iran, and Turkey. In 1976, *P. pseudomallei* was isolated from animals in the Paris zoo just behind Notre Dame. In Madrid, horses kept for serum died from melioidosis. Human melioidosis has been described only rarely in the western hemisphere (Panama, Ecuador)—a neonatal case in Hawaii, a case in Georgia, and a possible case in Oklahoma. With these exceptions, confirmed melioidosis has occurred in United States or European residents only when they have traveled in endemic areas. As of January 1973, when all American forces had been withdrawn from Vietnam, there had been 343 cases with 36 deaths reported in United States Army personnel who were or had been in Vietnam.

Pseudomonas pseudomallei is a saprophyte which can be isolated from soil, stagnant streams, ponds, rice paddies, and market produce in endemic areas. Its ubiquitous nature is illustrated by its isolation as a laboratory contaminant. *Pseudomonas pseudomallei* is capable of causing disease in epizootic form among sheep, goats, swine, and horses. Outbreaks have occurred in dolphins in oceanariums in Paris and Hong Kong. Occasional isolates have also been reported from cows, rodents, dogs, cats, wallabies, and birds. Although animals are susceptible to the disease, they apparently do not represent a reservoir for human disease. Attempts to culture *P. pseudomallei* from the urine and feces of a large variety of healthy animals have been unsuccessful. Arthropod-borne infection does not occur naturally. Humans contract melioidosis by soil contamination of skin abrasions. Ingestion, nasal instillation, and inhalation are other probable methods of spread. In contrast to glanders, infections have been uncommon, but can occur, in laboratory workers. *P. pseudomallei* has been recovered from urine specimens from two patients, both diabetic, who had urethral catheters, while hospitalized in an endemic area. Person-to-person transmission of melioidosis is rare. Venereal transmission from a patient with chronic prostatitis with *P. pseudomallei* isolated from prostatic secretions to his wife, who had never been in an endemic area and who had a hemagglutination titer of 1:10,240, has been recorded. Also, the development of melioidosis in a 2-day-old newborn in Hawaii and demonstration of a significant antibody titer in a nurse who had never been in an endemic area but who had worked on wards with melioidosis patients raise the question of spread from person-to-person within a hospital.

Pathology   In acute infections, the majority of lesions occur in the lungs, with occasional abscesses in other organs. In subacute infections, lung abscesses tend to be more extensive, and lesions are found throughout the body, in the skin, subcutaneous tissue, meninges, brain, eye, heart, liver, kidney, spleen, bone, prostate, synovial membranes, and lymph nodes. The acute abscesses are characterized by an outer border of hemorrhage, a medial zone heavily infiltrated with polymorphonuclear leukocytes, and an inner core of necrotic debris containing large histiocytes with two or three nuclei that have been termed giant cells. A striking histologic feature has been the marked karyorrhexis. In chronic infections, the lesion consists of a central area of caseation necrosis, mononuclear and plasma cells, and granulation tissue. Calcification does not occur.

Melioidosis is associated with impaired cellular immunity; total lymphocyte counts are usually less than 1000 per cubic millimeter; the percentage of total T cells is less than 50 percent due to a decrease in T helper cells; and skin tests with dinitrochlorobenzene are negative. The number of T suppressor cells is normal, as is the number of B cells.

Clinical manifestations   The clinical manifestations of melioidosis are variable. The illness can present as an acute, subacute, or chronic process. The incubation period has not been defined; however, judging by the lapse of time between injury and the development of infection, it may be as short as 2 days. Following a laboratory accident, an incubation period of 3 days ensued. Clinically inapparent infections may remain latent for a number of years after an individual leaves an endemic area, with an interval of 26 years reported in one patient. Men are more often affected than women, a finding which is thought to represent occupational exposure. Melioidosis may be recognized as inapparent infection, asymptomatic pulmonary infiltration, acute localized suppurative infection, acute pulmonary infection, acute septicemic infection, or chronic suppurative infection.

INAPPARENT INFECTION   In Thailand, Vietnam, and Malaysia, 6 to 8 percent of healthy adult men have significant antibody titers against *P. pseudomallei*, with the prevalence reaching 20 percent in a group of Army recruits from the rice-growing states of western Malaysia. Only 1 percent of Thai women had positive reactions. None of the serums from a control group from the United States was positive. The prevalence of significant antibody titers has been reported as 2 percent for Europeans living in Vietnam and 1 to 9 percent in unselected patients in United States Army hospitals and in a group of normal uninjured soldiers who had served in Vietnam. Occasionally, asymptomatic infections have been discovered by routine chest x-ray. In northern Queensland, the prevalence of positive indirect hemagglutination titers (1:40 or higher) is as high as 10.6 percent, averages 5.7 percent, and is equal in men and women. Ten percent of serums from inhabitants of a village in Upper Volta were positive, yet melioidosis had never been recognized.

ACUTE LOCALIZED SUPPURATIVE INFECTION   Infection by inoculation of a break in the skin usually results in a nodule with an area of acute lymphangitis and regional lymphadenitis. There are usually fever and generalized malaise. This form of infection may rapidly progress to the acute septicemic form.

ACUTE PULMONARY INFECTION   The most common form of the disease has been pulmonary infection, which may represent a primary pneumonitis or hematogenous spread. The acute pulmonary infection can vary in severity from a mild bronchitis to overwhelming necrotizing pneumonia. The onset may be abrupt without prodromal symptoms or more gradual, with headache, anorexia, and generalized myalgia. Fever occurs in almost all patients, is often in excess of 38.9°C (102°F), and may be associated with rigors. Dull or pleuritic chest pain is common. Cough, with or without sputum, occurs. There may be mild pharyngitis. Tachypnea may be out of proportion to the fever and findings on physical or x-ray examination. Chest findings may be minimal but usually consist of rales in the area of pneumonitis. In the absence of dissemination, the spleen and liver are not palpable.

Laboratory findings include total leukocyte counts ranging from normal to 20,000 cells per cubic millimeter. Mild normochromic, normocytic anemia may appear during the illness. The pneumonia usually involves the upper lobes with the radiographic appearance of consolidation. Thin-walled cavities, usually 2 to 7 cm in diameter, frequently occur. Without specific therapy, the temperature may become normal within a few days; however, the upper lobe cavitation persists, resulting in a radiographic appearance of tuberculosis. While uncommon, pleural effusions, a pleural mass, and bilateral hilar adenopathy have been reported. Progressive pulmonary spread or hematogenous dissemination with the development of septicemic manifestations may ensue.

ACUTE SEPTICEMIC INFECTION   This is the form originally described primarily among narcotic addicts. Subsequent reports, however, have shown a predilection for debilitated patients with diabetes mellitus and alcoholism. The onset may be abrupt, with the dominant symptoms depending upon site of major involvement. In individuals with bacteremia complicating pneumonitis, symptoms may include disorientation, extreme dyspnea, severe headache, pharyngitis, watery diarrhea, and development of cutaneous pustular lesions on the head, trunk, or extremities. There is high fever, extreme tachypnea, a flushed skin, and cyanosis. Muscle tenderness may be striking. On examination of the chest, signs may be absent, or rales, rhonchi, and pleural rubs may be heard. The liver and spleen may be palpable. Signs of arthritis or meningitis may appear. Patients with the septicemic form usually have a rapidly progressive fatal course, which in many instances may be too fulminant to be altered by therapy. The leukocyte count may be normal or slightly increased. Chest radiographs most commonly show irregular nodular densities 4 to 10 mm in diameter disseminated throughout the lungs. These enlarge, coalesce, and often undergo cavitation as the disease progresses. Pleural effusion is rare. Other radiographic patterns include unilateral irregular mottled densities which become confluent.

CHRONIC SUPPURATIVE INFECTION   In some patients secondary abscesses develop which dominate the clinical picture. Organs involved include skin, brain, lung, myocardium, liver, spleen, prostate, bones, joints, lymph nodes, and even the eye. These patients may be afebrile.

RECRUDESCENT INFECTION   Activation of inapparent or quiescent infection may present as acute localized suppurative, acute pulmonary, acute septicemic, or chronic suppurative disease remote from the probable time of exposure (up to 26 years having been reported). Surgery, trauma, intercurrent illness such as severe influenzal pneumonia, diabetic ketoacidosis, alcoholic debauches, or radiation therapy appeared to act as triggering events. Since *P. pseudomallei* is an intracellular parasite and is associated with suppression of T helper lymphocytes, it is only a matter of time before melioidosis will be added to the list of infections which occur in individuals with HTLV-III virus infections and the acquired immunodeficiency syndrome (AIDS), especially in areas where *P. pseudomallei* is endemic.

Diagnosis   Melioidosis should be considered in the differential diagnosis of any febrile illness in an individual who has been in an endemic area, especially if the presenting features are those of fulminant respiratory failure, if multiple pustular or necrotic skin or subcutaneous lesions develop, or if there is a radiographic pattern of tuberculosis in a patient from whom tubercle bacilli cannot be isolated.

Microscopic examination of exudates will reveal poorly staining, small, gram-negative bacilli which show the characteristic staining irregularities and "safety pin" bipolar staining with methylene blue. *Pseudomonas pseudomallei* will grow on most laboratory media, including eosin methylene blue agar (EMB) or MacConkey's agar, in 24 to 48 h. The organisms can be differentiated from *P. mallei* and *P. aeruginosa* by standard bacteriologic procedures, although isolates may pose problems in identification with some commercial medium kits. The characteristic wrinkling of the colonies may require 72 h or longer. The hemagglutination, direct agglutination test, and complement fixation test are aids in diagnosis if a fourfold or greater rise in titer is demonstrated in paired serums. Single low titers are difficult to interpret because of nonspecific responses. The complement fixation test is said to be specific with titers above 1:8 during the acute illness, but may cross-react with *P. mallei*. A negative complement fixation test does not exclude disease. The hemagglutination and agglutination tests show more cross-reactions. Titers of 1:40 or more suggest infection. In one-third of patients, with both fulminating and subacute disease, the serology has been negative at the time the culture became positive.

Treatment The treatment regimen should vary with the form of the disease. Individuals with low-titer positive serologic tests but with no clinical evidence of infection do not require therapy. The choice of antibiotics in active infection should be based upon sensitivity studies, and therapy should be given for a minimum of 30 days. *Pseudomonas pseudomallei* is usually sensitive in vitro to the tetra-cyclines, chloramphenicol, novobiocin, kanamycin, amikacin, sulfadiazine or sulfisoxazole, trimethoprim-sulfamethoxazole, and the third-generation antipseudomonal cephalosporins, especially ceftazidime, and in most instances is resistant to penicillin G, ampicillin, carbenicillin, dicloxacillin, streptomycin, gentamicin, tobramycin, first- and second-generation cephalosporins, vancomycin, clindamycin, and rifampin. In patients with pneumonitis who are not too ill, effective therapy has included tetracycline, 2 to 3 g daily (40 mg/kg); chloramphenicol, 3 g daily (40 mg/kg); or trimethoprim-sulfamethoxazole (4 mg/kg trimethoprim, 20 mg/kg sulfamethoxazole) for 60 to 150 days. Ceftazidime, 6 g daily (100 mg/kg), has been reported to be effective. If the patient is severely ill, two of these antimicrobials in combination should be given for 30 days followed by another 30 to 120 days of trimethoprim-sulfamethoxazole alone. The mean interval for sputum cultures to become negative has been 6 weeks. If sputum cultures remain positive for 6 months, surgery with lobectomy should be considered. In patients with extrapulmonary suppurative lesions, therapy should be continued for 6 months to 1 year. The usual principles of surgical drainage should be followed. In desperately ill patients with severe pneumonitis or the septicemic form, multiple antibiotics should be administered by the parenteral route. Current recommendations for antibiotics in the septicemic form of melioidosis are tetracycline, 4 to 6 g per day (80 mg/kg); chloramphenicol, 4 to 6 g per day (80 mg/kg); and one of the following: trimethoprim-sulfamethoxazole (9 mg/kg trimethoprim, 45 mg/kg sulfamethoxazole), kanamycin (30 mg/kg), or novobiocin (60 mg/kg). In vitro studies have revealed antagonism between the following pairs of drugs: chloramphenicol-kanamycin, tetracycline-kanamycin, and sulfadiazine-chloramphenicol. Though the significance of such antagonism in clinical therapy has not been assessed, the data favor selection of trimethoprim-sulfamethoxazole or novobiocin as the third drug. The dosage should be tapered rapidly as clinical improvement occurs. Experience with the third-generation antipseudomonal cephalosporins is extremely limited; however, a combination of ceftazidime (in a dose of 100 mg/kg or 6 g daily) and trimethoprim-sulfamethoxazole is likely to emerge as the recommendation of choice. Levamisole[1] (150 mg twice per week) has been used as an adjunct to antibiotic therapy in several patients with results that suggest it may be beneficial in the treatment of relapses.

Prognosis Prior to antimicrobials, the mortality rate of apparent infection was 95 percent. With better diagnosis and more prolonged appropriate therapy, the mortality rate in all except the septicemic form is low. Even with vigorous appropriate antibiotics and supportive therapy, the mortality rate in patients with melioidosis septicemia is greater than 50 percent. Very few patients have had long-term follow-up, and the incidence of late relapses is approximately 20 percent.

Prevention There is no means of active immunization. In endemic areas, vigorous cleansing of abrasions and lacerations is recommended.

---

[1] *This drug has not been approved for this purpose by the Food and Drug Administration at the time of publication.*

GLANDERS **Definition** Glanders is a serious infection of equine animals caused by *P. mallei*, which is transmitted occasionally to other domestic animals and to human beings.

Etiology *Pseudomonas mallei* is a small, slender, nonmotile, gram-negative bacillus. When it is stained with methylene blue, marked irregularities in staining are observed. Organisms grow on most common meat infusion media but require glycerol for optimum growth.

Epidemiology Glanders was at one time widespread throughout Europe, but owing to the introduction of control measures, its incidence has decreased steadily in most countries. The disease still occurs in Asia, Africa, and South America, but not in the United States and western Europe. Glanders has never been common in humans; the occasional infection, however, may be very serious. There have been no naturally acquired infections in the United States since 1938.

Glanders is primarily a disease of horses, mules, and donkeys, although goats, sheep, cats, and dogs sometimes naturally contract the disease. Infection of lions at a safari park in Italy attributed to feeding imported horse meat has been reported. Pigs and cattle are resistant. In horses, the disease may be systemic, with prominent pulmonary involvement (*glanders*) or may be characterized by subcutaneous ulcerative lesions, and lymphatic thickening with nodules (*farcy*). Inhalation, ingestion, and inoculation through breaks in the skin have been suggested as routes of infection in animals. In humans, the disease occurs primarily in individuals with close contact with horses, mules, or donkeys through inoculation of or a break in the skin or by exposing the nasal mucosa to contaminated discharges. A number of instances of airborne infection have been reported in laboratory workers.

Pathology The acute lesion is characterized by nodules consisting of polymorphonuclear leukocytes surrounded by a zone of congestion. A characteristic histologic feature is a peculiar nuclear degeneration known as chromatotexis which occurs early and is extensive. Small foci of deeply staining detritus within the abscess result from this degeneration. In older nodules, the reaction is characterized by epithelioid cells surrounding an area of central necrosis. Giant cells may be present. Virtually any organ may be involved.

Clinical manifestations The manifestations which frequently overlap may be categorized as (1) acute localized suppurative infection, (2) acute pulmonary infection, (3) acute septicemic infection, and (4) chronic suppurative infection. Nearly 60 percent of patients have been between the ages of 20 and 40 years. The disease has been rare in women, probably because there is opportunity for contact.

Infection acquired by inoculation through an abrasion in the skin usually results in a nodule with an area of acute lymphangitis. The incubation period is probably 1 to 5 days. In all types of acute glanders, there are usually fever, generalized malaise, and prostration.

Infection of the mucous membranes may result in a mucopurulent discharge involving the eye, nose, or lips followed by extensive ulcerating granulomatous lesions which may or may not be associated with systemic reactions. With systemic invasion, a generalized papular eruption which may become pustular is frequent. This septicemic form of disease is usually fatal in 7 to 10 days.

Infection by inhalation is followed by an incubation period of 10 to 14 days. The more common symptoms include fever, occasionally associated with rigors, generalized myalgia, fatigue, headache, and pleuritic chest pain. Other symptoms consist of photophobia, lacrimation, and diarrhea. Findings on physical examination are usually normal except for fever and occasional lymphadenopathy, especially in the cervical chain, and splenomegaly. Laboratory findings include mild leukocytosis with 60 to 80 percent neutrophilic leukocytes, but leukopenia with relative lymphocytosis has been recorded. In the acute pulmonary form, chest radiographs characteristically reveal circumscribed densities which suggest early lung abscesses. Other findings may include lobar or bronchopneumonia. In the chronic suppurative form of the disease, the most frequent finding consists of multiple subcutaneous and intramuscular abscesses which most often involve the arms or legs. Approximately one-half the patients will have associated fever, lymphadenopathy, and nasal discharge or ulceration. Visceral involvement including pulmonary or pleural, ocular, skeletal, hepatic, splenic, and meningeal or intracranial involvement occurs in some patients.

Diagnosis Microscopic examination of exudates may reveal small gram-negative bacilli which stain irregularly with methylene blue; however, organisms generally are very scanty. *Pseudomonas mallei* and *P. pseudomallei* cannot be distinguished morphologically. Culturing is often avoided because of the hazard to laboratory personnel; however, if cultures are made, growth occurs on most meat infusion nutrient media. The material is often contaminated with other microorganisms, and incubation with penicillin G (1000 units per milliliter) prior to culturing may be helpful. Subcutaneous inoculation of material into a guinea pig or hamster affords an alternative means of isolation. Blood cultures are usually negative except in the terminal stages of disease. Serologic tests show a rapidly rising agglutination titer, which reaches levels of 1:640 within 2 weeks. Serum from normal persons has been reported to show agglutination titers in dilutions up to 1:320. The complement fixation test is less sensitive but more specific and usually becomes positive during the third week; it is considered positive in dilutions of 1:20 or greater.

Treatment The limited number of recent infections in human beings has precluded evaluation of most of the antibiotic agents. Sulfadiazine has been found to be an effective agent in experimental animals and in humans. The dosage utilized has been approximately 100 mg/kg administered in divided doses. In experimental infections, 3 weeks of therapy gave better results than 1 week. Penicillin is ineffective. Tetracycline, chloramphenicol, the antipseudomonal aminoglycosides, carbenicillin, the third-generation antipseudomonal cephalosporins, and trimethoprim-sulfamethoxazole have not been evaluated. In the absence of clinical experience and pending in vitro susceptibility studies, it would seem most reasonable to utilize the regimens appropriate for patients with melioidosis. In the acute infections, appropriate supportive measures are essential, and in chronic suppurative infections, the usual principles of surgical drainage should be followed.

Prognosis The prognosis depends upon the type of infection. The acute septicemic form has been uniformly fatal. The localized or chronic forms have a much better prognosis.

Prevention Next to acquisition from diseased horses, the commonest source of natural disease in human beings has been contact with human glanders. Isolation is indicated.

REFERENCES

ASHDOWN LR, GUARD RW: Prevalence of human melioidosis in northern Queensland. Am J Trop Med Hyg 33:474, 1984

DODIN A, FERRY R: Recherche epidemiologique du bacille de Whitmore en Afrique. Bull Soc Pathol Exot 67:121, 1974

———, GALIMAND M: Whitmore's bacillus. Rec Med Vet 152:323, 1976

EICKHOFF TC et al: *Pseudomonas pseudomallei:* Susceptibility to chemotherapeutic agents. J Infect Dis 121:95, 1970

EVERETT ED, NELSON R: Pulmonary melioidosis, observations in 39 cases. Am Rev Resp Dis 112:331, 1975

GUARD LR et al: Melioidosis in far north Queensland. Am J Trop Med Hyg 33:467, 1984

HOWE C, MILLER WR: Human glanders: Report of six cases. Ann Intern Med 26:93, 1947

JACKSON AE et al: Recrudescent melioidosis associated with diabetic ketoacidosis. Arch Intern Med 130:268, 1972

MCCORMICK JB et al: Human–to–human transmission of *Pseudomonas pseudomallei.* Ann Intern Med 83:512, 1975

MAYS EE, RICKETS EA: Melioidosis: Recrudescence associated with bronchogenic carcinoma twenty-six years following initial geographic exposure. Chest 68:261, 1975

SANFORD JP: Melioidosis: Another great imitator, in *Infectious Diseases: Current Topics in Diagnosis and Treatment,* DN Gilbert, JP Sanford (eds). New York, Grune & Stratton, 1978

SCHLECH WF III et al: Laboratory-acquired infection with *Pseudomonas pseudomallei* (melioidosis). N Engl J Med 305:1133, 1981

TANPHAICHITRA D, SRIMUANG S: Cellular immunity in tuberculosis, melioidosis, pasteurellosis, penicilliosis and role of levamisole and isoprinosine. Dev Biol Stand 57:117, 1984

WALL RA et al: A case of melioidosis in West Africa. J Infect Dis 152:424, 1985

WILKINSON L: Glanders: Medicine and veterinary medicine in common pursuit of a contagious disease. Med Hist 25:363, 1981

ZAJTCHUK R et al: Surgical treatment of melioidosis. J Thorac Cardiovasc Surg 66:838, 1973

---

107 SALMONELLA INFECTIONS

RICHARD L. GUERRANT

The genus *Salmonella* consists of three species which include more than 2000 different serologic types. Striking variation in pathogenicity of serotypes occurs, but almost all are pathogenic for animals and humans. Specific host preferences characterize certain serotypes, such as *S. typhi*, which under natural conditions of transmission produces disease only in humans. *Salmonella* infections in humans present a spectrum of clinical syndromes, which sometimes overlap. The syndromes are (1) enteric fever (typhoid or paratyphoid fever), (2) acute gastroenteritis, (3) bacteremia, and (4) localized infection which may occur at almost any site. In addition, *asymptomatic intestinal infections* and *transient convalescent intestinal carrier* states are common. Occasionally, a focus of infection persists in the gallbladder or urinary tract to produce a *chronic carrier* state.

ETIOLOGY Salmonellae are motile gram-negative bacilli that ferment glucose but do not ferment lactose or sucrose. *S. typhi* and *S. cholerae-suis* can usually be distinguished from most other serotypes by biochemical means. *S. typhi* does not produce gas and is ornithine-negative, which distinguishes it from almost all other *Salmonella* serotypes. *S. cholerae-suis* is almost uniquely trehalose-negative and is often dulcitol-negative. The many serotypes are identified by highly specific O (somatic) and H (flagellar) antigens. A given serotype will contain a specific combination of multiple O and H antigens. Identification by serotype is accomplished routinely only in major salmonella typing centers, which have the necessary collection of antiserums required for such work. Salmonellae are also divided into groups on the basis of O antigen composition. Most isolates from natural sources fall into five groups, A to E.

The species *S. typhi* and *S. cholerae-suis* consist of only one serotype each (in groups D and C, respectively). Considerable overlap in antigenic composition is responsible for the cross-reactivity which is commonly seen in serologic tests with salmonellae.

While *S. typhi* infections in the United States have declined to around 500 isolations per year (most of which are imported from abroad), non-*typhi* *Salmonella* infections appear to be increasing steadily, especially in patients who are immunocompromised or who are taking antibiotics.

Despite its passive, laboratory-based system of reporting, the Centers for Disease Control report a steady increase from less than 20,000 isolations of salmonellae annually from humans in the United States in 1968 to nearly 40,000 in 1983. This near doubling in frequency contrasts with the infrequency of *Salmonella* infections in developing countries and suggests, with increasing resistance to antimicrobial agents, that human salmonellosis is increasing, perhaps in association with agricultural practices in industrialized countries. It is estimated that over 2 million cases of human *Salmonella* infections occur each year in the United States.

In descending order, the most frequently isolated serotypes in 1983 were *S. typhimurium, S. heidelberg, S. enteritidis, S. newport, S. agona, S. infantis, S. saint-paul, S. montevideo, S. oranienburg,* and *S. typhi.* The 10 most frequently isolated serotypes account for over 70 percent of the total isolates from humans. *Salmonella typhimurium* perennially accounts for 25 to 35 percent of the isolates. *S. agona*, an organism apparently introduced indirectly via animals fed Peruvian fish meal in 1971, continues to increase. There is increasing appreciation of the association of *Salmonella* infections with raw milk consumption (especially *S. dublin*), and with antibiotic use in humans.

Typhoid fever, the classic example of enteric fever, is considered separately from other *Salmonella* infections because of its historical importance, the host specificity of *S. typhi*, and the extensive clinical experience with the disease.

TYPHOID FEVER

DEFINITION Typhoid fever is an acute systemic disease resulting from infection with *S. typhi*. The disease is unique to humans. It is characterized by malaise, fever, abdominal discomfort, transient rash, splenomegaly, and leukopenia. The most prominent major complications are intestinal hemorrhage and perforation. The disease is the classic example of enteric fever caused by salmonellae. However, enteric fever, similar to typhoid, can also be caused by other *Salmonella* serotypes and is termed *paratyphoid fever*.

EPIDEMIOLOGY *Salmonella typhi* gains access to the body by the oral route in almost all cases as a consequence of the ingestion of contaminated food, water, or milk. Humans are the only true reservoir of *S. typhi* in nature, and persons with typhoid fever, or convalescent or chronic carriers, always serve as the ultimate source of infection. Infected individuals can excrete millions of viable typhoid bacilli in the feces, which are the usual source of contamination of food or drink. Patients with active disease also occasionally have organisms in respiratory secretions, vomitus, or other body fluids. Flies or other insects can carry organisms from feces or other infected material to food or drink and have been implicated in a few outbreaks. The fact that *S. typhi* may survive freezing or drying enhances the possibility of spread by contaminated ice, dust, foods, and sewage. Oysters or other shellfish are contaminated at times in polluted waters and occasionally serve as sources of typhoid.

The incidence of typhoid fever has steadily decreased in the United States during the past century to the present relatively low level of less than 600 cases per year. The decrease in incidence has been coincident with improvement in socioeconomic conditions and is specifically related to development of pure water supplies, effective sewage disposal, pasteurization of milk, and methods to detect and control spread of organisms from persons with active disease or from carriers. Typhoid continues to occur on a large scale in countries where sanitation is suboptimal. Over 60 percent of the patients with typhoid fever in the United States have acquired their infections in areas where the disease is endemic, with 65 percent of these being from Mexico and India. However, fatalities are more common with domestically acquired cases, probably because the diagnosis is not suspected early. About 4 percent of cases in the United States are laboratory-acquired.

Typhoid can be eradicated ultimately because the infection is confined to humans and both the disease and the carrier state can be controlled with appropriate drugs. The importance of sewage disposal, a pure water supply, and control of carriers is highlighted repeatedly by the occurrence of outbreaks which develop when defects in sanitation occur such as failure of adequate water chlorination or during natural disasters such as flood.

The sex distribution of patients with typhoid fever in the United States shows no significant predilection. In recent years, about 75 percent of cases have occurred in persons less than 30 years of age. In contrast, the chronic carrier state is much more common in females than males (the female/male ratio is 3:1) and in older individuals (88 percent are over 50 years of age).

There is no seasonal variation in incidence of typhoid fever in the United States. However, in areas of the world where the disease is endemic, the incidence increases in the summer months.

PATHOGENESIS The outcome of the interaction between the typhoid bacillus and humans is determined during the early hours after ingestion of the organisms. Typhoid bacilli reach the small intestine shortly after ingestion and may multiply there. The organisms may then penetrate the mucosa with minimal epithelial destruction and enter intestinal lymphatics, perhaps via Peyer's patches, to be carried to the bloodstream. This initial early bacteremia apparently occurs within 24 to 72 h after ingestion of organisms and is rarely detected in natural infections because patients are usually asymptomatic at this early stage. The bacteremia is transient and is rapidly terminated as bacilli are phagocytized by cells of the reticuloendothelial system. Nevertheless, viable bacilli are disseminated throughout the body and apparently persist within reticuloendothelial cells. After intracellular multiplication takes place, organisms reenter the bloodstream, producing a continuous bacteremia for days or weeks. The reappearance of bacteremia corresponds with the onset of manifestations of the disease. The intracellular organisms are eventually destroyed as manifestations of disease subside and recovery ensues. Enhanced intracellular killing and recovery appear to be related to the onset of delayed hypersensitivity. Recovery is unrelated to the appearance, even in high titer, of agglutinins against the somatic, flagellar, or Vi antigens of the typhoid bacillus.

The number of organisms ingested is an important determinant of whether typhoid fever results from exposure to *S. typhi*. Studies in volunteers have shown that about 10^7 typhoid bacilli of the Quailes strain must be taken orally to produce typhoid fever in 50 percent of normal volunteers. The number of organisms ingested also influences the incubation period, and short incubation periods, in general, correspond to large doses of organisms. The volunteer studies have also demonstrated that different strains of typhoid bacilli vary considerably in their capacity to produce disease in humans.

The normal flora of the upper intestinal tract is an important protective mechanism against invasion by *S. typhi*. Volunteer studies have demonstrated that antimicrobial therapy a day or so before oral challenge with *S. typhi* markedly decreases the number of viable bacilli required to produce disease. It is possible that certain factors known to be associated with typhoid outbreaks, such as malnutrition, enhance susceptibility to typhoid infection by alterations in the intestinal flora or other host defenses.

During the phase of persistent bacteremia, all organs are repeatedly exposed to typhoid bacilli. Abscess formation may occur but is unusual. However, localization does occur in the gallbladder in almost all cases. Organisms multiply in the bile to high titer, usually without manifestations of cholecystitis, and are excreted with bile into the intestinal tract. Stool cultures, which are usually negative for *S. typhi* during the incubation period and early phases of the disease, become positive in a large proportion of cases during the third or fourth week of the disease, when excretion of organisms in the bile reaches a peak.

The factors responsible for the fever, leukopenia, and other manifestations of typhoid fever have been inadequately defined. Typhoid bacilli contain biologically active lipopolysaccharides or endotoxins which produce fever, leukopenia, thrombocytopenia, and hyperplasia of reticuloendothelial cells when injected into animals or humans. It is assumed that endotoxins play an important role in the pathogenesis of the signs and symptoms of typhoid fever. However, the evidence regarding the role of endotoxin in causing the manifestations of typhoid is inconclusive. For example, tolerance to the pyrogenic effects of endotoxins can be demonstrated during convalescence from typhoid fever, which suggests release of endotoxins during infection. While laboratory evidence for low-grade, subclinical disseminated intravascular coagulation can often be demonstrated in patients with typhoid fever, endotoxemia is usually not detectable. Other studies show that typhoid fever follows a normal course in volunteers rendered tolerant to endotoxins prior to challenge, indicating that more complex mechanisms than endotoxemia alone are responsible for the sustained fever and toxemia. It has been suggested that endogenous pyrogens released by local inflammatory effects of *S. typhi* endotoxin may sustain the pyrexia in typhoid fever.

PATHOLOGY The most prominent microscopic lesion in typhoid fever is proliferation of large mononuclear cells in many different tissues. Mononuclear hyperplasia leads to lymphadenopathy, splenomegaly, and impressive enlargement of lymphoid tissues in the intestines, especially in the terminal ileum (Peyer's patches). Proliferating mononuclear cells may also be observed in bone marrow, liver, and lung. Studies in volunteers using ^{131}I-tagged aggregated albumin have shown increased phagocytic activity of the reticuloendothelial system by the third to fifth day after onset of symptoms. Necrosis in hyperplastic Peyer's patches may be associated with erosion of blood vessels in the lesions in the intestinal tract, which leads to oozing of blood or massive hemorrhage. Lesions may extend deep into the intestinal wall and cause perforation, usually in the distal ileum, an event which characteristically occurs late in the disease, most often in the third febrile week.

The gallbladder and bile ducts are routinely infected during the disease. As a rule, this biliary infection is asymptomatic, although acute cholecystitis may occur occasionally. Biliary infection terminates spontaneously during convalescence in the vast majority of patients within 12 months, but about 3 percent of adults continue to harbor organisms in the gallbladder and become chronic carriers of the typhoid bacillus.

MANIFESTATIONS The incubation period averages about 10 days but may vary from extremes of 3 to 60 days depending on the infecting dose.

The clinical manifestations and duration of illness vary markedly from one patient to another. Mild forms of the disease, characterized primarily by fever, may last only a week, or illness may be prolonged, lasting 8 weeks or more if untreated.

In a typical patient not treated with antimicrobials, the illness lasts about 4 weeks. The onset is insidious with headache, malaise, anorexia, and fever. Headache may be the first manifestation of disease and is usually generalized and severe. Chilly sensations are common, and frank chills may be observed. The fever is remittent, frequently increasing in a steplike manner from day to day as the illness develops. Abdominal discomfort, bloating, and constipation are common during the early phase of illness. A dry cough is observed in about two-thirds of the patients and occasionally may be so prominent as to direct attention away from the generalized nature of the infection. Nosebleeds may occur during the early phase of illness.

The temperature gradually increases for 5 to 7 days and then plateaus as a continuous or mildly remittent fever in the range of 39 to 40°C. The temperature may be sustained at these levels with little variation for 2 or 3 weeks. A relative bradycardia occurs in 30 to 40 percent of the patients. The prolonged persistent fever leads to general debility; patients are weak and anorectic. Mental dullness is common and delirium may occur. Abdominal pain and marked distention are usual. Constipation during the early phase of illness may give way to diarrhea later in the course of the disease.

The characteristic rash (rose spots) is most often observed during the second week of the disease. The lesions are small, 2- to 4-mm, erythematous macules which occur in small numbers on the upper abdomen and anterior thorax. The lesions blanch on pressure and last only 2 to 3 days. Some reports describe rose spots in as many as 90 percent of patients, whereas other reports indicate a frequency of only 10 percent or even less. The evanescent nature of the rash and the difficulties encountered in detecting lesions in highly pigmented individuals probably account for the marked variation in incidence reported in the literature.

The liver and spleen are frequently enlarged and palpable after the first week of illness. The spleen is palpable in about three-quarters of the patients. The liver may be tender, and occasionally a friction rub is audible over the spleen.

Abdominal tenderness is frequent and distention occurs in the

majority of cases. Marked abdominal pain with signs of peritonitis should call attention to the possibility of perforation of the bowel.

After the third week, the symptoms slowly abate, and the temperature returns to normal over a period of days.

Jaundice secondary to extensive mononuclear cell infiltration in the liver and hepatic cell necrosis is a rare complication of typhoid. Acute renal failure also is observed rarely; the pathogenesis of this so-called typhoid nephritis has not been adequately defined. Disseminated intravascular coagulation may develop in severe typhoid and lead to additional clinical manifestations secondary to thrombosis or hemorrhage.

Complications Prior to the introduction of chloramphenicol, the prolonged febrile course of typhoid often led to profound debility, weight loss, and multiple nutritional deficiencies. Intestinal hemorrhage and bowel perforation, the most feared complications, were common causes of death in 12 to 32 percent of cases. The frequency of complications in typhoid fever has been reduced to 2 percent or less since the advent of effective chemotherapy.

INTESTINAL HEMORRHAGE Erosion of blood vessels in hyperplastic and necrotic Peyer's patches or in other mononuclear cell accumulations in the wall of the intestine leads to bleeding into the intestinal tract. Occult blood in feces is quite common during the course of the disease, occurring in 20 percent or more of patients. Gross blood is present in feces in about 10 percent of patients, and massive hemorrhage occurs occasionally. Major hemorrhage is usually a late complication, occurring most often during the second or third week of disease. A sudden drop in blood pressure or temperature may be the first manifestation of hemorrhage.

INTESTINAL PERFORATION The pathologic process in the lymphoid tissues of the intestine may also involve the muscular and serosal layers of the bowel and lead to perforation. Prior to the advent of chloramphenicol, perforation occurred in about 3 percent of patients with typhoid. The incidence has been reduced by antimicrobial therapy to about 1 percent. Perforation is most common in the distal 60 cm of ileum and is observed most frequently during the third week of the disease. The onset of perforation may be quite unexpected during an otherwise uncomplicated convalescence. Pain in the right lower quadrant of the abdomen is the most frequent initial manifestation, but signs of localized or generalized peritonitis develop rapidly.

OTHER COMPLICATIONS Typhoid bacilli may localize in any tissue in the body with the production of localized suppurative infection. Meningitis, chondritis, periostitis, osteomyelitis, arthritis, and pyelonephritis are examples of localized infections that may be observed occasionally. Pneumonia is not unusual and may be caused by the typhoid bacillus or by a secondary bacterial invader, such as the pneumococcus. Severe deep thrombophlebitis may occur during the febrile period. Late complications also include peripheral neuritis, deafness, and alopecia. Hemolytic anemia may be observed, especially in infected individuals deficient in glucose 6-phosphate dehydrogenase.

Relapse After illness has subsided for a variable period, usually about 2 weeks, all the manifestations which characterized the initial infection may recur. Blood cultures, negative during convalescence, may become positive again. Although relapse may be severe, it is usually milder and of shorter duration than the original illness. The incidence of relapse was about 5 to 10 percent prior to the introduction of effective chemotherapy. Chloramphenicol has not decreased the frequency of relapse; in fact, the relapse rate in chloramphenicol-treated patients is higher than in patients not receiving the drug. Periods of antimicrobial therapy longer than 2 weeks do not seem to alter the incidence of relapse. Relapse cannot be correlated with the titer of agglutinins against the flagellar, somatic, or Vi antigens of the typhoid bacillus.

Chronic carriers Although the vast majority of patients with typhoid fever eradicate the site of infection in the gallbladder during convalescence, about 3 percent of adults do not, and these individuals become chronic typhoid carriers who continue to excrete organisms in feces for years, usually for life. A chronic carrier is defined as a person documented to have been excreting typhoid bacilli in the stool for a period of at least 1 year. In the United States, almost all chronic carriers have a persistent site of infection in the gallbladder from which organisms reach the intestinal tract in bile. Chronic carriers may be detected by follow-up of patients with typhoid fever, but many carriers give no history of typhoid. In these patients, it is assumed that the initial illness was so mild as to go unrecognized or undiagnosed. Once organisms have been demonstrated in the stools for as long as a year, it is unlikely that the focus of infection in the gallbladder will terminate spontaneously. The chronic carrier state is rare in children and occurs more commonly with increasing age and is about three times more common in women than men. It is possible that these age and sex characteristics are related to the greater prevalence of gallbladder disease in older women, a factor which would favor persistence of organisms in the biliary tract.

The chronic biliary carrier is usually asymptomatic. Despite millions of organisms entering the intestine in each milliliter of bile, patients show no systemic manifestations. Gallstones and dysfunction of the gallbladder on cholecystogram can be demonstrated in a large proportion of chronic carriers, and carriers occasionally develop acute cholecystitis.

In areas of the world where *Schistosoma haematobium* infections are common, a chronic urinary carrier state results from localization of typhoid bacilli or other *Salmonella* serotypes in the obstructed urinary tract or adjacent lesions resulting from the schistosomiasis. These chronic urinary carriers not only excrete *Salmonella* in the urine but also may have intermittent bacteremic episodes which are not necessarily accompanied by fever.

LABORATORY FINDINGS Leukopenia of 3000 to 4000 cells per cubic millimeter is characteristic of the febrile phase of typhoid fever. A sudden increase in leukocyte count to 10,000 cells per cubic millimeter or higher should suggest the possibility of intestinal perforation, hemorrhage, or a pyogenic complication, but these complications may occur in the absence of leukocytosis. A normocytic normochromic anemia develops during the course of the disease and may be aggravated by blood loss from intestinal lesions. Occult blood and a mononuclear leukocytosis in feces is common from the second week of disease. Urine is usually normal except for transient albuminuria during the febrile period.

The most dependable way to establish a definitive diagnosis of typhoid fever is by blood culture. Organisms can be recovered by culture of blood in 70 to 90 percent of patients during the first week of disease. Bacteremia is continuous and prolonged. Positive blood cultures are obtained in as many as 30 or 40 percent of patients during the third week of disease, but the incidence of bacteremia rapidly decreases after this time. Blood cultures frequently are positive during relapse. Recent evidence in partially treated cases suggests that culture of bone marrow may yield the organism when other cultures are negative, especially after antibiotics have been given.

Only about 10 to 15 percent of patients have positive stool cultures during the first week of disease. However, the frequency of positive stool cultures increases as the disease progresses, reaching a maximum of about 75 percent during the third or fourth week of illness. The frequency of positive cultures then begins to decline so that only about 10 percent of patients have positive stool cultures 8 weeks after onset of illness. Most of these patients' cultures become negative over the next several weeks or months, but about 3 percent of adults continue to excrete organisms even after 1 year. Persistent excretion in these chronic carriers is secondary to infection in the gallbladder and biliary tract.

The incidence of positive urine cultures varies markedly during the course of typhoid fever and parallels the frequency of positive stool cultures. At least some of the positive cultures represent contamination of urine with feces harboring typhoid bacilli.

The majority of patients, but certainly not all, develop a fourfold or greater rise in serum agglutinins against the somatic or O antigens of the typhoid bacillus during the course of the disease. Detection of *S. typhi* Vi, D, or d antigens in the urine of patients with typhoid fever may be even more sensitive. A fourfold or greater increase in serum titer in the absence of recent typhoid immunization is compatible with infection with *S. typhi* but is by no means specific. All the group D organisms, one of which is *S. typhi*, as well as organisms in groups A and B, have certain common antigens which can evoke the formation of antibodies reactive with the O antigen used in the Widal test. Agglutinins against flagellar or H antigens also appear, frequently in higher titer than agglutinins against the O antigens. However, the H agglutinins are even more subject to nonspecific variation than O agglutinins and are of no value in diagnosis. Agglutinins begin to appear after about 1 week of illness and reach a peak titer during the fifth or sixth week. Early antimicrobial therapy may dampen the immunologic response in patients with typhoid fever. Relapse bears no relation to agglutinin titer. Rheumatoid factor activity in high titer can be detected in a large proportion of patients with typhoid or paratyphoid fever.

DIFFERENTIAL DIAGNOSIS The clinical features of typhoid fever, while characteristic and suggestive of the diagnosis, are certainly not pathognomonic. Many other diseases give a clinical picture which may be confused with typhoid; these include the rickettsioses, brucellosis, tularemia, leptospirosis, psittacosis, infectious hepatitis, infectious mononucleosis, primary atypical pneumonia, miliary tuberculosis, malaria, lymphoma, and rheumatic fever. Typhoid should be considered in any patient with unexplained fever, especially if there is a history of recent foreign travel to endemic areas.

TREATMENT Antimicrobial therapy Chloramphenicol is the antibiotic of choice for the treatment of typhoid fever caused by sensitive organisms. Despite the fact that a number of antimicrobial agents show excellent in vitro activity against *S. typhi*, chloramphenicol has consistently been shown to be more effective in terminating the febrile toxic course of the disease in the greatest proportion of patients in the shortest period of time. Nevertheless, the response to chloramphenicol is not dramatic or rapid. Subjective improvement usually occurs within about 48 h after beginning therapy, but the temperature usually does not return to normal for 2 to 5 days after initiating treatment. Bacteremia usually clears within hours after therapy is instituted, but occasionally organisms can be recovered from the blood 24 to 48 h after beginning treatment. The dose of chloramphenicol should be 50 mg per kilogram of body weight per day divided into three or four equal doses given orally at intervals of 6 to 8 h. After the patient has become afebrile, the dose may be reduced to 30 mg/kg per day. Therapy should be continued for 2 weeks. If chloramphenicol cannot be given by the oral route, comparable doses should be given parenterally.

Ampicillin in doses of 80 mg/kg per day or 6 g per day for adults divided into four or six doses given parenterally or a combination of trimethoprim and sulfamethoxazole is effective in the treatment of typhoid, but the response is not as predictable or as prompt as with chloramphenicol. If there is a contraindication to therapy with chloramphenicol, ampicillin, amoxicillin, or trimethoprim-sulfamethoxazole is recommended.

Occasional patients with typhoid without evidence of suppurative complications do not respond clinically even after 4 or 5 days of antimicrobial therapy, even though blood cultures become negative. Delayed responses of this type occur in only about 1 percent of patients treated with chloramphenicol, in contrast to 5 or 10 percent of patients treated with ampicillin.

Chloramphenicol-resistant strains have been reported since 1972 from many areas of the world, predominantly Mexico, southeast Asia, and India. Resistance is due to a transferable R factor which also codes for resistance to sulfonamides, tetracycline, and streptomycin. *Salmonella typhi* resistant to both chloramphenicol and ampicillin have been isolated from a few patients, and the in vivo acquisition of resistance to chloramphenicol, and sulfonamide/trimethoprim, in a patient treated with these drugs, has been reported. If chloramphenicol resistance is encountered, then ampicillin, amoxicillin, or trimethoprim-sulfamethoxazole should be used.

Adrenal hormones The administration of dexamethasone, prednisone, or steroids with similar activity can terminate within a matter of hours the severe febrile toxemic state seen in some patients. Because of the lag in time between institution of antimicrobial therapy and evidence of response, patients with life-threatening toxemia, hypotension, or clouded sensorium should be treated with a brief course of corticosteroids in addition to chloramphenicol. While 300 mg of cortisone (or 60 mg prednisone) have been effective, very high doses of dexamethasone (3 mg/kg) have been shown to reduce mortality in very severe typhoid fever. In any case, steroids should be rapidly tapered over 24 to 48 h. Hypothermia and hypotension occasionally occur within hours after initiation of steroids.

Supportive treatment Nursing care and attention to nutritional requirements are important. Laxatives and enemas should be avoided despite constipation because of the danger of precipitating hemorrhage or perforation. Salicylates should not be used, because in addition to their effects on blood platelets and irritating action on the bowel, these compounds can induce wide swings in temperature with very uncomfortable chills and sweats. Hypothermia and hypotension occur in some patients after administration of salicylates.

Hemorrhage and perforation Patients should be observed carefully to detect these complications at an early stage. Typing and cross matching should be carried out at the time of initial diagnosis of typhoid, and transfusion is indicated in the event of significant hemorrhage. Patients with typhoid are poor surgical risks. If perforation is suspected, emphasis should be placed on efforts to combat shock and decompress the bowel. Additional antimicrobials may have to be added to control peritonitis. Small perforations may localize and can be managed without surgical intervention. However, if evidence of localization does not develop, prompt surgical intervention may be required.

Relapse The therapy of relapse is identical to that for the primary episode.

Chronic carriers Chronic carriers should be investigated for the presence of gallstones or a nonfunctioning gallbladder. Carriers without evidence of gallstones or gallbladder disease on cholecystogram or with ultrasound usually can be cured with a prolonged course of ampicillin. One program which has been found to be effective consists of 6 g ampicillin divided into four equal oral doses each day with probenecid for a period of 6 weeks. If gallstones or a nonfunctioning gallbladder are demonstrated, antimicrobial therapy is unlikely to be effective in terminating the carrier state. These patients should have cholecystectomy, which cures the chronic carrier state in about 85 percent of patients. Ampicillin may be used in conjunction with cholecystectomy. Therapy should be started a few days prior to the procedure and continued for 2 or 3 weeks. One study has reported success of sulfamethoxazole-trimethoprim and rifampin in the treatment of chronic *Salmonella* carriers.

PREVENTION AND CONTROL Control of typhoid fever involves improved sanitation, sewage control, and water supplies, and identification and cure or control of chronic carriers. Although immunization with typhoid vaccine affords significant protection against typhoid infection, the degree of immunity is not great and can be readily overcome with a large dose of organisms. Nevertheless, immunization is recommended for individuals living or traveling in areas where the disease is endemic and for persons working with the organism in laboratories. Adults should receive 0.5 mL vaccine on two occasions separated by a period of 1 or 2 weeks. A booster is recommended every 3 years to maintain immunity. Immunization with typhoid vaccine causes a transient elevation for several months

in titer of agglutinins against typhoid O antigens and a persistently elevated titer for H antigens. A live, attenuated vaccine is being developed that shows promising efficacy in initial field trials.

All typhoid patients should be reported to local health authorities, and stool specimens should be cultured during convalescence. Three consecutively negative stool cultures obtained at weekly intervals indicate that a carrier state has not developed.

Caution should be observed to prevent spread of infection from persons with active disease or from carriers. Chronic or convalescent carriers should not be allowed to prepare food until clear documentation shows that at least three or more stool cultures are negative for typhoid bacilli. Carriers should be cautioned regarding routine sanitary techniques.

PROGNOSIS The mortality rate from typhoid fever prior to the introduction of chloramphenicol was about 12 percent. Death was associated with toxemia, inanition, pneumonia, bowel perforation, and intestinal hemorrhage. The mortality rate is still about 2 percent; deaths are observed primarily in infants, the aged, or individuals with malnutrition or other underlying diseases, or in those in whom the diagnosis is not suspected early.

SALMONELLA INFECTIONS OTHER THAN TYPHOID FEVER

DEFINITION Bacteria of the genus *Salmonella* may produce asymptomatic infection of the intestinal tract in humans or several different clinical syndromes including acute gastroenteritis (or enterocolitis), bacteremia, paratyphoid fever, or localized infections ranging from osteomyelitis to endocarditis. The clinical syndromes resulting from infection with *Salmonella* cannot always be sharply differentiated and sometimes overlap.

Salmonella infections are among the most prevalent recognized communicable diseases caused by bacteria in the United States today. These infections are transmitted in the vast majority of cases from animals to humans and occasionally from person to person and, in normal hosts, are usually brief, self-limited, and mild.

EPIDEMIOLOGY Salmonellae can be isolated from the intestinal tracts of humans and many lower animals. The prevalence of asymptomatic excretors of these organisms in the general population has been estimated to be about 0.2 percent (with probably over 2 million cases annually in the United States), but the most important reservoir of salmonellae is in domestic and wild animal species in which infection rates vary from less than 1 to more than 20 percent. An incomplete list of animals from which *Salmonella* species have been isolated includes chickens, turkeys, ducks, pigs, cows, dogs, cats, rats, parakeets, as well as certain cold-blooded animals and insects. Animals sold as pets, especially baby chicks, ducks, and turtles, may also harbor *Salmonella* and serve as sources of infection.

Salmonella infection is almost always acquired by the oral route, usually by ingestion of contaminated food or drink. Rare exceptions are *Salmonella* infections acquired by intravenous platelet transfusions or contaminated fiberoptic instruments. Any food product is a potential source of human infection. The source of contamination of food or drink may be asymptomatic human carriers or persons with active clinical disease, but the greatest single source of human infection in the United States is the vast reservoir of *Salmonella* in lower animals. The high incidence of infection in domestic animals used as a source of food for humans and present methods of processing foods and food products in bulk result in the availability of foods for human consumption with a potentially high incidence of contamination with *Salmonella*. For example, a significant proportion varying from 1 to more than 50 percent of raw meats purchased in retail markets is contaminated with *Salmonella*. Meat is contaminated by many routes, but the most common are natural infection of the animal used as a source of meat and contamination of the carcass during slaughter and processing. Eggs or egg products, including dried or frozen eggs, are also common sources of *Salmonella* infection. Of the various animal species, domestic fowl, including chickens, turkeys, ducks, and eggs and egg products, constitute the single largest reservoir of infection and the source most often responsible for infection of humans. Adequate cooking of food prior to human consumption serves to decrease the possibility of infection. However, salmonellae may survive cooking at low temperature, or food may be recontaminated after cooking by organisms from kitchen equipment or personnel. Raw or inadequately pasteurized milk is increasingly recognized as a potential vehicle of *Salmonella* infections, especially with *S. dublin,* that may cause more severe or bloodstream infections.

Food or drink may also be contaminated by rats, mice, insects, or other vermin harboring these organisms. Cross infection occurs occasionally by the airborne route from dried foods such as egg whites or dust which contain viable *Salmonella. Salmonella* contamination of a large variety of processed foods has also been documented. Some of these foods contain ingredients of animal origin such as eggs, whereas others contain contaminated products of vegetable origin such as coconut or yeast. A variety of pharmaceutical products of animal origin have been shown to be responsible for *Salmonella* infections of humans; these products include carmine dye, pancreatin, bile salts, and extracts of various organs such as thyroid, adrenal, and stomach.

Pet turtles are an important source of *Salmonella* infection in humans, especially in children, accounting for perhaps as many as 10 to 20 percent of reported *Salmonella* infections in certain areas. Turtles are infected on breeding farms and continue to excrete organisms in feces into tank water for long periods of time. Although knowledge of the manner of transmission to humans is incomplete, it is likely that turtle feces or tank water harboring salmonellae contaminates the hands of handlers, from which organisms are passed to the mouth or to food or drink.

Salmonella species may also be transmitted directly or via fomites from humans to humans or from animals to humans without the intervention of contaminated food or drink, but this method of spread is not common. However, cross infection of this type has been shown to be responsible for a number of outbreaks of salmonellosis among patients in nurseries and hospitals. Nosocomial salmonellosis poses a particular threat to newborns, immunosuppressed patients, patients in burn units, and those receiving multiple broad-spectrum antibiotics, who may be infected by relatively few organisms. Multiply drug-resistant salmonellae are often found in this setting. Nursery outbreaks have been traced to newborn infants from mothers with recent *Salmonella* infections.

Fish meal, meat meal, bone meal, and other by-products of the meat-packing industry are often contaminated with *Salmonella* organisms. These products are incorporated in animal and poultry feeds and apparently play an important role in the perpetuation of infection among domestic animals that can be spread to humans.

The true incidence of *Salmonella* infection is difficult to determine. The reported isolations of salmonellae from humans in the United States represent about 10 cases per 100,000 population per year. However, reported cases represent only a small proportion of the actual number because bacteriologic studies are usually performed only on patients with severe or protracted diarrhea, and many outbreaks are not investigated. It is estimated that over 2 million cases probably occur each year, affecting nearly 1 percent of the population in the United States. Although *Salmonella* infection occurs throughout the year, the Salmonella Surveillance Unit of the National Communicable Disease Centers has observed a distinct seasonal pattern with the greatest number of isolations reported from July through November for each year.

A close correlation exists between the *Salmonella* serotypes most often responsible for human infection and those isolated from animals in any specific geographic area. The similarities document the importance of nonhuman reservoirs of *Salmonella* in the epidemiology of *Salmonella* infection in humans.

PATHOGENESIS The course of events after salmonellae have gained access to the gastrointestinal tract is determined by the dose, serotype, and invasive potential of the organism, and by the resistance of the host. Different *Salmonella* serotypes show marked variation in invasive potential and capacity to produce disease in humans. For example, *S. anatum* characteristically produces asymptomatic intestinal infection and rarely invades the bloodstream. In contrast, *S. cholerae-suis,* the most invasive serotype, frequently produces bacteremia and metastatic infection. Bloodstream invasion may occur as a complication of gastroenteritis but usually develops without preceding intestinal symptoms. Bacteremia with any serotype may be transient or prolonged, and may be accompanied by recurrent chills and fever or manifestations of paratyphoid fever. Bloodborne bacteria may localize at any site and lead to suppuration in bone, joints, meninges, pleura, or other tissues.

Multiplication of ingested organisms in the intestinal tract may be followed by symptoms of gastroenteritis. The intestinal irritation and inflammation are produced by a true infection deep in the mucosa as evidenced by polymorphonuclear leukocytes typically found in the diarrheal stool. However, studies in animals have shown that mucosal invasion alone is not sufficient to account for the intestinal fluid observed in experimental infections. The secretory effects of certain strains of *S. typhimurium* can be abolished in animals by indomethacin without altering the invasive process. This has led to the hypothesis of a possible enterotoxin-like effect on upper intestinal transport. An enterotoxin-like effect has also been shown with culture filtrates of *Salmonella* in animals and tissue culture models used to study *Escherichia coli* and cholera enterotoxins.

Studies in human volunteers indicate that large numbers of viable organisms must be ingested to produce clinically apparent disease. However, a transient carrier state can be produced with doses 10 or 100 times smaller than those required to evoke symptoms of infection. The minimal infectious dose varies markedly among different serotypes.

Many host factors influence the frequency and nature of *Salmonella* infections. The minimal infectious dose varies considerably among different individual hosts and can be reduced by antacids, antimotility drugs, or antimicrobial agents in experimental animals. Some have reported the precipitation of severe systemic disease following antimotility therapy for mild gastroenteritis.

The bacterial flora of the intestine is important in determining the fate of ingested salmonellae. Increasingly impressive epidemiologic and experimental data show that antibiotics increase the susceptibility to *Salmonella* infections. Symptomatic infections in outbreaks are often associated with recent antibiotic consumption. Administration of certain antibiotics by the oral route to mice results in a 10,000-fold increase in susceptibility to infection with *S. enteritidis.* In experimental typhoid fever in volunteers, the dose of *S. typhi* required to initiate infection by the oral route in humans can also be reduced sharply by giving certain antimicrobials orally prior to challenge. Epidemiologic studies have also shown that prior antimicrobial therapy alters the capacity of the human intestinal tract to eradicate *Salmonella* acquired naturally. The effect of antibiotic therapy may be related to a marked diminution in the number of *Bacteroides* or other organisms which produce substances such as short-chain fatty acids that inhibit the growth of *Salmonella.* Alteration in intestinal flora also has been suggested as a mechanism of the increased susceptibility of patients with previous major gastric surgery, especially gastrectomy and gastroenterostomy, to intestinal infection with salmonellae. However, reduced acidity or rapid emptying time consequent to gastric surgery may also play a role by increasing the number of viable organisms reaching the small intestine.

Cell-mediated immune mechanisms are also important in host resistance to infection with salmonellae. About one-third of patients who are hospitalized because of salmonellosis have some type of major underlying disease, such as leukemia, lymphoma, lupus erythematosus, or aplastic anemia. Several reports describe an increased frequency of persisting or recurring *Salmonella* infections in patients with the acquired immunodeficiency syndrome (AIDS). In a few other diseases there is evidence to indicate a particular predisposition to infection by salmonellae that exceeds susceptibility to other bacterial species. Patients with sickle cell anemia and other hemolytic processes are unusually susceptible to bloodstream invasion by salmonellae. In patients with sickle hemoglobinopathies there is a strong tendency for localization in bone, and salmonellae, not staphylococci, are the most common cause of osteomyelitis in patients with sickle cell diseases. *Salmonella* bacteremia is also an unusually frequent complication of the acute hemolytic phase of bartonellosis (see Chap. 116).

Infants are more susceptible to *Salmonella* infection and remain convalescent carriers for a longer period of time than adults. The mortality rate from the disease is also higher in infants and in the elderly than in young adults.

CLINICAL MANIFESTATIONS Gastroenteritis Although gastroenteritis often occurs in large epidemics among individuals who have eaten the same contaminated food, family outbreaks and sporadic cases are even more common. After an incubation period of 8 to 48 h, there is sudden onset of colicky abdominal pain and loose, watery diarrhea, occasionally with mucus or blood. Nausea and vomiting are frequent but are rarely severe or protracted. Fever of 38 to 39°C is common, and there may be an initial chill. Patients usually have mild to moderate abdominal tenderness on palpation, but severe tenderness, even with rebound, occurs in occasional patients. Peristalsis is usually hyperactive. Abdominal findings may be prominent in some patients and lead to confusion with certain intraabdominal emergencies, such as acute appendicitis or acute cholecystitis. Colonic involvement with tenesmus and with mucosal friability and crypt abscess may also occur. Symptoms usually subside promptly within 2 to 5 days and recovery is uneventful. However, the illness is occasionally more protracted, with persistence of diarrhea and low-grade fever for 10 to 14 days. Fatalities rarely exceed 1 percent of the affected population and are limited almost entirely to infants, the aged, and debilitated patients.

The causative organism can often be isolated from the suspected food and from feces during the acute illness. Stool cultures usually become negative for salmonellae within 1 to 4 weeks, but occasional patients continue to excrete organisms for months. Organisms tend to persist in the stools of infants and young children for longer periods than in older children or adults. The blood leukocyte count is usually normal. The blood culture is usually negative.

Enteric or paratyphoid fever Certain species can produce an illness clinically indistinguishable from typhoid fever, with prolonged fever, rose spots, splenomegaly, leukopenia, gastrointestinal symptoms, and positive blood and stool cultures. The organisms most likely to produce this picture are *S. cholerae-suis* and *S. enteritidis*, serotypes *paratyphi A* and *paratyphi B*. Occasionally a typical attack of food poisoning is followed in a few days by manifestations of paratyphoid fever. Generally, paratyphoid fevers tend to be milder than *S. typhi* infections, but differentiation on clinical grounds is not possible in the individual case. Recovery may be followed by continued excretion of the causative organism in the stools for several months, but the chronic carrier state is less frequent than in typhoid fever.

Bacteremia *Salmonella* species may produce a syndrome characterized primarily by prolonged fever and positive blood cultures. Although symptoms of gastroenteritis can precede bacteremia, they are usually lacking, and most cases arise sporadically. In many instances, the only manifestations are prolonged fever, which is usually spiking and is accompanied by repeated rigors, sweats, aching, anorexia, and weight loss. The characteristic features of typhoid and paratyphoid fever, such as rose spots, persistent leukopenia, and sustained fever, are absent. Stool cultures are usually negative. In contrast to the constant bacteremia of typhoid fever, discharge of organisms into the bloodstream is intermittent, and repeated blood cultures may be required to demonstrate the causative

organism. At some time in the course of the illness, localizing signs of infection appear in about one-fourth of the cases. Pulmonary infection in the form of bronchopneumonia or abscess, pleurisy, empyema, pericarditis, endocarditis, pyelonephritis, meningitis, osteomyelitis, and arthritis is relatively common. The blood leukocyte count is usually normal, but with the development of focal lesions, polymorphonuclear leukocytosis as high as 20,000 to 25,000 cells per cubic millimeter occurs. *Salmonella* bacteremia can be a very puzzling disorder, especially before localization takes place, and should be considered in cases of fever of unknown origin.

A prolonged febrile illness lasting weeks or months and characterized by weight loss, marked anemia, hepatosplenomegaly, and bacteremia with *Salmonella* has been described in Brazil and other areas of the world in patients with hepatosplenic schistosomiasis due to *Schistosoma mansoni*. Intermittent bacteremia with *Salmonella* also occurs in patients with *Schistosoma haematobium* infection who are also urinary carriers of *Salmonella*.

Local pyogenic infections *Salmonella* organisms can produce abscesses in almost any anatomic site, and these can occur independently of previous symptoms of gastroenteritis or other systemic illness, or as complications of bacteremias. There is nothing characteristic about the suppurative lesions, and the correct etiologic diagnosis is rarely made on the basis of clinical findings alone. There is a strong tendency for salmonellae to localize in tissues that are the site of preexisting disease. Localization has been described in aneurysms, bone adjacent to aortic aneurysms, hematomas, and many different tumors, including hypernephroma, ovarian cyst, and pheochromocytoma. Meningeal localization of infection is common in newborns and infants, and occasional small outbreaks of *Salmonella* infection in nurseries have consisted almost entirely of meningitis. In addition to suppurative joint disease, a chronic aseptic polyarthritis has been described.

DIAGNOSIS Febrile gastroenteritis produced by presumed viral agents, *Campylobacter jejuni* or *Shigella* sp., can be distinguished from *Salmonella* gastroenteritis only by appropriate stool cultures, especially in sporadic cases. Polymorphonuclear fecal leukocytes are frequently present in *Salmonella* gastroenteritis and in bacillary dysentery (shigellosis), but not in viral, giardial, or enterotoxin-induced gastroenteritis. Staphylococcal food poisoning usually is not associated with fever, and vomiting is a more prominent feature than in most *Salmonella* infections. Systemic manifestations are usually much less striking in patients with gastroenteritis caused by enterotoxigenic *E. coli* and *Clostridium perfringens*. Many toxic agents and drugs can produce diarrhea, nausea, and abdominal pain, but fever is rarely a feature of these disorders, and the diagnosis depends upon a history of exposure or ingestion. The diagnosis of paratyphoid fever or *Salmonella* bacteremia depends upon isolation of the causative organism. Agglutination tests with acute and convalescent serums as performed in the usual clinical laboratory are not very helpful. The possibility of an underlying disease should be considered in every patient with a severe *Salmonella* infection.

TREATMENT The treatment of *Salmonella* gastroenteritis is supportive. Dehydration should be corrected by parenteral administration of fluids and electrolytes. Abdominal cramps and diarrhea often are much improved if the patient takes nothing by mouth for 8 to 12 h. Antimicrobial therapy does not shorten the clinical course of *Salmonella* gastroenteritis, but actually prolongs the duration of excretion of organisms in the stool and may increase the clinical relapse rate. Unless there is documented bacteremia or a protracted febrile course suggesting the diagnosis of enteric fever, antibiotics are *not* indicated in uncomplicated *Salmonella* gastroenteritis. Because of the predilection of *Salmonella* bacteremia to colonize endovascular foci, it has been suggested that patients over 50 years old, especially those with atherosclerotic arterial aneurysms, prosthetic vascular prostheses or valves, or even underlying valvular or coronary disease, who develop febrile *Salmonella* enteritis and suspected bacteremia should be considered for early antimicrobial therapy. Certainly, persons with documented bacteremia or those who relapse with these actual or potential intravascular foci should receive effective antimicrobial therapy.

There has been a steady increase in the frequency of antimicrobial resistance due to transferable resistance factors among *Salmonella* isolates from humans. This may be due in part to the widespread use of antibiotics in animals and in humans.

Chloramphenicol in doses of 3 g daily in adults is the antibiotic of choice in systemic infections including *Salmonella* bacteremia, metastatic infection, and paratyphoid fever. The response is characteristically slow, and the temperature rarely returns to normal until 3 to 4 days after beginning therapy. Therapy should be continued for at least 2 weeks, but in certain infections, such as osteomyelitis or meningitis, the duration may have to be extended. As resistance to multiple antibiotics is increasing, antibiotic sensitivity of the organism should be tested in cases of bacteremia, metastatic infection, or enteric fever.

Because of the hematologic toxicity of chloramphenicol, some prefer ampicillin to treat systemic infections caused by sensitive *Salmonella* strains, and ampicillin is preferred over chloramphenicol for suspected intravascular infection as noted above. However, a significant proportion of *Salmonella* strains are highly resistant to ampicillin in vitro. For this reason, ampicillin should not be used in therapy of serious infections unless it is known that the causative organism is sensitive. As in cases of typhoid fever, the combination of trimethoprim and sulfamethoxazole holds promise in the therapy of *Salmonella* infection when the organism is resistant to chloramphenicol and ampicillin. The tetracycline derivatives have sometimes appeared to exert a beneficial effect, but streptomycin, polymyxin, neomycin, kanamycin, and the sulfonamides are generally ineffective.

Antimicrobial therapy is usually not indicated in convalescent or asymptomatic transient carriers of *Salmonella* species. The carrier state will cease spontaneously in 1 to 3 months in the vast majority of individuals.

The chronic carrier state with localization of infection in the gallbladder and positive stool cultures for a period of time exceeding 1 year is rarely caused by *Salmonella* serotypes other than *S. typhi* and *S. paratyphi* A and B. Its treatment has been discussed. Surgically accessible suppurative lesions should be drained.

PREVENTION AND CONTROL Continuous surveillance and careful reporting of all *Salmonella* isolates improve awareness of new strains, common sources, antibiotic resistance, and the carrier state. Because of the great number of specific serotypes, surveillance and serotyping have occasionally brought attention to widespread occurrence of relatively rare serotypes traced to single sources. Adequate cooking of meat and egg products and careful surveillance of poultry products and persons who handle food have been only moderately successful in controlling salmonellosis. Probably most important, besides food surveillance, is personal hygiene, including handwashing. Transient or permanent carriers should be warned to take these precautions and, as much as possible, to avoid food preparation. Minimizing the time that foods are allowed to stand at room temperature (as between cooking and refrigeration) should reduce the chances of bacterial growth to infectious inocula.

Careful obstetrical histories for any diarrheal illness at the time a woman enters for delivery should always be obtained, and mothers and infants so affected should be isolated until cultures rule out *Salmonella* carriage. Finally, because of the increasing antibiotic resistance, the indiscriminate use of unnecessary or "prophylactic" antimicrobial agents should be avoided.

REFERENCES

ALVAREZ-ELCORO S et al: *Salmonella* bacteremia in patients with prosthetic heart valves. Am J Med 77:61, 1984

BAINE WB et al: Institutional salmonellosis. J Infect Dis 128:357, 1973

BLASER MJ et al: *Salmonella typhi:* The laboratory as a reservoir of infection. J Infect Dis 142:934, 1980

BUTLER T et al: Typhoid fever: Studies of blood coagulation, bacteremia and endotoxemia. Arch Intern Med 138:407, 1978

COHEN PS et al: The risk of endothelial infection in adults with *Salmonella* bacteremia. Ann Intern Med 89:931, 1978

FREERKSEN E et al: Treatment of chronic salmonella carriers. Chemotherapy 23:192, 1977

HOFFMAN SL et al: Reduction of mortality in chloramphenicol-treated severe typhoid fever by high-dose dexamethasone. N Engl J Med 310:82, 1981

HOLMBERG SD et al: Drug-resistant *Salmonella* from animals fed antimicrobials. N Engl J Med 311:617, 1984

HOOK EW: Typhoid fever today. N Engl J Med 310:82, 1981

HORNICK RB, GRIESMAN S: On the pathogenesis of typhoid fever. Arch Intern Med 138:357, 1978

Human *Salmonella* isolates—United States, 1980. Morb Mort Week Rep 30:377, 1981

JACOBS JL et al: *Salmonella* infections in patients with the acquired immunodeficiency syndrome. Ann Intern Med 102:186, 1985

KAYE D et al: Treatment of chronic enteric carriers of *Salmonella typhosa* with ampicillin. Ann NY Acad Sci 145:429, 1967

LEVY SB: Playing antibiotic pool: Time totally the score. N Engl J Med 311:617, 1984

MANDAL BK: Typhoid and paratyphoid fever. Clin Gastroent 8:715, 1979

POTTER ME et al: Unpasteurized milk. The hazards of a health fetish. JAMA 252:2048, 1984

QUE JU, HENTGES DJ: Effect of streptomycin administration on colonization resistance to *Salmonella typhimurium* in mice. Infect Immun 48:169, 1985

RYDER RW et al: Increase in antibiotic resistance among isolates of *Salmonella* in the U.S. J Infect Dis. 142:485, 1980

TAUXE RV et al: Turtle-associated salmonellosis in Puerto Rico. JAMA 254:237, 1985

TAYLOR DN et al: Typhoid in the United States and the risk to the international traveler. J Infect Dis 148:599, 1983

TURNBULL PCB: Food poisoning with special reference to *Salmonella*—Its epidemiology, pathogenesis and control. Clin Gastroent 8:663, 1979

---

108 SHIGELLOSIS

RICHARD D. PEARSON / RICHARD L. GUERRANT

DEFINITION Shigellosis refers to an acute bacillary infection of the intestinal tract produced by one of four *Shigella* species. The spectrum of disease ranges from mild, watery diarrhea to severe dysentery characterized by crampy abdominal pain, tenesmus, fever, and signs of systemic toxicity.

ETIOLOGY The genus *Shigella* of the family Enterobacteriaceae is composed of a group of closely related species which are nonmotile, nonencapsulated, nonsporulating, gram-negative rods. They are aerobes or facultative anaerobes and grow best at 37°C. The species differ in their ability to ferment carbohydrates. All strains produce acid, but not gas, from glucose and either fail to ferment lactose or do so slowly. The four species are further subdivided into a total of approximately 40 serotypes. Four species or groups are separated on the basis of major somatic (O) antigens and fermentation patterns: *S. dysenteriae* (group A), *S. flexneri* (group B), *S. boydii* (group C), and *S. sonnei* (group D). In developing countries, *S. dysenteriae* type 1 and *S. flexneri* are the most common isolates. They predominated in the United States and Europe prior to 1940, but *S. sonnei* has been the most frequent isolate since that time.

Shigella species have lipopolysaccharide endotoxin which is chemically and biologically similar to the endotoxins of other Enterobacteriaceae. *Shigella dysenteriae* type 1 (Shiga bacillus) also produces an exotoxin. The exotoxin has since been shown to have enterotoxin activity which may cause intestinal secretion as well as cytotoxic properties directed against intestinal epithelial cells. It may also account for the neurotoxicity observed in children with shigellosis. *S. flexneri* and *S. sonnei* produce a similar exotoxin although in smaller amounts.

EPIDEMIOLOGY Shigellosis is worldwide in distribution and remains a major problem in countries which lack effective sanitation and where malnutrition is common. In 1983, approximately 15,000 cases of shigellosis were reported in the United States; *S. sonnei* was responsible for 66 percent. Children under 10 years of age accounted for the greatest number of cases. In the United States, shigellosis is particularly common among children in day-care centers and among male homosexuals. In emerging nations, *S. flexneri* and *S. dysenteriae* type 1 remain the most important pathogens.

Humans and other primates are the only known reservoirs of *Shigella* species. The portal of entry is the gastrointestinal tract. Shigellosis is one of the most communicable of the bacterial diarrheal diseases; ingestion of fewer than 100 organisms can produce disease among healthy volunteers. Spread of *Shigella* is primarily person-to-person through contaminated hands or objects or by consumption of contaminated food or water. Poor sanitation, low standards of personal hygiene, crowded conditions, and a high proportion of children in the population favor spread of infection in the developing world. Outbreaks of shigellosis in the United States have tended to occur in confined populations where there are poor sanitary conditions or hygiene such as day-care centers, cruise ships, Indian reservations, mental institutions, geriatric wards, or other custodial care centers. Secondary transmission in industrialized countries frequently follows acquisition of shigellosis by children in day-care centers. Fecal-oral transmission of *Shigella* among male homosexuals has been increasingly recognized. *Shigella* species have caused traveler's diarrhea in visitors to Russia and other areas of the world. Laboratory-acquired cases are also well-documented.

Common source outbreaks have involved food contaminated by careless handlers who are *Shigella* carriers. Outbreaks associated with drinking water have occurred, and swimming in contaminated water has led to infection. However, food- and waterborne transmission appear to be less important in shigellosis than in cholera or typhoid fever, in which larger inocula are usually necessary to produce disease.

In developing countries where spread of disease is primarily person-to-person, carriers may be the important reservoir. In patients who receive no antibiotic treatment, fecal excretion of *Shigella* usually lasts 1 to 4 weeks, but in a small percentage of cases shedding persists for much longer periods. Prolonged carriage seems to be more common among the malnourished.

PATHOGENESIS AND PATHOLOGY After ingestion, the organism is thought to colonize and multiply in the upper small bowel where it may cause secretion early in illness. The colon rapidly becomes the principal site of pathology in *Shigella* dysentery. *Shigella* penetrate epithelial cells, multiply intracellularly, and spread laterally to cause cell death. Superficial microulcers and inflammation result.

The multiple factors which contribute to the virulence of *Shigella* are under polygenic control. There is a strong correlation between invasiveness and gastrointestinal virulence. Virulent *Shigella* produce an exotoxin that has cytotoxic, enterotoxic, and neurotoxic properties. It is composed of active and binding subunits, binds to a glycoprotein membrane receptor on epithelial cells, is transported into the cell by an energy-dependent mechanism, and inhibits protein synthesis by catalytic inactivation of the 60S ribosomal subunit. Roles for enterotoxin activity in causing secretion, cytotoxin activity in causing cell damage, and neurotoxin activity in producing the neurologic manifestations of shigellosis have been postulated but not proven. A 120–140 Mcal plasmid encoding translucent colony morphology, smooth lipopolysaccharide, and antigenic peptides is necessary, but not sufficient for invasiveness. Necessary chromosomal traits include somatic antigens, intestinal survival, invasiveness as assessed by the Serény test, and possibly exotoxin production.

Innate and acquired host defenses against *Shigella* are not completely understood. Gastric acidity and bile do not appear to provide effective barriers. Increased intestinal motility during infection may contribute to clearance of the organism. Normal intestinal flora may impede the growth of *Shigella*. Humoral immunity is thought to be important in acquired host defense against *Shigella*, protection deriving mainly from coproantibodies (IgA). After natural infection, serotype-specific antibodies and enterotoxin-neutralizing antibodies are identified in serum within 1 to 2 weeks. Serotype-specific vaccine efficacy has also been demonstrated. Breast-feeding appears to be protective in newborns. This may be mediated by maternal antibodies against *Shigella* or nonspecific factors. Cellular immune responses during or following shigellosis in humans have not been thoroughly characterized, but in vitro studies indicate that Fc receptor–bearing lymphocytes, monocytes, and granulocytes can kill *Shigella* in the presence of anti-*Shigella* antisera.

CLINICAL MANIFESTATIONS The spectrum of shigellosis ranges from mild diarrhea to severe dysentery with crampy abdominal pain, tenesmus, fever, and systemic toxicity. Symptoms usually begin abruptly 1 to 7 days after exposure. Patients initially have watery stools accompanied by fever (as high as 41°C), diffuse abdominal pain, nausea, and vomiting. Other symptoms include myalgias, chills, backache, and headache. Dysentery develops after the first few days of illness and is associated with tenesmus and frequent, small, bloody, mucoid stools. Fever subsequently decreases, and abdominal pain may localize to the lower quadrants. Diarrhea peaks at about 7 days. Bloody dysentery is more common and appears earlier in infection with *S. dysenteriae* type 1 than with other serotypes. Neonatal infection, which is uncommon even in endemic areas, may present with weight loss, poor feeding, diarrhea, and occasionally jaundice.

The physical examination is normal in mild cases, or there may be signs of severe dehydration. Diffuse or localized lower abdominal tenderness is often present, but there is seldom evidence of peritoneal irritation. Bowel sounds are usually hyperactive. Diffuse mucosal edema, hyperemia, and superficial ulceration are seen on proctosigmoidoscopy.

Shigellosis is generally a self-limited disease, but in certain patients, particularly infants and the elderly, severe dehydration or even malnutrition may be precipitated by fluid and electrolyte loss, anorexia, and fever. In normal hosts who do not receive antibiotics, fever usually resolves after 3 or 4 days, but diarrhea and abdominal cramps may continue for 1 to 2 weeks. The overall mortality rate associated with shigellosis in the United States is less than 0.1 percent, but the illness is often more severe and the prognosis poorer among children and the elderly. *S. dysenteriae* type 1 produces more severe infection than other *Shigella* species, and mortality rates in epidemics in the developing world have been high, particularly in malnourished children.

Extraintestinal complications of *Shigella* infection are uncommon. In addition to headache, meningismus or seizures may occur. Seizures are most common in children under 5 years of age and are not always associated with marked temperature elevation. The cerebrospinal fluid is usually normal. Transient peripheral neuropathy has followed *S. dysenteriae* type 1 infection, and the Guillain-Barré syndrome has followed by 1 week an outbreak of *S. boydii* gastroenteritis. *Shigella* species are infrequently recovered from the bloodstream, possibly because *Shigella* are susceptible to complement-mediated lysis in serum. Hematogenous dissemination is relatively infrequent except in malnourished infants, and *Shigella* abscesses and meningitis have been reported. Respiratory symptoms are rare. Cough, chest pain, pulmonary infiltrates, and pleural effusions may occur, but *Shigella* species are seldom isolated from sputum. As with other types of inflammatory colitis, Reiter's syndrome with arthritis, sterile conjunctivitis, and urethritis may follow shigellosis, usually within 1 to 4 weeks after the onset of diarrhea in patients with HLA-B27 histocompatibility antigens (see Chap. 268). Some *Shigella* isolates have antigens that immunologically cross-react with the B27 locus. Isolated, nonsuppurative monoarticular or oligoarticular arthritis may also follow shigellosis. This condition is usually self-limited and resolves within several months without deformity. Urinary tract infections due to *Shigella* species have been reported but are rare. A hemolytic-uremic syndrome has been observed with shigellosis in children. It tends to occur in association with leukemoid reactions, severe colitis, and circulating endotoxin but usually without demonstrable bacteremia. Culture-positive, purulent keratoconjunctivitis occasionally results from direct autoinoculation of the eye by contaminated fingers.

DIAGNOSIS AND LABORATORY FINDINGS

Shigellosis should be considered in every febrile illness associated with diarrhea. The stool is usually watery and contains variable amounts of mucus, blood, or pus. There is no consistent alteration in the peripheral blood white count during shigellosis. Occasionally a leukemoid reaction with 50,000 or more polymorphonuclear cells per cubic millimeter is encountered. An increase in band forms is frequent. Anemia is uncommon. Serum electrolyte abnormalities may result from vomiting and diarrhea.

The finding of fecal leukocytes and erythrocytes in a fresh stool specimen indicates inflammatory enteritis. A definitive diagnosis is established when a *Shigella* species is isolated from stool culture. The organisms are relatively fastidious and easily destroyed in fecal specimens which have been allowed to stand or dry. Cultures should be immediately plated from freshly passed stool or a rectal swab, or if that is not possible, placed into transport media. An enteric agar medium (MacConkey or *Shigella-Salmonella,* SS), a moderately selective agar (xylose-lysine-desoxycholate, XLD), and an enrichment broth (gram-negative or selenite broth) should be used. The stool culture is usually positive during acute shigellosis. During the postacute phase, multiple stool cultures may be necessary to isolate the organism. Antibodies develop in the serum of the majority of patients with positive cultures, but are not detectable until after the patient has recovered. Although not useful in the acutely ill patient, serology may be helpful in identifying endemic serotypes or in documenting the occurrence of an epidemic.

The differential diagnosis of inflammatory colitis characterized by fever, gross or microscopic blood in the stool, and fecal leukocytes includes infection with *Shigella* species, *Campylobacter jejuni, Salmonella* species, enteroinvasive *Escherichia coli, Yersinia* species, *Vibrio parahemolyticus,* cytotoxigenic *Clostridium difficile,* and *Entamoeba histolytica* (see Chap. 89). These pathogens cannot be clearly distinguished on clinical grounds. The onset of amebic colitis is often more gradual than that of shigellosis, the diarrhea less voluminous, and fecal leukocytes are pyknotic or absent. In viral gastroenteritis, fever is uncommon and the stool does not usually contain blood or pus. The bacterial causes of inflammatory colitis can be differentiated with certainty only be microbiologic studies. Shigellosis occasionally causes more prolonged, intermittent diarrhea resulting in a clinical picture that mimics ulcerative colitis. The extraintestinal manifestations of shigellosis may initially suggest acute meningitis, infectious arthritis, or other diseases.

TREATMENT

Correction of fluid and electrolyte loss is a mainstay of therapy and can be accomplished with an oral glucose-electrolyte solution and ad libitum fluids if the patient is mild to moderately dehydrated, not vomiting, and able to drink. Otherwise, intravenous fluids may be necessary. The clinical state of hydration must be monitored especially closely in infants and the elderly. Once appetite returns, regular food or breast-feeding of infants should be offered to replace the acute protein-calorie deficit.

Although shigellosis is usually a self-limited disease, chemotherapy is effective in reducing the duration of fever and in shortening the period of *Shigella* carriage. Stool cultures become negative within 48 h after initiation of antibiotic treatment for susceptible strains, and clinical relapses after therapy are rare. Emergence of antibiotic resistance has been an important problem throughout the world. Resistance is usually mediated by R factors. In the United States, 90 percent of *Shigella* isolates are resistant to sulfonamides, and many are now resistant to ampicillin.

The treatment of choice for shigellosis when susceptibility is unknown or when ampicillin/tetracycline–resistant strains are encountered, is trimethoprim-sulfamethoxazole (trimethoprim 160 mg plus sulfamethoxazole 800 mg) every 12 h orally for 5 to 6 days. Ampicillin 50 mg/kg per day in four equally divided doses for 5 days is considered the treatment of choice for sensitive strains. Clinical failures have been observed with amoxicillin, and it should not be used. A single dose of 2.5 g of oral tetracycline has been used

successfully in some adult patients. Tetracycline should be avoided in children under 10 years of age because of its deposition in growing teeth and bone. Other antibiotics which are active against *Shigella* in vitro have not been effective in vivo. These include cefamandole, cephalexin, cefaclor, and kanamycin. Experience in widely scattered areas around the world indicates that trimethoprim-sulfamethoxazole resistance is now emerging among *Shigella* species. Newer drugs such as bicozamycin or quinoline compounds including nalidixic acid or ciprofloxacin may be necessary to treat infections with these strains. Antimotility drugs such as paregoric, loperamide, and diphenoxylate hydrochloride with atropine (Lomotil) are contraindicated because they may worsen the clinical illness and prolong excretion of *Shigella.*

PREVENTION

Preventive measures should be aimed both at the individual and the community. Good personal hygiene with hand washing after defecation is important. Infected patients should not prepare food, and toilets should be adequately disinfected. In the future, immunologic control may become possible given the relatively limited number of serotypes of *Shigella* which cause disease. Serotype-specific protection has been shown with orally administered live, attenuated *Shigella* vaccines in humans, but a completely stable, nonreverting vaccine strain capable of producing long-lasting immunity is not available.

Community measures include the development of adequate sewage disposal systems and safe water supplies. Hospitalized patients should be placed on stool isolation precautions, not allowed to contact others, and have their linen and clothing isolated. Attending personnel must wash their hands and instruments after patient contact. Patients who have recovered from shigellosis should not prepare food until their stool culture is negative.

REFERENCES

BARRETT-CONNOR E, CONNOR JD: Extraintestinal manifestations of shigellosis. Am J Gastroenterol 53:234, 1970

DRITZ SK et al: Patterns of sexually transmitted enteric diseases in a city. Lancet 2:3, 1977

DUPONT HC: *Shigella* species (bacillary dysentery), in *Principles and Practice of Infectious Diseases 2,* GL Mandell et al (eds). New York, Wiley, 1985, pp 1269–1273

KEUSCH GT: The epidemiology and pathophysiology of invasive bacterial diarrheas with a note on biological considerations in control strategies, in *Diarrhea and Malnutrition: Interactions, Mechanisms and Interventions,* LC Chen, NS Scrimshaw (eds). New York, Plenum, 1983, pp 45–72

PICKERING LK et al: Diarrhea caused by *Shigella,* rotavirus, and *Giardia* in day-care centers: Prospective study. J Pediatr 99:51, 1981

SANSONETTI PJ et al: Genetics of virulence in enteroinvasive *Escherichia coli,* in *Microbiology—1985,* L Leive et al (eds). Am Soc Microbiol, 1985, pp 74–77

SHIGELLOSIS— United States, 1983. Morb Mort Week Rep 33:616, 1984

STRUELENS MJ et al: *Shigella* septicemia: Prevalence, presentation, risk factors, and outcome. J Infect Dis 152:784, 1985

TACKETT CO, COHEN ML: Shigellosis in day care centers: Use of plasmid analysis to assess control measures. Pediatr Infect Dis 2:127, 1983

---

109 *HAEMOPHILUS* INFECTIONS

RALPH D. FEIGIN / FREDERICK M. MURPHY[1]

Haemophilus influenzae was isolated by Pfeiffer in 1892 from the sputum of individuals afflicted during an influenza pandemic. The requirement of blood for in vitro growth and its presumptive role in the pandemic prompted the designation. Other species have since been classified as members of the *Haemophilus* genus on the basis of morphology and physiology: small, pleomorphic, aerobic or

[1] The editors wish to acknowledge the contribution of David H. Smith, M.D. It is on his chapter in the tenth edition of Principles of Internal Medicine that this revision is based.

facultatively anaerobic, nonmotile, non-spore-forming, gram-negative bacilli that require enriched media containing blood or certain preformed growth factors present in blood.

There are 16 species belonging to the genus *Haemophilus*. The single most important member is *H. influenzae*. Other important pathogenic species include *H. aegypticus*, *H. ducreyi*, *H. parainfluenzae*, *H. aphrophilus*, and *H. paraphrophilus*. Previously included in the genus *Haemophilus* were *H. vaginalis* and *H. pertussis*. Neither of these two species has a strict requirement for either growth factor X or V; therefore, they are excluded from this genus. *H. vaginalis* is now classified as *Gardnerella vaginalis* and is considered in Chap. 143. *H. pertussis* is now classified as *Bordetella pertussis* and is included in this chapter.

HAEMOPHILUS INFLUENZAE

Etiology *H. influenzae* is distinguished by its growth requirement of a heat-labile V factor and a heat-stable X factor found in erythrocytes and its inability to hemolyze erythrocytes during growth. V factor can be replaced by coenzyme I (DPN), coenzyme II (TPN), or nicotinamide nucleoside, and X factor by hematin. X factor is not required for anaerobic growth. Fermentation reactions and tests of other metabolic activities are variable and not useful in identification but may help in ''biotyping'' individual isolates. Based upon indole production and ornithine decarboxylase and urease activities, seven biotypes (I to VII) have been described.

Optimal growth of *H. influenzae* is realized with media in which erythrocytes are disrupted to release the growth factors, e.g., chocolate or Levinthal agar. ''Satellism,'' growth around colonies of hemolytic *Staphylococcus aureus* which release growth factors, is often used to identify *H. influenzae*. Some strains grow best in 5 to 10% carbon dioxide; many laboratories therefore incubate specimens suspected of containing *H. influenzae* in a candle jar or an incubator purged with carbon dioxide. Since viability of this bacterium is lost rapidly on drying or heating, clinical specimens should be inoculated without delay.

The organism exists with or without a polysaccharide capsule. Colonies of nonencapsulated isolates are usually 0.5 to 1.5 mm in diameter and appear granular after overnight incubation on solid agar; those of encapsulated isolates are usually 3 to 4 mm in diameter and initially appear mucoid or glistening. *H. influenzae* grown on enriched media appear microscopically as relatively uniform, small coccobacilli $(1 \times 0.3 \ \mu m)$; under less than optimal growth conditions, long filaments or short chains are common. Because *H. influenzae* in clinical specimens often have variable morphology and do not always react with safranin dye, gram-stained smears of infected material are frequently misdiagnosed.

The outer membrane of *H. influenzae*, like that of other gram-negative bacilli, is composed of a lipopolysaccharide (endotoxin)-containing cell wall and a number of proteins, some of which are common to all isolates. Determination of the composition of *H. influenzae* outer membrane proteins has been useful for epidemiologic studies. The antigenic activity of *H. influenzae* endotoxin and these outer membrane proteins has not been defined. Only a small percentage of isolates recovered from the respiratory tract are encapsulated. Six antigenically distinguishable capsular types, designated a to f, have been identified. Each is a complex carbohydrate. Type a, b, and c capsules share antigenic determinants with those of certain pneumococci. In addition, type b capsule, polyribose ribitol phosphate (PRP), cross-reacts immunologically with the capsules or cell walls of several species of gram-positive bacteria and enteric bacilli.

Strains with decreased or absent capsular antigen arise spontaneously from encapsulated strains. This variation proceeds M (fully encapsulated) → S (partially encapsulated) → R (nonencapsulated). The genetic basis of this variation and the natural existence of its converse, i.e., R→S→M, remain undescribed. DNA purified from an M strain can transform an R strain to the serotype of the donor M strain. Transformation of *H. influenzae* in the host has not been studied, but the demonstration of pneumococcal transformation in experimentally infected mice supports the possibility that this occurs.

Transformation between *H. aegypticus* and *H. influenzae* and between *H. influenzae* and *H. parainfluenzae* demonstrates the close genetic relation of these species.

The physiologic release by *H. influenzae* b of its capsular antigen (PRP) during growth in vitro and in the host provides the basis for clinically useful immunologic detection systems, e.g., countercurrent immunoelectrophoresis or agglutination of latex particles to which antibody is absorbed.

H. influenzae was previously susceptible to many antibiotics, but a significant percentage of strains is now resistant to ampicillin, and resistance to tetracycline has been increasing. Ampicillin-resistant strains are widely but variably distributed and are as pathogenic and transmissible as antibiotic-sensitive strains. Ampicillin resistance, which is plasmid-mediated, occurs in 25 percent of isolated strains of *H. influenzae* type b, and higher resistance rates have been reported. Chloramphenicol-resistant and multiple-resistant (chloramphenicol, tetracycline, and/or ampicillin) strains have been isolated with increasing frequency.

Epidemiology *H. influenzae* infects only humans and primarily in the upper respiratory tract. It can be recovered from the nasopharynx of up to 90 percent of healthy individuals with the frequency of infection related inversely to age. The colonization rate of type b organisms averages 5 percent. Asymptomatic nasopharyngeal infection lasts days to a few months, is not eradicated by systemic antibody, and often is not eliminated by antibiotic therapy adequate to cure type b meningitis.

H. influenzae diseases occur worldwide and for the most part are endemic. Systemic *H. influenzae* diseases have a marked age relationship: children of 6 to 48 months are highly susceptible; newborns, older children, and adults are uncommonly affected. Systemic type b diseases occur at an attack rate up to 6000 times normal among children of susceptible ages who have intimate contact with primary cases and among persons with certain diseases that increase their susceptibility, e.g., sickle cell disease, splenectomy, agammaglobulinemia, and treated Hodgkin's disease. Alcoholic adults appear to be at modestly increased risk of *H. influenzae* pneumonia. Increased risk also is noted among blacks, the poor, urban dwellers, and members of large families. In temperate climates, systemic *H. influenzae* diseases occur most commonly during the late winter and spring.

The incidence of systemic *H. influenzae* b diseases has increased fourfold during the past 3 to $4\frac{1}{2}$ decades, and more adults are being affected. The basis for this increased attack rate is not understood, but improved diagnostic laboratories and diminution in the prevalence of type-specific immunity due to excessive use of antibiotics have been suggested as possible mechanisms. Changes in antigenic composition and/or virulence of the organism and the prevalence of cross-reactive antibodies also may be responsible for this change.

Pathogenicity The relatively common asymptomatic nasopharyngeal infection occasionally develops into symptomatic disease which may spread contiguously to involve the sinuses, middle ear, or bronchi, or may invade local tissues, causing epiglottitis, pneumonia, or pericarditis. The frequent bacteremia associated with local invasion may lead to metastatic disease such as facial cellulitis, meningitis, or septic arthritis. Nonencapsulated strains produce luminal diseases, while systemic diseases are caused almost entirely by encapsulated *H. influenzae*, of which at least 95 percent are type b.

The pathogenicity of invasive strains is related directly to the inhibition of phagocytosis by the capsule. The basis for the disproportionate virulence of type b strains is under study, as is the role of outer membrane proteins and other constituents. Animal studies indicate that, unlike other bacteria, piliated strains have no apparent advantages over nonpiliated *H. influenzae* for colonization or invasion. Synergy between *H. influenzae* and certain respiratory viruses has been demonstrated in studies of human disease and experimental models.

Immunity Susceptibility to *H. influenzae* is correlated inversely with age and with anticapsular antibody titer. Antibodies to the PRP capsule of *H. influenzae* b promote phagocytosis and bacteriolysis in vitro, protect animals from lethal concentrations of *H. influenzae* b, and are responsible for the efficacy of the anti–*H. influenzae* b serum used in the preantibiotic era. The genesis of naturally occurring anti-PRP antibody is not known but may result from nasopharyngeal carriage of *H. influenzae* b or from infection with cross-reacting bacteria such as *E. coli* K100, which also has a capsule composed of PRP. Antibodies to strain-specific, noncapsular protein antigens also protect against lethal inocula of *H. influenzae* b in animals, increase the clearance rate of bacteria administered intravenously, and may be protective in humans. Immunity may result from a composite effect of anticapsular and antisomatic antibodies as well as from cellular immunity.

Studies of patients recovering from systemic *H. influenzae* b disease and those immunized with PRP have revealed that infants respond infrequently and poorly, younger children have intermediate reactivity, while older children and adults develop marked, nonboostable responses. A few children fail to produce anti-PRP antibody (measured by radioimmunoassay) following systemic disease and subsequently develop a second distinct episode of invasive type b disease. Although these children appear to have been "immunologically nonreactive" for periods up to months, all subsequently raised anti-PRP antibody activity. These observations indicate the need for further study and close follow-up of young children recuperating from invasive *H. influenzae* b disease. Likewise, survivors of intensive therapy for Hodgkin's disease—chemotherapy, splenectomy, and/or radiation—produce transient, infantlike anti-PRP antibody responses, even following systemic *H. influenzae* b disease.

Clinical manifestations *H. influenzae* can cause local respiratory tract or invasive diseases. Surveys of hospitalized children indicate that *H. influenzae* b is now the most common cause of bacteremic disease and that about one-half of children with *H. influenzae* disease have meningitis, one-sixth pneumonia, about 10 percent bacteremia without a primary focus, facial cellulitis, or epiglottitis, and 1 percent pyarthrosis. Adults may develop *H. influenzae* bacteremia, meningitis, and, less commonly, epiglottitis; however, bronchitis, due to nonencapsulated strains, and pneumonia are more common.

H. influenzae diseases are generally acute with symptoms reflecting the pyogenic process; however, the clinical course of certain of these diseases may be surprisingly prolonged.

MENINGITIS *H. influenzae* is the most common cause of bacterial meningitis, primarily affecting children 9 months to 4 years of age. The signs and symptoms depend on the patient's age and the time in the course of the disease when medical care is sought. Young children and those early in the disease generally have a nonspecific clinical picture: preceding upper respiratory tract symptoms, fever, anorexia, lethargy, vomiting, and, with older children and adults, headache. A history of stiff neck or back may be elicited. Mental confusion, paresis of cranial nerves, coma, convulsions, opisthotonus, and shock occur with more prolonged and serious disease. The clinical findings are identical to those of other bacterial causes. Age and certain types of concurrent disease, e.g., cellulitis, pyarthrosis, or epiglottitis, suggest *H. influenzae*, but the diagnosis depends on bacteriologic studies. Demonstration of PRP in cerebral spinal fluid by latex agglutination or CIE (counterimmunoelectrophoresis) permits rapid diagnosis.

PNEUMONIA *H. influenzae* may cause either a broncho- or lobar pneumonia. Up to 75 percent of the children with lobar pneumonia have an associated empyema. Purulent pericarditis may develop in up to 5 percent of cases. Concomitant otitis media due to *H. influenzae* is frequent. Lobar disease, particularly with pleural involvement, is most often confused with pneumococcal or *S. aureus* pneumonia, but the course can be prolonged enough to suggest tuberculosis. Elderly patients, particularly those with primary lung disease and/or alcoholism, are being infected increasingly by *H. influenzae*.

BACTEREMIA WITHOUT LOCALIZED DISEASE Children, particularly those 6 to 24 months of age, may develop bacteremia without evidence of localized disease. This condition most often occurs in those with a temperature greater than 102°F and an elevated circulating neutrophil count. Persons with sickle cell disease, previous splenectomy, or chemotherapy for Hodgkin's disease are at increased risk of bacteremia without localized disease. Although pneumococci are the most common cause of this syndrome, *H. influenzae* b is the second most common etiologic agent. Fever, chills, anxiety, anorexia, and lethargy dominate the clinical picture. Among highly susceptible persons, this disease can progress to shock and death within a few hours.

CELLULITIS *H. influenzae* causes a cellulitis, particularly among children 6 to 24 months of age. It is characterized as a raised, warm, tender area of distinctive reddish-blue hue, usually located on one cheek or, less commonly, the periorbital area. The child is moderately febrile and toxic and has a history of preceding rhinorrhea, fever, and, at times, ipsilateral otitis media. The cellulitis develops and spreads within a few hours. *H. influenzae* cellulitis on the limbs or hands is seen rarely and usually in older children. The distinctive color, location, and clinical course suggest the etiology. Bacteremia is almost always present, and a secondary focus is present in 10 percent of cases.

EPIGLOTTITIS *H. influenzae* b is the leading cause of this potentially lethal disease. The mean age in children is 4 years with males outnumbering females. Caucasians predominate. Bacteremia is detected in 90 percent of cases, but extraepiglottic foci are rare. The disease is characterized by the rapid onset of fever, dysphagia, toxicity, anxiety, stridor, retractions, and drooling. Patients assume a typical position of sitting forward with protrusion of the mandible and hyperextension of the neck to maximize airway diameter. The dramatic clinical presentation is usually sufficient to justify direct laryngoscopy and, if epiglottitis is present, endotracheal intubation. This should be performed in a setting where emergency tracheostomy can be performed if attempted intubation is unsuccessful. Lateral neck radiographs can be helpful if the diagnosis is not obvious and the patient is stable. Examination of the oropharynx utilizing a tongue depressor may precipitate complete airway obstruction and respiratory arrest and probably should not be attempted.

Acute epiglottitis in adults most often has a viral etiology and a more indolent clinical course of dysphagia and sore throat and less often requires intubation or tracheostomy. When due to *H. influenzae*, the clinical course approximates that in children but is less severe.

PYARTHROSIS *H. influenzae* b joint disease occurs during a septic invasion with or without other systemic disease usually in children under 2 years of age. Single, large, weight-bearing joints are usually involved, and concomitant osteomyelitis is present in up to 22 percent of cases. Response to systemic antibiotics without surgical drainage is dramatic and curative, but long-term follow-up reveals some joint dysfunction in a significant number of children.

PERICARDITIS *H. influenzae* b causes purulent pericarditis usually associated with pneumonia. The clinical signs and symptoms are generally similar to those caused by other pyogenic bacteria, but the course is often more prolonged.

OTHER RESPIRATORY TRACT DISEASE *H. influenzae* is the second leading cause of childhood otitis media and often causes sinusitis. Nearly all the etiologic strains are nonencapsulated. These diseases cannot be distinguished clinically from those produced by other microbial agents, nor can the disease caused by encapsulated or nonencapsulated *H. influenzae* be differentiated clinically. Fever, local pain, irritability, and, in sinusitis, foul breath, postnasal drip, and cough predominate. Chronic bronchitis, particularly among adults and those with agammaglobulinemia, is often caused by nonencapsulated *H. influenzae* or mixed bacterial species among which *H. influenzae* predominates. Cough productive of purulent sputum, dyspnea with prolonged expiration, and anorexia dominate the clinical picture, which is aggravated by smoking and by inhalation of respiratory pollutants.

OTHER DISEASES   H. influenzae can cause endocarditis and brain abscess, but such cases are rare and are usually associated with a primary underlying disease. H. influenzae endophthalmitis, pyelonephritis, and osteomyelitis have been reported. Pharyngitis is only rarely caused by H. influenzae, and this organism plays no role in bronchiolitis.

Diagnosis   The etiology of many H. influenzae diseases, especially facial cellulitis and epiglottitis, can generally be suspected on the basis of the history and clinical findings. Chemical analysis of infected fluids is consistent with any pyogenic etiology. Leukocytosis is common, and children often have a significant anemia. Gram stains of infected body fluids correlate with culture results in 70 percent of cases. Among the remainder of culture-positive specimens, 15 percent have negative smears, while another 15 percent have misinterpreted smears. Staining such specimens with methylene blue generally does not improve these results. Quellung reactions are even less accurate.

PRP can be detected in the serum, CSF, or concentrated urine of up to 95 percent of patients with meningitis by countercurrent electrophoresis, the enzyme-linked immunosorbent assay (ELISA) technique, latex agglutination, or coagglutination. Several studies have compared these various techniques. CIE is the least sensitive, and the ELISA technique requires too much time to be clinically practical. Despite the apparent widespread distribution of immunologically cross-reactive antigens among bacteria in nature, false-positive reactions are unusual. PRP is generally detected in infected pericardial fluid or joint fluid but is found infrequently in the serum of children with epiglottitis, presumably due to the fulminant course of this disease and the time required for antigen release from invasive bacteria. Detection of antigen in the supernatant of liquid cultures can expedite laboratory diagnosis. Since antigen often persists after antibiotic therapy, its detection is helpful in the diagnosis of patients with systemic H. influenzae diseases who have received antibiotics.

Positive nasopharyngeal cultures are not meaningful because of the high carriage rate of H. influenzae by healthy individuals. Needle aspiration of the edge of the site of cellulitis or of diseased lung markedly increases the rate of bacterial isolation and is recommended, particularly in patients who are critically ill or who have a complicated course. Cultures of empyema, pericardial and joint fluid, and an inflamed epiglottis are diagnostic. Blood cultures are positive in up to 80 percent of patients with H. influenzae septic arthritis, facial cellulitis, epiglottitis, and meningitis prior to the onset of antibiotic therapy. Even if antibiotic therapy has been initiated, the yield is sufficiently great to recommend that blood cultures be taken. It has been suggested that H. influenzae pneumonia, in which 30 percent of persons have a positive blood culture, is underdiagnosed. The role of PRP detection in this diagnosis deserves further evaluation.

Treatment   Without treatment, systemic H. influenzae disease, particularly meningitis and epiglottitis, has a very high, if not uniform, mortality. Chloramphenicol therapy yields very high concentrations of antibiotic in joint and cerebrospinal fluid relative to serum and produces excellent clinical results. The potential toxicity of chloramphenicol and the excellent results obtained with ampicillin made this agent the antibiotic of choice for H. influenzae diseases for many years. However, the current prevalence of ampicillin-resistant strains requires that all systemic diseases that might be due to H. influenzae be treated with chloramphenicol, 100 mg/kg per day for children, 4 g per day for adults, given intravenously in divided doses at 6-h intervals until the etiologic agent is proved to be sensitive to ampicillin. Some, including the American Academy of Pediatrics, recommend that ampicillin also be added to the initial chloramphenicol therapy. If the etiologic strain is sensitive, ampicillin is given intravenously in doses of 200 to 400 mg/kg per day for children and 6 g per day for adults, divided into six infusions given at 4-h intervals.

Chloramphenicol given orally yields higher serum levels of the antibiotic than identical doses given intravenously; administration of chloramphenicol by intramuscular injection yields variable and unpredictable blood levels and is contraindicated. Routine sensitivity testing of H. influenzae in invasive disease has become increasingly important, and the increasing frequency of ampicillin- and chloramphenicol-resistant strains of H. influenzae has stimulated a search for new antimicrobial agents for the treatment of meningitis.

In one excellent prospective randomized study moxalactam was shown to be as effective and safe as ampicillin or chloramphenicol in the treatment of meningitis. Other agents that have been employed successfully for the treatment of multiply resistant H. influenzae diseases in a small number of patients include ceftriaxone, ceftazidime, cefotaxime, and cefuroxime.

Amoxicillin is recommended for outpatient therapy of disease caused by H. influenzae. Alternative antibiotics when the organism is resistant to ampicillin or the patient is allergic to penicillin include cefaclor, trimethoprim-sulfamethoxazole, erythromycin-sulfasoxazole, cefaclor plus a sulfonamide, or chloramphenicol. Although chloramphenicol is an excellent antibiotic for oral therapy of serious H. influenzae infections, its routine use on an outpatient basis is not recommended because of its hematologic toxicities and the potential for accelerating the emergence of chloramphenicol resistance. Tetracycline can be used in adults to treat bronchitis and other respiratory diseases caused by sensitive strains.

The duration of chemotherapy for H. influenzae disease depends on the disease and the status of the individual patient. All systemic diseases should be treated with intravenous drugs at least until cultures of the infected area are sterile and the patient is afebrile and without clinical and laboratory evidence of active infection for 3 to 5 days. Patients with meningitis are therefore usually treated for 10 to 14 days. Occasionally, ampicillin does not clear the bacteria from the CSF, and relapses follow the cessation of therapy. Most therapeutic failures with ampicillin have been associated with antibiotic courses that are too brief, employ too low a dose, or are given otherwise than by the intravenous route; some result from localized disease that was not completely eradicated with standard treatment. In treatment failures, re-treatment according to the above guidelines should be undertaken, usually with chloramphenicol.

Patients with endocarditis or pericarditis should receive 3 to 6 weeks of intravenous therapy. Ampicillin and chloramphenicol diffuse well into inflamed joint spaces, and there is no indication for local instillation of antibiotics. Children with otitis media may be treated orally with amoxicillin in dosage of 50 mg/kg per day (adults 2 g per day in four divided doses) until their symptoms are alleviated plus 3 to 4 days; hence, the usually total course is 7 to 10 days. Sinusitis requires therapy of 3 or more weeks; therapy of bronchitis may need to be prolonged even longer.

Antibiotic therapy is only one facet of the management of the patient with a systemic H. influenzae disease. Careful evaluation of the airway, consideration of oxygen therapy and transfusion, vigorous treatment of shock and disseminated intravascular coagulation, conservative fluid replacement, anticonvulsant therapy, and medical management of cerebral edema are often critical. Repeated aspirations of an infected joint or empyema may be needed, but installation of a surgical drain is rarely required. The creation of a pericardial "window" for drainage in patients with pericarditis is preferable to repeated aspirations.

Prevention   A large, prospective study coordinated by the Centers for Disease Control has shown that secondary cases of invasive H. influenzae diseases occur at significantly increased rates among young, household contacts. Specifically, the risk in household contacts was as follows: for those less than 6 years of age, 0.5 percent; less than 4 years, 2.1 percent; and less than 1 year, 6 percent. Several studies have shown that attack rates in day care center contacts less than 4 years of age range from 0 to 1 percent.

Several antibiotic regimens were studied between 1978 and 1984 to determine their efficacy in eradicating H. influenzae b from the nasopharynx. The only reliably effective regimen proved to be rifampin in a 20 mg/kg dose (maximum 600 mg per day) provided once daily for 4 days. This regimen is not only effective in eliminating nasopharyngeal carriage of *H. influenzae,* but also appears to be efficacious in preventing secondary cases of disease among household contacts.

The American Academy of Pediatrics currently recommends that rifampin be given orally once each day for 4 days in a 20 mg/kg dose (maximum 600 mg per day) to all household contacts (including adults) in households where there are children other than the index case younger than 4 years of age. Prophylaxis of contacts should begin as soon as possible after the diagnosis is established in the index case. Prophylaxis of day-care center or nursery school contacts is no longer recommended unless two or more cases of invasive disease have occurred among attendees within a 60-day period. It is also important to provide the same prophylactic regimen for all children with invasive disease prior to discharge from the hospital since they may still harbor the organism in their nasopharynx despite appropriate antibiotic therapy.

The increased attack rate and the constant mortality (5 to 10 percent) and neurologic morbidity (30 percent) during the past two decades for *H. influenzae* meningitis in children and the prevalence of ampicillin-resistant strains have stimulated an attempt to produce a vaccine to prevent *H. influenzae* diseases. Because of the primacy of the type b capsule in pathogenicity and the efficacy of anticapsular serum, attention was focused initially on a vaccine composed of purified capsular PRP. Such a vaccine has been found to be nontoxic and immunogenic for older children and adults. A single dose protects children older than 18 months from septic diseases for at least 4 years; however, the vaccine is not immunogenic or protective for children less than 18 months of age. This PRP vaccine is now licensed, and it is recommended for children 2 to 5 years of age and is suggested beginning at 18 months of age for those at high risk of invasive disease, such as the Alaskan Inuit, Navajo Indians, sickle cell disease patients, and day-care center attendees. Efforts have been made to investigate the immunogenicity of several vaccines in which PRP has been linked to a protein carrier such as pertussis, tetanus toxoid, or diphtheria. Such combinations have improved immunogenicity in infants compared to PRP alone (particularly the PRP-diphtheria vaccine), but further studies are needed to establish their efficacy.

Oral ingestion of nonpathogenic species of *Escherichia coli* which have an immunologically cross-reactive capsule may elevate systemic anti-PRP antibody activity. However, the observation in one center of an unusually high incidence of intestinal carriage of such *E. coli* among children with *H. influenzae* b meningitis has precluded further studies. Other studies are evaluating the role of *H. influenzae* outer membrane proteins either as a primary vaccine or a polysaccharide carrier, with the hope that such a vaccine might be protective against diseases caused by nonencapsulated as well as encapsulated *H. influenzae.*

HAEMOPHILUS AEGYPTICUS
H. aegypticus, also known as the Koch-Weeks bacillus, causes conjunctivitis in humans. Morphologically and biochemically, this organism closely resembles an unencapsulated *H. influenzae.* Moreover, *H. aegypticus* and *H. influenzae* share certain antigens and can be transformed by DNA of the other species.

The conjunctivitis, which primarily affects children, occurs worldwide, often in epidemics, and in some areas seasonally. It must be distinguished from trachoma-inclusion conjunctivitis (TRIC) agents, adenoviruses, and other bacterial agents such as pneumococcus, *S. aureus,* and *Neisseria gonorrhoeae.* Therapy consists of local instillation of antibiotic drops or ointment, such as sulfonamide, polymyxin B, or gentamicin five or six times daily, and moist soaks to keep the eyelids clean.

HAEMOPHILUS APHROPHILUS
H. aphrophilus is a small, nonmotile, aerobic, gram-negative coccobacillus which requires factor X (but not V) and high concentrations of CO_2 (5 percent is optimal) for growth. It is part of the normal oral flora, and although uncommon,

is being recognized increasingly as a cause of many types of infection, particularly bacteremia, endocarditis, and brain abscess. Other reported infections due to *H. aphrophilus* include acute and chronic sinusitis, pneumonia, empyema, osteomyelitis, septic arthritis, otitis media, peritonitis, cholecystitis, periapical dental abscess, meningitis, deep tissue abscess, wound infection, and necrotizing fasciitis.

H. aphrophilus by itself can cause disease in otherwise normal individuals, but most cases are associated with predisposing conditions such as malignancy, immunosuppression, rheumatic or congenital heart disease, recurrent otitis media, and asthma.

Most strains are sensitive to the majority of commonly used antibiotics including penicillin, cephalosporins, aminoglycosides, tetracycline, and chloramphenicol.

HAEMOPHILUS DUCREYI
H. ducreyi causes a localized venereal disease, chancroid (see Chap. 110). This disease is uncommon in the United States, but is endemic throughout the tropics, and accounts for 50 percent of genital ulcers in Kenya. The organism requires X but not V factor for growth. In clinical specimens and colonies grown on solid medium, the organism appears as small ovoid rods arranged in pairs, groups, or parallel chains. The disease is characterized by painful, nonindurated ulceration of the genitalia with enlarged, and often suppurative, regional lymph nodes. Chancroid must be distinguished from primary syphilis; not infrequently the two diseases occur simultaneously. Isolation on special selective media is successful in only 50 to 70 percent of cases, even in the best equipped laboratories. Because of the increasing incidence of sulfa and tetracycline resistance, which is usually plasmid-mediated, the recommended therapy is now trimethoprim-sulfamethoxazole or erythromycin.

HAEMOPHILUS PARAINFLUENZAE
This species differs from *H. influenzae* by requiring V but not X factor for growth. Since *H. influenzae* does not require X factor for anaerobic growth, diagnostic confusion can arise, especially in stabbed cultures. This phenomenon may have played a role in certain systemic infections allegedly caused by *H. parainfluenzae* which, on further testing, were found to be due to *H. influenzae.*

Acute upper respiratory disease, e.g., otitis media, and less commonly meningitis, pneumonia, and brain abscess have been ascribed to *H. parainfluenzae.* Rarely, in less than 1 percent of cases, it is the infecting agent in endocarditis, and its isolation in this disease is often delayed (mean of 6 to 8 days) due to fastidious growth requirements and need for blind subculturing onto chocolate agar. *H. parainfluenzae* may be confused with *H. paraphrophilus,* which causes clinically identical endocarditis and from which it is very difficult to differentiate biochemically. A small but significant percentage of *H. parainfluenzae* carries plasmids mediating β-lactamase production and ampicillin resistance.

BORDETELLA PERTUSSIS
Bordetella pertussis causes an acute infection of the respiratory tract that is most serious in infants and young children and is characterized by a repetitious, paroxysmal cough and prolonged, inspiratory stridor. The word *pertussis* means intensive cough, and this designation is preferable to "whooping cough" since not all patients with pertussis whoop.

Etiology The vast majority of cases of pertussis syndrome are caused by *B. pertussis;* however, *B. parapertussis, B. bronchiseptica,* and several adenoviruses can produce an identical illness.

B. pertussis is a minute, nonmotile, non-spore-forming, aerobic, gram-negative coccobacillus with extremely fastidious growth requirements. This organism is inhibited by many factors present in routine bacteriologic media. The classic medium for the primary isolation of *B. pertussis* (Bordet-Gengou) contains blood and starch. Addition of penicillin inhibits the growth of other organisms. The absence of an antigenic relation and with it the ability to transform *B. pertussis* with *H. influenzae* DNA or vice versa suggests that these species are not closely related. *B. pertussis* does not require X or V factors for growth; therefore, it cannot be included in the genus *Haemophilus. B. pertussis* is related closely, however, to *B. para-*

pertussis, which can cause a milder, similar disease in humans, and *B. bronchiseptica,* which causes respiratory disease in animals but rarely in humans. They have similar growth requirements and morphologic appearance and can be distinguished from each other by specific agglutination reactions.

Freshly isolated *B. pertussis* is in phase I, the virulent, morphologically uniform, encapsulated, and piliated form. Passage in culture may induce nonvirulent forms (phase II, III, or IV). Phase I organisms are required for transmission of disease and for the production of vaccine.

Epidemiology   *B. pertussis* exists worldwide and naturally affects only humans, although nonhuman primates and mice can be infected experimentally. Pertussis is one of the most contagious infectious diseases because it is transmitted by aerosolized droplets. (The infectivity of respiratory secretions and contact transmission is not well studied.) Up to 90 (and in some reports 100) percent of exposed, susceptible persons develop the disease. Asymptomatic infection is rare. Although pertussis occurs endemically, it produces epidemics in a susceptible population. There is little seasonal variation in the incidence of pertussis. Females are affected more frequently than males, and this difference is accentuated with increasing age.

More than 50 percent of *B. pertussis* disease occurs in infants, presumably owing to deficient maternal immunity and possibly the lack of transplacental transfer of a protective bacteriologic antibody. Although adults were thought to be resistant to pertussis, neither the disease nor active immunization provides lifelong immunity; in fact, pertussis is not an uncommon cause of bronchitis in adults. More than 5 percent of cases now occur in individuals 15 years of age or older. Hospital personnel also are at increased risk, as evidenced by reports of epidemics involving hospital staff and patients.

About 3000 cases of pertussis are reported each year in the United States, but most observers think this number is falsely low because of the difficulty in bacteriologic confirmation. Reported cases probably represent 15 to 25 percent of the number of actual cases. Prior to widespread active immunization initiated in the 1940s, pertussis was a major cause of morbidity and mortality with the vast majority of deaths occurring in children less than 1 year of age. Since 1944, the pertussis mortality rate has decreased over 85-fold, although it has remained relatively constant since 1974. Pertussis remains a very significant health problem in developing countries, particularly in areas of poor nutrition and immunization. The limitation in the rate of immunization to pertussis in Great Britain to 30 percent of children has been accompanied by an epidemic affecting as many persons as in the prevaccine era. Certain adenoviruses can cause a clinical picture identical to that of pertussis, but there can be little doubt that *B. pertussis* is a primary pathogen.

Pathogenesis   Inhaled phase I *B. pertussis* organisms attach to the ciliated respiratory epithelium by pili; the organisms multiply on the surface of the airways, but do not invade the bloodstream. Acute inflammation results: epithelial cell ciliary action is inhibited and mucous secretions are stimulated. The subsequent necrosis results in patchy ulceration of respiratory epithelium. The bronchi and bronchioles are primarily affected; the trachea, larynx, and nasopharynx may be involved, but less severely. The mucopurulent exudate can compromise the diminutive airway of the infant or small child. Focal atelectasis and emphysema and peribronchial infiltration by inflammatory cells, particularly lymphocytes, are common, and bronchopneumonia may develop.

Pertussis is mediated by a surface protein toxin which is composed of histamine-sensitizing factor (HSF), lymphocytosis-promoting factor (LPF), islet-activating protein (IAP), beta-adrenergic blockadelike effect, adjuvant effect, and mitogenicity. A heat-stable lipopolysaccharide endotoxin is also present on the surface of the organism but probably is not important in the pathogenesis of the disease. Additional biologically active components include a cytoplasmic heat-labile toxin (HLT), a tracheal cytotoxin (TCT), an intracellular adenylate cyclase, cell surface filamentous hemagglutinin (FHA), and surface agglutin-

ogens. The capsule of *B. pertussis* is antiphagocytic. Antibody against capsular antigen is not protective.

Antipertussis secretory IgA is protective and specifically inhibits bacterial adherence to cilia. Antitoxin antibodies also are protective and either inhibit fixation of toxin to receptor cells or neutralize toxin. The role played by cell-mediated immunity in pertussis remains unclear.

Clinical manifestations   Following an incubation period of 6 to 20 days (mean 7 days), sneezing, mild fever, rhinorrhea, anorexia, and a mild cough become evident (catarrhal period) and last 1 to 2 weeks, after which the cough increases in frequency and intensity. Paroxysms of cough are followed, particularly in infants, by a prolonged, often distressing, inspiratory gasp (the whoop). The cough occurs at variable intervals, often every few minutes, for 2 to 4 weeks (paroxysmal period). The disease is much more severe in the infant. The cough inhibits oral intake, and swallowed mucus may provoke vomiting, resulting in significant dehydration and weight loss. The cough can provoke venous congestion with hemoptysis, epistaxis, and small blood vessel hemorrhage. Hypoxia is more common and severe than is usually appreciated clinically and may be responsible for seizures, hypoxic encephalopathy, or coma. The contribution of toxin to neurologic complications is unclear. Adults and older children are less ill and have symptoms of a severe, prolonged bronchitis. The paroxysmal period is followed by a recovery period that lasts 1 to 6 weeks, during which the cough decreases in frequency and intensity. Spasms can be provoked during recovery, however, particularly by smoke or irritating inhalants.

Pneumonia, either caused by *B. pertussis* itself or more likely by secondary bacterial pathogens, is the most frequent complication of pertussis and is responsible for more than 90 percent of deaths in children under 3 years of age. Mucous plugging may result in atelectasis. Apnea is frequent. Other complications include activation of latent tuberculosis, otitis media (frequently due to *Streptococcus pneumoniae*), subarachnoid or intraventricular hemorrhage, severe alkalosis secondary to persistent vomiting, epistaxis, subdural hematomas, rupture of the diaphragm, umbilical or inguinal hernia, rectal prolapse, and meningoencephalitis.

Diagnosis   The clinical diagnosis is suggested by a history of contact, the classic cough, and a marked absolute lymphocytosis. The diagnosis depends on the identification of *B. pertussis* in respiratory secretions. Success of isolation is favored by the immediate culture of a deep nasopharyngeal (NP) specimen in a freshly prepared selective medium. Because the characteristic pearllike colonies cannot be appreciated for 4 to 6 days, inhibitors of normal NP flora, e.g., methicillin, are added to the medium to prevent overgrowth of *B. pertussis.* The recovery rate on "cough plates" is too low to recommend this technique. *B. pertussis* can be isolated from as many as 90 percent of patients during the catarrhal stage of the disease but from no greater than 50 percent during the paroxysmal stage. Fluorescent-labeled antibody can detect *B. pertussis* in NP smears, but false-positive results may be obtained with up to 40 percent of specimens and false-negative tests in 10 to 20 percent. Serologic studies are of little value. Blood cultures are sterile and are not recommended; chest radiographs may show peribronchial thickening, atelectasis, or emphysema, but are not diagnostic. Dual infection with adenoviruses occurs, and positive viral cultures do not exclude *B. pertussis* as an etiologic agent.

An enzyme-linked immunosorbent assay (ELISA) can be used to detect IgM, IgA, and IgG antibodies in serum and may be useful in patients with negative cultures. The ELISA technique also can be used to detect IgA against *B. pertussis* in nasopharyngeal secretions beginning in the second or third week of illness up to at least 3 months. This antibody is induced by infection but not by vaccination. Pertussis may be distinguished from viral, mycoplasmal, and other bacterial causes of tracheobronchitis by a history of contact, the character and duration of symptoms, and the laboratory findings. The results of cultures are definitive.

Spasmodic coughing also may be associated with bronchiolitis; bacterial, mycoplasmal, and viral pneumonia; tuberculosis; cystic fibrosis; foreign bodies; and disease causing airway compression such as malignancy or chronic obstructive pulmonary disease. These diseases can be distinguished by their clinical and laboratory findings and by the course of the illness.

Treatment General supportive care is critical: careful nursing, avoidance of stimuli that provoke paroxysms, oxygen, suctioning of respiratory secretions, and attention to caloric needs and fluid and electrolyte balance. A single controlled study reporting beneficial effects of steroids in severely ill infants deserves attention.

B. pertussis is sensitive to many antibiotics in vitro. Antibiotics can eliminate infection and, if given in the catarrhal phase, prevent disease. Since the pathologic process is well-developed by the time paroxysms occur, antibiotic therapy given thereafter does not affect the clinical course. Erythromycin is preferred and should be used to prevent interpersonal transmission. Tetracycline and chloramphenicol are almost as effective as erythromycin but are not recommended because of potential toxicity, particularly for infants. Ampicillin appears to be relatively ineffective in eradicating nasopharyngeal infection. Antibiotic therapy may reduce the frequency and morbidity of secondary bacterial infection. Hyperimmune, antibacterial rabbit serum has no effect on bacterial shedding or clinical manifestations and is not recommended.

Prevention Patients suspected of having pertussis should be isolated until the diagnosis is disproved or the infection is eradicated by antibiotics. Exposed susceptibles should be vaccinated to prevent disease (see below) and treated with erythromycin to prevent infection and retransmission.

Prior to the availability of a vaccine, pertussis caused as many deaths in the United States as all other contagious diseases of children *combined*. In order to prevent the disease, a vaccine composed of a chemical extract of bacterial cells was developed. Because of the risk of pertussis to infants, the proposal was made to start immunization as early in life as possible. Unfortunately, pertussis immunization at 7 days of age produced a limited antibody response in only a small percentage of infants and resulted in reduced booster responses at 1 year. This vaccine is now mixed with diphtheria and tetanus toxoids, for convenience and because pertussis enhances the antibody responses to the toxoids, and is given five times during the first 6 years of life, with three doses being given at 2-month intervals starting at 8 weeks of age.

Although the vaccine was 70 to 80 percent effective in preventing disease among intimately exposed children, its effectiveness and toxicity have been questioned. Completely immunized children may develop pertussis, although the disease is milder than among the unimmunized. Furthermore, the protection provided by the vaccine is transient, with minimal resistance being evident a decade or later following the last immunization. Indeed, improved housing, hygiene, and nutrition are cited by some as responsible for the dramatic decline in pertussis during the past several decades. However, available data indicate that the rate of decline in the attack rate of pertussis in the United States has been positively affected by the vaccine. The association of an epidemic of pertussis in Great Britain with a decline in pertussis immunization also strongly supports the efficacy of the vaccine.

Pertussis vaccine provokes local reactions in up to 50 percent of recipients; neurologic complications, including uncontrollable screaming fits, convulsions, and encephalopathy, are a rare but real risk. However, the efficacy of the vaccine far outweighs the risk of significant neurologic complications. Convulsions, alteration of consciousness, shock, persistent screaming for 3 h or more, high-pitched cry, focal neurologic signs, temperature of 40.5°C or greater, and anaphylaxis following pertussis vaccination are contraindications to further doses. Immunization of infants residing in the United States should be deferred if they previously have had a seizure. Such individuals may be more prone to experience a convulsion after

receipt of pertussis vaccine. There is no convincing evidence that isolated seizures either produce permanent neurologic disease or aggravate existing neurologic conditions. Children with neurologic disorders such as inherited defects that may be associated with seizures could be at increased risk of seizures following receipt of pertussis vaccine. Immunization of these children may be deferred, but such deferral is suggested on a case-by-case basis; the situation should be reevaluated at each visit to a physician.

Prematurity is not believed to increase the likelihood of seizures following pertussis immunization. Children with developmental delay or cerebral palsy who are not otherwise predisposed to seizures generally are not considered to be at increased risk of seizures following pertussis immunization. Because toxic reactions are more common in older persons, the vaccine is rarely given to those over 6 years of age. However, older persons with chronic pulmonary disease and exposed hospital personnel may be candidates for an absorbed pertussis vaccine (0.1 to 0.25 mL).

REFERENCES

Haemophilus aphrophilus

BIEGER RC et al: *Haemophilus aphrophilus:* A microbiologic and clinical review and report of 42 cases. Medicine 57:345, 1978

ELSTER SK et al: *Hemophilus aphrophilus* endocarditis: A review of 23 cases. Am J Cardiol 35:72, 1975

Haemophilus influenzae

BAND JD et al: Prevention of *Haemophilus influenzae* type b disease. JAMA 251:2381, 1984

FLEMING DW et al: Secondary *Haemophilus influenzae* type b in day-care facilities. Risk factors and prevention. JAMA 254:509, 1985

KAPLAN SL et al: Prospective comparative trial of moxalactam versus ampicillin or chloramphenicol for treatment of *Haemophilus influenzae* type b meningitis in children. J Pediatr 104:447, 1984

LEVIN DC et al: Bacteremic *Haemophilus influenzae* pneumonia in adults: Report of 24 cases and review of the literature. Am J Med 62:219, 1977

MUSTOE T, STROME M: Adult epiglottitis. Am J Otolaryngol 4:393, 1983

PELTDA H et al: *Haemophilus influenzae* type b capsular polysaccharide vaccine in children: A double-blind field study of 100,000 vaccines 3 months to 5 years of age in Finland. Pediatrics 60:730, 1977

ROTBART HA, GOLDE MP: *Haemophilus influenzae* type b septic arthritis in children: Report of 23 cases. Pediatrics 75:254, 1985

SMITH AL: Antibiotic resistance in *Haemophilus influenzae.* Pediatr Infect Dis 2:352, 1983

SMITH DH et al: Responses of children immunized with the capsular polysaccharide of *Haemophilus influenzae* type B. Pediatrics 52:637, 1973

TODD JK, BRUHN FW: Severe *Haemophilus influenzae* infections. Am J Dis Child 129:607, 1975

Update: *Haemophilus influenzae* b polysaccharide vaccine: Morb Mort Week Rep 35:144, 1986

WARD JI et al: *Haemophilus influenzae* meningitis: A national study of secondary spread in household contacts. N Engl J Med 301:122, 1979

Haemophilus parainfluenzae

CHUNN CJ et al: *Haemophilus parainfluenzae* infective endocarditis. Medicine 56:99, 1977

FRAZIER JP: Meningitis due to *Haemophilus parainfluenzae:* Report of three cases and review of the literature. Pediatr Infect Dis 1:119, 1983

Haemophilus aegipticus

ALBRITTON WL: Infections due to *Haemophilus* species other than *H. influenzae.* Ann Rev Microbiol 36:199, 1982

Haemophilus ducreyi

PLUMMER FA et al: Antimicrobial therapy of chancroid: Effectiveness of erythromycin. J Infect Dis 148:726, 1983

Bordetella pertussis

AMERICAN ACADEMY OF PEDIATRICS COMMITTEE ON INFECTIOUS DISEASES: Pertussis vaccine. Pediatrics 74:303, 1984

BASS JW et al: Antimicrobial treatment of pertussis. J Pediatr 75:768, 1969

BUCHANAN RD, GIBBONS NE (eds): *Bergey's Manual of Determinative Bacteriology,* 9th ed. Baltimore, Williams & Wilkins, 1984

CHERRY JD: The epidemiology of pertussis and pertussis immunization in the United Kingdom and the United States: A comparative study. Curr Probl Pediatr 14(2):1, 1984

DONALDSON P, WHITAKER J: Diagnoses of pertussis by fluorescent antibody staining of nasopharyngeal smears. Am J Dis Child 99:423, 1960

KOPLAN JP et al: Pertussis vaccine—An analysis of benefits, risks and costs. N Engl J Med 301:906, 1979

NELSON JD: The changing epidemiology of pertussis in young infants: The role of adults as reservoirs of infection. Am J Dis Child 132:371, 1978

110　CHANCROID

ALLAN R. RONALD / FRANCIS A. PLUMMER

DEFINITION　Chancroid, or soft chancre (ulcer molle), is an acute sexually transmitted infection characterized by painful genital ulcerations often associated with inflammatory inguinal adenopathy which may progress to suppuration. The diagnosis is established by isolation of *Haemophilus ducreyi* from the lesion or a suppurative node and by exclusion of syphilis, genital herpes, and other specific causes of genital ulceration.

ETIOLOGY　The isolation of *H. ducreyi* from ulcers proves the microbial etiology of chancroid. Gram-positive cocci and anaerobic gram-negative rods are often also present. However, there is no evidence that these organisms are independent pathogens or require specific therapy, and the clinical response to antimicrobial therapy parallels the susceptibility of *H. ducreyi*. In areas where chancroid is common, *H. ducreyi* can be isolated from up to 90 percent of ulcers that clinically appear to be chancroid. The organism is a gram-negative facultative aerobe which requires hemin (X factor) but not nicotinamide adenine dinucleotide (V factor) for growth. Many strains also require serum. Although no unique biochemical or immunologic features are known, the colonial morphology of *H. ducreyi* is distinct in that the yellow-gray colonies can be moved intact across the agar surface. Some strains demonstrate a typical streptobacillary "chaining" appearance on Gram stain, but this feature is variable and cannot be used as a taxonomic criterion.

EPIDEMIOLOGY　The incidence of chancroid is unknown, owing to inaccurate diagnosis and incomplete reporting. It is common in southeast Asia and Africa, and is more prevalent than syphilis in many countries. Less than 1000 cases are reported annually in the United States. However, localized outbreaks do occur; for example, hundreds of cases involving predominantly migrant workers occurred in southern California in 1981 and 1982. The sex ratio of reported cases in the United States is five males to one female. Uncircumcised

FIGURE 110-1　*The classic chancroid.*

males are more susceptible to the disease. Prostitution plays a major role in transmission, and among merchant seamen and military troops whose sexual contacts are prostitutes, chancroid is more common than syphilis. The role of cervical carriage in the transmission of *H. ducreyi* is uncertain. Over one-half of the secondary sex partners of men with chancroid develop clinical chancroid. Asymptomatic carriage without disease has not been proven to occur.

CLINICAL MANIFESTATIONS　After an incubation period of 3 to 10 days, a small inflammatory papule appears which ulcerates within 2 to 3 days. The classic chancroidal ulcer (Fig. 110-1) is superficial, ranging in size from a few millimeters to several centimeters in diameter. The edge is ragged and undermined. The ulcer base is covered by a necrotic exudate. The ulcers are often multiple and may merge to form giant or serpiginous ulcers. Occasionally, the lesions remain pustular and resemble folliculitis or pyogenic infection. In contrast to syphilis, the chancroidal ulcer in males is painful and not indurated. The most frequent areas of localization are the preputial orifice, the internal surface of the prepuce, and the frenulum in men, and the labia, fourchette, and perianal region in women. The lesions in females tend to be more superficial and less painful. Extragenital ulcers are rare.

Acute, painful, tender inflammatory inguinal adenopathy occurs in almost 50 percent of patients and is frequently unilateral. If the patient is untreated, the involved nodes become matted, forming a unilocular suppurative bubo. The overlying skin becomes erythematous and tense and finally ruptures, forming a deep single ulcer.

DIAGNOSIS　The morphologic diagnosis of genital lesions is fraught with error, and many lesions diagnosed as chancroid are actually genital herpes or syphilis. In the United States, one study of 100 consecutive men with penile ulceration disclosed genital herpes in 22, syphilis in 17, and traumatic lesions in 8. Classic chancroidal ulcers were noted in 12, only 2 of whom had ulcers that yielded *H. ducreyi*. In another study, two patients with suspected granuloma inguinale had positive cultures for *H. ducreyi*. These lesions have been termed *pseudogranuloma inguinale chancroid*. In contrast, in Kenya, of 97 consecutive men with penile ulceration, 60 were infected with *H. ducreyi*, 11 had syphilis, and only 4 had genital herpes.

Primary genital infection with herpes simplex virus produces tender inguinal adenopathy, but can be distinguished by the history of onset with vesicular lesions or of recent exposure to herpes and the presence of systemic symptoms such as fever and myalgia. Chancroid rarely causes systemic symptoms.

The chancre of primary syphilis is indurated, and the associated adenopathy is bilateral, nontender, and nonsuppurative. To exclude syphilis, all patients with genital ulcers should have two dark-field examinations performed on separate days, together with monthly serologic tests for syphilis for 3 months.

Lymphogranuloma venereum (LGV) differs from chancroid in that the adenopathy develops after the ulcer is healed. It is indolent, often bilateral and nontender, and develops multilocular suppuration and fistulas.

The diagnosis of chancroid is confirmed by the isolation of *H. ducreyi* from an ulcer or bubo. Exudate should be directly plated onto chocolate agar enriched with 1% Isovitalex and 5% sheep serum, plus 3 µg/mL of vancomycin. Colonies usually appear within 48 h of incubation in 5% CO_2 with 100% humidity but may require 4 to 5 days. No serologic tests are available for the diagnosis of chancroid.

TREATMENT　Untreated chancroidal ulcers persist for long periods of time and often progress. Small lesions may heal within 2 to 4 weeks. Although sulfonamides and tetracyclines have been considered effective for chancroid, the emergence of multiresistant strains has resulted in many failures with both agents. Many isolates of *H. ducreyi* possess plasmids which mediate resistance to sulfonamides, tetracyclines, chloramphenicol, ampicillin, and kanamycin. Trimethoprim/sulfamethoxazole 320/1600 mg daily or erythromycin 2 g daily, each for 1 week are the regimens recommended by the Centers for

Disease Control. Trimethoprim/sulfamethoxazole will not interfere with the dark-field examination for *Treponema pallidum* or with the development of a positive serologic test for syphilis. The usual time to healing after onset of therapy is about 9 days. Several single-dose regimens including trimethoprim 640 mg/sulfonamide 3200 mg, spectinomycin 2 g IM, and ceftriaxone 250 mg IM have proved very effective for chancroid in Kenya. Fluctuant buboes should be aspirated to prevent rupture. Lymph node suppuration may progress despite otherwise effective therapy. Buboes larger than 5 cm in diameter almost always require aspiration.

Sexual contacts of patients with chancroid should be examined for ulcers, and treatment of contacts is recommended. Although the epidemiology of chancroid suggests that effective control measures, specifically designed for limited target populations such as prostitutes and known sexual contacts, could halt the spread of this disease, further prospective epidemiologic studies to demonstrate this are required.

REFERENCES

BLACKMORE CA et al: An outbreak of chancroid in Orange County, California: Descriptive epidemiology and disease-control measures. J Infect Dis 151:840, 1985

CHAPEL T et al: How reliable is the morphologic diagnosis of penile ulcers? Sex Trans Dis 4:150, 1977

FAST M et al: Treatment of chancroid by clavulanic acid with amoxicillin in patients with beta-lactamase-positive *Haemophilus ducreyi* infection. Lancet 2:509, 1982

HAMMOND GW et al: Comparison of specimen collection and laboratory techniques for isolation of *Haemophilus ducreyi*. J Clin Microbiol 7:39, 1978

——— et al: Epidemiologic, clinical, laboratory and therapeutic features of an urban outbreak of chancroid in North America. Rev Infect Dis 2:867, 1980

HANDSFIELD HH et al: Molecular epidemiology of *Haemophilus ducreyi* infection. Ann Intern Med 95:315, 1981

KRAUS SJ et al: Pseudogranuloma inguinale caused by *Haemophilus ducreyi*. Arch Dermatol 118:494, 1982

MCNICOL PJ et al: The plasmids of *Haemophilus ducreyi*. J Antimicrob Chemother 14:561, 1984

NSANZE H et al: Genital ulcers in Kenya: A clinical and laboratory study of 97 patients. Br J Vener Dis 57:378, 1981

PLUMMER FA et al: Short course of single-dose antimicrobial therapy of chancroid in Kenya: Reports of studies with rifampin-trimethoprim and rifampin alone. Rev Infect Dis 5:S565, 1983

——— et al: Single-dose therapy of chancroid with trimethoprim-sulfametrole. N Engl J Med 309:67, 1983

——— et al: Epidemiology of chancroid and *Haemophilus ducreyi* in Nairobi. Lancet 2:1293, 1983

RONALD AR et al: Chancroid and *Haemophilus ducreyi*, in *Sexually Transmitted Diseases*, KK Holmes et al (eds). New York, McGraw-Hill, 1984

———, PLUMMER FA. Chancroid and *Haemophilus ducreyi*. Ann Intern Med 102:705, 1985

111 DONOVANOSIS (GRANULOMA INGUINALE)

KING K. HOLMES

DEFINITION Donovanosis (granuloma inguinale) is a mildly contagious, chronic, indolent, progressive, autoinoculable, ulcerative disease involving the skin and lymphatics of the genital or perianal areas. The disease may be sexually transmitted and is associated with the presence in affected tissues of an intracellular microorganism, identified morphologically as the Donovan body.

ETIOLOGY Donovanosis was described by McLeod in India in 1882, and in 1905 Donovan described the intracellular bodies which are thought to cause the disease. Encapsulated bacteria resembling Donovan bodies have been recovered from lesions and pseudobuboes of granuloma inguinale by inoculation of chick embryo yolk sacs or yolk-agar medium. These bacteria, which are known as *Calymmatobacterium granulomatis,* measure 1.5 by 0.7 μm. They are antigenically related to *Klebsiella* species but do not reproduce the disease when inoculated intradermally in humans. It is uncertain whether these isolates are responsible for the disease. Electron microscopic studies of Donovan bodies confirm their morphologic resemblance to gram-negative bacteria.

EPIDEMIOLOGY Donovanosis is endemic in the tropics, particularly in New Guinea and among Hindus in India, and in parts of the Caribbean and Africa. In the United States the disease is rare. Most cases occur in the southeastern states and involve homosexual men. In reported cases the sex ratio of males to females is nearly 10:1. The disease is uncommon in Caucasians. The reported frequency of donovanosis in conjugal partners of chronically infected patients ranges from 1 to 64 percent. Evidence for sexual transmission includes the age-specific incidence, which corresponds to that of other sexually transmitted diseases, the frequent concomitant presence of syphilis, and the predilection for genital involvement in heterosexuals and for anorectal infection in homosexually active men.

CLINICAL MANIFESTATIONS The incubation period ranges from 8 days to 12 weeks, but most lesions appear within 30 days after sexual exposure.

Donovanosis begins as a papule, which ulcerates and develops into a painless elevated zone of clean, beefy-red, friable granulation tissue. The edges are irregular and spread by continuity or by autoinoculation of approximated skin surfaces. Secondary anaerobic infection may produce pain and a foul-smelling exudate. Less common complications of the disease include deep ulcerations, chronic cicatricial lesions, phimosis, lymphedema, and exuberant epithelial proliferation which grossly resembles carcinoma. In men, the lesions are usually located on the glans, prepuce, or shaft of the penis (Fig. 111-1A) or the perianal area, while infection of the labia is most common in women. Lesions in women often arise at the fourchette and progress anteriorly in a V shape along the vulva. Extragenital lesions may occur, involving the face, neck, mouth, and other sites. The chronicity of the disease is of diagnostic importance, since several months often elapse before patients seek treatment. Extension to the inguinal region by autoinoculation, by continuity, or via the lymphatics results in diffuse intradermal and subcutaneous swelling or suppuration, known as "pseudobubo," because involvement of the underlying lymph nodes is minimal. Locally destructive lesions and secondary infection may produce severe morbidity or death. Fatal disseminated disease, involving the bones, joints, or liver, has been reported after several years of chronic local infection. The relationship of donovanosis to subsequent carcinoma of the genitalia is uncertain.

DIAGNOSIS Early donovanosis may be mistaken for the primary chancre or condyloma latum of syphilis. Epithelial proliferation resembling carcinoma in the genital or perianal region in a young individual should always raise the suspicion of donovanosis if unnecessary destructive surgery is to be avoided. Chronic ulcerative or cicatricial changes may resemble lymphogranuloma venereum.

Amebiasis can produce penile lesions resembling donovanosis. In the United States, *Haemophilus ducreyi* has frequently been isolated from lesions resembling donovanosis; this has been termed *pseudogranuloma inguinale–chancroid*. Histologic studies in donovanosis reveal marked acanthosis and pseudoepitheliomatous hyperplasia. The dermis contains an inflammatory infiltrate consisting mainly of plasma cells and histiocytes. Because Donovan bodies are seldom detectable in sections stained with hematoxylin and eosin, these changes may lead to an erroneous diagnosis of carcinoma and to unnecessary destructive surgery. Although silver impregnation techniques are useful for demonstration of Donovan bodies in sections, the diagnosis is best made by examination of impression smears prepared from specimens obtained by punch biopsy of granulation tissue from the periphery of a lesion; the deep portion of the specimen is removed, crushed between two slides which are air-dried and fixed in methanol, and stained with Wright-Giemsa stain. With this method, Donovan bodies appear as very rounded coccobacilli, 1 by 2 μm in size, which lie within cystic spaces in the cytoplasm of large mononuclear cells (Fig. 111-2). The capsule stains as a dense acidophilic zone surrounding the bacterium, which resembles a closed

FIGURE 111-1 *A. Extensive granuloma inguinale, extending along the scrotum and involving both inguinal areas, with elevated, clean, exuberant granulation tissue. B. Same patient, following treatment. (Courtesy of A Brathwaite.)*

FIGURE 111-2 *Biopsy from granuloma inguinale ulcer, showing mononuclear cells containing Donovan bodies. Wright-Giemsa stain.*

intramuscularly every 12 h for 10 to 15 days. In New Guinea, chloramphenicol, 500 mg every 8 h orally, or gentamicin, 1 mg/kg twice daily, is used for cases which appear resistant to tetracycline. Co-trimoxazole (trimethoprim 160 mg, sulfamethoxazole 800 mg) twice daily for 10 days is also reported to be effective. In pregnant women, erythromycin, 500 mg every 6 h, may be effective. Treatment is reviewed in more detail in the chapter by Hart (1984).

REFERENCES

DAVIS CM: Granuloma inguinale. A clinical, histological, and ultrastructural study. JAMA 211:632, 1970

DODSON RF et al: Donovanosis: A morphologic study. J Invest Dermatol 62:611, 1974

GARG BR et al: Efficacy of cotrimoxazole in donovanosis. Br J Vener Dis 54:348, 1978

HART G: Chancroid, donovanosis, lymphogranuloma venerum. US Department of Health, Education, and Welfare Publication (CDC) 75-8302, 1975

————: Donovanosis, in *Sexually Transmitted Diseases*, KK Holmes et al (eds). New York, McGraw-Hill, 1984, pp 393–397

JOFRE ME et al: Granuloma inguinale simulating advanced pelvic cancer. Med J Aust 2:869, 1976

KRAUS SJ et al: Pseudogranuloma inguinale caused by *Haemophilus ducreyi*. Arch Dermatol 118:494, 1982

KUBERSKI T: Granuloma inguinale (donovanosis). Sex Transm Dis 7:29, 1980

———— et al: Ultrastructure of *Calymmatobacterium granulomatis* in lesions of granuloma inguinale. J Infect Dis 142:744, 1980

LAL S, NICHOLAS C: Epidemiological and clinical features in 165 cases of granuloma inguinale. Br J Vener Dis 46:461, 1970

SOWMINI CN: Donovanosis, in *International Perspectives on Neglected Sexually Transmitted Diseases: Impact on Venereology, Infertility, and Maternal and Infant Health*, KK Holmes, PA Mardh (eds). Washington, DC, Hemisphere Publishing, 1982, pp 205–217

safety pin because of bipolar condensation of chromatin. The pathognomonic mononuclear cell is 25 to 90 μm in diameter and has many cystic areas containing Donovan bodies.

Perianal donovanosis may resemble condylomata lata of secondary syphilis. Other venereal diseases, particularly syphilis, very frequently coexist with donovanosis. Repeated dark-field examinations of lesions before treatment and a serologic test for syphilis should therefore be performed. In countries where donovanosis is endemic, the persistence of suspected condylomata lata after appropriate penicillin therapy for syphilis is highly suggestive of donovanosis.

TREATMENT The treatment of choice is tetracycline, 2 g daily, for at least 10 days. The risk of relapse is reduced if treatment is continued until healing is complete. Healing is usually apparent within 3 weeks, as the lesions become pale and flatter and develop peripheral reepithelialization (Fig. 111-1B). Donovan bodies disappear from lesions within a few days after onset of therapy. If tetracycline cannot be given, streptomycin may be used in a dose of 1 g

---

112 BRUCELLOSIS

DONALD KAYE / ROBERT G. PETERSDORF

DEFINITION Brucellosis (undulant fever, Malta fever, Mediterranean fever) is an infection caused by microorganisms of the genus *Brucella*, which are usually transmitted to humans from domestic animals. The illness is characterized by fever, sweats, weakness, malaise, and weight loss, often without localized findings.

ETIOLOGY Human brucellosis is an infection caused by one of four species: *B. melitensis* (goats), *B. suis* (hogs), *B. abortus* (cattle), and *B. canis* (dogs). Relatively few cases of *B. canis* infection have been reported, but it is probably much more prevalent than is recognized. Although infections are usually confined to the major animal host, infections of swine with *B. abortus* or of cattle with *B. suis* may occur, and *Brucella* infection has been reported in other animals. The species of *Brucella* are separated from one another by biochemical and serologic reactions. The organisms are small, nonmotile, nonspore-forming, gram-negative coccobacilli which grow best at 37°C in trypticase soy broth or tryptose phosphate broth with a pH of 6.6 to 6.8 under increased CO_2 tension.

EPIDEMIOLOGY The natural reservoir of brucellosis is in domestic animals, particularly cattle, swine, goats, and sheep. Brucellosis in the natural host is very contagious. However, spread may occur to secondary hosts such as human beings. Person-to-person spread is rare. Animal-to-animal transmission is usually venereal or by ingestion of infected tissue or milk. Human infection most commonly results from ingestion of infected animal tissues or milk products, or directly through abraded skin.

On the average, approximately 200 cases of brucellosis are reported in the United States every year. However, it has been estimated that only about 4 percent of cases are recognized and reported. On a worldwide basis, the prevalence of the disease correlates closely with the extent of animal brucellosis in a given country. Brucellosis has nearly been eradicated in several European countries, where the incidence of animal brucellosis is also very low. In the United States, areas in which cattle-raising is an important industry generally have a higher incidence of brucellosis.

Brucellosis most frequently occurs in individuals who are exposed to *Brucella*-infected tissues and milk or milk products, including slaughterhouse workers, butchers, farmers, livestock producers, veterinarians, and individuals who ingest unpasteurized milk products. In most of the instances in which brucellosis has been acquired from unpasteurized dairy products, these products were purchased in other countries, particularly in Mexico, the Mediterranean basin, the Far East, and South America. In the United States, brucellosis occurs mainly in males of working age, more than half of them slaughterhouse workers. Fortunately, isolation of *Brucella* from infected meat decreases following refrigeration, but the high rates of accidental cuts and exposure to blood and lymph of freshly killed animals make abattoir workers particularly susceptible to this infection. In Alaska, a number of cases have been transmitted via raw meat from caribou and moose.

In the United States, *B. abortus* is the most frequent cause of brucellosis followed by *B. suis*. *B. melitensis* and *B. canis* are rare causes. Approximately 2 to 3 percent of cases acquired in this country occur in laboratories, often in veterinarians who are accidentally inoculated (via needle or the conjunctival or airborne routes) with live vaccine. The vaccine-induced disease is usually mild.

PATHOGENESIS AND PATHOLOGY *Brucella* invade the body through abraded skin and, less commonly, through the oropharynx, conjunctivae, or respiratory passages. They interact with polymorphonuclear leukocytes (PMN) and tissue macrophages. Many organisms are phagocytized, but if the inoculum is sufficiently large, they spread via the lymphatics to the regional lymph nodes, most commonly in the axillary, cervical, and supraclavicular regions. If localization does not occur there, the organisms spread via the bloodstream to other reticuloendothelial tissues such as the bone marrow, liver, and spleen, but visceral organs such as kidneys, bones, testes, and endocardium are involved as well. *Brucella* can multiply within PMN, tissue macrophages, and cells of the reticuloendothelial system and destroy them. In their intracellular location, *Brucella* are protected both from antibody and from many antibiotics.

The characteristic but nonspecific reaction of tissues to *Brucella* is the appearance of epithelioid cells, giant cells of the foreign body and Langhans' types, and lymphocytes and plasma cells with formation of granulomas. Although many *Brucella* are killed by PMNs, the macrophage is the ultimate cell that destroys *Brucella*. *B. abortus* causes mild disease with noncaseating granulomas in liver and other reticuloendothelial organs. *B. suis* causes more severe disease with local suppurative complications and granulomas that may caseate. *B. melitensis* causes the most severe acute disease with symptoms that may be disabling. *B. canis* causes mild disease similar to that seen with *B. abortus*. Granulomas in brucellosis eventually heal with fibrosis and often calcification.

Although brucellosis is a common cause of abortion in cattle, swine, and goats, there is no evidence that human abortions occur any more frequently with this disease than with other bacteremias.

MANIFESTATIONS Brucellosis may be asymptomatic with only serological evidence of infection. The manifestations of symptomatic brucellosis may be divided into acute brucellosis, localized disease, and chronic brucellosis.

Acute brucellosis The incubation period of acute brucellosis usually varies between 7 and 21 days, but may be months. The onset may be acute with a toxic course, especially when caused by *B. melitensis*. However, the onset is often insidious. Patients frequently have a low-grade fever with no localizing complaints but only malaise, fatigue, headache, weakness, sweats, chills, backache, and myalgias. Most patients are anorectic and lose weight. Some have cough or arthralgias.

Typically there are a multitude of complaints but a paucity of physical findings. When physical findings occur, the major manifestations are splenomegaly (which occurs in 10 to 20 percent of patients), lymphadenopathy (15 percent of patients), and hepatomegaly (less than 10 percent).

Localized brucellosis Localized disease may occur at almost any anatomic location, but osteomyelitis, splenic abscess, genitourinary tract localization, pulmonary involvement, and endocarditis are among the more common sites of involvement. Osteomyelitis usually occurs in the vertebrae, with the lumbosacral area as the most frequent site. There is a disc space infection with involvement of both adjacent vertebrae. Bone scans are positive early, followed by roentgenographic evidence of osteoporosis, anterior vertebral plate erosion, and formation of "parrot-beaked" osteophytes. Arthritis, which is much less common than osteomyelitis, most often involves the knee. Splenic abscesses may occur and result in areas of calcification. Epididymoorchitis and less often clinically apparent prostatic or renal infection may be observed. Meningoencephalitis, myelitis, radiculitis, or neuropathy are the neurologic complications. Pleural effusion and pneumonia are occasional manifestations.

Bacterial endocarditis is the most common cause of death among patients with brucellosis. It has been reported predominantly in males, follows an indolent course, is accompanied by a high rate of congestive heart failure and arterial embolization, and has required both valve replacement and antibiotic therapy to achieve cure.

Chronic brucellosis Chronic brucellosis is defined as ill health for more than 1 year following onset of brucellosis. Included in this group have been patients with relapsing illness with no localized infection, those with localization of infection in one or more organs, and those who have no objective signs of infection (e.g., no fever) and no evidence of active brucellosis (i.e., by serologic methods or by culture). It is doubtful that this last group has active brucellosis; it is more likely their complaints, fatigue and weakness, are psychoneurotic in nature.

An unusual complication that occurs in veterinarians removing placentas from infected animals consists of an erythematous macular, papular, or pustular rash on the hand and arms which is presumed to be a hypersensitivity reaction to *Brucella* antigens.

DIAGNOSIS Brucellosis is a relatively rare disease, and there are many common illnesses that mimic it. Among them are influenza, infectious mononucleosis, toxoplasmosis, viral hepatitis, disseminated gonococcal infection, rheumatic fever, systemic lupus erythematosus, tuberculosis, leptospirosis, and typhoid fever. The clinical suspicion that the patient has brucellosis should be higher in farmers, abattoir workers, and others exposed to infected tissues or animal products.

The definitive evidence of *Brucella* infection consists of isolating the *Brucella* organisms from the patient. However, culturing *Brucella* organisms may be dangerous to laboratory personnel. *All cultures should be clearly marked "possible brucellosis" and should be processed employing sterile techniques in a biohazard hood certified for handling class III infectious agents.* It is recommended that laboratories not having these facilities not undertake *Brucella* cultures.

Cultures Up to half the patients whose blood is submitted for culture early in the course of infection, and who have not received antibiotics, will have *Brucella* organisms in the blood when a culture is grown in trypticase soy broth for 1 to 3 weeks in the presence of 5 to 10% CO_2. However, many laboratories discard blood cultures after 10 days' incubation. This is another reason for the clinician to communicate any suspicion of brucellosis to the laboratory and to urge the laboratory to hold these cultures for at least 4 weeks. Sometimes, bone marrow cultures may be positive in acute brucellosis when blood cultures are not. Later in the course of illness, bacteremia is less frequent and organisms may then be isolated from infected lymph nodes or granulomas involving the spleen, liver, and bone. Altogether, only 15 to 20 percent of cases of brucellosis are confirmed by culture. In localized brucellosis, biopsy and isolation of *Brucella* may be necessary for diagnosis. In the majority of cases of brucellosis, the diagnosis is made serologically.

Serology IgM antibody titers rise early (usually in the first week of infection), peak at about 3 months, and then fall over a period of months. Titers may persist for several years. IgG antibodies appear 2 to 3 weeks after onset of illness, rise to peak titers in about 8 weeks, and persist as long as the infection is active. Therefore, the persistence of IgG antibody indicates continuing active infection. With treatment, IgG antibody titers decrease rapidly and usually disappear within 1 year. With relapse, both IgM and IgG titers increase. The most reliable serologic test is the standard tube *Brucella* agglutination test (STA) which measures antibodies directed primarily at *Brucella* lipopolysaccharide antigens. A fourfold or greater rise in titer of serum specimens drawn 1 to 4 weeks apart is indicative of recent exposure to *Brucella* or *Brucella*-like antigens. The specimen should be tested on the same day, in the same laboratory, under identical conditions. Using this test, most patients develop a rise in titer to *Brucella* antigens within 1 to 2 weeks of illness, and within 3 weeks virtually all patients will show seroconversion. False-positive tests may be due to *Brucella* skin tests, cholera vaccination, and infection with *Vibrio cholerae, Francisella tularensis,* or *Yersinia enterocolitica.* These cross-reactive causes of seroconversion are usually readily eliminated.

Significance of serologic findings A single STA titer of 160 or higher indicates past or present exposure to *Brucella* organisms or antigens that cross-react with *Brucella* species. If there is strong clinical suspicion of brucellosis, dilutions as high as 1:1280 should be made, because false-negative tests due to blocking antibodies have been reported in titers as high as 1:640. Virtually all patients with brucellosis have STA titers ≥ 1:160. Lower titers are of no diagnostic significance.

IgG-agglutinating antibodies can be recognized in the STA by extraction with 2-mercaptoethanol (2-ME). This procedure destroys the agglutinating activity of IgM antibodies and allows recognition of only the IgG-agglutinating antibody. Existence of a single elevated titer (≥ 1:160) in the 2-ME *Brucella* agglutination test is good objective evidence of either current or recent infection and the need for treatment. Many patients maintain elevated IgM-agglutinating antibodies for several years, even after presumed complete cure of their infection. For this reason, a 2-ME *Brucella* agglutination test that measures only IgG-agglutinating antibodies is the most useful indicator of whether the patient has been cured.

Other serologic tests are of no additional value. The *Brucella* skin test is of no more significance than a positive tuberculin test in patients suspected of having tuberculosis. Moreover, the test may interfere with interpretation of serologic tests by causing a rise in titer. For this reason, a skin test should not be performed.

Standard agglutination tests for antibodies to *Brucella* use *B. abortus* antigens. Antibodies to *B. melitensis* and *B. suis* cross-react with *B. abortus* but not with *B. canis.* To test for *B. canis* the antigen must be prepared from *B. canis*; these tests are not routinely available.

Other laboratory tests An occasional patient will develop anemia. The white blood cell count is normal or low, and the erythrocyte sedimentation rate may be normal or high.

TREATMENT It is generally accepted that the combination of tetracycline 500 mg orally four times daily for 3 to 6 weeks plus streptomycin 1 g every 12 h intramuscularly for the first 2 weeks will result in cure of brucellosis. This regimen has produced lower relapse rates than has treatment with tetracycline alone. With this program, relapses have occurred in only 2 percent of patients, and these have responded to retreatment. Tetracycline should not be used in pregnant women or children below the age of 8 because of the danger of staining developing teeth. Streptomycin may cause ototoxicity, and the dose must be decreased in patients with renal insufficiency.

A variety of other drugs, including gentamicin in lieu of streptomycin, doxycycline instead of tetracycline, or trimethoprim-sulfa or rifampin have been tried, but none has been found clearly superior to the tetracycline-streptomycin combination. When tetracycline plus streptomycin cannot be used, trimethoprim/sulfamethoxazole (480/2400 mg per day) for 4 weeks is a reasonable substitute. Addition of rifampin (900 mg per day) to the basic tetracycline-streptomycin or trimethoprim-sulfamethoxazole regimen may improve results when response is poor. Despite apparent in vitro activity against strains of *Brucella,* the role of the third-generation cephalosporins, if any, in brucellosis remains to be determined.

Abscesses should be drained when indicated. Splenectomy has been performed in some patients with splenomegaly and multiple relapses and has apparently been successful in preventing further relapses.

Febrile patients with either acute or subacute brucellosis characterized by severe anorexia, depression, and generalized debilitation may be given a short course of steroids. Prednisone in an oral dose of 60 mg a day tapered rapidly over a 5- to 7-day period can be administered and may be helpful. However, it is not necessary in most patients.

Therapeutic use of *Brucella* vaccine is of questionable value and is not recommended. Headache, backache, and generalized aches and pains should be treated with analgesics.

PROGNOSIS Even before antimicrobial treatment, the mortality rate of brucellosis was low, and only 15 percent of patients had an illness exceeding 3 months in duration. With chemotherapy, long illnesses have become quite rare, as have complications. When the morbidity exceeds 1 to 2 months, other causes of illness, previously unsuspected underlying disease, or a complication of brucellosis should be considered. The mortality rate of acute brucellosis is less than 2 percent.

The diagnosis of chronic brucellosis, continued active brucellosis, or a complication of brucellosis can best be made by demonstrating a titer of 1:160 or greater in the 2-ME agglutination test. If the titer is less than 1:40 on this test, it is highly unlikely that persistent illness or relapse is due to brucellosis.

Most patients who develop brucellosis in the course of their work can be permitted to return to their place of work. Immunity to reinfection appears to follow the first *Brucella* infection in most cases, but reinfection can occur.

PREVENTION Prevention of brucellosis in cattle can be achieved with live attenuated *Brucella* vaccine. No vaccine is available for humans in the United States. The risk of acquiring brucellosis can be reduced by decreasing exposure to freshly killed animal tissue from potentially infected animals and by drinking pasteurized milk and using pasteurized milk products. Slaughterhouse workers, meat inspectors, veterinarians, and others who examine a large number of cattle and hogs can mitigate the risk of infection by wearing protective gloves or goggles and by avoiding hand or arm cuts that could provide a portal of entry for *Brucella*. However, brucellosis will not be eliminated in humans unless it is first eliminated in animals.

REFERENCES

BUCHANAN TM et al: Brucellosis in the United States, 1960–1972: An abattoir-associated disease: I. Clinical features and therapy; II. Diagnostic aspects; III. Epidemiologic evidence for acquired immunity. Medicine 53:403, 415, 427, 1974

———, FABER LC: 2-Mercaptoethanol *Brucella* agglutination test: Usefulness for predicting recovery from brucellosis. J Clin Microbiol 11:691, 1980

CERVANTES F et al: Liver disease in brucellosis: A clinical and pathological study of 40 cases. Postgrad Med J 58:346, 1982

COHEN PS et al: Infective endocarditis caused by gram-negative bacteria. Prog Cardiovasc Dis 22:205, 1980

HEIBIG J et al: *Brucella* aortic endocarditis corrected by prosthetic valve replacement. Am Heart J 106:594, 1983

HEWITT WG, PAYNE DJ: Estimation of IgG and IgM *Brucella* antibodies in infected and non-infected persons by a radioimmune technique. J Clin Pathol 37:692, 1984

LARBRISSEAU A et al: The neurological complications of brucellosis. Can J Neurol Sci 5:369, 1978

LLORENS-TEROL J, BUSQUETS RM: Brucellosis treated with rifampicin. Arch Dis Child 55(6):486, 1980

POLT SS et al: Human brucellosis caused by *Brucella canis*: Clinical features and immune response. Ann Intern Med 97:717, 1982

SPINK WW: *The Nature of Brucellosis*. Minneapolis, University of Minnesota Press, 1956

YOUNG EJ: Human brucellosis. Rev Infect Dis 5:821, 1983

113 TULAREMIA

DONALD KAYE

DEFINITION Tularemia (rabbit fever, deer fly fever) is an infection caused by *Francisella tularensis*. *F. tularensis* is found in many animals and is transmitted to human beings by direct contact or via an insect vector. The illness is characterized by an ulcerative lesion at the site of inoculation with regional lymphadenopathy, by pneumonia, or by fever without localizing findings.

ETIOLOGY *F. tularensis* is a small, nonmotile, pleomorphic, gram-negative aerobic coccobacillus. It grows poorly in many media but will grow well in glucose-cysteine blood agar, thioglycolate broth, and other media supplemented with cysteine. *F. tularensis* is found only in the northern hemisphere. There are two types of *F. tularensis*. Jellison type A is distributed solely in North America, is virulent for humans and rabbits, produces citrulline ureidase, and ferments glycerol. Type B is found in North America, Europe, and Asia, causes no or mild disease in humans and rabbits, does not produce citrulline ureidase, and does not ferment glycerol. *F. tularensis* cross-reacts serologically with *Brucella* species and *Yersinia pestis*. It contains an endotoxin similar to endotoxins of other gram-negative bacilli.

EPIDEMIOLOGY *F. tularensis* has been found in many mammals including rabbits, squirrels, muskrats, beavers, deer, cattle, and sheep, in birds, in amphibians, and in fish. Tularemia can result from skin contact with any of these species. Tularemia has also been transmitted by cat bite. Ticks, deer flies, and mosquitoes can transmit the bacterium. Ticks transmit *F. tularensis* to their offspring through transovarian passage. In the United States the disease can be carried by *Dermacentor andersoni* (Rocky Mountain wood tick), *Dermacentor variabilis* (American dog tick), *Dermacentor occidentalis* (Pacific Coast dog tick), and *Amblyomma americanum* (Lone Star tick). *F. tularensis* has also been recovered from streams.

In the United States most cases of tularemia result from skin contact with infected wild rabbits (especially cottontail rabbits) or the bite of a tick or deer fly. Infection occasionally results from ingestion or inhalation of infected material. The highest risk groups are hunters and trappers. Therefore, tularemia is most likely to occur in adult males. Person-to-person transmission rarely, if ever, occurs.

Tularemia has been reported from all parts of the United States, but mostly from Arkansas, Missouri, Oklahoma, Texas, and Utah. About 300 cases are reported each year in the United States. Arthropod-borne disease occurs mainly in the spring and summer, and rabbit-produced infection mainly in the winter.

PATHOGENESIS AND PATHOLOGY In human infection, the most common portal of entry is through the skin or mucous membranes. This may be direct through inapparent abrasions or via the bite of a tick or other arthropod. Inhalation or ingestion of *F. tularensis* can also result in infection. Fewer than 50 organisms will result in infection when injected into the skin or inhaled, whereas more than 10^8 are usually required to produce infection via the oral route.

Following inoculation into the skin, the bacteria multiply locally and after 2 to 5 days (occasionally 1 to 10 days) produce an erythematous, tender, or pruritic papule. The papule rapidly enlarges and forms an ulcer with a black base. The bacteria spread to regional lymph nodes producing lymphadenopathy, and further spread with bacteremia may occur. With bacteremia, organisms are cleared from the blood by phagocytic cells of the reticuloendothelial system (mainly in the liver and spleen) and may survive intracellularly for long periods of time.

Affected organs (liver, spleen, lymph nodes) demonstrate areas of focal necrosis initially surrounded mainly by polymorphonuclear leukocytes. Subsequently granulomas form with epithelioid cells and lymphocytes and sometimes multinucleated giant cells surrounding the areas of necrosis which may resemble caseation necrosis. Coalescence of granulomas can lead to formation of abscesses. Nodes may occasionally become fluctuant and even rupture. Healing occurs with fibrosis and calcification of the granulomas.

Contamination of the conjunctiva can result in infection of the eye with regional lymph node enlargement. Aerosolization of *F. tularensis* with inhalation can result in pneumonia. Pneumonia can also occur via the hematogenous route. There is an inflammatory reaction with foci of alveolar necrosis and initially polymorphonuclear leukocytic and later mononuclear cell infiltration with granuloma formation. Chest roentgenograms usually reveal bilateral patchy infiltrates rather than large areas of consolidation. Mediastinal or other regional lymphadenopathy may occur.

Pharyngitis with cervical lymphadenopathy or gastrointestinal tularemia with mesenteric lymphadenopathy may follow ingestion of large numbers of *F. tularensis*. The portal of entry is unknown in typhoidal tularemia, an uncommon form, but may be the skin, lung, or gastrointestinal system. There is fever with no localizing symptoms.

CLINICAL MANIFESTATIONS Tularemia usually has an incubation period of 2 to 5 days after which there is onset of one of a number of syndromes (listed below), all of which are usually associated with fever and chills. Headache, myalgias, and malaise are also often present. Hepatosplenomegaly, which may be tender, is a common finding. About 20 percent of patients develop a generalized maculopapular rash which may occasionally become pustular.

Ulceroglandular tularemia Most patients with tularemia (75 to 85 percent) develop infection secondary to inoculation of the skin. In cases related to rabbits the portal of entry is usually on the finger or hand. In tick-related cases, the site of inoculation is usually on the lower extremities, inguinal or axillary areas, scalp, abdomen, or chest.

At time of onset of illness there is usually an erythematous papule that may be tender or pruritic, or there is already an ulcer present at the portal of entry of the organism. If there is a papule, it evolves over a period of several days to form a punched out ulcer with sharply demarcated edges and a yellow exudate. The ulcer gradually develops a black base. There is very tender, large regional lymphadenopathy (usually axillary or epitrochlear with tularemia from rabbits, and inguinal or femoral lymphadenopathy with tick-borne disease). The nodes may become fluctuant and may drain spontaneously. In 5 to 10 percent of cases of tularemia, the skin lesion may be inapparent and the lymphadenopathy the only physical finding. This has been called "glandular tularemia."

Oculoglandular tularemia In a small percent of patients (about 1 percent), the conjunctiva serves as the portal of entry for the organism. There is purulent conjunctivitis with regional lymphadenopathy (preauricular, submandibular, or cervical). Corneal perforation may occur.

Oropharyngeal tularemia A rare form of tularemia (less than 1 percent of cases) which may occur after ingestion of *F. tularensis* (usually in undercooked meat) is acute exudative or membranous pharyngitis associated with cervical lymphadenopathy.

Gastrointestinal tularemia Rarely following ingestion of *F. tularensis* there may be ulcerative intestinal lesions with associated mesenteric lymphadenopathy. In addition to fever, the patient has diarrhea, abdominal pain, nausea and vomiting, and gastrointestinal bleeding.

Pulmonary tularemia Involvement of the lung can result from inhalation of *F. tularensis* or as a part of the bacteremia caused by tularemia at another site. Inhalation pulmonary disease occurs most often in laboratory workers and is a serious infection with high mortality. Pulmonary involvement occurs in 10 to 15 percent of patients with ulceroglandular tularemia and in about half of the patients with typhoidal tularemia. There is cough, which is usually nonproductive, and there may be dyspnea or pleuritic chest pain. The physical examination is usually normal. Roentgenograms of the chest usually reveal bilateral patchy infiltrates which have been described as "ovoid densities." Lobar pneumonia may occur, and pleural effusion(s) may be present.

Typhoidal tularemia In about 10 percent of cases of tularemia there is fever without apparent skin lesion or lymphadenopathy. In the absence of a history of possible contact with a vector of the disease, diagnosis is extremely difficult.

Other manifestations Meningitis, pericarditis, peritonitis, endocarditis, and osteomyelitis have all been reported. The meningitis causes a lymphocytic response in the spinal fluid.

DIAGNOSIS Differential diagnosis In patients with fever and large, tender lymphadenopathy the possibility of tularemia should be strongly considered, and an attempt should be made to determine if there was an appropriate animal or arthropod vector contact. The suspicion of tularemia should be especially high in hunters, trappers, game wardens, veterinarians, and laboratory workers. However, in up to 40 percent of patients with tularemia, no history of epidemiologic contact with an animal or arthropod vector can be elicited.

Ulceroglandular tularemia is often so characteristic that it does not present a problem in differential diagnosis, but on occasion it must be differentiated from other diseases. The skin lesion may resemble those seen in sporotrichosis, skin infection with coagulase-positive staphylococci or group A streptococci, syphilis, anthrax, rat bite fever (caused by *Spirillum minor*), rickettsial infections (such as scrub typhus) and *Mycobacterium marinum* infection. However, the regional lymphadenopathy in these diseases is usually not as impressive as in tularemia.

The lymphadenopathy of tularemia must be differentiated from that of plague (Chap. 114), lymphogranuloma venereum (Chap. 150), and cat scratch fever (Chap. 118). However, in these infections there is usually no local lesion resembling the ulcer of tularemia.

Typhoidal tularemia may resemble typhoid fever, other *Salmonella* bacteremias, rickettsial infections (such as Rocky Mountain spotted fever), brucellosis, infectious mononucleosis, toxoplasmosis, miliary tuberculosis, sarcoid, or hematologic malignancies. Tularemia pneumonia may resemble pneumonias caused by other bacteria as well as viral or *Mycoplasma* pneumonia.

Laboratory diagnosis The diagnosis of tularemia is usually made serologically by agglutination methods. A significant rise in titer (i.e., fourfold or greater) in paired serum specimens over a 2- to 3-week period is diagnostic. Agglutinating antibody appears after 1 to 2 weeks of illness. Fifty percent of patients have antibody in the second week, and the rest develop antibody later in the course. Titers peak at 4 to 8 weeks and may remain elevated for years. A single agglutinating titer of $\geq$ 1:160 in a patient who has been ill for at least 2 weeks is highly suggestive of tularemia but may only indicate old infection. Antibodies to *F. tularensis* may cross-react with *Brucella*, but the titers to *Brucella* are usually much lower than the titers to *F. tularensis*.

F. tularensis is rarely observed on Gram stains of skin lesions, sputum, or aspirates of nodes. While cultures of these materials or blood may be positive if processed on appropriate media, there is a major risk of infection in laboratory personnel. Cultivation of *F. tularensis* should only be attempted in laboratories with adequate isolation techniques and experienced personnel.

Isolation of *F. tularensis* can be achieved by inoculation intraperitoneally into guinea pigs, which will die within 10 days, and by direct plating onto glucose-cysteine blood agar. Agents such as cycloheximide, polymyxin B, and penicillin are frequently added to media to suppress other organisms in specimens that may overgrow *F. tularensis*.

A delayed-type skin test (similar to the tuberculin test) with *F. tularensis* antigen or killed whole bacilli has been used. It turns positive during the first week of illness, prior to the appearance of agglutinating antibody, and persists for years. A positive skin test may be helpful in early diagnosis, but the skin test antigen is not available commercially. The skin test can boost titers of agglutinating antibodies.

There are no other helpful laboratory tests in the diagnosis of tularemia. The white blood cell count is usually normal, and the erythrocyte sedimentation rate may be normal as well.

TREATMENT Streptomycin, in a dose of 7.5 to 10 mg/kg every 12 h intramuscularly, is considered the drug of choice in treatment of tularemia. In severe infections, 15 mg/kg every 12 h may be used for the first 48 to 72 h. Therapy is continued for 7 to 10 days. Gentamicin, in a dose of 1.7 mg/kg, intramuscularly or intravenously, every 8 h, is also effective. Virtually all strains are susceptible to streptomycin and gentamicin. Temperature response occurs within 2 days, but skin lesions and lymph nodes may take 1 to 2 weeks to heal. When therapy is not initiated until several weeks of illness have elapsed, the temperature response may be delayed. Relapses are very uncommon with streptomycin therapy.

Tetracycline or chloramphenicol, 30 mg/kg per day in four divided doses for 14 days, has also been used to treat tularemia. While response to these agents is good, the relapse rate is unacceptably high, occurring in up to 20 percent of patients.

If fluctuant nodes require aspiration or drainage, at least several days of antibiotic therapy should be given first to avoid exposure of medical personnel to aerosolization of infected material.

PREVENTION Prevention of tularemia is based on avoidance of exposure and vaccination of high-risk populations. Avoidance of skinning wild mammals, especially rabbits, will decrease the frequency of transmission. Wearing gloves while handling rabbit carcasses will decrease the risk of transmission. Use of insect repellents and prompt removal of ticks will help prevent transmission by ticks in tick-infested areas.

A multiple-puncture intradermal vaccine (used in a fashion similar to vaccinia) made from live attenuated *F. tularensis* and available from the Centers for Disease Control, Atlanta, Georgia, is effective in decreasing the frequency and severity of disease, but will not totally prevent tularemia. Protection is long-lasting. The vaccine induces agglutinins to *F. tularensis* and skin test reactivity. It is effective by stimulating cellular immunity, as circulating antibodies do not seem to be protective.

Veterinarians, hunters, trappers, game wardens, and others who are likely to come in contact with infected wild mammals are candidates for immunization. Laboratory workers who handle specimens containing *F. tularensis* should be immunized.

Prophylactic treatment with streptomycin will prevent development of clinical disease in patients who are incubating *F. tularensis*.

PROGNOSIS If untreated, symptoms of tularemia usually last 1 to 4 weeks but may continue for months. The mortality of severe untreated infection (which includes all tularemia pneumonia) can be as high as 30 percent. However, the overall mortality rate for untreated tularemia is less than 8 percent. Mortality is rare with appropriate therapy. Following tularemia there is usually lifelong immunity.

REFERENCES

BUCHANAN TM et al: The tularemia skin test. 325 skin tests in 210 persons: Serologic correlation and review of the literature. Ann Intern Med 74:336, 1971

KOSKELA P, HERVA E: Cell-mediated and humoral immunity induced by a live *Francisella tularensis* vaccine. Infect Immunol 36:983, 1982

MASON WL et al: Treatment of tularemia, including pulmonary tularemia, with gentamicin. Ann Rev Resp Dis 121:39, 1980

SANDSTROM G et al: Antigen from *Francisella tularensis:* Nonidentity between determinants participating in cell-mediated and humoral reactions. Infect Immunol 45:101, 1984

SANFORD JP: Landmark perspective: Tularemia. JAMA 250:3225, 1983

SCHMID GP: Clinically mild tularemia associated with tick-borne *Francisella tularensis.* J Infect Dis 148:63, 1983

Tularemia. Morb Mort Week Rep 31:39, 1982

YOUNG LS et al: Tularemia epidemic: Vermont 1968. Forty-seven cases linked to contact with muskrats. N Engl J Med 280:1253, 1969

114 PLAGUE AND OTHER *YERSINIA* INFECTIONS

DARWIN L. PALMER

DEFINITION Plague is an acute infectious illness of human beings, wild rodents, and their ectoparasites which is caused by the gram-negative bacillus *Yersinia pestis*. The disease persists because of its firm entrenchment in sylvatic rodent-flea ecosystems throughout the world. Wild rodent contact leads to sporadic human disease; the historically explosive urban epidemics resulted from transmission of disease into rats. Human bubonic plague follows bites by rodent fleas; after several days painful local adenopathy (the bubo) and sepsis spread to other organ systems, and death occurs. Primary plague pneumonia is transmitted between humans by cough-generated aerosols, has a fulminant course, and is almost universally fatal if untreated.

EPIDEMIOLOGY Sylvatic plague involves more than 200 species of wild rodents and is concentrated in the southwestern United States, the southern Soviet Union, India, Indochina, and South Africa. In the United States, ground squirrels, mice, voles, marmots, wood rats, prairie dogs, and chipmunks are potential carriers. Rodent disease is characterized by occurrence in the spring and summer, year-to-year variations in disease activity, chronicity in the populations involved, slow regional spread, and rare geographic regression. The disease dies off in some populations in cyclical fashion, leaving both resistant survivors and infected fleas seeking another host. Disease also persists in natural foci because of latent infection during animal

hibernation, by prolonged viability of *Y. pestis* in soil of rodent burrows, by survival of infected fleas, and by persistent infection in relatively resistant rodents. Rodent predators may also spread plague; felines, such as domestic cats, generally die when infected with *Y. pestis*, while canines, such as foxes, coyotes, and dogs, often recover and may serve as serologic sentinels of wild rodent disease. Human disease can be readily acquired from domestic pets when the pets catch and return plague-infected rodents or their fleas to rural homes. Hares and rabbits are occasional nonrodent sources of the disease in humans, especially during the winter hunting season.

Rodent fleas are critical to the natural plague cycle and are implicated in about 85 percent of human cases. After infection, fleas develop obstruction of the foregut, causing regurgitation of plague bacilli during the next blood meal. The rat flea, *Xenopsylla cheopsis*, is an especially efficient plague vector both between rats and between rodents and humans. Transmission without fleas may occur by ingestion of infected carcasses by predators, possibly by contact with infected tissue through an open wound, or by inhalation of infected aerosols. Human body lice as well as ticks are also capable of inter-human or person-to-person transmission.

In the last three decades there has been a rising incidence of sporadic human plague originating in the western United States, with a death rate of 15 percent. This rate, double that seen in large outbreaks, reflects delay in the diagnosis or incorrect therapy due to travel during the incubation period out of plague endemic areas, or failure to elicit a history of animal exposure. Sporadic human plague occurs most frequently in the spring and summer, especially in children or youths under 20 and in adult males, reflecting their increased risk of wild rodent contact. While urban rat–related human outbreaks are now rare, they represent a continued threat; spread from sylvatic rodents into urban rats was documented as recently as 1983 in Los Angeles. Primary plague pneumonia arises as a secondary infection during bubonic/septicemic disease, with subsequent person-to-person spread via infectious aerosols. In closed quarters it is rapidly transmitted. A primary pneumonic plague outbreak in the United States last occurred in 1919, when 13 cases with 12 deaths (including two physicians and one nurse) developed before the disease was recognized and halted by case isolation. Cases of primary human pneumonic plague have also been acquired from domestic cats dying of plague pneumonia.

ETIOLOGY *Yersinia pestis* is a member of the family Enterobacteriaceae. It is a pleomorphic, gram-negative, nonmotile, aerobic bacillus which grows optimally at 28°C. The organism grows readily but slowly on routine media, and cultures should not be discarded before 72 h. Although weakly gram-negative, *Y. pestis* stains best with Giemsa's or Wayson's stains, with which it shows prominent bipolar "safety pin" microscopic morphology. The organism is a facultative intracellular parasite which maintains its virulence by the production of V and W antigens, enabling the organism to resist phagocytic intracellular killing, while production of capsular fraction 1 antigen partially protects the organism from phagocytosis by polymorphonuclear leukocytes. Other virulence factors include pesticin, fibrinolysin, coagulase, and a lipopolysaccharide endotoxin. The production of V and W antigens is plasmid-mediated, dependent on calcium, and may reflect the response of *Y. pestis* to its frequent intracellular location. No separate serotypes are recognized, but biotypes *antigua, orientalis,* and *mediaevalis* have geographic distributions which presumably mark previous epidemic spread. The organism is relatively resistant to drying and may maintain its viability in cool, moist conditions, such as the soil of an animal burrow, for many months. Antibiotic resistance can be developed in the laboratory, and both streptomycin- and tetracycline-resistant strains have been isolated from clinical specimens.

PATHOGENESIS After *Y. pestis* is inoculated into the skin by a flea bite, bacteria migrate to local lymph nodes, where they are taken up but not killed by mononuclear cells. Intracellular multiplication results in development of capsular envelopes containing fraction 1 protein; other toxins are elaborated. An acute inflammatory response is provoked in the lymph node in 2 to 6 days. At this stage the organisms are relatively resistant to phagocytosis by polymorphonuclear leukocytes because of the protection by capsules containing fraction 1 antigen and the lack of specific opsonic antibody. Characteristically, hemorrhagic necrosis of lymph nodes next occurs from which large numbers of bacteria gain access to the bloodstream and other organs. Extension along lymphatics involves both superficial nodes at the site of inoculation, the spleen, and nodes in the abdomen, mediastinum, or perihilar areas. The lung is secondarily infected in 10 to 20 percent, generally as a rapidly progressive, multilobar pneumonia, often with pleural exudate. The early acute inflammatory reaction is followed by lobar consolidation and hemorrhagic necrosis, and if death does not intervene, may progress to abscess formation. Fibrin thrombi may be extensive in the pulmonary vessels as well as in glomeruli and vessels of skin and other organs. Secondarily, the adult respiratory distress syndrome or a rise in pulmonary artery pressure may be seen. Pericarditis with a small amount of seropurulent exudate is frequent, and meningitis may occur late in untreated bacteremic plague. In 5 to 15 percent, the skin, predominantly of the extremities, is involved early on with petechiae and hemorrhages due to thrombocytopenia and vasculitis. Late in the disease, buboes may become fluctuant and occasionally may become superinfected with other bacteria. Endotoxemia can be detected during plague sepsis. It may result in both endotoxin shock and disseminated intravascular coagulation.

MANIFESTATIONS Bubonic plague has an incubation period of 2 to 7 days from flea bite to onset of illness. Although many patients do not remember an insect contact, a small eschar may be found at the bite site. Patients present with a painful bubo and fever accompanied by headache, prostration, and abdominal distress. The bubo, a tender enlarged lymph node or nodes, ranges in size from 1 to 10 cm and is found in the groin in 70 percent; alternatively, buboes may develop in axillary or cervical nodes or in several lymphatic chains simultaneously. Buboes are extremely tender, not fixed to skin or underlying structures, and the overlying skin is often erythematous. Fever and rigors are prominent and occasionally precede appearance of a bubo by 1 to 3 days. Gastrointestinal symptoms are present in more than half the patients, with abdominal pain often extending from the groin bubo and accompanied by anorexia, nausea, vomiting, and diarrhea, which may be bloody. Cutaneous petechiae and hemorrhages occur in 5 to 50 percent, and may be extensive late in the disease. Disseminated intravascular coagulation occurs in subclinical form in as many as 86 percent of patients, 5 to 10 percent of whom have clinical manifestations, including gangrene of the skin, fingers, toes, and penis. If untreated, bubonic disease may proceed without other organ system involvement to generalized sepsis, prostration, hypotension, and death within the next 2 to 10 days. Some patients have very prominent signs of sepsis with no demonstrable bubo. This represents a form of bubonic plague in which lymphatic involvement is limited to deep structures or where the buboes are so small as to be overlooked in the presence of overwhelming signs of infection. Septicemic disease may progress rapidly with chills, fever, rapid pulse, severe headache, nausea, vomiting, delirium, and death within 48 h. In such fulminant sepsis, bacteremia is so prominent that blood buffy coat may readily show *Y. pestis* on Gram stain.

Other than the lymphatics, the lung is the organ most commonly involved, with development of secondary pneumonia in 10 to 20 percent of all patients. Cough, fever, and tachypnea appear on days 2 to 3 of illness, accompanied by minimal pulmonary infiltrates. Later, or less commonly from the start, symptoms worsen rapidly with marked dyspnea, bloody sputum, and evidence of respiratory failure. There may be multilobar involvement, with variable degrees of consolidation, and the sputum may teem with *Y. pestis* and is highly contagious when disseminated by cough-generated aerosols. Primary plague pneumonia is a fulminant illness; time from the initial contact to death ranges from 2 to 6 days. The adult respiratory distress

syndrome (ARDS), characterized by noncardiac pulmonary edema, anoxia, and respiratory failure, also occurs as a manifestation of plague sepsis and may be indistinguishable from plague pneumonia except for the absence of bacteria in respiratory secretions. Both *Y. pestis* pneumonia and the ARDS form of illness have a mortality in excess of 75 percent, despite appropriate antimicrobial and supportive therapy. Less commonly, marked perihilar adenopathy may present alone or accompany pneumonia.

Plague meningitis, as a late complication in fewer than 5 percent of untreated patients, is characterized by nuchal rigidity, headache, confusion, and coma, and is often preceded or accompanied by bacteremia.

Rarely, patients with plague have a very mild illness manifested chiefly by low-grade fever and adenopathy. In this group are patients with tonsillar plague, who have positive throat cultures, serologic conversion, and minimal illness. Other less common late complications include persistent hectic fever despite appropriate therapy; fluctuance and spontaneous drainage from buboes; and pulmonary cavitation with abscess formation.

LABORATORY FINDINGS With the exception of definitive microbiologic studies, laboratory tests are of little diagnostic help. A polymorphonuclear leukocytosis of 15,000 to 20,000 cells per cubic millimeter is common, and the white cells may show toxic changes. Rarely, a marked leukemoid reaction with more than 100,000 white cells is seen. Modest elevations of serum glutamic oxaloacetic transaminase are common, but otherwise liver function studies are normal. Evidence of disseminated intravascular coagulation with low platelet counts, prolonged partial thromboplastin times, and positive fibrin degradation products is common. The electrocardiogram is usually normal but may show right axis deviation and peaked P waves indicative of acute cor pulmonale. The chest x-ray will show infiltrates, often with pleural effusion, in secondary or primary plague pneumonia or show evidence of pulmonary edema in patients with the adult respiratory distress syndrome. In meningitis, examination of cerebrospinal fluid demonstrates polymorphonuclear pleocytosis, low sugar, elevated protein, and gram-negative coccobacillary organisms, although culture may demonstrate *Y. pestis* more reliably.

Confirmation of the clinical suspicion of bubonic plague may be obtained by needle-aspiration of a bubo with direct staining of the aspirated material. With either Wayson's or Giemsa's stain, the characteristic bipolar-staining, "safety pin" forms are seen. By fluorescent antibody staining, a presumptive diagnosis may be specifically confirmed in about 80 percent of cases. Cultures of aspirated material, as well as sputum, pleural fluid, and blood, will be positive in a high percentage of patients. Microscopic examination of buffy coat smear may show *Y. pestis* in septicemic cases. A serologic response with a fourfold or greater rise is detected in the second week of illness by complement fixation, hemagglutination or indirect immunofluorescent antibody.

DIAGNOSIS Bubonic plague must be suspected in any febrile patient with painful adenopathy who has a history of wild animal exposure in a plague endemic area, but may be confused with other illnesses. Presentation with fever and a painful groin bubo can mimic granuloma venereum or syphilis or, when more severe, an acute abdominal crisis such as incarcerated inguinal hernia, appendicitis, or a ruptured viscus. Abdominal pain and bloody diarrhea can be mistaken for shigellosis or other acute diarrheal processes. With an axillary or cervical bubo, acute streptococcal or staphylococcal lymphadenitis, tularemia, cat-scratch fever, granuloma venereum, or syphilis may be considered. Bubonic/septicemic disease with an absent or minimal bubo, suggests typhoid fever or bacteremia due to other causes. Primary or secondary pneumonic plague may mimic bacterial pneumonia from any cause.

When plague is suspected, diagnostic maneuvers must include aspiration of buboes with appropriate stains and cultures, as well as blood cultures and cultures from other sources. Cultures should not be discarded early because the organism grows slowly and may only appear in 48 to 72 h. A serologic rise by passive hemagglutination is evident by day 5 and peaks by day 14. Newer serologic methods such as enzyme-linked immunosorbent assay compare well in sensitivity to standard passive hemagglutination tests and are more rapid.

TREATMENT If plague is strongly suspected on clinical and/or epidemiologic grounds, therapy must be started immediately, prior to completion of diagnostic studies. Antibiotic and supportive treatment should reduce the 40 to 100 percent mortality of untreated bubonic or pneumonic plague to 5 to 10 percent. Effective antibiotics include streptomycin, tetracycline, and chloramphenicol. Streptomycin should be given initially at a dosage of 7.5 to 15 mg/kg every 12 h intramuscularly; tetracycline, given intravenously at 5 to 10 mg/kg every 6 h, may be started concurrently and streptomycin discontinued when the patient becomes afebrile. Larger doses, even in those with severe illness, offer no benefit. Tetracycline should be continued for a total of 3 to 4 days after the fever has disappeared. In less severely ill patients, tetracycline alone at 5 to 10 mg/kg every 6 h may be given either by mouth or intravenously. Chloramphenicol in a dose of 12.5 to 25 mg/kg given intravenously every 6 h should be substituted for tetracycline in patients with meningitis due to its better central nervous system penetration. While antibiotic-resistant organisms have appeared only rarely, gentamicin is as effective as streptomycin. Tetracycline or trimethoprim-sulfamethoxazole are effective for the prophylaxis of case contacts and should be given orally for 5 days. Local treatment of the bubo is not indicated unless fluctuance or spontaneous drainage occurs, when cultures should be obtained to detect staphylococci. Ventilatory support for patients with plague pneumonia or adult respiratory distress syndrome may be necessary and lifesaving.

PREVENTION AND CONTROL Individuals working in high-risk occupations in plague endemic areas or conducting laboratory work with *Y. pestis* should consider use of the formalin-killed whole-bacteria vaccine; however, the vaccine must be readministered every 6 months due to rapidly waning immunity. Alternatively, individuals briefly visiting a plague endemic area may take tetracycline or trimethoprim-sulfamethoxazole prophylaxis. Following the presumptive diagnosis of pneumonic plague, patients should be placed in respiratory isolation; simple hand-washing precautions suffice for bubonic cases. Contacts of a patient with plague pneumonia should be given oral tetracycline prophylaxis, at 250 mg four times daily by mouth, and should be advised to seek medical attention upon the development of respiratory symptoms or fever. Possibly due to such precautions, transmission of primary plague pneumonia has not occurred in this country for many years.

The potential for spread of plague into urban rat populations from sylvatic rodent sources is an ever-present risk. Prevention depends on control of urban rat populations and their exclusion from dwellings as well as surveillance of sylvatic rodents and of their local predators. Picnickers, hikers, and others traveling into plague endemic regions during the spring-summer season should be warned that plague is a potential danger. They should avoid touching carcasses or sick rodents and should restrain and treat pets with flea-repellent powders. No practical measures exist for eliminating plague from wild rodent sources. Reducing rodent harborage around rural homes in endemic regions is important. Killing rodents around rural dwellings with rodenticides should be preceded by insect control to prevent displaced rodent fleas from seeking humans or domestic pets.

OTHER *YERSINIA* INFECTIONS (*Y. PSEUDOTUBERCULOSIS* AND *Y. ENTEROCOLITICA*)

ETIOLOGY *Y. enterocolitica* and *Y. pseudotuberculosis* are both non-lactose-fermenting, gram-negative, aerobic bacilli related to one

another and to *Y. pestis* and are members of the Enterobacteriaceae. Both organisms grow slowly on media used for the detection of other enteric bacteria, and their detection can be enhanced by cold enrichment incubation at 20 to 25°C. Cold enrichment, however, requires refrigeration for several weeks and is of little use in diagnosis of any one patient. Strains can be distinguished from one another and from *Y. pestis* on the basis of serologic and biochemical reactions as well as by antibiotic sensitivities. As in *Y. pestis*, both organisms elaborate W and V virulence factors and, with *Y. pseudotuberculosis*, virulence is also related to its ability to survive intracellularly. Both organisms produce an endotoxin and *Y. enterocolitica* elaborates a heat-stable enterotoxin which may be of significance in foodborne illness. A large number of serotypes of both organisms exist causing disease in many animal species, but most human infections are caused by a limited number of strains.

MANIFESTATIONS Although recognized most commonly in northern Europe and North America, *Y. enterocolitica* causes enteric infection worldwide and accounts for approximatley 1 to 3 percent of all cases of acute bacterial enteritis. Although the origin of the disease is often unclear, outbreaks traced to both food and water have been reported; person-to-person as well as animal-to-person transmission is common. Manifestations of the disease vary with age. In infants and young children the predominant symptom is acute watery diarrhea lasting 3 to 14 days; 5 percent of children have blood in the stool. In older children and young adults, a syndrome of right lower quadrant pain accompanied by fever and moderate leukocytosis indistinguishable from acute appendicitis occurs. In adults, especially in women over age 40, erythema nodosum often follows enteritis by 1 to 2 weeks. Adults may develop a monoarticular arthritis of the knee, foot, or hand with or without preceding enteritis. Rarely, a severe, disabling suppurative arthritis is seen. Among patients with arthritis, 65 percent have histocompatibility group HLA-B27. *Y. enterocolitica* also causes bacteremia, mostly in individuals with underlying illness such as diabetes mellitus, severe anemia, cirrhosis, or malignancy. Septicemic patients complain of headache, fever, and abdominal pain with or without diarrhea and frequently develop abscesses in multiple organs. Exudative pharyngitis with *Y. enterocolitica* was found in adult patients during the course of an outbreak of milkborne yersiniosis.

Pseudotuberculosis is a rare illness acquired from humans or domestic and wild animals, presumably by fecal-oral contact. Most cases are sporadic and occur in the young, with males more commonly affected than females and with a peak in the winter months corresponding to the peak occurrence in animals. After ingestion, the organisms apparently penetrate the ileal mucosa, localize in the ileocecal lymph nodes, and produce an acute mesenteric adenitis, which is generally accompanied by vomiting, abdominal pain, and diarrhea. Fever is usually high and leukocytosis common. At laparotomy the appendix appears normal, but enlarged mesenteric lymph nodes and inflammation of the terminal ileum may be seen. Complications appear in adults less commonly than with *Y. enterocolitica* but include arthritis, erythema nodosum, and septicemia.

DIAGNOSIS *Y. enterocolitica* and *Y. pseudotuberculosis* cause similar signs and symptoms but may have different reservoirs; the first is characterized primarily by diarrhea and the second by mesenteric adenitis. Therefore *Y. enterocolitica* causes disease similar to other bacterial diarrheas and must be distinguished from them by microbiologic means. Laboratory detection of the organism depends on special cultural techniques. The diagnosis is made best by isolation of the organism from stool in patients with enteritis, or atypical cases of appendicitis, erythema nodosum, or reactive arthritis. Cultures of the pharyngeal exudate, peritoneal fluid, and other body fluids should be obtained where clinically indicated. Hemagglutination titers peak in 8 to 10 days and remain elevated for 18 months after infection. Cross-reactivity with some *Brucella*, *Salmonella*, and *Vibrio cholerae* antigens occurs. The diagnosis of *Y. pseudotuberculosis* is also made by culture of stool and mesenteric lymph nodes.

THERAPY AND PREVENTION *Y. enterocolitica* organisms are susceptible in vitro to aminoglycosides, chloramphenicol, tetracycline, trimethoprim-sulfamethoxazole, and the third-generation cephalosporins but are generally resistant to the penicillins and first-generation cephalosporins. However, the value of antimicrobial therapy is unclear, because most cases of enteritis are self-limited. Patients with very severe illness or septicemia should be treated, because treatment may shorten both the duration of disease and the shedding of organisms. *Y. pseudotuberculosis* is usually sensitive to ampicillin, tetracycline, choramphenicol, and cephalosporins. No controlled clinical trials demonstrate efficacy of treatment, although patients with septicemic disease should receive ampicillin or tetracycline, because severe infection has a high mortality. Prevention depends on hygienic measures such as careful food handling, availability of clean drinking water, and hand washing to prevent spread within families or other human contacts.

PASTEURELLA MULTOCIDA INFECTION

Pasteurella multocida is a small, aerobic, gram-negative, bipolar-staining coccobacillus, distantly related to *Yersinia* species but differing from them in microbiologic characteristics and clinical disease patterns. Three related species (*P. haemolytica, P. pneumotropica,* and *P. ureae*) cause occasional disease in human beings. All grow well on routine media (but not MacConkey's agar), possess endotoxin, and are sensitive to penicillins, late-generation cephalosporins, tetracyclines, and chloramphenicol, but are variably resistant to aminoglycosides and erythromycin. *P. multocida* is a member of the normal flora of the digestive and respiratory tract of many wild and domestic mammals and birds; carriage in dogs and cats ranges from 50 to 90 percent.

The organism causes septicemia and pneumonia in domestic animals and most frequently results in human infections following animal bites or scratches, especially of cats and dogs. Skin wound infections typically develop rapidly (1 to 2 days) with severe pain, fever, suppuration, and surrounding cellulitis and adenitis. Complications include abscess formation, tendonitis, osteomyelitis, and septic arthritis. Pulmonary infections are next most common, and consist of pneumonia, acute and chronic bronchitis, and sinusitis. Infections occur in those with underlying respiratory disease and may not be associated with animal contact. Bacteremia may accompany pulmonary infection but may also originate from or accompany abdominal abscesses, meningitis, endocarditis, and genitourinary infection.

The diagnosis should be suspected following animal bites. Neither wound nor other organ site infections are clinically unique, often resembling infection due to staphylococci, streptococci, or cat-scratch fever. The diagnosis should be confirmed by laboratory identification of *Pasteurella* species. Therapy of infection with parenteral penicillin or tetracycline is usually effective, but the value of prophylaxis of bite wounds has not been proved.

REFERENCES

Plague

BARNES AM, POLAND JD: Plague in the United States, 1983, Centers for Disease Control Surveillance Summaries, Publication 33 (no 1SS), 1984

BUTLER T: A clinical study of bubonic plague: Observations on the 1970 Vietnam epidemic with emphasis on coagulation studies, skin histology, and electrocardiograms. Am J Med 53:268, 1972

KAUFMAN AF et al: Public health implications of plague in domestic cats. Am J Vet Assoc 179:875, 1981

REED WP et al: Bubonic plague in the Southwestern United States—A review of recent experience. Medicine 49:465, 1970

TOMICH PQ et al: Evidence for the extinction of plague in Hawaii. Am J Epidemiol 119: 261, 1984

P. multocida

WEBER DJ et al: *Pasteurella multocida* infections. Report of 34 cases and review of the literature. Medicine 63:133, 1984

Yersinia

BOYCE JM: *Yersinia* species, in *Principles and Practice of Infectious Diseases*, 2d ed, GL Mandell, et al (eds). New York, Wiley, 1985, pp 1296–1301

BRUBAKER RR: The Vwa+ virulence factor of yersiniae: The molecular basis of the attendant nutritional requirement for Ca++. Rev Infect Dis 5(Suppl 4):S748, 1983

TACKET CO et al: *Yersinia enterocolitica* pharyngitis. Ann Intern Med 99:40, 1983

TERTTI R et al: An outbreak of *Yersinia pseudotuberculosis* infection. J Infect Dis 149:245, 1984

115 CHOLERA

CHARLES C. J. CARPENTER

DEFINITION Cholera is an acute illness which results from colonization of the small intestine by *Vibrio cholerae*. The disease is characterized by its epidemic occurrence and the production in the more severe cases of massive diarrhea with rapid depletion of extracellular fluid and electrolytes.

ETIOLOGY AND EPIDEMIOLOGY *Vibrio cholerae* is a curved, aerobic, gram-negative bacillus with a single polar flagellum. It is rapidly motile and possesses both O and H antigens. Serologic identification is based on differences in the polysaccharide O antigens.

Cholera has been endemic for a century and a half in the Gangetic Delta of West Bengal and Bangladesh and is often epidemic throughout south and southeast Asia. The seventh and most recent pandemic spread of this disease, from 1961 to 1981, extended from the Celebes northward to Korea and westward to the whole of Africa and southern Europe. The last major epidemic of cholera in the western hemisphere occurred from 1866 to 1867. However, since 1978, over 40 persons have developed cholera, serotype Inaba, in coastal Texas or Louisiana. Sporadic cases have occurred after ingestion of inadequately cooked seafood caught in lakes or coastal Gulf waters of Louisiana, and one large (14 cases) common-source outbreak resulted from contamination of drinking water on a Gulf Coast oil rig. Only one other documented case of cholera has been acquired in any other western hemisphere country since 1900.

The majority of epidemics have clearly been waterborne, but direct contamination of food by infected feces also contributes to spread within affected households. Poor sanitation is primarily responsible for the continuing presence of cholera, but host factors, such as relative or absolute achlorhydria, also play an important role in the susceptibility of the individual to infection. In endemic areas, cholera is predominantly a disease of children; in rural Bangladesh, attack rates are 10 times greater in the 1- to 5-year-old age group than in those above 14 years of age. However, when the disease spreads to previously uninvolved areas, the attack rates are initially at least as high in adults as in children.

A chronic gallbladder carrier state has been observed in a small percentage of elderly convalescent cholera patients. The basis for the annual cholera epidemics throughout the Gangetic Delta, for the periodic outbreaks throughout the remainder of south and southeast Asia, and for the occasional global pandemics is, however, not known.

PATHOGENESIS *Vibrio cholerae* produce a protein enterotoxin which is responsible for all known pathophysiologic aberrations in cholera. This enterotoxin, which has a molecular weight of 84,000, stimulates adenylate cyclase in the intestine epithelial cells, and the resultant increase in intracellular cyclic adenosine $3',5'$-monophosphate leads to secretion of isotonic fluid by all segments of the small intestine. The enterotoxin-induced electrolyte secretion occurs in the absence of any demonstrable damage to intestine epithelial cells or to the capillary endothelial cells of the lamina propria. The stool of the adult cholera patient is nearly isotonic, with sodium and chloride concentrations slightly less than those of plasma, a bicarbonate concentration approximately twice that of plasma, and a potassium concentration three to five times that of plasma. The pathophysiologic defect in cholera is extracellular fluid depletion with resultant hypovolemic shock, base-deficit acidosis, and progressive potassium depletion. *Vibrio cholerae* does not invade the gut wall, nor has the enterotoxin been shown, in human disease, to have any direct effect on any organ other than the small intestine.

MANIFESTATIONS The incubation period generally lasts from 12 to 48 h. This is followed by the abrupt onset of watery, generally painless diarrhea. In the more severe cases, the initial diarrheal stool may be in excess of 1000 mL, and several liters of isotonic fluid may be lost within hours, leading rapidly to profound shock. Vomiting generally follows, but occasionally precedes, the onset of diarrhea; the vomiting is characteristically effortless and not preceded by nausea. As saline depletion progresses, severe muscle cramps, commonly involving the calves, occur.

When first seen, the typical severely ill cholera patient is cyanotic, with pinched facies, scaphoid abdomen, poor skin turgor, and thready or absent peripheral pulses. The voice is faint, high-pitched, and often inaudible, and there are tachycardia, hypotension, and varying degrees of tachypnea. In all epidemics there are many subclinical or mild cases in which gastrointestinal fluid loss is not severe enough to require hospitalization. With the *el tor* strain of *V. cholerae*, which has been responsible for the most recent pandemic, the ratio of subclinical infections to clinical cholera cases is greater than 10:1.

The disease runs its course in 2 to 7 days, and subsequent manifestations depend on the adequacy of electrolyte repletion therapy. With prompt fluid and electrolyte repletion, physiologic recovery is remarkably rapid, and mortality exceptionally rare. The important causes of death, in inadequately treated patients, are hypovolemic shock, metabolic acidosis, and uremia resulting from acute tubular necrosis.

LABORATORY FINDINGS In epidemics or in endemic areas, the clinical picture should arouse strong suspicion immediately. The most reliable technique for identification of *V. cholerae* consists of direct plating of a sample of cholera stool on bile salt, gelatin-tellurite-taurocholate (GTT), or thiosulfate–citrate–bile salt–sucrose (TCBS) agar. On bile salt or GTT agar the organisms appear as typical translucent colonies within 24 h. On TCBS agar, *V. cholerae* appear at 24 h as distinct, large, flat yellow colonies. Further classification requires agglutination with type-specific antiserums. In mild or convalescent cases, recovery of vibrios may be enhanced by initial enrichment for 6 h in alkaline peptone water followed by subculture on bile salt, GTT, or TCBS agar. Rapid presumptive diagnosis is possible either by directly observing immobilization of vibrios by type-specific antiserums, by using dark-field or phase microscopy, or by identifying the organisms with immunofluorescent methods.

TREATMENT Successful therapy requires only prompt and adequate replacement of gastrointestinal losses of saline and alkali. A uniformly satisfactory solution for intravenous fluid therapy can be simply prepared by the addition of 5 g sodium chloride, 4 g sodium bicarbonate, and 1 g potassium chloride to 1 liter of pyrogen-free distilled water. If commercially prepared fluids are available, lactated Ringer's solution is generally satisfactory. The intravenous fluids are initially infused at 50 to 100 mL/min, until a strong pulse has been restored. The same fluids should subsequently be infused in quantities equal to the gastrointestinal losses. If losses cannot be measured accurately, intravenous fluids should be given at a rate sufficient to maintain a normal radial pulse and normal skin turgor. Overhydration can be avoided by careful observation of neck venous filling and auscultation of the lungs. Close observation is mandatory during the acute phase of the illness, because the cholera patient can lose as much as 1 liter of isotonic fluid per hour during the first 24 h of the disease. Inadequate or delayed restoration of fecal fluid losses may result in a high incidence of acute renal failure. Serious hypokalemic symptoms are rare in adults, and potassium repletion can be carried out orally if potassium-containing intravenous fluids are not available. Hypokalemia may contribute significantly, however, to the morbidity

in inadequately treated pediatric patients, and potassium, 10 to 13 meq per liter, should be included in the intravenous fluids administered to children.

Although adequate intravenous saline and alkali repletion alone results in rapid recovery of virtually all cholera patients, a dramatic reduction in the duration and volume of the diarrhea and early eradication of vibrios from the stool may be effected by antibiotic therapy. Oral tetracycline, 500 mg every 6 h for the first 48 h of treatment, has been most successful. Other antibiotics, including chloramphenicol and furazolidone, are also of value, but both appear to be slightly less effective than tetracycline.

Oral therapy Since the cholera enterotoxin does not alter glucose-facilitated sodium absorption, fluid repletion can be effected by the oral administration of glucose-containing electrolyte solutions. Since the limiting factor in treatment of cholera in both epidemic and endemic situations is often the lack of adequate quantities of intravenous fluids, the availability of an oral treatment regimen has greatly reduced the mortality from cholera outbreaks during the most recent pandemic. An oral rehydration solution (ORS) containing glucose 20 g per liter (or sucrose 40 g per liter), sodium bicarbonate 2.5 g per liter, sodium chloride 3.5 g per liter, and potassium chloride 1.5 g per liter can be readily prepared and should be satisfactory for treatment of all age groups. Roughly, 41 million packets of the salts contained in ORS were distributed by the World Health Organization to a total of 87 countries in 1981 and 1982. ORS, administered orally at a rate equal to the stool losses, can be given to patients with milder cholera throughout the course of illness and is also satisfactory in the more severe cases, once the hypovolemic shock has been corrected by intravenous fluid therapy. Oral therapy does not decrease the rate of intestinal fluid loss but provides an electrolyte solution which can be absorbed at a rate sufficient, in most cases, to counterbalance the continuing fluid losses. Therefore, successful management of the cholera patient with oral therapy requires just as close supervision, with careful monitoring of pulse volume, skin turgor, and neck veins, as does management with intravenous solutions. Supplemental intravenous fluids must be administered whenever clinical signs of saline depletion recur.

PROGNOSIS Under ideal conditions and with prompt and adequate fluid replacement, mortality approaches zero, and significant sequelae are rare. Unfortunately, death rates as high as 60 percent still occur, especially during the initial phases of outbreaks. This high mortality reflects lack of pyrogen-free intravenous fluids in remote areas, the difficulties of initiating treatment promptly when large numbers of cases are occurring in poverty-striken populations, and the compromises which may have to be made under emergency conditions.

PREVENTION Immunization by standard commercial vaccine, containing 10 billion killed organisms per milliliter, provides only limited (40 to 60 percent) protection for a relatively short (4- to 6-month) period in endemic areas. Vaccination, therefore, is not recommended for Americans who are traveling abroad. Careful hygiene provides the only sure protection against cholera.

REFERENCES

CARPENTER CCJ et al: Clinical studies in Asiatic cholera, I–VI. Bull Johns Hopkins Hosp 118:165, 1966

FISHMAN PH: Mechanism of action of cholera toxin: Events on the cell surface, in *Secretory Diarrhea*, M Field *et al* (eds). Bethesda, American Physiological Society, 1980, pp 85–106

GANGAROSA EF et al: The nature of the gastrointestinal lesion in Asiatic cholera and its relation to pathogenesis: A biopsy study. Am J Trop Med Hyg 9:125, 1960

HIRSCHHORN N et al: The treatment of cholera, in *Cholera*, D Barua, W Burrows (eds). Philadelphia, Saunders, 1974, p 235

JOHNSON JM et al: Cholera on a Gulf Coast oil rig. N Engl J Med 309:523, 1983

MAHALANOBIS D et al: Oral fluid therapy of cholera among Bangladesh refugees. Johns Hopkins Med J 132:197, 1973

MORRIS JG JR et al: Non-O group 1 *Vibrio cholerae* gastroenteritis in the United States: Clinical, epidemiologic, and laboratory characteristics of sporadic cases. Ann Intern Med 94:656, 1981

116 BARTONELLOSIS

JAMES J. PLORDE

DEFINITION Bartonellosis (Carrión's disease) is an infection with *Bartonella bacilliformis*. Two well-defined clinical stages occur: an acute febrile anemia of rapid onset and high mortality, designated *Oroya fever*, and a benign eruptive form with chronic cutaneous lesions, called *verruga peruana*. Either of these types may be mild, and asymptomatic cases constitute the greatest epidemiologic hazard.

ETIOLOGY *Bartonella bacilliformis* is a small, motile, aerobic, pleomorphic, gram-negative coccobacillus which stains reddish violet with Giemsa's stain. It can be cultured on enriched media and does not produce a hemolysin. The organisms are sensitive to several antibiotics in vitro.

EPIDEMIOLOGY The disease is limited to certain valleys in the Andes Mountains comprising parts of Peru, Ecuador, and Colombia. It occurs in regions between the altitudes of 2400 and 8000 ft where the phlebotomine sandfly vector, *Lutzomyia*, propagates. Although *L. verrucarum* is the principal vector of the disease, other species are involved in Colombia as well. Asymptomatic cases and convalescent carriers are the only known reservoir of infection. A low-grade bacteremia may persist for years following resolution of symptoms, and *B. bacilliformis* can be recovered from the blood of 5 to 10 percent of the apparently normal population in an endemic area. Epidemics often coincide with immigration of workers from uninfected areas.

PATHOLOGY AND PATHOGENESIS The manifestations of the disease are thought to reflect the immune status of the host. In nonimmune individuals Oroya fever develops. Large numbers of the *Bartonella* bacteria enter the bloodstream, adhere to erythrocytes, and invade the endothelial cells of the capillaries and lymphatics where they multiply. Subsequent invasion and multiplication within erythrocytes results in their phagocytosis and destruction by the liver and spleen. The red blood cell life span is greatly shortened, and anemia develops. This is accentuated by a defective erythropoietic response early in the course of infection. The pathogenesis of the hemolytic anemia remains unknown. Agglutinins and hemolysins have not been found, and tests for mechanical fragility of red blood cells have given variable results. Invasion and swelling of capillary endothelial cells may lead to vascular occlusion and tissue infarcts. It is possible that an impairment of reticuloendothelial function secondary to massive phagocytosis of red blood cells is responsible for the frequency with which *Salmonella* and other coliform bacteremias are seen in Oroya fever.

With developing immunity, the bacteria nearly disappear from the peripheral blood and capillary endothelium. After a latent period they reappear in the skin and subcutaneous tissue where they are apparently responsible for the development of the hemangioid lesions of verruga peruana. Second attacks of Carrión's disease are unusual. When they occur, they almost invariably present as verruga.

CLINICAL MANIFESTATIONS The incubation period is approximately 3 weeks but may be longer. The initial symptoms are fever and pains in the bones, joints, and muscles. At this point the disease often resembles influenza or malaria, but blood cultures are positive. After these prodromes, the patient usually develops one of the two classic forms of the infection.

Oroya fever This form is characterized by sudden onset of high fever, extreme pallor, weakness, and a precipitous drop in the number of red blood cells. The count may fall from normal to 1 million per cubic millimeter within 4 or 5 days. The anemia is characterized by normochromic macrocytes in the peripheral blood, striking polychromasia and polychromatophilia, nucleated red blood cells, Howell-Jolly bodies, Cabot rings, and basophilic stippling. There may also be a mild leukocytosis with a shift to the left. Organisms are numerous in the blood, and stained smears may show 90 percent of the erythrocytes heavily invaded. Salmonellosis, malaria, amebiasis, tuberculosis, and other intercurrent infections may occur and are an important factor in fatal cases.

Muscle and joint pain and headache are severe, and insomnia, delirium, and coma are the terminal manifestations. In untreated patients, the mortality rate may exceed 50 percent; death occurs within 10 days to 4 weeks. With treatment, or sometimes spontaneously, recovery results if the organisms decrease and fever abates. The red blood cell count stabilizes and approaches normal values in about 6 weeks, when convalescence begins.

Verruga peruana This form of the disease, characterized by a profuse skin eruption, may follow the anemic form or may occur in patients without previous symptoms. The verrugas vary in color from red to purple. They may be miliary, nodular, or eroding, and they range in size from 2 to 10 mm up to 3 or 4 cm in diameter. The three types of verruga may occur together; since eruption takes place in successive crops, verrugas of all types and in all stages of development may be found on the same patient. The chief sites involved are the limbs and face, and less frequently the genitalia, scalp, and mucosa of the mouth and pharynx. They may persist for 1 month to 2 years. The eruption is accompanied by pain, fever, and moderate anemia. Bartonellas may be demonstrated in the lesions and cultured from the blood.

DIAGNOSIS A clinical diagnosis of verruga peruana can be made with accuracy in endemic areas. It is confirmed by demonstrating the Giemsa-stained organism in biopsy specimens from representative lesions. During Oroya fever the organism is easily seen on peripheral blood smears. It may be recovered from blood cultures in all stages of the disease.

TREATMENT Oroya fever responds dramatically to a number of antibiotics including tetracycline and chloramphenicol. The latter in a dose of 2 g per day for 7 days is often preferred because of the frequency with which *Salmonella* infections complicate this disease. Fever disappears within 48 h, and the patient recovers rapidly. Transfusions may be required when the anemia is severe. Antibiotic therapy of the verrugal stage may hasten the involution of these lesions. The use of DDT in both the interior and exterior of human dwellings is highly effective in controlling the night-biting sandflies. Insect repellents and bed netting afford personal protection.

REFERENCES

CAUDRA MC: Salmonellosis complication in human bartonellosis. Tex Rep Biol Med 14:97, 1956
DOOLEY JR: Haemotropic bacteria in man. Lancet 2:1237, 1980
KAYE D et al: Factors influencing host resistance to *Salmonella* infections: The effects of hemolysis and erythrophagocytosis. Am J Med Sci 254:205, 1967
RICKETTS WE: Clinical manifestations of Carrión's disease. AMA Arch Intern Med 84:751, 1949
SCHULTZ MG: Daniel Carrión's experiment. N Engl J Med 278:1323, 1968

117 LEGIONELLA INFECTIONS

HARRY N. BEATY / A. WILLIAM PASCULLE

DEFINITION *Legionella* infections are acute respiratory infections caused by species of bacteria within the genus *Legionella*. The type species of the genus is *L. pneumophila*, and Legionnaires' disease, the common name for pneumonia caused by this bacterium, is still the prototype for infections with this group of organisms. Collectively, these infections often are referred to as legionellosis. While the various species within the genus *Legionella* are quite distinctive microbiologically, multiple characteristics of the various forms of legionellosis differ inconsequentially from those of Legionnaires' disease and other clinical expressions of *L. pneumophila* infection. Therefore, much of what is known concerning legionellosis is derived, sometimes by inference, from what has been learned about Legionnaires' disease.

HISTORY In July of 1976, an explosive outbreak of severe respiratory illness occurred in Philadelphia—chiefly among delegates of an American Legion Convention. Initial investigation failed to document a familiar infective or toxic etiology, and so a comprehensive, coordinated effort was undertaken to define the epidemiology and cause of the outbreak. As the ensuing saga unfolded, it became apparent that at least 220 cases of pneumonia—34 of which were fatal—resulted from a common source of airborne infection that was present for several days inside and in the immediate vicinity outside one of the convention hotels. The infective agent was proved to be a previously unknown gram-negative bacterium that ultimately was named *Legionella pneumophila.*

Using serologic techniques, it has been shown that the same organism, or antigenically related species, has caused other outbreaks of respiratory illness. One of these occurred among attendees at a convention of Oddfellows, which took place in 1974 at the same Philadelphia hotel that was involved in the outbreak of Legionnaires' disease. The organism also was found to be responsible for nosocomial infections when an outbreak of pneumonia that occurred in 1965 in a psychiatric hospital in Washington, D.C., and involved 81 patients with 14 fatalities was retrospectively attributed to *L. pneumophila* infection. The earliest outbreak of Legionnaires' disease that has been identified occurred in 1957 among employees of a meat packing plant in Austin, Minnesota. Seventy-eight persons were infected, and there were two fatalities.

A second form of disease due to *L. pneumophila* was recognized when it was shown that a brisk epidemic of nonpneumonic, influenza-like illness that occurred in 1968 among employees and visitors of the county health department building in Pontiac, Michigan, had been caused by *L. pneumophila.*

The use of techniques developed for the isolation and characterization of *L. pneumophila* resulted in the subsequent recognition of several closely related organisms, some of which caused human disease. In 1978 and 1979 two outbreaks of nosocomial pneumonia among patients in hospitals in Pittsburgh, Pennsylvania, and Charlottesville, Virginia, were attributed to an organism that was isolated initially by the Pittsburgh workers from the lung tissue of one patient. This "Pittsburgh pneumonia agent," as it was first called, ultimately was shown to be phenotypically similar to but genetically distinct from *L. pneumophila* and was named *Legionella micdadei* in honor of Joseph McDade who first isolated *L. pneumophila.*

Subsequently, a linkage was established between a group of rickettsia-like bacteria first isolated decades ago and the newly recognized genus, *Legionella.* Many of these isolates resembled *L. pneumophila* phenotypically, but were "atypical" antigenically and genetically. Initially these organisms were referred to as "atypical *Legionella*-like organisms'" (ALLO), but all are now recognized species in the genus. Currently there are 22 distinct species of *Legionella* consisting of 35 antigenically different organisms (Table 117-1).

ETIOLOGY The legionellae are gram-negative aerobic rods that do not grow on commonly used bacteriologic media. In clinical specimens, the bacteria appear as 0.5-μm rods while organisms from artificial media may be highly pleomorphic and even include filamentous forms many times longer. Most species are motile and contain one or two polar flagella that appear to be antigenically identical among all the species.

Legionellae have complex growth and pH requirements. The medium of choice for their isolation from clinical specimens is buffered charcoal yeast extract agar supplemented with alpha-ketoglutarate (BCYE-alpha). BCYE agar is a very rich culture medium and is in no way selective for legionellae. Many common bacterial species, including *Francisella tularensis,* are capable of growth on this medium as are many fungi, such as *Coccidioides immitis.* The addition of cefamandole, polymyxin, and anisomycin to BCYE-alpha results in a semiselective medium which can be used for the isolation of at least some *Legionella* species from normally contaminated clinical specimens such as sputum. Biochemically, the legionellae do not appear highly diverse and cannot be identified by metabolic testing. When only a few species were known, the legionellae could be rapidly classified by serologic testing with antibody conjugates prepared against the known species. Serologic cross reactions among the first ten species identified were very minor and did not interfere with the production of relatively specific reagents. Several of the recently recognized species, however, cross-react significantly with other species, and specific antisera are not yet available for serologic identification of all *Legionella* species.

At the present time, the definitive identification of an isolate at the species level requires DNA homology studies. It is on the basis of these determinations that the legionellae have been divided into the 22 currently recognized species. Their classification in the genus *Legionella* is based upon their phenotypic similarity.

ECOLOGY AND EPIDEMIOLOGY Legionellosis occurs worldwide, and the legionellae are ubiquitous microorganisms that appear to be part of the natural microbial community of many natural and artificial aquatic ecosystems. They have been isolated from a variety of moist habitats ranging from alpine lakes to the hot springs of Yellowstone National Park.

The ecologic niche of these organisms that has the most direct clinical importance is the warm moist areas of the mechanical systems of large buildings, particularly hotels and hospitals. Legionellae have been found in the evaporative coolers of large air conditioning systems, and aerosols from these cooling towers can carry the organisms significant distances before they are inhaled by a susceptible host. The outbreak of Legionnaires' disease in Philadelphia and of Pontiac fever in Michigan almost certainly arose from contaminated air conditioning systems. Air handling equipment also has been incriminated as a source of nosocomial outbreaks of Legionnaires' disease in Burlington, Vermont, and Memphis, Tennessee, to name only a few.

Potable water distribution systems are a frequent source of these bacteria, particularly in association with nosocomial legionellosis. Overwhelming evidence indicates that the legionellae can thrive in

TABLE 117-1 Recognized species and serotypes of *Legionella*

Organism	Number of serotypes	Human isolation	Environmental isolation
L. pneumophila	10	Yes	Yes
L. micdadei	1	Yes	Yes
L. bozemanii	2	Yes	Yes
L. dumoffii	1	Yes	Yes
L. gormanii	1	Yes	Yes
L. feeleii	2	Yes	Yes
L. longbeacheae	2	Yes	Yes
L. jordanis	1	Yes	Yes
L. oakridgensis	1	Yes	Yes
L. wadsworthii	1	Yes	Yes
L. hackeliae	1	Yes	No
L. maceachernii	2	Yes	Yes
L. sainthelensi	1	No	Yes
L. spiritensis	1	No	Yes
L. jamestownensis	1	No	Yes
L. santicrucis	1	No	Yes
L. anisa	1	No	Yes
L. cherrii	1	No	Yes
L. steigerwaltii	1	No	Yes
L. paresiensis	1	No	Yes
L. rubrilucens	1	No	Yes
L. erythra	1	No	Yes

the hot water distribution system of some buildings. Organisms live and multiply in the sludge of hot water tanks in association with other bacterial species. From there, the organisms can be disseminated throughout the plumbing systems in hospitals, hotels, and even a small number of private homes. Water passing through contaminated fixtures such as shower heads and faucet valves produces an effective aerosol of bacteria.

Medical devices utilizing unsterilized tap water also can become contaminated with legionellae. For example, *L. micdadei* has been isolated from an ultrasonic nebulizer and from room humidifiers. Outbreaks also have been linked to contaminated whirlpools and hot tubs.

The mere presence of legionellae in a water distribution system does not always predict the presence of disease among those potentially exposed. The reasons for this are not yet understood, but one intriguing hypothesis is that not all *Legionella* strains are equally virulent. Virulence, in turn, may be related to the presence of a plasmid.

Infection appears to be acquired by the respiratory route. In the case of Legionnaires' disease, the usual incubation period is 2 to 10 days. While organisms have been identified in the sputum of patients with Legionnaires' disease, person-to-person spread has not been documented. Common-source outbreaks have received the greatest public attention, but hundreds of sporadic cases of legionellosis occur each year. Incidence may increase in the summer and early fall, but these infections occur year-round.

Although Legionnaires' disease has been reported in children, most patients with legionellosis are middle-aged or older. Cigarette smokers and individuals with serious underlying diseases such as chronic renal failure, malignancy, and immunosuppression have increased susceptibility to infection. The mortality rate of Legionnaires' pneumonia that is serious enough to require hospitalization is around 15 percent; among immunocompromised patients it may exceed 50 percent.

Serologic surveys using the indirect fluorescent-antibody technique have shown that less than 5 percent of healthy individuals from around the United States have reciprocal antibody titers to *L. pneumophila* of 128 or higher. However, some more geographically restricted surveys have shown that 15 to 25 percent of the population has similar serologic evidence of significant exposure to *L. pneumophila* or antigenically related organisms. This suggests that the infection may be endemic in some regions.

PATHOLOGY AND PATHOGENESIS Most pathologic features ascribable directly to infection with legionellae are limited to the lungs. Those associated with Legionnaires' disease have been studied most extensively and are representative of changes seen in infections with other organisms in the genus. Apparent lobar involvement almost always represents confluent bronchopneumonia. Prominent microscopic features include extensive exudation of proteinaceous fluid and inflammatory cells into the alveoli. In most cases, the cellular component of the exudate is a mixture of polymorphonuclear neutrophils and macrophages. Extensive lysis of inflammatory cells, with accumulations of nuclear debris and fibrin, is a distinctive feature of this pneumonia. Alveolar septa usually are edematous and infiltrated with inflammatory cells; hyaline membranes are seen in about half the cases. Terminal bronchioles are routinely involved, but larger bronchioles and bronchi are unaffected. None of these changes is unique to pulmonary infection with legionellae, but the histopathologic alterations are sufficiently distinctive to suggest the diagnosis.

Bacteria usually can be demonstrated in the inflammatory exudate with the Dieterle stain or by using direct fluorescent-antibody conjugates. Other stains are less reliable although *L. micdadei* may be demonstrated by acid-fast stains of tissue. Many bacilli appear to be intracellular, and an increase in the number of organisms is associated with lysis of inflammatory cells.

Little is known about the pathogenesis of legionellosis. The fact that cigarette smokers are more susceptible to infection than non-

smokers suggests that the defective alveolar macrophage function plays a role in the development of disease. Experimental evidence indicates that legionellae can survive and proliferate in normal macrophages and other cells, a characteristic that has important pathogenetic implications. The extensive lysis of inflammatory cells and the edema of the interstitium raise the possibility that a toxin is produced by the infecting organism. Such a toxin might be responsible for some of the clinical features seen with this infection.

CLINICAL MANIFESTATIONS The total spectrum of clinical manifestations of legionellosis is not known. Mild respiratory illness has been recognized, but asymptomatic infection has not been excluded as a possible explanation for elevated antibody titers among healthy individuals. The outbreak in Pontiac, Michigan, was characterized by the acute onset and short duration of a moderately severe influenza-like syndrome of fever, myalgia, and headache. Legionellosis with this presentation is referred to as "Pontiac fever" and until an outbreak associated with *L. feeleii* was described, was thought to be caused exclusively by *L. pneumophila* infection.

The more typical patient with legionellosis has pneumonia that is severe enough to require hospitalization. No clinical features distinguish between infections caused by the different species of *Legionella* or between legionellosis and other forms of pneumonia. The most characteristic patients with Legionnaires' disease have malaise and a slight headache, which precedes a rapidly rising fever by less than a day. Within 24 to 48 h, temperatures reach 40°C in about half the patients, and shaking chills are common. A modest, nonproductive cough frequently is present early; it progresses in severity over the first few days of illness and usually becomes productive of variable amounts of mucoid to mucopurulent sputum. Minimal hemoptysis is seen in about 20 percent of patients. Additional symptoms that occur less frequently include dyspnea, pleuritic chest pain, and myalgia. About 25 percent of patients have various combinations of gastrointestinal symptoms which include nausea and vomiting, diarrhea, and abdominal pain. In a few patients, these manifestations predominate despite the presence of pneumonia. In some individuals, the onset of legionellosis is more protracted and the clinical expression less distinctive. These cases are likely to be missed unless the epidemiologic setting or subtle clinical clues stimulate physicians to suspect the diagnosis. The findings on physical examination are not specific for legionellosis, and they are affected by patients' associated diseases. High fever, tachypnea, and tachycardia are common. Patients frequently are flushed, mildly diaphoretic, and appear moderately to severely prostrated. Examination of the chest shows moist rales, but signs of consolidation usually are absent. Chest roentgenograms characteristically show more involvement of the lungs than is suspected on clinical grounds.

During the first 4 to 6 days, the disease becomes progressively worse. An additional 4 to 5 days may pass before dramatic clinical improvement begins, even though appropriate antimicrobial therapy is given. The average duration of fever in one large series was 13 days. Clearing of pulmonary infiltrates lags significantly behind improvement of other manifestations of infection, and minor residual scarring is not uncommon. Many patients experience weakness and easy fatigability for weeks after the acute stages of the illness.

The major complication of legionellosis is respiratory failure. Twenty to thirty percent of patients sick enough to require hospitalization have hyperventilation and hypoxemia. In about half of these patients, progression of disease leads to intubation and mechanical ventilation. The mortality rate among patients with respiratory failure is high. Hypotension and shock, with secondary acute renal failure, are additional complications that may be encountered.

LABORATORY FINDINGS Most patients have a modest granulocytosis, or even neutropenia, but about 20 percent have leukocyte counts in excess of 20,000 per cubic millimeter. The erythrocyte sedimentation rate is elevated, and there is moderate proteinuria. Reversible renal insufficiency and mild changes in liver function have been reported, but it is not always possible to attribute these abnormalities to the infection.

Chest roentgenograms show unilateral pulmonary parenchymal infiltrates in about 65 percent of cases early in the illness. By the time of maximal involvement, the pneumonia has progressed to involve both sides in most cases. Nonspecific poorly marginated rounded opacities or diffuse patchy lobar shadows predominate. Small pleural effusions are seen in about a third of cases.

Routine bacteriologic studies including blood and sputum cultures are negative. Lower respiratory tract secretions obtained by transtracheal aspiration or other suitable techniques show many granulocytes and alveolar macrophages but may show no organisms on Gram's stain and are sterile on routine culture media.

DIAGNOSIS The diagnosis of legionellosis is most firmly established by the demonstration of legionellae in the respiratory secretions of patients by either culture or immunofluorescent staining. Since colonization with these organisms is not known to occur, their demonstration in sputum is confirmation of their role in the infection. Culture of respiratory secretions is somewhat more sensitive than immunofluorescent staining for the detection of these organisms. The highest yields have been achieved when samples of respiratory secretions have been collected without contamination by oral flora. Such specimens include transtracheal aspirates, percutaneous fine-needle aspirates, and bronchoalveolar lavages. The sensitivity of culture for these specimens approaches 90 percent because of the lack of interference from contaminating flora.

When expectorated sputum is employed, two factors reduce the sensitivity of cultural techniques. The first is that contaminating microorganisms may inhibit the growth of the legionellae on nonselective media. In addition, selective media contain antimicrobial agents to which several species are sensitive. For instance, *L. micdadei* does not grow well on these media because it is susceptible to cefamandole, and cultures from patients with this infection may be falsely negative.

Immunofluorescent staining is less sensitive than culture. The antigenic diversity of the genus contributes to the difficulty in making diagnoses by immunofluorescent staining because antibody conjugates are routinely available only for *L. pneumophila*, *L. micdadei*, *L. bozemanii*, *L. dumoffii*, *L. gormanii*, and *L. longbeacheae*. While it is true that the great majority of cases of legionellosis are caused by *L. pneumophila*, the possibility that a particular patient's disease may be due to a known but undetected species must be kept in mind when evaluating a negative direct fluorescent antibody (DFA) test. Patients with Legionnaires' disease have been shown to shed antigens of the organism in urine. This antigen(s) is detectable in the urine within the first 3 days of illness, which makes the test potentially useful for rapid diagnosis. This test suffers from the same limitation as other serologic tests that might be used to diagnose all forms of legionellosis, in that a large number of reagents will be required to detect all species and serotypes.

Because of the plethora of antigens that must be employed and the vagaries of the immune response to the legionellae, serologic testing is more of epidemiologic than clinical value.

TREATMENT AND PREVENTION Although in vitro sensitivity tests indicate that a number of antibiotics might be effective in the treatment of Legionnaires' disease, clinical experience has shown that the lowest case-fatality ratio is achieved with erythromycin in a dose of 0.5 to 1 g every 6 h for adults and 15 mg/kg every 6 h for children. Tetracycline is less effective. Rifampin has shown promise in laboratory testing, but its propensity to induce resistance may limit its potential usefulness. Certainly, it should not be used alone. With increasing frequency, the combination of rifampin and erythromycin is being used for critically ill patients. It has not been documented, however, that this combination is more effective than erythromycin alone.

Although the case-fatality ratio of patients treated with erythro-

mycin is low, response to treatment frequently is not dramatic. If therapy is continued for at least 14 days, relapses are uncommon. When they occur, they usually respond to a second course of erythromycin. Because Legionnaires' disease can cause pneumonia in patients not sick enough to be hospitalized and who are assumed to have either *Mycoplasma* infection or early pneumococcal infection, erythromycin should be considered the drug of choice for the treatment of pneumonia in an ambulatory care setting.

There is more to treatment of Legionnaires' disease than administration of antibiotics. High fever, diaphoresis, and tachypnea produce excessive fluid loss, and volume replacement with intravenous fluids may be needed. Hypoxic patients should receive supplemental oxygen.

Prevention of legionellosis depends upon identifying contaminated environmental reservoirs and eradicating the organisms from them. These organisms are so ubiquitous, however, that routine surveillance of the environment is of limited value in the absence of disease. A more productive activity for hospitals is active surveillance, involving both the laboratory and infection control personnel, for *Legionella* infections. Attempts should be made to determine if nosocomial cases cluster in time and space so that environmental samples for culture are collected rationally. All possible contacts, such as respiratory therapy equipment and potable water, must be evaluated epidemiologically to determine their relative contribution to patients' risk of developing nosocomial legionellosis.

PROGNOSIS The overall mortality rate of legionellosis is unknown. Among patients with pneumonia who are sick enough to require hospitalization, the mortality rate is around 15 percent. The presence of complicating associated illnesses may raise that figure two- or threefold. Individuals who recover from pulmonary infection with legionellae usually have no significant residua. It is not known whether they are immune to reinfection with the same or related organisms.

REFERENCES

BERNARDINI DL et al: Neurogenic bladder. New clinical finding in Legionnaires' disease. Am J Med 78:1045, 1985

BRENNER DJ et al: Ten new species of *Legionella*. Int J Sys Bacteriol 35:50, 1985

GARBE PL et al: Nosocomial Legionnaires' disease. Epidemiologic demonstration of cooling towers as a source. JAMA 254:521, 1985

HERWALDT LA et al: A new *Legionella* species, *Legionella feeleii* species nova, causes Pontiac fever in an automobile plant. Ann Intern Med 100:333, 1984

MEYER RD: *Legionella* infections: A review of five years of research. Rev Infect Dis 5:258, 1983

RUDIN JE, WING EJ: A comparative study of *Legionella micdadei* and other nosocomial acquired pneumonia. Chest 86:675, 1984

THORNSBERRY C et al (eds): *Legionella, Proceedings of the 2d International Symposium.* Washington, American Society for Microbiology, 1984

WINN WC JR et al: The pathology of the *Legionella* pneumonias. Human Pathol 12:401, 1981

118 CAT-SCRATCH DISEASE

LAWRENCE COREY

DEFINITION Cat-scratch disease is an infection characterized by indolent, occasionally suppurative, regional lymphadenitis usually occurring following a scratch or a close contact with a cat. A cutaneous lesion at the site of inoculation is often present, and 90 percent of patients report cat scratches or close contact with cats.

ETIOLOGY The etiology of cat-scratch disease remains undefined. Agents incriminated in the past included atypical acid-fast bacteria, *Chlamydia*-like organisms, and viruses. The current candidate is a small, pleomorphic, presumably gram-negative bacillus identified by Warthin-Starry silver impregnation stain in lymph nodes of 25 of 34 patients who fulfilled the clinical and histologic criteria for cat-scratch disease. The organism was identified most frequently in capillary walls and macrophages lining the sinuses or germinal centers, and rarely from areas of suppuration or microabscess formation. The organism has also been identified in biopsies of cutaneous lesions from patients with the disease. A second group of workers isolated a similarly sized organism from a lymph node of a patient with cat-scratch disease. The putative pathogen is pleomorphic and gram-variable on Gram's stain and may be related to the *Rothia* genus of bacteria. This genus commonly is part of the oropharyngeal flora. The organism is sensitive in vitro to penicillin, erythromycin, cotrimoxazole, cephalosporins, and clindamycin. Koch's postulates have not been fulfilled for this organism.

EPIDEMIOLOGY   The disease has been reported in numerous geographic areas; it is most common in fall and winter, and 75 percent of cases occur in children. Reactivity to the skin test antigen is seen in 3 to 20 percent of the population. Persons who have frequent contact with cats, such as veterinarians and family contacts of index cases, have a higher prevalence of past infection as detected by a positive reaction to the skin test antigen. Cats appear to act only as vectors of the disease. The animals are usually not ill and have negative skin tests. Familial occurrence of several infections interspersed by months or years suggests that cats are intermittent or long-term carriers. A compatible syndrome has been described following monkey scratches and injuries due to inanimate objects.

PATHOLOGY   The histopathologic appearance of lymph nodes is not specific. Three stages have been described: (1) early lesions show reticulum-cell hyperplasia; (2) intermediate lesions show granuloma formation; and (3) late lesions show microabscesses. These histologic changes are similar to those seen with atypical mycobacterial infections, lymphogranuloma venereum, toxoplasmosis, sarcoidosis, brucellosis, tularemia, and even Hodgkin's disease.

MANIFESTATIONS   The incubation period ranges from 3 days to several weeks, usually 3 to 10 days. In a typical case, a primary lesion consisting of a raised, slightly tender, nonpruritic papule. The papule may progress through a small vesicle or eschar over a 2- to 3-day period. Multiple primary lesions have been described. The lesion is often felt to be an insect bite and usually does not cause the patient to present to the physician. In about 40 percent of cases no primary lesion is present, and in some patients no history of inciting trauma is elicited.

Regional lymphadenopathy becomes evident in a few days or as long as 6 weeks after infection. Adenopathy is usually confined to a single region and is usually unilateral and asymmetric; in most instances only one node is involved. The axillary, cervical, preauricular, submandibular, inguinal, femoral, or epitrochlear nodes (in decreasing order of frequency) on one side become visibly swollen and tender, often with redness of the overlying skin. The nodes occasionally suppurate, soften, and drain spontaneously; fistulas heal completely with only slight scarring. Usually the tenderness subsides gradually, and nontender, firm, enlarged nodes remain palpable for some weeks or even months. With rare exceptions, there is no generalized glandular enlargement, and the spleen is not palpable.

Systemic symptoms are usually mild and consist of headache, fever, and malaise, which subside within a few days. Shaking chills and fever with temperatures as high as 104°F can occur but are unusual. Many patients are entirely symptom-free. During the early stages of illness a transient macular or vesicular rash which subsides within 48 h may occur. Erythema nodosum and multiforme and thrombocytopenic purpura have also been reported.

Other clinical forms of this disease include: (1) encephalitis characterized by fever, convulsions, alterations in consciousness, mild cerebrospinal fluid pleocytosis, and elevation in protein (this usually resolves with complete recovery); (2) Parinaud's oculoglandular syndrome characterized by granulomatous conjunctivitis and enlargement of the homolateral preauricular node; (3) mesenteric lymphadenitis; (4) osteolytic bone lesions, which subside spontaneously; and (5) thrombocytopenic and nonthrombocytopenic purpura. In all these syndromes the diagnostic criteria for cat-scratch disease must be present before the illness can be ascribed to this disease.

DIAGNOSIS   The following criteria should be fulfilled before a diagnosis of cat-scratch disease is established: (1) history of contact with cats, (2) presence of a primary lesion, (3) regional lymphadenopathy, (4) positive intradermal skin test, (5) biopsy of lymph node with demonstration of histopathologic changes consistent with cat-scratch disease (this may not be necessary if the skin test is positive), (6) demonstration of the presumptive causative bacillus from the primary lesion or lymph node, and (7) failure to demonstrate other causative agents.

The specific diagnosis is made by means of a skin test. In the United States standardized skin test antigen is not commercially available. Antigen for skin tests is prepared by mixing one part pus aspirated from infected lymph nodes with three parts saline solution and inactivating the mixture by heating or by irradiation. A positive reaction is of the delayed tuberculin type, consisting of 5 mm induration and 10 mm erythema, that appears in 24 to 48 h. Although batches of antigen vary in potency, in general patients reacting to one batch react to another. Skin test material can be preserved by freezing. The test becomes positive within 30 days after infection and may persist for many years. Each batch of antigen must be tested against patients known to have had the disease. False-negative reactions have been reported. Approximately 5 percent of normal individuals will have positive reactions.

Other laboratory abnormalities include mild leukocytosis (up to 15,000 cells per cubic millimeter), occasional mild eosinophilia, and an elevated sedimentation rate.

Cat-scratch disease is a benign illness, and the prognosis is uniformly good. Its main clinical importance lies in its possible confusion with other, more serious diseases of the lymphatics. Diseases to be considered are tularemia, lymphatic tuberculosis, sporotrichosis, histoplasmosis, coccidioidomycosis, toxoplasmosis, and bacterial adenitis. Because of the indolent character of the adenopathy, Hodgkin's disease or other lymphomas may be suspected. Cat-scratch disease must be differentiated from tularemia, which occasionally can be transmitted by cats. Neck masses may be confused with thyroglossal duct cysts, cleft cysts, dermoids, cystic hygromas, thyroid and parathyroid adenomas, salivary gland tumors, carotid body tumors, aneurysms, pharyngeal or esophageal diverticula, and mesodermal tumors, as well as lymphomas. Appropriate serologic and cultural tests serve to rule out other infections; biopsy may be needed to exclude tumor. A positive skin test with cat-scratch antigen may obviate the necessity for biopsy.

TREATMENT   The disease is self-limited and symptoms resolve spontaneously in 1 to 2 months. Occasionally aspiration of suppurative nodes affords relief of pain. Antibiotics and steroids are ineffective.

REFERENCES

CARITHERS HA et al: Cat-scratch disease; its natural history. An overview based on a study of 1200 patients. Am J Dis Child 135:1124, 1985
————: Cat-scratch skin test antigen: Purification by heating. Pediatrics 60:928, 1977
ELLIOT DL et al: Pet-associated illness. N Engl J Med 313:985, 1985
GERBER MA et al: The aetiological agent of cat-scratch disease. Lancet 1:1236, 1985
LYON LW: Neurologic manifestations of cat-scratch disease. Arch Neurol 25:23, 1971
MARGILETH AM: Cat-scratch disease: Bacteria in skin at the primary inoculation site. JAMA 252:928, 1984
————, MARCY SM: Cat-scratch disease: Safety of cat-scratch skin test material. Pediatr Infect Dis 3:281, 1984
WEAR DJ et al: Cat-scratch disease: A bacterial infection. Science 221:1403, 1983

section 4 Mycobacterial diseases

119 TUBERCULOSIS

THOMAS M. DANIEL

DEFINITION Tuberculosis is a chronic bacterial infection caused by *Mycobacterium tuberculosis* and characterized by the formation of granulomas in infected tissues and by florid cell-mediated hypersensitivity. The usual site of disease is the lungs, but other organs may be involved. In the absence of effective treatment, a chronic wasting course is usual and death ultimately supervenes in most cases.

ETIOLOGY *Mycobacterium tuberculosis*, the tubercle bacillus, is one of more than 30 well-characterized and many unclassified members of the genus *Mycobacterium*. Along with the closely related *M. bovis*, it causes tuberculosis. *M. leprae* is the etiologic agent of leprosy (Chap. 120), and a number of other mycobacterial species produce less common human diseases (Chap. 121). Most mycobacteria are not pathogenic for human beings, and many are readily isolated from environmental sources.

Mycobacteria are distinguished by their surface lipids which render them acid-fast. That is, these organisms cannot be decolorized with acid alcohol after staining. Because of this lipid, heat or detergents are usually necessary to accomplish primary staining.

Important to understanding the pathogenesis of tuberculosis is recognition that *M. tuberculosis* contains many immunoreactive substances. Surface lipids of mycobacteria and water-soluble components of cell wall peptidoglycan are important adjuvants that may exert their effects through their primary actions on host macrophages. *M. tuberculosis* survives the intracellular milieu of macrophages, and this intracellular persistence may be facilitated by cell wall lipids which inhibit phagosome-lysosome fusion. Mycobacteria contain an array of protein and polysaccharide antigens, some probably species-specific but others clearly sharing their antigenicity broadly throughout the genus. Tuberculous infection results in the presentation of antigens to the host in the presence of adjuvants; cell-mediated hypersensitivity is characteristic of tuberculosis and is an important determinant of the disease's pathogenesis.

EPIDEMIOLOGY There is little doubt that tuberculous disease was widely prevalent in ancient times. Tuberculosis was portrayed by European physicians and lay writers of the eighteenth and nineteenth centuries, and early public health data indicate that as many as one-quarter to one-third of all deaths in European cities in the mid-nineteenth century may have been due to tuberculosis. Today tuberculosis is disappearing rapidly from Europe and North America, but in the rest of the world it continues as an important cause of death.

In 1984, a total of 22,255 cases of tuberculosis were reported in the United States, a new case rate of 9.4 per 100,000 per year. In recent years this case rate has been falling at a rate of 5 to 6 percent per year. In 1982, there were 1,807 deaths due to tuberculosis in the United States. It is estimated that 10,000,000 Americans have a positive tuberculin test but that fewer than 1 percent of American children are tuberculin reactors. Tuberculosis in North America tends to be a disease of the elderly urban poor and of minority groups. At all ages case rates among nonwhites tend to be twice those in whites. Hispanic, Haitian, and southeast Asian immigrants may have case rates as high as those of the countries from which they come, and in these individuals the frequency of disease among younger persons reflects its occurrence in those countries. Increasingly, tuberculosis in the United States is being seen in microepidemics, often centered in families.

In the United States tuberculosis has become a disease of the elderly. It is frequently seen in nursing homes. Although transmission of infection can occur at any age, most disease in older persons represents a legacy of previous times. The elderly of today were children when transmission of tubercle bacilli occurred much more frequently. Of those who were infected, many developed disease in young adulthood. Some, especially males, did not and are only now developing reactivation disease in their late years. However, an increasing portion of elderly persons has never been infected, and nosocomial new infection has been recognized as a problem in nursing homes.

Worldwide, tuberculosis case rates are decreasing, but this decrease is not as rapid as the increase in population, so that the number of new cases is rising and will continue to rise. In much of the world transmission of tuberculous infection is declining, but in many impoverished nations this is not true. In some countries estimated new case rates are as high as 400 per 100,000 per year. As in North America and Europe, poverty and tuberculosis go hand in hand. In high-prevalence areas, tuberculosis is seen with equal prevalence in rural and urban settings, and this disease afflicts chiefly young adults. A reasonable estimate of the magnitude of tuberculosis in the world is that half of the population of the world is infected with *M. tuberculosis*, that there are 30 million cases of active tuberculosis in the world, that 10 million new cases occur annually, and that 3 million die of tuberculosis each year. Tuberculosis probably causes 6 percent of all deaths worldwide.

TRANSMISSION *M. tuberculosis* is transmitted from person to person via the aerial route. Although other routes of transmission are possible and have been documented on occasion, none is of major importance. Tubercle bacilli in respiratory secretions form nuclei for water droplets expelled during coughing, sneezing, and vocalizing. Small droplets evaporate within a short distance from the mouth, and thereafter desiccated bacilli remain airborne for long periods. Infection of a susceptible host occurs when a few of these bacilli are inhaled. The number of bacilli excreted by most infected persons is not large; typically, household contact of many months is required for transmission. However, patients with laryngeal tuberculosis, endobronchial disease, recent transbronchial spread of tuberculosis, and extensive cavitary pulmonary disease are often highly contagious. Infectiousness correlates with number of organisms in the expectorated sputum, extent of pulmonary disease, and frequency of cough. Mycobacteria are susceptible to ultraviolet irradiation, and transmission of infection rarely occurs out-of-doors in daylight. Adequate ventilation is the most important measure which can be employed to reduce the infectiousness of the environment. Fomites are not important in the transmission of tuberculosis. Most patients become noninfectious within 2 weeks after the institution of appropriate chemotherapy because of decrease in the number of organisms excreted and decrease in cough.

Transmission of infection with *M. bovis* has long been associated with the consumption of contaminated cow's milk. This organism is no longer a major cause of human disease in much of the world.

PATHOGENESIS The initial entry of tubercle bacilli into the lungs or other site of a previously uninfected individual elicits a nonspecific acute inflammatory response which is rarely noted and is usually accompanied by few or no symptoms. The usual infecting inoculum is no more than one to three organisms which reach the pulmonary alveoli directly via the airborne route. They are then ingested by macrophages and transported to the regional lymph nodes. If spread of the organism is not contained at the level of regional lymph nodes, then tubercle bacilli reach the blood stream and widespread dissemination ensues. Most lesions of disseminated tuberculosis heal, as do most primary pulmonary lesions, although they remain potential foci of later reactivation. Dissemination may result in miliary or meningeal tuberculosis—illnesses with potential for major morbidity and mortality, especially in infants and young children.

During the 2 to 8 weeks after primary infection, while bacilli continue to multiply in their intracellular environment, cell-mediated hypersensitivity develops in the infected host. Immunologically competent lymphocytes enter areas of infection. They elaborate chemotactic factors, interleukins, and lymphokines. In response, monocytes enter the area and undergo transformation into macrophages and subsequently into specialized histiocytic cells which are organized into granulomas. Mycobacteria may persist within macrophages despite increased lysozyme production within these cells, but their further multiplication and spread is usually confined. Healing then occurs, often with late calcification of the granulomas, which sometimes but not always leaves a residual lesion visible on chest radiograph. The combination of a calcified peripheral lung lesion and calcified hilar lymph node is known as a Ghon complex.

In the United States, 95 percent of individuals undergo complete healing of their primary tuberculous lesions with no subsequent evidence of disease. In other populations, where infective inocula may be higher and where nutritional status and other host factors may be less propitious, failure of complete healing may occur in more than 5 percent of individuals. Famine and many intercurrent diseases adversely affect healing and threaten the stability of healed tuberculous lesions.

Tuberculosis—the clinical disease—develops in the minority who do not successfully contain their primary infections. In some individuals tuberculosis develops within weeks after primary infection; in most, organisms lie dormant for many years before entering a phase of logarithmic multiplication leading to disease. Among many factors, age can be identified as a significant factor determining the course of tuberculosis. In infants tuberculous infection frequently progresses rapidly to disease, and the risk of disseminated disease including meningitis and miliary tuberculosis is high. In children older than 1 or 2 years up to about the age of puberty, primary tuberculous lesions almost always heal; most of those destined to develop tuberculosis do so during adolescence or young adulthood. Individuals infected in adulthood are at greatest risk of developing tuberculosis within approximately 3 years following infection. Tuberculous disease is more common in young adult women, whereas it is more common in men later in life.

IMMUNOLOGY Immunity Human beings display native immunity to tuberculosis, with substantial individual variation. Twin studies have demonstrated that tuberculosis is more likely to occur in both members of monozygotic sibships than in dizygotic sibships or other family relationships. Attempts to link susceptibility to tuberculosis to HLA phenotype have produced conflicting data. Although susceptibility to tuberculosis has been associated with race, the evidence is largely anecdotal and is not convincing. As noted, age is an important determinant of native immunity to tuberculosis. Although specific data on nutrition and tuberculosis immunity are lacking, the association of tuberculosis with famine is clear.

Acquired immunity follows primary tuberculous infection. Disease due to exogenous reinfection is probably rare in North America and Europe; it may be more frequent in populations of high prevalence where risk of repeated exposure is great. It is useful to recall that *immunity* in the classic use of the word refers to resistance to infection, whereas *hypersensitivity* describes a state of altered host reactivity. In this sense, immunity may also result from infection with other species of mycobacteria, whether through bacillus Calmette-Guérin (BCG) vaccination or by naturally acquired infection with environ-

mental species of mycobacteria. Studies with BCG in mice have provided substantial evidence that nonspecific immunity extends across generic lines. As an example, BCG protects animals against infection with *Listeria* and *Salmonella*, which are nonrelated intracellular murine pathogens. This nonspecific acquired immunity may reflect primarily macrophage activation.

Antigen-specific immunity is T-lymphocyte-dependent and can be transferred adoptively with lymphocytes. It closely parallels delayed hypersensitivity in its development. It may be an independent phenomenon but is most usefully considered as a functional expression of cellular hypersensitivity.

Tuberculin hypersensitivity Tuberculin hypersensitivity is antigen-specific in nature and follows primary infection. It is chiefly or perhaps entirely directed against protein antigens. It is mediated by T lymphocytes through secretion of lymphokines which act upon effector monocytes.

Mycobacterial antigens have been subjected to extensive immunochemical study. It is clear that there is no single dominant antigen, and that infected and artificially sensitized hosts develop hypersensitivity to an array of mycobacterial proteins. Tuberculin purified protein derivative (PPD), the antigen preparation most frequently employed clinically and epidemiologically to demonstrate tuberculin hypersensitivity, is a crude mixture of largely denatured antigens and is a poor representative of native antigens. Nevertheless, its use has yielded much information.

Mycobacteria are rich in adjuvants. Trehalose dimycolate is the principal adjuvant of chloroform-methanol lipid extracts, wax D, and cord factor. Cell wall arabinogalactan complexed to the underlying peptide constitutes a potent water-soluble adjuvant. Muramyl dipeptide, which lies between the structural polysaccharide arabinogalactan and the cytoplasmic membrane in the cell wall, is a small, soluble, and potent adjuvant. In infection the protein antigens of mycobacteria are always presented to the host in the company of this battery of adjuvants. Purified arabinogalactan has been shown in in vitro studies to be a potent immunosuppressive agent.

Antigen recognition by the sensitized host follows processing by macrophages and depends upon expression by the macrophage at its surface of antigen-specific epitopes in association with Ia antigen, a gene product of the major histocompatability locus. This complex is recognized by specific T lymphocytes. Macrophage synthesis and secretion of interleukin 1 is also necessary for T lymphocyte response to the presented antigen.

Following antigen presentation, T-lymphocyte clonal expansion occurs. Specific subsets of T lymphocytes develop which have antigen-specific immunoregulatory functions and which modulate the immune response. These functions are associated with surface expression of lymphocyte antigens recognizable with monoclonal antibody reagents. Reactivity with monoclonal antibody OKT4 is characteristic of T lymphocytes with helper function, and reactivity with monoclonal antibody OKT8 is characteristic of suppressor T lymphocytes.

Immunoreactive lymphocytes secrete mediators, and in response macrophages become activated and serve as the principal effector cells of tuberculin hypersensitivity. Peripheral blood monocytes from tuberculous patients have been shown to have several features characteristic of activated macrophages, including increased hexose monophosphate shunt activity, augmented surface adhesiveness, expression of characteristic membrane structures, and increased bactericidal activity. Animal studies have demonstrated that these features are T-lymphocyte-dependent. Activated monocytes/macrophages are important immunoregulatory cells possessing suppressor functions.

In tuberculosis, aberrations of this carefully modulated state of hypersensitivity occur with some frequency and are recognizable in 15 percent of acutely ill patients. This has given rise to the suggestion that tuberculosis may present with an immunologic spectrum similar to that seen in leprosy but more subtly expressed. At one pole are patients with chronic cavitary disease, relatively chronic courses, and florid expression of tuberculin hypersensitivity. At the other pole are the less frequently seen patients with cutaneous anergy, a few of whom have absence of granuloma formation and all other manifestations of cellular hypersensitivity and have pancytopenia, widely disseminated disease, and a progressive downhill course. Although the delayed tuberculin skin reaction is the best known manifestation of tuberculin hypersensitivity (see below), granuloma formation is probably its central and most important expression. Granuloma formation is important in containing the spread of infection. Studies with tuberculin antigens on the surface of bentonite or agarose particles have shown that granuloma formation in response to antigen presented in particulate fashion has all of the characteristics of an immunologic hypersensitivity response.

B-lymphocyte-mediated production of antibodies to protein and polysaccharide antigens of mycobacteria is readily demonstrated in tuberculosis. There is no evidence that these antibodies play any role in immunity, hypersensitivity, or pathogenesis of tuberculosis.

CLINICAL MANIFESTATIONS **Primary tuberculosis** Primary tuberculous infection is usually asymptomatic. A nonspecific pneumonitis typically occurs in the lower or midlung zones. Hilar lymph node enlargement is usual and in children is sometimes sufficient to produce bronchial obstruction. In low-prevalence areas primary infection now occurs frequently in adults. It may progress directly to clinical disease which has the pathologic features of reactivation disease. In these persons such perplexing presentations as subapical pneumonias are common.

Reactivation tuberculosis Reactivation tuberculosis is a chronic wasting disease, and constitutional manifestations are often more prominent than respiratory symptoms in patients with pulmonary tuberculosis. Weight loss and low-grade fever are common. Many patients present with typical drenching night sweats over the upper half of the body several times a week.

Pulmonary tuberculosis Pulmonary tuberculosis has a predilection for the apical posterior segments of the upper lobes and the superior segments of the lower lobes of the lungs. The location has been attributed both to posture and to higher intraalveolar oxygen concentration in the uppermost portions of the lung. The extent of disease varies from minimal infiltrates that produce no clinical illness and that are barely discernible on chest radiograph to massive involvement with extensive cavitation and debilitating constitutional and respiratory symptoms. In the absence of effective therapy, pulmonary tuberculosis pursues a chronic and progressive course. There are often periods of long stability and relative well-being, but in most patients these give way to episodes of disease progression with involvement of more and more lung parenchyma.

The onset of pulmonary tuberculosis is usually insidious, and illness may not be noted by the patient for some time. However, it is incorrect to view this onset as one of slow progression. In fact, pulmonary tuberculosis usually reaches its full extent within a few weeks. About one-third of patients will live long lives with chronic illness interspersed with periods of relative well-being. However, the overall death rate of untreated pulmonary tuberculosis probably approaches 60 percent, and the median course to death is about $2\frac{1}{2}$ years.

As pulmonary lesions progress, central necrosis occurs with development of caseation, so named because of the cheesy nature of necrotic material which only partly liquifies in the absence of proteolytic enzymes common in other forms of suppuration. Satellite lesions grow concomitantly. They can usually be recognized on chest radiograph and are often helpful in distinguishing tuberculosis from pulmonary neoplasms. Necrotic material may empty into bronchi resulting in cavitation of the nodular disease. Other parts of the lung may be seeded transbronchially with the development of exudative lesions. In some patients tuberculous pneumonia develops in a lobar or segmental pulmonary distribution. Occasionally transbronchial spread following rupture of a tuberculous peribronchial lymph node

into a bronchus leads to tuberculous pneumonia in the absence of other obvious disease. With the progression of pulmonary tuberculosis, the normal pulmonary architecture is lost. Fibrosis, volume loss, and upward contraction are typical. However, recently diseased areas may heal with relatively little destruction when effective chemotherapy is administered.

Pulmonary cavities may persist even though effective chemotherapy has resulted in apparent cure. In the absence of therapy, persistence of cavities is to be expected. Cavities may be a source of major hemoptysis, especially in the presence of continued active disease. Rasmussen's aneurysm consists of a persistent terminal pulmonary artery within such a cavity and may be a source of bleeding. An important cause of bleeding is the presence of an aspergilloma in a chronic tuberculous cavity, and bleeding in this instance may occur without persisting tuberculous disease. Rupture of a tuberculous cavity into the pleural space may lead to tuberculous empyema and bronchopleural fistula.

Chronic cough is the principal respiratory symptom. Sputum is usually scant and nonpurulent. Hemoptysis is frequent and is usually limited to blood streaking of the sputum. Massive, life-threatening hemoptysis is rare.

Findings on physical examination of the lung in patients with pulmonary tuberculosis are typically few and generally can be appreciated only in the presence of extensive disease. Rales which are accentuated or heard only posttussively are characteristic of apical disease. With extensive cavitation, amphoric breath sounds may be present. Dullness to percussion may sometimes be recognized in Krönig's isthmus and at the clavicles, reflecting extensive apical disease.

Contemporary classification of tuberculosis in the United States is based primarily on bacteriologic status, reflecting concern with infectivity. Previously, pulmonary tuberculosis was classified by the extent of disease that was apparent on the posteroantero chest radiograph. *Minimal lesions* are those which are noncavitary and do not exceed in total extent the area of one lung above the second chondrosternal junction and the spine of the fourth or body of the fifth vertebra. *Moderately advanced* disease is that which does not exceed the area of one lung and which has total cavitation diameter of less than 4 cm. Greater extensiveness of disease is termed *far advanced*.

Extrapulmonary tuberculosis PLEURISY WITH EFFUSION Pleurisy with effusion results when the pleural space is seeded with *M. tuberculosis*. Following a peripheral primary infection, the pleural space may be contaminated by organisms that are transported lymphogenously to the pleura and hence across the surface of the lung to the hilum. Pleural effusion occurs, sometimes massively, usually with substantial pleuritic pain. The onset of symptoms is often abrupt. The effusion is most frequently, but not invariably, unilateral. Classically, tuberculous pleurisy with effusion occurs in younger individuals in the absence of pulmonary tuberculosis. However, in current North American experience this disease presents in many individuals past the age of 35 and simultaneous pulmonary tuberculosis is present in about one-third of patients with tuberculous pleurisy. The effusion is exudative in nature, and a protein concentration greater than 3.0 g/dL is the most characteristic feature of the pleural fluid. Lymphocytes usually, but not invariably, predominate among the pleural fluid cells. Mesothelial cells are rare. Needle biopsy of the parietal pleura may reveal granulomas, and such a finding confirms the diagnosis of tuberculous pleurisy. The tuberculin skin test is negative in one-third of patients, sometimes because the disease presents early before tuberculin reactivity develops, and sometimes because this form of tuberculosis is particularly prone to aberrations of immunoregulation. Untreated, tuberculous pleurisy usually remits, but active pulmonary tuberculosis develops within 5 years in two-thirds of cases. Response to chemotherapy is good. Complete removal of pleural fluid is not necessary. There is rarely a need for surgical decortication.

Bronchopleural fistula and tuberculous empyema are catastrophic complications of untreated tuberculosis resulting from rupture of a pulmonary lesion into the pleural space. The diagnosis is usually not difficult, and acid-fast bacilli are usually readily demonstrated in the pleural exudate. Treatment consists of adequate surgical drainage and chemotherapy.

TUBERCULOUS PERICARDITIS AND PERITONITIS The pericardium and peritoneum are serosal surfaces which are not infrequently the sites of tuberculosis. Pericarditis sometimes occurs in association with pleurisy and may represent an extension of that process. More commonly the pericardium is seeded by drainage from an infected lymph node. Exudative effusion occurs and patients present with fever and pericardial pain. A friction rub may be present. Cardiac tamponade occasionally occurs. Chronic constrictive pericarditis is a late sequel. The diagnosis of tuberculous pericarditis is often difficult and sometimes requires thoracotomy for pericardial biopsy.

Tuberculous peritonitis results from hematogenous seeding of the peritoneum or entry of bacilli from an abdominal lymphatic or genitourinary organ source. As with other serositis, an exudative effusion occurs. The onset is usually insidious, and the disease is often mistaken for hepatic cirrhosis in alcoholic patients. As with tuberculous pericarditis, the diagnosis is often difficult, and recovery of the organism from paracentesis fluid is possible only in a minority of cases. Surgical biopsy may be necessary for diagnosis.

LARYNGEAL AND ENDOBRONCHIAL TUBERCULOSIS Tuberculosis of the larynx is usually seen in association with far-advanced pulmonary disease. Occasionally it occurs with only minimal pulmonary involvement. It results from seeding of the mucosal surface during expectoration. The disease progresses from a superficial laryngitis to ulceration and granuloma formation. The epiglottis and hypopharynx are occasionally involved. Hoarseness is the principal symptom of tuberculous laryngitis. In a similar fashion the bronchial mucosa may be seeded, causing tuberculous bronchitis. Indeed, localized bronchitis in segmental bronchi leading to diseased portions of lung is common. Cough and minor hemoptysis are the chief clinical manifestations. Patients with tuberculous laryngitis and extensive bronchitis are usually highly infectious. These forms of disease respond rapidly to chemotherapy and have a favorable prognosis with treatment.

TUBERCULOUS ADENITIS Scrofula is chronic tuberculous lymphadenitis of the cervical lymph nodes. Any of the cervical nodes may be involved, but those high in the neck just below the mandible are the most frequent site of disease. Tuberculous nodes are usually rubbery to palpation and not tender. With progression, they become harder and matted. Chronic draining fistulas may develop, but these are rare, and the course of this form of tuberculosis is usually indolent. The diagnosis is commonly established by surgical biopsy. Lymph node biopsy specimens obtained for this purpose should always be submitted for culture as well as histologic examination, and chemotherapy should be instituted at or before the time of surgery to avoid postoperative fistulas in the surgical wound site. Lymph nodes other than those in the cervical regions are less commonly involved in tuberculosis and account for about 35 percent of tuberculous adenitis. When it was an important cause of disease, M. bovis had a predilection for causing scrofula.

In children, M. scrofulaceum and M. intracellulare are frequently the cause of scrofula. The onset of this disease is usually before 5 years of age. As with tuberculosis, lymph nodes high in the neck are most frequently involved. A single enlarged node is commonly the presenting manifestation. Constitutional symptoms are absent, and the adenitis is usually not tender. Progression is common, with necrosis of the node and the development of fistulous sinus tracts. The organisms involved are usually not susceptible to drugs, and treatment, if necessary, is surgical excision. Spontaneous resolution is usual after puberty.

SKELETAL TUBERCULOSIS Bone and joint disease is a not infrequent manifestation of tuberculosis. Pott's disease, tuberculosis of the spine, usually involves the midthoracic spine. Tubercle bacilli reach the spine hematogenously or through lymphatic channels from the pleural space to paravertebral lymph nodes. Anterior erosion of vertebral bodies leads to collapse. The result is a sharply angulated kyphosis without scoliosis (gibbus deformity). Paraplegia may result. If there is no neurologic compromise, Pott's disease can be treated with chemotherapy. If the spine is unstable, surgical stabilization may be necessary. In the face of new paraparesis, immediate orthopedic consultation should be obtained. Paravertebral "cold abcesses" are a frequent concomitant of tuberculous spondylitis. They usually do not need to be drained, if adequate chemotherapy is given, unless they are very large. They may extend along fascial planes and point in the inguinal region or in other remote sites.

Tuberculosis of joints most frequently affects large weight-bearing joints such as the hips and knees. It responds well to immobilization and chemotherapy. Tuberculous synovitis may occur alone or in association with tuberculous arthritis. In prior years bone and joint tuberculosis was frequently caused by M. bovis, an organism that is now rare.

GENITOURINARY TUBERCULOSIS Genitourinary tuberculosis may involve any part of either the male or female genitourinary system. Renal tuberculosis usually presents initially as microscopic pyuria and hematuria with a sterile urine culture. The diagnosis may be established by finding tubercle bacilli on culture of the urine. As the disease progresses, cavitation of the renal parenchyma occurs. In the past, nephrectomy was often performed for renal tuberculosis. However, with adequate chemotherapy surgical removal of a kidney is almost never necessary. The ureters and bladder may be infected by tubular spread of the organism, and ureteral stricture may result.

Tuberculous salpingitis often results in female sterility. Genital tuberculosis in the male most commonly involves the prostate, seminal vesicles, and epididymis. Prostatic and epididymal tuberculosis are characterized by nontender nodular induration detectable by physical examination. The presentation of genital tuberculosis in both males and females is insidious, with chronic or subacute symptoms. The diagnosis is usually made by culture of acid-fast bacilli.

MENINGEAL TUBERCULOSIS The leptomeninges are relatively frequently seeded by organisms which disseminate during primary infection. In young children, tuberculous meningitis may develop at this time. This chronic infection is manifested not only by meningeal signs but also by frequent cranial nerve signs, reflecting a tendency for basilar distribution of the infection. High protein content, low glucose, and lymphocytosis are characteristic of the cerebrospinal fluid. Prior to the advent of effective chemotherapy, this disease was almost always fatal. Chemotherapy with isoniazid, rifampin, and ethambutol is effective. Intrathecal drug administration is not necessary. Late reactivation of meningeal tuberculous foci may produce disease in adults who have no evidence of pulmonary tuberculosis. Tuberculomas of the meninges or brain may become evident in adult life many years after primary infection, and seizures are often their major clinical manifestation.

OCULAR TUBERCULOSIS Tuberculosis may involve almost any part of the eye. Chorioretinitis and uveitis are the most common manifestations. The diagnosis of tuberculosis of the eye is extremely difficult to establish, and most diagnoses are presumptive. The manifestations cannot be distinguished clinically from sarcoidosis or systemic mycoses, but phlyctenular keratitis strongly suggest tuberculosis. Phlyctenular lesions are thought to represent manifestations of tuberculin hypersensitivity rather than bacterial infection. Choroid tubercles are often present in patients with miliary tuberculosis, and their recognition may be helpful in the diagnosis of miliary tuberculosis. Ocular tuberculosis responds well to standard chemotherapeutic agents.

GASTROINTESTINAL TUBERCULOSIS The stomach is extremely resistant to tuberculous infection, and a large number of virulent tubercle bacilli can be swallowed without establishing an infection. Rarely, usually concomitantly with extensive cavitary pulmonary disease and severe debility, swallowed organisms reach the terminal ileum and cecum and tuberculous ileitis develops. Chronic diarrhea and fistula development are the principal manifestations, and the disease is difficult to distinguish from Crohn's disease. Tuberculosis of the liver can occur as an isolated event, but it is usually a manifestation of miliary tuberculosis.

ADRENAL TUBERCULOSIS Hematogenous seeding of the adrenal gland is probably fairly common, but disease due to this infection is rare and usually seen only in association with long-standing and extensive pulmonary tuberculosis. The cortex is most frequently involved. It may lead to adrenal insufficiency. In contrast, carcinomatous involvement of the adrenal cortex, even though very extensive, rarely produces clinical adrenal insufficiency.

CUTANEOUS TUBERCULOSIS Tuberculous infection of the skin is rare in the absence of long-standing, untreated disease elsewhere. Lupus vulgaris is a granulomatous disease of the skin, and it responds well to treatment. Diagnosis is made by skin biopsy. Tuberculin hypersensitivity manifestations are common. Erythema nodosum may be present, although it much more commonly results from other granulomatous diseases including sarcoidosis and systemic mycoses. Tuberculids are poorly understood papular lesions of tuberculin hypersensitivity.

MILIARY TUBERCULOSIS Miliary tuberculosis results from widespread hematogenous dissemination. It often presents as a perplexing fever, sometimes with a double quotidian curve, often accompanied by anemia and splenomegaly, in a patient with a relatively preserved sense of well-being. Miliary tuberculosis is apt to be more fulminating in children than in adults.

Classically, miliary tuberculosis develops following hematogenous dissemination at the time of primary infection, and patients present no antecedent history of tuberculosis. Lesions develop synchronously throughout the body. The appearance of these lesions suggested millet seeds; hence the name miliary tuberculosis. Patients become ill before radiographic changes appear on the chest radiograph; these take 4 to 6 weeks to become recognizable. The typical radiologic findings are soft, uniformly distributed, fine nodules throughout both lung fields. They often can be recognized first on a lateral chest film or an underpenetrated posteroantero radiograph. The diagnosis is difficult, and expectorated sputum rarely contains organisms. Transbronchial biopsy and liver biopsy are usually but not invariably positive. Bone marrow biopsy is positive in approximately two-thirds of patients.

When hematogenous dissemination occurs in a previously diseased individual, a much more fulminant course results. Prostration is common. Diffuse but ragged nodular infiltrates develop within a few weeks, and the sputum is often positive. The diagnosis is rarely difficult.

The subacute form and the rare chronic form of miliary tuberculosis often present major problems in diagnosis. This type of disease is usually attributed to repeated seeding of the blood stream from a tuberculous focus. A very rare form of disseminated tuberculosis occurs with widespread dissemination of disease, a massive number of bacteria in tissues, complete absence of granuloma formation, and pancytopenia. It is termed disseminated nonreactive tuberculosis. It has a poor prognosis, even with chemotherapy.

Tuberculin anergy is common in miliary tuberculosis, and a negative skin test should not be a deterrent to the consideration of this diagnosis. Anergy may extend to other delayed hypersensitivity antigens as well, but it does not always do so. In vitro cultured leukocyte studies also demonstrate hyporesponsiveness, and they suggest that this anergy is mediated by monocytes with suppressor function. With treatment and stabilization of patients with miliary tuberculosis, tuberculin hypersensitivity is restored.

Without treatment, the prognosis for miliary tuberculosis is grave. This disease responds well to chemotherapy, however, and can be treated with the same drug regimens employed for other forms of tuberculosis.

SILICOTUBERCULOSIS Tuberculosis occurs with increased frequency in patients with silicosis and possibly in patients with some other pneumoconioses. The diagnosis is often difficult because of confounding radiographic changes due to the underlying pneumoconiosis. Even with therapy, the prognosis is less favorable than in other patients. Experimental animal work has shown that silica exposure increases susceptibility to infection, and work in both animals and humans has demonstrated that silica impairs macrophage function. Patients with silicotuberculosis should be treated for longer than customary periods. Patients with silicosis who are tuberculin-positive should be considered for isoniazid prophylaxis even when they do not meet other criteria for this form of therapy. It is likely that isoniazid prophylaxis is somewhat less effective in persons with silicosis.

DIAGNOSIS Bacteriology The diagnosis of tuberculosis is established when tubercle bacilli are identified in the sputum, urine, body fluids, or tissues of the patient. For the majority of patients who have pulmonary tuberculosis, the diagnosis can be most readily established by sputum examination. The staining characteristics of *M. tuberculosis* allow its ready identification in clinical specimens, although it is usually present in small numbers so that prolonged study of stained slides is necessary. A slender (less than 0.5 μm diameter), curved, often polychromatically beaded rod, it frequently presents in clinical specimens as pairs or clumps of a few organisms lying side by side. When stained with fluorescent auramine-rhodamine, tubercle bacilli can be seen under usual high-dry (100×) microscope magnification, but the morphology of organisms is often indistinct with this stain and at this magnification. A more definitive stain is accomplished using carbol fuchsin, and this stain requires meticulous scanning with oil immersion (1000×) microscopy. Sputum culture adds to the diagnostic yield and also permits the specific identification of acid-fast bacilli and the study of drug susceptibility of the organisms. However, the generation time of mycobacteria is 20 to 24 h. Primary isolation from clinical specimens usually requires 4 to 8 weeks on classical media. Radiometric techniques using highly selective media allow cultivation in 1 or 2 weeks, but confirmation of the identity of an isolated organism may require additional time. Mycobacteria are aerobes. Modern culture techniques are excellent, and there is no longer reason to inoculate guinea pigs for primary isolation. Niacin production characterizes *M. tuberculosis* and helps to distinguish it from other species.

If expectorated sputum is not readily available for examination, expectoration may be induced or samples obtained by nasotracheal aspiration. Early morning gastric aspiration provides excellent material for culture and for smear examination. Although nonpathogenic mycobacteria are occasionally found in gastric aspirates, their number is so small as to preclude their appearance in smears of gastric aspirates. Bronchoscopy has a high yield in the diagnosis of tuberculosis, but in the absence of other considerations it should not be undertaken unless multiple attempts by simpler means have failed and the diagnosis remains obscure.

The diagnostic yield of sputum smear and culture is directly related to the extent of pulmonary disease. Overall, about two-thirds of patients in whom a positive culture can be obtained will have a positive direct sputum smear. However, only about one-third of patients with minimal pulmonary tuberculosis will have a positive sputum smear, even after multiple examinations. If there is no lesion visible on the chest radiograph, then there is usually little reason to obtain sputum examinations for tubercle bacilli. Conversely, if a patient with extensive cavitary disease or an exudative pneumonic process has a negative sputum smear, diagnoses other than tuberculosis should be sought. If an initial sputum smear is negative, repeated smears should be obtained on separate days. There is rarely indication for obtaining more than five sputum examinations.

It is clear that both the sensitivity and specificity of sputum examinations for tubercle bacilli depend on the experience of those performing the examination. False-positive and false-negative sputum smears occur with distressing frequency in laboratories in which cases of tuberculosis are rarely encountered, and sputum smears performed by medical students and house officers in teaching hospitals are often unreliable. False-positive sputum cultures also have been well documented. Laboratory identification of mycobacteria poses difficult problems for many clinical laboratories, and use of reference laboratories is desirable to confirm speciation.

Serology Serologic tests for the diagnosis of tuberculosis remain experimental and are not routinely available. The most specific serologic tests have used highly purified antigens. Enzyme-linked immunosorbent assay (ELISA) techniques offer the potential for readily applied serologic tests for tuberculosis, and should have great value in the diagnosis of tuberculosis in children and in extrapulmonary disease where sputum examination is not available.

Radiology The chest radiograph is an important tool for both the diagnosis and evaluation of tuberculosis. Healed primary lesions may leave a small peripheral nodule which may calcify with the passing of years. When calcified and present together with a calcified hilar lymph node, this is known as a Ghon complex. Similar lesions result from histoplasmosis, and it is not possible to distinguish between healed primary lesions of these two diseases radiologically. Calcification of right paratracheal lymph nodes is more commonly seen in histoplasmosis.

Multinodular infiltration in the apical posterior segments of the upper lobes and superior segments of the lower lobes is the most typical lesion of pulmonary tuberculosis. Cavitation is frequently present and is usually accompanied by substantial amounts of infiltration in the same pulmonary segments. Laminagrams are often helpful in recognizing satellite nodular lesions, which are characteristic of tuberculosis and not usually seen in carcinoma. Lordotic views may be of help in evaluating disease obscured by the intersection of the third or fourth posterior rib, second anterior rib, and clavicle. They are of little use in evaluating disease located elsewhere. As tuberculosis becomes inactive or heals, fibrotic scarring becomes apparent on the chest radiograph. There is frequently volume loss in the involved upper lobes, and upward and medial retraction of hilar markings is common. Fibrotic lesions may develop calcifications. The activity of tuberculosis may be judged from serial films. It is never wise to judge tuberculosis to be inactive on the basis of a single radiographic examination.

Clinical pathology Other than bacteriologic examinations, clinical laboratory tests contribute relatively little to the diagnosis of tuberculosis. Peripheral blood monocytosis in the range of 8 to 12 percent is common. The erythrocyte sedimentation rate is usually elevated.

Tuberculin test The intracutaneous tuberculin skin test is a reliable means of recognizing prior mycobacterial infection. Its correct interpretation requires some thought and knowledge. The preferred antigen is tuberculin purified protein derivative (PPD). For all routine use the intermediate-strength dose should be used. In North America this is 5 tuberculin units of material which is standardized by bioassay (bioequivalent) against reference antigen designated PPD-S. In other parts of the world, PPD lot RT-23, prepared in Denmark and widely distributed by the World Health Organization, is available. A gravimetric unit has been assigned to this material, and 2 units of this PPD are equivalent to 5 units of PPD-S. Diluents for PPD should contain polysorbate 80, which decreases loss of potency due to adsorption onto glass and plastic surfaces. Multiple puncture devices offer much convenience, but do so at the cost of decreased specificity. They can be recommended only as screening tests, and positive tests should be repeated using intracutaneous PPD.

The tuberculin test is usually applied on the forearm. Reactions should be read by measuring the transverse diameter of induration as detected by gentle palpation at 48 to 72 h. Patients with tuberculosis have normally distributed reaction sizes with the mean and mode at 17 mm. Infected but healthy, nondiseased individuals have similarly

distributed reactions. Hence, a reaction to PPD is presumptive evidence of prior mycobacterial infection.

Tuberculin hypersensitivity may result from contact with nonpathogenic, environmental mycobacteria, and this nonspecific reactivity may seriously confound the interpretation of tuberculin tests. The magnitude of this problem varies substantially geographically. Nonspecific tuberculin reactivity is rarely found in northern climates, and in such areas all reactivity to PPD can be considered to reflect infection with *M. tuberculosis*. In many warm and humid climatic zones, including all of the coastal areas of the southeastern United States, nonspecific tuberculin reactivity is common. In such regions it is customary to consider reactions smaller than 10 mm as not significant and attribute them to cross reactivity with environmental mycobacterial antigens. However, considering smaller reactions as not significant always incurs the cost of missing some reactions which bespeak infection with *M. tuberculosis*.

Repeated skin testing may boost reaction size, whether the primary reactivity was directed to *M. tuberculosis* or was nonspecific. Caution must be used in attributing a small increase in reactivity to new infection. It is well-established, however, that repeated skin testing with PPD does not lead to positive reactions in uninfected persons. Positive reactions do not occur as a result of allergy to components of the diluent. Tuberculin reactivity wanes with advancing age, and the booster phenomenon may be useful in this situation. For example, if an older person fails to react to initial testing, repeat testing with intermediate strength PPD may be done after 7 to 10 days. A reaction at this time should be accepted as significant.

PPD is also available in a second strength which contains 50 times the amount of PPD in intermediate-strength material. Except as a test for anergy, this product has little use. Because PPD at this strength so readily elicits nonspecific reactivity, a positive reaction to second-strength PPD is much more apt to give misinformation than to contribute to the correct diagnosis. A first-strength PPD is also available. It contains one-fifth the amount of PPD of intermediate PPD. It has not been adequately standardized for clinical use.

Anergy is the paradoxical absence of dermal tuberculin reactivity in infected persons. It occurs in association with a number of disease states and in immunosuppressed individuals. It also occurs in as many as 15 percent of tuberculous patients with newly active pulmonary disease. In these persons tuberculin reactivity reappears with stabilization of the disease process. One-half of patients with miliary tuberculosis and one-third of patients with newly diagnosed tuberculous pleurisy have negative tuberculin tests. It has become common practice in many medical centers to use a battery of delayed hypersensitivity antigens to serve as controls for tuberculin tests in demonstrating anergy. However, antigens standardized for this purpose are not available, and tuberculin anergy may be antigen-specific. False-negative tuberculin tests may result from technical errors including subcutaneous injection, use of outdated PPD, and permitting PPD to stand in syringes before use. Such errors should not be mistaken for anergy.

TREATMENT The modern treatment of tuberculosis is based on the administration of effective drugs. In the presence of adequate chemotherapy, hospitalization, rest, and improved diet do not contribute to achieving cures. In order to prevent the emergence of drug-resistant mutants which are present initially in very small numbers, two effective drugs are always required. Because of the slow generation time of mycobacteria and because these organisms can be metabolically inactive for long periods of time, prolonged courses of drug therapy are always necessary. Treatment regimens do not differ for pulmonary and extrapulmonary tuberculosis.

Table 119-1 presents dosage and toxicity information on drugs currently in use for the treatment of tuberculosis. Table 119-2 describes several effective treatment regimens. Daily therapy with isoniazid and rifampin for 9 to 12 months represents the most effective regimen available and is capable of achieving a favorable outcome in 99 percent of patients. At this level of success, it probably will be impossible ever to mount a controlled clinical trial sufficiently large to demonstrate that any other regimen is significantly better. Certainly, the addition of a third drug does not offer anything to a patient with drug-sensitive organisms. However, many experts add ethambutol initially until the results of sensitivity tests become available. Daily therapy with isoniazid and ethambutol for 18 months is 90 to 95 percent effective, and it is probably the equal of isoniazid and rifampin in patients with minimal disease. In developing countries where drug costs are a limiting factor, the extremely low cost combination of isoniazid and thioacetazone for 12 to 18 months provides a regimen which can achieve 80 to 90 percent cure rates.

General acceptance has been given to a hypothesis which states that tubercle bacilli exist in tuberculous patients in three pools—a metabolically active extracellular pool and relatively metabolically inactive intracellular and necrotic caseum pools. Only rifampin is thought to be bactericidal for all of these pools, and hence it may not be necessary to continue rifampin-containing regimens for as long as other regimens which rely upon organisms entering the metabolically active pool to achieve sterilization. Isoniazid and streptomycin are both bactericidal against extracellular, metabolically active organisms. Against intracellular organisms, isoniazid and pyrazinamide are bactericidal and streptomycin is inactive. In clinical trials, pyrazinamide has been found to be particularly useful during the first 2 months of treatment. Ethambutol is only bacteriostatic.

The major problem in tuberculosis treatment programs today is patient default. It is unusual for any tuberculosis clinic to achieve a default rate of less than 15 percent, and default rates of 40 to 60 percent are common. Unfortunately, these rates tend to be highest in those parts of the world where high tuberculosis prevalence is coupled with limited resources. Default not only leads to treatment failure but also leads to the emergence and transmission of drug-resistant organisms. This situation has led to an emphasis on short-course therapeutic regimens. However, since most patient defaults occur within the first 6 months of the treatment program, short-course therapy is likely to have a meaningful impact only if the resources conserved by shortening treatment are used to strengthen those components of the program responsible for maintaining patient compliance. Completely supervised regimens are successful for noncompliant patients, but their widespread use is costly. Twice weekly drug administration is effective and facilitates patient supervision.

Short-course treatment programs are best considered as consisting of two phases. An initial 2-month intensive phase of daily therapy should include isoniazid, rifampin, pyrazinamide, and either streptomycin or ethambutol. A consolidation phase of daily therapy with isoniazid and one other drug should be given for at least 4 months, with a 6-month course duration perhaps being superior. In the United States, success has been achieved with a regimen of isoniazid 300 mg and rifampin 600 mg daily for 1 month, followed by isoniazid 900 mg and rifampin 600 mg twice weekly for 8 months.

Relapses after successful therapy should be fewer than 1 percent. Since these few relapses usually present with symptoms and are almost never found by routine x-rays, patients may be discharged from follow-up at the completion of therapy. Relapses are more frequent after short-course therapy, usually occurring within the first year, and follow-up for such patients for 1 or 2 years is justified.

The physician following a patient being treated for tuberculosis should expect symptomatic improvement within the first 2 to 3 weeks in most patients. Clearing of infiltrates on the chest radiograph may not occur within the first month but usually is readily recognized between the second and fourth months. Most patients reach a point of radiologic stability between 4 and 6 months. Although it has become customary to continue drug therapy for arbitrary periods, there is logic in continuing therapy for 6 months after this point of stability is reached, even if this means prolonging the planned period of treatment. Sputum conversion occurs in most patients within the first 2 months. The fact that an individual patient responds more slowly than the norm should not necessarily be a cause for concern, provided the patient is taking effective drugs.

Since there are alternative effective drug regimens, toxicity becomes a factor in choice of therapy. Major individual drug toxicities are listed in Table 119-1; the toxicity of greatest concern is hepatitis. Toxicity sufficient to require change in regimen occurs in 3 to 5 percent of patients taking isoniazid and rifampin and in about 1.5 percent of patients taking isoniazid and ethambutol. The toxicity of isoniazid and thioacetazone appears to vary with racial characteristics of the patient population. It reaches about 30 percent in oriental groups but is only 2 to 5 percent in other populations. Routine monitoring of serum enzymes or other blood test values reflecting liver disease is of little use and is not recommended. Normal values

TABLE 119-1 Drugs used in the treatment of tuberculosis

Drug	Usual daily adult dose	Major toxicity
Isoniazid	300 mg	Hepatitis, peripheral neuropathy, drug fever
Rifampin	600 mg	Hepatitis, influenza-like syndrome, thrombocytopenia (rare)
Streptomycin	0.75–1 g	Deafness, loss of vestibular function, loss of renal function
Pyrazinamide	1.5–2 g	Hepatitis, hyperuricemia
Ethambutol	15 mg/kg	Optic neuritis (extremely rare at this dose)
p-Aminosalicylic acid	12 g	Diarrhea, hepatitis, hypersensitivity reactions
Ethionamide	1 g	Hepatitis
Cycloserine	1 g	Depression, personality changes, psychosis, convulsions
Thioacetazone	150 mg	Exfoliative dermatitis, hepatitis
Kanamycin	1 g	Deafness, loss of renal function, loss of vestibular function (rare)
Capreomycin	1 g	Deafness, loss of vestibular function, loss of renal function
Viomycin	1 g	Deafness, loss of vestibular function, loss of renal function

TABLE 119-2 Effective drug regimens for the treatment of tuberculosis

Regimen (adult drug dose)	Comment
Isoniazid (300 mg) and rifampin (600 mg) daily for 9–12 months	The usual regimen for initial treatment of all patients unless drug resistance is suspected, in which case ethambutol 15 mg/kg should be added.
Isoniazid (300 mg) and ethambutol (15 mg/kg) daily for 12–18 months	The least toxic effective regimen. Suitable for patients with minimal disease. The regimen of choice in pregnant women.
Isoniazid (300 mg) and thioacetazone (150 mg) daily for 12–18 months	The least expensive effective regimen. Streptomycin (0.75–1 g) may be added daily for the first 8 weeks to increase effectiveness, but this doubles both cost and toxicity.
Isoniazid (300 mg), rifampin (600 mg), pyrazinamide (2 g), and streptomycin (1 g) or ethambutol (15 mg/kg) daily for 2 months followed by one of the following: a Isoniazid (300 mg) and rifampin (600 gm) daily for 4 months b Isoniazid (300 mg) and thioacetazone (150 mg) daily for 6 months c Isoniazid (300 mg), rifampin (600 mg), and streptomycin (1 g) twice weekly for 6 months	Initial intensive phase for short course regimens. Short course regimens have only been demonstrated to be effective under conditions of close patient supervision. Inexpensive. Suitable for fully supervised therapy.
Isoniazid (300 mg) and rifampin (600 mg) daily for 1 month followed by isoniazid (900 mg) and rifampin (600 mg) twice weekly for 8 months	Effectiveness demonstrated in ambulatory treatment programs in Arkansas. Has not been compared with other regimens in clinical trials.

do not predict absence of toxicity, and serum enzymes in patients taking isoniazid may rise transiently to three times normal values without the subsequent development of hepatitis. A well-educated patient and an alert treatment supervisor are the principal available safeguards against drug hepatitis. If medication is discontinued during the prodromal phase or promptly with the onset of jaundice, drug hepatitis can be expected to resolve without untoward incident. Isoniazid toxicity is probably due to toxic metabolites of acetyl isoniazid. Induction of cytochrome P-450 enzymes by alcohol or long-acting barbiturates predisposes to isoniazid hepatitis. Isoniazid also causes a peripheral neuropathy which is preventable and reversible by the administration of pyridoxine. Patients with such predisposing factors as old age, diabetes, alcoholism, and malnutrition should be given pyridoxine concomitantly with isoniazid; the usual dose is 50 mg/day.

Isoniazid is known to be safe in pregnant patients. Data are less complete for other drugs but suggest that ethambutol is the companion drug of choice. Rifampin should be used if the tuberculosis is disseminated or very extensive. Streptomycin should not be used in pregnancy because of the risk of fetal ototoxicity. Tuberculosis often pursues an unfavorable course during and just after pregnancy, and treatment of a pregnant woman should never be deferred. It is reasonable to postpone isoniazid prophylaxis until just after delivery.

Patients with chronic renal failure also present special treatment problems, and these patients have tuberculosis case rates approximately 10 times those of the general population. Isoniazid is acetylated to an inactive form by the liver and then excreted by the kidney. Acetyl isoniazid is the precursor of hydrazines which are probably hepatotoxic. Both isoniazid and acetyl isoniazid are not bound by plasma proteins and are dialyzable. The usual daily dose of isoniazid should be given to patients with renal failure at intervals of two or three times weekly. Patients on dialysis should receive the drug following each dialysis. Ethambutol behaves like isoniazid, except that it is excreted by the kidney as the active drug. As with isoniazid, the usual daily dose should be given at longer intervals, and administration should follow dialysis. Optic nerve toxicity of ethambutol appears to be related not to intermittent high drug levels but to sustained high drug levels. Patients with renal failure who are receiving ethambutol should have their color vision and visual acuity monitored regularly. Rifampin is protein-bound, nondialyzable, and excreted in the bile by the liver. No change in dose or interval is necessary in the presence of renal failure. Caution should be exercised in using rifampin in patients with hepatic failure.

Faced with relapse in a previously treated patient, a major concern should be the possibility of drug resistance, and resistance studies of the organism should be obtained in a competent reference laboratory. In fact, in one-third of patients who relapse after adequate drug therapy taken regularly, the relapse is caused by drug-resistant organisms. If, however, the patient took the drug sporadically or the previous regimen was inadequate, then the likelihood of drug resistance having developed is about two chances in three. Therapy for presumed drug-resistant tuberculosis should be instituted with two drugs which the patient has not taken previously, provided that one of these two new drugs is isoniazid or rifampin. Otherwise, four drugs should be used, including as many new drugs as possible. When resistance studies become available, the regimen should be modified appropriately. Data from studies conducted before rifampin became available suggest that it is beneficial to continue isoniazid even when laboratory studies indicate drug resistance. In general, all re-treatment regimens should be closely supervised and directed by physicians with special experience with this problem.

Primary drug resistance should be suspected in patients who appear to have contracted their infection from patients with known drug resistance or with known noncompliance and in patients who come from areas where drug resistance is common. This group includes immigrants from Haiti, southeast Asia, and many areas of Latin America. While laboratory resistance studies are pending, drug therapy should be dictated by the prior treatment of the suspected index case.

In immigrant populations, most of the drug resistance of concern is to isoniazid. In this circumstance, therapy should be initiated with isoniazid, rifampin, and ethambutol. One of these drugs may be discontinued when resistance studies become available.

PREVENTION Chemoprophylaxis In one of the largest controlled clinical trials ever conducted, 1 year of isoniazid has been shown to be effective in reducing the incidence of tuberculosis in tuberculin-positive individuals presumed to have been infected with *M. tuberculosis*. The benefit of isoniazid prophylaxis has been demonstrated so clearly that the question of its use now hinges primarily on the risk of drug toxicity, chiefly hepatitis.

In administering isoniazid prophylaxis, highest priority should be assigned to treating household contacts of persons with active tuberculosis and to persons known to have become infected within the preceding year. The risks of developing tuberculosis in these two groups are, respectively, 0.5 percent per year and 3 percent during the first year. Particular attention should be given to treating children in these categories. Prophylaxis of childhood household contacts with isoniazid should be started immediately. After 3 months of therapy, the child should be skin-tested with intermediate-strength PPD. If the skin test is negative at that time, isoniazid may be discontinued. If it is positive, 12 months of prophylaxis should be completed.

In general, younger individuals benefit most from isoniazid prophylaxis because the drug is most effective when the infection is recent and because older individuals have often already outlived a substantial part of their risk. The risk of hepatitis rises with age, reaching approximately 2 percent by the seventh decade. Cost-benefit analyses with large data bases have shown that there is a 1:1 ratio of cases of tuberculosis prevented and hepatitis caused at age 45 when individuals without added risks are considered. Based on this calculation, there is a general consensus that all persons younger than age 35 with a positive tuberculin reaction should receive isoniazid 300 mg per day for 1 year.

It is also possible to develop criteria for the prophylactic use of isoniazid in older persons with remote tuberculosis, either known historically or evident radiographically, who have never received adequate chemotherapy. The annual risk of tuberculosis in such persons is at least 0.5 percent, and isoniazid prophylaxis will prevent 70 percent of the cases. Assuming an isoniazid hepatitis risk of 2 percent, a 1:1 ratio of tuberculosis prevented and hepatitis caused is reached in 5.7 years. Isoniazid 300 mg per day should be given for 1 year to all persons in this category who have a life expectancy greater than 10 years. Other individuals at high risk for the development of tuberculosis include tuberculin-positive persons who have such diseases as the acquired immunodeficiency syndrome (AIDS) and Hodgkin's disease, which alter T-lymphocyte-mediated immunity; patients with silicosis, which alters macrophage function; patients who are receiving adrenocortical steroids chronically; patients with renal failure; and patients receiving immunosuppressive agents. One year of isoniazid prophylaxis should be given to tuberculin-positive persons in these categories regardless of age. As with therapy for active tuberculosis, monitoring serum enzymes is not useful in patients receiving isoniazid prophylaxis.

BCG vaccination Baccillus Calmette-Guérin (BCG) is an attenuated strain of *M. bovis* which has been given to hundreds of millions of persons as a vaccine against tuberculosis. It is clearly safe, but its efficacy is in some dispute. In controlled studies in North America and Britain, it was found to offer greater than 80 percent protection. In well-designed studies in Georgia and Puerto Rico, it offered little or no protection. In a large study carried out in south India, no protection was observed. There may be unusual aspects to the host-parasite relationship in that population that make it hazardous to extrapolate the results from south India to other populations. Even in those studies where no protection was observed, the disseminated forms of tuberculosis which have such high mortalities among children were virtually eliminated. While final judgment on the efficacy of

BCG is reserved, its continued use in high-prevalence areas appears justified.

BCG vaccination induces tuberculin hypersensitivity. However, the dermal reaction to PPD is usually not as large as that which follows natural infection, usually does not persist as long, and varies from strain to strain of vaccine. Individuals with large PPD reactions persisting for many years after vaccination should be viewed as infected and considered for isoniazid prophylaxis.

CONTROL PROGRAMS Tuberculosis control programs must be mounted in varying situations. In most low-prevalence areas, such as those which exist in North America, resources are relatively abundant and disease occurrence is mostly sporadic. Increasingly, tuberculosis is being seen in microepidemics, often centered in family groups. High-risk groups can be identified, immigrant groups and residents and employees of nursing homes being among the most important. Central to any program is an efficient case-reporting and registry system. Contact investigation must be carried out effectively and is especially important when index cases occur in children. The major effective tool for decreasing the spread of infection is chemotherapy for all infectious patients. Chemoprophylaxis also has an important role.

At the other end of the spectrum are high-prevalence areas with few or no resources for tuberculosis control. The single, most effective measure in this situation is the establishment of a network of ambulatory tuberculosis treatment centers providing diagnosis by direct sputum smear and standardized drug therapy. Hospital beds, chest radiographs, sputum cultures, and individualized treatment regimens are all luxuries until basic treatment is available to all. Success has only followed the assumption of responsibility for providing treatment, and this usually means treatment at no cost to the patient. Tuberculosis diagnostic and treatment programs should be integrated into national health programs, but categoric and expert supervision is always necessary. Treatment records should be maintained, but complex registries are of little value.

In high-prevalence areas, BCG vaccine should be offered to every individual under 15 or 20 without prior tuberculin testing. Older individuals can be assumed to have been infected already. Before a mass BCG campaign is initiated, planning should begin for continuing vaccination of newborns or young school children. Community-wide isoniazid prophylaxis programs have not proved to be successful.

REFERENCES

AMERICAN THORACIC SOCIETY: Diagnostic standards and classification of tuberculosis and other mycobacterial diseases (14th ed). Am Rev Respir Dis 123:343, 1981
————: Treatment of tuberculosis and other mycobacterial diseases. Am Rev Respir Dis 128:336, 1983
COMSTOCK GW, EDWARDS PQ: The competing risks of tuberculosis and hepatitis for adult tuberculin reactors. Am Rev Respir Dis 111:573, 1975
———— et al: The tuberculin skin test. Am Rev Respir Dis 124:356, 1981
————: Epidemiology of tuberculosis. Am Rev Respir Dis 125(suppl):8, 1982
DUTT AK et al: Short-course chemotherapy for extrapulmonary tuberculosis. Ann Intern Med 104:7, 1986
EDWARDS LB et al: An atlas of sensitivity to tuberculin, PPD-B, and histoplasmin in the United States. Am Rev Respir Dis 99(suppl):1, 1969
FOX W: The chemotherapy of pulmonary tuberculosis: A review. Chest 76(suppl):785, 1979
GLASSROTH J et al: Tuberculosis in the 1980s. N Engl J Med 302:1441, 1980
GOREN MB: Immunoreactive substances of mycobacteria. Am Rev Respir Dis 125(suppl):50, 1982
GROSSET J: Bacteriologic basis of short-course chemotherapy for tuberculosis. Clin Chest Med 1:231, 1980
GRZYBOWSKI S, ENARSON DA: The fate of cases of pulmonary tuberculosis under various treatment programmes. Bull Int Union Tuberc 53:70, 1978
SNIDER DE, JR: The tuberculin skin test. Am Rev Respir Dis 125(suppl):108, 1982
STEAD WW et al: Tuberculosis as an endemic and nosocomial infection among the elderly in nursing homes. N Engl J Med 312:1483, 1985
TENDAM HG et al: Present knowledge of immunization against tuberculosis. Bull WHO 54:255, 1976

120 LEPROSY (HANSEN'S DISEASE)

RICHARD A. MILLER[1]

DEFINITION Leprosy (Hansen's disease) is a chronic granulomatous infection of humans which attacks superficial tissues, especially the skin and peripheral nerves. Accounts of leprosy extend back to the earliest historical records and document a stigmatization of leprosy patients which transcends cultural and religious boundaries. The clinical and immunologic manifestations of disease form a continuum extending from polar *tuberculoid* leprosy to polar *lepromatous* leprosy. The borderline portion of the spectrum lies between these two extremes, and is usually subdivided into *borderline tuberculoid*, *borderline*, and *borderline lepromatous* classes. In addition, an early indeterminate form is seen, which may spontaneously remit or develop into overt leprosy.

ETIOLOGY *Mycobacterium leprae*, or Hansen's bacillus, is the causal agent of leprosy. It is an acid-fast rod assigned to the family Mycobacteriaceae on the basis of morphologic, biochemical, antigenic, and genetic similarities to other mycobacteria. Although it has not been cultivated in artificial media or tissue culture, it can be consistently propagated in the foot pads of mice. Systemic infections with manifestations similar to those of human disease can be induced in armadillos and mangabey monkeys. The bacillus multiplies exceedingly slowly, with an estimated optimal doubling time of 11 to 13 days during logarithmic growth in mouse foot pads. The mouse model has been used extensively for the study of antileprosy drugs, and the high bacterial yield from armadillos has been crucial for immunologic studies.

Lepromin is a suspension of killed *M. leprae* prepared from heavily infected human or armadillo tissue. Intradermal injection elicits, somewhat variably, a tuberculin-like reaction at 48 h (Fernandez's reaction) and more consistently, a papular reaction at 3 to 4 weeks (Mitsuda's reaction). The Mitsuda reaction is usually positive in tuberculoid patients and is always negative in lepromatous patients. However, because it is also positive in nearly all normal adults, even those residing in areas free of endemic leprosy, it has no diagnostic value. Lepromin is not commercially available.

EPIDEMIOLOGY There are probably 10 to 20 million persons affected with leprosy in the world. The disease is more common in tropical countries, in many of which the prevalence rate is 1 to 2 percent of the population. A warm environment is not critical for transmission, as leprosy also occurs in certain regions with cooler climates, such as Korea and central Mexico. Distribution of infected individuals within countries is very nonhomogeneous, and districts in which 20 percent of the population is affected can be found. The distribution of cases across the spectrum of leprosy also varies between countries, with lepromatous disease predominating in some countries, such as Mexico, and tuberculoid disease in other areas, including India. Ninety percent of the approximately 270 cases per year diagnosed in the United States have occurred in immigrants from leprosy-endemic countries. Indigenous transmission occurs primarily in Hawaii, the Pacific Island territories, and sporadically along the Gulf coast.

Leprosy can present at any age, although cases in infants less than 1 year of age are extremely rare. The age-specific incidence peaks during childhood in most developing countries, with up to 20 percent of cases occurring in children under 10. Since leprosy is most prevalent in poorer socioeconomic groups, this may simply reflect the age distribution of the high-risk population. The sex ratio of leprosy presenting during childhood is essentially 1:1, but males predominate by a 2:1 ratio in adult cases.

[1] *Dr. Charles C. Shepard (deceased) contributed significantly to the text on which this revision was based.*

Direct human-to-human transmission is believed responsible for most cases of leprosy. Animal reservoirs exist among feral armadillos and possibly among nonhuman primates, but there is little evidence that they have an important role in the epidemiology of human disease. Familial spread is facilitated by the indolence of the clinical illness and the potential for transmission prior to the development of symptoms. Among close family contacts (spouse-spouse or spouse-child) of untreated lepromatous patients the risk of disease is increased approximately eightfold, and the attack rate can be as high as 10 percent. Development of clinical disease in contacts of tuberculoid patients is less common, although sensitive immunologic tests suggest that most of these contacts have been sensitized to *M. leprae*. The site of entry remains a matter of conjecture, but is probably either the skin or the mucosa of the upper respiratory tract. The chief portal of exit is thought to be the nasal mucosa of untreated lepromatous patients. Transmission is theoretically possible from infected breast milk or via hematophagous arthropod vectors, but the importance of these alternative modalities appears to be minor.

The incubation period is frequently 3 to 5 years, but has been reported to range from 6 months to several decades.

PATHOGENESIS   The early events following the entry of *M. leprae* into the body have not been described in humans. The bacilli are surrounded by a dense, nearly inert lipid capsule, produce no exotoxins, and engender little inflammatory response. The factors which determine the nature and efficacy of the host response to *M. leprae* are unknown. Immunologic and epidemiologic studies suggest that only a small fraction, possibly 10 to 20 percent, of those exposed to viable bacilli will develop signs of indeterminate leprosy and that only about 50 percent of those with indeterminate disease will progress to full-blown clinical leprosy.

The intensity of the specific cell-mediated immune response to *M. leprae* correlates with the clinical and histologic disease class. Individuals with polar tuberculoid disease have an intense cellular response to *M. leprae* and a low bacillary load, whereas patients with lepromatous leprosy have no detectable cellular immunity to the leprosy bacillus. There is evidence from sibling studies that specific HLA-associated genes may be linked to different classes of disease. HLA-DR3 was inherited preferentially by children with polar tuberculoid disease, whereas HLA-MT1 was associated with polar lepromatous disease. The effect of the HLA-associated genes was limited to influencing the type of leprosy which developed. There was no association between HLA haplotypes and overall susceptibility to leprosy. These findings are analogous to those made in mice infected with *Mycobacterium lepraemurium* or *Leishmania donovani*. In the mouse, innate susceptibility or resistance to these intracellular pathogens is controlled by non-H-2 genes (the H-2 locus in mice is the analogue of the human HLA system), but H-2-linked genes subsequently influence the severity of infection which develops in susceptible mice.

The defect in cell-mediated immunity in lepromatous patients is extremely specific. They do not suffer increased morbidity following infection by pathogens such as viruses or parasites for which cellular immunity is important, and they do not have an increased risk of neoplasia. Tuberculin reactivity may be suppressed in untreated lepromatous disease, but usually returns with treatment, unlike the lepromin response, which remains negative. Patients with lepromatous leprosy have been shown to have an increased number of circulating OKT8 ("suppressor") lymphocytes which can be specifically activated by *M. leprae* antigens, and the lymphocytes present in their cutaneous granulomas are almost exclusively OKT8-positive. In contrast, OKT4-positive ("helper") cells predominate among the T cells in the cutaneous lesions of tuberculoid patients. In lepromatous leprosy, cells of the monocyte-macrophage family become engorged with *M. leprae* and are unable to kill or digest the organisms. However, when studied in vitro, monocytes from these patients respond normally to lymphokines and display normal phagocytic and microbicidal activity. These results suggest that an underlying defect

in regulation of T-lymphocyte subpopulations is responsible for the immunologic tolerance characteristic of lepromatous leprosy.

Intense bacillemia is very common in lepromatous leprosy, and organisms can often be seen in stained smears of peripheral blood or buffy coats, but high fever and signs of systemic toxicity are absent. Even in the most advanced cases, destructive lesions are limited to the skin, peripheral nerves, anterior portions of the eyes, upper respiratory passages above the larynx, testes, and structures of the hands and feet. The trophism of *M. leprae* for these tissues may be due to the fact that they are all usually several degrees cooler than 37°C. Two sites of preferential involvement are the ulnar nerves near the elbow and the peroneal nerves where they pass around the head of the fibula; above and below these areas where these nerves take deeper courses, they are much less severely involved. In patients with lepromatous leprosy, collections of bacilli are also found in the liver, spleen, and bone marrow. No visceral organ system dysfunction has been associated with the presence of these bacilli, and it is unclear whether they are capable of reproduction at core body temperatures.

CLINICOPATHOLOGIC CLASSIFICATION   As is true of other chronic infections, such as syphilis and tuberculosis, the manifestations of leprosy are many and variable. The classification in general use is based on clinical and histopathologic findings.

Lepromatous leprosy is one of the polar forms. The cutaneous involvement is extensive, diffuse, and bilaterally symmetric. Even apparently normal skin will usually contain bacilli demonstrable by staining. Peripheral nerves are heavily infected but often better preserved than in the tuberculoid form. Histologically, there is a diffuse granulomatous reaction with macrophages, large foam (Virchow's) cells, and many intracellular bacilli, frequently in spheroidal masses (globi). Epithelioid cells and giant cells are not found.

Tuberculoid leprosy is the other polar type. Skin lesions are single or few and are sharply demarcated. Neurologic involvement is relatively pronounced and may occur in the absence of cutaneous lesions (pure neural leprosy). The histologic picture consists of lymphocytes, epithelioid cells, and perhaps giant cells; bacilli are frequently absent or difficult to demonstrate.

Classification within the borderline region of the spectrum is less precise. Lesions tend to increase in number and heterogeneity, but decrease in individual size as the lepromatous pole is approached. The histopathology of the granulomas also changes from an epithelioid cell predominance to a macrophage predominance. The presence and number of lymphocytes is variable and correlates poorly with the disease class. Bacilli are present in large numbers in the skin granulomas of borderline and borderline lepromatous patients. For this reason, these groups, together with polar lepromatous leprosy, are referred to as "multibacillary leprosy." Borderline tuberculoid, polar tuberculoid, and indeterminate classes are grouped together as "paucibacillary leprosy." The borderline disease states are unstable and may shift toward the lepromatous form in the untreated patient or toward the tuberculoid pole during treatment. Slight discrepancies between the clinical appearance and histopathologic findings are also common. Change of either polar type to the other is exceedingly rare.

In all forms of leprosy peripheral nerve involvement is a constant feature. In any histologic section involvement of nerves will tend to be more severe than involvement of other tissues. Much of the neural destruction appears to result from the granulomatous reaction of the host, rather than from an innate neurotoxic property of the bacillus.

CLINICAL MANIFESTATIONS   Early leprosy   The first signs of leprosy are usually cutaneous. One or more hypopigmented or hyperpigmented macules or plaques may be seen. Often an anesthetic or paresthetic patch is the first symptom noted by the patient, but on careful examination skin involvement can also be found. When contacts are examined, a single skin lesion is often noted, especially in children; usually, this is a hypesthetic macule that may clear spontaneously in a year or two, but specific treatment is usually recommended. Sensation is often preserved in early lesions, particularly those on the face.

Tuberculoid leprosy Early tuberculoid leprosy is frequently manifested by a hypopigmented macule, sharply demarcated and hypesthetic. Later the lesions are larger, and the margins are elevated and circinate or gyrate. There is peripheral spread and central healing. Fully developed lesions are densely anesthetic and have lost the normal skin organs (sweat glands and hair follicles). The lesions appear singly or are few in number and are not symmetric. Nerve involvement occurs early, and the superficial nerves leading from the lesions may be enlarged. The larger peripheral nerves (especially the ulnar, peroneal, and greater auricular nerves) may be palpably and visibly enlarged, particularly those closest to the skin lesion. There may be severe neuritic pain. Neural involvement leads to muscle atrophy, especially of the small muscles of the hand. Contractures of the hand and foot are frequent. Trauma, especially from burns and splinters and from excessive pressure, leads to secondary infection of the hands and to plantar ulcers. Later, resorption and loss of phalanges may supervene. When the facial nerves are involved, there may be lagophthalmos, exposure keratitis, and corneal ulceration leading to blindness.

Lepromatous leprosy The skin lesions are macules, nodules, plaques, or papules. The macules are often hypopigmented. The borders of the lesions are ill defined and the centers of raised lesions are indurated and convex (rather than concave as in tuberculoid disease). There is also diffuse infiltration between the lesions. The sites of predilection are the face (cheeks, nose, brows), ears, wrists, elbows, buttocks, and knees. Involvement with infiltration and little or no nodulation may progress so subtly that the disease goes unnoticed. Loss of the eyebrows, especially the lateral portions, is common. Much later the skin of the face and forehead becomes thickened and corrugated (leonine facies), and the earlobes become pendulous.

Nasal symptoms (nasal "stuffiness," epistaxis, and obstructed breathing) are common early symptoms. Complete nasal obstruction, laryngitis, and hoarseness are also frequent. Septal perforation and nasal collapse lead to saddlenose. Invasion of the anterior portion of the eye leads to keratitis and iridocyclitis. Painless inguinal and axillary lymphadenopathy occurs. In adult males infiltration and scarring of the testes lead to sterility. Gynecomastia is common.

Involvement of major nerve trunks is less prominent in the lepromatous form, but diffuse hypesthesia involving the peripheral portions of the extremities is common in advanced disease.

Borderline leprosy The skin lesions of borderline tuberculoid leprosy generally resemble those of tuberculoid disease, but are greater in number and have more poorly defined borders. Involvement of multiple peripheral nerve trunks is more common than in polar tuberculoid disease. Increasing variability in the appearance of the skin lesions is characteristic of borderline leprosy (sometimes referred to as "dimorphic" leprosy). Papules and plaques may coexist with macular lesions. Anesthesia is less prominent than in tuberculoid disease. Borderline lepromatous disease is characterized by very heterogeneous and relatively symmetric skin lesions. The earlobes may be slightly thickened, but the eyebrows and nasal regions are spared.

REACTIONAL STATES The general course of leprosy is indolent, but it may be interrupted by two types of reaction. Both forms of reactions can occur in untreated patients, but more often emerge as complications of chemotherapy.

Erythema nodosum leprosum Erythema nodosum leprosum (ENL), or type 2 lepra reaction, occurs in lepromatous and borderline lepromatous patients, most frequently in the latter half of the initial year of treatment. Tender, inflamed subcutaneous nodules develop, usually in crops. Each nodule lasts a week or two, but new crops may appear. ENL may last only a week or two, or it may continue for long periods. Low-grade fever, lymphadenopathy, and arthralgias

can accompany severe ENL. Histologically, ENL is characterized by polymorphonuclear infiltration and deposits of IgG and complement; hence, it resembles an Arthus reaction.

Reversal reaction Reversal reaction, or type 1 lepra reaction, can complicate all three borderline categories. Existing skin lesions develop erythema and swelling, and new lesions may appear. An early influx of lymphocytes into existing lesions is followed by edema and a shift toward tuberculoid histology. Cellular immunity increases. Reversal reactions can be differentiated from disease progression or relapse by mouse inoculations to test bacillary viability and by histologic studies. Downgrading reactions, which clinically mimic reversal reactions, are most common in untreated patients and in women during the third trimester of pregnancy. Skin biopsies reveal a shift toward lepromatous histology and reflect a decrease in cellular immunity.

COMPLICATIONS Leprosy is probably the most frequent cause of crippling of the hand in the world. Trauma and secondary chronic infections can lead to loss of digits or distal extremities. Blindness is also common.

The *Lucio phenomenon* is limited to patients with a diffuse, infiltrative, nonnodular lepromatous disease; it is seen most often in Mexico and central America. Arteritis leads to ulceration of the skin in a characteristic angular pattern, and subsequently to angular thin scars. Severe cases clinically resemble other forms of necrotizing vasculitis and are associated with a high mortality rate.

Amyloidosis is a complication of severe lepromatous disease, especially when complicated by chronic ENL.

DIAGNOSIS The demonstration of acid-fast bacilli in skin smears made by the scraped-incision method is strong evidence for leprosy, but in tuberculoid disease bacilli may not be demonstrable. Wherever possible, a skin biopsy specimen from the affected area should be sent to a pathologist knowledgeable in leprosy. The histologic involvement of peripheral nerves is pathognomonic, even in the absence of bacilli.

The lepromin test has no diagnostic value. Hematologic and blood chemistry tests are likewise of little help. Lepromatous patients frequently have mild anemia, elevated erythrocyte sedimentation rate, and hyperglobulinemia. Between 10 and 40 percent of lepromatous patients have false-positive serologic tests for syphilis or autoantibodies directed against nuclear or cellular antigens.

Major advances in the search for a specific serodiagnostic test for leprosy have been made. A surface glycolipid antigen unique to *M. leprae,* referred to as phenolic glycolipid I, has been purified and its chemical structure determined. Assay systems to detect antibody directed against this antigen have been developed and have a sensitivity of over 95 percent in polar lepromatous disease and about 50 percent in polar tuberculoid cases. The specificity is excellent, even when testing serums from patients with tuberculosis or other mycobacterial diseases. When perfected, these assays may be useful for confirming the diagnosis of leprosy, for monitoring the response to therapy, and for screening contacts of leprosy patients for subclinical disease.

The differential diagnosis includes conditions such as lupus erythematosus, lupus vulgaris, sarcoidosis, yaws, dermal leishmaniasis, and a host of banal skin diseases. The skin lesions of leprosy, especially of turberculoid disease, are characterized by hypesthesia, and peripheral nerve involvement can always be demonstrated. Peripheral neuropathy from other causes and syringomyelia may be confused with leprosy, although skin involvement is not a feature of other diseases causing peripheral neuropathy. The combination of a chronic skin disease and peripheral nerve involvement should always lead to the consideration of leprosy.

TREATMENT The management of leprosy involves a broad, multidisciplinary approach, including consultative services such as orthopedic surgery, ophthalmology, and physical therapy in addition to antimicrobial chemotherapy.

Specific chemotherapy *Dapsone* (4,4'-diaminodiphenylsulfone, DDS, diphenylsulfone), a folate antagonist, is the mainstay of therapy. The daily dosage is 50 to 100 mg in adults. Dapsone is very inexpensive, safe in pregnancy, and has a long serum half-life of about 24 h, allowing once daily administration. Major side effects are relatively uncommon, but include hemolysis, agranulocytosis, hepatitis, and potentially fatal exfoliative dermatitis. In lepromatous disease enough bacilli are killed during the first 10 to 12 weeks of dapsone monotherapy to render mouse foot pad inoculations negative. However, in this form of the disease nonviable bacilli disappear slowly and may be found in the tissues for 5 to 10 years. Moreover, a few viable bacilli (persisters) may survive in the tissues for many years and cause a relapse if treatment is discontinued.

Dapsone resistance is a problem of increasing concern. Secondary resistance is most common in lepromatous patients and presents as a clinical and bacteriologic relapse after several years of apparently successful, regular therapy. Sulfone resistance can be demonstrated by mouse foot pad inoculation. The frequency of this secondary resistance has been 2 to 30 percent in different countries, depending on the sulfone used and the regularity of its administration. Primary dapsone resistance in as many as 30 percent of previously untreated patients has complicated empiric therapy in many parts of the world, but has remained uncommon in newly diagnosed patients in the United States. Because of the problems of dapsone-resistant bacilli and of persister bacilli, multiple drug therapy is now recommended for all multibacillary disease.

Rifampin is the most rapidly mycobactericidal drug known for *M. leprae*. The viability of skin bacilli falls to undetectable levels within 5 days following a single 1500-mg dose of oral rifampin. The usual dosage is 600 mg per day. The high cost of rifampin has limited its use in the developing world, and has led to regimens in which it is given at a dosage of 600 or 900 mg once per month. These intermittent regimens are based on animal studies but have not been extensively evaluated in human disease. Until more clinical experience has been accumulated, many leprologists prefer to treat with daily or twice weekly rifampin. Rare cases of rifampin-resistant *M. leprae* have been reported. Rifampin has not been approved for this purpose by the Food and Drug Administration.

Clofazimine is a compound derived from a phenazine dye. It is highly lipophilic and accumulates in the skin, the gastrointestinal tract, and in macrophages and monocytes. Its pharmacokinetics are poorly understood, but it is usually given in a dosage of 50 to 200 mg per day and has an apparent half-life of over 70 days. Major toxicity is restricted to the skin and the intestinal tract. The reddish skin pigmentation, often accompanied by ichthyosis, is unacceptable to many light-skinned patients, and can lead to poor compliance. The intestinal toxicity is also dose-related and is reflected in diarrhea and cramping abdominal pain. Clofazimine has not been shown to be safe for use during pregnancy. Clofazimine is an investigational drug in the United States and is available for protocol use through the National Hansen's Disease Center, Carville, Louisiana.

Several other agents, including ethionamide, prothionamide, thiambutosine, and amithiozone, have limited activity against *M. leprae* and may be of value in multiple drug regimens. None of these drugs have been approved for this purpose by the Food and Drug Administration.

Therapy for multibacillary disease should consist of three drugs, usually dapsone, rifampin, and clofazimine. If the organism is known to be dapsone-sensitive, the combination of dapsone and rifampin may be adequate for borderline and borderline lepromatous cases, but the likelihood of secondary dapsone resistance makes the addition of a third drug advisable in lepromatous disease. Objective measures of response to therapy, including skin scrapings and biopsies, should be monitored and therapy continued at least until they are consistently negative. The optimal duration of therapy is unknown, but a minimum of 2 years is recommended. Indefinite therapy may be required for lepromatous disease.

Therapeutic regimens containing two drugs, usually dapsone and rifampin, are adequate for paucibacillary leprosy. The World Health Organization recommends a 6-month course, which can be repeated if relapse occurs. Standard practice in the United States is to treat with dapsone and rifampin for the first 6 to 12 months (depending on the clinical response), followed by dapsone alone to complete a total of 24 months of therapy.

Objective evidence of clinical improvement should be visible by the second or third month of treatment. The clinical response to adequate therapy may be confused by intercurrent reactional states, but the disease stops progressing and the skin lesions gradually improve. Recovery from neurologic impairment is limited.

Treatment of reactional states Mild ENL is managed with antipyretics and analgesics. Severe cases can be rapidly controlled with high dosages of prednisone (60 to 120 mg per day). Antimicrobial therapy should be continued as corticosteroid therapy promotes the viability of *M. leprae* in mice not given antileprosy drugs. Rifampin enhances the metabolism of corticosteroids by the liver, necessitating administration of larger doses to achieve a given therapeutic effect. Thalidomide is the most effective drug for ENL. The usual initial dosage is 200 mg twice a day, which can be gradually tapered to a maintenance dosage of 50 to 100 mg per day for patients with chronic ENL. Thalidomide is absolutely contraindicated in women of childbearing age because of its teratogenicity, but has proved relatively free of major side effects in other leprosy patients. This drug has not been approved by the Food and Drug Administration but is available through the National Hansen's Disease Center as an investigational agent. Clofazimine has anti-inflammatory properties as well as antimycobacterial activity and can be valuable in the treatment of chronic ENL, but requires at least 3 to 4 weeks to reach effective levels, making it of little use in acute attacks. Other classes of anti-inflammatory agents including antimalarials such as chloroquine and cytotoxic drugs have been used in difficult cases; in general these unusual situations should be managed in consultation with a leprosy specialist.

Reversal reactions are often acute and can lead to rapid and irreversible neurologic damage. Corticosteroids are indicated for severe reversal reactions. Clofazimine is of some use in chronic situations, but it is generally necessary to continue corticosteroids as well. Reversal reactions do not respond to thalidomide.

Other measures Many of the deformities and disabilities of leprosy are preventable. Plantar ulcers, which are very common, may be prevented by rigid-soled footwear or walking plaster casts, and contractures of the hand may be prevented by physical therapy and application of casts. Reconstructive surgery is sometimes helpful. Nerve and tendon transplants and release of contractures can give patients more functional ability. Vocational retraining is often necessary for those with permanent disability. Plastic repair of facial deformities assists acceptance of patients in society. The psychological trauma which resulted from prolonged segregation is now minimized by home therapy in virtually all cases.

Control Case finding and chemotherapy form the present basis of control because infectiousness is quickly suppressed, as is the development of deformity. Early detection of cases is especially important. In endemic countries this means the establishment of clinics or traveling teams. Family and other close contacts need regular examinations for leprosy. In the United States patients are eligible for treatment by the Public Health Service, and special clinics are located in several major cities, as well as an inpatient facility at the National Hansen's Disease Center in Carville, Louisiana. Risk of transmission is very low, even in untreated patients, and no unusual infection control precautions are required when patients are hospitalized. Chemoprophylaxis with lowered dosages of dapsone is effective, but contact screening by yearly physical examinations is preferred to empiric therapy in most situations. Field trials of bacillus Calmette-Guérin (BCG) vaccination in endemic areas have given conflicting results, but even the most optimistic reports have shown only modest efficacy. A vaccine which combines viable BCG and heat-killed *M. leprae* has shown promise in pilot studies and is now undergoing field trials.

REFERENCES

BLOOM BR, GODAL T: Selective primary health care: Strategies for control of disease in the developing world. V. Leprosy. Rev Infect Dis 5:765, 1983

BULLOCK WE: Rifampin in the treatment of leprosy. Rev Infect Dis 5:S606, 1983

————: *Mycobacterium leprae* (leprosy), in *Principles and Practice of Infectious Diseases*, 2 ed, GL Mandell et al (eds). New York, Wiley, 1985, pp 1406–1413

DUNCAN ME et al: Pregnancy and leprosy: The consequences of alterations of cell-mediated and humoral immunity during pregnancy and lactation. Int J Lepr 50:425, 1982

NEILL MA et al: Leprosy in the United States, 1971–1981. J Infect Dis 152:1064, 1985

RIDLEY DS, JOPING WH: Classification of leprosy according to immunity: A five-group system. Int J Lepr 34:255, 1966

SANSONETTI P, LAGRANGE PH: The immunology of leprosy: Speculations on the leprosy spectrum. Rev Infect Dis 3:422, 1981

VAN EDEN W et al: HLA-linked control of predisposition to lepromatous leprosy. J Infect Dis 151:9, 1985

VAN VOORHIS WC et al: The cutaneous infiltrates of leprosy: Cellular characteristics and the predominant T-cell phenotypes. N Engl J Med 307:1593, 1983

WHO STUDY GROUP: Chemotherapy of leprosy for control programs. WHO Tech Rep Ser 675:7, 1982

YOUNG DB, BUCHANAN TM: A serological test for leprosy with a glycolipid specific for *Mycobacterium leprae*. Science 221:1057, 1983

121 OTHER MYCOBACTERIAL INFECTIONS

STANLEY D. FREEDMAN[1]

INTRODUCTION Myobacteria other than the tubercle bacilli were shown to be agents of human disease in the 1950s. A classification of these organisms based upon colonial morphology and growth characteristics was provided by Runyon. These bacteria are widely distributed in nature as saprophytes, primarily in soil and water. Animals can be infected and serve as reservoirs for infection of humans. Person-to-person transmission has not been documented. Epidemiologic studies using tuberculins from the various species demonstrated the extent of infection in the United States and other countries, as well as notable geographic differences. These organisms have been referred to as atypical mycobacteria or anonymous mycobacteria. Although the organisms are not always anonymous, the frequency with which they are found in the environment demands repeated isolation from a diseased area before they can be accepted as the etiologic agent. With the steady improvement of laboratory techniques including radiometric cultures, species designations are now increasingly familiar and preferred in the study of these pathogens (Table 121-1). With increasing sophistication of medical practice and the emergence of newly recognized diseases, additional syndromes associated with different species have emerged and have assumed major importance.

MYCOBACTERIUM ULCERANS *M. ulcerans* is the etiologic agent of the Buruli or Bairnsdale ulcer. It grows only at 30 to 33°C. Colonies require 7 weeks to appear; isolation is enhanced by inoculation of mouse foot pads. A disease of the tropics, it is concentrated in Australia and Africa. The first sign of infection with *M. ulcerans* is a small painless nodule developing into an extensive granulomatous ulceration usually affecting the extensor surfaces of the extremities. Characteristically, the ulcer is deep with a necrotic base and undermined edges. Wide surgical excision with skin grafting is curative; there are no clear data regarding chemotherapy.

MYCOBACTERIUM MARINUM This organism, previously called *M. balnei*, is a psychrophilic (30°C) photochromogen which inhabits fresh and salt water and causes disease in fish. Human infections are usually associated with some aquatic activity, like working in aquaria and swimming. The organism enters abraded skin and either forms a nodule, which can spread along lymphatics suggesting sporotrichosis, causes verrucous lesions, or, less commonly, ulcerates. The pathology consists of a granulomatous lesion usually without caseation—the so-called swimming pool or fishtank granuloma. Infection is frequently associated with a positive tuberculin test reflecting shared antigens with *M. tuberculosis*. Because the differential diagnosis includes sporotrichosis as well as other mycobacterial infections, appropriate cultures (30 to 32°C incubation) are critical. Infections of tendon sheaths and synovia have been described in association with penetrating injuries. Ulcerations similar to those caused by *M. ulcerans*, as well as disseminated skin lesions, have been reported in immunocompromised patients. Minor lesions can resolve spontaneously. The organism is often sensitive in vitro to rifampin and ethambutol, and these drugs have been curative. Tetracycline, especially minocycline, and trimethoprim/sulfamethoxazole have also been used with favorable results.

MYCOBACTERIUM KANSASII *M. kansasii* produces pigment upon exposure to light, grows at 37°C, and is a long, thick, acid-fast organism with prominent transverse banding. Infections are more common in the central United States, Texas, England, and Wales. The reasons for these geographic variations are unknown, but likely relate to subtle ecologic properties of these organisms. Person-to-person spread is not recognized. Reported cases reflect a preponderance of white adult men.

Pulmonary disease is the commonest expression of this organism, and the clinical picture closely resembles pulmonary tuberculosis although signs and symptoms are milder. Pneumoconiosis and chronic obstructive pulmonary disease (COPD) are considered predisposing conditions. Thin-walled cavities with minimal inflammatory reaction are characteristic. The usual situation, without treatment, is slow progression.

Disseminated disease is now recognized as an important manifestation of *M. kansasii* infections. Such hematogenous spread is associated with pancytopenia, hairy cell leukemia, malignancies, and

[1] Dr. Charles C. Shepard (deceased) contributed significantly to the text on which this revision was based.

TABLE 121-1 Human mycobacterial pathogens other than *M. tuberculosis* and *M. leprae*

Mycobacterium	Pigmentation of culture*	Usual site of disease	Usual source of infection	Response to drugs
M. marinum	P	Skin	Swimming pools, aquaria, fish	Good
M. ulcerans	N	Skin	Tropical environment	Variable
M. avium-intracellulare	N	Lungs	Environment, animals?	Poor
M. kansasii	P	Lungs	Environment?	Good
M. xenopi	S	Lungs	Water, animals?	Variable
M. szulgai	S†	Lungs	?	Good
M. scrofulaceum	S	Lungs, lymph nodes	Water, soil	Good
M. fortuitum	N	Skin (abscesses), lungs	Soil, dirt, water	Poor
M. chelonei	N	Skin (abscesses), lungs	Soil, dirt, water	Poor

* P = photochromogenic (develops yellow-orange pigment only when exposed to light); N = nonpigmented; S = scotochromogenic (develops yellow-orange pigment in the dark).
† Scotochromogenic at 37°C, photochromogenic at 25°C.

bone marrow and renal transplantations. Fever, anemia, and signs and symptoms referrable to multiple organ system involvement occur. The diagnosis is confirmed by appropriate cultures of involved tissues. Skin and soft tissue involvement is seen and may mimic *M. marinum* infections. Tenosynovitis, osteomyelitis, lymphadenitis, pericarditis, and genitourinary tract infections have been reported.

Diseases due to *M. kansasii* respond well to treatment. Rifampin appears to be the most effective drug and should be used in all initial regimens. Ethambutol and isoniazid are usually the other drugs administered. Over 95 percent of patients respond to this combined regimen. Retreatment programs should be guided by in vitro sensitivity testing, and rifampin used if the organism is sensitive.

MYCOBACTERIUM SCROFULACEUM This scotochromogenic bacillus is a major cause of lymphadenitis in children. Cervical nodes are usually involved, and associated systemic symptoms are rare. Definitive diagnosis requires culture, and definitive therapy requires total excision of the node and sinus tract, if present. There are a few reports of pulmonary disease and osseous and soft tissue infections; dissemination usually is associated with serious underlying conditions. Sensitivity patterns vary, and multiple-drug regimens have been used.

MYCOBACTERIUM SZULGAI At 37°C this organism is scotochromogenic and can be confused with more common tap water contaminants. It was initially recognized as an uncommon pulmonary pathogen; there are also reports of bursitis, lymphadenitis, and tenosynovitis. Most isolates are sensitive to rifampin and ethambutol.

MYCOBACTERIUM XENOPI *M. xenopi* is a slow-growing scotochromogen which infrequently causes tuberculosis-like pulmonary disease in humans. However, reports of disseminated disease are becoming more common and include an association with the acquired immunodeficiency syndrome (see below). Unlike a number of nontuberculous mycobacteria it is sensitive to most of the antituberculous drugs.

MYCOBACTERIUM AVIUM-INTRACELLULARE Although seroagglutination, thin-layer chromatography, and enzyme-linked immunoabsorbent assays can distinguish *M. avium* from *M. intracellulare*, distinction is difficult and they are considered as a complex (MAI). These ubiquitous organisms are particularly prevalent in the southeastern United States and, overall, are the most commonly isolated mycobacteria other than *M. tuberculosis*. Colonization and inapparent infection are common; knowledge of transmission is limited. The lungs are most commonly involved, and the clinical picture is similar to pulmonary tuberculosis. Underlying pulmonary disease, a possible genetic predilection, and age are risk factors. Solitary pulmonary nodules are not uncommon. It is important to be certain of the etiology and the pathogenic role of the organism isolated, because chemotherapy is often associated with morbidity.

Skin involvement and musculoskeletal infections including vertebral osteomyelitis resembling Pott's disease have been described. MAI is a major cause of lymphadenitis in children. Disseminated disease is also recognized in children, and in adults in association with severe underlying diseases. Fever, anemia, leukocytosis, hypergammaglobulinemia, and hepatosplenomegaly are prominent features.

These organisms have been added to the list of opportunistic infections complicating the acquired immunodeficiency syndrome (AIDS). They represent one of the most common life-threatening infections in this syndrome. The manifestations are unique and basically reflect overwhelming infection in these hosts with impaired cellular immunity. There is mycobacteremia, and organisms abound in most organs and body secretions. There is a minimal cellular response, granulomatous or otherwise. Profound diarrhea with intestinal pathology that strikingly resembles Whipple's disease, due to macrophages packed with MAI, is recognized. In other organs these macrophages resemble lepra cells.

Treatment is difficult and unsatisfactory. The organisms are usually resistant to most of the antimycobacterial agents. Yet multiple-drug therapy is recommended with some demonstrable benefit possibly reflecting synergy which is difficult to prove in vitro. Drugs chosen should include those antimicrobials to which the organism is sensitive. Three to six drugs are used concurrently, chosen from among isoniazid, ethambutol, rifampin, ethionamide, pyrazinamide, cycloserine, streptomycin, kanamycin, and capreomycin. Of these, ethambutol, ethionamide, and cycloserine appear more effective. Surgical excision is the treatment of choice for lymphadenitis and is a reasonable alternative for a few other localized infections. The experimental drugs clofazimine and rifabutine have been used along with immunomodulators in patients with MAI infections complicating AIDS (see Chap. 257).

MYCOBACTERIUM FORTUITUM AND CHELONEI The unique feature of these acid-fast bacteria is their rapid growth; initial growth may take 1 to 5 weeks, but subsequent subcultures grow within 5 days. Reflecting their meager nutritional requirements, they are readily cultured on most media. These two species account for virtually all the reported infections due to rapid growers. *M. fortuitum* is more frequently associated with posttraumatic and postsurgical skin and soft tissue infection. *M. chelonei* is a more common cause of pulmonary infections and disseminated disease. Subspeciation is not necessary for clinical purposes. Widespread in nature and in hospital environments, and highly resistant to drugs, antiseptics, and disinfectants, rapid growers are important nosocomial pathogens.

Most human infections are associated with interruption of the integument and injury or alteration of the soft tissues. Inhalational pulmonary disease complicates underlying lung disease. Although a chronic granulomatous reaction with caseation may occur, the distinguishing feature is a suppurative process with microabscesses, and diphtheroid-like organisms on Gram stain. Infections have followed cardiothoracic surgery, augmentation mammoplasty, arthroplasty, injections, ocular surgery, and dialysis. Clinical manifestations include lymphadenitis, keratitis, osteomyelitis, meningitis, and endocarditis involving porcine, prosthetic, and natural valves. Hematogenous dissemination is uncommon, and affects those with impaired host defenses.

Adequate debridement and drainage with removal of foreign bodies is indicated whenever possible. Many of these organisms are highly resistant to all antimicrobial agents. However, reflecting their growth characteristics, antimicrobial sensitivity testing is more reliable in determining appropriate chemotherapy. Amikacin is most often effective, but other drugs of proven value include gentamicin, cefoxitin, doxycycline, erythromycin, sulfonamides, rifampin, and ethambutol. Sulfonamides are more active against *M. fortuitum*, and erythromycin inhibits some *M. chelonei*. Because of the emergence of resistant organisms, two or three drugs may be preferable to one.

OTHER MYCOBACTERIA *M. haemophilum* has emerged as a skin pathogen. It is psychrophilic, but requires iron supplements for growth. Virtually all reported cases have been in immunosuppressed patients. Ulcerating skin lesions with acid-fast bacilli that could not be grown have been described in individuals living in Minnesota and the adjacent Canadian border. The disease is self-limited. Unclassified mycobacterial species are being sought as etiologic agents in inflammatory bowel disease; these might be similar to *M. paratuberculosis*, the agent of Johne's disease, an intestinal disease of ruminants.

With increasing laboratory and clinical sophistication, the list of diseases caused by nontuberculous mycobacteria may lengthen.

REFERENCES

COLLINS CH, GRANGE JM: *Mycobacterium marinum* infections in man. J Hyg Camb 94:135, 1985

GREENE JB, SIDHU GS: *Mycobacterium avium-intracellulare:* A cause of disseminated life-threatening infection in homosexuals and drug abusers. Ann Intern Med 97:539, 1982

LICHTENSTEIN IH, MACGREGOR RR: Mycobacterial infections in renal transplant recipients: Report of five cases and review of the literature. Rev Infect Dis 5:216, 1983

ROTH RI, OWEN RL: Intestinal infection with *Mycobacterium avium* in acquired immune deficiency syndrome (AIDS). Dig Dis Sci 30:497, 1985

RUNYON EH: Anonymous mycobacteria in pulmonary disease. Med Clin North Am 43:273, 1959

SANDERS WE: Other *Mycobacterium* species, in *Principles and Practice of Infectious Diseases*, 2d ed, GL Mandel et al. (eds). New York, Wiley, 1985

WALLACE RJ, SWENSON JM: Spectrum of disease due to rapidly growing mycobacteria. Rev Infect Dis 5:657, 1983

————: Treatment of nonpulmonary infections due to *Mycobacterium fortuitum* and *Mycobacterium chelonei* on the basis of in vitro susceptibilities. J Infect Dis 152:500, 1985

WEINBERG JR, GERTNER D: Disseminated *Mycobacterium xenopi* infection. Lancet 1:1033, 1985

WOLINSKY E: Nontuberculous mycobacteria and associated diseases. Am Rev Resp Dis 119:107, 1979

WONG B, EDWARDS FF: Continuous high-grade *Mycobacterium avium-intracellulare* bacteremia in patients with the acquired immune deficiency syndrome. Am J Med 78:35, 1985

section 5 Spirochetal diseases

122 SYPHILIS

KING K. HOLMES / SHEILA A. LUKEHART

DEFINITION Syphilis is a chronic systemic infection caused by *Treponema pallidum* subspecies *pallidum*, is usually sexually transmitted, and is characterized by an incubation period averaging 3 weeks, followed by a primary lesion associated with regional lymphadenopathy; a secondary bacteremic stage associated with generalized mucocutaneous lesions and generalized lymphadenopathy; a latent period of subclinical infection lasting many years; and, in about one-third of untreated cases, a tertiary stage characterized by progressive destructive mucocutaneous musculoskeletal or parenchymal lesions, aortitis, or central nervous system disease.

ETIOLOGY The discovery of *Treponema pallidum* in syphilitic material was made by Schaudinn and Hoffman in 1905. *Treponema pallidum* is one of the many spiral-shaped microorganisms which propel themselves by spinning around their longitudinal axis. The Spirochaetales include three genera which are pathogenic for humans and for a variety of other animals: the *Leptospira*, which cause human leptospirosis; the *Borrelia*, including *B. recurrentis* and *B. vincentii*, which cause relapsing fever and Vincent's angina, respectively, as well as *B. burgdorferi*, the causative agent of Lyme disease; and the *Treponema*, responsible for the diseases known as treponematoses. The *Treponema* include *T. pallidum* subspecies *pallidum* (hereafter called *T. pallidum*) which causes syphilis; *T. pallidum* subspecies *pertenue*, *T. pallidum* subspecies *endemicum*, and *T. carateum*, the organisms which cause yaws, endemic syphilis, and pinta (see Chap. 123); and *T. paraluiscuniculi*, the cause of rabbit syphilis. Other treponema include nonpathogenic species found in the human mouth and several species of anaerobic saprophytic genital treponemes of low pathogenicity which often coexist with anaerobic gram-negative rods in ulcerative genital lesions (so-called fusospirochetal infections). These can also be confused with *T. pallidum* on dark-field examination.

Treponema pallidum is a thin, delicate organism with 6 to 14 spirals and tapered ends, measuring 6 to 15 μm in total length and 0.2 μm in width. The cytoplasm is surrounded by a trilaminar cytoplasmic membrane, which in turn is surrounded by a delicate inner mucopeptide layer, the periplast, thought to be composed of alternating molecules of *N*-acetyl glucosamine and *N*-acetyl muramic acid, and which provides some structural rigidity, while an outer lipoprotein membrane is selectively permeable and osmotically sensitive. The spiral structure of *T. pallidum* is maintained by six fibrils, three arising at each end of the organism, which wind around the cell body in a space between the inner cell wall and the outer cell membrane, and may be the contractile elements responsible for motility. None of the four pathogenic treponemes has yet been cultured in vitro in quantities sufficient to permit detailed comparisons of the organisms, and no convincing morphologic, serologic, or metabolic differences between them have been discerned. They are distinguished primarily according to the clinical syndrome they produce. Limited animal inoculation studies also indicate some differences in host range and virulence, even among different strains of *T. pallidum*. The only known natural host for *T. pallidum* is the human. Many mammals can be infected with *T. pallidum*, but only humans, higher apes, and a few laboratory animals regularly develop syphilitic lesions. Virulent strains of *T. pallidum* are maintained in rabbits.

HISTORY The first clear descriptions of syphilis were recorded at the end of the fifteenth century, when a pandemic known as the great pox, as distinguished from smallpox, swept over Europe and Asia. Severe morbidity or death often occurred during the secondary stage, indicating an unexplained virulence then which is almost unknown today, except in congenital syphilis. The sexual mode of transmission of syphilis was recognized early during the European pandemic, and description of the primary and secondary stages of the disease followed. The major cardiovascular and neurologic complications of late syphilis were recognized during the eighteenth and nineteenth centuries. Gummas were not recognized as being syphilitic in origin until this century.

A rapid series of important advances began in 1903 with the successful inoculation of syphilis into primates. The discovery of *Treponema pallidum* in serum from secondary lesions was made in 1905. In 1910, the complement fixation test for the diagnosis of syphilis and an arsenic derivative, arsphenamine (Compound 606, Salvarsan), which was effective in treatment, were introduced.

EPIDEMIOLOGY Nearly all cases of syphilis are acquired by sexual contact with infectious lesions (i.e., the chancre, mucous patch, skin rash, or condyloma latum). Less common modes of transmission include nonsexual personal contact and infection in utero or following blood transfusions.

In the United States, infant deaths due to syphilis, and new admissions of patients with syphilitic psychoses, have fallen by 99 percent since 1940. The total reported number of cases of late and late latent syphilis has fallen almost every year since 1943. The 7.4 cases per 100,000 population reported in 1983 represent a decrease of over 98 percent since 1943. Only 239 cases of congenital syphilis were reported in 1983, a decrease of 98 percent since 1941; however, 321 cases were reported in 1984, an increase of 34 percent over the previous year. The number of new cases of infectious syphilis reached a peak in 1947, then fell steadily to about 6000 in 1957, but then began to increase again in the late 1970s. In 1984, there were 28,559 cases of primary and secondary syphilis and 23,117 cases of early latent syphilis reported; the number of unreported cases was estimated to be greater.

The peak incidence of syphilis occurs in the age group 15 to 34. In the United States, the male/female ratio of reported early cases (<1 year) increased from 0.8:1 in 1950 to 3.2:1 in 1980, and dropped to 2.6:1 in 1983. The high male/female ratio results from the disproportionate representation of syphilis in male homosexuals. Of all men with primary, secondary, or early latent syphilis interviewed in the United States during 1980, one-half were homosexual or bisexual. It has been speculated that the AIDS epidemic has caused a decrease in new sexual exposure in the homosexual population and that this change is largely responsible for the decreasing overall incidence of sexually transmitted diseases, including syphilis, observed since 1983. There are few data to support this hypothesis for syphilis, however. Although there was a 12.7 percent decrease in the total number of reported cases of primary and secondary syphilis from 1983 to 1984, the number of reported cases of primary and secondary syphilis in women also decreased by 12.2 percent during that same period, indicating that the incidence in homosexual men was not decreasing more rapidly than in heterosexuals.

Although the reported incidence of syphilis appears higher in nonwhites than in whites, and is higher in urban than in rural areas, these differences partly reflect the fact that urban racial groups are treated at public clinics, where case reporting is complete. The case rates of early syphilis are highest in the south and southwest, and in those states with large urban populations.

Of patients with reported early syphilis in 1983, 52 percent were self-referred, 24 percent were contact referrals, and 23 percent were identified by serologic screening. Interviews of patients with early syphilis disclose an average of 1.98 sexual contacts at risk per patient. Approximately one of two individuals named as contacts of infectious syphilis becomes infected. Many contacts will have already developed manifestations of syphilis when they are first seen, and about 30 percent of apparently uninfected contacts of infectious syphilis who are examined within 30 days of exposure will actually be in the incubation stage and will themselves develop infectious syphilis if not treated. Because of this, the identification and "epidemiologic" treatment of all recently exposed contacts has become an important aspect of syphilis control. Also important is the identification of syphilitics by serologic testing of pregnant women, hospital admissions, military inductees, and persons undergoing examination in physicians' offices. Of 45 million blood specimens examined during 1980 in the United States, 1.4 million tests were reactive, representing untreated syphilis, previously treated syphilis, or false-positive tests. Of all reported early syphilis cases of less than 1 year's duration in 1983, 47 percent were detected as a direct result of either contact tracing or serologic testing. More controversial are laws and regulations requiring routine premarital serologic testing for syphilis. Of 3.8 million premarital serologies performed in 1978, only 1 in 8461 was positive for infectious syphilis; the number positive for latent syphilis requiring treatment is probably larger, though national data are not available. Each state should review its own data on the yield of premarital testing; in general, the yield is currently highest in certain southern states, Texas, and the District of Columbia.

NATURAL COURSE AND PATHOGENESIS OF UNTREATED SYPHILIS

Treponema pallidum can rapidly penetrate intact mucous membranes or abraded skin and within a few hours enters the lymphatics and blood to produce systemic infection and metastatic foci long before and after the appearance of a primary lesion. Blood from a patient with incubating syphilis is infectious. The generation time of *T. pallidum* in vivo is estimated to be 30 to 33 h, and the incubation period of syphilis is inversely proportional to the number of organisms inoculated. The concentration of treponemes generally reaches at least 10^7 per gram of tissue before the appearance of a clinical lesion. In experimental infection in rabbits or humans, very low numbers of

treponemes can initiate infection which leads to a discernible lesion only after several weeks, although histopathologic changes are evident earlier; intradermal injection of 10^6 organisms usually produces a lesion within 72 h. The number of organisms required for production of symptomatic infection in humans was determined by intradermal injection of three graded doses of *T. pallidum* simultaneously at separate inoculation sites into each of eight volunteers. While lesions developed at all sites infected with 10^3 organisms, chancres appeared at 63 and 38 percent of sites inoculated with 10^2 and 10 *T. pallidum*, respectively, with incubation periods ranging from 20 to 42 days for the lowest dose. Based upon these results, the infectious dose 50 (ID_{50}) was calculated to be 57 organisms. The median incubation period in humans is about 21 days, suggesting an average inoculum of 500 to 1000 infectious organisms for naturally acquired disease. Although the incubation period is traditionally stated as ranging from 9 to 90 days, experimental inoculations of humans and rabbits show that the period from inoculation until the primary lesion is discernible rarely exceeds 6 weeks. Subcurative therapy during the incubation period may delay the onset of the primary lesion, but it is not certain that this reduces the probability of ultimate development of symptomatic disease.

The primary lesion appears at the site of inoculation, usually persists for 2 to 6 weeks, and then heals spontaneously. Histopathology of primary lesions shows perivascular infiltration, chiefly by lymphocytes, plasma cells, and histiocytes, with capillary endothelial proliferation, and subsequent obliteration of small blood vessels. At this time *T. pallidum* is demonstrable in the chancre in spaces between epithelial cells as well as within invaginations or phagosomes of epithelial cells, fibroblasts, plasma cells, and the endothelial cells of small capillaries, within lymphatic channels, and in the regional lymph nodes. Macrophages can be seen taking up treponemes into phagocytic vacuoles where the organisms are destroyed.

The generalized parenchymal, constitutional, and mucocutaneous manifestations of secondary syphilis usually appear about 6 to 8 weeks after healing of the chancre, although 15 percent of patients with secondary syphilis have persisting or healing chancres. In other patients, secondary lesions may appear only several months after the chancre has healed, and some patients may enter the latent stage without ever developing secondary lesions. Secondary maculopapular skin lesions show histopathologic features of hyperkeratosis of the epidermis, capillary proliferation with endothelial swelling in the superficial corium, and dermal papillae with transmigration of polymorphonuclear leukocytes, and in the deeper corium, perivascular infiltration by monocytes, plasma cells, and lymphocytes. Treponemes are found in many tissues including the aqueous humor of the eye and the cerebrospinal fluid. Cerebrospinal fluid abnormalities are detected in as many as 40 percent of patients during the secondary stage. Hepatitis and immune complex–induced glomerulonephritis are relatively rare but recognized manifestations of early syphilis. Generalized lymphadenopathy is present in 85 percent of patients with secondary syphilis, and is characterized by marked follicular hyperplasia, with histiocytic infiltration and lymphocyte depletion of the paracortical areas, where treponema are present in greatest numbers. The reason for the paradoxical appearance of secondary manifestations in the face of high titers of humoral antibody (including immobilizing antibody) to *T. pallidum* is unknown. The secondary lesions subside within 2 to 6 weeks, and the patient enters the latent stage, which is detectable only by serologic testing. In the preantibiotic era, up to 25 percent of untreated patients experienced one or more subsequent generalized or localized mucocutaneous relapses at some time during the first 2 to 4 years after infection. Since 90 percent of such infectious relapses occur during the first year, identification and examination of sexual contacts are most important for patients with syphilis of less than 1 year's duration.

The World Health Organization now arbitrarily divides latent syphilis into early latent (less than 1 year's duration) and late latent (over 1 year's duration) stages. However, because infectious relapse can occur during the first 2 years, and because the risk of congenital syphilis continues to be high during the first 2 years after acquisition of infection, the International Classification of Diseases defines early latent syphilis as less than 2 years' duration and late latent as over 2 years' duration. In the preantibiotic period, about one-third of patients with untreated latent syphilis developed clinically apparent tertiary disease; today, in medically advanced societies, specific and coincidental therapy of early and latent syphilis have greatly reduced the incidence of tertiary disease. In the past, the most common type of tertiary disease was the gumma, a usually benign granulomatous lesion. Today, gummas are very uncommon, perhaps because they respond to very low doses of antitreponemal drugs. The remaining tertiary lesions are caused by obliterative small vessel endarteritis which usually involves the vasa vasorum of the ascending aorta and, less often, the central nervous system. Factors which determine development of tertiary disease are unknown.

The course of untreated syphilis has been studied retrospectively in a group of nearly 2000 patients with primary or secondary syphilis diagnosed clinically, before the dark-field and Wasserman tests came into use (the Oslo Study, 1891–1951); prospectively in 431 black men with seropositive latent syphilis of 3 or more years' duration (the Tuskegee Study, 1932–1972); and retrospectively in a review of 198 autopsies of patients with untreated syphilis.

In the Oslo Study, 24 percent of the patients developed relapsing secondary lesions within 4 years, and 28 percent eventually developed one or more manifestations of late syphilis. Cardiovascular syphilis, including aortitis, was detected in 10 percent, with no cases occurring in those infected before age 15; symptomatic neurosyphilis occurred in 7 percent, and 16 percent developed benign tertiary syphilis (gumma of the skin, mucous membranes, and skeleton). Syphilis was the primary cause of death in 15 percent of males and 8 percent of the females. However, many patients alive when the Oslo Study was completed remained at risk for developing complications, while tuberculosis and other infections prematurely eliminated others before complications of syphilis occurred, so the Oslo figures probably represent minimum estimates of the risk of late complications. Cardiovascular syphilis was found in 35 percent of men and 22 percent of women who eventually underwent autopsy. In general, serious late complications were nearly twice as common in men as in women.

The Tuskegee Study showed that the death rate of untreated syphilitic black men, 25 to 50 years of age, was 17 percent greater than in nonsyphilitics, and 30 percent of all deaths were attributable to cardiovascular or central nervous system syphilis. The ethical issues raised by this study, begun in the preantibiotic era but continuing into the early 1970s, had a major influence on development of current guidelines for human medical experimentation. By far the most important factor in increased mortality was cardiovascular syphilis. Anatomic evidence of aortitis was found in 40 to 60 percent of autopsied syphilitics (versus 15 percent of controls), while central nervous system lues was found in only 4 percent. Hypertension was also increased in the syphilitics. The incidence of cardiovascular syphilis was higher and central nervous system syphilis lower in the prospective Tuskegee Study than in the Oslo Study. These studies each show that about one-third of patients with untreated syphilis develop clinical or pathologic evidence of tertiary syphilis; about one-fourth die as a direct result of tertiary syphilis; and additional excess mortality not directly attributable to tertiary syphilis is also seen. Untreated syphilis may make people more susceptible to other diseases, or individuals who get syphilis coincidentally may be more susceptible to other diseases, perhaps because of socioeconomic factors.

MANIFESTATIONS   Primary syphilis   The typical primary chancre
usually begins as a single painless papule which rapidly becomes eroded and usually, but not always, is indurated, with a characteristic cartilaginous consistency on palpation of the edge and base of the ulcer (Fig. 122-1). Histologic examination of the ulcer shows mononuclear and histiocytic infiltrates with obliterative endarteritis

and periarteritis of small vessels. *Treponema pallidum* is seen by electron microscopy to lie in interstitial perivascular spaces and within invaginations or phagosomes of macrophages, neutrophils, endothelial cells, and plasma cells.

In heterosexual men, the chancre is usually located on the penis. In homosexual men, the chancre is often found in the anal canal or rectum, within the mouth, or on the external genitalia. It may occur on any site of the body. In women, common primary sites are the cervix and labia. Primary syphilis is often overlooked in women or in homosexual men. For example, during 1974 in the United States, 42 percent of cases of early syphilis in heterosexual men were detected in the primary stages, whereas only 23 percent of early cases in homosexual men and 11 percent of early cases in women were detected in the primary stages. Anorectal chancres account for only 15 percent of primary syphilis among homosexuals in the United States, suggesting that anorectal chancres are most often asymptomatic or are not sought by clinicians evaluating men with suspected syphilis, or that the clinician fails to consider syphilis in the evaluation of anal lesions in men.

Regional lymphadenopathy accompanies the primary lesion, appearing within 1 week of the onset of the lesion. The nodes are firm, nonsuppurative, and painless. Inguinal lymphadenopathy is bilateral and may occur with anal as well as with genital chancres, since lymphatic drainage of the anus involves inguinal nodes. The chancre heals within 4 to 6 weeks (range 2 to 12 weeks), but the lymphadenopathy may persist for months.

Atypical primary lesions are common. The clinical appearance depends upon the number of treponemes inoculated and upon the preinfection immune status of the patient. A large inoculum produces a dark-field–positive ulcerative lesion in nonimmune human volunteers, but in individuals with a previous history of syphilis may produce either a small dark-field–negative papule, an asymptomatic but seropositive latent infection, or no response at all. A small inoculum usually produces only a papular lesion, even in nonimmune humans. Therefore, syphilis should be considered even in the evaluation of trivial or atypical, dark-field–negative, genital lesions. The most common genital lesions which must be differentiated from primary syphilis include traumatic superinfected lesions, genital herpes simplex virus infection (see Chap. 136), and chancroid (see Chap. 110). *Primary genital herpes* may produce inguinal adenopathy, but the nodes are tender and associated with multiple painful vesicles which later ulcerate, and with systemic symptoms including fever; *recurrent genital herpes* typically begins with a cluster of painful vesicles, usually without associated adenopathy. *Chancroid* produces painful, superficial exudative, nonindurated, more often multiple ulcers; adenopathy is either unilateral or bilateral, is tender, and may suppurate.

FIGURE 122-1   *Primary chancre on the penis. (Reprinted, with permission, from Sexually Transmitted Diseases, Prof. Dr. E. Stolz, Rotterdam, ©Boehringer Ingelheim International, 1977.)*

Secondary syphilis The manifestations of the secondary stage are protean but usually include localized or diffuse symmetric mucocutaneous lesions and generalized nontender lymphadenopathy. The healing primary chancre is still present in 15 percent of cases. The skin rash consists of macular, papular, papulosquamous, and occasionally pustular syphilides, often with one or more forms present simultaneously. The eruption may be very subtle, and approximately 25 percent of patients with a discernible rash of secondary syphilis may be unaware that they have dermatologic manifestations. Initial lesions are bilaterally symmetric, pale red or pink, nonpruritic, discrete, round macules, 5 to 10 mm in diameter, distributed on the trunk and proximal extremities (Fig. 122-2). After 1 to 2 months, red, papular lesions 3 to 10 mm in diameter also appear. These may progress to necrotic lesions (resembling pustules) in association with increasing endarteritis and perivascular mononuclear infiltration. These lesions are distributed widely and may occur on the palms, soles (Fig. 122-3), face, and scalp. Tiny papular *follicular syphilides* involving hair follicles may result in patchy alopecia (alopecia areata) and loss of scalp hair, eyebrows, or beard. Nonpatchy hair loss (telogen effluvium) also occurs in secondary syphilis, as in other systemic diseases. Progressive endarteritis obliterans and ischemia result in superficial scaling of papules (*papulosquamous syphilides*) and eventually may lead to central necrosis (*pustular syphilide*). In warm, moist, intertriginous areas, including the perianal area, vulva, scrotum, and inner thighs, axillae, and the skin under pendulous breasts, papules enlarge and become eroded, to produce broad, moist, pink or gray-white highly infectious lesions called *condylomata lata*, which are seen in 10 percent of patients with secondary syphilis. Superficial mucosal erosions, called *mucous patches*, occur in up to one-third of patients and may involve lips, oral mucosa, tongue (Fig. 122-4), palate, pharynx, vulva and vagina, glans penis, or inner prepuce. The typical mucous patch is a silver-gray erosion surrounded by a red periphery and is usually painless.

FIGURE 122-3 *Secondary rash on palms and soles. (From Ronald Roddy; reprinted, with permission, from Gynecology and Obstetrics, JW Sciarra (ed), New York, Harper & Row, 1985.)*

During relapses of secondary syphilis, condylomata lata are particularly common, and skin lesions tend to be asymmetrically distributed and more infiltrated, resembling skin lesions of late syphilis, perhaps reflecting increasing cellular immunity.

Constitutional symptoms which may accompany or precede secondary syphilis include sore throat (15 to 30 percent), fever (5 to 8 percent), weight loss (2 to 20 percent), malaise (25 percent), anorexia, headache (10 percent), and meningismus (5 percent). *Acute meningitis* occurs in only 1 to 2 percent of patients, but increased cells and protein have been found in the cerebrospinal fluid in 30 percent or more. *Treponema pallidum* has also been recovered by rabbit inoculation from cerebrospinal fluid during secondary syphilis in up to 40 percent of patients; this is often correlated with other cerebrospinal fluid (CSF) abnormalities, but may also be seen in patients with normal CSF.

Gastrointestinal involvement can be found with surprising frequency during secondary syphilis and may include hypertrophic syphilitic gastritis suggestive of linitis plastica or lymphosarcoma of the stomach, patchy proctitis, or an ulcerative or mass lesion resembling a rectosigmoid neoplasm.

Other less common complications of secondary syphilis include hepatitis, nephropathy, arthritis and periostitis, and iridocyclitis. Ocular findings which suggest secondary syphilis include otherwise unexplained pupillary abnormalities, optic neuritis, and a retinitis pigmentosa syndrome, as well as the classic iritis (especially granu-

FIGURE 122-2 *Maculopapular rash of secondary syphilis. (Reprinted, with permission, from Sexually Transmitted Diseases, Prof. Dr. E. Stolz, Rotterdam, ©Boehringer Ingelheim International, 1977.)*

FIGURE 122-4 *Mucous patches on the tongue. (From Ronald Roddy; reprinted, with permission, from Sexually Transmitted Diseases, KK Holmes et al (eds), New York, McGraw-Hill, 1984.)*

lomatous iritis) or uveitis. The diagnosis of secondary syphilis is often considered only after failure to respond to steroid therapy. *Syphilitic hepatitis* is distinguished by an unusually high serum alkaline phosphatase and by a nonspecific histologic appearance which is unlike viral hepatitis and includes moderate inflammation with polymorphonuclear leukocytes and lymphocytes, some hepatocellular damage, and no cholestasis. The *renal involvement* is associated with proteinuria, an acute nephrotic syndrome, or rarely with hemorrhagic glomerulonephritis and is characterized by subepithelial electron-dense deposits and glomerular immune complexes, suggesting that this complication is a form of immune complex glomerulonephritis. Anterior uveitis has been reported in 5 to 10 percent of patients with secondary syphilis, and *T. pallidum* has been demonstrated in the aqueous humor in such cases.

Latent syphilis A diagnosis of latent syphilis is established by the finding of a positive specific treponemal antibody test for syphilis, together with a normal cerebrospinal fluid examination, the absence of clinical manifestations of syphilis on physical examination and chest films, and a history of primary or secondary lesions, history of exposure to syphilis, or delivery of an infant with congenital syphilis. *Early latent* syphilis encompasses the first year after infection, while *late latent* syphilis, beginning 1 year after infection, in the untreated patient, is associated with relative immunity to infectious relapse and with increasing resistance to reinfection. *Treponema pallidum* may still intermittently seed the bloodstream during this stage, pregnant women with latent syphilis may infect the fetus in utero, and transfusion syphilis has been transmitted from patients with latent syphilis of many years' duration. Until recently, it was thought that untreated late latent syphilis had three possible outcomes; (1) it could persist throughout the life of the infected individual; (2) it could end in development of late syphilis; or (3) it could end with spontaneous cure of infection, with reversion of serologic tests to negative. It is now apparent, however, that the more sensitive treponemal antibody tests rarely if ever become negative. Fifty to seventy percent of untreated patients with latent syphilis never develop clinically evident late syphilis, but the occurrence of spontaneous cure is in doubt.

Late syphilis The onset of slowly progressive inflammatory disease of the aorta or central nervous system begins early during the pathogenesis of syphilis. Evidence of early syphilitic aortitis is present soon after the secondary lesions subside, and it is patients who develop CSF abnormalities during the early stages of syphilis who appear to be at risk of late neurologic complications.

ASYMPTOMATIC NEUROSYPHILIS In patients with untreated latent syphilis, if the CSF is normal 2 years or more after infection, there is probably no future risk of subsequent development of neurosyphilis, except for the purely vascular type. The diagnosis of asymptomatic neurosyphilis is made in patients with no clinical manifestations of neurosyphilis who have cerebrospinal fluid abnormalities, including pleocytosis, elevated protein, or positive cerebrospinal fluid Wasserman or Venereal Disease Research Laboratory (VDRL) tests. One or more of these findings are present in 20 to 30 percent of patients with untreated syphilis after 2 years, and spontaneous regression to normal is rare. The risk of progression to symptomatic neurosyphilis is two or three times greater in whites than in blacks and is twice as common in men as in women. The risk of parenchymal neurosyphilis (tabes dorsalis or general paresis) is five times greater in men than in women. In patients with untreated asymptomatic neurosyphilis, the overall cumulative probability of progression to clinical neurosyphilis is about 20 percent in the first 10 years, but increases with passing time, and is highest in those who show the greatest degree of pleocytosis or protein elevation. The evaluation of CSF for treponemal antibody is controversial and complex and is discussed below under "Laboratory Diagnosis."

SYMPTOMATIC NEUROSYPHILIS Although mixed features are common, the major clinical categories of symptomatic neurosyphilis include meningovascular and parenchymatous syphilis. The latter category includes general paresis and tabes dorsalis. The interval from infection to onset of symptoms is a few months to 12 years (average 7 years) for meningovascular syphilis, 20 years for general paresis, and 25 to 30 years for tabes dorsalis. However, many patients with symptomatic neurosyphilis, particularly in the antibiotic era, do not present a classic picture, but have mixed and subtle or incomplete syndromes. *Meningovascular syphilis* is associated with diffuse inflammation of the pia and arachnoid, together with evidence of focal or widespread arterial involvement of small, medium, or large vessels. The most common presentation is a stroke syndrome in a relatively young adult, involving the middle cerebral artery; however, unlike the usual thrombotic or embolic stroke syndrome of sudden onset, meningovascular syphilis often presents after a subacute encephalitic prodrome with headaches, vertigo, insomnia, and psychologic abnormalities followed by a gradually progressive vascular syndrome. The manifestations of *general paresis* reflect widespread parenchymal damage and include abnormalities corresponding to the mnemonic *paresis* [*p*ersonality, *a*ffect, *r*eflexes (hyperactive), *e*ye (e.g., Argyll Robertson pupils), *s*ensorium (illusions, delusions, hallucinations), *i*ntellect (decreased recent memory orientation, calculations, judgment, insight), and *s*peech]. *Tabes dorsalis* presents symptoms and signs of demyelinization of the posterior column, dorsal roots, and dorsal root ganglia. Symptoms include ataxic, wide-based gait and footslap, paresthesias, bladder disturbances, impotence, areflexia, and loss of position, deep pain, and temperature sensation. Trophic joint degeneration (Charcot's joints) and perforating ulceration of the feet can result from loss of pain sensation. The Argyll Robertson pupil, seen in both tabes dorsalis and paresis, is a small, irregular pupil which reacts to accommodation but not to light. *Optic atrophy* also occurs frequently in association with tabes.

CARDIOVASCULAR SYPHILIS Cardiovascular manifestations are limited to the large vessels in which the blood supply is provided by vasa vasorum. Endarteritis obliterans of the vasa vasorum produces medial necrosis with destruction of elastic tissue, particularly in the ascending and transverse segments of the aortic arch, resulting in uncomplicated aortitis, aortic regurgitation, saccular aneurysm, or coronary ostial stenosis. Until recently, these complications had not been described following congenital syphilis or syphilis acquired before age 14, suggesting some unexplained resistance of the large blood vessels in youth to invasion by *T. pallidum*. The onset of symptoms occurs from 10 to 40 years after infection. Cardiovascular complications are more common and occur at an earlier age in men than in women, and in blacks than in whites. The incidence of symptomatic cardiovascular complications in late untreated syphilis is approximately 10 percent, with aortic regurgitation being two to four times as common as aneurysm. However, syphilitic aortitis can be demonstrated at autopsy in about one-half of black males with untreated syphilis.

Asymptomatic syphilitic aortitis may be suspected in life if linear calcification of the ascending aorta is demonstrated on chest x-ray films, since arteriosclerotic disease seldom produces this sign. Aortic dilatation and a tambour quality of the sound of aortic closure are unreliable signs of aortitis. Syphilitic aneurysms are usually saccular, occasionally fusiform, and do not lead to dissection. Approximately 1 in 10 aortic aneurysms of syphilitic origin may involve the abdominal aorta, but tend to occur above the renal arteries, whereas arteriosclerotic abdominal aneurysms usually are found below the renal arteries. With increasing age, the nervous system is also affected in up to 40 percent of patients with cardiovascular syphilis.

LATE LESIONS OF THE EYES Iritis associated with pain, photophobia, and dimness of vision or chorioretinitis occurs not only during secondary syphilis, but also as a relatively common manifestation of late syphilis. Adhesions of the iris to the anterior lens may produce a fixed pupil, not to be confused with Argyll Robertson pupil.

LATE BENIGN SYPHILIS (GUMMA) Gummas may be multiple or diffuse, but are usually solitary lesions which range from microscopic size to several centimeters in diameter, and histologically consist of granulomatous inflammation with central necrosis surrounded by mononuclear, epithelioid, and fibroblastic cells, occasional giant cells, and perivasculitis. Although *T. pallidum* is rarely demonstrated microscopically, it has reportedly been recovered from the lesions by rabbit inoculation. The most commonly involved sites are the skin and skeletal systems, mouth and upper respiratory tract, larynx, liver, and stomach. Virtually any organ may be involved. Gummas of skin produce painless nodular, papulosquamous, or ulcerative lesions, which are indurated, and form characteristic circles or arcs, with peripheral hyperpigmentation. The lesions are usually indolent, and may heal spontaneously with scarring, but may also be explosive in onset and are often destructive. These lesions may resemble many other chronic granulomatous conditions, including tuberculosis and sarcoidosis, leprosy, and deep fungal infections. Skeletal gummas involve long bones of the legs with greatest frequency, although any bone may be affected. Trauma may predispose to involvement of a specific site. Presenting symptoms usually include focal pain and tenderness. When sufficiently advanced to produce radiographic abnormalities, the findings may include periostitis or destructive or sclerosing osteitis. Gummas of the upper respiratory tract can lead to perforation of the nasal septum or palate. Gummatous hepatitis may produce epigastric pain and tenderness and low-grade fever, and may be associated with splenomegaly and anemia.

The histopathology and extensive tissue necrosis associated with gummas suggest that delayed hypersensitivity to *T. pallidum* produces these lesions. Certain individuals appear to develop an exaggerated delayed hypersensitivity response to *T. pallidum*, presumably mediated by sensitized T lymphocytes and macrophages. In areas where syphilis is endemic in childhood, reinfection may result in gummas; when one member of a household acquires a fresh infection, other members of the household who then become reinfected develop gummas. Experimental inoculation of *T. pallidum* into individuals with latent or late syphilis also sometimes results in gumma formation at the site of inoculation.

Since the histologic changes may be suggestive but are nonspecific, the diagnosis of late benign syphilis is confirmed by serologic testing and by therapeutic trial. Treatment with penicillin results in rapid healing of active gummatous lesions.

Congenital syphilis Transmission of *T. pallidum* from a syphilitic mother to her fetus across the placenta may occur at any stage of pregnancy, but the lesions of congenital syphilis develop only after the fourth month of gestation, when immunologic competence begins to develop. This suggests that the pathogenesis of congenital syphilis may depend upon the immune response of the host rather than upon a direct toxic effect of *T. pallidum*. The risk of infection of the fetus during untreated early maternal syphilis is estimated to be 75 to 95 percent, decreasing to about 35 percent for maternal syphilis of longer than 2 years' duration, with the risk of fetal infection apparently continuing during late latent maternal syphilis. Adequate treatment of the mother before the sixteenth week of pregnancy should prevent fetal damage. During the past decade, the number of reported cases of congenital syphilis in infants less than 1 year of age in the United States has remained steady at about 2 cases per 100 reported cases of primary and secondary syphilis in women. However, the dramatic rise in the number of reported cases of primary and secondary syphilis in women between 1978 and 1983, from 5331 to 9082 cases, was consequently accompanied by a striking 48 percent increase in reported congenital syphilis in infants, from 107 to 158 cases. In 1984, 240 infants with congenital syphilis were reported, a 120 percent increase over the 1978 low figure. A study of 50 cases reported in 1982 showed that 56 percent of the mothers of infected children had not sought prenatal examination, but had reactive serologic tests at delivery, 14 percent had negative or no serologic test performed during prenatal care, and 14 percent were serologically nonreactive at delivery and were presumably infected late in pregnancy. Laboratory error and physicians' delay in therapy only contributed to 2 and 6

percent, respectively, of the cases, and 8 percent represented treatment failure. Syphilis acquired during pregnancy may remain subclinical in the mother while nearly always causing serious fetal infection. Untreated maternal infection may result in up to 40 percent fetal loss (stillbirth is more common than abortion, because of the late onset of fetal pathology), prematurity, neonatal death, or nonfatal congenital syphilis. Of mothers with untreated syphilis of <2 years' duration, 21 percent aborted or had a stillbirth, 13 percent had infants who died within 2 months, 43 percent had infants with syphilis alive at 2 months, and 23 percent had nonsyphilitic infants. Therefore, routine serologic testing in early pregnancy as well as at delivery and repeat serologic testing of "high-risk" pregnant women in the third trimester are fully justified.

Only fulminant cases of congenital syphilis are clinically apparent in live infants at birth, and these babies have a very poor prognosis. The most common clinical problem is the healthy appearing baby born to a mother who has a positive serologic test.

The manifestations of congenital syphilis can be divided into (1) early manifestations, which appear within the first 2 years of life, often between 2 and 10 weeks of age, are infectious, and resemble severe secondary syphilis in the adult; (2) late manifestations, which appear after 2 years, and are noninfectious; and (3) the residual stigmata of congenital syphilis. During 1984, 75 percent of reported cases of congenital syphilis were diagnosed during the first year of life.

The earliest sign of congenital syphilis is usually rhinitis ("snuffles") soon followed by other mucocutaneous lesions. These may include bullae (syphilitic pemphigus), vesicles, superficial desquamation, petechiae, and later, papulosquamous lesions, mucous patches, and condylomata lata. The most common early manifestations are osteochondritis and osteitis, particularly involving the metaphyses of long bones, progressing in severity during the first 6 months of life, then spontaneously subsiding; and periostitis, which continues to progress after the first 6 months. Hepatosplenomegaly, lymphadenopathy, anemia, jaundice, thrombocytopenia, and leukocytosis are common. The anemia is usually hypoproliferative but may be hemolytic (paroxysmal cold hemoglobinuria). The nephrotic syndrome in early congenital syphilis, as in adult secondary syphilis, represents an immune complex–induced glomerulonephritis.

Neonatal congenital syphilis must be differentiated from other generalized congenital infections, including rubella, cytomegalovirus or herpes simplex virus infection, and toxoplasmosis, and also from erythroblastosis fetalis. Neonatal death is usually due to pulmonary hemorrhage, secondary bacterial infection, or severe hepatitis. Pathologic findings include interstitial and perivascular inflammation followed by variable fibroblastic proliferation, involving skin, bones, liver, kidneys, pancreas, spleen, lungs, and intestines, and by extramedullary hematopoiesis.

Late congenital syphilis is defined as congenital syphilis which remains untreated after 2 years of age. In perhaps 60 percent of cases, the infection remains latent, while the clinical spectrum in the remainder differs in certain respects from that of acquired late syphilis in the adult. For example, cardiovascular syphilis rarely develops in late congenital syphilis, whereas interstitial keratitis is much more common and occurs between ages 5 and 25. The onset is acute with photophobia, pain, and circumcorneal injection, followed by superficial and deep vascularization of the cornea, which progresses despite antibiotic therapy, and eventually becomes bilateral. The symptoms and signs may be suppressed with corticosteroid therapy. Although treponemes have occasionally been demonstrated in aqueous humor in interstitial keratitis, the pathogenesis is obscure and is ascribed to "hypersensitivity." Other manifestations associated with interstitial keratitis are eighth-nerve deafness and recurrent arthropathy. Bilateral knee effusions are known as *Clutton's joints*. Examination of CSF discloses asymptomatic neurosyphilis in about one-third of untreated patients without other late clinical manifestations, and clinical neurosyphilis occurs in a quarter of untreated individuals with congenital syphilis over 6 years of age. The clinical manifestations of congenital neurosyphilis correspond to those seen in adult neurosyphilis. Gummatous periostitis occurs between ages 5 and 20 and, as in nonvenereal endemic childhood syphilis, tends to cause destructive lesions of the palate and nasal septum.

Characteristic stigmata include Hutchinson's teeth, the centrally notched, widely spaced, peg-shaped upper central incisors, and "mulberry" molars, sixth-year molars which have multiple, poorly developed cusps, rather than the usual four. The abnormal facies, which includes frontal bossing, saddlenose, and poorly developed maxilla, may also be seen in congenital ectodermal dysplasia. Saber shins, or anterior tibial bowing, are rare but were probably more common in the past when syphilitic periostitis of the anterior tibia was associated with vitamin D deficiency. *Rhagades* are linear scars at the angles of the mouth and nose caused by secondary bacterial infection of the early facial eruption. Other stigmata include unexplained nerve deafness, old chorioretinitis, optic atrophy, and corneal opacities due to past interstitial keratitis.

LABORATORY EXAMINATIONS Dark-field examination technique Dark-field examination is essential in evaluating cutaneous lesions, such as the chancre of primary syphilis, or condylomata lata of secondary syphilis. Although it is often difficult to demonstrate *T. pallidum* in dry maculopapular lesions in secondary syphilis by dark-field examination, the organism may be demonstrated by saline aspiration of lymph nodes during this stage. The surface of the suspected ulcerated lesion should be cleaned with saline and gauze, then gently abraded further with dry gauze, without production of bleeding. The lesion is then squeezed to express a serous transudate, and a drop of the transudate is picked up on the surface of a glass slide. A drop of saline (without bacteriostatic additives) may be mixed with the transudate if necessary, and this is then covered with a coverslip and examined immediately for *T. pallidum* with a dark-field or phase contrast microscope by an experienced individual. A single negative examination does not exclude syphilis, since at least 10^4 treponemes per milliliter transudate must be present to be detected, and prior use of topical antiseptic or cleansing by the patient may obfuscate the examination. Cleansing or use of topical medication should, therefore, be avoided, and the dark-field examination should be repeated on three successive days before being considered negative.

Direct Immunofluorescence Most syphilis is diagnosed in private physicians' offices where dark-field microscopy is not available, and alternative methods for the identification of *T. pallidum* in exudate are needed. The direct fluorescent antibody *T. pallidum* (DFA-TP) test, available at central laboratories, uses fluorescein-conjugated polyclonal antitreponemal antibody for detection of *T. pallidum* in fixed smears prepared from suspect lesions. Because of cross-reactive antibodies which will also stain commensal nonpathogenic spirochetes, the antiserum is extensively absorbed with cultured treponemes in an effort to produce a specific reagent.

A refinement of this technique using a monoclonal antibody which is specific for only the pathogenic treponemes has been developed. It has been shown in clinical trials to be as sensitive and specific as dark-field microscopy for examination of suspicious lesions.

Demonstration of *T. pallidum* in tissue It is often necessary to demonstrate *T. pallidum* in tissue when clinical or histopathologic features suggest the diagnosis of syphilis. Although the organism can be found in tissue by appropriate silver stains, these should be interpreted with caution, because artifacts resembling *T. pallidum* are often seen. Treponemes can be demonstrated more reliably in tissue by immunofluorescence, using specific monoclonal or polyclonal antibodies against *T. pallidum*.

Serologic tests for syphilis The profusion of serologic tests for syphilis causes much unnecessary confusion. Syphilitic infection produces two types of antibodies, the nonspecific *reaginic* antibody and specific antitreponemal antibody, which are measured by the nontreponemal and treponemal tests, respectively (Table 122-1). The treponemal tests, as well as the nontreponemal tests, are reactive in persons with any treponemal infection, including yaws, pinta, and endemic syphilis.

The nontreponemal antibodies produced in syphilis contain both IgG and IgM immunoglobulins directed against a lipoidal antigen that results from the interaction of *T. pallidum* with host tissues, and possibly against a lipoidal antigen of *T. pallidum* itself. The term *reagin* is unfortunate, since the unrelated IgE antibody involved in certain allergic phenomena is also known as reagin.

The most widely used nontreponemal or reagin antibody tests are the rapid plasma reagin (RPR) test, which can be automated (ART), and the VDRL slide test. Other less frequently used nontreponemal tests include the unheated serum reagin (USR) and the reagin screen test (RST). In these tests, antibody is detected by the microscopic (VDRL, USR) or macroscopic (RPR, RST) flocculation of the antigen suspension (Table 122-1).

The RPR is often more expensive than the VDRL test but is easier to perform and uses unheated serum; it is the test of choice for rapid serologic diagnosis in a clinic or office setting. The VDRL reagents are less expensive, but must be prepared fresh daily. Although the development of the simpler macroscopic tests has resulted in the replacement of the VDRL by the RPR for examination of serum in many laboratories, the VDRL test remains the standard test for use with cerebrospinal fluid.

RPR and VDRL tests are equally sensitive and may be used for initial screening or for quantitation of serum reagin antibody titer. The reagin titer reflects the activity of the disease: a fourfold or greater rise in titer may be seen during the evolution of primary syphilis; VDRL titers usually reach 1:32 or higher in secondary syphilis; a persistent fall in titer following treatment of early syphilis provides essential evidence of an adequate response to therapy. VDRL titers do not correspond directly to RPR titers, and sequential quantitative testing (as for response to therapy) must employ a single test.

There are three standard treponemal tests: the fluorescent treponemal antibody-absorption (FTA-ABS), the microhemagglutination assay for antibodies to *T. pallidum* (MHA-TP), and the hemagglutination treponemal test for syphilis (HATTS). A third hemagglutination test, the TPHA, is widely used in Canada and Europe, but is not available in the United States.

For the FTA-ABS test, the patient's serum is first diluted with a substance containing nonpathogenic treponemal antigens (sorbent) to bind group-specific antibodies which may be produced against saprophytic oral and genital treponemes. The patient's absorbed serum is then placed on a slide which contains fixed *T. pallidum*. If specific antibody to *T. pallidum* is present in the patient's serum, it is bound to the dried treponemes, and then is detected by the addition of fluorescein-labeled antihuman gamma globulin and subsequent examination of the slide by fluorescence microscopy. The *T. pallidum* hemagglutination tests (MHA-TP, HATTS, and TPHA) also use a sorbent-like diluent for binding treponemal group antibodies. *T. pallidum*–specific antibody is detected by agglutination of *T. pallidum*–coated sheep or turkey erythrocytes. The *T. pallidum* immobilization (TPI) test, in which immobilization of live *T. pallidum* is produced by immune serum plus complement, is the most specific treponemal test, but is more laborious, and in the United States is available only

TABLE 122-1 Common serologic tests for syphilis

NONTREPONEMAL (REAGIN) TESTS

Microscopic flocculation: Venereal Disease Research Laboratory (VDRL)
Macroscopic flocculation: rapid plasma reagin (RPR)

TREPONEMAL TESTS

Immunofluorescence: fluorescent treponemal antibody-absorption (FTA-ABS)
Hemagglutination: *T. pallidum* hemagglutination assay (MHA-TP, HATTS, TPHA)
Immobilization: *Treponema pallidum* immobilization (TPI)

in research laboratories. Both the hemagglutination and FTA-ABS tests are very specific and, when used for confirmation of positive reaginic antibody tests, have a very high positive predictive value for the diagnosis of syphilis. However, even these tests give false-positive rates as high as 1 to 2 percent when used for screening normal populations.

The relative sensitivities of the VDRL, FTA-ABS, and MHA-TP tests in the various stages of syphilis are shown in Table 122-2. The nontreponemal tests are nonreactive in nearly one-third of patients with primary or late syphilis. In early primary syphilis, the detection of antibody can be maximized either by performing an FTA-ABS test or simply by repeating a VDRL test after 1 to 2 weeks if the initial VDRL was negative. However, obtaining a reagin antibody test alone is not sufficient in evaluating late symptomatic syphilis; the more sensitive FTA-ABS test should be obtained routinely in suspected late syphilis. The hemagglutination tests are even less sensitive than the reagin tests in primary syphilis, but are as sensitive as the FTA-ABS in other stages. All treponemal and nontreponemal tests are reactive during secondary syphilis, and a nonreactive result virtually excludes syphilis in a patient with otherwise compatible mucocutaneous lesions. (An estimated 1 to 2 percent of patients with secondary syphilis have a nonreactive or weakly reactive VDRL test with undiluted serum which becomes positive in higher dilutions—the *prozone* phenomenon.)

False-positive serologic tests for syphilis Because the antigen used in the nontreponemal tests is found in other tissues, the tests may be reactive in persons without treponemal infection, although rarely in titers exceeding 1:8. Of all reactive reagin tests, an estimated 20 to 40 percent are false-positive, but the percentages vary widely depending upon the population being examined. In a population which has been selected for screening because of clinical suspicion, history of exposure, or increased risk for sexually transmitted infections, the percentage of reactive tests which is falsely positive is much lower. False-positive reagin tests are classified as acute if they become negative within 6 months. Acute false-positive reagin tests occur during a variety of acute infections, such as viral diseases, mycoplasma pneumonia, and malaria, and following certain immunizations. Chronic reactions, which persist 6 months or longer, occur in addiction, autoimmune diseases, and aging. False-positive reagin tests occur in 25 percent of narcotics addicts, and in 10 to 20 percent of patients with active systemic lupus erythematosus. The autoimmune nature of the false-positive reagin test is suggested by the occurrence of systemic lupus erythematosus or other connective tissue diseases in 15 to 45 percent of chronic false-positive reactors. Other antibodies which have been found with great frequency in serums from chronic false-positive reactors include antinuclear, antithyroid, and antimitochondrial antibodies, as well as rheumatoid factor and cryoglobulins. The Donath-Landsteiner antibody responsible for paroxysmal cold hemoglobinuria is a hemolysin which appears in syphilis. The prevalence of false-positive reagin tests increases with advancing age, and 10 percent of people over 70 years of age have false-positive reactions. Other diseases associated with hyperglobulinemia, such as leprosy, may also produce chronic false-positive reactions.

In the patient with a false-positive reagin test, syphilis is excluded

by obtaining a nonreactive treponemal test. The results of the FTA-ABS test are reported as negative, borderline, or reactive. *Borderline* results are more common in patients who are pregnant or have diseases associated with abnormal or increased globulins, and are frequently not associated with either clinical, historical, or other serologic evidence of syphilis. Borderline results should, therefore, always be repeated in questionable cases and interpreted with caution. A typical *reactive* FTA-ABS occurs infrequently in conditions other than syphilis. Although false-positive FTA-ABS tests have been reported in 15 percent of patients with active systemic lupus erythematosus, the fluorescent staining is "borderline" or has an atypical "beaded" appearance in most cases (thought to be due to attachment of antinuclear antibody to treponemal DNA or nucleoprotein leaked through breaks in the outer treponemal membranes). However, because of the occasional occurrence of false-positive FTA-ABS tests, only a positive TPI provides conclusive proof of past or present treponemal infection.

For practical purposes, most clinicians need to be familiar with the three uses of serologic tests for syphilis: (1) for testing large numbers of serums for screening or diagnostic purposes (e.g., RPR or VDRL); (2) for quantitative measurement of reaginic antibody titer in order to assess the clinical activity of syphilis, or to follow the reagin titer in response to therapy (e.g., VDRL or RPR); and (3) for confirmation of the diagnosis of syphilis in a patient with a positive reagin antibody test or with a suspected clinical diagnosis of syphilis (e.g., FTA-ABS, MHA-TP, HATTS).

Evaluation for asymptomatic neurosyphilis Asymptomatic involvement of the central nervous system is detected by examination of cerebrospinal fluid (CSF). CSF abnormalities are very infrequent in the primary stage, but pleocytosis or elevated protein can be demonstrated in CSF from up to 40 percent of patients with secondary or latent syphilis. *T. pallidum* has been recovered by rabbit inoculation from up to 40 percent of those with secondary syphilis, but rarely from those with latent syphilis. The demonstration of *T. pallidum* in CSF is often associated with other CSF abnormalities; however, organisms can be recovered from patients without pleocytosis or elevated protein. In the prepenicillin era, the risk of developing clinical neurosyphilis was roughly proportional to the intensity of spinal fluid changes in early syphilis. CSF examination is essential in any seropositive patient with neurologic signs and symptoms and is recommended in all patients with untreated syphilis of unknown duration or of greater than 1 year's duration. The possibility that asymptomatic neurosyphilis is present in some patients with secondary and early latent disease is not addressed by these recommendations. Because standard therapy for early syphilis fails to achieve treponemicidal levels in the CSF, some experts currently advise lumbar puncture in secondary and early latent syphilis, with follow-up examinations for patients with abnormalities.

CSF is examined for pleocytosis, increased protein concentration, and VDRL reactivity. The CSF-VDRL is very specific if the fluid is not contaminated with blood. The CSF-VDRL is relatively insensitive, however, and may be nonreactive even in progressive symptomatic neurosyphilis. The unabsorbed FTA test on cerebrospinal fluid is reactive far more often than the VDRL test in all stages of syphilis, but may reflect passive transfer of serum antibody into the CSF. Most specialists do not recommend performing an FTA test on spinal fluid. Similarly, the finding of a reactive CSF-FTA-ABS test without other cerebrospinal fluid abnormalities in a patient with nonspecific neurologic findings does not prove a diagnosis of "atypical" neurosyphilis. However, even in the absence of confirmatory CSF examination, a therapeutic trial of penicillin in doses adequate for neurosyphilis is warranted in any patient with a positive serum treponemal antibody test who also has neurologic findings consistent with neurosyphilis.

Attempts to identify a more sensitive and specific marker for neurosyphilis have included CSF oligoclonal banding and measurement of intrathecal production of antitreponemal IgM and IgG. CSF

TABLE 122-2 Reactivity of serodiagnostic tests in untreated syphilis

Test	Stage of disease, % positive*			
	Primary	Secondary	Latent	Tertiary
VDRL	59–87	100	73–91	37–94
FTA-ABS	86–100	99–100	96–99	96–100
MHA-TP	64–87	96–100	96–100	94–100

* Percentage figures provided should not be interpreted as absolute values because there are small numbers in certain categories and test results vary from study to study.
SOURCE: *Modified (with permission) from H Jaffe, Management of the reactive serology, in Sexually Transmitted Diseases, KK Holmes et al (eds), New York, McGraw-Hill, 1984.*

from 80 percent of patients with multiple sclerosis and approximately 40 percent of patients with other inflammatory CNS diseases (including neurosyphilis, bacterial meningitis, viral encephalitis, subacute sclerosing panencephalitis) have discrete oligoclonal immunoglobulin bands in the gamma globulin region following agarose gel electrophoresis of CSF. These antibodies are thought to be intrathecally produced and have specificity for the etiologic agent (e.g., *T. pallidum* in syphilis and measles virus in subacute sclerosing panencephalitis); however, an oligoclonal banding pattern per se is not specific for neurosyphilis in a seropositive patient. The intrathecal production of specific anti-*T. pallidum* IgG and IgM antibodies has been estimated by several techniques which are still investigational.

TREATMENT OF ACQUIRED SYPHILIS Penicillin G is the drug of choice for all stages of syphilis. *Treponema pallidum* is killed by very low concentrations of penicillin G, although a long period of exposure to penicillin is required for treatment because of the unusually slow rate of multiplication of the organism. The efficacy of penicillin for syphilis remains undiminished after 40 years of use. Other antibiotics which are effective in syphilis include the tetracyclines, erythromycin, and the cephalosporins. Aminoglycosides inhibit *T. pallidum* only in very large doses, and the sulfonamides are inactive. The optimal dose and duration of therapy have not been established for any antimicrobial for any stage of syphilis. The U.S. Public Health Service recommendations are based on limited therapeutic trials and should be interpreted in light of the considerations noted below.

Recurrence rates for a given regimen increase as infection progresses from incubating syphilis to seronegative primary to seropositive primary to secondary to late syphilis. Therefore it is probable, but unproved, that a longer duration of therapy is required to effect cure as the infection progresses. For these reasons some authorities use more prolonged penicillin therapy than that recommended by the U.S. Public Health Service when treating secondary, latent, or late syphilis.

The optimal dose and duration of therapy have not been carefully evaluated in well-controlled studies. A variety of data suggests that it is necessary to achieve serum levels of penicillin G of 0.03 μg/mL or more for at least 7 days to cure early syphilis. Other tentative

conclusions which can be gleaned from published studies include the following: (1) extending therapy with aqueous procaine penicillin G beyond 2 weeks does not improve cure rates for primary or secondary syphilis; (2) studies of experimental syphilis show that *T. pallidum* begin to regenerate if penicillinemia is allowed to fall to subinhibitory levels for periods of 18 to 24 h; (3) in human beings, increases in the dosage of crystalline penicillin G administered over 9 h from 0.03 to 0.6 mg/kg progressively increased the rate of disappearance of *T. pallidum* from chancres, but further increases in dosage did not further speed the disappearance of treponemes; and (4) the serum concentration of penicillin G achieved after one injection of 2.4 million units of benzathine penicillin G probably does not kill *T. pallidum* at the maximum rate.

The treatment regimens currently recommended for syphilis by the Centers for Disease Control are summarized in Table 122-3 and described below.

Early syphilis In very early incubating syphilis, treatment of concurrently acquired gonorrhea with 4.8 million units of procaine penicillin G (plus 1.0 g probenecid) aborts the syphilis. The ampicillin-probenecid and tetracycline regimens recommended for gonorrhea are probably also effective against incubating syphilis, although proof is not available. Follow-up serologic testing for syphilis is considered unnecessary in patients treated for gonorrhea with the recommended dose of procaine penicillin G, ampicillin, or tetracycline. Preventive (abortive, "epidemiologic") treatment is recommended for seronegative individuals without signs of syphilis who were exposed to infectious syphilis within the previous 6 weeks. Before treatment is given, every effort should be made to establish a diagnosis by examination and serologic testing. *The regimens recommended for preventive treatment are the same as those recommended for early syphilis.*

Benzathine penicillin G is the most widely used form of treatment for early syphilis, including primary, secondary, and early latent syphilis, although it is more painful on injection than procaine penicillin G. A single dose of 2.4 million units cures over 95 percent of cases of primary syphilis. Because efficacy for secondary syphilis may be slightly lower, some physicians administer a second dose of 2.4 million units 1 week after the initial dose for secondary syphilis.

TABLE 122-3 Recommended therapy for syphilis

Stage of syphilis	Patients without penicillin allergy	Patients with penicillin allergy
Primary, secondary, or early latent	Benzathine penicillin G, 2.4 million units single dose IM (1.2 million units in each hip).	Tetracycline hydrochloride, 2 g daily for 15 days.
Late latent or latent of uncertain duration	Lumbar Puncture *CSF normal:* Benzathine penicillin G, 2.4 million units IM weekly for 3 weeks. *CSF abnormal:* Treat as neurosyphilis.	Lumbar Puncture *CSF normal:* Treat as neurosyphilis. *CSF abnormal:* Treat as neurosyphilis.
Neurosyphilis* (asymptomatic or symptomatic)	Aqueous procaine penicillin G, 2.4 million units IM daily plus probenecid 500 mg, by mouth, 4 times a day, both for 10 days, followed by benzathine penicillin G, 2.4 million units IM weekly for 3 doses. *Or* aqueous penicillin G, 12 to 24 million units per day IV for at least 10 days, followed by benzathine penicillin G, 2.4 million units IM weekly for 3 doses.	Tetracycline hydrochloride, 2 g daily for 30 days.
Late cardiovascular or benign tertiary	Benzathine penicillin G, 2.4 million units IM weekly for 3 weeks.	Treat as for neurosyphilis.
Congenital (see text)	Aqueous procaine penicillin G, 50,000 units/kg, IM daily for at least 10 days. *Or* aqueous crystalline penicillin G, 50,000 units/kg per day, IM or IV, in two divided daily doses for at least 10 days. *Or, only if CSF normal:* benzathine penicillin G, 50,000 units/kg, IM, in a single dose.	Antibiotics other than penicillin should not be used.
Syphilis in pregnancy	According to stage.	See text.

* *Benzathine penicillin G has given inferior results for treatment of symptomatic neurosyphilis. Although tetracycline was recommended by the CDC Syphilis Therapy Advisory Committee for CNS Syphilis in penicillin-allergic patients, there is minimal experience with this drug (which does not achieve high CSF levels) in CNS syphilis. Doxycycline has higher theoretical efficacy than tetracycline hydrochloride for neurosyphilis because of better CSF penetration, although controlled studies have not been performed. Many patients who give a history of penicillin allergy prove negative when skin-tested for immediate hypersensitivity to penicillin and could be given aqueous crystalline penicillin G for CNS syphilis under close supervision in the hospital. Certain third-generation cephalosporins (e.g., ceftriaxone, cefotaxime) have some promise for penicillin-allergic patients with CNS syphilis but require further evaluation.*

SOURCE: *Sexually transmitted diseases treatment guidelines 1985. Morb Mort Week Rep Suppl 34(4S), 1985*

Late latent and late syphilis Recommended treatment for late latent syphilis with normal CSF, for cardiovascular syphilis, and for late benign syphilis (gumma) is benzathine penicillin G, 2.4 million units intramuscularly once a week for 3 successive weeks (7.2 million units total). Lumbar puncture should be performed in the evaluation of latent syphilis of more than 1 year's duration, in suspected neurosyphilis, and also in late complications other than symptomatic neurosyphilis, since asymptomatic neurosyphilis may coexist with other late complications. Abnormal cerebrospinal fluid findings can then be followed serially as a guide to therapy. No studies of benzathine penicillin G for cardiovascular syphilis have been reported, and the efficacy of penicillin therapy in any form for cardiovascular syphilis has not been proved. The response of cardiovascular syphilis to penicillin is seldom dramatic because aortic aneurysm and aortic regurgitation cannot be reversed by antibiotic treatment, although further progression of these lesions may be arrested.

In contrast, the response of benign tertiary syphilis and of meningovascular syphilis to penicillin G is usually impressive. The response of parenchymal neurosyphilis has been variable. In a cooperative study of the treatment of 1086 general paretics with penicillin, the frequency of clinical improvement or termination of progression ranged from 38 percent of those with severe involvement to 81 percent of those with mild involvement. All patients who relapsed following initial improvement in cerebrospinal fluid pleocytosis had received less than 6 million units of penicillin, and all had improvement of CSF pleocytosis with subsequent therapy. Tabes dorsalis or optic atrophy responds less often. In general, treatment of inactive neurosyphilis in which neurologic damage has already occurred may not produce any clinical change, and retreatment of such cases is not warranted. However, persistence of cerebrospinal fluid pleocytosis, or recurrence of pleocytosis following initial response to treatment, indicates continuing active infection, which should respond to additional treatment. The optimal dose and duration of penicillin for neurosyphilis has not been determined, but administration of 600,000 to 900,000 units of procaine penicillin G daily for 10 days has been about 90 percent effective. The 1985 Centers for Disease Control treatment guidelines for neurosyphilis are presented in Table 122-3. Since benzathine penicillin G given in single doses of 2.4 million units to adults or 50,000 units per kilogram to infants does not produce detectable concentrations of penicillin G in cerebrospinal fluid, this form of penicillin is unreliable for the treatment of neurosyphilis in the adult or infant, and asymptomatic neurosyphilis has been found to relapse in up to one-quarter of patients treated with 2.4 million units of benzathine penicillin. Many authorities therefore do not advocate use of benzathine penicillin alone for treatment of neurosyphilis. On the other hand, administration of intravenous penicillin G in doses of 12 million units or more per day for 10 days or longer ensures treponemicidal concentrations of penicillin G in cerebrospinal fluid, and occasionally cures patients who failed to respond to conventional therapy. There are no data to support the use of antibiotics other than penicillin G for the treatment of neurosyphilis; however, some of the third-generation cephalosporins (e.g., ceftriaxone, cefotaxime) may deserve further evaluation.

Management of syphilis in pregnancy Every pregnant woman should be tested with a nontreponemal test at her first prenatal visit, and women who are at high risk for acquiring sexually transmitted diseases should have a repeat test in the third trimester. In the pregnant patient with presumed syphilis, evidenced by a reactive serology, with or without clinical manifestations, and with no history of treatment for syphilis, expeditious evaluation and initiation of treatment is essential. Therapy should be administered according to stage of the disease, as for nonpregnant patients. Because of the risk of Jarisch-Herxheimer reaction, some experts advise that women with syphilis who are several months pregnant be hospitalized for treatment, to permit early administration of tocolytic therapy if premature labor should occur during the reaction.

If the patient has well-documented penicillin allergy, and this is confirmed by demonstration of an immediate wheal-and-flare response to skin testing with penicilloyl polylysine or penicillin G minor determinant mixture, no satisfactory and proven alternative to penicillin therapy is available. Erythromycin, the commonly recommended alternative in penicillin-allergic pregnant patients, crosses the placenta poorly, with fetal blood levels varying from 0 to 20 percent of maternal levels. The birth of infected infants has been reported following therapy for syphilis in several women treated during pregnancy with recommended doses of erythromycin. Erythromycin estolate is often associated with liver toxicity in pregnancy. Doxycycline, 100 mg twice daily for 15 days, or certain cephalosporins (e.g., ceftriaxone) may be preferable alternatives, although doxycycline has potential toxicity in pregnancy and cephalosporins may produce allergic reactions in some penicillin-allergic patients. After treatment, a quantitative reagin test should be repeated monthly throughout pregnancy, and if a fourfold rise in titer occurs, treatment should be repeated. Treated women who do not show a fourfold decrease in titer in a 3-month period should also be retreated.

Evaluation and management of congenital syphilis Newborn infants of mothers with reactive VDRL or FTA-ABS tests will themselves have reactive tests, whether or not they have become infected, because of transplacental transfer of maternal IgG antibody. Neonatal IgM antibody can be detected in cord or neonatal serums in a modified FTA-ABS test, employing fluorescein-labeled antihuman IgM to detect antitreponemal IgM antibody. However, the specificity of this test is questionable because of evidence that infants with a variety of congenital infections may produce IgM antibody to maternal allotypes of IgG (rheumatoid factor). IgM antibody detected in the IgM-FTA-ABS test may then be directed against maternal IgG antibody bound specifically to *T. pallidum,* rather than against *T. pallidum* itself. Because of the questionable sensitivity and specificity of this test, the IgM-FTA-ABS is not currently recommended. Instead, monthly quantitative reagin tests are performed on asymptomatic infants born to women who were treated adequately with penicillin during pregnancy. Rising or persistent titers indicate infection, and the infant should be treated. If the seropositive mother received inadequate penicillin treatment or treatment other than penicillin, or her treatment status is unknown, or if the infant may be difficult to follow, the infant should be treated at birth. It is unwise to require proof of diagnosis before treatment in such cases. The CSF should be examined as a baseline before treatment of such infants. The calculation of penicillin dosage for treatment of late congenital syphilis is the same as for that used in the infant, until dosage based upon body weight reaches that used for adult neurosyphilis.

Jarisch-Herxheimer reaction A dramatic reaction consisting of fever (average temperature elevation, 1.5°C), chills, myalgias, headache, tachycardia, increased respiratory rate, increased circulating neutrophil count (average total white blood cell count, 12,500 per cubic millimeter), and vasodilatation with mild hypotension, may occur following initiation of treatment of syphilis. This reaction occurs in approximately 50 percent of patients with primary syphilis, 90 percent with secondary, and 25 percent with early latent syphilis. The onset occurs within 2 h of treatment, the peak temperature occurs at about 7 h, and defervescence takes place within 12 to 24 h. The reaction is more delayed in neurosyphilis, with peak fever occurring after 12 to 14 h. In patients with secondary syphilis, an increase in erythema and edema of the mucocutaneous lesions occurs; occasionally subclinical or early mucocutaneous lesions may first become apparent during the reaction. The pathogenesis of this reaction is controversial. Patients should be warned to expect such symptoms, which can be managed by bed rest and aspirin. The Jarisch-Herxheimer reaction in neurosyphilis or cardiovascular syphilis has, on very rare occasions, been associated with acute progression of irreversible organ damage.

Follow-up evaluation of responses to therapy for all stages of syphilis The response of early syphilis to treatment should be determined by following the quantitative VDRL titer 1, 3, 6, and 12 months after treatment. Because the FTA-ABS and hemagglutination tests remain positive in nearly all patients treated for seropositive early syphilis, these tests are not useful in following the response to therapy. After successful treatment of seropositive primary or secondary syphilis, the VDRL titer progressively declines, becoming negative within 3 to 12 months in about 75 percent of seropositive primary cases and 40 percent of secondary cases. Two years after treatment for primary syphilis, nearly all patients have a negative VDRL, although 25 percent of secondary cases and a higher proportion of those treated for early latent syphilis maintain low reagin titers. If the VDRL becomes negative or reaches a fixed low titer within 1 or 2 years, performing a lumbar puncture is unnecessary at that time, since the spinal fluid examination is almost invariably normal and there is little risk of subsequent neurosyphilis. However, if a VDRL titer of 1:8 or more fails to fall at least fourfold within 12 months, if the VDRL titer rises fourfold, or if clinical symptoms persist or recur, retreatment is indicated. Every effort should be made to differentiate treatment failure from reinfection, and the CSF should be examined. Suspected treatment failures, especially those with abnormal CSF, should be treated as described for neurosyphilis. If the patient remains seropositive but asymptomatic after such retreatment, no further therapy is necessary. Patients treated for late latent syphilis frequently have a low-titered VDRL prior to therapy and may not demonstrate a fourfold drop following therapy with penicillin; 56 percent of these patients remain seropositive in low titer for years following therapy. Retreatment is not warranted unless the titer rises or signs and symptoms of syphilis recur.

The activity of neurosyphilis correlates best with the degree of cerebrospinal fluid pleocytosis. Changes in the cerebrospinal fluid cell count, and to a lesser extent, in cerebrospinal fluid protein concentration, provide the most sensitive index of response to treatment. Spinal fluid examination should be performed every 3 to 6 months for 3 years after treatment of asymptomatic neurosyphilis. An elevated cerebrospinal fluid cell count falls to 10 or less per cubic millimeter within 3 to 12 months in 95 percent of adequately treated cases, and becomes normal in all cases within 2 to 4 years. Elevated levels of cerebrospinal fluid protein fall more slowly, and the CSF reagin titer declines slowly over a period of several years.

Persistence of treponemal forms   The persistence of *T. pallidum* in the aqueous humor, cerebrospinal fluid, lymph nodes, brain, inflamed temporal arteries, and other tissues following "adequate" penicillin treatment of latent or late syphilis has been suggested by dark-field microscopy and by immunofluorescent antibody and silver staining techniques. It is not surprising that *T. pallidum* might persist in the aqueous humor or cerebrospinal fluid despite penicillin treatment, because of poor penetration of the antibiotic, but persistence in lymph nodes and other sites remains unexplained. Limited evidence indicates no increase in resistance to penicillin of such persistent treponemes. Since the data on persisting treponemes are scanty, no modification of the treatment recommendations for latent or late syphilis seems warranted.

IMMUNITY AND PREVENTION OF SYPHILIS   Only about 50 percent of the named contacts of primary and secondary syphilis become infected. The actual risk of infection from a single exposure is probably much lower. The relative importance of variations in sexual and hygienic practices, inoculum size, body and environmental temperature, and other local and systemic factors affecting transmissibility of syphilis remains undefined. There is some interest in the possible efficacy of intravaginal contraceptive gels as prophylactics against venereal diseases including syphilis, since many available preparations have bacteriostatic as well as spermicidal properties. Humans have no natural resistance to infection by pathogenic treponemes. The rate of development of acquired resistance to *T. pallidum* following natural or experimental infection is quantitatively related to the amount of the antigenic stimulus, which depends upon both the size of the infecting inoculum and the duration of infection prior to treatment. Resistance of human beings to reinfection

by intradermal inoculation of *T. pallidum* was studied in volunteers. Those who had previously been treated for *early* syphilis developed a primary lesion and a serologic response, while the majority of those who had previously been treated for *late latent* syphilis and all those with *untreated latent* syphilis developed neither primary lesions nor serologic response following inoculation. Two patients treated for late latent or late congenital syphilis developed gummas at the site of inoculation.

The role of serum antibody in conferring immunity to syphilis remains controversial. Reagin antibody is not protective. Passively administered antibody from rabbits recovering from experimental syphilis prevents or delays appearance of clinical manifestations of syphilis; it does not prevent infection. Evidence for the importance of cellular immunity includes histopathologic studies in experimental rabbit syphilis, which demonstrates clearance of treponemes from primary lesions soon after peak infiltration of the lesion by T lymphocytes and macrophages. The histopathology of gummas suggests that the cellular immune response is involved in the pathogenesis of these lesions.

Inability to cultivate pathogenic treponemes in vitro has hindered analysis, purification, and concentration of treponemal antigens, and attempts to induce immunity to syphilis by vaccination have shown limited promise. However, repeated injection of rabbits with gamma-irradiated motile strains has conferred immunity to a rechallenge with 10^5 organisms. Currently, the prevention of syphilis depends upon use of mechanical or antiseptic prophylactic agents, and upon detection and treatment of infectious cases.

REFERENCES

BRYCESON ADM: Clinical pathology of the Jarisch-Herxheimer reaction. J Infect Dis 133:696, 1976

CAMPISI D, WHITCOMB C: Liver disease in early syphilis. Arch Intern Med 139:365, 1979

CHAPEL T: The signs and symptoms of secondary syphilis. Sex Trans Dis 7:161, 1980

CLARK EG, DANBOLT N: The Oslo study of the natural course of untreated syphilis. Med Clin North Am 48:613, 1964

FISCHER A et al: Tertiary syphilis in Denmark 1961–1970, a description of 105 cases not previously diagnosed or specifically treated. Acta Derm Venereol 56:485, 1976

FIUMARA NJ: Treatment of primary and secondary syphilis: Serologic response. JAMA 243:2500, 1980

GREENE BM et al: Failure of penicillin G benzathine in the treatment of neurosyphilis. Arch Intern Med 140:1117, 1980

HOOK EW III et al: Detection of *Treponema pallidum* in lesion exudate with a pathogen-specific monoclonal antibody. J Clin Microbiol 22:241, 1985

HOTSON JR: Modern neurosyphilis: A partially treated chronic meningitis. West J Med 135:191, 1981

IDSOE O et al: Penicillin in the treatment of syphilis. Bull WHO 47(Suppl):1, 1972

JAFFE HW: The laboratory diagnosis of syphilis: New concepts. Ann Intern Med 83:846, 1975

JOHNSON RC (ed): *The Biology of the Parasitic Spirochetes.* New York, Academic, 1976

LUGER A et al: Diagnosis of neurosyphilis by examination of the cerebrospinal fluid. Br J Vener Dis 57:232, 1981

LUKEHART SA et al: Characterization of lymphocyte responsiveness in early experimental syphilis: II. Nature of cellular infiltration and *Treponema pallidum* distribution in testicular infection. J Immunol 124:461, 1980

MAGNUSON HJ et al: Inoculation studies in human volunteers. Medicine 35:33, 1956

MASCOLA L et al: Congenital syphilis. Why is it still occurring? JAMA 252:17, 1984

MOHR JA et al: Neurosyphilis and penicillin levels in cerebrospinal fluid. JAMA 236:2208, 1976

MOORE JE, HOPKINS HH: Asymptomatic neurosyphilis. VI. The prognosis of early and late asymptomatic neurosyphilis. JAMA 95:1637, 1930

MULLER F, MOSKOPHIDIS M: Estimation of the local production of antibodies to *Treponema pallidum* in the central nervous system of patients with neurosyphilis. Br J Vener Dis 59:80, 1983

PALEY SS: Syphilis in pregnancy. NY State J Med 37:585, 1937

QUINN TC et al: Rectal mass caused by *Treponema pallidum:* Confirmation by immunofluorescent staining. Gastroenterology 82:135, 1982

REIMER CB et al: The specificity of fetal IgM: Antibody or anti-antibody? NY Acad Sci 254:77, 1975

ROSAHN PD: *Autopsy Studies in Syphilis.* CDC Publication 433, US Department of Health, Education, and Welfare, 1960

ROSS WH, SUTTON HFS: Acquired syphilitic uveitis. Arch Ophthalmol 98:496, 1980

Sexually transmitted diseases treatment guidelines 1985. Morb Mort Week Rep Suppl 34(4S), 1985

SIMON RP: Neurosyphilis. Arch Neurol 42:606, 1985

TURNER DR, WRIGHT DJM: Lymphadenopathy in early syphilis. J Pathol 110:305, 1973

ZOLLER M et al: Detection of syphilitic hearing loss. Arch Otolaryngol 104:63, 1978

123 NONVENEREAL TREPONEMATOSES: YAWS, PINTA, AND ENDEMIC SYPHILIS

PETER L. PERINE

GENERAL CONSIDERATIONS   Nonvenereal treponematoses occur in remote, impoverished areas of the world. Yaws, pinta, and endemic syphilis are distinguished from venereal syphilis solely by clinical and epidemiologic features. Yaws and pinta are caused by treponemes which are conventionally designated as unique species (*Treponema pertenue* causes yaws, and *T. carateum* pinta), but no convincing morphologic or antigenic differences have yet been demonstrated among *T. pertenue*, *T. carateum*, and *T. pallidum*. The etiologic agent of endemic syphilis is generally held to be identical with *T. pallidum* and is sometimes designated as *T. pallidum endemicum*. Pinta involves the skin alone; yaws affects skin and bones; and endemic syphilis involves the skin, bone, and mucous membranes. Each disease tends to progress by stages, but these are neither as distinct nor as predictable as in syphilis. Congenital infections and cardiovascular and central nervous system involvement occur rarely, if ever, in the nonvenereal treponematoses but are common in syphilis. It is unclear whether the clinical and epidemiologic differences among yaws, pinta, endemic syphilis, and venereal syphilis are solely determined by environmental and host factors or are attributable to undefined biologic differences among the causal treponemes. The relationship of the treponematoses is summarized in Table 123-1.

EPIDEMIOLOGY   Treponemal antibodies are demonstrable in some proportion of nonhuman primates in regions of Africa where human yaws and endemic syphilis are common, and pathogenic treponemes have been found in skin lesions and lymph nodes of seropositive animals. These treponemes have produced yaws-like lesions in susceptible monkeys and hamsters.

Yaws and endemic syphilis are diseases of young children. Yaws occurs throughout the world between the tropics of Cancer and Capricorn, in humid, warm environments. Transmission of yaws among children is favored by scanty clothing, poor hygiene, and frequent skin trauma. Spread occurs by direct contact with infected lesions and perhaps by passive transfer of treponemes by insects. Endemic syphilis occurs in arid subtropical or temperate climates in Africa, the eastern Mediterranean, the Arabian peninsula, and central Asia. It is not observed in the western hemisphere. Skin-to-skin transmission is less important than in yaws; instead, infection of mucous membranes results from direct mouth-to-mouth contact or from contaminated fomites, such as shared drinking or eating utensils. Venereal syphilis can spread by nonvenereal contact among children

and cause household outbreaks in modern cities when crowding and poverty favor transmission of *T. pallidum*.

Although cutaneous pigmentary changes resembling late stages of pinta occur in yaws or endemic syphilis, pinta is a separate, more benign disease which occurs only in the western hemisphere. The onset is typically later than in yaws or endemic syphilis, usually when the person is between 10 and 20 years of age. Pinta is not very contagious, and its mode of transmission is not well defined.

The WHO/UNICEF-assisted mass campaign for eradication of endemic nonvenereal treponematosis from 1948 to 1969 was an unusually successful public health campaign. Over 160 million people were examined in 46 countries, and approximately 50 million cases, contacts, and latent infections were treated. The impact of this program was remarkable. The prevalence of active yaws lesions was reduced from over 20 percent to less than 1 percent in many rural areas. In Bosnia, Yugoslavia, endemic syphilis was eradicated—the only example of eradication of an endemic treponematosis.

Relaxation of active surveillance activities after the mass campaigns has led to a resurgence of yaws, particularly in Africa. Yaws has not been eradicated in any large area. The Ivory Coast, Ghana, Togo, and Benin have large reservoirs of yaws and account for over 90 percent of cases reported to WHO since 1982. North of these countries, the Sahelian nations of Mali, Niger, Burkina Faso, and Senegal have prevalence rates in some areas of 10 to 15 percent for endemic syphilis. These rates exceed those reported before the mass treatment campaigns. Seroactivity and late manifestations of endemic syphilis continue to occur among nomads in Saudi Arabia. The resurgence of yaws and endemic syphilis has led to a new yaws campaign in Ghana in 1980, and other national campaigns are planned to control resurgent yaws and endemic syphilis in Africa.

Antitreponemal and reaginic seroreactivity has been detected in a small percentage of children without clinical disease born after the mass campaigns in some areas (e.g., Nigeria, New Guinea, and Bosnia). This may represent attenuated or asymptomatic infection, or may simply reflect the decreased predictive value of serologic tests (probability that disease is present if the test is positive) when the prevalence of disease is sharply reduced.

In the Americas, foci of yaws persist in Haiti; Dominica, St. Lucia, and St. Vincent; Peru, Colombia, and Ecuador; a few areas of Brazil; and Guyana and Surinam. Pinta is confined to Central America and northern South America, where it appears to have regressed to remote Indian villages. Its prevalence today is probably less than 1 percent of that found 20 years ago.

BIOLOGIC RELATIONSHIPS   Specific humoral antibodies to *T. pallidum* are produced in individuals with yaws, pinta, or endemic syphilis, but the time of appearance of antibodies after onset of infections is variable. The fluorescent treponemal antibody absorption (FTA-ABS) test, the *T. pallidum* hemagglutination test (TPHA), and

TABLE 123-1   Etiology, epidemiology, and clinical manifestations of the treponematoses

	Venereal syphilis	Endemic syphilis	Yaws	Pinta
Organism	*T. pallidum*	*T. pallidum endemicum*	*T. pertenue*	*T. carateum*
Transmission	Sexual, transplacental*	Household contacts: mouth-to-mouth or via drinking, eating utensils	Skin-to-skin ? Insect vector	Skin-to-skin ? Insect vector
Usual age	Adult	Early childhood	Early childhood	Adolescent
Primary lesion	Cutaneous ulcer (chancre)	Rarely seen	Framboise (raspberry), or "mother yaw"	Nonulcerating papule with satellites
Secondary lesion	Mucocutaneous; occasional periostitis	Florid mucocutaneous lesions (mucous patch, split papule, condyloma latum); osteoperiostitis	Cutaneous papulosquamous lesions; osteoperiostitis	Pintides
Tertiary	Gumma, cardiovascular, and CNS lues	Destructive cutaneous osteoarticular gummas	Destructive cutaneous osteoarticular gummas	Dyschromic, achromic macules

* *Since the nonvenereal treponematoses are usually acquired in childhood and treponemal bacteremia ceases with time, only in adult-onset venereal syphilis is there any likelihood of a mother giving birth to an infected child.*

the *T. pallidum* immobilization (TPI) test cannot differentiate among the treponematoses.

In addition to the clinical and epidemiologic differences among the treponematoses in humans, the range of susceptible animal hosts and some manifestations of experimental infection are also different. In particular, *T. carateum* has produced an infection in chimpanzees which resembles pinta, but attempts to infect other experimental animals have been unsuccessful. Differences between *T. pallidum* and *T. pertenue* have been reported for infections produced in the rabbit and golden hamster, and experimental rabbit infection with one species conferred greater immunity to reinfection with the homologous species than with the heterologous species. However, these interspecies differences in superinfection immunity are no greater than intraspecies differences among different strains of *T. pallidum*. Individuals who have had yaws or pinta are considered relatively immune to syphilis, and persons with active pinta or syphilis cannot be superinfected with *T. pertenue* by experimental inoculation.

CLINICAL MANIFESTATIONS Yaws

Also known as pian, framboesia, or bubas, yaws is a chronic infectious disease of childhood caused by *T. pertenue*. The disease is characterized by an initial skin lesion(s) followed by relapsing, nondestructive, secondary lesions of skin and bone. In the late stages, destructive lesions of skin, bone, and joints occur.

The incubation period following experimental inoculation of susceptible human beings is 3 to 4 weeks. Disruption of the skin by insect bites, abrasions, or injuries promotes acquisition of natural infection from infected contacts, most likely by fingers contaminated directly or indirectly with material from early yaws lesions. The initial early lesion is a single papule which is usually located on a leg. The lesion enlarges and becomes papillomatous. This lesion is known as a framboesioma (raspberry) or "mother yaw." It becomes superficially eroded and covered by a thin yellow crust of serous exudate containing *T. pertenue*. Erythema and induration do not occur. The lesion is mildly pruritic, and regional lymphadenopathy occurs. The initial lesion usually heals in 6 months. As a result of treponemal bacteremia and autoinoculation, a generalized secondary eruption of similar lesions appears either before or after the initial lesion has healed and is most extensive on the exposed surfaces of the body. These early cutaneous lesions of yaws have a variety of forms, including desquamative macular and papular as well as papillomatous types (Fig. 123-1). Painful papillomata on the soles of the feet result in a crablike gait referred to as *crab yaws*. Early lesions are infectious and heal slowly; they may result in scarring, hyperpigmentation, or depigmentation, resembling the pigmentary changes seen in pinta. Histologic findings are mononuclear-cell infiltration, acanthosis (Fig. 123-2), hyperkeratosis, and the presence of many treponemes. Other manifestations of early yaws include lymphadenopathy and nocturnal bone pain and polydactylitis due to periostitis. Fever and other constitutional symptoms are rare, however, unless lesions become secondarily infected. Infectious cutaneous relapses are characteristic during the first 5 years after infection. Late yaws lesions occur in about 10 percent of cases, starting 5 years or more after infection, and differ histologically from early lesions in showing endarteritis. Late lesions include gummas of the skin and long bones, particularly of the legs, hyperkeratoses of the soles and palms, osteitis, periostitis, juxtaarticular fibromatous nodes, and hydrarthrosis.

Late lesions of yaws are characteristically extensive and usually destructive. Destruction of the nose, maxilla, palate, and pharynx, termed *gangosa*, or *rhinopharyngitis mutilans*, occurs in late yaws, as well as in leprosy and leishmaniasis. Hypertrophic paranasal maxillary osteitis produces distinctive facies known as *goundou*.

The clinical features of yaws have become less reliable for diagnosis

FIGURE 123-1 *Recrudescent yaws lesions of the left arm with subcutaneous juxtaarticular nodules.*

FIGURE 123-2 *Secondary yaws ulceropapillomata on the right leg.*

as the prevalence of yaws has decreased, necessitating the use of easily performed serologic tests, such as the rapid plasma reagin (RPR) card test, by paramedical field workers engaged in the consolidation phase of yaws surveillance.

T. pertenue can be demonstrated by dark-field examination in early cutaneous lesions but should not be confused with other spirochetes found in tropical ulcers. The serum reagin antibody tests become positive after 1 month, and the FTA-ABS test is also positive.

Endemic syphilis Synonyms for endemic syphilis are Bejel, Siti, Dichuchwa, Njovera, Belesh, and Skerljevo. It is a chronic nonvenereal, treponemal infection of childhood, characterized by early mucous membrane or mucocutaneous lesions, a latent period of indeterminate duration, and late complications including gummas of bone and skin. The causative organism is indistinguishable from *T. pallidum.* Endemic syphilis differs from congenital syphilis in that dental changes, interstitial keratitis, and neurosyphilis rarely, if ever, occur. Cardiovascular complications are considered rare in both endemic and congenital syphilis.

Primary cutaneous lesions are infrequent and when present are extragenital. The earliest manifestation of endemic syphilis is usually an intraoral mucous patch or mucocutaneous lesion resembling the split papules or condylomata of secondary syphilis. Periostitis is common. Regional lymphadenopathy occurs, but generalized lymphadenopathy is unusual. Treponemes are abundant in the moist early lesions and in aspirates from regional lymph nodes. After a variable latent period, late lesions may develop and are the most frequent clinical manifestations. These resemble the lesions of late benign syphilis and include osseous or cutaneous gummas. Destructive gummas, osteitis, and periostitis of nasopharyngeal structures are more common than in late yaws. Gummas occur on the nipples of mothers who have themselves previously had endemic syphilis who breastfeed infants with oral lesions. Both early and late forms of endemic syphilis thus may coexist in the same family. The tertiary lesions of endemic syphilis sometimes may be a consequence of repeated reexposure of a previously sensitized host to reinfection.

Pinta Also known as mal del pinto, carate, azul, or purupuru, pinta is an infectious disease of the skin caused by *T. carateum.* This disease has three cutaneous stages characterized by marked changes in the skin color, does not involve osseous tissue or viscera, and causes no disability other than that associated with cosmetic disfigurement.

The initial lesion is a small papule which appears 7 to 30 days after exposure and is located most often on the extremities, face, neck, or buttocks. It increases in size slowly by peripheral extension and by coalescing with smaller satellite papules. Regional lymphadenopathy occurs. A secondary eruption not associated with generalized lymphadenopathy appears 1 month to 1 year after the appearance of the initial lesion. The secondary lesions are termed *pintides,* may be numerous, and evolve into a psoriatic or circinate configuration. Pintides are initially red but become deeply pigmented, reaching a slate-blue color after a period of time which is related to exposure to sun. Pigmentation occurs most rapidly on the exposed parts of the body. These pigmented lesions are known as dyschromic macules and contain treponemes which are located principally in the epidermis in older lesions. Histologically there is deposition of pigment in the dermis with decreased melanin pigment in the basal cell layer. Within 3 months to a year, most of the pintides show varying degrees of depigmentation, becoming brown and finally white and giving the skin a mottled appearance. The porcelain-white achromic lesions represent the "late" stage of the disease in which the epidermis is atrophic, and melanocytes and melanin are absent. *T. carateum* can be demonstrated in transudates from initial, early secondary, or dyschromic lesions. Serologic reaginic and antitreponemal antibody tests are positive, but may take four times longer to become positive in pinta than in venereal syphilis.

TREATMENT Treatment is similar for all the endemic treponematoses. Intramuscular injection of 1.2 million units of benzathine

penicillin G in adults and half this dose in children results in rapid resolution of lesions and prevents recurrence. Procaine penicillin G in oil and 2% aluminum monostearate (PAM) has been used extensively. In persons who are allergic to penicillin, tetracycline hydrochloride in a dose similar to that used for infectious syphilis (see Chap. 122) is effective. In areas where less than 5 percent of the population has active disease, cases are managed on an individual basis, and all contacts of infected persons are treated with antibiotics.

PREVENTION Although the nonvenereal treponematoses are less amenable to eradication than smallpox, the resurgence of yaws has led some authorities to suggest that the application of *selective epidemiologic control* as used in smallpox eradication be applied to yaws control. This strategy would emphasize ongoing active surveillance, investigation of outbreaks, and treatment of active cases and their contacts rather than mass treatment.

REFERENCES

BURKE JP et al (eds): International symposium on yaws and other endemic treponematoses. Rev Infect Dis 7:S217, 1985

Editorial: Yaws again. Br Med J 2:1090, 1980

GRIN EI, GUTHE T: Evaluation of a previous mass campaign against endemic syphilis in Bosnia and Herzogovina. Br J Vener Dis 49:1, 1973

GUTHE T: Clinical, serological and epidemiological features of framboesia tropica (yaws) and its control in rural communities. Acta Derm Venereol 49:343, 1969

HOPKINS DR: Yaws in the Americas, 1950–1975. J Infect Dis 136:548, 1977

PERINE PL et al: *Handbook of Endemic Treponematoses.* WHO, Geneva, 1984

Treponematoses Research: Report of a WHO Scientific Group, WHO Technical Report Series 455, 1970

WORLD HEALTH ORGANIZATION: Endemic treponematoses. Week Epidem Rec 56:241, 1981

---

124   LEPTOSPIROSIS

JAY P. SANFORD

DEFINITION *Leptospirosis* is a term applied to disease caused by all leptospiras regardless of specific serotype. Correlation of clinical syndromes with infection by differing serotypes leads to the conclusion that a single serotype of *Leptospira* may be responsible for a variety of clinical features; conversely, a single syndrome, e.g., aseptic meningitis, may be caused by multiple serotypes. Hence there is a preference for the general term leptospirosis rather than the synonyms such as Weil's disease and canicola fever.

ETIOLOGY The genus *Leptospira* contains only one species, *L. interrogans,* which may be subdivided into two complexes, interrogans and biflexa. The interrogans complex includes the pathogenic strains, while the biflexa complex includes saprophytic strains. Within each complex the organisms show antigenic variations that are stable and allow them to be classed as serotypes (serovars). Serotypes with common antigens are arranged in serogroups (varieties). Despite contrary common usage, an example of the correct designation of *Leptospira* is as follows: Pomona serogroup of *L. interrogans* or *L. interrogans* var. pomona, not *L. pomona.* The interrogans complex now contains about 170 serotypes arranged in 18 serogroups (the number in parentheses refers to number of serotypes within the serogroup): Icterohemorrhagiae (18), Hebdomadis (30), Autumnalis (17), Canicola (12), Australis (12), Tarassovi (17), Pyrogenes (12), Bataviae (10), Javanica (8), Pomona (8), Ballum (3), Cynopteri (3), Celledoni (3), Grippotyphosa (5), Panama (2), Shermani (1), Ranarum (2), and Bufonis (1). At least 27 serotypes of *Leptospira* occur naturally in the United States.

EPIDEMIOLOGY Leptospirosis is thought to be the most widespread zoonosis in the world. Cases are regularly reported from all continents hemolysis. Antibodies detected by ELISA, FIA, and RIA tend to parallel the hemagglutination-inhibiting antibodies, while the appearance of CF antibody lags behind the others by a period of 3 to 7 days and often does not disappear until 1 or 2 years after infection. The PHA antibody first appears even later (14 to 21 days after rash onset), but persists thereafter. The presence of IgM-specific antibodies suggests recent rubella infection (within 2 months); however, they have been known to persist as long as 1 year in some cases. There are no other laboratory findings helpful in the diagnosis of rubella, although lymphocytosis with atypical lymphocytes may occur.

Patients with the congenital rubella syndrome may lose hemagglutination-inhibiting antibodies at age 3 or 4 years. Therefore a negative serologic test in a child over 3 years does not exclude the possibility of congenital rubella. Congenital rubella should be differentiated by appropriate serologic tests from congenital syphilis (see Chap. 122), toxoplasmosis (see Chap. 157), and cytomegalic inclusion virus disease (see Chap. 137). IgM-specific antibodies are often found early in the first year of life in infants with congenital rubella, but virus isolation is the most reliable way to confirm the diagnosis.

PREVENTION In adults and children rubella is usually a mild disease with infrequent complications. However, the severity of congenital infection has prompted efforts to prevent the disease. Administration of gamma globulin to exposed persons can abort the clinical disease, but seroconversion and transmission of the disease from mother to fetus may occur despite the administration of large amounts of gamma globulin soon after exposure.

Active immunization with live attenuated rubella vaccines has been practiced in this country since 1969, especially among young children. The aim has been to decrease the frequency of the infection in the population and to decrease the chance that susceptible pregnant women will be exposed. Because of concern for a possibly enlarging pool of susceptible adolescents and adults, there has been increasing enthusiasm for serologic screening of pubertal females with no history of immunization, followed by selective immunization of those who are seronegative. Such immunization must of course be done with appropriate precautions, as noted below. Persons working in hospitals or clinics who might contract rubella from infected patients or who, if infected, might transmit the infection to pregnant patients should all be required to have proof of immunity (either documented immunization or presence of serum antibody).

The attenuated virus can be detected in the respiratory secretions of vaccinees for as long as 4 weeks after immunization, but transmission to other susceptible individuals rarely, if ever, occurs, even in households where susceptible pregnant women are in contact with children who are being vaccinated. The vaccine induces detectable antibodies in about 95 percent of recipients, but the degree and duration of protection are still being evaluated. After heavy exposure in closed populations, vaccinated individuals sometimes develop subclinical infections (diagnosed by antibody rises and virus isolation). However, viremia has not been demonstrated in immunized persons, which suggests that previously vaccinated pregnant women will not infect their fetuses even if they acquire subclinical rubella.

Side effects of fever, rash, lymphadenopathy, polyneuropathy, or arthralgias occur very seldom in vaccinated children, but joint pain and swelling or paresthesias were seen in more than 25 percent of women who were immunized with the earlier vaccines. This risk has been reduced to less than 2 percent with the advent of vaccines prepared in human embryonic fibroblast cell cultures (RA 27/3 vaccine). The joint symptoms usually begin 2 to 10 weeks after vaccination, and they may be confused with other forms of arthritis. *Rubella vaccine must never be given to pregnant women or to those who may become pregnant within 3 months of immunization.* Although no infant with the congenital rubella syndrome has been reported to have been born to a woman inadvertently vaccinated during pregnancy, the theoretical risk of vaccine virus–induced fetal damage remains. In addition, vaccine is contraindicated in patients with immune-deficiency diseases or who are taking immunosuppressive drugs.

OTHER VIRAL EXANTHEMS

In addition to the diseases such as measles, rubella, and chickenpox which historically have been associated with prominent skin lesions there are other virus infections in which skin manifestations may occur. Table 133-1 lists the other most commonly recognized causes of maculopapular eruptions. Some of them, particularly the enteroviruses, can also occasionally cause papulovesicular or petechial rashes; others are capable of provoking erythema multiforme–like eruptions. One helpful aspect of the physical examination is the observation that viral-caused maculopapular (not vesicular) exanthems usually *relatively* spare the palms and soles. This is in contrast to eruptions associated with drug reactions, bacteria, *Mycoplasma*, and *Rickettsia*, in which a prominent palmar or plantar eruption is often noted.

EXANTHEM SUBITUM (ROSEOLA INFANTUM) Exanthem subitum is a benign disease of infants 6 to 24 months of age that is characterized by a high fever and rash. The disease can be transmitted to humans and monkeys by the transfer of blood obtained from a patient during the first few days of illness. The infectious agent is probably a virus, although it has not been isolated. The first manifestations of disease, after an estimated incubation period of 5 to 15 days, are the abrupt onset of irritability and fever, which last for 3 to 5 days; the temperature may be as high as 105°F. There may be mild pharyngitis and slight lymph node enlargement; convulsions may occur during the height of the fever. On the fourth to fifth day of illness, there is a sudden drop in temperature to normal or below normal; several hours before or after defervescence the rash suddenly and surprisingly appears. It is characterized by faint 2- to 3-mm macules or maculopapules over the neck and trunk and may extend to the thighs and buttocks; it may last for only a few hours or may be present for a day or two. Leukopenia is frequently noted later in the febrile period. The disease is benign and not associated with complications, although rarely an infant may show sequelae as a result of febrile convulsions. In the early, preeruptive phase, the disease may be difficult to differentiate from an acute bacteremia, particularly from one associated with *Streptococcus pneumoniae*. Though a leukocytosis with an increase in band forms is often seen in bacteremias presenting in this fashion, blood cultures are necessary to make the diagnosis.

ERYTHEMA INFECTIOSUM (FIFTH DISEASE) Erythema infectiosum is a mild febrile exanthematous disease with little or no prodrome. The mean incubation period is estimated as approximately 4 to 12 days (median 7 days). The first manifestations are low-grade fever with varying degrees of conjunctivitis, upper respiratory complaints, cough, myalgia, itching, nausea, and diarrhea, followed in many cases by the appearance of indurated, confluent erythema over the cheeks, giving a "slapped face" appearance. A day or so later, a bilaterally symmetric eruption is seen on the arms, legs, and trunk, but rarely on the palms or soles. The lesions are maculopapular and tend to be confluent, forming slightly raised blotchy areas and reticular or lacy patterns. When it occurs, the rash usually lasts about a week, and during this time it may disappear, only to reappear in the same areas a few hours later. The waxing and waning eruption may

TABLE 133-1 Causes of maculopapular eruptions

Viral	Other
Measles	*Mycoplasma pneumoniae*
Rubella	Syphilis
Exanthem subitum	Typhoid fever
Erythema infectiosum	Bacterial toxins:
Enteroviruses: coxsackievirus,	streptococci and staphylococci
echovirus	Rat-bite fever
Infectious mononucleosis	*Rickettsia*
Adenoviruses	Live-virus vaccines
Reoviruses	Drug eruptions
Arboviruses	Mucocutaneous lymph node
	syndrome

occasionally persist for several weeks, and can be brought on by fever, heat, exercise, sunlight exposure, or emotional stress. Mild joint pain and swelling have been observed in a large proportion of adults with the disease, and some have had symptoms lasting from a few months to over 4 years. Erythema infectiosum affects all ages but is most common in children of school age and may occur in epidemic form. The etiologic agent has now been identified as a human parvovirus (B19) which also is considered to be the primary cause of aplastic crises in patients with chronic hemolytic anemias such as sickle cell disease and hereditary spherocytosis. The route of transmission of the natural disease is probably respiratory. Subclinical infection is common. Antibody to the virus has been demonstrated in 30 to 50 percent of healthy adults. Specific diagnosis is accomplished by detection of the virus particles in early acute-phase serum by electron microscopy, by demonstration of specific viral DNA in serum or pharyngeal secretions, or more commonly by detection of IgM-specific antibodies in serums collected in the acute or early convalescent phase of illness. However, these methods are not yet routinely available in the United States. A clinical diagnosis of this disease must sometimes be made with caution, since rubella and some enteroviruses have also been shown at times to cause a nearly identical syndrome.

ENTEROVIRAL EXANTHEMS   Many individual enteroviruses have been associated with rash. Of these, polioviruses are rarely implicated. More commonly, echovirus serotypes 1 through 7, 9, 11, 12, 14, 16, 18, 19, 20, 25, and 30, coxsackievirus serotypes A4, A5, A6, A9, A10, A16, and B2, B3, and B5 have all been implicated. With the exception of hand-foot-and-mouth disease, usually associated with coxsackievirus A16 or enterovirus 71 infection (see Chap. 139), there is no set of clinical or epidemiologic features that aids in differentiating the specific enteroviral agent involved in a specific case. All are capable of producing maculopapular rashes which vary in intensity and duration, and can also occasionally produce petechial or papulovesicular exanthems and enanthems. In community and household outbreaks, younger children and infants are usually more likely to have exanthems, while other features of enteroviral infection, such as fever, myalgia, and aseptic meningitis, are more prominent among older children and young adults. Two enterovirus infections which have been frequently associated with rashes and have been studied extensively are described as examples of epidemic enteroviral infections.

Boston exanthem (infections with echovirus 16)   Echovirus 16 infection was described first and most extensively during an epidemic in Boston in 1951. Children who were infected usually had a disease characterized by exanthem and low-grade fever, while adult family contacts often developed high fever, prostration, and signs of aseptic meningitis with absent or fleeting rash. The first manifestation of the disease in children was fever of 101 to 102°F, lasting for a day or two, pharyngitis with small ulcerated lesions resembling herpangina, and slight enlargement of the cervical and postauricular lymph nodes. The rash appeared during fever or after defervescence and consisted of small pink maculopapules on the face, upper part of the chest, and occasionally on the whole body, including the palms and soles. The rash lasted for 1 to 5 days, and there were no important complications or sequelae. The disease resembled exanthem subitum but occurred in children of all ages and in adults.

Infection with echovirus 9   Infection with this virus in children and adults has been characterized by a febrile illness with a high incidence of aseptic meningitis. The incubation period is 5 to 8 days. About 30 percent of patients have a rash, which may occur with or without meningitis. It is usually maculopapular, developing at the onset of fever. The exanthem appears first on the face and neck, spreads to the trunk and extremities, may involve the palms and soles, although slightly, and persists for 3 to 5 days. Petechiae with or without maculopapules have been recognized; when they are seen in association with meningitis, there may be confusion with meningococcal

meningitis. This can be a point of some concern, since concurrent outbreaks of echovirus 9 and meningococcal disease have been observed. A vesicular eruption with crusting lesions has been seen occasionally. An exanthem on the buccal mucosa and soft palate occurs in about 30 percent of patients and consists of small red areas with white centers which resemble Koplik's spots. The disease is usually benign but rarely has been associated with permanent central nervous system damage. Acute rhabdomyolysis with myoglobinuria has also been associated with echovirus 9 infection, and can be severe.

REFERENCES

ANDERSON MJ et al: Experimental parvoviral infection in humans. J Infect Dis 152:257, 1985

CHONMAITREE T et al: Enterovirus 71 infection: Report of an outbreak with two cases of paralysis and a review of the literature. Pediatrics 67:489, 1981

CLARKE WL et al: Autoimmunity in congenital rubella syndrome. J Pediatr 104:370, 1984

Current trends: Rubella and congenital rubella syndrome—United States, 1984–1985. Morb Mort Week Rep 35:129, 1986

HALL CB et al: The return of Boston exanthem. Echovirus 16 infections in 1974. Am J Dis Child 131:323, 1977

HERRMANN KL: Available rubella serologic tests. Rev Infect Dis 7:S108, 1985

HILL HR, RAY CG: The differential diagnosis of viral exanthems and enanthems, in Infections in Children, RJ Wedgwood et al (eds). Philadelphia, Harper & Row, 1982, p 235

IMMUNIZATION PRACTICES ADVISORY COMMITTEE: Rubella prevention. Ann Intern Med 101:505, 1984

JOSSELSON J et al: Acute rhabdomyolysis associated with an echovirus 9 infection. Arch Intern Med 140:1671, 1980

NEVA FA et al: Clinical epidemiological features of an unusual epidemic exanthem. JAMA 155:544, 1954

ORENSTEIN WA et al: The opportunity and obligation to eliminate rubella from the United States. JAMA 251:1988, 1984

PLUMMER FA et al: An erythema infectiosum-like illness caused by human parvovirus infection. N Engl J Med 313:74, 1985

PREBLUD SR: Some current issues relating to rubella vaccine. JAMA 254:253, 1985

REID DM et al: Human parvovirus-associated arthritis: A clinical and laboratory description. Lancet 1:422, 1985

SEVER JL et al: Rubella epidemic, 1964: Effect on 6,000 pregnancies. Am J Dis Child 110:395, 1965

TINGLE AJ et al: Failed rubella immunization in adults: Association with immunologic and virological abnormalities. J Infect Dis 151:330, 1985

TOWNSEND JJ et al: Progressive rubella panencephalitis: Late onset after congenital rubella. N Engl J Med 292:990, 1975

WHITE DG et al: Human parvovirus arthropathy. Lancet 1:419, 1985

134   SMALLPOX, VACCINIA, AND OTHER POXVIRUSES

C. GEORGE RAY

Poxviruses are a group of large (200 to 320 nm), brick-shaped, DNA-containing viruses that have a predilection for skin. Many of the poxviruses, such as myxoma and fowl pox agents, cause disease mainly in lower animals. Smallpox (variola major), alastrim (variola minor), vaccinia, and cowpox agents are closely related members of the poxvirus group that cause human disease.

SMALLPOX (VARIOLA)

DEFINITION   Smallpox is a severe, contagious, febrile disease characterized by a vesicular and pustular eruption. Alastrim is a similar but milder illness, with a lower mortality rate. Though the difference in severity between these diseases is apparent, the agents of variola major and variola minor are biologically and immunologically indistinguishable from each other in the laboratory.

Smallpox (both variola major and variola minor) is considered to no longer exist in nature. In 1967, the World Health Organization launched an ambitious program aimed at total eradication of smallpox.

Two important epidemiologic factors which suggested that this was possible were the absence of nonhuman reservoirs of the virus and the apparent nonexistence of completely asymptomatic human carriers. As a result of this astonishing effort, the last recorded case of naturally acquired smallpox occurred in Somalia in 1977. After 2 more years of worldwide surveillance with no further infections, global eradication of smallpox was confirmed in 1979 and accepted by the World Health Organization in May 1980. This was followed by destruction of laboratory stocks of virus, with the exception of two laboratories: one in Atlanta, the other in Moscow. Surveillance continues, including studies of poxviruses of animals which are antigenically somewhat similar to smallpox. Some virologists remain legitimately concerned that an animal poxvirus (e.g., monkeypox, whitepox) could undergo mutation and become virulent for humans, although the chance of such an occurrence seems remote. Also, the possibility of "escape" of virus from a laboratory, although unlikely, must be considered.

Because the disease appears to be eradicated, the following description may be more of historical than practical interest. However, the disease might reappear unexpectedly, and a discussion of its features and prevention is still warranted.

PATHOGENESIS AND PATHOLOGY The virus gains access to the body by the respiratory tract and multiplies in unidentified sites, probably in lymph nodes or liver. After several days, during which there is no evidence of infection, viremia ensues, with swelling of the endothelium of blood vessels in the corium and perivascular inflammation. Loculated vesicles are the result of cellular destruction and exudation of serum. The infected epithelial cells are swollen and contain intracytoplasmic inclusions surrounded by a halo (Guarnieri bodies). The extent of skin involvement is greater in smallpox than in chickenpox and reaches into the corium. Pitting, most commonly seen on the face, is said to result from destruction of sebaceous glands, which are abundant in this area. The liver, spleen, and lymph nodes may be enlarged and may show focal accumulations of large mononuclear cells.

EPIDEMIOLOGY Smallpox is not as contagious as measles or influenza, and ordinarily face-to-face contact with an infected person is required to transmit the disease; however, airborne dissemination from contaminated fomites has also been shown to occur. A patient with smallpox is infectious from a day before the rash appears until all lesions have healed and the scabs have fallen off. During the early phase of the illness, the virus is transmitted in nasopharyngeal secretions; when the eruption is fully formed, the lesions themselves are a major source of infectious material. Variola virus may contaminate clothing, bedding, dust, or other inanimate objects and remain infectious for months, necessitating disinfection of articles in the patient's environment.

MANIFESTATIONS The incubation period of smallpox, from the time of exposure to the onset of the prodrome, is about 12 days, with extremes of 4 to 17 days. The disease can be divided into a prodrome, an early eruptive phase, and a period of vesiculation and pustule formation. The prodrome is characterized by a temperature of 102 to 106°F, headache, myalgia especially in the back, abdominal pain, vomiting, and in some patients by a transient, blotchy, erythematous eruption. After 3 or 4 days the fever subsides, the symptoms decrease, and the patient seems to recover. It is at this time, when the patient is afebrile, that the focal eruption begins. Early manifestations are painful ulcers on the buccal mucosa and macules which appear first on the face and forearms, and rapidly become firm, shotty papules. The papules increase in number and spread from the face and distal extremities to involve the trunk. The individual lesions may remain discrete and scattered, or they may become confluent and involve most of the body. They are most concentrated on the face and distal extremities, including the palms and soles, and are relatively sparse in the axilla. On the third or fourth day after the appearance of the focal rash, the papules progress to vesicles containing clear fluid, which, over the next few days,

becomes cloudy because of infiltration by pus cells and desquamated epithelial cells; hemorrhage into the vesicles and surrounding skin may also be seen. During the course of smallpox, the lesions at any one time, in one area, are all at the same stage of evolution. At the time the vesicles become pustular, there is recurrence of fever, which may persist until healing occurs. The pustules umbilicate and form crusts and scabs which usually fall off 3 weeks after the beginning of illness, leaving small scars or deep pits.

The above description applies to disease of moderate severity. A milder illness may occur in previously immunized persons or in some who have no history of vaccination. It is characterized by the usual incubation period and prodrome, but is followed either by focal eruption of fewer than 100 papules, or by a rash resembling chickenpox. Smallpox with prodrome but with no eruption of any kind has been recognized (variola sine eruptione). The disease may also occur in a rapidly fulminating form ("sledgehammer" smallpox). After the usual incubation period, the patient develops an initial illness characterized by severe prostration, fever, bone marrow depression, hemorrhagic skin lesions, and bleeding. The disease progresses from inception to death within 3 or 4 days without evidence of the typical focal skin lesions.

Alastrim is similar to mild and moderate forms of variola major in that it has the same incubation period and prodromal illness, but the skin eruption is less extensive, and fatalities are rare.

COMPLICATIONS Bacterial superinfections of the lesions, usually with *Staphylococcus aureus,* may occur in the late pustular stage. Bacterial pneumonia and sepsis may be seen in severe forms of smallpox. Mild conjunctivitis is quite common, and iritis and keratitis have been recognized. Encephalomyelitis may occur in the late stage of the disease and is similar to other postinfectious encephalitides. Osteomyelitis and joint effusions may complicate the disease, and orchitis has also been reported.

LABORATORY FINDINGS Leukopenia is present during the prodromal illness, and there is usually leukocytosis during the pustular stage. Rapid diagnosis of poxvirus infection can be made by the finding of characteristic brick-shaped particles in preparations of vesicle fluid examined by electron microscopy. Specific precipitation in agar by use of antigen prepared from lesions and antivariola or antivaccinia immune serum may also allow detection of poxvirus within a few hours. For definitive identification the virus must be grown in cell culture or on the chorioallantoic membrane and neutralized with specific antiserum.

DIFFERENTIAL DIAGNOSIS The major problem in differential diagnosis is in distinguishing smallpox from chickenpox. Smallpox is preceded by a longer prodrome than chickenpox, and the eruption vesiculates over a period of days instead of hours. The smallpox lesions are all characteristically in the same stage of development, whereas those of chickenpox may, in one area, display all stages of evolution. Electron microscopy and agar precipitation techniques (see above) are especially useful in distinguishing between smallpox and chickenpox. Cytologic examination of scrapings of the base of a vesicle can also be helpful in the differential diagnosis. The presence of multinucleated giant cells and/or intranuclear inclusions strongly suggests a herpes group infection (varicella-zoster or herpes simplex); such findings are not seen with poxvirus infections.

Other conditions which are sometimes confused with smallpox include eczema vaccinatum, eczema herpeticum, rickettsialpox, drug eruptions, some cases of contact dermatitis, and Stevens-Johnson syndrome. The fulminant, hemorrhagic smallpox may closely resemble meningococcemia, typhus, and hemorrhagic fevers.

PREVENTION Smallpox may be prevented among the patient's contacts by vaccination. Because this procedure is most successful if carried out during the early part of the incubation period, all exposed persons, regardless of previous immunization, should be vaccinated immediately upon recognition of exposure. Large, controlled, clinical trials have demonstrated that oral administration of N-methylisatin 3-thiosemicarbazone (methisazone), a drug which interferes with poxvirus multiplication, can prevent smallpox and alastrim in patients exposed to the diseases. The use of a drug together with prompt vaccination results in greater chance of protection than either measure alone. A drawback to the use of methisazone is its tendency to induce vomiting. The combined use of vaccination and parenteral administration of vaccinia immune globulin early in the incubation period is also effective in the prevention of smallpox in exposed individuals.

TREATMENT There is no specific therapy for smallpox. Thiosemicarbazone, although effective in prophylaxis, has not been shown to be of value in the treatment of established cases. Fluid deficits should be replaced by the administration of appropriate solutions. During the vesicular and pustular phases of the disease, an attempt should be made to prevent bacterial infection by the use of sterile sheets and aseptic nursing procedures. Antihistamines may be helpful in decreasing pruritus. Application of lotions or ointment should be avoided. Later in the course of the illness, when desquamation has begun, showers or baths may be helpful in removing desquamating tissue. If bacterial infection develops, an antibiotic active against the infecting organism should be given by the parenteral route. Topical antibiotics should be avoided.

VACCINIA

Vaccinia is a virus disease of the skin which is induced by inoculation for the prevention of smallpox. The exact origin of the vaccinia virus is obscure. The material first used by Jenner in 1796 was propagated for many years by successive passage from person to person through use of exudate from fresh skin lesions.

VACCINATION Use of vaccinia virus is now indicated *only* for a few laboratory workers directly involved with smallpox or closely related animal poxviruses, such as monkeypox. A few countries in Asia and Africa still require an up-to-date certification of smallpox vaccination as a condition of entry, even though there is no medical reason to do so. It has been suggested that travelers to these areas obtain smallpox vaccination–waiver letters indicating that vaccination is contraindicated for health reasons, rather than undergo the risk of complications from the vaccine. Many United States military personnel are still routinely vaccinated, representing a continued source for complications and spread of the virus to civilian contacts.

In the past, vaccinia virus has also been occasionally used for the treatment of diseases such as recurrent herpes simplex infection or warts. There is *no* evidence of therapeutic efficacy in these situations, and the use of the virus for these purposes is strictly contraindicated. Live, lyophilized vaccinia virus prepared from vesicle fluid of infected calves maintains potency for 18 months at 46°F. It is dissolved in a diluent solution just prior to use. The usual method for vaccination is to apply a small drop of vaccine to the skin over the deltoid muscle and to press a sterile needle through the vaccine several times in such a way that only the superficial layer of skin is entered, or by simultaneous puncture utilizing a plastic tine device. Vaccination should always induce some form of skin reaction; complete absence of any kind of lesion indicates that the vaccine was not viable or was not administered properly. The reaction which occurs in nonimmune individuals is characterized by a red papule at the site of inoculation 3 to 5 days after vaccination. The papule becomes vesicular on about the fifth or sixth day and pustular by the ninth or eleventh day after inoculation. The vesicle and pustule may be surrounded by a large area of erythema. About 2 weeks after vaccination, the pustule dries and develops a crust which falls off by the end of the third week, leaving a scar. Fever, malaise, and irritability are common in children during the vesicular and pustular phases, and axillary lymphadenopathy may develop and persist for several months. In the partially immune person, a modified reaction develops without fever or constitutional symptoms. A papule appears on the skin within 3 days, vesiculates in 5 to 7 days, and heals without much scarring. The so-called immune reaction described by some, where a papule and/or erythema appears in a few days, then recedes without vesiculation, is an "equivocal" reaction, and may simply represent allergy to the components of an inadvertently inactivated vaccine. A successful vaccination is defined as the presence of a Jennerian vesicle (vesicular, pustular, or crusted) 7 days after inoculation. If the criterion is not met, the patient should be revaccinated, preferably with vaccine from a different lot.

Revaccination every 3 years is required to ensure protection. *Absolute contraindications* to vaccination include individuals with congenital or acquired immune deficiencies, lymphoma, leukemia or other blood dyscrasias, patients being treated with steroids, antimetabolites, alkylating agents, irradiation, and individuals with a history of vaccinia encephalitis. *Relative contraindications* include patients or household contacts with eczema or a history of eczema, severe acne, or other similar dermatologic problems, pregnancy, and infants under 12 months of age. If the necessity to vaccinate any individual in this latter group is great, simultaneous administration of vaccinia immune globulin (VIG), 0.3 mL/kg, is suggested, to be given at a separate site intramuscularly at the time of immunization.

COMPLICATIONS Healing of the primary vaccinal lesion may not occur, and some patients go on to develop slowly progressive necrosis with destruction of large areas of skin, subcutaneous tissue, and underlying structures *(vaccinia gangrenosum)*. In addition to the local destruction, there may be metastatic lesions on other parts of the skin surface and in bone and viscera. Vaccinia gangrenosum occurs most frequently in persons with disorders of immunity and, if untreated, is nearly always fatal. *Eczema vaccinatum* is a serious complication that is seen in persons with eczema or other types of chronic skin conditions. Widespread infection in the previously affected areas, as well as in normal skin, may result from direct vaccination of an eczematous patient or from exposure to a recently vaccinated individual. *Generalized vaccinia* in patients without preexisting skin disease is characterized by a few satellite lesions surrounding the inoculation site or by widely disseminated pox resembling the primary vaccination lesion. This condition is usually mild with generally complete recovery. Vaccinia virus may be transferred from the primary inoculation site to the eye or other sites by scratching. *Postvaccinal encephalomyelitis* appears from 2 to 25 days after vaccination. The patient suddenly becomes severely ill with nuchal rigidity, drowsiness, vomiting, convulsions, coma, and signs suggesting disease of the spinal cord. The period of coma lasts for a few days, and in those who recover there are usually no permanent sequelae. Death occurs in about 30 to 40 percent of the patients with encephalomyelitis. *Erythema multiforme bullosum,* or *diffuse blotchy erythema,* may occur in vaccinated patients 7 to 10 days after vaccination, and is thought to be an allergic reaction to the virus or other components of the vaccine.

The rates of adverse effects per million primarily vaccinated persons were vaccinia gangrenosum, 0.9; eczema vaccinatum, 10.4; generalized vaccinia, 23.4; vaccinal lesions resulting from accidental implantation of virus, 25.4; postvaccinal encephalitis, 2.9; other complications, 11.8; the death rate was 1 per million.

Active treatment of vaccinia complications, aside from control of bacterial superinfection and treatment of any underlying defects, is limited. VIG is of possible value in accidental inoculation into secondary sites such as the eye, vaccinia gangrenosum, eczema vaccinatum, and generalized vaccinia. Dosage is usually 0.6 mL/kg intramuscularly, although much larger doses are sometimes used in severe cases. VIG is of no use in erythema multiforme or postvaccinal encephalitis. Thiosemicarbazone has been used in some cases of progressive vaccinia gangrenosum, and 5-Iodo-2'-deoxyuridine is suggested for topical treatment of vaccinial keratitis and conjunctivitis; however, the evidence supporting their efficacy is equivocal.

COWPOX

Cowpox is primarily a disease of the teats and udders of cows. Humans are almost always infected by milking, but occasional spread to contacts may occur from an infected person. The human disease is characterized by low-grade fever and by small papules on the fingers and hand, which go through vesicular and pustular stages resembling the course of vaccinia infection. The lesions may be ruptured by trauma and spread to immediately adjacent areas on the hand and continue to ulcerate for several weeks. Edema, lymphangitis, and axillary lymph node enlargement are common. Very rare cases of post-cowpox encephalitis and serious infections of eczematous persons have been reported. In general, the disease is benign, heals without scarring, and is uncomplicated.

PARAVACCINIA (MILKERS' NODULES)

Paravaccinia is a poxvirus which is antigenically unrelated to cowpox, but produces similar lesions in humans. It is primarily a disease of calves and milk cows, producing lesions on the teats of the cows and oral lesions in the suckling calf. Humans acquire infection through the skin by direct contact. The lesion is usually solitary, beginning as a macule on the finger, hand, or wrist, and progressing to a firm nodule, 1 to 2 cm in diameter, in 10 days. It then crusts and heals without scarring in 2 to 3 weeks. Occasionally, there is associated lymphadenitis. The lesion and its evolution are closely similar to ecthyma contagiosum (orf), a poxvirus of sheep, or bovine papular stomatitis which can also infect humans by direct inoculation.

MOLLUSCUM CONTAGIOSUM

Molluscum contagiosum is spread by direct contact with infected cells. In children, the lesions are commonly seen on the face, trunk, and limbs as a result of skin-to-skin or fomites-to-skin spread. The adult form most commonly occurs in the genital, lower abdomen, and inner thigh areas as a result of sexual contact.

After an incubation period of 2 to 8 weeks, pale, firm, pearllike nodules 2 to 10 mm in diameter develop in the epidermis. The lesions are painless, umbilicated, and not associated with systemic symptoms. A cheesy material can often be expressed from the pore at the center of each. Local spread can occur if the lesions and surrounding skin are traumatized. Pathologic findings include epidermal hyperplasia, ballooning degeneration, and acanthosis. The diagnosis is usually made on clinical grounds, but can be confirmed by demonstration of large, eosinophilic cytoplasmic inclusions (molluscum bodies) in the affected epithelial cells.

If left alone, the lesions disappear in 2 to 12 months. Specific treatment, if desired, is often by curettage or careful removal of the central core by expression with forceps.

REFERENCES

Bowman KF et al: Cutaneous form of bovine papular stomatitis in man. JAMA 246:2813, 1981
Breman JG, Arita I: The confirmation and maintenance of smallpox eradication. N Engl J Med 303:1263, 1980
Dixon CW: Smallpox. London, Churchill, 1962
Goldstein JA et al: Smallpox vaccination reactions, prophylaxis, and therapy of complications. Pediatrics 55:342, 1975
Moore RM: Human orf in the United States, 1972. J Infect Dis 127:731, 1973
Nakano JH: Poxviruses, in Manual of Clinical Microbiology, 4th ed, EH Lennette et al (eds). Washington, DC, American Society for Microbiology, 1985, p 733
Rockoff AS: Molluscum dermatitis. J Pediatr 92:945, 1978
White PJ, Shackelford PG: Edward Jenner MD, and the scourge that was. AM J Dis Child 137:864, 1983

135 VARICELLA-ZOSTER VIRUS INFECTIONS

RICHARD J. WHITLEY

DEFINITION   Varicella-zoster virus (VZV) causes two distinct clinical entities: varicella, or chickenpox, and herpes zoster, or shingles. Chickenpox, a ubiquitous and extremely contagious infection, is usually a benign illness of childhood characterized by an exanthematous, vesicular rash. With reactivation of latent VZV, more common after the sixth decade of life, the disease presents as a dermatomal, vesicular rash which is usually associated with severe pain.

ETIOLOGY   A clinical association between varicella and herpes zoster has been recognized for nearly 100 years. Early in the twentieth century, similarities in the histopathologic findings of skin lesions resulting from varicella and herpes zoster were demonstrated. Isolation of VZV in 1952 permitted a definition of the biology of this virus. Viral isolates from patients with chickenpox and herpes zoster demonstrated similar alterations in tissue culture, specifically the appearance of eosinophilic intranuclear inclusions and multinucleated giant cells, suggesting that the viruses were biologically similar. Later studies proved their identity by rigorous biochemical methods. Restriction endonuclease analysis of viral DNA from a patient with chickenpox who subsequently developed herpes zoster verified the molecular identity of the two viruses responsible for these differing clinical presentations. Varicella-zoster virus is a member of the herpesvirus family, sharing such similar structural characteristics as a lipid envelope, surrounding a nucleocapsid with icosahedral symmetry, a total size of approximately 150 to 200 nm, and centrally located double-stranded DNA with a molecular weight of approximately 80 million. Only enveloped virions are infectious; this may, in part, account for the lability of VZV.

PATHOGENESIS AND PATHOLOGY   Primary infection   The pathogenesis of chickenpox may evolve in a fashion similar to that proposed by Fenner for mousepox. Transmission is likely by the respiratory route, followed by localized replication at an undefined site, and leading to seeding of the reticuloendothelial system with, ultimately, viremia. The occurrence of viremia in patients with chickenpox is supported by the diffuse and scattered nature of the skin lesions and can be verified in selected cases by the recovery of virus from the blood. Vesicles involve the corium and dermis with degenerative changes characterized by ballooning, multinucleated giant cells, and eosinophilic intranuclear inclusions. Infection may involve localized blood vessels of the skin, resulting in necrosis and epidermal hemorrhage. With disease evolution, vesicular fluid becomes cloudy with the recruitment of polymorphonuclear leukocytes, degenerated cells, and fibrin. Ultimately, the vesicles rupture and release their fluid contents which include infectious virus or are gradually reabsorbed.

Recurrent infection   The mechanism of reactivation of VZV that results in herpes zoster is unknown. It is presumed that virus infects the dorsal root ganglia during chickenpox where it remains latent until reactivated. Histopathologic examination of the representative dorsal root ganglia during active herpes zoster demonstrates hemorrhage, edema, and lymphocytic infiltration.

Involvement with active VZV replication in other organs, such as the lung or brain, can occur during either chickenpox or herpes zoster but is uncommon in the immune-competent host. Lung involvement is characterized by interstitial pneumonitis, multinucleated giant cell formation, intranuclear inclusions, and pulmonary hemorrhage. Central nervous system (CNS) infection leads to histopathologic evidence of perivascular cuffing similar to that encountered with measles and other viral encephalitides. Focal hemorrhagic necrosis of the brain, characteristic of herpes simplex virus encephalitis, is uncommon with VZV infection.

EPIDEMIOLOGY AND CLINICAL PRESENTATION Chickenpox

Humans are the only known reservoir for VZV. Chickenpox is highly contagious with an attack rate of at least 90 percent among susceptible or seronegative individuals. Both sexes and individuals of all races are infected equally. The virus is endemic in the population at large; however, it becomes epidemic among susceptible individuals during seasonal periods, namely, late winter and early spring in the temperate zone. Children between the ages of 5 and 9 are most commonly affected and account for 50 percent of all cases. Most other cases occur between the ages of 1 to 4 and 10 to 14. Over the age of 15, approximately 10 percent of the population of the United States is susceptible to infection.

The incubation period of chickenpox ranges between 10 and 21 days but is usually between 14 and 17 days. Secondary attack rates in susceptible siblings within a household are defined as between 70 and 90 percent. Patients are infectious approximately 48 h prior to the onset of the vesicular rash, during the period of vesicle formation, generally 4 to 5 days, and until all vesicles are crusted.

Clinically, chickenpox presents with a rash, low-grade fever, and malaise, although a few patients will develop a prodrome 1 to 2 days prior to the onset of the exanthem. In the immune-competent child, this is usually a benign illness that is associated with lassitude and fever from 100 to 103°F of 3 to 5 days' duration. The skin manifestations, the hallmark of the infection, consist of maculopapules, vesicles, and scabs in varying stages of evolution. The evolution of lesions from maculopapules to vesicles occurs over a matter of hours to days. The lesions appear on the trunk and face and rapidly involve other areas of the body. Most lesions are small and have an erythematous base with a diameter of 5 to 10 mm. Successive crops of lesions appear over a 2- to 4-day period. Lesions can also be found on the mucosa of the pharynx or the vagina. The severity of skin lesions varies from individual to individual. Some individuals have very few lesions, while others can have as many as 2000. Younger children tend to have fewer vesicles compared to older individuals. Immunocompromised children, particularly those with leukemia, have more numerous lesions, often with a hemorrhagic base. Healing takes nearly three times longer in this population. These children are at greater risk for visceral complications, which occur in 30 to 50 percent of cases and which are fatal in 15 percent of cases.

The most common infectious complication of varicella is secondary bacterial superinfection of the skin, which is usually caused by *Streptococcus pyogenes* or *Staphylococcus aureus*. This may result from excoriation of skin lesions following scratching. Gram's stain of skin lesions should help clarify the etiology of unusually erythematous and pustulated lesions.

The most common extracutaneous site of involvement in children is the central nervous system and consists of acute cerebellar ataxia. Cerebellar ataxia generally appears approximately 21 days after the onset of the rash and rarely occurs in the preeruptive phase. The most prominent clinical finding is ataxia and meningeal irritation. The cerebrospinal fluid contains lymphocytes and elevated levels of protein. This is a benign complication of VZV infection in children and does not generally require hospitalization. In addition, aseptic meningitis, encephalitis, transverse myelitis, and Reye's syndrome can also occur. Encephalitis is reported in 0.1 to 0.2 percent of children with chickenpox. No specific therapy is available at this time for patients with central nervous system involvement caused by VZV.

Varicella pneumonitis is the most serious complication following chickenpox, occurring more commonly in adults (up to 20 percent) than in children. It usually appears 3 to 5 days into the course of illness and is associated with tachypnea, cough, dyspnea, and fever. Cyanosis, pleuritic chest pain, and hemoptysis are frequent physical findings. Roentgenographic evidence of disease consists of nodular infiltrates and an interstitial pneumonitis. Resolution of pneumonitis parallels improvement of skin rash; however, patients may have persistent fever and compromised pulmonary function for weeks.

Other complications of chickenpox include myocarditis, corneal lesions, nephritis, arthritis, bleeding diatheses, acute glomerulonephritis, and hepatitis. Hepatic involvement, distinct from Reye's syndrome, is extremely common in chickenpox and is usually characterized by an elevation of liver enzymes, particularly serum glutamic oxaloacetic transaminase (SGOT) and serum glutamic pyruvic transaminase (SGPT). Hepatic involvement is usually asymptomatic, although a few patients report nausea and vomiting.

Perinatal varicella is associated with a high mortality rate when maternal disease develops within 5 days before delivery or 48 h post partum. Because the newborn does not receive protective transplacental antibodies and has an immature immune system, illness may be exaggerated. The mortality rate has been reported as high as 30 percent in this group. Congenital varicella with clinical manifestations at birth is extremely uncommon. It is characterized by skin scarring, hypoplastic extremities, eye abnormalities, and usually evidence of central nervous system impairment.

Herpes zoster   Herpes zoster, a sporadic disease, is the consequence of reactivation of latent virus from the dorsal root ganglia. It is a disease which occurs at all ages but mainly among the elderly. Most patients who develop herpes zoster have no history of exposure to other individuals with VZV infection at that time. The highest incidence of disease ranges between 5 and 10 cases per 1000 persons for individuals in the sixth through the eighth decades of life. Approximately 2 percent of herpes zoster patients who do not receive immunosuppressive therapy will develop a second episode of infection. This figure is at least fivefold higher in immunocompromised individuals.

Herpes zoster, or "shingles," is characterized by a unilateral vesicular eruption within a dermatome, often associated with severe pain. The dermatomes from T3 to L3 are frequently involved. Unique complications are encountered if the ophthalmic branch of the trigeminal nerve is involved, resulting in zoster ophthalmicus. The factors responsible for reactivation of virus are not known. In the child, reactivation is usually benign, whereas in the adult, acute neuritis and postherpetic neuralgia can be particularly debilitating. The onset of disease is heralded by pain within the dermatome that may precede lesions by 48 to 72 h, followed by an erythematous maculopapular rash which evolves rapidly to vesicular lesions. In the normal host, these lesions may remain few in number and continue to form only for a period of 3 to 5 days. The total duration of disease is generally between 7 and 10 days; however, it may take as long as 2 to 4 weeks before the skin returns to normal. In a very few patients, characteristic localization of pain to a dermatome with serologic evidence of herpes zoster has been reported without skin lesions ever appearing. When branches of the trigeminal nerve are involved, lesions may appear on the face, in the mouth, in the eye, or on the tongue. The ear canal and tongue may be involved as part of the involvement of the sensory branch of the facial nerve (Ramsay Hunt syndrome).

The most debilitating complication of herpes zoster, both in the normal and in the immunocompromised host, is pain associated with acute neuritis and postherpetic neuralgia. Postherpetic neuralgia is extremely uncommon in young individuals; however, at least 50 percent of patients over age 50 with zoster will report pain in the involved dermatome months after resolution of cutaneous disease. Changes in sensation within the dermatome, resulting in either hypo- or hyperesthesia, have been reported.

Central nervous system involvement following localized herpes zoster may be more common than has been reported. Many patients without signs of meningeal irritation will have cerebrospinal fluid (CSF) pleocytosis and moderately elevated levels of CSF protein. Symptomatic meningoencephalitis is characterized by headache, fever, photophobia, meningitis, and vomiting. A rare manifestation of CNS involvement by herpes zoster is granulomatous angiitis with contralateral hemiplegia, which can be diagnosed by cerebral arteriography. Other neurologic manifestations include transverse myelitis with or without motor paralysis.

As with chickenpox, herpes zoster in the immunocompromised host is more severe than in the normal individual. Lesion formation continues for over a week, and total scabbing does not develop in the majority of patients until 3 weeks into the disease's course. Therefore, the natural history of the disease is extended approximately twofold. Patients with Hodgkin's disease and non-Hodgkin's lymphoma are at greatest risk for progressive herpes zoster because cutaneous dissemination develops in about 40 percent of these patients. Among patients with cutaneous dissemination, there is a 5 to 10 percent increased risk of pneumonitis, meningoencephalitis, hepatitis, and other serious complications. However, even in immunocompromised patients disseminated zoster is rarely fatal.

DIFFERENTIAL DIAGNOSIS   Chickenpox is a clinical diagnosis which is certainly less confusing now than 20 to 30 years ago when smallpox or disseminated vaccinia could easily be confused with varicella. The characteristic rash of chickenpox and the epidemiologic history of recent exposure should lead to prompt diagnosis. Other viral infections which can mimic chickenpox include disseminated herpes simplex virus infection in patients with atopic dermatitis, and the disseminated vesiculopapular lesions sometimes associated with coxsackievirus, echovirus, or atypical measles infections. These rashes are more commonly morbilliform with a hemorrhagic component rather than vesicular or vesiculopustular. Rickettsialpox can be confused with chickenpox; however, it can be easily distinguished by finding the "herald spot" at the site of the mite bite and a more pronounced headache. The serologic test is also useful in differentiating rickettsialpox from varicella.

Unilateral vesicular lesions in a dermatomal pattern should lead rapidly to the diagnosis of herpes zoster. Both herpes simplex virus infections and coxsackievirus infections can be a cause of dermatomal vesicular lesions. In such situations, a Tzanck smear with supportive diagnostic virology will be helpful in assuring the proper diagnosis. In the prodromal stage of herpes zoster, the diagnosis can be exceedingly difficult and may only be achieved once lesions have appeared, or by retrospective serologic assessment.

LABORATORY FINDINGS   The diagnosis of chickenpox or shingles can often be made by history and physical examination. Unequivocal confirmation of the diagnosis is possible only through the isolation of virus in susceptible tissue culture cell lines or by the demonstration of seroconversion or a fourfold or greater antibody rise when comparing acute and convalescent specimens. A rapid impression can be obtained by a Tzanck smear, performed by scraping the base of the lesions in an attempt to demonstrate multinucleated giant cells. Direct immunofluorescent staining of cells from the skin base or detection of viral antigens by other assays (immunoperoxidase) can also be utilized, although such tests are not yet commercially available. The most frequently employed serologic tools for assessing host response are immunofluorescent detection of antibodies to VZV membrane antigens, fluorescent antibody to membrane antigen (FAMA) test, immune adherence hemagglutination, or enzyme-linked immunoabsorbent assay (ELISA). The FAMA and ELISA tests appear to be the most sensitive.

PROPHYLAXIS   In the normal host, prophylaxis and treatment of chickenpox are of little relevance since the disease is usually benign. However, because the immunocompromised child is at significant risk for developing progressive varicella, modalities of prevention include passive immunization or experimental administration of a live attenuated vaccine. Immune prophylaxis can be accomplished by the administration of specific zoster immune globulin (ZIG), derived from patients with herpes zoster, varicella-zoster immune globulin (VZIG), or the intravenous formulation of zoster immune

plasma (ZIP). Both ZIG and VZIG should be given within 96 h, but preferably within 72 h, of exposure in order to be effective. It is likely that ZIP can be given somewhat later. Indications for the administration of ZIG or VZIG are summarized in Table 135-1. VZIG should be administered to immunodeficient patients under 15 who have a negative or unknown history of chickenpox, who have not been vaccinated against VZV, and who have had a contact in a household, with a playmate for more than 1 h indoors, or in a shared hospital room. It should also be administered to the newborn whose mother had an onset of chickenpox less than 5 days before delivery or 48 h post partum. The use of VZIG for susceptible individuals over 15 must be evaluated on an individual basis. There is no evidence that VZIG is useful for adults with chickenpox, including pregnant women.

An alternative approach to prophylaxis evolved from the development of a live attenuated vaccine for administration to high-risk and normal individuals. Clinical trials performed in Japan and the United States demonstrated efficacy both in normal individuals and in the immunocompromised host. A live attenuated VZV vaccine may be licensed in the United States in the near future, particularly for use in the immunocompromised child.

TREATMENT   Medical management of chickenpox in the normal host is directed toward preventing avoidable complications. Obviously, good hygiene including daily bathing, astringent soaks, and closely cropped fingernails are the key to avoiding this complication. Secondary bacterial infection of the skin can be avoided by meticulous skin care, particularly with close cropping of fingernails. Pruritus can be decreased with topical dressings or the administration of antipruritic drugs. Tepid water baths and wet compresses are better than drying lotions for the relief of itching. Domeboro soaks for the management of herpes zoster can be both soothing and cleansing. Administration of antipyretics should be approached with care, especially for the child suffering from chickenpox because of the recent association between aspirin derivatives and the development of Reye's syndrome.

Patients with varicella pneumonia will require excellent supportive nursing care including removal of bronchial secretions and ventilatory support, as needed. Zoster ophthalmicus should be referred promptly and immediately to an ophthalmologist. Therapy consists of administration of analgesics for severe pain and the use of atropine. The role of parenteral administration of antivirals for the management of zoster ophthalmicus remains unknown at this time, although both acyclovir and vidarabine have been utilized.

The treatment of both chickenpox and herpes zoster in the immunocompromised host can be successfully accomplished with intravenous administration of vidarabine or acyclovir. When the former drug is administered to patients with either disease, healing of skin lesions is accelerated and visceral complications are likely to be decreased. For patients with herpes zoster, intravenous vidarabine therapy will also accelerate resolution of acute neuritis and decrease both the duration of postherpetic neuralgia and the frequency of

TABLE 135-1   Recommendations for VZIG utilization

I Exposure:
  A Both exposure to person with chickenpox or zoster as:
    1 Continuous household contact
    2 Playmate of >1-h duration indoors
    3 Hospital contact (same room or prolonged face-to-face)
    4 Newborn exposure whereby mother had onset of chickenpox <5 days before delivery or 48 h post partum
  B And time elapsed ≤96 h (preferably sooner)
II Candidates should:
  A Have significant exposure (see *I* above)
  B Be susceptible to VZV infection
  C Be <15 years of age (older immunocompromised patients require individual decision)
  D Have one of the following conditions:
    1 Leukemia or lymphoma
    2 Congenital or acquired immune deficiency
    3 Immunosuppressive treatment
    4 Newborn defined above (see *IA4*)

cutaneous dissemination. The dosage is 15 mg/kg per day once daily intravenously over 12 h at a concentration of 0.5 mg of standard intravenous fluids. Acyclovir is not yet approved for this indication by the Food and Drug Administration. The administration of intravenous acyclovir leads to the decreased occurrence of visceral complications but with no effect, demonstrable at this time, on healing of skin lesions or pain. While high-dose intramuscular human leukocyte interferon has been beneficial in a limited number of immunocompromised patients, the more readily available and genetically produced recombinant interferons have not been shown to be effective for treating either varicella or herpes zoster. Concomitant with the administration of an intravenous antiviral to the immunosuppressed host, it is desirable to attempt to wean patients from immunosuppressive treatment.

Management of acute neuritis and/or postherpetic neuralgia can be particularly difficult. In addition to the judicious use of analgesics, ranging from nonnarcotic to narcotic derivatives, supplementation with such drugs as amitriptyline hydrochloride and fluphenazine hydrochloride has been reported to be beneficial for pain relief. Corticosteroids have been reported in some studies to be useful when administered early in the course for prevention of postherpetic neuralgia. Large-scale controlled studies remain to be performed to address the utility and potential complications of such an approach.

Over the next decade, it is likely that significant advances will be achieved in the area of prevention and treatment of varicella-zoster virus infections both in the normal and the immunocompromised host, both with drugs and vaccines.

REFERENCES

BRUNELL PA et al: Prevention of varicella by zoster immune globulin. N Engl J Med 280:1191, 1969

GERSHON AA et al: Live attenuated varicella vaccine. JAMA 252:355, 1984

HOPE-SIMPSON RE: The nature of herpes zoster: A long-term study and a new hypothesis. Proc R Soc Med 58:9, 1965

PROBER CG et al: Acyclovir therapy of chickenpox in immunosuppressed children—a collaborative study. J Pediatr 101:622, 1982

ROSS HA: Modification of chickenpox in family contacts by administration of gamma globulin. N Engl J Med 267:369, 1962

WEIBEL RE et al: Live attenuated varicella versus vaccine: Efficacy trial in healthy children. N Engl J Med 310:1409, 1984

WELLER TH: Varicella and herpes zoster: Changing concepts of the natural history, control, and importance of a not-so-benign virus. N Engl J Med 309:1362, 1434, 1983

WHITLEY RJ et al: Early vidarabine therapy to control the complications of herpes zoster in immunosuppressed patients. N Engl J Med 307:971, 1982

———: Vidarabine therapy of varicella in immunosuppressed patients. J Pediatr 1:125, 1982

———: Varicella-zoster virus infections, in Antiviral Agents and Viral Diseases of Man 2, GJ Galasso et al (eds). New York, Raven Press, 1984, pp 517–542

ZAIA JA et al: Evaluation of varicella-zoster immune globulin: Protection of immunosuppressed children after household exposure to varicella. J Infect Dis 147:737, 1983

136 HERPES SIMPLEX VIRUSES

LAWRENCE COREY

DEFINITION Herpes simplex viruses (HSV-1, HSV-2) (*Herpesvirus hominis*) produce a variety of infections involving mucocutaneous surfaces, the central nervous system, and occasionally visceral organs. The advent of effective antiviral chemotherapy for HSV infections has made prompt recognition of these syndromes of clinical importance.

HISTORY The word *herpes* from the Greek "to creep" was utilized to describe fever blisters by Herodotus in 100 A.D. In the early 1960s it was demonstrated that HSV could be divided by neutralization tests into two antigenic types (HSV-1 and HSV-2) and that there was

an association between the antigenic type and the site of viral recovery.

ETIOLOGY The genome of herpes simplex virus is a linear, double-stranded DNA molecule (about 100×10^6 in molecular weight) large enough to encode in excess of 60 to 70 gene products. The structure of the genome is unusual among DNA viruses because two unique nucleotide sequences are flanked by inverted repeated sequences. The two components can invert relative to each other, so that DNA isolated from the virus consists of four isomers differing in their orientation of the two components. About 50 percent of the HSV-1 and HSV-2 genomes are homologous. The homologous sequences are distributed over the entire genome map, and most (if not all) of the polypeptides specified by one viral type are antigenically related to polypeptides of the other viral type. Restriction endonuclease analysis of viral DNA can be utilized to distinguish between the two subtypes and among strains of the two subtypes. The variability of nucleotide sequences from clinical strains of HSV-1 and HSV-2 are such that for practical purposes HSV isolates obtained from two individuals can be differentiated by restriction enzyme patterns unless the isolates are from epidemiologically related sources such as sexual partners, mother-infant pairs, or common source outbreaks.

The viral genome is packaged within a regular icosahedral protein shell (capsid) composed of 162 capsomers. The outer covering of the virus is a lipid-containing membrane (envelope) derived from modified cell membrane, acquired as the DNA-containing capsid buds through the inner nuclear membrane of the host cell. Between the capsid and lipid bilayer of the envelope is the tegument, composed of a number of viral proteins whose properties and functions are largely unknown. Viral replication has both nuclear and cytoplasmic phases. The initial steps of replication include attachment, fusion between the viral envelope and a cell membrane to liberate the nucleocapsid into the cytoplasm of the cell, and disassembly of the nucleocapsid to release the viral DNA. Three classes of HSV genes have been defined. The genes designated α are expressed earliest in infection without any requirement for prior viral protein synthesis. The second class of HSV genes, designated β, require prior synthesis of an α protein but not viral DNA replication. The β proteins include regulatory proteins and enzymes required for DNA replication. Most current antiviral drugs interrupt β proteins such as the viral DNA polymerase enzyme. The third class of HSV genes, designated γ, require viral DNA replication for expression, and most of the structural proteins specified by the virus are γ proteins.

Following replication of the viral genome and synthesis of structural proteins, nucleocapsids are assembled in the nucleus of the cell. Envelopment occurs as the nucleocapsids bud through the inner nuclear membrane into the perinuclear space. In some cells, viral replication within the nucleus forms two types of inclusion bodies, type A basophilic Feulgen-positive bodies that contain viral DNA, and an eosinophilic inclusion body which is devoid of viral nucleic acid or protein, representing a "scar" of viral infection. Virions are then transported via the endoplasmic reticulum and the Golgi apparatus to the cell surface.

HSV infection of certain cells (neurons in particular) does not result in virus replication and cell death. Instead, viral genomes are maintained by the cell in a repressed or largely repressed state compatible with survival and normal activities of the cell, a process called *latency*. Subsequently, activation of the viral genome may occur resulting in viral replication and, in some cases, the redevelopment of herpetic lesions, a process termed *reactivation*. Whereas infectious virus rarely can be recovered from sensory or autonomic nervous system ganglia dissected from cadavers, maintenance and growth of the neural cells in tissue culture results in production of infectious virions, a process called explantation, and subsequent permissive infection of susceptible cells, a process called *cocultivation*. Virus replication was first detected in neurons during reactivation in vitro suggesting that the neuron harbors the latent virus in vivo. Subsequently, viral DNA has been found in neural tissue at times when infectious virus cannot be isolated. HSV DNA extracted from latently infected neural tissue differs from HSV DNA in cells actively replicating virus. Current data suggest that the HSV DNA in latently infected cells may exist in circular or concatameric form.

PATHOGENESIS Exposure to virus at mucosal surfaces or abraded skin permits entry of virus and initiation of replication in cells of the epidermis and dermis. Whether or not clinically apparent lesions develop, sufficient viral replication to permit infection of either sensory or autonomic nerve endings may occur. Whether latency always results from peripheral mucosal infection is unclear. Virus, or more likely, nucleocapsid, is then thought to be transported intraaxonally to the nerve cell bodies in ganglia. In humans, the time from inoculation of virus in peripheral tissue to spread to the ganglia is unknown. During the initial phase of infection, viral replication occurs in ganglia and contiguous neural tissue. Virus then spreads to other mucosal skin surfaces through centrifugal migration of infectious virions via peripheral sensory nerves. This centrifugal spread of virus to the skin from peripheral sensory nerves helps explain the large surface area, and the high frequency of new lesions distant from the initial crop of vesicles which are characteristic in patients with primary genital or oral-labial HSV and the recovery of virus from neural tissue distant from neurons innervating the inoculation site. Contiguous spread of locally inoculated virus may also occur and allow further mucosal extension of disease.

Following resolution of primary disease, infectious virus can no longer be recovered in the ganglia, and the surface viral proteins are not expressed in detectable amounts. The mechanisms by which latency is maintained and by which various stimuli cause reactivation of HSV infection are unknown. Ultraviolet light, immunosuppression, and trauma to the skin or ganglia are associated with reactivation.

Analysis of the HSV DNA from sequentially isolated strains of HSV or from multiple infected ganglia from any one individual has revealed identical restriction endonuclease patterns in most persons. Occasionally, and more frequently in immunocompromised persons, multiple strains of the same viral subtype can be detected in the same person, suggesting that exogenous infection with different strains of the same subtype is possible.

IMMUNITY Host responses to infection influence the acquisition of disease, severity of infection, resistance to development of latency, maintenance of latency, and frequency of HSV recurrences. Both antibody-mediated and cell-mediated reactions are clinically important. Immunocompromised patients with defects in cell-mediated immunity experience more severe and extensive HSV infections than those with deficits in humoral immunity such as agammaglobulinemia. In mice experimental ablation of lymphocytes indicates that T cells play a major role in preventing lethal disseminated disease, although antibodies help reduce virus titers in neural tissue. Some aspects of the pathogenesis of disease may also be related to the host immune response, e.g., stromal opacities associated with recurrent herpetic keratitis. The surface viral glycoproteins have been shown to be antigens recognized by antibodies mediating neutralization and immune-mediated cytolysis (antibody-dependent cell-mediated cytotoxicity, ADCC). Monoclonal antibodies specific for each of the known viral glycoproteins have, in experimental infections, conferred protection against subsequent neurologic disease or ganglionic latency. Multiple cell populations including natural killer (NK) cells, macrophages, a variety of T-lymphocyte populations, and lymphokines generated by these cells play a role in host defenses to HSV infections. In animals passive transfer of primed lymphocytes confers protection from subsequent challenge. Maximum protection usually requires the activation of multiple T-cell subpopulations. Both class I MHC-restricted and class II MHC-restricted responses appear important. Effector cells involved in containing virus include cytotoxic T cells and T cells responsible for delayed hypersensitivity. The latter cells may confer protection by the antigen-stimulated release of lymphokines (e.g., interferons) which may have a direct antiviral effect or activate other nonspecific effector cells.

EPIDEMIOLOGY HSV infections are found worldwide. Standard complement fixation (CF) antibody assays do not distinguish between HSV-1 and HSV-2 infection. However, several serologic assays such as neutralization, indirect immunofluorescence (IFA), passive hemagglutination (PHA), radioimmunoassay (RIA), and enzyme-linked immunosorbent assay (ELISA) can measure the relative selectivity of serum antibodies to the two subtypes. Much of the humoral immune response to HSV is to type common antigenic determinants, making it difficult to detect HSV-2 antibody in persons with prior HSV-1 infection and HSV-1 infection in those with prior HSV-2.

Seroepidemiologic studies performed in the 1940s and 1950s demonstrated that in almost all populations studied, over 90 percent of persons had antibodies to HSV by the fourth decade. In developing countries, similar patterns still prevail. In many western industrialized middle-class populations, however, the age-specific prevalence rates of HSV-1 infection appear to be decreasing, and serosurveys of middle-class populations in the United States indicate only 40 percent of persons between 25 and 29 possessed antibodies to HSV with antibody prevalence increasing by about 1.5 percent per year.

Antibodies to HSV-2 are not routinely detected until puberty, and antibody prevalence rates correlate with past sexual activity. HSV-2 antibodies have been detected in 80 percent of female prostitutes, up to 60 percent of adults of lower, and 20 to 40 percent of middle to higher socioeconomic status, and 0 to 3 percent of nuns. Only about one-third of persons who possess HSV-2 antibody give a history of a prior or current genital ulceration. Consultations with private practitioners for genital herpes increased ninefold in the United States between 1966 and 1981.

HSV infections occur throughout the year. The incubation period ranges from 1 to 26 days (median 6 to 8 days). Contact with active ulcerative lesions or asymptomatically excreting patients can result in transmission. Asymptomatic salivary excretion of HSV-1 has been reported in 2 to 9 percent of adults and 5 to 8 percent of children. HSV-2 has been isolated from the genital tract of from 0.3 to 5.4 percent of males and 1.6 to 8 percent of females attending sexually transmitted disease clinics. The titer of HSV in cultures from lesions is 100 to 1000 times higher than from salivary or genital tract secretions from asymptomatically excreting persons. The efficiency of transmission is likely to be greater during symptomatic versus asymptomatic periods of viral excretion.

CLINICAL SPECTRUM HSV has been isolated from nearly all visceral or mucocutaneous sites. The clinical manifestations and course of HSV depend on the anatomic site of the infection, the age and immune status of the host, and the antigenic type of the virus. First episodes of HSV disease, especially primary infection (that is, first infections with either HSV-1 or HSV-2 in which the host lacks HSV antibodies in acute phase serums), are frequently accompanied by systemic signs and symptoms, involve both mucosal and extramucosal sites, have a longer duration of symptoms, a longer time from which virus is isolated from lesions, and a higher rate of complications than recurrent episodes of disease. Both viral subtypes can cause genital and oral-facial infections, and these infections are clinically indistinguishable. However, the frequency of future reactivations of infection is influenced by the anatomic site and virus type. Genital HSV-2 infection is twice as likely to reactivate and will recur 8 to 10 times more frequently than genital HSV-1 infection. Conversely oral-labial HSV-1 infections will recur more frequently than oral-labial HSV-2 infections.

Oral-facial HSV infections Gingivostomatitis and pharyngitis are the most frequent clinical manifestations of first-episode HSV-1 infection, while recurrent herpes labialis is the most frequent clinical manifestation of reactivation HSV infection. HSV pharyngitis and gingivostomatitis usually result from primary infection and are most commonly seen in children and young adults. Clinical symptoms and signs include fever, malaise, myalgias, inability to eat, irritability, and cervical adenopathy, which may last from 3 to 14 days. Lesions may involve the hard and soft palate, gingiva, tongue, lip, and facial area. HSV-1 or HSV-2 infection of the pharynx usually results in exudative or ulcerative lesions of the posterior pharynx and/or tonsillar pillars. Concomitant lesions of the tongue, buccal mucosa, or gingiva may occur later in the course in one-third of cases. Fever lasting from 2 to 7 days and cervical adenopathy are common. The clinical differentiation of HSV pharyngitis from bacterial pharyngitis, *Mycoplasma pneumoniae* infections, and noninfectious causes of pharyngeal ulcerations such as Stevens-Johnson syndrome may be difficult. No substantial evidence suggests that reactivation oral-labial HSV infection is associated with symptomatic recurrent pharyngitis.

Reactivation of HSV from the trigeminal ganglia may be associated with asymptomatic excretion in the saliva, development of intraoral mucosal ulcerations, or herpetic ulcerations on the vermillion border of the lip or external facial skin. About 50 to 70 percent of seropositive patients undergoing trigeminal nerve root decompression and 10 to 15 percent of those undergoing dental extraction will develop oral-labial HSV infection a median of 3 days after these procedures.

In immunosuppressed patients extension of the infection into mucosal and deep cutaneous layers may occur. Friability, necrosis, bleeding, severe pain, and inability to eat or drink may result. HSV mucositis is clinically similar to mucosal lesions due to cytotoxic drug therapy, trauma, or fungal or bacterial infections. Concomitant HSV and *Candida* infection may also occur commonly. Systemic acyclovir therapy speeds the rate of healing and relieves the pain of mucosal HSV infections in immunosuppressed patients. Patients with atopic eczema may also develop severe oral-facial HSV infections (eczema herpeticum) which may rapidly involve extensive areas of skin and occasionally disseminate to visceral organs. Prompt resolution of extensive eczema herpeticum has been achieved with the administration of intravenous acyclovir. Erythema multiforme (EM) may also be associated with HSV infections, and some evidence suggests that it is the precipitating event in about 75 percent of cases of cutaneous EM. HSV antigen has been demonstrated in both circulatory immune complexes and in skin lesion biopsy of these patients. Patients with severe HSV-associated erythema multiforme may be candidates for chronic suppressive oral acyclovir therapy.

Genital HSV infections   First-episode primary genital herpes is characterized by fever, headache, malaise, and myalgias. Pain, itching, dysuria, vaginal and urethral discharge, and tender inguinal adenopathy are the predominant local symptoms. Characteristically widely spaced bilateral distributed lesions of the external genitalia are seen. Lesions may be present in varying stages including vesicles, pustules, or painful erythematous ulcers. Involvement of the cervix and urethra are seen in over 80 percent of women with first-episode infections. First episodes of genital herpes in patients who have had prior HSV-1 infection are associated with less frequent systemic symptoms and faster healing than primary genital herpes. The clinical courses of acute first-episode genital herpes among patients with HSV-1 and HSV-2 infections are similar. However, the recurrence rates of genital disease differ. Over 80 percent of patients with first-episode HSV-2 infection will have a recurrence within 12 months (median number of recurrences, four) compared to 55 percent of those with primary HSV-1 infections (median number of recurrences, less than one). Recurrence rates of genital HSV-2 infections vary greatly between individuals and over time within the same individual. HSV has been isolated from the urethra and urine from men and women without concomitant external genital lesions. A clear mucoid discharge and dysuria are characteristic of symptomatic HSV urethritis. HSV has been isolated from the urethra of 5 percent of women with the dysuria-frequency syndrome. Occasionally, genital tract disease manifested by HSV endometritis and salpingitis in women and HSV prostatitis in men may occur.

Rectal and perianal HSV infections due to HSV-1 and HSV-2 may be seen, especially among homosexual men and/or heterosexual women who engage in anorectal intercourse. Symptoms of HSV proctitis include anorectal pain, anorectal discharge, tenesmus, and constipation. Sigmoidoscopy reveals ulcerative lesions of the distal 10 cm of the rectal mucosa. Rectal biopsies show mucosal ulceration,

necrosis, polymorphonuclear and lymphocytic infiltration of the lamina propria, and occasionally multinucleated intranuclear inclusion–bearing cells. Autonomic nervous system dysfunction manifested by burning sacral paresthesias, impotence, and urinary retention may also accompany symptomatic HSV proctitis. Perianal herpetic lesions are also seen in immunosuppressed patients receiving cytotoxic therapy. HSV-1 strains, usually identical to those found in the oropharynx, are obtained from these lesions, suggesting the mode of spread is autoinoculation of the perianal area from HSV-infected saliva and/or finger lesions. Extensive perianal herpetic lesions and/or HSV proctitis may occur in patients with the acquired immunodeficiency syndrome (AIDS). Anecdotal observations suggest healing of these lesions can be achieved with the use of systemic acyclovir.

Herpetic whitlow   Herpetic whitlow, HSV infection of the finger, is most often seen in medical practitioners, although it may occur as a complication of primary oral or genital herpes by inoculation of virus via a break in the epidermal surface. Clinical signs and symptoms include the abrupt onset of edema, erythema, and localized tenderness of the infected finger. Vesicular or pustular lesions of the fingertip indistinguishable from pyogenic bacterial infection are seen. Fever, lymphadenitis, and epitrochlear and axillary lymphadenopathy are common. Recurrences may occur. Prompt diagnosis to avoid unnecessary and potentially exacerbating surgical therapy and/or transmission to patients is necessary.

Herpetic eye infections   HSV infection of the eye is the most frequent cause of corneal blindness in the United States. HSV keratitis presents with acute onset of pain, blurring of vision, chemosis, conjunctivitis, and characteristic dendritic lesions of the cornea. Use of topical corticosteroids may exacerbate symptoms and lead to involvement of deep structures of the eye. Debridement, topical antiviral, and/or interferon therapy hasten healing. However, recurrences are common and immunopathologic injury of the deeper structures of the eye may occur. Chorioretinitis, usually as a manifestation of disseminated HSV infection, may occur in neonates or those with AIDS. Acute necrotizing retinitis due to HSV is also an uncommon but severe manifestation of HSV infection.

Central and peripheral nervous system infections with HSV-1 and HSV-2   HSV encephalitis is the most common identified cause of acute, sporadic viral encephalitis in the United States, comprising 10 to 20 percent of all cases. The estimated incidence is about 2.3 cases per million persons per year. Cases are distributed throughout the year, and the age distribution appears biphasic with peaks at between 5 and 30 and greater-than-50 years of age. HSV-1 accounts for more than 95 percent of cases. The pathogenesis of HSV encephalitis is varied. In children and young adults primary HSV infection may result in encephalitis; presumably exogenously acquired virus enters the CNS by neurotropic spread from the periphery via the olfactory bulb. However, most adults with HSV encephalitis have clinical or serologic evidence of mucocutaneous HSV-1 infection prior to the onset of the CNS symptoms. In about 25 percent of the cases examined, the HSV-1 strains from the oropharynx and brain tissue from the same patient differ, suggesting that some cases may result from reinfection with another strain of HSV-1 that reached the CNS. Two theories have been proposed to explain the development of actively replicating HSV in localized areas of the CNS in persons from whom the ganglionic and CNS isolates are similar. Reactivation of latent trigeminal or autonomic nerve root HSV-1 infection may be associated with extension of virus into the CNS via nerves innervating the middle cranial fossa. HSV DNA has been demonstrated by DNA hybridization in human autopsy brain tissue. As such, reactivation of long-standing latent CNS infection may be another potential mechanism for the development of HSV encephalitis.

The clinical hallmark of HSV encephalitis has been the acute onset of fever and focal neurologic, especially temporal lobe, symptoms. To date no reliable noninvasive radiologic or virologic technique has been developed to diagnose HSV encephalitis during its early clinical stages, and differentiation of HSV encephalitis from

REFERENCES

COREY L et al: A trial of topical acyclovir in genital herpes simplex infections. N Engl J Med 306:1313, 1982

———: Genital herpes simplex virus infection: Clinical manifestations, course and complications. Ann Intern Med 98:958, 1983

———, SPEAR P: Infections with herpes simplex viruses. N Engl J Med 314:686, 749, 1986

DOUGLAS JM et al: A double-blind study of oral acyclovir for suppression of recurrences of genital herpes simplex virus infection. N Engl J Med 310:1551, 1984

HILL TJ: Herpes simplex virus latency, in The Herpesviruses, 3, B Roizman (ed). New York, Plenum, 1984, pp 175–240

HIRSCH MS, SCHOOLEY RT: Drug therapy: Treatment of herpesvirus infections. N Engl J Med 309(16):963 and 309(17):1035, 1983

MERTZ GJ et al: Double-blind placebo-controlled trial of oral acyclovir in first episode genital herpes simplex virus infection. JAMA 242:1147, 1984

RAMSEY PG et al: Herpes simplex virus pneumonia. Ann Intern Med 97:812, 1982

SHEPP DH et al: Oral acyclovir therapy for mucocutaneous herpes simplex virus infections in immunocompromised marrow transplant recipients. Ann Intern Med 102:783, 1985

STRAUSS SE et al: Acyclovir for chronic mucocutaneous herpes simplex virus infection in immunosuppressed patients. Ann Intern Med 96(3):270, 1982

——— et al: Herpes simplex virus infection: Biology, treatment and prevention. Ann Intern Med 103:404, 1985

WADE JC et al: Intravenous acyclovir to treat mucocutaneous herpes simplex virus infection after marrow transplantation. Ann Intern Med 96:265, 1982

WHITLEY RJ et al: Vidarabine therapy of neonatal herpes simplex virus infection. Pediatrics 66:495, 1980

——— et al: Vidarabine versus acyclovir therapy in herpes simplex encephalitis. N Engl J Med 314:144, 1986

137 CYTOMEGALOVIRUS INFECTION

MARTIN S. HIRSCH

DEFINITION Cytomegalovirus (CMV), which was initially isolated from patients with congenital cytomegalic inclusion disease, is now recognized as an important pathogen in all age groups. In addition to inducing severe birth defects, CMV causes a wide spectrum of disorders in older children and adults, ranging from an asymptomatic, subclinical infection to a mononucleosis syndrome in healthy individuals to disseminated disease in the immunocompromised. Human CMV is one of several related species-specific viruses that cause similar diseases in various animals. All are associated with the production of characteristic enlarged cells; hence the name cytomegalovirus.

ETIOLOGY CMV is a member of the herpesvirus group and thus contains double-stranded DNA, a protein capsid, and a lipoprotein envelope. Like other members of the herpesvirus group, CMV demonstrates icosahedral symmetry, replicates in the cell nucleus, and can cause either a lytic and productive or a latent infection. CMV can be distinguished from other herpesviruses by certain biologic properties such as host range and the type of cytopathology induced. Virus replication is associated with the production of large intranuclear inclusions and smaller cytoplasmic inclusions. The virus appears to replicate in a variety of cell types in vivo; in tissue culture it grows preferentially in fibroblasts. It is unclear whether CMV is oncogenic in vivo. However, the virus can rarely transform fibroblasts and genomic transforming fragments have been identified.

EPIDEMIOLOGY CMV has a worldwide distribution. Approximately 1 percent of newborns in the United States are infected with CMV, and the percentage is higher in many less-developed countries. Communal living and poor personal hygiene facilitate early spread. Perinatal and early childhood infections are common. Virus may be present in milk, saliva, feces, and urine. Transmission of CMV has been identified among young children in day-care centers.

The virus is not readily spread by casual contact but requires repeated or prolonged intimate exposure for transmission. In late adolescence and young adulthood, CMV is often transmitted venereally, and asymptomatic viral carriage in semen or cervical secretions is common. CMV antibody titers approach 100 percent in female prostitutes and in sexually active homosexual men. Transfusion of whole blood or certain blood products containing viable leukocytes may also transmit CMV with a frequency of 2 to 10 percent per unit transfused.

Once infected, an individual probably carries the virus for life. Most commonly these infections remain latent. However, with compromise of T-lymphocyte-mediated immunity, as occurs following organ transplantation or in association with lymphoid neoplasms and certain acquired immunodeficiencies, CMV reactivation syndromes develop frequently.

PATHOGENESIS Congenital CMV infection can follow either primary or reactivation infection of the mother. However, clinical disease in the fetus or newborn is almost exclusively limited to primary maternal infections. Factors determining the severity of congenital infection are unknown; a deficient capacity to produce precipitating antibodies and to mount T-cell responses to CMV are associated with more severe disease.

Primary infection in late childhood or adulthood is often associated with a vigorous T-lymphocyte response that may contribute to the development of a mononucleosis syndrome similar to that observed following Epstein-Barr virus infection (see Chap. 138). The hallmarks of such infections are the appearance of atypical lymphocytes in the peripheral blood; these cells are predominantly activated T lymphocytes of cytotoxic-suppressor phenotype. Polyclonal activation of B cells by the virus contributes to the development of rheumatoid factors and other autoantibodies during CMV mononucleosis.

Once acquired during symptomatic or asymptomatic primary infection, CMV persists indefinitely in tissues of the host. The sites of persistent or latent infection are unclear, but probably involve multiple cell types and various organs. Transmission following blood transfusion or organ transplantation points to silent infections in these tissues. Autopsy studies suggest that lungs, salivary glands, and bowel may also be areas of latent infection.

If T-cell responses of the host become compromised by disease or by iatrogenic immunosuppression, latent virus can be reactivated to cause a variety of syndromes. Chronic antigenic stimulation, as occurs following tissue transplantation, in the presence of immunosuppression, appears to be an ideal setting for CMV activation and CMV-induced disease. Certain particularly potent suppressants of T-cell immunity such as antithymocyte globulin are associated with a high rate of clinical CMV syndromes which may follow either primary or reactivation infection. CMV may itself contribute to further T-lymphocyte hyporesponsiveness which often precedes superinfection with other opportunistic pathogens, such as Pneumocystis carinii. CMV and pneumocystis are frequently found together in immunosuppressed patients with severe interstitial pneumonia.

PATHOLOGY Cytomegalic cells in vivo are presumed to be infected epithelial cells. They are two to four times larger than surrounding cells and often contain an 8- to 10-µm intranuclear inclusion that is eccentrically placed and surrounded by a clear halo, resulting in an "owl's eye" appearance. Smaller granular cytoplasmic inclusions may also be demonstrated occasionally. Cytomegalic cells are found in a wide variety of organs including salivary glands, lung, liver, kidney, intestines, pancreas, adrenal glands, and the central nervous system.

The cellular inflammatory response to infection consists of plasma cells, lymphocytes, and monocyte-macrophages. Granulomatous reactions are occasionally observed, particularly in the liver. Immunopathologic reactions may contribute to CMV disease. Immune complexes have been described in infected infants, sometimes associated with CMV-related glomerulopathies. Immune complex glomerulopathy has been observed in some CMV-infected patients following renal transplantation.

CLINICAL MANIFESTATIONS **Congenital CMV infection** Fetal infections range from inapparent to severe and disseminated. Cytomegalic inclusion disease develops in approximately 5 percent of infected fetuses and is seen almost exclusively in infants born to mothers who develop primary infections during pregnancy. Petechiae, hepatosplenomegaly, and jaundice are the most common presenting features (60 to 80 percent). Microcephaly with or without cerebral calcifications, intrauterine growth retardation, and prematurity are noted in 30 to 50 percent of patients. Inguinal hernias and chorioretinitis are observed less commonly. Laboratory abnormalities in decreasing order of frequency include increased serum IgM (>20 mg/dL), atypical lymphocytosis, elevated liver transaminases, thrombocytopenia, hyperbilirubinemia, and increased cerebrospinal fluid protein (>20 mg/dL). Prognosis among severely infected infants is poor with mortality rates of 20 to 30 percent; few patients escape intellectual or hearing difficulties in later years. Differential diagnoses of cytomegalic inclusion disease in infants include syphilis, rubella, toxoplasmosis, herpes simplex or enterovirus infection, and bacterial sepsis.

Most congenital CMV infections are clinically inapparent at birth. Between 5 to 25 percent of asymptomatically infected infants develop significant psychomotor, hearing, ocular, or dental abnormalities over the next several years.

Perinatal CMV infection   The newborn may acquire CMV at the time of delivery by passage through an infected birth canal or by postnatal contact with maternal milk or other secretions. Approximately 40 to 60 percent of infants who are breast-fed for over 1 month by seropositive mothers will become infected. Iatrogenic transmission can also result from neonatal blood transfusion. Screening of blood products prior to transfusion to eliminate CMV-positive blood will decrease the risk of infection. The great majority of infants infected at or after delivery will remain asymptomatic. However, protracted interstitial pneumonitis has been associated with perinatally acquired CMV infection, particularly in premature infants, occasionally associated with *Chlamydia trachomatis, P. carinii,* or *Ureaplasma urealyticum* infections. Poor weight gain, adenopathy, rash, hepatitis, anemia, and atypical lymphocytosis may also be present, and CMV excretion often persists for months to years.

CMV mononucleosis   The most common clinical manifestation of CMV infection in normal hosts beyond the neonatal period is a heterophil-antibody negative mononucleosis syndrome. This may occur spontaneously or following the transfusion of leukocyte-containing blood products. Although the syndrome occurs at all ages, sexually active young adults are most often involved. Incubation periods range from 20 to 60 days, and the illness generally lasts 2 to 6 weeks. Prolonged high fevers, sometimes accompanied by chills, profound fatigue, and malaise characterize this disorder. Myalgias, headache, and splenomegaly are frequent, but exudative pharyngitis and cervical lymphadenopathy are rare, in contrast to infectious mononucleosis caused by Epstein-Barr virus. Occasional patients will develop rubelliform rashes, often after exposure to ampicillin. Less commonly observed are interstitial or segmental pneumonia, myocarditis, pleuritis, arthritis, or encephalitis. Rarely, Guillain-Barré syndrome may complicate CMV mononucleosis. The characteristic laboratory abnormality is a peripheral blood relative lymphocytosis with greater than 10 percent atypical lymphocytes. Total leukocyte counts may be low, normal, or markedly elevated. Although significant jaundice is uncommon, moderately elevated serum transaminase and alkaline phosphatase levels are often present. Heterophil antibodies are absent; however, transient immunologic abnormalities are common. These may include the presence of cryoglobulins, rheumatoid factors, cold agglutinins, and antinuclear antibodies. Rarely, hemolytic anemia, thrombocytopenia, and granulocytopenia complicate recovery.

Most patients recover without sequelae, although postviral asthenia may persist for months. CMV excretion in urine, genital secretions, or saliva often continues for months to years. Rare patients have recurrent episodes of fever and malaise, sometimes associated with autonomic nervous system dysfunction, e.g., attacks of sweating or flushing.

CMV infection in the immunocompromised host   CMV appears to be the most frequent and important viral pathogen complicating organ transplantation. In renal, cardiac, and liver transplant recipients, CMV induces a variety of syndromes including fever and leukopenia, hepatitis, pneumonitis, colitis, and retinitis. The maximal period of risk appears between 1 to 4 months after transplantation, although retinitis is often a later complication. The relative risk of disease appears greater following primary infection than after reactivation. However, reactivation infection is much more common since the population of seronegative recipients of organs from seropositive donors is relatively small. Therefore, the overall morbidity rate from reactivation infection may be equally as high as that after primary infection. Clinical disease is related to the degree of immunosuppression; patients receiving certain immunosuppressive agents, such as antithymocyte globulin, appear more likely to have severe infections than those receiving other agents, such as cyclosporin A.

CMV pneumonia occurs in nearly 20 percent of bone marrow transplant recipients, with a case fatality rate of 88 percent. The risk is greatest between 5 to 13 weeks after transplant, and several risk factors have been identified. These include degree of immunosuppression, acute graft-versus-host disease, older age, seropositivity before transplantation, and granulocyte transfusions.

CMV has become recognized as an important pathogen in patients with the acquired immunodeficiency sydrome (AIDS). CMV infection is nearly ubiquitous in this disorder and often causes disseminated disease, contributing to death. CMV-induced immunosuppression probably also contributes to the T-lymphocyte deficiency initiated by the etiologic retrovirus.

CMV syndromes in the immunocompromised host often begin with prolonged fever, malaise, anorexia, fatigue, night sweats, and arthralgias or myalgias. Liver function abnormalities, leukopenia, thrombocytopenia, and atypical lymphocytosis may be observed during these episodes. The development of tachypnea, hypoxia, and unproductive cough signals respiratory involvement. Radiologic examination of the lung often demonstrates bilateral interstitial or reticulonodular infiltrates, beginning in the periphery of the lower lobes and spreading centrally and superiorly; localized segmental, nodular, or alveolar patterns are less commonly observed. Diagnosis requires lung biopsy, since neither peripheral virus excretion nor high antibody titers provides sufficient information to prove etiology. The differential diagnoses include *P. carinii,* other viral, bacterial, or fungal pathogens, pulmonary hemorrhage, and injury secondary to radiation or cytotoxic drugs.

Gastrointestinal CMV involvement may be localized or extensive and occurs almost exclusively in compromised hosts. Ulcers of the esophagus, stomach, small intestine, or colon may result in bleeding or perforation. CMV infection may lead to exacerbations of underlying ulcerative colitis. Hepatitis frequently occurs, and CMV-associated acalculous cholecystitis has been described.

CMV rarely causes meningoencephalitis in otherwise healthy individuals. However, in patients with AIDS, it has been associated with chronic encephalitis and with subacute encephalopathy which presents as lethargy and social withdrawal and progresses to dementia over weeks to months. Although CMV inclusions have been observed in patients dying of AIDS-encephalopathy, the role of CMV in this disorder is unclear (see Chap. 257).

CMV retinitis is an important cause of blindness in immunocompromised patients, including patients with AIDS and organ transplant recipients. Early lesions consist of small, opaque, white areas of granular retinal necrosis that spread in a centrifugal manner and are later accompanied by hemorrhages, vessel sheathing, and retinal edema (see Fig. A4-14). CMV must be distinguished from other causes of retinopathy including toxoplasmosis, candidiasis, and herpes simplex virus.

Fatal infections are often associated with persistent viremia and multiple organ system involvement. Progressive pulmonary infiltrates, pancytopenia, hyperamylasemia, and hypotension are characteristic, often with a terminal bacterial, fungal, or protozoan superinfection. Extensive adrenal necrosis with CMV inclusions is present at autopsy, as well as CMV involvement of many other organs.

In the renal transplant recipient, CMV also contributes to graft dysfunction by mechanisms other than direct viral cytopathic effects. An immune complex glomerulopathy may accompany CMV infection and should be differentiated from true graft rejection, since the former does not respond well to increased immunosuppression. Kidney biopsy is often necessary to distinguish the two, although CMV viremia and abnormal inverted ratios of T-lymphocyte subsets strongly suggest CMV glomerulopathy.

DIAGNOSIS The diagnosis of CMV infection cannot be made reliably on clinical grounds alone. Virus isolation from appropriate clinical specimens, together with demonstration of a fourfold or greater antibody rise or persistently elevated antibody titers, are the preferred diagnostic approaches. Virus excretion or viremia is readily detected by culture of appropriate specimens on human fibroblast monolayers. If virus titers are high, as is frequently the case in congenital disseminated infection or in patients with AIDS, characteristic cytopathic effects may be detected within a few days. However, in some situations, e.g., CMV mononucleosis, virus titers are low and cytopathic effects may take several weeks to appear. Virus isolation from urine or saliva by itself does not necessarily imply acute infection since excretion from these sites may continue for months to years following illness. Detection of CMV viremia is a better predictor of acute infection.

Advances in molecular biology have allowed DNA-DNA hybridization techniques to be used for rapid detection of CMV in urine and buffy coat specimens with a sensitivity and specificity of approximately 90 percent. To date, these techniques are experimental and require the use of ^{32}P-labeled probes. The use of nonradioactive stable probes will allow this promising technique to become more generally available. Another rapid technique that will be employed increasingly is detection of CMV antigens in specimens by immunofluorescence of immunoperoxidation using monoclonal antibodies directed against CMV-specific antigens.

A variety of serologic assays (complement fixation, immunofluorescence, indirect hemagglutination, enzyme-linked immunosorbent assay) are available to detect antibody rises to CMV antigens. Antibody rises may not be detectable for up to 4 weeks after primary infection, and titers often remain high for years after infection. For this reason, single-sample antibody determinations are of no value in assessing the acuteness of infection. Detection of CMV-specific IgM is sometimes useful in the early diagnosis of infection, particularly in infants with congenital infection; circulating rheumatoid factors may result in occasional false-positive IgM tests.

PREVENTION AND TREATMENT Although no specific therapy is available for CMV infections, prophylactic measures may be useful in certain situations. The use of blood from seronegative donors or blood that was frozen, thawed, and deglycerolized greatly decreases transfusion-associated transmission of CMV. Similarly, matching of kidney transplants by CMV serology, using only organs from seronegative donors for seronegative recipients, reduces primary infections following transplantation. CMV immune globulin has been reported to be useful in certain seronegative bone marrow transplant recipients and is under study in kidney transplant patients. A live, attenuated CMV vaccine is undergoing trial among renal transplant patients. Prophylactic interferon alpha has been demonstrated to prevent reactivation CMV syndromes and to delay CMV excretion in high-risk kidney transplant recipients, i.e., those receiving cadaver organs and antithymocyte globulin. Its use in transplant recipients susceptible to primary infection is under investigation.

Treatment of ongoing CMV syndromes has been largely unsuccessful to date in transplant recipients and in patients with AIDS. Interferons, vidarabine, and acyclovir have failed, whether used alone or in combination. Newer nucleoside derivatives, such as 9-(1,3-dihydroxy-2-propoxymethyl)guanine (DHPG), show considerable activity against CMV in vitro. DHPG also shows promise in early clinical trials against CMV retinitis, colitis, and pneumonitis.

REFERENCES

ADLER S: Transfusion-associated cytomegalovirus infections. Rev Infect Dis 5:977, 1983

BRADY MT et al: Use of deglycerolized red blood cells to prevent posttransfusion infection with cytomegalovirus in neonates. J Infect Dis 150:334, 1984

CHOU S, MERIGAN TC: Rapid detection and quantitation of human cytomegalovirus in urine through DNA hybridization. N Engl J Med 308:921, 1983

GLENN J: Cytomegalovirus infections following renal transplantation. Rev Infect Dis 3:1151, 1981

COHEN JI, COREY GR: Cytomegalovirus infection in the normal host. Medicine 64:100, 1985

FELSENSTEIN D et al: Treatment of cytomegalovirus retinitis with 9-[2-hydroxy-1-(hydroxymethyl)ethoxymethyl] guanine (BWB759U). Ann Intern Med 103:377, 1985

HANDSFIELD HH et al: Cytomegalovirus infection in sex partners: Evidence for sexual transmission. J Infect Dis 151:344, 1985

HIRSCH MS et al: Effects of interferon-alpha on cytomegalovirus reactivation syndromes in renal-transplant recipients. N Engl J Med 308:1489, 1983

HO M: *Cytomegalovirus: Biology and Infection.* New York, Plenum, 1982

JORDAN MC et al: Spontaneous cytomegalovirus mononucleosis: Clinical and laboratory observations in nine cases. Ann Intern Med 79:153, 1973

KLEMOLA E et al: Cytomegalovirus mononucleosis in previously healthy adults. Ann Intern Med 71:11, 1969

MEYERS JD et al: Nonbacterial pneumonia after allogeneic marrow transplantation: review of ten years' experience. Rev Infect Dis 4:1119, 1982

——— et al: Prevention of cytomegalovirus infection by cytomegalovirus immune globulin after marrow transplantation. Ann Intern Med 98:442, 1983

ONORATO IM et al: Epidemiology of cytomegaloviral infections: Recommendations for prevention and control. Rev Infect Dis 7:479, 1985

PASS RF et al: Cytomegalovirus infection in a day-care center. N Engl J Med 307:477, 1982

PLOTKIN S et al (eds): CMV: *Pathogenesis and Prevention of Human Infection.* New York, Alan R Liss, 1984.

SCHOOLEY RE et al: Association of herpesvirus infections with T-lymphocyte subset alterations, glomerulopathy, and opportunistic infections after renal transplantation. N Engl J Med 308:307, 1983

SPECTOR SA et al: Detection of human cytomegalovirus in clinical specimens by DNA-DNA hybridization. J Infect Dis 150:121, 1984

VOLPI A et al: Rapid diagnosis of pneumonia due to cytomegalovirus with specific monoclonal antibodies. J Infect Dis 147:1119, 1983

138 EPSTEIN-BARR VIRUS INFECTIONS, INCLUDING INFECTIOUS MONONUCLEOSIS

ROBERT T. SCHOOLEY

DEFINITION Epstein-Barr virus (EBV) is a B lymphotropic human herpesgroup virus which is worldwide in distribution. Primary infection with EBV during childhood is usually subclinical. Between 25 and 70 percent of adolescents and adults who undergo a primary EBV infection develop the clinical syndrome of infectious mononucleosis. Infectious mononucleosis is defined by the clinical triad of fever, lymphadenopathy, and pharyngitis combined with the transient appearance of heterophil antibodies and an atypical lymphocytosis. EBV is also associated with nasopharyngeal carcinoma and certain B-cell lymphomas.

EPIDEMIOLOGY OF EBV INFECTIONS EBV is a ubiquitous agent that has been found in all population groups surveyed to date. The virus was initially described by Epstein, Achong, and Barr who noted, by electron microscopy, the presence of particles similar in morphology to herpes simplex virus in continuous cell lines which had arisen from tumor tissue obtained from patients with Burkitt's lymphoma. The perceptive observation by the Henles that antibodies to this agent developed in conjunction with infectious mononucleosis in one of their laboratory personnel was followed quickly by large-scale serologic surveys at Yale which confirmed EBV as the etiologic agent for infectious mononucleosis.

EBV is transmitted primarily in saliva, although infections can also be transmitted by blood transfusion. Primary infection tends to occur at an earlier age among lower socioeconomic groups and in developing countries. In industrialized countries approximately 50 percent of individuals have experienced a primary EBV infection by adolescence. These early infections are usually mild and non-specific or clinically inapparent. A second wave of seroconversions to EBV occurs with the onset of the social activity associated with adolescence and young adulthood. Primary EBV infection among this age group accounts for most cases of infectious mononucleosis. The peak incidence of infectious mononucleosis occurs between 14 and 16 years of age for girls, and between 16 and 18 years of age for boys. By adulthood most individuals are EBV-seropositive.

EBV is shed from the oropharynx for up to 18 months following primary infection; thereafter it is shed intermittently by all EBV-seropositive individuals in the absence of a clinical illness. EBV can be isolated from the oropharyngeal washings of 15 to 25 percent of healthy EBV-seropositive individuals on any given day. Immunosuppressed individuals shed the virus more frequently. EBV can be isolated from 25 to 50 percent of the oropharyngeal washings obtained from renal allograft recipients and from virtually all patients with the acquired immunodeficiency syndrome (AIDS). Asymptomatic shedding of EBV by healthy individuals accounts for most of the spread to uninfected members of the population despite the fact that it is not highly contagious. Transmission is largely dependent on salivary contact (e.g., kissing). It is not likely to be transmitted by aerosol or fomites. Thus, isolation restrictions on patients with mononucleosis or individuals likely to be shedding EBV are not appropriate. EBV infection can also be transmitted by blood transfusion.

ETIOLOGY AND PATHOGENESIS OF INFECTIOUS MONONUCLEOSIS   By electron microscopy the EB virus appears as an icosahedral nucleocapsid surrounded by a complex envelope and is indistinguishable from other members of the human herpesvirus group. The double-stranded EBV DNA has a molecular weight of approximately 101×10^6 and encodes for at least 30 polypeptides. At present, there is no convincing evidence that there are strain differences among EBV isolates which account for the wide range of clinical conditions associated with EBV infection.

When EBV is transmitted by saliva, the initial site of replication is the oropharynx. B lymphocytes support a productive infection by EBV and are the only cells known to have surface receptors for the virus. However, recent studies have documented the presence of the virus within oropharyngeal epithelial cells of patients with infectious mononucleosis. During the acute phase of the illness, EBV antigens can be demonstrated within the nuclei of up to 20 percent of circulating B lymphocytes. After the infection subsides, the virus can be isolated from a small number of B lymphocytes of EBV-seropositive individuals and may also reside within nasopharyngeal epithelial cells.

Virus-host interactions   EBV infection has both direct and indirect effects on the cellular and humoral immune responses. Understanding the interactions between EBV and the host provides an insight into the clinical manifestations and complications of EBV infection. Within 18 to 24 h after entry of EBV into B lymphocytes by means of the C3d receptor, Epstein-Barr nuclear antigens (EBNA) are detectable within the nucleus of the infected cell. Expression of EBNA corresponds to the acquisition of the transformed or immortalized phenotype. EBV-infected B lymphocytes also express lymphocyte-determined membrane antigens (LYDMA) which serve as the putative target for the cellular immune response to virus-infected B lymphocytes. Immortalized B lymphocytes can be propagated continuously in vitro and are polyclonally stimulated by EBV to produce immunoglobulin. Antibodies reactive with sheep red blood cells (heterophil) and antibodies with several other specificities are the in vivo correlate of the polyclonal immunoglobulin production demonstrable in vitro and may mediate several of the complications of infectious mononucleosis. A minority of EBV-infected B lymphocytes enter the lytic cycle (production of mature, progeny virus and death of the host cell) and produce EBV antigens that are detected during virus replication. These are divided into the early antigen complex (EA) and viral capsid antigens (VCA). The early antigen complex consists of two groups of antigens; (1) diffuse (EA-D), which are detectable in both the cytoplasm and the nucleus of cells in the lytic cycle, and (2) restricted (EA-R), which are demonstrable only in the cytoplasm. EBV-induced membrane antigens are also produced during productive infection. These antigens serve as markers of infection at the cellular level; the pattern of the antibody response to these antigens is useful diagnostically in the identification of EBV-associated disease states (Table 138-1). After the appearance of VCA the host cell dies and whole virions are released, which can infect and transform additional B lymphocytes.

TABLE 138-1   EBV-specific antibodies

Antibody specificity	Time of appearance in IM	Persistence	Percent of IM patients with antibody	Comments
VCA:				
IgM	At clinical presentation	1–2 months	100	Best indicator of primary infection; not present with reactivation; technically difficult to perform
IgG	At clinical presentation	Lifelong	100	Standard "EBV titer" reported by most commercial and state labs; major utility is as a marker for prior or current infection in epidemiologic studies
EA:				
EA-D	Peaks 3–4 weeks after onset	3–6 months	70	Presence correlates with more severe disease in patients with IM; present in nasopharyngeal carcinoma; IgA anti-EA-D antibodies useful for prediction of NPC in high-risk populations
EA-R	Several weeks after onset	Months to years		Present in high titer in African Burkitt's lymphoma; may be useful as an indicator of reactivation of EBV in immunosuppressed patients
EBNA	3–6 weeks after onset	Lifelong	100	Late appearance of anti-EBNA antibodies in IM makes seroconversion a useful marker for primary infection if IgM anti-VCA antibody studies are not available

NOTE: *IM = infectious mononucleosis; VCA = viral capsid antigen; EA = early antigens; EA-D = diffuse early antigens; EA-R = restricted early antigens; EBNA = Epstein-Barr nuclear antigens; NPC = nasopharyngeal carcinoma.*

An effective immune response to EBV involves humoral and cellular components. Neutralizing antibodies which inactivate cell-free virus and antibodies to VCA and EBNA appear during primary infection in all patients; antibodies to EA-D appear in most patients. The cellular immune response is largely responsible for controlling B-cell proliferation and polyclonal immunoglobulin production triggered by EBV and is composed primarily of T lymphocytes having functional and surface phenotypic characteristics of activated, suppressor-cytotoxic T lymphocytes (T8$^+$, Ia$^+$). As the illness progresses, memory T lymphocytes capable of limiting proliferation of autologous EBV-infected B lymphocytes are demonstrable. These memory T lymphocytes persist for life. However, latent EBV remains in a small proportion of B lymphocytes and perhaps also in epithelial cells in the oropharynx.

During the primary immune response to EBV, global cellular immune hyporesponsiveness is readily demonstrable. This resolves after resolution of the illness, but reactivation of EBV is facilitated by conditions which interfere with the cellular immune response (immunosuppressive drugs, especially cyclosporin A, and disorders associated with cellular immunodeficiency, e.g., AIDS). EBV and cytomegalovirus (CMV) reactivation in immunosuppressed patients are frequently associated with a return of the immunoregulatory abnormalities characteristic of the primary immune response to these viruses. In the case of CMV, particularly, this hyporesponsiveness may contribute to many of the superinfections which frequently accompany CMV infections in immunocompromised hosts. The cellular hyporesponsiveness associated with EBV reactivation is generally less intense and less prolonged than that associated with CMV but may also contribute to morbidity in immunocompromised individuals.

CLINICAL MANIFESTATIONS Symptoms and signs

After an incubation period of 4–8 weeks, prodromal symptoms of malaise, anorexia, and chills frequently precede the onset of pharyngitis, fever, and lymphadenopathy by several days. Severe pharyngitis is the symptom which most frequently prompts patients to seek medical attention. Occasionally patients will note only fever or lymphadenopathy or will present with one of the complications of infectious mononucleosis discussed below. Most patients also complain of headache and malaise. Abdominal pain is infrequent in the absence of splenic rupture.

Physical examination Fever is present in 90 percent of patients with infectious mononucleosis and is generally higher in the late afternoon, and may reach 39 to 40°C. Periorbital edema was frequently noted in early series of cases of mononucleosis but has been commented upon less frequently recently. The pharyngitis is usually diffuse; an exudate is observed in one-third of the cases. Palatine petechiae may also be observed. Posterior and/or anterior cervical adenopathy is noted in 90 percent of patients with infectious mononucleosis. Individual nodes are rarely painful and may be moderately tender to palpation. Hepatomegaly is infrequently noted, although mild hepatic tenderness is present in up to half the patients. Approximately half of all patients will have splenomegaly, which is usually maximal in the second or third week of illness. In 5 percent of patients a macular, petechial, scarlatiniform, urticarial, or erythema multiforme-like rash may appear. Administration of ampicillin results in a pruritic, maculopapular eruption in 90 to 100 percent of patients.

Clinical course Infectious mononucelosis is a self-limiting illness in the vast majority of cases. The pharyngitis is maximal for 5 to 7 days and then resolves over the subsequent 7 to 10 days. Fever usually persists for 7 to 14 days, but occasionally may continue somewhat longer. The course of the lymphadenopathy is variable, but rarely exceeds 3 weeks. The most persistent symptom is malaise. Most patients are well enough to return to work or school within 3 to 4 weeks, but occasional patients remain exhausted, have difficulty concentrating, and are unable to return to full activities for months. This subgroup is often found among those who present with a more subacute onset without severe pharyngitis and high fever.

Occasional patients have been reported in which recurrent pharyngitis and fever is accompanied by persistent or resurgent heterophil antibodies. More recently a group of patients has been described with nonspecific symptoms which may include malaise, fatigue, pharyngitis, fever, lymphadenopathy, and difficulty with higher cognitive function. These patients are usually heterophil-negative. The demonstration that some of these patients have anti-VCA and EA-R titers which are higher, and anti-EBNA titers which are lower, than median titers for the general population has led to the speculation that this symptom complex may be a manifestation of ongoing replication of EBV. However, healthy members of the general population not infrequently have antibodies to EA-R antigens, and one should be cautious about applying the diagnosis of chronic active EBV infection to patients with these nonspecific symptoms simply on the basis of the presence of anti-EA-R antibodies. At present, no specific therapy is available for these patients.

Complications Complications of infectious mononucleosis occur infrequently but may be so dramatic as to be the predominant manifestation of the illness (Table 138-2). Hematologic complications include autoimmune hemolytic anemia, which may be mediated by IgM antibodies with anti-i specificity. Hemolytic anemia usually subsides over a 1- to 2-month period. Mild thrombocytopenia occurs in up to 50 percent of cases; profound thrombocytopenia is a rare, but well-recognized, complication and is frequently antibody-mediated. Mild granulocytopenia is frequently observed in uncomplicated infectious mononucleosis, and severe granulocytopenia associated with infection or death has been reported. Antibodies which react with granulocytes have been detected in up to 80 percent of patients and may contribute to the profound granulocytopenia which is occasionally observed. Both the thrombocytopenia and the granulocytopenia are usually self-limited and resolve over 3 to 6 weeks. Corticosteroids have been advocated for treatment of both hemolytic anemia and thrombocytopenia associated with infectious mononucleosis, but efficacy has not been proved in controlled studies. Splenic rupture is an infrequent complication of infectious mononucleosis, often accompanied by the insidious or abrupt onset of abdominal pain, and is usually observed during the second or third week of illness. Surgery, which usually includes splenectomy, is the only effective management.

Neurologic complications of infectious mononucleosis may be the presenting or sole manifestation of the illness. Heterophil antibodies may be absent, and atypical lymphocytes may not be present at the onset of the neurologic event. The most frequent neurologic complications are cranial nerve palsies and encephalitis which may initially present with cerebellar findings. The onset of the encephalitis is usually abrupt. Cerebrospinal fluid findings are not diagnostic, and localization by noninvasive neurodiagnostic studies may suggest

TABLE 138-2 Complications of infectious mononucleosis

Hematologic complications:
  Autoimmune hemolytic anemia
  Thrombocytopenia
  Granulocytopenia
Splenic rupture
Neurologic complications:
  Encephalitis
  Cranial nerve palsies, especially Bell's palsy
  Meningoencephalitis
  Guillain-Barré syndrome
  Seizures
  Mononeuritis multiplex
  Transverse myelitis
  Psychosis
Hepatic complications:
  Hepatitis
Cardiac complications:
  Pericarditis
  Myocarditis
Pulmonary complications:
  Airway obstruction
  Interstitial pneumonitis

herpes simplex encephalitis. Eighty-five percent of patients with EBV-associated neurologic findings recover spontaneously.

Hepatitis is a common component of infectious mononucleosis. Almost 90 percent of patients have mild elevation of hepatic transaminases. Although more serious hepatic sequellae have been reported, severe or permanent hepatic dysfunction is exceedingly rare.

Cardiac abnormalities are uncommon but may include pericarditis, myocarditis, coronary artery spasm, or electrocardiographic abnormalities.

Airway obstruction from pharyngeal or paratracheal adenopathy can occur. This may require surgical intervention but is usually quite sensitive to corticosteroid therapy. Pulmonary parenchymal abnormalities such as interstitial infiltrates are noted infrequently and appear to be more common among children.

Infectious mononucleosis is rarely fatal. Neurologic complications, airway obstruction, and splenic rupture are the most frequent causes of death in previously healthy individuals with primary EBV infection. Sporadic or X-linked cases of overwhelming EBV infection accompanied by lymphoproliferation and hepatic dysfunction have been reported. The X-linked condition, known as X-linked lymphoproliferative (XLP) or Duncan's syndrome, results in the death of 40 percent of affected males during primary EBV infection. In addition to overwhelming lymphoproliferation, XLP patients may manifest severe immunologic or hematologic sequellae such as agammaglobulinemia, aplastic anemia, or lymphocytic lymphoma. The pathophysiology of the XLP syndrome has not yet been completely elucidated, but an X-linked defect in the immune response to EBV may result in failure to control EBV replication or in disordered immunoregulation which leads to the other immunologic sequellae observed in this syndrome.

LABORATORY MANIFESTATIONS **Heterophil antibodies** Antibodies to sheep erythrocytes which can be removed by prior absorption with beef red blood cells, but not with guinea pig kidney, are termed heterophil antibodies. Heterophil antibodies are demonstrated in 50 percent of children and 90 to 95 percent of adolescents and adults with mononucleosis. Although the classic tube heterophil titer is still performed in many laboratories, the "monospot" test using a commerical kit is a sensitive, specific, easily performed substitute. The frequency of heterophil positivity associated with infectious mononucleosis depends upon the test used, the age of the patient population, and the time during the illness at which the test is performed. Monospot tests may be slightly more sensitive than heterophil titers. Ten to fifteen percent of patients with mononucleosis may be heterophil-negative if tested only during the first week of the illness. If the clinical suspicion of mononucleosis is high enough, retesting for heterophil antibodies during the second or third week of illness is warranted. Heterophil antibodies decline in titer after the acute illness is resolved but may be detectable for up to 9 months after the onset of the illness.

Atypical lymphocytosis A relative and absolute lymphocytosis is present in about 75 percent of cases of infectious mononucleosis. The lymphocytosis usually peaks in the second or third week of illness and is characterized by cells with atypical morphology. These atypical lymphocytes, which are primarily activated T lymphocytes, are larger than mature lymphocytes and often contain eccentrically placed lobulated nuclei with nucleoli, and vacuolated cytoplasm with rolled up edges. As noted above, mild neutropenia and thrombocytopenia are frequently observed. Other laboratory abnormalities include a mild polyclonal increase in immunoglobulins of the IgM, IgG, and IgA classes, and mild elevations of hepatocellular enzymes.

EBV-specific antibody response Antibodies to several EBV-specific antigens arise during primary EBV infection (Table 138-1) Proper utilization of EBV-specific antibody studies may facilitate the diagnosis of primary EBV infection in clinically atypical or heterophil-negative cases. IgM antibodies to the VCA are diagnostic of a primary EBV infection. Unfortunately this study is technically difficult to perform and available only in certain reference laboratories. IgG anti-VCA antibodies are present at clinical presentation in almost all patients and remain detectable for life. IgG anti-VCA antibodies are, thus, useful mainly as a test for susceptibility to EBV and are not useful for the diagnosis of primary infection. Approximately 70 percent of patients with infectious mononucleosis make antibodies to EA-D. Anti-EA-D antibodies usually peak 3 to 4 weeks after the onset of illness and usually disappear after recovery. Antibodies to EBNA appear 6 to 8 weeks into the illness and persist for life. The presence of IgM anti-VCA antibodies, and seroconversion to EBNA is diagnostic of a primary EBV infection. Patients with defects in cellular immunity may fail to make antibodies to EBNA.

DIAGNOSIS The diagnosis of infectious mononucleosis is not difficult in the vast majority of cases. The constellation of fever, pharyngitis, and lymphadenopathy coupled with an atypical lymphocytosis and heterophil antibodies is virtually always due to primary EBV infection and requires no further laboratory studies. Certain patients with EBV-induced mononucleosis, particularly preadolescents, or those with neurologic complications may be heterophil-negative or may lack an atypical lymphocytosis. Primary EBV infection can be diagnosed with certainty in these patients with the proper use of EBV-specific serologic studies (see above). Culturing EBV from oropharyngeal washings or peripheral blood mononuclear cells is laborious, and because of the ubiquity of the virus among EBV-seropositive individuals, it is not diagnostic of primary EBV infection.

Primary CMV infection is the illness most frequently confused with EBV-induced infectious mononucleosis. About two-thirds of adults with heterophil-negative mononucleosis have CMV-induced mononucleosis. Patients with CMV mononucleosis are, on the average, slightly older than those with EBV-induced infectious mononucleosis and usually manifest an illness characterized predominantly by fever and malaise. Pharyngitis and lymphadenopathy are less common than with infectious mononucleosis. CMV-induced mononucleosis is usually more insidious in onset and slower to resolve than EBV-induced mononucleosis. The diagnosis can be made by the isolation of CMV from the peripheral blood, and the demonstration of seroconversion or a fourfold or greater rise in antibody titer to CMV. Although CMV is also shed in saliva and urine by patients with CMV mononucleosis, demonstration of the agent in the blood is a more specific, but less sensitive, indicator of CMV-induced morbidity.

Severe pharyngitis may also be caused by another virus (e.g., herpes simplex) or by group A beta-hemolytic streptococci. Since group A beta-hemolytic streptococci can be isolated from the throat of up to 30 percent of patients with infectious mononucleosis, isolation of this organism does not rule out the diagnosis of infectious mononucleosis. Atypical lymphocytes may also be observed in a number of other conditions including rubella, hepatitis, toxoplasmosis, mumps, and drug reactions. These conditions rarely pose major differential diagnostic problems when careful attention is paid to the other clinical and laboratory features of these illnesses.

MANAGEMENT Infectious mononucleosis usually requires only supportive management. Although patients should be advised to obtain adequate rest, there is no evidence that forced bed rest hastens recovery. Fever and pharyngitis are usually ameliorated by acetaminophen. Because of the infrequent complication of splenic rupture, patients should be advised to avoid contact sports for 6 to 8 weeks after the onset of illness. The timing of return to school or work is determined solely by symptomatology. Patients with mild illness may not require any major changes in routine. Occasional patients with protracted illness may not return to a full school or work schedule for several months. It is important to emphasize to patients that recovery from mononucleosis is often gradual and that the malaise may wax and wane for some time.

Although corticosteroids may hasten defervescence and the resolution of pharyngitis, they are indicated only for certain specific complications of mononucleosis; airway obstruction usually responds dramatically to parenteral corticosteroids. Corticosteroids may also hasten the recovery of patients with severe hemolytic anemia or thrombocytopenia. There is no evidence that corticosteroids are beneficial for the neurologic complications of the illness. Occasional selected patients with protracted illness may benefit from a short course of prednisone, but corticosteroids should be avoided in the majority of patients with infectious mononucleosis.

Acyclovir, interferon alpha, and 9-[2-hydroxy-1-(hydroxy-methyl)ethoxy]methyl guanine are active inhibitors of EBV replication in vitro. Their role in the management of EBV infections is currently under evaluation. Interferon alpha has antiviral activity and can decrease shedding of EBV by renal allograft recipients treated with antithymocyte globulin.

EBV-ASSOCIATED MALIGNANCY Since the initial description of EBV in patients with African Burkitt's lymphoma, the virus has been detected in association with several other malignancies. Its role in the pathogenesis of these malignancies remains the subject of intense discussion. EBV DNA sequences have been detected in tumor tissue from more than 90 percent of patients with African Burkitt's lymphomas. American Burkitt's lymphoma, which often affects older children, and more often presents as an intraabdominal tumor, is EBV-associated in only 15 percent of cases. Anaplastic nasopharyngeal carcinoma, a common neoplasm in southeast China, is highly associated with EBV; virtually all adequately studied patients with this malignancy have evidence of EBV in tumor tissue.

There is increasing evidence that implicates EBV in the pathogenesis of certain cases of lymphocytic lymphoma in the immunoincompetent host. B-cell lymphoma is greatly overrepresented among malignancies developing in immunosuppressed individuals such as organ allograft recipients, patients with ataxia telangiectasia, and patients with AIDS. Immunologically privileged areas such as the central nervous system also appear to be particularly susceptible to B-cell lymphomas. Cardiac allograft recipients treated with cyclosporin A appear to be particularly susceptible to B-cell lymphoma. EBV sequences are detectable in up to half of the B-cell malignancies encountered in immunosuppressed individuals. Controversy exists as to whether the B-cell lymphoproliferation, which is initially polyclonal and may be driven by EBV reactivated in the setting of cellular immunodeficiency, is the first step in the development of these malignancies. The process, which is thought to be polyclonal initially, becomes oligoclonal or monoclonal with a second-step chromosomal translocation made more likely by the increased number of proliferating B lymphocytes. The biologic behavior of these tumors does not always correlate with clonality as defined by conventional techniques. Patients have been described who have succumbed to lymphoproliferative processes which appear to be polyclonal by surface immunoglobulin studies. More sensitive techniques of defining clonality, such as that utilizing immunoglobulin gene rearrangement, may reveal that a larger proportion of the polyclonal lymphomas are in fact oligo- or monoclonal. The response of these B-cell lymphomas to conventional chemotherapy is often disappointing. Some have advocated acyclovir therapy; others feel many of these lymphoproliferative syndromes are reversible if the immunosuppression is decreased. Studies of larger numbers of these patients for the presence of EBV sequences and for the progression from a polyclonal to an oligoclonal or monoclonal disorder will shed more light on the role of EBV in oncogenesis in both immunoincompetent and immunologically normal hosts.

REFERENCES

ANDIMAN W et al: Use of cloned probes to detect Epstein-Barr viral DNA in tissues of patients with neoplastic and lymphoproliferative diseases. J Infect Dis 148:967, 1983
EPSTEIN MS et al: Virus particles in cultured lymphoblasts from Burkitt's lymphoma. Lancet 1:702, 1964
GROSE C et al: Primary Epstein-Barr virus infections in acute neurologic diseases. N Engl J Med 292:392, 1975

HANTO DW et al: Epstein-Barr virus induced B-cell lymphoma after renal transplantation. Acyclovir therapy and transition from polyclonal to monoclonal B-cell proliferation. N Engl J Med 306:913, 1982
HAYNES BF et al: Emergence of suppressor cells of immunoglobulin synthesis during acute Epstein-Barr virus-induced infectious mononucleosis. J Immunol 123:2095, 1979
HENLE G et al: Immunofluorescence in cells derived from Burkitt lymphoma. J Bacteriol 91:1248, 1966
HENLE W et al: Epstein-Barr virus specific diagnostic tests in infectious mononucleosis. Hum Pathol 5:551, 1974
HOAGLAND RJ: Infectious mononucleosis. Am J Med 13:158, 1952
JONES JF et al: Evidence for active Epstein-Barr virus infection in patients with persistent, unexplained illnesses: Elevated anti-early antigen antibodies. Ann Intern Med 102:1, 1985
PURTILO DT et al: Epstein-Barr virus infections in the X-linked recessive lymphoproliferative syndrome. Lancet 1:798, 1978
REINHERZ EL et al: The cellular basis for viral-induced immunodeficiency: Analysis by monoclonal antibodies. J Immunol 125:1269, 1980
SCHOOLEY RT et al: Antineutrophil antibodies in infectious mononucleosis. Am J Med 76:85, 1984
SIXBEY JW et al: Epstein-Barr virus replication in oropharyngeal epithelial cells. N Engl J Med 310:1225, 1984
THORLEY-LAWSON DA et al: Suppression of in vitro Epstein-Barr virus infection: A new role for the adult human T lymphocyte. J Exp Med 146:495, 1977

139 ENTEROVIRUSES AND REOVIRUSES

C. GEORGE RAY

GENERAL CONSIDERATIONS

Enteroviruses consist of a major subgroup of picornaviruses that include the polioviruses, coxsackieviruses, echoviruses, and more recently discovered agents that are simply designated enteroviruses. The number of serotypes that infect humans is nearly 70, and more are likely to be found in the future. Their name is derived from their ability to infect intestinal tract epithelial and lymphoid tissues and to be shed into the feces.

Enteroviruses can cause paralytic disease, encephalitis and acute aseptic meningitis syndromes, pleurodynia, exanthems, pericarditis, myocarditis, nonspecific febrile illness, and occasional fulminant disease in the newborn. The spectrum of disease may be even broader. Some infections can lead to permanent damage, and others may trigger chronic, active disease processes.

Since these viruses have many features in common, they will first be considered as a group. Some of the special features of important serotypes will be discussed in detail later in this chapter.

CHARACTERISTICS OF ENTEROVIRUSES As a group, the picornaviruses are extremely small (17 to 28 nm in diameter), single-stranded RNA viruses with icosahedral symmetry. In contrast to the rhinoviruses, the enterovirus subgroup is resistant to ether, acid pH (4.0), and bile. Another feature is cationic stability; in the presence of magnesium sulfate, the viruses become more resistant to thermal inactivation. They can survive for prolonged periods in sewage and even in chlorinated water if sufficient organic debris is present. Although some of the enterovirus serotypes share antigens, there are no significant serologic relationships between the major classes listed in Table 139-1. Definitive identification of isolates usually requires neutralization tests.

Most of these agents can be isolated in primate (human or simian) cell cultures; however, some strains, such as several coxsackievirus group A serotypes, are grown with difficulty in cell cultures, and inoculation of newborn mice may be necessary for detection. Inoculation of newborn mice was one basis for the original classification of group A and B coxsackieviruses. After the mice have been inoculated, at 24 h of age or less, and observed for 2 to 12 days, group A viruses primarily have a widespread, inflammatory, necrotic effect on skeletal muscle, leading to flaccid paralysis and usually death; similar inoculation of group B viruses causes encephalitis, resulting in spasticity and occasionally convulsions. Other organs are variably affected, and histopathologic examination is sometimes helpful in distinguishing the two. Echoviruses and polioviruses rarely have an adverse effect on mice, unless special adaptation procedures are employed. The higher-numbered enteroviruses (types 68 to 72), which have overlapping growth and host characteristics, have been classified separately. Hepatitis A virus has been classified as enterovirus 72 and is discussed in Chap. 247.

Humans are the major natural host for the polioviruses, coxsackieviruses, and echoviruses. There are enteroviruses of other animals with a limited host range that does not appear to extend to humans. Conversely, viruses thought to be identical or related to human enteroviruses have been isolated from dogs and cats. Whether these agents cause disease in these animals is debatable, and there is no evidence of spread from animals to humans.

EPIDEMIOLOGY   The enteroviruses have a worldwide distribution, and asymptomatic infection is common. The proportion of infected individuals who will develop illness varies from 2 to 100 percent, depending upon the serotype or strain involved, prior immune status, and the age of the patient. Secondary infections in households are common and range as high as 40 to 70 percent, depending upon factors such as family size, crowding, and sanitary conditions.

There is a seasonal predilection; epidemics are usually observed during the summer and fall. In subtropical and tropical climates, the duration of greatest transmission sometimes extends into the winter. In some years, certain serotypes emerge as dominant strains; they then may wane, only to reappear in epidemics years later. The emergence of dominant serotypes is unpredictable from year to year.

Direct or indirect fecal-oral transmission is considered the most common mode of spread. After infection, the virus persists in the oropharynx for 1 to 4 weeks, and it can be shed in the feces for 1 to 18 weeks. Sewage-contaminated water, contaminated foods, or insect vectors (flies, cockroaches) may occasionally be the source of infection. More commonly, however, spread is directly from person to person. Approximately two-thirds of all isolates are from children 9 years of age or younger.

Incubation periods vary, but relatively short intervals (2 to 10 days) are the rule. Illness is often seen concurrently in more than one family member, and the clinical features may vary within the household.

PATHOGENESIS AND PATHOLOGY   After primary replication in the epithelial cells and lymphoid tissues in the upper respiratory and gastrointestinal tracts, viremic spread to other sites can occur. Potential target organs vary according to the virus strain and its tropism, but may include the central nervous system, heart, vascular endothelium, liver, pancreas, gonads, lungs, skeletal muscles, synovial tissues, skin, and mucous membranes. Histopathologic findings include cell necrosis and mononuclear cell inflammatory infiltrates; in the central nervous system, the inflammatory cells are localized most prominently in perivascular sites. The initial tissue damage is thought to result from the lytic cycle of virus replication. Viremia is usually undetectable by the time symptoms appear, and termination of virus replication commences with the appearance of circulating interferon,

neutralizing antibody, and mononuclear cell infiltrations of infected tissue. The early antibody response is mediated by immunoglobulin M, which usually wanes 6 to 12 weeks after onset to be replaced by IgG-specific antibodies. The important role of antibodies in the termination of infection is supported by the observation of persistent enterovirus replication in patients with antibody-deficiency diseases.

Although initial acute tissue damage may be caused by the lytic effects of the virus on the cell, many of the secondary sequelae appear to be immunologically mediated. Enterovirus-caused poliomyelitis, disseminated disease of the newborn, aseptic meningitis, encephalitis, exanthems, and acute respiratory illnesses, thought to represent primary lytic infections, can usually be identified through routine methods of virus isolation and determination of specific antibody titer changes. On the other hand, syndromes such as myopericarditis, nephritis, and myositis have been associated with enteroviruses primarily by serologic and epidemiologic evidence. In many of these cases, viral isolation is the exception. The pathogenesis of these infections is not clear; however, it seems likely that the acute phase of the infection may be mild or subclinical and often subsides by the time the clinical illness becomes evident. Illness probably represents a host immunologic response to tissue injury by the virus or to viral or virus-induced antigens that persist in the affected tissues. Experiments with coxsackieviruses in murine models tend to support this hypothesis.

Infection by a specific serotype in an immunologically normal host is followed by a humoral antibody response, which can often be detected by neutralization methods for many years thereafter. There is relative immunity to reinfection by the same serotype; however, reinfection has been reported, usually resulting in subclinical infection or mild illness. Although there is some antigenic sharing between serotypes in some of the enterovirus classes (for example, group B coxsackieviruses), there is no evidence of significant heterotypic immunity to infection by different serotypes.

LABORATORY DIAGNOSIS   In acute enteroviral infections, the diagnosis is most readily established by virus isolation from throat swabs, stool or rectal swabs, body fluids, and occasionally tissues. Except in young infants, viremia is usually undetectable by the time symptoms appear. When there is central nervous system involvement, cerebrospinal fluid cultures taken during the acute phase of the disease may be positive in 10 to 85 percent of cases (except in poliovirus infections, in which virus recovery from this site is rare), depending upon the stage of illness and the serotype involved. Direct isolation of virus from affected tissues or body fluids in enclosed spaces (for example, pleural, pericardial, or cerebrospinal fluid) usually confirms the diagnosis. Isolation of an enterovirus from the throat is suggestive of an etiologic association, as the virus is usually detectable at this site for only 2 days to 2 weeks after infection; isolation of virus from fecal specimens only must be interpreted more cautiously, as asymptomatic shedding from the bowel may persist for as long as 4 months.

The diagnosis may be further supported by fourfold or greater neutralizing antibody titer changes between paired acute and convalescent serum samples. This method is expensive and cumbersome, requiring careful selection of serotypes for use as antigens. Serodiagnosis is generally reserved for critical situations in which the etiology is questionable, such as isolation of a virus only from a peripheral source such as the feces, or in illnesses such as myopericarditis, in which the yield on routine culture is low and the number of serotypes that might be expected to be involved is limited. Quantitative interpretations of antibody titers on single serum samples are rarely helpful because of the high prevalence and wide range of titers to different serotypes that can be found in groups of healthy individuals. In acute poliovirus infections, complement-fixing antibody titer determinations on acute and convalescent sera can aid in diagnosis.

White blood cell counts and the erythrocyte sedimentation rates are usually only mildly elevated. If there is necrosis (e.g., liver, lung), a neutrophilic reaction may be noted. Hyperbilirubinemia and elevated transaminase and alkaline phosphatase levels may be seen

TABLE 139-1   Enteroviruses that infect humans

Class	Number of serotypes
Poliovirus	3
Coxsackievirus	
Group A	23*
Group B	6
Echovirus	31
Enterovirus	Types 68–72†

* Includes several subtypes; coxsackievirus A23 is the same as echovirus 9.
† The classification of the more recently described enteroviruses is based on overlapping biologic characteristics. These are identified numerically. Enterovirus 72 is hepatitis A virus.

in patients with hepatitis. Albuminuria often occurs transiently, but hematuria is rare.

PROPHYLAXIS AND TREATMENT Vaccines, which are available only for the prevention of poliovirus infections, will be discussed in detail below. Although proper disposal of feces and careful personal hygiene are recommended, the usual quarantine or isolation measures are relatively ineffective in controlling the spread of enteroviruses in the family or community.

None of the currently available antiviral agents or immune serum globulins has been shown effective in treatment or prophylaxis of enterovirus infections. The only exception to this may be the use of high-titered immunoglobulin in the treatment of chronic enteroviral encephalitis in antibody-deficient patients. Otherwise, treatment is entirely symptomatic and supportive. Glucocorticosteroids are usually considered contraindicated; they are sometimes employed, however, in the management of severe myocarditis, but only as a last resort.

POLIOVIRUS INFECTIONS

The most important enteroviruses are the three poliovirus serotypes (types 1, 2, and 3). They first emerged as important causes of disease in developed temperate-zone countries during the latter part of the nineteenth century, and they continue to be a serious public health problem in developing countries.

The particular tropism of polioviruses for the central nervous system (CNS), which they usually reach by passage across the blood-CNS barrier, is perhaps favored by reflex dilatation of capillaries supplying the affected motor centers of the anterior horn of the brainstem or spinal cord. An alternate pathway is via the axons or perineural sheaths of peripheral nerves. Motor neurons are particularly vulnerable to infection and variable degrees of destruction. The histopathologic findings in the brainstem and spinal cord include necrosis of neuronal cells and perivascular "cuffing" by infiltration with mononuclear cells, primarily lymphocytes.

CLINICAL MANIFESTATIONS Most infections (perhaps 90 percent) are either subclinical or extremely mild. When disease does result, the incubation period can be from 4 to 35 days, but is usually between 7 and 14 days. The disease falls into three classes: The first, abortive poliomyelitis, is a nonspecific febrile illness of 2- to 3-day duration with no signs of CNS localization. A second group of patients will additionally develop aseptic meningitis. Recovery is rapid and complete, usually within a few days. The third class, paralytic poliomyelitis, is the major possible outcome of infection and is often preceded by a period of fever and "minor illness." Classically, after several days, symptoms disappear. In 5 to 10 days fever recurs, and signs of meningeal irritation and asymmetric flaccid paralysis ensue. Cramping muscle pain and spasm as well as coarse twitching in affected parts follows. The maximum extent of involvement is apparent within a few days after first paralysis. In children younger than 5 years, paralysis of one leg is most common. In patients 5 to 15 years of age, weakness of one arm or paraplegia is frequent, while in adults quadriplegia is more likely to occur. Urinary bladder and respiratory muscle dysfunction are also frequent in adults. Inoculations of vaccines are associated with involvement of the muscles around the site of injection.

Tendon reflexes are diminished or absent. Sensation is intact, separating poliomyelitis from the usually symmetric paralysis of the Guillain-Barré syndrome. Paralysis due to heavy metal poisoning may also be difficult to distinguish clinically from poliomyelitis.

Among paralytic cases, 6 to 25 percent may be bulbar. Myocarditis, hypertension, pulmonary edema, shock, nosocomial gram-negative or staphylococcal pneumonias, urinary tract infections, and emotional problems are among the complications of severe paralytic disease. Treatment is supportive. About 2 to 5 percent of children and 15 to 30 percent of adults with paralyzing infection die. As temporarily damaged neurons regain their function, recovery begins and may continue for as long as 6 months. Paralysis persisting beyond that time is permanent, and may be associated with complaints of severe pain in the affected areas which sometimes recur years after the illness.

PREVENTION Two types of poliovirus vaccines are currently licensed in the United States: inactivated polio vaccine and live, oral, attenuated virus vaccine. Each contains the three serotypes of poliomyelitis virus.

Inactivated polio vaccine (IPV) was introduced in 1955; it remains the only vaccine used in some countries, notably Sweden, Finland, and the Netherlands, and its efficacy has been excellent. Primary vaccination with four doses (three doses 4 to 8 weeks apart and the fourth 6 to 12 months later) produces antibody responses in more than 95 percent of recipients. The current product is considered safe, with no significant deleterious side effects.

Oral polio vaccine (OPV) is composed of live, attenuated viruses. It was first licensed in the United States in 1963. The vaccine is given as a primary series of three doses (the first two doses usually 6 to 8 weeks apart, and the third 8 to 12 months later) and produces antibodies to all three serotypes in more than 95 percent of recipients. As with IPV, recall boosters are recommended to maintain adequate antibody levels. Like wild poliovirus, OPV viruses infect and replicate in the oropharynx and intestinal tract, and may be shed into the feces for 6 weeks or longer.

One disadvantage of OPV is the remote risk of vaccine-associated paralytic disease in some recipients, such as immunocompromised persons; susceptible adults are at a slightly higher risk than children. There is speculation that some instances of vaccine-associated paralytic disease may also be related to reversion of attenuated virus to more virulent characteristics in vivo after passage from person to person. The incidence of vaccine-associated paralytic poliomyelitis is estimated at approximately 1 per 3.7 million doses distributed. Of the 76 cases reported in the United States during 1969 to 1978, 18 were in otherwise healthy vaccine recipients, 47 in healthy close contacts of vaccine recipients, and 11 in persons with immune-deficiency conditions.

The major advantages of OPV include ease of administration and secondary immunization of nonimmune contacts through shedding of vaccine virus into the intestinal tract, resulting in more widespread immunity in the population. It is also theorized that during outbreaks, transient vaccine virus colonization results in the induction of mucosal immunity (primarily through secretory IgA), which may interfere with subsequent acquisition and spread of wild poliovirus.

The choice between IPV and OPV for routine primary immunization is widely debated; however, it is clear that both are highly effective vaccines, and that routine immunization with one or the other is important in the prevention of disease. Ideally, immunization should commence in infancy. A susceptible adult at risk of exposure to infection because of travel to an endemic area should receive complete immunization. Persons with immunodeficiency or altered immune status should not be exposed to OPV, either directly or by household contact, because of the increased risk of vaccine-associated paralysis.

Although there are no currently recognized areas of wild poliovirus prevalence in the United States, importation of these strains can readily occur from endemic areas in contiguous countries as well as from developing nations abroad. Once introduced into a community, the virus can spread rapidly among susceptible individuals. For this reason, continuing immunization programs are of utmost importance in preventing spread of this disease.

COXSACKIEVIRUSES AND ECHOVIRUSES

The coxsackieviruses and echoviruses are widespread throughout the world. The basic features of their epidemiology and pathogenesis appear to be the same as those of the polioviruses. Unlike polioviruses, they have a greater tendency to affect the meninges and occasionally the cerebrum, and only rarely do they affect anterior horn cells.

The consequences of infection with these agents are highly variable and related only in part to virus subgroup and serotype. Up to 60 percent of infections are subclinical. The main interest in these agents stems from their ability to cause more serious illness, which becomes most evident during epidemics.

Inapparent infection is common, but varies with the infecting strain and the host involved. The manifestations of illness range from mild to lethal and from acute to chronic. Table 139-2 lists the major syndromes and serotypes commonly associated with each. Considerable overlap occurs, however, and it is not surprising to find an enteroviral serotype associated with a specific syndrome which differs from that most often encountered. The group B coxsackieviruses generally appear to have the greatest latitude with regard to tissue tropism.

ASEPTIC MENINGITIS (See Chap. 347) In terms of relative frequency, aseptic meningitis is the most important illness associated with enterovirus infections. This syndrome can be mild and self-limiting; however, it is occasionally accompanied by encephalitis, which can lead to permanent sequelae, particularly in infants. Overall, enteroviruses cause the majority of all nonbacterial CNS infections now observed in the United States.

There may be a mild prodromal malaise, but major illness usually begins with fever, headache, and stiff neck. Kernig's and Brudzinski's signs may be present. Localizing sensory or motor deficits are unusual. Confusion and delirium are common. These acute findings may persist for 4 to 7 days. Cerebrospinal pleocytosis is usually less than 500 cells per cubic millimeter. Early, there may be as many as 90 percent polymorphonuclear leukocytes, but within 48 h the cellular response becomes completely mononuclear. Persistence of polymorphonuclear leukocytes in the cerebrospinal fluid suggests pyogenic meningitis or intracerebral, subdural, or epidural abscess. Gram's stain and appropriate spinal fluid cultures must be done to exclude bacterial meningitis, tuberculosis, or mycotic meningitis. Protein concentration in the cerebrospinal fluid is moderately elevated, but glucose is usually normal. Early in the illness enteroviruses may be isolated from spinal fluid, even in the absence of significant pleocytosis. It usually takes several weeks before the cerebrospinal fluid reverts to normal. An occasional patient may develop a transient syndrome of inappropriate secretion of antidiuretic hormone. In hypo- or agammaglobulinemic syndromes echoviruses have persisted in CSF for months to years, producing a progressive encephalitis.

For attempts at virus isolation, throat, stool, and cerebrospinal fluid specimens should be collected as early in the course as possible. Acute and convalescent serums can also be studied for rises in type-specific neutralizing antibodies in patients in whom viral isolation results are negative or equivocal.

It is not possible to distinguish clinically between aseptic meningitis due to various enteroviruses, arboviruses, Epstein-Barr virus, and mumps. Localizing findings, hemiplegia, oculogyric crises, coma, and bloody spinal fluid favor the diagnosis of type 1 herpes simplex virus encephalitis (see Chap. 136). Although enterovirus aseptic meningitis most often is self-limited and recovery in persons afflicted after the first year of life is usually complete, about 10 percent of patients have more serious involvement of the central nervous system. Minor muscle weakness with reflex changes may persist for weeks to months, but over 90 percent of patients recover completely within a year. Occasionally, choreiform movements, ataxia, nystagmus, transverse myelitis, Guillain-Barré syndrome, poliomyelitis-like symptoms, coma, bulbar involvement, and death result.

OTHER ENTEROVIRAL ILLNESSES *Generalized disease of the newborn* is a highly lethal expression of enteroviral infection, in which the infant may be overwhelmed by simultaneous virus infection of the heart, liver, adrenals, brain, and other organs.

Acute myocarditis and/or pericarditis can be caused by a variety of viral agents; however, it is estimated that as many as 50 percent of cases are associated with infection by coxsackie B viruses. Such infections are usually self-limited, but can lead to a fatal outcome (arrhythmia or heart failure) or cause chronic heart disease (see Chaps. 192 and 194).

The exanthems may or may not be associated with CNS inflammation (see Chap. 133). The observed rashes usually resemble rubella, roseola infantum, or adenovirus macular or maculopapular exanthems, but may also appear as vesicular or hemangioma-like lesions. Hand-foot-and-mouth disease usually affects children and is characterized by a vesicular eruption over the extremities and the anterior oral cavity. Coxsackievirus A16 is the specific agent most frequently implicated, but others, such as enterovirus 71, can cause a similar illness.

Herpangina is an enanthematous (mucous membrane) disease characterized by the acute onset of fever and sore throat. Characteristic small vesicles or white papules (lymphonodules) surrounded by a red halo are seen over the posterior half of the palate, pharynx, and tonsillar areas. This mild, self-limiting (1 to 2 weeks) illness has usually been associated with infection by several different group A coxsackievirus serotypes.

Epidemic myalgia (pleurodynia, or Bornholm disease) is characterized by fever and sudden onset of intense upper abdominal or lower thoracic pain, often accompanied by a frontal headache. The pain may be aggravated by movement, such as breathing or coughing, and usually persists for 3 to 14 days. Coxsackie B viruses are most frequently implicated.

A variety of other illnesses may also result from infections by this subgroup. Epidemic acute hemorrhagic keratoconjunctivitis associated with enterovirus 70 has been reported in Asia and the United States, and disease resembling paralytic poliomyelitis caused by enterovirus 71 infection has occurred in Bulgaria and the United States. In addition, there is some evidence that certain enteroviruses may participate in the pathogenesis of at least some cases of insulin-dependent diabetes mellitus, acute arthritis, polymyositis, hemolytic-

TABLE 139-2   Clinical syndromes reported to be commonly associated with enterovirus serotypes

Syndrome	Coxsackievirus Group A	Group B	Echovirus and enterovirus (E)
Aseptic meningitis, encephalitis	2,4,7,9,10	1,2,3,4,5	4,6,9,11,16,30;E70,E71
Muscle weakness and paralysis (poliomyelitis-like disease)	7,9	2,3,4,5	2,4,6,9,11,30;E71
Cerebellar ataxia	2,4,9	3,4	4,6,9
Generalized disease (infants)	—	1,2,3,4,5	3,6,9,11,14,17,19
Exanthems and enanthems	4,5,6,9,10,16	2,3,4,5	2,4,5,6,9,11,16,18,25;E71
Pericarditis, myocarditis	4,16	2,3,4,5	1,6,8,9,19
Epidemic myalgia (pleurodynia), orchitis	9	1,2,3,4,5	1,6,9
Respiratory symptoms	9,16,21,24	1,3,4,5	4,9,11,20,25
Conjunctivitis	24	1,5	7;E70

uremic syndrome, and idiopathic acute nephritis. However, the associations between these viruses and the diseases mentioned have not been clearly elucidated.

REOVIRUS INFECTIONS

The reoviruses (respiratory enteric orphans) are naked virions that contain double-stranded RNA. They are extremely ubiquitous and have been found in humans, simians, cattle, rodents, and a variety of other hosts. Three serotypes are known to infect humans; however, their role and relative importance in human disease remains uncertain. Sporadic cases of febrile upper respiratory infections, exanthems, pneumonia, hepatitis, encephalitis, and gastroenteritis have all been reported to be associated with these viruses. Reovirus type 3 has also been implicated as a possible cause of biliary atresia and neonatal hepatitis. Asymptomatic shedding of reoviruses also occurs, which makes it difficult to prove association with disease. Reoviruses have been used as models in the laboratory for the study and understanding of viral pathogenesis.

Reoviruses can be isolated in cell cultures, particularly primary monkey kidney or human kidney monolayers.

REFERENCES

BARRETT-CONNOR E: Is insulin-dependent diabetes mellitus caused by coxsackievirus B infection? A review of the epidemiologic evidence. Rev Infect Dis 7:207, 1985

BOWEN GS et al: Epidemic of meningitis and febrile illness in neonates caused by ECHO type 11 virus in Philadelphia. Pediatr Infect Dis 2:359, 1983

CHEMTOB S et al: Syndrome of inappropriate secretion of antidiuretic hormone in enteroviral meningitis. Am J Dis Child 139:292, 1985

ERLENDSSON K et al: Successful reversal of echovirus encephalitis in X-linked hypogammaglobulinemia by intraventricular administration of immunoglobulin. N Engl J Med 312:351, 1985

GLASER JH et al: Role of reovirus type 3 in persistent infantile cholestasis. J Pediatr 105:912, 1984

HORSTMANN DM: Control of poliomyelitis: A continuing paradox. J Infect Dis 146:540, 1982

JEHN UW, FINK MK: Myositis, myoglobinemia, and myoglobinuria associated with enterovirus echo 9 infection. Arch Neurol 37:457, 1980

JENISTA JA et al: Epidemiology of neonatal enterovirus infection. J Pediatr 104:685, 1984

JOSSELSON J et al: Acute rhabdomyolysis associated with an echovirus infection. Arch Intern Med 140:1671, 1980

KAPLAN MH et al: Group B coxsackievirus infections in infants younger than three months of age: A serious childhood illness. Rev Infect Dis 5:1019, 1983

KEREIAKES DJ, PARMLEY WW: Myocarditis and cardiomyopathy. Am Heart J 108:1318, 1984

SHARPE AH, FIELDS BN: Pathogenesis of viral infections: Basic concepts derived from the reovirus model. N Engl J Med 312:486, 1985

WOLFE JL et al: Intestinal M cells: A pathway for entry of reovirus into the host. Science 212:471, 1981

140 VIRAL GASTROENTERITIS

HARRY B. GREENBERG

INTRODUCTION In less developed countries, acute infectious diarrheal disease is a leading cause of morbidity in all age groups, and of mortality in infants and young children. In developed countries, acute diarrheal illness remains an important cause of morbidity among both children and adults. Two distinct groups of viruses—the rotaviruses and the Norwalk viruses (Fig. 140-1)—as well as a variety of bacterial pathogens (see Chap. 89) have emerged as important etiologic agents of gastroenteritis. The rotaviruses are primarily pathogens of young children. The Norwalk and related small round viruses affect predominantly older children and adults.

ROTAVIRUS Classification and characterization Rotaviruses are members of the Reoviridae family. The rotavirus virion consists of a 70-nm double-shelled icosahedral capsid which surrounds a genome composed of 11 segments of double-stranded RNA. The virus has two surface proteins which are both involved with viral neutralization. Because rotaviruses have a segmented genome, they are capable of undergoing gene reassortment at very high frequency. The role of gene reassortment in generating rotavirus antigenic diversity is not known. In humans, rotavirus infection is characterized by replication that is localized exclusively in the small intestinal epithelial cells.

Epidemiology Rotavirus infection occurs worldwide. By the age of 3, virtually every individual has been infected by rotaviruses at least once. In areas with a temperate climate, rotavirus infection is seasonal, occurring in the cooler winter months. In tropical areas rotavirus infection tends to occur throughout the year, with some increase in incidence during the cooler rainy season. Rotaviruses are the single most important cause of severe dehydrating diarrhea in infants and young children under 3 in both developed and less developed countries, and account for between 30 and 50 percent of all cases of diarrhea requiring hospitalization or intensive rehydration therapy. Although rotavirus infections are primarily confined to infants and small children, they are frequently associated with diarrhea in adults, particularly family members of affected infants, geriatric patients, and immunocompromised hosts. They account for up to 25 percent of traveler's diarrhea (see Chap. 89). Subclinical infections or mild gastrointestinal illnesses which do not require hospitalization account for the majority of rotavirus infections. Subclinical infections have also been documented in neonates; these infections were shown to protect against severe rotavirus gastroenteritis for up to 3 years. At least four distinct serotypes of human rotavirus have been described. The relationship of the frequency of infection with these serotypes to host immune status is unclear. A large variety of other mammals and avian species can be infected by rotavirus, but it does not appear that these animal rotavirus strains cause disease in humans under natural conditions. Rotaviruses are shed in very large numbers (up to 10^{10} particles per gram of feces) in the stool; it is presumed that transmission occurs via fecal-oral spread.

Pathophysiology Rotavirus infects and kills the mature villus tip cells of the small intestine. The mature epithelial cells are replaced by immature absorptive cells that cannot absorb carbohydrate or other nutrients efficiently. Rotavirus infection leads to an osmotic diarrhea due to nutrient malabsorption. Changes in intracellular cyclic adenosine monophosphate or guanosine monophosphate are not involved in the etiology of rotavirus diarrhea.

Manifestations These range from subclinical infections to mild diarrhea to severe, occasionally fatal, illness. Most information concerning the signs and symptoms of rotavirus infection has been derived from studies of hospitalized young children. The onset of illness is usually abrupt. Vomiting, followed by diarrhea, occurs in over 80 percent of affected children. About one-third of hospitalized children will have a temperature greater than 39°C. Gastrointestinal symptoms usually last between 2 and 6 days. Mucus is commonly found in the stool but white blood cells and red blood cells are present in less than 15 percent of cases. Rotavirus infection frequently occurs in conjunction with respiratory tract symptoms, but there is little evidence to indicate that rotavirus replicates in the repiratory tract. Rotavirus infection has been observed in association with a wide variety of other clinical syndromes, including sudden infant death syndrome, Reye's syndrome, encephalitis, aseptic meningitis, pneumonia, exanthem subitum, Kawasaki's syndrome, necrotizing enterocolitis, gastroenteritis, which may be accompanied by hemorrhage, intussusception, Henoch-Schönlein purpura, hemolytic uremic syndrome, disseminated intravascular coagulation, and Crohn's disease. The etiologic relationship between these clinical syndromes and rotavirus infection is probably coincidental rather than causal. Rotavirus infection may be especially severe, and even fatal, in immunocompromised children.

Clinical immunity Relative immunity to rotavirus illness is acquired following infection early in childhood. Immunity is not complete, and adults with low levels of antibody can be symptomatically infected. Local immunity appears to be the critical determinant in protection.

Diagnosis   Because rotavirus is shed in large amounts in the stool, detection is relatively easy. A variety of specific commercial immunoassays are available to detect rotavirus antigen in fecal specimens. There are no pathognomonic signs or symptoms of rotavirus infection, but rotavirus infection is more frequently associated with severe dehydration than other enteric bacterial or viral pathogens.

Treatment and prevention   Despite the fact that rotavirus diarrhea is caused by intestinal epithelial cell lysis and death, it can be adequately treated by standard oral rehydration therapy. Only rarely is intravenous rehydration required. Since rotavirus infections have persisted in developed countries with advanced sanitation facilities and widely available clean water, it is unlikely that the viral infection will be preventable by hygienic measures alone. Progress with a number of candidate live attenuated vaccines suggests that prevention through vaccination may be feasible in the next decade.

NORWALK AND RELATED SMALL ROUND VIRUSES   Classification and characterization   A variety of round 27- to 32-nm particles, most of which have a poorly defined ultrastructure, have been identified in the stools of individuals with acute nonbacterial gastroenteritis.

FIGURE 140-1   *A. A group of Norwalk virus particles observed in the stool of a volunteer. (From AZ Kapikian et al, J Virol 10:1075, 1972.) B. Human rotavirus particle observed in a stool filtrate. (Reprinted with permission from AZ Kapikian et al. Copyright 1974 by the AAAS.) Bars = 100 nm.*

These agents have not been definitely classified because they are shed in the stool in small amounts for only a few days, and they have not been adapted to cell culture or to animal models. The Norwalk virus represents the most extensively studied and best characterized member of this group of agents, which also includes such serologically distinct viruses as the Hawaii agent, the Snow Mountain agent, the W-Ditchling agent, the Marin agent, and a number of agents described as either astrovirus-like or calicivirus-like. The Norwalk virus and the Snow Mountain virus appear to have a protein structure similar to typical caliciviruses, and it is likely that most of these 27-nm gastroenteritis agents will prove to be plus-stranded RNA viruses.

Epidemiology   Norwalk infection occurs year round, not seasonally. Infection with Norwalk virus is common. From 58 to 70 percent of adults in both developed and less developed countries have antibodies to this virus. Norwalk antibody acquisition occurs at a considerably younger age in children in less developed countries than in those in developed areas, consistent with the presumption that Norwalk virus is spread by the fecal-oral route. In developed countries, Norwalk virus is responsible for approximately one-third of all epidemics of nonbacterial gastroenteritis. Norwalk virus has been incriminated in a variety of food-borne epidemics, and transmission vehicles have included oysters, green salad, and chocolate icing. The virus is a common cause of water-borne epidemics of gastroenteritis and has been shown to be the etiologic agent in nursing home, cruise ship, and institutional (summer camps and schools) outbreaks.

In less developed countries, the role of Norwalk virus infection in the etiology of diarrhea has not been thoroughly investigated.

Preliminary studies indicate that Norwalk virus can cause mild diarrhea in young children, but it does not appear to cause severe illness in infants in either developed or less developed countries. The other serologically distinct small round gastroenteritis viruses must be studied in more detail before their epidemiology can be distinguished from Norwalk infection.

Pathophysiology Following infection with Norwalk or Hawaii viruses, the proximal small intestinal architecture is altered with villus shortening, crypt hyperplasia, and lamina propria infiltration by polymorphonuclear and mononuclear cells. Changes are not observed in the stomach or colon. The cells in which viral replication occurs have not been identified. The histologic alterations are accompanied by mild steatorrhea, carbohydrate malabsorption, and decreased levels of some brush border enzymes. Changes in adenylate cyclase activity have not been observed.

Manifestations Norwalk illness has an incubation period of between 18 and 72 h. Disease is characterized by the abrupt onset of nausea and abdominal cramps followed by vomiting and/or diarrhea. Vomiting occurs more frequently in children than adults. Low-grade fever (above 37.5°C) is seen in about half of affected individuals. Headache, myalgias, and abdominal pain are common. The white blood cell count is normal; rarely there is leukocytosis with a relative lymphopenia. Red and white cells are not found in the stool. The illness is usually mild and self-limited, lasting 24 to 48 h.

Clinical immunity For most people long-term (2 years or greater) resistance to Norwalk reinfection does not occur. In volunteers, there is a paradoxical relationship between the level of antibody to Norwalk virus and susceptibility to illness. Low levels of Norwalk antibody in the serum and intestine are associated with clinical resistance to illness. It appears, therefore, that immune mechanisms are not the primary determinants of protection from Norwalk virus.

Diagnosis, treatment, and prevention Radioimmunoassays and ELISA have been developed for Norwalk virus and several other 27- to 30-nm gastroenteritis agents. These tests are not yet available commercially. Norwalk illness is acute and self-limited; treatment is not usually required. In the rare case of severe vomiting or diarrhea, oral or intravenous rehydration is indicated. Because long-term immunity to Norwalk illness does not usually follow natural infection, it seems unlikely that a vaccine will be developed.

MISCELLANEOUS ENTERIC VIRAL PATHOGENS Enteric adenoviruses are a minor (~10 percent) cause of diarrheal illness in infants and children. These viruses differ from other adenovirus strains in a variety of ways including neutralization serotype, restriction endonuclease digestion pattern, and their ability to grow in tissue culture. The role of enteric adenovirus illness in adults or in less developed countries is not known.

Several strains of antigenically distinct rotaviruses, presently called "atypical rotaviruses" (or pararotaviruses) have been identified as the cause of occasional episodes of diarrhea in humans and animals. One strain of atypical rotavirus caused a very large water-borne outbreak of diarrheal disease in adults in China. From the scanty data available, it can be concluded that the atypical rotaviruses are not frequent causes of diarrheal illness in humans.

Corona viruses are frequent causes of diarrheal disease in a variety of animals. Several investigators, using electron microscopy, have identified putative corona virus–like particles in the stools of patients with diarrhea. In most cases, however, these particles do not have the typical morphologic features of corona viruses and may represent bacterial breakdown products or cellular fragments. A serologically distinct corona virus has been shown to cause necrotizing enterocolitis in newborn infants.

REFERENCES

BLACK RE et al: A two-year study of bacterial, viral and parasitic agents associated with diarrhea in rural Bangladesh. J Infect Dis 142:660, 1980

BRANDT CD et al: Pediatric viral gastroenteritis during eight years of study. J Clin Microbiol 18:71, 1983

ESTES MK et al: Rotaviruses: A review, in Current Topics in Microbiology and Immunology, M Cooper et al (eds). New York, Springer-Verlag, 1983, p 123

GREENBERG HB et al: Proteins of Norwalk virus. J Virol 37:994, 1981

KAPIKIAN AZ et al: Visualization by immune electron microscopy of a 27-nm particle associated with acute infectious non-bacterial gastroenteritis. J Virol 10:1075, 1972

——— et al: Reovirus-like agent in stools: Association with infantile diarrhea and development of a serologic test. Science 185:1049, 1974

KAPLAN JE et al: Epidemiology of Norwalk gastroenteritis and the role of Norwalk virus in outbreaks of acute non-bacterial gastroenteritis. Ann Intern Med 96:756, 1982

MORSE DL et al: Widespread outbreaks of clam- and oyster-associated gastroenteritis. Role of Norwalk virus. N Engl J Med 314:678, 1986

RESTA S et al: Isolation and propagation of a human enteric coronavirus. Science 229:978, 1985

TYRELL DA, KAPIKIAN AZ (eds): Virus Infections of the Gastrointestinal Tract. New York, Dekker, 1982

VESIKARI T et al: Protection of infants against rotavirus diarrhea by RIT 4237 attenuated bovine rotavirus strain vaccine. Lancet 1:977, 1984

141 MUMPS

C. GEORGE RAY

DEFINITION Mumps is an acute communicable disease of viral origin characterized by painful enlargement of the salivary glands and sometimes by involvement of the gonads, meninges, pancreas, and other organs.

ETIOLOGY The causative agent of mumps is a paramyxovirus of intermediate size (120 to 200 nm in diameter). It has a tight helical inner core (RNA) enclosed in an outer envelope of lipid and protein. The virus of mumps has two components capable of fixing complement. These are the soluble, or S, antigens derived from the nucleocapsid, and the V antigen derived from the surface hemagglutinin. The virus can be cultivated in chick embryos and in a variety of mammalian cell cultures.

EPIDEMIOLOGY Human beings are the only natural host for mumps. The disease is worldwide and is endemic in urban communities. Epidemics are relatively infrequent and are confined to closely associated groups who live in orphanages, army camps, or schools. The disease is most frequent in the spring, particularly during April and May. Although mumps is generally considered less "contagious" than measles and chickenpox, this difference may be more apparent than real because many mumps infections (at least 25 percent) tend to be inapparent clinically. In some surveys, 80 to 90 percent of an adult population had serologic evidence of previous infection with mumps. The incidence of mumps in the United States has reached its lowest point since reporting began in 1922.

Infections are rare before the age of 2 years and then increase in frequency, reaching a peak at ages 5 to 9. Clinical mumps may be more common in males than in females. The virus is transmitted in infected salivary secretions, although its isolation from urine suggests that the virus may also spread via this route. Mumps virus is rarely isolated from stools. The saliva is infectious for approximately 6 days prior to the onset of parotitis, and virus has been recovered from this site for as long as 2 weeks after onset of parotid swelling. Viruria also persists for 2 to 3 weeks in some patients. Despite this prolonged secretion of virus, the peak of infectivity occurs a day or two before onset of parotitis and subsides rapidly after the appearance of glandular enlargement.

One attack of clinical or subclinical mumps confers lasting immunity, and second attacks are most unusual. Unilateral parotitis affords protection just as effectively as does bilateral disease.

PATHOGENESIS The virus enters via the respiratory route; during the incubation period of 15 to 21 days it presumably replicates in the upper respiratory tract and cervical lymph nodes, from which it is disseminated via the bloodstream to other organs, including the meninges, gonads, pancreas, breasts, thyroid, heart, liver, kidneys, and cranial nerves. The salivary adenitis is thought by many to be secondary to viremia, but primary spread from the respiratory tract has not been ruled out as an alternative mechanism.

MANIFESTATIONS   **Salivary adenitis**   The onset of typical parotitis is usually sudden, although it may be preceded by a prodromal period of malaise, anorexia, chilly sensations, feverishness, sore throat, and tenderness at the angle of the jaw. In many cases, however, parotid swelling is the first indication of illness. The glands enlarge progressively over a period of 1 to 3 days, and the swelling resolves within a week after maximal enlargement. The swollen gland extends from the ear to the lower portion of the mandibular ramus and to the inferior portion of the zygomatic arch, often displacing the ear upward and outward. The skin over the gland is usually not warm or erythematous, in contrast to what happens in bacterial parotitis. There may be reddening and pouting of the orifice of Stensen's duct. Usually, pain and tenderness are marked, although at times they are absent. The edema of mumps has been described as "gelatinous," and when the involved gland is tweaked, it rolls like jelly. Swelling may involve only the submaxillary and sublingual glands and may extend over the anterior part of the chest, producing *presternal edema*. Involvement of submaxillary glands alone can cause difficulty in distinguishing mumps from acute cervical adenitis. Swelling of the glottis occurs rarely but may require tracheostomy. Parotitis is bilateral in two-thirds of cases and remains confined to one side in the remainder. The second gland tends to swell as the first is subsiding, usually 4 to 5 days after onset. In general, parotitis is accompanied by a temperature of 100 to 103°F, malaise, headache, and anorexia, but systemic symptoms may be virtually absent, particularly in children. In most patients, the chief complaints refer to difficulty in eating, swallowing, and talking.

Epididymoorchitis   Mumps is complicated by orchitis in 20 to 35 percent of postpubertal males. Testicular involvement usually appears 7 to 10 days after onset of parotitis, although it may precede it or appear simultaneously. Occasionally, orchitis occurs in the absence of parotitis. Gonadal involvement is bilateral in 3 to 17 percent of patients. Orchitis is heralded by recrudescence of malaise and appearance of chilly sensations, headache, nausea, and vomiting. Shaking chills and high fevers, with temperatures between 103 and 106°F, are frequent. The testicle becomes greatly swollen and acutely painful. The epididymis is often palpable as a swollen tender cord. Occasionally there may be epididymitis without orchitis. Swelling, pain, and tenderness persist for 3 to 7 days and gradually subside; lysis of fever usually parallels abatement of swelling. Occasionally, the temperature falls by crisis. Mumps orchitis is followed by progressive atrophy of the testicle in one-half the cases. Even after bilateral orchitis, sterility is unusual, provided no significant atrophy has taken place. However, if bilateral testicular atrophy occurs after mumps, sterility or subnormal sperm counts are quite common. Plasma testosterone levels are depressed during acute orchitis but return to normal with recovery. *Pulmonary infarction* has been noted to follow mumps orchitis. This may be the result of thrombosis of the veins in the prostatic and pelvic plexuses in association with the testicular inflammation. Priapism is a rare but painful complication of mumps orchitis.

Pancreatitis   Pancreatic involvement is a potentially serious manifestation of mumps, which may rarely be complicated by shock or pseudocyst formation. It should be suspected in patients with abdominal pain and tenderness together with clinical or epidemiologic evidence of mumps. It is difficult to document, since hyperamylasemia, the hallmark of pancreatitis, is also often present in parotitis. Many times the symptoms resemble those of gastroenteritis. Although diabetes or pancreatic insufficiency rarely follows mumps pancreatitis, several children have developed "brittle" diabetes a few weeks after mumps.

Central nervous system involvement   Nearly half the patients with mumps have an increased number of cells, usually lymphocytes, in the cerebrospinal fluid (CSF), although symptoms of meningitis, stiff

neck, headache, and drowsiness are less common. In typical cases, the onset of overt central nervous system signs and symptoms occurs 3 to 10 days after the onset of parotitis; however, the onset has also been noted to develop prior to the parotitis or 2 to 3 weeks later. In approximately 30 to 40 percent of laboratory-proven cases, there is *no* associated salivary gland involvement at any time in the course of illness. The CSF protein is moderately elevated, and CSF glucose tends to be normal, although in as many as 10 percent of patients low CSF glucose concentrations, in the range of 20 to 50 mg/dL, may be seen. True encephalitis is unusual, although it is responsible for most of the central nervous system sequelae, including behavioral disturbances, headaches, seizures, deafness (usually unilateral), and visual disturbances. At least seven cases of aqueductal stenosis and hydrocephalus have been reported as possible late sequelae to mumps encephalitis, but the association remains unproven. Mumps should also be recognized as capable of presenting a picture of mild paralytic poliomyelitis; definition of the cause depends on isolation of virus or serologic confirmation of mumps in the absence of changing antibody titers to poliomyelitis viruses. Rarely, mumps may produce a transverse myelitis, cerebellar ataxia, or the Guillain-Barré syndrome. Mumps meningitis, without clinical encephalitis, is generally thought to be benign.

Other manifestations   Mumps virus tends to involve glandular tissues; inflammation of the lacrimal glands, thymus, thyroid, breasts, and ovaries occurs occasionally. *Oophoritis* may be recognized by persistence of pain in the lower part of the abdomen and fever. It does not result in sterility. Mumps virus has been implicated in the causation of subacute thyroiditis; the diagnosis can be made serologically, and occasionally the virus can be isolated from the thyroid gland. Myxedema following mumps thyroiditis has been reported. Ocular manifestations of mumps include dacryoadenitis, optic neuritis, keratitis, iritis, conjunctivitis, and episcleritis. Although these conditions may transiently interfere with vision, complete resolution is the rule. Mumps *myocarditis*, evidenced primarily by transient abnormalities in the electrocardiogram, is relatively common. On rare occasions it can be fatal but it does not usually produce symptomatic disease or impair cardiac function. Similarly, *hepatic* involvement may be manifested by mild abnormalities in liver function, but icterus and other clinical signs of hepatic damage are extremely rare. *Thrombocytopenic purpura* as a complication of mumps has been described, and an occasional patient has a leukemoid reaction involving predominantly lymphocytes. Tracheobronchitis and interstitial pneumonia have also been associated with mumps infection, particularly among young children.

A rare but interesting manifestation of mumps is *polyarthritis* which is often migratory. It is most common in males between the ages of 20 and 30. Joint symptoms begin 1 to 2 weeks after subsidence of parotitis; usually the large joints are involved. The illness lasts 1 to 6 weeks, and complete recovery is the rule. It is not clear whether arthritis is due to viremia or whether it is a "hypersensitivity reaction."

Acute hemorrhagic glomerulonephritis in the absence of streptococcosis has been reported after mumps. The relationship of these two diseases is not clear.

Late complications   With the exception of the rare central nervous system complications, and occasional patients who become sterile following bilateral testicular involvement, mumps leaves no sequelae. There is no firm evidence that stillbirths and offspring with congenital defects are more common among mothers who have mumps during pregnancy. Likewise, the causal relationship between intrauterine mumps infection and endocardial fibroelastosis has not been clearly established.

LABORATORY FINDINGS   In uncomplicated parotitis, the blood leukocyte count is normal, although there may be mild leukopenia with relative lymphocytosis. Patients with mumps orchitis, however, may have a marked leukocytosis with a shift to the left. In meningoencephalitis, the white blood cell count is usually within normal limits. The erythrocyte sedimentation rate is usually normal but may rise with testicular or pancreatic involvement. The serum amylase level is elevated both in pancreatitis and in salivary adenitis. It may also be elevated in some patients in whom the sole evidence of mumps is meningoencephalitis, and probably reflects subclinical involvement of the salivary glands. In contrast to the amylase, the serum lipase level is elevated only in pancreatitis, in which hyperglycemia and glucosuria also may occur. The cerebrospinal fluid contains 0 to 2000 cells per cubic millimeter, almost all mononuclear, although occasionally polymorphonuclear cells will predominate in the early stages. The pleocytosis in mumps meningitis tends to be greater than in aseptic meningitides caused by the polio-, coxsackie-, and echoviruses. There is no relationship between the cell count and the severity of central nervous system involvement. Transient hematuria and mild reversible abnormalities in renal function, including inability to concentrate the urine maximally and to clear creatinine, occur in association with the viruria of mumps.

DIAGNOSIS The definitive diagnosis of mumps depends on isolation of the virus from blood, throat swabs, secretions from Stensen's duct, cerebrospinal fluid, or urine. Immunofluorescence methods can detect positive cell cultures in 2 to 3 days rather than the 6 days required with standard methods. In addition, immunofluorescence can be utilized to rapidly detect the viral antigen directly in oropharyngeal cells. Serologic determination of acute infection or susceptibility can be done by a variety of methods. The usual test of choice is the enzyme-linked immunosorbent assay (ELISA). Immunofluorescent assays are also commonly available, and can be used for identification of IgM- and IgG-specific antibody responses. The complement fixation test can also be employed to quantitate antibody responses to the S and V antigenic components for the diagnosis of acute or recent mumps infection. Antibodies to the S antigen develop rather rapidly, often reaching a peak within 1 week after the onset of symptoms, and usually disappear in 6 to 12 months. Complement-fixing antibodies to the V antigen follow a more typical pattern, reaching a peak titer within 2 to 3 weeks after onset, remaining elevated for at least 6 weeks, and then persisting at lower levels for years afterward. Paired serums obtained 2 to 3 weeks apart are recommended. A fourfold increase in titer by any standard assay confirms recent infection. In cases where an acute serum is not obtained until later in the course of illness, an elevation of antibodies to the S antigen which exceeds the V antibody titer or the presence of IgM-specific antibody suggests recent infection. The *skin test* consists of intradermal injection of killed mumps virus; previous exposure will result in a delayed reaction of the tuberculin type and an anamnestic antibody titer rise to mumps. The skin test is unreliable when used alone in determining the immune status of an individual, is useless in the diagnosis of acute mumps, and is no longer commercially available in the United States.

The diagnosis of mumps during an epidemic is usually obvious. Sporadic cases, however, must be distinguished from other causes of parotid enlargement. Parotitis may be caused by other viruses, notably parainfluenza, influenza, and coxsackieviruses. *Bacterial parotitis* usually occurs in debilitated patients with severe underlying diseases, such as uncontrolled diabetes mellitus, cerebrovascular accidents, or uremia. It may also follow surgical operations. The parotid glands are swollen, warm, and tender, and pus can be expressed from the orifices of Stensen's ducts. Marked polymorphonuclear leukocytosis is present. The disease is usually acquired in the hospital, and *Staphylococcus aureus* is the usual causative organism. Dehydration followed by inspissation of secretions in the salivary ducts is an important predisposing factor. *Calculus* in a salivary duct is usually detectable by palpation or by injection of radiopaque media into Stensen's duct. *Drug reactions* may produce tender swelling of the parotid and other salivary glands. "Iodine mumps" is the commonest type; it may follow such procedures as intravenous urography. Mercurialism and the antihypertensive agent guanethidine may also cause parotid enlargement and tenderness. A careful history usually serves to clarify the cause of these reactions. *Cervical adenitis* caused by streptococci, "bullneck" diphtheria,

infectious mononucleosis, cat-scratch disease, sublingual cellulitis (Ludwig's angina), and cellulitis of the external auditory canal are usually easy to distinguish from mumps by careful examination. Parotid tumors and chronic infections such as actinomycosis tend to follow a more indolent course, with slowly progressive swelling. The common "mixed tumor" of the parotid is well-circumscribed, nontender, and very firm, almost cartilaginous on palpation. Parotid swelling and fever, often accompanied by lacrimal adenitis and uveitis (Mikulicz's syndrome), may occur in tuberculosis, leukemia, Hodgkin's disease, and lupus erythematosus. The onset may be sudden, but the process is usually painless and of long duration. "Uveoparotid fever" of similar type may be the first manifestation of sarcoidosis; in this disease parotid swelling is frequently accompanied by single or multiple palsies of cranial nerves, particularly the facial nerve, and is referred to as Heerfordt's syndrome. Presternal edema may also be a manifestation of malignant lymphoma involving retrosternal lymph nodes. Bilateral painless parotid swelling unassociated with fever is found in patients with Laennec's cirrhosis, chronic alcoholism, malnutrition, diabetes mellitus, pregnancy and lactation, and hypertriglyceridemia.

Sjögren's syndrome (see Chap. 266) is a chronic inflammation of the parotid and other salivary glands which is often associated with atrophy of the lacrimal glands and occurs most commonly in women past the menopause. With cessation of lacrimal and salivary function, there may be striking dryness of the conjunctiva and the cornea (keratoconjunctivitis sicca) and of the mouth (xerostomia). These patients may also have a variety of systemic manifestations, including arthritis of the rheumatoid type, splenomegaly, leukopenia, and hemolytic anemia. The chronicity of the process and its occurrence in elderly women make confusion with mumps unlikely. Finally, benign hypertrophy of both masseter muscles, presumably due to habitual clenching and grinding of teeth, may be confused with painless parotid swelling.

The causes of aseptic meningitis are discussed in Chap. 347.

Orchitis occurring in the absence of parotitis is likely to remain undiagnosed. Serologic testing may later confirm the diagnosis of mumps. Orchitis may occur in association with acute bacterial prostatitis and seminal vesiculitis. It is a rare complication of gonorrhea. Occasionally testicular inflammation accompanies pleurodynia, leptospirosis, melioidosis, tuberculosis, relapsing fever, chickenpox, brucellosis, and lymphocytic choriomeningitis.

TREATMENT There is no specific treatment for infections with the mumps virus. Patients with parotitis should receive mouth care, analgesics, and a bland diet. Bed rest is advisable only as long as the patient is febrile; contrary to popular belief, physical activity has no influence on the development of orchitis or other complications. Patients with epididymoorchitis may be acutely ill and in great pain. Many forms of treatment, including surgical decompression of the testicle, infiltration of the spermatic cord with local anesthetics, estrogens, convalescent serum, and broad-spectrum antibiotics, have not been regularly effective. Despite failure to document their effectiveness in controlled studies, adrenal steroids have been of considerable benefit in diminishing fever, as well as testicular pain and swelling, and in restoring the sense of well-being in a number of patients. It is important to give a large initial daily dose corresponding to 300 mg cortisone or 60 mg prednisone. Subsequently, administration of the hormone can be tapered off over 7 to 10 days. Adrenal steroids have not exerted an adverse effect on concomitant pancreatitis or meningitis, although they have not benefited patients with meningeal involvement, and their withdrawal has usually been accompanied by a recrudescence of symptoms. Adrenal steroids have not prevented the appearance of parotid involvement on the contralateral side. Mumps arthritis is usually mild and requires no treatment. Mumps thyroiditis may subside spontaneously, but excellent relief has been obtained with adrenal hormones.

PREVENTION A live attenuated mumps virus vaccine (Jeryl Lynn strain) has been highly effective in producing significant rises in mumps antibody in individuals who are seronegative prior to vaccination, and has afforded 75 to 95 percent protection to individuals subsequently exposed to mumps. The vaccine also has boosted antibody levels in vaccinated individuals who are seropositive. The vaccine produces an inapparent, noncommunicable infection. Parotitis after vaccination has been reported only rarely, and central nervous system dysfunction has not been proved to be a complication. It has conferred excellent protection for at least 12 years and has not interfered with vaccines against measles, rubella, and poliomyelitis or with smallpox vaccination given simultaneously. Protection has been demonstrated in both children and adults.

Live mumps vaccine can be administered at any time after 1 year of age, and should be particularly considered for children approaching puberty, adolescents, and adult males who have not had clinical mumps or live mumps vaccine in the past. Individuals living in groups or in institutions should be vaccinated, particularly because it has been shown that physical isolation of mumps patients does not effectively prevent transmission of the infection.

Vaccination is contraindicated in babies under the age of 1 year because of the interfering effect of maternal antibody; in individuals with a history of hypersensitivity to vaccine components; in patients with febrile illnesses, leukemia, lymphoma, or generalized malignancies; in those receiving steroids, alkylating drugs, antimetabolites, or irradiation; and during pregnancy.

It is not known whether the vaccine will prevent infection when administered after exposure, but no contraindication to its use in this situation exists. Neither mumps immune globulin nor ordinary gamma globulin has been shown to be efficacious in postexposure prophylaxis, and therefore neither is recommended.

REFERENCES

Beard CM et al: The incidence and outcome of mumps orchitis in Rochester Minnesota 1935 to 1974. Mayo Clin Proc 52:3, 1977

Gordon SC, Lauter CB: Mumps arthritis: Unusual presentation as adult Still's disease. Ann Intern Med 97:45, 1982

Immunization Practices Advisory Committee: Mumps vaccine. Ann Intern Med 98:192, 1983

Koplan JP, Preblud SR: A benefit-cost analysis of mumps vaccine. Am J Dis Child 136:362, 1982

Koskiniemi M et al: Clinical appearance and outcome in mumps encephalitis in children. Acta Paediatr Scand 72:603, 1983

Levitt LP et al: Central nervous system mumps: A review of 64 cases. Neurology 20:829, 1970

Shehab ZM et al: Epidemiological standardization of a test for susceptibility to mumps. J Infect Dis 149:810, 1984

142   RABIES AND OTHER RHABDOVIRUSES

LAWRENCE COREY

RABIES

DEFINITION   Rabies is an acute viral disease of the central nervous system that affects all mammals and that is transmitted by infected secretions, usually saliva. Most exposures to rabies are through the bite of an infected animal, but on occasion a virus aerosol or the ingestion or transplantation of infected tissues may initiate the disease process.

ETIOLOGY   The rabies virus is a bullet-shaped, enveloped, single-stranded ribonucleic acid (RNA) virus of 75 to 80 nm diameter belonging to the rhabdovirus group. Glycoprotein excrescences, 6 to 7 nm long, each with a knoblike structure at the distal end, cover the surface of the virion. The viral glycoproteins are capable of

binding to acetylcholine receptors and contribute to the neurovirulence of rabies virus. These surface structures elicit neutralizing and hemagglutination-inhibiting antibodies, while a nucleocapsid antigen induces a complement-fixing antibody. Neutralizing antibodies to the surface glycoproteins appear to be protective. Antirabies antibodies used in diagnostic immunofluorescent assays are generally directed against the nucleocapsid antigens. Isolates of rabies virus from different animal species and locales have different biologic properties. Antigenic variations in strains have also been documented and may account for differences in virulence and lack of response to some types of rabies vaccination regimens. Interferon is induced by rabies virus, particularly in those tissues with high virus concentrations, and may play some role in retarding progressive infection.

EPIDEMIOLOGY   Rabies exists in two epidemiologic forms: *urban*, propagated chiefly by unimmunized domestic dogs and/or cats, and *sylvatic*, propagated by skunks, foxes, raccoons, mongooses, wolves, and bats. Infection in domestic animals usually represents a "spillover" from sylvatic reservoirs of infection, and human beings can be infected by either. Hence, human infection tends to occur in locales where rabies is enzootic or epizootic, where there is a large population of unimmunized domestic animals, and where human contact with the outdoors is common. While only about 800 rabies deaths are reported to the World Health Organization (WHO) each year, the worldwide incidence of rabies is approximated at 15,000 cases per year. Southeast Asia, the Philippines, Africa, and the Indian subcontinent are areas where the disease is especially common. Increased spread of terrestrial rabies and increased travel to countries where urban rabies is present has made recognition of clinical rabies and its prevention of increasing importance. In the United States human rabies is still exceedingly rare, and 0 to 5 cases are reported yearly.

In most areas of the world, the dog is the important vector of rabies virus for humans. However, the wolf (eastern Europe, arctic regions), the mongoose (South Africa, the Caribbean), the fox (western Europe), and the vampire bat (Latin America) may also be prominent vectors of the disease. Rodents and lagomorphs are rarely infected with rabies. In the United States the most important sources of human disease have been skunks, bats, and raccoons. In the United States, rabies in wildlife accounts for about 85 percent of the reported animal rabies, with dogs and cats comprising only about 2 and 3 percent, respectively. However, most of the reported cases of postexposure prophylaxis are associated with dog bites. Many human cases of rabies in U.S. citizens have resulted from domestic animal bites that occurred outside the country.

Several cases of human-to-human transmission of rabies through corneal transplantation have been documented.

PATHOGENESIS   The first event is the introduction of live virus through the epidermis or onto a mucous membrane. Initial viral replication appears to occur within striated muscle cells at the site of inoculation. The peripheral nervous system is exposed at the neuromuscular and/or neurotendinal spindles. The virus then spreads centripetally up the nerve to the central nervous system, probably via peripheral nerve axoplasm. Experimentally, viremia has been shown to occur, but is not thought to play a role in naturally acquired disease. Once the virus reaches the central nervous system, it replicates almost exclusively within the gray matter and then passes centrifugally along autonomic nerves to reach other tissue—the salivary glands, adrenal medulla, kidney, lung, liver, skeletal muscle, skin, and heart. Passage into the salivary glands facilitates further transmission of the disease via infected saliva. The incubation period of rabies is exceedingly variable, ranging from 10 days to over 1 year (mean 1 to 2 months). The time period appears to depend upon the amount of virus introduced, the amount of tissue involved, host defense mechanisms, and the actual distance that the virus has to travel from the site of inoculation to the central nervous system. Studies in animals have shown that host immune responses and viral strains may also influence disease expression. Attenuated strains of rabies virus produce high cytotoxic responses compared with wild "street virus." Animals which develop paralytic rabies (dumb rabies) appear to have a more marked immune response to infection than those which develop fulminant encephalitis.

The neuropathology of rabies resembles other viral diseases of the central nervous system: hyperemia, varying degrees of chromatolysis, nuclear pyknosis, and neuronophagia of the nerve cells; infiltration by lymphocytes and plasma cells of the Virchow-Robin space; microglial infiltration, and parenchymal areas of nerve cell destruction. The pathognomonic lesion of rabies is the Negri body. This eosinophilic mass, approximately 10 nm in size, is made up of a finely fibrillar matrix and rabies virus particles. Negri bodies are distributed throughout the brain, particularly in Ammon's horn, the cerebral cortex, the brainstem, the Purkinje cells of the cerebellum, and the dorsal spinal ganglia. Negri bodies are not demonstrated in at least 20 percent of rabies, and their absence in brain material does not rule out the diagnosis.

MANIFESTATIONS

The clinical manifestations of rabies can be divided into four stages: (1) a nonspecific prodrome, (2) an acute encephalitis similar to other viral encephalitides, (3) a profound dysfunction of brainstem centers which produces the classic features of rabies encephalitis, and (4) rarely, recovery.

The prodromal period usually persists for 1 to 4 days and is marked by fever, headache, malaise, myalgias, increased fatigability, anorexia, nausea and vomiting, sore throat, and a nonproductive cough. The prodromal symptom suggestive of rabies is the complaint of paresthesias and/or fasciculations at or about the site of inoculation of virus. This symptom is present in 50 to 80 percent of patients.

The encephalitic phase is usually ushered in by periods of excessive motor activity, excitation, and agitation. Quickly, confusion, hallucinations, combativeness, bizarre aberrations of thought, muscle spasms, meningismus, opisthotonic posturing, seizures, and focal paralysis appear. Characteristically, the periods of mental aberration are interspersed with completely lucid periods, but as the disease progresses, the lucid periods get shorter until the patient lapses into coma. Hyperesthesia, with excessive sensitivity to bright light, loud noise, touch, and even gentle breezes, is very common. On physical examination the temperature may be found to be as high as 40.6°C (105°F). Abnormalities of the autonomic nervous system include dilated, irregular pupils, increased lacrimation, salivation, perspiration, and postural hypotension. Evidence of upper motor neuron paralysis with weakness, increased deep tendon reflexes, and extensor plantar responses is the rule. Paralysis of the vocal cords is common.

The manifestations of brainstem dysfunction begin shortly after the onset of the encephalitic phase. Cranial nerve involvement causes diplopia, facial palsies, optic neuritis, and the characteristic difficulty with deglutition. The combination of excessive salivation and difficulty in swallowing produces the traditional picture of "foaming at the mouth." Hydrophobia, the painful, violent involuntary contraction of the diaphragm, accessory respiratory, pharyngeal, and laryngeal muscles initiated by swallowing liquids, is seen in about 50 percent of cases. Involvement of the amygdaloid nucleus may result in priapism and spontaneous ejaculation. The patient lapses into coma, and involvement of the respiratory center produces an apneic death. The prominence of early brainstem dysfunction distinguishes rabies from other viral encephalitides and accounts for the rapid downhill course. The median survival after the onset of symptoms is 4 days, with a maximum of 20, unless artificial supporting measures are instituted.

If intensive respiratory support is used, a number of late complications may appear and include inappropriate secretion of antidiuretic hormone, diabetes insipidus, cardiac arrythmias, vascular instability, adult respiratory distress syndrome, gastrointestinal bleeding, thrombocytopenia, and paralytic ileus. Recovery is very rare and when it occurs has been gradual. There have been only three well-documented nonfatal cases of rabies in humans. Two of these survivors received partial postexposure prophylaxis and the third, a case of laboratory-associated rabies, probably from an aerosol exposure, had received preexposure prophylaxis.

Occasionally, rabies may present as an ascending paralysis resembling the Landry-Guillain-Barré syndrome (dumb rabies, *rage tranquile*). This clinical pattern occurs most frequently in those bitten by vampire bats or who have received postexposure rabies prophylaxis.

The difficulty of suspecting rabies when it is associated with ascending paralysis is illustrated by the documentation of person-to-person transmission of the virus by tissue transplantation. Corneal transplants from donors who died of presumed Landry-Guillain-Barré syndrome have produced clinical rabies and death in the recipient. Retrospective pathologic examinations of the brains of both patients demonstrated Negri bodies, and rabies virus was subsequently isolated from each donor's frozen eye.

LABORATORY FINDINGS

Early in the disease the hemoglobin and routine blood chemistries are normal, but abnormalities occur as hypothalamic dysfunction, gastrointestinal bleeding, and other complications ensue. The peripheral white blood cell count is usually slightly elevated (12,000 to 17,000 per cubic millimeter) but may be normal or as high as 30,000 per cubic millimeter.

As in any viral infection, the specific diagnosis of rabies depends upon (1) the isolation of virus from infected secretions [saliva, rarely cerebrospinal fluid (CSF), or tissue (brain)], (2) the serologic demonstration of acute infection, or (3) the demonstration of viral antigen in infected tissue, e.g., corneal impression smears, skin biopsies, or brain. Samples of brain obtained either on postmortem examination or from brain biopsy should be subjected to (1) mouse inoculation studies for virus isolation, (2) fluorescent-antibody (FA) staining for viral antigen, and (3) histologic and/or electron microscopic examination for Negri bodies. While the mouse inoculation studies for virus isolation and direct FA staining for viral antigen are quite reliable and sensitive, if the patient's life has been prolonged and high levels of neutralizing antibody are present in serum and CSF, "autosterilization" may occur, and these tests may be negative. The use of FA staining of skin biopsies, corneal impression smears, and saliva for evidence of rabies antigen has been helpful in diagnosing rabies during life. Confirmation of these findings either serologically or by demonstration of virus in brain should be sought.

If the patient has not received antirabies immunization, then a fourfold rise in neutralizing antibody to rabies virus in serial serum samples is diagnostic. If the patient has received rabies vaccination, then a clue to the diagnosis may be obtained from the absolute titers of serum-neutralizing antibody and the presence of neutralizing antibody to rabies in CSF. Postexposure rabies prophylaxis rarely produces CSF-neutralizing antibody to rabies. If present, it is usually in low titer, e.g., less than 1:64, whereas CSF titers in human rabies may vary from 1:200 to 1:160,000.

DIFFERENTIAL DIAGNOSIS

There is little to distinguish rabies from other viral encephalitides, and the most helpful point in diagnosis is the history of exposure. Other problems to be considered include hysterical reactions to animal bites (pseudohydrophobia), Landry-Guillain-Barré syndrome, poliomyelitis, and allergic encephalomyelitis to rabies vaccine. The latter occurs most commonly after use of nerve tissue–derived vaccine and usually begins 1 to 4 weeks after vaccination.

PREVENTION AND TREATMENT

Each year more than 1 million Americans are bitten by animals. In each instance, a decision must be made whether to initiate postexposure rabies prophylaxis. When deciding whether to institute rabies prophylaxis, the following considerations apply: (1) whether the individual came into physical contact with saliva or another substance likely to contain rabies virus; (2) whether rabies is known or suspected in the species and area associated with the exposure (e.g., all persons within the continental United States bitten by a bat that then escapes should receive postexposure prophylaxis); (3) the circumstances surrounding the exposure; and (4) the treatment alternative and complications. A guide for postexposure rabies prophylaxis is illustrated in Fig. 142-1.

If rabies is known to be present or suspected to be present in the animal species involved in a human exposure, the animal should be captured, if possible. Captured wild animals or any ill, unvaccinated, or stray domestic animal involved in a rabies exposure, particularly any animal involved in an unprovoked bite, exhibiting abnormal behavior, or suspected of being rabid, should be captured and killed, and the head should be sent immediately to an appropriate laboratory for rabies FA examination. If examination of the brain by the FA technique is negative for rabies, it can be assumed that the saliva contains no virus, and the exposed person need not be treated. Persons exposed to escaped wild animals capable of carrying rabies (bats, skunks, coyotes, foxes, raccoons, etc.) in an area where rabies is known or suspected to be present should receive both passive and active immunization against rabies.

If a healthy dog or cat bites a person, the animal should be captured, confined, and observed for 10 days. If any illness or abnormal behavior develops in the animal during the observation period, it should be killed for FA examination.

Postexposure prophylaxis   Once a decision regarding the necessity to initiate postexposure rabies prophylaxis has been made, the general principle of postexposure therapy is to minimize the amount of virus at the site of inoculation with local treatment of the wound and to establish an early and long-lasting neutralizing antibody titer to rabies virus. In most instances, this includes administration of globulin and vaccines. The following therapeutic regimen is recommended:

1 Local wound therapy with generous scrubbing with soap and then flushing the wound with water is recommended. Both mechanical and chemical cleansing are important. Quaternary ammonium compounds such as 1 to 4% benzalkonium chloride or 1% cetrimonium bromide are also useful. However, 0.1% benzalko-

nium solutions are less effective than 20% soap solutions. Usually tetanus toxoid and antibiotics (generally penicillin) should be administered.

2 Passive immunization with antirabies antiserum of either equine or human origin. Human rabies immune globulin (RIG) is preferred because of the high incidence of serum sickness (20 to 40 percent) with the equine product. Fifty percent of the total dose of 20 units per kilogram for RIG and 40 units per kilogram for the equine antiserum is given by local infiltration of the wound, and the rest is administered intramuscularly.

3 Active immunization with antirabies vaccine. Human diploid cell vaccine (HDCV) is now the only available antirabies vaccine in the United States. HDCV is an inactivated vaccine prepared from a laboratory strain of rabies virus grown in human diploid cell cultures. The vaccine developed in Europe (Merieux Institute) is a whole-virus preparation. The HDCV developed in the United States is a subunit vaccine dissolved with tri-*n*-butyl phosphate and then inactivated with β-propiolactone. The Merieux product appears more immunogenic, and the Wyeth vaccine was recalled from the U.S. market in February 1985.

Severe reactions to HDCV are uncommon. Immediate hypersensitivity responses such as urticaria have been reported in approximately 1 in 650 recipients. Systemic reactions such as fever, headache, and nausea are generally mild and are reported in 1 to 4 percent of recipients. Local reactions such as swelling, erythema, and induration at the injection site occur in 15 to 20 percent of vaccinees.

Five 1-mL doses of HDCV are given intramuscularly (IM) as soon as possible after exposure. The first dose (day 0) should also be accompanied by antirabies serum (RIG) given in the opposite arm. Subsequent doses of HDCV are given on days 3, 7, 14, and 28. The WHO also recommends a 21- and 90-day dose.

To date, follow-up evaluation of over 575 persons with bites from confirmed rabid animals has shown that no person who has received HDCV in combination with RIG has developed rabies. All persons

FIGURE 142-1 *Postexposure rabies prophylaxis algorithm.*

*Livestock exposure and normally behaving unvaccinated dogs or cats should be
considered individually and local and state public health officials should be consulted.

treated with RIG and five 1.0-mL IM doses of HDCV have developed an adequate titer ($\geq$1:5 by the rapid fluorescent focus inhibition test). The combination of RIG plus 0.1-mL intradermal doses at eight sites on day 0, four sites on day 7, and one site on days 28 and 91 also produces good antibody responses.

Preexposure prophylaxis Individuals with a high risk of contact with rabies virus—veterinarians, spelunkers, laboratory workers, and animal handlers—should have preexposure prophylaxis with rabies vaccine. HDCV is the preferred vaccine for preexposure prophylaxis; three IM injections on days 0, 7, and 21 to 28 should be administered. Alternatively, three 0.1-mL doses intradermally in the skin overlying the deltoid region can be administered on the same days. A neutralizing antibody titer should be checked after vaccination. Booster doses may be administered either as a single 1-mL IM or 0.1-mL intradermal injection. Postexposure prophylaxis in individuals previously given preexposure therapy consists of HDCV vaccine alone (two IM doses of HDCV on days 0 and 3 are usually adequate).

Routine booster doses of vaccine at 2-year intervals have been recommended, but up to 6 percent of persons receiving IM booster doses of HDCV have developed an immune complex–like reaction characterized by urticaria, arthritis, nausea, vomiting, and, occasionally, angioedema. While these reactions have been self-limited in patients who develop them, consideration should be given to periodic measurement of antibodies. Booster doses are still recommended for those with low antibody titers who are at continued risk of exposure.

MARBURG VIRUS DISEASE

DEFINITION Marburg virus causes an acute systemic febrile illness characterized by the abrupt onset of headache, myalgias, pharyngitis, rash, and hemorrhagic manifestations. It was recognized first in 1967 when it caused simultaneous outbreaks in the Federal Republic of Germany and Yugoslavia among laboratory workers exposed to imported African green monkeys (*Cercopithecus aethiops*). More recent outbreaks have been reported from Kenya. The clinical manifestations are similar to other hemorrhagic fevers of the arenavirus class or flavivirus group (Argentina and Bolivian hemorrhagic fever, Chap. 144). The high case fatality rate and demonstrated ability for nosocomial spread has made recognition of this rare agent an important worldwide public health concern.

ETIOLOGY The Marburg virus has been isolated in guinea pig and various cell culture systems such as vervet monkey kidney. The virus particle contains lipid and RNA, and under the electron microscope the virus appears as an 80- to 100-nm elongated filamentous particle with occasional "blister-like excrescences." The Marburg virus exhibits some morphologic relationship to other members of the rhabdoviruses, e.g., rabies and Mokola viruses. However, physico-chemical studies indicate that the Marburg and Ebola agents (see below) appear unique. A proposal has been made to include them in a new family of agents (Filoviridae).

EPIDEMIOLOGY The initial outbreaks affected 31 patients in Marburg and Frankfurt, Germany, and Belgrade, Yugoslavia, and was epidemiologically linked to monkeys imported from the same source in Uganda. Virus was isolated from the blood and tissue of these monkeys. Of the 25 primary infections, there were seven deaths. Six secondary cases, involving two physicians, one nurse, a postmortem attendant, and the wife of a veterinarian, occurred. Person-to-person transmission was felt to take place via accidental needle sticks or abrasions, although respiratory and conjunctival infection could not be ruled out. The wife of one patient developed Marburg virus disease. Marburg virus was demonstrated in semen of the original patient, despite the presence of circulating antibody, and this secondary case is believed to have been acquired through sexual intercourse. The natural reservoir of Marburg virus is unknown. Serologic examination of a large number of primates in Uganda suggests that monkeys appear to be susceptible but incidental hosts.

PATHOLOGY Marburg virus appears "pantropic" and produces lesions in almost all organs including lymphoid tissue, liver, spleen, pancreas, adrenals, thyroid, kidney, testes, skin, and brain. In lymphoid tissue focal necrosis with degeneration of lymphoid tissue is apparent. In the liver, eosinophilic cytoplasmic bodies resembling the Councilman bodies of yellow fever have been noted. The lungs may show interstitial pneumonitis, as well as vascular lesions in small arterioles indicative of endarteritis. Neuropathologic changes consist of multiple small hemorrhagic infarcts with glial proliferation.

CLINICAL MANIFESTATIONS After an incubation period of 3 to 9 days, patients develop the abrupt onset of frontal and temporal headache, malaise, myalgias, especially in the lumbar area, nausea, and vomiting. Fever of 39.4 to 40°C (103 to 104°F) is characteristic, and about half the patients have conjunctivitis. Between 1 and 3 days after onset, watery diarrhea, which is often severe, lethargy, and a change in mentation are noted. An enanthem of the palate and tonsils, and cervical lymphadenopathy may also be noted during the first week of illness. The most reliable clinical feature is the appearance of nonpruritic maculopapular rash which begins on the fifth to seventh day on the face and neck and spreads centrifugally to involve the extremities. A fine desquamation of the affected skin, especially the palms and soles, appears 4 to 5 days later. Hemorrhagic manifestations, including gastrointestinal, renal, vaginal, and/or conjunctival hemorrhages, generally develop between days 5 and 7 of disease.

During the first week, the temperature continues in the vicinity of 40°C (104°F), falling by lysis during the second week, to increase again between the twelfth and fourteenth days. Other clinical signs apparent in the second week of disease include splenomegaly, hepatomegaly, facial edema, and scrotal or labial reddening. Complications include orchitis, which may lead to testicular atrophy, myocarditis with irregular pulse and electrocardiographic abnormalities, and pancreatitis. The overall case fatality rate has been about 25 percent, with death usually occurring during the eighth to sixteenth days of illness. Recovery is often protracted over a 3- to 4-week period, and during this period loss of hair, intermittent abdominal pain, poor appetite, and prolonged psychotic disturbances have been noted. Late sequelae including transverse myelitis and uveitis have been reported. Marburg virus has been isolated from the anterior eye chamber and semen nearly 3 months after onset of disease.

LABORATORY FINDINGS Abnormalities in granulocyte function are found, and leukopenia is detected as early as the first day, with leukocyte counts as low as 1000 per cubic millimeter, and a neutrophilia by the fourth day. Subsequently, atypical lymphocytes, as well as neutrophils exhibiting the characteristic of the Pelger-Huet anomaly, may appear. Thrombocytopenia appears early and is most marked, often less than 10,000 cells per cubic millimeter, between the sixth and twelfth days. In fatal cases, evidence of disseminated intravascular coagulation can be demonstrated. Hypoproteinemia, proteinuria, and azotemia may occur. Elevations in serum glutamic oxaloacetic transaminase (SGOT) and alanine aminotransferase (SGPT) are usual. Lumbar puncture may be normal or reveal a minimal pleocytosis. The erythrocyte sedimentation rate is usually low.

DIAGNOSIS The characteristic clinical course and epidemiologic features are the basis of the diagnosis. Specific diagnosis requires isolation of the virus or serologic evidence of infection in paired serum samples. Viremia coincides with the febrile state of disease, and virus has been isolated from tissue as well as urine, semen, throat, and rectal swabs. Attempts to isolate virus must be carried out only in *specialized high-security laboratories*. All patients should be kept in strict isolation, and all specimens should be handled and shipped according to World Health Organization guidelines.

TREATMENT Patients have received a multiplicity of drugs without apparent influence on the course of the illness. Convalescent serum was administered to four patients, whose subsequent disease followed a mild course. However, similarly benign outcomes were observed in patients who did not receive serum.

EBOLA VIRUS

Between July and November 1976 simultaneous outbreaks of an acute febrile hemorrhagic disease occurred in southern Sudan and northern Zaire. "Secondary and tertiary" spread of infection, particularly among hospital staff, was noted. In the Sudan over 300 cases with 151 deaths and in Zaire 237 cases with 211 fatalities were reported. The virus isolated from these patients was morphologically similar to but antigenically distinct from the Marburg agent. The name Ebola virus, after the river in Zaire located near the epidemic, has been proposed. Biologic and antigenic differences between strains of Ebola viruses isolated in Zaire and Sudan may account for the differences in mortality between the two outbreaks. Sporadic cases of disease also appear to occur, and a serosurvey revealed a prevalence rate of 7 percent for antibodies to Ebola virus in endemic areas. As with other hemorrhagic fevers, neutrophil leukocytosis, hypofibrinogine-mia, thrombocytopenia, and microangiopathic hemolytic anemia are features of the illness.

Ebola virus has been propagated in tissue culture (Vero cells) and in suckling mice and guinea pigs. The source of the outbreak in both the Sudan and Zaire is unknown; however, as with other viral hemorrhagic fevers, peridomestic rodents are suspected as being a reservoir of the infection, and serologic evidence of Ebola virus infection was detected in a domestic guinea pig trapped in Zaire. Once established, nosocomial as well as community-acquired cases occur, especially among those with close and prolonged contact. Parenteral exposure to the virus through disinfected rather than sterilized needles may have played a role in transmission. Barrier nursing and strict isolation precautions using protective clothing appeared to decrease the number of nosocomial cases.

CLINICAL MANIFESTATIONS   Clinically, the disease is similar to Marburg virus disease. The incubation period ranges from 4 to 6 days (mean is 7 days). Patients usually present on the fifth day of illness with a history of abrupt onset of headache, malaise, myalgias, high fever, diarrhea, abdominal pain, dehydration, and lethargy. Pleuritic chest pain, a dry hacking cough, and a pronounced pharyngitis were also noted. A maculopapular eruption develops between days 5 to 7 of illness. On black skins the rash is often faint and not recognized until desquamation occurs. Hematemesis, melena, and bleeding from the nose, gums, and vagina are common. Abortion and massive metrorrhagia was a frequent complication among pregnant women. Death usually occurs in the second week of illness and is preceded by severe blood loss and shock.

TREATMENT   Patients should be isolated until virologic studies indicate they are free of virus, usually 21 days from onset of illness. Malaria parasites were frequently found in blood films of patients with Ebola virus infection in the Sudan indicating that the presence of parasitemia does not rule out concomitant viral illness. Treatment with plasma containing Ebola virus–specific antibodies has resulted in diminished levels of viremia; however, further tests are required to establish the effectiveness of this form of therapy. Requests for viral isolation as well as convalescent plasma should be addressed to WHO Regional Centers in Atlanta or Geneva.

MOKOLA VIRUS

Mokola virus was first isolated from wild shrews captured in Nigeria and subsequently was shown to be related morphologically and serologically to rabies. However, neither of the two reported cases of human disease (both children) demonstrated classic clinical features of rabies. One patient had a nonfatal illness characterized by fever, pharyngitis, and convulsions. Mokola virus was recovered from her cerebrospinal fluid. The second patient initially had fever, cough, and vomiting, followed in several days by drowsiness, confusion, and generalized flaccid weakness. Her cerebrospinal fluid was normal. She progressed to deep coma and died within 10 days of onset.

Mokola virus was isolated from her brain, and histopathologic sections revealed finely granular cytoplasmic inclusions that were distinguishable from Negri bodies in many neurons.

VESICULAR STOMATITIS VIRUS

Vesicular stomatitis is a viral illness of animals which can occasionally infect humans. It presents as an acute self-limited influenza-like disease. The disease in animals is found in the United States and South America and affects chiefly domestic cattle, horses, swine, and wild deer, raccoons, skunks, and bobcats.

In animals, vesicular stomatitis is characterized by the development of vesicles on the oral mucosa, particularly the tongue, udders, and heels. The mode of spread is probably by direct contact; however, epidemics tend to occur in warm weather, and the virus has been isolated from *Phlebotumus* sandflies in Panama and *Äedes* species in New Mexico, suggesting these as possible vectors. Two distinct serotypes, New Jersey and Indiana, have been recognized, and most of the outbreaks in North America have been attributed to the New Jersey strain. The disease is most common in laboratory workers, and in one report three-fourths of laboratory personnel handling experimentally infected animals or manipulating the virus developed neutralizing antibodies. The disease is transmissible, however, under natural conditions among workers having direct contact with infected animals, especially cattle. The incubation period ranges from 1 to 6 days. This is followed by the sudden onset of fever, up to 40°C (104°F), chills, profuse sweating, myalgias, malaise, headache, and pain on ocular movement. One-third to one-half of patients have sore throat and cervical and/or submandibular adenopathy. Small raised vesicular lesions may appear on the buccal mucosa. Conjunctivitis and coryza are present in about 20 percent of cases. Occasionally, small subcorneal, intraepithelial vesicles may appear on the fingers, usually associated with direct inoculation of the virus. Symptoms generally last 3 to 4 days, but occasionally a diphasic course may occur. Inapparent infection is common, and among laboratory workers with serologic evidence of infection, only about one-half reported clinical symptoms. In some areas of Panama, 17 to 35 percent of the population have neutralizing antibodies against vesicular stomatitis virus.

The differential diagnosis includes hand-foot-and-mouth disease, herpangina, primary herpetic pharyngitis and other mucocutaneous syndromes, and influenza. Viral isolation from patients is not common; however, a rise in complement fixation and/or neutralizing antibodies to vesicular stomatitis virus between acute and convalescent serums will help to confirm the diagnosis. Treatment is nonspecific.

REFERENCES

Marburg virus

GEAR JSS et al: Outbreak of Marburg virus disease in Johannesburg. Br Med J 4:489, 1975
SIMPSON DIH: Marburg and ebola virus infections: A guide for their diagnosis, management and control. WHO Offset Publication no 36, Geneva, 1977
SMITH DH et al: Marburg-virus disease in Kenya. Lancet 1:816, 1982

Mokola virus

FAMILUSI JB: Fatal human infection with Mokola virus. Am J Trop Med Hyg 21:959, 1972

Rabies

ANDERSON LJ: Human rabies in the United States, 1960 to 1979. Epidemiology, diagnosis and prevention. Ann Intern Med 100:728, 1984
BAER GM: *The Natural History of Rabies*. New York, Academic, 1975
BAHMANYAR M: Successful protection of humans exposed to rabies: Post exposure treatment with the new human diploid cell rabies vaccine and antirabies serum. JAMA 236:2751, 1976
Compendium of Animal Rabies Vaccines, 1986. Morb Mort Week Rep 34:770, 1986
HATTWICK MA et al: Recovery from rabies: A case report. Ann Intern Med 76:931, 1972
HOUGH SA et al: Human-to-human transmission of rabies virus by a corneal transplant. N Engl J Med 300:603, 1979

PLOTKIN SA: Rabies vaccine prepared in human cell culture: Progress and perspectives. Rev Infect Dis 2:433, 1980

Rabies Prevention, United States, 1984. Morb Mort Week Rep 33:393, 1984

WARRELL MJ et al: Economical multiple site intradermal immunization with human diploid-cell-strain vaccine. Lancet 1:1059, 1985

Ebola virus

McCORMICK JB et al: Biologic differences between strains of Ebola virus from Zaire and Sudan. J Infect Dis 147:264, 1983

STANSFIELD SK: Antibody to Ebola virus in guinea pigs: Tandala, Zaire. J Infect Dis 146:483, 1982

143 ARBOVIRUS INFECTIONS

JAY P. SANFORD

Most viral infections in humans are either asymptomatic or present as undifferentiated illnesses characterized by fever, malaise, headache, and generalized myalgia. The similarities in clinical features between infections caused by viruses as dissimilar as the myxoviruses (e.g., influenza), the enteroviruses (e.g., poliovirus, coxsackievirus, echovirus), some of the herpesviruses (e.g., cytomegalovirus), and the arboviruses usually preclude an etiologic diagnosis based entirely on clinical manifestations without ancillary information regarding epidemiologic features and serologic findings. The purpose of this chapter is to direct attention to the ever-expanding list of viruses which produce febrile disease in humans. Because the number of agents is large, mention will be made of those which have been best documented, have demonstrated unusual features, or seem to be of greatest potential public health importance.

DEFINITION AND CLASSIFICATION The earliest efforts to classify viruses were based on common pathogenic properties (e.g., hepatitis viruses), common tropisms (e.g., respiratory viruses), or common ecologic characteristics (e.g., arboviruses). The definition of an arthropod-borne virus (arbovirus) was published in 1967 by the World Health Organization:

Arboviruses are viruses which are maintained in nature principally, or to an important extent, through biological transmission between susceptible vertebrate hosts by hematophagous arthropods; they multiply and produce viremia in the vertebrates, multiply in the tissues of arthropods, and are passed on to new vertebrates by the bites of arthropods after a period of extrinsic incubation.

From this definition it can be appreciated that the term *arbovirus* is used in the ecologic sense. Transmission by vectors is not correlated with virus architecture. Current approaches to taxonomy are based upon viral morphology, structure, and function. As a result, for taxonomic purposes, the term *arbovirus* has been eliminated.

The more than 250 antigenically distinct "arboviruses" are now grouped into five families (Table 143-1). The majority of agents contain single-stranded RNA, although some, such as the Reoviridae contain double-stranded RNA.

"Arboviruses" are of importance in both temperate and tropical zones. Representative viruses have been isolated in almost every geographic area outside the polar regions.

"Arbovirus" infection of vertebrates is usually asymptomatic. The viremia stimulates an immune response which sharply limits the duration of the viremia. In "arbovirus" infections other than urban yellow fever, phlebotomus fever, chikungunya, o'nyong-nyong, mayaro, oropouche, dengue, and possibly Ross River virus, infection of humans represents an incidental occurrence which is tangential to the basic maintenance cycle of the virus. Hence, the isolation of virus from arthropod vectors or the detection of infection in the natural vertebrate host may provide a means for early detection and enable control of epizootic infection before significant spread to humans occurs.

TABLE 143-1 Virus taxonomy and arboviruses-arenaviruses*

Family	Genus	Virus "English vernacular name"†
Reoviridae	Orbivirus	Colorado tick fever‡ Orongo Kemerovo

Togaviridae	Alphavirus (group A)	Eastern equine encephalitis‡
		Venezuelan encephalitis‡
		Western equine encephalitis‡
		Sindbis
		Semliki Forest complex
		  Chikungunya‡
		  O'nyong-nyong
		  Ross River‡
		  Mayaro

	Flavivirus (group B)	*Associated with encephalitis*
		St. Louis encephalitis‡
		Japanese encephalitis‡
		Murray Valley encephalitis‡
		Tick-borne encephalitis complex‡
		  Russian spring-summer encephalitis
		  Central European encephalitis
		  Negishi
		  Powassan‡
		  Louping-ill
		Rocio
		
		Associated with fever-arthralgia-rash
		Dengue fever‡
		West Nile fever‡
		Nine other agents–not of major public health importance
		
		Associated with hemorrhagic fever
		Yellow fever‡
		Dengue fever‡
		Omsk hemorrhagic fever
		Kyasanur Forest disease

Rhabdoviridae	Vesiculovirus	Vesicular stomatitis Indiana‡ Vesicular stomatitis New Jersey‡ Cocal Chandipura Piry Isfahan
	Lyssavirus	Rabies‡ Mokola Duvenhage
Filoviridae		Marburg‡ Ebola‡

Bunyaviridae	Bunyavirus (16 serogroups)	Twenty-four agents may cause fever, fever-rash. None cause death. None in United States.
		California serogroup
		  LaCrosse‡
		  Snowshoe hare
		  Jamestown Canyon
		  California encephalitis
		  Tahyna
		  Inkoo

	Phlebovirus	Thirty-seven phleboviruses isolated from human beings; none cause death except Rift Valley fever virus. Sandfly fever–Naples‡ Sandfly fever–Sicilian‡ Rift Valley fever‡
	Nairovirus	Crimean-Congo hemorrhagic fever‡
	Not yet established	Hantaan‡ Puumala‡ Prospect Hill‡ Tchoupitoulas‡
Arenaviridae	Arenavirus	Lymphocytic choriomeningitis‡ Lassa‡ Machupo‡ Junin‡

* Only agents which have been shown to naturally infect humans are tabulated.
† Virus species have not yet been designated formally. The International Committee on Taxonomy of Viruses lists species under the term "English vernacular name."
‡ Viruses found in the United States and/or of major public health importance.

Most human "arbovirus" infections are asymptomatic. When disease is produced, the spectrum of clinical illness is varied both in predominant features and in severity. Most commonly, disease is self-limited with symptoms of fever, headache, malaise, and myalgia. Associated lymphadenopathy may be a feature. "Arboviruses" which may cause three major clinical syndromes—arthralgia-arthritis, encephalitis–aseptic meningitis, or hemorrhagic disease—are tabulated in Table 143-2.

TABLE 143-2   Major clinical syndromes, associated arboviruses-arenaviruses, and major geographic distribution

Clinical syndrome*	Virus	Geographic distribution
Fever, arthralgia, rash	Chikungunya	Africa, southeast Asia
	O'nyong-nyong	East Africa
	Ross River	Australia, Fiji, Samoa, Cook Islands, New Guinea
	Sindbis	Africa, U.S.S.R., Finland, Sweden
	Mayaro	South and Central America
	Dengue fever	Tropical Asia, Oceania, Africa, Australia, Americas
	West Nile fever	Africa, Middle East, U.S.S.R., France, India, Indonesia
	Lymphocytic choriomeningitis	United States, Germany, Hungary, Argentina
Encephalitis/aseptic meningitis	Kemerovo	Central Europe
	Eastern equine encephalitis	Atlantic, Gulf coasts, United States, upper New York, Caribbean, western Michigan
	Venezuelan equine encephalitis	Northern South America, Central America, Mexico, Florida
	Western equine encephalitis	United States, Canada, Central and South America
	Semliki Forest	Africa
	St. Louis encephalitis	United States, Caribbean
	Japanese encephalitis	Japan, Korea, China, India, Philippines, southeast Asia, eastern U.S.S.R.
	Murray Valley encephalitis	Australia
	Rocio	Brazil
	Omsk hemorrhagic fever	U.S.S.R.
	Kyasanur Forest disease complex	India
	Negishi	Japan
	Powassan	New York, eastern Canada
	Louping ill	United Kingdom, Ireland
	Russian spring-summer encephalitis	U.S.S.R.
	Central European encephalitis	Eastern Europe, Scandinavia, France, Switzerland
	California group	North America
	Tahyna	Europe
	Inkoo	Europe
	Phlebotomus fever	Mediterranean basin, Balkans Near and Middle East, east Africa, central Asia, Pakistan, parts of India, southern China, Panama, Brazil
	Rift Valley fever	South and east Africa
	Lymphocytic choriomeningitis	United States, Germany, Hungary, Argentina
Hemorrhagic fever	Yellow fever	South America, Africa
	Dengue	Caribbean, southeast Asia
	Chikungunya	Southeast Asia
	Kyasanur Forest disease	India
	Omsk hemorrhagic fever	U.S.S.R.
	Crimean-Congo hemorrhagic fever	Africa, eastern Europe, Middle East, Asia
	Hantaan	Korea, Japan, Scandinavia, U.S.S.R., central Europe
	Marburg	Uganda, Kenya, Zimbabwe
	Ebola	Zaire, Sudan
	Lassa fever	West Africa
	Machupo	Bolivia
	Junin	Argentina

* Most agents are more often associated with undifferentiated febrile illness than with the specific syndrome. See text for exceptions.

"ARBOVIRUS" INFECTIONS PRESENTING CHIEFLY WITH FEVER, MALAISE, HEADACHE, AND MYALGIA Phlebotomus fever

Phlebotomus (sandfly, pappataci, or 3-day) fever is an acute, relatively mild, self-limited infection caused by at least five immunologically distinct phleboviruses (Naples, Sicilian, Punta Toro, Chagres, and Candiru). Serologic evidence of human infection has been demonstrated for four additional agents (Bujaru, Cacao, Karimabad, and Salehabad). Humans, the only known host, probably serve as a dead-end host. Voles are suspected of being an endemic host in the Middle East.

PREVALENCE   The disease occurs throughout the Mediterranean basin, the Balkans, the Near and Middle East, the eastern part of Africa, the Soviet republics of central Asia, Pakistan, parts of India, and possibly certain parts of southern China. Recently, sandfly fever has been recognized in Panama and Brazil. In the Middle East and central Asia native populations acquire the disease at an early age and develop and maintain high levels of immunity. Cases in Panama and Brazil are sporadic, occurring mainly in persons entering the forest. The apparent absence of phlebotomus fever in indigenous adult populations residing in areas where sandflies are abundant may present a deceptive picture of the actual risk to susceptible persons.

EPIDEMIOLOGY   In the Middle East and central Asia, the disease occurs during the hot, dry season (summer or autumn months) and is transmitted to human beings by the bite of infected sandflies (Phlebotomus papatasii), which are small (2- to 3-mm) urban flies that can penetrate ordinary house screens. Only the female bites and usually does so during the night. In persons who are not sensitive, there is neither pain nor local irritation after the bite; hence only about 1 percent of patients will remember having been bitten. In contrast, most of the human-biting sandflies (Lutzomyia sp.) of tropical America are sylvan in their habits. Transovarial and transstadial transmission of the virus has been demonstrated and in view of the low-titered and transient viremia in humans suggests the phlebotomine fly is both vector and reservoir. In humans, the incubation period averages 3 to 5 days. Viremia is present for at least 24 h before the onset of fever, but is not detectable for more than 2 days after the onset of illness.

CLINICAL MANIFESTATIONS   The onset of symptoms is abrupt in over 90 percent of patients, with the temperature rapidly rising to its highest point, which may vary from 37.8 to 40.1°C (100 to 105°F). Headache is nearly always present and often is accompanied by pain on moving the eyes and by retroorbital pain. Myalgia is common and may be localized to the chest, resembling pleurodynia, or to the abdomen. Other symptoms may include vomiting, photophobia, giddiness, neck stiffness, alteration or loss of taste, and arthralgia. Conjunctival injection is present in approximately one-third of patients. Small vesicles may be seen on the palate, and macular or urticarial rashes occur. The spleen is rarely palpable, and lymphadenopathy is absent. The pulse rate may be elevated in proportion to the temperature on the first day; thereafter bradycardia is often present. The fever persists 3 days in most patients, with gradual defervescence. Giddiness, weakness, and feelings of depression are frequently encountered during convalescence. Second attacks 2 to 12 weeks after the first occur in 15 percent of cases.

In common with other "arbovirus" infections, phlebotomus fever may be associated with aseptic meningitis. In one series, 12 percent of patients had symptoms and signs sufficient to warrant a lumbar puncture. Findings in these patients included pleocytosis, with an average cell count of 90 per cubic millimeter and a predominance of either polymorphonuclear or mononuclear leukocytes. Spinal fluid protein concentration ranged from 20 to 130 mg/dL. In another series mild papilledema was observed in a few patients with severe illness.

LABORATORY FINDINGS   The changes in leukocyte count constitute the only positive laboratory findings. Total leukocyte counts of less than 5000 per cubic millimeter are observed in 90 percent of patients if daily counts are done during the febrile period and convalescence.

The leukopenia may not appear until the last day of fever or even after defervescence. The differential leukocyte count will reveal an absolute decrease in lymphocytes on the first day, accompanied by an increase in nonsegmented neutrophils. During the second or third day, the number of lymphocytes begins to return to normal and may constitute 40 to 65 percent of the total count. Concurrently, there is a reversal in proportion of segmented and band neutrophils. The differential count usually returns to normal within 5 to 8 days after defervescence. Erythrocyte values and urinalyses are usually normal.

DIAGNOSIS In the absence of a specific serologic test, the diagnosis must be made on clinical and epidemiologic grounds.

TREATMENT The disease is self-limited, and no specific therapy is available. Symptomatic care, including bed rest, adequate fluid intake, and analgesia with aspirin, is recommended. Convalescence may require a week or longer.

PROGNOSIS No fatalities have been recorded among the tens of thousands of cases.

Colorado tick fever Colorado tick fever is one of the two tick-transmitted virus diseases of human beings recognized in the United States and Canada, Powassan virus being the other. Though "mountain fever" had been described ever since the advent of immigrants to the Rocky Mountain region, it must be differentiated from mild Rocky Mountain spotted fever. Once the clinical picture of disease had been established, it was renamed Colorado tick fever. A second serotype of the Colorado tick fever serogroup (Eyach virus) was isolated from *Ixodes ricinus* ticks near the village of Eyach in West Germany.

ETIOLOGY Colorado tick fever virus is grouped as an "arbovirus" because it replicates in ticks. It is a double-stranded RNA virus belonging to the orbivirus genus of the Reoviridae family (see Table 143-1).

PREVALENCE The disease has been contracted in Colorado, Idaho, Nevada, Wyoming, Montana, Utah, the eastern portions of Oregon, Washington, California, and northern portions of Arizona and New Mexico, and Alberta and British Columbia. The virus of Colorado tick fever has been isolated from the dog tick, *Dermacentor variabilis*, obtained from Long Island. This observation has not been confirmed, but suggests the possibility that Colorado tick fever may occur over a wider geographic area. Mild and clinically inapparent forms of the disease occur. Up to 15 percent of perennial campers have neutralizing antibodies. The number of cases of Colorado tick fever reported in Colorado is 20 times greater than that of Rocky Mountain spotted fever. In fact, almost one-half of the patients diagnosed as having Rocky Mountain spotted fever in Utah were subsequently shown to have Colorado tick fever.

EPIDEMIOLOGY Colorado tick fever is transmitted to humans by the adult hard-shelled wood tick, *Dermacentor andersoni*. The virus has been found in as many as 14 percent of this species of ticks collected in endemic areas. Transovarial transmission of the virus in the tick has been established. Illness occurs from late March through September, mostly in May and June. Virus can be recovered from blood for 2 weeks in most patients, for at least 1 month in nearly one-half, and from spinal fluid during the acute illness. The virus persists within erythrocytes of convalescent patients for as long as 120 days. Virus can be readily isolated from washed erythrocytes 100 days following infection. Transfusion-associated Colorado tick fever has been reported.

CLINICAL MANIFESTATIONS The incubation period is usually 3 to 6 days, and in 90 percent a history of tick contact within 10 days of onset of illness can be obtained. Failure to obtain such a history militates against the diagnosis. Persons affected usually are those whose occupational or recreational activities bring them in contact with ticks. The disease may occur at any age, although 40 percent in one series were 20 to 29 years of age. The clinical picture is characterized by the sudden onset of severe aching of the muscles of the back and legs, chilliness without true rigors, a rapid increase in temperature, which usually reaches 38.9 to 40°C (102 to 104°F), headache with pain on ocular movement, retroorbital pain, and photophobia. Abdominal pain and vomiting occur in one-fourth of patients; diarrhea is rare. The physical findings are not specific. Tachycardia in proportion to the temperature, flushed facies, and variable conjunctival injection may be present. Occasionally the spleen is palpable. Rash occurs in only 5 percent of patients, but on occasion a petechial rash involving primarily the arms and legs or a maculopapular rash over the entire body may occur. Rarely, punched-out ulcers may form at the site of tick bite. The fever with the associated symptoms lasts about 2 days, then abruptly lyses to normal or subnormal, leaving the patient very weak. After an afebrile period of about 2 days, the fever recurs, may be higher than in the first phase, and may last as long as 3 days. One-half of patients show this saddleback pattern of temperature. Rarely there may be three febrile phases. Convalescence of more than 3 weeks is reported in 70 percent of patients over age 30, while symptoms last less than 1 week in 60 percent of patients under 20. Prolonged convalescence has no relationship to persistent viremia.

Evidence of central nervous system involvement has been recorded in a few patients. The findings are those of either an aseptic meningitis with stiffness of the neck or encephalitis with clouding of the sensorium, delirium, and coma. Single instances of reported complications include epididymoorchitis and patchy pneumonitis.

The clinical manifestations of Eyach virus infection have not been elucidated. Antibodies to Eyach virus were found in patients with various neuropathies.

LABORATORY FINDINGS The most important laboratory feature is moderate to marked leukopenia, although in one-third of confirmed cases leukocyte counts remain about 4500 per cubic millimeter. On the first day of illness, the total leukocyte count may be at normal levels, but usually by the fifth or sixth day there has been a decrease to 2000 to 3000 per cubic millimeter. Characteristically there is a proportionate decrease in lymphocytes and granulocytes. Toxic changes in neutrophils are often conspicuous, and "virocyte" types of lymphocytes are frequently observed. Bone marrow examination reveals "maturation arrest" in the granulocytic series. Erythrocyte values remain normal. Thrombocytopenia has been recorded in an isolated case report. The blood picture returns to normal within a week after the fever subsides.

DIAGNOSIS The diagnosis of Colorado tick fever is suspected on the basis of the epidemiologic history and clinical findings. Because of the infrequency of rash, patients who develop fever and rash after tick bites should be suspected of having Rocky Mountain spotted fever. The usual methods for confirming Colorado tick fever are mouse inoculation and fluorescent antibody (FA) staining of patients' erythrocytes; a combination of the two is best. Special handling of blood is not necessary for the FA test which remains positive for several weeks after clinical illness.

TREATMENT Treatment is entirely symptomatic.

PROGNOSIS The prognosis is excellent.

PREVENTION Only one patient has been reported as having the disease twice. Active immunity with an attenuated virus has been produced, but the immunization itself frequently produced mild disease. Colorado tick fever is best prevented by avoiding contact with the wood tick. Convalescent individuals should be excluded as blood donors for at least 6 months.

Venezuelan equine encephalitis Venezuelan equine encephalitis (VEE) was first noted in equines in Colombia in 1935.

ETIOLOGY Like other alphaviruses, the causative agent of VEE is a 40- to 45-nm, single-stranded RNA virus. Based on serologic tests and oligonucleotide fingerprints a complex of Venezuelan encephalitis viruses has been established: VE subtypes IA to IE, II (Everglades),

III (Mucambo), and IV (Pixuna). IA was the original epidemic strain which occurred in Venezuela, and IB, which was recognized in Ecuador in 1963, spread through Central America into Mexico and was responsible for the epidemic in Mexico in 1971 which spread into southern Texas, with the occurrence of at least 76 laboratory-confirmed human cases. In early 1973, almost 4000 cases occurred in Peru.

EPIDEMIOLOGY   VEE has been primarily a disease of equines and other mammals, although occasionally the agent has infected humans. Evidence of human infection (virus isolation or specific neutralizing antibodies) has been found in Colombia, Ecuador, Panama, Surinam, Guyana, French Guiana, Mexico, Brazil, Curaçao, Trinidad, Argentina, Peru, Florida, and Texas. Each subtype of VE virus is unique to its enzootic vector and does not replicate well in other vectors. Most common is an enzootic cycle between *Culex* mosquitoes and forest rodents. Enzootic VEE infects people who enter the rain forest or swamps, rubber tappers, forestry workers, and military personnel on jungle maneuvers. During an epizootic, many species of mosquitoes can transmit virus, especially *Aëdes*, *Mansonia*, and *Psorophora*. The virus has a wide host range in wild mammals, with at least 20 genera, including capuchin monkeys, rats, mice, opossum, jackrabbit, fox, and bats, being naturally infected. Domestic animals other than equines which have been shown to be infected include cattle and pigs in Mexico and goats and sheep in Venezuela. VEE appears to multiply well in mammals with high titers of virus in the blood; e.g., infected horses may have titers of up to $10^{7.5}$ mouse intraperitoneal lethal doses per milliliter of blood. Though 29 species of wild birds have been shown to be naturally infected with VEE (20 percent of which are colonial nestling herons and related species), whether the VEE-viremia levels in birds are high enough to infect vector mosquitoes is not known. During the initial 3 days of illness, viremia has been detected in approximately two-thirds of patients. The levels of viremia are sufficiently high that humans could serve as a reservoir. VEE virus also has been isolated by pharyngeal swab in a few patients, suggesting the potential for person-to-person transmission. The available observations make it reasonable to consider that the natural vector is a mosquito, with the primary reservoir being either wild or domestic terrestrial mammals. However, natural infection can probably take place without an arthropod vector. Laboratory infections have occurred and are probably due to inhalation of aerosols.

CLINICAL MANIFESTATIONS   In humans, infection with VEE virus usually results in a mild acute febrile illness without neurologic complications. No age is spared, and there is no sex preponderance. The incubation period is 2 to 5 days, followed by the abrupt onset of headache, fever often associated with rigors, malaise, and myalgia. Other common symptoms may include nausea, vomiting, diarrhea, and sore throat. Uncommon features include photophobia, seizures, mental confusion, coma, tremors, and diplopia. Lymphadenopathy occurs in one-third of patients. On laboratory examination initial leukocyte counts are normal with 80 percent neutrophils. By the third day leukopenia occurs in two-thirds of patients. The cerebrospinal fluid may reveal pleocytosis with modest increases in protein concentration and normal glucose concentration. Virus may be isolated both from blood and from cerebrospinal fluid. The symptoms usually last 3 to 5 days in mild cases and up to 8 days in more severe cases, although one patient reported from Florida was febrile for 3 weeks. A biphasic course of illness may be encountered, with recrudescence of symptoms at the sixth to the ninth day. In one case report, palatine petechiae were noted and the patient vomited "coffee-grounds" material. In an epidemic in Venezuela in 1962, almost 16,000 cases of acute disease were evaluated; 38 percent were classified as encephalitis, but only 3 to 4 percent had severe neurologic abnormalities: convulsions, nystagmus, drowsiness, delirium, or meningitis. The mortality rate was estimated to be less than 0.5 percent, and nearly all deaths occurred in young children.

Rift Valley fever   Rift Valley fever is an acute disease principally of livestock, sheep, goats, cattle, and camels which is widespread throughout east and South Africa. It was first described in humans during an extensive epizootic of hepatitis in sheep in the Rift Valley in Kenya. During an epizootic in South Africa in 1950–1951, an estimated 20,000 humans became infected. Fatal human disease, four cases of hemorrhagic illness and hepatitis, was first reported during an epizootic in South Africa in 1975. In 1977 Rift Valley fever jumped the Sahara to Egypt with a major outbreak. Cases occurred in subsequent years until 1980; an estimated 200,000 cases with 598 reported deaths occurred in 1977. At least one case has been reported in a Canadian tourist.

Virus has been found in several species of mosquitoes: *Culex pipiens*, *Eretmapodites chrysogaster*, *Aëdes caballus*, *Aëdes circumluteolus*, and *Culex theileri*. *Culex pipiens* has been suggested as the vector in Egypt. While antibodies to Rift Valley fever have been found in wild field rats in Uganda, the reservoir is unknown. It has been suggested that the virus may be maintained by transovarial transmission in floodwater *Aëdes*. Although humans presumably can be infected by arthropods, many infections occur as a result of handling infected animal tissues. In addition, laboratory-acquired infections have been common, suggesting a respiratory route of transmission.

The incubation period is usually 3 to 6 days. The onset is abrupt, with malaise, chilly sensation or rigors, headache, retroorbital pain, and generalized aching and backache. The temperature rises rapidly to 38.3 to 40°C (101 to 104°F). Later complaints include anorexia, loss of taste, epigastric pain, and photophobia. Findings on examination are usually unremarkable except for flushing of the face and conjunctival injection. The temperature curve is often saddleback in type, with an initial elevation lasting 2 to 3 days, followed by a remission and second febrile period. Convalescence is typically rapid. Prior to the outbreak in Egypt, Rift Valley fever was a benign illness with almost no fatalities. In Egypt, approximately 1 percent of patients developed severe complications, such as encephalitis, retinopathy, or hemorrhagic manifestations. Encephalitis appeared as the acute infection waned and was severe with serious residua in some survivors. Hemorrhagic manifestations appeared as the disease evolved with generalized hemorrhages and icterus. Deaths from massive hepatic necrosis occurred 7 to 10 days after onset of illness. The fatality rate in severely ill patients may exceed 50 percent. Visual loss, including light perception, occurred 2 to 7 days after the onset of fever. Macular edema, hemorrhage, vasculitis, retinitis, and vascular occlusion were noted. One-half of patients had some permanent loss of visual acuity. A characteristic finding is an initial normal total leukocyte count followed by leukopenia with a decrease in neutrophils associated with an increase in band forms. The diagnosis is made by isolating the virus from the blood by inoculation of mice. Three-fourths of patients are viremic (up to 10^8 mouse intraperitoneal lethal doses per milliliter blood) when first seen. Neutralizing antibodies have been demonstrated as early as 4 days after onset. There is no specific treatment. A killed vaccine which had been stockpiled in the United States is being utilized.

Zika virus   Zika virus was first isolated from a captive rhesus monkey in Uganda and subsequently from wild mosquitoes. Serologic surveys reveal a prevalence of human infection up to 50 percent in central Africa and parts of Asia (Indonesia), but human disease is rarely reported. During investigation in eastern Nigeria of an outbreak of jaundice that was suspected of being yellow fever, physicians isolated Zika virus from one patient and noted that two others had a rise in neutralizing antibodies. The symptoms in these patients included fever, arthralgia, and headache with retroorbital pain. Jaundice was present in one, and bile was demonstrated in the urine of another. Albuminuria was noted in one patient. Prothrombin times were normal. The clinical syndrome appears to simulate mild yellow fever.

Bunyaviruses   The family Bunyaviridae consists almost entirely of viruses transmitted to vertebrate animals by arthropods. There are more than 200 viruses in the family, classified into five genera: Bunyavirus (formerly the Bunyamwera supergroup), Uukuvirus, Nairovirus, phlebovirus, Hantaan virus (Table 143-1). The majority of Bunyaviruses were isolated in exploratory surveys of tropical ecosystems in South America, southeast Asia, and Africa. Most Bunyaviruses have not been associated with human infection or disease. Currently, 24 Bunyaviruses have been associated with febrile human disease which may or may not be associated with rashes. This includes the C group, Bunyamwera and Oropouche. The geographic distribution of C-group viruses includes Brazil, Trinidad, and Panama. Isolates have been obtained mostly from forest workers and laboratory technicians. Epidemics have not been recognized. The disease begins with headache, fever [with temperature up to 40.6°C (105°F)], and myalgia. Additional symptoms include malaise, photophobia, vertigo, and nausea. Illness is generally mild, lasting 2 to 4 days, and is occasionally followed by a relapse. No fatalities have been reported. Occasionally a prolonged period of convalescence ensues. Leukopenia, with total leukocyte counts as low as 2600 per cubic millimeter, is a common finding. Diagnosis has been established mainly by virus isolation.

Representative viruses of the Bunyamwera group are found in all inhabited continents except Australia. Only five viruses of the group—Bunyamwera itself, Germiston, Ilesha, Guaroa, and Wycomyia—have been associated with clinical disease. Serologic surveys give evidence of a high prevalence of inapparent infection in some areas. Clinical illness is characterized by low-grade fever, headache, and myalgia which last several days, and may be followed by weakness during convalescence. Infection due to Bunyamwera virus is associated often with arthralgia and sometimes with a rash. Since 1962 seven epidemics of Oropouche disease involving thousands of persons in Brazil, in the populated regions south of the Amazon River, have occurred. Outbreaks occurred during the rainy season. The epidemic vector is the midge of *Culicoides paraensis*. The incubation period is 4 to 8 days. Clinical features include abrupt onset of fever, usually to 39 to 40°C (102 to 104°F), with rigors. Symptoms, which include headache, photophobia, dizziness, myalgia, anorexia, nausea, and vomiting, last 2 to 5 days. Lymphadenopathy, splenomegaly, or rash have not been features. Laboratory findings include leukopenia with relative lymphocytosis. Urinalyses are normal. Mild elevations of transaminase may occur. Fatalities have not been reported.

"ARBOVIRUS" INFECTIONS PRESENTING CHIEFLY WITH FEVER, MALAISE, ARTHRALGIA, AND RASH Chikungunya

In 1952 an epidemic of a disease occurred in Tanzania, which was given the name *chikungunya* ("that which bends up") because of the sudden onset of joint pains. An alphavirus of the Semliki Forest complex was isolated in 1956 both from serum of patients ill with the disease and from a pool of *A. aegypti* mosquitoes.

Chikungunya virus is responsible for a dengue-like illness in Africa, India, southeast Asia, New Guinea, and Guam, as well as for a rather mild form of hemorrhagic fever in Asiatic children. Outbreaks have been associated with high attack rates, with as many as 80 percent of inhabitants in some settlements becoming ill. In large epidemics, *Aëdes aegypti* is the vector. In Africa, virus is transmitted among monkeys and baboons by forest *Aëdes* mosquitoes, *A. africanus*. The cycle in southeast Asia has not been clearly defined, but humans may be the host.

After an incubation period of 3 to 12 days, the onset is typically abrupt, with a rapid rise in temperature to 38.9 to 40.6°C (102 to 105°F), often associated with a rigor and headache. Pain in large joints occurs early, incapacitating some individuals within a few minutes of onset. The arthralgia is often associated with objective arthritis. Sites of involvement include knees, ankles, shoulders, wrists, or proximal interphalangeal joints. Myalgia, especially backache, and malaise occur frequently. In 60 to 80 percent of patients a maculopapular eruption, which may appear at any time during the febrile course, is noted on the trunk or on the extensor surfaces of the extremities. Mild lymphadenopathy, predominantly in the axillary

or inguinal areas, may be evident. Pharyngitis and conjunctival suffusion may be observed in a few patients. Fever continues for 1 to 10 days, and in some patients an afebrile interval of 1 to 3 days is followed by a secondary rise in temperature. The joint pains may continue after the temperature has returned to normal. In a few individuals joint pains have persisted for up to 4 months. Hematocrit values remain normal. Total leukocyte counts may be less than 5000 per cubic millimeter in some patients, while in others they remain normal. Urinalyses are normal. There is no specific antiviral treatment. Anti-inflammatory agents such as aspirin or indomethacin have been utilized. No second attacks have been recognized, and in the absence of the hemorrhagic fever syndrome, no deaths have been described.

Mayaro virus disease Outbreaks involving a number of persons have occurred in Brazil and Bolivia. Survey for antibodies in serums obtained from residents in Rio de Janeiro showed that almost one-third were positive. Mayaro virus has been isolated from a wild mosquito, *Mansonia venezuelansis*, and can be maintained serially in *A. aegypti* and *Anopheles quadrimaculatus*.

The incubation period has not been clearly defined but is about 1 week. Ages of patients have ranged from 2 to 62 years, with both sexes involved. Illness begins abruptly with fever, chills, severe frontal headache, myalgia, and dizziness. Temperatures usually exceed 40°C (104°F). Arthralgia occurs uniformly and is very prominent, occasionally incapacitating, and in some patients precedes the fever by a few hours. Involvement of the wrists, fingers, ankles, and toes predominates. Other initial symptoms (in less than one-third of patients) include nausea, vomiting, and diarrhea. Initial examination reveals inguinal lymphadenopathy (one-half of cases), swelling of affected joints (one-quarter of cases), and occasional conjunctival congestion. The initial clinical features last 3 to 5 days except the arthralgia, which may persist for 2 months. On about the fifth day a maculopapular rash develops over the chest, back, arms, and legs. Rash appeared in 90 percent of children and in one-half of adults and lasted about 3 days.

Laboratory findings include leukopenia with leukocyte counts as low as 2500 per cubic milliliter during the first week. Urinalysis revealed albuminuria (2+) in one-fourth of patients. Some patients showed slight elevations in serum glutamic oxaloacetic transaminase levels.

In Brazil, no relapses were observed and no deaths have been recognized. In Bolivia, more severe illness and several fatalities have been reported.

O'nyong-nyong fever O'nyong-nyong fever was first noted as an epidemic illness characterized by joint pains, rash, and lymphadenopathy in the northern province of Uganda in 1959. The agent is an alphavirus which shows close antigenic relationships with chikungunya viruses. The original outbreak was associated with an explosive epidemic which spread to Tanzania and other areas in east Africa. By 1961, 2 million cases were recorded. In some areas, 91 percent of the population had either clinical disease or inapparent infection. Local outbreaks extended over the entire year. All age groups were affected. The most likely vector is *Anopheles funestus*. The clinical features are similar to those of chikungunya virus infection. The disease disappeared in 1962. While the virus was isolated from *A. funestus* in Kenya in 1978, no further outbreaks have been recognized.

Sindbis virus Sindbis virus, once thought rarely to present as clinical disease, has been recognized in Africa (Uganda, Republic of South Africa), Australia, and Europe (U.S.S.R., Finland, and Sweden). In the U.S.S.R. it is known as Karelian fever, in Sweden as Okelbo disease, and in Finland as Pogosta disease. Clinically, fever is low-grade and accompanied by malaise, myalgia, and arthralgia involving joints and tendons. The most striking feature is a maculopapular rash appearing on the trunk and extremities but usually sparing the face. Unlike the rash of chikungunya or o'nyong-nyong, the rash often becomes vesicular, especially on the feet and hands.

Ross River virus Epidemics of polyarthritis associated with rashes have been observed in Australia since 1928. Outbreaks occur almost entirely in the period December to June. Ross River virus infection was limited to Australia, New Guinea, and the Solomon Islands until 1979 when a major outbreak occurred in Fiji which spread to the Samoan, Cook, and some Melanesian Islands. In the Fiji outbreak in 1979, infection rates were equal at all ages and in both sexes, but clinical attack rates were 4 percent in patients under 20 years of age and 42 percent in adults, and the clinical attack rate of males to females was 1:1.7. The onset is characterized by headache, mild catarrh, and occasionally tenderness of the palms and soles. Initially fever may be absent or minimal [highest 38°C (100.4°F)]. In about one-half of patients, arthritis, involving mainly the small joints, wrists, and ankles and sometimes associated with swelling, and paresthesias precede a rash by 1 to 15 days. In the other half, the rash precedes the arthralgia. The rash, which lasts 2 to 10 days, is usually maculopapular, appears on the cheeks and forehead, occasionally spreads to the trunk, or may be restricted to the limbs. The rash may be pruritic. Vesicles occur rarely. Tender lymphadenopathy occurs in one-fifth of the patients. Joint symptoms persist for 3 weeks to 3 months. The presence of antibody early in the clinical course suggests an immunopathogenesis. Infection has not been associated with fetal loss or congenital anomalies in children. The virus has been isolated from *Culex annulirostris* and *Aëdes vigilax*. Animals may serve as reservoir hosts in Australia. In the Pacific, person-mosquito-person transmission seems likely.

Other "arboviruses" Bunyamwera viruses occasionally have been associated with the syndrome of rash and arthralgia.

"ARBOVIRUS" INFECTIONS PRESENTING CHIEFLY WITH FEVER, MALAISE, LYMPHADENOPATHY, AND RASH Dengue fever

Dengue is endemic over large areas of the tropics and subtropics, southeast Asia, the South Pacific, and Africa. Outbreaks of dengue have occurred in the Caribbean including Puerto Rico and the U.S. Virgin Islands since 1969. Approximately 3000 cases were reported in Mexico in 1979. Indigenous infection occurred in the United States for the first time in 35 years in the fall of 1980. Eleven cases have been recognized in residents of the Rio Grande valley of Texas. In the summer of 1981, 79,000 cases of dengue-like illness with 31 deaths were reported from Cuba. *Aëdes aegypti*, the vector, has reappeared along the U.S. Gulf Coast; hence, the threat of dengue along the Gulf Coast is real.

ETIOLOGY There are four distinct serogroups of dengue viruses, types 1, 2, 3, and 4, all of which are flaviviruses. In the Caribbean, type 1 was associated with the 1977–1978 outbreak, type 2 in 1968–1969, type 3 in 1963–1964, and type 4 was documented in the western hemisphere for the first time in 1981.

EPIDEMIOLOGY Dengue infections in nature involve primarily human beings and *Aëdes* mosquitoes. Dengue transmission involving monkeys and forest *Aëdes* spp. has been documented in Malaysia and West Africa. *Aëdes aegypti* is the most important worldwide vector species. This species, as well as the less common vector species, is peridomestic, biting humans readily or even preferentially and breeding in small collections of water such as cisterns and backyard litter. Surveys in Texas have revealed containers with water in which *A. aegypti* were breeding in up to 25 percent of premises. They fly during the day. Humans appear to be uniformly susceptible, and susceptibility is not influenced by age, sex, or race. During outbreaks, attack rates may be very high; in Puerto Rico and the U.S. Virgin Islands, the overall rate of clinical illness was 20 percent, with infection rates as determined by serologic survey as high as 79 per 100.

CLINICAL MANIFESTATIONS Dengue viruses frequently produce inapparent infections in humans. When symptoms develop, three broad clinical patterns may be encountered: classic dengue, hemorrhagic fever (see below), and a mild atypical form. Classic dengue (breakbone

fever) occurs primarily in nonimmune individuals, specifically nonindigenous adults and children. The usual incubation period is 5 to 8 days. Prodromal symptoms such as mild conjunctivitis or coryza may occur, followed in hours by the abrupt onset of a severe splitting headache, retroorbital pain, backache, especially in the lumbar area, and leg and joint pains. The headache is aggravated by movement. At least three-fourths of patients have ocular soreness, with pain on moving the eyes. A few have mild photophobia. Though true rigors are common during the course, they are usually not present at the onset. Additional symptoms include insomnia, anorexia with loss of taste or bitter taste, and weakness. Mild transient rhinopharyngitis occurs in as many as one-quarter of the individuals. Cough is almost never seen. Epistaxis has been observed. Examination reveals scleral injection (90 percent), tenderness upon pressure on the ocular globe, and nontender posterior cervical, epitrochlear, and inguinal lymphadenopathy. Over one-half of patients have an enanthem characterized initially by pinpoint-sized vesicles over the posterior half of the soft palate. The tongue is often coated. Skin rashes, varying from diffuse flushing to scarlatiniform and morbilliform, are frequently present over the thorax and inner aspects of the arms. These are transient and fade, only to be followed by a more definite maculopapular rash which appears on the trunk on the third to the fifth day and spreads peripherally. The rash may be pruritic and generally terminates with desquamation. Extreme bradycardia is not observed. Within 2 to 3 days after the onset, the temperature may decrease to nearly normal and other symptoms disappear. The remission typically lasts 2 days and is followed by return of fever and the other symptoms, although they are generally less severe than during the initial phase. This "saddleback" diphasic febrile course is considered characteristic, but often is not encountered. The febrile illness usually lasts 5 to 6 days and terminates abruptly. Complaints of fatigue for several weeks after infection are common.

In addition to this "classic" syndrome, an atypically mild illness may occur. Symptoms include fever, anorexia, headache, and myalgia. On examination, evanescent rashes may be seen, but lymphadenopathy is usually absent. The course is usually less than 72 h in duration.

At the onset both in classic and in mild dengue, the leukocyte counts may be low or normal; however, by the third to the fifth day, leukopenia, usually with counts of less than 5000 leukocytes per cubic millimeter, and neutropenia are usually seen. Occasionally albuminuria of moderate degree occurs.

DIAGNOSIS Inoculation of blood obtained within the first 3 to 5 days onto mosquito tissue cell cultures or inoculation into mosquitoes is used for primary viral isolation. Diagnosis can be made by serologic tests employing paired serums for hemagglutination inhibition tests and complement fixation tests. IgM antibodies are produced in primary dengue infections. Specific serologic diagnosis is complicated by cross-reactions with other flavivirus antibodies such as those following immunization with yellow fever vaccine.

TREATMENT Treatment is entirely symptomatic.

PROGNOSIS In the absence of the dengue hemorrhagic fever or dengue shock syndrome, mortality is nil.

PREVENTION An attenuated vaccine for dengue type 2 is undergoing early experimental evaluation. Control depends upon mosquito abatement.

West Nile fever West Nile virus is distributed throughout Africa, the Middle East, parts of Europe (Camargue, France), U.S.S.R., India, and Indonesia. It produces a clinical picture closely resembling dengue. Outbreaks of disease involving several hundred patients occurred in Israel in 1950 to 1952. In one outbreak, over 60 percent of the population developed overt disease.

EPIDEMIOLOGY The disease is highly endemic in Egypt but goes largely unrecognized. Presumably most of the adult population is immune, and the infection in childhood is an undifferentiated mild febrile illness, whereas in Israel it mainly affects adults. The infection occurs in the summer both in Israel and in Egypt. The transmission cycle in the Middle East is bird-to-mosquito-to-bird, with *Culex univittatus* and *Culex pipiens molestus* being the principal vectors. *Culex tritaeniorhynchus* is an important vector in Asia. Although humans and a variety of other vertebrates are infected by the virus, their involvement is tangential.

CLINICAL MANIFESTATIONS The incubation period is 1 to 6 days. Most of the patients in Israel have been young adults, with neither sex predominating. The onset is usually abrupt and without prodromal symptoms. The temperature quickly rises to 38.3 to 40°C (101 to 104°F), with chills occurring in one-third of patients. Symptoms include drowsiness, severe frontal headache, ocular pain, and pain in the abdomen and back. A small number of patients have anorexia, nausea, and dryness of the throat. Cough is uncommon. Signs observed include flushing of the face, conjunctival injection, and coating of the tongue. The prominent finding is general enlargement of lymph nodes, which are of moderate size but are not hard and are only slightly tender. Occipital, axillary, and inguinal nodes are usually involved. The spleen and liver are slightly enlarged in a small proportion of patients. In one-half the patients a rash may appear from the second to the fifth day of illness and may persist for several hours or until defervescence. The rash occurs predominantly over the trunk and consists of pale roseolar maculopapular lesions. The illness is self-limited and lasts 3 to 5 days in 80 percent of patients.

In a few patients, transitory meningeal involvement may be encountered. Spinal fluid examinations may reveal a pleocytosis and some increase in protein concentration.

Leukopenia occurs in the majority of patients, and total leukocyte counts are lower than 4000 per cubic millimeter in one-third. Differential counts vary from a moderate shift to the left to a slight lymphocytosis.

Convalescence is often prolonged, lasting 1 to 2 weeks, with prominent symptoms of fatigue. Enlargement of lymph nodes subsides over several months. Only rarely have complications, sequelae, or fatalities been seen in natural infections, although in one outbreak in a group of elderly patients a high proportion of patients developed meningoencephalitis, and four fatalities ensued.

Accurate diagnosis rests on virus isolation, which can be accomplished because viremia persists for as long as 6 days, or the demonstration of a rising specific antibody titer.

The treatment is symptomatic.

"ARBOVIRUS" INFECTIONS PRESENTING CHIEFLY WITH CENTRAL NERVOUS SYSTEM INVOLVEMENT

Four "arboviruses" are presently recognized as numerically important causes of central nervous system disease in the United States: St. Louis encephalitis virus (SLE), eastern equine encephalitis virus (EEE), western equine encephalitis virus (WEE), and the California serogroup (CE) viruses. The spectrum of infection caused by these agents includes inapparent infection, fever with headache, aseptic meningitis, and encephalitis. Some 1500 to 2000 cases of encephalitis are reported in the United States each year. In the absence of epidemics, 5 to 10 percent of these (75 to 200 cases) are confirmed as "arboviral" in etiology. In nonepidemic years, California serogroup viruses (predominantly LaCrosse virus) represent two-thirds to three-fourths of the cases. Because of epidemics of St. Louis and western equine encephalitis, which contribute larger numbers of cases, the overall distribution in the 30 years between 1955 and 1984 has been: SLE 65 percent, CE 20 percent, WEE 13 percent, and EEE 2 percent.

ETIOLOGY Despite the diversity of specific viral etiologies (see Table 143-2), in individual patients the clinical manifestations of aseptic meningitis and encephalitis are very similar, and preclude an etiologic diagnosis without ancillary information regarding epidemiologic and serologic features (see Table 143-3). The clinical features of aseptic meningitis due to "arboviruses" are indistinguishable from those due to the more prevalent enteroviruses. Since transmission to humans in the United States and Canada involves arthropods, specifically mosquitoes, except for Powassan and Colorado tick fever, indigenously acquired disease occurs at times when mosquitoes are prevalent, such as late spring through early fall. The broad clinical picture of "arbovirus" encephalitis will be discussed; then the specific epidemiologic and prognostic features which characterize the major types will be presented.

CLINICAL MANIFESTATIONS The clinical features of "arbovirus" encephalitis differ among age groups. In infants under 1 year of age, the only consistently noted symptoms are sudden onset of fever, which is often accompanied by convulsions. Convulsions may be either generalized or focal. Typically the fever ranges between 38.9 and 40°C (102 and 104°F). Other physical findings may include bulging of the fontanelle, rigidity of the extremities, and abnormalities in reflexes.

In children between 5 and 14 years of age, subjective symptoms are more easily elicited. Headache, fever, and drowsiness of 2 to 3 days' duration before medical attention is sought are common. The symptoms may then subside or become more intense and may be associated with nausea, vomiting, muscular pain, photophobia, and, less frequently, convulsions (less than 10 percent except in California encephalitis). On examination, the child is found to be acutely ill, febrile, and lethargic. Nuchal rigidity and intention tremors are often present, and on occasion muscular weakness can be demonstrated.

In adults, the initial symptoms commonly include the fairly abrupt onset of fever, nausea with vomiting, and severe headache. The headache is most often frontal but may be occipital or diffuse in location. Mental aberrations, represented by confusion and disorientation, usually appear within the subsequent 24 h. Other symptoms may include diffuse myalgia and photophobia. The abnormalities found on physical examination predominantly relate to the neurologic examination, although conjunctival suffusion is frequently seen and skin rashes may occur. Disturbances in mentation are among the most outstanding clinical features. These range from coma through severe disorientation to subtle abnormalities detected only by cerebral function tests such as the subtraction of serial 7s. A small proportion

TABLE 143-3 Features of arboviral encephalitides common in the United States

Etiology	Geographic predominance in the United States	Urban/ rural	Age, years	Sex	Unique clinical features	Mortality, %	Residua
California encephalitis	Midwest	Rural	5–10	M	Seizures	2	Seizures (one-fourth who had them in acute phase), behavioral problems (15%)
Eastern equine encephalitis	Eastern seaboard	Both	<5 >55	=	CSF may have >1000 WBC/ mm³	50	Children <10 years have emotional lability, retardation, convulsions
St. Louis encephalitis	Eastern and midwest	Both	>35	=	Dysuria	2–12	Ataxia, speech difficulties (5%)
Western equine encephalitis	Entire	Both	<1 >55	=	None	3	Children <3 months have behavioral problems, convulsions

of patients show only lethargy, lying quietly, apparently asleep unless stimulated. Tremor is common and is observed more frequently in individuals over 40 years of age. The tremors vary in location and may be continuous or intention in type. Cranial nerve abnormalities resulting in oculomotor muscle paresis and nystagmus, facial weakness, and difficulty in deglutition may occur and are usually present within the initial several days. Objective sensory changes are unusual. Hemiparesis or monoparesis may occur. Reflex abnormalities are also common; these include exaggerated palmomental reflexes, and suck and snout reflexes. Superficial abdominal and cremasteric reflexes are usually absent. Changes in the tendon reflexes are variable and inconstant. The plantar response may be extensor and fluctuates almost hourly. Dysdiadochokinesia often exists.

The duration of the fever and neurologic symptoms and signs varies from several days to a month but usually ranges from 4 to 14 days. Clinical improvement generally follows the subsidence of the fever within several days unless irreversible anatomic changes have occurred.

LABORATORY FINDINGS   Erythrocytes are usually normal. Total leukocyte counts often reveal both a slight to moderate leukocytosis (occasionally greater than 20,000 leukocytes per cubic millimeter) and neutrophilia. Examination of the cerebrospinal fluid usually reveals several hundred cells per cubic millimeter, but on occasion cloudy cerebrospinal fluid with cells in excess of 1000 per cubic millimeter may be seen. Within the first several days of illness, polymorphonuclear neutrophils may predominate. The initial cerebrospinal fluid protein is usually only slightly elevated but on occasion may exceed 100 mg/dL. The level of spinal fluid sugar is normal; a significant decrease should raise serious consideration of an alternative diagnosis. As the illness progresses, mononuclear cells in the cerebrospinal fluid tend to increase so that they predominate and the protein concentration may increase. Other laboratory studies have been performed only sporadically, but abnormalities may include hyponatremia, often due to the inappropriate secretion of antidiuretic hormone, and elevations in serum creatine phosphokinase.

DIAGNOSIS   Specific diagnosis requires the isolation of the virus or detection of antibodies with a rising titer between the acute phase of disease and convalescence. Antibodies can be detected by hemagglutination inhibition, complement fixation, or virus neutralization techniques.

TREATMENT   Treatment is entirely supportive and requires meticulous attention in the comatose patient.

LaCrosse encephalitis   A previously undescribed virus was isolated in 1943 from mosquitoes in Kern County, California. Since 1963, a large number of agents now designated as the California group of viruses have been isolated (Table 143-1). LaCrosse, snowshoe hare, Jamestown Canyon, and California encephalitis viruses cause human encephalitis in North America. Tahyna and Inkoo viruses are associated with febrile and, rarely, encephalitic disease in Europe.

Since 1966 in the midwest United States, LaCrosse virus (California) encephalitis has been incriminated in 5 to 6 percent of cases of acute central nervous system disease, ranking above all agents except the enteroviruses.

EPIDEMIOLOGY   LaCrosse virus infection occurs in the north central states, New York, in wooded areas of eastern Texas and Louisiana, and along the eastern seaboard. The virus is maintained by transovarial transmission in woodland mosquitoes, *Aëdes triseratus,* which breed in tree holes in hardwood forests and have adapted to discarded tires. The virus is present in seminal fluid of male mosquitoes and transmitted to the female. The virus overwinters in eggs of *A. triseratus.* Chipmunks and gray squirrels serve as amplifier hosts. LaCrosse virus (California) encephalitis occurs during the summer months (June to October), most often involving boys (60 percent) 5 to 10 years of age (60 percent) who live in rural areas.

CLINICAL MANIFESTATIONS   Two clinical patterns of LaCrosse virus disease have been defined. One is a mild form with a 2- to 3-day prodrome of fever, headache, malaise, and gastrointestinal symptoms. About the third day the temperature increases to 40°C (104°F), and the patient becomes lethargic and develops meningeal signs. These findings abate gradually over a 7- to 8-day period without overt sequelae. The second pattern, a severe form which occurs in at least one-half of the patients, begins abruptly with fever, headache, and vomiting, followed shortly by lethargy and disorientation. During the first 2 to 4 days the course is rapidly progressive with the occurrence of seizures (50 to 60 percent), focal neurologic signs (20 percent), pathologic reflexes (10 percent), and coma (10 percent). Focal neurologic signs may include asymmetric flaccid paralysis. Uncommon findings have included arthralgia and rash. Clinical laboratory features include peripheral leukocyte counts ranging from 7000 to 30,000 per cubic millimeter (median 16,000 per cubic millimeter) with neutrophilia. Cerebrospinal fluid examination reveals 10 to 500 cells per cubic millimeter, usually with a predominance of mononuclear cells, protein concentrations of less than 100 mg/dL, and normal sugar concentrations. Electroencephalograms (EEGs) are abnormal in at least 80 percent of patients, revealing slow deltawave activity. In one-half of the patients the abnormality is asymmetric, suggesting focal destructive lesions. Brain scans using [⁹⁹Tc]pertechnetate and computerized tomography (CT) also may be abnormal, and temporal lobe localization has been observed. Beginning about the fourth day and proceeding over the next 3 to 7 days, there is progressive improvement, with almost all patients becoming afebrile, seizure-free, and ready for discharge from the hospital within 2 weeks after onset.

DIAGNOSIS   Serum and CSF should be tested for LaCrosse virus IgM antibodies. Serum capture IgM ELISA tests detected 83 percent on admission in LaCrosse encephalitis. Early specific diagnosis eliminates the need for brain biopsy to exclude herpes encephalitis which is suggested by the temporal lobe localization.

TREATMENT   Initial seizure activity is frequently prolonged and difficult to control. The most effective anticonvulsant medication has been parenteral diazepam. Patients with the severe form of disease should be discharged on anticonvulsants such as phenobarbital for 6 to 12 months.

PROGNOSIS   The case fatality ratio is low (2 percent or less); however, one-third of patients may have abnormal neurologic findings at the time of discharge. During the early convalescent period, emotional lability and irritability are common. In one series, recurrent seizures occurred in one-quarter of the patients who had seizures during the acute phase. In this same series EEGs were abnormal in one-third of patients evaluated 1 to 8 years after their acute illness. In another series, 15 percent had sequelae, predominantly personality or behavioral problems.

Other California group encephalitides   Jamestown Canyon encephalitis is uncommon, but in contrast to LaCrosse encephalitis usually occurs in adults. Snowshoe hare virus has been isolated from mosquitoes throughout Canada and from Alaska. Encephalitis has been reported from the eastern provinces. Clinical features of Tahyna virus disease, which has been seen in children in Europe, include fever, pharyngitis, pneumonitis, gastrointestinal symptoms, and aseptic meningitis. Neither mortality nor sequelae are reported.

Eastern equine encephalitis   Eastern equine encephalitis (EEE), an alphavirus, was first isolated in 1933 from the brain tissue of horses during an outbreak of equine illness in New Jersey. The first recognized human outbreak occurred in Massachusetts in 1938.

EPIDEMIOLOGY   The virus is distributed along the eastern coast of the Americas from northeastern United States to Argentina. Foci have been found in the Syracuse region of New York, Ontario, Canada, western Michigan, and South Dakota. Viral isolations also have been reported in the Philippines, Thailand, Czechoslovakia, Poland, and the U.S.S.R., but the question of type specificity has not been resolved. In the northeastern United States, epidemics occur in the late summer and early fall. Epizootics in horses precede the occurrence of human cases by 1 to 2 weeks. The disease affects mainly infants, children, and adults over 55 years of age. There is no sex preponderance. Inapparent infection occurs in all age groups, suggesting that the decreased likelihood of developing overt infection in the 15- to 54-year age group is not the result of decreased exposure. The ratio of inapparent infection to overt encephalitis approximates 25:1.

The transmission of EEE involves *Culiseta melanura* mosquitoes and swamp-dwelling birds, e.g., red-winged blackbirds, sparrows, pheasants. Transmission by pecking has been shown in domestic pheasant flocks. *C. melanura* rarely feed on horses or humans, and other mosquitoes, especially *Aëdes sollicitans,* a salt-marsh mosquito which is an avid human feeder, have been postulated as the epidemic vector. The epidemiology of overwintering and maintenance between outbreaks remains unknown. Equine animals and human beings are "dead ends" in the transmission cycle, and infection in them is accidental.

CLINICAL MANIFESTATIONS Though human infections have been thought usually to result in serious, if not fatal, central nervous system involvement, the detection of inapparent infection as well as relatively mild disease establishes the occurrence of milder forms. In many patients, the cerebrospinal fluid is cloudy and contains in excess of 1000 cells per cubic millimeter.

DIAGNOSIS Enzyme-linked immunosorbent assay (ELISA) tests for the detection of specific IgM antibodies in CSF or serum enable early diagnosis, although absence of IgM does not exclude infection. Confirmation can be obtained by a fourfold or more rise or fall in complement fixation (CF), hemagglutination inhibition, or virus neutralization tests.

PROGNOSIS The mortality rate in clinical infection exceeds 50 percent. In the most severe cases, death occurs between the third and fifth days. Children under 10 years of age have a greater likelihood of surviving the acute illness, but they also have a greater likelihood of developing severe disabling residuals: mental retardation, convulsions, emotional lability, blindness, deafness, speech disorders, and hemiplegia.

St. Louis encephalitis St. Louis encephalitis (SLE) was first recognized as an entity during a major outbreak in St. Louis, Missouri, and the surrounding area in 1933. Subsequently, sporadic, unpredictable outbreaks have occurred, for example, in Houston, 1964, Dallas, 1966, Memphis, 1974, northern Mississippi and Illinois, 1975. The attack rate in Greenville, Mississippi, in 1975 was the highest which has been encountered, 10 per 10,000 population.

EPIDEMIOLOGY In the United States, epidemics of SLE fall into two epidemiologic patterns. One pattern is found in the west, where mixed outbreaks of western equine encephalitis and SLE have occurred primarily in irrigated rural areas. The vector has been *Culex tarsalis.* The second pattern occurred in the original St. Louis outbreak and the numerous subsequent epidemics in the midwest, Texas, New Jersey, and Florida. These outbreaks have been more urban in location and are characterized by occurrence of encephalitis in older persons. In such urban-suburban epidemics, the epidemic vectors have been mosquitoes of the *Culex pipiens-quinquefasciatus* complex with the exception of the Florida epidemic, in which *Culex nigripalpus* was incriminated. The presence of SLE virus outside the United States has been proved by isolations in Trinidad, Panama, Jamaica, Brazil, and Argentina. However, except for Jamaica, SLE has not been reported outside the United States. The basic transmission cycle is that of wild bird–mosquito–wild bird. The virus survives the winter in female mosquitoes which ingest a blood meal from a viremic bird before overwintering. The disease in humans usually appears in midsummer to early fall. In urban epidemics, there is no sex predominance while among sporadic cases in the west, men predom-

inate 2:1 due to greater occupational exposure. The human represents an accidental host and plays no role in the basic transmission cycle. Serologic studies following most urban epidemics indicate that infection rates are similar in all age groups, and that the increasing age-specific attack rate for clinical encephalitis which is typical of urban St. Louis encephalitis is probably due to age differences in host susceptibility to overt disease rather than to a higher rate of infection.

CLINICAL MANIFESTATIONS Infection with SLE virus most commonly results in an inapparent infection. Of the patients with confirmed disease, approximately three-fourths have clinical encephalitis; the remainder present with aseptic meningitis, febrile headaches, or nonspecific illness. Virtually all patients over 40 years of age have encephalitic manifestations. Urinary frequency and dysuria have been symptoms in approximately 20 percent of patients despite sterile routine aerobic urine cultures. SLE virus antigen has been demonstrated in urine; this may account for the occurrence of urinary tract symptoms.

DIAGNOSIS The occurrence of either encephalitis or aseptic meningitis as manifested by febrile illness with cerebrospinal fluid pleocytosis in the months of June through September in an adult, especially over 35 years of age, should raise the suspicion of St. Louis encephalitis. Because approximately 40 percent of patients with SLE have antibodies detectable by hemagglutination inhibition at the onset of illness, acute serum for serologic studies should be submitted promptly to a competent laboratory. ELISA tests for the detection of specific IgM antibodies in CSF or serum provide a means of early specific diagnosis.

PROGNOSIS The case fatality ratio in the original St. Louis epidemic was 20 percent. In most subsequent outbreaks the mortality rate has varied from 2 to 12 percent. Subjective nervous complaints, including nervousness, headaches, and easy fatigability and excitability, appear to be the most common residuals. Late organic defects such as speech defects, difficulty in walking, and disturbances in vision were demonstrated in approximately 5 percent of patients 3 years following infection.

Western equine encephalitis Western equine encephalitis (WEE) virus is an alphavirus which was isolated in 1930 in California from horses with encephalitis. In 1938 it was recovered from a fatal human infection.

EPIDEMIOLOGY WEE virus has been isolated in the United States, Canada, Brazil, Guyana, and Argentina. Human disease has been diagnosed in the United States, Canada, and Brazil. In the United States, the virus is found in virtually all geographic areas. The central valley of California represents an important endemic area. The disease occurs mainly in early summer and midsummer. Wild birds, which develop viremia of sufficiently high titer to be able to infect mosquitoes that feed on them, are the basic reservoir. *Culex tarsalis* is the principal vector in the western United States. In areas east of the Appalachian Mountains, another vector must be operative. The virus has been repeatedly isolated from *Culiseta melanura;* however, the importance of this species has been questioned, since it is not primarily a human-biting mosquito. The overwintering mechanism is not known. The ratio of inapparent infection to disease, as evidenced by serologic survey studies, varies from 58:1 in children to 1150:1 in adults. Approximately one-fourth of patients are less than 1 year of age. The highest attack rates occur in persons 55 years or older.

PROGNOSIS The fatality rate approximates 3 percent in laboratory-confirmed cases. The incidence and severity of sequelae are related to age. Sequelae among very young infants are frequent (appearing in 61 percent of a group of patients less than 3 months old) and severe; they consist of upper motor neuron impairment, involving the pyramidal tracts, extrapyramidal structures, and cerebellum, and result in behavioral problems and convulsions. Both the incidence and severity of sequelae diminish rapidly after 1 year of age. Adults may complain of nervousness, irritability, easy fatigability, and tremulousness for 6 months or longer after the acute illness. Probably not more than 5 percent of adults have sequelae which are sufficiently severe to be of practical significance. Postencephalitic seizures are rare.

Japanese encephalitis   The name Japanese B encephalitis was employed during an epidemic which occurred in 1924 to distinguish it from von Economo's disease, which was designated as type A encephalitis. The designation as Japanese B no longer seems useful, and the term Japanese encephalitis (JE) will be employed.

EPIDEMIOLOGY   Japanese encephalitis virus infection is known to occur in eastern Siberia, China, Korea, Taiwan, Japan, Malaya, Vietnam, Thailand, Singapore, Guam, and India. Since the late 1960s JE has declined in Japan and China. JE remains a major problem in northern Thailand. In temperate climates, the disease shows a late-summer early-fall seasonal incidence. In tropical climates there is no seasonal variation. The mosquito *Culex tritaeniorhynchus* is the major vector species. It is a rural mosquito which breeds in rice fields and preferentially bites large domestic animals, such as pigs, but also feeds on birds and humans. The human is an accidental host in the transmission cycle. In endemic areas, children ages 3 to 15 are primarily affected. Epidemics in nonendemic areas have affected all age groups, but young children and older adults predominate. The ratio of inapparent infection, as evidenced by a serologic survey study of Australian troops in Vietnam, was 210:1.

CLINICAL MANIFESTATIONS   The incubation period is 5 to 15 days. As with SLE, illness may present as encephalitis, aseptic meningitis, or febrile headache. The occurrence of severe rigors at the onset has been noted in almost 90 percent of patients. On admission, most patients are alert, but deterioration of mental status occurs in about three-fourths of patients within 3 to 4 days. Localized paresis is found more often than with other ''arboviral'' encephalitides, e.g., in 31 percent of cases, with predominantly upper extremity involvement; however, it resolves rapidly with defervescence. Convulsions are frequent in children, but occur in less than 10 percent of adults. Severe hyperthermia may occur and require treatment. A peripheral leukocytosis with 50 to 90 percent neutrophils is common. Weight loss has been very striking. The failure of the temperature to lyse, appearance of diaphoresis, tachypnea, and the accumulation of bronchial secretions are grave prognostic signs.

PROGNOSIS   The immediate mortality rate has varied from 7 to 33 percent or higher. The rate of occurrence of sequelae varies inversely with the fatality rate; in those series with high fatality rates (33 percent), sequelae occurred in 3 to 14 percent. In another series with a fatality rate of 7.4 percent, the rate of adverse sequelae was 32 percent. Individuals who had neurologic abnormalities during the acute phase but survived have no more than an 80 percent chance for complete recovery. Sequelae consist of seizures, persistent paralysis, ataxia, mental retardation, and behavioral disorders.

Other ''arboviruses'' with central nervous system involvement   A large group of additional ''arboviruses'' have been associated with encephalitis or aseptic meningitis. Some of these agents are listed in Table 143-2. Though the epidemiologic picture of each of these agents is unique, the general features are sufficiently similar to require laboratory support for their differentiation.

''ARBOVIRUS'' DISEASES PRESENTING CHIEFLY WITH HEMOR-RHAGIC MANIFESTATIONS   For 300 years, yellow fever was the only epidemic viral disease known to be accompanied by grave hemorrhagic manifestations. Since the 1930s diverse viral etiologies of the hemorrhagic fever syndrome have been recognized (Table 143-2). Additional agents include members of several families and genera: flavivirus, Filoviridae, phlebovirus, Nairovirus, the Hantaan group of viruses, and arenavirus (Chap. 144). Despite diverse etiologies, there are many similar clinical manifestations. The onset is usually sudden, with headache, backache, generalized myalgia,

conjunctivitis, and prostration. From approximately the third day, the initial stage is followed by hypotension, and hemorrhagic manifestations may occur; these are characterized by bleeding gums, epistaxis, hemoptysis, hematemesis, melena, petechiae, ecchymoses, and hemorrhages into most visceral organs. Mild leukopenia develops early, but with the appearance of hemorrhagic manifestations, leukocytosis may occur. The pathophysiology of the cardinal signs is attributable to hematopoietic and capillary damage, with variable localization of lesions. On the basis of limited confirmatory observations, variable degrees of disseminated intravascular coagulation may be in part responsible for the pathophysiology of the hemorrhagic fever syndromes. Death usually occurs in the second week of disease, at which time a high titer of antibody has developed and the patient may have become afebrile. Death is usually associated with coma, which is due not to encephalitis but to an encephalopathy. The pathologic changes may be similar despite diverse viral etiologies, with midzonal hepatic necrosis and acidophilic cytoplasmic inclusions similar to the Councilman bodies of yellow fever.

Yellow fever   Yellow fever is an acute infectious disease of short duration and extremely variable severity; it is caused by a flavivirus and is followed by lifelong immunity. The classic triad of symptoms—jaundice, hemorrhages, and intense albuminuria—is present only in severe infections, which make up only a small proportion of the total.

PREVALENCE   For more than 200 years, after the first identifiable outbreak occurred in Yucatan in 1648, yellow fever was one of the great plagues of the world. As late as 1905, New Orleans and other southern United States ports experienced at least 5000 cases and 1000 deaths. Because of the existence of the sylvatic form of the disease, protective measures must be maintained against human disease, as demonstrated by outbreaks in Central America from 1948 to 1957. In southern Ethiopia from 1962 to 1964 there were over 100,000 cases with some 30,000 deaths. From 1978 to 1980 there have been outbreaks in Bolivia, Brazil, Colombia, Ecuador, Peru, and Venezuela. In 1979, yellow fever reappeared in Trinidad. During the same time period extensive epidemics were seen in Nigeria, Ghana, Senegal, and Gambia. In Gambia the attack rate was 2.6 to 4.4 percent with a case fatality rate of 19 percent. In 1983, epidemics occurred in Burkino Faso (formerly Upper Volta) and Ghana.

EPIDEMIOLOGY   Human infection results from two basically different cycles of virus transmission, urban and sylvatic. The urban cycle is human-mosquito-human, i.e., *Aëdes aegypti*–transmitted yellow fever. After a 2-week extrinsic incubation period, mosquitoes can transmit infection. Sylvan yellow fever differs under various ecologic circumstances. In the rain forests of South and Central America, species of treetop *Haemagogus* or *Sabethes* mosquitoes maintain transmission in wild primates. Once infected, the mosquito vector remains infectious for life; hence it may serve as a reservoir as well as a vector. When humans come into proximity with the forest-canopy mosquitoes, sporadic cases or focal outbreaks may occur. With sylvan yellow fever, males predominate. Focal outbreaks may be quite extensive; in Brazil in 1973 at least 21,000 persons out of 1.5 million (1.4 percent) were infected. In east Africa, the mosquito-primate cycle is maintained by the forest-canopy mosquito, *A. africanus,* which seldom feeds on humans. The peridomestic mosquito *A. simpsoni* feeds upon primates entering the village gardens and can then in turn transmit the virus to humans. Once yellow fever is reintroduced into urban areas, the urban cycle can be reinitiated, with the potential for epidemic disease. Why yellow fever has never invaded Asia despite widespread distribution of human-biting *A. aegypti* mosquitoes has never been satisfactorily explained.

CLINICAL MANIFESTATIONS   The incubation period is usually 3 to 6 days. In accidental laboratory- or hospital-acquired infections longer incubation periods (10 to 13 days) have been reported. In considering the clinical features, it is advantageous to classify the illness as to severity: inapparent, mild, moderately severe, and malignant. In mild yellow fever the only symptoms may be the abrupt onset of fever and headache. Additional symptoms may include nausea, epistaxis, relative bradycardia known as Faget's sign [e.g., with a temperature of 38.9°C (102°F) the pulse may be only 48 to 52 beats per minute], and slight albuminuria. The mild illness lasts only 1 to 3 days and resembles influenza except that coryzal symptoms are lacking.

Moderately severe and malignant attacks of yellow fever are characterized by three distinct clinical periods: the period of infection, the period of remission, and the period of intoxication. Prodromal symptoms are usually absent. The onset is characteristically sudden, with headache, dizziness, and temperature elevations to 40°C (104°F) without a relative bradycardia. Young children may have febrile convulsions. The headache is followed quickly by pains in the neck, back, and legs. Often there is nausea with vomiting and retching. Examination reveals a flushed face and injection of the conjunctivae. The congestion of the eyes persists until the third day. The tongue characteristically shows bright-red margins and tip and a white furred center. Faget's sign appears by the second day. Epistaxis and gingival bleeding are common. On the third day of illness, the fever may fall by crisis and the patient enters remission, or, in the malignant form, copious hemorrhages, anuria, or delirium may occur. The stage of remission lasts from several hours to several days. In the third stage, the "classic" symptoms develop; the fever returns but the pulse remains slow. Jaundice becomes detectable about the third day; however, jaundice often is not prominent even in fatal illnesses. Increased epistaxis, melena, and uterine hemorrhages are common, but gross hematuria is rare. Of the classic signs, "black vomit" is more characteristic than is jaundice. Hematemesis usually does not occur before the fourth day and is often associated with a fatal outcome. Albuminuria, which rarely develops before the third day, occurs in 90 percent of patients and may be quite marked (3 to 20 g albumin per liter). In spite of this massive albuminuria, edema or ascites has not been reported. In malignant infections, coma frequently occurs 2 to 3 days before death. Shortly before death, which usually occurs between the fourth and the sixth days, the patient commonly becomes delirious and wildly agitated. Though the duration of fever in the third stage is usually 5 to 7 days, the period of intoxication is the most variable of the stages and may last up to 2 weeks. Clinical yellow fever is relatively free from complications, suppurative parotitis being the most striking of those which do occur. Clinical relapses are not characteristic of yellow fever.

LABORATORY FINDINGS Early in the disease, progressive leukopenia may occur. By the fifth day, total leukocyte counts of 1500 to 2500 per cubic millimeter often are found, the decrease being due mostly to a decrease in neutrophils. Total leukocyte counts return to normal by the tenth day, and in fatal cases there may be a marked terminal leukocytosis. Hemoglobin values remain normal except terminally, when hemoconcentration or bleeding may occur. Platelet counts are normal or decreased. Prolongation of clotting, prothrombin, and partial thromboplastin times is marked in patients with jaundice. Increases in total and conjugated bilirubin occur. In icteric patients, marked elevations of serum glutamic oxaloacetic transaminase occur. Hypoglycemia has been seen in patients with severe hepatic damage. Electrocardiograms may show T-wave changes. Clinical examinations of cerebrospinal fluid have not revealed abnormalities.

DIAGNOSIS Inoculation onto mosquito cell cultures or intrathoracically into mosquitoes are methods of choice for virus isolation from blood. Isolation is most likely from specimens obtained during the first 3 days of illness. Serologic methods include plaque reduction neutralization tests on paired serums and detection of yellow fever IgM antibodies, and antigen usually by ELISA methods. The ELISA method enables confirmation in the field within 3 h.

TREATMENT The management has been symptomatic and supportive and should be based upon assessment and correction of the circulatory abnormalities. If evidence of disseminated intravascular coagulation is present, the administration of heparin should be considered. Close attention to fluids and electrolytes is essential.

PROGNOSIS The overall fatality rate in yellow fever is between 5 and 10 percent of clinical cases; it may be even less since many infections are mild or inapparent.

PREVENTION Effective control measures are available. Immunization has been effective in the prevention of outbreaks. With the occurrence of sylvatic outbreaks, work in the area of epizootic activity should be discontinued and intensive mosquito abatement measures should be instituted. These measures may provide the time necessary for a mass immunization program.

Dengue hemorrhagic fever All four dengue virus serotypes can cause dengue hemorrhagic fever (DHF) and dengue shock syndrome (DSS). Infection with dengue 1, 3, or 4 followed within a few years by dengue 2 may be especially important in the pathogenesis. There is consensus that DHF is an immunologically mediated disease. Enhanced growth of dengue 2 virus occurs in peripheral blood mononuclear phagocytes obtained from dengue immune donors or in cells from normal donors in the presence of subneutralizing concentrations of dengue or cross-reacting heterotypic flavivirus antibodies. Infectious virus-antibody complexes attach and enter mononuclear phagocytes by way of Fc receptors. Increased replication of virus in these cells may be followed by a secondary set of reactions: complement activation, mast cell degranulation, and activation of the kinin system.

PREVALENCE The reasons for the apparent sudden "appearance" of the syndrome in the past 30 years are completely obscure. However, during the 1922 epidemic of dengue fever in Louisiana, hemorrhagic manifestations, including epistaxis, bleeding gums, melena, menorrhagia, and even "black vomit," were observed. DHF is now a leading cause of morbidity and mortality in tropical Asia. During the past 5 years, over 500,000 cases of DHF have been officially reported with major epidemics in the People's Republic of China, Vietnam, Indonesia, Thailand, and Cuba. In the Cuban outbreak in 1981, almost 350,000 persons developed dengue, approximately 10,000 had hemorrhagic manifestations, and 158 died (1.6 percent mortality). DHF in Asia is a disease of childhood with one peak observed in children under 1 year, and a second in children ages 3 to 5. The disease in infants is associated with primary infection in the presence of maternal antibody. Studies in Thailand have estimated the frequency of DSS as 11 cases per 1000 secondary dengue infections. DSS occurs more frequently in girls than boys. Dengue hemorrhagic fever occurs almost exclusively in indigenous populations; it has been observed only rarely in whites of European descent despite the frequent occurrence of classic dengue in this group.

CLINICAL MANIFESTATIONS Illness begins abruptly with a minor stage characterized by fever, cough, pharyngitis, headache, anorexia, nausea, vomiting, and abdominal pain which is often severe. This continues for 2 to 4 days. In contrast to classic dengue, myalgia, arthralgia, and bone pain are unusual. Physical signs include fever varying from 38.3 to 40.6°C (101 to 105°F), injection of the tonsils and pharynx, and palpable lymph nodes and liver. The initial state is followed by abrupt deterioration, with the rapid onset of lassitude and weakness (Table 143-4). On examination the child is found to

TABLE 143-4 World Health Organization's clinical classification of dengue hemorrhagic fever

Grade		Clinical features	Laboratory findings
DHF* {	I	Fever, constitutional symptoms, positive tourniquet test	Hemoconcentration Thrombocytopenia
	II	Grade I plus spontaneous bleeding (e.g., skin, gums, gastrointestinal tract)	Hemoconcentration Thrombocytopenia
DSS* {	III	Grade II plus circulatory failure, agitation	Hemoconcentration Thrombocytopenia
	IV	Grade II plus profound shock (blood pressure = 0)	Hemoconcentration Thrombocytopenia

* DHF, dengue hemorrhagic fever; DSS, dengue shock syndrome.

be restless and to have cold clammy extremities with a warm trunk and a pallid face with circumoral cyanosis. Petechiae, most frequently located on the forehead and distal extremities, are seen in half the cases. Occasionally there may be a macular or maculopapular rash. The extremities are frequently cyanotic. Hypotension, with narrowing of the pulse pressure, and tachycardia occur. Pathologic reflexes may be observed. Most fatalities occur in the fourth or fifth day of illness, melena, hematemesis, coma, or unresponsive shock being poor prognostic signs. Cyanosis, dyspnea, and convulsions are terminal manifestations. Following this critical period, survivors show steady and quite rapid improvement.

LABORATORY FINDINGS   In one study, hemoconcentration was found in one-fifth of the children. The majority had leukocyte counts between 5000 and 10,000 per cubic millimeter, with one-third showing a leukocytosis. Only 10 percent of children had a true leukopenia. The most characteristic findings were thrombocytopenia, rarely with blood platelets under 75,000 per cubic millimeter, positive tourniquet test, and prolonged bleeding time. Prothrombin time and partial thromboplastin times were usually near normal values. Depression of clotting factors V, VII, IX, and X may be present. Bone marrow examination may reveal maturation arrest of megakaryocytes. In Manila or Bangkok, hematuria has been infrequent even with other serious bleeding manifestations; however, in Tahiti, gross hematuria was common. Cerebrospinal fluid examinations are usually normal. Other abnormal laboratory findings may include hyponatremia, acidosis, elevated blood urea nitrogen levels, elevation in serum glutamic oxalacetic transaminase levels, mild hyperbilirubinemia, and hypoproteinemia. Electrocardiograms may reveal diffuse myocardial abnormalities. Two-thirds of patients have radiologic evidence of bronchopneumonia, with many showing pleural effusions.

DIAGNOSIS   The World Health Organization (WHO) has established criteria for the diagnosis of DHF: fever—acute onset, high, continuous, and lasting for 2 to 7 days; hemorrhagic manifestations including at least a positive tourniquet test and any of the following: petechiae, purpura, ecchymoses, epistaxis, bleeding gums, hematemesis, or melena; enlargement of the liver; thrombocytopenia, ≤100,000 per cubic millimeter; hemoconcentration, hematocrit increased by ≥20 percent. Criteria for DSS are a rapid, weak pulse with narrowing of the pulse pressure (≤20 mmHg) or hypotension with cold, clammy skin and restlessness. The WHO classification includes a grading of severity (Table 143-4). Minor hemorrhagic manifestations may be seen during the course of classic dengue fever without meeting WHO criteria for DHF. These cases should be termed dengue fever with hemorrhage, not DHF. For specific viral diagnosis, see "Dengue Fever."

TREATMENT   The mainstay is correction of circulatory collapse while avoiding fluid overload. Administration of 5% glucose in 0.5 N saline at a rate of 40 mL/kg restored blood pressure within 1 to 2 h in one-half of patients. When stable, the rate of administration of intravenous fluids was slowed to 10 (mL/kg)/h. If improvement did not occur, plasma or a plasma expander (20 mL/kg) was administered. Transfusion of whole blood is not recommended. Oxygen should be administered. Glucocorticosteroids have been used, but doses of 25 mg/kg have not resulted in significant improvement. Since the evidence for severe disseminated intravascular coagulation is questionable, use of heparin is not clear-cut, although in a group of Filipino children with type 3 dengue virus, administration of heparin (1 mg sodium heparin per kilogram) was associated with a dramatic rise in number of platelets and level of plasma fibrinogen. Antibiotics are not indicated; sympathomimetic amines and salicylates are contraindicated. Recovery from vascular collapse usually occurs within 24 to 48 h, at which time diuretics and digitalis may be necessary. An uncontrolled trial of interferon was conducted during the 1981 epidemic in Cuba with some indication of efficacy.

PROGNOSIS   Mortality has varied from 1 to 23 percent. Deaths have been most common in infants under 1 year of age.

PREVENTION   At present, vector control is the only method available to prevent hemorrhagic fever.

Tick-borne hemorrhagic fevers

CRIMEAN-CONGO HEMORRHAGIC FEVER   At the close of World War II, a new disease entity was recognized in the Crimea region of the U.S.S.R. Retrospective studies demonstrated that an almost identical syndrome had been recognized in the south central Asian republics of the U.S.S.R. for many years. Soviet workers repeatedly isolated virus strains during 1967 to 1969.

The virus of Crimean hemorrhagic fever (CHF) is antigenically identical with Congo virus, which was isolated from patients, cattle, and ticks in Africa (Kenya, Uganda, Congo, and Nigeria). Crimean-Congo hemorrhagic fever (CCHF) virus is now known from South Africa, throughout most of subSaharan Africa, eastern Europe, the Middle East, and Asia as far as the Xinjiang province of China. CCHF occurs where *Hyalomma* ticks are found.

Approximately 30 cases of CCHF have been recorded annually in each of the known areas of occurrence in the U.S.S.R. The cases occur between April and September. The sex distribution of CCHF is equal, and 80 percent of the cases occur in the 20- to 60-year age group, with the majority occurring in dairy and agricultural workers. The major arthropod vectors for transmission to humans are ticks which belong to the genus *Hyalomma*. Cattle and wild hares appear to be important reservoirs, and rooks and other birds have been implicated. Once a case of human CCHF occurs, person-to-person transmission is possible. Nosocomial outbreaks have occurred in the U.S.S.R., Pakistan, India, and Iraq. Transmission is presumed to occur through direct contact with infected blood. There are no data to suggest airborne transmission.

After an incubation period of 3 to 6 days, the onset is abrupt, with temperatures to 40°C (104°F), dizziness, headache, and diffuse myalgia. The course of fever is occasionally biphasic, with an average duration of 8 days. Physical signs include flushing of the face, conjunctival injection, vomiting, and, on occasion, epigastric pain. Hepatomegaly is found in half the patients. Splenomegaly has been reported in 2 to 25 percent of patients. Respiratory symptoms or signs are unusual. Hemorrhagic manifestations generally begin on the fourth day with petechiae on the oral mucosa and skin, epistaxis, gingival bleeding, hematemesis, and melena. Neurologic abnormalities, seen in 10 to 25 percent of patients, include nuchal rigidity, excitation, and coma. Laboratory findings show leukopenia, with the number of white blood cells falling as low as 1000 per cubic millimeter, and thrombocytopenia, which is often severe. Proteinuria and microscopic hematuria are common, but azotemia and oliguria are not. Convalescence may be prolonged. Death is usually attributed to shock or intercurrent infection. Sequelae include transient alopecia and mono- or polyneuritis.

The major approach to therapy has been supportive. Convalescent immune serum has shown promise if administered during the first 3 days of illness. Patients should be isolated with contact restricted to hospital staff and immediate family. Masks and gowns should be worn, and blood and body fluids handled as infectious. The reported mortality rate has shown variation between 9 and 50 percent.

OMSK HEMORRHAGIC FEVER   Omsk hemorrhagic fever (OHF) is an acute febrile disease which occurs in the Omsk and Novosibirsk oblasts in the U.S.S.R. and is caused by a flavivirus. The seasonal occurrence of OHF shows a biphasic pattern with peaks in May and August. The transmission cycle is uncertain. OHF is transmitted to humans either by the bite of infected ticks, *Ixodes apronophorus,* or by the handling of infected muskrats. The natural reservoir includes muskrats, other rodents, especially water voles, and ticks. Epidemics occurred from 1945 to 1948, but recently the disease has been less prevalent.

Following an incubation interval of 3 to 8 days, illness begins abruptly with fever, headache, and hemorrhagic manifestations, which include epistaxis and gastrointestinal and uterine bleeding. Rarely, neurologic abnormalities may occur. Laboratory features include leukopenia. In contrast to many of the other hemorrhagic fevers, OHF has a low case fatality rate (0.5 to 3.0 percent).

KYASANUR FOREST DISEASE Kyasanur Forest disease was first recognized in south India in 1957 as a discrete clinical entity shown to be due to a flavivirus. Kyasanur Forest disease occurs following occupational exposure to *Haemaphysalis spinigera* ticks in the tropical forests of western Mysore in southern India. The silent reservoir cycle which infects the primate- and bird-feeding *Haemaphysalis* ticks is now believed to be *Ixodes* ticks transmitted among small forest mammals, especially the shrew. Laboratory-associated infections have been common.

The major symptoms include abrupt onset of fever, headache, fatigue, myalgia (especially of the lumbar area and calf muscles), and retroorbital pain. Cough and abdominal pain occur in half the patients. Additional symptoms may include photophobia and polyarthralgia. Epistaxis and hematemesis are observed in some patients. On examination, findings include relative bradycardia, conjunctival injection, and generalized lymphadenopathy. Fine and coarse rales are frequently heard. Hepatosplenomegaly has been encountered occasionally. During the initial phase, generalized hyperesthesia of the skin occurs occasionally. The fever usually lasts from 6 to 11 days. After an afebrile period of 9 to 21 days, approximately half the patients may develop a second phase, which lasts from 2 to 12 days. This is manifested by recurrence of fever, severe headache, neck stiffness, mental disturbance, coarse tremors, giddiness, and abnormalities in reflexes, as well as by recurrence of many of the initial symptoms. No sequelae have been observed, but convalescence is often prolonged.

Only limited laboratory studies have been performed. During the initial phase, leukopenia is a constant feature, with a total leukocyte count of fewer than 3000 per cubic millimeter by the fourth to sixth day. The leukopenia is associated with neutropenia. During the second phase there is a mild leukocytosis. Lumbar puncture during the second phase has shown a pattern of aseptic meningitis. Diagnosis is based upon virus isolation from blood; this is readily accomplished, since viremia is prolonged. Serologic tests of paired serums also can be performed. The management is supportive. The mortality rate is approximately 5 percent.

HEMORRHAGIC FEVER WITH RENAL SYNDROME
Synonyms for this disease (HFRS) include Korean hemorrhagic fever, far eastern hemorrhagic fever, endemic or epidemic nephrosonephritis, Manchurian epidemic hemorrhagic fever, Songo fever, and Churilov's disease. A similar but milder disease in Scandinavia has been called nephropathica epidemica or epidemic nephritis (EN).

In 1932, the Russians first observed HFRS in southeastern Siberia. In April 1951, a previously unknown illness, subsequently recognized as HFRS, broke out among the United Nations forces in Korea.

Etiology In 1976, the antigen of HFRS was reported in the lungs of the rodent *Apodemus agrarius coreae*. Diagnostic increases in immunofluorescent antibodies were demonstrated in 113 of 116 cases of severe HFRS. The agent designated Hantaan virus is a single-stranded RNA virus belonging to the family Bunyaviridae. It has been proposed as a separate genus (Table 143-1). The Hantaan group consists of at least four agents: Hantaan virus (Korean hemorrhagic fever), Puumala virus (nephropathica epidemica), and two viruses from the United States (Prospect Hill virus and Tchoupitoulas virus) which have not been associated with disease.

Prevalence In Korea between April 1951 and January 1953, 2070 cases of EHF were reported among United Nations personnel. The disease usually occurs as an isolated event; hence, overall attack rates have relatively less meaning. With this reservation, attack rates in two United States Army divisions stationed in Korea varied between 1.9 and 2.9 cases per 1000 persons per epidemic season. Approximately 800 cases per year have continued to occur; however, most cases are now seen in Korean civilians and military with less than 10 cases per year in U.S. military personnel. During the past decade

the disease has increased in prevalence in Korea, urban Japan, and in China. The People's Republic of China reported 30,000 hospitalized cases in 1980 and 42,000 in 1981. Hundreds of cases of nephropathica epidemica have occurred annually in Finland and other Scandinavian countries since the 1930s. In 1953 a severe form of HFRS was recognized in the Balkan countries, and in 1982 in Greece and France. Antibody studies indicate worldwide distribution. Antibodies in human serums have been found in Argentina, Brazil, Colombia, Belgium, Canada, the United States, including Hawaii and Alaska, southeast Asia, Egypt, and central Africa.

Epidemiology The majority of cases occur in May to June and in October to November. These peaks coincide with rodent density population. Hantaan virus is present in rodent urine, feces, and saliva in high titer. Transmission from rodent to rodent is primarily respiratory, with transmission to people through inhalation of virus-containing dried excreta. There is no evidence for person-to-person transmission. The urban reservoir appears to be the house rat. Laboratory outbreaks have occurred in the U.S.S.R., Korea, Japan, France, and Belgium with Wistar rats implicated in Korea and Japan.

Clinical manifestations There are two forms of disease, a mild illness characteristically diagnosed in Scandinavia as nephropathica epidemica (NE) and the more severe far eastern form (EHF).

Nephropathica epidemica (NE) is characterized by sudden onset of high fever, backache, headache, and abdominal pain. On the third or fourth day, hemorrhagic manifestations may occur and conjunctival hemorrhages, palatine petechiae, and a petechial rash appear on the trunk. About one patient in five is "toxic" and mentally obtunded. Oliguria and azotemia develop. Urinalysis reveals proteinuria, hematuria, and leukocyturia. After about 3 days the rash subsides, the patient develops polyuria, and recovers over several weeks.

EPIDEMIC HEMORRHAGIC FEVER The incubation period in epidemic hemorrhagic fever (EHF) is usually 10 to 25 days, with possible extremes of 7 and 36 days. Visitors who contract the disease in an endemic area may not develop illness until after their return home.

The clinical course of EHF may be divided into phases on the basis of the underlying physiologic aberrations: febrile, hypotensive, oliguric, diuretic, and convalescent. There is considerable variation among patients in the severity of the illness. In one study two-thirds of the 264 cases studied were classified as mild, while 14 percent were termed severe. The illness in most patients was of comparable severity in each phase.

Febrile (invasive) phase From 10 to 20 percent of patients describe vague prodromal symptoms resembling mild upper respiratory infections. The onset is then usually abrupt, often initiated by a chill and accompanied by fever, headache, backache, abdominal pain, and generalized myalgia. Anorexia and thirst are almost universal, while nausea and vomiting are common although not constant symptoms. The headache is most commonly frontal or retroorbital. Eye symptoms, especially mild photophobia and pain on movement of the eyes, are characteristic. Diarrhea is not a feature. Fever is present in almost all patients; the temperature ranges from 37.8 to 41.1°C (100 to 106°F), reaches a peak on the third or fourth day after onset, and falls by lysis on the fourth to seventh day. There is a relative bradycardia. Initially the blood pressure is normal. One of the most typical early findings is a diffuse reddening of the skin, most marked over the face and V area of the neck that may resemble a severe sunburn. The erythema blanches on pressure. Dermographism can be demonstrated in over 90 percent of patients at the same time as the flush. Slight edema of the upper eyelids causes a bleary-eyed appearance. Bulbar and palpebral conjunctivas show injection. Conjunctival petechiae may develop by the third or fifth day of illness. Subconjunctival hemorrhages may be striking. Intense pharyngeal reddening without significant sore throat is typical. The first location for petechiae is usually the palate, where they occur in half the patients. Within 12 to 24 h, petechiae appear at pressure areas such as the axillary folds, lateral chest wall, belt line, hips, and thighs.

Retinal hemorrhages occur rarely. Cervical, axillary, and inguinal nodes are moderately enlarged but nontender. Abdominal and costovertebral tenderness is almost a constant finding. Splenomegaly is unusual and in Korea was generally attributable to malaria with which EHF coexisted in about 1 percent of patients. The degree of flush, fever, and conjunctival injection and the number of petechiae correlate quite well with the overall severity of illness.

Laboratory studies during this phase are often not striking. Initial hemoglobin and hematocrit values are usually normal. Prior to the fourth day, leukocyte counts range from 3600 to 6000 per cubic millimeter but are associated with neutrophilia. Early in the course urine specific gravity may be high. Albuminuria, which is an almost universal finding, appears, often abruptly, between the second and fifth days of illness. The urinary sediment reveals microscopic hematuria and hyaline, granular, red blood cell casts, and/or white blood cell casts. Erythrocyte sedimentation rates are normal during the first week. Capillary fragility tests are usually positive at the time of admission and become most abnormal by the ninth day. Electrocardiographic abnormalities may be seen in 15 to 30 percent of patients; these include sinus bradycardia and low or inverted T waves. Lumbar punctures may reveal gross blood in the spinal fluid.

Hypotensive phase   On about the fifth day of illness, during the last 24 to 48 h of the febrile phase, hypotension or shock may occur. In mild cases, only a transient fall in blood pressure occurs; among moderately and severely ill patients shock may persist for 1 to 3 days. In 828 patients, 16.5 percent had clinical shock, and another 14 percent had hypotension without shock. Headache often diminishes, but thirst persists. In the beginning of the hypotensive phase, most patients have warm, dry skin and extremities. As the hypotensive phase progresses and the systolic blood pressure decreases and pulse pressure narrows, the skin becomes cool and moist. Tachycardia replaces the relative bradycardia.

At this stage, an increase in hematocrit with no change in total serum protein level is found. This is thought to reflect a loss of plasma through damaged capillaries. On about the fifth day, all patients develop marked proteinuria. The previously normal urine specific gravity begins to fall and in 2 to 3 days is usually around 1.010. Blood urea nitrogen concentrations begin to increase. Other laboratory findings include leukocytosis with white blood cell counts of 10,000 to 56,000 per cubic millimeter with neutrophilia and toxic granulation. The number of platelets often decreases to less than 70,000 per cubic millimeter.

Oliguric phase (*hemorrhagic or toxic phase*)   About the eighth day of illness, blood pressure returns to the normal range and in some instances increases to hypertensive levels. While oliguria may have appeared during the shock phase, it now becomes a prominent feature. Oliguria develops even though hypotension was not recognized. Symptomatically patients continue to feel weak and thirsty and have more severe backache. Protracted vomiting and hiccups may ensue.

Blood urea nitrogen levels increase rapidly and are associated with hyperkalemia, hyperphosphatemia, and hypocalcemia. Metabolic acidosis is rarely severe. Although platelets begin to return to normal, hemorrhagic manifestations become more prominent and include petechiae, hematemesis (analogous to "black vomit" in yellow fever), melena, hemoptysis, gross hematuria, and hemorrhages into the central nervous system. The enlarged lymph nodes may now become tender.

With the onset of diuresis on about the seventh day in moderately ill patients and the ninth to eleventh day in severely ill patients, symptoms of fluid and electrolyte abnormalities and central nervous system or pulmonary complications may appear. Central nervous system symptoms include disorientation, extreme restlessness, lethargy, paranoid delusions, and hallucinations. Grand mal seizures, pulmonary edema, and pulmonary infection occur in some patients.

Diuretic phase   With the onset of diuresis, progressive improvement is the rule. Most patients begin to eat and regain their strength. In fatal cases the diuretic phase is associated with a daily urine output of less than 4 liters and often less than 2 liters, in contrast to larger volumes in surviving patients.

Convalescent phase   The convalescent phase lasts 3 to 6 weeks. Weight is regained slowly. Complaints include muscular weakness, intention tremor, and lack of stamina. Hyposthenuria and polyuria are present; however, within 2 months most patients are able to concentrate their urine to a specific gravity of 1.023 or greater after a 12-h period of water deprivation.

Diagnosis   Diagnosis is based on demonstration of specific IgM antibodies by ELISA or a fourfold change in immune adherence hemagglutination titers in paired serums.

Treatment   Clinical management primarily revolves around meticulous supportive care. Trials with a variety of agents including antibiotics, adrenocortical steroid hormones, antihistamines, and convalescent serum were without significant beneficial effect during the Korean epidemics.

Prognosis   The Soviet experience indicates a mortality rate of 3 to 32 percent; in China, the case fatality ratio was 7 to 15 percent. Between April 1951 and December 1976 the overall case fatality ratio in Korea was 6.6 percent.

Residua are uncommon. Of 783 surviving patients cared for at the Hemorrhagic Fever Center in Korea between April and December 1952, only 16 were unable to return to duty within a period of 4 months. Fifteen of these individuals still had hyposthenuria. Follow-up studies on former EHF patients 3 to 5 years later showed that they had many more subsequent hospital admissions for urologic problems than did a control group and that the relative frequency correlated with the severity of the acute episode of EHF. Asymptomatic residual renal tubular dysfunction may be more common than has been appreciated.

REFERENCES

"Arboviruses": Definition and classification

FIELDS BN et al (eds): *Virology*. New York, Raven, 1985

"Arbovirus" infections characterized by fever, malaise, headaches, and myalgia

BECKER FE: Tick-borne infections in Colorado. Col Med 27:36, 1930

BOWEN GS et al: Clinical aspects of human Venezuelan equine encephalitis in Texas, 1971. Bull Pan Am Health Org 10:46, 1976

BRICENO ROSSIE AL: Rural epidemic encephalitis in Venezuela caused by a group A arbovirus (VEE). Prog Med Virol 9:176, 1967

CALISHER CH et al: Rio Grande—a new phlebotomus fever group virus from south Texas. Am J Trop Med Hyg 26:997, 1977

DIETZ WH JR et al: Ten clinical cases of human infection with Venezuelan equine encephalomyelitis virus, subtype I-D. Am J Trop Med Hyg 28:329, 1979

FLEMING J et al: Sandfly fever. Review of 664 cases. Lancet 1:443, 1947

GOODPASTURE HC et al: Colorado tick fever: Clinical, epidemiologic and laboratory aspects of 228 cases in Colorado in 1973–1974. Ann Intern Med 88:303, 1978

HUGHES LE et al: Persistence of Colorado tick fever virus in red blood cells. Am J Trop Med Hyg 23:530, 1974

LAUGHLIN LW et al: Epidemic Rift Valley fever in Egypt: Observations of the spectrum of human illness. Trans R Soc Trop Med Hyg 73:630, 1979

LENNETTE EH, KOPROWSKI H: Human infection with Venezuelan equine encephalomyelitis virus. JAMA 123:1088, 1943

SCHERER WF et al: Ecologic studies of Venezuelan encephalitis virus in Southeastern Mexico: VII. Infection of man. Am J Trop Med 21:79, 1972

SIAM AL et al: Rift Valley fever ocular manifestations: Observations during 1977 epidemic in Egypt. Br J Ophthalmol 64:366, 1980

SPRUANCE SL, BAILEY A: Colorado tick fever. A review of 115 laboratory confirmed cases. Arch Intern Med 131:288, 1973

VAN VELDEN et al: Rift Valley fever affecting humans in South Africa: A clinicopathologic study. S Afr Med J 29:867, 1977

"Arbovirus" infections presenting chiefly with fever, malaise, arthralgia, and rash

AASKOV JG et al: An epidemic of Ross River virus infection in Fiji, 1979. Am J Trop Med Hyg 30:1053, 1981

CLARK JA et al: Annually recurrent epidemic polyarthritis and Ross River virus activity in a coastal area of New South Wales. I. Occurrence of the disease. Am J Trop Med Hyg 22:543, 1973

DELLER JJ JR, RUSSELL PK: Chikungunya disease. Am J Trop Med 17:107, 1968

MALHERBE H et al: Sindbis virus infection in man. Report of a case with recovery of virus from skin lesions. S Afr Med J 37:547, 1963

PINHEIRO FP et al: An outbreak of Mayaro virus disease in Belterra, Brazil: I. Clinical and virological findings. Am J Trop Med Hyg 30:674, 1981

ROBINSON MC: An epidemic of virus disease in Southern Province, Tanganyika territory in 1952–53: I. Clinical features. Trans R Soc Trop Med Hyg 49:28, 1955

SHORE H: O'nyong-nyong fever: An epidemic virus disease in East Africa: III. Some clinical and epidemiological observations in the Northern Province of Uganda. Trans R Soc Trop Med Hyg 55:361, 1961

"Arbovirus" infections presenting chiefly with fever, malaise, lymphadenopathy, and rash

ALVAREZ MD, RAMÍREZ-RONDA CH: Dengue and hepatic failure. Am J Med 79:670, 1985

CENTERS FOR DISEASE CONTROL: Dengue in the United States, 1983–1984. CDC Surveillance Summaries 34(255):555, 1985

MARBERG K et al: The natural history of West Nile fever: I. Clinical observations during an epidemic in Israel. Am J Hyg 64:259, 1956

MICKS DW, MOON WB: Aëdes aegypti in a Texas coastal county as an index of dengue fever receptivity and control. Am J Trop Med Hyg 29:1382, 1980

PERELMAN A, STERN J: Acute pancreatitis in West Nile fever. Am J Trop Med Hyg 23:1150, 1974

TAYLOR RM et al: A study of the ecology of West Nile virus in Egypt. Am J Trop Med 5:579, 1956

"Arbovirus" infections presenting chiefly with central nervous system involvement

BALFOUR HH JR et al: California arbovirus (LaCrosse) infections. Pediatrics 52:680, 1973

CENTERS FOR DISEASE CONTROL: Arboviral infections of the central nervous system— United States, 1984. Morb Mort Week Rep 34:283, 1985

DICKERSON RB et al: Diagnosis and immediate prognosis of Japanese B encephalitis. Observations based on more than 200 patients with detailed analysis of 65 serologically confirmed cases. Am J Med 12:277, 1952

EDELMAN R, PARYANONDA A: Human immunoglobulin M antibody in the serodiagnosis of Japanese encephalitis virus infections. Am J Epidemiol 98:29, 1973

FINLEY KH et al: Western equine and St. Louis encephalitis. Preliminary report of a clinical follow-up study in California. Neurology 5:223, 1955

GRABOW JD et al: The electroencephalogram and clinical sequelae of California arbovirus encephalitis. Neurology 19:394, 1969

HILTY MD et al: California encephalitis in children. Am J Dis Child 124:530, 1972

KETEL WB, OGNIBENE AJ: Japanese B encephalitis in Vietnam. Am J Med Sci 261:271, 1971

LUBY JP et al: The epidemiology of St. Louis encephalitis (SLE): A review. Ann Rev Med 20:329, 1969

———: Antigenemia in St. Louis encephalitis. Am J Trop Med Hyg 29:265, 1980

SCHNEIDER RJ et al: Clinical sequelae after Japanese encephalitis: One year follow-up study in Thailand. Southeast Asian J Trop Med Public Health 5:560, 1974

WEAVER OM et al: Japanese encephalitis: Sequelae. Neurology 8:887, 1958

"Arbovirus" diseases presenting primarily with hemorrhagic manifestations

BURNEY MI et al: Nosocomial outbreak of viral hemorrhagic fever caused by Crimean hemorrhagic fever—Congo virus in Pakistan, January 1976. Am J Trop Med Hyg 29:941, 1980

CASALS J et al: A current appraisal of hemorrhagic fevers in the USSR. Am J Trop Med 15:751, 1966

CENTERS FOR DISEASE CONTROL: Viral hemorrhagic fever. Initial management of suspected and confirmed cases. Ann Intern Med 101:73, 1984

DENNIS LH et al: The original hemorrhagic fever: Yellow fever. Blood 30:858, 1967

HALSTEAD SB, O'ROURKE EF: Dengue viruses and mononuclear phagocytes: I. Infection enhancement by non-neutralizing antibody. J Exp Med 146:201, 1977

———: Dengue hemorrhagic fever—a public health problem and a field for research. Bull WHO 58:1, 1980

———: The pathogenesis of dengue: Molecular epidemiology in infectious disease. Am J Epidemiol 114:632, 1981

KIRK R: An epidemic of yellow fever in the Nuba Mountains, Anglo-Egyptian Sudan. Ann Trop Med Parasitol 35:67, 1941

LEE HW et al: Isolation of the etiologic agent of Korean hemorrhagic fever. J Infect Dis 137:298, 1978

MONATH TP et al: Yellow fever in the Gambia, 1978–1979: Epidemiologic aspects with observations on the occurrence of Orongo virus infections. Am J Trop Med Hyg 29:912, 1980

———: Pathophysiologic correlations in a monkey model of yellow fever with special observations on the acute necrosis of B cell areas of lymphoid tissues. Am J Trop Med Hyg 30:431, 1981

NELSON ER: Hemorrhagic fever in children in Thailand: Report of 69 cases. J Pediatr 56:101, 1960

PINHEIRO FP et al: An epidemic of yellow fever in Central Brazil 1972–1973: I. Epidemiological studies. Am J Trop Med Hyg 27:125, 1978

Technical guide for diagnosis, treatment, surveillance, prevention and control of dengue hemorrhagic fever. Geneva, World Health Organization, 1982

WORLD HEALTH ORGANIZATION: Hemorrhagic fever with renal syndrome: Memorandum from a WHO meeting. Bull WHO 61:269, 1983

144 ARENAVIRUS INFECTIONS

JAY P. SANFORD

DEFINITION AND CLASSIFICATION The term *arenavirus* is the proposed designation for a group of RNA viruses which have unique morphology. The virions are round, oval, or pleomorphic, with diameters between 60 and 350 nm, and contain an electron-dense membrane with projections and 2 to 10 inclusion-like dense particles (resembling ribosomes) that give the virion an appearance of having been sprinkled with sand (Latin *arenaceus*, "sandy"). Eleven distinct arenaviruses have been described (Table 144-1). All except Tacaribe are parasites of rodents, and most are unique to tropical America. A special property of arenaviruses that cause disease in humans, especially Machupo and lymphocytic choriomeningitis, is their capacity to induce persistent infection in their reservoir hosts with no ill effects and in the absence of an immune response.

LYMPHOCYTIC CHORIOMENINGITIS The first-recognized arenavirus was lymphocytic choriomeningitis (LCM) virus. It was recognized early that LCM was carried by apparently healthy laboratory mice. Clinically LCM has been considered primarily in the context of aseptic meningitis; however, it is associated with at least two clinical syndromes in humans: central nervous system and influenza-like illness which may be associated with rash, arthritis, or orchitis. LCM virus has provided a valuable model for the study of chronic, persistent, and generally symptomless viral infections in laboratory animals.

Prevalence In the United States human infection with LCM virus is rare; however, seroepidemiologic studies on specimens obtained in 1935 to 1940 from persons with no history of central nervous system disease from all parts of the United States revealed neutralizing antibodies in 10 to 28 percent. In recent years, the prevalence of infection seems to have decreased markedly.

Epidemiology The virus of LCM is worldwide in distribution. Foci of LCM virus have been defined in Germany, Hungary, and elsewhere in Europe. Scandinavia appears to be LCM virus–free as are most of the Americas except Argentina. Although infection can be induced

TABLE 144-1 Classification of arenaviruses

Virus	Clinical disease	Reservoir	Known geographic range
Lymphocytic choriomeningitis	Aseptic meningitis, meningoencephalitis, influenzal syndrome, orchitis, arthritis	Mice, hamsters	Worldwide except Australia
Tacaribe		Bats	Trinidad
Junin	Argentinian hemorrhagic fever	*Calomys musculinus*	Argentina
Machupo	Bolivian hemorrhagic fever	*Calomys callosus*	Northeast Bolivia
Amapari			Brazil
Latino			Bolivia
Parana			Paraguay
Pichinde			Colombia
Tamiami			Florida
Lassa	Lassa fever	*Mastomys natalensis*	Nigeria, Liberia, Sierra Leone, Republic of Guinea, Central African Republic
Flexal		*Orzomys* sp.	Brazil

in a variety of animals, mice are the major natural reservoir as well as the primary host in which latent, asymptomatic infection occurs. The latency of infection in the mouse depends upon immunologic tolerance. Animals infected in utero or shortly after birth excrete LCM virus for life without overt disease. Human infections are secondary to contact with an infected rodent. The mode of transmission is thought to be via airborne spread or contact with excrement from infected animals. In the past, most cases have arisen in persons living in rodent-infested houses, but lately outbreaks of LCM virus disease in humans have been reported from Germany and from the United States in which the source of infection was traced to laboratory animals and household pets, specifically hamsters which, like mice, can shed LCM virus in urine and stool. LCM occurs throughout the year but has been more frequent in the colder months when "the mice come in from the fields." Person-to-person transmission has not been demonstrated.

Pathogenesis   In natural infection, the portal of entry of the LCM virus is probably through the respiratory tract. Virus multiplication occurs initially in the respiratory epithelium, and an influenza-like illness develops. Dissemination of virus to extrapulmonary sites, presumably to reticuloendothelial cells with multiplication, and viremia occur. LCM virus crosses the blood-brain barrier. In mice, the resulting meningitis is attributed to a cell-mediated immune reaction. Support for this hypothesis derives from observations that disease but not infection can be prevented in experimental animals by neonatal thymectomy, irradiation, or immunodepressant drugs such as cyclophosphamide. Similar pathogenetic mechanisms may operate in humans, although isolation of LCM virus from the CSF of patients with aseptic meningitis is quite common.

Clinical manifestations   The exact incubation period is not known. Following experimental inoculation of LCM virus into volunteers, fever occurred in $1\frac{1}{2}$ to 3 days, while an influenza-like constellation of symptoms developed 5 to 10 days after exposure. An influenza-like illness is the commonest clinical pattern. In some patients, up to one-half in some series, the illness may be biphasic with subsequent aseptic meningitis or encephalomyelitis. Fever, usually from 38.3 to 40°C (101 to 104°F), associated with rigors, is uniformly noted. Other symptoms which are encountered in over one-half of patients include malaise, weakness, myalgia (especially lumbar aching), retroorbital headache, photophobia, anorexia, nausea, and light-headedness. Other prominent symptoms which occur in one-fourth to one-half of patients include sore throat, vomiting, and dysesthesias. Later arthralgias, especially in the hands, occur. Less common complaints (up to one-quarter of patients) include aching pain in the chest, associated with pneumonitis; increased hair loss progressing to generalized alopecia, 2 or 3 weeks after the onset of illness; testicular pain or frank orchitis, usually unilateral, again 1 to 3 weeks after onset; and parotid pain, which may lead to a misdiagnosis of mumps. Physical findings in the first week of illness are few. Patients often have a relative bradycardia. Pharyngeal injection without exudate is commonly seen (60 percent). Mild nontender cervical or axillary lymphadenopathy may occur. The initial phase lasts from 5 days to 3 weeks followed by improvement. After a remission of 1 to 2 days many patients relapse with recurrent fever and more prominent headache. Physical signs may include skin rashes, swelling of metacarpophalangeal and proximal interphalangeal joints, meningeal signs, orchitis, parotitis, and alopecia. Convalescence generally is of 1 to 4 weeks' duration, characterized by easy fatigability, an excessive need for sleep, dysesthesias, and occasional dizziness. Patients with aseptic meningitis almost always recover without sequelae. With encephalitis, 25 to 30 percent of patients have neurologic residua.

Laboratory findings   Leukopenia and thrombocytopenia are almost uniform during the first week of illness. Although leukocyte counts usually vary between 2000 and 3000 per cubic millimeter, counts as low as 600 per cubic millimeter have been recorded. Differential counts generally show slight relative lymphocytosis. Platelet counts are usually between 50,000 and 100,000 per cubic millimeter. Anemia is not encountered. The erythrocyte sedimentation rate often is normal. Mild elevations of serum glutamic oxaloacetic transaminase (SGOT) and lactic dehydrogenase (LDH) may occur. Chest radiographs may suggest basilar pneumonias. In patients with meningeal signs examination of the cerebrospinal fluid usually reveals several hundred cells per cubic millimeter, although cell counts in excess of 1000 per cubic millimeter are reported in half the patients in some series. Lymphocytes predominate (greater than 80 percent) even early. The initial cerebrospinal fluid protein is usually slightly elevated, but on occasion levels may exceed 150 mg/dL. Although a normal cerebrospinal fluid glucose level is considered the hallmark of viral meningitides, hypoglycorrhachia has been observed in up to 27 percent of patients with LCM, glucose values as low as 15 mg/dL with normal simultaneous blood sugar levels having been reported.

Diagnosis   The diagnosis of LCM can be established with certainty by recovery of the virus from blood or spinal fluid. Complement-fixing antibodies are usually detectable 1 to 2 weeks after the onset of infection, peak at 5 to 8 weeks, and are gone by 6 months. Neutralizing antibodies appear after 6 to 8 weeks, increase in titer slowly, and remain high for years. Immunofluorescent studies have detected antibody to LCM virus earlier in the course of illness, and its appearance seems to parallel the development of the neurologic phase. The clinical manifestations of LCM cannot be differentiated from those produced by numerous other viruses.

Treatment   There is no specific treatment.

ARGENTINIAN AND BOLIVIAN HEMORRHAGIC FEVERS   The first cases of a new American hemorrhagic disease were seen near the Argentinian town of Junin near Buenos Aires in 1953. A virus was isolated from patients' blood and from local rodents and their mites. In 1959, cases of a disease thought to resemble severe epidemic typhus were noted among rural workers in northeastern Bolivia. The similarity between these syndromes was recognized. In 1963, the causal virus was isolated from patients and rodents and named the Machupo virus. Machupo virus is serologically related to but distinct from Junin virus.

Prevalence   Junin virus infections have occurred in epidemic form since 1958 with between 100 and 3500 cases reported annually. The hemorrhagic disease in Bolivia has been particularly severe. Of a total population of 4000 to 6000 in the endemic area, 750 persons were affected between 1959 and 1963.

Epidemiology   Argentinian hemorrhagic fever (AHF) occurs in sharply endemic seasonal form (February to August), mostly among male rural workers, especially those exposed to fields at the time of the maize harvest. Virus is transmitted in the urine of rodents with chronic infection and viruria. Humans acquire the virus through contact with items or foodstuffs which have been contaminated with infected rodent urine. The main reservoir is two species of cricetidae, *Calomys laucha* and *C. musculinus*.

Bolivian hemorrhagic fever (BHF) is similarly transmitted by the urine of *C. callosus* (a mouselike rodent) chronically infected with Machupo virus. Direct person-to-person transmission is possible and may have occurred in the outbreak in Cochabamba. Disease has not occurred in medical personnel attending infected patients.

Clinical features   Argentinian hemorrhagic fever presents manifestations of renal, cardiovascular, and hematologic involvement. Inapparent infections are rare. The incubation period is estimated to be 7 to 16 days, followed by a gradual onset of chills, fever, headache, malaise, myalgia, anorexia, nausea, and vomiting. The temperature reaches 38.9 to 40°C (102 to 104°F), facial flushing may be prominent, and there is a painless enanthem of the pharynx. Lymphadenopathy and splenomegaly are not present. From 3 to 5 days after the onset, the signs and symptoms worsen, with the appearance of signs of dehydration, hypotension to 50 to 100 mmHg, oliguria, and relative bradycardia. In the more severe cases, hemorrhagic manifestations, including bleeding from the gums, hematemesis, hematuria, and melena, occur. Progressive oliguria and tremor of the tongue and extremities may develop. Some patients develop psychic manifestations, with agitation, delirium, or stupor. Progressive shock, hypothermia, gallop rhythm, or gastrointestinal bleeding may occur from the seventh to tenth days. In fatal cases, pulmonary edema usually is the cause of death. During convalescence temporary alopecia has been noted. Erythrocyte counts are normal or elevated. The total leukocyte count drops to 1200 to 3400 blood cells per cubic millimeter. Thrombocytopenia may occur. Disseminated intravascular coagulation does not seem to be the mechanism responsible for the hemorrhagic manifestations. Complement components C2, C3, and C5 are decreased. The urine is dark and may approach the color of mahogany, with intense albuminuria. Blood urea nitrogen levels rise rapidly.

The clinical picture of Bolivian hemorrhagic fever is similar to Argentinian, although epistaxis and hematemesis at the onset is more common.

Diagnosis Antibody responses, including IgM antibodies, do not occur before 10 to 20 days.

Treatment Treatment consists of supportive measures, including peritoneal dialysis or hemodialysis-filtration to correct both the azotemia and the pulmonary edema. In AHF, a double-blind trial of administration of immune plasma reduced mortality from 16 to 1 percent. However, fever and cerebellar signs occurred in patients treated with immune plasma. Preliminary studies suggest that ribavirin may be effective in experimental BHF in rhesus monkeys.

Prognosis The mortality rate among patients with Argentinian hemorrhagic fever is usually 3 to 15 percent, while that in Bolivian hemorrhagic fever is 5 to 30 percent.

Prevention In Bolivia, rodent control measures directed primarily against *C. callosus* populations in the houses has resulted in a prompt and dramatic cessation of human cases. In Argentina, the wide dispersal of infected hosts renders rodent control measures futile.

LASSA FEVER A virus disease which is both highly contagious and virulent occurred in a missionary nurse in Lassa, a town in northeast Nigeria, in 1969.

Epidemiology Since the initial outbreak at Lassa in 1969, during which one of the patients was transferred to New York City, there have been other outbreaks near Jos in northern Nigeria in 1970 (32 suspected cases with 10 deaths), in Zorzor, Liberia, in 1972 (11 cases with 4 deaths), and in the eastern province of Sierra Leone with 63 suspected cases admitted to two hospitals between 1970 and 1972. Lassa fever occurs as an endemic disease in eastern Sierra Leone. Population surveys showed more than one-half of older adults had antibodies. Other countries in west Africa having clinical or serologic evidence of Lassa fever include Senegal, Gambia, Guinea, Ghana, Burkina Faso (formerly Upper Volta), Mali, and Ivory Coast. Lassa-related viruses (Mopeia, Mobala) have been isolated from rodents in Mozambique, Zimbabwe, and the Central African Republic; however, they have not yet been associated with human illness. In Jos and Zorzor, outbreaks apparently resulted from person-to-person nosocomial spread from the index case to hospital workers or other patients. In Sierra Leone, the great majority of cases were acquired outside the hospital, although hospital workers were at risk. *Mastomys natalensis,* a multimammate rat widespread in Africa, is the animal reservoir, and primary human cases result from contamination of foodstuffs with rodent urine. Human-to-human transmission may occur through contact with urine, feces, vomitus, or saliva through droplets, and particularly through wounds contaminated with blood. Intrafamilial outbreaks have occurred around several cases. There are a number of cases which have been acquired through accidental autoinoculation with needles while starting intravenous fluids. At least one laboratory-acquired infection has occurred. In Sierra Leone 6 percent of the population surveyed had complement-fixing antibody against Lassa virus, while only 0.2 percent had recognized disease,

suggesting mild disease or inapparent infection. In Liberia 10 percent of hospital personnel had antibodies.

Clinical features The incubation period is 1 to 24 days, and was 10 days following accidental inoculation. Patients have ranged from 5 months to 46 years of age; approximately two-thirds are women. Three of eight women in one series were 22 to 28 weeks pregnant during their illness. The apparent predilection for women may relate to exposure to contaminated food or work in hospitals rather than to differences in susceptibility. The onset of illness was described by most patients as insidious. The most frequent initial symptoms were fever (100 percent), chilliness and true rigors, headache (50 percent), malaise (100 percent), and myalgia (50 percent). Most patients did not seek medical attention for 4 to 9 days after onset. Symptoms of a systemic viral illness then developed with anorexia, nausea, vomiting, myalgia, and pain in the chest, epigastrium, and lumbar area. Headache was usually present. Early examination revealed fever and flushing of the face and V area of the neck. Pharyngitis developed early and became progressively more severe during the first week; examination in some cases revealed raised patches of whitish exudate occurring on the palatine arches which occasionally coalesced into a pseudomembrane. Oral ulcerations have been noted in up to one-half of cases. Generalized nontender lymphadenopathy occurred in one-half of patients. During the second week severe lower abdominal pain and intractable vomiting were common, and facial and neck swelling with conjunctival edema and infection frequently developed. Occasionally patients had tinnitus, epistaxis, bleeding from the gums and venipuncture sites, maculopapular rashes, cough, and dizziness. During the acute stage, systolic blood pressures of less than 90 mmHg, with pulse pressures less than 20 mmHg, occurred in 60 to 80 percent of patients. Initially, relative bradycardia was common. During the second week, the patients who recovered defervesced, while the patients who died often developed signs of shock, clouding of the sensorium, rales, signs of pleural effusion, agitation and, on occasion, grand mal seizures. The duration of illness in surviving patients ranged from 7 to 31 days (average 15 days), while that in fatal cases was 7 to 26 days (average 12 days). The mortality rates in Jos and Zorzor were 52 percent and 36 percent, respectively, while in Sierra Leone the rate was 8 percent. During convalescence occasional flurries of rapid involuntary eye movements (oculogyric crises) occurred. Late sequelae include deafness in a number of patients (two of six in one series) and alopecia in one patient.

Laboratory features The hematologic findings include relatively normal hematocrit values and early leukopenia (less than 4000 cells per cubic millimeter in 36 percent) with a relative neutrophilia and immature forms of leukocytes. In two cases in which it was recorded, the erythrocyte sedimentation rate was normal. Urinalyses revealed proteinuria, which was often massive. Chest radiographs may suggest basilar pneumonitis and pleural effusions. Electrocardiographic abnormalities compatible with diffuse myocardial disease have been encountered. Levels of serum enzymes, SGOT, creatinine phosphokinase (CPK), and LDH have been elevated. Lassa virus has been recovered from cerebrospinal fluid in two patients.

Diagnosis Diagnosis can be made by demonstrating a fourfold rise in antibody titer to Lassa virus between acute phase and convalescent phase serum specimens with the indirect fluorescent antibody technique or with Lassa IgM antibodies. The diagnosis is unlikely if IgM antibodies are absent by the fourteenth day of illness.

Treatment The management has been supportive. Infusion of immune plasma from convalescent patients resulted in a dramatic effect in three of four patients. Because of the self-limited nature of the disease, these results cannot be assessed easily. In a study of the antiviral agent ribavirin, 19 of 20 patients treated intravenously within 6 days of onset with a 2.0-g loading dose, followed by 1.0 g every 6 h for 4 days, then 0.5 g every 8 h for another 6 days, survived, whereas 11 of 18 who received no therapy, and 10 of 16 who received convalescent plasma died. In view of the hospital association and the presence of virus in pharyngeal secretions and urine, respiratory and enteric isolation and blood precautions are required. With reasonable isolation practices, nosocomial spread need not be as feared as previously.

OTHER HEMORRHAGIC FEVERS   Ebola hemorrhagic fever and Marburg virus disease are caused by members of the family Filoviridae and are discussed in Chap. 142 and summarized in Table 143-1.

REFERENCES

BAUM SG et al: Epidemic non-meningitic lymphocytic-choriomeningitis virus infection. N Engl J Med 274:934, 1966

CASALS J: Arenaviruses. Yale J Biol Med 48:115, 1975

CENTERS FOR DISEASE CONTROL: Viral hemorrhagic fever. Initial management of suspected and confirmed cases. Ann Intern Med 101:73, 1984

FARMER TW, JANEWAY CA: Infections with the virus of lymphocytic choriomeningitis. Medicine 21:1, 1942

FIELDS BN et al (eds): *Virology*. New York, Raven, 1985

FRAME JD et al: Lassa fever, a new virus disease of man from West Africa: I. Clinical description and pathological findings. Am J Trop Med Hyg 19:670, 1970

JOHNSON KM et al: Hemorrhagic fever of Southeast Asia and South America. A comparative approach. Prog Med Virol 9:105, 1967

McCORMICK JB et al: Lassa fever: Effective therapy with ribavirin. N Engl J Med 314:20, 1986

MacKENZIE RB et al: Epidemic hemorrhagic fever in Bolivia: 1. A preliminary report of the epidemiologic and clinical findings in a new epidemic area in South America. Am J Trop Med Hyg 13:620, 1964

MAIZTEGUI JI et al: Efficacy of immune plasma in treatment of Argentine hemorrhagic fever and association between treatment and a late neurological syndrome. Lancet 2:1216, 1979

MERTENS PE et al: Clinical presentation of Lassa fever cases during the hospital epidemic at Zorzor, Liberia, March–April 1972. Am J Trop Med Hyg 22:780, 1973

MONATH TP et al: Lassa fever in the Eastern Province of Sierra Leone, 1970–1972: II. Clinical observations and virological studies on selected hospital cases. Am J Trop Med Hyg 23:1140, 1974

VANZEE BE et al: Lymphocytic choriomeningitis in University hospital personnel. Clinical features. Am J Med 58:803, 1975

145   VIRAL WARTS

RICHARD C. REICHMAN

DEFINITION   Warts are epithelial tumors that result from papillomavirus (PV) infection of skin or mucous membranes.

ETIOLOGY   PV, members of the A genus of the family Papovaviridae, are nonenveloped viruses, 50 to 55 nm in diameter, with icosahedral capsids composed of 72 capsomeres. They contain a double-stranded, circular DNA genome of about 8000 base pairs. PV appear to be species specific, and human papillomaviruses (HPV) have not been propagated in tissue culture or in experimental animals. Significant quantities of virus are difficult to obtain, and HPV are incompletely characterized. Suitable HPV antigens have not been available and work on the epidemiology, pathogenesis, immunology,

TABLE 145-1   Correlation of human papillomavirus (HPV) type with disease

Virus type	Disease
1	Plantar and palmar warts
2	Common warts
3, 10, 28, 29	Flat warts
4	Plantar and common warts
5, 8, 9, 12, 14, 15, 17, 19–25, 36, 39, 40	Epidermodysplasia verruciformis
6,11	Condyloma acuminatum, respiratory papillomatosis
7	Common warts in meat and animal handlers
13, 32	Focal epithelial hyperplasia (Heck's disease)
16, 18, 31, 33, 35	Genital dysplasias and carcinomas
26, 27	Warts in immunosuppressed patients
30, 34, 37, 38	Isolated cases of benign and malignant neoplasms

and treatment of HPV-induced disease has been difficult to carry out. Structural viral proteins make up 88 percent of the mass of PV virions. A major capsid protein with a molecular weight of 55,000 and as many as 10 additional polypeptides have been identified by sodium dodecyl sulfate polyacrylamide gel electrophoresis. Four cellular histones are associated with the viral DNA. Type-specific antigenic determinants appear to be located on the virion surface and genus-specific determinants internally. Antisera produced by immunization of experimental animals with disrupted PV virions are broadly cross-reactive.

The genomic organization of all PV is similar. Types and subtypes are defined by degree of polynucleotide sequence homology under stringent conditions. DNA of a distinct PV type has a maximum of 50 percent homology with that of other classified viruses. Viruses with greater than 50 percent but less than 100 percent homology constitute subtypes. More than 40 types of HPV are recognized. Individual types are associated with specific kinds of warts (Table 145-1).

EPIDEMIOLOGY   Seroepidemiologic studies of HPV infections have been hampered severely by lack of appropriate antigens, and there are few good studies of the incidence or prevalence of human warts in well-defined populations. Common warts are found in as many as 25 percent of some groups, and are most prevalent among young children. Plantar warts are also widely prevalent and occur most commonly among adolescents and young adults. The incidence of venereal warts (condylomata acuminata) has risen dramatically in the last 10 to 15 years, and condyloma acuminatum is one of the most common sexually transmitted diseases in the United States.

CLINICAL MANIFESTATIONS   Until the mid-1970s, it was generally believed that there was only one HPV and that clinical and pathologic differences among warts were a function of the nature of the squamous epithelium at the site of infection. With the discovery of multiple HPVs, it has become clear that the specific HPV is an important determinant of the nature of the lesion. Thus, clinical manifestations of HPV infection depend upon location of lesions and virus type. Common warts (verrucae vulgaris) usually occur on the hands, and are flesh-colored to brown, exophytic, hyperkeratotic papules. Plantar warts (verrucae plantaris) differ from most other warts by growing inward. They may be quite painful, and can be differentiated from callus by paring the surface to reveal thrombosed capillaries that bleed easily. Flat warts (verrucae plana) are most common among children and occur on the face, neck, chest, and flexor surfaces of forearms and legs.

Anogenital warts (condylomata acuminata, or venereal warts) occur on skin and mucosal surfaces of external genitalia and perianal areas. The differential diagnosis of anogenital warts includes condylomata lata of secondary syphilis, molluscum contagiosum, pearly penile papules, fibroepitheliomas, and a variety of mucocutaneous malignancies. Anogenital warts are sexually transmitted, and have an incubation period of 1 to 6 months. In men, condylomata are found most frequently at the frenum or coronal sulcus, but they may affect any part of the penis. They occur commonly at the urethral meatus, and may extend proximally. Perianal warts are common among homosexual men, but appear in heterosexual men as well. In women, warts appear first at the posterior introitus and adjacent labia. They then spread to other parts of the vulva and commonly involve the perineum and anus. Condylomata frequently involve the vagina and cervix. These lesions may be present in the absence of external warts. Laryngeal papillomatosis is uncommon, occurs predominantly in preschool children, and may result from acquisition of virus at the time of delivery through an infected birth canal. These lesions are typically multiple and may produce life-threatening airway obstruction. Disease in adults may be acquired by orogenital sexual contact.

Immunosuppressed patients, particularly those undergoing organ transplantation, often develop pityriasis rosea–like lesions from which DNA of several HPV types has been extracted. Occasionally, such lesions appear to undergo malignant transformation.

Epidermodysplasia verruciformis is a rare, autosomal recessive disease characterized by the inability to terminate HPV infection and later development of cutaneous squamous cell malignancies. Lesions resemble flat warts or macules similar to those of pityriasis rosea.

Complications of warts include itching and occasionally bleeding. Rarely, they may become secondarily infected with bacteria or fungi. Large masses of warts may produce mechanical problems such as obstruction of the birth canal. Epidemiologic, cytopathologic and histologic data suggest an association of HPV infection with dysplasia and carcinoma of the uterine cervix. HPV nucleic acid sequences have been detected in cervical scrapings and biopsy specimens from patients with these pathologic findings. Sequences homologous to HPV types 16 and 18 have been found in 70 to 80 percent of specimens of cervical cancer tissue from patients in certain geographic areas. Other genital tract malignancies have also been associated with these viruses.

PATHOGENESIS HPV infection is transmitted by close personal contact and is facilitated by minor trauma at the site of inoculation. It may result from direct contact with another individual, by autoinoculation, or via fomites. All types of squamous epithelium may be infected by HPV, and gross and histologic appearances of individual lesions vary with site of infection and virus type. Exophytic warts are characterized by papillomatosis, hyperkeratosis, and elongation of dermal papillae. Acanthosis, an increase in cellularity, occurs in the prickle cell layer in association with viral DNA synthesis. Late gene expression, manifested by appearance of structural proteins and assembled virions, is evident within nuclei of cells in the granular layer, where koilocytosis develops. Koilocytes are large round cells with pyknotic nuclei and large areas of perinuclear vacuolization surrounded by a ring of dense amphophilic cytoplasm.

Host defense responses to HPV infection are poorly understood. Most immunologic studies are difficult to interpret because crude and poorly characterized preparations have been employed as antigens. The potential importance of type-specific responses has not been adequately evaluated because the recognition that there are multiple HPV types is new, and appropriate antigenic materials are not widely available. Virus-specific IgM and IgG antibodies have been demonstrated in patients with and without clinical evidence of active infection. Cell-mediated immune responses to HPV antigens have also been measured, and patients with defects in cell-mediated immunity appear to be more susceptible than normals to HPV infections. Such patients occasionally develop extensive HPV disease.

DIAGNOSIS Most warts that are visible to the naked eye can be diagnosed correctly by history and physical examination alone. Colposcopy is invaluable in assessing vaginal and cervical lesions, and may prove to be helpful in the diagnosis of oral and cutaneous HPV disease as well. Papanicolaou smears prepared from cervical scrapings often show cytologic evidence of HPV infection. Persistent or atypical lesions should be biopsied and examined by routine histologic methods. In addition, the genus-specific capsid antigen can be identified in tissue sections using immunologic techniques, and virus type can be determined by restriction endonuclease analysis of DNA extracted from infected tissues and by hybridization with nucleic acid probes.

TREATMENT Therapy should be initiated with the knowledge that no treatment of proven safety and efficacy is currently available, and that many warts resolve spontaneously. Frequently used therapies include application of caustic agents, cryosurgery, electrodesiccation, surgical excision, and ablation with laser. Topical antimetabolites such as 5-fluorouracil have been used also. Failure as well as recurrence have been well-documented following all these methods of treatment. The high frequency of recurrence may be explained by the presence of HPV DNA in normal-appearing tissue adjacent to lesions, and in previously involved areas during periods of remission. For many years, topically applied podophyllum preparations have been used in treatment of condyloma acuminatum. However, use of these compounds is associated with resolution rates of less than 50 percent, and initial treatment of venereal warts with cryosurgery may be preferable. Promising preliminary results have been observed in the treatment of laryngeal papillomatosis and condyloma acuminatum with different interferon preparations.

At the present time, no effective methods of prevention are available for warts other than avoiding contact with infectious lesions. Barrier methods of contraception may be helpful in preventing transmission of condyloma acuminatum.

REFERENCES

Crum CP et al: Human papillomavirus type 16 and early cervical neoplasia. N Engl J Med 310:880, 1984

Durst M et al: A papillomavirus DNA from a cervical carcinoma and its prevalence in cancer biopsy samples from different geographic regions. Proc Natl Acad Sci USA 80:3812, 1983

Ferenczy A et al: Latent papillomavirus and recurring genital warts. N Engl J Med 313:784, 1985

Jenson AB et al: Human papillomaviruses, in *Textbook of Human Virology*, RB Belshe (ed). Littleton, Mass, Wright-PSG Publishing, 1984, pp 951–968

Lutzner MA et al: Clinical observations, virologic studies, and treatment trials in patients with epidermodysplasia verruciformis, a disease induced by specific human pipillomaviruses. J Invest Dermatol 83:18s, 1984

Oriel JD: Genital warts, in *Sexually Transmitted Diseases*, KK Holmes et al (eds). New York, McGraw-Hill, 1984, chap 46

Pfister H: Biology and biochemistry of papillomaviruses, in *Reviews of Physiology, Biochemistry and Pharmacology*, vol 99, RH Adrian et al (eds). New York, Springer-Verlag, 1984, pp 111–210

Shah KV: Papovaviruses, in *Virology*, BN Fields et al (eds). New York, Raven, 1985

Steinberg BM et al: Laryngeal papillomavirus infection during clinical remission. N Engl J Med 308:1261, 1983

Vance JC et al: Intralesional recombinant alpha-2 interferon for the treatment of patients with condyloma acuminatum or verruca plantaris. Arch Dermatol (in press)

146 FUNGAL INFECTIONS

JOHN E. BENNETT

INTRODUCTION Actinomycetes and fungi are considered together in this section, but this should not obscure profound differences between these two groups of organisms. The agents of actinomycosis, nocardiosis, and actinomycetoma are actinomycetes. These organisms are gram-positive higher bacteria which branch but have the diameter, antibiotic susceptibility, and ability to induce a neutrophilic inflammatory response in common with other bacteria. Actinomycetes resemble fungi in causing infections which may be extremely chronic and which are poorly transmissible from person to person. Few other similarities exist between fungi and actinomycetes. This introductory section will concern mycoses.

The diagnosis of a mycosis requires demonstration of the pathogenic fungus in appropriate patient specimens. Visualization of the fungus by smear or histology is a less precise and less sensitive diagnostic method than culture but is more rapid. Culture allows definitive identification of the pathogen and can detect a small number of organisms. False-positives occur with both methods. Artifacts may be mistaken for fungi in smears or histologic sections. *Candida albicans* can be isolated from the mouth, vagina, sputum, urine, or stool in the absence of candidiasis. *Aspergillus* and, occasionally, *Cryptococcus neoformans* appear in sputum of patients without a mycosis. Histology has the uniquely valuable potential of demonstrating the fungus within the area of inflammation. Only this method can show whether *Aspergillus* in the lung or paranasal sinus tissue exists as a pathogen or merely as a saprophyte growing in pooled secretions. Demonstration of fungi in tissue section usually requires special stains, such as methenamine silver.

Skin testing with fungal antigens has little diagnostic value in active infection. Serologic testing is very helpful in diagnosing coccidioidomycosis and cryptococcosis, as well as in following response to therapy of these mycoses. In histoplasmosis, and paracoccidioidomycosis, serologic tests are useful in adding some support to the clinical diagnosis. A positive serology may provide the impetus for more aggressive diagnostic maneuvers. Serologic results differ enough between laboratories that the physician must know the individual laboratory's experience and expertise.

Topical therapy of a mycosis can be very effective if the fungus is confined to the epidermis or squamous mucosa. Ringworm of the glabrous skin, tinea versicolor, and candidiasis of the skin and mucosa often respond to topical therapy, whereas infection of the skin's deeper layers, such as occurs in sporotrichosis, chromomycosis, mycetoma, and blastomycosis, fails to improve with topical drugs. Allergic bronchopulmonary aspergillosis is presented in Chap. 203.

ANTIFUNGAL AGENTS

TOPICAL AGENTS Imidazoles and triazoles These synthetic compounds act by inhibiting ergosterol synthesis in the fungal cell wall and also probably by direct damage to the cytoplasmic membrane. Drug resistance rarely arises in the previously sensitive strains. Agents of this class include three topical drugs already on the market in the United States: miconazole, clotrimazole, and econazole. Ketoconazole

cream will soon be on the market. Compounds currently available elsewhere or undergoing trial include tioconazole, bifonazole, terconazole, isoconazole, and sulconazole. Miconazole is available without prescription. As yet, no substantial difference in efficacy or local intolerance between these agents has appeared. All are effective in treatment of cutaneous candidiasis, tinea versicolor, and mild to moderately severe ringworm of the glabrous skin. Vaginal formulations are effective in vulvovaginal candidiasis. Clotrimazole is poorly absorbed from the gastrointestinal tract, but the oral troche is useful as a topical treatment for oral and esophageal candidiasis.

Polyene macrolide antibiotics These broad-spectrum antifungal agents combine with sterol in the fungal cytoplasmic membrane, increasing membrane permeability. Topically they are not active against ringworm but are effective against candidiasis of the skin and mucous membranes. Nystatin suspension is effective in oral thrush, and vaginal troches are effective in vulvovaginal candidiasis. Both nystatin and amphotericin B are available in topical preparations for cutaneous candidiasis. Natamycin ophthalmic suspension is marketed in some countries for mycotic keratitis and conjunctivitis.

Other topical antifungals Ciclopirox olamine and haloprogin have the same clinical spectrum among the cutaneous mycoses as the imidazoles. Tolnaftate and undecylenic acid are effective against ringworm but not candidiasis. Keratolytic agents, such as salicyclic acid, are helpful as accessory drugs for some hyperkeratotic skin lesions. Many other topical antifungal preparations are available.

SYSTEMIC ANTIFUNGALS Griseofulvin Griseofulvin is a useful drug in treating certain kinds of ringworm; however, it is ineffective in treating candidiasis. The microcrystalline and ultramicrocrystalline preparations differ in dose but not in efficacy. Absorption of both is enhanced when drug is ingested with fat-containing foods. Griseofulvin metabolism interacts with phenobarbital and coumarin-type anticoagulants.

Imidazoles and triazoles Ketoconazole is the only systemically absorbed oral drug of this class that is currently available, though similar drugs are now undergoing clinical trial. Absorption of ketoconazole is variable between individuals, not affected by food, and poor in patients taking cimetidine or ranitidine. Simultaneous administration of antacids can also impair absorption. Metabolism is chiefly hepatic, although substantial liver disease has minimal effect on blood ketoconazole concentrations. Ketoconazole blood levels are decreased in patients takin rifampin and also possibly isoniazid. Ketoconazole administration can elevate cyclosporin blood levels and, occasionally, can enhance the anticoagulant effect of warfarin. Neither renal disease nor hemodialysis affects the metabolism of ketoconazole. The most common toxicity of ketoconazole is dose-related nausea, anorexia and, occasionally, vomiting. Hepatotoxicity is idiosyncratic and usually mild. Serious hepatotoxicity is rare but can be fatal. Several dose-related, temporary endocrine effects have been observed: decreased adrenal reserve; gynecomastia; decreased serum testosterone, libido, and potency in males; and menstrual irregularity in females. Pruritus or rash may also occur. Ketoconazole is effective in blastomycosis, histoplasmosis, paracoccidiomycosis, chronic mucocutaneous candidiasis, esophageal candidiasis, and some forms of disseminated coccidioidomycosis and pseudallescheriasis. Partial improvement may be seen in cutaneous sporotrichosis and chromomycosis. Although vulvovaginal candidiasis, ringworm, and tinea versicolor are responsive to the drug, the toxicity of oral ketoconazole makes topical imidazoles or other drugs preferable for these indications. Miconazole is available as both a topical and an intravenous preparation. The latter is rarely indicated.

Amphotericin B A colloidal preparation of this drug is available for intravenous or intrathecal administration. The drug cannot be given intramuscularly and is not absorbed orally. Sodium or potassium salts must not be added to the infusion solutions because the colloidal drug will precipitate out of solution. In-line filters with 0.22-μm pore diameter may trap some of the colloid. Within the bloodstream, the drug binds first to plasma lipoproteins and then transfers to tissues throughout the body. The tissue-bound drug slowly elutes back into the blood. Catabolism is extremely slow and is not influenced by renal failure, hepatic failure, or hemodialysis. Penetration into cerebrospinal fluid and vitreous humor is poor; however, concentrations in pleural, peritoneal, and articular exudates are adequate for many mycoses. Histoplasmosis, blastomycosis, paracoccidioidomycosis, candidiasis, and cryptococcosis are the most responsive mycoses. Coccidioidomycosis, extraarticular sporotrichosis, aspergillosis, and mucormycosis are less responsive; chromomycosis, mycetoma, and pseudallescheriasis show little if any response. The usual course is 8 to 10 weeks of 0.4 to 0.6 mg/kg daily. Infusions are generally given in 5% dextrose over 2 to 4 h. Severe febrile reactions to initial doses generally prompt use of an initial test dose with 1 mg, followed by escalating doses based upon the gravity of the patient's infection and tolerance of the drug. Essentially all patients show substantial toxic reactions that are related to the dose and duration of therapy. These side effects include azotemia, anemia, hypokalemia, nausea, anorexia, weight loss, phlebitis and, occasionally, hypomagnesemia. Intrathecal amphotericin B is indicated in coccidioidal meningitis and refractory cryptococcal meningitis, though this therapy is associated with formidable toxicity. Doses of 0.1 to 0.5 mg are given three times per week initially, then with decreasing frequency.

Flucytosine Flucytosine (5-fluorocytosine) is a synthetic oral drug useful in cryptococcosis, candidiasis, and chromomycosis. Within the fungal cell, flucytosine is converted to the antimetabolite 5-fluorouracil. Drug resistance appears rather rapidly when flucytosine is used alone. For this reason the drug is used frequently in combination with amphotericin B, permitting a lower dose of the latter. The usual regimen is amphotericin B 0.3 mg/kg daily and flucytosine 37.5 mg/kg every 6 h. Flucytosine is well absorbed from the gastrointestinal tract, even in the presence of food. The drug penetrates well into the cerebrospinal fluid and is excreted unchanged in the urine. Hemodialysis results in significant drug removal. Even modest reductions in renal function may elevate flucytosine blood levels into the toxic range, meaning more than 100 or 125 μg/mL. Elevated levels are associated with a significant incidence of neutropenia and thrombocytopenia. Elevated flucytosine blood levels also seem to predispose to colitis, the other major toxicity of this drug. Hepatotoxicity is idiosyncratic and uncommon. An allergic rash may also occur.

THE DEEP MYCOSES

CRYPTOCOCCOSIS Etiology Cryptococcosis is an infection caused by the yeastlike fungus *Cryptococcus neoformans*. *C. neoformans* reproduces by budding and forms round, yeastlike cells 4 to 6 μm in diameter. Within the host and on certain culture media, a large polysaccharide capsule surrounds each yeast cell. The fungus grows well as smooth, creamy white colonies on Sabouraud's or other simple media at 20 to 37°C. Certain culture media for ringworm contain cycloheximide, which inhibits *C. neoformans*. Identification is based on gross and microscopic appearance, biochemical tests, and growth at 37°C. The fungus has four capsular serotypes, designated A, B, C, and D, and a perfect state called *Filobasidiella neoformans*.

Pathogenesis and pathology Infection is thought to be acquired by inhalation of fungus into the lungs. Pulmonary infection has a tendency toward spontaneous resolution and is frequently asymptomatic. Silent hematogenous spread to the brain leads to clusters of cryptococci in the perivascular areas of cortical gray matter, basal ganglia, and, to a lesser extent, other areas of the central nervous system. Inflammatory response around these foci is usually scant. In the more chronic cases, a dense basilar arachnoiditis occurs. Lung lesions show an intense granulomatous inflammation. Cryptococci are best seen in tissue by staining with methenamine silver or periodic acid Schiff. A strongly positive mucicarmine stain of the organism in tissue is diagnostic, but staining varies from intense to absent.

Cryptococcus neoformans has been isolated from several sites in nature, particularly weathered pigeon droppings. Patients are usually unaware of any unusual exposure to pigeon droppings. No significant case clustering, highly endemic areas, or racial or occupational predisposition is known. Infection before puberty is uncommon. The male/female ratio is about 2:1. Approximately half the patients have a predisposing condition, such as lymphoma or sarcoidosis, or are receiving supraphysiological doses of adrenal corticosteroids. Patients with the acquired immunodeficiency syndrome (AIDS) are prone to develop rapidly progressive cryptococcosis that is difficult to cure. Neither neutropenia nor hypogammaglobulinemia seems to increase susceptibility to cryptococcosis. Cryptococcosis occurs in animals, especially the cat family. Transmission from animals to humans or from person to person has not been documented.

Clinical manifestations The majority of patients have *meningoencephalitis* at the time of diagnosis. This form of the infection is invariably fatal without appropriate therapy, and death occurs anywhere from 2 weeks to several years from onset of symptoms. Early manifestations include headache, nausea, staggering gait, dementia, irritability, confusion, and blurred vision. Both fever and nuchal rigidity are often mild or absent. Papilledema is present in one-third of the patients at the time of diagnosis. Cranial nerve palsies, typically asymmetric, occur in about one-fourth of the patients. Other lateralizing signs are rare. With progression of the infection, deepening coma and signs of brainstem compression appear. Autopsy often reveals cerebral edema in the more acute cases or hydrocephalus in more chronic cases.

Pulmonary cryptococcosis causes chest pain in about 40 percent of patients and cough in 20 percent. Chest x-ray shows one or more dense infiltrates, which are often well circumscribed. Cavitation, pleural effusions, or hilar adenopathy are infrequent. Calcification is not present, and fibrotic stranding is rarely noticeable.

Skin lesions are present in 10 percent of patients with cryptococcosis. These appear to be hematogenously disseminated because the vast majority of patients will be found to have disseminated infection. One or a few asymptomatic tiny papular lesions appear, slowly enlarge, and tend to show central softening leading to ulceration. Osteolytic bone lesions occur in 4 percent of patients and usually present as a cold abscess. Rare manifestations of cryptococcosis include prostatitis, endophthalmitis, hepatitis, pericarditis, endocarditis, and renal abscess.

Diagnosis Cryptococcal meningoencephalitis must be distinguished from tuberculosis, neoplasm, coccidioidomycosis, histoplasmosis, candidiasis, viral meningitis, and sarcoidosis. Focal lesions are virtually never demonstrable in cryptococcosis by technetium brain scan, cerebral angiography, or electroencephalogram. Computerized tomography (CT) scan will occasionally show one or two areas of decreased density with contrast-enhancing margins. Lumbar puncture is the single most useful test. An india ink smear of centrifuged spinal fluid sediment reveals encapsulated yeast in one-half the cases, but artifacts resembling cryptococci may cause confusion. Cerebrospinal fluid glucose is reduced in half the cases, protein concentration is usually increased, and 20 to 600 leukocytes per cubic millimeter are typically present and consist predominantly of lymphocytes. Approximately 90 percent of patients with cryptococcal meningoencephalitis, including all those with a positive cerebrospinal fluid smear, will have capsular antigen detectable in cerebrospinal fluid or serum by latex agglutination. False-positive tests occur occasionally, making culture the definitive diagnostic test. *C. neoformans* is often present in urine in patients with meningoencephalitis. Fungemia occurs in 10 percent of patients.

Pulmonary cryptococcosis mimics malignancy by x-ray and symptoms. Sputum culture is positive in only 10 percent, and serum antigen tests are positive in only a third. Occasionally, *C. neoformans* appears in one or multiple sputum specimens as an endobronchial saprophyte. Biopsy is usually required for diagnosis of pulmonary cryptococcosis. Cutaneous cryptococcosis may be mistaken for a comedo, basal-cell carcinoma, or sarcoidosis. Biopsy reveals a myriad of cryptococci. Osseous cryptococcosis resembles tuberculosis.

Treatment   Cryptococcal meningoencephalitis may be treated either with amphotericin B alone or in combination with flucytosine. Amphotericin B is given as 0.5 to 0.6 mg/kg per day when used alone or as 0.3 mg/kg per day in combination therapy. With either regimen, double-dose therapy on alternate days may be employed. Flucytosine is given as 150 mg/kg per day divided into four doses, 6 h apart. Reduction of the dose is required in patients with compromised renal function. Lesser nephrotoxicity and more rapid culture conversion with the combination have led to its general acceptance. With either regimen, approximately 50 to 70 percent of patients can be cured. Treatment with either regimen is continued for at least 6 weeks and until at least four weekly cultures of 2 to 4 mL cerebrospinal fluid are sterile. Intrathecal amphotericin B is usually reserved for treatment of patients refractory to conventional therapy. Permanent sequelae include dementia, personality change, hydrocephalus, and blindness.

Patients with extraneural cryptococcosis most often require intravenous amphotericin B, with or without flucytosine. Observation or excision of lesions may suffice for some patients who are previously normal, who have a single focus in lung, skin, or bone, and who have no cryptococci in the cerebrospinal fluid, urine, or blood. All too often, however, patients who present with a presumed single focus of extracranial cryptococcosis are discovered to have early asymptomatic meningoencephalitis or dissemination to other organs.

BLASTOMYCOSIS Etiology   *Blastomyces dermatitidis* is a dimorphic fungus, growing at room temperature as a white or tan mold but growing within the host or at 37°C as budding, round yeastlike cells. The fungus is identified by its appearance, its dimorphism, and the appearance of small spores borne on hyphae of the mold form. When isolates of the two opposite mating types are grown closely together on specialized culture media, sporulating structures appear which characterize the perfect form, *Ajellomyces dermatitidis*.

Pathogenesis and pathology   The infection is restricted by geography and age. Blastomycosis is uncommon in any locality, but the majority of cases occur in the southeast, central, and midatlantic areas of the United States, with occasional cases in other localities in the United States and Canada. Cases have also been encountered in Africa, Mexico, Central America, and, rarely, South America. Most patients are between 20 and 69 years old. The male/female ratio is about 10:1. There is no occupational predisposition.

Infection appears to be acquired by inhalation of the fungus from nature, but the reservoir remains unknown. The fungus has been isolated only rarely from sources other than infected humans or animals. No carrier state or transmission from animal to human or from person to person has been observed. The initial pulmonary infection may heal spontaneously or become chronic. Spread to other portions of the lung, cavitation, or endobronchial lesions may appear in chronic cases. Whether or not the lung lesion resolves spontaneously, infection commonly spreads hematogenously to skin, subcutaneous tissue, bone, prostate, epididymis, or mucosa of the nose, mouth, or larynx. Less commonly, infection spreads to the brain, meninges, liver, lymph nodes, or spleen. Dissemination may not be evident for weeks or years after the appearance of the lung lesion. Progressive infection is only rarely attributable to an underlying

disease or immunosuppressive treatment. The inflammatory response includes lymphocytes, giant cells, and neutrophils. Pseudoepitheliomatous hyperplasia may be striking and lead to a mistaken diagnosis of squamous-cell carcinoma.

Clinical manifestations   A small number of patients have an acute, self-limited pneumonia. Fever, productive cough, myalgia, and malaise usually have resolved within a month. Pulmonary infiltrates have cleared slowly as *B. dermatitidis* disappeared from the sputum. Laboratory exposure or case clusters in certain geographic sites have suggested the diagnosis in many of these cases. In one such case cluster, the incubation period appeared to be 4 weeks. In none of these case clusters has the exact activity leading to exposure been identified.

The vast majority of patients with blastomycosis have an indolent onset and a chronically progressive course. Fever, cough, weight loss, lassitude, skin lesions, and chest ache are common symptoms. Skin lesions favor exposed areas and enlarge over many weeks from a pimple to a well-circumscribed, verrucous, crusted, or ulcerated lesion. Pain and regional lymphadenopathy are minimal. Large chronic lesions may show central healing with scarring and contracture. Mucous membrane lesions resemble squamous-cell carcinoma. Chest x-ray is abnormal in two-thirds of cases, with one or more pneumonic or nodular infiltrates. Calcification, hilar adenopathy, and large pleural effusions are rare. Osteolytic lesions may occur in nearly any bone and present as cold abscess or a draining sinus. Extension to a contiguous joint may cause indolent swelling, pain, and restricted motion. Prostatic and epididymal lesions resemble tuberculosis clinically.

Diagnosis   The diagnosis is made by demonstrating the fungus in culture of sputum, pus, or urine. In experienced hands, diagnosis by appearance of the organism in wet smear or histopathologic section is adequate. The fungus may be visible in a sputum cytology smear but is easily overlooked. Skin tests and serologic tests lack sufficient sensitivity and specificity to be useful.

Treatment   A few patients have been observed with transitory lung lesions, but no guidelines are known to distinguish these patients from those who will progress locally or disseminate. Therefore, every patient should receive treatment. Intravenous amphotericin B is the most established drug and is the drug of choice for patients with rapidly progressive infections, severe illness, or meningitis. Skin and noncavitary lung lesions should be treated for about 8 to 10 weeks. The recommended total dose for an adult is about 2.0 g. Cavitary lung disease or infection beyond the lung and skin should be treated for about 10 to 12 weeks with 2.5 g or more. Ketoconazole is an effective drug in patients with indolent nonmeningeal blastomycosis of mild to moderate severity and who take the drug reliably. The initial adult dose is 400 mg once daily, raised after a month to 600 or 800 mg daily if improvement is suboptimal. Therapy is continued for 6 to 12 months. Iodide therapy is ineffective. The mortality rate in appropriately treated cases is 15 percent or less.

HISTOPLASMOSIS Etiology   *Histoplasma capsulatum* is a dimorphic fungus that grows in nature or on Sabouraud's agar at room temperature as a mold. Hyphae bear both large and small spores that are used for identification. *H. capsulatum* grows as a small budding yeast in host tissue and on enriched agar, such as blood cysteine glucose, at 37°C. Despite the name, the fungus is unencapsulated. When two isolates of the opposite mating type, both in mold form, are grown closely together on an appropriate culture medium, specialized spore-bearing structures are formed which characterize the perfect state, *Emmonsiella capsulata*.

Pathogenesis and pathology   Infection with *H. capsulatum* has been encountered in many areas of the world but is much more frequent in certain areas. Within the United States infection is most common in the southeastern, midatlantic, and central states. Endemic areas are probably determined by the availability of proper conditions in nature for growth of the fungus. *H. capsulatum* prefers moist surface soil, particularly when it is enriched by droppings of certain birds and bats. The fungus has not only been isolated repeatedly from such sites but many case clusters have occurred 5 to 18 days after groups were exposed to such dust, for example, by raking, cleaning dirt-floored chicken coops, bulldozing, or cave exploring. In many endemic areas, 80 percent or more of residents over age 16 have been exposed, judging by skin test reactivity.

Microconidia, or small spores, of *H. capsulatum* are small enough to reach the alveoli on inhalation and are transformed to budding forms. With time, an intense granulomatous reaction occurs. Caseation necrosis or calcification may mimic tuberculosis. The primary infection in children usually heals completely but may leave spotty calcification in the hilar nodes or lung. Transient dissemination may leave calcified granulomas in the spleen. In adults, a rounded mass of scar tissue, with or without central calcification, may remain in the lung. This has been called a *histoplasmoma*. Previous exposure is thought to confer some protection against reinfection, but infection of persons with prior positive skin tests clearly has occurred.

In a small proportion of patients, histoplasmosis becomes a progressive, potentially fatal infection. The disease occurs either as chronic fibrocavitary pneumonia or, less commonly, as disseminated infection. Patients with either form lack a history of acute primary pulmonary histoplasmosis. Chronic pulmonary infection favors otherwise healthy males over the age of 40. A history of cigarette use can be elicited from nearly all patients with chronic progressive pulmonary histoplasmosis. An acute, rapidly fatal course is most likely to be encountered in young children and immunosuppressed patients, including those with AIDS. A more chronic but equally lethal disseminated infection is more common in previously healthy adults.

Clinical manifestations The vast majority of infections are either asymptomatic or mild, and the diagnosis is elusive. Cough, fever, malaise, and chest x-ray findings of hilar adenopathy with or without one or more areas of pneumonitis occur. Erythema nodosum and erythema multiforme have been reported in a few outbreaks. Hilar adenopathy may cause temporary compression of the right middle lobe bronchus in children and young adults. Subacute pericarditis may occur, probably by extension from contiguous lymph nodes. Rarely, hilar nodes undergo a caseous, granulomatous reaction with perinodal fibrosis. Mediastinal structures become encased by progressive fibrosis, and, over many years, compression of the pulmonary veins, superior vena cava, pulmonary arteries, and esophagus may occur. Late in mediastinal disease only rare nonviable histoplasma can be found in caseous residua of lymph nodes.

Patients with *chronic pulmonary histoplasmosis* have a gradual onset over weeks or months of increasing productive cough, weight loss, and sometimes night sweats. Chest x-ray reveals uni- or bilateral fibronodular apical infiltrates. Approximately one-third of cases will stabilize or improve spontaneously early in the course. The remainder have insidious progression. Retraction and cavitation of the upper lobes occur with spread to the apex of the lower lobes and other areas of the lung. Emphysema and bullae formation further compromise pulmonary function. Death from cor pulmonale, bacterial pneumonia, or histoplasmosis occurs after months or years.

Acute disseminated histoplasmosis may be mistaken for miliary tuberculosis (see Chap. 119). Common findings include fever, emaciation, hepatosplenomegaly, lymphadenopathy, jaundice, anemia, leukopenia, and thrombocytopenia. All these features may occur in chronic dissemination as well, but the disease tends to be more localized. Indurated ulcers of the mouth, tongue, nose, or larynx occur in about a fourth of patients. Other focal findings include granulomatous hepatitis, Addison's disease, gastrointestinal ulceration, endocarditis, and chronic meningitis. Chest x-ray abnormalities occur in half the cases and show discrete nodules or a miliary pattern.

The presumed *ocular histoplasmosis* syndrome is a distinct clinical form of uveitis. Although a positive histoplasmin skin test is a requisite for diagnosis, none of these patients has had active histoplasmosis.

Diagnosis Histoplasmosis may be suspected by serologic tests and clinical manifestations, but definitive diagnosis requires demonstration of the organism by culture or histology. Serologic tests are performed with either a culture filtrate called histoplasmin or with whole yeast form cells. The results are interchangeable. Complement fixation is quantifiable and is the best test. Agar gel diffusion with histoplasmin is a useful but not quantifiable test. An H band on agar gel testing is more diagnostic of active histoplasmosis than an M band. Frequent false-negatives and false-positives limit all current serologic tests. Serologic conversion is helpful but occurs rarely except in acute pulmonary histoplasmosis. Higher complement fixation titers, such as 1:32 or greater, are most suggestive of the diagnosis, but no titer is diagnostic. Cross-reactions with serologic tests for blastomycosis are very common. A 5-mm or more diameter area of induration 24 to 48 h after skin testing with histoplasmin has been very helpful in identifying prior exposure to *Histoplasma,* but false-negatives and false-positives are so frequent that skin testing has little value in the study of ill patients. Further, approximately one-fifth of normal volunteers with a positive skin test will convert their histoplasmin serology from negative to positive after skin testing.

Culture of *H. capsulatum* from sputum is difficult but is the procedure of choice in chronic pulmonary histoplasmosis. Digestion by proteolytic enzymes and centrifugation of sputum are helpful. In disseminated histoplasmosis, cultures of bone marrow, blood, centrifuged urine sediment, and biopsy specimens are most often positive. Cultures should be performed on agar surfaces of enriched media at room temperature. Growth occurs in 2 to 6 weeks. Histologic sections of bone marrow, liver, lymph node, lung, and mucosal lesions may yield the diagnosis.

Treatment Acute pulmonary histoplasmosis requires no therapy. Mediastinal fibrosis may benefit by surgery, but the ultimate prognosis is poor. All patients with disseminated or chronic fibronodular pulmonary histoplasmosis should receive chemotherapy. The indications for using ketoconazole, as well as the treatment regimen, are the same as those given in the section on "Blastomycosis." Amphotericin B is given as 0.4 to 0.5 mg/kg per day or double that on alternate days, continued for at least 10 weeks. In chronic pulmonary histoplasmosis, chest x-ray abnormalities improve somewhat, but pulmonary function improves very little. Successful therapy prevents progression. Addisonian crisis is a preventable cause of death in disseminated histoplasmosis.

African histoplasmosis Patients have been encountered in Africa who seem to be infected with *H. capsulatum* except that the yeast form is larger. Clinical manifestations resemble blastomycosis more than histoplasmosis because skin and bone lesions are very common.

COCCIDIOIDOMYCOSIS Etiology *Coccidioides immitis* has two forms, growing as a white fluffy mold on most culture media but as a nonbudding spherical form, a spherule, in host tissue or under specialized conditions. Reproduction in the host tissue is by formation of small endospores within mature spherules. After rupture of the spherule, the released endospores enlarge, become spherules, and repeat the cycle. The fungus is identified by its appearance and by formation of thick-walled, barrel-shaped spores, called *arthrospores,* in the hyphae of the mold form.

Pathogenesis and pathology *C. immitis* is a soil saprophyte in certain arid regions of the United States, Mexico, Central America, and South America. Within the United States, most cases are acquired in California, Arizona, West Texas, and New Mexico. A few cases are acquired in bordering areas and by exposure to fomites from endemic areas, such as cotton bales.

Infection in humans and animals results from inhalation of windborne arthrospores arising from soil sites. This primary pulmonary infection is symptomatic in only 40 percent of individuals, with symptoms ranging from a mild, influenza-like illness to severe pneumonia. Mild, self-limited infections may come to medical attention because of case clusters or hypersensitivity reactions:

erythema nodosum, erythema multiforme, toxic erythema, arthralgia, arthritis, conjunctivitis, or episcleritis. Case clusters occur 10 to 14 days after a group of susceptible individuals is exposed to dust in an endemic area through such activities as unearthing Indian relics, rock hunting, military maneuvers, or construction. Wind storms can carry spores to adjacent nonendemic areas and cause case clusters. The usual course of primary pulmonary infection is complete healing, though an area of pneumonitis on x-ray may heal by forming a coinlike lesion, or coccidioidoma. Less commonly, a single thin-walled cavity remains as a chronic sequela in the area of consolidation. Also, the consolidation may persist as a chronic pneumonia or progress to fibronodular, cavitary disease.

Pleural effusion may be the only manifestation of primary infection. Self-healing of this form is common.

An uncommon but dreaded complication of coccidioidomycosis is dissemination beyond the lung and hilar lymph nodes. Dissemination is more frequent in blacks, Filipinos, Native Americans, Mexican-Americans, and pregnant or immunosuppressed patients, including those with AIDS.

C. immitis incites a chronic granulomatous reaction in host tissue, often with caseation necrosis. Lung and hilar node lesions may show calcification. Both IgM and IgG antibodies against *C. immitis* are induced by infection but neither appears protective. The amount of specific IgG antibody is a rough measure of the antigenic mass, i.e., of the amount of infection, making a high titer a poor prognostic sign. Appearance of delayed hypersensitivity to antigens of *C. immitis* is most common in those clinical forms of disease with a good prognosis, such as self-limited primary pulmonary disease. Negative skin tests to *Coccidioides* antigens occur in roughly half the patients with disseminated disease and portend a poor prognosis.

Clinical manifestations   Symptomatic primary pulmonary infection is manifested by fever, cough, chest pain, malaise, and sometimes hypersensitivity reactions. Chest x-ray may show an infiltrate, hilar adenopathy, or pleural effusion. Peripheral blood may show a mild eosinophilia. Spontaneous improvement begins after several days to 2 weeks of illness and usually culminates in complete recovery.

The symptoms of a chronic thin-walled cavity include cough or hemoptysis in half the cases; the other patients are asymptomatic. Chronic progressive pulmonary coccidioidomycosis produces cough, sputum, variable degrees of fever, and weight loss. The first indications of dissemination usually appear during the primary infection. Reactivation with dissemination in later years occurs occasionally, especially if Hodgkin's disease, non-Hodgkin's lymphoma, renal transplantation, or other immunosuppression has supervened. Dissemination should be suspected when fever, malaise, hilar or paratracheal lymphadenopathy, and elevated sedimentation rate show abnormal persistence in patients with primary pulmonary coccidioidomycosis. High complement fixation titers support this concern. With time, lesions appear in the bone, skin, subcutaneous tissue, meninges, joints, and other sites. Without therapy, dissemination may progress rapidly to death or wax and wane for years.

Diagnosis   When coccidioidomycosis is suspected, sputum, urine, and pus should be examined for *C. immitis* by wet smear and culture. *The laboratory request should indicate clearly that coccidioidomycosis is suspected because the mold form must be handled with extreme care to prevent infection of laboratory personnel.* On biopsy, smaller spherules must be distinguished from nonbudding forms of *Blastomyces* and *Cryptococcus*, but appearance of the mature spherule is diagnostic.

Serologic tests are very helpful in coccidioidomycosis. Latex agglutination and agar gel diffusion tests are useful in screening serums for antibody to *Coccidioides*. The complement fixation test is used on cerebrospinal fluid and to confirm and quantitate serum antibody detected by screening tests. The number of cases with a positive complement fixation test will depend upon the severity of disease and upon the laboratory performing the test. Positive tests are least common in patients with solitary pulmonary cavities or primary pulmonary infection, while serums from patients with multiorgan disseminated disease are nearly all positive. Seroconversion is helpful in primary pulmonary coccidioidomycosis but may not occur for up to 8 weeks after onset. A positive complement fixation test in unconcentrated cerebrospinal fluid is diagnostic of meningitis. Rarely, a parameningeal focus will cause a positive CSF serology.

Conversion of the skin test from negative to positive (≥ 5 mm induration at 24 or 48 h) with either coccidioidin or spherulin, the two commercially available antigens, may be observed between the third and twenty-first days of symptoms in primary pulmonary coccidioidomycosis. Skin testing can also be helpful in epidemiologic studies, such as investigation of case clusters or definition of endemic areas. The utility of skin testing as a diagnostic tool is limited by the presence of persistent positive tests resulting from remote exposures to *Coccidioides* and by the frequency of negative skin tests in many patients with either thin-walled cavities or disseminated coccidioidomycosis.

Treatment   Primary pulmonary coccidioidomycosis usually resolves spontaneously. Some physicians give a few weeks of intravenous amphotericin B when patients show an unusually severe or protracted primary infection, hoping to abort disseminated or chronic pulmonary disease. There is no solid evidence to support this practice, but the stronger the suspicion of dissemination becomes in any given patient, the more logical this approach appears. Once evidence for dissemination becomes incontrovertible, amphotericin B may be palliative rather than curative. Incomplete recovery and relapse after apparent cure with amphotericin B have been distressingly common in both disseminated and chronic progressive pulmonary infection. The low toxicity and possibility of long-term oral therapy with ketoconazole have encouraged study of this drug in nonmeningeal coccidioidomycosis. Doses of 200 to 400 mg per day have improved some patients with skin, bone, and lung coccidioidomycosis. Patients failing to respond to this dose should have the dose escalated gradually in the 10 to 20 mg/kg per day range to assess clinical response and toxicity. Treatment is continued 12 months or more. A seriously ill or rapidly deteriorating patient should not be treated with this drug. Such patients are given intravenous amphotericin B 0.5 to 0.7 mg/kg daily or a double dose on alternate days until infection appears relatively quiescent, often 10 or 12 weeks. More prolonged courses may be changed to 1.0 mg/kg three times a week. Surgical debridement of bone lesions and drainage of abscesses contribute to cure. Resection of chronic progressive pulmonary lesions is a helpful adjunct to chemotherapy when infection is confined to the lung and in one lobe. A single thin-walled cavity tends to close spontaneously, and ordinarily is not resected. Such a cavity responds poorly to chemotherapy. Coccidioidal meningitis is treated with long-term intrathecal amphotericin B. Hydrocephalus, a frequent complication, renders this therapy less effective. The prognosis in all forms of chronic progressive coccidioidomycosis must be guarded.

THE OPPORTUNISTIC DEEP MYCOSES

CANDIDIASIS   Etiology   *Candida albicans* is the most common cause of candidiasis, but *C. tropicalis, C. parapsilosis, C. guilliermondii, C. krusei,* and a few other species can cause candidiasis and may even be fatal. *C. parapsilosis* is particularly notable for its ability to cause endocarditis. All *Candida* species pathogenic for humans are also encountered as commensals of humans, particularly in the mouth, stool, and vagina. These species grow rapidly at 25 to 37°C on simple media as oval budding cells. In specialized culture media, hyphae or elongated branching structures called *pseudohyphae* are formed. *C. albicans* can be identified presumptively by its ability to form germ tubes in serum or by the formation of thick-walled large spores, called *chlamydospores*. Final identification of all species requires biochemical tests.

Pathogenesis and pathology Either local or systemic factors may lead to tissue invasion by *Candida*. Chronic maceration predisposes to cutaneous candidiasis, as in diaper rash, intertrigo in obese patients, or paronychia in bartenders or cannery workers. Age is important because neonatal colonization often leads to oral candidiasis (thrush). Women in the third trimester of pregnancy are prone to vulvovaginal thrush. Patients with diabetes mellitus, AIDS, or hematologic malignancy, or who are receiving broad-spectrum antibiotics or high doses of adrenal corticosteroids, are especially susceptible to candidiasis. Breaks in the integrity of the skin or mucous membranes may provide access to deeper tissues. Examples include perforation of the gastrointestinal tract by trauma, surgery, and peptic ulceration; indwelling catheters for intravenous alimentation, peritoneal dialysis, and urinary tract drainage; severe burns; and intravenous drug abuse.

Candida grows within tissues in both yeast and pseudohyphal forms. Rarely, only one form is present. Visceral lesions are characterized by necrosis and a neutrophilic inflammatory response. Neutrophils kill *Candida* yeast cells and damage segments of pseudohyphae in vitro, suggesting a major role for the neutrophil in host defense against this fungus. Visceral lesions show a preference for kidney, brain, spleen, heart, and liver.

Clinical manifestations *Oral thrush* presents as discrete and confluent adherent white plaques on the oral and pharyngeal mucosa, particularly in the mouth and tongue. These lesions are usually painless, but fissuring at the corners of the mouth can be painful. *Cutaneous candidiasis* presents as red, macerated intertriginous areas, paronychia, balanitis, or pruritus ani. Candidiasis of the perineal and scrotal skin may be accompanied by discrete pustular lesions on the inner aspects of the thighs. *Chronic mucocutaneous candidiasis* or *Candida granuloma* typically presents as circumscribed hyperkeratotic skin lesions, crumbling dystrophic nails, partial alopecia in areas of scalp lesions, and both oral and vaginal thrush. Systemic infection is very rare, but disfigurement of the face and hands can be severe. Other findings may include chronic epidermophytosis, dental dysplasia, and hypofunction of the parathyroid, adrenal, or thyroid glands. A variety of defects in T-cell function have been described in these patients. Vulvovaginal thrush causes pruritus, discharge, and sometimes pain on intercourse or urination. Speculum examination reveals an inflamed mucosa and a thin exudate, often with white curds.

From one to multiple small shallow ulcerations due to *Candida* may appear in the esophagus or gastrointestinal tract. Esophageal lesions favor the distal third and may cause dysphagia or substernal pain. Other such lesions tend to be asymptomatic but assume importance in the leukemic patient as a portal for disseminated candidiasis. Within the urinary tract, the most common lesions are either hematogenous renal abscesses, which can cause azotemia, or bladder thrush. Bladder invasion usually follows catheterization or instrumentation of a patient with diabetes mellitus or who is receiving broad-spectrum antibiotics. This lesion generally is asymptomatic and benign. Rarely, retrograde invasion of the renal pelvis leads to renal papillary necrosis.

Hematogenous dissemination of Candida presents with fever and toxicity but with few localizing findings. One or more retinal abscesses may appear and extend slowly into the vitreous humor. The patient may note orbital pain, blurred vision, scotoma, or opacities floating across the visual field. Pulmonary candidiasis is almost always hematogenous and is visible on chest x-ray only when the abscesses are numerous enough to cause a diffuse, vaguely nodular infiltrate. Candidiasis of the endocardium or around intracardiac prostheses resembles bacterial infection of these sites. Chronic *Candida* meningitis or arthritis may occur, from either disseminated disease or insertion of a prosthesis in the case of arthritis. Rare focal manifestations of disseminated disease include osteomyelitis, pustular skin lesions, myositis, and brain abscess.

Diagnosis Demonstration of pseudohyphae on wet smear with confirmation by culture is the procedure of choice for diagnosing superficial candidiasis. Scrapings for the smear may be obtained from skin, nails, and oral and vaginal mucosa. Culture alone is not diagnostic.

Deeper lesions of *Candida* may be diagnosed by histologic section of biopsy specimens or by culture of cerebrospinal fluid, blood, joint fluid, or surgical specimens. Blood cultures in vented bottles or concentrated by lysis-centrifugation are very useful in *Candida* endocarditis and intravenous catheter-induced sepsis but are positive less often in other forms of disseminated disease. The utility of serodiagnosis remains controversial.

Treatment Cutaneous candidiasis of macerated areas responds to measures which reduce moisture and chafing plus a topically applied antifungal agent in a nonocclusive base. Nystatin, ciclopirox, and the imidazole creams such as clotrimazole and miconazole appear roughly equivalent. Nystatin and some imidazoles are available also for vaginal application. Oral candidiasis should be treated with clotrimazole troches or a nystatin suspension. Swallowing nystatin suspension, sucking on clotrimazole troches, or taking ketoconazole, 200 to 400 mg per day, may improve symptoms of esophageal candidiasis. When esophageal symptoms are pronounced, a 5- to 10-day course of intravenous amphotericin B, 0.3 mg/kg per day, may be beneficial. Bladder thrush responds to bladder irrigations with amphotericin B, 50 μg/mL for 5 days. In all forms of skin and mucosal candidiasis, relapse after successful treatment is common.

Intravenous amphotericin B is the drug of choice in disseminated candidiasis. The drug is usually given as 0.4 to 0.5 mg/kg every day or as a double dose on alternate days for several weeks. In patients with no contraindication to the use of flucytosine, administration of that drug in dosage of 100 to 150 mg/kg per day plus amphotericin B, 0.3 mg/kg per day, is an effective alternative. Ketoconazole in an adult dose of 200 mg daily is probably the drug of choice for chronic mucocutaneous candidiasis.

Candida isolated from a properly obtained blood culture should be considered significant, for true false-positives are rare. Whether a patient with candidiasis should receive antifungal therapy will depend on the degree of illness and the likelihood of spontaneous recovery. For example, a febrile, severely immunosuppressed patient with one positive blood culture should receive prompt therapy because a rapidly fatal course is common. A nonimmunosuppressed patient acquiring candidiasis from an indwelling intravenous plastic catheter may recover spontaneously if the catheter is removed promptly. The species of *Candida* is irrelevant to this decision. Patients with candidiasis in whom antifungal therapy is withheld should be observed carefully for the development of endophthalmitis, endocarditis, arthritis, osteomyelitis, or other visceral lesions that require therapy.

ASPERGILLOSIS **Etiology** *Aspergillus fumigatus* is the most common pathogen, but *A. flavus, A. niger,* and several other species can cause disease. *Aspergillus* is a mold with septate hyphae about 2 to 4 μm in diameter. Sporulating structures, called *conidial heads,* may be seen when the fungus is growing in nature, on an artificial medium, or within air-containing spaces of the body. The appearance of the colonies and of conidial heads is used for identification.

Pathogenesis and pathology All the common species of *Aspergillus* which cause disease in humans are ubiquitous in the environment, growing on dead leaves, stored grain, compost piles, hay, and other decaying vegetation. Inhalation of *Aspergillus* spores must be extremely common, but disease is rare. Invasion of lung tissue is almost entirely confined to immunosuppressed patients. Roughly 90 percent will have two of these three conditions: less than 500 granulocytes per cubic millimeter of peripheral blood, supraphysiologic doses of adrenal corticosteroids, and a history of cytotoxic drugs such as azathioprine. Infection in such patients is characterized by hyphal invasion of blood vessels, thrombosis, necrosis, and hemorrhagic infarction. Chronic granulomatous disease of childhood also predisposes to invasive pulmonary aspergillosis, but here the inflammatory response is granulomatous. Blood vessel invasion is rare.

Massive inhalation of *Aspergillus* spores by normal persons can lead to an acute, diffuse, self-limited pneumonitis. Epithelioid granulomas with giant cells and central pyogenic areas containing hyphae are seen. Spontaneous recovery taking several weeks is the usual course.

Aspergillus can colonize the damaged bronchial tree, pulmonary cysts, or cavities of patients with underlying lung disease. Balls of hyphae within cysts or cavities may reach several centimeters in diameter and be visible on chest x-ray. Tissue invasion does not occur. The term *allergic bronchial aspergillosis* denotes the condition of patients with preexisting asthma who have eosinophilia, IgE antibody to *Aspergillus,* and fleeting pulmonary infiltrates from bronchial plugging (see Chap. 203).

Clinical manifestations *Endobronchial pulmonary aspergillosis* presents as chronic productive cough and often hemoptysis in a patient with prior chronic lung disease, such as tuberculosis, sarcoidosis, bronchiectasis, or histoplasmosis. *Aspergilloma* refers to a ball of hyphae within a lung cyst or cavity, usually in the upper lobe. *Aspergillus* may be spread from its endocavitary or endobronchial site to the pleura during the course of bacterial lung abscess or surgery.

Invasive aspergillosis in the immunosuppressed host presents as an acute pneumonia. Infection progresses by hematogenous spread as well as extension to surrounding lung and other contiguous structures. Occasionally the portal of infection in the immunosuppressed host is the paranasal sinus, gastrointestinal tract, skin, or palate.

Aspergillus sinusitis in nonimmunosuppressed patients may take two forms. A ball of hyphae may form in a chronically obstructed paranasal sinus, without tissue invasion. Much less commonly, a chronic, fibrosing granulomatous inflammation with *Aspergillus* hyphae within tissue may begin in the sinus and spread slowly to the orbit and brain.

Growth of *Aspergillus* on cerumen and detritus within the external auditory canal is termed *otomycosis.* Trauma to the cornea may cause chronic *Aspergillus* keratitis. Endophthalmitis follows introduction of *Aspergillus* into the globe by trauma or surgery. *Aspergillus* may infect intracardiac or intravascular prostheses.

Diagnosis Repeated isolation of *Aspergillus* from sputum or demonstration of hyphae in sputum or bronchial brushing specimens suggests endobronchial colonization or infection. Fungus ball of the lung is usually detectable by chest x-ray. Antibody of the IgG class to *Aspergillus* antigens is demonstrable in the serum of many colonized patients and of virtually all patients with fungus ball.

Biopsy is usually required to diagnose invasive aspergillosis of the lung, paranasal sinus, or sites of dissemination. Blood cultures are rarely positive, even in patients with infected cardiac prosthetic valves. *Aspergillus* hyphae can be identified presumptively by histology, but culture is required for confirmation and determination of species. Serologic and skin tests have not proved helpful in invasive aspergillosis.

Treatment Patients with severe hemoptysis due to fungus ball of the lung may benefit by lobectomy. Poor pulmonary function in residual lung and dense pleural adhesions around the lesion can complicate the resection. Systemic chemotherapy is of no value in endobronchial or endocavitary aspergillosis.

Intravenous amphotericin B has resulted in arrest or cure of invasive aspergillosis when immunosuppression is not severe. Combined flucytosine–amphotericin B may be useful in nonneutropenic patients with invasive aspergillosis.

MUCORMYCOSIS (ZYGOMYCOSIS, PHYCOMYCOSIS) Etiology

Rhizopus and *Mucor* species are the principal pathogens, though *Cunninghamella* and *Absidia* species are occasionally encountered. These molds have broad, rarely septate hyphae of uneven diameter, ranging from 6 to 50 μm. The fungus is inexplicably difficult to grow from infected tissue. When it occurs, growth is rapid and profuse on most media at room temperature. Identification is based upon gross and microscopic appearance of the mold.

Pathogenesis and pathology *Rhizopus* and *Mucor* species are ubiquitous, appearing on decaying vegetation, dung, and foods of high sugar content. Infection is uncommon and largely confined to patients with serious preexisting diseases. Mucormycosis originating in the paranasal sinuses and nose occurs predominantly in patients with poorly controlled diabetes mellitus. Mucormycosis in patients with hematologic malignancy or organ transplantation more often originates in the lung than in the nose and paranasal sinuses. Gastrointestinal mucormycosis occurs in a variety of conditions, including uremia, severe malnutrition, and diarrheal diseases. Infection is acquired from nature, with no person-to-person spread. Elastic bandages contaminated with *Rhizopus* species have caused several postoperative skin and subcutaneous infections.

In all forms of mucormycosis, vascular invasion by hyphae is prominent. Ischemic or hemorrhagic necrosis is the predominant histologic finding.

Clinical manifestations Mucormycosis originating in the nose and paranasal sinuses produces a characteristic clinical picture. Low-grade fever, dull sinus pain, and sometimes nasal congestion or a thin, bloody nasal discharge are followed in a few days by double vision, increasing fever, and obtundation. Examination reveals a unilateral generalized reduction of ocular motion, chemosis, and proptosis. The nasal turbinates on the involved side may be dusky red or necrotic. A sharply delineated area of necrosis, strictly respecting the midline, may appear in the hard palate. The skin of the cheek may become inflamed. Fungal invasion of the globe or ophthalmic artery leads to blindness. Opacification of one or more sinuses is found on x-ray. Carotid arteriogram may show invasion or obstruction of the carotid siphon. Coma is due to direct invasion of the frontal lobe. Early symptoms mimic bacterial sinusitis. Clouding of the sensorium may be attributed to diabetic acidosis. Cavernous sinus thrombosis may be considered when orbital invasion occurs. Without treatment, death may occur in a few days to a few weeks.

Pulmonary mucormycosis is a progressive severe pneumonia, accompanied by high fever and toxicity. The necrotic center of large infiltrates may cavitate. Hematogenous spread to other areas of the lung, as well as to brain and other organs, is common. Survival beyond 2 weeks is unusual. Gastrointestinal invasion presents as one or more ulcers which tend to perforate. Hematogenous dissemination can originate from the gastrointestinal tract, lung, or paranasal sinuses. Sometimes no portal of entry can be found.

Diagnosis Lesions of the lung and craniofacial structures are best diagnosed by biopsy and histologic section. Cultural confirmation should be attempted. Wet smear of crushed tissue can provide rapid diagnosis. Cultures of blood and cerebrospinal fluid are negative. Smear and culture of sputum may be positive during cavitation of a lung lesion. Serologic tests are of little assistance.

Treatment Regulation of diabetes mellitus and decreasing immunosuppressive drugs aid in the treatment. Extensive debridement of craniofacial lesions appears to be very important. Orbital exenteration may be required. Intravenous amphotericin B is clearly of value in craniofacial mucormycosis and should be employed in the other forms of mucormycosis as well. Maximum tolerated doses are given until progression is halted. The drug is continued for a total of 10 to 12 weeks. Appropriate management results in cure of about half of the craniofacial infections. Survival of patients with pulmonary, gastrointestinal, or disseminated mucormycosis is rare.

SPOROTRICHOSIS Etiology *Sporothrix schenckii* lives as a saprophyte on plants in many areas of the world. In nature and on culture at room temperature the fungus grows as a mold, but within host tissue or at 37°C on enriched media it grows as a budding yeast. Identification is by appearance of the fungus in mold and yeast forms. Small spores with a hairlike attachment to hyphae give the fungus the name *Sporothrix.*

Pathogenesis and pathology Infection results when minor trauma inoculates the fungus into subcutaneous tissue. Nursery workers, florists, and gardeners acquire the illness from roses, sphagnum moss, and other plants. Infection may be limited to the site of inoculation (plaque sporotrichosis) or extend along proximal lymphatic channels (lymphangitic sporotrichosis). Spread on an extremity, the usual site, even as far as inguinal or axillary nodes is rare, and hematogenous dissemination from the skin remains unproven. The portal for osteoarticular, pulmonary, and other extracutaneous forms of sporotrichosis is unknown but is likely the lung.

Untreated sporotrichosis shows little evidence of self-healing and is capable of extreme chronicity. The inflammatory response contains both clusters of neutrophils and a marked granulomatous response with epithelioid cells and giant cells.

Clinical manifestations Lymphangitic sporotrichosis, by far the most common manifestation, forms a nearly painless red papule at the site of inoculation. Over the next several weeks, similar nodules form along proximal lymphatic channels. Nodules intermittently discharge small amounts of pus. Ulceration may occur. The proximal extension of these lesions, often with skip areas, is quite distinctive but may be mimicked by lesions of *Nocardia brasiliensis, Mycobacterium marinum,* or, on rare occasions, by *Leishmania brasiliensis* or *M. kansasii.*

Plaque sporotrichosis is a nontender red maculopapular granuloma confined to the site of inoculation. Osteoarticular sporotrichosis presents as mono- or polyarticular arthritis of indolent onset and progression over months or years, involving the elbows, knees, wrists, ankles, and, rarely, smaller joints of the extremities. Periarticular bone gradually appears "moth-eaten," and draining sinuses may appear over joints and bursas. Hematogenous spread to the skin may be observed during polyarticular disease, but none of the skin lesions shows lymphangitic spread. Immunosuppression predisposes to such spread. Pulmonary sporotrichosis usually presents as a single chronic cavitary upper-lobe lung lesion.

Diagnosis Culture of pus, joint fluid, sputum, or skin biopsy specimen is the preferred method of diagnosis. Appearance of *S. schenckii* in tissue is quite variable. In skin lesions, organisms are hard to find.

Treatment Cutaneous sporotrichosis can be cured with oral administration of a saturated solution of potassium iodide, given in increasing divided daily doses up to 4.5 to 9 mL per day for adults, as tolerated. Gastrointestinal disturbance or acneform rash over the cape area and face are common, but therapy should be continued for 1 month after resolution of all lesions. Patients with serious allergic reactions to iodides may respond to local heat, particularly when plaque sporotrichosis is the only form of disease. Extracutaneous sporotrichosis rarely responds to iodides, but cures have been obtained in over half such patients with prolonged courses of intravenous amphotericin B.

RARER DEEP MYCOSES

PARACOCCIDIOIDOMYCOSIS Etiology Formerly called *South American blastomycosis,* this is the mycosis caused by *Paracoccidioides brasiliensis.* A dimorphic fungus, *P. brasiliensis* grows as a budding yeast but may be grown as either yeast or mold on a culture medium. Identification is by gross and microscopic appearance. A superficial resemblance to *Blastomyces dermatitidis* may cause misdiagnosis.

Pathogenesis and pathology Infection is thought to be acquired by inhalation of spores from environmental sources, but the reservoir in nature remains obscure. Pulmonary infection produces few symptoms initially. Hematogenous spread to the mucous membranes of the mouth and nose, the lymph nodes, and other sites brings the patient to medical attention. Fatal cases show spread to the adrenal, the gastrointestinal tract, and many other viscera.

Clinical manifestations Common symptoms include indurated ulcers of the mouth, oropharynx, larynx, and nose, enlarged and draining lymph nodes, lesions of the skin and genitalia, productive cough, weight loss, dyspnea, and sometimes fever. Acquisition of infection is restricted to South America, Central America, and Mexico, but the extreme indolence of this infection may lead to recognition many years after the patient has left the endemic area. Chest x-ray most often shows a bilateral patchy pneumonia.

Diagnosis Cultures of sputum, pus, and mucosal lesions are often diagnostic. The diagnosis can be made by smear or histologic section, though confirmation by culture is preferable. Serologic tests are useful in suggesting the diagnosis and monitoring therapy.

Treatment Milder cases may be cured by one year's treatment with oral ketoconazole, 200 to 400 mg daily. More advanced cases are given intravenous amphotericin B, followed by ketoconazole.

PSEUDALLESCHERIASIS Etiology Also called *Petriellidium boydii, Pseudallescheria boydii* is a mold frequently found in soil. When the fungus is isolated in the imperfect state, it is called *Seedosporium apiospermum.*

Pathogenesis and pathology Wind-borne spores of *P. boydii,* arising in soil, are the presumed source of infection. The fungus grows as a mold within tissue, causing necrosis and abscess formation.

Clinical manifestations *P. boydii* resembles *Aspergillus* in its ability to colonize the endobronchial tree, to form fungus balls in the lung or paranasal sinuses, to invade the cornea or globe following trauma or surgery, and by its propensity to invade the immunosuppressed host. Hyphae of *P. boydii* in tissue may be difficult to distinguish from *Aspergillus.* Infection with *P. boydii* is much less common than with *Aspergillus. P. boydii* is the single most common cause in the United States of mycetoma. Intravascular hyphae, a hallmark of invasive aspergillosis, also can be found in pseudallescheriasis. Occasional normal patients have developed necrotizing pneumonia or abscesses in brain or other organs due to *P. boydii.*

Diagnosis Demonstration of hyphae in tissue and culture confirmation are required for diagnosis.

Treatment Intravenous miconazole or ketoconazole is recommended, but therapeutic response to all drugs has been poor.

TORULOPSOSIS Etiology *Torulopsis glabrata (Candida glabrata)* is a small yeast-like fungus, the same size as the yeast form of *Histoplasma capsulatum. T. glabrata* does not form hyphae or pseudohyphae. Identification is by biochemical tests.

Pathogenesis and pathology *T. glabrata* is a normal inhabitant of the human gastrointestinal tract and vagina. Within tissue, *T. glabrata* causes abscess formation with a neutrophilic inflammatory response. In immunosuppressed patients, a scanty or mononuclear inflammatory response may be seen.

Clinical manifestations Torulopsosis mimics many of the manifestations of candidiasis, but infection is less common and often less severe. Clinical entities include intravenous catheter–induced sepsis or endocarditis, gastrointestinal and disseminated infection in immunosuppressed patients, and retrograde infection of the urinary tract.

Diagnosis *Torulopsis* may be difficult to distinguish from yeast cells of *Candida* in histologic section. Culture is the most reliable diagnostic tool.

Treatment Therapeutic measures used in candidiasis appear appropriate for torulopsosis.

MYCETOMA Etiology *Actinomycetoma* refers to infection by actinomycetes of the genera *Nocardia, Streptomyces,* and *Actinomadura. Eumycetoma* is caused by true fungi of many different genera. The most common agent varies with the locality.

Pathogenesis and pathology The pathogens live in the soil and enter the skin through minor trauma. The most common site of infection is the foot. Infection runs a relentless course over many years, with destruction of contiguous bone and fascia. Grains are found in purulent foci, surrounded by fibrosis and a mononuclear cell inflammatory response.

Clinical manifestations *Mycetoma* is a chronic suppurative infection originating in subcutaneous tissue and characterized by the presence of grains, which are tightly clumped colonies of the causative agent. The infected site shows painless swelling, woody induration, and sinus tracts which discharge pus intermittently. Systemic symptoms and spread to distant sites in the body are not seen.

Diagnosis The clinical picture is characteristic, but confusion with chronic osteomyelitis or botryomycosis may occur. The diagnosis requires demonstration of grains in pus from the draining sinus or in biopsy sections. Many histologic sections may need to be examined to locate a grain.

Treatment Actinomycetoma may respond to prolonged therapy with sulfonamides, trimethoprim-sulfamethoxazole, or other antibacterial agents. Eumycetoma does not respond reliably to any drug. Amputation may be required.

CHROMOMYCOSIS Etiology The five species of fungi currently recognized as causing this syndrome have received a bewildering number of different names. Using Emmons' classification, these fungi are called *Phialophora verrucosa*, *P. pedrosoi*, *P. compacta*, *P. dermatitidis*, and *Cladosporium carrionii*.

Pathogenesis and pathology Infection occurs in tropical and subtropical areas where workers acquire many small puncture wounds from thorns or splinters. Histopathologic section of the skin lesion shows pseudoepitheliomatous hyperplasia and a granulomatous dermal infiltrate. Microabscesses with neutrophils also occur. Clumps of the pathogenic organism are found in these abscesses or elsewhere in the dermis as rounded, thick-walled brown cells. The epidermis and superficial crusts may contain branching brown hyphae.

Clinical manifestations *Chromomycosis* is characterized by chronic verrucoid, ulcerated, or crusted skin lesions. The site of the lesion depends upon the area of trauma but is usually the foot or leg. The lesion begins as a pimple, pustule, or ulcer with slow progression over many years. Lesions may remain flat or become pedunculated. Pain is minimal, but itching is common. Infection usually remains confined to the same extremity, but a few cases have spread hematogenously to cause brain abscess.

Diagnosis Demonstration of the characteristic organisms in histologic sections of skin biopsy is the best diagnostic method. Positive cultures are obtained readily, but accurate identification may require the service of a reference laboratory.

Treatment Prolonged therapy with oral flucytosine appears helpful. Relapse with secondary drug resistance has been encountered with sufficient frequency to make flucytosine plus low-dose intravenous amphotericin B appear preferable for large lesions.

DERMATOPHYTOSIS

Definition Dermatophytosis, also known as ringworm or tinea, is a chronic fungal infection of the skin, hair, or nails.

Etiology Species of *Trichophyton*, *Microsporum*, and *Epidermophyton* are called *dermatophytes*. They grow in and remain confined to the keratinous structures of the body. Other mycoses can show fungal invasion of keratinous structures, such as candidiasis, pityriasis versicolor, and tinea nigra, but are traditionally not termed *dermatophytoses*.

Pathology and pathogenesis Dermatophyte species are called anthropophilic, zoophilic, or geophilic, depending on whether their usual reservoir within nature appears to be humans, animals, or soil. Infectivity of all those sources is low, and group outbreaks are largely confined to an occasional case clustering of scalp infections in children. Acquisition of a dermatophytosis appears to be favored by minor trauma, maceration, and poor hygiene of the skin. Infection does not seem to confer solid immunity. Repeated infection with the same species is commonplace, particularly with anthropophilic species. Infrequency of scalp infection in adults has been attributed to local factors rather than immunity.

Invasion of the stratum corneum by dermatophytes may cause little inflammation, or, particularly with zoophilic fungi, inflammation can be intense. Shedding of the stratum corneum is increased by inflammation. To the extent that fungal growth cannot keep up with shedding, inflammation may help terminate infection. Conversely, infection is probably favored when shedding is reduced by corticosteroids and cytotoxic drugs. Antifungal drugs interfere with the ability of fungal growth to keep up with shedding.

Clinical manifestations The disease varies with the site of infection and fungal species. Foot infection (athlete's foot, tinea pedis) may present as fissuring of the toe webs, scaling of the plantar surfaces, or vesicles around the toe webs and soles. Interdigital lesions may be pruritic or, when bacterial superinfection occurs, may be painful. Hand infection is less common but resembles foot infection. Scalp dermatophytosis (tinea capitis) is characterized by areas of alopecia and scaling. In so-called endothrix infection, the hair shaft breaks off at the skin surface, leaving the hairs visible as black dots in the scalp. With some forms of scalp infection an intense boggy suppuration occurs, called a *kerion*. Dermatophytosis of the glabrous skin (tinea corporis) presents as circumscribed lesions with a wide variety of appearances. Scales, vesicles, or pustules may appear. Inflammation may be minimal or intense. Central healing of less inflamed lesions may be seen. The serpiginous border of inflammation is the source of the name *ringworm*. Dermatophytosis of the bearded area (tinea barbae) appears as a pustular folliculitis. Onychomycosis (tinea unguium) presents as white discolored nails or thickened, chalky crumbling nails. Peeling and fissuring of the perinychia or keratotic debris under the nail edge may also be seen.

Diagnosis Discolored hairs, scales, and keratotic debris under infected nails should be collected for KOH smear and culture. In the scraping of skin lesions, a drop of water on the skin site may keep the removed scales from flying off and aid in their collection. Culture is important in distinguishing dermatophytes from *Candida* and fungal saprophytes growing in keratinaceous debris.

Treatment Mild or moderately severe lesions of the trunk, groin, and feet often respond to topical therapy with an imidazole or one of the other agents mentioned earlier in this chapter. Hyperkeratotic lesions of the palms and soles respond less well. Ringworm that is moderately severe or severe, that is unresponsive to topical therapy, or that involves the scalp, nails, or bearded area should be treated systemically. The drug of choice is griseofulvin. Either 500 mg of the microcrystalline form or 375 mg of the ultramicrocrystalline form is given once daily or divided into two doses, given with meals. Double this amount has been recommended for refractory infections. Treatment must be continued until all infected keratin is gone. Cutting of infected hair, epilating nails, and cleansing interdigital webs can expedite cure. Secondary bacterial infection of the foot may require soaks or antibacterial agents. Relapse of dermatophyte foot infections may be decreased by measures to keep the feet clean and dry. Griseofulvin-resistant cases may respond to oral ketoconazole, 200 to 400 mg daily.

REFERENCES

Therapy

AMA DEPARTMENT OF DRUGS: Antifungal agents for systemic mycoses, in *AMA Drug Evaluations*, 5th ed. Chicago, American Medical Association, 1983, pp 1779–1788

BENNETT JE: Treatment of cryptococcal, candidal and coccidioidal meningitis, in *Current Clinical Topics in Infectious Diseases*, JS Remington, M Swartz (eds). New York, McGraw-Hill, 1980, vol 2, pp 54–67

Drugs for treatment of systemic fungal infections. The Medical Letter 24:35, 1982

EMMONS CW: *Medical Mycology*. Philadelphia, Lea & Febiger, 1977

HEIDEMANN HT et al: Amphotericin B nephrotoxicity in humans decreased by salt repletion. Am J Med 75:476, 1983

KERRIDGE D: Present status of antimycotics. Microbiol Sci 2:83, 1985

MEDOFF G, KOBAYASHI GS: Strategies in the treatment of systemic fungal infections. N Engl J Med 302:145, 1980

NIAID MYCOSES STUDY GROUP. Treatment of blastomycosis and histoplasmosis with ketoconazole. Ann Intern Med 103:861, 1986

RIPPON JW: *Medical Mycology. The Pathogenic Fungi and the Pathogenic Actinomycetes*. Philadelphia, Saunders, 1982

Cryptococcosis

BENNETT JE et al: A comparison of amphotericin B alone and combined with flucytosine in treatment of cryptococcal meningitis. N Engl J Med 301:126, 1979

KHOURY MB et al: Thoracic cryptococcosis: Immunologic competence and radiologic appearance. Am J Radiol 141:893, 1984

PERFECT JR et al: Cryptococcemia. Medicine 62:98, 1983

Blastomycosis

EDSON RS, KEYS TF: Treatment of primary pulmonary blastomycosis. Results of long term follow-up. Mayo Clin Proc 56:683, 1981

HABTE-GABR E, SMITH IM: North American blastomycosis in Iowa. Review of 34 cases. J Chronic Dis 26:523, 1973

HALVORSEN RA et al: Pulmonary blastomycosis: Radiologic manifestations. Radiology 150:1, 1984

KLEIN BS et al: Isolation of *Blastomyces dermatitidis* in soil associated with a large outbreak of blastomycosis in Wisconsin. N Engl J Med 314:529, 1986

SAROSI GA, DAVIES SF: Blastomycosis. Am Rev Respir Dis 120:911, 1979

Histoplasmosis

GOODWIN RA et al: Histoplasmosis in normal hosts. Medicine 60:231, 1981

WHEAT LJ et al: Cavitary histoplasmosis occurring during two large urban outbreaks. Analysis of clinical, epidemiologic, roentgenographic, and laboratory features. Medicine 63:201, 1984

——— et al: Histoplasmosis in the acquired immune deficiency syndrome. Am J Med 78:203, 1985

Coccidioidomycosis

BOUZA E et al: Coccidioidal meningitis. An analysis of thirty-one cases and review of the literature. Medicine 60:139, 1980

DRUTZ DJ, CATANZARO A: Coccidioidomycosis. Am Rev Respir Dis 117:559, 727, 1978

———: Amphotericin B in the treatment of coccidioidomycosis. Drugs 26:337, 1983

EINSTEIN HE (ed): Proceedings of the 4th International Conference on Coccidioidomycosis. Washington, DC, National Foundation for Infectious Diseases, 1984

SALOMON NW et al: Surgical manifestations and results of treatment of pulmonary coccidioidomycosis. Ann Thorac Surg 30:433, 1980

Candidiasis

DUPONT B, ROUHET E: Cutaneous, ocular, and osteoarticular candidiasis in heroin addicts: New clinical and therapeutic aspects in 38 patients. J Infec Dis 152:577, 1985

LEVINE MS et al: *Candida* esophagitis; accuracy of radiographic diagnosis. Radiology 154:581, 1985

LEWIS JH et al: The spectrum of hepatic candidiasis. Hepatology 2:479, 1982

ROSE HD, SHETH NK: Pulmonary candidiasis. A clinical and pathological correlation. Arch Intern Med 138:964, 1978

SOLOMKIN JS et al: The role of *Candida* in intraperitoneal infections. Surgery 88:524, 1980

Aspergillosis

FAULKNER SL et al: Hemoptysis and pulmonary aspergilloma: Operative versus non-operative treatment. Ann Thorac Surg 25:389, 1978

RINALDI MG: Invasive aspergillosis. Rev Infect Dis 5:1061, 1983

WEILAND D et al: Aspergillosis in 25 renal transplant patients. Epidemiology, clinical presentation, diagnosis and management. Ann Surg 198:622, 1983

YOUNG RC et al: Aspergillosis: Spectrum of the disease in 98 patients. Medicine 49:149, 1970

Mucormycosis

BARTRUM RJ et al: Roentgenographic findings in pulmonary mucormycosis. Am J Roentgenol 117:810, 1973

LEHRER RI et al: Mucormycosis. Ann Intern Med 93:93, 1980

MANIGLIA AL et al: Cephalic phycomycosis: A report of eight cases. Laryngoscope 92:755, 1982

MEYERS BR et al: Rhinocerebral mucormycosis. Premortem diagnosis and therapy. Arch Intern Med 139:557, 1979

Sporotrichosis

BULLPITT P, WEEDON D: Sporotrichosis: A review of 39 cases. Pathology 10:249, 1978

CROUT JE et al: Sporotrichosis arthritis. Clinical features of seven patients. Ann Intern Med 86:294, 1977

ENGLAND DM, HOCHHOLZER L: Primary pulmonary sporotrichosis. Am J Surg Path 9:193, 1985

FRIEDMAN SJ, DOYLE JA: Extracutaneous sporotrichosis. Int J Dermatol 22:171, 1983

LYNCH PJ et al: Systemic sporotrichosis. Ann Intern Med 73:23, 1970

Paracoccidioidomycosis

CASTANEDA OJ et al: *Paracoccidioides brasiliensis* arthritis. Report of a case and review of the literature. J Rheumatol 12:356, 1985

LONDERO AT, SEVERO LC: The gamut of progressive pulmonary paracoccidioidomycosis. Mycopathologia 75:65, 1981

RESTREPO A et al: The gamut of paracoccidioidomycosis. Am J Med 61:33, 1976

——— et al: Ketoconazole in paracoccidioidomycosis: Efficacy of prolonged therapy. Mycopathologia 72:35, 1980

SUGAR AM et al: Paracoccidioidomycosis in the immunosuppressed host: Report of a case and review of the literature. Am Rev Respir Dis 129:340, 1984

Pseudallescheriasis

BAKERSPIGEL A, SCHAUS D: Petrielliodiosis (pseudallescheriasis) in southwestern Ontario, Canada. Sabouraudia 22:247, 1984

GALGIANI JN et al: *Pseudallescheria boydii* infections treated with ketoconazole. Chest 86:219, 1984

TRAVIS LB et al: Clinical significance of *Pseudallescheria boydii*: A review of 10 years' experience. Mayo Clin Proc 60:531, 1985

WINSTON DJ et al: *Allescheria boydii* infections in the immunosuppressed host. Am J Med 63:830, 1977

Torulopsosis

KAUFFMAN CA, TAN JS: *Torulopsis glabrata* renal infection. Am J Med 57:217, 1974

VALDIVIESO M et al: Fungemia due to *Torulopsis glabrata* in the compromised host. Cancer 38:1750, 1976

Mycetoma

GREEN WO, ADAMS TE: Mycetoma in the United States. Am J Clin Pathol 42:75, 1964

MAHGOUB ES: Medical management of mycetoma. Bull WHO 54:303, 1976

TARALAKSHMI VV et al: Mycetomas caused by *Streptomyces pelletieri* in Madras, India. Arch Dermatol 114:204, 1978

Chromomycosis

LONDERO AT, RAMOS DC: Chromomycosis: A clinical and mycologic study of thirty-five cases observed in the hinterland of Rio Grande Do Sul, Brazil. Am J Trop Med Hyg 25:132, 1976

LOPES CF: Recent developments in the therapy of chromoblastomycosis. Bull Pan Am Health Organ 15:58, 1981

Dermatophytosis

COX FW et al: Oral ketoconazole for dermatophyte infections. Am Acad Dermatol 6:445, 1982

ROBERTSON MH et al: Ketoconazole in griseofulvin-resistant dermatophytosis. J Am Acad Dermatol 6:224, 1982

147 ACTINOMYCOSIS AND NOCARDIOSIS

JOHN E. BENNETT

ACTINOMYCOSIS

DEFINITION Actinomycosis is an indolent suppurative infection caused by certain anaerobic actinomycetes. The microorganisms grow within the tissue as grossly visible tightly knit clusters, called *grains*.

ETIOLOGY *Actinomyces israelii* is the usual pathogen, with occasional cases due to other species of *Actinomyces* (*A. naeslundii, A. viscosus, A. odontolyticus, A. meyeri*) or *Arachnia propionica*. All can form branching gram-positive hyphae, are the same width as bacteria, and grow best in an atmosphere which is either anaerobic or contains 6 to 10% CO_2. Isolation of the causal agent is rendered difficult by the usual presence of mixed flora in actinomycotic abscesses.

PATHOLOGY AND PATHOGENESIS All agents of actinomycosis are commensals in the mouth and gastrointestinal tract of humans. The portal of entry appears to be either a break in the integrity of the mucosa or aspiration into the lung. Poor dental hygiene and dental abscess predispose to cervicofacial lesions. Within the gastrointestinal tract, the appendiceal area is the most common site. Infection presents as a chronic suppurative inflammation, usually in the cervicofacial, thoracic, or abdominal area. In histopathologic section, each grain is typically surrounded by polymorphonuclear neutrophils. The adjacent tissue shows subacute or chronic inflammation with extensive fibrosis and formation of sinus tracts. Giant cells are infrequent. The grain stains variably with hematoxylin and eosin, and may have an eosinophilic coating composed of human proteins. Hyphal filaments cannot be seen on hematoxylin and eosin stain but may be demonstrated in the periphery of the grain by tissue Gram stain (such as Brown and Brenn) or by a heavily stained Gomori methenamine silver. These stains may be useful if there is chance for confusion with the grains of eumycetoma or staphylococcal botryomycosis. The grains are a few millimeters in diameter, making them difficult to miss if they are present in the histologic section being examined. Several sections may have to be searched to find a grain. Grains may be observed grossly in pus or on bandages covering draining sinuses. These pale yellow, cheeselike particles can be crushed on a microscope slide, and the gram-positive branching filaments demonstrated on Gram stain.

Infection spreads by direct extension and hematogenously. Direct extension through the skin causes one or more chronic draining sinuses to appear in the abdomen, chest, or cervicofacial area. Hematogenous foci may appear in bone, brain, liver, or other organs.

CLINICAL MANIFESTATIONS *Cervicofacial actinomycosis* presents as a red or purplish firmly indurated subcutaneous mass, typically in the submandibular area or in the anterior cervical triangle near the angle of the mandible. One or more draining sinuses may be present. Tenderness is slight or absent. Lethargy, weight loss, variable low-grade fever, anemia, and leukocytosis are infrequent in cervicofacial actinomycosis but common in *thoracic* and *abdominal actinomycosis*. Localizing findings in the latter forms include draining sinuses and, in thoracic actinomycosis, cough and purulent sputum. Pulmonic lesions may extend through the chest wall and present as an indolent subcutaneous abscess. Pain or a palpable mass may appear in abdominal actinomycosis. *Pelvic actinomycosis*, once rare, is now being seen in women with intrauterine devices. The indolent onset, variable low-grade fever, abdominal pain, and adnexal mass may lead to an erroneous diagnosis of pelvic inflammatory disease or tumor. In all forms of actinomycosis, disease typically has been present for weeks or months at time of diagnosis.

Chest x-ray may reveal an area of dense pneumonitis. Fibrosis, empyema, or cavitation may be seen. Periappendiceal abscess may appear as an extrinsic mass on barium enema.

DIAGNOSIS Laboratory tests other than culture or histologic section are not helpful. Blood cultures are rarely positive. Isolation of *Actinomyces* or *Arachnia* species from the mouth, sputum, stool, or feculent draining sinuses is not diagnostic. Demonstration of a grain in pus or deep tissue is diagnostic, if botryomycosis and mycetoma can be excluded. Nocardiosis can be distinguished by the absence of grains, identification of the organism in culture, and, usually, by the weak acid-fast staining of *Nocardia*.

TREATMENT Milder cases of actinomycosis, including most cervicofacial infections, respond well to oral tetracycline or penicillin V, an adult dose being 500 mg qid of either drug. Oral erythromycin would be second choice. More severe cases, including most thoracic and abdominal infections, should receive parenteral penicillin G for roughly 6 weeks (in adults 2 to 6 million units per day) followed by prolonged therapy with oral penicillin V or tetracycline. The likelihood of relapse is reduced if the total duration of therapy is 2 to 4 months in mild cases and up to 6 to 12 months in severe forms. Drug resistance has not been encountered in relapses. Curettage of bone lesions, surgical resection of necrotic tissue, and drainage of empyema, brain abscess, or other large collections of pus facilitate recovery but are usually not curative by themselves.

It is common in actinomycosis to isolate microbes other than actinomycetes from pus. In general, the antibiotic susceptibility of

these secondary organisms does not have to be considered in the selection of therapeutic agents.

NOCARDIOSIS

DEFINITION Nocardiosis is an acute, subacute, or chronic infection, most often beginning in the lung.

ETIOLOGY *Nocardia asteroides, N. brasiliensis,* and *N. caviae* are the etiologic agents of two different diseases, nocardiosis and mycetoma. In the latter infection, the organism enters the skin by trauma, forms grains within tissue, and spreads slowly to contiguous tissue (see Chap. 146). While nocardiosis can result from local trauma, the organism usually enters via the lung, does not form grains, and is prone to hematogenous spread. Even though the etiologic agents of these diseases do overlap, *N. asteroides* causes most cases of nocardiosis and *N. brasiliensis* is the species usually isolated from mycetoma. *Nocardia caviae* is a rare cause of either disease. *Nocardia brasiliensis* can also cause a lymphocutaneous disease closely resembling sporotrichosis; this infection differs from mycetoma by its lymphangitic spread and by the absence of grains.

Nocardia species are aerobic actinomycetes with branching hyphae the same width as bacteria. Hyphae are weakly gram-positive and weakly acid-fast. Growth appears in 2 to 5 days on blood agar, Sabouraud's agar, or other simple media. Incorporation of antibiotics into the media to inhibit bacterial growth usually inhibits *Nocardia* as well. Colonies become rough and chalky with an orange or yellow hue. Identification of *Nocardia* species, including distinction between *Streptomyces, Actinomadura,* and *Nocardia,* is difficult and best assigned to a reference laboratory.

PATHOGENESIS AND PATHOLOGY *Nocardia* is a soil saprophyte widely distributed throughout the world. Infection is acquired from sites in nature, never from infected persons or animals. Males are infected two to three times more commonly than females. No age or exposure is known to predispose to nocardiosis. Many patients have serious preexisting conditions, such as adrenal corticosteroid therapy, cancer, pulmonary alveolar proteinosis, or chronic granulomatous disease of childhood.

Lesions of nocardiosis show suppuration, necrosis, and abscess formation. Neutrophils are the predominant inflammatory cell. Hyphae are scattered throughout the lesion without formation of grains. Tissue Gram stain or overstained methenamine silver demonstrates the hyphae best. A modified Fite-Faraco stain of histologic sections can be used to demonstrate acid-fastness.

CLINICAL MANIFESTATIONS *Nocardia* pneumonia presents with fever and productive cough of several days' or up to several months' duration. The initial illness may resemble a bacterial pneumonia, but slow radiologic progression continues despite antibiotic therapy, often with cavitation of radiodense central areas. Hematogenous dissemination to brain and subcutaneous tissue is frequent in nocardiosis. A pulmonary portal is usually but not always detectable clinically. Brain lesions are typically multiple abscesses. Purulent meningitis may result from rupture of an abscess into the ventricle. The subcutaneous lesion typically consists of one or a few indolent abscesses. Hematogenous dissemination to other organs occurs but is rarely detectable clinically.

DIAGNOSIS *Nocardia* is difficult enough to detect in sputum culture on Gram stain or in histologic section so that the diagnosis is readily missed. A progressive pneumonia with purulent sputum should suggest the diagnosis, particularly if cavitation or spread to brain or subcutaneous tissue occurs. Sputum, pus, bronchial brushing, or bronchial washing specimens should be examined by Gram stain and modified acid-fast stain. On Gram stain the hyphae are usually branching, beaded, and refractile. They are not strongly gram-positive but take the red counterstain even less well. Conventional acid-fast staining procedures such as Ziehl-Neelsen or a fluorochrome often do not stain *Nocardia*. Identification of branching, weakly acid-fast organisms in histologic section or smear of pus or sputum, is sufficient to establish the diagnosis of nocardiosis. Cultural confirmation is highly desirable, but isolation of *Nocardia* from heavily contaminated specimens is difficult. Isolation of *Nocardia* from otherwise sterile pus is readily accomplished. *Nocardia* is rarely isolated from blood, but diphasic culture media are said to facilitate isolation.

When *Nocardia* is isolated from sputum, the diagnosis of nocardiosis should be suspected, but occasionally no disease can be detected. Rarely, *Nocardia* is an airborne contaminant.

TREATMENT Surgical drainage of empyema and abscesses in brain or subcutaneous tissue is helpful but not sufficient to achieve cure. Virtually all patients should receive prolonged chemotherapy. The treatment of choice is sulfisoxazole or trimethoprim-sulfamethoxazole. Sulfadiazine had been regarded as the drug of choice because of favorable clinical experience and excellent penetration into the cerebrospinal fluid. The poor availability of intravenous solutions and the danger of oliguria with crystalluria has restricted the use of sulfadiazine. Sulfisoxazole therapy is begun orally or intravenously at 100 mg/kg per day in four divided doses. The dose is then adjusted downward to achieve a peak blood concentration of 10 to 15 mg/dL (100 to 150 µg/mL). Alternatively, trimethoprim-sulfamethoxazole can be given orally or intravenously as 50 mg/kg per day of the sulfamethoxazole component, divided into two doses per day. With either regimen, therapy is continued for 6 to 12 months, depending on the severity of the infection and the presence of immunosuppression. Addition of other antibiotics to sulfa drugs may be indicated in patients who show continued deterioration. Ampicillin 150 mg/kg per day is preferred. High doses of minocycline or erythromycin also have been advocated. Parsimonious use of other drugs during sulfa therapy of nocardiosis minimizes the probability that a drug allergy will necessitate discontinuance of sulfa.

Survival has been reported in 92 percent of cases with isolated pulmonary nocardiosis compared to 52 percent in cases with brain abscess. Concomitant use of immunosuppressive therapy seems to impair therapeutic response in nocardiosis.

REFERENCES

Actinomycosis

BARTELS LJ, VRABEC DP: Cervicofacial actinomycosis—A variable disorder. Arch Otolaryngol 104:705, 1978

BENHOF DF: Actinomycosis: Diagnostic and therapeutic considerations and a review of 32 cases. Laryngoscope 94:1198, 1984

DAVIES M, KEDDIE NC: Abdominal actinomycosis. Br J Surg 60:18, 1973

DUGUID HL et al: *Actinomyces*-like organisms in cervical smears from women using intrauterine contraceptive devices. Br Med J 23:534, 1980

FRADIS M et al: Actinomycosis of the face and neck. Arch Otolaryngol 102:87, 1976

LUDMERER KM et al: Draining inguinal ulcer in a middle-aged woman. Am J Med 77:537, 1984

WEESE WC, SMITH IM: A study of 57 cases of actinomycosis over a 36-year period. Arch Intern Med 135:1562, 1975

Nocardiosis

CURRY WA: Human nocardiosis. Arch Intern Med 140:818, 1980

DEWSNUP DH, WRIGHT CN: In vitro susceptibility of *Nocardia asteroides* to 25 antimicrobial agents. Antimicrob Agents Chemother 25:165, 1984

GALLIS HA: The clinical spectrum of *Nocardia brasiliensis* infection in the United States. Rev Infect Dis 6:164, 1984

GEISELER PJ, ANDERSEN BR: Results of therapy in nocardiosis. Am J Med Sci 278:188, 1979

SMEGO RA et al: Trimethoprim-sulfamethoxazole therapy for *Nocardia* infections. Arch Intern Med 143:711, 1983

section 8 Rickettsia, *Mycoplasma,* and *Chlamydia*

148 RICKETTSIAL DISEASES

THEODORE E. WOODWARD

Introduction The rickettsial diseases of humans consist of a variety of clinical entities caused by microorganisms of the family Rickettsiaceae. The rickettsias are obligate intracellular parasites about the size of bacteria and are usually seen microscopically as pleomorphic coccobacilli. Each of the rickettsias pathogenic for humans is capable of multiplying in one or more species of arthropod as well as in animals and humans. Indeed, the majority of the rickettsias are maintained in nature by a cycle which involves an insect vector and an animal reservoir, and infection of humans is unimportant in the cycle. Epidemic typhus presents a number of points of dissimilarity to most of the other rickettsioses. Until recently, the natural cycle of infection was thought to involve only humans and lice. The finding of a sylvatic reservoir in flying squirrels associated with a human illness which resembles classic typhus emphasizes that there are other mechanisms.

A compendium of information of the rickettsial diseases is given in Table 148-1. Because each of the rickettsioses responds therapeutically to tetracyclines or chloramphenicol, the table mentions no therapy. Procedures for diagnostic isolation of the rickettsias are omitted because they generally are less useful than serologic methods, and the techniques which they require are highly specialized and hazardous. Information on isolation may be found in textbooks devoted to viral and rickettsial diseases.

Of all the afflictions of the human race the rickettsial diseases, particularly epidemic typhus, rank among the foremost as a cause of suffering and death. The record of deaths from epidemic typhus in this century in the Balkan countries and in Poland and Russia reached astounding figures. Typhus ravaged Russia and eastern Poland from 1915 to 1922, infecting 30 million of the inhabitants and causing an estimated 3 million deaths.

The past two decades have seen the development of excellent methods for the prevention and treatment of rickettsioses. In fact, these measures have been so successful that the rickettsioses have become of minor importance in the United States and in many other countries. Although conquered, the rickettsioses have not been eliminated, and they could again become rampant if the will to control them, the present high standards of sanitation, and the necessary industrial capacities for production of effective insecticides and therapeutic agents should be decreased through war or disaster.

Pathogenesis Rickettsial diseases develop after infection through the skin or the respiratory tract. Agents of the typhus and spotted fever group are introduced through the bite of the infected arthropod vector. Ticks and mites, which transmit the agents of spotted fever and scrub typhus, inoculate the rickettsias directly into the dermis during feeding. The louse and flea, which transmit epidemic and murine typhus, respectively, deposit infected feces on the skin; infection occurs when organisms are rubbed into the puncture wound made by the arthropod. The rickettsias of Q fever gain entry through the respiratory tract when infected dust is inhaled; moreover, the respiratory route is occasionally implicated in epidemic typhus when infection results from inhalation of dried infected louse feces.

Although organisms probably multiply at the original site of entry in all instances, local lesions appear with regularity only in certain diseases, namely, the initial cutaneous lesions of scrub typhus, rickettsialpox, and boutonneuse fever, and the pneumonitis which develops in about half the persons infected with Q fever.

Volunteers infected with either scrub typhus or Q fever develop rickettsemia late in the incubation period, often some hours before the onset of fever. Similar events probably occur in all the rickettsial diseases; circulating rickettsias can be detected during the early febrile period in practically all patients. Little is known about the pathogenesis of infection during the midportion of the incubation period. However, it is reasonable to assume that during this time, in patients with typhus or spotted fever, a transient low-grade rickettsemia results from release of organisms multiplying at the initial site of infection and that this seeds infection in the endothelial cells of the vascular tree. Vascular lesions developing at such sites account for the pathologic changes, including the rash.

Rickettsias apparently invade and proliferate in the endothelial cells of small blood vessels. Endothelial cell destruction occurs from the proliferation of organisms and eventual disruption. Rickettsias may exert a cytotoxic effect on endothelial cells; in mice the rickettsial toxin causes remarkable increase in capillary permeability, independent of proliferation. The anatomic localization of multiple microscopic-sized lesions and the numerous foci of rickettsial vascular changes with rickettsias present coincide well for organs carefully examined such as the kidney, lung, heart, and liver. Current observations along these lines confirm Wolbach's original conclusion that "the lesions of the blood vessel are due to the presence of the parasite." Absence of inflammatory cell reactions in fulminant Rocky Mountain spotted fever tends to exclude several host-mediated pathogenic mechanisms. A delayed type of hypersensitivity does occur during infection. The entire process, however, is not explainable by immunopathologic mechanisms.

The underlying cause of the toxic-febrile state which characterizes the rickettsial diseases remains unknown. Several rickettsial species contain type-specific toxins which are lethal for mice; these may play a role.

Pathologic physiology Peripheral vascular collapse results in death in fulminating cases during the first week, with capillary dilatation and pooling of blood without increased capillary permeability or loss of fluid into extravascular spaces. As proliferative and thrombotic lesions develop in small vessels, anoxia occurs in the areas supplied, resulting in necrosis and increased capillary permeability, with loss of water, electrolytes, proteins, and erythrocytes. This in turn results in a decrease in blood volume, together with an increase in the

TABLE 148-1 Rickettsial diseases

Disease Type	Agent	Geographic distribution	Natural cycle — Arthropod	Natural cycle — Mammal	Principal means of transmission to humans	Serologic diagnosis — Weil-Felix reaction	Serologic diagnosis — CF, MA, and IFA reactions*
SPOTTED FEVER GROUP							
Rocky Mountain spotted fever	R. rickettsii	Western hemisphere	Ticks	Wild rodents, dogs	Tick bite	Positive OX-19 OX-2	Positive group- and type-specific
Boutonneuse fever	R. conorii	Africa, Europe, Middle East, India					
Queensland tick typhus	R. australis	Australia		Marsupials, wild rodents			
North Asian tick-borne rickettsiosis	R. sibirica	Siberia, Mongolia		Wild rodents			
Rickettsialpox	R. akari	United States, Russia, Africa(?)	Blood-sucking mite	House mouse, other rodents	Mite bite	Negative	
TYPHUS GROUP							
Endemic (murine)	R. typhi	Worldwide	Flea	Small rodents	Infected flea feces into broken skin	Positive OX-19	Positive group- and type-specific
Epidemic	R. prowazekii	Worldwide	Body louse	Humans Flying squirrels	Infected louse feces into broken skin	Positive OX-19	
	R. Canada	North America	Ticks			Positive OX-19	
Brill-Zinsser disease	R. prowazekii	Worldwide	Recurrence years after original attack of epidemic typhus			Usually negative	
Scrub	R. tsutsugamushi	Asia, Australia, Pacific islands	Trombiculid mites	Wild rodents	Mite bite	Positive OX-K	Positive in about 50% of patients
OTHER RICKETTSIAL DISEASES							
Q fever	R. burnetii	Worldwide	Ticks	Small mammals, cattle, sheep, goats	Inhalation of dried infected material	Negative	Positive
Trench fever	R. quintana†	Europe, Africa, North America	Body louse	Humans	Infected louse feces into broken skin	Negative	None available

* CF = complement fixation; MA = microscopic agglutination; IFA = immunofluorescent antibody.
† Some authorities no longer place the agent in the genus Rickettsia because it can be cultured on artificial media.

extravascular space and clinical edema. Edema, anoxia of the myocardium, and histologic evidence of myocarditis are disclosed by electrocardiographic abnormalities, including serious arrhythmias. Liver function is impaired. The azotemia which develops in seriously ill patients appears to be prerenal. Clinical manifestations resulting from the peripheral vascular collapse are oliguria and anuria, azotemia, anemia, hypoproteinemia, hyponatremia, edema, and coma. In spotted fever and typhus patients with hemorrhagic skin lesions, consumptive coagulopathy is present. All these alterations are absent or minimal in mild cases or in those who are given specific treatment early.

Pathology The basic changes in the spotted and typhus fever groups are vascular, with resultant widespread lesions in adjacent parenchymatous tissues throughout the body. They are most common in the skin, muscles, heart, lung, and brain. The most conspicuous and diverse are found in Rocky Mountain spotted fever. Here swelling, proliferation, and degeneration of the endothelial cells occur, frequently with thrombus formation which partially or completely occludes the lumen. The muscle cells of the arterioles undergo swelling and fibrinoid changes. The adventitial tissues are infiltrated with mononuclear leukocytes, lymphocytes, and plasma cells. The vascular damage is scattered along the arteries, veins, and capillaries, with normal architecture prevailing throughout most of the vascular bed. The changes in murine, epidemic, and scrub typhus fevers resemble those in Rocky Mountain spotted fever, but thrombosis is uncommon and involvement of the musculature is rare.

Interstitial myocarditis occurs in each of these diseases but is usually most extensive in Rocky Mountain spotted fever and in scrub typhus. In the brain glial nodules are found in all members of the group, but microinfarcts in the brain tissue or in the myocardium are most often observed in spotted fever.

A rickettsial pneumonitis occurs, at least to some extent, in many patients with spotted or typhus fever and is the characteristic pathologic change in patients with Q fever. The process is patchy and consists microscopically of areas of congestion and edema. Within the consolidated areas the alveoli are filled with compact fibrinocellular exudate containing lymphocytes, plasma cells, large mononuclear cells, and erythrocytes, but few, if any, polymorphonuclear leukocytes.

Rickettsias can occasionally be observed microscopically in sections of tissue. Failure to demonstrate them is of no diagnostic significance. They are readily identifiable by the immunofluorescent technique.

Laboratory diagnosis Diagnostic procedures which depend on isolation of the etiologic agent from blood or other clinical material are expensive, time-consuming, and hazardous to laboratory personnel. Primary isolation of rickettsias by inoculation in the yolk sac of the chick embryo or tissue cells usually fails because of the small number of organisms in the patient's blood. Rickettsias have been identified in stained cultured monocytes of infected monkeys and by direct or indirect immunofluorescence of tissues of animals infected with R. rickettsii. Except in unusual circumstances, however, currently available serologic tests are adequate for laboratory confirmation of the clinical diagnosis in each of the rickettsial diseases. The demonstration of a rise in titer of specific antibody during convalescence is of prime importance in establishing the laboratory confirmation. Table 148-2 summarizes the serologic results usually encountered in persons who have rickettsial diseases in the United States. The Weil-Felix test employing Proteus strains OX-19 and OX-2 gives positive results in patients with spotted fever and murine typhus and negative results in those with rickettsialpox and Q fever. It is useful as a screening procedure but cannot be relied upon to differentiate spotted fever from murine typhus. In patients with Brill-Zinsser disease the Proteus OX-19 reaction is usually negative or low in titer.

Serologic tests employing group-specific rickettsial antigens provide data which clearly differentiate the most common infections, i.e., epidemic typhus, murine typhus, Rocky Mountain spotted fever, and Q fever. Moreover, if type-specific rickettsial antigens are employed, it is generally possible to distinguish rickettsialpox from spotted fever and Brill-Zinsser disease from murine typhus.

Utilizing better antigens, other serologic procedures for rickettsial diseases not only distinguish between specific rickettsioses but help to determine the type of immunoglobulin in acute (IgM) and late or recurrent (IgG) illness, such as in recrudescent typhus (Brill-Zinsser disease). The Weil-Felix and complement fixation tests are useful for routine diagnosis; microscopic agglutination, immunofluorescent antibody, and hemagglutination reactions are valuable for specific identification.

Specific antibiotic therapy has little effect on the time of appearance of antibodies or on their ultimate titer, provided treatment is instituted some days after onset of the illness. However, if the illness is cut short by early and vigorous treatment, antibody production may be delayed for a week or so, and also the maximal titers attained may be below those illustrated in Table 148-2. Under these circumstances a sample of blood taken 4 to 6 weeks after onset of illness should also be tested.

The immunofluorescent antibody test is a very useful procedure for detecting rickettsia in the tissues of patients with the typhus group of rickettsioses, the spotted fevers, and Q fever. Identifiable rickettsias have been visualized in skin lesions of patients with Rocky Mountain spotted fever as early as the fourth day of illness and as late as the tenth day. Rickettsias may be visualized in human tissues several days after administration of chloramphenicol or tetracycline. The technique also visualizes rickettsias in ticks and the tissues of animals. This test is useful with paraffin-fixed tissues.

Normochromic anemia occurs in patients severely ill with rick-

TABLE 148-2 Serologic diagnosis of rickettsial diseases in the United States

Group	Disease	Proteus	Weil-Felix reaction Illustrative titer 10th day	20th day	Cases with diagnostic titer	Rickettsial antigen	Complement fixation tests with type-specific antigen Illustrative titer 10th day	20th day	30th day	Cases with diagnostic titer
Spotted fever	Rocky Mountain spotted fever	OX-19 OX-2	40 20	320 160	Most	R. rickettsii	20	160	80	Most
	Rickettsialpox	OX-19 OX-2	0 0	0 0	None	R. akari	0	64	128	Most
Typhus	Murine typhus	OX-19 OX-2	160 10	640 40	Most	R. typhi	0	160	160	Most
	Epidemic typhus squirrel related	OX-19 OX-2	160 10	640 40	Most	R. prowazekii	0	160	160	Most
	Brill-Zinsser disease	OX-19 OX-2	160 0	20 0	Infrequent	R. prowazekii	1280	640	320	Most
	Q fever	OX-19 OX-2	0 0	0 0	None	R. burnetii	10	80	160	Most

ettsial diseases. The white blood cell count in Rocky Mountain spotted fever, rickettsialpox, murine and epidemic typhus, Brill-Zinsser disease, Q fever, and other rickettsial diseases is usually within the normal range; 6000 to 10,000 cells per cubic millimeter. Leukopenia is occasionally observed, and in the presence of complications, such as superimposed infections and extensive vascular lesions, moderate leukocytosis occurs. The differential blood cell count is usually normal.

Thrombocytopenia occurs in severely ill spotted and scrub typhus fever patients with extensive vascular lesions; hypofibrinogenemia, prolonged prothrombin and partial thromboplastin times, and other clotting abnormalities occur.

Treatment   Certain physiochemical changes occurring in the patient seriously ill with one of the diseases of the typhus–spotted fever group should be understood before a therapeutic regimen is outlined. These changes are circulatory collapse, coma, oliguria and anuria, azotemia, anemia, hypoproteinemia, hypochloremia and hyponatremia, and edema. These alterations are often absent in the mildly ill, and in them management is much less complicated. The therapeutic principles necessary for treatment of all rickettsioses are (1) specific chemotherapy and (2) supportive care. Attention to both is mandatory for the seriously ill patient first recognized late in the disease. During the first week in the moderately ill patient, supportive therapy may need to be less energetic, because specific chemotherapy usually suffices. The early mild case may be successfully treated at home; more severely ill patients should receive hospital care.

Therapeutic measures advisable for all the rickettsioses will be described in detail. Variations of this regimen which apply to the individual rickettsioses are described in subsections covering those diseases.

SPECIFIC THERAPY   Specific therapy is most effective when initiated during the early stages of disease coincident with the appearance of the rash. When therapy is delayed until the rash has become hemorrhagic and widespread, the response is less dramatic. The antibiotics of choice are chloramphenicol and the tetracyclines, which are effective because of their rickettsiostatic properties. They are not rickettsiocidal.

The following antibiotic regimen is considered optimal: for chloramphenicol, an initial dose of 50 mg per kilogram of body weight, and for tetracycline, 25 mg/kg. Subsequent daily doses are the same as the initial loading dose, with the requirement divided equally and given at 6- to 8-h intervals. Antibiotic treatment is continued until the patient has improved and has been afebrile approximately 24 h. In patients too ill to take oral medication, an intravenous preparation of one of the antimicrobials should be employed.

Adrenal cortical hormones may be needed for their antitoxemic effects in patients first observed late in the course of severe illness. Large doses for brief periods of about 3 days, in combination with specific antibiotics, are recommended in critically ill patients.

Therapy with antibiotics is continued until the toxemia has abated, the general condition has markedly improved, and the temperature has remained at normal levels for 24 h. In uncomplicated cases of spotted fever, there is symptomatic improvement within 24 h and the temperature becomes normal in 60 to 72 h.

SUPPORTIVE CARE   Frequent turning of the patient relieves pressure from prominent bony parts and also militates against the development of aspiration pneumonia. Proper mouth care, with frequent swabbing of the oral cavity, may avert the development of parotitis and gingivitis. Sucking of the juice of a lemon or the oral use of glycerin or mineral oil is helpful.

A generous intake of protein should be provided by frequent feedings as soon as the disease is suspected, in order to avoid subsequent protein deficiency. Usually food is well tolerated by patients with rickettsial disease, and the daily diet should provide 1 to 2 g protein per kilogram of normal body weight, with adequate carbohydrate and fat to make it palatable. When the patient is uncooperative, the diet may be supplemented by hourly liquid protein feedings via stomach tube, provided that there is no abdominal distention.

At the critical stage, when hypoproteinemia is present and changes in capillary permeability lead to edema and vascular embarrassment, careful attention must be given to parenteral hyperalimentation with high concentration of glucose and amino acids. When indicated by hematologic studies, whole-blood transfusions given slowly are helpful. The judicious administration of one of the plasma expanders at this stage may have a definite favorable effect upon impending circulatory collapse. If the patient is anuric and azotemia is pronounced, overloading the circulation with fluids should be governed by clinical judgment and very careful laboratory studies. Frequent determinations of hemoglobin, hematocrit, electrolytes, and protein, sometimes at intervals of a few hours during crucial periods, are necessary in order to ascertain abnormalities and to permit institution of corrective measures. Dialysis is indicated when there is clear-cut evidence of acute renal failure.

ROCKY MOUNTAIN SPOTTED FEVER   **Definition**   Rocky Mountain spotted fever is an acute febrile illness caused by *Rickettsia rickettsii*. It is transmitted to humans by ticks. The disease is characterized by sudden onset with headache and chills and by fever which persists for 2 to 3 weeks. A characteristic exanthem appears on the extremities and trunk about the fourth day of illness. Delirium, shock, and renal failure occur in severely ill patients.

Etiology and epidemiology   The causative microbe, *R. rickettsii*, is the prototype for the rickettsial group of agents. The minute organisms are purple when stained by Giemsa's method or red by Macchiavello's technique; most of them are gram-negative. These organisms often occur in pairs and possess a cell wall similar in structure and chemical composition to that of gram-negative bacteria; there are a cell membrane, cytoplasmic granules corresponding to ribosomes, and prokaryotic organization of nuclear material. The cell membrane is selectively permeable; the cell wall is the focus of important antigens and an endotoxin-like substance.

The rickettsias grow in the nucleus and the cytoplasm of infected cells of ticks, mammals, and embryonated eggs; the intranuclear situation of the organisms is shared by the other members of the spotted fever group, but not by rickettsias of the typhus group. *Rickettsia rickettsii* is readily distinguishable from the agents of the typhus fevers by cross-immunity tests in guinea pigs and by complement fixation tests employing antigens prepared from infected yolk sac tissues. The differentiation of *R. rickettsii* from closely related members of the spotted fever group frequently requires elaborate procedures. Strains of the agent of Rocky Mountain spotted fever vary considerably in their virulence for humans and animals.

The first reports of spotted fever in Idaho and Montana during the final decade of the last century led to the name Rocky Mountain spotted fever. However, the disease has been reported from all states (except Maine, Alaska, and Hawaii), as well as from Canada, Mexico, Colombia, and Brazil. Although related diseases are found on other continents, this particular infection is limited to the western hemisphere. In the years 1981, 1982, 1983, and 1984 there were 1176, 976, 1126, and 848 cases reported, respectively. The mortality rate was about 20 percent in the days before specific therapy but has decreased to about 7 percent. More than half the cases occur in the south Atlantic and south central states, with the greatest number of these in North Carolina, Virginia, Georgia, Maryland, Tennessee, and Oklahoma.

A number of species of ticks are found infected with *R. rickettsii* in nature, but only two are important in transmitting spotted fever to humans. These are *Dermacentor andersoni*, the wood tick, which is the principal vector in the west, and *D. variabilis*, the dog tick, which assumes this role in the east. *Amblyomma americanum*, the lone star tick, and *D. variabilis* are the common vectors in the west south central states. Infected female ticks transmit the agent transovarially to at least some of their offspring. Ticks which become infected, either through the egg or at one of the stages during their development cycle by feeding on an infected mammal, harbor the rickettsias throughout their lifetime, which may be several years, making the tick a reservoir as well as a vector. Small wild mammals are suspected of playing an important role in spreading the rickettsias in nature by infecting ticks which feed on them during rickettsemia.

Disease in humans is generally acquired from the bite of an infected tick. Transmission is unlikely unless the tick remains attached for a number of hours. Infection may also be acquired through abrasions in the skin which become contaminated with infected tick feces or tissue juices; hence, the hazard associated with crushing ticks between the fingers when removing them from persons or animals. The agent of Rocky Mountain spotted fever has been transmitted accidentally to humans by transfusion of blood taken from a donor just before onset of illness.

There are seasonal variations in the incidence of cases of spotted fever, as well as differences in age and sex distribution of cases. In each instance these differences are related to exposure to ticks. Most cases are seen during the period of maximal tick activity, i.e., April to September, and 60 percent of cases occur in individuals under 20 years of age. This age distribution is undoubtedly influenced by propinquity to the wood and dog ticks. The mortality rate increases with the age of the patient.

Rocky Mountain spotted fever has been acquired by laboratory workers via aerosol transmission, and special precautions are necessary when the agent is handled in the laboratory.

Clinical manifestations INCUBATION PERIOD AND PRODROMATA A history of tick bite is elicited in approximately 80 percent of patients. The incubation period varies between 3 and 12 days with a mean of 7 days. A short incubation period usually indicates a more serious infection.

ONSET In nonvaccinated persons, the onset is usually abrupt, with severe headache, a sudden shaking rigor, prostration, generalized myalgia, especially in the back and leg muscles, nausea with occasional vomiting, and fever which reaches 103 to 104°F within the first 2 days. Pain in the abdominal muscles may be severe, and arthralgia is not uncommon. Deep muscle palpation often elicits tenderness. Occasionally the debut of illness in children and adults is mild, accompanied by lethargy, anorexia, headache, and low-grade fever. These symptoms are similar to those of many acute infectious diseases, making specific diagnosis difficult during the first few days.

PYREXIA Fever continues for approximately 15 to 20 days in untreated cases. The febrile course in children may be shorter. Hyperthermia of 105°F or greater is of unfavorable prognostic significance, although fatalities may occur when the patient is hypothermic, with concurrent vasomotor collapse. Fever generally terminates by lysis over a period of several days, but rarely does so by crisis. Recurrent fever is uncommon except in the presence of secondary pyogenic complications.

The *headache* is generalized and excruciating, and frequently most intense over the frontal area. It persists throughout the first and second weeks of illness in untreated cases. Occasionally headache is mild. Malaise continues for the first week; irritability is notable, and the patient shuns distractions such as questioning and examination.

CUTANEOUS MANIFESTATIONS The rash which is present in practically all cases is the most characteristic and helpful diagnostic sign. It usually appears on the fourth febrile day; the range is 2 to 6 days. Faint-pink macules which fade on pressure have been noted on the first febrile day. The initial lesions are on the wrists, ankles, palms, soles, and forearms. The first lesions are macular, nonfixed, pink, irregularly defined, and measure 2 to 6 mm. A warm compress applied to the extremity accentuates the rash in the early stages. The exanthem is most prominent when the temperature is elevated. After 6 to 12 h, the rash extends centripetally to the axilla, buttocks, trunk, neck, and face. (This is in contrast to the eruption of typhus fever,

which begins on the trunk and spreads centrifugally, rarely involving the face, palms, or soles.) The rash becomes maculopapular after 2 to 3 days (it may be felt by light palpation) and assumes a deeper red hue. By about the fourth day it is petechial and fails to fade on pressure. Not uncommonly, the hemorrhagic lesions coalesce to form large ecchymotic blemishes; these lesions tend to form over bony prominences and may ultimately slough to form indolent, slow-healing ulcers. Patients who have had the typical rash show brownish discolorations at the site for several weeks during convalescence. In milder cases, the rash does not become purpuric and may disappear within a few days. Antibiotic therapy may abort the early exanthem; the later fixed lesion fades less rapidly with specific therapy. Occasionally, a rash does not occur or is unnoticed, particularly in dark-skinned patients.

The application of tourniquets for several minutes, or the occasional taking of the blood pressure may provoke additional petechiae (Rumpel-Leede phenomenon), further evidence of capillary abnormalities.

CARDIOVASCULAR AND RESPIRATORY FEATURES During the early stages, the pulse is full and regular and is accelerated in proportion to the height of the temperature, and the blood pressure is well sustained. During the peak of illness in seriously ill patients, the pulse is rapid and feeble, and hypotension of 90 mmHg or less is common. If circulatory failure is sustained, the resultant hypoxia and shock lead to agitation and delirium and contribute to the formation of ecchymoses and gangrene of fingers, toes, genitalia, buttocks, earlobes, and nose. Cyanosis of the peripheral parts of the body is common. Venous pressure determinations show no elevation. A reduction of the total blood volume is occasionally found. The ECG shows low voltage of ventricular complexes, minor ST-segment deflections, and occasionally delay in atrioventricular conduction. These changes are transient and nonspecific. Severely ill patients have a puffy appearance of the face, hands, ankles, feet, and lower parts of the sacrum. Occasionally a severe arrhythmia associated with myocarditis results in sudden death.

Respirations are either normal or slightly accelerated. Cough may be harassing and nonproductive, and localized pneumonitis may occur, but pulmonary consolidation is extremely rare. Pulmonary edema may develop after injudicious use of intravenous fluids.

HEPATIC AND RENAL MANIFESTATIONS In the majority of patients, there is little alteration in renal or hepatic function. The liver may be enlarged, but jaundice is unusual. Oliguria commonly occurs in the seriously ill, and anuria may mark the critically ill patient. Azotemia is common; when marked, it is a very unfavorable sign. Abnormalities in liver function include hypoproteinemia, with reduction in the albumin fraction.

NEUROLOGIC MANIFESTATIONS The principal neurologic manifestations are headache, restlessness, and varying degrees of insomnia. Stiffness of the back is common. The cerebrospinal fluid (CSF) is clear, with normal dynamics and normal chemical constituents. Occasionally, the CSF pressure is elevated; there may be a slight increase in mononuclear cells. Coma and muscular rigidity may occur. Athetoid movements, convulsive seizures, and hemiplegia are grave manifestations. Deafness during the active stages of the disease is not uncommon. As a rule, all neurologic signs abate without residua. Findings based upon follow-up examinations and electro-encephalograms may be interpreted as indicative of minor residual brain damage for a year or more following recovery of certain patients from Rocky Mountain spotted fever.

OTHER PHYSICAL MANIFESTATIONS Patients become dehydrated, with extreme dryness of lips, gums, tongue, and pharynx. The skin is hot and dry, the conjunctivas are frequently injected, and the eyes suffused. Photophobia is common in the early stages of illness. Petechial hemorrhages may be noted in the conjunctivas or in the retina. The spleen is enlarged in approximately one-half the cases and is firm and nontender. Abdominal distention is frequent, and occasionally some degree of intestinal ileus is observed. Constipation is usual.

Course   In patients with mild and moderately severe cases who are given no specific antibiotic therapy, the disease abates within 2 weeks, and convalescence is rapid. In fatal cases death usually occurs during the latter part of the second week as a result of toxemia, vasomotor collapse and shock, or renal failure. In a few patients, the course is fulminant with death occurring as early as the sixth day of illness.

In vaccinated individuals who contract the disease, the illness is mild, with a short febrile course and an atypical rash.

Prognosis   If the serious manifestations of spotted fever mentioned above are regarded as intrinsic parts of the disease, then complications are uncommon and consist mainly of secondary bacterial infections, namely, bronchopneumonia, otitis media, and parotitis. Thrombosis of major blood vessels may result in gangrene of a portion of an extremity. Hemiplegia and peripheral neuritis are rare sequelae.

The overall mortality rate for spotted fever was formerly about 20 percent. Death occurred in more than half of persons over 40 years of age, but the mortality rate was much lower in children and young adults. Since the introduction of the broad-spectrum antibiotics and the development of more precise knowledge regarding correction of the physiologic abnormalities which develop during the disease, fewer deaths occur. Some of the fatalities can be attributed to failure to consider spotted fever in the differential diagnosis and resultant delay in instituting appropriate treatment.

Differential diagnosis   During the early stages of infection before the rash has appeared, differentiation from other acute infections is difficult. History of tick bite while living or traveling in wooded or bushy sites known to be in a highly endemic area is helpful. The rash of meningococcemia (see Chap. 103) resembles Rocky Mountain spotted fever in certain aspects, because it is macular, maculopapular, or petechial in the chronic form, and petechial, confluent, or ecchymotic in the fulminant type. The meningococcal skin lesion is tender and develops with extreme rapidity in the fulminant form, whereas the rickettsial rash occurs on about the fourth day of disease and gradually becomes petechial. *Spotted fever is often confused with measles.* The exanthem of rubeola rapidly becomes confluent, while that of rubella *usually remains discrete.*

Murine typhus is a milder disease than Rocky Mountain spotted fever; the rash is less extensive, nonpurpuric, and nonconfluent, and renal and vascular complications are uncommon. Not infrequently differentiation of these two rickettsial infections must await the results of specific serologic tests. Epidemic typhus fever is capable of causing all the pronounced clinical, physiologic, and anatomic alterations seen in patients with Rocky Mountain spotted fever, i.e., hypotension, peripheral vascular collapse, cyanosis, skin necrosis and gangrene of digits, renal failure and azotemia, and neurologic manifestations. However, the rash of classic typhus is noted initially in the axillary folds of the trunk and later extends peripherally, rarely involving the palms, soles, or face. The serologic patterns in these two diseases are distinctive when specific rickettsial antigens are employed. Moreover, louse-borne typhus is now recognized in the United States as a flying squirrel–related illness which occurs sporadically and as Brill-Zinsser disease (recrudescent typhus fever). Rickettsialpox, although caused by a member of the spotted fever group is usually readily differentiated from Rocky Mountain spotted fever by the initial lesion, the relative mildness of the illness, and the early vesiculation of the maculopapular rash. The Weil-Felix reaction is positive in Rocky Mountain spotted fever and in murine and epidemic typhus, but is negative in rickettsialpox. Agglutinins against *Proteus* OX-19 and OX-2 appear in the serum of patients with spotted fever, but only those against OX-19 are generally found in murine and epidemic typhus.

Complications   *Pyogenic complications,* including otitis media and parotitis, are encountered in patients severely ill with Rocky Mountain

spotted fever and other rickettsioses. These localized infections respond to therapy with appropriate antibiotics combined with surgical measures.

Pneumonitis usually develops as a result of specific rickettsial action. The sputum is scant but should be examined to determine whether superimposed bacterial infection is present. Specific therapy is guided by the results of these laboratory studies. The pneumonitis generally responds to the antibiotic therapy the patient is receiving, but if staphylococcal pneumonia is suspected, a penicillinase-resistant penicillin should be added to the broad-spectrum drug.

Circulatory failure of peripheral or central origin is combated by careful administration of plasma expanders and fluids. Heart failure may develop from the disease or as a result of overzealous intravenous therapy and is recognized by rapid pulse, gallop rhythm, and increase in venous pressure. When the clinical signs reveal unmistakable evidence of cardiac failure, digitalis and diuretics should be employed. Oxygen therapy improves the cardiac and circulatory status and is helpful in hypoxemic patients with involvement of the central nervous system.

Prevention   Prevention is attained primarily by avoidance of tick-infested areas. When this is impractical, prophylactic measures include (1) spraying the ground with dieldrin or chlordane for area control of ticks (though there are environmental objections to the use of residual insecticides in area control of ticks, under special conditions such procedures may be warranted); (2) application of repellents such as diethyltoluamide or dimethylphthalate to clothing and exposed parts of the body, or in very heavily infested areas the wearing of clothing which interferes with the attachment of ticks, i.e., boots and a one-piece outer garment, preferably impregnated with repellent; and (3) daily inspection of the entire body, including the hairy parts, to detect and remove attached ticks. In removing attached ticks great care should be taken to avoid crushing the arthropod with resultant contamination of the bite wound; touching the tick with gasoline or whisky encourages detachment but gentle traction with tweezers applied close to the mouth parts may be necessary; the skin area should be disinfected with soap and water or other antiseptics. Similarly, precautions should be employed in removing engorged ticks from dogs and other animals, because infection through minor abrasions on the hands is possible. Improved vaccines containing inactivated *R. rickettsii* are under development and when available commercially should be used for those at great risk, namely, persons frequenting highly endemic areas and laboratory workers exposed to the agent. Because the broad-spectrum antibiotics are such excellent therapeutic agents in spotted fever, there has been less impetus for vaccination of persons who run only a minor risk of infection.

After tick bite in a known endemic area an exposed person should be observed for signs of fever, headache, prostration, and rash; therapy is very effective early in the infection.

MURINE (ENDEMIC) TYPHUS FEVER   Definition   Murine typhus fever is an acute febrile disease caused by *Rickettsia typhi (mooseri)* and transmitted to humans by fleas. The clinical illness is characterized by fever of 9 to 14 days, headache, a maculopapular rash appearing on the third to fifth day, and myalgia.

Etiology and epidemiology   *R. typhi* resembles other rickettsias in morphologic properties, staining characteristics, and intracellular parasitism. Under the electron microscope *R. typhi* is seen to contain dense masses of nuclear material in a less dense homogeneous protoplasmic substance, the whole of which is surrounded by a limiting membrane. It differs from *R. rickettsii* in that it always multiplies within the cytoplasm of cells, in contrast to the intranuclear and cytoplasmic positions of spotted fever rickettsias.

Invasion of the body by *R. typhi* provokes specific and nonspecific immunologic responses. Utilizing highly purified antigens, specific antibodies may be demonstrated readily by complement fixation, microscopic agglutination, and immunofluorescent antibody reactions. The positive Weil-Felix reaction which occurs in this disease is nonspecific, because it is attributable to the presence of a common carbohydrate antigen in *Proteus* OX-19 and *R. typhi* and because the reaction is also positive in epidemic typhus and spotted fever. Group-specific rickettsial antigens are common to both *R. typhi* and *R. prowazekii*.

The common vector of *R. typhi* for rats and humans is the rat flea (*Xenopsylla cheopis*). In nature, the rat louse (*Polypax spinulosis*) may transmit the agent among rodents. Customarily, rat fleas become infected on ingestion of blood from diseased rats; the rickettsias multiply within the intestinal cells of the arthropod and are excreted in the feces. Infection in humans occurs after the flea bite and contamination of the broken skin by rickettsia-laden feces. Dried flea feces may also infect via the conjunctivas or the upper part of the respiratory tract.

Rats and mice are naturally infected with murine typhus, and although the rodent disease is nonfatal, viable rickettsias persist in the brain for variable periods.

Murine typhus is one of the most benign and widespread of the rickettsioses in the United States. Prevalent in the southeastern and Gulf Coast states, it has been identified in most of the other states and in harbor centers throughout the world wherever rats and fleas abound. In the early 1940s, 2000 to 5000 cases of murine typhus were reported annually. This contrasts to 61 and 58 cases reported in the United States in 1981 and 1982, respectively. This sharp reduction was achieved by control of rats and their fleas in known areas of high prevalence. In urban areas the disease is more prevalent during the summer and fall months and occurs predominantly among persons working in proximity to granaries or food depots. There has been an extension to certain rural areas when changing agricultural practices have provided rats with ready access to adequate food supplies. A small cluster of five cases occurred in late 1982 in a rural area in north central Texas. Conceivably, use of rat poison several weeks before the illness forced infected fleas to seek an alternative human host. All five patients recovered; four were treated with tetracycline. Endemic typhus has been reported in laboratory workers. This emphasizes the importance of taking special precautions when working with rickettsial organisms in the laboratory.

Clinical manifestations INCUBATION PERIOD AND PRODROMATA The incubation period ranges from 8 to 16 days, with a mean of 10 days. Common prodromata are headache, backache, arthralgia, and chilly sensations. Nausea, malaise, and transient temperature rises may precede the true onset of disease.

ONSET AND GENERAL SYMPTOMS A frank shaking chill and repeated rigors are present at the onset, associated with a severe frontal headache and fever. This triad of headache, chill, and pyrexia is usually followed within a few hours by nausea and vomiting. Prostration, malaise, and weakness are sufficient to enforce cessation of activity in adults, in contrast to children, whose illness is less severe. Occasionally, mild symptoms make it difficult to define the actual onset.

PYREXIA The usual febrile course in murine typhus lasts for about 12 days in adults; the temperature ranges from 102 to 104°F but may reach 105 to 106°F in children. The temperature may reach high levels abruptly after onset or ascend in a stepwise manner during the first few days. With the appearance of the rash, fever is usually sustained, with partial daily remissions which occasionally reach normal levels in the morning. Defervescence is generally by lysis over several days but sometimes occurs by crisis. Transient mild fever of 100°F is not uncommon during early convalescence. A few patients experience only low-grade fever throughout, but this does not necessarily connote a mild illness.

CUTANEOUS MANIFESTATIONS The early lesions, which are sparse and discrete, are hidden in the axillae and inner surface of the arm. Most patients then develop with surprising suddenness a generalized, dull-red macular rash of the upper part of the abdomen, shoulders, chest, arms, and thighs. The individual lesions are discrete and pea size, with an ill-defined border, and fade on pressure during the first 24 h. They later become maculopapular, in contrast to the exanthem of epidemic typhus, which is persistently macular. The distribution over the trunk with sparse involvement of the extremities, palms, soles, and face differs from the peripheral distribution and facial involvement of Rocky Mountain spotted fever. The murine rash generally appears initially on the fifth febrile day, but rarely it is seen concurrently with the onset of fever or develops as late as the seventh day.

Eighty percent of patients develop a rash which persists for 4 to 8 days and fades before defervescence. The cutaneous manifestations vary greatly in intensity and duration and may be fleeting. They are readily overlooked in dark-skinned patients, in whom they should be sought by light palpation and indirect lighting.

CARDIOVASCULAR AND RESPIRATORY FEATURES An irritating, nonproductive cough is frequent and is occasionally associated with moderate hemoptysis. Early in the second week, rales may be detected in the basilar lung areas. These changes are generally rickettsial rather than bacterial in origin and respond to the broad-spectrum antibiotics. Pulmonary congestion occurs in extremely ill and elderly patients.

Accelerated pulse, hypotension, and general circulatory weakness occur, although less frequently than in patients with epidemic typhus or Rocky Mountain spotted fever.

NEUROLOGIC MANIFESTATIONS Headache is the most common neurologic manifestation of murine typhus and may dominate the clinical picture. It is frontal and continues into the second week of illness. Stupor and prostration may occur in the second week, and in severe cases, there may be delirium, extreme agitation, or coma. Coma in elderly patients after 2 weeks of illness presages death. Nuchal rigidity and general spasticity often suggest meningitis, although the spinal fluid is normal except for slight increases in pressure and lymphocytes (5 to 30 per cubic millimeter). Transient partial deafness occurs occasionally, but rarely is there localized neuritis or hemiplegia. Neurologic sequelae are unusual. Children experience minimal neurologic changes.

OTHER PHYSICAL MANIFESTATIONS During the first 2 days of illness the patient may be nauseated and vomit, but vomiting later in the illness should arouse suspicion of an intercurrent complication. Abdominal pain is bothersome; when associated with diarrhea, it responds to intravenous alimentation. Hepatomegaly and jaundice are unusual. There is splenomegaly in approximately 25 percent of patients.

Photophobia, retroocular pain, and suffusion of the conjunctivas are common but are less severe than in the other typhus and spotted fevers.

Renal function is usually unaltered except in elderly patients with prolonged hypotension. Under these circumstances, azotemia may develop to the degree observed in epidemic typhus. In severe murine typhus, as in the epidemic typhus, hyponatremia and hypoalbuminemia are encountered.

Course After defervescence, murine typhus patients recover rapidly. Fatalities occur between the ninth and twelfth days in elderly or debilitated patients, usually as a result of circulatory and renal failure or intercurrent bacterial infection.

Prognosis The mortality rate in murine typhus was low even before the introduction of modern specific therapy. Only one death occurred in 114 cases studied by Maxcy and none in the 180 reported by Stuart and Pullen.

Differential diagnosis Because murine typhus and Rocky Mountain spotted fever occur in many of the same states, the problem of differential diagnosis often arises. Flea-borne murine typhus, which is predominantly an urban disease, is more likely to occur in late summer and autumn. In contrast, spotted fever is a rural and suburban disease in which exposure to ticks is important. Most cases occur in the spring and summer.

Treatment and prevention Both chloramphenicol and the tetracycline antibiotics have controlled the disease (see above).

Prevention of murine typhus in humans is attained by reducing the natural reservoir and vector by applying measures for eliminating rodents and employing appropriate insecticides in rat-infested areas to control fleas. Spraying of rat burrows with DDT effectively reduces the population of the vector.

EPIDEMIC (LOUSE-BORNE) TYPHUS FEVER **Definition** The classic epidemic form of typhus is a severe, febrile disease caused by *R. prowazekii* and transmitted to humans by the body louse. Intense headache, continuous pyrexia of about 2 weeks, a macular skin eruption appearing on about the fifth febrile day, malaise, and vascular and neurologic disturbances represent the principal clinical features. Confirmation of the diagnosis is made by demonstration of *Proteus* OX-19 agglutinins and of specific complement-fixing antibodies in convalescence. The broad-spectrum antibiotics are specific therapeutic agents.

Etiology and epidemiology The causative microbe, *R. prowazekii*, is closely related to *R. typhi*, which causes murine typhus; indeed, the two have a number of common antigens.

Human beings generally are infected when rickettsia-laden louse feces are rubbed into the broken skin; scratching the louse bite facilitates this process. *Pediculus humanus corporis*, which is peculiarly adapted to humans, is the only important vector of epidemic typhus. It dies of its infection and fails to transmit rickettsias to its offspring. *R. prowazekii* has been isolated from flying squirrels, and the organism probably infests their ectoparasites. Generally, however, the organism is maintained by a cycle involving human-louse-human. New epidemics apparently originate from patients with Brill-Zinsser disease (recurrent epidemic typhus). Flying squirrels can serve as a potential host to initiate an outbreak of epidemic typhus provided an avid human vector, such as the body louse, is prevalent. Pathogenic rickettsias reside for long periods in patients with epidemic typhus as well as Rocky Mountain spotted fever and scrub typhus. Lice readily become infected when fed on patients with recurrent typhus. Inhalation of dust containing dried louse feces may cause infection. An established nonhuman reservoir such as flying squirrels poses a serious threat.

If uncontrolled, epidemic typhus behaves as a cyclic disease in a susceptible population, extending over a 3-year period. During the first year there is a gradual seeding of cases throughout the group; during the second there is epidemic spread; and during the third the epidemic tapers off, because the majority of persons have become immune. Outbreaks of epidemic typhus last occurred in the United States in the nineteenth century, and its presence is now recognized in the form of Brill-Zinsser disease and flying squirrel–related typhus.

Clinical manifestations Epidemic typhus resembles murine typhus but is more severe. After an incubation period of about 7 days an abrupt onset of headache, chill, and rapidly mounting fever ushers in the illness. Headache, malaise, and prostration continue unabated until the rash appears on the fifth febrile day. It is initially macular in the axillary folds but ultimately invades the trunk and extremities as a pink, irregular macular lesion, which becomes fixed, petechial, and confluent in the later stages.

Neurologic features range from headache and general spasticity to extreme agitation, stupor, and coma. Circulatory disturbances consisting of tachycardia, hypotension, and cyanosis are more profound than those observed in murine typhus and are almost as severe as in Rocky Mountain spotted fever. Ultimately, in untreated cases azotemia often reaches high levels as a result of vascular and renal failure, and death occurs late in the second week of illness. Furthermore, thrombosis of major blood vessels and cutaneous gangrene develop in a manner similar to that seen in the virulent form of Rocky Mountain spotted fever.

The complications and sequelae of epidemic typhus are more severe than those in murine typhus, but not as severe as those in Rocky Mountain spotted fever. However, during certain outbreaks, epidemic typhus was fatal in 60 percent of those infected, and convalescence in survivors was prolonged. Broad-spectrum antibiotics have almost eradicated mortality in this dread disease, provided therapy is instituted before irreversible changes have been established in the tissues.

Differential diagnosis Differentiation of epidemic typhus from the various rickettsioses and other diseases with which it may be confused was described above. The disease is not known to occur in epidemic form in the absence of lousiness in the general population. Under the conditions in which typhus epidemics are likely to occur, other diseases which may cause confusion include malaria, relapsing fever, pneumonia, and tuberculosis. Classic typhus contracted by a previously vaccinated person is usually mild and may be clinically indistinguishable from murine typhus except by serologic methods. An illness simulating Rocky Mountain spotted fever is caused by *R. canada*, a member of the typhus group.

Treatment and prevention Both chloramphenicol and the tetracycline antibiotics have been found to be highly efficient therapeutic agents in epidemic typhus. Usually the patient becomes afebrile after 2 days of treatment. Under field conditions, 100 mg doxycycline in a single oral dose resulted in abatement of clinical manifestations and defervescence in epidemic typhus.

The most effective measures for controlling epidemic typhus are those which eliminate lousiness. DDT or lindane powder when dusted into clothing is suitable for this purpose. If resistant lice are found, malathion or carbaryl may prove effective.

A commercially available vaccine prepared from formalin-treated suspensions of infected yolk sac tissue is an effective immunizing agent. A viable vaccine utilizing an attenuated strain of *R. prowazekii* is effective but is not available commercially.

BRILL-ZINSSER DISEASE (RECRUDESCENT TYPHUS) Brill-Zinsser disease is a recrudescent episode of epidemic typhus fever which occurs years after the initial attack, in persons who had recovered from the epidemic disease acquired while residing in countries where it was prevalent. *R. prowazekii* have been isolated from lice fed on patients during the active stages of illness.

The clinical entity, not always mild, resembles epidemic typhus in the character of the rash, circulatory disturbances, and hepatic, renal, and nervous system changes. Recovery is the rule. The Weil-Felix reaction with the various *Proteus* antigens is usually negative, or positive in very low titer. The specific complement fixation, microscopic agglutination, and immunofluorescent antibody reactions are valuable in establishing the diagnosis. In Brill-Zinsser disease the specific complement-fixing antibodies appear as early as the fourth day after the onset of illness; antibodies are of the IgG class, and the peak response is attained by the eighth to tenth days. Specific antibody titers in the primary attack of epidemic typhus begin later, about the eighth to twelfth day, with maximum titers on about the sixteenth day after onset. Treatment is the same as for other rickettsial infections.

SCRUB TYPHUS **Definition** Scrub typhus is limited to eastern and southeastern Asia, India, northern Australia, and the adjacent islands. It is caused by *R. tsutsugamushi* and is characterized by a primary lesion at the site of the bite of an infected mite, a fever of about 2 weeks' duration, a cutaneous rash which develops about the fifth day, and the appearance late in the second week of agglutinins against the OX-K strain of *Proteus* bacillus. The broad-spectrum antibiotics are specific therapeutic agents.

Etiology The agent of scrub typhus resembles other rickettsias in its physical properties but differs from them in antigenic structure, vector, and reservoir. The disease is transmitted by larvae of several species of mites, especially *Leptotrombidium* (*Trombicula*) *akamushi* and *L. deliense*. These tiny chiggers attach themselves to the skin and during the process of obtaining a meal of tissue juice may acquire infection from the host or transmit rickettsias to the vertebrate. The infection is maintained in nature by a cycle involving mites and small rodents and by transovarial transmission in mites; human infection represents an accident attributable to propinquity.

Clinical manifestations About 10 to 12 days after infection, illness begins abruptly with chilliness, severe headache, fever, conjunctival injection, and moderate generalized lymphadenopathy, which is most prominent in the nodes draining the area of the primary lesion. The initial lesion at the beginning of fever is evidenced by an erythematous indurated area 1 cm in diameter, surmounted by a multiloculated vesicle; within a few days the vesicle ulcerates and becomes covered with a black crust.

Fever increases progressively during the first week, generally reaching 104 to 105°F, but the pulse remains relatively slow, 70 to 100 beats per minute. The red macular rash, which begins on the trunk about the fifth day and spreads to the extremities, sometimes becomes maculopapular but usually fades in a few days. The course of the disease and the complications resemble those of endemic and epidemic typhus; however, interstitial myocarditis is more prominent than in the other typhus fevers.

Prognosis Before the introduction of the broad-spectrum antibiotics the mortality rate varied from 1 to 60 percent, depending on the geographic area and the virulence of the local strains of *R. tsutsugamushi,* and convalescence was prolonged. With modern therapeutic methods, deaths are rare and convalescence is short.

Differential diagnosis Scrub typhus is to be differentiated from the other members of the typhus and the spotted fever group of diseases as well as from measles, typhoid fever, and the meningococcal infections. The geographic localization of scrub typhus, the primary lesion, and the occurrence of OX-K agglutinins are especially useful in establishing the diagnosis.

Treatment and prevention Chloramphenicol and the tetracycline antibiotics are extremely effective in scrub typhus. Scrub typhus is more amenable to drugs than are the other rickettsial infections, and patients with this disease regularly become afebrile and are decidedly improved within 24 to 36 h after beginning treatment, irrespective of the stage of disease. Antibiotic treatment may be discontinued after several afebrile days.

Relapse of clinical illness is unusual unless specific treatment is initiated early, such as before the fifth febrile day. Under these circumstances, recrudescence is obviated by giving the antibiotic for several days and resuming treatment about 5 days after cessation of the initial course of therapy.

Prevention of disease in the individual is accomplished by the application of miticidal chemicals (dibutyl phthalate, benzyl benzoate, diethyltoluamide, and others) to clothing and the skin. There is no satisfactory vaccine. Chemoprophylactic studies conducted in highly endemic infested areas of scrub typhus showed that single oral doses of chloramphenicol or tetracycline given every 5 days for a total of 35 days (seven doses with 5-day nontreatment intervals) prevents scrub typhus and results in active immunity. This procedure is recommended under special circumstances. A long-acting tetracycline (doxycycline) serves the same purpose.

TRENCH FEVER Definition Trench fever is a febrile disease transmitted between humans by the body louse, *Pediculus humanus corporis.* It is characterized by a sudden onset with headache and severe pain in the muscles, bones, and joints. In most cases, the fever and other symptoms assume a relapsing character. Fatalities are rare. The disease is also known as shin bone fever, Volhynia fever, His-Werner disease, and quintan fever.

Etiology and epidemiology *R. quintana,* the etiologic agent, grows extracellularly in the louse gut, in contrast to other pathogenic rickettsias which can multiply only within cells. A European strain

of *R. quintana* has been cultivated on blood agar, and typical trench fever has been induced in volunteers.

Humans are the only known reservoir of infection. The louse does not transmit the organism transovarially but acquires its infection by ingesting the blood of a person with rickettsemia. The organisms multiply extracellularly in the louse gut, without injury to this host, and are excreted in large numbers with the feces. Humans become infected by the inoculation of the contaminated feces into abraded skin or conjunctivas. *R. quintana* may be recovered periodically from human blood for several years after convalescence from an acute attack. Trench fever is known to exist in Mexico, Tunisia, Eritrea, Poland, the U.S.S.R., and possibly China, and there is serologic evidence for its occurrence in Bolivia, Burundi, and Ethiopia.

Pathology Since there have been no recorded fatalities, histologic examination has been confined to excised macules of the skin, which have shown nonspecific perivascular infiltrates without the involvement of the vessel walls that is seen in typhus fever.

Clinical manifestations Clinical manifestations range from a mild afebrile disease to a debilitating illness with a protracted clinical course involving numerous relapses. Following an incubation period of 10 to 30 days the onset may be insidious or dramatically abrupt. The acute disease is characterized by malaise, headache, fever, and bone and body pain, especially severe in the shins. In some cases only one fever peak occurs; in others the fever continues for 5 to 7 days; and in others there is an initial febrile episode lasting 1 to 3 days followed by relapses which characteristically occur at 4- to 5-day intervals. In some cases the fever and symptoms are continuous for 2 or 3 weeks. Enlargement of the spleen and a red macular rash occur in 70 to 80 percent of the cases. Pain and soreness in the muscles usually recur with each febrile relapse.

The disease is marked by a persistent rickettsemia, which is present during the initial attack and which continues during the relapses, throughout the asymptomatic periods between relapses, and for months or even years after cessation of physical symptoms. A relapse has been reported 10 years after the original attack.

Prognosis The disease causes no known deaths, but its duration is variable. About 85 percent of patients are able to return to work within 2 months of onset, but about 5 percent of all cases become chronic. Recovery is even more delayed in the aged and debilitated.

Differential diagnosis During epidemics, typical cases are easily diagnosed on the basis of symptoms. The disease may be differentiated from influenza, typhoid, typhus, dengue, and relapsing fever by the specific laboratory tests available for the diagnosis of each of these diseases.

Treatment and prevention *R. quintana* is highly sensitive in vitro to the broad-spectrum antibiotics, but no reliable information has been obtained about the value of these drugs in treating trench fever. The treatment is symptomatic. Aspirin is used to control pain and discomfort, but codeine may be necessary. Patients should remain in bed for a week or more after complete cessation of subjective and objective evidence of infection. They should be kept under observation for several months.

The methods employed to control epidemic typhus should be equally efficacious in controlling trench fever. These are based on the elimination of lousiness and the improvement of living conditions with provision for frequent bathing and washing of clothing. DDT or lindane powder should be applied by hand or power duster at appropriate intervals to clothes and persons living under conditions favoring lousiness. If resistant lice are found, malathion or other effective lousicides may be substituted as a dusting powder.

RICKETTSIALPOX Definition Rickettsialpox is a mild, nonfatal, self-limited, febrile illness caused by *R. akari,* which is transmitted from mouse to humans by mites. It is characterized by an initial skin lesion at the site of the mite bite, a week's febrile course, and a papulovesicular rash.

Etiology and epidemiology   Rickettsialpox was first recognized in New York City in 1946, and about 180 cases were reported annually for several years thereafter. It has been diagnosed in several other areas of the United States, and outbreaks have been reported in European Russia. The vector is a small, colorless mite, *Allodermanyssus sanguineus* (Hirst), which infests small mice and rodents. House mice serve as the reservoir of infection.

R. akari is morphologically and biologically similar to other rickettsias and is antigenically related to, but distinct from, *R. rickettsii*, the cause of Rocky Mountain spotted fever.

Clinical manifestations   The initial skin lesion appears about 7 to 10 days after the mite bite as a firm red papule 1 to 1.5 cm in diameter. In a few days, the center vesiculates, and the papule is surrounded by an area of erythema. The regional lymph glands are moderately enlarged. The primary lesion, which is never painful, becomes covered with a black scab; it heals slowly, and a small scar is visible on separation of the crust.

The febrile phase begins 3 to 7 days after the initial lesion, and an exanthem may accompany the fever or begin several days later. The onset of fever is sudden, with chilly sensations or frank chills, headache, sweats, myalgia, anorexia, and photophobia. The pyrexia ranges from 103 to 104°F and continues for about a week, occasionally with morning remissions.

The exanthem is maculopapular-vesicular, generalized in distribution, and may be abundant or scant. The lesions may involve the oral cavity but not the palms or soles. In a week, the vesicles dry and form scabs which eventually scale but leave no scar.

The constitutional symptoms are generally mild, and the course of illness is uncomplicated. No fatal cases have been reported.

The disease may be confused with chickenpox, which is different because it occurs usually in childhood and has no initial lesion and the papular cutaneous lesion is entirely transformed into a vesicle. Variola (smallpox) is accompanied by a more severe constitutional reaction, and the vesicles become pustules. The skin lesions of the other rickettsioses differ in their lack of vesiculation. The Weil-Felix reaction is usually negative in this rickettsial disease, but specific complement fixation, microscopic agglutination, and immunofluorescent antibody reactions are useful diagnostic aids even though there is considerable antigenic crossing with materials from Rocky Mountain spotted fever.

Treatment and prevention   Chloramphenicol and the tetracycline antibiotics are all effective for treating patients with rickettsialpox. The temperature reaches normal levels in about 2 days, and recovery is rapid.

Control measures should be directed toward elimination of house mice and the vector mites responsible for transmitting the disease.

OTHER TICK-BORNE RICKETTSIAL DISEASES   Definition   Boutonneuse fever, North Asian tick-borne rickettsiosis, and Queensland tick typhus, three diseases occurring in the eastern hemisphere, are caused by rickettsias closely related to one another and to the agent of Rocky Mountain spotted fever. Each is transmitted by the bite of an ixodid tick. These mild to moderately severe illnesses are characterized by an initial lesion (called *tache noire* in boutonneuse fever), a fever of several days to 2 weeks, and a generalized maculopapular erythematous rash which appears on about the fifth day and usually involves the palms and soles. Specific complement-fixing antibodies appear in the patients' serums during convalescence, but agglutinins to *Proteus* OX-19 (Weil-Felix reaction) are frequently found only in low titer.

Etiology and epidemiology   The etiologic agents of these three diseases are all members of the spotted fever group of rickettsias. Together with *R. rickettsii* and *R. akari* they possess common group antigens which are readily demonstrated by agglutination, complement fixation, microscopic agglutination, and immunofluorescent antibody reactions.

Boutonneuse fever, which may be regarded as the prototype of the three, is caused by *R. conorii*. Modern serologic methods employing specific rickettsial antigens have shown this rickettsia to be the causative agent for a single widely disseminated disease known by various local names. Information on the distribution and etiology of the various tick-borne rickettsial diseases is contained in Table 148-1.

In general, the epidemiology of these tick-borne rickettsioses resembles that of spotted fever in the western hemisphere. Ixodid ticks and small wild animals maintain the rickettsias in nature; if humans intrude accidentally into the cycle, they become a dead end in the transmission chain. In certain areas, the cycle of boutonneuse fever involves domiciliary environments, with the brown dog tick *Rhipicephalus sanguineus* as the dominant vector.

Clinical manifestations   These three tick-borne rickettsioses, which occur in different parts of the eastern hemisphere, resemble one another closely. The clinical course is usually milder than that of spotted fever, with a shorter febrile period and fewer severe complications; fatalities are rare and generally limited to the aged and debilitated. The initial lesion, which is present in most cases at the onset of fever, heals slowly; the regional lymph nodes are enlarged. The rash usually remains papular and only in severe cases becomes hemorrhagic.

The clinical picture (including the primary lesion), the geographic location, and epidemiologic considerations are helpful in establishing the diagnosis. The typhus fevers, meningococcal infections, leptospirosis, and measles must be considered in the differential diagnosis; the serologic reactions, i.e., Weil-Felix and complement fixation tests, are of value here.

Treatment and prevention   Chloramphenicol and the tetracyclines are effective therapeutic agents for boutonneuse fever. Patients generally become afebrile after 2 to 3 days of treatment, and recovery is rapid. Presumably these measures are also applicable to North Asian tick-borne rickettsiosis and Queensland tick typhus.

The major effective methods of control are concerned with avoidance of tick bites; these include application of new repellents and prompt removal of attached ticks. Effective vaccines are not available commercially.

Q FEVER   Definition   Q fever is an acute infectious disease caused by *Coxiella burnetii* and characterized by a sudden onset of fever, malaise, headache, weakness, anorexia, and interstitial pneumonitis. Rickettsemia occurs during the febrile period, and specific complement-fixing antibodies are present during convalescence. In contrast to the other rickettsioses, the disease is not associated with a cutaneous exanthem or agglutinins for the *Proteus* bacteria (Weil-Felix reaction).

Etiology and epidemiology   *C. burnetii* possesses the general properties of other rickettsias but is somewhat more resistant to inactivation in unfavorable environments and more pleomorphic than the others. Its infectivity after drying under natural conditions is of importance in the spread of infection to humans. *C. burnetii* has a wide host range in nature, but guinea pigs and embryonated eggs are the common laboratory hosts employed for its propagation.

Human cases of Q fever are contracted by inhalation of infected dusts, by handling infected materials, possibly by drinking milk contaminated with *C. burnetii* and, in one instance, by blood transfusion. The disease in Australia is enzootic in animals, especially bandicoots, and is transmitted in nature by ticks. Rickettsia-laden tick feces may contaminate cattle hides, and inhalation of this material has caused infection in humans. In the United States, a number of species of ticks are naturally infected, among them *Dermacentor andersoni* and *Amblyomma americanum,* and in North Africa transovarial transmission of the agent in indigenous ticks has been demonstrated. Sheep, goats, and cows have been found to be naturally infected in North America and in Europe, and *C. burnetii* has been recovered from the milk of such animals. Milk, as well as infected excretions from livestock, probably accounts for certain outbreaks of human disease following inhalation by cows of infected dust from barns and pens. The airborne route of dried contaminated material is the most likely method of spread. A number of epidemics have occurred among laboratory workers engaged in studies on *C. burnetii*. The disease is not transmitted between humans.

Clinical manifestations After incubation of approximately 19 days (the range is 14 to 26 days), the disease begins with headache, chilly sensations, fever, malaise, myalgia, and anorexia. For several days, the temperature ranges from 101 to 104°F; the entire course rarely exceeds 2 weeks and usually ranges from 3 to 6 days. There may be wide fluctuations in the fever. Respiratory and gastrointestinal symptoms are not conspicuous in the early stages. Headache and fever predominate. A dry cough and chest pain occur after about 5 days, when rales are usually audible. Roentgenographic findings indistinguishable from those of primary atypical pneumonia are present usually by the third to fourth day of disease, first as patchy areas of consolidation involving a portion of one lobe, giving a homogeneous ground-glass appearance. Occasionally, a homogeneous localized infiltration may resemble a tumor mass. These manifestations persist beyond the febrile period and may appear in patients who are unaware of pulmonary involvement. Complications are rare, and coincident with defervescence the appetite begins to return. Convalescence progresses slowly for several weeks, during which time the principal disability is weakness. It is not uncommon for patients to lose 7 to 9 kg during the active stages of disease. The disease may be protracted in approximately 20 percent of cases, with fever persisting for longer than 4 weeks, particularly in elderly patients. Occasionally relapse occurs, especially in patients treated with antibiotics during the first several days of disease.

Hepatitis, with the development of clinically detectable icterus, occurs in approximately one-third of patients with the protracted form. This form of Q fever is characterized by fever, malaise, absence of headache or respiratory signs, and hepatomegaly with right upper quadrant pain. Liver biopsy specimens show diffuse granulomatous changes with multinucleated giant cells and scattered infiltrations of polymorphonuclear leukocytes, lymphocytes, and macrophages. *C. burnetii* may be demonstrated in such specimens with the fluorescent antibody technique. Therefore, Q fever must be included in the differential diagnosis of patients with hepatitis and those with hepatic granulomas such as tuberculosis, sarcoidosis, histoplasmosis, brucellosis, tularemia, syphilis, and others.

Endocarditis also has been reported, and *C. burnetii* has been identified by smear and isolation in vegetations on the heart valves obtained at operation or autopsy. The aortic valve is most commonly involved, often with large vegetations. It is important, therefore, to suspect the possibility of Q fever in cases of apparent subacute bacterial endocarditis with persistently negative blood cultures. Operative intervention with replacement of damaged valves is usually necessary for recovery because the available antibiotics are not rickettsicidal. In some selected instances long-term antibiotic therapy has been successful.

A high complement-fixing antibody titer to phase I antigen is present in patients with endocarditis and granulomatous hepatitis.

Prognosis Few fatalities have been recorded and, except for the patient with protracted illness and hepatic involvement or endocarditis, the course of disease is generally uncomplicated and benign.

Treatment and control The tetracycline antibiotics and chloramphenicol are effective in the treatment of patients with Q fever. Most patients, when treated early in the course of disease, respond promptly and recover without relapses. The therapeutic procedures are comparable to those used in spotted fever.

Control of Q fever depends primarily on immunization of susceptible persons with specific vaccines. Vaccines made from phase I rickettsias are potent and afford considerable protection to slaughterhouse and dairy workers, herders, rendering-plant workers, woolsorters, tanners, laboratory workers, and others at risk. Measures should be taken to avoid exposure to infected aerosols; milk from infected domestic livestock must be pasteurized or boiled.

REFERENCES

Andrew R et al: Tick typhus in North Queensland. Med J Aust 2:253, 1946

Bozeman FM et al: Serologic evidence of *Rickettsia canada* infection in man. J Infect Dis 121:367, 1970

——— et al: Epidemic typhus rickettsiae isolated from flying squirrels. Nature 255:545, 1975

Centers for Disease Control: Epidemic typhus—Georgia. Morb Mort Week Rep 33:618, 1984

Derrick EH: The epidemiology of Q fever: A review. Med J Aust 1:245, 1953

DeShazo RD et al: Early diagnosis of Rocky Mountain spotted fever. Use of primary monocyte culture technique. JAMA 235:1353, 1976

Ferguson IC et al: Clinical, virological and pathological findings in a fatal case of Q fever endocarditis. Br J Clin Pathol 15:235, 1962

Gambrill MR, Wisseman CL Jr: Mechanisms of immunity in typhus infections. Infect Immun 8:519, 1973

Harrell GT: Rickettsial involvement of the nervous system. Med Clin North Am 37:395, 1953

Hattwick MAW et al: Rocky Mountain spotted fever: Epidemiology of an increasing problem. Ann Intern Med 84:732, 1976

Hazard GW et al: Rocky Mountain spotted fever in the Eastern United States. N Engl J Med 280:57, 1969

Koster FT et al: Cellular immunity in Q fever: Specific lymphocyte unresponsiveness in Q fever endocarditis. J Infect Dis 152:1283, 1985

Moulton FR (ed): *The Rickettsial Diseases of Man.* Washington, DC, American Association for the Advancement of Science, 1948

Murray ES et al: Brill's disease: I. Clinical and laboratory diagnosis. JAMA 142:1059, 1950

———, Snyder JC: Brill's disease: II. Etiology. Am J Hyg 53:22, 1951

Ormsbee RA et al: The influence of phase on the protective potency of Q fever vaccine. J Immunol 92:404, 1964

——— et al: Serologic diagnosis of epidemic typhus fever. Am J Epidemiol 105:261, 1977

Oster CN et al: Laboratory acquired Rocky Mountain spotted fever: The hazard of aerosol transmission. N Engl J Med 297:859, 1977

Pedersen CE et al: Demonstration of *Rickettsia rickettsii* in Rhesus monkeys by immune fluorescence microscopy. J Clin Microbiol 2:121, 1975

Philip RN et al: A comparison of serologic methods for diagnosis of Rocky Mountain spotted fever. Am J Epidemiol 105:56, 1977

Rocky Mountain spotted fever—United States, 1985. Morb Mort Week Rep 35:247, 1986

Rose HM: The clinical manifestations and laboratory diagnosis of rickettsialpox. Ann Intern Med 31:871, 1949

Smadel JE: Influence of antibiotics on immunologic responses in scrub typhus. Am J Med 17:246, 1954

——— (ed): *Symposium on Q Fever,* Medical Science Publication 6. Washington, DC, Walter Reed Army Institute of Research, 1959

———, Jackson EB: Rickettsial infections, in *Diagnostic Procedures of Viral and Rickettsial Diseases,* 3d ed. New York, American Public Health Association, 1964, p 743

Somenshine DE et al: Epizootiology of epidemic typhus (*Rickettsia prowazekii*) in flying squirrels. Am J Trop Med Hyg 27:339, 1978

Vinson JW: Etiology of trench fever in Mexico, in *Industry and Tropical Health,* vol V. Boston, Harvard School of Public Health, 1964, p 109

Walker DH, Cain BG: A method for specific diagnosis of Rocky Mountain spotted fever on fixed, paraffin-embedded tissue by immunofluorescence. J Infect Dis 137:206, 1978

———, Bradford WD: Rocky Mountain spotted fever in childhood, in *Perspectives in Pediatric Pathology,* vol 6, HS Rosenberg, J Bernstein (eds). New York, Masson Publishing, 1981, pp 35–61

Wolbach SB: Studies on Rocky Mountain spotted fever. J Med Res 41:1, 1919

Woodward TE: Rickettsial diseases in the United States. Med Clin North Am 43:1507, 1959

———: A historical account of the rickettsial diseases with a discussion of unsolved problems. J Infect Dis 127:583, 1973

———: Identification of *Rickettsia* in skin tissues. J Infect Dis 134:297, 1976

149 *MYCOPLASMA* INFECTIONS

WALLACE A. CLYDE, JR.[1]

The mycoplasmas, formerly called pleuropneumonia-like organisms (PPLO) after the organism that causes a highly contagious form of bovine pneumonia and pleurisy, are now designated class Mollicutes, with three families and four genera.

The mycoplasma of chief importance in human disease is *M. pneumoniae,* a respiratory pathogen. Others include *M. hominis* and *Ureaplasma urealyticum,* which involve the genitourinary tract.

[1] *The editors wish to acknowledge the contribution of Vernon Knight. It is on his chapter in the 10th edition of* Principles of Internal Medicine *that this revision is based.*

M. pneumoniae grows on peptone-enriched beef-heart infusion as small round colonies partially buried in the agar without the "fried egg" periphery characteristic of growth of *M. hominis* and many mycoplasmas. *Ureaplasma urealyticum* requires anaerobic incubation and special media of acid pH.

Mycoplasmas are resistant to penicillin and antibiotics known to interfere with polymerization of cell wall precursors, and they do not retain the dye-iodine complex of Gram stain. They are inhibited by tetracyclines and, in selected instances, erythromycin. Like bacteria, they grow outside the cell, possess ribonucleic and deoxyribonucleic acids, and reproduce by fission.

MYCOPLASMA PNEUMONIAE

DEFINITION Pneumonia caused by *M. pneumoniae* is characterized by fever, pharyngitis, cough, and pulmonary infiltration, in which roentgenographic signs are more extensive than indicated by physical examination. Synonyms are primary atypical pneumonia, Eaton agent pneumonia, and cold agglutinin–positive pneumonia. This organism also commonly causes upper respiratory illness without pneumonia and asymptomatic infection.

ETIOLOGY *M. pneumoniae* is distinguished from other mycoplasmas by rapid hemolysis of sheep or guinea pig erythrocytes and utilization of glucose and other sugars. It may be identified serologically by fluorescent antibody, complement fixation, growth inhibition, and indirect hemagglutination tests, all of which are useful for serologic diagnosis of human infection.

EPIDEMIOLOGY In the general population *M. pneumoniae* infection is characterized by intrafamilial spread. In most cases the infection is introduced into the family by a schoolchild. Once it is introduced, most family members become infected. In family outbreaks, pneumonia occurs with greatest frequency among school-age children, with a predominance in males. The disease is less common above age 40. *M. pneumoniae* pneumonia occurs throughout the year, although prolonged wintertime outbreaks may occur in college groups or communities. The total incidence of *M. pneumoniae* pneumonia in a study in Seattle was 1.3 per 1000 per year, which constituted about 15 to 20 percent of pneumonia from all causes. At intervals of several years, epidemics of *M. pneumoniae* pneumonia may occur with about double the usual incidence of disease.

Certain populations are at high risk for acquisition of *M. pneumoniae* infections. This mycoplasma is the leading cause of pneumonia among college students, accounting for 50 percent of all cases. Another group having a high incidence of infections is military recruits; 20 to 50 percent of pneumonia in this setting is caused by *M. pneumoniae*.

M. pneumoniae is probably spread by means of infected respiratory secretions. The organisms can be cultured from sputum of naturally occurring cases and from volunteers infected artificially. In volunteers naturally acquired antibody is associated with a high degree of resistance to infection. However, this immunity is not permanent since second episodes of pneumonia have been documented within 4 to 10 years.

CLINICAL MANIFESTATIONS The incubation period is from 9 to 12 days in experimental infections, but the interval between cases in families is approximately 3 weeks. Illness usually begins with symptoms of upper respiratory infection, which in some patients progresses to bronchitis and pneumonia. Four syndromes of respiratory disease have been identified: pneumonia, tracheobronchitis, pharyngitis, and bullous myringitis. About one-third of cases in family members will develop pneumonia, up to one-half will have tracheobronchitis, 10 percent exhibit only pharyngitis, and 10 percent will be asymptomatic. Children 5 to 10 years old have the greatest incidence of disease. Ear involvement and nondescript skin rashes are common in children, while sinusitis is present in half of adults.

Cough is almost universal in pneumonia and is frequent in cases without pulmonary involvement. Blood-flecked sputum may occur in the more severe cases, but gross hemoptysis is rare. A variety of other respiratory and systemic complaints may occur. Fever, nasal congestion, and sore throat are common. In pneumonia, harsh or diminished sounds are frequent but bronchial breathing is uncommon. Fine inspiratory rales are found in most patients but are not impressive. Pleural rubs and pleural effusion are infrequent. Studies on the distribution of pneumonia in one large series showed that more than one-half of cases were multilobular and slightly less than one-half were bilateral. Lower-lobe pneumonia was appreciably more frequent than upper-lobe pneumonia. Pulmonary infiltrates may occur as an isolated area in the lung periphery but more often spread from the hilum.

The disease is variable in severity, but high fever may persist for 1 to 2 weeks in untreated cases. X-ray changes last for as long as 3 weeks in untreated cases, but for 7 to 10 days in treated cases. Even in untreated cases, complications are rare and consist of occasional purulent sinusitis, persistent cough, and, rarely, pleurisy. Prolonged weakness and malaise follow the untreated illness in adults.

Rare complications include meningoencephalitis, polyneuritis, monoarticular arthritis, Stevens-Johnson syndrome, pericarditis, myocarditis, hepatitis, diffuse intravascular coagulation, noncardiogenic pulmonary edema, and hemolytic anemia.

LABORATORY FINDINGS During acute illness leukocytosis in the range of 10,000 to 15,000 leukocytes per cubic millimeter occurs in about 25 percent of cases. Increase in sedimentation rate above 40 mm/h occurs in at least two-thirds of cases. Urinalysis, electrocardiograms, and fluid and electrolyte and liver function studies show no characteristic changes. The complement fixation, fluorescent antibody, indirect hemagglutination, and growth inhibition tests yield specific diagnostic information. The simplicity of the complement fixation test recommends it for general use, although it is less sensitive and specific than the other tests. Fourfold rises in titer often occur within 2 weeks, and maximum rise is achieved in 4 weeks. A nonspecific test for *M. pneumoniae* infection in use for many years is the detection of cold agglutinins. The end point is the dilution of the patient's serum which agglutinates human type O red blood cells at 4°C. The test depends on the presence of a macroglobulin antibody to the I antigen of red blood cells. In *M. pneumoniae* infection, cold agglutinins appear at the end of the first week of illness and can serve as a rapid diagnostic test; they disappear in 2 to 6 weeks. The test is positive in about half the patients, more commonly in those who are severely ill. The cold agglutinin reaction occurs with other red blood cell antigens in infectious mononucleosis, lymphoproliferative diseases, and in several respiratory infections, particularly in children younger than 5 years.

New information about perturbations of host immune response in *M. pneumoniae* infections dictates caution in interpreting serologic data. Due to polyclonal B-cell activation "nonspecific" antibody rises to diverse agents can occur; coupled with T-lymphocyte suppression, this also may explain the appearance of various host tissue autoantibodies and transient anergy. Since other infectious agents, including cytomegalovirus, Epstein-Barr virus, and measles, produce similar effects, diagnostic confusion can result. *M. pneumoniae* serologic tests never should be included in panels of studies for illness of unknown cause.

DIFFERENTIAL DIAGNOSIS Pneumonia due to *M. pneumoniae* needs to be distinguished from pneumonia of all other types. It is usually less severe, is associated with less dense pulmonary infiltration than pneumococcal and other bacterial pneumonias, and occurs throughout the year. Pulmonary infiltrates in the absence of symptoms or physical signs may initially suggest acute pulmonary tuberculosis. In military populations adenoviral pneumonia must be excluded. Pneumonic involvement as a direct result of influenza viral infection or its complication by pneumococcal, streptococcal, staphylococcal, or *Haemophilus influenzae* infection may cause difficulty in diagnosis.

Q fever, psittacosis, and tularemia are less frequent causes of pneumonia that may be difficult to distinguish from *M. pneumoniae* infection. In children, especially young infants, pneumonia due to respiratory syncytial, parainfluenza, adenovirus, and influenza viruses may resemble *M. pneumoniae* infection. Legionnaires' disease (see Chap. 117) resembles severe cases of *M. pneumoniae* pneumonia.

TREATMENT Erythromycin and tetracycline derivatives are effective in treating *M. pneumoniae* disease. For adults, erythromycin (0.5 g every 8 h orally) or tetracycline (250 mg every 6 h orally) for 10 to 14 days usually is prescribed. In severe illnesses the dose may be increased and given for 21 days; intravenous erythromycin at times is useful, but tetracycline is not recommended by this route. For children below age 8, erythromycin is the primary antibiotic at doses of 30 to 50 mg/kg per day orally for 10 to 14 days. Tetracycline is an effective alternative in older patients.

Treatment temporarily reduces the frequency of positive cultures from the respiratory tract, but shedding may continue for several weeks after treatment, a finding similar to that in psittacosis pneumonia. Relapse of *M. pneumoniae* pneumonia occurs occasionally, but such cases respond to re-treatment. In cases in which there is doubt between the diagnosis of *M. pneumoniae* and *Legionella* or pneumococcal infection, erythromycin should be used in preference to a tetracycline. No vaccines are available.

OTHER *MYCOPLASMA* INFECTIONS

A growing body of literature documents evidence of other human *Mycoplasma* infections, particularly in the perinatal period, and a variety of genitourinary syndromes in both sexes. *Mycoplasma* should be suspected in suppurative processes that are bacteriologically sterile, such as urethritis, salpingitis, amnionitis, neonatal meningitis, and pneumonia and pyelonephritis. *Mycoplasma* abscesses and arthritis may occur in immunocompromised hosts. Sexually transmitted *Mycoplasma* diseases are considered elsewhere (see Chap. 91).

Mycoplasmas most commonly encountered are *M. hominis* and *U. urealyticum*. *M. hominis* hydrolyzes arginine in liquid media, producing ammonia which results in an alkaline pH shift. Ureaplasmas are so-named because they cleave urea, again producing ammonia. Selective, differential media have been described which allow demonstration of the unique urease activity on primary isolation within 24 to 48 h.

Very few diagnostic microbiology laboratories perform *Mycoplasma* cultures, and serodiagnosis remains a research tool for species other than *M. pneumoniae*. Specimens should be transported on wet ice (within 24 h or less) or dry ice (greater than 24 h) to reference laboratories for assistance. Generally, *M. hominis* is sensitive to tetracycline and clindamycin but not erythromycin, while ureaplasmas are sensitive to tetracyclines and erythromycin. Since antibiotic sensitivity patterns of these species vary widely, laboratory guidance may be required for effective therapy.

REFERENCES

CASSELL GH, COLE BC: Mycoplasmas as agents of human disease. N Engl J Med 304:80, 1981

CHERRY JD et al: *Mycoplasma pneumoniae* infections and exanthems. J Pediatr 87:369, 1975

CLYDE WA, FERNALD GW: Mycoplasmas: The pathogens' pathogen. Cell Immunol 82:88, 1983

COUCH RB: *Mycoplasma pneumoniae*, in *Principles and Practice of Infectious Diseases*, G Mandell et al (eds). New York, Wiley, 1985, pp 1065–1076

FOY HM et al: Viral and mycoplasmal pneumonia in a prepaid medical care group during an eight year period. Am J Epidemiol 97:93, 1973

KALB RE et al: Stevens-Johnson syndrome due to *Mycoplasma pneumoniae* in an adult. Am J Med 79:541, 1985

MCDADE JE et al: Legionnaires' disease. Isolation of a bacterium and demonstration of its role in other respiratory disease. N Engl J Med 297:1197, 1978

ROIFMAN CM et al: Increased susceptibility to *Mycoplasma* infection in patients with hypogammaglobulinemia. Am J Med 80:590, 1986

150 CHLAMYDIAL INFECTIONS

WALTER E. STAMM / KING K. HOLMES

The genus *Chlamydia* contains two species, *C. psittaci* and *C. trachomatis*. *C. psittaci* is widely distributed in nature, producing genital, conjunctival, intestinal, or respiratory infections in many mammalian and avian species. Genital infections with *C. psittaci* have been well characterized in several species and cause complications such as abortion and infertility. Although mammalian strains of *C. psittaci* are not known to infect humans, avian strains do occasionally infect humans, causing pneumonia.

C. trachomatis is exclusively a human pathogen and was first recognized as the cause of trachoma in the 1940s. Since then, *C. trachomatis* has been recognized as a major sexually transmitted and perinatal infection. Chlamydiae are obligate, intracellular parasites that were originally considered large viruses. However, they possess both DNA and RNA, have a cell wall and ribosomes similar to those of gram-negative bacteria, and can be inhibited by antibiotics such as tetracycline. Therefore, chlamydiae are now classified as bacteria belonging to their own order (Chlamydiales) and genus (*Chlamydia*).

A unique feature of all chlamydia is their complex reproductive cycle. Two forms of the microorganism—the extracellular elementary body and the intracellular reticulate body—participate in this cycle. The elementary body is adapted for extracellular survival and is the infective form transmitted from one person to another. Elementary bodies attach to susceptible target cells (usually columnar or transitional epithelial cells) via specific receptors and enter the cell within a phagosome. Within 8 h, the elementary bodies reorganize into reticulate bodies. These forms are adapted to intracellular survival and multiplication. They undergo binary fission, eventually producing numerous replicates contained within the membrane-bound "inclusion body" which occupies much of the infected host cell. Chlamydial inclusions resist lysosomal fusion until late in the developmental cycle. After 24 h, the reticulate bodies condense and form elementary bodies still contained within the inclusion. The inclusion then ruptures, releasing elementary bodies from the cell to initiate infection of adjacent cells.

C. psittaci and *C. trachomatis* share a genus-specific or group antigen. Antibody against this antigen is measured in the complement-fixation serologic test available in most state health departments. *C. trachomatis* strains can be further characterized serologically on the basis of antibody produced against their major outer membrane protein. These antigens serve as the basis for the serovar classification of Wang and Grayston. Using this system, strains associated with trachoma have generally been those of the A, B, Ba, and C serovars, while serovars D through K have been largely associated with sexually transmitted and perinatally acquired infections. Serovars L_1, L_2, and L_3 produce lymphogranuloma venereum (LGV) and hemorrhagic proctocolitis. These strains demonstrate unique biologic behavior in that they are more invasive than the other serovars, produce disease in lymphatic tissue, grow readily in cell culture systems and macrophages, and are fatal when inoculated intracerebrally in mice and monkeys. Non-LGV strains of *C. trachomatis* characteristically produce superficial infections involving the columnar epithelium of the eye, genitalia, and respiratory tract.

C. psittaci and *C. trachomatis* can be differentiated in the laboratory by inclusion type and sensitivity to sulfonamide. While *C. trachomatis* is sensitive to sulfa, *C. psittaci* is resistant. *C. trachomatis* inclusions contain glycogen and stain with iodine, while *C. psittaci* inclusions do not.

SEXUALLY TRANSMITTED AND PERINATAL *C. TRACHOMATIS* INFECTIONS

SPECTRUM OF *C. TRACHOMATIS* GENITAL INFECTIONS Genital infections caused by *C. trachomatis* are now recognized as the most common sexually transmitted disease (STD) in the United States. An estimated 3 to 4 million cases occur each year. In adults the clinical spectrum of sexually transmitted *C. trachomatis* infections is easily understood because it parallels closely the spectrum of gonococcal infections (Table 150-1). Both agents have been associated with urethritis in both sexes, with epididymitis, mucopurulent cervicitis, acute salpingitis, bartholinitis, proctitis, and the Fitz-Hugh–Curtis syndrome (perihepatitis), and both can be associated with systemic complications, particularly with arthritis. Simultaneous infection with *C. trachomatis* occurs in 30 to 50 percent of women with cervical gonococcal infection and in 25 percent of heterosexual men with gonococcal urethritis.

EPIDEMIOLOGY   Genital infections other than LGV are caused by *C. trachomatis* serovars D through K. Although data are lacking, the incidence of genital *C. trachomatis* infection is probably increasing, because the incidence of nongonococcal urethritis (NGU) has risen dramatically over the last two decades, and *C. trachomatis* has consistently been isolated from 30 to 50 percent of men with NGU. The peak age incidence of genital *C. trachomatis* infections is in the late teens and early twenties, resembling other sexually transmitted infections. Further evidence for sexual transmission is the rising prevalence of serum antibody to *C. trachomatis* in proportion to an increasing number of sex partners. The prevalence of chlamydial urethral infection in young men ranges from 3 to 5 percent of men seen in general medical settings, to over 10 percent of asymptomatic soldiers undergoing routine physical examination, to 15 to 20 percent of men seen in STD clinics. Among homosexual men, urethral infection appears less common (4 to 5 percent of homosexual men in STD clinics) than in heterosexual men, but rectal infections occur with a prevalence of 4 to 7 percent in homosexual male STD clinic patients. Cervical infection in women has ranged from 5 percent or more of asymptomatic college students or prenatal patients in the United States, to over 10 percent of women seen in family planning clinics, to over 20 percent of women seen in STD clinics. In the United States, the prevalence of *C. trachomatis* in the cervix of pregnant women is 5 to 10 times higher than that of *N. gonorrhoeae*. The prevalence of genital infection with either agent is highest in individuals who are single, nonwhite, unmarried, and between ages 18 and 24. The ratio of chlamydial to gonococcal urethritis is highest for heterosexual men and those with high socioeconomic status, and lowest for homosexual men and indigent populations. The proportion of infections that are asymptomatic appears to be higher for *C. trachomatis* than for *N. gonorrhoeae*, and symptomatic *C. trachomatis* infections are clinically less severe. It is suspected that mild or

asymptomatic chlamydial infections of the fallopian tubes may nonetheless cause ongoing tubal damage and infertility. Furthermore, because the total number of *C. trachomatis* infections exceeds that of *N. gonorrhoeae* infections in industrialized countries, the total morbidity caused by *C. trachomatis* genital infections is comparable with that caused by *N. gonorrhoeae*. The prevalence of *C. trachomatis* is higher than that of *N. gonorrhoeae* in industrialized countries, in part because measures such as treatment of sex partners and routine cultures for case detection in asymptomatic individuals are being applied much more effectively for gonorrhea than for control of *C. trachomatis* infection.

CLINICAL MANIFESTATIONS   Nongonococcal and postgonococcal urethritis   Nongonococcal urethritis is a diagnosis of exclusion that is applied to men with symptoms and/or signs of urethritis who do not have gonorrhea. Postgonococcal urethritis (PGU) refers to nongonococcal urethritis which develops 2 to 3 weeks after treatment of gonococcal urethritis in men. *C. trachomatis* causes 30 to 50 percent of the cases of NGU and PGU in heterosexual men but is less commonly isolated from homosexual men with these syndromes. The cause of the remainder is uncertain, although considerable evidence suggests that *Ureaplasma urealyticum* causes some of these infections.

In current practice, NGU is diagnosed by documentation of a leukocytic urethral exudate and by exclusion of gonorrhea by Gram's stain or culture. *C. trachomatis* urethritis is generally less severe than gonococcal urethritis, although in an individual patient these two forms of urethritis cannot be differentiated solely on clinical grounds. Symptoms include urethral discharge, dysuria (often whitish and mucoid rather than frankly purulent), and urethral itching. The examination may show meatal erythema and tenderness and a urethral exudate which is often demonstrable only by stripping the urethra. About one-third of male STD patients who have *C. trachomatis* urethral infection have no demonstrable signs or symptoms of urethritis. Such patients frequently have first-glass pyuria (15 leukocytes per $400\times$ microscopic field in the sediment of first-voided urine) or an increased number of leukocytes on gram-stained smear prepared from a urogenital swab inserted 1 to 2 cm into the anterior urethra. The smear is first scanned at low power to identify areas of the slide containing the highest concentration of leukocytes. These areas are then examined under oil immersion ($1000\times$). An average of four or more leukocytes in five $1000\times$ (oil immersion) fields is indicative of urethritis and correlates with recovery of *C. trachomatis*. To differentiate between true urethritis and functional symptoms among symptomatic patients, or to make a presumptive diagnosis of *C. trachomatis* infection in asymptomatic men (e.g., male patients in STD clinics, sex partners of women with nongonococcal salpingitis or mucopurulent cervicitis, fathers of children with inclusion conjunctivitis), the examination of an endourethral specimen for increased leukocytes is useful if specific diagnostic tests are not available.

Epididymitis   *C. trachomatis* is the major cause of epididymitis in sexually active males. In one study, *C. trachomatis* infection was found by cultures of the urethra, urine, semen, or epididymal aspirate or by serology in 17 of 34 men under 35 years of age who presented with epididymitis, while 7 had gonorrhea; of 16 men over 35 with epididymitis, only 1 had chlamydial infection, and none had gonorrhea. Coliform bacteria and *Pseudomonas aeruginosa* are the most common causes of epididymitis in men over 35. The presence of a urethral discharge or a history of recent urethritis in association with unilateral scrotal pain, swelling, and tenderness suggests the diagnosis of chlamydial or gonococcal epididymitis. However, the presence of midstream pyuria and bacteriuria in an older patient without urethral discharge, but with a history of genitourinary instrumentation or bacterial urinary tract or prostatic infection, suggests coliform or *Pseudomonas* infection. Testicular torsion should be promptly excluded by radionuclide scan, Doppler flow study, or surgical exploration in a teenager or young adult who presents with acute unilateral testicular pain without urethritis. Testicular tumor or chronic infection

TABLE 150-1   Clinical parallels between sexually transmitted infections due to *Neisseria gonorrhoeae* and *Chlamydia trachomatis*

Site of infection	Resulting clinical syndrome	
	N. gonorrhoeae	*C. trachomatis*
MEN		
Urethra	Urethritis	NGU, PGU
Epididymis	Epididymitis	Epididymitis
Rectum	Proctitis	Proctitis
Conjunctiva	Conjunctivitis	Conjunctivitis
Systemic	Disseminated gonococcal infection (DGI)	Reiter's syndrome
WOMEN		
Urethra	Acute urethral syndrome	Acute urethral syndrome
Bartholin's gland	Bartholinitis	Bartholinitis
Cervix	Cervicitis	Cervicitis
Endometrium	Endometritis	Endometritis
Fallopian tube	Salpingitis	Salpingitis
Conjunctiva	Conjunctivitis	Conjunctivitis
Liver capsule	Perihepatitis	Perihepatitis
Systemic	DGI	Reiter's syndrome

(e.g., tuberculosis) should be excluded in the patient with unilateral intrascrotal pain and swelling who does not respond to appropriate antimicrobial therapy.

Reiter's syndrome *C. trachomatis* has been recovered from the urethra of up to 70 percent of men with untreated nondiarrheal Reiter's syndrome and associated urethritis. The syndrome consists of conjunctivitis, urethritis, arthritis, and characteristic skin lesions (see Chap. 268). In the absence of overt urethritis, it is important to exclude subclinical urethritis as discussed above.

Proctitis *C. trachomatis* of either the genital immunotypes D through K or the LGV immunotype L₂ causes proctitis in homosexual men and heterosexual women who practice anal intercourse. Either asymptomatic infection or mild proctitis not unlike gonococcal proctitis results from infection with immunotypes D through K. Clinically, these patients present with mild rectal pain, mucus discharge, tenesmus, and, occasionally, bleeding. Nearly all have polymorphonuclear leukocytes in their rectal Gram stain. Sigmoidoscopy in these non-LGV cases of chlamydial proctitis reveals mild, patchy mucosal friability and the disease process is limited to the distal rectum. LGV strains produce a more severe ulcerative proctitis or proctocolitis which histologically resembles Crohn's disease in that giant-cell formation and granulomas are seen (see Chap. 238). The differential diagnosis of proctitis limited to the distal rectum in homosexual men includes gonococcal or herpes simplex virus infection, in addition to *C. trachomatis* infection.

Mucopurulent cervicitis *C. trachomatis* has been isolated from the cervix of 30 to 60 percent of women with gonorrhea or a history of contact with gonorrhea, from 30 to 70 percent of women whose male partners have nongonococcal urethritis, and from 10 to 20 percent of women attending STD clinics who do not have a history of contact with a partner with urethritis. Women who have cervical ectopy or who use oral contraceptives appear to have an increased prevalence of cervical infection with *C. trachomatis*.

Although some women with *C. trachomatis* infection of the cervix have no symptoms or signs, careful speculum examination shows that many have mucopurulent cervicitis. As discussed more fully in Chap. 91, mucopurulent cervicitis is associated with yellow mucopurulent discharge from the endocervical columnar epithelium, and with ≥10 polymorphonuclear (PMN) leukocytes per 1000× microscopic field within strands of cervical mucus on a thinly smeared, Gram-stained preparation of endocervical exudate. Pap smear also shows increased PMN leukocytes, as well as a characteristic pattern of mononuclear inflammatory cells, including plasma cells, transformed lymphocytes, and histiocytes. Cervical biopsy shows predominantly a mononuclear infiltrate, often with a follicular cervicitis (i.e., lymphoid aggregates with germinal centers containing transformed lymphocytes.)

Pelvic inflammatory disease (PID) *C. trachomatis* plays an important causative role in salpingitis. *C. trachomatis* infection has been demonstrated in laparoscopically verified salpingitis, recovered from the fallopian tubes in the absence of other pathogens, and serologic evidence of *C. trachomatis* infection has been adduced in women with PID. In the United States *C. trachomatis* has been identified in the fallopian tubes or endometrium in up to 50 percent of women with PID, and its role as an important etiologic agent in this syndrome is now well accepted. The ability of *C. trachomatis* to cause salpingitis has been confirmed in animal models.

Pelvic inflammatory disease occurs via ascending intraluminal spread of *C. trachomatis* from the lower genital tract, and mucopurulent cervicitis is followed by endometritis, endosalpingitis, and finally pelvic peritonitis. Evidence of mucopurulent cervicitis is usually present in women with laparoscopically verified salpingitis. Similarly, endometritis, demonstrated by endometrial biopsy showing plasma cell infiltration of the endometrial epithelium, is present in nearly all women with laparoscopically verified chlamydial (or gonococcal) salpingitis. Chlamydial endometritis also occurs in the absence of clinical evidence of salpingitis: approximately 40 percent of women with mucopurulent cervicitis were found to have plasma cell endometritis in one study. Histologic evidence of endometritis was correlated with an "endometritis syndrome," consisting of vaginal bleeding, lower abdominal pain, and uterine tenderness in the absence of adnexal tenderness, and with peripheral blood leukocytosis. Since laparoscopy was not performed in these patients, it is not known what proportion of those with chlamydial endometritis without adnexal tenderness nonetheless had salpingitis. However, chlamydial salpingitis apparently produces milder symptoms then does gonococcal salpingitis and is associated with less marked adnexal tenderness. The presence of mild adnexal or uterine tenderness in sexually active women with cervicitis should suggest PID.

Infertility associated with fallopian tube scarring has been strongly linked to antecedent *C. trachomatis* infection in serologic studies. Since not all infertile women with tubal scarring and antichlamydial antibody in these studies gave a history of prior PID, subclinical tubal infection may produce scarring. Ectopic pregnancy, which occurs in over 60,000 women in the United States annually, is also thought to be related to chlamydia-induced tubal scarring in many cases.

Perihepatitis, or the Fitz-Hugh–Curtis syndrome, was originally described as a complication of gonococcal PID. However, cultural and/or serologic evidence of *C. trachomatis* infection in most women with this syndrome has come to light. *C. trachomatis* has also been cultured from exudate on the hepatic capsule in laparoscopically verified cases. This syndrome should be suspected whenever a young, sexually active woman presents with an illness resembling cholecystitis (fever and right upper quadrant pain of subacute or acute onset). Symptoms and signs of salpingitis may be minimal.

Urethral syndrome in women *C. trachomatis* has been found to be the most common pathogen isolated from college women with acute dysuria, frequency, and pyuria, together with the absence of uropathogens such as coliforms or *Staphylococcus saprophyticus* in *any* concentration in a clean-catch midstream urine specimen (see Chap. 225). *Chlamydia* can also be isolated from the urethra of women without symptoms of urethritis, and up to 25 percent of female STD clinic patients have had positive *C. trachomatis* cultures from the urethra only.

***C. trachomatis* infection in pregnancy** *C. trachomatis* in pregnancy has been associated in some studies (but not in others) with premature delivery and with postpartum endometritis. Whether these complications are in part attributable to *C. trachomatis* requires further investigation.

PERINATAL INFECTIONS: INCLUSION CONJUNCTIVITIS AND PNEUMONIA

EPIDEMIOLOGY Studies in the United States have demonstrated that 5 to 25 percent of pregnant women have *C. trachomatis* infections of the cervix. In these studies, approximately one-half to two-thirds of the children who were exposed during birth eventually showed laboratory evidence of *C. trachomatis* infection. Roughly half of the infants who developed laboratory evidence of infection (or 25 percent of the group exposed) developed clinical inclusion conjunctivitis. In addition to eye infection, *C. trachomatis* was isolated frequently and persistently from the nasopharynx and the rectum. Pneumonia occurs in about 10 percent of children infected perinatally, and otitis media may in some cases result from perinatally acquired chlamydial infection.

INCLUSION CONJUNCTIVITIS OF THE NEWBORN (NEONATAL CHLAMYDIAL CONJUNCTIVITIS) In the newborn, chlamydial conjunctivitis generally has a longer incubation period than gonococcal conjunctivitis (usually 5 to 14 days vs. 1 to 3 days), but this is not reliable in the individual patient. The other common causes of conjunctivitis in newborns include *Staphylococcus aureus, Haemophilus influenzae, Streptococcus pneumoniae,* and herpes simplex virus. Neonatal chlamydial conjunctivitis has an acute onset and often produces a profuse mucopurulent discharge. However, it is impossible to differentiate *Chlamydia* conjunctivitis from other forms of neonatal bacterial conjunctivitis clinically, and laboratory diagnosis is required. Inclusions within epithelial cells often can be demonstrated in Giemsa-stained conjunctival smears, but these smears are less sensitive than cultures or antigen detection tests. Similarly, Gram-stained smears may show gonococci, or occasional small gram-negative coccobacilli in *Haemophilus* conjunctivitis, but smears should be accompanied by cultures for these agents. Very rarely a trachoma-like eye disease with chlamydial infection occurs in children living in areas that do not have endemic trachoma. This probably is the late result of neonatally acquired infection. If neonatal chlamydial conjunctivitis is not treated appropriately with oral antimicrobials, it may be followed by chlamydial pneumonia.

INFANT PNEUMONIA   There is a distinctive pneumonia syndrome in infants infected with *C. trachomatis* which occurs in two to six cases per 1000 live births. The diagnosis of *C. trachomatis* pneumonia has been confirmed by isolation of the organism from lung biopsy and by development of high titers of specific IgM antibody to *C. trachomatis.* This pneumonia has been found in infants from 1 to 4 months of age. The onset is gradual and the course protracted, but the child is usually afebrile. Radiographically, there is diffuse interstitial involvement of the lungs. Most of the infants have a distinctive cough (a series of closely spaced staccato coughs, each separated by a brief inspiration), tachypnea, rales, hyperinflation, slight eosinophilia, and elevated serum immunoglobulins. Clinical illness lasts several weeks, while inspiratory rales and radiologic signs may persist for months. About half of the infants with pneumonia also have conjunctivitis. While many infants with pneumonia have recovered without therapy, a few in whom the illness has been associated with apnea have been severely ill.

LYMPHOGRANULOMA VENEREUM

DEFINITION   Lymphogranuloma venereum (LGV) is a sexually transmitted infection caused by *C. trachomatis* strains of the L_1, L_2, or L_3 serovars. Most cases are caused by L_2 infections. The acute disease in heterosexual men is characterized by a transient primary genital lesion followed by multilocular suppurative regional lymphadenopathy. Women, homosexual men, and, occasionally, heterosexual men may develop hemorrhagic proctitis with regional lymph-

FIGURE 150-1 *Lymphogranuloma venereum. Bilateral inguinal buboes, with the ''sign of the groove,'' caused by adenopathy above and below Poupart's ligament. (Courtesy of A Brathwaite.)*

adenitis. Acute LGV is almost always associated with systemic symptoms such as fever and leukocytosis and rarely with systemic complications such as meningoencephalitis. After a latent period of years, late complications include genital elephantiasis, strictures, and fistulas of the penis, urethra, and rectum.

EPIDEMIOLOGY   LGV is usually sexually transmitted, but occasional transmission by nonsexual personal contact, fomites, or laboratory accidents has been documented. Laboratory work involving creation of aerosols of this organism (e.g., sonication, homogenization) must be conducted with appropriate biologic containment.

The peak incidence of LGV corresponds to the age of greatest sexual activity, the second and third decades of life. The worldwide incidence of LGV is falling, but the disease is still endemic and a major cause of morbidity in Asia, Africa, and South America. Only 235 cases were reported in the United States in 1982.

The frequency of infection following exposure is believed to be much less than that associated with gonorrhea and syphilis. Early manifestations are recognized far more often in men than in women, who usually present with late complications. In the United States, where the reported sex ratio is 3.4 males to 1 female, most cases involve homosexually active men; travelers, seamen, and military personnel returning from abroad; and individuals of low socioeconomic status living in areas of low endemicity in the southeast. The main reservoir of infection is presumed to be asymptomatically infected individuals, although this has not been directly demonstrated.

CLINICAL MANIFESTATIONS   In heterosexuals, a *primary genital lesion* occurs from 3 days to 3 weeks after exposure. It is a small, painless vesicle or nonindurated ulcer or papule located on the penis in men or on the labia, posterior vagina, or fourchette in women. The primary lesion is noticed by less than one-third of men with LGV and only rarely by women. It heals in a few days without scarring and even when noticed is usually not recognized as LGV except in retrospect. LGV strains of *C. trachomatis* have occasionally been recovered from genital ulcers, and also from the urethra of men and the endocervix of women who present with inguinal adenopathy, suggesting that these areas may be the primary site of infection in some cases.

In women and homosexual men, *primary anal or rectal infection* occurs following rectal intercourse. In women, rectal infection with LGV (or non-LGV) strains of *C. trachomatis* presumably can also arise either via contiguous spread of infected secretions along the perineum (as with rectal gonococcal infection in women) or perhaps by spread to the rectum via the pelvic lymphatics. From the site of the primary urethral, genital, anal, or rectal infection, the organism spreads via the regional lymphatics. Penile, vulvar, and anal infection can lead to inguinal and femoral lymphadenitis. Rectal infection produces hypogastric and deep iliac lymphadenitis. Upper vaginal or cervical infection results in enlargement of the obturator and iliac nodes. The most common presenting picture in heterosexual men is the *inguinal syndrome,* which is characterized by painful inguinal lymphadenopathy beginning 2 to 6 weeks after presumed exposure; rarely the onset occurs after a few months. The inguinal adenopathy is unilateral in two-thirds of cases, and palpable enlargement of the iliac and femoral nodes is often present on the same side as the enlarged inguinal nodes. The nodes are initially discrete, but progressive periadenitis results in a matted mass of nodes which become fluctuant and suppurative. The overlying skin becomes fixed, inflamed, and thinned and finally develops multiple draining fistulas. Extensive enlargement of chains of inguinal nodes above and below the inguinal ligament (''the sign of the groove'') is common but is not specific, and is present in only a minority of cases (Fig. 150-1). Histologically, infected nodes initially show characteristic small stellate abscesses surrounded by histiocytes. These abscesses coalesce to cause large, necrotic, suppurative foci. Spontaneous healing usually occurs after several months, leaving inguinal scars or granulomatous masses of varying size which persist for life. Massive pelvic lymphadenopathy in women or homosexual men may lead to exploratory laparotomy.

As cultures and serology for *C. trachomatis* are being used more often, increasing numbers of cases of LGV proctitis are being recognized in homosexual men. Such patients present with anorectal pain and mucopurulent, bloody rectal discharge. Although patients may complain of diarrhea, this usually represents frequent, painful unsuccessful attempts at defecation (tenesmus). Sigmoidoscopy reveals ulcerative proctitis or proctocolitis, with purulent exudate and mucosal bleeding. Since the LGV agent is an obligate intracellular pathogen, the histopathologic findings in the rectal mucosa include granulomas with giant cells, along with crypt abscesses and extensive inflammation. These clinical, sigmoidoscopic, and histopathologic findings may closely resemble Crohn's disease of the rectum (Fig. 150-2).

Constitutional symptoms are common during the state of regional lymphadenopathy and, in the presence of proctitis, may include fever, chills, headache, meningismus, anorexia, myalgias, and arthralgias. These findings in the presence of lymphadenopathy are sometimes mistaken for malignant lymphoma. Other systemic complications are infrequent but include arthritis with sterile effusion, aseptic meningitis, meningoencephalitis, conjunctivitis, hepatitis, and erythema nodosum. Chlamydiae have been recovered from the cerebrospinal fluid, and in one case from the blood in a patient with severe constitutional symptoms, indicating the occurrence of disseminated infection. Laboratory infections due to suspected inhalation of aerosols have been associated with mediastinal lymphadenitis, pneumonitis, and pleural effusion.

Associated laboratory findings during the acute stage of infection include leukocytosis and slight elevation of the sedimentation rate. Abnormal liver function tests, hyperglobulinemia, mixed cryoglobulinemia, rheumatoid factor activity, and elevated IgG, IgA, and IgM have been reported in subacute and chronic LGV. False-positive serologic tests for syphilis are rare, and syphilis should be suspected if these tests are positive, as is often the case.

Complications of untreated anorectal infection include perirectal abscess, fistula in ano, and rectovaginal, rectovesical, and ischiorectal fistulas. Secondary bacterial infection probably contributes to these complications. Rectal stricture is a late complication of anorectal infection and usually occurs 2 to 6 cm from the anal orifice, within reach on digital rectal examination. The stricture may extend proximally for several centimeters, leading to a mistaken clinical and radiographic diagnosis of carcinoma.

A small percentage of cases of LGV in men presents with chronic progressive infiltrative, ulcerative, or fistular lesions of the penis, urethra, or scrotum. Urethral stricture may occur and usually involves the posterior urethra, causing incontinence or difficulty with micturition.

An uncommon late complication of LGV is *genital elephantiasis*, a chronic induration and edema of the penis or vulva caused by lymphatic obstruction. Polypoid swelling of the skin and large stellate hyperplastic keloidal scars of the genitalia may be associated with vulvar induration or lymphedema and are difficult to distinguish clinically from granuloma inguinale and genital tuberculosis. Chronic ulcerations of the vulva (esthiomene) and smooth pedunculated perianal growths (lymphorrhoids) also occur. The significance of reports of malignant changes associated with chronic anorectal or genital LGV is uncertain.

DIAGNOSIS Although LGV is uncommon, it frequently enters the differential diagnosis of common conditions such as inguinal lymphadenopathy; vesicular, papular, or ulcerative genital lesions; and perirectal abscess, fistula in ano, or proctitis.

The most reliable method of diagnosis is isolation of an LGV strain of *Chlamydia* from aspirated bubo pus, from the rectum, or from the urethra, endocervix, or other infected tissue. Isolation has been possible from bubo pus in about 30 percent of cases with inguinal lymphadenopathy and from the rectum in most homosexual men who have proctitis. The most widely used immunodiagnostic tests in the past have been the LGV complement fixation (CF) test and the Frei skin tests. An LGV CF titer ≥1:64 is suggestive of

LGV and can be found in most patients after the bubo has appeared. The titer may not increase in paired serums since most patients have already been infected for several weeks when first seen. The LGV CF test can also become positive during infections with non-LGV strains of *C. trachomatis*, and high titers of CF antibody can be seen in patients who have had severe infections with such non-LGV strains. The Frei skin test is less sensitive than the LGV complement fixation test and is no longer available.

The microimmunofluorescent antibody test detects antibody to *C. trachomatis* in nearly all patients with culture-proven LGV. Serum microimmunofluorescent antibody titers from patients with LGV are usually ≥1:512, exceeding the highest titers that occur in chlamydial NGU and can usually be shown to have a characteristic broad pattern of reactivity against many immunotypes of *C. trachomatis*. The histopathology of excised nodes or of rectal biopsy specimens is seldom definitive, but suggestive findings (e.g., stellate abscesses in lymph nodes or granulomas on rectal biopsy) may raise the question of LGV and lead to more specific tests. Fluorescein-conjugated monoclonal antibodies against *C. trachomatis*, and against the L₂ strain of *C. trachomatis*, may prove useful for identification of the agent in properly fixed specimens from lymph nodes or other tissue, and monoclonal antibody to L₂ can be used for rapid identification of L₂ strains isolated in tissue cell culture.

TREATMENT The LGV and non-LGV strains of *C. trachomatis* have similar antimicrobial susceptibilities. Antimicrobial therapy does not have a dramatic effect on the duration and healing of inguinal buboes, but acute constitutional symptoms are often terminated abruptly, and LGV proctitis improves rapidly after antimicrobial therapy has been instituted. Antibiotics are usually not helpful in improving late complications such as rectal stricture or genital elephantiasis unless secondary infection is also present. Genital

FIGURE 150-2 *Histopathologic findings in LGV proctitis in a homosexually active man. Note granulomatous changes, with giant cells, and crypt abscess with adjacent giant cell (insert). These changes resemble those seen in Crohn's disease of the rectum. (From TC Quinn et al, N Engl J Med 305:195, 1981.)*

elephantiasis and rectal, penile, and urethral strictures and fistulas usually require surgical correction, although sometimes urethral and even rectal strictures can be managed by repeated mechanical dilation.

The recommended treatment regimen is tetracycline hydrochloride, 0.5 g four times a day for 3 weeks. A sulfonamide preparation, 4 g per day for 3 weeks, can also be used, but occasional isolates have been resistant to sulfonamides in vitro. Fluctuant buboes should be aspirated through normal skin with a syringe and 18-gauge needle as often as necessary to prevent spontaneous rupture. It is not unusual for buboes to increase in size or to develop at another site after initiation of treatment. Although these seldom progress to fistula formation, they should be aspirated if fluctuant. A fourfold or greater fall in CF titer or microimmunofluorescent antibody titer eventually occurs over several months in most treated patients, and LGV *Chlamydia* cannot be isolated from lesions after the initiation of antibiotic treatment.

TRACHOMA AND ADULT INCLUSION CONJUNCTIVITIS[1]

DEFINITION   Trachoma is a chronic conjunctivitis associated with infection by *C. trachomatis* serovars A, B, and C. It has produced an estimated 20 million cases of blindness throughout the world and remains an important preventable cause of blindness. Inclusion conjunctivitis is an acute ocular infection caused by sexually transmitted *C. trachomatis* strains (usually serovars D through K) in adults exposed to infected genital secretions and in their newborn offspring.

EPIDEMIOLOGY   Epidemiologically, two types of eye disease are caused by *C. trachomatis*. In trachoma-endemic areas where the classic eye disease is seen, transmission is from eye to eye, via hands, towels, flies, and other fomites, and usually involves serovars A, B, or C. In nonendemic areas, organisms of serovars D through K can be transmitted from the genital tract to the eye, usually causing only the inclusion conjunctivitis syndrome with or without keratitis. Rarely the eye disease acquired in this way progresses with the development of pannus and scars similar to endemic trachoma. These cases may be referred to as *paratrachoma* to differentiate them epidemiologically from eye-to-eye transmitted endemic trachoma.

The worldwide incidence and severity of trachoma have decreased dramatically during the past 30 years in areas with improving hygienic and economic conditions. Endemic trachoma is still the major cause of preventable blindness in north Africa, sub-Saharan Africa, the Middle East, and parts of Asia. Transmission of the endemic disease occurs primarily through close personal contact, particularly among young children in rural communities. In endemic areas, trachoma is associated with repeated exposure, but the infection can also be latent. In the United States a mild form of endemic trachoma still occurs in Mexican Americans as well as in immigrants from areas where trachoma is endemic. Acute relapse of old trachoma may be seen occasionally following treatment with cortisone eye ointment or in very old persons exposed in their youth.

CLINICAL MANIFESTATIONS   Both endemic trachoma and adult inclusion conjunctivitis present initially as a conjunctivitis characterized by small lymphoid follicles in the conjunctiva. In regions with hyperendemic classic blinding trachoma, the disease usually starts insidiously before the age of 2 years. Reinfection is common and probably contributes to the pathogenesis of trachoma. In experimental primate models, repeated reinfection of the eye at regular intervals produces trachoma-like scarring.

The cornea becomes involved with inflammatory leukocytic infiltration and superficial vascularization (pannus formation). As the inflammation continues, there is conjunctival scarring that eventually distorts the eyelids, causing them to turn inward so that the inturned lashes constantly abrade the eyeball (trichiasis and entropion); even-

tually the corneal epithelium is abraded and may then develop a bacterial corneal ulcer with subsequent corneal scarring and blindness. Destruction of the conjunctival goblet cells, lacrimal ducts, and lacrimal gland may produce a "dry-eye" syndrome with resultant corneal opacity due to drying (xerosis) or secondary bacterial corneal ulcers.

Communities with blinding trachoma often experience seasonal epidemics of bacterial conjunctivitis with *Haemophilus influenzae* (biotype III or the Koch-Weeks bacillus), which contribute to the intensity of the inflammatory process. In such areas the active infectious process usually resolves spontaneously in affected persons between 10 and 15 years of age, but the conjunctival scars continue to shrink, producing trichiasis and entropion and subsequent corneal scarring in adult life. In areas with milder and less prevalent disease the process may be much slower, with active disease continuing into adulthood; blindness is rare in these cases.

Eye infection with genital *C. trachomatis* strains, usually in sexually active young adults, presents with acute onset of unilateral follicular conjunctivitis and preauricular lymphadenopathy similar to acute adenovirus or herpes virus conjunctivitis. If untreated, the disease may persist for 6 weeks to 2 years. It is frequently associated with corneal inflammation in the form of discrete opacities ("infiltrates"), punctate epithelial erosions, and minor degrees of superficial corneal vascularization. Very rarely conjunctival scarring and eyelid distortion occur, particularly in patients treated for many months with topical corticosteroids. Recurrent eye infections occur most often in patients whose sexual consorts are not treated with antimicrobials.

DIAGNOSIS   The clinical diagnosis of classic trachoma can be made if two of the following signs are present:

1 Lymphoid follicles on the upper tarsal conjunctiva
2 Typical conjunctival scarring
3 Vascular pannus
4 Limbal follicles or their sequelae, Herbert's pits

The clinical diagnosis of endemic trachoma should be confirmed by laboratory tests in children with more marked degrees of inflammation. Intracytoplasmic chlamydial inclusions occur in 10 to 60 percent of Giemsa-stained conjunctival smears in such populations, but isolation in cell cultures is more sensitive. Follicular conjunctivitis in adult Europeans or Americans living in trachomatous regions is rarely trachoma.

Sporadic cases of adult inclusion conjunctivitis must be differentiated from adenovirus and herpes simplex virus keratoconjunctivitis during the first 15 days after onset, and later from other forms of chronic follicular conjunctivitis. Demonstration of chlamydial infection by Giemsa- or immunofluorescent-stained smears or by isolation in cell cultures constitutes definitive evidence of infection. Serum antibody does not constitute evidence of chlamydial eye infection since many sexually active adults have serum antibody. A practical diagnostic procedure in cases with chronic follicular conjunctivitis is treatment for 6 days with an oral tetracycline or erythromycin; a marked symptomatic response within 3 to 4 days is highly suggestive of inclusion conjunctivitis, and treatment should be continued for at least 3 weeks.

DIFFERENTIAL DIAGNOSIS   The eye and its adnexa may be infected during the course of many cutaneous and systemic viral diseases. Sometimes these ocular infections produce minor manifestations, such as the transient loss of accommodation of dengue and the milder forms of conjunctivitis in systemic adenovirus infections. Other virus infections, however, such as herpes simplex (see Chap. 136), herpes zoster (see Chap. 135), measles (see Chap. 132), and vaccinia (see Chap. 134), occasionally produce serious and permanent visual loss. In addition, congenital viral infections are an important cause of blindness, particularly rubella, which leads to cataracts, microphthalmus, and cytomegalic inclusion disease with retinal involvement.

Among the viral infections limited to the outer eye and manifested as a follicular conjunctivitis are epidemic keratoconjunctivitis (EKC),

---

[1] *Much of this section is based on the separate chapter on this topic by Doctors Grayston and Dawson in the previous (tenth) edition of this book.*

herpes simplex keratoconjunctivitis, Newcastle disease virus (NDV) conjunctivitis, and acute hemorrhagic conjunctivitis. Adenovirus types 8 and 19 are the usual cause of epidemics of EKC, although milder cases may be associated with other adenovirus types. The most common method for transmission of adenovirus type 8 is through manipulation of the eye by medical personnel, e.g., for foreign-body removal or during an ophthalmologic examination. The virus, which is unusually resistant to inactivation, is transmitted on the fingers, by instruments, or in solutions. One of the rarer causes of EKC, adenovirus type 19, appears to be transmitted person-to-person during small community outbreaks.

Following an incubation period of 5 to 12 days, EKC presents a moderate to very severe follicular conjunctivitis with preauricular lymphadenopathy that is usually unilateral at onset. Severe cases may have subconjunctival hemorrhages and conjunctival membrane formation with subsequent conjunctival scarring. In adults, the associated systemic manifestations are minimal with little if any fever, headache, or malaise, but in children adenovirus type 8 infections may present as febrile upper respiratory disease, or otitis media, with only a minor conjunctivitis; such children may be a source of infection for adults. In EKC, the usual onset of focal corneal involvement is 7 days after onset of conjunctivitis when there is a severe foreign-body sensation, photophobia, and lacrimation. As the conjunctivitis subsides during the second week of the disease, subepithelial corneal opacities 1 to 2 mm in diameter appear, and these opacities may persist for 2 years or longer.

Occasionally herpes simplex virus produces an acute follicular conjunctivitis that is usually accompanied by one or multiple herpetic skin vesicles on the eyelids. In children this may be the primary herpetic infection, but in adults the conjunctivitis is often a recurrent herpetic infection at a new site. The skin lesions may be inconspicuous, misdiagnosed as a sty, or even not present, so that the disease is indistinguishable from early EKC. The cornea may have focal epithelial lesions, a typical linear, branching (dendritic) ulcer, or no involvement at all. The conjunctivitis usually resolves in 2 weeks.

Human infection with Newcastle disease virus, which is related to influenza, occurs mainly in poultry workers, veterinarians, and virologists. In humans, accidental introduction of contaminated material from naturally infected animals or from live virus (e.g., vaccines) is followed in 24 to 72 h by conjunctivitis, edema of the lids, and tearing. Systemic symptoms occur very rarely, and recovery is complete in 10 to 14 days. The diagnosis may be confirmed by virus isolation in embryonated eggs.

Acute hemorrhagic conjunctivitis (AHC) presents as an acute conjunctivitis with numerous punctate hemorrhages on the bulbar conjunctiva which become confluent within 24 h. There is also minor involvement of the cornea. The inflammation subsides in 4 to 5 days, but the hemorrhages do not resolve for 7 to 10 days. The only reported complication has been the rare occurrence of lumbar radiculomyelitis with resultant flaccid paralysis like poliomyelitis. Enterovirus 70 (a member of the picornavirus group) has been identified as the etiologic agent in most epidemics, but some outbreaks have been caused by coxsackievirus A24, another picornavirus. Epidemics of AHC have occurred in the crowded urban populations of developing countries, affecting all age groups and social classes. Occasional outbreaks in Europe have been centered around eye clinics. Community-wide epidemics of AHC have occurred in the United States and Central America.

TREATMENT *C. trachomatis* strains are susceptible to the tetracyclines, erythromycin, and the sulfonamides. Public health control programs for endemic trachoma have consisted of the mass application of tetracycline or erythromycin ointment to the eyes of all children in affected communities for 21 to 60 days or on an intermittent schedule. These programs also include surgical correction of inturned eyelids by a mobile surgical team that visits each locality. Oral erythromycin, but not oral tetracyclines, offers a useful alternative method of mass antibiotic treatment for trachoma of young children and pregnant women.

Adult inclusion conjunctivitis responds well to treatment with full doses of systemic tetracycline or erythromycin for 3 weeks. Treating all sexual consorts of the patient simultaneously is also necessary to prevent ocular reinfection and to avoid the genital diseases due to chlamydial infection. Topical antibiotic treatment is not required in patients treated with systemic antibiotics.

PREVENTION Efforts to develop a practical trachoma vaccine have not been successful. General hygienic measures associated with improved living standards are effective in the elimination of endemic trachoma. Adequate water supply for personal cleanliness may be a key factor. In some areas the reduction of flies in the household is important.

OTHER INFECTIONS CAUSED BY *C. TRACHOMATIS* IN ADULTS *C. trachomatis* has been reported as an infrequent cause of subacute endocarditis and may cause respiratory infections in older children and adults. Serologic evidence supporting a role for *Chlamydia* in community-acquired pneumonia and in acute pharyngitis has been gathered, but the agent has not been isolated from such cases. Immunosuppressed patients with pneumonia have had, in some cases, either serologic or cultural evidence of *C. trachomatis* infection, but more data are necessary to define the role of *Chlamydia* in these patients. Many infections caused by *C. trachomatis* produce few or no symptoms, or symptoms that are nonspecific and thus not diagnostic of *C. trachomatis* infection. These considerations, plus the limited availability and high cost of culture tests for chlamydial infection have markedly hampered confirmation of infection in individual patients and have limited public health control efforts.

PSITTACOSIS

DEFINITION Psittacosis is primarily an infectious disease of birds caused by *Chlamydia psittaci*. Transmission of infection from birds to humans results in a febrile illness characterized by pneumonitis and systemic manifestations. Inapparent infections or mild influenza-like illnesses may also occur. The term *ornithosis* is sometimes applied to infections contracted from birds other than parrots or parakeets, but *psittacosis* is the preferred generic term for all forms of the disease. A previously unrecognized *C. psittaci* strain, the TWAR strain, has been serologically linked with human respiratory illness. This strain appears to cause a mild pneumonitis and/or upper respiratory tract infection in young adults.

EPIDEMIOLOGY Almost any avian species can harbor *C. psittaci*. Psittacine birds (parrots, parakeets, budgerigars) are most commonly infected, but human cases have been traced to contact with pigeons, ducks, turkeys, chickens, and many other birds. Psittacosis may be considered an occupational disease of pet-shop owners, poultry raisers, pigeon fanciers, taxidermists, and zoo attendants. The incidence of human infection in the United States rose steadily from 1930, owing in large measure to the increasing popularity of parrots and parakeets as pets and, as subsequently recognized, transmission of infection by barnyard fowl and pigeons. The number of reported cases reached a peak in 1956 and gradually declined thereafter. By 1963, with acceptance of control measures such as incorporation of tetracyclines in poultry feed, the disease had again become relatively uncommon. However, since 1973, there has been a steady increase in incidence, with cases occurring primarily among employees of poultry processing plants. In 1983, about 150 cases of psittacosis were reported to the Centers for Disease Control. It is suspected that many cases are undiagnosed and not reported. The disease appears to be more common in England, where budgerigars are popular household pets and where restrictions on the importation of these birds have been eased.

The agent is present in nasal secretions, excreta, tissues, and feathers of infected birds. Although the disease can be fatal, infected birds frequently show only minor evidence of illness, such as ruffled feathers, lethargy, and anorexia. Asymptomatic avian carriers are common, and complete recovery may be followed by continued shedding of the organism for many months.

Psittacosis is almost always transmitted to humans by the respiratory route. On rare occasions the disease may be acquired from the bite of a pet bird. Prolonged contact is not essential for transmission of the disease; a few minutes spent in an environment previously occupied by an infected bird has resulted in human infection. The severity of the disease in humans bears no apparent relationship to closeness or duration of contact, although sick birds are more likely to transmit infection than healthy ones. Transmission of a psittacosis-like agent between humans has occurred among hospital personnel, with severe and sometimes fatal infections. There is evidence that these "human" strains are more virulent than native avian organisms. There is no record of infection acquired by eating poultry products.

PATHOGENESIS The psittacosis agent gains entrance to the body through the upper part of the respiratory tract, spreads via the bloodstream, and eventually localizes in the pulmonary alveoli and in the reticuloendothelial cells of the spleen and liver. Invasion of the lung probably takes place by way of the bloodstream rather than by direct extension from the upper air passages. A lymphocytic inflammatory response occurs on both the interstitial and respiratory surfaces of the alveoli as well as in the perivascular spaces. The alveolar walls and interstitial tissues of the lung are thickened, edematous, necrotic, and occasionally hemorrhagic. Histologically, the affected areas show alveolar spaces filled with fluid, erythrocytes, and lymphocytes. The picture is not pathognomonic of psittacosis unless macrophages containing characteristic cytoplasmic inclusion bodies (LCL bodies) can be identified. The respiratory epithelium of the bronchi and bronchioles usually remains intact.

CLINICAL MANIFESTATIONS The clinical manifestations and course of psittacosis are extremely variable. After an incubation period of 7 to 14 days or longer, the disease may start abruptly with shaking chills and fever ranging as high as 40.5°C (105°F), but the onset is often gradual with increasing fever over a 3- to 4-day period. Headache is almost always a prominent symptom; it is usually diffuse and excruciating and often the patient's chief complaint.

Many patients present with a dry hacking cough which is usually nonproductive, but small amounts of mucoid or bloody sputum may be raised as the disease progresses. Cough may appear early in the course of the disease or as late as 5 days after the onset of fever. Chest pain, pleurisy with effusion, or a friction rub may all occur but are rare. Pericarditis and myocarditis have been reported. Most patients have a normal or slightly increased respiratory rate; marked dyspnea with cyanosis occurs only in severe psittacosis with extensive pulmonary involvement. In psittacosis, as in most nonbacterial pneumonias, the physical signs of pneumonitis tend to be less prominent than symptoms and x-ray findings would suggest. The initial examination may reveal fine, sibilant rales, or clinical evidence of pneumonia may be completely lacking. Rales usually become audible and more numerous as the illness progresses. Signs of frank pulmonary consolidation are usually absent. Symptoms of upper respiratory tract infection are not prominent, although mild sore throat, pharyngeal infection, and cervical adenopathy are often present; on occasion they may be the only manifestations of illness. Epistaxis is encountered early in the course of nearly one-fourth of the cases. Photophobia is also a common complaint.

There is commonly a complaint of generalized myalgia, and spasm and stiffness of the muscles of the back and neck may lead to an erroneous diagnosis of meningitis. Lethargy, mental depression, agitation, insomnia, and disorientation have been prominent features of the illness in some epidemics, but not in others; delirium and stupor occur near the end of the first week in severe cases. Occasional patients are comatose when first seen, and the diagnosis of psittacosis may be missed. Gastrointestinal complaints such as abdominal pain, nausea, vomiting, or diarrhea are present in some cases; constipation and abdominal distention sometimes occur as late complications. Icterus, the result of severe hepatic involvement, is a rare and ominous

finding. A faint, macular rash (Horder's spots) simulating the rose spots of typhoid fever has been described.

Patients without cough or other clinical evidence of respiratory involvement come to the physician with fever of unknown origin. The pulse rate is slow in relation to the fever. When splenomegaly is present in a patient with acute pneumonitis, psittacosis should be considered; the reported incidence of splenomegaly ranges from 10 to 70 percent. Nontender hepatic enlargement also occurs, but jaundice is rare. Thrombophlebitis is not unusual during convalescence; indeed, pulmonary infarction is sometimes a late complication and may be fatal.

In untreated cases of psittacosis, sustained or mildly remittent fever persists for 10 days to 3 weeks, or occasionally as long as 3 months. Over this period, the respiratory manifestations gradually abate. Psittacosis contracted from parrots or parakeets is more likely to be a severe, prolonged illness than infections acquired from pigeons or barnyard fowl. Relapses occur but are rare. Occasional patients develop endocarditis, and C. psittaci infection should be considered in cases of culture-negative endocarditis. Secondary bacterial infections are uncommon. Immunity to reinfection is probably permanent.

LABORATORY FINDINGS The chest x-ray in psittacosis mimics that in a great variety of pulmonary diseases. The pneumonic lesions are usually patchy in appearance but can be hazy, diffuse, homogeneous, lobar, atelectatic, wedge-shaped, nodular, or miliary. The white blood cell count is normal or moderately decreased in the acute phase of the disease but may rise in convalescence. The erythrocyte sedimentation rate is frequently not elevated. Transient proteinuria is common. The cerebrospinal fluid sometimes contains a few mononuclear cells but is otherwise normal. Despite hepatomegaly, liver function tests are generally normal.

The diagnosis can be confirmed only by isolation of the causative microorganism or by serologic studies. The agent is present in the blood during the acute phase of the disease and in the bronchial secretions for weeks or sometimes years after infection, but it is difficult to isolate. Psittacosis is most readily diagnosed by the demonstration of a rising titer of complement-fixing antibody in serum. An acute and convalescent specimen should always be tested. Even a low titer of antibody during the acute febrile phase constitutes presumptive evidence of psittacosis. The prompt initiation of treatment with tetracycline has been shown to delay antibody rise in convalescence for several weeks or months. Interpretation of a single complement fixation test may sometimes be difficult because of the antigenic cross reaction between C. psittaci and C. trachomatis.

DIFFERENTIAL DIAGNOSIS A history of exposure to birds may be the only clinical basis for differentiating psittacosis from a great variety of infectious and noninfectious febrile disorders. A partial list of pneumonic disease that may be confused with psittacosis includes Mycoplasma pneumonia, Q fever, coccidioidomycosis, tuberculosis, enteroviral infection, carcinoma of the lung with bronchial obstruction, and bacterial pneumonias. In the early stages, before pneumonitis appears, psittacosis may be mistaken for influenza, typhoid fever, miliary tuberculosis, infectious mononucleosis, and Legionnaires' disease.

TREATMENT The tetracyclines are consistently effective in the treatment of psittacosis. Defervescence and alleviation of symptoms usually occur in 24 to 48 h after instituting therapy with 2 g daily in four divided doses. To avoid relapse, treatment should probably be continued for at least 7 days after defervescence. In severe cases, oxygen and other supportive measures are indicated.

APPROACH TO THE DIAGNOSIS AND TREATMENT OF C. TRACHOMATIS INFECTIONS

Traditionally, three types of laboratory procedures have been used to confirm C. trachomatis infection. These include direct microscopic examination of tissue scrapings for typical intracytoplasmic inclusions, isolation of the organism, and detection of antibody in the serum or in local secretions. Direct microscopic examination of Giemsa-stained cell scrapings has an unacceptably low sensitivity, and false-positive interpretations by inexperienced observers are common. Cell culture techniques have replaced the yolk sac of embryonated eggs for isolation of *C. trachomatis*. The cell cultures are much more convenient and sensitive, particularly for strains from the genital tract. While LGV strains grow well in many cell lines, the other *C. trachomatis* strains are much more difficult to culture. The most common cell lines used are McCoy cells and HeLa 229 cells. Both cell lines require special pretreatment and centrifugation of the inoculum onto the monolayer for efficient isolation of genital or ocular trachoma strains. Positive cultures are identified by visualizing typical intracytoplasmic inclusions stained by Giemsa stain, by iodine stain, or by using fluorescein-conjugated monoclonal antibodies.

Although culture remains the "gold standard" for diagnosis of chlamydial infection, it is expensive, technically demanding, and not widely available. Therefore, antigen detection methods have been developed that can be used instead of cultures. In the immunofluorescent slide test, potentially infected genital or ocular secretions are smeared on a slide, fixed, and stained with fluorescein-conjugated monoclonal antibody. When viewing the slide using a fluorescence microscope, the presence of fluorescing elementary bodies confirms the diagnosis. Compared with culture, this test is 85 to 90 percent sensitive and quite specific when used for confirmation of urethral, cervical, or ocular infection in high-risk patients with suspected *C. trachomatis* infection. Its value as a screening test has not been widely assessed. An enzyme-linked immunosorbent assay (ELISA) technique for chlamydial antigen detection has also been developed and provides another alternative to culture. Reported sensitivity and specificity of this test for genital infections has been 67 to 95 percent and 92 to 97 percent in populations studied to date.

Serologic tests have limited usefulness in chlamydial diagnosis. A complement fixation (CF) test with the heat-stable group-reactive antigen has been used to diagnose psittacosis and LGV with some success. It is insensitive in non-LGV *C. trachomatis* infections. The microimmunofluorescence (micro-IF) test with *C. trachomatis* antigens is more sensitive but remains available only in research laboratories. The test measures antibodies by serovar specificity and by immunoglobulin class (IgM, IgG, IgA, secretory IgA) in both serum and local secretions. Serologic diagnosis using the micro-IF test may be useful in several specific instances. In infant pneumonia, a high antibody titer is nearly always present and, since a definite clinical syndrome may bring the infant to the physician early in the course of disease, high-titer IgM antibody and/or fourfold titer rises can often be demonstrated. For similar reasons, serodiagnosis has been used in a research setting in women with chlamydial salpingitis, especially with Fitz-Hugh–Curtis syndrome. In LGV the micro-IF antibody titer against *C. trachomatis* is high ($\geq$1:512) and usually has a characteristic pattern of broad reactivity against all immunotypes of *C. trachomatis* (since LGV strains induce broadly reactive antibody).

Table 150-2 summarizes the diagnostic tests of choice for patients with suspected chlamydial infection. With few exceptions, the most

TABLE 150-2 Diagnostic tests in *C. trachomatis* infection

Infection	Suggestive signs/symptoms	Presumptive diagnosis*	Confirmatory test of choice
ADULT MALES			
Nongonococcal urethritis, postgonococcal urethritis	Discharge, dysuria	Gram stain with more than four polymorphonuclear (PMN) leukocytes per oil immersion field, no gonococci	Urethral culture or antigen detection test for *C. trachomatis*
Epididymitis	Unilateral intrascrotal swelling, pain, tenderness; fever; nongonococcal urethritis	Gram stain with more than four PMN leukocytes per oil immersion field, no gonococci	Urethral culture or antigen detection test for *C. trachomatis*
ADULT FEMALES			
Cervicitis	Mucopurulent cervical discharge, cervical edema, ectopy, bleeding	Cervical Gram stain with $\geq$10 PMNs per oil immersion field in cervical mucus	Cervical culture or antigen detection test for *C. trachomatis*
Salpingitis	Evidence of pelvic inflammatory disease on examination	*C. trachomatis* should always be suspected in salpingitis	Cervical culture or antigen detection test for *C. trachomatis*
Urethritis	Dysuria and frequency without urgency or hematuria	Mucopurulent cervicitis, sterile pyuria, negative routine urine culture	Urethral and cervical cultures or antigen detection test for *C. trachomatis*
ADULTS OF EITHER SEX			
Proctitis	Rectal pain, discharge, diarrhea, blood; homosexual patient	Negative gonococcal culture and Gram stain; $\geq$1 PMN leukocytes in rectal Gram stain	Rectal culture or direct immunofluorescence test for *C. trachomatis*
Reiter's syndrome	Nongonococcal urethritis, arthritis, conjunctivitis, typical skin lesions	Gram stain with more than four PMN leukocytes per oil immersion field, no gonococci	Urethral culture or antigen detection test for *C. trachomatis*
LGV	Regional adenopathy, primary lesion, proctitis, systemic symptoms	None	Isolation of LGV strain from node, rectum, occasionally from urethra or cervix; LGV CF-titer $\geq$1:64; micro-IF titer $\geq$1:512
NEONATES			
Conjunctivitis	Purulent conjunctival discharge 6 to 18 days postdelivery	Negative cultures and gram stains for gonococci, *Haemophilus* sp., pneumococci, staphylococci	Conjunctival culture or antigen detection test for *C. trachomatis*; Giemsa-stained scraping of conjunctival material can provide more rapid diagnosis but is less sensitive
Infant pneumonia	Afebrile, staccato cough, diffuse rales, bilateral hyperinflation, interstitial infiltrates	None	Chlamydial culture of sputum, pharynx, eye, rectum; micro-IF antibody to *C. trachomatis*—fourfold change in IgG or IgM antibody

* *Although a presumptive diagnosis of chlamydial infection is often made in the syndromes listed when gonococci are not found, a positive test for* Neisseria gonorrhoeae *does not exclude* C. trachomatis, *which is very often also present in patients with gonorrhea.*

suitable method for diagnosis is demonstration of the agent in tissue-cell culture or by antigen detection methods. Selection of the most appropriate of these tests depends upon local availability and expertise. Since *C. trachomatis* is an intracellular pathogen, adequate specimens for chlamydial culture must include epithelial cells. Cultures of pus result in fewer isolations of the organism. In urethritis, a thin-shafted urogenital swab should be inserted at least 2 cm into the urethra to obtain an appropriate specimen. When a cervical culture is taken, the external os should first be cleaned of debris and purulent material, and a plastic-shafted swab then inserted into the cervix, rotated slowly several times, and withdrawn. When conjunctival specimens are sought, the epithelium should be swabbed to remove cells, rather than simply purulent material. All specimens for chlamydial culture should be placed immediately into a transport medium and then either refrigerated if they will reach the laboratory within 12 to 18 h or frozen at $-70°C$ if longer storage is anticipated. A major advantage of antigen detection techniques is their less rigid transport requirements.

From a public health viewpoint, the most effective use of chlamydia diagnostic testing has not been established and will vary depending upon clinical population, local resources, and laboratory expertise. The Centers for Disease Control have recommended empiric treatment (without diagnostic testing if resources are not available for testing) of selected high-risk groups. These include men with NGU or sexually transmitted epididymitis; women with mucopurulent cervicitis (MPC) or PID; asymptomatic sexual partners of patients with these syndromes; women and heterosexual men with gonorrhea (because of the high proportion of these patients who will also have *C. trachomatis* infection); and contacts of men or women with gonorrhea. Where funds for diagnostic testing are limited (e.g., in public clinics serving indigent patients), it is rationalized that these groups will receive empiric therapy in any event, and hence diagnostic testing is not absolutely essential. However, where available, diagnostic testing has several potential benefits in these patients, including confirmation of infection (especially in women with MPC and PID), enhancement of sex partner referral, determination of prognosis, and education of physicians (ability to correlate signs and symptoms with culture results). Where diagnostic testing must be rationed because of limited resources, highest priority should be given to screening asymptomatic high-risk women, especially those seen in high-risk settings (i.e., STD clinics, abortion clinics, family planning clinics), or individuals with a high-risk profile (young, multiple sexual partners, lower socioeconomic status).

ANTIMICROBIAL SUSCEPTIBILITY   In laboratory tests, death of inoculated mice and chick embryos, as well as growth in cell cultures, is prevented or inhibited by tetracyclines, erythromycin, and rifampin; sulfonamides and cycloserine are active against *C. trachomatis* but not *C. psittaci;* bacitracin and polymyxin B are less effective; penicillin and ampicillin suppress *Chlamydia* multiplication but do not eradicate the organism in vitro. The cephalosporins also appear relatively ineffective against *C. trachomatis*. Streptomycin, gentamicin, neomycin, kanamycin, vancomycin, ristocetin, spectinomycin, and nystatin are not effective at concentrations inhibitory for most bacteria and fungi. For treatment of human infection, the tetracyclines, erythromycin, and sulfonamides are most useful.

TREATMENT   In general, chlamydial infections cannot be eradicated by single-dose or short-term antimicrobial regimens. In most situations, at least 7 days and sometimes 2 to 3 weeks of antibiotic should be given. Treatment failure after treatment of genital infections with a tetracycline usually indicates inadequate therapy, poor compliance, or reinfection. Tetracycline-resistant strains of *C. trachomatis* have not been described.

Therapy of *C. trachomatis* urethritis is more effective than therapy of other forms of NGU. *C. trachomatis* is eradicated from the urethra by treatment with tetracycline hydrochloride, 500 mg four times daily for 7 days, or doxycycline, 100 mg by mouth bid for 7 days. An effective alternative regimen is erythromycin, 500 mg four times daily for 7 days.

Eradication of *C. trachomatis* from the cervix has been demonstrated with similar doses and durations of tetracycline, doxycycline, and erythromycin. Erythromycin base, 500 mg four times daily for 10 to 14 days, is the regimen of choice for pregnant women with *C. trachomatis* infection. Tetracycline hydrochloride, 500 mg four times daily for 14 days, produces clinical and microbiologic cure of epididymitis associated with *C. trachomatis* infection. Treatment of PID is discussed in Chap. 91. Treatment of gonorrhea should include an effective antichlamydial drug (see Chap. 104).

Treatment of sex partners   Genital *C. trachomatis* infections have continued to increase in incidence from the mid-1970s to the mid-1980s, whereas gonococcal infections have steadily fallen in incidence over the same period. The increase in chlamydial infection probably is due to the inability of clinicians to diagnose asymptomatic infection and also failure to diagnose and treat *C. trachomatis* infections in symptomatic patients or their sexual partners. Cases of NGU, epididymitis, Reiter's syndrome, and mucopurulent endocervicitis are sometimes not treated with antimicrobials, and sex partners are treated even less often. *C. trachomatis* urethral or cervical infection has been well documented in a high proportion of the sex partners of patients with NGU, epididymitis, Reiter's syndrome, salpingitis, or endocervicitis. This is analogous to the problem of asymptomatic gonococcal infection in sex partners of patients with gonorrhea. Confirmatory laboratory tests for *Chlamydia* should be obtained if possible, but antigen detection tests may be less sensitive in asymptomatic carriers. Even those without evidence of clinical disease who have been recently exposed to proven or possible chlamydial infection (for example, NGU) should be offered therapy.

In neonates with conjunctivitis or infants with pneumonia, erythromycin ethylsuccinate or estolate can be given orally in a dose of 50 mg/kg per day, preferably as 12.5 mg/kg four times daily, for 2 weeks. Careful attention must be given to compliance with therapy—a frequent problem. Relapses of eye infection are common following treatment with topical erythromycin or tetracycline ophthalmic ointment and may occur after oral erythromycin therapy also, so that follow-up cultures should be obtained after treatment. Both parents should be examined for *C. trachomatis* infection and, if diagnostic tests are not readily available, should also be treated with a tetracycline.

REFERENCES

ALEXANDER ER, HARRISON ER: Role of *Chlamydia trachomatis* in perinatal infection. Rev Infect Dis 5:713, 1983

BRUNHAM RC et al: Mucopurulent cervicitis—the ignored counterpart in women of urethritis in men. N Engl J Med 311:1, 1984

CENTERS FOR DISEASE CONTROL: Morb Mort Week Rep 31:65, 1983

————: Morb Mort Week Rep 32:27SS, 1984

COUTTS II et al: Clinical and radiographic features of psittacosis infection. Thorax 40:530, 1985

JONES RB et al: *Chlamydia trachomatis* in the pharynx and rectum of heterosexual patients at risk for genital infection. Ann Intern Med 102:757, 1985

MÄRDH PA et al: *Chlamydial Infections.* Amsterdam: Elsevier Biomedical Press, 1982

SCHACHTER J: Chlamydial infection. N Engl J Med 298:428, 490, 540, 1973

————— et al: Experience with the routine use of erythromycin for chlamydial infections in pregnancy. N Engl J Med 314:276, 1986

STAMM WE et al: Causes of the acute urethral syndrome in women. N Engl J Med 303:309, 1980

—————: Use of antigen detection methods for the diagnosis *Neisseria gonorrhoeae* and *Chlamydia trachomatis* infections. Diagn Micro Infect Dis, in press

THOMPSON SE, WASHINGTON AE: Epidemiology of sexually transmitted *C. trachomatis* infections. Epidemiol Rev 5:96, 1983

WORLD HEALTH ORGANIZATION: *Guide to the Laboratory Diagnosis of Trachoma.* Geneva, WHO, 1975

151 THE DIAGNOSIS AND THERAPY OF PARASITIC INFECTIONS

JAMES J. PLORDE

Parasitic diseases such as malaria, trypanosomiasis, leishmaniasis, schistosomiasis, and filariasis remain among the major causes of human sickness and death in the world today. A number of technical, social, economic, and political phenomena have combined to produce a dramatic increase in the prevalence of some of these illnesses. This has been most devastating in the case of malaria. Growing resistance of the mosquito vector to insecticides, development of drug-resistant strains of *Plasmodium falciparum,* and cutbacks in many malaria control programs have led to a worldwide resurgence of this disease. At present, over 1 billion people reside in endemic areas; between 125 and 200 million of these are infected at any given time. In Africa, where the intensity of parasite transmission defies current control measures, malaria kills over 1 million children annually. The resurgence of malaria together with an increase in international travel has resulted in an upsurge in the number of infected patients who enter the United States. From 1969 to 1980 civilian malaria cases reported annually to the Centers for Disease Control have increased from 151 to 1864; in the four subsequent years, the number has averaged 1000 cases annually. Over the same 15-year period, the number of infections involving U.S. citizens has climbed steadily from 90 to 360.

In Africa, from the Sahara in the north to the Kalahari Desert in the south, human strains of *Trypanosoma brucei* cause one of the most lethal of all human diseases, sleeping sickness. Animal strains of this species limit food supply in the same area through their impact on animal husbandry. In South America, a related organism, *T. cruzi*, infects several million people, leaving many with severe heart and gastrointestinal lesions (Chagas' disease).

Leishmaniasis is found in parts of Europe, Asia, Africa, and South and Central America where it may present as a chronic, highly lethal infection of the reticuloendothelial system (kala azar), a mutilating mucocutaneous infection (espundia), or a self-limiting skin ulcer (oriental sore).

Schistosomiasis is the most serious of the helminthic infections, affecting an estimated 200 million individuals living between the tropics of Cancer and Capricorn. In many it produces bladder, intestinal, and/or liver disease which can eventually result in death. In many countries irrigation schemes have resulted in the dissemination of the disease to previously uninvolved areas, mitigating the economic gains of these development projects. Although not transmitted in the continental United States, exogenously acquired schistosomiasis involves nearly a half million people now residing in this country.

Wuchereria bancrofti and *Brugia malayi,* two closely related filarial worms, obstruct lymphatic circulation and produce grotesque swellings of the legs, arms, and genitals in tropical populations. Onchocerciasis, another filarial infection, affects millions of people in Africa, leaving thousands blind.

Toxoplasmosis, pneumocystosis, giardiasis, and trichomoniasis are four cosmopolitan protozoan infections well known in the United States. The first infects perhaps one-third of the world's population. Although it is usually asymptomatic, congenital toxoplasmosis may result in abortion, stillbirth, prematurity, or severe neurologic defects. Even when there are no obvious signs at birth, chorioretinitis with visual impairment may occur years later. Asymptomatic toxoplasma and pneumocystis infections can both result in fatal illness later in life during periods of immunosuppression.

In contrast, giardiasis and trichomoniasis seldom result in severe disability; nevertheless their morbidity can be attested to by millions of otherwise healthy individuals. Both appear to be increasing in incidence, apparently the result of changing American lifestyles. Giardiasis is particularly frequent among day-care center attendees, hikers and campers in our western states, and male homosexuals who practice anilingus, while the incidence of trichomoniasis is closely tied to the level of promiscuous heterosexual activity.

DIAGNOSIS Although some of the diseases mentioned above are uncommon in the United States, the continuous arrival of travelers and immigrants from endemic areas of the world makes it necessary to consider them in the differential diagnosis of many illnesses. Typically, neither the clinical manifestations nor the general laboratory findings observed in patients suffering from parasitic infections are sufficiently unique to raise this possibility in the mind of the clinician. Although eosinophilia has long been recognized as a clue to the presence of a hidden parasite, this phenomenon is characteristic only of helminthic infections. Even here its absence does not preclude this diagnosis. The eosinophilia presumably reflects an immunologic response to the complex foreign proteins of the worm and is most marked during the early stages of tissue migration and invasion. Once migration ceases and the worm matures to adulthood, eosinophilia may diminish or disappear.

Unless a careful travel, transfusion, and socioeconomic history is taken, the correct diagnosis may never be entertained. Once considered, however, the presence of a parasitic disease is easily confirmed. Most commonly, this is accomplished by the recovery and morphologic identification of the parasite in the stool, urine, sputum, blood, or tissues of the patient.

In intestinal infections, examination of a wet-mount and/or stained smear of the stool is usually adequate. Because many parasites are passed intermittently or in fluctuating numbers, the examination of a single stool specimen may detect only one-third to one-half of involved patients. The testing of three such specimens collected at intervals of 2 or 3 days will improve this yield substantially. Alternatively, a saline cathartic may be administered to evacuate the cecal area where many protozoa are concentrated, and the entire purge examined. The stool must be free of interfering substances such as antidiarrheal or contrast agents, antacids, and antibiotics. If the appropriate specimens cannot be obtained prior to administration of such substances, testing should be performed 1 week or, in the case of antimicrobial agents, 3 weeks after their discontinuation. Occasionally, specimens other than stool must be examined. In small-bowel infections such as giardiasis and strongyloidiasis, the diagnosis, at times, can be established only by sampling the duodenal contents or by performing a jejunal biopsy. Similarly, eggs of *Enterobius* (pinworm) and *Taenia* (tapeworm) are frequently found on the perianal skin when absent from the feces. Recovery of large-bowel parasites such as *Entamoeba histolytica* and *Schistosoma mansoni* may require colonic intubation with aspiration or biopsy of suspect lesions. Whenever intestinal aspirates or soft to watery fecal specimens are collected, they should be immediately placed in a preservative such as polyvinyl alcohol (PVA) to prevent rapid disintegration of fragile protozoan trophozoites and allow the preparation of permanently stained smears. Protozoan cysts and helminthic ova found in formed stool will survive for 1 to 2 days at room temperature and indefinitely if placed in 5% formaldehyde.

Direct examination of the blood is useful for the detection of malaria parasites, leishmania, trypanosomes, and microfilaria. Preferably, fresh capillary blood should be used to prepare thin and thick blood smears and, when appropriate, wet mounts. Only specially prepared glass slides should be used as traces of soda lime or potash on uncleaned slides may alter the pH of the stain, making recognition of parasites difficult. If an experienced technologist is not available to assist in the bedside preparation of smears, it is preferable to collect venous blood in an EDTA Vacutainer and send it to the laboratory. As in the case of intestinal parasites, organisms in the peripheral blood may fluctuate, requiring the collection of multiple specimens over a period of several days.

Parasites dwelling within the tissues of the host are more difficult to identify. Some discharge their offspring into the sputum (lung flukes) where they can be found with appropriate concentration procedures. In others, larvae can be recovered with skin (*Onchocerca volvulus*) or muscle (*Trichinella spiralis*) biopsies. In some diseases, however, parasite recovery is uncommon. Reliable immunodiagnostic tests have been developed for a few of these. Unfortunately, serologic tests for parasites often lack the sensitivity and specificity of those developed for viral and bacterial agents. This is particularly true for helminths which are broadly cross-reactive with one another. With the use of molecular technologies, more highly specific antigens are being developed. Table 151-1 lists the serologic tests available through the Centers for Disease Control (CDC). In Table 151-2 the diagnostic titer, sensitivity, and specificity of the most frequently requested CDC procedures are given.

Soluble antigens have been detected in the blood, body fluids, tissues, and excreta of a number of protozoan and helminthic diseases, including amebiasis, primary amebic meningoencephalitis, giardiasis, malaria, toxoplasmosis, filariasis, trichinosis, and schistosomiasis. The diagnostic usefulness of such procedures is being explored; at present none are commercially available. Similarly, diagnostic DNA probes have been described for falciparum malaria and cutaneous leishmaniasis. Highly sensitive and specific, these tests may revolutionize the diagnosis of parasitic diseases in the near future, but are not currently commercially available.

TREATMENT   Over the past decade, a number of new chemotherapeutic agents have been introduced for the treatment of parasitic diseases. A few, such as praziquantel and nifurtimox, represent the first effective agents available for the treatment of previously refractory diseases (i.e., clonorchiasis, Chagas' disease). Others, such as mebendazole, possess activity against a broad spectrum of helminths, allowing single-drug therapy of multiple intestinal infections. Many of the new agents are better tolerated than the ones they are destined to replace, permitting them to be used in mass therapy programs.

Despite these gains, however, treatment of parasitic diseases remains unsatisfactory. For a number of infections, including cryptosporidiosis, cysticercosis, echinococciasis, and trichinosis, satisfactory anthelmintics are not available. Drug resistance, a phenomenon so common to bacterial pathogens, also threatens the usefulness of some antiparasitic agents. This is particularly serious among the antimalarials. Chloroquine-resistant *P. falciparum*, long present in southeast Asia and Latin America, has now spread to Africa, the continent most devastated by this disease. Some Asian strains of this same organism have now developed resistance to the pyrimethamine-sulfadoxine regimen that has been used so successfully to suppress chloroquine-resistant infections.

Yet another problem relates to the availability of antiparasitic agents in the United States. Many of the drugs recommended in the following chapters have not been approved by the U.S. Food and Drug Administration either for use in this country or for the particular disease indicated. Those available as investigational agents through the Centers for Disease Control are listed in Table 151-3. Others, such as DL-α-difluoromethylornithine (DFMO), must be obtained

TABLE 151-1   Parasitic diseases for which serology is available

Taxonomic group	Diagnostic usefulness	
	High	Marginal
Protozoan	Amebiasis*	Malaria*
	Babesiosis*	Giardiasis
	Chagas' disease*	Pneumocystosis
	Leishmaniasis*	
	Toxoplasmosis*	
Helminthic	Cysticercosis*	Ascariasis
	Echinococcosis*	Clonorchiasis*
	Paragonimiasis*	Dracunculiasis*
	Toxocariasis*	Filariasis*
	Trichinosis*	Schistosomiasis*
		Strongyloidiasis

* Available at the Centers for Disease Control, Atlanta, Ga.

TABLE 151-2   Interpretation of tests frequently performed at the Centers for Disease Control

Disease	Test*	Diagnostic titer	Sensitivity %†	Specificity %†	Comments
Invasive amebiasis	IHA	≥:256	70[1], 95[2]	90[3]	1 Intestinal. 2 Extraintestinal. 3 Titers may persist for years.
Cysticercosis	ELISA	≥1:32	50[1], 70[2], 95[3]	83–95[4]	1 Intracranial calcifications, seizures. 2 Meningitis. 3 ↑ Intracranial pressure. 4 Cross-reacts with echinococcosis.
Echinococcosis	IHA	≥1:256	10[1], 88[2]	90–95[3,4]	1 Lung or calcified cyst. 2 Liver or peritoneal. 3 Cross-reacts with cysticercosis. 4 Titer may persist for years.
	IEP	Arc 5	Very high	—[5]	5 Arc 5 indicates echinococcosis.
Toxocariasis Visceral	ELISA	≥1:32	78	92[1,2]	1 Cross-reacts with ascariasis but eliminated by preabsorption. 2 In children.
Ocular	ELISA	≥1:8	90	91[3]	3 Patients with ocular disease.
Trichinosis	BFT	≥1:5	97[1]	90[2]	1 Detected after third week of illness. 2 Titers may persist for years.

* IHA = indirect hemagglutination; ELISA = enzyme-linked immunosorbent assay; BFT = bentonite flocculation; IEP = immunoelectrophoresis.
† Superscript numbers refer to comments at right.
SOURCE: Adapted from data provided by Kenneth W. Walls, Ph.D., December 1985.

TABLE 151-3 Agents available through the parasitic diseases division, CDC*

Infection	Therapeutic agent
Amebiasis	Dehydroemetine
	Diloxanide furoate
Chagas' disease (*Trypanosoma cruzi*)	Nifurtimox
Dracunculosis	Niridazole
Fascioliasis	Bithionol
Leishmaniasis	Sodium antimony gluconate (stibogluconate sodium)
Malaria	Parenteral chloroquine hydrochloride
	Parenteral quinine dihydrochloride
Onchocerciasis	Suramin
Paragonimiasis	Bithionol
Schistosomiasis	Metrifonate
	Niridazole
Sleeping sickness (*Trypanosoma brucei*)	Melarsoprol
	Suramin

* *Parasitic Diseases Division, Centers for Disease Control, Atlanta, GA 30333. Day telephone: (404) 329-3670.*

TABLE 151-4 Fecal egg counts associated with illness

Worm	Approximate egg output per female worm per day	Minimum egg output usually associated with illness
Necator americanus	25,000	>2000/mL
Trichuris trichiura	7500	>3000/g
Schistosoma mansoni	60–300	>200/g

SOURCE: *After DP Stevens, Clin Gastroenterol 7:236, 1978.*

directly from the manufacturer. When a clinician prescribes such an agent, the patient should be informed of the drug's investigational status and potential side effects.

Finally, the toxicity of many agents is such that the benefit of treatment must be carefully weighed against its potential side effects. This is particularly true in helminthic infections. Since most worms do not multiply within the body and because disability is usually related to the intensity of infection, treatment is directed primarily at reducing the worm burden of moderately to heavily infected patients. Total eradication is often unnecessary and may be unwise considering the toxicity of many anthelmintics. Light infections should be treated only when (1) small numbers of worms may be dangerous as in the case of strongyloidiasis, (2) the chance of reinfection is slight, and/or (3) the anthelmintic agent in question is without serious side effects. The intensity of many intestinal infections can be determined by enumerating the eggs found in stool (Table 151-4). Multiplying the total seen on direct smear by 750 provides a rough estimate of the number present per gram of feces. The Stoll dilution and the various modifications of the Kato thick-smear technique provide more precise results.

REFERENCES

Drugs for parasitic infections. Med Lett 26:27, 1984

Health Information for International Travel 1981. US Department of Health, Education, and Welfare Publication (CDC) 81-8280. Morb Mort Week Rep 1981;30 (August Suppl)

PLORDE JJ: Introduction to pathogenic parasites, in *Medical Microbiology: An Introduction to Infectious Diseases*, JC Sherris (ed). New York, Elsevier North-Holland, 1982

SMITH JW, BARTLETT MS: Diagnostic parasitology: Introduction and methods, in *Manual of Clinical Microbiology*, 4th ed, EH Lennette et al (eds). Washington, Am Soc Microbiol, 1985, pp 595–611

WALLS KW: Serodiagnosis of parasitic diseases, in *Manual of Clinical Microbiology*, 4th ed, EH Lennette et al (eds). Washington, Am Soc Microbiol, 1985, chap 97, pp 945–984

152 THE IMMUNOLOGY OF PARASITES

JOHN R. DAVID

During the past decade interest in parasitic diseases of humans and in new approaches to their control has increased steadily. One reason for this is the enormous scope of the problem. Over a billion people in the world are affected by parasitic diseases. Although accurate statistics are difficult to obtain, it is estimated that over 200 million people have malaria, the most serious protozoan disease of humans, and that more than a million children die of malaria each year in Africa alone. Schistosomiasis, a disease caused by helminths that are transmitted by snails, affects 200 to 300 million persons. Filarial parasites affect an equal number of people, and one of these, *Onchocerca volvulus,* is the second major cause of blindness in the world. *Trypanosoma cruzi,* another protozoan, is the major cause of heart disease in South America, and hookworm infects over 800 million persons.

With the modernization of developing countries, many of these diseases are becoming more prevalent. For example, the pressure to provide energy for industrialization leads to building dams which have brought about profound changes in the local environment; the lake behind the Volta Dam has increased the coastline by 4000 miles, and the snails on its banks infected with schistosomes have increased the prevalence of schistosomiasis in people living on the lake's borders from a few percent to almost 100 percent. Improvement schemes for agriculture often involve extension of irrigation as is necessary for the cultivation of rice. Some of these projects have been associated with increases in transmission of malaria by mosquitoes, which breed in the irrigation ditches. Another example of the unanticipated effects of progress can be seen in the Amazon basin, where the clearing of the forests in order to reclaim the land for industry and agriculture has greatly increased human contact with sandflies which live in these areas and transmit leishmaniasis.

Another reason for the increasing focus on these diseases by scientists and physicians is that the classic control measures are less than adequate. The most telling example of this is malaria. After World War II, there was great optimism that this disease could be eradicated by spraying homes with DDT and by treating the disease in humans with chloroquine. After an extensive eradication program was instituted in the early 1960s in Sri Lanka, only 18 cases of malaria were reported in that country. However, 5 years later there were over a half million cases. The failure of malaria eradication was due to at least three factors: (1) the surveillance stage of the eradication effort was not maintained; (2) mosquitoes became resistant to DDT; and (3) the parasite became resistant to chloroquine. Moreover, the cost of these control measures proved to be enormous.

The large number of people affected by parasitic diseases, the increasing environmental changes in the developing world, and the failure of classic control programs have stimulated the search for new approaches for the control of these disorders. One of these approaches is immunologic. Currently, immunologists are studying several aspects of parasites' interaction with the host. They are trying to delineate the mechanisms that parasites have evolved to evade the immune response of the host, to define which immune mechanisms they do not escape, and to learn which immune responses are the basis for the pathologic lesions. Immunology is also providing diagnostic tests and ultimately, it is hoped, will provide effective vaccines for some of these diseases. At present, there is not a single vaccine available to protect humans against parasites, despite the availability of several effective vaccines against animal parasitic diseases. For the purposes of this discussion, the most useful way to present the problems of vaccine development in these complex diseases is to give a relatively detailed description of what is being done in one disease, malaria, rather than a cursory summary of many.

MALARIA VACCINE Although investigators are trying to produce vaccines to many parasites, especially intensive work is under way on vaccines for *Plasmodium falciparum,* the most malignant malaria parasite. In order to understand the various approaches that are being pursued, it is necessary to review briefly the life cycle of the malaria parasite (see Chap. 154). When an infected mosquito bites a human, it injects the motile sporozoite, which is in the salivary gland. In less than half an hour, the sporozoite leaves the blood and invades the liver. It then goes through the exoerythrocytic cycle, undergoing asexual division by schizogeny and producing many merozoites. These burst out of the liver cells into the blood and invade erythrocytes. Here, they differentiate into trophozoites, undergo division by schizogony, and burst, liberating more merozoites which reinvade erythrocytes and continue the cycle. Some of the merozoites develop into the sexual stages, the gametocytes. When a mosquito bites an infected person, the gametocytes are taken up in the blood meal and rapidly come out of the erythrocytes. The male microgametes then fertilize the female macrogametes, forming the ookinete and then the oocyst. Further division within the oocyst leads to the infective stage, the sporozoite. Several of these stages can be targeted for immunologic attack by a vaccine.

Sporozoite vaccine   Persons can become immune to *P. falciparum* via the sporozoite stage. This has been shown by allowing irradiated infected mosquitoes (containing irradiated sporozoites which cannot divide) to bite humans. Investigations have resulted in the characterization of a single sporozoite antigen. Monoclonal antibodies to this antigen can passively transfer resistance to malaria in rodents and monkeys. Using recombinant DNA technology, the gene coding for the protective sporozoite antigen of *P. falciparum* has been cloned. The protective epitope is made up of four amino acids repeated 23 times. This repeated sequence can be synthesized for the development of a vaccine. The advantages of a sporozoite vaccine are that it might be effective without an adjuvant and that it may protect against different strains of *P. falciparum*. The disadvantage is that immunity is an all-or-none phenomenon; if a few sporozoites evade the immune response, the person will get malaria.

Merozoite vaccine   The host encounters merozoites for short periods, as they leave one erythrocyte and invade another. Erythrocytes infected by parasites develop new antigens, probably of parasite origin, on their surface. Both the merozoite and the infected erythrocyte could be targets for a vaccine. Monoclonal antibodies to merozoites and infected erythrocytes of rodent malaria transferred passively can confer partial protection. These monoclonal antibodies have been used to isolate antigens which can induce protective immunity. This vaccine would have the advantage of acting against stages of the parasite that interact with the host for a longer time period than the sporozoites. The disadvantages are that adjuvants are required for effective protection and that the vaccine may be strain-specific.

Gamete vaccine   If an animal is made immune to gametes, a state that does not usually occur in nature because the gamete is isolated from the immune apparatus by the erythrocyte membrane, the antigamete antibodies, when taken up with the gametes in the mosquitoes' blood meal, will neutralize the gametes when they leave the erythrocyte. It appears as if at least two antigens are involved in this process because neutralization will occur when two different monoclonal antigamete antibodies act in concert but not when they act alone. A vaccine aimed at gametes would not protect the vaccinated individual from malaria but might be effective in reducing its transmission. It could be useful, therefore, if it were incorporated into a multivalent vaccine.

IMMUNE EVASION BY PARASITES   Parasites have developed a variety of ingenious ways of evading the immune response of the host. Some of these are listed in Table 152-1. The most fascinating mechanism is that of antigenic variation by African trypanosomes, the flagellated protozoa transmitted by the tsetse fly that is the cause of sleeping sickness. The trypanosome has a thick surface coat, which is made up of many molecules of a single antigenic glycoprotein. When cloned organisms, all having the same surface antigen, are injected into certain animals, successive waves of parasitemia ensue similar to those seen when a human is bitten by an infected tsetse fly. Each peak consists of organisms expressing a single variant surface glycoprotein antigen (VSG), and this VSG is different from all other VSGs expressed by organisms in previous peaks of parasitemia in the same animal. A cloned organism can produce waves of parasites with over 100 different VSGs! Each peak of parasitemia induces soluble antibody directed at the major VSG. Presumably the antibody eliminates the organism with that specific VSG, but trypanosomes which can switch to another VSG escape. Analysis of the amino acid sequence of a number of VSGs indicates that they do not differ by only a few substitutions which could be explained by point mutations; on the contrary, the amino acid sequence of each VSG is quite different.

Studies on the genes encoding the VSGs have shown that each VSG is encoded by a distinct gene. Every trypanosome, regardless of the VSG it is expressing, contains a copy of each VSG gene. Trypanosomes have several mechanisms for expressing a VSG. For example, the organism expressing a particular VSG gene may have an additional, duplicate copy of that gene; this is referred to as the expression-linked copy. Studies using restriction enzymes indicate that the expression-linked copy is moved to a new site in the trypanosome that is gene-specific for expression. If each gene is visualized as a tape cassette in a library, to express the VSG the cassette is duplicated, the duplicate is removed from the library and inserted into a genetic tape deck, and expressed.

Although it was thought initially that the driving force for antigenic variation was antibody to that antigen, it has been shown that antigenic variation can be triggered in the absence of antibody both in vitro and in vivo.

Some organisms have developed multiple ways of evading the immune response. Schistosomes, for instance, can lose surface antigens after they enter the host, can take up host antigens and masquerade as host tissue, can develop certain intrinsic membrane changes making them resistant to attack even when surface antigens are present, and can shed antigens which may block effector cells and antibodies. A number of parasites, *Toxoplasma* being one example, when engulfed by a macrophage, prevent the fusion of the phagosome with the lysosomes. Others, such as *Leishmania,* do not prevent fusion when engulfed but are resistant to toxic substances in the lysosomes of the macrophage. And still others, such as *Trypanosoma cruzi,* escape from the lysosomes into the cytoplasm.

A number of parasites such as filaria, *Leishmania,* and *Plasmodium* induce strong suppressor mechanisms, including T suppressor cells, which dampen or eliminate the host's effective immune response. Some parasites can destroy mediators of inflammation involved in an effective immune response. For example, *Taenia* destroys complement components, and amoebae produce factors which neutralize chemotactic factors for macrophages. Other parasites such as *Ascaris* appear to have a surface coat that is antigenic and can induce an immune response but is, nevertheless, resistant to its effect. Against these parasites, there is no effective protective immune response.

Although some parasites can evade the immune response, they can induce an effective protective immune response to a subsequent

TABLE 152-1   Some mechanisms of immune evasion

Parasite	Mechanism
Trypanosoma brucei	Antigenic variation
Toxoplasma	Lysosome-phagosome fusion prevented
Malaria, *Babesia*	Escape into host cells
Schistosomes	Host molecule acquisition
	Loss of surface antigens
	Intrinsic membrane changes
	Immune complex blockade
Filaria, *Leishmania*	Specific T-cell suppression
Taenia, amoeba	Inactivation of mediators of inflammation

infection by the same species. This is called *concomitant immunity* or *premunition*.

EFFECTOR MECHANISMS AGAINST PARASITES Mechanisms that may be effective against parasites include the following: antibodies, cells including cytotoxic T cells, T-cell–induced activated macrophages, natural killer cells, and a variety of cells that mediate antibody-dependent cell-mediated cytotoxicity. Amplifiers of the immune system such as lymphokines and complement are also involved.

Immunity against several parasites such as malaria, schistosomes, and *Trypanosoma cruzi* can be transferred by antibodies. Nevertheless, evidence obtained in a number of animal models suggests that cell-mediated immunity is also involved against these and other parasites, including the organisms causing malaria, leishmaniasis, toxoplasmosis, schistosomiasis, filariasis, and trichinosis. It is less clear whether protective immunity develops against amoebae, African trypanosomes, or hookworm. There appears to be no naturally acquired immunity to *Ascaris,* guinea worm, or pinworm.

Two immune mechanisms have been described which appear to be unique for helminths. These involve eosinophils in one case and IgE in the other.

EOSINOPHILS AND ANTIBODY-DEPENDENT CELL-MEDIATED CYTOTOXICITY (ADCC) It has been known for over 100 years that eosinophils are associated with helminth infections, but only in the past few years has it become known that these cells can function as killer cells. Specifically, highly purified preparations of eosinophils, when mixed with antibody-coated schistosomula of *Schistosoma mansoni* in vitro, killed the larvae. The antibody formed is of the IgG class, and the eosinophils attach to the Fc portion of the IgG by the cells' Fc receptor. Immune complexes or staphylococcal protein A which can interfere with the binding of esosinophils to the Fc portion of the antibody inhibit the reaction. Incubation at 37°C makes the interaction between eosinophils and antibody-coated schistosomula become irreversible. This is associated with degranulation and the release of major basic protein (MBP), the most abundant protein in the eosinophil granule and eosinophil cationic protein (ECP) over the surface of the schistosomula. MBP and ECP, in turn, are toxic to the larvae. Eosinophils can also kill other helminths such as *Trichinella spiralis,* presumably by a similar mechanism.

Eosinophils from patients with eosinophilia exhibit an enhanced ability to kill antibody-coated schistosomula in vitro; they act as if they were activated. Moreover, a number of soluble substances can enhance the killing capacity of eosinophils in vitro. These include eosinophil stimulator promoter (ESP), ECF-A, a soluble substance similar or identical to eosinophil colony stimulating factor, and a soluble mediator produced by blood monocytes and lymphocytes in culture.

PROTECTIVE ROLE FOR IgE The observation that IgE levels are elevated in some persons in the tropics, notably those infected with helminths, suggests that IgE may act to protect the host against parasites. The mediators released by triggered mast cells could affect the parasites directly or, by increasing vascular permeability and releasing eosinophil chemotactic factors, they could lead to the accumulation of necessary antibodies (IgG) and cells to attack the parasite. IgE-immune complexes can induce macrophage-mediated cytotoxicity to schistosomula. Rats made specifically IgE-deficient by the repeated injection of antiepsilon chain antibodies show markedly impaired resistance to *Trichinella* infection.

IMMUNOPATHOLOGY Immune mechanisms play a major role in the pathology induced by many parasites. Such mechanisms are the cause of the granulomatous reaction to eggs of *S. mansoni* which is the basis of the immunopathology of this disease; immune complex renal disease in malaria and visceral leishmaniasis; heart disease due to *T. cruzi;* the obstructive and ocular disease in filariasis and onchocerciasis; the muscle pathology in trichinosis; the allergic reactions to ruptured hydatid cyst fluid; and the pulmonary compli-

cations to migrating nematode larvae. Just as suppressor mechanisms are involved in damping protective immunity, they are also involved in modulating the immunopathology. An example of this is the modulation of *S. mansoni* granulomas by T suppressor cells.

MONOCLONAL AND ANTI-IDIOTYPIC ANTIBODIES Monoclonal antibodies to various stages of malaria parasites have been used to detect antigens that can induce protective immunity. In addition, passive protection has been demonstrated with monoclonal antibodies to the promastigote stage of *Leishmania mexicana* and to schistosomula of *S. mansoni.* Because of their specificity, monoclonal antibodies can also be used for diagnosis because they can be selected not to show the multiple cross-reactions with other parasites that are frequently found with serums from infected animals. For example, species-specific monoclonal antibodies have been developed which can distinguish between five different species of South American *Leishmania* without cross-reacting with *T. cruzi.* Antibodies in the serum of an infected patient will usually cross-react with all these parasites. Diagnostic tests using these antibodies are being developed.

An antibody to an antigen has a specific antigen unique to itself on the immunoglobulin. This antigen is called the *idiotype,* which is the unique amino acid sequence and configuration of the antigen-binding site of that antibody. For instance, it is possible to make an antibody to a particular monoclonal antibody; that antibody will then recognize the idiotype and is called an *anti-idiotypic antibody.* The monoclonal antibody will bind to the anti-idiotype or to the original antigen. If a monoclonal antibody to a parasite were used to induce an anti-idiotypic antibody, it should be possible to induce protective immunity with this anti-idiotype instead of using the antigen. This would have the advantage of bypassing the need to purify antigens and then to produce them in large quantities. This novel strategy for the production of a vaccine is under study.

The rapidly accelerating pace of discovery and definition of the regulatory systems of the immune response, together with the revolution in technology, may soon make it possible to induce stronger protective immunity artificially than that which is acquired naturally, and the prediction that vaccines can be produced against the diseases caused by a number of parasites is based on this assumption.

REFERENCES

Bloom BR: Games parasites play: How parasites evade immune surveillance. Nature 279:21, 1979

Cohen S, Warren K (eds): *Immunology of Parasitic Infections,* 2d ed. London, Blackwell Scientific, 1982

———, Cross GAM (eds): Towards the immunological control of human protozoal diseases: A symposium. Phil Trans Roy Soc London B 307:1, 1984

Donelson JE, Turner MJ: How the trypanosome changes its coat. Sci Am 252(2):44, 1985

Hommell M: Antigenic variation in malaria parasites. Immunology Today 6:28, 1985

Mahmoud AF, Austen KF (eds): *The Eosinophil in Health and Disease.* New York, Grune & Stratton, 1981

Marchalonis JJ (ed): *Contemporary Topics in Immunobiology,* vol 12: *Immunobiology of Parasites and Parasitic Infections.* New York, Plenum Press, 1984

Moller G (ed): *Immunoparasitology.* Immunological Reviews 161. Copenhagen, Munksgaard, 1982, pp 5–269

---

153 AMEBIASIS

JAMES J. PLORDE

DEFINITION Amebiasis is an infection of the large intestine produced by *Entamoeba histolytica.* It is an asymptomatic carrier state in most individuals, but diseases ranging from chronic, mild diarrhea to fulminant dysentery may occur. Among extraintestinal complications, the commonest is hepatic abscess, which may rupture into peritoneum, pleura, lung, or pericardium.

ETIOLOGY There are seven species of ameba that naturally parasitize the human mouth and intestine, but of these only *E. histolytica* causes disease. *Entamoeba coli* and *E. hartmanni* are the two species with which it is most likely to be confused in examination of stools.

Entamoeba histolytica exists in two forms: the motile trophozoite and the cyst. The trophozoite is the parasitic form and dwells in the lumen and/or wall of the colon, divides by binary fission, grows best under anaerobic conditions, and requires the presence of either bacteria or tissue substrates to satisfy its nutritional requirements. When diarrhea occurs, the trophozoites are passed unchanged in the liquid stool, where they can be distinguished by their size (10 to 20 μm in diameter), directional motility, sharply demarcated clear ectoplasm with slender finger-like pseudopodia, and finely granular endoplasm. In dysentery, the trophozoites are larger (up to 50 μm in diameter), and often contain ingested erythrocytes. In the absence of diarrhea, the trophozoites usually encyst before leaving the gut. The cysts have a chitinous wall which renders them highly resistant to environmental changes, chlorine concentrations found in water purification systems, and gastric acid. With rare exception they are responsible for transmission of disease. Young cysts have a single nucleus, a glycogen vacuole, and sausage-shaped collections of ribosomes known as chromatoid bodies. As the cyst matures, it absorbs its cytoplasmic inclusions and becomes quadrinucleate. The cysts of *E. histolytica* can be distinguished from those of *E. hartmanni* by their larger diameter (10-μm) and from those of *Entamoeba coli* by the presence of one to four nuclei with small centric karyosomes and fine peripheral chromatin and by their thick chromatoid bodies with round ends.

The electrophoretic mobility patterns of four enzymes found in trophozoites have been used to define 22 *E. histolytica* zymodemes. Amebas recovered from patients with invasive disease belong to just 9; all are characterized by the presence of advanced, paired hexokinase bands and/or a beta phosphoglucomutase without an accompanying alpha-phosphoglucomutase band. The zymodemes are highly stable, and transitions between the invasive and commensal isoenzyme patterns have not been observed. Further studies will be required to determine whether the biologic differences between the two groups of organisms are sufficient to warrant the division of *E. histolytica* into separate pathogenic and nonpathogenic species.

Entamoeba histolytica can be cultivated in artificial media, a procedure that is essential for the determination of isoenzyme patterns and preparation of the purified antigens used in serologic testing. Its diagnostic value remains uncertain.

EPIDEMIOLOGY Although *E. histolytica* can sometimes infect rats, cats, dogs, and primates, humans are the principal hosts and reservoir. Because trophozoites die rapidly after leaving the intestine, the asymptomatic cyst passer is the source of new infections; a chronic carrier may excrete several million organisms daily. The infective dose usually exceeds 10^3, but infection has followed the ingestion of a single cyst. These structures are transmitted by the fecal-oral route, usually through direct person-to-person contact. Poverty, ignorance, mental retardation, and other factors which impair personal hygiene facilitate the spread of the parasite. Oral-anal sexual contact produces high infection rates in male homosexuals. Food- and waterborne transmission occur in poorly sanitated areas of the world, including certain southern rural communities, Indian reservations, and migrant farm camps in the United States. Occasionally this results in common source outbreaks; these epidemics, however, are never as explosive as those produced by pathogenic intestinal bacteria. Symptomatic amebiasis is unusual below the age of 10 years in temperate climates, and both intestinal and hepatic lesions predominate in adult males to an extent that is not readily explainable on the basis of different rates of exposure to infection.

It has been estimated that 50 percent of inhabitants of some less well-developed nations, 10 percent of the world's population as a whole, and 1 percent of Americans are infected with *E. histolytica*. Invasive amebiasis, which produces an estimated 30,000 deaths annually, is concentrated in comparatively few parts of the world, most notably Mexico, western South America, south Asia, and west and southeastern Africa. This is presumably related to the concurrent presence in these geographic areas of virulent strains of *E. histolytica* and the hygienic and sanitary conditions necessary for their transmission. Even in areas endemic for invasive disease, however, only 10 percent of infected patients harbor virulent zymodemes of *E. histolytica*. A minority of these experience clinical disease. In the United States the incidence of invasive amebiasis dropped sharply in the four decades preceding the 1970s. Between 1971 and 1974, an average of 3500 cases were reported annually to the Centers for Disease Control; since then the numbers have steadily increased. Isoenzyme studies of *E. histolytica* strains isolated from male homosexuals and inmates of mental hospitals in Great Britain indicate the overwhelming majority belong to nonpathogenic zymodemes, suggesting that virulent strains are now uncommon in the developed nations. Although patients with dysentery and liver abscess can still be found in the impoverished segments of the American population, the bulk of the invasive disease diagnosied in the United States is now acquired outside the country.

IMMUNITY There are both animal and human data suggesting the presence of protective immunity. However, repeated infections are common, and there is no correlation between the presence of circulating antibodies and immunity to infection. It is likely that immunity is incomplete, serves to limit rather than prevent disease, and is cell mediated.

PATHOGENESIS AND PATHOLOGY After ingestion, cysts undergo further nuclear division. In the small intestine, the cyst wall disintegrates, and trophozoites are released. The immature amebas are carried to the large intestine, where they live in the lumen of the gut feeding on bacteria and debris. Experimental and epidemiologic evidence indicates that organisms belonging to nonpathogenic zymodemes, although capable of inducing transient, focal epithelial damage, are seldom responsible for sustained tissue invasion and destruction. In contrast, the almost universal presence of specific humoral antibodies in carriers of pathogenic zymodemes suggests that tissue invasion by these strains is the rule. Only in the minority, however, is this sufficiently extensive to produce symptoms. The factors modulating invasion are not completely understood, but the state of the host and the virulence of the infecting organism both play roles. High iron and carbohydrate intake, corticosteroids, protein malnutrition, and pregnancy all render the host more susceptible. Trophozoite virulence is enhanced by rapid animal passage; presumably, a similar phenomenon occurs in epidemiologic settings conducive to rapid spread of the protozoan from human to human. Direct association with certain strains of bacteria may also enhance the virulence of pathogenic strains, possibly by protecting the ameba from oxidant stress or through the exchange of genetic material.

The precise pathogenic mechanisms responsible for tissue invasion are not fully understood. The invasiveness of a strain correlates well with its phagocytic prowess, production of collagenase and an immunogenic cytotoxic protein, resistance to the host's inflammatory response, and, perhaps most importantly, its capacity to induce histolysis following direct cell-to-cell contact with host tissue. The latter phenomenon is initiated by a lectin-mediated adherence of the trophozoite to a target cell. Cytolysis, which appears to require both intact microfilament function and amebic phospholipase A enzymes, rapidly follows.

Amebic ulceration of the intestinal wall is characteristic. A small mucosal defect overlies a larger, burrowing area of necrosis in the submucosa and muscularis, producing a bottle-shaped lesion. There is little acute inflammatory response, and in contrast to the picture in bacillary dysentery, the mucosa between ulcers is normal. The sites of involvement in order of frequency are cecum and ascending colon, rectum, sigmoid, appendix, and terminal ileum. In the cecum and sigmoid, chronic infection may lead to the formation of large masses of granulation tissue or *amebomas*. Amebas can enter the portal circulation and lodge in venules; liquefaction necrosis of liver tissue leads to the formation of an abscess cavity. Rarely, embolization results in lung, brain, or splenic abscess.

CLINICAL MANIFESTATIONS Asymptomatic cyst passer
In the majority of patients with this common form of amebiasis, *E. histolytica* probably lives as a commensal in the bowel lumen. Individuals infected in temperate climates are unlikely to harbor virulent strains. However, as invasion can occasionally occur, treatment of all cyst passers is warranted.

Symptomatic intestinal amebiasis In some patients there is intermittent diarrhea consisting of one to four foul-smelling loose or watery stools daily. The stools sometimes contain mucus and blood. Loose stools alternate with periods of relative normality and may persist for months or years. Flatulence and abnormal cramping are frequent. The only physical findings are occasional tender hepatomegaly and slight pain when the cecum and ascending colon are palpated. Sigmoidoscopy sometimes reveals typical ulcerations with areas of normal mucosa interspersed. The diagnosis depends upon finding the organism in the feces or in ulcers.

Fulminating attacks of amebic dysentery are less common. Waterborne outbreaks may occur, but fulminating dysentery is more likely to occur spontaneously in debilitated individuals. Attacks may be precipitated by pregnancy or corticosteroids. The onset in half the cases is abrupt with high fever, between 40 and 40.6°C (104 and 105°F), severe abdominal cramps, and profuse, bloody diarrhea with tenesmus. There is diffuse abdominal tenderness, often so severe that peritonitis is suspected. Hepatomegaly is very frequent, and sigmoidoscopy almost always demonstrates extensive rectosigmoid ulceration. Trophozoites are numerous in stools and in material obtained directly from the ulcers.

In some cases there may be extensive destruction of the colonic mucosa and submucosa, massive hemorrhage or perforation of the bowel wall, with resultant peritonitis. Repeated severe attacks of intestinal amebiasis can lead to an ulcerative postdysenteric colitis. Amebas can usually not be demonstrated in this condition, but serologic tests are strongly positive. Invasion of the appendix may lead to a clinical picture of *appendicitis*. Penetration of trophozoites through the muscle wall of the bowel may result in the development of large masses of granulation tissue. When the entire circumference of the intestine is involved, there may then be partial obstruction, and a movable, tender, sausage-shaped mass is often palpable. This lesion or ameboma is most frequently seen in the cecum where a palpable mass and radiologic demonstration of a ragged encroachment of the lumen may lead to a mistaken diagnosis of adenocarcinoma.

Hepatic amebiasis The term *amebic hepatitis* is used for a syndrome of tender hepatomegaly, right upper quadrant pain, fever, and leukocytosis in patients with amebic colitis. Hepatic biopsy reveals nonspecific periportal inflammation. The absence of ameba within the areas of inflammation, the rarity with which the syndrome is followed by an amebic liver abscess, and the resolution of the liver signs following treatment of the intestinal disease with luminal amebicides indicate that these manifestations are not secondary to spread of trophozoites from the intestine, but are rather a nonspecific accompaniment of amebic colitis. As such, the syndrome does not merit the appellation of "amebic hepatitis."

Hepatic abscess may develop insidiously, with fever, sweats, weight loss, and no local signs other than painless or slightly tender hepatomegaly. In immunologically naive patients, there is more often an abrupt onset, with chills, fever to 40.6°C (105°F), nausea, vomiting, severe upper abdominal pain, and polymorphonuclear leukocytosis. Initially, cholecystitis, perforated ulcer, or acute pancreatitis may be suspected. Over 80 percent of patients with an insidious onset and half of those presenting with acute manifestations have a single abscess. Most commonly, this is localized in the posterior portion of the right lobe of the liver, because this lobe receives most of the blood draining the right colon through the "streaming" effect in portal vein flow. This location is responsible for several features that

aid in diagnosis. *Point tenderness* in the posterolateral portion of a lower right intercostal space is frequent even in the absence of diffuse liver pain. Most abscesses enlarge upward, producing a bulge in the diaphragmatic dome, obliteration of the costophrenic gutter, small hydrothorax, basilar atelectasis, and pain referred to the right shoulder.

Liver function tests may be mildly to moderately disturbed and provide little diagnostic aid; the level of the serum glutamic oxaloacetic transaminase (SGOT), however, is of clinical value as it directly reflects the severity of disease. Jaundice is uncommon, and when present implies a grave prognosis. Radiologically, unruptured abscesses do not show a fluid level, and calcification of the liver parenchyma is very rare. Isotope liver scan utilizing two, or preferably three, projections is invaluable in confirming the presence and location of a liver abscess. It becomes positive within the first days of illness, often prior to other imaging techniques. Presumably these early changes reflect either a focal decrease in blood supply or injury to the Kupffer cells rather than liquefaction necrosis. Ultrasonic scanning and computerized tomography, although becoming positive slightly later in the course of the disease, are ultimately as sensitive as isotopic scanning and provide confirmation of the cystic nature of the lesion. The defect seen on imaging commonly persists for several months after the complete recovery of the patient. Serologic tests are positive in over 90 percent of cases.

Needle puncture results in the withdrawal of "pus" which consists of liquefied, necrotic liver. Typically, it is thick and odorless, resembling "chocolate syrup" or "anchovy paste." It may, however, be thin in consistency and yellow or green in color. The pus contains no polymorphonuclear leukocytes (barring secondary bacterial infection) and, usually, no amebas. The parasites are localized in the cyst wall and may be demonstrated in the terminal portion of the aspirate or, at times, by a Vim-Silverman needle biopsy of the cyst wall following aspiration of the abscess.

Hepatic abscess complicates asymptomatic infection of the colon more often than symptomatic intestinal disease, another factor making recognition difficult. Trophozoites or cysts are demonstrable in the feces of only about one-third of patients with abscess, and fewer than one-half can recall significant diarrheal illness.

Pleuropulmonary amebiasis The right pleural cavity and lung are involved by direct extension from the liver in 10 to 20 percent of patients with liver abscess. Rarely, amebic lung abscess has resulted from embolization rather than direct extension.

Manifestations are those of a consolidating pneumonia or lung abscess. If perforation into a bronchus occurs, patients expectorate large amounts of the typical exudate, some patients even commenting that the sputum "tastes like liver." Cough, pleural pain, fever, and leukocytosis are the rule, and secondary bacterial infection is frequent. Rupture into the free pleural space results in a massive pleural effusion; aspiration of "chocolate" fluid is diagnostic.

Other extraintestinal lesions Extension of an abscess from the left lobe of the liver to the pericardium is the most dangerous complication of hepatic abscess. It may be mistaken for tuberculous pericarditis or congestive cardiomyopathy. Less frequently, rapid cardiac tamponade occurs with ensuing dyspnea, shock, and death. *Peritonitis* is a result of perforation of colonic ulcer or rupture of liver abscess. Painful ulcers or condylomata of the genitalia, perianal skin, or abdominal wall (draining sinuses) are unusual complications which may be mistaken for syphilitic, tuberculous, or neoplastic lesions. They usually result from direct extension of intestinal disease; some are thought to result from sexual transmission. Metastatic brain abscess is rare, and an etiologic diagnosis is seldom made clinically. Splenic abscess has been reported but is very unusual.

DIFFERENTIAL DIAGNOSIS Intestinal amebiasis
Patients with nondysenteric amebiasis are often misdiagnosed as having irritable bowel syndrome, diverticulitis, or regional enteritis. Ameboma may mimic colonic carcinoma or granulomatous disease, while the clinical spectrum of amebic dysentery overlaps those of shigellosis, salmo-

nellosis, ulcerative colitis, and, in endemic areas, schistosomiasis. The invasive bacterial infections are usually more acute, severe, and self-limited than amebiasis. Stools from patients with shigellosis, salmonellosis, and ulcerative colitis contain large numbers of polymorphonuclear leukocytes, while those in amebic infection do not. Nevertheless, amebiasis may closely resemble any of the above diseases both clinically and radiologically and must be considered in the differential diagnosis of any chronic diarrhea or dysentery.

The identification of *E. histolytica* in the stool, however, does not eliminate other diagnostic possibilities. Amebic infection is often superimposed on or exacerbated by other colonic disease including schistosomiasis and cecal carcinoma. For this reason, patients with intestinal amebiasis and abdominal complaints still require stool culture, sigmoidoscopy, and a barium enema.

Hepatic abscess   Once a filling defect has been demonstrated by isotope liver scanning, the differential diagnosis includes hepatic neoplasm, hydatid cyst, and pyogenic abscess. Neoplasms can usually be differentiated on the basis of their ultrasonic scanning characteristics, while the lack of constitutional manifestations and presence of an appropriate epidemiologic history is helpful in recognizing echinococcosis. The most difficult problem lies in the exclusion of a pyogenic abscess. An insidious onset in an adult male, a history of chronic diarrhea, significant pleuritic chest pain, and a single right lobe lesion favors the diagnosis of amebiasis. High fever, hyperbilirubinemia, multiple hepatic filling defects, and foul-smelling hepatic aspirate are more suggestive of pyogenic disease. Ultimately, the separation of the two diseases rests upon laboratory procedures.

LABORATORY DIAGNOSIS   The diagnosis of intestinal amebiasis depends upon *identification of the organism in the stool or tissues.* Formed stools are microscopically examined initially in saline and iodine mounts for amebic cysts; concentration methods such as the formalin-ether technique increase the yield two- to threefold. Liquid or semiformed stools should be examined immediately in saline solution for the presence of motile hematophagous trophozoites. The addition of a supravital stain such as buffered methylene blue to the saline enhances nuclear detail and minimizes the possibility of confusing fecal leukocytes with amebic trophozoites. If there is any delay in examination of the stool, a portion of the specimen may be refrigerated for a few hours at 4°C, or placed in polyvinyl alcohol and 10% formalin. Definitive identification of *E. histolytica* requires the examination of permanently stained slides prepared from the material preserved with polyvinyl alcohol. An ocular micrometer is necessary to separate *E. hartmanni* from its larger relative. Four to six stool specimens may be required for diagnosis. If possible, the stool should be examined before the administration of antimicrobial, antidiarrheal, or antacid preparations, because all these agents may interfere with the recovery of amebas. Likewise, enemas and radiographic procedures utilizing barium sulfate are best postponed until after a thorough search for *E. histolytica* has been made. A simple, sensitive, and specific enzyme-linked immunosorbent assay has been developed for the detection of *E. histolytica* antigen in the stool. If commercially developed, it could provide a useful alternative to microscopic examination.

Sigmoidoscopy is of value in symptomatic cases. The mucosal lesions should be aspirated and the material examined for trophozoites as described above. Biopsy material obtained from such lesions and stained with periodic acid Schiff solution also will frequently reveal trophozoites.

The diagnosis of extraintestinal amebiasis is difficult. The parasite usually cannot be recovered from stool or tissue. Cultivation of amebas from feces or pus is possible but is not practical in most laboratories. *Serologic tests* employing purified antigens are positive in nearly all patients with proven amebic liver abscess and in a great majority of those with acute amebic dysentery. They are generally negative in asymptomatic cyst passers, suggesting that tissue invasion is required for antibody production. The persistence of significant antibody titers for months to years after complete cure makes serology,

particularly in endemic areas, of more value in excluding the diagnosis than in confirming it. Some authors recommend the routine screening of all patients thought to have inflammatory bowel disease for serologic evidence of amebiasis. Steroid therapy could then be withheld in patients with positive tests pending the outcome of parasitological examination. Of the available tests, the indirect hemagglutination and enzyme-linked immunosorbent assays appear to be the most sensitive; average time to positivity is 3 and 2 weeks, respectively. Indirect immunofluorescence, countercurrent electrophoresis, and agar gel diffusion are also highly reliable. A number of these testing procedures are now available as commercial kits, making serologic testing feasible for most laboratories.

TREATMENT   Treatment should be aimed at relief of symptoms, replacement of fluid, electrolyte, and blood losses, and eradication of the organism. Amebas may be found in the lumen of the bowel, in the intestinal wall, or extraintestinally. Most amebicides are not effective at all sites or when used alone, and a combination of drugs is often necessary to achieve cure. The available drugs based on their site of action fall into two categories.

Luminal amebicides   These oral agents act by direct contact with trophozoites dwelling in the bowel lumen but are ineffective against amebas in tissue. Of the large number of available drugs, diloxanide furoate is one of the most effective and well tolerated but is presently available in the United States only through the Centers for Disease Control. A response rate of 80 to 85 percent has been noted; flatulence appears to be the only major side effect.

Iodoquinol has been effective in 60 to 70 percent of cases. As with its analogue iodochlorhydroxyquin, myelooptic neuropathy has been reported after long-term use. However, no such case has been noted when the dosage was limited to that given in Table 153-1. The drug should not be used in patients with thyroid disease or preexisting optic neuropathy.

Tissue amebicides   *Chloroquine phosphate* is a systemic amebicide which is useful in hepatic disease because of its high concentration in the liver. It has little activity elsewhere.

Emetine is an alkaloid derivative of ipecac. When given intramuscularly, it is highly effective in destroying trophozoites in tissue including those in the wall of the intestine. It is ineffective against luminal amebas. Emetine is relatively toxic and may produce vomiting, diarrhea, abdominal cramping, weakness, muscle pain, tachycardia, hypotension, precordial pain, and electrocardiographic abnormalities. The common ECG changes include T-wave inversion and prolongation of the QTc interval. Rarely arrhythmias and prolongation of the QRS complex are seen. A synthetic derivative, dehydroemetine, is thought to be less toxic by virtue of its more rapid excretion and lower concentration in myocardial tissue. It is not free of toxicity, however, and patients treated with either drug should be at bed rest with ECG monitoring. Neither drug should be used in patients with renal, cardiac, or muscle disease, during pregnancy, or in children, unless other drugs fail.

Metronidazole is unique because it is effective against trophozoites at all sites, intestinally and extraintestinally. For intestinal amebiasis it is given in dosage of 750 mg three times daily for 5 to 10 days. Smaller doses are effective in hepatic amebiasis. Metronidazole has an Antabuse-like action, and alcohol should be avoided during its administration. The evidence that this drug is carcinogenic and possibly teratogenic in animals when given in large doses is disturbing. The potential risk in human beings must be weighed against the severity of the disease; it should not be given in the first trimester of pregnancy.

Specific antiprotozoal therapy is outlined in Table 153-1.

In extraintestinal amebiasis including hepatic abscess, metronidazole is the drug of choice. In cases of relapse, impending rupture of an abscess, or in situations where the patient is unable to take oral medication, therapy with dehydroemetine or emetine should be instituted, and oral chloroquine added as soon as possible. Diagnostic trials should employ the chloroquine-emetine regimen because pyogenic liver abscesses may temporarily respond to metronidazole. Most authors prefer to add luminal amebicides to both the metronidazole and chloroquine-emetine programs. Treatment failures have been reported for both emetine-chloroquine and metronidazole. They appear to be unrelated to the organism's resistance.

There is debate over the value of routine aspiration of amebic liver abscesses. Certainly, if there is localized swelling over the liver, marked elevation of the diaphragm, severe localized liver tenderness, and failure to respond to systemic amebicides within 72 h, it should be done. Adequate drainage can usually be accomplished by needle alone, and surgical drainage is rarely necessary. The greatest hazard in needling an abscess is secondary bacterial infection.

PROGNOSIS Intestinal amebiasis usually responds readily and completely to appropriate drugs. Parasitologic relapses sometimes occur, and posttreatment stools should be checked monthly for 6 months. Repeated relapses, however, are usually a manifestation of reinfection, complicating illness, inadequate therapy, or incorrect diagnosis. The fatality rate is less than 5 percent.

Hepatic and pulmonary amebiasis are still accompanied by an appreciable mortality, but no reliable figures are available.

PREVENTION For the individual, avoidance of contaminated food and water, scalding of vegetables, and the use of iodine-releasing tablets in drinking water (chlorine, in the form of halazone, is ineffective) are important measures. Globaline tablets, containing tetraglycine hydroperiodide, are convenient and effective.

Improvements in general sanitation and the detection of cyst passers and their removal from food-handling duties are general measures in prophylaxis, but such segregation of carriers is rarely practiced. Community control of amebic disease by periodic mass treatment with metronidazole and diloxanide furoate has been successful in some areas. Personal chemoprophylaxis for travelers is not recommended.

TABLE 153-1 Drug therapy of amebiasis

	Dosage
ASYMPTOMATIC INTESTINAL CARRIER	
Iodoquinol*	650 mg tid for 20 days
or diloxanide furoate†	500 mg tid for 10 days
MILD TO MODERATE INTESTINAL DISEASE	
Metronidazole	750 mg tid for 5–10 days
plus iodoquinol	As above
or diloxanide furoate	As above
or tetracycline	500 mg qid for 5 days
SEVERE INTESTINAL DISEASE	
Above regimen	
plus dehydroemetine†	1.0–1.5 mg/kg IM per day (maximum 90 mg per day) for up to 5 days
or emetine	1 mg/kg IM per day (maximum 60 mg per day) for up to 5 days
EXTRAINTESTINAL DISEASE	
Metronidazole	As above
plus iodoquinol	
or chloroquine phosphate	1 g per day for 2 days, then 500 mg per day for 4 weeks
plus dehydroemetine†	As above for 10 days
or emetine	As above for 10 days

* Glenwood Laboratories, Inc., 83 North Summit St., Tenafly, NJ 07670.
† Investigational drug available through the Parasitic Drug Service, Centers for Disease Control, Atlanta, Ga., (404) 633-3311, nights and weekends 633-2176.

PRIMARY AMEBIC MENINGOENCEPHALITIS

Primary amebic meningoencephalitis is caused by free-living amebas of the genus *Naegleria* or *Acanthamoeba*. The former most often affects children and young adults, appears to be acquired by swimming in fresh, warm water, and is almost invariably fatal. *Acanthamoeba* infections involve older immunocompromised individuals, and spontaneous recovery is sometimes seen.

Free-living amebas are ubiquitous in nature where they are commonly found in soil and water. Although generally considered harmless, some varieties are clearly pathogenic for the central nervous system of mammals. In those instances of human meningoencephalitis where the responsible organism has been isolated and cultured, it has, with few exceptions, been identified as an amoeboflagellate, *Naegleria fowleri*.

Over 100 *Naegleria* cases have been reported from different parts of the world including Australia, Belgium, Brazil, Czechoslovakia, Great Britain, Ireland, New Zealand, Zambia, and the United States. Serologic studies suggest that inapparent infections are much more common. Most of the 50 cases recognized in the United States have occurred in the southeastern states, particularly Florida, Georgia, and Virginia. Characteristically the patients have fallen ill during the summer months approximately 1 week after swimming in fresh or brackish water. The 16 Czechoslovakian cases followed swimming in an indoor pool with chlorinated water maintained at 24°C, and 6 cases have been acquired apparently after bathing in hot mineral water. In sub-Saharan Africa, cases appear to follow inhalation of airborne cysts during the dry, windy harmattan season. Histologic evidence suggests that the amebas reach the central nervous system directly via the nasal mucosa at the level of the cribriform plate. Clinically, the illness is rapid in onset, brief in duration, and inexorable in course. The initial symptom is a severe, persistent, frontal headache followed by nausea, vomiting, fever, and nuchal rigidity. Unusual tastes or smells may be noted. Later, drowsiness, confusion, convulsions, and coma appear. Focal neurologic findings may occur late in the course of the illness.

A more benign, chronic form of meningoencephalitis is produced by organisms of the genus *Acanthamoeba*. They appear to be disseminated to the brain and other organs from the skin or respiratory tract. Patients with this clinical syndrome are frequently older, are immunocompromised, lack a history of freshwater swimming, and may recover spontaneously. Pathologically, the disease can be distinguished from *Naegleria* infections by the granulomatous nature of the inflammatory reaction and the presence of both trophozoites and cysts in the tissues. Unfortunately, the identification of the responsible organisms remains in some doubt as they have seldom been recovered by culture. It is possible that the free-living amebas of several species are involved. Approximately a dozen cases of *Acanthamoeba* keratitis have been reported.

A careful examination of the cerebrospinal fluid is the single most helpful diagnostic procedure. In *Naegleria* infections the fluid is usually bloody or sanguinopurulent and demonstrates an intense neutrophilic response. The protein is elevated and the glucose diminished. No organisms are demonstrated on Gram's stain or routine culture. Early examination of a wet preparation of unspun spinal fluid will usually reveal viable trophozoites. They are 10 to 20 μm in diameter, possess a granular cytoplasm, a distinct ectoplasm, and bulbous pseudopodia. If the specimen is allowed to cool, the trophozoites may become immobile and more difficult to recognize. The diagnosis is confirmed with direct fluorescent antibody (DFA) stains. Although the amebas may be easily grown on ordinary culture media which have been seeded with coliform bacteria, this is not helpful in clinical management, so rapidly progressive is the disease. In contrast, the spinal fluid in *Acanthamoeba* infections usually demonstrates a mononuclear response. Trophozoites have been neither cultured nor seen on wet mounts. A positive DFA stain has been seen in a few cases. Treatment with standard antiprotozoal agents seems completely ineffective. *Naegleria*, however, is highly sensitive to amphotericin B, miconazole, tetracycline, and rifampin. To date only four patients have survived a *Naegleria* infection. All were diagnosed early and treated, three with amphotericin B and the other with amphotericin B, miconazole, and rifampin. Intracisternal, as well as intravenous, administration of amphotericin is probably essential to rapidly obtain effective levels in the cerebrospinal fluid. The intraventricular dose is 0.5 to 1 mg for the first few days. The intravenous dose is similar to that for cryptococcal meningitis (see Chap. 146). *Acanthamoeba* are sensitive to sulfanilamides, clotrimazole, 5-FC, and polymyxin B, but no clinical studies have been done.

If the source of the infection can be determined, further *Naegleria* cases might be prevented by closing the area to bathing.

REFERENCES

Amebiasis

ADAMS EB, MACLEOD IN: Invasive amebiasis. Medicine 56:315, 1977

BARBOUR GL, JUNIPER K JR: A clinical comparison of amebic and pyogenic abscess of the liver in sixty-six patients. Am J Med 53:323, 1972

JACKSON TFHG, GATHIRAM V: Seroepidemiological study of antibody responses to the zymodemes of *Entamoeba histolytica*. Lancet 1:716, 1985

KATZENSTEIN D et al: New concepts of amebic liver abscess derived from hepatic imaging, serodiagnosis, and hepatic enzymes in 67 consecutive cases in San Diego. Medicine 61:237, 1982

KNOBLOCH J, MANNWEILER E: Development and persistence of antibodies to *Entamoeba histolytica* in patients with amebic liver abscess: Analysis of 216 cases. Am J Trop Med Hyg 32:727, 1983

MARTINEZ-PALOMO A, MARTINEZ-BAEZ M: Selective primary health care: Strategies for control of disease in the developing world. X. Amebiasis. Rev Infect Dis 5:1093, 1983

McGOWAN K et al: *Entamoeba histolytica* cytotoxin: Purification, characterization, strain virulence, and protease activity. J Infect Dis 146:616, 1982

RAVDIN JI, GUERRANT RL: A review of the parasite cellular mechanisms involved in the pathogenesis of amebiasis. Rev Infect Dis 4:1185, 1982

THOMPSON JE et al: Amebic liver abscess: A therapeutic approach. Rev Infect Dis 7:171, 1985

TRISSL D: Immunology of *Entamoeba histolytica* in human and animal hosts. Rev Infect Dis 4:1154, 1982

UNGER BLP et al: Use of a monoclonal antibody in an enzyme immunoassay for the detection of *Entamoeba histolytica* in fecal specimens. Am J Trop Med Hyg 34:465, 1985

Primary amebic meningoencephalitis

JOHN DT: Primary amebic meningoencephalitis and the biology of *Naegleria fowleri*. Ann Rev Microbiol 36:101, 1982

MA PE et al: A case of keratitis due to *Acanthamoeba* in New York, New York, and features of 10 cases. J Infect Dis 143:662, 1981

SEIDEL JS et al: Successful treatment of primary amebic meningoencephalitis. N Engl J Med 306:346, 1982

154 MALARIA

JAMES J. PLORDE / NICHOLAS J. WHITE

DEFINITION Malaria is a protozoan disease transmitted to humans by the bite of *Anopheles* mosquitoes. It is characterized by *fever, rigors, splenomegaly, anemia,* and a *chronic relapsing course.* Despite the impressive results of the World Health Organization–sponsored malaria eradication program initiated in 1956, technical and socioeconomic difficulties have led to a resurgence of the disease in many areas of the world. Consequently, malaria remains today, as it has been for centuries, one of the most serious infectious disease problems in the world. In the United States and Europe, several thousand imported cases are seen annually in travelers from endemic areas.

ETIOLOGY *The causative organisms are protozoa of the genus Plasmodium.* The four species known to infect human beings are *P. vivax, P. ovale, P. malariae,* and *P. falciparum.* Human infection begins when a female anopheline inoculates plasmodial *sporozoites* into the lymphohematogenous system while feeding. After a brief

passage in the peripheral blood, these organisms invade hepatocytes where they initiate the preclinical hepatic (exoerythrocytic) phase of disease. By a process of asexual multiplication referred to as *schizogony,* a single sporozoite eventually produces 2000 to 40,000 hepatic *merozoites.* In most cases, these daughter cells rupture back into the circulatory system within 1 to 6 weeks. In infections produced by some northern strains of *P. vivax,* release of hepatic merozoites occurs some 10 months after initial infection, a time which coincides with the short mosquito breeding period of the following year. In *P. falciparum* and *P. malariae* infections, the hepatic phase terminates at this point. In the other species, liver forms (*hypnozoites*) persist and produce new episodes of bloodstream invasion months to years later.

The erythrocytic or clinical phase of malaria starts with the attachment of a released merozoite to a specific receptor site on the red blood cell surface. This site appears to differ for each species of malaria; in the case of *P. vivax,* it is related to the Duffy blood group antigens (Fy^a or Fy^b). Duffy-negative (FyFy) individuals, who include the majority of people of West African extraction, are resistant to vivax malaria, presumably for this reason. Glycophorin, a red blood cell membrane sialoglycoprotein, has been implicated as the attachment site for the *P. falciparum.* Following attachment, the merozoite invaginates the cell surface and is slowly interiorized. The intracellular parasite first appears as a ring-shaped trophozoite which later enlarges and assumes an irregular or ameboid shape. Its nucleus then divides into several portions to form a multinucleated *schizont.* Eventually, cytoplasm condenses around each daughter nucleus to form a new generation of merozoites. Forty-eight hours after its original invasion (72 h in the case of *P. malariae*) the erythrocyte ruptures, releasing 6 to 24 merozoites, each of which is capable of initiating a new red blood cell cycle. With repetition of this cycle, some of the red blood cells become filled with morphologically distinct *sexual forms* (gametocytes); these do not induce cell lysis and are unable to undergo further development unless ingested by an appropriate mosquito during a blood meal. In the gut of the mosquito fertilization occurs, and the resulting *zygote* encysts on the outer surface of the gut and releases myriads of *sporozoites.* These migrate to the salivary glands and are inoculated into a human subject at the next feeding.

EPIDEMIOLOGY Malaria survives only in areas of the world where both the anopheline and infected human population remain above certain *critical densities* required for the sustained transmission of disease. Control measures are directed toward reducing both populations to levels that are too low for the infection to survive. Important procedures include drainage or filling of breeding areas, use of residual insecticide sprays, screening, use of skin repellents, effective treatment of cases, and large-scale suppressive drug programs in some human populations.

An active international cooperative program aimed at the eradication of malaria resulted in a significant decline in the incidence of the disease between 1956 and 1968. In over three-quarters of the original malarial areas of the world, the disease was eradicated, or active eradication programs were instituted. Presently, however, malaria still infects between 250 and 300 million inhabitants of 104 countries throughout Africa, Latin America, South America, Asia, and Oceania. Tropical Africa alone harbors 200 million of these afflicted individuals and contributes most of the estimated 1 million deaths that occur annually from this terrible disease. The presence of mobile populations, outdoor-biting mosquitoes, and high levels of disease transmission make successful eradication in these remaining areas unlikely. Furthermore, the emergence of insecticide-resistant mosquitoes as well as a variety of administrative and socioeconomic problems has produced serious setbacks to several previously successful eradication programs. Added to these difficulties has been the continuing spread of drug-resistant *P. falciparum* throughout southern Asia, the western Pacific, Central America, and South America. Resistant strains have been discovered in east and central Africa and the Indian subcontinent, areas previously free of this problem.

Endemic malaria did not disappear from the United States until the 1950s. Imported cases and occasional outbreaks of malaria acquired by mosquito transmission from imported infections (*introduced malaria*) have continued to occur, but until 1966 the total never exceeded 200 cases a year. This number rapidly increased with the return of infected military personnel from southeast Asia, reaching a peak of over 4000 in 1970. Associated with this wave of imported malaria was a smaller increase in the number of infections induced by blood transfusion and intravenous heroin use. Although this epidemic has waned, the incidence of malaria in the civilian population has not (Fig. 154-1). From 1970 to 1979, the number of cases reported annually among tourists, businesspeople, teachers, students, and other civilians rose from 151 to 825; in 1984 and 1985, approximately 1000 cases of malaria diagnosed in this country were reported annually. With rare exceptions, malaria was acquired abroad: approximately 40 percent in Asia, 30 percent in Africa, and 20 percent in the Caribbean or Latin America. Forty percent of the recent infections have involved U.S. citizens; over half of these had been acquired in Africa. Most infections involving foreign civilians occurred in émigrés from southeast Asia. Surveillance studies suggest that 2 to 5 percent of this population are infected at the time of entry to this country. Clinical manifestations usually develop within 6 months of arrival in the United States, but in one-third of the vivax cases they are delayed beyond that point. In 1983, one-fourth of the cases and all three of the deaths were caused by the virulent *P. falciparum*. Most of these cases could have been prevented with appropriate chemoprophylaxis. Until travelers are more fully informed of dangers inherent in traveling unprotected to malarious areas, the number of cases seen in this country each year will continue to increase.

PATHOGENESIS AND PATHOLOGY The invasion, alteration, and destruction of red blood cells by malaria parasites, local and systemic circulatory changes, and the related metabolic abnormalities are all important in the pathophysiology of malaria.

Red blood cell changes Malaria species differ significantly in their ability to invade red blood cells. *Plasmodium vivax* and *P. ovale* attack only immature erythrocytes; *P. malariae*, only senescent ones. During infection with these species, therefore, no more than 1 or 2 percent of cells are involved at any one time. *Plasmodium falciparum*, although preferring younger erythrocytes, invades red blood cells of all ages and may cause extremely high levels of parasitemia, a factor contributing to the lethality of this disease. The presence of certain erythrocytic abnormalities, however, appears capable of limiting the intensity of the parasitemia and its attendant morbidity and mortality. This has been most convincingly demonstrated in patients with sickle cell trait. Parasite growth is retarded in AS cells exposed to conditions of reduced oxygen tension such as that present in the visceral capillary bed. The tactoids formed during sickling of AS cells may also directly damage the parasite and render the deformed erythrocyte more susceptible to phagocytosis. Although not well documented, a similar protective effect may be exerted in thalassemia and in glucose 6-phosphate (G6PD) or pyridoxal-kinase deficiency, since these abnormalities are found more commonly in malarious areas. The protection, if present, may be related in part to the increased susceptibility of such erythrocytes to oxidant damage. In thalassemia and related hemoglobinopathies, the persistent production of fetal hemoglobin may also contribute since maturation of *P. falciparum* is retarded in cells containing hemoglobin F. In subjects with melanesian ovalocytosis, protection is afforded by the rigidity of the erythrocytic wall which prevents merozoite penetration.

Once parasitized, the cells undergo a number of changes. Up to 75 percent of the hemoglobin content is ingested and metabolized by the plasmodia as they begin to grow. In falciparum infections, electron-dense "knobs" form on the eyrthrocytic membrane where it overlays accumulations of parasitic antigen. These structures appear to mediate the attachment of the involved cells to the capillary and postcapillary venous endothelium of the deep tissues, resulting in intravascular agglutination and sludging. Infection with any of the four plasmodium species renders the red blood cell less deformable and hence susceptible to removal by the spleen. With the stimulation of the immune system, circulation of erythrocytes through the splenic cords increases, splenic trapping is enhanced, and parasitized erythrocytes are forced into intimate contact with activated macrophages. Here the intracellular parasite is damaged or destroyed by macrophage-secreted cytotoxins, and/or the erythrocyte itself is phagocytosed. Parasitized cells escaping splenic removal are destroyed at the time of sporulation, a process which elicits fever in the host. The specific mechanism responsible remains obscure, but is presumably related to the release of an intracellular pyrogen.

The severity of the anemia in acute malaria often exceeds that which would be predicted from the loss of parasitized cells alone. Several factors account for this discrepancy; sequestration results in

FIGURE 154-1 *Cases of malaria in civilians and foreigners in the United States (including Puerto Rico, the Virgin Islands, and Guam), 1970–1983. (From Malaria Surveillance: Annual Summary, 1984, Atlanta, GA., Centers for Disease Control, 1985.)*

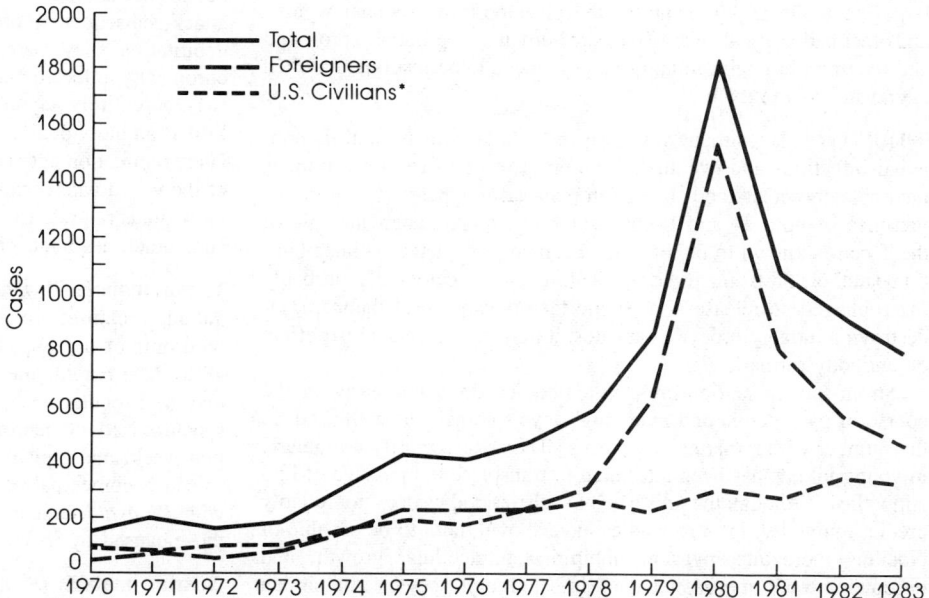

*Includes 5 cases acquired in the United States

an underestimation of the total number of infected erythrocytes, erythropoiesis is dampened, and nonparasitized as well as parasitized cells are removed from the circulation. The most unusual and profound example of this process is blackwater fever, in which there is massive intravascular hemolysis. More commonly, the red blood cells are destroyed in the reticuloendothelial system of the liver and spleen. The Coombs test is occasionally positive. These phenomena are reflected in other blood components as well. Thrombocytopenia, the result of both splenic pooling and a shortened platelet life span, is common. Disseminated intravascular coagulation occurs in severe falciparum malaria, but is clinically significant in less than 5 percent of cases. The leukocyte and differential white blood cell counts are generally normal.

Circulatory changes   Except for the periods of cutaneous vasoconstriction that accompany malarial rigor, the febrile patient is usually warm and well-perfused with low or normal blood pressure and a rapid pulse. In severe falciparum malaria, this vasodilatory state may be exaggerated with hypotension and a decreased central venous pressure. An increase in the radioiodinated serum albumin space and the secretion of aldosterone and antidiuretic hormone suggests a decrease in effective circulating blood volume due to enhanced vascular capacitance. Myocardial function remains surprisingly good despite sequestration of parasitized erythrocytes in the small vessels of the heart. Fluid replacement must be carefully managed if the twin dangers of acute tubular necrosis and pulmonary edema are to be avoided. Occasionally severe shock develops without apparent cause; this has been called *algid malaria* and may be secondary to spontaneous gram-negative rod bacteremia.

Almost all deaths in malaria result from the occlusion of the visceral microcirculation with *P. falciparum*–infected erythrocytes, a reflection of that organism's ability to invade a large proportion of the nonimmune patient's red blood cells and the selective adhesion of these cells to the vascular endothelium of capillaries and postcapillary venules. Although the process involves all deep tissues, it is most intense in the brain. Infants, children, pregnant women, travelers to endemic regions, and other nonimmune or immunocompromised subjects in whom the parasitemia rate may exceed 100,000 per cubic millimeter are most commonly involved.

Metabolic changes   Local tissue hypoxia in the regions of abnormal microcirculatory flow is presumed to mediate most pathologic events seen in severe falciparum malaria. Lactic acidosis resulting from anaerobic glycolysis in both host and parasite may be lethal. The large metabolic requirements of the plasmodia in pregnant women and other patients with a large parasite burden may produce a profound and recurrent hypoglycemia; quinine-induced hyperinsulinemia often aggravates this problem.

IMMUNITY   The immune response to malaria, which controls nonlethal infections and eventually confers protection to reinfection, is incompletely understood. In simian malaria, it appears to require the presence of both T- and B-cell lymphocytes. Although the role of the T cell is known to be vital, its mechanism of action is uncertain. Some authors have suggested that it stimulates effector cells, probably macrophages, to release nonspecific factors capable of damaging or destroying intraerythrocytic parasites; it may also have a helper effect on antibody formation.

Strain-specific antiplasmodial antibodies do occur early in the course of parasitemia and reach high levels coincident with a fall in the number of circulating organisms. The relative rarity of malaria in young infants has been attributed to transplacental passage of IgG antibodies. Although the presence of such antibodies does not reliably predict immunity, in vitro studies have shown them to be capable of blocking merozoite invasion, inhibiting intracellular growth, and opsonizing both merozoites and infected erythrocytes. In simian malaria, antigenic change in the parasite results in cycles of recrudescent parasitemia and production of variant-specific antibodies. It seems probable that similar changes occur in humans, leading to the eventual disappearance of erythrocytic forms. In falciparum malaria,

this results in cure. In vivax and ovale infections, the intracellular hepatic forms escape the humoral immune defenses and may later discharge fresh merozoites into the bloodstream to maintain the infection for a period of 3 to 5 years. *Plasmodium malariae* produces chronic disease of extremely long duration, up to 53 years in one case, despite the lack of a persistent exoerythrocytic focus. This effect is presumably due to long-term survival of circulating parasites in concentrations too low to be detected on routine blood films. How these parasites escape immunologic destruction is unknown. In a closely related simian malaria, however, splenectomy rapidly leads to termination of infection, suggesting that suppressor T cells in the spleen may play a protective role.

MANIFESTATIONS   General   The incubation period between the bite of the mosquito and onset of symptoms is usually 10 to 14 days in vivax and falciparum malaria and 18 days to 6 weeks in malariae infections. This period may be prolonged in certain vivax infections acquired in temperate climates and in persons who have taken antimalarial suppressants. In the United States, the interval between entry into the country and onset of disease exceeds 6 months in one-quarter of the patients developing vivax infections; it exceeds 1 month in a similar proportion of falciparum cases. There is some variation in clinical manifestations produced by the different plasmodia in nonimmune hosts, but in all, chills, fever, headache, muscle pains, splenomegaly, and anemia are common. Herpes labialis is frequent and usually appears after the infection is well established. Hepatomegaly, mild icterus, and edema are often observed, especially in falciparum infections. Urticaria is common in patients with chronic malaria.

The hallmark of the disease is the malarial *paroxysm*, which recurs regularly in all but falciparum infections. The typical paroxysm begins with a rigor that lasts 20 to 60 min—the "cold stage"—followed by a "hot stage" of 3 to 8 h with temperature of 40 to 41.7°C (104 to 107°F). The "wet stage" consists of defervescence with profuse diaphoresis and leaves the patient exhausted.

First attacks are often severe, and, if untreated, may persist for weeks. The paroxysms eventually become more irregular and less frequent and finally, with the disappearance of parasites from the blood, cease altogether, marking the end of the primary attack. Relapses occur when hypnozoites persisting in the liver reinvade the bloodstream. In hyper- and holoendemic areas (e.g., West Africa), where parasite transmission is intense and constant, individuals first acquire malaria at approximately 6 months of age following the decline of maternal antibody. If the infected child survives the primary attack, subsequent reinfections become progressively milder, although debilitation may persist and become progressive; by adulthood chronically infected individuals are usually afebrile and, at times, may be entirely asymptomatic. This hard-won immunity is readily lost. If an individual leaves an endemic area and returns several years later, reinfection again results in symptomatic disease. In those areas of the world where transmission is intermittent, or when nonimmune individuals migrate from nonendemic to endemic areas, symptomatic and sometimes fatal infections develop in adult life.

Tertian malaria (*P. vivax* or *P. ovale*)   This infection is rarely fatal, although relapses are common, and it is the most difficult to cure. A prodrome of myalgia, headache, chilliness, and low-grade fever for 48 to 72 h heralds the onset of the acute illness. Initially, the fever may be irregular because the maturation cycle of the parasite is not synchronized. Synchronization usually occurs toward the end of the first week, and typical paroxysms then occur on alternate days. The spleen becomes palpable at the end of the second week. Infections with *P. ovale* tend to be milder, and primary attacks shorter than those caused by *P. vivax*.

Quartan malaria (*P. malariae*)   Paroxysms occur every third day and tend to be regular. The disease is usually the mildest and most chronic of the malarias but responds well to treatment. Edema, albuminuria, and hematuria (*not* hemoglobinuria), a clinical state similar to acute hemorrhagic nephritis, occasionally appear during the course. This complication should not be confused with *blackwater fever*. Chronic *P. malariae* infection may be associated with a clinically and histologically unique nephrosis. Granular deposits of IgG, IgM, C3 component of complement, and *P. malariae* antigens have been noted along the glomerular basement membrane, establishing this as an immune-complex nephropathy. The prolonged duration of asymptomatic parasitemia characteristic of the species helps to explain the frequency with which it is implicated in transfusion-induced malaria. There appears to be positive association between *P. falciparum* and *P. malariae* parasitemias in Africa. Within a given individual, the former is more frequent during the dry season and the latter during the wet season.

Falciparum malaria (*P. falciparum*) Because of an asynchronous cycle of multiplication, the onset may be insidious and fever continuous, remittent, or irregular. Typical paroxysms occur in a minority of patients. Splenomegaly appears rapidly, and headache, mental confusion, postural hypotension, edema, and gastrointestinal symptoms are common. If the acute attack is treated rapidly, the disease is usually mild and recovery uneventful. If left untreated in a nonimmune individual, sequestration of infected red blood cells in the deep tissues can give rise to serious complications. This should be anticipated if the intensity of parasitemia exceeds 100,000 organisms per cubic millimeter. Clinical warning signs include severe anemia, jaundice, hyperventilation, and evidence of central nervous system dysfunction such as delirium, stupor, or coma. Depending upon the organ system involved, one or more of the following *pernicious syndromes* may develop:

Cerebral malaria, the most important complication of falciparum malaria, is a symmetric encephalopathy that presents as unarousable coma in a patient without focal neurologic findings. Convulsions occur in half of all adults and the majority of children. Disturbances in conjugate gaze, alterations in tone, and extensor plantar responses are common; abdominal reflexes are invariably absent. Abnormal posturing may occur. Retinal hemorrhages are found in 13 percent of adults. The cerebrospinal fluid is usually under normal pressure and papilledema is rare. The mortality rate in adults is 20 percent. Most deaths occur within 3 days of admission and are associated with multiorgan dysfunction. Poor prognostic signs include deep coma, infection of more than 5 percent of all red blood cells, a total white blood cell count over 10,000 per cubic millimeter, and evidence of renal impairment. The major differential diagnoses include viral and bacterial meningoencephalitis, postictal states following febrile convulsions in children, and the obtundation and delirium commonly found with high fever. These conditions are relatively easy to exclude in a nonimmune adult. However, because asymptomatic malarial infections are common in endemic areas, the finding of *P. falciparum* in the blood smear of an immune, comatose patient does not definitively establish the diagnosis of cerebral malaria.

Unlike most of the life-threatening complications of falciparum malaria which typically are present on admission, *acute pulmonary insufficiency* may not develop until the third or fourth day of therapy. Nevertheless, it is highly lethal, killing approximately 80 percent of those involved. Pulmonary distress frequently accompanies cerebral malaria; pregnant women and patients with intense parasitemia are also at increased risk. Although overhydration is responsible for this syndrome in some patients, the pulmonary capillary wedge pressure is normal in most. This suggests that the major pathogenic mechanism is a malaria-induced change in the pulmonary capillary bed, not unlike that found in the adult respiratory distress syndrome (ARDS). Pathologic studies performed in patients dying with respiratory distress have demonstrated marked swelling of the pulmonary endothelial cells with narrowing of the capillary lumen, septal edema, and the presence of interstitial macrophages harboring phagocytized malaria pigment.

The splanchnic capillaries can become obstructed with consequent vomiting, abdominal pain, diarrhea, or melena. Such patients are sometimes thought to have bacillary dysentery or cholera. Hepatic dysfunction leads to a reduction in clotting factor synthesis, reduced

clearance of antimalarial drugs, and impaired gluconeogenesis, and contributes to the jaundice seen in severe falciparum malaria. Marked dysfunction resulting in "liver failure" seldom occurs. Fever in patients with predominantly gastrointestinal manifestations may be low or absent.

The blood urea nitrogen (BUN) is commonly elevated in severe falciparum malaria. Dehydration, increased protein catabolism, and transient renal impairment all contribute. The BUN and serum creatinine fall to normal levels in most patients following appropriate rehydration and antimalarial treatment. A serum creatinine level of more than 3 μg/mL on admission, urine output of less than 400 mL in the first 24 h of hospital stay, and the presence of another *pernicious syndrome* strongly suggest the patient has developed acute tubular necrosis. Recovery of renal function is usual provided the patient survives the acute phase of the disease and there are facilities for intensive care management and dialysis.

Blackwater fever This is a disorder that occurs in association with malaria, particularly and perhaps only with *P. falciparum* infections. The usual attack begins with a rigor and fever followed by massive intravascular hemolysis, icterus, hemoglobinuria, collapse, and often acute renal failure and uremia. The pathologic findings in the kidney are necrosis of tubules and occasionally hemoglobin casts. The mortality is 20 to 30 percent, and survivors are very likely to experience hemolytic episodes with subsequent malarial infections.

Although blackwater fever is often classified as one of the "pernicious" complications of falciparum malaria, its cause is obscure. In many patients, parasitemia is absent at the time hemolysis occurs. In the past blackwater fever has usually occurred in nonimmune or partially immune patients with falciparum infections who received quinine intermittently, suggesting that the hemolysis results from an autoimmune reaction to the red blood cells that have been altered by the drug, parasite, or both. However, blackwater fever can occur in patients with glucose 6-phosphate dehydrogenase (G6PD) deficiency who have received oxidant antimalarial therapy and in those with severe malaria prior to the initiation of treatment. The institution of an appropriate regimen for acute renal failure will reduce the fatality rate considerably.

Miscellaneous complications Rupture of the spleen is relatively rare, but malaria is by far the commonest cause of spontaneous rupture and predisposes to traumatic rupture of this organ. It is most commonly seen in vivax infections.

Chronic malaria or repeated infection in an endemic area leads to anemia, debility, cachexia, and macrophage and T cell–mediated immunosuppression. These manifestations are particularly severe in children under the age of 3. Falciparum malaria during pregnancy is extremely dangerous to both mother and fetus. The immunosuppression of pregnancy enhances parasite multiplication. Intense parasitemia with its associated complications, particularly hypoglycemia and acute pulmonary insufficiency, is common. Sequestration of parasitized erythrocytes in the placental circulation may lead to fetal distress and death. Surviving children have low birth weights and a high neonatal mortality. Congenital malaria, although rare, does occur; it is probably most common in the offspring of nonimmune individuals. Secondary bacterial infection is frequent and is often the immediate cause of death. Bacillary dysentery, cholera, and pyogenic pneumonia are common. Tuberculous foci often extend in malarial patients, and miliary tuberculosis is occasionally observed.

Patients living in endemic malarious areas commonly present with chronic hepatosplenomegaly of unknown cause. In some of these, there is infiltration of hepatic sinusoids by lymphocytes, very high levels of serum IgM, and high malaria antibody titers. This condition, which is known as the *tropical splenomegaly syndrome,* is seldom seen before the age of 8. It differs from the ordinary hepatosplenomegaly of malaria in that parasitemia is rare. It has been suggested that the condition results from defective T-cell control of immunoglobulin production, leading to excessive macroglobulin production and immune-complex formation. Long-term antimalarial therapy leads to a decrease in spleen size and a disappearance of hepatic sinusoidal lymphocytosis. The epidemiologic evidence implicating malaria as a contributory factor in the etiology of Burkitt's lymphoma has increased. It has been suggested that continuous stimulation of the lymphoid system in chronic malaria makes it more susceptible to neoplastic transformation in the presence of Epstein-Barr virus.

LABORATORY FINDINGS The blood leukocyte count is low or normal. The platelet count is often reduced, especially in falciparum malaria. The erythrocyte sedimentation rate is very high. Plasmodia are demonstrable in smears of peripheral blood from the vast majority of patients with symptomatic malaria. When the disease is suspected, appropriately stained blood films should be examined diligently. For the inexperienced examiner, a thin smear of fingertip blood on a clean glass slide should be stained with Wright's or Giemsa's stain. Parasitized erythrocytes are most frequent at the edges of a smear; extracellular parasites are not found. Thick smears should be thoroughly dried and stained with diluted Giemsa's or Field's stain. This method has the advantage of concentrating the parasites, but artifacts are numerous, and correct interpretations of these preparations require much experience.

The morphology of the four species of plasmodia that infect humans is specific enough to allow identification in blood smears. The parasitized red blood cells in *P. vivax* infections are enlarged and pale and may contain diffuse bright-red dots (Schüffner's dots), and the parasite presents in a wide variety of shapes and sizes; in *P. ovale* infections, the red blood cells containing parasites are oval but otherwise resemble those in *P. vivax;* in *P. malariae* the red blood cells are of normal size and do not contain dots. The parasites often present in "band" forms, and the merozoites are arranged in a rosette around central pigment; in *P. falciparum* infections the rings are very small, may contain two rather than one chromatin dot, and often are found lying flat against the margin of the cell. Only the ring stages of the asexual forms are found in the peripheral smear, and there may be more than one ring in a single red blood cell. The gametocytes are distinctively large and banana-shaped. A parasitemia of more than 2 percent is strongly suggestive of *P. falciparum* infection.

There is no advantage of blood over material obtained by splenic or sternal puncture. Serologic tests are used primarily for epidemiologic rather than diagnostic purposes but are also helpful in screening potential blood donors. The indirect immunofluorescent test seems to be the most sensitive and specific. Monoclonal antibodies and DNA probes have been shown to be capable of detecting extremely low levels of parasitemia. Their ultimate role in clinical diagnosis, epidemiologic studies, and blood screening remains to be determined.

DIAGNOSIS The most important diagnostic test is a careful medical history. The diagnosis must be considered in any febrile patient who has resided in or traveled to Haiti, Latin America, Asia, or Africa within the previous 12 months. History of previous attacks of malaria, typical malarial paroxysms, or some artificial exposure (blood transfusion, narcotic injections in an addict) should also suggest the disease. Splenomegaly is a very common finding during the second week of illness. Leukocytosis is *not* a feature of malaria. The diagnosis is confirmed by demonstrating the parasites in the peripheral blood. Because the intensity of parasitemia varies greatly from hour to hour, particularly in *P. falciparum* infections, blood smears should be examined repeatedly over 2 or 3 days before the diagnosis is abandoned.

While final cure of malaria may be difficult, particularly in *P. vivax* infections, almost all cases will respond symptomatically to quinine or one of the newer antimalarial drugs, and failure of response to a therapeutic trial argues strongly against the diagnosis.

TREATMENT The use of appropriate chemotherapy can suppress symptoms in individuals exposed in endemic areas or cure malarial infection completely. However, the emergence of drug-resistant falciparum malaria in southeast Asia, including Burma, Indonesia, and the Philippines, in the Indian subcontinent, South America, and east and central Africa necessitates the use of drug combinations in the treatment of this infection.

Treatment of acute attack Treatment of an acute attack can be accomplished with chloroquine for all types of malaria except drug-resistant falciparum infection (Table 154-1). The drug usually produces complete subsidence of symptoms and destruction of the erythrocytic forms of the parasite. If vomiting is present, chloroquine hydrochloride should be given intramuscularly or, in the case of shock, by slow intravenous infusion. Oral therapy should be resumed as soon as possible. Although side effects are uncommon, this agent may produce nausea, epigastric distress, agranulocytosis, and neurotoxicity, including involuntary movements and convulsion. Pruritus occurs in up to 50 percent of dark-skinned patients.

If patients have transfusion-induced malaria or have contracted the disease in an area known to harbor drug-resistant *P. falciparum,* they should be treated with quinine administered in combination with one or more additional antimalarial agents. In uncomplicated infections, quinine sulfate, an extremely bitter, unpleasant oral medication is given in a dose of 650 mg three times daily for 3 days. If nausea and vomiting, shock, or one of the pernicious syndromes preclude oral therapy, quinine dihydrochloride diluted in saline or glucose should be administered by slow intravenous therapy. This intravenous drug is no longer commercially available in the United States and must be obtained from the Centers for Disease Control. However, another cinchona alkaloid, the readily available antiarrhythmic agent quinidine gluconate, has proved to be a highly satisfactory substitute. Although roughly four times more cardiotoxic than quinine, quinidine

TABLE 154-1 Malaria treatment

Purpose	Drug	Dosage
Cure chloroquine-resistant *P. falciparum* infection	Quinine sulfate*	650 mg PO tid for 10–14 days
	or quinine dihydrochloride†	600 mg in 300 mL normal saline IV over 1 h; repeat in 6–8 h; maximum 1800 mg per day‡
	plus pyrimethamine	25 mg PO bid for 3 days
	plus sulfadiazine	500 mg PO bid for 5 days
	or quinine as above	
	plus tetracycline	250 mg qid for 7 days
	or quinine as above	
	plus clindamycin	900 mg tid for 3 days
Cure *P. malariae* and chloroquine-sensitive *P. falciparum* infection	Chloroquine phosphate	1 g (600-mg base) PO, then 500 mg in 6 h, then 500 mg per day for 2 days
	or chloroquine hydrochloride†	250 mg (200-mg base) IM or IV every 6 h; administer IV dose as for quinine dihydrochloride above; maximum 900 mg per day
Cure *P. vivax* and *P. ovale* infection	Same as for *P. malariae*	
	plus primaquine phosphate	26.3 mg (15-mg base) PO qd for 14 days

* *If quinine is not immediately available, begin with chloroquine and switch when quinine arrives.*
† *For use when patient cannot take oral drug. Switch to oral therapy as soon as possible. If quinine dihydrochloride is unavailable, quinidine gluconate can be used in the dose of 800 mg, administered as described for quinine. See text.*
‡ *In southeast Asia, loading dose should be 20 mg/kg.*

can be used safely in the treatment of malaria if careful electrocardiographic monitoring is employed. It should be started if quinine dihydrochloride is not immediately available. In critical situations, the initial dose of either drug should be doubled to achieve parasiticidal blood levels as rapidly as possible. Oral therapy should be instituted as soon as possible. Because only 20 percent of the drugs are cleared by the kidney, acute renal failure does not require immediate dose reduction. After the third day of therapy, however, the maintenance dose should be reduced by one-third if renal failure is established or the patient has failed to demonstrate clinical improvement. Even in the absence of overt kidney failure, concentrations of both quinine and quinidine may be high in severe malaria due to a decrease in the total apparent volume of distribution. When plasma concentrations exceed 5 µg/mL, tinnitus and then nausea, dysphonia, and occasionally deafness result. However, this symptom complex, known as "cinchonism," is seldom dose-limiting. Quinine-induced hyperinsulinemia with hypoglycemia may develop in pregnant women. Thrombocytopenic purpura, neuromuscular blockade, and fever are rare adverse effects. The appearance of a Coombs-positive hemolytic anemia requires the immediate withdrawal of the drug. Mefloquine, a quinoline methanol structurally related to quinine, has proved to be effective in chloroquine-resistant falciparum malaria, but is not licensed for use in the United States

Pyrimethamine plus one of the sulfonamides is the most commonly used supplemental agent. It is given orally in dosage of 25 mg two times daily for 3 days. Because pyrimethamine is an antifolate agent, it may cause megaloblastic anemia; folate supplementation should be provided for pregnant and poorly nourished patients. Sulfisoxazole or sulfadiazine, 2.0 g initially and then 0.5 g every 6 h for 5 days, should be given concurrently with the pyrimethamine and quinine. A variety of other combinations of antifolate agents and sulfonamides have also been used with quinine to good effect. Fansidar, a fixed drug combination containing 25 mg pyrimethamine and 500 mg sulfadoxine has been particularly effective. Tetracycline 250 mg qid for 7 days or clindamycin 900 mg tid for 3 days plus quinine are also acceptable combinations.

Patients with uncomplicated disease who are capable of taking oral medications do not require hospital admission unless pregnant, poorly nourished, or very young. All should be followed for 1 month to detect recrudescence of the infection. If there are circulating asexual erythrocytic forms, retreatment with pyrimethamine and a sulfonamide should be instituted. The presence of gametocytes is not, however, an indication for retreatment.

Radical cure *Plasmodium vivax* and *P. ovale* persist in the liver in the exoerythrocytic stage and in this form are not affected by drugs used in the treatment of the acute attack. Unless destroyed, they will eventually reinvade the bloodstream. Primaquine base, 15 mg by mouth daily for 14 days, will effect a radical cure in most cases. If relapse occurs after primaquine therapy, a second course of the drug at twice the dosage should be given. Alternatively, 45 mg primaquine base can be given in combination with 300 mg chloroquine once weekly for 8 weeks. Primaquine may cause oxidant hemolysis in patients with G6PD deficiency; this is less likely to occur if the drug is administered once weekly.

Treatment of severe falciparum malaria Patients with severe malaria require intensive monitoring and nursing care. Immediately after the diagnosis has been confirmed and the parasitemia quantitated, the patient should be weighed and an intravenous infusion of quinine, quinidine, or chloroquine begun. Blood should be drawn for culture, type and cross match, hematocrit, blood glucose, BUN, and creatinine. Arterial blood gases are also obtained if the patient shows evidence of hyperventilation, cyanosis, or postictal aspiration pneumonia. Unconscious patients should have a lumbar puncture to exclude bacterial meningitis.

Comatose patients should be nursed on their side, because vomiting and convulsion are common. Although their value has not been determined in severe malaria, prophylactic anticonvulsants are employed by some experts. Rectal temperature is kept below 38.5°C with tepid sponging, fanning, and nonaspirin antipyretics. Urine output should be monitored hourly. If there is any doubt as to the state of hydration or fluid balance, a central venous catheter is inserted and the patient cautiously rehydrated to maintain urine output. Because overly enthusiastic fluid administration can precipitate pulmonary edema, central venous pressure should be maintained below 5 cmH₂O. Patients whose oliguria advances to acute renal failure can be managed with either peritoneal or hemodialysis. Hemodialysis is preferred because there is some evidence that peritoneal solute clearance is decreased in falciparum infections; dialysis-induced peritonitis is also common in the rural tropics. Indications for dialysis are the same as those in any other hypercatabolic infection complicated by renal failure. If acute pulmonary insufficiency develops, it should be managed as ARDS, although if there is any possibility of volume overload, intravenous diuretics should be given. Blood transfusion is indicated when the hematocrit falls below 20 percent; whole fresh blood is preferable. There have been several case reports documenting the dramatic clinical recovery of patients with severe falciparum malaria and hyperparasitemia following exchange transfusion. This form of therapy should be considered if the parasite count exceeds 10 percent. Gastrointestinal bleeding may occur in severe disease, but the incidence appears to have decreased since use of heparin and corticosteroids has been discontinued. Although thrombocytopenia is usual, clinically significant disseminated intravascular coagulation is uncommon, occurring in less than 5 percent of cases of cerebral malaria. Dexamethasone, mannitol, urea, and heparin have been shown to be either deleterious or unhelpful in the treatment of cerebral malaria and should be avoided.

The response to treatment is assessed by resolution of abnormal physical signs (such as recovery of consciousness in cerebral malaria), defervescence, and clearance of parasitemia. Parasite counts should be checked at least twice daily until negative, and rechecked if fever recurs. Hypoglycemia or bacteremia should be suspected in any severely ill patient who fails to improve or suddenly deteriorates on treatment. The management of hypoglycemia is often difficult, as it tends to recur, particularly in the presence of quinine-induced hyperinsulinemia.

PREVENTION   General   In areas of the world such as Africa where eradication is presently impractical, limited residual insecticides plus chemoprophylaxis for pregnant women and children are recommended. The long-term hope for eradication depends on the introduction of new technologies. Until recently, the development of a practical and effective vaccine has been hampered by the lack of a suitable in vitro culture system for plasmodia, difficulty in identifying the parasitic antigens responsible for the induction of protective immunity, and the wide antigenic differences found between malaria species, strains, and even life cycle stages. The achievement of continuous culture of *P. falciparum* in red blood cells and the application of monoclonal antibody and recombinant DNA procedures to the characterization of plasmodial antigens has permitted identification of short repeated amino acid sequences in the polypeptide surface coat of all falciparum sporozoites that are capable of stimulating the production of protective antibodies. These peptides have now been artificially synthesized and coupled with a carrier molecule to produce a "sporozoite" vaccine; it is anticipated that field trials will be conducted in the near future. Work on merozoite and gametocyte-based vaccines continues.

Personal protection   The traveler to malarious areas should attempt to reduce the frequency of mosquito bites by avoiding exposure at peak feeding times (usually early morning or evening), use of house screens, bed netting, insect repellents, pyrethrum-containing insect spray, and appropriate clothing. In addition, chemoprophylaxis should be utilized as described below.

Chemoprophylaxis (Table 154-2)   Although it is not possible to prevent infection with chemotherapeutic agents, it is possible to

TABLE 154-2 Malaria chemoprophylaxis

Purpose	Drug	Dosage
To suppress clinical malaria in areas *without* chloroquine-resistant strains	Chloroquine phosphate	500 mg (300 mg base) PO once weekly, continued 6 weeks after leaving malarious area
	or amodiaquine dehydrochloride	520 mg (400 mg base) PO once weekly, continued 6 weeks after leaving malarious area
To suppress clinical malaria in areas *with* chloroquine-resistant strains	Same as above	
	plus pyrimethamine-sulfadoxine* (Fansidar, Hoffmann-LaRoche)	25 mg pyrimethamine and 500 mg sulfadoxine PO once weekly, continued 6 weeks after leaving malarious area
	or mefloquine	250 mg PO once weekly, continued 6 weeks after leaving malarious area
To prevent relapses of *P. vivax* and *P. ovale* infection	Primaquine phosphate†	26.3 mg (15-mg base) PO daily for 14 days or 79 mg (45-mg base) for 8 weeks; start during last 2 weeks of suppressive therapy or immediately upon its completion

* Given only in areas of intense exposure as described in the text.
† Recommended only for travelers without G6PD deficiency who have had heavy exposure.

suppress symptoms while the patient is residing in an endemic area with the use of appropriate drugs. Because of its safety and efficacy, chloroquine remains the drug of choice for travelers to all malarious areas. Cases of retinopathy have been reported in patients who have taken this agent in prophylactic dosage over periods of 5 to 20 years. This, however, is rare, and the danger to individuals planning shorter stays in malarious areas is probably nonexistent. It is recommended that chloroquine be initiated 1 or preferably 2 weeks prior to departure for an endemic area. This allows time for the early adverse effects to develop and for therapeutic blood concentrations to be achieved. If this is not possible, the prophylactic dose should be doubled for the first few weeks in the malarious zone. Travelers must be warned that protection is not complete, and that malaria should be considered in the differential diagnosis of any febrile illness developing during the stay in an endemic area. Following departure from an endemic area, chloroquine should be continued for an additional 6 weeks. This will eradicate *P. malariae* and sensitive strains of *P. falciparum*. The hepatic forms of *P. ovale* and *P. vivax* will not be affected, however, and may produce relapse with clinical manifestations some weeks or months after chloroquine is discontinued. This can be circumvented by administration of primaquine during the final 2 weeks of chloroquine administration.

Chloroquine is not effective in suppressing chloroquine-resistant *P. falciparum* (CRPF) infections. Nevertheless, it should be used by travelers to malarious areas with CRPF because malaria caused by other plasmodium species that remain sensitive to chloroquine are also present in such areas. Fansidar, a fixed-combination tablet containing 25 mg of pyrimethamine and 500 mg of sulfadoxine, may be combined with the chloroquine for the suppression of CRPF. This is contraindicated in pregnant women, persons allergic to sulfonamides, and children under 2 months. Leukopenia and megaloblastic anemia is a hazard of long-term pyrimethamine therapy. Several cases of severe cutaneous reactions (erythema multiforme, Stevens-Johnson syndrome, and toxic epidermal necrolysis) have been documented among American travelers using pyrimethamine-sulfadoxine prophylaxis. Because of the potential untoward effects related to the prophylactic administration of this agent, it should be reserved for individuals planning prolonged visits to areas of intense CRPF transmission. These include the CRPF areas of Africa, Oceania (Papua, New Guinea, Irian Jaya, the Solomon Islands, and Vanuatu) and certain rural areas of China, southeast Asia, and South America. For visits of 3 weeks or less to these areas, a therapeutic dose of Fansidar can be carried with the traveler for presumptive treatment of any febrile illness occurring during travel when professional medical care is not readily available. The serious cutaneous side effects reported during Fansidar prophylaxis have not been seen with single-dose therapy.

Of the several alternatives to Fansidar for CRPF prophylaxis, mefloquine, the methanol quinoline mentioned in the treatment section above, holds the most promise. Both safe and effective, it has been used extensively in southeast Asia where Fansidar-resistant falciparum

malaria is common. It has not yet been approved for use in the United States and its availability in other areas of the world is still limited. Amodiaquine, a 4-aminoquinoline related to chloroquine, may provide somewhat more protection than chloroquine against African strains of CRPF. Although not marketed in the United States, it is widely available in Africa.

Transfusions Transfusion malaria continues to occur in the United States; *P. malariae* and *P. falciparum* have been the most common causes. Adherence to recommendations of the American Association of Blood Banking will prevent most of these cases.

REFERENCES

Bruce-Chwatt LJ: Man against malaria; conquest or defeat. Trans R Soc Trop Med Hyg 73:517, 1979

Drugs for parasitic infections. Med Lett 26:27, 1984

Galbraith RM et al: The human materno-faetal relationship in malaria. Trans R Soc Trop Med Hyg 74:52 and 61, 1980

Guerrero IC et al: Transfusion malaria in the United States, 1972–1981. Ann Intern Med 99:221, 1983

Harinasuta T et al: Trials of mefloquine in vivax and of mefloquine plus "Fansidar" in falciparum malaria. Lancet 1:885, 1985

Lobel HO et al: Recent trends in the importation of malaria caused by *Plasmodium falciparum* into the United States from Africa. J Infect Dis 152:613, 1985

Looareesuwan S et al: Quinine and severe falciparum malaria in late pregnancy. Lancet 2:4, 1985

Luzzatto L: Genetics of red cells and susceptibility to malaria. Blood 54:961, 1979

Macpherson GG et al: Human cerebral malaria: A quantitative ultrastructural analysis of parasitized erythrocyte sequestration. Am J Pathol 119:385, 1985

McLaughlin GL et al: Detection of *Plasmodium falciparum* using a synthetic DNA probe. Am J Trop Med Hyg 34:837, 1985

Miller LH: Hypothesis on the mechanism of erythrocyte invasion by malaria merozoites. Bull WHO 55:157, 1977

Molineaux L, Gramiccia G: *The Garki Project. Research on the Epidemiology and Control of Malaria in the Sudan Savanna of West Africa.* Geneva, WHO, 1980

Nielson RL et al: The use of exchange transfusions: A potentially useful adjunct in the treatment of fulminant falciparum malaria. Am J Med Sci 277:325, 1979

Phillips RE et al: Intravenous quinidine for the treatment of severe falciparum malaria: Clinical and pharmacokinetic studies. N Engl J Med 312:1273, 1985

Revised recommendations for preventing malaria in travelers to areas with chloroquine-resistant *Plasmodium falciparum.* Morb Mort Week Rep 34(14):185, 1985

Stilma JS: Chloroquine retinopathy in a rural hospital in Ghana. Trop Geogr Med 32:221, 1980

Warrell DA et al: Dexamethasone proves deleterious in cerebral malaria: A double blind trial in 100 comatose patients. N Engl J Med 306:313, 1982

Watkins WM et al: Effectiveness of amodiaquine as treatment for chloroquine-resistant *Plasmodium falciparum* infections in Kenya. Lancet 1:357, 1984

Wyler DJ: Malaria—resurgence, resistance and research. N Engl J Med 308:875 and 934, 1983

Zavala F et al: Rationale for development of a synthetic vaccine against *Plasmodium falciparum* malaria. Science 228:1463, 1985

155 LEISHMANIASIS

RICHARD M. LOCKSLEY / JAMES J. PLORDE

DEFINITION Four major clinical syndromes are caused by protozoa of the genus *Leishmania*—visceral leishmaniasis (kala azar), cutaneous leishmaniasis of the old and new world, mucocutaneous leishmaniasis (espundia), and diffuse cutaneous leishmaniasis. These parasites of canines and rodents are transmitted from animal to human and occasionally from person to person by the bite of phlebotomine sandflies.

ETIOLOGY A large number of *Leishmania* species may infect humans. Morphologically these different organisms appear identical and are generally distinguished by clinical and geographic characteristics. Definitive speciation may require determination of isoenzyme patterns, kinetoplast DNA buoyant densities, or specific phlebotomine vectors. Newer methods using monoclonal antibodies, DNA hybridization, and DNA restriction endonuclease fragment analysis are being evaluated.

In the sandfly and in culture media, *Leishmania* exist as motile, spindle-shaped promastigotes (1.5 to 4 μm by 14 to 20 μm) with a single anterior flagellum. On inoculation into a mammalian host the organisms enter mononuclear phagocytes, lose their flagella, and multiply as small (2 by 5 μm), oval, intracellular amastigotes (Leishman-Donovan bodies). In stained preparations a dark, slightly flattened nucleus and rod-shaped kinetoplast may be discerned.

EPIDEMIOLOGY Leishmaniasis is a zoonotic infection which involves the rodents and canines of every inhabited continent except Australia. The prevalence varies; 4 to 10 percent of dogs in the Mediterranean littoral and 80 to 95 percent of the gerbils in the southern U.S.S.R. are infected, many subclinically. The disease is spread when female sandflies of the genus *Phlebotomus* (old world) or *Lutzomyia* (new world) ingest amastigotes while taking a blood meal from an infected mammal. These transform into promastigotes within the insect's gut, migrate to the proboscis, and are deposited on the skin of the new host when the insect next engorges. Phlebotomines breed in warm, humid microclimates and are typically found in rodent burrows, termite hills, and rotting vegetation. Humans may acquire the disease when they encroach upon this sylvatic cycle. Establishment of infection in the domestic dog provides an important urban reservoir of leishmaniasis. Person-to-person transmission is infrequent except in the Indian form of kala azar. Rarely, transmission can occur by blood transfusion, contact inoculation, and coitus. It is estimated that worldwide over 12 million people are infected with these parasites.

PATHOGENESIS Promastigotes are deposited on the skin into a small pool of blood drawn by the probing sandfly. The organisms fix complement onto their surface by the alternative pathway, and rapidly enter macrophages via the type 3 complement receptor (CR3) and the mannosyl/fucosyl receptor. The promastigotes transform into amastigotes within phagolysosomes and replicate by binary fission. They eventually rupture the cell and invade adjacent macrophages.

The course of the subsequent disease is determined by the host's cellular immunity as well as the species of the parasite. In cutaneous leishmaniasis, there is a marked lymphocytic infiltration associated with a reduction in the number of parasites, the development of a delayed skin (leishmanin) reaction, and, frequently, spontaneous cure. In mucocutaneous disease, the complete or partial resolution of the primary lesion may be followed by metastatic mucocutaneous lesions at some later date. The destructiveness of the metastatic lesions is attributed to the development of hypersensitivity to parasite antigens. An exception to the general pattern in cutaneous disease is diffuse cutaneous leishmaniasis in which there is no infiltration of lymphocytes and plasma cells or reduction in the number of parasites, the leishmanin reaction remains negative, and the skin lesions become chronic, progressive, and disseminated. The patients appear to have a selective anergy to leishmania antigens which is mediated at least in part by adherent suppressor cells. In visceral leishmaniasis, the cellular changes are similar, but the parasites spread to macrophages throughout the body, perhaps due to the greater resistance of *L. donovani* to the spontaneous cidal activity present in normal serum. Although antibodies are present, they are nonprotective. The ability of the organism to cause progressive disease may be related to the development in the host of suppressor T lymphocytes. Cure of leishmaniasis confers immunity to the infecting strain.

DIAGNOSIS Establishing a diagnosis of leishmaniasis requires demonstrating the organism by smear or culture of aspirates or tissue. Although Novy-MacNeal-Nicolle (NNN) medium traditionally has been used to culture *Leishmania,* several commercially available liquid media offer improved storage capability and enhanced recovery of organisms. Cultures are maintained at 22 to 28°C for 21 days and examined microscopically for the presence of the motile promastigotes. Inoculation of hamsters with infected clinical material results in infections after a period of months.

Species-specific diagnosis of human cutaneous new world isolates has been achieved by hybridization of tissue touch blots with radiolabeled kinetoplast DNA probes, but the method is not readily available.

Antibodies are detectable in all forms of leishmaniasis. The direct agglutination test[1] detects IgM antibody and is a sensitive indicator of acute disease. The test is group-specific, but the titer is generally greatest to the homologous strain. A positive test (>1:32) varies from 97 percent in visceral leishmaniasis to 81 percent in new world cutaneous leishmaniasis. Other serologic tests, including complement fixation, hemagglutination, microenzyme-linked immunoabsorbent assays, and indirect immunofluorescence, are less commonly available. Direct agglutination antibodies decline and may disappear with cure.

VISCERAL LEISHMANIASIS (KALA AZAR) *Leishmania donovani* causes kala azar, a disease that may be endemic, epidemic, or sporadic. Although the characteristics of the disease are similar throughout the world, certain local peculiarities in its behavior justify the classification of visceral leishmaniasis into three main types. These differences are attributed principally to the length of time that the disease has been endemic in a population.

African kala azar is found in the eastern half of Africa from the Sahara in the north to the equator in the south. Sporadic cases have been reported from west Africa. It is a disease of older children and young adults (10 to 25 years); males are involved more commonly than females. It is endemic in dogs and several wild carnivores in many areas and is more resistant to therapy with antimony compounds than the forms of kala azar found in the rest of the world.

Mediterranean, or infantile, kala azar, is seen primarily in the Mediterranean area, China, U.S.S.R., and Latin America. It is a disease of children under the age of 4, but adults, particularly travelers to endemic areas, are not spared. Dogs, jackals, and foxes serve as reservoirs. Rats have been identified as a potential reservoir in Italy. The strains responsible for the Eurasian and American disease are sometimes referred to as *L. infantum* and *L. chagasi,* respectively.

Indian kala azar has an age and sex distribution similar to African kala azar. Humans are the only known reservoir, and transmission is carried out by anthropophilic sandflies.

Manifestations The incubation period is generally about 3 months (3 weeks to 18 months). A primary cutaneous lesion (leishmanioma) is not uncommon in Africa. The onset of disease may be insidious or abrupt; the latter occurs more frequently in individuals from nonendemic areas. Fever, typically nocturnal and occasionally double-quotidian, is almost universal and is accompanied by tachycardia without signs of toxemia. Daily fever progresses to recurrent febrile

---

[1] *The leishmanin skin test (Montenegro test), performed by the intradermal injection of promastigote antigens, is nonstandardized and generally unavailable.*

waves. Diarrhea and cough are frequent. Nontender splenomegaly becomes dramatic by the third month. The liver enlarges less conspicuously. Cirrhosis and portal hypertension occur in about 10 percent of patients. Lymphadenopathy accompanies some cases of African kala azar. Atypical forms, including isolated tonsillar infections and cervical adenopathy, have been reported. Asymptomatic or subclinical disease has been suspected.

Pancytopenia is characteristic. Anemia is multifactorial: autoimmune hemolysis, splenomegaly, and gastrointestinal blood loss all contribute. The latter is exacerbated by thrombocytopenia. Agranulocytosis, cancrum oris, and superinfections complicate untreated cases. Extensive leishmanial infiltration of the gastrointestinal tract may lead to malabsorption. Hypoalbuminemia and polyclonal hypergammaglobulinemia (IgG and IgM) are constant features. Circulating immune complexes are frequently present. Immune-complex glomerulonephritis and interstitial nephritis have been described. Amyloidosis may occur in patients with chronic infections. Edema, cachexia, and hyperpigmentation (kala azar means ''black fever'') are late manifestations. Without treatment death occurs within 3 to 20 months in 90 to 95 percent of adults and 75 to 85 percent of children, usually due to superinfections or gastrointestinal hemorrhage.

After successful treatment, 3 percent of African cases and up to 10 percent of Indian cases develop post-kala azar dermal leishmaniasis (PKDL), characterized by a spectrum of lesions ranging from depigmented macules to wartlike nodules over the face and extensor surfaces of the limbs. PKDL appears shortly after symptoms subside in African cases and typically disappears after several weeks. In the Indian disease, PKDL appears after a latent period of 1 to 2 years and may last for years, creating a persistent human reservoir.

Diagnosis Buffy coat preparations may demonstrate the parasite, particularly in Indian kala azar (90 percent). Bone marrow aspirate and biopsy are positive in over 85 percent of cases. In Kenya, splenic aspiration (95 percent) has proved quite safe and has been used serially to assess the response to therapy. In general, however, aspiration of the spleen or liver (75 percent) is not recommended because of the risk of fatal hemorrhage. Aspirates or biopsy of enlarged lymph nodes will show parasites in 60 percent of cases. Suspicious skin lesions should be biopsied as well. The direct agglutination test is positive early in the disease. The leishmanin skin test becomes positive 6 to 8 weeks after recovery. Other causes of fever in the tropics, including malaria, brucellosis, tuberculosis, typhoid, and hepatic abscess, can be distinguished by appropriate testing. PKDL must be differentiated from leprosy, syphilis, and yaws.

Treatment Transfusions and treatment of complicating superinfections must supplement specific therapy. Pentavalent antimonials are highly effective against leishmania and are relatively nontoxic. Sodium antimony gluconate (Pentostam;[2] 100 mg Sb^{5+} per milliliter) is given intravenously or intramuscularly in a single daily dose of 10 mg/kg for adults and 20 mg/kg for patients under 18 years of age. Treatment should be given for at least 20 days in Indian kala azar and 30 days in other forms. Meglumine antimoniate (Glucantime; 85 mg Sb^{5+} per milliliter) can also be used. Therapy should be repeated using 20 mg/kg for 40 to 60 days in patients with relapses or incomplete responses. The addition of oral allopurinol (20 to 30 mg/kg per day in three divided doses) has been effective. Resistant cases must be treated with intravenous amphotericin B (0.5 to 1 mg/kg on alternate days) or pentamidine (3 to 4 mg/kg three times per week for 5 to 25 weeks, depending on the response). Adjunctive splenectomy has been successful in some cases of drug-resistant kala azar. Mortality remains 15 to 25 percent in advanced cases, although the cure rate is over 90 percent when therapy is given early. Follow-up at 3 and 12 months is recommended to detect relapses. PKDL should be treated in the same fashion as the initial illness.

[2] *Available from the Centers for Disease Control, Atlanta, Georgia.*

Prevention Preventive measures include early treatment of human cases, elimination of diseased dogs, and the use of DDT against sandflies. Application of insect repellents and the use of fine netting are important for travelers. There are no useful prophylactic agents.

CUTANEOUS AND MUCOCUTANEOUS LEISHMANIASIS This form of leishmaniasis is caused by a number of species in both the old world and the new world. Disease is characterized by the development of single or multiple localized lesions on exposed areas of skin that typically ulcerate. Although spontaneous healing is the rule for old world cutaneous leishmaniasis, this is less common in new world disease.

Old world cutaneous leishmaniasis *L. tropica* causes anthroponotic (urban, chronic, dry) cutaneous leishmaniasis, an endemic disease of children and young adults in areas bordering the Mediterranean, the Middle East, the southern U.S.S.R., and India. The principal reservoirs are humans, although domestic dogs are synanthropic hosts. The incubation period ranges from 2 to 24 months. Usually the lesion begins as a single, red pruritic papule on the face (oriental sore). The central area ulcerates and slowly enlarges centrifugally, reaching a size of approximately 2 cm. Lymphadenopathy is unusual. Healing occurs over 1 to 2 years and leaves a small depigmented scar. The disease can be complicated by the development of leishmaniasis recidiva, a condition marked by persistent facial lesions containing a scant number of parasites, and by an exaggerated delayed hypersensitivity response to parasite antigens. Rarely, the organism may spread to the viscera.

L. major causes zoonotic (rural, acute, moist) cutaneous leishmaniasis, which is endemic to the desert areas of the Middle East, the southern U.S.S.R., and Africa. The reservoir is maintained in burrowing rodents. The incubation period ranges from 2 to 6 weeks. The initial lesions are often multiple and located on the lower extremities. Regional lymphadenopathy and satellite lesions are common. Healing with scarring occurs within 3 to 6 months. *L. major* has been implicated in cases of mucocutaneous leishmaniasis in Saudi Arabia. Although *L. major* confers immunity to *L. tropica*, the converse is not true.

L. aethiopica, maintained in rock hyraxes of the Ethiopian and Kenyan highlands, causes cutaneous leishmaniasis which may pursue a relatively prolonged course and can be complicated by the development of diffuse cutaneous leishmaniasis (see below).

DIAGNOSIS Lesions should first be cleansed with alcohol to reduce bacterial contamination, which hinders recovery of the organisms. Aspirates should be obtained from the outer edge of the ulcer. If the aspirated smears are negative, full-thickness skin biopsies from the ulcer margin should be taken for touch smears, histology, and culture. The direct agglutination test and the leishmanin skin test become positive within 4 to 6 weeks.

TREATMENT Specific therapy should be withheld in endemic areas until ulceration takes place, thereby conferring immunity. Exceptions include disfiguring or disabling lesions and lesions persisting for longer than 6 months. Treatment is with antimonials as described for kala azar, although shorter courses (10 days) are effective. Higher doses of antimony may be required for *L. aethiopica* infections (20 mg/kg twice a day for 30 days). Ulcers should be covered to prevent infection of vectors and other canine and human hosts.

New world cutaneous and mucocutaneous leishmaniasis Leishmania causing new world cutaneous disease is divided into subspecies within the *L. mexicana* and *L. braziliensis* groups. The natural reservoirs for these organisms include a wide variety of mammals inhabiting the forests of South and Central America. Organisms are transmitted to humans entering the jungle to gather chicle or to clear land for new settlements. Disease is most prevalent in the Amazon basin but occurs in most countries of the area. *L. mexicana* species are endemic in south-central Texas.

L.m. mexicana causes chiclero's ulcer, or bay sore. Chicle gatherers who work in forests during the rainy season when sandflies of Rhodesian disease. A severalfold increase in IgM globulins in the serum is of confirmatory value. Complement fixation, indirect fluorescent antibody, indirect hemagglutination, and enzyme-linked immunosorbent assay (ELISA) tests utilizing stable antigens are useful for screening patients in endemic areas. A card agglutination test for trypanosomiasis (CATT) can be performed on finger-stick blood within a few minutes. Positive serologic results must be confirmed by the direct demonstration of the parasite.

TREATMENT *Suramin* (Bayer 205, Antrypol) is the most effective agent before central nervous system involvement has occurred. The initial dose should be limited to 0.2 g intravenously because of possible idiosyncrasy. If there is no evidence of sensitivity, a full course of therapy can be instituted the following day. One gram (10 mL fresh 10% solution) is given intravenously on the first, third, seventh, fourteenth, and twenty-first days for a total of 5 g. If red blood cells, casts, or significant amounts of protein occur in the urine, therapy should be discontinued. Pentamidine given in water intramuscularly each day for 10 injections is also effective in early disease. The dose is 3 to 4 mg pentamidine base per kilogram for each injection. When the agent is given too rapidly by the intravenous route, it may cause hypotension.

Lumbar puncture should always be performed in patients who are about to undergo therapy for trypanosomiasis. If the central nervous system is involved, agents that will penetrate the blood-brain barrier must be used; for this purpose the most effective is *melarsoprol* (Mel B). This drug, an arsenic derivative of British antilewisite (BAL), is effective at all stages of the disease but is more toxic than suramin. It is given intravenously in the dose of 1.8 to 3.6 mg/kg on 3 consecutive days. This 3-day course is repeated in 7 days and again after 10 to 21 days. In frail patients the initial dose should be limited to 18 mg; subsequent doses are progressively increased to the daily maximum described above. If signs of arsenic toxicity occur, the drug should be discontinued. A reactive encephalopathy, probably due to the release of trypanosomal antigen, occurs early in the course of treatment in 5 to 10 percent of patients; it is fatal in 1 to 5 percent. Pretreatment with suramin may help avert this complication. A hemorrhagic encephalopathy, a direct arsenic toxic reaction, may also occur and is usually fatal. BAL may be of some use in this situation. An experimental ornithine decarboxylase inhibitor, DL-α-difluoromethylornithine (DFMO), is undergoing clinical trial in Africa. It appears effective in acute trypanosomiasis and, when used in combination with suramin, curative in CNS infection. It appears free of serious side effects.

PROGNOSIS The disease is probably always fatal if untreated. If the infection is treated with suramin prior to central nervous system involvement, the cure rate is high and recovery is rapid and complete. When the nervous system becomes involved, the prognosis is less bright, and in far-advanced disease the survivors may suffer neurological damage. Relapses may occur, particularly following treatment with suramin, if the central nervous system was already involved at the time therapy was instituted. Less commonly they may be the result of drug resistance. Examination of the spinal fluid 6 and 12 months after therapy, or earlier if symptoms recur, is helpful in detecting relapse. Such patients must be re-treated with a second therapeutic agent.

PREVENTION Personal protection is achieved by the use of repellents and protective clothing. A single intramuscular injection of pentamidine in a dosage of 3 to 4 mg base per kilogram (maximum 300 mg) will protect against the Gambian form of disease for 6 months or more. Because of the danger of cryptic infections occurring during chemoprophylaxis, it has been generally restricted to populations or work groups at particularly high risk. Wide-scale disease control projects employ active surveillance and treatment of infected individuals to decrease the size of the human reservoir. Use of insecticide-impregnated traps after an initial application of a residual insecticide to resting sites of flies has proved effective in controlling tsetse fly densities. During acute outbreaks of disease, aerosol application of insecticides from aircraft can temporarily interrupt transmission.

CHAGAS' DISEASE

DEFINITION American trypanosomiasis is an infection caused by *T. cruzi* that is characterized by an acute, often asymptomatic illness followed, after a latent period that may span decades, by chronic cardiac and gastrointestinal sequelae.

ETIOLOGY *Trypanosoma cruzi* circulates in the blood as a slender, fusiform trypomastigote measuring 20 μm in length. In stained preparations, its narrow undulating membrane, large kinetoplast, and characteristic C shape are easily recognized. Unlike the trypanosomes of sleeping sickness, it does not multiply within the bloodstream. After invading tissue cells, it loses its undulating membrane and flagellum, assumes its amastigote form, and divides by binary fission. Eventually, new flagellated forms are produced which reenter the general circulation to initiate another cycle.

Strains of *T. cruzi* vary widely in their host preference, geographic distribution, virulence, and tissue tropism. They may be distinguished by specific antiserum, zymotype, and DNA restriction pattern.

EPIDEMIOLOGY This infection is found in scattered foci from Chile and Argentina to Mexico. Within these endemic areas it affects 15 to 20 million people and is the leading cause of heart disease, responsible for one-quarter of all deaths in the 25- to 44-year age group. *Trypanosoma cruzi* has been found in insect vectors and wild animals in several areas of the southern United States, and serologic studies have documented that acquisition of human infection occurs within this country. There are to date, however, only a handful of clinically apparent autochthonous cases reported from Texas and California.

The disease is transmitted to humans by reduviid ("assassin" or "kissing") bugs, primarily those of the genera *Triatoma, Panstrongylus,* and *Rhodnius.* These winged, hematophagous insects can be found in the burrows of animals and in the cracks and thatch of poorly constructed rural dwellings. The insect attacks human beings at night, usually biting the face at the mucocutaneous junction (most frequently the lip or outer canthus of the eye). The flagellated trypanosomes are ingested by the bug while feeding, and after multiplying and developing in the midgut of the insect for 8 to 10 days, are discharged in the feces following a subsequent feeding; human infection occurs through contamination of the bite wound. This is referred to as transmission by the "posterior station." The reduviid may remain infected as long as 2 years.

Human beings, domestic animals (cats and dogs), and wild animals, especially the opossum and armadillo, may serve as reservoirs for the infection. The close association of human beings, domestic animals, and the vector within human dwellings is of prime epidemiologic importance, but the disease is also transmitted by a blood transfusion and via the placenta to newborn infants. Occasional laboratory infections have also been reported.

PATHOGENESIS AND CLINICAL MANIFESTATIONS Only one-third of newly infected patients have clinical manifestations. In them a local inflammatory reaction, manifested clinically as an erythematous nodule or *chagoma,* appears within 1 to 3 weeks at the site of inoculation of the protozoan. If the portal of entry has been the conjunctiva, the presenting manifestations are a unilateral, painless conjunctivitis, palpebral edema, and preauricular lymphadenopathy (Romaña's sign). This primary complex may persist for 1 to 2 months during which parasites can be demonstrated in the lesion.

Following an incubation period of 2 weeks, trypanosomal forms reach the general circulation, producing a parasitemia and initiating the acute phase of the illness. After circulating in the blood for some time, the trypanosomes invade tissue cells of mesenchymal origin, assume the amastigote form, and multiply, producing intracellular pseudocysts. In 4 to 6 days these pseudocysts rupture, releasing both amastigotes and newly formed trypomastigotes. The amastigotes disintegrate, eliciting an intense inflammatory reaction, while the flagellated forms regain the bloodstream to maintain the infection and invade new tissues, particularly the heart, skeletal muscle, smooth muscle, and nervous system. *Trypanosoma cruzi* antigens can absorb to the surface of both normal and infected cells, possibly rendering them susceptible to destruction by the host's hormonal and cellular immune response.

Clinically, the patient experiences a continuous or recurrent fever, generalized lymphadenopathy, hepatosplenomegaly, and in some cases extensive gelatinous edema of the face and trunk. A transient morbilliform or urticarial skin eruption may occur early in the acute phase. Although trypanosomes frequently can be demonstrated in the cerebrospinal fluid at this time, acute meningoencephalitis is relatively rare; newborn infants and young children are affected most commonly. Myocarditis characterized by tachycardia and nonspecific electrocardiographic changes is very common. In severe cases, there may be conduction disturbances, cardiac dilatation, and heart failure. The duration of the acute illness is variable. In 5 to 10 percent of cases, meningoencephalitis or severe heart disease results in a fatal outcome within a few days or weeks. Most often, the disease, in response to the development of humoral antibody, resolves slowly over a period of several weeks. Parasites become extremely scanty in both the tissues and blood, the patient appears well, and the persistent infection is detectable only by serological means. Rarely, in the face of leukemia or immunosuppression, parasitemia and acute manifestations reappear. In the overwhelming majority of patients, however, the infection remains latent for the remainder of life. In approximately 10 percent, progressive immunologic destruction of mesenchymal tissue eventually leads to the development of chronic organ damage. Most patients presenting with late manifestations deny a history of acute illness, suggesting that subclinical infections often result in chronic disease. It has been suggested that host cell antigens released during the acute phase of the illness initiate an autoimmune inflammatory reaction, and antibodies reactive with endocardium, striated muscle, and vascular tissues have been described. Self-reactive cytotoxic lymphocytes have also been demonstrated in experimental animals, and lymphocytic infiltrates are commonly seen in patients dying of chagasic cardiopathy. Some authors have suggested that the late manifestations of disease are primarily due to neuropathies caused by the destruction of ganglionic nerve cells during this phase of the disease, resulting in the dilatation and malfunction of the affected organs.

The most important late manifestation is heart disease. Symptoms and signs range from precordial pain, arrhythmias, and heart block to chronic congestive heart failure (predominantly right-sided). Thromboembolic phenomena and sudden cardiac arrest are relatively common. Right bundle branch block and left anterior hemiblock, premature ventricular contractions, and inverted T waves are frequently seen on ECG. Echocardiography has been shown to be of value both in screening patients with infection for evidence of cardiac involvement and in following the progress of those with established cardiomyopathy. At autopsy the hearts of patients with Chagas' disease may show a peculiar herniation of the endocardium through the apical muscle bundles. Megacolon and megaesophagus are sequelae seen in southern South America. In patients with megaesophagus, regurgitation and aspiration pneumonia are common; the incidence of esophageal cancer is increased. Neurologic manifestations including mental deficiency and cerebellar symptoms also have been reported in chronic Chagas' disease.

DIAGNOSIS   The diagnosis depends on the demonstration of *T. cruzi* in the patient or upon serologic tests. In the acute phase of the disease the parasite may be seen in the peripheral blood by means of the same direct methods described for African trypanosomiasis. A microhematocrit concentration procedure has proved useful. If these are negative, blood may be cultured in a variety of artificial media, or inoculated into rats, mice, or guinea pigs.

Trypanosoma cruzi is easily grown in blood broth and incubated at 28°C. The technique of *xenodiagnosis* is often used in endemic areas; a laboratory-reared vector, known to be parasite-free, is allowed to feed on subjects with suspected cases, and 2 weeks later, the insect's intestinal contents are examined for parasites. Confusion sometimes arises from the finding of trypanosomes in blood. Many children in Venezuela and other South American countries are infected with a harmless species, *T. rangeli*, which produces no symptoms but may be present in the blood for many months. By utilization of both culture and xenodiagnosis repeatedly, organisms can be recovered from most acute cases and from up to 40 percent of chronic ones. Biopsy of an involved lymph node or calf muscle may reveal the organism during the initial illness when the parasites cannot be recovered from the blood. The Machado-Guerreiro test (a complement fixation reaction) is most helpful in the diagnosis of chronic cases and in survey work. Fluorescent antibody and hemagglutination inhibition tests appear more sensitive, but less specific. Rapid slide agglutination tests have been developed for use in blood banks. Most of these serologic tests employ crude epimastigote antigens which cross-react with serums from patients with leishmaniasis or *T. rangeli* infection. A new enzyme-linked immunosorbent assay utilizing a purified glycoprotein antigen eliminates these false-positive results.

TREATMENT AND PREVENTION   There is no satisfactory treatment for Chagas' disease. Several drugs shorten the period of parasitemia, prevent seroconversion, and decrease both the duration of symptoms and the mortality in acute Chagas' disease; there is some doubt whether any have the capacity to destroy intracellular parasites at tolerable doses. Nifurtimox, a nitrofurazone derivative given in the dose of 10 mg/kg per day in four divided doses for 3 or 4 months, shows the greatest promise, but is frequently associated with serious side effects. Benznidazole, a nitroimidazole not presently available in the United States, is similar in efficacy. Ketoconazole has shown significant effectiveness against intracellular amastigotes in experimental infections but has not been tested in humans. Chronic organ damage is generally thought irreversible.

Prevention consists of using residual insecticides on the walls and roofs of houses, the main habitat of the vectors. The addition of latex to the insecticide creates a colorless paint which significantly prolongs the activity of the insecticide. The use of fumigant canisters can prevent reinfestation. Patching wall cracks, cementing over dirt floors, and moving firewood piles away from human habitations will also dramatically decrease the concentration of reduviid vectors within the home. Transfusion infections can be prevented by adding gentian violet or one of its analogues to the blood. Leukemia patients from endemic areas should be serologically screened before immunosuppressive therapy is initiated.

REFERENCES

Sleeping sickness

CLARKSON AB et al: New drug combination for experimental late-stage African trypanosomiasis: DL-α-difluoromethylornithine (DFMO) with suramin. Am J Trop Med Hyg 33:1073, 1984

DONELSON JE, TURNER MJ: How the trypanosome changes its coat. Sci Am 252:44, 1985

MOLYNEUX DH: Selective primary health care: Strategies for control of disease in the developing world. VIII. African trypanosomiasis. Rev Infect Dis 5:945, 1983

SEED JR et al: A physiologic mechanism to explain pathogenesis in African trypanosomiasis. Contrib Microbiol Immunol 7:83, 1983

WERY M et al: Hematologic manifestations, diagnosis, and immunopathology of African trypanosomiasis. Semin Hematol 19:83, 1982

Chagas' disease

APT W et al: Natural history of chagasic cardiopathy in Chile. Follow-up of 71 cases after 4 years. J Trop Med Hyg 86:217, 1983

HAMMERMEISTER KE et al: Left ventricular wall motion in patients with Chagas' disease. Br Heart J 51:70, 1984

LORCA M et al: *Trypanosoma cruzi* in blood banks of 12 Chilean hospitals. Bull Pan Health Organ 17:269, 1983

MARSDEN PD: Selective primary health care: Strategies for control of disease in the developing world. XVI. Chagas' disease. Rev Infect Dis 6:855, 1984

MARTINI-CAMPOS JV, TAFURI WL: Chagas' enteropathy. Gut 14:910, 1973

MILES MA: The epidemiology of South American trypanosomiasis—biochemical and immunological approaches and their relevance to control. Trans R Soc Trop Med Hyg 55:5, 1983

Status of Chagas' disease in the region of the Americas. Epidemiol Bull 5:5, 1984

157 TOXOPLASMOSIS

RIMA McLEOD / JACK S. REMINGTON

DEFINITION The term *toxoplasmosis* refers to disease caused by the obligate intracellular protozoan *Toxoplasma gondii* and must be differentiated from the more common asymptomatic infection caused by this organism. The infection and disease in older children and adults are discussed below. The reader is referred to the reference by Remington and Desmonts for information on congenital toxoplasmosis.

ETIOLOGY *Toxoplasma gondii* is classified among the coccidia and exists in three forms: tachyzoite, cyst, and oocyst.

Tachyzoites *Tachyzoites* are crescent or oval, approximately 3 by 7 μm in size, and stain well with either Wright's stain or Giemsa's stain. Tachyzoites invade all mammalian cells except nonnucleated erythrocytes and are found in tissues during the acute stage of infection.

Cysts Tissue cysts are formed within host cells and may contain thousands of organisms. They are 10 to 100 μm in size and stain well with periodic acid Schiff stain; the cyst wall stains with silver stain. Cysts are important in transmission, as they may be present in animal tissues ingested by carnivores. They may persist in virtually every organ, but skeletal and heart muscle and the central nervous system appear to be the most common sites of chronic (latent) infection.

Oocysts Oocysts are oval and 10 to 12 μm in diameter. They are formed only in the mucosal cells of the intestines of members of the cat family and are subsequently excreted in the feces. The cat is the only animal in which the organism has a sexual cycle in the intestine, and cats have systemic infection with *T. gondii* as well. The time of appearance of oocysts in the feces depends on the form of the organism with which the cat becomes infected and varies from 3 to 24 days. Excretion continues for 7 to 20 days, and as many as 10 million oocysts are shed in the feces in a single day. Except under unusual conditions, once a cat has been infected and has excreted oocysts, it will not shed oocysts again. When a cat becomes infected with *Isospora felis,* renewed oocyst excretion has been reported to occur. Sporulation, which occurs from 2 to 3 days (at 24°C) after the oocysts are excreted, is required for the oocysts to become infectious and does not occur below 4°C or above 37°C. Oocysts may remain infectious for more than 1 year under favorable conditions (e.g., in warm, moist soil). They presumably play a major role in transmission by the oral route since their ingestion has been shown to transmit infection.

EPIDEMIOLOGY *Toxoplasma gondii* is ubiquitous and infects herbivorous, omnivorous, and carnivorous animals, including mammals, birds, and reptiles. Prevalence of infection varies with locale; prevalence of positive serologic reaction increases with age. In the United States, approximately 5 to 30 percent of individuals 10 to 19 years old and 10 to 67 percent of individuals over 50 years old have serologic evidence of infection. Generally, less infection occurs in cold regions, in hot and arid areas, and at high elevations. No particular genetic susceptibility has been documented for humans. Epidemics of toxoplasmosis have occurred in humans and in domestic animals. Simultaneous occurrence of infection in multiple members of the same household has been reported to occur commonly.

The natural mechanism of infection is by ingestion of cysts or oocysts or by transplacental transmission. Infection may also be acquired through blood transfusion, leukocyte transfusion, organ transplantation, and laboratory accident. Clinical illness due to reinfection from an exogenous source has not been reported.

Oral transmission Cysts are present in approximately 10 percent of lamb and 25 percent of pork used for human consumption; cysts have been isolated from beef, but their prevalence in beef has not been defined. Direct contact with any material contaminated by infected cat feces may result in ingestion of oocysts, and this form can be transmitted to food by insects. When humans or other animals (including cats) eat infected tissues (from any animal) or mature oocysts (excreted only by cats), the life cycle is completed. Approximately 1 percent of cats have been found to be excreting oocysts in their feces.

Transplacental transmission Accumulated data support the concept that *Toxoplasma* is transmitted to the fetus in utero when the pregnant woman acquires infection during the current pregnancy. Most often, when a mother is infected during pregnancy, the outcome is a normal uninfected infant, but spontaneous abortion, stillbirth, or delivery of a premature or full-term infected infant may result. Congenital infection will occur in approximately one-third of infants born to mothers who acquire their infection during the current pregnancy. In infants born to mothers infected during the first trimester, congenital infection is least common (approximately 17 percent) but disease is most severe; in infants born to mothers infected during the third trimester, congenital infection is most common (approximately 65 percent) but is usually asymptomatic. The fetus is at risk whether or not the infection is symptomatic in the mother.

The following are general guidelines for ascertaining the risk of transmission of the organism to the fetus of a woman who is known to have been infected *prior to the pregnancy in question.* If a woman acquires *Toxoplasma* infection more than 6 months before gestation, she will not deliver an infected infant. When conception occurs less than 6 months after acquisition of *Toxoplasma,* the risk to the fetus is exceedingly low, but transplacental transmission has been documented in this setting. *Toxoplasma* has been isolated on rare occasions from abortuses of women with chronic (latent) infection. The frequency of chronic *Toxoplasma* infection as a cause of abortion has not been defined and is the subject of considerable controversy.

Transmission by blood or leukocyte transfusion or organ transplantation *Toxoplasma* may be transmitted by blood or leukocyte transfusion. The organism has been isolated from leukocytes of individuals without recognized clinical evidence of *Toxoplasma* infection, and parasitemia has been reported to persist in otherwise normal individuals for as long as 1 year after acquisition of infection. The high incidence of isolation of the organism from the blood of patients who have chronic myelogenous leukemia and high antibody titers to *Toxoplasma* is particularly noteworthy. The organism has survived for 50 days in whole citrated blood stored at 4°C. Immunodeficient patients who require multiple blood transfusions may be particularly at risk for transmission of infection by this route. *Toxoplasma* has also been transmitted by transplantation of hearts from acutely infected donors to recipients who were not previously infected with *Toxoplasma.*

PATHOGENESIS Organisms released from cysts or oocysts enter cells of the gastrointestinal tract, multiply, cause cell disruption, and then infect neighboring cells. Extracellular organisms or organisms within leukocytes are transported throughout the body via the lymphatic system and bloodstream and are capable of invading every organ and tissue. Proliferation of tachyzoites usually leads to death of invaded cells, resulting in foci of necrosis, surrounded by an intense cellular reaction. The immune response of the host primarily governs the outcome of the acute process. Both humoral and cell-mediated immunity are important. In some apparently normal individuals and in immunodeficient patients, the acute infection may progress with acute necrotizing encephalitis, pneumonitis, or myocarditis which may be fatal. Tachyzoites disappear from the tissues with development of the normal immune response. Organisms may continue to proliferate and to cause destruction in the central nervous system and eye while they are disappearing from extraneural tissues because of the barrier to transfer of antibody in the eye and central nervous system.

A unique aspect of the infection is that organisms persist in cysts in many organs during the life span of the host. Either persistence of viable tachyzoites within cells of the reticuloendothelial system or disruption of cysts may be the source of the recurrent parasitemias that occur in some asymptomatic individuals with chronic infection. Cysts are the probable origin of the organisms that cause recrudescent disease in immunocompromised patients or chorioretinitis in older children and adults with congenital toxoplasmosis.

PATHOLOGY The histopathologic changes in toxoplasmic lymphadenitis are characteristic and consist of reactive follicular hyperplasia with irregular clusters of epithelioid histiocytes that have vesicular nuclei and abundant eosinophilic cytoplasm and that encroach upon and blur the margins of germinal centers; numerous mitoses in the germinal centers; many necrotic cells and an associated focal distention of subcapsular and trabecular sinuses with monocytoid cells. Tachyzoites or cysts are only rarely observed in conventionally stained sections.

Single or multiple foci of necrosis occur as the earliest manifestations of involvement of the eye. Infiltrates are composed largely of lymphocytes, plasma cells, and mononuclear phagocytic cells. There are intra- and extracellular tachyzoites and cysts in the retinal lesions. Granulomatous inflammation of the choroid occurs secondary to necrotizing retinitis. Iridocyclitis, glaucoma, and cataracts may be complications of the chorioretinitis.

In cases of acute central nervous system infection, there is a focal or diffuse meningoencephalitis with necrosis and microglial nodules. In immunodeficient adults other than those with acquired immunodeficiency syndrome (AIDS), the major finding is necrotizing encephalitis. Often these lesions are multiple, small, and diffusely distributed, although large single lesions also occur. Margins of areas of necrosis may be infiltrated with monocytes, lymphocytes, and plasma cells. Perivascular mononuclear inflammation frequently is present contiguous to areas of necrosis, and occasionally there is necrosis of vessel walls. Intra- and extracellular tachyzoites are usually found at the periphery of areas of necrosis, and these areas of necrosis may mimic mass lesions. Cysts may be present after the first week of infection. In patients with AIDS, cysts are often found in normal brain adjacent to areas of necrosis in autopsy specimens. Cysts are seen less frequently in biopsy specimens. Polymorphonuclear leukocytes are present in addition to lymphocytes, plasma cells, and histiocytes in the toxoplasmic central nervous system lesions of patients with AIDS and mononuclear leukocytes in the toxoplasmic central nervous system lesions of other immunocompromised adults. The size of lesions and extent and location of central nervous system involvement vary considerably.

In cases of disseminated infection, pathologic changes occur in the heart, lungs, kidney, and multiple other organs. They consist of necrosis and the presence of tachyzoites, cysts, and inflammatory cells alone or in combination. Glomerulonephritis with deposits of gamma-M globulin (IgM), fibrinogen, and *Toxoplasma* antigen and antibody has been reported. Involvement of the pancreas has been a prominent finding in infection in immunocompromised patients. Findings in skeletal muscle vary from parasitized fibers without pathologic changes to focal areas of infiltration to widespread myositis with necrosis.

There are prolonged and marked changes in T-lymphocyte subpopulations associated with *T. gondii* infection. These changes can be correlated with particular disease syndromes but not with disease outcome: Some patients with prolonged fever and malaise have lymphocytosis, elevation in number of suppressor T cells, and depression of the ratio of helper to suppressor cells. Significant depression in the number of helper cells may persist when the patient is clinically asymptomatic. The number of helper cells may be significantly decreased in some patients with lymphadenopathy. Depression in the number of helper cells has persisted for more than 6 months after the onset of infection. T-cell subpopulations are normal in patients with asymptomatic infection. There is a marked reduction in the number of T cells and a marked depression of the ratio of helper to suppressor lymphocytes in some patients with disseminated disease.

CLINICAL MANIFESTATIONS **Lymphadenopathy and other manifestations in the immunocompetent individual** Lymphadenopathy is the most commonly recognized clinical manifestation of acute acquired toxoplasmosis. Cervical nodes are involved most frequently. Nodes may be single or multiple, and involvement may be symptomatic or asymptomatic. Asymptomatic lymphadenopathy may mimic lymphoma, and involvement of a pectoral node has been suspected to be carcinoma of the breast. Suboccipital, supraclavicular, axillary, inguinal, and mediastinal nodes may be involved. When mesenteric or retroperitoneal nodes are involved, abdominal pain and significant temperature elevation (e.g., up to 40°C) may occur. Involved lymph nodes vary in firmness, may be tender, do not suppurate, and are usually discrete. Confusion, malaise, fever, stiff neck, myalgias, arthralgias, headache, sore throat, maculopapular rash (which spares the palms and soles), urticaria, hepatosplenomegaly, hepatitis, or reactive lymphocytes may occur. In one epidemic, 35 of 37 individuals with serologic evidence of acute acquired *Toxoplasma* infection had signs or symptoms of infection. Although 25 individuals sought medical advice from physicians, only 3 were correctly diagnosed as having toxoplasmosis. Lymphadenopathic toxoplasmosis is self-limited, but malaise and/or lymphadenopathy may persist or recur for months. Recrudescent lymphadenopathy has also been described.

Individuals who appear to be normal immunologically rarely may present with any of the following, alone or in combination: pneumonitis, myocarditis, pericarditis, pericardial effusion, hepatitis, polymyositis, encephalitis, or meningoencephalitis. Signs or symptoms of involvement of these organs are nonspecific. Significant morbidity has occurred, and some of these patients have died of the infection.

Ocular involvement *Toxoplasma* has been estimated to be the cause of approximately 35 percent of cases of chorioretinitis in children and adults. Although chorioretinitis has been estimated to occur in approximately 1 percent of patients with the acute acquired infection, ocular disease is most often a consequence of congenital *Toxoplasma* infection. Chorioretinitis is usually unilateral with the acute acquired infection and as a sequel of congenital infection which occurs in adolescents or adults. Blurred vision, scotomas, pain, photophobia, or epiphora may be due to active chorioretinitis. If the macula is involved, impairment or loss of central vision may occur. In children, strabismus may be an early sign of chorioretinitis. Associated signs of systemic infection occur only rarely. Vision improves, but frequently visual acuity recovers only partially as inflammation subsides. Commonly, episodic flares of chorioretinitis cause destruction of irreplaceable retinal tissue. The peak incidence of symptomatic disease is in the second and third decades, and it is uncommon for clinically apparent reactivation to occur after the age of 40. These multiple recurrences may result in glaucoma or loss of vision and ultimately may necessitate enucleation. The acute lesions appear as yellowish-white, cotton-like patches that have elevated, indistinct margins surrounded by a zone of hyperemia. Papillitis is usually associated with overt central nervous system disease. Inflammatory exudate in the vitreous may obscure the fundus. Older lesions characteristically appear as atrophic, whitish-gray plaques with distinct borders and black spots of choroidal pigment. Lesions usually are located near the posterior pole of the retina, although they may be peripheral. They may be single but are more commonly multiple, and lesions of varying age may be seen simultaneously. Panuveitis and papillitis with optic atrophy occur less commonly. Isolated anterior uveitis due to *Toxoplasma* infection has never been proved. The typical ocular lesion of congenital toxoplasmosis in the newborn consists of bilateral congenital chorioretinitis.

Toxoplasmosis in the immunocompromised patient (non-AIDS)

All forms of toxoplasmosis that occur in normal individuals may also occur in immunocompromised individuals. Patients receiving immunosuppressive therapy for lymphoproliferative disorders (especially Hodgkin's disease), for hematologic malignancy, or for prevention of organ graft rejection have the greatest predilection for life-threatening toxoplasmosis. Individuals who have not been infected previously with *T. gondii* and who receive a cardiac transplant from an infected individual have developed signs and symptoms of toxoplasmosis. The untreated infection in these patients is frequently fulminant and rapidly fatal. Central nervous system involvement, present in greater than 50 percent of documented cases, is the most characteristic clinical feature of toxoplasmosis in immunocompromised patients. Therefore, the diagnosis of toxoplasmosis must be excluded in any immunosuppressed patient with symptoms or signs referable to the central nervous system. Symptoms and signs are manifestations of diffuse encephalopathy, meningoencephalitis, or cerebral mass lesions and include changes in mental status, headache, focal neurologic deficits, and seizures. Brain involvement has been established by demonstration of tachyzoites in material from brain biopsy or in material aspirated from mass lesions that may have the characteristic appearance of a brain abscess on computerized tomography (CT) scan. CT scan may detect multiple, diffusely distributed or single lesions. Delayed (30 min or 1 h after infusion of contrast material) films may be important for detection of such lesions. Typically, the cerebrospinal fluid shows a mononuclear pleocytosis, a moderate elevation in protein, and a normal glucose. Some patients have had hypoglycorrhachia. Immunocompromised patients also may have other nonspecific manifestations of the infection which are reflections of inflammation and necrosis of the organs involved, particularly the heart and lungs. Toxoplasmosis may simulate rejection of a transplanted heart. Tachyzoites have been seen in endomyocardial biopsy, which established the diagnosis of toxoplasmosis.

Toxoplasmic encephalitis and AIDS

Toxoplasmic encephalitis is a major cause of morbidity and mortality in patients with AIDS. The incidence of toxoplasmic encephalitis in patients with AIDS who have antibody to *T. gondii* has been reported to be between 6 and 12 percent. Based on this observation, an estimate is that there have been approximately 170 cases of toxoplasmic encephalitis among the 7000 patients with AIDS reported by 1984 and another 170 cases would be expected to develop in the 7000 patients projected to develop AIDS in 1985. The incidence of *T. gondii* as a cause of encephalitis in patients with AIDS and encephalitis has been reported to be between 25 and 80 percent. The diagnosis of toxoplasmic encephalitis should be considered in individuals who have central nervous system disease but who do not have the usual risk factors for AIDS, since heterosexual transmission of human T-cell leukemia virus (HTLV III) has resulted in AIDS in individuals who are not the usual high-risk groups.

Prominent signs and symptoms of toxoplasmic encephalitis in patients with AIDS include chills, fever, headache, seizures, depressed mental status, and neurologic findings; these may occur in conjunction with chorioretinitis. The majority of patients with AIDS and toxoplasmic encephalitis fail to produce a serum antibody response indicative of acute infection with *T. gondii*. Demonstration of a rising titer of antibody to *T. gondii* present in cerebrospinal fluid but not present in serum has been associated with toxoplasmic encephalitis in a patient with AIDS.

Cerebrospinal fluid abnormalities have included pleocytosis, elevated protein content, and hypoglycorrhachia; tachyzoites have been seen in cytocentrifuge preparations of cerebrospinal fluid. When cerebrospinal fluid (or brain) is cultured for viruses, tissue cultures should also be examined for *T. gondii*, which may form plaques or widespread cytopathic effects. The cultures can be stained with Giemsa stain.

On CT scans of the brain, findings include diffuse encephalitis and/or one or more mass lesions. Contrast infusion may produce ring, nodular, target, or no enhancement of the lesions. Lesions may be in the cortex or white matter, and there is some proclivity for these lesions to be deep within the basal ganglia. Initially, no abnormalities may be observed on CT scan of the brain of symptomatic individuals; abnormalities may first appear several weeks later. One-hour delayed, double-dose contrast studies have detected lesions which were isodense on plain scans.

Brain biopsy of lesions seen in CT scan of brain should be performed when feasible because the differential diagnosis of these lesions includes encephalitis due to *Candida* species, *Aspergillus* species, *Mycobacterium*, and *Cryptococcus neoformans*, as well as multifocal leukoencephalopathy and lymphoma. When conventional stains are used, *T. gondii* is seen in only 50 percent of brain biopsies from such patients with toxoplasmic encephalitis. When specific immunohistologic stains are used, however, the presence of *T. gondii* tachyzoites, cysts, and/or antigens are found in brain biopsies obtained from most infected patients (see under "Pathology").

If the CT scan of brain is normal or without focal lesions in a patient with AIDS who has neurologic signs or symptoms, and the patient has either a positive Sabin-Feldman dye test, or an IgG indirect fluorescent antibody (IFA) level that is high, empiric therapy for toxoplasmic encephalitis seems warranted. If there is a focal abnormality on CT scan, serology positive for antibodies to *Toxoplasma*, and the lesion is inaccessible for biopsy or the patient's clinical condition contraindicates biopsy, presumptive therapy for *T. gondii* should be instituted. In patients who are started on presumptive therapy, a therapeutic response within 7 to 10 days supports the diagnosis of toxoplasmic encephalitis. If the patient is being treated with corticosteroids, radiographic improvement does not provide reliable evidence of a therapeutic response.

If the standard therapy with 25 mg per day of pyrimethamine and 6 to 8 g per day of trisulfapyrimidines or sulfadiazine is not effective, the daily dose of pyrimethamine should be increased to 50 mg. If therapy is limited by adverse reactions to the sulfonamide, pyrimethamine (50 mg per day) alone may be used. Folinic acid dosage may need to be as high as 15 mg per day, especially when there is marrow depression caused by pyrimethamine. However, the mechanism for the marrow suppression in patients with AIDS may be immunologic, and prophylactic folinic acid may not reverse the leukopenia. Optimal duration of therapy is not known (see "Therapy"), but relapse of toxoplasmic encephalitis is frequent in patients with AIDS when therapy is discontinued, and treatment for the duration of the patient's life may be warranted.

Toxoplasmosis and *Toxoplasma* infection in the pregnant woman

Toxoplasma infection acquired by the mother during pregnancy is symptomatic in only about 10 to 20 percent of cases. See also "Transplacental Transmission" above.

DIAGNOSIS Acute infection with *Toxoplasma* may be diagnosed by isolation of *T. gondii* from body fluids or blood (see qualification under "Isolation Procedures" below), demonstration of tachyzoites in histologic sections or in impression smears of tissue or body fluids, demonstration of characteristic lymph node histology, and serologic tests.

Isolation of the organism

The organism can be isolated by inoculation of leukocytes, body fluids, or tissue specimens into tissue culture or by subcutaneous or intraperitoneal inoculation into mice. Body fluids should be processed and inoculated immediately, but blood and tissues may be stored at 4°C overnight. Freezing or treatment of specimens with formalin kills the organism. Mice should be examined for organisms in the peritoneal fluid 6 to 10 days after inoculation, or earlier if they die. Mice that survive 6 weeks should be tested for *Toxoplasma* antibody in serum. When antibody is present, visualization of *Toxoplasma* cysts in the mouse brain establishes the diagnosis. If cysts are not demonstrable in brains of mice with *Toxoplasma* antibody, portions of brain, liver, and spleen should be inoculated into other mice.

Isolation of *T. gondii* from body fluids reflects the acute stage of infection, as does isolation from blood in most patients. Although persistent parasitemia has been described in asymptomatic individuals with latent infection, this appears to be a rare occurrence, except, perhaps, in patients with chronic myelogenous leukemia. Isolation from tissues (e.g., skeletal muscle, lung, brain, or eye) obtained by biopsy or at autopsy may reflect the presence of tissue cysts and does not prove that infection is acute.

Histologic diagnosis Demonstration of tachyzoites in tissue sections (e.g., endomyocardial biopsy in cardiac transplant recipients) or smears (e.g., brain biopsy, bone marrow aspirate) or in body fluids (e.g., cerebrospinal fluid, amniotic fluid) establishes the diagnosis of the acute infection. It is difficult to identify tachyzoites by ordinary staining methods; direct and indirect immunofluorescent antibody techniques and a peroxidase-antiperoxidase (PAP) immunohistochemical staining technique have been used successfully for this purpose. Demonstration of tissue cysts does not differentiate between acute or chronic infection. When there are numerous cysts in any organ, infection is usually of recent onset. Characteristic histologic criteria establish toxoplasmic lymphadenitis (see ''Pathology'' above).

Serologic tests Methods most widely used to establish the diagnosis of acute *Toxoplasma* infection are the Sabin-Feldman dye test, indirect fluorescent antibody (IFA) test, and indirect hemagglutination (IHA) test. Measurement of antibodies by enzyme-linked immunosorbent assay (ELISA) or radioimmunoassay is potentially valuable because these techniques may be automated.

The dye test, which measures primarily IgG antibodies, is sensitive and specific. The World Health Organization has recommended that dye test titers be expressed in international units (IU/mL) and will supply a standard reference serum.

The IFA test appears to measure the same antibodies as the dye test and is the most widely available procedure. In both tests, titers tend to be parallel. Dye test IgG-neutralizing antibody and IFA test antibodies usually appear 1 to 2 weeks after infection, reach high titers ($\geq$1:1000) in 6 to 8 weeks, and gradually decline over months to years; low titers (e.g., 1:4 to 1:64) commonly persist for life. The magnitude of the antibody titer does not correlate with severity of illness.

The agglutination test is available commercially in Europe (Bio-Merieux, Lyons, France). It detects IgG antibody. Formalin-preserved whole parasites are used. Because the test is very sensitive to IgM antibodies, ''natural'' IgM antibodies frequently cause nonspecific agglutination in serum of individuals who are negative when tested in the dye and IFA tests. Including 2-mercaptoethanol in the test obviates this problem. This method should not be used for measurement of IgM antibodies. The method is simple, accurate, inexpensive, excellent for screening sera of pregnant women, and useful in detection of antibodies to *T. gondii* in patients with AIDS.

The IgM–fluorescent antibody (IgM-IFA) test is useful in establishing the diagnosis of acute infection with *T. gondii* because IgM antibodies appear early (as early as 5 days after infection) and disappear early as contrasted with gamma-G globulin (IgG) antibodies. In most cases, IgM-IFA test antibodies rise rapidly (to levels of 1:80 to $\geq$1:1000) and fall to low titers (1:10 or 1:20) or disappear within a few weeks or months. However, in some patients they are present at low titer for several years. Some immunodeficient patients with acute toxoplasmosis and most patients with only active ocular toxoplasmosis may not have IgM *Toxoplasma* antibodies. Rheuma-

toid factor may cause false-positive reactions in the IgM-IFA test. Removal of rheumatoid factor (e.g., by absorption) will eliminate false-positive test results in the IgM-IFA test. Antinuclear antibodies may cause false-positive reactions in both the IFA and IgM-IFA tests.

The double-sandwich enzyme-linked immunosorbent assay (DS-IgM-ELISA) is more sensitive and specific than the IgM-IFA test for detection of IgM antibodies. Antinuclear antibodies and rheumatoid factor do not cause false-positive test results. As a guideline in adults, a serum level of IgM antibodies against *T. gondii* of 6 to 10 in this test indicates that *T. gondii* infection has most likely been acquired recently (i.e., within the prior 5 months); levels of 2 or 3 indicate infection has been acquired several months or more in the past; levels of 4 or 5 are intermediate; and levels of 0 or 1 are negative.

The DS-IgM-ELISA is a more specific and sensitive test that the IgM-IFA test to establish the diagnoses of congenital and acute acquired toxoplasmosis: The DS-IgM-ELISA detects approximately 75 percent of babies with congenital *Toxoplasma* infection whereas the IgM-IFA test detects only 25 percent of infants with proven congenital infection. The DS-IgM-ELISA avoids false-positive results due to the presence of rheumatoid factor (which the infant can produce in utero) and false-negative results due to competition from high levels of maternal IgM antibody (which occur in the IgM-IFA test).

The IgM-immunosorbent assay (IgM-ISA) combines trapping of the patient's IgM to a solid surface and formalin-fixed organisms or antigen-coated latex particles to detect the IgM antibodies. It is specific, sensitive, does not require use of an enzyme conjugate, and is simple to perform.

The antibodies measured in the IHA test may persist for years and are different than those measured in the IFA and dye tests. The IHA test may be helpful when titers in the IFA or dye test have stabilized since IHA test titers rise later. However, the rise in titer may occur so late that it is not helpful in diagnosis of the acute infection. Because of the frequency of false-negative results, the IHA test should not be used in infants with suspect congenital infection or in screening to determine if the infection has been acquired during pregnancy, since the test may be negative for too long a period early in the infection.

Titers in the complement fixation (CF) test also may appear several weeks later than those measured in the IFA and dye tests and also may persist for years. A negative CF test titer does not exclude acute or chronic infection, and a single positive CF test titer does not prove acute infection. A significant rise in CF test titer (i.e., of two serial dilutions performed at the same time on serums obtained several weeks apart) establishes recent infection.

Acute acquired *Toxoplasma* infection in the immunocompetent individual In settings in which acute acquired infection is suspected in an immunocompetent individual, a negative dye test or IFA test virtually excludes the diagnosis. The diagnosis of recent acute acquired infection is confirmed if there is a serial two-tube rise in titer when serums drawn at 3-week intervals are run at the same time or if there is seroconversion from a negative to a positive titer (in the absence of transfer of antibody by transfusion). A single high titer in any test does not prove the presence of active infection.

Guidelines for interpretation of test results are presented below and in Table 157-1. Exceptions to these generalizations may occur.

A dye test or IFA test titer of $\geq$1:1000, a high IgM-IFA test titer ($\geq$1:80), or high DS-IgM-ELISA or IgM-ISA titer ($\geq$6, as a guideline) are probably diagnostic of recent acute infection whether or not symptoms are present. In an individual with a positive titer in the dye test or IFA test, absence of IgM-IFA test or DS-IgM-ELISA or IgM-ISA antibodies almost always excludes very recent infection.

Ocular toxoplasmosis The diagnosis of ocular toxoplasmosis in older children and adults may be difficult because the level of antibody titer in serum does not necessarily correlate with presence of active lesions in the fundus. A patient with active *Toxoplasma* chorioretinitis usually has low serologic test titers (1:4 to 1:64). If a serologic test is negative when performed on undiluted serum, toxoplasmic chorioretinitis is excluded. If retinal lesions are characteristic and serologic tests are positive (see also "Serologic Tests" above), the diagnosis can be made with a high degree of confidence. If retinal lesions are atypical and serologic tests are positive, the diagnosis of toxoplasmosis is only presumptive; the high prevalence of *Toxoplasma* antibodies in the normal population precludes assumption of a causal relationship.

Active infection in the immunocompromised patient Because antibody formation may be deficient in immunocompromised patients, available serologic methods, including the IgM-IFA, DS-IgM-ELISA, and IgM-ISA tests, are at times insufficient for detection of active infection. For example, in patients with AIDS, dye test antibody titers are <1:1000 in many cases, and IgM antibody is rarely demonstrable. These patients do make IgG antibody when measured by other methods, such as in the IFA and agglutination tests. Serologic tests to screen for *Toxoplasma* infection are useful in asymptomatic immunocompromised individuals in order to identify those patients who are at risk for primary infection or reactivation of latent infection (see also "Prevention" below). Detection of *Toxoplasma* antigen in serum and possibly in cerebrospinal fluid by an ELISA appears to be promising as an adjunct method for establishing the diagnosis of disseminated *Toxoplasma* infection in immunocompromised individuals.

Toxoplasmosis and *Toxoplasma* infection in the pregnant woman It seems advisable to perform serology in any woman considering becoming pregnant to determine whether she has *Toxoplasma* infection prior to pregnancy and to provide essential information when tests are performed during pregnancy (see "Transplacental Transmission" above).

In the absence of a routine screening program in which *Toxoplasma* serology is performed frequently during pregnancy, an IgM-IFA, DS-IgM-ELISA, or IgM-ISA test should be performed if any other serologic test is found to be positive in any titer at any time during gestation. If the IgM-IFA test, DS-IgM-ELISA, or IgM-ISA is not available, a repeat serologic test should be obtained in 3 weeks to determine if the titer is stable or rising. No further evaluation is necessary if the IgM-IFA, DS-IgM-ELISA, or IgM-ISA test is negative and an IFA or dye test titer is stable and <1:1000 (<300 IU). If the dye test or IFA test is ≥1:1000 (≥300 IU) and stable (regardless of titer in the IgM-IFA test), the infection should be considered to have been acquired *at least* 4 weeks earlier and probably more than 8 weeks before the serum was obtained. For practical purposes, risk to the fetus is very low if the dye test or IFA test titer is ≥ 1:1000 and stable in the first 2 months of pregnancy.

Whereas titers in the dye test or IFA test may have peaked and stabilized by 8 weeks after onset of infection, titers in the CF or IHA test may continue to rise for 4 to 6 months or longer after acquisition of infection. Therefore, rises in these latter two tests may not be helpful in defining when infection occurred relative to the time of conception and should not be used as the sole test for this purpose.

A common problem arises when an asymptomatic woman is tested for *Toxoplasma* antibody late in the first trimester or in the second trimester of pregnancy and her IFA or dye test titer is found to be in the vicinity of 1:2000, her IgM-IFA, DS-IgM-ELISA or IgM-ISA test titer is found to be negative, and no significant rise in titer in any test is demonstrable. It is not possible to establish whether infection occurred before, at, or after conception in this situation. Detection of *Toxoplasma* antigen in amniotic fluid may become a useful adjunct in determining whether the fetus of a woman who acquired *Toxoplasma* during the current pregnancy is infected. Its use in this setting is experimental at this time, however.

THERAPY **Therapy in specific clinical settings** The need for and duration of therapy are determined by the clinical severity of illness and by the underlying medical problem.

Most immunologically normal patients with lymphadenopathic toxoplasmosis do not require specific treatment. Indication for treatment in these cases is severe and persistent symptoms. Evidence of serious damage to vital organs is also an indication for therapy. Infections acquired via transfusions or in laboratory accidents may be more severe than naturally acquired infections and probably should be treated.

TABLE 157-1 **Guidelines for interpretation of commonly employed serologic tests in the diagnosis of toxoplasmosis***

	IgG Sabin-Feldman dye test	Indirect fluorescent antibody (IFA) test	Indirect fluorescent antibody test for IgM *Toxoplasma* antibodies (IgM-IFA)	DS-IgM-ELISA or IgM-ISA	Indirect hemagglutination (IHA) test	Complement fixation (CF) test	Direct agglutination
Positive titer	1:4, undiluted†	1:10‡	1:2 infants‡ 1:10 adults‡	≥2	1:16‡	1:4‡	≥1:20
Titer in acute infection	≥1:1000	≥1:1000	≥1:80	≥6	≥1:1000	Varies among laboratories	Relatively low, usually <1:1000
Titer in chronic (latent) infection	1:4–1:2000	1:8–1:2000	Negative to 1:20	0–1	1:16–1:256	Negative to 1:8	Later may be ≥1:6000
Duration of elevation of titer	Years	Years	Weeks to months; occasionally years	Unknown, often >1 year	Years	Years	
Special considerations	1 No known cross-reactions or false-positive results in humans.	1 Antibody measured is same as that measured in dye test. 2 Antinuclear antibodies may cause false-positive results.	1 Either antinuclear antibodies or rheumatoid factor (IgM) may cause false-positive results. Rheumatoid factor may be absorbed from serum.	1 Limited experience with this new test. 2 No cross-reaction with rheumatoid factor or antinuclear antibody if Fab$_2$ conjugate used.	1 Not useful for diagnosis of congenital toxoplasmosis. 2 IHA antibodies rise later than in dye test and IFA. May be especially useful if rising IHA titer can be demonstrated.	1 Antigen preparations have not been standardized. 2 CF antibodies also rise later than dye test and IFA; see special consideration 2 under IHA.	1 Measures IgG. 2 Titer more often less than dye test in early weeks of acute infection. 3 Titer more often higher than dye test in older infection and much greater in chronic infection.

* These guidelines are useful in the interpretation of test results, but exceptions to these generalizations may occur.
† In some cases of eye disease, the dye test may be positive only in undiluted serum.
‡ These values are representative, but normal values for each laboratory may differ significantly.

Patients with active chorioretinitis should be treated with specific therapy. When there is potential for serious visual impairment secondary to macular or optic nerve involvement, corticosteroids are added to the regimen. For treatment of active ocular toxoplasmosis, pyrimethamine and sulfadiazine should be administered for 1 month. Within 10 days, the borders of retinal lesions should become sharper and the vitreous haze should disappear. In 60 to 70 percent of cases, there is a favorable clinical response. If the response is not favorable, repeated courses of pyrimethamine and sulfadiazine are needed. If vision is endangered by lesions involving the macula, optic nerve head, or papillomacular bundle, systemic corticosteroids should be added. Since the majority of new lesions appear contiguous to old ones, photocoagulation has been used to treat active lesions and to prevent spread of lesions. Occasionally, vitrectomy and removal of the lens may be needed to restore visual acuity.

Because of the high mortality rate associated with toxoplasmosis in patients whose resistance to infection is compromised by underlying disease or by therapy (e.g., corticosteroids or cytotoxic drugs), toxoplasmosis should be treated in all immunocompromised individuals. In immunocompromised patients, serologic evidence of acute infection (with or without signs and symptoms of infection) or demonstration of tachyzoites in tissue (with or without serologic test titers or signs and symptoms) is an indication for therapy. Improvement has been reported to occur in the majority of patients to whom specific therapy was administered. Considering the diagnosis early enough to institute treatment is the major problem.

When a pregnant woman who acquired infection at any time during pregnancy is treated, the chance of congenital infection in her infant is decreased but not eliminated. Pyrimethamine is a potential teratogen; therefore, sulfadiazine (which is highly effective in animal models when used alone) should be used alone if a decision is made to treat during the first trimester of pregnancy. When infection occurs during the first trimester, some authorities have recommended therapeutic abortion because of the high probability of severe damage when infection occurs early in fetal life. Other authorities recommend treatment rather than abortion because the risk of transmission of the infection to the fetus is low (approximately 15 percent) in the first trimester and because the incidence of congenital toxoplasmosis can be reduced significantly by intrapartum therapy.

Pyrimethamine plus sulfadiazine or trisulfapyrimidines In vivo, pyrimethamine and sulfadiazine act synergistically against *Toxoplasma*. Clinical experience confirms the efficacy of this combination. Comparative tests have shown that sulfapyrazine, sulfamethazine, and sulfamerazine are about as effective as sulfadiazine. In general, other sulfonamides are much less effective.

Pyrimethamine In adults, a loading dose of 100 to 200 mg pyrimethamine is given orally in two divided doses on the first 2 days of treatment. In young children, a loading dose of 2 mg per kilogram of body weight (not to exceed adult loading dose) is given for the first 2 to 3 days of treatment. The maintenance dose is 1 mg per kilogram of body weight (with a usual maximum of 25 mg) in a single dose. The dosage may be raised to 50 mg per day to treat severe disease in immunodeficient patients. In view of the drug's half-life of 4 to 5 days, administration of the maintenance dose at 3- to 4-day intervals has been suggested. Daily administration is recommended for the patient who is very ill, since there are no data concerning absorption of the drug in this situation. Daily therapy is also recommended for active ocular infection. Pyrimethamine is available only in tablet form.

Pyrimethamine is a folic acid antagonist and produces a dose-related, usually gradual, and reversible depression of the bone marrow. Anemia, leukopenia, and thrombocytopenia may occur. Platelet and peripheral blood cell counts should be evaluated twice weekly in any patient receiving pyrimethamine.

Folinic acid To prevent suppression of the bone marrow, folinic acid (calcium leucovorin) is administered in conjunction with pyri-

methamine therapy. Optimal frequency for administration of folinic acid has not been established. A single oral dose of 5 to 20 mg daily is recommended. If folinic acid is not available, bakers' yeast (three to four cakes daily) may be used to prevent toxicity due to pyrimethamine. Neither folinic acid nor bakers' yeast inhibits the action of pyrimethamine on *T. gondii*, whereas folic acid does.

Sulfadiazine and trisulfapyrimidines The loading dose is 50 to 75 mg per kilogram of body weight; thereafter, a total daily dose of 75 to 100 mg per kilogram of body weight is administered in four divided doses at intervals of approximately 6 h. Tablet and liquid oral forms as well as an intravenous form of sulfadiazine are available. The potential toxicities of sulfonamides (e.g., crystalluria, hematuria, and rash) must be carefully monitored. Hypersensitivity reactions to sulfonamides are a particular problem in patients with AIDS. In this case, 50 mg per day of pyrimethamine has been administered alone. If standard therapy with 25 mg per day of pyrimethamine and 6 to 8 g per day of trisulfapyrimidines or sulfadiazine is not effective, the daily dose of pyrimethamine should be increased to 50 mg. If therapy is limited by adverse reaction to the sulfonamide, pyrimethamine (50 mg per day) may be used alone.

Other drugs Trimethoprim alone or in combination with a sulfonamide has not been proved to be effective in treatment of toxoplasmosis in humans, but the activity of this combination in vitro and in vivo in animal models warrants carefully designed and controlled clinical trials. This combination is significantly less active than the combination of pyrimethamine with sulfadiazine.

Spiramycin is less active and less toxic than the combination of pyrimethamine and sulfadiazine. This antibiotic can be obtained through the Food and Drug Administration in the United States and is available in most other countries in North America and Europe. The usual dose of 2 to 4 g per day for adults is administered orally in two to four divided dosages. Spiramycin can reduce the incidence of congenital transmission. Clindamycin is concentrated in the choroid and has been used to treat ocular toxoplasmosis, but efficacy has not been demonstrated in controlled clinical trials.

Duration of therapy Optimal duration of specific therapy has not been defined for any form of toxoplasmosis. Specific therapy should be continued for 4 to 6 weeks in a patient who appears to be immunologically normal but who requires treatment for severe and persistent symptoms or evidence of damage to vital organs (e.g., chorioretinitis, myocarditis). Longer treatment may be necessary.

It seems advisable to treat an immunocompromised patient for at least 4 to 6 weeks *beyond* complete resolution of all signs and symptoms of active disease. Careful follow-up of these patients is imperative because relapse may occur and requires prompt reinstitution of therapy. Relapse of central nervous system disease is frequent in patients with AIDS. There are no data as to whether prolonged therapy or prophylaxis should be used. Pyrimethamine plus sulfadoxine administered once or twice a week has been used in attempts to prevent relapse after therapy, but no controlled data are available to determine whether this is useful. Although therapy may be effective against *T. gondii* tachyzoites and may induce a beneficial clinical response, it does not eradicate cysts from the central nervous system.

Desmonts and Couvreur suggest that an acutely infected pregnant woman should be treated with spiramycin and use a total dose of 2 to 3 g daily, administered orally in four divided doses. A 3-week course of treatment is alternated with 2 weeks without treatment from the time of diagnosis until term.

PREVENTION Measures for prevention of infection involve intervention in the cycle of transmission and are most important for immunodeficient patients and seronegative pregnant women. It is important that patients at high risk be educated concerning the avoidance of cysts (in undercooked meat) and contact with sporulated oocysts (from cats). To kill cysts, meat should be heated to 60°C or frozen at −20°C. (Commercial freezers do not reach or maintain this temperature reliably.) Hands should be washed after touching uncooked meat, and fruits and vegetables that may be contaminated with oocysts should be washed. Dry heat (66°C) or boiling water renders oocysts noninfectious. Contact with cat feces should be avoided.

There are no definitive data to allow for a firm recommendation regarding the use of whole blood, leukocyte transfusions, or organ transplants when a donor is seropositive for *Toxoplasma* antibodies. It seems reasonable, however, not to use blood or blood products donated by an individual with *Toxoplasma* antibody in an immuno-suppressed individual, and an organ transplanted to a seronegative recipient should be from an individual without serologic evidence of *Toxoplasma* infection.

No effective vaccine to prevent infection with *Toxoplasma* has been developed.

REFERENCES

ARAUJO FG, REMINGTON JS: Antigenemia in recently acquired acute toxoplasmosis. J Infect Dis 141:144, 1980

CONLEY FK, REMINGTON JS: *Toxoplasma gondii* infection of the central nervous system. Use of the PAP method to demonstrate *Toxoplasma* in formalin-fixed paraffin-embedded tissue sections. Hum Pathol 12:690, 1981

DESMONTS G, COUVREUR J: Congenital toxoplasmosis: A prospective study of 378 pregnancies. N Engl J Med 290:1110, 1974

DORFMAN RF, REMINGTON JS: Value of lymph node biopsy in the diagnosis of acute acquired toxoplasmosis. N Engl J Med 289:878, 1973

DUBEY JP et al: Characterization of the new fecal form of *Toxoplasma gondii*. J Parasitol 56:447, 1970

KIMBALL AC et al: Congenital toxoplasmosis: A prospective study of 4048 obstetric patients. Am J Obstet Gynecol 111:211, 1971

LUFT BJ et al: Primary and reactivated *Toxoplasma* infection in patients with cardiac transplants. Ann Intern Med 99:27, 1983

———— et al: Toxoplasmic encephalitis in patients with acquired immune deficiency syndrome. JAMA 252:913, 1984

————, REMINGTON JS: Acute *Toxoplasma* infection among family members of patients with acute lymphadenopathic toxoplasmosis. Arch Intern Med 144:53, 1984

————, ————: Toxoplasmosis of the central nervous system, in *Current Clinical Topics in Infectious Diseases 6*, JS Remington, MN Swartz (eds). New York, McGraw-Hill, 1985, pp 315–358

NAOT Y, REMINGTON JS: An enzyme-linked immunosorbent assay for detection of IgM antibodies to *Toxoplasma gondii:* Use for diagnosis of acute acquired toxoplasmosis. J Infect Dis 142:757, 1980

O'CONNOR GR: Manifestations and management of ocular toxoplasmosis. Bull NY Acad Med 50:192, 1974

REMINGTON JS, DESMONTS G: Toxoplasmosis, in *Infectious Diseases of the Fetus and Newborn Infant*, 2d ed. JS Remington, JO Klein (eds). Philadelphia, Saunders, 1983

RUSKIN J, REMINGTON JS: Toxoplasmosis in the compromised host. Ann Intern Med 84:193, 1976

TOWNSEND JJ et al: Acquired toxoplasmosis. Arch Neurol 32:335, 1975

158 PNEUMOCYSTIS CARINII PNEUMONIA

PETER D. WALZER

DEFINITION *Pneumocystis carinii* is an opportunistic pathogen whose natural habitat is the lung. The organism is an important cause of pneumonia in the compromised host.

ETIOLOGY The taxonomy of *P. carinii* is unsettled, but the generally accepted view is that it is a protozoan. The organism exists in two basic forms: the small (1 to 4 μm), pleomorphic, more numerous trophozoites; the 5- to 7-μm cyst, which has a thick wall and contains up to eight daughter forms, termed *sporozoites*. The sporozoites excyst and appear to develop into trophozoites. The life cycle of *P. carinii* is poorly understood, but may involve different forms of reproduction for the trophozoite and cyst stages; an intracellular phase in the life cycle of *P. carinii* has not been identified. *P. carinii* of animal origin has been grown in tissue culture. Ultrastructurally, *P. carinii* has a primitive organelle system, but little is known about its metabolism.

EPIDEMIOLOGY *P. carinii* has a worldwide distribution among humans and has been found in a variety of animals. Organisms for these hosts are morphologically identical, but species or strain differences probably exist. Data about environmental sources of *P. carinii* are lacking. Serologic surveys indicate that most normal children have been exposed to the organism by 3 to 4 years of age. Animal model experiments have demonstrated that *P. carinii* is transmitted by the airborne route. Human-to-human transmission has been suggested by the occurrence of outbreaks of pneumocystis pneumonia among institutionalized debilitated infants and in hospitals caring for immunosuppressed patients. Based on animal studies, the incubation period is thought to be 4 to 8 weeks.

PATHOGENESIS *P. carinii* pneumonia occurs in the following hosts: premature, malnourished infants; children with primary immunodeficiency diseases; patients receiving immunosuppressive therapy (particularly corticosteroids) for cancer, organ transplantation, and other disorders; and patients with the acquired immunodeficiency syndrome (AIDS). AIDS is currently the most common underlying disease for *P. carinii;* conversely, *P. carinii* is the most common opportunistic infection in AIDS and the leading cause of death (see Chap. 257).

Available data suggest that impaired cellular immunity is the major host predisposing factor in the development of pneumocystis pneumonia. Antibodies are produced locally and systemically in response to exposure to *P. carinii,* but do not appear to have a protective role. Pneumocystis pneumonia which develops with the use of immunosuppressive drugs probably represents reactivation of latent infection. At some institutions the incidence of the disease has been related to the intensity of the immunosuppression. *P. carinii* pneumonia which develops in patients with primary immunodeficiency diseases and AIDS could arise from latent infection with the progressive breakdown of host defenses, or could be acquired by contagion.

PATHOLOGY The histopathologic features of *P. carinii* pneumonia in humans and experimental animals are identical. Early in the infection the organisms line up along walls of alveoli in close apposition to the type I pneumocyte. The interaction of *P. carinii* with this alveolar cell plays a major role in the host-parasite relationship in the infection. The organisms slowly propagate and, as seen on methenamine silver–stained lung sections, gradually fill the alveolar spaces. With hematoxylin and eosin staining there is the typical foamy, vacuolated alveolar exudate which consists of organisms, host serum proteins, debris, and surfactant. On electron microscopy in the animal model there is a series of changes in alveolar microenvironment which culminate in damage to the type I cell. Very rarely, *P. carinii* has been found in tissue beyond the lungs.

The host inflammatory changes are mild and nonspecific, even with extensive infection. Hypertrophy of alveolar type II cells can frequently be found and has been interpreted as a reparative response. Alveolar macrophages are present but usually not prominent in phagocytosis of the organism. In most compromised hosts there is a mild mononuclear cell interstitial cell infiltrate. However, malnourished infants display an intense interstitial plasma cell infiltrate which was responsible for the disease's early name of "interstitial plasma cell pneumonia."

CLINICAL FEATURES Patients with *P. carinii* pneumonia complain of dyspnea, fever, and nonproductive cough. When corticosteroids have been administered, symptoms frequently begin after the dose has been tapered. The duration of illness until diagnosis is typically 1 to 2 weeks, although considerable variation exists, particularly among patients with AIDS in whom this time span may be much longer (see Chap. 257). Physical findings include tachypnea, tachycardia, and cyanosis but lung auscultation reveals few abnormalities. The white blood count is variable and usually governed by the patient's underlying disease. Arterial blood gases demonstrate hypoxemia, increased alveolar-arterial oxygen gradient, and respiratory alkalosis. Alterations in pulmonary function tests (e.g., vital capacity, diffusing capacity) are also present. The classic findings on chest radiograph consist of bilateral diffuse infiltrates beginning in the perihilar regions; with time, air bronchograms develop. Variants (e.g., nodular densities, unilateral infiltrates) to this picture have also been reported. Some patients may have a normal chest radiograph early in the course of the disease but demonstrate increased uptake on gallium scan.

P. carinii pneumonia in AIDS follows a more chronic and indolent course. The average duration of pulmonary symptoms is about 4 weeks, but some patients may be ill for several months. The cough and shortness of breath may be overlooked unless a careful history is taken, and fever may be present with other infectious complications of AIDS. Objective measurements (e.g., respiratory rate and arterial oxygenation) are also less severely impaired in AIDS patients.

DIAGNOSIS   Since the clinical picture of *P. carinii* can be produced by many different infectious and noninfectious agents, diagnosis must be made by specific identification of the organism. Culture of human *P. carinii* is not yet feasible, and serology, whether based on antibody or antigen detection, is not reliable. Definitive diagnosis is made by histopathologic staining. Stains which selectively stain the cell wall of *P. carinii* cysts are the most popular. Methenamine silver is the prototype; toluidine blue and cresyl echt violet are simpler, more rapid alternatives. Stains such as Giemsa's or Diff Quik stain both the trophozoite and cyst forms of *P. carinii;* these stains also stain host tissues, and hence require a greater degree of experience for proper interpretation. Recently, *P. carinii* has been observed in Wright's and Gram's stains.

P. carinii is present rarely in sputum, and infrequently in transtracheal aspiration, so a more invasive procedure is usually necessary to obtain adequate specimens. This is best performed early in the patient's hospitalization according to an organized protocol with close cooperation between clinicians and laboratories. In recent years, fiberoptic bronchoscopy with bronchoalveolar lavage and/or transbronchial biopsy has become the most widely used procedure in adults with a diagnostic yield of ≥90 percent in patients with AIDS and about 40 percent in other immunocompromised hosts. The reasons for higher diagnostic efficacy in AIDS patients are unclear but may possibly reflect a higher organism burden. Open lung biopsy is generally performed when bronchoscopy is nondiagnostic or when infection with an additional organism is suspected.

COURSE AND PROGNOSIS   According to current concepts, *P. carinii* causes an asymptomatic infection in the normal host but an almost invariably fatal pneumonia in the compromised host unless treatment is given. In premature infants the mortality of *P. carinii* pneumonia is 50 percent, and in the animal model the disease is reversible with removal of corticosteroids. The prognosis of *P. carinii* pneumonia in response to therapy is influenced by such factors as the status of the underlying disease, host nutrition, degree of abnormalities in respiratory function, prior lung damage (e.g, radiation), and total leukocyte and lymphocyte counts. Concomitant infection with other opportunistic pathogens frequently occurs and may adversely affect treatment of *P. carinii*.

TREATMENT   The two major drugs used in the treatment of *P. carinii* pneumonia have been trimethoprim-sulfamethoxazole (TMP-SMX) and pentamidine isethionate. These drugs are equally effective, with success rates of 50 to 80 percent in different series. TMP-SMX inhibits folic acid synthesis, and pentamidine affects several different systems in cell replication; however, their mode of action against *P. carinii* is unknown. TMP-SMX is administered orally or intravenously in a dose of 20 mg/kg per day TMP and 100 mg/kg per day SMX in four divided doses for 14 days. Optimal serum levels in adults are ≥5 μg/mL TMP and 100 to 150 μg/mL SMX; these guidelines can be used to adjust the dose of TMP-SMX in renal insufficiency. TMP-SMX is preferred over pentamidine in non-AIDS patients because it is much better tolerated.

Pentamide is given intramuscularly or by slow intravenous infusion in a dose of 4 mg/kg per day for 14 days. Side effects occur in about 50 percent of patients and include painful induration at injection sites and systemic reactions, such as hypoglycemia, hyperglycemia, hypocalcemia, azotemia, and hepatic dysfunction.

Response to TMP-SMX or pentamidine begins on the average after 4 days of treatment and is characterized by improvement in fever, respiratory symptoms, and blood gases; chest radiograph findings usually lag behind. If a response fails to occur with one drug within 5 to 7 days, it is best to substitute the other agent. The combination of TMP-SMX and pentamidine does not appear to improve efficacy and may increase the risk of toxicity. General supportive measures including maintenance of adequate oxygenation, fluid and electrolyte balance, and nutrition are also important. Corticosteroids and other immunosuppressive drugs should be tapered to as low a dose as permitted by the patient's underlying disease. Except for patients with AIDS, recurrence of *P. carinii* pneumonia is generally uncommon, but has occurred in about 10 percent of pediatric patients at selected institutions.

Success rates for the treatment of the initial episode of *P. carinii* pneumonia in AIDS are similar to those for other immunocompromised hosts. However, AIDS patients respond more slowly and appear to require longer duration of therapy. Organisms can be found in the lungs even after 4 to 6 weeks of treatment. *P. carinii* pneumonia recurs in 20 to 30 percent of AIDS patients and is usually refractory to any form of therapy. AIDS patients have a high frequency (60 to 80 percent) of adverse reactions (rash, leukopenia, fever) to TMP-SMX which often requires discontinuation of the drug. The mechanism of these effects is unclear, and treatment with folinic acid has not been helpful. AIDS patients may also be somewhat more prone to developing leukopenia with pentamidine.

The experience in the treatment of *P. carinii* infection in AIDS has stimulated a search for alternative drugs. Pyrimethamine and sulfadiazine appear to be effective but have the same potential problems as TMP-SMX. Dapsone and difluoromethylornithine (DFMO), an inhibitor of polyamine biosynthesis, are undergoing clinical evaluation.

PREVENTION   Controlled studies have shown that TMP-SMX in a dose of 5 mg/kg per day TMP and 25 mg/kg per day SMX can prevent *P. carinii* pneumonia in selected high-risk populations. Although chronic administration of TMP-SMX is well-tolerated in non-AIDS patients, a high incidence of side effects has limited its use in patients with AIDS. TMP-SMX is not lethal to *P. carinii*, and hence is only effective as long as it is being taken. Since *P. carinii* may be communicable, patients with the disease should be separated from direct contact with other susceptible hosts.

REFERENCES

CUSHION MT et al: *Pneumocystis carinii:* Growth variables and estimates in the A549 and WI-38 VA 13 cell lines. Exper Parasitol 60:43, 1985

GORDIN FM et al: Adverse reactions to trimethoprim-sulfamethoxazole in patients with the acquired immunodeficiency syndrome. Ann Intern Med 100:495, 1984

HAVERKOS HW: Assessment of therapy for *Pneumocystis carinii* pneumonia. Am J Med 76:501, 1984

HELMICK CG, GREEN JK: Pentamidine-associated hypotension and route of administration. Ann Intern Med 103:480, 1985

HUGHES WT: Natural mode of acquisition for de novo infection with *Pneumocystis carinii.* J Infect Dis 145:842, 1982

———: Trimethoprim-sulfamethoxazole therapy for *Pneumocystis carinii* pneumonitis in children. Rev Infect Dis 4:602, 1982

KOVACS JA et al: *Pneumocystis carinii* pneumonia: A comparison between patients with the acquired immunodeficiency syndrome and patients with other immunodeficiencies. Ann Intern Med 100:663, 1984

MURRAY JF et al: Pulmonary complications of the acquired immunodeficiency syndrome: Report of a National Heart, Lung and Blood Institute workshop. N Engl J Med 310:1682, 1984

SHELHAMER JH et al: Persistence of *Pneumocystis carinii* in lung tissue of acquired immunodeficiency syndrome patients treated for *Pneumocystis* pneumonia. Am Rev Resp Dis 130:1161, 1984

WALZER PD et al: Lymphocyte changes during chronic administration and withdrawal of corticosteroids: Relevance to *Pneumocystis carinii* pneumonia. J Immunol 133:2502, 1984

——— et al: *Pneumocystis carinii* pneumonia in the United States: Epidemiologic, clinical and diagnostic features. Ann Intern Med 80:83, 1974
———, YOUNG LS: The clinical relevance of animal models of *Pneumocystis carinii* pneumonia. Diag Microbiol Infect Dis 2:1, 1984
YOUNG LS (ed): *Pneumocystis carinii Pneumonia: Pathogenesis, Diagnosis, Treatment.* New York, Dekker, 1984

159 BABESIOSIS

JAMES J. PLORDE

DEFINITION AND HISTORY Known since biblical times, this cosmopolitan infection of domestic and wild animals is caused by protozoa of the genus *Babesia*. These organisms are transmitted by ticks, multiply in red blood cells, and produce an acute febrile hemolytic anemia, the most prominent manifestation of which is hemoglobinuria.

EPIDEMIOLOGY AND CLINICAL MANIFESTATIONS The first human infection was described in Yugoslavia by Skrabalo in 1957. This and six other European cases were particularly severe with high fever, hemoglobinuria, jaundice, and renal failure. Both in their clinical presentation and in the presence of small intraerythrocytic parasites they closely resembled falciparum malaria with which they were originally confused. All seven occurred in splenectomized patients and five ended fatally. The causative agents were bovine parasites (*B. bovis, B. divergens*). Some 100 cases have now been documented in the United States. Two California cases resembled the European infections and were thought to be caused by equine babesia. The remaining cases have been acquired during the summer months on Cape Cod and the offshore islands lying between New York and Massachusetts, including Long Island, Fire Island, Shelter Island, Nantucket, and Martha's Vineyard. All were caused by a rodent parasite, *B. microti,* and approximately 80 percent occurred in patients with intact spleens. The patients experienced a prolonged illness characterized by the insidious onset of fever, chills, sweating, myalgia, and mild to moderate hemolytic anemia presumably caused by direct, parasite-induced damage to the erythrocytic membrane. The physical examination was usually negative except for occasional splenomegaly. In general, clinical manifestations have been more severe in asplenic subjects. Most patients were over 50 years of age and all but one recovered. The carrier state persisted for weeks to months in some patients and in three resulted in subsequent transfusion-induced infections. Two of the three recipients were asplenic; the third was an elderly individual who represents the only fatality in the series. Serologic studies suggest that most patients infected with *B. microti* are asymptomatic; seroconversion rates of nearly 6 percent and point prevalence rates of 2 to 4.4 percent have been noted in endemic areas. All age groups seem equally susceptible. Like their symptomatic counterparts, patients with subclinical infections may remain parasitemic for several months.

B. microti has been found in field moles and deer mice in New York State, Utah, and California. On the offshore islands of New England, however, the principal reservoir is the white-footed mouse. The northern deer tick, *Ixodes dammini,* which also serves as the vector in Lyme disease, is responsible for the transmission of *B. microti.* This hard-bodied tick takes a blood meal during each of its three developmental stages: larva, nymph, and adult. Rodents are the principal hosts of the first two stages while deer host the adult ticks. Only the nymphs, which feed from May through September, are capable of transmitting *B. microti* to humans. Since the engorged nymph measures 2 mm in diameter, infested patients may be oblivious to its presence. Transovarial transmission does not occur.

DIAGNOSIS The diagnosis depends on the demonstration of the intraerythrocytic parasite in Giemsa-stained peripheral blood smears. Like malaria parasites, these organisms measure 2 to 3 μm in diameter and demonstrate red-staining nuclear material with blue cytoplasm. In contrast to malaria parasites, however, neither gametocytes nor pigment are seen. As the parasites multiply by a nonsynchronous budding process, the organism displays marked pleomorphism; a single red cell may contain multiple parasites in different developmental stages. Unique basket shapes, tetrads, and trophozoites with multiple chromatin dots are helpful distinguishing features. In heavy infections, organisms can be seen outside red blood cells. Serologic diagnosis can be made with the indirect fluorescent antibody test or enzyme-linked immunosorbent assay. Because the disease is insidious in onset, most infected patients have titers $\geq$1024 at the time they present for medical care. There is no correlation between disease severity and the titer level; cross reactions with other *Babesia* species and malaria may be seen, but titers with homologous antigens are generally higher. Active infections have been demonstrated in smear-negative, serology-positive infections by inducing infection in experimental animals.

TREATMENT Mild disease should be managed symptomatically with antipyretics. If significant hemolysis ensues, transfusion may be warranted. In more severe infections specific therapy should be attempted. Although chloroquine provides symptomatic improvement, it appears to have little activity against this parasite. Quinine and clindamycin therapy has been successful in several patients. Antitrypanosomal agents also appear effective, and, in life-threatening infections, pentamidine should be considered. This agent appears to be effective in controlling the clinical manifestations of babesiosis and decreasing parasitemia; it may not eradicate the organism. Exchange transfusions are helpful in fulminant infections.

PREVENTION The prevention of *B. microti* infections in humans is difficult. Individuals summering on the offshore islands of New England should consider the use of insect repellents containing diethyltoluamide and examine themselves daily for the presence of the 2- to 3-mm nymphs. A pilot tick control program has been initiated on one of the islands. Asplenic patients should be advised to avoid endemic areas. To avoid transfusion-transmitted babesiosis, blood donors should be screened serologically for evidence of *B. microti* infection.

REFERENCES

CHISHOLM ES et al: *Babesia microti* infection in man: Evaluation of an indirect immunofluorescent antibody test. Am J Med Hyg 27:14, 1978
DAMMIN GJ et al: Babesiosis, in *Seminars in Infectious Diseases,* L Weinstein, J Fields (eds). New York, Stratton, 1978, pp 169–199
———: The rising incidence of clinical *Babesia microti* infections. Hum Pathol 12:398, 1981
FRANCIOLI PB et al: Response of babesiosis to pentamidine therapy. Ann Intern Med 94:326, 1981
JACOBY GA et al: Treatment of transfusion-transmitted babesiosis by exchange transfusion. N Engl J Med 303:1098, 1980
ROSNER F et al: Babesiosis in splenectomized adults: Review of 22 reported cases. Am J Med 76:696, 1984
RUEBUSH TK II et al: Development and persistence of antibody in persons with *Babesia microti.* Am J Trop Med Hyg 30:291, 1981
——— et al: Epidemiology of human babesiosis on Nantucket Island. Am J Trop Med Hyg 30:937, 1981
STEKETEE RW et al: Babesiosis in Wisconsin: A new focus of disease transmission. JAMA 253:2675, 1985
SUN T et al: Morphologic and clinical observations in human infection with *Babesia microti.* J Infect Dis 148:239, 1983
WITTER M et al: Successful chemotherapy of transfusion babesiosis. Ann Intern Med 96:601, 1982

160 GIARDIASIS

JAMES J. PLORDE

ETIOLOGY AND EPIDEMIOLOGY *Giardia lamblia* is a pear-shaped multiflagellar protozoan that parasitizes the human duodenum and jejunum of humans and other animals where it multiplies by longitudinal fission. Under a microscope, its pyriform shape, two nuclei, and central parabasal body give the organism the appearance of a face with two large eyes. It may actively browse the unstirred mucous layer at the bases of the microvilli or attach to the intestinal mucosa by means of a large ventral sucking disk. Unattached trophozoites may be carried in the fecal stream to the large bowel. If their passage through the gut is hurried, they will exit unchanged in the liquid stool and perish rapidly. With normal colonic transit times, however, the organisms retract their flagella, envelop themselves in a protective membrane, and undergo nuclear division. The resulting quadrinucleate cysts are infectious and may be transmitted to new hosts by a number of fecal-oral routes. Cysts deposited in cold water can survive for more than 2 months and have been shown to be resistant to chlorine concentrations (0.4 mg per liter) routinely used in community purification systems. The ingestion of water contaminated with as few as 10 cysts is sufficient to establish human infection. Not surprisingly, waterborne outbreaks in humans have been documented repeatedly during the past two decades. In fact, *G. lamblia* is now the single most frequently defined cause of waterborne outbreaks of diarrhea in the United States. They have involved campers who have drunk from remote surface waters, skiers who have used well water, and ordinary citizens served by chlorinated municipal systems. Contamination of the water supply with raw sewage has been found in several outbreaks. In others, *G. lamblia*–infected beavers were located within the watershed, suggesting that these mammals may serve as alternate reservoirs. Waterborne cysts are also thought to be responsible for the high incidence of giardiasis in travelers returning from third-world countries. Food may also serve as a transmission vehicle in these areas as well.

Direct person-to-person spread occurs with some frequency. This is most dramatically evident among male homosexuals practicing anilingus and groups of ambulatory, non-toilet-trained children. It also appears to be responsible for the secondary cases seen in families of infected children.

Giardiasis is a cosmopolitan infection that is particularly common in areas with poor sanitation and among populations unable to maintain adequate levels of hygiene. In developing countries, the prevalence of giardiasis often exceeds 10 percent. In the United States, *G. lamblia* is the most frequently identified intestinal parasite, being found in over 4 percent of stools submitted for parasitologic examination. Young children are three times more likely to be involved than adults; the prevalence may be particularly high among toddlers attending day-care centers and the institutionalized retarded, in whom rates exceeding 50 percent have been reported. Giardiasis is also frequent in individuals with immunoglobulin deficiencies and may be a major cause of intestinal abnormalities in this population. It has been suggested that the parasite is able to persist in such patients because of a relative deficiency of secretory IgA. Similarly, the immune deficiencies accompanying protein-calorie malnutrition are thought to enhance the susceptibility of involved individuals to parasitization with *G. lamblia*.

Among adults, parasitism is common in parents of infected children, travelers, and campers, but the precise prevalence in these populations is unknown. Achlorhydric individuals may be more susceptible to infection. Several studies have emphasized the association between male homosexuality and intestinal parasitosis; infection rates for *G. lamblia* and/or *Entamoeba histolytica* have ranged from 11 to 40 percent. In a New York study, all nontraveled immunocompetent males with giardiasis were homosexual.

PATHOLOGY AND PATHOGENESIS Clinical manifestations appear to be caused by an impairment of the absorptive capacity of the gut, particularly for fat and carbohydrates. The mechanism responsible for these changes is unknown. Mechanical blockage of the intestinal mucosa by large numbers of trophozoites, competition for essential nutrients, altered jejunal mobility with or without overgrowth of enteric bacteria or yeasts, pancreatic or biliary dysfunction, and organism-induced deconjugation of bile salts have been implicated. None, however, correlates well with disease severity, and eradication of associated microorganisms does not uniformly result in clinical improvement. Disaccharidase deficiency with lactose intolerance, altered levels of peptide hydrolyase and enteropeptidase, and decreased vitamin B_{12} absorption indicate that *G. lamblia* produces direct or indirect damage to the microvillar structure of the small bowel. Mechanical irritation to the fuzzy coat by the trophozoite's sucking disk might induce an accelerated turnover of the mucosal epithelium, resulting in functional immaturity of the transport systems. Excretion of a soluble toxin that interacts with the epithelial cell has been hypothesized, but never documented. Mucosal invasion may provoke a T cell–mediated insult to the jejunal mucosa. In experimentally infected nude mice immunologic reconstitution with lymphoid cells from previously infected animals results in marked mucosal changes including cellular infiltration and a decreased villus/crypt ratio. Similar pathologic findings have been reported in humans with giardial malabsorption. Both the structural changes and the malabsorption are reversible with specific therapy.

Although reinfection is common, the frequent occurrence of giardiasis in patients with immunologic defects, and the rarity with which it is seen in older adults, suggest that protective immunity, albeit incomplete, does develop with time. Animal experiments suggest humoral, secretory, and cellular mechanisms are all involved. The diversity of surface antigens, secretory products, and DNA banding patterns in *Giardia* isolates could influence the effectiveness of the host immune response in preventing reinfection.

CLINICAL MANIFESTATIONS In endemic situations, over two-thirds of infected patients may be asymptomatic. This ratio is usually reversed in point-source outbreaks. From 1 to 3 weeks after exposure, the patient notes the explosive onset of watery diarrhea. The stool is foul smelling, greasy in appearance, and floats. There is neither blood nor mucus. Abdominal cramping is present and is epigastric in location. The formation of large quantities of intestinal gas produces distention, sulfuric eructation, and flatulence. Anorexia, nausea, vomiting, and low-grade fever may be present. Typically, acute symptoms continue for at least 5 to 7 days. In an occasional patient, they may persist for months, leading to significant malabsorption and weight loss. More commonly, the illness resolves spontaneously in 1 to 4 weeks or lapses into a chronic phase characterized by intermittent bouts of flatulence, epigastric pain, and the passage of mushy stools. It is not unusual for patients to present in this fashion without having experienced the more acute manifestations described above. Chronic giardiasis is associated with reduced growth in preschool children. Eventually, both parasites and symptoms disappear. Lactose intolerance, however, may persist, producing a clinical picture easily confused with the parasitologic disease and subjecting the patient to unnecessary therapy.

DIAGNOSIS The diagnosis is made by identifying the cyst in formed feces or the trophozoite in diarrheal stools, duodenal secretions, or jejunal biopsies. In the majority of acute cases, the parasite can be demonstrated easily in a series of stool specimens collected and examined in the manner described for amebiasis (see Chap. 153). In acute illness, the onset of clinical manifestations may antedate the excretion of organisms by 5 to 7 days while in chronic infections the discharge of parasites is often scanty or intermittent, making laboratory confirmation more difficult. Purgation does not improve the yield. Many of these patients, however, can be diagnosed by examining specimens collected at weekly intervals for a period of 4 to 5 weeks. Alternatively, the duodenal contents can be sampled with a nylon string (Enterotest) or gastric tube and cultured by direct wet-mount preparation. Occasionally, jejunal biopsy is required to establish the diagnosis in patients with typical clinical manifestations. Immuno-diagnostic methods for the rapid detection of *Giardia* antigen in feces appear both highly sensitive and specific, but are not commercially available. Enzyme-linked immunosorbent and indirect fluorescent serologic tests using axenically cultured *G. lamblia* have been developed. Their diagnostic usefulness remains to be established.

TREATMENT Treatment is usually carried out with quinacrine hydrochloride or metronidazole. Tinidazole, a more effective agent, is presently not available in the United States. Quinacrine, 0.1 g given three times daily for 5 days, eliminates the organisms in 70 to 95 percent of cases. Although the drug is usually well tolerated, it may produce gastrointestinal disturbances, exacerbate psoriasis, and, rarely, produce toxic psychosis. Metronidazole appears to be better tolerated and equally effective. A single oral dose of 2.0 g given on 3 consecutive days, 750 mg tid for 5 days, and 250 mg tid for 5 days give cure rates of 95, 95, and 70 percent, respectively. However, this drug is not currently licensed for giardiasis, and there is concern over its mutagenicity. Household contacts and sexual partners of infected patients should be examined; individuals harboring the parasite should be treated even if asymptomatic to prevent the spread to others. Pregnant women, however, should receive therapy only if severely symptomatic and never in the first trimester. Because parasitologic and clinical relapse can occur up to 7 weeks after the completion of therapy, long-term follow-up is essential.

PREVENTION Chemoprophylactic drugs are not effective in pre-venting the acquisition of giardiasis. Individuals visiting endemic areas should avoid the ingestion of potentially contaminated food and water. The latter may be made potable by boiling or by treating with a suitable halogen disinfectant. Most of the commercially available tablets appear effective when appropriate concentrations and contact times are utilized; they are temperature-dependent, and their dose should be increased when dealing with cold water. Custodial insti-tutions for children should screen new admissions for the presence of *G. lamblia* and treat those found to be positive. Handwashing by children and staff must be emphasized. Community water purification systems should provide for adequate filtration as well as disinfection. Breast feeding appears to protect infants from giardiasis; this may be related to the known presence of antigiardial substances, including specific IgA antibodies, in breast milk.

REFERENCES

BLACK RE et al: Giardiasis in day-care centers—Evidence of person to person transmission. Pediatrics 60:486, 1977

DYKES AC et al: Municipal waterborne giardiasis: An epidemiologic investigation. Ann Intern Med 93:165, 1980

GUPTA MC, URRUTIA JJ: Effect of periodic antiascaris and antigiardia treatment on nutritional status of preschool children. Am J Clin Nutr 36:79, 1982

JARROLL EL JR et al: *Giardia* cyst destruction: Effectiveness of six small-quantity water disinfection methods. Am J Trop Med Hyg 29:8, 1980

OSTERHOLM MT et al: An outbreak of foodborne giardiasis. N Engl J Med 304:24, 1981

SOLOMONS NW: Giardiasis: Nutritional implications. Rev Infect Dis 4:859, 1982

SPEELMAN P: Single-dose tinidazole for the treatment of giardiasis. Antimicrob Ag Chemother 27:227, 1985

STEVENS DP: Giardiasis: Host-pathogen biology. Rev Infect Dis 4:851, 1982

————: Selective primary health care: Strategies for control of disease in the developing world. XIX. Giardiasis. Rev Infect Dis 7:530, 1985

UNGER LP et al: Enzyme-linked immunosorbent assay for the detection of *Giardia lamblia* in fecal specimens. J Infect Dis 149:90, 1985

161 CRYPTOSPORIDIOSIS AND OTHER PROTOZOAN INFECTIONS

JAMES J. PLORDE

CRYPTOSPORIDIOSIS

DEFINITION Cryptosporidiosis is a diarrheal disease of vertebrates produced by protozoa of the genus *Cryptosporidium*. These parasites inhabit the microvillous border of the intestinal epithelium, where they produce clinical illness ranging from an acute, self-limited, watery diarrhea in normal individuals to chronic, severe, life-threatening gastroenteritis in the immunocompromised. Unknown as human pathogens prior to 1976, cryptosporidia now rank with *Salmonella, Shigella, Campylobacter,* enterotoxigenic *Escherichia coli,* rotavirus, and *Giardia lamblia* as major enteric pathogens of humans.

ETIOLOGY Regardless of animal host, all strains of this tiny (2- to 6-μm) parasite appear morphologically identical. In the absence of firm evidence for host specificity, they can reasonably be regarded as a single species. Cryptosporidia exhibit alternating cycles of sexual and asexual reproduction and are thereby classified as sporozoan protozoa. As is true for *Toxoplasma, Isospora,* and other members of the sporozoan subgroup known as Coccidia, both cycles are completed within the gastrointestinal tract of a single host. The infective forms or oocysts are shed into the intestinal lumen of the parasitized animal. Unlike those of *Toxoplasma* and *Isospora,* cryp-tosporidia oocysts are fully mature and immediately infective upon passage in the feces. Following ingestion by another animal, *sporozoites* are released from the oocyst, attach themselves to the epithelial surface, and begin a series of developmental changes. Although excluded from the cytoplasm of the epithelial cell, *trophozoites* and all subsequent developmental stages are surrounded by a double membrane of host origin and are, by definition, intracellular parasites. The trophozoites divide asexually by a process of multiple fission (*schizogony*) to form *schizonts* containing eight daughter cells known as type I *merozoites.* Upon release from the schizont, each merozoite attaches itself to another epithelial cell, where it repeats the schizogony cycle, producing another generation of type I merozoites. Eventually, schizonts containing only four daughter cells are seen. Incapable of continued asexual reproduction, these type II merozoites are trans-formed into male (*microgamete*) and female (*macrogamete*) sexual forms. Following fertilization, the resulting *zygote* develops into an oocyst. The majority possess a thick protective cell wall which ensures their intact passage in the feces and survival in the external environ-ment. Approximately 20 percent of the oocysts, however, fail to develop such a wall. Their thin cell membrane ruptures, releasing infective sporozoites directly into the intestinal lumen and initiating a new "autoinfective" cycle within the original host. In the normal host, the presence of innate or acquired immunity dampens both the cyclic production of type I merozoites and the formation of thin-walled oocysts, halting further parasite multiplication and terminating the acute infection. In the immunocompromised both presumably continue, explaining why such individuals develop severe, persistent infections in the absence of repeated reinfections.

EPIDEMIOLOGY Cryptosporidiosis appears to involve most verte-brate groups; the available prevalence studies demonstrate that although rare in adult animals, infection rates can be high in immature pets and farm stock. Experimental transmission of human *Crypto-sporidium* strains to rodents, kittens, and puppies, and an outbreak of infection in human handlers of infected calves clearly suggest that domestic animals constitute an important reservoir of disease for humans. Disease outbreaks in day-care centers, hospitals, and urban family groups, however, indicate that most human infections result from person-to-person transmission rather than zoonotic spread. As in animals, human disease is more common in the young. In western countries, 1.4 to 4.1 percent of small children presenting to medical centers with gastroenteritis have been shown to harbor cryptosporidia oocysts; in third world countries the rates have varied from 4 to 11 percent. Up to 63 percent of children attending day-care centers during outbreaks of diarrhea have had oocysts detected in their stool. Infection rates in adults suffering from gastroenteritis are approximately one-third those reported for children and have been highest in family members of infected children, medical personnel caring for patients with cryptosporidiosis, male homosexuals, and travelers to foreign countries. Asymptomatic carriage is uncommon; other enteric pathogens, particularly *Giardia lamblia,* are recovered from a significant minority of infected patients. Since oocysts are found almost exclusively in stool, the principal transmission route is undoubtedly fecal-oral. In day-care centers and among male homosexual groups the spread is probably direct. The hardy nature of the oocysts makes it likely that there is also indirect transmission via contaminated food, water, and fomites. The increase in infection rates seen during the summer months is compatible with this hypothesis. On rare occasions oocysts have been recovered from the pharynx or found in expectorated sputum, raising the possibility that cryptosporidiosis may be acquired through contact with the respiratory secretions of infected patients.

PATHOGENESIS AND PATHOLOGY　Although the jejunum is most heavily involved, cryptosporidia have been found in the pharynx, esophagus, stomach, duodenum, gallbladder, ileum, appendix, colon, and rectum of immunocompromised subjects. They appear as small, basophilic, spherical structures arranged in rows or clusters along the brush border of the epithelial cells. They color readily with Giemsa and hematoxylin-eosin, but not with acid-fast stains; they may be mistaken for epithelial blebs. Electron microscopy reveals the entire gamut of developmental forms including trophozoites, schizonts, merozoites, and macrogametes. All are covered by a double membrane derived from the reflection, fusion, and attenuation of the microvilli over the parasite. The attachment site is electron dense. Multiple, dense, membrane-bound bodies located within the apexes of the epithelial cells can be seen in the immediate vicinity. Some resemble degenerating parasites, raising the possibility that cryptosporidia can, in fact, invade the epithelial cytoplasm. By light microscopy, bowel changes appear minimal, consisting of mild-to-moderate villous atrophy, crypt enlargement, and a mononuclear infiltrate of the lamina propria.

The pathophysiology of the diarrhea that accompanies cryptosporidiosis is unknown, but its nature and intensity suggest a cholera-like enterotoxin. The vital role played by the host's immune status in the pathogenesis of the disease is indicated by both the enhanced susceptibility of the young to infection and the prolonged, severe clinical disease seen in immunocompromised patients. Animal studies with related coccidian parasites suggest that resistance to reinfection is mediated by T lymphocytes while the severity and duration of the primary infection are influenced by both cellular and humoral mechanisms.

CLINICAL MANIFESTATIONS　Immunocompetent hosts　Following an incubation period of 4 to 14 days, the patient notes the onset of an explosive, profuse, watery diarrhea accompanied by abdominal cramping. Typically, these manifestations persist for 5 to 11 days before rapidly abating; rarely, purging may continue for up to 4 weeks. When this happens, mild malabsorption with weight loss may be seen. Its shorter duration, more prominent abdominal pain and relative lack of flatulence help to distinguish cryptosporidiosis from the clinically similar *Giardia lamblia* infection. A small percentage of patients describe nausea, anorexia, low-grade fever, or vomiting. Routine laboratory work is unremarkable. Radiographic and endoscopic examinations of the gut either are normal or demonstrate mild, nonspecific abnormalities. Recovery is complete, and neither relapse nor reinfection has been reported.

Immunocompromised hosts　Cryptosporidiosis has been described in patients with a broad range of immunodeficiencies. In third world countries, marasmus and other forms of childhood malnutrition have been most common. In the United States, the acquired immunodeficiency syndrome (AIDS), congenital hypogammaglobulinemia, cancer chemotherapy, and immunosuppressive management of organ transplantation patients have been the abnormalities noted most frequently. In patients with these conditions, cryptosporidiosis is usually indolent in onset and prolonged in duration. The abdominal cramping and systemic manifestations are similar to those seen in normal hosts. The diarrhea, however, is characteristically more severe; fluid losses of 1 to 17 liters a day have been described. Unless the patient's immunologic defect is reversed, the disease usually continues in a persistent or remittent fashion for the duration of life. In two-thirds, the diarrhea has lasted for more than 4 months; in a few it has persisted unabated for a number of years. Weight loss is often prominent. The prognosis depends upon the nature of the underlying immunologic abnormality; the 6-month survival rate in patients with AIDS is 50 percent. Although other intercurrent infections are usually the direct cause of death, malnutrition and complications of parenteral nutrition are often thought to play a contributory role.

DIAGNOSIS　The diagnosis of cryptosporidiosis must be pursued in any immunocompromised patient who develops diarrhea. Before 1978, the diagnosis required small-bowel biopsy. The development of effective concentration and staining techniques, as well as the growing experience of clinical laboratories with this parasite, have made the recovery and identification of cryptosporidia oocysts from the stool the procedure of choice. Oocyst excretion is most intense during the first 4 or 5 days of illness, tapers during the second week, and generally stops within 2 or 3 days of the cessation of diarrhea; oocysts are rarely recovered from solid stool. Specimens should be examined immediately after passage or preserved in 2.5% potassium dichromate or 10% buffered formalin. Fresh and dichromate-preserved specimens are infectious and must be handled with care. The specimen may contain small amounts of mucus, but fecal erythrocytes or white cells are uncommon. Initially, an iodine wet mount can be made from the unconcentrated specimen and examined microscopically; the spherical 5-μm oocysts are differentiated from yeasts, which they resemble in size and morphology, by their failure to take up the iodine. As cryptosporidia oocysts are one of the few acid-fast particles found in feces, identification can be confirmed with any one of the many acid-fast staining procedures developed for mycobacteria. If the direct examinations are negative, the stool should be concentrated using either Sheather's sugar flotation or Ritchie's formalin-diethylacetate sedimentation procedure. The two are equally sensitive; use of both will improve yield in specimens with few oocysts. Supernatant from the former is examined by light or phase microscopy for the typical pink-tinged, refractile oocysts. Sediment from the formalin-diethylacetate procedure is acid-fast–stained before examination.

A highly sensitive and specific indirect immunofluorescent test has been described. Seroconversion occurs within 60 days of acute infection in both immunocompetent patients and those with AIDS; antibodies persist for at least 1 year. The usefulness of such tests for the diagnosis of acute infection remains undetermined.

TREATMENT AND PREVENTION　In the immunocompetent patient, the disease is self-limited, and attempts at specific antiparasitic therapy are not warranted. Oral, and occasionally parenteral, rehydration may be required in small children. In the immunocompromised host, the severity and chronicity of the diarrhea warrants therapeutic intervention. The only uniformly successful approach has been the reversal of underlying immunologic abnormalities. Withdrawal of cancer chemotherapy agents, discontinuation of immunosuppressive drugs, and successful bone marrow transplantation have all resulted in cure. Specific anticryptosporidial therapy has been attempted with a large number of drugs; most have been ineffective. Some patients have experienced an amelioration or complete resolution of symptoms following treatment with spiramycin, furazolidone, or alpha-difluoromethylornithine (DFMO); however, clinical failures have been common, and parasitologic cures have been reported in few. In patients who responded clinically but continued to excrete oocysts, relapses have followed discontinuation of the therapeutic agent. Because spontaneous remissions can occur, the value of these drugs in the treatment of cryptosporidiosis remains uncertain.

The stools of patients with cryptosporidiosis are infectious. Stool precautions should be instituted at the time the diagnosis is first suspected; for the immunosuppressed patient this should be whenever diarrhea, regardless of presumed etiology, is first noted. This is particularly important in cancer chemotherapy and transplantation units, where spread of the disease, directly or indirectly, from a symptomatic patient to other immunosuppressed patients can have life-threatening consequences.

TRICHOMONIASIS

Trichomoniasis is a venereal infection caused by the protozoan *Trichomonas vaginalis*. Of the many members of the genus *Trichomonas*, three are parasites of human beings: *T. hominis* in the intestine, *T. tenax* in the oral cavity, and *T. vaginalis*, the only established pathogen, in the vagina, urethra, and prostate. All three exist only in the trophozoite stage and resemble one another morphologically. *Trichomonas vaginalis* is the largest, however, and confusion in diagnosis is rare because of the anatomic specificity of their habits. Strains varying in size, growth rates, virulence, and antigenic characteristics have been described.

Trichomonas vaginalis is transmitted by sexual intercourse. Although the organism is viable for up to 24 h in urine, semen, and water and may survive on moist washcloths for a few hours, transmission by fomites is probably uncommon. Approximately 5 percent of children born to infected mothers acquire the infection. The parasite is cosmopolitan in its distribution. It is estimated that 3 million women in the United States and 180 million worldwide are infected annually; 30 to 70 percent of their male sexual partners are parasitized, at least transiently. Prevalence correlates directly with the number of sexual contacts. The incidence in adult virgins is zero; rates as high as 70 percent have been seen in prostitutes, individuals with other venereal disease, and sexual partners of infected patients. Women with trichomoniasis are, on the average, a decade older than those with gonorrhea. Although the peak incidence is between 16 and 35 years, there is a relatively high prevalence among the 30- to 40- and 40- to 50-year-old age groups.

In the female, trichomoniasis usually presents as a persistent vaginitis. It is estimated that half of women with *Trichomonas* are asymptomatic when first diagnosed. A significant proportion, however, go on to develop clinical manifestations within 6 months. In approximately two-thirds a discharge is present and is frequently accompanied by vulvar itching (50 percent), dyspareunia (50 percent), odor (10 percent), and dysuria. This acute stage may persist for a week or months, often fluctuating in intensity; it may worsen following menstruation. Eventually the discharge and other symptoms subside and may actually disappear completely, even though the patient still harbors trichomonads. Examination shows inflammation ranging from mild hyperemia of the vaginal vault and endocervix to extensive erosion, petechial hemorrhages, and perianal intertrigo. The finding of a granular, friable, reddened endocervix (strawberry cervix) is a highly characteristic, although uncommon, finding. A discharge, typically thin, gray to yellow, and frothy in nature, is found pooled in the posterior vaginal fornix.

The prostate and urethra are the usual sites of infection in the male. Most commonly the infection is completely asymptomatic, but may present as persistent or recurring nonspecific urethritis. Approximately 5 percent of all episodes of nongonococcal urethritis in males is caused by *T. vaginalis*. The prevalence is higher among those failing tetracycline therapy. Acute purulent urethritis occurs rarely.

The diagnosis is made by examining vaginal, prostatic, or urethral secretions for the presence of *Trichomonas*. The organism may also be found in the sedimented urine. A wet mount reveals squamous epithelial cells, polymorphonuclear nucleocytes, and *T. vaginalis* with its characteristic twitching motility; although highly specific when positive, it is often negative in asymptomatic women and in patients who have douched in the previous 24 h. Stained smears provide little additional help. Culture is more sensitive but is not generally available.

Trichomonas is sometimes responsible for confusing changes in the cytologic pattern of exfoliated vaginal cells. Moreover, ordinary Papanicolaou preparations are not well suited to the diagnosis, and when trichomoniasis is suspected, fresh material should be looked at immediately.

Oral metronidazole (Flagyl), given either in dosage of 250 mg three times daily for 7 days or in a single 2-g dose, is an extremely effective therapeutic agent. Concurrent treatment of sexual partners is very important, particularly when single-dose therapy is given, if recurrent infection is to be avoided. A small number of *T. vaginalis* strains with high levels of resistance to metronidazole have been isolated from patients failing multiple courses of therapy.

The evidence that metronidazole is carcinogenic in rodents and mutagenic in bacteria mandates that the drug should not be used in the first trimester of pregnancy until further information on its teratogenicity is available. Because of the agent's antabuse-like action, alcohol consumption is contraindicated during therapy and for 24 h following its completion. Topical therapy with clotrimazole, an imidazole antifungal agent, can be employed in situations where systemic metronidazole therapy is contraindicated. The drug is applied intravaginally, in a dose of 100 mg daily for 6 days.

ISOSPORIASIS

This is an infrequently recognized disease characterized by fever, diarrhea, abdominal pain, and weight loss which results from ingestion of the oocysts of coccidia belonging to the genus *Isospora*. These sporozoan protozoa are widespread in the animal kingdom. *I. hominis* and *I. belli* have been shown to infect humans. Parasitization is much more common in children and is worldwide in distribution, particularly in tropical areas. In this country, a disproportionately large percentage of reported cases have occurred in male homosexuals.

Like the related plasmodia, there is both an asexual and sexual stage of multiplication in *I. belli* infections. However, both occur within a single host. Following the ingestion of an oocyst, *sporozoites* are released which invade the epithelial cells of the intestine to become trophozoites. These multiply asexually producing a large number of *merozoites*, which in turn invade other epithelial cells to continue the cycle. In some cells sexual gametocytes are produced. With the fertilization of the female gametocyte, an oocyst is formed which is then passed in the stool. Transmission is by the fecal-oral route. Volunteers develop symptoms about 1 week after the ingestion of viable oocysts. The illness usually has an acute onset with fever, headache, abdominal cramps, and diarrhea. Stools are often fatty and weight loss is common. Isosporiasis may be associated with a malabsorption syndrome and abnormalities of the mucosa in the small bowel. Symptoms, which presumably continue as long as the asexual cycle of multiplication continues, usually subside spontaneously within a few weeks. In the immunocompromised host, however, they are often severe, and may persist for months or even years, eventually resulting in death.

A peripheral eosinophilia occurs in approximately half of the infected patients. The diagnosis can be made by examination of stool for oocysts. These are often scanty, and concentration techniques such as zinc sulfate flotation or the formol-ether method must usually be employed. Incubation of the stool for 2 days at room temperature improves the recovery rate. Duodenal aspiration and jejunal biopsy are less cumbersome and more reliable. The oocysts stain well with the acid-fast techniques described for the closely related *Cryptosporidium* species (see above). *Isospora belli* infections have been successfully treated with combinations of pyrimethamine-sulfonamide and trimethoprim-sulfamethoxazole. The dose for the latter combination is 160/800 mg qid for 10 days, then bid for 3 weeks.

Isospora hominis is probably identical with *Sarcocystis fusiformis*. Its oocysts are believed to be infectious only for pigs and cattle in which it produces tissue sarcocysts. Humans become infected by eating undercooked pork or beef containing the cysts. These liberate trophozoites which invade intestinal epithelial cells to undergo gametogony with the formation of new oocysts. The disease in humans is usually asymptomatic, but mild self-limited gastrointestinal manifestations have been described. Therapy is not required.

BALANTIDIASIS

Balantidium coli, the largest protozoan of human beings, inhabits the large intestine. In addition to producing an asymptomatic carrier state, it elicits disease ranging from mild recurrent diarrhea to fulminant ulceration with perforation and death. In many respects the disease is similar to amebiasis in its range of manifestations, exclusive of spread to the liver.

The illness has been reproduced by feeding the organism to volunteers. The diagnosis is made by finding the trophozoite or cyst in the stool, but repeated examinations may be required because shedding of *Balantidium* is intermittent. The disease is more likely to occur in tropical areas, but at least 60 cases have been reported in the United States. Swine and rats are frequent carriers of *B. coli* and may play an important role in the spread of the disease to humans. Outbreaks have been noted in mental institutions where coprophagy implicated direct person-to-person transmission.

The tetracyclines in ordinary doses are highly effective in treatment, as is iodoquinol given in the dosage of 650 mg three times daily for 20 days. Metronidazole in the dosage used for amebiasis has also been effective (see Chap. 153).

DIENTAMEBIASIS

Dientamebiasis is an intestinal infection produced by a flagellated ameba, *Dientamoeba fragilis*. The genus and species names derive, respectively, from the binucleate nature of the trophozoite and the fragmented appearance of its nuclear chromatin. Like the related *Trichomonas* genus, the protozoan lacks a cyst stage. By virtue of its location in the large bowel, it has been thought to be spread from person to person by the fecal-oral route. However, the prevalence of the organism does not parallel that of other intestinal protozoa, its incidence in homosexual men does not correlate with the frequency of oral-anal sex, and the trophozoite is rapidly destroyed in both water and gastric juice. A mechanism of transmission compatible with these facts was suggested when *D. fragilis*–like structures were noted inside the eggs of pinworms. Several studies have now demonstrated that coinfection with these two intestinal parasites is 9 to 20 times higher than that expected by random occurrence, reinforcing the possibility that the helminth eggs may serve as a vector for the protozoan trophozoite. *D. fragilis* is a cosmopolitan parasite. Studies in this country report prevalence rates ranging from 1.4 to 18.6 percent. Rates are highest among children between 0 and 10 years of age, institutionalized individuals, communal groups, and missionaries serving in tropical areas. While *D. fragilis* was thought to be a harmless commensal of the colonic mucosal crypts, and probably is not capable of tissue invasion, it may act as a chronic irritant producing excess mucous secretion and hypermotility. Pathologic studies of surgically removed appendices shown to harbor *D. fragilis* demonstrated fibrosis that encroached upon the mucosal lymphoid tissue. Patients free of intestinal pathogens other than

D. fragilis have reported a variety of clinical manifestations including diarrhea (58 percent) with blood or mucus (11 percent), abdominal pain (54 percent), and anal pruritus (11 percent).

The diagnosis is established by the identification of the parasite in stool. As the number of organisms varies greatly from day to day, at least three stool samples should be collected over a period of 3 to 6 days. Because the trophozoites are rapidly destroyed in the external environment, the stool should be examined immediately or preserved in polyvinyl alcohol. The use of permanent stains increases both the yield and identification accuracy of the examination. Tetracycline, iodoquinol, or metronidazole in the doses recommended for *E. histolytica* infections have all been used. There is little data available on their relative efficacy.

BLASTOCYSTIS HOMINIS INFECTION

Previously considered a commensal yeast, it now appears that *Blastocystis hominis* is a protozoan that, at least on occasion, may act as an agent of human disease. Evidence of its protozoan nature includes the lack of a cell wall, the capacity for pseudopod formation and particulate matter ingestion, multiplication by binary fission or sporulation, and possession of a well-demarcated smooth and rough endoplasmic reticulum, membrane-bound central body, and protozoan-like mitochondria and Golgi apparatus. Physiologically the organism is a strict anaerobe that requires the presence of bacteria for growth; it grows best at a neutral pH and a temperature of 37°C. The organism is resistant to high concentrations of amphotericin B.

Evidence of pathogenicity rests on the experimental induction of diarrhea in guinea pigs, its assocation with diarrhea in nonhuman primates, and a small number of reports describing human diarrheal disease, one fatal, for which no other cause could be established. A retrospective study designed to evaluate the pathogenicity and clinical relevance of *B. hominis* found the organism in 12 percent of all stools submitted for parasitologic examination; in 90 percent the numbers of *Blastocystis* were judged to be few or moderate. In approximately two-thirds of the positive stools, *B. hominis* was the only parasite present. An evaluation of case histories of a subset of patients whose stools were also known to be free of bacterial pathogens revealed that 67 percent had gastrointestinal complaints including nausea, vomiting, abdominal pain, and diarrhea, most for a period of 3 to 10 days. Only a single patient had received therapy; in none had the stools been screened for viral agents. Over half of the patients had an underlying, immunosuppressive disease.

Routine stool examinations utilizing concentration and permanent staining procedures are adequate for the identification of *B. hominis*. Some authorities recommend treating symptomatic patients shown to have more than five organisms per oil immersion field if other causes of disease cannot be identified. Metronidazole, used in the dose described for *E. histolytica* appears to be a suitable agent.

REFERENCES

Balantidiasis

KNIGHT R: Giardiasis, isosporiasis and balantidiasis. Clin Gastroenterol 7:31, 1978
NICHOLSON NW: Case report of *Balantidium coli* infection. East Afr Med J 55:133, 1978
WALZER PD et al: Balantidiasis outbreak in Truk Islands. Am J Trop Med Hyg 22:33, 1973

Blastocystis hominis infection

CALLAGHER PG et al: *Blastocystis hominis* enteritis. Pediatr Infect Dis 4:556, 1985
GARCIA LS et al: Clinical relevance of *Blastocystis hominis*. Lancet 1:1233, 1984
ZIERDT CH: *Blastocystis hominis,* A protozoan parasite and intestinal pathogen of human beings. Clin Microbiol Newsletter 5:57, 1983

Cryptosporidiosis

D'ANTONIO RG et al: A waterborne outbreak of cryptosporidiosis in normal hosts. Ann Intern Med 103:886, 1985

KOCH KL et al: Cryptosporidiosis in hospital personnel. Evidence for person-to-person transmission. Ann Intern Med 102:593, 1985

LEFKOWITCH JH et al: Cryptosporidiosis of the human small intestine: A light and electron microscopic study. Hum Pathol 15:746, 1984

NAVIN TR, JURANEK DD: Cryptosporidiosis: Clinical, epidemiologic, and parasitologic review. Rev Infect Dis 6:313, 1984

PORTNOY D et al: Treatment of intestinal cryptosporidiosis with spiramycin. Ann Intern Med 101:202, 1984

SOAVE R et al: Cryptosporidiosis in homosexual men. Ann Intern Med 100:504, 1984

WOLFSON JS et al: Cryptosporidiosis in immunocompetent patients. N Engl J Med 312:1278, 1985

Dientamebiasis

SHEIN R, GELB A: Colitis due to *Dientamoeba fragilis*. Am J Gastroenterol 78:634, 1983

SPENCER MJ et al: *Dientamoeba fragilis*. Gastrointestinal protozoan infection in adults. Am J Gastroenterol 77:565, 1982

YANG J et al: *Dientamoeba fragilis*: A review with notes on its epidemiology, pathogenicity, mode of transmission and diagnosis. Am J Trop Med Hyg 26:16, 1977

Isosporiasis

FORTHAL DN, GUEST SS: *Isospora belli* enteritis in three homosexual men. Am J Trop Med Hyg 33:1060, 1984

NG E et al: Demonstration of *Isospora belli* by acid-fast stain in a patient with acquired immune deficiency syndrome. J Clin Microbiol 20:384, 1984

TRIER JS: Chronic intestinal coccidiosis in man: Intestinal morphology and response to treatment. Gastroenterology 66:923, 1974

WESTERMAN EL, CHRISTENSEN RP: Chronic *Isospora belli* infection treated with co-trimoxazole. Ann Intern Med 91:413, 1980

Trichomoniasis

FOUTS AC, KRAUS SF: *Trichomonas vaginalis*: Reevaluation of its clinical presentation and laboratory diagnosis. J Infect Dis 141:137, 1980

KRIEGER JN et al: Geographic variation among isolates of *Trichomonas vaginalis*: Demonstration of antigenic heterogeneity by using monclonal antibodies and the indirect immunofluorescence technique. J Infect Dis 152:979, 1985

REIN MF, MÜLLER M: *Trichomonas vaginalis*, in *Sexually Transmitted Diseases*, KK Holmes et al (eds). New York, McGraw-Hill, 1984, pp 525–536

WAITKINS SA, THOMAS DJ: Isolation of *Trichomonas vaginalis* resistant to metronidazole. Lancet 2:590, 1981

162 TRICHINOSIS

JAMES J. PLORDE

DEFINITION Trichinosis is an intestinal and tissue infection of humans and other mammals caused by the nematode *Trichinella spiralis*. The disease is characterized by diarrhea during the development of the adults in the intestine and by myositis, fever, prostration, periorbital edema, eosinophilic leukocytosis, and, occasionally, evidence of myocarditis, pneumonitis, or encephalitis during the stage of larval migration in tissue.

ETIOLOGY Trichinosis in humans is contracted by ingestion of meat containing the encysted larvae of *T. spiralis*. The meat has almost always been pork, but for the past several years about 10 percent of cases reported in this country have been attributed to feral meat, usually bear or walrus. This has been particularly frequent in the northern and western states including Alaska, California, and Idaho. There are no intermediate hosts, and both the adult and larval stages develop in the same animal. Infection has been produced or observed in the bear, wild boar, wolf, coyote, fox, muskrat, horse, cow, dog, cat, rabbit, guinea pig, mouse, and marine mammals, in addition to the rat and the pig. Humans are particularly susceptible; most fowl are resistant. Among pigs, infection is contracted following feeding of the uncooked scraps, less often by eating infected rats. The incidence of infection in pigs has been reduced by laws requiring that garbage be cooked thoroughly before being fed. Rats also feed on uncooked pork scraps and, in addition, maintain a high incidence of infection by their cannibalism.

Soon after ingestion, the larvae are liberated from their cysts by gastric digestion and migrate into the intestinal mucosa, where copulation takes place. The male dies, and within a week, the viviparous female is discharging larvae (100 by 6 μm), which enter vascular channels and are distributed throughout the body. Larviposition continues for about 4 to 16 weeks, each female producing approximately 1500 offspring. The larvae enter skeletal muscle, grow, and begin encysting within 3 weeks; calcification of cysts begins in 6 to 18 months. The life span of the encysted organism has been estimated at 5 to 10 years. The muscles of the diaphragm, tongue, and eye, and the deltoid, pectoral, gastrocnemius, and intercostal muscles are most often affected. Larvae carried to sites other than skeletal muscles do not encyst but disintegrate, often stimulating a granulomatous inflammatory reaction. The life cycle can be carried further only if a new host ingests the encysted larvae.

The description of a fatal case of trichinosis in an immunosuppressed patient emphasizes the importance of the immune response in limiting the intensity of infection. Apparently, it does so by acting directly on circulating larvae, inhibiting the reproduction of the female worms, and accelerating the expulsion of the adult parasites from the intestine. Eosinophils as well as B- and T-cell lymphocytes are involved in the response. The T cells appear to have a "helper" function in promoting the production of IgG and IgM antibodies which, in collaboration with eosinophils, induce fracture of the larval cuticle and disintegration of its internal structures. Once safely encysted in striated muscle, the larvae appear resistant to immunologic attack.

EPIDEMIOLOGY Trichinosis is particularly common in Europe and North America, but with the exception of Australia it is found worldwide. In the United States its prevalence as measured by finding cysts in human diaphragms at autopsy has declined from 16.1 to 4.2 percent over the past 30 years. This decline has been accompanied by a similar reduction of trichinosis in pigs. The prevalence appears highest in the New England states, New Jersey, Louisiana, Hawaii, and Alaska. It is estimated that 1.5 million Americans carry live trichinae in their musculature and that somewhere between 150,000 and 300,000 acquire new infections annually. The overwhelming majority of these infections are asymptomatic, and many of those that become clinically manifest are never correctly diagnosed. In 1982 only 95 cases were officially reported in the United States; over the last 5 years the case fatality rate has been 0.6 per 1000. Large outbreaks are usually caused by consumption of ready-to-eat pork sausage prepared in noninspected facilities or at home. The incidence appears highest among Americans of Italian, German, Polish, or Portuguese descent, presumably because of their inclination to make and eat pork sausage over the holiday season. Although pork products are not currently inspected for trichinosis, U.S. Department of Agriculture–inspected "ready-to-eat" products are processed in a manner designed to destroy trichina larvae. Outbreaks have been reported among southeast Asian refugees living in the United States following the ingestion of undercooked pork obtained from private farms. Notable epidemics have also followed the ingestion of trichinae-infected wild pig in Hawaii and California and walrus in Alaska. The latter is the first reported outbreak caused by this host in North America. Each year, a few cases are acquired from ground beef, attesting to the frequency with which this meat is adulterated with pork.

PATHOLOGY The most striking lesions are in the skeletal muscles, where there is a severe myositis with basophilic granular degeneration of the invaded muscle fiber. Adjacent fibers exhibit hyalin or hydropic degeneration, and the focus becomes infiltrated with neutrophilic and eosinophilic leukocytes, some lymphocytes, and mononuclear macrophages. Hyperemia, edema, and hemorrhages are constant features.

Larvae do not encyst in cardiac muscle, but an intense myocarditis has been observed in fatal cases.

In cases of central nervous system involvement, there may be granulomatous nodules, and vasculitis involving small arterioles and capillaries of the brain and meninges. Encystment of larvae in the brain is unusual.

CLINICAL MANIFESTATIONS The severity of the clinical manifestations generally relates to the number of larvae disseminated to the tissues of the host; patients with severe disease usually harbor 50 to 100 larvae per gram of muscle, while those with 10 or less are often asymptomatic. The first symptoms usually appear within 1 to 2 days after ingestion of the uncooked or undercooked meat containing encysted larvae. At that time diarrhea, abdominal pain, nausea, and sometimes prostration and fever develop. Although generally brief, the intestinal phase may be prolonged in infections produced by arctic strains of trichina (*T. spiralis* var. *nativa*). The next stage, that of muscular invasion, typically begins about the end of the first week and may last as long as 6 weeks. During this period, patients have fever, periorbital edema, conjunctivitis and subconjunctival hemorrhages, muscle pain and tenderness, and often severe weakness. There may be a maculopapular rash which lasts for several days and subungual "splinter hemorrhages." More serious manifestations accompany lung, heart, or central nervous system invasion. Lung involvement is manifested by hemoptysis and consolidation on chest x-rays. Central nervous system involvement may be evident as polyneuritis, poliomyelitis, myasthenia, meningitis, encephalitis, focal or diffuse pareses, delirium, psychosis, and coma. Despite the severity of central nervous system involvement in some patients, the cerebrospinal fluid remains normal.

Myocarditis is characterized by persistent tachycardia or development of congestive heart failure. There are marked electrocardiographic alterations, including ST-T wave changes and conduction abnormalities in 20 percent of patients. High levels of circulating eosinophils may produce damage to the ventricular endothelium with superimposed thrombosis.

A causal relationship between trichinosis and polyarteritis nodosa has been reported, presumably related to the presence of circulating immune complexes.

LABORATORY FINDINGS The most constant finding, and one of significance early in the course of the disease, is the eosinophilic leukocytosis (over 500 eosinophilic leukocytes per cubic millimeter) which generally appears before the end of the second week. In cases of moderate severity, the proportion of eosinophilic leukocytes ranges between 15 and 50 percent. In severe cases, particularly terminally, the eosinophilic leukocytosis may disappear entirely.

The skin test to larval antigen becomes positive early in the third week of infection and may remain so for up to 20 years. The usual positive response is a wheal of 5 mm or more appearing within 30 min. Unfortunately, the commercially available skin test preparations are not reliable and should not be used.

There are a variety of serologic tests for trichinosis, including the countercurrent electrophoresis test, the complement fixation test, the indirect fluorescent antibody test, and the bentonite flocculation test, which is probably the most widely used. A commercially available latex agglutination test appears as sensitive but is somewhat less specific. These serologic tests all become positive during the third week of the disease and may remain positive for a few years. A newly introduced, highly sensitive enzyme-linked immunosorbent test is able to detect specific antibody in the first week of infection. Since each may occasionally be falsely negative, two or more tests should be used. The serologic tests are most valuable if they are negative initially and then in turn positive or if there is a change in titer.

Muscle biopsy when carried out during the third week of infection remains the most useful test for demonstration of larvae or cysts. The deltoid or gastrocnemius muscles are the most useful sites for biopsy. A 1-g portion of the excised muscle should be compressed between glass slides and examined under a low-power microscope for the presence of larvae. Calcified cysts or larvae represent an old infection. The remainder of the biopsy should be submitted for routine processing because myositis is a significant finding even in the absence of larvae or cysts.

In severe trichinosis there may be marked hypoalbuminemia, probably because of protein leakage from damaged capillaries. During the fourth, fifth, and sixth weeks of the disease, concomitant with a rise in antibody, diffuse hypergammaglobulinemia occurs. Elevated levels of circulating IgE have been reported. There may be moderate rises in serum glutamic oxaloacetic transaminase, serum aldolase, and creatine phosphokinase, probably related to myositis; electromyography may show evidence of altered motor function. Typically the sedimentation rate is slow.

DIFFERENTIAL DIAGNOSIS Trichinosis must be differentiated from diseases which are characterized by eosinophilia (such as Hodgkin's disease, eosinophilic leukemia, and periarteritis nodosa) and from entities which are characterized by myopathy, such as dermatomyositis. When the central nervous system is involved, the diagnosis may be very difficult.

TREATMENT Thiabendazole, in dosage of 25 mg/kg bid for 5 to 7 days, has resulted in apparent improvement in a number of patients, with relief of muscle pain and tenderness and with lysis of fever. The results have not been uniform, however, and the use of this drug in trichinosis has been associated with nausea, vomiting, abdominal discomfort, dermatitis, and drug fever. Mebendazole, given in the dosage of 400 mg tid for 2 weeks, has also been employed; its role in human disease has not been established.

Patients with "allergic" manifestations of trichinosis, including angioedema and urticaria as well as myocardial or central nervous system involvement, should be treated with prednisone in dosage of 20 to 60 mg per day. Response to steroids usually has been prompt, particularly in central nervous system trichinosis. Not all focal lesions have resolved, however.

Other measures should be directed at relief of pain and maintenance of adequate caloric and fluid intake.

PROGNOSIS The prognosis in trichinosis has improved markedly, and even when the central nervous system is involved, the mortality rate has fallen to under 10 percent. The overall mortality rate is now less than 1 percent.

PREVENTION The responsibility for control rests with the consumer. Adequate cooking of pork involves heating all portions of the meat to 170°F (77°C). Freezing procedures to kill porcine larvae require a temperature of −15°C for 20 days or −18°C for 24 h. Larvae isolated from arctic animals appear much more resistant to freezing. Proper smoking and pickling will also destroy the larvae. Important in control is the cooking of garbage fed to hogs. The enzyme-linked immunosorbent procedure described above is sufficiently sensitive, specific, and simple to be used for the routine inspection of pork. To date, however, such screening tests have not been made mandatory.

REFERENCES

Barrett-Connor E et al: An epidemic of trichinosis after ingestion of wild pig in Hawaii. J Infect Dis 133:473, 1976

Campbell WC (ed): *Trichinella and Trichinosis.* New York, Plenum, 1983

Frayha RA: Trichinosis-related polyarteritis nodosa. Am J Med 71:307, 1981

Kazura JW, Aikawa M: Host defense mechanisms against *Trichinella spiralis* infection in the mouse: Eosinophil mediated destruction of newborn larvae *in vitro.* J Immunol 124:355, 1980

Kolata G: Testing for trichinosis: A new serological test should make it quick and easy to detect trichinosis in meat—a feat of no small economic importance. Science 227:621, 1985

Levin ML: Treatment of trichinosis with mebendazole. Am J Trop Med Hyg 32:980, 1983

Margolis HS et al: Trichinosis: Two Alaskan outbreaks from walrus meat. J Infect Dis 139:102, 1979

Metzler MH et al: Second-degree atrioventricular block in acute trichinosis. Am J Dis Child 124:598, 1972

Most H: Current concepts in parasitology. Trichinosis—preventable yet still with us. N Engl J Med 298:1178, 1978

Pun KK et al: The first documented outbreak of trichinellosis in Hong Kong Chinese. Am J Trop Med Hyg 32:772, 1983

163 FILARIASIS

JAMES J. PLORDE

DEFINITION Filariasis is a group of disorders produced by infection with the threadlike nematodes of the superfamily Filarioidea. These worms invade the lymphatics and subcutaneous and deep tissues of humans producing reactions ranging from acute inflammation to chronic scarring. The viviparous female discharges microfilariae into the blood or subcutaneous tissues where they live for weeks or months until taken up by hematophagous arthropods. Within these vectors they are transformed into filariform larvae which then infect a new host when the arthropod takes another blood meal. The clinical pictures produced by various species in this group are more or less specific. The term *lymphatic filariasis* is commonly used to designate the disease produced by *Wuchereria bancrofti*, *Brugia malayi*, and *Brugia timori*, the organisms responsible for lymphatic blockade and elephantiasis. *Loa loa* causes loiasis, a disease characterized by transient subcutaneous (Calabar) swellings, and *Onchocerca volvulus* produces the blindness and pruritic skin rash typical of onchocerciasis. *Mansonella ozzardi*, *M. perstans*, and *M. streptocerca* cause infections of questionable clinical significance to humans.

These parasites are identified by the location, periodicity, and morphologic characteristics of their microfilariae. Those of *W. bancrofti*, *B. malayi*, *B. timori*, *L. loa*, *M. perstans*, and *M. ozzardi* are all found in the blood, and, with the exception of the last, all display nocturnal or diurnal periodicity. *Onchocerca volvulus* and *M. streptocerca* are found in the subcutaneous tissues and are nonperiodic. Morphologically, the microfilariae are distinguished by the presence or absence of a sheath and by the distribution of their deeply staining column of nuclei. The sheath, which is an elongation of the original eggshell, can be seen extending beyond the head and tail only in the microfilariae of *W. bancrofti*, *B. malayi*, *B. timori*, and *L. loa*. The nuclear column extends to the very tip of the microfilariae of *B. malayi*, *B. timori*, *L. loa*, *M. perstans*, and *M. streptocerca*.

Skin and serologic tests are group-specific, lack sensitivity, and may be falsely positive in other nematode infections. In the absence of microfilariae and other helminthic infections, however, they may be helpful in establishing a diagnosis in clinically suspect cases.

LYMPHATIC FILARIASIS (BANCROFTIAN AND MALAYAN) Etiology and epidemiology

The threadlike adult worms live coiled together in human lymphatics. The male *W. bancrofti* measures 35 mm and the female 80 to 100 mm. The *Brugia* adults are about one-half as long. Gravid females release microfilariae in large numbers into the lymphatics. These embryos, which are sheathed, measure approximately 200 to 300 μm. They eventually reach the peripheral blood, where further development depends on their ingestion by a proper mosquito vector. Species of *Culex*, *Aëdes*, and *Anopheles* transmit Bancroftian filariasis; *Mansonia*, *Anopheles*, and *Coquillettidia* serve as vectors in Brugian disease. After further development in the vector, larvae migrate to the mouthparts. If the mosquito feeds on a human host, they penetrate the puncture site and reach maturity in about a year. In the absence of reinfection, humans harbor microfilariae for 5 to 10 years, the reproductive life of the adult worms. In most *W. bancrofti* and *Brugia* infections, the microfilariae are found in the blood in greatest numbers between 9 P.M. and 2 A.M. During the day, apparently in response to changes in oxygen tension, they accumulate in the pulmonary vessels and disappear from the peripheral blood. However, in Polynesia and New Caledonia there is an *Aëdes*-transmitted variety of *W. bancrofti* (*W. pacifica*) in which microfilaria circulate for 24 h with a peak concentration at midday (diurnal subperiodicity). A nocturnally subperiodic form of *B. malayi* is present in Malaysia, Thailand, and Indonesia. Periodicity is of epidemiologic significance because it determines which species of mosquito serves as the vector. The human is the only known vertebrate host for *W. bancrofti* and the periodic strains of *B. malayi*; subperiodic *B. malayi* is found in monkeys and cats as well as humans.

It has been estimated that 100 million persons throughout the world are infected, and both the prevalence and distribution of the disease seem to be increasing in many parts of Africa and Asia.

Wuchereria bancrofti infection is endemic between latitudes 41°N and 30°S involving primarily Africa, the Pacific Islands, and southeastern Asia from Korea on the north to India in the west. The West Indies, Central America, and the eastern coastal plains of South America are also involved. Distribution is irregular, and there are many peculiar "skip areas" in this geographic pattern, presumably because the endemic disease can be maintained only where human infection and mosquitoes are prevalent. *B. malayi* infection is much more restricted in its distribution and occurs in India, Burma, Thailand, Vietnam, China, South Korea, Japan, Malaysia, Indonesia, Borneo, New Guinea, and the Philippines. The parasite has disappeared from Sri Lanka. *B. timori* is limited to the eastern Indonesian archipelago.

Pathogenesis Pathologic changes are caused primarily by the presence of the adult worm in the lymphatics and may be divided into inflammatory and obstructive. The inflammatory response, thought to be due to an immediate-type hypersensitivity reaction to molting larvae, consists of infiltration with lymphocytes, plasma cells, and eosinophils. There are hyperplasia of lymphatic endothelium, acute lymphangitis, and thrombosis. Obstructive phenomena are thought to be caused by a granulomatous reaction to dead or dying adults which may lead to reversible lymphatic obstruction. Repetition of this process over a period of years leads to permanent lymphatic blockade. The tissues become edematous, thickened, and fibrotic. Secondary streptococcal infections are common and may contribute to lymphatic blockade. Dilated lymphatics may rupture into surrounding tissue. Elephantiasis is actually a relatively unusual complication of filarial infections and is actually more common in immigrants to endemic areas. Apparently, exposure to filarial antigens early in life provides some protection against elephantiasis. If repeated reinfections do not occur, the disease is self-limited.

Manifestations The clinical manifestations vary with the geographic area, species of parasite, immune response of the infected patient, and intensity of infection. Light infections may be completely asymptomatic. Symptoms may occur within 3 months of infection, but ordinarily the incubation period is 8 to 12 months. The clinical findings closely reflect the pathological changes, with inflammation early in the disease followed by obstruction later. Inflammatory filariasis consists of a series of brief febrile attacks occurring over a period of weeks. Fever is usually low grade but may reach 40.6°C (105°F) and be accompanied by chills and sweats. Other symptoms include headache, nausea and vomiting, photophobia, and muscle pain. If the involved lymphatics lie close to the surface, the local symptoms dominate the clinical picture. Lymphangitis is very common, involving the legs more frequently than the arms. It often begins as a tender spot in the region of the malleoli or femoral area and spreads centrifugally. The involved vessels are palpably tender and painful. The overlying skin is red and swollen. When abdominal lymphatics are involved, the picture may simulate that of an acute abdomen. In Bancroftian filariasis the vessels of the spermatic cord and testes may be involved, resulting in painful orchitis, epididymitis, or funiculitis. Lymphadenitis almost always accompanies and may sometimes precede lymphangitis. The inguinal, femoral, and epitrochlear nodes are involved. Abscesses which may form about involved lymphatics and lymph nodes may discharge to the surface, resulting in persistently draining sinus tracts. The acute manifestations last only a few days and then subside spontaneously, only to recur at irregular intervals over a period of weeks or months. Recovery finally ensues. With repeated infections, slowly progressive lymphatic obstruction may develop in areas where the inflammatory reactions have occurred previously. Edema, ascites, lymph scrotum, hydrocele, pleural effusion, or joint effusion may appear as a result of interference with lymphatic drainage. Lymphadenopathy persists. The lymphatic vessels become palpably enlarged as tense elastic masses beneath the skin, especially in the femoral, inguinal, and scrotal areas. They may rupture and form draining sinuses. Internal rupture of lymphatics may give rise to chylous ascites or chyluria. In a small percentage of cases elephantiasis develops. This complication is rare below the age of 20 even in natives of heavily infested areas. The chronic obstructive phase of the disease often is punctuated by acute inflammatory episodes.

TROPICAL EOSINOPHILIA   Attention has been focused on an aberrant type of filariasis which is characterized by the presence of hypereosinophilia, circulating filarial antibodies, microfilariae in tissue but *not in the blood*, and a chronic, clinical course that can be terminated with specific antifilarial treatment. These amicrofilaremic forms were originally thought to be caused by zoonotic parasites, but it is more likely that they represent an atypical host response to various filariae including *W. bancrofti* and *B. malayi*. The syndrome is most commonly seen in India, Indonesia, Sri Lanka, Pakistan, and southeast Asia, all areas of intense transmission for these organisms. Involved patients lack the IgG-blocking antibodies present in the patients with circulating microfilariae. Animal models suggest that microfilariae are removed from the peripheral circulation and trapped in various tissue sites by an IgG-dependent cell-mediated effector mechanism. Antigens released when the parasites are destroyed initiate an immediate IgE-mediated reaction. The eosinophilic inflammatory reaction, in time, progresses to granuloma formation and fibrosis. Clinically there may be marked enlargement of the lymph nodes and spleen (Meyers-Kouwenaar syndrome) and/or chronic cough, nocturnal bronchospasm, and miliary pulmonary infiltrates (Weingarten syndrome). The former syndrome is most frequently seen in children, and the latter in young male adults. Only one-quarter of the patients with pulmonary manifestations demonstrate obstructive defects on pulmonary function testing. All show restrictive disease, and irreversible pulmonary hypertension has been described in a few. A number of diseases characterized by pulmonary infiltration and eosinophilia (PIE) must be considered in the differential diagnosis of this disease. They include other helminthic infections, Loeffler's syndrome, chronic eosinophilic pneumonia, allergic aspergillosis, vasculitis, idiopathic hypereosinophilia, and drug allergies.

Diagnosis   A history of exposure, the long incubation period, the occurrence of typical inflammatory episodes, and the finding of regional lymphadenopathy, thickening of the spermatic cord, or swelling of an extremity should suggest the diagnosis. There is usually eosinophilia during acute episodes. Lymphangiography may reveal dilated afferent and small efferent lymphatics. The definitive diagnosis depends on demonstration of the parasite. Although adult worms can be demonstrated in biopsied lymph nodes, biopsy is not recommended because it may interfere further with lymphatic drainage. Microfilariae are found in the blood during intermediate stages but not early or late in the disease. As they are motile, they can often be seen in a wet mount. Definite identification, however, requires staining with Giemsa. As in malaria, both thin and thick smears should be prepared. Either the Knott concentration, counting chamber, or membrane filtration technique should be employed if the parasite is not found in thick smears. Because the appearance of microfilariae in peripheral blood is periodic, it is essential to obtain blood at appropriate times. When this proves difficult, the oral administration of 100 mg diethylcarbamazine usually produces positive blood specimens within 30 to 60 min. Microfilariae may also be found in lymphatic fluid, hydrocele fluid, ascites, and pleural fluid. Indirect hemagglutination, bentonite flocculation, and soluble antigen fluorescent antibody tests are available and, although not completely reliable, are helpful when microfilariae cannot be demonstrated. An indirect immunofluorescent test utilizing adult *B. malayi* as the source of antigen is both more sensitive and specific than previously developed procedures. Filarial antigens are present in the blood and urine of most microfilaremic and in some seropositive–microfilaremic-negative

patients, suggesting antigen detection may provide a more definitive indicator of active diseases than do standard serologic procedures. At present, such techniques are available only in research laboratories.

The diagnosis of *tropical eosinophilia* is confirmed by (1) a history of prolonged residence in an endemic area, (2) lack of microfilariae in the peripheral blood despite examination of both day and night specimens by concentration techniques, (3) peripheral eosinophilia in excess of 3000 cells per milliliter, (4) high titers of filarial antibodies, (5) IgE levels of at least 1000 units per milliliter, and (6) response to diethylcarbamazine within 7 to 10 days of initiating therapy. Recovery of microfilariae from the tissues is uncommon, and biopsy is not warranted.

Treatment   Diethylcarbamazine rapidly eliminates microfilariae from the blood. It probably also kills or injures adult worms, impairing their ability to reproduce, and clears microfilariae permanently from the bloodstream of many patients. The drug is given in doses of 2 mg/kg three times a day for 3 or 4 weeks. Treatment with this agent is often followed by allergic reactions to the dying parasite. These reactions may be quite severe, especially in Malayan filariasis. They can be controlled with aspirin, antihistamines, or corticosteroids. In heavy infections, it may be desirable to begin treatment with antihistamines before administration of diethylcarbamazine.

Reassurance of the patient is very important in this disease. Effective and safe vaccines are presently not available. Pressure bandages and surgery sometimes benefit elephantiasis. The prognosis for life is excellent, particularly if infected individuals leave endemic areas or otherwise avoid reinfections. Disease control is accomplished by combining mass treatment with mosquito control measures.

ONCHOCERCIASIS ("RIVER BLINDNESS")   Definition   Onchocerciasis is a cutaneous filariasis caused by *Onchocerca volvulus*. It is characterized by subcutaneous nodules, a pruritic skin rash, sclerosing lymphadenitis, and ocular lesions.

Etiology and epidemiology   The disease is found in focal areas within Mexico, Guatemala, Colombia, Venezuela, Ecuador, Surinam, Brazil, Saudi Arabia, and Yemen, and throughout tropical Africa. It is estimated that at least 40 million individuals in Africa and 200,000 in the new world are infected and that about 5 percent of these are blind as a result of the disease.

The infection is transmitted by black flies of the genus *Simulium*, which breed along turbulent, fast-moving streams. An inoculated larva matures into a single male or female in approximately 1 year. Since larvae do not multiply within the human host, heavy parasite loads are the result of repeated infections. The adult worms are found coiled together in fibrous subcutaneous nodules. The gravid females, which may live as long as 15 years, release thousands of unsheathed microfilariae daily. These migrate in the skin, subcutaneous tissue, and eye for up to 30 months until they either degenerate or are ingested by a feeding *Simulium*.

Pathogenesis and clinical manifestations   The subcutaneous nodules which enclose the adult worms are usually 2 to 3 cm in diameter when fully developed. Generally found over the bony prominences, they are firm, nontender, and freely movable, although occasionally they may be adherent to underlying tissue. Their location on the body is related to the biting habits of the vector. In Central America, where the fly bites on the upper part of the body, the nodules are frequently over the head; in Africa they are primarily on the trunk and thighs. They usually number less than 10, but more than 100 have been reported in a single patient.

The important pathologic changes occur as a result of an immediate hypersensitivity reaction to the dead or dying microfilariae. Specific antibody, complement, and eosinophils are all thought to be involved. Pruritus is often severe and constant. The skin lesion may appear as an erysipelas-like reaction over the face or a papular rash over one extremity. In chronic cases thickening, lichenification, and depigmentation may be present. In Africa microfilariae produce a fibrosing obstructive lymphadenitis, possibly by stimulating the deposition of immune complexes. This lesion is frequently associated with large folds of skin called *hanging groins* and with elephantiasis. Children living in endemic areas may not demonstrate these changes for decades even though microfilariae are present. The most serious complications of onchocerciasis are eye lesions which are usually found in patients repeatedly infected on the upper part of the body. A punctate and later sclerosing keratitis, iridocyclitis, optic atrophy, or chorioretinitis may eventually lead to blindness.

Diagnosis The diagnosis is made by demonstrating microfilariae in a skin snip taken from an involved area. A thin sliver of superficial skin is removed with a razor or punch. Care must be taken to prevent bleeding and possible contamination with blood microfilariae. The skin is weighed and is then placed in saline, teased with a pair of sharp dissecting needles, and observed for emerging microfilariae over the next hour. The results should be expressed in microfilariae per milligram of tissue. Multiple skin snips may be necessary. In patients with eye lesions, microfilariae can sometimes be seen in the anterior chamber with a slit lamp. If organisms cannot be detected by the above methods, the patient may be given 50 mg diethylcarbamazine orally. The occurrence of a pruritic rash within 24 h strongly suggests the presence of cutaneous microfilariae (Mazzotti's test). Several filarial serologic tests are available. Most use crude antigen preparations and lack specificity. The anticipated availability of more specific antigens in the near future may ameliorate this problem. Techniques for the detection of onchocercal antigens in blood and urine require further development.

Treatment and prevention Diethylcarbamazine is effective in destroying microfilariae but has little effect on the adult worm. The drug must be used with great care as rapid destruction of the parasites may cause a severe allergic reaction. If the eye is involved, this can result in further ocular damage. The initial adult dose is 50 mg orally. It is increased to 50 mg three times daily on the second day, 100 mg three times daily on the third day, and finally 200 mg three times a day for an additional 7 days. Antihistamines, or in rare cases corticosteroids, can be used to control allergic reactions. In ocular reactions, the pupil should be dilated and topical steroids applied.

The adult worms may be eliminated by excision of nodules on the head and neck, a procedure which is useful in preventing ocular complications, or by chemotherapy with suramin. Details of the administration and toxicity of this drug are given in Chap. 156. The dosage is 0.1 g given intravenously to detect drug idiosyncrasy, followed by 1.0 g intravenously once weekly for five to six doses.

Ivermectin, a macrocyclic antibiotic, is a slightly more effective microfilaricidal agent, and its administration does not appear to induce the severe allergic reactions seen with diethylcarbamazine. Although further studies are required to establish optimum dosage, it appears that this agent may be suitable for use in mass treatment programs.

Chemoprophylaxis is not practical, and personal protection depends upon the use of protective clothing. Insecticides, mass therapy, and nodulectomies have been used but have not been very satisfactory. A massive control project in west Africa utilizing insecticides dropped by airplane and helicopter has been more successful.

LOIASIS This form of filariasis is produced by *Loa loa* and is prevalent in west and central Africa. The infection is transmitted by deerflies of the genus *Chrysops*. The adult worms, which like the other filariae may live for 10 to 15 years, migrate continuously through the subcutaneous tissue. The resulting localized areas of allergic inflammation, *Calabar swellings,* are the hallmark of the disease. Occasionally the adult worms may be seen crossing the eye subconjunctivally. This usually results in intense lacrimation, pain, and anxiety. Infestation may, however, be completely asymptomatic. An association between loiasis, the nephrotic syndrome, and endomyocardial fibrosis has been reported; these conditions are considered autoimmune disorders. The diagnosis can be made by finding the adult worm or by demonstrating the distinctive sheathed microfilariae in contents of the Calabar swellings or in the bloodstream during the daytime. Microfilariae are often not found. In these cases, there are usually marked eosinophilia and a positive filarial complement fixation test. Diethylcarbamazine, administered for 2 to 3 weeks in the manner described for onchocerciasis, will kill both adult worms and microfilariae. This drug must be used with great care as it may induce a severe meningoencephalitis in patients with intense microfilaremia; this presumably reflects an allergic reaction to dead or dying parasites. It is taken in a dose of 200 mg twice daily for 3 days each month and is also effective as a chemoprophylactic agent.

MANSONELLIASIS PERSTANS *Mansonella perstans* (*Dipetalonema perstans, Acanthocheilonema perstans*) is a filarial parasite of humans and other primates inhabiting the tropical areas of Africa and Latin America. The adult worm lives encysted in the subserosal tissues of the pericardium, pleura, and peritoneum, particularly the mesentery. The unsheathed microfilariae, which can be found in the peripheral blood throughout the day, measure 200 μm in length and have four to six nuclei in their tail. They are transmitted from host to host by blood-sucking gnats of the genus *Culicoides*. Most infections are asymptomatic, and their principal significance lies in the fact that they may be confused with other, more serious, forms of filariasis. Nevertheless, some patients complain of fever, pruritus, Calabar swellings, erysipelas-like rashes, and abdominal pain. Although microfilariae are frequently seen in the cerebrospinal fluid, neurologic manifestations are rare. Peripheral eosinophilia is common, but filarial complement fixation tests are generally negative. The diagnosis is made by finding the characteristic microfilariae in the peripheral blood. Treatment with diethylcarbamazine is of doubtful benefit.

MANSONELLIASIS STREPTOCERCA *Mansonella streptocerca* (*Dipetalonema streptocerca*) is found in equatorial Africa where it inhabits the dermis and subcutaneous tissues of chimpanzees and humans. Like *M. perstans*, it is transmitted by *Culicoides*. The microfilariae inhabit the dermal collagen where they elicit a lymphocytic and eosinophilic inflammatory response, fibrosis, lymphatic dilatation, pruritus, hypopigmented macules, and a papular rash. The diagnosis is made by recovering the nonperiodic microfilariae from skin snips as described for onchocerciasis above. They are unsheathed and possess a sharply crooked tail with nuclei. Diethylcarbamazine, as described for Bancroftian filariasis above, is effective. Treatment often provokes a reaction similar to the Mazzotti reaction described for onchocerciasis.

MANSONELLIASIS OZZARDI *Mansonella ozzardi* are found as adult worms in the mesentery and visceral fat of people living in the tropical areas of Latin America and the Caribbean. This species is thought to be transmitted by flies of the genus *Simulium* and gnats of the genus *Culicoides*. The nonperiodic microfilariae are released into the peripheral blood where they can be identified by their lack of a sheath or caudal nuclei. Occasionally, they may also be found in skin snips, producing confusion with onchocerciasis. This common infection is thought to be asymptomatic, but reports of patients presenting with fever, pruritus, lymphadenopathy, hydroceles, and chronic arthritis have been published. There are conflicting reports on the efficacy of diethylcarbamazine therapy.

DIROFILARIASIS *Dirofilaria immitis* (canine heartworm) is a large, cosmopolitan filaria of dogs which lives in their right ventricle and pulmonary arteries and releases its microfilariae into the peripheral blood. It is transmitted by several types of mosquitoes. Human infections are increasingly reported, particularly from the eastern and southern United States, the Mississippi Valley, and California. The worm does not mature in humans, and hence microfilaremia is not present. Although cardiac infections have been noted at autopsy, most human infections present as well-defined pulmonary nodules, the result of an embolic infarct produced by an immature worm. The patients are most frequently asymptomatic and are discovered to have a "coin lesion," 2 cm or less in diameter, on pulmonary roentgenography. Less commonly they complain of cough and chest pain or, rarely, of hemoptysis, fever, chills, and myalgia. The diagnosis is usually made by the microscopic examination of excised pulmonary nodules. Eosinophilia is mild or absent and serologic tests are not helpful.

Other *Dirofilariae* may rarely invade humans producing subcutaneous eosinophilic granulomas of the eyelid, trunk, or extremities. The nodules, which measure 1 to 2 cm in diameter, may be painful or completely asymptomatic. In the southern United States, the filaria most frequently involved is *D. tenuis*, a parasite of raccoons. The nodules are removed by surgical excision.

REFERENCES

CHERNIN E: Sir Patrick Manson's studies on the transmission and biology of filariasis. Rev Infect Dis 5:148, 1983

CIFERRI F: Human pulmonary dirofilariasis in the United States: A critical review. Am J Trop Med Hyg 31:302, 1982

CONNOR DH et al: Pathologic changes of human onchocerciasis: Implications for future research. Rev Infect Dis 7:809, 1985

GREENE BM et al: Comparison of ivermectin and diethylcarbamazine in the treatment of onchocerciasis. N Engl J Med 313:133, 1985

GROVE DI: Selective primary health care: Strategies for the control of disease in the developing world. VII. Filariasis. Rev Infect Dis 5:933, 1983

HAWKING F: The 24-hour periodicity of microfilariae: Biological mechanisms responsible for its production and control. Proc R Soc Lond [Biol] 169:59, 1967

KOCHAR AS: Human pulmonary dirofilariasis. Report of three cases and brief review of the literature. Am J Clin Pathol 84:19, 1985

MEYERS WM et al: Human streptocerciasis. A clinico-pathological study of 40 Africans (Zaireans) including identification of the adult filaria. Am J Trop Med Hyg 21:528, 1972

NEGESSE Y et al: Loiasis: "Calabar" swellings and involvement of deep organs. Am J Trop Med Hyg 34:537, 1985

NEVA FA, OTTESON EA: Current concepts in parasitology. Tropical (filarial) eosinophilia. N Engl J Med 298:1129, 1978

ONKEL TC: Infections with *Dipetalonema perstans* and *Mansonella ozzardi* in the aboriginal Indians of Guyana. Am J Trop Med Hyg 16:628, 1967

OTTESEN EA: Immunologic aspects of lymphatic filariasis and onchocerciasis in man. Trans R Soc Trop Med Hyg 78(suppl):9, 1984

RAO CK, KUMAR S: Role of filariasis in endomyocardial fibrosis. J Commun Dis 14:91, 1982

THYLEFORS B: Ocular onchocerciasis. Bull WHO 56:63, 1978

WELLER PF et al: Tourism-acquired *Mansonella ozzardi* microfilaria in a regular blood donor. JAMA 240:858, 1978

WORLD HEALTH ORGANIZATION: Lymphatic filariasis. Fourth report of the WHO Expert Committee on Filariasis. Technical Report Series 702, Geneva:WHO, 1984

YANGCO BG et al: A survey of filariasis among refugees in south Florida. Am J Trop Med Hyg 33:246, 1984

164   SCHISTOSOMIASIS

THEODORE E. NASH

INTRODUCTION   Three major schistosome species, *Schistosoma mansoni*, *Schistosoma haematobium*, and *Schistosoma japonicum*, and a number of less prevalent species of the genus *Schistosoma* infect humans. Both *Schistosoma mansoni* and *Schistosoma japonicum* adults reside in the venules of the intestine, and the major disease manifestations of these parasites are hepatic. *S. mansoni* is found in parts of South America (Brazil, Venezuela, and Surinam), some Caribbean islands, Africa, and the Middle East while infections with *S. japonicum* occur in the Far East, mostly in China and the Philippines. *S. haematobium* adults are found mostly in the venules of the urinary tract and cause disease primarily of the ureters and bladder. Infections with this species occur in Africa and the Middle East. Of lesser importance are *Schistosoma mekongi*, a newly recognized parasite related to *S. japonicum* which is found along the Mekong River in Indochina, and *Schistosoma intercalatum*, found in certain areas of central West Africa. Worldwide, as many as 200 million persons may be infected, and infection of entire communities

is common. However, most infected persons experience few, if any, signs and symptoms, and only a small minority develop significant disease.

LIFE CYCLE   The schistosome species infecting humans all share the same basic life cycle but are unique in a number of important ways which account for some of the different clinical and pathologic findings. Important differences include the length of time before egg laying begins (prepatent period), location of the adult worms, number of eggs produced by each pair of worms, response by the host to the ova, and eventual fate of retained eggs. The morphology of the various stages of the parasites and the types of intermediate host snail are also distinct. Humans become infected after contact with water containing the infective stage of the parasite, called a cercaria, which is a microscopic form of the schistosome possessing a forked tail used for swimming and a head which is the anlage of the future worm. Cercariae penetrate the unbroken skin, with the help of secreted enzymes, and in the skin transform into schistosomules or developing schistosomes. After 2 to 3 days the schistosomules migrate to the lungs and then to the portal vein, probably by an intravascular route. In the portal vein the maturing male and female schistosomes pair and migrate to the venules of the mesentery, bladder, or ureters, depending on the species of schistosome, and begin to deposit eggs. The time spent in migration and maturation differs. *S. mansoni* and *S. japonicum* begin depositing eggs around 4 to 5 weeks after infection, while egg deposition begins after 2 to 3 months for *S. haematobium*. Adult worms are about 1 to 2 cm in length and migrate in the blood vessels without eliciting a local inflammatory reaction. Adult worms do not multiply in humans, and immunosuppressive therapy does not result in increased numbers of worms. Once released, eggs are either retained in the tissues at the site of deposition or swept back, mostly to the liver, by way of the venous portal system in the case of the intestinal schistosomes. Eggs are deposited mainly in the bladder and ureters by *S. haematobium*. A portion of the mature schistosome ova are extruded into the lumen of the intestines, bladder, or ureters and after contact with water hatch, releasing a miracidium. This free-swimming ciliated stage seeks out the proper intermediate snail vector and burrows into the soft tissues of the snail. After 1 to 2 months, depending on the species of parasite, the miracidium develops into a primary and then secondary sporocyst which, after further development, begins releasing cercariae into the surrounding water. Thousands of cercariae can be released daily from each infected snail. Therefore one miracidium produces many cercariae, and this amplifies the number of infective parasites and the risk of infection. Cercariae are most infectious immediately after shedding and are not viable 48 h after release so storing water for 48 h before contact prevents exposure and infection. Unlike most other trematodes the sexes are separate in schistosomes, but this is only evident in the adult stage. Ova are laid only when males and females infect the same individual.

PATHOPHYSIOLOGY   There are a number of factors which determine the disease manifestations of the host. These include the duration and intensity of infection, location of egg deposition, host genetics, concurrent infections, and other still undefined factors.

In individuals from endemic areas initial infection goes unnoticed. There are a number of possible reasons for this, including age of initial exposure, manner of exposure, and transfer of maternal immunity. However, in visitors to endemic areas initial infection with schistosomes commonly results in an acute febrile illness (Katayama fever or acute schistosomiasis) which is a manifestation of the immune response to the developing schistosomes and eggs. There is a good immune response which becomes suppressed. These individuals have elevated levels of eosinophils and immune complexes and react markedly to schistosome antigens as measured by lymphocyte blastogenesis. Despite ongoing infection, symptoms subside, as do blastogenic responses to antigens but not to unrelated antigens such as purified protein derivative of tuberculin (PPD). The exudative acute granulomatous response to schistosome eggs is also suppressed.

A major factor in determining the development of disease in humans is the worm burden of the host, which determines the number of eggs produced. It is the inflammatory and fibrotic response to these eggs which is responsible for most of the morbidity and mortality associated with schistosomiasis. Those factors which limit parasite survival will limit the development of disease. In human schistosome infections it is not known if protective immunity develops, but immunity clearly exists in experimental animals. In the first few days after infection the schistosomule is relatively susceptible to immune attack. A number of systems employing antibody and/or eosinophils, neutrophils, macrophages, and complement have been used to kill schistosomules in vitro. However, as the schistosomules mature, they become refractory to these immune responses. In addition, schistosomes coat their tegument with host proteins and evade recognition by the host. A number of pertinent schistosomule and adult antigens have been defined with the hope of developing vaccines; the administration of murine monoclonal antibodies to some of these antigens has reduced worm burdens in challenge infections by about 50 percent, and immunization with one antigen has produced similar levels of protection. Successful vaccination with anti-idiotypes has also been reported.

All schistosome eggs elicit a granulomatous response which is best understood in *S. mansoni* infections. The host becomes sensitized to the egg proteins by a T-cell-mediated mechanism which induces a larger granuloma. However, with continued infection the granuloma decreases in size due to the recruitment of suppressor T cells, while antibody has no effect on granuloma size. The regulation of granulomas due to *S. japonicum* eggs differs from that of granulomas from *S. mansoni* eggs. Immune modulation is mediated by serum factors, at least in the chronic stage of infection. Both eggs and granulomas release factors which induce fibroblast proliferation in vitro. The early cellular response induced by granulomas is followed by fibrosis in vivo; however, liver fibrosis in humans probably involves more than simple fusion of fibrotic granulomas. After years of continued infection, a minority of heavily infected individuals develop end-stage fibrotic lesions; mainly portal fibrosis (Symmers's fibrosis), esophageal varices, and splenomegaly in *S. mansoni, S. japonicum,* and *S. mekongi* infections and fibrosis of the ureters and bladder in *S. haematobium* infections. After the development of portal fibrosis eggs are shunted to the lungs via portal-systemic collateral veins resulting in cor pulmonale. Immune complexes shunted to the systemic circulation cause glomerulonephritis.

Host genetic factors have been found to influence the development of Symmers's fibrosis although there is no general agreement as to which factors are important. Schistosomes even of the same species are also genetically diverse, as shown by endonuclease restriction analysis, but the effect of this on disease in humans is unknown.

CLINICAL SYNDROMES Acute schistosomiasis

Acute schistosomiasis, or Katayama fever, occurs following initial exposure and infection with *S. mansoni* and *S. japonicum*. It rarely follows infection with *S. haematobium*. Acute schistosomiasis is seldom recognized in endemic populations and therefore is noted primarily in visitors to endemic areas. Immediately following exposure patients frequently complain of intense transient itching. From 2 to 6 weeks or longer after exposure the patient may complain of a variety of symptoms including fever, chills, headache, hives or angioedema, weakness, weight loss, nonproductive cough, abdominal pain, and diarrhea. Sometimes symptoms abate but return with increased intensity about the time egg laying commences. These symptoms gradually diminish but may last as long as 2 to 3 months. Other newly infected individuals may be asymptomatic or have only minimal symptoms. In these individuals the diagnosis is established only after further evaluation prompted by suggestive laboratory test results or exposure history. More severe symptoms occur with heavier infections, but light infections may cause severe illness. Central nervous system lesions may occur during acute schistosome infection. The diagnosis of acute schistosomiasis is suggested by the clinical findings and the presence

of eosinophilia, which is sometimes greater than 50 percent. Leukocytosis, increased immune complexes, and elevated IgM, IgG, and IgE immunoglobulins are found commonly. Although immune complexes have been suggested to play a role in the pathophysiology of acute schistosomiasis, glomerulonephritis and vasculitis are not present. The specific diagnosis can be established even before the shedding of ova by the detection of antibodies to adult schistosome gut antigens, or after egg excretion (5 to 6 weeks following exposure) by appropriate serologic testing and the finding of eggs in the stool or rectal biopsy. Clinically, acute schistosomiasis is frequently misdiagnosed as typhoid fever but can be confused with any prolonged febrile illness. Although these patients seem to tolerate chemotherapy well, it is unclear if therapy shortens the course of disease or decreases symptoms. Corticosteroids may be useful, but this has not been demonstrated in controlled studies.

Liver fibrosis The most important complication of intestinal schistosome infection is the development of periportal or Symmers's fibrosis and portal hypertension (hepatosplenic schistosomiasis). This pathognomonic finding occurs in *S. mansoni, S. japonicum,* and *S. mekongi* infections but has been best studied in *S. mansoni* infections, where it normally develops after 10 to 15 years of prolonged exposure and infection. The liver is usually but not always enlarged, firm, and nodular, and the left lobe is characteristically prominent. Macroscopically, finger-sized bands of fibrosis ("pipe-stem" fibrosis) encompass the portal tracts. The portal venous tracts are replaced with fibrous tissue leading to presinusoidal blockage, portal hypertension, splenomegaly, and esophageal and gastric varices. The intrahepatic pressure is normal. Hepatic function is generally well preserved, and patients commonly present with hematemesis and/or signs and symptoms of splenomegaly. Ascites, hepatic coma, edema, spider angiomas, gynecomastia, and other signs of liver failure occur less frequently than in alcoholic and postnecrotic cirrhosis. Despite repeated episodes of hematemesis, patients may do reasonably well.

The diagnosis of periportal fibrosis is established by wedge biopsy of the liver; needle biopsy specimens are inadequate. Ultrasonograms of the liver show characteristic findings. The fibrotic bands appear as dense echogenic areas surrounding the portal vein and its tributaries. Further studies of the correlation between the pathologic and ultrasound findings are necessary to establish the sensitivity and specificity of this technique.

Patients with periportal fibrosis may not have schistosome eggs in their feces because of previous treatment and/or attrition of adult worms without subsequent reinfection. Since schistosome infections are practically universal in many populations, the mere presence of schistosome eggs in the feces of a patient does not establish the diagnosis of schistosomal periportal fibrosis; other liver diseases may be present. It is not clear whether there is any benefit from shunting procedures or splenectomy although these procedures are used commonly. The mortality of patients with portal fibrosis has not been well studied but in one group was 8.2 percent after 3.6 years.

Glomerulonephritis and pulmonary hypertension These two complications occur almost exclusively in patients with periportal fibrosis and portal hypertension, probably as a result of eggs and circulating antigens or immune complexes bypassing the liver. Pulmonary hypertension appears to be due to obliteration of pulmonary arterioles by granulomatous inflammation induced by shunted and embolized schistosome eggs. This is most frequently recognized with *S. mansoni* and *S. japonicum* infections but also occurs with *S. haematobium.* The association of glomerulonephritis and schistosomiasis has been noted in humans and in experimentally infected animals. This complication is manifested clinically as proteinuria and/or renal failure. Schistosome-specific antibodies and antigens have been detected in the glomeruli of infected patients.

Other complications Focal dense deposits of eggs of *S. mansoni* in the large intestine (and less commonly of *S. haematobium* and probably of *S. japonicum*) incite an exudative granulomatous response resulting in the formation of inflammatory polyps. Histologically, these consist of masses of eggs, inflammatory cells, and fibrosis. The major clinical presentation is bloody diarrhea, sometimes associated with protein-losing enteropathy and anemia. This type of involvement of the bowel is recognized primarily in Egypt and the Sudan. However, gastrointestinal symptoms are not increased in most chronically infected patients compared to control populations. In addition, granulomatous masses involving the bowel wall may mimic carcinoma of the bowel. Central nervous system (CNS) involvement with *S. mansoni* and *S. haematobium* has a predilection for the spinal cord while the brain is involved more commonly in *S. japonicum* infections.

Patients infected with the three major species of schistosomes and subsequently infected with salmonella may develop a prolonged intermittent febrile illness. In *S. haematobium* infections prolonged excretion of salmonella in the urine is common. Many times treatment of the salmonella infection alone is not effective, and specific antischistosomal chemotherapy is also required. Salmonella may be protected from host immune responses by residing in schistosome gut or by adhering to the surface tegument of the schistosome.

SCHISTOSOMA MANSONI Epidemiology and manifestations

S. mansoni is found in South America and certain islands of the Caribbean Sea, Africa, and the Middle East. The prepatent period is about 4 to 5 weeks. The intermediate hosts are various species in the genus *Biomphalaria*.

S. mansoni is the most common schistosome species infecting humans, and more is known about this parasite and human infection and disease than about the other schistosome species. Although infection is frequent and sometimes universal in endemic areas, the development of disease is relatively uncommon and depends on a number of factors which include the duration and intensity of infection. In endemic populations chronic infections are usual, many times lasting decades, and disease manifestations develop in a predictable manner. For the most part, the initial infection of persons living in endemic areas goes unnoticed. In endemic populations, throughout the first decade of life the intensity of infection as measured by the number of eggs excreted in the feces increases, and prevalence rates

often approach 100 percent in highly endemic communities. Few if any symptoms are attributable to schistosomiasis during this time. The liver, particularly the left lobe, gradually enlarges and becomes firm in consistency. Between 10 and 15 years of age, some heavily infected persons develop splenomegaly which partly reflects the presence of portal fibrosis and portal hypertension. At about the same time, the number of eggs in the feces decreases, and there is some evidence to suggest that immune factors as well as decreased water contact are responsible for this. During the next three decades, persons with portal fibrosis and hypertension may experience repeated bouts of hematemesis secondary to esophageal varices or symptoms secondary to a massively enlarged spleen. Not infrequently, either because of prior chemotherapy, decreased exposure, or increased host immunity, patients with end-stage portal fibrosis no longer excrete viable eggs. Adult schistosomes can survive 20 years or more in the human host but usually live 5 to 8 years. The prognosis and the potential for reversing complications of infection after appropriate chemotherapy depend on the stage of disease. End-stage fibrotic lesions are not reversible after chemotherapy. Glomerulonephritis and cor pulmonale secondary to schistosomiasis occur exclusively in patients with portal fibrosis. Central nervous system (CNS) involvement can occur in any stage of the infection and is not related to the intensity of infection. Other complications are noted in Table 164-1 and in the pathophysiology section.

Diagnosis The diagnosis of schistomiasis mansoni is established by identification of *S. mansoni* ova in the feces or tissues. The ova are 114 to 175 μm in length and 45 to 68 μm in width and have a prominent lateral spine. In light infections with less than 50 eggs per gram of feces, ova may not be detectable in the stool without the use of techniques which sample large quantities of stool. Even in light infections, ova can usually be detected in rectal biopsies and are best identified by squashing a small amount of tissue between two glass slides and searching for ova microscopically.

Many serologic tests have been employed in the diagnosis of schistosomiasis. These tests are not standardized and differ in sensitivity and specificity. In general, most currently employed tests have greater than 90 percent sensitivity, and a positive serology is indicative of a present or past infection. An immunofluorescent antibody test employing sections of adult schistosomes to determine the presence of antibodies to schistosome gut antigens has been extremely useful in identifying recently infected expatriates and persons with acute schistosomiasis.

Treatment In previous years, chemotherapy was offered to more heavily infected individuals who were more likely to develop disease. Although the risks of continued infection have not been clearly defined, with the availability of easily administered and safe drugs, most infected persons are likely to benefit from treatment. Patients with active infections have live eggs which can be identified microscopically by experienced parasitologists or by the presence of flame cells, or by their ability to hatch after contact with water. Although a number of drugs are available for the treatment of schistosomiasis mansoni, praziquantel and oxamniquine are the drugs of choice (Table 164-2). Both drugs are equally safe and effective in schistosomiasis mansoni found in the Caribbean and South America. Because some strains of *S. mansoni* in Africa are relatively resistant to oxamniquine, praziquantel is the better drug in treating these individuals. Both drugs can be used in patients with portal fibrosis. The side effects of praziquantel and oxamniquine are frequent but transient and mild. For praziquantel they include abdominal pain, lethargy, diarrhea, and fever and for oxamniquine, dizziness, tiredness, nausea and vomiting, neuropsychiatric manifestations, and rarely convulsions.

SCHISTOSOMA JAPONICUM Epidemiology and clinical manifestations

Schistosoma japonicum is found in southeast Asia and is an important health concern in areas of China and the Philippines. The intermediate hosts are amphibious snails of the genus *Oncomelania*. Besides humans, numerous mammals such as cattle and water

TABLE 164-1 Clinical manifestations of schistosomiasis from various *Schistosoma* species*

Manifestation	S. mansoni	S. japonicum	S. haematobium
Acute toxemic schistosomiasis	+	+	+
Chronic asymptomatic schistosomiasis	+	+	+
Hepatosplenic schistosomiasis	+	+	0
Cor pulmonale	+	+	±
Glomerulonephritis (clinically significant)	+	+	0†
Colonic polyposis	+	+	±
Ectopic lesions			
Brain	±	+	±
Spinal cord	+	±	+
Skin	+	+	+
Chronic cystitis and ureteritis	0	0	+
Mass lesions, bladder and ureters	0	0	+
Bladder cancer	0	0	+
Association with salmonella	+	+	+
Prolonged fever	+	+	+
Urinary carrier stage	?	?	+
Swimmer's itch‡	+	+	+

* + = recognized complications of infections by this species; ± = findings much less prominent in individuals infected by this species; 0 = complications not present in infections by this species.
† Except with associated salmonella infections.
‡ Usually from schistosomes that do not infect humans.

buffalo are naturally infected and serve as reservoirs of infection. The prepatent period is about 4 weeks.

The course of infection and clinical manifestations of *S. japonicum* are similar to those of *S. mansoni*, but the epidemiology and disease manifestations are less well studied. Experimental infections are more virulent, probably because each worm pair produces 10 times as many eggs as *S. mansoni*. The granulomas contain clusters of eggs and are larger and frequently show central necrosis. As in *S. mansoni* infections, periportal fibrosis is the major clinical manifestation. The other clinical syndromes described in *S. mansoni* also occur as complications of this infection (see above). However, there are some notable differences in disease manifestations, particularly CNS involvement. In acute schistosomiasis associated with *S. japonicum* infections, about 2 to 3 percent of patients experience CNS symptoms and signs that mimic acute encephalitis or a focal neurologic process. Computerized axial tomography shows multiple enhancing lesions. In chronic infections, patients may present with focal lesions of the brain which mimic brain tumors. These lesions contain masses of eggs and granulomas. Uncontrolled studies suggest that treatment with antischistosomal drugs and corticosteroids is effective.

Diagnosis The principles of diagnosis are similar to those of *S. mansoni* and require the demonstration of the typical ova in the tissues or feces of infected individuals. The eggs are oval in shape, 70 to 100 μm by 50 to 65 μm, and have a vestigial spine. Old, calcified, dead eggs are commonly retained in the tissues for long periods of time and do not indicate active infection (see *S. mansoni*).

Treatment Most infected persons should be treated. The only safe and effective therapy for *S. japonicum* infections is praziquantel (Table 164-2).

SCHISTOSOMA MEKONGI *Schistosoma mekongi* occurs in the Mekong River in Indochina (Laos, Cambodia, and Thailand). The intermediate host is an aquatic snail, *T. aperta*. The eggs are similar to *S. japonicum's* but are slightly smaller and round, about 56 μm by 64 μm. Dogs and human beings are frequently naturally infected. The prepatent period is about 5 weeks. The disease manifestations appear to be similar to those of *S. japonicum* but are not fully documented. Praziquantel is effective therapy for this infection (Table 164-2).

SCHISTOSOMA HAEMATOBIUM Epidemiology and clinical manifestations *S. haematobium* infections occur in extensive areas of Africa and in the Middle East. The intermediate hosts are of the genus *Bulinus*. The prepatent period is 2 to 3 months. Natural infection is primarily limited to human beings.

As in *S. mansoni* infections, the prevalence and intensity of infection in endemic areas increases until 10 to 15 years of age. Thereafter, the intensity decreases markedly while the prevalence rate falls moderately. The signs and symptoms due to *S. haematobium*, owing to its predilection for the veins of the urinary tract, result from involvement of the ureters and bladder. In contrast to the asymptomatic period following initial infection with the intestinal schistosomes, dysuria and hematuria are frequently noted 2 to 3 months after infection. These findings may continue throughout the course of active infection. Initially, the eggs invoke an intense inflammatory and granulomatous response which may cause anatomic and/or functional obstruction, hydroureter and hydronephrosis, and masses in the bladder or ureters. Cystoscopic examination may reveal friable masses extending into the bladder, ulceration, petechiae, and granulomas. These early lesions are reversible after antischistosomal chemotherapy. Eggs shed into the urine are usually easily demonstrable. As the infection progresses, the inflammatory component lessens, possibly due to a modulating effect of the host's immune response, and fibrosis increases, most likely due to the accumulation of many old and some new lesions. Still later, a majority of the lesions consist of masses of dead and calcified eggs in fibrous tissue. When the concentration of calcified eggs in the tissues is large enough, radiographic opacification of the affected areas of the urinary tract becomes evident. Old fibrotic lesions which cause hydroureter and hydronephrosis are not reversible by antischistosomal chemotherapy. Renal failure occurs in a surprisingly small proportion of infected individuals.

Portal fibrosis and clinically significant glomerulonephritis are not complications of this infection, but passage of eggs into the lungs may result in pulmonary hypertension. Prolonged excretion of salmonella in the urine and intermittent bacteremias are well documented. Urinary tract infections with other bacteria do not appear to be increased in frequency unless there is instrumentation of the urinary tract; however, they may be difficult to eradicate once established. Central nervous system infection most commonly involves the spinal cord, as in *S. mansoni* infections. Although eggs of *S. haematobium* are frequently detected in the feces in low numbers and are often found in rectal biopsies, intestinal polyposis is uncommon. In certain geographic areas squamous cell cancer of the bladder is felt to be associated with *S. haematobium* infection and is a significant cause of morbidity and mortality.

Diagnosis The diagnosis of *S. haematobium* is established by demonstrating the characteristic eggs in the tissues or urine. These are 112 to 170 μm by 40 to 70 μm, have a prominent terminal spine, and are easily seen in the urine. An increased number of eggs is excreted around midday, and microscopic examination of a centrifuged urine specimen collected at this time usually reveals ova. In light infections, examination of increased quantities of urine is sometimes required. Gross or microscopic hematuria is common in endemic populations, and its presence should always suggest the diagnosis in exposed individuals. Antibodies to *S. haematobium* can be detected using *S. mansoni* antigen preparations.

Treatment Infected persons should be treated. Dead and calcified eggs are common in tissue, are often seen in urine specimens, and

TABLE 164-2 Treatment of schistosomiasis

Species	Drug	Total dose* (mg per kilogram body weight)	Regimen
S. haematobium	Praziquantel	40	Single dose or two 20 mg/kg doses
	Metrifonate†	22.5–30	Single dose of 7.5 to 10 mg per kilogram body weight administered every other week × 3
S. mansoni			
Americas and Caribbean	Oxamniquine	15	Single oral dose with food
	Praziquantel	40	Single or two 20 mg/kg doses 4 h apart with food
Africa and Middle East	Oxamniquine	60	15 mg per kilogram body weight twice a day for 2 days with food
	Praziquantel	40	Single dose or two 20 mg/kg doses 4 h apart with food
S. japonicum or S. mekongi	Praziquantel	60	20 mg per kilogram body weight every 4 h with food

* All recommended drugs are given orally.
† Available from the Parasitic Diseases Division, Centers for Infectious Diseases, Centers for Disease Control, Atlanta, GA 30333.

should be differentiated from viable eggs. Although a number of drugs have been used to treat *S. haematobium* in the past, praziquantel is the treatment of choice (Table 164-2). Metrifonate, a safe, orally administered agent, is also effective. Its major advantage is low cost, and the major disadvantage is that it is optimally given in three doses 2 weeks apart.

SCHISTOSOMA INTERCALATUM *Schistosoma intercalatum* infection is limited to areas of West Africa. Eggs, 140 to 240 μm by 50 to 85 μm, are found in the stool and have a terminal spine. Few symptoms can be attributable to this infection, and no cases of portal fibrosis have been reported. Praziquantel is effective treatment (Table 164-2).

SCHISTOSOME DERMATITIS (SWIMMER'S ITCH) When cercariae penetrate the skin, they may provoke a reaction known as schistosome dermatitis. Symptoms occur most commonly after penetration of nonhuman schistosomes of birds and mammals. In previously unexposed persons, the initial invasion causes transient itching and uncommonly urticaria followed by the development of macules within 24 h and papules after 24 h. Following repeated exposures, the signs and symptoms increase dramatically and occur earlier. Large pruritic, erythematous papules and uncommonly vesicles develop within 24 h. The lesions are most intense 2 to 3 days following exposure and subside after a few days. These lesions represent a delayed hypersensitivity reaction to the invading schistosome. Nonhuman schistosomes do not fully develop in humans, and the signs and symptoms are limited to the skin. A similar dermatitis also occurs after infection with human schistosomes.

Schistosome dermatitis occurs in many freshwater areas of the world but is particularly common in the north central and western United States. A dermatitis following seawater exposure (clam digger's itch) has also been described.

Treatment is symptomatic. Since cercariae need some time to invade the skin (15 min or less), rapid removal of cercariae-containing droplets after water contact will decrease exposure. Limiting the numbers of the intermediate host snail in frequented areas can effectively control exposure.

CONTROL OF SCHISTOSOMIASIS Theoretically, schistosome infections can be controlled by a variety of methods, but their application has generally been only partially successful. Simple and effective health education measures such as the elimination of indiscriminate urination and defecation are difficult to implement in endemic areas. Elimination of the intermediate molluscan host can be accomplished with the use of molluscicides or by destroying the habitat of the snail. Both methods require dedication of resources and personnel often not readily available. Mass chemotherapy of populations has been tried, and repeated treatments will be needed depending on the degree of reinfection. Some advocate the treatment of those likely to develop serious disease (e.g., those heavily infected). The methods employed will depend on the nature of the endemic area and the resources available.

REFERENCES

Cheever AW, Andrade ZA: Pathological lesions associated with *Schistosoma mansoni* infection in man. Trans R Soc Trop Med Hyg 61:626, 1968

Davis A, Wegner DHG: Multicenter trials of praziquantel in human schistosomiasis: Design and techniques. Bull WHO 57:767, 1979

Forsyth DM: A longitudinal study of endemic urinary schistosomiasis in a small East African community. Bull WHO 40:771, 1969

Hiat RA et al: Factors in the pathogenesis of acute schistosomiasis mansoni. J Infect Dis 139:659, 1979

Kolata G: Avoiding the schistosome's tricks. Science 227:285, 1985

Lehman JS et al: Urinary schistosomiasis in Egypt: Clinical, radiological, bacteriological, and parasitological correlations. Trans R Soc Trop Med Hyg 67:384, 1973

McCutchan TF et al: Differentiation of schistosome by species, strain, and sex by using cloned DNA markers. Proc Natl Acad Sci 81:889, 1984

Nash TE et al: Schistosome infections in humans: Perspective and recent findings. Ann Intern Med 97:740, 1982

——— et al: Treatment of *Schistosoma mekongi* with praziquantel: A double-blinded study. Am J Trop Med Hyg 3:977, 1982

Schistosomiasis, Epidemiology, Treatment and Control, P Jordan, G Webbe (eds). London, Heinemann Medical, 1982

165 TISSUE NEMATODES

JAMES J. PLORDE

ANGIOSTRONGYLIASIS CANTONENSIS Definition *Angiostrongylus cantonensis*, the rat lungworm, is the etiologic agent of the common form of *eosinophilic meningitis* found in southeast Asia and the tropical areas of the Pacific.

Etiology The delicate filariform adults (20 mm in length) reside and lay their eggs in the pulmonary arterioles of rats and certain other rodents. After hatching, the larvae break into the alveoli, migrate up the respiratory tract, are swallowed, and pass in the feces. They develop into infective third-stage larvae within snails and slugs, their natural intermediate host. Viable third-stage organisms may also be found in land planarians, crabs, and freshwater prawns. These carriers appear to acquire the larvae by feeding on the tissues of infected mollusks. Humans, like rodents, become parasitized when they ingest raw intermediate or carrier hosts containing the infective stage. In rodents the larvae migrate to the brain where they grow into young adults. After a period of further maturation, the worms travel to the lungs and begin to deposit eggs. The nematode does not complete its life cycle in humans and dies after reaching the central nervous system.

Epidemiology The majority of human infections with *A. cantonensis* have been found in Thailand, Vietnam, Cambodia, Indonesia, the Philippines, Taiwan, Hawaii, and several smaller Pacific islands from Okinawa in the north to New Caledonia, American Samoa, and Tahiti in the south. Cases have been described in Cuba, Egypt, and the Ivory Coast. In addition, rodent infections have been found in the islands of East Africa, Sri Lanka, India, and China. The rat lungworm may have been spread from Madagascar to Asia and to the Pacific by the recent dispersal of the giant African land snail, *Achatina fulica*.

Pathology and pathogenesis The nematode can produce extensive tissue damage by moving through the brain when alive and provokes a marked inflammatory reaction when dead. The pathologic lesions are characterized by (1) marked lymphocyte and eosinophilic infiltration of the meninges, (2) hemorrhagic and nonhemorrhagic worm tracts through the brainstem and spinal cord, (3) granuloma formation around dead parasites and necrotic debris which sheathes the worm, and (4) engorgement of almost all blood vessels, particularly the veins. Necrosis of vessel walls, aneurysmal dilatation of arteries, and perivascular hemorrhages have been noted. Living worms have been removed from the eyes of patients without central nervous system involvement.

Clinical manifestations The eosinophilic meningitis usually presents as an acute severe headache. Fever is usually mild or absent, and only 15 percent of patients show signs of meningeal irritation. Patients frequently complain of visual impairment and, in a majority of these, visual defects or blurring of the optic disk can be demonstrated. Paresthesias and exquisite pains of the trunk and lower extremities are a common complaint, and paralysis of the sixth and seventh nerves is seen in 3 to 7 percent of cases. Paralysis of the limbs, convulsions, and loss of consciousness are rare. Although some patients have experienced significant neurologic residua, the disease usually ends in complete spontaneous recovery. Death is rare. The cerebrospinal fluid contains several hundred cells per cubic millimeter and many eosinophils, and the cerebrospinal fluid protein is elevated. There may or may not be an eosinophilia in the peripheral blood.

A second clinically distinct form of eosinophilic meningitis has been reported. This presents as a radiculomyeloencephalitis with limb pain, paresis, and bowel and bladder dysfunction. This syndrome may be more common in heavy infections. In Thailand, this syndrome is thought to be caused by the nematode *Gnathostoma spinigerum*. The cerebrospinal fluid eosinophilic leukocytosis is less marked than in the meningitic form of the disease. The fluid is often xanthochromic. Death may occur from cerebral hemorrhage or destruction of vital centers.

Diagnosis The diagnosis is made on the basis of the clinical manifestations in an endemic area. Rarely, the adult worm is found in the cerebrospinal fluid. Angiostrongyliasis must be differentiated from other ectopic worm infections of the central nervous system including strongyloidiasis, filariasis, paragonimiasis, hydatid disease, schistosomiasis japonicum, trichinosis, cysticercosis, toxocariasis, and gnathostomiasis. A case of visceral larva migrans with eosinophilic meningitis has been described, in which the raccoon ascarid, *Baylisascaris procyonis*, was implicated.

Treatment and prevention There is no known effective treatment. Anthelmintic therapy has been thought by some authors to be dangerous since the simultaneous death of many worms might produce a severe inflammatory reaction. Steroids may be beneficial in severe cases. Prevention depends upon avoidance or proper cooking of such foods as snails, prawns, and crabs. Raw vegetables should be carefully inspected for the presence of planarians and mollusks before they are eaten. Freezing of crustaceans and mollusks at −15°C for 12 h will destroy infective larvae of *A. cantonensis*.

ANGIOSTRONGYLIASIS COSTARICENSIS *Angiostrongylus costaricensis* is a nematode that dwells in the mesenteric arteries of Central American rats. Larvae pass in the stool and develop in slugs, the intermediate hosts. Rats, and incidentally humans, are infected when they ingest slugs or vegetables contaminated with third-stage larvae deposited in the mucous trail of these mollusks. The larvae mature in the lymphatics and move to the mesenteric radicals of the cecum. Here they may cause arterial thrombosis, ischemic necrosis, ulceration, and eosinophilic granuloma formation. Infected patients present with fever, eosinophilic leukocytosis, abdominal pain, and a right lower quadrant mass. Occasionally perforation of the bowel and generalized peritonitis occur. The fever may persist for up to 2 months. Children are more frequently involved than adults. Neither larvae nor eggs are seen in the stool of the human host. No specific therapy is available.

GNATHOSTOMIASIS Definition Gnathostomiasis is a tissue infection of humans caused by *Gnathostoma spinigerum*, an intestinal nematode of carnivores. Clinically it is manifest as migratory subcutaneous swellings, creeping eruption, or a lethal eosinophilic meningitis.

Etiology and epidemiology The parasite, which is found throughout the Far East, lives encysted in the gastric mucosa of dogs, cats, and wild felines. The ova are passed to the external environment via the feces, hatch in water, and are ingested by *Cyclops*, the first intermediate hosts. These in turn are eaten by freshwater fish, frogs, snakes, and eels in whose flesh the infective third-stage larvae develop. Ducks and chickens fed on these second intermediate hosts may also come to harbor infective larvae. Human infections, which are most commonly seen in Thailand and Japan, occur when humans ingest infected uncooked fish (somfak, sashimi), duck, or chicken.

Pathogenesis and manifestations The parasite cannot complete its cycle in humans, and the immature worms migrate through the abdominal and thoracic organs producing localized areas of inflammation and hemorrhage. Clinically, this is manifest as fever, eosinophilic leukocytosis, urticaria, and pain. Typically, the systemic manifestations subside within a month as the worms make their way to the subcutaneous tissues. Here, their continued migration results in the production of transient serpiginous pruritic swellings, subcutaneous tunnels, and abscesses. If the worm invades the epidermis, the resulting lesions closely resemble those of cutanea larva migrans. Rarely the eye may be involved with orbital cellulitis, iritis, or uveitis. Migration into the central nervous system results in a lethal

eosinophilic meningitis (see "Angiostrongyliasis Cantonensis" above). This presents as a radiculomyeloencephalitis with limb pain and paresis. The cerebrospinal fluid eosinophilic leukocytosis is present but less marked than in *Angiostrongylus* infections. The fluid is often xanthochromic. Death may occur from cerebral hemorrhage or destruction of vital centers.

Diagnosis and treatment Painless, recurrent migratory subcutaneous swellings and eosinophilic leukocytosis occurring in an endemic area make the diagnosis likely. It must be differentiated from cutanea larva migrans, however, and from angiostrongyliasis cantonensis when the central nervous system is involved. Definitive diagnosis depends upon the removal and identification of the worm. Other than excision, there is no specific therapy. The disease can be prevented by the adequate cooking of fish, chicken, and duck in endemic areas.

DRACUNCULIASIS Definition Dracunculiasis is an infection of human connective and subcutaneous tissues by the guinea worm, *Dracunculus medinensis*. The gravid female produces symptoms when she ruptures the skin to discharge her eggs.

Etiology and epidemiology Dracunculiasis affects about 50 million people in west, central, and northeast Africa, the Middle East, Iran, Pakistan, India, northeastern South America, and the Caribbean islands. Humans acquire the parasite when they ingest raw drinking water containing infected copepods (*Cyclops* spp.) which serve as the intermediate host. Shallow ponds, cisterns, and wells are the usual habitat of these crustaceans. In the stomach the copepod is digested and the larvae are released. The larva penetrates the intestinal wall and matures in the connective tissue of the retroperitoneal space. The adult male is small, seldom seen, and presumably dies after mating. In contrast, the female *Dracunculus* is one of the largest nematodes known—1 to 2 mm in diameter and 300 to 800 mm in length. The female reaches gravidity in approximately one year and then migrates to the subcutaneous tissue of the lower extremities. When the anterior end of the worm approaches the skin, a blister forms. This breaks down in a few days, forming a superficial ulcer. When the protruding portion of the worm comes in contact with water, the uterus prolapses through the body and discharges large numbers of motile rhabditiform larvae. Following ingestion by one of several species of *Cyclops*, the larvae undergo further development, becoming infective in 10 to 12 days. Mammals other than humans may be infected, but their importance as a disease reservoir is uncertain.

Pathogenesis and manifestations The infection is asymptomatic until the gravid female appears in the subcutaneous tissues, where it may, on occasion, be palpable. A few days before the formation of the blister, the patient frequently has fever, generalized urticaria, periorbital edema, and wheezing. Blister formation is accompanied by intense local pain and pruritus; like the systemic manifestations, this is thought to represent an allergic reaction to prematurely liberated larvae. The local lesion is usually found over the feet and ankles but may occur on the trunk or the upper extremities. Multiple infections are common. With the rupture of the blister and the release of embryos, the systemic manifestations abate, and the worm is slowly extruded over a period of 4 to 5 weeks. Secondary infection and cellulitis are common, particularly if the worm is ruptured during the process of extraction. In Nigeria, guinea worm ulcers are a common portal of entry for the spores of *Clostridium tetani*. The female worm often fails to reach the surface and discharge her larvae. In most of these cases, it dies without producing symptoms. The calcified appearance on roentgenograms is characteristic. Occasionally the worm may invade the deep tissues, causing serious symptoms, and sterile abscesses may follow the release of embryos. Invasion of joint spaces by the adult worm or larvae results in arthritis.

Diagnosis The clinical picture is characteristic. Placing a small amount of water on the worm results in discharge of larvae which can then be examined microscopically. A fluorescent antibody test may permit the diagnosis to be made prior to emergence of the gravid female.

Treatment and prevention   If the outline of the worm can be clearly seen or palpated, it may sometimes be completely removed with a single incision. The gradual extraction of the worm can be accomplished by winding a few centimeters onto a stick each day. Administration of niridazole (Ambilhar) results in prompt remission of symptoms. The dose is 25 mg per kilogram of body weight given in three divided doses for 7 days. Thiabendazole in dosage of 25 mg/kg twice daily for 2 days or metronidazole 250 mg three times a day for 7 days is also effective in the relief of symptoms. At present, there is serious question whether any of the above agents hasten worm extrusion or death. Some authorities suggest the rapid symptomatic improvement induced by these agents is secondary to their anti-inflammatory rather than anthelmintic properties. Dracunculiasis can be prevented by the chemical treatment of drinking water or the provision of piped water.

REFERENCES

Editorial: After smallpox, guineaworm? Lancet 1:61, 1983
Fox AS et al: Fatal eosinophilic meningoencephalitis and visceral larva migrans caused by the raccoon ascarid *Baylisascaris procyonis*. N Engl J Med 312:1619, 1985
Kliks MM et al: Eosinophilic radiculomyeloencephalitis: An angiostrongyliasis outbreak in American Samoa related to ingestion of *Achatina fulica* snails. Am J Trop Med Hyg 31:1114, 1982
Loria-Cortes R, Lobo-Sanahuja JF: Clinical abdominal angiostrongylosis. A study of 116 children with intestinal eosinophilic granuloma caused by *Angiostrongylus costaricensis*. Am J Trop Med Hyg 29:538, 1980
Pascual JE et al: Eosinophilic meningoencephalitis in Cuba caused by *Angiostrongylus cantonensis*. Am J Trop Med Hyg 30:960, 1981
Punyagupta S et al: Eosinophilic meningitis in Thailand. Am J Trop Med 24:921, 1975

166   INTESTINAL NEMATODES

JAMES J. PLORDE

ENTEROBIASIS   Definition   Enterobiasis (pinworm, seatworm, or threadworm infection, oxyuriasis) is an intestinal infection of humans caused by *Enterobius vermicularis* and characterized by perianal pruritus. Eggs of this parasite have been found in a 10,000-year-old coprolith, making it the oldest demonstrated infection of humans. It has been estimated that the worm infects 200 million people, 30 to 40 million of them in the United States and Canada.

Etiology   The female averages 10 mm in length, the male 3 mm. They live with their heads attached to the mucosa of the cecum, appendix, and adjacent parts of the bowel. The gravid female migrates through the anal canal at night, deposits her 10,000 eggs on the perianal skin, and dies. In female patients the worm may enter the vagina and occasionally gain access to the peritoneal cavity through the fallopian tubes. Each egg contains an embryo which, within a few hours, develops into an infective larva. After the egg has been ingested, the larva is released in the small intestine and migrates down the bowel lumen to the cecum. In less than 1 month from the time of ingestion, newly developed gravid females are again discharging eggs. They are planoconvex and measure approximately 20 by 50 μm. The shell is clear and doubly contoured.

Epidemiology   Humans are usually infected by the direct transfer of eggs from the anus to the mouth by way of contaminated fingers. Retroinfection, which is seen primarily in adults, may occasionally take place when eggs hatch in the perianal area and the larvae migrate back into the bowel to mature. The eggs, which are relatively resistant to desiccation, also contaminate nightclothes and bed linen, where they remain viable and infective for 2 to 3 weeks. Airborne trans-

mission is possible, and spread within family and children's groups occurs readily. Enterobiasis is found in all climates and is probably the most common helminthic infection of humans. Its low incidence in some tropical areas, however, is not fully explained.

Clinical manifestations   The most common symptom is pruritus ani, which is most troublesome at night, being related to the migration of the gravid female worms. Irritability, insomnia, enuresis, and other minor complaints are probably secondary to the pruritus. Scratching may lead to perianal eczema or pyogenic infection. Vaginal discharge has been reported, and rarely a chronic granulomatous salpingitis or endometritis results from the presence of ectopic adults. An association between enterobiasis and cystitis in young females has been reported. This, it is suggested, results from the transport of enteric bacteria into the bladder by the migrating worm. Other rare ectopic locations include the lung, liver, and peritoneum. Probably the worms can penetrate the bowel wall only if its continuity has been compromised by some other disease.

Laboratory findings   Examination for ova of material obtained from the perianal skin by means of a Scotch brand cellophane tape swab is the preferable method for the detection of enterobiasis. The tape is folded sticky-side out over the end of a tongue blade, pressed firmly against the perianal area, and then spread on a glass slide and examined under the lower power of a microscope. The swab should be taken at home by the patient on three to five consecutive mornings prior to bathing and brought to the laboratory for examination. Searching for ova in the feces is rarely helpful, but scrapings from under the nails may reveal ova. The diagnosis is sometimes made by finding adult worms in the perianal area or in the feces following a laxative or an enema. Eosinophilic leukocytosis may occur but is not a typical finding.

Treatment   All infected individuals in a family or communal group should be treated simultaneously. The frequently recommended sanitary measures aside from daily bathing and hand washing before meals and after stools are of dubious benefit. It is relatively easy to eradicate the worms, but reinfection is frequent. Retreatment does not appear necessary unless symptoms recur.

Two highly satisfactory drugs are available. Pyrantel pamoate given in a single oral dose of 11 mg/kg (maximum 1.0 g) is probably the drug of choice. Alternatively, a single 100-mg oral dose of mebendazole can be used. This drug is not recommended for infants or pregnant women. Pyrvinium pamoate is equally effective but less convenient. It is given orally as a single dose of 5 mg/kg in tablet or liquid form. This compound turns the stool red and may stain bedclothes or undergarments. In heavily contaminated environments, treatment with the above drugs may be repeated after an interval of 2 weeks to eliminate any new infections.

Prevention   Methods of preventing autoinfection and dissemination within a group involving children are extremely difficult to enforce. Personal environmental hygiene should be stressed, and anthelmintic and symptomatic treatment of pruritus ani should be instituted. To control infection within a group, simultaneous treatment of all cases is mandatory.

TRICHURIASIS   Definition   Trichuriasis (whipworm infection, trichocephaliasis) is an intestinal infection of humans caused by *Trichuris trichiura* and is characterized by invasion of the colonic mucosa by the adult trichuris. Five hundred million persons are thought to be infected with this parasite including 2 million in the United States. It may be the most commonly encountered helminthic infection in Americans returning from tropical areas.

Etiology   The adult whipworms are found in the large intestine with their anterior ends deeply embedded in the mucosa. They are 30 to 50 mm in length and possess a threadlike anterior two-thirds with a stouter posterior third, giving them a whiplike structure. The female produces about 5000 eggs each day. They are characteristically barrel-shaped (20 to 50 μm), brown, thick-walled, and translucent with knoblike ends. The eggs, like those of *Ascaris*, must incubate at least 3 weeks in soil before they become infective. After ingestion, the eggs hatch in the small intestine and the larvae become embedded in the intestinal villi. After several days they migrate to the large intestine where they mature in about 3 months. The adult worms may live for 4 to 8 years. Occasionally, *T. vulpis*, the whipworm of dogs, may infect humans. The eggs are larger (35 by 75 μm) but otherwise identical to those of the human parasite.

Epidemiology Whipworm is a cosmopolitan parasite but is most commonly found in the tropics where the level of sanitation is low and environmental conditions necessary for the incubation of the eggs are optimal. In the United States, it is found throughout the rural areas of the southeast. Its distribution is similar to that of *Ascaris* and hookworm, but the eggs are less resistant than those of *Ascaris* to sunlight and drying. Because of their general lack of sanitary habits, children and the mentally retarded have the highest incidence of infection. For example, 13 percent of patients confined to hospitals for the mentally subnormal were found to harbor *Trichuris*.

Pathogenesis and clinical manifestations Symptomatic infection generally requires the presence of large numbers of adult whipworms and may be correlated in part with the degree of mucosal involvement. Heavy infections usually occur only in children and may be accompanied by finger clubbing, nausea, abdominal pain, diarrhea, and dysentery. It has been estimated that infected patients lose 0.005 mL blood per worm per day. Infections with more than 800 worms often result in anemia. In heavier infections, the distribution of worms throughout the colon and rectum may result in rectal prolapse while straining at stool. Some investigators also feel that *Trichuris* infections predispose to amebic dysentery and bacterial gastroenteritis.

Laboratory findings In symptomatic infection, large numbers of eggs are present in the feces, and there may be eosinophilic leukocytosis and anemia. In light infections, concentration techniques may be necessary to recover the eggs. Quantitation of egg output is helpful since only counts above 3000 eggs per gram of feces are likely to be associated with symptoms. Stools should be cultured for bacterial pathogens and examined for the presence of *Entamoeba histolytica*.

Treatment Treatment is unsatisfactory. Mebendazole in the oral dose of 100 mg twice daily for 3 days is the drug of choice. Its cure rate is 60 to 70 percent, and it achieves a 90 percent reduction in egg burden. The dose may have to be repeated in patients with heavy infections. It is not recommended for children under the age of 2 or pregnant women.

Prognosis Whipworm infection, unless characterized by severe diarrhea, blood loss, and systemic reaction, usually responds well to treatment. Serious infections may require supportive treatment as well as chemotherapy.

Prevention Measures recommended for ascariasis apply also to trichuriasis.

ASCARIASIS Definition Ascariasis is an infection of humans caused by *Ascaris lumbricoides* and characterized by an early pulmonary phase related to larval migration and a later, prolonged intestinal phase. It is estimated that 25 percent of the world's population, including 4 million Americans, are infected with this nematode.

Etiology The adult ascarids are large (15 to 40 cm in length), cylindric worms with blunt ends which maintain themselves in the lumen of the jejunum by virtue of their muscular activity. Despite a life span of only 6 to 18 months, the female releases millions of eggs, both fertile and infertile, into the fecal stream; the daily output is estimated to be 200,000 per worm. Fertilized eggs are elliptic (30 to 40 μm by 50 to 60 μm) with an irregular, dense outer shell and a regular, translucent inner shell. They require a period of soil

incubation before they become infective. Under optimum conditions of warmth and moisture this occurs in 2 to 3 weeks. The eggs may then remain viable for up to 6 years in temperate climates and may survive freezing. When an infective egg is ingested, the larva is liberated in the small intestine. It migrates through the wall and is carried by the bloodstream or lymphatics to the lung. After about 10 days in the pulmonary capillaries and alveoli, the larvae pass in turn up the bronchioles, bronchi, trachea, and epiglottis, are swallowed, and return to the jejunum. There they develop into mature adult worms within 2 to 3 months of ingestion. *Ascaris suum*, a roundworm of pigs, may occasionally complete a similar life cycle in humans.

Epidemiology Infection follows the ingestion of the embryonated eggs contained in contaminated food, or, more commonly, the introduction of the eggs into the mouth by the hands after contact with contaminated soil. Geophagia may produce massive infections. In endemic areas, the infection is maintained primarily by small children who defecate indiscriminately in the area of the home. In dry, windy climates, eggs may become airborne, get into the mouth, and be swallowed. Since the eggs are relatively resistant to desiccation and wide variations in temperature, the disease is worldwide. In the developing areas of the world where the lack of sanitary facilities exposes populations to the greatest risk, the prevalence of infection may be as high as 80 to 90 percent. Children are almost universally infected in these areas, with peak infection rates achieved by age 5. In temperate areas, the infection occurs in family clusters.

Pathogenesis and clinical manifestations Because of the extensive migration of which both the larvae and adults are capable, the manifestations may be diverse. Bronchopneumonia characterized by fever, cough, dyspnea, wheeze, eosinophilic leukocytosis, and migratory pulmonary infiltrates may occur during the passage of the larvae through the lung. This is most commonly seen in communities where *Ascaris* transmission is seasonal. The severity of symptoms is apparently related to both intensity of infection and the degree of sensitization resulting from previous exposures. Significant arterial oxygen desaturation and, rarely, death may occur. Adult worms may produce no symptoms if the infection is light and may be detected accidentally when the adult worm is vomited or passed in the stool. Heavier infections may cause abdominal pain and malabsorption of fat, protein, carbohydrate, and vitamins. In marginally nourished children this may produce growth retardation. Occasionally a bolus of worms may result in volvulus, intussusception, or intestinal obstruction in the iliocecal area. Children are most likely to have these complications because of their anatomically smaller intestine and larger worm loads. Up to 2000 worms have been found in children, although the usual load is less than 20. In the United States where worm loads are usually modest, the incidence of obstruction is 2 per 1000 infected children per year. It often follows a febrile illness or drug therapy which stimulates the worms to increase motility. Rarely, an adult worm will migrate into the appendix, bile ducts, or pancreatic ducts, causing obstruction and inflammation of these organs. Biliary tract obstruction may be associated with bacterial cholangitis and liver abscess. Worms may also penetrate the intestinal wall, particularly at a site of surgical anastomosis, and patients should be dewormed prior to elective surgery. Migration of the worms into the oral pharynx and mouth may lead to acute respiratory distress.

Laboratory findings The diagnosis is usually made by finding the ova in the feces. The fertilized eggs are usually numerous, characteristic, and not easily confused with those of other helminths. The occasional unisexual infection may pose diagnostic problems. The male produces no eggs, and the unfertilized ova produced by a single female may be atypical and difficult to recognize. Occasionally the worms may be seen after a barium meal, either as negative images or after ingesting barium themselves. In biliary ascariasis an intravenous cholangiogram will often demonstrate dilatation of the common duct and/or the negative image of the parasite. *Ascaris* pneumonia may be diagnosed by finding larvae and eosinophils in the sputum or gastric aspirate. Eggs will usually not be found until after the larvae have matured in the intestine. Eosinophilic leukocytosis is usually noted during larval migration, but diminishes and often disappears during the chronic intestinal phase of infection.

Treatment   Only symptomatic treatment can be used during the period of pulmonary involvement by the migrating larvae. For removal of the adult worms from the intestines, either pyrantel pamoate or mebendazole should be used. Pyrantel is given as a single oral dose of 11 mg/kg (maximum 1.0 g). Mebendazole is given as described for trichuriasis and is the preferred agent if both *Ascaris* and *Trichuris* are present. An older agent, piperazine citrate, is highly effective, less expensive, but slightly more toxic than the above two agents. It is given as a flavored syrup administered in a single dose after breakfast on two successive days and will cure the majority of cases. The drug acts by paralyzing the ascarids, which are then passed in the stool. The dose of piperazine is 75 mg/kg with a maximum of 3.5 g. No particular dietary regulation is necessary. The drug must be administered with caution to patients with renal insufficiency, because impaired elimination may produce neurotoxic signs. In intestinal obstruction, nasogastric suction should be initiated. After vomiting is controlled, piperazine should be given through the nasogastric tube every 12 to 24 h in dosage of 65 mg/kg (maximum 1.0 g) for six doses. Surgery usually is not required.

Prognosis   The prognosis in intestinal infection is generally good. When acute or chronic obstruction of ducts or hollow viscera has occurred, the immediate prognosis is determined by the promptness of diagnosis and treatment. The case fatality rate of intestinal obstruction in the United States is 3 percent.

Prevention   Ascariasis is primarily a household infection of rural areas. All infections should be treated, personal hygiene stressed, and adequate toilet facilities provided. Mass therapy administered at 6-month intervals may be effective in controlling ascariasis in small communities.

TOXOCARIASIS (VISCERAL LARVA MIGRANS)   Definition   This is a human infection with *Toxocara canis.* The animal ascarid is usually unable to complete its life cycle in humans, but they may be widely disseminated in the body, producing a variety of clinical manifestations, collectively referred to as *visceral larva migrans.*

Etiology and epidemiology   The large adult toxocaral worms live in the intestine of dogs. Their eggs must be passed in the stool and incubate in soil for 2 to 3 weeks before they become infective. When ingested by a mammal, larvae are liberated in the intestine, penetrate the wall, and are carried in the blood to the liver, where most remain, and lung. If the host is a young puppy, the larvae burst into the alveoli and complete their life cycle in a manner analogous to *A. lumbricoides* in humans. In humans and fully grown dogs, *Toxocara* larvae, which are approximately one-half the size of those of *A. lumbricoides,* pass through the pulmonary capillaries to reach the systemic circulation. Larvae leave the circulatory system when their gradually increasing size approaches the diameter of the vessel through which they are traveling. They migrate extensively in the surrounding tissue; some may become dormant for years, only to resume migration at a later time. *Toxocara* infections of dogs are common and widespread. Transplacental and transmammary migration of larvae account for infection rates of 80 percent or more in young puppies; they can shed a large number of ova within 4 weeks of birth. Viable ova were found in 25 percent of soil samples taken from public parks in the United States and Great Britain. Although most of the 2000 documented human infections have occurred in the United States and Europe, cases have been reported from 48 countries around the world. Children from the age of 2 to 5 years, because of their sanitary habits, predilection to geophagia, and intimate association with domestic pets, are most frequently involved. The seroprevalence of human *Toxocara* infection in the United States is approximately 3 percent; the rates are highest in the south and northeast.

Pathogenesis and clinical manifestations   The larvae migrate freely in tissues, causing hemorrhage, necrosis, eosinophilic inflammatory reaction, and eventually granuloma formation. The most frequently involved organs are the liver, lungs, brain, eye, heart, and skeletal muscles. Symptoms and signs are related to the number and location of the granulomas as well as sensitization to the parasite antigen. Commonly, only asymptomatic eosinophilia marks the presence of infection. Symptomatic patients most frequently present with fever and tender hepatomegaly. Splenomegaly, skin rash, and recurrent pneumonitis with wheezing respirations may occur in more severe infections. Respiratory failure with death has been reported. Most fatalities, however, result from involvement of the myocardium or central nervous system; the latter may result in convulsions, behavior disorders, or focal neurological defects. There is often a history of dirt eating and contact with puppies. Leukocytosis with eosinophilia to high levels (over 60 percent) and hypergammaglobulinemia with raised levels of IgG, IgM, and IgE are common. These manifestations may persist for months or years. At surgery or autopsy the liver may be studded with small granulomas. A granulomatous endophthalmitis, which may be mistaken for retinoblastoma, may be observed in older children and adults. Typically, this is unilateral and occurs in the absence of other clinical manifestations of visceral larva migrans. Decreased visual acuity or strabismus brings the patient to the attention of the physician.

Diagnosis   The diagnosis can usually be made on the basis of clinical findings. Infections with *A. lumbricoides,* hookworm, and *Strongyloides stercoralis,* as well as other nonhuman nematodes, may also on occasion present as visceral larva migrans, making the etiologic diagnosis difficult. Eosinophilic leukemia, trichinosis, trematode infections, and periarteritis nodosa must be ruled out. Isoagglutinin, particularly anti-A, titers of 1:1024 or greater are present in 85 percent of patients with visceral but in very few with ocular disease. The adaption of larval antigens to the enzyme-linked immunosorbent assay has, for the first time, provided clinicians with a serologic test of diagnostic value. In one study, the sensitivity and specificity were 78 and 92 percent, respectively. A definitive diagnosis depends on the identification of the larvae in sputum or tissue granuloma. Biopsy of the liver with serial sections of the specimen may reveal eosinophilic granulomas or a *Toxocara* larva.

Treatment   No uniformly effective therapy is available. Diethylcarbamazine as used in Bancroftian filariasis (see Chap. 163) is probably the drug of choice. Thiabendazole in dosage of 25 to 50 mg/kg for 7 to 10 days may be helpful. Adrenocortical steroids may be beneficial when respiratory difficulty is pronounced. Control measures are directed toward preventing ingestion of eggs. Removal and repeated worming of infected dogs must be considered. Animals less than 6 months of age should be wormed monthly; older ones every 2 or 3 months.

ANISAKIASIS   Ascarids belonging to family Anisakidae infect seals, dolphins, porpoises, whales, and other large sea mammals. Their larval stages are found in the flesh of squid and several marine fish including cod, mackerel, salmon, herring, and various rock fishes, including "Pacific red snapper." Humans are infected by eating raw, pickled, or slightly salted fish delicacies such as "green herring," sushi, sashimi, sunomono, ceviche, and gravlax which contain the third-stage larvae. The infection may be asymptomatic and noted only when the worm is coughed or vomited up. More characteristically, the larvae burrow into the mucosa of the stomach, small intestine, or more rarely the colon. Here they produce eosinophilic granulomatous tumors with edema, thickening, and induration of the bowel wall which may be mistaken for gastric carcinoma or regional enteritis. Occasionally, larvae may penetrate the intestinal wall to involve other abdominal organs. Perforations of the bowel with peritonitis have also been described. The pathologic changes are thought to be the result of a hypersensitivity reaction. In the acute gastric syndrome common in Japan, the patient may develop epigastric pain, nausea, and vomiting within a few hours of ingesting infected fish. With a gastroscope 2- to 4-cm larvae can be seen penetrating the mucosa and can sometimes be removed. In Europeans, the small intestine has been the site most frequently involved. The clinical picture may be severe enough to simulate an acute surgical abdomen. More commonly, colicky pain, diffuse abdominal tenderness, fever, and leukocytosis develop a week or more after the ingestion of fish. Peripheral eosinophilia is not always present, and a definitive diagnosis can be made only by the identification of larvae in tissue. Serologic tests are being developed, but are neither highly reliable nor generally available. The disease usually subsides spontaneously with conservative therapy. Occasionally, a chronic illness develops which requires surgical resection of the lesion.

Over 1000 cases have been recognized in the Netherlands and Japan, and several cases have been reported from North America. The disease can be prevented by storing marine fish at $-20°C$ for a single day or by cooking it at normal cooking temperatures.

HOOKWORM DISEASE   Definition   Hookworm disease is a symptomatic infection caused by *Necator americanus, Ancylostoma duodenale*, or, less commonly, *A. ceylanicum*. Asymptomatic infection may be termed simply *hookworm infection*, and the individual with such infection is called a *carrier*.

Etiology   *Ancylostoma duodenale*, also known as the "old world" hookworm, possesses four prominent hooklike teeth in its adult stage. The adults are about 1 cm long and inhabit the upper part of the human small intestine, where they attach to the mucosa by means of the mouth parts and suck blood. Each adult extracts approximately 0.20 mL blood daily. The adults migrate within the small intestine, and each site of attachment persists temporarily as a bleeding point. Following fertilization, the female liberates approximately 20,000 eggs per day. They measure about 40 by 60 μm and are usually in the two- to four-celled stage when discharged in the feces.

Necator americanus, the "new world" hookworm, has a buccal capsule containing dorsal and ventral plates rather than teeth. It is slightly smaller, deposits fewer eggs, and causes much less blood loss than *A. duodenale* (0.03 mL per worm daily). *Ancylostoma ceylanicum*, a hookworm of cats found in the Far East, may occasionally reach maturity in humans.

The life cycles of the hookworms are similar. Under appropriate conditions, the eggs hatch in 24 to 48 h, releasing free-living or rhabditiform larvae. Within a few days, these develop into infective or filariform larvae which may remain viable in the soil for several weeks. These, in turn, penetrate the skin to enter vessels which carry them to the lungs. The larvae leave the alveolar capillaries, enter the alveoli, ascend the respiratory tree, enter the pharynx, and are swallowed. They reach the intestine about 1 week after penetration of the skin and mature within 5 weeks. Larval development of *Ancylostoma* may be arrested or retarded in the human host. This may result in a prolonged latent period between the onset of infection and the appearance of gravid females in the intestine. Adults have been known to survive in the human intestine for as long as 14 years, but *A. duodenale* seldom persists beyond 6 to 8 years, and most *N. americanus* infections are eliminated within 2 to 4 years.

Epidemiology   It has been estimated that hookworms infect 700 million people and cause the loss of 7 million liters of blood daily throughout the world from 45°N to 30°S latitude. *Necator americanus* is found predominantly in the tropical areas of Africa, Asia, and the Americas, while *A. duodenale* occurs in the Mediterranean Basin, the Middle East, northern India, China, and Japan. In many areas both species are found. In general, *Ancylostoma* presents a greater public health hazard than *N. americanus*, the species which is most prevalent in the southern United States, because it is more persistent in the environment, more harmful to the host, and less amenable to treatment. Conditions conducive to the development of the hookworm egg into infective filariform larvae are a mean temperature between 23 and 33°C, abundant rainfall, shade, and well-drained sandy soil.

Hookworm infection occurs where there is opportunity for direct contact of the skin with soil contaminated by promiscuous defecation. The disease may also be acquired by oral ingestion of infective larvae, particularly those of *A. duodenale*. Lactogenic transmission may also occur with this species; presumably this results from the activation of larvae whose development within the tissues of the host has been arrested or retarded. Probably because of greater exposure, males show a higher incidence of infection than females. Infections are particularly common in closed, heavily populated communities such as coffee or tea plantations.

Repeated infections of hookworm in dogs result in immunity and elimination of the parasite. It seems probable that a similar phenomenon occurs in human infections. When the possibility of reinfection is eliminated, the majority of worms is eliminated spontaneously within 1 or 2 years.

Pathogenesis and clinical manifestations   During the invasion of the exposed skin by the larvae, there may be an erythematous maculopapular skin rash and edema with severe pruritus. These manifestations, which may persist for several days, are more marked in *N. americanus* infection. The lesions are most common about the feet, particularly between the toes, and have been termed "ground itch."

During migration through the lungs, cough, pneumonia, and, in severe infections, fever may occur. Usually, however, pulmonary involvement does not give rise to clinical symptoms.

Various gastrointestinal symptoms, ranging from vague epigastric distress and pica to typical ulcer pain, have been reported in association with hookworm infection. Roentgenographic studies may reveal nonspecific changes such as excessive peristalsis and "puddling," particularly in the proximal jejunum. However, gross and microscopic examination of the bowel itself reveals conspicuously little damage. Previous reports of absorptive abnormalities in hookworm infection have not been supported.

The major clinical manifestations of hookworm disease clearly are those of iron-deficiency anemia and hypoalbuminemia consequent to chronic intestinal blood loss. Whether anemia develops and how severe it becomes depends on the balance between iron lost in the gut and iron absorbed from the diet. In many endemic areas, dietary iron is largely of vegetable origin and is absorbed poorly. General dietary deficiency also may lower resistance to parasitic infections. The severity of the disease and the prognosis depend on such factors as the age of the patient, the magnitude of the worm burden, the duration of the disease, and diet. Young children often have extreme anemia, with cardiac insufficiency and anasarca. These conditions may precipitate kwashiorkor. Those who survive to puberty show retarded physical, mental, and sexual development. Milder degrees of the disease, as seen in older children and adults, are characterized by lassitude, dyspnea, palpitation, tachycardia, constipation, and pallor of the skin and mucous membranes.

Asymptomatic infections outnumber symptomatic infections, considering all age groups, 20 to 40 times in endemic areas. The worm burden is small in asymptomatic infections, and the carrier state may be indicative of some degree of acquired host resistance.

Laboratory findings   In symptomatic infection, hookworm eggs are usually numerous enough to be detected by microscopic examination of a direct or concentrated fecal smear. A quantitative egg count, using the Stoll or Beaver technique, allows an estimation of the intensity of infection. If a stool specimen is allowed to stand for several hours before examination, the eggs may hatch, releasing larvae which are easily confused with those of *Strongyloides*. The eggs must be differentiated from those of *Trichostrongylus* and *Ternidens diminutus*, which are larger and in a later stage of maturation when observed in a fresh fecal specimen than are those of *Necator* or *Ancylostoma*. Abdominal and pulmonary symptoms appear before the eggs are discharged, although a presumptive diagnosis may be made on the basis of the clinical history and the eosinophilic leukocytosis. The feces seldom contain gross blood in hookworm disease, although tests for occult blood are usually positive.

Generally, the leukocyte count is normal. However, in some early cases, leukocytosis may be marked, with an eosinophilia as high as 70 or 80 percent. The anemia is characteristically hypochromic and microcytic.

The species of hookworm may be determined by the identification of the adult worm passed in the stool following treatment or by culturing the feces and identifying the third-stage larvae. This is seldom important in clinical practice.

Differential diagnosis   Since hookworm disease occurs in areas in which beriberi and malaria are also common, these diseases must be differentiated from hookworm disease, or their coexistence must be established.

Treatment   Therapy specific for the infection and directed toward the improvement of nutrition and the anemia should be considered simultaneously. In areas where reinfection is likely, administration of anthelmintics to patients with light infections (less than 2000 eggs per milliliter of feces) is probably not beneficial. In most cases requiring specific therapy, anthelmintics may be administered immediately, followed by iron and a high-protein diet. A number of satisfactory anthelmintic agents are available, but two, pyrantel pamoate (see ''Ascariasis'' above) and mebendazole (see ''Trichuriasis'' above) are currently favored. Where expense remains a major consideration, the drug of choice is tetrachloroethylene (TCE). It is highly effective, nontoxic, inexpensive, and ideal for mass treatment. (The USP tetrachloroethylene available to veterinarians may be used.) In most instances a single dose of this agent will decrease the worm load substantially. Complete cure may require several courses of treatment but is not necessary in endemic areas; the aim of therapy is reduction of the worm load to an asymptomatic level. Tetrachloroethylene is administered as a single 5-mL oral dose. Children should receive 0.12 ml/kg (to a maximum of 5 mL) by the same route. The night before treatment, the patient is permitted a light fat-free meal. The following morning, breakfast is omitted and the drug is administered. No food is permitted for 4 h and no alcohol for 24 h. Treatment can be repeated in a week if complete cure is desired and has not been accomplished.

The anemia requires iron replacement. When anemia is severe and there is malnutrition with anasarca, blood transfusions and a high-protein diet should be given before drug treatment is begun. Blood should be given in an amount sufficient to raise the hemoglobin level to 10 g/dL. In advanced cases it may be necessary to delay drug treatment for 2 to 3 weeks.

Prognosis   The immediate prognosis is good. When opportunity for reinfection persists and nutrition cannot be maintained, a state of chronic debility develops. Maturation of children is impaired, and intercurrent disease is a serious problem in adults.

Prevention   Many of the measures required are obvious but difficult to apply on a large scale. Even if facilities for proper disposal of feces are provided, it is no simple matter to educate the population in their use. Soil pollution must be eliminated. Avoidance of direct skin contact with the soil (by wearing shoes) is often not practical in endemic areas. Periodic mass treatment of the population has been used in some hookworm control programs.

CUTANEOUS LARVA MIGRANS (CREEPING ERUPTION)
Definition   Creeping eruption is an infection of human skin caused by the larvae of the dog and cat hookworm, *A. brasiliense*. The other dog hookworms, *A. caninum* and *Uncinaria stenocephala*, as well as the human parasites, *Strongyloides stercoralis* and *Necator americanus*, may also produce the disease. The larvae of *Gnathostoma spinigerum*, a nematode found in the Orient, and *Gasterophilus*, the horse botfly, may produce a similar cutaneous infection.

Etiology   *Ancylostoma brasiliense* reaches adulthood regularly only in the dog and cat. The larvae emerging from eggs discharged in the feces develop to the filariform stage and then are capable of penetrating the skin. In humans, the larvae usually remain in the skin and migrate, producing an irregular erythematous tunnel visible on the skin surface.

Epidemiology and distribution   Transmission to humans requires environmental temperature and humidity appropriate for development of the egg to the infective filariform larva stage. Beaches and other moist, sandy areas are hazardous, because animals choose such areas for defecation, and the *A. brasiliense* eggs develop well in such soil. In the United States infection is found in the southern Atlantic and Gulf states.

Pathogenesis and clinical manifestations   The site of penetration of the skin by the larvae becomes apparent in a few hours. The migration of the larvae in the skin is accompanied by severe itching. Scratching may lead to bacterial infection. In the course of 1 week, the initial red papule develops into an irregular, erythematous, linear lesion which may attain a length of 15 to 20 cm. The larvae may persist for weeks to months without treatment.

Loeffler's syndrome has been observed in 26 of 52 cases of creeping eruption. Transient, migratory pulmonary infiltrations associated with an increased number of eosinophils in the blood and sputum were interpreted as an allergic reaction to the helminthic infection but may have reflected pulmonary migration of the larvae.

Laboratory findings   Eosinophils occur in the lesion, but eosinophilic leukocytosis is slight, except when Loeffler's syndrome appears. The percentage of eosinophils in the blood may then rise to 50 percent and in the sputum to 90 percent. Only rarely are larvae found on skin biopsy.

Treatment   Thiabendazole is the drug of choice; it should be given orally in the dosage suggested for strongyloidiasis (see below). It may be repeated if necessary. Alternatively, it may be applied topically as a 10% aqueous suspension. Topical administration avoids systemic toxicity. Superficial bacterial infections are improved by the application of wet dressing and elevation of the extremity. For intense itching, oral antihistaminics may be of aid.

Prognosis   Untreated infections last several months. Treatment, which is usually sought because of severe pruritus, is usually successful.

Prevention   Dogs and cats should be prevented from contaminating recreation areas and children's sandboxes.

TRICHOSTRONGYLIASIS   **Definition**   Trichostrongyliasis is an intestinal infection of herbivorous animals throughout the world. Humans are incidental hosts.

Etiology   Almost a dozen species of *Trichostrongylus* are known to have infected humans. The disease is common in Asia, the Middle East, and South America, but few human infections have been reported in the United States. In view of the high frequency of animal infections here, the low incidence of human infections is difficult to understand. The possibility exists that some such infections are mistaken for hookworm infections.

The ova resemble those of the hookworm but are larger, have more pointed ends, and, when observed in a fresh fecal specimen, show a more advanced stage of segmentation (16- to 32-cell stage).

Pathogenesis   Infection is acquired by ingestion of green leafy plants contaminated with third-stage larvae. On reaching the small intestine, they attach themselves to the mucosa and develop into adult worms within 4 weeks. The adult at that time sucks blood and maintains residence in the intestine for long periods. Sandground, who infected himself, observed infection to last more than 8 years.

Manifestations   Most infections are asymptomatic, but massive infections may result in epigastric distress and anemia. The parasite owes its importance primarily to the resemblance of its ova to those of the hookworms. Moreover, because the trichostrongylidae do not respond to some of the anthelmintics effective in hookworm infection, it may be assumed incorrectly that refractory hookworm infection is present.

Laboratory diagnosis   The diagnosis depends on the finding of the ova in the feces. Since they are few, they are usually found only when a concentration method is used. In symptomatic infections, there may be leukocytosis with marked eosinophilia (for example, 80 percent).

Treatment   These infections do not respond to tetrachloroethylene. Thiabendazole 25 mg/kg twice daily for 2 or 3 days, or pyrantel pamoate as used in hookworm infections, is effective in symptomatic infections. Both are considered investigational drugs for this condition by the U.S. Food and Drug Administration.

Prevention   Leafy vegetables should be cooked before ingestion in endemic areas.

STRONGYLOIDIASIS   Definition   Strongyloidiasis is an intestinal infection of humans caused by *Strongyloides stercoralis* or, on occasion, the primate species, *S. fuelleborni*. Extraintestinal involvement may occur in severe cases.

Etiology   The tiny (2 mm in length) adult female resides and lays her eggs in the mucosa of the upper part of the jejunum. In heavy infections, the biliary and pancreatic ducts, the entire small bowel, and the colon may be parasitized. The eggs quickly hatch, releasing rhabditiform larvae which enter the lumen of the bowel and are passed in the feces. On reaching the soil, the larvae develop into the infective filariform stage. There, as in the case of the filariform larvae of hookworm, they penetrate the skin and small blood vessels of humans. They are then carried to the lungs where they leave the alveolar capillaries, ascend the respiratory tree, enter the pharynx, and are swallowed. On reaching the small intestine, they mature and copulate. The fertilized female burrows into the jejunal mucosa, while the male is excreted in the stool. Oviposition (up to 40 eggs per day) begins 17 to 28 days after the initial infection. It is likely that the females also reproduce parthenogenetically. In addition to the *direct* host-soil-host cycle, *Strongyloides* has two alternative cycles. In the first, or *indirect*, cycle, the rhabditiform larvae, after passing from the host, develop into free-living adults which reside and reproduce in the soil, thus creating a reservoir of infection independent of the human host. Under certain environmental conditions, the free-living larvae are capable of transforming back into filariform larvae which initiate a new cycle in humans. In the second, or *autoinfection*, cycle, the rhabditiform larvae develop into filariform larvae before they are passed in the stool. They may then invade the intestinal mucosa or perianal skin of the same host without first going through a soil phase. This may explain the long persistence (20 to 30 years) of strongyloidiasis in patients who have left endemic areas and may also account for the extremely heavy worm loads in some individuals. The early transformation of the filariform larvae is probably also responsible for the frequency with which strongyloidiasis is seen in crowded, unsanitary institutions for the mentally retarded. It appears to occur frequently in patients with achlorhydria, delayed intestinal transit time, and blind loops or diverticula.

Epidemiology   The usual mode of infection is the penetration of the skin by larvae. Some infections may result from ingestion of contaminated food and drink, and some are believed to be transmitted by contact. Transmission between sexual partners, however, appears to be uncommon. Transmammary passage in humans has been demonstrated for *S. fuelleborni*. This disease is endemic in the tropics, where the warmth, moisture, and lack of sanitation favor its spread. Sporadic cases appear among Puerto Ricans and throughout the rural south of the continental United States. Former British and American soldiers imprisoned in southeast Asia during World War II were examined for the presence of this parasite. Over one-quarter were found infected nearly four decades after exposure; the majority were

symptomatic. Chronic stronglyoidiasis has been reported in Vietnam veterans.

Pathogenesis and clinical manifestations   The initial cutaneous penetration of the filariform larvae usually produces no symptoms. However, *larva currens,* transitory skin eruptions characterized by blotchy erythema, serpiginous lesions, and urticaria, may be seen. These may recur at irregular intervals thereafter and are particularly common following recovery from an acute febrile illness. In these situations the lesions are generally found over the lower back and buttocks and are related to episodes of autoinfection. Cough, dyspnea, gross hemoptysis, and bronchospasm may accompany migration through the lungs. Chest x-rays may show pulmonary infiltration at this time. The intestinal infestation is usually asymptomatic or productive only of vague abdominal complaints. In heavier infections, epigastric pain and tenderness, nausea, flatulence, vomiting, and diarrhea alternating with constipation may be observed. Peptic ulcer may be simulated, but food often aggravates the pain. The mucosal inflammation may be severe enough to produce subacute obstruction, segmental ileus, and impaired absorption. Chronic, relapsing intestinal and pulmonary manifestations have been noted in a few patients. A severe form of ulcerative colitis, accompanied by intestinal perforation and peritonitis, has also been encountered. In debilitated, immuno-depressed, steroid-treated, alcoholic, and hemodialyzed patients, massive autoinfection with widespread dissemination of larvae to the extraintestinal organs including the central nervous system may occur. This hyperinfection is often associated with pulmonary manifestations, severe enterocolitis, persistent gram-negative bacteremia, and occasionally gram-negative meningitis. Unrecognized, it usually leads to death. Disseminated strongyloidiasis should be considered in any compromised host with unexplained gram-negative bacteremia, abdominal complaints, and pulmonary infiltrates with or without eosinophilia.

Laboratory findings   Although clinical findings may be suggestive, the definitive diagnosis can be made only in the laboratory. Fresh fecal specimens should be examined to avoid confusion with hookworm infection; generally, fresh specimens contain *larvae* in strongyloidiasis infections, while in hookworm infection they contain *eggs*. Since the number of larvae in the stool is small and varies from day to day, several samples should be checked, using concentration and culture techniques. If pulmonary involvement is present, the sputum should be examined for larvae. Microscopic examination of the duodenal aspirates and jejunal biopsies may also establish the diagnosis. Alternatively, a weighted string can be passed into the duodenum, allowed to remain for a short time, and then withdrawn. The bile-stained section of the string is stripped of fluid which is then examined for the presence of larvae. An enzyme-linked immunosorbent assay utilizing *S. stercoralis* larval antigens was shown to be positive in approximately 80 percent of patients and may have some diagnostic utility.

Eosinophilic leukocytosis is common, except in very severe cases. When eosinophilia occurs in association with peptic ulcer symptoms, strongyloidiasis should be suspected.

Treatment   All infected patients should be treated to prevent the occurrence of severe invasive disease. The drug of choice is thiabendazole, which should be given orally in dosage of 25 mg/kg twice a day for 2 or 3 days. In disseminated strongyloidiasis, treatment should be continued for 7 days or more. Lightheadedness, nausea, and vomiting are common accompaniments of therapy with this agent. Delayed aminophylline excretion may result in toxicity. Hypersensitivity reactions may occur but usually respond to treatment with antihistamines. The stools should be rechecked at intervals of 3 months because the parasite is not easily eradicated and retreatment may be necessary.

Prognosis   In the usual case, the prognosis is good. Since the occurrence of hyperinfection is unpredictable, every effort should be made to eradicate the infection in each case. In severe cases with hyperinfection, the prognosis is poor.

Prevention   In general, the measures are those for the control of hookworm infection. In addition, it is well to remember that infection may be contracted by ingestion of contaminated food (especially uncooked vegetables) or of contaminated drinking water and by contact. Patients who have a history of residence in an endemic area should be carefully checked for the presence of the parasite prior to the initiation of steroid or immunosuppressive therapy. Because the larvae may not appear in the stool for several weeks after the initiation of such therapy, repeated examinations of stool and upper intestinal aspirates are indicated. Since sputum, vomitus, stool, and body fluids of patients with disseminated disease may contain infective filariform larvae, gloves and gowns should be worn by hospital personnel caring for such patients.

INTESTINAL CAPILLARIASIS   Definition   Intestinal capillariasis is an infection of humans caused by the roundworm *Capillaria philippinensis*. This species of *Capillaria* was first discovered in 1963 from a fatal human infection occurring in the Philippines. The infection results in intractable diarrhea with a high mortality rate. Clinical studies have shown a severe protein-losing enteropathy and malabsorption of fats and sugars.

Etiology   *Capillaria* are nematodes of the family Trichuroidea and are closely related to comembers *Trichuris* and *Trichinella*. Adult *C. philippinensis* are small, measuring 2 to 4 mm in length. The peanut-shaped eggs have flattened bipolar plugs and an average size of 42 by 20 μm. The adults inhabit the mucosa of the small intestine, especially the jejunum. Adults, larval forms, and eggs are found in the stool.

Epidemiology   The infection has been found almost exclusively in persons residing along the north and west coastal areas of Luzon, Philippines. Several cases from Thailand have also been reported. Since 1966 the disease has occurred in epidemic form, and more than 2000 cases and 100 deaths have been reported. Males are infected more frequently than females, perhaps because of occupational exposure. Prior to the discovery of an effective chemotherapeutic agent, the mortality rate in untreated cases was about 30 percent. With chemotherapy, the case fatality rate has been reduced to 6 percent.

The mode of transmission and life cycle of the parasite are incompletely understood. First-stage larvae have been found in several species of freshwater fish. When these fish or the larvae are fed to gerbils, they develop to adulthood within their intestinal lumina. These adults rapidly produce new larvae which mature to a second generation of adults. Most of the females from this generation are oviparous, the resulting eggs passing in the gerbil's stool. Some, however, remain larviparous, leading to another generation of intestinal adults. Eggs must presumably embryonate in fresh water before being ingested by the fish host. No naturally infected mammal other than humans has been found, but both birds and rats can be experimentally infected. The presence of many adult worms, larviparous females, embryonated eggs, and all larval stages in human intestinal contents suggests that the parasitic cycles in gerbils and humans are the same. The mechanism by which humans originally became infected remains unproven. However, it is known that many of the naturally infected lagoon fish, particularly "bagsit" or *Hypselotris bipartita*, are eaten raw by the people of Luzon.

Pathogenesis and manifestations   Adult worms in large numbers invade the small-intestinal mucosa and cause a severe protein-losing enteropathy and malabsorption. Hypokalemia, hypocalcemia, and hypoproteinemia are the rule. Autopsy studies have failed to show extraintestinal spread of the parasite. Initial symptoms of intestinal "gurgling" (borborygmi) and recurrent vague abdominal pain are followed, usually within 2 to 3 weeks, by a voluminous watery diarrhea. Other findings, consistent with the basic pathophysiologic process, are anorexia, vomiting, weight loss, muscle wasting and weakness, hyporeflexia, and edema. Abdominal tenderness and distention may occur. The period between onset of symptoms and death is usually 2 to 3 months. Subclinical infection has not been noted.

Diagnosis   The diagnosis is made by finding ova in the stool. The ova of *C. philippinensis* must be differentiated from those of *T. trichiura*, which are similar. Care must be taken that capillaria are not overlooked in patients with *Trichuris* infections because in the endemic area most patients with capillariasis have coexistent *Trichuris* infection.

Treatment   Administration of mebendazole combined with fluid and electrolyte replacement leads to dramatic improvement; 400 mg per day in divided dosage should be given for 20 days to prevent relapse.

REFERENCES

Banwell JG, Schad GA: Hookworm. Clin Gastroenterol 7:129, 1978

Cross JH, Basaca-Sevilla V: Experimental transmission of *Capillaria philippinensis* to birds. Trans R Soc Trop Med Hyg 77:511, 1983

Embil JA et al: Prevalence of *Ascaris lumbricoides* infection in a small Nova Scotian community. Am J Trop Med Hyg 33:595, 1984

Fishman JA, Perrone TL: Colonic obstruction and perforation due to *Trichuris trichiura*. Am J Med 77:154, 1984

Gilles HM: Selective primary health care: Strategies for control of disease in the developing world. XVII. Hookworm infection and anemia. Rev Infect Dis 7:111, 1985

Glickman LT, Schantz PM: Epidemiology and pathogenesis of zoonotic toxocariasis. Epidemiol Rev 3:230, 1981

Irga-Siegman Y et al: Syndrome of hyperinfection with *Stronglyoides stercoralis*. Rev Infect Dis 3:397, 1981

Kliks MM: Anisakiasis in the western United States: Four new case reports from California. Am J Trop Med Hyg 32:526, 1983

Little MD et al: *Ancylostoma* larva in a muscle fiber of man following cutaneous larva migrans. Am J Trop Med Hyg 32:1285, 1983

Milder JE et al: Clinical features of *Strongyloides stercoralis* infection in an endemic area of the United States. Gastroenterology 80:1481, 1981

Neva FA et al: Comparison of larval antigens in an enzyme-linked immunosorbent assay for strongyloidiasis in humans. J Infect Dis 144:427, 1981

Pawlowski Z: Ascariasis. Clin Gastroenterol 7:157, 1978

Pelletier LL Jr: Chronic strongyloidiasis in World War II Far East ex-prisoners of war. Am J Trop Med Hyg 33:55, 1984

Smith B et al: Pulmonary strongyloidiasis. Diagnosis by sputum Gram stain. Am J Med 79:663, 1985

Stephenson LS: The contribution of *Ascaris lumbricoides* to malnutrition in children. Parasitology 81:221, 1980

Wagner ED, Eby WC: Pinworm prevalence in California elementary school children, and diagnostic methods. Am J Trop Med Hyg 32:998, 1983

Wolfe MS: *Oxyuris*, *Trichostrongylus* and *Trichuris*. Clin Gastroenterol 7:201, 1978

World Health Organization: Intestinal protozoan and helminthic infections. WHO Tech Rep Ser 1981, no 666

Worley G et al: *Toxocara canis* infection: Clinical and epidemiological association with seropositivity in kindergarten children. J Infect Dis 149:591, 1984

167   OTHER TREMATODES OR FLUKES

JAMES J. PLORDE

The trematodes of humans are long-lived parasites which produce progressive damage to the tissues of their hosts. With the exception of schistosomes, they are similar in morphology and life cycle. The adult flukes are flat, leaflike hermaphrodites that vary in length from a few millimeters to several centimeters. Their digestive tract, unlike that of the nematodes, ends blindly. As their name indicates, they have two "holes" in the form of oral and ventral suckers which are used as organs of attachment and locomotion. The operculated eggs, which are passed in the feces or sputum, hatch in the water to produce a ciliated, free-swimming *miracidium*. The miracidium reaches and penetrates the tissue of an intermediate snail host to undergo a period of development, eventuating in the release of thousands of swarms of free-living *cercariae* from the snail. These thousands of tail-bearing larvae must, in turn, reach a second intermediate host, usually an aquatic animal or vegetation, where they encyst forming *metacercariae*. The definitive host is infected when he or she ingests the parasitized second intermediate host. The distribution of flukes is usually limited by the location of their molluscan intermediate host. With the exception of *Opisthorchis* and *Fasciola*, most hermaphroditic flukes are found only in tropical or subtropical areas.

PARAGONIMIASIS **Definition** Paragonimiasis (endemic hemoptysis) is a chronic infection of the lung caused by trematodes of the genus *Paragonimus*. Clinically, the disease is characterized by cough and hemoptysis. Ectopic worms may cause a variety of other manifestations. Geographically, it is probably the most widely distributed disease caused by hermaphroditic flukes.

Etiology and epidemiology Although *P. westermani*, which is widely distributed in the far east, is the most common cause of human paragonimiasis, a number of other species, including *P. skrjabini*, *P. heterotremus* (China), *P. africanus*, *P. uterobilateralis* (central and west Africa), *P. kellicotti* (North America), *P. mexicanus*, *P. ecuadoriensis*, and *P. caliensis* (Central and South America), may cause the disease. Approximately 1 percent of Indochinese immigrants to the United States harbor *P. westermani*. The short, plump adults (7 to 12 mm in length, 4 to 6 mm in width) have a life span of 4 to 5 years which they typically spend encysted in the lung parenchyma of the host. Their golden-brown operculated eggs (50 by 90 μm) reach the bronchioles from where they are coughed up and excreted in the sputum or swallowed and passed in the feces. They must embryonate several weeks in fresh water before hatching to release the miracidia.

The infection is acquired by ingestion of cysts in the second intermediate host, a freshwater shrimp, crab, or crayfish. The metacercariae excyst in the duodenum, burrow through the intestinal wall into the peritoneal cavity, and then usually migrate through the diaphragm and into the lung. The worms also may be found in the intestinal wall, liver, pancreas, kidney, epididymis, mesentery, skeletal muscle, subcutaneous tissues, and central nervous system, particularly the brain. The dog, cat, pig, rat, and wild carnivores are definitive hosts for the parasite in addition to humans. In some of these, very young adults can be found in their striated muscles. Human infection has been reported following the ingestion of this undercooked flesh.

The incidence of paragonimiasis is often affected by food shortages or local customs. The metacercariae survive in vinegar, and lightly pickled or inadequately cooked food usually serves as the source of infection in the far east. Fresh crab juice used for the treatment of measles in Korea and for infertility in the Cameroons may also transmit the parasite. Children may acquire the disease in endemic areas while handling or eating raw crabs during play.

Pathogenesis and clinical manifestations An eosinophilic granuloma forms about the adult worm, eventually leading to the formation of a fibrous cyst. The pulmonary lesions which measure up to 1 cm in diameter frequently communicate with a bronchiole, resulting in secondary bacterial infection. Small, fibrous nodules representing reaction around deposited eggs also occur. Clinically the picture is one of chronic bronchitis and bronchiectasis with production of brownish sputum and hemoptysis. A poorly resolving pulmonary infiltrate, lung abscess, or pleural effusion may be present in heavy infections. Effusions are often large, may occur in the absence of parenchymal disease, and are typically exudative with eosinophils and cholesterol crystals. The roentgenographic findings vary with the stage of infection. Initially diffuse or segmental infiltrates, with or without pleural effusions, may be seen in lower or midlung fields. These are then gradually replaced by round 2- to 4-cm nodules which not infrequently cavitate. Eventually, cystic rings, fibrosis, and calcification occur, presenting a picture closely resembling tuberculosis, a disease which often coexists with paragonimiasis.

An abdominal mass, pain, and dysentery characterize intestinal or peritoneal infections. Various types of paralysis and epilepsy occur in cerebral involvement. Homonymous hemianopsia, optic atrophy, and papilledema are common. The cerebrospinal fluid usually shows an eosinophilic leukocytosis and elevated protein. Cerebral calcifications are seen on x-ray in 50 percent of cases. *Paragonimus skrjabini* and, perhaps, *P. ecuadoriensis* infections are characterized by migratory subcutaneous nodules that contain adult flukes.

Laboratory findings Eosinophilia is a constant finding. Definitive diagnosis depends upon finding the characteristic operculated ova in the sputum, stool, pleural fluid, or tissue. Eggs may be rare or totally absent from the sputum during the first 3 months of infection but are eventually found in 75 to 85 percent of infected patients. Their presence correlates well with the roentgenographic appearance of cavities. Even later, however, repeated examinations using concentration techniques may be required for their recovery. Ziehl-Neelsen staining, often carried out for suspected tuberculosis, usually will not demonstrate the eggs. In fact, the sputum concentration techniques for tuberculosis may destroy the eggs that are present. Since many patients have concomitant tuberculosis, the diagnosis may be overlooked. Stool examination is frequently helpful in children. A complement fixation test is available, and the results correlate well with active infection. It usually becomes negative within 6 months of successful therapy. The skin test does not distinguish present and past infections and is used primarily for epidemiologic purposes.

Treatment and prevention Praziquantel is the drug of choice. A total of 75 mg/kg is given in three divided doses for 1 or 2 days. Alternatively, bithionol may be administered. From 30 to 40 mg/kg in divided doses should be given every other day for a total of 10 to 15 treatment days. The symptoms disappear rapidly, and most infiltrates resolve within 3 months. Side effects are minor and consist of nausea, vomiting, and urticaria. Concomitant bacterial infection must be treated. Prevention of superinfection by the same parasite is important, because the disease is self-limiting.

The most practical control measure is the adequate cooking of all shellfish before they are eaten.

CLONORCHIASIS **Definition** Clonorchiasis is an infection of the biliary passages caused by *Clonorchis sinensis*, the most important liver fluke of humans. Although the infection is usually asymptomatic, heavy worm loads may produce manifestations of biliary obstruction.

Etiology and epidemiology *Clonorchis sinensis* is a small fluke (5 by 15 mm) that lives as long as 50 years in the biliary tree of its host. Here the flukes feed on mucosal secretions and pass operculated eggs into the feces. On reaching fresh water, the eggs are ingested by the intermediate snail host. After multiplication and development within the snail, the cercariae are released and penetrate freshwater fish. Infections result from ingestion of the raw, dried, salted, or pickled flesh of freshwater fish containing encysted metacercariae. The larva is released in the duodenum. It enters the common bile duct and migrates to the second-order bile ducts, where it develops into the adult form in about 1 month. In addition to humans, dogs, cats, pigs, and rats serve as disease reservoirs. The main endemic areas are Korea, Japan, Taiwan, Hong Kong, southern China, and Vietnam where, in previous years, clonorchiasis was perpetuated by the practice of fertilizing fish ponds with manure and human feces. Improvements in the disposal of human feces have dramatically decreased transmission in most areas, but the infection rate has remained high due to the prolonged life span of the adult worm. Twenty-five percent of the population of Hong Kong and a small proportion of Chinese immigrants to this country have been shown to be infected. The disease may also be acquired in the United States by the ingestion of infected, dried, frozen, or pickled fish imported from the far east. Clinically apparent cases are restricted to the adult population in whom the accumulated worm load eventually produces pathologic effects.

Pathogenesis and clinical manifestations Light infections are usually asymptomatic, but worm loads of 500 to 1000 flukes often result in clinical manifestations. During the migration of the larvae, the patient may have fever, chills, tender hepatomegaly, mild jaundice, and eosinophilia. The mature worm causes proliferation of the biliary epithelium, increased mucin production, adenoma formation, chronic pericholangitis, and periductal fibrosis. Hepatic parenchymal damage and portal hypertension are not seen in uncomplicated infections. Recurrent attacks of suppurative cholangitis with or without intrahepatic choledocholithiasis may follow biliary obstruction with dead flukes. These occasionally present as hypoglycemic coma. The occurrence of biliary stones in clonorchiasis is associated with an increased incidence of chronic *Salmonella typhi* carriage. Cholangiocarcinoma may occur in patients with severe, long-standing infections. The adult worms may infest the pancreatic ducts, where they can cause squamous metaplasia, periductal fibrosis, and acute pancreatitis.

Laboratory diagnosis Clinical and epidemiologic findings often suggest the diagnosis. There may be elevation of the alkaline phosphatase and hyperbilirubinemia. Eosinophilia is variable. Occasionally, a plain film of the abdomen will demonstrate intrahepatic calcification. Liver scan is usually negative in asymptomatic infections but may show multiple areas of diminished uptake in acute symptomatic disease. Percutaneous transhepatic cholangiography in such patients often reveals dilatation of the peripheral intrahepatic bile ducts. The adult worms appear as round filling defects several millimeters in diameter. Definitive diagnosis depends on the demonstration of the eggs in the feces or the duodenal contents. They measure 29 by 16 μm, possess a conspicuous opercular rim as well as a posterior knob, and can be distinguished from the eggs of *Metagonimus, Heterophyes,* and *Opisthorchis* only with difficulty. An antigen extracted from adult worms can be used in a complement fixation or enzyme-linked immunosorbent test for the detection of the host's antibody response.

Treatment and prevention The introduction of praziquantel has provided an effective chemotherapeutic agent for clonorchiasis. It is administered in a dosage of 25 mg/kg tid for a single day. Thorough cooking of freshwater fish will prevent infection.

OPISTHORCHIASIS Opisthorchiasis is caused by *Opisthorchis felineus* or *O. viverrini* and is characterized by hepatic lesions produced by adult worms in the larger bile ducts. The life cycle resembles that of *C. sinensis.* The geographic distribution differs in that *O. felineus* is endemic in eastern and central Europe and in Siberia and occurs in some parts of Asia, while *O. viverrini* is found in Thailand and Laos. Cats and wild carnivores act as the principal reservoir hosts, and the infection is found most commonly along rivers and lakes which harbor an abundant fish life. Up to 90 percent of inhabitants of some villages in northeastern Thailand are purported to carry the parasite. The clinical lesions are similar to those seen in clonorchiasis except that gallstones are rare. Cholangiocarcinoma occurs in approximately 50 percent of infected patients who come to autopsy. The diagnosis usually is based on the finding of the eggs in the feces or duodenal contents. Treatment as recommended for clonorchiasis may be used. Infection can be prevented by eating only well-cooked fish.

FASCIOLIASIS Fascioliasis is caused by *Fasciola hepatica,* which, like *Clonorchis,* inhabits the bile ducts of the definitive host. When fully matured, the adult measures about 3 by 1 cm and discharges large operculate eggs 140 by 70 μm which must embryonate in fresh water before hatching.

Fascioliasis produces so-called liver rot in sheep, the principal definitive host. The disease is most common in sheep- and cattle-raising countries but has been reported from many parts of the world. In North America it occurs in the southern and western United States, Central America, and in the Caribbean Islands, including Puerto Rico.

Infection is contracted by ingestion of the encysted forms of the fluke attached to edible aquatic plants such as watercress. The larvae excyst in the duodenum, migrate through the intestinal wall, pass into the peritoneal cavity, penetrate the liver capsule, and finally reach the bile ducts, where they mature. Occasionally larvae may migrate to and mature in ectopic locations including the pancreas, subcutaneous tissue, chest cavity, or brain.

Early clinical manifestations are related to the migration of the larval form to and within the liver. Epigastric pain, fever, diarrhea, jaundice, urticaria, pruritus, arthralgia, and eosinophilia may be observed during this stage. Fibrosis of the liver similar to that found in clonorchiasis appears only after prolonged residence of many adult worms in the bile ducts. Obstruction of the bile duct occurs frequently and may be the presenting manifestation of disease. A pharyngeal form of the disease, called *halzoun,* can result from eating infected raw liver, the young adults attaching themselves to the pharyngeal mucosa, occasionally interfering with respiration.

The diagnosis usually is based on the finding of the eggs in the feces or in the duodenal contents. It is difficult to distinguish the eggs from those of *Fasciolopsis buski.* Complement fixation, hemagglutination, and precipitin tests have been reported to be helpful. A skin test is also available.

Treatment is as described above for clonorchiasis.

To prevent infection, aquatic plants such as watercress should not be eaten, vegetables grown in fields irrigated with polluted water should be boiled, and safe drinking water should be provided.

FASCIOLOPSIASIS Fasciolopsiasis is caused by the large intestinal fluke *F. buski,* which inhabits the upper part of the intestine of its definitive host. The principal definitive host is the pig. China, Thailand, India, and other areas in the far east are the major endemic loci. Infection of humans occurs following ingestion, or peeling with the teeth, of water chestnuts, water lotus, and other edible aquatic plants. The large adults attach themselves to the intestinal mucosa, and these sites may later ulcerate. The infection is usually asymptomatic. In heavy infections, diarrhea, abdominal pain, gastrointestinal hemorrhage, and intestinal obstruction may appear early. Later, asthenia with ascites and anasarca occurs. Diagnosis is based upon the history and the finding of eggs in the feces. The eggs resemble those of *Fasciola hepatica.* The prognosis in untreated heavy infections, especially in children, is poor. Praziquantel as given for clonorchiasis is the treatment of choice. Tetrachloroethylene as given for hookworm infections may also be used.

HETEROPHYIASIS AND METAGONIMIASIS *Heterophyes heterophyes* and *Metagonimus yakagawa* are small intestinal flukes of humans and other fish-eating mammals. They are found in the far east and, in the case of *Heterophyes,* in India, Egypt, and Tunisia. Both are acquired by ingesting the raw or undercooked flesh of metacercarial-infected freshwater fish. The 2- to 3-mm adults attach themselves to the mucosa of the small intestine. If present in sufficient numbers, they may cause abdominal pain and/or diarrhea. Rarely the eggs have been found in sites such as the brain, spinal cord, or heart where they produce granulomatous lesions. Most commonly, they are passed in the stool where they very closely resemble those of *Clonorchis.* Both species can be treated with praziquantel as described for clonorchiasis or tetrachloroethylene as outlined in Chap. 166 for hookworm. As the life span of these trematodes is limited to a year or less, treatment is not indicated unless the patient is symptomatic.

REFERENCES

FLAVELL DJ: Liver-fluke infection as an aetiologic factor in bile-duct carcinoma of man. Trans R Soc Trop Med Hyg 75:814, 1981

HOOVER R et al: Seasonal transmission of *Fasciola hepatica* to cattle in northwestern United States. J Am Vet Med Assoc 184:695, 1984

JOHNSON RJ, JOHNSON JR: Paragonimiasis in Indochinese refugees: Roentgenographic findings with clinical correlations. Am Rev Resp Dis 128:534, 1983

—— et al: Paragonimiasis: Diagnosis and the use of praziquantel in treatment. Rev Infect Dis 7:200, 1985

JONES EA et al: Massive infection with *Fasciola hepatica* in man. Am J Med 63:842, 1977

JONG EC et al: Praziquantel for the treatment of *Clonorchis/Opisthorchis* infections. Report of a double-blind, placebo-controlled trial. J Infect Dis 152:637, 1985

KOENIGSTEIN RP: Observations on the epidemiology of infections with *Clonorchis sinensis*. Trans R Soc Trop Med Hyg 42:503, 1949

KOOMPIROCHANA C et al: Opisthorchiasis: A clinicopathologic study of 154 autopsy cases. Southeastern Asian J Trop Med 9:60, 1978

McFADZEAN AJS, YEUNG RTT: Hypoglycemia in suppurative pancholangitis due to *Clonorchis sinensis*. Trans R Soc Trop Med Hyg 59:179, 1965

PACHUCKI CT et al: American paragonimiasis treated wtih praziquantel. N Engl J Med 311:582, 1984

PLANT AG et al: A clinical study of *Fasciolopsis buski* in Thailand. Trans R Soc Trop Med Hyg 63:470, 1969

UPATHAM ES et al: Morbidity in relation to intensity of infection in *Opisthorchiasis viverrini*: Study of a community in Khon Kaen, Thailand. Am J Trop Med Hyg 31:1156, 1982

YOKOGAWA M: *Paragonimus* and paragonimiasis, in *Advances in Parasitology*, B Dawes (ed). London, Academic, 1969, vol 7, p 375

168 CESTODE (TAPEWORM) INFECTIONS

PAUL G. RAMSEY / JAMES J. PLORDE

The tapeworms, or cestodes, are ribbon-shaped segmented hermaphroditic worms which inhabit the intestinal tract of many vertebrates. Unlike other helminths, they lack a digestive tract but absorb food through their entire surface. Tapeworms have a primitive nervous system, a muscular system, and excretory canals. Attachment to the host's intestinal mucosa is accomplished by sucking cups or grooves located on the head, or *scolex*. In some species, attachment is aided by hooklets located on the scolex. Behind the globular scolex lies a short, narrow neck from which segments or *proglottides* develop to form the chainlike *strobila* of the worm. The proglottides progressively mature as they are displaced further from the neck by new segments. As each section becomes gravid, eggs are released either through a uterine pore, by splitting open, or by disintegrating. Because the eggs of many tapeworms appear identical, species identification depends on the morphological characteristics of the scolex or gravid proglottides.

Except for *Hymenolepis nana* the human tapeworms require one or more intermediate hosts for larval development. After ingestion by a susceptible intermediate host, the eggs develop into larvae or *oncospheres* which are capable of penetrating the intestinal mucosa, migrating in tissues, and developing into encysted forms. If the cyst contains a single scolex, it is called a *cysticercus*, or *cysticercoid* in the case of *H. nana*. A *coenurus* is a cyst which contains several scolices, and a *hydatid* is a structure with daughter cysts each containing several scolices. Ingestion of tissues containing cysts with viable scolices by a definitive host allows development of the larval stage into an adult tapeworm. Cestodes in the *Diphyllobothrium* genus have a more complex life cycle involving two intermediate hosts (see below).

Human tapeworm infections may be divided into two major clinical groups. In the first, humans act as the definitive host and harbor the adult tapeworm in their intestines. The important species in this group include *Taenia saginata*, *Diphyllobothrium latum*, *Hymenolepis* species, and *Dipylidium caninum*. In the second group, humans are intermediate hosts and harbor the larval forms in their tissues. This is exemplified by echinococcosis, sparganosis, and coenurosis. *Taenia solium* is unique because humans may act as both the definitive and intermediate hosts.

TAENIASIS SAGINATA Definition Taeniasis saginata is an intestinal infection of humans caused by the beef tapeworm.

Epidemiology Infection with *Taenia saginata* occurs in all countries where raw or undercooked beef is eaten. It is particularly prevalent in Ethiopia, Kenya, Yugoslavia, the Middle East, Mexico and parts of South America, and the U.S.S.R. Indigenously acquired infection is uncommon in the United States except in areas where cattle and humans are concentrated such as around feedlots in the southwest.

Etiology and pathogenesis Humans are the only definitive host for the adult stage of *T. saginata* which inhabits the upper jejunum for as long as 25 years. The cestode is 5 to 10 m long and has a small, unarmed scolex with four prominent suckers and 1000 to 2000 proglottides. The gravid segments are longer than they are wide (5 by 20 mm) and have 15 to 30 lateral uterine branches (*T. solium* has 8 to 12). The eggs, which are indistinguishable from *T. solium* eggs, measure 30 by 40 μm, have a thick brown radially striated shell, and contain a fully developed embryo with three pairs of hooklets. After the egg-containing proglottides are deposited on soil or vegetation, they are ingested by cattle or other herbivores. The embryo is released in the intestine, invades the intestinal wall, and is carried by vascular channels to striated muscle in the hind limbs, diaphragm, and tongue where it is transformed over a period of 3 to 4 months into an ovoid bladder worm, or cysticercus. This form, which may be viable for 1 to 3 years, measures about 5 by 10 mm and consists of one scolex suspended in a fluid-filled sac. After ingestion of the cyst in raw or undercooked beef by humans, the adult worm develops in the intestine in about 2 months.

Clinical manifestations Most patients have minimal or no symptoms. Mild epigastric discomfort, nausea, and hunger sensations may occur. Weight loss, diarrhea, irritability, and an increase in appetite are more unusual. Movements of the worm are sometimes apparent, and occasionally proglottides may crawl through the anus, appearing in the bed linen or underclothing of the distraught host. Rarely segments become impacted in the appendix or cystic or pancreatic duct producing obstruction and inflammation of these organs.

Diagnosis After the adult tapeworm has been established for 2 to 3 months, several proglottides are shed daily in the stool and can be detected readily. Eggs may be distributed in the stool or on the perianal area if a proglottid ruptures during defecation and should be looked for in the absence of segments. The perianal region may be examined as for pinworm infection, using a Scotch brand cellophane tape swab. By this method 85 to 95 percent of infections may be detected, whereas by stool examination only 50 to 75 percent are recognized. Since egg morphology is not diagnostic, examination of mature proglottides or the scolex is necessary to identify the tapeworm species correctly. Reliable serologic tests are not available.

Treatment Niclosamide (Yomesan) is a highly effective taenicide which kills the scolex and immature segments of the worm on contact. Four 0.5-g tablets are thoroughly chewed at one time and swallowed with a small amount of water. No preparation or purge is necessary, and few side effects have been reported. As the worm is digested before it is passed in the stool, no attempt should be made to recover the scolex. Stool should be examined at 3 and 6 months for test of cure. Paromomycin (Humatin), 1.0 g orally every 15 min for four doses, is an alternative drug. Mebendazole in a dose of 300 mg twice daily for 3 days or a single dose of praziquantel (10 mg/kg) is effective, but these agents have not been approved for treating taeniasis in the United States.

Prevention Thorough cooking of beef is the major means of preventing taeniasis saginata. Temperatures as low as 56°C for as little as 5 min will destroy cysticerci. Refrigeration and salting for prolonged periods or freezing at −10°C for 9 days also destroys the cysticercus. General preventive measures include adequate meat inspection and proper disposal of human feces.

TAENIASIS SOLIUM AND CYSTICERCOSIS Definition *Taenia solium*, the pork tapeworm, inhabits the intestinal lumen of humans, its only definitive host. The hog is the usual intermediate host, although humans, dogs, cats, and sheep may harbor the larval form. When human tissue is invaded by the larval form, the condition is referred to as *cysticercosis*.

Epidemiology Taeniasis solium is worldwide but is most common in Mexico, Africa, southeast Asia, eastern Europe, and South America. *T. solium* has been found in swine in Colorado and New

Mexico, but autochthonously acquired human disease is rare in the United States. Cysticercosis has been recognized more frequently in industrialized nations due to migration of infected persons from endemic areas.

Etiology and pathogenesis   The adult worm is about 3 m in length, resides in the upper jejunum, and may live for decades. The globular scolex contains a rostellum with two rows of hooklets. There are usually fewer than 1000 proglottides. The gravid proglottid is about 6 by 12 mm and contains a uterus with 8 to 12 lateral branchings. The eggs are infective for both human and hog. Infection usually occurs by the fecal-oral route, but humans may be autoinfected when gravid segments are returned to the stomach by reverse peristalsis. In the intermediate host, the embryo is released from the egg, penetrates the intestinal wall, and is carried by vascular channels to all parts of the body. Localization with development over 60 to 70 days to the encysted larval stage (''bladder worm'') occurs primarily in striated muscle of the tongue, neck, and trunk. The cysticerci are ovoid, gray-white opalescent structures about 1 cm in diameter. They can survive for 5 years. Humans become infected with the adult stage following ingestion of undercooked pork containing cysticerci.

Clinical manifestations   Clinical manifestations of adult worm infestation resemble those with *T. saginata*. When humans serve as the intermediate host (cysticercosis), the clinical picture is entirely different. Cysticerci develop in the subcutaneous tissues, in muscles, in viscera, and, most importantly, in the eye and brain. Only a moderate tissue reaction occurs while the scolex is viable, but the dead larvae invoke a marked tissue response with muscular pains, weakness, fever, and eosinophilia. Brain cysts are usually located in the cerebrum, ventricles, or subarachnoid space. The cerebral cysts are often less than 2 cm in diameter but may rarely be as large as 5 cm. If the cysticerci are widely distributed, the patient has signs and symptoms of meningoencephalitis. Epilepsy, brain tumors, and other types of neurologic or psychiatric disorders may also be simulated. Clinical findings may change during the course of infection due to changes in the inflammatory response.

Diagnosis   Infection with the adult worm can be detected by finding eggs in perianal scrapings or in the feces. However, to differentiate *T. solium* from *T. saginata*, proglottides or the scolex must be examined. Cysticercosis should be suspected in an individual who has lived in a hyperendemic area and who develops neurologic findings. Subcutaneous cysts may be found in approximately 50 percent of patients, and roentgenograms of soft tissue may show typical calcifications later in the course of cysticercosis. Contrast-enhanced computerized tomography (CT) scans are valuable for identifying brain lesions, which may appear as solid nodules or cystic or calcified lesions. In some patients, only hydrocephalus may be seen. Cerebrospinal fluid is often abnormal but not diagnostic. Enzyme-linked immunosorbent assay (ELISA) provides a sensitive serologic test for diagnosis of cysticercosis, but cross-reactive antibodies occur in some patients with other infections. Brain, subcutaneous nodule, or skin biopsy specimens are needed to establish a specific diagnosis.

Treatment   The stage and location of the parasite determine the prognosis and treatment. For removal of the adult worm in the human intestine, niclosamide, paromomycin, mebendazole, or praziquantel may be given as for *Taeniasis saginata*. However, because these drugs cause maceration of the proglottides with release of ova, cysticercosis could theoretically occur. To prevent this, some authorities recommend that a saline purge be administered 1 h after the medication. Treatment of ocular cysticercosis should be surgical.

Praziquantel has been used to treat cerebral cysticercosis with promising results. A dose of 50 mg of praziquantel per kilogram given daily in three divided doses for 15 days has been recommended. Corticosteroids have been used with praziquantel to treat fever, headache, and meningismus which presumably occur secondary to an inflammatory response to dying cysticerci. The optimal dose and duration of praziquantel, the long-term side effects, and the need for concomitant corticosteroid treatment have not been studied adequately.

HYMENOLEPIASIS NANA   Definition   Hymenolepiasis nana is an intestinal infection of humans, rats, and mice by *Hymenolepis nana*, the dwarf tapeworm. The life cycle is unique in that both the larval and adult phases occur in the same host.

Epidemiology   Dwarf tapeworm infection has been reported in temperate and tropical regions around the globe. It is the most common autochthonously acquired tapeworm in the United States, most of the infections occurring in the southern states. The infection is spread by the direct fecal-oral route and is particularly common in children and institutional populations.

Etiology and pathogenesis   The adult worm is small, about 2 cm, and lives for only a few weeks in the proximal ileum. Its proglottides are very small and are rarely seen in the stool. The gravid segments break apart in the fecal stream releasing spherical eggs. These measure 30 to 44 μm in diameter and have a double membrane enclosing the embryo which has six hooklets. The inner vitelline membrane has four to eight slender filaments arising from each pole. The eggs are immediately infective, and when ingested by a new host, the freed oncospheres penetrate the intestinal villi, becoming cysticercoids. Larvae migrate back into the intestinal lumen, attach to the mucosa, and mature into adult worms. The eggs may also hatch before passing in the stool, causing internal autoinfection with gradually increasing numbers of worms in the host.

Clinical manifestations   Dwarf tapeworm infection may be asymptomatic even with many adult worms in the intestine. When infection is massive, abdominal cramps and diarrhea occur. Rarely, dizziness or seizures have been seen in children and have been attributed to a neurotoxic product of the worms.

Treatment   Niclosamide, 2 g per day, must be given for 5 to 7 consecutive days. The dosage for children must be adjusted for body weight. The longer treatment course is necessary because niclosamide is not effective against the cysticercoid stage, and the encysted larvae continue to release organisms for 4 days. A repeat treatment course may be required in 2 weeks for patients with heavy infections. Paromomycin, 45 mg/kg daily for 5 to 7 days, may also be effective.

Prevention   With a single host involved and the eggs being immediately infective, eradication of the disease presents problems similar to those encountered with enterobiasis. Personal hygiene is imperative. In an institution, epidemics can be avoided by proper screening programs.

HYMENOLEPIASIS DIMINUTA   *Hymenolepis diminuta* is a cestode of rats and mice that occasionally infects small children. Larval development occurs in a wide variety of insects including fleas and mealworms. Humans become infected with the adult worm when they ingest uncooked cereal foods contaminated by these insects. Infection is usually asymptomatic, and the diagnosis is made only when characteristic eggs are found in the stool. The eggs resemble those of *H. nana* but are longer and lack polar filaments. Niclosamide, as prescribed for *H. nana*, results in approximately a 90 percent cure rate.

DIPYLIDIASIS   *Dipylidium caninum* is the common tapeworm of cats and dogs. The orange-brown proglottid, which resembles a pumpkin seed, is often passed intact in the stool or migrates through the anal canal. This may cause animals harboring the parasite to drag their buttocks across the floor. The characteristic egg packets are then expelled by the proglottides and ingested by fleas to develop into infective larval forms. The definitive host becomes infected by swallowing involved fleas. Human infections occur primarily in small children who ingest fleas while playing with their pets. The diagnosis is made by recovering the characteristic proglottid or egg packet. Treatment is the same as for *T. saginata* described above. Periodic deworming of pets provides the best prevention.

DIPHYLLOBOTHRIASIS **Definition** *Diphyllobothrium latum* and other *Diphyllobothrium* species, the fish or broad tapeworms, produce an intestinal infection in the definitive host (including humans).

Epidemiology Diphyllobothriasis is common in the Baltic and Scandinavian countries, Japan, U.S.S.R., Switzerland, Italy, Chile, and central Africa. It occurs in the north central United States, Florida, and with increased frequency along the Pacific coast. The prevalence of infection is enhanced by the disposal of raw sewage into freshwater lakes. Anadromous Alaskan salmon have been implicated in an outbreak along the west coast. The popularity of raw fish dishes such as Japanese sushi and sashimi may lead to increased prevalence of the disease in the United States.

Etiology and pathogenesis The adult worm lies attached to the mucosa of the ileum and occasionally the jejunum by a pair of sucking grooves located on the scolex. It can live 20 years and achieve a length of more than 10 m. The 3000 to 4000 proglottides are wider than they are long. Unlike *Taenia*, the gravid segments are retained by the worm, and each day a million operculated ova are passed directly in the stool. On reaching water, the egg hatches, releasing a free-swimming embryo. This is eaten by small freshwater crustaceans belonging to the species *Cyclops* or *Diaptomus*, in which it develops into a *procercoid*. When the infected crustacean is swallowed by a fish, the larva migrates into the flesh and grows into a *plerocercoid*, or *sparganum*, larva. Humans acquire disease by ingesting raw infected fish. In 3 to 5 weeks the tapeworm matures in the intestine into an adult capable of discharging eggs. Several *Diphyllobothrium* species can infect humans, and *D. latum* cannot be distinguished from other species by its eggs or proglottides. Species determination requires examination of the scolex.

Clinical manifestations Most infections are asymptomatic or produce slight, transient abdominal discomfort. Rarely, there may be severe cramping abdominal pain, diarrhea or constipation, vomiting, weakness, and loss of weight. Intestinal obstruction has been reported in multiple infections. In 0.1 to 2 percent of infected patients, an anemia develops, and about 40 percent of fish tapeworm carriers will have low serum vitamin B_{12} levels. The anemia appears to result from the ability of the tapeworm to compete successfully with its host for vitamin B_{12} and resembles pernicious anemia including central nervous system involvement. A worm located high in the jejunum may take up 80 to 100 percent of labeled vitamin B_{12} ingested by a patient with anemia. These patients tend to be elderly, have diminished production of intrinsic factor, and have worms located in the proximal small bowel. Folate absorption may also be decreased and contribute to the anemia. Lysolecithin, a product of the tapeworm, may contribute to the severity of the disease. Neurologic manifestations are more common than in pernicious anemia and may occur in the absence of hematologic findings. Typically, they include paresthesias, impaired vibration sense, numbness, weakness, and, less commonly, central scotomas secondary to optic atrophy. These findings are reversible with proper treatment.

Diagnosis The characteristic eggs are present in the stool in large numbers, making the diagnosis easy. They measure 55 to 76 by 41 to 56 μm and possess a single shell with an operculum at one end and a knob on the other. Mild eosinophilia may be present.

Treatment Niclosamide or paromomycin as prescribed for taeniasis saginata will cure most infections. In the presence of macrocytic anemia, parenteral vitamin B_{12} should be given.

Prevention Fish tapeworm infection can be prevented by cooking to a temperature of at least 56°C for 5 min. Freezing at −10°C for 72 h or placing the fish in a brine solution with appropriate salt concentration and exposure time can also prevent disease. Commercially prepared lox is usually brined appropriately before smoking.

SPARGANOSIS The *sparganum*, or plerocercoid larva, of *Diphyllobothrium*-related tapeworms belonging to the genus *Spirometra* will develop in humans following ingestion (usually in drinking water) of a *Cyclops* bearing the procercoid larva. Sparganosis also follows ingestion of infected frogs or application of infected fresh frog flesh as a poultice. The frog tissues contain the sparganum, which is capable of invading human tissues. The dog and cat are definitive hosts for *Spirometra*. The infection often presents as a painful subcutaneous swelling. The periorbital tissues may be involved with marked palpebral edema and destruction of the globe. A marked eosinophilia is usually present. The location of the larvae determines the prognosis of the infection in humans. Surgery and injection of ethyl alcohol with epinephrine-free procaine to kill worms is the preferred method of treatment.

COENUROSIS This is a rare infection of humans by the larval stage, or coenurus, of the dog tapeworm *Taenia multiceps*. As in cysticercosis, the subcutaneous tissue, eye, and central nervous system may be involved. In tropical areas the brain has often been invaded, and the cases have been fatal. The clinical presentation is that of a slowly growing space-occupying lesion. Diagnosis and treatment both rely on surgical excision of the lesion. Treatment with drugs including mebendazole has not been effective.

ECHINOCOCCIASIS **Definition** Echinococciasis is a tissue infection of humans caused by the larval stage of *Echinococcus granulosus* or *E. multilocularis*. These species of echinococcus are distinct morphologically and biologically. In humans, *E. granulosus* produces cystic lesions primarily involving the liver and lungs, whereas *E. multilocularis* causes multilocular (alveolar) lesions that are locally invasive. A "sylvatic" form of *E. granulosus* differs significantly in clinical findings from a "pastoral" form.

Epidemiology Canines are the definitive hosts for *E. granulosus*. Sheep, cattle, and, in the Middle East, camels are the common intermediates for the pastoral form. This form of the disease has its highest incidence in countries where sheep and cattle raising is carried out with the help of dogs, particularly in the Middle East, Australia, New Zealand, east and south Africa, South America, and central Europe. Approximately 200 cases per year of echinococciasis are diagnosed in the United States, but most are imported. Autochthonously acquired cases have been reported from a few well-defined populations, including Basque sheep farmers in California, southwestern Indians, and sheep raisers in Utah.

The sylvatic focus of *E. granulosus* exists primarily in Alaska and western Canada, where wolves act as the definitive host and caribou and moose as the intermediate. A second sylvatic cycle involving deer and coyotes has been reported from California. A domestic cycle can be established when humans kill the herbivores and feed their viscera to dogs.

In *E. multilocularis* infections, rodents such as deer mice are the natural intermediate hosts, while wolves, foxes, coyotes, and domestic dogs and cats may serve as definitive hosts. An urban cycle involving the cat and common house mouse has been described. Human infection in the United States is most common in Alaska but has also been described in Minnesota. Large series of patients with *E. multilocularis* have been reported from Siberia and Switzerland.

Etiology The adult *E. granulosus* is a small worm measuring 5 mm in length which resides in the jejunum of canines for 5 to 20 months. In addition to the scolex and neck, it has three proglottides, one immature, one mature, and one gravid. The gravid segment splits, either before or after passage in the stool, to release eggs which appear identical with those of *T. saginata*. When ingested by an appropriate intermediate host, the embryos escape from the eggs, penetrate the intestinal mucosa, and enter the portal circulation. Most are filtered out by the liver or lung, but some escape into the general circulation to involve brain, kidney, bones, and other tissues. The larvae that are not phagocytosed and destroyed develop into hydatid cysts which are unilocular and consist of an external laminated cuticula and an inner germinal layer. The laminated membrane in the sylvatic form may be semitranslucent in appearance and more fragile than in the pastoral type. Fluid fills and distends the cyst. Brood capsules and second- or third-generation daughter cysts develop from the germinal layer. "Hydatid sand" found in the cyst consists of scolices liberated from ruptured brood capsules. The cysts grow slowly over a period of years. In the pastoral type cysts often reach a diameter of over 10 cm, while cysts in the sylvatic form are usually only 3 to 5 cm. When the hydatid cyst is ingested by a canine, the cycle is complete.

The life cycle of *E. multilocularis* is similar except that small rodents serve as the natural intermediate host. However, the cyst is quite different. The larval stage of *E. granulosus* develops normally in humans, and the unilocular cyst remains unattached to host tissue. In contrast, humans do not provide optimal conditions for development of *E. multilocularis,* and the larval form remains in the proliferative phase. The hydatid cyst is always multilocular or alveolar in type. Its vesicles progressively invade the host tissue, usually the liver, by extension of processes from the germinal layer. In general, the growth pattern is like a neoplasm, and the lesions may metastasize when growth extends into blood vessels.

Clinical manifestations   Echinococciasis is usually acquired in childhood, but a latent period of 5 to 20 years occurs before diagnosis. In one patient the latent period of a hepatic cyst was 75 years. Enlarging cysts usually produce tissue damage by mechanical means. The resulting symptoms depend upon the site, type, and rate of growth of the cystic lesions.

Patients with the sylvatic form of *E. granulosus* are usually asymptomatic at the time of diagnosis. Approximately 60 percent of the cysts are found in the lung and 40 percent in the liver. The cysts are diagnosed as an incidental finding on routine x-ray. Rarely, a patient may present with hemoptysis or a palpable mass in the liver. Morbidity and mortality are almost never seen.

With the pastoral type the ratio of pulmonary to liver cysts is reversed, and the hydatids may reach enormous size. In as many as 20 percent of patients, the pulmonary hydatid may rupture producing cough, chest pain, or hemoptysis. Hepatic lesions often present as abdominal pain or a palpable mass. Rupture through the diaphragm or into the peritoneal cavity can occur. Intrabiliary extrusion of calcified hepatic cysts has been reported in 5 to 15 percent of affected patients and mimics recurrent cholecystitis. Obstruction of the bile duct may result in jaundice. Rupture of a hydatid into the bile duct, peritoneal cavity, lung, pleura, or bronchus may produce fever, pruritus, urticarial rash, or an anaphylactoid reaction which may be fatal. Release of the numerous scolices leads to disseminated infection. Most patients initially have one or more hydatids in a single site, but in about 10 percent other tissues are involved. In bone, the cysts are semisolid, invade the medullary cavity, and slowly erode bone, producing pathologic fractures. Central nervous system involvement may produce epilepsy or blindness. Cardiac cysts can lead to conduction blocks, pericarditis, and ventricular rupture. Hydatid antigen has been shown by fluorescent antibody in the glomerulus and has been related to membranous glomerulonephritis. Many other sites can be involved including spleen, ovary, prostate, and thyroid.

The alveolar cyst of *E. multilocularis* usually presents as a slowly growing hepatic tumor, with a minority of patients having metastatic disease to lung, brain, or other tissues. The natural course is one of malignant growth with massive destruction of the liver and extension into vital structures. If untreated, the disease is fatal in 70 percent of cases, but there is considerable individual variation in the course of the disease.

Diagnosis   If a hydatid cyst ruptures or leaks fluid, an anaphylactoid reaction associated with eosinophilia and increased IgE levels may suggest the diagnosis. However, the clinical picture is usually not characteristic, and eosinophilia is seen in fewer than 25 percent of cases. Echinococciasis is most commonly discovered by routine x-ray. Pulmonary lesions usually are round, somewhat irregular masses of uniform density. They do not calcify. In contrast, hepatic cysts of *E. granulosus* show a smooth rim of calcification in about

50 percent of cases. Diffuse radiolucencies (2 to 4 mm) outlined by calcific densities may be seen in the liver with *E. multilocularis.* CT can be useful in demonstrating more details of the hydatid. In some cases of *E. granulosus,* simple, fluid-filled cysts indistinguishable from benign hepatic cysts are seen. In others, the findings of daughter cysts and hydatid sand strongly suggest echinococciasis. Thin eggshell calcification may indicate active disease. With alveolar hydatids, CT reveals indistinct solid masses, often with central necrosis, and plaque-like calcification. Ultrasound can also be helpful in distinguishing hydatid structure, and angiography may be necessary prior to surgical therapy.

Specific diagnosis is best accomplished by histologic examination. However, diagnostic aspiration should not be attempted because of potential anaphylactoid reactions to leakage of cyst fluid. Occasionally scolices may be found in sputum, stool, or urine and are best shown by Ziehl-Neelsen stain. The skin test (Casoni's test) is sensitive but gives 40 percent false-positive results. Serologic tests including indirect hemagglutination and latex agglutination are more useful if positive, but many cyst carriers will not develop an immune response. Indirect hemagglutination should be positive in 90 percent of patients with hepatic cysts but in only 50 to 60 percent of those with pulmonary hydatids. The presence of "arc 5" in the immunoelectrophoresis test provides the most specific serologic diagnosis of hydatid disease, and the adaptation of this technique to an enzyme-linked immunoelectro-diffusion assay may provide a more sensitive, rapid test. Following surgical removal of cysts, serologic tests may be helpful in screening for residual or recurrent disease. The Clq assay has also been employed for this purpose.

Treatment   Surgical treatment remains the standard therapy. Patients with small calcified hepatic cysts and pulmonary hydatids of the sylvatic type need to be operated on only if the cysts are symptomatic or enlarge dramatically over time. All others should have their cysts excised if possible, or sterilized and drained. With a large cyst, the contents should be sterilized with hypertonic saline before an attempt is made to open it. The entire endocyst should then be removed if possible, and all biliary or bronchial fistulas carefully closed. The residual space must be obliterated to prevent postoperative infection or prolonged drainage. Aspergillomas have been seen in residual cavities of pulmonary cysts.

Medical therapy with "high-dose" mebendazole (40 mg/kg per day) may be considered in patients with other medical problems that preclude surgery or in patients with extensive disease that makes surgical cure impossible. In selected patients, it may also be considered in conjunction with definitive surgery to reduce the risk of metastatic spread of viable organisms. In animal models, mebendazole is larvacidal for *E. granulosus* but not for *E. multilocularis.* In human trials, all forms of echinococciasis appear to respond to the agent, although the experience with *E. multilocularis* is limited. Significant side effects including neutropenia have been reported. At present, the agent should be used only with the patient's informed consent. The absorption is erratic and drug levels should be followed. The drug is contraindicated in pregnancy.

Prevention   The incidence of echinococciasis can be reduced by appropriate control measures as demonstrated in Iceland. Contact with infected dogs must be avoided, infected carcasses and offal should be burned or buried, and infected dogs should be treated.

REFERENCES

BEAVER PC et al: *Clinical Parasitology,* 9th ed. Philadelphia, Lea and Febiger, 1984

BENGER A et al: A human coenurus infection in Canada. Am J Trop Med Hyg 30:638, 1981

DE GHETALDI et al: Cerebral cysticercosis treated biphasically with dexamethasone and praziquantel. Ann Intern Med 99:179, 1983

GAMBLE WG et al: Alveolar hydatid disease in Minnesota: First human case acquired in the contiguous United States. JAMA 241:904, 1979

GHARBI HA et al: Ultrasound examination of the hydatidic liver. Radiology 139:459, 1981

GROLL E: Praziquantel for cestode infections in man. Acta Trop 37:293, 1980

JONES TC: Cestodes. Clin Gastroenterol 7:105, 1978

JONES WE: Niclosamide as a treatment for *Hymenolepis diminuta* and *Dipylidium caninum* infection in man. Am J Trop Med Hyg 28:300, 1979

KATZ R et al: Pulmonary echinococcosis: A pediatric disease of the southwestern United States. Pediatrics 65:1003, 1980

LOO L, BRAUDE A: Cerebral cysticercosis in San Diego. A report of 23 cases and a review of the literature. Medicine 61:341, 1982

MOHAMMED IN et al: Enzyme-linked immunosorbent assay for the diagnosis of cerebral cysticercosis. J Clin Microbiol 20:775, 1984

NASH TE, NEVA FA: Recent advances in the diagnosis and treatment of cerebral cysticercosis. N Engl J Med 311:1492, 1984

PINON JM et al: Immunological study of hydatidosis. Am J Trop Med Hyg 28:318, 1979

PORAT S, JOSEPH KN: Hydatid disease of bone. Israel J Med Sci 14:223, 1978

TAYLOR RL: Sparganosis in the United States. Report of a case. Am J Clin Pathol 66:560, 1976

WERCZBERGER A et al: Disseminated echinococcosis with repeated anaphylactic shock treated with mebendazole. Chest 76:482, 1979

WILSON JF et al: Cystic hydatid disease in Alaska. Am Rev Resp Dis 98:1, 1968

———, RAUSCH RL: Alveolar hydatid disease. A review of clinical features of 33 indigenous cases of *E. multilocularis* infection in Alaskan Eskimos. Am J Trop Med Hyg 29:1340, 1980

XANTHAKIS D et al: Hydatid disease of the chest. Report of 91 cases surgically treated. Thorax 27:517, 1972

section 10 Disorders caused by environmental agents

169 SCABIES, CHIGGERS, AND OTHER ECTOPARASITES

JAMES J. PLORDE

SCABIES Scabies is a cosmopolitan skin infection commonly referred to as the "seven-year itch." It is caused by a burrowing mite, *Sarcoptes scabiei* var. *hominis,* and is transmitted from person to person by close bodily contact, particularly among family members and bed partners. Although the disease is more common in the poor and unclean, sporadic cases involve individuals of all socioeconomic groups. Children under 15 years of age have the highest prevalence of scabies and are usually the first members of families to contract the disease. Those who spend nights with friends or exchange clothing with others are at increased risk. Institutional outbreaks in hospitals, nursing homes, mental institutions, and aboard naval vessels have been reported. There has been a worldwide resurgence of this infection over the past 20 years, and in the United States it currently involves 2 to 4 percent of patients seen in dermatologists' offices.

The turtle-shaped female measures 0.4 mm in length and possesses four pairs of legs. With the help of the two anterior pairs and her mouth, she burrows into the superficial layer of the epidermis. Here she deposits two or three enormous eggs daily until she dies 30 to 60 days later. The newly hatched larvae mature to adulthood on the skin surface within 2 weeks to continue the cycle of infection. Although an involved person may harbor thousands or occasionally millions of adult mites, the average number of adult females per infection is 11.

Two-thirds of the burrows are found in the upper extremities, particularly on the interdigital spaces of the hands and the flexor surface of the wrists. In heavy infections, other sites are typically involved. These include the dorsal surfaces of the elbows, anterior axillary folds, female breasts, periumbilical area, penis, scrotum, and buttocks. In bedridden patients, lesions are often concentrated over pressure points. The face, head, palms, and soles are seldom involved in adults; in infants, any area of the skin can be involved. Characteristically, a burrow appears as a short dark wavy line which may end in a small vesicle, the site of the adult female.

Sensitization (type IV) to the mites and their products begins approximately 1 month after infection and results in a papular or eczematous reaction at the sites of involvement. Itching is often severe and tends to be more marked at night or after a hot bath. Scratching frequently leads to secondary infection with pustulation; acute glomerulonephritis has followed infection with nephritogenic strains of streptococci. Occasionally, reddish pruritic nodules are seen in the groin and axillary regions. Infected individuals with good personal hygiene usually have few lesions, and burrows may be difficult to identify. In mentally retarded, debilitated, or immunosuppressed patients, a particularly virulent infection known as *Norwegian scabies* is sometimes seen. Millions of mites may be present, producing a highly infectious exfoliative dermatitis; itching is often mild or absent. Scabies usually terminates spontaneously in a few months, but chronic cases do occur.

The diagnosis should be considered in any patient presenting with a pruritic eruption, particularly if it involves several members of a living group. The occurrence of symmetric lesions at the sites of predilection should initiate a search for the characteristic burrows. These should be vigorously scraped with a sterile needle or scalpel blade, and the scrapings transferred to a drop of 10% potassium hydroxide on a glass slide. A coverslip is placed over the top, and the preparation examined for adults, larvae, and eggs. The diagnosis can also be made on histologic sections prepared from a punch biopsy. Considering the mode of disease transmission, adults shown to have scabies should also be checked for venereal disease.

All sexual contacts and household members should be treated simultaneously with the patient to prevent the occurrence of "ping-pong infections." The therapeutic agents are applied topically, covering the skin thinly but completely from the neck down. Although the patient is rendered noninfectious within 24 h, up to 2 months may be required for the clinical manifestations of the disease to disappear completely. Needless retreatment during this period can lead to contact dermatitis. Bed linen and clothes used by the patient the day prior to therapy should be washed in hot water.

A number of effective agents are available for use. Gamma benzene hexachloride (Gamene, Kwell) is left on for 12 h and then thoroughly washed off. Care must be taken to keep it away from eyes and mucous membranes. It should not be used in infants or pregnant adults. Benzyl benzoate (25%) is administered in a similar fashion. Crotamiton (Eurax) is massaged into the skin, and a second dose applied 24 h later. Antihistamines or salicylates are helpful in counteracting pruritus. Topical steroids may potentiate the infection and should not be used. Antibiotics are required occasionally when there is a significant bacterial superinfection.

CHIGGER MITES The term *chigger* is used to refer to larvae of harvest mites belonging to the family Trombiculidae. The cosmopolitan adults feed on vegetable matter and deposit their eggs upon the ground. The tiny (0.4 mm) emergent larvae crawl along the ground and upward onto vegetation. Here, they await the passage of a vertebrate host, upon which they must feed before again dropping to the ground and molting. In humans, the chigger usually attaches about the ankles, but some advance along the skin until they are stopped by tight-fitting clothing. It then pierces the skin, releases a digestant to liquefy tissue cells, and feeds for 3 or 4 days. Within a few hours, the chigger's secretions have produced an intensely pruritic papule 0.5 to 2 cm in diameter. This usually vesiculates, resulting in a chickenpox-like lesion. Occasionally, subcutaneous bleeding results in a surrounding area of ecchymosis. The lesion and itching may persist for several weeks. In the United States, most clinical cases are seen during the summer months; in warm climates, the seasonal pattern is missing. Treatment is directed at the relief of itching and the prevention of secondary infections. Insect repellants are highly effective prophylactic agents.

FLEAS Fleas are small wingless laterally compressed ectoparasites of humans and other warm-blooded animals. They tend to be found on the hairy portions of the host where they feed and deposit their eggs. The active larvae which hatch in 3 days can be found on the host, in its nest, or in dust. They eventually pupate and may remain dormant for weeks or months before completing their development to adults.

Medically, fleas serve as both vectors and agents of disease. Rodent fleas of the genus *Xenopsylla* are the most important. They are responsible for the transmission of both plague (*Yersinia pestis*) and murine typhus (*Rickettsia mooseri*) from animal reservoirs to humans. Humans may also acquire the rat tapeworm *Hymenolepis diminuta* by swallowing fleas containing the cysticeroid. The dog tapeworm *Dipylidium caninum* may be transmitted in a similar fashion. The bites of these and other species of fleas belonging to the family Pulicidae can induce an irritating dermatitis. In addition, the tungidae (*Tunga penetrans*) may burrow into the subcutaneous tissues, producing a painful and debilitating disease.

Flea dermatitis The fleas of humans (*Pulex irritans*), cats and dogs (*Cetenocephalides*), and rodents (*Xenopsylla*) may all induce dermatitis. In many individuals, the bites seem completely innocuous, but in sensitive persons, the saliva induces an erythematous raised pruritic papule. Repeated scratching may result in secondary infection with pustulation or ulceration. The intense pruritus, the ability of the flea to escape capture by virtue of its prodigious jumping ability, and the difficulty involved in crushing their hard chitinous bodies has led to many a frustrating nocturnal safari dedicated to the destruction of this unwanted bed partner. Control is effected by the use of frequent vacuuming to remove eggs, larvae, pupae, and adults from the environment. Insecticide sprays are also of help, but fleas have developed resistance to many of these. Dogs and cats should be washed, flea collars should be applied, and kennels should be dusted or sprayed with DDT or malathion. If rat runs can be located, they should also be dusted.

Tunga penetrans, sometimes referred to as a *jigger* or *chigoe flea*, is a burrowing flea found in the tropical areas of South America and Africa. These small (1 mm) free-living insects reside in sandy soil. The fertilized female burrows into the skin of the first warm-blooded animal encountered. In humans, they usually embed on the sole of the foot or under a toenail with only their anal pore exposed to the outside. Multiple infections are common. As the female becomes engorged with blood and eggs, a painful and pruritic pea-sized swelling is produced. Eventually, the overlying skin ulcerates, the flea dies, and the eggs are extruded. Secondary bacterial infections including tetanus and gas gangrene occur commonly. Autoamputation of the toes has been reported from Africa. The intact flea can usually be extracted by gently enlarging the entrance hole with a sterile needle and then applying pressure from the side. Alternatively, the lesion can be soaked in Lysol, the flea penetrated with a needle, and the lesion resoaked to kill the eggs and sterilize the wound. Antibiotics may be required to treat secondary bacterial infections.

PEDICULOSIS Lice are obligate human ectoparasites that complete their entire 30- to 40-day life cycle on the body of the host. *Pediculus humanus* var. *capitis* infests the head, *P. humanus* var. *corporis* the

body and clothing, and *Phthirius pubis* (crab lice) the genital and occasionally other hairy areas of the body. All three are flattened dorsoventrally and measure 2 to 3 mm in length. The crab louse is broader and flatter than *Pediculus* and possesses powerful claws on its second and third legs with which it clings to the pubic hair. The females lay five or six eggs daily which they firmly attach to the hairs or, in the case of the body louse, the clothing of the host. These clearly visible tiny white nits hatch in 8 to 10 days. The resulting nymph matures to adulthood in an additional 2 weeks. Both the larvae and adults take two blood meals daily, leaving behind a small purpuric puncture site. With repeated exposure, the host develops an inflammatory hypersensitivity reaction manifested as a small red papule at each new feeding site. Pruritus results in scratching, a weeping dermatitis, and secondary infection. Chronic infections of the scalp may result in a fetid mass of matted hair and exudate. On the body and genital areas, the lesions may become pigmented—so-called vagabond disease. Heavy infections with *P. pubis* may involve the eyebrows and eyelids leading to blepharitis.

Lice can be transferred from person to person by direct contact or via discarded clothing in which the body louse can survive for up to a week. Migration is stimulated by fever, making *P. humanus* var. *corporis* an efficient vector of relapsing fever (*Borrelia recurrentis*), typhus (*R. prowazekii*), and trench fever (*R. quintana*). *Phthirius pubis* is not known to be a vector of human disease.

Pediculosis corporis is typically seen in the poor and transient who are unable to maintain even minimal levels of personal hygiene. In contrast, head and pubic lice are found on patients of all socioeconomic classes and are currently enjoying a resurgence in the United States. *P. capitis* most frequently infests white schoolchildren; blacks are seldom involved. Pubic lice are more common among the sexually active; their presence should stimulate a search for venereal disease.

The diagnosis is suggested by the typical dermatitis and confirmed by finding the adults or nits on the hair or clothing of the patient. Treatment may be carried out with pyrethrins with piperonyl butoxide (RID) or 1% gamma benzene hexachloride (lindane, Kwell). The latter agent may be absorbed through the skin, resulting in central nervous system toxicity if inappropriately applied. It should not be used in infants and pregnant women. In head infections, the hair should first be shampooed with ordinary soap. RID is then rubbed in for at least 10 min (Kwell shampoo, 4 min), the hair is rinsed, dried, and combed with a fine-tooth comb to remove the nits. The process should be repeated in 7 days. Combs and brushes should be heated in water to 65°C for 5 min or soaked in 2% Lysol. The clothing and bedding of the patient with body lice are heat-sterilized. The patient's body should be lathered for 10 min with RID or 4 min with Kwell and then rinsed thoroughly. The therapy may be repeated in 7 days. In crab louse infestations, RID or Kwell cream or lotion should be used on the involved areas and left for 24 h. In hirsute individuals, the treatment can be repeated in 1 week. If the eyelashes are involved, 0.25% physostigmine ophthalmic ointment is applied twice daily for 10 days. Lice and nits are carefully removed with a cotton-tipped applicator. Narrow-angle glaucoma should be ruled out before the physostigmine is used.

MYIASIS Infections with maggots or fly larvae are seen worldwide in a variety of animals. Human involvement occurs most frequently where people live in close contact with domestic animals. Many different species of flies are involved. In some, an animal host is required for larval development; in these, the larvae are capable of invading normal tissue or enter the body through the nose, mouth, or ears. Others are opportunists, depositing their eggs or larvae in the open wounds of debilitated patients. The clinical manifestations vary with the species of fly and site of involvement. Four of the more common clinical syndromes are described below.

Localized cutaneous myiasis In tropical America the lesions are produced by *Dermatobia hominis*, the human botfly. This remarkable forest-dwelling Diptera captures a mosquito or other blood-feeding insect on which to deposit its packet of eggs. When this unwilling vector then lands on a warm-blooded animal to feed, the eggs hatch and penetrate the feeding site. Within the skin of the host, the larva develops for 2 or 3 months. Finally, it emerges, drops to the ground, and pupates. The lesions are most frequently seen on unprotected areas of the body including the hands, feet, head, and neck. During the first week of infection, the pruritic lesion closely resembles a mosquito bite. As the larva grows and begins to move, it produces severe pain and itching. Tissue destruction and inflammation results in the development of a furuncle-like lesion. Generally, a central opening is present through which the posterior end of the larva protrudes. A dark serosanguinous discharge containing the feces of the insect may be noted.

In Africa, a similar lesion is produced by *Cordylobia anthropophaga* (tumbu fly). These flies deposit their eggs on sandy soil or laundry laid out to dry. The larvae hatch and invade the unbroken skin of humans or wild rodents, where they mature in 8 or 9 days. In either case, the larvae can be surgically extracted without difficulty. In tumbu fly infections, letting the larvae mature and drop off spontaneously may be appropriate. This process can occasionally be hastened by applying mineral oil to the central opening. This results in the suffocation of the larva and stimulates its early exodus.

Cutanea larva migrans This is usually caused by the large (1 to 2 cm) horse botflies belonging to the genus *Gasterophilus*. When the larvae hatch on the skin, they penetrate to the lower epidermis. Because they do not mature in humans, they may migrate in the skin for several months. Clinically, the infection presents as a pruritic serpiginous band of erythema closely resembling cutanea larva migrans produced by *Ancylostoma braziliense*. The diagnosis can be made by placing a small drop of mineral oil on the skin just in advance of the worm tract. This allows visualization of black backward-directed spines on its body segments. The parasite can be easily removed with a sharp needle. Occasionally, the larvae may penetrate the eye. A similar clinical picture is sometimes produced by the larvae of *Hypoderma* spp. (cattle botfly). These, however, often penetrate deeply into the subcutaneous tissue and produce more pain and less pruritus than *Gasterophilus* larvae.

Deep-tissue myiasis Screwflies of several genera can deposit large batches of eggs on unbroken skin or in wounds, ears, or the nose. After hatching, the larvae burrow into the tissues and develop for 2 or 3 weeks. The mature 1- to 2-cm larvae then drop to the ground and pupate. At times, they penetrate deep tissues, including the eye, nasal sinuses, and cranium, where they produce destructive foul-smelling lesions. Bacterial superinfection is common. In India and Africa, the flies are usually of genus *Chrysomyia*. In the western hemisphere, *Callitroga* spp. are involved. The occurrence of human cases in the United States often accompanies epizootics of screwworm activity. Flesh flies of the family Sarcophagidae have also been implicated in deep-tissue myiasis both in the United States and elsewhere. In all the above infections, the lesions should be surgically incised and debrided, the larvae removed, and secondary infections treated.

Intestinal myiasis When humans ingest food contaminated with the eggs or larvae of several genera of flies, some survive passage through the stomach and later mature in the intestine before they are extruded in the stool. In the United States, *Tubifera tenax* is the most frequently implicated species. Invasion of the intestinal mucosa may occur with *Sarcophaga* infections.

REFERENCES

BARKIN JS: Intestinal myiasis. Am J Gastroenterol 78:560, 1983

BURKHART CG: Scabies: An epidemiologic reassessment. Ann Intern Med 98:498, 1983

Drugs for parasitic infections. Med Lett 26:27, 1984

LEIBOWITZ M et al: Keratotic scabies (Norwegian scabies): Case reports and literature review. S Afr Med J 57:363, 1980

MAGNARELLI LA, ANDREADIS TG: Human cases of furuncular, traumatic and nasal myiasis in Connecticut. Am J Trop Med Hyg 30:894, 1981

STRICKLAND GT: Hunter's Tropical Medicine, 6th ed. Philadelphia, Saunders, 1984

170 DISORDERS CAUSED BY VENOMS, BITES, AND STINGS

JAMES F. WALLACE

Humans have the propensity to come into contact with a great variety of venomous animals. These contacts occur with many zoologic classes including snakes, lizards, sea animals, spiders, scorpions, and numerous species of insects. In general two types of injuries result: those due to the direct effect of venom on the victim, as exemplified in snakebite, and those due to indirect effects of the poison, of which hypersensitivity reaction to bee stings is an example. Each year in the United States at least 50 persons die as the result of venomous injuries. Three groups of animals—hymenopterous insects, snakes, and spiders—account for over 90 percent of the fatalities. Of even greater public health significance is the loss in economic productivity and human potential resulting from the many serious, nonfatal envenomations which occur annually in otherwise healthy children or working adults.

SNAKE BITE Epidemiology Fewer than one-tenth of the nearly 3500 known species of snakes are venomous. These poisonous varieties belong to five families or subfamilies: Elapidae (cobras, kraits, mambas, and coral snakes) found in all parts of the world except Europe; Viperidae (true vipers) found in all parts of the world except the Americas; Hydrophidae (sea snakes); Crotalidae (pit vipers) found in Asia and the Americas; and Colubridae (boomslangs, bird snakes) of the African continent. The poisonous varieties of the United States, with the single exception of the coral snake, are pit vipers and include rattlesnakes, the water moccasin, and the copperhead. Although this discussion centers around these species, most of the therapeutic measures outlined are applicable to snakes in all parts of the world.

The number of individuals bitten by poisonous snakes in the United States is estimated to be about 8000 per year, with a relatively large number occurring in the southeastern and Gulf states, particularly Texas. Deaths are not reported separately but are undoubtedly rare, numbering fewer than 20 per year, and most are due to bites of various species of rattlesnake. In many European countries deaths from snakebite have averaged only one every 3 to 5 years for the last half-century. In contrast, the estimate of annual deaths from snakebite throughout the world is between 30,000 and 40,000 with the largest number occurring in the countries of Burma and Brazil, where 2000 deaths are estimated to occur each year.

Etiology The *coral snake* is found in the southern states from Florida to Arizona. It is usually marked by alternating red and black bands separated by yellow rings; however, black and albino forms exist. Coral snakes are generally nocturnal in their activities, shy and elusive, and rarely bite humans. Their fangs are short and permanently erect; the highly toxic venom is injected into multiple puncture wounds produced by a series of chewing movements.

The *pit vipers* are so named because of a small pit between the eye and the nostril. Large venom glands in the temporal regions give the head a triangular appearance. They are generally aggressive and likely to strike if disturbed. The fangs are long and hinged, folding posteriorly when the mouth is closed. Pit vipers strike suddenly with a forward thrust of the head. The instant that the erect fangs make contact, venom is expressed by sudden muscular contraction.

The *rattlesnakes,* recognized by the horny rattle on the tail, which buzzes when the snake is disturbed, are widely distributed. The diamondbacks (*Crotalus adamanteus* in the southeast and *C. atrox* in the southwest) are the largest and most dangerous snakes in this country. Others include the prairie rattler (*C. confluentus*), the timber rattler (*C. horridus*), and the pigmy rattlers.

The *water moccasin,* or cottonmouth (*Agkistrodon piscivorus*), is found in swampy areas or along the banks of streams. It is a strong swimmer and can bite under water. This snake is notorious for inflicting severe facial bites when disturbed in the branches of small trees. The copperhead, or highland moccasin (*A. mokasen*), is a closely related species. Its bite is painful but rarely fatal.

Pathogenesis SNAKE VENOMS The venoms of most species which have been analyzed have been found to be mixtures of several toxic proteins and enzymes with diversified and complicated pharmacologic effects. As an example, the venom of the Indian cobra (*Naja naja*) contains these distinct and separate substances: a neurotoxin, a hemolysin, a cardiotoxin, a cholinesterase, at least three phosphatases, a nucleotidase, and a potent inhibitor of cytochrome oxidase. Several venoms, including those of the pit vipers, contain hyaluronidase and numerous proteolytic enzymes. Although the exact roles of these components in toxicity are incompletely understood, the venom of a given species is usually predominantly neurotoxic or necrotizing and is frequently associated with hemolysis, abnormalities of blood coagulation, changes in cardiac dynamics, and alterations in vascular resistance. Venoms of elapids, including the coral snake, are neurotoxic, with death resulting from respiratory paralysis probably caused by damage to brain centers and a curariform interference with transmission at the neuromuscular junction. Venoms of crotalid snakes produce local tissue injury, hemorrhage, and hemolysis. Death is often preceded by circulatory collapse associated with a marked fall in circulating blood volume resulting from pooling of blood in the microcirculation, and loss of plasma due to increased capillary permeability. Systemic absorption of venom occurs through the lymphatics, and therapeutic measures designed to reduce lymphatic function are helpful in controlling symptoms.

FACTORS AFFECTING SEVERITY OF SNAKE BITE Several factors affect the outcome of snake bite:

1 The age, size, and health of the patient. Envenomation in children is usually serious, and a fatal outcome is more likely, since a relatively large dose of poison is injected into a small victim.
2 Location of bite. Bites on extremities or into adipose tissue are less dangerous than those on the trunk, face, or directly into a blood vessel. A direct strike of the fangs is more dangerous than a scratch, a glancing blow, or one hitting a bone. The discharge orifice of a fang is well above its tip so that the point of the fang can penetrate the skin without envenomation; even a thin layer of clothing may afford great protection. Because of the superficial nature of the wound as many as one-fifth of patients bitten by venomous snakes will have no evidence of envenomation, even though the fangs have penetrated the skin.
3 The size of the snake (a large pit viper can inject over 1000 mg venom, six times a lethal dose for an adult), the extent of its anger or fear (if hurt it may inject a larger amount of venom), the condition of the fangs (broken or recently renewed), and the condition of the venom glands (recently discharged or full). All these factors are important. Contrary to popular belief, the bite of a snake which has recently killed and fed is not necessarily less venomous for humans; the snake usually does not exhaust its venom in a single bite.
4 The presence of various bacteria, particularly clostridia and other anaerobic organisms, in the mouth of the snake or on the skin of the victim. This may lead to serious infection in the necrotic tissues at the local site.
5 Exercise or exertion, such as running, immediately after the bite. This speeds systemic absorption of toxin.

Manifestations Following the bite of a pit viper, severe burning pain develops within a few minutes at the site of the wound. Local swelling rapidly develops and spreads in all directions, accompanied by the appearance of ecchymoses and bullae over the involved area. As the edema spreads, serosanguinous fluid oozes from the puncture wounds. Later gangrene of the skin and subcutaneous tissues may develop. Systemic effects resulting from the absorption of venom and local tissue destruction may include fever, nausea and vomiting,

circulatory collapse, bleeding into the skin and from all body orifices, low-grade jaundice, neuropathic muscle cramping, pupillary constriction, disorientation, delirium, and convulsions. Death may occur after 6 to 48 h. Survival may be attended by massive local tissue loss from gangrene or secondary infection, or may be complicated by acute renal failure, secondary to disseminated intravascular clotting and cortical necrosis, or by tubular necrosis following circulatory collapse.

The bite of the coral snake causes little pain and local swelling. There are usually multiple fang marks. Within 10 to 15 min numbness and weakness begin in the region of the bite, followed by ataxia, ptosis, pupillary dilatation, palatal and pharyngeal paralysis, slurring of speech, salivation, and occasionally nausea and vomiting. The patient becomes comatose, develops respiratory paralysis and seizures, and dies within 8 to 72 h.

Cobra bites are painful and are often accompanied by severe hemolysis, local necrosis, and sloughing in addition to their neurotoxic effects. There is little pain and no edema at the site of a sea snake bite. Symptoms of systemic envenomation follow a latent period which may vary from 15 min to 8 h. Although the venom is both myotoxic and neurotoxic, the injury to skeletal muscle is most prominent and is characterized by generalized muscle pain, weakness, and myoglobinuria. Hemorrhagic manifestations predominate following envenomation by colubrids (boomslangs and bird snakes) and many pit vipers including certain species of rattlesnake.

Laboratory abnormalities In severe cases, laboratory abnormalities may include progressive anemia, polymorphonuclear leukocytosis of 20,000 to 30,000 cells per cubic millimeter, thrombocytopenia, hypofibrinogenemia, disordered tests of coagulation, proteinuria, and azotemia.

Treatment An attempt should be made to determine with certainty that the patient has been bitten by a poisonous snake. Absence of distinct fang punctures and failure of local pain, edema, numbness, or weakness to appear within 20 min are strong evidence against snake venom poisoning. If the species of snake is not known, the offending reptile should be killed for the purpose of identification.

FIRST AID This consists of reassuring and calming the victim, instituting measures to retard the absorption of venom and to remove it from the tissues as quickly as possible after the bite, and arranging for transportation to the nearest hospital. The patient should be promptly placed at rest and the bitten extremity immobilized to reduce the rate of spread of the venom. If anatomically feasible, a wide constriction band should be placed a few centimeters above the bite and made tight enough to allow one finger to pass beneath with difficulty. The purpose is to impede lymph flow; it is not necessary to obstruct venous return. The band should be loosened and moved proximally when local swelling causes it to tighten. If the victim is more than 30 min from the hospital and is seen within 5 min following the bite, incision and suction of the wound should be started prior to evacuation. By use of whatever antisepsis is available, 1.0-cm *linear* (not cruciate) incisions about 0.3-cm deep should be carefully made through each fang mark and suction applied. A rubber bulb, breast pump, or heated jar are all preferable to mouth suction, but if other means are not available and no oral lesions are present, this method may be employed. Suction should be continued for up to 1 h following the bite, or until antivenin has been administered. The practice of making multiple incisions along the advancing edge of edema as swelling progresses has not been found to be beneficial and is no longer advised. *Incision and suction are extremely important and should be diligently carried out.* When begun promptly, they may result in the removal of up to 50 percent of subcutaneously injected venom.

While the patient is being transported to a hospital, immobilization of the affected part is important in controlling lymph flow. This is best achieved by splinting. Although ice packs relieve pain and slow lymphatic drainage, they do not neutralize venom, and even a small amount of cooling may result in irreparable damage to already injured tissues by causing ischemia. For this reason, it is recommended that no form of cryotherapy be used.

IMMEDIATE HOSPITAL CARE This should include appropriate treatment for shock and respiratory difficulty, antivenin, measures to combat infection, and general supportive care. Initial laboratory studies in a patient with obvious crotalid envenomation should include blood typing and cross-matching, a complete blood count, urinalysis, coagulation screening tests, blood urea nitrogen (BUN), blood glucose, and serum electrolytes. In severe envenomations it is also advisable to obtain an electrocardiogram. None of these tests are particularly helpful in the initial evaluation of a patient with a coral snake bite.

Antivenin is the only specific treatment of snake venom poisoning, and its use in severe bites is vital. In the United States polyvalent crotaline antivenin effective against all American pit vipers and antivenin for North American coral snake poisoning are commercially available. Both products are a lyophilized powder of refined horse serum. Kits are available containing antivenin powder (reconstituted by diluting with water to 10 mL per vial), syringe, normal horse serum for prior sensitivity testing of the patient, and detailed instructions. Intravenously administered antivenin leads to the most rapid and effective response. It is not advisable to infiltrate antivenin at the local site. The initial dose should depend upon an estimate of the amount of envenomation. For pit viper bites accompanied by progressive local swelling but no systemic symptoms (minimal envenomation), 5 vials (50 mL) are usually sufficient. When swelling has progressed beyond the site of the bite, and mild systemic symptoms and/or hematologic and coagulation abnormalities are present, moderate envenomation has occurred, and initial treatment should be 5 to 10 vials (50 to 100 mL). For severe poisonings, associated with rapidly progressive and extensive local effects as well as systemic symptoms and evidence of hemolysis or coagulopathy, 10 to 20 vials (100 to 200 mL) or more should be administered. Up to 50 percent greater doses of antivenin should be given to children or small adults to neutralize the relatively higher venom concentrations. Reconstituted antivenin is diluted in 500 mL of intravenous fluid and administered as rapidly as tolerated over 1 to 2 h. Additional infusions containing 5 to 10 vials (50 to 100 mL) should be repeated hourly until progressive swelling in the bitten part ceases and systemic signs and symptoms have disappeared. When an adequate dose has been achieved, improvement in the victim's clinical signs is often extremely rapid.

If *any* evidence of envenomation appears during the first several hours following a coral snake bite, antivenin should be given without waiting for systemic manifestations to develop. Three vials of antivenin should be given intravenously for bites associated only with minimal swelling and/or local paresthesias. If evidence of a bite is more definitive, particularly if there was initial pain, 5 vials of antivenin should be given as soon as possible.

In the patient with severe envenomation who is allergic to horse serum, the relative risks of death from anaphylaxis rather than from venom poisoning should be carefully weighed before undertaking desensitization with small doses of diluted horse serum.

No antivenin for other snakes is manufactured in the United States, but antiserum for various types is usually kept on hand at large zoos all over the world. A national antivenin index is maintained by the Oklahoma Poison Information Center in cooperation with the Oklahoma City Zoo [(405) 271-5454], and provides 24-h telephone consultation service for physicians needing advice in handling snakebite accidents.

Maintaining *respiration* by mechanical or other means is important. In patients bitten by elapid snakes, respiratory failure is usually reversible. *Tetanus toxoid* or *tetanus immune globulin* of human origin should be given. If wound infections appear, antibiotics should be used with the knowledge that the predominant microorganisms in the mouths of snakes are gram-negative pathogens. Treatment should

be preceded by appropriate aerobic and anaerobic cultures. *Fasciotomy* occasionally may be necessary to prevent further ischemic injury to a massively swollen limb. Whenever possible, intracompartmental tissue pressures should be monitored, with surgical decompression undertaken only if pressure exceeds 30 to 40 mmHg. *Surgical debridement* of vesicles and superficial necrotic tissue should be instituted near the end of the first week following the bite. *Relief of pain* with salicylates or meperidine, moderate sedation, maintenance of fluid balance, measures to combat shock and hemorrhagic diathesis, and appropriate management of coma or convulsions are all important.

The usefulness of corticosteroids to prevent tissue damage or systemic intoxication has not been convincingly demonstrated. However, these drugs may be of value in the management of severe shock associated with envenomation and for allergic reactions, particularly serum sickness, following the administration of antivenin.

Prevention In snake-infested regions long trousers, high shoes, boots, or leggings, and gloves should be worn. Most important of all is to look where one steps or reaches. A sharp knife or lancet, constriction band, suction bulb, and antiseptic suffice for an emergency kit, and in inaccessible areas, antivenin should also be carried.

POISONOUS LIZARD BITE Of the nearly 3000 species of lizard in the world, only two are venomous: the Gila monster (*Heloderma suspectum*) of the arid southwestern United States and the closely related Mexican beaded lizard (*H. horridum*) which inhabits the lowland forests of western Mexico. These reptiles are not aggressive, and virtually every instance of their attacking a human has involved teasing or handling the animals in captivity. The venom is elaborated in eight glands in the floor of the mouth and secreted directly into the oral cavity, where it bathes the teeth, which are grooved posteriorly. The lizard clings tenaciously and is often dislodged only after considerable effort; envenomation occurs by contamination of the wound. The venom contains a potent neurotoxin which is undoubtedly responsible for its lethal effect on experimental animals. Death in humans following a bite is extremely rare. Most often, human envenomation results in tissue injury, excruciating pain, massive edema, and patchy erythema. Acute systemic symptoms may last for 3 to 4 days and include nausea, vomiting, hematemesis, blurred vision, dyspnea, dysphonia, and profound weakness. Intense hyperesthesia of the bitten extremity may persist for several weeks. There is no antivenin available. Treatment should consist of constriction band, incision, suction, cooling of the bitten area, measures to prevent or combat infection, including tetanus, and supportive measures. Parenteral meperidine (Demerol) or infiltration of local anesthetic around the bite may be necessary to relieve pain.

SPIDER BITES The bite of many spiders is locally irritating, and several species can cause severe, even fatal systemic poisoning in humans. In North America, only two types of spiders are of medical importance: the widow spiders (*Latrodectus* species) and the recluse spiders (*Loxosceles* species).

Widow spider bite The most numerous and important of the venomous spiders are members of the genus *Latrodectus*, widely distributed throughout the world. In the United States and Canada, *L. mactans*, the black widow or show-button spider, causes a majority of clinically significant arachnidism. In Florida, *L. bishopi*, the red-legged widow spider, has been reported to produce human poisoning resembling mild black widow bite.

It is the female *L. mactans*, the black widow, that bites humans. She is glossy black with a body 1 cm in diameter, a leg span of 5 cm, and a characteristic red hourglass mark on her abdomen. She spins her web in woodpiles, sheds, basements, or outdoor privies, is very aggressive, and will bite on slight provocation. The venom produces diffuse central and peripheral nervous excitement, autonomic activity, muscle spasm, hypertension, and vasoconstriction.

In the United States, most black widow bites occur between April and October, and many patients are males bitten on the genitalia or buttocks while using a privy. After a momentary sharp pain at the site, there is cramping pain that begins locally within 15 to 60 min and gradually spreads. It may involve all extremities and the trunk. The abdomen is boardlike, and the waves of pain become excruciating, causing the patient to turn, toss, and cry out. Respirations are often labored and grunting. There are also nausea, vomiting, headache, sweating, salivation, hyperactive reflexes, twitching, tremor, paresthesias of the hands and feet, and occasionally, systolic hypertension. A mild polymorphonuclear leukocytosis is usual, and many patients have slight fever. After several hours, the pains subside, although mild recurrences for 2 or 3 days are common. It may be a week before well-being is restored. Deaths due to cardiac or respiratory failure have occurred, mostly in children and the aged.

Because the bite itself is not prominent, patients are often thought to have some abdominal catastrophe such as perforated ulcer, pancreatitis, or appendicitis. Renal colic, myocardial infarction, tetanus, strychnine poisoning, tabetic crisis, lead colic, and porphyria are other conditions to be ruled out. The abdomen is not tender to palpation in arachnidism, and pains in the extremities are not typical of most of these other disorders.

Treatment For *Latrodectus* poisoning, treatment consists of measures to relieve pain and administration of antivenin. Initial treatment should include a hot tub bath which affords prompt, although temporary, relief. A vial (10 mL) of 10% calcium gluconate slowly injected intravenously over 10 to 20 min usually produces dramatic, but transient, cessation of cramps. A solution of 10% methocarbamol administered intravenously also may be effective in treatment of muscle spasms. Opiates are sometimes necessary. When symptoms are severe or when the patient is a small child or is at special risk due to other associated medical problems, treatment with *Latrodectus* antivenin is indicated. An intravenous injection of 1 vial (2.5 mL) diluted in 50 mL of saline and administered over a 15-min period is usually quite effective within a few hours and can be repeated if symptoms recur. Since the antivenin is prepared from horse serum, appropriate testing for hypersensitivity should be undertaken prior to its administration.

***Loxosceles* spider bite** During the past 30 years in the United States, there have been increasing numbers of reports of severe necrotizing bites due to *Loxosceles* spiders. Originally thought to be a problem only in the midwestern states and associated only with the brown recluse spider, necrotic arachnidism has now been seen in many of the southern and southwestern states as well as in California and has been attributed to at least six species of *Loxosceles* spider. The bite of these spiders may initially produce only a mild stinging discomfort. In severe bites, intense local pain appears within 2 to 8 h, accompanied by bullae formation and erythema at the site of the wound. Subsequently, ischemic necrosis occurs leaving a deep ulcer with a necrotic base. The pathogenetic mechanism for the local reaction is not completely understood but is thought to involve complement-activated tissue damage. Some patients also experience a systemic reaction characterized by fever, myalgias, and a morbilliform rash 24 to 48 h after the bite. Intravascular hemolysis is seen occasionally, and in severe cases hemoglobinuria and acute renal failure may occur. Fatalities have been reported, mostly in children.

Treatment depends upon the severity of the bite. If bullae formation, intense pain, and signs of rapidly progressing ischemic necrosis do not appear within the first 6 to 8 h, the bite is probably not severe and treatment is unnecessary. When symptoms of more serious local reaction are present, the parenteral use of corticosteroids within the first 24 h following a bite has been advocated to prevent progression of the lesion, but convincing evidence that this is effective is lacking. Dapsone has been reported to prevent extensive ulceration in rapidly progressing *Loxosceles* spider bites. However, use of the drug in this setting should be considered experimental. Other therapeutic measures consist mainly of local wound care, timely surgical debridement, and treatment of secondary infection, if it occurs. The ulcer usually heals spontaneously, although skin grafting may be

required on occasion. Patients with systemic loxoscelism should be hospitalized and monitored closely for signs of hemolysis, disseminated intravascular coagulation and acute renal failure. Although of unproven efficacy, systemic corticosteroids are usually given for the duration of the acute phase of the illness, which lasts 2 to 4 days. Renal failure should be treated as advised in Chap. 219.

SCORPION STING Scorpions are eight-legged arthropods. Glands in the terminal segment produce venom, which is injected into the victim by a stinger located on the tip of the tail. Scorpions often enter dwellings. During the day they retreat into crevices; emerging at night, they often get into shoes and clothing and even into bedding. They do not deliberately attack humans, but accidental contact results in a sting.

Of about 650 species, roughly 40 occur in the United States, distributed over three-fourths of the nation. They are most numerous in the south from Florida to California, but the only dangerous species, *Centruroides exilicauda*, is limited to Arizona, New Mexico, southern California, parts of Texas, and northern Mexico. This species reaches a maximal length of about 7 cm. Their sting may be fatal to young children or old people, but seldom to a healthy adult.

Most of the nonlethal species of scorpions in the United States cause only minor reactions, like a bee sting. Some in the southwest, however, produce local edema and ecchymosis, with burning pain. In contrast, many species whose venom has potentially lethal systemic effects, including the Arizona *Centruroides*, evoke little or no visible reaction at the site of the sting. There is an immediate burning sensation followed by local paresthesia (''pins and needles''), hyperesthesia, or numbness. These sensations spread to involve the whole extremity, and within an hour or two, malaise, restlessness, neurologic hyperexcitability, lacrimation, rhinorrhea, salivation, perspiration, nausea, and vomiting may appear.

The patient passes from an agitated state with hyperactive reflexes into coma; convulsions follow. Release of catecholamines may result in tachycardia, various arrhythmias, and hypertension. Myocarditis and pancreatitis have also been reported. Death usually occurs within 12 h, but sometimes as late as 2 days after the sting.

Treatment Despite the reputation for lethality associated with envenomation by *C. exilicauda*, most often the symptoms consist only of pain and paresthesias lasting less than 4 h. These patients can be treated at home with cold compresses and mild analgesics. There is no clear consensus on the management of more severe envenomations. Although constriction bands, incision, and suction as in the treatment of snake bite have been recommended, the amount of venom is minute; it produces no local necrotizing effect and is absorbed very rapidly.

Specific antivenin, reconstituted from lyophilized goat serum, is available in some areas and should be considered if the victim develops signs of central nervous system or cardiac involvement. Supportive therapy is directed at combating shock and dehydration. Diazepam or phenobarbital are useful in reducing restlessness, and adrenergic blockers in managing symptoms secondary to catecholamine release.

Prevention This depends upon alertness in avoiding contact with scorpions in infested areas. Clothing and shoes should be well shaken before being put on in the morning. Towels and bedclothes should be inspected. A house infested with scorpions can in time be rid of them by closing all obvious ways of ingress; picking up debris in the environment, such as piles of brush, logs, stones; introducing a mixture of fuel oil or kerosene, containing a small amount of creosote, between the earth and the house foundation; and spraying with a mixture of 2% chlordane, and 0.2% pyrethrins in an oil base.

HYMENOPTERA STINGS Each year in the United States, nearly twice as many people die as a result of bites by hymenopterous insects (including bees, wasps, hornets, yellow jackets, and fire ants) as from poisonous snake bites. Occasionally, multiple stings in enormous numbers (500 to 1000) are the cause of death. However, the majority of systemic reactions and deaths are due to allergic reactions to the venoms of these insects.

Hymenoptera venoms contain many nonallergenic amines and peptides such as histamine and various kinins which contribute to the local sting reaction through their inflammatory and vasoactive properties. The allergenic venom proteins, which elicit an IgE antibody response in those who are stung, include phospholipases, hyaluronidases, acid phosphatases, and melittin. Venoms are distinctly different for each of the three genera of hymenoptera capable of causing allergic sting reactions: Apidae (various species of bees), Vespidae (hornets, yellowjackets, and wasps), and *Solenopsis* (fire ants).

The usual reaction to a single bee or wasp sting is sharp pain, which lasts for several minutes, local wheal and erythema, followed by intense itching. All signs of the sting normally subside within a few hours. Only in the rare case when a bee is swallowed or inhaled and edema of the laryngopharynx or glottis develops is there danger. A sting directly into a peripheral nerve can destroy its function for a time, much as does an injection of alcohol. Bell's palsy has followed a sting into the trunk of the facial nerve. Unusual reactions such as optic neuritis, generalized polyneuropathy, and myasthenia gravis may follow a sting. The etiology of these reactions is unknown.

In hypersensitive individuals, the response to a single sting may vary from an exaggerated local reaction, unassociated with systemic symptoms, to serious anaphylaxis with urticaria, nausea, abdominal or uterine cramps, bronchospasm, massive edema of the face and glottis, dyspnea, cyanosis, hypotension, coma, and death. These symptoms usually appear within a few minutes of the sting. Other patients may experience delayed reactions of the serum-sickness type occurring 10 to 14 days after envenomation. Sensitization is usually the result of previous stings although may fatalities have occurred in individuals who experienced no apparent allergic reaction to earlier envenomation. It has been estimated that 10 to 15 percent of the general population in this country has hymenoptera venom allergy. Those who have experienced a previous systemic allergic reaction to a sting, such as respiratory difficulty, hypotension, or generalized urticaria, are at greatest risk for serious reactions if stung again by the same type of insect.

Many species of ant can produce stinging bites with local redness and swelling. The most notorious of these are the fire ants (*Solenopsis*), particularly two "imported" South American species (*S. invicta* and *S. richteri*). The *invicta* species is now found in thirteen southern states and has largely supplanted all others, including several domestic species. In addition to being a major agricultural pest, fire ants, whose bites may result in extensive vesiculation and skin necrosis or cause serious hypersensitivity reactions, have become a significant health hazard to humans. Unlike other hymenoptera venoms, fire ant venom is mostly a simple insoluble alkaloid rather than a complex mixture of proteins. Although associated with life-threatening allergic reactions of the type seen with IgE-mediated immediate hypersensitivity, there is limited cross-sensitivity between fire ant venom and the venoms of bees, wasps, hornets, and yellowjackets.

Treatment The wound site should be examined for a stinger which, if present, should be carefully removed in order to prevent further envenomation from the attached gland. The local reaction to the usual sting is treated by local cool application and antipruritic lotions or oral antihistamines. Fire ant stings, which are frequently multiple, should be thoroughly cleaned with soap and water. Secondary bacterial infection is common and should be anticipated and treated promptly. Epinephrine, 0.3 to 0.5 mL of a 1:1000 aqueous solution subcutaneously repeated every 20 to 30 min, may be lifesaving in patients with an anaphylactic reaction to a sting. A tourniquet to slow the absorption of venom and ice packs to relieve pain may be used. Oxygen, endotracheal intubation, vasopressors, and other supportive measures should be used as needed. In addition, corticosteroids should be employed in severe cases, although their maximum effect is not achieved until several hours after administration.

Prevention Allergic persons should make every effort to avoid contact with these insects, including wearing shoes when outside and not wearing perfumes or bright colors which may attract them. In addition, they should keep epinephrine readily available for immediate use in case of a sting, without waiting for symptoms to develop. Sting kits containing premeasured doses of 1:1000 epinephrine in disposable syringes, tourniquets, and antihistamine tablets are commercially available. Careful instruction in their use should be provided by the person's physician.

Immunotherapy Desensitization by injection of preparations containing venom of the specific insect has long been recommended for any patient who has had a systemic or generalized reaction to hymenopterous insect sting. For many years, the only products available for this purpose were extracts of the crushed whole bodies of the stinging insect. However, skin testing with whole-body extracts was frequently unreliable in identifying persons at risk for systemic reactions, and immunization with these materials did not increase IgG-blocking antibodies to venom proteins, a response felt to be essential for protection against insect allergy. In contrast, purified hymenopterous venoms, which were approved for clinical use in the United States in 1979, have proved to be highly accurate in the diagnosis of sting allergy by skin testing. In addition, venom immunotherapy has been shown consistently to stimulate production of circulating venom-specific IgG antibodies, and to provide much better protection than whole-body extracts. The purified venoms have not been associated with a greater number of adverse reactions than treatment with whole-body extracts or with desensitization for pollinosis. These venom antigens are the materials of choice for diagnosis and immunotherapy of high-risk patients, those who have had previous systemic sting reactions and who have positive venom skin tests.

TICK BITE Although ticks may be vectors for such serious diseases as Rocky Mountain spotted fever, Q fever, tularemia, borreliosis, human babesiosis, and Lyme disease, the local reaction to the bite of a tick may be nothing more than an itching papule which subsides within a few days unless there is secondary bacterial infection. However, incomplete removal of a tick, with retention of the mouthparts, may result in the local formation of a nodule which continues to grow and is sometimes annoyingly pruritic. The definitive treatment is surgical excision of the nodule. Histologically, the nodule is a granuloma, but the inflammatory response is sometimes so bizarre and changes in the overlying epithelium are so striking that, in the absence of a history of tick bite, a mistaken diagnosis of malignant tumor may be made.

Ticks should always be removed intact, using gentle, steady traction. Application of a drop of oil, petrolatum, nail polish, or other organic solvent may facilitate removal without leaving embedded remnants. However, touching with a hot object such as a glowing cigarette should be discouraged because of the likelihood of injuring the host.

Tick paralysis A progressive, ascending, flaccid paralysis, acute ataxia, or a combination of both sometimes develops in humans and certain other mammals while a tick is engorging upon them. Human cases have most frequently been reported from the northwestern United States and western Canada, where the wood tick, *Dermacentor andersoni* Stiles, is responsible. The dog tick, *D. variabilis* Say, has been identified in a number of cases occurring in the southeastern states. *Amblyomma americanum*, the Lone Star tick, *A. maculatum*, the Gulf Coast tick, and *Ixodes scapularis*, the black-legged deer tick, have also been incriminated.

This disorder is caused by a neurotoxin secreted in the saliva of the engorging tick which acts upon spinal and bulbar nuclei, slowing motor nerve conduction without affecting neuromuscular transmission. The tick must feed for several days before symptoms develop.

Most human cases occur in children, generally in young girls. The tick is usually attached to the scalp and hidden by the hair, but may be found on any part of the body, especially the ear, axilla, groin, vulva, or popliteal region.

The patient may be irritable or restless for up to 24 h before frank motor involvement appears. Weakness usually is noted first in the distal muscles of the lower extremities, progressing over the next 24 to 48 h to flaccid paralysis, which may extend to involve the trunk, arms, neck, tongue, pharynx, and bulbar centers. Sensory changes are typically absent, and there is little or no fever unless a secondary infection is present. Results of routine laboratory tests including cerebrospinal fluid examination are normal. Nerve conduction studies may reveal decreased velocities and compound action potentials of nerves and their corresponding muscles.

Tick paralysis is apt to be confused with poliomyelitis, the more so because ticks are active in warm weather when poliomyelitis is most prevalent. Among other diseases which might be considered in differential diagnosis are diphtheritic polyneuropathy, transverse myelitis, the Guillain-Barré syndrome, myasthenia gravis, the Eaton-Lambert syndrome, and botulism.

Definitive treatment is removal of the tick, including any mouthparts retained in the skin. After this is done, there is striking improvement of motor function within a few hours and complete recovery within 48 h.

The patient should be observed until the recovery trend is established, because if other ticks or retained mouthparts have been overlooked, the paralysis may progress. When bulbar or respiratory paralysis is present, death may occur if the tick is not removed in time. The mortality rate is 10 percent; nearly all who die are children.

OTHER ARTHROPOD BITES AND ENVENOMATIONS   Flea bite
There are many fleas that attack humans, including *Pulex irritans* and chicken fleas. In sensitive individuals, the salivary secretion of these bloodsuckers produces large, itching papules. It is thought that much of the papular urticaria of children is probably due to flea bites. Treatment is symptomatic only. Elimination of fleas from the environment may be very difficult, but persistent treatment of animals and of premises with appropriate insecticides is usually successful.

Centipede bite   The giant desert centipede, which reaches 15 cm in length, is responsible for most centipede bites in the United States. It is capable of inflicting an intensely painful bite, associated with erythema, edema, and sometimes with regional lymphangitis. Rhabdomyolysis and acute renal failure have occurred following the bite of this arthropod. Pain usually disappears within a few hours, but may require oral or parenteral analgesics. The wound should be washed well with soap and water to help prevent secondary infection.

Caterpillar rash   Contact with the early larval or caterpillar stage of several species of moth produces irritation of skin and mucous membranes resulting in a pruritic, erythematous rash, occasionally accompanied by urticaria and bullae. Symptoms come on rapidly after direct contact with caterpillars, after handling cocoons, or on being exposed to windblown fuzz. The pathogenesis is thought to be due to the direct irritant effects of insect hairs or appendages, although other mechanisms, including intracutaneous injection of toxins or hypersensitivity to insect antigens, have been suggested. The symptoms usually subside within a few days. Local soaks and oral antihistamines are often indicated.

Bedbug bite   Members of the genus *Cimex* inflict bites that leave reactions varying from a simple puncture to large urticarial lesions, apparently depending on the sensitivity of the bitten individual. There is no specific treatment.

Kissing bug bite   Of the many species of true bugs, those in the family Reduviidae are relatively commonly associated with severe bite reactions. The most important reduviid bug in this country is the kissing bug (genus *Triatoma*), which is found throughout the southern crescent of the United States. The bites of this bug, which is a nocturnal feeder, are characteristically inflicted in multiple groups. Reactions which follow are thought to be allergic in nature and may

include intensely pruritic and painful papules with a central punctum, grouped vesicles with moderate swelling and redness but no central lesions, giant urticaria, generalized allergic reactions, including systemic anaphylaxis, and hemorrhagic nodular-to-bullous lesions on a hand or foot, appearing several days after the bite. These may be confused with necrotizing spider bites or with erythema multiforme. However, the former are usually single lesions and the latter rarely has a unilateral distribution. The possibility of kissing bug bites should be considered in patients who awaken in the middle of the night with intense itching, hives, and other signs of a systemic allergic reaction.

Treatment of the local reaction is symptomatic. More severe reactions should be managed similarly to other allergic sting reactions. Patients who have had accelerated reactions to reduviid bites should be provided with sting kits and instructions in their use.

Chiggers or redbugs   These are tiny mites which are commonly found in foliage or grass in many parts of the world. In the United States, the larval form of *Eutrobicula alfreddugesi* attacks the skin by secreting a substance which digests tissue, creating a red papule that itches intensely. The tiny reddish larva can be seen in the center of the lesion. Treatment is palliative and consists of antipruritic applications. The use of insect repellents, appropriate protective clothing, and prompt bathing after exposure reduce the risk of infestation considerably.

Bloodsucking-fly bite   Many species of flies, particularly the horsefly and the deerfly, viciously attack and feed upon warm-blooded animals, including humans. Occasionally, transmission of diseases such as anthrax, tularemia, loiasis, and trypanosomiasis has been attributed to horseflies and deerflies. More commonly in North America, however, their bites are responsible for painful, intensely pruritic cutaneous lesions which may be followed by delayed localized allergic reactions characterized by erythema, edema, and urticaria. Treatment should include thorough cleaning of the bite sites, topical corticosteroids, and oral antihistaminics for severe itching. Antibiotics may be necessary if the wounds become secondarily infected.

MARINE ANIMAL VENOM DISEASES   The venoms of certain marine animals are known to cause illness in humans after injection or inoculation under naturally occurring conditions. Information concerning these toxins is limited; most appear to be composed of proteins and peptides as well as other substances that are pharmacologically active. Although probably less complex than the venoms of reptiles, many marine animal venoms are capable of causing several pathologic effects including neurotoxicity as well as local necrosis.

Portuguese man-of-war and jellyfish stings   The burning discomfort induced by contact with sea nettles or jellyfish is familiar to most surf bathers. Contact with the tentacles of the colorful Portuguese man-of-war (*Physalia* species), which is found mainly in or near the Gulf of Mexico, or the more toxic jellyfish (*Chiropsalmus* of the Indian Ocean and *Rhizostoma* of the Atlantic) is followed by burning pain, swelling, and erythema. Severe, generalized muscular cramps, nausea, vomiting, and pulmonary edema may occur. Victims have died as a result of jellyfish stings, sometimes within minutes after contact. In nonfatal cases, systemic symptoms usually subside within several hours. Treatment consists of bathing the wound in salt water, taking care not to rub the area of the sting. Next, any tentacles still clinging to the skin should be scraped off after first inactivating any remaining nematocysts to prevent discharge of additional venom into the victim. This can be done by sprinkling baking soda over the wound to form a slurry for sea nettle stings or by bathing with vinegar or isopropyl alcohol for man-of-war stings. Rinsing with fresh water or household ammonia, or rubbing with sand are not recommended since these measures may actually cause nematocysts to discharge. Analgesics should be used for pain control, and antihistaminics if there is an accompanying pruritic rash. Severe envenomations may require advanced life support measures. Corticosteroids may be helpful in these cases. An antivenin is now available for treatment of stings by the highly lethal Australian sea wasp, *Chironex fleckeri*.

Coral wounds and stings The colorful structures known as coral are composed of thousands of small marine animals of the coelenterate phylum, surrounded by a stony exoskeleton of calcium carbonate. Several species, including the fire coral, found in many parts of the world, contain microscopic nematocysts capable of producing painful stings similar to those caused by jellyfish. Often more serious are wounds resulting from abrasions and cuts by the sharp edges of the outer skeleton. These frequently contain small pieces of animal protein and skeletal material which act as foreign bodies, and may lead to chronic, suppurative wound infections if not promptly and adequately debrided.

Sea anemone sting ("sponge diver's disease") Contact with certain sea anemones (especially *Sargatia elegans*) in Mediterranean and African waters produces extensive dermatitis with chronic ulceration. Occasionally, especially during August and September, systemic symptoms of headache, sneezing, nausea, chills, fever, and collapse are noted. Rare fatalities have occurred. No specific therapy is known; symptomatic treatment with topical steroids or oral antihistaminics may provide temporary relief.

Cone shell poisoning The colorful cone shells are highly prized by collectors. However, many species in the Pacific are venomous, a great danger to unwary hobbyists who pick them up. The poison, a neurotoxin, is delivered into a wound inflicted by pointed hollow teeth resembling darts in the long proboscis of the animal. Local manifestations include sudden intense pain, followed by swelling and numbness which may persist for several days. Symptoms of serious poisoning include muscular incoordination and weakness progressing to respiratory paralysis. Death may occur within 3 to 6 h, but recovery within 24 h is the rule. There is no specific therapy; recommended treatment is the use of tourniquet, incision, and suction (as for snake bite), and supportive measures which may include artificial respiration and administration of oxygen.

Sponge dermatitis Direct contact with several species of sponge results in a painful dermatitis, which may persist for several weeks. The lesions appear to be caused by mechanical irritation from the exoskeleton of the sponge as well as by toxins within its tissues. Delayed hypersensitivity reactions may also occur. Antihistaminics provide relief from the pruritus; dilute acetic acid ameliorates local pain, while alkali will intensify it. The lesions are self-limited.

Sea urchin wounds and stings Contact with the spines of some species of sea urchin results in painful erythema and ulceration, occasionally accompanied by neurotoxic symptoms of weakness and frank paralysis of lips, tongue, and face lasting for several hours. Treatment is purely symptomatic and supportive. The toxins isolated from sea urchins have produced paralysis in animals and are notably resistant to heat. Deaths from paralysis and drowning have been reported. Occasionally, fragments of sea urchin spines may remain in the skin, leading to granulomatous reactions, or they may migrate into a joint or lodge against a nerve, causing intractable pain. Treatment of these complications is surgical.

Paralytic and neurotoxic shellfish poisoning Certain dinoflagellates, which make up part of the marine phytoplankton, elaborate a potent neurotoxin. Occasionally, conditions in coastal waters become favorable for the growth of excessive numbers of these organisms, causing the water to develop an amber appearance termed the "red tide" and killing massive numbers of fish by exhausting their oxygen supply. When humans ingest shellfish which have themselves ingested toxic dinoflagellates, an illness occurs that is characterized by paresthesias of the face and extremities, dysphonia, and generalized muscular weakness, often accompanied by nausea, vomiting, and diarrhea and occasionally by paralysis and respiratory arrest. The more severe syndrome, known as paralytic shellfish poisoning, is encountered along the Pacific northwest and New England coasts. A milder form, not associated with paralysis in humans, is seen along the Gulf and Atlantic coasts of Florida. Treatment should include induced emesis and purgation to remove unabsorbed toxin from the gastrointestinal tract and whatever additional supportive measures are necessary. Spontaneous recovery usually takes place within 24 h. There is a standardized mouse bioassay procedure for demonstrating and quantitating toxin in shellfish but no diagnostic test for detecting toxin in clinical specimens.

Venomous fish injuries The dorsal fins or spines of bullhead sharks, dogfish, and ratfish and the dorsal and other fins of the lionfish, weeverfish, toadfish, and catfish are grooved, and at their bases are found venom glands. Little is known of the venoms involved except that they contain highly unstable proteins of variable molecular weights and are capable of causing toxic as well as allergic reactions.

Envenomation results in immediate, severe local pain and edema which, if untreated, reaches greatest intensity in 60 to 90 min and resolves within 8 to 12 h. Local necrosis with extensive tissue loss may occur, particularly following lionfish and catfish stings. Systemic reactions, including cardiac arrhythmias, hypotension, muscular weakness, seizures, and paralysis, have been reported and attributed to the effects of the venom.

Treatment should be immediate immersion of the wound in water as hot as the patient can stand for at least 1 h or until symptoms subside. The venoms are extremely heat labile, accounting for the usefulness of this procedure. Although rarely needed, an antivenin is available for patients with severe systemic reactions from stonefish envenomation. It can be obtained from the Health Services Department, Sea World of San Diego [(619) 222–0411]. Tetanus prophylaxis should be given as needed. Narcotics may be required to control pain. Secondary pyogenic infection is a frequent complication.

Probably the most frequent type of fish envenomation in the United States is that produced by the lashing tail of the stingray of the California coast (*Urobatis halleri*). The bony spine is encased in a sheath of epithelial cells containing venom which is expressed into the puncture wound. The wound may be several centimeters deep; portions of the bony spine may break off in it, or, more often, the integumentary sheath remains in the wound. The venom is a circulatory depressant in animals, but local injury predominates in humans. Severe pain and blanching followed by erythema and edema occur immediately. Symptoms due to systemic absorption of venom are infrequent but may include salivation, muscle cramps and weakness, cardiac arrhythmias, seizures, and death. Treatment consists of application of a constriction band (the vast majority of these injuries occur on the legs) and copious syringing of the wound with salt water to remove fragments of sheath. Additional therapeutic measures are the same as for other fish envenomations, including immersion of the injured area in hot water for up to 1 h.

REFERENCES

Hymenoptera stings

GOLDEN DBK, VALENTINE M: Insect sting allergy. Ann Allergy 53:444, 1984
LIGHT WC et al: Unusual reactions following insect stings. J Allergy Clin Immunol 59:391, 1977
PATTERSON R, VALENTINE M: Anaphylaxis and related allergic emergencies including reactions due to insect stings. JAMA 248:2632, 1982
PAULL BR: Imported fire ant allergy: Perspectives on diagnosis and treatment. Postgrad Med 76:155, 1984

Marine animal venoms

AUERBACH PS, HALSTEAD BW: Hazardous marine life, in *Management of Wilderness and Environmental Emergencies*, PS Auerbach, HR Gee (eds). New York, Macmillan, 1983
BURNETT JW et al: First aid for jellyfish envenomation. South Med J 76:870, 1983
GUESS HA et al: Hemolysis following a Portuguese man-of-war sting. Pediatrics 70:979, 1982
HUGHES JM, MERSON MH: Fish and shellfish poisoning. N Engl J Med 295:1117, 1976
KIZER KW et al: Scorpaenidae envenomation: A 5-year poison center experience. JAMA 253:807, 1985
SCOGGIN CH: Catfish stings. JAMA 231:176, 1975

Other arthropod bites and stings

FRAZIER CA: *Insect Allergy: Allergic and Toxic Reactions to Insects and Other Arthropods.* St Louis, Grace, 1969

HILLIER FF, WARM RP: Caterpillar dermatitis. Br Med J 1:346, 1967

HUNT GR: Bites and stings of uncommon arthropods: 2. Reduviids, fire ants, puss caterpillars, and scorpions. Postgrad Med 70:107, 1981

LOGAN JL, OGDEN DA: Rhabdomyolysis and acute renal failure following the bite of the giant desert centipede *Scolopendra heros.* West J Med 142:549, 1985

SHELLEY ED et al: The diagnostic challenge of non-burrowing mite bites. JAMA 251:2690, 1984

WIRTZ RA: Allergic and toxic reactions to non-stinging arthropods. Ann Rev Entomol 29:47, 1984

Scorpion stings

LIKES K et al: *Centruroides exilicauda* envenomation in Arizona. West J Med 141:634, 1984

RIMSZA ME et al: Scorpion envenomation. Pediatrics 66:298, 1980

Snake and lizard bites

GARFIN SR et al: Rattlesnake bites and surgical decompression: Results using a laboratory model. Toxicon 22:177, 1984

KITCHENS CS, VANMIEROP LHS: Mechanisms of defibrination in humans after envenomation by the eastern diamondback rattlesnake. Am J Hematol 14:345, 1983

LOPRINZI CL et al: Snake antivenin administration in a patient allergic to horse serum. South Med J 76:501, 1983

MINTON SA JR: *Venom Diseases.* Springfield, Ill, Charles C Thomas, 1974

MITRAKUL C, DHAMKRONG A: Clinical features of neurotoxic snake bite and response to antivenom in 47 children. Am J Trop Med Hyg 33:1258, 1984

RUSSELL FE: *Snake Venom Poisoning.* New York, Scholium International, 1983

STAHNKE HL et al: Bite of the Gila monster. Rocky Mt Med J 67:25, 1970

Spider bites

HUNT GR: Bites and stings of uncommon arthropods: 1. Spiders. Postgrad Med 70:91, 1981

KING LE JR, REES RS: Dapsone treatment of a brown recluse bite. JAMA 250:648, 1983

KOBERNICK M: Black widow spider bite. Am Fam Physician 29:241, 1984

REES RS et al: Management of the brown recluse spider bite. Plast Reconstr Surg 68:768, 1981

Tick bite and tick paralysis

GOTHE R et al: The mechanism of pathogenicity in the tick paralysis. J Med Entomol 16:357, 1979

SPIELMAN A: How to diagnose and treat tick and mite infestations. Drug Therapy 11:77, 1981

---

171   POISONING AND ITS MANAGEMENT

PAUL A. FRIEDMAN

GENERAL PRINCIPLES

In the United States accidental poisoning by chemical agents causes about 5000 deaths each year while suicides by chemical agents annually number more than 6000. In addition to the victims of fatal poisoning there is a much greater number of persons who are made seriously ill by chemical agents but recover after appropriate therapy. Unfortunately, some such patients are left with permanent sequelae of their intoxication.

Accidental poisonings occur far more frequently in the home than through industrial exposure and are usually acute; industrial intoxication is more often the result of chronic exposure. Accidental poisoning results most commonly from ingestion of toxic substances and involves children in the majority of cases. Each year 1 to 2 million American children accidentally swallow toxic materials, and approximately 1 ingestion in 1000 is fatal. Medicines are involved in 50 percent of all ingestions. Cleaning and polishing agents are ingested by 15 percent, while cosmetics, pesticides, petroleum products, and turpentine paints account for 20 percent.

Despite all precautions, accidental, suicidal, and criminal poisonings will remain an important problem which every physician must be prepared to treat promptly and effectively. Besides their immediate therapeutic responsibilities, physicians have legal obligations in cases of attempted suicide, homicide, criminal abortion, and industrial exposure. The physician should also obtain psychiatric care for any patient who has attempted suicide by poison.

DIAGNOSIS OF CHEMICAL POISONING

Optimal management of the poisoned patient requires a correct diagnosis. Although the toxic effects of some chemical substances are quite characteristic, most poisoning syndromes can simulate other diseases.

Poisoning usually is included in the differential diagnosis of coma, convulsions, acute psychosis, acute hepatic or renal insufficiency, and bone marrow depression. Although it should be, poisoning may not be considered when the major manifestation is a mild psychiatric disturbance or neurologic disorder, abdominal pain, bleeding, fever, hypotension, pulmonary congestion, or skin eruption. Furthermore, the patient may be unaware of exposure to poison, as in chronic, insidious intoxications, or, as after attempted suicide or abortion, may be unwilling to admit it. Physicians always should remember the variegated manifestations of poisoning and maintain a high index of suspicion.

In every case of poisoning, identification of the toxic agent should be attempted. Specific antidotal therapy is obviously impossible without such identification. In cases of homicide, suicide, or criminal abortion the identity of the poison may be of legal importance. When poisoning results from industrial exposure or therapeutic mishap, accurate knowledge of the responsible agents is essential for future prevention.

In acute accidental poisoning the offending substance may be known to the patient. In many other cases information can be obtained from relatives or acquaintances, by a search for containers at the scene of the poisoning, or by questioning the patient's physician or pharmacist. Frequently such efforts yield only the trade name of a product, which gives no clue to its component chemicals. A number of books which identify the active ingredients of household products, agricultural compounds, proprietary medicines, and poisonous plants are listed in the references to this chapter. A small handbook of this type should be carried in every physician's bag. Poison control centers and manufacturers' representatives are other useful sources of such information. When poisoning is chronic, rapid identification of the toxic agent from the history is often impossible. The lesser therapeutic urgency of such cases usually permits the required painstaking exploration of the patient's habits and environment.

Some poisons can produce clinical features characteristic enough to strongly suggest the diagnosis. Careful examination of the patient may reveal the unmistakable odor of cyanide; the cherry-colored flush of carboxyhemoglobin in skin and mucous membranes; the pupillary constriction, salivation, and gastrointestinal hyperactivity produced by cholinesterase-inhibitor insecticides; or the lead line and extensor paralyses of chronic lead poisoning. Unfortunately, these features are not always present, and in any case telltales are the exception in chemical poisonings.

Chemical analysis of body fluids provides the most definite identification of the intoxicating agent. Some common poisons, such as aspirin and barbiturates, can be identified and even quantitated by relatively simple laboratory procedures. Others require more complex toxicologic techniques, such as gas or high-performance chromatography, which are carried out only in specialized laboratories. Furthermore, the results of toxicologic determinations are rarely available in time to guide the initial treatment of acute poisoning. Nevertheless, specimens of vomitus, gastric aspirate, blood, urine, and feces should be saved for toxicologic study if diagnostic or legal questions are likely to arise. Chemical analyses of body fluids or tissues are of particular value in the diagnosis and evaluation of chronic intoxications. Finally, they are useful in following the success of some forms of therapy.

TREATMENT OF CHEMICAL POISONING

Correct treatment of the poisoned patient requires knowledge of both the general principles of management and the details of therapy for specific poisons. Treatment involves four steps: (1) prevention of further absorption of the poison, (2) removal of absorbed poison from the body, (3) symptomatic supportive therapy or symptomatic treatment of circulatory, respiratory, neurologic, and renal function, and (4) administration of systemic antidotes (Table 171-1). The first three are applicable to most types of poisoning. The fourth is most often used only when the toxic agent is known and a specific antidote is available. However, naloxone is given sometimes if the index of suspicion is high that the patient has had an overdose of an opiate. It should be recognized both that most poisons do not have a specific antidote and that essential supportive care does not require knowledge of the toxic agent. Thus, although the physician should always try to identify the poison, such attempts must never delay vital therapeutic measures.

PREVENTION OF ABSORPTION OF INGESTED POISONS
If appreciable amounts of a poison have been ingested, one should attempt to minimize its absorption from the gastrointestinal tract. The success of such endeavors depends upon the time elapsed since ingestion and upon the site and speed of absorption of the poison.

Evacuation of the stomach Attempts to empty the stomach are always worthwhile unless specifically contraindicated. They can be highly successful if made soon after ingestion. Significant amounts of poison still may be recovered from the stomach hours after ingestion because gastric emptying may be delayed by gastric atony or pylorospasm. Such is the case with phenothiazines, antihistamines, and tricyclic antidepressants.

Emesis occurs spontaneously after the ingestion of many poisons. In a minority of instances it may be induced in the home by mechanical stimulation of the posterior pharynx. The emetic action of syrup of ipecac (not the 14 times more concentrated fluid extract) in 15- to 30-mL dosage is more effective and is safe enough for home use. Its action has an average latent period of 20 min and depends in part on gastrointestinal absorption, so that concurrent administration of charcoal, to which it adsorbs, is to be avoided. A second dose of ipecac should be given if the patient fails to vomit after 20 min (90 to 95 percent of patients will vomit after two doses). If ipecac is not available at home, every effort should be made to locate some, even if this requires taking the patient to the hospital. Apomorphine, 0.06 mg/kg intramuscularly, acts within 5 min but may cause prolonged vomiting. When given intravenously in doses of 0.01 mg/kg, apomorphine tends to produce almost immediate vomiting which is not followed by any other central nervous system effects. On occasion it is impossible to induce vomiting, and valuable time should not be lost with hopeful waiting. Induction of vomiting should not be attempted in convulsing patients, in patients with severe central nervous system depression, or (because of the danger of gastroesophageal perforation or tracheal aspiration of vomitus) in patients who have ingested strong caustics or small amounts (<100 mL) of liquid hydrocarbons which are potent lung irritants (e.g., kerosene, furniture polish).

In comparison with emesis, *gastric lavage* is more predictably and immediately active but usually no more effective in removing poison from the stomach. It can be employed in unconscious patients, and removal of gastric contents reduces the risk of aspiration of vomitus in such patients. It is, however, contraindicated after the ingestion of strong corrosives because of danger of perforating injured tissues. When properly performed, gastric lavage carries little risk of aspiration of gastric contents into the lungs. The patient should be prone, with head and shoulders lowered. A mouth gag is placed, and a gastric tube of sufficient diameter to permit withdrawal of particulate matter (size 30) is passed into the stomach. If central nervous system function is depressed, if introduction of the tube produces retching, or if pulmonary irritants have been ingested, it is wise to place a *cuffed endotracheal tube* before performing lavage. Gastric contents are withdrawn with a large syringe and usually contain most of the poison that will be removed. Thereafter 200 mL (less in children) of warm water or dilute solution alternately is instilled and withdrawn until the aspirate becomes clear.

Interference with gastrointestinal absorption Since neither emesis nor gastric lavage empties the stomach completely, one should attempt to minimize absorption by administering substances which trap ingested poisons. Many poisons are adsorbed by powdered, activated charcoal. A good grade of activated charcoal can adsorb as much as half its weight of many common poisons. A slurry of activated charcoal (20 to 50 g in 100 to 200 mL) should be administered after evacuation of the stomach.

Adsorption by charcoal is reversible, and the effectiveness of adsorption of many poisons varies with the pH. Acidic substances are adsorbed better in acid solutions and therefore may be released in the small intestine. It is desirable to speed the charcoal with its adsorbed poison through the intestine as quickly as possible. This will also decrease intestinal absorption of any unadsorbed poison which has passed beyond the pylorus. In patients with good renal and cardiac function this is best accomplished by oral or gastric administration of an osmotic cathartic such as magnesium or sodium sulfate (10 to 30 g given in solution at a concentration of 10% or less).

PREVENTION OF ABSORPTION OF POISON FROM OTHER SITES
Most topically applied poisons can be removed by copious flushing with water. In certain instances weak acids or bases or alcohol plus soap or detergent are more effective, but rapid and voluminous washing with water should always proceed while they are being obtained. Chemical antidotes can be hazardous because tissue injury may result from the heat of the chemical reaction.

The systemic distribution of injected poisons can be slowed by the application of cold to the injection site or by the proximal application of a tourniquet.

Following inhalation of toxic gases, vapors, or dusts, the victim should be moved to clean air and adequate ventilation should be maintained. If the patient cannot be moved, a protective mask should be applied.

REMOVAL OF ABSORBED POISON FROM THE BODY
Unlike prevention or retardation of absorption, measures to speed removal of the toxic agent from the body rarely have much influence on the peak poison concentration. However, they can significantly abbreviate the time during which the concentration of many poisons remains above any given level and may thereby reduce morbidity, avoid

TABLE 171-1 Treatment of acute chemical poisoning

I Prevention of further absorption of poison
  A Poisoning by ingestion
    1 Emptying the stomach
      a Induction of vomiting
      b Gastric lavage
    2 Minimizing gastrointestinal absorption
      a Adsorption
      b Catharsis
  B Poisoning by other routes
II Removal of absorbed poisons from body
  A Detoxification—enzyme induction?
  B Biliary excretion—interruption of enterohepatic circulation
  C Urinary excretion
    1 Forced diuresis
    2 Alteration of urinary pH
  D Dialysis
    1 Peritoneal dialysis
    2 Hemodialysis
  E Charcoal or resin hemoperfusion
  F Exchange transfusion
  G Chelation and chemical binding
III Supportive therapy
IV Administration of systemic antidotes
  A Chemical agents
  B Pharmacologic antagonists

complications, and save lives. In judging the need for such measures, one must consider the patient's clinical state, the properties and metabolic fate of the poison, and the amount absorbed as judged by the history and the blood level. Removal of some poisons can be accelerated by several methods; selection depends on the clinical urgency, the amount in the body, and the skills and equipment available.

Biliary excretion   Certain organic acids and active drugs are secreted into the bile against large concentration gradients. This process takes time and cannot be accelerated. However, the intestinal resorption of substances already secreted into the bile, such as glutethimide, can be decreased by the administration of charcoal every 6 h. The organochlorine pesticide chlordecone is eliminated slowly from the body (blood half-life 165 days). Cholestyramine (16 g per day) significantly accelerates elimination (blood half-life 80 days).

Urinary excretion   Acceleration of renal excretion is applicable to a much larger number of poisons. Renal excretion of toxic substances depends on glomerular filtration, active tubular secretion, and passive tubular resorption. The first two processes should be protected by maintenance of adequate circulation and renal function, but for practical purposes they cannot be accelerated. On the other hand, passive tubular resorption of many poisons plays an important role in the prolongation of their action and can frequently be decreased by readily available methods. The effectiveness of forced diuresis by administration of large volumes of electrolyte solutions together with intravenous furosemide in increasing renal excretion has been demonstrated for drugs such as salicylates and long-acting barbiturates.

Alteration of the urinary pH can also inhibit passive back-diffusion of some poisons and increase their renal clearance. The renal tubular epithelium is more permeable to uncharged molecules than to ionized solutes. Weak organic acids and bases readily diffuse out of the tubular fluid in their un-ionized form but are trapped in it when ionized. Acidic poisons are ionized only at pHs above their pK_a. Alkalinization of the urine greatly increases the ionization in the tubular fluid of such organic acids as phenobarbital and salicylate. In contrast, the pK_a of pentobarbital (8.1) and secobarbital (8.0) are so high that renal clearance is not increased greatly by raising the urinary pH into the physiologic alkaline range. Alkalinization of the urine is achieved by the infusion of sodium bicarbonate at a rate determined by the urinary and blood pH. Excessive systemic alkalosis or electrolyte disturbances must be prevented. A combination of forced diuresis and alkalinization of the urine can raise the renal clearance of some acidic poisons tenfold or more and has been found highly effective in poisoning by salicylate, phenobarbital, barbital, and 2,4-dichlorophenoxyacetic acid. Conversely, depression of the urinary pH below its usual range has been shown to augment the clearance of amphetamines, phencyclidines, fenfluramine, and quinine.

Finally, the renal excretion of certain poisons can be increased in a highly specific fashion. An example is the removal of bromide by administration of chloride and chloriuretics. Such methods are discussed with the individual poisons.

Dialysis and hemoperfusion   Dialysis has been found effective in the removal of many compounds, including barbiturates, borate, chlorate, ethanol, glycols, methanol, salicylate, sulfonamides, theophylline, and thiocyanate. Theoretically, it should accelerate the removal from the body of any dialyzable toxin which is not bound irreversibly to tissues. Its effectiveness does not extend to large-molecule, nondialyzable poisons and is decreased by a high degree of protein binding or lipid solubility of the toxic substance.

Peritoneal dialysis can be performed easily in any hospital and may be continued for long periods. It is valuable for the removal of poisons only if renal function is impaired, hemodialysis or hemoperfusion is not possible, or forced diuresis cannot be carried out.

Hemodialysis is unquestionably a more effective procedure for removing large amounts of dialyzable poisons. For barbiturates dialysance rates of 50 to 100 mL/min have been achieved, a removal rate 2 to 10 times faster than during peritoneal dialysis or forced diuresis. Perfusion of blood through activated charcoal or exchange resin achieves even higher clearance rates than hemodialysis for most poisons. Extracorporeal dialysis and hemoperfusion are clearly the procedures of choice for the rapid removal of poisons from patients who have absorbed amounts which make survival unlikely even with the best supportive care. Since the required equipment and skilled personnel are not available in every hospital, the possibility of transfer of such patients to an institution with these capabilities should be considered.

Chelation and chemical binding   The removal of some poisons is accelerated by chemical interaction with other substances followed by renal excretion. These substances are considered systemic antidotes and are discussed with the individual poisons.

SUPPORTIVE THERAPY   Most chemical poisonings are reversible, self-limited disease states. Skillful supportive therapy can keep many seriously poisoned patients alive and their detoxifying and excretory mechanisms functioning until the concentration of poison in the body has fallen to safe levels. Symptomatic measures are especially important when the poison is one of the many compounds for which no specific antidote is known. Even when an antidote is available, disturbances of vital functions must be prevented or controlled by appropriate supportive care.

The poisoned patient may suffer a variety of physiologic disturbances. Most of these are not peculiar to chemical intoxications, and their therapeutic management is described elsewhere in this text. Only those aspects of supportive therapy specially relevant to poisonings are discussed briefly here.

Central nervous system depression   Specific therapy directed against the depressant effects of poisons on the central nervous system is usually both unnecessary and difficult. Most poisoned patients will emerge from coma as from a prolonged anesthesia. During the period of unconsciousness, meticulous nursing care and close observation are essential. If depression of medullary centers results in circulatory or respiratory failure, these vital functions must be immediately and vigorously supported by chemical or mechanical means. The use of analeptics in the treatment of poison-induced central nervous system depression has been largely abandoned. Certainly these agents should never be employed to restore consciousness, and it is doubtful whether their use to hasten the restoration of spontaneous breathing and active reflexes is ever justified. By contrast, the narcotic antagonist naloxone administered intravenously in adequate doses generally will reverse central nervous system depression secondary to narcotic overdosage.

Convulsions   Many poisons (e.g., chlorinated hydrocarbons, insecticides, strychnine) cause convulsions by their specific excitatory effects. Poisoned patients also may have convulsions because of hypoxia, hypoglycemia, cerebral edema, or metabolic disturbances. In such cases these abnormalities should be corrected as far as possible. Regardless of the cause of the convulsions, anticonvulsant drugs often are required. Intravenously administered diazepam, phenobarbital, or phenytoin is usually effective.

Cerebral edema   Intracranial hypertension due to cerebral edema is also a characteristic effect of some poisons and a nonspecific result of other chemical intoxications. For example, cerebral edema is seen in poisoning by lead, carbon monoxide, and methanol. Symptomatic treatment consists of use of adrenocortical steroids and, when necessary, the intravenous administration of hypertonic solutions of mannitol or urea.

Hypotension   The causes of hypotension and shock in the poisoned patient are legion, and often several of them coexist. Poisons can depress the medullary vasomotor centers, block autonomic ganglia or adrenergic receptors, directly depress the tone of arterial or venous smooth muscle, reduce myocardial contractility, or induce cardiac arrhythmias. Less specifically, the poisoned patient may be in shock because of tissue hypoxia, extensive tissue destruction from corrosives, loss of blood or fluids, or metabolic disturbances. When possible, these abnormalities should be corrected. If the central venous pressure is low, fluid replacement should be the first therapeutic approach. Vasoactive drugs are often helpful and sometimes essential in the hypotensive poisoned patient, particularly in shock resulting from central depression. As in shock from other causes, choice of the most appropriate agent requires an analysis of the hemodynamic disturbance which goes beyond determination of the arterial pressure.

Cardiac arrhythmias Disturbances of cardiac impulse generation or conduction in the poisoned patient arise from the effects of certain poisons on the electrical properties of cardiac fibers or from myocardial hypoxia or metabolic disturbances. The latter should be corrected, and antiarrhythmic agents administered as indicated by the nature of the arrhythmia (see Chap. 184).

Pulmonary edema The poisoned patient may develop pulmonary edema because of depressed myocardial contractility or because of alveolar injury from irritant gases or aspirated fluids. The latter type of edema is less responsive to treatment and may be associated with laryngeal edema. Therapeutic measures include suctioning, administration of high concentrations of oxygen under positive pressure, aerosols of surface-active agents, bronchodilators, and adrenocortical steroids (see Chap. 26).

Hypoxia Poisoning may cause tissue hypoxia by various mechanisms, and several of these may operate in one patient. Inadequate ventilation can result from central respiratory depression, from muscular paralysis, or from airway obstruction by retained secretions, laryngeal edema, or bronchospasm. Alveolar-capillary diffusion may be impaired by pulmonary edema. Anemia, methemoglobinemia, carboxyhemoglobinemia, or shock can interfere with oxygen transport. Cellular oxidation may be inhibited (e.g., cyanide, fluoroacetate). Maintenance of an adequate airway is essential to treatment. The clinical situation and the site of obstruction may indicate frequent suctioning, insertion of an oropharyngeal airway or of an endotracheal tube, or a tracheotomy. If, despite a clear airway, ventilation remains inadequate, as judged by clinical appearance or by measurement of minute volume or blood gases, artificial ventilation by appropriate mechanical means is imperative. Administration of high concentrations of oxygen is indicated whenever tissue hypoxia occurs. When the central nervous system is severely depressed, oxygen administration often results in apnea and must be combined with artificial ventilation.

Acute renal insufficiency Renal failure with oliguria or anuria may occur in the poisoned patient because of shock, dehydration, or electrolyte disturbances. More specifically, it may be due to the nephrotoxic potential of some poisons (e.g., mercury, phosphorus, carbon tetrachloride, bromate), many of which are concentrated and excreted by the kidney. Renal damage due to poisons is usually reversible. The management of acute renal insufficiency is outlined in Chap. 219.

Electrolyte and water disturbances Imbalances of fluid and electrolytes are common features of chemical poisoning. They may result from vomiting, diarrhea, renal insufficiency, or therapeutic maneuvers such as catharsis, forced diuresis, or dialysis. These disturbances are corrected or, ideally, prevented by appropriate therapy. Certain poisons produce more specific defects, such as metabolic acidosis (e.g., methanol, phenol, salicylate) or hypocalcemia (e.g., fluoride, oxalate). These abnormalities and any specific treatment are described under the individual poisons.

Acute hepatic insufficiency The primary manifestation of some poisonings (e.g., chlorinated hydrocarbons, phosphorus, cinchophen, certain mushrooms) is acute hepatic failure. Its management is described in Chap. 247.

ADMINISTRATION OF SYSTEMIC ANTIDOTES Specific antidotal therapy is available for only a few poisons. Some systemic antidotes are chemicals which exert their therapeutic effect by reducing the concentration of the toxic substance. They may do this by combining with the poison (e.g., ethylene diaminetetraacetate with lead, dimercaprol with mercury, sulfhydryl-containing reagents with a toxic metabolite of acetaminophen) or by increasing its excretion (e.g., chloride or mercurial diuretics in bromide poisoning). Other systemic antidotes compete with the poison for its receptor site (e.g., atropine with muscarine, naloxone with morphine; physostigmine reverses some of the anticholinergic effects of the tricyclic antidepressants, as well as those of the antihistamines, belladonna, and other atropinic substances). Specific antidotes are discussed with the individual poisons.

COMMON POISONS

The poisons discussed in this section are some of those encountered by the general population such as commonly used nonprescription drugs, household products, solvents, pesticides, and poisonous plants. It has been necessary to disregard many uncommon toxic materials and products to which exposure occurs only in specialized industrial environments. Details concerning poisoning by such compounds may be found in some of the references to this chapter. In addition, toxic effects of many drugs are considered throughout this text in conjunction with their therapeutic and illicit uses as well as with overdose (see especially Chaps. 364 to 367). Manifestations of hypersensitivity to chemicals are described in Chap. 65. The following discussions of specific poisons stress those details of their action which are pertinent to the recognition or treatment of clinical poisoning.

ACETAMINOPHEN Termed *paracetamol* in the United Kingdom, acetaminophen, a popular alternative to salicylates as an analgesic and antipyretic, is a frequent cause of poisoning. While the toxic and lethal doses of acetaminophen may vary from patient to patient, hepatic damage may be expected if an adult has taken more than 8 g as a single dose. A plasma concentration of greater than 200 μg/mL at 4 h after ingestion is also cause for concern. Clinical manifestations of acetaminophen poisoning are nonspecific. In the first few hours after ingestion lethargy, pallor, nausea, vomiting, and diaphoresis may occur; there are no acid-base derangements like those which may accompany aspirin overdose. Hepatic damage, the most important manifestation of acetaminophen toxicity, becomes evident 1 to 2 days after ingestion. While some patients show only elevation of serum transaminase and others show tender hepatomegaly and jaundice, more severe damage can lead to hyperammonemia, asterixis, mental confusion, coma, bleeding, and death from acute liver failure. Acute tubular necrosis, pancreatitis, hypoglycemia, cardiac damage, and hypersensitivity reactions sometimes are seen. Damage to tissue (especially liver) is caused by metabolites of acetaminophen and not the drug itself. At therapeutic doses acetaminophen is eliminated mainly conjugated to sulfate or glucuronic acid. After an overdose, the pathways of conjugation to the sulfate and glucuronic acid become saturated, an increasing fraction of the drug is activated by the P_{450} system, glutathione stores are depleted, and the reactive intermediates then become free to bind covalently to liver macromolecules and cause necrosis.

Treatment should begin with induction of emesis or gastric lavage followed by administration of activated charcoal. Since endogenous glutathione appears to have a protective effect, the administration of one of several other sulfhydryl compounds has been studied for protection against acetaminophen hepatotoxicity. When administered orally within 10 h of ingestion, either N-acetylcysteine or cysteamine is effective in decreasing hepatotoxicity. A potentially toxic dose (>7.5 g) ingested within the previous 24 h is an indication for N-acetylcysteine therapy. Since early treatment is paramount, a patient suspected of having ingested a potentially hepatotoxic dose should be started on sulfhydryl therapy while awaiting the plasma acetaminophen level. A 5% solution of N-acetylcysteine in a cola beverage or fruit juice is given with a loading dose of 140 mg/kg and a maintenance dose of 70 mg/kg every 4 h for 3 days. If sulfhydryl therapy is to be instituted, charcoal and osmotic cathartic administration are contraindicated since both may reduce absorption of the antidote. In a mixed poisoning, charcoal may be removed by lavage prior to administration of the antidote.

ACIDS   Corrosive acids are used widely in industry and laboratories. Ingestion is almost always with suicidal intent. Toxic effects are due to their direct chemical action. Ingestion of acids may produce irritation, bleeding, and sloughing in the mouth and esophagus with more severe burns occurring in the stomach, particularly in the pylorus. Perforations with peritonitis, though uncommon, may occur. Mouth and pharynx may be brownish black and may have a charred appearance. Yellow staining is seen after ingestion of nitric and picric acids. Severe pain in mouth, pharynx, chest, and abdomen is the rule and soon is followed by hematemesis and bloody diarrhea. Frequently profound shock develops and may be fatal. Survivors can develop mediastinitis or peritonitis from early or delayed esophageal or gastric perforation. Recovery from acid ingestion can be associated with stricture formation which most commonly involves the pylorus.

Ingested acid should be diluted immediately with large amounts of water or milk (when possible, in a hundredfold excess). The danger of perforation contraindicates the use of emesis or gastric lavage. Diagnostic esophagoscopy, if performed, should be done in the first 24 h after ingestion. Following the emergency measures, appropriate supportive therapy is administered for the relief of pain and the treatment of shock, perforation, and infection.

ALKALIES   Strong alkalies such as ammonium hydroxide, potassium hydroxide (potash), potassium carbonate, sodium hydroxide (lye, Clinitest tablets), and sodium carbonate (washing soda) are used widely in industry and in cleansers and drain cleaners. Sodium and potassium phosphates find use as water softeners. Strong alkalies form soaps with fats and proteinates with proteins, resulting in penetrating necrosis of tissues. Fatalities have occurred from the ingestion of 5 to 30 g of such compounds.

The toxic effects of alkalies are due to irritation and destruction of local tissues. Ingestion is followed by severe pain in mouth, pharynx, chest, and abdomen. Vomiting of blood and sloughed mucosa and diarrhea are common. Reflex loss of vascular tone frequently leads to profound shock. Perforation of the esophagus or stomach may be immediate or delayed for several days. Mouth and pharynx show erythema and gelatinous necrotic areas. After ingestion of water softeners profound reduction in serum calcium may be seen and lead to tetany and hypotension. Survivors usually suffer from esophageal strictures.

Treatment consists of immediate administration of large amounts of water or milk. Because of the danger of perforation, both induction of emesis and gastric lavage are contraindicated. Esophagoscopy should be done within the first 24 h in patients with significant esophageal or gastric burns. Steroids usually are administered for about 3 weeks to decrease the incidence of stricture formation, although definitive evidence of efficacy is lacking. After the ingestion of water softeners (phosphates), calcium gluconate should be administered intravenously as needed. Treatment is otherwise symptomatic and directed at the relief of pain, respiratory obstruction due to edema of the hypopharynx, fluid loss, and shock.

Inhalation of ammonia, which is used as a refrigerant, results in irritation of the upper and lower parts of the respiratory tract. Laryngeal and pulmonary edema may occur and must be treated symptomatically.

ANILINE   This substance is used in printing and clothmarking inks, paints, and paint removers. Both aniline and its derivatives, such as toluidine, nitroaniline, and nitrobenzene, are widely used in industrial synthesis. Aniline is absorbed from the gastrointestinal tract and through the lungs or skin. Ingestion of 1 g has been fatal. Methemoglobinemia is the most important manifestation. Headache, dizziness, hypotension, convulsions, and coma may occur. If the acute period is survived, jaundice and anemia may appear. Treatment consists of correction of methemoglobinemia (see Chap. 288) and supportive measures.

Antihistamines   The common and unprescribed use of antihistamines makes them readily available for accidental overdosage and suicide attempts. There is wide variation among patients in tolerance to these drugs and in the manifestations of poisoning. Manifestations of poisoning are central nervous system excitement or depression. In adults drowsiness, stupor, and coma predominate, but convulsions followed by further depression may occur.

Treatment is supportive and directed toward removal of the unabsorbed drug and maintenance of vital functions. Convulsions may be controlled with phenobarbital or diazepam. Some antihistamines have prominent atropine-like properties. Patients poisoned with these drugs may show manifestations of atropine poisoning and are treated accordingly (see below).

ANTIMUSCARINIC COMPOUNDS   Atropine, related belladonna alkaloids (hyoscyamine and scopolamine), and synthetic substitutes (e.g., benztropine, cyclopentolate, homatropine, methantheline, propantheline) are widely prescribed drugs and occur in many proprietary mixtures.

Individual sensitivity to the toxic effects of belladonna alkaloids varies widely; fatalities have occurred from as little as 10 mg atropine, but doses of 500 mg have been nonfatal. Young children are particularly susceptible to poisoning with belladonna alkaloids. Older persons appear to be more sensitive to the central nervous system effects of these drugs. Since atropine is both hydrolyzed in the liver and excreted unchanged in the urine, hepatic or renal insufficiency may lead to poisoning with otherwise therapeutic doses.

The most characteristic manifestations of atropine poisoning are those of parasympathetic blockade: dryness of mucous membranes, thirst, dysphagia, hoarseness, xerophthalmia, dilated pupils, blurring of vision, rise in intraocular tension, flushing, dryness and increased temperature of the skin, fever, tachycardia, hypertension, urinary retention, and abdominal distention. This widespread parasympatholysis is almost diagnostic of belladonna poisoning, but the diagnosis can be strengthened further by the reversal of blockade by physostigmine (2 mg administered intravenously over several minutes).

Central nervous system symptoms are also very common; atropine and scopolamine produce similar toxic psychoses. Restlessness, excitation, confusion, and incoordination precede mania, hallucinations, and delirium. Patients intoxicated by scopolamine not infrequently show lethargy and somnolence rather than excitement. In severe intoxication, central nervous system depression and coma are the rule. When death results, it is because of circulatory collapse and respiratory failure.

In the *treatment* of belladonna poisoning, emesis or gastric lavage should be followed by the administration of activated charcoal. Symptomatic treatment is directed at the reduction of body temperature, the moistening of mucous membranes, and urethral catheterization in the presence of urinary retention. Excitement or convulsions may require appropriate pharmacotherapy. Patients with deep coma, life-threatening cardiac arrhythmias, severe hallucinations, or severe hypertension have been treated with physostigmine with some reversal of these effects. It has not been established whether physostigmine reduces mortality.

Death occurs in fewer than 1 percent of cases of atropine or scopolamine poisoning. No permanent sequelae have been observed, but manifestations may persist for several days.

BENZENE, TOLUENE   These solvents are used in paint removers, dry-cleaning solutions, and rubber or plastic cements. Benzene is also present, to some extent, in most gasolines. Poisoning may result from ingestion or from the breathing of concentrated vapors. Toluene is an ingredient in some cement used by glue sniffers.

Acute poisoning by these compounds causes central nervous system manifestations. With sufficient exposure, symptoms progress from an initial period of restlessness, excitement, euphoria, and dizziness to coma, convulsions, and respiratory failure. Ventricular arrhythmias may occur. Renal tubular acidosis can occur following repeated inhalation of toluene. Chronic poisoning by benzene or toluene results from repeated exposure to their vapors in low concentration. Central nervous system symptoms include irritability, insomnia, headache, tremors, and paresthesias. Anorexia and nausea are also common. Fatty degeneration of the heart, liver, and kidneys may occur. By far the most important manifestation of chronic exposure to benzene is bone marrow depression, which may progress to aplastic anemia and complete aplasia of the bone marrow. Individual susceptibility to this effect varies greatly and may not become apparent for months after the initial exposure to the poison.

Treatment of both acute and chronic poisoning is symptomatic. Neurologic, pulmonary, or cardiovascular problems are treated as in poisoning by petroleum distillates.

BLEACHES Industrial strength bleaching solutions contain 10% or more sodium hypochlorite, while household products (e.g., Clorox, Purex, Sanichlor) contain 3 to 6%. The solution used for chlorinating swimming pools is 20%. Their corrosive action in mouth, pharynx, and esophagus is similar to that of sodium hydroxide. Acid gastric juice releases hypochlorous acid from such solutions. This compound is very irritating to mucous membranes, and inhalation of its fumes causes severe pulmonary irritation and pulmonary edema. However, the systemic toxicity of hypochlorous acid is low. Perforation and stricture formation are rare after the ingestion of household bleaching solutions.

Treatment consists of dilution of the ingested bleach with water or milk. The usual household bleaching solutions do not cause enough corrosive injury to the esophagus to preclude the induction of emesis or gastric lavage, but one should be wary of this possibility if one of the more concentrated solutions has been ingested. Although sodium thiosulfate (100 mL of a 1 to 2.5% solution by lavage), which will reduce hypochlorite to nontoxic products, has been administered routinely to these patients, there is great doubt that it is of any use except very early after ingestion of very large quantities of bleach.

CARBON MONOXIDE (CO) Carbon monoxide is a colorless, odorless, tasteless, and nonirritating gas produced by the incomplete combustion of carbonaceous materials. Almost any flame or combustion device emits carbon monoxide. The gas is present in the exhaust of internal combustion engines in a concentration of 3 to 7 percent. Much higher concentrations are generated during the burning of most illuminating and heating gases, but normally not in the burning of natural gas. However, if gas appliances are defective, incomplete combustion of natural gas and the generation of toxic amounts of carbon monoxide can occur. CO annually is responsible for about 3500 accidental and suicidal deaths in the United States.

The toxic effects of CO are the result of tissue hypoxia. CO combines with hemoglobin to form carboxyhemoglobin. Since CO and O_2 react with the same group in the hemoglobin molecule, and since the affinity of hemoglobin for CO is 200 times greater than for O_2, carboxyhemoglobin is incapable of carrying O_2. (At equilibrium 1 part of CO in 1500 parts of air will result in 50 percent conversion of hemoglobin to carboxyhemoglobin.) Carboxyhemoglobin also interferes with the release of O_2 from oxyhemoglobin. This further reduces the amount of O_2 available to the tissues and explains why tissue anoxia appears in the CO-poisoned person at levels of arterial oxyhemoglobin concentration well tolerated by the anemic patient.

The extent of saturation of hemoglobin with CO depends on the concentration of the gas in inspired air and on the time of exposure. The severity of hypoxic symptoms depends further on an individual's state of activity, tissue O_2 needs, and hemoglobin concentration. As a general rule, no symptoms will develop at a concentration of 0.01% CO in inspired air, since this will not raise blood saturation above 10%. Exposure to 0.05% for 1 h during light activity will produce a blood concentration of 20% carboxyhemoglobin and result in a mild

or throbbing headache. Greater activity or longer exposure to the same concentration causes a blood saturation of 30 to 50%. At this point headache, irritability, confusion, dizziness, visual disturbances, nausea, vomiting, and fainting on exertion may be observed. After exposure for 1 h to concentrations of 0.1% in inspired air, the blood will contain 50 to 80% carboxyhemoglobin, which results in coma, convulsions, respiratory failure, and death. On inhalation of high concentrations of CO, saturation of the blood proceeds so rapidly that unconsciousness may occur suddenly and without warning. When poisoning is more gradual, the individual may notice decreased exercise tolerance and dyspnea on exertion or even at rest. Patients with such subacute or chronic exposure can present with vague "flu-like" symptoms. Excessive sweating, fever, hepatomegaly, skin lesions, leukocytosis, bleeding diathesis, albuminuria, and glycosuria also have been described. Cerebral edema and intracranial hypertension may result from the increased permeability of hypoxic capillaries. Myocardial hypoxia is reflected by electrocardiographic abnormalities.

The most characteristic sign of severe CO poisoning is the cherry color of skin and mucous membranes, which results from the bright red carboxyhemoglobin. If the characteristic flush is not present and CO poisoning is suspected, 1 mL of the patient's blood can be diluted with 10 mL water; when 1 mL of 5% sodium hydroxide is added to this dilution, an oxyhemoglobin solution will turn brown. If significant amounts of carboxyhemoglobin are present, the solution will turn straw yellow (<20% carboxyhemoglobin) or will remain pink (>20% carboxyhemoglobin).

Treatment of CO poisoning requires effective ventilation in the presence of high O_2 tensions and in the absence of CO. If necessary, ventilation should be supported artificially. Pure O_2 should be administered. This will result not only in the replacement of CO by O_2 in the hemoglobin molecule but also in the partial relief of tissue hypoxia by O_2 dissolved in the plasma. For the same reasons hyperbaric O_2 is helpful in seriously poisoned patients. Transfusion of blood or packed cells is also of value. In order to reduce tissue needs for O_2, the patient must be kept absolutely quiet. Induction of hypothermia is not indicated. Cerebral edema should be treated with diuretics and steroids.

If severe tissue hypoxia has obtained too long, neurologic symptoms such as tremors, mental deterioration, and psychotic behavior may persist. Histologic changes characteristic of hypoxia may be observed in cerebral cortex, medulla, myocardium, and other organs.

CHLORINATED INSECTICIDES These compounds are ingredients of dusts, sprays, and solutions used as insecticides. The great majority of these compounds are chlorinated diphenyls (e.g., DDT, TDE, DFDT, DMC, Neotran) or chlorinated polycyclic compounds (e.g., aldrin, chlordane, dieldrin, endrin, hepatochlor). Lindane is a hexachlorobenzene. Their toxicity has led to their greatly diminished use in recent years, and many are banned in certain locales, including the United States. The chlorinated insecticides are soluble in lipid and organic solvents but not in water. They are poorly absorbed unless dissolved in a vehicle such as kerosene, petroleum distillates, or other organic solvents and can readily enter the body through the skin, lungs, or gastrointestinal tract. These compounds vary considerably in toxicity, and the toxicity of the dissolving vehicle must also be considered. The effects of the solvent may overshadow or modify those of the insecticide.

The initial symptoms of acute poisoning are nausea, vomiting, headache, dizziness, apprehension, excitement, and muscular tremors and weakness. These symptoms progress to generalized central nervous system hyperexcitability and delirium and clonic or tonic convulsions. This stage is in turn followed by progressive depression with paralysis, coma, and death. Except for endrin, which is strongly hepatotoxic, liver toxicity occurs only at extreme dosage levels. *Treatment* consists of induction of emesis or gastric lavage, activated charcoal administration, catharsis, anticonvulsive therapy, artificial ventilation, and other supportive measures. Sympathomimetic compounds should be avoided, since chlorinated insecticides apparently increase susceptibility to ventricular fibrillation. Cholestyramine accelerates the excretion of the chlorinated hydrocarbon chlordecone by preventing reabsorption following biliary excretion, and it may well have a similar effect on the excretion of pesticides such as DTT, dieldrin, chlordane, and heptachlor which remain in the body for prolonged periods.

CHOLINESTERASE INHIBITOR INSECTICIDES   Many substances used in agriculture for control of soft-bodied insects are potent inhibitors of cholinesterase. Most of these compounds are organic phosphates (e.g., Parathion, Malathion, Guthion), others are carbamates (e.g., Carbaryl, Mactacil). The toxicity of these compounds varies widely. Usually they are prepared for use by dilution with powders, organic solvents, or water. Formulations containing 1 to 95 percent of the active ingredient are available. The cholinesterase inhibitor insecticides are absorbed rapidly through the intact skin and after inhalation or ingestion.

The toxicity of these agents results from inactivation of acetylcholinesterase which allows accumulation of excessive amounts of acetylcholine at a number of sites: central nervous system, autonomic ganglia, parasympathetic nerve endings, and motor nerve endings. In the central nervous system coma and respiratory depression and, less commonly, seizures can occur. Toxic muscarinic effects include nausea, vomiting, diarrhea, involuntary defecation and urination, blurring of vision due to miosis, sweating, lacrimation, and salivation. Nicotinic effects include muscle twitching, fasciculations, weakness, and flaccid paralysis. Cardiac arrhythmias and pulmonary edema, as well as EEG abnormalities, also occur.

Treatment consists of emesis or lavage, charcoal instillation, catharsis, and washing of contaminated skin with soap and water. Atropine should be given immediately to block the parasympathetic and central nervous system effects. A dose of 2 mg is injected intramuscularly and repeated every 10 min until parasympathetic manifestations are controlled and signs of atropinization appear. The same dosage must be repeated frequently to maintain xerostomia and mild tachycardia. Fatal respiratory failure or pulmonary edema may occur quickly upon cessation of atropine therapy, and the drug should be withdrawn judiciously. Atropine is virtually ineffective against the autonomic ganglionic actions of acetylcholine and against the peripheral neuromuscular paralysis. Relief of muscle weakness, in particular respiratory paralysis, can be achieved with certain oximes which can reactivate cholinesterase by reversing the phosphate ester bond formed by the organic phosphate at the enzyme active site. Pralidoxime is useful in the treatment of organic phosphate cholinesterase inhibition but should not be used if the inhibition is due to a carbamate. A dose of 1 g pralidoxime in aqueous solution is administered intravenously over a 5-min period, and this dose is repeated up to four times every 8 to 12 h. Supportive therapy includes administration of oxygen with artifical ventilation if necessary, removal of pulmonary secretions by suction, and treatment of convulsions with diazepam and phenobarbital. Energetic therapy with artificial ventilation, atropine, and pralidoxime allows survival after doses of organic phosphate esters vastly exceeding the usual fatal dose.

CYANIDE   The cyanide ion is an exceedingly potent and rapid-acting poison, but one for which specific and effective antidotal therapy is available. Cyanide poisoning may result from the inhalation of hydrocyanic acid or from the ingestion of soluble inorganic cyanide salts or cyanide-releasing substances such as cyanamide, cyanogen chloride, and nitroprusside. Parts of many plants also contain substances such as amygdalin which release cyanide on digestion. Among these are the seeds of certain stone fruits (chokecherry, pin cherry, wild black cherry, peach, apricot, bitter almond), cassava roots, the berries of the jet berry bush, the leaves and shoots of elderberry, and all parts of hydrangea. The controversial drug Laetrile, composed in part of an extract of apricot kernels, has been responsible for fatal cyanide poisoning. Cyanides are widely used in industry and for fumigation and may reach the home in photographic chemicals or silver polishes. As little as 300 mg potassium cyanide may cause death.

The extreme toxicity of cyanide is due to its ready reaction with the trivalent iron of cytochrome oxidase. Formation of the cytochrome oxidase—cyanide complex blocks electron transport, thus inhibiting oxygen utilization. This results in cellular dysfunction and death. Inhalation of hydrogen cyanide may cause death within a minute. Oral doses act more slowly, requiring several minutes for the appearance of symptoms and up to several hours for death. The first effect is an increase in ventilation because of the blockade of oxidative metabolism in the chemoreceptor cells. As more cyanide is absorbed, there are headache, dizziness, nausea, drowsiness, hypotension, profound dyspnea, characteristic electrocardiographic changes, coma, and convulsions.

Cyanide poisoning is a true medical emergency. However, *treatment* is highly effective if given rapidly. The chemical antidotes should be immediately available wherever emergency medical care is dispensed. The diagnosis may be made by the characteristic "bitter almond" odor on the breath of the victim, and physicians should familiarize themselves with this smell. Since the saturation of hemoglobin is not disturbed by cyanide, cyanosis is not seen until respiratory depression supervenes. The objective of treatment is the production of methemoglobin by the administration of nitrite. The trivalent iron of methemoglobin competes with cytochrome oxidase for the cyanide ion. The cytochrome oxidase—cyanide complex dissociates, and enzymatic function and cell respiration are restored. Further detoxification then is achieved by the administration of thiosulfate. The enzyme rhodanese catalyzes the reaction of thiosulfate with cyanide liberated by the dissociation of cyanmethemoglobin; thiocyanate, which is relatively nontoxic, is formed and readily excreted in the urine.

Since speed is of the essence, nitrite should be immediately administered by inhalation of amyl nitrite perles, one every 2 min unless blood pressure is below 80 mmHg. This is followed as soon as possible by the intravenous injection of 10 mL of 3% sodium nitrite over a 3-min period. An intravenous infusion of norepinephrine may be necessary to maintain blood pressure during this injection period. After the administration of sodium nitrite, 50 mL of 25% sodium thiosulfate should be administered intravenously over a 10-min period. Supportive measures, especially artificial respiration with 100% O_2, should be instituted as soon as possible, but unless methemoglobinemia is produced promptly, other forms of treatment are of no value. Administration of sodium nitrite and sodium thiosulfate may have to be repeated. Ideally, dosage should be based on methemoglobin determinations, and the methemoglobin should not exceed 40%. If the patient survives 4 h, recovery is likely but residual cerebral symptoms may persist.

DETERGENTS AND SOAPS   These substances fall into the three groups of anionic, nonionic, and cationic detergents. The first group contains common soaps and household detergents. They may cause vomiting and diarrhea but have no serious effects, and no treatment is required. However, some laundry compounds contain phosphate water softeners whose ingestion may cause hypocalcemia. The ingestion of nonionic detergents also requires no treatment.

Cationic detergents, such as benzalkonium chloride and many others, are commonly used for bactericidal purposes in hospitals and homes. These compounds are well absorbed from the gastrointestinal tract and interfere with cellular functions. The fatal oral dose is approximately 3 g. Concentrated preparations (>20% detergent) are corrosive to mouth and esophagus. Ingestion produces nausea and vomiting, and shock, coma, convulsions, and death may occur in a few hours. Treatment after ingestion of dilute preparations consists of minimizing gastrointestinal absorption by emesis and gastric lavage with ordinary soap solution, which rapidly inactivates cationic detergents. Emesis and lavage are contraindicated in the presence of esophageal injury which is unlikely to occur except after ingestion of concentrated preparations. Activated charcoal and an osmotic cathartic should be administered. If significant absorption has occurred, intensive supportive therapy may be required.

FLUORIDES Fluoride salts are used in insecticides. The gases fluorine and hydrogen fluoride are used in industry; the latter is a strong corrosive. Fluorine and fluorides are cellular poisons which inhibit a number of enzymatic reactions, probably the most important of which is the glycolytic degradation of glucose. Fluorides also form an insoluble precipitate with calcium and cause hypocalcemia. Finally, in an acid medium fluorides form the corrosive hydrofluoric acid. Ingestion of 1 to 2 g sodium fluoride may be fatal.

Inhalation of fluorine or hydrogen fluoride produces coughing and choking. After an asymptomatic period of a day or two, fever, cough, cyanosis, and pulmonary edema may develop. Ingestion of fluoride salts is followed by nausea, vomiting productive of corroded tissues, diarrhea, and abdominal pain. Consequent to the decrease in serum calcium the victim develops muscular hyperirritability, fasciculations, tremors, spasms, and convulsions. Death results from respiratory paralysis or circulatory collapse. If the patient survives the acute period, jaundice and oliguria may appear. Chronic fluoride poisoning (fluorosis) is characterized by weight loss, weakness, anemia, brittle bones, and stiff joints. Mottling of teeth is seen when exposure occurs during enamel formation.

Treatment of acute fluoride poisoning consists of immediate administration of milk, lime water, calcium gluconate, or calcium lactate solution to precipitate calcium fluoride. After lavage or emesis and charcoal instillation, calcium (e.g., calcium gluconate, 10 g) can be given again followed by an osmotic cathartic. Then 10% calcium gluconate or 1% calcium chloride should be slowly injected intravenously and repeated as needed to prevent a positive Chvostek's sign. Symptomatic and supportive therapy is administered as indicated.

FORMALDEHYDE This gas is available as 40% solution (formalin) which is used as a disinfectant, fumigant, or deodorant. Poisoning by formalin may be diagnosed by the characteristic odor of formaldehyde. Formaldehyde reacts chemically with cellular constituents, depresses cellular functions, and causes cell death. The fatal dose of formalin is about 60 mL. Ingestion of formalin immediately causes severe abdominal pain, nausea, vomiting, and diarrhea. This may be followed by collapse, coma, severe metabolic acidosis, and anuria. Death is usually the result of circulatory failure.

Since any organic material can inactivate formaldehyde, milk, bread, soup, etc., should be administered immediately unless activated charcoal is available. Formaldehyde is a corrosive, and emesis and lavage are not recommended. Parenteral administration of sodium bicarbonate is indicated to combat acidosis. The treatment is otherwise supportive.

GLYCOLS Ethylene glycol and diethylene glycol are used in antifreeze solutions. The more than 50 annual deaths from these compounds usually result from intentional drinking of antifreeze by alcoholics. The fatal dose of ethylene glycol is about 100 g while that of diethylene glycol is somewhat lower. Glycols are metabolized by alcohol dehydrogenase to the aldehyde, which is ultimately converted to oxalate. It is the metabolites of the glycols (particularly the aldehyde and oxalate) which are most responsible for toxicity after glycol ingestion.

The initial symptoms of acute poisoning by these glycols resemble those of alcoholic intoxication. They may progress to vomiting, stupor, coma with absent reflexes and anisocoria, and convulsions. Tachypnea, bradycardia, and hypothermia are seen commonly, as are metabolic acidosis and hyocalcemia. After massive ingestion death may occur from respiratory failure within a few hours or from pulmonary edema within a day or two. If the patient survives this stage, acute tubular necrosis often develops.

Intravenous infusion of ethanol to maintain a blood level of 100 mg/dL is effective in competing for alcohol dehydrogenase, thus slowing the conversion of glycol to the more toxic aldehyde. Pyridoxine (100 mg daily administered intravenously) and thiamine (100 mg daily administered intravenously) are given to stimulate conversion of glyoxalate, the immediate metabolic precursor of oxalate, to the nontoxic metabolites, glycine and α-hydroxy-β-ketoadipate, respectively. However, the effectiveness of these latter procedures has not been established. Dialysis is highly effective in the removal of ethylene and diethylene glycol from the body. Acidosis and hypocalcemia must be treated vigorously.

HALOGENATED HYDROCARBONS Halogenated hydrocarbons (carbon tetrachloride, ethylene chlorohydrin, ethylene dichloride, methyl halides, trichloroethane, trichloroethylene) find wide industrial use as solvents, refrigerants, and fumigants, and in chemical synthesis. They enter the home in household cleaners, floor waxes, fire extinguishers, and rubber or plastic cements. These compounds are highly fat-soluble and produce cell damage either directly or after conversion in the body to other compounds. Individual halogenated hydrocarbons differ considerably in the degree and the exact manifestations of their toxicity, but in sufficient concentration all these compounds are capable of inducing central nervous system depression and varying amounts of hepatic and renal toxicity. Myocardial depression, vascular damage, and pulmonary edema also may occur.

The most important halogenated hydrocarbon is carbon tetrachloride, which still is employed widely as a nonflammable solvent and fire extinguisher fluid but which largely has been replaced in products intended for household use by the less toxic trichloroethane. Poisoning may occur from inhalation of the vapor, ingestion, or, rarely, percutaneous absorption. An oral dose of as little as 4 mL may be fatal. Absorption from the gastrointestinal tract is slow and unpredictable but is increased by the presence of fats and alcohol. Abdominal pain, hematemesis, and hepatic damage are more common and severe after ingestion than when the poison is inhaled. Inhalation may lead to irritation of the upper part of the respiratory tract.

Acute systemic absorption of carbon tetrachloride results in nausea, dizziness, confusion, and headache within a few minutes. Depending upon the quantity absorbed, the symptoms may quickly progress to stupor, coma, convulsions, respiratory failure, hypotension, or ventricular fibrillation. The patient may recover from these immediate manifestations until evidence of hepatic or renal toxicity appears several hours to several days after the exposure. Liver and kidney damage also may occur in the absence of any severe early central nervous system effects. Initially tender hepatomegaly may be present, jaundice may be rapidly progressive, and death due to severe centrilobular necrosis may occur within days. The renal lesion has the characteristics of acute tubular necrosis, and manifests itself by proteinuria, hematuria, oliguria, or anuria. Uremia, acidosis, hypertension, and pulmonary edema may develop as complications of renal failure. Optic neuritis, pancreatitis, and adrenal cortical necrosis are less common manifestations of carbon tetrachloride intoxication.

Chronic poisoning may occur after repeated exposures to low concentrations of carbon tetrachloride and may also lead to liver or kidney damage. Usually it manifests itself by vague symptoms of fatigue, weakness, mental confusion, abdominal pain, anorexia, nausea, blurring of vision, and paresthesias.

Treatment of acute poisoning by halogenated hydrocarbons includes vigorous efforts at minimizing gastrointestinal absorption by lavage or emesis and catharsis. Treatment is otherwise symptomatic. Sympathomimetic drugs should be avoided because of the danger of inducing ventricular arrhythmias in the sensitized myocardium. Acute renal and hepatic failure must be managed carefully. Often, hemodialysis is required and may be lifesaving until kidney function returns 3 or more weeks after poisoning. Both hemodialysis and hemoperfusion will effectively remove carbon tetrachloride and trichloroethane from the body but are potentially useful in preventing severe toxicity and death only when begun early in the postingestion period.

IODINE The traditional antiseptic iodine tincture is an alcoholic solution of 2% iodine and 2% sodium iodide. Strong iodine solution (Lugol's solution) is an aqueous solution of 5% iodine and 10% potassium iodide. The fatal dose of tincture of iodine is approximately

2 g. Iodides are very much less toxic, and no fatalities have been reported.

The diagnosis of iodine poisoning is suggested by the brown staining of the oral mucous membranes. The effects largely result from the corrosive effects of the compound on the gastrointestinal tract. Burning abdominal pain, nausea, vomiting, and bloody diarrhea may occur soon after ingestion. If the stomach contained starch, the vomitus is blue or black. Tissue trauma from corrosive gastroenteritis and fluid loss by vomiting and diarrhea may result in shock. Severe edema of the glottis, fever, delirium, stupor, and anuria also have been observed.

Treatment consists of the immediate administration of milk, starch, bread, etc., or activated charcoal to provide a source other than human tissue with which the iodine can react. Catharsis should be induced. Sodium thiosulfate will reduce iodine to less toxic iodide; 100 mL of a 5% solution should be given orally followed by an osmotic cathartic. A 10-mL dose of a 10% thiosulfate solution also should be given intravenously every 4 h. Induction of emesis and lavage should not be attempted if esophageal injury is suspected. With appropriate treatment most patients poisoned by iodine survive, but esophageal strictures may complicate their recovery.

IRON SALTS (See Chap. 172)

ISOPROPYL ALCOHOL This compound is used as a sterilizing agent or as rubbing alcohol. Ingestion produces gastric irritation and raises the danger of vomiting with aspiration. The systemic effects of isopropyl alcohol are similar to those of ethyl alcohol, but it is approximately twice as potent as the latter. Coma is produced readily but rarely lasts longer than 12 h. About 15 percent of an ingested dose of isopropanol is metabolized to acetone; transient acetonuria is common, but significant acidosis does not occur. Emesis should be induced, or gastric lavage should be performed. Supportive therapy is required only after ingestion of massive amounts, and there are no sequelae other than transient gastritis.

MAGNESIUM Magnesium sulfate is used intravenously as a hypotensive agent and orally as a cathartic. The magnesium ion is a profound depressant of the central nervous system and of neuromuscular transmission. Poisoning after oral or rectal administration is unlikely in the presence of normal renal function, because the kidney removes magnesium more rapidly than it is absorbed by the gastrointestinal tract. In the presence of impaired renal function an oral dose of 30 g may be fatal. Symptoms begin at a serum magnesium level of 4 meq per liter, and concentrations of over 12 meq per liter may be fatal. Oral ingestion of concentrated solutions may cause gastrointestinal irritation. Manifestations of systemic poisoning are depression of reflexes, flaccid paralysis, hypotension, hypothermia, coma, and respiratory failure. Respiratory death usually precedes significant myocardial depression. The actions of magnesium on neurologic and neuromuscular function are antagonized by calcium. *Treatment* of magnesium poisoning therefore includes the intravenous administration of 10 mL of a 10% solution of calcium gluconate, which may be repeated as necessary.

METHYL ALCOHOL This simplest of alcohols, also called wood alcohol or methanol, is used as a solvent, antifreeze, paint remover, and as a denaturant in ethyl alcohol. Denatured ethyl alcohol preparations, such as Sterno or Solox, contain 5 to 15% methyl alcohol as well as other denaturants. Methyl alcohol poisoning results almost entirely from its ingestion as a substitute for ethanol or to the drinking of denatured ethyl alcohol. The toxic dose is quite variable: death has occurred after a dose of 20 mL, but 250 mL has been ingested with survival. As little as 15 mL methanol has caused permanent blindness.

Methanol is less inebriating than ethyl alcohol, and inebriation is not a prominent symptom of methyl alcohol intoxication. Methanol is oxidized in the body by alcohol dehydrogenase first to formaldehyde and then to formic acid; these metabolites cause the toxic mainfestations of methanol poisoning. At equivalent concentrations the rate of its metabolism is only 15 percent that of ethanol for which alcohol dehydrogenase has a greater affinity and which can inhibit competitively the rate of metabolism of methanol. Formic acid and especially formaldehyde have toxic actions on many cells; the retina and optic nerve are damaged specifically. The toxic metabolites of methyl alcohol are also responsible for the severe acidosis which is the most prominent feature of methyl alcohol poisoning. This acidosis results partly from the accumulation of formic acid, but formate also appears to exert an inhibitory effect upon enzymes involved in the oxidation of carbohydrate with consequent accumulation of acid intermediates.

Symptoms of methanol poisoning usually do not appear until 12 to 24 h after ingestion, when sufficient toxic metabolites have accumulated. Manifestations include headache, dizziness, nausea, vomiting, vasomotor disturbances, central nervous system depression, and respiratory failure. Visual disturbance is almost universal and ranges from mild blurring of vision to total blindness. Impairment of vision may be transient, but permanent blindness may follow survival of the acute intoxication. The pupils are dilated and nonreactive, and there is hyperemia of the optic disc and retinal edema. Acidosis is commonly severe.

In the *treatment* of methyl alcohol intoxication emesis and gastric lavage are of use only within the first 2 h after ingestion. Intravenous administration of large amounts of sodium bicarbonate combats acidosis. Return of acidosis is frequent after initial correction, and additional alkali must be administered as indicated by close observation of the patient and laboratory determinations. It is most useful to obtain a blood methanol level as soon as possible. At any time after ingestion, levels between 20 and 50 mg/dL are associated with acidosis and significant symptomatology and are an indication for intravenous ethanol therapy (1 g ethanol per kilogram of body weight in 5% dextrose in water over 30 min to load, then 7 to 10 g/h in adults to maintain the blood ethanol level at about 100 mg/dL). Severely symptomatic patients should be treated even if a methanol level cannot be obtained. A methanol level exceeding 50 mg/dL is an indication for hemodialysis as well as ethanol therapy; dialysis also is indicated in the presence of severe acidosis with lower blood levels.

MUSHROOMS There are many species of poisonous mushrooms, but in the United States most poisoning is due to the *Amanita*. More than 100 deaths result each year from consumption of wild poisonous mushrooms, 90 percent being due to *A. phalloides* (death cap) or closely related species. Fatalities have occurred after ingestion of only part of one mushroom.

A usually less severe poisoning follows ingestion of *A. muscaria* (fly agaric) which contains the parasympathomimetic alkaloid muscarine, as well as variable amounts of a substance active on the central nervous system and a parasympatholytic alkaloid. Symptoms are largely those of parasympathetic stimulation: lacrimation, pupillary constriction, perspiration, salivation, nausea, vomiting, diarrhea, abdominal pain, bronchorrhea, wheezing, dyspnea, bradycardia, and hypotension. Muscular tremors, confusion, excitement, and delirium are common in severe poisoning. Very rarely symptoms of atropine poisoning have predominated. After ingestion of *A. muscaria,* symptoms appear within minutes to 2 h. The patient may die within a few hours, but with appropriate therapy complete recovery in 24 h is the rule.

A. phalloides, A. virosa (destroying angel), some other *Amanita* species, and *Galerina venenata* contain heat-stable cyclopeptide cytotoxins which are rapidly bound to tissues. The principal toxin is α-amanitin, which binds to and inhibits specifically the mammalian RNA polymerase responsible for messenger RNA synthesis. Severe cell damage and fatty degeneration may occur in liver, kidneys, striated muscle, and brain. Ingestion of these dangerous mushrooms is followed by a latent period of 6 to 20 h. Manifestations of cytotoxicity then may appear suddenly and consist of severe nausea, violent abdominal pain, bloody vomiting and diarrhea, and cardiovascular collapse. Headache, mental confusion, coma, or convulsions are common. Painful and tender hepatomegaly, jaundice, hypoglycemia, dehydration, and oliguria or anuria frequently appear on the first or second day after ingestion. The victim may die from acute hepatic necrosis (yellow atrophy) within 4 days. About one-half of all poisonings with *A. phalloides* have a fatal outcome in 5 to 8 days. Recovery tends to be slow.

Ingestion of other poisonous mushrooms may cause gastrointestinal symptoms, visual disturbances, ataxia, disorientation, convulsions, coma, fever, hemolysis, and methemoglobinemia.

Treatment of mushroom poisoning depends upon the species ingested. If parasympathomimetic manifestations are prominent, atropine in doses of 1 to 2 mg is given intramuscularly and repeated every 30 min until symptoms are controlled. Poisoning by cytotoxic mushrooms is treated mainly symptomatically. Fluid and electrolyte balance must be carefully maintained. Hypoglycemia should be avoided; large quantities of carbohydrate may exert some protective effect on the liver. Excitement, convulsions, pain, hypotension, and fever may need symptomatic therapy. Early intensive hemoperfusion can remove α-amanitin from the body and probably is indicated in *A. phalloides* poisoning. Both thioctic acid (α-lipoic acid) and cytochrome c have been advocated as antidotes for α-amanitin poisoning, but convincing data as to their efficacy are lacking.

NAPHTHALENE Poisoning by this substance almost always results from ingestion of moth repellents. An oral dose of 2 g has been fatal. Nausea, vomiting, and diarrhea are the initial symptoms. Larger doses may produce hepatic damage with jaundice and renal toxicity which may progress to hematuria, oliguria, or anuria. Depending upon the amount ingested, central nervous system manifestations may range from headache, mental confusion, and excitement to coma and convulsions. In persons with glucose 6-phosphate dehydrogenase-deficient red blood cells the ingestion of naphthalene will produce hemolysis. *Treatment* consists of emesis or gastric lavage, catharsis, and supportive measures.

NICOTINE This alkaloid is an exceedingly potent and rapidly acting poison. It is a component of many insecticides. Nicotine is absorbed readily from the oral and gastrointestinal mucosa, from the respiratory tract, and through the skin. The lethal dose for an adult is approximately 50 mg, the quantity contained in two cigarettes. However, tobacco is much less toxic than would be anticipated on the basis of its nicotine content. Nicotine is poorly absorbed from ingested tobacco, and on smoking, most of the nicotine is burned. Nicotine acts on chemoreceptors, on synapses in the central nervous system and in autonomic ganglia, on the adrenal medulla, and on neuroeffector junctions. Furthermore, its transient initial stimulant effects are followed by a more persistent depressant phase of action. It is not surprising that the manifestations of nicotine poisoning are highly complex and somewhat unpredictable.

Small doses of nicotine produce nausea, vomiting, diarrhea, headache, dizziness, and neurologic stimulation manifested by tachycardia, hypertension, hyperpnea, tachypnea, sweating, and salivation. Larger doses also cause cortical irritability, progressing to convulsions, and myocardial arrhythmias. Finally coma, respiratory depression and arrest, and cardiac arrest or fibrillation may supervene. Severe poisoning may cause death from respiratory failure within a few minutes.

Treatment consists of induction of emesis or gastric lavage, followed by the instillation of activated charcoal and the administration of an osmotic cathartic. Potassium permanganate will oxidize nicotine, and a 1:10,000 solution can be used for lavage. Atropine, 2 mg, and phentolamine, 5 mg, may be given intramuscularly or intravenously and repeated as often as required to control signs and symptoms of parasympathetic or sympathetic hyperactivity. These compounds are ineffective in preventing paralysis of the respiratory muscles and disturbances in cardiac rhythm. Careful attention must be given to artificial ventilation with oxygen and to therapy of catecholamine-induced cardiac tachyarrhythmias. Propranolol is the drug of choice for the latter purpose. Nicotine is rapidly detoxified in the liver, and

recovery will be prompt if the patient can be tided over the initial period.

NITRITES Poisoning by the nitrite ion may result from the ingestion of large amounts of drugs such as amyl, butyl, isobutyl, or sodium nitrite. Ingested nitrates may be reduced to nitrite by intestinal bacteria, especially *Escherichia coli*. Except after the ingestion of very large amounts, adults usually absorb all nitrate before this reduction takes place. However, in children nitrite poisoning may result from the ingestion of nitrates or nitrate-containing well water. Fatalities have occurred from the oral ingestion of 2 to 4 g nitrites.

Acute nitrite poisoning may lead to severe headache, flushing, dizziness, hypotension, and syncope. Usually the patient only need be positioned to facilitate venous return to the heart. Pressor agents seldom are required. The most important toxic effect of the nitrite ion is its ability to oxidize hemoglobin to methemoglobin (Chaps. 53 and 288).

PARAQUAT Paraquat is a dipyridilium compound which is used in 5 to 20% aqueous solutions as a herbicide. An oral dose of 5 mg/kg may be fatal. Some victims die within 24 h in respiratory failure, often with refractive pulmonary edema. In others a serious toxic effect is the delayed (3 days to 2 weeks postingestion) development of progressive pulmonary fibrosis. The lungs selectively accumulate paraquat from the blood over several days until a critical concentration is reached, after which pulmonary edema and fibrosis ensue. Progressive respiratory failure is the usual cause of death. The metabolism of paraquat by lung tissue leads to the production of radical intermediates as well as the superoxide radical; the latter appears to be at least partly responsible for the toxicity of the compound.

Prolonged absorption (up to several days) of paraquat from the gastrointestinal tract is common. After gastric emptying, diluted bentonite (Fuller's earth) or activated charcoal should be administered followed by an osmotic cathartic twice daily for 48 h. Forced diuresis, hemodialysis, and hemoperfusion significantly augment clearance of paraquat. Oxygen administration to animals experimentally poisoned with paraquat is associated with increased mortality; it would seem prudent to avoid, if possible, oxygen-enriched breathing mixtures in patients poisoned with paraquat. Intravenous administration of superoxide dismutase has been reported to decrease lung toxicity from paraquat in animals, but no beneficial effect has been demonstrated yet in humans.

PETROLEUM DISTILLATES Petroleum distillates (diesel oil, gasoline, kerosene, paint thinner, solvent distillate) are liquids with a boiling point between 50 and 325°C. They contain variable amounts of branched or straight-chain aliphatic and aromatic hydrocarbons. Kerosene is used widely as a fuel and as a vehicle for cleaning agents, furniture polishes, insecticides, and paint thinners. Not surprisingly, each year petroleum distillates cause about 100 accidental deaths in the United States, 90 percent of these in young children. Furthermore, these products are annually responsible for almost 20,000 hospitalizations. Ingestion of 10 mL kerosene has been fatal, but adults have recovered from as much as 250 mL. Petroleum distillates are central nervous system depressants; they damage cells by dissolving cellular lipids. Pulmonary damage manifested by pulmonary edema or pneumonitis is a common and serious complication.

Inhalation of gasoline or kerosene vapors induces a state resembling alcoholic intoxication. Headache, nausea, tinnitus, and a burning sensation in the chest may also be present. When aliphatic hydrocarbons are inhaled, these symptoms may progress to profound drowsiness or coma with absence of deep reflexes. If the distillate contains a high proportion of aromatic hydrocarbons, the coma is characterized by tremors, muscle jactitations, hyperactive reflexes, and convulsions. Death usually results from respiratory depression, rarely from ventricular fibrillation.

The oral ingestion of petroleum distillates causes irritation of the mucous membranes of the upper part of the intestinal tract. When large amounts have been ingested, the same manifestations as after inhalation may appear. Frequently eructation or vomiting results in aspiration of petroleum distillates into the trachea. Because of their low surface tension, minute amounts of these substances then may spread widely throughout the lungs and produce pulmonary edema and pneumonitis. Pulmonary damage also may arise because of absorption of ingested petroleum distillates from the gastrointestinal tract. However, kerosene is at least 100 times more toxic by the intratracheal route than when ingested.

In the *treatment* of poisoning by petroleum distillates extreme care must be used to prevent aspiration. If the patient is coughing when seen, aspiration is likely already to have occurred. When large amounts (>100 mL) have been ingested, gastric emptying is indicated. In the alert patient emesis may be induced; when vomiting occurs, the head of the patient should be lower than the hips. Otherwise, gastric lavage should be performed but only after insertion of an endotracheal tube with an inflatable cuff. A saline cathartic may be administered. All victims of kerosene poisoning should be hospitalized for at least 24 h for observation. If signs or symptoms of pulmonary irritation appear, oxygen should be given. Steroids do not appear useful in treatment of this pulmonary lesion and may be detrimental. Prophylactic antibiotics are not indicated. Symptomatic therapy for central nervous system depression or treatment of convulsions may be necessary. Sympathomimetic amines should be avoided because of the danger of inducing ventricular fibrillation in the hydrocarbon-sensitized heart.

PHENOL Phenol and related compounds (creosote, cresols, hexachlorophene, hydroquinone, Lysol, resorcinol, tannic acid) are used as antiseptics, caustics, and preservatives. These substances poison all cells by denaturing and precipitating cellular proteins. The approximate fatal oral dose ranges from 2 mL for phenol and cresols to 20 mL for tannic acid.

Ingestion of phenolic compounds produces erosion of mucosa from mouth to stomach. The corroded areas may have a characteristic dead-white appearance. Hematemesis and bloody diarrhea may occur. After an initial phase of hyperpnea due to stimulation of the respiratory center, stupor, coma, convulsions, pulmonary edema, and shock are seen. The initial respiratory alkalosis is soon followed by a profound acidosis which results from the renal excretion of base during the alkalotic stage, from the acidic nature of phenol, and from disturbances in carbohydrate metabolism, presumably the result of defects in enzymatic function. If the patient survives the acute stage, acute tubular necrosis may lead to oliguria or anuria and hepatic toxicity to jaundice. Poisoning by phenolic compounds often may be diagnosed by their characteristic odor. Development of a violet or blue color of the urine after addition of a few drops of ferric chloride indicates the presence of a phenolic compound.

Emesis and lavage are indicated for *treatment* in the absence of significant corrosive injury to the esophagus. Activated charcoal should be administered. Although definitive proof of efficacy is lacking, olive oil or castor oil, which dissolve phenol and are reputed to retard its absorption, may be given, followed by an osmotic cathartic. Supportive therapy consists of correction of the acidosis, the control of shock and convulsions, and the maintenance of a patent airway in the face of glottal edema by intubation or tracheotomy.

PHOSPHORUS Phosphorus occurs in two forms: a red, nonpoisonous form and a yellow, fat-soluble, highly toxic form. The latter is used in rodent and insect poisons and in fireworks. Yellow phosphorus and phosphides cause fatty degeneration and necrosis of tissues, particularly of the liver. The lethal ingested dose of yellow phosphorus is approximately 50 mg.

Ingestion of yellow phosphorus is followed within 1 h by burning pain in the upper part of the gastrointestinal tract, vomiting, diarrhea, and a garlic odor of the breath and excreta. The patient may die in coma during the first day or two, or symptoms may subside after a few hours. Then, 1 to 2 days later, the victim may develop tender hepatomegaly, jaundice, hypocalcemia, hypotension, and oliguria

and may die following convulsions and coma. Death from acute hepatic necrosis may occur in a few days.

Treatment consists of induction of emesis or gastric lavage, instillation of activated charcoal, and administration of an osmotic cathartic. Calcium gluconate is given intravenously to maintain the serum calcium level. Treatment is otherwise supportive.

SALICYLATES Each year 30 million pounds of aspirin is consumed in the United States, and salicylates can probably be found in most American households. Aspirin is found in many compound analgesic tablets. Methyl salicylate (oil of wintergreen) is present in most skin liniments, and salicylic acid is used in ointments and corn plasters. The ingestion of 10 to 30 g aspirin or sodium salicylate may be fatal to adults, but survival has been reported after an oral dose of 130 g aspirin.

Salicylate intoxication may result from the cumulative effect of therapeutic administration of high doses. There is considerable individual variation: toxic symptoms may begin at dosages of 3 g per day or may not appear when 10 g per day is given. Toxic symptoms are also poorly correlated with the serum salicylate concentration, but few patients become intoxicated at levels less than 15 mg/dL and most at levels over 35 mg/dL. Therapeutic salicylate intoxication is usually mild and is called *salicylism*. The earliest symptoms are vertigo, tinnitus, and impairment of hearing. Further overdosage causes nausea, vomiting, sweating, diarrhea, fever, drowsiness, headache, dimness of vision, and mental aberrations. The latter may be characterized by confusion, excitement, restlessness, and talkativeness; this "salicylate jag" resembles alcoholic intoxication without the euphoria. The central nervous system effects may progress to hallucinations, convulsions, and coma. Toxic doses of salicylates also have a direct stimulant effect on the respiratory center, resulting in hyperventilation, loss of carbon dioxide, and respiratory alkalosis. Renal excretion of bicarbonate may compensate partially for this.

In acute salicylate poisoning due to accidental or suicidal ingestion of massive amounts, the same manifestations may be seen in more rapid succession. However, they usually are overshadowed by severe disturbances in the acid-base balance which follow a definite sequence. Early in the course of intoxication there may be only hyperpnea, and the seriousness of the poisoning may not be appreciated at that time. The hyperventilation causes a fall in blood P_{CO_2} and an increase in pH. Renal excretion of bicarbonate, sodium, and potassium will bring the pH back toward normal and produce a compensated respiratory alkalosis. At that point the buffering capacity of the extracellular fluid will have been decreased significantly. In young children and after large doses in adults further developments may then produce a combination of respiratory acidosis and metabolic acidosis which stems from a number of factors. High concentrations of salicylate depress the respiratory center and cause CO_2 retention. Renal function becomes impaired because of dehydration and hypotension, and inorganic metabolic acids accumulate. Furthermore, salicylic acid derivatives may displace several milliequivalents of blood bicarbonate. Finally, salicylates impair carbohydrate metabolism and cause accumulation of acetoacetic, lactic, and pyruvic acids. Severe acidosis and disturbances in electrolyte balance are seen most commonly in febrile young children.

Blood salicylate levels are of value in the estimation of the severity of poisoning. Serious poisoning is rare at levels less than 50 mg/dL but usual at levels between 50 and 100 mg/dL. Levels above 100 mg/dL during the first 6 h after poisoning signify severe intoxication and may be fatal. Excretion of salicylates is renal, and in the presence of normal renal function about 50 percent will be excreted in 24 h. Addition of a few drops of ferric chloride solution to 5 mL boiled acidified urine containing salicylate yields a violet color and may aid in diagnosis.

Treatment of salicylate poisoning consists initially of inducing emesis or of gastric lavage after which activated charcoal and then an osmotic cathartic are administered. Disturbances of acid-base or electrolyte balance and hypoglycemia are corrected by the intravenous administration of appropriate solutions. Respiratory depression may require artificial ventilation with oxygen. Convulsions may be treated with diazepam or phenobarbital. The renal clearance of salicylate is enhanced ten- to twentyfold if the pH of the urine can be kept between 7 and 8. In addition to intravenous bicarbonate and a diuretic to raise the pH above 7, it may be necessary to give potassium to prevent paradoxical aciduria. Peritoneal dialysis and hemodialysis are also highly effective in removing salicylate from seriously poisoned patients, but forced alkaline diuresis is so effective in clearing salicylate that these maneuvers most often are not required.

SMOKE Poisoning by smoke is usually due to carbon monoxide inhalation. However, burning material may also release irritant fumes. Many irritant gases combine with water to form corrosive acids or alkalies and cause chemical burns of exposed skin and of the upper part of the respiratory tract. Such gases (and the corrosives formed) are ammonia (ammonium hydroxide), nitrogen oxide (nitric acid), sulfur dioxide (sulfurous acid), and sulfur trioxide (sulfuric acid). These irritating gases as well as hydrogen sulfide also may be present in smog. Another highly toxic gas which may be inhaled by firefighters or victims is phosgene. This compound is formed by the high-temperature decomposition of chlorinated hydrocarbons and is released when carbon tetrachloride from fire extinguishers comes into contact with hot surfaces.

After inhalation of irritant gases the victim may notice burning pain in the throat and chest and severe coughing. These symptoms may subside completely, but from several hours to a day after exposure dyspnea and cyanosis may appear and progress rapidly to severe pulmonary edema and death from respiratory and circulatory failure. Treatment consists of administration of oxygen and adrenal steroids and appropriate therapy of pulmonary edema, should that develop.

REFERENCES

General

ARENA JM: *Poisoning: Toxicology, Symptoms, Treatments,* 4th ed. Springfield, Ill, Charles C Thomas, 1979
ARLEFF AL et al: Coma following nonnarcotic drug overdosage—management of 208 adult patients. Am J Med Sci 266:405, 1973
BOURNE PG: *Acute Drug Abuse Emergencies.* New York, Academic, 1976
Casarett and Doull's Toxicology: The Basic Science of Poisons, 2d ed, J Doull, CD Klaasen, MO Amdur (eds). New York, Macmillan, 1980
DREISBACH RH: *Handbook of Poisoning: Prevention, Diagnosis and Treatment,* 11th ed. Los Altos, CA, Lange, 1983
HADDAD LM, WINCHESTER JF: *Clinical Management of Poisoning and Drug Overdose.* Philadelphia, Saunders, 1983
LOOMIS TA: *Essentials of Toxicology,* 3d ed. Philadelphia, Lea & Febiger, 1978
LOVEJOY FH JR: Acute poisoning, in *Current Pediatric Therapy,* 9th ed, SS Gellis, BM Kegan (eds). Philadelphia, Saunders, 1980, p 654
TURK MH: *Occupational Medicine: Surveillance, Diagnosis and Treatment.* Cambridge, MA, Ballinger, 1982
WINCHESTER JF et al: Dialysis and hemoperfusion of poisons and drugs—update. Trans Am Soc Artif Intern Organs 23:762, 1977

Toxic product information

BILINGS NF, BILLINGS SM: *American Drug Index,* Philadelphia, Lippincott, 1984
GOODMAN and GILMAN: *The Pharmacological Basis of Therapeutics,* 7th ed, AG Gilman et al (eds). New York, Macmillan, 1985
GOSSELIN RE: *Clinical Toxicology of Commercial Products: Acute Poisoning,* 5th ed. Baltimore, Williams & Wilkins, 1984
HAYES WJ: *Pesticides Studies in Man.* Baltimore, Williams & Wilkins, 1982
The Merck Index, 9th ed. Rahway, NJ, Merck & Co, 1976
Poisonous Plants and Fungi. Philadelphia, Rittenhouse, 1976
SCHERZ RG: The history of poison control centers in the United States. Clin Toxicol 12:291, 1978

COMMON POISONS

Acetaminophen

PRESCOTT LF et al: Treatment of paracetamol poisoning with *N*-acetylcysteine. Lancet 2:432, 1977
RUMACK LF et al: Acetaminophen overdose: 662 cases with evaluation of oral acetyl-cysteine therapy. Arch Intern Med 141:380, 1981
ZIEVE L et al: Acetaminophen liver injury: Sequential changes in two biochemical indices

of regeneration and their relationship to histologic alterations. J Lab Clin Med 105:619, 1985

Antimuscarinic compounds

RUMACK BH: Anticholinergic poisoning: Treatment with physostigmine. Pediatrics 52:449, 1973

Benzene, toluene

HAYDEN JW: The clinical toxicology of solvent abuse. Clin Toxicol 9:169, 1976
STREICHER HZ et al: Syndromes of toluene sniffing in adults. Ann Intern Med 94:758, 1981

Carbon monoxide

DOLAN MC: Carbon monoxide poisoning. Can Med Assoc J 133:392, 1985
REMICK RA, MILES JE: Carbon monoxide poisoning: Neurologic and psychiatric sequelae. Can Med Assoc J 117:654, 1977
TURINO GM: Effect of carbon monoxide on the cardiorespiratory system. Circulation 63:253A, 1981

Caustics

CAMPBELL GS et al: Treatment of corrosive burns of the esophagus. Arch Surg 112:495, 1977
RUMACK BH, BURLINGTON JD: Caustic ingestions: A rational look at diluents. Clin Toxicol 11(1):27, 1977

Chlorinated insecticides

BOYLAN JJ et al: Cholestyramine: Use of a new therapeutic approach for chlordecone (Kepone) poisoning. Science 199:893, 1978
STARR GH, CLIFFORD NJ: Acute lindane intoxication. Arch Environ Health 25:374, 1972
TAYLOR JR, CALABRESE VP: Organochlorine and other insecticides. Handbook Clin Neurol 36:391, 1979

Cholinesterase inhibitor insecticides

LUZHNIKOR EA et al: Plasma perfusion through charcoal in methylparathion poisoning. Lancet 1:38, 1977
MILBY TH: Prevention and management of organophosphate poisoning. JAMA 216:2131, 1971
WYCKOFF W et al: Diagnostic and therapeutic problems of parathion poisonings. Ann Intern Med 68:875, 1968

Cyanide

BRAICO KT et al: Laetrile intoxication: Report of a fatal case. N Engl J Med 300:238, 1979
UITTI RJ et al: Cyanide-induced parkinsonism: A clinicopathologic report. Neurology 35:921, 1985
VICK JA, FROEHLICH HL: Studies of cyanide poisoning. Arch Int Pharmcodyn Ther 273:314, 1985
WESSON DE et al: Treatment of acute cyanide intoxication with hemodialysis. Am J Nephrol 5:121, 1985

Detergents

TEMPLE AR, VELTRI JC: Outcome of accidental ingestions of soaps, detergents, and related household products. Vet Hum Toxicol 21:9, 1979
WILSON, JT, BURR, IM: Benzalkonium chloride poisoning in infant twins. Am J Dis Child 129:1208, 1975

Fluorides

BAYLESS JM, TINANOFF N: Diagnosis and treatment of acute fluoride toxicity. J Am Dent Assoc 110:209, 1985
SMITH GE: Toxicity of fluoride-containing dental preparations: A review. Sci Total Environ 43:41, 1985

Glycols

CATCHINGS TT et al: Adult respiratory distress syndrome secondary to ethylene glycol ingestion. Ann Emerg Med 14:594, 1985
DAROZA R et al: Acute ethylene glycol poisoning. Crit Care Med 12:1003, 1984

Halogenated hydrocarbons

BAERG RD, KIMBERG DV: Centrilobular hepatic necrosis and acute renal failure in "solvent sniffers." Ann Intern Med 73:713, 1970
RECHNAGEL RO: Carbon tetrachloride hepatotoxicity. Pharmacol Rev 19:145, 1967
SCHWARZBECK A, KOSTERS W: Extracorporeal hemoperfusion in acute carbon tetrachloride intoxication. Arch Toxicol 35:207, 1976

Isopropyl alcohol

LACOUTURE PG et al: Acute isopropyl alcohol intoxication. Diagnosis and management. Am J Med 75:680, 1983

Methyl alcohol

BENNET H JR et al: Acute methyl alcohol poisoning: A review based on experiences in an outbreak of 323 cases. Medicine 32:431, 1953
KAPLAN K: Methyl alcohol poisoning. Am J Med Sci 244:170, 1982
RAVICHANDRAN R et al: Methyl alcohol poisoning. J Postgrad Med 30:69, 1984

Mushrooms

CURRY SC, ROSE MC: Intravenous mushroom poisoning. Ann Emerg Med 14:900, 1985

HANRAHAN JP, GORDON MA: Mushroom poisoning. Case reports and a review of therapy. JAMA 251:1057, 1984

VESCONI S et al: Therapy of cytotoxic mushroom intoxication. Crit Care Med 13:402, 1985

Naphthalene

HAGGERTY RJ: Naphthalene poisoning. N Engl J Med 255:919, 1956

Nicotine

GEHLBACH SH et al: Nicotine absorption by workers harvesting green tobacco. Lancet 1:478, 1975

Nitrites

KEATING JP et al: Infantile methemoglobinemia caused by carrot juice. N Engl J Med 288:824, 1973

Paraquat

GAUDREAULT P et al: Efficacy of activated charcoal and magnesium citrate in the treatment of oral paraquat intoxication. Ann Emerg Med 14:123, 1985

VANDENBOGAERDE J et al: Paraquat poisoning. Forensic Sci Int 26:103, 1984

Petroleum distillates

BROWN J et al: Experimental kerosene pneumonia: Evaluation of some therapeutic regimens. J Pediatr 84:396, 1974

PEARLSON GD: Psychiatric and medical syndromes associated with phencyclidine (PCP) abuse. Johns Hopkins Med J 1:25, 1981

SHIRKEY H: Treatment of petroleum distillate ingestion. Mod Treat 8:580, 1971

TAUSSIG LN et al: Pulmonary function 8 to 10 years after hydrocarbon pneumonitis. Clin Pediatr 16:57, 1977

Phosphorus

SIMON FA, PICKERING LK: Acute yellow phosphorus poisoning. JAMA 235:1343, 1976

TALLEY RC et al: Acute elemental phosphorus poisoning in man: Cardiovascular toxicity. Am Heart J 84:139, 1972

WINEK CL et al: Yellow phosphorus ingestions: Three fatal poisonings. Clin Toxicol 6:541, 1973

Salicylates

ANDERSON RJ et al: Unrecognized adult salicylate intoxication. Ann Intern Med 85:745, 1976

BUSCHANUN N, RABINOWITZ L: Infantile salicylism: A reappraisal. J Pediatr 84:391, 1974

DONE AK, TEMPLE AR: Treatment of salicylate poisoning. Mod Treat 8:528, 1971

HILL JB: Salicylate intoxication. N Engl J Med 288:1110, 1973

PROUDFOOT AT, BROWN SS: Acidaemia and salicylate poisoning in adults. Br Med J 2:537, 1969

SEGAR WE, HOLLIDAY MA: Physiologic abnormalities of salicylate intoxication. N Engl J Med 259:1191, 1958

172   HEAVY METAL POISONING

JOHN W. GRAEF / FREDERICK H. LOVEJOY, JR.

ARSENIC

SOURCE   Inorganic arsenic compounds such as arsenic trioxide and arsenic pentoxide as well as sodium and potassium arsenite and arsenate are found in insecticides, rodenticides, fungicides, wood preservatives, and herbicides, and in glass manufacturing. Organic arsenic compounds are present in the environment. Arsine gas poisonings have occurred in industry in the smelting and refining of metals, in galvanizing and etching, in lead plating, and in the silicon microchip industry. Historically, organic arsenical compounds have been used in the treatment of syphilis, epilepsy, psoriasis, and amebiasis. Currently, acute toxicity is encountered following accidental ingestion, industrial accidents, or suicidal or homicidal intoxications. Chronic exposures occur most commonly following low-dose exposure in industry or chronic consumption of contaminated food, water, or medications.

METABOLISM   Arsenic is absorbed through the skin, lungs, and gastrointestinal tract. Inorganic compounds are absorbed more readily than organic. Arsine is efficiently absorbed through the lungs. Arsenic is distributed from blood to liver, kidney, lung, and spleen within 24 h of ingestion and within 2 weeks to skin, hair, and bone. Inorganic arsenic compounds are found in high levels in leukocytes. Inorganic arsenic does not cross the blood-brain barrier but does cross the placenta. Five to ten percent is excreted in feces and 90 to 95 percent in the urine. Arsenic may be detected in urine for 7 to 10 days following a single dose.

CLINICAL TOXICOLOGY   Arsine gas combines with hemoglobin in red blood cells to produce severe hemolysis with anemia, hemoglobinuria, and subsequent gross hematuria occurring within 3 to 4 h of ingestion. Subsequent jaundice may be severe. Signs and symptoms of toxicity include nausea, vomiting and diarrhea, apprehension and malaise, tachycardia, and dyspnea. Acute renal failure is common and often fatal.

Manifestations of acute toxicity following arsenic ingestion include in the gastrointestinal tract—burning in the throat, difficulty swallowing, nausea, vomiting, diarrhea, abdominal pain, and a garlic odor on the breath; in the cardiovascular system—cyanosis, difficulty breathing, hypotension; in the central nervous system—delirium, coma, seizures; in the kidney—acute tubular necrosis; in the hematologic system—hemolysis, eosinophilia, and rarely bone marrow depression. Manifestations of chronic arsenic poisoning occurring 2 to 8 weeks following ingestion include in the skin and nails—erythroderma, hyperkeratosis, hyperpigmentation, exfoliative dermatitis, Aldrich-Mees lines in the nails; in the mucous membranes—laryngitis, tracheitis, bronchitis; in the central nervous system—polyneuritis (sensory and motor) occurring 1 to 3 weeks following ingestion. Skin basal cell carcinomas, squamous cell carcinomas, and Bowen's disease as well as lung carcinomas have been associated with chronic arsenic exposure.

Arsenic produces its toxicity by binding with tissue sulfhydryl groups. Other effects include capillary injury and direct toxic effects on large organs. Of lesser importance is uncoupling of oxidative phosphorylation. Pathologic findings include necrosis of the stomach and small bowel and vasculature and degenerative changes in the liver and kidneys.

LABORATORY FINDINGS   Arsenic is radiopaque and is demonstrable on x-ray of the abdomen. It may also be detected in hair and nails for months following exposure. With specific organ system involvement the following may be seen: abnormal liver function tests; in the blood—anemia, leukocytosis, leukopenia, hemoglobinemia; in the urine—proteinuria, hematuria, hemoglobinuria, and urinary casts. Normal blood arsenic levels should not exceed 3 µg/dL or 100 µg per liter in urine.

TREATMENT   Acute ingestion should be treated by inducing vomiting with ipecac syrup if the patient is alert. Gastric lavage is indicated if the patient is obtunded. Activated charcoal is ineffective, and cathartics are contraindicated. Cardiovascular stabilization is critical. Dimercaprol chelates arsenic by producing insoluble complexes that are excreted by the kidneys. For mild symptoms and elevated serum or urinary levels, 2 to 3 mg/kg per dose is given every 6 h for 24 h and then every 12 to 24 h for 10 days. Adequacy of urinary mobilization is confirmed by measurement of serum levels. Toxic manifestations of dimercaprol (increased blood pressure, tachycardia, nausea, vomiting, headache, burning sensation in the lips, mucous membrane irritation, coma, and convulsions) occur with increasing doses. For patients with severe symptoms and significantly elevated arsenic levels 3 to 5 mg/kg per dose of dimercaprol is administered in a similar regime.

D-Penicillamine has been successfully used in chronic poisoning, administered orally, up to 1 g per day in four divided doses for 5 days. Side effects of penicillamine include rashes, leukopenia, eosinophilia, thrombocytopenia, and nephrotoxicity. Hemodialysis removes arsenic with a clearance of 80 to 90 mL/min and is indicated if renal failure occurs.

Exchange transfusion and, if renal failure develops, hemodialysis are the preferred treatments for arsine poisoning. Dimercaprol does not appear to be useful.

CADMIUM

SOURCE Exposure to cadmium is usually occupational or via pollution from mining or smelting operations. Commercially produced as a by-product of copper and lead or zinc smelting, cadmium is used in the manufacture of batteries, in ceramics, in electroplating, and as a pigment in paints and plastics. In contaminated areas, high concentrations may be found in shellfish.

METABOLISM Absorption occurs via ingestion or inhalation. The normal range of daily oral intake is 2 to 200 μg with an estimated mean of 20 to 40 μg per day. Only 5 to 10 percent of this is absorbed, although like lead, absorption may be increased in the presence of calcium and iron deficiency. Similarly, about 5 percent of inhaled cadmium is absorbed depending on particle size. Small, highly soluble particles are absorbed at a rate of 25 to 50 percent.

About 50 percent of absorbed cadmium is concentrated in the liver and kidneys. In erythrocytes and soft tissues cadmium is bound to metallothionein, a low-molecular-weight protein containing a large number of available sulfhydryl groups which thereby exert a protective effect. With large single cadmium exposures saturation of the protein may be exceeded with loss of protective effect. Cadmium does not pass the placenta and gradually accumulates in the body with age. Biologic half-life has been estimated at more than 20 years except in the presence of kidney damage when urinary excretion is increased. In the kidney, metallothionein-bound cadmium is filtered at the glomerulus and is then reabsorbed by the proximal tubules into the renal cortex. The daily urinary excretion rarely exceeds 0.5 μg.

CLINICAL TOXICOLOGY Acute cadmium intoxication may occur after either ingestion or inhalation. Ingestion of water containing concentrations of 15 mg per liter or foods containing as little as 30 mg of cadmium can induce vomiting, abdominal pain, and severe diarrhea. Shock may ensue. Acute inhalation produces dyspnea, weakness, chest pain, shortness of breath, and cough. A chemical pneumonitis produces pulmonary edema and respiratory failure. Clinical symptoms may occur with air exposure as low as 1 mg/m^2 over 8 h. During the same time period inhalation of 5 mg/m^2 may be fatal. A latent period of 4 to 24 h from exposure to onset of symptoms may complicate accurate diagnosis. Death usually occurs in 5 to 10 days. Chemical pneumonitis may continue for several months, and pulmonary function can be abnormal for longer than 1 year after exposure.

Chronic intoxication usually occurs by industrial inhalation and produces emphysema and characteristic renal tubular damage with proteinuria and increased excretion of beta$_2$ microglobulin. Cadmium's inhibitory effect on alpha$_1$ antitrypsin may be the explanation for cadmium-induced emphysema. Relatively minor changes in liver function, a microcytic hypochromic anemia unresponsive to iron therapy, and hypertension are associated findings. Chronic oral intake of contaminated food and drinking water has produced a syndrome in Japan called *itai-itai* (ouch-ouch) disease wtih renal tubular damage and osteomalacia.

LABORATORY FINDINGS Measurement of blood cadmium levels are not useful because of preferential deposition of cadmium in the kidney. Urinary cadmium excretion exceeding 10 μg per liter is associated with renal tubular damage especially when accompanied by elevated urinary beta$_2$ microglobulin and metallothionein levels. Kidney cadmium content obtained by renal biopsy can be assessed by neutron activation analysis. A renal cadmium concentration exceeding 200 μg per gram of net weight is associated with renal disease.

TREATMENT Treatment is controversial. Although chelating agents bind cadmium, they may effectively shift cadmium to the kidney, where further damage can occur. In acute exposure, ethylenediaminetetraacetic acid (EDTA) in a dose of 1 g/m^2 daily can be beneficial. Dimercaprol has not been effective. A new investigational oral chelating agent, dimercaptosuccinic acid, appears promising. Acute inhalation pneumonitis should be treated with steroids and diuretics. Itai-itai disease appears to respond to large doses of vitamin D in the presence of adequate dietary calcium and phosphate. Long-term sequelae of chronic cadmium exposure include emphysema and chronic renal insufficiency.

IRON

SOURCE Iron preparations are used in the treatment of iron-deficiency anemia, as a dietary supplement during pregnancy, and in conjunction with multivitamin preparations. They are accidentally ingested with high frequency by children and occasionally purposefully by adults. They are available by prescription or over the counter.

PATHOPHYSIOLOGY Iron is essential for the synthesis of hemoglobin and myoglobin and is contained in cytochrome systems throughout the body. Of the total content of iron in the body, 70 percent is present in hemoglobin, 20 percent as ferritin or hemosiderin, 5 percent as myoglobin, and 5 percent coupled with enzymes in multiple tissues. Iron in its ferrous state is absorbed through the gastrointestinal mucosa and is carried in the blood in its ferric state bound to transferrin, a specific beta$_1$ globulin. Ferric iron is either transferred to specific sites in the bone marrow for use in erythropoiesis or is stored in ferritin or hemosiderin pools. Each day 1 mg is lost from the body through the intestine, skin, and urine. In overdose, binding sites in the blood are exceeded and free iron is available to cause toxicity. Iron injures cells through peroxidation leading to mitochondrial injury and alteration in oxidative enzymes of the Krebs cycle.

Pathologic findings in fatal cases include necrosis and inflammation of stomach and small bowel, fatty degeneration of hepatocytes, myocardial cells, and renal tubules, and pulmonary atelectasis and emphysema. Iron deposition is demonstrable histologically in intestines, liver, and spleen.

CLINICAL TOXICOLOGY Ingested doses of greater than 30 mg/kg are toxic; greater than 250 mg/kg may be fatal. Signs of poisoning occur within 6 h of ingestion, and the subsequent course of illness follows four stages. Stage I includes injury to the gastrointestinal mucosa with resultant vomiting and diarrhea. A consequent decrease in plasma volume leads to hemoconcentration and decreased cardiac output. Vasodilation from high iron levels and ferritin release augment hypovolemia with resultant clinical evidence of shock. Decreased cerebral perfusion and a possible direct effect of excess iron on the central nervous system cause lethargy and coma. Stage II may involve a quiescent period in milder cases of variable duration, but generally 6 to 24 h. Stage III includes shock, evidence of liver injury with jaundice and elevated liver enzymes, renal failure, and evidence of pulmonary injury. Stage IV occurs several months following the initial insult and involves pyloric scarring with subsequent intestinal obstruction.

LABORATORY FINDINGS Iron is radiopaque and is demonstrable on a flat plate of the abdomen. Efficacy of gastrointestinal decontamination may be confirmed by a follow-up x-ray. A white blood cell count greater than 150,000 per cubic millimeter or a blood sugar of greater than 120 mg/dL are correlated with a serum iron level in excess of 300 μg/dL, a figure associated with clinical evidence of serious systemic toxicity. A provocative chelation challenge test using deferoxamine may be used to determine when the serum iron level has exceeded the iron-binding capacity. Deferoxamine in a dose of 25 mg/kg (not to exceed 1 g) is given intramuscularly. If the serum iron has exceeded the iron-binding capacity, free circulating unbound iron is chelated to deferoxamine. The complex ferrioxamine is excreted as a *"vin rosé"* color in the urine. The most accurate index of severity of iron overdose is the serum iron level. Serum iron levels peak 2 to 4 h after ingestion in most patients. Levels less than 500 μg/dL are associated with a 6 percent risk of shock and coma; levels of 500 to 1000 μg/dL with a 20 percent risk of shock and coma, levels of greater than 1000 μg/dL with a 60 percent risk of shock and coma. Levels exceeding 5000 μg/dL are usually fatal.

TREATMENT Ingested doses of elemental iron greater than 30 mg/kg are best removed with syrup of ipecac (if the patient is alert) or gastric lavage with a large orogastric tube (if the patient is unconscious). Lavage should be carried out with half-normal saline followed by instillation of 50 to 100 mL of 1% bicarbonate to form the ferrous carbonate salt which is less irritating than iron and is poorly absorbed. If an x-ray of the stomach shows presence of iron tablets following gastrointestinal decontamination, repetition of this procedure is recommended. Activated charcoal is ineffective. Calcium phosphate salts, which precipitate iron in the gastrointestinal tract, are associated with significant systemic toxicity, and thus should not be used. Oral deferoxamine forms a ferrioxamine complex which is poorly absorbed and is a useful adjunct to therapy in cases of a large overdose.

Colloid or blood products should be used to correct hypotension. Intravenous sodium bicarbonate may be needed to correct metabolic acidosis. Correction of coagulation defects secondary to hepatic injury may require administration of vitamin K or fresh frozen plasma.

Deferoxamine, the chelating agent of choice, binds free iron in the plasma resulting in excretion of the ferrioxamine complex through the urine. Deferoxamine does not bind iron in ferritin or hemosiderin pools or iron bound to hemoglobin or cytochrome oxidase systems. If the patient is normotensive, deferoxamine 50 mg/kg per dose, up to a total of 1 to 2 g per dose, may be given intramuscularly every 4 to 6 h. If the patient is hypotensive, deferoxamine should be given intravenously at an infusion rate not to exceed 15 mg/kg per hour. A lessening in the *vin rosé* color of the urine and a decline in serum iron levels are used to document the efficacy of therapy. Adverse reactions to deferoxamine include flushing, blotchy erythema, or urticaria; hypotension may occur if the infusion rate is excessively rapid. Therapy should be continued until serum iron levels are less than the iron-binding capacity.

The intensity of therapy with deferoxamine is determined by the serum iron level. A patient with a level of less than 300 μg/dL will require only general supportive care. A level between 300 to 500 μg/dL will require brief chelation therapy, while a level greater than 500 μg/dL will require vigorous chelation therapy. Levels in excess of 1000 μg/dL may require continuous intravenous deferoxamine treatment coupled with close monitoring of serum iron and deferoxamine concentrations. Neither exchange transfusion nor hemodialysis is effective since they remove only a small portion of the total ingested dose (total-body burden) of iron.

LEAD

SOURCE Lead constitutes about 2 percent of the earth's crust and is ubiquitous throughout the world. The increased use of lead during the Industrial Revolution caused extensive disease among lead workers; the addition in the 1870s of lead salts to paints as coloring agents and stabilizers set the stage for what is now the largest epidemic of lead poisoning in history, that of childhood plumbism. This syndrome, caused by ingestion by small children of lead from paint, soil, or household dust, affects an estimated 2,000,000 preschool children annually in the United States alone. Evidence of permanent neurologic sequelae from levels of lead previously thought to be safe has raised fears of possible damage to the fetus and newborn as well. The nature of this epidemic has forced prohibition against the addition of organic lead salts to gasoline as well as extensive prohibitions against the use of lead in consumer products.

METABOLISM Inorganic lead salts are absorbed through ingestion or inhalation. Organic lead salts may also be absorbed through the skin. Gastrointestinal absorption is enhanced by deficiency of iron, calcium, and zinc. Generally, gastrointestinal absorption is about 10 percent of an ingested dose. Absorption through the lung varies with tidal volume and particle size. Particles smaller than 1 μm may be absorbed if they reach the alveoli. Adults may ingest up to 150 μg per day of lead from normal exposure to food and drinking water. Positive lead balance may occur at these levels since renal excretion normally does not exceed 80 to 100 μg per day. In children, no more than 5 μg per kilogram of body weight is tolerated without increasing the body lead burden.

Under steady state conditions, 5 to 10 percent of ingested lead may be found in blood; 95 percent of that fraction is associated with the erythrocyte. Up to 80 to 90 percent is taken up by bone and incorporated into hydroxyapatite crystals where it is relatively inactive. The remainder is found in soft tissues, principally the kidneys and brain. The principal route of excretion is stool (80 to 90 percent), and the remainder is found in the urine (10 percent). The half-life of lead in blood and soft tissues is 24 to 40 days, while that in bone is 104 days.

Lead is a poison of enzymes, binding to the disulfide groups of protein. In high concentration, lead alters the tertiary structure of intracellular proteins, denaturing them and causing cell death with resultant tissue inflammation.

CLINICAL TOXICOLOGY The toxic effects of lead differ between children and adults. The adult form is generally characterized by abdominal pain, anemia, renal disease, headache, peripheral neuropathy with demyelination of long neurons, ataxia, and memory loss. Symptoms are usually associated with prolonged elevation of lead levels above 80 to 100 μg per deciliter of whole blood. A subclinical form is recognized in adults, and affects primarily the peripheral nervous system and the kidneys. A linear association between hypertension and elevated lead levels (i.e., greater than 30 μg/dL) has been reported. Encephalopathy is rare in adults.

Childhood lead poisoning is manifested by anemia and abdominal pain, but the central nervous system effects are most important. As an enzymatic poison, lead affects susceptible developing tissues more than tissues with stable metabolism. Hence, a subclinical form of lead poisoning is most dangerous to children because its effects emerge without associated symptoms that bring the victim to medical attention. In the acute clinical form, signs and symptoms are thought to reflect both the direct effect of high concentrations of lead (i.e., blood lead greater than 80 to 100 μg/dL) and consequent severe alterations in porphyrin synthesis. Signs and symptoms include pallor (anemia), abdominal pain, irritability followed by lethargy, anorexia, ataxia, and slurred speech. In severe cases, convulsions, coma, and death are usually due to severe generalized cerebral edema and renal failure. Almost always associated with this syndrome is a "high-dose" exposure to lead (usually paint chips), pica (the ingestion of nonfood substances) and malnutrition (iron, calcium, and zinc deficiency).

The subclinical form of childhood plumbism is associated with elevated blood lead and increased erythrocyte protoporphyrin. However, no symptoms are usually detected. The syndrome is widespread, and its effects on the developing central nervous system are irreversible. These include mental retardation and selective deficits in language, cognitive functions, and behavior, depending on the age and duration of exposure.

LABORATORY FINDINGS Laboratory abnormalities include blood lead levels greater than 25 μg/dL associated with free erthrocyte protoporphyrin (FEP) greater than 35 μg/dL when determined by ethylacetate extraction. Although a hemolytic anemia is associated with acute plumbism, chronic plumbism produces a microcytic hypochromic anemia with associated or secondary iron deficiency. Other heme prescursors are increased in plasma and urine (e.g., coproporphyrin, delta aminolevulinic acid).

Renal abnormalities include pyuria, the Fanconi syndrome, and azotemia. In plumbism, 24-h urinary excretion of lead exceeds 80 to

100 μg. In adults, demyelination of long nerves produces prolonged nerve conduction time and subsequent paralysis of extensor muscles with atrophy (wrist drop or foot drop). While slight prolongation of nerve conduction can be seen in children, it is clinically evident only in those with sickle cell disease. This observation is not completely understood but may be due to an associated zinc deficiency. Abnormalities of cardiac, thyroid, and hepatic function have been observed in adults. In children, a characteristic laboratory finding is increased density at the metaphyseal plate of growing long bones, so-called lead lines. These are generally seen in association with prolonged blood lead levels greater than 50 μg per deciliter of whole blood. They are not seen in adults.

TREATMENT The *sine qua non* of treatment is removal of the source of exposure. Cases of industrial lead poisoning should be reported to the Occupational Safety Hazards Administration (OSHA). Cases of childhood plumbism should be reported to the local board of health to initiate examination of housing for sources of lead.

Reduction of the body burden of lead is accomplished by use of chelating agents, principally the calcium salt of EDTA, dimercaprol, and D-penicillamine (Cuprimine). A new oral chelating agent, dimercaptosuccinic acid (DMSA), is undergoing clinical trials. The lead mobilization test is used to determine the size of the "chelatable" pool of lead. In this test, administration of a calculated dose of chelating agent, usually EDTA, induces a lead diuresis which is then compared to the dose of chelating agent. The test is positive when greater than 1 μg lead is excreted per milligram of chelating agent administered per 24 h. The mobilization test can be useful in determining the utility of chelation therapy in patients with borderline lead levels or in those patients who have been previously treated.

In acute encephalopathy, double therapy (dimercaprol and EDTA) is used until blood lead levels are less than 40 μg/dL. Urine flow must be established, and even in the presence of cerebral edema, fluids must be sufficient to produce a lead diuresis. Mannitol and dexamethasone can reduce cerebral edema, but removal of the metal is essential. In symptomatic adults and children, double therapy should be used for 5 days at EDTA doses of 0.5 to 1 g/m² up to 1.5 g/m² daily. If further chelation is required, a minimum interval of 48 to 72 h should intervene between courses of therapy. The D-penicillamine dose is 20 to 40 mg/kg per day, not to exceed 1 g. Adverse effects, particularly allergy, may be reduced by beginning therapy with one-quarter of the total dose for 1 week, then doubling and redoubling the dose until full dose is reached. D-Penicillamine can be administered for 3 to 6 months until the body lead burden is depleted. Only D-penicillamine and, to a lesser extent, EDTA remove lead directly from bone. If EDTA is indicated, as many separate 5-day courses as are needed may be given provided that the total safe dose is not exceeded and proper intervals between courses are observed.

MERCURY

SOURCE Human beings may encounter mercury in an inorganic (elemental or mercuric salt) or an organic (usually methyl) form. All three are toxic, but organic mercury is most widespread and potentially dangerous. Elemental mercury is used in thermometers, sphygmomanometer, and dental amalgams. It is volatile at room temperature and rapidly oxidized to mercuric mercury when exposed to oxygen. Toxicity usually occurs from inhalation of mercury vapor during industrial exposure. Mercuric salts are found in topical medicines, as catalytic agents in the manufacture of plastics, as cathartics (e.g., Calomel), and in foodstuffs. Toxicity is usually through gastrointestinal exposure. Organic mercury is found in paints, fungicides, seeds, foods, medicines, and cosmetic agents. Because mercuric salts are methylated by bacteria in the environment, large amounts of methyl mercury are formed from inorganic mercury waste as occurred in the methyl mercury epidemic in Minamata Bay, Japan, following ingestion of mercury-laden fish.

METABOLISM Elemental mercury is absorbed primarily as vapor through the lungs, where 80 to 100 percent of inhaled mercury enters the bloodstream through the alveoli. Gastrointestinal absorption of elemental mercury is low. Volatilization of ingested elemental mercury is reduced by oxidation of surface mercury to mercuric sulphide, preventing vapor formation from the residual metallic mass. Absorbed mercury vapor is lipid-soluble and readily crosses the blood-brain barrier and the placenta. However, it is rapidly oxidized to the mercuric form, which combines readily with sulfhydryl groups of proteins and has limited mobility. Thus, an acute single exposure contributes to brain mercury levels more than similar doses ingested chronically. Excretion is similar to that of mercuric salts. Small amounts of mercury vapor may be excreted via the lungs. In humans, the half-life of elemental mercury is approximately 60 days.

Inorganic mercury is absorbed through the gastrointestinal tract and percutaneously. High intake produces corrosive effects on the gastrointestinal tract with consequent increased absorption. Normal uptake is less than 10 percent of an intravenous dose. Mercuric salts accumulate primarily in the kidney, but are distributed to the liver, erythrocytes, bone marrow, spleen, lung, intestine, and skin. Excretion is via the urine and feces. The half-life of inorganic mercury is approximately 40 days.

Organic (methyl) mercury is readily absorbed through the intestines and the skin. Short-chain alkyl and methyl mercury penetrate the erythrocyte membrane and bind to hemoglobin. The ratio of red blood cell to plasma methyl mercury may be as high as 9:1. Because of its high lipid solubility, methyl mercury freely passes the placenta and blood-brain barrier and enters breast milk. Organic mercury also concentrates in the kidneys and the central nervous system. Metallothionein synthesis is induced by mercury exposure, the augmented protein concentrations exerting a protective effect against tissue damage. Excretion is complex. A portion is excreted through renal tubules into urine, but this represents only 1 percent of the body burden. Methyl mercury is also acetylated in the liver or may be conjugated with cysteine or glutathione. The N-acetyl-homocysteine–methyl mercury complex then enters the enterohepatic circulation and is ultimately excreted in the urine. The half-life of organic mercury in humans is about 70 days.

CLINICAL TOXICOLOGY Mercury is a poison of enzymes with an affinity for thiol groups. Acute metallic mercury (vapor) poisoning causes inflammation of large and small airways with interstitial pneumonitis leading to respiratory failure. The rapid uptake of mercury vapor into the central nervous system produces associated symptoms including tremor and increased excitability. Chronic mercury vapor poisoning primarily affects the central nervous system. Initial symptoms include lassitude, anorexia, weight loss, and gastrointestinal disturbances. Increasing exposure produces the characteristic intention tremor of mercury poisoning. Initially peripheral, the tremor may become generalized and is accompanied by mercurial *erethism* (timidity, memory loss, insomnia, excitability, and, in severe cases, delirium). This neurologic picture in felt-hat workers exposed to mercury vapor and mercuric salts led to the phrase "mad as a hatter."

While chronic inorganic mercury poisoning also produces the above neurologic constellation, excessive salivation, loosening of the teeth, gingivitis, and stomatitis are also seen. When applied to the skin, mercuric salts may cause hypersensitivity reactions ranging from mild erythema to full-blown exfoliative dermatitis. Acrodynia, or pink disease, occurs in young children and may be mistaken for Kawasaki's disease. Symptoms include generalized rash, irritability, photophobia, hypertrichosis, and profuse perspiration associated with desquamation of the feet and hands. There may be hyperkeratosis of the skin and swelling of the hands and feet.

Acute inorganic mercury poisoning is characterized by the corrosive effect of mercuric salts on the gastrointestinal tract. Mild or, more often, severe gastrointestinal inflammation produces nausea, vomiting, hematemesis, and abdominal pain followed by tenesmus, bloody diarrhea, and necrosis of intestinal mucosa. Acute fluid loss in massive overdose can produce shock and death. Acute inorganic mercury poisoning causes acute tubular necrosis, while chronic inorganic mercury poisoning produces a nephrotic syndrome.

Acute organic mercury poisoning cannot be distinguished from the chronic form. Rather, the long half-life coupled with a latent period before onset of symptoms due to acute exposure produce a syndrome which varies more with species and gestational age than with duration of exposure. Prenatal poisoning produces cerebral palsy due to cortical and cerebellar atrophy. Postnatal poisoning causes paresthesias, headache, pain, visual, hearing, and speech disorders, neurasthenia, loss of memory and coordination, erethism, spasticity, paralysis, stupor, coma, and death. These neurologic abnormalities are often permanent.

The daily intake of methyl mercury should not exceed 100 parts per billion. In several studies of normal blood and urinary mercury levels, more than 90 percent of samples showed urinary mercury below 10 μg per liter. Blood mercury levels were below 20 ng/mL in 89 percent of samples. Thus, blood mercury levels above 35 ng/mL and urine mercury levels above 150 μg per liter are abnormal. Abnormalities may, of course, be associated with somewhat lower concentrations depending on when exposure occurred. Symptoms may be seen with blood mercury levels above 500 ng/mL and urine mercury levels above 600 μg per liter.

TREATMENT Treatment is aimed at reducing the absorption of mercury, protecting susceptible tissues from distribution of absorbed mercury, and eliminating absorbed mercury. In the case of ingestion of mercuric salts, initial treatment consists of removing mercury from the stomach by inducing emesis or by gastric lavage. Polythiol resins have been shown effective in binding mercury in the gastrointestinal tract. Activated charcoal, however, does not bind metals.

Generally, chelation therapy is indicated in mercury poisoning when high urine or blood mercury levels are present. Chelating agents with active mono- or dithiol groups are most effective. These include dimercaprol and D-penicillamine. The experimental oral chelating agent dimercaptosuccinic acid shows promise. Because D-penicillamine and dimercaprol form a toxic complex, they should not be used together. In acute inorganic mercury poisoning, dimercaprol should be used at a dose not exceeding 24 mg/kg per 24 h intramuscularly, in divided doses. Generally, therapy should not exceed 5 days at a time but can be reinstituted after a suitable rest period. D-Penicillamine can be used in the treatment of inorganic mercury poisoning but N-acetyl-DL-penicillamine is recommended as equally effective, stable, and less toxic. The dose is 30 mg/kg per day in two to three divided doses. Peritoneal dialysis and hemodialysis have also been used with some success. Neither is as effective as chelation therapy but may be useful in the presence of renal failure.

In chronic inorganic mercury poisoning, the use of dimercaprol does not appear to be beneficial in reducing the mercury burden and either N-acetyl-DL-penicillamine or D-penicillamine are the drugs of choice. N-acetyl-DL-penicillamine also appears to have an advantage in organic mercury poisoning and is more effective than either dimercaprol or EDTA. The goal of therapy is the reduction of symptoms and enhanced urinary excretion of mercury.

THALLIUM

SOURCE Thallium has been used as an insecticide and rodenticide, as a catalyst in fireworks, in optical lenses, in industry as an alloy, and in cardiac perfusion imaging. Accidental as well as purposeful ingestions of thallium occur. Epidemic poisoning has followed the ingestion of grain impregnated with thallium. Thallium is available as iodide, sulfate, and nitrate salts.

METABOLISM Thallium is absorbed percutaneously, by inhalation, and by oral ingestion. It has a large volume of distribution of 10

liters per kilogram with distribution to body organs including kidney, pancreas, spleen, liver, lung, muscles, and brain. Thallium is bound to sulfhydryl groups on mitochondrial membranes at intracellular sites. The elimination half-life is variable ranging from 3 to 15 days. The major pathway of elimination in human beings is through the urine, conforming to first-order pharmacokinetics; 3 percent of a dose is eliminated per day.

Thallium interferes with oxidative phosphorylation by inhibition of ATPase. Pathologic findings at postmortem include cerebral edema, loss of myelin in peripheral nerves, fatty infiltration of the liver, and degenerative changes in the myocardium.

CLINICAL TOXICOLOGY Severe poisoning occurs following a single ingested dose greater than 1 g or 8 mg/kg. Death has occurred following an ingested dose of 15 mg/kg.

Immediate signs and symptoms (occurring within 3 to 4 h of ingestion) include nausea and vomiting, abdominal pain, diarrhea, and hematochezia. Intermediate manifestations (within 1 week of ingestion) include involvement of the central nervous system with confusion, psychosis, choreoathetosis, organic brain syndrome, convulsions, and coma. Peripheral neurologic involvement is both motor and sensory and includes paresthesias, myalgias, weakness, tremor, and ataxia. Autonomic manifestations are less common and include tachycardia, hypertension, and salivation. Ophthalmologic abnormalities include neuritis, ophthalmoplegia, ptosis, strabismus, and cranial nerve palsies. Late manifestations (occurring 2 to 4 weeks after ingestion) include diffuse hair loss (with sparing of pubic and body hair and the lateral one-third of the eyebrows) with regrowth occurring as body burden decreases over time. Residual effects include memory loss, ataxia, tremor, and foot drop.

LABORATORY FINDINGS Thallium is radiopaque and is evident on an x-ray of the abdomen. Thallium levels with severe ingestion range from 30 to 200 μg/dL, and thallium excretion in excess of 10 to 20 μg per 24 h. The electroencephalogram (EEG) is diffusely abnormal, and peripheral nerve conduction may be delayed.

TREATMENT Therapeutic modalities include gastrointestinal decontamination, enhanced renal excretion by potassium chloride, hemodialysis, and the antidote diethyldithiocarbamate (Dithiocarb). Gastric lavage or ipecac syrup is indicated within 4 to 6 h of acute ingestion. Adequacy of removal of thallium can be documented by follow-up abdominal x-ray. Prussian blue absorbs thallium in the gastrointestinal tract by exchanging potassium for thallium on its crystal lattice network thereby preventing absorption. The oral dose is 250 mg/kg, administered once. Mannitol or magnesium citrate are used as a laxative to enhance gastrointestinal removal. The efficacy of this treatment has been demonstrated by a 50 percent shortening in serum half-life.

Potassium chloride–induced renal excretion of thallium occurs through the exchange of potassium for thallium thereby releasing thallium from tissue sites into blood and augmenting urinary excretion. Two- to threefold increases in urinary excretion of thallium have been demonstrated with quantitative thallium excretion rates of 20 to 30 mg per day. Efficacy of this method has been documented by shortening half-life in human studies, but this therapy has risks, and the amount of thallium removed as compared to the total ingested dose is small. Peritoneal dialysis removes 15 to 20 mg of thallium per day and hemodialysis 8 mg for each 8 h of dialysis. Prolonged hemodialysis can remove up to 25 mg of thallium per day, and while an increase over endogenous clearance, the total amount removed is relatively small. Hemoperfusion with activated charcoal may be useful.

Diethyldithiocarbamate has been advocated for early use in overdose because it leads to increased thallium blood levels and a two- to threefold increase in thallium excretion. However, Dithiocarb-thallium complexes diffuse into the brain with subsequent clinical and EEG worsening; therefore diethyldithiocarbamate is contraindicated in thallium intoxication.

CHELATING AGENTS

Chelating agents are used to bind toxic metals in stable, cyclic compounds with relatively low toxicity and enhanced renal excretion.

DIMERCAPROL (BAL) Dimercaprol was first developed during World War II as an antidote for the arsenical war gas lewisite; its chelating capacity is due to its four sulfhydryl groups which bind in a complex to polyvalent metal ions. Affinity of dimercaprol for metals is strong enough to reverse a significant portion of toxic metal enzyme binding. Dimercaprol diffuses well into erthrocytes and enhances fecal as well as urinary metal excretion. It is given intramuscularly in oil every 4 to 8 h in a dose of 12 to 24 mg/kg per 24 h. Toxicity includes mild febrile reactions, nausea, headache, lacrimation, conjunctivitis, salivation, and rhinorrhea. The drug emits a strong sulfide odor, and patients may complain of metallic taste. Contraindications to dimercaprol include glucose 6-phosphate dehydrogenase deficiency, allergy to peanut oil, and concurrent use of medicinal iron, which forms a toxic complex with dimercaprol.

ETHYLENEDIAMINETETRAACETATE (EDTA) Because the sodium salt of EDTA can produce profound hypocalcemia, only the calcium disodium salt should be used in therapy of metal poisoning. EDTA forms a sexadentate complex with divalent cations exchanging one atom of calcium for each metal ion. It enhances urinary excretion of lead twenty- to fiftyfold but also increases excretion of zinc and, to a lesser extent, iron. It does not enter the erythrocytes but removes metals from the extracellular compartment. Oral administration is contraindicated because it enhances absorption of metals from the gastrointestinal tract. The drug is given parenterally either by constant intravenous infusion or intramuscular injection in a dose of 500 to 1000 mg/m² per day. The drug can be used safely in conjunction with other chelating agents. Toxicity increases after 4 to 5 days of administration with concomitant reduction in metal excretion; as a consequence, the drug is given for several "courses" of from 3 to 5 days each.

Toxicity is principally renal, dose-related, and usually reversible. It can be reduced by maintaining adequate urine flow. During treatment renal function should be carefully monitored.

D-PENICILLAMINE D-Penicillamine (Cuprimine) is the only commercially available oral chelating agent. Not presently licensed by the Federal Drug Administration for treatment of lead poisoning, it is licensed for use in the treatment of rheumatoid arthritis, Wilson's disease, and cystinuria. Nevertheless, there is extensive experience in its use in chelation of other metals. The N-acetyl form is particularly helpful in the treatment of inorganic mercury poisoning.

Penicillamine enhances excretion of heavy metals in the urine by an unclear mechanism. The drug is given orally in a dose of 20 to 40 μg/kg per day. By initiating therapy at low doses (usually 25 percent of the anticipated maximum dose) and gradually increasing the dose, the frequency of side effects can be reduced substantially.

Side effects may be seen in up to 20 percent of patients receiving D-penicillamine. The most common resemble penicillin hypersensitivity and include rash, fevers, thrombocytopenia, and leukopenia. Rare side effects include autoimmune hemolytic anemia and Stevens-Johnson syndrome. Anorexia, nausea, sleep disturbances, and urinary frequency may be seen occasionally. Nephrotoxicity is reported in adults receiving large doses and in one case has been reported in a child. Patients receiving D-penicillamine should, therefore, be carefully monitored for signs of renal, hematologic, or allergic side effects.

DEFEROXAMINE Deferoxamine (Desferal) binds iron in a 9:1 molar ratio. It exerts its effect primarily on free iron in the plasma. It does not chelate iron bound to hemoglobin in red blood cells, iron present in hemosiderin or ferritin, or, finally, iron in myoglobin or the cytochrome oxidase systems of the body. The complex ferrioxamine, stable and resistant to dissociation in water, is soluble and readily excreted in the urine. The dose may be given intramuscularly or intravenously at a dose of 50 mg/kg (up to 2 g per dose) or 1 to 2 g per dose in an adult not to exceed 6 to 8 g total dose per day. Intravenous deferoxamine should be administered slowly not exceeding 15 mg/kg per hour, thereby preventing hypotension.

REFERENCES

Arsenic

FOWLER BA, WEISSBERG JB: Arsine poisoning. N Engl J Med 291:1171, 1974
HEYMAN A et al: Peripheral neuropathy caused by arsenical intoxication. N Engl J Med 254:402, 1956
MASSEY EW et al: Arsenic: Homicidal intoxication. South Med J 77:848, 1984
PETERSON RG, RUMACK BH: D-Penicillamine therapy of acute arsine poisoning. J Pediatr 91:661, 1977

Cadmium

FRIBERG L et al: Cadmium in the environment, 2d ed. Cleveland, CRC Press, 1974
—— et al: Handbook on the Toxicology of Metals. Amsterdam, Elsevier, 1979
MORGAN WD: New ways of measuring cadmium in man. Nature 282:673, 1979

Iron

LACOUTURE PG et al: Emergency assessment of severity in iron overdose by clinical and laboratory methods. J Pediatr 99:89, 1981
PROPPER R, NATHAN D: Clinical removal of iron. Ann Rev Med 35:509, 1982
ROBOTHAM JL, LIETMAN PS: Acute iron poisoning. Am J Dis Child 134:874, 1980
WHITTEN CF et al: Studies in iron poisoning: Parts I and II. Pediatrics 36:322, 1965, 38:102, 1966

Lead

BYERS RK: Lead poisoning: Review of the literature and report on 45 cases. Pediatrics 23:585, 1959
CANTAROW A, TRUMPER M: Lead Poisoning. Baltimore, Williams & Wilkins, 1944
CARNOW B (ed): Health Effects of Occupational Lead and Arsenic Exposure, A Symposium. Chicago, US Department of Health, Education, and Welfare, 1976
CDC: Preventing Lead Poisoning in Young Children, US Department of Health and Human Services, 1985
CHISOLM JJ JR: The use of chelating agents in the treatment of acute and chronic lead intoxication in childhood. J Pediatr 73:1, 1968
NATIONAL ACADEMY OF SCIENCES: Lead in the Human Environment, A Report Prepared by the Committee on Lead in the Human Environment, Environmental Studies Board, Commission on Natural Resources, National Research Council, Washington, DC, 1980
KEHOE RA: The metabolism of lead in man in health and disease. The Harben Lectures, 1960. J R Inst Pub Health 24:1, 101; 129; 177, 1961
WALDRON HA, STOFEN D: Sub-Clinical Lead Poisoning. New York, Academic, 1974

Mercury

FRIBERG L, VOSTAL J (eds): Mercury in the Environment. Cleveland, CRC Press, 1972
NATIONAL ACADEMY OF SCIENCES: An Assessment of Mercury in the Environment, Washington, DC, 1978
WHO Environmental Health Criteria, Mercury, Geneva, World Health Organization, 1976

Thallium

BANK WJ et al: Thallium poisoning. Arch Neurol 26:456, 1972
SADDIQUE A, PETERSON CD: Thallium poisoning. Vet Hum Toxicol 25:1, 1983
VAN KESTEREN RG et al: Thallium intoxication: An evaluation of therapy. Intensivmed 17:293, 1980

173   TOBACCO

JOHN H. HOLBROOK

Tobacco smoke is a ubiquitous personal and environmental pollutant. Although tobacco has been used in western culture for more than 400 years, human inhalation of cigarette smoke is a twentieth century phenomenon with major medical and economic consequences. In industrialized nations cigarette smoking is the principal cause of preventable disease, disability, and premature death. In the United States the estimated costs for smoking-related medical care and loss of productivity exceed $55 billion per year.

Important changes in smoking trends are occurring in the United States. In general, there is less smoking. For example, annual per capita cigarette consumption in adults declined from its 1963 peak of 4345 cigarettes to a 1984 estimate of 3454 cigarettes. Between 1965 and 1983, the proportion of adult cigarette smokers in the United States declined from 52 to 36 percent of men and 34 to 29 percent of women (Table 173-1). There are 51 million current adult smokers and 36.1 million former smokers in the United States; the distribution of smokers between the sexes is approximately equal with 26.4 million men and 24.5 million women. Among teenagers, smoking is slightly more prevalent in females than in males. While consumption of cigar and pipe tobacco has decreased, use of smokeless tobacco has increased.

CIGARETTE SMOKE Large prospective epidemiologic studies have shown a strong association between cigarette smoking and several diseases. More than 4000 substances have been identified in cigarette smoke, including some that are pharmacologically active, antigenic, cytotoxic, mutagenic, and carcinogenic; these diverse biologic effects provide a framework for understanding the adverse consequences of smoking.

Cigarette smoke is a heterogeneous aerosol produced by incomplete combustion of the tobacco leaf. It is composed of gases and uncondensed vapors in which droplets are dispersed. Mainstream smoke emerges from the mouthpiece during puffing. Sidestream smoke is emitted between puffs at the burning cone and from the mouthpiece. The composition of the smoke is influenced by several factors including type of tobacco, temperature of combustion, length of the cigarette, porosity of the paper, additives, and filters. The major tobacco leaf constituents are carbohydrates, nonfatty organic acids, nitrogen-containing compounds, and resins. Cigarette temperatures vary greatly from $30°C$ at the mouthpiece to $900°C$ at the burning cone. In the presence of intense heat some tobacco constituents undergo thermic decomposition (pyrolysis). Volatile substances are distilled directly into the smoke. Unstable molecules recombine to generate new compounds (pyrosynthesis). Concentration of smoke constituents occurs as the smoke is filtered by unburnt tobacco and is redistilled by the burning cone. Some substances found in tobacco pass unchanged into cigarette smoke.

Approximately 92 to 95 percent of the total weight of mainstream smoke is present in a gas phase. Nitrogen, oxygen, and carbon dioxide account for 85 percent of the smoke's weight. The remaining gases, uncondensed vapors, and particulate matter are the substances of medical importance (Table 173-2). Mainstream smoke contains 0.3 to 3.3 billion particles per milliliter; the mean particle size is 0.2 to 0.5 μm, which is within the respirable range.

Because a pack-a-day cigarette smoker puffs more than 70,000 times a year, the membranes of the mouth, nose, pharynx, and tracheobronchial tree are exposed repetitively to tobacco smoke. Some constituents act directly on the membranes, while others are absorbed into the blood or are dissolved in saliva and swallowed.

PHARMACOLOGY Tissue and organ system responses to cigarette smoke inhalation are multiple and complex. Most studies in humans have dealt with exposure to whole smoke or to selected constituents thought to pose the greatest risk to health, such as nicotine and carbon monoxide. Relatively little is known about the individual effects and interactions of other potentially toxic smoke constituents that are present in low concentrations.

Nicotine, the component most characteristic of tobacco, is a highly toxic alkaloid that is both a ganglionic stimulant and depressant. Many of its complex effects are mediated by catecholamine release. Acute cardiovascular responses to nicotine observed in normal smokers include increases in systolic and diastolic blood pressure, heart rate, force of myocardial contraction, myocardial oxygen consumption, coronary artery blood flow, myocardial excitability, and peripheral vasoconstriction. Nicotine has also been shown to increase serum concentrations of glucose, cortisol, free fatty acids, and antidiuretic hormone and to increase platelet aggregation. Nicotine plays an important but not exclusive role in maintaining the smoking habit.

Carbon monoxide is a toxic gas that interferes with oxygen transport and utilization. Because cigarette smoke contains 2 to 6 percent carbon monoxide, smokers inhale concentrations as high as 400 parts per million (ppm) and develop elevated carboxyhemoglobin (COHb) levels. While the range of COHb found in smokers is 2 to 15 percent, levels for nonsmokers are near 1 percent. The average COHb level of moderate cigarette smokers is 5 percent. Carbon monoxide produces its adverse effects by reducing the amount of available oxyhemoglobin and myoglobin, and displacing the oxygen-hemoglobin dissociation curve to the left. Chronic, mild elevations of COHb due to smoking are a common cause of mild polycythemia and may produce subtle impairment of central nervous system function.

Cigarette smoke and its condensate are carcinogenic in several species of animals. The major identified carcinogens in cigarette smoke are polynuclear aromatic hydrocarbons, aromatic amines, and nitrosamines (Table 173-2). Cocarcinogens present in cigarette smoke, such as catechol, greatly enhance its carcinogenicity. The sister chromatid exchange rate, a sensitive indicator of mutagenic effects, is higher in the lymphocytes of smokers than in nonsmokers. Cigarette smoke condensate is also mutagenic in a microbial test system.

Potent pulmonary irritants and ciliotoxins are found in cigarette smoke (Table 173-2). These substances increase bronchial mucus secretion and mediate acute and chronic decreases in pulmonary and mucociliary function. Cigarette smoke also increases lung epithelial permeability.

EPIDEMIOLOGY Data from large prospective studies of populations in several countries show that cigarette-smoking men have 70 percent higher death rates than nonsmokers. This excess male mortality is present in all groups over the age of 35, but it is proportionately greatest in the age group 45 to 54. In a study of British physicians it was shown that 40 percent of 35-year-old men who smoked more than 25 cigarettes per day died before the age of 65, compared with 15 percent of nonsmokers in the same category. The excess mortality of female smokers has been somewhat less than that of male smokers, but recent trends suggest it is increasing. Smoking is responsible for an estimated 350,000 premature deaths each year in the United States. Coronary heart disease (CHD) is the chief contributor to smoking-related excess mortality. In the United States cigarette smokers experience more disability due to chronic illness and report 45 percent more days absent from work than do nonsmokers.

A strong dose-response relationship exists between tobacco exposure and excess mortality, as measured by age at onset of smoking, cigarette consumption, and smoke inhalation. Cessation of smoking is associated with a decrease in the excess mortality. These observations together with clinical, experimental, and pathologic studies indicate that smoking, per se, causes the excess mortality.

CHARACTERISTICS OF SMOKERS Demographic, anthropometric, physiologic, and laboratory features which distinguish cigarette smokers from nonsmokers are due both to baseline differences between these groups and to the effects of smoking. Smokers drink more alcohol, coffee, and tea than do nonsmokers. Their weight and blood pressure are slightly less and their heart rate is slightly faster than those of nonsmokers. In women the menopause comes earlier in smokers than in nonsmokers. Smokers have impaired maximum exercise performance and impaired immune systems. A markedly

TABLE 173-1 Estimated percentage of current cigarette smokers in the United States

Year	Percent current smokers 20 years of age and over		
	Females	Males	Both sexes
1965	34.1	52.4	42.7
1976	32.0	41.9	36.4
1980	29.4	38.3	33.6
1983	29.1	35.7	32.0

increased number of pulmonary alveolar macrophages is present in smokers, and the function and metabolism of these cells are abnormal. Serum thiocyanate concentrations are much higher in smokers. When compared with nonsmokers, smokers show small increases in the total white blood cell count and serum IgE levels as well as small decreases in leukocyte vitamin C levels, serum uric acid, and albumin. In smokers, the ratio of high-density lipoprotein cholesterol to low-density lipoprotein cholesterol is reduced. Smokers also show reduced levels of prostacyclin (PGI$_2$).

CLINICAL CORRELATIONS   Individual patient risks due to cigarette smoking vary widely. Factors which influence these risks include the duration, intensity, and type of smoke exposure; genetically mediated susceptibility; occupational and environmental exposures; use of medication; and coexisting risk factors and diseases.

Cardiovascular disease   Premature CHD is the most important medical consequence of cigarette smoking (see Chap. 189). Approximately 25 percent of the more than 500,000 CHD deaths occurring each year in the United States is attributable to smoking. Cigarette smoking is the most important modifiable CHD risk factor, acting both independently of and synergistically with other CHD risk factors. There is a dose-response relationship between CHD risk and cigarette smoking. The risk of CHD is 60 to 70 percent greater in male smokers than nonsmokers. Sudden death may be the first manifestation of CHD, and it is two to three times more likely to occur in 35- to 54-year-old male cigarette smokers than in nonsmokers. Women cigarette smokers are also at greater risk of developing CHD than nonsmokers, and the use of both cigarettes and oral contraceptives increases this risk approximately tenfold. Cessation of smoking is associated with decreased CHD mortality, an effect which is measurable within 1 year. Those who continue to smoke after an acute myocardial infarction are more likely to die from CHD than are those who quit smoking. Smokers who undergo coronary artery bypass surgery have increased perioperative mortality compared to nonsmokers. Cigarette smoking produces an imbalance between myocardial oxygen supply and demand, a decrease in the threshold for ventricular fibrillation, and an increase in platelet aggregation; avoidance of these effects may explain the prompt cardiac benefits of quitting smoking. Coronary atherosclerosis and intimal thickening of intramyocardial arteries and arterioles are more frequent in smokers than in nonsmokers.

Cigarette smoking is the most powerful risk factor for arteriosclerosis obliterans (see Chap. 195) and thromboangiitis obliterans (see Chap. 198). It also aggravates peripheral ischemia and may adversely affect peripheral bypass grafts. The mortality rate for atherosclerotic aortic aneurysm is greater in male smokers than nonsmokers. Cigarette smoking is not a risk factor for the development of hypertension; however, hypertensives who smoke appear to be at greater risk to develop malignant hypertension and renal artery stenosis. Cigarette smoking decreases cerebral blood flow and appears to increase the risk for cerebrovascular disease. Among women, subarachnoid hemorrhage is more likely to occur in smokers than nonsmokers, and the use of both cigarettes and oral contraceptives greatly increases this risk. Because of the association with chronic obstructive lung disease, cigarette smoking is an important factor leading to chronic pulmonary heart disease.

Cancer   Cigarette smoking is the single most important cause of cancer mortality in the United States, accounting for 30 percent of all cancer deaths. In spite of the well-documented cause-and-effect relationship between cigarette smoking and lung cancer, more Americans continue to die from this cancer than from any other tumor (see Chap. 213). In 1985 an estimated 107,000 lung cancer deaths occurred in the United States; approximately 85 percent of these deaths were attributable to cigarette smoking. The risk of developing lung cancer is quantitatively related to cigarette smoke exposure. Men who smoke one pack a day increase their risk tenfold compared with nonsmokers; men who smoke two packs a day may increase their risk more than 25 times compared with nonsmokers. Asbestos workers who smoke

cigarettes are at especially high risk for developing lung cancer. Cigarette consumption by women increased rapidly in the United States during the past 50 years, and lung cancer mortality is currently increasing at a faster rate in women than in men. Lung cancer has become the leading cause of cancer death among American women. Because 5-year survival rates for lung cancer are less than 10 percent, emphasis must be placed on prevention. Giving up cigarettes is associated with a gradual decline in the risk of developing lung cancer.

Cigarette smoking is causally associated in men and women with cancer of the larynx, oral cavity, and esophagus; alcohol consumption acts synergistically with cigarette smoking to increase the risk for these neoplasms. Carcinoma of the bladder, kidney, pancreas, stomach, and uterine cervix is also associated with cigarette smoking.

Respiratory disease   Cigarette smoking is the major cause of chronic obstructive lung disease (COLD), that is, chronic bronchitis and emphysema (see Chap. 208). Of the estimated 60,000 deaths from COLD that occurred in the United States in 1983, approximately 85 percent were attributable to smoking, and many of these deaths were preceded by prolonged respiratory disability. There is a dose-response relationship between COLD death rates and cigarette smoking. Depending upon the extent of smoke exposure, male cigarette smokers experience from 4 to 25 times higher mortality secondary to COLD than do nonsmokers. Although the death rate from COLD among female smokers is somewhat lower than among male smokers, it is increasing much more rapidly in female than in male smokers. Chronic cough, sputum production, and breathlessness are much more common in smokers. Smokers are more likely than nonsmokers to show abnormalities in a number of pulmonary function tests including measurements of elastic recoil, airflow in large and small airways, and diffusing capacity. Mild airflow obstruction in small airways may be present even in teenage smokers. When compared with continuing smokers, ex-smokers experience a decrease in mortality from COLD, a decrease in prevalence of pulmonary symptoms, and a slowing of the rate of decline of lung function to approximately that seen in age-matched nonsmokers. Chronic inhalation of pulmonary irritants and ciliotoxins (Table 173-2) may contribute to the development of COLD. Studies of the pathogenesis of emphysema suggest that smoking results in an excess of pulmonary

TABLE 173-2   Selected cigarette smoke constituents

Substance	Effect
PARTICULATE PHASE	
"Tar"*	Carcinogen
Polynuclear aromatic hydrocarbons	Carcinogens
Nicotine	Ganglionic stimulator and depressor, cocarcinogen
Phenol	Cocarcinogen and irritant
Cresol	Cocarcinogen and irritant
β-Naphthylamine	Carcinogen
N-Nitrosonornicotine	Carcinogen
Benzo[a]pyrene	Carcinogen
Trace metals (e.g., nickel, arsenic, polonium 210)	Carcinogens
Indole	Tumor accelerator
Carbazole	Tumor accelerator
Catechol	Cocarcinogen
GAS PHASE	
Carbon monoxide	Impairs oxygen transport and utilization
Hydrocyanic acid	Ciliotoxin and irritant
Acetaldehyde	Ciliotoxin and irritant
Acrolein	Ciliotoxin and irritant
Ammonia	Ciliotoxin and irritant
Formaldehyde	Ciliotoxin and irritant
Oxides of nitrogen	Ciliotoxin and irritant
Nitrosamines	Carcinogen
Hydrazine	Carcinogen
Vinyl chloride	Carcinogen

The aggregate of particulate matter in cigarette smoke after subtracting nicotine and moisture.

proteases, which may produce pulmonary damage. The damage is apparently mediated via release of elastase from increased numbers of lung leukocytes and partial inactivation of pulmonary antiproteases by oxidants present in smoke. For most people in the United States cigarette smoking is a more important cause of COLD than are occupational or environmental factors; however, factors such as cotton dust exposure may act independently or conjointly with smoking to produce COLD. In a rare disorder, homozygous α_1-antitrypsin deficiency, smoking greatly accelerates the tendency to panacinar emphysema; furthermore, smoking may play an additive role in individuals heterozygous for this state.

Cigarette smoking has been associated with an increased incidence of respiratory infections and deaths from pneumonia and influenza. Postoperative respiratory complications and spontaneous pneumothorax are also more common in smokers. Because tobacco smoke may increase airway obstruction, asthmatics should be urged not to smoke. Chronic stomatitis and chronic laryngitis occur more frequently in smokers than in nonsmokers.

Pregnancy Smoking may delay conception, and smoking during pregnancy may affect the fetus adversely. Infants whose mothers smoked during pregnancy weigh, on an average, 170 g less than infants whose mothers did not smoke. This effect probably results from impaired uteroplacental circulation. Maternal smoking during pregnancy increases the risk of spontaneous abortion, fetal death, neonatal death, and the sudden infant death syndrome. This increased risk may be much greater in pregnancies already at high risk due to other factors. Smoking by a woman during pregnancy may also adversely affect the long-term physical growth and intellectual development of the child.

Gastrointestinal disorders Gastric and duodenal ulcer disease is more prevalent in male than female cigarette smokers and causes more deaths in male smokers than in nonsmokers. Smoking impairs spontaneous and drug-induced healing of peptic ulcers, increases the likelihood of duodenal ulcer recurrence, inhibits pancreatic bicarbonate secretion, and decreases the pressure of esophageal and pyloric sphincters. Histamine-2-receptor antagonist inhibition of nocturnal gastric secretion is also prevented by smoking.

Involuntary smoke inhalation Indoor atmospheres and other confined spaces are often contaminated by tobacco smoke which is inhaled involuntarily by both smokers and nonsmokers. Most of the atmospheric pollutants arise from sidestream smoke. It contains greater concentrations of many smoke constituents than does mainstream smoke, but since sidestream smoke is diluted in a large volume of air, the smoke exposure from involuntary inhalation is less than that associated with smoking.

Initially, involuntary or passive smoking was thought to cause primarily an irritant effect such as ocular burning. It is now recognized as an important cause of air pollution. Approximately two-thirds of the adults in one survey reported some involuntary smoke exposure. The levels of smoke constituents or their metabolites measured in nonsmokers may be comparable to those found in "light" smokers. Parental smoking in the home is associated with an increased risk of respiratory illness in infants and impaired development of lung function in children. Asymptomatic nonsmokers who are chronically exposed to smoke-contaminated air may develop small-airways dysfunction. Several studies suggest that passive smoking increases the risk for lung cancer. In addition, patients with symptomatic CHD or COLD may experience exacerbation of symptoms when exposed to smoke-contaminated air.

Drug interactions Tobacco smoke constituents induce hepatic microsomal enzyme systems that are important in the metabolism of many drugs. For example, cigarette smoking increases the metabolism of propranolol, propoxyphene, and theophylline. Smokers may also demonstrate decreased insulin absorption compared to nonsmokers. With smoking cessation, adjustment of drug dose may be necessary.

TYPES OF SMOKING During the past 20 years the amount of tar and nicotine delivered by cigarettes made in the United States decreased by more than 50 percent. In 1980 the average American cigarette delivered 1 mg nicotine and 14 mg tar. The paucity of scientific data concerning the relative risks of lower-tar and -nicotine cigarettes compared with higher-tar and -nicotine cigarettes is of concern, because filter-tipped cigarettes and lower-tar and -nicotine cigarettes now account for more than 90 and 50 percent of sales, respectively. Lung cancer and laryngeal cancer are the only tobacco-related diseases for which the use of lower-tar and -nicotine cigarettes has been shown to result in risk reduction, compared with the use of higher-tar and -nicotine cigarettes; however, compared with not smoking or quitting, the benefits are minimal. Consumers who choose lower-tar and -nicotine cigarettes and then smoke a larger number of cigarettes or inhale more frequently or deeply may actually increase their exposure to harmful substances. There is also concern because unidentified flavoring agents are added to these cigarettes to enhance consumer acceptance. Their presence represents an undefined risk for both active and passive smokers.

Cigar and pipe smokers usually inhale less smoke than cigarette smokers, presumably because the alkaline pH of cigar and pipe tobacco makes it more irritating to the respiratory tract. The smoke exposure and overall mortality rates of pipe and cigar smokers in the United States are substantially less than those of cigarette smokers. Death rates of cigarette, cigar, and pipe smokers are approximately equal for carcinoma of the oral cavity, larynx, and esophagus, sites where exposures to cigarette, cigar, and pipe smoke are similar. The mortality rates of most cigar and pipe smokers for cancer at other sites, CHD, and COLD are not greatly elevated above the rates of nonsmokers, but cigar and pipe smokers who inhale consistently may experience adverse health effects comparable with those of cigarette smokers. The use of smokeless tobacco increases the risk for oral and pharyngeal cancer and may produce plasma nicotine levels comparable to those of smokers.

CESSATION OF SMOKING Psychosocial forces lead to initiation of smoking, especially among teenagers. Later, drug addiction and psychological factors help maintain dependence on tobacco. It is estimated that more than 36 million people in the United States have stopped smoking; 95 percent of these succeeded without formal assistance. Many long-term smokers quit because of smoking-related health problems. This seems to explain the observation that the death rate of men smoking more than 20 cigarettes a day was somewhat higher in the months immediately after quitting than that of continuing smokers. Thereafter, a gradual decline in death rates was observed in ex-smokers. Ten or more years after quitting, the death rate of those who had smoked more than 20 cigarettes a day decreased about two-thirds, and the death rate of individuals who had smoked 20 cigarettes a day or less was about the same as that of nonsmokers. Ex-smokers usually experience prompt symptomatic improvement. On the average they also gain approximately 5 lb.

In the United States more than 80 percent of cigarette smokers would like to stop smoking. Many self-care and organized programs are available to assist these individuals. Organized programs employ several techniques including instruction, counseling, withdrawal clinics, behavioral modification, hypnosis, aversive conditioning, self-monitoring, and drug therapy. In these programs 1-year abstinence rates of 20 to 30 percent are common. Relapse usually occurs during the 3-month interval after quitting. Successful programs emphasize maintenance of the nonsmoking state during this critical period.

Although only 10 percent of physicians smoke, a minority of patients report receiving advice from their physician to quit. Controlled trials have shown that physician counseling increases long-term smoking cessation rates. Polls also show that patients are inadequately informed about the hazards of smoking. All smokers should be encouraged to quit, especially those in high-risk groups with chronic pulmonary disease, coronary artery disease, and pregnancy. Physicians can help their smoking patients in the following manner:

1 Obtain a quantitative smoking history.
2 Explain the health risks in a personally relevant fashion.
3 Emphasize the benefits associated with cessation.
4 Advise and assist the patient to quit smoking.
5 Provide self-help reading materials.
6 Consider referring the patient to a formal treatment program.
7 Support the patient in a maintenance program.

A nicotine-containing chewing gum, which helps alleviate withdrawal symptoms, may be a useful adjunct in medically supervised programs. Patients who are unable or unwilling to stop cigarette smoking should be assisted to reduce their smoke exposure by smoking fewer cigarettes, inhaling less, taking fewer puffs, and leaving a longer stub.

Political, social, and cultural forces play a critical role in the individual decision to start or stop smoking. For this reason, physicians should lead and support efforts to increase tobacco excise taxes, to eliminate all tobacco advertisements and promotional activities, and to ban smoking in public places.

Ultimately, primary smoking prevention in the pediatric and adolescent age groups may be the most effective program. Young people who have been trained to resist social pressures, who understand the consequences of smoking to their health, and who appreciate the difficulty of quitting are less likely to start smoking.

REFERENCES

HOLBROOK JH et al: Cigarette smoking and cardiovascular disease. A statement for health professionals by a Task Force appointed by the Steering Committee of the American Heart Association. Circulation 70:1114A, 1984
LOEB LA et al: Smoking and lung cancer: An overview. Cancer Res 44:5940, 1984
REPACE JL, LOWREY AH: A quantitative estimate of nonsmoker's lung cancer risk from passive smoking. Environ Int 11:3, 1985
US DEPARTMENT OF HEALTH, EDUCATION, AND WELFARE: Smoking and Health: A Report of the Surgeon General. DHEW(PHS) Publication no 79-50066, 1979
US DEPARTMENT OF HEALTH AND HUMAN SERVICES: The Health Consequences of Smoking: Cancer. A Report of the Surgeon General. DHHS(PHS) Publication no 82-50179, 1982
————: The Health Consequences of Smoking: Cardiovascular Disease. A Report of the Surgeon General. DHHS(PHS) Publication no 84-50204, 1983
————: The Health Consequences of Smoking: Chronic Obstructive Lung Disease. A Report of the Surgeon General. DHHS(PHS) Publication no 84-50205, 1984

174   ELECTRICAL INJURIES

JAMES F. WALLACE

EPIDEMIOLOGY Since the first human fatality from accidental electrocution was reported in 1879, electrical injury has become progressively more common. In recent years, nearly 4000 electricity-related injuries have occurred annually in the United States, and major electrical burns have constituted nearly 5 percent of all admissions to burn centers. There are approximately 1000 deaths each year from electric current accidents, while another 200 persons die as a result of being struck by lightning. Electrical injuries occur most commonly among agricultural workers, utility pole linemen, crane and heavy equipment operators, and construction workers who come into contact with high-tension current, but nearly a third result from accidents in the home or other settings including the hospital with its many electrically powered instruments and appliances.

PATHOGENESIS For an electric current to flow, there must be a closed pathway or circuit, and a difference in potential or voltage must exist between two points in this completed circuit. The flow of current is directly related to the voltage difference and inversely proportional to the electrical resistance between two points in the circuit (Ohm's law). High-resistance paths allow relatively small currents to flow, while low resistances permit large currents to flow.

When the voltage is very high, the flow of current will likewise be relatively great, unless the resistance is increased proportionally to the voltage; however, if the potential difference between the two points can be minimized, the current flow can also be minimized regardless of resistance.

Although the end result of passage of an electric current through the human body is unpredictable in the individual case, many factors are known to influence the nature and severity of electrical injuries. Body tissues vary considerably in their resistance to the flow of current, with conductivity being roughly proportional to water content. Bone and skin offer relatively high resistance, while blood, muscle, and nerve are good conductors. The resistance of normal skin can be lowered by moisture, and this factor alone can convert what might ordinarily be a mild injury to a fatal shock. Of importance at the time of contact is grounding which, if effective, can minimize the voltage difference between two points in the electric circuit and lower the intensity of current passing through the body. The pathway of the current through the body is also crucial. An accident involving passage of a current between a point of contact on the leg and the ground is less likely to be injurious than one between the head and the foot, in which the heart lies between the two poles of the circuit. Similarly, a small current leak which would be innocuous when applied to the surface of the intact body may result in a fatal arrhythmia when conducted directly to the heart via a low-resistance intracardiac catheter. Duration of contact also influences the outcome of electrical injury. Alternating current is much more dangerous than direct current, partly because of its ability to produce tetanic muscular contractions which prevent the victim from being able to release contact with the circuit. This is usually accompanied by sweating, which lowers skin resistance, allowing current of still greater intensity to pass into the body until fatal cardiac arrhythmia results.

In general, when sudden death occurs following low-voltage shock, it is due to the direct effect of relatively small amounts of current upon the myocardium resulting in ventricular fibrillation. With high-tension injury (greater than 1000 V), cardiac asystole and respiratory arrest occur probably as a result of injury to the medullary centers of the brain.

In addition, contact with high-intensity current may cause three types of thermal injuries. Current coursing externally to the body from the contact point to the ground may generate temperatures as high as 10,000°C and cause extensive carbonification of skin and immediately underlying tissues termed *arc* or *flash burns*. Such burns often ignite surrounding clothing or nearby objects which result in *flame burns*. Finally, there is injury due to the *direct heating* of tissues by electric current. As it traverses the skin, energy from current is converted into heat which produces coagulation necrosis at the points where it enters and exits from the skin as well as in striated muscle and blood vessels through which it passes. The associated vascular injury results in thromboses, often at sites distant from the body surface, and accounts for the observation that a greater amount of tissue destruction characteristically occurs in an electrical injury than is apparent on first inspection.

PATHOLOGY In patients who die immediately, autopsy findings are limited to burns and generalized petechial hemorrhages. If patients survive for a period of days or longer, postmortem examination reveals focal necrosis of bone, large blood vessels, muscle, peripheral nerves, spinal cord, or brain. Renal tubular necrosis may also be seen when acute renal failure follows extensive tissue destruction.

CLINICAL MANIFESTATIONS Immediately after a severe electrical shock, patients are usually comatose, apneic, and in circulatory collapse from ventricular fibrillation or cardiac standstill. If they survive this stage, they often are disoriented, combative, and frequently have seizures. Often they will be found to have fractures of bone caused either by convulsive muscular contractions accompanying the shock or from falls at the time of the accident. Hypovolemic shock often appears soon after high-tension electrical injury and is due to the rapid loss of fluid into areas of tissue damage, and from body surface burns. Hypotension, direct injury to the kidneys by the electric current, and renal tubular damage from myoglobin and hemoglobin pigments liberated during massive muscle necrosis and hemolysis may lead to acute renal failure.

Besides the extensive destruction of tissue occurring instantly in electrical burns, additional injury from ischemia produced by swelling of damaged tissues may appear later and is often accompanied by severe metabolic acidosis. Other serious complications are gastrointestinal hemorrhage from preexisting or acute Curling-type ulcers, neurogenic pulmonary edema, disseminated intravascular coagulation, and both anaerobic and aerobic infections originating in inadequately debrided necrotic muscle masses. Lightning injury may result in cerebral edema with coma lasting from several minutes to several days. Rupture of one or both tympanic membranes is seen in over half of lightning victims.

Late effects include various neurologic disabilities, visual disturbances, and the residual damage left by burns. Nervous system injuries are frequent and include peripheral neuropathies, incomplete transection of the spinal cord, and reflex sympathetic dystrophies, as well as late convulsive disorders and intractable headache. Psychological effects, particularly disturbances in memory and mood, are common in survivors of lightning strikes and may last for several months. The development of cataracts of one or both eyes has been reported to occur up to 3 years following electrical injury.

LABORATORY FINDINGS　Immediately following major electrical injury the hematocrit is elevated and the plasma volume reduced, reflecting sequestration of fluid in the wound. Unless extensive flame burns are also present, serial determinations of either of these parameters provide a good means of monitoring the adequacy of fluid replacement therapy. Myoglobinuria is seen frequently in association with severe shocks, and when it persists following establishment of urine flow, usually indicates massive muscle injury. In many patients arterial blood pH determinations will indicate the presence of metabolic acidosis. Lumbar puncture may show elevated pressure associated with cerebral edema or bloody spinal fluid as a result of intracerebral hemorrhage. The electrocardiogram not infrequently shows tachycardia and minor ST-segment alterations which can persist for several weeks following injury. Unexplained acute hypokalemia leading to respiratory arrest and cardiac arrhythmias has developed in some patients between the second and fourth weeks following injury.

TREATMENT　Removal of victims from contact with the current should be accomplished immediately without touching them directly. Rescuers should use a rubber sheet, a leather belt applied as a sling, a wooden pole, or other nonconductive material to detach them, and this should be preceded by cutting off the source of current when possible. If the victim is not breathing, mouth-to-mouth ventilation should be instituted at once. Although most cases who survive develop spontaneous respiration within half an hour, complete recovery after longer periods occurs often enough that respiratory support should be continued for at least 4 h. If there is no evidence of heartbeat, external cardiac massage should accompany ventilatory resuscitation. Persons struck by lightning frequently have cardiac asystole which responds to a manual blow to the chest, or which spontaneously resolves after several minutes of closed-chest cardiac massage and mouth-to-mouth resuscitation, while victims of low-voltage shocks will usually require defibrillation to restore heart action. During cardiopulmonary resuscitation and evacuation to the hospital, attention should be paid to possible broken bones and spinal cord injuries incurred at the time of the accident.

Subsequent hospital management of patients with electrothermal injuries requires considerable specialized care; whenever feasible, they should be referred to an appropriate burn or trauma unit.

Rapid institution of fluid and electrolyte therapy for hypovolemic shock and acidosis is essential, with guidelines being the patient's urine output, hematocrit, osmolality, central venous pressure, and arterial blood gases. Standard burn formulas should not be used to estimate fluid therapy since these are based only upon extent of body surface area injury and do not take into account the extensive damage to muscle which is usually present. Instead, fluid replacement principles used in the treatment of crush injury, which electrical injury closely resembles, should be followed. Large volumes of fluid, preferably lactated Ringer's solution, should be administered in order to maintain urine output greater than 50 mL/h. If myoglobinuria persists after adequate urine flow has been established, the use of furosemide or an osmotic diuretic such as mannitol along with alkalinization of the urine is indicated. Management of the electrical wound should include adequate debridement of necrotic tissue and often will require fasciotomy to prevent further ischemic injury. Anticlostridial prophylaxis, including tetanus toxoid and high doses of penicillin, should be administered to all severely injured patients, while topical antimicrobial chemotherapy with mafenide acetate or silver sulfadiazine may be useful in preventing or delaying infections in extensive surface burns. Survivors of the acute episode often require extensive treatment for infection, visceral injury, and delayed hemorrhage as devitalized tissues slough. If acute renal failure occurs, it should be managed as described in Chap. 219. Patients who remain comatose after being struck by lightning should undergo monitoring of intracranial pressure and cerebral perfusion and be treated for cerebral edema if it should develop.

PREVENTION　Proper installation of appliances, grounding of telephone lines and radio and television aerials, and the use of rubber gloves and dry shoes when working with electric circuits should be routine. Unused wall sockets should be kept plugged and live extension cords not left unattended, particularly in households where there are young children. Electrical appliances used in bathrooms should be disconnected when not in use and never used in wet bathtubs. During a severe thunderstorm, refuge near hilltops, riverbanks, hedges, telephone poles, and trees should be avoided. The safest shelter is the closed house, while a closed automobile, cave, ditch, or even lying on the ground curled up with hands close together is relatively secure. In hospitalized patients, the hazard of ventricular fibrillation precipitated by minute current leaks conducted directly to the myocardium from monitoring equipment via pacemakers or intravascular manometric catheters should be more widely appreciated. Hospital personnel should be aware that, in addition to medical instruments, patient contact with two or more other power line–operated devices such as television sets, radios, electric razors, lamps, and especially electric beds can also result in electrocution if the heart lies within the current path through the patient. These hazards can be minimized by proper grounding of equipment *before* a patient is connected to the instrument, periodic measurement for leakage of current supplied by each device, and by instruction in the principles of electrical safety for hospital personnel who use the complex and dangerous equipment that is so much a part of modern medical practice.

REFERENCES

AMY BW et al: Lightning injury with survival in 5 patients. JAMA 253:243, 1985

APFELBERG DB et al: Pathophysiology and treatment of lightning injuries. J Trauma 14:453, 1974

BUDNICK LD: Bathtub-related electrocutions in the US, 1979–1982. JAMA 252:918, 1984

HUNT J et al: Acute electric burns: Current diagnostic and therapeutic approaches to management. Arch Surg 115:434, 1980

SAFFLE JR et al: Cataracts: Long-term complication of electrical injury. J Trauma 25:17, 1985

SOLEM L et al: The natural history of electrical injury. J Trauma 17:487, 1977

175 DROWNING AND NEAR-DROWNING

JAMES F. WALLACE

EPIDEMIOLOGY In the United States, drowning accounts for approximately 7000 fatalities per year and is the third leading cause of accidental death among all age groups, and the second among individuals aged 5 to 44 years. Although no national statistics are available, it has been estimated that as many as 48,000 persons annually are near-drowning victims: those who live at least temporarily following an immersion incident. Children and young adults are most often the victims, and nearly 80 percent are males. Other risk factors are epilepsy, mental retardation, and alcohol abuse. With the increasing popularity of boating and water sports in this country nearly half the population is at risk of drowning each year, especially during the summer months.

PATHOPHYSIOLOGY Ten to twenty percent of drowning victims have no evidence of water aspiration in their lungs at autopsy ("dry drowning"). Death is due to asphyxia secondary to reflex laryngospasm and glottic closure. It is probable that a similar number of near-drowning victims also do not aspirate. If ventilation is reestablished before they sustain irreversible anoxic brain damage, prompt and complete recovery can be anticipated.

When aspiration accompanies drowning ("wet drowning"), the clinical situation is further complicated by the amount of surrounding water that is introduced into the respiratory tract as well as by the solutes and solids contained in it. A severe pulmonary injury often occurs, resulting in persistent arterial hypoxia and metabolic acidosis even after ventilation has been restored.

In the past, an important distinction was made between the pathophysiology of saltwater and freshwater drowning with respect to changes in blood volume, serum electrolyte concentrations, and cardiovascular function. However, it has been established that the most important problem in human near-drowning is hypoxia and that the other disturbances are of considerably less significance in determining survival.

The mechanisms by which hypoxia develops in near-drowning with aspiration are often multiple: laryngospasm, bronchospasm, airway obstruction secondary to aspirated particulate matter, and pulmonary edema following prolonged hypoxia can take place regardless of the composition of the water aspirated, while other types of lung injury causing hypoxia depend upon the osmolar and chemical characteristics of the immersion fluid. Aspiration of seawater, which is hypertonic compared with blood and chemically irritating to the pulmonary alveolocapillary membrane, causes a rapid shift of plasma proteins and water from the circulation into the alveolar lumen. Continued perfusion of these nonventilated, edema-filled alveoli results in an intrapulmonary right-to-left shunt and arterial hypoxia. When hypotonic fresh water is aspirated, fluid is rapidly absorbed from the lung into the circulation. Injury to alveolar lining cells takes place, altering or destroying the properties of pulmonary surfactant that maintains surface tension, and leading to alveolar collapse. Ventilation-perfusion ratios change in these atelectatic areas of lung, and hypoxia is the result. Metabolic acidosis, which is present in as many as 70 percent of near-drowning victims, is a consequence of tissue hypoxia and may be severe.

Although changes in electrolyte concentrations occur, depending upon the type and volume of fluid aspirated, these disturbances are rarely life-threatening. Most persons who aspirate sufficient quantities to produce marked electrolyte abnormalities do not survive the immersion incident. Similarly, profound changes in circulating blood volume are unusual. However, hypovolemia requiring treatment may be seen in massive saltwater aspiration accompanied by shifts of fluid from the vascular space into the lung.

Although rarely of clinical significance, some hemolysis of red blood cells often takes place, especially with freshwater aspiration.

Free hemoglobin may be found in the urine and blood, but the abnormality requires no specific therapy. Disseminated intravascular coagulation has been reported as a complication of freshwater near-drowning. It is thought that with extensive pulmonary injury, "tissue factor" in lung parenchyma and plasminogen activator from pulmonary endothelium are released, triggering the extrinsic clotting and fibrinolytic systems. Other pathophysiologic events in near-drowning include the development of renal failure secondary to acute tubular necrosis, probably due to the combined effects of hypoxia and hypotension, and neurologic deficits secondary to cerebral anoxia. Although the extent of the central nervous system injury tends to correlate with the duration of hypoxia, hypothermia accompanying the incident may be a moderating factor by reducing cerebral oxygen requirements. Complete neurologic recovery has been reported in victims submerged as long as 40 min in water temperatures less than 20°C.

CLINICAL MANIFESTATIONS The clinical features in near-drowning are variable and depend upon many factors including the amount and type of water aspirated and the promptness and effectiveness of treatment. Pulmonary and neurologic abnormalities usually predominate. Patients may present with mild cough and tachypnea, or with fulminant pulmonary edema. At least a third will require endotracheal intubation and some type of ventilatory therapy for the management of pulmonary injury. Instead of gradual recovery during the first 48 to 72 h of treatment, some patients will develop the adult respiratory distress syndrome, associated with progressive respiratory failure and reduction in lung compliance (see Chap. 216). Other pulmonary complications often include regional atelectasis due to aspirated particulate matter; secondary bacterial pneumonia; lung abscess; empyema; and injuries such as pneumothorax or pneumomediastinum sustained during resuscitation or related to ventilator therapy.

Early neurologic manifestations include seizures, especially during resuscitative efforts, and altered mental status, ranging from normal alertness to agitation, combativeness, or coma. Patients may present with speech, motor, or visual abnormalities or with more diffuse organic brain syndromes. Some of these neurologic deficits will improve gradually and resolve over several months. However, 5 to 20 percent of patients will have permanent sequelae, many of which prove ultimately fatal. Neurologic status usually does not continue to worsen after a near-drowning victim is admitted to the hospital unless there has been a preceding deterioration in pulmonary status. The possibility of unrecognized head trauma coincident with the drowning episode or a subdural hematoma should be considered as well.

Near-drowning victims often require treatment for cardiac as well as respiratory arrest during resuscitation. If this is successfully accomplished, most patients experience few additional cardiovascular problems. Supraventricular arrhythmias are common but usually resolve promptly when acidosis and hypoxia are treated. Heart failure secondary to myocardial ischemia or acutely expanded blood volume is unusual. Instead, pulmonary edema and low cardiac output states are usually due to the pulmonary injury from water aspiration with extravasation of fluid into the lung, resulting in hypovolemia.

Fever, frequently greater than 38°C, is seen in most patients within the first 24 h following significant aspiration. Its appearance later in the hospital course usually indicates a complicating infection. Vomiting is common during and after resuscitation. This often is associated with gastric distention by large quantities of fluid and air swallowed during the near-drowning episode and may result in additional aspiration. Other rare, but clinically important, features which may be encountered include acute renal failure and a severe hemorrhagic diathesis.

LABORATORY FINDINGS Arterial blood gas and pH determinations on admission reveal varying degrees of hypoxia and acidosis; follow-up values are the most reliable indicators of the effectiveness of ventilatory therapy. In 25 percent of near-drowning victims the initial chest x-ray film may be normal; however, this finding does not exclude the possibility that the patient has significant hypoxia. In the remainder of cases, radiologic findings range from fine, symmetric, perihilar infiltrates with relative sparing of apexes, bases, and lateral lung fields to massive bilateral pulmonary edema with little or no areas of sparing. Marked clearing of these abnormalities usually takes place within 72 to 96 h.

Alterations in serum sodium and potassium are generally mild and require no corrective treatment. Although leukocytosis up to 40,000 white blood cells per cubic millimeter is common during the first 24 to 48 h following near-drowning, significant changes in hematocrit and hemoglobin are rare, irrespective of the type of fluid aspirated. A *falling* hematocrit should raise the possibility of bleeding, not hemolysis, which, if it has occurred, should be apparent at the time of initial evaluation. Thrombocytopenia, prolonged prothrombin and partial thromboplastin times, hypofibrinogenemia, and elevated fibrin degradation products may be seen if disseminated intravascular coagulation takes place (see Chap. 281).

THERAPY   The primary objective of therapy is to correct hypoxia and acidosis as rapidly as possible. On-the-scene efforts should include immediate institution of mouth-to-mouth breathing and, if necessary, closed-chest cardiac massage. Time should not be wasted with attempts to drain water from the victim's lungs. However, it is important to establish and maintain a clear airway at the onset of resuscitation in order to avoid accidental overdistention of the stomach which might result in regurgitation and aspiration. One hundred percent oxygen should be administered by inhalation as soon as possible, and other necessary resuscitative efforts continued during evacuation to the hospital. Even if spontaneous ventilation returns and the patient seems coherent, high concentrations of oxygen should be continued, since severe hypoxia and acidosis may be present even in persons who are alert and without cyanosis.

All near-drowning victims should be taken to a hospital for further evaluation. Initial diagnostic studies should include arterial blood gas and pH determinations, hemogram, serum electrolytes, and chest x-ray. Patients who are alert, have normal chest x-rays, and show no evidence of hypoxia or acidosis usually require no further therapy. Nevertheless they should be observed for several hours for evidence of deterioration in blood gas and acid-base status prior to discharge. Metabolic acidosis should be treated by intravenous administration of sodium bicarbonate ($NaHCO_3$), and hypoxia with supplemental oxygen. If bronchospasm is present, aerosol inhalation of a bronchodilator may be given. Patients with pulmonary edema or hypoxia which fails to respond to increasing inspired oxygen tensions up to 40 percent should be intubated endotracheally and have positive end-expiratory pressure (PEEP) applied to the airways. When respiratory failure is present, lung compliance is markedly reduced, or the patient is unable to breathe spontaneously, mechanical ventilatory support should be used in addition to PEEP. Arterial blood gas tensions and pH should be determined frequently to assess the adequacy of respiratory therapy. Treatment with PEEP should be continued long enough for the lung injury to stabilize before it is withdrawn. This may take 48 to 72 h or even longer. Monitoring the magnitude of the intrapulmonary shunt, the pulmonary wedge pressure, and cardiac output by means of a Swan-Ganz intraarterial catheter is often very helpful in weaning patients from PEEP as well as in managing cases complicated by low cardiac output and hypotension.

Comatose near-drowning victims frequently are found to have elevated intracranial pressure, which is caused by cerebral edema and loss of cerebrovascular autoregulation. Prolonged elevations over 15 to 20 mmHg lead to reductions of cerebral blood flow, adding ischemic injury to already damaged brain tissue. In order to preserve cerebral function in such patients, aggressive therapy termed *cerebral resuscitation,* and including controlled hyperventilation, deliberate hypothermia, and the use of barbiturates, corticosteroids, and osmotic and loop diuretics, has been advocated while the intracranial pressure is closely monitored via subarachnoid bolts and intraventricular catheters. Although several investigators have reported that there are fewer major neurologic sequelae, particularly in children treated in this manner, the need for such aggressive and potentially hazardous therapy requires further study before it can be recommended for all patients in deep coma following near-drowning.

Other therapeutic measures are largely supportive. Patients should be observed closely for evidence of pulmonary infection and treated with appropriate antibiotics on the basis of results of cultures of respiratory secretions. Prophylactic use of antibiotics and corticosteroids has been of no benefit in near-drowning victims. Fluid and electrolyte balance should be carefully maintained. If hypovolemia is associated with low urinary output or hypotension, plasma expanders may be required. Transfusion with packed red blood cells or whole blood, depending upon circulating blood volume status, may be used for significant anemia. Acute renal failure should be managed as described in Chap. 219.

PROGNOSIS   The prognosis depends largely upon the extent and duration of the hypoxic episode. In addition, such factors as the temperature of the submersion medium, the availability and appropriate application of specific treatment, and coexisting medical illness or trauma are often important in determining the outcome. In general, patients who are alert and have normal chest x-rays upon arrival at the hospital can be expected to recover fully. Those who are obtunded but arousable and have normal respirations have nearly as good a prognosis, while approximately two-thirds of those who present in coma or cardiopulmonary arrest die or are left with significant neurologic deficits. Prediction of outcome on the basis of other presenting neurologic features or laboratory abnormalities is unreliable. The fact that nearly 90 percent of victims who live long enough to receive definitive hospital care will survive should serve to emphasize that extensive resuscitative efforts are advisable in all cases of near-drowning.

REFERENCES

CENTERS FOR DISEASE CONTROL: Drownings—Georgia, 1981–1983. Morb Mort Week Rep 34:281, 1985

CONN AW et al: Cerebral salvage in near-drowning following neurologic classification by triage. Can Anaesth Soc J 27:201. 1980

DAVIS S et al: Drownings of children and youth in a desert state. West J Med 143:196, 1985

FRATES RC JR: Analysis of predictive factors in the assessment of warm-water near-drowning in children. Am J Dis Child 135:1006, 1981

MARTIN TG: Near-drowning and cold water immersion. Ann Emerg Med 13:263, 1984

MODELL JH: Biology of drowning. Ann Rev Med 29:1, 1978

OAKES DD et al: Prognosis and management of victims of near-drowning. J Trauma 22:544, 1982

PFENNINGER J, SUTTER M: Intensive care after freshwater immersion accidents in children. Anesthesia 37:1157, 1982

YOUNG RSK et al: Neurological outcome in cold water drowning. JAMA 244:1233, 1980

section 1 Disorders of the heart

176 APPROACH TO THE PATIENT WITH HEART DISEASE

EUGENE BRAUNWALD

The symptoms caused by heart disease result most commonly from myocardial ischemia, from disturbance of the contractile activity of the myocardium, or from an abnormal cardiac rhythm or rate. Ischemia is manifest most frequently as chest discomfort, while reduction of the pumping ability of the heart commonly leads to weakness and fatigability or, when severe, produces cyanosis, hypotension, syncope, and elevated intravascular pressure behind a failing ventricle; the latter results in abnormal fluid accumulation, which in turn leads to dyspnea, orthopnea, and edema. Cardiac arrhythmias often develop suddenly, and the resulting signs and symptoms—palpitation, dyspnea, angina, hypotension, and syncope—generally occur abruptly and may disappear as rapidly as they develop.

A cardinal principle useful in the evaluation of the patient with suspected heart disease is that myocardial or coronary function which may be adequate at rest may be inadequate during exertion. Thus, a history of chest discomfort and/or dyspnea which appears only during activity is characteristic of heart disease, while the opposite pattern, i.e., the appearance of these symptoms at rest and their remission during exertion, is rarely observed in patients with organic heart disease.

Patients with cardiocirculatory disease may also be entirely asymptomatic, both at rest and during exertion, but may present an abnormal physical finding, such as a heart murmur, elevated systemic arterial pressure, or an abnormality of the electrocardiogram or of the cardiac silhouette on the chest roentgenogram.

Diseases of the heart and circulation are so common and the laity is so well acquainted with the major symptoms resulting from these disorders that patients, and occasionally physicians, erroneously attribute many complaints to organic cardiovascular disease. Furthermore, the combination of the widespread fear of heart disease in the western world with the deep-seated emotional connotations concerning this organ's function results in the frequent development in persons with normal cardiovascular systems of symptoms which mimic those of organic disease. Sometimes it is difficult to interpret correctly the symptoms of patients with recognized organic cardiovascular disturbances. Such patients, in addition to having symptoms resulting from their disease, may also develop functional complaints referable to the cardiovascular system. The unraveling of symptoms and signs due to organic heart disease from those which are not directly related is an important and challenging task in these patients.

It must be recognized that dyspnea, one of the cardinal manifestations of diminished cardiac reserve, is not limited to disease of the heart, but is also characteristic of conditions as diverse as pulmonary disease, marked obesity, and anxiety (Chap. 26). Similarly, chest discomfort (Chap. 4) may result from a variety of causes other than myocardial ischemia. Whether heart disease is responsible for these symptoms can frequently be determined by carrying out a detailed clinical examination. Noninvasive testing using electrocardiography at rest and during exercise (Chap. 178), roentgenography, and echocardiography (Chap. 179) usually provide important additional information to permit the correct interpretation of symptoms; more specialized invasive examinations (catheterization and angiography) are occasionally necessary.

DIAGNOSIS In every branch of medicine the establishment of the prognosis and development of a rational plan of management are based on a correct diagnostic appraisal. In patients with disorders of the cardiocirculatory system, particular care must be taken to establish not only a correct but also a *complete* diagnosis. As outlined by the New York Heart Association, the elements of a complete cardiac diagnosis include consideration of:

1 *The underlying etiology.* Is the disease congenital, rheumatic, hypertensive, or arteriosclerotic in origin?
2 *The anatomic abnormalities.* Which chambers are enlarged? Which valves are affected? Is there pericardial involvement? Has there been a myocardial infarction?
3 *The physiologic disturbances.* Is an arrhythmia present? Is there evidence of congestive heart failure or of myocardial ischemia?
4 *The extent of functional disability.* How strenuous is the physical activity required to elicit symptoms?

Two simple examples may serve to illustrate the importance of establishing a complete diagnosis. The identification of myocardial ischemia as the cause of exertional chest discomfort is of great clinical importance. However, this diagnosis is insufficient to develop either a strategy of specific treatment or prognosis until the underlying disease process, e.g., coronary atherosclerosis or aortic stenosis, which is responsible for the myocardial ischemia, is identified and a judgment made as to whether severe anemia, thyrotoxicosis, or supraventricular tachycardia plays a contributory role. Similarly, determining that heart disease is congenital provides an important starting point, but the decision about whether surgical treatment is advisable depends upon the specific anatomic defect present and often upon the nature of the physiologic disturbance and the functional impairment as well.

The establishment of a correct and complete cardiac diagnosis often requires the use of six different methods of examination: (1) history, (2) physical examination (Chap. 177), (3) electrocardiogram (Chap. 178), (4) chest roentgenogram (Chap. 179), (5) noninvasive graphic examinations (echocardiogram, radionuclide scanning techniques, and other "noninvasive" tests, Chap. 179), and occasionally (6) specialized "invasive" examinations, such as cardiac catheterization or angiocardiography (Chap. 180). In order to be most effective, the results obtained from each of these six modalities should be analyzed independently of one another as well as with the information derived from the other methods clearly in mind. Only in this way can one avoid overlooking a subtle, though extremely significant, finding. For example, an electrocardiogram should be obtained in every patient suspected of having heart disease. It may provide the critical clue in establishing the correct diagnosis, e.g., the finding of an atrioventricular conduction disturbance in a patient with unexplained syncope, even when all other methods of examination reveal no abnormal findings. On the other hand, when combined intelligently with the results of other methods of examination, the electrocardiogram may provide essential confirmatory data. Thus, the knowledge that a patient has an apical diastolic rumbling murmur may direct particular attention to the P waves, and the recognition of left atrial enlargement electrocardiographically supports the suggestion that the murmur is caused by mitral stenosis. Under these circumstances the additional finding on the electrocardiogram of right ventricular hypertrophy suggests that pulmonary hypertension is present and that the mitral stenosis is severe.

Although the electrocardiogram is an invaluable aspect of every cardiovascular examination, with the exception of the identification of arrhythmias it rarely permits establishment of a specific diagnosis. In the absence of any other abnormal findings, electrocardiographic changes must not be overinterpreted. The range of normal electrocardiographic findings is wide, and the tracing can be affected significantly by many noncardiac factors, such as age, body habitus, and serum electrolyte concentrations.

In obtaining the history of the patient with known or suspected cardiovascular disease, particular attention should be directed to the family history. Familial clustering is common in many forms of heart disease. Genetic transmission may occur, as in hypertrophic cardiomyopathy (Chap. 192) or Marfan's syndrome (Chap. 319). In patients with essential hypertension or coronary atherosclerosis the genetic component may be less obvious but also of considerable importance. Familial clustering of cardiovascular diseases may not only occur on a genetic basis but may also be related to familial, dietary, or behavior patterns.

When an attempt is made to ascertain the severity of functional impairment in a patient with heart disease, it is essential to determine the precise extent of activity and the rate at which it is performed before symptoms develop. Thus, breathlessness which occurs after running up two long flights of stairs denotes far less functional impairment than similar symptoms occurring after taking a few steps on the level. Also, the degree of customary physical activity at work and during recreation should be considered. The development of two-flight dyspnea in a marathon runner may be more significant than the development of dyspnea on far less exertion in a previously sedentary person. Similarly, the history must include a detailed consideration of the patient's therapeutic regimen. For example, the persistence or development of edema in a patient whose diet is rigidly restricted in sodium content and who is receiving optimum doses of diuretics must be interpreted quite differently from the finding of edema in the absence of these measures. In an effort to ascertain the rate of progression of symptoms, and thereby of the severity of the underlying illness, it may be useful to ascertain what, if any, specific tasks the patient could carry out 1 year earlier which he or she cannot carry out now.

PITFALLS IN CARDIOVASCULAR MEDICINE Increasing subspecialization in internal medicine and the perfection of advanced diagnostic techniques in cardiology may sometimes be accompanied by several undesirable consequences, which can be summarized as follows:

1 Failure by the *noncardiologist* to recognize cardiac manifestations of systemic illnesses. The latter include but are by no means limited to (a) the Down syndrome (associated with endocardial cushion defect); (b) gonadal dysgenesis, i.e., Turner's syndrome (associated with a variety of congenital defects, particularly coarctation of the aorta); (c) bony abnormalities of the upper extremities (associated with atrial septal defect); (d) muscular dystrophies (associated with

cardiomyopathy); (e) hemochromatosis and glycogen storage disease (associated with myocardial infiltration); (f) congenital deafness (associated with serious cardiac arrhythmias); (g) Raynaud's disease (associated with primary pulmonary hypertension and coronary vasospasm); (h) connective tissue disorders, i.e., Marfan's syndrome, Ehlers-Danlos syndrome, Hurler's syndrome, and related disorders of mucopolysaccharide metabolism (aortic dilatation, prolapsed mitral valve, a variety of arterial abnormalities); (i) chronic hemolytic anemia (cardiac dilatation); (j) Refsum's disease (myocardial failure and conduction defects); (k) acromegaly (accelerated coronary atherosclerosis, conduction defects, cardiomyopathy); (l) hyperthyroidism (heart failure, atrial fibrillation); (m) rheumatoid arthritis (pericarditis, aortic valve disease); (n) Whipple's disease (pericarditis and endocarditis); (o) scleroderma (cor pulmonale, myocardial fibrosis, pericarditis); (p) systemic lupus erythematosus (valvulitis, myocarditis); (q) polymyositis (pericarditis, myocarditis); (r) sarcoidosis (arrhythmias, cardiomyopathy); (s) Fabry's disease (myocardial ischemia, heart failure); (t) exfoliative dermatitis (high-output heart failure). In patients in whom these and other systemic disorders in which cardiovascular involvement may occur, a detailed cardiovascular examination should be carried out.

2 Failure by the cardiac specialist to recognize an underlying systemic illness, such as those listed above, among patients with a cardiac disorder. Patients known or suspected of having heart disease require a detailed general assessment and a search for the frequent noncardiac manifestations of systemic disorders with cardiovascular manifestations. Indeed, the cardiovascular abnormality may provide the clue critical to the recognition of these systemic disorders. Closely related is the failure to appreciate the profound effects of stress, such as that resulting from an intercurrent infection, of pregnancy, or from emotional disturbances, on cardiovascular performance and symptoms.

3 Overreliance on and overutilization of laboratory tests, particularly specialized invasive techniques for the examination of the cardiovascular system. Catheterization of the right and left sides of the heart, selective angiography, and coronary arteriography (Chap. 180), provide precise diagnostic information under many circumstances. For example, they aid in establishing a specific anatomic diagnosis and in determining the physiologic consequences of the abnormalities in patients with congenital heart disease, in patients with chest pain of uncertain etiology in whom coronary artery disease is suspected, and in determining the functional significance of valvular abnormalities in patients with rheumatic heart disease being considered for surgical treatment. Although a great deal of attention has been lavished on the newer specialized laboratory examinations, it should be recognized that they serve to *supplement*, not *supplant*, a careful examination carried out by clinical and noninvasive examination. There is an unfortunate tendency to carry out procedures such as coronary arteriography, in patients with chest pain suspected of having coronary artery disease, instead of taking a detailed and thoughtful history; although it may be established whether the coronary arteries are obstructed, the results often do not provide a definite answer to the question of whether a patient's complaint of chest pain is clearly attributable to coronary arteriosclerosis. Coronary arteriography is often carried out unnecessarily in patients with mild symptoms and signs of myocardial ischemia during exertion with normal left ventricular function who are not likely to be candidates for coronary bypass surgery. Similarly, catheterization of the left side of the heart is all too frequently employed to determine whether operative treatment of valvular disease is indicated, even before the patient has had a trial of medical therapy. Despite their enormous value, it must not be overlooked that these specialized examinations entail some small risk to the patient, involve discomfort and substantial cost, and place a strain on existing medical facilities. Therefore, *they should be carried out not as part of a "fishing expedition" or as evidence to the patient and the family that "everything is being done," but*

only if, after detailed clinical examination and assessment by noninvasive tests, the results of the invasive examination can be expected to modify or aid in the patient's management.

Treatment After a complete diagnosis has been established, a number of therapeutic options are usually available. Several examples may be used to demonstrate some of the principles of modern cardiovascular therapeutics:

1 In the absence of evidence for the existence of heart disease a clear, definitive statement to that effect should be made and the patient should *not* be asked to return at intervals for repeated examinations. If there is no evidence for disease, such attention may lead to the patient developing an abnormal fixation on the heart.

2 If there is no evidence of cardiovascular disease but the patient has one or more risk factors for the development of ischemic heart disease (Chap. 195), a plan for their reduction should be developed and the patient should be retested at intervals to assess that he or she is complying and that these risk factors are in fact being reduced.

3 Asymptomatic or mildly symptomatic patients with established organic heart disease, e.g., valvular heart disease, should be evaluated periodically, e.g., every 6 to 12 months, by clinical and noninvasive examinations (Chap. 179). Early warning signs of deterioration of ventricular function can be detected in this manner and in appropriate patients may signify the need for surgical treatment despite the absence of disabling symptoms (Chap. 187).

4 It is critical for the physician to establish clear criteria for deciding on the form of treatment (medical, angioplasty, or surgical revascularization) in patients with ischemic heart disease (Chap. 189). Surgical treatment represents a major therapeutic advance in the treatment of this most common form of heart disease, but operation has probably been employed too widely in the United States; the mere presence of angina pectoris and/or the demonstration of coronary arterial narrowing at angiography should not reflexly evoke a decision to treat the patient surgically. Instead, this form of treatment should be limited to those patients with ischemic heart disease in whom it has been demonstrated that surgical treatment is superior to medical treatment.

REFERENCES

BRAUNWALD E (ed): *Heart Disease*, 2d ed. Philadelphia, Saunders, 1984

FOWLER NO: *Cardiac Diagnosis and Treatment*, 3d ed. Hagerstown, Harper & Row, 1980

HORWITZ LD, GROVES BM (eds): *Signs and Symptoms in Cardiology*. Philadelphia, Lippincott, 1985

HURST JW et al (ed): *The Heart*, 6th ed. New York, McGraw-Hill, 1986

NEW YORK HEART ASSOCIATION, INC, CRITERIA COMMITTEE: *Nomenclature and Criteria for Diagnosis of Diseases of the Heart and Great Vessels*, 8th ed. Boston, Little, Brown, 1981

PERLOFF JK (ed): *Physical Examination of the Heart and Circulation*. Philadelphia, Saunders, 1982

177 PHYSICAL EXAMINATION OF THE HEART

ROBERT A. O'ROURKE / EUGENE BRAUNWALD

The general examination of a patient with cardiac disease often provides important information concerning the status of the cardiovascular system. The general physical appearance should first be assessed. The patient may appear tired because of a persistently low cardiac output; the respiratory rate may be increased, indicating pulmonary venous congestion. Central cyanosis, often associated with clubbing of the fingers and toes, indicates right-to-left shunting

of blood in the heart or great vessels or inadequate oxygenation of blood by the lungs. Cyanosis in the distal extremities, cool skin, and increased sweating result from vasoconstriction in patients with severe heart failure (Chap. 27). Noncardiovascular details can be equally important. For example, the diagnosis of infective endocarditis is highly likely in patients with petechiae, Osler's nodes, and Janeway lesions (Chap. 188).

The blood pressure should be taken in both arms and with the patient supine and upright; the heart rate should be timed for 1 min. Orthostatic hypotension and tachycardia may indicate a reduced blood volume, while resting tachycardia may be a clue to the presence of severe heart failure.

Careful examination of the optic fundi is essential (Chap. 196), and the retinal vessels may show evidence of systemic hypertension, arteriosclerosis, or embolism. The latter may result from atherosclerosis in larger arteries (e.g., carotid) or may represent a complication of valvular heart disease (e.g., endocarditis).

Palpation of the peripheral arterial pulses in the upper and lower extremities is necessary to define the adequacy of systemic blood flow and to detect the presence of occlusive arterial lesions. It is also important to examine both legs for evidence of edema, varicose veins, or thrombophlebitis (Chap. 198). The cardiovascular examination includes careful evaluation of both the carotid arterial and the jugular venous pulses, as well as deliberate precordial palpation and attentive cardiac auscultation. An understanding of the events of the cardiac cycle (Fig. 179-1, page 882) is vital to performing an accurate cardiovascular examination.

ARTERIAL PRESSURE PULSE The normal central aortic pulse wave is characterized by a fairly rapid rise to a somewhat rounded peak (Fig. 177-1). The anacrotic shoulder, present on the ascending limb, occurs at the time of peak rate of aortic flow just before maximum pressure is reached. The less steep descending limb is interrupted by a sharp downward deflection, synchronous with aortic valve closure, called the *incisura*. As the pulse wave is transmitted peripherally, the initial upstroke becomes steeper, the anacrotic shoulder becomes less apparent, and the incisura is replaced by the smoother dicrotic notch. Accordingly, palpation of a peripheral pulse (e.g., the radial arterial) frequently gives less information than examination of a more central pulse (e.g., the carotid arterial) regarding alterations in left ventricular ejection or aortic valve function. However, certain findings such as the bounding pulses of aortic regurgitation or pulsus alternans are more readily evident in peripheral than in central arteries (Fig. 177-2). The carotid pulse usually is best examined with the sternocleidomastoid muscle relaxed

FIGURE 177-1 *A. Schematic representation of electrocardiogram, aortic pressure pulse (AOP), phonocardiogram recorded at the apex, and apexcardiogram (ACG). On the phonocardiogram, S_1, S_2, S_3, and S_4 represent the first through fourth heart sounds; OS represents the opening snap of the mitral valve, which occurs coincident with the O point of the apexcardiogram. S_3 occurs coincident with the termination of the rapid-filling wave (RFW) of the ACG, while S_4 occurs coincident with the a wave of the ACG. B. Simultaneous recording of electrocardiogram, indirect carotid pulse (CP), phonocardiogram along the left sternal border (LSB), and indirect jugular venous pulse (JVP). ES, ejection sound; SC, systolic click.*

and with the head rotated slightly toward the examiner. In examining the brachial arterial pulse, the examiner can support the subject's relaxed elbow with his or her right arm while compressing the brachial pulse with the thumb. The usual technique for palpating the pulse is to compress the artery with the thumb or forefinger until the maximum pulse is sensed. The examiner should apply varying degrees of pressure while concentrating on the separate phases of the pulse wave. This method, referred to as *trisection*, is useful for assessing the sharpness of the upstroke, systolic peak, and diastolic slope of the arterial pulse. In most normal persons a dicrotic wave is not palpable.

A small weak pulse, *pulsus parvus*, is frequently present in conditions with a diminished left ventricular stroke volume, a narrow pulse pressure, and increased peripheral vascular resistance (Fig. 177-2). A hypokinetic pulse may be due to hypovolemia, to left ventricular failure secondary to myocardial disease or myocardial infarction, to restrictive pericardial disease, or to mitral valve stenosis. In aortic valve stenosis the delayed systolic peak, *pulsus tardus*, is the result of mechanical obstruction to left ventricular ejection and is often accompanied by the transmission of a coarse systolic thrill. In contrast, a large bounding pulse is usually associated with an increased left ventricular stroke volume, a wide pulse pressure, and a decrease in peripheral vascular resistance. This occurs characteristically in patients with abnormally elevated stroke volumes as in complete heart block, hyperkinetic circulation due to anxiety, anemia, exercise, or fever, or in patients with an abnormally rapid runoff of blood from the arterial system (patent ductus arteriosus, peripheral arteriovenous fistula). Patients with mitral regurgitation or a ventricular septal defect may also have a bounding pulse, since vigorous left ventricular ejection produces a rapid upstroke in the arterial pulse even though the duration of systole and the forward stroke volume may be diminished. In aortic regurgitation the rapidly rising, bounding arterial pulse results from increased left ventricular stroke volume and the associated increased rate of ventricular ejection.

The *bisferiens pulse*, which consists of two systolic peaks, is characteristic of aortic regurgitation (with or without accompanying stenosis) and of hypertrophic cardiomyopathy (Chap. 192). In the latter the pulse wave upstroke rises rapidly and forcefully, producing the first systolic peak ("percussion wave"). A brief decline in pressure follows because of the sudden decrease in the rate of left ventricular ejection during midsystole, when severe obstruction often develops. This pressure trough is followed by a smaller and more slowly rising positive pulse wave ("tidal wave") produced by continued ventricular ejection and by reflected waves from the periphery. The *dicrotic pulse* has two palpable waves, one in systole and one in diastole. It occurs most frequently in patients with a very low stroke volume, particularly in those with dilated (congestive) cardiomyopathy.

Pulsus alternans refers to a pattern in which there is regular alteration of the pressure pulse amplitude, despite a regular rhythm (Fig. 177-2). It is due to alternating left ventricular contractile force, usually denotes severe left ventricular decompensation, and commonly occurs in patients who also have a loud third heart sound. Pulsus alternans may also occur during or following paroxysmal tachycardia

or for several beats following a premature beat in patients without heart disease. In *pulsus bigeminus* there is also regular alteration of pressure pulse amplitude, but it is caused by a premature ventricular contraction that follows each regular beat. *Pulsus paradoxus* is an accentuation of the decrease in systolic arterial pressure accompanying the reduced amplitude of the arterial pulse which normally occurs during inspiration. In patients with pericardial tamponade, airway obstruction, or superior vena cava obstruction, the decrease in systolic arterial pressure frequently exceeds the normal of 10 mmHg and the peripheral pulse may disappear completely during inspiration.

Simultaneous palpation of the radial and femoral arterial pulses, which normally are virtually coincident, is important to rule out aortic coarctation, in which the latter is weaker and delayed (Chap. 185).

JUGULAR VENOUS PULSE (JVP)   The two main objectives of the bedside examination of the neck veins are inspection of their waveform and estimation of the central venous pressure (CVP). In most patients, the right internal jugular vein is superior for both purposes, but occasionally examination of the left internal jugular vein, the external jugular veins, or the venous pulsations in the supraclavicular fossae may yield more information. In most normal subjects, maximum pulsation of the internal jugular vein is observed when the trunk is inclined by less than 30°. In patients with elevated venous pressure it may be necessary to elevate the trunk further, sometimes to as much as 90°. When the neck muscles are relaxed, shining a beam of light tangentially across the skin overlying the vein exposes the pulsations of the internal jugular vein. Simultaneous palpation of the left carotid artery aids the examiner in deciding which pulsations are venous and in relating the venous pulsations to their timing in the cardiac cycle.

The normal JVP reflects phasic pressure changes in the right atrium and consists of two or sometimes three positive waves and two negative troughs (Fig. 177-1). The positive presystolic *a* wave is produced by venous distention consequent to right atrial contraction and is the dominant wave in the JVP, particularly during inspiration. Large *a* waves indicate that the right atrium is contracting against an increased resistance (Fig. 177-3), such as occurs with obstruction at the tricuspid valve (tricuspid stenosis) or more commonly with increased resistance to right ventricular filling (pulmonary hypertension or pulmonic stenosis). Large *a* waves also occur during dysrhythmias whenever the right atrium contracts while the tricuspid valve is closed by right ventricular systole. Such "cannon" *a* waves may occur regularly (as during junctional rhythm) or irregularly (as in atrioventricular dissociation with ventricular tachycardia or complete heart block). The *a* wave is absent in patients with atrial fibrillation, and there is an increased temporal delay between the *a* wave and the carotid arterial pulse in patients with first-degree atrioventricular block.

The *c* wave, often but not invariably observed in the JVP, is a positive wave produced by the bulging of the tricuspid valve into the right atrium during right ventricular isovolumetric systole and by the impact of the carotid artery adjacent to the jugular vein. The *x* descent is due to a combination of atrial relaxation and the downward displacement of the tricuspid valve during ventricular systole. In

A. Hypokinetic Pulse

B. Parvus et Tardus Pulse   C. Hyperkinetic Pulse

D. Bisferiens Pulse   E. Dicrotic Pulse + Alternans

FIGURE 177-2   *Schematic representation of arterial pulse waveforms that occur with alterations in cardiac hemodynamics which may result from normal physiologic responses or may be due to cardiac disease S, systole; D, diastole.*

A. Tricuspid Stenosis   B. Constrictive Pericarditis   C. Tricuspid Regurgitation

D Complete AV Block   E. Atrial Fibrillation

FIGURE 177-3 *Abnormal jugular venous pulse waveforms commonly present in patients with cardiac disease and/or arrhythmias. See text.*

patients with constrictive pericarditis (Fig. 177-3), there is often increased prominence of the x descent wave during systole, but this wave is reduced with right ventricular dilatation and may even be reversed in tricuspid regurgitation. The positive, late systolic v wave results from the increasing volume of blood in the venae cavae and right atrium during ventricular systole when the tricuspid valve is closed. With mild tricuspid regurgitation the v wave becomes more prominent, and when tricuspid regurgitation becomes severe, the prominent v wave and the obliteration of the x descent result in a single large positive systolic wave ("ventricularization"). After the peak of the v wave is reached, the right atrial pressure diminishes because of the decreased bulging of the tricuspid valve into the right atrium as right ventricular pressure declines and the tricuspid valve opens (Fig. 177-3).

Following the summit of the v wave there is a negative descending limb, referred to as the y descent or "diastolic collapse," which is produced mainly by the tricuspid valve opening and the rapid inflow of blood into the right ventricle. A rapid, deep y descent in early diastole occurs with severe tricuspid regurgitation. A venous pulse characterized by a sharp y descent, a deep y trough, and a rapid ascent to the baseline is seen in patients with constrictive pericarditis or with severe failure of the right side of the heart and a high venous pressure. A slow y descent in the JVP suggests an obstruction to right ventricular filling, as occurs with tricuspid stenosis or right atrial myxoma.

For accurate estimation of the CVP, the right internal jugular vein is best utilized, with the sternal angle as the reference point, since in the average patient the center of the right atrium lies approximately 5 cm below the sternal angle, regardless of body position. The patient is examined at the optimum degree of trunk elevation for visualization of venous pulsations. The vertical distance between the top of the oscillating venous column and the level of the sternal angle is determined and generally found to be less than 3 cm (3 cm + 5 cm = 8 cm blood). The most common cause of an elevated venous pressure is an elevated right ventricular diastolic pressure. In patients suspected of having right ventricular failure who have a normal CVP at rest, the abdominojugular reflux test may be helpful. The palm of the hand is placed over the abdomen and firm pressure is applied for 30 to 60 s. Normally, the jugular venous pressure is not significantly altered, but with impaired function of the right side of the heart the upper level of venous pulsation usually increases. Also, abdominal compression may elicit the typical JVP of tricuspid regurgitation when the resting pulse wave is normal. Kussmaul's sign, an increase rather than the normal decrease in the CVP during inspiration, is most commonly caused by severe right-sided heart failure; it is a frequent finding in patients with constrictive pericarditis or right ventricular infarction.

PRECORDIAL PALPATION The location, amplitude, duration, and direction of the cardiac impulse can usually be best appreciated by using the fingertips. The normal left ventricular apex impulse is located at or medial to the left midclavicular line in the fourth or fifth intercostal space and is a tapping, early systolic outward thrust localized to a point not more than 3 cm in diameter. It is due primarily to recoil of the heart as blood is ejected and should be evaluated with the patient supine and in the left lateral decubitus position. Left ventricular hypertrophy results in an exaggerated amplitude and duration of the normal left ventricular thrust. The impulse may be displaced laterally and downward into the sixth or seventh interspace, particularly in patients with a left ventricular volume load such as occurs in aortic regurgitation.

Additional abnormal features of the left ventricular apex include marked presystolic distention of the left ventricle, often accompanying a fourth heart sound in patients with an excessive left ventricular pressure load or myocardial ischemia/infarction, and a prominent early diastolic rapid-filling wave, often accompanying a third heart sound in patients with left ventricular failure or mitral valve regurgitation (Fig. 177-1). A double systolic impulse is frequently palpable in patients with hypertrophic cardiomyopathy.

Right ventricular hypertrophy results in a sustained systolic lift at the lower left parasternal area which starts in early systole and is synchronous with the left ventricular apical impulse. In patients with chronic obstructive pulmonary disease a right ventricular impulse may often be detected by sliding the fingers up under the rib cage just beneath the sternum. The enlarged right ventricle strikes the ends of the fingertips as an inferiorly directed movement.

Abnormal precordial pulsations occur during systole in patients with abnormal left ventricular wall motion due to ischemic heart disease or to diffuse myocardial disease from some other cause. These pulsations often occur in patients with a recent transmural myocardial infarction and may be present in some patients only during episodes of anginal pain. They are most commonly felt in the left midprecordium one or two interspaces above and/or 1 to 2 cm medial to the left ventricular apex. When a systolic bulge occurs in the region of the apex, it is difficult to distinguish it from the impulse of left ventricular hypertrophy.

A left parasternal lift is present frequently in patients with severe mitral regurgitation. This pulsation occurs distinctly later than the left ventricular apical impulse, is synchronous with the v wave in the left atrial pressure curve, and is due to anterior displacement of the right ventricle by an enlarged, expanding left atrium. A similar impulse occurring to the right of the sternum has been noted in some patients with severe tricuspid regurgitation and a giant right atrium. Pulsation of the right sternoclavicular joint may indicate a right-sided aortic arch or aneurysmal dilatation of the ascending aorta. Pulmonary artery pulsation is often visible and palpable in the second left intercostal space and may be normal in children or thin young adults. However, this pulsation usually denotes pulmonary hypertension, increased pulmonary blood flow, or poststenotic pulmonary artery dilatation.

Thrills are palpable, low-frequency vibrations associated with heart murmurs. The diastolic rumble of mitral stenosis and the systolic murmur of mitral regurgitation may be palpated at the cardiac apex. When the palm of the hand is placed over the precordium, the thrill of aortic stenosis crosses the palm of the hand toward the right side of the neck, while the thrill of pulmonic stenosis radiates more often to the left side of the neck. The thrill due to a ventricular septal defect is usually located in the third and fourth intercostal spaces near the left sternal border.

Percussion should be performed in each patient to identify normal or abnormal position of the heart, stomach, and liver. However, in patients with a normal cardiac situs, percussion adds little to careful inspection and palpation in the recognition of cardiac enlargement.

CARDIAC AUSCULTATION

To obtain maximal information from cardiac auscultation, the observer should keep in mind several principles: (1) This portion of the examination should be carried out in a quiet room to avoid the distractions caused by the noises of normal activity. (2) In order to hear a faint heart sound or murmur, it is necessary to focus attention on that phase of the cardiac cycle during which the auscultatory event may be expected to occur. (3) The accurate timing of a heart sound or murmur necessarily involves ascertaining its relation to other observable events in the cardiac cycle—the carotid arterial pulse, the JVP, or the apical impulse. (4) To determine the significance of a cardiac sound or murmur, it is often necessary to observe alterations in its timing or intensity during various physiologic and/or pharmacologic interventions (Table 177-1).

HEART SOUNDS The major components of heart sounds are vibrations associated with the abrupt acceleration or deceleration of blood within the cardiovascular system, but there is continuing controversy regarding the relative significance of the vibrations of valves, muscles, vessels, and supporting structures in the production of the heart sounds. Recent studies using simultaneous echocardiographic-phonocardiographic recordings indicate that the first and second heart sounds are produced primarily by the closure of the AV and semilunar valves and the events that accompany these closures. The intensity of the *first heart sound* (S_1) is influenced by (1) the position of the mitral leaflets at the onset of ventricular systole, (2) the rate of rise of the left ventricular pressure pulse, (3) the presence or absence of structural disease of the mitral valve, and (4) the amount of tissue, air, or fluid between the heart and the stethoscope. S_1 is increased in intensity if diastole is shortened because of tachycardia, if atrioventricular flow is increased because of high cardiac output or prolonged because of mitral stenosis, or if atrial contraction precedes ventricular contractions by a short PR interval. The loud S_1 in mitral stenosis usually signifies that the valve is pliable and that it remains open at the onset of isovolumetric contraction because of the elevated left atrial pressure. A reduction in the intensity

of S_1 may be due to poor conduction of sound through the chest wall, a slow rise of the left ventricular pressure pulse, a long PR interval, or imperfect closure due to reduced valve substance, as in mitral regurgitation. S_1 is also soft when the anterior mitral leaflet is immobile because of rigidity and calcification even in the presence of predominant mitral stenosis.

Splitting of the two high-pitched components of S_1 by 10 to 30 ms is a normal phenomenon (Fig. 177-1). The first component of S_1 normally is attributed to mitral valve closure and the second to tricuspid valve closure. A widened split of S_1 is most often due to complete right bundle branch block and the resulting delay in onset of the right ventricular pressure pulse. Reversed splitting of the S_1 with the mitral component following the tricuspid component has occasionally been noted in complete left bundle branch block and frequently is present in patients with severe mitral stenosis or a left atrial myxoma.

Splitting of S_2 into audibly distinct aortic (A_2) and pulmonic (P_2) components occurs normally during inspiration when augmented inflow into the right ventricle increases its stroke volume and ejection period and delays closure of the pulmonic valve. P_2 is coincident with the incisura of the pulmonary artery pressure curve, which is separated from the right ventricular pressure tracing by an interval termed the "hangout time." The absolute value of this interval reflects the resistance to pulmonary blood flow and the impedance characteristics of the pulmonary vascular bed. This interval is prolonged, and physiologic splitting of S_2 is accentuated in conditions associated with right ventricular volume overload and a distensible pulmonary vascular bed. However, in patients with an increase in pulmonary vascular resistance, the "hangout time" is markedly reduced and narrow splitting of S_2 is present. Splitting that persists with expiration, heard best at the pulmonic area or left sternal border, is usually abnormal when the patient is in the upright position. Such splitting may be due to delayed activation of the right ventricle (right bundle branch block), to prolongation of right ventricular contraction with an increased right ventricular pressure load (pulmonary embolism or pulmonic stenosis), or to delayed pulmonic valve closure because of right ventricular volume overload associated with diminished impedance of the pulmonary vascular bed and a prolonged "hangout time" (atrial septal defect). In pulmonary hypertension, P_2 is increased in intensity and splitting of the second heart sound may be diminished, normal, or accentuated, depending on the cause of the pulmonary hypertension, the pulmonary vascular resistance, and the presence or absence of right ventricular decompensation. Early aortic valve closure, occurring with mitral regurgitation or a ventricular septal

TABLE 177-1 Effects of physiologic and pharmacologic interventions on the intensity of heart murmurs and sounds*

Intervention	Changes in heart murmurs and sounds
Respiration	Systolic murmurs due to TR or pulmonic blood flow through a normal or stenotic valve and diastolic murmurs of TS or PR generally increase with inspiration or the Mueller maneuver as do right-sided S_3 and S_4. Left-sided murmurs and sounds usually are louder during expiration.
Valsalva maneuver	Most murmurs decrease in length and intensity. Two exceptions are the systolic murmur of HCM, which usually becomes much louder, and that of MVP, which becomes longer and often louder. Following release of the Valsalva, right-sided murmurs tend to return to control intensity earlier than left-sided murmurs.
Post VPB or AF	Murmurs originating at normal or stenotic semilunar valves increase in the cardiac cycle following a VPB or in the cycle after a long cycle length in AF. By contrast, systolic murmurs due to AV valve regurgitation do not change, diminish (papillary muscle dysfunction), or become shorter (MVP).
Positional changes	With *standing* most murmurs diminish, two exceptions being the murmur of HCM, which becomes louder, and that of MVP, which lengthens and often is intensified. With *squatting* most murmurs become louder but those of HCM and MVP usually soften and may disappear.
Exercise	Murmurs due to blood flow across normal or obstructed valves (e.g., PS, MS) become louder with both isotonic and submaximal isometric (handgrip) exercise. Murmurs of MR, VSD, and AR also increase with handgrip exercise. However, the murmur of HCM often decreases with near maximum handgrip exercise. Left-sided S_4 and S_3 are often accentuated by exercise, particularly when due to ischemic heart disease.
Pharmacologic interventions	During the initial relative hypotension following amyl nitrite inhalation, murmurs of MR, VSD, and AR decrease while murmurs of aortic stenosis or sclerosis increase. During the later tachycardia phase, murmurs of MS and right-sided lesions also increase. The response in MVP often is biphasic (softer then louder than control). The arterial constrictor phenylephrine tends to produce the opposite effects.
Transient arterial occlusion	Transient external compression of both arms by bilateral cuff inflation to 20 mmHg > peak systolic pressure augments the murmurs of MR, VSD, and AR but not murmurs due to other causes.

* TR, tricuspid regurgitation; TS, tricuspid stenosis; PR, pulmonic regurgitation; HCM, hypertrophic cardiomyopathy; MVP, mitral valve prolapse; PS, pulmonic stenosis; MS, mitral stenosis; MR, mitral regurgitation; VSD, ventricular septal defect; AR, aortic regurgitation; VPB, ventricular premature beat; and AF, atrial fibrillation.

defect, may also produce splitting that persists during expiration. It may also occur with constrictive pericarditis. In patients with large atrial septal defects the proportion of right atrial filling contributed by the left atrium and the venae cavae varies reciprocally during the respiratory cycle so that right atrial inflow remains relatively constant. Therefore, the volume and duration of right ventricular ejection are not significantly increased by inspiration, and there is little inspiratory exaggeration of the splitting of S_2. This phenomenon, termed "fixed splitting" of the second heart sound, is of considerable diagnostic value.

A delay in aortic valve closure causing P_2 to precede A_2 results in so-called reversed (paradoxic) splitting of S_2. Splitting is then maximal in expiration, and decreases during inspiration with the normal delay of pulmonic valve closure. The commonest causes of reversed splitting of S_2 are left bundle branch block and delayed excitation of the left ventricle from a right ventricular ectopic beat. Mechanical prolongation of left ventricular systole, resulting in reversed splitting of S_2, may be caused by severe aortic outflow obstruction, a large aorta-to-pulmonary artery shunt, systolic hypertension, and ischemic heart disease or cardiomyopathy with left ventricular failure. P_2 is normally softer than A_2 in the second left intercostal space; when P_2 is greater than A_2 in this area, it suggests pulmonary hypertension, except in patients with atrial septal defect.

The *third heart sound* is a low-pitched sound produced in the ventricle 0.14 to 0.16 s after A_2, at the termination of rapid filling. This sound is frequent in normal children and in patients with high cardiac output. However, in patients over 40 years of age, an S_3 usually indicates ventricular decompensation, AV valve regurgitation, or other conditions which increase the rate or volume of ventricular filling. The left-sided S_3 is best heard with the bell piece of the stethoscope at the left ventricular apex during expiration and with the patient in the left lateral position. The right-sided S_3 is best heard at the left sternal border or just beneath the xiphoid and is increased with inspiration. Often it is accompanied by the systolic murmur of functional tricuspid regurgitation. Third heart sounds often disappear with treatment of heart failure.

An earlier (0.10 to 0.12 s after A_2), higher-pitched third heart sound (pericardial knock) often occurs in patients with constrictive pericarditis; its presence is dependent upon the restrictive effect of the adherent pericardium, which halts diastolic filling abruptly.

The opening snap (OS) is a brief, high-pitched, early diastolic sound which is usually due to stenosis of an AV valve, more commonly the mitral valve. It is usually heard best at the lower left sternal border and radiates well to the base of the heart. The A_2-OS interval during exercise is inversely related to the height of the mean left atrial pressure, and ranges from 0.04 to 0.12 s. At the base an OS is often confused with P_2. However, careful auscultation at the upper left sternal border will reveal both components of the second heart sound, followed by the opening snap. The OS of tricuspid stenosis occurs later in diastole than the mitral OS. Since most patients with tricuspid stenosis also have severe mitral valve disease, the tricuspid OS is often overshadowed by the diastolic rumble and OS originating in the stenotic mitral valve. An OS also may occur when there is increased flow across an AV valve, such as exists with left-to-right intracardiac shunts and mitral or tricuspid regurgitation.

The *fourth heart sound* is a low-pitched, presystolic sound produced in the ventricle during the ventricular filling associated with an effective atrial contraction, and is heard best with the bell piece of the stethoscope. The sound is absent in patients with atrial fibrillation. The S_4 occurs when diminished ventricular compliance increases the resistance to ventricular filling, and it is present frequently in patients with systemic hypertension, aortic stenosis, hypertrophic cardiomyopathy, coronary artery disease, and acute mitral regurgitation. Most patients with an acute myocardial infarction and sinus rhythm have an audible S_4. The fourth heart sound is frequently accompanied by visible and palpable presystolic distention of the left ventricle. It is maximal in intensity at the left ventricular apex with the patient in the left lateral position, and is accentuated by mild supine exercise.

The right-sided S_4 is present in patients with right ventricular hypertrophy, secondary to either pulmonic stenosis or pulmonary hypertension, and frequently accompanies a prominent presystolic a wave in the JVP.

Audible fourth heart sounds also may be present during increased ventricular filling and normal ventricular compliance such as occurs in patients with severe anemia, thyrotoxicosis, or a peripheral arteriovenous fistula. An S_4 frequently accompanies delayed AV conduction even in the absence of clinically detectable heart disease. The incidence of an audible S_4 increases with increasing age. Whether an audible S_4 in adults without other evidence of cardiac disease is abnormal remains controversial.

The *ejection sound* is a sharp, high-pitched event occurring in early systole closely following the first heart sound. Ejection sounds occur in the presence of semilunar valve stenosis, i.e., opening snaps of the aortic or pulmonic valves, and in conditions associated with dilatation of the aorta or pulmonary artery. The aortic ejection sound is usually heard best at the left ventricular apex and the second right interspace; the pulmonary ejection sound is of maximal intensity at the upper left sternal border. The latter, unlike most other right-sided acoustical events, is heard better during expiration.

Nonejection systolic clicks, occurring with or without a late systolic murmur, often denote prolapse of one or both leaflets of the mitral valve. They may also be caused by tricuspid valve prolapse (Chap. 187). They probably result from functional unequal length of the chordae tendineae of either or both AV valves and are heard best along the lower left sternal border and at the left ventricular apex. Systolic clicks may be single or multiple, and they may occur at any time in systole but usually later than the systolic ejection sound. Frequently the midsystolic click is misinterpreted as S_2, and the actual second heart sound is called an OS or S_3.

HEART MURMURS Cardiac murmurs result from vibrations set up in the bloodstream and the surrounding heart and great vessels as a result of turbulent blood flow, the formation of eddies, and cavitation (bubble formation as a result of sudden decrease in pressure).

The intensity or loudness of murmurs may be graded from I to VI. A grade I murmur is so faint that it can be heard only with special effort, and a grade VI murmur is audible with the stethoscope removed from contact with the chest. The configuration of a murmur may be crescendo, decrescendo, crescendo-decrescendo (diamond-shaped), or plateau. The precise time of onset and time of cessation of a murmur depend on the instant in the cardiac cycle at which an adequate pressure difference between two chambers appears and disappears (Fig. 177-4).

FIGURE 177-4 *Schematic representation of ECG, aortic pressure (AOP), left ventricular pressure (LVP), and left atrial pressure (LAP). HSM is a holosystolic murmur; PSM, a presystolic murmur; MDM, a middiastolic murmur; MSM, a midsystolic murmur; EDM, an early diastolic murmur; LSM, a late systolic murmur; and CM, a continuous murmur.*

The location on the chest wall where the murmur is best heard and the areas to which it radiates can be helpful in identifying the cardiac structure from which the murmur originates. For example, the murmur of aortic valve stenosis is loudest usually in the second right intercostal space and radiates to the carotid arteries. By contrast, the murmur of mitral regurgitation is most often loudest at the cardiac apex and may radiate to the left sternal border and base of the heart when the posterior mitral leaflet is predominantly involved or to the axilla and back when the anterior leaflet is more severely affected. In the former case, the regurgitant blood is directed toward the posterior left atrial wall.

Many times it is difficult to classify with certainty a cardiac murmur based on its timing, configuration, location, radiation, pitch, or intensity. However, by noting changes in the characteristics of the murmur during maneuvers which alter cardiac hemodynamics, the auscultator often can identify its correct origin and significance (Table 177-1).

Accentuation of a murmur during inspiration with the augmentation of systemic venous return implies that it originates on the right side of the circulation; expiratory exaggeration has less significance. Prolonged expiratory pressure against a closed glottis, the Valsalva maneuver, reduces intensity of most murmurs by diminishing both right and left ventricular filling. The systolic murmur associated with *hypertrophic cardiomyopathy* and the late systolic murmur due to a *mitral valve prolapse* are exceptions and may be accentuated during the Valsalva maneuver. Murmurs due to flow across a normal or obstructed semilunar valve increase in intensity in the beat following a premature ventricular beat or a long RR interval in atrial fibrillation. In contrast, murmurs due to AV valve regurgitation or a ventricular septal defect do not change appreciably during the beat following a prolonged diastole. Standing, which decreases heart size, accentuates the murmur of hypertrophic cardiomyopathy and occasionally the murmur due to a prolapse of the mitral valve. Squatting, which increases both venous return and systemic arterial resistance, increases most murmurs, except those due to hypertrophic cardiomyopathy and mitral regurgitation due to a prolapsed mitral valve, which often decrease. Sustained handgrip exercise, which increases the systemic arterial pressure and heart rate, often accentuates the murmurs of mitral regurgitation, aortic regurgitation, and mitral stenosis but usually diminishes those due to aortic stenosis or hypertrophic cardiomyopathy. Pharmacologic interventions include inhalation of amyl nitrite, which reduces systemic arterial pressure and increases blood flow, thereby increasing the intensity of murmurs due to valvular stenosis while diminishing those due to aortic or mitral regurgitation (Table 177-1). Transient external arterial occlusion by the inflation of bilateral arm cuffs to 20 mmHg above systolic blood pressure for 5 s has been shown to intensify murmurs due to left-sided regurgitant lesions; this method is applicable to almost all patients and does not require administration of any drug.

Systolic murmurs   *Holosystolic (pansystolic) murmurs* are generated when there is a flow between two chambers which have widely different pressures throughout systole, such as the left ventricle and either the left atrium or the right ventricle. The pressure gradient is established early in contraction and lasts until relaxation is almost complete. Therefore, holosystolic murmurs begin before aortic ejection, and at the area of maximal intensity they begin with S_1 and end after S_2. Holosystolic murmurs accompany mitral or tricuspid regurgitation, ventricular septal defect, and under certain circumstances, aorta-pulmonary shunts. Although the typical high-pitched murmur of mitral regurgitation usually continues throughout systole, the shape of the murmur may vary considerably. The holosystolic murmurs of mitral regurgitation and ventricular septal defect are augmented by raising the arterial pressure with intravenous phenylephrine and are diminished by lowering the left ventricular systolic pressure by inhalation of amyl nitrite. The murmur of tricuspid regurgitation associated with pulmonary hypertension is holosystolic and frequently increases during inspiration, a feature of diagnostic importance. Not all patients with mitral or tricuspid regurgitation or ventricular septal defect have holosystolic murmurs (Chap. 187).

Midsystolic murmurs, often crescendo-decrescendo in shape, occur when blood is ejected across the aortic or pulmonic outflow tracts. The murmur starts shortly after S_1 when the ventricular pressure rises sufficiently to open the semilunar valve. Ejection then begins and with it the onset of the murmur; as ejection increases, the murmur is augmented, and as ejection declines, it diminishes. The murmur ends before the ventricular pressure falls enough to permit closure of the aortic or pulmonic leaflets. In the presence of normal semilunar valves and increased flow rate, as may occur in states of elevated cardiac output, ejection into a dilated vessel beyond the valve, or increased transmission of sound through a thin chest wall may be responsible for the production of this murmur. Most benign, functional murmurs are midsystolic and originate from the pulmonary outflow tract. Valvular or subvalvular obstruction to either ventricle may also cause such a midsystolic murmur, the intensity being related to the flow.

The murmur of aortic stenosis is the prototype of the left-sided midsystolic murmur. The location and radiation of this murmur appear to be influenced by the direction of the high-velocity jet within the aortic root. In *valvular aortic stenosis* the murmur is usually maximal in the second right intercostal space, with radiation into the neck. In *supravalvular aortic stenosis* the murmur is occasionally loudest even higher, with disproportionate radiation into the right carotid artery. In hypertrophic cardiomyopathy, the murmur originates within the left ventricular cavity, and is usually maximal at the lower left sternal edge and apex, with relatively little radiation to the carotids. When the aortic valve is immobile (calcified), the aortic closure sound (A_2) may be soft and inaudible so that the length and configuration of the murmur are difficult to determine. Midsystolic murmurs also occur in patients with mitral regurgitation or, less frequently, tricuspid regurgitation resulting from papillary muscle dysfunction. Murmurs due to mitral regurgitation are often confused with those originating in the aorta, particularly in elderly patients.

The patient's age and the area of maximal intensity aid in determining the significance of midsystolic murmurs. Thus, in a young adult with a thin chest and high velocity of blood flow, a faint or moderate midsystolic murmur heard only in the pulmonic area is usually without clinical significance, while a somewhat louder murmur in the aortic area may indicate congenital aortic stenosis. In elderly patients pulmonic flow murmurs are rare, while aortic systolic murmurs are frequent and may be due to aortic dilatation, to a significant degree of valvular aortic stenosis, or to nonstenotic deformity of the aortic valve. Midsystolic aortic and pulmonic murmurs are intensified by amyl nitrite inhalation and during the cardiac cycle following a premature ventricular contraction, while those due to mitral regurgitation are unchanged or softer. Aortic systolic murmurs are diminished by interventions which increase systemic arterial resistance, such as intravenous phenylephrine. Echocardiography or cardiac catheterization may be necessary to separate a prominent and exaggerated functional murmur from one due to congenital semilunar valve stenosis.

Early systolic murmurs begin with the first heart sound and end in midsystole. They may be due to a very small *ventricular septal defect, a large defect with pulmonary hypertension,* or *severe acute mitral* or *tricuspid regurgitation.* In large ventricular septal defects with pulmonary hypertension, the shunting at the end of systole may be small or absent, resulting in an early systolic murmur. A similar murmur may occur with very small muscular ventricular septal defects, the shunt being interrupted in late systole. An early systolic murmur is a feature of tricuspid regurgitation occurring in the absence of pulmonary hypertension. This lesion is common in drug addicts with infective endocarditis, in whom a tall regurgitant right atrial *v* wave reaches the level of the normal right ventricular pressure in late systole, confining the murmur to early systole. In patients with acute mitral regurgitation and a large *v* wave in a noncompliant left atrium, a loud early systolic murmur is frequently heard which diminishes as the pressure gradient between left ventricle and left atrium decreases in late systole (Chap. 187).

Late systolic murmurs are faint or moderately loud high-pitched apical murmurs, which start well after ejection and do not mask either heart sound. They are probably related to papillary muscle dysfunction caused by infarction or ischemia of these muscles or to their distortion by left ventricular dilatation. They may appear only during angina but are common in patients with myocardial infarction or diffuse myocardial disease. Late systolic murmurs following mid-systolic clicks are associated with late systolic mitral regurgitation caused by prolapse of the mitral valve into the left atrium (Chap. 187).

Diastolic murmurs *Early diastolic murmurs* begin with or shortly after the second heart sound as soon as the corresponding ventricular pressure falls sufficiently below that in the aorta or pulmonary artery. The high-pitched murmurs of aortic regurgitation or pulmonic regurgitation due to pulmonary hypertension are generally decrescendo, since there is a progressive decline in the volume or rate of regurgitation during diastole. Faint, high-pitched murmurs of aortic regurgitation are difficult to hear unless they are specifically sought by applying firm pressure with the diaphragm over the left midsternal border while the patient sits, leans forward, and holds a breath in full expiration. The diastolic murmur of aortic regurgitation is enhanced by an acute elevation of the arterial pressure such as occurs with handgrip exercise; it diminishes with a decrease in arterial pressure which may be induced during amyl nitrite inhalation. The diastolic murmur of congenital pulmonic regurgitation in the absence of pulmonary hypertension is low- to medium-pitched. The onset of this murmur is delayed because at the onset of pulmonic valve closure the regurgitant flow is minimal, since the reverse pressure gradient responsible for the regurgitation is negligible at this time.

Middiastolic murmurs usually arise from the AV valves, occur during early ventricular filling, and like most midsystolic murmurs, are due to disproportion between valve orifice size and flow rate. Such murmurs may be loud despite only slight AV valve stenosis when there is normal or increased blood flow. Conversely, the murmur may be soft or even absent despite severe obstruction if the cardiac output is markedly reduced. When stenosis is marked, the diastolic murmur is prolonged and the duration of the murmur is more reliable than its intensity as an index of the degree of valve obstruction.

The low-pitched, middiastolic murmur of mitral stenosis characteristically follows the opening snap. It should be specifically sought by placing the bell of the stethoscope at the site of the left ventricular impulse, which is best localized with the patient on the left side. Frequently the murmur of mitral stenosis is present only at the left ventricular apex, and it may be increased in intensity by mild supine exercise or by inhalation of amyl nitrite. In tricuspid stenosis the middiastolic murmur is localized to a relatively limited area along the left sternal edge and may increase in intensity during inspiration.

Middiastolic murmurs may be generated across the mitral valve in ventricular septal defect, patent ductus arteriosus, or mitral regurgitation, and across the tricuspid valve in atrial septal defect or tricuspid regurgitation. These murmurs are related to the torrential flow across an AV valve, usually follow a third heart sound, and tend to occur with large left-to-right shunts or severe AV valve regurgitation. A soft middiastolic murmur may sometimes be heard in patients with acute rheumatic fever (Carey-Coombs murmur). It has been attributed to inflammation of the mitral valve cusps or excessive left atrial blood flow as a consequence of mitral regurgitation.

In acute aortic regurgitation, the left ventricular diastolic pressure may exceed the left atrial pressure, resulting in a middiastolic murmur due to "diastolic mitral regurgitation." In severe chronic aortic regurgitation a murmur is frequently present which may be either middiastolic or presystolic (Austin Flint murmur). This murmur appears to originate at the anterior mitral valve leaflet when blood

simultaneously enters the left ventricle from both the aortic root and the left atrium.

Presystolic murmurs begin during the period of ventricular filling that follows atrial contraction and therefore occur in sinus rhythm. They are usually due to AV valve stenosis and have the same quality as the middiastolic filling rumble but are usually crescendo, reaching peak intensity at the time of a loud S_1. The presystolic murmur corresponds to the AV valve gradient, which may be minimal until the moment of right or left atrial contraction. It is the presystolic rather than the middiastolic murmur which is most characteristic of tricuspid stenosis and sinus rhythm. A right or left *atrial myxoma* may occasionally cause either middiastolic or presystolic murmurs that resemble the murmurs of mitral or tricuspid stenosis.

Continuous murmurs begin in systole, peak near S_2, and continue into all or part of diastole. These murmurs signify continuous flow due to communication between high- and low-pressure areas which persists through the end of systole and the beginning of diastole. A *patent ductus arteriosus* causes a continuous murmur as long as the pressure in the pulmonary artery is much below that in the aorta. The murmur is intensified by elevation of the systemic arterial pressure and is reduced by amyl nitrite inhalation. When pulmonary hypertension is present, the diastolic portion may disappear, leaving the murmur confined to systole. A continuous murmur is uncommon in aortopulmonary septal defects, since this malformation is generally associated with severe pulmonary hypertension. Surgically produced aortopulmonary connections and the subclavian–pulmonary artery anastomosis result in murmurs similar to that of a patent ductus.

Continuous murmurs may result from congenital or acquired *systemic arteriovenous fistula, coronary arteriovenous fistula,* anomalous origin of the left coronary artery from the pulmonary artery, and communications between the *sinus of Valsalva and the right side of the heart.* Continuous murmurs may also occur when high left atrial pressure results in continuous flow across a small defect in the atrial septum. Murmurs associated with *pulmonary arteriovenous fistulas* may be continuous but are usually only systolic. Continuous murmurs may also be due to disturbances of flow pattern in constricted systemic (e.g., renal) or pulmonary arteries when marked pressure differences between the two sides of the narrow segment persist; a continuous murmur in the back may be present in *coarctation of the aorta; pulmonary embolism* may cause continuous murmurs in partially occluded vessels.

In nonconstricted arteries continuous murmurs may be due to rapid flow through a tortuous bed. Such murmurs typically occur within the bronchial arterial collateral circulation in cyanotic patients with severe pulmonary outflow obstruction. The "mammary souffle," an innocent murmur heard during late pregnancy and early postpartum, may be systolic or continuous. The innocent cervical venous hum is a continuous murmur usually heard over the medial aspect of the right supraclavicular fossa with the patient upright. The hum is usually louder during diastole and can be instantaneously abolished by digital compression of the ipsilateral internal jugular vein. Transmission of a loud venous hum to the area below the clavicles may result in a mistaken diagnosis of patent ductus arteriosus.

The *pericardial friction rub,* which may have presystolic, systolic, and early diastolic scratchy components, may be confused with a murmur or extracardiac sound when heard only in systole. It is best appreciated with the patient upright and leaning forward and may be accentuated during inspiration.

REFERENCES

BARAGAN J et al (eds): *Dynamic Auscultation and Phonocardiography.* Maryland, Charles Press Publishers, 1979

BRAUNWALD E: Physical examination, in *Heart Disease,* 2d ed, E Braunwald (ed). Philadelphia, Saunders, 1984, p 14

CRAIGE E: Echophonocardiography and other noninvasive techniques to elucidate heart murmurs, in *Heart Disease,* 2d ed, E Braunwald (ed). Philadelphia, Saunders, 1984, p 68

————: Heart Sounds: Phonocardiography pulse tracings; and systolic time intervals, in *Heart Disease*, 2d ed, E Braunwald (ed). Philadelphia, Saunders, 1984, p 40

DELL ITALIA LJ et al: Physical examination for exclusion of hemodynamically important right ventricular infarction. Ann Intern Med 99:608, 1983

EILEN SD, CRAWFORD MH, O'ROURKE RA: Accuracy of precordial palpation for detecting increased left ventricular volume. Ann Intern Med 99:628, 1983

FOWLER NO: Cardiac auscultation, in *Cardiac Diagnosis and Treatment*, 3d ed, NO Fowler (ed). Hagerstown, Harper & Row, 1980, p 62

LEATHAM A: *Auscultation of the Heart and Phonocardiography*, 2d ed. New York, Churchill Livingstone, 1976

PERLOFF JK (ed): *Physical Examination of the Heart and Circulation*. Philadelphia, Saunders, 1982

REDDY PS, SALERNI R, SHAVER JA: Normal and abnormal heart sounds in cardiac diagnosis, Part II: Diastolic sounds. Curr Probl Cardiol 10(4):1, 1985

ROTHMAN A, GOLDBERGER AL: Aids to cardiac auscultation. Ann Intern Med 99:346, 1983

SHAVER JA, SALERNI R, REDDY PS: Normal and abnormal heart sounds in cardiac diagnosis, Part I: Systolic sounds. Curr Probl Cardiol 10(3):1, 1985

TAVEL ME: *Clinical Phonocardiography and External Pulse Recordings*, 4th ed. Chicago, Year Book, 1985

178 ELECTROCARDIOGRAPHY

ROBERT J. MYERBURG

INTRODUCTION The electrocardiogram (ECG) is a graphic description of the electrical activity of the heart, recorded from the body surface by electrodes positioned to reflect activity from a variety of spatial perspectives. The source of cardiac electrical activity resides within the working (contracting) myocardial cells as well as within the automatic and specialized cells as described in Chap. 183.

The magnitude and direction of the electrical activity recorded on the body surface are an average of the numerous cell depolarizations or repolarizations occurring at a given instant. Although much of the electrical activity from individual cells is canceled out before reaching the body surface by opposing forces from other cells, the resultant recording is a reasonably reproducible and accurate approximation of net cardiac electrical activity. However, the signals recorded at the body surface do not identify sites of origin because a given vector at the body surface can be accounted for by innumerable combinations of cellular signals at their source in the heart.

Early in the development of the ECG, Einthoven popularized the concept that the human body represents a large volume conductor having the source of cardiac electrical activity at its center. While this theory is not strictly accurate, it provides the clinician with a practical point from which to work. As an extension of this concept, the *net* electrical activity at any instant in the cardiac cycle may be viewed as originating from a polarized point source at a theoretical "electrical center" of the heart. Since this "equivalent dipole" would have direction and magnitude, one might then extend the pattern into a sequence of instantaneous vectors recordable from the body surface. The application of this concept to ECG analysis is discussed below.

LEAD SYSTEMS The ECG lead system is composed of five electrodes, one on each of the four limbs and one placed at various sites on the precordium. Each lead is a continuous recording of the change in electrical potential during the cardiac cycle between two of the electrodes, or between one electrode and a combination of the others. The right-leg electrode is an inactive ground electrode in all leads.

The original lead system developed by Einthoven is based on assumptions of (1) the homogeneity of the body volume conductor, (2) the symmetry of the leads, and (3) a single equivalent dipole at the center of the volume conductor. The *standard limb leads* (I, II, and III) are composed of three permutations of the right arm (RA), left arm (LA), and left leg (LL) electrodes [Fig. 178-1A (1)]. Lead I records the potential difference between the LA and the RA, the positive electrode on the LA, and the negative electrode on the RA [Fig. 178-1A (2)]. Lead II records the potential difference between the electrodes on the RA and the LL, the positive electrode on the LL. Lead III records the potential difference between the LA and the LL, with the positive electrode on the LL. It is likely that Einthoven

arbitrarily selected the relationships between positive and negative electrodes in the three leads in order to have the major deflection of the QRS complex (see below) moving in an upward (positive) direction in most normal individuals.

The central terminal of Wilson (CTW) is constructed by connecting the RA, LA, and LL electrodes through 5000-Ω resistances, in order to cancel out the potentials from these three points. With the forces canceled out, the CTW theoretically remains inactive during the entire cardiac cycle, and an exploring electrode will function as a unipolar lead [Fig. 178-1B (1)]. The selection of the positions for the six *unipolar chest leads* [Figs. 178-1B (2) and 178-2] was based on the concept that the proximity of the heart to the anterior chest wall resulted in the unipolar chest leads functioning as "semidirect" leads, being influenced primarily by the tissue immediately beneath the electrode. While this concept does not have the quantitative signifi-

FIGURE 178-1 *Lead systems. A. Standard limb leads, showing (1) electrode positions, (2) the equilateral triangle of Einthoven, and (3) the conversion of the triangle to a triaxial reference system with positive (+) and negative (−) polarity. B. The unipolar chest leads, showing (1) the central terminal of Wilson (CTW) (or the indifferent electrode −i) and the chest electrode (C) (or the exploring electrode −E). The 5000 Ω between CTW and each limb electrode is not shown. The relationship between CTW and V_1 to V_6 in the horizontal plane is shown in B (2). C. The augmented unipolar limb leads, using the modified CTW. D. The hexaxial frontal plane reference system. Normal ranges are described in the text, and applications are derived in Figs. 178-5 and 178-6. RA, right arm; LA, left arm; LL, left leg; RL, right leg.*

Standard Limb Leads (I, II, and III)

Unipolar Chest Leads (V_1 - V_6)

Augmented Unipolar Limb Leads (aVR, aVL, aVF)

FIGURE 178-2 *The unipolar chest leads. A. The position of the chest electrode for V₁ to V₆. B. The relationship between the CTW and the chest electrode (C) in the horizontal plane.*

FIGURE 178-3 *Standardization of the ECG. Standard time calibration is 1 mm = 0.04 s or 5 mm = 0.20 s. Standard voltage is 0.1 mV/mm. A repetitive event occurring every 5 mm (A) on time axis (0.20 s) is occurring at 300 per minute. A repetitive event occurring every 10 mm (B) (0.40 s) is occurring at 150 per minute. C, D, and E indicate that repetitive events at 0.60, 0.80, and 1.00 s are occurring at rates of 100, 75, and 60 per minute, respectively.*

cance originally assumed, and the recordings do reflect the activity of the total heart, there is weighting of the voltages recorded by the tissue closest to the exploring electrode. The six standard chest leads (V₁ to V₆) are recorded by positioning the exploring chest electrode as follows: V₁ in the fourth intercostal space (4ICS) at the right sternal border; V₂ in the 4ICS at the left sternal border; V₄ in the 5ICS at the midclavicular line; V₃ midway between V₂ and V₄; V₅ at the left anterior axillary line at the level of V₄ horizontally; and V₆ at the left midaxillary line at the level of V₄ horizontally (Fig. 178-2). The CTW is the indifferent electrode, and the exploring chest electrode is the active electrode.

Unipolar limb leads may be recorded by a system in which the CTW constitutes the indifferent electrode and the exploring electrode is one of the three active limb electrodes. These leads are referred to as VR, VL, and VF. By disconnecting the input to the CTW from the extremity being explored, the voltage of the unipolar limb leads is augmented by as much as 50 percent. This modification is universally used for clinical ECGs, and the leads are labeled aVR, aVL, and aVF (Fig. 178-1C).

In recent years, the clinical value of chest wall mapping has been studied by a number of investigators. Multiple electrodes (32 to 192) are used for simultaneous recording, and computer processing for data reduction and display. This procedure yields information not available from the standard 12-lead ECG. New insights into normal and abnormal depolarization and repolarization patterns are evolving, and the value of sequential changes in ST segments during acute myocardial infarction is being studied.

ELECTROCARDIOGRAPHIC WAVEFORMS, DURATIONS, AND INTERVALS
Clinical ECGs are recorded on paper having a graphic background (Fig. 178-3) to permit rapid measurement of standardized time intervals and voltages. Time lines are 1 mm apart, with every fifth line intensified. Standard paper speed is 25 mm/s. Thus, 1 mm = 0.04 s (lighter lines), and 5 mm = 0.20 s (heavier lines). The horizontal lines, 1 mm apart, permit calibration of the voltage deflections of the ECG. Usual standardization is ↑ 10 mm = +1 mV (Fig. 178-3).

The P wave reflecting atrial depolarization is normally the initial wave of activity during the cardiac cycle (Fig. 178-4). Ventricular muscle depolarization is represented by the *QRS complex*. A Q wave is an initial negative wave; an R wave is an initial positive wave or a positive wave following a Q wave; and an S wave is a negative deflection following an R wave (Fig. 178-4). A QRS complex having a Q wave which returns to the baseline but does not produce a positive wave is labeled a QS complex, and the second R wave in a QRS complex having more than one R wave is labeled R′. The T wave represents ventricular muscle repolarization and is sometimes followed by a small wave, the U wave, the mechanism of which remains uncertain. Repolarization of atrial muscle is represented by the Tₐ (or T_p) wave, which occurs during the PR interval and QRS complex, and is usually difficult to identify. The interval between

the end of the QRS complex and the onset of the T wave is the ST segment, representing the period of time between depolarization of the ventricles and the period of rapid repolarization of ventricular muscle.

The interval between the P wave and the QRS complex is the PR (or PQ) interval, measured from the *onset* of atrial depolarization (P) to the *onset* of ventricular depolarization (Q or R) (Fig. 178-4). The duration is 0.12 to 0.20 s in the adult. Since AV nodal activation begins before the end of depolarization of atrial muscle, the PR interval may be used as a rough approximation of AV conduction time.

The duration of the QRS complex (0.04 to 0.10 s) reflects the time required for depolarization of ventricular muscle. It may be slightly prolonged by regional block in a portion of the intraventricular SCT or by delayed conduction in a region of ventricular muscle. Block in a bundle branch prolongs the QRS to a greater extent. An approximation of the refractory period of the ventricles may be obtained by measuring the QT interval (from the onset of the QRS to the end of the T wave) (Fig. 178-4). The QT interval is rate-dependent, and may be altered by numerous pathophysiologic or pharmacologic influences.

FIGURE 178-4 *The waves of the electrocardiogram—P, QRS, T, and U—are indicated. The measurements of the PR interval, QRS complex, ST segment, and QT interval are identified on the right.*

THE VECTOR CONCEPT AND ELECTRICAL AXIS The representation of a force by a graphic description of its direction and magnitude is referred to as a *vector*. In specific reference to cardiac electrical activity, a vector may be projected onto a two-dimensional plane as a scalar vector (Fig. 178-5A to D), or considered in three dimensions as a spatial vector (Fig. 178-5E to H). It may be used to represent instantaneous forces in the sequence of the cardiac electrical cycle (Fig. 178-5A and E), or it may represent either the mean or maximum axis during the cardiac cycle (Fig. 178-5H). Mean, maximum, and instantaneous vectors are most commonly applied to the analysis of the QRS complex, but the same principles may be applied to the P wave, ST segment, or T wave.

When an instantaneous electrical force recorded from the body surface is oriented in a direction perpendicular (or nearly so) to one of the leads (Fig. 178-5C, vector 6), the potential recorded by that lead at that instant will be minimum or isoelectric (Fig. 178-5D, point 6). Conversely, if the lead system is oriented parallel to the direction of an instantaneous electrical force (Fig. 178-5C, vector 4), the potential recorded by that lead will be maximum (Fig. 178-5D, point 4). An intermediate direction will record an intermediate voltage (for example, Fig. 178-5C and D, vector 2). If the instantaneous electrical force is oriented to the positive side of the lead, the deflection will be positive (4 in Fig. 178-5C and D); if the direction is oriented to the negative side, the deflection will be negative (1 in Fig. 178-5C and D). These general considerations may be applied to either instantaneous vectors occurring at any point during the inscription of the QRS complex, or the mean vector produced by total ventricular depolarization.

In Fig. 178-5E to H, seven instantaneous vectors are represented in three dimensions, indicating the spatial sequence of ventricular depolarization. In panel E, the mean spatial QRS vector, representing the net vector of all instantaneous forces, is shown. If the principles described above were applied, the QRS voltage would be large in lead I and small in aVF in the frontal plane (limb leads), and oriented posteriorly in the horizontal plane (chest leads).

When a triaxial system representing the augmented unipolar limb leads is superimposed on the triaxial system of Einthoven, a hexaxial system is obtained which is convenient for estimating the mean QRS axis, or any of the instantaneous vectors, in the frontal plane (Fig. 178-1D). When the appropriate positive and negative voltage orientations are assigned to each of the leads, the hexaxial reference system becomes a simple means of scalar vector analysis, requiring a minimum of two leads for estimation of the mean axis. An ECG which reveals a maximum positive QRS deflection in lead I and an isoelectric deflection in aVF would be oriented at 0°. Conversely, if the QRS voltage is positive and maximum in lead II and isoelectric in aVL, it would be oriented at +60°. The mean QRS axis in the frontal plane in normal adults ranges from −30 to +110°. Overlap between normal and abnormal occurs in the range of +90 to +110°. Generally, an axis > +90° is referred to as *right axis deviation*, and more negative than −30° as *abnormal left axis deviation*. The determination of the mean QRS axis in the horizontal plane (Fig. 178-2B) is similarly derived, normal orientation being to the left and posteriorly.

Three normal ECGs are shown in Fig. 178-6. Analysis of the mean QRS axis in the *frontal plane* (I, II, III, aVR, aVL, aVF) reveals the axis of A to be oriented horizontally, of C to be oriented vertically, and of B to be oriented in an intermediate range. In A the net voltage of the QRS complex is largest in lead I, almost isoelectric in lead III, and low in aVF, placing the mean axis in a direction almost perpendicular to lead III. In B, the voltages in lead I and aVF are almost identical, and maximum in lead II and aVR. The mean QRS axis is between lead II (+) and aVR (−). In C, net voltage is largest in leads II and aVF and almost isoelectric in lead I, placing the mean QRS axis almost perpendicular to lead I. A similar approach is applied to QRS axis determination in the *horizontal plane*. In C, the lead in which the net forces are isoelectric is V₃. Therefore, as shown in the axial representation of the horizontal plane of tracing C, the QRS is oriented to the left and posteriorly. If this information is added to that obtained from the frontal plane axis, it is apparent that the mean QRS vector of electrocardiogram C is oriented inferiorly, to the left, and posteriorly. Similar principles may be applied to the analysis of the mean T-wave axis, which is normally oriented in the same general direction as the QRS axis. An angle between the QRS and T axes >45° in the frontal plane, or >60° in the horizontal plane, is abnormal.

ELECTRICAL ACTIVITY OF THE ATRIA The mean P-wave vector is normally directed to the left, inferiorly, and slightly anteriorly; the frontal plane P axis is usually oriented between +30 and +60°. Right atrial enlargement causes tall, peaked P waves (≥0.25 mV), most prominent in standard leads II and V₁ (Fig. 178-7). Left atrial enlargement causes broad, notched P waves in lead II, and inverted or biphasic P waves (with the inverted portion of the biphasic P wave broader and deeper than the upright portion) in lead V₁. The upper limit of normal for P-wave duration is 0.11 s, and the broad P wave of left atrial enlargement usually is ≥0.12 s. However, criteria for left atrial enlargement are nonspecific, similar changes occurring in

FIGURE 178-5 *A. Frontal plane scalar projection of six instantaneous QRS vectors. B. Vectors originating from a point source at the electrical center of the heart. C. Projection of the vectors on the lead I axis. D. Lead I QRS produced by the instantaneous vectors in panel C (see text). E. Spatial representation of ventricular depolarization. Seven instantaneous vectors in the sequence of depolarization indicated in spatial orientations. F. Spatial vectors originating from the electrical center of the heart. G. A line drawn through the terminations of the spatial vectors produces a spatial QRS loop (vector loop). H. The mean spatial QRS vector, average of all the instantaneous vectors—to the left, slightly inferiorly, and posteriorly. (See text.) (From JW Hurst, RJ Myerburg, Introduction to Electrocardiography, 2d ed, New York, McGraw-Hill, 1973; modified and reproduced by permission of the publisher.)*

FIGURE 178-6 *Three normal ECGs demonstrating: (A) horizontal, (B) intermediate, and (C) vertical mean frontal plane QRS axes constructed on the hexaxial system. In addition, the horizontal plane vector in C is constructed on an axial system and is posteriorly oriented. T-wave vectors are similarly constructed.*

intraatrial conduction disturbances (Fig. 178-7), and the two must be distinguished on clinical grounds.

ABNORMALITIES OF VENTRICULAR DEPOLARIZATION: QRS COMPLEX

Since the QRS complex is the ECG representation of the sequence, time, and synchronization of total ventricular muscle depolarization, focal or diffuse abnormalities in ventricular muscle or in the SCT may cause changes in QRS form. Abnormalities may be confined to initial depolarization (Fig. 178-8B), terminal depolarization (Fig. 178-8C), or mid and late depolarization (Fig. 178-8D), or they may be diffuse (Fig. 178-8E to G).

The normal earliest site of activation is in the midportion of the left side of the interventricular septum, followed closely by a site on the lower portion of the right side of the interventricular septum and the adjacent free wall endocardium. The dominant wavefront is that one arising on the left septum, which results in a small initial R wave in V_1 (anterior movement), and a small initial Q wave in I, aVL, and/or V_6 (rightward movement). Small initial Q waves in II, III, and aVF may be observed as an indication of a small superior movement of the initial wavefront. Normal septal Q waves are ≤0.02 s and of low amplitude. A normal R in V_1 is ≤0.4 mV.

After septal depolarization has been initiated, rapid endocardial propagation occurs through both ventricles. In the normal heart, the greater mass of the left ventricle predominates, and the magnitude and direction of the electrical vectors reflect this fact (Fig. 178-6). During normal depolarization, the sequence of instantaneous vectors rotates from rightward and anterior to leftward, posterior, and superior, as illustrated in Fig. 178-5E to G. Most individuals will have maximum QRS duration (i.e., the lead having the longest measurable QRS) of 0.05 to 0.08 s (normal range is 0.04 to 0.10 s). A QRS duration of 0.09 or 0.10 s may be a normal variant or may represent a conduction delay to limited regions of either ventricle. QRS durations ≥0.12 s represent left or right bundle branch block or severe degrees of diffuse intraventricular conduction delay (see Fig. 178-13).

Abnormal initial Q waves or an abnormal initial R in V_1 usually represents (1) a loss of muscle mass; (2) abnormal sequence of depolarization; or (3) a change in the relative muscle mass in the two ventricles.

The *intrinsicoid deflection* of the QRS complex is the major

deflection *returning* to the baseline in a left (for example, 2→3 in Fig. 178-8D) or a right (S wave→2, Fig. 178-8E) precordial lead. Its *onset* should not exceed 0.035 s from the *onset* of the QRS complex in V_1, or 0.055 s from the *onset* of the QRS in V_5 or V_6. Delayed onset of the intrinsicoid deflection may indicate hypertrophy or conduction abnormalities (see Fig. 178-8).

The AV node and His bundle constitute the one normal pathway for impulse conduction from atria to ventricles. However, *accessory pathways* are present in some hearts. These are bands of muscle parallel to the AV junction, named Kent bundles, which form the

FIGURE 178-7 *P waves of right atrial enlargement (RAE) and left atrial enlargement (LAE).*

FIGURE 178-8 *QRS complexes. The lead is indicated above each example. A. Normal. B. Prolongation due to initial QRS delay between arrows (1→2) in Wolff-Parkinson-White syndrome (see Chap. 183). C. Prolongation due to terminal delay (1→2) in right bundle branch block. D. Prolongation due to mid (1→2) and late (2→3) delay in left bundle branch block. E. Minor uniform prolongation (1→2) in left ventricular hypertrophy. F. Distortion of total QRS pattern (1→2) in a cardiomyopathy. G. Uniform prolongation (1→2) in an electrolyte abnormality. H. Pathologic Q wave (1→2) in myocardial infarction. Intrinsicoid deflection = 2→3 in D and S→2 in E.*

anatomic substrate for the Wolff-Parkinson-White syndrome (see Chap. 184). The ECG manifestation is the *delta wave* (Fig. 178-8*B*).

ABNORMALITIES OF VENTRICULAR REPOLARIZATION: ST SEGMENT, T WAVE, AND U WAVE In the normal ECG, the ST segment is "isoelectric," resting at the same potential as the interval between the T wave and the next P wave. Deviations of the ST segment from the baseline may occur as a result of injury to cardiac muscle, changes in the synchronization of ventricular muscle depolarization, or drug or electrolyte influences. Elevations of the ST segment, in association with an elevation of the takeoff point of the ST segment from the QRS complex (the J point), may occur as a normal variant, especially in young individuals (Fig. 178-9*A*). The most common pathologic causes of ST-segment elevation are acute myocardial infarction and pericarditis (Fig. 178-9*B* to *F*), and the normal variant must be differentiated from these. Horizontal depression or a downsloping ST segment merging into the T wave occurs as a result of ischemia, ventricular strain, changes in the pattern of ventricular depolarization, or drug effects (Fig. 178-9*H, I, M, N, Q,* and *R*).

Since the sequence of ventricular muscle *de*polarization is from endocardium to epicardium, and *re*polarization represents an electrical current opposite in direction to depolarization, the T wave would be in the opposite direction to the QRS complex if the sequence of repolarization were in the same direction as depolarization. However, T waves generally assume the same direction as the major deflection of the QRS complex (see Fig. 178-6). It is assumed, therefore, that the direction of normal repolarization is opposite to the wave of depolarization—from epicardium to endocardium. T waves are considered abnormal when they are of low voltage, flat, or inverted in leads in which they are normally upright, or when they are abnormally tall and peaked. T-wave inversions are reflected vectorially by a widening of the angle between the QRS vector and the T vector (Fig. 178-6). Common causes of abnormalities of the T waves include ischemic heart disease, ventricular hypertrophy and strain, primary muscle disease, abnormal sequences of depolarization, electrolyte abnormalities, and drug influences (see Fig. 178-9*C, D, F, I, K, L,* and *N* to *R*). However, T-wave changes are often not specific.

The U wave is usually positive in leads in which the QRS complex is positive. The abnormal U wave is manifested as either an exaggeration of normal U-wave voltage, the appearance of a U wave in leads in which it is not normally seen, or inversion of a U wave. U-wave abnormalities occur in ischemic heart disease, left ventricular strain, and electrolyte disturbances. Unfortunately, the information they provide is usually nonspecific.

ECG MANIFESTATIONS OF VENTRICULAR HYPERTROPHY The normal dominance of the left ventricle on the features of the QRS complex is decreased or reversed in right ventricular hypertrophy (RVH) and exaggerated in left ventricular hypertrophy (LVH) (Fig. 178-10). RVH causes a shift of the net forces of depolarization from the left and posterior toward the right and anteriorly. On the ECG, this produces tall R waves in V_1 (≥ 0.5 mV), with an abnormal S wave in V_5 or V_6 (≥ 0.7 mV). In the frontal plane, the mean QRS axis shifts to the right of vertical (usually $>110°$). Less extreme degrees of RVH may result in preservation of a moderately deep S wave in V_1, with an R-wave voltage exceeding the S-wave voltage, or a normal R wave with a shallow S wave and prominent terminal S waves in V_5 and V_6. The primary QRS manifestation of LVH is an increase in voltage in those leads which reflect the electrical activity of the left ventricle. R waves in the standard limb leads may increase beyond the normal limit of 2.0 mV. Concomitantly, there is a tendency for a shift of the frontal plane QRS axis to the left. It is not likely that LVH alone will cause a shift in the QRS axis beyond $-30°$, but it commonly causes a shift in the range of 0 to $-30°$ (Fig. 178-10). LVH causes a deep S wave in lead V_1 or V_2 (>2.5 mV) or an abnormal R wave in lead V_5 or V_6 (>2.5 mV). When T waves are normal, the presence of voltage criteria for LVH must be interpreted in terms of body habitus of an individual. Young, healthy, thin-chested individuals will frequently exceed the QRS voltage criteria for LVH in its absence. However, when the ST-segment and T-wave changes associated with "strain" are present (Figs. 178-9*Q* and 178-10), the diagnosis of LVH is clarified. Similarly, borderline voltage criteria are more specific for LVH when associated with the ST-segment and T-wave changes of left ventricular strain.

ACUTE MYOCARDIAL INFARCTION Three pathophysiologic events occur, either in sequence or simultaneously, in an acute myocardial infarction—ischemia, injury, and infarction. The ECG manifestations

FIGURE 178-9 *ST-segment and T-wave changes. Arrows in each panel indicate the major features of each complex. A. Early repolarization (J-point elevation), normal variant. B. Acute pericarditis: (1) depressed T_a; (2) elevated ST; (3) normal T. C. Early acute myocardial infarction (AMI): (1) elevated ST; (2) tall, peaked T wave; steep angle between 1 and 2. D. AMI: (1) small Q wave; (2) elevated ST segment; (3) tall, peaked T wave with steep 2→3 angle. E. AMI: (1) pathologic Q wave; (2) elevated ST segment. F. AMI: (1) Q wave; (2) elevated ST segment; (3) terminal T-wave inversion. G. Angina pectoris (Prinzmetal variant) with ST elevation during pain. H and I. Angina pectoris (usual form) with horizontal or downward sloping ST* *segment during pain or exercise. J. J-point depression with upsloping ST segment during exercise, normal response. K. Primary T-wave inversion (2) in ischemia or primary muscle disease. L. Myocardial infarction (healed): (1) pathologic Q; (2) ST returning to baseline; (3) symmetrically inverted T wave. M. Digitalis effect: (1) downward coving of ST segment, merging into (2) an upright T wave. N to P. Nonspecific ST-segment and T-wave changes often seen in chronic ischemic heart disease. Q. Left ventricular strain pattern with (1) downsloping ST segment and (2) asymmetrically inverted (secondary) T wave. R. Downsloping ST segment merging into a deeply inverted T wave in ventricular conduction abnormality.*

of these processes include changes in the T waves (ischemia), ST segments (injury), and QRS complexes (infarction). The earliest T-wave changes of acute myocardial ischemia are tall, peaked T waves ("hyperacute") (Fig. 178-9C and D), followed later by symmetrically inverted T waves (Fig. 178-9F and K). When the electrical integrity of the cell membranes is affected, currents of injury develop. The injury pattern on ECG during evolution of a transmural infarction is an elevation of the ST segments in the leads facing the infarcting area (Fig. 178-9C and F). The combination of ischemia and injury causes elevated ST segments, followed by either tall, peaked T waves (in the very early stages) or inverted T waves (Fig. 178-11). In leads opposite the region of the acute infarction, reciprocal changes occur: depressed ST segments and upright or isoelectric T waves (Figs. 178-11 and 178-12). There is some controversy about the distinction between "reciprocal changes" and nearly identical changes reflecting coexistent ischemia in a vascular bed remote from the infarction, i.e., "ischemia at a distance." It is likely that remote ST depressions

could be due to either. As the period of active injury resolves, the ST segments return to the baseline, but the inverted T waves may persist for months or years (Fig. 178-9L). Pathologic Q waves are the QRS manifestation of a transmural myocardial infarction. Q waves are pathologic when they appear in a lead in which Q waves were previously not present, or when the Q waves of normal septal depolarization become exaggerated (>20 ms; >0.2 mV).

The ECG in an acute inferior wall myocardial infarction is shown in Fig. 178-11. Leads II, III, and aVF, which face the inferior surface of the left ventricle (see Fig. 178-1D), demonstrate the direct patterns of infarction (pathologic Q waves), injury (elevated ST segments), and ischemia (inversion of the T waves). Reciprocal changes (depressed ST, tall T) are demonstrated in aVL. The evolution of an acute anterior myocardial infarction is demonstrated in Fig. 178-12. The most obvious direct changes occur in aVL, V_2, and V_3, and reciprocal changes in II, III, and aVF. In the tracing of 4/11, ST elevations (most prominent in aVL, V_2, and V_3) are accompanied by

FIGURE 178-10 *Ventricular hypertrophy. Left ventricular hypertrophy and strain with R wave >2.0 mV in limb leads; R >2.5 mV in V_5 and V_6, and S in V_1 >2.5 mV. The sum of S-V_1 or S-V_2 and R-V_5 or R-V_6 exceeds 3.5 mV. Strain is indicated by the downsloping ST segments and asymmetrically inverted T waves, especially in the lateral chest leads. The QRS-T vector angle is abnormally wide. Right ventricular hypertrophy is indicated by right axis deviation in the frontal plane and abnormal anterior forces in the horizontal plane. The former is indicated by a small R and deep S wave in lead I, and the latter by tall R waves in V_1 and V_2 with deep S waves in V_5 and V_6. The QRS-T angle is wide (strain).*

"hyperacute" peaked T waves in V_2 and V_3. On 4/12, deeper Q waves are present in aVL and V_1 to V_3, and T waves have inverted in aVL and V_2 to V_5. ST elevations persist but less prominently. On 4/25, the pattern of a healing infarction—pathologic Q waves and ischemic T waves—is present. Eventually, the T waves might become partially or completely normal, with persistence of the Q waves. An infarction of the true posterior wall of the left ventricle causes ECG changes opposite to those of an anterior infarction. Instead of Q waves, ST elevation, and T-wave inversion in the anterior precordial leads (V_1 and V_2), true posterior infarction is characterized by tall R waves, ST depression, and upright T waves in these leads. These infarctions usually occur in combination with inferior wall infarctions. Right ventricular myocardial infarction occurs infrequently and is almost always associated with inferior and/or posterior infarction of the left ventricle. Right ventricular infarction has no specific pattern on the standard 12-lead ECG; however, ST elevations on special right-sided precordial leads (V_4R to V_6R) may identify acute RV infarcts.

FIGURE 178-11 *Acute inferior wall myocardial infarction. The ECG of 11/29 shows minor nonspecific ST-segment and T-wave changes. On 12/5 an acute myocardial infarction occurred. There are pathologic Q waves (1), ST-segment elevation (2), and terminal T-wave inversion (3) in leads II, III, and aVF indicating the location of the infarct on the inferior wall (see text). Reciprocal changes in aVL (small arrow). Increasing R-wave voltage with ST depression and increased voltage of the T wave in V_2 is characteristic of true posterior wall extension of the inferior infarction.*

A nontransmural (subendocardial or subepicardial) myocardial infarction may cause persistent ST-segment and T-wave changes similar to those seen in transmural infarctions. However, abnormal Q waves do not appear in the QRS complex, although R-wave and/or S-wave voltages may change. The Q-wave criterion for distinguishing transmural and subendocardial infarctions is a useful ECG tool, but pathologic data have shown that exceptions do occur. The ST-segment and T-wave changes of nontransmural infarction are common in leads I, II, III, aVL, aVF, and/or V_4 to V_6. Similar, but transient, changes may occur during the pain of angina pectoris, in shock, after pulmonary embolism, and secondary to acute central nervous system lesions.

CHRONIC ISCHEMIC HEART DISEASE   The ECG in chronic ischemic heart disease is often nonspecific. The patterns of chronic myocardial ischemia are intrinsically variable, and this is compounded by the problem of coexistent ECG changes related to pharmacologic interventions and/or LVH. Chronic ischemic heart disease causes a broad range of ST-segment and T-wave changes (Fig. 178-9G to I, K, L, and N to P). There may be moderate degrees of horizontal ST-segment depression or a downward sloping ST segment, flattening of inversion of T waves, and prominent U waves. It is difficult to define an abnormal ST-segment depression in precise quantitative terms. However, if the J point is more than 0.5 mm below the isoelectric line, the ST segment is horizontal or downsloping, and

FIGURE 178-12 *Acute anterior wall myocardial infarction. On 4/11, changes of a very early acute myocardial infarction in leads I, aVL, V_2, and V_3, with reciprocal changes in II, III, and aVF. On 4/12, ST segments remain elevated in the anterior leads, but T waves are inverted. On 4/25, a completed large anterior myocardial infarction is recorded—Q in I, aVL, V_1 to V_4.*

there is an associated T-wave abnormality, myocardial ischemia should be considered. The common clinical expression of chronic ischemic heart disease, angina pectoris, may be accompanied by a normal resting ECG or nonspecific ST-segment and T-wave changes. However, during spontaneous or exercise-induced pain, the ECG may demonstrate the horizontal or downward sloping ST-segment depressions shown in Fig. 178-9*H* and *I*, or rarely the variant pattern of spontaneous transient ST elevations (Prinzmetal variant) (Fig. 178-9*G*).

INTRAVENTRICULAR CONDUCTION DISTURBANCES
The complex anatomy of the specialized conducting system of the ventricles, in conjunction with the focal nature of most cardiac diseases, is reflected in the multiplicity of ECG patterns which result from disorders of the sequence of activation of the ventricles. Disease of both the SCT and ventricular myocardium plays a role in the various patterns. The universal feature of ventricular conduction disturbances is a prolongation of the time required for depolarization of a portion of a ventricle, an entire ventricle, or both ventricles. Delayed or slow conduction may be diffuse or may be confined to a portion of the QRS complex (Fig. 178-8). Prolongation of the QRS may be modest, as in left ventricular hypertrophy, or extreme, as in cardiomyopathies or metabolic abnormalities (Fig. 178-8).

The classic bundle branch block patterns are associated with specific lesions in the left or right bundle branch in the majority of cases. Complete right bundle branch block (RBBB) (Fig. 178-13) is characterized by prolongation of the QRS complex ($\geq$0.12 s) with the delayed activation of the right ventricle accounting for a terminal delay on the ECG. Since septal activation from the left bundle branch system normally precedes right ventricular activation, *the initial forces of ventricular depolarization are not disturbed in RBBB*, and the ability to identify coexistent pathologic Q waves is not hindered. The delayed activation of the right ventricle is reflected by the presence of terminal forces directed anteriorly and to the right.

The rightward direction of the slow terminal forces is indicated by the broad terminal S wave in leads I, aVL, and V$_6$ (Fig. 178-13). The anterior orientation of these forces is indicated by a large terminal R wave (R') in V$_1$. Since initial forces are not disturbed, the normal initial R wave in V$_1$ persists, followed by an S wave. Incomplete RBBB is present when the waveform criteria for RBBB (rSR') are present, but the QRS duration is <0.12 s.

Left bundle branch block (LBBB) is also characterized by a QRS duration $\geq$0.12 s. However, since normal initial ventricular depolarization is dependent upon the LBB to deliver the impulses of initial depolarization to the left septum, the patterns produced by LBBB are more complex. Normal septal depolarization is disturbed, and delay of the normally dominant left ventricular forces produces a more generalized disturbance of QRS morphology. The septal Q wave in standard leads I, aVL, and V$_6$ is typically lost. In addition, the initial anterior force reflected by the small R wave in lead V$_1$ may be lost because of a less anterior orientation of the initial forces. The delay in left ventricular activation produces the greatest degree of slowing in the mid and late portion of the QRS complex. This often results in notching at the peak of the upstroke in leads I and V$_6$ (see Figs. 178-8*D* and 178-14), with a late intrinsicoid deflection (>0.055 s) in V$_5$ and V$_6$. Most cases of LBBB produce secondary T-wave abnormalities as demonstrated in Fig. 178-14. Because of the changes in the initial forces, and the secondary ST-segment and T-wave changes, it is usually difficult to evaluate the QRS-complex, ST-segment, and T-wave changes of coexistent ischemic heart disease. When the intrinsicoid deflection is delayed in leads V$_5$ or V$_6$, but the QRS duration is <0.12 s, incomplete LBBB may be present. LBBB may be associated with either a normal QRS axis (Fig. 178-13) or left axis deviation.

In recent years a great deal of attention has been given to the ECG patterns referred to as the *left hemiblocks*. As the name implies, *left anterior hemiblock* (LAH) has been proposed to result from disease in the anterior radiation of fibers referred to as the anterior division of the LBB. *Left posterior hemiblock* (LPH) has been

FIGURE 178-13 *Intraventricular conduction abnormalities. Illustrated are right bundle branch block (RBBB); left bundle branch block (LBBB); left anterior hemiblock (LAH); right bundle branch block with left anterior hemiblock (RBBB + LAH); and right bundle branch block with left posterior hemiblock (RBBB + LPH) (see text).*

assumed to result from disease in the left posterior radiation. The complex nature of the LBB system has thus far defied a determination of whether focal proximal disease or diffuse distal disease in the distribution of these portions of the LBB is the mechanism responsible for the hemiblock patterns, although it is known that the pathologic process tends to be diffuse in those cases studied at autopsy.

LAH results in a moderate delay of activation of the superior portion of the left ventricular free wall, causing a modest prolongation of the QRS complex and shift of the front plane axis to the left. Initial septal depolarization is undisturbed (Fig. 178-13), and the QRS complex rarely exceeds 0.09 to 0.10 s. The differentiation between LAH and left ventricular hypertrophy (LVH) may occasionally be difficult. In general, LVH alone will not produce a left axis shift beyond $-30°$, and LAH will often produce left axis deviation $\geq -60°$. The key QRS features in left anterior hemiblock include small Q waves in leads I and aVL, with small initial R waves and deep S waves in leads II, III, and aVF.

LPH results in a moderate delay of activation of the posterior-inferior portion of the left ventricular free wall. Again, there is a modest prolongation of the QRS complex, but a shift of the frontal plane QRS axis to the *right*. Thus, the initial septal forces, though generally undisturbed, may be oriented more superiorly, producing small initial Q waves in leads II, III, and aVF. Since the specificity

FIGURE 178-14 *A. Acute pericarditis with ST-segment elevations in all leads except III, aVR, and V$_1$. B. Myocarditis: diffuse ST-segment and T-wave changes, with low-voltage T waves in the limb leads and primary T-wave changes in the chest leads. C. Cardiomyopathy: gross distortion of the QRS complex.*

of the ECG manifestations of LPH is not very reliable, many clinicians will not make a diagnosis of isolated LPH without demonstrating a right axis shift on serial ECGs, plus definite exclusion of other causes of right axis shift. Of all the intraventricular conduction disturbances, isolated LPH is the most difficult to diagnose.

The hemiblocks frequently coexist with disease in the RBB system. The combination of RBB, plus LAH or LPH, is referred to as *bifascicular block*—implying that two fascicles of the trifascicular model of the intraventricular SCT are diseased. This probably represents a pathophysiologic oversimplification, but it is useful for clinical purposes. Since RBBB alone does not produce abnormal axis deviation either to the left or to the right, the coexistence of RBBB with abnormal left axis deviation (Fig. 178-13) is usually interpreted as LAH plus RBBB. Similarly, abnormal right axis deviation in association with RBBB is usually interpreted as the coexistence of LPH with RBBB, when the QRS criteria for LPH are met (Fig. 178-13). As is the case in isolated LPH, the diagnosis of LPH plus RBBB is difficult because a number of clinical settings may cause abnormal right axis deviation in conjunction with RBBB.

Trifascicular block describes abnormal conduction in all three divisions of the intraventricular SCT. The ECG diagnosis can be made only by inference when a patient has bifascicular block and a prolonged PR interval. Confirmation can be achieved only with His bundle electrocardiography (Chap. 183).

PERICARDITIS, MYOCARDITIS, AND THE CARDIOMYOPATHIES

Acute pericarditis causes elevation of the ST segments in many leads without the reciprocal changes seen in acute myocardial infarction (Fig. 178-14A). ST-segment elevation may occur in all leads except aVR and rarely involves V_1. After a period of days, the diffuse ST elevations return to the baseline, and T-wave inversions may occur. Coexistent ST elevations and T-wave inversions do not occur as often as they do in myocardial infarction (compare Figs. 178-11 and 178-14A). T-wave abnormalities may persist for weeks or months after the acute episode of pericarditis. If the pericarditis is accompanied by significant degrees of pericardial effusion, electrical alternans may occur. On alternate beats, ECG voltage shifts in magnitude. There also may be low voltage of the QRS complexes and T waves in all leads. Finally, the T_a waves may be transiently depressed because of atrial involvement by the inflammatory process [see Fig. 178-9B (1)].

The ECG changes of myocarditis (Chap. 192 and Fig. 178-14B) are often difficult to differentiate from the late phase of pericarditis, in which symmetric T-wave inversions are present. However, myocarditis may occur in many other settings, and an appreciation of the range of the ECG changes is important. Almost all systemic infections may produce minor myocardial involvement. Measles, mumps, influenza, hepatitis, infectious mononucleosis, and scarlet fever, just to name a few diseases, may be associated with ECG abnormalities and with histopathologic evidence of myocardial inflammation. When the myocardial involvement is subclinical, the ECG changes are usually subtle and nonspecific. There are minor T-wave changes, manifested as flattening or perhaps shallow inversion of the T waves in multiple leads (Fig. 178-9O and P). The conducting system may be involved, and prolongation of the PR interval may be noted.

In clinically evident myocarditis, the ECG demonstrates symmetrically inverted T waves in most of the standard limb leads and in the lateral precordial leads (Fig. 178-14B). When the specialized conducting system is involved, bundle branch block or patterns of nonspecific intraventricular conduction defects may occur.

The ECG may be helpful in distinguishing types of cardiomyopathies (Chap. 192). In the hypertrophic cardiomyopathies, the most common ECG pattern is LVH and strain (Fig. 178-10). When asymmetric septal hypertrophy is present, abnormal septal depolarization may be indicated by the presence of deep abnormal Q waves in leads I, aVL, V_5, and/or V_6, and a tall initial R wave in V_1. In the congestive cardiomyopathies, nonspecific intraventricular conduction abnormalities, indicated by broad, notched QRS complexes without a specific bundle branch block pattern, are common (Fig. 178-14C). Nonspecific ST-segment and T-wave abnormalities are almost universal in congestive cardiomyopathies. In the restrictive cardiomyopathies, intraventricular conduction defects, low-voltage QRS complexes, or loss of R-wave progression across the precordium may occur.

ECG ABNORMALITIES IN METABOLIC AND ELECTROLYTE DISTURBANCES

The electrically active tissues of the heart are particularly sensitive to changes in the extracellular concentration of K^+, and dramatic ECG changes may accompany abrupt changes in K^+. The initial effect of acute *hyper*kalemia is the appearance of tall, peaked T waves (Figs. 178-15 and 41-1). As the severity of hyperkalemia increases, the QRS complex widens and blends into the tall, peaked T waves, P-wave voltage decreases and may disappear entirely, and the PR interval is prolonged. As these changes evolve, there is marked prolongation of the QRS complex (Fig. 178-15) with the evolution of continuity between the S wave and T wave, ultimately producing a sine wave configuration. This pattern is a very late and ominous manifestation of hyperkalemia. Equally dangerous is the occurrence of severe *hypo*kalemia, which also produces characteristic ECG changes. Instead of the tall, peaked T waves of hyperkalemia, hypokalemia produces a flattening or inversion of the T wave with concomitant prominence of the U wave. In its fully developed state, the ECG gives the appearance of a very long QT interval. Careful analysis reveals that the QT interval is not so prolonged, and the U wave has assumed the appearance of the T wave (Fig. 178-15). Thus, the major prolongation is a "QU" prolongation. This ECG manifestation of hypokalemia may forewarn of the occurrence of serious ventricular arrhythmias, especially in the presence of digitalis. One must be careful to differentiate the ECG effects of hypo*calc*emia from hypo*kalemia*. Whereas hypokalemia may produce the appearance of a long ST segment and late T wave because of flattening of the T

FIGURE 178-15 *Electrolyte disturbances. Hyperkalemia ($K^+ = 6.8$) with tall, peaked T waves. Severe hyperkalemia ($K^+ = 9.1$) with (1) flattening of the P wave, and ↑ PR interval (1→2), (2) marked widening of the QRS complex (2→3), and (3) merging of the S wave into the T wave. Hypokalemia produces flat or inverted T waves with prominent U waves, causing prolonged "QU" interval, while hypocalcemia produces true prolongation of the ST segment with marked QT prolongation.*

Hyperkalemia

V_3

$K^+ = 6.8$

II

$K^+ = 9.1$

Hypokalemia

II

ST-T   U

Hypocalcemia

II

ST   T

wave and prominence of the U wave, hypocalcemia does, in fact, produce prolongation of the ST segment with a late T wave (Fig. 178-15). Hypocalcemia is not as immediately ominous as hypokalemia in regard to potentially serious ventricular arrhythmias. Most of the other electrolyte imbalances produce ECG changes too nonspecific to be clinically useful.

Abnormalities of metabolism, such as hyper- or hypothyroidism, Addison's disease, diabetic ketoacidosis, and infiltrative diseases, such as amyloidosis and hemochromatosis, all may produce ECG abnormalities which may be helpful in the recognition of the disease process but are often nonspecific.

Many drugs, especially the antiarrhythmics and psychotropics, can influence the ECG. The most common effects are on the AV node (prolonged PR interval) and on repolarization (ST-T wave changes and prolonged QT intervals).

VECTORCARDIOGRAPHY

A vectorcardiogram (VCG) is a continuous loop representing the sequence of instantaneous electrical vectors in a two-dimensional plane (shown diagrammatically in Fig. 178-5G). This form of recording, requiring simultaneous voltage information from two leads, is achieved by recording one ECG lead on the vertical axis and replacing time by a second lead on the horizontal axis. The resulting loop is photographed on an oscilloscope screen. Most VCG systems today employ an XYZ lead system in which X is analogous to lead I (left-right), Y is analogous to lead aVF (superoinferior), and Z represents a lead in the anteroposterior orientation, most closely analogous to lead V_2. The XY plane records a vectorial loop in the frontal plane, projected on the hexaxial reference in Fig. 178-1D. The XZ plane records the horizontal loop in which the left-right orientation is plotted against the anteroposterior orientation on a reference system similar to that in Fig. 178-2B. In the YZ plane, the loop is in the sagittal orientation—the anteroposterior orientation (Z) plotted against the superoinferior orientation (Y). Recording in three planes provides information about spatial vectors, as in Fig. 178-5F. Loops consist of comma-shaped dots, the orientation of the comma indicating the direction of rotation, and the frequency of interruption providing a measurement of time. Closely grouped dots indicate a slow change in the magnitude and direction of the vector, while widely spread dots indicate rapid changes. Vectorial information of P waves, QRS complexes, ST segments, and T waves may be obtained.

The greatest value of the VCG today lies in the analysis of Q waves of uncertain significance and of certain intraventricular conduction abnormalities. When normal septal Q waves are absent in lead I or V_6, and no other evidence of septal infarction is present, the VCG may demonstrate either that the normal Q loop in the horizontal plane is absent, indicating a septal infarction or scarring, or conversely that the Q loop in the horizontal plane is morphologically normal but oriented directly anteriorly, accounting for the absence of the initial rightward forces. Similarly, the VCG can be helpful in assessing confusing initial forces or poor R-wave progression in the anterior precordial leads.

The VCG is particularly useful in identifying inferior wall myocardial infarctions. When the ECG is equivocal, the VCG may show the superior displacement of initial forces in the frontal plane and the clockwise rotation that is characteristic of inferior wall myocardial infarction. Furthermore, the difficulty in differentiating inferior wall infarctions from left anterior hemiblock on ECG, or recognizing their coexistence, may be aided by a VCG. In left anterior hemiblock, the initial forces are often normal, but there is superior displacement of the major portion of the frontal plane loop. However, the rotation is counterclockwise, in contrast to the clockwise rotation of inferior wall myocardial infarction. When the combination of inferior wall myocardial infarction and left anterior hemiblock is present, the infarction may be masked on the ECG; but the VCG may show the

distinctly abnormal superiorly displaced initial forces of inferior wall myocardial infarction plus the counterclockwise rotation in the frontal plane characteristic of left anterior hemiblock.

REFERENCES

BERNE RM (ed): Electrophysiology of the heart, in *Handbook of Physiology*, sec 2: *The Cardiovascular System*, vol 1: *The Heart*. Washington, DC, American Physiological Society, 1979, pp 187–428

CASTELLANOS A, MYERBURG RJ: The resting electrocardiogram, in *The Heart*, 6th ed, JW Hurst et al (eds). New York, McGraw-Hill, 1986, p 206

COOKSEY JD et al: *Clinical Vectorcardiography and Electrocardiography*, 2d ed. Chicago, Year Book, 1977

FISCH C (ed): *Cardiovascular Clinics*, vol 5, no 3: *Complex Electrocardiography I*. Philadelphia, Davis, 1973

————: Electrocardiography and vectorcardiography, in *Heart Disease*, 2d ed, E Braunwald (ed). Philadelphia, Saunders, 1984, p 195

GOLDMAN MJ: *Principles of Clinical Electrocardiography*, 12th ed. Los Altos, California, Lange Medical Publishers, 1986

HOFFMAN BF, CRANEFIELD PF: *Electrophysiology of the Heart*. New York, McGraw-Hill, 1960

SILVERMAN ME et al: *Electrocardiography: Basic Concepts and Clinical Application*. New York, McGraw-Hill, 1983

---

179 NONINVASIVE METHODS OF CARDIAC EXAMINATION
Roentgenography, phonocardiography, echocardiography, radionuclide techniques, and magnetic resonance imaging

PATRICIA C. COME / JOSHUA WYNNE / EUGENE BRAUNWALD

ROENTGENOGRAPHY

The chest roentgenogram provides pathoanatomic information about the size and configuration of the heart and great vessels and pathophysiologic information about pulmonary arterial and venous pressures and flow. Chamber dilatation usually produces changes in cardiac size and contour. Myocardial hypertrophy, in contrast, often results in wall thickening at the expense of cavity size, producing only a slight alteration of the cardiac silhouette. Although standard 6-ft posteroanterior (PA) and lateral chest roentgenograms are routinely obtained, a cardiac series (Fig. 179-1) permits better assessment of chamber sizes and shapes. Image-intensification fluoroscopy may be used to detect calcification, recognize pericardial effusion or thickening if epicardial fat can be identified, assess movement of radiopaque valvular prostheses, or define further the size and motion of cardiac chambers and great vessels.

CARDIAC SILHOUETTE The *right atrium* is the most difficult chamber to evaluate. Enlargement, however, may cause bulging of the heart to the right and an increased curvature of the right heart border on PA and left anterior oblique views. The *right ventricle* is best seen on the lateral view, where its anterior wall lies behind the lower third of the sternum. As it enlarges, it displaces lung tissue, filling in the upper retrosternal space. Further dilatation may passively displace other chambers, particularly the left ventricle.

Enlargement of the *left atrial appendage* may be suspected by a bulge beneath the pulmonary artery on the PA film. Dilatation of the body of the *left atrium* is best demonstrated by posterior displacement of the barium-filled esophagus in the lateral or right anterior oblique view. As the left atrium dilates further, its right border contacts right lung posteriorly, forming a second border or "double density" adjacent to the right atrial wall. The left bronchus may be displaced posteriorly and superiorly. The *left ventricle* enlarges inferiorly, posteriorly, and to the left, often increasing the cardiothoracic ratio

FIGURE 179-1 *Posteroanterior (A,B), lateral (C,D), right anterior oblique (E,F), and left anterior oblique (G,H) views of the heart, demonstrating the positions of the cardiac chambers, valves, and interatrial and interventricular septa. AV = azygos vein; SVC = superior vena cava; RA = right atrium; IVC = inferior vena cava; TV = tricuspid valve; RV = right ventricle; MPA = main pulmonary artery; RPA = right pulmonary artery; LPA = left pulmonary artery; AO = aorta; LA = left atrium; LAA = left atrial appendage; LV = left ventricle; MV = mitral valve; IVS = interventricular septum; IAS = interatrial septum; RAA = right atrial appendage. [From PC Come (ed): Diagnostic Cardiology. Reprinted with permission of Robert E. Dinsmore, M.D., and J.B. Lippincott Company.]*

(maximal cardiac diameter divided by maximal internal thoracic diameter, normally less than 0.50). The chest roentgenogram is a useful screening or initial test, but other imaging techniques, such as echocardiography, provide more definitive assessment of individual cardiac chambers.

PULMONARY VASCULATURE Since pulmonary vessel size is proportional to flow, vessels normally taper from central to peripheral and from dependent to nondependent portions of the lungs. Increased flow, as with left-to-right shunts, results in enlargement and tortuosity of all vessels. Regional or global reduction of flow, due to pulmonary emboli, emphysematous blebs, or a right-to-left shunt, results in decreased vessel caliber.

Increases in pulmonary venous pressure produce perivascular edema in the dependent portions of the lungs, causing loss of vessel wall definition and redistribution of flow to nondependent areas. Further increases cause interstitial edema, with peribronchial cuffing, perihilar and peripheral lung haziness, and linear densities (Kerley B lines) perpendicular to the pleura. They represent fluid collection in the dependent interlobular septa. Alveolar pulmonary edema, with air bronchograms, may ultimately develop. There may be considerable temporal delay between hemodynamic changes and roentgenographic findings.

Pulmonary artery hypertension produces dilatation of the main pulmonary artery and its central branches. When associated with conditions increasing pulmonary arteriolar resistance, such as primary pulmonary hypertension, the distal pulmonary arteries often appear small ("pruned").

SPECIALIZED RADIOGRAPHIC METHODS *Digital subtraction angiography* (DSA) uses computer processing to digitize high-resolution fluoroscopic images. An image of the region of interest is subtracted from images obtained following intravenous, intracardiac, or intraarterial injection of contrast medium. Elimination of radiographic densities resulting from soft tissues and bone permits excellent definition of vascular structures using a concentration of contrast medium lower than that necessary for routine angiography. Vascular applications include recognition of vascular tumors, pulmonary emboli, and abnormalities of the aorta or of peripheral, cerebral, and renal arteries. Study of the heart permits assessment of ventricular function, intracardiac shunts, other congenital abnormalities, and bypass graft patency.

Computed tomography provides thin, cross-sectional images of the body by measuring attenuation of x-rays passing through the bodily planes of interest. The x-rays, generated by a rotating source, are detected by an array of detectors surrounding the patient. Digitized data accrued from contiguous, horizontal planes can subsequently be used to construct multiple two-dimensional projections. Contrast enhancement and electronic gating permit high-resolution images of the beating heart. Regions of infarction and ischemia, ventricular aneurysms, intracardiac thrombi, diseases of the aorta and pericardium, and patency of bypass grafts have been recognized.

PHONOCARDIOGRAPHY, SYSTOLIC TIME INTERVALS, AND PULSE TRACINGS

Although imaging techniques have largely replaced phonocardiography and pulse tracings as diagnostic tests, the latter may be useful, especially in combination with M-mode echocardiography, in clarifying the origin and timing of abnormalities noted on auscultation and palpation. The indirect recordings of the jugular, carotid, and apex pulses resemble the right atrial, central aortic, and left ventricular obstruction. The systolic time intervals consist of electromechanical systole (QS_2), measured from the onset of the QRS complex to the aortic component of S_2; the left ventricular ejection time (LVET), which begins with the upstroke of the carotid pulse and ends with the dicrotic notch; and the preejection period (PEP = $QS_2 -$ LVET) (Fig. 179-2). In left ventricular failure, the PEP lengthens (reflecting primarily a decrease in rate of ventricular pressure generation) and the LVET shortens (reflecting a reduced stroke volume), increasing the PEP/LVET ratio. In fixed left ventricular outflow obstruction (e.g., valvular aortic stenosis) the carotid upstroke may be slow, while in dynamic obstruction (hypertrophic obstructive cardiomyopathy) it is brisk due to unimpeded early systolic flow. In the absence of concomitant heart failure, the LVET is generally prolonged in both forms of outflow obstruction.

ECHOCARDIOGRAPHY

Echocardiography uses ultrasound to image the heart and great vessels. A transducer containing a piezoelectric ceramic, which interconverts electrical and mechanical (i.e., sound) energy, functions both as the transmitter of sound and as the receiver of reflected waves. Three types of studies are performed: M-mode, two-dimensional, and Doppler. In *M-mode echocardiography,* a single transducer, emitting 1000 to 2000 pulses per second along a single line, provides an "ice-pick" view of the heart, with excellent *temporal* resolution. When beam direction is changed, the heart can be scanned from the ventricles to the aorta and left atrium (Fig. 179-3). *Two-dimensional*

FIGURE 179-2 *Diagrammatic representation of intracardiac and aortic pressure tracings correlated with the ECG and phonocardiogram (Phono). The striped and cross-hatched areas labeled IsoV represent the isovolumetric phases of contraction and relaxation of the left and right ventricles, respectively; M_1, T_1, A_2, and P_2, sounds produced by closure of the mitral, tricuspid, aortic, and pulmonary valves, respectively; OT and OM, sounds produced by tricuspid and mitral opening. The QS_2 interval includes the preejection period (PEP) and the left ventricular ejection time (LVET), all of which can be measured noninvasively (see text).*

pressure tracings, respectively. The phonocardiogram provides a graphic display of heart sounds and murmurs.

The *carotid pulse morphology* and derived *systolic time intervals* may provide information about left ventricular function and outflow

FIGURE 179-3 *Schematic diagrams of an M-mode echocardiographic scan through a normal heart. A long-axis section of the heart is depicted in the upper diagram. The echocardiographic movement patterns that arise from the corresponding anatomic structures are illustrated in the bottom diagram. CW = chest wall; T = echocardiographic transducer; S = sternum; RV = right ventricle; LV = left ventricle; AO = aortic root; AMV = anterior mitral leaflet; PMV = posterior mitral leaflet; LA = left atrium; RVW = right ventricular wall; AV = aortic valve; PPM = posterior papillary muscle; LVW = left ventricular wall. [From Come PC: Echocardiography in diagnosis and management of cardiovascular disease. Compr Ther 6(5):58, 1980. Courtesy The Laux Company, Inc., Ayer, MA.]*

echocardiography (Figs. 179-4 and 179-5) produces an image in two distance dimensions by steering the sound beam through an arc of up to 90° some 30 times per second. It provides excellent *spatial* resolution, permitting analysis of structural movement in real time, from multiple transducer positions.

Doppler echocardiography detects blood flow velocity and turbulence. When sound encounters moving red blood cells, the frequency of its reflected signal is altered. The magnitude of the change *(Doppler shift)* indicates the velocity *V* of blood flow with respect to the sound beam:

$$V = \frac{C \times (\text{Doppler shift})}{(2 \times \text{emitted frequency}) \cos \theta}$$

where *C* is the speed of sound in tissue, and θ is the angle between the Doppler beam and the mean axis of blood flow. An upward shift (increased frequency of the reflected sound) indicates blood motion toward the transducer and a downward shift, motion away. High-flow velocities, such as across stenotic semilunar valves, can be measured, enabling calculation of transvalvular pressure gradients *(P)* using the modified Bernoulli equation, $P = 4V^2$. Recording of flow signals from small, preselected areas permits spatial localization of turbulence resulting from valvular stenosis and regurgitation and from shunts. Combined Doppler and imaging techniques permit calculation of cardiac output. Unfortunately, not all patients can be successfully studied by echocardiography. Sound penetration may be suboptimal in many elderly, obese, and emphysematous patients.

VALVULAR HEART DISEASE Imaging echocardiography can detect abnormalities of valve thickness and movement responsible for stenosis and regurgitation. In addition, the heart's response to pressure or volume overload can be assessed in terms of chamber dilatation, hypertrophy, and wall movement. Doppler techniques permit evaluation of regurgitation and stenosis. (See also Chap. 187.)

Mitral stenosis The echocardiographic appearance of a restricted valve opening, due to leaflet thickening and commissural fusion, and of shortened, thickened chordae is virtually diagnostic (Fig. 179-4).

Planimetry of the mitral area in the diastolic short axis view and evaluation of the rate of falloff of the estimated transmitral diastolic pressure gradient by Doppler permit quite reliable estimation of valve area. Other causes of inflow obstruction, such as atrial myxoma (Fig. 179-4, right) or thrombus, massive annular calcification, supravalvular ring, cor triatriatum, and parachute mitral valve may also be detected.

Mitral regurgitation Systolic mitral competence depends upon normal function of the mitral leaflets and their supporting structures, including the annulus, chordae tendineae, papillary muscles, and surrounding myocardium. Two-dimensional techniques are preferable to M-mode in recognizing etiologies of mitral regurgitation, which include rheumatic disease, prolapse, flail leaflets resulting from chordal or papillary muscle rupture, annular calcification, atrioventricular canal defects, myxomas, endocarditis, hypertrophic cardiomyopathy, and ventricular dysfunction. Doppler mapping of the extent of systolic turbulence within the atrium provides a gross estimate of the severity of regurgitation.

Aortic stenosis Subvalvular, valvular, and supravalvular obstruction can generally be detected by two-dimensional echocardiography. Systolic leaflet doming and an unusual number or size of cusps (two in a bicuspid valve) suggest congenital valve disease. Acquired fibrosis and calcification cause valve thickening. Normal leaflet separation excludes critical acquired aortic stenosis, but decreased separation is not specific for stenosis. Doppler detection of high-flow velocity across the valve supports stenosis. Lesser flow velocities do not, however, exclude stenosis because both reduced stroke volume and inability to position the Doppler beam parallel to flow may appreciably decrease measured velocities.

Aortic regurgitation Aortic root dilatation and dissection can be distinguished from valve abnormalities causing regurgitation, including congenital disease, sclerosis, endocarditis, prolapse, and flail cusps. Two-dimensional techniques best define structural pathology, but M-mode techniques more readily detect both diastolic vibrations of the anterior mitral leaflet, a very sensitive sign of aortic regurgi-

FIGURE 179-4 *Two-dimensional long- and short-axis views in diastole from patients with marked reduction of effective mitral valve orifice area (MVO) due to mitral stenosis (MS) and left atrial (LA) myxoma (MYX). In the MS patient, the valve leaflets are thickened, particularly at their tips, and there is markedly reduced diastolic separation of the anterior and posterior leaflets. The LA is enlarged. The LA MYX is seen to prolapse into the MVO during diastole, causing obstruction. RV = right ventricle; LV = left ventricle; AoV = aortic valve.*

FIGURE 179-5 *Long-axis parasternal views of the left ventricle in diastole and systole in a normal individual and in patients with dilated cardiomyopathy (CM) and hypertrophic cardiomyopathy (HCM). Normal diastolic wall thicknesses and normal systolic wall thickening and excursion are illustrated in the left panels. In the patient with dilated CM, left ventricular (LV) and left atrial (LA) diameters are increased, and there is markedly reduced systolic thickening and excursion of the septum (SEP) and posterior wall (PW). In the patient with HCM, the SEP is abnormally thick and highly echogenic. The LV cavity is small in diastole and almost disappears during systolic contraction. RV = right ventricle; MV = mitral valve; AoV = aortic valve.*

tation, and premature mitral closure, produced by the marked elevation of left ventricular diastolic pressure which may accompany severe, acute regurgitation.

Tricuspid and pulmonary valve disease Two-dimensional scanning has improved visualization of right-sided valves. Changes in structure and movement may permit detection of rheumatic deformity, Ebstein's malformation, prolapse, flail cusps, endocarditis, congenital dysplasia, and thickening due to carcinoid, amyloid, Loeffler's endocarditis, or endocardial fibrosis. Systolic doming of the pulmonic valve is characteristic of pulmonic stenosis.

Prosthetic valves Mechanical prostheses are difficult to evaluate, because their intrinsically high echogenicity interferes with the recognition of vegetations and thrombi. Abnormal timing of valve opening and closure, best assessed using combined phonocardiography and M-mode techniques, and abnormalities on Doppler study may suggest dysfunction, but angiography and hemodynamic assessment are often necessary for full evaluation. Abnormalities of bioprostheses, including fibrosis, calcification, vegetations, and tears, are more easily recognized.

Endocarditis Valvular vegetations, characterized by masses of shaggy-appearing echoes, are evident in over half of patients with endocarditis. While their detection is associated with an increased risk of complications, many patients recover uneventfully with antibiotic therapy alone. (See also Chap. 188.)

Left ventricle M-mode echocardiography is widely used to measure left ventricular size, wall thickness, and function. The rate of wall thinning in diastole may permit assessment of diastolic function, and the percentage of shortening of the minor axis, normally greater than 28 percent, and the mean velocity of circumferential fiber shortening are useful measurements of systolic performance. These indexes of systolic performance are influenced, however, by preload and afterload

as well as by myocardial contractility. Analyses of end-systolic pressure-dimension relations, which are independent of preload and incorporate afterload, provide better information regarding contractile function. Estimates of global ventricular performance, based on ice-pick M-mode views, are useful, however, only when ventricular shape is normal and systolic movement relatively symmetric in extent and timing. Two-dimensional echocardiography, which images the ventricle in a number of different planes, improves assessment of volumes and function, particularly in patients with asymmetric contraction resulting from ischemic heart disease. The left ventricular apex, the most common site of wall movement abnormalities and thrombi, can be adequately visualized only by two-dimensional techniques.

Echocardiography permits recognition of *cardiomyopathy* and classification into dilated, hypertrophic, and restrictive-obliterative types (Fig. 179-5). In dilated cardiomyopathy, both ventricles are generally enlarged and poorly contracting, and wall thicknesses are normal or only slightly increased. In contrast, appreciable ventricular hypertrophy, usually involving the septum asymmetrically, small ventricular size, enhanced systolic performance and impaired diastolic relaxation, characterize hypertrophic cardiomyopathy. Systolic anterior movement of the mitral valve to abut the septum and partial midsystolic closure of the aortic valve correlate with dynamic obstruction. Increased wall thickness also characterizes infiltrative disorders. In amyloidosis, the thick walls are often "speckled" in appearance and are associated with diminished voltage on electrocardiogram (ECG).

Pericardial effusion Echocardiography can detect effusions as small as 15 to 20 mL. While certain findings, such as diastolic compression of the right atrium and ventricle, may suggest tamponade, decisions regarding therapy are best based on clinical and hemodynamic observations.

Cardiac masses Most masses involving the heart and pericardium are easily recognized. They include myxomas (Fig. 179-4), other primary and secondary tumors, and thrombi.

Congenital heart disease Since valvular abnormalities and relationships of atria, valves, ventricles, and great vessels can easily be recognized by two-dimensional echocardiography, this technique has revolutionized the diagnosis of congenital heart disease. Contrast and Doppler echocardiography facilitate detection of shunts and of valvular stenosis and regurgitation.

RADIONUCLIDE IMAGING OF THE HEART

There are four major clinical indications for radionuclide study of the heart: (1) assessment of systolic and diastolic ventricular function using radionuclide ventriculography; (2) identification and quantification of intracardiac shunts using radioangiocardiography; (3) assessment of myocardial perfusion using ionic tracers, principally thallium 201; and (4) detection of acute myocardial infarction with infarct-avid radionuclides.

VENTRICULAR PERFORMANCE Radionuclide ventriculography (RVG) uses a radioactive intravascular indicator to delineate heart chambers and great vessels (Fig. 179-6). The radionuclide, usually technetium 99m, is generally attached to red blood cells. RVGs may be performed using two different methods. In the *first-pass* technique, radiotracer is injected intravenously, and a scintillation camera tracks its transit through the right heart, lungs, and left heart. In the *equilibrium,* or *gated, method,* counts are recorded from several hundred cardiac cycles following uniform distribution of radiotracer throughout the blood pool. The scintigraphic information in each cycle is divided into multiple frames (often 30 or more), using the ECG as a timing reference. Counts from corresponding frames of each cycle are then summed by computer to provide images of the spatial distribution and density of counts over time. Images are generally obtained in at least two views [anterior and left anterior oblique (LAO)]. Gated scans are frequently obtained after first-pass scans, since no additional injection of radionuclide is required. Because detected counts, after background subtraction, are proportional to blood volume, equilibrium studies permit estimation of chamber volumes, enabling calculation of left and right ventricular ejection fractions, left-to-right ventricular stroke volume ratios, and rates of ventricular ejection and filling. Agreement with standard catheterization methods has been excellent. Repeated scans can be obtained up to 20 h after injection, permitting assessment of the effects of interventions, such as exercise and medications, on ventricular performance.

RVG may be used to detect patients with chronic ischemic heart disease. Since resting function may be normal, exercise is often used to provoke ischemia. Scans are obtained at rest and at peak exercise. Failure to increase left ventricular ejection fraction by at least 5 percent and development of one or more regional wall movement abnormalities have a sensitivity and specificity of approximately 90 and 60 percent, respectively, for detection of significant coronary disease. The test is most helpful in patients with an intermediate pretest probability of disease. Low resting ejection fractions after acute infarction have been correlated with increased short- and long-term morbidity and mortality. Mitral regurgitation, septal rupture, and aneurysms resulting from infarction may also be detected. RVG can assess systolic and diastolic function in patients with cardiomyopathy (Fig. 179-6) or volume overload. A reduced resting ejection fraction correlates with a poor prognosis in patients with mitral or aortic regurgitation, even after valve replacement. The added value of exercise RVG in detecting reduced myocardial reserve due to volume overload remains controversial. Thrombi and other tumors may be recognized, but RVG is less sensitive than echocardiography.

SHUNT SCINTIGRAPHY Assessment of left-to-right shunts utilizes a modification of the first-pass RVG in which the "region of interest" is focused over an area of lung. Following rapid injection of radiotracer

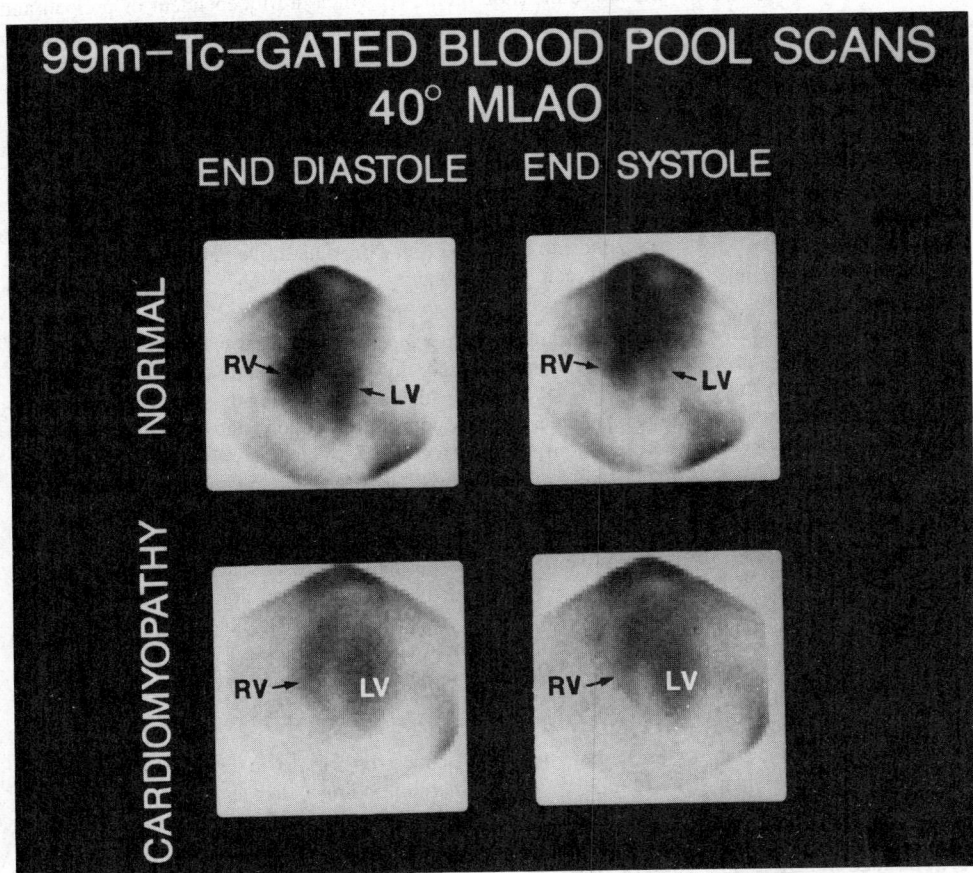

FIGURE 179-6 *End-diastolic and end-systolic gated blood pool images from a normal individual (with estimated left and right ventricular ejection fractions of 69 and 45 percent, respectively) and from a patient with idiopathic dilated cardiomyopathy and marked, global reduction of left ventricular systolic function (left ventricular ejection fraction of 23 percent). In the patient with cardiomyopathy, there is very little change in left ventricular cavity size or count density from diastole to systole. The right ventricle, however, shows normal function, with an ejection fraction of 57 percent. RV = right ventricle; LV = left ventricle.*

into a large vein, usually the external jugular, the pulmonary time-activity curve is recorded by a gamma camera-computer system. Normally, counts increase sharply as the bolus reaches the lung underlying the detector. Following peak activity, there is a smooth descent and a later, smaller increase in counts representing normal recirculation of the radiotracer following systemic circulation. Left-to-right shunts cause premature interruption of the descent, due to early reappearance of radioactivity within the lung. Computer analysis of the areas under the curve permits reliable determination of the ratio of pulmonic-to-systemic blood flow. Right-to-left shunts may also be recognized and quantified.

MYOCARDIAL PERFUSION IMAGING Certain radiolabeled mono-valent cations, especially the potassium analogue thallium 201 (half-life of 72 h), are widely used to assess myocardial perfusion since their active uptake by normal myocardial cells is proportional to regional blood flow. Areas of myocardial necrosis, fibrosis, and ischemia show reduced thallium accumulation ("cold spots") on images obtained soon after injection. Following its initial accumulation within cells, however, thallium 201 continues to exchange with the systemic pool. After several hours, all viable myocardial cells with intact membrane function will contain nearly equal concentrations.

Thallium 201 scintigraphy is most commonly used to detect exercise-induced ischemia (Fig. 179-7). Thallium is injected intra-venously at peak exercise, and images are obtained in several projections 5 to 10 min later. Normal scans show relatively homogeneous distribution of activity, while those of patients with infarction or ischemia typically demonstrate one or more "cold spots." Due to continued exchange of thallium between viable cells and the systemic pool, however, initial defects due to ischemia "fill in" on repeat imaging several hours later. Areas of infarction demonstrate persistent reduction of uptake. Compared to routine exercise electrocardiography, exercise thallium scintigraphy increases the sensitivity for detection of coronary disease from approximately 60 to 80 percent and increases specificity slightly from about 80 to 90 percent. It is most useful in patients with atypical chest pain in whom the exercise ECG is nondiagnostic or uninterpretable due to left bundle branch block, ventricular hypertrophy, or drug and electrolyte effects; in patients who fail to achieve 85 percent of predicted maximal heart rate; and in patients with a high likelihood of a false-positive exercise ECG study. Thallium scanning improves localization of ischemia and provides prognostic information, since the presence and number of redistributing defects correlate with the incidence of future cardiac events. Thallium scintigraphy has also been used to detect ischemia during pacing, dipyridamole-induced coronary vasodilatation, or spontaneous pain.

Thallium scanning does not distinguish new from old infarcts and is less accurate than serum enzyme analysis in detecting acute necrosis. It does, however, offer prognostic information. Patients with smaller defects have better survival rates. On submaximal exercise thallium tests following infarction, the presence of multiple or redistributing defects or increased lung uptake of thallium (probably representing transudation into the lung during periods of high pulmonary capillary pressure) identifies patients at higher risk for postinfarction morbidity and mortality.

Computed tomography using positron-emitting isotopes of potassium analogues permits quantitative assessment of radiotracer uptake. The short half-lives of such isotopes permit multiple studies over short periods of time, allowing assessment of changes in myocardial perfusion induced by therapeutic interventions.

ACUTE INFARCT SCINTIGRAPHY Pyrophosphate appears to bind to calcium and organic macromolecules in irreversibly damaged myocardial cells. If coronary flow is sufficient for its delivery to necrotic myocardium (10 to 40 percent of normal flow is required), technetium 99m stannous pyrophosphate will bind there, producing an image with increased uptake ("hot spot"). Scans are most likely to be positive when injections are performed 48 to 72 h after suspected infarction, when the elevated creatine kinase activity has often returned to normal. The major clinical indication is the detection of acute infarction in patients in whom traditional diagnostic methods cannot be interpreted or have provided equivocal results. Sensitivity and specificity for transmural infarcts are both about 90 percent. Uptake is often fainter and more poorly localized in subendocardial infarcts, and myocardial damage from causes other than coronary disease may result in a positive scan.

MAGNETIC RESONANCE IMAGING (MRI)

Certain atomic nuclei, which possess an odd number of either protons or neutrons (or both), absorb and reemit electromagnetic energy when they are placed in a strong magnetic field and have their net magnetization vector deflected by application of a radiofrequency pulse. Signals emitted during return of the magnetization vector to its equilibrium position can be analyzed to provide spectral and imaging information. Since blood flowing at normal velocities produces virtually no MR signal, there is a high natural contrast between the walls of the heart and great vessels and the moving blood. ECG gating of signals from ^{1}H has permitted excellent structural definition of myocardial, pericardial, great vessel, and congenital cardiac abnormalities. Advantages of MR imaging relative to computed

FIGURE 179-7 *Serial thallium 201 scintigrams obtained in the 45° LAO projection in a patient undergoing exercise testing for evaluation of chest pain. The immediate post-exercise image* (left) *demonstrates decreased perfusion of the septum. The 1- and 2-h delayed images* (middle and right) *demonstrate "filling in" of the defect, reflecting redistribution. The computer-derived time-activity curves* (bottom) *confirm the significant reduction in initial counts in the septum, relative to the posterolateral wall, and demonstrate near equalization of activity by 2 h. S = septum; PL = posterolateral wall. [From PC Come (ed): Diagnostic Cardiology. Reprinted with permission of George A. Beller, M.D., and J.B. Lippincott Company.]*

tomography include the lack of both ionizing radiation and the need for contrast administration. Advantages relative to echocardiography include the ability to image in any desired plane, the capability for transmission of signals through bone and air, a wider field of view, and improved spatial resolution. Disadvantages include the relatively long duration of the imaging procedure, the greater sensitivity of MR imaging to body movement, and the high cost and lack of portabililty of the required equipment. ^{1}H imaging also provides potential for tissue characterization. Areas of acute myocardial ischemia and infarction in experimental animals and in humans have been identified as locations of high signal intensity relative to normal myocardium, probably reflecting the greater number of hydrogen nuclei in areas of myocardial edema. Conversely, areas of fibrosis produce signals of lesser intensity. ^{31}P MR spectroscopy permits quantification of high-energy phosphate compounds and of intracellular pH. It is therefore a powerful research tool for evaluation of intracellular metabolism.

REFERENCES

BERGER HJ, ZARET BL: Nuclear cardiology. N Engl J Med 305:799; 305:855, 1981

COME PC (ed): *Diagnostic Cardiology: Noninvasive Imaging Techniques.* Philadelphia, Lippincott, 1985

FEIGENBAUM H: *Echocardiography,* 4th ed. Philadelphia, Lea & Febiger, 1986

HIGGINS CB et al: Magnetic resonance imaging of the cardiovascular system. Am Heart J 109:136, 1985

KISSLO J et al (eds): *Basic Doppler Echocardiography,* vol 17. New York, Churchill Livingstone, 1986

McNAMARA MT, HIGGINS CB: Magnetic resonance imaging of chronic myocardial infarcts in man. AJR 146:315, 1986

NANDA NC (ed): *Doppler Echocardiography.* New York, Igaku-Shoin, 1985

180 CARDIAC CATHETERIZATION AND ANGIOGRAPHY

KIRK L. PETERSON / JOHN ROSS, JR.

Catheterization of the right and left sides of the heart and selective injection of contrast media into the coronary arteries and cardiac chambers during exposure of high-speed x-ray motion pictures (cineangiography) remain the most reliable methods for defining the dynamic physiology and anatomy of the heart in the normal state and a variety of cardiac disorders. When performed after the application of noninvasive or atraumatic techniques of cardiac diagnosis, the great majority of disorders of the heart can be accurately and fully defined and a rational decision made for medical or surgical therapy. In addition, in the past half-decade, cardiac catheterization techniques have been developed which provide therapeutic benefit and are now being applied on a broad scale.

DIAGNOSTIC INDICATIONS

The types of problems for which diagnostic catheterization studies (see Table 180-1) are commonly performed may be summaried as follows:

1 In patients with valvular heart disease, hemodynamic measurements and determination of angiographic pathoanatomy often are required to determine whether the mechanical valvular defect(s) is amenable to surgical correction and whether its severity warrants it. In these same patients, coronary angiography is often performed in order to search for or exclude associated coronary artery disease.

2 In patients with congenital heart disease, hemodynamic studies and angiography usually are necessary to characterize the type and

TABLE 180-1 Diagnostic information that can be obtained by cardiac catheterization and angiography

1 Intracardiac and intravascular pressure measurements and determination of pressure gradients across the cardiac valves
2 Cardiac output, pulmonary vascular resistance, and systemic vascular resistance
3 Radiographic anatomy of the cardiac chambers and great vessels (aorta, pulmonary artery)
4 Radiographic anatomy of the coronary arteries and detection of coronary artery spasm
5 Detection and quantification of intracardiac shunts
6 Intracardiac electrograms, His bundle electrograms, electrical pacing studies, and intracardiac phonocardiograms
7 Acute effects (hemodynamic and electrophysiologic) of cardioactive drugs
8 Quantification of coronary blood flow
9 Histology of myocardium from endomyocardial catheter biopsies

severity of the primary defect and to determine whether associated lesions are present.

3 In patients with known coronary artery disease, angiographic visualization of the coronary arteries may be indicated to obtain useful prognostic information and help determine whether operative treatment is feasible. In other patients with a chest pain syndrome of undetermined cause, coronary angiography may be indicated to define the presence or absence of atherosclerotic coronary disease or coronary artery spasm.

4 In patients who have undergone cardiac operations, cardiac catheterization and angiography may be indicated to evaluate the success of the operation, particularly when residual symptoms are present. Such studies may reveal malfunction of a prosthetic valve, residual obstruction or regurgitation of a surgically reconstructed native valve, loss of patency of a coronary artery bypass graft, inadequate correction of a congenital defect, or residual disease of the ventricular myocardium.

5 In patients with suspected myocardial or pericardial disease, hemodynamic and angiographic information may be needed to detect or exclude lesions potentially amenable to surgical treatment, such as mitral regurgitation, coronary heart disease, constrictive pericarditis, or obstructive hypertrophic cardiomyopathy.

6 In patients with evidence of pulmonary hypertension, cardiac catheterization is needed to search for possible mitral stenosis, pulmonary venous obstruction, left-to-right shunts, multiple pulmonary emboli, or peripheral pulmonary artery stenosis, or to establish, by exclusion, the diagnosis of primary pulmonary hypertension.

7 In some patients in an intensive care setting (e.g., for hypotension or heart failure following acute myocardial infarction), catheterization of the right side of the heart by means of a balloon-tipped flotation catheter (Swan-Ganz catheter) often is employed to measure the pulmonary artery pressure, the pulmonary artery wedge pressure (as a measure of the left ventricular filling pressure), and the cardiac output. Such studies permit proper diagnosis, and repeated measurements allow accurate assessment of the effects of treatment.

8 In patients with known myocardial failure, or in the transplanted human heart, an endomyocardial biopsy specimen(s) is used to detect histologic evidence of inflammation, an infiltrative process (e.g., amyloidosis, hemochromatosis, granuloma, neoplasm), or immune rejection.

9 In patients with rhythm disturbances, recordings of intracardiac electrograms via electrode catheters provide insight into the anatomic locus of a conduction abnormality (e.g., accessory pathway), or stimulation of the right atrium or ventricle to produce extrasystoles over a spectrum of coupling intervals is used to test the efficacy of antiarrhythmic therapy for controlling repetitive tachycardias (Chap. 184).

THERAPEUTIC INDICATIONS

These are the major categories of cardiac problems for which catheterization techniques are applied for therapeutic benefit:

1 In patients with obstructive single- or multi-vessel coronary heart disease, passage of a balloon-dilation catheter (transluminal coronary angioplasty) is performed when judged feasible (Chap. 189).

2 In patients with recent (generally less than 6 h) myocardial infarction due to coronary thrombosis, selective coronary artery infusion of a thrombolytic agent (streptokinase or tissue plasminogen activator) serves to lyse the offending clot and reperfuse the jeopardized area of myocardium (Chap. 190). In some instances, successful clot lysis is followed by balloon angioplasty in order to relieve the atherosclerotic obstruction responsible for the thrombosis.

3 In some patients, particularly children with coarctation of the aorta or congenital aortic or pulmonic stenosis, a large balloon-dilation catheter can be utilized to relieve an anatomic obstruction to blood flow (Chap. 185).

4 In patients with congenital heart disease and inadequate pulmonary blood flow, balloon atrial septostomy (enlargement of an existing interatrial communication) serves to improve delivery of desaturated blood to the lungs (Chap. 185).

5 In patients with pulmonary arteriovenous fistulas, selective embolization of the artery with beads can serve to close off a right-to-left shunt.

6 In patients with knotted or fragmented intracardiac or intravascular catheters (due to iatrogenic manipulation), "snare" or "basket" devices can be used to uncurl and extract the offending segments of catheter.

TECHNIQUES

CATHETERIZATION OF THE RIGHT SIDE OF THE HEART   Catheterization of the right side of the heart is now a safe and well-standardized procedure. With the patient under local anesthesia an antecubital or saphenous vein is isolated and a long, flexible radiopaque catheter is introduced. Alternatively, the percutaneous approach is employed, in which a needle is positioned in the vessel, a small, flexible wire is passed through the needle, and with a vein dilator, a sheath is then passed over the dilator into the femoral, internal jugular, or other vein. The guidewire is removed, leaving the sheath in place, and through it a catheter is guided sequentially into the right atrium, right ventricle, the pulmonary artery, and pulmonary arterial wedge positions. When fluoroscopy is not available (e.g., at the bedside, operating room, intensive care unit) a balloon-flotation catheter may be passed through the sheath, or directly into an exposed vein, and advanced by tactile sense until it is considered to be near the right atrium. Then while intracardiac pressure is being monitored, the balloon is inflated and the catheter advanced further, whereupon it is usually carried by the bloodstream directly into the right ventricle, the pulmonary artery, and into a second- or third-order pulmonary artery branch, from which a pulmonary arterial wedge tracing is obtained. Also, with a thermistor-tipped balloon catheter, cardiac output can be measured serially by using the indicator-dilution principle discussed subsequently in this chapter.

The course of the catheter in the right side of the heart on fluoroscopy or cineangiography may provide a clue to the diagnosis of certain congenital malformations. The catheter may enter an anomalous pulmonary vein or left superior vena cava; it may directly traverse a patent ductus arteriosus or an atrial septal defect; inability to cross the tricuspid valve may indicate tricuspid atresia; and passage of the catheter from the right ventricle to the aorta may indicate a ventricular septal defect or a form of transposition of the great vessels.

CATHETERIZATION OF THE LEFT SIDE OF THE HEART   Various methods for catheterization of the left side of the heart have been devised, and each has found application under certain circumstances. Currently, the *retrograde arterial* approach is used most widely for entrance into the ascending aorta, left ventricle, and, less frequently, the left atrium; the catheter usually is inserted via the femoral artery by the percutaneous method, or through a small incision directly into the exposed brachial artery. The *transseptal* approach may be

employed to gain access to the left atrium and left ventricle, particularly when severe obstruction of the aortic valve, obstructive hypertrophic cardiomyopathy, or a mechanical aortic prosthesis are present or suspected. With this method, a catheter is inserted via the right saphenous or femoral vein, and its tip positioned in the right atrium. A long needle, curved at its tip, is introduced through the catheter and employed to puncture the intact interatrial septum in the region of the fossa ovalis. The catheter then is advanced over the needle into the left atrium; preshaping of the catheter also allows ready entrance across the mitral valve into the left ventricle.

Other methods of catheterization of the left side of the heart are used less commonly; e.g., with the *anterior percutaneous* approach a needle is introduced directly into the left ventricle in the region of the cardiac apex. This procedure is occasionally useful for measuring the left ventricular pressure in patients with valvular aortic stenosis, or in postoperative patients with prosthetic valves in both the aortic and mitral positions.

CARDIAC ANGIOGRAPHY   Right side of heart   Selective injection of radiopaque contrast media at various sites within the right side of the heart also may be performed during cardiac catheterization. Injections into the superior or inferior vena cava are useful for detecting the thickened right atrial wall of constrictive pericarditis and for defining certain congenital lesions such as Ebstein's malformation of the tricuspid valve and tricuspid atresia (Chap. 185). Selective right ventriculography is used to detect tricuspid regurgitation and to delineate congenital cardiac lesions such as pulmonic stenosis and tetralogy of Fallot. Injection into the main pulmonary artery permits visualization of pulmonary thromboemboli, congenital pulmonary arterial branch stenoses, and anomalous pulmonary venous connections, and during the levophase of contrast passage may be useful in the detection of tumor or thrombus within the left atrium.

Left side of heart   Selective left ventriculography is employed to define congenital and acquired lesions affecting the mitral valve and the left ventricular outflow tract and to assess the adequacy of left ventricular function. Mitral stenosis may be detected by left ventriculography as thickening and/or calcification of the valve leaflets, shortening of the chordal subvalvular apparatus, and reduced excursion and delayed closure of the leaflets. Mitral regurgitation may be detected and its degree estimated by noting the amount and density of contrast agent which enters the left atrium after left ventricular injection (Fig. 180-1). In addition systolic prolapse into the left atrium of one or both of the mitral valve leaflets, secondary to either chordal malfunction or primary myxomatous degeneration, and redundancy of the leaflets themselves may be identified. The site of discrete subvalvular, valvular, or supravalvular aortic stenosis may be visualized, and the abnormal apposition of the ventricular septum and the anterior mitral valve leaflet in hypertrophic cardiomyopathy can be defined.

Both regional and global left ventricular function can be determined from analysis of the silhouette of the left ventricular cavity on the left ventriculogram. Regions of absent contraction (akinesis), reduced contraction (hypokinesis), or paradoxical systolic expansion (dyskinesis), as well as frank aneurysm formation, can thereby be detected and assessed as to severity (Fig. 180-2). Mural thrombi also may be visualized within such areas where wall motion is disordered. In addition, by determination of a magnification factor, the area of the left ventricular cavity can be measured accurately, and by assumption of a geometric model of an ellipse, the volume of the chamber at end diastole and end systole can be determined (Fig. 180-1), and the total stroke volume can be calculated. The total stroke volume minus the forward stroke volume (calculated by an independent method for determining cardiac output, as discussed below) can then be used to derive the amount of aortic or mitral regurgitation per beat.

Values for end-diastolic volume greater than 90 mL per square meter of body surface area (average normal, plus 1 SD) generally indicate left ventricular dilatation due to heart failure, or to a volume overload such as occurs in aortic or mitral regurgitation. The ejection

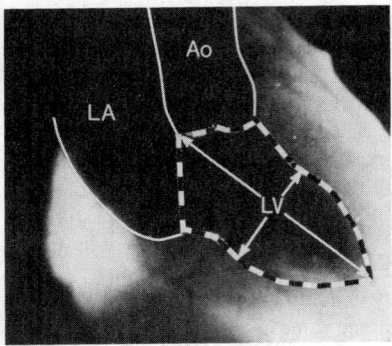

FIGURE 180-1 *Cineangiogram with injection of contrast medium into the left ventricle (LV). End diastole is on the left and end systole on the right. Study is performed in the right anterior oblique projection in a patient with severe mitral regurgitation in whom the left atrium (LA) is densely opacified simultaneously with the aorta (Ao) during ventricular systole.*

Volume (V) and LV is determined by planimetry of chamber area (enclosed by dashed line) and measurement of longest length (solid line between base and apex), using a geometric model of an ellipsoid. Thus, $D = 4A/\pi L$ and $V = \pi(D^2L/6)$, where D = calculated diameter, L = longest measured length, A = area, and V = LV volume. Mean velocity of circumferential fiber shortening (mean V_{cf}, normalized to per unit circumference) can also

be calculated by direct measurement of the minor axis (indicated by line with arrows) perpendicular to the midpoint of the long axis, and determination of the ejection time from cine frame rate and number of frames exposed from the beginning to the end of ejection.

$$Ejection\ fraction = \frac{end\text{-}diastolic\ V - end\text{-}systolic\ V}{end\text{-}systolic\ V}$$

$$Mean\ V_{cf} = \frac{end\text{-}diastolic\ D - end\text{-}systolic\ D}{end\text{-}diastolic\ D \times ejection\ time}$$

where V = ventricular volume, D = minor axis diameter

fraction, the ratio of stroke volume to end-diastolic volume, reflects the percent shortening of the left ventricular myocardium (normal range of ejection fraction = 0.56 to 0.78). When the ejection fraction is reduced, the presence of depressed left ventricular contractile function is suggested. A further useful index of myocardial function is the mean velocity of circumferential fiber shortening (mean V_{cf}), the fractional shortening per unit time of the minor axis of the left ventricular chamber (Fig. 180-1). Mean V_{cf} values below 1.2 end-diastolic circumferences per second in the basal state are considered indicative of depressed myocardial contractility. (Other measures of depressed contractility are discussed below in "Measurement of Intravascular and Intracardiac Pressures.")

Selective ascending aortography is used for assessing the severity

FIGURE 180-2 *Diagrammatic representation of end-diastolic (solid line) and end-systolic (dashed line) silhouettes of left ventricular cineangiograms in various forms of localized wall motion disorder in patients with coronary heart disease. Normal patient exhibits relatively symmetrical contraction; patient with hypokinesis exhibits reduced contraction over anterior and apical surfaces; patient with dyskinesis exhibits paradoxic, outward movement over anterior surface during systole.*

Normal   Hypokinesis

Akinesis   Dyskinesis

of aortic regurgitation, for determining the size and location of aortic aneurysms, and for visualizing less common congenital or acquired malformations such as sinus of Valsalva aneurysm, paraaortic sinus tract or aortic valvular vegetation (infective endocarditis), or dissection of the aorta due to cystic medial necrosis. Direct injection of contrast medium into the left atrium has been used to study left atrial function or the movement of the mitral valve, and to detect thrombi or tumor (myxoma, rhabdomyoma, rhabdomyosarcoma) within that chamber.

CORONARY ARTERIOGRAPHY   Selective angiographic visualization of the coronary arterial tree is one of the most commonly applied diagnostic procedures in the cardiac catheterization laboratory. Accurate visualization of coronary artery atherosclerotic lesions has significantly increased understanding of the pathogenesis and natural history of ischemic heart disease. Moreover, this procedure has contributed in large measure to the advent of surgical procedures for bypassing obstructive lesions within the coronary arteries. Visualization of coronary artery anatomy is useful, likewise, for defining congenital abnormalities such as anomalous origin of the coronary arteries, or coronary arteriovenous fistula. Administration of ergonovine maleate during coronary arteriography is useful for inducing focal coronary artery spasm, particularly in patients with chest pain at rest in whom Prinzmetal's variant angina is suspected.

Coronary arteriography is performed by selective injection of 5 to 10 mL of contrast medium directly into each coronary artery orifice with cinefilming in multiple oblique and angulated projections at 30 to 60 frames per second and/or large film or photospot exposures at 4 to 6 frames per second, thereby obtaining dynamic as well as high-resolution images of the coronary arterial tree (Fig. 180-3). Specially designed catheters are used: one type, which has an open, tapered tip and multiple side holes, is inserted via a brachial arteriotomy (Sones technique); another type is advanced over a guidewire inserted percutaneously via the femoral artery and is preshaped to allow ready access to the right or left coronary artery orifices (Judkins technique). Both techniques provide diagnostic visualization of obstructive lesions within the main branches of the coronary vessels (Fig. 180-4*A* and *B*). In addition, collateral vessels, or new vascular pathways which serve to carry blood around a significant obstruction, can often be seen, and the vessel beyond a complete obstruction thereby visualized (Fig. 180-4*A*). The latter finding has obvious importance in determining the site for implantation of the distal end of a bypass graft.

DIGITAL ANGIOGRAPHY   Digital computer processing of fluoroscopic or cineangiographic images is now being used to provide

RAO

Sinus Node A.
Conus Branch
Rt. Coronary
Acute Marginal Branch
A.V. Node A.
Post. Descending
Obtuse Marginal Branch
Ant. Descending
Lt. Circumflex
Septal Branch

LAO

S.A. Node A.
Rt. Coronary
Conus Branch
Septal Branch
Post. Descending
Lt. Atrial Circumflex
Intermediate Branch
Ant. Descending
Lt. Circumflex
A.V. Node

FIGURE 180-3 *Diagram of the coronary arterial tree as viewed in two projections commonly used in coronary arteriography, the right anterior oblique (RAO) and left anterior oblique (LAO) projections. A., artery; Ant., anterior, A.V., atrioventricular; Lt., left; Post., posterior; Rt., right; S.A., sinoatrial.*

visual enhancement of structures on both the right and left sides of the heart. In many of these studies the radiopaque contrast material is injected into a peripheral or central vein, obviating the need for a direct left-sided injection. This new approach to cardiac angiography has to date revealed the following advantages: (1) it allows definition of cardiac chamber size and geometry while using less contrast agent; (2) it facilitates computer generation of quantitative indexes of left ventricular function; (3) premature systoles generally are not induced during the recording of the angiographic images; (4) so-called functional or parametric images can be readily constructed which portray visually in one frame a physiologic or pathophysiologic parameter, e.g., regional wall motion (Fig. 180-2), global shortening of the left ventricle, rapidity of contrast wash-in and wash-out through the coronary arteries or into the myocardium.

COMPLICATIONS   Catheterization of the right side of the heart is rarely associated with morbidity or mortality when performed under proper laboratory or bedside conditions. However, catheterization and angiography of the left side of the heart are procedures which unavoidably, although uncommonly, can lead to serious complications. Diagnostic cardiac catheterization procedures nevertheless have been increasingly applied in recent years, primarily in response to the need for precise functional and anatomic information prior to carrying out cardiac operations. In the pediatric age group great attention has been paid to preventing metabolic disorders (hypoxia and acidemia) and pulmonary difficulties, utilization of small amounts of contrast agents, and use of flexible catheters; such precautions have significantly reduced the incidence of major complications and

markedly decreased the overall mortality rate in infants. In adults, the advent of coronary artery bypass graft surgery has brought about a predominance in the application of coronary arteriography and left ventriculography by retrograde aortic catheterization compared with other catheterization procedures. A prospective survey in 7553 patients of complications due to coronary arteriography reported in 1979 by the Collaborative Study of Coronary Artery Surgery (CASS) reported an overall mortality rate of 0.2 percent, an incidence of myocardial infarction of 0.025 percent, and an incidence of systemic embolization and vascular injury of 0.09 and 0.74 percent, respectively (all figures apply to 0 to 48 h after completion of the procedure). The brachial artery (Sones) technique increased the risk of death 3.6 times compared with the femoral approach, but this excess risk did not apply if a given laboratory performed greater than 80 percent of its procedures via the arm approach.

It seems clear that specialized invasive cardiac procedures in any age group should be performed only in well-equipped laboratories by highly experienced personnel, and the risks of cardiac catheterization and angiography should be weighed carefully in relation to the potential therapeutic benefits to be derived from an accurate anatomic and functional diagnosis.

MEASUREMENT OF INTRAVASCULAR AND INTRACARDIAC PRESSURES

The upper limits of normal for intracardiac pressures and certain other hemodynamic variables are shown in Table 180-2. In under-

FIGURE 180-4 *Selective coronary arteriograms obtained in the right anterior oblique projection. A and B show a normal subject, and C, a patient with severe stenosis of the right coronary artery. LMCA, left main coronary artery; CCA, circumflex coronary artery; LADCA, left anterior descending coronary artery; RCA, right coronary artery. In C, arrow 1 indicates the* area of narrowing in the right coronary artery, and arrow 2 shows retrograde filling of the anterior descending coronary artery via collateral vessels, indicating that a severe obstruction is present in that vessel as well. (Courtesy of MP Judkins.)

TABLE 180-2 Normal hemodynamic values*

	a wave	*v* wave	Mean	S/D
Right atrium	8	7	6	
Right ventricle				30/7
Left ventricle				145/12
Pulmonary artery			17	30/14
Pulmonary artery wedge or left atrium	10	15	12	

Cardiac index = 2.4–3.8 (liters/min)/m² body surface area
AV O_2 difference = 3.5–5.0 mL/dL
Pulmonary vascular resistance = 250 (dyn·s)/cm⁵ (3 resistance units)

* The figures shown indicate the upper limits of pressure (mmHg) in normal adult subjects. The values for the pressure waves, the mean pressures, and the systolic and diastolic pressures (S/D) are shown; in the ventricles, D = end-diastolic pressure. The ranges for cardiac index and arterial–mixed venous (AV) O_2 differences are shown.

standing the contours of the intracardiac pressure pulses, thorough knowledge of the temporal relations between the electrical and mechanical events of the cardiac cycle is important (Fig. 179-2).

The amplitude of the *a* wave in the right atrium normally is larger than the *v* wave, whereas in the left atrium the *v* wave is dominant

(Table 180-2). Therefore, when the *v* wave in the right atrial pressure pulse exceeds the *a* wave, abnormal filling of the right atrium during ventricular systole, as occurs in tricuspid regurgitation or atrial septal defect, should be suspected. A characteristic right atrial pressure pulse also may be seen in the presence of tricuspid stenosis, the contour resembling that in the left atrium in mitral stenosis (see below), as well as in constrictive pericarditis, when an early diastolic "dip" and "plateau" elevation of pressure in mid and late diastole occur.

In many patients, the mean level of pressure in the left atrium is reflected with reasonable accuracy by the pulmonary artery wedge pressure (also sometimes termed the pulmonary "capillary" pressure), although the excursions of the wedge tracing often do not coincide with those measured directly within the left atrium. The characteristic contours of the left atrial pressure pulse in a normal subject and in patients with several forms of mitral valve disease are shown in Fig. 180-5. In the normal pressure pulse, or in the presence of mitral regurgitation without stenosis, there is a rapid fall in pressure during early diastole (the *y* descent), and a slow rise in pressure occurs during late diastole (diastasis), reflecting equilibration between the atrial and ventricular pressures during this slow phase of ventricular filling (Fig. 180-5A). In contrast, in patients with mitral stenosis

FIGURE 180-5 *Simultaneously recorded left ventricular (LV) and left atrial (LA) pressure tracings in a normal subject (A) and in patients with various forms of mitral valve disease (B to D). The tracings are recorded at high sensitivity (0 to 40 mmHg), and therefore the top portion of the left ventricular pressure tracing is cut off. The electrocardiogram is recorded in the upper portion of each panel.*

A. In the normal heart, diastole is initiated by a rapid-filling wave, which is followed by a period of slow ventricular filling, or diastasis (bracket D), in which atrial and ventricular pressure rise together slowly. This period of diastasis is followed by the atrial contraction (a), which precedes the onset of isometric contraction in the ventricle, the end-diastolic pressure. The c wave occurs during the phase of isometric ventricular contraction and is followed by the x descent. The v wave occurs during late systole, and the downslope of the v wave, constituting the y descent, occurs immediately after opening of the mitral valve.

B. Tracings obtained in a patient with mitral stenosis and atrial fibrillation. The pressure gradient from left atrium to left ventricle during diastole is indicated by the diagonally shaded area. The a wave is absent, and the c-v wave is prominent, and the y descent is slowed.

C. Tracings from a patient with mitral stenosis and normal sinus rhythm. The pressure gradient is indicated by the diagonally shaded area. A large pressure gradient occurs at the time of atrial contraction. No pressure rise during the period of diastasis is evident in the left atrial pressure tracings of panels B and C.

D. Tracings from a patient with isolated, severe mitral regurgitation and atrial fibrillation. The c wave is not evident, and the giant v wave in the left atrial pressure is nearly 70 mmHg. There is a small pressure gradient during the phase of rapid ventricular filling, because of the large volume of antegrade flow across the mitral valve.

(Chap. 187) the y descent is slow and prolonged; pressure in the left atrium continues to fall throughout diastole, and evidence of diastasis on the left atrial pressure pulse is absent because of the persistent atrioventricular pressure gradient (Fig. 180-5B). When mitral stenosis is present with normal sinus rhythm (Fig. 180-5C), the a wave is present, and a large pressure gradient accompanies atrial contraction. In patients with pure mitral regurgitation, the v wave is prominent, and the descending limb of this wave (the y descent) is rapid (Fig. 180-5D).

The left ventricular end-diastolic pressure immediately precedes the onset of isometric contraction in the left ventricular pressure pulse. This pressure point therefore follows the a wave and precedes the c wave, and the coincident pressure point in time in the left atrial tracing is termed the z point (Fig. 180-5A). The left ventricular end-diastolic pressure may be elevated in several situations: (1) in the presence of myocardial failure, (2) when the ventricle bears a high flow load (as in aortic or mitral regurgitation), (3) when the ventricle is hypertrophied and/or relatively noncompliant (restrictive myocardial disease), (4) in the presence of constrictive pericarditis, and (5) with cardiac tamponade secondary to a pericardial effusion.

The systolic pressure in the left ventricle exceeds that in the aorta in any of the forms of aortic stenosis which produce significant obstruction to ventricular outflow (Chap. 187). In patients with severe valvular aortic stenosis, the left ventricular pressure pulse resembles that of an isometric contraction, the contour being more symmetric and the pressure peak more delayed than normal (a similar phenomenon is observed in the right ventricle in patients with pulmonic stenosis). The characteristics of the peripheral arterial pressure tracing also may be distinctive in patients with different types of aortic stenosis. Thus, when valvular stenosis is present, a slow and delayed rise of the peripheral arterial pulse wave is seen, while in hypertrophic obstructive cardiomyopathy an initially sharp upstroke is followed first by a rapid decline in pressure and then by a secondary positive wave, which reflects the development of the obstruction during systole (Chap. 192).

Derivatives of pressure pulses The rate of change, or slope, of the isovolumetric phase of the right or left ventricular pressure pulse, called the first derivative, or dp/dt, frequently is used in addition to ejection phase measures mentioned above (ejection fraction, mean V_{cf}) to characterize the contractile behavior of the ventricular myocardium. The dp/dt may be measured manually by determining the slope of the pressure rise, but it is recorded more accurately by means of an electronic circuit or by digital computer processing. The peak of this derivative tracing (maximum dp/dt) as well as the maximum value of the ratio of dp/dt to the corresponding instantaneous ventricular pressure [peak $(dp/dt)/p$] provide indexes of the speed of contraction of the ventricle and therefore can help to define the level of the inotropic or contractile state of the heart. These measures tend to be below 1200 mmHg/s and 32 per second, respectively, in the left ventricles of patients with disease of the myocardium, and they may be augmented strikingly by agents which improve the contractility of the heart, such as digitalis or catecholamines.

MEASUREMENT OF CARDIAC OUTPUT

The direct Fick and indicator-dilution methods presently are widely used in patients for the determination of volume blood flow, or the cardiac output. In general, the equations used with these techniques are derived from the principle proposed by Adolf Fick, which states that the rate at which a substance distributed in a fluid is delivered to an area by the moving fluid stream is equal to the product of the flow rate and the difference between the concentration of the substance at sites proximal and distal to the area. Thus,

$$Q = F(C_a - C_v)$$

where Q = quantity of substance delivered per unit time
F = flow rate

$C_a - C_v$ = concentrations of the substance at proximal and distal sampling sites, respectively

(The same equation is applicable to the measurement of the removal rate, or clearance, of a substance.) When flow is the quantity to be derived, the equation is rearranged to

$$F = \frac{Q}{C_a - C_v}$$

DIRECT FICK METHOD In this method for measuring the cardiac output it is assumed that at rest the oxygen uptake in the lungs is equal to that used by the tissues, and systemic flow, i.e., left ventricular output, is equated with blood flow through the lungs. It is essential to this method that a sample of mixed venous blood be obtained, because blood samples in the venae cavae and the coronary sinus have widely different oxygen concentrations, and therefore the venous blood sample generally is withdrawn from the right ventricular outflow tract or preferably the pulmonary artery. In practice, arterial and venous blood samples $(C_a - C_v)$ are obtained during the measurement of oxygen consumption Q over a 3-min period by spirometry and subsequent chemical analysis of the expired gas. Flow F, or cardiac output, is then calculated. The subject must be in a steady state throughout the period of measurement to avoid transient changes in systemic blood flow or in the rate of ventilation that can negate the assumption that oxygen uptake in the lungs equals that taken up in the tissues.

INDICATOR-DILUTION METHOD This is a special application of Fick's principle. A variety of relatively nondiffusible indicators have been employed, the indicator substance being injected into the circulation and its concentration measured at a downstream sampling site by a suitable detector. For example, the dye indocyanine green is injected intravenously and blood is withdrawn from an artery at a constant rate through a calibrated densitometer, which provides direct measurement of the dye concentration. Generally, a single bolus of the indicator is injected rapidly and is thoroughly mixed in one of the vascular spaces, such as a ventricular chamber; the concentration versus time curve then provides a measure of the rate at which indicator is washed out of the mixing site. Prior to recirculation of the indicator, the downslope of this curve is exponential, and therefore extrapolation of the curve using semilog paper permits the elimination of recirculated indicator. The mean concentration c of the dye is determined from the area of this corrected curve and its duration. The rate of blood flow F then is directly related to the quantity of indicator injected i and is inversely related to the mean concentration of the indicator c and the duration of the curve t (in seconds) by the formula $F = 60\ i/ct$. A simple example will serve to illustrate this principle: if 8 mg dye is injected and a mean concentration of 2 mg per liter is recorded, and if the indicator takes 60 s to pass the sampling site, then the flow is 4 liters per minute.

Cold saline is another indicator which is used commonly when a thermodilution catheter is situated in the pulmonary artery. A standard amount of saline is injected at the junction of the superior or inferior vena cava with the right atrium, and the resultant change in temperature (analogous to concentration) is measured in the pulmonary artery by a small thermistor located 2 to 5 cm from the tip of the catheter. The thermodilution technique has demonstrated empirically an excellent correlation with other methods of measuring cardiac output. Cardiac output can also be computed by continuous infusion. Single thermodilution curves provide certain advantages: (1) no arterial entry is required, (2) the indicator is inexpensive, (3) recirculation is minimal, and (4) the analogue signal is well suited to rapid calculation of the cardiac output by computer analysis.

MEASUREMENT OF PULMONARY AND SYSTEMIC VASCULAR RESISTANCE The formula for calculation of pulmonary vascular resistance in simplified form (omitting consideration of vessel length and blood viscosity) states that resistance is directly proportional to the pressure drop across the bed and inversely proportional to the rate of blood flow. This ratio of mean pressure difference (expressed in dynes per square centimeter) to volume flow (expressed in cubic centimeters per second) is expressed in units of dyne-seconds per centimeter to the fifth power [(dyn·s)/cm⁵]; e.g., the mean pressure difference across the pulmonary bed is obtained by subtracting the mean left atrial or pulmonary artery wedge pressure from the mean pulmonary artery pressure:

$$\text{Resistance} = \frac{[P_{pa}(\text{mmHg}) - P_{la}(\text{mmHg})] \times 1332 \text{ dyn/cm}^2}{\text{cardiac output (mL/s)}}$$

where P_{pa} and P_{la} = mean pulmonary artery and left atrial pressures, respectively

1 mmHg = 1.36 cmH₂O
1 cmH₂O = 980 dyn/cm² force

The resistance unit (i.e., the pressure difference in millimeters of mercury divided by the cardiac output in liters per minute and expressed in arbitrary units) also has been employed as an index of arteriolar resistance (Table 180-2). Estimation of the pulmonary vascular resistance, which normally is about 15 percent of that in the systemic vascular bed, is of particular importance in patients with congenital heart disease and circulatory shunts, as well as in certain forms of acquired cardiac and pulmonary diseases. Its calculation provides a useful means of interpreting the level of pulmonary arterial pressure relative to pulmonary blood flow, high pressure and high flow obviously bearing a different connotation than high pressure and low flow.

VALVE ORIFICE SIZE AND VALVULAR REGURGITATION When the cardiac output is normal, the severity of a stenotic valve lesion may be estimated from the magnitude of the pressure gradient across the valve. When the cardiac output is elevated or reduced, however, reliance on the pressure gradient alone may lead to an erroneous estimate of the degree of mechanical obstruction. In addition, it is of importance to consider the heart rate in assessing the significance of a pressure gradient. When the heart rate is rapid, systole occupies a disproportionate amount of time in each cardiac cycle, diastolic filling time is limited, and a large pressure gradient across an atrioventricular valve may exist in the face of relatively mild stenosis. The application of the hydraulic formulas devised by Gorlin and Gorlin to the calculation of valve orifice size has proved helpful in analyzing the degree of valve stenosis in these situations. These formulas state that

$$\text{Aortic valve area (cm}^2) = \frac{F/\text{systolic s}}{44.5\sqrt{\Delta P}}$$

$$\text{Mitral valve area(cm}^2) = \frac{F/\text{diastolic s}}{38.0\sqrt{\Delta P}}$$

where F = flow across the orifice
ΔP = the mean pressure gradient across the orifice

These formulas state that the area of a short-bore orifice is directly proportional to the rate of blood flow across the orifice and inversely proportional to the square root of the pressure gradient. For example, if the flow rate across a narrowed valve orifice of fixed size doubles, as occurs frequently when the cardiac output increases during exertion, the pressure gradient will quadruple, often leading to a striking elevation of pressure in the chamber upstream to the stenotic valve. Conversely, when the flow rate is reduced, as in patients with heart failure, a small pressure gradient may exist in the presence of a severe degree of valve stenosis. This relationship differs from the general resistance equation discussed above and reflects the fact that the kinetic energy losses across a stenotic valve are high, a large pressure head being expended in developing the rapid flow velocity across the narrowed orifice.

The use of the above orifice formulas is not valid when significant valvular regurgitation is present and forward (systemic) cardiac output alone is measured, since an unknown volume of blood is regurgitated and recrosses the valve during the subsequent cardiac cycle. Application of the formulas under these circumstances leads to an underestimation of the valve orifice area, since forward flow across the valve is underestimated. However, when regurgitant flow is determined, generally by angiographic techniques, and total flow across the stenotic orifice is calculated, these orifice formulas may be applied.

DETECTION AND QUANTIFICATION OF CIRCULATORY SHUNTS
When a communication exists between the left and the right sides of the heart, and when pulmonary vascular resistance and right ventricular stiffness are lower than systemic vascular resistance and left ventricular stiffness, respectively, a left-to-right shunt of oxygenated blood will occur. Conversely, when the resistance in the pulmonary bed is higher than that in the systemic circuit, or an obstruction such as pulmonic stenosis exists distal to an intracardiac communication, and right ventricular diastolic stiffness has increased, a right-to-left shunt of venous blood may occur.

Many types of indicators have been employed for the detection of circulatory shunts. The indicator may be the oxygen in room air, blood samples being withdrawn from various sites in the systemic venous bed, right heart, and pulmonary arteries, and analyzed for oxygen concentration manometrically or by an oximeter. A foreign, inert gas such as hydrogen may also be employed; this, like oxygen, is "injected" into the pulmonary circulation by inhalation and sampled from the right side of the heart by a catheter-tip sensor placed sequentially in the pulmonary artery, right ventricle, right atrium, and venae cavae. An inappropriate increase in concentration or early appearance of these indicators indicates the site of entry of a left-to-right shunt. Sometimes indicator-dilution curves are obtained by injecting indocyanine green into the right side of the circulation sampling through a densitometer from a peripheral artery; an early appearance of the indicator indicates a right-to-left shunt beyond (downstream to) the site of dye injection. Thereafter, sequential repeat injections into right atrium, right ventricle, and pulmonary artery until early appearance of contrast at the sampling site is no longer detected allow localization of the site of shunting. In most patients, however, the sites of shunting can be readily visualized and localized by exposure of cineangiograms during selective injections of contrast medium.

For quantification of left-to-right and right-to-left shunts, the oxygen content or saturation of the blood samples taken from the inferior and superior vena cava, the chambers of the right heart, pulmonary veins, left heart chambers, ascending aorta, and peripheral artery are used within the Fick equation to calculate the relative magnitude of pulmonary and systemic flow rates and the absolute amounts of right-to-left and left-to-right shunting. Generally, a pulmonary to systemic flow ratio of 1.5 to 1.0 or greater is considered to indicate a left-to-right shunt of clinical importance.

TRANSLUMINAL CORONARY ANGIOPLASTY

Following his development of a balloon catheter system for transluminal dilatation of peripheral arterial stenoses, Gruentzig designed a similar system for the coronary arterial tree and first applied it to a lesion of the anterior descending artery in 1977. This technique is now being used instead of surgery to treat coronary arterial obstruction in approximately 10 to 30 percent of those patients who, following diagnostic coronary angiography, are considered potential candidates for coronary artery bypass graft surgery (Chap. 189). The relief of obstruction is brought about by several mechanisms including (1) splitting of the plaque with development of a localized, partial circumferential dissection, (2) compression of the surrounding media and adventitia, and (3) remodeling of the "injured" artery over time as the small area of dissection heals (Fig. 180-6). The procedure is performed by passing a small, inflatable balloon-dilation catheter through a larger guiding catheter into the coronary artery ostium (Fig. 180-7B). A flexible guidewire passed through the balloon-dilation

FIGURE 180-6 *Diagrammatic representation of the currently proposed mechanism by which angioplasty increases the luminal diameter of an atherosclerotic vessel is shown in two planes. A corresponds to the original stenosis, B to the introduction of the deflated balloon catheter, C to inflation of the balloon, and D to the final vessel appearance. Note extensive cracking of the intimal plaque, stretching of the media and adventitia, and expansion of the outer diameter of the vessel. (From W Castaneda-Zuniga, The mechanism of balloon angioplasty, Radiology 135:565–571, 1980.)*

catheter is then advanced down the appropriate coronary artery branch and across the stenosis until it reaches close to the cardiac apex. Thereafter, the deflated dilation catheter is advanced over the guidewire until it is situated within the stenotic segment of coronary artery, and the balloon is inflated with several atmospheres of pressure and for as long as 30 to 40 s. After two or more sequential inflations, the result is assessed by measuring the transstenotic gradient and by repeat coronary angiography (Fig. 180-7C).

The most comprehensive analysis of the results of transluminal coronary angioplasty has come from the Registry of the National Heart, Lung, and Blood Institute, which encompassed data from 105 centers in 3079 patients. The procedure was considered successful in approximately 66 percent of the total procedures attempted with a decrease in the degree of stenosis from approximately 80 to 30 percent by angiographic measurement. Emergency coronary artery bypass graft surgery was necessary in 6.6 percent of the patients analyzed, and the incidences of acute myocardial infarction and mortality were found to be 5.0 percent and 0.9 percent, respectively. Approximately 20 percent of patients later developed symptoms or signs of restenosis; many of this subgroup later underwent a successful redilation of the obstructed segment. With improvement in equipment design, patient selection, and operator experience, the primary (initial) success rate has now reached approximately 90 percent in many centers, and the need for emergency coronary bypass surgery and the incidence of infarction have each fallen to the neighborhood of 3 percent. Successful

FIGURE 180-7 *Cine coronary arteriographic frames in right anterior oblique projection in patient undergoing percutaneous transluminal coronary angioplasty of the proximal left anterior descending branch of the left coronary artery.*

coronary angioplasty has been shown to result in enhanced myocardial perfusion, improvement in global left ventricular function, loss of electrocardiographic signs of ischemia during exercise, and an overall improvement in exercise capacity.

OTHER SPECIAL CARDIAC CATHETERIZATION TECHNIQUES

Miniaturization of electronics has permitted the construction and application of cardiac catheters with special measuring devices mounted on, or close to, the tip. For example, a catheter-tip micromanometer permits the measurement of intracardiac pressure free of the artifacts produced by fluid-filled manometer systems and catheter motion. Accurate high-fidelity pressure measurements are of particular utility in the assessment of the contractile and distensibility properties of the left ventricle. Micromanometer-tipped catheters also can be used for highly sensitive recordings of intracardiac sounds and murmurs. Electromagnetic or ultrasonic catheter-tip velocity probes also are available and have proved useful for study of phasic blood flow patterns in the venae cavae and pulmonary artery in patients with constrictive pericarditis and cardiac tamponade, and for analysis of the pattern and velocity of left ventricular ejection into the ascending aorta in patients with disorders of left ventricular function.

Other special catheters have been designed to record the intracardiac electrocardiogram and have made it possible to record selective potentials from the right atrium, right ventricle, and along the bundle of His. Recordings from the latter area are useful, for example, in determining whether a conduction delay or block on the surface electrocardiogram is located at or below the atrioventricular junction. His bundle recordings also have improved understanding of the mechanisms underlying paroxysmal atrial tachycardia and the pre-excitation syndromes. Electrophysiologic studies with cardiac pacing are now being used in the diagnosis and selection of therapy for refractory cardiac tachyarrhythmias (Chap. 184). Electrode catheters have also been utilized to deliver a localized, high-intensity electrical discharge in order to ablate the atrioventricular node or an accessory pathway.

Transvenous intracardiac biopsy The subendocardium of the right and left ventricles may be biopsied safely by specially designed catheters. The specimens have proved to have some value from a diagnostic standpoint in uncommon varieties of infiltrative cardiomyopathy, e.g., those due to amyloid, iron, glycogen, granuloma, and neoplasm, and for identifying histologically differing patterns of inflammation. Endomyocardial biopsy is particularly useful in the detection of early cardiac rejection following cardiac transplantation.

REFERENCES

BAIM DS: Percutaneous transluminal angioplasty, in *Treatment Modalities. Harrison's Principles of Internal Medicine*, RG Petersdorf et al (eds), New York, McGraw-Hill, 1985, p 133

A. Before balloon dilation. B. During inflation of the contrast-filled balloon on the dilation catheter which has been passed over a tiny guidewire. C. After balloon catheter is withdrawn, demonstration of significant relief of stenosis.

BARRY W, GROSSMAN W: Cardiac catheterization, in *Heart Disease,* 2d ed, E Braunwald (ed). Philadelphia, Saunders, 1984, p 279

BREDLAU CE et al: In-hospital morbidity and mortality in patients undergoing elective coronary angioplasty. Circulation 72:1044, 1985

DAVIS K et al: Complications of coronary arteriography from the Collaborative Study of Coronary Artery Surgery (CASS). Circulation 59:1105, 1979

FOWLES RE, MASON JW: Role of cardiac biopsy in the diagnosis and management of cardiac disease. Prog Cardiovasc Dis 27:153, 1984

GROSSMAN W (ed): *Cardiac Catheterization and Angiography,* 3d ed. Philadelphia, Lea & Febiger, 1986

KENT KM, MULLIN SM, PASSAMANI ER: Proceedings of the National Heart, Lung, and Blood Institute Workshop on the Outcome of Percutaneous Transluminal Coronary Angioplasty. Am J Cardiol 53(12):1C–146C, 1984

RACKLEY CE: Quantitative evaluation of left ventricular function by radiographic techniques. Circulation 54:862, 1976

181   NORMAL AND ABNORMAL MYOCARDIAL FUNCTION

EUGENE BRAUNWALD

CELLULAR BASIS OF CARDIAC CONTRACTION

The *myocardium* is composed of individual striated muscle cells (fibers), normally 10 to 15 μm in diameter and 30 to 60 μm in length (Fig. 181-1A). Each fiber contains multiple cross-banded strands (myofibrils), which run the length of the fiber and are composed of a serially repeating structure, the sarcomere. The remainder of the cytoplasm, lying between the myofibrils, contains other cell constituents, such as the single centrally located nucleus, numerous mitochondria, and intracellular membrane systems.

The *sarcomere,* the structural and functional unit of contraction, is delimited by two adjacent dark lines, the Z lines (Fig. 181-1). The distance between Z lines varies with the degree of contraction or stretch of the muscle and ranges between 1.6 and 2.2 μm. Within the confines of the sarcomere, alternating light and dark bands are seen, giving the myocardial fibers their striated appearance under the light microscope. At the center of the sarcomere is a broad dark band of constant width (1.5 μm), the A band, which is flanked by two lighter bands, the I bands, which are of variable width. The sarcomere of heart muscle, like that of skeletal muscle, is made up of two sets of myofilaments. Thicker filaments, composed principally of the protein myosin, traverse and are limited to the A band. They are about 100 Å in diameter, with tapered ends, and measure 1.5 to 1.6 μm in length. Thinner filaments, composed primarily of actin, course from the Z line through the I band into the A band. They are approximately 50 Å in diameter and 1.0 μm in length. Thus, there is overlapping of thick and thin filaments only within the A band, while the I band contains only thin filaments (Fig. 181-1). On electron-microscopic examination, bridges may be seen to extend between the thick and thin filaments within the A band.

The contractile process   The "sliding" model for muscle rests on the fundamental observation that both the thick and thin filaments are constant in overall length, both at rest and during contraction. With activation of the sarcomere, repetitive interactions take place at the bridges between the actin and myosin filaments, and the actin filaments are propelled further into the A band. In the process, the A band remains constant in width, whereas the I band becomes more narrow and the Z lines move toward one another.

The myosin molecule is a complex, asymmetric fibrous protein with a molecular weight of about 500,000; it has a rod-like portion that is about 1500 Å in length with a globular portion at its end. This globular portion of the myosin contains adenosine triphosphatase (ATPase) activity and also forms the bridges between the myosin and actin. In forming the thick myofilament, the rod-like portions of the myosin molecules are laid down in an orderly, polarized manner,

leaving the globular portions projecting outward so that they can interact with actin to generate force and shortening (Fig. 181-2A). Actin has a molecular weight of 47,000. The thin filament is composed of a double helix of two chains of actin molecules wound about each other, intimately associated with two regulatory proteins, tropomyosin and troponin (Fig. 181-2B); the latter can be separated into three components, troponins C, I, and T (Fig. 181-2C). In contrast to myosin, actin has no intrinsic enzymatic activity, but it has the ability to combine reversibly with myosin in the presence of ATP and Mg^{2+}, which activates the myosin ATPase. In relaxed muscle this interaction is inhibited by tropomyosin. During activation Ca^{2+} becomes attached to troponin C which results in a conformational change exposing the actin cross-bridge interaction sites. Physical changes in the cross-bridges result in sliding of the actin along the myosin filaments, ultimately causing muscle shortening or the development of tension. The splitting of ATP then dissociates the myosin cross-bridge from the actin. Linkages between actin and myosin filaments are made and broken cyclically as long as sufficient Ca^{2+} is present; these linkages are broken when Ca^{2+} concentration falls below a critical lead, and the troponin-tropomysin complex once more prevents interactions between the myosin cross-bridges and the actin filaments. Ionic calcium is a principal mediator of the inotropic state of the heart; most positive inotropic drugs, including the digitalis glycosides and catecholamines, act by increasing delivery of Ca^{2+} to the myofilament.

The *sarcoplasmic reticulum,* (Fig. 181-1B), a complex network of anastomosing, membrane-lined intracellular channels, which invests the myofibrils and which is less profuse in cardiac than in skeletal muscle, consists of a series of interconnecting longitudinally disposed membrane tubules closely applied to the surfaces of the individual sarcomeres; it has no direct continuity with the outside of the cell. Closely related, both functionally and structurally, are the transverse tubules or T system, formed by tubelike invaginations of the sarcolemma, which extend into the myocardial fiber, along the Z lines, i.e., the ends of the sarcomeres.

Cardiac activation   At rest, the cardiac cell is polarized; i.e., the interior has a negative charge relative to the outside of the cell, with a transmembrane potential of -80 to -100 mV (Chap. 183). The sarcolemma, which in the resting state is largely impermeable to Na^+ and has a Na^+- and K^+-stimulated pump requiring adenosine triphosphate (ATP) which extrudes Na^+ from the cell, plays a critical role in establishing this resting potential. Thus, the inside of the cell has relatively large quantities of K^+ with far less Na^+, while the extracellular milieu is high in $[Na^+]$ and low in $[K^+]$. At the same time, in the resting state, the extracellular $[Ca^{2+}]$ greatly exceeds the free intracellular $[Ca^{2+}]$.

During the plateau of the action potential (phase 2) there is a slow inward current which reflects primarily a movement of Ca^{2+} into the cell (Fig. 181-3), although the absolute quantity of Ca^{2+} that crosses the surface membrane is relatively small and in and of itself appears to be incapable of bringing about full activation of the contractile apparatus. However, the depolarizing current not only extends across the surface of the cell but penetrates deeply into the cell by way of the ramifying T system. As a consequence of the transsarcolemmal movement of Ca^{2+}, much larger quantities of Ca^{2+} are released from the sarcoplasmic reticulum, a process termed "regenerative release" of Ca^{2+}.

The Ca^{2+} then diffuses toward the sarcomere, and as already described, combines with troponin, and, by repressing the inhibitor of contraction, activates the myofilaments to produce contraction. The sarcoplasmic reticulum then reaccumulates Ca^{2+}, thereby lowering its concentration in the myofibril to a level that inhibits the actin-myosin interaction which is responsible for contraction, and in this manner leads to relaxation. Thus, the cell membrane, transverse tubules, and the sarcoplasmic reticulum, with their ability to transmit an action potential, to release and then reaccumulate Ca^{2+}, appear to play a fundamental role in the rhythmic contraction and relaxation of heart muscle.

The ATP formed from substrate oxidation is the principal source

FIGURE 181-1 *Microscopic structure of heart muscle. A. Myocardium as seen under the light microscope. Branching of fibers is evident. Each fiber, or cell, contains a centrally located nucleus. B. Myocardial cell, reconstructed from electron micrographs. Each cell is composed of multiple parallel fibrils. Each fibril is composed of serially connected sarcomeres (N, nucleus). C. Sarcomere from a myofibril, with diagrammatic representation of myofilaments. Thick filaments (1.5 μm long, composed of myosin) form the A band, and thin filaments (1 μm long, composed primarily of actin) extend from the* Z line through the I band into the A band. The overlapping of thick and thin filaments is seen only in the A band. D. Cross sections of the sarcomere indicate the specific lattice arrangements of the myofilaments. In the center of the sarcomere only the thick, or myosin, filaments arranged in a hexagonal array are seen. In the distal portions of the A band, both thick and thin, or actin, filaments are found, with each thick filament surrounded by six thin filaments. In the I band only thin filaments are present. (From Braunwald et al, 1976.)

of energy for almost all of the mechanical work of contraction performed by the myocardial cell. The high-energy phosphate stores in ATP are in equilibrium with those in the form of creatine phosphate. The activity of the myosin ATPase determines the rate of forming and breaking the actin-myosin cross-bridges and ultimately the velocity of muscle contraction.

The role of muscle length In all forms of striated muscle, including cardiac muscle, the force of contraction depends on initial muscle length. The sarcomere length associated with the most forceful contraction is 2.2 μm. It is at this length that the two sets of myofilaments of the sarcomere are most ideally situated to provide

the greatest area for their interaction. In support of the sliding-filament hypothesis, force development diminishes in direct proportion to the decrease in the overlap between thick and thin filaments, and the resultant reduction in the number of reactive sites. The length of the sarcomere also appears to regulate the extent of activation of the contractile system, i.e., its sensitivity to Ca^{2+}, which is greatest at 2.2 μm. When sarcomere length is increased to 3.65 μm, developed tension falls to zero, and it is at this point that the thin filaments are entirely withdrawn from the A band. Similarly, when the sarcomeres are shorter than 2.0 μm, the thin filaments bypass one another, producing a double overlap of the thin filaments, a reduction of sensitivity of the contractile sites to Ca^{2+}, and force also falls.

FIGURE 181-2 *Contractile protein interactions and the role of calcium as activator messenger are shown schematically: (A) Contractile proteins (myosin and actin) and regulatory proteins (troponin complex and tropomyosin) are shown in relative positions on myofilaments. (B) Contraction takes place when the heads of myosin molecules, which form cross-bridges of thick filament, bind to actin, followed by shift in orientation of cross-bridge that pulls thin filament toward center of sarcomere. Activation requires calcium binding to troponin complex, reversing inhibition of interaction between myosin and actin. In the cycle of chemical reactions underlying contraction, hydrolysis of ATP produces the cross-bridge motion. Relaxation occurs when calcium becomes dissociated from troponin. (C) Molecular rearrangements at the level of the thin filament involve regulatory proteins (tropomyosin and troponins C, I, T) in an allosteric effect. Calcium binding to troponin C loosens bond linking troponin I to actin; resulting dissociation of troponin T from actin backbone of thin filament displaces tropomyosin, exposing active sites for interaction with myosin. (Reproduced by permission, from AM Katz, VE Smith, Hosp Prac, 19(1):69, 1984. Illustration by Bunji Tagawa.)*

The relation between the initial length of the muscle fibers and the developed force is of prime importance for the function of heart muscle. This forms the basis of the Frank-Starling relation (Starling's law of the heart), which states that, within limits, an augmentation of initial volume of the ventricle, which is a function of the initial length of the muscle, results in an increase in the force of ventricular contraction. It has been shown for heart muscle that sarcomere length is directly proportional to muscle length along the ascending limb of the length–active tension curve. As muscle length decreases to the point at which developed tension approaches zero and at which sarcomere length approaches 1.5 μm, the I bands at first narrow, then disappear while the A band remains constant in length. At this latter point, the Z lines abut on the edges of the A bands. Thus, the sarcomere length–active tension curve forms the ultrastructural basis of Starling's law of the heart.

MYOCARDIAL MECHANICS

The mechanical activity of all muscle may be expressed externally in two ways: shortening and the development of tension. Hill showed in skeletal muscle that the velocity of shortening is inversely related to the magnitude of tension development, an expression of the so-called force-velocity relation, now acknowledged to be a fundamental property of muscle. Expressed simply, the greater the load the muscle

is called upon to lift, the lower the velocity of shortening and vice versa. The force-velocity relation also applies to cardiac muscle. However, in this respect there is a basic difference between skeletal and cardiac muscle. Skeletal muscle has a single, essentially fixed, force-velocity curve; i.e., at any given muscle length, force and velocity are always related to each other in the same manner. The contractile activity of skeletal muscle is increased by the recruitment of additional muscle fibers, i.e., motor units, and by increasing the frequency of nerve impulses, while the contractile properties of each individual fiber remain constant. Although resting length also influences the characteristics of contraction, this variable remains essentially fixed in vivo because of the skeletal muscles' attachment to bone. In contrast, the number of cardiac cells and within them the myofibrils and sarcomeres which become activated during each contraction is constant. However, the contractile activity of the myocardium may be readily altered under physiologic conditions by changes in resting fiber length and by changes in the inotropic state, i.e., the contractility, both of which shift the myocardial force-velocity curve.

Variations in myocardial contractile activity may be expressed as displacements of the force-velocity curve in two fundamental ways. Figure 181-4A shows a family of force-velocity curves obtained from an isolated cardiac muscle; each curve was obtained at a different preload, i.e., with a different degree of stretch on the muscle. Note that changing the preload alters the intercept of the force-velocity curve on the horizontal axis; i.e., it increases the isometric force developed by the muscle. However, within limits, these alterations in preload do not appear to alter the velocity of shortening, since all the curves extrapolate to the same intercept on the vertical axis. Thus, a change in initial length of heart muscle shifts the force-velocity curve primarily by altering the total force which can be developed by the muscle, as illustrated by the isometric length-tension curve, shown in the insert of Fig. 181-4A.

This type of shift in the force-velocity curve may be contrasted with that obtained when a positive inotropic agent, such as Ca²⁺, digitalis, or norepinephrine (which act ultimately, by increasing either the concentration of Ca²⁺ in the vicinity of the myofilaments and/or their sensitivity to Ca²⁺) is added to the muscle while the initial length is held constant (Fig. 181-4B). These agents not only increase the force which the muscle is capable of developing, i.e., the intercept of the force-velocity curve on the horizontal axis, therefore shifting the isometric length-tension curve upward, but they also increase the velocity of shortening of the unloaded muscle, i.e., the extrapolated intercept on the vertical axis.

It has been postulated that an increase in initial muscle length up to an optimal length brings about an increase in the number of effective force-generating sites as a consequence of a more advantageous overlap of interdigitating contractile filaments within the sarcomere and in the extent of activation of the contractile sites, i.e., their sensitivity to Ca²⁺. A change in the inotropic state, characterized

by an increase in the velocity of shortening of the unloaded muscle, can also result from an increase in the rate of cyclic force-generating processes at the contractile sites, without a change in the number of these sites, i.e., at a constant muscle length. Increased contractility appears to be related primarily to an increased availability of Ca²⁺ within the cell.

CONTRACTION OF THE INTACT VENTRICLE

Analysis of the heart as a pump has classically centered upon the relation between the filling pressure, or diastolic volume, of the ventricle (length of the muscle fibers) and its stroke volume (the Frank-Starling relation). In the heart-lung preparation the stroke volume is a function of diastolic fiber length, and the failing heart delivers a smaller-than-normal stroke volume from a normal or elevated end-diastolic volume. The relation between the mean atrial or the ventricular end-diastolic pressure and the stroke work of the corresponding ventricle (the ventricular function curve) provides a useful definition of the level of the contractile, or inotropic, state of the ventricle. Significant increases in the level of ventricular contractility are accompanied by shifts of the ventricular function curve upward and to the left, while depression of contractility is identified by downward and rightward displacement of this relation.

It has been observed that during the adrenergic stimulation of the

FIGURE 181-3 *Calcium fluxes that activate contraction are downhill, and those that cause relaxation are uphill. As depicted in heart muscle at rest, calcium channels in the sarcolemmal membrane are closed, and intracellular calcium is stored in the sarcoplasmic reticulum. With excitation and membrane depolarization, voltage-sensitive sodium channels (not shown) and calcium channels in the sarcolemma open to allow rapid entry of extracellular sodium and calcium. Entry of calcium is now believed to cause release of calcium from the sarcoplasmic reticulum that initiates contraction. Reuptake of calcium by the sarcoplasmic reticulum by an ATP-dependent calcium pump is essential for the heart to relax. Importantly, contraction is activated mainly by passive calcium fluxes from the sarcoplasmic reticulum. By contrast, during diastole* calcium must be pumped actively out of the cytosol to accomplish relaxation. *Energy also must be expended during diastole to restore sodium and calcium gradients across the sarcolemma, which provide for the depolarizing ionic currents that generate the action potential. Sodium transport is accomplished by the sarcolemmal sodium pump (Na⁺-K⁺-ATPase), which utilizes ATP to pump sodium out of the cell in exchange for potassium. The resultant sodium gradient is largely responsible for active transport of calcium out of the cell during relaxation, via sodium-calcium exchange. (Reproduced by permission from AM Katz, VE Smith, Hosp Prac, 19(1):69, 1984. Illustration by Bunji Tagawa.)*

FIGURE 181-4 *A. Effects of increasing initial muscle length on the force-velocity relation of cat papillary muscle. Initial velocity of shortening has been plotted as a function of load for five different muscle lengths. The maximum velocity of shortening is essentially unchanged, whereas the maximum force of contraction is augmented. The insert shows the places* *along the length-tension curves at which these force-velocity curves were determined. B. Effects of norepinephrine on the force-velocity relation of the cat papillary muscle. Both the maximum velocity of shortening and the force of contraction are increased. (From Braunwald et al, 1976.)*

myocardium accompanying a stress such as exercise, relatively little change in ventricular end-diastolic size occurs, while cardiac output, aortic flow velocity, stroke work, and the rate of ventricular pressure development are all greatly augmented. Thus, neural and humorally mediated changes in myocardial contractility, heart rate, venous return, and peripheral vascular resistance may be of greater importance in circulatory adaptation than changes in ventricular end-diastolic volume and the operation of the Frank-Starling mechanism.

The important influence of the neurotransmitter substance norepinephrine on the mechanical properties of the myocardium has long been recognized. Direct stimulation of the cardiac sympathetic nerves augments ventricular function as a consequence of the release of norepinephrine from sympathetic nerve endings in the heart. These adrenergic effects are evidenced by tachycardia, a reduction in cardiac dimensions, increased velocity of ejection, and an enhanced rate of tension development.

CONTROL OF CARDIAC PERFORMANCE AND OUTPUT

The extent of shortening of mammalian heart muscle and, therefore, the stroke volume of the intact ventricle are, in the final analysis, determined by three influences: (1) the length of the muscle at the onset of contraction, i.e., the preload; (2) the inotropic state of the muscle, i.e., the position of its force-velocity-length relation; and (3) the tension which the muscle is called upon to develop during contraction, i.e., the afterload. Heart rate determines the cardiac output at any stroke volume as long as ventricular filling is maintained.

VENTRICULAR END-DIASTOLIC VOLUME (PRELOAD) At any level of its inotropic state, the performance of the myocardium is influenced profoundly by ventricular end-diastolic fiber length and therefore by diastolic ventricular volume. The following are the major determinants of ventricular preload in the intact organism:

Total blood volume When depleted, as in hemorrhage or prolonged vomiting, venous return to the heart declines (Chap. 29) and ventricular end-diastolic volume falls, as does ventricular performance, as reflected in ventricular work.

Distribution of blood volume At any given total blood volume, the ventricular end-diastolic volume is influenced by the distribution of blood between the intra- and extrathoracic compartments. This distribution in turn is influenced by the following:

1 *Body position.* Gravitational forces tend to pool blood in dependent portions. The upright posture augments extrathoracic at the expense of intrathoracic blood volume, and reduces ventricular work.
2 *Intrathoracic pressure.* Normally, mean intrathoracic pressure is negative, a factor which acts to increase thoracic blood volume and ventricular end-diastolic volume and to enhance the return of blood to the heart, particularly during inspiration. Elevation of intrathoracic pressure, as occurs in a tension pneumothorax, during the Valsalva maneuver, in prolonged bouts of coughing, or with positive-pressure ventilation, tends to impede venous return to the heart, diminish intrathoracic blood volume, and ultimately reduce stroke volume and ventricular work.
3 *Intrapericardial pressure.* When elevated, as in pericardial tamponade (Chap. 194), there is interference with cardiac filling, and the resultant reduction in ventricular diastolic volume lowers stroke volume and ventricular work.
4 *Venous tone.* The venous system is not a simple system of passive conduits between the systemic capillary bed and the right atrium. Instead, the smooth muscle in the walls of the venules and veins responds to a variety of neural and humoral stimuli. Venoconstriction occurs during muscular exercise, deep respiration, fright, or marked hypotension, tending to diminish extrathoracic and to augment intrathoracic blood volume, venous return to the heart, and ventricular performance.
5 *The pumping action of skeletal muscle.* During exercise the contracting skeletal muscles squeeze blood out of the venous bed

and, with the aid of the venous valves, displace it centrally, thereby increasing intrathoracic blood volume, ventricular end-diastolic volume, and ventricular work.

Atrial contraction Vigorous, appropriately timed atrial contraction augments ventricular filling and end-diastolic volume. The atrial contribution to ventricular filling is of particular importance in patients with ventricular hypertrophy, in whom the loss of atrial systole (as in atrial fibrillation) tends to reduce ventricular end-diastolic pressure and volume, ultimately lowering myocardial performance.

INOTROPIC STATE (MYOCARDIAL CONTRACTILITY)

A number of factors determine the level of ventricular performance at any given ventricular end-diastolic volume, i.e., the position of the ventricular function curve. These influences may be considered to operate by modifying myocardial force-velocity-length relations.

Sympathetic nerve activity The quantity of norepinephrine released by sympathetic nerve endings in the heart is, under ordinary circumstances, dependent on the sympathetic nerve impulse traffic, and alterations in the frequency of nerve impulses modify the quantity of norepinephrine released and acting upon the beta-adrenergic receptors in the myocardium. This mechanism is the most important one which acutely modifies the position of the force-velocity and ventricular function curves under physiologic conditions.

Circulating catecholamines The adrenal medulla and other sympathetic ganglia outside the heart, when stimulated by sympathetic nerve impulses, release catecholamines, which, when they reach the heart, augment the inotropic state.

The force-frequency relation The position of the myocardial force-velocity curve is influenced by the rate and rhythm of cardiac contraction; e.g., ventricular extrasystoles result in post-extrasystolic potentiation, presumably by increasing the Ca^{2+} which enters the cardiac cell.

Exogenously administered inotropic agents The cardiac glycosides, isoproterenol and other sympathomimetic agents, calcium, caffeine, theophylline, and their derivatives, all improve the myocardial force-velocity relation and therefore may be used therapeutically to augment ventricular performance at any given ventricular end-diastolic volume.

Physiologic depressants Included among these are severe myocardial hypoxia, hypercapnea, ischemia, and acidosis. Acting either singly or in combination, these influences exert a depressant effect on the myocardial force-velocity curve and lower the level of the left ventricular work at any given ventricular end-diastolic volume.

Pharmacologic depressants These include quinidine, procainamide, barbiturates, and other local and general anesthetics, as well as many other drugs.

Loss of ventricular substance When a portion of ventricular myocardium becomes nonfunctional or necrotic, as occurs temporarily during ischemia (Chap. 189), and permanently in myocardial infarction (Chap. 190), total ventricular performance at any given level of end-diastolic volume is depressed, even if the remaining myocardium functions normally.

Intrinsic myocardial depression Although the fundamental mechanisms responsible for depression of myocardial contractility in chronic congestive heart failure still remain to be elucidated, it is now apparent that in this condition the inotropic state of each unit of myocardium is depressed and that the level of ventricular performance at any ventricular end-diastolic volume is thereby lowered.

VENTRICULAR AFTERLOAD

The stroke volume is ultimately a function of the extent of ventricular fiber shortening. As in isolated cardiac muscle, the velocity and extent of shortening of ventricular muscle fibers at any given level of diastolic fiber length and myocardial inotropic state are inversely related to the afterload imposed on the muscle. The afterload on the intact heart is dependent on the level of aortic pressure, but it may be defined as the tension or stress developed in the wall of the ventricle during ejection. Therefore, the afterload on the ventricular muscle fibers also is dependent on the size of the heart, according to Laplace's law, which indicates that the tension of the myocardial fiber is a function of the product of the intracavitary ventricular pressure and ventricular radius divided by the wall thickness. Thus, at the same level of aortic pressure, the afterload faced by a dilated left ventricle is higher than that encountered by a ventricle of normal size. Furthermore, at any level of aortic pressure and left ventricular volume the afterload placed on any wall fiber varies inversely with wall thickness. The aortic pressure, in turn, is influenced largely by the peripheral vascular resistance, the physical characteristics of the arterial tree, and the volume of blood it contains at the onset of ejection. At any given ventricular end-diastolic volume and level of the inotropic state, the left ventricular stroke volume is a function of the afterload.

The critical role played by the ventricular afterload in cardiovascular regulation is summarized in Fig. 181-5. As already noted, increases in both preload and contractility increase myocardial fiber shortening, while increases in afterload reduce it. The extent of myocardial fiber shortening and left ventricular size are the determinants of stroke volume. Arterial pressure, in turn, is related to the product of cardiac output and systemic vascular resistance, while afterload is a function of left ventricular size and arterial pressure. An increase in arterial pressure induced by vasoconstriction, for example, augments afterload, which through a negative feedback depresses myocardial fiber shortening, stroke volume, and cardiac output; this in turn tends to restore arterial pressure to its previous level.

When left ventricular function becomes impaired, and the chamber dilates, i.e., when there is no preload reserve, left ventricular afterload

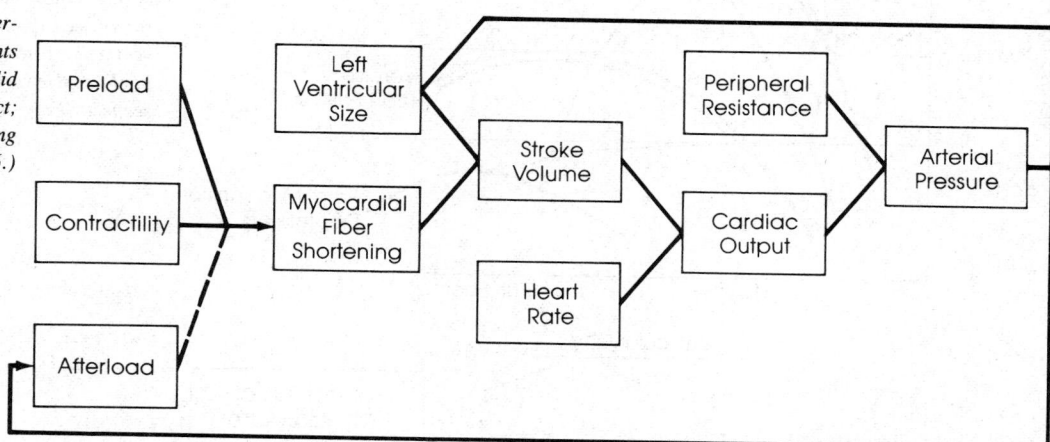

FIGURE 181-5 *Scheme of interactions among various components that regulate cardiac activity. Solid lines indicate an augmenting effect; broken line represents an inhibiting effect. (From Braunwald et al, 1976.)*

becomes increasingly important in determining cardiac performance. Increases in afterload may result from the influence on the arterial bed of neural, humoral, or structural changes which can occur in response to a fall in cardiac output. This increased afterload may further reduce cardiac output while myocardial oxygen requirements are increased. Treatment with vasodilators (Chap. 182) has the opposite effect. In this way, alterations in the peripheral vascular bed probably play an important role in the hemodynamic and metabolic events which usually are attributed to progressive impairment of the myocardium.

All of the influences acting on cardiac performance enumerated above interact in a complex fashion to maintain cardiac output at a level appropriate to the requirements of the metabolizing tissues, and in a normal person interference with one of these mechanisms may not influence the cardiac output. For example, a moderate reduction of blood volume or the loss of the atrial contribution to ventricular contraction can ordinarily be sustained without a reduction in the resting cardiac output. Presumably other factors, such as an increase in the frequency of sympathetic nerve impulses to the heart and an increase in heart rate, will, in the normal person, augment contractility and sustain cardiac output. Mechanisms are also available which prevent elevation of the cardiac output when there is no physiologic demand for augmented flow. For example, augmentation of myocardial contractility by means of cardiac glycosides does not increase the cardiac output in normal humans. Thus, in analyzing the effect of an intervention on cardiac output, it is important to recognize that it is the preload, which in turn is related to the volume of blood available for filling the heart, rather than the inotropic state of the myocardium or the afterload which limits cardiac output in the normal individual and that an improvement of myocardial contractility by a drug such as digitalis or the reduction of afterload with nitroprusside would not be expected to elevate the output in a normal subject. On the other hand, in the presence of congestive heart failure, the cardiac output usually is limited by the depressed contractile state of the myocardium, and a positive inotropic drug or reduction of afterload would be expected to raise cardiac output, and, indeed, does so.

EXERCISE   The hemodynamic changes which normally occur during exercise in the upright position are complex (Fig. 181-6). The hyperventilation, the pumping action of the exercising muscles, and the venoconstriction which occur all tend to augment venous return

and hence ventricular filling and preload. Simultaneously, the increase in the sympathetic nerve impulses to the myocardium, the increased concentration of circulating catecholamines, and the tachycardia which occur during exercise all combine to augment the contractile state of the myocardium (Fig. 181-6, curves 1 and 2) and lead to an elevation of stroke volume, with no change or even a decrease of end-diastolic pressure and volume (Fig. 181-6, points A and B). Vasodilatation occurs in the exercising muscles, thus tending to offset the marked increase in arterial pressure which would otherwise occur as cardiac output rises. This ultimately allows the achievement of a greatly elevated cardiac output during exercise, at an arterial pressure usually only slightly higher than in the resting state.

THE FAILING HEART

Though heart failure may be readily described as a clinical syndrome, characterized by well-known symptoms and physical signs, a precise physiologic or biochemical definition is far more difficult. However, from the clinical point of view, heart failure may be considered to be the condition in which *an abnormality of cardiac function is responsible for the inability of the heart to pump blood at a rate commensurate with the requirements of the metabolizing tissues or can do so only from an abnormally elevated filling pressure.* Abnormalities during systole and/or diastole may be present in heart failure (Fig. 181-7). In so-called *systolic heart failure,* i.e., classical heart failure, an impaired inotropic state leads to weakened systolic contraction, which leads, ultimately, to a reduction in stroke volume and cardiac dilatation. Idiopathic dilated cardiomyopathy is the prototype of systolic heart failure. In *diastolic heart failure* the principal abnormality involves impaired relaxation of the ventricle and leads to an elevation of ventricular diastolic pressure at a normal diastolic volume. Failure of relaxation can be functional, i.e., as during transient ischemia, or it can be caused by a stiffened, thickened ventricle. Typical conditions in which diastolic failure occurs are restrictive cardiomyopathy secondary to infiltrative conditions, such as amyloidosis or hemochromatosis (Chap. 192). In many patients with cardiac hypertrophy and dilatation, systolic and diastolic failure coexist; the ventricle both empties and fills abnormally. There may be cardiac dilatation, but the ventricle's pressure-volume relation is shifted, raising the ventricular diastolic pressure at any given volume.

FIGURE 181-6 *Diagram showing the interrelations among influences on ventricular end-diastolic volume (EDV) through stretching of the myocardium and the contractile state of the myocardium. Levels of ventricular EDV associated with filling pressures that result in dyspnea and pulmonary edema are shown on the abscissa. Levels of ventricular performance required when the subject is at rest, while walking, and during maximal activity are designated on the ordinate. The dotted lines are the descending limbs of the ventricular-performance curves, which are rarely seen during life but which show the level of ventricular performance if end-diastolic volume could be elevated to very high levels. For further explanation see text. (From Braunwald et al, 1976.)*

FIGURE 181-7 *Relationship between left ventricular end-diastolic volume and (1) end-diastolic pressure (top), describing the* compliance *of the left ventricle, i.e., its* diastolic properties; *and (2) left ventricular stroke work (bottom), describing the ventricle's systolic function curve. The normal left ventricle (left) reaches an end-diastolic pressure of 30 mmHg (pulmonary edema level) when its end-diastolic volume is elevated to 200 mL. The concentrically hypertrophied left ventricle (center), exhibits normal systolic function since the relation between left ventricular end-diastolic volume and stroke work is unchanged, but there is "diastolic failure" in that end-diastolic pressure reaches pulmonary edema level (i.e., 30 mmHg) at a lower level than normal (i.e., 130 mL). The dilated ventricle (right) exhibits "systolic failure" in that the maximal stroke work and the stroke volume at any level of end-diastolic volume are depressed. The left ventricle displays increased diastolic compliance, i.e., distensibility, with a higher than normal end-diastolic volume (280 mL) required to reach the pulmonary edema level. (Reprinted with permission from Gorlin R, Prim Cardiol 6:84, 1980.)*

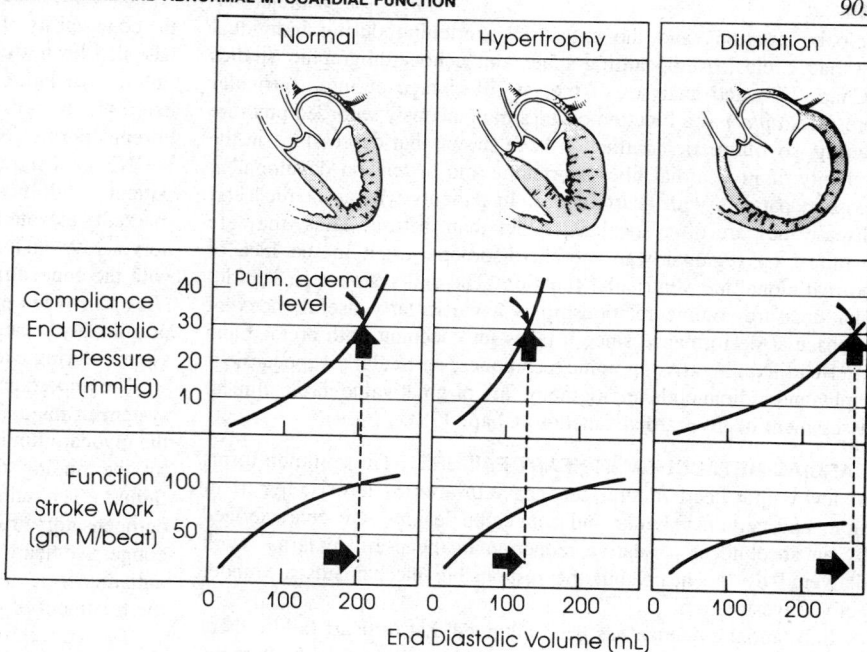

Though a defect in myocardial contraction is characteristic of systolic heart failure, this defect may result from a primary abnormality in the heart muscle, as in cardiomyopathy, or it may be secondary to a chronic excessive work load as in hypertension and valvular heart disease, as well as in many forms of congenital heart disease. In ischemic heart disease systolic heart failure results from a loss in the quantity of normally contracting cells. It is important to distinguish heart failure from (1) states of circulatory insufficiency in which myocardial function is not primarily impaired, such as cardiac tamponade or hemorrhagic shock, (2) conditions in which there is circulatory congestion because of abnormal salt and water retention but in which there is no serious disturbance of the heart's function, and (3) conditions in which a normally contracting myocardium is suddenly presented with a load which exceeds its capacity, e.g., accelerated hypertension or rupture of a valve cusp secondary to infective endocarditis.

The intrinsic contractile state of myocardium removed from normal, hypertrophied, and failing animal hearts has been evaluated, and both ventricular hypertrophy and heart failure were shown to reduce the maximum isometric tension and velocity of shortening to subnormal levels; the changes are more marked in the myocardium of animals in which heart failure had been present than in those with hypertrophy alone. However, ventricular hypertrophy, in the absence of heart failure, also appears to be associated with a depression of the inotropic state per unit of myocardium, although the absolute increase of total muscle mass maintains overall cardiac compensation. Papillary muscles removed from the left ventricles of patients with heart failure have also shown a depression of the maximum degree of active tension which they can develop. Electron-microscopic analysis of failing cat papillary muscles fixed at the apexes of the length–active tension curves revealed sarcomere lengths averaging 2.2 μm. Thus, the abnormalities of contractility do *not* appear to be produced by an alteration in the overlap of filaments within the sarcomere.

The failing ventricle may still eject a normal or nearly normal stroke volume despite considerable depression of function, when its end-diastolic volume increases, i.e., through the operation of the Frank-Starling mechanism. As outlined above, an increase in the initial volume of the ventricle is associated with stretching of the sarcomere, a process which augments the number of sites at which the actin and myosin filaments can interact and/or which increases their sensitivity to Ca^{2+}. Furthermore, the development of ventricular hypertrophy may be considered to provide additional contractile units,

and thereby constitutes an important compensatory mechanism when the myocardium's intrinsic inotropic state is depressed.

ASSESSMENT OF CARDIAC PERFORMANCE Several techniques are available for defining impaired cardiac performance in intact humans. With the patient at rest, the cardiac output and stroke volume may be depressed, but not uncommonly these variables are within normal limits. A more sensitive index is the ejection fraction, i.e., the ratio of stroke volume to end-diastolic volume, which may be estimated by standard radiologic or radionuclide angiography (Chaps. 179 and 180), and which is frequently depressed in heart failure even when the stroke volume itself is normal. A limitation of the ejection fraction (and of cardiac output) in the assessment of cardiac function is that these variables are influenced by ventricular loading conditions. Thus, a depressed ejection fraction and lowered cardiac output may be observed in patients with normal ventricular function but reduced preload, as occurs in hypervolemia, or with acutely elevated arterial pressure. An even more sensitive method for detecting impaired ventricular performance is based on the measurement of the circulatory changes occurring during stresses such as exercise or increased afterload. Thus, left ventricular performance may be estimated accurately by measuring the left ventricular end-diastolic pressure, cardiac output, and total body O_2 consumption at rest and during exercise. In normal persons, the cardiac output rises by more than 500 mL/min for each 100-mL increase in minute O_2 consumption. The left ventricular end-diastolic pressure at rest is less than 12 mmHg and rises slightly, remains unchanged, or decreases slightly during exercise, while stroke volume usually rises. The failing left ventricle, on the other hand, is characterized by an elevation of end-diastolic pressure during exercise, which reaches a value exceeding 12 mmHg, accompanied by either no change or a fall in stroke volume and a subnormal increase in cardiac output related to the increase in minute O_2 consumption. Various degrees of impairment intermediate between the normal response and that of the failing left ventricle during the stress of exercise also have been described.

The potential value of stressing the left ventricle is emphasized by the fact that the basal values for left ventricular end-diastolic pressure, cardiac index, and ventricular stroke work may be in the same range in patients with depressed ventricular function as in normal persons. The response to stress may prove useful not only in the detection of the impairment of myocardial function, but also in expressing the severity of this impairment quantitatively.

The performance of the left ventricle in humans may also be characterized by examining the instantaneous myocardial force-velocity relations and the extent of shortening during individual cardiac cycles. Angiocardiographic and echocardiographic studies (Chap. 179) and analyses of the rate of change of intraventricular pressure (*dp/dt*) as a function of the simultaneously recorded pressure during isovolumetric contraction have shown that depressions in the velocity of myocardial fiber shortening and of tension development exist in patients with heart failure. In patients with ischemic heart disease they are often localized rather than diffuse. Thus, they are manifest by regional wall motion disorders, often in the face of normal global left ventricular function. The end-systolic left ventricular pressure-volume relationship is a particularly useful index of ventricular performance since it takes into account both preload and afterload. Noninvasive, graphic techniques, particularly echocardiography and radionuclide angiography, are of great value in the clinical assessment of myocardial function (Chap. 179).

CARDIAC METABOLISM IN HEART FAILURE   The common forms of low-output heart failure, secondary to arteriosclerosis, hypertension, and certain valvular and congenital lesions, are characterized by an absolute or a relative reduction in the useful external work delivered by the heart, but the responsible mechanisms are under active investigation.

Substantial evidence has been obtained that in heart failure there is an *abnormality of excitation-contraction coupling,* which alters the delivery of Ca^{2+} to the contractile sites, thereby impairing cardiac performance. The molecular basis of this abnormality, indeed its site, i.e., the sarcolemma, T tubules, and/or sarcoplasmic reticulum, has yet to be defined.

Considerable attention has also been directed to the question of whether cardiac failure is due to a defect in the production of energy, its conservation, or its utilization. Only in isolated instances of heart failure, such as those associated with beriberi, are there clear-cut disturbances of myocardial energy production. The major pathway by which pyruvate enters the citric acid cycle and some reactions within the cycle itself are dependent on the presence of adequate concentrations of thiamine (Chap. 76). Thiamine deficiency results in diminished pyruvic acid utilization by heart slices, and in abnormally low pyruvate extraction coefficients in intact dogs and in humans.

In the second phase of cardiac metabolism, energy conservation, the energy of substrate oxidation is converted into the terminal-bond energy of creatine phosphate (CP) and of ATP, the immediate source of chemical energy utilized by heart muscle. This process, known as oxidative phosphorylation, occurs in the mitochondria. The effectiveness of the combined energy production-conservation mechanisms may be studied by measuring the stores of ATP and CP existing in the myocardium, while energy conservation may be evaluated by determining (1) the P/O ratio, i.e., the ratio of high-energy phosphate produced to oxygen consumed in the mitochondria, and (2) the degree of coupling between electron transport and the generation of high-energy phosphate compounds. Although lively controversy exists concerning the status of this phase of metabolism in heart failure, it now appears that severe impairment of myocardial performance may occur *without* disturbances of mitochondrial function or reduction of high-energy phosphate stores, although abnormalities in these processes do occur in some forms of experimental heart failure.

In the absence of a definitive abnormality of energy liberation or conservation in the failing myocardium, attention has naturally been directed to the possibility that energy *utilization* is abnormal. An abnormality of energy liberation could certainly occur if the contractile proteins themselves were altered. A cardiac myosin isoenzyme characterized by immunologic and electrophoretic properties exhibiting a lower Ca^{2+}-dependent ATPase activity has been shown in some forms of experimentally produced heart failure, particularly those produced by mechanical overloading. It is possible that this depression may be responsible for a defect in the breakdown of ATP, the process which leads to contraction.

THE ADRENERGIC NERVOUS SYSTEM IN HEART FAILURE   In view of the importance of the adrenergic nervous system in stimulating the contractility of the normal myocardium, the activity of this system has also been studied intensively in patients with congestive heart failure. An index of the activity of this system, at rest and during exercise, is provided by measurements of the concentration of norepinephrine (NE) in arterial blood. Relatively small increases in the NE concentration occur during exercise in normal subjects. In patients with heart failure the levels of circulating NE may be markedly elevated at rest, indicating that the activity of the adrenergic nervous system is augmented at rest, and the prognosis varies inversely with the concentration. Also, much greater increments in circulating NE occur when patients with congestive heart failure exercise, again presumably because of an increased activity of the adrenergic nervous system during exercise in these patients.

The importance of the increased activity of the adrenergic nervous system in maintaining ventricular contractility when the function of the myocardium is depressed in congestive heart failure also is shown by the finding that beta-adrenergic blockade may intensify heart failure. The adrenergic nervous system thus plays an important compensatory role in the circulatory adjustments of patients to congestive heart failure, and caution must be exercised in the use of antiadrenergic drugs, particularly beta-adrenergic blocking agents, in the treatment of patients with limited cardiac reserve (Chap. 182).

The concentration and content of the NE in cardiac tissue of patients with heart failure are reduced, sometimes to only 10 percent of normal. The mechanism responsible is not entirely clear, but a prolonged increase in cardiac sympathetic tone appears to play a critical role and to interfere in some manner with the biosynthesis of NE. Also, there is evidence that the beta-adrenergic receptor density and myocardial cyclic AMP concentration are reduced in chronic, severe heart failure.

In view of the strongly positive inotropic effect exerted by the NE released from these nerves, the adrenergic nervous system may be considered to provide an important potential source of support to the failing myocardium. However, the increments of heart rate and contractile force which occur in animals with experimental heart failure and cardiac NE depletion are abolished or markedly reduced with stimulation of the cardiac sympathetic nerves. Thus, it is likely that when congestive heart failure is accompanied by depletion of cardiac NE stores, the quantity of NE released by the sympathetic nerve endings in the heart is deficient relative to the impulse traffic along these nerves. Furthermore, whatever NE is released may not elicit a normal effect due to reduction of myocardial adrenergic receptor-effector mechanisms.

Cardiac stores of NE are not fundamentally necessary for maintaining the intrinsic contractile state of the myocardium. However, since the reduction of NE stores in heart failure is associated with a diminished release of neurotransmitter, this depletion of NE may be responsible for loss of the much-needed adrenergic support in the failing heart. In the later stages of heart failure, when the levels of circulating catecholamines are elevated and the cardiac NE stores depleted, the myocardium is largely dependent on a more generalized adrenergic stimulation derived from extracardiac sources, presumably the adrenal medulla; this would explain the deterioration of cardiac performance which may occur in patients with heart failure who are treated with beta-adrenergic blocking drugs. This generalized adrenergic stimulation resulting from circulating catecholamines may, however, also exert undesirable side effects, because it elevates vascular resistance and may present the heart with an afterload which is higher than optimal.

In the final analysis, in heart failure, the fundamental abnormality resides in depressions of the myocardial force-velocity relationship and of the length-active tension curve, reflecting reductions in the contractile state of the myocardium (Fig. 181-6, curves 1 to 3). In many instances, cardiac output and external ventricular performance at rest are within normal limits but are maintained at these levels only by an increased end-diastolic fiber length and an elevated ventricular end-diastolic volume, i.e., through the operation of the Frank-Starling mechanism (Fig. 181-6, points A to D). The elevation of left ventricular preload is associated with similar changes in the pulmonary capillary pressure, contributing to the dyspnea experienced by patients with heart failure. The normal improvement of contractility due to augmented sympathetic activity during exercise is attenuated or even prevented by norepinephrine depletion which occurs in severe heart failure (Fig. 181-6, curves 3 and 3'). The factors which tend to augment ventricular filling during exercise in the normal subject push the failing myocardium even farther along its flattened length-active tension curve, and although the left ventricle may perform somewhat better, this occurs only as a consequence of an inordinate elevation of ventricular end-diastolic volume and pressure and, therefore, of the pulmonary capillary pressure. The elevation of the latter intensifies dyspnea and therefore plays an important role in limiting the intensity of exercise which the patient can perform. Left ventricular failure becomes fatal when the myocardial length-active tension curve is depressed (Fig. 181-6, curve 4) to the point at which cardiac performance fails to satisfy the requirements of the peripheral tissues even at rest, and/or the left ventricular end-diastolic and pulmonary capillary pressures are elevated to levels which result in pulmonary edema (Fig. 181-6, point E).

REFERENCES

BRAUNWALD E et al (eds): *Congestive Heart Failure: Current Research and Clinical Applications.* New York, Grune & Stratton, 1982

———, et al: *Mechanisms of Contraction of the Normal and Failing Heart,* 2d ed. Boston, Little, Brown, 1976

———, SONNENBLICK EH, ROSS J: Contraction of the normal heart, in *Heart Disease,* 2d ed, E Braunwald (ed). Philadelphia, Saunders, 1984, p 409

BRISTOW MR et al: Decreased catecholamine sensitivity and beta-adrenergic-receptor density in failing human hearts. N Engl J Med 307:205, 1982

COHN, JN et al: Plasma norepinephrine as a guide to prognosis in patients with chronic congestive heart failure. N Eng J Med 311:819, 1984

GROSSMAN W: Evaluation of systolic and diastolic function of the myocardium, in W Grossman (ed): *Cardiac Catheterization and Angiography,* 3d ed. Philadelphia, Lea & Febiger, 1986, p 301

KASS DA et al: Determination of left ventricular end-systolic pressure-volume relationships by the conductance (volume) catheter technique. Circulation 73:586, 1986

LOMPRE AM et al: Myosin isoenzyme redistribution in chronic heart overload. Nature 282:105, 1979

MORGAN JP et al: Intracellular calcium transients in human working myocardium as detected with aequorin. J Am Coll Cardiol 3:410, 1984

SPIRITO P et al: Noninvasive assessment of left ventricular diastolic function: Comparative analysis of Doppler echocardiographic and radionuclide angiographic techniques. J Am Col Cardiol 7:518, 1986

182 HEART FAILURE

EUGENE BRAUNWALD

Heart failure may be defined as the pathophysiologic state in which an abnormality of *cardiac* function is responsible for the failure of the heart to pump blood at a rate commensurate with the requirements of the metabolizing tissues or can do so only from an abnormally elevated filling pressure. Heart failure is frequently, but not always, caused by a defect in myocardial contraction, and then the term *myocardial failure* is appropriate. The latter may result from a primary abnormality in the heart muscle, as occurs in the cardiomyopathies (Chap. 192). Myocardial failure may also result from extramyocardial abnormalities, such as coronary atherosclerosis which leads to myocardial ischemia, as well as from abnormalities of the heart valves in which the heart muscle is damaged by the long-standing excessive hemodynamic burden imposed by the valvular abnormality, and/or by the rheumatic process (Chap. 187). In patients with chronic constrictive pericarditis, myocardial damage resulting from infiltration of the heart muscle by pericardial inflammation and calcification is common (Chap. 194).

In other patients with heart failure, however, a similar clinical syndrome is present, but without any detectable abnormality of *myocardial* function. In these patients the normal heart is suddenly presented with a load that exceeds its capacity, such as an acute hypertensive crisis, rupture of an aortic valve cusp, or massive pulmonary embolism. Heart failure, in the presence of normal myocardial function, also occurs in chronic conditions in which there is impairment of filling of the ventricles due to tricuspid and/or mitral stenosis, constrictive pericarditis without myocardial involvement, and endocardial fibrosis.

Heart failure should be distinguished from (1) conditions in which there is circulatory congestion consequent to abnormal salt and water retention but in which there is no disturbance of cardiac function per se (the latter syndrome, termed the *congested state,* may result from the abnormal salt and water retention of renal failure, or from excess parenteral administration of fluids and electrolytes), and (2) from noncardiac causes of inadequate cardiac output, including shock due to hypovolemia and redistribution of blood volume (Chap. 29).

The ventricles respond to a chronically increased hemodynamic burden with the development of hypertrophy. With volume overload when the ventricle is called upon to deliver an elevated cardiac output, as in valvular regurgitation, it develops *eccentric* hypertrophy, i.e., cavity dilatation, with an increase in muscle mass so that the ratio between wall thickness and ventricular cavity size remains constant. With pressure overload when the ventricle is called upon to develop increased pressure, as in valvular aortic stenosis, it develops *concentric* hypertrophy, in which the ratio between wall thickness and ventricular cavity size increases. In both conditions, a stable hyperfunctioning state may exist for many years but myocardial function may ultimately deteriorate, leading to heart failure.

CAUSES OF HEART FAILURE

In evaluating patients with heart failure, it is important to identify not only the *underlying cause* of the heart disease but the *precipitating cause* of heart failure as well. The cardiac abnormality produced by a congenital or acquired lesion such as valvular aortic stenosis may exist for many years and produce no or only trivial disability. Frequently, however, the manifestations of clinical heart failure appear for the first time in the course of some acute disturbance which places an additional load on a myocardium that chronically is excessively burdened and while compensated has no additional reserves, resulting in further deterioration of cardiac function. Identification of such precipitating causes is of critical importance because their prompt alleviation may be lifesaving. However, in the absence of underlying heart disease these acute disturbances do not usually, by themselves, lead to heart failure.

PRECIPITATING CAUSES

1 *Pulmonary embolism.* Patients with low cardiac output and physical inactivity are at increased risk of developing thrombi in the veins of the lower extremities or the pelvis. Pulmonary embolization may result in further elevation of pulmonary arterial pressure, which in turn may produce or intensify failure of the right ventricle. In the presence of pulmonary vascular congestion, such emboli may also cause infarction of the lung (Chap. 211).

2 *Infection.* Patients with pulmonary vascular congestion are also more susceptible to pulmonary infections, but any infection may precipitate heart failure. The resulting fever, tachycardia, hypoxemia, and the increased metabolic demands may place a further burden on the overloaded, but compensated, myocardium of a patient with chronic heart disease.

3 *Anemia.* In the presence of anemia the oxygen needs of the metabolizing tissues can be satisfied only by an increase in the cardiac output (Chap. 53); though such an increase in the cardiac output might be sustained by a normal heart, a diseased, overloaded, but otherwise compensated heart may be unable to augment sufficiently the volume of blood which it delivers to the periphery. In this manner the combination of anemia and heart disease can lead to inadequate oxygen delivery and precipitate heart failure.

4 *Thyrotoxicosis and pregnancy.* As in anemia and fever, in these

conditions adequate tissue perfusion requires an increased cardiac output. The development or intensification of heart failure may actually be one of the first clinical manifestations of hyperthyroidism in a patient with underlying heart disease (Chap. 324). Similarly, heart failure not infrequently occurs for the first time during pregnancy in women with rheumatic valvular disease in whom cardiac compensation may return following delivery.

5 *Arrhythmias.* These are among the most frequent precipitating causes of heart failure in patients with underlying but compensated heart disease for a variety of reasons: (*a*) tachyarrhythmias reduce the time period available for ventricular filling; (*b*) the dissociation between atrial and ventricular contractions characteristic of many arrhythmias result in the loss of the atrial booster pump mechanism, thereby tending to raise atrial pressures; (*c*) in any arrhythmia associated with abnormal intraventricular conduction, myocardial performance may become further impaired because of the loss of normal synchronicity of ventricular contraction; (*d*) the marked bradycardia associated with complete atrioventricular block requires a greatly elevated stroke volume if a marked reduction in cardiac output is to be prevented.

6 *Rheumatic and other forms of myocarditis.* Acute rheumatic fever and a variety of infectious or inflammatory processes affecting the myocardium may further impair myocardial function in patients with preexisting heart disease (Chaps. 186 and 192).

7 *Infective endocarditis.* The additional valvular damage, anemia, fever, and myocarditis which often occur as a consequence of infective endocarditis may, singly or in concert, precipitate heart failure (Chap. 188).

8 *Physical, dietary, environmental, and emotional excesses.* The augmentation of sodium intake, the discontinuation of medications to treat heart failure, physical overexertion, excessive environmental heat or humidity, and emotional crises may all precipitate cardiac decompensation.

9 *Systemic hypertension.* Rapid elevation of arterial pressure, as may occur in some instances of hypertension of renal origin or upon discontinuation of antihypertensive medication, may result in cardiac decompensation (Chap. 196).

10 *Myocardial infarction.* In patients with chronic but compensated ischemic heart disease, a fresh infarct, sometimes otherwise silent clinically, may further impair ventricular function and precipitate heart failure (Chap. 190).

A systematic search for these precipitating causes should be made in every patient with heart failure, particularly if it is refractory to the usual methods of therapy. If properly recognized, the precipitating cause of heart failure can usually be treated more effectively than the underlying cause. Therefore, the prognosis in patients with heart failure in whom a precipitating cause can be identified, treated, and eliminated is more favorable than in patients in whom the underlying disease process has advanced to the point of producing heart failure.

FORMS OF HEART FAILURE

Heart failure may be described as *high-output* or *low-output, acute* or *chronic, right-sided* or *left-sided, forward* or *backward,* and *systolic* or *diastolic.* These descriptors are often useful in a clinical setting, particularly early in the patient's course, but they do not signify fundamentally different disease states, and late in the course the differences between some of these forms become blurred.

HIGH-OUTPUT VERSUS LOW-OUTPUT HEART FAILURE It is useful to classify patients with heart failure into those with a low cardiac output, i.e., *low-output heart failure,* and those with an elevated cardiac output, i.e., *high-output heart failure.* The cardiac output is often depressed in patients with heart failure secondary to ischemic heart disease, hypertension, cardiomyopathy, valvular and pericardial disease, but tends to be elevated in patients with heart failure and hyperthyroidism, anemia, arteriovenous fistulas, beriberi,

and Paget's disease. In clinical practice, however, it is not always easy to distinguish between low-output and high-output heart failure. The normal range of cardiac output is wide [2.5 to 3.8 (liters/min)/ m²], and in many patients with so-called low-output heart failure the cardiac output may actually be just within the normal range at rest, although it is lower than it had been previously and fails to rise normally during exertion. On the other hand, in patients with so-called high-output heart failure the output may not be excessive, although it would have been found to be so had it been measured before heart failure supervened, but rather may be close to the upper limit of normal, particularly when heart failure is severe. Regardless of the absolute level of the cardiac output, however, cardiac failure may be said to be present when the characteristic clinical manifestations described below are accompanied by a depression of the curve relating ventricular end-diastolic volume to cardiac performance (Fig. 181-6, p. 902).

An integral part of systolic heart failure (p. 903) is evidence that the heart does not deliver the quantity of oxygen required by the metabolizing tissues. In the absence of peripheral shunting of blood, such inadequate delivery of oxygen to the metabolizing tissues is reflected in an abnormal widening of the normal arterial–mixed venous oxygen difference (3.5 to 5.0 mL/dL in the basal state), relative to the total-body oxygen consumption. In mild cases, such an abnormality may not be present at rest but becomes evident only during exertion or other hypermetabolic states. In patients with the high-output cardiac states associated with arteriovenous fistula, beriberi, thyrotoxicosis, Paget's disease, etc., the arterial–mixed venous oxygen difference is normal or low. The mixed venous oxygen saturation is raised by the admixture of blood which has been diverted from the metabolizing tissues, and it may be presumed that even in these patients the delivery of oxygen to the latter is reduced despite the normal or even elevated mixed venous oxygen saturation. When heart failure occurs in such patients, the arterial–mixed venous oxygen difference, regardless of the absolute value, still exceeds the level which existed prior to the development of heart failure, and therefore the cardiac output, though normal or elevated, is lower than before heart failure occurred.

The mechanisms responsible for the development of heart failure in patients whose cardiac outputs are initially high are complex and depend on the underlying disease process. In most of these conditions the heart is called upon to pump abnormally large quantities of blood in order to deliver the normal quota of oxygen to the metabolizing tissues. The burden placed on the myocardium by the increased flow load resembles that produced by regurgitant valvular lesions. In addition, thyrotoxicosis and beriberi may impair myocardial metabolism directly, while severe anemia may interfere with myocardial function by producing myocardial anoxia.

ACUTE VERSUS CHRONIC HEART FAILURE The prototype of acute heart failure develops in patients with large myocardial infarctions or valve rupture, while chronic heart failure is typically observed in patients with slowly progressive dilated cardiomyopathy or multivalvular heart disease. In acute failure, the sudden reduction in cardiac output often results in systemic hypotension without peripheral edema, while in chronic heart failure, arterial pressure tends to be well maintained, but there is accumulation of edema. Despite these differences in clinical presentation, there is no fundamental distinction between acute and chronic failure. For example, intensive efforts to prevent expansion of blood volume by means of dietary sodium restriction and the administration of diuretics will frequently delay the development of exertional dyspnea and edema in patients with chronic valvular heart disease, i.e., it will mask the clinical manifestations of chronic heart failure, until an acute episode, such as an arrhythmia or infection precipitates acute heart failure. Without intensive efforts to restrict blood volume the same patients would have been considered to have been suffering from chronic heart failure, even though their underlying myocardial disease was no further advanced.

RIGHT-SIDED VERSUS LEFT-SIDED HEART FAILURE Many of the clinical manifestations of heart failure result from the accumulation of excess fluid behind one or both ventricles (Chaps. 26 and 28). This fluid usually localizes upstream to the specific cardiac chamber which is initially affected. For example, patients in whom the left ventricle is mechanically overloaded (e.g., aortic stenosis) or weakened (e.g., postmyocardial infarction) develop dyspnea and orthopnea as a result of pulmonary congestion, a condition referred to as *left-sided heart failure.* In contrast, when the underlying abnormality affects the right ventricle primarily, e.g., valvular pulmonic stenosis or pulmonary hypertension secondary to pulmonary thromboembolism, symptoms resulting from pulmonary congestion such as orthopnea or paroxysmal nocturnal dyspnea are less common, and edema, congestive hepatomegaly, and systemic venous distention, i.e., clinical manifestations of *right-sided heart failure,* are more prominent. However, when heart failure has existed for months or years, such localization of excess fluid behind the failing ventricle may no longer exist. For example, patients with long-standing aortic valve disease or systemic hypertension may have ankle edema, congestive hepatomegaly, and systemic venous distention late in the course of their disease, even though the abnormal hemodynamic burden initially was placed on the left ventricle, in part because of the secondary pulmonary hypertension and resultant right-sided heart failure, but also because of the persistent retention of salt and water. It is also useful to recall that the muscle bundles composing both ventricles are continuous and both ventricles share a common wall, the interventricular septum. Also, biochemical changes which occur in heart failure and which may be involved in the impairment of myocardial function, such as norepinephrine depletion and alterations in the activity of myosin ATPase, occur in the myocardium of both ventricles, regardless of the specific chamber on which the abnormal hemodynamic burden is placed.

BACKWARD VERSUS FORWARD HEART FAILURE For many years a controversy has revolved around the question of the mechanism of the clinical manifestations resulting from heart failure. The concept of *backward heart failure,* propounded by James Hope in 1832, contends that when heart failure occurs, one or the other ventricle fails to discharge its contents normally, the end-diastolic volume of the ventricle rises, the pressures and volumes in the atrium and venous system behind the failing ventricle become elevated, and retention of sodium and water occurs as a consequence of the elevation of systemic venous and capillary pressures and the resultant transudation of fluid into the interstitial space (Chap. 28). In contrast, the proponents of the *forward heart failure* hypothesis, expounded by MacKenzie in 1913, maintain that the clinical manifestations of heart failure result directly from an inadequate discharge of blood into the arterial system. Salt and water retention, then, is a consequence of diminished renal perfusion and excessive proximal tubular sodium reabsorption and of excessive distal tubular reabsorption, through activation of the renin-angiotensin-aldosterone system.

A rigid distinction between *backward* and *forward heart failure* is artificial, since both mechanisms appear to operate to varying extents in most patients with heart failure. However, the rate of onset of heart failure often influences the clinical manifestations. For example, when a large portion of the left ventricle is suddenly destroyed, as in myocardial infarction, acute pulmonary edema may develop rapidly, and although stroke volume is reduced, the patient may die of acute pulmonary edema, a manifestation of backward failure, before the reduced cardiac output can be responsible for the renal retention of salt and water. However, if the patient survives the acute insult, clinical manifestations resulting from the abnormal retention of fluid within the systemic vascular bed might develop. Similarly, the right ventricle may dilate and the systemic venous pressure may rise to high levels immediately following acute massive pulmonary embolism, but this state may have to be maintained for some days before sodium and water retention sufficient to produce peripheral edema occurs.

SYSTOLIC VERSUS DIASTOLIC FAILURE The distinction between these two forms of heart failure, described on page 903 and in Fig. 181-7, relates to whether the principal abnormality is the inability to expel sufficient blood (systolic failure) or to relax and fill normally (diastolic failure). The major clinical manifestations of systolic failure relate to an inadequate cardiac output with weakness, fatigue, and other symptoms of hypoperfusion, while in diastolic failure they relate principally to an elevation of filling pressures. In many patients, particularly those who have both ventricular hypertrophy *and* dilatation, abnormalities both of contraction and relaxation coexist.

REDISTRIBUTION OF CARDIAC OUTPUT The redistribution of cardiac output also serves as an important compensatory mechanism when flow is reduced. This redistribution is most marked when a patient with heart failure exercises, but as heart failure advances, redistribution occurs even in the basal state. Blood flow is redistributed so that the delivery of oxygen to vital organs, such as the brain and myocardium, is maintained at normal or near-normal levels, while flow to less critical areas, such as the cutaneous and muscular beds and splanchnic viscera, is reduced. Vasoconstriction mediated by the sympathetic nervous system is largely responsible for this redistribution, which in turn may be responsible for many of the clinical manifestations of heart failure, such as fluid accumulation (reduction of renal flow), low-grade fever (reduction of cutaneous flow), and fatigue (reduction of muscle flow).

SALT AND WATER RETENTION (See also Chap. 28)

When the volume of blood pumped by the left ventricle into the systemic vascular bed is chronically reduced, and when one or both ventricles fail to expel the normal fraction of their end-diastolic volumes, a complex sequence of adjustments occurs which ultimately results in the abnormal accumulation of fluid. Though, on the one hand, many of the clinical manifestations of heart failure are secondary to this excessive retention of fluid, on the other hand, this abnormal fluid accumulation and the expansion of blood volume which accompanies it also constitute an important compensatory mechanism which tends to maintain cardiac output and therefore perfusion of the vital organs. Except in the terminal stages of heart failure, the ventricle operates on an ascending, albeit depressed and flattened function curve (Fig. 181-6), and the augmented ventricular end-diastolic volume and pressure characteristic of heart failure must be regarded as aiding the maintenance of cardiac output, despite causing pulmonary and systemic venous congestion.

In the presence of heart failure, effective filling of the systemic arterial tree is reduced, a condition which initiates the complex hemodynamic, renal, and hormonal adjustments that interact to promote reduced renal sodium and water excretion. Patients with severe heart failure may exhibit a reduced capacity to excrete a water load, which may result in dilutional hyponatremia. These abnormalities may be caused, in part, by excess antidiuretic hormone activity and/or factors that prevent sodium reabsorption in the distal tubule, such as avid proximal tubular reabsorption of sodium or the action of a diuretic acting on the distal tubule.

The importance of elevated systemic venous pressure and of the alterations of renal and adrenal function characteristic of heart failure vary in their relative importance in the production of edema in different patients with heart failure. The renin-angiotensin-aldosterone axis is activated most intensely by acute heart failure, and its activity tends to decline as heart failure becomes chronic. In patients with tricuspid valve disease or constrictive pericarditis the elevated venous pressure and the transudation of fluid from systemic capillaries appear to play the dominant role in edema formation. On the other hand, severe edema may be present in patients with ischemic or hypertensive heart disease, in whom systemic venous pressure is within normal limits or is only minimally elevated. In such patients, the retention of salt and water is probably due primarily to a redistribution of cardiac output and a concomitant reduction in renal perfusion, as well as activation of the renin-angiotensin-aldosterone axis. Regardless of the mechanisms involved in fluid retention, untreated patients with chronic congestive heart failure have elevations of total blood volume, interstitial fluid volume, and body sodium. These abnormalities diminish after clinical compensation has been achieved by treatment.

CLINICAL MANIFESTATIONS OF HEART FAILURE

Dyspnea   Respiratory distress which occurs as the result of increased effort in breathing is the most common symptom of heart failure (Chap. 26). In early heart failure, dyspnea is observed only during activity, when it may simply represent an aggravation of the breathlessness which normally occurs under these circumstances. As heart failure advances, however, it appears with progressively less strenuous activity. Ultimately, breathlessness is present even when the patient is at rest. The principal difference between exertional dyspnea in normal persons and in cardiac patients is the degree of activity necessary to induce the symptom. Cardiac dyspnea is observed most frequently in patients with elevations of pulmonary venous and capillary pressures. Such patients have engorged pulmonary vessels and interstitial pulmonary edema, which reduces the compliance of the lungs and thereby increases the work of the respiratory muscles required to inflate the lungs. The activation of receptors in the lungs results in the rapid, shallow breathing of cardiac dyspnea. The oxygen cost of breathing is increased by the excessive work of the respiratory muscles. This is coupled with the diminished delivery of oxygen to these muscles, which occurs as a consequence of the reduced cardiac output, and which may contribute to fatigue of the respiratory muscles and the sensation of shortness of breath.

Orthopnea   Dyspnea in the recumbent position occurs in part because of the redistribution of fluid from the abdomen and lower extremities into the chest causing an increase in the pulmonary capillary hydrostatic pressure. Patients with orthopnea generally elevate their heads on several pillows at night and frequently awaken short of breath if their heads slip off the pillows. The sensation of breathlessness usually is relieved by sitting bolt upright, since this position reduces venous return and pulmonary capillary pressure, and many patients report that they find relief from sitting in front of an open window. As heart failure advances, orthopnea may be so severe that patients cannot lie down at all and must spend the entire night in a sitting position. On the other hand, in other patients with long-standing, severe left ventricular failure, symptoms of pulmonary congestion may actually diminish with time as the function of the right ventricle becomes impaired.

Paroxysmal (nocturnal) dyspnea   This term refers to attacks of severe shortness of breath which generally occur at night and usually awaken the patient from sleep. Though simple orthopnea may be relieved by sitting upright at the side of the bed with legs dependent, in the patient with paroxysmal nocturnal dyspnea coughing and wheezing often persist even in this position. The depression of the respiratory center during sleep may reduce ventilation sufficiently to lower arterial oxygen tension, particularly in patients with interstitial lung edema and reduced pulmonary compliance. Also, ventricular function may be further impaired at night because of reduced adrenergic stimulation of myocardial function. Acute pulmonary edema (Chap. 26) is a severe form of cardiac asthma due to further elevation of pulmonary capillary pressure leading to alveolar edema, associated with extreme shortness of breath, rales over the lung fields, and the transudation and expectoration of blood-tinged fluid. If not treated promptly acute pulmonary edema may be fatal.

Cheyne-Stokes respiration   Also known as *periodic* or *cyclic respiration*, Cheyne-Stokes respiration is characterized by diminished sensitivity of the respiratory center. There is an apneic phase, during which the arterial P_{O_2} falls and the arterial P_{CO_2} rises. These changes in the arterial blood stimulate the depressed respiratory center, resulting in hyperventilation and hypocapnia, followed in turn by

apnea. Cheyne-Stokes respiration occurs most often in patients with cerebral atherosclerosis and other cerebral lesions, but the prolongation of the circulation time from the lung to the brain which occurs in heart failure, particularly in patients with hypertension and coronary artery disease and associated cerebral vascular disease, also appears to precipitate this form of breathing.

Fatigue and weakness   These nonspecific but common symptoms of heart failure are related to the reduction of perfusion of skeletal muscle. Anorexia and nausea associated with abdominal pain and fullness are frequent complaints which may be related to the congested liver and portal venous system.

Cerebral symptoms   In severe heart failure, particularly in elderly patients with accompanying cerebral arteriosclerosis, arterial hypoxemia, and reduced cerebral perfusion, there may be alterations in the mental state characterized by confusion, difficulty in concentration, impairment of memory, headache, insomnia, and anxiety.

PHYSICAL FINDINGS   In moderate heart failure the patient appears to be in no distress at rest except that it may be uncomfortable to lie flat for more than a few minutes. In more severe heart failure the pulse pressure may be diminished, reflecting a reduction in stroke volume, and occasionally the diastolic arterial pressure may be elevated as a consequence of generalized vasoconstriction. There may be cyanosis of the lips and nail bed and sinus tachycardia. *Systemic venous pressure* is often abnormally elevated in heart failure and may be recognized most readily by observing the extent of distention of the jugular veins. In the early stages of heart failure the venous pressure may be normal at rest but may become abnormally elevated during and immediately after exertion as well as with sustained pressure on the abdomen (positive abdominojugular reflux).

Third and fourth heart sounds (Chap. 177) are often audible but are not specific for heart failure, and *pulsus alternans,* i.e., a regular rhythm in which there is alternation of strong and weak cardiac contractions and therefore alternation in the strength of the peripheral pulses, may be present. Pulsus alternans may be detected by sphygmomanometry and in more severe instances by palpation; it frequently follows an extrasystole and is observed most commonly in patients with cardiomyopathy or with hypertensive or ischemic heart disease. It is caused by a reduction in the number of contractile units during weak contractions and/or by alternation in the ventricular end-diastolic volume.

Basal pulmonary rales   Moist, inspiratory, crepitant rales and dullness to percussion over the posterior lung bases are common in patients with heart failure and elevated pulmonary venous and capillary pressures. In patients with pulmonary edema, rales may be heard widely over both lung fields; they are frequently coarse and sibilant and may be accompanied by expiratory wheezing. Rales may, however, be caused by many conditions other than left ventricular failure.

Cardiac edema   Cardiac edema is usually dependent, occurring in the legs symmetrically, particularly in the pretibial region and ankles in ambulatory patients, and in the sacral region of individuals at bed rest. Pitting edema of the arms and face occurs rarely and only late in the course of heart failure.

Hydrothorax and ascites   Pleural effusion in congestive heart failure results from the elevation of pleural capillary pressure and transudation of fluid into the pleural cavities. Since the pleural veins drain into both the systemic and pulmonary veins, hydrothorax occurs most commonly with marked elevation of pressure in both venous systems, but may also be seen with marked elevation of pressure in either venous bed. It is more frequent in the right pleural cavity than the left. *Ascites* also occurs as a consequence of transudation and results from increased pressure in the hepatic veins and the veins draining the peritoneum (Chap. 39). Marked ascites occurs most frequently in patients with tricuspid valve disease and with constrictive pericarditis.

Congestive hepatomegaly An enlarged, tender, pulsating liver also accompanies systemic venous hypertension and is observed not only in the same conditions in which ascites occurs, but also in milder forms of heart failure from any cause. With prolonged, severe hepatomegaly, as in patients with tricuspid valve disease or chronic constrictive pericarditis, enlargement of the spleen may also occur.

Jaundice This is a late finding in congestive heart failure and is associated with elevations of both the direct- and indirect-reacting bilirubin levels; it results from impairment of hepatic function secondary to hepatic congestion and the hepatocellular hypoxia associated with central lobular atrophy. Serum enzyme concentrations, particularly SGOT and SGPT, are frequently elevated. If hepatic congestion occurs acutely, the jaundice may be severe and the enzymes strikingly raised.

Cardiac cachexia With severe chronic heart failure there may be serious weight loss and cachexia because of (1) elevation of the metabolic rate, which results in part from the extra work performed by the respiratory muscles, the increased oxygen needs of the hypertrophied heart, and the discomfort associated with severe heart failure; (2) anorexia, nausea, and vomiting due to central causes, to digitalis intoxication, or to congestive hepatomegaly and abdominal fullness; (3) some impairment of intestinal absorption due to congestion of the intestinal veins; and (4) rarely, in patients with particularly severe failure of the right side of the heart, a protein-losing enteropathy.

Other manifestations With reduction of blood flow the extremities may be cold, pale, and diaphoretic. Urine flow is depressed, and the urine contains protein and has a high specific gravity and a low concentration of sodium. In addition, prerenal azotemia may be present. In patients with long-standing severe heart failure impotence and depression are common.

ROENTGENOGRAPHIC FINDINGS In addition to the enlargement of the particular chambers characteristic of the lesion responsible for heart failure, vascular changes in the lung fields are common in patients with heart failure and elevated pulmonary vascular pressures (Chap. 179). Also, pleural effusions may be present and associated with interlobar effusions.

DIFFERENTIAL DIAGNOSIS The diagnosis of congestive heart failure may be established by observing some combination of the clinical manifestations of heart failure, enumerated above, together with the findings characteristic of one of the etiologic forms of heart disease. Since chronic heart failure is often associated with cardiac enlargement, the diagnosis should be questioned, but is by no means excluded, when all chambers are normal in size. Heart failure may be difficult to distinguish from pulmonary disease, and the differential diagnosis is discussed in Chap. 26. Pulmonary embolism also presents many of the manifestations of heart failure, but hemoptysis, pleuritic chest pain, a right ventricular lift, and the characteristic mismatch between ventilation and perfusion on lung scan should point to this diagnosis (Chap. 211).

Ankle edema may be due to varicose veins, cyclic edema, or gravitational effects (Chap. 28), but in these patients there is no jugular venous hypertension at rest or with pressure over the abdomen. Edema secondary to renal disease can usually be recognized by appropriate renal function tests and urinalysis and is rarely associated with elevation of the venous pressure. Enlargement of the liver and ascites occur in patients with hepatic cirrhosis, but may also be distinguished from heart failure by normal jugular venous pressure and absence of a positive abdominojugular reflux.

TREATMENT OF HEART FAILURE

The treatment of heart failure may be divided into three components: (1) removal of the precipitating cause, (2) correction of the underlying cause, and (3) control of the congestive heart failure state. The first two are discussed together in subsequent chapters with each specific disease entity or complication. In many instances surgical treatment will correct or at least improve the underlying cause. The third component of the treatment of heart failure may, in turn, also be divided into three categories: (1) reduction of cardiac work load, including afterload; (2) control of excessive salt and water retention; and (3) enhancement of myocardial contractility. The vigor with which each of these measures is pursued in any individual patient should depend upon the severity of the heart failure state. Following effective treatment, recurrence of the clinical manifestations of heart failure can often be prevented by continuing those measures that were originally effective. While a simple rule for the treatment of all patients with heart failure cannot be formulated because of the varied etiologies, hemodynamic features, and clinical manifestations of heart failure, insofar as the treatment of chronic congestive failure is concerned, simple measures such as moderate restriction of activity and sodium intake should be tried first. If these are insufficient, therapy with a thiazide and/or a glycoside is then begun. The next step is more rigorous restriction of salt intake and a loop diuretic in place of the thiazide. If heart failure persists, then a vasodilator is added. Hospitalization with rigid salt restriction, bed rest, intravenous vasodilators, and positive inotropic agents comes next. In some patients the order in which these measures are applied may be altered.

REDUCTION OF CARDIAC WORK LOAD This consists of reducing physical activity, instituting emotional rest, and reducing afterload. The latter is generally instituted *after* the use of diuretics and cardiac glycosides. Modest restriction of physical activity in mild cases and rest in bed or in a chair in severe failure remain cornerstones in the treatment of heart failure. Meals should be small in quantity, and every effort should be made to diminish the patient's anxiety. Physical and emotional rest tend to lower arterial pressure, and reduce the load on the myocardium by diminishing the requirements for cardiac output. These influences act in concert to diminish the need for redistribution of the cardiac output, and in many patients, particularly those with mild heart failure, simple bed rest and mild sedation often result in an effective diuresis.

Rest at home or in the hospital should be maintained for 1 to 2 weeks in patients with overt congestive failure and should be continued for several days after the patient's condition has stabilized. The hazards of phlebothrombosis and pulmonary embolism which occur with bed rest may be reduced with anticoagulants, leg exercises, and elastic stockings. In any event, absolute bed rest rarely is required, and the patient should be encouraged to sit in a chair and be given toilet privileges unless heart failure is extreme. Heavy sedation should be avoided, but small doses of tranquilizers may be helpful in calming the emotionally disturbed patient through the first few days of therapy and in permitting much-needed sleep. In patients with chronic, mild heart failure, bed rest on weekends will frequently allow continuation of gainful employment. Following recovery from heart failure, the patient's activities must be carefully assessed, and often his or her professional, family, and/or community responsibilities must be reduced. Intermittent rest during the day and the avoidance of strenuous exertion are often helpful once compensation has been restored. Weight reduction by restriction of caloric intake in the obese patient with heart failure also diminishes cardiac work load and is an essential component of the therapeutic program.

ENHANCEMENT OF MYOCARDIAL CONTRACTILITY—DIGITALIS The improvement of myocardial contractility by means of cardiac glycosides is the second of the cornerstones in the control of heart failure. The basic molecular structure of the digitalis glycosides is a steroid nucleus to which an unsaturated lactone ring is attached at C-17. These two elements together are called *aglycone* or *genin*, and it is this portion of the molecule which is responsible for the cardiotonic activity. The addition of sugar residues to this basic structure determines water solubility and pharmacokinetic properties for individual glycosides.

Pharmacokinetics In the absence of severe malabsorption, most digitalis glycosides are adequately absorbed from the intestinal tract even in the presence of vascular congestion secondary to heart failure. Oral absorption is close to complete within 2 h. The bioavailability (i.e., percent of intravenous dose) of orally administered glycoside varies. Considerable variability of bioavailability has been found in different commercial preparations of digoxin. The bioavailability of Lanoxin elixir is 70 to 85 percent, Lanoxin tablets 60 to 80 percent, and Lanoxicaps 90 to 100 percent. Digitoxin tablets have a bioavailability of virtually 100 percent. Cholesterol-lowering resins, antidiarrheal agents containing pectin and kaolin, nonabsorbable antacids, and neomycin can reduce the absorption of digoxin and digitoxin. Varying degrees of protein-binding of glycosides occur in the bloodstream (for example, 97 percent for digitoxin and 25 percent for digoxin), and though these differences may account in part for the varying durations of the effect of different glycosides, they are not related to the speed of action of these drugs. The plasma contains only approximately 1 percent of the body stores of digoxin; therefore, digoxin is not effectively removed from the body by dialysis, exchange transfusions, or during cardiopulmonary bypass, presumably because of tissue binding. The major fraction of the glycosides is directly bound by various tissues including the heart, in which the concentration is approximately 30 times that in the plasma for digoxin and 7 times for digitoxin; the latter is less polar and more lipid-soluble than digoxin.

Digoxin, which has a half-life of 1.6 days, is filtered in the glomeruli and secreted by the renal tubules; 85 percent is excreted in the urine, most in unchanged form; only 10 to 15 percent of digoxin is eliminated in the stool through biliary excretion in the presence of normal renal function. The ratio of digoxin clearance to endogenous creatinine clearance is 0.8, and the percentage of the body's total stores of digoxin lost per day can be calculated as $(14 \pm 0.2) \times$ creatinine clearance in milliliters per minute. In patients with normal renal function a plateau concentration in the blood and tissue is reached after 5 days of daily maintenance treatment without a loading dose (Fig. 64-2). Therefore, significant reductions of the glomerular filtration rate reduce the elimination of digoxin (but not of digitoxin) and, therefore, may prolong digoxin's effect, allowing it to accumulate to toxic levels if it is administered as in patients with normal renal function. The administration of most diuretics does not alter the excretion of digoxin significantly, but spironolactone can inhibit tubular secretion of digoxin, resulting in significant accumulation of the drug. Serum levels and pharmacokinetics are essentially unchanged by massive weight loss. In about 10 percent of patients receiving digoxin, large amounts of digoxin reduction products are formed by bacterial flora in the gastrointestinal tract. Antibiotic therapy that alters gut flora reverses this tendency to metabolize digoxin to cardioinactive products and can result in striking alterations in the state of digitalization. *Digitoxin,* with a half-life of approximately 5 days, is metabolized chiefly in the liver; only 15 percent is excreted in the urine unchanged and an equal fraction in the stool. Drugs such as phenobarbital and phenylbutazone that increase the activity of hepatic microsomal enzymes accelerate the metabolism of digitoxin. To reach a steady state, digitoxin requires maintenance doses for 3 to 4 weeks. *Ouabain* is very rapidly acting, exhibiting an onset of action in 5 to 10 min and a peak effect within 60 min following intravenous injection. It is poorly absorbed from the gastrointestinal tract and, therefore, is not suitable for oral use; it is excreted by the kidneys, has a half-life of 21 h, and is useful in emergencies.

Mechanism of action The cardiac actions of all digitalis glycosides are alike. The clinical effects result from augmenting contractility and from slowing heart rate and atrioventricular conduction.

The most important effect of digitalis on cardiac muscle is to shift its force-velocity relation upward (Chap. 181). This positive inotropic effect is exhibited in normal, nonfailing hypertrophied as well as in failing hearts. In the absence of heart failure, however, when cardiac output is not limited by cardiac contractility, the drug does not elevate the output. The finding that digitalis increases the contractility of the nonfailing heart has led to its use (1) in patients with heart disease but without heart failure prior to operation or other stressful situations such as serious infections, and (2) in the presence of a chronically increased load, such as hypertension without heart failure. However, definitive evidence of its efficacy in these circumstances is not available.

Excitation-contraction coupling is the membrane and intracellular process most likely involved in producing the positive inotropic effect of digitalis glycosides. These drugs inhibit transmembrane sodium and potassium movement by inhibition of the monovalent cation transport enzyme–coupled Na^+,K^+-ATPase. The latter, localized to the sarcolemma, appears to be the receptor for cardioactive glycosides whose action results in an increase in intracellular sodium content, and this in turn increases intracellular calcium concentration through a Na^+-Ca^{2+} exchange carrier mechanism. The increased myocardial uptake of calcium augments calcium released to the myofilaments during excitation and, therefore, invokes a positive inotropic response. There is a correlation between the degree of enzyme inhibition and the inotropic potency of the glycoside.

Cardiac glycosides also produce alterations in the electrical properties of both the contractile cells and the specialized automatic cells. While low concentrations of glycosides produce little effect on the action potential, high concentrations result in a reduction in the resting potential (phase 4, see Fig. 183-1, p. 916) and an augmented rate of diastolic depolarization. The reduction in the resting potential brings the cell closer to the threshold for depolarization. These two effects lead to increased automaticity and ectopic impulse activity. With the lowering of the resting potential, the rate of rise of the action potential is reduced, resulting in a slowing of conduction velocity, which is conducive to the development of reentry. Thus, the known electrophysiologic effects of digitalis glycosides are capable of explaining the development of both reentry and ectopic foci and the resultant arrhythmias associated with digitalis intoxication.

The glycosides also prolong the effective *refractory period* of the atrioventricular node, largely as a result of an enhanced vagal effect. Digitalis also shortens the refractory period of the atrial and ventricular muscle. Small action potentials are propagated in a decremental fashion in the atrioventricular junction. Most do not reach the ventricles but leave some of the atrioventricular junctional cells in a refractory state. This helps to explain the slowing of ventricular rate produced by digitalis in supraventricular tachycardias. In atrial fibrillation, the slowing of ventricular rate is explained by prolongation of the effective refractory period of the atrioventricular node and increased concealed conduction with fewer impulses penetrating the atrioventricular junction owing to both vagal and possibly direct effects of glycosides on junctional tissue.

Digitalis exerts a clinically significant negative chronotropic action, usually only in the setting of ventricular failure. In heart failure, slowing of the sinus rate following the administration of digitalis results also from withdrawal of sympathetic activity secondary to general improvement in circulatory status due to the positive inotropic effect of the glycoside. In the nonfailing heart the slowing effect is negligible, and digitalis should not be used for the treatment of sinus tachycardia unless heart failure is present. The apparent suppression of pacemaker activity which may take place following large doses of digitalis is probably due not to arrest of the pacemaker but rather to a sinoatrial block related to a depression of conduction of impulses out of the sinus node.

In addition, the digitalis glycosides also exert an action on the peripheral vasculature, causing venous and arterial constriction in normal individuals and reflex dilatation resulting from withdrawal of sympathetic constrictor activity in patients with congestive heart failure.

Use in heart failure By stimulating the contractile function of the heart, digitalis improves ventricular emptying; i.e., it augments the ejection fraction, increases cardiac output, promotes diuresis, and reduces the elevated diastolic pressure and volume and end-systolic volume of the failing ventricle with consequent reduction of symptoms resulting from pulmonary vascular congestion and elevated systemic venous pressure. It is most beneficial in patients in whom ventricular contractility is impaired secondary to chronic ischemic heart disease, or when hypertensive, valvular, or congenital heart disease imposes an excessive volume or pressure load. It is helpful in slowing the rapid ventricular rate of patients with atrial flutter and fibrillation. It is of relatively little value in most forms of cardiomyopathy, myocarditis, beriberi with heart failure, mitral stenosis, thyrotoxicosis and sinus rhythm, cor pulmonale when the lung disease is not being treated concurrently (Chap. 191), and chronic constrictive pericarditis (Chap. 194). Nonetheless, when used in proper doses, it is not contraindicated in these disorders and is frequently used since it may exert a beneficial effect, albeit not a striking one.

Digitalis intoxication Although digitalis is one of the cornerstones of the treatment for heart failure, it is a two-edged sword, because intoxication due to digitalis excess is a common, serious, and potentially fatal complication of its use. The therapeutic-to-toxic ratios are identical for all cardiac glycosides. In most patients with heart failure the lethal dose of most glycosides is probably 5 to 10 times the minimal effective dose and only about twice the dose which leads to minor toxic manifestations. In addition, old age, acute myocardial infarction or ischemia, hypoxemia, magnesium depletion, renal insufficiency, hypercalcemia, electrical cardioversion, and hypothyroidism all may reduce the tolerance of the patient to the digitalis glycosides or provoke latent digitalis intoxication. The most common precipitating cause of digitalis intoxication, however, is depletion of potassium stores, which often occurs as a result of diuretic therapy and secondary hyperaldosteronism. Since it is not necessary for a patient to receive a maximally tolerated dose of digitalis to derive a beneficial effect, even small doses provide some therapeutic action; this point should be considered if these drugs are to be used in patients prone to toxicity.

Anorexia, nausea, and vomiting, which are among the earliest signs of digitalis intoxication, are caused by direct stimulation of centers in the medulla and are not of gastrointestinal origin. The most frequent disturbance of cardiac rhythm caused by digitalis is premature ventricular beats, which may take the form of bigeminy because of increased myocardial irritability or facilitation of reentry. Atrioventricular block of varying degrees of severity may occur. Nonparoxysmal atrial tachycardia with variable atrioventricular block is quite characteristic of digitalis intoxication. Sinus arrhythmia, sinoatrial block, sinus arrest, and atrioventricular junctional and multifocal ventricular tachycardia may also occur. These arrhythmias are due to action of the glycoside both on cardiac tissues and on the central nervous system. Chronic digitalis intoxication may be insidious in onset and characterized by exacerbations of heart failure, weight loss, cachexia, neuralgias, gynecomastia, yellow vision, and delirium. Digitalis-toxic cardiac arrhythmias precede extracardiac (gastrointestinal or central nervous system) toxicity in about one-half of cases.

Digitalis intoxication has been reported to occur in as many as 20 percent of hospitalized patients receiving a cardiac glycoside, which emphasizes the importance of the ability to diagnose this condition. The administration of quinidine to patients receiving digoxin raises the serum concentration of the latter by reducing both the renal and nonrenal elimination of digoxin and by reducing its volume of distribution and thereby increasing the propensity to digitalis intoxication. The calcium channel antagonist verapamil and the experimental antiarrhythmic agent amiodarone also appear to raise serum digoxin levels. Therefore, serum digoxin concentrations and electrocardiograms should be followed carefully when these drugs are administered to digitalized patients. The radioimmunoassays for digoxin and digitoxin make possible the correlation of serum glycoside levels with the presence of toxicity. In patients receiving standard maintenance doses of digoxin and digitoxin and in whom no sign of intoxication is present, serum concentrations approximate 1 to 1.5 and 20 to 25 ng/mL, respectively. When signs of intoxication are present, serum levels of more than 2 and 30 ng/mL, respectively, of these glycosides are often found. Since many factors other than the serum concentration determine digitalis intoxication, and since there is overlap in serum glycoside concentrations in patients with and without toxicity, it is clear that these levels cannot be used as a sole guide to digitalis dosage. However, when taken together with findings on the clinical examination and electrocardiogram, they add useful information to the clinical evaluations of digitalis intoxication. In addition they will indicate whether a patient for whom the history of digitalis intake is in doubt has, in fact, been receiving the drug.

Treatment of digitalis intoxication When tachyarrhythmias result from digitalis intoxication, withdrawal of the drug and treatment with potassium, phenytoin, propranolol, or lidocaine are indicated. Potassium should be administered cautiously and by the oral route whenever possible if hypokalemia is present, but small doses may also be helpful when serum potassium levels are normal; *potassium must not be employed in the presence of atrioventricular block or hyperkalemia.* Propranolol should not be used to treat digitalis toxicity in the presence of severe heart failure or atrioventricular block but may be useful otherwise; lidocaine is effective in the treatment of digitalis-induced ventricular tachyarrhythmias in the absence of preceding atrioventricular block. A cardiac pacemaker may be required in digitalis-induced atrioventricular block. Electrical conversion may not only be ineffective in treating these arrhythmias but may induce more serious arrhythmias. However, it may be lifesaving in digitalis-induced ventricular fibrillation. Quinidine and procainamide are of only limited value in the treatment of digitalis intoxication. Fab fragments of purified, intact digitalis antibodies represent a potentially lifesaving approach to the treatment of severe intoxication.

SYMPATHOMIMETIC AMINES (See also Chap. 66) Four sympathomimetic amines which act largely on beta-adrenergic receptors—epinephrine, isoproterenol, dopamine, and dobutamine—improve myocardial contractility in various forms of heart failure. The latter two agents appear to be most effective; they must be administered by constant intravenous infusion and are useful in patients with intractable heart failure, particularly in those with a reversible component, such as exists in patients who have undergone cardiac surgery, and in some instances of myocardial infarction and shock or pulmonary edema. While they improve the hemodynamics in that condition, it is not clear that they improve survival. Their administration must be accompanied by careful and continuous monitoring of the electrocardiogram, intraarterial pressure, and if possible pulmonary artery wedge pressure, in an intensive care unit.

Dopamine, the naturally occurring immediate precursor of norepinephrine, has a combination of actions which make it particularly useful in the treatment of a variety of hypotensive states and congestive heart failure. At very low doses, that is, 1 to 2 (μg/kg)/min, it dilates renal and mesenteric blood vessels through stimulation of specific dopaminergic receptors, thereby augmenting renal and mesenteric blood flow and sodium excretion. In the range of 2 to 10 (μg/kg)/min, dopamine stimulates myocardial beta receptors but induces relatively little tachycardia, while at higher doses it also stimulates alpha-adrenergic receptors and elevates arterial pressure.

Dobutamine is a synthetic catecholamine which acts on $beta_1$, $beta_2$, and alpha receptors. It exerts a potent inotropic action, has only a modest cardioaccelerating effect, and lowers peripheral vascular resistance, but since it raises cardiac output, it has little effect on systemic arterial pressure. Dobutamine, given in continuous infusions of 2.5 to 10 (μg/kg)/min, is useful in the treatment of acute heart failure without hypotension. Like the other sympathomimetic amines it may be particularly valuable in the management of patients requiring relatively short-term inotropic support—up to 1 week—in conditions which are reversible, such as the cardiac depression which sometimes follows open-heart surgery, or in patients with acute heart failure who are being prepared for operation. Adverse effects include sinus tachycardia, tachyarrhythmias, and hypertension.

A major problem with all sympathomimetics is the loss of responsiveness, apparently due to "downregulation" of adrenergic receptors, which becomes evident within 8 h of continuous administration.

Amrinone This bipyridine, a noncatecholamine, nonglycoside exerts both positive inotropic and vasodilator actions by inhibiting a specific phosphodiesterase. It is suitable for intravenous use only, and by simultaneously stimulating cardiac contractility and dilating the systemic vascular bed it reverses the major hemodynamic abnormalities associated with heart failure. Milrinone, a derivative of amrinone, and several other active phosphodiesterases are under active investigation for chronic oral administration.

CONTROL OF EXCESSIVE FLUID RETENTION Many of the clinical manifestations of heart failure result from hypervolemia and expansion of the interstitial fluid volume. By the time fluid retention due to heart failure first becomes clinically evident, considerable expansion of the extracellular space has already occurred, and heart failure usually is already advanced. Treatment aimed at reducing extracellular fluid volume is dependent primarily on lowering total body sodium stores, while fluid restriction is of less importance. A negative sodium balance can be achieved by reducing the dietary intake and increasing the urinary excretion of this ion with the aid of diuretics. In severe heart failure mechanical removal of extracellular fluid by means of thoracentesis, paracentesis, and rarely hemodialysis or peritoneal dialysis may also be employed.

Diet In patients with mild heart failure, considerable improvement in symptoms may result from simply reducing the sodium intake, particularly if accompanied by periods of rest. In patients with more severe heart failure the sodium intake must be controlled more rigidly, and other measures, such as diuretics and glycosides, are used. Even following recovery from a bout of heart failure, at least moderate sodium restriction should be maintained. The normal diet contains approximately 6 to 10 g sodium chloride; this intake can be reduced by half simply by excluding salt-rich foods and salt which is added at the table. Reduction of the ordinary dietary intake to approximately one-fourth of normal may be achieved if, in addition, all salt is omitted from cooking. In patients with severe heart failure, in whom the daily sodium chloride intake should be reduced to between 500 and 1000 mg, milk, cheese, bread, cereals, canned vegetables and soups, some salted cuts of meat, and some fresh vegetables, including spinach, celery, and beets, must be eliminated. A variety of fresh fruit, green vegetables, specially processed breads and milk, and salt substitutes are permissible, but such diets are difficult to keep palatable. Water intake may be ad libitum in all but the most severe forms of congestive heart failure. However, late in the course of heart failure, dilutional hyponatremia may develop in patients who are unable to excrete a water load, sometimes because of excessive secretion of antidiuretic hormone. In such cases water intake as well as sodium intake must be restricted.

Attention must also be directed to the caloric content of the diet. Substantial improvement can result from caloric restriction in obese patients with heart failure, in whom weight loss will reduce the load placed on the myocardium. On the other hand, in individuals with severe heart failure and cardiac cachexia, an attempt must be made to maintain nutritional intake and to avoid caloric and vitamin deficiencies.

Diuretics A variety of diuretic agents is available, and in patients with mild heart failure almost all are effective. However, in the more severe forms of heart failure, the selection of diuretics is more difficult, and any existing abnormalities in serum electrolytes must be taken into account. Overtreatment must be avoided, since the resultant hypovolemia may reduce cardiac output, interfere with renal function, and produce profound weakness and lethargy.

THIAZIDE DIURETICS These agents are widely used in clinical practice because of their effectiveness when administered orally. In patients with chronic heart failure of mild or moderate severity the continued administration of chlorothiazide or one of its many analogues abolishes

or diminishes the need for very rigid dietary sodium restriction, although salty foods and table salt should still be avoided. Thiazides are well absorbed following oral administration; chlorothiazide and hydrochlorothiazide reach their peak action in 4 h, and diuresis persists for approximately 12 h. Thiazide diuretics reduce the reabsorption of sodium and chloride in the first half of the distal convoluted tubule and a portion of the cortical ascending limb of the loop of Henle, and water follows the unreabsorbed salt. Thiazides fail to increase free water clearance, and in some instances reduce it, supporting the hypothesis that these drugs inhibit selective sodium chloride reabsorption in the distal cortical diluting segment, at a site where the urine is normally diluted (Chap. 218). This may result in the excretion of a hypertonic urine and may contribute to dilutional hyponatremia. As a consequence of increased delivery of sodium to the distal nephron, sodium-potassium ion exchange is enhanced and kaliuresis results. The weak carbonic anhydrase–inhibiting properties of the thiazides are of limited importance and need not be invoked to account for most of the diuretic action. In contrast to the loop diuretics which enhance calcium excretion, the thiazides have the opposite effect. These drugs are effective and useful in the treatment of heart failure as long as the glomerular filtration rate exceeds 50 percent of normal.

Chlorothiazide is administered in doses of up to 500 mg every 6 h. Many derivatives of this compound are available but differ principally in dosage and duration of action and therefore offer few, if any, significant advances over the parent compound, except for chlorthalidone which may be administered once daily. Potassium depletion and metabolic alkalosis (the latter due to increased H^+ secretion as a substitute for the depleted intracellular stores of potassium and increased proximal tubular reabsorption of filtered HCO_3^- when there is relative depletion of the extracellular fluid volume) are the chief adverse metabolic effects following prolonged administration of the thiazides (as well as of metozalone and of the loop diuretics), and may seriously enhance the dangers of digitalis intoxication and induce fatigue and lethargy. Hypokalemia may be prevented by the oral supplementation of potassium chloride. However, the solution is not palatable and may be hazardous in patients with renal failure. Therefore, to control potassium depletion, intermittent dosage schedules, e.g., omitting the diuretic every third day, and the addition of a potassium-retaining diuretic, such as a spironolactone or triamterene, may be preferable. Other side effects of thiazides include reduction of the excretion of uric acid, which may lead to hyperuricemia, and a hyperglycemic effect, which rarely may precipitate hyperosmolar coma in the poorly regulated diabetic. Skin rashes, thrombocytopenia, and granulocytopenia have also been reported.

METOZALONE This quinethazone derivative has a site of action and potency similar to that of the thiazides, but has been reported to be effective in the presence of moderate renal failure. The usual dose is 5 to 10 mg/day.

FUROSEMIDE, BUMETANIDE, AND ETHACRYNIC ACID These "loop" diuretics are similar physiologically but differ chemically. These extremely powerful diuretics reversibly inhibit the reabsorption of sodium, potassium, and chloride in the thick ascending limb of Henle's loop, apparently by blocking a cotransport system in the luminal membrane. These agents may induce renal cortical vasodilatation and can produce rates of urine formation which may be as high as one-fourth of the glomerular filtration rate. While other diuretics lose their effectiveness as blood volume is restored to normal levels, the loop diuretics remain effective despite the elimination of excessive extracellular fluid volume. The major side effects of these agents are due to this marked diuretic potency, which on rare occasions may result in contraction of the plasma volume, circulatory collapse, reductions in the renal blood flow and glomerular filtration rate, and the development of prerenal azotemia. Metabolic alkalosis is produced by a large increase in the urinary excretion of chloride, hydrogen, and potassium ions. Hypokalemia (see discussion of thiazides, above) and hyponatremia may occur, and hyperuricemia and hyperglycemia are observed occasionally, as with thiazide diuretics. The reabsorption of free water is decreased.

All three drugs are readily absorbed orally and are excreted in the bile and urine. They are usually effective by mouth and intravenously. Weakness, nausea, and dizziness may complicate the administration of all three loop diuretics; ethacrynic acid has been associated with skin rash and granulocytopenia, as well as with transient or permanent deafness.

These extremely effective diuretics are useful in all forms of heart failure, particularly in otherwise refractory heart failure and pulmonary edema. They have been shown to be effective in patients with hypoalbuminemia, hyponatremia, hypochloremia, hypokalemia, and reductions in the glomerular filtration rate, and to produce a diuresis in patients in whom thiazide diuretics and aldosterone antagonists, alone and in combination, are ineffective.

In patients with refractory heart failure the action of furosemide, bumetanide, and ethacrynic acid may be potentiated by intravenous administration and the addition of thiazide diuretics, carbonic anhydrase inhibitors, osmotic diuretics, and the potassium-sparing diuretics—spironolactone, triamterene, and amiloride. These latter agents act on the cortical collecting ducts, are relatively weak, and therefore are rarely indicated as sole agents. However, their potassium-sparing properties make them particularly useful in conjunction with the more potent kaliuretic agents, the loop diuretics and thiazides. These agents fall into two classes, as noted below.

ALDOSTERONE ANTAGONISTS The 17-spironolactones resemble aldosterone structurally and act on the distal half of the convoluted tubule and the cortical portion of the collecting duct by competitive inhibition of aldosterone, thereby blocking the exchange between sodium and both potassium and hydrogen in the distal tubules and collecting ducts. These agents produce a sodium diuresis, and, in contrast to the thiazides, ethacrynic acid, and furosemide, they result in potassium retention. Although secondary hyperaldosteronism exists in some patients with congestive heart failure, the spironolactones are effective even in patients in whom the serum aldosterone concentration is within normal limits. Aldactone A may be administered in doses of 25 to 100 mg three to four times daily by mouth. The maximal effect of this regimen is not observed for approximately 4 days. Spironolactones are most effective when administered in combination with thiazide and loop diuretics. The opposing action of these drugs on urine and serum potassium makes possible a sodium diuresis without either hyper- or hypokalemia when spironolactone and one of these other agents are administered in combination. Also, since spironolactone (as well as triamterene and amiloride) acts on the distal tubule, it is particularly effective when used in combination with one of these other diuretics which acts more proximally.

Spironolactone should not be administered alone to patients with hyperkalemia, renal failure, or hyponatremia. Reported complications include nausea, epigastric distress, mental confusion, drowsiness, gynecomastia, and erythematous eruptions.

TRIAMTERENE AND AMILORIDE These two drugs exert renal effects similar to those of the spironolactones; i.e., they block sodium reabsorption and secondarily inhibit potassium secretion in the distal tubules. However, their fundamental mechanism of action differs from those of the spironolactones, since they are active in adrenalectomized animals and their action does not depend on the presence of aldosterone. The effective dose of triamterene is 100 mg once or twice daily and that of amiloride is 5 mg daily. Side effects include nausea, vomiting, diarrhea, headache, granulocytopenia, eosinophilia, and skin rash. Both triamterene and the chemically unrelated diuretic amiloride resemble Aldactone A in that their diuretic potency is not great, and they are effective in preventing the hypokalemia characteristic of the administration of thiazides, furosemide, and ethacrynic acid. A number of diuretic preparations contain a combination of a thiazide and either triamterene or amiloride in a single capsule. They may be useful in patients who develop hypokalemia with a thiazide

but should not be used in patients with impaired renal function and/or hyperkalemia.

CHOICE OF DIURETICS Orally administered thiazides or metozalone are the agents of choice in the treatment of chronic cardiac edema of mild to moderate degree in patients without hyperglycemia, hyperuricemia, or hypokalemia. Spironolactones, triamterene, and amiloride are not potent diuretics when used alone, but they potentiate other diuretics, particularly the thiazides and loop diuretics. However, in patients with heart failure and severe secondary hyperaldosteronism, spironolactone may be quite effective. Ethacrynic acid, bumetanide, or furosemide, given alone or with spironolactone or triamterene, are the agents of choice in patients with severe heart failure refractory to other diuretics. In very severe heart failure the combination of a thiazide, a loop diuretic (ethacrynic acid or furosemide), and a potassium-sparing diuretic (spironolactone, triamterene, or amiloride) is required.

VASODILATOR THERAPY In many patients with heart failure, left ventricular afterload is increased as a consequence of the several neural and humoral influences which act to constrict the peripheral vascular bed. These include increased activity of the adrenergic nervous system, elevation of circulating catecholamines, and activation of the renin-angiotensin system, and perhaps of increased circulating antidiuretic hormone as well. In addition to the vasoconstriction, the ventricular end-diastolic volume rises and as a consequence of the operation of Laplace's law, which relates myocardial wall tension to the product of intraventricular pressure and radius, the aortic impedance, i.e., the force which opposes left ventricular ejection, or the ventricular afterload, rises. The maintenance or even the elevation of arterial pressure is generally considered to be a useful compensatory mechanism that allows blood flow to vital organs to persist in the presence of hypovolemia, despite inadequacy of the total cardiac output. While this is the case in many forms of shock (Chap. 29), when there is no preload reserve in the presence of severely impaired cardiac function, the increase in afterload may reduce cardiac output and elevate myocardial oxygen consumption further.

As shown in Fig. 181-5, afterload is a major determinant of cardiac function. When cardiac function is normal, a moderate elevation in afterload does not alter stroke volume, because the resultant increase in left ventricular end-diastolic volume, i.e., preload, can be tolerated easily. However, when myocardial function is impaired, such an increase in preload evoked by an elevation of afterload may raise ventricular end-diastolic and pulmonary capillary pressures to levels that may produce severe pulmonary congestion or pulmonary edema. In many patients with heart failure, the ventricle is already operating at the peak, flat portion of its Frank-Starling curve (Fig. 181-6), and any additional increase in aortic impedance (afterload) will reduce stroke volume (page 902). Conversely, a reduction of afterload will tend to restore hemodynamics to normal by elevating the stroke volume of the failing ventricle, and may reduce the elevated ventricular filling pressure.

The pharmacologic reduction of impedance to left ventricular ejection with vasodilator drugs represents an important adjunct in the management of heart failure. This approach may be particularly helpful in patients with acute heart failure due to myocardial infarction (Chap. 190), valvular regurgitation, elevated systemic vascular resistance and/or arterial pressure, and marked cardiac dilatation. The reduction of afterload by means of a variety of vasodilators reduces left ventricular end-diastolic pressure, volume, and oxygen consumption, while raising stroke volume and cardiac output and causing only modest reduction in aortic pressure. Vasodilators should not be used in patients with hypotension.

In patients with both acute and chronic heart failure secondary to coronary artery disease, cardiomyopathy, or valvular regurgitation who are treated with vasodilators, cardiac output increases, the pulmonary wedge pressure falls, the signs and symptoms of heart failure are relieved, and a new steady state is achieved in which cardiac output is higher and afterload lower with no or only mild

FIGURE 182-1 *Effects of various vasodilators on the relationship between left ventricular end-diastolic pressure (LVEDP) and cardiac index or stroke volume in normal (N) and failing (F) hearts. H represents hydralazine or any other pure arterial dilator. It produces only a minimal increase in cardiac index in the normal subject (A' → H') or in the patient with heart failure with normal LVEDP (C → H''). In contrast, it elevates output in the patient with heart failure and elevated LVEDP (A → H). P represents a balanced vasodilator, such as sodium nitroprusside or prazosin. It reduces filling pressure in all patients, elevates cardiac output in patients with heart failure and elevated LVEDP (A → P), lowers cardiac output in normal subjects (A' → P'), and has little effect on cardiac output in heart failure patients with normal filling pressures (C → P''). (Reprinted with permission from TW Smith, E Braunwald, in Heart Disease: A Textbook of Cardiovascular Medicine, 2d ed. Philadelphia, Saunders, 1984.)*

reduction of arterial pressure (Fig. 182-1). Furthermore, the reduction of elevated left end-diastolic pressure may improve subendocardial perfusion.

Vasodilator therapy is particularly useful in the treatment of acute pulmonary edema, which, if not precipitated by myocardial infarction, is often associated with hypertension. Also, vasodilator therapy is often helpful in refractory congestive heart failure; when heart failure is acute, the addition of an inotropic agent such as dobutamine may be required.

The several available vasodilators vary in their hemodynamic effects, locus and duration of action, and mode of administration (Table 182-1). Some vasodilators, such as hydralazine, minoxidil,

TABLE 182-1   Spectrum of vasodilators used for the treatment of heart failure*

	Principal site of action	Mode of administration	Duration of action
Phentolamine	Arterial	Continuous intravenous	Minutes
Hydralazine	Arterial	Oral	Hours
Minoxidil	Arterial	Oral	Hours
Captopril, enalapril	Arterial and venous	Oral	Hours
Nitroprusside	Arterial and venous	Continuous intravenous	Minutes
Prazosin	Arterial and venous	Oral	Hours
Nitroglycerin	Venous	Intravenous or sublingual	Minutes
		Ointment, patch	Hours
Isosorbide dinitrate	Venous	Sublingual	Minutes to hours

* Although all these drugs have been demonstrated to be effective vasodilators in the treatment of heart failure, only captopril has been approved for this use in the United States at the time of this writing.

and the alpha-adrenergic blocking agents, act predominantly on the arterial bed and primarily increase stroke volume while others, such as nitroglycerin and isosorbide dinitrate, act almost entirely on the venous side of the circulation; the latter agents cause pooling of blood in the venous bed and act primarily to reduce ventricular filling pressures. Captopril, prazosin, and sodium nitroprusside are "balanced vasodilators" which act on both the arterial and venous beds. Some agents, such as sodium nitroprusside, must be administered by continuous intravenous infusion, nitroglycerin requires administration in ointment or patch form when a prolonged effect is desired, while isosorbide dinitrate is most effective when it is administered by the sublingual route.

The ideal vasodilator for the treatment of *acute* heart failure should have a rapid onset and brief duration of action when administered by intravenous infusion; sodium nitroprusside qualifies as such a drug, but its use requires careful monitoring of the intraarterial pressure and electrocardiogram, and if possible of the pulmonary artery wedge pressure, in an intensive care unit. For the treatment of chronic congestive heart failure, the agent should be effective on oral administration, and its action should persist for at least 6 h. Captopril (an angiotensin-converting enzyme inhibitor), hydralazine (a smooth muscle dilator), prazosin (an alpha-adrenergic blocking agent), and hydralazine (a direct relaxant of vascular smooth muscle) satisfy these requirements. It is advisable to commence therapy with very low doses in order to avoid hypotension and gradually increase them as needed and tolerated.

In view of the spectrum of actions of available vasodilators, the selection of the specific agent or combinations of agents for any given patient should depend on the pathophysiologic state. For example, when the primary defect is a reduction of cardiac output and/or mitral regurgitation, an arterial vasodilator such as hydralazine or minoxidil is the drug of choice; when pulmonary congestion is the principal problem, a venodilator would be preferable. When it is desired both to elevate cardiac output and to reduce pulmonary vascular pressures, an agent which acts both on the arterial and venous beds, such as captopril or prazosin, or the combination of hydralazine and a nitrate is indicated. Vasodilators are potent and effective in acutely improving the deranged hemodynamics of heart failure and there is some evidence in favor of a beneficial chronic effect as well. Some studies with captopril have demonstrated a favorable long-term reduction of symptoms and enhancement of exercise tolerance. It has been reported that the combination of hydralazine and isosorbide dinitrate prolong survival of patients with heart failure.

Vasodilators are ineffective, indeed they may even exert a deleterious action, in patients without heart failure (Fig. 182-1). Arterial dilators may produce postural hypotension with little effect on cardiac output. Venodilators lower arterial pressure and cardiac output in patients with normal cardiac function, and in patients with heart failure whose ventricular filling pressures have previously been restored to normal by diuretic therapy.

REFRACTORY HEART FAILURE   When the response to ordinary treatment is inadequate, heart failure is considered to be refractory. Before assuming that this state simply reflects advanced, perhaps preterminal, myocardial depression, careful consideration must be given to several possibilities: (1) an underlying and overlooked cause of the heart disease that may be amenable to specific surgical or medical therapy, such as silent aortic or mitral stenosis, constrictive pericarditis, infective endocarditis, hypertension, or thyrotoxicosis; (2) one or a combination of the precipitating causes of heart failure, such as pulmonary or urinary tract infection, recurrent pulmonary emboli, arterial hypoxemia, anemia, or arrhythmia; and (3) complications of overly vigorous therapy, such as digitalis intoxication, hypovolemia, or electrolyte imbalance.

Recognition and proper treatment of the aforementioned complications are likely to make the patient responsive to therapy again. Perhaps the most common complication results from overzealous treatment with diuretics. When administered too rapidly, these drugs can produce sudden hypovolemia before edema fluid can be mobilized to replace the loss of blood volume, the result being a shocklike state with evidence of systemic hypoperfusion in the presence of edema. The chronically excessively diuresed patient has exchanged the hazards of pulmonary edema and the inconvenience of systemic edema for a persistently depressed cardiac output with its associated weakness, lethargy, prerenal azotemia, and sometimes cardiac cachexia. Temporarily easing up on salt restriction and diuretic administration may overcome this difficulty, but as heart failure worsens, this course of action may lead to increased pulmonary congestion which is equally unacceptable.

Hyponatremia is a late manifestation of refractory heart failure. It, too, may be a complication of overaggressive diuresis leading to reduced glomerular filtration rate and decreased delivery of NaCl to the diluting sites in the distal tubule. Hyponatremia may also result from nonosmotic stimuli for the continued secretion of antidiuretic hormone. Therapy involves improvement of the cardiovascular status, if possible, as well as temporary cessation of diuretic therapy particularly of thiazides, and restriction of oral water intake. Hypertonic saline is very rarely indicated because total body sodium is usually elevated, not depressed.

The combination of an intravenously administered vasodilator, such as sodium nitroprusside, along with a potent sympathomimetic amine, such as dopamine or dobutamine, often results in an additive effect, raising cardiac output and lowering filling pressure. Intravenous amrinone, sometimes accompanied by oral captopril, may also be useful in patients with refractory heart failure. Once compensation is established, therapy can be continued with the combination of oral hydralazine or captopril to reduce afterload and one of the orally active nonglycoside inotropic agents, such as milrinone, a derivative of amrinone, which is available only for clinical investigation at the time of this writing.

Cardiac transplantation When patients with heart failure become unresponsive to a combination of all of the aforementioned therapeutic measures, are in New York Heart Association class IV, and are deemed unlikely to survive 1 year, they should be considered for cardiac transplantation. To qualify for this procedure, patients should be under 55 years of age, be stable psychologically, and possess a strong family support system. Contraindications include severe pulmonary hypertension, parenchymal lung disease, recent pulmonary emboli, active infection, insulin-requiring diabetes mellitus, and other diseases which may limit survival. As in renal transplantation (Chap. 221) the principal problem is graft rejection and the combination of cyclosporin A and corticosteroids has been helpful in reducing the severity of this complication; a second serious problem is infection as a consequence of the immunosuppression. In the hands of a skilled, experienced team, the 1-year survival rate is approximately 80 percent with a subsequent attrition of approximately 3 percent per year. The shortage of donor hearts and the enormous expense associated with this procedure have limited its application.

TREATMENT OF ACUTE PULMONARY EDEMA Pulmonary edema secondary to left ventricular failure or mitral stenosis is described in Chap. 26. It is life-threatening and must be considered a medical emergency. As is the case for the more chronic forms of heart failure, in the treatment of pulmonary edema, attention must be directed to identifying and removing any precipitating causes of decompensation, such as an arrhythmia or infection. However, because of the acute nature of the problem, a number of additional nonspecific measures are necessary. When possible, and if it does not delay treatment unduly, recording pulmonary vascular pressures through a Swan-Ganz catheter and intraarterial pressure directly is advisable. The first six measures listed below are ordinarily applied simultaneously.

1 Morphine is administered intravenously repetitively, as needed in doses from 2 to 5 mg. This drug reduces anxiety, reduces adrenergic vasoconstrictor stimuli to the arteriolar and venous beds, and thereby helps to break a vicious cycle. Naloxone should be available in case respiratory depression occurs.

2 Because the alveolar fluid interferes with oxygen diffusion, resulting in arterial hypoxemia, 100% oxygen should be administered, preferably under positive pressure. The latter increases intraalveolar pressure and therefore reduces transudation of fluid from the alveolar capillaries and impedes venous return to the thorax, reducing pulmonary capillary pressure.

3 The patient should be maintained in the sitting position, with the legs dangling along the side of the bed, if possible, which also tends to reduce venous return.

4 Intravenous loop diuretics, such as furosemide or ethacrynic acid (40 to 100 mg), or bumetanide (1 mg) will, by rapidly establishing a diuresis, reduce circulating blood volume and thereby hasten the relief of pulmonary edema. In addition when given intravenously, furosemide also exerts a venodilator action, reduces venous return, and reduces pulmonary edema even before the diuresis commences.

5 Afterload reduction is achieved with intravenous sodium nitroprusside at 20 to 30 μg/min in patients whose systolic arterial pressures exceed 100 mmHg.

6 If digitalis has not been administered previously, three-fourths of a full dose of a rapidly acting glycoside, such as ouabain, digoxin, or lanatoside C, should be administered intravenously.

7 Sometimes, aminophylline (theophylline ethylenediamine), 240 to 480 mg intravenously, is effective in diminishing bronchoconstriction, increasing renal blood flow and sodium excretion, and augmenting myocardial contractility.

8 If the above mentioned measures are not sufficient, rotating tourniquets should be applied to the extremities.

After these emergency therapeutic measures have been instituted, and the precipitating factors treated, the diagnosis of the underlying cardiac disorder responsible for the pulmonary edema must be established if it is not already known. After stabilization of the patient's condition a long-range strategy for prevention of future episodes of pulmonary edema must be established, and this may require surgical treatment.

PROGNOSIS

The prognosis in heart failure depends primarily on the nature of the underlying heart disease and on the presence or absence of a precipitating factor which can be treated. Also, the long-term prognosis for heart failure is most favorable when the underlying forms of heart disease can be treated. When one of the latter can be identified and removed, the outlook for immediate survival is far better than if heart failure occurs without any obvious precipitating cause. In the latter situation, median survival ranges between 6 months and 5 years depending on the severity of the heart failure. The prognosis can also be estimated by observing the response to treatment. When clinical improvement occurs with only modest dietary sodium restriction and small doses of diuretics or digitalis, then the outlook is far better than if, in addition to these measures, intensive diuretic therapy and vasodilators are necessary.

REFERENCES

ARNOLD SB et al: Long-term digitalis therapy improves left ventricular function in heart failure. N Engl J Med 303:1443, 1980

BERGER BE, WARNOCK DG: Mechanisms of action and clinical use of diuretics, in *The Kidney*, 3d ed, BM Brenner, FC Rector (eds). Philadelphia, Saunders, 1986, p 433

BRAUNWALD E (ed): Newer positive inotropic agents. Circulation 73(Suppl III):1, 1986

——— et al (eds): *Congestive Heart Failure: Current Research and Clinical Applications.* New York, Grune & Stratton, 1982

BRISTOW MR: The adrenergic nervous system in heart failure. N Engl J Med 311:850, 1984

CHERNIACK NS, LONGOBARDO GS: Cheyne-Stokes breathing: An instability in physiologic control. N Engl J Med 288:952, 1973

CREAGER MA et al: The acute and long-term effects of enalapril on the cardiovascular response to exercise tolerance in patients with congestive heart failure. J Am Coll Cardio 6:163, 1985

DZAU VJ et al: Angiotensin converting enzyme inhibition in the treatment of congestive heart failure and hypertension, in *Update IV: Harrison's Principles of Internal Medicine*, KJ Isselbacher et al (eds). New York, McGraw-Hill, 1982, p 137

FISCH C (guest ed): An account of the foxglove and some of its medical uses: 1785–1985. J Am Coll Cardiol 5 (Suppl A):1A, 1985

GOODMAN LS, GILMAN A (eds): Cardiovascular drugs, in *The Pharmacological Basis of Therapeutics,* 7th ed. New York, Macmillan, 1985, pp 716, 887

HUMPHREYS MH, RECTOR FC JR: Pathophysiology of edema formation, in *The Kidney: Physiology and Pathophysiology,* 2d ed, DW Seldin, G Giebisch (eds). New York, Raven Press, 1985, p 1163

ISKANDRIAN AS, HAKKI A-H, MATTLEMAN SJ: Predicting left ventricular function: Bedside examination. Prim Cardiol (Suppl) 10:3A, 1984

LEE WH, PACKER M: Prognostic importance of serum sodium concentration and its modification by converting-enzyme inhibition in patients with severe chronic heart failure. Circulation 73:257, 1986

MAKABALI C et al: Dobutamine and other sympathomimetic drugs for the treatment of low cardiac output failure. Semin Anesth 1:63, 1982

SMITH TW (ed): *Digitalis Glycosides.* New York, Grune & Stratton, 1986

——, BRAUNWALD E: Management of heart failure, in *Heart Disease,* 2d ed, E Braunwald (ed). Philadelphia, Saunders, 1984, p 503

SUKI WN et al: Physiology of diuretic action, in *The Kidney: Physiology and Pathophysiology,* 2d ed, DW Seldin, G Giebisch (eds). New York, Raven Press, 1985, p 2127

---

183   THE BRADYARRHYTHMIAS

MARK E. JOSEPHSON / ALFRED E. BUXTON / FRANCIS E. MARCHLINSKI

ANATOMY OF THE CONDUCTING SYSTEM   Under normal conditions the pacemaker function of the heart resides in the sinoatrial node which lies at the junction of the right atrium and superior vena cava. The node is approximately 1½ cm long and 2 to 3 mm wide and is supplied by the sinus node artery, which arises from either the right coronary artery (60 percent of cases) or the left circumflex coronary artery (40 percent). Once the impulse exits the sinus node and perinodal tissue, it traverses the atrium until it reaches the atrioventricular (AV) node, whose blood supply is derived from the posterior descending coronary artery in 90 percent of cases and which lies at the base of the interatrial septum just above the tricuspid annulus and anterior to the coronary sinus. The electrophysiologic properties of the AV node result in slow conduction, which is responsible for the normal delay in AV conduction, i.e., the PR interval.

The bundle of His emerges from the AV node, enters the fibrous skeleton of the heart, and courses anteriorly across the membranous interventricular septum. It has a dual blood supply from the AV nodal artery and a branch of the anterior descending coronary artery. The branching (distal) portion of the bundle of His gives rise to a broad sheet of fibers which course over the left side of the interven-

tricular septum to form the left bundle branch and a narrow, cablelike structure on the right side to form the right bundle branch. The arborization of both the right and left bundle branches gives rise to the distal His-Purkinje system, which ultimately extends throughout the endocardium of the right and left ventricles.

The sinus node, atrium, and AV node are significantly influenced by autonomic tone. Vagal influences depress automaticity of the sinus node, depress conduction, and prolong refractoriness in the perinodal tissue surrounding the sinus node and prolong AV nodal conduction and refractoriness. Sympathetic influences exert the opposite effect.

ELECTROPHYSIOLOGIC PRINCIPLES

In the resting state, the interior of most cardiac cells, with the exception of the sinus and AV nodes, is approximately 80- to 90-mV negative with respect to a reference extracellular electrode. The resting membrane potential is primarily determined by the concentration gradient of potassium across the cell membrane. Activation of cardiac cells results from movement of ions across the cell membrane, causing a transient depolarization known as the *action potential.* The ionic species responsible for the action potential vary among the cardiac tissues, and the configuration of the action potential is therefore unique to each tissue (Fig. 183-1).

The action potential of the bundle of His–Purkinje system and ventricular myocardium has five phases (Fig. 183-2). The rapid depolarizing current (phase 0) is mainly determined by an influx of sodium into myocardial cells with a secondary, slower, influx of calcium. The repolarization phases of the action potential (phases 1 to 3) are primarily related to outward potassium flux. The resting membrane potential is phase 4.

The bradyarrhythmias result from abnormalities either of impulse formation, i.e., automaticity, or of conduction. *Automaticity,* which is normally observed in the sinus node, the specialized fibers of the His-Purkinje system, and some specialized atrial fibers, is the property of a cardiac cell to depolarize spontaneously during phase 4 of the action potential, leading to the generation of an impulse. To exhibit automaticity the resting membrane potential must decrease spontaneously until threshold potential is reached and an all-or-none regenerative response occurs. The ionic components producing spontaneous diastolic depolarization appear to involve the inward current of either sodium or calcium. The velocity of conduction, i.e., impulse propagation through cardiac tissues, is influenced by the rate of rise and amplitude of phase 0 of the action potential. The more positive the threshold potential and the slower the rate of depolarization

FIGURE 183-1 *Action potential configurations in different regions of the mammalian heart. (From AM Katz:* Physiology of the Heart, *New York, Raven Press, 1977.)*

FIGURE 183-2 *Schematic representation of the action potential in normal ventricle depicting the direction, strength, and period of flow of the ionic currents underlying the action potential. The arrows' direction and size indicate whether current is inward- or outward-directed and the approximate current strength, respectively, of the ion identified at the arrow's base. The horizontal position of the arrow corresponds to the same moment in the time course of action potential (see text). The five phases of the action potential are indicated by the numerals placed next to the corresponding portion of the waveform. (Originally published in Ten Eick et al: Ventricular dysrhythmia: Membrane basis or currents, channels, gates, and cables, in Progress in Cardiovascular Diseases, vol XXIV, no 2, pp 157–188. New York, Grune & Stratton, 1981, by permission.)*

toward threshold, the slower the rate of rise of phase 0 of the action potential and the slower the conduction velocity. Disease states or drugs may result in lower rates of rise of phase 0 at any given membrane potential.

Refractoriness is a property of cardiac cells which defines the period of recovery that cells require before they can be reexcited by a stimulus after being discharged. The *absolute refractory period* is defined by that portion of the action potential during which no stimulus, regardless of its strength, can evoke another response. The *effective refractory period* is that part of the action potential at which time a stimulus can only evoke a local nonpropagated response. The *relative refractory period* extends from the end of the effective refractory period to the time that the tissue is fully recovered. During this time a stimulus of greater than threshold strength is required to evoke a response which is propagated more slowly than normal. After completion of the action potential, excitability recovers and evoked responses have characteristics similar to the spontaneous normal response.

INTRACARDIAC RECORDINGS OF THE SPECIALIZED CONDUCTING SYSTEM Electrode catheters allow the recording of activation of portions of the specialized conducting system including the bundle of His. To obtain a recording from the bundle of His the electrode catheter is positioned across the tricuspid valve (Fig. 183-3). The interval from local atrial depolarization in the His bundle recording to the onset of depolarization of the His bundle deflection is called the AH interval (normal = 60 to 125 ms) and represents an indirect method of assessing AV nodal conduction time. The interval from the beginning of the His bundle deflection to the earliest onset of ventricular activation, as measured from any of the multiple-surface electrocardiogram (ECG) leads or the intracardiac ventricular electrogram (the HV interval, normal = 35 to 55 ms), represents conduction time through the His-Purkinje system. Electrode catheters can be positioned in the area of the sinus node to record high right atrial activity. Left atrial activity may be recorded directly via a catheter placed across a patent foramen ovale, or indirectly using a catheter inserted into the coronary sinus. The atrial activation sequence may be ''mapped,'' and sites of intra- and interatrial conduction abnormalities may be ascertained.

SINUS NODE DYSFUNCTION

The sinus node is normally the dominant cardiac pacemaker because its intrinsic discharge rate is the fastest of all potential cardiac pacemakers. Its responsiveness to alterations in autonomic nervous

system tone is responsible for the normal acceleration of heart rate during exercise and the slowing which occurs during rest and sleep. Increases in sinus rate normally result from an increase in sympathetic tone acting via beta-adrenergic receptors and/or a decrease in parasympathetic tone acting via muscarinic receptors; slowing of the heart rate is normally due to opposite alterations. In adults, the normal sinus rate under basal conditions is 60 to 100 beats per minute. Sinus bradycardia is said to exist when the sinus rate is less than 60 beats

FIGURE 183-3 *Normal intracardiac recording. Surface ECG leads I, II, and V_1 are displayed with intracardiac ECGs from the high right atrium (HRA), left atrium from the coronary sinus (CS), and AV junction to obtain a His bundle electrogram (HBE). T = time lines. Atrial activation begins in the high right atrium and spreads inferiorly to the low atrial septum as recorded in the HBE and left atrium as recorded in the CS. The AH and HV intervals represent AV nodal and His-Purkinje conduction time, respectively. Vertical lines = 0.10 s. (From Josephson and Seides.)*

per minute, and sinus tachycardia when it exceeds 100 per minute. However, there is wide variation among individuals, and rates less than 60 per minute do not necessarily indicate pathologic states. For example, trained athletes often exhibit resting rates under 50 per minute due to increases in vagal tone. Elderly patients may also show marked sinus bradycardia at rest consequent to decreases in the intrinsic heart rate with age.

ETIOLOGY Sinus node dysfunction most often is found in the elderly as an isolated phenomenon. Although interruption of the blood supply to the sinus node may produce dysfunction, the correlation between sinus node artery obstruction and clinical sinus node dysfunction is poor. Specific disease states associated with sinus node dysfunction include senile amyloidosis and other conditions associated with infiltration of the atrial myocardium. Sinus bradycardia is associated with hypothyroidism, advanced liver disease, hypothermia, typhoid fever, and brucellosis. Sinus bradycardia occurs during episodes of hypervagotonia (vasovagal syncope), severe hypoxia, hypercapnia, acidemia, and acute hypertension. However, in most cases of sinus node dysfunction a specific cause cannot be identified.

MANIFESTATIONS Although marked sinus bradycardia (<50 beats per minute) may cause fatigue and other symptoms due to inadequate cardiac output, more commonly sinus node dysfunction is manifested as paroxysmal dizziness, presyncope, or syncope. These symptoms usually result from abrupt, prolonged sinus pauses caused by failure of sinus impulse formation (sinus arrest) or block of conduction of sinus impulses to the surrounding atrial tissue (sinus exit block). In either case, the ECG manifestation is a prolonged period (>3 s) of atrial asystole. In some patients sinus node dysfunction is accompanied by abnormalities in AV conduction. In addition to the absence of atrial activity, lower pacemakers fail to emerge during the sinus pauses, resulting in periods of ventricular asystole and syncope. Occasionally, sinus node dysfunction is manifested initially by the failure of the sinus rate to accelerate in response to conditions such as exercise or fever, which normally cause increases in the sinus rate. In some people sinus node dysfunction may become manifest only in the presence of certain cardioactive drugs: cardiac glycosides, beta-adrenergic blocking drugs, quinidine and other antiarrhythmic agents, and verapamil or diltiazem. These agents, which do not cause sinus node dysfunction in otherwise normal people, may unmask evidence of sinus node dysfunction in susceptible individuals.

The *sick-sinus syndrome* refers to a combination of symptoms (dizziness, confusion, fatigue, syncope, and congestive heart failure) caused by sinus node dysfunction and manifested by marked sinus bradycardia, sinoatrial block, or sinus arrest. Because these symptoms are nonspecific and because ECG manifestation of sinus node dysfunction are not infrequently intermittent, it may be difficult to prove that such symptoms are actually caused by sinus node dysfunction.

Atrial tachyarrhythmias such as atrial fibrillation, flutter, or atrial tachycardia may be accompanied by sinus node dysfunction. The *bradycardia-tachycardia syndrome* refers to the combination of paroxysmal atrial arrhythmias which upon termination is followed by prolonged sinus pauses (Fig. 183-4) or in which there are alternating periods of tachyarrhythmias and bradyarrhythmias. Syncope or pre-

syncope may result from failure of the sinus node to recover function following suppression of automaticity by atrial tachyarrhythmias.

DIAGNOSIS AND EVALUATION First-degree *sinoatrial exit block* denotes a prolonged conduction time from the sinus node to the surrounding atrial tissue. It cannot be recognized on a standard (surface) ECG but requires invasive intracardiac recordings (see below). Second-degree sinoatrial exit block denotes the intermittent failure of conduction of sinus impulses to the surrounding atrial tissue; it is manifested as the intermittent absence of P waves (Fig. 183-5). Third-degree, or complete, sinoatrial block is characterized by a lack of atrial activity or by an ectopic subsidiary atrial pacemaker. On the standard ECG, it cannot be distinguished from sinus arrest, but direct intracardiac recordings of sinus node activity permit this distinction. The bradycardia-tachycardia syndrome is manifested on the standard ECG as inappropriate (>3 s) pauses in sinus activity following spontaneous cessation of tachyarrhythmias (Fig. 183-4). Most often these are atrial flutter or fibrillation, although any tachycardia with retrograde conduction to the atria may cause overdrive suppression of the sinus node, resulting in clinical appearance of this syndrome.

The most important step in the diagnosis is to correlate symptoms with ECG evidence of sinus node dysfunction. While ambulatory ECG (Holter) monitoring remains a mainstay in evaluating sinus node function, most episodes of syncope are paroxysmal and unpredictable. Single and even multiple 24-h Holter monitor recordings may fail to include a symptomatic episode. Therefore, noting the response to carotid sinus pressure and pharmacologic autonomic "denervation" of the heart is frequently helpful. Carotid sinus pressure is particularly useful in patients in whom paroxysmal dizziness or syncope is compatible with the hypersensitive carotid sinus syndrome (see Chap. 12). In such patients, the response can be dramatic, and sinus pauses in excess of 5 s may occur. Normally a sinus pause of ≤3 s results from 5 s of unilateral carotid sinus massage. If atropine can prevent the effects of carotid sinus pressure, autonomic dysfunction, not primary sinus node dysfunction, is responsible. The other noninvasive test of sinus node function involves the use of pharmacologic agents to manipulate the autonomic nervous system and assess the balance of parasympathetic and sympathetic activity on the sinus node. Vagomimetic (Valsalva maneuver or phenylephrine-induced hypertension) and vagolytic (atropine) agents as well as sympathomimetic (isoproterenol or hypotension by nitroprusside) and beta-adrenergic blocking agents can be utilized, singly and in combination. These studies are designed to test the response of the sinus node to autonomic stimulation and inhibition and thereby characterize the status of autonomic regulation of the sinus node. Abnormalities of the autonomic control of sinus function are particularly common in patients in whom the only presenting arrhythmias are sinus bradycardia.

Intrinsic heart rate This is a manifestation of the primary activity of the sinus node, and its determination requires chemical denervation of the heart. Complete autonomic blockade is achieved with 0.2 mg/kg propranolol intravenously, followed after 10 min by 0.04 mg/kg of atropine sulfate intravenously. Normal values of intrinsic heart rate = 118.1 − (0.57 × age) beats per min. The use of autonomic blockade can separate patients with asymptomatic sinus bradycardia into a group with primary sinus node dysfunction (slow intrinsic heart rate) and a group with autonomic imbalance (normal intrinsic heart rate). Autonomic blockade is particularly useful when combined with invasive assessment of sinus node function (see below). Autonomic blockade may depress conduction in patients with intrinsic disease of the conduction system and should be carried out only in a setting where arrhythmias can be monitored and rapidly treated.

FIGURE 183-4 *Tachycardia-bradycardia syndrome. Rhythm strip of ECG lead II showing spontaneous cessation of supraventricular tachycardia followed by a 5.6-s pause prior to resumption of sinus activity. The patient was asymptomatic during supraventricular tachycardia, but the sinus pause caused severe lightheadedness.*

FIGURE 183-5 *Second-degree sinoatrial exit block. Surface ECG denoting abrupt absence of P wave during sinus rhythm. Prior to the pause the sinus rate is regular. The interval of the pause is exactly twice the basal sinus cycle length.*

Sinus node recovery time Sinus node recovery time is evaluated by assessing the response of the sinus node to rapid atrial pacing (Fig. 183-6). When atrial pacing is discontinued, a pause, the *sinus node recovery time,* occurs prior to resumption of spontaneous sinus rhythm. When the sinus recovery time is prolonged, the results of this test mimic the prolonged sinus pauses seen following termination of atrial tachyarrhythmias in the bradycardia-tachycardia syndrome (see Fig. 183-4). The corrected sinus node recovery time (sinus recovery time − sinus cycle length) normally is less than 550 ms, and the uncorrected sinus node recovery time less than 150 percent of the spontaneous cycle length. In patients with sinus node dysfunction, prolongation of the sinus node recovery time is often observed. Marked prolongation of the sinus node recovery time is rare in the absence of symptoms. Patients with abnormally slow intrinsic heart rates usually have abnormal sinus node recovery times, while those with normal intrinsic heart rates have normal recovery times.

Sinoatrial conduction time Determination of the conduction time from the sinus node to the atrium allows for the differentiation of abnormalities of sinoatrial conduction from abnormalities of sinus impulse formation. The conduction time equals one-half of the pause following termination of brief periods of pacing, minus the sinus cycle length. Alternatively, the sinus node electrogram can be recorded directly by a catheter electrode placed near the sinoatrial node.

EVALUATION Electrophysiologic investigation of sinus node dysfunction should be undertaken in patients who have had symptoms compatible with sinus node dysfunction and in whom no documentation of the arrhythmia responsible for these symptoms has been obtained by prolonged Holter monitoring. Asymptomatic patients with sinus bradycardia need not be tested since no therapy is indicated. Similarly, symptomatic patients with ECG documentation of asystole, sinoatrial block or arrest, or the bradycardia-tachycardia syndrome do not require electrophysiologic tests for diagnosis. However, in symptomatic patients *without* documentation of an arrhythmia, elec-

trophysiologic assessment of sinus node function can yield information which may be used to guide appropriate therapy. Electrophysiologic studies may also be useful in assessing the effects of pharmacologic therapy. If a pacemaker is indicated, the site of pacemaker implantation for maximum hemodynamic effects can be guided by the results of electrophysiologic investigation. However, the results of tests of sinus node function must be interpreted with caution. Sinus node dysfunction coexists frequently with other disorders such as AV conduction disturbances or ventricular tachycardia which may cause symptoms such as syncope. Thus, electrophysiologic evaluation of patients with symptoms such as undiagnosed syncope must not stop with the demonstration of abnormalities of sinus node dysfunction or carotid sinus hypersensitivity. Instead, complete evaluation, including programmed atrial and ventricular stimulation (see Chap. 184) is necessary to search for additional electrophysiologic abnormalities which could be responsible for symptoms.

TREATMENT Permanent pacemakers (page 922) are the mainstay of therapy for patients with symptomatic sinus node dysfunction. Patients with intermittent paroxysms of bradycardia or sinus arrest and with the cardioinhibitory form of the hypersensitive carotid sinus syndrome are usually adequately treated by demand ventricular pacemakers. These devices are reliable, relatively inexpensive, and suffice to prevent episodic symptoms due to abrupt bradycardia. Patients with symptomatic chronic sinus bradycardia or frequent prolonged episodes of sinus node dysfunction may do better with dual-chamber pacemakers that preserve the normal AV activation sequence. Although theoretically an atrial demand pacemaker should be adequate for patients with sinus node dysfunction, the frequent accompaniment of dysfunction in other portions of the cardiac conduction system and its progressive nature usually mandates placement of a pacemaker capable of ventricular pacing.

FIGURE 183-6 *Example of sinus node recovery time in a patient with symptomatic sinus node dysfunction. Cessation of atrial pacing at 150 beats per minutes (cycle length, 400 ms) results in a prolonged sinus pause. Surface ECG leads I, II, III, V_1, and V_6, are shown in addition to intracardiac recordings at the high right atrium (A) and His bundle (H). T = time lines.*

AV CONDUCTION DISTURBANCES

The specialized cardiac conducting system normally assures synchronous conduction of each sinus impulse from the atria to the ventricles. Abnormalities of conduction of the sinus impulse to the ventricles may portend the development of heart block, which can ultimately lead to syncope or cardiac arrest. In order to evaluate the clinical significance of conduction abnormalities the physician must determine (1) the site of conduction disturbance, (2) the risk of progression to complete block, and (3) the probability that a subsidiary escape rhythm arising distal to the site of block will be electrophysiologically and hemodynamically stable. This latter point is perhaps the most important since the rate and stability of the escape pacemaker determine what symptoms result from heart block. The escape pacemaker following AV nodal block is in the His bundle, which generally has a stable rate of 40 to 60 beats per minute and is associated with a QRS complex of normal duration (in the absence of a preexisting intraventricular conduction defect). This contrasts with escape rhythms arising in the distal His-Purkinje system, which have lower intrinsic rates (25 to 40 beats per minute), manifest QRS complexes with prolonged duration, and are unstable. Although prolonged QRS complexes are invariable when the distal His-Purkinje pacemakers form the escape mechanism, wide QRS complexes can

also coexist with AV nodal block and a His bundle rhythm. Therefore, QRS morphology alone may not be adequate to identify the site of block.

ETIOLOGY   The AV node is heavily supplied by the parasympathetic and sympathetic nervous systems and is sensitive to variations in autonomic tone. Chronic AV nodal dysfunction may be seen in highly trained athletes with hypervagotonia. A variety of diseases can also influence AV nodal conduction. These include acute processes, such as myocardial infarction (particularly inferior); coronary spasm (usually of the right coronary artery); digitalis intoxication; excesses of beta and/or calcium blockers; acute infections such as viral myocarditis; acute rheumatic fever; infectious mononucleosis; and miscellaneous disorders such as Lyme disease, sarcoidosis, amyloidosis, and neoplasms, particularly cardiac mesotheliomas. AV nodal block may also be congenital.

Two degenerative diseases are commonly responsible for damage to the specialized conducting system and produce AV block usually associated with bundle branch block (see Chap. 178). In *Lev's disease,* there is calcification and sclerosis of the fibrous cardiac skeleton, which frequently involves the aortic and mitral valves, the central fibrous body, and the summit of the ventricular septum. *Lenegre's disease* appears to be a primary sclerodegenerative disease

FIGURE 183-7 *A. Mobitz type I second-degree AV block. Intracardiac recordings of AV Wenckebach demonstrate that the PR prolongation (320, 615 ms) is localized to the AV node (AH 240, 535 ms, respectively). HBE = His bundle electrogram; A = atrium; H = His; V = ventricle. (Adapted*

from Josephson and Seides.) B. Mobitz type II second-degree AV block. Intracardiac recordings document block below the His bundle. HBE = His bundle electrogram; A = atrium; H = His; V = ventricle.

within the conducting system itself without involving the myocardium or fibrous skeleton of the heart. These latter two diseases are probably the most common causes of isolated chronic heart block in adults. Hypertension and aortic and/or mitral stenosis are specific disorders which either accelerate the degeneration of the conducting system or have a direct effect by calcification and fibrosis of the conducting system.

First-degree AV block, more properly termed prolonged AV conduction, is characterized by a PR interval >0.20 s. Since the PR interval is determined by atrial, AV nodal, and His-Purkinje activation, delay in any one or more of these structures can contribute to a prolonged PR interval. In the presence of a QRS complex of normal duration, a PR interval >0.24 s almost invariably is due to a delay within the AV node. If the QRS is prolonged, delays may be present at any of the levels mentioned above. Delay within the His-Purkinje system is always accompanied by prolonged QRS duration in addition to a prolonged PR interval. However, as indicated below, it is only with intracardiac recordings that the exact site of delay can be determined.

Second-degree heart block (intermittent AV block) is present when some trial impulses fail to conduct to the ventricles. Mobitz type I second-degree AV block (AV Wenckebach block) is characterized by progressive PR-interval prolongation prior to block of an atrial impulse (Fig. 183-7A). The pause that follows is less than fully compensatory (i.e., is less than two normal sinus intervals), and the PR of the first conducted impulse is shorter than the last conducted atrial impulse prior to the blocked P wave. This type of block is almost always localized to the AV node and associated with a normal QRS duration. It is most often seen as a transient abnormality with inferior wall infarction or with drug intoxication, particularly digitalis, beta blockers, and occasionally calcium channel antagonists. This type of block can also be observed in normal individuals with heightened vagal tone. Although Mobitz type I block can progress to complete heart block, this is uncommon. Even when it does, however, the heart block is usually well tolerated because the escape pacemaker usually arises in the proximal His bundle and provides a stable rhythm. As a result, the presence of Mobitz type I second-degree AV block usually does not mandate aggressive therapy. Therapeutic decisions depend upon the ventricular response and the symptoms of the patient. If the ventricular rate is adequate and the patient is asymptomatic, observation is sufficient.

In Mobitz type II second-degree AV block, conduction fails suddenly and unexpectedly without a preceding change in PR intervals (Fig. 183-7B). It is usually due to disease of the His-Purkinje system and is most often associated with a prolonged QRS complex. It is important to recognize this type of block since it has a high incidence of progression to complete heart block with an unstable, slow, lower

escape pacemaker. Therefore, pacemaker implantation is necessary in this condition. Mobitz type II block may occur in the setting of anteroseptal infarction or in the primary or secondary sclerodegenerative or calcific disorders of the fibrous skeleton of the heart.

In 2:1 block, intracardiac recordings are necessary in order to ascertain the site of the conduction disturbance because the typical ECG features of Mobitz type 1 or Mobitz type 2 block cannot be discerned during a 2:1 pattern of AV conduction on the surface ECG. In so-called high-degree AV block there are periods of two or more consecutively blocked P waves. Regardless of the site of origin of the escape rhythm, if it is slow and the patient is symptomatic, a cardiac pacemaker is mandatory.

Third-degree AV block is present when no atrial impulse propagates to the ventricles. If the QRS complex of the escape rhythm is of normal duration and occurs at a rate of 40 to 55 beats per minute and increases with atropine or exercise, AV nodal block is probable. Congenital complete AV block is usually localized to the AV node (Fig. 183-8). If the block is within the His bundle, the escape pacemaker usually is less responsive to these perturbations. If the escape rhythm of the QRS is wide and associated with rates ≤40, block is usually localized in, or distal to, the His bundle and mandates a pacemaker since the escape rhythm in this setting is unreliable.

AV DISSOCIATION AV dissociation exists whenever the atria and ventricles are under the control of two separate pacemakers and, while present in complete AV block, can occur in the absence of a primary conduction disturbance. AV dissociation *unrelated* to heart block may occur under two circumstances: (1) an AV junctional rhythm in response to severe sinus bradycardia. When the sinus rate and the escape rate are similar and the P waves occur just before, in, or following the QRS, *isorhythmic AV dissociation* is said to be present. Treatment usually consists of removal of the offending cause of sinus bradycardia (i.e., discontinuation of digitalis, beta blockers, or calcium antagonists), accelerating the sinus node by vagolytic agents, or insertion of a pacemaker if the escape rhythm is slow and results in symptoms. (2) AV dissociation can be caused by an enhanced lower (junctional or ventricular) pacemaker which competes with normal sinus rhythm and frequently exceeds it. This has been called *interference AV dissociation* because the rapid lower pacemaker results in bombardment of the AV node in a retrograde fashion, rendering it refractory to the normal sinus impulses. Thus failure of antegrade conduction is a physiologic response in this circumstance, which commonly occurs during ventricular tachycardia, digitalis intoxication, myocardial ischemia and/or infarction, or local irritation

FIGURE 183-8 *Third-degree AV block. Complete heart block with a slow, wide complex escape rhythm is present. Block in this instance is usually intra-His. See text.*

following cardiac surgery. The accelerated rhythm should be treated with either antiarrhythmic drugs (see Chap. 184), removal of the offending drug, or correction of the metabolic abnormality.

INTRACARDIAC ELECTROCARDIOGRAPHIC RECORDINGS IN DIAGNOSIS AND MANAGEMENT   The main therapeutic decision in patients with AV conduction disturbance is whether or not a permanent pacemaker is required, and a number of circumstances exist in which His bundle electrocardiography can provide a useful diagnostic tool upon which to base this decision. It is unquestionable that patients with symptomatic second- or third-degree AV block should be paced, and therefore these patients do not require electrophysiologic study. However, intracardiac ECG recordings can be useful in at least the following four groups of patients:

1 Patients with syncope and bundle branch block without documentation of AV block. In such patients the demonstration of marked infra-His conduction disturbances, i.e., a prolonged HV interval (>80 ms) may usually be taken as an indication of the need for the insertion of a permanent pacemaker. With intervals ranging from 55 to 80 ms, the indications for pacing are equivocal. In this group observation appears most reasonable for those patients with normal HV intervals (<55 ms).

2 Patients with bundle branch block and second-degree AV block. When such patients are symptomatic, intracardiac recordings may demonstrate that AV nodal block, intra-His block, infra-His block, or combinations of block may be responsible. A finding that suggests an infra-His lesion is the presence of alternating bundle branch block associated with changing PR intervals. Intracardiac recordings in such patients show that when block is present in these patients, it is almost always in the His-Purkinje system. The finding of infra-His block in patients with asymptomatic second-degree AV block mandates pacemaker therapy because of the high likelihood of their developing symptomatic high-grade AV block and syncope.

3 Asymptomatic patients with third-degree AV block. In such patients electrophysiologic studies may be useful in assessing the stability of the junctional pacemaker. Pacing is indicated when the His bundle escape pacemaker is shown to be unstable by an inadequate response to excercise, atropine, or isoproterenol or by a prolonged junctional recovery time following ventricular pacing.

4 Patients with bundle branch block, particularly bifascicular block (see Chap. 178). Intracardiac recordings may be helpful in predicting whether these patients are at increased risk of developing AV block. HV intervals, even in excess of 80 ms, are not predictive of subsequent intra-His block. However, patients who have *extremely prolonged* HV intervals, i.e., >100 ms, and those in whom alternating bundle branch block is associated with changing HV intervals frequently develop complete AV block; therefore, these findings necessitate insertion of a pacemaker. Block below the His bundle developing during atrial pacing at rates of less than 150 beats per minute and the development of an infra-His block or HV prolongation >100 ms following 1 g procainamide intravenously also signify that the patient is at high risk for the development of subsequent AV block and that a pacemaker is indicated. The frequency of these findings is low so their widespread use may not be cost effective.

PACEMAKERS IN THE MANAGEMENT OF BRADYARRHYTHMIAS

External energy sources can be used to stimulate the heart when disorders in impulse formation and/or transmission occur, leading to symptomatic bradyarrhythmias. Pacer stimuli can be applied to the atria and/or ventricles.

TEMPORARY PACING   This is usually instituted to provide immediate stabilization prior to permanent pacemaker placement or to provide pacemaker support when a bradycardia is precipitated by a transient event such as ischemia or drug toxicity. Temporary pacing is usually achieved by the transvenous insertion of an electrode catheter with the catheter positioned in the right ventricular apex and attached to an external generator. This procedure is associated with a small risk of cardiac perforation, infection at the insertion site, and thromboembolism; the risk of the latter two complications increases markedly after 48 h. The development of an entirely external transthoracic cardiac pacing system may preclude the need for transvenous pacing in selected patients. However, occasional failure of venticular capture and significant discomfort related to the large current required for effective transthoracic ventricular stimulation precludes the uniform use of this approach.

PERMANENT PACING   This mode of pacing is instituted for persistent or intermittent symptomatic bradycardia not related to a self-limiting precipitating factor or for documented infranodal second- or third-degree AV block. Permanent pacing leads are usually inserted transvenously through the subclavian vein with the leads positioned in the right atrial appendage for atrial pacing and the right ventricular apex for ventricular pacing. The leads are then attached to the pulse generator, which is inserted into a subcutaneous pocket below the clavicle. Epicardial lead placement is used when: (1) transvenous access cannot be obtained; (2) the chest is already open, i.e., in the course of a cardiac operation; and (3) if adequate endocardial lead placement cannot be achieved. Two separate leads must be placed if both atrial and ventricular chambers are to be sensed and/or paced.

Most pacemaker generators are powered by lithium batteries. The life expectancy of the generator is related to (1) current output required for capture; (2) requirements for incessant or intermittent pacing; and (3) the number of cardiac chambers paced. Life expectancy of the simple ventricular demand pacemaker can exceed 10 years.

PACING CODE   A code consisting of three to five letters has been developed for describing pacemaker type and function. The first letter indicates the chamber(s) paced and is designated V for ventricular pacing, A for atrial pacing, or D for dual chamber (both atrial and ventricular) pacing. The second letter indicates the chamber in which electrical activity is sensed and is also indicated by A, V, or D. An additional designation, O, has been used when pacemaker discharge is not dependent on a sensed electrical activity. The third letter refers to the response to a sensed electrical signal: O represents no response to an underlying electrical signal, usually related to the absence of associated sensing function; I represents inhibition of pacing function; T represents triggering of pacing function; and D indicates a dual response, i.e., spontaneous atrial and ventricular activity inhibiting atrial and ventricular pacing and atrial activity triggering a ventricular response. Additional fourth and fifth letters of the pacing code have been recommended to indicate whether the pacemaker is programmable and whether special antitachycardia functions are available. It follows from the described code that the standard VVI (ventricular demand pacemaker) can sense the ventricle, pace the ventricle, and be inhibited by sensed spontaneous ventricular activity, while the DDD pulse generator is capable of sensing and pacing both the atrium and ventricle and has a dual response to sensed atrial and ventricular activity.

Selection of the appropriate pacemaker and pacing mode depends on the clinical condition and the type of bradyarrhythmia being treated. The two most common pacing mode selections are DDD and VVI. DDD, or so-called universal pacing, provides AV sequential pacing which is ideally suited for the relatively young and active patient who has intact sinus node function or intermittent dysfunction and high-grade persistent or intermittent AV block. The DDD mode will allow physiologic atrial sensed and ventricular paced rates and improved exercise tolerance. AV synchrony and dual chamber pacing may also be desirable in patients with borderline hemodynamic reserve who are dependent on the atrial contribution to cardiac output and in those patients who develop the pacemaker syndrome (see below) in response to ventricular demand pacing. The DDD pacing mode is contraindicated in chronic atrial fibrillation or flutter and

TABLE 183-1   Programmable pacemaker functions

Rate*
Energy output
Sensitivity
Lead polarity
Hysteresis
Refractory period
Mode of function
AV Delay

* Lower-end upper rate limits apply to dual-chamber pacing.

atrial asystole. In these situations, ventricular demand (VVI) pacing is indicated. The DDD pacing mode may also be contraindicated in patients with intermittent or persistent ventriculoatrial (VA) conduction, who may develop pacemaker-mediated tachycardia (see below).

PROGRAMMABILITY OF PACEMAKERS   This allows for modification of pacing function after implantation and thereby for adaptation to changes in clinical needs. Pacemaker programming is accomplished by activation of the programming head positioned over the implanted pulse generator after making the desired changes in programmable parameters (Table 183-1). A radiofrequency system is routinely used to communicate the program to the pacemaker.

COMPLICATIONS   Adverse effects of permanent pacing are usually associated with failure or malfunction of the pacing system. These problems are usually secondary to over- or undersensing, output failure, and/or lead fracture or displacement. Two other problems may occur. The *pacemaker syndrome* consists of fatigue, dizziness, syncope, and distressing pulsations in the neck and chest and can be related to adverse hemodynamic effects of ventricular pacing. The pathophysiologic contributors to the pacemaker syndrome include (1) loss of atrial contribution to ventricular systole; (2) vasodepressor reflex initiated by cannon *a* waves; (3) systemic and pulmonary venous regurgitation due to atrial contraction against a closed AV valve. The symptoms associated with the pacemaker syndrome can be obviated by maintaining AV synchrony by dual chamber pacing or, in the case of a ventricular demand pacemaker, by programming an escape rate 15 to 20 beats per minute below that of the paced rate. The second major problem peculiar to dual chamber pacemakers is the development of *pacemaker-mediated tachycardia*, which is caused by ventriculoatrial conduction. In this instance, retrograde depolarization of the atria, resulting from a premature ventricular depolarization or a paced ventricular complex, is sensed and leads to subsequent triggering of ventricular pacing. This, in turn, can result in repetition of the phenomenon of ventriculoatrial conduction with the development of an endless-loop, pacemaker-mediated tachycardia. It may be corrected by programming the atrial refractory period.

REFERENCES

AUSTIN JL et al: Analysis of pacemaker malfunction and complications of temporary pacing in the coronary care unit. Am J Cardiol 49:301, 1982

BECKER AE et al: Functional anatomy of the cardiac conducting system, in *Cardiac Arrhythmias, A Decade of Progress*, DC Harrison (ed). Boston, G.K. Hall, 1981

CHUNG EK: Sick sinus syndrome: Current views. Mod Concepts Cardiovasc Dis 49:61, 1980

FURMAN S: Newer modes of cardiac pacing: Description of pacing modes. Mod Concepts Cardiovasc Dis 52:1, 1983

JOSEPHSON ME, SEIDES SF: *Clinical Cardiac Electrophysiology: Techniques and Interpretations*. Philadelphia, Lea & Febiger, 1979

LUDMER PL, GOLDSCHLAGER N: Cardiac pacing in the 1980's. N Engl J Med 311:1671, 1984

NARULA OS, SHANTHA N: Atrioventricular block: Clinical concepts and His bundle electrocardiography, in *Cardiac Arrthythmias*, WJ Mandel (ed). Philadelphia, Lippincott, 1980

PARSONETT V et al: Indications for dual chamber pacing. PACE 7:318, 1984

TONKIN AM, HEDDLE WF: Electrophysiological testing of sinus node function. PACE 7:735, 1984

ZOLL PM et al: External noninvasive temporary cardiac pacing: Clinical trials. Circulation 71:937, 1985

184   THE TACHYARRHYTHMIAS

MARK E. JOSEPHSON / ALFRED E. BUXTON / FRANCIS E. MARCHLINSKI

MECHANISMS OF TACHYARRHYTHMIAS

Tachyarrhythmias may be divided into disorders of impulse propagation and disorders of impulse formation. Disorders of impulse propagation (reentry) are generally considered to be the most common mechanism of sustained paroxysmal tachyarrhythmias. The requirements to initiate reentry include: (1) electrophysiologic inhomogeneity (i.e., differences in conduction and/or refractoriness) in two or more regions of the heart connected with each other to form a potentially closed loop; (2) unidirectional block in one pathway; (3) slow conduction over an alternative pathway, allowing time for the initially blocked pathway to recover excitability; and (4) reexcitation of the initially blocked pathway to complete a loop of activation. Repetitive circulation of the impulse over this loop can produce a sustained tachyarrhythmia. While anatomic obstacles may underlie reentry and provide an inexcitable center around which the impulse can circulate, they are not essential. Reentrant arrhythmias can be initiated as well as terminated by premature complexes and can be interrupted by rapid stimulation (overdrive suppression), which can help distinguish them from arrhythmias caused by triggered activity.

Disorders of impulse formation can be subdivided into tachyarrhythmias caused by enhanced automaticity and those caused by triggered activity. In addition to the sinus node, automatic pacemaker activity can be observed in specialized atrial fibers, fibers of the atrioventricular (AV) junction, and Purkinje fibers (see Chap. 183). Myocardial cells do not normally possess pacemaker activity. *Enhancement of normal automaticity* in latent pacemaker fibers or the development of abnormal automaticity due to partial depolarization of the resting membrane occurs as a consequence of a variety of pathophysiologic states, which include (1) increased endogenous or exogenous catecholamines; (2) electrolyte disturbances (e.g., hypokalemia, hypercalcemia); (3) hypoxia or ischemia; (4) mechanical effects (e.g., stretch); and (5) drugs (e.g., digitalis). Tachycardia caused by abnormal automaticity cannot be started or stopped by pacing.

Triggered activity has been observed in atrial, ventricular, and His-Purkinje tissue under conditions such as increased local catecholamine concentration, hyperkalemia, hypercalcemia, and digitalis intoxication. All of these conditions produce an accumulation of intracellular calcium which causes depolarizations following the action potential, termed *afterdepolarizations*. With increasing amplitude of the afterdepolarizations, threshold can be reached and repetitive activity produced. In contrast to automatic rhythms, triggered activity requires preceding activity for initiation and therefore can be initiated by pacing. In contrast to tachyarrhythmias caused by automaticity and reentry, the response of triggered activity to overdrive pacing is acceleration.

The use of electrophysiologic (EP) studies, i.e., intracardiac recordings and programmed stimulation, has greatly expanded our understanding of the mechanisms of tachyarrhythmias. In addition to helping in the diagnosis of arrhythmias, these techniques may be of value in determining the most appropriate types of therapy. EP studies of tachycardias require the positioning of multiple electrode catheters at critical areas within the heart; these electrodes must be capable of both stimulating and recording from multiple sites in the atria and/or ventricles.

PREMATURE COMPLEXES

ATRIAL PREMATURE COMPLEXES (APCs)   APCs can be found on 24-h Holter monitoring in over 60 percent of normal adults. APCs are usually asymptomatic and benign, although at times they may be associated with palpitations. In susceptible patients, they can initiate paroxysmal supraventricular tachycardias. APCs may originate from any location in either atrium, and they are recognized on the ECG as early P waves with a morphology which differs from the sinus P wave. While APCs conduct to the ventricles normally when they occur late in the cardiac cycle, those appearing relatively early may reach the AV conduction system while it is still in its relative refractory period, resulting in a conduction delay manifested by a prolonged PR interval following the premature P wave (Fig. 184-1A). Very early APCs may even block in the AV node if this structure is encountered during its effective refractory period. APCs, whether conducted or not, are usually followed by a pause before a return to sinus activity. Most commonly, an APC enters and resets the sinus node, so that the sum of the pre- and postextrasystolic PP intervals is less than the sum of two sinus PP intervals (Fig. 184-1A). In this

FIGURE 184-1   *A. Atrial premature complex. Lead I. Following a third sinus beat an atrial premature complex (APC) occurs which conducts slowly (prolonged PR interval) to the ventricles. The pause that follows the APC is less than compensatory. B. Complex ventricular ectopy. Lead II. Multiformed ventricular premature complexes (VPCs) and a couplet are shown (see dots). C. Atrial fibrillation. AF is characterized by an undulating baseline with an irregular ventricular response. D. Atrial flutter. Lead II. Note the sawtooth configuration of the flutter waves (arrows). E. AV nodal reentrant supraven-* *tricular tachycardia. Lead II is shown during supraventricular tachycardia (SVT) and normal sinus rhythm (NSR). The characteristic findings during SVT are pseudo S waves in lead II, which represent retrograde atrial activation. F. Proxysmal atrial tachycardia with block due to digitalis intoxication. A V₁ rhythm strip is shown at a paper speed of 50 mm/s. Atrial tachycardia is present at a rate of approximately 170 beats per minute. Every other P wave conducts to the ventricles, producing a ventricular response of 85 beats per minute.*

case the pause is said to be less than fully compensatory. The QRS complex following most APCs is normal, although early APCs may be followed by aberrantly conducted QRS complexes.

Since most APCs are asymptomatic, treatment is not required. When they cause palpitations or trigger paroxysmal supraventricular tachycardias (see below), treatment may be useful. Factors which precipitate APCs such as alcohol, tobacco, or adrenergic stimulants should be identified and eliminated, and in their absence mild sedation or the use of a beta blocker may be tried. If this fails, quinidine, procainamide, or a similar agent (Table 184-2) may be used.

AV JUNCTIONAL COMPLEXES The site of origin of these complexes is thought to be in the bundle of His, since the AV node itself possesses no automaticity (page 916). AV junctional complexes are less common than either atrial or ventricular premature complexes and are more often associated with cardiac disease or digitalis intoxication. Junctional premature impulses can conduct both antegradely to the ventricles and retrogradely to the atrium and, on rare occasions, may fail to conduct in either direction. Premature AV junctional complexes can be recognized by normal-appearing QRS complexes that are not preceded by a P wave. Retrograde P waves (inverted in leads II, III, and aV_F) may be observed after the QRS complex.

While often asymptomatic, junctional premature complexes may be associated with palpitations and cause cannon *a* waves which may result in distressing pulsations in the neck. When symptomatic, they should be treated like APCs.

VENTRICULAR PREMATURE COMPLEXES (VPCs) These are among the most common arrhythmia's and occur in patients with or without heart disease. Of adult males ≥60 percent will exhibit VPCs during a 24-h Holter monitoring. In patients without heart disease, VPCs have not been shown to be associated with any increased incidence in mortality or morbidity. VPCs may occur in up to 80 percent of patients with previous myocardial infarction, and in this setting, if frequent (>10 per hour) and/or complex (occurring in couplets or triplets), they have been associated with increased mortality. However, cardiac mortality in such patients usually occurs in association with significantly impaired ventricular function. While frequent and complex ventricular ectopy is an independent risk factor, it is not as strong a risk factor as is impaired ventricular function. Morever, even though ventricular tachycardia and/or fibrillation may be the basis for the sudden death in these patients, this does not a priori establish a cause-and-effect relation between spontaneous ectopy and life-threatening ventricular fibrillation. Very early VPCs have been stated by some to increase the risk of sudden death. Although this has been observed during acute ischemia and in the setting of QT prolongation, frequently ventricular tachycardia or fibrillation is precipitated by VPCs which occur after the T wave of the prior beat.

VPCs are recognized by wide (usually >0.14 s), bizarre QRS complexes that are not preceded by P waves (Fig. 184-1B). Often they bear a relatively fixed relationship to the preceding sinus complex and are thus considered *fixed coupled* VPCs. When fixed coupling is not present and the interval between VPCs has a common denominator, *ventricular parasystole* is said to be present. Under these circumstances the VPCs are a manifestation of abnormal automaticity of a ventricular focus which is protected so that it is not penetrated by sinus impulses which therefore do not reset this parasystolic focus, thereby allowing the interectopic intervals to remain fixed.

VPCs may occur singly in patterns of bigeminy, in which every sinus beat is followed by a VPC; trigeminy, in which two sinus beats are followed by a VPC; quadrigeminy, etc. Two successive VPCs are termed *pairs* or *couplets,* while three or more consecutive VPCs are termed *ventricular tachycardia.* Morphologically, VPCs may have a similar morphology (monomorphic) or may have different morphologies (multiformed or polymorphic) (Fig. 184-1B).

Most commonly VPCs are not conducted retrogradely to the atrium and the sinoatrial node and produce a fully compensatory pause, so that the interval between conducted beats which bracket the VPC

equals two basic RR intervals. Ventricular impulses may also manifest retrograde conduction to the atrium and cause inverted P waves in leads II, III, and aV_F. The pause that results may therefore be less than compensatory. In many instances, the QRS complex will not be associated with retrograde ventriculoatrial (VA) conduction but may block in the AV node. This renders the AV node refractory to the subsequent sinus beat and causes a block of the sinus P wave or conduction with a markedly prolonged PR interval. This prolonged PR interval is said to be a manifestation of *concealed retrograde conduction* of the ventricular impulse into the AV node. A VPC which does not produce any manifestation of retrograde concealed conduction and fails to influence the oncoming sinus impulse is termed an *interpolated VPC.*

VPCs can cause palpitations or neck pulsations secondary to either the occurrence of cannon *a* waves or the increased force of contraction due to post extrasystolic potentiation of ventricular contractility. Patients with frequent VPCs or bigeminy may develop syncope because the VPCs do not result in an adequate stroke volume and the cardiac output is reduced.

Management In the absence of cardiac disease, isolated asymptomatic VPCs, regardless of configuration and frequency, need no treatment. When arrhythmias are symptomatic, the symptoms should first be addressed by either allaying the patient's anxiety with reassurance, or if this is not successful, reducing the frequency of the VPCs with antiarrhythmic agents. Beta-adrenergic blockers (page 366) may be successful in managing VPCs which occur primarily in the daytime or under stressful situations and in specific settings such as mitral valve prolapse and thyrotoxicosis. Quinidine or quinidine-like agents may be tried should this be unsuccessful. In patients with cardiac disease, frequent VPCs are often associated with an increased risk of sudden and nonsudden cardiac death, and many physicians attempt to eliminate or reduce the frequency of these VPCs in an attempt to reduce this risk. However, the cause-and-effect relationship of the VPCs to fatal events has not been established, and it has not been shown definitively that the suppression of VPCs with antiarrhythmic drugs prevents sudden death. In addition, it is important to recognize that the antiarrhythmic agents can also produce the lethal arrhythmias which they are given to prevent. Thus, therapy directed toward VPCs in the setting of chronic cardiac disease may result in an inappropriate and costly use of agents without proven efficacy and with potential side effects in many patients. The high incidence of side effects and the frequent exacerbation of arrhythmias caused by all antiarrhythmic drugs by them makes it mandatory for one to monitor patients being treated with such agents.

In the presence of acute myocardial infarction the greatest incidence of primary ventricular fibrillation occurs within the first 24 h. Temporary prophylactic antiarrhythmic therapy has therefore been recommended for all patients with this condition, regardless of the presence and/or degree of spontaneous ectopy (see Chap. 190).

TACHYCARDIAS

Tachycardias refer to arrhythmias with three or more complexes at rates exceeding 100 beats per minute and occur more often in structurally diseased than in normal hearts. Those paroxysmal tachycardias that are initiated by APCs or VPCs are considered to be due to reentry. Some of the digitalis-induced tachyarrhythmias are due to triggered activity (see below).

If the patient is hemodynamically stable, an attempt should be made to determine the mechanism and origin of the tachycardia since this will usually lead to an appropriate therapeutic decision. It is useful first to compare the ECG during the tachycardia with one recorded during sinus rhythm, and it is often desirable to record long rhythm strips using surface leads with the largest P waves, usually lead II or V_1. One can also utilize electrodes situated at the end of a flexible pacing catheter inserted into the esophagus behind the left atrium to record atrial activity. Information to be obtained from the ECG includes (1) the presence, frequency, morphology, and regularity of P waves and QRS complexes; (2) the relationship between atrial and ventricular activity; (3) a comparison of the QRS morphology during sinus rhythm and during the tachycardia; and (4) the response to carotid sinus massage or other vagal maneuvers.

Carotid sinus pressure should only be performed while the patient is electrocardiographically monitored with resuscitative equipment available to manage the rare episode of asystole and/or ventricular fibrillation. Carotid sinus massage should not be performed in patients with carotid arterial bruits. The patient should be positioned flat with the neck extended. Massage of one carotid bulb at a time should be performed by applying firm pressure just underneath the angle of the jaw for up to 5 s. Alternative vagomimetic maneuvers include the Valsalva maneuver, immersion of the face in cold water, and the administration of 5 to 10 mg edrophonium.

Observation of the jugular venous pulse can provide clues to the presence of atrial activity and its relationship to ventricular ectopy. Intermittent cannon a waves suggest AV dissociation, while persistent cannon a waves suggest 1:1 VA conduction. Flutter waves may be seen or no atrial activity may be apparent, as in the presence of atrial flutter and fibrillation, respectively. The arterial pulse may also manifest AV dissociation by demonstrating variations in amplitude. A first heart sound of variable intensity during a regular rhythm also suggests AV dissociation.

SINUS TACHYCARDIA   In the adult sinus tachycardia is said to be present when the heart rate exceeds 100 beats per minute; sinus tachycardia does not usually exceed 200 beats per minute and is not a primary arrhythmia; instead, it represents a physiologic response to a variety of stresses, such as fever, volume depletion, anxiety, exercise, thyrotoxicosis, hypoxemia, hypotension, or congestive heart failure. Sinus tachycardia has a gradual onset and offset. The ECG demonstrates P waves with sinus contour preceding each QRS complex. Carotid sinus pressure usually produces modest slowing with a gradual return to the previous rate upon cessation. This contrasts with the paroxysmal supraventricular tachycardias which may slow slightly and terminate abruptly.

Sinus tachycardia should not be treated as a primary arrhythmia, since it is always a physiologic response to a demand placed on the heart. As such, the therapy should be directed to the primary disorder. This may involve institution of digitalis and/or diuretics for heart failure, oxygen for hypoxemia, treatment of thyrotoxicosis, volume repletion, aspirin for fever, or tranquilizers for emotional upset.

ATRIAL FIBRILLATION (AF)   This common arrhythmia may occur in paroxysmal and persistent forms. It may be seen in normal subjects, particularly during emotional stress or following surgery, exercise, or acute alcoholic intoxication. It may also occur in patients with heart or lung disease who develop acute hypoxia, hypercapnia, or metabolic or hemodynamic derangements. Persistent AF usually occurs in patients with cardiovascular disease, most commonly rheumatic heart disease, nonrheumatic mitral valve disease, hypertensive cardiovascular disease, chronic lung disease, atrial septal defect, and a variety of miscellaneous cardiac abnormalities. AF may be the presenting finding in thyrotoxicosis. So-called lone AF, which occurs in elderly patients without underlying heart disease, is considered to represent the tachycardiac phase of the bradycardia-syndrome (page 918).

The morbidity associated with AF is related to (1) excessive rate of the ventricular response, which in turn may lead to hypotension or angina pectoris in susceptible individuals; (2) the pause following cessation of AF (page 918), which can cause syncope; (3) systemic embolization, which occurs most commonly in patients with rheumatic heart disease; (4) loss of the contribution of atrial contraction to cardiac output, which may cause fatigue; and (5) anxiety secondary to palpitations. In patients with severe cardiac dysfunction, particularly those with hypertrophied, noncompliant ventricles, the combination of the loss of the atrial contribution to ventricular filling and the abbreviated filling period due to the rapid ventricular rate in AF can produce marked hemodynamic embarrassment, syncope, or heart failure. In patients with mitral stenosis in whom filling time is critical, development of AF with a rapid ventricular rate may precipitate pulmonary edema (see Chap. 187).

AF is characterized by disorganized atrial activity without discrete P waves on the surface ECG (Fig. 184-1C). Atrial activation is manifested by an undulating baseline or by more sharply inscribed atrial deflections of varying amplitude and frequency ranging from 350 to 600 per minute. The ventricular response is irregularly irregular. This results from the large number of atrial impulses which penetrate the AV node, making it partially refractory to subsequent impulses. This effect of nonconducted atrial impulses to influence the response to subsequent atrial impulses is termed concealed conduction. As a result, the ventricular response is relatively slow, considering the actual atrial rate. If AF converts to atrial flutter, which has a slower atrial rate, the effect of concealed conduction may be diminished and a paradoxic increase in the ventricular response may occur. The main factor determining the rate of the ventricular response is the functional refractory period of the AV node or the most rapid paced rate at which 1:1 conduction through the AV node can be observed.

If, in the presence of AF, the ventricular rhythm becomes regular and slow (e.g., 30 to 60 beats per minute), complete heart block is suggested, and if the rhythm is regular and rapid (≥ 100 beats per minute), a tachycardia arising in the AV junction or ventricle should be suspected. Digitalis intoxication is a common cause of both of these phenomena.

Patients with AF exhibit a loss of a waves in the jugular venous pulse and variable pulse pressures in the carotid arterial pulse. The first heart sound usually varies in intensity. On echocardiography, the left atrium is frequently enlarged, and in patients in whom the left atrial diameter exceeds 4.5 cm, it may not be possible to convert AF to sinus rhythm or to maintain the latter despite therapy.

Management   In acute AF, a precipitating factor such as fever, pneumonia, alcoholic intoxication, thyrotoxicosis, pulmonary emboli, or pericarditis should be sought. When such a factor is present, therapy should be directed toward the primary abnormality. If the patient's clinical status is severely compromised, electrical cardioversion is the treatment of choice. In the absence of severe cardiovascular compromise, slowing of ventricular rate becomes the initial therapeutic goal. This may be accomplished with digitalis, calcium channel antagonists, or beta-adrenergic blockers, all of which prolong the refractory period of and slow conduction in the AV node. Conversion to sinus rhythm may then be attempted, using quinidine or quinidine-like (type IA) agents (Table 184-1). It is important to slow AV node conduction prior to administering such drugs because their vagolytic effect and ability to convert AF to atrial flutter may reduce the concealed conduction and lead to an excessively rapid

---

TABLE 184-1 Classification of antiarrhythmic drugs

Type I   Drugs that reduce maximal velocity of phase 0 depolarization ($\dot{V}_{max}$) due to block of inward Na^+ current in tissue with fast response action potentials
  A $\downarrow \dot{V}_{max}$ at all heart rates and $\uparrow$ action potential duration e.g., quinidine, procainamide, disopyramide
  B   Little effect at slow rates on $\dot{V}_{max}$ in normal tissue; $\dot{V}_{max}$ in partially depolarized cells with fast response action potentials
        Effects increased at faster rates
        No change or $\downarrow$ in action potential duration, e.g., lidocaine, phenytoin, tocainide, mexiletine
  C $\downarrow \dot{V}_{max}$ at normal rates in normal tissue
        Minimal effect on action potential duration, e.g., encainide, lorcainide, flecainide
Type II   Antisympathetic agents, e.g., propranolol and other beta-adenergic blockers; automaticity, AV nodal refractoriness, and conduction velocity
Type III Agents that prolong action potential duration in tissue with fast response action potentials, e.g., bretylium, amiodarone
Type IV   Calcium (slow) channel blocking agents—decrease conduction velocity and increase refractoriness in tissue with slow response action potentials, e.g., verapamil, diltiazem

ventricular response. Beta-adrenergic blockers are especially useful in this regard. If medical therapy fails to convert AF, electrical cardioversion is useful; it generally requires 100 to 200 W·s of energy. Anticoagulation should be started at least 2 weeks prior to and continued for 2 weeks following any attempt at electrical cardioversion, either pharmacologic or electrical, in patients with long-standing AF. Anticoagulation appears to decrease the incidence of systemic embolization associated with cardioversion. It is less likely for chronic AF to convert to or remain in sinus rhythm in the presence of long-standing rheumatic heart disease and/or when the atria are markedly enlarged. It is also unlikely for patients with lone AF to be converted to and maintained in sinus rhythm.

If sinus rhythm is restored electrically or pharmacologically, quinidine or related agents may be used to prevent recurrence. In patients in whom cardioversion is unsuccessful or in whom AF is likely to recur, it is probably wisest to allow the patient to remain in AF and to control the ventricular response with calcium antagonists, beta-adrenergic blockers, or digitalis. Since they are always at risk of systemic embolization, chronic anticoagulation must be considered for such patients.

ATRIAL FLUTTER This arrhythmia occurs almost invariably in patients with organic heart disease. Flutter may be paroxysmal, in which case there is usually a precipitating factor, such as pericarditis or acute respiratory failure, or it may be persistent. Trial flutter (as well as AF) is very common during the first week following open heart surgery. Atrial flutter is usually less long-lived than is AF, although on occasion it may persist for months to years. Most commonly, if it lasts for more than a week, atrial flutter will convert to AF. Systemic embolization is less common in atrial flutter than AF.

Atrial flutter is characterized by an atrial rate between 250 and 350 beats per minute. Typically, the ventricular rate is half the atrial rate, i.e., approximately 150 beats per minute. If the atrial rate is slowed to <220 per minute by antiarrhythmic agents such as quinidine, which also possess vagolytic properties, the ventricular rate may rise suddenly because of the development of 1:1 AV conduction. Classically, flutter waves are seen as regular sawtooth-like atrial activity, most prominent in the inferior leads (Fig. 184-1D). When the ventricular response is regular and not a simple fraction of the atrial rate, AV block is present. Activation mapping suggests that atrial flutter is a form of atrial reentry localized to the low right atrium.

Management The most effective treatment of atrial flutter is dc cardioversion, which can be accomplished with low energy (10 to 50 W·s) under mild sedation. In patients who develop atrial flutter following open heart surgery or recurrent flutter in the setting of acute myocardial infarction, particularly when they are being treated with digitalis, atrial pacing (using temporary pacing wires implanted at the time of operation or using a pacing lead inserted into the atrium pervenously) at rates of 115 to 130 percent of the atrial flutter rate can usually convert the atrial flutter to sinus rhythm. Atrial pacing may also result in the conversion of atrial flutter into AF, which allows for easier control of the ventricular response. If immediate conversion of atrial flutter is not mandated by the patient's clinical status, the ventricular response should first be slowed by blocking the AV node with a beta blocker, calcium antagonist, or digitalis; the latter drug occasionally converts atrial flutter into AF. Once AV nodal conduction is delayed with any of these drugs, an attempt to convert flutter to sinus rhythm using quinidine or quinidine-like agents should be made. Increasing doses of the drug selected are administered until the rhythm converts or side effects occur.

Quinidine, quinidine-like drugs, and amiodarone, an experimental drug, (Table 184-2) are useful in preventing recurrences of both atrial flutter and fibrillation.

PAROXYSMAL SUPRAVENTRICULAR TACHYCARDIAS (PSVT) In most cases functional differences in conduction and refractoriness in the AV node or the presence of an AV bypass tract provide the substrate for the development of PSVT (previously termed paroxysmal atrial tachycardia). Electrophysiologic studies have demonstrated that *reentry* is the mechanism responsible for the vast majority of PSVT. Reentry has been localized to the sinus node, atrium, AV node, or to a macroreentrant circuit involving normal conduction in the antegrade direction through the AV node and retrograde conduction through an AV bypass tract. Such a bypass tract may also conduct antegradely, in which case the Wolff-Parkinson-White (WPW) syndrome is said to be present. More frequently, however, the bypass tract manifests only retrograde conduction, and therefore it is termed a *concealed* bypass tract. In the absence of the WPW syndrome, reentry through the AV node or through a *concealed* bypass tract makes up more than 90 percent of all PSVTs.

AV nodal reentrant tachycardia There is no age, sex, or disease predisposition for the development of AV nodal reentrant tachycardia, the most common cause of supraventricular tachycardia. This usually presents as a narrow QRS complex with regular rates ranging from 120 to 250 per minute. APCs which initiate the arrhythmia are almost always associated with a prolonged PR interval. Retrograde P waves may be absent, buried in the QRS complex, or appear as distortions at the terminal parts of the QRS complex.

AV nodal reentrant PSVT (Fig. 184-1E) can be reproducibly initiated and terminated by appropriately timed atrial premature extra stimuli. The onset of the tachycardia is almost always associated with prolongation of the PR interval due to marked AV nodal conduction delay (prolonged AH interval) that is critical for the genesis of the arrhythmia. The sudden prolongation of the AH interval is consistent with the concept of dual AV nodal pathways as the substrate for AV nodal reentry. This concept (Fig. 184-2) assumes that the AV node is longitudinally dissociated into two functionally different pathways: (1) a beta pathway which exhibits rapid conduction and a long refractory period (fast pathway), and (2) an alpha pathway which has a short refractory period but conducts slowly (slow pathway). During sinus rhythm the atrial impulse travels over the beta pathway to produce a single QRS complex with a normal PR interval. The impulse which simultaneously conducts down the slow pathway reaches the His bundle after it has been depolarized and is therefore refractory. Atrial extra stimuli are blocked in the beta pathway because of its longer refractory period and are conducted slowly through the alpha pathway. If conduction down the alpha pathway is slow enough to allow the previously refractory beta pathway time to recover excitability, a single atrial echo or sustained tachycardia ensues. A critical balance between conduction velocity and refractoriness within the node is required to sustain AV nodal reentry. Atrial and ventricular activation occur simultaneously, explaining why no P waves may be apparent on the surface ECG.

CLINICAL FEATURES AV nodal reentry may produce palpitations, syncope, and heart failure, depending on the rate and duration of the arrhythmia and the presence and severity of any underlying heart disease. Hypotension and syncope may occur because of the sudden loss of the atrial contribution to ventricular filling; this can also lead to a marked increase in atrial pressure, acute pulmonary edema, and a reduction in ventricular filling. Simultaneous atrial and ventricular contraction produces cannon *a* waves with each heart beat.

TREATMENT In patients without hypotension, vagal maneuvers, particularly carotid sinus massage, can terminate the arrhythmia in 80 percent of cases. If hypotension is present, raising the blood pressure by the cautious use of phenylephrine may terminate the arrhythmia alone or may aid termination with carotid sinus pressure. If these maneuvers are unsuccessful, verapamil (2.5 to 10 mg intravenously) is the agent of first choice. Propranolol (0.05 to 0.2 mg/kg, intravenously) or other beta blockers may be used. Digitalis glycosides have a slower onset of action. When these drugs fail to terminate the tachycardia or when the tachycardia is recurrent, pacing via a temporary pacemaker inserted pervenously may be used to terminate the arrhythmia.

AV nodal reentry can usually be prevented by the use of drugs

TABLE 184-2 Electrophysiologic effects

Drug	Sinus node	Atrium and ventricle	AV node	His-Purkinje system	Atrioventricular bypass tracts
Digoxin and other cardiac glycosides (also see p. 910)	No change; patients with sinus node disease may develop sinus exit block or arrest	Controversial	Increase in ERP; decreased conduction velocity	No change	No change or decrease in ERP
Propranolol and other beta-adrenoreceptor blockers (also see p. 980)	Decreased sinus rate; increased sinus node recovery time	No change	Increase in ERP; decreased conduction velocity	No change	No change
Verapamil	Decreased sinus rate; sinus exit block in patients with sinus node disease	No change	Increase in ERP; decreased conduction velocity	No change	Indirect effects may decrease ERP when given IV
Quinidine	No change; may suppress sinus node in patients with underlying sinus node disease	Increase in ERP; decreased conduction velocity	Decrease or no change in ERP, no change in conduction velocity	Decreased automaticity; decreased conduction velocity; increased ERP	Increase in ERP
Procainamide	No change	Increase in ERP; decreased conduction velocity	Decrease or no change in ERP; decrease or no change in conduction velocity	Decreased automaticity; decreased conduction velocity; Increased ERP	Increase in ERP
Disopyramide	No change	Increase in ERP; decreased conduction velocity	Decrease or no change in ERP; no change in conduction velocity	Decreased automaticity; increased ERP; decreased conduction velocity	Increase in ERP
Lidocaine	No change	No change in ERP	No change or decrease in ERP	No change or decrease in ERP	No change, decrease, or increase in ERP
Phenytoin	No change	No change in ERP	No change or decrease in ERP; no change or increased conduction velocity	Decrease in ERP; decreased automaticity	
Tocainide	No change	No change	No change	No change; decreased automaticity	Increase in ERP
Bretylium	Initial increase in sinus rate followed by decrease	Increase in ERP	No change	No change	
Amiodarone*	Decreased sinus rate	Increase in ERP	Increase in ERP; decreased conduction velocity	Increase in ERP; decreased conduction velocity	Increase in ERP
Mexiletine*	No change; patients with sinus node disease may develop sinus arrest	No change	Variable and inconsistent effects on conduction and refractoriness	Increase in ERP; no change or decreased conduction velocity	

* Investigation.

NOTE: *AV = atrioventricular, ERP = effective refractory period, IV = intravenous, SVT = supraventricular tachycardia, VT = ventricular tachycardia, AF = atrial fibrillation, VF = ventricular fibrillation.*

which act primarily on the antegrade slow pathway (such as digitalis, beta blockers, or calcium antagonists) or on the fast pathway (such as quinidine). Drugs most likely to prevent recurrences prevent induction of the arrhythmias by programmed stimulation. This technique utilizes temporary pacemaker catheters connected to a physiologic stimulator capable of variable rate pacing and stimulation with one or more precisely timed premature impulses. If episodes of PSVT are frequent and produce disabling symptoms, therapy based on electrophysiologic studies is preferable to empiric drug trials. Antitachycardia pacemakers can be used to terminate PSVT due to AV nodal reentry when these arrhythmias occur infrequently. Ablation of the AV junction (page 937) has been developed as a method of controlling AV nodal reentry, but this approach should only be considered as a last resort since it usually mandates insertion of a permanent pacemaker.

AV reentrant tachycardia PSVT due to AV reentry incorporates an AV bypass tract which conducts only retrogradely as part of the tachycardia circuit. Thus, the impulse passes antegradely from the atria through the AV node and His-Purkinje system to the ventricles, then retrogradely through the (concealed) bypass tract back to the atrium. Patients with this disorder manifest the same type of PSVT as do patients with the WPW syndrome (see below), but the bypass tract does not conduct in an antegrade direction in AV reentry tachycardia.

AV reentrant tachycardia can be initiated and terminated by either APCs or VPCs. Alternation of the QRS complexes and/or T wave occurs in approximately one-third of such tachycardias. Since atrial activation must follow ventricular activation during AV reentry, the P wave usually occurs after the QRS complex.

Atrial activation mapping is of major value in evaluating the origin

Indications	Side effects and toxicity
Slowing of ventricular rate during AF, atrial flutter, and other atrial tachycardias in the absence of preexcitation; SVT due to AV nodal reentry and AV reentry utilizing bypass tracts	Atrial tachycardia, VT, AV nodal block, accelerated junctional rhythms, atrial and ventricular premature depolarizations, VT, ventricular fibrillation, anorexia, nausea, vomiting; acceleration of ventricular rate during atrial fibrillation/flutter in the presence of preexcitation causing ventricular fibrillation
Slowing of ventricular rate during AF, atrial flutter, and other atrial tachycardias in the absence of preexcitation; SVT due to AV nodal reentry, reentry utilizing bypass tracts; arrhythmias induced by exercise, arrhythmias occurring in the presence of hyperthyroidism; polymorphic VT associated with congenital long QT syndrome	Sinus bradycardia, AV nodal block, congestive heart failure, bronchospasm, masking symptoms of hypoglycemia
Same as digoxin	Sinus arrest in patients with sinus node dysfunction; AV nodal block in patients with AV nodal dysfunction; exacerbation of congestive heart failure (may be potentiated in presence of beta-adrenergic blocking agents); elevation of digoxin levels; hypotension following IV administration; IV administration during AF/flutter in the presence of preexcitation may cause acceleration of ventricular response rate and VF or hemodynamic collapse; IV administration to patients with VT may cause hemodynamic collapse
Atrial and ventricular extrasystoles; atrial and ventricular tachyarrhythmias; all types of SVT; control of ventricular rate in patients with preexcitation and AF and flutter	Anorexia, nausea, vomiting, diarrhea; cinchonism: tinnitus, confusion, hearing and visual changes; thrombocytopenia, hemolytic anemia, rash; drug interactions: elevation of digoxin levels; phenytoin and phenobarbital will decrease quinidine levels; QT prolongation associated with polymorphic VT (torsade de pointes); conversion of nonsustained to sustained VT; acceleration of ventricular response to atrial flutter and fibrillation
Same as quinidine	Anorexia, nausea, confusion, hallucinations; agranulocytosis; lupus erythematosus-like syndrome; QT prolongation associated with polymorphic VT (torsade de pointes); marked elevations in the primary metabolite (NAPA) may be more likely to cause polymorphic VT; conversion of nonsustained into sustained VT; acceleration of ventricular response to atrial flutter and fibrillation
Same as quinidine	Anticholinergic actions including dry mouth, blurred vision, urinary retention or hesitancy, constipation, narrow angle glaucoma; congestive heart failure, especially in patients with abnormal ventricular function; QT prolongation associated with polymorphic VT (torsade de pointes)
VT and VF especially during acute ischemia and myocardial infarction	Dizziness, paresthesias, confusion, delirium, seizures, coma; may depress sinus node in patients with underlying sinus node disease; may suppress escape foci in patients with complete heart block; congestive heart failure or liver disease increase risk of side effects
Tachyarrhythmias induced by digitalis; occasionally effective for ventricular tachyarrhythmias not induced by digitalis alone or in combination with other antiarrhythmic agents; polymorphic VT associated with increased QT	Gingival hypertrophy, rash, blood dyscrasias, nystagmus, ataxia, stupor coma, lupus erythematosis syndrome; lymph node hyperplasia, peripheral neuropathy, hypocalcemia, hyperglycemia; phlebitis and hypotension during IV administration
VT, VF, frequent VPCs	Ataxia, tremor, paresthesias, lightheadedness, nausea, rash, lupus erythematosus syndrome, pulmonary fibrosis, bone marrow suppression; may exacerbate heart failure in patients with ventricular dysfunction
Refractory ventricular VT and VF, especially due to acute ischemia	Initially, transient hypertension; subsequently, hypotension increased in the upright position; the hypotensive effect can be prevented by tricyclic drugs; nausea, vomiting
Refractory atrial and ventricular tachyarrhythmias; refractory SVT due to AV nodal reentry and AV reentry utilizing bypass tracts	Marked sinus bradycardia, complete heart block; IV administration may cause hypotension; increased QT associated with polymorphic VT; increased T_4, hypo- and hyperthyroidism; peripheral neuropathy, proximal myopathy; pulmonary fibrosis; increased liver enzymes, hepatitis; photodermatitis, blue-gray skin discoloration; corneal microdeposits; elevation of digoxin levels; potentiation of oral anticoagulants
Ventricular tachyarrhythmias	Nausea, vomiting, ataxia, tremor, gait disturbances, rash

of these tachycardias. Most concealed bypass tracts are left-sided. Thus, during supraventricular tachycardia or during ventricular pacing, the earliest activation sequence is recorded in the left atrium, usually via a catheter in the coronary sinus (Fig. 184-3). This eccentric trial activation is quite distinct from the normal retrograde activation sequence in which the earliest activation of the atria is in the area of the AV junction. The ability of a ventricular stimulus to conduct to the atrium at a time when the bundle of His is refractory and termination of the tachycardia by a ventricular stimulus which does not reach the atrium are diagnostic of retrograde conduction over a concealed bypass tract.

Treatment is similar to that for AV nodal reentry tachycardia.

Sinus node reentry and other atrial tachycardias Reentry in the region of the sinus node or within the atria is invariably initiated by APCs. These arrhythmias are less common than AV nodal or AV reentry and are more often associated with underlying cardiac disease. During sinus node reentry the P-wave morphology is identical to that occurring in sinus rhythm, and the PR interval is prolonged. This is in contrast to sinus tachycardia, in which the PR interval tends to shorten. With intraatrial reentry the P-wave configuration differs from that during sinus rhythm, but the PR interval is prolonged.

TREATMENT Sinus node and atrial reentrant arrhythmias are managed like other reentrant PSVTs.

NONREENTRANT ATRIAL TACHYCARDIAS These may be a manifestation of digitalis intoxication or may be associated with severe pulmonary or cardiac disease, with hypokalemia, or with the administration of theophylline or adrenergic drugs. The digitalis-induced arrhythmias may be caused by triggered activity and/or enhanced automaticity. In such atrial tachycardias with AV block secondary to

FIGURE 184-2 *Mechanism of AV nodal reentry. The atrium, AV node (AVN), and His bundle are schematically shown. The AV node is longitudinally dissociated into two functionally different pathways, alpha and beta (see text). During sinus rhythm the impulse conducts down the beta pathway to produce a normal PR interval. Conduction down the alpha pathway cannot be completed because the His bundle is refractory. With a premature atrial impulse, block occurs in the fast beta pathway and slow conduction occurs to the ventricle over the slow alpha pathway. The impulse can then return to the chamber of* origin (atrium) to produce an atrial echo. This is schematically shown on the bottom, which is dissociation of a long PR interval with an atrial echo. In the tracing on the far right a more premature atrial impulse will again block in the fast pathway, but this time conduction will be so slow down the slow pathway that it will be able to recover to maintain a sustained circus movement within the AV node. This is schematically shown on the bottom where a premature atrial impulse associated with a PR interval of 0.39 s is followed by the initiation of supraventricular tachycardia (SVT).

digitalis intoxication (Fig. 184-1*F*), the atrial rate rarely exceeds 180 per minute, and typically 2:1 block is present. Atrial arrhythmias precipitated by digitalis can usually be treated by withdrawal of the drug.

Automatic trial tachycardias not caused by digitalis are difficult to terminate, and in such cases the main goal of therapy should be to control the ventricular response, either by drugs which affect the

AV node, such as digitalis, beta blockers, or calcium channel antagonists, or by ablation techniques. Surgery has been employed in resistant cases.

PREEXCITATION (WPW) SYNDROME The most frequently encountered type of ventricular preexcitation is that associated with AV bypass tracts. These connections are composed of strands of atrial-

FIGURE 184-3 *Intracardiac recordings during supraventricular tachycardia using a left-sided AV bypass tract. Intracardiac recordings during sinus rhythm (NSR) in supraventricular tachycardia (SVT) are shown. ECG leads I, aVF, and V₁ are displayed with electrograms from the high right atrium (HRA), coronary sinus (CS), His bundle (HBE), and right ventricle (RV). During NSR, the QRS complex and the AH and HV intervals are normal. During SVT the retrograde atrial activation sequence is abnormal. The earliest* site of atrial activation is in the CS, which is followed by activation in the HBE and HRA. This activation sequence is diagnostic of a left-sided AV bypass tract conducting retrogradely from ventricle to atrium. [From ME Josephson, in Update IV, Harrison's Principles of Internal Medicine, KJ Isselbacher et al (eds). New York, McGraw-Hill Book Company, 1983, by permission.]

like muscle which may occur almost anywhere around the AV rings. The term WPW syndrome is applied to patients with both preexcitation on the ECG and paroxysmal tachycardias. AV bypass tracts can be associated with certain congenital abnormalities, the most important of which is Ebstein's anomaly (see Chap. 185).

AV bypass tracts which conduct in an antegrade direction produce a typical ECG pattern of a short PR interval (<0.12 s), a slurred upstroke of the QRS complex (delta wave), and a wide QRS complex. This pattern results from a fusion of activation of the ventricles over both the bypass tract and the AV nodal His-Purkinje system (Fig. 184-4). The relative contribution of activation over each system determines the amount of preexcitation.

During PSVT in WPW the impulse is usually conducted antegrade along the normal AV system and retrograde through the bypass tract. The characteristics are identical to those described on page 928 under "AV Reentrant Tachycardia." Rarely (approximately 5 percent) tachycardias occurring in patients with WPW will exhibit a reverse pattern with antegrade conduction through the bypass tract and retrograde conduction through the normal AV system. This produces a tachycardia with a wide QRS complex in which the ventricles are totally activated by the bypass tract. Atrial flutter and AF also occur commonly in patients with the WPW syndrome. Since the bypass tract does not have the same decremental conducting properties as the AV node, the ventricular responses during atrial flutter or fibrillation may be unusually rapid and may cause ventricular fibrillation.

The goals of electrophysiologic evaluation in patients suspected of having the WPW syndrome are to (1) confirm the diagnosis; (2) localize the bypass tract; (3) demonstrate the role of the bypass tract in the genesis of the arrhythmias; (4) determine the refractory period of the bypass tract and its role in the development of potential life-threatening rates during atrial flutter or fibrillation; and (5) evaluate therapeutic options, such as specific pharmacologic agents, pacing therapy, and surgery.

Management This should be aimed at (1) decreasing the occurrence of the APCs and VPCs responsible for the initiation of the tachycardia;

(2) increasing the refractory period of the bypass tract (refractory periods <220 ms are associated with rapid ventricular responses during AF); and (3) blocking conduction down the normal AV conduction system. Specific antiarrhythmic therapy can be assessed by electrophysiologic studies, as described on page 935.

In patients with the WPW syndrome and AF, dc cardioversion should be carried out if there is a life-threatening, rapid ventricular response. Alternatively, lidocaine (2 to 4 mg/kg) or procainamide (15 mg/kg) administered intravenously over 15 to 20 min will usually slow the ventricular response. Caution should be employed when using digitalis, verapamil, or beta blockers in patients with the WPW syndrome and AF, since these drugs can shorten the refractory period of the accessory pathway and can increase the ventricular rate, thereby placing the patient at increased risk for ventricular fibrillation. Although atrial or ventricular pacing can almost always terminate PSVT in patients with the WPW syndrome, they can induce AF. Successful surgical ablations of bypass tracts is possible in more than 90 percent of cases (page 938) and offers a permanent cure.

ACCELERATED AV CONDUCTION IN THE ABSENCE OF MANIFEST PREEXCITATION The ECG pattern of a short PR interval (≤0.12 s) and a normal QRS complex is due to a partial or complete bypass of the AV node. Such patients may develop PSVT due to reentry in the AV node or through a concealed AV bypass tract (the *Lown-Ganong-Levine syndrome*). Treatment should be the same as for patients with normal PR intervals and these arrhythmias. Serial drug testing using the response to programmed stimulation can be utilized to tailor treatment specifically for those patients in whom initial empiric therapy fails.

NONPAROXYSMAL JUNCTIONAL TACHYCARDIA This rhythm usually results from conditions which produce enhanced automaticity or triggered activity in the AV junction and is most common due to digitalis intoxication, inferior wall myocardial infarction, myocarditis, endogenous or exogenous catecholamine excess, acute rheumatic fever, or following valve surgery.

The onset of nonparoxysmal junctional tachycardia is usually

FIGURE 184-4 *ECG in WPW syndrome. There is a short PR interval (0.11 s), a wide QRS complex (0.12 s), and slurring on the upstroke of the QRS produced by early ventricular activation over the bypass tract (delta wave, d in lead I). The negative delta waves in V_1 are diagnostic of a right-sided bypass tract.*

FIGURE 184-5 *Ventricular tachycardia with AV dissociation. P waves which are totally dissociated from the underlying ventricular rhythm can be noted (arrows). AV dissociation is highly suggestive of ventricular tachycardia.*

gradual with a "warm-up" period prior to stabilization of the rate, which can range from 70 to 150 per minute with faster rates usually being associated with digitalis intoxication. Nonparoxysmal junctional tachycardia is recognized by a QRS complex identical to that in sinus rhythm. The rate can be influenced by autonomic tone and can be increased by catecholamines, vagolytic agents, or exercise and can be slowed somewhat by carotid sinus pressure. When this rhythm is due to digitalis intoxication, it usually is associated with AV block and/or disassociation. Early after cardiac surgery, retrograde conduction is more likely to be present due to heightened sympathetic state.

Management This is directed toward elimination of the underlying etiologic factors. Since digitalis is the most common cause of this rhythm, discontinuation of this drug is indicated. If the rhythm is associated with other serious manifestations of digitalis intoxication, such as ventricular or atrial irritability, active intervention with lidocaine or a beta blocker may be useful, and in some instances use of digitalis antibodies (Fab fragments) should be considered. Cardioversion of this rhythm should *not* be attempted, particularly in the setting of digitalis intoxication. When AV conduction is intact, atrial pacing can capture and override the junctional focus and provide the AV synchrony necessary to maximize cardiac output. Nonparoxysmal junctional tachycardia usually is not a chronic recurrent problem and attention to the acute precipitating events often resolves the tachycardia.

VENTRICULAR TACHYCARDIA (VT) *Sustained* VT is defined as one which persists for more than 30 s or requires termination because of hemodynamic collapse. VT generally accompanies some form of structural heart disease, most commonly chronic ischemic heart disease associated with a prior myocardial infarction. Sustained VT may also be associated with nonischemic cardiomyopathies, metabolic disorders, drug toxicity, or prolonged QT syndrome, and it occurs occasionally in the absence of heart disease or other predisposing factors. Nonsustained VT (3 beats to 30 s) is also associated with cardiac disease but occurs in its absence more often than the sustained arrhythmia. While nonsustained VT usually does not produce symptoms, sustained VT is almost always symptomatic and is often associated with marked hemodynamic embarrassment and/or the development of myocardial ischemia. A fixed anatomic substrate, not acute ischemia, is responsible for most recurrent episodes of sustained VT. Acute ischemia appears to have little role in the genesis of sustained uniform VT associated with chronic infarction but may play a role in the degeneration of stable VT into ventricular fibrillation (VF). Most episodes of VF in fact begin with VT.

The ECG diagnosis of VT is suggested by a wide complex tachycardia at a rate exceeding 100 per minute. While the rhythm is usually quite regular, slight irregularity may exist. Atrial activity may be dissociated from ventricular activity (Fig. 184-5) or the atria may be depolarized retrogradely. The onset of the tachycardia is generally abrupt, but in nonparoxysmal tachycardias it can be gradual. The QRS configuration during any episode of VT may be uniform (monomorphic) (Fig. 184-6), or it may vary from beat to beat (polymorphic). *Bidirectional tachycardia* refers to VT which shows

A

B

FIGURE 184-6 *A. Ventricular tachycardia with right bundle branch block morphology. ECG characteristics compatible with ventricular tachycardia are wide QRS complexes ($\geq$0.14 s), superior axis, monophasic R waves in lead V_1, and R:S ratio <1 in lead V_6. B. Ventricular tachycardia with left bundle branch block morphology. ECG characteristics of ventricular tachycardia with a left bundle branch block morphology are the broad, slowly inscribed R waves in leads I and V_6.*

an alternation in QRS amplitude and direction. *Paroxysmal* VT is usually initiated by a VPC.

It is important to distinguish supraventricular tachycardia with aberration of intraventricular conduction from VT since the clinical implications and management of these two arrhythmias are totally different. It is always useful to have a 12-lead ECG recorded during sinus rhythm for comparison with that during the tachycardia. When the tracing obtained during sinus rhythm demonstrates a bundle branch block pattern with the same morphologic features as those during the tachycardia, the diagnosis of supraventricular tachycardia is favored. In addition, an infarction pattern on the sinus rhythm tracing suggests the presence of the anatomic substrate necessary for VT. Characteristics of the 12-lead ECG during the tachycardia which support a ventricular origin for the arrthymia are (1) a QRS complex >0.14 s in the absence of antiarrhythmic therapy; (2) AV dissociation or variable retrograde conduction; (3) a superior QRS axis; (4) concordance of the QRS pattern in all precordial leads (i.e., all positive or all negative deflections); and (5) other QRS patterns with prolonged duration but inconsistent with typical right or left bundle branch block patterns. A wide, complex, bizarre tachycardia that is very irregular suggests AF with conduction over an AV bypass tract (page 930). Similarly, a QRS complex in excess of 0.20 s is uncommon during VT in the absence of drug therapy and is more common with preexcitation.

The diagnosis of VT can be made by analyzing the relationship between the electrogram recording His bundle and ventricular activity. In three-fourths of the cases of VT, no consistent His deflection is observed (Fig. 184-7). Occasionally one may identify His bundle activity either just preceding or following the QRS, due to retrograde activation over the His-Purkinje system. In patients with a wide, complex tachycardia the diagnosis of VT is confirmed when atrial pacing produces normalization of the QRS complex with a normal HV interval. Regardless of QRS morphology [left or right bundle branch block patterns (Fig. 184-6)] VT due to ischemic heart disease arises from the *left* ventricular endocardium.

It has been possible to replicate sustained VT in more than 95 percent of patients with this arrhythmia using programmed stimulation. In most patients the tachycardia is initiated with ventricular premature stimuli. A sustained monomorphic VT with a morphology identical to that of the spontaneous arrhythmia is the rule. The clinical significance of polymorphic VT initiated by programmed stimulation is not clear. It has been shown that when more aggressive stimulation is performed (i.e., the use of three or four extra stimuli), polymorphic

VT and even VF can be induced in some normal subjects and in patients who have never had a clinical arrhythmia.

Sustained uniform VT can be terminated by programmed stimulation or rapid pacing in at least 75 percent of patients; the remainder require cardioversion. The ability to initiate and terminate a sustained, uniform VT reproducibly permits assessment of pharmacologic and electric therapy of these arrhythmias. Serial testing of antiarrhythmic agents over a period of several days can be accomplished and predicts the likelihood of success of the agents or devices tested (page 936).

The reproducible termination of VT by programmed stimulation permits evaluation of the effectiveness of antitachycardia pacemakers for long-term therapy of paroxysmal episodes of arrthythmia. Unfortunately, rapid pacing, which is the most effective form of therapy, can cause acceleration of the tachycardia and/or produce ventricular fibrillation.

Clinical features Symptoms resulting from VT depend on the ventricular rate, duration of the tachycardia, and presence and extent of underlying cardiac disease. When the tachycardia is rapid and associated with severe myocardial dysfunction and cerebrovascular disease, hypotension and syncope are common. The loss of the atrial contribution to ventricular filling and an abnormal sequence of ventricular activation are important factors producing a decreased cardiac output during VT.

The *prognosis* of VT depends on the underlying disease state. If sustained VT develops within the first 6 weeks following acute myocardial infarction, the prognosis is poor, with an 85 percent mortality rate at 1 year. Nonsustained VT following myocardial infarction is associated with a threefold risk of death over a comparable group of patients without this arrhythmia. However, a cause-and-effect relationship between the nonsustained tachycardia and subsequent sudden death has not been established.

Management The risk/benefit ratio of treating each specific type of VT should be considered before beginning therapy. This is important because antiarrhythmic agents can produce or exacerbate the very arrhythmias which they are given to prevent. In general, patients with VT but without organic heart disease have a benign course; such patients with asymptomatic, nonsustained VT need not be treated since their prognosis will not be affected. Patients with sustained VT in the absence of heart disease usually require therapy because the arrhythmia causes symptoms. These tachycardias may respond to beta blockers, verapamil, or quinidine-like agents. Among patients with VT and organic heart disease, if marked hemodynamic embar-

FIGURE 184-7 *Intracardiac recordings distinguishing supraventricular tachycardia from ventricular tachycardia. ECG leads I, aVF, and V₁ are shown with a His bundle electrogram (HBE) and time line (TL). Wide QRS complex tachycardias with a right bundle branch block morphology are shown on the left and right panels. On the left, supraventricular tachycardia is diagnosed by the presence of His deflection (H) preceding each QRS complex with a normal HV interval. During ventricular tachycardia no His bundle deflections can be seen (arrow) and AV dissociation is observed [note single atrial deflection (A)]. (From JA Kastor et al. Reprinted by permission of The New England Journal of Medicine 304:1004, 1981.)*

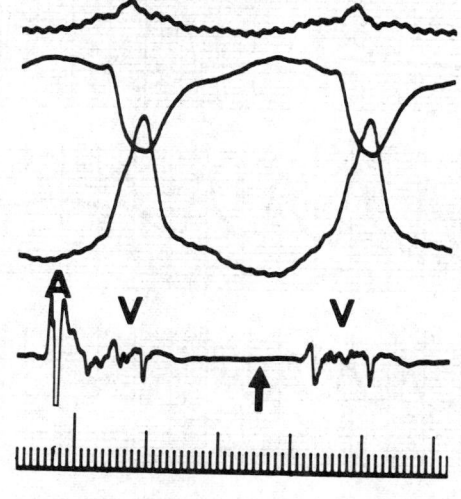

rassment is present or if there is evidence of ischemia, congestive heart failure, or central nervous system hypoperfusion, the rhythm should be promptly terminated by dc cardioversion (see below). If the patient with organic heart disease tolerates the VT well, pharmacologic therapy may be tried. Procainamide is probably the most effective agent. It may or may not terminate the tachycardia, but almost always slows the rate. In stable patients in whom these drugs do not terminate the arrhythmia, a pacing catheter can be inserted pervenously into the right ventricular apex, and the tachycardia can be terminated by rapid pacing.

Therapy guided by programmed stimulation is probably the most efficacious method for selecting the appropriate antiarrhythmic agent to prevent recurrent, sustained VT. In this controlled situation, drugs can be serially studied, and the drug which prevents initiation of the tachycardia can be selected and long-term successful prevention of the arrhythmia can be expected (see Pharmacologic Antiarrhythmic Therapy, page 936).

Antitachycardia pacing has been used as a means to terminate drug-resistant tachycardia. This usually requires that the tachycardia be stable and slow and the patient be aware of it. No automatic antitachycardia device has been approved for the therapy of VT at the time of this writing. Radiofrequency pacemakers which are best activated by a physician have been used in occasional patients.

The advent of endocardial catheter and intraoperative mapping has led to the development of new surgical techniques in the management of VT. In centers in which expertise in mapping is available, operation has been successfully employed to cure tachycardias in the majority of patients in whom it has been undertaken. Even though most patients with VT and ischemic heart disease have markedly impaired left ventricular function and multivessel coronary artery disease, the operative mortality rate has ranged between 8 and 15 percent. Following operation 85 to 90 percent of survivors are controlled either off (two-third of patients) or on (one-third) antiarrhythmic agents which were previously ineffective in controlling these rhythms.

Specific types of VT   TORSADE DE POINTES ("twisting of the points") (Fig. 184-8)   This refers to VT characterized by polymorphic QRS complexes which change in amplitude and cycle length, giving the appearance of oscillating around the baseline. This rhythm is by definition associated with QT prolongation. The latter may result from electrolyte disturbances (particularly hypokalemia and hypomagnesemia), use of a variety of antiarrhythmic drugs (especially quinidine), phenothiazines and tricyclic antidepressants, liquid protein diets, intracranial events, and bradyarrhythmias, particularly third-degree AV block.

The electrocardiographic hallmark is polymorphic VT preceded by marked QT prolongation, often in excess of 0.60 s. These patients often have multiple episodes of nonsustained polymorphic VT associated with recurrent syncope, but they may also develop VF and sudden cardiac death.

Therapy should be directed at removing the precipitating factors, i.e., correcting metabolic abnormalities and removing drugs which have induced the prolonged QT interval. In the setting of drug-induced torsade de pointes, atrial or ventricular pacing and the administration of magnesium have also been useful in terminating and preventing the arrhythmia. For patients with the congenital prolonged QT interval syndrome, beta-adrenergic blocking agents have been the mainstay of therapy; agents which shorten the QT interval may also be useful. Cervicothoracic sympathectomy has been proposed as a form of therapy for congenital prolonged QT syndrome, but it is not often effective as the sole therapy.

Polymorphic tachycardias associated with *normal QT intervals* in patients with ischemic heart disease which are initiated by "R on T" VPCs are probably caused by reentry, and their treatment is totally different. These are not true "torsade de pointes." In such cases, quinidine-like agents are the most effective form of therapy and should be administered in full antiarrhythmic doses.

ACCELERATED IDIOVENTRICULAR RHYTHM (Fig. 184-9)   This arrhythmia, also termed *slow VT*, with a rate which ranges from 60 to 120 per minute, usually occurs in acute myocardial infarction. It may also be seen following cardiac operations, in patients with cardiomyopathy or rheumatic fever or with digitalis intoxication as well as in patients with no evidence of heart disease. The rhythm is usually transient and in and of itself rarely causes significant hemodynamic compromise.

Regardless of whether accelerated idioventricular rhythm occurs in the setting of acute myocardial infarction, in which case the rates are generally slow, or during exercise when it may be more rapid, the arrhythmia is usually transient, rarely causes symptoms and the prognosis is generally excellent.

Treatment is rarely necessary and should usually be considered only if symptoms arise due to impaired hemodynamics, most commonly due to AV dissociation. In most cases, atropine can accelerate the sinus rate to overdrive the ventricular rhythm.

VENTRICULAR FLUTTER AND VENTRICULAR FIBRILLATION (VF) (Fig. 184-9, also see Chap. 30),   Ventricular flutter and VF occur

FIGURE 184-8 *Torsade de pointes. During sinus rhythm a markedly prolonged QR interval (0.74 s) was present. The arrhythmia commences with ventricular bigeminy (aVL) followed by progressively longer runs of polymorphic ventricular tachycardia (V₁, lead I).*

most often in patients with ischemic heart disease. They also occur following administration of antiarrhythmic drugs, particularly those which induce prolonged QT intervals and torsade de pointes (see above), with severe hypoxia or ischemia, and in patients with WPW who develop AF with an extremely rapid ventricular response (page 931). Electrical accidents frequently cause cardiac arrest due to the development of VF. The onset of these arrhythmias is rapidly followed by loss of consciousness and, if untreated, death. Episodes of cardiac arrest recorded during Holter monitoring reveal that approximately three-fourths of the patients have VT or VF producing the sudden cardiac death.

In patients with VF, the onset almost always begins with a short run of rapid VT, which is initiated by a relatively late coupled VPC. In patients with acute myocardial infarction or ischemia, however, VF is usually precipitated by a single early ventricular complex beat falling on the T wave (the vulnerable period), which produces a rapid VT which degenerates into VF (Fig. 184-9).

The clinical setting in which VF occurs is important, since most patients who have primary VF associated with an acute infarction have a good prognosis with a very low recurrence rate of sudden cardiac death. In contrast, most patients who experience VF unassociated with the development of acute myocardial infarction have a recurrence rate of 20 to 30 percent in the year following the event (see Chap. 30).

Ventricular flutter usually appears as a sine wave with rates between 150 and 300 beats per minute. These oscillations make it impossible to assign a specific morphology to the arrhythmia and in some cases to distinguish it from rapid VT. VF is recognized by grossly irregular undulations of varying amplitudes, contours, and rates (Fig. 184-9). Electrophysiologic studies have demonstrated that regardless of the apparent gross irregularity on the surface ECG, VF usually starts out with the rapid repetitive sequence of VT which ultimately breaks down into multiple wavelets of reentry.

Electrophysiologic studies have been useful in patients who have been resuscitated from cardiac arrest. Programmed stimulation has demonstrated that in approximately 70 percent of such patients one can reproducibly initiate a sustained VT. Treatment is discussed in Chap. 30.

PHARMACOLOGIC ANTIARRHYTHMIC THERAPY

Prior to initiation of pharmacologic antiarrhythmic therapy, potential aggravating factors such as transient metabolic abnormalities, congestive heart failure, or acute ischemia must be corrected and in some cases may suffice to control arrhythmias. In addition, the potential role of drugs as a cause or exacerbating factor in the development of the arrhythmia must be considered.

Antiarrhythmic drugs are used in three principal situations: (1) to terminate an acute arrhythmia, (2) to prevent recurrence of an arrhythmia, and (3) to prevent a life-threatening arrhythmia for which the patient is perceived to be at risk, but which has never occurred.

Most currently available antiarrhythmic agents have a relatively low toxic/therapeutic ratio; all can exert proarrhythmic effects, and therefore they may exacerbate underlying arrhythmias. Serum levels can be determined for most currently available antiarrhythmic agents. Standards for therapeutic and toxic levels can serve only as a rough guide for selecting the appropriate dose in any individual patient. In the final analysis, the therapeutic level in a given patient is that concentration which achieves the desired antiarrhythmic effect, and the toxic level for each patient is that at which undesirable side effects occur. Since many adverse effects are directly related to drug concentrations, the minimal serum level which achieves an effective antiarrhythmic response should be chosen.

In order to determine the therapeutic level for a patient, one must have a standard to judge drug efficacy. For a patient with an incessant arrhythmia, antiarrhythmic drugs may be administered empirically until the arrhythmia is suppressed. If a reproducible precipitating factor such as exercise can be identified, serial drug testing during such a provocative maneuver may be performed. Unfortunately, most arrhythmias are sporadic and occur unpredictably without identifiable precipitating factors. In these cases, assessment of drug efficacy may require months, if one waits to observe spontaneous recurrences on each antiarrhythmic drug. This type of assessment of efficacy may be adequate for arrhythmias which are not life-threatening. However, this mode of assessment is inadequate for arrhythmias which compromise hemodynamic stability, result in syncope, or are potentially life-threatening. In such cases two methods for determination of antiarrhythmic drug efficacy have been utilized. The first, which consists of continuous ECG monitoring in the control state and then in the presence of antiarrhythmic drugs, has been used in order to determine the effect which each drug has on spontaneous atrial or ventricular ectopy. This method presupposes that the mechanism responsible for sustained arrhythmias is the same as that causing isolated premature depolarizations (which may or may not be true) and that therefore eradication of isolated ectopy will correlate with prevention of sustained arrhythmias. This method has a number of limitations. First, patients frequently show marked degrees of spontaneous variation in frequency of ectopy, which may mimic antiarrhythmic drug effects. Second, 25 to 30 percent of patients with

FIGURE 184-9 *Top: Accelerated idioventricular rhythm. The lead II strip demonstrates the gradual onset and offset of a wide complex rhythm that is slightly faster than the sinus rhythm. Middle and bottom: Ventricular fibrillation. In a patient with coronary disease ventricular fibrillation is* *initiated by a VPC which produces a rapid polymorphic ventricular tachycardia which rapidly degenerates to ventricular fibrillation (note the undulating baseline with the inability to distinguish systole and diastole).*

sustained ventricular arrhythmias such as VT or VF demonstrate only rare spontaneous ectopy. Finally, many patients demonstrate a dissociation between the effects of antiarrhythmic agents on spontaneous ectopy and the effects of the same agent on sustained arrhythmias.

An alternative method to assess drug efficacy is programmed stimulation. Numerous studies have demonstrated that most clinically occurring supraventricular and ventricular tachyarrhythmias may be reproducibly initiated and terminated safely using this technique. Studies are performed initially in a control state in the absence of antiarrhythmic drugs (Fig. 184-10). If the patient's clinical arrhythmia can be reproducibly initiated, then the ability of individual antiar-

FIGURE 184-10 *Selection of an effective antiarrhythmic drug for ventricular tachycardia by programmed stimulation. From top to bottom, the effects of programmed stimulation during the control state and following administration of several antiarrhythmic agents. During the control state two ventricular extrastimuli initiate the ventricular tachycardia at a rate of 230 per minute. Lidocaine, phenytoin, and disopyramide at the plasma levels shown failed to prevent induction of the tachycardia. Both procainamide and quinidine at the plasma levels shown prevented initiation of sustained tachycardia. Chronic oral quinidine therapy effectively prevented recurrences of the arrhythmia. (From JA Kastor et al. Reprinted by permission of The New England Journal of Medicine 304:1004, 1981.)*

rhythmic drugs to prevent reinduction of the arrhythmia can be assessed after the drug is administered either intravenously or after several days of oral loading in order to achieve a steady-state serum concentration, and induction of the arrhythmia is attempted once again. Use of this method assumes that (1) the induced and spontaneous arrhythmias are identical, and (2) prevention of induction of arrhythmias will correlate with prevention of recurrent spontaneous tachycardias on the same drug regimen. This technique has been validated in patients with a variety of PSVTs secondary to reentry, as well as VT and VF. The technique is safe when carefully performed, the potential complications being those of any intravascular catheterization. Appropriate interpretation of the results of programmed stimulation is critically dependent on correlating the patient's spontaneous arrhythmias with those induced in the laboratory, with regard to rate and morphology.

A number of classifications of antiarrhythmic drugs have been proposed, the most frequently used of which is a modification of that proposed by Vaughn-Williams (Table 184-1). This classification is based in part on the ability of antiarrhythmic drugs to modify the cardiac cellular (1) excitatory currents (Na^+ or Ca^{2+}), (2) action potential duration, and (3) automaticity (phase 4 depolarization). These effects of the drugs on isolated cardiac cells are thought to account for some of the antiarrhythmic effects of the drugs. Thus, depression of excitatory currents in so-called type I and type IV antiarrhythmics results in slowing of conduction velocity and may interrupt arrhythmias by blocking conduction in areas of marginal excitability, where conduction velocity is already slow. Type III antiarrhythmics exert their action by increasing refractoriness through prolongation of the action potential duration. However, such classifications are limited in that the electrophysiologic effects of these drugs in vivo may differ from their effects on isolated cells. The uses and actions of currently available antiarrhythmic drugs are summarized in Tables 184-2 and 184-3.

ELECTRICAL THERAPY OF TACHYARRHYTHMIAS

PACEMAKERS Cardiac pacing can be used to terminate and in selected cases prevent recurrent supraventricular and ventricular arrhythmias. Because many tachyarrhythmias appear to be due to a reentrant mechanism with the impulse traveling in a circuit, a properly timed paced impulse can penetrate and prematurely depolarize part of the circuit, rendering it refractory to the next circulating wavefront, thereby interrupting the circus movement. Pacing therapy for arrhythmias is generally reserved for patients whose arrhythmias are refractory to drug therapy. All forms of pacing therapy require repeated demonstration of their effectiveness and reliability in terminating the arrhythmias during electrophysiologic testing prior to implantation of the pacing device.

The type of pacing device and modality selected for arrhythmia termination depend on (1) the rate of the tachycardia (rates >160 per minute are rarely terminated by a single premature stimulus); (2) the type of the arrhythmia (atrial flutter and VT are rarely terminated by single extrastimuli); and (3) concomitant drug therapy. Underdrive pacing, i.e., pacing at a rate slower than the tachycardia, can be used when a single premature stimulus has been demonstrated to reproducibly terminate a tachycardia. Implanted devices using underdrive pacing commence pacing at a fixed rate when the heart rate exceeds a preset limit. Such pacemakers, termed dual-demand pacemakers, may also discharge when the heart rate falls below a preset critical level.

Because many tachycardias cannot be terminated by single premature stimuli, pacemakers have been developed which allow for multiple extrastimuli (burst pacing) to be introduced. In reentrant tachycardias involving an accessory AV connection, sequential, near simultaneous activation of the heart from both the atria and the ventricle using a dual-chamber pacemaker will increase the likelihood of bidirectional block and termination of the tachycardia.

TABLE 184-3 Dose, serum half-life ($t_{\frac{1}{2}}$) following oral administration, and route of metabolism of drugs used in the treatment of arrhythmias

Drug	Mode of administration	$t_{\frac{1}{2}}$ (oral), h	Route of metabolism
Digoxin	IV 0.75–1.5 mg Oral, 0.75–1.5 mg loading dose over 12–24 h Maintenance, 0.25–0.50 mg/day	36	Renal
Propranolol	IV, 0.5–1 mg/min to total dose of 0.15–0.2 mg/kg Oral, 10–200 mg every 6 h	3–6	Hepatic
Verapamil	IV, 2.5–10 mg over 1–2 min to total 0.15 mg/kg Oral, 80–120 mg every 6–8 h	3–8	Hepatic
Quinidine	IV, 20 mg/min to total 10–15 mg/kg Oral, 200–400 mg every 6 h	5–9	Hepatic
Procainamide	IV, 40–50 mg/min to total 10–20 mg/kg Oral, 500–1000 mg every 4 h	3–5	Hepatic-renal
Disopyramide	Oral, 100–300 mg every 6–8 h	8–9	Renal
Lidocaine	IV, 20–50 mg/min to total dose of 5 mg/kg loading followed by 1–4 mg/min	1–2	Hepatic
Phenytoin	IV, 20 mg/min total dose to 1000 mg Oral, 1000-mg loading over 24 h Maintenance, 100–400 mg/day	18–36	Hepatic
Tocainide	Oral, 400 to 600 mg every 8–12 h	10–17	Hepatic-renal
Bretylium	IV, 1–2 (mg/kg)/min to total load, 5–10 mg/kg Maintenance, 0.5–2 mg/min	8–14	Renal
Amiodarone*	IV, 5–10 mg/kg Oral, load 800–1400 mg/day for 1–2 weeks Maintenance, 100–600 mg/day	Unknown	Hepatic
Mexiletine*	Oral, 100–300 mg every 6–8 h	9–12	Hepatic

* Investigational.

Cardiac pacing has also been used to prevent ventricular tachyarrhythmias. Polymorphic VT associated with a long QT interval and bradycardias (torsade de pointes, page 934) is most likely to respond. Pacing the atrium and/or ventricle at rates between 90 and 120 per minute appears to increase the homogeneity of electrical recovery and markedly reduces the propensity for a recurrence of arrhythmias. Regardless of the arrhythmia being treated and the pacing mode selected, the potential for alterations in pacing requirements for termination of tachycardia and therefore programmability of pacing modes (e.g., underdrive, dual-demand, dual-chamber, burst) as well as rate and coupling interval of introduced extrastimuli are probably essential features for pacemakers used to terminate tachycardias.

Pacemakers may be self-contained or energized by an external radiofrequency source. The self-contained pacemaker may function automatically [i.e., it incorporates an arrhythmia recognition program (circuit) or it is activated by an external magnet]. The major advantage of a fully automatic system is that there is no need for the patient to recognize the arrhythmia in order for termination to occur. The advantages of the externally activated system include (1) the decreased risk of unnecessary treatment because of faulty sensing; and (2) the opportunity to initiate monitoring at the time of attempted arrhythmia termination. This type of monitoring is frequently helpful if pacing techniques are employed to terminate VT, given the risk of acceleration of the arrhythmia by pacing.

The limitations of pacing therapy are primarily related to (1) the changes in the characteristics of the arrhythmia over time such that programmed pacing parameters no longer terminate the tachycardia; and (2) the risk of acceleration of the tachycardia with the development of AF when stimulating the atrium and the development of rapid VT and VF when stimulating the ventricles. In the future, pacing generators which can also deliver a larger amount of energy and perform cardioversion and defibrillation of accelerated arrhythmias are likely to increase the applicability of pacing therapy for the treatment of arrhythmias.

CARDIOVERSION AND DEFIBRILLATION Electrical cardioversion and defibrillation remain the most reliable method for terminating arrhythmias. By depolarizing all or at least a large portion of excitable myocardium in a near homogeneous fashion, the electric shock can interrupt reentrant arrhythmias. External cardioversion is routinely performed by placing two paddles 12 cm in diameter in firm contact with the chest wall, with one paddle usually located to the right of the sternum at the level of the second rib and the other in the left midclavicular line in the fifth intercostal space. If the patient is conscious, a short-acting barbiturate to act as an anesthetic or an amnesic drug such as diazepam should be administered to prevent patient discomfort. A person skilled in maintaining an airway should be present. Energy is delivered synchronously with the QRS complex for all arrhythmias except ventricular flutter and VF; sinoasynchronous shocks can produce VF. The amount of energy used will vary with the type of tachycardia being treated. With the exception of AF, supraventricular tachycardias can frequently be terminated with energy levels in the range of 25 to 50 W·s, while AF usually requires ≥100 W·s for termination. For terminating VT, energy levels ≥100 W·s should probably be employed. While energies as low as 25 W·s may be successfully used, they also have a higher incidence of producing VF. At least 200 W.s of energy should be used for initial attempts at terminating VF. All repeated attempts at defibrillation should be with the maximum energy that the defibrillator is capable of delivering (320 to 400 W·s).

Indications for cardioversion depend upon the clinical setting and the patient's general condition. Any tachycardia (except sinus tachycardia) that produces hypotension, myocardial ischemia, or heart failure warrants consideration of prompt termination using external cardioversion. Arrhythmias that fail to terminate with pharmacologic therapy may also be terminated by electrical cardioversion. Transient bradycardias and supraventricular and ventricular irritability following cardioversion are common and usually do not warrant antiarrhythmic intervention.

AUTOMATIC INTERNAL DEFIBRILLATION An automatic implanted cardioverting-defibrillating device has been developed to allow for prompt recognition and termination of life-threatening ventricular arrhythmias. The device delivers 25 to 33 W·s of energy. Clinical trials testing the function of the device in patients with drug refractory ventricular arrhythmias have demonstrated survival from sudden death at 1 year ranging between 92 and 100 percent. Based on the results of the initial trials, it appears that an automatic sensing, implanted cardioverter-defibrillator will play an important role in arrhythmia management. At the time of this writing, use of this device should be reserved for patients with VT which is not hemodynamically tolerated or for patients with VF whose arrhythmias are refractory to drug therapy and who are not candidates for surgical intervention (see below). The most frequent problem with the device has been its inappropriate discharge in the absence of sustained ventricular arrhythmias.

CATHETER ABLATION FOR ARRHYTHMIAS Catheter ablation of tachyarrhythmias, a technique which involves the delivery of large amounts of energy (25 to 400 W·s) through a catheter to effect closed-chest electroablation of the bundle of His has been primarily used to interrupt AV conduction and prevent a rapid ventricular response to supraventricular arrhythmias. Although not yet approved by the Food and Drug Administration, catheter ablation of the AV junction has become the procedure of choice for creating AV block to control supraventricular arrhythmias. However, the introduction of complete heart block necessitating a pacemaker following His bundle ablation and the small risk of sudden death associated with the procedure make catheter ablation a procedure of "last resort" at this time.

SURGICAL TREATMENT OF ARRHYTHMIAS

Programmed stimulation and endocardial activation mapping have provided a better understanding of the mechanisms and sites of origin of many supraventricular and ventricular tachyarrhythmias, so that in selected patients surgical treatment may be considered.

WPW SYNDROME   Surgery may be preferable to other forms of therapy in some patients, particularly those with the WPW syndrome and recurrent arrhythmias. Advances made in the localization and surgical ablation of bypass tracts now allow for an extremely high success rate with minimal morbidity. As a result, surgery can now be considered not only in patients with drug-refractory arrhythmias but also as a reasonable alternative in (1) patients with symptomatic arrhythmias who require long-term drug therapy; (2) patients with AF and a life-threatening rapid ventricular response; and (3) patients undergoing cardiac surgery for other reasons in whom a bypass tract is present.

SUPRAVENTRICULAR TACHYCARDIA AND OTHER ATRIAL ARRHYTHMIAS   Although atrial flutter, AF, and PSVT are usually not life-threatening, they may be refractory to pharmacologic or pacing interventions. In such cases surgery may be considered as a method of removing the abnormal focus, interrupting the reentry circuits, and curing the tachycardia or controlling the ventricular response by creating AV block. In atrial flutter and AF the pathophysiologic substrate cannot be identified; thus, the only surgical option is to destroy the AV node–His bundle region by cryosurgery or transvenous catheter electroablation (page 936). Similarly, surgery, cryoablation, or electrode catheter ablation for the treatment of AV nodal reentrant tachycardia usually results in the production of AV block and requires concomitant implantation of a permanent pacemaker. Focal atrial tachycardias have been treated surgically by discrete resection or ablation by cryothermal injury. Mapping the tachycardia is mandatory if a primary direct approach on the arrhythmia is to be performed.

Surgery should only be performed for patients with arrhythmias refractory to other treatment modalities and should only be performed for tachycardias in whom the tachycardia has been localized.

VENTRICULAR TACHYCARDIA   The demonstration that VT due to ischemic heart disease can often be reliably induced by programmed stimulation and that the arrhythmia is localized to a small region of endocardium in the area of prior infarction has permitted the development of specific surgical techniques for the cure of the arrhythmia.

Preoperatively all morphologically distinct tachycardias which occur spontaneously are induced by programmed stimulation and their respective sites of origin are determined by catheter activation mapping. Catheter mapping may be supplemented by intraoperative mapping, involving similar techniques. These studies have shown that tachycardias arise in the scar tissue near the endocardium.

Subendocardial resection and endocardial encircling ventriculotomy, the surgical techniques that have been applied to the management of ventricular tachycardia, are aimed at removing or isolating the pathophysiologic substrate of the arrhythmia, as identified by mapping. The major factor responsible for surgical success is the ability to localize the site from which the arrhythmias arise. These procedures are associated with a 10 percent operative mortality rate

but have prevented recurrences of VT and VF in 85 to 90 percent of survivors without drugs or with drugs that had been previously ineffective.

REFERENCES

BHANDARI AK, SCHEINMAN M: The long QT syndrome. Mod Concepts Cardiovasc Dis 54:45, 1985
BOINEAU JP: Atrial flutter: A synthesis of concepts. Circulation 72:249, 1985
———, COX JL: Rationale for a direct surgical approach to control ventricular arrhythmias. Relation of specific intraoperative techniques for mechanism and location of arrhythmia circuit. Am J Cardiol 49:381, 1982
CHAROS GS et al: A theoretically and practically more effective method for interruption of ventricular tachycardia: Self-adapting autodecremental overdrive pacing. Circulation 73:309, 1986
ECHT DS et al: Clinical experience, complications and survival in 70 patients with the automatic implantable cardioverter defibrillator. Circulation 71:289, 1985
FRAME LN, HOFFMAN BF: Mechanisms of tachycardia. In *Tachycardias*, B Surawicz (ed). Boston, Martinus Nijhoff, 1984
GALLAGHER JJ et al: The preexcitation syndromes. Prog Cardiovasc Dis 20:285, 1978
JOSEPHSON ME: Paroxysmal supraventricular tachycardia: An electrophysiologic approach. Am J Cardiol 41:1123, 1978
———, SEIDES SF: *Clinical Cardiac Electrophysiology: Techniques and Interpretations.* Philadelphia, Lea & Febiger, 1979
———, WELLENS HJJ (eds): *Tachycardias: Mechanisms, Diagnosis, Treatment.* Philadelphia, Lea & Febiger, 1984
ROSEN MR, HOFFMAN BF (eds): *Cardiac Therapy.* Boston, Martinus Nijhoff, 1983
SCHEINMAN MM, EVENS-BELL T: Catheter ablation of the atrioventricular junction: A report of the percutaneous mapping and ablation registry. Circulation 70:1024, 1984
TORRES V et al: QT prolongation and the antiarrhythmic efficacy of amiodarone. J Am Coll Cardiol 7:142, 1986
WALDECKER B et al: Dysrhythmias after direct-current cardioversion. Am J Cardiol 57:120, 1986
WIT AL, ROSEN MR: Cellular electrophysiology of cardiac arrhythmias. Mod Concepts Cardiovasc Dis 50:1, 1981

185   CONGENITAL HEART DISEASE

WILLIAM F. FRIEDMAN

GENERAL CONSIDERATIONS

INCIDENCE   Approximately 1 percent of all live births have a cardiovascular malformation. If recognized early, the anomalies can now be diagnosed accurately, and most patients can be salvaged by medical and surgical management.

Congenital heart disease shows an overall male preponderance, but specific defects may exhibit a specific sex preponderance; patent ductus arteriosus and atrial septal defect are common in females, whereas valvular aortic stenosis, congenital aneurysms of the sinus of Valsalva, coarctation of the aorta, tetralogy of Fallot, and transposition of the great arteries are more common in males.

ETIOLOGY   Congenital cardiovascular malformations are generally the result of aberrant embryonic development of the heart or a failure of such a structure to progress beyond an early stage. Malformations are due to complex multifactorial genetic and environmental causes; only rarely may a single causal factor be identified (Table 185-1).

A single gene mutation (Chap. 57) may be causal in the familial forms of atrial septal defect, mitral valve prolapse, ventricular septal defect, congenital heart block, situs inversus, the combination of supravalvular aortic stenosis and peripheral pulmonary arterial stenosis, idiopathic hypertrophic subaortic stenosis, and the syndromes of Noonan, Holt-Oram, Ellis–van Creveld, and Kartagener. Table 185-1 provides a partial list of syndromes in which cardiovascular anomalies are due to the pleiotropic effects of single genes or examples of gross chromosomal defects. Recognized chromosomal aberrations and mutations of single genes account for less than 10 percent of all cardiac malformations.

The fact that only one of a pair of monozygotic twins may be affected by congenital heart disease indicates that the majority of cardiovascular malformations are not inherited in a simple manner. Family studies indicate a two- to fivefold increase in the incidence of congenital heart disease in the siblings of affected patients. The malformations are concordant or partially concordant in at least half of such cases. Nonetheless, the incidence of congenital heart disease in the siblings of an index patient is only 2 to 5 percent. Most patients with isolated heart defects have a negative family history for malformations and a normal chromosome pattern, and it is rarely wise to discourage the parents of one affected child from having additional children. The low recurrence rate and the increasing possibilities for effective therapy for most cardiac lesions usually justify a positive approach to family counseling. If, however, two or more members of a family are affected, the recurrence risk may be quite high, and a detailed family history should be obtained prior to further counseling. If a dominant or recessive mendelian pattern is present, the risk of recurrence in each pregnancy can be predicted (Chap. 57).

PREVENTION The feasibility of preventive programs will depend upon what is learned in the future about the cause of the majority of cardiovascular anomalies for which no cause is known. An effective rubella vaccine is available, and immunization of children with this vaccine may lessen maternal rubella and its cardiac consequences. Strict testing in animals of new drugs that can be teratogenic when taken early in pregnancy may reduce the chances of another thalido-mide tragedy. In this regard, no medications should be taken during pregnancy without prior consultation with a physician. Physicians should be aware of known teratogens, as well as of drugs for which inadequate information exists as to teratogenic potential. Similarly, appropriate use of radiologic equipment and techniques for reducing gonadal and fetal radiation exposure may reduce the hazards of this likely cause of birth defects.

The presence of a cardiac malformation as one component of a multiple system involvement in Down's, Turner's, and the trisomy 13-15 (D_1) and 17-18 (E) syndromes (see Chap. 60) may be anticipated in occasional pregnancies at risk by fetal cells obtained from amniotic fluid or chorionic villus biopsy. Similarly, identification in such cells of the enzyme disorders characteristic of Hurler's syndrome, homo-cystinuria, or type II glycogen storage disease may allow one to predict cardiac disease.

THE FETAL AND TRANSITIONAL CIRCULATIONS

The fetus has a single circulation in which the pulmonary vasculature exists in parallel, not in series, with the systemic circulation. Prenatal survival is not endangered by severe cardiac anomalies as long as one side of the heart can drive blood from the great veins to the aorta. Inferior vena caval blood is deflected across the foramen ovale into the left atrium. Most of the blood that reaches the right ventricle bypasses the high-resistance, unexpanded lungs and passes through the ductus arteriosus into the descending aorta. In fetal life, pulmonary arteries and arterioles are surrounded by a fluid medium, have relatively thick walls and small lumens, and resemble comparable arteries in the systemic circulation.

Normally, at birth this single circulation is divided into two separate circulations in series. Inflation of the lungs at the first inspiration produces a reduction in pulmonary vascular resistance. Fetal pulmonary vessels, heretofore supported by fluid media, are suddenly suspended in air, reducing extravascular pressure. New vessels are opened, and already patent vessels enlarge. Pulmonary arterial pressure falls, and pulmonary blood flow increases, primarily because pulmonary arteriolar vasodilatation results from the increase in oxygen tension to which these vessels are exposed. The systemic vascular resistance rises because clamping the umbilical cord removes the low-resistance placental circulation. Increased pulmonary blood flow increases the return of blood to the left atrium and raises left atrial pressure, which in turn closes the foramen ovale. The shift in oxygen dependence from the placenta to the lungs produces a sudden increase in arterial blood oxygen tension, which, in concert with alterations in the local prostaglandin milieu, initiates constriction of the ductus arteriosus, and total anatomic closure follows within a few days.

PULMONARY HYPERTENSION Pulmonary hypertension is a common accompaniment of many congenital cardiac lesions, and the status of the pulmonary vascular bed is often the principal determinant of the clinical manifestations, the course, and the feasibility of surgical repair. Increases in pulmonary arterial pressure result from elevation of pulmonary blood flow and/or resistance, the latter due sometimes to an increase in vascular tone but usually the result of obstructive, obliterative structural changes within the pulmonary vascular bed. Fortunately, most patients with congenital heart disease are suitable for surgical repair because only a few isolated or combined malformations remain physiologically or anatomically uncorrectable by cardiovascular surgery. Moreover, there has been a remarkable advance in surgical techniques for infants and very young children and an enhanced awareness of the need to operate early on patients at risk for pulmonary vascular obstructive disease. These developments will reduce the number of older children and adults whose pulmonary vascular obstructive disease is the consequence of delayed operation or progression of pulmonary vascular obstruction after complete closure of the defect in childhood.

As in the other vascular beds, the pressure in the pulmonary artery is determined by the product of the volume of blood flow per unit of time and of the resistance to that flow. Equalization of pressures in the systemic and pulmonary circulations occurs if a large communication exists between the two great arteries or between the two ventricles in the absence of semilunar valve obstruction. Pulmonary vascular resistance is calculated as the transpulmonary pressure difference per unit of pulmonary blood flow (Chap. 180). When blood flow increases, existing patent vessels are distended, and additional vessels are opened, so that calculated vascular resistance diminishes. Therefore, in a normal pulmonary vascular bed, pressure rises substantially only if flow is greatly increased. In most patients with congenital heart disease and elevated pulmonary vascular resistance, the pulmonary arterioles are the principal locus of this abnormal resistance.

The causes of pulmonary vascular obstructive disease are unknown, although increased pulmonary blood flow, increased pulmonary arterial blood pressure, elevated pulmonary venous pressure, poly-cythemia, systemic hypoxia, acidosis, and the bronchial circulation have been implicated. In many patients with pulmonary vascular obstruction the cardiac anomaly places them at risk early in life, precluding survival to adulthood. Patients at particular risk for significant pulmonary vascular obstruction are those with cyanotic congenital heart disease, such as complete transposition of the great arteries, single ventricle, and double-outlet right ventricle without pulmonary stenosis and truncus arteriosus. Other conditions in which pulmonary vascular obstruction progresses rapidly include a large ventricular septal defect and the less common conditions of complete atrioventricular canal defects and congenital left-to-right shunts in an environment of high altitude or in association with Down's syndrome.

Variability among patients whose cardiac lesions have the same or similar time of appearance exists in the rate of progression of the pulmonary vascular obstructive process. Although genetic influences may be operative (witness the apparent acceleration of pulmonary vascular disease in patients with congenital heart disease and trisomy 21), important pre- and postnatal modifiers of the pulmonary vascular bed appear, at least in part, to be lesion-dependent. Thus, a quantitative variability exists in the pulmonary vascular bed as to the number, not just the size and wall structure, of arterial vessels within the pulmonary circulation. Modeling of the blood vessels proximal to and within terminal bronchioles (preacinar and intraacinar vessels, respectively) occurs continuously from before birth. The intraacinar vessels, in particular, increase in size and number from late fetal life throughout childhood with minimal muscularization of the walls. The

TABLE 185-1 Syndromes with associated cardiovascular involvement

Syndrome	Major cardiovascular manifestations	Major noncardiac abnormalities
HERITABLE AND POSSIBLY HERITABLE		
Ellis–van Creveld	Single atrium or atrial septal defect	Chondrodystrophic dwarfism, nail dysplasia, polydactyly
TAR (thrombocytopenia-absent radius)	Atrial septal defect, tetralogy of Fallot	Radial aplasia or hypoplasia, thromocytopenia
Holt-Oram	Atrial septal defect (other defects common)	Skeletal upper limb defect, hypoplasia of clavicles
Kartagener	Dextrocardia	Situs inversus, sinusitis, brochiectasis
Laurence-Moon-Biedl-Bardot	Variable defects	Retinal pigmentation, obesity, polydactyly
Noonan	Pulmonary valve dysplasia, cardiomyopathy (usually hypertrophic)	Webbed neck, pectus excavatum, cryptorchidism
Tuberous sclerosis	Rhabdomyoma, cardiomyopathy	Phacomatosis, bone lesions, hamartomatous skin lesions
Multiple lentigines (leopard) syndrome	Pulmonic stenosis	Basal-cell nevi, broad facies, rib anomalies
Rubenstein-Taybi	Patent ductus arteriosus (others)	Broad thumbs and toes, hypoplastic maxilla, slanted palpebral fissures
Familial deafness	Arrhythmias, sudden death	Sensorineural deafness
Osler-Rendu-Weber	Arteriovenous fistuals (lung, liver, mucous membranes)	Multiple telangiectasia
Apert	Ventricular septal defect	Craniosynostosis, midfacial hypoplasia, syndactyly
Incontinentia pigmenti	Patent ductus arteriosus	Irregular pigmented skin lesions, patchy alopecia, hypodontia
Alagille (arteriohepatic dysplasia)	Peripheral pulmonic stenosis, pulmonic stenosis	Biliary hypoplasia, vertebral anomalies, prominent forehead, deep-set eyes
DiGeorge	Interrupted aortic arch, tetralogy of Fallot, truncus arteriosus	Thymic hypoplasia or aplasia, parathyroid aplasia or hypoplasia, ear anomalies
Friedreich's ataxia	Cardiomyopathy and conduction defects	Ataxia, speech defect, degeneration of spinal cord dorsal columns
Muscular dystrophy	Cardiomyopathy	Pseudohypertrophy of calf muscles, weakness of trunk and proximal limb muscles
Cystic fibrosis	Cor pulmonale	Pancreatic insufficiency, malabsorption, chronic lung disease
Sickle cell anemia	Cardiomyopathy, mitral regurgitation	Hemoglobin SS
Conradi-Hünermann	Ventricular septal defect, patent ductus arteriosus	Asymmetric limb shortness, early punctate mineralization, large skin pores
Cockayne	Accelerated atherosclerosis	Cachectic dwarfism, retinal pigment abnormalities, photosensitivity dermatitis
Progeria	Accelerated atherosclerosis	Premature aging, alopecia, atrophy of subcutaneous fat, skeletal hypoplasia
CONNECTIVE TISSUE DISORDERS		
Cutis laxa	Peripheral pulmonic stenosis	Generalized disruption of elastic fibers, diminished skin resilience, hernias
Ehlers-Danlos	Arterial dilatation and rupture, mitral regurgitation	Hyperextensible joints, hyperelastic and friable skin
Marfan	Aortic dilatation, aortic and mitral incompetence	Gracile habitus, arachnodactyly with hyperextensibility, lens subluxation
Osteogenesis imperfecta	Aortic incompetence	Fragile bones, blue sclera
Pseudoxanthoma elasticum	Peripheral and coronary arterial disease	Degeneration of elastic fibers in skin, retinal angioid streaks
INBORN ERRORS OF METABOLISM		
Pompe's disease	Glycogen storage disease of heart	Acid maltase deficiency, muscular weakness
Homocystinuria	Aortic and pulmonary arterial dilatation, intravascular thrombosis	Cystathionine synthetase deficiency, lens subluxation, osteoporosis
Mucopolysaccharidosis:		
Hurler, Hunter	Multivalvular and coronary and great artery disease, cardiomyopathy	Hurler: Deficiency of α-L-iduronidase, corneal clouding, coarse features, growth and mental retardation Hunter: Deficiency of L-iduranosulfate sulfatase, coarse facies, clear cornea, growth and mental retardation
Morquio, Scheie, Morateaux-Lamy	Aortic incompetence	Morquio: Deficiency of *N*-acetylhexosamine sulfate sulfatase, cloudy cornea, normal intelligence, severe bony changes involving vertebrae and epiphyses Scheie: Deficiency of α-L-iduronidase, cloudy cornea, normal intelligence, peculiar facies Morateaux-Lamy: Deficiency of arylsulfatase B, cloudy cornea, osseous changes, normal intelligence
CHROMOSOMAL ABNORMALITIES		
Trisomy 21 (Down's syndrome)	Endocardial cushion defect, atrial or ventricular septal defect, tetralogy of Fallot	Hypotonia, hyperextensible joints, mongoloid facies, mental retardation
Trisomy 13 (D)	Ventricular septal defect, patent ductus arteriosus, double-outlet right ventricle	Single midline intracerebral ventricle with midfacial defects, polydactyly, nail changes, mental retardation
Trisomy 18 (E)	Congenital polyvalvular dysplasia, ventricular septal defect, patent ductus arteriosus	Clenched hand, short sternum, low-arch dermal-ridge pattern on fingertips, mental retardation
Cri-du-chat (short-arm delection-5)	Ventricular septal defect	Cat cry, microcephaly, antimongoloid slant of palpebral fissures, mental retardation

the left ventricle include congenital valvular aortic stenosis, the discrete form of congenital subaortic stenosis, congenital narrowing of the supravalvular ascending aorta, and hypertrophic cardiomyopathy with outflow tract obstruction (Chap. 192).

Valvular aortic stenosis Valvular aortic stenosis is a relatively rare congenital cardiovascular defect that occurs three to four times more often in males than in females. However, the congenital bicuspid aortic valve, which is not necessarily stenotic, may actually be the most common congenital malformation of the heart, although it may go undetected in early life. Because bicuspid valves may become stenotic with time or be the site of infective endocarditis, the lesion may be difficult to distinguish in adults from acquired rheumatic aortic stenosis. Commonly associated anomalies include patent ductus arteriosus and coarctation of the aorta.

The dynamics of blood flow associated with a congenitally deformed, rigid aortic valve commonly lead to thickening of the cusps and, in later life, to calcification. Hemodynamically significant obstruction causes concentric hypertrophy of the left ventricular wall and dilatation of the ascending aorta.

The hemodynamic abnormalities are discussed in Chap. 187. A peak systolic pressure gradient exceeding 70 mmHg, in association with a normal cardiac output, or an effective aortic orifice less than 0.6 cm² per square meter of body surface, is considered to represent critical obstruction to left ventricular outflow. In children and young adults, the resting cardiac output is generally normal but often fails to rise normally during muscular exercise.

Most children with congenital aortic stenosis are asymptomatic. Usually, a murmur is detected on a routine examination. Moderately severe obstruction should be suspected if there is a history of fatigability and exertional dyspnea. With severe obstruction, the inability of the left ventricle to increase its output and maintain cerebral flow during exercise may result in exertional syncope, and the disparity between the oxygen supply and myocardial oxygen requirements may cause angina. The symptomatic patient with valvular aortic stenosis generally has critical stenosis, although a lack of symptoms does not preclude the presence of moderately severe obstruction. Sudden death occurs in patients with critical stenosis, and ventricular arrhythmias, perhaps initiated by acute myocardial ischemia, may be responsible.

Hemodynamically significant obstruction is associated with a left ventricular lift and a precordial systolic thrill over the base of the heart, with transmission to the jugular notch and along the carotid arteries. Presystolic expansion is often palpable. A systolic aortic ejection sound, signifying opening of the aortic valve, is typical at the cardiac apex when the valve is mobile, particularly with mild to moderate stenosis. Delayed closure of the stenotic aortic valve leads to a single or a closely split second heart sound, and paradoxic splitting may be present. A fourth heart sound is generally associated with severe obstruction. The systolic murmur starts after the completion of left ventricular isometric contraction, is rhomboid-shaped, loud, harsh, and best heard at the base of the heart. The murmur, like the thrill, radiates to the jugular notch and carotid vessels and to the apex. An early diastolic blowing murmur of aortic regurgitation may be present, but unless the valve has been eroded by infective endocarditis, the regurgitation is usually not hemodynamically significant; occasionally, in patients with a congenital bicuspid valve, severe aortic regurgitation may be the dominant hemodynamic lesion.

The electrocardiographic evidence of left ventricular hypertrophy tends to reflect the severity of obstruction, although a *normal or near-normal electrocardiogram does not exclude severe aortic stenosis*. The left ventricular "strain pattern" generally indicates that severe aortic stenosis is present.

The overall heart size is most often normal or only slightly enlarged. Left atrial enlargement and concentric left ventricular hypertrophy accompany moderate or severe obstruction. Poststenotic dilatation of the ascending aorta is common. Echocardiographic findings include multiple eccentric diastolic closure lines in the aortic

lumen, thickening of the left ventricular posterior wall and septum, reduced separation of thickened aortic valve leaflets, and aortic dilatation. Two-dimensional echocardiography demonstrates the aortic valve morphology; Doppler echocardiography is the most accurate means of noninvasively estimating the magnitude of obstruction. Cardiac catheterization is indicated when the clinical diagnosis of aortic stenosis has been established and when the history, clinical examination, roentgenogram, electrocardiogram, or echocardiogram suggests severe obstruction. The site and severity of obstruction are established, and any associated malformations are identified. With mild or moderate obstruction repeat left-sided heart catheterization should be carried out every 5 to 10 years because stenosis may progress.

The medical management of congenital valvular aortic stenosis includes prophylaxis against infective endocarditis and, in patients with diminished cardiac reserve, the administration of digitalis and diuretics and sodium restriction while awaiting operation. If severe aortic stenosis is present, strenuous physical activity should be avoided even when the patient is asymptomatic, and participation in competitive sports should probably be restricted in patients with milder degrees of obstruction. The decision concerning the advisability of operation depends on the severity of obstruction rather than on the symptoms. Operation is carried out under direct vision with the aid of cardiopulmonary bypass, and in children without valvular calcification the fused commissures are opened. Commissurotomy may result in aortic regurgitation that can progress to require prosthetic valve replacement. Moreover, since the valves remain deformed after valvulotomy, further degenerative changes, including calcification, may lead to significant stenosis later. The treatment of congenital aortic stenosis in the adult is described in Chap. 187.

Subaortic stenosis The most common form of subaortic stenosis is the *idiopathic hypertrophic* variety, also termed *hypertrophic cardiomyopathy*, which occurs in a congenital form in about one-third of the patients and is discussed in Chap. 192. Both clinically and physiologically, the *discrete* form of subaortic stenosis resembles valvular aortic stenosis. The lesion usually consists of a membranous diaphragm or fibrous ring encircling the left ventricular outflow tract just beneath the base of the aortic valve. It is less common than isolated valvular obstruction and occurs more frequently in males than in females. There are no reliable clinical criteria to distinguish the two forms of obstruction, although a systolic ejection sound is rare and the diastolic murmur of aortic regurgitation is more common in patients with discrete subvalvular aortic stenosis than with valvular aortic stenosis. Valvular calcification does not occur with subaortic stenosis. Echocardiography often demonstrates the subaortic obstruction; Doppler echocardiography demonstrates turbulence proximal to the aortic valve and may also detect aortic regurgitation. Definitive differentiation between valvular and subvalvular obstruction is accomplished at cardiac catheterization by recording pressure tracings as a cardiac catheter is withdrawn across the outflow tract and by left ventricular angiocardiography.

Because of the likelihood of progressive obstruction and aortic regurgitation, the presence of even mild or moderate subaortic stenosis warrants consideration of elective surgery to excise the membrane or fibrous ridge.

Occasionally, valvular and subvalvular aortic stenosis coexist in the same patient, producing a tunnel-like narrowing of the left ventricular outflow tract. Common associated findings are a small ascending aorta, hypoplasia of the aortic valve ring, and thickened valve leaflets. It may be recognized by angiography. Operative treatment frequently involves prosthetic replacement of the aortic valve, as well as enlarging the aortic annulus, proximal aorta, and left ventricular outflow tract, or the interposition of a valved conduit between the left ventricular apex and the aorta.

Supravalvular aortic stenosis Supravalvular aortic stenosis is a localized or diffuse narrowing of the ascending aorta, originating just above the level of the coronary arteries at the superior margin of the sinuses of Valsalva. In contrast to other forms of aortic stenosis, the coronary arteries are subjected to the elevated pressures that exist within the left ventricle and are often dilated and tortuous. Adherence of the free edges of the aortic cusps to the sites of supravalvular stenosis may interfere with coronary arterial inflow.

William's or the *supravalvular aortic stenosis syndrome* is the coexistence of the cardiovascular lesion and idiopathic infantile hypercalcemia, which is probably due to deranged cholecalciferol metabolism. Other manifestations include mental retardation, a peculiar "elfin facies," craniosynostosis, strabismus, narrowing of peripheral systemic and pulmonary arteries, inguinal hernias, cryptorchidism (in males), premature development of secondary sexual characteristics in females, auditory hyperacusis, and abnormalities of dental development. Supravalvular aortic stenosis and peripheral pulmonary arterial stenosis are also seen in familial and sporadic forms unassociated with the other features of the syndrome. The familial disorder is transmitted as an autosomal dominant trait with variable expressivity.

The physical findings resemble those in valvular aortic stenosis, except that the sound of aortic valve closure is accentuated, ejection sounds are infrequent, and transmission of the thrill and murmurs into the jugular notch and along the carotid vessels is more prominent; the systolic pressure in the right arm is characteristically higher than in the left. Poststenotic dilatation of the ascending aorta is rare.

The electrocardiogram reveals left ventricular hypertrophy. The diagnosis is confirmed by the demonstration at retrograde aortic catheterization of a pressure gradient just above the aortic valve, and a constriction at this level as revealed by aortography.

Surgical treatment consists of widening the lumen of the aorta by the insertion of a fabric prosthesis, and operative treatment is indicated if the obstruction is severe and discrete without generalized hypoplasia of the ascending aorta and arch.

Coarctation of the aorta   Narrowing or constriction of the lumen of the aorta may occur anywhere along its length but is most common distal to the origin of the left subclavian artery near the insertion of the ligamentum arteriosum. Coarctation occurs in about 7 percent of patients with congenital heart disease and is twice as common in males as in females, although the lesion occurs frequently in patients with gonadal dysgenesis (Chap. 331). Clinical manifestations depend on the site and extent of obstruction and the presence in the majority of associated cardiac anomalies. These include bicuspid aortic valve, congenital aortic stenosis, patent ductus arteriosus, ventricular septal defect, and mitral regurgitation. When diffuse narrowing of the aorta is proximal to the ductus arteriosus, right ventricular hypertrophy develops in utero, and pulmonary hypertension and congestive heart failure are common in early life. *Differential cyanosis* may result from preferential shunting of unsaturated pulmonary arterial blood through a patent ductus to the lower part of the body.

More commonly, the coarctation is at or just distal to the attachment of the ductus or ligamentum arteriosus. The majority of children and young adults with isolated juxta- or postductal coarctation are asymptomatic. Headache, epistaxis, cold extremities, and claudication with exercise may occur, and attention is usually directed to the cardiovascular system when a heart murmur or hypertension in the upper extremities is detected on physical examination. In childhood, mechanical rather than renal factors play the primary role in hypertension.

Absence, marked diminution, or delayed pulsations in the femoral arteries and a low or unobtainable arterial pressure in the lower extremities with hypertension in the arms are clues to diagnosis. In adults, enlarged and pulsatile collateral vessels may be palpated in the intercostal spaces anteriorly, in the axillae, or posteriorly in the interscapular area. The upper extremities and thorax may be more developed than the lower extremities. A midsystolic murmur over the anterior part of the chest, back, and spinous processes may become continuous if the lumen is narrowed sufficiently to result in

a high-velocity jet across the lesion throughout the cardiac cycle. Additional systolic and continuous murmurs over the lateral thoracic wall may reflect increased flow through dilated and tortuous collateral vessels. The *electrocardiogram* reveals left ventricular hypertrophy of varying degree, depending on the height of the arterial pressure proximal to the obstruction and the patient's age; predominant right or combined ventricular hypertrophy in infants and children usually implies a complicated lesion. *Roentgenograms* may show a dilated left subclavian artery high on the left mediastinal border and a dilated ascending aorta. Indentation of the aorta at the site of coarctation and pre- and poststenotic dilatation (the "3" sign) along the left paramediastinal shadow are almost pathognomonic. Notching of the ribs, an important radiographic sign, is due to erosion by dilated collateral vessels, increases with age, and usually becomes apparent between the sixth and twelfth years of life. Two-dimensional echocardiography from para- or suprasternal windows usually identifies the site and length of coarctation. Cardiac catheterization and aortography may be indicated to localize the site of obstruction, determine the length of the coarctation, and identify associated malformations.

The *treatment* of uncomplicated coarctation of the aorta is surgical; resection and end-to-end anastomosis or subclavian flap angioplasty can usually be accomplished with excellent results, although it may be necessary to use a tubular graft or patch if the narrowed segment is long. Paradoxic hypertension of short duration is common in the immediate postoperative period, and necrotizing panarteritis of the small vessels of the gastrointestinal tract of uncertain cause may complicate the recovery. In those who survive the first 2 years of life complications are uncommon before the second or third decade; operation on asymptomatic patients is recommended between the ages of 3 and 6. The chief hazards result from severe hypertension and include the development of cerebral aneurysms and hemorrhage, rupture of the aorta, left ventricular failure, and infective endocarditis. Systemic hypertension in the absence of residual coarctation postoperatively appears to be related to the duration of preoperative hypertension; lifelong observation is desirable because of the late onset of hypertension in some postoperative patients.

Pulmonary stenosis with intact ventricular septum   Obstruction to right ventricular outflow is relatively common; it may be localized to the supravalvular, valvular, or subvalvular levels or occur at a combination of these sites. Multiple sites of narrowing of the peripheral pulmonary arteries are a feature of rubella embryopathy and may occur with both the familial and sporadic forms of supravalvular aortic stenosis. Valvular pulmonic stenosis is the most common form of isolated right ventricular obstruction.

The severity of the obstructing lesion, rather than the site of narrowing, is the most important determinant of the course. In the presence of a normal cardiac output, a peak systolic transvalvular pressure gradient between 50 and 80 mmHg is considered to be moderate stenosis; levels below and above that range are classified as mild and severe, respectively. Patients with mild pulmonic stenosis are generally asymptomatic and demonstrate little or no progression in the severity of obstruction with age. In patients with more significant stenosis, the severity may increase with time. Atresia of the pulmonary valve is commonly associated with a hypoplastic right ventricle and interatrial communications. Symptoms vary with the degree of obstruction. Infants with pulmonary atresia often die from hypoxia. Fatigue, dyspnea, right ventricular failure, and syncope may limit the activity of older patients, in whom moderate or severe obstruction may prevent an augmentation of pulmonary blood flow with exercise.

In patients with severe obstruction, the systolic pressure in the right ventricle may exceed that in the left ventricle, since the ventricular septum is intact. Right ventricular ejection is prolonged with moderate or severe stenosis, and the sound of pulmonary valve closure is delayed and soft. Right ventricular hypertrophy reduces the compliance of that chamber, and a forceful right atrial contraction is necessary to augment right ventricular filling. A fourth heart sound, prominent *a* waves in the jugular venous pulse, and occasionally, presystolic pulsations of the liver reflect the vigorous atrial contraction. The clinical diagnosis is supported by a right parasternal lift and harsh systolic ejection murmur and thrill at the upper left sternal border, typically preceded by a systolic ejection sound if the obstruction is valvular. The systolic murmur becomes louder, and its crescendo occurs later in systole, and more severe degrees of valvular obstruction result in a greater prolongation of right ventricular systole. The holosystolic decrescendo murmur of tricuspid regurgitation may accompany severe pulmonic stenosis, especially in the presence of congestive heart failure. Cyanosis usually reflects venoarterial shunting through a patent foramen ovale or atrial septal defect. In patients with supravalvular or peripheral pulmonary arterial stenosis, the murmur is systolic or continuous and is best heard over the area of narrowing, with radiation to the peripheral lung fields.

The electrocardiogram may be helpful in assessing the degree of obstruction to right ventricular output. In mild cases, the electrocardiogram is often normal, whereas moderate and severe stenoses are associated with right axis deviation and right ventricular hypertrophy. A ventricular strain pattern, as well as high-amplitude P waves in leads II and V_1, indicating right atrial enlargement, is associated with severe stenosis. The chest roentgenogram with mild or moderate pulmonic stenosis often shows a heart of normal size and normal vascularity of the lungs. In the presence of valvular stenosis, poststenotic dilatation of the main and left pulmonary arteries may be evident. With severe obstruction and resultant right ventricular failure, right atrial and right ventricular enlargement are generally evident. The pulmonary vascularity may be reduced with severe stenosis, right ventricular failure, and/or a venoarterial shunt at the atrial level.

Two-dimensional echocardiographic visualization of pulmonary value morphology from a parasternal window is usually possible. The outflow tract pressure gradient can usually be estimated by Doppler ultrasonography. Cardiac catheterization and angiocardiography with right ventricular injection localize the site of obstruction, establish its severity, and document the coexistence of additional cardiac malformations. Catheter techniques are also available for therapeutic balloon valvuloplasty. Treatment of moderate and severe degrees of pulmonary valvular and subvalvular stenosis is usually surgical. Direct surgical relief of the obstruction is accomplished at a low risk. Multiple stenoses of the peripheral pulmonary arteries are usually inoperable, but narrowing of a single branch or at the bifurcation of the main pulmonary trunk may be corrected.

CYANOTIC—INCREASED PULMONARY BLOOD FLOW Complete transposition of the great arteries The aorta arises from the right ventricle to the right of and anterior to the pulmonary artery, which emerges from the left ventricle. This results in two separate and parallel circulations, and some communication between the two circulations must exist after birth to sustain life. Most patients have an interatrial communication, two-thirds have a patent ductus arteriosus, and about one-third have an associated ventricular septal defect. Transposition is more common in males and occurs more frequently in the offspring of diabetic mothers. It is a leading cause of death due to congenital heart disease in the first 2 months of life and accounts for approximately 10 percent of cyanotic heart disease.

The course is determined by the degree of tissue hypoxia, the ability of each ventricle to sustain an increased work load in the presence of reduced coronary arterial oxygenation, the nature of the associated cardiovascular anomalies, and the status of the pulmonary vascular bed. Severe morphologic alterations develop in the pulmonary vascular bed by 1 to 2 years of age in most patients who also have an associated large ventricular septal defect or large patent ductus arteriosus in the absence of obstruction to left ventricular outflow.

The usual manifestations are dyspnea and cyanosis from birth, retardation of growth, and congestive heart failure. The roentgenographic findings are often highly suggestive and consist of (1) progressive cardiac enlargement in early infancy, (2) characteristic oval or egg-shaped cardiac configuration in the anteroposterior view

and a narrow vascular pedicle, and (3) increased pulmonary vascular markings. In the absence of dextrocardia, two-dimensional echocardiography provides the diagnosis by demonstrating that the anterior great artery (aorta) is to the right of the posterior greater artery (pulmonary). Angiocardiography is also diagnostic and demonstrates that the anteriorly placed aorta arises from the right ventricle and that the posteriorly placed pulmonary artery in continuity with the mitral valve arises from the left ventricle.

The creation or enlargement of an interatrial communication is the simplest procedure for providing increased intracardiac mixing of systemic and pulmonary venous blood; it may be achieved surgically or, preferably, by rupturing the valve of the foramen ovale with a balloon catheter during cardiac catheterization (Rashkind's procedure). Systemic-pulmonary artery anastomosis may be indicated in the patient with severe obstruction to left ventricular outflow and diminished pulmonary blood flow. Intracardiac repair may be accomplished by rearranging the venous return so that the systemic venous blood is directed to the mitral valve and thence to the left ventricle and pulmonary artery, while the pulmonary venous blood is diverted through the tricuspid valve and right ventricle to the aorta (Mustard or Senning operation). For those patients with a ventricular septal defect in whom it is necessary to bypass a severely obstructed left ventricular outflow tract, corrective operation employs an intracardiac ventricular baffle and extracardiac prosthetic conduit to replace the pulmonary artery (Rastelli's procedure). The management of patients with a large ventricular septal defect is a subject of debate. In some centers pulmonary artery banding is advocated early in life, followed by definitive intracardiac repair at 1 to 2 years of age. In others, a one-stage operation is utilized to close the ventricular septal defect, transpose both coronary arteries to the posterior artery, and transect, contrapose, and anastomose the aorta and pulmonary arteries (Jatene or arterial switch operation).

Total anomalous pulmonary venous connection When all the pulmonary veins connect either to the right atrium directly or to the systemic veins or their tributaries, the condition is called total anomalous pulmonary venous connection (TAPVC). Because all venous blood returns to the right atrium, an interatrial communication is an integral part of this malformation. Most infants with TAPVC fail to thrive, are subject to repeated respiratory infections, and have congestive heart failure by the age of 6 months. Cyanosis is not prominent in the absence of congestive failure unless the patient survives long enough to acquire secondary pulmonary vascular changes and a reduction in pulmonary blood flow.

A characteristic finding is the presence of multiple heart sounds, consisting of a first sound followed by an ejection click, a fixed, widely split second heart sound with an accentuated pulmonic component, and a third, and often a fourth, heart sound. The electrocardiogram shows right axis deviation, as well as right atrial and ventricular hypertrophy. Roentgenograms of the chest reveal increased pulmonary blood flow; the right atrium and ventricle are dilated and hypertrophied, and the pulmonary artery segment is enlarged. Echocardiography demonstrates marked enlargement of the right ventricle and may reveal the course and level of entry of the anomalous pulmonary venous channels. Selective pulmonary arteriography is helpful in determining the drainage pathways of the pulmonary veins.

Balloon atrial septostomy may provide dramatic palliation for the infant in whom the small size of the interatrial communication limits the amount of blood reaching the left side of the heart and systemic circulation. Unless serious pulmonary vascular disease is present, results of operation for TAPVC in patients more than 1 year of age are good. The procedure consists of creating an anastomosis between the common pulmonary venous channel and the left atrium and of closing the atrial defect and the anomalous venous pathway.

CYANOTIC—DECREASED PULMONARY BLOOD FLOW Tetralogy of Fallot Tetralogy is responsible for about 10 percent of all forms of congenital heart disease and is the most common cause of cyanosis after 1 year of age. The four components of the tetralogy of Fallot are ventricular septal defect, obstruction to right ventricular outflow, aortic override (straddle) of the ventricular septal defect, and right ventricular hypertrophy. The basic anomaly results from an anterior deviation of the infundibular ventricular septum away from its usual location in the heart between the limbs of the trabecular septum. The ventricular defect is typically large and located just below the right cusp of the aortic valve, separated from the pulmonic valve by the crista supraventricularis. The aortic root may be displaced anteriorly, overriding the septal defect but, as in a normal heart, to the right of the pulmonary artery. In most cases, the overriding of the aorta is due to the subaortic location of the ventricular septal defect.

The severity of obstruction to right ventricular outflow determines the clinical presentation. The degree of hypoplasia of the outflow tract of the right ventricle varies from mild to complete (pulmonary atresia). Pulmonary valve stenosis and supravalvular and peripheral pulmonary arterial obstruction may coexist, and unilateral absence of the pulmonary artery (usually the left) occurs rarely. Circulation to the abnormal lung is by systemic arterial collaterals. Atresia of the pulmonic valve, infundibulum, or main pulmonary artery is occasionally referred to as *pseudotruncus arteriosus*. True truncus arteriosus with absent pulmonary arteries (truncus type 4) differs from tetralogy of Fallot in which pulmonary artery branches are present and are perfused by systemic arterial collaterals or a patent ductus arteriosus. A right-sided aortic arch and descending aorta occur in about 25 percent of patients with tetralogy. The coronary arteries may have variations that are surgically important. The anterior descending artery sometimes originates from the right coronary artery, which may also give rise to a left branch coursing anterior to the infundibulum; a single left coronary artery may give rise to a branch that crosses the outflow tract of the right ventricle. Associated cardiac anomalies occur in about 40 percent, and noncardiac anomalies are present in 20 to 30 percent of patients.

When right ventricular outflow obstruction is severe, the pulmonary blood flow is markedly reduced, and a large volume of unsaturated systemic venous blood is shunted from right to left across the ventricular septal defect, severe cyanosis and polycythemia occur, and symptoms of systemic anoxia are prominent. The term *pink,* or *acyanotic, tetralogy of Fallot* is used often to describe an interventricular communication and a milder degree of obstruction to right ventricular outflow with no appreciable venoarterial shunting. In many patients the obstruction to right ventricular outflow is mild but progressive, so that early in life pulmonary exceeds systemic blood flow, and the symptoms resemble those produced by a simple ventricular septal defect.

Most children with tetralogy of Fallot are cyanotic from birth or develop cyanosis before 1 year of age. Dyspnea with exertion, retarded growth and development, clubbing, and polycythemia are common. When resting after exertion, infants with tetralogy characteristically assume a squatting posture. Spells of severe anoxia and cyanosis (see ''Hypoxic Spells'' above) constitute a major threat to survival.

Physical examination reveals variable degrees of underdevelopment and cyanosis. Clubbing of the digits may be prominent after the first year of life. A right ventricular impulse and systolic thrill may be palpable along the left sternal border; there is no generalized cardiomegaly. The second heart sound is single, and the pulmonic component is rarely audible. A systolic ejection murmur is produced by flow across the narrowed right ventricular outflow tract or pulmonic valve. The intensity and duration of the murmur vary inversely with the severity of obstruction, the opposite of the relation existing in patients with an intact ventricular septum and pulmonary stenosis. Polycythemia, decreased systemic vascular resistance, and increased obstruction to right ventricular outflow may all be responsible for a decrease in the intensity of the murmur. A continuous murmur over the paravertebral area may indicate collateral circulation to the lungs through bronchial arteries.

The electrocardiogram ordinarily shows right ventricular and, less often, right atrial hypertrophy. Radiologic examination characteristically reveals a normal-sized, boot-shaped heart (*coeur en sabot*) with prominence of the right ventricle and a concavity in the region of the pulmonary conus. The pulmonary vascular markings are typically diminished, and the aortic arch and knob may be on the right side. Two-dimensional echocardiography from the parasternal or subcostal windows demonstrates the malalignment of the ventricular septal defect and the subpulmonary stenosis. The presence or absence of stenoses at the origins of the branch pulmonary arteries can also be assessed. Selective angiocardiography with right ventricular injection is necessary to confirm the diagnosis and to evaluate the architecture of the right ventricular outflow tract, pulmonary valve and annulus, and caliber of the main branches of the pulmonary artery.

Factors that may complicate the management of patients with tetralogy include infective endocarditis, paradoxic embolism, polycythemia, coagulation defects, and cerebral infarction or abscess. The paroxysmal cyanotic spells may respond to oxygen, placing the child in the knee-chest position, and morphine. If the spell persists, metabolic acidosis will develop from prolonged anaerobic metabolism, and infusion of sodium bicarbonate may be necessary to interrupt the attack. Vasopressors, beta-adrenergic blockade, or general anesthesia may occasionally be necessary.

In infants with pulmonary atresia cardiac catheterization is often done as an emergency. Because survival in this setting usually depends on patency of the ductus arteriosus, intravenous infusion of prostaglandin E_1 (0.1 mg per kilogram of body weight per minute) may dramatically reverse clinical deterioration and improve arterial blood gases and pH.

Primary correction is advisable at some point for almost all patients who have tetralogy of Fallot. Early intracardiac repair, even in infancy, is advocated in most centers properly equipped for infant cardiac operations. Successful early correction avoids progressive infundibular obstruction, acquired pulmonary atresia, delayed growth, and complications due to hypoxemia and polycythemia. The size of the pulmonary arteries rather than the age or size of the infant or child is the most important determinant in establishing candidacy for primary repair. Pronounced hypoplasia of the pulmonary arteries is a relative contraindication for an early corrective surgical procedure. When this problem is present, a palliative operation, such as creation of a systemic arterial–pulmonary arterial shunt, is carried out and is usually followed by complete correction, which can be carried out at a lower risk later in childhood.

Ebstein's anomaly   In this anomaly there is abnormal morphogenesis of the tricuspid valve, with redundancy of tricuspid valve tissue, and the attachment of portions of the septal and posterior leaflets of the tricuspid valve is lower than normal; the leaflets originate from the right ventricular wall rather than from the atrioventricular ring. Hence, the portion of the right ventricle that lies between the atrioventricular ring and the origin of the valve is continuous with the right atrial chamber. The tricuspid valve is usually incompetent, the foramen ovale is patent, and the right ventricle exhibits varying degrees of hypoplasia. The clinical manifestations of Ebstein's anomaly are variable, depending on the severity of the anatomic changes in the tricuspid valve. Ultimately, however, progressive cyanosis resulting from the right-to-left shunt across the interatrial communication, symptoms resulting from right ventricular dysfunction, and/or paroxysmal arrhythmias develop.

A prominent systolic pulsation of the liver and a large v wave in the jugular venous pulse accompany the systolic thrill and murmur of tricuspid regurgitation. Wide splitting of the first and second heart sounds and prominent third and fourth heart sounds may produce a characteristically rhythmic auscultatory cadence. The electrocardiogram shows giant P waves, a prolonged PR interval, and complete or incomplete right bundle branch block. Roentgenography usually demonstrates an enlarged right atrium and a small right ventricle and pulmonary artery and reduced pulsations; the pulmonary vascularity may be reduced if a large right-to-left shunt is present. The principal echocardiographic findings include a large anterior tricuspid leaflet with delayed tricuspid valve closure with respect to mitral closure. Two-dimensional echocardiography best demonstrates the morphologic features. At cardiac catheterization the intracavitary electrocardiogram recorded just proximal to the tricuspid valve shows a right ventricular type of complex, while the pressure recorded is that of the right atrium.

Most patients survive to the third decade at least. In some disabled patients moderate improvement has resulted from anastomosis of the superior vena cava to the right pulmonary artery to divert systemic venous return from the right atrium and to increase pulmonary blood flow. Patients beyond early childhood have occasionally benefited from prosthetic replacement of the tricuspid valve; at all ages, however, patients with Ebstein's anomaly are poor surgical risks.

Tricuspid atresia Atresia of the tricuspid valve, an interatrial communication, and, frequently, hypoplasia of the right ventricle and pulmonary artery exist in this malformation. The clinical picture is usually dominated by severe cyanosis as a result of greatly diminished pulmonary blood flow.

Blood atrial septostomy and palliative operations consisting of increasing pulmonary blood flow, often by systemic arterial or venous–pulmonary artery anastomosis, may allow survival to the age of 10 to 20 years; functional correction of the anomaly can then be accomplished in those with normal or low pulmonary arterial pressure by anastomosis of the right atrial appendage to the right ventricle with the aid of a pericardial patch or by insertion of a prosthetic conduit or direct anastomosis between the right atrium and pulmonary artery and closure of the interatrial communication.

REFERENCES

General

ADAMS FH, EMMANOUILIDES GC: *Moss' Heart Disease in Infants, Children and Adolescents*, 3d ed. Baltimore, Williams and Wilkins, 1983

BOROW KM et al: Congenital heart disease in the adult, in *Heart Disease*, 2d ed, E Braunwald (ed). Philadelphia, Saunders, 1984, p 1024

ENGLE MA, PERLOFF JK (eds): *Congenital Heart Disease After Surgery*. New York, Yorke, 1983

FREEDOM RM: *Angiocardiography of Congenital Heart Disease*. New York, Macmillan, 1984

FRIEDMAN WF: Congenital heart disease in infancy and childhood, in *Heart Disease*, 2d ed, E Braunwald (ed). Philadelphia, Saunders, 1984, p 941

———, HIGGINS CB: *Pediatric Cardiac Imaging*. Philadelphia, Saunders, 1984

STARK J, deLEVAL M: *Surgery for Congenital Heart Defects*. New York, Grune and Stratton, 1983

Specific malformations

BARBER G et al: Pulmonary atresia with ventricular septal defect. J Am Coll Cardiol 7:630, 1986

BEHL P: Ebstein's anomaly: 16 years experience with valve replacement without plication of the right ventricle. Thorax 39:8, 1984

BISSET GS: Aortic valve replacement in childhood: Evaluation of left ventricular function by electrocardiography, echocardiography and graded exercise testing. Am J Cardiol 52:568, 1983

DiSESSA TG et al: Systemic venous and pulmonary arterial flow patterns after Fontan's procedure for tricuspid atresia or single ventricle. Circulation 70:898, 1984

DOTY DB et al: Aortic pulmonary septal defect: Hemodynamics, angiography and operation. Ann Thorac Surg 32:244, 1981

FOSTER ED: Reoperation for aortic coarctation. Ann Thorac Surg 38:81, 1984

FREED MD et al: Repair of secundum and sinus venosus atrial septal defects. J Am Coll Cardiol 4:333, 1984

FRIEDMAN WF: Patent ductus arteriosus in respiratory distress syndrome: A historical review. Pediatr Cardiol 4:3, 1983

———, GEORGE BL: Medical progress—Treatment of congestive heart failure by altering loading conditions of the heart. J Pediatr 106:697, 1985

HAWKINS JA: Total anomalous pulmonary venous connection. Ann Thorac Surg 36:548, 1983

HENZE A et al: Ruptured sinus of Valsalva aneurysms. Scand J Thorac Cardiovasc Surg 17:249, 1983

KIRKLIN JW: Surgical results and protocols in the spectrum of tetralogy of Fallot. Ann Surg 198:251, 1983

MACRI R et al: Congenital coronary artery fistula. Thorac Cardiovasc Surg 30:167, 1982

MARX GR et al: Transposition of the great arteries with intact ventricular septum. J Am Coll Cardiol 1:476, 1983

MOODIE DS et al: Anomalous origin of the left coronary artery from the pulmonary artery in adult patients; long term follow-up after surgery. Am Heart J 106:381, 1983

POLANSKI DB: Pulmonary stenosis in infants and young children. Ann Thorac Surg 39:159, 1985

ROSENTHAL A: Long-term prognosis (15 to 26 years) after repair of tetralogy of Fallot. Ann Thorac Surg 38:151, 1984

STARK J: Transposition of the great arteries: Which operation? Ann Thorac Surg 38:429, 1984

TENORIO A et al: The spectrum of atrioventricular discordance: A clinical study. Br Heart J 51:498, 1984

VAN PRAAGH R: Diagnosis of complex congenital heart disease: A morphologic-anatomic method and terminology. Cardiovasc Intervent Radiol 7:115, 1984

WRIGHT GB et al: Subaortic stenosis in the young: Medical and surgical course in 83 patients. Am J Cardiol 52:830, 1983

---

186 RHEUMATIC FEVER

GENE H. STOLLERMAN

DEFINITION Rheumatic fever is an inflammatory disease which occurs as a delayed sequel to pharyngeal infection with group A streptococci. It involves principally the heart, joints, central nervous system, skin, and subcutaneous tissues. The usual manifestations in the acute form are migratory polyarthritis, fever, and carditis. Sydenham's chorea, subcutaneous nodules, and erythema marginatum may occur as other typical manifestations. No single symptom, sign, or laboratory test is pathognomonic of rheumatic fever, although several combinations of them are diagnostic. Although the name *acute rheumatic fever* emphasizes involvement of the joints, rheumatic fever owes its importance to the involvement of the heart, which can be fatal during the acute stage of the disease or can lead to rheumatic heart disease, a chronic condition due to scarring and deformity of the heart valves.

ETIOLOGY AND PATHOGENESIS The etiologic relationship of group A streptococci to rheumatic fever can be summarized briefly, as follows. (1) Numerous clinical and epidemiologic studies have shown a close association of group A streptococcal infections and rheumatic fever. (2) Antecedent streptococcal infection can almost always be demonstrated immunologically in the acute stage of rheumatic fever by increased titers of antibodies to streptococcal antigens. Moreover, in long-term prospective follow-up studies, rheumatic fever recurs only as a result of intercurrent streptococcal infections. (3) Both primary and secondary attacks of the disease can be prevented by prompt treatment or prevention of streptococcal infections with antimicrobial therapy. The pharyngeal route of infection is necessary to initiate the rheumatic process. Streptococcal skin infections do not do so. Furthermore, throat infections with some group A strains appear to produce rheumatic fever rarely or not at all.

The mechanism by which the group A streptococcus initiates the disease process remains unknown. A relatively small percentage of persons who suffer from streptococcal sore throats subsequently develop rheumatic fever. The organism is not demonstrable in the lesions when rheumatic fever appears several days or weeks after the acute streptococcal infection. No one product of the streptococcus has been incriminated as a cause of the lesions, either as a direct tissue toxin or as an antigen inducing hypersensitivity. Several streptococcal antigens have demonstrated cross-reactivity with cardiac and other tissues. Their direct relationship to pathogenesis is, however, unproven, and streptococcus-induced autoimmunity as a mechanism to explain the rheumatic process remains a popular but unestablished pathogenetic concept.

INCIDENCE AND EPIDEMIOLOGY Although rheumatic fever may occur at any age, it is extremely rare in infancy; it appears most commonly between the ages of 5 and 15 years, when streptococcal infection is most frequent and intense. Similarly, the geographic distribution, incidence, and severity of rheumatic fever are, in general, a reflection of the frequency and severity of streptococcal pharyngitis. The attack rate of rheumatic fever following exudative streptococcal pharyngitis in epidemics averages approximately 3 percent. When streptococcal pharyngitis is sporadic and mild or due to strains of lesser rheumatic potential, the attack rate of rheumatic fever may be very much lower. Strains of group A streptococci that cause epidemics of streptococcal pharyngitis are most likely to be rheumatogenic. Following such infections, the attack rate of rheumatic fever is directly correlated with the magnitude of the streptococcal immune response. Analysis of reported epidemics of acute rheumatic fever caused by a variety of serotypes shows some, such as type 5, to be overrepresented, and others to be conspicuously absent. In some populations, such as in Trinidad, strains responsible for rheumatic fever and acute glomerulonephritis are serotypically distinct.

Environmental, bacterial, and host factors which appear to play a role in the development of rheumatic fever are important primarily as they are related to the incidence and severity of preceding streptococcal infection. Such factors as latitude, altitude, dampness, economic factors, and age all affect the incidence of rheumatic fever because they are related to the incidence of streptococcal infection in general. Crowding is, however, the major environmental factor relating to the occurrence of this disease because, regardless of other variables, it promotes interpersonal spread of the most virulent group A streptococcal strains. Such crowding as occurs in military barracks, closed institutions, large families in small quarters, and those massed in the densely populated core of major urban centers is most likely to be associated with an increase in incidence of rheumatic fever.

The attack rate of rheumatic fever following streptococcal infections in patients who have had previous attacks of rheumatic fever is increased to as high as 5 to 50 percent and is also related to the virulence of the reactivating infection. Furthermore, the frequency of rheumatic recurrences following streptococcal infection is consistently greater in those with rheumatic heart disease than in those who escaped cardiac injury during prior attacks. The tendency to suffer recurrences of rheumatic fever following streptococcal infections declines with the passage of years since the preceding attack. It appears, therefore, that certain host variables, as well as probable qualitative and quantitative differences in the nature of the antecedent streptococcal infection, also influence the development of rheumatic fever. To what extent such variables are genetic or acquired has not been settled. It is common to obtain a family history of rheumatic fever as well as to encounter multiple cases among siblings of a single family. However, the concordance of rheumatic fever in identical twins is approximately 20 percent, suggesting only a limited penetrance of genetic predisposition to rheumatic fever. Although investigations of the distribution of haplotypes in rheumatic hosts have been limited in scope and number, there has been so far no consistent association of rheumatic fever, or any of its major manifestations, with any predominant histocompatibility locus antigens.

The mortality of acute rheumatic fever has been declining steadily for the past 30 years. It is still, however, a major cause of death and disability in children and adolescents in socioeconomically depressed areas of the world. The incidence of rheumatic fever has been decreasing for several years in countries where housing and economic conditions have been improving steadily. The rate of decrease may have been accelerated by the wide use of antimicrobial therapy. The decrease also may be due to a change in the prevalence of rheumatogenic streptococcal strains. Rheumatic fever remains, however, a worldwide disease having its greatest incidence wherever poor economic conditions, overcrowding, and substandard housing are most common.

PATHOLOGY The lesions of rheumatic fever are disseminated widely throughout the body, with special predilection for connective tissues. Focal inflammatory lesions occur particularly around small blood vessels.

Cardiovascular lesions The heart is the site of the most characteristic and consequential involvement, and all its layers—endocardium, myocardium, and pericardium—may be involved. This generalized involvement gives rise to the term *rheumatic pancarditis*. The most characteristic and specific pattern of rheumatic inflammation is found in the *myocardial Aschoff body*, a submiliary granuloma. This lesion, when present in its classic form, is generally considered to be pathognomonic of rheumatic fever. In many areas the inflammatory lesion is accompanied by swelling and fragmentation of the collagen fibers and alteration in the staining properties of the ground substances of the connective tissues. This change is described as *fibrinoid degeneration of collagen,* but its chemical basis has not been established. Aschoff bodies with less exudative and more productive changes may persist for many years as the lingering traces of chronic rheumatic inflammation in patients with rheumatic heart disease, long after rheumatic fever has become clinically quiescent. The persistence of such lesions is most common in patients who develop severe mitral stenosis. Eventually the Aschoff body is converted into a spindle-shaped or triangular scar lying between the muscle bundles and surrounding blood vessels.

Rheumatic endocarditis produces the verrucous valvulitis of acute rheumatic fever which leads to the most serious permanent cardiac damage. It may heal with fibrous thickening and adhesion of the valve commissures and chordae tendineae, leading to variable degrees of valvular regurgitation and stenosis. Deformity resulting in functional impairment of the heart occurs most commonly in the mitral and aortic valves, less frequently in the tricuspid, and almost never in the pulmonic valves. *Rheumatic pericarditis* (Chap. 194) produces a serofibrinous effusion, with the deposit of shaggy elements of fibrin on the surface of the heart. The pericardium may become calcified, but pericardial constriction does not occur.

Extracardiac lesions Involvement of the *joints* is characterized by exudative rather than proliferative changes, and healing of these structures occurs without significant scarring or deformity. *Subcutaneous nodules,* seen during the acute phase of the disease, are composed of granulomas with localized areas of "fibrinoid" swelling of subcutaneous collagen bundles, and perivascular collections of large cells with pale nuclei and prominent nucleoli. Synovitis is usually mild and nonspecific. *Pulmonary* and *pleural* lesions are less definite and less characteristic. Fibrinous pleurisy and rheumatic pneumonitis may occur with exudative and proliferative lesions but without definite Aschoff bodies. Patients with active *chorea* rarely die. The pathologic findings which have been reported in the central nervous system are not consistent, and no characteristic lesion has been reported to explain this clinical manifestation. During active chorea the spinal fluid remains normal, being free of cells, with no increase in total protein and no change in the relative concentration of various proteins.

CLINICAL FEATURES The major clinical manifestations by which rheumatic fever can be recognized are polyarthritis, carditis, chorea, erythema marginatum, and subcutaneous nodules.

Arthritis The classic attack of rheumatic fever appears as an acute migratory polyarthritis accompanied by signs and symptoms of an acute febrile illness. The large joints of the extremities are most frequently affected, but no joint is impervious to the inflammatory process; one may find arthritis of the hands and feet but only rarely of the spine or of the sternoclavicular or temporomandibular joints. Joint effusions occur but are not persistent. As pain and swelling subside in one joint, others tend to become involved. Although such "migratory" involvement is characteristic, it is not invariable, and several large joints may be inflamed at one time. To be acceptable as a criterion for the diagnosis of rheumatic fever, the polyarthritis should involve two or more joints, should be associated with at least two minor manifestations such as fever and elevation of sedimentation rate, and should be associated with high titer of antistreptolysin O or some other streptococcal antibody (Table 186-1). There is nothing

TABLE 186-1 Jones criteria (revised)

Major manifestations	Minor manifestations
Carditis	Fever
Polyarthritis	Arthralgia
Chorea	Previous rheumatic fever or rheumatic heart disease
Erythema marginatum	Elevated ESR or positive CRP
Subcutaneous nodules	Prolonged PR interval

Two major criteria or one major and two minor criteria indicate a high probability of the presence of rheumatic fever with supporting evidence of preceding streptococcal infection: history of recent scarlet fever; positive throat culture for group A streptococcus; increased ASO titer or other streptococcal antibodies.

SOURCE: *American Heart Association, 1965.*

distinctive about the arthritis of rheumatic fever, and other causes of migratory polyarthritis that may be associated only fortuitously with high streptococcal antibody levels must, of course, be excluded.

Acute rheumatic carditis Acute rheumatic carditis first manifests itself by the appearance of the heart murmurs of either mitral or aortic regurgitation, the former most frequently. Signs and symptoms of pericarditis and of congestive heart failure may supervene in more severe cases. Death may result from heart failure during the acute stage of the disease, or permanent valvular damage may be sustained which results ultimately in serious disability. Carditis may vary from a fulminating, fatal course to a low-grade, inapparent inflammation. *It is well to bear in mind that the vast majority of patients with carditis do not have symptoms referable to the heart.* The latter occur only in more severe cases when heart failure or pericardial effusions produce characteristic symptoms. For this reason, unless extracardiac manifestations, such as polyarthritis and chorea, are present, patients whose rheumatic fever is manifested only by carditis are frequently not diagnosed and in later life may be discovered to have rheumatic heart disease without a definite history of rheumatic fever.

When carditis is manifest, there is usually tachycardia disproportionate to the degree of fever, gallop rhythms are often heard, and the heart sounds may become fetal or "tic-tac" in quality. Occasionally, arrhythmias and/or a pericardial friction rub may be present. Prolongation of the conduction time may lead to dropped beats with varying degrees of heart block. Prolongation of the PR interval and other changes in the electrocardiogram are very common, but these findings, in the absence of clinical manifestations of carditis, have a benign prognosis. Therefore, changes in the electrocardiogram alone, unassociated with significant murmurs or cardiac enlargement, do not by themselves constitute an acceptable criterion for the diagnosis of rheumatic carditis. Pericarditis may cause precordial pain, and a friction rub may be audible.

A definite clinical diagnosis of carditis can be made if one or more of the following can be demonstrated: (1) the appearance of, or change in the character of, organic heart murmurs; (2) definite increase in heart size demonstrated by radiogram or fluoroscopy; (3) pericardial friction rub or effusion best demonstrated by echocardiography; or (4) signs of congestive heart failure. Rheumatic carditis is almost always associated with a significant murmur.

Subcutaneous nodules These are usually small, pea-sized, painless swellings over bony prominences and therefore frequently go unnoticed by the patient. The skin moves freely over them. Characteristic locations are the extensor tendons of the hands and feet, the elbows, margins of the patellae, the scalp, over the scapulae, and over the spinous processes of the vertebrae.

Chorea (Sydenham's chorea, chorea minor, Saint Vitus' dance) This is a disorder of the central nervous system characterized by sudden, aimless, irregular movements, often accompanied by muscle weakness and emotional instability. Chorea is a delayed manifestation of rheumatic fever, and other manifestations may or may not still be present at the time it appears. Polyarthritis, when part of the same

attack, always subsides before chorea appears. Carditis is often discovered for the first time when the presenting feature of rheumatic fever is chorea. Chorea usually appears after a long latent period (up to several months) from the antecedent streptococcal infection and at a time when all other manifestations of rheumatic fever have abated. When no previous rheumatic manifestations are noted, such cases are called *pure chorea.*

The clinical onset of chorea is often gradual. Patients may be unusually nervous and fidgety and may have difficulty in writing, drawing, and handiwork. They may stumble or fall, drop things, and grimace. As symptoms become more severe, spasmodic movements extend to all parts of the body, and muscular weakness may become so marked that patients cannot walk, talk, or sit up. Often the weakness is severe enough to simulate paralysis. The irregular, jerky, spasmodic movements may become so violent that cribs and beds must be padded to prevent injury. Symptoms are exaggerated by excitement, effort, or fatigue but subside during sleep. Emotional instability is almost invariable in patients with chorea. All degrees of speech disturbance are seen. Central nervous stimulants exacerbate and sedatives suppress choreiform activity.

Erythema marginatum This evanescent pink rash is characteristic of rheumatic fever. The erythematous areas often have clear centers and round or serpiginous margins. They vary greatly in size and occur mainly on the trunk and proximal part of the extremities, never on the face. The erythema is transient, migratory, and may be brought out by the application of heat; it is nonpruritic, not indurated, and blanches on pressure.

Minor clinical criteria These are clinical features which occur frequently in rheumatic fever but are also common to many other diseases and are therefore of minor diagnostic value. They include fever, arthralgia, abdominal pain, tachycardia, and epistaxis.

LABORATORY FINDINGS There is no specific laboratory test to indicate the presence of rheumatic fever. The appraisal of rheumatic activity by laboratory findings is, however, of value, since various tests may indicate *continued* rheumatic inflammation when clinical features are not apparent.

Streptococcal antibody tests to disclose preceding streptococcal infection Streptococcal antibody titers differentiate preceding streptococcal from other acute respiratory infections and are increased following asymptomatic as well as symptomatic streptococcal infections. These antibody levels are increased in the early stages of acute rheumatic fever. They may be declining, or low, if the interval between the acute streptococcal infection and the detection of rheumatic fever has been longer than 2 months, a situation which occurs most often in patients whose presenting rheumatic manifestation is chorea. However, patients whose only major manifestation is rheumatic carditis also may have low antibody titers when first seen. Their rheumatic attack may have been in progress several months before becoming symptomatic and recognized. Except in these two instances, *one should be reluctant to make the diagnosis of acute rheumatic fever in the absence of serologic evidence of a recent streptococcal infection.* The antistreptolysin O test (ASO) is the most widely used and best-standardized streptococcal antibody test. In general, single titers of at least 250 Todd units in adults and at least 333 units in children over 5 years of age are considered to be increased. Depending on the general prevalence of streptococcal infections, a varying percentage of the normal population may show titers of this magnitude.

About 20 percent of patients in the early stages of acute rheumatic fever, and most patients who present with chorea, have a low or borderline ASO titer. In these instances, it is advisable to obtain a different streptococcal antibody test such as anti-DNase B, or antihyaluronidase (AH). The antistreptozyme test (ASTZ) is a hemagglutination reaction to a concentrate of extracellular streptococcal antigens absorbed to red blood cells. It is a very sensitive indicator of recent streptococcal infection; virtually all patients with acute rheumatic fever have titers greater than 200 units per milliliter. The real value of the ASTZ test is in *ruling out* rheumatic fever when the titer is low in patients with isolated polyarthritis. To date, the specific antigens involved in the ASTZ test remain unidentified and therefore the test has not yet been adequately standardized. A rise in titer of two dilution tubes or more can be demonstrated for at least one of the streptococcal antibodies in almost all recurrent as well as primary attacks of rheumatic fever (Table 186-2). Increased streptococcal antibodies, however, do not reflect rheumatic activity per se, and their rate of decline is independent of the course of the rheumatic attack.

Isolation of group A streptococci   Some patients continue to harbor group A streptococci at the onset of acute rheumatic fever, but these organisms are usually present in small numbers and may be difficult to isolate by a single throat culture. The administration of penicillin or other antibodies may also result in failure to isolate the infecting organism. In addition, a significant number of *normal* individuals, particularly children, may harbor group A streptococci in the upper respiratory tract. For these reasons, throat cultures are less satisfactory than antibody tests as supporting evidence of recent streptococcal infection.

Acute phase reactants   These tests offer objective but nonspecific confirmation of the presence of an inflammatory process. *The erythrocyte sedimentation rate* (ESR) and the test for *C-reactive protein* (CRP) in serum are used most commonly. Unless the patient has received corticosteroids or salicylates, these reactions are almost always abnormal in patients presenting with polyarthritis or acute carditis, whereas they are often normal in patients with chorea. Other laboratory findings which reflect inflammation include reactions such as leukocytosis, and increases in serum complement, mucoproteins, and alpha$_2$ and gamma globulins. Prolongation of the PR interval of the electrocardiogram, although neither specific for rheumatic fever nor diagnostic of serious cardiac involvement, is frequent in acute rheumatic fever (about 25 percent of all cases), and other nonspecific electrocardiographic changes are also common. Anemia, due to the suppression of erythropoiesis characteristic of chronic inflammatory diseases, is another feature of rheumatic activity.

COURSE AND PROGNOSIS   The course of rheumatic fever varies greatly and is impossible to predict at the onset of the disease. In general, however, approximately 75 percent of acute rheumatic attacks subside within 6 weeks, 90 percent within 12 weeks, and less than 5 percent persist more than 6 months. These last usually consist of severe, intractable forms of rheumatic carditis or stubborn, prolonged attacks of Sydenham's chorea, both of which may persist for as long as several years. Once acute rheumatic fever has subsided and more than 2 months has elapsed after withdrawal of treatment with salicylates or adrenal corticosteroids, rheumatic fever does not recur in the absence of new streptococcal infections. Recurrences are most common within the first 5 years of the initial attack and tend to decline with increasing duration of freedom from rheumatic activity. The frequency of recurrences is dependent upon the frequency and

TABLE 186-2   Serologic results in patients with streptococcal disease

Patient group (no.)	Percent of patients whose serums were "positive"				
	ASO	AH	Anti-DNase B	At least 1 of 3	ASTZ
Acute rheumatic fever (20)	90	65	85	95	100
Acute glomerulo-nephritis (22)	50	63	72	91	95
Convalescent pharyngitis (11)	81	54	54	91	91
Convalescent pyoderma (23)	35	35	91	96	91
Total (76)	61	54	79	93	95

SOURCE: *AL Bisno, I Ofek, Am J Dis Child 127:676, 1974.*

severity of streptococcal infection, the presence or absence of rheumatic heart disease following an attack, and the duration of freedom from the last attack.

Approximately 70 percent of patients who develop carditis do so within the first week of the disease, 85 percent within the first 12 weeks of the disease, and almost all within 6 months from the onset of the acute attack. Thereafter, if significant murmurs have not appeared, the prognosis for a patient in whom recurrences are prevented is excellent.

Chronic rheumatic carditis and the course of rheumatic heart disease   The remarkable variability in the course of rheumatic carditis and rheumatic valvular disease stems from several factors: (1) the variability in the duration and severity of the rheumatic inflammation; (2) the amount of scarring of the valves and myocardium following the abatement of the acute inflammation; (3) the location and severity of the hemodynamic lesion due to valvular insufficiency or stenosis; (4) the frequency of recurrent bouts of carditis; and (5) the progression of valvular calcification and sclerosis, which occurs as a secondary phenomenon in a deformed or injured valve without recurrent or persistent rheumatic inflammation (as seen in congenital valvular disease or following healed acute bacterial endocarditis). These factors, and possibly others not yet appreciated, produce striking variations in the clinical syndromes of rheumatic heart disease.

Chronic rheumatic myocarditis   In this syndrome, the presenting picture is one of chronic heart failure in a patient with a markedly dilated heart and with physical, roentgenographic, and electrocardiographic findings of mitral regurgitation. The differentiation of this syndrome from other forms of chronic myocarditis may be very difficult, if not impossible, when the associated extracardiac features of rheumatic fever (chorea, polyarthritis, and so forth) are not present (Chap. 192). Although rheumatic fever does not produce *isolated* myocarditis, and is almost invariably a pancarditis, the pericardial inflammation may not be clearly evident, and the mitral valvulitis may not be distinguishable from mitral regurgitation due to dilation of the mitral ring. In such cases one must search diligently for an evanescent friction rub, evidence of pericardial effusion, appearance of a soft aortic regurgitation murmur, and extracardiac clues such as fever responding promptly to salicylates, arthralgias, transient subcutaneous nodules, evanescent erythema marginatum, and subtle signs of chorea.

The course of chronic rheumatic carditis may be intractable and end fatally after months or even several years. Often, however, the patient improves rather suddenly and even recovers cardiac reserve dramatically in association with the disappearance of systemic manifestations of the inflammatory process. The heart may remain large, may decrease somewhat in size, or in occasional instances may return to normal size with varying degrees of residual valvular deformity. Such a course signals the termination of the "toxic" phase of the rheumatic process, and thereafter the course of rheumatic heart disease depends on the variables in healing cited above.

DIFFERENTIAL DIAGNOSIS   Early cases of rheumatic fever may be confused with other diseases which begin with acute polyarthritis. It is wise to exclude *bacteremia* by blood cultures, particularly because such infections may be masked by penicillin given for presumed acute rheumatic fever. Polyarthritis due to *infective endocarditis* in a patient with preexisting rheumatic heart disease may be mistaken for a recurrence of acute rheumatic fever. If streptococcal antibodies are not increased, polyarthritis should be attributed to some cause other than rheumatic fever. Gonococcal polyarthritis may be distinguished from rheumatic fever by the dramatic response of the former to a therapeutic trial of penicillin. In rheumatoid arthritis, joint involvement will persist and characteristic joint deformities may appear. The latter are not seen in rheumatic fever. The rheumatoid factor so characteristic of rheumatoid arthritis is not present in rheumatic fever. Antibodies against nuclear components and other autoantibodies are absent in rheumatic fever. Rheumatic pericarditis and myocarditis, associated with cardiac enlargement and heart failure, are both almost invariably associated with valvular lesions which produce significant murmurs.

Overdiagnosis of rheumatic fever should be avoided. Unless ill-defined febrile syndromes are clearly associated with a major manifestation of rheumatic fever, the diagnosis of rheumatic fever should not be made. A common error is the premature, vigorous administration of corticosteroids or salicylates before the signs and symptoms of rheumatic fever are unmistakable. In the absence of a curative agent, one should not suppress the signs and symptoms of rheumatic fever until they are clearly expressed.

Particularly confusing in the differential diagnosis of rheumatic fever is the drug sensitivity with fever and polyarthritis which may occur after administration of penicillin for a previous pharyngitis. Urticaria or angioneurotic edema, if present, helps identify penicillin sensitivity in such cases. The abdominal pain of rheumatic fever may be mistaken for appendicitis, and the crisis of sickle cell anemia may also be associated with joint pain, enlargement of the heart, and cardiac murmurs. The rapidity with which the arthritis symptoms of rheumatic fever are controlled with salicylates is characteristic of this disease. Dramatic response to salicylates does not in itself, however, establish a diagnosis of rheumatic fever.

In order to help clarify the diagnosis of rheumatic fever, the American Heart Association has accepted and modified criteria usually referred to as the *Jones criteria* (Table 186-1). They are not to be used as a substitute for good medical judgment but are recommended as a guide for careful study of questionable cases. The finding of two major criteria, or of one major and two minor criteria, indicates a high probability of the presence of rheumatic fever if supported by evidence of a preceding streptococcal infection. The absence of the latter should always make the diagnosis questionable, except in the situation in which rheumatic fever is first discovered after a long latent period from the antecedent infection (Sydenham's chorea or low-grade carditis). Because the prognosis may differ according to the major manifestations, for recording purposes the diagnosis of rheumatic fever should be followed by a list of the major manifestations present, e.g., rheumatic fever manifested by polyarthritis and carditis. An indication of the severity of carditis in terms of presence or absence of congestive heart failure and cardiomegaly is also advisable.

TREATMENT There is no specific cure for rheumatic fever, and no known measures change the course of the attack. Good supportive therapy, however, can reduce the mortality and morbidity of the disease.

Chemotherapy After rheumatic fever is first diagnosed, a course of penicillin should be given to eliminate group A streptococci. This course is advisable even if bacteriologic examination yields throat cultures negative for streptococci, since the organisms may be present in areas inaccessible to swabs. It is preferable to administer penicillin parenterally. An effective course is a single injection of 1.2 million units of benzathine penicillin intramuscularly or 600,000 units of procaine penicillin intramuscularly daily for 10 days. Attempts to reduce ultimate heart damage by administering penicillin early in the acute rheumatic attack in larger doses have not been successful. After completion of the therapeutic course of penicillin, continuous protection from reinfection with streptococci should be provided by instituting one of the prophylactic regimens described below.

Suppressive therapy For patients without carditis treatment with adrenal corticosteroids is unnecessary. Acute arthritis can be relieved with codeine or with salicylate, the latter being preferable to reduce fever and joint inflammation. When salicylate is used in the therapy of rheumatic fever, the dosage should be increased until the drug produces either a clinical effect or systemic toxicity characterized by tinnitus, headache, or hyperpnea. A starting dose of 100 to 125 mg/kg per day in children and 6 to 8 g in adults given in four or five divided doses is recommended. Of the various salicylate preparations ordinary aspirin is cheapest and most effective.

Many physicians prefer corticosteroids to salicylates for the treatment of carditis, despite the lack of a demonstrated advantage

of these adrenal hormones in controlled clinical trials. Corticosteroids are more potent anti-inflammatory agents but are more likely to be followed by posttherapeutic "rebounds," and they have the additional disadvantage of more frequent side effects, particularly acne, hirsutism, and cushingoid changes in facies and habitus. For this reason it is preferable to begin treatment of patients who have carditis with salicylates; if these drugs fail to reduce fever and to ameliorate heart failure, therapy with corticosteroids may be initiated promptly. Prednisone is administered in doses of 60 to 120 mg or higher when necessary in four divided doses daily. After the inflammation has been brought under control by either salicylates or corticosteroids, treatment should be continued until the sedimentation rate approaches near-normal values and should be maintained for several weeks thereafter. To prevent poststeroid rebounds, an "overlap" course of salicylate therapy may be added when steroids are tapered off over a 2-week period. A useful method for tapering steroids is outlined in Chap. 325. Salicylates may then be continued for an additional 2 to 3 weeks. Rebounds of rheumatic activity are usually of short duration and, when mild, are best managed without resuming anti-inflammatory treatment, because a second or even a third rebound may occur when suppressive therapy is discontinued. About 5 percent of rheumatic attacks persist for 6 months or longer, either in the form of spontaneous acute recrudescences or as posttherapeutic rebounds. These "chronic" attacks are most likely to occur in patients with cardiac damage and with previous rheumatic episodes. Weekly tests for C-reactive protein in blood and for erythrocyte sedimentation rate are useful in following the healing process, particularly while treatment with corticosteroids or salicylates is gradually withdrawn.

Treatment of chorea The signs and symptoms of chorea usually do not respond well to treatment with antirheumatic agents. Because the patient with chorea is frequently emotionally unstable and because the manifestations of chorea may be exaggerated by emotional trauma, complete mental and physical rest is essential. Patients with chorea should be kept in a quiet room and cared for by sympathetic attendants. Corticosteroids or salicylates have little or no effect on chorea. Sedatives and tranquilizers, particularly diazepam and chlorpromazine, are useful. Chorea, no matter how severe, disappears during sleep, which should therefore be ensured by adequate sedation. Padded sideboards for the bed may be necessary to avoid injury to the patient. In the absence of other evidence of acute rheumatic disease, it is advisable to allow gradual resumption of physical activity when improvement is apparent rather than waiting for all choreiform movements to disappear, which may require many months.

Because of the great variability in the course of chorea, evaluating the effectiveness of various therapeutic measures is difficult. It is well to remember that chorea is a self-limited disease which is usually not followed by significant neurologic sequelae and that good results are almost invariably obtained by patient, attentive nursing care and by conservative medical management.

PREVENTION OF RECURRENCE The most efficient regimen for continuous prophylaxis against group A streptococci is a monthly intramuscular injection of 1.2 million units of benzathine penicillin. The disadvantages and discomfort of this regimen have to be weighed against the individual patient's susceptibility to recurrences. Those with rheumatic heart disease, recent rheumatic fever, and exposure to an environment in which the incidence of streptococcal infection is frequent deserve the most effective protection. As a second choice, prophylaxis may be administered orally with either 1 g sulfadiazine daily in a single dose or 200,000 units of penicillin given twice daily on an empty stomach. The duration of continuous prophylaxis cannot be fixed arbitrarily. Certainly, those under the age of 18 years should receive a continuous prophylactic regimen. A minimum period of 5 years is recommended for patients who develop rheumatic fever without carditis over the age of 18 years. The decision to continue prophylaxis beyond this period should take into account a number of variables. Patients with rheumatic heart disease are more susceptible to reactivation of rheumatic fever if they contract a streptococcal infection. Moreover, patients who have had carditis in a previous attack are much more likely to suffer carditis again in a subsequent attack. Climate, age, occupation, household situation, cardiac status, and length of time since the previous attack are all significant variables which influence the risk of recurrence. The decline in recurrence rates with increasing age is due to (1) decreased rate of streptococcal infection and (2) decrease in the rate of rheumatic reactivation following streptococcal infection in older rheumatic subjects. Despite this decreased rate, however, the risk of rheumatic recurrence in adults remains relatively high when the streptococcal disease encountered is severe or epidemic.

PREVENTION OF INITIAL RHEUMATIC ATTACKS Early and adequate treatment of pharyngeal infection due to group A streptococci will prevent initial attacks of rheumatic fever. If clinical streptococcal disease were properly detected by throat cultures and adequately treated, the spread of infection in a given population would be prevented, the epidemiology of streptococcal disease would be modified markedly, and the incidence of rheumatic fever in the community would be diminished. In communities where group A streptococcal disease has been diagnosed early and treated well and where socioeconomic standards are high, the group A organisms cultured frequently from schoolchildren's throats may be of relatively low virulence and may cause rheumatic fever less frequently than do more virulent strains prevalent in many epidemics.

Streptococcal pharyngitis is adequately treated by a single intramuscular injection of 600,000 units of benzathine penicillin in children less than 10 years of age or 1.2 million units in older children and adults. Any alternate plan of parenteral therapy or combined parenteral and oral therapy should provide for treatment over a period of 10 days. If oral penicillin is employed, at least 800,000 units per day in four divided doses must be given for no less than 10 days to achieve results comparable with a single injection of benzathine penicillin. Erythromycin in daily doses of 1 g for 10 days may be substituted in penicillin-sensitive individuals. Tetracycline is not recommended because some strains of group A streptococci have acquired resistance to it. All group A streptococci have so far remained extremely sensitive to penicillin.

REFERENCES

AMERICAN HEART ASSOCIATION: Jones criteria (revised) for guidance in the diagnosis of rheumatic fever. Circulation 69:204A, 1984

AYOUB EM: The search for host determinants of susceptibility to rheumatic fever: The missing link. Circulation 69:197, 1984

BISNO AL: Acute rheumatic fever: Current concepts and controversies, in *Current Clinical Topics in Infectious Diseases*, JS Remington, MN Swartz (eds). New York, McGraw-Hill, 1984

JOINT REPORT OF UK-US COOPERATIVE STUDY: The natural history of rheumatic fever and rheumatic heart disease. 10 year report of a cooperative clinical trial of ACTH, cortisone and aspirin. Circulation 32:457, 1965

LAND MA, BISNO AL: Acute rheumatic fever: A vanishing disease in suburbia. JAMA 249:895, 1983

McDANALD EC, WEISMAN MH: Ventricular manifestations of rheumatic fever in adults. Ann Intern Med 89:917, 1978

PERSELLIN RH: Acute rheumatic fever: Changing manifestations. Ann Intern Med 89:1002, 1978

READ S, ZABRISKIE JB (eds): *Streptococcal Diseases and the Immune Response*. New York, Academic, 1980

STOLLERMAN GH: *Rheumatic Fever and Streptococcal Infection*. New York, Grune & Stratton, 1975

———: Global changes in group A streptococcal diseases and strategies for their prevention, in *Advances in Internal Medicine* 27:373. Chicago, Year Book Medical Publishers, 1982

187   VALVULAR HEART DISEASE

EUGENE BRAUNWALD

The role of physical examination in the evaluation of patients with valvular disease is considered in Chap. 177; of roentgenography, echocardiography, phonocardiography and other indirect graphic techniques in Chap. 179; of electrocardiography in Chap. 178; and of cardiac catheterization and angiography in Chap. 180.

MITRAL STENOSIS

PATHOPHYSIOLOGY In normal adults the mitral valve orifice is 4 to 6 cm². In the presence of significant obstruction, i.e., when the orifice is less than one-half of normal, blood can flow from the left atrium to the left ventricle only if propelled by an abnormally elevated left atrioventricular pressure gradient, the hemodynamic hallmark of mitral stenosis. When the mitral valve opening is reduced to 1 cm², a left atrial pressure of approximately 25 mmHg is required to maintain a normal cardiac output. The elevated left atrial pressure·in turn raises pulmonary venous and capillary pressures, reducing pulmonary compliance and causing exertional dyspnea. The first bouts of dyspnea are usually precipitated by clinical events which increase the rate of blood flow across the mitral orifice, which results in further elevation of the left atrial pressure (see below). In order to assess the severity of obstruction, it is essential to measure both the transvalvular pressure gradient and the flow rate. The latter is dependent not only on the cardiac output but on the heart rate as well. An increase in heart rate shortens diastole proportionately more than systole, and diminishes the time available for flow across the mitral valve. Therefore, at any given level of cardiac output tachycardia augments the transvalvular gradient and elevates further the left atrial pressure.

The left ventricular diastolic pressure is normal in isolated mitral stenosis; coexisting mitral regurgitation, aortic valve disease, the residua of damage produced by rheumatic myocarditis, systemic hypertension, or ischemic heart disease may be responsible for elevations which reflect impaired left ventricular function and/or reduced left ventricular compliance. Left ventricular dysfunction, as reflected in reduced ejection fraction and circumferential fiber shortening rate, occurs in about one-fourth of patients with mitral stenosis, as a consequence of chronic reduction of preload and extension of the scarring from the valve into the adjacent myocardium. In pure mitral stenosis and sinus rhythm, the mean left atrial and pulmonary artery wedge pressures are usually elevated and the pressure pulse shows a prominent atrial contraction (*a* wave), and a gradual pressure decline after mitral valve opening (*y* descent). In patients with mild to moderate mitral stenosis without elevation of the pulmonary vascular resistance, the pulmonary arterial pressure may be normal at rest and may rise only with exercise. In severe mitral stenosis and whenever the pulmonary vascular resistance is significantly increased, the pulmonary arterial pressure is elevated even when the patient is at rest, and in extreme cases it may exceed the systemic arterial pressure. Further elevations of left atrial, pulmonary capillary, and pulmonary arterial pressures occur during exercise. When the pulmonary arterial systolic pressure exceeds approximately 50 mmHg in patients with mitral stenosis, or for that matter with any valvular lesion, the increased right ventricular afterload impedes the emptying of this chamber, and right ventricular end-diastolic pressure and volume usually rise as a compensatory mechanism.

The cardiac output at rest varies considerably in patients with mitral stenosis. Thus, the hemodynamic response to a given degree of mitral obstruction may be characterized by a normal cardiac output and a high left atrioventricular pressure gradient or, at the opposite end of the hemodynamic spectrum, by a reduced cardiac output and low transvalvular pressure gradient. In a small fraction of patients with moderately severe mitral stenosis, the cardiac output is normal at rest and rises normally during exertion; under these circumstances, the high atrioventricular pressure gradient elevates the left atrial and pulmonary capillary pressures markedly, and this elevation is responsible for symptoms of relatively severe pulmonary congestion. In the majority of patients, however, the cardiac output is normal at rest but rises subnormally during exertion. In patients with severe stenosis, particularly those in whom the pulmonary vascular resistance is strikingly elevated, the cardiac output is subnormal at rest and may fail to rise or may even decline during activity. The depressed cardiac output in patients with mitral stenosis is related primarily to the obstruction of the mitral orifice but may also be due to the impairment of the function of either ventricle.

The clinical and hemodynamic features of mitral stenosis are dictated largely by the level of the pulmonary artery pressure. Pulmonary hypertension results from (1) the passive backward transmission of the elevated left atrial pressure, (2) pulmonary arteriolar constriction, which presumably is triggered by left atrial and pulmonary venous hypertension (reactive pulmonary hypertension), and (3) organic obliterative changes in the pulmonary vascular bed. The elevation of pulmonary vascular resistance may be considered to be a complication of long-standing and severe mitral stenosis; in time, the resultant severe pulmonary hypertension results in tricuspid and pulmonary incompetence as well as right-sided heart failure. However, the changes in the pulmonary vascular bed may also be considered to exert a protective effect; the elevated precapillary resistance reduces the likelihood of symptoms of pulmonary congestion by reducing the surge of blood into the pulmonary capillary bed which then dams up behind the stenotic mitral valve during activity. However, this protection occurs at the expense of a decreased cardiac output.

ETIOLOGY AND PATHOLOGY Mitral stenosis is generally rheumatic in origin. Pure or predominant mitral stenosis occurs in approximately 40 percent of all patients with rheumatic heart disease; two-thirds of all patients with mitral stenosis are females. The valve leaflets are diffusely thickened by fibrous tissue and/or calcific deposits. The mitral commissures fuse, the chordae tendineae fuse and shorten, the valvular cusps become rigid, and these changes in turn lead to narrowing at the apex of the funnel-shaped valve. While the initial insult to the mitral valve is rheumatic, the later changes may be a nonspecific process resulting from trauma to the valve caused by altered flow patterns due to the initial deformity. Calcification of the stenotic mitral valve immobilizes the leaflets and narrows the orifice. Thrombus formation and arterial embolization may arise from the calcific valve itself. Rarely, mitral stenosis is congenital in origin.

SYMPTOMS In temperate climates the latent period between the initial attack of rheumatic carditis, in the rare circumstances in which a history of one can be elicited, and the development of symptoms due to mitral stenosis is generally on the order of two decades; most patients begin to experience disability in the fourth decade. Once a patient with mitral stenosis becomes seriously symptomatic, continuous progression of the disease to death usually occurs in 2 to 5 years unless the stenosis is relieved by operation. In economically deprived areas, particularly on the Indian subcontinent, in Central America, and the Middle East, mitral stenosis tends to progress more rapidly and frequently causes serious symptoms before the age of 20 years. On the other hand, slowly progressive mitral stenosis in the elderly is also being recognized with increasing frequency in the United States and western Europe.

When valvular obstruction is mild, many of the physical signs of mitral stenosis may be present in the absence of any symptoms. However, even in those patients whose mitral orifices are large enough to accommodate a normal blood flow with only mild elevations of left atrial pressure, extreme exertion, excitement, fever, severe anemia, paroxysmal tachycardia, sexual intercourse, pregnancy, and thyrotoxicosis all may precipitate elevations of pulmonary capillary pressure and lead to dyspnea and cough. As stenosis progresses, the stresses that precipitate dyspnea become less severe, and the patient becomes limited in his or her daily activities. Redistribution of blood from the dependent portions of the body to the lungs, which occurs when the recumbent position is assumed, leads to orthopnea and paroxysmal nocturnal dyspnea. *Pulmonary edema* develops when there is a sudden increase in flow rate across a markedly narrowed mitral orifice (Chap. 26). When moderately severe mitral stenosis has existed for several years, *atrial arrhythmias*—premature contractions, paroxysmal tachycardia, flutter, and fibrillation—occur with increasing frequency. The rapid ventricular rate associated with untreated or inadequately treated atrial fibrillation is frequently responsible for acute exacerbations of dyspnea. The development of permanent atrial fibrillation often marks a turning point in the patient's course and is generally associated with acceleration of the rate at which symptoms progress.

Hemoptysis (Chap. 25) results from rupture of pulmonary-bronchial venous connections secondary to pulmonary venous hypertension. It occurs most frequently in patients who have elevated left atrial pressures without markedly elevated pulmonary vascular resistances and is almost never fatal. True hemoptysis must be distinguished from the bloody sputum that occurs with pulmonary edema, pulmonary infarction, and bronchitis, three conditions that occur with increased frequency in the presence of mitral stenosis.

When the pulmonary vascular resistance rises or when tricuspid stenosis or regurgitation develops, symptoms secondary to pulmonary congestion may diminish, and the episodes of acute pulmonary edema and hemoptysis become reduced in frequency and severity. Elevation of pulmonary vascular resistance further increases right ventricular systolic pressure, leading to right ventricular failure, fatigue, weakness, abdominal discomfort due to hepatic congestion, and edema.

Recurrent pulmonary emboli with infarction (Chap. 211) are an important cause of morbidity and mortality late in the course of mitral stenosis, occurring most frequently in patients with right ventricular failure. *Pulmonary infections,* i.e., bronchitis, bronchopneumonia, and lobar pneumonia, commonly complicate untreated mitral stenosis. *Infective endocarditis* (Chap. 188) is rare in pure mitral stenosis but is not uncommon in patients with combined stenosis and regurgitation. *Chest pain* occurs in about 10 percent of patients with severe mitral stenosis; it may be due to pulmonary hypertension, or myocardial ischemia secondary to coronary atherosclerosis; often the cause cannot be discovered.

In addition to the aforementioned changes in the pulmonary vascular bed, fibrous thickening of the walls of the alveoli and pulmonary capillaries occurs commonly in mitral stenosis. The vital capacity, total lung capacity, maximal breathing capacity, and oxygen uptake per unit of ventilation are reduced, and in patients with severe stenosis the latter fails to rise normally during exertion. The reduction of pulmonary compliance that occurs generally correlates directly with the severity of the dyspnea and with the heightened pulmonary capillary pressure, and these changes are intensified during exercise. In some patients airway resistance is abnormally increased. These alterations in pulmonary mechanics contribute to an increase in the work of breathing and play an important role in the genesis of dyspnea. The changes in the lungs are due, in part, to increased transudation of fluid from the pulmonary capillaries into the interstitial and alveolar spaces as a consequence of the elevated pulmonary capillary pressure. The distribution of blood flow and ventilation may be uneven; as in other conditions in which left atrial pressure is elevated, pulmonary blood flow in the erect position is displaced from the basal to the superior segments of the lung (Chap. 200). The diffusing capacity may be reduced, particularly during exertion, as a result of structural changes in the diffusing surface and reduction of the pulmonary capillary blood volume. The thickening of the alveolar and capillary walls impedes the transudation of fluid into the alveoli and the development of pulmonary edema at times when the pulmonary capillary pressure exceeds the plasma oncotic pressure. The increased capacity of the pulmonary lymphatic system to drain excess fluid also retards the development of pulmonary edema.

Thrombi may form in the left atria, particularly in the enlarged atrial appendages of patients with mitral stenosis. When they embolize, they do so most commonly to the brain, kidneys, spleen, and extremities. This complication occurs much more frequently in patients with atrial fibrillation or unstable rhythms, in older patients, and in those with a reduced cardiac output, but it is also seen in patients with relatively mild as well as severe obstruction. Thus, systemic embolization may be the presenting complaint in otherwise asymptomatic patients with mild mitral stenosis. At operation, thrombi are not found more frequently in the left atria of patients with past history of embolization than in those without this complication, indicating that it is usually the freshly formed clots that dislodge. Patients who have had one or more systemic emboli have the predilection to have further embolic episodes more often than patients with stenosis of comparable severity without previous embolization. Rarely, a large pedunculated thrombus or a free-floating clot may suddenly obstruct the stenotic mitral orifice. Such "ball valve" thrombi produce syncope, angina, and changing auscultatory signs with alterations in position, findings that resemble those produced by a left atrial myxoma (Chap. 193).

PHYSICAL FINDINGS (See also Chap. 177)   Peripheral and facial *cyanosis* may occur in patients with extremely severe mitral stenosis. In advanced cases there is a malar flush and the facies appear pinched and blue. The jugular venous pulse reveals prominent *a* waves due to vigorous right atrial systole in patients with sinus rhythm who have severe pulmonary hypertension or associated tricuspid stenosis. When atrial fibrillation is present, the jugular pulse reveals only a single expansion during systole (*c-v* wave). The systemic arterial pressure is usually normal or slightly low. A right ventricular tap is present along the left sternal border, signifying an enlarged right ventricle. The first heart sound may be palpable in patients with pliable valve leaflets. In patients with pulmonary hypertension, the impact of pulmonary valve closure can usually be felt in the second and third left intercostal spaces just left of the sternum; the left ventricle is not palpable in severe, pure mitral stenosis. A diastolic thrill is frequently present at the cardiac apex, particularly if the patient is turned into the left lateral recumbent position.

The first heart sound is generally accentuated and snapping, and since the mitral valve does not close until the left ventricular pressure reaches the level of the elevated left atrial pressure, this sound is often slightly delayed on phonocardiography, particularly in patients with severe stenosis. In patients with pulmonary hypertension, the pulmonary component of the second heart sound is often accentuated, and the two components of the second heart sound are closely split. A pulmonary systolic ejection click may be heard in patients with severe pulmonary hypertension and marked dilatation of the pulmonary artery. The opening snap of the mitral valve is most readily audible in expiration at, or just medial to, the cardiac apex but may also be easily heard along the left sternal edge or at the base of the heart. This sound generally follows the sound of aortic valve closure by 0.06 to 0.12 s, that is, it follows the pulmonic valve closure sound. Since the opening snap of the mitral valve occurs at the instant at which the left ventricular pressure falls below the left atrial pressure, the time interval between aortic closure and the opening snap varies inversely with the severity of the mitral stenosis. It tends to be short, that is, 0.06 to 0.07 s, in patients with severe obstruction and long, that is, 0.10 to 0.12 s, in patients with mild mitral stenosis. The intensities of the opening snap and the first heart sound correlate with the mobility of the anterior mitral leaflet.

The opening snap usually ushers in a low-pitched, rumbling, diastolic murmur, heard best at the apex with the patient in the left lateral recumbent position, and often accentuated by exercise carried out just before auscultation. In general, the duration of this murmur correlates with the severity of the stenosis. In patients with sinus rhythm the murmur often reappears or becomes reaccentuated during

atrial systole, as atrial contraction reelevates the rate of blood flow across the narrowed orifice. Soft (grade I or II/VI) systolic murmurs are commonly heard at the apex or along the left sternal border in patients with pure mitral stenosis and do not necessarily signify the presence of mitral regurgitation. Hepatomegaly, ankle edema, ascites, and pleural effusion, particularly in the right pleural cavity, may occur in patients with mitral stenosis and right ventricular failure.

Associated lesions   With severe pulmonary hypertension a loud pansystolic murmur produced by functional tricuspid regurgitation may be audible along the left sternal border. This murmur may be accentuated by inspiration, diminishes during forced expiration or during performance of the Valsalva maneuver, diminishes or disappears as compensation is restored, and must not be confused with the apical pansystolic murmur of mitral regurgitation, since management is quite different if mitral regurgitation is present.

The recognition of associated mitral regurgitation is of considerable clinical importance in patients with mitral stenosis. A presystolic murmur and an accentuated first heart sound speak against the presence of serious associated mitral regurgitation, but when the first heart sound and/or the opening snap are soft or absent in a patient with mitral valve disease, it is likely that significant mitral regurgitation and/or serious calcification of the deformed mitral valve leaflets are present. A third heart sound at the apex often signifies that the mitral regurgitation is serious; this sound is generally duller and lower pitched and follows the opening snap. Occasionally, in patients with pure mitral stenosis, physical signs may falsely suggest mitral regurgitation. Thus, in the presence of severe pulmonary hypertension and right ventricular failure, a third heart sound may originate from the right ventricle. The enlarged right ventricle may rotate the heart in a clockwise direction and form the cardiac apex, giving the examiner the erroneous impression of left ventricular enlargement. Under these circumstances the rumbling diastolic murmur and the other auscultatory features of mitral stenosis become less prominent or may even disappear and be replaced by the systolic murmur of functional tricuspid regurgitation. When cardiac output is markedly reduced in a patient with mitral stenosis, none of the typical auscultatory findings may be detectable, but they may reappear as compensation is restored. Associated tricuspid stenosis also tends to obscure many of the physical signs of mitral stenosis.

The Graham Steell murmur of pulmonary regurgitation, a high-pitched, diastolic, decrescendo blowing murmur along the left sternal border, results from dilatation of the pulmonary valve ring and occurs in patients with mitral valve disease and severe pulmonary hypertension. This murmur may be indistinguishable from the more common murmur produced by mild aortic regurgitation except that it is rarely audible at the second right intercostal space, and may disappear following successful surgical treatment of the mitral stenosis.

Electrocardiogram   In mitral stenosis and sinus rhythm the P wave usually suggests left atrial enlargement (Chap. 178). It may become tall and peaked in lead II and upright in lead V_1 when severe pulmonary hypertension or tricuspid stenosis complicates mitral stenosis and right atrial enlargement occurs. The QRS complex may be normal, even in patients with critical mitral stenosis. However, with severe pulmonary hypertension, right axis deviation and right ventricular hypertrophy are usually found. When left ventricular hypertrophy is present in patients with mitral stenosis, it generally indicates that an additional lesion which places a burden on the left ventricle, such as mitral regurgitation, aortic valve disease, or hypertension, is present.

Echocardiogram (see also Chap. 179)   The echocardiogram is the most sensitive and specific noninvasive method for diagnosing mitral stenosis. The M-mode tracing reveals that the anterior and posterior mitral leaflets do not separate widely in early diastole (i.e., less than 15 mm) and they maintain a fixed relation to each other throughout diastole. A reduction in the EF slope reflects failure of the anterior leaflet of the mitral valve to float back to midposition in middiastole.

Calcification and thickening of the mitral valve are detected as multilayered echoes or a thickening of the echo pattern. Mitral orifice area may be estimated with cross-sectional (two-dimensional) echocardiography. The left atrium is usually enlarged. Doppler studies reveal increased turbulence and transvalvular flow velocity and may be used both in the diagnosis of mitral stenosis and in estimating the transvalvular gradient.

Roentgenographic features (Chap. 179) The earliest changes are straightening of the left border of the cardiac silhouette, prominence of the main pulmonary arteries, dilatation of the upper lobe pulmonary veins, and backward displacement of the esophagus by an enlarged left atrium. In patients with mild or moderate stenosis, the heart is not grossly enlarged. In severe mitral stenosis, however, all chambers and vessels upstream to the narrowed valve are prominent, including the two atria, the pulmonary arteries and veins, right ventricle, and superior vena cava. Kerley B lines are fine, dense, opaque, horizontal lines which are most prominent in the lower and midlung fields and which result from distention of interlobular septa and lymphatics with edema when the resting mean left atrial pressure exceeds approximately 20 mmHg. As the pulmonary arterial pressure rises, the smaller pulmonary arteries become attenuated, at first in the lower, then in the mid-, and finally in the upper lung fields. Deposits of hemosiderin occur in the lungs of patients who have had multiple hemoptyses; the hemosiderin-containing macrophages fill the air spaces, and if they become confluent result in a fine, diffuse nodulation most prominent in the lower lung fields.

DIFFERENTIAL DIAGNOSIS Significant[i] mitral regurgitation may be associated with a prominent diastolic murmur at the apex, but this murmur commences slightly later than in patients with stenosis, and there is often clear-cut evidence of left ventricular enlargement on physical examination, roentgenography, and electrocardiography. In addition, an apical pansystolic murmur of at least grade III/VI intensity as well as a third heart sound should arouse the suspicion of significant associated regurgitation. Similarly, the apical middiastolic murmur associated with aortic regurgitation (Austin Flint murmur) may be mistaken for mitral stenosis. However, in a patient with aortic regurgitation the absence of an opening snap or of presystolic accentuation if sinus rhythm is present points to the absence of mitral stenosis. Tricuspid stenosis, a valvular lesion that occurs very rarely in the absence of mitral stenosis, may mask many of the clinical features of mitral stenosis. Echocardiography is particularly useful in detecting mitral stenosis in patients who have or are suspected of having other valve lesions.

Exertional dyspnea and recurrent pulmonary infections may be falsely ascribed to pulmonary emphysema in patients with both *chronic lung disease* and mitral stenosis. Careful auscultation, however, will generally reveal the characteristic opening snap and rumbling diastolic murmur. Similarly, the hemoptysis that occurs in many otherwise asymptomatic patients with mitral stenosis may be improperly attributed to bronchiectasis or tuberculosis. Actually, the latter condition is uncommon in patients with significant mitral obstruction.

Primary pulmonary hypertension (Chap. 210) results in a number of the clinical and laboratory features observed in mitral stenosis. It occurs most frequently in young women; however, the opening snap and diastolic rumbling murmur are absent, there is no left atrial enlargement, and the pulmonary artery wedge and left atrial pressures are *normal*. *Atrial septal defect* (Chap. 185) may also be mistaken for mitral stenosis; in both conditions there is often clinical, electrocardiographic, and roentgenographic evidence of right ventricular enlargement and accentuation of the pulmonary vascularity. The widely split second heart sound of atrial septal defect may be confused with the mitral opening snap, and the diastolic flow murmur across the tricuspid valve mistaken for the mitral diastolic murmur. However, the absence of left atrial enlargement and of Kerley B lines and the demonstration of fixed splitting of the second heart sound all favor atrial septal defect over mitral stenosis. *Cor triatriatum* is an unusual congenital malformation that consists of a fibrous ring within the left atrium (Chap. 185). It results in elevation of the pulmonary venous, capillary, and arterial pressures. This lesion can be recognized most readily by means of left atrial angiography.

Left atrial myxoma (Chap. 193) may obstruct left atrial emptying, resulting in dyspnea, a diastolic murmur, and hemodynamic changes resembling those of mitral stenosis. However, patients with left atrial myxoma often demonstrate findings suggestive of a systemic disease, with weight loss, fever, anemia, systemic emboli, and elevated erythrocyte sedimentation rate and serum gamma-globulin concentration. Usually an opening snap is not audible, there is no clinical evidence of associated aortic valve disease, and the auscultatory findings frequently change with body position. The diagnosis can be established by demonstrating a characteristic echo-producing mass in the left atrium by echocardiography and a lobulated filling defect by angiocardiography.

Specialized techniques Catheterization of the left side of the heart (Chap. 180) is extremely helpful in deciding whether valvulotomy is necessary in patients in whom it is difficult to estimate the severity of obstruction by clinical means and noninvasive tests. When combined with aortography and left ventricular angiocardiography, this procedure serves as the ultimate method for detecting and estimating associated mitral regurgitation and coexisting lesions such as aortic stenosis and regurgitation as well as left ventricular dysfunction. Left atrial thrombi and tumors may be detected or excluded by angiocardiography, particularly when the contrast medium is injected directly into the left atrium. These ''invasive'' methods are also helpful in the detection of accompanying conditions, such as coronary artery disease, that impair left ventricular function and would thereby contraindicate or reduce the effectiveness of mitral valvulotomy. Catheterization and left ventricular angiography are indicated in most patients who have undergone previous mitral valve operations and who have redeveloped serious symptoms; in such patients clinical assessment may be particularly difficult, and the hemodynamic studies allow determination of the severity of the lesion, intelligent planning of the operative procedure when it is indicated, and a more accurate estimate of the risk.

MANAGEMENT In the asymptomatic adolescent with mitral valve disease, penicillin prophylaxis of beta-hemolytic streptococcal infections (Chap. 186), prophylaxis for infective endocarditis (Chap. 188), and vocational counseling are particularly important; physically strenuous occupations should be avoided so that premature retirement will not be necessary should symptoms develop later. In symptomatic patients some improvement usually occurs with restriction of sodium intake and maintenance doses of oral diuretics. Digitalis glycosides do not alter the hemodynamics and usually do not benefit patients with pure stenosis and sinus rhythm, but they are necessary for slowing the ventricular rate of patients with atrial fibrillation and for reducing the manifestations of right-sided heart failure in the advanced stages of the disease. Small doses of beta blockers (e.g., atenolol 25 to 50 mg qd) may be added when cardiac glycosides fail to control ventricular rate in patients with atrial fibrillation or flutter. Particular attention should be directed to detecting and treating any accompanying anemia and infections. Hemoptysis is treated by measures designed to diminish pulmonary venous pressure, including bed rest, the sitting position, salt restriction, and diuresis. Anticoagulants should be administered for at least 1 year in patients with mitral stenosis who have suffered systemic and/or pulmonary embolization and those with intermittent atrial fibrillation.

If atrial fibrillation is of relatively recent origin in a patient whose mitral stenosis is not severe enough to warrant surgical treatment, reversion to sinus rhythm, pharmacologically or by means of electrical countershock is indicated. Usually this should be undertaken following 4 weeks of anticoagulant treatment. Conversion to sinus rhythm is rarely helpful in patients with severe mitral stenosis, particularly those in whom the left atrium is especially enlarged or in whom atrial fibrillation has been present for more than 1 year, since reversion to atrial fibrillation is common.

Surgical treatment Unless there is a specific contraindication, operative treatment is indicated in the symptomatic patient with pure mitral stenosis whose effective orifice is less than approximately 1.2 cm². Operation not only usually results in striking symptomatic and hemodynamic improvement but also prolongs survival. In uncomplicated cases, the surgical mortality rate should be 0 to 2 percent. However, there is no evidence that surgical treatment improves the prognosis of patients with slight or no functional impairment. Therefore, unless recurrent systemic embolization has occurred, valvulotomy is *not* recommended for patients who are entirely asymptomatic, regardless of hemodynamic findings. When there is little symptomatic improvement following valvulotomy, it is likely that the procedure was ineffective, that it induced mitral regurgitation, or that associated valvular or myocardial disease was present. The recurrence of symptoms several years after what appeared to be a satisfactory initial result is usually due to an inadequate valvulotomy, but progression of other valvular lesions, the development of myocardial disease, restenosis of the mitral valve, or some combination of these conditions may also be responsible. In the *pregnant patient* with mitral stenosis operative treatment should be carried out if pulmonary congestion occurs despite intensive medical treatment.

An "open" operation using cardiopulmonary bypass is usually preferable for patients with pure mitral stenosis who have not been operated upon previously. In addition to opening the valve commissures, it is important to loosen any subvalvular fusion of papillary muscles and chordae tendineae and to remove large deposits of calcium, thereby improving valvular function, and to remove atrial thrombi. In patients with significant associated mitral regurgitation, those in whom the valve has been severely distorted by previous operative manipulation, or those in whom the surgeon does not find it possible to improve valve function significantly, the valve may have to be replaced with a prosthesis or a heterograft. Since the operative mortality of replacement of the mitral valve is still approximately 5 to 10 percent and since there are long-term complications of valve replacement, patients in whom preoperative evaluation suggests the possibility that replacement may be required should be operated on only if they have *critical* mitral stenosis, i.e., an orifice <1.0 cm², and are in the New York Heart Association class III, i.e., symptomatic with ordinary activity, despite optimal medical therapy.

VALVE REPLACEMENT The results of replacement of any valve are dependent primarily on (1) the patient's myocardial function at the time of operation, (2) the technical abilities of the operative team and the quality of the postoperative care, and (3) the durability, hemodynamic characteristics, and thrombogenicity of the prosthesis. Increased operative mortality is associated with the degree of preoperative functional disability and pulmonary hypertension. Late complications of replacement of any valve, which fortunately are declining in incidence, include paravalvular leakage, thromboemboli, bleeding due to anticoagulants, mechanical dysfunction of the prosthesis, and infective endocarditis.

The considerations regarding the choice between a bioprosthetic and artificial mechanical valve are similar in the mitral and aortic positions and in the treatment of stenotic, regurgitant, or mixed lesions. All patients who have undergone replacement of any valve with a mechanical prosthesis must be maintained permanently on anticoagulants. The primary advantage of bioprostheses (tissue valves) over mechanical prostheses is the reduction of thromboembolic complications and, except for patients with chronic atrial fibrillation, few such instances have been associated with their use. Bioprosthetic valves are contraindicated in younger patients (<35 years) because of accelerated deterioration and are particularly useful in the elderly (>65 years) in whom there is more concern about chronic anticoagulation than about long-term (>15 years) valve durability. These valves are also indicated in women who expect to become pregnant as well as others in whom anticoagulation may be contraindicated.

In patients without such contraindications, particularly those under 60 years, a mechanical prosthesis may be preferable. Many surgeons now select the St. Jude prosthesis, a double-disk tilting prosthesis, for replacement of both aortic and mitral valves because of somewhat more favorable hemodynamic characteristics and a suggestion of lower thrombogenicity.

The overall 9-year survival of operative survivors following mitral valve replacement is approximately 60 percent. Long-term prognosis is worse in subgroups of older patients and those with marked disability and striking depression of the cardiac index preoperatively.

MITRAL REGURGITATION

PATHOPHYSIOLOGY The regurgitant mitral orifice may be considered to be in parallel with the aortic orifice, and therefore the resistance to left ventricular emptying is reduced in patients with mitral regurgitation. As a consequence, the left ventricle decompresses itself into the left atrium during ejection, and with the reduction in left ventricular size there is a rapid decline in left ventricular tension, allowing a greater proportion of the contractile activity of the left ventricle to be expended in shortening. Thus, the initial compensation to mitral regurgitation consists of more complete systolic emptying of the left ventricle. However, a progressive increase in left ventricular end-diastolic volume occurs as the severity of the regurgitation increases and the function of the left ventricle deteriorates. The atrial contraction wave in the left atrial pressure pulse (*a* wave) is usually not as prominent as it is in mitral stenosis, but the *v* wave is often much taller, since it is inscribed during ventricular systole, when the left atrium fills from the pulmonary veins as well as from the left ventricle. During early diastole, as the distended left atrium suddenly empties, there is a particularly rapid *y* descent as long as there is no associated mitral stenosis. Left ventricular end-diastolic pressure may be slightly elevated. However, in chronic mitral regurgitation, there is often an increase in left ventricular compliance, so that ventricular volume may be greatly increased with little elevation in end-diastolic pressure. The effective cardiac output usually declines in seriously symptomatic patients. Although a left atrioventricular pressure gradient persisting throughout diastole signifies the presence of significant associated mitral stenosis, a brief, early diastolic gradient may occur in patients with pure regurgitation as a result of the torrential flow of blood across a normal-sized mitral orifice.

The prompt appearance of contrast material in the left atrium following its injection into the left ventricle signifies the presence and can be useful in the diagnosis of mitral regurgitation. The regurgitant volume can be measured by determining the difference between the total left ventricular stroke estimated angiocardiographically and the effective forward stroke volume determined by the Fick method. The results of such studies suggest that the regurgitant volume may be of the same magnitude as the effective forward stroke volume or may even exceed it in patients with severe regurgitation. Qualitative, but clinically useful, estimates of the severity of regurgitation may be made by Doppler echocardiography and by observation on cineangiograms of the degree of left atrial opacification following the injection of contrast material into the left ventricle.

Patients with severe mitral regurgitation may be divided into several subgroups, depending on the compliance, i.e., the pressure-volume relationship, of the left atrium and pulmonary venous bed. Among patients with severe mitral regurgitation, three major groups have been identified:

1 Normal or reduced compliance. These patients usually have *acute* mitral regurgitation. There is little enlargement of the left atrium, but marked elevation of the mean left atrial pressure, particularly of the *v* wave. In these patients severe mitral regurgitation has usually developed suddenly, as when it follows rupture of chordae tendineae, infarction of one of the heads of a papillary muscle, or tear of a mitral leaflet. Pulmonary edema is common. After several months the pulmonary vascular resistance may become markedly elevated, presumably as a consequence of the left atrial hypertension, and right-sided heart failure may also occur; sinus rhythm is usually present.

2 *Marked increase in compliance.* At the opposite end of the spectrum from group 1 are those patients with severe long-standing mitral regurgitation, massive enlargement of the left atrium, and normal or only slightly elevated left atrial pressure. The pulmonary artery pressure and pulmonary vascular resistance are also normal or only slightly elevated at rest. Clinically, these patients usually complain of severe fatigue and exhaustion secondary to a low cardiac output, while symptoms resulting from pulmonary congestion are less prominent; atrial fibrillation is almost invariably present. The association of a near-normal left atrial pressure with a markedly enlarged, thin-walled left atrium indicates that this chamber is far more compliant than normal. Thus, long-standing mitral regurgitation may, in some instances, alter the physical properties of the left atrial wall and thereby displace the atrial pressure-volume curve, allowing a normal pressure to exist in a greatly enlarged left atrium.

3 *Moderate increase in compliance.* By far the most common group are patients whose clinical and hemodynamic features are between those in the other two groups with variable degrees of enlargement of the left atrium and with significant elevation of the left atrial pressure. Symptoms are secondary to both reduced cardiac output and pulmonary congestion.

ETIOLOGY In about half the patients mitral regurgitation is caused by chronic *rheumatic heart disease,* but in contrast to mitral stenosis, pure or predominantly rheumatic mitral regurgitation occurs more frequently in males. The rheumatic process produces rigidity, deformity, and retraction of the valve cusps, and commissural fusion, as well as shortening, contraction, and fusion of the chordae tendineae. Mitral regurgitation may also occur as a congenital anomaly (Chap. 185), most commonly as (1) a defect of the endocardial cushions or in association with (2) corrected transposition, (3) endocardial fibroelastosis, and (4) the "parachute" mitral valve deformity. Mitral regurgitation may occur with fibrosis of a papillary muscle in patients with healed myocardial infarction as well as in patients with a ventricular aneurysm involving the base of a papillary muscle. Transient regurgitation may also occur during periods of ischemia involving a papillary muscle or the adjacent myocardium and may accompany bouts of angina pectoris. Mitral regurgitation may occur with marked left ventricular enlargement of any cause in which dilatation of the mitral annulus and lateral displacement of the papillary muscles interfere with coaptation of the valve leaflets. In hypertrophic cardiomyopathy the anterior leaflet of the mitral valve is displaced anteriorly during systole, leading to regurgitation (Chap. 192). Massive calcification of the mitral annulus of unknown cause, which occurs most commonly in elderly women, can also be responsible for significant mitral regurgitation. Systemic lupus erythematosus, rheumatoid arthritis, and ankylosing spondylitis are less common causes. *Acute* mitral regurgitation may occur secondary to infective endocarditis involving the valve or chordae tendineae, in acute myocardial infarction with rupture of a papillary muscle or one of its heads as a consequence of trauma, or as a complication of cardiac surgery.

Abnormal elongation of chordae tendineae and/or redundant posterior cusps of the mitral valve with prolapse of the cusps into the left atrium, the so-called floppy valve, leading to the syndrome of midsystolic click and midsystolic murmur, also referred to as the *prolapsing mitral valve leaflet syndrome* (see below), is another important cause of mitral regurgitation.

Regardless of etiology, serious mitral regurgitation tends to be progressive since enlargement of the left atrium places tension on the posterior mitral leaflet, pulling it away from the mitral orifice, thereby aggravating the valvular dysfunction. Similarly, the dilatation of the left ventricle increases the regurgitation, which in turn further enlarges the left atrium and ventricle, resulting in a vicious cycle; hence the aphorism, "mitral regurgitation begets mitral regurgitation."

SYMPTOMS Only a fraction of patients with chronic mitral regurgitation ever experience any reduction of cardiac reserve, but in those who do become symptomatic, fatigue, exertional dyspnea, and orthopnea may be prominent complaints. Symptoms resulting from pulmonary congestion tend to be less episodic in nature in patients with chronic severe mitral regurgitation than mitral stenosis, since fluctuations of the mean pulmonary capillary pressure are less marked. Indeed, acute paroxysmal pulmonary edema is quite rare in patients with chronic mitral regurgitation. Hemoptysis and systemic embolism also occur far less frequently in mitral regurgitation than in stenosis. On the other hand, fatigability, weakness, exhaustion, weight loss, and even cachexia are more prominent and occur most frequently in patients with marked reduction of cardiac output. Right-sided heart failure, with painful hepatic congestion, ankle edema, distended neck veins, ascites, and tricuspid regurgitation, may be observed in patients with mitral regurgitation who have associated pulmonary vascular disease. In patients with *acute* severe mitral regurgitation, left ventricular failure with acute pulmonary edema and/or cardiovascular collapse is common.

PHYSICAL FINDINGS The arterial pressure is usually normal, and the arterial pulse is often characterized by a sharp upstroke. The jugular venous pulse shows abnormally prominent *a* waves in patients with sinus rhythm and marked pulmonary hypertension. A systolic thrill is often palpable at the cardiac apex, the left ventricle is hyperdynamic with a brisk systolic impulse and a palpable rapid-filling wave, and the apex beat is often displaced laterally. When the left atrium is markedly enlarged, it may extend anteriorly, and its expansion may be palpable along the sternal border late during ventricular systole, resembling a right ventricular lift. The combination of the retraction of the left ventricle and expansion of the left atrium during systole may produce a characteristic rocking motion of the chest with each cardiac cycle. A right ventricular tap and the shock of pulmonary valve closure may be palpable in patients with marked pulmonary hypertension.

The first heart sound is generally absent, soft, or buried in the systolic murmur, and an accentuated mitral closure sound is useful in excluding severe regurgitation. A pulmonary ejection sound is often audible in patients with associated pulmonary hypertension. Splitting of the second heart sound is usually normal, but in patients with severe regurgitation, the aortic valve may close prematurely, resulting in wide splitting of the second heart sound. An opening snap indicates associated mitral stenosis but does not exclude predominant regurgitation. A low-pitched third heart sound, occurring 0.12 to 0.17 s after the aortic valve closure sound, at the completion of the rapid-filling phase of the mitral valve, is believed to be caused by the sudden tensing of the papillary muscles, chordae tendineae, and valve leaflets and is an important auscultatory feature of severe mitral regurgitation. The absence of a third heart sound indicates that if mitral regurgitation exists, it may not be severe. The third heart sound may be followed, often after a brief interval, by a short, rumbling, diastolic murmur, even in the absence of mitral stenosis. A fourth heart sound is often audible in patients with acute severe regurgitation of recent onset who are in sinus rhythm. A presystolic murmur is not ordinarily heard in patients with pure regurgitation and sinus rhythm but is present when there is significant associated mitral stenosis.

A systolic murmur, grade III/VI in intensity or louder, is the most characteristic auscultatory finding in severe mitral regurgitation. It is usually holosystolic (Chap. 177), but it may be decrescendo because the tall *v* wave in the left atrial pressure pulse results in a reduced late systolic left ventricular–atrial pressure gradient in patients with acute severe mitral regurgitation. Although the systolic murmur usually radiates into the axilla, in a minority of patients, particularly those with ruptured chordae tendineae or primary involvement of the posterior mitral leaflet, the regurgitant jet strikes the left atrial wall adjacent to the aortic root, and the systolic murmur is referred to the base of the heart and therefore may be confused with the murmur of aortic stenosis. In patients with ruptured chordae tendineae the systolic murmur may have a cooing or "sea gull" quality; in patients with a flail leaflet the murmur may have a musical quality.

Electrocardiogram　In patients with sinus rhythm there is evidence of left atrial enlargement, but right atrial enlargement may also be present when pulmonary hypertension is extreme. Chronic, severe mitral regurgitation with left atrial enlargement is generally associated with atrial fibrillation. In many patients there is no clear-cut electro-cardiographic evidence of enlargement of either ventricle. In severe regurgitation the signs of left ventricular hypertrophy are often present, although in patients with pulmonary hypertension combined ventricular hypertrophy or rarely pure right ventricular hypertrophy may be present.

Echocardiogram　The left atrium is usually enlarged and/or exhibits increased pulsations; the left ventricle may be hyperdynamic. With ruptured chordae tendineae or a flail leaflet coarse, erratic motion of the involved leaflets may be noted. Two-dimensional echocardiography usually shows incomplete coaptation of the anterior and posterior mitral leaflets. Annular calcification can be readily identified, as can left ventricular dilatation, aneurysm, or dyskinesis, which may be causally associated. Doppler echocardiography is the most accurate noninvasive technique for the detection and estimation of mitral regurgitation. The echocardiogram in patients with mitral valve prolapse is described below.

Roentgenographic features　The left atrium and left ventricle are the dominant chambers; in chronic cases the latter may be enlarged to aneurysmal proportions and forms the right border of the cardiac silhouette. On fluoroscopy the left ventricle is hyperdynamic and the left atrium exhibits vigorous systolic expansions. Marked calcification of the mitral leaflets occurs commonly in patients with long-standing combined regurgitation and stenosis but is uncommon in patients with pure regurgitation. Contrast left ventriculography is useful in the detection and quantification of mitral regurgitation.

TREATMENT　The nonsurgical management of mitral regurgitation is directed toward restricting those physical activities which regularly produce extreme fatigue and dyspnea, reducing sodium intake, and enhancing sodium excretion with the appropriate use of diuretics (Chap. 182). Digitalis glycosides and vasodilators increase the output of the failing left ventricle. The same considerations as in patients with mitral stenosis apply to the reversion of atrial fibrillation to sinus rhythm. In the late stages anticoagulants and leg binders are used to diminish the likelihood of venous thrombi and pulmonary emboli. Effective surgical treatment of rheumatic mitral regurgitation generally requires valvular replacement with a suitable prosthesis or tissue valve. Though most patients who survive operation appear to be greatly improved, some degree of myocardial dysfunction may persist.

When surgical treatment is contemplated, right- and left-sided heart catheterization and selective left ventricular angiocardiography are generally indicated. These studies are helpful in confirming the presence of severe regurgitation and aid in the identification of patients with primary myocardial disease and relatively mild, functional mitral regurgitation, who usually do not benefit from operation. Hemodynamic studies are also helpful in detecting and assessing the severity of any associated valve lesions, which may have to be dealt with at the time of operation or which might limit the patient's ultimate improvement if they are left untreated.

Surgical treatment of mitral regurgitation usually requires replacement of the valve with a prosthesis, although in selected patients, particularly those with severe annular dilatation, flail leaflets, or ruptured chordae, mitral annuloplasty or reconstruction of the mitral valve apparatus may be possible.

In the selection of patients for surgical treatment, the chronic, often slowly progressive nature of the disease must be balanced against the immediate risks and long-term uncertainties attendant upon valve replacement. Patients with mitral regurgitation who are asymptomatic or who are limited only during strenuous exertion are not considered to be candidates for surgical treatment, since they may live for many years with little deterioration. On the other hand, unless there are contraindications, surgical treatment should be offered to patients with severe mitral regurgitation whose limitations do not allow them to work full time or carry out normal household activities despite optimal medical management. The risks of valve replacement rise sharply, the recovery of impaired left ventricular function is incomplete, and the long-term survival is reduced in patients with congestive heart failure. However, conservative management has little to offer these patients, so that operative treatment may be indicated even at these advanced stages of the disease, and occasionally the clinical and hemodynamic improvement following surgical treatment is dramatic. It is likely that the immediate results of surgical treatment will continue to improve considerably and will lead to recommendations of operative treatment for selected patients with mitral regurgitation before they become severely disabled.

MITRAL VALVE PROLAPSE　This is also variously termed the *systolic click-murmur syndrome, Barlow's syndrome, floppy-valve syndrome,* and *billowing mitral leaflet syndrome,* a common, but highly variable, clinical syndrome resulting from diverse pathogenic mechanisms of the mitral valve apparatus. Among these are excessive or redundant mitral leaflet tissue, which is commonly involved with myxomatous degeneration and greatly increased concentration of acid mucopolysaccharide. This is a frequent finding in patients who have the typical features of Marfan's syndrome or cystic medial necrosis (Chap. 197), although in most patients myxomatous degeneration is confined to the mitral valve leaflets without other clinical or pathologic manifestations of disease; the posterior leaflet is usually more affected than the anterior, and the mitral valve annulus is often greatly enlarged. In many patients, elongated redundant chordae tendineae have been identified. There are probably several subsets of these patients, who differ in regard to the etiology and hemodynamic and clinical sequelae of abnormal mitral valve function. In the majority of patients, the etiology is unknown, but mitral valve prolapse may be a genetically determined collagen tissue disorder. It may be associated with thoracic skeletal deformities similar to but not as severe as those in Marfan's syndrome, including a high arched palate, and alterations of the chest and thoracic spine. Mitral valve prolapse may also occur in acute rheumatic fever, chronic rheumatic heart disease, and following mitral valvulotomy, in ischemic heart disease, and cardiomyopathies as well as in 20 percent of patients with ostium secundum atrial septal defect.

Mitral valve prolapse is usually a benign abnormality that may progress to a stage involving significant regurgitation and ventricular dilatation in some individuals. In these, prolapse of the valve leads to excessive stress on the papillary muscles, which in turn leads to dysfunction and ischemia of the papillary muscles and subjacent ventricular myocardium; rupture of chordae tendineae and progressive annular dilatation also contribute to valvular regurgitation. The electrocardiographic changes (see below) and ventricular arrhythmias appear to result from regional ventricular dysfunction related to increased stress placed on the papillary muscles.

Mitral valve prolapse is more common in females and occurs in a wide age range but most commonly between the ages of 14 and 30. Echocardiographic surveys have suggested that it may occur in as many as 7 percent of this group. There is an increased familial incidence suggesting an autosomal dominant form of inheritance. In many patients the echocardiographic abnormality is not accompanied by any other clinical manifestation of cardiac disease, and the significance of this finding is uncertain.

Most of the patients are asymptomatic and remain so for their entire lives. Although severe mitral regurgitation is an uncommon complication of mitral valve prolapse, the latter has become the most common cause of isolated severe mitral regurgitation. Arrythmias, most commonly ventricular premature contractions and paroxysmal supraventricular and ventricular tachycardia, have been reported. Patients with arrhythmias complain of palpitations, light-headedness, and syncope. Sudden death is a very rare complication. Many patients have chest pain which is difficult to evaluate. It is often substernal, prolonged, poorly related to exertion, and rarely resembles typical angina pectoris. Transient cerebral ischemic attacks secondary to emboli from the roughened surface of the valve have been reported. Infective endocarditis may occur in patients with mitral regurgitation associated with mitral valve prolapse.

Physical examination The most common finding is the mid- or late (nonejection) systolic click, which occurs 0.14 s or more after the first heart sound, and is thought to be generated by the sudden tensing of slack, elongated chordae tendineae or by the prolapsing mitral leaflet when it reaches its maximum excursion; systolic clicks may be multiple and are often followed by a high-pitched late systolic crescendo-decrescendo murmur, occasionally "whooping" or "honking," which is heard best at the apex. The click and murmur occur earlier with standing, the Valsalva maneuver, or inhalation of amyl nitrate, interventions which decrease left ventricular volume, exaggerating the propensity of mitral leaflet prolapse. Conversely, squatting or isometric exercise, which increases left ventricular end-diastolic volume, diminish the propensity for the mitral valve leaflets to prolapse, and the click-murmur complex is delayed and may even disappear. Some patients have a midsystolic click without the murmur; others have the murmur without a click.

Laboratory examination The *electrocardiogram* most commonly shows biphasic or inverted T waves in leads II, III, and aVF. The *echocardiogram* characteristically shows an abrupt posterior displacement of the posterior or sometimes of both mitral valve leaflets in mid- to late systole, immediately after the click, and during the systolic murmur. Two-dimensional echocardiography is particularly useful in identifying the abnormal position of the mitral valve leaflets, and Doppler studies are helpful in revealing and evaluating accompanying mitral regurgitation. *Angiocardiography* generally shows prolapse of the posterior and sometimes of both mitral valve leaflets and, rarely, severe mitral regurgitation. Many patients have bulging of the posteroinferior wall of the left ventricle into the left ventricular cavity during systole and/or hypokinesis of the anterolateral left ventricular wall. Others display prolapse of other valves, particularly the tricuspid, as well.

Treatment The management of patients with mitral valve prolapse is directed toward reassurance of the asymptomatic patient, the prevention of infective endocarditis with antibiotic prophylaxis, and the relief of the atypical chest pain; beta blockers have been found to be helpful in this regard, although their use is empiric. Antiarrhythmic agents are administered if frequent ventricular premature contractions are present or if tachyarrhythmias have occurred. If mitral regurgitation is severe, mitral valve replacement is indicated. Antiplatelet aggregation agents (aspirin and dipyridamole) should be given to patients with transient ischemic attacks, and if these are not effective, anticoagulants should be employed.

AORTIC STENOSIS

This lesion occurs in about one-fourth of all patients with chronic valvular heart disease; approximately 80 percent of adult patients with symptomatic valvular aortic stenosis are male.

PATHOPHYSIOLOGY The primary hemodynamic abnormality is obstruction to left ventricular outflow which leads to a systolic pressure gradient between the left ventricle and aorta. When severe obstruction is suddenly produced experimentally, the left ventricle responds by dilatation and reduction of stroke volume. However, in patients the obstruction may be present at birth or it increases gradually over the course of many years, and left ventricular output is maintained by the presence of left ventricular hypertrophy, which serves as a useful compensatory mechanism since it reduces toward normal the systolic stress developed by each segment of myocardium. A large transaortic valvular pressure gradient may exist for many years without a reduction of cardiac output, left ventricular dilatation,

or the development of any symptoms. As aortic stenosis progresses in severity, the left ventricular systolic pressure continues to rise, but rarely exceeds 300 mmHg.

A peak systolic pressure gradient exceeding 50 mmHg in the face of a normal cardiac output or an effective aortic orifice less than 0.5 cm^2 per square meter of body surface area, i.e., less than approximately one-third of the normal orifice, is generally considered to represent critical obstruction to left ventricular outflow. The left ventricular pressure pulse exhibits a rounded summit as the contraction of this chamber becomes progressively more isometric. The elevated left ventricular end-diastolic pressure observed in many patients with severe aortic stenosis does not necessarily signify the presence of left ventricular dilatation or failure, but may instead reflect diminished compliance of the hypertrophied left ventricular wall.

A large *a* wave in the left atrial pressure pulse is usually present with severe stenosis, because of enhanced atrial contraction and diminished ventricular compliance. Atrial contraction tends to raise left ventricular end-diastolic pressure without producing a similar elevation of mean left atrial pressure. This "booster pump" function of the left atrium prevents the pulmonary venous and capillary pressures from rising to levels which would produce pulmonary congestion, while at the same time maintaining left ventricular end-diastolic pressure at the elevated level necessary for effective left ventricular contraction. Loss of an appropriately timed, vigorous atrial contraction, as occurs in atrial fibrillation or atrioventricular dissociation, may result in a rapid aggravation of symptoms.

Although the cardiac output at rest is within normal limits in the majority of patients with severe aortic stenosis, it may fail to rise normally during exercise. Late in the disease the cardiac output and left ventricular–aortic pressure gradient decline, and the mean left atrial, pulmonary artery wedge, pulmonary arterial, and right ventricular pressures become elevated.

The hypertrophied left ventricular muscle mass elevates myocardial oxygen requirements. In addition, even in the absence of obstructive coronary artery disease, there may be interference with coronary blood flow, because the pressure compressing the coronary arteries exceeds the coronary perfusion pressure. Metabolic evidence of myocardial ischemia, i.e., lactate production, can be demonstrated in patients with aortic stenosis both in the presence and in the absence of coronary arterial narrowing, when myocardial oxygen needs are stimulated by isoproterenol.

A significant fraction of patients with rheumatic aortic stenosis has associated mitral valve disease. Aortic stenosis intensifies the severity of mitral regurgitation by increasing the pressure driving blood from the left ventricle to the left atrium.

Etiology Aortic stenosis may be congenital in origin, secondary to rheumatic inflammation of the aortic valve, or due to degenerative calcification of the aortic cusps of unknown cause. The *congenitally affected valve* may already be stenotic at birth and may gradually become calcified during the first three decades of life, becoming progressively more stenotic. In others, the valve may also be congenitally bicuspid without serious narrowing of the aortic orifice during childhood; its abnormal architecture makes its leaflets susceptible to otherwise ordinary hemodynamic stresses, which ultimately lead to valvular calcification, increased rigidity, and narrowing of the aortic orifice.

Rheumatic endocarditis of the aortic leaflets produces commissural fusion, resulting, sometimes, in a bicuspid valve. This, in turn, also makes the leaflets more susceptible to trauma, and ultimately leads to calcification and further narrowing. By the time the obstruction to left ventricular outflow causes serious clinical disability, the valve is usually a rigid calcified mass, and careful examination may make it difficult or even impossible to determine whether the underlying process was rheumatic or congenital. Rheumatic aortic stenosis is almost always associated with rheumatic involvement of the mitral valve. A rheumatic etiology is also favored by a history of active rheumatic fever and by associated severe aortic regurgitation. *Idiopathic calcific aortic stenosis* occurs most often in the elderly and is occasionally associated with fibrosis and fusion of the valve cusps; the pathologic process is considered to be a degenerative one—a "wear-and-tear" phenomenon. It may produce many of the characteristic physical signs of aortic stenosis. The valvular obstruction is usually relatively mild and of little if any hemodynamic significance; it may, however, on occasion, produce critical obstruction.

OTHER FORMS OF OBSTRUCTION TO LEFT VENTRICULAR OUTFLOW   Besides valvular aortic stenosis, three other lesions may be responsible for obstruction to left ventricular outflow.

1 *Hypertrophic cardiomyopathy.* This is the most important of these conditions numerically. It is characterized by marked hypertrophy of the left ventricle, involving in particular the interventricular septum of the left ventricular outflow tract, and may cause subaortic obstruction, as described in Chap. 192.
2 *Discrete congenital subvalvular aortic stenosis.* This condition is produced by either a membranous diaphragm or a fibrous ridge just below the aortic valve (Chap. 185).
3 *Supravalvular aortic stenosis.* This uncommon congenital anomaly is produced by narrowing of the ascending aorta or by a fibrous diaphragm with a small opening just above the aortic valve (Chap. 185).

SYMPTOMS   Aortic stenosis is rarely of hemodynamic or clinical importance until the valve orifice has narrowed to approximately one-third of normal. In contrast to mitral stenosis, which results in symptoms as soon as the obstruction becomes severe because the chamber just proximal to the narrowed valve, i.e., the left atrium, provides little compensation, severe aortic stenosis may exist for many years without producing any clinical disability because of the ability of the hypertrophied left ventricle to generate the elevated intraventricular pressures and the presence of a competent mitral valve behind the left ventricle.

Most patients with pure or predominant aortic stenosis have gradually increasing obstruction for years but do not become symptomatic until the fifth to seventh decades. Exertional dyspnea, angina pectoris, and syncope are the three cardinal symptoms. Often there is a history of insidious progression of fatigue and dyspnea associated with gradual curtailment of activities. Dyspnea results primarily from elevation of the pulmonary capillary pressures, which in turn is caused by elevations of left atrial and left ventricular end-diastolic pressures. Angina pectoris usually develops somewhat later and reflects an imbalance between the augmented myocardial oxygen requirements and reduced oxygen availability; the former results from the increased myocardial mass and intraventricular pressure, while the latter may result from accompanying coronary artery disease which is not uncommon in patients with aortic stenosis, as well as from compression of the coronary vessels by the hypertrophied myocardium. Therefore, angina may occur in severe aortic stenosis without organic coronary obstruction, but the *absence* of angina usually signifies that severe coronary obstructive disease is unlikely. Exertional syncope may result from a decline in arterial pressure caused by vasodilatation in the exercising muscles and inadequate vasoconstriction in nonexercising muscles in the face of a fixed cardiac output, or from a sudden fall in cardiac output produced by an arrhythmia.

Since the cardiac output is usually well maintained at rest until late, marked fatigability, weakness, peripheral cyanosis, and other clinical manifestations of a low cardiac output are usually not prominent until this stage is reached. Orthopnea, paroxysmal nocturnal dyspnea, and pulmonary edema, i.e., symptoms of left ventricular failure, also occur only in the advanced stages of the disease. Severe pulmonary hypertension leading to right ventricular failure and systemic venous hypertension, hepatomegaly, atrial fibrillation, and tricuspid regurgitation are usually preterminal findings.

When aortic stenosis and mitral stenosis coexist, the latter lesion masks many of the clinical findings of the former. The reduction of cardiac output induced by mitral stenosis lowers the pressure gradient across the aortic valve, diminishes the frequency of anginal episodes, and retards the development of severe left ventricular hypertrophy. On the other hand, symptoms considered more characteristic of mitral stenosis, such as pulmonary congestion and hemoptysis, may be present. Physical, electrocardiographic, radiologic, and echocardiographic examinations in patients with aortic and mitral stenosis generally reveal more evidence of left ventricular enlargement than in patients with pure mitral stenosis, and catheterization of the left side of the heart is helpful in defining the relative importance of each valvular abnormality.

PHYSICAL FINDINGS AND GRAPHIC TRACINGS   The systemic arterial pressure is usually within normal limits. In the late stages, however, when stroke volume declines, the systolic pressure may fall and the pulse pressure narrow. Systemic hypertension is unusual in patients with marked aortic stenosis, and a basal systolic arterial pressure exceeding 200 mmHg practically excludes severe narrowing of this valve. The peripheral arterial pulse, as palpated in the carotid or brachial arteries, rises slowly to a delayed sustained peak. Indirect recordings of the carotid pulse exhibit a gradually ascending limb, often with a prominent anacrotic notch or shoulder on the upstroke, as well as a delayed peak, with coarse systolic vibrations. The left ventricular ejection period is prolonged, the preejection period is abbreviated, and the ratio of these two, i.e., the preejection period/ systolic ejection period, is characteristically reduced (Chap. 179). Late in the course of the disease, in the presence of heart failure, the ratio may be normal. A palpable double systolic arterial pulse, the so-called bisferiens pulse, excludes pure or predominant aortic stenosis and signifies dominant or pure aortic regurgitation or obstructive hypertrophic cardiomyopathy (Chap. 192). In the late stages of valvular aortic stenosis, when the pulse pressure is reduced, the pulse amplitude may be so small that the anacrotic nature of the pulse and the delay in its upstroke may become more difficult to appreciate. The jugular venous pulse may be normal, although in many patients the *a* wave is accentuated. This results from the diminished distensibility of the right ventricular cavity caused by the bulging, hypertrophied interventricular septum and/or the presence of pulmonary hypertension.

The apex beat is usually active and displaced inferiorly and laterally, reflecting the presence of left ventricular hypertrophy. A double apical impulse may be appreciated, particularly with the patient in the left lateral recumbent position; the first outward expansion occurs during atrial systole and reflects the important contribution made by atrial contraction to ventricular systole, while the second occurs during ventricular systole, usually is forceful and sustained during ejection. The right ventricle is usually palpable only when pulmonary hypertension develops in the late stages of the disease. A systolic thrill is generally present at the base of the heart, in the jugular notch, and along the carotid arteries, but occasionally it is palpable only during expiration and with the patient leaning forward. In patients who do not have marked pulmonary emphysema, a thick chest wall, thoracic deformity, or heart failure, the absence of a systolic thrill suggests that the aortic stenosis is relatively mild.

The rhythm is generally regular until very late in the course; at other times, atrial fibrillation should suggest the possibility of associated mitral valve disease. An early systolic ejection sound, actually the opening snap of the aortic valve, is frequently audible in children and adolescents with congenital noncalcific valvular aortic stenosis. This sound usually disappears when the valve becomes calcified and rigid. The sound of aortic valve closure can also be identified most frequently in patients with aortic stenosis who have pliable valves, and calcification diminishes the intensity of this sound as well. As aortic stenosis increases in severity, left ventricular systole may become prolonged so that the aortic valve closure sound no longer precedes the pulmonic valve closure sound, and the two components may become synchronous, or aortic valve closure may even follow pulmonic valve closure, causing paradoxic splitting of the second heart sound (Chap. 177). In patients with aortic stenosis without a left intraventricular conduction defect, this finding usually signifies severe obstruction to left ventricular outflow. A fourth heart sound is audible at the apex in many patients with severe aortic stenosis, and reflects the presence of left ventricular hypertrophy and an elevated left ventricular end-diastolic pressure; a third heart sound generally occurs when the left ventricle dilates and fails.

The murmur of aortic stenosis is characteristically an ejection systolic murmur which commences shortly after the first heart sound, increases in intensity to reach a peak toward the middle of the ejection period, and diminishes progressively thereafter to end just before aortic valve closure (Chaps. 177 and 179). The murmur is usually low-pitched, rough, and rasping in character and is loudest at the base of the heart, most commonly in the second right intercostal space. It is transmitted to the jugular notch and upward along the carotid arteries. In patients with mild degrees of obstruction or in those with severe stenosis with heart failure in whom the stroke volume and therefore the transvalvular flow rate is reduced, the murmur may be relatively soft and brief. However, in almost all patients with severe obstruction, the murmur is at least grade III/VI. Occasionally, the murmur is transmitted downward and to the apex and may be confused with the systolic murmur of mitral regurgitation. However, the latter is usually holosystolic (Chap. 177).

Electrocardiogram This reveals left ventricular hypertrophy in the majority of patients with severe aortic stenosis (Chap. 178). In advanced cases, ST-segment depression and T-wave inversion in standard leads I and aVL and in the left precordial leads are evident. However, there is no close correlation between the electrocardiogram and the hemodynamic severity of obstruction, and the absence of electrocardiographic signs of left ventricular hypertrophy does not exclude severe obstruction. Left bundle branch block or the presence of intraventricular conduction defects suggests diffuse fibrotic involvement of the myocardium. The presence of left atrial enlargement should suggest the possibility of associated mitral valve disease.

Echocardiogram This reveals left ventricular hypertrophy, and in patients with valvular calcification, multiple, bright, thick, echoes from within the aortic root. While cusp calcification does not necessarily indicate significant valve stenosis, its absence can usually be used to exclude such a diagnosis after the age of 25. Eccentricity of the aortic valve cusps is characteristic of congenitally bicuspid valves (Chap. 179). Left ventricular dilatation and reduced systolic shortening reflecting impairment of left ventricular function can be recognized. The severity of aortic stenosis can be estimated from the ratio of end-systolic wall thickness to ventricular diameter on an M-mode study, from the degree of aortic leaflet separation on a two-dimensional echocardiogram, and most accurately by estimating the transvalvular pressure gradient using Doppler techniques. Echocardiography is particularly useful for identifying valvular abnormalities such as mitral stenosis and aortic regurgitation which sometimes accompany aortic stenosis, and for differentiating valvular from obstructive hypertrophic cardiomyopathy.

Roentgenographic features The chest roentgenogram may show no or little overall cardiac enlargement for many years, since the development of concentric left ventricular hypertrophy is the initial response to obstruction to left ventricular outflow. Hypertrophy without dilatation may produce some rounding of the cardiac apex in the frontal projection and slight backward displacement in the lateral view; critical aortic stenosis is often associated with poststenotic dilatation of the ascending aorta. Aortic calcification is usually readily apparent on fluoroscopic examination with an image intensifier or by echocardiography; *the absence of valvular calcification in an adult suggests that severe valvular aortic stenosis is not present.* In later stages of the disease as the left ventricle dilates, there is progressively more evidence of left ventricular enlargement, and there may also be roentgenologic signs of pulmonary congestion, as well as enlargement of the left atrium, pulmonary artery, right ventricle, and right atrium.

Catheterization and angiocardiography Catheterization of the left side of the heart should generally be carried out in patients suspected

of having severe aortic stenosis, particularly before a final decision concerning operative treatment is made. The goals are to assess (1) the severity of the aortic obstruction, (2) the status of left ventricular function, and (3) the location of left ventricular outflow obstruction. These investigations are especially indicated in the following:

1 Young, asymptomatic patients with noncalcific congenital aortic stenosis (Chap. 185), in order to define the severity of obstruction to left ventricular outflow, since operation may be indicated in them even in the absence of symptoms if severe aortic stenosis is present.
2 Patients in whom it is suspected that the obstruction to left ventricular outflow may not be at the aortic valve, but rather in the sub- or supravalvular regions.
3 Patients with clinical signs of aortic stenosis and symptoms of myocardial ischemia, in whom associated coronary artery disease is suspected. An effort should be made to determine whether aortic stenosis or coronary atherosclerosis is primarily responsible for the symptoms, and coronary arteriography should be carried out in addition to catheterization of the left side of the heart.
4 Patients with multivalvular disease, in whom the role played by each valvular deformity must be defined before operative treatment is planned.

Angiographic studies are helpful in defining the size of the left ventricular cavity, the thickness of the wall, the site of obstruction, the degree of deformity and mobility of the aortic valve cusps, the diameter of the ascending aorta, and the presence and degree of accompanying mitral and aortic regurgitation and of obstructive coronary disease. In patients with severe narrowing, a jet of contrast substance passing through the aortic orifice is readily visualized.

NATURAL HISTORY Death in patients with severe aortic stenosis occurs most commonly in the seventh decade. Based on analysis of data obtained at postmortem examination, the average duration of various symptoms was as follows: angina pectoris, 3 years; syncope, 3 years; dyspnea, 2 years; and congestive heart failure, 1.5 to 2 years. Moreover, in more than 80 percent of patients who died with aortic stenosis, symptoms had existed for less than 4 years. Congestive heart failure was considered to be the cause of death in one-half to two-thirds of patients. Among adults dying with valvular aortic stenosis, sudden death, which presumably results from an arrhythmia, occurred in 10 to 20 percent, and at an average age of 60 years (Chap. 30).

TREATMENT Strenuous physical activity should be avoided even in the asymptomatic stage in patients with *severe* aortic stenosis. Digitalis glycosides, sodium restriction, and diuretics are indicated in the treatment of congestive heart failure. While nitroglycerin is helpful in relieving angina pectoris, vasodilator therapy for heart failure is usually of little value. The most critical decision in the management of aortic stenosis, indeed of any valvular lesion, concerns the advisability of surgical treatment. The indications and results of operation, as well as the techniques, differ considerably, depending on the patient's age and the nature of the valvular deformity.

In children and adolescents with noncalcific congenital aortic stenosis, considerable hemodynamic improvement can be anticipated from simple commissural incision under direct vision (Chap. 185). When carried out by an experienced surgical team, this procedure may be expected to be hemodynamically effective and to be associated with a mortality rate of less than 2 percent. This operation is recommended not only for symptomatic patients but also for asymptomatic children and adolescents with hemodynamic evidence of severe obstruction to left ventricular outflow, with a peak systolic pressure gradient exceeding 50 mmHg when the cardiac output is normal, or a calculated effective orifice less than 0.6 cm² per square meter of body surface area. Though this procedure can be expected to result in complete or almost complete relief of obstruction in the majority of patients, the valve cannot be rendered entirely normal anatomically, and it may become deformed, calcified, and stenotic again, and may require valve replacement at some later date.

In the majority of adults with calcific aortic stenosis, satisfactory valve function cannot be restored, even by deliberate sculpturing procedures carried out under direct vision, and replacement of the valve is necessary. In most instances, it is prudent to postpone operation in patients with severe calcific aortic stenosis who are asymptomatic, since their future course is difficult to predict and they may continue to do well for many years. However, they should be followed carefully by clinical examination for the development of symptoms and by the various noninvasive tests, such as echocardiograms and/or radionuclide angiograms (Chap. 179), for evidence of deteriorating left ventricular function. It is likely that as the results of surgical replacement of the aortic valve continue to improve, many of these patients will become candidates for operation before their disease reaches the symptomatic stage. At the present, replacement of the aortic valve should be undertaken in patients with symptoms, even when relatively mild, that are believed to result primarily from aortic stenosis and who have hemodynamic evidence of severe obstruction. In such patients the operative risk is relatively low (<5 percent) in centers with experience.

When angina pectoris, syncope, or left ventricular decompensation develops in adults with valvular aortic stenosis, the outlook, despite medical treatment, is very poor and can be improved significantly by replacement of the aortic valve with a mechanical or bioprosthetic valve. Therefore, the risk entailed by operation in this group of patients is considerably lower than the risk involved by nonoperative treatment; moreover, the symptomatic improvement in many survivors of operation has been remarkable.

Operation should, if possible, be carried out before frank left ventricular failure supervenes; at this late stage, the operative risk is high (approx. 15 percent), and evidence of myocardial disease may persist even when the operation is technically successful. Furthermore, long-term postoperative survival also correlates inversely with preoperative functional disability. Nonetheless, in view of the very poor prognosis of such patients when they are treated medically, there is usually little choice but to advise immediate surgical treatment. In patients in whom severe aortic stenosis and coronary artery disease coexist, relief of the aortic stenosis and revascularization of the myocardium by means of aortocoronary bypass grafting may result in striking clinical and hemodynamic improvement. Since many patients with calcific aortic stenosis are elderly, particular attention must be directed to the adequacy of hepatic, renal, and pulmonary function before valve replacement is recommended. The mortality rate depends to a substantial extent on the patient's preoperative clinical and hemodynamic state. The 9-year survival rate of operative survivors following aortic valve replacement is approximately 67 percent. Approximately 15 percent of bioprosthetic valves evidence primary valve failure in 10 years, requiring re-replacement, and an approximately equal percentage of patients with mechanical prostheses develop significant hemorrhagic complications as a consequence of treatment with anticoagulants. Fortunately, there is evidence that regression of left ventricular hypertrophy may occur following relief of obstruction.

AORTIC REGURGITATION

PATHOPHYSIOLOGY The total stroke volume expelled by the left ventricle (i.e., the sum of the effective forward stroke volume and the volume of blood which regurgitates back into the left ventricle) is increased in aortic regurgitation. In patients with free aortic regurgitation the volume of regurgitant flow may be of the same order of magnitude as the effective forward stroke volume. In contrast to mitral regurgitation, in which a fraction of the left ventricular stroke volume is delivered into the low-pressure left atrium, in aortic regurgitation the entire left ventricular stroke volume must be ejected into a high-pressure zone, the aorta. Although the low aortic diastolic pressure facilitates ventricular emptying during early systole, an increase of the left ventricular end-diastolic volume constitutes the major hemodynamic compensation to aortic regurgitation. The dilatation of the left ventricle allows this chamber to expel a larger stroke volume without requiring any increase in the relative shortening of each myofibril. Therefore, severe aortic regurgitation may occur with a normal effective forward stroke volume and a normal ejection fraction [total (forward plus regurgitant) stroke volume/end-diastolic volume], together with an elevated left ventricular end-diastolic pressure and volume. On the other hand, through the operation of Laplace's law (which indicates that myocardial wall tension is the product of intracavitary pressure and left ventricular radius), left ventricular dilatation increases the left ventricular systolic tension required to develop any given level of systolic pressure. As left ventricular function deteriorates, the end-diastolic volume increases without further elevation of the aortic regurgitant volume; the ejection fraction and forward stroke volume decline. Deterioration of left ventricular function often precedes the development of symptoms. Considerable thickening of the left ventricular wall also occurs with chronic aortic regurgitation, and at autopsy the hearts of these patients may be among the largest encountered, occasionally exceeding 1000 g in weight.

The reduction of the aortic diastolic pressure in aortic regurgitation shortens the left ventricular isometric contraction period, which is advantageous since it prolongs the left ventricular ejection period. The reverse pressure gradient from aorta to left ventricle, which is responsible for the aortic regurgitant flow, falls progressively during diastole, accounting for the decrescendo nature of the diastolic murmur. Equilibration between aortic and left ventricular pressures may occur toward the end of diastole, particularly when the heart rate is slow, and the left ventricular end-diastolic pressure may be elevated, occasionally to extremely high levels (>40 mmHg). Rarely, the left ventricular pressure exceeds the left atrial pressure toward the end of diastole, and this reversed pressure gradient closes the mitral valve prematurely, or may cause diastolic mitral regurgitation.

In patients with free aortic regurgitation the effective forward cardiac output usually is normal or only slightly reduced at rest, but often it fails to rise normally during exertion. Early signs of left ventricular dysfunction include reductions of the fraction of systolic shortening and of the ejection fraction determined by echocardiography or radionuclide or contrast angiography. In advanced stages there may be considerable elevation of the left atrial, pulmonary artery wedge, pulmonary arterial, and right ventricular pressures, and lowering of the forward cardiac output at rest.

Myocardial ischemia occurs in patients with aortic regurgitation because both left ventricular dilatation and the elevated left ventricular systolic pressure tend to augment myocardial oxygen requirements. However, the major portion of coronary blood flow occurs during diastole, when arterial pressure is subnormal, thereby reducing coronary perfusion pressure. The result is a combination of increased oxygen demand and reduced supply.

ETIOLOGY Approximately three-fourths of all patients with pure or predominant regurgitation are males; however, females predominate among patients with aortic regurgitation who have associated mitral valve disease. In approximately two-thirds of patients with aortic regurgitation the disease is rheumatic in origin, resulting in a chronic form of the disorder with thickening, deformation, and shortening of the individual aortic valve cusps, changes which prevent their proper closure during diastole. A rheumatic etiology is less common in patients with isolated aortic regurgitation. Acute aortic regurgitation may also result from infective endocarditis, which may attack a valve previously affected by rheumatic disease, a congenitally deformed valve, or rarely a normal aortic valve, and may result in the perforation or erosion of one or more of the leaflets. Patients with discrete membranous subaortic stenosis may develop thickening of the aortic valve leaflets, which in turn leads to mild or moderate degrees of aortic regurgitation and makes these valves particularly susceptible to endocarditis. Aortic regurgitation may also occur in patients with congenital bicuspid aortic valves. Prolapse of an aortic cusp, resulting in progressive chronic aortic regurgitation, occurs in approximately 15 percent of patients with ventricular septal defect (Chap. 185). Congenital fenestrations of the aortic valve occasionally produce mild aortic regurgitation. Although traumatic rupture of the aortic valve is an uncommon cause of acute aortic regurgitation, it does represent the most frequent serious lesion observed in patients surviving nonpenetrating cardiac injuries. In patients with aortic regurgitation due to primary valvular disease, dilatation of the aortic annulus may occur secondarily and intensify the regurgitation.

Aortic regurgitation, both acute and chronic, may also be due entirely to marked aortic dilatation, without primary involvement of the valve leaflets; widening of the aortic annulus and separation of the aortic leaflets are responsible for the aortic regurgitation. Syphilis and ankylosing rheumatoid spondylitis may be associated with cellular infiltration and scarring of the media of the thoracic aorta, leading to aortic dilatation, aneurysm formation, and severe regurgitation. In syphilis of the aorta (Chap. 197), the involvement of the intima may narrow the coronary ostia, which in turn may be responsible for myocardial ischemia. Cystic medial necrosis of the ascending aorta, which may or may not be associated with other manifestations of the Marfan syndrome (Chap. 197), idiopathic dilatation of the aorta, and severe hypertension all may also widen the aortic annulus and lead to progressive aortic regurgitation. Occasionally, retrograde dissection of the aorta involving the aortic annulus produces aortic regurgitation.

The coexistence of hemodynamically significant aortic stenosis with aortic regurgitation usually excludes all of the rarer forms of aortic regurgitation because it occurs almost exclusively in patients whose aortic regurgitation is on a rheumatic or congenital basis.

HISTORY A family history may frequently be elicited from patients with the Marfan syndrome, and a history of a heart murmur heard early in life may be obtained from patients with congenital aortic regurgitation. Patients with aortic regurgitation of obscure cause should also be questioned about a positive serologic test for syphilis, and about prior chest trauma; a history compatible with infective endocarditis may sometimes be elicited from patients with rheumatic or congenital involvement of the aortic valve, and the infection often precipitates or seriously aggravates preexisting symptoms. Ankylosing spondylitis is usually self-evident.

The interval between the first episode of acute rheumatic fever and the development of hemodynamically significant aortic regurgitation averages approximately 7 years, and this period is followed by an asymptomatic interval of approximately 10 to 20 years, during which the severity of the aortic regurgitation usually increases. Thus, asymptomatic severe aortic regurgitation may exist for many years.

In chronic severe aortic regurgitation, uncomfortable awareness of the heartbeat, especially on lying down, is often an early complaint. Sinus tachycardia during exertion or with emotion, or premature ventricular contractions, may produce particularly uncomfortable palpitations, as well as head pounding. These complaints may persist for many years before the development of exertional dyspnea, usually the first symptom of diminished cardiac reserve. This is followed by orthopnea, paroxysmal nocturnal dyspnea, and excessive diaphoresis. Chest pain occurs frequently, even in younger patients, and it is not necessary to invoke the presence of coronary artery disease to explain this symptom in patients with aortic regurgitation. It may be due to myocardial ischemia, or it may originate from excessive cardiac pounding on the chest wall. Anginal pain may develop at rest as well as during exertion. Nocturnal angina may be a particularly troublesome symptom and is frequently accompanied by marked diaphoresis. The anginal episodes may be prolonged and often do not respond satisfactorily to sublingual nitroglycerin. Late in the course of the disease, evidence of systemic fluid accumulation, including congestive hepatomegaly, ankle edema, and ascites, may develop. Patients with severe aortic regurgitation tolerate high fevers, infections, or cardiac arrhythmias poorly, and may die in pulmonary edema as a result of one of these complications.

In patients with acute severe aortic regurgitation, as may occur in trauma or infective endocarditis, the left ventricle rapidly exhausts its ability to dilate, and left ventricular diastolic pressure rises rapidly with associated elevations of left atrial and pulmonary capillary pressures.

PHYSICAL FINDINGS The examination should be directed toward the detection of causes predisposing to aortic regurgitation, such as the Marfan syndrome, rheumatoid spondylitis, syphilis, essential hypertension, and ventricular septal defect. Even prior to the examination of the heart of the patient with free aortic regurgitation, the jarring of the entire body and the bobbing motion of the head with each systole can be appreciated, and the abrupt distention and collapse of the larger arteries are easily visible. A rapidly rising "water-hammer" pulse, which collapses suddenly as arterial pressure falls rapidly during late systole and diastole (Corrigan's pulse), and capillary pulsations (Quincke's pulse), an alternate flushing and paling of the skin at the root of the nail while pressure is applied to the tip of the nail, are characteristic of free aortic regurgitation. A booming, "pistol-shot" sound can be heard over the femoral arteries, and a to-and-fro murmur (Duroziez's sign) is audible if the femoral artery is lightly compressed with a stethoscope.

The arterial pulse pressure is widened, with an elevation of the systolic pressure, sometimes to as high as 300 mmHg, and a depression of the diastolic arterial pressure. The measurement of arterial diastolic pressure with a sphygmomanometer may be complicated by the fact that systolic sounds are frequently heard with the cuff completely deflated. However, the level of cuff pressure at the time of muffling of the Korotkoff sounds generally corresponds fairly closely to the true intraarterial diastolic pressure. The severity of aortic regurgitation does not always correlate directly with the arterial pulse pressure, and severe regurgitation may exist in patients with arterial pressures in the range of 140/60. As the disease progresses, and the left ventricular end-diastolic pressure becomes markedly elevated, the arterial diastolic pressure may actually rise since the aortic diastolic pressure cannot fall below the left ventricular end-diastolic pressure.

The apex beat is displaced laterally and inferiorly. The left ventricle is hyperdynamic in patients with free regurgitation, and the systolic expansion and subsequent retraction of the apex are prominent and contrast sharply with the sustained systolic thrust characteristic of severe aortic stenosis. A diastolic thrill is often palpable along the left sternal border, and a prominent systolic thrill may be palpable in the jugular notch and transmitted upward along the carotid arteries. This thrill and the accompanying systolic murmur are due to the markedly increased blood flow across the aortic orifice, and do not necessarily signify the coexistence of aortic stenosis. In many patients with pure aortic regurgitation, or with combined stenosis and regurgitation, palpation, or indirect recording of the carotid arterial pulse, reveals it to be bisferiens, i.e., with two systolic waves separated by a trough.

In patients with severe regurgitation the aortic valve closure sound is usually diminished or absent, and the indirectly recorded carotid arterial pulse does not usually show a clear-cut incisura. A third heart sound is common, and occasionally a fourth heart sound may also be heard. A loud systolic ejection sound is frequently audible; presumably it results from the sudden dilatation of the aorta by a greatly increased stroke volume.

The murmur of aortic regurgitation is typically a high-pitched, blowing, decrescendo diastolic murmur which is usually heard best in the third left intercostal space. In patients with mild regurgitation this murmur is brief, but as the severity increases, the murmur generally becomes louder and longer, and in patients with free aortic regurgitation it is usually holodiastolic. When the murmur is soft, it can be heard best with the diaphragm of the stethoscope and with the patient sitting up, leaning forward, and with the breath held in forced expiration. As it increases in intensity it tends to radiate widely, particularly down the lower sternal edge. In patients in whom the regurgitation is caused by primary valvular disease, the diastolic murmur is usually louder along the left than the right sternal border. However, when the decrescendo diastolic murmur is heard best along the right sternal border, it suggests that the aortic regurgitation is caused by dilatation or an aneurysm of the aortic root. "Cooing" or musical diastolic murmurs suggest eversion of an aortic cusp vibrating in the regurgitant stream. A diastolic blowing murmur along the left sternal border is much more commonly caused by aortic than by pulmonic regurgitation. Unless it is trivial in magnitude, the aortic regurgitation is usually accompanied by peripheral signs such as a widened pulse pressure or a collapsing pulse. On the other hand, with the Graham Steell murmur of pulmonary regurgitation there usually is clinical evidence of severe pulmonary hypertension, including a loud and palpable pulmonary component of the second heart sound. In addition, the phonocardiogram reveals that the murmur of aortic regurgitation begins with the aortic second sound and therefore commences somewhat before the murmur of pulmonary regurgitation.

A midsystolic ejection murmur is generally heard best at the base of the heart and is transmitted to the jugular notch and along the carotid vessels. This murmur may be as loud as grade V/VI without indicating the presence of organic obstruction; it is often higher pitched, shorter, and less rasping in quality than the ejection systolic murmur heard in patients with predominant aortic stenosis. A third murmur which is frequently heard in patients with aortic regurgitation is the Austin Flint murmur, a soft, low-pitched, rumbling middiastolic or presystolic bruit. It is probably produced by the displacement of the anterior leaflet of the mitral valve by the aortic regurgitant stream but does not appear to be associated with hemodynamically significant obstruction to left ventricular filling; earlier onset of and longer Austin Flint murmurs correlate with more severe aortic regurgitation. Both the Austin Flint murmur and the rumbling diastolic murmur of mitral stenosis are loudest at the apex, but the murmur of mitral stenosis is usually accompanied by a loud first heart sound and immediately follows the opening snap of the mitral valve, while the Austin Flint murmur is often shorter in duration than the murmur of mitral stenosis, and in patients with sinus rhythm the latter more frequently is characterized by presystolic accentuation. The auscultatory features of aortic regurgitation are intensified by isometric exercise such as strenuous handgrip, which augments systemic resistance, and reduced by inhalation of amyl nitrite, which evokes the opposite effect. A blowing holosystolic murmur at the apex, which is transmitted to the axilla, may also be heard in patients with aortic regurgitation who have marked left ventricular dilatation and functional mitral regurgitation.

In *acute* severe aortic regurgitation, the elevation of left ventricular end-diastolic pressure may lead to early closure of the mitral valve, an associated middiastolic sound, a soft or absent S_1, a pulse pressure that is not particularly wide, and a soft, short diastolic murmur.

Electrocardiogram In patients with mild aortic regurgitation there may be no electrocardiographic abnormalities, but as the severity of chronic aortic regurgitation increases, so do the electrocardiographic signs of left ventricular hypertrophy (Chap. 178). In addition to the abnormally tall R waves over the left precordium and deep S waves over the right precordium, patients with severe aortic regurgitation frequently exhibit ST-segment depressions and T-wave inversions in leads I, aVL, V_5, and V_6. Left axis deviation and/or QRS prolongation denote diffuse myocardial disease, generally associated with patchy fibrosis, and usually denote a poor prognosis.

Echocardiogram This reveals increased systolic excursion of the posterior left ventricular wall; the extent and velocity of wall motion is supernormal or normal, until myocardial contractility declines. A rapid, high-frequency fluttering of the anterior mitral leaflet produced by the impact of the aortic regurgitant jet is a characteristic finding. The echocardiogram is also useful in detecting dilatation of the aortic annulus, and of the left atrium. Thickening of the aortic valve and failure of coaptation of the leaflets may be noted in patients with primary valve disease. Doppler studies are most sensitive, both in detecting aortic regurgitation and in quantifying it.

Roentgenogram Moderate or severe degrees of chronic aortic regurgitation are associated with varying degrees of left ventricular enlargement. The apex is displaced downward and to the left in the frontal projection, and frequently the cardiac shadow extends below the left diaphragm. Left ventricular enlargement may also be apparent in the left anterior oblique and lateral projections, in which the left ventricle is displaced posteriorly and encroaches on the spine. On fluoroscopic examination the aorta and left ventricle pulsate vigorously and in opposite directions. In patients in whom primary valvular disease is responsible for the aortic regurgitation, the ascending aorta and aortic knob may be moderately dilated. When aortic regurgitation is caused by primary disease of the aortic wall, aneurysmal dilatation of the aorta may be noted roentgenographically, and the aorta may fill the retrosternal space in the lateral view.

TREATMENT In deciding upon the advisability and proper timing of surgical treatment, two points should be kept in mind: (1) patients with chronic aortic regurgitation usually do not become symptomatic until *after* the development of myocardial dysfunction; and (2) surgical treatment often does not restore normal left ventricular function. Therefore, careful clinical follow-up and noninvasive testing, preferably with echocardiography, at approximately 6-month intervals, are necessary if operation is to be undertaken at the optimal time, i.e., with the onset of left ventricular dysfunction but prior to the development of severe symptoms. Operation can be deferred as long as the patient remains asymptomatic *and* retains normal left ventricular function.

Replacement of the aortic valve with a suitable mechanical or tissue prosthesis is generally necessary in patients with rheumatic aortic regurgitation and in many patients with other forms of regurgitation. Rarely, when a leaflet has been perforated during an episode of infective endocarditis, or torn from its attachments to the aortic annulus, surgical repair may be possible. When aortic regurgitation is due to aneurysmal dilatation of the annulus and ascending aorta, rather than to primary valvular involvement, it may be possible to reduce the regurgitation by narrowing the annulus or by excising a portion of the aortic root without replacing the valve. More frequently, however, regurgitation can be eliminated only by replacing the aortic valve, excising the aneurysm responsible for the regurgitation, and replacing the latter with a graft. This formidable procedure entails a higher risk than aortic valve replacement alone.

As in patients with aortic stenosis, both the operative risk of aortic valve replacement and late mortality are largely dependent on the stage of the disease and on myocardial function at the time of operation; patients with marked cardiac enlargement and prolonged left ventricular dysfunction have a late mortality of approximately 5 percent per year despite a technically satisfactory operation.

Although operation constitutes the principal treatment of aortic regurgitation, and should be carried out before the development of heart failure, the latter usually does respond initially to treatment with digitalis glycosides, salt restriction, and diuretics. Digitalis may also be indicated in patients with severe regurgitation and dilated left ventricles without symptoms of frank left ventricular failure. Cardiac arrhythmias and infections are poorly tolerated in patients with free aortic regurgitation, and must be treated promptly and vigorously. Although nitroglycerin and long-acting nitrates are not as helpful in relieving anginal pain as in patients with coronary artery disease or aortic stenosis, they are worth a trial. Patients with syphilitic aortitis should receive a full course of penicillin therapy (Chap. 122).

ACUTE AORTIC REGURGITATION Infective endocarditis, aortic dissection, and trauma are the most common causes of severe, acute aortic regurgitation. Since the left ventricle has not had time to dilate, stroke volume declines and ventricular diastolic pressure rises markedly; the arterial pulse pressure is often not markedly widened and the physical signs characteristic of severe chronic regurgitation may be absent. Premature closure of the mitral valve is common and can be recognized by echocardiography. The first heart sound is soft or absent; the aortic diastolic murmur is characteristically brief. Patients present with pulmonary congestion and edema, and cardiovascular collapse secondary to a low cardiac output. Acute, severe regurgitation requires prompt surgical treatment, which may be lifesaving.

TRICUSPID STENOSIS

Tricuspid stenosis, a relatively uncommon valvular lesion, is generally rheumatic in origin and is much more common in women than in men. It does not usually occur as an isolated lesion or in patients with pure mitral regurgitation, but most commonly is observed in association with mitral stenosis, and sometimes with combined mitral and aortic stenosis. Hemodynamically significant tricuspid stenosis occurs in 5 to 10 percent of patients with severe mitral stenosis; rheumatic tricuspid stenosis is commonly associated with some degree of regurgitation.

PATHOPHYSIOLOGY A diastolic pressure gradient between the right atrium and ventricle is present. This gradient can be recorded most accurately and conveniently with a double-lumen cardiac catheter. It is augmented when the transvalvular blood flow increases during inspiration, and reduced during expiration. A mean diastolic pressure gradient exceeding 5 mmHg is usually sufficient to elevate the mean right atrial pressure to levels which result in systemic venous congestion and, unless sodium intake has been restricted or diuretics have been given, is associated with ascites and edema. In patients with sinus rhythm, the right atrial a wave may be extremely tall and may even approach the level of the right ventricular systolic pressure. The resting cardiac output is usually quite low and fails to rise during exercise. The low cardiac output is responsible for the normal or only slightly elevated left atrial, pulmonary arterial, and right ventricular systolic pressures despite the presence of even moderately severe mitral stenosis.

SYMPTOMS Since mitral stenosis generally precedes the development of tricuspid stenosis, many patients initially have symptoms of pulmonary congestion. Amelioration of the latter should raise the possibility that tricuspid stenosis may be developing. Characteristically, patients complain of relatively little dyspnea for the degree of hepatomegaly, ascites, and edema which they present. Weakness secondary to a low cardiac output and discomfort due to refractory edema, ascites, and marked hepatomegaly are common in patients with tricuspid stenosis and/or regurgitation. In some patients tricuspid stenosis may be suspected for the first time when symptoms of right ventricular failure persist after an adequate mitral valvulotomy.

PHYSICAL FINDINGS The diagnosis is often missed unless it is specifically considered and searched for. Severe tricuspid stenosis is associated with marked hepatic congestion, often resulting in cirrhosis, jaundice, serious malnutrition, severe edema, and ascites. Congestive hepatomegaly and, in cases of severe tricuspid valve disease, splenomegaly are present. The jugular veins are distended, and in patients with sinus rhythm there may be giant a waves. The v waves are less conspicuous, and since tricuspid obstruction impedes right atrial emptying during diastole, there is a slow y descent. In patients with sinus rhythm there may be prominent presystolic pulsations of the enlarged liver as well.

The right ventricle and the shock of pulmonary valve closure are usually not easily palpable. Indeed, a giant a wave in the jugular venous pulse without palpatory evidence of pulmonary hypertension or right ventricular enlargement suggests the possibility of tricuspid stenosis. The pulmonic closure sound is not accentuated on auscultation, and occasionally an opening snap of the tricuspid valve may be heard or recorded phonocardiographically approximately 0.06 s after pulmonary valve closure. The diastolic murmur of tricuspid stenosis has many of the qualities of the mitral diastolic murmur, and since tricuspid stenosis almost always occurs in the presence of mitral stenosis, the less-common valvular lesion may be missed. However, the tricuspid murmur is generally heard best along the left

lower sternal margin and over the xiphoid process and is most prominent during presystole in sinus rhythm. In patients with sinus rhythm the presystolic component is often loudest. It is augmented during inspiration, and it is reduced during expiration and particularly during the Valsalva maneuver, when tricuspid blood flow is reduced. This finding (Carvallo's sign) is often most easily elicited when the patient is in the erect position. The diastolic murmur is reduced in amplitude as the stethoscope is inched laterally, only to intensify or reappear as the mitral murmur at the apex.

Noninvasive examinations The features of right atrial enlargement (Chap. 178) include tall, peaked P waves in lead II, as well as prominent, upright P waves in lead V_1. The *absence* of electrocardiographic evidence of right ventricular hypertrophy in a patient with right-sided heart failure who is believed to have mitral stenosis should suggest associated tricuspid valve disease. The chest roentgenograms in patients with combined tricuspid and mitral stenosis show particular prominence of the right atrium and superior vena cava without much enlargement of the pulmonary artery and with less evidence of pulmonary vascular congestion than occurs in patients with pure mitral valve disease. On echocardiographic examination the tricuspid valve is usually thickened with reduction of the EF slope.

TREATMENT Patients with tricuspid stenosis generally exhibit marked systemic venous congestion; intensive salt restriction and diuretic therapy are required during the preoperative period. Such a prolonged preparatory period may diminish hepatic congestion and thereby improve hepatic function sufficiently so that the risks of operation are diminished. Surgical treatment of the tricuspid valve is not ordinarily indicated at the time of mitral valve surgery in patients with mild tricuspid stenosis. On the other hand, definitive surgical relief of the tricuspid stenosis should be carried out, preferably at the time of mitral valvulotomy, in patients with moderate or severe tricuspid stenosis who have mean diastolic pressure gradients exceeding 5 mmHg and tricuspid orifices less than 1.5 to 2.0 cm². Tricuspid stenosis is almost always accompanied by significant tricuspid regurgitation. Open-heart operations utilizing cardiopulmonary bypass may permit substantial improvement of tricuspid valve function. If this cannot be accomplished, the tricuspid valve may have to be replaced with a prosthesis, preferably a tissue valve.

TRICUSPID REGURGITATION

Most commonly, tricuspid regurgitation is functional and secondary to marked dilatation of the right ventricle and the tricuspid valve ring. Functional tricuspid regurgitation may complicate right ventricular failure of any cause, including inferior wall infarcts that involve the right ventricle, and is commonly seen in the late stages of heart failure due to rheumatic or congenital heart disease with severe pulmonary hypertension, as well as in ischemic heart disease, cardiomyopathy, and cor pulmonale. It is in part reversible if pulmonary hypertension is relieved. Rheumatic fever may produce organic tricuspid regurgitation, often associated with tricuspid stenosis. Less commonly, regurgitation results from congenitally deformed tricuspid valves, and it occurs with defects of the atrioventricular canal, as well as with Ebstein's malformation of the tricuspid valve (Chap. 185). Infarction of right ventricular papillary muscles, tricuspid valve prolapse, carcinoid heart disease, endomyocardial fibrosis, infective endocarditis, and trauma may also produce tricuspid regurgitation.

As is the case for tricuspid stenosis, the clinical features of tricuspid regurgitation result primarily from systemic venous congestion and reduction of cardiac output. With the onset of tricuspid regurgitation in patients with pulmonary hypertension, as cardiac output declines, symptoms of pulmonary congestion diminish, but the clinical manifestations of right-sided heart failure become intensified. The neck veins are distended, with prominent v waves, and marked hepatomegaly, ascites, pleural effusions, edema, systolic pulsations of the liver, and positive hepatojugular reflux are common. A prominent right ventricular pulsation along the left parasternal region and a blowing holosystolic murmur along the lower left sternal margin which is generally intensified during inspiration and reduced during expiration or the Valsalva maneuver are characteristic findings; atrial fibrillation is usually present.

The electrocardiogram may show changes characteristic of the lesion responsible for the enlargement of the right ventricle which leads to this form of valvular dysfunction. In the rare instances of isolated tricuspid regurgitation the electrocardiogram often shows incomplete right bundle branch block. Roentgenographic examination usually reveals enlargement of both the right ventricle and right atrium, and the latter chamber expands during systole. Echocardiography may be helpful by demonstrating right ventricular dilatation and prolapsing or flail tricuspid leaflets; the diagnosis of tricuspid regurgitation can be made by contrast echocardiography.

The cardiac output is usually markedly reduced, and the right atrial pressure pulse may exhibit no *x* descent during early systole, but a prominent *c-v* wave, with a rapid *y* descent. The mean right atrial and the right ventricular end-diastolic pressures are often elevated.

Isolated tricuspid regurgitation, without pulmonary hypertension, such as that occurring as a consequence of infective endocarditis or trauma, is usually well tolerated and does not require operation. Indeed, even total excision of an infected tricuspid valve is often well tolerated. Treatment of the underlying cause of heart failure usually reduces the severity of functional tricuspid regurgitation. In patients with mitral valve disease and tricuspid regurgitation due to pulmonary hypertension and massive right ventricular enlargement, effective surgical correction of the mitral valvular abnormality results in lowering of the pulmonary vascular pressures and gradual reduction or disappearance of the tricuspid regurgitation without direct treatment of the tricuspid valve. However, recovery may be much more rapid in patients with severe secondary tricuspid regurgitation if, at the time of mitral replacement, tricuspid annuloplasty or, if necessary, tricuspid valve replacement is performed. Surgical treatment of the tricuspid regurgitation, consisting of either valve replacement or narrowing of the annulus, should be carried out in patients with severe regurgitation secondary to deformity of the tricuspid valve due to rheumatic fever, particularly those without severe pulmonary hypertension.

PULMONIC VALVE DISEASE

The pulmonic valve is affected by rheumatic fever far less frequently than the other valves and is uncommonly the seat of infective endocarditis. The most common acquired abnormality affecting the pulmonic valve is regurgitation secondary to dilatation of the pulmonary valve ring as a consequence of severe pulmonary hypertension of any cause. This produces the Graham Steell murmur, a high-pitched, decrescendo, diastolic blowing murmur along the left sternal border, which is difficult to differentiate from the far more common murmur produced by aortic regurgitation. It is of little hemodynamic significance; indeed surgical removal or destruction of the pulmonic valve by infective endocarditis does not produce heart failure unless serious pulmonary hypertension is also present.

Congenital pulmonic stenosis is discussed in Chap. 185.

REFERENCES

BRAUNWALD E: Valvular heart disease, in *Heart Disease,* 2d ed, E Braunwald (ed). Philadelphia, Saunders, 1984, p 1063

COHN LH et al: Early and late risk of aortic valve replacement: A 12-year concomitant comparison of the porcine bioprosthetic and tilting disc prosthetic aortic valves. J Thorac Cardiovasc Surg 88:695, 1984

COME PC: Echocardiographic evaluation of valvular heart disease, in *Diagnostic Cardiology: Noninvasive Imaging Techniques,* PC Come (ed). Philadelphia, Lippincott, 1985, p 407

FRANKL WS, BREST AN (eds):*Valvular Heart Disease: Comprehensive Evaluation and Management.* Philadelphia, FA Davis, 1986

GREENBERG BH et al: Arterial dilators in mitral regurgitation: Effects on rest and exercise, hemodynamics and long-term clinical follow-up. Circulation 65:181, 1982

GROSSMAN W: Aortic and mitral regurgitation: How to evaluate the condition and when to consider surgical intervention. JAMA 252:2447, 1984

IONESCU MI, COHN LH (eds): *Mitral Valve Disease: Diagnosis and Treatment.* London, Butterworths, 1985

JERESATY RM: Mitral valve prolapse: An update. JAMA 254:793, 1985

KIRKLIN JW, BARRATT-BOYES BG: Part III. Acquired valvular heart disease, in *Cardiac Surgery,* JW Kirklin, BG Barratt-Boyes (eds). New York, Wiley, 1986, p 323

LINGAMENI R et al: Tricuspid regurgitation: Clinical and angiographic assessment. Cath Cardiovasc Diag 5:7, 1979

MAHAPATRA RK et al: Rheumatic tricuspid stenosis. Indian Heart J 30:1381, 1978

MASUYAMA T et al: Noninvasive evaluation of aortic regurgitation by continuous-wave Doppler echocardiography. Circulation 73:460, 1986

MORGANROTH J et al: Acute severe aortic regurgitation. Ann Intern Med 87:223, 1977

OHLSSON J, WRANNE B: Noninvasive assessment of valve area in patients with aortic stenosis. J Am Coll Cardiol 7:501, 1986

RICHARDS KL: Doppler echocardiographic diagnosis and quantification of valvular heart disease. Curr Probl Cardiol 10:7, 1985

ROSS J JR: Left ventricular function and the timing of surgical treatments in valvular heart disease. Ann Intern Med 94:498, 1981

SAGAR KB et al: Doppler echocardiographic evaluation of Hancock and Bjork-Shiley prosthetic valves. J Am Coll Cardiol 7:681, 1986

188   INFECTIVE ENDOCARDITIS

LAWRENCE L. PELLETIER, JR. / ROBERT G. PETERSDORF

DEFINITION Infective endocarditis is a microbial infection of the heart valves or of the endocardium in proximity to congenital or acquired cardiac defects. A similar clinical illness develops when there is infection of arteriovenous fistulas or aneurysms. The infection may develop abruptly or insidiously, may pursue a fulminant or prolonged course, and is fatal unless treated. Infection caused by indigenous microorganisms with low pathogenicity is ordinarily subacute, whereas infection by microorganisms with high pathogenicity is often acute. Fever, cardiac murmurs, splenomegaly, anemia, hematuria, mucocutaneous petechiae, and embolic manifestations are characteristic of the disease. Valve destruction may result in acute mitral or aortic regurgitation requiring urgent surgical intervention. Mycotic aneurysms may develop in the aortic root, cerebral artery bifurcations, or other remote sites.

ETIOLOGY AND EPIDEMIOLOGY In the preantimicrobial era 90 percent of infections were due to *Streptococcus viridans* acquired as a consequence of transient bacteremias originating from the upper respiratory tract, most often in young patients with rheumatic valvular heart disease. These individuals were usually seen after prolonged infection and possessed most of the classic physical manifestations of infective endocarditis. In contrast, patients with infective endocarditis today are more likely to be older, male, have other forms of congenital or valvular heart disease, have acquired the infection in hospital or from drug abuse, and have infections with organisms other than the *S. viridans.* Patients often present early in the course of infection without clubbing of the digits, splenomegaly, Osler's nodes, or Roth's spots.

Certain clinical settings are associated with specific etiologic agents as outlined in Table 188-1. Parenteral drug addicts may have sepsis without any evident portal of entry, but often will have signs of phlebitis, septic pulmonary emboli, and tricuspid regurgitation. The use of intravascular devices for prolonged periods has increased the incidence of nosocomial endocarditis. Patients with prosthetic heart valves are at risk of acquiring infection from organisms implanted at the time of surgery, or from transient bacteremias that colonize the heart valves months or years after operation.

PATHOGENESIS Hemodynamic events are important in the development of infective endocarditis. Bacteria in the circulation are often deposited on the endothelium at sites at high flow rates distal to an obstruction where lateral pressure is decreased, such as the pulmonary side of a ventricular septal defect (in the absence of pulmonary hypertension and reversal of the shunt) or patent ductus arteriosus. Alterations in blood flow at such sites or other areas of structural change or abnormality may cause changes in the endothelial surface resulting in the formation of a sterile vegetation consisting of platelets and fibrin. This vegetation becomes the nidus on which microorganisms are implanted.

Most often, endocardial infections are initiated by transient bacteremias that seed abnormal endothelial surfaces. Transient *S. viridans* bacteremias are common following dental manipulation or extraction, tonsillectomy, use of a water jet, or chewing of food. Bacteremia is increased in the presence of gingival disease or dental infection. Enterococcal bacteremia may result from manipulation of an infected genitourinary tract, such as urinary catheterization or cystoscopy. Bacteremia may occur spontaneously or as a result of manipulation of localized infections at other sites. Although gram-negative rod bacteremia occurs frequently, gram-negative rod endocarditis is relatively rare. The low incidence of gram-negative rod endocarditis may be due to protection offered by nonspecific complement-fixing antibodies, or the relative lack of adherence of gram-negative bacteria to fibrin-platelet aggregates and fibronectin-coated endothelial surfaces.

Infective endocarditis occurs most often in persons with preexisting heart disease, but virulent organisms can seed normal cardiac valves. Infection most commonly involves the left side of the heart with the mitral, aortic, tricuspid, and pulmonary valves involved in decreasing order of frequency. Congenital bicuspid aortic valves, mitral and aortic valves damaged by rheumatic fever, calcific mitral and aortic valves in the elderly with arteriosclerosis, mitral valve prolapse, mechanical and bioprosthetic heart valves, Marfan's syndrome, idiopathic hypertrophic subaortic stenosis, coarctation of the aorta, arteriovenous shunt, ventricular septal defect, and a patent ductus arteriosus all predispose to the development of endocarditis. Infective endocarditis rarely involves interatrial septal defects.

Prolonged intravascular infection results in high titers of antibodies against the infecting microorganisms. Circulating antigen-antibody complexes are commonly found, and are sometimes associated with immune-complex glomerulonephritis and cutaneous vasculitis.

Intravascular organisms adherent to endothelium are rapidly covered with a coat of fibrin and platelets, forming a vegetation. Large numbers of organisms within a vegetation exhaust available nutrients producing a static growth phase less susceptible to antimicrobial agents that inhibit cell wall development and require rapidly proliferating organisms for maximal killing. Highly pathogenic microorganisms often cause rapid valvular destruction and ulceration associated with valvular regurgitation. Less pathogenic microorganisms usually cause less valvular destruction or ulceration but can lead to the development of large polypoid vegetations that may obstruct the valve or become dislodged, producing emboli. The infection may extend from the valve to the surrounding mural endocardium or penetrate the valve ring to produce a mycotic aneurysm, myocardial abscess, or cardiac conduction defect. Involvement of the chordae tendineae may lead to rupture and acute valvular insufficiency. Infected vegetations are poorly vascularized and heal by granulation tissue forming on the surface of the vegetation, sometimes trapping within the vegetation viable organisms that may be grown months after successful treatment if the valves are cultured after removal at surgery.

The microbemia of intravascular infections is usually continuous unless interrupted by antimicrobial therapy. For this reason, few blood cultures are required to demonstrate the microorganisms. The microorganisms are primarily cleared from the blood by the reticuloendothelial cells of the liver and spleen, often producing splenomegaly. There is no reduction in the number of bacteria in the blood during circulation through the extremities, so that arterial blood cultures are no more likely to show bacteremia than venous blood cultures.

Embolization is a characteristic feature of infective endocarditis. The friable fibrin vegetations may separate from the site of infection and be propelled into the systemic or pulmonary circulation, depending on whether the endocarditis involves the left or right side of the heart. Emboli vary in size and most often involve the brain, spleen, kidney, gastrointestinal tract, heart, or extremities. Emboli in fungal endocarditis tend to be large and occlude major vessels. Pulmonary infarction or abscess is common in right-sided endocarditis. Septic infarction is uncommon in endocarditis caused by organisms of low pathogenicity, such as *S. viridans*, although osteomyelitis has been described as a complication of viridans streptococcal and enterococcal endocarditis. *Staphylococcus aureus* and other virulent microorganisms often produce septic infarction with metastatic abscesses and may result in meningitis. Involvement of major arteries by emboli produces mycotic aneurysms, which may rupture. Focal myocarditis may be due to emboli. Myocardial infarction may develop after coronary embolization. Three types of renal lesions may be produced: segmental infarction due to large emboli, focal glomerulitis from small emboli, and a diffuse glomerulonephritis indistinguishable from other types of immune-complex disease most commonly seen with group A streptococcal endocarditis. Petechial skin lesions characterized histologically by acute vasculitis are probably immunologic in origin. Other skin lesions associated with pain, tenderness, and cellulitis may be embolic.

MANIFESTATIONS Subacute infective endocarditis Infections are commonly caused by organisms with lesser virulence, *S. viridans* in patients with native valves, and diphtheroid organisms or *Staphylococcus epidermidis* in individuals with prosthetic valves. Enterococci and numerous other microorganisms also can produce the syndrome. Even *S. aureus* may on occasion follow a subacute course. Symptoms usually begin insidiously, and patients find it difficult to date the onset of infection. In some individuals the onset of infection can be related to a recent dental extraction, urethral instrumentation, tonsillectomy, acute respiratory infection, or abortion.

Weakness, fatigability, weight loss, feverishness, night sweats, anorexia, and arthralgia are the usual symptoms of subacute bacterial endocarditis. Emboli may produce paralysis, chest pain due to myocardial or pulmonary infarction, acute vascular insufficiency with pain in the extremities, hematuria, acute abdominal pain, or sudden blindness. Painful fingers or toes and painful skin lesions may also be important symptoms. Chills are not common. Transient cerebral ischemic attacks, toxic encephalopathy, headache, brain abscess, subarachnoid hemorrhage from rupture of a mycotic aneurysm, or purulent meningitis may develop.

Physical examination may reveal a variety of findings, none of which alone is pathognomonic of subacute infective endocarditis. Physical examination may be normal early in the course of infection. The association of the different manifestations, however, usually provides a characteristic picture of the disease. The patient usually appears chronically ill and pale and has an elevated temperature. The fever is most often remittent, with afternoon or evening peaks. The pulse is usually rapid, and if cardiac failure complicates the infection, it may be greater than expected with the degree of fever.

Mucocutaneous lesions are common and vary in type. Petechiae are most frequent and may be found in the mucosa of the mouth, pharynx, or conjunctivas. These small, red, hemorrhagic-appearing lesions do not blanch on pressure and are not tender or painful. On the mucous membranes or conjunctivas these petechiae may have a pale center. Petechiae may be found anywhere on the skin but are most common over the upper part of the trunk anteriorly. They are frequently difficult to distinguish from angiomas, but they gradually become brownish and disappear. Frequently, petechiae continue to appear, even during convalescence. Linear hemorrhages (splinter hemorrhages) may be found under the nails, but these are difficult to differentiate from traumatic lesions, particularly in manual laborers. These mucocutaneous lesions are not specific for bacterial endocarditis but may be found in patients with other conditions such as profound anemia, leukemia, trichinosis, and sepsis without endocarditis. Erythematous or purple, painful, tender nodules (Osler's nodes) may develop on the palms of the hands, soles of the feet, pulp of the fingers, or other sites. These are probably embolic lesions. Emboli to larger peripheral arteries may result in gangrene of the fingers, toes, or larger portions of the extremities. Clubbing of the fingers is observed in long-standing or prolonged infective endocarditis. Mild jaundice is found occasionally.

Findings in the heart are usually those of underlying heart disease. Major changes in cardiac murmurs, primarily development of a new diastolic murmur, may be attributable to ulceration of a valve, dilatation of the heart or valve ring, rupture of chordae tendineae, or development of a very large vegetation. Minor changes in systolic bruits are usually of little significance. In rare instances, no cardiac murmurs are detected. In this situation, right-sided endocarditis or an infected mural thrombus, or pulmonary, or peripheral arteriovenous fistula should be suspected.

Splenomegaly is common in subacute infective endocarditis. Rarely is the spleen tender, but a friction rub may be heard over it when there is infarction. Hepatomegaly is not characteristic unless heart failure develops.

Arthralgia is relatively common, and arthritis resembling acute rheumatic fever may occur.

Embolic phenomena may precipitate awareness of the infection. Sudden development of hemiplegia, flank pain with hematuria, abdominal pain with melena, pleuritic pain and hemoptysis, left upper abdominal pain with splenic friction rub, blindness, or monoplegia in a patient with fever and cardiac murmurs makes infective endocarditis suspect. Pulmonary emboli in right-sided endocarditis may be confused with pneumonia.

Acute bacterial infective endocarditis   Suppurative infection commonly antedates the onset of endocarditis. For example, infection of the heart may develop as a complication of pneumococcal meningitis, septic thrombophlebitis, group A streptococcal cellulitis, or staphylococcal abscesses. The source of cardiovascular infection, therefore, is often evident.

Acute endocarditis often involves the normal heart, in contrast to the subacute infection, which almost invariably involves the abnormal

heart. It is particularly common in intravenous drug users and individuals with previously undetected abnormalities of the aortic valve. The acute infection is fulminant and pursues a rapid course. Fever is often greater, may be intermittent, and in certain instances (as in gonococcal endocarditis) may be characterized by a twice daily temperature elevation. Chills are common. Petechiae may be numerous, and embolic phenomena are prominent. Small, occasionally flame-shaped hemorrhages that may have pale centers (Roth's spots) are found in the retina. Osler's nodes are uncommon, but the pulp of the fingers may show nontender subcutaneous erythematous maculopapular lesions (Janeway's spots) that may ulcerate. Hematuria is seen with embolic lesions of the kidney, and diffuse glomerulonephritis may occur. Destruction of the cardiac valves can be complicated by rupture of chordae tendineae or perforation of cusps, leading to rapidly progressing cardiac failure. Metastatic abscesses following septic emboli are frequent.

Right-sided endocarditis   Tricuspid valve and rarely pulmonary valve endocarditis or pulmonary artery mycotic aneurysm are seen in parenteral drug addicts with skin cellulitis or septic phlebitis. Infected peripheral or central venous catheters or transvenous pacing wires may also result in right-sided infective endocarditis. The infecting organisms originate from the skin (*S. aureus, Candida albicans*) or presumably from injected materials (*Pseudomonas aeruginosa, Serratia marcescens*). *S. aureus* is the most frequently isolated organism, and the tricuspid valve the most common site of involvement in parenteral drug addicts. The clinical presentation is that of acute endocarditis with pulmonary infarction and abscess formation. The most frequent symptoms are high fever of several weeks' duration, pleuritic chest pain, hemoptysis and sputum production, dyspnea on exertion, malaise, anorexia, and fatigability. A tricuspid valve regurgitant murmur accentuated by inspiration with pulsatile neck veins and liver may be present, but more often there is no audible murmur at all or the murmur is difficult to detect. Two-dimensional echocardiogram may be required to confirm the presence of endocardial vegetations. Blood cultures are as likely to be positive in right-sided endocarditis as in left-sided lesions. The chest roentgenograph usually shows peripheral wedge-shaped pulmonary infiltrates with cavitation. Due to the absence of emboli to vital organs, acute hemodynamic decompensation secondary to valve destruction, and a generally younger, healthier patient population, and perhaps because of a better response to antimicrobial agents, patients with right-sided endocarditis have a better prognosis. Large (greater than 1-cm diameter) vegetations or infection caused by resistant microorganisms may require valve debridement or excision in conjunction with antimicrobial therapy to eradicate the infection.

Prosthetic valve endocarditis   Prosthetic valve infections develop in 2 to 3 percent of patients the first year following prosthetic valve placement, and 0.5 percent per year subsequently. About one-third of infections in the first year develop *within 2 months of surgery* and are probably due to colonization of the prosthesis or suture sites during surgery. Organisms that cause early infections (Table 188-1) are often resistant to antimicrobial agents; such infections are associated with a high mortality due to septic shock, valve dehiscence, and myocardial invasion. Gram-negative bacteremia in the immediate postoperative period may originate from the urinary tract, wound, pulmonary infections, or septic phlebitis and is often not associated with prosthetic valve infection.

Prosthetic valve infections that occur *more than 2 months after surgery* (Table 188-1) may result from implantation at surgery or colonization of the prosthesis or its site of attachment during transient bacteremias. Patients with prosthetic valves should receive prophylactic antimicrobial agents when undergoing procedures known to produce bacteremia, and minor infections that might produce bacteremia should be treated promptly. Late onset infections caused by streptococci have a better prognosis than early infections and may be controlled with antibiotics alone.

Prosthetic valve infections often produce symptoms and signs

TABLE 188-1   Organisms causing infective endocarditis

Predisposing condition	Organism	Comment
Dental manipulations	Viridans streptococci	
Parenteral drug addicts	*S. aureus* Group A streptococcus Gram-negative rods *Candida* spp.	Septic phlebitis and right-sided endocarditis are common.
Prosthetic valve recipients		
< 2 months after surgery	*S. epidermidis* Diphtheroids Gram-negative rods *Candida* spp. Enterococcus *S. aureus*	Early-onset infections tend to be resistant to prophylactic antimicrobials administered at surgery.
> 2 months after surgery	*Streptococcus* spp. *S. epidermidis* Diphtheroids Enterococcus *S. aureus*	Some low-virulence infections implanted at surgery are slow to develop.
Urinary tract infections	Enterococcus Gram-negative rods	Associated in older males with prostatism and in women with genitourinary tract infections.
Catheter-related phlebitis	*S. aureus* *S. epidermidis* *Candida* spp. Gram-negative rods	An increasingly common source of endocarditis in hospitalized patients.
Alcoholism	Pneumococcus	May be associated with simultaneous pneumonia and meningitis.
Colon cancer	*Streptococcus bovis*	

indistinguishable from infections on natural valves, but there is a greater frequency of valve ring infection that may involve part or all of the circumference producing valve dehiscence or penetration into the myocardium or surrounding tissues. Myocardial abscess, conduction disturbances, sinus of Valsalva aneurysm, or fistulas into the right side of the heart or pericardium may result. Prolongation of the PR interval, a new left bundle branch block, or right bundle branch block with left anterior hemiblock should suggest involvement of the ventricular septum in aortic valve infections. Extension of infection from the mitral valve annulus may be associated with nonparoxysmal junctional tachycardia, or second- or third-degree heart block with a narrow QRS complex. Prosthetic valve stenosis due to vegetations narrowing the orifice or interfering with valve excursion may be detected by auscultation or echocardiography. A postoperative regurgitant murmur or abnormal position or movement of the valve on fluoroscopic examination or echocardiogram may indicate partial dehiscence of the prosthesis. Prosthetic valve infections complicated by valve stenosis, valve dehiscence with congestive heart failure, recurrent emboli, resistance to antimicrobial therapy, or evidence of myocardial invasion require early surgical intervention. Patients receiving anticoagulants to prevent embolism who develop endocarditis should continue to take the medication if the risk of embolization without anticoagulation is high and accept a 36 percent risk of intracranial hemorrhage with 80 percent consequent mortality. Relapse following appropriate antimicrobial treatment or fungous infections also requires early surgical removal of the infected prosthesis.

LABORATORY FINDINGS Leukocytosis with neutrophilia is the rule but is by no means invariable. Macrophages (histiocytes) may be found in the blood, particularly in the first drop obtained from the earlobe. Normocytic, normochromic anemia is almost always found in subacute infective endocarditis but may not be present early in acute bacterial endocarditis. The erythrocyte sedimentation rate is rapid. Serum immunoglobulins are increased but return to normal during convalescence. The anti-gamma globulin latex fixation test is commonly positive due to IgM and IgA factors. Circulating immune complexes are usually present and titers often decline with successful antimicrobial therapy, but may remain elevated in bacteriologic cures when associated with arthritis, glomerulitis, or drug reactions. Mild bilirubinemia is detected occasionally. Proteinuria is common, and microscopic hematuria is frequently present. Serum total hemolytic complement and the third component of complement may be decreased. Antiteichoic acid antibody titers in *S. aureus* endocarditis are usually 1:4 or greater after 2 weeks of antimicrobial therapy.

An echocardiogram may identify high-risk patients with large vegetations or unsuspected preexisting valvular lesions, or it may provide an indication for early operation in patients with acute aortic insufficiency and severe volume overload of the left ventricle. The echocardiogram does not detect vegetations smaller than 2 mm, nor does it differentiate active from healed lesions. Two-dimensional scanners are more sensitive than M-mode echocardiography but demonstrate vegetations in only 43 to 80 percent of patients with endocarditis. Degenerative bioprosthetic valve changes may mimic echocardiographic changes of infective endocarditis.

Blood cultures are positive in the majority of cases. Three to five cultures of 20 to 30 mL of blood, taken at intervals determined by the patient's clinical status, are usually adequate to demonstrate the bacteremia, if it is demonstrable at all. Blood cultures may not become positive for several days, if at all, in patients who have received antibiotics prior to the time when cultures are obtained. Failure to demonstrate bacteremia or delayed growth in blood cultures also may be due to infection by unusual microorganisms such as *Hemophilus parainfluenzae*, *Cardiobacterium hominis*, *Corynebacterium* spp., *Histoplasma capsulatum*, *Brucella*, *Pasteurella*, or anaerobic streptococci that require special nutrient media or extended (up to 4 weeks) incubation. Thiol-requiring streptococcal variants may require pyridoxine- or cysteine-supplemented broth. Castañeda-type culture bottles assist in the recovery of fungi and *Brucella*.

Aspergillus endocarditis is seldom associated with positive blood cultures. *Coxiella burnetii* endocarditis and *Chlamydia psittaci* endocarditis are diagnosed by serologic tests, since blood cultures are always negative. Bone marrow cultures and serologic testing for *Candida*, *Histoplasma*, and *Brucella* may be helpful in culture-negative endocarditis.

DIFFERENTIAL DIAGNOSIS When several of the manifestations of infective endocarditis occur together, the diagnosis is not difficult. In particular, the presence of fever, petechiae, splenomegaly, microscopic hematuria, and anemia in a patient with cardiac murmurs is most suggestive of infection. When only a few manifestations are present, however, the diagnosis is not simple. Prolonged fever in a patient with rheumatic heart disease is particularly troublesome, but the diagnosis of bacterial endocarditis should be considered in every patient with fever and a heart murmur. The diagnosis becomes even more difficult when blood cultures show no growth.

Acute rheumatic fever with carditis is often difficult to distinguish from infective endocarditis, and in a few instances, active rheumatic fever has been found to coexist with the valvular infection. The diagnosis of rheumatic carditis hinges on a combination of clinical and laboratory criteria (see Chap. 186).

Subacute infective endocarditis is no longer a common cause of "fever of undetermined origin" (see Chap. 9). However, occasionally it may be mistaken for a hidden neoplasm, systemic lupus erythematosus, periarteritis nodosa, poststreptococcal glomerulonephritis, and intracardiac tumors such as myxoma of the atrium. Aortic dissection with acute aortic regurgitation also may mimic bacterial endocarditis. Postoperative endocarditis should be suspected in patients who develop fever, anemia, and leukocytosis after cardiovascular surgery. In these postoperative patients, the various postthoracotomy and postcardiotomy syndromes must also be considered.

PROGNOSIS Recovery from untreated infective endocarditis is rare. With appropriate antibiotic therapy, however, over 70 percent of the patients with infection on endogenous valves and 50 percent with infection on prosthetic valves survive the infection. Intravenous drug users with right-sided staphylococcal endocarditis generally have a good prognosis. Factors that suggest a less favorable outcome are the presence of congestive heart failure, extreme age of the patient, involvement of the aortic valve or multiple heart valves, polymicrobial bacteremia, failure to identify the etiologic agent owing to negative blood cultures, antimicrobial resistance to nontoxic bactericidal drugs, and delay in initiating therapy. Prosthetic valve, gram-negative bacillus, and fungal endocarditis are associated with the poorest prognosis.

The commonest cause of death in treated endocarditis is congestive heart failure, attributable either to valve destruction or to myocardial damage. Additionally, death may be precipitated by embolization to vital organs, by renal insufficiency, by rupture of a mycotic aneurysm, or by complications following cardiac surgery. Many patients recover completely without apparent worsening of the underlying cardiovascular disease. When recurrent endocarditis develops, it usually involves the same valve and is due to failure to kill microorganisms in an environment of suboptimal host resistance.

Further reduction in the mortality rate of infective endocarditis will depend primarily on the increased use of cardiac surgery in combination with antimicrobial therapy to eliminate refractory infections, and the early replacement of damaged valves in patients with congestive heart failure.

PROPHYLAXIS Patients with suspected congenital or acquired valvular heart disease, prosthetic heart valves, ventriculoseptal patches, or prior history of infective endocarditis should receive antimicrobial prophylaxis for viridans streptococci immediately before any dental manipulation that causes bleeding, oral surgery, and tonsillectomy or adenoidectomy. Likewise, patients with similar cardiac risks undergoing urinary catheterization, cystoscopy, prostatectomy, obstetrical or gynecologic manipulation of infected tissues, or rectal or colon surgery should receive prophylaxis directed against the enterococcus. Patients with mitral valve prolapse, asymmetric septal hypertrophy, and tricuspid or pulmonary valve lesions are at lower risk of developing endocarditis but should also receive antimicrobial prophylaxis. Prophylaxis is not required for atherosclerotic arterial plaques, coronary artery bypass grafts, systolic clicks, isolated atrial septal defects, or transvenous pacemakers. The high-risk patients mentioned above undergoing surgical manipulation of infected tissues at other sites should receive an antimicrobial active against the most likely infecting organism.

The rationale for antimicrobial prophylaxis is that when these patients develop bacteremia, they are more likely to develop endocarditis. The best experimental evidence available holds that for prevention of endocarditis caused by viridans streptococci with penicillin, both a high concentration and relatively prolonged duration of action are necessary. It has been shown that penicillin and streptomycin act synergistically in killing viridans streptococci. These data suggest a regimen consisting of a single dose of 1.2 million units of aqueous procaine penicillin G plus 1.0 g streptomycin administered intramuscularly within 30 min of dental surgery, followed by penicillin V 0.5 g orally at 6-h intervals for four doses, is effective. A single oral preoperative dose of 3 g amoxicillin is probably equally effective. Patients who are allergic to penicillin should receive vancomycin, 1.0 g intravenously over 30 min, 1 h before the procedure or erythromycin, 1.0 g orally 1 h before the procedure. Either antibiotic should be followed with erythromycin, 0.5 g orally every 6 h for four doses. The best regimen for preventing enterococcal endocarditis is ampicillin plus gentamicin. Ampicillin,

1 g, plus gentamicin, 1.0 mg/kg (not over 80 mg), should be given intramuscularly or intravenously 30 to 60 min before the procedure, and both agents should be repeated every 8 h for two doses. Penicillin-allergic patients should receive vancomycin, 1.0 g intravenously, and gentamicin 1.0 mg/kg intramuscularly, 30 to 60 min before the procedure; administration of both agents is repeated 12 h later. Antistaphylococcal prophylaxis is indicated during surgery associated with implantation of prosthetic heart valves, intracardiac materials, or vascular prostheses. Cefazolin, 1.0 g intravenously, every 6 h should be given 30 min prior to surgery and continued no longer than 24 h.

The prophylactic doses of penicillin used to prevent group A streptococcal infection and recurrent rheumatic fever will not prevent bacterial endocarditis. The dose of benzathine penicillin given for rheumatic fever prophylaxis does not predispose to bacterial endocarditis caused by penicillin-resistant microorganisms, whereas oral penicillin V does promote the emergence of penicillin-resistant oral flora. All high-risk patients should be cautioned to maintain a high level of oral hygiene, avoid the use of a water jet in the mouth, and seek prompt treatment of infections that occur at any site.

TREATMENT   Intravascular infections must be treated with antimicrobial agents that kill microorganisms at concentrations attainable in serum because organisms within endocardial vegetations are protected by surrounding fibrin and platelet aggregates against the bactericidal action of host neutrophils, complement, and antibodies. Infective endocarditis is the prototype infection for which bacteriostatic agents that inhibit but do not kill organisms are ineffective, and bactericidal drugs are necessary for cure. The best results occur when a microbicidal agent active against the infecting organism is administered early in the course of the infection in high dosage, and treatment is continued for a relatively long period of time. When a prosthetic valve is infected, the microorganism is relatively resistant to available agents; or when a mycotic aneurysm or myocardial abscess develops, surgery in addition to antimicrobial therapy is often required to eliminate the infection.

The initial step in selecting the correct antimicrobial agent begins with obtaining blood cultures before empiric antimicrobial therapy is begun so that the organism can be isolated and identified, and antimicrobial susceptibilities determined. It is generally advisable to obtain macrotube or microtube dilution minimum inhibitory concentration measurements for therapeutic agents, although this is not always necessary for microorganisms with large zones of inhibition on disc diffusion susceptibility tests. Penicillin-susceptible *Streptococcus bovis* group D organisms should be differentiated from enterococci; and methicillin-resistant *S. aureus* and *S. epidermidis* separated from methicillin-susceptible strains. Determination of the bactericidal activity of antimicrobial agents against the infecting organism would be desirable, but since there is no standardized reproducible laboratory measurement of bacterial killing, routine use of minimum bactericidal concentration (MBC) tests to select antimicrobial agents or serum bactericidal activity (SBA) tests to adjust dosage is usually not recommended.

Table 188-2 outlines recommended treatment programs for the most common causes of endocarditis. Two weeks of penicillin and streptomycin are as effective as 4 weeks of penicillin alone in the treatment of penicillin-susceptible *S. viridans* infections. When streptomycin is administered, the minimum inhibitory concentration (MIC) of streptomycin should be determined, and gentamicin used instead of streptomycin if the streptomycin MIC is greater than 2000 μg/mL. Elderly patients and individuals with deafness or renal insufficiency are likely to have increased aminoglycoside renal and ototoxicity and should be treated with penicillin alone for 4 weeks. If 2 weeks of parenteral penicillin are followed by 2 weeks of oral therapy, then serum levels of the oral agent should be measured to demonstrate adequate absorption. Amoxicillin provides better oral absorption than penicillin V. In patients allergic to penicillin, cefazolin may be administered with caution if the reaction was a mild drug

TABLE 188-2   Recommended treatment for infective endocarditis

S. viridans and nonenterococcal group D streptococci (penicillin G MIC < 0.1 μg/mL)	Penicillin G 10–20 million units per day IV in divided doses every 4–6 h × 4 weeks
	Penicillin G 10–20 million units per day IV with streptomycin 7.5 mg/kg IV or IM every 12 h or gentamicin 1 mg/kg IV every 8 h × 2 weeks
	Penicillin G 10–20 million units per day IV × 2 weeks, followed by amoxicillin 1 g PO every 6 h × 2 weeks
	Cefazolin 2 g IV every 6–8 h × 4 weeks if allergic to penicillin
	Vancomycin 15 mg/kg IV every 12 h × 4 weeks if allergic to penicillin
Enterococcus or relatively penicillin-resistant viridans streptococci (penicillin G MIC > 0.1 μg/mL)	Penicillin G 15–24 million units per day IV in divided doses every 4–6 h with gentamicin 1 mg/kg IV every 8 h × 4–6 weeks
	Ampicillin 2 g IV every 6 h possible substitute for penicillin G
	Streptomycin 7.5 mg/kg IV or IM possible substitute for gentamicin if the MIC for streptomycin is < 2000 μg/mL
	Vancomycin 15 mg/kg IV every 12 h with gentamicin 1 mg/kg IV every 8 h × 4–6 weeks, if allergic to penicillin
Pneumococcus or group A streptococcus	Penicillin G 6–12 million units per day IV in divided doses every 4–6 h × 4 weeks
	Cefazolin 2 g IV every 6–8 h × 4 weeks if allergic to penicillin
Methicillin-susceptible *S. aureus* or *S. epidermidis*	Nafcillin 2 g IV every 4 h × 4–6 weeks or longer
	Cefazolin 2 g IV every 6 h × 4–6 weeks or longer, if allergic to penicillin
	Vancomycin 15 mg/kg IV every 12 h × 4–6 weeks or longer, if allergic to penicillin
Methicillin-resistant *S. aureus*, *S. epidermidis*, or *Corynebacterium* spp.	Vancomycin 15 mg/kg IV every 12 h × 4–6 weeks or longer
	Vancomycin in combination with rifampin 900–1200 mg PO once daily for 4–6 weeks or longer with gentamicin 1 mg/kg IV every 8 h × 2 weeks

rash or fever. If there is a history of a life-threatening anaphylaxis to penicillin, then vancomycin should be given. Skin testing with major and minor penicillin antigens may be used to guide antimicrobial selection in patients with an unclear history of penicillin allergy. In view of the availability of effective alternative drugs, penicillin desensitization by frequent sequential administrations of increasing concentrations of penicillin under close supervision with readiness to treat anaphylactic reactions is seldom required.

Penicillin alone is not bactericidal against enterococcal organisms (*Streptococcus fecalis, S. faecium, S. durans*), and requires combination with an aminoglycoside to cure endocarditis. The combination of penicillin and gentamicin is synergistic against almost all enterococci, whereas 30 to 40 percent of enterococci are resistant to penicillin and streptomycin. Resistance to penicillin and streptomycin synergy is predicted by a streptomycin MIC greater than 2000 μg/mL. Ampicillin may be substituted for penicillin G. Lower doses of gentamicin (3 mg/kg per day) are as effective as higher doses and are less toxic. Cephalosporin antimicrobials are not active against the enterococcus and should not be used to treat enterococcal endocarditis. Vancomycin and gentamicin or streptomycin should be used to treat patients allergic to penicillin. Many patients can be treated for 4 weeks, but those with prosthetic valves, mitral valve involvement, or symptoms for longer than 3 months should be treated for 6 weeks.

Nafcillin should be used to treat *S. aureus* bacteremia while waiting for antimicrobial susceptibility results unless methicillin-resistant *S. aureus* is epidemic, in which case vancomycin should be administered instead. The addition of gentamicin to a penicillinase-resistant penicillin or cephalosporin results in enhanced killing of methicillin-susceptible staphylococci in the test tube and in animal models, but does not seem to improve the clinical outcome for most patients. Combination therapy for staphylococcal endocarditis is controversial and should not be used routinely except in the treatment of methicillin-resistant *S. epidermidis* prosthetic valve endocarditis. In staphylococcal endocarditis in particular, attention must be given to possible metastatic abscesses requiring surgical drainage and especially prolonged antimicrobial therapy to prevent relapse.

Prosthetic valve infections should be treated for 6 to 8 weeks, and patients should be monitored closely for signs of valve dysfunction and embolism. Mechanical valves are more likely to require placement than bioprostheses.

Patients with suspected endocarditis but negative blood cultures present a difficult clinical decision since treatment must be based on a guess about the likely organism. Patients with a native valve and no obvious portal of entry should be treated for enterococcal endocarditis with penicillin G and gentamicin. Parenteral drug addicts should be treated for staphylococcal and gram-negative bacilli endocarditis with nafcillin, ticarcillin, and gentamicin. The extended-spectrum penicillin should be adapted to gram-negative organisms usually encountered locally in drug addicts. Culture-negative prosthetic valve infections should be treated for methicillin-resistant *S. epidermidis* and enterococcal endocarditis with vancomycin and gentamicin.

Usually, fever begins to disappear within 3 to 7 days after the start of treatment of infective endocarditis. Embolic complications of the disease, heart failure, phlebitis, and infection with resistant microorganisms, however, may delay defervescence. If a drug fever or rash to penicillin develops during the course of therapy, antihistamines or corticosteroids may be used to alleviate the manifestations of the reaction; or more commonly, penicillin is discontinued and an alternative agent initiated. When attempting to discern the cause of a fever, cessation of all therapy for 72 h is not hazardous and may identify such a drug reaction readily. Sterile emboli or late valve rupture occurs occasionally up to 12 months after cessation of therapy.

Many patients with arteriovenous fistulas, valve ring abscess, recurrent embolization, endocarditis produced by resistant organisms, or infected cardiac prostheses require surgical intervention before the infection can be controlled. In addition, early valve replacement should be considered in patients who develop congestive heart failure

associated with marked valve damage (particularly aortic or mitral regurgitation) as a consequence of infective endocarditis. Valve replacement may be lifesaving and must be undertaken before intractable heart failure ensues. Whether operation can be based entirely on cardiac ultrasound results or whether cardiac catheterization always needs to be performed remains controversial.

Fungal endocarditis is usually fatal. However, a few survivors have been reported after surgical debridement and replacement of infected valves combined with amphotericin B therapy.

When infective endocarditis recurs, it usually develops within 4 weeks after treatment is terminated. Reinstitution of antimicrobial therapy is required, and the sensitivity of the microorganisms should be reevaluated. Relapse may indicate inadequate or inappropriate treatment, or the need for surgical intervention. Recrudescence of infective endocarditis more than 6 weeks after cessation of treatment usually connotes a new infection.

REFERENCES

DINUBILE MJ: Surgery in active endocarditis. Ann Intern Med 96:650, 1982

FREEDMAN LR: *Infective Endocarditis and other Intravascular Infections.* New York, Plenum, 1982

KARCHMER AW et al: *Staphylococcus epidermidis* causing prosthetic valve endocarditis: Microbiologic and clinical observations as guides to therapy. Ann Intern Med 98:447, 1983

KAYE D (ed): *Infective Endocarditis.* Baltimore, University Park Press, 1976

————: Prophylaxis for infective endocarditis: An update. Ann Intern Med 104:419, 1986

KORZENIOWSKI O et al: Combination antimicrobial therapy for *Staphylococcus aureus* endocarditis in patients addicted to parenteral drugs and in non-addicts. Ann Intern Med 97:496, 1982

PETERSDORF RG, PELLETIER LL: Prevention of infective endocarditis, in *Cardiology 2: Preventive Cardiology,* DG Julian, JO Humphries (eds). London, Butterworth, 1983, pp 86–122

SHULMAN ST et al: Prevention of bacterial endocarditis. Circulation 70:1123A, 1984

VON REYNE CF et al: Infective endocarditis: An analysis based on strict case definitions. Ann Intern Med 94:505, 1981

WEINSTEIN L: Infective endocarditis, in *Heart Disease: A Textbook of Cardiovascular Medicine,* E Braunwald (ed). Philadelphia, Saunders, 1984, pp 1136–82

WEINSTEIN MP et al: Multicenter collaborative evaluation of a standardized serum bactericidal test as a prognostic indicator in infective endocarditis. Am J Med 78:262, 1985

WILSON WR et al: Short-term therapy for streptococcal infective endocarditis. JAMA 245:360, 1981

———— et al: Treatment of streptomycin-susceptible and streptomycin-resistant enterococcal endocarditis. Ann Intern Med 100:816, 1984

WOLFSON JS, SWARTZ MN: Serum bactericidal activity as a monitor of antibiotic therapy. N Engl J Med 312:968, 1985

189 ISCHEMIC HEART DISEASE

ANDREW P. SELWYN / EUGENE BRAUNWALD

Ischemia refers to a lack of oxygen due to inadequate perfusion. *Ischemic heart disease* is a condition of diverse etiologies all having in common a disturbance of cardiac function due to an imbalance between oxygen supply and demand.

ETIOLOGY AND PATHOPHYSIOLOGY

The most common cause of ischemia is atherosclerotic disease of epicardial coronary arteries, which by reducing the lumen of these vessels causes an absolute decrease in myocardial perfusion in the basal state or limits appropriate increases in perfusion when demand for flow is augmented. Coronary blood flow can also be limited by arterial thrombi, spasm, and rarely coronary emboli, arteritis, and ostial narrowing due to luetic aortitis. Congenital abnormalities, such as anomalous origin of the left anterior descending coronary artery from the pulmonary artery (Chap. 185), may cause myocardial ischemia and infarction in infancy but this is a very rare cause in adults. Myocardial ischemia can also occur if myocardial oxygen demands are abnormally increased, as in severe ventricular hypertrophy due to hypertension or aortic stenosis. The latter can present with angina that is indistinguishable from that caused by coronary atherosclerosis. Myocardial ischemia occurs rarely if the oxygen-carrying capacity of the blood is reduced, as in extremely severe anemia or in the presence of carboxyhemoglobin. Not infrequently, two or more causes of ischemia will coexist, such as an increase in oxygen demand due to left ventricular hypertrophy and a reduction in oxygen supply secondary to coronary atherosclerosis.

The normal coronary circulation is dominated and controlled by the myocardial requirements for oxygen. This need is met by the ability to vary considerably the coronary vascular resistance (and therefore blood flow) while the myocardium extracts a high and relatively fixed percentage of oxygen (Chap. 4). Normally, intramyocardial resistance arterioles demonstrate an immense capacity for dilation. With exercise and emotional stress, the changing oxygen needs affect coronary vascular resistance and in this manner regulate the supply of blood and oxygen (metabolic regulation). These same vessels adapt to physiologic alterations in blood pressure in order to maintain coronary blood flow at levels appropriate to myocardial needs (autoregulation). Although the large epicardial coronary arteries are capable of constriction and relaxation, in healthy persons they serve as conduits, and are referred to as *conductance vessels,* while the intramyocardial arterioles normally exhibit striking changes in tone and are therefore referred to as *resistance vessels.*

CORONARY ATHEROSCLEROSIS (See also Chap. 195) Epicardial coronary arteries are a major site of atherosclerotic disease. Subintimal collections of abnormal fat, cells, and debris, i.e., atherosclerotic plaques, develop at irregular rates in different segments of the epicardial coronary tree and lead eventually to segmental reductions in cross-sectional area. The relationship between pulsatile flow and luminal stenosis is complex, but experiments have shown that when a stenosis reduces the cross-sectional area by approximately 75 percent, a maximal increase in flow to meet increased myocardial demand is not possible. When the luminal area is reduced by more than approximately 80 percent, blood flow at rest may be reduced and minor further reductions of the stenotic orifice can cause dramatic limitations of coronary flow and myocardial ischemia.

Segmental atherosclerotic narrowing of epicardial coronary arteries is caused most commonly by the formation of a plaque, which is subject to fissuring, hemorrhage, and thrombosis. Any of these events can temporarily worsen the obstruction, reduce coronary blood flow, and cause clinical manifestations of myocardial ischemia, as described below. In addition, the location of the stenosis will influence the quantity of myocardium rendered ischemic and this will determine the severity of the clinical manifestations. Severe coronary narrowing and myocardial ischemia are frequently accompanied by the development of collateral vessels, especially when the narrowing develops gradually. When well developed, such vessels can provide sufficient blood flow to sustain the viability of the myocardium at rest, but not during circumstances of increased demand.

Once severe stenosis of a proximal epicardial artery has reduced the cross-sectional area by more than ~70 percent the distal resistance, vessels will dilate to reduce vascular resistance to maintain coronary blood flow. A pressure gradient develops across the proximal stenosis, poststenotic pressure falls, and when the resistance vessels are maximally dilated, myocardial blood flow becomes dependent on the pressure in the coronary artery distal to the obstruction. Once the resistance vessels are maximally dilated, alterations in myocardial oxygenation can be caused by changes in myocardial oxygen demand, by alterations in the caliber of the stenosed coronary artery caused by physiologic vasomotion, by pathologic spasm, or by small platelet plugs. All of these transient events can upset the critical balance between oxygen supply and demand and thus precipitate myocardial ischemia.

EFFECTS OF ISCHEMIA The inadequate oxygenation induced by coronary atherosclerosis may cause transient disturbances of the mechanical, biochemical, and electrical function of the myocardium. The abrupt development of ischemia usually affects a segment of left ventricular myocardium with almost instantaneous failure of normal muscle relaxation and contraction. The relatively poor perfusion of the subendocardium causes more intense ischemia of this portion of the wall. Ischemia of large segments of the ventricle will cause transient left ventricular failure and if the papillary muscles are involved, mitral regurgitation can complicate this event. When ischemic events are transient, they may be associated with angina pectoris, but if prolonged they can lead to myocardial necrosis and scarring with or without the clinical picture of acute myocardial infarction. Coronary atherosclerosis is a focal process that causes nonuniform ischemia. The resulting focal disturbances of ventricular contractility cause segmental bulging or dyskinesia and can greatly reduce the efficiency of myocardial pump function.

Underlying these mechanical disturbances are a wide range of abnormalities in cell metabolism, function, and structure. When oxygenated, the normal myocardium metabolizes fatty acids and glucose to carbon dioxide and water. With severe oxygen deprivation, fatty acids cannot be oxidized and glucose is broken down to lactate; intracellular pH becomes reduced as do the myocardial stores of high-energy phosphates, adenosine triphosphate (ATP), and creatine phosphate. Impairment of cell membrane function leads to leakage of potassium and uptake of sodium by myocytes. The severity and duration of the imbalance between myocardial oxygen supply and demand will determine whether the damage is reversible or whether it is permanent with the development of myocardial necrosis.

Ischemia also alters the electrical properties of the heart. The most characteristic early electrocardiographic changes represent repolarization abnormalities, as evidenced by inversion of the T wave and later by displacement of the ST segment (Chap. 178). Transient ST-segment depression often reflects subendocardial ischemia, while transient ST-segment elevation is thought to be caused by more severe transmural ischemia. Another important consequence of myocardial ischemia is electrical instability, since this may lead to ventricular tachycardia or ventricular fibrillation (Chap. 184). Most patients who die suddenly from ischemic heart disease do so because of the occurrence of ischemia-induced malignant ventricular arrhythmias (Chap. 30).

CLINICAL MANIFESTATIONS

ASYMPTOMATIC VERSUS SYMPTOMATIC CORONARY ARTERY DISEASE Postmortem studies on accident victims and military casualties in western countries have shown that coronary atherosclerosis often starts prior to age 20 and is widespread among adults who were asymptomatic during life. In addition, exercise stress tests in asymptomatic persons may show evidence of silent myocardial ischemia, i.e., exercise-induced electrocardiographic changes not accompanied by angina, and coronary angiography in such persons frequently reveal obstructive coronary artery disease. Postmortem studies in patients with obstructive coronary artery disease who had no history of myocardial ischemia frequently show macroscopic scars of myocardial infarction in regions supplied by diseased coronary arteries. In addition, population studies have shown that approximately 25 percent of patients with acute myocardial infarctions may not reach medical attention and that these carry the same adverse prognosis as those in whom the classic clinical syndrome (Chap. 190) develops. *Sudden death* may be unheralded and is a common presenting manifestation of coronary disease (Chap. 30). Patients can also present with cardiomegaly and heart failure secondary to ischemic damage to left ventricular myocardium that caused no symptoms prior to the development of heart failure, a condition referred to as *ischemic cardiomyopathy.* In contrast to the asymptomatic phase of ischemic heart disease, the *symptomatic* phase presents with chest pain due either to angina pectoris or acute myocardial infarction (Chap. 190). Once having entered the symptomatic phase, the patient may exhibit a stable or progressive course, revert to the asymptomatic stage, or die suddenly.

Angina pectoris This is an episodic clinical syndrome resulting from transient myocardial ischemia. Various diseases that result in myocardial ischemia as well as the numerous pain syndromes with which it may be confused are discussed in Chap. 4. Approximately 80 percent of patients with angina pectoris, and an even greater fraction of those younger than 50 years of age, are male. The typical patient with angina is a 50- to 60-year-old man who seeks medical help for troublesome or frightening chest discomfort, usually described as heaviness, pressure, squeezing, smothering, or choking, and only rarely as frank pain. When the patient is asked to localize the sensation, he or she will typically press on the sternum, sometimes with a clenched fist, to indicate a squeezing central, substernal site of the discomfort. This symptom is usually crescendo-decrescendo, lasting 1 to 5 min. Angina can radiate to the left shoulder and to both arms, and especially to the ulnar surfaces of the forearm and hand. It can also arise in or radiate to the back, neck, jaw, teeth, and epigastrium.

Although angina is typically caused by exertion (e.g., exercise, hurrying, or sexual activity) or emotion (e.g., stress, anger, fright, or frustration) and is relieved by rest, it may also occur at rest and at night while the patient is recumbent (angina decubitus). The patient may be awakened at night distressed by typical chest discomfort and dyspnea. The pathophysiology of nocturnal angina may be similar to that of paroxysmal nocturnal dyspnea (Chap. 182) with the development of transient left ventricular failure due to expansion of the intrathoracic blood volume that occurs with recumbency and a resultant increase in cardiac size and myocardial oxygen demand.

The threshold for the development of angina pectoris may vary with the time of day and the patient's emotional state. The typical patient may have to stop because of symptoms at exactly the same spot on the way to work each morning, yet by midday may be able to cover many times that distance without symptoms. After experiencing chest discomfort while shaving in the morning, a man might be able to perform moderately heavy manual labor later in the day after he has "warmed up." Angina is frequently precipitated by unfamiliar tasks, by a heavy meal, or by exposure to cold.

Sharp fleeting chest pain or prolonged dull aches localized to the left submammary area are rarely due to myocardial ischemia. However, angina pectoris may be atypical in location and may not be strictly related to provoking factors. This symptom can also exacerbate and remit over days, weeks, or months, and its occurrence can be seasonal.

Systematic questioning of the patient with suspected ischemic heart disease is important to uncover a positive family history of ischemic heart disease, diabetes, hyperlipidemia, hypertension, cigarette smoking, and other risk factors for coronary atherosclerosis.

In *variant (Prinzmetal's) angina,* the chest discomfort characteristically occurs at rest or awakens the patient from sleep. It can be accompanied by palpitations or severe shortness of breath, may be explosive in onset, severe, and frightening. It may also be brought on by effort, although the workload at which it is precipitated usually varies considerably. Variant angina is caused by focal spasm of proximal epicardial coronary arteries; in approximately three-fourths of the patients atherosclerotic coronary artery obstruction is present, and in them the vasospasm occurs near the stenotic lesion.

PHYSICAL EXAMINATION The physical examination is usually normal. The patient's general appearance may reveal signs and risk factors associated with coronary atherosclerosis such as xanthelasma, xanthomas (Chap. 195), or diabetic skin lesions. There may also be signs of anemia, thyroid disease, and nicotine stains on the fingertips from cigarette smoking. Palpation can reveal thickened or absent peripheral arteries, signs of cardiac enlargement, and abnormal contraction (akinesia or dyskinesia) of the cardiac impulse. Examination of the fundi may reveal increased light reflexes and arteriovenous nicking as evidence of hypertension, while auscultation can uncover arterial bruits, a third and/or fourth heart sound, and when acute ischemia or previous infarction impairs papillary muscle function, a late apical systolic murmur due to mitral regurgitation. These ausculatory signs are best appreciated with the patient in the left decubitus position. Aortic stenosis, aortic regurgitation (Chap. 187), and hypertrophic cardiomyopathy (Chap. 192) must be excluded, since these disorders may cause angina even in the absence of coronary artery disease. Examination during an anginal attack is useful, since ischemia can cause transient left ventricular failure with the appearance of a third and/or fourth heart sound, a dyskinetic cardiac apex, mitral regurgitation, and even pulmonary edema.

LABORATORY EXAMINATION Although the diagnosis of ischemic heart disease can be made with confidence from a typical history, a number of simple laboratory tests can be most helpful. The urine should be examined for evidence of diabetes mellitus and renal disease, since both of these conditions may accelerate atherosclerosis. Similarly, examination of the blood should include measurements of lipids (cholesterol and high-density lipoproteins), glucose, creatinine, hematocrit, and, if indicated from the physical examination, thyroid function. The chest x-ray is an important test, since the consequences of ischemic heart disease, i.e., cardiac enlargement, ventricular aneurysm, or signs of heart failure, may be evident. Calcification of the coronary arteries can sometimes be identified by chest fluoroscopy. These signs can provide confirmation of the diagnosis of coronary artery disease and are important in assessing the degree of cardiac damage and the effects of treatment.

ELECTROCARDIOGRAM A normal ECG does not exclude the diagnosis of ischemic heart disease; however, certain characteristic abnormalities in tracings obtained at rest can confirm it. A 12-lead ECG recorded at rest is normal in about half of the patients with typical angina pectoris, but there may be signs of old myocardial infarction (Chap. 178). Serial tracings are particularly useful to look for evolving signs of infarction. Repolarization abnormalities, i.e., T-wave and ST-segment changes and intraventricular conduction disturbances at rest, are suggestive of ischemic heart disease but they are nonspecific, since they can also occur in pericardial, myocardial, and valvular heart disease or with anxiety, changes in posture, drugs, or esophageal disease. Typical ST-segment and T-wave changes which accompany episodes of angina pectoris and which disappear thereafter are more specific. The most characteristic changes include displacement of the ST segment that is similar in every way to that induced during a stress test (see below). The ST segment is usually depressed during angina but may be elevated, sometimes strikingly so, as in the early stages of myocardial infarction and in Prinzmetal's angina.

STRESS TESTING The most widely used test in the diagnosis of ischemic heart disease involves recording the 12-lead ECG before, during, and after exercise on a treadmill or using a bicycle ergometer. The patient undergoes a standardized incremental increase in external workload while the ECG, symptoms, and arm blood pressure are continuously monitored. The test is usually symptom-limited, and is discontinued with the onset of chest discomfort, severe shortness of breath, dizziness, fatigue, ST-segment depression of greater than 2 mm, a fall in systolic blood pressure exceeding 15 mmHg or the development of ventricular tachyarrhythmias. This test seeks to establish the relationship between chest discomfort and the typical electrocardiographic signs of myocardial ischemia. The ischemic ST-segment response is generally defined as flat depression of the ST segment of *more* than 0.1 mV below the baseline (i.e., the PR segment) and lasting *longer* than 0.08 s. This type of depression is designated a square wave or "plateau" type and is flat or downsloping. Upsloping or junctional ST-segment changes are not considered characteristic of ischemia and do not constitute a positive test. T-wave abnormalities, conduction disturbances, and ventricular arrhythmias developing during exercise should be noted but are also not diagnostic.

Based on the above criteria, the rate of false-positive diagnoses, using the coronary arteriogram as the "gold standard," is approximately 15 percent, and an approximately equal percentage of patients with severe, multivessel coronary artery will not have a positive test (false-negative). The incidence of false-negative tests is higher in young women without angina and much lower in men over 45 years with typical angina pectoris. There is an increased incidence of false-positive tests in women, in patients taking cardioactive drugs such as digitalis and quinidine, or in those with conduction disturbances, resting abnormalities of the ST segment and the T wave, myocardial hypertrophy, or abnormal serum potassium levels. It should be noted that the posterior surface of the heart is less accessible to the electrocardiogram and therefore more silent clinically. Negative exercise tests in which the target heart rate (85 percent of maximal heart rate for age and sex) is not achieved are considered to be nondiagnostic. It is important to emphasize that according to Bayes' theorem the probability that ischemic heart disease exists in the population under study (pretest probability) must be considered in accord with the diagnostic features of the test in order to interpret a positive or negative test result (Fig. 2-2). For example, a positive exercise result indicates that the likelihood of coronary artery disease is 98 percent in patients with typical angina pectoris, 88 percent in those with atypical chest pain, 44 percent in those patients with nonanginal chest pain, and 33 percent in asymptomatic persons.

The physician should be present throughout the exercise test, and it is important to measure total duration of exercise, the external work performed, and the internal cardiac work performed, as represented by the heart rate–blood pressure product with the time to the onset of ischemic ST-segment change and chest discomfort. It is also important to note the depth of the ST-segment depression and the time for recovery of these electrocardiographic changes. Because the risks of exercise testing are small but real, equipment for resuscitation should be available. The risks are estimated at one fatality and two nonfatal complications per 10,000 tests. Modified (heart rate–limited rather than symptom-limited) exercise tests can be performed safely in patients as early as 10 days after myocardial infarction.

The normal response to exercise includes a progressive increase in heart rate and blood pressure. Failure of the blood pressure to increase or an actual decrease in blood pressure during the test is an important adverse prognostic sign, since it may reflect ischemia-induced global left ventricular dysfunction. The presence of pain or severe ST-segment depression at a low workload and ST-segment depression persisting for more than 5 min after the termination of exercise all increase the specificity of the test and point to the presence of severe ischemic heart disease.

The exercise test can be enhanced by the intravenous administration of a radioisotope such as thallium 201 to assess regional myocardial perfusion by means of a gamma camera, with images recorded immediately after exercise (to identify acute ischemia) and 2 to 4 h later to discriminate between reversible ischemia and infarction (Fig. 179-7). Another radioisotope, most often technetium 99m, can be used to label the blood pool for gated radioisotope angiography. This technique (Fig. 179-6) can provide a measure of ventricular volume, ejection fraction, and regional ventricular wall motion at rest and during exercise, and can identify transient global and regional left ventricular dysfunction due to myocardial ischemia. A reduction in ejection fraction during exercise with the appearance of regional wall motion abnormalities represent important signs of myocardial ischemia and suggests the presence of severe ischemia and/or multivessel coronary disease.

The two-dimensional echocardiogram records cross-sectional images of the left ventricle and can identify regional wall motion abnormalities resulting from myocardial infarction (Chap. 179). In this way this test too can be used as an aid in the diagnosis of ischemic heart disease.

CORONARY ARTERIOGRAPHY (Chap. 180) This invasive diagnostic method outlines the coronary anatomy and can provide important evidence of coronary atherosclerosis or can exclude this condition. The severity of obstructive lesions and the global and regional function of the left ventricle can be assessed. Coronary arteriography is indicated in (1) patients with chronic stable or unstable angina pectoris who are refractory to medical therapy and who are being considered for revascularization, i.e., percutaneous transluminal coronary angioplasty or coronary artery bypass graft surgery; (2) patients with troublesome symptoms that present diagnostic difficulties and in whom there is need to establish or rule out coronary artery disease; and (3) patients suspected of having left main stem or three-vessel coronary artery disease, regardless of the presence or severity of symptoms.

Examples of other particular clinical situations include:

1 Patients with chest discomfort suggestive of angina pectoris but a negative exercise test who require a definitive diagnosis for guiding medical management, alleviating psychological stress, career or family planning, or for insurance purposes.

2 Patients who have been admitted to the hospital several times for suspected acute myocardial infarction but in whom this diagnosis has not been established and in whom the presence or absence of coronary artery disease should be determined.

3 Patients with responsible careers that involve the safety of others (e.g., airline pilots) who have questionable symptoms and suspicious or positive noninvasive tests and in whom there are reasonable doubts about the state of the coronary arteries.

4 Patients with aortic stenosis or hypertrophic cardiomyopthy and angina in whom the pain could be due to coronary artery disease.

5 Patients after myocardial infarction who are at high risk because of an unstable state characterized by angina, heart failure, or frequent ventricular premature contractions.

6 Patients with angina pectoris, regardless of severity, in whom noninvasive testing reveals signs of severe ischemia [e.g., marked (>2 mm) ST-segment depression], development of one large or multiple perfusion defects in thallium-201 scintigrams during exercise, and/or global left ventricular dysfunction at rest or precipitated by exercise.

PROGNOSIS The three principal prognostic indicators in patients with ischemic heart disease are the functional state of the left ventricle, the location and severity of coronary arterial narrowing, and the severity or activity of myocardial ischemia. Compromise of left ventricular function may be indicated by symptoms and signs of heart failure, roentgenographic evidence of cardiac enlargement, and by angiographic evidence of elevated left ventricular end-diastolic pressure and ventricular volume, and reduced ejection fraction. Patients with chest discomfort but normal left ventricular function and normal coronary arteries have an excellent prognosis. In patients with normal left ventricular function, mild angina, and critical (>70 percent luminal diameter) stenoses of one, two, or three epicardial coronary arteries, the 5-year mortality rates are approximately 2, 8, and 11 percent, respectively. Critical stenosis of the left main coronary artery is accompanied by a mortality of about 15 percent per year. With any degree of obstructive coronary artery disease, mortality is greatly increased when left ventricular function is impaired; conversely at any level of left ventricular function, prognosis is influenced importantly by the quantity of myocardium perfused by critically obstructed vessels. In addition, at any level of left ventricular function and degree of obstructive coronary artery disease the mortality is related to the rate of progression of the underlying atherosclerotic process. The development of unstable angina and severe ischemia in an exercise stress test reflects rapid progression.

It is useful to consider coronary atherosclerosis to be a process that destroys myocardial tissue, thereby reducing cardiac reserve at an unpredictable rate. The larger the amount of myocardial necrosis, the less the ability to tolerate additional damage and the poorer the prognosis. In this light, the various indexes of ischemic damage, such as an ECG showing evidence of old infarction or symptoms or signs of heart failure or cardiac enlargement, should be taken as indications of myocardial damage. Obstructive lesions of the proximal left anterior descending coronary artery are associated with a greater risk than are lesions of the right or left circumflex coronary artery since they usually perfuse a greater quantity of myocardium.

Frequent angina pectoris that is difficult to control with medical therapy, angina following myocardial infarction, a fall in ejection fraction associated with the development of regional wall motion abnormalities during exercise, and a strongly positive exercise test for myocardial ischemia at low workloads (>2 mm ST segment depression) all indicate that myocardial ischemia is severe and reflect a poor prognosis.

The segmental atherosclerotic plaques in epicardial arteries show phases of cellular activity, degeneration, endothelial instability, vasomotion, platelet aggregation, and fissuring or hemorrhage. These factors could also temporarily cause worsening of the stenosis and abnormal reactivity of the vessel and thus exacerbate the manifestations of ischemia.

MANAGEMENT

Each patient must be evaluated individually with respect to life patterns, risk factors, control of symptoms, and prevention of damage to left ventricular myocardium. The degree of the patient's disability and the specific physical and emotional stresses that precipitate pain must all be carefully recorded in order to set the proper goals for treatment. The management plan should consist of (1) explanation and reassurance, (2) reduction of risk factors in an attempt to slow the progression of coronary atherosclerosis, (3) treatment of coexisting conditions capable of aggravating angina, (4) sensible adaptations of activities to minimize anginal attacks, (5) a program of drug therapy, and (6) definition of end points that will indicate the need to consider mechanical revascularization.

EVALUATION AND REASSURANCE Patients with ischemic heart disease need to understand their condition as best they can and to realize that a long and useful life is possible even though they suffer from angina pectoris or have experienced and recovered from an acute myocardial infarction. Offering case histories of persons in public life who have lived with coronary disease can be of great value when encouraging patients to resume or maintain activity and return to their occupation.

REDUCTION OF RISK FACTORS (See also Chap. 195) Although there is no definitive proof that the lesions of coronary atherosclerosis in human beings can be made to regress, extrapolation from animal experiments makes this appear possible. Even more likely, the rate of progression of coronary atherosclerosis may be retarded by reduction of risk factors, which is important in the management of patients with coronary atherosclerosis. Ideal weight should be attained and maintained, hypertension treated if present, and cigarette smoking forbidden. Diabetes and hyperlipidemia, when present, should be treated. Unless angina is provoked, the patient should be encouraged to engage in steady dynamic exercise such as walking; isometric exercise may be hazardous. By maintaining good physical condition, the patient will be able to perform physical work more efficiently and at a lower pulse rate, thus reducing the frequency of anginal episodes. Patients in good physical condition may also have a better chance of surviving a myocardial infarction.

ELIMINATION OF COEXISTING ILLNESS A number of illnesses that are not primarily cardiac in nature may either increase oxygen demand or decrease oxygen supply to the myocardium and may precipitate or exacerbate angina. In the former category, hypertension and hyperthyroidism may be treated successfully in order to reduce anginal frequency. Decreased myocardial oxygen supply may be due to reduced oxygenation of the blood (e.g., with intrinsic pulmonary disease or carboxyhemoglobin due to cigarette or cigar smoking) or decreased oxygen-carrying capacity (e.g., in anemia). Correction of these abnormalities, if present, may reduce or even eliminate angina pectoris.

ADAPTATION OF ACTIVITIES Therapy of ischemic heart disease consists of eliminating the discrepancy between the demand of the heart muscle for oxygen and the ability of the coronary circulation to meet this demand. Most patients will understand this fundamental concept and utilize it in the rational programming of activity. Many tasks that ordinarily evoke angina may be accomplished without symptoms simply by reducing the speed at which they are performed. Patients must appreciate the diurnal variation in their tolerance of certain activities and should reduce their energy requirements in the morning and immediately after meals. It is sometimes helpful to alter the eating pattern and take small and more frequent meals.

It may be necessary to recommend a change in employment or residence to avoid physical stress; however, with the exception of manual laborers, most patients with ischemic heart disease can usually continue to function merely by allowing more time to complete each task. In some patients, anger and frustration may be the most important factors precipitating myocardial ischemia. If these cannot be avoided, tranquilizing and sedative drugs should be used, although caution is necessary when prescribing any of these agents for a prolonged time. A treadmill exercise test to determine the approximate heart rate at which ischemic electrocardiographic changes or symptoms develop may be helpful in the development of a specific exercise program. Ambulatory electrocardiography during daily activities may also be helpful in this regard.

DRUG THERAPY   Nitrates This is the most valuable class of drugs in the management of angina pectoris. These drugs act by causing systemic venodilatation, thereby reducing myocardial wall tension and oxygen requirements, as well as by dilating the epicardial coronary vessels and increasing blood flow in collateral vessels. The activity of these agents depends on their absorption, which is most rapid and complete through the mucous membranes. For this reason, nitroglycerin is administered sublingually in tablets of 0.4 or 0.6 mg. Patients with angina should be instructed to take the medication both to relieve an attack and also in anticipation of stress that is likely to induce an attack. When the patient experiences discomfort on exertion, he or she should cease activity and place a tablet under the tongue. The discomfort generally disappears more rapidly with nitroglycerin than would be expected if the drug were not administered. Walking up a flight of stairs or up a hill or sexual intercourse may produce angina consistently, and this can often be prevented by the anticipatory use of nitroglycerin. The value of this *prophylactic* use of the drug cannot be overemphasized.

The dose of nitroglycerin should be sufficient to relieve discomfort but not so large as to produce hypotension, headache, or a feeling of pulsating fullness in the head. The latter is the most common side effect of nitroglycerin and fortunately only rarely becomes disturbing at a dose required to relieve or prevent angina. Nitroglycerin deteriorates with exposure to air, moisture, and sunlight, so that if it produces neither relief of discomfort nor headache, nor a slight sensation of burning at the sublingual site of absorption, the preparation may be inactive and a fresh supply should be obtained. If relief is not attained with the first dose of nitroglycerin, a second or third dose may be given, but the patient should be instructed not to continue to take the medication if the first few doses prove unsuccessful. If discomfort continues for more than 7 to 10 min despite nitroglycerin, the patient should consult the physician or report promptly to a hospital emergency room for evaluation of possible acute myocardial infarction (Chap. 190).

Asking the patient with recently diagnosed angina pectoris to keep a diary of the time of occurrence of pain relative to activity and other precipitating factors with nitroglycerin consumption is often helpful to the physician attempting to tailor a management program. A diary may also be valuable for detecting changes in the frequency or severity of discomfort that may signify the development of unstable angina pectoris (p. 981) and/or herald an impending myocardial infarction.

Unfortunately, none of the long-acting nitrates is as effective as sublingual nitroglycerin for the relief of angina. These preparations can be swallowed, chewed, or administered as a patch or paste by the transdermal route. They can provide effective plasma levels for up to 24 h, but the therapeutic response is highly variable, and tolerance often develops. Different preparations and increased dosage should be used in an attempt to relieve discomfort in the individual patient while avoiding side effects. Useful preparations include isosorbide dinitrate (5 to 20 mg sublingual every 3 h or 5 to 40 mg PO tid), nitroglycerin ointment (0.5 to 2.0 in qid), or sustained-release transdermal patches (5 to 25 mg per day). Individual dose titration is important in order to avoid headache and dizziness. Long-acting nitrates are relatively safe and can be used together with intermittent sublingual nitroglycerin to relieve discomfort and prevent attacks of angina.

Beta-adrenoceptor blockade (see also Chap. 66)   Beta-adrenoceptor blockade represents an important component of the pharmacologic treatment of angina pectoris. These drugs reduce myocardial oxygen demand by inhibiting the increases in heart rate and myocardial contractility caused by adrenergic activity. Beta blockade reduces these variables most strikingly during exercise while causing only small reductions in heart rate, cardiac output, and arterial pressure at rest. Propranolol is usually administered in an initial dose of 20 to 40 mg four times a day and is increased as tolerated to 320 mg per day in divided doses; sometimes higher doses are required. Long-acting beta-blocking drugs (atenolol 50 to 100 mg per day and nadolol, 40 to 80 mg per day) offer the advantage of once-a-day dosage (see Table 66-1). The therapeutic aims include relief of angina and effective inhibition of exercise-induced increases in heart rate. These drugs can produce fatigue, impotence, cold extremities, intermittent claudication, and bradycardia, and can worsen disturbed cardiac conduction, left ventricular failure, bronchial asthma, or intensify the hypoglycemia produced by oral hypoglycemic agents and insulin. Reducing the dose or even discontinuation of the drug may be necessary if these side effects develop and persist.

Calcium channel antagonists   Nifedipine (10 to 40 mg qid), verapamil (80 to 120 mg tid), and diltiazem (30 to 90 mg qid) are all coronary vasodilators that produce a variable and dose-dependent reduction in myocardial oxygen demand, contractility, and arterial pressure. These combined pharmacologic effects are of advantage and make these agents quite effective in the treatment of angina pectoris. Verapamil and diltiazem can produce symptomatic disturbances in cardiac conduction and bradyarrhythmias and all three of these agents can cause left ventricular failure, particularly when used in combination with beta-adrenergic blockers in patients with underlying left ventricular dysfunction. Although useful effects are usually achieved when calcium channel antagonists are combined with beta-adrenoreceptor blockers and nitrates, individual titration of doses is essential with these potent combinations. Variant (Prinzmetal's) angina responds particularly well to calcium channel antagonists, supplemented when necessary by nitrates.

Treatment of angina and heart failure   Patients with angina pectoris may also have evidence of cardiac enlargement and elevated ventricular diastolic pressures and volume. This increases left ventricular wall tension and thereby raises myocardial oxygen demand. Agents that are useful in the treatment of congestive heart failure, such as digitalis and diuretics (Chap. 182), may also be useful in the management of patients with angina and heart failure since they decrease heart size, wall tension, and myocardial oxygen demands. Nocturnal angina can often be favorably affected by these agents; however, there is no benefit and possibly aggravation of angina when these drugs are used in patients with a normal heart size and no evidence of heart failure. The nitrates can also have beneficial effects on angina and heart failure.

MECHANICAL REVASCULARIZATION   It is important to appreciate that the basic management of patients with a lifelong condition such as ischemic heart disease is medical. The years of medical management may be punctuated by mechanical revascularization, as described below, but these important interventions do not replace the continuing need to ease symptoms and modify risk factors.

Percutaneous transluminal coronary angioplasty (PTCA)   PTCA is a widely used method to achieve revascularization of the myocardium in patients with symptomatic ischemic heart disease and suitable proximal stenoses of epicardial coronary arteries. Whereas patients with stenosis of the left main coronary artery and those with distal three-vessel coronary artery disease who require revascularization are best treated by coronary artery bypass surgery (CAS), the use of PTCA in patients with symptomatic proximal stenoses of one or two vessels, and even selected cases with three-vessel disease, is widely employed and may have many advantages over CAS.

The method is described in Chap. 180 and illustrated in Figs. 180-6 and 180-7. After a flexible guidewire is advanced into a coronary artery and across the stenosis to be dilated, a miniature balloon catheter is advanced over the guidewire and into the stenosis followed by repeated inflations until the stenosis is decreased or relieved. The development of a range of guiding catheters, steerable guidewires, and low-profile balloon catheters and the use of high inflation pressures have all helped to decrease complications, reach more distal lesions, and dilate more complex stenoses.

INDICATIONS AND PATIENT SELECTION   The most common clinical indication is angina pectoris, stable or unstable, which should be accompanied by evidence of ischemia in an exercise test. This symptom should be sufficiently severe to warrant the consideration of bypass graft surgery. Some physicians will perform angioplasty on asymptomatic or mildly symptomatic patients with suitable stenosis of the left anterior descending coronary artery and severe ischemia on an exercise stress test. PTCA can also be used to dilate stenoses in native coronary arteries and in bypass grafts in patients who have recurrent angina following CAS. This is an important indication when considering the technical difficulties and the increased mortality that accompanies reoperation. Angioplasty has also been carried out in patients with recent total occlusion (within 3 months) of a coronary artery and severe angina; in this group the primary success rate is decreased to approximately 50 percent.

RISKS   Two and three vessels can be dilated in sequence with a modest increase in risk. Female gender, the presence of left ventricular damage, a stenosis of an artery which perfuses a large segment of myocardium without collaterals, long eccentric or irregular stenoses, and calcified plaques all increase the likelihood of complications. The major complications are usually due to dissection or thrombosis with vessel occlusion, uncontrolled ischemia, and ventricular failure. In the most experienced hands, the overall mortality rate should be less than 1 percent, the need for emergency coronary surgery is 3 to 5 percent, and myocardial infarction occurs in approximately 3 percent of cases. Minor complications occur in 5 to 10 percent of patients and include occlusion of a branch of a coronary artery, and complications of arterial catheterization.

EFFICACY   Primary success, i.e., adequate dilation with relief of angina, occurs in 85 to 90 percent of cases. Recurrent stenosis of the dilated vessels occurs in 15 to 40 percent of cases within 6 months of the procedure, and angina will recur within 6 to 12 months in 25 percent of cases. This recurrence of symptoms and restenosis is more common in patients with unstable angina and with incomplete dilatation of the stenosis. It is usual clinical practice to administer aspirin, persantine, and a calcium blocker for months after the procedure; however, there are no controlled clinical trials that prove that these medications reduce the incidence of restenosis.

If patients do not develop restenosis or angina during the first year following angioplasty, the prognosis for maintenance of improvement for the subsequent 4 years is excellent. If restenosis occurs, the success rate of repeat PTCA is marginally better than the first procedure.

Between 15 and 30 percent of patients with symptomatic coronary artery disease who require revascularization can be treated by PTCA and need not undergo CAS. Successful angioplasty is less invasive and expensive than CAS, requires only 2 to 3 days in the hospital, and permits considerable savings in the cost of care. Successful PTCA also allows earlier return to work and the resumption of an active life.

Coronary artery surgery (CAS) A section of a vein (usually the saphenous) is used to form a connection between the aorta and the coronary artery distal to the obstructive lesion. Alternatively, anastomosis of the left internal mammary artery to the coronary artery distal to the obstructive lesion may be employed.

Some indications for CAS are controversial, but certain areas of agreement exist:

1 The operation is relatively safe, with mortality rates less than 1 percent when it is performed by an experienced surgical team in selected patients with normal left ventricular function.

2 Intraoperative and postoperative mortality increase with ventricular dysfunction and surgical inexperience. The effectiveness and risk of CAS vary widely depending on the skill and experience of the surgical team. Therefore the selection of patients must take into account the results of the team which will perform the procedure.

3 Occlusion is observed in 10 to 20 percent of vein grafts during the first year, the incidence is ~2 percent per year during 5 to 7 year follow-up and ~5 percent per year thereafter. Long-term patency rates are higher for internal mammary artery implantations, and in patients with left anterior descending coronary artery obstruction coronary bypass with an internal mammary artery results in better survival than venous bypass grafting.

4 Angina is abolished or unequivocally reduced in 85 percent of patients following complete revascularization. Although this is usually associated with graft patency and restoration of blood flow, the pain may also be improved as a result of infarction of the ischemic segment or a placebo effect.

5 CAS does not appear to reduce the incidence of myocardial infarction in patients with chronic ischemic heart disease; perioperative myocardial infarction occurs in 5 to 10 percent of cases but in most instances these infarcts are small.

6 Mortality is reduced by operation in patients with stenosis of the left main coronary artery. Some reduction in mortality also occurs in patients with three-vessel coronary artery disease and impaired left ventricular function. There is no evidence that CAS reduces mortality in patients with one- or two-vessel disease who have chronic stable angina and normal left ventricular function or in patients with one-vessel disease and impaired left ventricular function. There is conflicting evidence concerning the effects of operation on survival in patients with impaired left ventricular function and obstructive disease of two coronary arteries, one of which is the proximal left anterior descending artery.

7 Other important considerations which affect the outcome include the age of the patient as well as accompanying medical problems such as diabetes mellitus, obesity, and renal disease.

Indications for CAS are usually based on the severity of symptoms, coronary anatomy, and ventricular function. The ideal candidate is less than 70 years of age, has no other complicating disease, has troublesome or disabling symptoms which are not adequately controlled by medical therapy, wants to lead a more active life, and has severe stenoses of several epicardial coronary arteries with objective evidence of myocardial ischemia as a cause of the chest discomfort. Great symptomatic benefit can be anticipated in such patients. When disturbance of left ventricular function coexists, CAS may, in addition, prolong life.

UNSTABLE ANGINA PECTORIS

This condition includes four groups of patients: (1) patients with angina pectoris of recent onset (within 6 weeks) that is troublesome and frequent; (2) patients with angina of any duration that occurs at rest; (3) patients with chronic stable angina with a recent increase in intensity, frequency, or duration of pain; and (4) patients with angina pectoris developing or becoming more severe within days or weeks of acute myocardial infarction. Unstable angina, particularly groups 2 and 4 defined above, carries an adverse prognosis, with a high risk of acute myocardial infarction, sudden death, and the development of intractable chronic stable angina. In short, the course tends to be unstable in these patients—hence its name. When unstable angina is accompanied by objective electrocardiographic evidence of transient myocardial ischemia, it is almost always associated with critical stenoses in one or more major epicardial coronary arteries. Less than 10 percent of such patients have normal coronary arteries at arteriography. The atherosclerotic lesions may have a complicated morphology with evidence of superimposed thrombosis in approximately one-fourth of cases. Segmental spasm in the vicinity of atherosclerotic plaques may also play a role in the development of unstable angina. The diagnosis of unstable angina is made on the basis of the history and transient ST-segment changes, most commonly depressions, and/or T-wave inversions occurring during episodes of chest pain.

Management The patient should be admitted promptly to the hospital for observation, further diagnosis, and treatment. It is important immediately to identify and treat concomitant conditions which can intensify ischemia such as uncontrolled hypertension and diabetes, cardiomegaly, heart failure, arrhythmias, and any acute febrile illness. Acute myocardial infarction should be ruled out using serial electrocardiograms and measurements of plasma cardiac enzyme activity.

Continuous elecrocardiographic monitoring should be carried out and the patients should receive reassurance and sedation. Beta-adrenergic blocking drugs and calcium channel antagonists should be administered, but with caution, noting all of the side effects discussed above. Dosages must be titrated to avoid bradycarida, heart failure, and hypotension. Nitroglycerin should be given by the sublingual route. In addition, intravenous nitroglycerin is quite effective, but requires continuous monitoring of intraarterial pressure. It is begun at a dosage of 5 μg/min and raised in 5-μg/min increments to a level at which chest pain is abolished, but systolic arterial pressure is maintained or reduced only slightly and other side effects are avoided. Thrombus formation frequently complicates the atheromatous narrowing of coronary arteries in this condition. Therefore, intravenous heparin should be given for 3 to 5 days to maintain the partial thromboplastin time at 2 to 2.5 times control, followed by oral coumadin and aspirin at a dose of 325 mg per day.

The majority of patients will improve on this treatment. However, the clinical outcome is highly variable. If angina and objective evidence of ischemia do not diminish within 24 to 48 h of treatment in patients in whom there are no obvious contraindications for revascularization, then cardiac catheterization and coronary arteriography should be performed. If the anatomy is suitable, PTCA can be performed with surgical standby. If this cannot be done, CAS should be considered to relieve symptoms and myocardial ischemia and as a means of preventing myocardial damage. If the patient's symptoms and signs are controlled on medical therapy, a diagnostic exercise electrocardiogram should be obtained at the time of discharge from hospital, and the patient can be managed as outlined above for chronic stable angina pectoris. However, it should be recognized that among those patients with unstable angina who respond to medical therapy, severe coronary artery disease is usually present, and although angina may become stable, it often remains severe and ultimately mechanical revascularization is necessary.

ASYMPTOMATIC ISCHEMIA

Both obstructive coronary artery disease and myocardial ischemia are frequently asymptomatic. During continuous ambulatory electrocardiographic (Holter) monitoring, the majority of patients with typical chronic stable angina are found to have objective evidence of myocardial ischemia (ST-segment deviation) during episodes of chest discomfort while they are active outside of the hospital, but most of these patients also appear to have more frequent episodes of asymptomatic ischemia. In addition, there is a large, but as yet unknown, number of totally asymptomatic people with severe coronary atherosclerosis who exhibit ST-segment changes during activity.

The widespread use of exercise electrocardiography during routine examinations has defined some of these heretofore unrecognized patients with asymptomatic coronary artery disease. Longitudinal studies of young military personnel have demonstrated an increased incidence of coronary events (sudden death, myocardial infarction, and angina) in asymptomatic patients with positive exercise tests. In addition, patients who are asymptomatic after suffering a myocardial infarction are nonetheless at far greater risk for a second coronary event than is the general population. Patients with asymptomatic ischemia should be subjected to a detailed noninvasive examination, utilizing stress electrocardiography and radionuclide scintigraphy.

Management of patients with asymptomatic ischemia must be individualized. Thus, the physician should consider the following: (1) the degree of positivity of the exercise test, the stage of exercise at which electrocardiographic signs of ischemia appear, and/or the magnitude of the perfusion defect on thallium scintigraphy; (2) the electrocardiographic leads showing a positive response, with changes in the anterior precordial leads indicating a less favorable prognosis than changes in the inferior leads; (3) the patient's age and occupation. Most would agree that an asymptomatic 45-year-old commercial airline pilot with 4-mm ST-segment depression in leads V_1 to V_4 during mild exercise should undergo coronary arteriography, while the asymptomatic, sedentary 75-year-old retiree with 1-mm ST-segment depression in leads II and III during maximal activity need not. However, there is no consensus about the appropriate procedure in the majority of patients for whom the situation is less extreme. Patients with evidence of severe ischemia on noninvasive testing should be subjected to coronary arteriography and depending on the findings should be considered for revascularization. Thus, asymptomatic patients with three-vessel coronary disease and impaired left ventricular function and asymptomatic patients with left main coronary artery disease may be considered appropriate candidates for CAS.

While the incidence of asymptomatic ischemia can be reduced by treatment with beta blockers and calcium antagonists, it is not clear whether this is necessary or desirable in patients who have not suffered a myocardial infarction. However, there is evidence that beta-adrenoceptor blockade begun 7 to 35 days after acute myocardial infarction improves survival. This therapy is recommended in asymptomatic patients as long as there are no contraindications such as heart failure, bradycardia, heart block, and asthma.

REFERENCES

AMBROSE JA et al: Angiographic evolution of coronary artery morphology in unstable angina. J Am Coll Cardiol 7:472, 1986

BRAUNWALD E (ed): Symposium on experimental and clinical aspects of coronary vasoconstriction. Am J Cardiol 56(Suppl):1E, 1985

———— et al (eds): Surgery in the treatment of coronary artery disease. Circulation 72(Suppl):V1, 1985

BREDLAU CE et al: In-hospital morbidity and mortality in patients undergoing elective coronary angioplasty. Circulation 72:1044, 1985

CHRISTIE LG et al: Systematic approach to evaluation of angina-like chest pain: Pathophysiology and clinical testing with emphasis on objective documentation of myocardial ischemia. Am Heart J 102:897, 1981

COHN PF, BRAUNWALD E: Chronic ischemic heart disease, in *Heart Disease*, 2d ed, E Braunwald (ed): Philadelphia, Saunders, 1984, p 1334

———— (ed): *Diagnosis and Therapy of Coronary Artery Disease*, 2d ed. Boston, Little, Brown, 1985

GOTTLIEB SO et al: Effect of the addition of propranolol to therapy with nifedipine for unstable angina pectoris: A randomized, double-blind, placebo-controlled trial. Circulation 73:331, 1986

HOMMA A et al: Usefulness of oral dipyridamole suspension for stress thallium imaging without exercise in the detection of coronary artery disease. Am J Cardiol 57:503, 1986

HULTGREN HN et al: Treatment of unstable angina. JAMA 253:2555, 1985

MADDAHI J et al: Noninvasive identification of left main and triple vessel coronary artery disease: Improved accuracy using quantitative analysis of regional myocardial stress distribution and washout of thallium-201. J Am Coll Cardiol 7:53, 1986

---

190   ACUTE MYOCARDIAL INFARCTION

RICHARD C. PASTERNAK / EUGENE BRAUNWALD / JOSEPH S. ALPERT

Myocardial infarction is one of the commonest diagnoses occurring in hospitalized patients in western countries. In the United States, approximately 1.5 million myocardial infarctions occur each year. Mortality with acute infarction is approximately 35 percent, with slightly more than half of the deaths occurring before the stricken individual reaches the hospital. An additional 15 to 20 percent of survivors die in the first year following myocardial infarction. Risk of excess mortality persists in patients who recover; indeed, the age-corrected risk of death is increased 3.5 times as long as 10 years after infarction.

CLINICAL PRESENTATION   *Pain* is the most common presenting complaint in patients with myocardial infarction. In some instances, the discomfort may be severe enough to be described as the worst pain the patient has ever experienced (Chap. 4). The pain of myocardial infarction is deep and visceral; adjectives commonly used to describe it are *heavy, squeezing,* and *crushing*. It is similar in character to the discomfort of angina pectoris but is usually more severe and lasts much longer. Typically the pain involves the central portion of the chest and/or epigastrium, and in about 30 percent of cases it radiates to the arms. Less common sites of radiation include the abdomen, back, lower jaw, and neck. The location of the pain beneath the xiphoid and patients' denial that they may be suffering a heart attack are chiefly responsible for the mistaken diagnosis of indigestion. The pain of myocardial infarction may radiate as high as the occipital area but not below the umbilicus. The pain is often accompanied by weakness, sweating, nausea, vomiting, giddiness, and anxiety. The discomfort usually commences with the patient at rest and more commonly in the morning than at any other time of day. However, when it begins during a period of exertion, in contrast to angina pectoris, it does not usually subside with cessation of activity.

Although pain is the most common presenting complaint, it is by no means always present; a minimum of 15 to 20 percent of myocardial infarcts are *painless*. The frequency of such silent infarcts is probably even higher than this estimate because patients without pain may not seek medical attention. The incidence of painless infarcts is greater in patients with diabetes mellitus, and it increases with age. In the elderly, myocardial infarction may present as sudden-onset breathlessness, which may progress to pulmonary edema. Other less common presentations, with or without pain, include sudden loss of consciousness, a confusional state, a sensation of profound weakness, the appearance of an arrhythmia, or merely an unexplained drop in arterial blood pressure.

PHYSICAL FINDINGS   In many instances the dominant feature of the patient's presentation is the reaction to the chest pain. Patients are typically anxious and restless, attempting to relieve the pain by moving about in bed, squirming, stretching, belching, or even inducing vomiting. This is in contrast to the discomfort of angina pectoris, which causes the patient to remain relatively immobile for fear of making the discomfort reappear. Pallor is common and is often associated with perspiration and coolness of the extremities. The combination of substernal chest pain persistent for more than 30 min and diaphoresis strongly suggests acute myocardial infarction. Although many patients have a normal pulse rate and blood pressure, within the first hour of infarction about one-fourth of patients with anterior infarction have manifestations of sympathetic nervous system hyperactivity (tachycardia and/or hypertension), and up to one-half with inferior infarction show evidence of parasympathetic hyperactivity (bradycardia and/or hypotension).

The precordium is usually quiet, and the apical impulse may be difficult to palpate. In about one-fourth of patients with anterior wall infarction, an abnormal systolic pulsation develops in the periapical area within the first days of the illness and then may resolve. Other physical signs of ventricular dysfunction that may be present include, in decreasing incidence, fourth (S₄) and third (S₃) heart sounds, decreased intensity of heart sounds, and, rarely, paradoxical splitting of the second sound (Chap. 177). A transient apical systolic murmur, presumably due to mitral regurgitation secondary to papillary muscle dysfunction during acute infarction, may be midsystolic or late systolic in timing. A pericardial friction rub is heard in many patients with transmural myocardial infarction at some time in their course if they are examined frequently. Jugular venous distention occurs commonly in patients with right ventricular infarction. The carotid pulse is often decreased in volume despite a normal upstroke. Temperature elevations in the range of 37 to 38°C may be observed during the first week following acute myocardial infarction; however, a temperature exceeding 38°C should prompt a search for other causes. The arterial pressure is variable; in most patients with transmural infarction systolic pressure declines approximately 10 to 15 mmHg from the preinfarction state.

LABORATORY DIAGNOSIS The laboratory tests of value in confirming the diagnosis of myocardial infarction may be divided into three groups: (1) nonspecific indexes of tissue necrosis and inflammation, (2) the electrocardiogram, and (3) serum enzyme changes.

The *nonspecific reaction* to myocardial injury is associated with polymorphonuclear leukocytosis, which appears within a few hours after the onset of pain, persists for 3 to 7 days, and often reaches levels of 12,000 to 15,000 leukocytes per cubic millimeter. The erythrocyte sedimentation rate rises more slowly than the white blood cell count, peaking during the first week, and sometimes remaining elevated for 1 or 2 weeks.

The *electrocardiographic manifestations* of acute myocardial infarction are described in Chap. 178. Although electrocardiographic/pathologic correlations are not excellent, transmural infarction is diagnosed if the electrocardiogram demonstrates Q waves or loss of R waves; nontransmural infarction is said to be present if the electrocardiogram shows only transient ST-segment and sustained T-wave changes. However, these changes are variable and nonspecific and should not form the sole basis for the diagnosis of infarction. Therefore, a more rational nomenclature for designating electrocardiographic infarction would be *Q-wave* or *ST-T-wave infarction* in place of the terms *transmural* or *nontransmural infarction*, respectively.

SERUM ENZYMES Enzymes are released in large quantities into the blood from necrotic heart muscle following myocardial infarction. The rate of liberation of specific enzymes differs following infarction, and the temporal pattern of enzyme release is of diagnostic importance. The time course of the serum concentration of the most commonly used enzymes is shown in Fig. 190-1. Levels of two of the enzymes, serum glutamic oxaloacetic transaminase (SGOT) and creatine phosphokinase (CK), rise and fall rapidly, while that of lactic dehydrogenase (LDH) rises later and remains elevated longer. SGOT has the disadvantage that it is also present in skeletal muscle, liver, and red blood cells and may be liberated from these extracardiac stores. SGOT is less widely used than heretofore because of its lack of specificity and because of its time course, which is intermediate between CK and LDH, making the information redundant in most

cases. The MB isoenzyme of CK has an advantage over SGOT in that it is not present in significant concentrations in extracardiac tissue, and therefore it is more specific than SGOT. Since rises in serum concentration of CK and SGOT are short-lived, they may be missed if initial blood samples are obtained more than 48 h after the infarct develops. MB-CK isoenzymes are particularly useful when skeletal muscle and/or brain damage are suspected since both tissues contain large quantities of the enzyme but none of the MB isoenzyme. The myocardial specificity of the MB isoenzyme determination depends on the technique used for measurement. Radioimmunoassay techniques are most specific, but the more commonly employed gel electrophoresis technique is significantly less specific and therefore prone to more frequent false positives. In myocardial infarction, the level of LDH rises during the first day, peaks at 3 to 4 days, and returns to normal in 14 days. Five common LDH isoenzymes may be separated by starch-gel electrophoresis. Tissues differ with respect to the specific isoenzyme patterns; the rapidly migrating isoenzyme which predominates in the heart is referred to as LDH₁, while the slowly migrating components predominate in liver and skeletal muscle. LDH₁ rises before total LDH in patients with myocardial infarction and may rise when there is no change in total LDH. Therefore, increased LDH₁ is a more sensitive indicator of myocardial infarction than total LDH; sensitivity exceeds 95 percent.

Of particular clinical importance is the fact that a two- to threefold elevation of total CK (not MB-CK) may follow an intramuscular injection. This may lead to the erroneous diagnosis of myocardial infarction in a patient who has been given an intramuscular injection of a narcotic for chest pain of noncardiac origin. Other potential sources of total CK elevation worthy of note are (1) muscular diseases including muscular dystrophy, myopathies, and polymyositis, (2) electrical cardioversion, (3) cardiac catheterization, (4) hypothyroidism, (5) stroke, (6) surgery, and (7) skeletal muscle damage secondary to trauma, convulsions, and prolonged immobilization. Cardiac surgery and electrical cardioversion often result in elevation of serum levels of MB isoenzyme.

It has long been recognized that the amount of enzyme released correlates with the size of the infarct. It has been demonstrated that the mass of heart muscle infarcted can be estimated from analysis of

FIGURE 190-1 *The time course of serum enzyme concentration changes following a typical myocardial infarction. CK, creatinine phosphokinase; LDH, lactic dehydrogenase; GOT, glutamic oxaloacetic transaminase.*

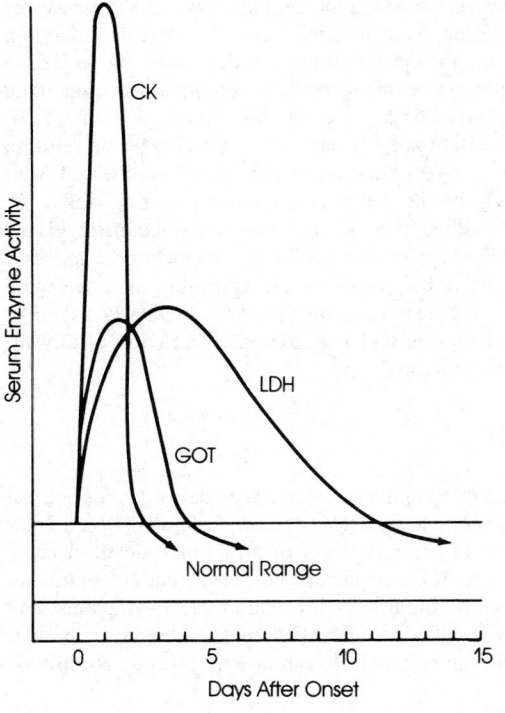

the concentration-time curve of the enzyme if the kinetics of the release, degradation, disposal, etc., of the enzyme are known. The size of an infarct in terms of grams of infarcted tissue can be estimated from an analysis of the MB-CK–time curve. While the *area* under the MB-CK–time curve is related to infarct size, the *absolute* value of the peak MB-CK and its time to peak are related to the kinetics of MB-CK washout from myocardium. The opening of a coronary artery occlusion (either spontaneously, or by mechanical or pharmacologic means) in the early hours of myocardial infarction will cause early peaking (at about 1 to 3 h following reperfusion) of the MB-CK–time curve. However, the total area under the curve may be smaller than without reperfusion, reflecting smaller overall infarction size.

Characteristic rises occur in serum enzyme concentration in more than 95 percent of patients with clinically proven myocardial infarction. CK, LDH, and SGOT levels generally do not rise in unstable angina. Many patients with suspected infarction have baseline enzyme levels which are normal and increase threefold in a pattern consistent with infarction, although the absolute level of enzyme in the blood never exceeds the upper limits of normal. This situation is most commonly observed in patients with small infarctions and, although not diagnostic, is highly suggestive of acute infarction. Isoenzyme studies are particularly helpful in this situation.

Several radionuclide imaging techniques are of value in the diagnosis or assessment of the patient with acute myocardial infarction (Chap. 179). Acute infarct scintigraphy ("hot-spot" imaging) is carried out with an infarct-avid imaging agent such as ^{99m}Tc stannous pyrophosphate. Scans are usually positive 2 to 5 days after infarction, particularly in patients with transmural infarcts; although they aid in *localizing* infarcts and provide a measure of infarct size (page 887), these scans are less accurate than CK determination for making the *diagnosis* of myocardial infarction. Myocardial perfusion imaging with thallium 201, which is taken up and concentrated by viable myocardium, reveals a defect ("cold spot") in most patients during the first few hours after development of a transmural infarct. This localized area of decreased radioactivity may fill in during the following hours (page 887). However, it is not possible to distinguish acute infarcts from chronic scars. Therefore, while thallium scanning is extremely sensitive for the detection of myocardial infarction, it is not specific for *acute* myocardial infarction. Radionuclide ventriculography, carried out with ^{99m}Tc-labeled red blood cells (page 886), frequently demonstrates wall motion disorders and reduction in ventricular ejection fraction in patients with acute myocardial infarction. While of value in assessing the hemodynamic consequences of infarction, and in aiding in the diagnosis of right ventricular infarction when the right ventricular ejection fraction is depressed, the technique is quite nonspecific, since many cardiac abnormalities other than myocardial infarction alter the radionuclide ventriculogram. Two-dimensional echocardiography (Chap. 179) can also be of value in patients with acute myocardial infarction. Abnormalities of wall motion, particularly of the septal and inferior-posterior walls, are readily detectable. Although acute infarction cannot be distinguished from old myocardial scar or from acute severe ischemia, the ease and safety of the procedure make its use appealing as a screening tool. Additionally, echocardiography may be particularly useful in the diagnosis of right ventricular infarction, ventricular aneurysm, and left ventricular thrombus.

MANAGEMENT

Two general classes of complications have been defined: (1) electrical (arrhythmias) and (2) mechanical ("pump failure"). Ventricular fibrillation is the most common form of arrhythmic death in acute myocardial infarction. The vast majority of deaths due to ventricular fibrillation occur within the first 24 h of the onset of symptoms, and of these deaths, over half occur in the first hour. Although ventricular premature beats or ventricular tachycardia may precede an episode

of ventricular fibrillation, the latter often occurs without warning arrhythmias. This observation has led to the use of lidocaine in the prophylactic treatment of ventricular ectopic activity in acute myocardial infarction. The focus of coronary care has shifted from resuscitation to prevention, and the incidence of primary ventricular fibrillation has diminished markedly in the last two decades. Reduction of in-hospital mortality for acute myocardial infarction from about 30 to less than 10 percent is in large measure the result of institution of measures such as rapid transfer of patients with acute myocardial infarction to facilities with ECG monitoring capability staffed by personnel (not necessarily physicians) knowledgeable in the recognition and immediate treatment of ventricular arrhythmias.

With sudden and unexpected in-hospital arrhythmic deaths essentially eliminated by the preventive approach to ventricular arrhythmias, attention has turned to the other major complication of acute myocardial infarction, i.e., pump failure. Although advances have been made in the treatment of pump failure, it remains the primary cause of in-hospital death from acute myocardial infarction. The extent of ischemic necrosis correlates well with the degree of pump failure and with mortality, both early, i.e., within 10 days of infarction, and later as well. A clinical classification dependent on the status of cardiac pump function originally proposed by Killip divides patients into four groups as follows: class I, no signs of pulmonary or venous congestion; class II, moderate heart failure as evidenced by rales at the lung bases, S_3 gallop, tachypnea, or signs of failure of the right side of the heart including venous and hepatic congestion; class III, severe heart failure, pulmonary edema; class IV, shock with systolic pressure less than 90 mmHg and evidence of peripheral constriction, diaphoresis, peripheral cyanosis, mental confusion, and oliguria. The expected hospital mortality rate of patients in these clinical classes has been established by a number of investigators as follows: class I, 0 to 5 percent; class II, 10 to 20 percent; class III, 35 to 45 percent; and class IV, 85 to 95 percent.

GENERAL CONSIDERATIONS Given the information summarized above, the principal objectives of management of the patient with myocardial infarction are to prevent death from arrhythmia and to minimize the mass of infarcted tissue.

Arrhythmias can usually be managed successfully if trained personnel and appropriate equipment are available when this complication develops. Since mortality from arrhythmia is greatest during the first few hours after infarction, it is obvious that the effectiveness of coronary care units relates directly to the speed with which patients come under medical observation. The biggest delay usually is not in transportation to the hospital but rather between the onset of pain and the patient's decision to call for help. This delay can best be reduced by education of the public concerning the significance of chest pain and the importance of seeking early medical attention.

A number of "common sense" rules in the management of acute myocardial infarction deserve particular emphasis. First and foremost, it is mandatory to maintain an optimal balance between myocardial oxygen supply and demand in order to salvage as much as possible of the jeopardized zone of myocardium surrounding the center of the infarct. Therapeutic strategies that help to attain this goal include rest, analgesia, mild sedation, and a quiet atmosphere in order to reduce anxiety and thereby lower heart rate, a major determinant of myocardial oxygen consumption.

Marked sinus bradycardia (heart rate less than approximately 45 beats per minute) should be treated by leg elevation and atropine or by electrical pacing, particularly if the bradycardia is associated with a fall in blood pressure or with worsening ventricular arrhythmias. However, routine administration of atropine, with resultant increase in heart rate, to patients without serious bradycardia is not recommended. Patients with acute myocardial infarction who have a hyperdynamic state, i.e., tachycardia and elevation of arterial pressure, should be treated with a beta-adrenergic blocking agent. Initially, 0.1 mg/kg propranolol or 15 mg metoprolol given intravenously in three divided doses is safe, if there are no contraindications, such as heart failure, AV block, or asthma. All forms of tachyarrhythmias require prompt and direct treatment. Drugs that exert a positive inotropic effect, such as digitalis glycosides and cardioactive sympathomimetics, should be administered only if there is evidence of pronounced heart failure; they should not be given prophylactically. Of the various sympathomimetic amines available, isoproterenol with its chronotropic and vasodilator effects is the least desirable. Dobutamine (page 911), which has less effect on heart rate and systemic vascular resistance, is more desirable when it is necessary to augment cardiac contractility. Dopamine (page 911) is useful in patients with left ventricular failure and systemic hypotension (systolic pressure <90 mmHg. Diuretics are indicated in the presence of heart failure and should, in fact, be used prior to cardiac stimulants unless the patient is hypovolemic or hypotensive.

All patients should inhale oxygen-enriched air (see below). Particular attention must be paid to preserving arterial oxygenation in patients with hypoxemia, as occurs in patients with chronic pulmonary disease, pneumonia, or left ventricular failure. Severe anemia, which can also extend the area of ischemic injury, should be corrected by cautious administration of packed red blood cells, sometimes accompanied by a diuretic. Associated conditions, particularly infections with accompanying tachycardia and elevated myocardial oxygen demand, require immediate attention. Systolic arterial pressure should not be allowed to deviate by more than 25 to 30 mmHg from the patient's usual level.

Coronary care units Coronary care units have resulted in improved care of patients with myocardial infarction, reduction in mortality rates, and major increases in knowledge about myocardial infarction. The coronary care unit is a specially designed *nursing unit,* the most important feature of which is a staff of highly trained nursing personnel with authority to take immediate action in emergency situations. The unit should be equipped with a system which permits continuous monitoring of the electrocardiogram of each patient and hemodynamic monitoring in selected patients. Defibrillators, respirators, and facilities for introducing pacing catheters and flow-directed balloon-tipped catheters should be available. However, equipment alone does not ensure an effective coronary care unit. Of prime importance is the organization of a highly trained team of nurses who can recognize arrhythmias, adjust the dosage of antiarrhythmic drugs, and perform cardiac resuscitation, including the application of electroshock, when necessary. A physician should be available at all times, but many lives have been saved because nurses have treated ventricular tachycardia or fibrillation before the physician's arrival.

The policies and procedures for admission to a coronary care unit should ensure that patients are admitted early in their illness when they may expect to derive maximum benefit from the care provided. In order to accomplish this, the threshold for admission of patients with suspected infarction should be low, and this is best monitored in terms of the fraction of total admissions in whom myocardial infarction is eventually proven. In the past, all patients with suspected myocardial infarction were admitted to the coronary care unit. Currently, however, several factors have led to a change in this rule. The availability of electrocardiographic monitoring and trained personnel in "intermediate care units" has allowed admission of lower-risk patients (e.g., those not hemodynamically compromised or without active arrhythmias) to such units. For economic reasons, and to utilize limited facilities optimally, many institutions have developed guidelines to aid in triaging patients with suspected myocardial infarction. While most such patients in the United States are admitted to the hospital, in other countries, such as the United Kingdom, the patients at lowest risk may be cared for at home. Once admitted to the hospital the fraction of patients actually admitted to the coronary care unit may depend on a balance between the clinical status of the patient and bed availability. In some units beds are utilized primarily for patients with a complicated course, particularly those who require hemodynamic monitoring. Mortality rates for myocardial infarction treated in coronary care units vary from 5 to 20 percent; this variation can be explained, in part, by variations in admission policies as regard age limitations, the type of population being served, the nature of the hospital (tertiary care referral center versus community hospital), and other as yet unidentified factors.

REPERFUSION An occlusive or near-occlusive thrombus overlying or adjacent to an atherosclerotic plaque in a coronary artery appears to be the cause of most transmural infarcts. Therefore, reperfusion of the ischemic zone by the prompt dissolution of the thrombus with a thrombolytic agent is a logical approach to the reduction of infarct size. There is considerable evidence that if reperfusion is to be effective in salvaging jeopardized myocardium, it must be carried out immediately after the onset of the clinical event; certainly within 4 h, and preferably within 2 h.

Streptokinase (SK), administered via a coronary catheter, has been approved by the Food and Drug Administration (FDA) in the treatment of acute myocardial infarction. While the administration of this agent is effective in lysing the offending thrombus in about 75 percent of cases, many questions, such as whether or not this therapy reduces mortality or morbidity, remain unanswered, and its role in therapy remains to be established. Intravenous administration of SK appears to be less effective than intracoronary administration, but has the advantage of not requiring cardiac catheterization. Tissue plasminogen activator (tPA), when administered intravenously, lyses approximately two-thirds of recent coronary thrombi; it has the theoretical advantage of causing fibrinolytic activity predominantly at the site of a fresh thrombus, and thus may be safer than SK by virtue of causing a less intensive systemic lytic state than that produced by intravenous SK. However, even while the ideal thrombolytic agent is sought, it remains unclear whether such therapy will be effective in routinely salvaging myocardium, whether mechanical revascularization by means of coronary angioplasty or coronary bypass surgery will be required following successful thrombolysis in the majority of patients, and whether the mortality and morbidity of acute myocardial infarction can actually be reduced by this intervention. Studies are underway to address these issues. At the time of writing, as tPA is not available for widespread clinical use or approved by the Bureau of Biologics, the very early (<4 h from the onset of chest pain) administration of intravenous or, if possible within this time interval, intracoronary SK, followed by percutaneous transluminal coronary angioplasty (PTCA) if a severe (>80 percent luminal diameter) obstruction persists appears to be a reasonable approach to therapy. The necessity of having a well-trained angiography team "stand by" at all times, will limit this approach to a small fraction of patients with acute myocardial infarction. However, if studies which are presently underway indicate that the intravenous infusion of tPA, followed by coronary arteriography within 1 or 2 days, and if necessary by PTCA, salvages substantial myocardium in the majority of patients, a practical approach for the treatment of acute myocardial infarction will have been found. The tPA would be given intravenously as soon as the diagnosis was established; it could be administered in an emergency room, ambulance, physician's office, even in the patient's home or work site. The patient would then be taken to a center where coronary arteriography or PTCA could be carried out within 2 days. This would not require standby of trained personnel and specialized facilities.

Acute primary PTCA, i.e., without preceding thrombolysis, has also been reported to be effective in restoring effective reperfusion in acute myocardial infarction, but this technique is very expensive in terms of personnel and facilities.

The amount of myocardial tissue which becomes necrotic secondary to a vascular occlusion is determined by factors other than just the site of occlusion. One such important factor is the status of collateral blood supply to ischemic tissue. Myocardium well supplied by collaterals clearly has the capacity to survive hours longer than poorly collateralized areas. Infarct size is now known to vary with time and be affected by a number of therapeutic agents currently in use. The balance between myocardial oxygen supply and demand in areas rendered ischemic determines the ultimate fate of these areas of jeopardized myocardium. While no routine therapeutic approach to reduce infarct size in all patients is currently recommended, the realization that infarct size may be increased by interventions which adversely alter the supply-demand balance has prompted the reevaluation of previously accepted therapeutic maneuvers in the management of patients with acute infarction.

TREATMENT OF THE PATIENT WITH AN UNCOMPLICATED INFARCT Analgesia

Since myocardial infarction usually presents with severe pain, one of the important initial therapeutic objectives is the relief of pain. Morphine, the agent traditionally used for this purpose, is an extremely effective analgesic for the pain associated with myocardial infarction. However, it may lower arterial pressure by reducing sympathetically mediated arteriolar and venous constriction. The resultant venous pooling may produce a reduction in cardiac output. This must be recognized but does not necessarily contraindicate its use. Hypotension associated with venous pooling usually responds promptly to elevation of the legs, but in some patients volume expansion with intravenous saline is required. The patient may experience diaphoresis and nausea, but these events usually pass and are replaced by a feeling of well-being associated with the relief of pain. It is important to recognize this syndrome as one attributable to morphine, rather than as a manifestation of the shock syndrome, so that inappropriate vasoconstrictor therapy is not initiated. Morphine also has a vagotonic effect and may cause bradycardia or advanced degrees of heart block, particularly in patients with posteroinferior infarction. These side effects of morphine usually respond to atropine (0.4 mg intravenously). Morphine is routinely administered by repetitive (every 5 min) intravenous injection of small doses of drug (2 to 4 mg) rather than by administration of a larger quantity by the subcutaneous route, by which absorption may be unpredictable. Meperidine hydrochloride or hydromorphone hydrochloride may be effectively employed in place of morphine.

Prior to administering morphine, sublingual nitroglycerin can be given safely to most patients with myocardial infarction. As long as hypotension does not occur, up to three 0.3-mg doses should be administered at about 5-min intervals. In addition to diminishing or abolishing chest discomfort, this form of therapy, once considered contraindicated in the setting of acute myocardial infarction, may be capable of both decreasing myocardial oxygen demand (by lowering preload) and increasing myocardial oxygen supply (by dilating infarct-related coronary vessels or collateral vessels). However, therapy with nitrates should be avoided in patients who present with a low systolic arterial pressure (<100 mmHg). The potential for an idiosyncratic reaction to nitrates, consisting of sudden marked hypotension and bradycardia, should be recognized. This problem, occurring more frequently in patients with inferior wall infarction, can usually be promptly reversed by the rapid administration of intravenous atropine.

Intravenous beta blockers are also useful in the control of the pain of acute myocardial infarction. These drugs have been shown to control pain effectively in some patients, presumably by diminishing ischemia consequent to lowering myocardial oxygen demand. More importantly, there is some evidence that intravenous beta blockers reduce in-hospital mortality, particularly in high-risk patients. Dosing similar to that used to treat the hyperdynamic state (see above) may be utilized.

Oxygen The routine use of oxygen is supported by the observation that the arterial P_{O_2} is reduced in many patients with myocardial infarction and that oxygen inhalation reduces the area of ischemic injury in experimental animals. Inhalation of oxygen increases arterial P_{O_2} and hence increases the concentration gradient responsible for the diffusion of oxygen into the ischemic myocardium from adjacent, better-perfused areas. Although oxygen therapy has been associated with theoretically deleterious effects such as elevation of systemic vascular resistance and slight reduction of cardiac output, the weight of evidence favors its administration. It should be administered by face mask or nasal prongs for the first day or two after infarction.

Activity Factors which increase the work of the heart may increase the size of the infarct. Circumstances in which heart size, cardiac output, or myocardial contractility are increased should be avoided. It has been demonstrated that 6 to 8 weeks are required for complete healing, i.e., replacement of the infarcted myocardium by scar tissue. The purpose of reduced physical activity is to provide the most favorable possible circumstances for this healing.

Most patients with myocardial infarction should be admitted to a coronary care unit or suitable monitoring facility and remain there for 2 to 4 days under constant observation by trained personnel utilizing continuous electrocardiographic monitoring. A catheter should be introduced into a peripheral vein, firmly fixed so that it is not easily dislodged, and be kept open either by the slow infusion of isotonic glucose solution or by a closed heparin lock. This provides a route of administration for antiarrhythmic or other drugs which may be necessary. In the absence of heart failure or other complications during the first 2 to 3 days, the patient should be in bed most of the day, with one or two periods of 15 to 30 min in a bedside chair. The patient may use a bedside commode and should be bathed but may eat unassisted. Bedside commode privileges are given to all hemodynamically stable patients with a stable rhythm from the first day. The bed should be equipped with a footboard, and the patient should push both feet against the footboard firmly 10 times during each waking hour to prevent venous stasis and thromboembolism and to maintain muscle tone in the legs.

By the third or fourth day the patient with an uncomplicated course should be spending at least 30 to 60 min in a chair twice a day. At this time the patient's blood pressure should be measured when standing in order to be aware of postural hypotension, which may be a problem when ambulation is begun. Standing and gradual ambulation are usually begun between the third and fifth days post infarction in patients with uncomplicated myocardial infarction. Initial walking is to the bathroom if it is in the patient's room or nearby. Ambulation is progressively increased, eventually including walks about the hospital floor. In many hospitals a cardiac rehabilitation program with progressive exercise is initiated in the hospital and continued after discharge. The total duration of hospitalization in uncomplicated cases is usually 7 to 12 days, but some physicians still hospitalize patients with Q-wave infarction for 3 weeks. Patients in clinical class II or higher may require 3 or more weeks of hospitalization, depending upon the rapidity with which heart failure resolves and the home situation to which the patient is returning. Many physicians perform a limited (heart rate–limited) exercise tolerance test just prior to discharge in selected patients with myocardial infarction. Such testing identifies high-risk patients as those who develop angina, ST-segment change, hypotension, or serious ventricular ectopic activity during or immediately following exercise. These patients require special attention, including measures such as antiarrhythmic drugs for ectopic activity, and beta-adrenergic blockers, long-acting nitrates, and/or calcium channel blocking agents for evidence of ischemia. If ischemia occurs at rest, or if during limited exercise ischemia and/or hypotension occur, coronary arteriography should be carried out. If a large quantity of viable myocardium, perfused by critically narrowed vessel(s), is found at angiography, then revascularization (either by operation or by angioplasty) may be required. Exercise tests also aid in formulating an individualized exercise prescription, which can be much more vigorous in patients who tolerate exercise without any of the above-mentioned adverse signs. Additionally, predischarge stress testing may provide an important psychological benefit related to building the patient's confidence through the demonstration of reasonable exercise tolerance. Furthermore, particularly when no arrhythmias or signs of ischemia are identified, the patient benefits by the physician's reassurance that objective evidence suggests no immediate jeopardy.

The remainder of the convalescent phase of myocardial infarction may be accomplished at home. From 3 to 8 weeks, the patient should be encouraged to increase activity by walking about the house and outdoors in good weather. Patients should still spend 8 to 10 h in bed each night. Additional rest periods in the morning and afternoon may be advisable for selected patients.

From 8 weeks onward, the physician must regulate the patient's activity on the basis of his or her exercise tolerance. It is during this period of increasing activity that the patient may become aware of profound fatigue. Postural hypotension may still be a problem. Most patients will be able to return to work after 12 weeks, and many patients much earlier. A maximal exercise test is frequently performed after 6 to 8 weeks or prior to returning to work. A trend toward earlier ambulation, hospital discharge, and resumption of full activity for patients recuperating from acute myocardial infarction has developed in recent years.

Diet During the first 4 or 5 days, a low-calorie diet divided into multiple small feedings is preferred. Cardiac output increases following ingestion of food, and therefore the quantity of individual feedings should be kept low. If heart failure is present, sodium intake should be restricted. Since constipation is common, it is reasonable to give average or even increased amounts of bulk in the diet. In addition, the ingestion of potassium-rich foods should be encouraged in patients receiving diuretics. During the second week, increasing amounts of food may be introduced into the diet. At this time, the importance of restriction of calories, cholesterol, and saturated fat may be explained to the patient, and he or she can be started on an appropriate diet. Willingness to accept dietary restriction and to discontinue cigarette smoking is usually never greater than it is during this early period of convalescence.

Bowels Bed rest of 3 to 5 days and the effect of the narcotics utilized for the relief of pain often lead to constipation. Most patients are not comfortable using a bedpan, which frequently results in excessive straining. A bedside commode, a diet rich in bulk, and the routine use of a stool softener such as dioctyl sodium sulfosuccinate, 200 mg daily, are recommended. If the patient remains constipated despite these measures, a laxative can be safely used. It is safe to perform a gentle rectal examination on patients with acute myocardial infarction.

Sedation Most patients require sedation during hospitalization in order to withstand the period of enforced inactivity with tranquillity. Diazepam 5 mg or oxazepam 15 to 30 mg given four times daily is usually effective. Appropriate sleeping medication may be given at night to ensure adequate sleep. Triazolam 0.25 to 0.5 mg is a rapid-onset, short-acting benzodiazepine ideal for inducing sleep. If maintenance of sleep is required, then temazepam 15 to 30 mg or flurazepam 15 to 30 mg can be used. Attention to this problem is especially important during the first few days in the coronary care unit, where the atmosphere of 24-h vigilance may interfere with the patient's sleep. Sedation is no substitute for reassuring, quiet surroundings.

Anticoagulants Few topics are more controversial than the use of anticoagulants in the routine treatment of acute myocardial infarction. The lack of a confirmed, statistically clear-cut demonstration of a lower mortality rate in the first few weeks following myocardial infarction suggests that the benefit of anticoagulant therapy, if any, is small. The use of anticoagulant therapy to retard the process of coronary occlusion during the initial phases of the illness, while not clearly justified, is undergoing renewed interest as a result of the recognition that thrombosis plays an important role in the pathogenesis of acute myocardial infarction. However, there is agreement that anticoagulant therapy does reduce the incidence of both arterial and venous thromboembolic complications. Since the incidence of venous thromboembolic disease is known to be increased in patients with heart failure, shock, and previous venous or thromboembolic disease, the routine, prophylactic use of anticoagulant drugs to prevent pulmonary embolism in the coronary care unit is recommended for those patients at high risk for this complication. Routine anticoagulation as prophylaxis against venous thromboembolism is not rec-

ommended in class I patients. Patients in classes III and IV are at greater risk for pulmonary embolism, and therefore systemic anticoagulation should be considered during the initial 10 to 14 days of hospitalization, or until they are ambulatory. This is best accomplished initially by the continuous intravenous administration of heparin with a constant infusion pump with measurement of the clotting time or partial thromboplastin time to define the need for increasing or decreasing the infusion rate. Once the patient is out of the intensive care area, oral anticoagulants may be substituted for heparin. Alternatively, small subcutaneous doses of heparin (5000 units every 8 to 12 h) can be employed. Controversy as to the need for anticoagulant therapy in class II patients persists. It seems appropriate to anticoagulate these patients if the signs of congestive heart failure persist for more than 3 or 4 days or if they have large anterior infarctions.

The incidence of arterial embolism from clot originating in the ventricle at the site of infarct is small but definite. Two-dimensional echocardiography allows for the early detection of left ventricular thrombi in about one-third of patients with anterior wall infarction but rarely in patients with inferior or posterior infarction. Arterial embolism often presents as a major complication, such as hemiparesis when the cerebral circulation is involved, or hypertension if the renal circulation is compromised. The low incidence of these complications, contrasted with their severity, renders it impractical to establish firm guidelines for the use of anticoagulant drugs as prophylaxis against arterial embolism in acute myocardial infarction. The likelihood of arterial embolism appears to increase with the extent of infarction and the resultant inflammation and endocardial stasis due to akinesis. Therefore, as is the case with venous thromboembolism, the indication for anticoagulation as prophylaxis against arterial embolism increases with the extent of infarction. When a thrombus has been clearly demonstrated by echocardiographic or other techniques, systemic anticoagulation should be undertaken (in the absence of contraindications), for the incidence of embolic complications appears to be markedly lowered by such therapy. The appropriate duration of therapy is unknown, but probably should be carried out for 3 to 6 months.

Beta-adrenergic blockers Use of intravenous beta-adrenergic blockers is discussed on page 986. The chronic routine use of oral beta-adrenergic blockers for at least 2 years following acute myocardial infarction is supported by several well-conducted placebo-controlled trials which have demonstrated reductions in total mortality, sudden death, and in some instances, the reinfarction rate. Patients are ordinarily begun on oral beta blockers 5 to 28 days following the acute event. Propranolol in a dose of 60 to 80 mg tid, or an equivalent dose of a more slowly acting beta blocker, is usually prescribed. Contraindications include congestive heart failure, bradyarrhythmias, heart block, hypotension, asthma, and "brittle" insulin-dependent diabetes mellitus.

TREATMENT Arrhythmias (see also Chaps. 183 and 184) The improved management of arrhythmias constitutes a most significant advance in the treatment of myocardial infarction.

VENTRICULAR PREMATURE SYSTOLES Infrequent, sporadic ventricular premature depolarizations occur in almost all patients with infarction and do not require therapy. Suggested indications for suppression of ventricular ectopic beats are generally considered to be the following: (1) the presence of more than five isolated ectopic beats per minute, (2) the occurrence of consecutive or multifocal ventricular extrasystoles, and (3) the occurrence of ectopic ventricular beats early in diastole and hence superimposed on the T wave of the preceding beat (the so-called R-on-T phenomenon). Intravenous lidocaine has become the treatment of choice for ventricular premature beats and ventricular arrhythmias, because it acts rapidly and side effects disappear soon (15 to 20 min) after its administration is discontinued. Lidocaine is given as an intravenous bolus of 1 mg/kg to establish adequate blood levels quickly. This initial dose usually eliminates the ectopic activity, if present, and is followed by an infusion of 2 to 4 mg/min. An additional bolus of 0.5 mg/kg is given 10 min after the initial bolus if ectopy is still present. The dose should be reduced by half in patients with congestive heart failure, shock, or hepatic disease. Usually, ventricular premature beats spontaneously disappear after 72 to 96 h. If significant ventricular ectopic activity persists past this time, chronic antiarrhythmic therapy is often initiated.

Procainamide, tocainide, and quinidine are commonly used for the treatment of persistent ventricular ectopic activity; beta-adrenergic blocking agents and disopyramide are also effective in abolishing ventricular ectopic activity in infarction patients. The latter agent should be used with great care in patients with left ventricular failure since it has a significant negative inotropic action. If the usual doses of these drugs (Chap. 184), singly or in combination, are not effective, blood levels should be measured to ensure that adequate blood concentrations are being obtained. Frequent clinical and electrocardiographic assessment of the patient for signs of drug toxicity is mandatory when higher doses of these agents are employed.

VENTRICULAR TACHYCARDIA AND VENTRICULAR FIBRILLATION Within the first 24 h of myocardial infarction, ventricular tachycardia and fibrillation often occur without prior warning arrhythmias. The occurrence of such primary arrhythmias can be materially reduced by prophylactic administration of intravenous lidocaine. The use of prophylactic antiarrhythmic drug therapy is particularly well suited to patients who cannot reach a hospital or those treated in hospitals that lack constant physician presence in the coronary care unit. Sustained ventricular tachycardia is treated first with lidocaine, and if it cannot be terminated by one or two 50- to 100-mg doses, electroconversion should be employed (Chap. 184). Electroshock is used immediately in patients with ventricular fibrillation, or when ventricular tachycardia causes hemodynamic deterioration. If fibrillation has persisted for more than a few seconds, the first shock may be unsuccessful, and in this situation it is advisable to administer closed-chest massage, mouth-to-mouth respiration, and intravenous sodium bicarbonate solution (40 to 90 meq) before attempting electroconversion again. Improvement of oxygenation and perfusion and correction of acidosis increase the likelihood of successful defibrillation (see also Chap. 30). Bretylium is useful in the treatment of both refractory ventricular fibrillation and ventricular tachycardia. For ventricular fibrillation, bretylium is given as a 5-mg/kg bolus and defibrillation is again attempted. If the latter fails, a second bolus of 10 mg/kg is given to facilitate electroconversion of ventricular fibrillation. Ventricular tachycardia can be treated with bretylium 5 to 10 mg/kg injected slowly over 10 min. In either situation, the initial dose of bretylium may be followed by a continuous infusion of 2 mg/min if the arrhythmia is recurrent. Severe postural hypotension occurs after intravenous bretylium administration; therefore, patients should always be supine when and immediately after the drug is given, and intravenous fluids should be available for rapid administration if needed.

Long-term survival is good in patients with *primary* ventricular fibrillation, i.e., ventricular fibrillation resulting as a primary response to acute ischemia and not associated with predisposing factors such as congestive heart failure, shock, bundle branch block, or ventricular aneurysm. In one series, 87 percent of patients with primary ventricular fibrillation left the hospital alive. This prognosis is in sharp contrast to that for patients who develop ventricular fibrillation *secondary* to severe pump failure. Only 29 percent of patients in this group survived.

In patients who develop ventricular tachycardia late in their hospital course, the mortality in 1 year may be as high as 85 percent. Such patients warrant electrophysiologic study (Chap. 184).

ACCELERATED IDIOVENTRICULAR RHYTHM Accelerated idioventricular rhythm (AIVR, "slow ventricular tachycardia"), a ventricular rhythm with a rate of 60 to 100 beats per minute, occurs in 25 percent of patients with myocardial infarction. It is especially frequent in inferoposterior infarction, where it is usually associated with sinus bradycardia. The rate of AIVR is usually similar to that of the sinus rhythm which precedes and follows it, and this similarity of rate and the relatively minor hemodynamic effects make this rhythm difficult to detect other than by electrocardiographic monitoring. The rhythm comes and goes spontaneously as fluctuation in sinus rate causes the atrial rate to fall below the accelerated escape level. For the most part, this rhythm is benign and does not presage the development of classic ventricular tachycardia. However, a number of cases have been documented wherein AIVR was associated with more dangerous forms of ventricular ectopic activity or where AIVR degenerated into a potentially fatal ventricular arrhythmia. Most AIVR does not require treatment if the patient is monitored carefully since degeneration into a more serious arrhythmias is rare, and if it occurs, the AIVR can generally be readily treated with a drug which decreases the ventricular escape rate, such as tocainide, and/or one that increases the sinus rate (atropine).

SUPRAVENTRICULAR ARRHYTHMIAS The common arrhythmias in this group are junctional rhythm and tachycardia, atrial tachycardia, atrial flutter, and atrial fibrillation. These rhythm disturbances are often secondary to left ventricular failure. The administration of digoxin is usually the treatment of choice. If the abnormal rhythm persists for more than 2 h with a ventricular rate in excess of 120 beats per minute, or at any time when tachycardia induces heart failure, shock, or ischemia (as manifested by recurrent pain or ECG changes), electroshock should be utilized.

Junctional arrhythmias are of diverse etiology, are not indicative of any specific abnormality, and from a therapeutic viewpoint must be considered on an individual basis. Digitalis excess must be ruled out as a cause of junctional tachycardia. In some patients with severely compromised left ventricular function, the loss of appropriately timed atrial systole results in a marked decrease in cardiac output. Right atrial or coronary sinus pacing is indicated in such instances. The hemodynamic effects of these two modes of pacing are identical, but coronary sinus pacing offers the advantage of better catheter stability.

SINUS BRADYCARDIA The significance of bradycardia as a factor predisposing to ventricular fibrillation in acute myocardial infarction is controversial. While the incidence of ventricular tachycardia in patients with sustained bradycardia is twice that observed in patients with normal heart rates, sinus bradycardia has also been identified in hospitalized patients as an index of a favorable prognosis. Experience with mobile coronary care units indicates that sinus bradycardia occurring within the first hour after infarction is more consistently associated with ventricular ectopic rhythms than that occurring later in the course of the illness. Treatment of sinus bradycardia is indicated if significant ventricular ectopic activity is present or if hemodynamic compromise results from the slow heart rate. Elevation of the legs and/or the foot of the bed is frequently helpful in the treatment of sinus bradycardia. Atropine is the most useful drug for increasing heart rate and should be given intravenously in doses of 0.4 to 0.6 mg. If the rate remains below 60 beats per minute, additional doses of 0.2 mg, up to a total of 2.0 mg, may be given in divided doses. Persistent bradycardia (< 40 beats per minute) despite atropine may be treated with electrical pacing. Isoproterenol should be avoided.

CONDUCTION DISTURBANCES Failure of conduction may develop at three different levels in the conduction system: the atrioventricular (AV) node, the bundle of His, or the more peripheral portions of the conduction system (Chap. 183). If the block occurs in the AV node, the escape rhythm usually originates in the AV junction, and the QRS complexes are usually of normal duration; but when the block occurs distal to the AV node, the escape site is ventricular, and the QRS configuration is abnormal and its duration is prolonged. Disturbances of conduction may occur in the three peripheral branches (fascicles) of the conduction system, and their recognition is of value in identifying patients at risk of developing complete heart block. When block occurs in any two of the three fascicles, bifascicular block is said to exist; complete AV block often develops in such patients. Thus, patients who develop the combination of right bundle branch block and either left anterior or left posterior hemiblock or patients with new left bundle branch block have a particularly high risk of progression to complete heart block.

The mortality rate of patients with complete AV block in association with anterior infarction (80 to 90 percent) is almost three times that of patients who develop AV block with inferior infarction (30 percent), and the risk of subsequent death in those who survive to leave the hospital is also increased in the former group. This difference is related to the fact that heart block in inferior infarction is usually caused by AV nodal ischemia. The AV node is a small discrete structure, and thus a small amount of ischemia or necrosis can result in AV nodal dysfunction. In anterior wall infarction, heart block is related to ischemic malfunction of all three fascicles of the conduction system and thus results only from extensive myocardial necrosis.

Electrical pacing provides an effective means of increasing the heart rate of patients with bradycardia due to AV block, but it is not possible to be sure that such acceleration is always beneficial. For example, in patients with anterior wall infarction and complete heart block, the large size of the infarct is the major factor determining the outcome, and correction of the conduction deficit does not clearly improve the poor prognosis in this group. Pacing does appear to be beneficial, however, in patients with inferoposterior infarction who have complete heart block associated with heart failure, hypotension, marked bradycardia, or significant ventricular ectopic activity. A subgroup of these patients, those with right ventricular infarction, often respond poorly to ventricular pacing because of the loss of the atrial "kick." In such patients, dual chamber, atrioventricular sequential pacing may be required.

Some cardiologists advocate the placement of a pacing catheter prophylactically in patients with conduction disturbances known to be precursors of complete heart block. Unanimity of opinion does not exist on this point. Permanent pacing has been advocated for patients who develop the combination of persistent bifascicular and transient third-degree heart block during the acute phase of myocardial infarction. Retrospective studies in small numbers of such patients suggest that the incidence of sudden death is decreased in those in whom permanent pacing was instituted.

Heart failure   Some degree of transient impairment of left ventricular function occurs in over half of patients with myocardial infarction. The most common clinical signs are pulmonary rales and S_3 and S_4 gallop rhythms. Pulmonary congestion is also frequently seen on chest roentgenogram. However, roentgenographic signs of pulmonary congestion often fail to parallel, temporally, clinical evidence of pulmonary congestion, i.e., the presence of rales and dyspnea. Elevation of left ventricular filling pressure and pulmonary artery pressure are the characteristic hemodynamic findings, but it should be appreciated that these findings may result from a reduction of diastolic ventricular compliance (diastolic failure) and/or a reduction of stroke volume with secondary cardiac dilatation (systolic failure) (Chap. 181). The therapy of heart failure in association with myocardial infarction is similar to that of heart failure secondary to other forms of heart disease, with a few exceptions (Chap. 182). The major difference concerns the use of cardiac glycosides. The benefit following the administration of digitalis in acute myocardial infarction is unimpressive. This is not surprising since the function of the noninfarcted tissue may be normal and digitalis would not be expected to improve the systolic or diastolic dysfunction of infarcted or ischemic tissue. On the other hand, diuretic agents are extremely effective in the treatment of heart failure following myocardial infarction, since they diminish pulmonary congestion in the presence of systolic and/or diastolic heart failure. A fall in left ventricular filling pressure and an improvement in orthopnea and dyspnea follow the intravenous administration of furosemide. This drug should be used with caution, however, as it can result in a massive diuresis with associated decrease in plasma volume, cardiac output, systemic blood pressure, and hence coronary perfusion. Nitrates in various forms may be used to decrease

preload and congestive symptoms. Oral isosorbide dinitrate or topical nitroglycerin ointment have the advantage over a diuretic of lowering preload through venodilatation without decreasing the total plasma volume. Additionally, nitrates may improve ventricular compliance if concurrent ischemia is present, since ischemia causes an elevation of left ventricular filling pressure. The patient with pulmonary edema is treated in the manner described in Chap. 182. Studies with vasodilators to reduce cardiac afterload indicate that the reduction in cardiac work, which results from the lowered afterload, may significantly improve left ventricular performance with a reduction of ventricular filling pressure and pulmonary congestion concomitant with an elevation of cardiac output.

Hemodynamic monitoring   Hemodynamic evidence of abnormal left ventricular function becomes apparent when contraction is seriously impaired in 20 to 25 percent of the left ventricle. Infarction of 40 percent or more of the left ventricle usually results in the syndrome of cardiogenic shock (see below). Pulmonary capillary wedge pressure and pulmonary artery diastolic pressure correlate well with left ventricular diastolic pressure and are therefore often referred to as left ventricular filling pressures. Positioning of a balloon flotation catheter in the pulmonary artery enables the physician to monitor left ventricular filling pressure constantly, a technique which is useful in patients who exhibit clinical evidence of hemodynamic abnormalities or instability. Cardiac output can also be determined with a pulmonary artery catheter. With the addition of intraarterial pressure monitoring, systemic vascular resistance can be calculated as a guide to adjusting vasopressor and vasodilator therapy. Some patients with acute myocardial infarction have markedly elevated left ventricular filling pressures (>22 mmHg) and normal cardiac outputs [>2.6 and <3.6 (liters/min)/m²], while others have relatively low filling pressures (<15 mmHg) and reduced cardiac outputs. The former usually benefit from diuresis, while the latter respond to volume expansion by means of intravenous administration of colloid-containing solutions.

Cardiogenic shock—power failure   With the development of effective methods for treating arrhythmias, cardiogenic shock has become the most important fatal complication of acute myocardial infarction for patients who reach the hospital. It occurs in approximately 10 percent of such patients and now accounts for about two-thirds of in-hospital deaths. Unfortunately, improvements in care have not affected the mortality rate in patients with acute myocardial infarction and cardiogenic shock (Killip class IV), which continues to be in the 85 to 95 percent range.

It is useful to consider cardiogenic shock as a form of severe left ventricular failure. This syndrome is characterized by marked hypotension with systolic arterial pressure <80 mmHg and a marked reduction of cardiac index [<1.8 (liters/min)/m²] in the face of elevated left ventricular filling (pulmonary capillary wedge) pressure >18 mmHg. Hypotension alone is not a basis for the diagnosis of cardiogenic shock, because many patients who make an uneventful recovery will have serious hypotension (systolic pressure <80 mmHg) for several days. Such patients often have low left ventricular filling pressures, and their hypotension usually resolves with intravenous administration of colloid-containing solutions. In cardiogenic shock hypotension is accompanied by other clinical signs of circulatory inadequacy. The following *clinical* criteria for cardiogenic shock define a population of patients with a mortality rate of >85 percent: (1) systolic arterial blood pressure <90 mmHg which has declined by at least 30 mmHg below the previous level; (2) clinical signs of peripheral circulatory insufficiency, e.g., cold, moist skin and cyanosis; (3) dulled sensorium; (4) oliguria with urine flow of less than 20 mL/h; and (5) failure of improvement following relief of pain and administration of oxygen. Specifically *excluded* are patients with hypotension secondary to vasovagal reaction, hypovolemia, arrhythmia, drug reaction, or sepsis.

PATHOPHYSIOLOGY OF PUMP FAILURE   Marked reduction in the quantity of contracting myocardium is the cause of cardiogenic shock in myocardial infarction, although all organ systems are ultimately involved. The function of the heart is impaired by the initial insult; this results in a decrease in arterial pressure and hence in coronary blood flow because of its dependence on aortic perfusion pressure (Fig. 190-2). The reduction in coronary perfusion pressure and myocardial blood flow further impairs myocardial function and may increase the size of the myocardial infarction. Arrhythmias and metabolic acidosis also contribute to this deterioration because they are the result of inadequate perfusion, and both tend to perpetuate the precipitating conditions. It is this positive feedback loop which accounts for the high mortality rate associated with the shock syndrome.

Arterial blood pressure is a function of two factors—cardiac output and systemic vascular resistance—and a decrease in either without a compensatory rise in the other will result in a fall in arterial blood pressure. Cardiac output is lower in a population of patients with myocardial infarction and shock. However many patients with myocardial infarction without shock have cardiac outputs in the same range as those in patients with shock, and therefore it is not possible to characterize these patients on the basis of reductions of cardiac output alone. Systemic vascular resistance, the other factor important in determining blood pressure, may be either normal or increased in myocardial infarction. Normally, a fall in cardiac output is accompanied by a compensatory rise in systemic vascular resistance, but in patients with shock due to myocardial infarction, the appropriate elevation in resistance may fail to occur. However, it is necessary to return to the heart itself as the site of the fundamental physiologic alteration in cardiogenic shock.

A simple schematic diagram depicting the relationship between left ventricular work and filling pressure is seen in Fig 190-3. The upper curve represents the familiar Frank-Starling relationship in the normal heart; the lower curve shows the relation which might be expected in the patient with shock secondary to myocardial infarction. It is obvious that, at all levels of end-diastolic pressure, the left ventricular work of the patient with myocardial infarction is depressed. At point C, the end-diastolic pressure is elevated, but at point B, it may be normal despite the fact that myocardial work is well below that expected of the normal heart at this diastolic pressure, as indicated by point A.

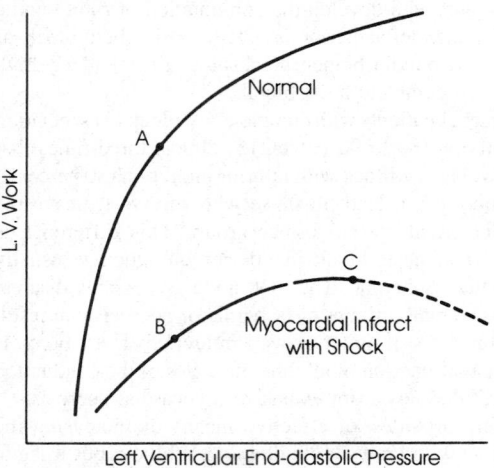

FIGURE 190-3 *Schematic representation of the Frank-Starling relationship as applied to patients with the shock syndrome in myocardial infarction.*

TREATMENT OF PUMP FAILURE   The physiology and ominous prognosis associated with this condition dictate that all patients with shock should, if possible, have continuous monitoring of arterial pressure and of left ventricular filling pressure (as reflected in the pulmonary capillary wedge pressure measured with a pulmonary artery balloon catheter) as well as frequent determinations of cardiac output. All patients with the shock syndrome should receive 100% oxygen continuously to help combat the hypoxemia which is universally present. When pulmonary edema coexists, endotracheal intubation may be necessary to ensure oxygenation. The relief of pain is important, as some vasodepressor reflex activity may be a response to severe pain. However, narcotics should be used cautiously in view of their propensity to lower arterial pressure.

Treatment is directed at the interruption of the feedback loop (Fig. 190-2), whereby impaired myocardial function leads to a reduction in arterial pressure, decreased coronary blood flow, and further depression of left ventricular function. This objective is approached by attempting to maintain coronary perfusion by raising the arterial blood pressure with vasopressors (see below), intraaortic balloon counterpulsation, and manipulation of blood volume to a level that ensures an optimum left ventricular filling pressure (approximately 20 mmHg). The latter may require either infusion of crystalloid or diuresis. In patients seen within the first 4 h of the onset of infarction, reperfusion by thrombolytic therapy and/or PTCA (page 985) may improve left ventricular function dramatically.

Hypovolemia   This is an easily corrected condition which may contribute to the hypotension and vascular collapse associated with myocardial infarction in some patients. Fluid loss may be secondary to previous diuretic use, to reduced fluid intake during the early stages of the illness, and/or to vomiting associated with pain or medications. In addition, a state of relative hypovolemia may exist; i.e., with the acute reduction in contractile function and ventricular compliance resulting from infarction an increase in vascular volume is needed to maintain cardiac output. Owing to the acute nature of the process, there is insufficient time for compensatory fluid retention to accommodate this need, and relative hypovolemia in a normally hydrated patient results. Consequently, hypovolemia should be identified and corrected in patients with acute myocardial infarction and hypotension before embarking upon more vigorous forms of therapy. If left ventricular filling pressure is in the normal range, fluid should be administered until the cardiac output is maximized. This usually occurs at a left ventricular filling pressure of approximately 20 mmHg. However, the optimal left ventricular filling or pulmonary artery wedge pressure may vary considerably among different patients. Each patient's ideal level is reached by cautious fluid administration during

FIGURE 190-2 *Diagram depicting the sequence of events in the vicious cycle in which coronary artery obstruction leads to cardiogenic shock and progressive circulatory deterioration.*

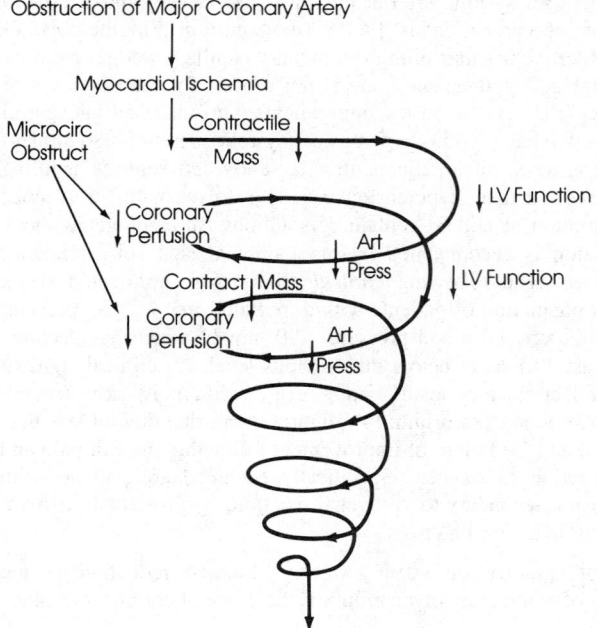

careful monitoring of oxygenation and cardiac output. When the cardiac output plateaus (Fig. 190-3, point C), further increases in left ventricular filling pressure will only increase congestive symptoms and decrease systemic oxygenation. Central venous pressure measurements reflect right rather than left ventricular filling pressure and are inadequate in this situation, since left ventricular function is almost always affected much more adversely than is right ventricular function in acute myocardial infarction.

VASOPRESSORS   A variety of intravenous drugs may be used to augment arterial pressure and cardiac output in patients with cardiogenic shock. Unfortunately, all have important disadvantages or problems associated with their use, and none have been shown to change the outcome in patients with established shock. *Isoproterenol* is a synthetic sympathomimetic amine which is now rarely used in the treatment of shock due to myocardial infarction. Although this agent increases contractility, it also produces peripheral vasodilatation and increases heart rate. The resultant increase in myocardial oxygen consumption and reduction of coronary perfusion pressure may extend the area of ischemic injury. *Norepinephrine* is a potent alpha-adrenergic agent with powerful vasoconstrictive properties. It also possesses beta-adrenergic activity and therefore enhances contractility. Norepinephrine can be effective in raising arterial pressure, but usually the increase in afterload and contractility associated with its use cause a marked increase in myocardial oxygen consumption as well. It should be reserved for relatively desperate situations or for patients with cardiogenic shock and lowered systemic vascular resistance. It should be used at the lowest dose possible (begin infusion at 2 to 4 µg/min) to maintain systolic blood pressure near 90 mmHg. If pressure cannot be maintained with a dosage of 15µg/min, it is unlikely that a further increase will be beneficial.

Dopamine (Chap. 66) is useful in many patients with power failure. At low doses [2 to 10 (µg/kg)/min] the drug has positive chronotropic and inotropic effects as a consequence of stimulation of beta receptors. At higher doses, a vasoconstrictive effect as a result of the stimulation of alpha receptors is also noted. Dopamine at lower doses [≤2 (µg/kg)/min] also has the unique effect of dilating the renal and splanchnic vascular beds and apparently has little effect on myocardial oxygen consumption. Intravenous dopamine is started at an infusion rate of 2 to 5 (µg/kg)/min with increments in dosage every 2 to 5 min up to a maximum of 20 to 50 (µg/kg)/min. Systolic arterial blood pressure should be maintained at approximately 90 mmHg. *Dobutamine* is a synthetic sympathomimetic amine with positive inotropic action and minimal positive chronotropic or peripheral vasoconstrictive activity in the usual dosage range [2.5 to 10 (µg/kg)/min]. It should not be employed when a vasoconstrictor effect is deemed desirable. However, in patients with less profound degrees of hypotension, dobutamine may be an extremely useful agent, particularly if positive chronotropy is to be avoided.

Amrinone (see page 912) is a positive inotropic agent without catecholamine structure or activity. It resembles dobutamine in its pharmacologic activity, although its vasodilating effect appears to be more potent. Initially a loading dose of 0.75 mg/kg is given. If effective, this is followed by an infusion of 10 (µg/kg)/min, followed if necessary 30 min later by an additional bolus of 0.75 mg/kg.

Patients with global left ventricular ischemia as the cause of power failure and profound hypotension, such as those with critical left main coronary artery obstructive disease, may benefit from brief treatment with a pure vasoconstrictor in preference to a positive inotropic agent. In such cases coronary perfusion may be improved by the vasoconstrictor-induced increase in arterial pressure, whereas a positive inotropic agent may only increase ischemic injury in muscle that is incapable of performing more work. In this situation a vasoconstrictor such as *neosynephrine,* 10 to 100 µg/min, should be used, as briefly as possible, usually only as interim therapy while preparations are made for counterpulsation with an interaortic balloon pump and/or emergency coronary artery surgery.

CARDIAC GLYCOSIDES (Chap. 182)   Consideration of the central role of impaired myocardial function in the shock syndrome leads to the conclusion that cardiac glycosides should be administered to patients with this condition. Controlled studies, however, have failed to demonstrate significant beneficial effects of glycoside therapy in the early phases (0 to 48 h) of acute myocardial infarction. Hemodynamic improvement has been documented at later times, but this effect, too, is marginal. Since cardiac glycosides cannot improve the function of necrotic myocardium and since pump failure is thought to be related to the total mass of infarcted tissue, digitalis therapy does not result in dramatic improvement in patients with acute myocardial infarction. Nonetheless, it may be useful to treat patients with signs and symptoms of left ventricular failure with digitalis. It has been demonstrated that when scrupulous attention is paid to the dosage, the incidence of arrhythmias and cardiac rupture is no higher in patients with myocardial infarction treated with digitalis than in a control group, and therefore digitalis can be administered with relative safety.

AORTIC COUNTERPULSATION   The basic defect in the shock syndrome is impaired myocardial function; therefore, mechanical assist devices have been developed to supplement the pumping action of the heart. The largest body of clinical experience has been obtained with the intraaortic balloon system of diastolic pressure augmentation. A sausage-shaped balloon at the end of a catheter is introduced into the aorta via the femoral artery, and the balloon is inflated during early diastole, thereby enhancing both coronary blood flow and peripheral perfusion. The balloon collapses in early systole, thereby reducing the afterload against which left ventricular ejection takes place. Improvement in hemodynamic status has been observed with balloon pumping in a large number of patients, but long-term survival following this mode of therapy in patients with cardiogenic shock is still disappointing. The balloon counterpulsation system may best be reserved for patients whose condition merits surgical intervention (e.g., continuing ischemia, ventricular septal rupture, or mitral regurgitation) and in whom a successful surgical result is likely to result in the reversal of cardiogenic shock.

There is reason to believe that results of therapy of the shock syndrome secondary to myocardial infarction, while improving gradually as a result of meticulous attention to the details of therapy outlined above, will continue to be disappointing overall because a large fraction of patients with the syndrome have large areas of infarcted myocardium with severe, diffuse coronary atherosclerosis. Although occasional dramatic results have been reported with emergency revascularization surgery alone, or in combination with infarctectomy, the overall results with this approach, too, have been disappointing. It is hoped that early thrombolytic therapy will reduce the amount of myocardium which becomes necrotic and thereby reduce the incidence of this syndrome.

Other complications   MITRAL REGURGITATION   Apical systolic murmurs of mitral regurgitation appear in more than one-fourth of patients during the first 5 days after the onset of a myocardial infarction, but mitral regurgitation is of hemodynamic importance in only a minority of these patients. In most patients the murmur is present during the acute phase of infarction, disappearing with recovery. The most common cause of mitral regurgitation following myocardial infarction is dysfunction of the papillary muscles of the left ventricle due to ischemia or infarction.

Mitral regurgitation may also be the result of alteration in the size or shape of the ventricle due to impaired contractility or to aneurysm formation. Either papillary muscle may rupture, the posterior one twice as frequently as the anterior. Left ventricular function may deteriorate dramatically with superimposition of mitral regurgitation. The differential diagnosis includes perforation of the ventricular septum (see below), and the differentiation from mitral regurgitation is conveniently made at the bedside with a flow-directed balloon catheter. Large *v* waves may be recorded in the pulmonary capillary wedge position in patients with hemodynamically significant mitral regurgitation, and there is no oxygen ''step up'' as the catheter is advanced from the right atrium to the right ventricle. Surgical replacement of the mitral valve may be followed by dramatic improvement in patients in whom acute heart failure results primarily from severe mitral regurgitation due to papillary muscle rupture or dysfunction and in whom myocardial function is relatively well maintained.

If aortic systolic pressure is lowered in patients with mitral regurgitation, a greater fraction of the left ventricular output will be ejected antegrade, thus lessening the regurgitant fraction. To this end, both intraaortic balloon counterpulsation, which lowers the aortic systolic pressure mechanically, and the infusion of sodium nitroprusside, 0.5 to 8.0 (μg/kg)/min, which reduces systemic vascular resistance, have been used with success for the interim management of patients with severe mitral regurgitation in the setting of acute myocardial infarction. Ideally, definitive operative treatment should be postponed for 4 to 6 weeks after the infarct. However, if the patient's hemodynamic and/or clinical condition does not improve and stabilize, surgical treatment should be undertaken, even in the acute stage.

CARDIAC RUPTURE Myocardial rupture is a dramatic complication of myocardial infarction most likely to occur during the first week after the onset of symptoms; its frequency increases with the age of the patient. First infarction, female sex, and hypertension are associated with a higher incidence of cardiac rupture. The clinical presentation may often be that of a sudden disappearance of the pulse, blood pressure, and consciousness while the electrocardiogram continues to show sinus rhythm (*apparent* electromechanical dissociation). The myocardium continues to contract, but forward flow is not maintained as blood escapes into the pericardium. Cardiac tamponade (Chap. 194) ensues, and closed-chest massage is ineffective. Although almost universally fatal, there have been a few instances in which cardiac rupture has been recognized and successfully treated by pericardiocentesis and emergency cardiac surgery.

SEPTAL PERFORATION The pathogenesis of perforation of the ventricular septum is similar to that of external rupture of the myocardium, but the therapeutic potential is greater. Patients with ventricular septal rupture present with severe heart failure in association with the sudden appearance of a pansystolic murmur, often accompanied by a parasternal thrill. It is often impossible to differentiate this condition from rupture of a papillary muscle with resultant mitral regurgitation, and a tall *v* wave in the pulmonary capillary wedge pressure in both conditions further complicates the differentiation. The diagnosis can be established by the demonstration of a left-to-right shunt (i.e., an oxygen step-up at the level of the right ventricle) by limited cardiac catheterization performed at the bedside using a flow-directed balloon catheter. Rupture of the ventricular septum is amenable to immediate surgical treatment, albeit at a relatively high mortality rate, but this form of therapy is ordinarily indicated on an urgent basis in patients whose condition cannot be stabilized rapidly. A prolonged period of hemodynamic compromise may produce end-organ damage and other complications that can be avoided by early intervention including nitroprusside infusion and intraaortic balloon counterpulsation. If stabilization occurs, surgical intervention can be postponed for 4 to 8 weeks, to allow for formation of scar tissue at the margins of the defect, rendering surgical closure easier. However, mortality is primarily a function of the overall extent of myocardial damage rather than the timing of surgical treatment.

The physiology of acute mitral regurgitation and acute ventricular septal perforation are similar in that the level of aortic systolic pressure determines in part the regurgitant volume, the principal difference being the chamber into which the regurgitant fraction is ejected. In septal perforation, a fraction of left ventricular output is ejected into the right ventricle. In a manner analogous to mitral regurgitation, lowering of aortic systolic pressure by mechanical (intraaortic balloon counterpulsation) and/or pharmacologic (nitroglycerin or nitroprusside) means can decrease the hemodynamic compromise caused by perforation.

VENTRICULAR ANEURYSM The term *ventricular aneurysm* is usually used to describe *dyskinesis* or local expansile paradoxical wall motion. Normally functioning myocardial fibers must shorten more if stroke volume and cardiac output are to be maintained in patients with ventricular aneurysm, and if they are unable to do so, overall ventricular function is impaired. Aneurysms are composed of scar tissue and neither predispose to nor are associated with cardiac rupture.

The complications of left ventricular aneurysm do not usually occur for weeks to months following myocardial infarction; they include congestive heart failure, arterial embolism, and ventricular arrhythmias. Apical aneurysms are the most common and the most easily detected by clinical examination. The physical finding of greatest value is a double, diffuse, or displaced apical impulse. The standard roentgenogram frequently reveals an abnormal bulge distorting the contour of the left heart border, but the roentgenogram may be entirely normal, especially with posterior aneurysms. The electrocardiographic finding of ST-segment elevation at rest is present in precordial leads in 25 percent of patients with either apical or anterior aneurysms. Ventricular aneurysms are readily detectable by two-dimensional echocardiography, which may also reveal a mural thrombus in aneurysms involving the anterior wall and/or apex. Ventricular aneurysms may cause sustained ventricular tachycardia which requires treatment with antiarrhythmic drugs or endocardial resection (Chap. 184).

RIGHT VENTRICULAR INFARCTION Approximately one-third of patients with inferoposterior infarction demonstrate at least a minor degree of right ventricular necrosis. An occasional patient with inferoposterior left ventricular infarction also has extensive right ventricular myocardial infarction. These patients often present with signs of severe right ventricular failure (jugular venous distention, hepatomegaly) with or without hypotension. ST-segment elevations of the right-sided precordial electrocardiographic leads, particularly lead V_4R, are present in the majority of patients with right ventricular infarction. Radionuclide ventriculography and two-dimensional echocardiography are also sensitive in the detection of right ventricular damage associated with acute myocardial infarction. Catheterization of the right side of the heart often reveals a distinctive hemodynamic pattern resembling cardiac tamponade or constrictive pericarditis (Chap. 194). Volume expansion is often successful in treating low cardiac output and hypotension associated with extensive right ventricular infarction.

THROMBOEMBOLISM Clinically apparent thromboembolism complicates myocardial infarction in approximately 10 percent of cases, but embolic lesions are found in 45 percent of patients in necropsy series, suggesting that thromboembolism is often clinically silent. Thromboembolism is considered to be at least an important contributing cause of death in 25 percent of infarct patients who die following admission to the hospital. Arterial emboli originate from left ventricular mural thrombi, but most pulmonary emboli arise in the leg veins. Thromboembolism most commonly occurs in association with large infarcts in the presence of heart failure. Thromboembolism occurs extremely commonly in patients with echocardiographic evidence of a left ventricular thrombus, but only rarely if a thrombus is not present on the echocardiogram. Although well-controlled trials do not exist, the incidence of embolization appears to be decreased by anticoagulation.

PERICARDITIS (see also Chap. 194) Pericardial friction rubs and/or pericardial pain are frequently encountered in patients with acute transmural myocardial infarction. This complication can usually be managed with aspirin (650 mg qid). It is important to diagnose the chest pain of pericarditis accurately, since failure to appreciate it may lead to the erroneous diagnosis of recurrent ischemic pain and/or infarct extension with resultant inappropriate use of anticoagulants, nitrates, beta blockers, or narcotics. No definite cause and effect relationship between administration of anticoagulants and pericarditis or tamponade has been proved. Nonetheless, the possibility that anticoagulants can cause tamponade in the presence of acute pericarditis is sufficiently high to contraindicate their use in patients with pericarditis, as manifested by either pain or persistent rub, unless there is a compelling indication.

POSTMYOCARDIAL INFARCTION SYNDROME—DRESSLER'S SYNDROME (see also Chap. 194) This syndrome, characterized by fever and pleuropericardial chest pain, is thought to be due to an autoimmune pericarditis, pleuritis, and/or pneumonitis. It may begin from a few days to 6 weeks after myocardial infarction. The occurrence of Dressler's syndrome may be etiologically related to the early use of anticoagulants and appears to have decreased markedly in the last decade as anticoagulants are used less frequently in acute myocardial infarction. The syndrome usually responds promptly to therapy with salicylates. On occasion, corticosteroids may be required to relieve discomfort of an unusual, refractory nature. Effusions associated with Dressler's syndrome may become hemorrhagic if anticoagulants are administered.

REFERENCES

ALPERT JS, FRANCIS GS: *Manuel of Coronary Care*, 3d ed. Boston, Little, Brown, 1984
———, BRAUNWALD E: Acute myocardial infarction: Pathological and clinical manifestations, in *Heart Disease*, 2d ed, E Braunwald (ed). Philadelphia, Saunders, 1984, p 1262

CALIFF RM, WAGNER GS (eds): *Acute Coronary Care: Principles and Practice*. Boston, Martinus Nijhoff, 1985

CHADDA K et al: Effect of propranolol after acute myocardial infarction in patients with congestive heart failure. Circulation 73:503, 1986

COHN PF: The role of noninvasive cardiac testing after an uncomplicated myocardial infarction. N Engl J Med 390:90, 1983

DAVIES MJ, THOMAS AC: Plaque fissuring—The cause of acute myocardial infarction, sudden ischaemic death, and cresendo angina. Br Heart J 53:363, 1985

DEBUSK RF et al: Stepwise risk stratification soon after acute myocardial infarction. Am J Cardiol 52:1161, 1983

FRIEDMAN LM et al: Effect of propranolol in patients with myocardial infarction and ventricular arrhythmia. J Am Coll Cardiol 7:1, 1986

FRISHMAN WH et al: Beta-adrenergic blockade for survivors of acute myocardial infarction. N Engl J Med 310:830, 1984

GOLD HK et al: Acute coronary reocclusion after thrombolysis with recombinant human tissue-type plasminogen activator: Prevention by a maintenance infusion. Circulation 73:347, 1986

HJALMARSON A (ed): Miami: Metoprolol in acute myocardial infarction. Am J Cardiol 56:1G, 1985

KEEFE DL et al: Prophylactic tocainide or lidocaine in acute myocardial infarction. Am J Cardiol 57:527, 1986

KRONE RJ et al and the Multicenter Postinfarction Research Group: Low-level exercise testing after myocardial infarction: Usefulness in enhancing clinical risk stratification. Circulation 71:80, 1985

LAFFEL GL, BRAUNWALD E: Thrombolytic therapy: A new strategy for the treatment of acute myocardial infarction. N Engl J Med 311:710, 770, 1984

PAPAPRETRO SE et al: Percutaneous transluminal coronary angioplasty after intracoronary streptokinase in evolving myocardial infarction. Am J Cardiol 55:48, 1985

SOBEL BE, BRAUNWALD E: Management of acute myocardial infarction, in *Heart Disease*, 2d ed, E Braunwald (ed). Philadelphia, Saunders, 1984, p 1301

The TIMI Study Group: The thrombolysis in myocardial infarction (TIMI) trial: Phase I findings. N Engl J Med 312:932, 1985

191 COR PULMONALE

ALFRED P. FISHMAN

Cor pulmonale denotes enlargement of the right ventricle secondary to malfunctioning lungs. However, the abnormal performance of the lungs is not always due to intrinsic lung disease: in some instances, an abnormal chest bellows or a depressed ventilatory drive from the respiratory centers (Table 191-1) is the cause. If the cause is intrinsic to the lungs, the disease will be diffuse, bilateral, and extensive, in most cases affecting airways as well as parenchyma. As a rule, hypertrophy and dilatation contribute to the right ventricular enlargement; in chronic cor pulmonale hypertrophy is more apt to predominate than in acute cor pulmonale.

Pulmonary arterial hypertension invariably precedes cor pulmo-

nale. In practice, cor pulmonale is synonymous with pulmonary hypertensive heart disease, even though hypoxemia and polycythemia, as well as pulmonary hypertension, often contribute to overloading the right ventricle. But before making the diagnosis of cor pulmonale, *primary disease of the left side of the heart* and *congenital heart disease* must be excluded. It is worth emphasizing that the term *cor pulmonale* does not automatically imply heart failure. However, it is understood that if the pulmonary hypertension that led to enlargement of the right ventricle is not relieved, cor pulmonale will become associated with right ventricular failure.

Hypertrophy and/or dilatation of the right ventricle are usually much more difficult to detect and to quantify, both clinically and at autopsy, than are left ventricular hypertrophy and dilatation. Moreover, in dealing with right ventricular enlargement it is essential to understand the mechanisms that operated during life to impose an abnormal hemodynamic load upon it.

The definitions and reservations above have several practical implications. By underscoring the critical role that is played by some abnormality of the respiratory system in the pathogenesis of cor pulmonale, they underscore that prognosis and treatment of cor pulmonale *depend more on relieving the respiratory disorder than on improving the performance of the right ventricle.* Moreover, by stressing *enlargement* of the right ventricle as the hallmark of cor pulmonale—without distinguishing between dilatation and hypertrophy—they stress that pulmonary hypertension is an antecedent of cor pulmonale and that right ventricular failure is a consequence of both.

TYPES OF COR PULMONALE By tradition, the designation *acute* is generally reserved for the dilatation of the right side of the heart which follows acute embolization of the lungs. The designation *chronic* is less specific. Usually chronicity is judged by the type and duration of the respiratory disorder that led to the cardiac enlargement (Table 191-1). Just how long, and to what degree, the heart remains enlarged will depend on fluctuations in its workload, i.e., primarily pulmonary arterial pressure, but also cardiac output, polycythemia, heart rate, and the level of arterial hypoxemia.

FREQUENCY Reliable estimates of the prevalence of chronic cor pulmonale are sparse. After the age of 50, cor pulmonale is the most common cardiac disorder except for coronary and hypertensive heart disease. Most instances are secondary to obstructive disease of the airways and the pulmonary hypertension that it elicits. Indeed, in parts of the world where cigarette smoking and air pollution have resulted in a high incidence of chronic bronchitis and emphysema (described in detail in Chap. 208), cor pulmonale may comprise up to one-quarter of all types of heart failure. Men are more often affected than women presumably because of greater exposure to air pollutants, including cigarette smoke. Chronic cor pulmonale is a

TABLE 191-1 Respiratory disorders predisposing to chronic cor pulmonale*

1 Intrinsic disease of the lungs and intrapulmonary airways
 a Chronic obstructive lung disease (COLD)
 b Diffuse pulmonary interstitial disease
 c Pulmonary vascular disease
2 Upper airways obstruction
 a Tracheal stenosis
 b Obstructive sleep apnea syndromes
 c Congenital anatomic abnormalities of oropharynx
3 Malfunctioning chest bellows
 a Kyphoscoliosis
 b Neuromuscular incompetence
 c Marked obesity ("Pickwickian syndrome")
4 Inadequate ventilatory drive from respiratory centers
 a Primary or idiopathic alveolar hypoventilation ("Ondine's curse")
 b Chronic mountain sickness
 c Central sleep apnea syndromes

* *The term* respiratory disorders *includes not only the diseases and disorders of the lungs, airways, and chest bellows, but also malfunctioning of the centers that control breathing and the support structures of the oropharynx. In essence, respiratory disorders refers to malfunctioning of any part or parts of the entire respiratory system and of the structures that impinge upon it.*

common sequel to cystic fibrosis (Chap. 207) but an unusual complication of allergic asthma.

Most diffuse pulmonary diseases are either too limited in extent or too circumscribed in their effects on alveolar-capillary gas exchange to set in motion the train of events leading to cor pulmonale. Even patients with extensive silicosis, emphysema, or diffuse fibrosis usually fail to develop appreciable pulmonary hypertension or cardiomegaly even though the disease may suffice to evoke breathlessness for years.

PATHOGENESIS

Pulmonary hypertension is a prerequisite for cor pulmonale. Although a high cardiac output, tachycardia, and an expanded blood volume may contribute to the pulmonary hypertension, the crux in the pathogenetic sequence is right ventricular overload due to an increase in pulmonary vascular resistance to blood flow through small muscular arteries and arterioles. The increase in vascular resistance may be anatomic or vasomotor in origin; often both mechanisms are involved (Table 191-2). In contrast to the situation in left ventricular failure, cardiac output is often normal or high, the peripheral pulses strong, and the extremities warm in the face of overt signs of systemic venous congestion. Peripheral edema complicating cor pulmonale is generally attributed to the heart failure, but the explanation is not entirely satisfying because pulmonary arterial pressures rarely exceed 65 to 80 kPa except during the acute exacerbation when hypoxia and acidosis are severe.

It has been noted above that the increase in the work of the right ventricle imposed by the pulmonary hypertension may cause it to fail. However, even in patients in whom the right ventricular stroke volume is decreased due to pulmonary hypertensive overloading, the myocardium of the right ventricle seems capable of responding normally when the overload is relieved.

ANATOMIC INCREASE IN PULMONARY VASCULAR RESISTANCE   In the normal resting individual, the pulmonary circulation is a highly distensible, low-resistance circuit, accommodating the same blood flow as the systemic circulation at approximately one-fifth the mean blood pressure; during moderate exercise, tripling the blood flow elicits only slight increments in pulmonary arterial pressure. Even after pneumonectomy, the residual pulmonary vascular bed accepts considerable increments in pulmonary blood flow with only a slight increase in pulmonary artery pressure as long as the lung is free of fibrosis, emphysema, or pulmonary vascular change. Similarly, amputation of large portions of the pulmonary capillary bed in emphysema generally fails to elicit pulmonary hypertension.

However, when pulmonary vascular reserve has been exhausted by progressive reduction in the extent and distensibility of the pulmonary vascular tree, even the modest increments in pulmonary blood flow associated with daily living may suffice to elicit marked pulmonary hypertension. For this to occur the cross-sectional area of the pulmonary resistance vessels must be considerably reduced. Restriction of the pulmonary vascular bed stems from widespread narrowing and obstruction of small pulmonary arteries and arterioles, usually accompanied by a decrease in the distensibility not only of the vessels but also of the adjacent lung.

VASOMOTOR INCREASE IN PULMONARY VASCULAR RESISTANCE (HYPOXIA AND ACIDOSIS)   The most potent stimulus for pulmonary vasoconstriction is alveolar hypoxia, which acts directly on adjacent small pulmonary arteries and arterioles; systemic arterial hypoxemia supplements the local effects of alveolar hypoxia indirectly by way of the sympathetic nerves to the pulmonary circulation. Experiments in dogs indicate that severe acidosis (pH < 7.2) also elicits pulmonary vasoconstriction. In humans, acidosis acts synergistically with hypoxia, whereas alkalosis diminishes the pressor response to hypoxia. The biologic basis for this interplay remains unclear. In chronic hypoxia, the effects of these pulmonary hypertensive stimuli are often intensified by increased viscosity of the blood arising from secondary polycythemia.

HYPERCAPNIA   In contrast to the effects of hypoxia and acidosis, the effects of CO_2 on the pulmonary circulation appear to be by way of the acidosis that it generates rather than by a direct action on pulmonary vessels. However, because heart failure in cor pulmonale is often associated with respiratory insufficiency, and because management of the respiratory insufficiency generally determines the outcome of the heart failure, the extracardiac effects of hypercapnia merit consideration.

Hypercapnia affects mainly the central nervous system, producing cerebral vasodilatation, increased cerebrospinal fluid pressure, and neurologic derangements ranging from weakness, irritability, lassitude, and cloudy sensorium to somnolence, confusion, and coma. These derangements are most apt to occur if hypercapnia is acute in onset and severe, or if chronic hypercapnia is acutely aggravated. In contrast, during chronic hypercapnia, the patient may be virtually free of central nervous system disturbances if respiratory acidosis is fully compensated. When severe hypoxemia and hypercapnia coexist, it may be impossible to distinguish between their neurologic effects because severe hypoxia causes anatomic damage to nervous tissues.

Carbon dioxide retention, with elevated CO_2 tensions in the blood and tissues, is self-perpetuating. On the one hand, hypercapnia from any cause blunts the responsiveness of the respiratory center to the

TABLE 191-2   Pathogenetic mechanisms in chronic pulmonary hypertension and cor pulmonale

Pathogenetic mechanism	Intermediaries	Examples
PRIMARY MECHANISMS		
Anatomic increase in pulmonary vascular resistance	Obliteration, obstruction, reduction, and stiffening of pulmonary vascular tree	*Vascular disease:* Primary pulmonary hypertension; recurrent pulmonary emboli *Extravascular disease:* Diffuse interstitial disease; fibrosing alveolitis; pneumoconiosis
Vasomotor increase in pulmonary vascular resistance	Pulmonary vasoconstriction by hypoxia and acidosis	*General alveolar hypoventilation with normal lungs:* 1 Disorders of chest bellows: neuromuscular; extreme obesity; kyphoscoliosis 2 Diminished ventilatory drive: primary alveolar hypoventilation; sleep; hypercapnia
Combined anatomic restriction and vasomotor	Combination of above	*Net alveolar hypoventilation with abnormal lungs:* Chronic obstructive lung disease: ''blue bloater''; cystic fibrosis of pancreas
SECONDARY MECHANISMS		
Increase in cardiac output	Increase in metabolic rate; acute hypoxia	Daily activities; acute respiratory infection
Increase in blood viscosity	Secondary polycythemia	Chronic hypoxia
Tachycardia	Aggravation of hypoxia	Heart failure

CO_2 stimulus; on the other, hypercapnia promotes retention of bicarbonate by the kidney. Not only the hypercapnia originating in disorders of the lungs or ventilation, but also the hypercapnia of metabolic alkalosis, such as that produced by powerful diuretics, causes ventilatory depression. This is why patients with chronic hypercapnia are particularly vulnerable to the effects of sedatives or oxygen breathing, both of which may cause calamitous increments in the degree of hypercapnia: sedatives by depressing further the respiratory centers in the brain, and oxygen by abolishing the hypoxic peripheral drive to ventilation. A large diuresis in which the loss of chloride is inordinate for the output of bicarbonate may be equally effective in depressing the ventilation. It is usually in the severely hypoxic, hypercapnic patient that right-sided heart failure occurs.

ALVEOLAR HYPOVENTILATION A large disparity commonly exists between the degree of pulmonary hypertension recorded during life and the anatomic changes in the lungs and pulmonary vessels at autopsy. This discrepancy is particularly marked in patients with obstructive disease of the airways, in whom the anatomic changes in the gas-exchanging parts of the lungs consistently appear to be inadequate to explain either the blood-gas abnormalities or the pulmonary arterial pressor response. Similarly, the most extensive emphysema may be associated with normal levels of blood gases and normal pulmonary arterial pressures. Much of this discrepancy disappears when account is taken of alveolar hypoventilation, an important functional disorder which cannot be quantified at autopsy. Recognizing that alveolar hypoventilation is an essential component in the pathogenesis of cor pulmonale is critical for two reasons: (1) elimination of the initiating mechanism (e.g., acute respiratory infection) usually reverses the alveolar hypoventilation, and (2) unless alveolar ventilation is improved, other therapeutic measures are apt to be ineffective.

The importance of alveolar hypoventilation in the pathogenesis of cor pulmonale has been underscored in recent years by observations of its occurrence in patients with sleep apnea syndromes in whom hypoxia is a consequence of inadequate ventilatory drive (central apnea) or of upper airways obstruction (peripheral apnea) whereas the lungs and chest bellows are normal. Dramatic improvements have often followed relief of the initiating mechanism, e.g., hypertrophied tonsils and adenoids, or bypass of an area of obstruction, e.g., tracheostomy for tracheal stenosis.

PULMONARY HYPERTENSION

Two distinct patterns characterize the natural history of cor pulmonale at sea level: (1) The pattern of *episodic* pulmonary hypertension, due to exacerbations of the underlying pulmonary disorder, is more common. Generally, each bout leaves its imprint and predisposes to continuing hypertension even though recovery from the *early* bouts frequently is associated with the return of pulmonary arterial pressures to normal. (2) The pattern of *progressive,* unremitting pulmonary hypertension and cor pulmonale leading inexorably to right-sided heart failure is generally a consequence either of progressive pulmonary vascular or interstitial disease or of unremitting hypoxia (as in continuing alveolar hypoventilation). Distinction between the two sequences tends to become blurred if intercurrent respiratory infections decrease the intervals between bouts of hypoxia and pulmonary hypertension. Also, each bout of pulmonary hypertension seems to predispose to a subsequent bout of cor pulmonale because of residual hypertrophy of the muscular pulmonary arteries or further curtailment of the extent and distensibility of the pulmonary vascular tree. Consequently, although relief of hypoxia may restore the pulmonary arterial pressure to normal or near-normal levels, with each attack the pulmonary vascular tree seems to lose some of its adaptability and the patient moves a little closer to the verge of persistent pulmonary hypertension and cor pulmonale.

As a general rule, pulmonary hypertension appears in a predisposed individual either when blood flow is increased (exercise, fever) or during a bout of acute hypoxia (bronchopulmonary infection). In time, pulmonary hypertension is present even at rest. The highest pulmonary artery pressures occur in pulmonary vascular and interstitial disease; the levels of pulmonary hypertension are neither as high nor as fixed in chronic obstructive diseases of the airways, even during an acute exacerbation.

The pulmonary hypertension that comes on only during exercise or hypoxia is associated with normal end-diastolic pressure in the right ventricle. However, as pulmonary hypertension becomes persistent and severe, abnormally high filling (end-diastolic) pressure develops in the right ventricle as a result either of incomplete emptying of the ventricle as it dilates or of the decrease in ventricular compliance associated with hypertrophy; cardiac output is still normal at rest and increases normally during exercise (cor pulmonale without heart failure). Finally, the onset of right-sided heart failure is identified by abnormally high end-diastolic pressures in the right ventricle. At this stage, the cardiac output, which may still be normal at rest, fails to increase normally during exercise; the systemic veins are engorged, reflecting the inability of the right ventricle to empty normally.

Interest is high in developing techniques to permit the diagnosis of pulmonary hypertension, using noninvasive techniques, especially echocardiography. Approaches to the problem have differed in that some aim to predict pulmonary arterial pressure whereas others attempt inferences based on right ventricular dimensions and hypertrophy and on the motions of the pulmonic valve. The diverse patient populations complicate extrapolation and generalization. But it does seem that some noninvasive procedures can detect pulmonary hypertension that is moderate or severe even though none are reliable or of sufficient accuracy to substitute for direct determinations by cardiac catheterization. Attention is currently shifting to a combination of approaches in the hope that indirect determinations of multiple aspects of right ventricular performance and of the pulmonary circulation will provide more accurate and reproducible measurements of the level of pulmonary hypertension than any single measure alone. It is perhaps worth reiterating that evaluations of accuracy require simultaneous determinations of cardiac output since in pulmonary hypertensive states the level of pulmonary blood flow strongly influences the level of pulmonary arterial pressure.

THE LEFT VENTRICLE IN COR PULMONALE Recent observations on the interplay between the two ventricles (''interdependence'') have served as a reminder that not only are both ventricles encased in common muscle bundles and pericardium, but they also have one wall in common, i.e., the ventricular septum. Increasing pressures in the right ventricle displace the septum into the left ventricle, thereby encroaching upon its lumen and modifying left ventricular pressures as well as volumes. However, the clinical significance of these changes is uncertain.

Except in the case of the few severely hypoxemic high-altitude dwellers who develop mountain sickness, the left ventricle does not seem to share in the cardiomegaly of high altitude. Consequently, *tolerable* levels of hypoxia do not exert serious noxious effects on the myocardium; nor are they associated with an inordinate hemodynamic load on the left ventricle. Conversely, severe, intolerable levels of hypoxia and arterial hypoxemia at altitude may impair myocardial function of both ventricles as well as produce right ventricular overload. The left ventricle then enlarges and fails, primarily because of inadequate oxygen delivery to the myocardium. These observations at high altitude suggest that right ventricular overload, per se, does not interfere with left ventricular function unless pulmonary hypertension is severe and accompanied by severe hypoxemia.

At sea level, cor pulmonale is not associated with left ventricular enlargement as long as the respiratory disorder is not long-standing and arterial hypoxemia is modest in degree. But in pulmonary disorders associated with chronic severe hypoxemia, left ventricular enlargement and malfunction may become evident, presumably due to independent disease of the left ventricle—particularly arteriosclerotic heart disease—aggravated by the direct effects of inadequate oxygen delivery to the myocardium plus the noxious effect of severe hypoxemia and acidosis on the myocardium. In turn, the consequences of respiratory insufficiency, which contributed to impaired myocardial performance by way of arterial hypoxemia and acidosis, are intensified by interstitial and alveolar pulmonary edema if the left ventricle should fail.

CLINICAL MANIFESTATIONS

The likelihood that a physician will recognize that a patient has cor pulmonale depends on his or her awareness that the underlying respiratory disorder can culminate in pulmonary hypertension. The diagnosis is generally straightforward in obliterative diseases of the pulmonary circulation, e.g., multiple pulmonary emboli. It is much more elusive in obstructive disease of the airways because chronic bronchitis and bronchiolitis may be more subtle in their clinical manifestations, and clinical indexes of pulmonary hypertension are not always reliable. Indeed, the first bout of pulmonary hypertension and cor pulmonale secondary to chronic bronchitis may be appreciated only retrospectively, i.e., after an episode of frank right ventricular failure. Detection may be particularly difficult if the systemic venous congestion and peripheral edema develop insidiously, over days to weeks, rather than suddenly in the course of an acute bronchopulmonary infection. Attention has recently been focused on the gradual onset of cor pulmonale and right ventricular failure by patients who develop alveolar hypoventilation as part of a sleep apnea syndrome rather than as a consequence of intrinsic pulmonary disease.

DIFFERENTIAL DIAGNOSIS Cor pulmonale is particularly important to recognize in the elderly patient who is old enough to have arteriosclerotic heart disease, has had cough and sputum for many years ("chronic bronchitis"), and clearly manifests right ventricular failure. Analyses of arterial blood gases are then most helpful in deciding whether the primary cardiac disorder is in the right or left ventricle, since appreciable arterial hypoxemia, hypercapnia, and acidosis are unusual in left-sided heart failure unless frank pulmonary edema is also present.

Support for the diagnosis of cor pulmonale may be adduced from roentgenographic and electrocardiographic evidence of right ventricular enlargement. Rarely is catheterization of the right side of the heart needed to settle the question, once suspicion of cor pulmonale is aroused. But, if necessary, cardiac catheterization will typically show pulmonary arterial hypertension, normal left atrial ("pulmonary wedge") pressures, and the classic hemodynamics of right ventricular failure.

The conventional signs of right ventricular enlargement include a cardiac thrust along the left sternal border, or immediately below the sternum, and a fourth heart sound arising in the hypertrophied ventricle. Concomitant pulmonary hypertension is suggested by a thrust in the second left interspace adjacent to the sternum, an unusually loud second component of the second heart sound in the

same area, and occasionally the murmur of pulmonary valvular insufficiency. If the right ventricle fails, tricuspid insufficiency and a right ventricular gallop sound are often added. Hydrothorax is uncommon, even after the advent of overt right ventricular failure. Permanent arrhythmias, such as atrial flutter or fibrillation, are unusual, but transitory arrhythmias are common during severe hypoxia or when respiratory alkalosis has been induced by mechanical hyperventilation.

The diagnostic value of the *electrocardiogram* in cor pulmonale depends on the underlying pulmonary or ventilatory disorder (Table 191-3). It is most valuable in pulmonary vascular or interstitial disease, particularly if unassociated with obstructive disease of the airways, or in alveolar hypoventilation with normal lungs. Conversely, because of the hyperinflated lungs and the episodic nature of the pulmonary hypertension and right ventricular overload, patterns diagnostic of right ventricular hypertrophy are uncommon in cor pulmonale secondary to chronic bronchitis and emphysema. Consequently, even if right ventricular enlargement in the course of chronic bronchitis and emphysema is marked, as during a bout of acute upper respiratory infection, electrocardiographic evidence may be inconclusive because of rotation and displacement of the heart, widened distances between electrodes and the cardiac surface, and the predominance of dilatation over hypertrophy in the cardiac enlargement. Thus a reliable diagnosis of right ventricular enlargement can be expected in one-third of patients with chronic bronchitis and emphysema whose hearts show right ventricular hypertrophy at autopsy, whereas the diagnosis is easily and reliably made in the great majority of patients with cor pulmonale originating in pulmonary disorders other than chronic bronchitis and emphysema. With these qualifications in mind, the more reliable criteria for right ventricular hypertrophy in a patient who has chronic bronchitis and emphysema have proved to be an S_1Q_3 pattern; right axis deviation $\geq 110°$; an $S_1S_2S_3$ pattern; and an R/S ratio in $V_6 \leq 1.0$. Combinations of these criteria enhance their diagnostic sensitivities.

Roentgenography has more diagnostic value in arousing suspicion of, or in confirming, enlargement of the right ventricle than in detecting it. Suspicion is aroused by evidences of an antecedent predisposing pulmonary disorder coupled with large central pulmonary arteries and a pruned peripheral arterial tree, i.e., evidence of pulmonary hypertension. Serial x-rays are generally more useful than a single examination for heart size, particularly in obstructive disease of the airways, where dramatic changes in heart size may occur between a bout of acute respiratory insufficiency and recovery.

Echocardiography has recently come into play as a tool for detecting pulmonary hypertension on the basis of movements of the pulmonic valve. The technique is not easy but is gaining in popularity.

CLINICAL FORMS OF COR PULMONALE AND THEIR TREATMENT

Regardless of the mechanism of initiation—anatomic, vasomotor, or both—chronic pulmonary hypertension tends to be self-perpetuating because of anatomic changes that cause continuing narrowing of small arteries and arterioles and obliteration of the pulmonary vascular bed by muscular hypertrophy, arteriosclerosis, and thrombosis. Often the impact of these anatomic changes is heightened by increased pulmonary vasomotor tone.

ANATOMIC INCREASE IN PULMONARY VASCULAR RESISTANCE These abnormalities may be sorted into two general categories (Table 191-2): vascular disease and extravascular disease, as described below.

Vascular disease; occlusive disease of the small pulmonary arteries In these disorders, widespread occlusion of the small pulmonary vessels takes place over months to years. Most often, the cause is multiple pulmonary emboli (Chap. 211); less common are multiple thromboses such as those which complicate sickle cell

---

TABLE 191-3 ECG patterns in chronic cor pulmonale

1 Chronic obstructive lung disease (suggestive, but not diagnostic, of right ventricular enlargement)*
  a "P pulmonale" (in leads II, III, aVF)
  b Right axis deviation $\geq 110°$
  c R/S ratio in $V_6 \leq 1$
  d rRS' in right chest leads
  e Right bundle branch block (partial or complete)
2 Pulmonary vascular or interstitial disease; general alveolar hypoventilation (diagnostic of right ventricular enlargement)
  a Classic pattern in V_1 or V_3R (dominant R or R' with inverted T waves in right chest leads)
  b Often associated with "suggestive" criteria above

* Among the "suggestive" criteria, it is difficult to distinguish right ventricular enlargement (hypertrophy and dilatation) from changes in the anatomic and electrical positions of the heart produced by the hyperinflated lungs. Consequently, the "suggestive" criteria are more useful as confirmatory, than as diagnostic, evidence.

anemia. A rare cause is primary (unexplained) pulmonary hypertension (Chap. 210).

Tachypnea, persisting during sleep, is an outstanding feature of multiple pulmonary emboli. This increase in respiratory frequency is associated with alveolar hyperventilation as indicated by characteristically low values for alveolar and arterial P_{CO_2} and for serum bicarbonate. Incapacitating breathlessness occurs on mild exertion. Precordial or thoracic pain is not uncommon: occasionally the pain mimics angina; at other times it is clearly pleuritic, intensifying during inspiration. The clinical roentgenographic and electrocardiographic signs of right ventricular enlargement are present. Cyanosis, which is rarely impressive before heart failure, usually becomes striking after the right ventricle fails. Objective evidence for pulmonary emboli is conventionally sought by photoscanning and pulmonary angiography (Chaps. 201 and 211).

Of all patients who develop cor pulmonale, those with multiple pulmonary emboli or primary pulmonary hypertension have the highest pulmonary arterial pressures; these may equal or even exceed systemic arterial pressures. The cardiac output tends to be low. Mild arterial hypoxemia is the rule and seems to arise from shunting within the lungs. Whether the shunts represent blood flow through recanalized vessels that divert mixed venous blood from contact with alveoli, or too-rapid passage of the entire cardiac output through unoccluded and dilated portions of the pulmonary vascular tree, or blood flow through anatomic pulmonary arteriovenous channels that are ordinarily inoperative is conjectural. During right-sided heart failure, these shunts cause profound arterial hypoxemia because the shunted (mixed venous) blood has an extremely low O_2 content.

Once pulmonary hypertension is fixed, treatment directed at the process in the lungs is rarely effective, since organization of emboli has led to irreversible occlusions of innumerable small arteries. Continuous administration of O_2-enriched mixtures is standard. Caution must be exercised to avoid oxygen toxicity by administering as little additional oxygen as possible. Unfortunately, compromises are often required, since arterial blood is not easily restored toward normal levels of oxygenation because of the magnitude of the venous shunts.

The grim outlook for treating the cor pulmonale of multiple pulmonary emboli, as well as the ever-present prospect of catastrophic pulmonary embolization, has emphasized the need for prophylactic measures in patients judged to be candidates for pulmonary emboli (Chap. 211). Heart failure is treated by the usual cardiotonic measures in conjunction with measures directed at improving arterial oxygenation. Rarely does it respond dramatically as long as the hemodynamic overload persists.

Diffuse interstitial fibrosis and granuloma Among the diverse entities included in this category are (1) sarcoidosis, berylliosis, and the "nonspecific" granulomatoses (Chap. 209); (2) scleroderma of the lung (Chap. 209); (3) the various interstitial or alveolar-septal fibroses such as "fibrosing alveolitis," radiation fibrosis, or pulmonary asbestosis, and the special progressive form of interstitial disease known as the Hamman-Rich syndrome (Chap. 209); (4) immuno-pathologic disease of the lungs, exemplified by "farmer's lung" (Chap. 203); and (5) diffuse carcinomatous infiltration of the lung, such as "alveolar cell" or lymphangitic carcinoma (Chap. 213).

Clinically, the respiratory difficulty is often manifested by an acute respiratory illness that fails to resolve. Tachypnea persists. The roentgenogram shows fine nodular or fibrotic lesions widely disseminated throughout both lung fields. In the resting subject, the arterial P_{O_2} is sustained at near-normal levels by chronic hyperventilation; during exercise, it drops precipitously. The arterial P_{CO_2} is normal or slightly low, reflecting the balance between the augmented ventilation, the oxygen consumption, which is often increased, and the partition of the augmented ventilation between the alveoli and the dead space.

As long as hypoxemia is mild, pulmonary hypertension is modest. But as the disease progresses and as hypoxemia increases—in part because of ventilation-perfusion abnormalities—the level of pulmo-

nary hypertension also increases, and cor pulmonale begins to evolve. Right ventricular failure generally occurs late in the course of the disease. At first, it responds well to oxygen mixtures and the usual forms of treatment of heart failure (Chap. 182). Oxygen therapy is quite useful since it affords relief of dyspnea and improves oxygenation without threat of carbon dioxide retention. However, oxygen dependence may become marked, and the hazards of oxygen toxicity increase pari passu with the increasing concentrations of inspired oxygen and the duration of exposure.

Relief of heart failure is usually transient unless the initiating mechanism is controlled. Rarely is the underlying lesion in the lung reversible, even though steroids occasionally have been associated with dramatic benefit, especially in some of the granulomatoses and "fibrosing alveolitis." More apt to be rewarding is the successful treatment of superimposed respiratory infection which has toppled a stable patient into heart failure.

VASOMOTOR INCREASE IN PULMONARY VASCULAR RESISTANCE For convenience, alveolar hypoventilation, a prime cause of elevated pulmonary vascular resistance, can be identified by a value for arterial P_{CO_2} greater than 60 kPa; the disorder may be regarded as either "general" or "net."

Alveolar hypoventilation: general The critical importance of abnormal values for blood gases in the pathogenesis of cor pulmonale is illustrated by the syndrome of alveolar hypoventilation coexistent with normal lungs ("general alveolar hypoventilation"). In these patients, some abnormality, either in the regulation of ventilation or in the neuromuscular apparatus, rather than intrinsic pulmonary disease, is responsible for the hypoxia and hypercapnia. The syndrome may have diverse etiologies. Sleep apnea syndromes associated with alveolar hypoventilation are currently receiving considerable attention. These disorders and the pathways by which they lead to alveolar hypoventilation and cor pulmonale are considered in Chap. 215.

Alveolar hypoventilation: net The common denominator in this group of disorders is the imbalance between alveolar ventilation, blood flow, and diffusion, resulting in hypercapnia and hypoxemia. In contrast to *general* alveolar hypoventilation, in which the same abnormalities of arterial blood-gas levels occur despite normal lungs, intrinsic lung disease is the basis for the abnormal values for blood gases in *net* alveolar hypoventilation.

The assortment of obstructive airways diseases predisposing to cor pulmonale has been pictured as a spectrum of bronchopulmonary disorders, ranging from pure obstruction of the airways at one end to pure emphysema at the other; between the two ends are the mixtures which are most prevalent (Chap. 208). Most likely to develop cor pulmonale is the patient with bronchitis and bronchiolitis, usually with some emphysema, in whom obstructive disease of the airways has so deranged the balance between alveolar ventilation, blood flow, and diffusion as to cause the characteristic syndrome of cyanosis (hypoxemia), somnolence (hypercapnia), and right ventricular failure; these are the "blue bloaters." In contrast, the "pink puffers," with comparable degrees of airways obstruction by conventional tests, do not develop hypoxia in the course of their breathless existence; only during an intercurrent respiratory infection, as hypoxia is superimposed, do they become candidates for cor pulmonale. Emphysema without bronchitis is rarely associated with cor pulmonale since alveolar ventilation and capillary blood flow seem to be commensurately curtailed, as after pulmonary resection, so that neither hypoxia nor pulmonary hypertension becomes appreciable.

Treatment of the "blue bloater" with cor pulmonale is directed at relieving the bronchitis and bronchiolitis (Chap. 216); the mainstays are antibiotics for respiratory infection and bronchodilators for bronchoconstriction. Prolonged oxygen therapy (on the order of 15 h per day by nasal catheter) relieves pulmonary hypertension due to alveolar and arterial hypoxia. Cardiac glycosides are useless unless oxygenation is improved. If the patient succeeds in maintaining good oxygenation, digitalis and diuretics can usually be discontinued.

Relief of airways obstruction is more readily accomplished in some disorders than in others. For example, it is generally easier in chronic bronchitis than in cystic fibrosis, in which most of the airways remain plugged with abnormal thick, tenacious sputum despite heroic therapeutic efforts.

Cor pulmonale is uncommon in uncomplicated silicosis or tuberculosis. On the other hand, it is not uncommon when silicosis, anthrosilicosis, or long-standing fibrotic tuberculosis is complicated by extensive, conglomerate, massive fibrosis, distorted adjacent parenchyma, shrunken lobes, and bronchitis. The likelihood of cor pulmonale is increased further by chronic pleurisy, fibrothorax, or excisional surgery. In such cases, a combination of anatomic restriction of the vascular bed and disturbances in gas exchange is involved in the pathogenesis of the pulmonary hypertension. Indeed, the disturbances in gas exchange, often brought to clinical levels by an acute respiratory infection, are the most reversible element of this disorder.

Although it is convenient to separate "net" from "general" alveolar hypoventilation on pathogenetic grounds, the therapeutic principles are basically the same for both and are described in Chap. 216. The present section will deal only with the circulatory abnormalities.

Since the pulmonary hypertension in the most prevalent pulmonary disorders is rarely anatomically fixed but arises mainly from hypoxia and acidosis, relief of alveolar hypoventilation is usually remarkably successful in restoring the circulation to normal. Measures to improve alveolar ventilation vary considerably. In mild cases, simple measures, such as hydration, antibiotics, and bronchodilators, often suffice; in more severe degrees of hypoxemia and hypercapnia, in which heart failure is associated with respiratory insufficiency, mechanical aids to respiration are usually needed.

It has been noted above that treatment of right-sided heart failure is less important than restoring the blood gas values to tolerable levels. The usual therapeutic measures for heart failure (Chap. 182) apply: low-salt regimen, digitalis, diuretics. However, measures to decrease the circulating blood volume (and hematocrit) are of greater importance. Several phlebotomies, each draining 300 to 400 mL, may be needed within a period of 2 to 3 weeks to bring hematocrit and blood volume back to normal; repeated phlebotomies at monthly or bimonthly intervals may have to be instituted to prevent return of the hypervolemia. Diuretics have to be given with more care than usual because the metabolic alkalosis, which may complicate the use of potent diuretics such as ethacrynic acid, aggravates ventilatory insufficiency by depressing the effectiveness of the CO_2 stimulus on the respiratory centers.

The effects of vigorous therapy, directed mainly to the pulmonary disorder, are often dramatic in improving the blood gas abnormalities and heart failure. Other manifestations usually clear more slowly. Indeed, several weeks to a month may elapse before the arterial blood gases, hematocrit, cardiac output, and pulmonary arterial pressures return to optimal levels. But therapy throughout is guided by the fact that the final outcome in cor pulmonale usually depends on the ability to cope with the underlying respiratory disorder rather than with the changes in the heart and circulation.

Vasodilators in pulmonary hypertension and cor pulmonale In recent years, vasodilator agents, such as hydralazine, nitroprusside, prostaglandins, and nifedipine, have been given to patients with pulmonary hypertension of diverse etiologies. These trials have been undertaken with some trepidation, particularly in patients with intrinsic lung disease, in whom relaxation of vascular tone in diseased areas might exaggerate ventilation–blood flow abnormalities and, thereby, increase arterial hypoxemia. As a rule, in acute experiments pulmonary vasodilators do decrease pulmonary arterial pressures toward normal, and the fear of increasing arterial hypoxemia has not been realized. Instead, cardiac output and oxygen delivery to the tissues do increase at the same time that pulmonary arterial pressure decreases. Symptomatic improvement, at rest and during exercise, accompanies the increase in cardiac output and oxygen delivery to the tissues. However,

periods of observation have been brief, and long-term consequences of this therapy are still unknown. Moreover, as far as the work of the heart is concerned, the increase in cardiac output often nullifies the direct vasodilator effect of the agent, leaving pulmonary arterial pressure unchanged and occasionally increased; often, the heart rate increases concomitantly. The end result of increase in cardiac output, unchanged pulmonary arterial pressure, and tachycardia is an increase in the work of the heart, raising questions about the extent to which the evolution of cor pulmonale can be favorably influenced by the use of pulmonary vasodilators that also exert direct and reflex stimulatory effects on the heart. Finally, the proper place of pulmonary vasodilator agents in therapy remains to be defined since antibiotics, bronchodilators, and oxygen still remain the essential ingredients.

REFERENCES

FISHMAN AP: Chronic cor pulmonale: State of the art. Am Rev Resp Dis 114:775, 1976
——— (ed): *Pulmonary Diseases and Disorders*, 2nd ed. New York, McGraw-Hill, 1987
———, PIETRA GG: Vasodilator treatment of primary pulmonary hypertension, in *Update: Pulmonary Diseases and Disorders*, AP Fishman (ed). New York, McGraw-Hill, 1982, p 396
HEATH D, WILLIAMS DR: *Man at High Altitude*. Edinburgh, Churchill Livingstone, 1977
LUPI-HERRERA E et al: Hemodynamic effect of hydralazine in interstitial lung disease patients with cor pulmonale. Immediate and short-term evaluation at rest and during exercise. Chest 87:564, 1985
MATTHAY RA, BERGER HJ: Cardiovascular function in cor pulmonale. Clin Chest Med 4:269, 1983
McFADDEN ER, BRAUNWALD E: Cor pulmonale and pulmonary thromboembolism, in *Heart Disease*, 2d ed, E Braunwald (ed). Philadelphia, Saunders, 1984, p 1572
MIDGREN B et al: Nocturnal hypoxaemia and cor pulmonale in severe chronic lung disease. Bull Eur Physiopathol Respir 21:527, 1985
RUBIN LJ, PETER RH (eds): *Pulmonary Heart Disease*. Hingham, Mass, Martinus Nijhoff-MTP Press, 1984
STERN RC et al: Heart failure in cystic fibrosis. Am J Dis Child 134:267, 1980
WAGENVOORT CA, WAGENVOORT N: *Pathology of Pulmonary Hypertension*. New York, Wiley, 1977
WEIR EK, REEVES JT (eds): *Pulmonary Hypertension*. Mt Kisco, NY, Futura, 1984
WEITZENBLUM E et al: Long-term course of pulmonary arterial pressure in chronic obstructive lung disease. Am Rev Resp Dis 130:993, 1984

---

192   THE CARDIOMYOPATHIES AND MYOCARDITIDES

JOSHUA WYNNE / EUGENE BRAUNWALD

CARDIOMYOPATHY

The cardiomyopathies are diseases involving the myocardium primarily, not as the result of hypertension or of congenital, valvular, coronary, arterial, or pericardial abnormalities.[1] Although not a leading cause of heart disease in western countries, cardiomyopathy in some of the underdeveloped parts of the world may account for 30 percent or more of all deaths due to heart disease. When the cardiomyopathies are classified on an etiologic basis, two fundamental forms are recognized: (1) a primary type, consisting of heart muscle disease of unknown cause; (2) a secondary type, consisting of myocardial disease of known cause, or associated with a disease involving other organ systems (Table 192-1). In many cases it is not possible to arrive at an etiologic diagnosis on clinical grounds, and thus it is often more desirable to classify the cardiomyopathies on the basis of differences in their pathophysiology and clinical presentation (Tables 192-2 and 192-3). The distinction between the

[1] *Diffuse myocardial fibrosis secondary to multiple myocardial scars produced by extensive coronary arterial narrowing and occlusion can impair left ventricular function and is frequently referred to as ischemic cardiomyopathy. According to the definition given above, however, the term* cardiomyopathy *should be restricted to a condition primarily involving heart muscle. In ischemic cardiomyopathy the primary involvement is in the coronary vessels.*

TABLE 192-1 Etiologic classification of cardiomyopathies

I Primary myocardial involvement
  A Idiopathic (D,R,H)
  B Familial (D,H)
  C Eosinophilic endomyocardial disease (R)
  D Endomyocardial fibrosis (R)
II Secondary myocardial involvement
  A Infective (D)
    1 Viral myocarditis
    2 Bacterial myocarditis
    3 Fungal myocarditis
    4 Protozoal myocarditis
    5 Metazoal myocarditis
  B Metabolic (D)
  C Familial storage disease (D,R)
    1 Glycogen storage disease
    2 Mucopolysaccharidoses
  D Deficiency (D)
    1 Electrolytes
    2 Nutritional
  E Connective tissue disorders (D)
    1 Systemic lupus erythematosus
    2 Polyarteritis nodosa
    3 Rheumatoid arthritis
    4 Scleroderma
    5 Dermatomyositis
  F Infiltrations and granulomas (R,D)
    1 Amyloidosis
    2 Sarcoidosis
    3 Malignancy
    4 Hemochromatosis
  G Neuromuscular (D)
    1 Muscular dystrophy
    2 Myotonic dystrophy
    3 Friedreich's ataxia (H,D)
    4 Refsum's disease
  H Sensitivity and toxic reactions (D)
    1 Alcohol
    2 Radiation
    3 Drugs
  I Peripartum heart disease (D)
  J Endocardial fibroelastosis (R)

NOTE: *The principal clinical manifestation(s) of each etiologic grouping is denoted by D (dilated), R (restrictive), or H (hypertrophic) cardiomyopathy.*
SOURCE: *Adapted from the WHO/ISFC task force report on the definition and classification of cardiomyopathies, 1980.*

functional categories is not absolute, however, and there is often some overlap.

DILATED (CONGESTIVE) CARDIOMYOPATHY

Systolic pump function is impaired, leading to cardiac enlargement and often producing symptoms of congestive heart failure. Mural thrombi are often present, particularly in the left ventricular apex. Histologic examination reveals extensive areas of interstitial and perivascular fibrosis, with minimal necrosis and cellular infiltration. Although no

TABLE 192-2 Clinical classification of cardiomyopathies

1 Dilated (congestive): Left and/or right ventricular enlargement, impaired systolic function, congestive heart failure, arrhythmias, emboli
2 Restrictive: Endomyocardial scarring or myocardial infiltration resulting in restriction to left and/or right ventricular filling
3 Hypertrophic: Disproportionate left ventricular hypertrophy, typically involving septum more than free wall, with or without obstruction to ventricular outflow; usually of a nondilated left ventricular cavity

etiology is apparent in many cases, dilated cardiomyopathy (formerly called congestive cardiomyopathy) is probably the end result of myocardial damage produced by a variety of toxic, metabolic, or infectious agents. There is increasing evidence to suggest that in at least some patients dilated cardiomyopathy may be the late sequel of acute viral myocarditis, possibly mediated through an immunologic mechanism. Although most commonly a disease of middle-aged men, it may occur in any patient population. A reversible form of dilated cardiomyopathy may be found with selenium deficiency.

CLINICAL MANIFESTATIONS Symptoms of left- and right-sided congestive failure, manifested by dyspnea on exertion, fatigue, orthopnea, paroxysmal nocturnal dyspnea, peripheral edema, and palpitations, develop gradually in most patients. Some patients have left ventricular dilatation for months or even years before becoming symptomatic. Although vague chest pain may be present, typical angina pectoris is unusual and suggests the presence of concomitant coronary artery disease.

PHYSICAL EXAMINATION Variable degrees of cardiac enlargement and findings of congestive heart failure are noted. In patients with advanced disease, the pulse pressure is small, and the jugular venous pressure is elevated. Third and fourth heart sounds are common, and mitral or tricuspid regurgitation may occur. Diastolic murmurs, valvular calcification, hypertension, and changes of vascular disease in the optic fundi militate *against* the diagnosis of cardiomyopathy.

LABORATORY EXAMINATIONS The chest roentgenogram demonstrates left ventricular enlargement, although generalized cardiomegaly is often seen, sometimes due to a concomitant pericardial effusion. The lung fields may demonstrate evidence of pulmonary venous hypertension and interstitial or alveolar edema. The electrocardiogram often shows sinus tachycardia or atrial fibrillation, ventricular arrhythmias, left atrial enlargement, diffuse nonspecific ST-T-wave changes, and sometimes intraventricular conduction defects. Echocardiography and radionuclide ventriculography show left ventricular enlargement, with normal or minimally thickened or thinned walls, and systolic dysfunction (reduced ejection fraction); a pericardial

TABLE 192-3 Laboratory evaluation of the cardiomyopathies

	Dilated (congestive)	Restrictive	Hypertrophic
Chest roentgenogram	Moderate to marked cardiac enlargement Pulmonary venous hypertension	Mild cardiac enlargement	Mild to moderate cardiac enlargement
Electrocardiogram	ST-segment and T-wave abnormalities	Low-voltage Conduction defects	ST-segment and T-wave abnormalities Left ventricular hypertrophy Abnormal Q waves
Echocardiogram	Left ventricular dilatation and dysfunction	Increased left ventricular wall thickness Normal systolic function	Asymmetric septal hypertrophy (ASH) Systolic anterior motion (SAM) of the mitral valve
Radionuclide studies	Left ventricular dilatation and dysfunction (RVG)	Normal systolic function (RVG)	Vigorous systolic function (RVG) Asymmetric septal hypertrophy (RVG or ^{201}Tl)
Cardiac catheterization	Left ventricular dilatation and dysfunction Elevated left- and often right-sided filling pressures Diminished cardiac output	Normal systolic function Elevated left- and right-sided filling pressures	Vigorous systolic function Dynamic left ventricular outflow obstruction Elevated left- and right-sided filling pressures

NOTE: *RVG = radionuclide ventriculogram; ^{201}Tl = thallium 201.*

effusion is often noted. Radioisotopic imaging with gallium 67 may identify patients with dilated cardiomyopathy and myocarditis.

Hemodynamic studies reveal a cardiac output that is moderately or severely reduced at rest, and that does not increase normally with exercise. The left ventricular end-diastolic, left atrial, and pulmonary capillary wedge pressures usually are elevated; when failure of the right side of the heart supervenes, the right ventricular end-diastolic, right atrial, and central venous pressures are also elevated. Angiography reveals a dilated, diffusely hypokinetic left ventricle, often with some degree of mitral regurgitation; the coronary arteries are normal, thereby excluding so-called ischemic cardiomyopathy. Transvenous endomyocardial biopsy (Chap. 180) may be helpful in excluding certain conditions such as myocardial infiltration by amyloid; in some patients there is biopsy evidence of myocardial round cell inflammation, suggesting an inflammatory etiology and compatible with previous viral myocarditis.

TREATMENT   Most patients pursue an inexorably downhill course, and the majority, particularly those over 55 years of age, die within 2 years of the onset of symptoms. Death is due to either congestive heart failure or ventricular arrhythmia; sudden death, presumably arrhythmic in etiology, is a constant threat. Systemic embolization is common, and all patients without contraindications should receive anticoagulants. Since the cause of primary dilated cardiomyopathy is, by definition, unknown, specific therapy is not possible. Prolonged strict bed rest for up to 1 year or more has been advocated, but the effectiveness of this form of therapy remains controversial and such therapy is not feasible in most patients; strenuous exertion should, however, be interdicted. Treatment of heart failure in dilated cardiomyopathy should be considered palliative and directed toward improvement in symptoms; there is no convincing evidence that therapy alters prognosis. Standard therapy of heart failure with salt restriction, diuretics, digitalis, and vasodilators may produce symptomatic improvement, at least in the initial phases of the illness; however, these patients appear to be at increased risk of digitalis toxicity. Newer cardiotonic agents, such as amrinone and the related experimental agent milrinone, may provide additional clinical improvement (Chap. 182). Some patients with dilated cardiomyopathy who have evidence of myocardial inflammation have been treated with corticosteroids, often in association with azathioprine; others have been treated cautiously with gradually increasing doses of beta-adrenergic blockers. However, the indications and value of such experimental therapy remain controversial. Antiarrhythmic agents may be used to treat symptomatic or serious arrhythmias, although they may be extremely resistant to the usual as well as investigational agents. Because of this, alternative experimental therapies, such as surgical interruption of the arrhythmic circuit or implantation of an automatic internal defibrillator, have gained favor. In patients with advanced disease who are refractory to medical therapy and who have no contraindications to the procedure (Chap. 182), cardiac transplantation should be considered.

The preceding discussion emphasized clinical features of the dilated cardiomyopathies, regardless of whether they are primary or secondary in etiology. Many cases of dilated cardiomyopathy are primary (without a definable cause), but a number of specific conditions may also cause dilated cardiomyopathy secondarily. Since some of these conditions are reversible, features peculiar to these disorders will be considered in turn.

Alcoholic cardiomyopathy   Individuals who consume large quantities of alcohol over many years may develop a clinical picture identical to idiopathic dilated cardiomyopathy; indeed, alcoholic cardiomyopathy is the major form of secondary dilated cardiomyopathy in the western world. Ceasing alcohol consumption before severe heart failure has developed may halt the progression, or even reverse the course of this disease, unlike the idiopathic variety which is marked by progressive deterioration. Alcoholics with advanced heart failure have a poor prognosis, particularly if they continue to drink; less than one-quarter survive 3 years. The key to the treatment

of alcoholic cardiomyopathy is total and permanent abstinence. Although thiamine deficiency may be present in some of these patients, alcoholic cardiomyopathy is associated with a low cardiac output and systemic vasoconstriction. In contrast, beriberi heart disease (Chaps. 76 and 193) is characterized by elevated cardiac output and diminished peripheral vascular resistance, so that thiamine deficiency per se does not appear to cause alcoholic cardiomyopathy. A second presentation of alcoholic cardiotoxicity may be found in individuals without overt heart failure, and consists of recurrent supraventricular or ventricular tachyarrhythmias. Termed the "holiday heart syndrome," it typically appears after a drinking binge; atrial fibrillation is seen most frequently, followed by atrial flutter and ventricular premature depolarizations.

Peripartum cardiomyopathy   Cardiac dilatation and congestive heart failure of unexplained cause may develop during the last month of pregnancy or within the first few months after delivery. The etiology of this disorder is unknown but may relate to a preexisting cardiomyopathy that was not apparent prior to pregnancy. Necropsy shows cardiac enlargement, often with mural thrombi, along with histologic evidence of myocardial degeneration and fibrosis. The patient who develops peripartum cardiomyopathy is typically multiparous, black, and over the age of 30. While some patients are malnourished, there is no conclusive evidence that dietary deficiencies are etiologically involved. The symptoms, signs, and treatment are similar to those in patients with idiopathic dilated cardiomyopathy. The prognosis in these patients appears to be closely related to whether the heart size returns to normal after the first episode of congestive heart failure. If it does, subsequent pregnancies may sometimes be well tolerated; if the heart remains enlarged, however, further pregnancies frequently produce increasing myocardial damage, ultimately leading to refractory congestive heart failure and death. Those who recover should be encouraged to avoid further pregnancies, particularly if cardiomegaly persists.

Neuromuscular disease (see also Chap. 357)   Cardiac involvement is common in many of the muscular dystrophies. In *Duchenne's progressive muscular dystrophy,* myocardial involvement is most frequently indicated by a distinctive and unique electrocardiographic pattern consisting of tall R waves in right precordial leads with an R/S ratio greater than 1.0, often associated with deep Q waves in the limb and lateral precordial leads, and is not found in other forms of muscular dystrophy. These electrocardiographic abnormalities appear to result from selective transmural necrosis of the posterobasal left ventricle and associated papillary muscle. A variety of supraventricular and ventricular arrhythmias is frequently found. Rapidly progressive congestive heart failure may supervene after years of apparent circulatory stability during which the only detectable abnormalities are in the electrocardiogram. *Myotonic dystrophy* is characterized by a variety of electrocardiographic abnormalities, especially disorders of impulse formation and conduction, but other overt clinical evidence of heart disease is uncommon. Because of the abnormalities of impulse generation and conduction, syncope and sudden death are major hazards; in appropriate patients, insertion of a permanent pacemaker may be efficacious. In *limb-girdle* and *fascioscapulohumeral dystrophy,* cardiac involvement is uncommon and seldom severe. Involvement of the heart is very common in *Friedreich's ataxia,* with as many as half of the patients developing cardiac symptoms. It is now generally accepted that the heart disease in Friedreich's ataxia is similar to hypertrophic cardiomyopathy (page 1002), although typically of the concentric form (with symmetric hypertrophy of left ventricular septum and free wall) and without the cellular disarray found in the usual case of hypertrophic cardiomyopathy. The electrocardiogram may demonstrate inappropriate sinus tachycardia and a variety of arrhythmias, as well as ventricular hypertrophy and ST-segment and T-wave abnormalities. The echocardiogram usually demonstrates left ventricular hypertrophy, and dynamic left ventricular outflow tract obstruction is seen on occasion.

Drugs A variety of pharmacologic agents may damage the myocardium acutely, producing a pattern of inflammation (myocarditis), or they may lead to chronic damage of the type seen with idiopathic dilated cardiomyopathy. Certain drugs produce only electrocardiographic abnormalities, while others may precipitate fulminant congestive heart failure and death. The anthracycline derivatives, particularly *doxorubicin* (Adriamycin), are powerful antineoplastic agents, which, when given in high doses (more than 550 mg/m² for doxorubicin), may produce fatal heart failure. The incidence of heart failure is related not only to the dose of the drug but to the presence or absence of several risk factors (cardiac irradiation, age greater than 70 years, underlying heart disease, hypertension, treatment with cyclophosphamide); at any dose patients with these risk factors have an eight- to tenfold greater frequency of developing heart failure than do patients lacking them. Radionuclide ventriculography (Chap. 179) may document preclinical deterioration of left ventricular function and allow appropriate dose adjustments; half of asymptomatic patients treated with standard doses may demonstrate left ventricular dysfunction for years after treatment. Recent efforts to modify the dose schedule by giving the drug more slowly have reduced the risk of cardiotoxicity further. High-dose *cyclophosphamide* may produce congestive heart failure acutely or within 2 weeks of administration; a characteristic histopathologic feature is myocardial edema and hemorrhagic necrosis. Rarely, patients treated with *5-fluorouracil* will develop chest pain and electrocardiographic changes of myocardial ischemia or infarction. Electrocardiographic changes and arrhythmias may result from treatment with tricyclic antidepressants, the phenothiazines, emetine, lithium, and various aerosol propellants.

RESTRICTIVE CARDIOMYOPATHY

The hallmark of the restrictive cardiomyopathies is abnormal diastolic function; the ventricular walls are excessively rigid and impede ventricular filling. Myocardial fibrosis, hypertrophy, or infiltration secondary to a variety of etiologies is usually responsible. The infiltrative diseases, which represent important etiologies for secondary restrictive cardiomyopathy, may also show some impairment of systolic function. Myocardial involvement with *amyloid* is a common cause of secondary restrictive cardiomyopathy, although restriction is also seen in hemochromatosis, glycogen deposition, endomyocardial fibrosis, fibroelastosis, the eosinophilias, neoplastic infiltration, and myocardial fibrosis of diverse causes. In many of these conditions, particularly those with substantial concomitant endocardial involvement, partial obliteration of the ventricular cavity by fibrous tissue and thrombus contributes to the abnormally increased resistance to ventricular filling. As a result of persistently elevated venous pressure these patients commonly have dependent edema, ascites, and an enlarged, tender liver. The jugular venous pressure is elevated and does not fall normally, or it may rise with inspiration (Kussmaul's sign). The heart sounds may be distant, and third and fourth heart sounds are common. In contrast to constrictive pericarditis, which these diseases resemble, the apex impulse is usually easily palpable. The electrocardiogram shows low-voltage, nonspecific ST-T-wave changes and various arrhythmias. Pericardial calcification on x-ray, which would suggest constrictive pericarditis, is absent. Echocardiography typically reveals symmetrically thickened left ventricular walls and normal or slightly reduced systolic function. Cardiac catheterization shows a decreased cardiac output, elevation of the right and left ventricular end-diastolic pressures, and a dip-and-plateau configuration of the diastolic portion of the ventricular pressure pulse resembling that seen in constrictive pericarditis.

Differentiation from constrictive pericarditis, at the bedside and even after cardiac catheterization, may be difficult or impossible (Chaps. 180 and 194). This distinction is of importance because the latter condition is potentially curable by operation. Right ventricular transvenous endomyocardial biopsy may be helpful in the differentiation of these two diseases by revealing interstitial infiltration or fibrosis in restrictive cardiomyopathy, but exploratory thoracotomy is occasionally necessary to distinguish restrictive cardiomyopathy from chronic constrictive pericarditis.

Endomyocardial fibrosis This is a progressive disease of unknown etiology which occurs most commonly in children and young adults residing in tropical and subtropical Africa, particularly Uganda and Nigeria. The disease is characterized by fibrous endocardial lesions of the inflow portion of the right or left ventricle (or both) and often involves the atrioventricular valves, producing valvular regurgitation. The apex of the ventricles may be obliterated by a mass of thrombus and fibrous tissue. In many ways this disease resembles eosinophilic endomyocardial disease, although they occur in quite different geographic areas and age groups. Endomyocardial fibrosis is a frequent cause of heart failure in Africa, accounting for up to one-quarter of deaths due to heart disease.

The clinical picture depends upon which ventricle and atrioventricular valve show predominant involvement; left-sided involvement results in symptoms of pulmonary congestion, while predominant right-sided disease presents features of a restrictive cardiomyopathy. Medical treatment is often disappointing, and surgical excision of the fibrotic endocardium and replacement of the involved atrioventricular valve has led to substantial symptomatic improvement in a small number of patients.

Eosinophilic endomyocardial disease Also called *Loeffler's endocarditis* and *fibroplastic endocarditis*, this disease appears to be a subcategory of the hypereosinophilic syndrome in which the heart is predominantly involved. Typically, the endocardium of either or both ventricles thickens markedly, with involvement of the underlying myocardium. Large mural thrombi may develop in either ventricle, thereby compromising the size of the ventricular cavity and serving as a source of pulmonary and systemic emboli. Hepatosplenomegaly and localized eosinophilic infiltration of other organs are usually present. Once the disease becomes clinically evident, survival is usually brief, although recent reports have suggested a more benign course, with average survival exceeding 5 years. The reason for this improvement in prognosis is unclear but may be related to therapy with corticosteroids and immunosuppressive drugs.

Differential diagnosis Involvement of the heart is the most frequent cause of death in *primary amyloidosis* (Chap. 259), while clinically significant cardiac involvement is uncommon in the secondary form. Biopsy of the rectal mucosa, gingiva, liver, kidney, and myocardium permits the diagnosis to be made before death in over three-quarters of cases. The heart is firm, rubbery, and noncompliant, and four clinical presentations (alone or in combination) are seen: (1) diastolic dysfunction (restrictive cardiomyopathy); (2) systolic dysfunction; (3) arrhythmias; and (4) orthostatic hypotension. The two-dimensional echocardiogram may be helpful in making the diagnosis of amyloidosis and may show a thickened myocardial wall with a distinctive "speckled" appearance. *Hemochromatosis* (Chap. 310) should be suspected if cardiomyopathy occurs in the setting of diabetes mellitus, hepatic cirrhosis, and increased skin pigmentation. Phlebotomy may be of some benefit if employed early in the course of the disease. Continuous subcutaneous administration of desferrioxamine may reduce body iron stores in advanced cases, but whether this produces clinical improvement is unclear. Myocardial *sarcoidosis* (Chap. 270) is generally associated with other manifestations of systemic disease and may have restrictive as well as congestive features, since cardiac infiltration by sarcoid granulomata results not only in increased stiffness of the myocardium but also in diminished systolic contractile function. A variety of arrhythmias, including atrioventricular block, have been noted. *Endocardial fibroelastosis* is a disease seen in infants, characterized by a thickened endocardium that shows proliferation of elastic tissue. It is most unusual in adult patients, although small patches of it may be found in patients with endomyocardial fibrosis.

Transvenous biopsy of the endocardium (Chap. 180), usually right ventricular, has been used increasingly to obtain tissue specimens for histologic and electron-microscopic study. This relatively simple and safe technique is important in the diagnosis of myocardial disease, particularly in the recognition of infiltrative diseases such as amyloidosis, hemochromatosis, and sarcoidosis.

HYPERTROPHIC CARDIOMYOPATHY This disease is characterized by left ventricular hypertrophy, typically of a nondilated chamber, without obvious antecedent cause. The hypertrophy is thus not secondary to a cardiovascular or systemic disease, such as hypertension or aortic stenosis, that places a hemodynamic burden on the left ventricle. Two features of the disease which are common, but by no means universal, have attracted the greatest attention: (1) asymmetric septal hypertrophy (ASH), wherein the upper portion of the interventricular septum is preferentially hypertrophied in comparison to the thickness of the posterobasal left ventricular free wall; and (2) dynamic left ventricular outflow tract obstruction, due to narrowing of the subaortic area usually resulting from the midsystolic apposition of the anterior mitral valve leaflet against the hypertrophied septum, i.e., systolic anterior motion of the mitral valve (SAM). Initial studies of this disease emphasized the dynamic obstructive features, and it has been termed idiopathic hypertrophic subaortic stenosis (IHSS), hypertrophic obstructive cardiomyopathy (HOCM), and muscular subaortic stenosis. It has become clear, however, that many and perhaps most patients with hypertrophic cardiomyopathy do not, in fact, demonstrate outflow tract obstruction. The ubiquitous pathophysiologic abnormality is not systolic but rather *diastolic* dysfunction, characterized by increased stiffness of the hypertrophied muscle. This results in elevated diastolic filling pressures and is present despite a hypercontractile left ventricle.

The pattern of hypertrophy is distinctive in hypertrophic cardiomyopathy and differs from that seen in secondary hypertrophy (as in hypertension). Most patients demonstrate a ventricular septum whose thickness is disproportionately increased when compared with the free wall. Other patients may demonstrate disproportionate involvement of the apex or left ventricular free wall; 10 percent or more of patients have concentric involvement of the ventricle. All, however, show a bizarre and disorganized arrangement of cardiac muscle cells in the septum, whether or not obstruction is present. Patients without obstruction may demonstrate similar derangements of the left ventricular free wall.

At least half of all cases of hypertrophic cardiomyopathy appear to be transmitted as autosomal dominants with a high degree of penetrance; the remainder occur sporadically. Echocardiographic studies have confirmed that up to one-half the first-degree relatives (i.e., parents, siblings, and children) of patients with familial hypertrophic cardiomyopathy have evidence of septal hypertrophy, although many of these are without evidence of obstruction and are asymptomatic.

In contrast to the obstruction produced by a fixed narrowed orifice, such as valvular aortic stenosis, the obstruction in hypertrophic cardiomyopathy, when present, is dynamic and may change between examinations and even from beat to beat. Obstruction appears to result from further narrowing of an already small left ventricular outflow tract by systolic anterior motion of the mitral valve against the hypertrophied septum. While SAM may be found in a variety of other conditions besides hypertrophic cardiomyopathy, it is *always* found when obstruction is present in hypertrophic cardiomyopathy. Three basic mechanisms are involved in the production of dynamic obstruction: (1) increased left ventricular contractility, which reduces ventricular systolic volume and increases the ejection velocity of the blood moving through the outflow tract, thus drawing the anterior mitral valve leaflet against the septum as a result of reduced distending pressure; (2) decreased ventricular volume (preload), which reduces further the size of the outflow tract; and (3) decreased aortic impedance and pressure (afterload), which increases the velocity of flow through the subaortic area and also reduces ventricular systolic volume. Interventions that increase myocardial contractility, such as exercise, isoproterenol, and digitalis glycosides, and those that reduce ventricular volume, such as the Valsalva maneuver, sudden standing, nitroglycerin, amyl nitrite, or tachycardia, all may cause an increase in obstruction. Conversely, elevation of arterial pressure by phenyl-

ephrine, squatting, sustained handgrip, augmentation of venous return by raising the legs, and expansion of the blood volume all increase ventricular volume and ameliorate the obstruction. Sometimes the hypertrophied septum bulges into the outflow tract of the right ventricle, thereby impeding the ejection of blood from this chamber as well. Hypertrophic cardiomyopathy has been found in association with *lentiginosis* and other disorders of neural crest tissue. Similar gross anatomic and hemodynamic patterns may be found in the infants of diabetic mothers and in patients with *Friedreich's ataxia.*

CLINICAL FEATURES Many patients with hypertrophic cardiomyopathy are asymptomatic and may be relatives of patients with known disease. Unfortunately, the first clinical manifestation of the disease may be sudden death, frequently occurring in children and young adults, often during or after physical exertion. In symptomatic patients the most common complaint is dyspnea, largely due to increased stiffness of the left ventricular walls, which impairs ventricular filling and leads to elevated left ventricular diastolic and left atrial pressures. Other symptoms include angina pectoris, fatigue, syncope, and near syncope ("graying-out spells"). Symptoms are not related to the presence or severity of outflow obstruction. Most patients with obstruction demonstrate a double or triple apical impulse, a rapidly rising carotid arterial pulse, and a fourth heart sound. The hallmark of obstructive hypertrophic cardiomyopathy is a systolic murmur, which is typically harsh, diamond-shaped, and usually begins well after the first heart sound, since ejection is unimpeded early in systole. The murmur is best heard at the lower left sternal border as well as at the apex, where it is often more holosystolic and blowing in quality, no doubt due to the mitral regurgitation that usually accompanies obstructive hypertrophic cardiomyopathy.

LABORATORY EVALUATION The *electrocardiogram* commonly shows left ventricular hypertrophy and widespread, deep, broad Q waves that suggest an old myocardial infarction but apparently result from the abnormal electrophysiologic properties of the hypertrophied septum. Many patients demonstrate arrhythmias, both atrial (supraventricular tachycardia or atrial fibrillation) as well as ventricular (ventricular tachycardia) during ambulatory (Holter) monitoring. *Chest roentgenography* may be normal, although a mild to moderate increase in the cardiac silhouette is common. Aortic root enlargement and valvular calcification are not seen, helping to differentiate this condition from valvular aortic stenosis. The mainstay of the diagnosis of hypertrophic cardiomyopathy is the *echocardiogram*, which demonstrates left ventricular hypertrophy, typically with the septum 1.3 or more times the thickness of the high posterior left ventricular free wall. The septum may demonstrate an unusual ground-glass appearance, probably related to its abnormal cellular architecture and myocardial fibrosis. Systolic anterior motion of the mitral valve is found in patients with obstruction. The left ventricular cavity is typically small in hypertrophic cardiomyopathy, with vigorous posterior wall motion, but reduced septal excursion. A rare form of hypertrophic cardiomyopathy is characterized by massive apical hypertrophy, often associated with giant negative T waves on the electrocardiogram and a "spade-shaped" left ventricular cavity on angiography. The two-dimensional *echocardiogram* is particularly useful in identifying all of the characteristic changes, including the size and shape of the left ventricular cavity. The indirectly recorded *carotid arterial pulse* tracing rises unusually rapidly and often displays a "spike-and-dome" configuration when an outflow pressure gradient is present. *Radionuclide scintigraphy* with thallium 201 and blood pool scans permits visualization of the size and orientation of the interventricular septum.

The two typical *hemodynamic* features are an elevated left ventricular diastolic pressure due to diminished left ventricular compliance and, when obstruction is present, a systolic pressure gradient between the body of the left ventricle and the subaortic region. When a gradient is not present, it often can be induced by provocative maneuvers such as infusion of isoproterenol, inhalation of amyl nitrite, or the Valsalva maneuver.

TREATMENT Beta-adrenergic blockers are often used and may ameliorate to some degree the symptoms of angina pectoris and syncope. Resting intraventricular pressure gradients are usually unchanged, although these drugs may limit the increase in the gradient that occurs during exercise. However, there is no evidence that beta blockers protect against sudden death, which is presumably arrhythmic in origin. It is unestablished whether any antiarrhythmic agent is efficacious in this setting. However, the experimental agent amiodarone appears to be effective in reducing the frequency of supraventricular as well as life-threatening ventricular arrhythmias. The calcium channel blocking drugs, particularly verapamil and nifedipine, are promising agents that may reduce the stiffness of the ventricle, reduce the elevated diastolic pressures, increase exercise tolerance, and in some instances reduce the severity of outflow tract obstruction. Disopyramide has been used in some patients to reduce left ventricular contractility and the outflow gradient. Surgical myotomy/myectomy of the hypertrophied septum may result in lasting symptomatic improvement, but the mortality of approximately 10 percent limits the operation to severely symptomatic patients with high-grade obstruction unresponsive to medical management. Digitalis, diuretics, nitrates, and beta-adrenergic agonists are best avoided if possible, particularly in patients with known left ventricular outflow tract pressure gradients.

PROGNOSIS The natural history of hypertrophic cardiomyopathy is variable, although many patients demonstrate an improvement or stabilization of symptoms with time. Atrial fibrillation is common late in the course of the disease; its onset usually leads to a striking increase in symptoms, presumably due to loss of the atrial contribution to filling of the thickened ventricle. This rhythm, when sustained, is associated with a poor prognosis. Infective endocarditis occurs in less than 10 percent of patients, and endocarditis prophylaxis is indicated, particularly in patients with resting obstruction and mitral regurgitation. Progression of obstructive hypertrophic cardiomyopathy to left ventricular dilatation and dysfunction without an outflow gradient has been reported but is unusual. The major cause of mortality in hypertrophic cardiomyopathy is sudden death, which may occur in asymptomatic patients or interrupt an otherwise stable course in symptomatic ones. Paradoxically, younger patients and those with mild or no obstruction appear to be at particular risk of sudden death. Since sudden death often occurs during or just after physical exertion, strenuous exercise should be avoided in all patients, regardless of symptoms. Although hemodynamic factors may play a role, it is likely that most deaths, particularly those that are sudden, are due to ventricular arrhythmias. Beta-adrenergic blockade appears to be ineffective in preventing sudden death. The protective effect of calcium channel blockers or antiarrhythmic agents has not been established, but of the agents available, amiodarone appears to be the most promising in this regard.

MYOCARDITIS

Myocarditis is said to be present when the heart is involved in an inflammatory process. Most commonly the result of an infectious process, myocarditis may also be present in hypersensitivity states such as acute rheumatic fever (Chap. 186) or may be caused by radiation, chemicals, physical agents, and drugs. Myocarditis may be acute or chronic. In an unknown number of cases, acute myocarditis progresses to chronic dilated cardiomyopathy. While almost every infectious agent is capable of producing myocarditis, clinically significant acute myocarditis in the United States is caused most commonly by viruses. Coxsackie B is the most frequent etiologic agent of viral myocarditis, but Coxsackie A, poliomyelitis, influenza, adeno, echo, rubeola, and rubella viruses also cause the disease. In most cases, the presence of myocarditis is inferred only by the finding of transient electrocardiographic ST-T-wave abnormalities, but arrhythmias, heart failure, and death may occur in fulminant cases, particularly in infants and pregnant women. Myocarditis is frequently

associated with acute pericarditis, particularly when it is caused by Coxsackie B strains or echoviruses (Chap. 140).

Physical examination may be normal in patients who have only electrocardiographic abnormalities, although more severe cases may show a muffled first heart sound, along with a third heart sound and a murmur of mitral regurgitation. A pericardial friction rub may be audible in patients with associated pericarditis.

Experimental studies suggest that exercise may be deleterious in patients with myocarditis, and strenuous activity should be proscribed until the electrocardiogram has returned to normal. Prolonged bed rest has been advocated for more severe cases, although its efficacy remains to be established. Patients who develop congestive heart failure respond to the usual measures (digitalis, diuretics, salt restriction), but they appear to be unusually sensitive to digitalis. Arrhythmias are common and are occasionally difficult to manage. Deaths attributed to heart failure, tachyarrhythmias, and heart block have been reported, and it seems prudent to monitor the electrocardiogram of patients with arrhythmias, especially during the acute illness.

Though viral myocarditis is most often self-limited and without sequelae, active disease may recur, and it is likely that acute viral myocarditis occasionally progresses to a chronic form. Patients with viral myocarditis often give a history of a preceding upper respiratory febrile illness, and viral nasopharyngitis or tonsillitis may be evident clinically. The isolation of virus from the stool, pharyngeal washings, or other body fluids, and changes in specific antibody titers are helpful clinically. Many instances of apparent *idiopathic* dilated cardiomyopathy (page 999) appear to arise from mild or subclinical episodes of myocarditis. While corticosteroids may exacerbate heart damage in animals with acute viral myocarditis, a small number of humans with congestive heart failure and inflammatory myocarditis appear to respond to an experimental protocol utilizing immunosuppression with prednisone and azathioprine. Serial right ventricular endomyocardial biopsies have shown regression of inflammatory infiltrates in some patients so treated. However, the effects of this treatment program have not been rigorously compared to a comparable control group.

Bacterial myocarditis Bacterial involvement of the heart is uncommon, but when it does occur, it is usually as a complication of bacterial endocarditis (typically due to *Staphylococcus aureus* and enterococci). Myocardial abscess formation may involve the valve rings and interventricular septum. *Diphtheritic myocarditis* develops in over one-quarter of the patients with diphtheria, is one of the most serious complications, and is the most common cause of death due to diphtheria (Chap. 96). Cardiac damage is due to the liberation of a toxin that inhibits protein synthesis, and leads to a dilated, flabby, hypocontractile heart; the conducting system is frequently involved as well. Cardiomegaly and severe congestive heart failure typically appear after the first week of illness. ST-segment and T-wave abnormalities on the electrocardiogram are the rule, but atrial and ventricular arrhythmias, bundle branch block, and abnormalities of atrioventricular conduction are also common. Prompt therapy with antitoxin is crucial; antibiotic therapy is also indicated but is of less urgency.

Chagas' disease Chagas' disease, caused by the protozoan *Trypanosoma cruzi* (Chap. 156), produces an extensive myocarditis that typically becomes evident years after the initial infection. It is one of the most common causes of heart disease encountered in Central and South America; in rural areas up to 20 percent of the population may be affected. Although only a minority of infected individuals have an acute illness, upwards of one-third develop chronic myocardial damage, typically appearing 20 years after the initial infection. The chronic form is characterized by dilatation of several cardiac chambers, fibrosis and thinning of the ventricular wall, aneurysm formation in the areas of thinning (especially at the apex), and mural thrombi. Chronic progressive heart failure, often predominantly right-sided, is the rule. The electrocardiogram typically shows right bundle branch block and left anterior hemiblock, which may progress to complete atrioventricular block. The echocardiogram may reveal a unique pattern of hypokinesis of the posterior left ventricular wall and relatively preserved septal motion. Ventricular arrhythmias are common and are seen particularly during and after exertion; oral amiodarone appears to be particularly effective in treating ventricular tachyarrhythmias. The cause of death is either intractable congestive heart failure or an arrhythmia. Therapy is directed toward amelioration of the congestive heart failure and arrhythmias; the latter may require implantation of a pacemaker.

Toxoplasmic myocarditis (see also Chap. 157) This uncommon form of protozoal myocardial involvement occurs most frequently in immunosuppressed adults; congenital toxoplasmal infections are much more common, but myocardial is not a prominent feature. Myocardial involvement may lead to cardiac dilatation, pericarditis, and percardial effusion. Heart failure, arrhythmias, and conduction abnormalities may be seen. Because of the difficulty in diagnosing this condition, it may be a more common problem than is usually appreciated. Treatment is with pyrimethamine and sulfonamides, but the response to treatment is variable.

Giant cell myocarditis This rare myocarditis of unknown etiology is characterized by the presence of multinucleated giant cells in the myocardium. It usually causes rapidly fatal congestive heart failure and arrhythmia in young to middle-aged adults. At necropsy, the distinctive features include grossly visible serpiginous areas of myocardial necrosis in both ventricles and microscopic evidence of giant cells within an extensive inflammatory infiltrate. The cause of giant cell myocarditis remains obscure, although it occurs in association with thymoma, systemic lupus erythematosus, and thyrotoxicosis.

Lyme carditis (see also Chap. 127) Lyme disease is a newly described condition, caused by a tick-borne spirochete. Conduction abnormalities are the most common manifestations of cardiac involvement and may progress to complete atrioventricular block with syncope. Concomitant myopericarditis is not uncommon, and mild left ventricular dysfunction may occur. Prednisone may be efficacious in ameliorating the heart block; penicillin is used to treat the accompanying skin rash, arthritis, and neurologic abnormalities.

Radiation myocarditis A variety of acute and chronic cardiac complications may result from the use of ionizing radiation in the treatment of carcinoma of the lung or breast, lymphoma, or Hodgkin's disease. Only an occasional patient manifests acute cardiac abnormalities; typically such an abnormality consists of acute pericarditis. The most common presentation is that of chronic pericardial effusion or constriction occurring months or years after exposure (in rare cases up to 10 years) (Chap. 194). Myocardial fibrosis, resulting from damage to the microvasculature, often with formation of atherosclerotic plaques of the epicardial coronary arteries, is also common.

REFERENCES

ABELMANN WH: Classification and natural history of primary myocardial disease. Prog Cardiovasc Dis 27:73, 1984

BROSIUS FC III et al: Radiation heart disease. Am J Med 70:519, 1981

CUETO-GARCIA L et al: Echocardiographic findings in systemic amyloidosis: Spectrum of cardiac involvement and relation to survival. J Am Coll Cardiol 6:737, 1985

DALY K et al: Acute myocarditis: Role of histological and virological examination in the diagnosis and assessment of immunosuppressive treatment. Br Heart J 51:30, 1984

DEC GW JR et al: Active myocarditis in the spectrum of acute dilated cardiomyopathies: Clinical features, histologic correlates, and clinical outcome. N Engl J Med 312:885, 1985

FENOGLIO JJ JR et al: Diagnosis and classification of myocarditis by endomyocardial biopsy. N Engl J Med 308:12, 1983

FIGUILA HR et al: Spontaneous hemodynamic improvement or stabilization and associated biopsy findings in patients with congestive cardiomyopathy. Circulation 71:1095, 1985

GOTTDIENER JS et al: Doxorubicin cardiotoxicity: Assessment of late left ventricular dysfunction by radionuclide cineangiography. Ann Intern Med 94:430, 1981

GREENSPON AJ, SCHAAL SF: The "holiday heart": Electrophysiologic studies of alcohol effects in alcoholics. Ann Intern Med 98:135, 1983

HARTZ AJ et al: The association of smoking with cardiomyopathy. N Engl J Med 311:1201–1206, 1984

KNOCHEL JP: Cardiovascular effects of alcohol. Ann Intern Med 98:849, 1983

KOWEY PR et al: Sustained arrhythmias in hypertrophic obstructive cardiomyopathy. N Engl J Med 310:1566, 1984

LANGE RM et al: Adverse effects of acute alcohol ingestion in young adults. Ann Intern Med 102:742, 1985

MASON JW: Endomyocardial biopsy: The balance of success and failure. Circulation 71:185, 1985

McKENNA WJ: Arrhythmia and prognosis in hypertrophic cardiomyopathy. Eur Heart J 4:225, 1983

OLSEN EG, SPRY CJ: Relation between eosinophilia and endomyocardial disease. Prog Cardiovasc Dis 27:241, 1985

PARRILLO JE et al: The results of transvenous endomyocardial biopsy can frequently be used to diagnose myocardial diseases in patients with idiopathic heart failure: Endomyocardial biopsies in 100 consecutive patients revealed a substantial incidence of myocarditis. Circulation 69:93, 1984

POLL DS et al: Sustained ventricular tachycardia in patients with idiopathic dilated cardiomyopathy: Electrophysiologic testing and lack of response to antiarrhythmic drug therapy. Circulation 70:451, 1984

REGAN TJ: Alcoholic cardiomyopathy. Prog Cardiovasc Dis 27:141–152, 1984

REYES MP, LERNER AM: Coxsackie-virus myocarditis: With special reference to acute and chronic effects. Prog Cardiovasc Dis 27:373–394, 1985

SIEGEL RJ et al: Idiopathic restrictive cardiomyopathy. Circulation 70:451, 1984

STEERE AC et al: Lyme carditis: Cardiac abnormalities of Lyme disease. Ann Intern Med 93:8, 1980

TEN CATE FJ (ed): Hypertrophic Cardiomyopathy: Clinical Recognition and Management. Vol. 4, Basic and Clinical Cardiology. New York, Marcel Dekker, 1985

TORTI FM et al: Reduced cardiotoxicity of doxorubicin delivered on a weekly schedule: Assessment by endomyocardial biopsy. Ann Intern Med 99:745, 1983

VEILLE J-C: Peripartum cardiomyopathies: A review. Am J Obstet Gynecol 148:805, 1984

WYNNE J: Hypertrophic cardiomyopathy: A broadened concept of the disease and its management, in Update III: Harrison's Principles of Internal Medicine, KJ Isselbacher, et al (eds). New York, McGraw-Hill, 1982, p 129

———, BRAUNWALD E: The cardiomyopathies and myocarditides, in Heart Disease, 2d ed, E Braunwald (ed). Philadelphia, Saunders, 1984, p 1399

---

193   CARDIAC TUMORS, CARDIAC MANIFESTATIONS OF SYSTEMIC DISEASES, AND TRAUMATIC CARDIAC INJURY

WILSON S. COLUCCI / EUGENE BRAUNWALD

TUMORS OF THE HEART

PRIMARY TUMORS Primary tumors of the heart are rare and are often classified as "benign" histologically (Table 193-1). However, since all cardiac tumors have the potential for causing life-threatening complications, and many are now curable by surgery, it is important that this diagnosis be made whenever possible. Approximately three-quarters are *histologically* benign, and the remainder are malignant, in almost all cases sarcomas.

Clinical presentation Cardiac tumors may present with a wide array of cardiac and noncardiac manifestations. There may be signs and symptoms of all the more common forms of heart disease, including chest pain, syncope, heart failure, murmurs, arrhythmias, conduction disturbances, and pericardial effusion or tamponade. The specific signs and symptoms produced are most closely related to the location of the tumor.

Myxoma Myxomas are the most common type of primary cardiac tumor, accounting for one-third to one-half of all cases. They occur at all ages, show no sex preference, and may be familial. Most authorities consider the myxoma a true neoplasm, while others have suggested that it is formed by organization of an intracardiac thrombus attached to the endocardium. The large majority of myxomas are located in the atria, particularly the left, and arise from the interatrial septum in the vicinity of the fossa ovalis. Myxomas may also occur in the ventricles or be multiple in location. Most are pedunculated on a fibrovascular stalk and average 4 to 8 cm in diameter. The most common clinical presentation resembles that of mitral valve disease,

TABLE 193-1 Relative incidence of primary tumors of the heart

Type	Percent
BENIGN	
Myxoma	30.5
Lipoma	10.5
Papillary fibroelastoma	9.9
Rhabdomyoma	8.5
Fibroma	4.0
Hemangioma	3.5
Teratoma	3.3
Mesothelioma of the AV node	2.8
Other benign tumors	2.1
Total	75.1
MALIGNANT	
Sarcomas	18.6
Lymphoma	1.6
Other malignant tumors	4.7
Total	24.9

SOURCE: *Modified from HA McAllister, JJ Fenoglio, in Atlas of Tumor Pathology, Washington, Armed Forces Institute of Pathology, 1978, fasc 15, 2d series.*

either stenosis as a result of tumor prolapse into the mitral orifice during diastole or regurgitation as a consequence of injury to the valve by tumor-induced trauma. Ventricular myxomas may cause outflow obstruction and may therefore mimic subaortic or subpulmonic stenosis. Characteristically, the symptoms and signs are highly dependent on position, intermittent, and sudden in onset as a result of changes in tumor position with gravity. On auscultation, a characteristic low-pitched sound, termed a "tumor plop," is audible during early or middiastole and is thought to result from the tumor abruptly stopping as it strikes the ventricular wall. Myxomas may also present with peripheral or pulmonary emboli, or any of several noncardiac signs and symptoms including fever, weight loss, cachexia, malaise, arthralgia, rash, clubbing, Raynaud's phenomenon, hypergammaglobulinemia, anemia, polycythemia, leukocytosis, elevated erythrocyte sedimentation rate, thrombocytopenia, or thrombocytosis. Not surprisingly, myxomas are frequently misdiagnosed as endocarditis, collagen vascular disease, or noncardiac tumor.

Both M-mode and two-dimensional echocardiography are useful in the diagnosis of cardiac myxoma, the latter having the advantage of allowing determination of the site of tumor attachment and tumor size, important considerations in the planning of surgical excision. While cardiac catheterization and angiography are often performed prior to surgery, catheterization of the chamber from which the tumor originates is attended by the risk of dislodgment of tumor emboli. In many centers catheterization is no longer considered mandatory when adequate noninvasive information is available.

Surgical excision utilizing cardiopulmonary bypass is indicated in all patients and is generally curative. Occasional reports of tumor recurrence are most likely due to inadequate excision of multiple tumor sites.

Other benign tumors Cardiac *lipomas,* although relatively common, are usually incidental findings at postmortem examination and seldom result in symptoms. However, they may grow as large as 15 cm and present with symptoms due to mechanical interference with cardiac function, arrhythmias, or conduction disturbances, or as an abnormality of the cardiac silhouette on chest x-ray. *Papillary fibroelastomas,* similarly, are relatively common findings on cardiac valves or the adjacent endothelium but seldom result in clinical symptoms. Occasionally, these growths may cause mechanical interference with valvular function. *Rhabdomyomas* and *fibromas,* the most frequent tumors in infants and children, most commonly occur in the ventricles, and therefore produce signs and symptoms by mechanical obstruction which may mimic valvular stenosis, congestive heart failure, restrictive or hypertrophic cardiomyopathy, and pericardial constriction. Rhabdomyomas are probably hamartomatous growths, are multiple in about 90 percent of cases, and may be associated with tuberous sclerosis, adenoma sebaceum, and benign kidney tumors. *Heman-*

giomas and *mesotheliomas* are generally small tumors, most often intramyocardial in location, and may cause atrioventricular (AV) conduction disturbances and even sudden death as a result of their propensity for location in the region of the AV node.

Sarcomas Cardiac sarcomas may be of several histologic types, but in general are characterized by a rapidly downhill course leading to the patient's death in weeks to months from the time of presentation as a result of hemodynamic compromise, local invasion, or distant metastases. Sarcomas commonly involve the right side of the heart, and because of their rapid growth, invasion of the pericardial space and obstruction of the cardiac chambers or venae cavae are common. At the time of presentation these tumors have often spread too extensively for surgical excision. While there are scattered reports of palliation with surgery, radiotherapy, and chemotherapy, the overall experience with cardiac sarcomas is poor. The one exception to this appears to be cardiac lymphosarcomas, which may respond to a combination of chemo- and radiotherapy.

TUMORS METASTATIC TO THE HEART Tumors metastatic to the heart are several times more common than primary tumors, and as the life expectancy of patients with various forms of malignant neoplasms is extended by more effective therapy, it is likely that the frequency of cardiac metastases will also increase. Although cardiac metastases occur in all tumor types with an incidence ranging from 1 to 20 percent, the incidence is especially high in malignant melanoma, and to a somewhat lesser extent in leukemia and lymphoma. In absolute numbers, cardiac metastases are most common in carcinoma of the breast and lung, reflecting the high incidence of these cancers. Cardiac metastases almost always occur in the setting of widespread primary disease, and most often there is either primary or metastatic disease elsewhere in the thoracic cavity. Nevertheless, occasionally a cardiac metastasis may be the initial presentation of a tumor elsewhere in the body.

Cardiac metastases reach the heart via the bloodstream, lymphatics, or direct invasion and generally are small, firm nodules; although diffuse infiltrations may also occur, especially with sarcomas or hematologic neoplasms. The pericardium is most often involved, followed by myocardial involvement of any chamber, and, rarely, by involvement of the endocardium or cardiac valves.

Cardiac metastases result in clinical manifestations only about 10 percent of the time, and rarely are they the cause of death. In most patients they are *not* the cause of the presenting clinical features but occur in the setting of a previously recognized malignant neoplasm. While cardiac metastases may present a large number of nonspecific signs and symptoms, the most common are dyspnea, a new systolic murmur, signs of acute pericarditis, cardiac tamponade, a rapid increase in the cardiac silhouette on chest x-ray, the new onset of an ectopic tachyarrhythmia, AV block, and congestive heart failure. As with primary cardiac tumors, the clinical presentation is more closely related to the location and size of the tumor than to its histologic type. Many of these signs and symptoms may also occur with myocarditis, pericarditis, or cardiomyopathy resulting from radiotherapy or chemotherapy.

The electrocardiographic findings are entirely nonspecific and may include ST-T–wave changes, decreased QRS voltage, arrhythmias, and conduction disturbances. On chest roentgenography the cardiac silhouette is most often normal but may reveal a pericardial effusion or bizarre contour. Echocardiography is useful for the diagnosis of pericardial effusion and the visualization of larger metastases. Angiography may delineate discrete lesions, and pericardiocentesis can allow a specific cytologic diagnosis. Since most patients with cardiac metastases have widespread disease, therapy generally consists of pericardiocentesis when there is hemodynamic compromise, and treatment directed at the primary tumor. The removal of a malignant effusion by pericardiocentesis with or without concomitant instillation of a sclerosing agent (e.g., tetracycline) may palliate symptoms and delay or prevent reaccumulation of the effusion.

CARDIAC EFFECTS OF CANCER THERAPY See Chap. 192.

CARDIOVASCULAR MANIFESTATIONS OF SYSTEMIC DISEASES

DIABETES MELLITUS (see Chap. 327)   In patients with insulin-dependent diabetes mellitus there is an increased incidence of large-vessel atherosclerosis and myocardial infarction, and diabetics are more likely to have an abnormal or absent pain response to myocardial ischemia, probably as a result of generalized autonomic nervous system dysfunction. Diabetic patients may also have myocardial dysfunction characteristic of a restrictive cardiomyopathy in the absence of large-vessel coronary artery disease, as evidenced by elevated left ventricular filling pressures. Histologically, these patients have increased amounts of collagen, glycoprotein, triglycerides, and cholesterol in the myocardial interstitium, and in some cases intimal thickening, hyaline deposition, and inflammatory changes have been observed in small intramural arteries. While these changes alone seldom result in clinical heart failure, it is likely that they contribute to the excessive cardiovascular morbidity and mortality of diabetics. There is some evidence that insulin therapy results in an amelioration of the myocardial dysfunction.

MALNUTRITION AND THIAMINE DEFICIENCY (BERIBERI)
Malnutrition (see Chap. 72)   In patients whose intake of protein, calories, or both is severely deficient, the heart may become thin, pale, and flabby with myofibrillar atrophy and interstitial edema. The systolic pressure and cardiac output are low, and the pulse pressure narrow. Generalized edema is common and is due to a combination of factors, including reduced serum oncotic pressure and myocardial dysfunction. Such profound states of malnutrition, termed *marasmus* in the case of caloric deficiency, or *kwashiorkor* in the case of relative protein deficiency, are most common in underdeveloped countries. However, significant nutritional heart disease may also occur in developed nations, particularly in patients with severe cardiac failure in whom gastrointestinal hypoperfusion and venous congestion may cause anorexia and malabsorption. Open-heart surgery poses an increased risk in such patients, who may benefit from preoperative intensive hyperalimentation. Deficient nutrients and minerals should be replaced gradually since rapid expansion of the intravascular space may stress the weakened heart and result in overt congestive heart failure.

Thiamine deficiency (see Chap. 76)   In many cases, malnutrition is accompanied by thiamine deficiency, although this hypovitaminosis may also occur in the presence of an adequate protein and caloric intake, particularly in the far east, where polished rice deficient in thiamine is a major dietary component. The widespread use of thiamine-enriched flour in western nations confines this disease primarily to alcoholics and food faddists. Clinically, there is usually evidence of generalized malnutrition, peripheral neuropathy, glossitis, and anemia. The characteristic cardiovascular syndrome is that of high-output heart failure with tachycardia, increased cardiac output, and often elevated filling pressures in the left and right side of the heart. It appears that the major cause of the high-output state is vasomotor depression, the precise mechanism of which is not understood, but which leads to a reduced systemic vascular resistance. The cardiac examination reveals a wide pulse pressure, tachycardia, a third heart sound, and, frequently, a systolic murmur at the apex. The electrocardiogram may show decreased voltage, a prolonged QT interval, and T-wave abnormalities; the chest x-ray generally shows a large heart with signs of congestive heart failure. The response to thiamine is often dramatic, with diuresis and a reduction in heart size. Although the response to digitalis and diuretics may be poor prior to thiamine therapy, these agents may be important *after* thiamine is given since the left ventricle may not be capable of dealing with the increased workload presented by the return of vascular tone.

OBESITY (see Chap. 317)   Although not defined as a disease per se, severe obesity is associated with an increase in cardiovascular morbidity and mortality, due in part to hypertension, glucose intolerance, and atherosclerotic coronary artery disease, all of which are more prevalent in obese patients. In addition, these patients have a distinct abnormality of the cardiovascular system characterized by increases in total and central blood volumes, cardiac output, and left ventricular filling pressure. It appears that cardiac output is elevated in order to help supply the metabolic needs of the excessive adipose tissue. Left ventricular filling pressure is often at the upper limits of normal and rises excessively with exercise. As a result of chronic volume and pressure overload, abnormal ventricular function may develop. Pathologically, there is left and, in some cases, right ventricular hypertrophy and generalized cardiac enlargement, which is not due simply to fatty infiltration of the myocardium. Clinically, these patients may develop pulmonary congestion, peripheral edema, and exercise intolerance, findings which may be difficult to recognize in massively obese patients. Weight reduction is the most effective therapy and results in reduction in blood volume and in return of cardiac output toward normal. Digitalis, sodium restriction, and diuretics may also be useful. This form of heart disease should be distinguished from the Pickwickian syndrome (Chap. 215), which may share several of the cardiovascular features but, in addition, frequently has components of central apnea, hypoxemia, pulmonary hypertension, and cor pulmonale.

THYROID DISEASE (see Chap. 324)   Thyroid hormone exerts a major influence on the cardiovascular system by a number of direct and indirect mechanisms, and not surprisingly, cardiovascular effects are prominent in both hypo- and hyperthyroidism. Thyroid hormone causes increases in total-body metabolism and oxygen consumption which indirectly place an increased workload on the heart. In addition, although the exact mechanism has not been defined, thyroid hormone exerts direct inotropic and chronotropic effects which are similar to those seen with adrenergic stimulation (e.g., tachycardia, increased cardiac output). It has been shown that thyroid hormone increases the synthesis of myosin and of Na^+, K^+-ATPase, as well as the density of myocardial beta-adrenergic receptors.

Hyperthyroidism   Excess thyroid hormone results in increases in heart rate, cardiac output, and pulse pressure. Patients may present with palpitations, systolic hypertension, fatigue, or, in patients with underlying heart disease, angina, or heart failure. Sinus tachycardia is found in about 40 percent of patients, and atrial fibrillation in about 15 percent. Other findings include a hyperactive precordium, an increase in the intensity of the first heart sound and the pulmonic component of the second heart sound, a third heart sound, and, in some cases, a midsystolic murmur heard best at the left sternal border with or without a systolic ejection click. A systolic scratchy sound, the *Means-Lerman scratch,* may occasionally be heard at the left second intercostal space during expiration and is thought to result from the rubbing of the hyperdynamic pericardium against the pleura. Elderly patients with hyperthyroidism may present with only the cardiovascular manifestations of thyrotoxicosis, which may be resistant to therapy until the hyperthyroidism is controlled. Both angina pectoris and congestive heart failure are unusual, unless there is coexistent underlying heart disease, and in many cases will resolve with therapy of the hyperthyroidism.

Hypothyroidism   There is a reduction in cardiac output, stroke volume, heart rate, blood pressure, and pulse pressure. In about one-third of patients there is a pericardial effusion which only rarely results in tamponade. Clinically, there is cardiomegaly, bradycardia, weak arterial pulses, and distant heart sounds. Biochemical abnormalities, including elevations of creatine kinase (CK), serum glutamic oxaloacetic transaminase (SGOT), and lactic dehydrogenase (LDH), may lead to a mistaken diagnosis of myocardial infarction. The electrocardiogram generally shows sinus bradycardia and low voltage and may show prolongation of the QT interval, decreased P-wave voltage, prolonged AV conduction time, intraventricular conduction disturbances, and nonspecific ST-T–wave abnormalities. Chest x-ray shows cardiomegaly, often with a "water bottle" configuration, pleural effusions, and, in some cases, evidence of congestive heart failure. Pathologically, the heart is pale, dilated, and flabby, often with myofibrillar swelling, loss of striations, and interstitial fibrosis.

Patients with hypothyroidism frequently have elevations of cholesterol and triglycerides and severe atherosclerotic coronary artery disease. Prior to treatment with thyroid hormone, patients with hypothyroidism frequently do not have angina pectoris, presumably because of the low metabolic demands made by their condition. However, such patients, especially when elderly, are prone to angina and myocardial infarction during replacement of thyroid hormone, and this should always be done with extreme care, starting with very low doses which are increased gradually.

MALIGNANT CARCINOID (see Chap. 299)   These tumors elaborate a variety of vasoactive amines, kinins, indoles, and other substances which are believed to be responsible for the diarrhea, flushing, and labile blood pressure seen in these patients. The cardiac lesions due to gastrointestinal carcinoids are almost exclusively in the right side of the heart and occur only when there are hepatic metastases, suggesting that the substance responsible for the cardiac lesions is inactivated by passage through the liver and lungs. Similar lesions occur in the left side of the heart when there is a right-to-left shunt or the tumor is located in the lungs. Fibrous plaques are found on the endothelium of the cardiac chambers, valves, and great vessels. These plaques, which result in distortion of the cardiac valves, consist of smooth muscle cells imbedded in a stroma of acid mucopolysaccharide and collagen, and presumably result from healing of endothelial injury. The clinical syndrome is most often that of tricuspid regurgitation, pulmonic stenosis, or both. In some cases a high-output state may occur, presumably as a result of a decrease in systemic vascular resistance due to a vasoactive substance released by the tumor. Progression of the cardiac lesions does not appear to be affected by treatment with serotonin antagonists, and in some cases valve replacement is indicated. Coronary artery spasm, presumably due to a circulating vasoactive substance, may occur in patients with carcinoid syndrome.

PHEOCHROMOCYTOMA (see Chap. 326)   In addition to causing hypertension, which may be labile or sustained, the high circulating levels of catecholamines may also cause direct myocardial injury. Focal myocardial necrosis and inflammatory cell infiltration are seen in about 50 percent of patients who die with pheochromocytoma and may contribute to clinically significant left ventricular failure and pulmonary edema. In addition, hypertension results in left ventricular hypertrophy.

RHEUMATOID ARTHRITIS AND THE COLLAGEN VASCULAR DISEASES Rheumatoid arthritis (see Chap. 263)   There may be inflammation of any or all parts of the heart in patients with rheumatoid arthritis. *Pericarditis* is the most common cause of clinically apparent disease and may be found in 30 to 50 percent of all patients with rheumatoid arthritis, particularly those with subcutaneous nodules, if carefully searched for by echocardiography or at postmortem examination. However, only a small fraction of these patients will have clinical evidence of pericarditis, which usually follows a benign course, but occasionally may progress to cardiac tamponade or constrictive pericarditis. The pericardial fluid is generally an exudate, with decreased concentrations of complement and glucose and elevated cholesterol. Treatment is directed at the underlying rheumatoid arthritis and may include corticosteroids. Pericardiectomy is usually required in cases of tamponade or persistent effusion. *Coronary arteritis* with intimal inflammation and edema is present in about 20 percent of cases but only rarely results in angina pectoris or myocardial infarction. The cardiac valves, most often the mitral and aortic, may be involved by inflammation and granuloma formation which in some cases may cause clinically significant regurgitation due to valve deformity. Myocarditis rarely results in cardiac dysfunction.

Seronegative arthropathies   The seronegative arthropathies (Chaps. 267 and 276), ankylosing spondylitis, Reiter's syndrome, psoriatic arthritis, and the arthritides associated with ulcerative colitis and regional enteritis may be accompanied by a pancarditis with tachycardia, cardiomegaly, and prolongation of the AV conduction time. These patients are particularly likely to develop aortic regurgitation due to an aortitis and consequent dilatation of the aortic root and AV block, both of which are more common in patients with peripheral joint involvement and long-standing disease. Up to one-fifth of patients with peripheral joint involvement and disease for more than 30 years have significant aortic regurgitation. Occasionally, aortic regurgitation precedes the onset of arthritis, and, therefore, the diagnosis of a seronegative arthritis should be considered in young males with isolated aortic regurgitation.

Systemic lupus erythematosus (SLE) (see Chap. 262)   Pericarditis is common, occurring in about two-thirds of patients, and generally pursues a benign course, although rarely tamponade or constriction may result. The characteristic *endocardial lesions* of SLE, described by Libman and Sacks, consist of wartlike lesions most often located at the angles of the AV valves or on the ventricular surface of the mitral valve. Although arteritis of large coronary arteries may rarely result in myocardial ischemia, there is also an increased frequency of coronary atherosclerosis which may be related to hypertension or corticosteroid therapy.

TRAUMATIC HEART DISEASE

Cardiac damage may be due to both penetrating and nonpenetrating injuries. The most frequent cause of a *nonpenetrating injury* is impact of the chest against the steering wheel of an automobile. Serious injury of the heart may ensue even though no external sign of thoracic trauma is evident. Although the commonest injury is myocardial contusion, any structure of the heart may be affected by the trauma. If the valvular apparatus is ruptured, a loud heart murmur produced by valvular regurgitation may appear, followed by the development of rapidly progressive heart failure. The most serious consequence of nonpenetrating injury is rupture, either of the atria or of the ventricles, which is generally fatal. Hemopericardium may also follow tearing of a pericardial vessel or coronary artery.

Myocardial contusion may cause arrhythmias, bundle branch block, or electrocardiographic abnormalities resembling those of infarction, and so it is important to bear trauma in mind as a cause of otherwise unexplained electrocardiographic changes. Similarly, myocardial contusion may produce positive radionuclide scans and regional impairment of ventricular function, as occurs in patients with acute myocardial infarction (Chap. 179). Pericardial effusion may occur weeks or even months after the accident. In these cases, the pericardial effusion is a manifestation of the postcardiac injury syndrome, which resembles the postpericardiotomy syndrome (Chap. 194).

Acute myocardial failure resulting from rupture of a valve usually requires operative correction. Myocardial infarction due to trauma is treated similarly to that due to ischemic heart disease (Chap. 190). Pericardial hemorrhage often leads to constriction which must be treated by decortication.

Penetrating injuries of the heart, produced by bullets or stab wounds, usually result in immediate or very rapid death because of hemopericardium or massive hemorrhage. However, sometimes the patient survives the acute incident and presents with a cardiac murmur and congestive heart failure. A left-to-right shunt due to traumatic ventricular septal defect, aortopulmonary artery fistula, or coronary arteriovenous fistula may be suspected and confirmed by cardiac catheterization and angiocardiography. Operation is indicated if hemodynamically significant abnormalities are present or if a foreign body, e.g., a bullet, is lodged in the heart. Immediate thoracotomy should be carried out if there is cardiac tamponade and/or shock, whether the trauma was penetrating or nonpenetrating. Pericardiocentesis may be helpful in patients with tamponade, but usually only as a holding maneuver. Patients who suffer penetrating injuries of the heart should be carefully examined several weeks after the event to rule out a ventricular septal defect or mitral regurgitation which may have gone undetected at the time of emergency surgery.

Rupture of the aorta is a common consequence of chest trauma. Indeed, rupture of the aorta at the isthmus or just above the aortic valve is the most common vascular deceleration injury. The clinical presentation is similar to that in aortic dissection (Chap. 197). The arterial pressure and pulse amplitude may be increased in the upper extremities and decreased in the lower extremities, and on chest roentgenogram there may be widening of the mediastinum. Occasionally, the rupture is limited by the aortic adventitia and results in a silent false aneurysm which may be discovered months or years after the injury. When great vessel rupture is due to a penetrating injury, there is usually a hemothorax and, less often, a hemopericardium. Hematoma formation may compress major vessels, and arteriovenous fistulae may be formed, sometimes resulting in high-output congestive heart failure.

REFERENCES

AYZENBERG O et al: Beriberi heart disease. S Afr Med J 68:263, 1985

BRANCH CL JR, et al: Left atrial myxoma with cerebral emboli. Neurosurgery 16:675, 1985

BULKLEY BH, ROBERTS WC: The heart in systemic lupus erythematosus and the changes induced in it by corticosteroid therapy. A study of 36 necropsy patients. Am J Med 58:243, 1975

COHN PF, BRAUNWALD E: Traumatic heart disease, in *Heart Disease*, 2d ed, E Braunwald (ed). Philadelphia, Saunders, 1984, p 1528

COLUCCI WS, BRAUNWALD E: Primary tumors of the heart, in *Heart Disease*, 2d ed, E Braunwald (ed). Philadelphia, Saunders, 1984, p 1457

FEIN FS, SONNENBLICK EH: Diabetic cardiomyopathy. Progr Cardiovasc Dis 27:255, 1985

FYKE FE et al: Primary cardiac tumors: Experience with 30 consecutive patients since the introduction of two-dimensional echocardiography. J Am Coll Cardiol 5:1465, 1985

KLEIN I, LEVEY GS: New perspectives on thyroid hormone, catecholamines, and the heart. Am J Med 76:167, 1984

LOCKWOOD WB, BROGHAMER WL JR: The changing prevalence of secondary cardiac neoplasms as related to cancer therapy. Cancer 15:2659, 1980

PERLOFF JK: Cardiac rhythm and conduction in Duchenne's muscular dystrophy: A prospective study of 20 patients. J Am Col Cardiol 3:1263, 1984

ROBERTS WC, SJOERDSMA A: The cardiac disease associated with the carcinoid syndrome. Am J Med 36:5, 1969

SEMB RK et al: Angiographic and echocardiographic observations in surgical patients with atrial myxoma. Cardiovasc Intervent Radiol 8:119, 1985

STOLLERMAN E: Rheumatic fever, connective tissue disorders and heart disease, in *Heart Disease*, 2d ed, E Braunwald (ed). Philadelphia, Saunders, 1984, p 1641

SUTHERLAND GR et al: Hemodynamic adaptation to acute myocardial contusion complicating blunt chest injury. Am J Cardiol 57:291, 1986

194   PERICARDIAL DISEASE

EUGENE BRAUNWALD

NORMAL FUNCTIONS OF THE PERICARDIUM   The visceral pericardium is a serous membrane, separated by a small amount of fluid, an ultrafiltrate of plasma, from a fibrous sac, the parietal pericardium. The pericardium prevents sudden dilatation of the cardiac chambers during exercise and hypervolemia, and as the result of the development of a negative intrapericardial pressure during ejection it facilitates atrial filling during ventricular systole. The pericardium also restricts the anatomic position of the heart, minimizes friction between the heart and surrounding structures, prevents displacement of the heart and kinking of the great vessels, and probably retards the spread of infections from the lungs and pleural cavities to the heart. Notwithstanding the foregoing, total absence of the pericardium does not produce obvious clinical disease. In partial left pericardial defects the main pulmonary artery and left atrium may bulge through the defect; rarely herniation and subsequent strangulation of the left atrium may cause sudden death.

ACUTE PERICARDITIS

It is useful to classify the types of pericarditis both clinically and etiologically (Table 194-1), as this disorder is by far the most common pathologic process involving the pericardium.

Pain, a pericardial friction rub, electrocardiographic changes, and pericardial effusion with cardiac tamponade and paradoxic pulse are cardinal manifestations of many forms of acute pericarditis and will be considered prior to a discussion of the most common forms of the disorder.

Pain is an important but not invariable symptom in various forms of acute pericarditis; it is usually present in the acute infectious types and in many of the forms presumed to be related to hypersensitivity or autoimmunity. Pain is often absent in a slowly developing tuberculous, postirradiation, neoplastic or uremic pericarditis. The pain of pericarditis is often severe; its character and location have been described in Chap. 4. It is characteristically in the center of the chest, referred to the back and the trapezius ridge. Often the pain is pleuritic, i.e., sharp and aggravated by inspiration, coughing, and changes in body position, but occasionally it is a steady, constrictive pain, which radiates into either arm or both arms and resembles that

TABLE 194-1   Classification of pericarditis

I Clinical classification
  A Acute pericarditis (<6 weeks)
    1 Fibrinous
    2 Effusive (or bloody)
  B Subacute pericarditis (6 weeks to 6 months)
    1 Constrictive
    2 Effusive-constrictive
  C Chronic pericarditis (>6 months)
    1 Constrictive
    2 Effusive
    3 Adhesive (nonconstrictive)
II Etiologic classification
  A Infectious pericarditis
    1 Viral
    2 Pyogenic
    3 Tuberculous
    4 Mycotic
    5 Other infections (syphilitic, parasitic)
  B Noninfectious pericarditis
    1 Acute myocardial infarction
    2 Uremia
    3 Neoplasia
      a Primary tumors (benign or malignant)
      b Tumors metastatic to pericardium
    4 Myxedema
    5 Cholesterol
    6 Chylopericardium
    7 Trauma
      a Penetrating chest wall
      b Nonpenetrating
    8 Aortic aneurysm (with leakage into pericardial sac)
    9 Postirradiation
    10 Associated with atrial septal defect
    11 Associated with severe chronic anemia
    12 Infectious mononucleosis
    13 Familial Mediterranean fever
    14 Familial pericarditis
      a Mulibrey nanism*
    15 Sarcoidosis
    16 Acute idiopathic
  C Pericarditis presumably related to hypersensitivity or autoimmunity
    1 Rheumatic fever
    2 Collagen vascular disease
      a Systemic lupus erythematosus
      b Rheumatoid arthritis
      c Scleroderma
    3 Drug-induced
      a Procainamide
      b Hydralazine
      c Other
    4 Postcardiac injury
      a Postmyocardial infarction (Dressler's syndrome)
      b Postpericardiotomy

* *An autosomal recessive syndrome, characterized by growth failure, muscle hypotonia, hepatomegaly, ocular changes, enlarged cerebral ventricles, mental retardation, and chronic constrictive pericarditis.*

of myocardial ischemia; confusion with myocardial infarction is common. Characteristically, however, the pericardial pain is relieved by sitting up and leaning forward. This problem becomes even more perplexing when, with acute pericarditis, the serum transaminase level rises to about 80 units. However, the MB isoenzyme of creatine kinase does not rise in acute pericarditis.

The *pericardial friction rub* is the most important physical sign; it may have up to three components per cardiac cycle, as described in Chap. 177, and can sometimes be elicited only when firm pressure with the diaphragm of the stethoscope is applied to the chest wall. It is heard most frequently during expiration, but an independent pleural friction rub may be audible during inspiration, with the patient leaning forward or in the left lateral decubitus position. The rub is likely to be inconstant and transitory, and a loud to-and-fro leathery sound may disappear within a few hours, possibly to reappear the following day.

The *electrocardiogram* in acute pericarditis without massive effusion (see also Chap. 178) usually displays widespread elevation of the ST segments, involving two or three standard limb leads and V_2 to V_6, with reciprocal depressions only in aVR and V_1 and without significant changes in QRS complexes, except occasionally for some diminution in voltage. Several days later, the ST segments return to normal and the T waves *then* become inverted. In contrast, in acute myocardial infarction, reciprocal depression of ST segments is usually more prominent; QRS changes occur, particularly the development of Q waves, and notching and loss of the amplitude of R waves; and T-wave inversions usually occur *before* the ST segments have become isoelectric. Sequential electrocardiograms are useful in distinguishing acute pericarditis from acute myocardial infarction. Early repolarization is a normal variant and may also cause widespread ST-segment elevation, most prominent in left precordial leads. However, in this condition the T waves are usually tall and the ST/T ratio is under 0.25, but exceeds this number in acute pericarditis. Depression of the PR segment (below the TP segment) also is common in acute pericarditis. With large pericardial effusions, the QRS voltage is reduced. Atrial premature beats and atrial fibrillation are sometimes noted.

PERICARDIAL EFFUSION
Usually associated with one or more of the above-mentioned manifestations of pericarditis and an enlargement of the cardiac silhouette, pericardial effusion is especially important clinically when it develops within a relatively short time. Differentiation from cardiac enlargement may be difficult, but heart sounds tend to become faint; the friction rub may disappear or remain clearly audible, and the apex impulse may vanish, but sometimes it is palpable well medial to the left border of cardiac dullness. The chest roentgenogram may show a "water bottle" configuration of the cardiac silhouette, but it may also be normal or almost so. Lucent pericardial fat lines may be seen deep within the cardiopericardial silhouette. Fluoroscopic examination may show the ventricular pulsations to be diminished. When the effusion is large, an area of dullness and tubular breath sounds is often encountered at the angle of the left scapula, probably caused by compression of the lung (Ewart's sign).

Diagnosis of pericardial effusion
Echocardiography (Chap. 179) is the most effective laboratory technique available, since it is sensitive, specific, simple, innocuous, and noninvasive, and may be performed at the bedside. The presence of pericardial fluid is recorded as a relatively echo-free space between the posterior pericardium and the posterior left ventricular epicardium in patients with small effusions and such a space between the anterior right ventricle and the parietal pericardium just beneath the anterior chest wall with larger effusions (Fig. 194-1). In patients with large effusions the heart may swing freely within the pericardial sac; when severe, this motion may be associated with electrical alternans. While M-mode echocardiography is usually adequate for the diagnosis of pericardial effusion, two-dimensional echocardiography is often superior since it allows more precise localization and estimation of the quantity of pericardial fluid.

In tamponade, during inspiration, right ventricular diameter increases while left ventricular diameter and mitral valve opening decrease. Often there is late diastolic inward motion (collapse) of the right ventricular free wall, and of the right atrium. The diagnosis of pericardial fluid or thickening may be confirmed by one of the following:

1 *Cardiac catheterization.* A catheter is introduced into the right atrium and rotated so that its tip makes contact with the lateral right atrial wall. In the presence of an effusion, or pericardial thickening, the tip of the catheter is seen to be separated from the radiolucent lungs by an opaque band.
2 *Angiocardiography.* Contrast medium is injected rapidly into the right atrium; again the lateral wall is separated from the edge of the cardiac silhouette.

When it is deemed desirable to remove pericardial fluid for diagnostic and/or therapeutic purposes, a needle attached to a properly grounded electrocardiographic lead is inserted into the pericardial

FIGURE 194-1 *Two-dimensional (upper panel) and short-axis (lower panel) parasternal scans in systole in a patient with a large pericardial effusion surrounding the entire heart. Fluid is seen to extend behind the left atrium (white arrowhead) and anterior to the descending thoracic aorta (DA). AoV = aortic valve; LA = left atrium; LV = left ventricle; PE = pericardial effusion; RV = right ventricle. (Modified from PC Come (ed), Diagnostic Cardiology: Noninvasive imaging techniques, Philadelphia, Lippincott, 1985.)*

space, usually through a subxiphoid approach, and if possible using echocardiographic control. Intrapericardial pressure should be measured before fluid is withdrawn. When an effusion develops, the fluid nearly always has the physical characteristics of an exudate. Bloody fluid is commonly due to tuberculosis or tumor, but it may also be found in the effusion of rheumatic fever or in the post-cardiac injury syndrome (see below). Occasionally, bloody fluid may be found in the effusion of uremic pericarditis and in the hemopericardium following myocardial infarction, especially following the administration of anticoagulants.

CARDIAC TAMPONADE   The accumulation of fluid in the pericardium in an amount sufficient to cause serious obstruction to the inflow of blood to the ventricles results in cardiac tamponade. The amount of fluid necessary to produce this critical state may be as small as 250 mL, when the fluid develops rapidly; or it may be over 1000 mL in slowly developing effusions when the pericardium has had the opportunity to stretch and adapt to the increasing volume of fluid. The volume of fluid required to produce tamponade varies directly with the thickness of the ventricular myocardium and inversely with the thickness of the parietal pericardium. Tamponade results most often from bleeding into the pericardial space following cardiac operations, trauma (including cardiac perforation during diagnostic procedures), tuberculosis, and tumor (most commonly carcinoma of the lung and breast and lymphoma), but it may occur in acute viral or idiopathic pericarditis, postirradiation pericarditis, renal failure during dialysis, and hemopericardium which may result when a patient with any form of acute pericarditis is treated with anticoagulants.

The clinical manifestations are due to the fall in cardiac output and to systemic venous congestion. However, the classic findings of falling arterial pressure, rising venous pressure, and a small quiet heart with faint heart sounds usually are seen only with severe tamponade occurring within minutes, as happens with cardiac trauma. More frequently, tamponade develops more slowly and the clinical manifestations, resembling those of heart failure, include dyspnea, orthopnea, hepatic engorgement, and jugular venous hypertension. A high index of suspicion is required, since, in many instances, no obvious cause for pericardial disease is apparent, and tamponade should be considered in any patient with hypotension and elevation of jugular venous pressure with a prominent x descent; often the y descent is diminutive or absent. A widening of the area of flatness to percussion across the anterior aspect of the chest wall, a paradoxical pulse (see below), relatively clear lung fields, diminished pulsations of the cardiac silhouette on fluoroscopy, reduction in amplitude of the QRS complexes, and *electrical alternans* of the P, QRS, and T waves should raise the suspicion of cardiac tamponade. A positive Kussmaul's sign (see below) is rare in cardiac tamponade, as is a pericardial knock. Their presence suggests that the beginning of an organizing process and epicardial constriction are present in addition to effusion. Since immediate treatment may be lifesaving, prompt measures to establish the diagnosis definitely, i.e., echocardiography followed by cardiac catheterization, should be undertaken. The latter reveals elevation of the right atrial pressure with prominence of the x but not of the y descent. When measured, the pericardial pressure is also elevated and equal to the right atrial pressure. There is "equalization" of pressures, i.e., the pulmonary artery wedge is equal, or close, to right atrial, right ventricular, and pulmonary artery diastolic pressures. The "square root" sign in the ventricular pressure pulses and the prominent y descent in atrial and jugular venous pressure characteristic of constrictive pericarditis (see below) are usually absent.

Paradoxical pulse   This important clue to the presence of cardiac tamponade consists of *a greater than normal (10 mmHg) inspiratory decrease in systolic arterial pressure*. When severe, it may be detected by palpating weakness or disappearance of the arterial pulse during inspiration, but usually sphygmomanometric measurement of systolic pressure during slow respiration is required (Fig. 194-2).

The mechanism of paradoxical pulse in cardiac tamponade is complex. Normally, the inspiratory decline in intrathoracic pressure enhances right ventricular filling by virtue of the increased pressure gradient between the extrathoracic veins and the chambers of the right side of the heart. As a consequence right ventricular diastolic volume and stroke output increase, and this increase is transmitted to the left side of the heart several cardiac cycles later, leading to an increase in systemic arterial pressure during the following expiration. Therefore, normally a small pressure fall occurs during inspiration. Also, left ventricular afterload rises during inspiration as intrapericardial pressure falls, and left ventricular stroke volume and therefore arterial pressure decline slightly during inspiration. In cardiac tamponade, since both ventricles share a tight incompressible covering, the pericardial sac, the inspiratory increase in right ventricular volume compresses and reduces left ventricular volume; leftward bulging of the interventricular septum may further reduce the left ventricular cavity as the right ventricle enlarges during inspiration. Thus, in cardiac tamponade the inspiratory augmentation of right ventricular volume causes an exaggerated reciprocal reduction in left ventricular volume. Also, respiratory distress increases the fluctuations in intrathoracic pressure, which exaggerates the mechanism just described.

Low-pressure tamponade refers to mild tamponade in which the intrapericardial pressure is increased from its slightly subatmospheric levels to +5 to +10 mmHg; in some instances hypovolemia coexists. As a consequence the central venous pressure is slightly elevated while arterial pressure is unaffected. The patients are asymptomatic or complain of mild weakness and dyspnea. The diagnosis is aided by echocardiography, and both hemodynamic and clinical manifestations improve following mild pericardiocentesis.

Paradoxical pulse occurs in only approximately one-third of patients with *constrictive pericarditis*. It is important to bear in mind

FIGURE 194-2 *Simultaneous recording of electrocardiogram (ECG), blood flow velocity in the superior vena cava (SVC), brachial arterial pressure (BA), and the pneumogram (Pneumo) in a patient with cardiac compression and paradoxical pulse. A downward deflection of the pneumogram denotes inspiration, when SVC blood velocity rises and arterial pressure falls (paradoxical pulse). Arterial pressure is maintained during prolonged expiratory pause.*

that paradoxical pulse is not pathognomonic of pericardial disease because it may be observed in various forms of restrictive cardiomyopathies (Chap. 192) and, in some cases of hypovolemic shock, chronic obstructive airways disease, and severe bronchial asthma.

TREATMENT All patients with acute pericarditis should be observed frequently and carefully for the possibility of a developing effusion or, if effusion is already present, for signs of tamponade. In the presence of an effusion, arterial and venous pressures and heart rate should be monitored continuously or carefully followed and serial echocardiograms obtained. If manifestations of tamponade appear, pericardiocentesis must be carried out at once, since relief of the intrapericardial pressure may be lifesaving. A small catheter advanced over the needle inserted into the pericardial cavity may be left in place if fluid accumulation persists and allows draining of the pericardial space.

VIRAL OR IDIOPATHIC FORM OF ACUTE PERICARDITIS This disorder is an important clinical entity because of its frequency and because it may be confused with other more serious illnesses. In some cases an A or B coxsackievirus or the virus of influenza, echovirus type 8, mumps, herpes simplex, chickenpox, or adenovirus has been isolated from pericardial fluid and/or appropriate elevations in viral antibody titers have been noted; in other instances, acute pericarditis has occurred in association with illnesses of known viral origin and, presumably, was caused by the same agent. More commonly there is an antecedent infection of the respiratory tract, but in many patients such an association is not evident and viral isolation and serologic studies are negative. Most frequently, a viral causation cannot be established nor can it be excluded; the term *acute idiopathic pericarditis* is then appropriate. However, regardless of the specific causative factor, the clinical manifestations are similar. This form of acute pericarditis occurs at all ages but is more frequent in young adults; it is often associated with pleural effusions and pneumonitis. The appearance of fever and precordial pain at about the same time, often 10 to 12 days after a presumed viral illness, constitutes an important feature in the differentiation of acute pericarditis from myocardial infarction, in which pain precedes fever. The constitutional symptoms are usually mild to moderate, but occasionally the initial symptoms are stormy, the temperature rising to 40°C. The disease ordinarily runs its course in a few days to 2 weeks, but occasionally after the patient has apparently recovered he or she may have one or several recurrences, weeks or even months later. Tamponade is unusual, although accumulation of some pericardial fluid is common, and constrictive pericarditis develops rarely. A pericardial friction rub is often audible. The ST-T–wave alterations in the electrocardiogram are usually transitory, but the abnormal T waves may persist for several years or indefinitely and be a source of confusion in persons without a clear history of pericarditis. Pleuritis and pneumonitis frequently accompany pericarditis. The erythrocyte sedimentation rate is elevated. Granulocytosis followed by lymphocytosis is common.

There is no specific therapy, but anti-inflammatory treatment with aspirin, if necessary up to 900 mg qid, may be given. If this is ineffective, one of the nonsteroidal anti-inflammatory agents, such as indomethacin (25 to 75 mg qid) or a corticosteroid (e.g., prednisone, 20 to 80 mg daily) effectively suppresses the clinical manifestations of the acute illness and may be useful in patients in whom the purulent and tuberculous forms of pericarditis have been excluded. After the patient has been asymptomatic for 1 week, the dose of the anti-inflammatory agent is gradually tapered. Recurrences occur in about one-fourth of patients, but the tendency to relapse decreases within 2 years after the initial episode. When recurrences continue to occur beyond this period and are frequent and disabling, pericardiectomy may be effective in terminating the illness.

POST-CARDIAC INJURY SYNDROME During the past few years, it has been recognized that an acute form of pericarditis may appear under a variety of circumstances which have one common feature: previous injury to the myocardium, with blood in the pericardial cavity. The syndrome has been observed when the injury has been induced in the course of a cardiac operation (postpericardiotomy syndrome or, as it was originally designated, postcommissurotomy syndrome). It may also follow myocardial infarction (Dressler's syndrome) or develop after trauma of the heart (e.g., stab wound, contusions following a nonpenetrating blow to the chest, and following perforation of the heart with a pacemaker catheter).

The principal symptom is the pain of acute pericarditis, which usually develops after an interval of 1 to 4 weeks following the cardiac injury but sometimes appears only after a lapse of months. Recurrences are common and may occur up to 2 years or more after the injury. Fever up to 40°C, pericarditis, pleuritis, and pneumonitis are the outstanding features, the bout of illness usually subsiding in 1 or 2 weeks. The pericarditis, which appears to be the most constant lesion, may be of the fibrinous variety, or it may be a pericardial effusion, which is often serosanguineous and sometimes causes tamponade. Rarely, the pericarditis may be accompanied by arthralgias. Leukocytosis, an increased sedimentation rate, and electrocardiographic changes typical of acute pericarditis may also occur.

The mechanism whereby the clinical manifestations are induced is not certain, but there is a likelihood that they are the result of a hypersensitivity reaction in which the antigen originates from injured myocardial tissue and/or pericardium; the suggested designation of post-cardiac injury syndrome for this group of disorders implies that they may have a common pathogenetic mechanism. Circulating autoantibodies to myocardium occur frequently, but their precise role in this syndrome has not been defined. Viral infection may also play an etiologic role, since antiviral antibodies are often elevated in patients who develop this syndrome following cardiac surgery.

The clinical picture mimics acute viral or acute idiopathic pericarditis. Moreover, it is possible that the recurrences that occur so frequently in the latter condition are not always caused by an exacerbation of the original (presumably viral) infection, but that the original injury may have initiated the sequence of events that culminates in the post-cardiac injury syndrome.

Often no treatment is necessary aside from aspirin, nonsteroidal anti-inflammatory drugs, or analgesics. The management of pericardial effusion and tamponade has already been discussed. When the illness is severe and is followed by a series of disabling recurrences, therapy with a nonsteroidal anti-inflammatory agent or a corticosteroid is usually effective.

Differential diagnosis Differential diagnosis of *acute idiopathic pericarditis* is primarily one of exclusion, as there is no specific test for this disorder. Consequently all other disorders that may be associated with acute fibrinous pericarditis must be considered. When associated with *acute myocardial infarction,* acute fibrinous pericarditis may be confused with acute viral or idiopathic pericarditis; this complication of infarction, described on page 992, must be differentiated by the occurrence of fever, pain, and a friction rub in the first 4 days following the development of the infarct. Electrocardiographic abnormalities (such as the appearance of Q waves and earlier T-wave changes in myocardial infarction), the extent of the elevations of myocardial enzymes, and the total clinical picture are helpful in the identification of the pericarditis of acute myocardial infarction. A common error is assuming that acute viral or idiopathic pericarditis represents acute myocardial infarction.

Acute pericarditis occurring as a component of the *post-cardiac injury* syndrome is most likely to be confused with acute idiopathic pericarditis when it follows myocardial infarction or a nonpenetrating bruise to the chest. Such pericarditis is differentiated from acute idiopathic pericarditis chiefly by timing. If it occurs within a few weeks of an infarction or a chest blow, it may be justified to conclude that the two are probably related. If the infarct has been silent or the chest blow forgotten, the relationship to the pericarditis may not be recognized.

It is important to distinguish *pericarditis due to collagen disease* from acute idiopathic pericarditis. Most important in the differential diagnosis is the pericarditis due to systemic lupus erythematosus (Chap. 262). Sometimes the latter appears as an asymptomatic effusion; more often pain is present, and rarely tamponade develops. Very rarely, when pericarditis occurs in the absence of other evidence of any underlying disorder, differentiation from acute viral and idiopathic pericarditis or tuberculous pericarditis may be made on discovery of lupus erythematosus (LE) cells, a rise in antinuclear antibodies, or by the specific methods for diagnosing tuberculosis. Acute pericarditis is also an occasional complication of *rheumatoid arthritis*, *scleroderma*, and *periarteritis nodosa*, but again, other evidence of these diseases is usually obvious. Asymptomatic pericardial effusion is also frequent in these disorders. It is important to question every patient with acute pericarditis about the ingestion of procainamide, hydralazine, isoniazid, cromolyn, and minoxidil, since these drugs can cause this syndrome.

The pericarditis of *acute rheumatic fever* is generally associated with evidence of severe pancarditis and with cardiac murmurs (Chap. 186). *Pyogenic (purulent) pericarditis* is usually secondary to cardiothoracic operations, immunosuppressive therapy, rupture of the esophagus into the pericardial sac, and rupture of a ring abscess in a patient with infective endocarditis and with septicemia complicating aseptic pericarditis. It is now uncommonly due to pneumococcal pneumonia and pleuritis, previously the most common cause. *Tuberculous pericarditis* (see Chap. 119) may present as an acute pericarditis, associated with fever, weight loss, and other clinical manifestations of active systemic tuberculosis; the diagnosis may be aided by a positive tuberculin test and evidence of pulmonary or mediastinal tuberculosis. Tubercle bacilli can be cultured from the pericardial space only infrequently, and a biopsy of the pericardium with bacteriologic and histologic examination may be required. Alternatively, tuberculous pericarditis may present as a chronic asymptomatic effusion, as subacute effusive-constrictive pericarditis, or frank chronic constrictive pericarditis (see below). *Uremic pericarditis* (Chap. 220) occurs in up to one-third of patients with chronic uremia, and is seen most frequently in patients undergoing chronic hemodialysis. It may be fibrinous or associated with a bloody effusion. A friction rub is common, but pain is usually absent. Treatment with an anti-inflammatory agent and intensification of hemodialysis is usually adequate therapy. Occasionally, when tamponade occurs, pericardiocentesis is required. When pericarditis is recurrent or persistent, pericardiectomy is necessary. Pericarditis due to *neoplastic diseases* results from irradiation or extension of primary or metastatic tumors (most commonly carcinoma of the lung and breast, malignant melanoma, and lymphoma) to the pericardium or from invasion by a lymphomatous or leukemic process; pain, atrial arrhythmias, and tamponade are complications which occur occasionally. *Mediastinal irradiation* for neoplasm may cause pericarditis after eradication of the tumor. Unusual causes of acute pericarditis include syphilis, fungous infection (histoplasmosis, blastomycosis, aspergillosis, and candidiasis), and parasitic infestation (amebiasis, toxoplasmosis, echinococcosis, trichinosis).

CHRONIC PERICARDIAL EFFUSIONS Chronic pericardial effusions are often encountered in patients without an antecedent history of acute pericarditis. They may cause few symptoms per se, and may be suspected by finding an enlarged cardiac silhouette on chest roentgenogram which may be obtained in the course of the workup of a patient with symptoms related to the underlying illness.

Tuberculosis This is the most common cause of chronic pericardial effusion (Chap. 119). The symptoms are often those of a chronic, systemic illness in an individual with effusion. It is important to bear this condition in mind when a middle-aged or elderly person with fever has apparent enlargement of the heart of undetermined origin, with or without elevation of venous pressure. Weight loss, fever, and fatigability are sometimes observed. Inasmuch as effective specific methods of therapy have now reduced strikingly the mortality rate from the previous figures of about 70 percent, overlooking a tuberculous pericardial effusion is a serious error. Consequently, no method of examination should be omitted to establish this diagnosis. Included are chest roentgenograms for pulmonary tuberculosis and a search for tuberculosis in other organs; tuberculin skin tests, repeated after several weeks; cultures and smears of gastric washings and of pleural and pericardial fluid. Finally, if the diagnosis is still obscure, a pericardial biopsy, preferably by a limited thoracotomy, should be performed after 1 or 2 weeks of preliminary antituberculous chemotherapy. If definitive evidence is then still lacking, but the specimen shows caseation necrosis, antituberculous chemotherapy for at least 24 months is justified (Chap. 119). Pericardiectomy should be carried out in order to prevent the development of constriction if the biopsy specimen shows a thickened pericardium.

Other causes of chronic pericardial effusion *Myxedema* may be responsible for a pericardial effusion that is sometimes massive but rarely, if ever, causes cardiac tamponade. The other manifestations of myxedema should clarify the diagnosis, but unfortunately, even when they are present, the diagnosis is frequently overlooked. It is important, therefore, to carry out appropriate tests for thyroid function (Chap. 324) in patients with an enlarged cardiac outline of undetermined origin. The cardiac silhouette is markedly enlarged and an echocardiogram is necessary to distinguish cardiomegaly from pericardial effusion. *Cholesterol pericardial disease* produces large pericardial effusions with a high cholesterol content, which may induce an inflammatory response and constrictive pericarditis.

Neoplasms, systemic lupus erythematosus, rheumatoid arthritis, mycotic infection, radiation therapy, pyogenic infections, severe chronic anemia, and chylopericardium may also cause chronic pericardial effusion and should be considered and specifically looked for in such patients.

Aspiration and analysis of the pericardial fluid are often helpful in diagnosis. In infections the organism can often be identified by smear or culture. Grossly sanguineous pericardial fluid results most commonly from a neoplasm, tuberculosis, uremia, or slow leakage from an aortic aneurysm.

CHRONIC CONSTRICTIVE PERICARDITIS

This disorder results when the healing of an acute fibrinous or serofibrinous pericarditis is followed by obliteration of the pericardial cavity, with the formation of granulation tissue which gradually contracts and forms a firm scar, encasing the heart and interfering with filling of the ventricles. In some reports, a high percentage of all cases has been of tuberculous origin. In other series, particularly those reported in the United States in the last decade, tuberculosis has been an infrequent cause. The condition also may follow purulent infection, trauma, cardiac operation of any type, mediastinal irradiation, histoplasmosis, neoplastic disease, and acute viral or idiopathic pericarditis, rheumatoid arthritis, lupus erythematosus, and chronic renal failure with uremia treated by chronic dialysis. In many patients the cause of the pericardial disease is undetermined, and in them it is presumed that an asymptomatic or forgotten bout of acute pericarditis, acute or idiopathic, was the inciting event. Rarely, routine radiographic examination may reveal calcification of the pericardium in a person who is free of all symptoms referable to the heart.

The basic physiologic abnormality in symptomatic patients with chronic constrictive pericarditis, as in those with cardiac tamponade, is the inability of the ventricles to fill adequately during diastole because of the limitations imposed by the rigid, thickened pericardium or the tense pericardial fluid. Stroke volume is reduced, and the end-diastolic pressures in both ventricles, as well as the mean pressures in the atria, pulmonic veins, and systemic veins, are all elevated to about the same levels. Despite these hemodynamic changes myocardial function may be normal; instead, the ventricles may be considered to be underloaded. In constrictive pericarditis the central venous and right and left atrial pressure pulses display an M-shaped contour, with prominent *x* and *y* descents; the *y* descent is the most prominent deflection and is interrupted by a rapid rise in pressure during early diastole, when ventricular filling is impeded by the constricting pericardium. In cardiac tamponade the pressure contour differs in that the most prominent deflection is the *x* trough, while the *y* descent is usually absent. These characteristic changes are transmitted to the jugular veins, where they may be recognized by inspection or recorded. In constrictive pericarditis, both ventricular pressure pulses exhibit characteristic ''square root'' signs during diastole. These hemodynamic changes, although characteristic, are not pathognomonic of constrictive pericarditis but are also observed in cardiomyopathies characterized by restriction of ventricular filling, as discussed on page 1001.

CLINICAL FINDINGS Weakness, fatigue, weight loss, and anorexia are common. The patients often appear to be chronically ill with decreased muscle mass, a protuberant abdomen, and peripheral edema. Contrary to a widely held impression, dyspnea, though absent or slight at rest, is often present on exertion, and orthopnea is common in chronic constrictive pericarditis, although it is not severe. Attacks of acute left ventricular failure (acute pulmonary edema) practically never occur. The cervical veins are distended and may remain so even after intensive diuretic treatment, and venous pressure may fail to decline during inspiration (Kussmaul's sign). In about one-third of the cases a paradoxical pulse may be observed. Congestive hepatomegaly is pronounced and may impair hepatic function; ascites is common and is usually more prominent than dependent edema. In about half of the patients, the heart is normal in size; if it is enlarged, the enlargement is rarely extreme. The apical pulse is reduced in intensity. The heart sounds may be distant, an early third heart sound, i.e., a pericardial knock, occurring 0.06 to 0.12 s after aortic valve closure which coincides with a sudden deceleration in ventricular filling, is often conspicuous, and murmurs are usually absent. The apex beat is poorly defined, and cardiac pulsations under fluoroscopic examination are diminished. Because of the high sustained venous pressure, congestive splenomegaly may be sufficiently pronounced to make the spleen palpable. In the absence of infective endocarditis or tricuspid valve disease, splenomegaly in a patient with congestive heart failure should arouse suspicion of constrictive pericarditis. Protein-losing gastroenteropathy due to impaired lymphatic drainage from the small intestine, and the nephrotic syndrome, or sometimes only marked proteinuria or hypoalbuminemia, may complicate chronic constrictive pericarditis. The electrocardiogram frequently displays low voltage of the QRS complex and diffuse flattening or inversion of the T waves. P mitrale may be present in patients with sinus rhythm; atrial fibrillation is present in about one-third of these patients.

Systemic and/or pulmonary venous congestion is initially the result of impaired filling of the ventricles caused by the restrictive action of the inelastic pericardium. However, the fibrotic process may extend into the myocardium, and venous congestion may then be due to the combined effects of the myocardial and pericardial lesions. The interference with filling reduces the work of the heart and perhaps this leads to myocardial atrophy. The latter probably accounts for the delayed beneficial effects of operative treatment observed in some patients with advanced disease.

Inasmuch as the usual physical signs of cardiac disease (murmurs, cardiac enlargement) may be inconspicuous or absent, hepatic enlargement and dysfunction associated with intractable ascites may lead to a mistaken diagnosis of cirrhosis of the liver. This error should be avoided if the neck veins are inspected carefully in all patients with ascites and hepatomegaly. *Given a clinical picture resembling that of cirrhosis, but with the added feature of distended neck veins, careful search for calcification of the pericardium by chest roentgenograms, fluoroscopy, and echocardiography should be carried out and may disclose a curable or remediable form of heart disease.* Calcification occurs in only about one-half of these patients and usually in those with long-standing pericardial constriction. Most patients with chronic constrictive pericarditis show pericardial thickening on echocardiographic examination. Surgical exploration of the

pericardium is justifiable if the clinical picture and echocardiographic and cardiac catheterization findings are suggestive even in the absence of pericardial calcification.

DIFFERENTIAL DIAGNOSIS Like cor pulmonale (Chap. 191), chronic constrictive pericarditis may be associated with severe systemic venous hypertension but with little or no pulmonary congestion; the heart may not appear to be enlarged, and a striking inspiratory fall in arterial pressure may be present. However, in cor pulmonale advanced parenchymal pulmonary disease is usually evident and venous pressure *falls* during inspiration. *Tricuspid stenosis* may also simulate the picture of chronic constrictive pericarditis; congestive hepatomegaly and ascites may be equally prominent, and the manifestations of left-sided heart failure may be inconspicuous. However, in tricuspid stenosis, the characteristic murmur, the frequent coexistence of mitral stenosis, the absence of a paradoxic pulse, as well as the absence, in the jugular venous pulse, of the steep, deep *y* descent followed by a rapid ascent (manifested by the diastolic shock on palpation and its audible equivalent, the pericardial knock), should make the clinical differentiation possible.

It is of the greatest importance, though often difficult, to distinguish chronic constrictive pericarditis from various forms of heart disease which are characterized by a similar physiologic abnormality, i.e., restriction of ventricular filling, leading to a similar clinical picture. Described in Chap. 192, these include endomyocardial fibrosis, infiltrative cardiomyopathies such as amyloidosis, hemochromatosis, sarcoidosis, scleroderma and idiopathic myocardial hypertrophy, in which the marked thickening of the ventricular wall is responsible for the diminished compliance.

The features favoring the diagnosis of one of the above forms of cardiomyopathy are a well-defined apex beat, conspicuous enlargement of the heart, and pronounced orthopnea with attacks of acute left ventricular failure, left ventricular hypertrophy, gallop sounds, bundle branch block, and significant Q waves in the electrocardiogram. The echocardiogram shows ventricular thickening, sometimes with a granular sparkling appearance. At catheterization, patients with chronic constrictive pericarditis usually have left atrial or pulmonary arterial wedge pressure equaling right atrial pressure, the latter often exceeding 15 mmHg despite intensive medical treatment for heart failure; the pulmonary artery systolic pressure is often less than 50 mmHg, and the right ventricular end-diastolic pressure often reaches one-third of the systolic pressure; the cardiac output is slightly depressed. In contrast, in patients with cardiomyopathy, the left atrial usually exceeds the right atrial pressure by more than 5 mmHg, the mean right atrial pressure often falls to below 15 mmHg following intensive treatment, the pulmonary artery systolic pressure often exceeds 50 mmHg, and the right ventricular end-diastolic pressure is usually less than one-third of the systolic pressure, while the cardiac output is markedly depressed. The volumes of both ventricles, as determined by angiography or echocardiography, are characteristically reduced or normal in constrictive pericarditis, and the ejection fractions are normal; the left ventricular end-diastolic volume may be normal in some cardiomyopathies but is frequently elevated in others, in whom the ejection fraction is reduced; the latter finding militates strongly against the diagnosis of constrictive pericarditis. The echocardiogram in chronic constrictive pericarditis characteristically shows pericardial thickening, i.e., a distinct echo posterior to the left ventricular wall, and paradoxical septal motion. The left ventricular wall moves sharply outward in early diastole and then remains flat. The definitive diagnosis of restrictive cardiomyopathy, when it is due to an infiltrative disease such as amyloidosis, can often be established by endomyocardial biopsy.

It is important to emphasize that when a patient has progressive, disabling, and unresponsive congestive failure, and if he or she displays any of the phenomena of constrictive heart disease, the most careful and detailed clinical and laboratory studies must be carried out in order to detect or exclude constrictive pericarditis, which is potentially a curable condition. In many instances cardiac catheterization, selective angiocardiography, coronary arteriography, and endomyocardial biopsy may be required. However, when even these examinations do not yield a definitive diagnosis, surgical exploration of the pericardium is the only decisive method of determining whether constrictive pericarditis is responsible for the clinical manifestations of heart failure.

Occult constrictive disease   Patients with this condition may have unexplained fatigue, dyspnea, and chest pain. No overt manifestations of pericardial disease are present, but following the rapid intravenous infusion of 1 liter of saline solution, atrial and ventricular pressure pulses and diastolic equilibration of intracardiac pressures, as in overt constrictive pericarditis, occur. Although symptomatic improvement may follow pericardiectomy, this procedure should not be carried out in asymptomatic persons.

TREATMENT   Pericardial resection is the only definitive treatment of constrictive pericarditis, but diuretics and sodium restriction are useful during preoperative preparation. Digitalis may be beneficial in the prevention of heart failure when resection of the thickened pericardium permits an increased inflow into the ventricles and hence places an enhanced burden on an atrophic myocardium. The benefits derived from a complete cardiac decortication are often striking, and frequently the improvement, though slight at first, is progressive over a period of many months.

Many instances of constrictive pericarditis are of tuberculous origin. Antituberculous therapy during the phase of effusion may prevent the development of constriction, and such therapy should be carried out before and after operation, if a tuberculous origin is suspected or cannot be excluded in a patient with chronic constrictive pericarditis (Chap. 119).

SUBACUTE EFFUSIVE-CONSTRICTIVE PERICARDITIS   This form of pericardial disease is characterized by a combination of a tense effusion in the pericardial space, as well as constriction of the heart by thickened pericardium, and thus it shares a number of features both with pericardial effusion producing cardiac compression and with pericardial constriction. It may be caused by tuberculosis, multiple attacks of acute idiopathic pericarditis, radiation, traumatic pericarditis, uremia, and scleroderma. The heart is generally enlarged,

and there are a paradoxical pulse and a prominent *x* descent in the atrial pressure pulse. Following pericardiocentesis, the physiologic findings may change from those of cardiac tamponade to those of pericardial constriction, with a "square root sign" in the ventricular pressure pulse and a prominent *y* descent in the atrial and jugular venous pressures. In many patients the condition progresses to the chronic constrictive form of the disease. Wide excision of both the visceral and parietal pericardium is usually effective.

OTHER DISORDERS OF THE PERICARDIUM

Pericardial cysts appear as rounded or lobulated deformities of the cardiac silhouette, most commonly at the right cardiophrenic angle. They do not cause symptoms, and their major clinical significance lies in the possibility of confusion with a tumor, ventricular aneurysm, or massive cardiomegaly. *Tumors* involving the pericardium are most commonly secondary to malignant neoplasms originating in or invading the mediastinum, including carcinoma of the bronchus and breast, lymphoma, and melanoma. The most common *primary* malignant tumor is the mesothelioma. The usual clinical picture of malignant pericardial tumor is an insidiously developing, often bloody, pericardial effusion. Surgical exploration is required to establish a definitive diagnosis and to carry out definitive or, more commonly, palliative treatment.

REFERENCES

BOLTWOOD CM, SHAH PM: The pericardium in health and disease. Cur Probl Cardiol 9:1, 1984

BUSH CA et al: Occult pericardial disease. Circulation 56:924, 1977

HANCOCK EW: Subacute effusive-constrictive pericarditis. Circulation 43:183, 1971

LORELL B, BRAUNWALD E: Pericardial disease, in *Heart Disease*, 2d ed. Philadelphia, Saunders, 1984, p 1470

MCCAUHGAN BC et al: Early and late results of pericardiectomy for constrictive pericarditis. J Thorac Cardiovasc Surg 89:340, 1985

NISHIMURA RA et al: Constrictive pericarditis: Assessment of current diagnostic procedures. Mayo Clin Proc 60:397, 1985

REDDY et al (eds): *Pericardial Disease*. New York, Raven, 1982

RIBEIRO P et al: Constrictive pericarditis as a complication of coronary artery bypass surgery. Br Heart J 51:205, 1984

section 2 Disorders of the vascular system

195 ATHEROSCLEROSIS AND OTHER FORMS OF ARTERIOSCLEROSIS

EDWIN L. BIERMAN

Arteriosclerosis, a generic term for thickening and hardening of the arterial wall, is responsible for the majority of deaths in the United States and most westernized societies. One type of arteriosclerosis is *atherosclerosis,* the disorder of the larger arteries that underlies most *coronary artery disease, aortic aneurysm,* and *arterial disease of the lower extremities* and also plays a major role in *cerebrovascular disease.* Atherosclerosis is by far the leading cause of death in the United States, both above and below age 65 (Table 195-1).

Other types of arteriosclerosis include focal calcific arteriosclerosis (*Mönckeberg's sclerosis*) and *arteriolosclerosis.* The major arterial diseases other than arteriosclerosis include *congenital structural*

defects, inflammatory or granulomatous diseases (e.g., syphilitic aortitis), and disorders affecting mainly the smaller vessels, such as *hypersensitivity* or autoimmune diseases.

THE NORMAL ARTERY

STRUCTURE   The normal artery wall consists of three reasonably well-defined layers: the intima, the media, and the adventitia.

Intima   A single continuous layer of *endothelial cells* lines the lumen of all arteries. The intima is delimited on its outer aspect by a perforated tube of elastic tissue, the *internal elastic lamina.* This tube of elastic tissue is particularly prominent in the large elastic arteries and the medium-caliber muscular arteries, and it disappears in capillaries. The endothelial cells are attached to one another by a series of junctional complexes and are also attached, apparently somewhat tenuously, to an underlying meshwork of loose connective tissue, the *basal lamina*. These lining endothelial cells normally form a barrier that controls the entry of substances from the blood into the artery wall. Such substances usually enter the cells by specific transport systems. Normally, no other cell type is present in the intima of most arteries.

Media The media consists of only one cell type, the *smooth-muscle cell*, arranged in either a single layer (as in small muscular arteries) or multiple lamellae (as in elastic arteries). These cells are surrounded by small amounts of collagen and elastic fibers, which they elaborate, and usually take the pattern of diagonal concentric spirals through the vessel wall. They are closely apposed to one another and may be attached by junctional complexes. The smooth-muscle cell appears to be the major connective tissue–forming cell of the artery wall, producing collagen, elastic fibers, and proteoglycans. In that sense it is analogous to the fibroblast in skin, the osteoblast in bone, and the chondroblast in cartilage. The media is bounded on the luminal side by the internal elastic lamina and on the abluminal side by a less continuous sheet of elastic tissue, the *external elastic lamina*. In *elastic arteries*, like the aorta and the major pulmonary arteries, elastic lamellae are prominent. Such arteries expand and increase their elastic tension with the pulse of systole. In diastole, the elastic fibers recoil, helping to propel the blood distally and progressively damping the pulsatile character of flow toward more terminal vessels. In *muscular arteries*, in which smooth-muscle cells predominate, peripheral flow is regulated, particularly in arterioles, by contraction (vasoconstriction) and relaxation (vasodilatation). Located about midway through the media of most arteries is a "nutritional watershed." The outer portion is nourished from the small blood vessels (vasa vasorum) in the adventitia; the inner layers receive their nutrients from the lumen.

Adventitia The outermost layer of the artery is the adventitia, which is delimited on the luminal aspect by the external elastic lamina. This external coat consists of a loose interwoven admixture of collagen bundles, elastic fibers, smooth-muscle cells, and fibroblasts. This layer also contains the vasa vasorum and nerves.

METABOLISM AND FUNCTION The artery wall is a metabolically active organ that must meet a steady demand for energy to maintain smooth-muscle tension and endothelial cell function and to repair and replenish tissue constituents. The mechanical forces on the arterial wall are complex, and considerable tensile stresses are imposed on it, mainly by hydraulic force. Shear or frictional stresses are especially prominent near the entrance regions of branches. The form and manner in which these forces are dissipated depend upon flow, the amount of elastic tension developed, and the tethering or external support provided by surrounding structures. Arteries are also permeable pipes, which constantly exchange fluid and solutes with the blood they carry.

Maintenance of the endothelial cell lining is critical. Endothelial cell turnover occurs at a slow rate but may be accelerated in focal areas by changing patterns of flow along the vessel wall. When intact, these cells selectively control the passage of circulating substances by active transport (endocytosis and exocytosis) through their cytoplasm, and they elaborate connecting tissue components to form their own substratum. In addition, intact endothelial cells function to prevent clotting partly by elaboration of a particular prostaglandin (prostacyclin or PGI_2) that inhibits platelet function, thereby enhancing unimpeded flow of blood. When the lining is damaged, platelets adhere to it, in part as the result of production of a different class of prostaglandins, the thromboxanes, and form a clot; endothelial cells function in the clotting process by elaboration of key substances, including factor VIII.

The metabolism of arteries reflects the biochemistry of smooth-muscle cells. Arterial smooth-muscle cells form abundant collagen, elastic fibers, soluble and insoluble elastin, and glucosaminoglycans (mainly dermatan sulfate). Multiple anabolic and catabolic pathways are present. These cells metabolize glucose by both anaerobic and aerobic glycolysis. A variety of catabolic enzymes are present including fibrinolysins, mixed-function oxidases, and lysosomal hydrolases. Because of the prominence of lipids in atherosclerotic lesions, much attention has been directed to lipid metabolism in arteries. Arterial wall cells can synthesize fatty acids, cholesterol, phospholipids, and triglycerides from endogenous substrates to satisfy their structural needs (membrane replenishment), but smooth-muscle cells appear preferentially to utilize lipids from plasma lipoproteins transported into the wall. Circulating lipoproteins traverse endothelial cells in pinocytotic vesicles. Smooth-muscle cells possess specific high-affinity surface receptors for certain apoproteins on the surface of lipid-rich lipoproteins, thus facilitating the entry of lipoproteins into the cell by adsorptive endocytosis. As has been shown for cultured skin fibroblasts, in arterial smooth-muscle cells these vesicles fuse with lysosomes, resulting in catabolism of lipoprotein components (Chap. 315). Free cholesterol entering the cell in this manner inhibits endogenous cholesterol synthesis, facilitates its own esterification, and partially limits further entry of cholesterol by regulating the number of lipoprotein receptors. However, lipoprotein cholesterol can gain entry into arterial smooth muscle cells by non-receptor-mediated pathways, potentially causing cholesterol ester accumulation.

Thus, many complex and interrelated metabolic processes are present in arterial wall cells. Although some of these may play a role in the production of arteriosclerosis, no one biochemical reaction can be singled out as culpable. Physiologic factors, such as transfer processes across the endothelial lining, the flux of oxygen and substrates from both the luminal and adventitial sides of the wall, and the reverse flow of catabolic products, need to be considered as well. The ability of the arterial wall to maintain the integrity of its endothelium, prevent platelet aggregation, prevent adherence of blood mononuclear cells, and ensure the nutrition of its middle portion may be the critical determinants of the arteriosclerotic process.

CHANGES WITH AGING The major change that occurs with normal aging in the arterial wall in humans is a slow, apparently continuous, symmetric increase in the thickness of the intima. This intimal thickening results from a gradual accumulation of smooth-muscle cells (presumably resulting from migration of these cells from the media and their subsequent proliferation), surrounded by additional connective tissue. In the nondiseased artery wall, lipid content, mainly cholesterol ester and phospholipid (particularly sphingomyelin), also progressively increases with age. Phospholipid synthesis rises with aging (perhaps in response to the need for more membrane formation for plasma membranes, vesicles, lysosomes, and other intracellular organelles) followed by a compensatory increase in activity of all phospholipases except sphingomyelinase. While most of the phospholipid in the normal artery wall appears to be derived from in situ synthesis, the cholesterol ester that accumulates with aging appears to be derived from plasma, since it contains principally linoleic acid, the major plasma cholesterol ester fatty acid. Furthermore, low-density lipoproteins (LDL) are immunologically detectable in the intima of normal arteries in direct relation to their concentration in

TABLE 195-1 Deaths, by cause, in the United States, 1982

Causes of death	No. of deaths, thousands			
	Below age 65		Age 65 and above	
	Male	Female	Male	Female
All causes	396	224	660	695
All cardiovascular diseases	130	57	359	421
Ischemic heart disease	86	29	216	223
Cerebrovascular disease	11	11	52	84
Hypertensive disease*	1	1	3	4
All infectious disease	6	9	6	7
All cancer	85	75	149	125
Accidents	54	17	12	11

* *A substantial proportion of deaths of hypertensive persons occurs with ischemic heart disease or cerebrovascular disease; such deaths are classified in those categories.*
SOURCE: *National Center for Health Statistics, Vital Statistics Report, Final Mortality Statistics, 1982.*

plasma. It has been estimated that between the second and sixth decade, the normal intima accumulates approximately 10 mg cholesterol per gram of tissue. Thus, as the normal artery ages, smooth-muscle cells and connective tissue accumulate diffusely in the intima, leading to progressive thickening of this layer, coupled with progressive accumulation of sphingomyelin and cholesterol linoleate. This diffuse age-related intimal thickening is to be distinguished from focal discrete raised fibromuscular plaques, a characteristic feature of atherosclerosis.

Functionally, these changes with aging result in gradually increasing rigidity of vessels. The larger arteries may become dilated, elongated, and tortuous, and aneurysms may form in areas of an encroaching degenerating arteriosclerotic plaque. Such "wear-and-tear" changes are frequently proportional to the vessel diameter and correlated with branching, curvature, and anatomic points of attachment. The amount of external support also determines the ability of vessels, weakened by loss of elasticity, to withstand hydrostatic pressure. The unsupported cerebral arteries may be particularly vulnerable in this regard. Although senescence is accompanied by the intimal thickening that is a feature of localized atheromatosis, the changes of aging and arteriosclerosis appear to be separate and distinct processes.

NONATHEROMATOUS FORMS OF ARTERIOSCLEROSIS

Atherosclerosis involves primarily the intimal layer and occurs most commonly in the abdominal aorta and its large renal and lower extremity branches, the coronary arteries, and the cerebral vasculature. It may accompany or accelerate the other major forms of arteriosclerosis, *focal calcification* and *arteriolosclerosis* (Table 195-2).

FOCAL CALCIFICATION Not to be confused with atherosclerosis is focal calcification of the media, particularly in the medium-sized muscular arteries. This type of arteriosclerosis is called *Mönckeberg's sclerosis* and is common in the lower extremities, upper extremities, and the arterial supply of the genital tract in both sexes. This disorder is rare in individuals below age 50 and affects both sexes indiscriminately. The process involves degeneration of smooth-muscle cells, followed by calcium deposition. The vessels become hard and tortuous, so that palpable vessels such as the radial artery can be felt as rigid tubes. Its characteristic radiologic appearance consists of regular concentric calcifications, commonly seen in pelvic and femoral vessels. The medial changes alone do not narrow the lumen, have little effect on the circulation, and have relatively little clinical significance. However, in the lower extremities, medial sclerosis is often associated with atherosclerosis, leading to arterial occlusion.

TABLE 195-2 Disorders associated with early arteriosclerosis

ATHEROSCLEROSIS

Diabetes mellitus
Hypertension
Familial hypercholesterolemia
Familial combined hyperlipidemia
Familial dysbetalipoproteinemia
Hypothyroidism
Werner's syndrome
Cholesterol ester storage disease
Systemic lupus erythematosus

NONATHEROMATOUS ARTERIOSCLEROSIS

Diabetes mellitus
Chronic renal insufficiency
Chronic vitamin D intoxication
Pseudoxanthoma elasticum
Idiopathic arterial calcification in infancy
Aortic valvular calcification in the elderly
Werner's syndrome
Homocystinuria

These changes are common in the elderly, and in patients on long-term corticosteroid therapy, but in individuals with diabetes mellitus, focal calcification may be accelerated and severe. It is much more common in diabetics with neuropathy, and sympathetic denervation of medial smooth muscle has been implicated in its etiology.

Focal calcification also can produce the arteriosclerotic aortic valve in the elderly. Progressive calcium deposition occurs on the aortic surface of normal trileaflet aortic valves with age, resulting in a spectrum of clinical findings ranging from an innocent systolic murmur to severe calcific aortic stenosis (Chap. 187).

ARTERIOLOSCLEROSIS This disorder involves hyaline and degenerative changes affecting both the intima and media of small arteries and arterioles, particularly in the spleen, pancreas, adrenal, and kidney. In the kidney, but not necessarily elsewhere, arteriolosclerosis is almost invariably associated with hypertension. Lesser degrees of sustained hypertension characteristically cause *hyalinization* of renal arterioles; more severe or malignant hypertension produces a typical *fibrous and elastic hyperplasia,* and even necrosis, of the media and intima.

ATHEROSCLEROSIS

LESIONS Morbid anatomy Atherosclerosis is a patchy nodular type of arteriosclerosis. The lesions are commonly classified as *fatty streaks, fibrous plaques,* and *complicated lesions. Fatty streaks* may be the earliest lesions of atherosclerosis, but the evidence is very uncertain. They are characterized by an accumulation of lipid-filled smooth-muscle cells and macrophages (foam cells) and fibrous tissue in focal areas of the intima. They are stained distinctly by fat-soluble dyes but may be visible without staining as yellowish or whitish patches on the intimal surface. The lipid is mainly cholesterol oleate, partly derived from synthesis in situ. The fatty streak is usually sessile and causes little obstruction and no symptoms. The lesion is universal, appearing in various segments of the arterial tree at different ages beginning in the aorta in infancy. In all children, regardless of race, sex, or environment, fatty streaks are present in the aorta by age 10 and increase to occupy as much as 30 to 50 percent of the aortic surface by age 25, but they do not appear to extend further with aging. Despite a presumed relation between fatty streaks and fibrous atherosclerotic plaques, aortic fatty streaks are not correlated with the location and extent of fibrous lesions. In the coronary arteries, the extent of fatty streaks may be a better indicator of the development of clinically significant raised lesions later in life. They are usually observed by age 15 and continue to involve more surface area with increasing age. Fatty streaks in the cerebral arteries are also present in all populations, develop during the third and fourth decade, and are more extensive in those populations having a higher incidence of cerebrovascular disease. It is generally believed that fatty streaks may be reversible, but the evidence is inconclusive.

Fibrous plaques, also called raised lesions or pearly plaques, are palpably elevated areas of intimal thickening and represent the most characteristic lesion of advancing atherosclerosis. They do not share with fatty streaks the ubiquitous distribution among populations. These plaques first appear in the abdominal aorta, coronary arteries, and carotid arteries in the third decade and increase progressively with age. They appear in men before women, in the aorta before the coronary arteries, and much later in the vertebral and intracranial cerebral arteries. Reasons for the difference in susceptibility of various segments of the arterial tree and the nonuniform distribution of lesions are not known. Typically, the fibrous plaque is firm, elevated, and dome-shaped, with an opaque glistening surface that bulges into the lumen. It consists of a central core of extracellular lipid and necrotic cell debris ("gruel") covered by a fibromuscular layer or cap containing large numbers of smooth-muscle cells, macrophages, and collagen. Thus the plaque is much thicker than is normal intima. Although the lipid, like that of fatty streaks, is mainly cholesterol ester, the principal esterified fatty acid is linoleic rather than oleic. Thus plaque cholesterol ester composition differs from fatty streaks but resembles plasma lipoproteins.

The *complicated lesion* is a calcified fibrous plaque containing various degrees of necrosis, thrombosis, and ulceration. These are the lesions frequently associated with symptoms. With increasing necrosis and accumulation of gruel, the arterial wall progressively weakens, and rupture of the intima can occur, causing aneurysm and hemorrhage. Arterial emboli can form when fragments of plaque dislodge into the lumen. Stenosis and impaired organ function result from gradual occlusion as plaques thicken and thrombi form.

Localization Although the term *generalized atherosclerosis* is commonly used clinically, lesions are actually irregularly distributed; different vessels are involved at different ages and to varying degrees. The aorta, especially its abdominal portion, is involved earliest and most severely by atherosclerotic lesions, and it is the bellwether of lesions elsewhere. The *aorta* is usually most heavily involved in its abdominal portion, about the orifices of its branches (particularly at the level of the coronary and intercostal arteries), in the aortic arch, and frequently at its bifurcation into the iliac arteries. There is more atherosclerosis in the lower than in the upper limbs. In the legs, the incidence decreases peripherally, as the musculoelastic vessels give way to large muscular arteries and these become smaller vessels, such as the plantar or digital arteries. Plaques and thromboses are particularly common in the *femoral* artery, in Hunter's canal, and in the *popliteal* artery just above the knee joint. The *anterior* and *posterior tibial* arteries are often occluded together, but in different sites—the posterior where it rounds the internal malleolus and the anterior where it is superficial and becomes the dorsalis pedis artery. The peroneal artery, which is well embedded in muscle, often escapes when other major vessels are occluded, and it may be the main blood supply to the extremity (*peroneal leg*). Atherosclerosis in abdominal branches, except for the renal and mesenteric arteries, causes less difficulty than in coronary and cerebral vessels.

In the *coronary arteries,* raised lesions are most prominent in the main stems, the highest incidence being a short distance beyond the ostia. Atherosclerosis is nearly always found in the epicardial (extramural) portions of the vessels, while the intramural coronary arteries are spared. Coronary atherosclerosis is often diffuse. The degree to which the lumen is narrowed varies, but once the process is present, all the intima of the extramural portions of the vessel is usually involved. A single tiny plaque occluding an otherwise normal coronary artery is rare. Selective involvement of the coronary arteries may relate to the unique hemodynamic forces, unlike those of other major arteries, resulting from greater flow in diastole than systole. The implications of these flow patterns for atherogenesis are as yet unknown. Typical atheromatous fibrous plaques also develop in saphenous vein aortocoronary bypass grafts.

In the cervical and cerebral arteries the distribution of atherosclerosis is patchy, as it may be in other arteries. It first appears in the base of the brain in the carotid, basilar, and vertebral arteries. The proximal portion of the internal carotid artery in the neck is a site of special predilection. There is a concentration of lesions near bifurcations. Atherosclerosis in the *pulmonary artery* bears no relation to the severity of the disease in the aorta or other systemic arteries. There is some involvement in about half of adults over 50 years of age who have no reason to have pulmonary hypertension. Pulmonary hypertension per se, however, is associated with medial hypertrophy, intimal thickening, and great acceleration of atheroma formation.

THEORIES OF ATHEROGENESIS One generally accepted theory for the pathogenesis of atherosclerosis consistent with a variety of experimental evidence is the *reaction to injury* hypothesis. According to this idea the endothelial cells lining the intima are exposed to repeated or continuing insults to their integrity. The injury to the endothelium may be subtle or gross, resulting in a loss of the ability of the cells to function normally or to attach to one another and to the underlying connective tissue. In the extreme, the cells may

desquamate. Examples of types of "injury" to the endothelium include chemical injury, as in chronic hypercholesterolemia or homocystinemia, mechanical stress associated with hypertension, and immunologic injury, as may be seen after cardiac or renal transplantation. Loss of functional endothelial cells at susceptible sites in the arterial tree would lead to exposure of the subendothelial tissue to increased concentrations of plasma constituents and a sequence of events including platelet adherence, platelet aggregation and formation of microthrombi, and release of platelet granular components, including a potent mitogenic factor. This platelet factor, in conjunction with other plasma constituents, including lipoproteins and hormones such as insulin, could stimulate both the migration of medial smooth-muscle cells into the intima and their proliferation at these sites of injury. These proliferating smooth-muscle cells would deposit a connective tissue matrix and accumulate lipid, a process that would be particularly enhanced with hyperlipidemia. Macrophages derived from circulating blood monocytes can also accumulate lipid.

Adherence of monocytes and their migration into the arterial wall to become resident macrophages may be the earliest cellular abnormality in atherogenesis. Thus repeated or chronic injury could lead to a slowly progressing lesion involving a gradual increase in smooth-muscle cells, macrophages, connective tissue, and lipid. Areas where the shearing stress on endothelial cells is increased, such as branch points or bifurcation of vessels, would be at greater risk. As the lesions progress and the intima becomes thicker, blood flow over the sites will be altered and will potentially place the lining endothelial cells at even greater risk for further injury, leading to an inexorable cycle of events culminating in the complicated lesion. However, a single or a few injurious episodes may lead to a proliferative response that could regress, in contrast to continued or chronic injury. This hypothesis of reaction to injury thus is consistent with the known intimal thickening observed during normal aging, would explain how many of the etiologic factors implicated in atherogenesis might enhance lesion formation, might explain how inhibitors of platelet aggregation could interfere with lesion formation, and fosters some optimism regarding the possibility of interrupting progression or even producing regression of these lesions.

Other theories of atherogenesis are not mutually exclusive. The *monoclonal hypothesis* suggests, on the basis of single isoenzyme types found in lesions, that the intimal proliferative lesions result from the multiplication of single, individual smooth-muscle cells, as do benign tumors. In this manner, mitogenic, and possibly mutagenic, factors that might stimulate smooth-muscle cell proliferation would act on single cells. Focal *clonal senescence* may explain how intrinsic aging processes contribute to atherosclerosis. According to this theory, the intimal smooth-muscle cells that proliferate to form an atheroma are normally under feedback control by diffusible agents (mitosis inhibitors) formed by the smooth-muscle cells in the contiguous media, and this feedback control system tends to fail with age as these controlling cells die and are not adequately replaced. This is consistent with the recent observation that cultured human arterial smooth-muscle cells, like fibroblasts, show a decline in their ability to replicate as a function of donor age. If this loss of replicative potential applies to a controlling population of smooth-muscle cells, then cells that are usually suppressed would be able to proliferate.

The *lysosomal theory* suggests that altered lysosomal function might contribute to atherogenesis. Since lysosomal enzymes can accomplish the generalized degradation of cellular components required for continuing renewal, this system has been implicated in cellular aging and the accumulation of lipofuscin or "age pigment." It has been suggested that increased deposition of lipids in arterial smooth-muscle cells may be related in part to a relative deficiency in the activity of lysosomal cholesterol ester hydrolase. This would result in increased accumulation of cholesterol esters within the cells, perhaps accentuated by lipid overloading of lysosomes, eventually leading to cell death and extracellular lipid deposition. Consonant with this idea, patients with the rare cholesterol ester storage disease, caused by a defect in lysosomal cholesterol ester hydrolase, may have accelerated atherosclerosis. However, lipid droplets in foam cells are often cytoplasmic rather than lysosomal.

RECOGNITION OF ATHEROSCLEROSIS Angiographic visualization of deformity in the lumen of a vessel remains the best presumptive test of silent atherosclerosis. Coronary angiography now permits visualization and assessment of arteries as small as 0.5 mm in diameter. Several sophisticated noninvasive techniques have been developed for demonstrating its presence. Doppler probes for measuring velocity and amount of blood flow have been used noninvasively and adapted to determine vessel outlines. Ultrasonic techniques are not yet clinically useful for detection of plaques in the coronary arteries.

Functional tests based on pathophysiologic or metabolic effects of a narrowed arterial lumen often give indirect clues. Assessment of electrocardiographic changes induced after standardized exercise is a relatively simple noninvasive aid to the diagnosis of coronary atherosclerosis with significant narrowing. Similarly, myocardial perfusion defects demonstrable with imaging techniques using radionuclides are usually attributable to atherosclerosis (Chap. 179). Digit plethysmography with exercise often unmasks significant atherosclerotic involvement of lower extremity arteries.

Radiographic demonstration of calcification in the location of arteries does not always indicate the presence of atherosclerosis. Although calcified coronary vessels usually indicate atherosclerosis, complete luminal obstruction may occur in the absence of any calcification. Calcification or beading of peripheral arteries is not correlated directly with atherosclerosis. Abnormalities in retinal arterioles evident upon funduscopic examination are not well correlated with atherosclerosis in arteries. Thus despite the availability of a variety of tests, detection of atherosclerosis usually awaits one of the clinical complications attending a critical decrease of blood flow in an involved vessel. As yet there is no blood test for atherosclerosis. Knowledge of the prevalence and incidence of arteriosclerosis and most of the inferences concerning its causes are derived from tabulations of the appearance of its complications.

Ischemic heart disease (IHD), synonymous with *coronary heart disease* or *arteriosclerotic heart disease* (Chap. 189), is the most reliable indicator of atherosclerosis available today. Practically all patients with myocardial infarction, as defined by electrocardiographic and enzyme changes, have coronary atherosclerosis. Rare exceptions are due to congenital anomalies of the coronary vessels, emboli, or ostial occlusion due to other types of cardiac or vascular disease. Nontraumatic *sudden death* (Chap. 30) makes up a sizable portion of all deaths eventually certified as due to IHD. At autopsy, evidence of fresh myocardial infarction or of *coronary thrombosis* is usually absent. While ventricular fibrillation may have been due to sudden closure of a partially compromised vessel by a small thrombus or embolus, or to *spasm,* none of these need have preceded a fatal arrhythmia. The majority of victims of sudden death have had a previous diagnosis of IHD; the number who had diabetes or hypertension is also significant. In epidemiologic studies of IHD, *angina pectoris* and electrocardiographic changes attributable to ischemia

without infarction are considered "softer end points" and treated separately.

Cerebrovascular disease (stroke) is a less reliable criterion for the presence of atherosclerosis. It includes *cerebral hemorrhage* and *cerebral thrombosis* (Chap. 343). Cerebral thrombosis, including infarction or softening without evidence of embolus, is usually due to atherosclerosis. On the other hand, cerebral hemorrhage is most often the result of congenital aneurysms or of vascular defects peculiar to hypertension and diabetes. Dissections of the aorta (Chap. 197), *peripheral vascular disease* (Chap. 198), thrombosis of other major vessels, and ischemic renal disease (Chap. 227) likewise are not used to determine the prevalence of atherosclerosis in a population or as an index of atherosclerosis elsewhere. Therefore, from an epidemiologic standpoint, consideration of atherosclerosis focuses on IHD.

INCIDENCE AND PREVALENCE According to the National Health Examination Survey, about 5 million Americans have IHD. It is the leading cause of death in males after age 35 and in all persons after age 45. Premature deaths from IHD, arbitrarily defined as those appearing before age 65, occur preponderantly in men, and a third of all deaths from IHD in males occur before age 65. In fact nearly all the excess premature mortality in American males is due to IHD. Between the ages of 35 and 55 the death rate is five times higher in white men than in white women in the United States. The exceptions are women with hypertension, diabetes, hyperlipidemia, or premature (usually iatrogenic) menopause, who are at increased risk and often share the risk of the male. For both sexes, there is more than a fivefold increase in the average annual incidence of myocardial infarction between ages 40 and 60. A distressing higher mortality rate in younger nonwhite women is probably due mainly to a greater incidence of hypertension in blacks. There is less difference between men and women in the prevalence of angina pectoris than in that of myocardial infarction; after age 65 more women than men have angina without a history of infarction.

Changing death rates Death rates in the United States from IHD rose appreciably between 1940 and 1960. Mortality peaked in 1963 and started to decline, with the rate of decline accelerating in recent years for all ages, for both sexes, and for whites and nonwhites. This recent decline in mortality from coronary atherosclerosis (Table 195-3) is the first recorded in American history and is almost unique among industrialized countries. In other parts of the world, including the Soviet Union and many countries in Europe, IHD death rates are still climbing. In 1980 the reduction in IHD death rate averaged more than 20 percent for persons age 35 to 74. The trend remains unexplained, but there has been a concurrent change in living habits including reduced smoking among middle-aged males, decreased consumption of animal fats and cholesterol, better control of hypertension, and improved treatment of IHD.

International comparisons In most industrialized countries, IHD is the major single cause of premature cardiovascular deaths. There are, however, marked differences in premature death rates among them. The seven having the highest rates in males between 35 and 74 years of age are Finland, Scotland, Northern Ireland, Australia, New Zealand, England, and the United States. Much lower age-adjusted death rates from IHD are found in Latin America and Japan. The rates in Japan are about one-sixth of those in the United States. Subsamples obtained in many countries convey the strong impression that upper socioeconomic classes that have adopted the culture of western industrialized countries have far more IHD than do lower socioeconomic classes. Among the most obvious cultural differences between these groups are total calories, fat content of the diet, and amount of physical work. Extensive epidemiologic studies have not revealed the reasons for differences between cultures that are superficially similar. Migrants to the United States tend to have a higher risk of death from premature IHD than do age-matched relatives who remain at home. Although there are many instances in which different ethnic groups in the same locality have widely differing prevalences of IHD, the available data suggest that cultural factors are more

TABLE 195-3 Age-adjusted death rates by cause in the United States, 1968 and 1982

Cause of death	Rate per 100,000 population		
	1968	1982	Percent change
All deaths	744	554	−26
All cardiovascular diseases	362	238	−34
Ischemic heart disease	242	139	−42
Cerebrovascular disease	71	36	−50
Rheumatic heart disease	7	2	−69
Cancer	129	133	+3
Accidents and violence	77	58	−24

SOURCE: *The National Center for Health Statistics, Vital Statistics Report, Final Mortality Statistics, 1982.*

important than genetic determination of IHD. Nevertheless, genetic heterogeneity undoubtedly underlies many of the striking differences in susceptibility seen among individuals sharing the same ethnic and cultural setting.

ETIOLOGIC FACTORS A number of conditions and habits present more frequently in individuals who develop atherosclerosis than in the general population; these factors have been termed *risk factors*. The majority of people below age 65 afflicted with atherosclerosis have one or more identifiable risk factors other than aging per se (Table 195-4). The risk factor concept implies that a person with at least one risk factor is more likely to develop a clinical atherosclerotic event and is likely to do so earlier than a person with no risk factors. The presence of multiple risk factors further accelerates atherosclerosis. They vary in terms of importance in the population of the United States. There is general agreement from an epidemiologic perspective that hypercholesterolemia, hypertension, and cigarette smoking may be the most potent factors involved in causation of atherosclerosis. Risk factors also vary in terms of their potential reversibility with current techniques of preventive management.

Thus age, gender, and genetic factors are currently considered to be irreversible risk factors, whereas continually emerging evidence suggests that elimination of cigarette smoking and treatment of hypertension reverses the high risk for atherosclerosis attributable to those factors. A major multicenter trial has shown that reduction of hypercholesterolemia reduces the risk of IHD. Life insurance policy-holder data suggest that reduction of marked obesity reduces total mortality, presumably by diminishing the sequelae of atherosclerosis. Other potentially reversible factors are currently under study.

These factors are not mutually exclusive since they clearly interact. For example, obesity, particularly of the abdominal type (assessed by the waist/hip circumference ratio), appears to be causally associated with hypertension, hyperglycemia, hypercholesterolemia, and hypertriglyceridemia. Genetic factors may play a role by exerting direct effects on arterial wall cell structure and metabolism, or they may act indirectly via such factors as hypertension, hyperlipidemia, diabetes, and obesity. Aging appears to be one of the more complex factors associated with the development of atherosclerosis, since many of the risk factors in themselves are related to aging, e.g., elevated blood pressure, hyperglycemia, and hyperlipidemia. Thus in addition to the possible involvement of intrinsic aging in atherogenesis (perhaps through effects on arterial wall metabolism), a variety of associated metabolic factors are also age-dependent.

Hyperlipidemia Both *hypercholesterolemia* and *hypertriglyceridemia* appear to be important risk factors for atherosclerosis. While there is no absolute quantitative definition of hyperlipidemia, statistical definitions, based on the upper 5 or 10 percent of the distribution of plasma lipid levels within a population, are often used. Such definitions are likely to detect affected individuals from families with one of the familial hyperlipidemias or having hyperlipidemia associated with other diseases or drugs; they also are useful for prediction of emergence of premature atherosclerosis and institution of preventive measures. However, these upper limits of "normality" are too high for defining those cholesterol and triglyceride levels that are correlated with increasing risk of IHD in whole populations. Thus, correlations between the cholesterol concentrations in young men in North America and the incidence of premature IHD indicate that an increasing risk can be detected when the cholesterol level is higher than 220 mg/dL, a value close to the mean for men from 40 to 49 years of age in this population. Extrapolation of similar data from other populations suggests that a cholesterol level at birth averages 60 mg/dL. Within a month the average has risen to about 120 and by the first year to 175. A second rise begins in the third decade and continues to about age 50 in men and somewhat later in women.

A similar age-related increase in plasma triglyceride levels is also observed. The increases in cholesterol are associated mainly with a rise in *low-density lipoprotein* (LDL) concentrations, the increases in triglyceride with a rise in *very low density lipoproteins* (VLDL).

TABLE 195-4 Risk factors for atherosclerosis

1 Not reversible
  a Aging
  b Male sex
  c Genetic traits—positive family history of premature atherosclerosis
2 Reversible
  a Cigarette smoking
  b Hypertension
  c Obesity
3 Potentially or partially reversible
  a Hyperlipidemia—hypercholesterolemia and/or hypertriglyceridemia
  b Hyperglycemia and diabetes mellitus
  c Low levels of high-density lipoproteins (HDL)
4 Other possible factors
  a Physical inactivity
  b Emotional stress and/or personality type

Adiposity may play a key role in this age-associated rise in triglyceride and cholesterol levels since the increases in triglyceride, cholesterol, and body weight with age in whole populations occur concurrently. In primitive people who remain thin throughout adulthood, plasma lipids do not increase with age. Metabolic mechanisms have been postulated whereby obesity, which is associated with insulin resistance of peripheral tissues and compensatory hyperinsulinemia, promotes enhanced production of triglyceride- and cholesterol-rich lipoproteins by the liver. Current concepts of plasma lipoprotein transport suggest that accumulation of cholesterol in the circulation may in part be secondary to excessive production of triglyceride-rich lipoproteins.

Hypercholesterolemia is associated unequivocally with increased incidence of premature IHD; however, its importance varies in relation to age. In the Framingham Study, cholesterol levels in males below age 40 were closely related to the future development of IHD; this relation was much less pronounced in older individuals. For both sexes combined, the relative incidence of myocardial infarction in individuals between the ages of 30 and 49 with cholesterol levels greater than 260 mg/dL was three to five times that for individuals with cholesterol levels less than 220. There appears to be a continuous gradient of risk as the cholesterol level ascends. These data are supported by comparisons of the prevalence of IHD and cholesterol (or LDL) in many other populations. The relationship of triglycerides and VLDL to IHD is confounded by a rise in cholesterol as VLDL increases. Nevertheless, in several, but not all, population studies, increased triglycerides (or VLDL) are independently correlated with premature IHD.

Hypertriglyceridemia may be associated with premature atherosclerosis in some specific disorders; this association may not be apparent in studies of whole populations. Patients with high VLDL who come from families with familial combined hyperlipidemia appear to be at the same increased risk as those affected members of these families with elevated LDL levels. In contrast, patients with comparably elevated VLDL levels who come from families with pure monogenic familial hypertriglyceridemia do not appear to have an increased risk. In addition, high VLDL may increase the risk for premature atherosclerosis when associated with other risk factors for coronary artery disease, such as in diabetes, and in patients on chronic hemodialysis who smoke and are hypertensive. Individuals in whom remnant lipoproteins accumulate, with resulting elevations in both cholesterol and triglycerides (Chap. 315), also seem to be at risk for early development of atherosclerosis.

Some of these relationships were clarified in a comprehensive study in Seattle of the role of the genetics of hyperlipidemia in clinical atherosclerosis in which 500 consecutive survivors of myocardial infarction were tested. Hyperlipidemia was present in about one-third of the group. Approximately one-half of the males and two-thirds of the females below age 50 had either hypertriglyceridemia, hypercholesterolemia, or both. On the other hand, in individuals over age 70 the prevalence of atherosclerotic coronary disease was very high, yet virtually no males (and only about one-fourth of the females) had hyperlipidemia. Thus, in both sexes there appeared to be a progressive decline with age in the association of hyperlipidemia with myocardial infarction. More than half of the hyperlipidemic atherosclerotic survivors appeared to have simple monogenic familial disorders inherited as an autosomal dominant trait (*familial combined hyperlipidemia, familial hypertriglyceridemia,* and *familial hypercholesterolemia,* in descending order of frequency, Table 195-5). These simply inherited hyperlipidemias (particularly hypercholesterolemia) were more frequent in myocardial infarction survivors below age 60 than in those who were older. In contrast, nonmonogenic forms of hyperlipidemia occurred with equal frequency above and below age 60. Thus it appears that genes associated with the simply inherited hyperlipidemias accelerate changes seen with age, leading to atherosclerosis at an earlier age than usual. All studies indicate that hyperlipidemia is a more meaningful risk factor below age 50 and that it operates independently of, and in addition to, hypertension, diabetes, obesity, and other factors. For men and women over age 65, there is no evidence of a correlation between hyperlipidemia and atherosclerosis or its complications.

When the screening of individuals for hyperlipidemia occurs after a myocardial infarction, it is several decades too late. Screening at birth or in childhood for genetic hyperlipidemia is not practical or useful except in the instance of familial hypercholesterolemia, which may affect about 1 in 1000 children. This is detectable by LDL elevations in cord blood when one already knows that a parent is affected. Other genetic or nongenetic primary hyperlipidemia is often not apparent until the third decade. *Today, good health maintenance practice includes a test for detection of hyperlipidemia in all persons between 20 and 30 years of age. It is especially important in all young persons who have a family history of premature IHD.*

Hyperlipidemia is best detected by measurement of the concentration of cholesterol and triglycerides in serum or plasma in a sample obtained after an overnight fast. The measurements should be made by a reliable laboratory that follows a program of standardization. Routine use of lipoprotein electrophoresis provides little additional information, is nonspecific, and is not recommended for screening or for management. In adults less than 55 years of age, a cholesterol concentration (C) greater than 240 mg/dL or a triglyceride concentration (TG) greater than 250 mg/dL clearly indicates hyperlipidemia sufficient to require some attention by the physician to the items listed in Table 195-6. If hyperlipidemia is absent, the tests need not be repeated for several years in an adult who maintains body weight and does not otherwise change in health or life-style. Vigor in pursuing the "causative factors" in Table 195-6 should increase in proportion to the degree of hyperlipidemia. If causes of *secondary hyperlipidemia* or offending drugs are absent, attention to the origin of *primary hyperlipidemia* turns mainly to diet and genetic causes. Severe hyperlipidemia (C > 300 mg/dL or TG > 500 mg/dL) usually reflects a genetic disorder; when xanthomas are present, it practically always does. Diagnosis always includes examination of first-degree relatives and proceeds according to information contained in Chap. 315.

Reduction of hypercholesterolemia results in a decrease in progression of atherosclerosis in humans and other primates. Several controlled trials of different diets which have been accompanied by fall in mean cholesterol levels in small test populations have shown a favorable effect on incidence of the overall complications of IHD. The drug clofibrate given to a normal population reduced the incidence of nonfatal myocardial infarctions associated with a reduction of cholesterol levels; however, total mortality was not lowered. In the recent Lipid Research Clinics trial, the drug cholestyramine given to hypercholesterolemic asymptomatic men reduced morbidity and mortality from myocardial infarction in direct relation to the degree of cholesterol lowering; again, however, total mortality was not reduced. The weight of evidence strongly favors conservative measures to reduce cholesterol levels in patients through middle age and aggressive measures in patients who are frankly hypercholesterolemic.

The first step in treatment of primary hyperlipidemia is attention to diet. All patients with mild to moderate hyperlipidemia should first be brought to normal weight if they exceed it and then be maintained on a diet emphasizing decreases in intake of saturated fat and cholesterol. If hypertriglyceridemia is present, alcohol intake should be limited or eliminated. A single dietary approach to all forms of hyperlipidemia, including reduced intake of calories, cholesterol, and saturated fat, is appropriate for most patients. The degree of dietary restriction would be proportional to the degree and nature of the hyperlipidemia. The maximum effect of such a regimen will be observed within 2 months after body weight has stabilized. If at that time C is greater than 260 mg/dL, a 2-month trial of a bile acid–binding resin (cholestyramine or colestipol) should be considered. If TG remains greater than 300 mg/dL, a fibric acid derivative (clofibrate or bezafibrate) may be tried. These two types of drugs may be used simultaneously if both C and TG are high; their use remains empirical. In patients with familial hypercholesterolemia (Chap. 315) combined therapy with a resin and nicotinic acid has achieved dramatic normalization of LDL cholesterol levels. New cholesterol synthesis inhibitors (e.g., mevinolin), which are more specific and more effective than nicotinic acid, are currently being studied. Continued therapy with any hypolipidemic drug is dependent upon the demonstration that, when added to diet at stable weight, it is associated with at least a 15 percent further decrease in hyperlipidemia. However, further studies are needed to define the long-term efficiency of various hypolipidemic agents in the prevention of atherosclerosis and its sequelae in specific disorders. The long-term effects of these drugs used before puberty are unknown, and their use during pregnancy is not advocated.

High-density lipoproteins (HDL) HDL, a complex family of particles that carry about 20 percent of the total plasma cholesterol, is inversely associated with the development of premature atherosclerosis and therefore can be considered an "antirisk factor." HDL levels can be assessed simply by measurement of cholesterol in the supernatant fluid after the other lipoproteins in plasma have been

TABLE 195-5   Frequency of hyperlipidemia in survivors of myocardial infarction

Disorder	% of total myocardial infarction survivors		
	Under age 60	Over age 60	Ratio
1 Monogenic hyperlipidemias	20.6	7.5	—
a Familial hypercholesterolemia	4.1	0.7	6:1
b Familial hypertriglyceridemia	5.2	2.7	2:1
c Familial combined hyperlipidemia	11.3	4.1	3:1
2 Polygenic hypercholesterolemia	5.5	5.5	1:1
3 Sporadic hypertriglyceridemia	5.8	6.9	1:1

SOURCE: *Goldstein et al. 1973.*

TABLE 195-6   Factors to consider in patients with hyperlipidemia

1 Disorders to which hyperlipidemia is secondary
  a Uncontrolled diabetes mellitus (insulin deficiency)
  b Hypothyroidism
  c Uremia
  d Nephrotic syndrome (hypoproteinemia)
  e Obstructive liver disease
  f Dysproteinemia (multiple myeloma, lupus erythematosus)
2 Drugs producing or aggravating hyperlipidemia
  a Oral contraceptives
  b Estrogens
  c Glucocorticoids
  d Antihypertensives
3 Dietary factors
  a Caloric intake (recent weight gain)
  b Content of saturated fats and cholesterol
  c Alcohol intake
4 Genetic disorders (primary hyperlipidemias)
  a Family history of hyperlipidemia or xanthomas
  b History of pancreatitis or recurrent abdominal pain

precipitated. Thus individuals whose HDL cholesterol is elevated may be less likely to develop IHD; conversely, low HDL cholesterol is associated with increased risk of IHD. In the Framingham Study, low HDL cholesterol was a more potent lipid risk factor than was high cholesterol or LDL. At least five diverse population studies have confirmed a close correlation between IHD and low HDL, independent of other factors.

Consistent with differences in risk between the sexes, HDL cholesterol averages about 25 percent higher in women than in men. Estrogens tend to raise and androgens tend to lower HDL levels. In women, low HDL, particularly when associated with diabetes and obesity, markedly raises the risk of IHD. Octogenarians tend to have high HDL, which may be partly familial. Of interest for preventive measures, cigarette smoking decreases and regular strenuous exercise increases HDL cholesterol. Regular exercise increases HDL even in individuals after myocardial infarction. A small daily intake of alcohol has been associated with both reduced risk of IHD and high HDL levels. Mechanisms for these effects remain unknown.

HDL cholesterol measurements are usually not very helpful since the analytical error in most laboratories exceeds the differences in HDL levels associated with risk. HDL measurements are most helpful in individuals, especially women, with only a mild increase in plasma cholesterol and normal triglyceride levels to determine whether the increase is in HDL rather than in LDL. Because of the close inverse relationship between plasma triglycerides (or VLDL) and HDL, HDL in hypertriglyceridemic persons, with or without hypercholesterolemia, will be predictably low and gives little additional useful information.

Hypertension (see Chap. 196) High blood pressure is an important risk factor for atherosclerosis, mainly IHD and cerebrovascular disease. The risk increases progressively with increasing blood pressure; in the Framingham Study, IHD incidence in middle-aged men with blood pressures exceeding 160/95 was more than five times that in normotensive men (blood pressure 140/90 or less). Hypertensive men and women are both affected, with the diastolic pressure perhaps being more important. In industrialized populations, blood pressure appears to increase inexorably with age; however, the nature of this age relation varies among populations, since there are remote primitive populations that age without any changes in blood pressure levels. The age-associated blood pressure increase might be related to physical activity or dietary factors, particularly sodium and total caloric content. In contrast to the other age-related risk factors, hypertension appears to increase atherosclerosis throughout the age span. Thus, after the age of about 50, hypertension may be more potent than hypercholesterolemia as a risk factor.

Conversely, the risk for atherosclerosis appears diminished by therapeutic reduction of blood pressure. Recent intervention studies have shown convincingly that reduction of diastolic levels that had been greater than 105 mmHg significantly reduces the incidence of strokes, IHD, and congestive heart failure in men. Even when patients with diastolic pressures between 90 and 105 mmHg are similarly maintained on adequate treatment, the incidence of some of these complications may be reduced. Special urgency for relief of hypertension obtains when hyperlipidemia or other risk factors are present.

Cigarette smoking Not only is cigarette smoking one of the more potent risk factors for atherosclerosis, it is also one of the factors that when reduced or eliminated clearly decreases the risk of developing atherosclerosis. Ample statistical evidence supports a mean increase of about 70 percent in the death rate, and a three- to fivefold increase in risk of IHD, in men who smoke one pack of cigarettes per day compared with nonsmokers. In general, the increase in death rate is proportional to the amount smoked and decreases with age. Excess morbidity from myocardial infarction is also present in women smokers, but the relationship is somewhat less firm than in men. However, there is an impressive accentuation of IHD mortality in women over age 35 taking oral contraceptives who in addition smoke cigarettes. In some atherosclerosis-prone populations, such as patients maintained on long-term hemodialysis, cigarette smoking interacts with other risk factors, resulting in a marked enhancement of atherosclerosis mortality. Such interaction is also likely for diabetic and hypertensive populations.

The association of smoking and increased IHD remains unexplained. Pipe and cigar smokers have a lesser increase in risk of IHD, presumably because less smoke is inhaled. Smokers dying of causes other than IHD have been found at autopsy to have more coronary atherosclerosis than nonsmokers. The major influence of smoking is upon the incidence of sudden death, however. Those who stop smoking show a prompt decline in risk and may reach the risk level of nonsmokers as early as after 1 year of abstention.

Hyperglycemia and diabetes mellitus (see Chap. 327) Studies in a variety of populations have shown an association of hyperglycemia with clinically evident atherosclerotic disease, suggesting a role of hyperglycemia in atherogenesis. In known diabetics, both insulin-dependent and non-insulin-dependent types, there is at least a twofold increase in incidence of myocardial infarction compared with non-diabetics. This risk is markedly increased in younger diabetics, and diabetic women are even more prone to IHD than are diabetic men. There is an increased tendency toward cerebral thrombosis and infarction but not toward cerebral hemorrhage in diabetes. Gangrene of the lower extremities has been variously estimated to be from 8 to 150 times as frequent in diabetics as in nondiabetics and is most often found in diabetics who smoke. Diabetes is associated with an increase in atherosclerosis observed at autopsy in a variety of populations worldwide, whether the prevalence of atherosclerosis in a particular population is high or low. The approximately twofold increase in the frequency of hypertension among diabetics, particularly adult females, may accentuate the risk. This relationship is presumably associated with obesity.

The risk for atherosclerotic disease, however, does not appear to be grossly related to the degree of hyperglycemia among diabetics. Results in the University Group Diabetes Program Study have suggested that reduction of blood glucose by insulin does not appear to influence mortality from established atherosclerosis during a 5-year period. Thus, hyperglycemia and atherosclerosis are associated, since there is an increased prevalence of large-vessel disease in known diabetics and, conversely, an increased prevalence of hyperglycemia in association with atherosclerotic disease. These associations remain unexplained and reversibility undocumented. Clinical and experimental studies also support a role for high circulating insulin levels in IHD. The capillary microangiopathy, pathognomonic of diabetes and causing important dysfunction of the kidneys and retina, has unknown clinical significance in relation to atherosclerotic disease in larger arteries.

Obesity In general, morbidity and mortality from IHD are higher in direct relation to the degree of overweight beyond about 30 percent. Furthermore, from data obtained in the Framingham Study, it appears that obesity may accelerate atherosclerosis since its effect is more apparent before age 50. Nevertheless, some of the major epidemiologic studies of coronary heart disease have not demonstrated an independent relationship between this condition and anything less than very severe obesity. Recent studies have shown a close relation between type of obesity (i.e., abdominal) and IHD. Furthermore, obesity is a disorder closely associated with four other potent risk factors, i.e., hypertriglyceridemia, hypercholesterolemia, hyperglycemia, and hypertension. The relationship between obesity and atherosclerosis is thus multifaceted; since in practice obesity does not occur ''independently,'' it is of considerable importance as a risk factor.

Physical inactivity Study of the relationship of the prevalence of IHD to daily (occupational) physical activity is made difficult because so many variables are involved. Among prospective studies the Framingham data do indicate that the less sedentary an individual is, the less susceptible that individual is to sudden death. Physical work may be the major determinant of greatly differing incidences of IHD in southern black and white males in the United States and in populations that move from rural areas to urbanized environments. How physical activity may operate to decrease death from IHD, or possibly to decrease atherogenesis, is not known. Beyond the amelioration of hyperlipidemia by increasing caloric expenditure, no mechanism has been demonstrated. The meaning of the physical activity–induced increase in HDL, the antirisk factor for IHD, remains mysterious. Physical training has been shown to improve exercise performance in patients with IHD and angina pectoris. Regular physical activity is supported as a desirable element in a program of preventive health maintenance.

Stress and personality There is a valid clinical impression that psychic or emotional stress and anxiety are associated with precipitation of overt IHD and sudden death. Debate continues as to whether there may be distinct personality types prone to or relatively immune to premature IHD (the so-called personality types A and B), and whether the presumably more deleterious type is amenable to correction beyond elimination of cigarette smoking, adverse dietary patterns, and avoidance of stressful life situations. Many social and demographic analyses have so far failed to reach any agreement about the etiologic relationships of occupation and similar situational factors and the incidence of IHD.

Genetic factors Premature atherosclerosis often appears to be familial. In many instances this can be attributed to the inheritance of risk factors such as hypertension, diabetes mellitus, and hyperlipidemia. Occasionally, families with excessive premature vascular disease can be found in which none of the known risk factors appears to be operating. Genetic determinants of protective factors, such as HDL, need to be understood; undoubtedly other important determinants remain to be discovered. Nevertheless, family history is one of the more important factors to be weighed in assessment of risk in helping the physician to avoid missing treatable risk factors and in institution of appropriate preventive measures.

ROLE OF DIET IN RISK FOR ATHEROSCLEROSIS The relationship of diet to IHD remains an area of intense interest and persistent controversy. In epidemiologic studies, no population habitually subsisting on a diet low in saturated fat and cholesterol has an appreciable amount of IHD. These populations also tend to have lower plasma lipid concentrations. There is a general upward shift of average cholesterol and triglyceride levels in highly developed countries, which is an effect of change in total culture and life-style as well as in diet. Dietary changes in migrant populations who move from more primitive to more industrialized societies commonly include increased intake of total calories, animal fats, cholesterol, and salt, leading to a diet-accentuated emergence of risk factors such as obesity, hyperlipidemia, diabetes, and hypertension. There is no question that the plasma cholesterol (and LDL) level is sensitive to the amount of saturated fat and cholesterol in the diet. The "average" adult male in the United States eats about 140 g fat per day and about 500 mg cholesterol. The mixture of fats ingested usually contains about three times as much saturated fatty acids (mainly palmitic and stearic) as polyunsaturated fatty acids (mainly linoleic and linolenic). If a healthy young adult switches from this diet to one containing the same amount of total fat in which the ratio of polyunsaturates to saturates is closer to unity and the cholesterol content is less than 300 mg per day, the cholesterol concentration will usually drop by 10 to 15 percent within 2 weeks and remain depressed on continuation of the diet.

The average cholesterol level in most populations is most closely related to the amount of animal fats (meat, eggs, and milk products, major sources of long-chain saturated fatty acids and cholesterol) in the diet. Increased animal fat consumption also tends to be correlated with a greater proportion of dietary fats being saturated and with lesser intake of complex carbohydrates and vegetable fibers; these are dietary changes that may lead to a rise in plasma cholesterol levels. The average triglyceride level is more sensitive to total caloric balance and to alcohol intake. It is important to note that physical activity, emotional stress, smoking, and intake of coffee or tea have only weak or indirect influences on total cholesterol and triglyceride concentrations.

In experimental animals added dietary cholesterol and fat are essential for the production of atherosclerosis. Typical American diets fed to nonhuman primates produce aortic and coronary atherosclerosis which is reversible when a cholesterol-free diet is fed. Controlled metabolic studies in humans show a direct relation between dietary and plasma cholesterol below intakes of about 600 mg per day; no relation is observed at higher intakes when plasma cholesterol is already high. There appear to be marked genetic variations in the ability of dietary cholesterol to influence plasma cholesterol among individuals and among populations. The relation between dietary polyunsaturated/saturated fat ratio (P/S) and both cholesterol and triglyceride levels also has been amply established. The unique lipid-lowering effects of the particular long-chain polyunsaturated fatty acids in large ocean fish are currently under study.

A definitive prospective study of the effect of diet on IHD in the general population has never been undertaken. Nevertheless, preliminary reports of newer studies of alterations of diet in high-risk populations, coupled with published findings of studies in selected populations, provide strong evidence of a reversible relation among diet, plasma lipids, and IHD. On this basis, although without definite proof of effectiveness, numerous authoritative nutrition councils have recommended prudent dietary modifications for the general population of western countries to be instituted early in life and to include a caloric intake adjusted to achieve and maintain ideal body weight, a reduction in total fat calories to 30 to 35 percent of total calories achieved by a substantial reduction in dietary saturated fat to less than 10 percent of total calories, and a reduction in cholesterol intake to less than 300 mg per day. Although a causal relationship in humans between sodium intake and hypertension has not been firmly established, avoidance of excessive dietary sodium has also been recommended.

RISK FACTORS AND MECHANISMS OF ATHEROGENESIS *Adiposity* produces insulin resistance in peripheral tissues (mainly muscle and adipose), which leads to compensatory hyperinsulinemia. The liver is not resistant to some effects of insulin, and enhanced production of triglyceride-rich lipoproteins results, leading to elevated plasma triglyceride and cholesterol levels. Thus it has been demonstrated that body weight is related not only to triglyceride levels but also to cholesterol levels. Concomitantly, obesity is associated with increased total body cholesterol synthesis. Obesity produces higher circulating levels of insulin, both in the basal state and after stimulation with glucose or other secretagogues. Since obesity is related to atherosclerosis—both directly and via hypertension, hypertriglyceridemia, hypercholesterolemia, and hyperglycemia—it is not surprising that many studies show a relationship between serum insulin levels, particularly after oral glucose intake, and atherosclerotic disease of the coronary and peripheral arteries. A few studies, however, suggest that this association between insulin and atherosclerosis occurs independently of obesity. It has been postulated that insulin may directly affect arterial wall metabolism, leading to increased endogenous lipid synthesis and thus predisposing to atherosclerosis. Insulin has been shown in physiologic concentrations to stimulate proliferation of arterial smooth-muscle cells and enhance binding of LDL and VLDL to fibroblasts; it therefore may be one of the plasma factors involved in atheroma formation.

Hypertension may enhance atherogenesis by directly producing injury via mechanical stress on endothelial cells at specific high-pressure sites in the arterial tree. This would allow the sequence of events in the chronic injury hypothesis of atherogenesis to take place. In addition, hypertension might allow more lipoproteins to be transported through intact endothelial lining cells by altering permeability. Hypertension markedly increases lysosomal enzyme activity, presumably owing to stimulation of the cellular disposal system by the internalization of increased amounts of plasma substances. This might lead to increased cell degeneration and release of the highly destructive enzymes (within the lysosomes) into the arterial wall. Experimental hypertension also increases the thickness of the intimal smooth-muscle layer in the arterial wall and increases connective tissue elements. It is still not known if continued high pressure within the artery produces changes in the ability of smooth-muscle cells or stem cells to proliferate.

Diabetes could provide a unique contribution to atherogenesis. Although the fundamental genetic abnormality in human diabetes mellitus remains unknown, it has been suggested that genetic diabetes in humans represents a primary cellular abnormality intrinsic to all cells, resulting in a decreased life span of individual cells, which in turn results in increased cell turnover in tissues. If arterial endothelial and smooth-muscle cells are intrinsically defective in diabetes, accelerated atherogenesis can be readily postulated on the basis of any one of the current theories of pathogenesis. Platelet dysfunction in diabetes might also play a role.

The role of glucose in atheroma formation, if any, is poorly understood. Hyperglycemia is known to affect aortic wall metabolism. Sorbitol, a product of the insulin-independent aldose reductase pathway of glucose metabolism (the polyol pathway) accumulates in the arterial wall in the presence of high glucose concentrations, resulting in osmotic effects including increased cell water content and decreased oxygenation. Increased glucose also appears to stimulate proliferation of cultured arterial smooth-muscle cells.

The development of atherosclerosis accelerates in approximate quantitative relation to the degree of *hyperlipidemia*. A long-established theory suggests that the higher the circulating levels of lipoprotein the more likely they are to gain entrance to the arterial wall. By an acceleration of the usual transendothelial transport, large concentrations of lipoproteins within the arterial wall could overwhelm the ability of smooth-muscle cells to metabolize them. Lipoproteins have been immunologically identified in atheroma, and in humans there is a close relationship between plasma cholesterol and arterial lipoprotein cholesterol concentration. Chemically modified lipoproteins, possibly produced in hyperlipidemic disorders, could gain access to the scavenger arterial wall macrophages, leading to formation of foam cells as in xanthomas. It is possible that the lipid that accumulates in the arterial wall with increasing age results from infiltration of plasma lipoproteins. However, atheromatous lesions are associated with a more marked increase in arterial wall lipids, which may result in part from injury to the endothelium possibly produced by chronic hyperlipidemia, as demonstrated in cholesterol-fed monkeys. A further mechanism for accelerated atherogenesis in hyperlipidemia is related to the ability of LDL to stimulate proliferation of arterial smooth-muscle cells.

The effect of *chronic smoke inhalation* from cigarettes could result in repetitive injury to endothelial cells, thereby accelerating atherogenesis. Hypoxia stimulates proliferation of cultured human arterial smooth-muscle cells; thus, since cigarette smoking is associated with high levels of carboxyhemoglobin and low oxygen delivery to tissues, another mechanism for atherogenesis is suggested. Hypoxia could produce diminished lysosomal enzyme degradative ability, as evidenced by impaired degradation of LDL by smooth-muscle cells, causing LDL to accumulate in the cells. Consistent with this suggestion is the fact that aortic lesions that resemble atheroma have been produced in experimental animals by systemic hypoxia, and lipid accumulation in the arterial wall of cholesterol-fed rabbits and monkeys appears to be increased by hypoxia.

RISK FACTOR REVERSAL AND REGRESSION OF ATHEROSCLEROSIS
Although the emergence of clinical consequences of atherosclerosis can be lessened, no convincing instance of regression or interruption of progression of atherosclerosis, determined by direct or indirect examination of lesions, by removal or reversal of any single risk factor or group of risk factors has yet been proved in humans. Nevertheless, feasibility of such demonstrations is becoming established, and preliminary results are encouraging. Through mass-

media educational efforts, whole communities can be influenced to reduce smoking, change diet, and lower blood pressure levels. Adult males in the United States have lowered cigarette consumption, although increases among teenage girls have kept total usage high. There has been a trend toward lower cholesterol and saturated fat consumption in the United States, coupled with increasing attention to reducing overweight and the use of exercise programs. Concomitantly, and perhaps causally, there has been the noted decline in IHD mortality. Treatment of hyperlipidemia in some instances has been shown to reduce atherosclerotic involvement of peripheral vessels by both invasive and noninvasive measurement. There is also some encouraging evidence in animals, most notably in primates, that relatively complicated plaques induced by hyperlipidemia will regress, and that further progression of atherosclerosis will cease when hyperlipidemia is removed. Therefore efforts to prevent atherogenesis, to interrupt progression, and perhaps to promote regression of existing lesions by risk factor reduction seem warranted.

PREVENTION   Although premature IHD is overall the most costly and common of the untimely complications of atherosclerosis, preoccupation with IHD should not obscure the fact that angina pectoris and myocardial infarction are expressions of late-stage atherosclerotic lesions. Factors precipitating these clinical events may be independent of those leading to initiation of plaque formation or its progression to a complicated lesion. Steps taken to prevent recurrence of myocardial infarction or fatal arrhythmia, termed *secondary prevention*, will not necessarily be the same as those taken to delay or prevent formation of atherosclerosis (*primary prevention*). Since atherosclerotic plaques have been detected in the coronary arteries of American males as early as the second decade in autopsy studies of Korean and Vietnam war deaths, primary prevention of atherosclerosis must begin early in life, long before there is any suspicion of IHD.

Thus, *prevention of atherosclerosis, rather than treatment, is the goal*. Although an effective program has not been established with certainty, enough is known to act as a guide both in identification of those with a higher risk and in development of conservative measures that probably will reduce that risk. Thus prevention currently is equated with risk factor reduction.

The decline of American death rates from premature IHD today coincides with two trends in health practices. One is the increasing acceptance of the importance of detecting and attempting to correct some of the risk factors correlated with atherosclerosis. The other is a greater awareness of the dietary sources of cholesterol and saturated fats and a tendency of the public to restrict their intake somewhat. Whether these trends are causally related to the decline in death rate is not known. While a rigorous approach to changes in life-style for the general population may be debatable, it is desirable to continue finding and helping those most susceptible to early atherosclerosis. The physician's role in risk factor reduction involves treatment of hypertension and advice regarding diet, body weight, smoking, and exercise. Drug treatment of hyperlipidemia should be limited to those individuals at risk who do not respond adequately to dietary management. Although preliminary trials are encouraging, the long-term value of antiplatelet drugs in reducing either the mortality rate or incidence of myocardial infarction in individuals with IHD remains unproved, and trials are continuing.

TREATMENT   There is no agent proven to have any value in "treatment" of atherosclerosis unless it clearly reduces severe hyperlipidemia or obvious hypertension. In fact, there is no treatment of atherosclerosis, only of its complications. While end-stage treatment technology has reduced morbidity (Chap. 189), prevention remains the long-term goal of both research and health care practice.

REFERENCES

BIERMAN EL: Aging and atherosclerosis, in *Principles of Geriatric Medicine*, R. Andres et al (eds). New York, McGraw-Hill, 1985, p 42

BRUNZELL JD et al: Pathophysiology of lipoprotein transport. Metabolism 27:1109, 1978

GOLDSTEIN JL et al: Hyperlipidemia in coronary heart disease. J Clin Invest 52:1533, 1544, 1973

———— et al: Defective lipoprotein receptors and atherosclerosis. N Engl J Med 309:288, 1983

GORDON T et al: Diabetes, blood lipids, and the role of obesity in coronary heart disease risk for women. The Framingham Study. Ann Intern Med 87:393, 1977

———— et al: High density lipoprotein as a protective factor against coronary heart disease. The Framingham Study. Am J Med 62:707, 1977

KANNEL WB et al: Optimal resources for primary prevention of atherosclerotic diseases. Circulation 70:155A, 1984

LEVY RI: Declining mortality in coronary heart disease. Arteriosclerosis 1:312, 1981

McGILL HC: Persistent problems in the pathogenesis of atherosclerosis. Arteriosclerosis 4:443, 1984

PELL S, FAYERWEATHER WE: Trends in the incidence of myocardial infarction and in associated mortality and morbidity in a large employed population, 1957–1983. N Engl J Med 312:1005, 1985.

ROSS R: The pathogenesis of atherosclerosis—an update. N Engl J Med 314:488, 1986

STEINBERG D: Lipoproteins and atherosclerosis: A look back and a look ahead. Arteriosclerosis 3:283, 1983

196 HYPERTENSIVE VASCULAR DISEASE

GORDON H. WILLIAMS / EUGENE BRAUNWALD

An elevated arterial pressure is probably the more important public health problem in developed countries—being common, asymptomatic, readily detectable, usually easily treatable, and often leading to lethal complications if left untreated. As a result of extensive educational programs in the late 1960s and 1970s by both private and governmental agencies, the number of undiagnosed and/or untreated patients has been significantly reduced. This factor may be the most important one responsible for the decline in cardiovascular mortality which has taken place during the past 15 years (Chap. 195). Although our understanding of the pathophysiology of an elevated arterial pressure has increased, in 90 to 95 percent of cases the etiology (and thus potentially the prevention or cure) is still largely unknown.

DEFINITION

Since there is no dividing line between normal and high blood pressure, arbitrary levels have been established to define those who have an increased risk of developing a morbid cardiovascular event and/or will clearly benefit from medical therapy. These definitions should consider not only the level of diastolic pressure but also systolic pressure, age, sex, and race. For example, patients with a diastolic pressure greater than 90 mmHg will have a significant reduction in morbidity and mortality with adequate therapy. These, then, are patients who have hypertension and who should be considered for treatment.

The level of *systolic* pressure is also important in assessing arterial pressure's influence on cardiovascular morbidity. Males with normal diastolic pressures (<82 mmHg) but elevated systolic pressures (>158 mmHg) have a 2½-fold increase in their cardiovascular mortality rates when compared with individuals with similar diastolic pressures but whose systolic pressures are normal (<130 mmHg). Other significant factors which modify blood pressure's influence on the frequency of morbid cardiovascular events are age, race, and sex with young black males being most adversely affected by hypertension.

When hypertension is suspected, blood pressure should be measured at least twice on two separate examinations. In adults, a *diastolic* pressure below 85 mmHg is considered to be normal; between 85 and 89 is high normal; 90 to 104 is mild hypertension; 105 to 114 moderate hypertension; 115 or greater is severe hypertension. When the diastolic pressure is below 90 mmHg, a *systolic* pressure below 140 mmHg indicates normal blood pressure; between 140 and 159 is

borderline isolated systolic hypertension; 160 or higher is isolated systolic hypertension.

Arterial pressure fluctuates in most persons, whether they are normotensive or hypertensive. Those who are classified as having *labile* hypertension are patients who sometimes, but not always, have arterial pressures within the hypertensive range. These patients are often considered to have borderline hypertension.

Sustained hypertension can become accelerated or enter a malignant phase. Though a patient with *malignant hypertension* often has a blood pressure above 200/140, it is papilledema, usually accompanied by retinal hemorrhages and exudates, and not the absolute pressure level, that defines this condition. *Accelerated hypertension* signifies a significant recent increase over previous hypertensive levels associated with evidence of vascular damage on funduscopic examination but without papilledema.

FREQUENCY The prevalence of hypertension depends on both the racial composition of the studied population and the criteria used to define the condition. In a white suburban population as used in the Framingham Study, nearly one-fifth have blood pressures greater than 160/95, while almost one-half have pressures greater than 140/90. An even higher prevalance has been documented in the nonwhite population.

ETIOLOGY

The cause of elevated arterial pressure is unknown in most cases. The prevalence of various forms of secondary hypertension depends on the nature of the population studied and how extensive the evaluation is. There are no available data to define the frequency of secondary hypertension in the general population, although in middle-aged males it has been reported to be 6 percent. On the other hand, in referral centers where patients undergo an extensive evaluation, it has been reported to be as high as 35 percent. The various forms of hypertension are outlined in Table 196-1, and their relative frequencies are given in Table 196-2.

ESSENTIAL HYPERTENSION Patients with arterial hypertension and no definable cause are said to have *primary, essential,* or *idiopathic hypertension.* Undoubtedly, the primary difficulty in uncovering the mechanism(s) responsible for the hypertension in these patients is attributable to the variety of systems that are involved in the regulation of arterial pressure—peripheral and/or central adrenergic, renal, hormonal, and vascular—and to the complexity of the relationships of these systems to one another. Several abnormalities have been described in patients with essential hypertension, often with a claim that one or more of these are primarily responsible for the hypertension. While it is still uncertain whether these individual abnormalities are primary or secondary, varying expressions of a single disease process or reflective of separate disease entities, the accumulating data increasingly support the latter hypothesis. Thus, just as pneumonia is caused by a variety of infectious agents, even though the clinical picture observed may be similar, so essential hypertension likely has a number of distinct causes. Therefore, the distinction between primary and secondary hypertension has become blurred, and the approach to both the diagnosis and therapy of hypertensive patients have been modified. For example, as a group of patients with essential hypertension are separated into a distinct subset (e.g., low-renin essential hypertension), they have not been reclassified as a form of secondary hypertension but rather remain in the essential hypertensive group. In this chapter, we define those individuals with a specific organ defect responsible for hypertension as having a *secondary* form of hypertension. In contrast, individuals who may have generalized or functional abnormalities causing their hypertension are defined as having *essential* hypertension.

Heredity Genetic factors have long been assumed to be important in the genesis of hypertension. Data supporting this view can be found in animal studies as well as population studies in humans. One approach has been to assess the correlation of blood pressures within families (familial aggregation). From these studies the minimum size of the genetic factor can be expressed by a correlation coefficient of approximately 0.2. However, the variation in the size of the genetic factor in different studies reemphasizes the likely heterogeneous nature of the essential hypertensive population. Additionally, most studies support the concept that the inheritance is probably multifactoral.

Environment A number of environmental factors have been specifically implicated in the development of hypertension including salt intake, obesity, occupation, family size, and crowding. These factors have all been assumed to be important in the increase in blood pressure with age in more affluent societies, in contrast to the decline in blood pressure with age in more primitive cultures.

SALT-SENSITIVITY The environmental factor which has received the greatest attention is salt intake. Even this factor illustrates the heterogeneous nature of the essential hypertensive population in that the blood pressure in only approximately 60 percent of hypertensives is particularly responsive to the level of sodium intake. The etiologic basis for this special sensitivity to salt varies, with primary aldosteronism, bilateral renal artery stenosis, renal parenchymal disease, or low-renin essential hypertension accounting for about half of the patients. In the remainder, the pathophysiology is still uncertain, but recent postulated contributing factors include chloride, calcium, a generalized cellular membrane defect, and "nonmodulation" (vide infra).

Most studies assessing the role of salt in the hypertensive process have assumed that it is the sodium ion which is important. However,

some investigators have suggested that the chloride ion may be equally important. This suggestion is based on the observation that feeding chloride-free sodium salts to salt-sensitive hypertensive animals fails to increase arterial pressure. Calcium has also been implicated in the pathogenesis of some forms of essential hypertension. A low calcium intake has been associated with an increase in blood pressure in epidemiologic studies; an increase in leukocyte cytosolic calcium levels has been reported in some hypertensives; and finally calcium entry blockers are effective antihypertensive agents. Several studies have reported a potential link between the salt-sensitive forms of hypertension and calcium. It has been postulated that with salt loading and a defect in the kidney's ability to excrete it, a secondary increase in circulating natriuretic factors may occur. One of these, the so-called digitalis-like natriuretic factor, inhibits ouabain-sensitive sodium-potassium ATPase and thereby leads to intracellular calcium accumulation and a hyperreactive vascular smooth muscle.

A third postulated explanation for salt-sensitive hypertension is a generalized membrane defect. This hypothesis derives most of its data from studies on circulating blood elements, particularly red blood cells, in which abnormalities in the transport of sodium across the cell membrane have been documented. Since both increases and decreases in the activity of different transport systems have been reported, it is likely that some abnormalities are primary and some secondary processes. It has been assumed that this abnormality reflects a defect in the cellular membrane and that this defect occurs in many, perhaps all cells of the body, particularly the vascular smooth muscle. Because of this defect, there is then an abnormal accumulation of calcium within vascular smooth muscle, resulting in a heightened vascular responsivity to vasoconstrictor agents. This defect has been proposed to be present in 35 to 50 percent of the essential hypertensive population based on studies using red cells. Other studies suggest that the abnormality in the red cell sodium transport is not a fixed abnormality but can be modified by environmental factors. Finally, the mechanisms underlying salt sensitivity in some patients may be a defect in the kidney's ability to excrete sodium appropriately, secondary to an abnormality in the control of the renal circulation and aldosterone secretion with changes in sodium intake. Sodium intake normally modulates adrenal and renal vascular responses to angiotensin II. With dietary sodium restriction, the adrenal response is enhanced and the renal vascular response reduced. Sodium loading has the opposite effect. In this subset of hypertensives this adjustment is absent, thus leading to the term "nonmodulators" to describe those patients in whom the excretion of a sodium load is impaired.

Each of these hypotheses has as a common final pathway an increase in cytosolic calcium resulting in increased vascular reactivity. However, as described above, several mechanisms might produce the increase in calcium accumulation.

Factors modifying the course of essential hypertension Age, race, sex, smoking, serum cholesterol, glucose intolerance, weight, and perhaps renin activity may all alter the prognosis of this disease. The younger the patient when hypertension is first noted, the greater the reduction in life expectancy if left untreated. In the United States,

TABLE 196-1 Classification of arterial hypertension

I Systolic hypertension with wide pulse pressure
  A Decreased compliance of aorta (arteriosclerosis)
  B Increased stroke volume
    1 Aortic regurgitation
    2 Thyrotoxicosis
    3 Hyperkinetic heart syndrome
    4 Fever
    5 Arteriovenous fistula
    6 Patent ductus arteriosus
II Systolic and diastolic hypertension (increased peripheral vascular resistance)
  A Renal
    1 Chronic pyelonephritis
    2 Acute and chronic glomerulonephritis
    3 Polycystic renal disease
    4 Renovascular stenosis or renal infarction
    5 Most other severe renal disease (arteriolar nephrosclerosis, diabetic nephropathy, etc.)
    6 Renin-producing tumors
  B Endocrine
    1 Oral contraceptives
    2 Adrenocortical hyperfunction
      a Cushing's disease and syndrome
      b Primary hyperaldosteronism
      c Congenital or hereditary adrenogenital syndromes (17α-hydroxylase and 11β-hydroxylase defects)
    3 Pheochromocytoma
    4 Myxedema
    5 Acromegaly
  C Neurogenic
    1 Psychogenic
    2 "Diencephalic syndrome"
    3 Familial dysautonomia (Riley-Day)
    4 Poliomyelitis (bulbar)
    5 Polyneuritis (acute porphyria, lead poisoning)
    6 Increased intracranial pressure (acute)
    7 Spinal cord section (acute)
  D Miscellaneous
    1 Coarctation of aorta
    2 Increased intravascular volume (excessive transfusion, polycythemia vera)
    3 Polyarteritis nodosa
    4 Hypercalcemia
  E Unknown etiology
    1 Essential hypertension (>90% of all cases of hypertension)
    2 Toxemia of pregnancy
    3 Acute intermittent porphyria

TABLE 196-2 Prevalence of various forms of hypertension in the general population and in specialized referral clinics*

Diagnosis	General population, %	Specialty clinic, %
Essential hypertension	92–94	65–85
Renal hypertension:		
Parenchymal	2–3	4–5
Renovascular	1–2	4–16
Endocrine hypertension:		
Primary aldosteronism	0.3	0.5–12
Cushing's syndrome	<0.1	0.2
Pheochromocytoma	<0.1	0.2
Oral contraceptive–induced	2–4	1–2
Miscellaneous	0.2	1

* *Estimates based on a number of reports in the literature.*

urban blacks have about twice the prevalence rate for hypertension as whites and more than four times the hypertension-induced morbidity rate. At all ages and in both white and nonwhite populations, females with hypertension fare better than males. Yet, females with hypertension run the same relative risk of a morbid cardiovascular event compared with their normotensive counterparts as males do. Accelerated atherosclerosis is an invariable companion of hypertension. Thus, it is not surprising that independent risk factors associated with the development of atherosclerosis, e.g., an elevated serum cholesterol, glucose intolerance, and/or cigarette smoking, significantly enhance the effect of hypertension on mortality rates regardless of age, sex, or race (Chap. 195). There also is no question that there is a positive correlation between obesity and arterial pressure. A gain in weight is associated with an increased frequency of hypertension in subjects with normal pressures, and weight loss in obese subjects with hypertension lowers their arterial pressure and, if they are being treated, the intensity of therapy required to maintain them normotensive. However, there are no convincing data that obesity adversely affects the hypertension-associated mortality rate. Plasma renin activity has also been reported by some to influence and correlate with the development of morbid cardiovascular events in patients with hypertension.

Natural history Because essential hypertension is a heterogeneous disorder, variables in addition to the level of arterial pressure modify its course. Thus, the probability of developing a morbid cardiovascular event with a given arterial pressure may vary by as much as twentyfold depending on whether associated risk factors are present (Table 196-3). Although exceptions have been reported, most untreated adults with hypertension will develop further increases in their arterial pressure with time. Furthermore, both from actuarial data and from experience in the era prior to effective therapy, it has been documented that untreated hypertension is associated with a shortening of life by 10 to 20 years, usually related to an acceleration of the atherosclerotic process, with the rate of acceleration in part related to the severity of the hypertension. Even individuals with relatively mild disease, i.e., without evidence of end organ damage, left untreated for 7 to 10 years have a high risk of developing significant complications. Nearly 30 percent will exhibit atherosclerotic complications, and more than 50 percent will have end organ damage related to the hypertension itself, e.g., cardiomegaly, congestive heart failure, retinopathy, a cerebrovascular accident, and/or renal insufficiency. Thus, even in its mild forms, hypertension is a progressively lethal disease, if left untreated.

SECONDARY HYPERTENSION

As noted earlier, in only a small minority of patients with an elevated arterial pressure can a specific cause be identified. Yet, they should

TABLE 196-3 Factors indicating an adverse prognosis in hypertension

I Black race
II Youth
III Male
IV Persistent diastolic pressure >115 mmHg
V Smoking
VI Diabetes mellitus
VII Hypercholesterolemia
VIII Obesity
IX Evidence of end organ damage
   A Cardiac
     1 Cardiac enlargement
     2 ECG changes of ischemic or left ventricular strain
     3 Myocardial infarction
     4 Congestive heart failure
   B Eyes
     1 Retinal exudates and hemorrhages
     2 Papilledema
   C Renal: impaired renal function
   D Nervous system: cerebrovascular accident
X High-renin hypertension?

not be ignored for at least two reasons: (1) with correction of the cause their hypertension may be cured, and (2) the secondary forms may provide insight into the etiology of essential hypertension. Nearly all the secondary forms are related to an alteration in hormone secretion and/or renal function and are discussed in detail in other chapters.

RENAL HYPERTENSION (see also Chap. 227) Hypertension produced by renal disease is the result of either (1) a derangement in the renal handling of sodium and fluids leading to volume expansion or (2) an alteration in renal secretion of vasoactive materials resulting in a systemic or local change in arteriolar tone. The main subdivisions of renal hypertension are renovascular hypertension, including preeclampsia and eclampsia, and renal parenchymal hypertension. A simple explanation for *renal vascular hypertension* is that decreased perfusion of renal tissue due to stenosis of a main or branch renal artery activates the renin-angiotensin system, described in Chap. 325. Circulating angiotensin II elevates arterial pressure by direct vasoconstriction, by stimulation of aldosterone secretion with resultant sodium retention (Chap. 29), and/or by stimulating the adrenergic nervous system. In actual practice only about one-half of patients with renovascular hypertension have elevated absolute levels of renin activity in peripheral plasma, although when renin measurements are referenced against an index of sodium balance, a much higher fraction have inappropriately high values. The use of the competitive angiotensin antagonist, saralasin (1-sar, 8-ala angiotensin II), has further clarified the role of angiotensin in the genesis of the hypertension in this disease. Nearly all patients with surgically correctable disease have exhibited a reduction of arterial pressure when given this agent in the sodium- or volume-depleted state.

Activation of the renin-angiotensin system also has been offered as an explanation for the hypertension in both acute and chronic *renal parenchymal disease*. In this formulation the only difference between renovascular and renal parenchymal hypertension is that the decreased perfusion of renal tissue in the latter case results from inflammatory and fibrotic changes involving multiple small intrarenal vessels. There are enough differences between the two conditions, however, to suggest that there are other mechanisms active in renal parenchymal disease: (1) peripheral plasma renin activity is elevated far less frequently in renal parenchymal than in renovascular hypertension; (2) cardiac output is said to be normal in the renal parenchymal type (unless uremia and anemia are present), but slightly elevated in renovascular hypertension; (3) circulatory responses to tilting and to the Valsalva maneuver are exaggerated in the latter condition; and (4) blood volume tends to be high in patients with severe renal parenchymal disease and low in patients with severe renovascular hypertension. Alternate explanations for the hypertension in renal parenchymal disease include the possibilities that the damaged kidneys (1) produce an unidentified vasopressor substance other than renin, (2) fail to produce a necessary humoral vasodilator substance (perhaps prostaglandin or bradykinin), (3) fail to inactivate circulating vasopressor substances, and/or (4) are ineffective in disposing of sodium, and the retained sodium is responsible for the hypertension as outlined earlier. Though all these explanations, including participation of the renin-angiotensin system, probably have some validity in individual patients, the hypothesis involving sodium retention is particularly attractive. It is supported by the observation that those patients with chronic pyelonephritis or polycystic renal disease who are salt wasters do not develop hypertension, and by the observation that removal of salt and water by dialysis or diuretics is effective in controlling arterial pressure in the majority of patients with renal parenchymal disease.

A rare form of renal hypertension results from the excess secretion of renin by juxtaglomerular cell tumors or nephroblastomas. The initial presentation is similar to that of hyperaldosteronism with hypertension, hypokalemia, and overproduction of aldosterone. However, in contrast to primary aldosteronism, peripheral renin activity is *elevated instead of subnormal*. This disease can be distinguished from other forms of secondary aldosteronism by the presence of normal renal function and with unilateral increases in renal vein renin concentration without a renal artery lesion.

ENDOCRINE HYPERTENSION **Adrenal hypertension** Hypertension is a feature of a variety of adrenal cortical abnormalities. In *primary aldosteronism* (Chap. 325) there is a clear relationship between the aldosterone-induced sodium retention and the hypertension. Normal individuals given aldosterone develop hypertension only if they also ingest sodium. Since aldosterone causes sodium retention by stimulating renal tubular exchange of sodium for potassium, hypokalemia is a prominent feature in most patients with primary aldosteronism, and therefore the measurement of serum potassium provides a simple screening test. The effect of sodium retention and volume expansion in chronically suppressing plasma renin activity is critically important for the definitive diagnosis. In most clinical situations plasma renin activity and plasma or urinary aldosterone levels parallel each other, but in patients with primary aldosteronism, aldosterone levels are high and relatively fixed because of autonomous aldosterone secretion, while plasma renin activity levels are suppressed and respond sluggishly to sodium depletion. Primary aldosteronism may be secondary either to a tumor or bilateral adrenal hyperplasia. It is important to distinguish between these two conditions preoperatively, as usually the hypertension in the latter is not modified by operation.

The sodium-retaining effect of large amounts of glucocorticoids also offers an explanation for the hypertension in severe cases of Cushing's syndrome (Chap. 325). Moreover, increased production of mineralocorticoids also has been documented in some patients with Cushing's syndrome. However, the hypertension in many cases of Cushing's syndrome does not seem volume-dependent, leading investigators to speculate that it may be secondary to glucocorticoid-induced production of renin substrate (angiotensin-mediated hypertension) or a steroid-induced change in vascular reactivity. In the forms of the adrenogenital syndrome due to C-11 or C-17 hydroxylase deficiency (Chap. 325) deoxycorticosterone accounts for the sodium retention and the resultant hypertension, which is accompanied by suppression of plasma renin activity.

In patients with pheochromocytoma (Chap. 326) increased secretion of epinephrine and norepinephrine by a tumor most often located in the adrenal medulla causes excessive stimulation of adrenergic receptors, which results in peripheral vasoconstriction and cardiac stimulation. This diagnosis is confirmed by demonstrating increased urinary excretion of epinephrine and norepinephrine or their metabolites.

Acromegaly (see also Chap. 321) Hypertension, coronary atherosclerosis, and cardiac hypertrophy are frequent complications of this condition.

Hypercalcemia (see also Chap. 335) The hypertension which occurs in up to one-third of patients with hyperparathyroidism ordinarily can be attributed to renal parenchymal damage due to nephrolithiasis and nephrocalcinosis. However, increased calcium levels can also have a direct vasoconstrictive effect. In some cases, the hypertension disappears when the hypercalcemia is corrected. Thus, paradoxically the increased serum calcium level in hyperparathyroidism raises blood pressure, while epidemiologic studies suggest that a high calcium intake lowers blood pressure. To further confuse the issue, calcium entry blocking agents are effective antihypertensive agents. Additional studies are needed to resolve these seemingly conflicting observations.

Oral contraceptives The most common cause of endocrine hypertension is that resulting from the use of estrogen-containing oral contraceptives. Indeed, this may be the most common form of secondary hypertension. The mechanisms producing the hypertension is likely to be secondary to activation of the renin-angiotensin-aldosterone system. Thus, both volume (aldosterone) and vasonconstrictor (angiotensin II) factors are important. The estrogen component of oral contraceptive agents stimulates the hepatic synthesis of the renin substrate angiotensinogen, which in turn favors the increased production of angiotensin II and secondary aldosteronism. Women taking oral contraceptives have increased plasma concentrations of angiotensin II and aldosterone with some increase in arterial pressure. However, only about 5 percent actually have an increase in arterial pressure greater than 140/90, and in about half of these the hypertension will remit within 6 months of stopping the drug.

Why some women taking oral contraceptives develop hypertension and others do not is unclear but may be related to (1) increased vascular sensitivity to angiotensin II, (2) the presence of mild renal disease, (3) familial factors (over one-half have a positive family history for hypertension), (4) age (hypertension is significantly more prevalent in women over age 35), and/or (5) obesity. Indeed some investigators have suggested that the oral contraceptives are simply unmasking patients with essential hypertension.

COARCTATION OF THE AORTA (See also Chap. 185) The hypertension associated with coarctation may be caused by the constriction itself, or perhaps by the changes in the renal circulation which result in an unusual form of renal arterial hypertension. The diagnosis of coarctation is usually evident from physical examination and routine x-ray findings.

LOW-RENIN ESSENTIAL HYPERTENSION Approximately 20 percent of patients who by all other criteria have essential hypertension have suppressed plasma renin activity. This occurs more frequently in black than in white patients. Though these patients are not hypokalemic, they have been reported to have expanded extracellular fluid volumes, and it is tempting to implicate sodium retention and renin suppression due to excessive production of an unidentified mineralocorticoid. Involvement of the adrenal cortex is suggested by the observation that large doses of spironolactone, the mineralocorticoid antagonist, and the inhibition of steroidogenesis by aminoglutethimide can result in sodium loss and lowering of blood pressure in these patients. A search for other mineralocorticoids occasionally reveals increased secretion of 18-hydroxy-11-deoxycorticosterone or 16-hydroxydehydroepiandrosterone in some patients. However, the frequency of these abnormalities is no greater than in patients with normal renin hypertension. Some studies have suggested that many of these patients have an increased sensitivity of their adrenal cortex to angiotensin II which may be the underlying mechanism. Since this altered sensitivity has been reported even in patients with normal renin hypertension, it is likely that patients with low-renin hypertension are not a distinct subset but rather form part of a continuum of patients with essential hypertension.

HIGH-RENIN ESSENTIAL HYPERTENSION Approximately 15 percent of patients with essential hypertension have plasma renin levels elevated above the normal range. It has been suggested that plasma renin plays an important role in the pathogenesis of the elevated blood pressure in these patients. However, most studies have documented that saralasin significantly reduces blood pressure in less than half of these patients. This has led some investigators to postulate that the elevated renin levels and blood pressure may both be secondary to an increased activity of the adrenergic system. It has been proposed that, in those patients with angiotensin-dependent high-renin hypertension whose arterial pressures are lowered by saralasin, the mechanism responsible for the increased renin and, therefore, the hypertension is a compensatory hyperreninemia secondary to a decreased adrenal responsiveness to angiotensin II. Additional studies have documented that patients with high-renin hypertension are the same as the nonmodulators described on page 1025.

EFFECTS OF HYPERTENSION

Patients with hypertension die prematurely; the most common cause of death is heart disease, with stroke and renal failure also frequent, particularly in those with significant retinopathy.

EFFECTS ON HEART Cardiac compensation for the excessive work load imposed by increased systemic pressure is at first sustained by concentric left ventricular hypertrophy, characterized by an increase in wall thickness. Ultimately, the function of this chamber deteriorates, the cavity dilates, and the symptoms and signs of heart failure appear (Chap. 182). Angina pectoris may also occur because of the combination of accelerated coronary arterial disease and increased myocardial oxygen requirements as a consequence of the increased myocardial mass (Chap. 189). On physical examination the heart is enlarged and has a prominent left ventricular impulse. The sound of aortic closure is accentuated, and there may be a faint murmur of aortic regurgitation. Presystolic (atrial, fourth) heart sounds appear frequently in hypertensive heart disease, and a protodiastolic (ventricular, third heart) sound or summation gallop rhythm may be present. Electrocardiographic changes of left ventricular hypertrophy (Chap. 178) are common; evidence of ischemia or infarction may be observed late in the disease. The majority of deaths due to hypertension result from myocardial infarction or congestive heart failure.

NEUROLOGIC EFFECTS The neurologic effects of long-standing hypertension may be divided into retinal and central nervous system changes. Because the retina is the only tissue in which the arteries and arterioles can be examined directly, repeated ophthalmoscopic examination provides the opportunity to observe the progress of the vascular effects of hypertension (Table 196-4). The Keith-Wagener-Barker classification of the *retinal changes* in hypertension has provided a simple and excellent means for serial evaluation of hypertensive patients. Increasing severity of hypertension is associated with focal spasm and progressive general narrowing of the arterioles, as well as the appearance of hemorrhages, exudates, and papilledema. These retinal lesions often produce scotomata, blurred vision, and even blindness, especially in the presence of papilledema or hemorrhages of the macular area. Hypertensive lesions may develop acutely and, if therapy results in significant reduction of blood pressure, may show rapid resolution. Rarely, these lesions resolve without therapy. In contrast, retinal arteriolosclerosis results from endothelial and muscular proliferation, and it accurately reflects similar changes in other organs. Sclerotic changes do not develop as rapidly as hypertensive lesions, nor do they regress appreciably with therapy. As a consequence of increased wall thickness and rigidity, sclerotic arterioles distort and compress the veins as they cross within their common fibrous sheath, and the reflected light streak from the arterioles is changed by the increased opacity of the vessel wall.

Central nervous system dysfunction also occurs frequently in patients with hypertension. Occipital headaches, most often in the morning, are among the most prominent early symptoms of hypertension. Dizziness, lightheadedness, vertigo, tinnitus, and dimmed vision or syncope may also be observed, but the more serious manifestations are due to vascular occlusion, hemorrhage, or encephalopathy (Chap. 343). The pathogeneses of the former two disorders are quite different. *Cerebral infarction* is secondary to the increased atherosclerosis observed in hypertensive patients, while *cerebral hemorrhage* is the result of both the elevated arterial pressure and the development of cerebral vascular microaneurysms (Charcot-Bouchard aneurysms). Only age and arterial pressure are known to influence the development of the microaneurysms. Thus, it is not surprising that the association of arterial pressure with cerebral hemorrhage is much better than with either cerebral or myocardial infarction.

Hypertensive encephalopathy consists of the following symptom complex: severe hypertension, disordered consciousness, increased intracranial pressure, retinopathy with papilledema, and seizures. The pathogenesis is uncertain but probably not related to arteriolar spasm or cerebral edema. Focal neurologic signs are infrequent, and if present, suggest that infarction, hemorrhage, or transient ischemic attacks are more likely diagnoses. Although some investigators have suggested that prompt lowering of arterial pressure in these patients may adversely affect cerebral blood flow, most studies indicate that this is not the case.

RENAL EFFECTS (See also Chap. 227) Arteriolosclerotic lesions of the afferent and efferent arterioles and the glomerular capillary tufts are the most common renal vascular lesions in hypertension and result in decreased glomerular filtration rate and tubular dysfunction. Proteinuria and microscopic hematuria occur because of glomerular lesions, and approximately 10 percent of the deaths secondary to hypertension result from renal failure. Blood loss in hypertension occurs not only from renal lesions; epistaxis, hemoptysis, and metrorrhagia also occur frequently in these patients.

APPROACH TO THE PATIENT WITH HYPERTENSION

In evaluating patients with hypertension, the initial history, physical examination, and laboratory tests should be directed at (1) uncovering correctable secondary forms of hypertension (Table 196-1), (2) establishing a pretreatment baseline, (3) assessing factors which may influence the type of therapy or which may be adversely modified by therapy, and (4) determining whether other risk factors for the development of arteriosclerotic cardiovascular disease are present (Chap. 195). Ideally, this evaluation would also determine the

TABLE 196-4 Classification of hypertensive and arteriolosclerotic retinopathy

Degree	Hypertension					Arteriolosclerosis	
	Arterioles						
	General narrowing AV ratio*	Focal spasm†	Hemorrhages	Exudates	Papilledema	Arteriolar light reflex	AV crossing‡ defects
Normal	3:4	1:1	0	0	0	Fine yellow line, red blood column	0
Grade I	1:2	1:1	0	0	0	Broadened yellow line, red blood column	Mild depression of vein
Grade II	1:3	2:3	0	0	0	Broad yellow line, "copper wire," blood column not visible	Depression or humping of vein
Grade III	1:4	1:3	+	+	0	Broad white line, "silver wire," blood column not visible	Right-angle deviation, tapering, and disappearance of vein under arteriole. Distal dilatation of vein
Grade IV	Fine, fibrous cords	Obliteration of distal flow	+	+	+	Fibrous cords, blood column not visible	Same as grade III

* This is the ratio of arteriolar to venous diameters.
† This is the ratio of diameters of region of spasm to proximal arteriole.
‡ Arteriolar length and tortuosity increase with severity.

underlying mechanism(s) in essential hypertension, particularly if such information leads to a more specific therapeutic program. Unfortunately, at the present time this aspect of the evaluation is limited either by lack of knowledge of the underlying mechanisms, uncertainty as to the specificity of therapy for a distinct subset even if the underlying mechanisms are known, or the prohibitive expense in defining a subset of hypertensive patients even if specific therapy were available. However, with the accumulation of additional information a fifth component in the evaluation of patients with hypertension may become increasingly more important.

SYMPTOMS AND SIGNS The majority of patients with hypertension have no symptoms referable to their blood pressure elevation and will be identified only in the course of a physical examination. When symptoms do bring the patient to the physician, they fall into three categories. They are related to (1) the elevated pressure itself, (2) the hypertensive vascular disease, and (3) the underlying disease in the case of secondary hypertension. Though popularly considered a symptom of elevated arterial pressure, headache is characteristic only of severe hypertension; most commonly it is localized to the occipital region, is present when the patient awakens in the morning, and subsides spontaneously after several hours. Other possibly related complaints include dizziness, palpitations, and easy fatigability. Complaints referable to vascular disease include epistaxis, hematuria, blurring of vision owing to retinal changes, episodes of weakness or dizziness due to transient cerebral ischemia, angina pectoris, and dyspnea due to cardiac failure. Pain due to dissection of the aorta or to a leaking aneurysm is an occasional presenting symptom.

Examples of symptoms related to the underlying disease in secondary hypertension are polyuria, polydipsia, and muscle weakness secondary to hypokalemia in patients with primary aldosteronism, or weight gain and emotional lability in patients with Cushing's syndrome. The patient with a pheochromocytoma may present with episodic headaches, palpitations, diaphoresis, and postural dizziness.

CLINICAL EVALUATION History A strong family history of hypertension, along with the reported finding of intermittent pressure elevation in the past, favors the diagnosis of essential hypertension. Secondary hypertension often develops before the age of 35 or after the age of 55 years. The history of use of adrenal steroids or estrogens is of obvious significance. A history of repeated urinary tract infections suggests chronic pyelonephritis, although this condition may occur in the absence of symptoms; nocturia and polydipsia suggest renal or endocrine disease, while trauma to either flank or an episode of acute flank pain may be a clue to the presence of renal injury. A history of weight gain is compatible with Cushing's syndrome, and weight loss with pheochromocytoma. A number of aspects of the history aid in determining whether vascular disease has progressed to dangerous stages. These include angina pectoris and symptoms of cerebrovascular insufficiency, of congestive heart failure, and/or of peripheral vascular insufficiency. Other risk factors that should be elicited include cigarette smoking, diabetes mellitus, lipid disorders, and a family history of early deaths due to cardiovascular disease.

Physical examination The physical examination starts with the patient's general appearance. For instance, are the round face and trunkal obesity of Cushing's syndrome present? Is muscular development in the upper extremities out of proportion to that in the lower extremities, suggesting coarctation of the aorta? The next step is to compare the blood pressures and pulses in both upper extremities. Also, measurements in the supine position should be compared with measurements taken during standing. A rise in diastolic pressure when the patient goes from the supine to the standing position is most compatible with essential hypertension; a fall, in the absence of antihypertensive medications, suggests secondary forms of hypertension. Detailed examination of the ocular fundi is mandatory, since funduscopic findings provide one of the best indications of the duration of hypertension and of prognosis. The Keith-Wagener-Barker classification of funduscopic changes (Table 196-4) is useful; the specific changes in each fundus should be recorded and a grade assigned. Palpation and auscultation of the carotid arteries for evidence of stenosis or occlusion are important; narrowing of a carotid artery may be a manifestation of hypertensive vascular disease, and it may also be a clue to the presence of a renal arterial lesion, since these two lesions may occur together. In examination of the heart and lungs, one should search for evidence of left ventricular hypertrophy and cardiac decompensation. Is there a left ventricular lift? Are third and fourth heart sounds present? Are there pulmonary rales? Chest examination also includes a search for extracardiac murmurs and palpable collateral vessels that may result from coarctation of the aorta.

The most important part of the abdominal examination is auscultation for bruits originating in stenotic renal arteries. Bruits due to renal arterial narrowing nearly always have a diastolic component or may be continuous and are best heard just to the right or left of the midline above the umbilicus, or in the flanks; they are present in many patients with renal artery stenosis due to fibrous dysplasia and in 40 to 50 percent of those with functionally significant stenosis due to arteriosclerosis. The abdomen also should be palpated for abdominal aneurysm and for the enlarged kidneys of polycystic renal disease. The femoral pulses must be carefully felt, and, if they are decreased and/or delayed in comparison to the radial pulse, the blood pressure in the lower extremities must be measured. Even if the femoral pulse is normal to palpation, arterial pressure in the lower extremities should be recorded at least once in patients in whom hypertension is discovered before the age of 30 years. Finally, examination of the extremities for edema and a search for evidence of a previous cerebrovascular accident and/or other intracranial pathology should be performed.

Laboratory investigation Controversy exists as to what laboratory studies should be performed in patients presenting with hypertension. In general, the disagreement resides in how extensively to evaluate the patient for secondary forms of hypertension or subsets of essential hypertension. In the following discussion laboratory studies are divided into those which should be performed in all patients with sustained hypertension (basic studies) and those which should be added if (1) from the initial evaluation a secondary form of hypertension is suggested and/or (2) arterial pressure is not controlled after initial therapy (secondary studies).

BASIC STUDIES Renal status is evaluated by assessing the presence of protein, blood, and glucose in the urine and measuring serum creatinine and/or blood urea nitrogen (BUN). Microscopic examination of the urine is also helpful. A serum potassium level is needed both as a screen for mineralocorticoid-induced hypertension and as a baseline prior to initiating diuretic therapy.

Other blood chemistries may also be useful, particularly since they can often be ordered as a battery of automated tests at minimal cost to the patient. For example, a blood glucose is helpful both because diabetes mellitus may be associated with accelerated arteriosclerosis, renal vascular disease, and diabetic nephropathy in patients with hypertension, and because primary aldosteronism, Cushing's syndrome, and pheochromocytoma all may be associated with hyperglycemia. Furthermore, since antihypertensive therapy with diuretics, for example, can raise the blood glucose level, it is important to establish a baseline. The possibility of hypercalcemia may also be investigated. Serum uric acid is useful because of the increased incidence of hyperuricemia in patients with renal and essential hypertension and because, as with blood glucose, the level subsequently may be raised by treatment with diuretics. Serum cholesterol and triglycerides may be measured to identify other factors which predispose to the development of arteriosclerosis. An electrocardiogram should be obtained in all cases as an assessment of cardiac status, particularly if left ventricular hypertrophy is present, and as a baseline. The chest roentgenogram may also be helpful by providing the opportunity to identify aortic dilatation or elongation and the rib notching that occurs in coarctation of the aorta.

SECONDARY STUDIES (Table 196-5) Certain clues from the history, physical examination, and basic laboratory studies suggest an unusual cause for the hypertension and dictate the need for special studies. For example, the abrupt onset of severe hypertension and/or the onset of hypertension of any severity under the age of 25 or after the age of 50 years should lead to laboratory tests to exclude renovascular hypertension and pheochromocytoma. A history of headaches, palpitations, anxiety attacks, unusual sweating, hyperglycemia, and weight loss should also lead to tests to exclude pheochromocytoma. The presence of an abdominal bruit should lead to workup for renovascular hypertension, and the finding of bilateral upper abdominal masses on physical examination, consistent with polycystic renal disease, to the performance of an intravenous pyelogram. An elevated creatinine or blood urea nitrogen, associated with proteinuria and hematuria, should initiate a detailed workup for renal insufficiency (Chap. 218). Special studies for secondary hypertension are also indicated if there is therapeutic failure with the initial drug program. The specific diagnostic measures depend on the most likely causes of secondary hypertension.

Pheochromocytoma (see also Chap. 326). The easiest and best screening procedure for pheochromocytoma is the measurement of catecholamines or their metabolites in a 24-h urine collected during the time the patient is hypertensive. Measurement of plasma catecholamine levels may also be useful. These tests may be indicated even in patients who do not have episodic hypertension, since over half the patients with pheochromocytoma have fixed hypertension. Provocative tests are seldom if ever indicated, although occasionally a suppressive test may be useful.

Cushing's syndrome (see also Chap. 325). A 24-h urine test for cortisol or the administration of 1 mg dexamethasone at bedtime, followed by measurement of plasma cortisol at 7 to 10 A.M. is the best test for the presence of this condition. A urine cortisol less than 100 μg or suppression of the plasma cortisol level to below 5 μg/dL effectively rules out Cushing's syndrome.

Renovascular hypertension (see also Chap. 227). The standard screening test for renal vascular hypertension has been the rapid-sequence intravenous pyelogram (IVP). Features suggestive of renal ischemia include (1) unilateral delayed appearance and excretion of contrast material, (2) a difference in kidney size greater than 1.5 cm, (3) irregular contour of the renal silhouette, suggesting partial infarction or atrophy, (4) indentations on the ureter or renal pelvis, possibly due to dilated ureteral arteries (collateral notching), and (5) hyperconcentration of contrast medium in the collecting system of the smaller kidney. When these criteria are used, the false-positive rate is 11 percent and the false-negative rate 12 percent. The digital subtraction angiogram has been received with considerable enthusiasm as a more precise screening test for renal vascular disease. Its ultimate place as a screening test is unclear, however, because of its relatively high cost and as yet unproven greater sensitivity and specificity

relative to an IVP. The isotope renogram and saralasin infusion test, both enthusiastically endorsed in the past as screening procedures, are now used infrequently either because of lower sensitivity and specificity or limited availability.

The definitive test of surgically correctable renal disease is the combination of a renal angiogram and renal vein renin determinations. The renal arteriogram both establishes the presence of a renal arterial lesion and aids in determining whether the lesion is due to atherosclerosis or to one of the fibrous or fibromuscular dysplasias. It does not, however, prove that the lesion is responsible for the hypertension, nor does it permit prediction of the chances of surgical cure; it must be noted that (1) renal artery stenosis is a frequent finding by angiography and at postmortem in normotensive individuals, and (2) essential hypertension is a common condition and may occur in combination with renal arterial stenosis which actually may not be responsible for the hypertension. Bilateral renal vein catheterization for measurement of plasma renin activity is, therefore, used to assess the functional significance of any lesion noted on arteriography. When one kidney is ischemic and the other is normal, all the renin released comes from the involved kidney. In the most straightforward situation, the ischemic kidney has a significantly higher venous plasma renin activity than the normal kidney by a factor of 1.5 or more. Moreover, the renal venous blood draining the uninvolved kidney exhibits levels similar to those in the inferior vena cava below the entrance of the renal veins. Significant benefit from operative correction may be anticipated in at least 80 percent of patients with the findings described above if care is taken to prepare the patient properly prior to renal vein blood sampling, i.e., discontinuing renin-suppressing drugs, such as beta blockers, for at least 10 days, placing the patient on a low sodium intake for 4 days, and/or giving a converting enzyme inhibitor for 24 h. When obstructing lesions in the *branches* of the renal arteries are demonstrated by arteriography, an attempt to obtain blood samples from the main *branches* of the renal vein should be made in an effort to identify a localized intrarenal arterial lesion responsible for the hypertension.

Primary aldosteronism (see also Chap. 325). These patients almost always exhibit hypokalemia. Diuretic therapy often complicates the picture when the hypokalemia is first observed and needs to be assessed. Given hypokalemia, the relation between plasma renin activity and the aldosterone level becomes the key to the diagnosis of primary aldosteronism. The aldosterone concentration or excretion is high and plasma renin activity is low in primary aldosteronism, and these levels are relatively unaffected by changes in sodium balance. A critical part of the evaluation after primary aldosteronism has been established is to determine whether unilateral or bilateral disease is present since surgical removal of the lesion usually reduces arterial pressure only in those with unilateral disease.

Plasma renin activity measurements. Some studies have suggested that most hypertensive patients should have a plasma renin level measured and related to a 24-h urine sodium excretion rate to assess whether high, low, or normal levels are present. It has been proposed that this information may be important for both therapeutic and prognostic reasons. However, it is unclear, on the basis of presently available data and treatment programs, that these random measurements are really useful except in patients with findings suggestive of renal vascular disease or mineralocorticoid excess in whom lateralizing renal vein renin levels or suppressed peripheral renin levels may be of diagnostic and/or therapeutic significance.

TREATMENT

Virtually every patient with a diastolic arterial pressure which persistently exceeds 90 mmHg is a candidate for diagnostic studies and for subsequent treatment. Furthermore, at any given level of blood pressure elevation, the ultimate risk of developing hypertensive vascular complications is greater in men than in women, and in younger than in older persons. It may be argued, then, that it is hard

TABLE 196-5 Laboratory tests and special studies for evaluation of hypertension

I Basic studies
  A Always included
    1 Urine for protein, blood, and glucose
    2 Hematocrit
    3 Serum potassium
    4 Serum creatinine and/or blood urea nitrogen
    5 Electrocardiogram
  B Usually included, depending on cost and other factors
    1 Microscopic urinalysis
    2 White blood cell count
    3 Plasma/blood glucose, cholesterol, and triglycerides
    4 Serum calcium, phosphate, and uric acid
    5 Chest x-ray
II Special studies to screen for secondary hypertension
  A Renovascular: rapid sequence IVP or digital subtraction angiogram
  B Pheochromocytoma: 24-h urine for creatinine, metanephrines, and catecholamines or plasma catecholamines
  C Cushing's syndrome: overnight dexamethasone suppression test or 24-h urine cortisol

to justify producing the uncomfortable side effects of therapy in, for example, an asymptomatic woman over 70 years of age with a diastolic pressure of 90 mmHg. On the other hand, it is easy to justify side effects in a man of 30 with a diastolic pressure exceeding 110 mmHg, because such a person may be expected to receive the greatest benefit from therapy. Fortunately, the choice of treatment is such that a satisfactory program to control arterial pressure with minimal side effects can be developed for most patients. A reasonable guideline would be that all patients with diastolic pressure repeatedly above 90 mmHg should be treated unless specific contraindications exist. There is controversy regarding the advisability of treating isolated *systolic* hypertension. Until the results of a well-controlled prospective study provide evidence to the contrary, treatment of isolated systolic hypertension is not recommended. Patients with labile hypertension or isolated systolic hypertension who are not treated should have regular follow-up examinations at 6-month intervals, because of the frequent development of progressive and/or sustained hypertension.

The identification of an operable form of secondary hypertension does not automatically mean that surgical treatment is indicated. The decision depends upon the age and general health of the patient, the natural history of the lesion, and the response of the pressure to drug therapy. In patients with renovascular hypertension the feasibility of renal angioplasty, surgical repair versus nephrectomy, and the degree of overall renal function impairment must be considered. Age and general health are important in patients with renovascular hypertension due to arteriosclerosis, because there is no evidence that repair of the stenosis increases life expectancy in the elderly patient with other evidence of vascular disease. Knowledge of the natural history of the disease is especially important when approaching the decision in the young patient with renal-artery stenosis due to fibrous dysplasia. If the arteriographic appearance suggests that the stenosis is due to intimal or subadventitial fibroplasia, the lesion may be expected to progress and operation or angioplasty is required. Medial fibroplasia, on the other hand, often remains stable, and operation or angioplasty may not be necessary if pressure can be controlled by drug therapy. The decision regarding operation should also be considered carefully in patients with primary aldosteronism when bilateral adrenal venography does not demonstrate a tumor, because such patients may prove to have multinodular hyperplasia. This means that bilateral adrenalectomy would be required to eliminate the aldosterone excess, and, even then, hypertension usually persists. If hypokalemia can be controlled by spironolactone or other drug therapy, and arterial pressure lowered with antihypertensive agents, then it is reasonable to withhold operative treatment.

GENERAL MEASURES Nondrug therapeutic intervention is probably indicated in all patients with sustained hypertension and probably most with labile hypertension. The general measures employed include (1) relief of stress, (2) diet, (3) regular exercise, and (4) control of other risk factors contributing to the development of arteriosclerosis. Relief of emotional and environmental stress is one of the reasons for the improvement in hypertension that occurs when the patient is hospitalized. Though it is usually impossible to extricate the hypertensive patient from all internal and external stresses, he or she should be advised to avoid any unnecessary tensions. In rare instances, it may be appropriate to recommend a change of job or of life-style. Recently it has been suggested that relaxation techniques may also lower arterial pressure. However, it is uncertain that these techniques alone have much long-term effect.

Dietary management has three aspects:

1 Because of the documented efficacy of sodium restriction and volume contraction in lowering blood pressure, patients previously were instructed to curtail sodium intake drastically. Some investigators have suggested this is no longer necessary. They base their conclusion on two observations: (1) In many patients the blood pressure is not sensitive to the level of sodium intake, and (2) diuretics provide another method of decreasing body sodium stores

in those individuals whose blood pressure may be sodium-sensitive. However, a number of reports have documented that while mild sodium restriction has little, if any, direct action on blood pressure, it significantly potentiates the efficacy of nearly all antihypertensive agents and thereby by allowing blood pressure control with lower doses of drugs, side effects are reduced. In addition, it is quite clear that in some hypertensive patients, as noted above, the level of sodium intake does influence the blood pressure. Thus, since there is no apparent risk to mild sodium restriction, the most practical approach now is to advise mild dietary sodium restriction (up to 5 g NaCl per day), which can be achieved by eliminating all additions of salt to food which is prepared normally. Some studies have also reported lowering of arterial pressure by *increasing* calcium intake. While the advisability of this form of dietary alteration is still controversial, since a high calcium intake probably also reduces the extent of age-related osteoporosis, it is probably a useful adjunct.

2 Caloric restriction should be urged for the patient who is overweight. Some obese patients will show a significant reduction in pressure simply as a consequence of weight loss.

3 A restriction in intake of cholesterol and saturated fats is recommended on the suggestive evidence that such a diet may diminish the incidence of arteriosclerotic complications. Regular exercise is indicated within the limits of the patient's cardiovascular status. Not only is exercise helpful in controlling weight, but in addition there is evidence that physical conditioning itself may lower arterial pressure. Isotonic exercises (jogging, swimming) are better than isometric exercises (weight lifting) since, if anything, the latter raises arterial pressure. The dietary management outlined above is aimed at the control of other risk factors. Probably the most significant additional step that could be taken in this area would be to convince the smoker to give up cigarettes.

DRUG THERAPY (Table 196-6) To make rational use of antihypertensive drugs, the sites and mechanisms of their action must be understood. In general, there are four classes of drugs: diuretics, antiadrenergic agents, vasodilators, and angiotensin-converting enzyme (ACE) inhibitors.

Diuretics (see also Chap. 182) The thiazides are the most frequently used and most extensively investigated members of this group, and their early effect certainly is related to sodium diuresis and volume depletion. A reduction in peripheral vascular resistance also has been reported by some workers to be important in the long term. Traditionally, thiazide diuretics have formed the cornerstone of most therapeutic programs designed to lower arterial pressure and are usually effective within 3 to 4 days. However, in recent years increasing resistance to their routine use has occurred primarily because of their adverse metabolic effects, which include hypokalemia due to renal potassium loss, hyperuricemia due to uric acid retention, carbohydrate intolerance, and hyperlipidemia. The more potent diuretics, furosemide and ethacrynic acid, also have been shown to be antihypertensive but have been less extensively used for this purpose primarily because of their shorter duration of action. Spironolactone causes renal sodium loss by blocking the effect of endogenous mineralocorticoids, and therefore it may be more effective in patients whose mineralocorticoids are present in excess, e.g., primary or secondary aldosteronism. Although they do not compete directly with aldosterone, triamterene and amiloride act at the same site as spironolactone to impede sodium reabsorption and are effective in the same situations as spironolactone, except triamterene has little intrinsic antihypertensive effect. Their major disadvantage is that they can produce hyperkalemia, particularly in patients with impaired renal function. Any of these three potassium-sparing diuretics can also be given along with thiazide diuretics to minimize renal potassium loss.

Antiadrenergic agents (see also Chap. 66) These drugs act at one or more sites either centrally on the vasomotor center, in peripheral neurons modifying catecholamine release, or by blocking adrenergic

Site of action	Drug	Dosage	Indications	Contraindications	Frequent or peculiar side effects
DIURETICS					
Renal tubule	Thiazides: e.g., hydrochlo-rothiazide	Depends on specific drug Oral: 25 mg daily or twice daily	Mild hypertension as adjunct in treatment of moderate to severe hypertension	Diabetes mellitus, hyperuricemia, primary aldosteronism	Potassium depletion, hyperglycemia, hyperuricemia, dermatitis, purpura
	Loop acting: e.g., furosemide	Oral: 40–80 mg 2 or 3 times a day	Mild hypertension as adjunct in severe or malignant hypertension	Hyperuricemia, primary aldosteronism	Potassium depletion, hyperuricemia, nausea, vomiting, diarrhea
	Potassium-sparing: Spironolactone	Oral: 25 mg 2 to 4 times daily	Hypertension due to hypermineralocorticoidism, adjunct to thiazide therapy	Renal failure	Hyperkalemia, diarrhea, gynecomastia, menstrual irregularities
	Triamterene	Oral 50–100 mg 1 or 2 times daily	Hypertension due to hypermineralocorticoidism, adjunct to thiazide therapy	Renal failure	Hyperkalemia, nausea, vomiting, leg cramps, nephrolithiasis, hyperkalemia, GI disturbances
	Amiloride	Oral 5–10 mg daily			
ANTIADRENERGIC AGENTS					
Central	Clonidine	Oral: 0.1–0.6 mg twice daily	Mild to moderate hypertension, renal disease with hypertension		Postural hypotension, drowsiness, dry mouth, rebound hypertension after abrupt withdrawal, insomnia, lupuslike syndrome
	Guanabenz	Oral: 4–16 mg twice daily			
	Methyldopa (also acts by blocking sympathetic nerves)	Oral: 250–1000 mg twice daily IV: 250–1000 mg every 4–6 h (tolerance may develop)	Mild to moderate hypertension (oral), malignant hypertension (IV)	Pheochromocytoma, active hepatic disease (IV), during MAO inhibitor administration	Postural hypotension, sedation, fatigue, diarrhea, impaired ejaculation, fever, gynecomastia, lactation, positive Coombs tests (occasionally associated with hemolysis), chronic hepatitis, acute ulcerative colitis
Autonomic ganglia	Trimethaphan	IV: 1–6 mg/min	Severe or malignant hypertension	Severe coronary artery disease, cerebrovascular insufficiency, diabetes mellitus (on hypoglycemic therapy), glaucoma, prostatism	Postural hypotension, visual symptoms, dry mouth, constipation, urinary retention, impotence
Nerve endings	Rauwolfia alkaloids: Reserpine	Oral: 0.05–0.25 mg daily	Mild to moderate hypertension in young patient	Pheochromocytoma, peptic ulcer, depression, during MAO inhibitor administration	Depression, nightmares, nasal congestion, dyspepsia, diarrhea, impotence
	Guanethidine Guanadrel	Oral: 10–300 mg daily Oral 5–75 mg twice daily	Moderate to severe hypertension	Pheochromocytoma, severe coronary artery disease, cerebrovascular insufficiency, during MAO inhibitor administration	Postural hypotension, bradycardia, dry mouth, diarrhea, impaired ejaculation, fluid retention, asthma
Alpha receptors	Phentolamine	IV: 1–5 mg	Suspected or proved pheochromocytoma	Severe coronary artery disease	Tachycardia weakness, dizziness, flushing
	Phenoxybenzamine	Oral: 10–50 mg once or twice daily (tolerance may develop)	Proven pheochromocytoma		Postural hypotension, tachycardia, miosis, nasal congestion, dry mouth
	Prazosin	Oral: 1–10 mg twice daily	Mild to moderate hypertension		Sudden syncope, headache, sedation dizziness, tachycardia anticholinergic effect
Beta receptors	Propranolol	Oral: 10–120 mg 2 to 4 times daily	Mild to moderate hypertension (especially with evidence for hyperdynamic circulation), adjunct to hydralazine therapy	Congestive heart failure, asthma, diabetes mellitus (on hypoglycemic therapy), during MAO inhibitor administration	Dizziness, depression, bronchospasm, nausea, vomiting, diarrhea, constipation, heart failure
	Metoprolol	Oral: 25–150 mg twice daily			
	Nadolol	Oral: 20–120 mg daily			
	Atenolol	Oral 25–100 mg daily			
	Timolol	Oral: 10–30 mg twice daily			
	Pindolol	Oral: 5–30 mg twice daily			Less resting bradycardia than other beta blockers
	Labetalol	Oral: 100–600 mg twice daily			

Site of action	Drug	Dosage	Indications	Contraindications	Frequent or peculiar side effects
VASODILATORS					
Vascular smooth muscle	Hydralazine	Oral: 10–75 mg 4 times daily IV or IM: 10–50 mg every 6 h (tolerance may develop)	As adjunct in treatment of moderate to severe hypertension (oral), malignant hypertension (IV or IM), renal disease with hypertension	Lupus erythematosus, severe coronary artery disease	Headache, tachycardia, angina pectoris, anorexia, nausea, vomiting, diarrhea, lupus-like syndrome
	Minoxidil	Oral 2.5–50 mg twice daily	Severe hypertension	Severe coronary artery disease	Tachycardia, aggravates angina, marked fluid retention, hair growth on face and body, coarsening of facial features, possible pericardial effusions
	Diazoxide	IV: 1–3 mg/kg up to 150 mg rapidly	Severe or malignant hypertension	Diabetes mellitus, hyperuricemia, congestive heart failure	Hyperglycemia, hyperuricemia, sodium retention
	Nitroprusside	IV:0.5–8 (µg/kg)/min	Malignant hypertension		Apprehension, weakness, diaphoresis, nausea, vomiting, muscle twitching
ANGIOTENSIN-CONVERTING ENZYME INHIBITORS					
	Captopril	Oral: 12.5–75 mg twice daily	Mild to moderate and treatment-resistant hypertension, renal artery stenosis	Renal failure (reduction of dose)	Leukopenia, pancytopenia, proteinuria, nephrotic syndrome, membranous glomerulopathy, urticarial rash, fever, loss of taste, acute renal failure in bilateral renal artery stenosis
	Enalapril	Oral: 5–40 mg daily			Same as captopril, but no evidence for leukopenia, nephrotic syndrome, or taste loss

receptor sites on target tissue. Drugs that appear to have predominant *central actions* are *clonidine, methyldopa,* and *guanabenz.* These drugs and their metabolites are predominantly alpha-receptor agonists. Stimulation of alpha$_2$ receptors in the vasomotor centers of the brain *reduces* sympathetic outflow, thereby reducing arterial pressure. Usually a fall in cardiac output and heart rate also occurs, more commonly with clonidine and guanabenz, but the baroreceptor reflex is intact. Thus, postural symptoms are absent. However, rebound hypertension may rarely occur when these drugs, particularly clonidine and guanabenz, are stopped. This is probably secondary to the increase in norepinephrine release which had been inhibited by these agents secondary to their agonist effect on presynaptic alpha receptors.

Another class of antiadrenergic agents is the *ganglionic blocking* drugs, which have little effect when the patient is supine but prevent reflex vasoconstriction in the upright position. Ganglionic blocking agents interfere with parasympathetic as well as sympathetic function, and this results in such side effects as impairment of visual accommodation, paralytic ileus, retention of urine, and failure of erection and ejaculation. Because of these problems, ganglionic blocking agents are now usually reserved for the rapid lowering of arterial pressure by parenteral administration of the short-acting agent *trimethaphan* in patients with severe hypertension.

Various drugs act at *postganglionic adrenergic nerve endings.* The *rauwolfia alkaloids* such as reserpine are the oldest members of the group; their long-term effect results from their ability to inhibit the storage of norepinephrine within the vesicles in adrenergic nerve endings, thus leading to depletion of catecholamine stores. The frequent side effects including depression, nasal congestion, diarrhea, impairment of sexual function, and increased gastric secretion have limited the use of these drugs. *Guanethidine* and its shorter-acting

analogue guanadrel block the release of norepinephrine from adrenergic nerve endings. They have a greater postural effect than the other drugs that act at the nerve endings, and orthostatic hypotension is a frequent side effect. However, centrally mediated side effects (sedation, depression) are infrequently observed since they are poorly soluble in lipids and, therefore, do not readily enter the central nervous system.

The last group of drugs affecting the adrenergic system are those which block the *peripheral adrenergic receptors,* alpha, beta, or both (see also Chap. 66). *Phentolamine* and *phenoxybenzamine* block the action of norepinephrine at *alpha*-adrenergic receptor sites. While the above two compounds block both presynaptic (alpha$_2$) and postsynaptic (alpha$_1$) alpha receptors, the former action accounts for the tolerance which develops, while *prazosin* is more effective because it selectively blocks only *postsynaptic alpha* receptors, i.e., alpha$_1$ receptors. Thus, presynaptic alpha activity remains, suppressing norepinephrine release. Accordingly, prazosin produces less tachycardia but more postural hypotension than direct-acting vasodilators, e.g., hydralazine.

A variety of effective *beta-adrenergic receptor blocking agents* are available which block sympathetic effects on the heart and should be most effective in reducing cardiac output and in lowering arterial pressure when there is increased cardiac sympathetic nerve activity. In addition, they block the adrenergic nerve-mediated release of renin from the renal juxtaglomerular cells, and this action may be an important component of their blood pressure–lowering action. Beta-adrenergic blockers are particularly useful when employed in conjunction with vascular smooth-muscle relaxants, which tend to evoke a reflex increase in myocardial contractility, and with diuretics, the administration of which often results in an elevation of circulating renin activity. In practice, beta blockers appear to be effective even when there is no evidence of increased sympathetic tone with about one-half or more of all hypertensive patients showing a fall in pressure. However, these agents can precipitate congestive heart failure and asthma in susceptible individuals and must be used with caution in diabetics receiving hypoglycemic therapy because they inhibit the usual sympathetic responses to hypoglycemia. Cardioselective beta-blocking agents (so-called beta$_1$ blockers) have been developed (metoprolol, atenolol) which may be superior to nonselective beta blockers such as propranolol and timolol in patients with bronchospasm. Nadolol, a nonselective beta blocker, unlike other drugs of this class is excreted unchanged in the urine and has a half-life of 14 to 20 h. Therefore, only one dose a day is required. Atenolol also usually only needs to be given once a day. Pindolol is a nonselective beta blocker with partial agonist activity and, therefore, produces less bradycardia. Labetalol exerts both alpha- and beta-adrenergic blocking actions. Thus, it lowers arterial pressure by the same complex actions as do beta blockers, but also directly by reducing systemic vascular resistance.

Vasodilators *Hydralazine* is the most versatile of the drugs that cause direct relaxation of vascular smooth muscle; it is effective both orally and parenterally, acting mainly on arterial resistance, rather than on venous capacitance vessels, as evidenced by lack of postural changes. Unfortunately, the effect of hydralazine on peripheral resistance is partly negated by reflex increases in sympathetic discharges that raise heart rate and cardiac output. These limit the usefulness of hydralazine, especially in patients with severe coronary artery disease. However, the efficacy of hydralazine can be increased if it is given in conjunction with beta blockers or drugs such as methyldopa or clonidine, all of which block reflex sympathetic stimulation of the heart. A serious side effect of doses of hydralazine exceeding 300 mg per day has been the production of a lupus erythematosus-like syndrome.

Minoxidil is even more potent but unfortunately produces significant hirsutism and, therefore, is mainly limited to patients with severe hypertension and renal insufficiency.

Diazoxide, a thiazide derivative, is restricted in its application to acute situations. It is not a diuretic; in fact, it causes sodium retention. However, like other thiazides, it reduces carbohydrate tolerance. It must be given rapidly intravenously to guarantee effect. It begins to act immediately to lower blood pressure, and its effects may last for several hours. *Nitroprusside* given intravenously also acts as a direct vasodilator, with onset and offset of actions that are almost immediate. These latter two drugs are useful only for the treatment of hypertensive emergencies (Table 196-7).

Angiotensin-converting enzyme inhibitors Drugs from several of the categories discussed above have been shown to possess an additional action resulting in inhibition of renin secretion. These include clonidine, reserpine, methyldopa, and beta blockers. A second group of drugs in this class are those which inhibit the enzyme converting angiotensin I into angiotensin II, e.g., captopril and enalapril. These agents are useful because they not only inhibit the generation of a potent vasoconstrictor (angiotensin II) but also may retard the degradation of a potent vasodilator (bradykinin), alter prostaglandin production, and can modify the activity of the adrenergic nervous system. They are especially useful in renal or renovascular hypertension, as well as in accelerated and malignant hypertension. They are also effective in milder, uncomplicated hypertension with minimal side effects, although caution still needs to be exercised until their long-term safety is determined.

APPROACH TO DRUG THERAPY (Fig. 196-1) The aim of drug therapy is to use the agents just described, alone or in combination, to return arterial pressure to normal levels with minimal side effects. Ideally, one would choose a therapeutic program which specifically corrects the underlying defect resulting in the elevated blood pressure, e.g., spironolactone for patients with primary aldosteronism. As our knowledge of the mechanisms underlying the hypertension in individual patients increases, more specific drug programs will become available. This presumably will result in normalization of blood pressure with fewer side effects. In the absence of that information an empiric approach is used. When used in combination, drugs are chosen for their different sites of action. However, except for those individuals with severe hypertension (average diastolic blood pressure greater than 130 mmHg) in whom intensive therapy with several agents simultaneously usually is required, most patients should initially be treated with a single agent. Since many effective antihypertensive agents are available, a number of useful therapeutic regimens have been developed, with the ideal program still unclear. Previously, the step-care program suggested by the Joint National Committee on Detection, Evaluation and Treatment of High Blood Pressure was the primary approach. This program assumed that nearly all hypertensives should be treated similarly, beginning with a thiazide diuretic and adding other agents in a fixed pattern until the blood pressure was normalized. Recently, deviations from this standard approach have been advocated because of concern regarding the potential long-term adverse effects of thiazide diuretics and increasing evidence that other classes of drugs, e.g., beta blockers and angiotensin-converting enzyme inhibitors, may also be effective monotherapeutic agents. We believe that the first choice is between a beta blocker and a thiazide diuretic. The reason for choosing one over the other is empiric, although in general older individuals and blacks may be particularly responsive to diuretics while younger individuals and whites respond well to beta blockers.

The schema outlined in Fig. 196-1 takes into account the presently available data on effectiveness, adverse reactions, and cost in deciding when to use a given agent. This approach is applicable to all patients in whom an indication for a specific form of therapy is lacking. Because of its lower cost, low-dose thiazide therapy, e.g., 25 mg of hydrochlorothiazide or its equivalent, daily often is the first choice rather than a beta blocker. If a beta blocker is chosen, it also should be started at a low dose, e.g., equivalent to 25 mg of atenolol daily. If with either agent, seated blood pressure is lowered to less than 140/90, no further therapy is indicated. If not controlled, the next step is to combine these two agents in a low-dose program, e.g., 25

TABLE 196-7 Therapeutic agents used to treat malignant hypertension

| Drug | Route | Time course of action | | | Oral preparation available |
		Onset	Peak	Duration	
IMMEDIATE ONSET					
Diazoxide	IV bolus	1–3 min	2–4 min	4–12 h	No
Nitroprusside	Continuous IV	<1 min	1–2 min	2–5 min	No
Trimethaphan	Continuous IV	<1 min	1–2 min	2–5 min	No
DELAYED ONSET					
Hydralazine	IV, IM	10–20 min	20–40 min	2–6 h	Yes
Methyldopa	IV	1–3 h	3–5 h	2–12 h	Yes
Reserpine	IM	2–3 h	3–4 h	6–24 h	Yes

Low-Dose Beta Blocker or Low-Dose Thiazide

Continue Therapy ← **Controlled**

— Uncontrolled

Combine Low-Dose Beta Blocker and Thiazide

Discontinue Initial Drug ← **Controlled**

— Uncontrolled

Full-Dose Beta Blocker and Low-Dose Thiazide

Continue Therapy ← **Controlled**

— Uncontrolled

1. Assess Compliance and Search for Secondary Causes

2. Add Converting Enzyme Inhibitor

Sequential Withdrawal ← **Controlled**
of Beta Blocker then Thiazide

— Uncontrolled

1. Add Another Antiadrenergic Agent (e.g., clonidine), Peripheral Vasodilator (e.g., hydralazine), or Calcium Channel Blocker (e.g., nifedipine), or Combinations Thereof

2. When Controlled, Sequential Withdrawal of Drugs Initially Used

FIGURE 196-1 *Schematic approach to the treatment of the patient with hypertension in whom a specific form of therapy is unavailable or unknown.*

or 50 mg of atenolol (or its equivalent) and 25 mg of hydrochlorothiazide (or its equivalent) daily. Alternatively, the beta blocker could be increased to full dose, e.g., 100 mg of atenolol daily. Since the blood pressure response is often delayed, at least 8 weeks should elapse before changing the therapeutic program.

If combining low doses of a thiazide with a beta blocker does not achieve blood pressure control, the beta blocker is increased to a full dose. Rarely, increasing the thiazide to the equivalent of 50 mg of hydrochlorothiazide daily also may bring about control of the hypertension. However, thiazide doses higher than this are seldom, if ever, warranted since they almost invariably produce significant side effects, including reduction of serum potassium levels, hyperuricemia, and abnormalities in glucose metabolism with little increase in efficacy. If the hypertension is still uncontrolled despite treatment with a thiazide and full-dose beta blockers, then a detailed search for secondary causes of hypertension as outlined above is indicated. If none is found, then a converting enzyme inhibitor should be added. If control of blood pressure is achieved, then the beta blocker and/or thiazide is withdrawn or reduced in order to determine the minimum therapeutic program that will maintain the blood pressure at 140/90 mmHg or less.

Fewer than 5 percent of patients will still be hypertensive at this point. In them, one first should consider the reasons for therapeutic failure as shown in Table 196-8. If none can be identified, then one of the other agents such as a vasodilator listed in Table 196-6 (e.g., hydralazine) or an antiadrenergic agent (e.g., prazosin or clonidine) should be added. If blood pressure is controlled, previous drugs are sequentially withdrawn in order to determine the minimal therapeutic program that maintains a normal blood pressure.

While the recommendations outlined above are satisfactory for a large majority of patients, it is important to use a flexible approach since individual patients may respond differently to individual drugs and drug combinations. For those patients requiring multiple drugs,

once the appropriate combination has been found, the use of a single formulation with the appropriate combination of drugs may simplify the regimen and thereby increase compliance. Every effort should be made to reduce the number of times each day the patients must interrupt his or her schedule for the medication. Pharmacologic treatment of essential hypertension is usually lifelong, and since most patients are asymptomatic, compliance with a complex regimen may be a serious problem.

Special considerations Four groups of patients with hypertension require special consideration because of associated conditions.

RENAL DISEASE Reduction of arterial pressure in hypertensive patients with impaired renal function is often accompanied initially by an increase in serum creatinine. This change does not represent further structural renal damage and should not deter continuation of therapy, since achievement of blood pressure control may eventually reduce the value toward normal. However, if serum creatinine increases in patients treated with a converting enzyme inhibitor, care needs to be exercised since these patients may have bilateral renal artery disease. Their renal function will continue to deteriorate as long as the converting enzyme inhibitor is given. Thus, converting enzyme inhibitors should be used cautiously in patients with impaired renal function and renal function should be assessed frequently (every 4 to 5 days) for the first 3 weeks. While converting enzyme inhibitors are contraindicated in patients with bilateral renal artery stenosis, these are the drugs of choice in patients with unilateral renal artery stenosis and a normally functioning contralateral kidney.

CORONARY ARTERY DISEASE In these patients who may also be taking cardiac glycosides, thiazides should be used judiciously and a reduction in serum potassium levels should be looked for and if found, should be corrected rapidly. Beta blockers should be withdrawn carefully, if at all, in these patients. Finally, calcium channel antagonists and converting enzyme inhibitors may be particularly useful in these patients since they minimize a number of potential adverse reactions accompanying other therapeutic agents, particularly nonspecific vasodilators.

DIABETES MELLITUS The diabetic patient with hypertension is particularly challenging since many of the agents used to lower blood pressure can affect glucose metabolism adversely. Converting enzyme inhibitors may be particularly useful in these individuals. They have no known adverse effects on glucose or lipid metabolism and may actually minimize the development of diabetic nephropathy by reducing renal vascular resistance and renal perfusion pressure—the primary factor underlying renal deterioration in these patients.

PREGNANCY The patient who is pregnant and hypertensive or who develops hypertension during pregnancy (pregnancy-induced hypertension, preeclampsia, eclampsia) is particularly difficult to treat. Because it is uncertain that autoregulation of uterine blood flow occurs, lowering blood pressure in the pregnant hypertensive may result in reduced placental and fetal perfusion. Thus, a conservative approach to lowering blood pressure is usually indicated. In the second and third trimesters, antihypertensives often are not indicated unless the diastolic pressure exceeds 95 mmHg. In general, severe

TABLE 196-8 Reasons for poor therapeutic response in patients with hypertension

1 Inadequate patient compliance
2 Volume expansion
  a Excessive sodium intake
  b Secondary to nondiuretic antihypertensive agent
3 Excessive weight gain
4 Inadequate doses
5 Drug antagonism
  a Cold remedies
  b Sympathomimetics
  c Oral contraceptives (estrogens)
  d Adrenal steroids
6 Secondary forms of hypertension

salt restriction and/or diuretics are not given because of the associated increase in fetal wastage. Beta blockers need to be used cautiously, if at all, for similar reasons. Methyldopa and hydralazine are the most frequent antihypertensives used since they have no known adverse effects on the fetus. Little is known about the safety of other antihypertensives in pregnancy except that nitroprusside and converting enzyme inhibitors may cause adverse effects on the fetus and should be avoided.

Probably fewer than one-third of hypertensive patients in the United States are being treated effectively. Only a small number of these failures is related to drug unresponsiveness. The majority is related to (1) failure to detect hypertension, (2) failure to institute effective treatment of the asymptomatic hypertensive subject, and (3) failure of the asymptomatic hypertensive subject to adhere to therapy. In order to improve this deficiency, patients must be educated to continue treatment once an effective regimen has been identified. Side effects and inconveniences of treatment must be minimized or counteracted in order to obtain the patient's continued cooperation.

MALIGNANT HYPERTENSION

In addition to marked blood pressure elevation in association with papilledema and retinal hemorrhages and exudates, the full-blown picture of malignant hypertension may include manifestations of hypertensive encephalopathy, such as severe headache, vomiting, visual disturbances (including transient blindness), transient paralyses, convulsions, stupor, and coma. These have been attributed to spasm of cerebral vessels and to cerebral edema. In some patients who have died, multiple small thrombi have been found in the cerebral vessels. Cardiac decompensation and rapidly declining renal function are other critical features of malignant hypertension. Oliguria may, in fact, be the presenting feature. The vascular lesion characteristic of malignant hypertension is fibrinoid necrosis of the walls of small arteries and arterioles, and this can be reversed by effective antihypertensive therapy.

The pathogenesis of malignant hypertension is unknown. However, at least two independent processes, dilatation of cerebral arteries and generalized arteriolar fibrinoid necrosis, contribute to the associated signs and symptoms. The cerebral arteries dilate because the normal autoregulation of cerebral blood flow decompensates secondary to the markedly elevated arterial pressure. As a result, cerebral blood flow is excessive, producing the encephalopathy associated with malignant hypertension. Many patients also show evidence of a microangiopathic hemolytic anemia; this secondary phenomenon could contribute to the deterioration of renal function. Most patients also have elevated levels of peripheral plasma renin activity and increased aldosterone production, and these may be involved in causing vascular damage.

About 1 percent of hypertensive patients develop the malignant phase, which occurs in the course of both essential and secondary hypertension. Rarely it is the first recognized manifestation of the blood pressure problem. The average age at diagnosis is 40, and men are more often affected than women. Prior to the availability of effective therapy, life expectancy after diagnosis of malignant hypertension was less than 2 years, with most deaths being due to renal failure, cerebral hemorrhage, or congestive heart failure. With the advent of effective antihypertensive therapy, at least half of the patients survive for more than 5 years.

Malignant hypertension is a medical emergency and requires immediate therapy. The initial aim of therapy should be to reduce diastolic pressure toward, but not below, 90 mmHg. The drugs available for treatment of malignant hypertension can be divided into two groups on the basis of time of onset of action (Table 196-7). Those in the first group act within a few minutes but are not satisfactory for long-term management. If the patient is having convulsions, if arterial pressure must be reduced rapidly, then one from the immediate-acting group should be used. *Diazoxide* is the

easiest to administer, for no individual titration of dosage is required. A dose of 300 mg is given rapidly intravenously, and the antihypertensive effect is noted in 1 to 3 min. The same dose can be repeated when the pressure begins to rise, usually after several hours. In an occasional patient, pressure may drop below normal levels after diazoxide administration. Because of this, some physicians use a modified program, giving 150 mg rather than 300 mg initially, followed by a second 150-mg dose in 5 min if the blood pressure response has been minimal. It should not be used in patients in whom aortic dissection is suspected. The other two agents in this group require continuous infusion and close monitoring. *Nitroprusside* is given by continuous intravenous infusion at a dose of 0.5 to 8.0 (μg/kg)/min. It has the advantage over the ganglionic blockers of not being associated with the development of tachyphylaxis and can be utilized for days with few side effects. The dosage must be controlled with an infusion pump. *Trimethaphan*, a ganglionic blocker, is given at a rate of 1 to 15 mg/min. The patient should be in the sitting position, and the pressure should be monitored closely, preferably in an intensive care unit.

Patients given any of these agents should also receive other medications effective for long-term control. Those in the second group in Table 196-7 require 30 min or more to obtain full effect but have the advantage of being satisfactory for subsequent oral administration and for long-term management of the patient's hypertension. If such a delay in attainment of full effect is acceptable, intravenous *methyldopa* is an effective drug with which to begin therapy if symptoms of encephalopathy are absent. A dose of 500 mg in 100 to 200 mL 5% dextrose in water is given intravenously over 30 min; if the effect is inadequate in 2 to 4 h, a second dose of 500 to 1000 mg is given. Additional intravenous doses may then be given every 6 h until the pressure is stabilized. Intravenous *hydralazine* is effective in many patients within 10 min; an effective protocol involves giving 10-mg doses intravenously every 10 to 15 min until the desired effect has been obtained or until a total of 50 mg has been administered. The total required for response may then be repeated intramuscularly or intravenously every 6 h. Hydralazine should be used with caution in patients with significant coronary artery disease and should be avoided in patients evidencing myocardial ischemia or aortic dissection.

Furosemide is an important adjunct to the therapy just discussed. Given either orally or intravenously, it serves to maintain sodium diuresis in the face of a falling arterial pressure and thus will speed recovery from encephalopathy and congestive heart failure as well as maintain sensitivity to the primary antihypertensive drug. Digitalis (Chap. 182) also is indicated if there is evidence of cardiac decompensation.

In patients with malignant hypertension in whom the existence of pheochromocytoma is suspected, urine should be collected for measurement of the products of catecholamine metabolism, and drugs which might release additional catecholamines, such as methyldopa, reserpine, and guanethidine, must be avoided. The parenteral drug of choice in these patients is phentolamine, administered with care to avoid a precipitous reduction in arterial pressure.

There is hope even for patients who fail to respond sufficiently to any of the forms of therapy and who show progressive deterioration in renal function. In some, a period of peritoneal dialysis or hemodialysis to deplete extracellular fluid has resulted in better blood pressure control and eventual improvement in renal function. In other patients with refractory hypertension and renal failure who do not respond to volume depletion or hypotensive therapy, including minoxidil, particularly those with marked elevation of plasma renin activity, bilateral nephrectomy has resulted in amelioration of hypertension; subsequently these patients have been maintained on chronic dialysis or have received renal homografts. However, bilateral nephrectomy should be avoided where possible since (1) the loss of renal erythropoietin will contribute to the associated anemia, (2) vitamin D metabolism may be adversely affected, and (3) all residual renal function will be lost.

REFERENCES

AMERY A et al: Mortality and morbidity results from the European working party on high blood pressure in the elderly trial. Lancet 1:1349, 1985

BERGLUND G et al: Prevalence of primary and secondary hypertension: Studies in a random population sample. Br Med J 2:554, 1976

BLAUSTEIN MP: Role of a natriuretic factor in essential hypertension: An hypothesis. Ann Intern Med 98:785, 1983

BOUDOULAS H et al: Left ventricular mass and systolic performance in chronic systemic hypertension. Am J Cardiol 57:232, 1986

CAMPESE VM et al: Role of sympathetic nerve inhibition and body sodium-volume state in antihypertensive action of clonidine in essential hypertension. Kidney Int 18:351, 1980

CHALMERS MJ: The nervous system and the pathogenesis of essential hypertension, in Handbook of Hypertension: Clinical Aspect of Essential Hypertension, JIS Robertson (ed). Amsterdam, Elsevier, 1983, p 64

FUJITA I et al: Factors influencing blood pressure in salt-sensitive patients with hypertension. Am J Med 69:334, 1980

GENEST J: Personal views of the mechanisms of essential hypertension, in Hypertension, 2d ed, J Genest et al (eds). New York, McGraw-Hill, 1983

HOLME I et al: Treatment of mild hypertension with diuretics. The importance of ECG abnormalities in the Oslo study and in MRFIT. JAMA 251:1298, 1984

KAPLAN NM: Systemic hypertension: Therapy, in Heart Disease, E Braunwald (ed). Philadelphia, Saunders, 1984, p 902

KOTCHEN TA et al: Effect of chloride on renin and blood pressure responses to sodium chloride. Ann Intern Med 98:817, 1983

LINAS SL et al: Minoxidil. Ann Intern Med 94:61, 1981

McCARRON DA: Calcium in the pathogenesis and therapy of human hypertension. Am J Med 78:27, 1985

RAM CVS et al: Moderate sodium restriction and various diuretics in the treatment of hypertension. Arch Intern Med 141:1015, 1981

STRANDGAARD S: Autoregulation of cerebral blood flow in hypertensive patients. Circulation 53:720, 1976

THE 1984 REPORT OF THE JOINT NATIONAL COMMITTEE ON DETECTION, EVALUATION, AND TREATMENT OF HIGH BLOOD PRESSURE. Arch Intern Med 144:1045, 1984

VETERANS ADMINISTRATION COOPERATIVE STUDY ON ANTI-HYPERTENSIVE AGENTS: Racial differences in response to low-dose captopril are abolished by the addition of hydrochlorothiazide. Br J Clin Pharmacol 14:97S, 1982

VIDT DG, GIFFORD RW JR: A compendium for the treatment of hypertensive emergencies. Cleve Clin Q 51:421, 1984

VLASSES PH et al: Double-blind comparison of captopril and enalapril in mild to moderate hypertension. J Am Coll Cardiol 7:651, 1986

WILLIAMS GH, HOLLENBERG NK: Abnormal adrenal and renal responsiveness to angiotensin II, in Essential Hypertension as an Endocrine Disease, CRW Edwards, RMC Carey (eds). London, Butterworths, 1985

197 DISEASES OF THE AORTA

JAMES E. DALEN

The walls of the aorta must withstand the shearing effect of each systolic thrust of blood. With its large diameter, the aorta is under greater tension than the rest of the arterial system because wall tension is a direct function of both diameter and pressure. For this reason, the effects of hypertension are particularly deleterious. In addition, the aorta is subject to infection, trauma, necrosis of the media, and, most notably, arteriosclerosis, which has replaced syphilis as the disease most frequently affecting the aorta. Arising from these stresses are four major diseases of the aorta: aneurysm, dissection, arteriosclerotic occlusive disease, and aortitis. The number of deaths due to disease of the aorta is uncertain because other cardiovascular diseases, such as ischemic heart disease, hypertensive disease, and cerebrovascular disease, often coexist and take priority in the coding of death certificates.

ANEURYSMS A "true" aortic aneurysm is an abnormal widening that involves all three layers of its wall. The basic defect is destruction of elastic fibers in the media, which permits the remaining fibrous tissue to stretch and leads to an increase in diameter, which in turn raises wall tension. As this process leads to further enlargement, rupture becomes increasingly possible. "False" aneurysms, which are usually caused by trauma, are those disruptions of the inner and medial segments of the wall which permit expansion of the aorta so that the wall of the aneurysm consists of only adventitia and/or perivascular clot.

The commonest aneurysms are *fusiform,* in which a segment of the aorta becomes diffusely dilated, its total circumference being affected. In contrast, *saccular* aneurysms involve a portion of the circumference and consist of an outpouching with a mouth.

The commonest underlying cause of aneurysm is arteriosclerosis, but cystic medial necrosis, trauma, and syphilis and other infections must also be noted as causes.

Aneurysms of the abdominal aorta Three-fourths of all aortic aneurysms occur in the abdominal aorta, just below the renal arteries. Nearly all aneurysms in the abdominal aorta are caused by arteriosclerosis. Multiple aortic aneurysms occur in more than 10 percent of these patients. A familial occurrence of abdominal aortic aneurysms in males has recently been reported. The majority of victims are men older than age 60; more than one-half have associated hypertension. The incidence is increased in cigarette smokers.

The *diagnosis* is often made by physical examination, which reveals a pulsating mass in the midepigastrium. The diagnosis may first be suspected by x-ray of the abdomen, which demonstrates curvilinear calcification in the wall of the aneurysm. The diagnosis is confirmed by *ultrasound*. Continuous ultrasonic B scanning can visualize the abdominal aorta in longitudinal and transverse sections. This permits delineation of the size of the abdominal aorta and the thickness of its walls. It also allows detection of intraluminal clot (Fig. 197–1). Its noninvasive nature permits serial estimation of the size of the aneurysm. Abdominal aortic aneurysms increase their

FIGURE 197-1 *Aortic aneurysm. A. Longitudinal midline scan. B. Transverse scan just caudal to umbilicus. 1. Aortic aneurysm, 2. mural thrombus, 3. urinary bladder. [Reprinted with permission from HH Holm et al (eds): Abdominal Ultrasound: Static and Dynamic Scanning, 2d ed. Baltimore, University Park Press, 1980.]*

diameter at a rate of approximately 0.5 cm per year. Computed tomography can also accurately delineate abdominal aneurysms and may identify those that are at risk of rupture. Most patients are asymptomatic when the diagnosis is first made. When symptoms do occur, they consist of abdominal or low back pain.

The *prognosis* depends upon the size of the aneurysm and, very importantly, the presence of other arteriosclerotic cardiovascular diseases. The diameter of the normal abdominal aorta is 2.5 cm. When the diameter of the aneurysm is greater than 6 cm, the probability of rupture in a 10-year period is 45 to 50 percent, whereas it is only 15 to 20 percent when the diameter is less than 6 cm.

Ischemic arteriosclerotic heart disease, which is present in more than one-half of patients with abdominal aneurysm, has a profound impact on the prognosis. In one series of patients who did not have surgery, 5-year survival without clinically evident associated coronary disease was 50 percent. With ischemic heart disease, 5-year survival was only 20 percent. Follow-up of patients without surgery for abdominal aneurysms has shown that about one-third die of rupture of the aneurysm and one-third die of associated cardiovascular disease.

In properly selected patients operation prolongs life by preventing rupture. Symptomatic or expanding aneurysms and aneurysms more than 6 cm in diameter should have prompt surgical correction. The therapeutic decision for patients with asymptomatic aneurysms of moderate size (4 to 6 cm) is more difficult. Operative mortality with elective surgery, that is, before rupture, is about 5 to 10 percent. It is influenced by the size of the aneurysm but far more by the presence of associated cardiovascular disease. If there is no significant associated cardiovascular disease, small (4 to 6 cm) asymptomatic aneurysms should usually have surgical correction. With significant associated disease, it may be appropriate to follow the patient with serial ultrasound examinations. Surgery should be performed if symptoms occur, or if there is a significant increase in the size of the aneurysm.

Some patients with ruptured aneurysms survive long enough to become candidates for emergency surgical repair. They usually present in shock with severe pain in the abdomen, the lower back, or both. A tender pulsatile mass may be palpated. The salvage rate with emergency surgery in these circumstances is about 50 percent.

Aneurysms of the descending aorta   The second most frequent site of aortic aneurysms is in the descending aorta just distal to the origin of the left subclavian artery. These aneurysms are usually fusiform and due to arteriosclerosis. Many patients with an aneurysm of the descending aorta also have an aneurysm of the abdominal aorta. Most patients are asymptomatic when the diagnosis is first suspected by chest x-ray and then confirmed by computed tomography or aortography. Resection of thoracic aneurysms is more difficult than resection of abdominal aneurysms. The risk of operation is in large part determined by associated cardiovascular or pulmonary disease. Operative therapy to prevent rupture is indicated if the aneurysm is symptomatic, larger than 10 cm in transverse diameter, or enlarging rapidly, unless associated cardiovascular disease presents a prohibitive risk.

Traumatic, false aneurysms of the descending aorta may occur in patients who survive rupture of the aorta. The most frequent cause is deceleration injuries suffered in automobile accidents. Rupture usually occurs at the site of the ligamentum arteriosum. These patients usually note chest and back pain similar to that associated with dissection. Blood pressure may be increased in the upper extremities but absent or decreased in the lower extremities. Chest x-ray usually shows mediastinal widening. The diagnosis is confirmed by computed tomography or angiography. These patients are likely to be young and without associated cardiovascular disease. Surgical repair is indicated.

Less frequently, aneurysms of the descending aorta are saccular owing to *syphilis* or other *infection* (mycotic aneurysms). Saccular aneurysms are particularly likely to rupture and should be treated surgically.

Aneurysms of the ascending aorta   In a prior era, nearly all aneurysms of the ascending aorta were due to *syphilis*. They were readily recognized by x-ray by the presence of calcification in the wall of the ascending aorta. Luetic aneurysms can become huge, causing signs and symptoms by compression of adjacent structures. At the present time, the commonest cause of aneurysms of the ascending aorta is *cystic medial necrosis*, which may occur in association with Marfan's syndrome or as a response to hypertension and/or aging of the aorta, or may be of unknown etiology.

Aneurysms of the ascending aorta, particularly when they are due to cystic medial necrosis, may cause aortic regurgitation and lead to left ventricular failure. In this circumstance, resection of the aneurysm and replacement of the ascending aorta and aortic valve and coronary artery reimplantation are indicated.

The most common symptom of large aneurysms of the ascending aorta is chest pain, usually described as a deep, diffuse, aching sensation. The decision to resect an asymptomatic aneurysm to prevent rupture depends upon its size, the presence and severity of aortic regurgitation, and the presence of associated cardiovascular disease. More than half of these patients have additional aortic aneurysms.

Aneurysms of the aortic arch   These aneurysms—the least frequent of all—are the most likely to cause symptoms because they compress adjacent structures, thus causing dysphagia, dry cough, hoarseness, dyspnea, or pain. Arch aneurysms may be fusiform due to arteriosclerosis, or saccular due to syphilis or other infection. Surgical correction of aneurysms of the aortic arch carries an operative risk as high as 40 to 50 percent.

Management of concurrent hypertension   Hypertension, which is present in more than half of patients with aortic aneurysms, needs optimal management. Persistent systolic hypertension abets further enlargement of aneurysms and may predispose to their rupture. In addition to standard antihypertension medications, beta blockers are appropriate to help control hypertension and, in addition, decrease stress to the aortic wall by blunting myocardial contractility.

DISSECTION OF THE AORTA   This occurs when the intima is interrupted so that blood enters the wall of the aorta and separates its layers. Dissection is the most frequent and the most important acute disease involving the aorta and without treatment is almost always fatal. With prompt diagnosis and appropriate therapy, the majority of patients survive.

As with aneurysm of the aorta, the basic defect that permits dissection is disease of the media. The commonest risk factor for dissection is hypertension. In patients with dissection of the ascending aorta severe arteriosclerosis is uncommon, but severe medial degeneration (cystic medial necrosis) is present in about one-fifth of cases. Cystic medial necrosis may be associated with Marfan's syndrome, which is present in about 10 percent of dissections. This inheritable connective tissue disorder (Chap. 319) is characterized by ocular and skeletal abnormalities in addition to the cardiovascular complications of dissection, aortic aneurysm, and mitral or aortic valve regurgitation. The majority of patients with Marfan's syndrome die of these cardiovascular complications, often before age 40. Coarctation of the aorta and bicuspid aortic valves also increase the risk of dissection of the ascending aorta.

Dissection of the descending aorta is often associated with severe arteriosclerosis as well as hypertension. Cystic medial necrosis is less common in the descending aorta.

Nearly all aortic dissections begin as a tear in the intima at one of two sites: the ascending aorta (2 to 5 cm above the aortic valve) or the descending aorta, just distal to the origin of the left subclavian artery. The aorta is relatively fixed in each of these two positions, but is mobile on each side. Thus, at these two points, the hemodynamic stress of each systolic pressure wave is maximal, and the intima overlying diseased media may tear there, permitting blood to enter and separate the layers of the aorta.

The signs and symptoms and, importantly, the therapeutic implications are quite different when dissection involves the ascending aorta as opposed to the descending aorta only.

Dissection of the ascending aorta   Dissection usually begins as an intimal tear in the proximal ascending aorta. The so-called DeBakey type I dissection extends antegrade around the arch into the descending and abdominal aorta, while type II is confined to the ascending aorta. Dissection of the ascending aorta is the most common and the most lethal. In other cases, the intimal tear may occur in the aortic arch or descending aorta, and the dissection may progress retrograde to involve the ascending aorta. The majority of these patients are men under age 60. About one-half have hypertension.

Dissection of the ascending aorta is heralded by the abrupt onset of very severe chest pain. Unlike the pain of myocardial infarction, the pain is maximal at the onset. The pain is most frequent in the anterior chest, but may radiate to, or even be limited to, the midscapular area of the back. The pain is nearly always initially attributed to acute myocardial infarction. There are several ways that the appropriate diagnosis may be made. Since dissection of the ascending aorta involves the great vessels in the majority of cases, a discrepancy between the carotid pulses, or a difference in the blood pressure in the two arms, should lead to a search for other evidence of aortic dissection. Dissection involving the carotids can cause a sudden neurologic deficit that may be intermittent. If the dissection compromises the right coronary artery, arrhythmias may occur, and occasionally there may be electrocardiographic signs of acute inferior myocardial infarction. In approximately one-half of patients, the dissection causes acute aortic regurgitation. The presence of a new murmur of aortic regurgitation in the setting of apparent myocardial infarction should suggest the possibility of dissection of the ascending aorta. In the most severe cases, dissection causes hemopericardium. The appearance of a pericardial friction rub may be rapidly followed by pericardial tamponade.

Chest x-rays provide the most important clue to the presence of dissection of the ascending aorta. The most consistent finding is widening of the superior mediastinum. The ascending aorta may be enlarged out of proportion to the descending aorta. Once dissection is suspected by physical examination or chest x-ray, preparations for aortography to confirm the diagnosis should be made at once. Dissection of the ascending aorta can also be recognized by computed tomography or echocardiography. Unless hypotension is present, medical treatment, aimed at lowering blood pressure and depressing myocardial contractility, should be begun. This is most appropriately effected by beginning an infusion of nitroprusside, 20 to 400 ng/min, or trimethaphan, 1 to 2 mg/min, with intraarterial pressure monitoring in place.

Cineangiography of the aorta performed by the retrograde arterial technique will usually demonstrate a false lumen, and possibly an intimal flap separating the true and false lumina in the ascending aorta. If the blood in the false lumen has clotted, the principal finding will be an abnormal narrowing of the true lumen.

Once the diagnosis of dissection involving the ascending aorta has been established by aortography, the majority of patients should have surgical correction, which consists of resection of the portion of the aorta containing the intimal tear and replacement with a prosthetic graft. Concomitant aortic valve replacement may be required if severe aortic regurgitation is present. Surgical correction can be performed at a risk of about 20 percent. Although medical treatment is vital to stabilize the patient prior to operation, it rarely is definitive in patients with dissection involving the ascending aorta because the majority develop life-threatening complications, such as hemopericardium, hypotension, compromise of the carotid or coronary arteries, or aortic regurgitation. Without treatment, death is usually due to rupture into the pericardium.

Dissection of the descending aorta   (DeBakey type III dissection)   Dissection limited to the descending aorta is most likely to occur in elderly hypertensive patients with arteriosclerosis of the aorta. Dissection ordinarily begins with an intimal tear just beyond the origin of the left subclavian artery, and the hematoma proceeds distally to the diaphragm or into the abdominal aorta. Dissection of the descending aorta usually does not proceed in retrograde fashion. Therefore, aortic regurgitation and hemopericardium do not occur. The carotid pulses and blood pressure in the arms are usually not altered. The primary symptom is the sudden onset of chest pain, often interscapular, often radiating to the anterior chest. The prime supporting evidence of dissection is to be found in the chest roentgenogram, which usually shows a widening of the superior mediastinum and may show the descending to be larger than the ascending aorta. If there is intimal calcification in the aortic knob, its distance from the outer border of the aortic shadow may be increased.

The diagnosis of dissection of the descending aorta should be confirmed by aortography. As with dissection involving the ascending aorta, hypotensive treatment should begin when the diagnosis is first suspected. Nitroprusside or trimethaphan, in a continuous intravenous drip at an infusion rate sufficient to keep systolic pressure at 100 to 120 mmHg are the ideal first drugs. A beta blocker or reserpine should also be begun.

Patients with dissection of the descending aorta usually do not have urgent indications for surgical correction. Medical treatment to lower systolic pressure, and to depress myocardial contractility so as to blunt the force of systole, may control the dissection. If medical treatment does not relieve the pain, or if there is evidence of progression of the dissection by x-ray or the appearance of a left pleural effusion (due to hemothorax), surgical resection should be performed. Surgical correction of dissection of the descending aorta poses a higher risk than dissection of the ascending aorta because the patients are older and are more likely to have associated cardiovascular disease. Elective surgical correction may be indicated after the dissection is controlled with medical therapy.

Prolonged, optimal control of hypertension is essential in patients with dissection of the ascending or descending aorta. In the absence of overt or latent congestive heart failure, it is advisable to include beta blockers in the regimen to help prevent recurrent dissection. An important complication of aortic dissection is formation of aneurysms. Rupture of these aneurysms is the commonest cause of late death. Follow-up of patients treated for dissection should include periodic computerized tomography of the chest to detect the formation or enlargement of a thoracic aortic aneurysm.

ARTERIOSCLEROTIC OCCLUSIVE DISEASE   The majority of adults in the United States have some degree of arteriosclerosis of the aorta. However, the disease remains silent unless it causes aneurysm, or unless it is sufficiently advanced to cause occlusive disease. The mildest form of arteriosclerosis of the aorta, longitudinal fatty streaks of the intima, may be seen in children (Chap. 195). Elevated intimal plaques begin to appear in adult life. Occlusive disease of the aorta may occur if these plaques are complicated by hemorrhage, ulceration, calcification, or overlying thrombus formation.

Arteriosclerotic occlusive disease is most frequent in the abdominal aorta, where it involves the terminal part of the aorta and extends for a variable distance into the iliac and femoral arteries. Diabetes and cigarette smoking increase the severity of arteriosclerotic occlusive disease. Arteriosclerosis of the aorta may be complicated by superimposed thrombosis. Depending upon the adequacy of collateral circulation, arteriosclerotic occlusive disease may cause ischemia of the lower extremities.

The classic symptom is claudication, which is present in the buttocks and thighs or in the calves. If the occlusive disease is severe, or the collateral circulation is poor, severe ischemia may lead to pain at rest or tissue necrosis and gangrene. Impotence may also occur. The femoral pulses are absent or diminished in the majority of cases. The diagnosis of arteriosclerotic occlusive disease is confirmed by measuring segmental systolic pressure in the lower extremities with

Doppler ultrasound before and after exercise. Arteriography is needed to delineate the extent of the disease if surgical correction is indicated.

Surgical treatment consists of aortic-femoral bypass grafting. The results of operation are usually excellent; symptoms are relieved or decreased in more than 90 percent of the patients in some series. Patency rates of 80 to 90 percent at 10 years have been reported. Endarterectomy may be indicated when the disease is limited to the terminal aorta and proximal iliac arteries. Transluminal angioplasty performed by the percutaneous technique may also be effective in patients with iliac disease. As with aneurysms, operative and late death is usually due to associated ischemic heart disease, which is present in up to one-half of the patients. The status of the coronary and cerebrovascular circulations should be assessed prior to operation.

Symptomatic arteriosclerotic occlusive disease is rare in the ascending or descending thoracic aorta but may occur in the arch, where it becomes symptomatic by compromising the origin of one or more of the arch vessels. The carotid pulses, and/or pulses of the upper extremities, may be obliterated; thus, arteriosclerotic occlusive disease is one of the causes of the aortic arch syndrome. Other causes of this syndrome (also called ''pulseless disease'') include Takayasu's arteritis, syphilis, trauma, and neoplasm. Symptoms may include ischemia of the upper extremities or, more commonly, cerebrovascular ischemia, dependent upon the location of the disease. Surgical correction is usually feasible, utilizing a bypass graft; however, its appropriateness depends upon the extent of the disease, and the status of the coronary and cerebral circulations.

AORTITIS   Several different diseases may cause aortitis, i.e., an inflammatory process involving the wall of the aorta. The pathophysiology of aortitis depends on the severity of the process and upon its location. Aortitis becomes most evident when it involves the origins of the vessels of the aortic arch. Under these circumstances, it can, as noted above, cause the aortic arch syndrome.

The best understood cause of aortitis is *syphilis*. Only 10 percent of patients with luetic aortitis develop complications that permit its detection during life: saccular thoracic aneurysms, aortic valvulitis causing aortic regurgitation, and stenosis of the coronary ostia. Uncomplicated luetic aortitis is recognized at postmortem as a chronic panarteritis that causes patchy destruction of smooth muscle and elastic tissue of the media, endarteritis obliterans of the vasa vasorum, and intimal atherosclerosis. The process is most marked in the ascending aorta because of the predilection of treponemas for its rich lymphatic supply. The only clinical correlates of uncomplicated luetic aortitis are dilatation of the ascending aorta with or without calcification and a tambour-like aortic second sound.

TAKAYASU'S DISEASE   Takayasu's disease is a nonspecific obstructive arteritis that has a particular predilection for young females. It is more common in the orient than in the west. Although it is suspected to be an autoimmune disease, its exact etiology is unknown. In the majority of cases, the disease begins in the second or third decade of life. In its initial stage, constitutional symptoms may occur. These may include fever, malaise, anorexia, weight loss, night sweats, and at times arthralgias. The erythrocyte sedimentation rate is elevated.

These constitutional symptoms are then replaced by signs and symptoms secondary to involvement of the large arteries, particularly the aortic arch and its main branches. The pathologic lesion is a panarteritis that seems to begin with inflammation of the adventitia, with subsequent disruption and fibrotic changes in the media, and marked proliferation of the intima. Involvement of the arch vessels may be heralded by local pain and the presence of bruits. The activity of the disease is variable over time. Increased activity is usually associated with an increase in the erythrocyte sedimentation rate. Progression of the aortitis causes stenosis at, or obliteration of, the origins of the arch vessels, thereby causing the aortic arch syndrome. Obstruction of the carotid arteries causes ischemic retinopathy, blurred vision, syncope, and dizziness secondary to cerebral ischemia. Involvement of the subclavian arteries causes paresthesias, intermittent claudication, and loss of pulses of the upper extremities. In addition to segmental obstructions, aneurysms and aortic regurgitation may occur. The pulmonary arteries may be involved in some cases. Hypertension occurs in the majority of cases owing to involvement of the renal arteries or to suprarenal obstruction of the aorta. The presence of hypertension, with absent pulses in the upper extremities, has caused this syndrome to be called *reversed coarctation*. The diagnosis is confirmed by angiographic study of the aorta.

Although some studies have shown that corticosteroid therapy may alleviate some of the constitutional symptoms of this disease, there is no evidence that treatment improves life expectancy. Reconstructive vascular surgery may relieve symptoms; however, the disease follows a relentless course so that death from congestive failure or stroke usually occurs within 5 years of diagnosis.

REFERENCES

CRAWFORD ES, COHEN ES: Aortic aneurysm: A multifocal disease. Arch Surg 117:1393, 1982

DALEN JE et al: Dissection of the aorta: Pathogenesis, diagnosis, and treatment. Prog Cardiovasc Dis 23:237, 1980

DEBAKEY ME et al: Aneurysms of the thoracic aorta. Mod Concepts Cardiovasc Dis 10:53, 1975

———— et al: Dissection and dissecting aneurysms of the aorta: Twenty-year follow-up of five hundred twenty-seven patients treated surgically. Surgery 92:1118, 1982

DINSMORE RE et al: Magnetic resonance imaging of thoracic aortic aneurysms: Comparison with other imaging methods. AJR 146:309, 1986

GROSSMAN E et al: Clinical use of captopril in Takayasu's disease. Arch Intern Med 144: 95, 1984

HALL S et al: Takayasu arteritis. A study of 32 North American patients. Medicine 64:89, 1985

LARSON EW, EDWARDS WD: Risk factors for aortic dissection: A necropsy study of 161 cases. Am J Cardiol 53:849, 1984

LUPI-HERRERA E et al: Takayasu's arteritis: Clinical study of 107 cases. Am Heart J 93:94, 1977

MALONE JM et al: The natural history of bilateral aortofemoral bypass grafts for ischemia of the lower extremities. Arch Surg 110:1300, 1975

MILLER DC et al: Operative treatment of aortic dissections: Experience with 125 patients over a sixteen-year period. J Thorac Cardiovasc Surg 78:365, 1979

NORRGARD O et al: Familial occurrence of abdominal aortic aneurysms. Surgery 95:650, 1984

SLATER EE, DESANCTIS RW: Disease of the aorta, in *Heart Disease*, 2d ed, E Braunwald (ed). Philadelphia, Saunders, 1984, p 1540

SMUCKLER AL et al: Echocardiographic diagnosis of aortic root dissection by M-mode and two-dimensional techniques. Am Heart J 103:897, 1982

WHITE RD et al: Noninvasive evaluation of suspected thoracic aortic disease by contrast-enhanced computed tomography. Am J Cardiol 57:282, 1986

---

198   VASCULAR DISEASES OF THE EXTREMITIES

D. EUGENE STRANDNESS, JR.

The correct approach to patients with suspected peripheral vascular disease is to identify the system involved (arterial, venous, or lymphatic), estimate the degree of disability, and determine if special tests are required to clarify further the extent of the involvement. The therapy employed depends upon a knowledge of the natural history of the disorder as related to known risk factors, the potential for further complications, and the likelihood that available therapy will be successful.

ARTERIAL DISORDERS

ACUTE ARTERIAL OCCLUSION   Sudden interruption of the blood supply results in a spectrum of symptoms and signs which are dependent upon the location and extent of the occlusion and existing collateral circulation. The major causes are embolism, thrombosis, and injury. In the arm, the heart is the source of emboli in 95 percent of the patients. Less common causes include emboli from ulcerated plaques in the subclavian artery, aneurysms of the arch vessels, and paradoxical emboli via a patent foramen ovale.

In the leg, the heart is again the most common source of emboli, but they may also arise from ulcerated plaques and aneurysms of the thoracic, abdominal, femoral, and popliteal arteries. Over half of the large emboli from the heart lodge in the femoral or popliteal arteries. The iliac arteries are involved in approximately one-fifth, the abdominal aorta in one-sixth. The remainder will occlude the tibial or peroneal vessels.

When the heart is the source, the causes include mural thrombi from the left atrium or ventricle and the aortic or mitral valve. Mural thrombi arise secondary to atrial fibrillation or on the endocardial surface of the ventricle secondary to myocardial infarction. A prosthetic valve in either the aortic or mitral position may also be the source. While uncommon, the possibility of an atrial myxoma must always be kept in mind. When emboli arise from ulcerated plaques or aneurysms, they are often small and lodge in the small arteries of the distal limb. When they arise from the abdominal or thoracic aorta, bilateral involvement is the rule.

Arterial thrombosis occurs secondary to injury, arteriosclerosis obliterans, femoral or popliteal aneurysms, collagen vascular diseases, myeloproliferative disorders, disseminated intravascular coagulation, and the dysproteinemias.

Symptoms and signs Acute arterial occlusion results in symptoms and signs related to the site of involvement and the immediately available collateral circulation. If the pressure distal to the obstruction falls to below 40 mmHg, the clinical picture will be dramatic. The initial complaint is pain in the most distal part of the limb, followed by pallor, coldness, and a sensation of numbness. Cutaneous sensation is lost within the first hour. Within 6 h, ischemic muscular contracture develops associated with subcutaneous hemorrhage and focal areas of gangrene. Fixed staining of the skin is the most certain sign of irreversible tissue death.

If limb viability is not in question, pallor, a decrease in temperature, and numbness may be the only complaints. The appearance of rest pain in the digits and forefoot indicates that arterial inflow is marginal. Pulses are absent distal to the site of occlusion.

Though the diagnosis is rarely difficult when the extent of the ischemia is as outlined above, there are important variations in the clinical picture. If the immediately available collateral circulation is sufficient to maintain viability, the patient may complain only of a sensation of numbness, usually accompanied by a decrease in the temperature of the part. Under these circumstances, the circulation will nearly always improve, with these minor symptoms disappearing over the course of several hours.

Diagnosis The most important elements include a history of the sudden onset of pain, coldness, and numbness. If a combination of pain, pallor, and paralysis is noted, limb viability will be lost unless the responsible lesion can be corrected within a time frame of 6 h or less. If the limb remains viable, the only complaints may be coldness and numbness. Detection of a bruit is common when an arterial plaque or aneurysm is the source of the embolus.

When the leg is affected, it is important to determine if there is a history of intermittent claudication since under these circumstances, the acute ischemia may be due to thrombosis on an ulcerated plaque. When cholesterol emboli occur, the symptoms may be confusing depending upon the source. The most common situation is the "blue-toe" syndrome, which may be bilateral if the origin is the abdominal or thoracic aorta. Ischemic rest pain is often present and accompanied by prominent livedo reticularis of the feet. Peripheral pulses are nearly always present, since emboli rarely pass through collateral arteries in sufficient quantity to produce serious foot ischemia. When these tiny emboli originate from the thoracic aorta, abdominal pain and hematuria may also occur. Aneurysms of the femoral and popliteal arteries must always be kept in mind. The initial manifestation is often thrombosis or embolization. The diagnosis may be suspected by physical examination and verified by B-mode ultrasound.

Arteriography is rarely necessary to make the diagnosis of major artery occlusion and results in needless, dangerous delay when severe ischemia is present.

Treatment When limb viability is threatened, immediate operation is required for occlusion of the major arteries. Heparin should be given immediately. The occlusion may usually be removed under local anesthesia, but in some instances it may be necessary to bypass the obstructed area. If limb viability is not in doubt, streptokinase to urokinase should be considered, since lysis may be achieved by infusion of low doses directly into the thrombosis via an arterial catheter. When the acute occlusion is secondary to thrombosis in proximity to a stenosis, the underlying defect may be corrected by either transluminal angioplasty or bypass grafting after lysis of the thrombus. If the cause of the problem is embolic, long-term anticoagulation with coumadin should be employed. Chronic subcutaneous heparin, while also effective, should be used with caution since it may lead to the development of osteoporosis. Patients with microemboli should be treated expectantly with aspirin. On occasion it may be necessary to remove or bypass an ulcerated plaque responsible for the emboli, but usually surgery is reserved for those patients with aneurysms (particularly femoral and popliteal) that might be the source of emboli. Vasodilator drugs are not useful.

ARTERIOSCLEROSIS OBLITERANS The primary lesion of arteriosclerosis is the intimal plaque, which progressively narrows and, in many instances, leads to complete occlusion of large and medium-sized arteries (Chap. 195). In the abdomen the disease has its highest incidence in the aorta and common iliac arteries. The external iliac arteries are often spared. Distal to the inguinal ligament, occlusions are most common in the adductor canal, with the popliteal artery itself down to the level of its three major branches having a much lower incidence of involvement. In the lower leg, the posterior tibial artery at the ankle and the anterior tibial at its origin are most commonly diseased. Arteriosclerosis obliterans is usually a segmental disease, with marked variation from patient to patient in its extent.

Clinical features Unless complicated by thrombosis, the symptoms and signs that develop secondary to arteriosclerosis obliterans rarely have an abrupt onset, since the process is a gradual, progressive one. The most common symptom occurs with exercise and is termed *intermittent claudication,* i.e., the pain that occurs in a muscle(s) with an inadequate blood supply that is stressed by exercise. The patient often describes the discomfort as a cramp which disappears within 1 or 2 min after stopping the exercise. Occasionally, profound weakness will be noted as exercise progresses. The walk-pain-rest cycle is constant from day to day, which is the hallmark of this particularly troublesome complaint. The pain never occurs with standing or sitting. The pain is more severe and the walking distance is always shortened when the patient walks upstairs and up a hill.

A point not often appreciated is that, with arteriosclerosis obliterans, claudication does not occur with occlusions in the anterior tibial, posterior tibial, or peroneal arteries. The location of the involved muscle group(s) is useful in predicting the most proximal level of occlusion. For example, calf and thigh claudication suggests that the primary involvement is proximal to the origin of the thigh muscles, i.e., the profunda femoris artery. The combination of hip, thigh, and buttock claudication with impotence in a middle-aged male indicates terminal aortic occlusion, the *Leriche syndrome.*

The second important group of symptoms consists of those which occur at rest and are the result of either multiple levels of occlusion or involvement of a critical arterial segment where the major collaterals are also obstructed. Paresthesias and indeed numbness may occur but are less common than continuous pain in the toes or foot, which may be partially or completely relieved by dependency. Ulceration and gangrene of the toes and distal foot are a common occurrence when the disease reaches this advanced stage.

The patient with diabetes mellitus often presents variations in the clinical picture. Approximately 30 percent of patients with diabetes have a peripheral neuropathy which results in loss of deep pain sensation and sympathetic tone. When diabetics with a neuropathy develop ulcers with or without arterial occlusion, the lesions are typically painless. The combination of chronic arterial occlusion, peripheral neuropathy, and a nonhealing ulcer is a difficult therapeutic problem.

The physical examination is useful in substantiating the diagnosis and localizing the levels of disease. Patients with single occlusions in the aortoiliac or superficial femoral artery often have limbs which are normal in appearance. Patients with far-advanced disease secondary to multiple levels of disease often have ulcers, gangrene, loss of hair, trophic nail changes, and dependent rubor. Chronic arterial narrowing and occlusion lead to loss of pulses distal to the most proximal level of disease. The pulses should be examined in the groin, in the popliteal fossa, and at the level of the ankle. If the involvement results in narrowing only, bruits are commonly heard which are transmitted for varying distances downstream from the stenosis. Auscultation should be performed from the level of the midabdomen to the popliteal artery; one should listen for the characteristic sound which is diagnostic of arterial narrowing.

Special diagnostic tests The magnitude of the physiologic derangement can be assessed simply by measuring the ankle systolic blood pressure at rest and following exercise to the point of claudication. Since arterial occlusion forces the blood to follow alternate pathways (collaterals) whose resistance to flow exceeds that of the normal vessel, an abnormal pressure gradient develops which lowers the pressure recorded at the ankle. The pressure may be measured by a variety of plethysmographs or the ultrasonic velocity detector. In general, if the systolic pressure at the ankle is greater than one-half that recorded from the arm, occlusion of one segment is most likely. Ankle pressures less than one-half of the arm systolic pressure are most often observed with multiple levels of disease.

When the patient with intermittent claudication exercises to the point of pain, the postexercise ankle blood pressure falls, often to unrecordable levels, requiring several minutes to return to the prewalking level. With exercise there is a marked fall in arterial resistance in the muscle. The amount of inflow available through the collateral arteries is inadequate because of their high resistance to flow. As a consequence, distal arterial pressure falls and blood is shunted away from the foot. These changes explain the pallor in the foot which is so commonly observed during and immediately following exercise to the point of claudication. This test is most useful in following the progress of disease with and without therapy and is the most sensitive index of change available. Its great utility lies in the fact that each patient can serve as his or her own control.

Arteriography is essential prior to operation to localize precisely the disease and the extent of the involvement. With the introduction of ultrasonic duplex scanning, it is now feasible to scan the arterial system from the level of the celiac artery to the popliteal artery. Segments which are narrowed or occluded are readily identified. This method is useful in selecting patients for transluminal angioplasty and surgery and documenting the results of therapy.

Differential diagnosis It is rarely difficult to make the diagnosis of chronic arterial narrowing or occlusion when the clinical impression is combined with measurements of ankle blood pressure. However, there is a recognized subset of conditions, lumped under the title of "pseudoclaudication," that are not uncommon and may be a source of some confusion.

The features of the symptom complex which are useful in distinguishing it from true intermittent claudication include the following: (1) the exercise-pain-rest cycle is not constant; (2) the symptoms may include numbness, tingling, weakness, incoordination, and clumsiness; (3) patients with pseudoclaudication may have to sit down or even lie down for relief; and (4) the time required for the pain to disappear often exceeds the few minutes observed in claudication due to arterial occlusion. When it becomes clear that chronic arterial disease is not the basis for the leg pain, it is necessary to investigate the back and hip areas since diseases such as spinal stenosis, herniated nucleus pulposus, spinal cord tumors, and degenerative joint disease may be responsible for the patient's complaints.

Therapy Patients with mild or moderate intermittent claudication may benefit from a rigorous, daily exercise training program. The essential features of this program include (1) repetitive daily walks to 75 percent of the claudication distance with interspersed periods of rest (1 to 2 min); (2) weekly retesting of maximum walking time with readjustment of walking distance; and (3) continuation of the exercise program—this is essential, since evidence suggests that cessation of the daily walking periods will result in loss of improvement. A new drug, pentoxifylline, has become available which may improve muscle perfusion by decreasing blood viscosity. A multicenter trial in this country showed use of this drug resulted in a modest (59 percent) increase in the initial claudication distance over placebo in a group of patients with claudication. Vasodilator drugs are of no value.

Weight reduction can be useful in patients with intermittent claudication by simply reducing the workload involved. It is also important that *smoking be stopped* entirely. All patients with arteriosclerosis should have their serum lipid levels determined, since they may be found to have a treatable disorder (Chap. 195). Direct arterial surgery may be effective in bypassing or removing areas of occlusion but should be reserved for those patients with disabling claudication.

Transluminal angioplasty provides an excellent method of dealing with stenoses involving the aortoiliac segments, giving results comparable to those obtained by direct arterial surgery. The long-term patency below the groin is not as good as with the iliac arteries, but the procedure can be used when a short-term flow increase may be of benefit in providing the necessary increased blood flow to heal open, painful ulcers.

Most patients with ischemic rest pain, ulcers, or gangrene present serious problems which can be helped only by direct arterial surgery. Lumbar sympathectomy may be useful but should be used *only* in patients with mild rest pain. If the rest pain is controlled by nonnarcotic analgesics and transient dependency, about 50 percent of these patients can obtain permanent pain relief by lumbar sympathectomy.

The majority of patients with arteriosclerosis obliterans will never require surgical therapy even though they do suffer some disability. The nondiabetic will have a limb loss rate of about 2 percent per year; this rate increases to 7 percent per year if the patient has diabetes mellitus. Meticulous foot care, which includes properly fitting shoes, and immediate attention to cuts and blisters are critical in proper management. This is particularly true in patients with diabetes and a peripheral neuropathy who are unable to appreciate deep pain.

Selected patients with isolated stenoses of the iliac arteries or superficial femoral artery may be candidates for transluminal dilatation with a balloon catheter. The early results are promising, but performance of the procedure must be a joint decision between the radiologist and vascular surgeon.

THROMBOANGIITIS OBLITERANS (BUERGER'S DISEASE) In 1908 Buerger described a nonatheromatous lesion involving arteries, veins, and nerves occurring in young males and frequently leading to nonhealing ulcers and gangrene. The exact pathogenesis is obscure, but there appears to be a definite relationship with tobacco smoking or chewing. Recent studies have shown that patients with Buerger's disease may have abnormal cellular and humoral immune responses to type I and type III collagen. This provides further support for its existence as a distinct vascular disease and its diagnosis by means of immunologic testing.

The disease typically occurs in young males and has a characteristic location and set of clinical manifestations. Whereas arteriosclerosis obliterans is a segmental disease of large and medium-sized arteries, Buerger's disease starts in the smaller arteries of the hands and feet. There is usually an intense inflammatory component, which in later stages results in arterial and venous occlusion as well as fibrous encasement of the entire neurovascular bundle.

Clinical features   The diagnosis of Buerger's disease should be suspected when male patients in the 20- to 40-year age range give the following history: A superficial, migratory nodular phlebitis may occur early in the disease. These nodules are well localized, associated with cutaneous erythema, and tender to touch. Cold sensitivity of the Raynaud's type occurs in about one-half the patients and is frequently confined to the hands. The fingers turn white when exposed to cold, then blue, and finally red—the so-called triphasic color response.

One of the most characteristic and typical symptoms of Buerger's disease is *instep claudication*. Exercise results in pain in the instep, promptly relieved by rest. Calf claudication may occur but is unusual, since the disease does not commonly progress proximally to involve and occlude either the popliteal or superficial femoral artery. When there is hand involvement, the occlusions may be bilateral, are often symmetric, and may lead to the development of hand claudication and fingertip ulcers which are exquisitely painful and difficult to heal.

The following findings during *physical examination* should lead one to suspect Buerger's disease: (1) intense rubor of the feet; (2) absent foot pulses in the presence of a normal femoral and popliteal pulse; and (3) reduction or absence of the radial and/or ulnar pulses.

Therapy   There is only one effective treatment, and that is permanent, complete abstinence from tobacco. However, for some unknown reason, patients with Buerger's disease rarely discontinue smoking even though amputation is usually the inevitable consequence and the only method available of controlling the severe rest pain and ulceration which ultimately develop.

ARTERIOVENOUS FISTULAS   Acquired   Most acquired arteriovenous fistulas occur secondary to penetrating injuries; however, they may in certain circumstances occur secondary to blunt trauma. Malignancy, infection, and arterial aneurysms have also been responsible for the development of arteriovenous communications.

CLINICAL PICTURE   Patients with penetrating injuries of an extremity should all be suspected of having an arteriovenous fistula. Initially there are no distinguishing symptoms which alert the physician to the presence of the fistula. The diagnosis is made by noting a continuous murmur and palpable thrill over the abnormal communication. Compression of the feeding artery will obliterate the murmur and thrill. With large fistulas compression of the feeding artery results in an abrupt slowing of the heart rate (Branham's sign). In rare instances distal arterial perfusion may be so severely impaired that gangrene develops.

With chronic fistulas the clinical manifestations may mimic those of venous disease, with varicose veins, stasis pigmentation, and cutaneous ulcers. Cardiac enlargement with or without failure may be seen in long-standing fistulas. Infection (bacterial endarteritis) may complicate large fistulas.

THERAPY   The proper treatment of arteriovenous fistulas is division of the communication with maintenance of arterial continuity. Immediate operation may be indicated with large fistulas between such vessels as the abdominal aorta and inferior vena cava where cardiac failure may develop very quickly.

Congenital   The development of anomalous communications between arteries and veins can pose both diagnostic and therapeutic difficulties. When there is an arrest in the development of the circulation during the stage of an undifferentiated capillary network, a *cavernous hemangioma* results. There is at this period an interlacing system of blood spaces which contain mixed blood, and it is impossible to distinguish the arterial and venous components.

When the development is arrested at the stage of differentiation, intercommunicating arteriovenous channels may persist. If the fistulas are large enough to be visualized arteriographically, the term used is congenital *macrofistulous arteriovenous aneurysm*. When the fistulas

are too small to be visualized by arteriography, the term *microfistulous communication* should be used. This classification, based upon the size of the communications, is useful from a therapeutic standpoint.

CLINICAL MANIFESTATIONS   The clinical manifestations are extremely variable and largely depend upon the location and extent of the abnormal communications. The most common symptoms are (1) cosmetic changes due to the presence of the fistulas in the subcutaneous tissue and skin, (2) limb swelling and hypertrophy, (3) visible pulsations in some cases with macrofistulous communications, and (4) varicose veins in atypical locations. In long-standing cases stasis pigmentation and cutaneous ulcers may develop in response to the continued venous hypertension.

DIAGNOSIS   The presence of arteriovenous fistulas should be suspected when the following findings are presented: (1) unilateral leg or arm swelling, (2) cutaneous hemangioma of the ''port-wine'' variety, (3) varicose veins in atypical locations, and (4) an increase in temperature of the part. An important syndrome which may be confused with congenital arteriovenous fistulas is the *Klippel-Trénaunay* syndrome. The triad of this syndrome consists of varicose veins, ''port-wine'' hemangioma of the skin, and bone and soft-tissue hypertrophy. The arteriovenous communications are rarely demonstrable by arteriography.

THERAPY   The management of congenital arteriovenous fistulas depends entirely upon location, extent, and clinical manifestations. Treatment is largely conservative, with support stockings used to control the venous hypertension and valvular incompetence which often produce symptoms identical with those of the postthrombotic syndrome. If the fistulas are limited in extent, it may be possible to excise the lesions in their entirety, but this is usually not feasible.

THORACIC OUTLET SYNDROMES   The neurovascular bundle, by virtue of its course from the neck and thorax, is subject to compression by both muscular and skeletal structures. The symptoms which may develop include numbness and paresthesias (usually in the ulnar distribution) and pain which is brought on by a position of the arm that results in compression of the brachial plexus. From a diagnostic standpoint, obliteration of the radial pulse in a variety of arm positions has been considered the distinguishing feature of the underlying problem. This should no longer be considered the key diagnostic test since it frequently occurs in normal subjects. Further, the symptoms are generally due to compression of the brachial plexus and not the subclavian artery.

Those patients with the most prominent symptoms and signs will have cervical ribs with an associated fibrous band which attaches to the first rib producing compression of the neurovascular bundle. The key diagnostic features in these patients are (1) prompt appearance of paresthesias and numbness with the arm abducted to 90° and externally rotated, (2) appearance of a prominent bruit in the supraclavicular fossa, and (3) immediate disappearance of the symptoms when the arm is returned to the neutral position. There is little doubt that chronic arterial compression can lead to aneurysmal dilatation of the subclavian artery with occlusion and/or emboli, but this is rare.

In the absence of a *clear-cut* relationship between arm position and the symptoms, it is essential to rule out other causes for the clinical picture, which includes a cervical disc, degenerative joint disease, and the carpal tunnel syndrome. If cold sensitivity is also present, the vasospastic syndromes discussed in the next section must be ruled out. Removal of the first rib is performed too frequently and must be reserved for only those patients in whom the diagnosis is clear and other causes have been ruled out. The best results will be obtained in patients with cervical ribs in whom the relationship between arm position and neurovascular compression is easily demonstrated.

VASOSPASTIC DISORDERS   The diseases in this category include primary and secondary cold sensitivity of the Raynaud's type, livedo reticularis, and acrocyanosis. The challenge in dealing with these entities is not in making the correct diagnosis but rather in determining if there is an associated disease responsible for the symptoms and signs. Those that are primary, e.g., without underlying disease, are generally benign, rarely lead to digit ulcers, and never terminate fatally.

Cold sensitivity of the Raynaud's type To establish this diagnosis, it is necessary to determine if a "triphasic" color response occurs, i.e., pallor, cyanosis, and rubor in that sequence. The most important element is the pallor, during which the digits turn absolutely white.

Livedo reticularis Livedo reticularis presents with a persistent cyanotic mottling of the skin which has a typical "fishnet" appearance. In contrast to Raynaud's disease, a phenomenon which is confined to the digits, livedo reticularis may involve all parts of the extremities and trunk. This cutaneous pattern is often accentuated by exposure to cold.

Acrocyanosis The most uncommon of the vasospastic disorders is acrocyanosis, which is characterized by a persistent diffuse cyanosis of the fingers, hands, toes, and feet. This disease is benign and not associated with an underlying disorder. The involved parts are nearly always cold, with excessive perspiration being a common accompanying feature.

Diagnosis Primary cold sensitivity of the Raynaud's type is more common in women, often starting in the late teens, is bilateral and symmetric, and rarely leads to fingertip ulcers or gangrene. The hands are more commonly affected than the feet. Those factors which should lead the clinician to suspect an underlying disorder include (1) abrupt onset with rapid progression to tissue necrosis; (2) late onset in life (age greater than 50 years), particularly in men; (3) unilateral or asymmetric involvement; and (4) associated symptoms compatible with a systemic disease.

Sorting out the underlying causes is often difficult because of the wide variety of diseases which may have cold sensitivity as a part of their clinical picture. The following diseases must be kept in mind: (1) chronic arterial disease, most particularly thromboangiitis obliterans; (2) the collagen vascular disorders, with scleroderma being the most common; (3) occupational and industrial exposure to vibrating instruments; (4) poisoning with lead and arsenic; (5) ingestion of drugs, namely, the ergotamine preparations, methysergide, and propranolol; (6) hematologic disorders, namely, cryoglobulins, cold agglutinins, and dysproteinemias; (7) bilateral thoracic outlet syndromes; (8) late sequelae of bilateral cold injury; (9) primary pulmonary hypertension; and (10) occult carcinoma.

The secondary causes of livedo reticularis include (1) collagen diseases, in particular periarteritis nodosa and disseminated lupus erythematosus; (2) hematologic disorders, i.e., hyperviscosity syndrome, macroglobulinemia, and cryoglobulinemia; (3) cholesterol emboli arising from ulcerated plaques in the thoracic and abdominal aorta; (4) Cushing's syndrome; (5) drug ingestion, i.e., adrenal corticosteroids; (6) prolonged dependency or immobilization; (7) late result of cold injury; and (8) prolonged exposure to or the local application of heat.

Therapy The primary forms of cold sensitivity, i.e., livedo reticularis and acrocyanosis, rarely require treatment other than assurance and instruction relative to the dangers of prolonged exposure to cold. Sympathectomy has been widely applied, with inconsistent results, in the treatment of Raynaud's disease. Lumbar sympathectomy, probably because of the higher incidence of permanent denervation, is more likely to give good results than cervicodorsal sympathectomy. Sympathectomy, particularly in the upper extremity, should be performed only when conservative measures fail to control the symptoms. Vasodilator drugs have been used but with limited success. Nifedipine has been reported to be of benefit, but carefully controlled, randomized trials are not available. Biofeedback techniques may be used to lessen the severity of the attacks. When an underlying disease has been found, treatment is directed at the cause of the problem.

ERYTHROMELALGIA This rare disorder of unknown etiology expresses itself as burning, tingling, and often itching of the foot and lower leg which appears as the ambient temperature increases. There is usually a critical temperature for each patient above which the symptoms appear [usually in the range of 31.7 to 36.1°C (89 to 97°F)]. During the attack the patient's feet and lower legs become bright red. The patient quickly finds that the symptoms are related to temperature and will assiduously avoid those circumstances which bring out the symptoms. Characteristically, patients wear sandals, avoid stockings, sleep with their feet outside the bedcovers, and use fans to reduce skin temperature.

The *diagnosis* is established by the history and the examination of the extremities during an attack. The pedal pulses are intact, and the skin is warm and bright red. The disease is usually primary but has, in rare instances, been associated with myeloproliferative disorders.

Therapy is usually unsuccessful, but some patients have reported relief with aspirin or methysergide maleate.

VENOUS DISORDERS

VARICOSE VEINS Varicose veins are dilated, tortuous superficial veins with incompetent valves. The greater and lesser saphenous systems are most commonly involved, but it is not unusual for secondary branches of the superficial system of veins also to become dilated. They most often appear after the age of 20, but in women often develop in relation to puberty, during pregnancy, and with commencement of the menopause. In men there is a fairly even distribution in the onset of symptoms by decades up to age 70.

The etiology remains largely obscure, but varicose veins are known to be aggravated by hormonal factors in the female, increased intraabdominal pressure, and in rare instances, arteriovenous fistulas. Hereditary factors are important but have been poorly studied.

Classification It is important to classify varicose veins as either primary or secondary. Primary varicose veins occur in the absence of deep venous disease and generally have a benign course. Varicosities which occur secondary to obstruction and valvular incompetence of the deep venous system are much more serious.

Clinical features Primary varicose veins are brought to the attention of the patient first by the cosmetic deformity and second by the symptoms which develop with prolonged standing. The patient complains of a feeling of heaviness in the leg, combined with fatigue, that gets progressively worse toward the end of the day. Elevation of the legs will result in rapid and impressive relief from the symptoms. When the varicose veins are secondary to deep venous obstruction, loss of valves, and incompetent perforating veins, the symptoms are more severe and accompanied by swelling (see "Postthrombotic Syndrome" below).

Diagnosis The diagnosis of primary varicose veins is made largely by inspection of the legs in the upright position. The varicosities appear as dilated, often tortuous channels which are most commonly observed in the greater and lesser saphenous systems. When isolated clusters are observed in atypical locations, the possibility of an underlying incompetent perforating vein or arteriovenous fistula should be considered. To assess whether or not incompetent valves in the deep venous system and perforating veins are contributing factors, the Doppler velocity detector may be used. Valvular incompetence is detected by reflux (reversal of flow) in the vein when a Valsalva maneuver is performed.

Therapy The majority of patients with symptomatic primary varicose veins should be treated initially with compression stockings. It is rare for primary varicose veins to lead to stasis pigmentation and ulceration. In those rare instances in which treatment with compression stockings is inadequate, high ligation and stripping of the long and/or short saphenous veins may be required.

ACUTE VENOUS OCCLUSION Obstruction of superficial or deep veins occurs in two settings. The first is associated with an intense inflammatory component as usually observed with involvement of superficial veins. More common and potentially lethal is thrombosis of the deep veins where inflammation as either the inciting event or a clinical manifestation is uncommon. Thus, it is appropriate to separate these two entities since the clinical course and treatment are different.

Superficial thrombophlebitis Except for so-called chemical phlebitis secondary to direct intimal injury, the etiology remains obscure, but the clinical presentation is dramatic. The involved vein is exquisitely tender with surrounding erythema and edema. A fever is often present. While concern has been expressed regarding propagation of the thrombus into the deep venous system with subsequent pulmonary embolization, this rarely occurs. Treatment is directed at local measures to reduce the inflammation—application of heat, elevation of legs, and administration of anti-inflammatory agents such as indomethacin. It is important to be certain that the presenting symptoms are not signs due to a bacterial cellulitis or lymphangitis. The Doppler velocity detector is useful in making the distinction, since thrombophlebitis is always associated with thrombosis of the involved segment.

Acute venous thrombosis The most common in-hospital vascular disorder is thrombosis of the minor and major deep veins of the leg. In the initial stages, the soleus plexus of veins and sinus of the venous valve are the sites most commonly involved. When the thrombi remain confined to these areas, they are not detectable unless prospective screening with ^{125}I-labeled fibrinogen has been carried out (Chap. 211).

Upper extremity thrombosis is uncommon but may be associated with strenuous effort. The site of involvement is most commonly at the level of the axillary-subclavian vein as it enters the thorax.

ETIOLOGY There are definite known precipitating factors, which include trauma and bacterial infection, but these are not the most common causes. The much larger group of these patients develop this problem as a result of one or more of the following conditions or circumstances: (1) prolonged bed rest associated with a medical or surgical illness; (2) malignancy, particularly of the pancreas, lung, or gastrointestinal system; (3) administration of estrogens including oral contraceptives; (4) disseminated intravascular coagulation; (5) the postpartum period; and (6) paralysis.

CLINICAL FEATURES The most important factor concerning the symptoms and signs that develop is that they are not specific and may result from a variety of other diseases. Although edema and local tenderness with associated pain have been considered the most important findings, they are not sufficient to warrant either making the diagnosis of venous thrombosis or instituting therapy. Pulmonary embolization (Chap. 211) may, in fact, be the first clue that deep venous thrombosis is present.

DIAGNOSIS The bedside diagnosis of deep venous thrombosis is so inaccurate that it *must* be established by some independent means. The ^{125}I-labeled fibrinogen test is used for prospective studies but has limited application since it must be given prior to the initiation of the thrombosis. The most useful available noninvasive tests include Doppler ultrasound and plethysmography. Properly used, these tests have a rate of false-positive and false-negative results in the range of 5 to 10 percent. These methods are insensitive to thrombi confined to the muscular veins but can be used for sequential study to detect propagation into the major deep veins. If a vascular laboratory is present which has experience with these noninvasive tests, therapy can be based upon the results. However, if the tests are unavailable or the findings equivocal, contrast venography should be performed. A simpler test is radionuclide venography with simultaneous lung scanning. With this technique excellent visualization of the major deep veins from the popliteal to the vena cava can be obtained. The

procedure is of no value for evaluating the venous segments below the knee.

THERAPY The treatment is directed at control of the thrombotic process already initiated. There is agreement that intravenous heparin is the most effective therapy. The preferred method is continuous administration, starting with a loading dose of 5000 to 10,000 units and varying the dosage depending upon the partial thromboplastin time, which should be kept between two and three times the control time. The two major advantages of this approach are a more uniform level of anticoagulation and a lower incidence of hemorrhagic complications.

The duration of heparin therapy depends upon the degree of involvement and whether pulmonary embolization has occurred. With the latter, treatment must be continued for 10 to 14 days and even longer if the patient remains at risk. Oral therapy with one of the coumarin preparations should be started while the patient is still on heparin, which is discontinued only when a satisfactory level of anticoagulation has been achieved. The maintenance level varies considerably between 2 and 15 mg daily. It appears that adequate protection against recurrent episodes can be obtained by keeping the one-stage prothrombin time at 1.5 to 2.0 times the control level.

Fibrinolytic therapy may be of value in that small group of patients with spontaneous venous thrombosis not associated with surgery or trauma. Streptokinase may be effective in lysing thrombi that have been present for less than 10 days, but its efficacy in preserving valve function remains an open question.

The duration of oral anticoagulation is dependent upon the severity of the problem. For isolated calf vein thrombosis, therapy of 4 to 6 weeks is sufficient. However, for femoropopliteal or iliofemoral thrombosis, with or without pulmonary embolism, anticoagulation should be continued for 3 to 6 months.

PROPHYLACTIC MEASURES There is conflicting evidence that low-dose heparin (5000 units subcutaneously 2 h prior to operation, then three times daily) is effective in reducing the incidence of deep venous thrombosis as well as the occurrence of fatal and nonfatal pulmonary embolism.

Patients with pulmonary embolism that has occurred with adequate doses of heparin, or who have developed bleeding complications, should be considered for transvenous placement of an "umbrella" in the vena cava below the renal veins. This is effective and obviates the need for ligation of the inferior vena cava or for partial occlusion by the direct placement of a plastic clip.

POSTTHROMBOTIC SYNDROME Patients who have single or multiple episodes of deep venous thrombosis will frequently have irreversible changes in the veins which lead to further morbidity. The acute venous thrombosis often leads to residual chronic occlusion and destruction of the venous valves.

The loss of the valvular mechanism in the deep venous system forces the blood to follow abnormal pathways, particularly during exercise. In the standing position or during walking the muscle pump pushes the blood proximally, distally, and out through the perforating veins into the superficial system. By increasing venous and capillary pressures, this sequence of events, over a period of many years, leads to edema, and to rupture of small superficial veins in the vicinity of the perforating veins. The subcutaneous hemorrhage leads to deposition of hemosiderin pigment (stasis pigmentation), subcutaneous fibrosis, cutaneous atrophy, and lymphatic obstruction. These chronic changes lead to the development of stasis ulcers, which are difficult to manage.

Clinical features and diagnosis The important features of this disorder consist of swelling which is always worse at the end of the day, pain, cutaneous pigmentation (usually in the region of the medial malleolus), and nonhealing ulcers which develop secondary to minor trauma. Repeated trauma, subcutaneous hemorrhage, and cellulitis can produce changes in the skin and subcutaneous tissues that are indistinguishable from those of the postthrombotic state. In questionable cases venography is useful in establishing the cause of the problem.

Therapy The most important factor in the treatment of the post-phlebitic syndrome is to reduce the hydrostatic pressure and to prevent "high-pressure leaks" through the perforating veins when the patient is erect. This can best be accomplished by a tailored pressure-gradient stocking, which must be worn at all times that the patient is ambulatory, and by elevating legs when possible.

When an ulcer is present, healing may be accomplished by applying an impregnated gauze dressing from the base of the toes to below the knee. This is changed weekly and permits healing in 90 percent of patients. The remaining patients require excision of the ulcer with skin grafting. Support stockings must be worn regardless of the therapy directed at the ulcer, because the deep venous system remains incompetent and edema will continue to develop without adequate external support.

LYMPHATIC DISORDERS

LYMPHEDEMA Lymphedema, an abnormal accumulation of lymph in the extremities, occurs from multiple causes which include (1) lymphedema from organisms such as *Wuchereria bancrofti*; (2) infectious lymphedema resulting in thrombosis of lymphatics; (3) congenital lymphedema with arrest in lymph growth, which is apparent at birth or shortly thereafter; (4) traumatic lymphedema secondary to direct injury, burns, operations, and radiation; (5) essential lymphedema—so-called Milroy's disease, which appears at puberty and is most commonly observed in women; (6) allergic lymphedema occurring secondary to exposure to drugs and pollens; (7) postthrombotic lymphedema, which represents combined venous and lymphatic obstruction; and (8) malignant lymphedema, which occurs secondary to either direct invasion or obstruction of the lymphatics by tumor cells.

Clinical features Painless swelling of the involved extremity is the earliest and most common symptom and sign with most types of lymphedema. The swelling usually starts in the foot and ankle and then progresses proximally. Initially the swelling tends to subside somewhat at night, but as the process progresses, the swelling becomes permanent secondary to fibrosis of both the skin and subcutaneous tissues. Skin color and texture are normal until the late stages, when the skin becomes thickened and brown and has multiple papillary projections—so-called lymphostatic verrucosis.

Diagnosis The location and nature of the edema readily separate lymphedema from edema due to other causes. In the legs, the dorsa of the toes and foot are nearly always involved; this is uncommon in other causes of swelling. The edema is often brawny in character and pits only with difficulty. Though the other forms of edema often improve with bed rest, elevation, and diuretics, lymphedema, even in early stages, responds poorly to these measures. In later stages when fibrosis develops in the skin and subcutaneous tissues, these

conservative measures are of little, if any, value. Lymphangiography in selected cases may be of value in localizing and elucidating the cause of the lymphedema.

Therapy Therapy is directed at minimizing the amount of edema and preventing recurrent attacks of cellulitis when this is a problem. Pressure-gradient stockings and the use of intermittent-pressure devices at night are helpful in controlling the edema. Since recurrent attacks of cellulitis due to the beta-hemolytic streptococcus are not uncommon and always result in further lymphatic destruction, prophylactic penicillin should be used indefinitely. Excision of the edematous tissue is reserved for only the most advanced stage of the disease when there is marked, irreversible swelling and disfigurement.

ANTERIOR TIBIAL COMPARTMENT SYNDROMES

Acute swelling of the anterior tibial compartment may occur secondary to intensive exercise, increased capillary permeability (with ischemia), or hematoma in the enclosed space. When arterial revascularization has been successful for prolonged ischemia, muscular swelling resulting in an increase in compartment pressure may lead to nerve damage and muscle necrosis. This is recognized by the severe pain in the compartment, swelling, and local tenderness. If the anterior compartment is involved, there is anesthesia of a triangular area on the dorsum of the foot at the base of the first and second toes. *Immediate* fasciotomy is indicated, since a delay of even a few hours may result in irreversible changes.

REFERENCES

ADAR R et al: Cellular sensitivity to collagen in thromboangiitis obliterans. N Engl J Med 308:1113, 1983

BERNI GA et al: Streptokinase treatment of acute arterial occlusion. Ann Surg 198:185, 1983

BERNSTEIN EF (ed): *Noninvasive Diagnostic Techniques in Vascular Disease*, 3d ed. St Louis, Mosby, 1985

BROWSE NL: The diagnosis and management of primary lymphedema. J Vasc Surg 3:181, 1986

DAVL G et al: Inhibition of platelet function by ticlopidine in arteriosclerosis obliterans of the lower limbs. Throm Res 40:275, 1985

GERBRACHT DD et al: Evolution of primary Raynaud's phenomenon (Raynaud's disease) to connective tissue disease. Arthritis Rheum 28:87, 1985

HULL R et al: Adjusted subcutaneous heparin versus warfarin sodium on the long-term treatment of venous thrombosis. N Engl J Med 306:189, 1982

PORTER JM et al: Pentoxifylline efficacy in the treatment of intermittent claudication: Multicenter controlled double-blind trial with objective assessment of chronic occlusive arterial disease patients. Am Heart J 104:66, 1982

RICHMOND DM et al: Sequential pneumatic compression for lymphedema. A controlled trial. Arch Surg 120:1116, 1985

RUTHERFORD RF (ed): *Vascular Surgery*, 2d ed. Philadelphia, Saunders, 1984

STEININGER H: Thromboangiitis obliterans (Buerger's disease). Pathologe 6:204, 1985

STRANDNESS DE JR: The case against low-dose heparin, in *Current Controversies in Cardiovascular Disease*, E Rapaport (ed). Philadelphia, Saunders, 1980

———, THIELE BL: *Selected Topics in Venous Disorders*. New York, Futura, 1981

——— et al: Long-term sequelae of acute venous thrombosis. JAMA 250:1289, 1983

WESSLER SW: The case for low-dose heparin, in *Current Controversies in Cardiovascular Disease*, E Rapaport (ed). Philadelphia, Saunders, 1980

Harrison's
PRINCIPLES
OF INTERNAL
MEDICINE

APPENDIX
Pages A1–A10
INDEX
Pages I1–I130

APPENDIX

APPENDIX LABORATORY VALUES OF CLINICAL IMPORTANCE

INTRODUCTORY COMMENTS

Since *Principles of Internal Medicine* is a textbook used internationally, in preparing the Appendix the editors have taken into account the fact that the system of international units (SI, système international d'unités) has been adopted by many laboratories. To this end, where possible and appropriate, common laboratory values are expressed in terms of both traditional units and SI units. *Values in SI units appear in brackets* after values in traditional units. The use of SI units in medicine was endorsed by the Thirtieth World Health Assembly (May 1977) with the purpose of implementing an international language of measurement.[1] The SI *base* units, SI *derived* units, other units of measurement referred to in this Appendix, and SI prefixes are listed in Tables A-1 to A-3. These and other tables of laboratory values are to be found at the end of the Appendix.

ASCITIC FLUID

See Table 39-1, page 190.

BODY FLUIDS AND OTHER MASS DATA

Body fluid, total volume: 50 percent (in obese) to 70 percent (lean) of body weight
    Intracellular: 30 to 40 percent of body weight
    Extracellular: 20 to 30 percent of body weight
Blood:
    Total volume:
      Males: 69 mL per kilogram of body weight
      Females: 65 mL per kilogram of body weight
    Plasma volume:
      Males: 39 mL per kilogram of body weight
      Females: 40 mL per kilogram of body weight
    Red blood cell volume:
      Males: 30 mL per kilogram of body weight (1.15 to 1.21 liters per square meter of body surface area)
      Females: 25 mL per kilogram of body weight (0.95 to 1.00 liters per square meter of body surface area)

$$\text{meq/liter} = \frac{\text{mg/dL} \times 10 \times \text{valence}}{\text{atomic weight}}$$

$$\text{mg/dL} = \frac{\text{meq/liter} \times \text{atomic weight}}{10 \times \text{valence}}$$

CEREBROSPINAL FLUID[2]

Osmolarity	292–297 mosmol per liter

Electrolytes:

Sodium	137–145 meq per liter
Potassium	2.7–3.9 meq per liter
Calcium	2.1–3.0 meq per liter
Magnesium	2.0–2.5 meq per liter
Phosphorus	1.2–2.0 mg/dL
Chloride	116–122 meq per liter
Bicarbonate	20–24 meq per liter
P_{CO_2}	45–49 mmHg
pH	7.31–7.34
Glucose	40–70 mg/dL
Lactate	10–20 mg/dL
Pyruvate	0.078–0.081 meq per liter
Lactate/pyruvate ratio	26.0
Total protein:	20–45 mg/dL
Prealbumin	2–6%
Albumin	56–75%
Alpha$_1$ globulin	2–7%
Alpha$_2$ globulin	4–12%
Beta globulin	8–16%
Gamma globulin	3–12%
IgG	1.0–1.4 mg/dL
IgA	0.1–0.3 mg/dL
IgM	0.01–0.12 mg/dL
IgG synthesis rate	(−) 9.9 to (+) 3.3 mg per day
Ammonia	25–80 μg/dL
Urea	4.4–4.8 mmol per liter
Creatinine	0.5–1.9 mg/dL
Uric acid	0.23–0.27 mg/dL
Putrescine	130–230 pmol/mL
Spermidine	110–190 pmol/mL
Cyclic AMP	3–30 nmol per liter
HVA (homovanillic acid)	35–85 μg/mL
5-HIAA (5-OH indoleacetic acid)	0.03–0.05 μg/mL
MHPG (3-methoxy-4-hydroxy-phenylethyleneglycol)	13.0–17.0 mg/dL
Myelin basic protein	<4 ng/mL
CSF pressure	50–180 mmH$_2$O
CSF volume (adult)	100–160 mL
Leukocytes:	
Total	<4 per cubic millimeter
Differential:	
Lymphocytes	60–70%
Monocytes	30–50%
Neutrophils	1–3%

CHEMICAL CONSTITUENTS OF BLOOD

See also "Function Tests," especially "Metabolic and Endocrine."

Acetoacetate, plasma: <1.0 mg/dL [<0.1 mmol per liter]
Albumin, serum: 3.5 to 5.5 g/dL [35 to 55 g per liter]
Aldolase: 0 to 8 units per liter [0 to 130 nmol/s per liter]
Alpha$_1$ antitrypsin, serum: 85–213 mg/dL [0.85–2.13 g per liter]

[1] *The SI for the Health Professions, Geneva, World Health Organization, 1977.*

[2] *Since cerebrospinal fluid concentrations are equilibrium values, measurement of blood plasma obtained at the same time is recommended.*

α-Amino nitrogen, plasma: 3.0 to 5.5 mg/dL [2.1 to 3.9 mmol per liter]

Alpha fetoprotein (adult), serum: <30 mg/mL

Aminotransferases, serum:

Aspartate (AST, SGOT): 10 to 40 Karmen units per milliliter; 6 to 18 units per liter [100 to 300 μmol/s per liter]

Alanine (ALT, SGPT): 10 to 40 Karmen units per milliliter; 3 to 26 units per liter [50 to 430 μmol/s per liter]

Ammonia, whole blood, venous: 80 to 110 μg/dL [47 to 65 μmol per liter]

Amylase, serum: 60 to 180 Somogyi units per deciliters; 0.8 to 3.2 units per liter [13 to 53 nmol/s per liter]

Arterial blood gases:

[HCO₃⁻]: 21 to 28 meq per liter [21 to 28 mmol per liter]

P_{CO_2}: 35 to 45 mmHg [4.7 to 6.0 kPa]

pH: 7.38 to 7.44

P_{O_2}: 80 to 100 mmHg [11 to 13 kPa]

Ascorbic acid (vitamin C), serum: 0.4 to 1.0 mg/dL [23 to 57 μmol per liter]

Leukocytes: 25 to 40 mg/dL [1420 to 2270 μmol per liter]

Barbiturates, serum: nondetectable

Phenobarbital, ''potentially fatal'' level (Schreiner): approximately 9 mg/dL [390 μmol per liter]

Most short-acting barbiturates: 3.5 mg/dL [150 μmol per liter]

Base, total, serum: 145 to 155 meq per liter [145 to 155 mmol per liter]

β-Hydroxybutyrate, plasma: <3mg/dL [<0.3 mmol per liter]

Bilirubin, total, serum (Malloy-Evelyn): 0.3 to 1.0 mg/dL [5.1 to 17 μmol per liter]

Direct, serum: 0.1 to 0.3 mg/dL [1.7 to 5.1 μmol per liter]

Indirect, serum: 0.2 to 0.7 mg/dL [3.4 to 12 μmol per liter]

Bromides, serum: nondetectable

Toxic levels: >17 meq per liter; 150 mg/dL [17 mmol per liter]

Bromsulphalein, BSP (5 mg per kilogram of body weight, intravenously): 5 percent or less retention after 45 min

C-reactive protein, serum: 7–820 μg/dL

Calciferols (vitamin D), plasma:

1,25-dihydroxyvitamin D [1,25(OH)₂D]. 20 to 60 pg/mL [48 to 144 nmol per liter]

25-hydroxyvitamin D [25(OH)D]. 8 to 42 ng/mL [20 to 100 μmol per liter]

Calcium, ionized: 2.3 to 2.8 meq per liter; 4.5 to 5.6 mg/dL [1.1 to 1.4 mmol per liter]

Calcium, plasma: 4.5 to 5.5 meq per liter; 9 to 10.5 mg/dL [2.2 to 2.6 mmol per liter]

Carbon dioxide-combining power, serum (sea level): 21 to 28 meq per liter; 50 to 65 volume percent [21 to 28 mmol per liter]

Carbon dioxide content, plasma (sea level): 21 to 30 meq per liter; 50 to 70 volume percent [21 to 30 mmol per liter]

Carbon dioxide tension, arterial blood (sea level): 35 to 45 mmHg [4.7 to 6.0 kPa]

Carbon monoxide content, blood: nondetectable symptoms with over 20 percent saturation of hemoglobin

Carcinoembryonic antigen (CEA): 0 to 2.5 ng/mL (in healthy nonsmokers) [0 to 2.5 μg per liter]

Carotenoids, serum: 50 to 300 μg/dL [0.9 to 5.6 μmol per liter]

Ceruloplasmin, serum: 27 to 37 mg/dL [1.8 to 2.5 μmol per liter]

Chlorides, serum (as Cl⁻): 98 to 106 meq per liter [98 to 106 mmol per liter]

Cholesterol: see Table A-4

Complement, serum:

Total hemolytic (CH₅₀): 150 to 250 units per milliliter

C3: 55 to 120 mg/dL [0.55 to 1.20 g per liter]

C4: 20 to 50 mg/dL [0.20 to 0.50 g per liter]

Copper, serum (mean ± 1 SD): 114 ± 14 μg/dL [17.9 μmol per liter]

Creatine phosphokinase, serum (total):

Females: 10 to 70 units per millimeter [0.17 to 1.18 mmol/s per liter]

Males: 25 to 90 units per milliliter [0.42 to 1.51 mmol/s per liter]

Isoenzymes, serum: fraction 2 (MB) <5 percent of total

Creatinine, serum: <1.5 mg/dL [<133 μmol per liter]

Digoxin serum:

Therapeutic level: 1.2 ± 4 ng/mL [1.54 ± 0.5 nmol per liter]

Toxic level: >2.4 ng/mL [>3.2 nmol per liter]

Ethanol, blood:

Mild to moderate intoxication: 80 to 200 mg/dL [17 to 43 mmol per liter]

Marked intoxication: 250 to 400 mg/dL [54 to 87 mmol per liter]

Severe intoxication: >400 mg/dL [>87 mmol per liter]

Fatty acids, free (nonesterified), plasma: <18 mg/dL [<0.7 mmol per liter]

Ferritin, serum: 15 to 200 ng/mL [15 to 200 μg per liter]

Fibrinogen, plasma: see ''Platelets and Coagulation''

Fibrinogen split products: see ''Platelets and Coagulation''

Folic acid, serum: 6 to 15 ng/mL [14 to 34 nmol per liter]

Folic acid, red cell: 150 to 450 ng per milliliter of cells [340 to 1020 nmol per liter cells]

γ-Glutamyl transferase (transpeptidase), serum: 4 to 60 units per liter [0.07 to 1.00 μmol/s per liter]

Gastrin, serum: 40 to 200 pg/mL [40 to 200 ng per liter]

Globulins, serum: 2.0 to 3.0 g/dL [20 to 30 g per liter]

Glucose (fasting), plasma:

Normal: 75 to 115 mg/dL [4.2 to 6.4 mmol per liter]

Diabetes mellitus: >140 mg/dL (on more than one occasion) [>7.8 mmol per liter]

Glucose, 2 h postprandial, plasma:

Normal: <140 mg/dL [<7.8 mmol per liter]

Impaired glucose tolerance: 140 to 200 mg/dL [7.8 to 11.1 mmol per liter]

Diabetes mellitus: >200 mg/dL [>11.1 mmol per liter] (on more than one occasion)

Hemoglobin, blood (sea level):

Males: 14 to 18 g/dL [8.7 to 11.2 mmol per liter]

Females: 12 to 16 g/dL [7.4 to 9.9 mmol per liter]

Hemoglobin A₁c: up to 6 perrcent of total hemoglobin

Immunoglobulins, serum:

IgA: 90 to 325 mg/dL [0.9 to 3.2 g per liter]

IgD: 0 to 8 mg/dL [0 to 0.08 g per liter]

IgE: <0.025 mg/dL [<0.00025 g per liter]

IgG: 800 to 1500 mg/dL [8.0 to 15.0 g per liter]

IgM: 45 to 150 mg/dL [0.45 to 1.5 g per liter]

Iron, serum:

Males and females (mean ± 1 SD): 105 ± 35 μg/dL [19 ± 6 μmol per liter]

Iron-binding capacity, serum (mean ± 1 SD): 305 ± 32 μg/dL [55 ± 6 μmol per liter]

Saturation: 20 to 45 percent

Ketones, total: 0.5 to 1.5 mg/dL [5.0 to 15.0 mg per liter]

Lactate dehydrogenase, serum:

200 to 450 units per milliliter (Wrobleski)

60 to 100 units per milliliter (Wacker)

25 to 100 units per liter [0.4 to 1.7 μmol/s per liter]

Lactic dehydrogenase isoenzymes, serum (agarose):

Fraction 1 (% of total): 14–26

Fraction 2: 29–39

Fraction 3: 20–26

Fraction 4:   8–16

Fraction 5:   6–16

Lactate, venous plasma: 5 to 15 mg/dL [0.6 to 1.7 mmol per liter]

Lead, serum: <20 μg/dL [<1.0 μmol per liter]

Lipase, serum: 1.5 units (Cherry-Crandall)

Lipids: see Table A-4

Lipids, triglyceride, serum: see Table A-4

Lipoprotein: see Table A-4

Lithium, serum:

Therapeutic concentration: 0.6 to 1.2 mmol per liter

Toxic concentration: >2 mmol per liter [>2 mmol per liter]

Magnesium, serum: 1.3 to 2.1 meq per liter; 2 to 3 mg/dL [0.8 to 1.3 mmol per liter]

Nitrogen, nonprotein, serum: 15 to 35 mg/dL [0.15 to 0.35 g per liter]

5′-Nucleotidase, serum: 0.3 to 2.6 Bodansky units per deciliter [27 to 233 nmol/s per liter]

Osmolality, plasma: 285 to 295 mosmol per kilogram of serum water

Oxygen content:
   Arterial blood (sea level): 17 to 21 volume percent
   Venous blood, arm (sea level): 10 to 16 volume percent

Oxygen percent saturation (sea level):
   Arterial blood: 97 percent [0.97 mol/mol]
   Venous blood, arm: 60 to 85 percent [0.60 to 0.85 mol/mol]

Oxygen tension, blood: 80 to 100 mmHg ob11 to 13 kPa]

pH, blood: 7.38 to 7.44

Phenytoin, plasma:
   Therapeutic level: 10 to 20 μg/mL [40 to 79 μmol per liter]
   Toxic level: >30 μg/mL [>119 μmol per liter]

Phosphatase, acid, serum:
   Bessey-Lowry method: 0.10 to 0.63 units [28 to 175 nmol/s per liter]
   Bodansky method: 0.5 to 2.0 units
   Fishmann-Lerner (tartrate sensitive): <0.6 units per deciliter (up to 0.15 units per deciliter)
   Gutman method: 0.5 to 2.0 units
   International units: 0.2 to 1.8 [3 to 30 nmol/s per liter]
   King-Armstrong method: 1.0 to 5.0 units

Phosphatase, alkaline, serum:
   Bessey-Lowry method: 0.8 to 2.3 units (3.4 to 9 units[3])
   Bodansky method: 2.0 to 4.5 units (3.0 to 13.0 units[3]) [0.18 to 0.40 nmol/s per liter]
   Gutman method: 2.0 to 4.5 units (3.0 to 13.0 units[3])
   International units: 21 to 91 per liter at 37°C [0.4 to 1.5 μmol/s per liter]
   King-Armstrong method: 4.0 to 13.0 units (10.0 to 20.0 units[3])

Phospholipids, serum: 150 to 250 mg/dL (as lecithin) [48 to 81 mmol per liter]

Phosphorus, inorganic, serum: 1 to 1.5 meq per liter; 3 to 4.5 mg/dL [1.0 to 1.4 mmol per liter]

Potassium, serum: 3.5 to 5.0 meq per liter [3.5 to 5.0 mmol per liter]

Proteins, total, serum: 5.5 to 8.0 g/dL [55 to 80 g per liter]

Protein fractions, serum:
   Albumin: 3.5 to 5.5 g/dL (50 to 60 percent) [35 to 55 g per liter]
   Globulin: 2.0 to 3.5 g/dL (40 to 50 percent) [20 to 35 g per liter]
   Alpha$_1$: 0.2 to 0.4 g/dL (4.2 to 7.2 percent) [2 to 4 g per liter]
   Alpha$_2$: 0.5 to 0.9 g/dL (6.8 to 12 percent) [5 to 9 g per liter]
   Beta: 0.6 to 1.1 g/dL (9.3 to 15 percent) [6 to 11 g per liter]
   Gamma: 0.7 to 1.7 g/dL (13 to 23 percent) [7 to 17 g per liter]

Pyruvate, venous, plasma: 0.5 to 1.5 mg/dL [0.06 to 0.17 mmol per liter]

Quinidine, serum:
   Therapeutic range: 1.5 to 3 μg/mL [4.6 to 9.2 μmol per liter]
   Toxic range: 5 to 6 μg/mL [15.4 to 18.5 μmol per liter]

Salicylate, plasma: 0 mmol per liter
   Therapeutic range: 20 to 25 mg/dL [1.4 to 1.8 mmol per liter]
   Toxic range: >30 mg/dL [2.2 mmol per liter]

Sodium, serum: 136 to 145 meq per liter [136 to 145 mmol per liter]

Steroids: see "Metabolic and Endocrine" under "Function Tests"

Transaminase, serum glutamic oxaloacetic (SGOT, AST): 10 to 40 Karmen units per milliliter; 6 to 18 units per liter [100 to 300 μmol/s per liter]

Transaminase, serum glutamic pyruvic (SGPT, ALT): see Aminotransferases, serum

Transferase, γ-glutamyl, serum: 4 to 60 units per liter [0.07 to 1.00 μmol/s per liter]

Triglycerides: see Table A-4

Urea nitrogen, serum: 10 to 20 mg/dL [3.6 to 7.1 mmol per liter]

Uric acid, serum:
   Men: 2.5 to 8.0 mg/dL [0.15 to 0.48 mmol per liter]
   Women: 1.5 to 6.0 mg/dL [0.09 to 0.36 mmol per liter]

Vitamin A, serum: 20 to 100 μg/dL [0.7 to 3.5 μmol per liter]

Vitamin B$_{12}$, serum: 200 to 600 pg/mL [148 to 443 pmol per liter]

Zinc, serum (mean ± 1 SD): 120 ± 20 μg/dL [18 ± 3 μmol per liter]

FUNCTION TESTS

Circulation

Arteriovenous oxygen difference: 30 to 50 mL per liter

Cardiac output (Fick): 2.5 to 3.6 liters per square meter of body surface area per minute

Contractility indexes:
   Maximum left ventricular dp/dt: 1650 ± 300 mmHg/s
   Maximum $(dp/dt)/p$: 44 ± 8.4 s^{-1}
   $(dp/dt)/DP$ at DP = 40 mmHg: 37.6 ± 12.2 s^{-1} (DP = diastolic press.)
   Mean normalized systolic ejection rate (angiography): 3.32 ± 0.84 end-diastolic volumes per second
   Mean velocity of circumferential fiber shortening (angiography) 1.66 ± 0.42 circumferences per second

Ejection fraction, stroke volume/end-diastolic volume (SV/EDV):
   Normal range: 0.55 to 0.78; average: 0.67

End-diastolic volume: 75 ± 15 mL/m^2

End-systolic volume: 25 ± 8 mL/m^2

Left ventricular work:
   Stroke work index: 30 to 110 (g·m)/m^2
   Left ventricular minute work index: 1.8 to 6.6 [(kg·m)/m^2]/min
   Oxygen consumption index: 110 to 150 mL per liter

Pressures, intracardiac and intraarterial: see Table A-5

Pulmonary vascular resistance: 20 to 120 (dyn·s)/cm^5 [2 to 12 kPa·s per liter]

Systemic vascular resistance: 770 to 1500 (dyn·s)/cm^5 [77 to 150 kPa·s per liter]

Systolic time intervals: see Table A-6

Gastrointestinal See also "Stool."

Absorption tests:
   D-Xylose absorption test: After an overnight fast, 25 g xylose is given in aqueous solution by mouth. Urine collected for the following 5 h should contain 5 to 8 g [33 to 53 mmol] (or >20 percent of ingested dose). Serum xylose should be 25 to 40 mg per 100 mL 1 h after the oral dose [1.7 to 2.7 mmol per liter].
   Vitamin A absorption test: A fasting blood specimen is obtained and 200,000 units of vitamin A in oil is given by mouth. Serum vitamin A levels should rise to twice fasting level in 3 to 5 h.

Bentiromide test (pancreatic function): 500 mg bentiromide (chymex) orally; p-aminobenzoic acid (PABA) measured in plasma and/or urine
   Plasma: >3.6 (±1.1) μg/mL at 90 min
   Urine: >50 percent recovered as PABA in 6 h

Gastric juice:
   Volume:
      24 h: 2 to 3 liters
      Nocturnal: 600 to 700 mL
      Basal, fasting: 30 to 70 mL/h
   Reaction:
      As pH: 1.6 to 1.8
      Titratable acidity of fasting juice: 15 to 35 meq/h [4 to 10 μmol/s]
   Acid output:
      Basal:
         Females (mean ± 1 SD): 2.0 ± 1.8 meq/h [0.6 ± 0.5 μmol/s]
         Males (mean ± 1 SD): 3.0 ± 2.0 meq/h [0.8 ± 0.6 μmol/s]

---

[3] Values in parentheses are those found in children.

Maximal [after subcutaneous histamine acid phosphate 0.004 mg/kg and preceded by 50 mg promethazine (Phenergan); or after betazole (Histalog) 1.7 mg/kg or pentagastrin 6μg/mg]:

Females (mean ± 1 SD): 16 ± 5 meq/h [4.4 ± 1.4 μmol/s]

Males (mean ± 1 SD): 23 ± 5 meq/h [6.4 ± 1.4 μmol/s]

Basal acid output/maximal acid output ratio: 0.6 or less

Gastrin, serum: 40 to 200 pg/mL [40 to 200 ng per liter]

Secretin test (pancreatic exocrine function): 1 unit per kilogram of body weight, intravenously

Volume (pancreatic juice): >2.0 mL/kg in 80 min

Bicarbonate concentration: >80 meq per liter [>80 mmol per liter]

Bicarbonate output: >10 meq in 30 min [>10 mmol in 30 min]

Metabolic and endocrine

ACTH, plasma, 8 A.M.: <80 pg/mL [<80 ng per liter]

Adrenal cortex function tests: see Chap. 325

Adrenal medulla function tests: see Chap 326

Adrenal steroids, plasma:

Aldosterone, 8 A.M.: <8.5 ng/dL [<0.24 nmol per liter] (patient supine, 100 meq Na and 60 to 100 meq K intake)

Cortisol:

8 A.M.: 5 to 25 μg/dL [138 to 691 nmol per liter]

4 P.M.: 3 to 12 μg/dL [82 to 331 nmol per liter]

Dehydroepiandrosterone (DHEA): 0.2 to 0.9 μg/dL [7 to 31 nmol per liter]

Dehydroepiandrosterone sulfate (DHEA sulfate): 50 to 250 μg/dL [1.3 to 6.5 μmol per liter]

11-Deoxycortisol (compound S): <1 μg/dL [<30 nmol per liter]

17-Hydroxyprogesterone:

Women: follicular phase, 20 to 100 ng/dL [0.6 to 3 nmol per liter]; luteal phase, 50 to 350 ng/dL [1.5 to 10.6 nmol per liter]

Men: 6 to 300 ng/dL [1.8 to 9.0 nmol per liter]

Adrenal steroids, secretion rates:

Aldosterone: 50 to 250 μg per day [138 to 690 nmol per day]

Cortisol: 8 to 24 mg per day [22 to 69 μmol per day]

Adrenal steroids, urinary excretion:

Aldosterone: 5 to 19 μg per day [14 to 53 nmol per day]

Cortisol, free: 20 to 100 μg per day [54 to 276 nmol per day]

17-Hydroxycorticosteroids: 2 to 10 mg per day [5.4 to 28 μmol per day]

17-Ketosteroids:

Men: 7 to 25 mg per day [24 to 88 μmol per day]

Women: 4 to 15 mg per day [14 to 52 μmol per day]

Angiotensin II, plasma, 8 A.M.: 10 to 30 pg/mL [10 to 30 nmol per liter]

Arginine vasopressin (AVP), plasma:

Random fluid intake: 1 to 3 pg/mL [1 to 3 ng per liter]

Fluid deprivation, 18 to 24 h: 6 to 12 pg/mL [6 to 12 ng per liter]

Calcitonin, plasma: <50 pg/mL [<50 ng per liter]

Catecholamines, urinary excretion:

Free catecholamines: <100 μg per day [<590 nmol per day]

Epinephrine: <50 μg per day [295 nmol per day]

Metanephrines: <1.3 mg per day [<6.2 μmol per day]

Vanillylmandelic acid (VMA): <8 mg per day [<40 μmol per day]

Gastrin, plasma: <120 pg/mL [<120 ng per liter]

Glucagon, plasma: 50 to 100 pg/mL [14 to 29 pmol per liter]

Gonadal function tests: see Chaps. 330 and 331

Gonadal steroids, plasma:

Androstenedione:

Women: 110 to 190 ng/dL [3.9 to 6.6 nmol per liter]

Men: 80 to 130 ng/dL [2.9 to 4.6 mmol per liter]

Estradiol:

Women: 20 to 60 pg/mL [0.07 to 0.22 nmol per liter], higher at ovulation

Men: <50 pg/mL [<0.18 nmol per liter]

Progesterone:

Men, prepubertal girls, preovulatory women, and postmenopausal women: <2 ng/mL [<6 nmol per liter]

Women, luteal, peak: >5 ng/mL [>16 nmol per liter]

Testosterone:

Women: <100 ng/dL [<3.5 nmol per liter]

Men: 300 to 1000 ng/dL [10 to 35 nmol per liter]

Prepubertal boys and girls: 5 to 20 ng/dL [0.17 to 0.7 nmol per liter]

Gonadotropins, plasma:

Women, mature, premenopausal, except at ovulation:

FSH: 5 to 20 mU/mL [5 to 20 U per liter]

LH: 5 to 25 mU/mL [5 to 25 U per liter]

Ovulatory surge:

FSH: 12 to 30 mU/mL [12 to 30 U per liter]

LH: 25 to 100 mU/mL [25 to 100 U per liter]

Postmenopausal women:

FSH: >50 mU/mL [>50 U per liter]

LH: >50 mU/mL [>50 U per liter]

Men, mature:

FSH: 5 to 20 mU/mL [5 to 20 U per liter]

LH: 5 to 20 mU/mL [5 to 20 U per liter]

Children of both sexes, prepubertal:

FSH: <5 mU/mL [<5 U per liter]

LH: <5 mU/mL [<5 U per liter]

Growth hormone, after 100 g glucose by mouth: <5 ng/dL [<50 ng per liter]

Human chorionic gonadotropin, β subunit (β-hCG), plasma:

Men and nonpregnant women: <3 mIU/mL [<3 IU per liter]

Insulin, serum or plasma, fasting: 6 to 26 μU/mL [43 to 186 pmol per liter]

Insulin-like growth factor I (somatomedin C, IGF-1/SM C): see Chap. 322

Oxytocin, plasma:

Men and preovulatory women: 0.5 to 2 μU/mL [2 to 4 mU per liter]

Lactating women: 5 to 10 μU/mL [5 to 10 mU per liter]

Pancreatic islet function tests: Chap. 327

Parathyroid function tests: see Chap. 336

Pituitary function tests: see Chaps. 321 to 323

Pregnancy tests: see Chap. 331

Prolactin, serum: 2 to 15 ng/mL [2 to 15 μg per liter]

Renin-angiotensin function tests: see Chap. 325

Semen analysis: see Chap. 330

Thyroid function tests:

Dynamic tests of thyroid function: see Chap. 324

Radioactive iodine uptake, 24 h: 5 to 30 percent (range varies in different areas due to variations in iodine intake)

Resin T_3 uptake: 25 to 35 percent (varies among laboratories; for calculation of indexes of resin T_3 uptake, see Chap. 324)

Reverse triiodothyronine (rT_3), plasma: 10 to 40 ng/dL [0.15 to 0.61 nmol per liter]

Thyroid-stimulating hormone (TSH): <5 μU/mL [<5 mU per liter]

Thyroxine (T_4), serum radioimmunoassay: 5 to 12 μg/dL [64 to 154 nmol per liter]

Triiodothyronine (T_3), plasma: 70 to 190 ng/dL [1.1 to 2.9 nmol per liter]

Pulmonary   See Tables A-9 and A-10.

Arterial blood gas measurements in normal subjects (sea level):

P_{CO_2}, seated (mean ± 1 SD): 38.0 ± 2.9 mmHg (no change with age) [5.0 kPa]

P_{O_2}:

Seated (mean ± 1 SD): (104.2 ± 0.27 mmHg) × age in years [13.8 kPa]

Supine (mean ± 1 SD): (103.5 ± 0.42 mmHg) × age in years [13.8 kPa]

Renal

Clearances (corrected to 1.72 m² body surface area):
Measures of glomerular filtration rate:
Inulin clearance (C1):
Males (mean ± 1 SD): 124 ± 25.8 mL/min [2.1 ± 0.4 mL/s]
Females (mean ± 1 SD): 119 ± 12.8 mL/min [2.0 ± 0.2 mL/s]
Endogenous creatinine clearance: 91 to 130 mL/min [1.5 to 2.2 mL/s]
Urea: 60 to 100 mL/min [1.0 to 1.7 mL/s]
Measures of effective renal plasma flow and tubular function:
p-Aminohippuric acid clearance (Cl_PAH):
Males (mean ± 1 SD): 654 ± 163 mL/min [10.9 ± 2.7 mL/s]
Females (mean ± 1 SD): 594 ± 102 mL/min [9.9 ± 1.7 mL/s]
Concentration and dilution test:
Specific gravity of urine:
After 12-h fluid restriction: 1.025 or more
After 12-h deliberate water intake: 1.003 or less
Phenosulfonphthalein:
After intravenous injection:
Excretion in urine in 15 min: 25 percent or more
Excretion in urine in 2 h: 55 to 75 percent
Protein excretion, urine: <150 mg in 24 h [<0.15 g per day]
Males: 0 to 60 mg in 24 h [0 to 0.06 g per day]
Females: 0 to 90 mg in 24 h [0 to 0.09 g per day]
Specific gravity, maximal range: 1.002 to 1.028
Tubular reabsorption, phosphorus: 79 to 94 percent of filtered load

HEMATOLOGIC EXAMINATIONS

See also "Chemical Constituents of Blood."

Bone marrow   See Table A-11.

Erythrocytes and hemoglobin   See also Table A-12.

Carboxyhemoglobin:
Nonsmoker: 0 to 2.3 percent
Smoker: 2.1 to 4.2 percent
Erythrocyte "life span":
Normal survival: 120 days
Chromium-labeled, half-life ($t_{\frac{1}{2}}$): 28 days
Glucose 6-phosphate dehydrogenase: 12.1 ± 2 IU/gHb (WHO)
Ham's test (acid serum): negative
Haptoglobin, serum (mean ± 2 SD): 128 ± 15 mg/dL [1.3 ± 0.2 g per liter]
Heinz body stain: negative
Hemoglobin, plasma: 1 to 5 mg/dL [0.03 to 0.05 g per liter]
Hemoglobin A₂ (HbA₂): 1.5 to 3.5 percent
Hemoglobin, fetal (HbF): <2 percent
Hemoglobin H prep: negative
Methemoglobin: <1.7 percent
Nitroblue tetrazolium (chronic granulomatous disease): normal
Osmotic fragility:
Slight hemolysis: 0.45 to 0.39 percent
Complete hemolysis: 0.33 to 0.30 percent
Plasma iron turnover: 20 to 42 mg per 24 h [0.47 mg/kg]
Protoporphyrin, free erythrocyte (FEP): 16 to 36 μg per deciliter of red blood cells [0.28 to 0.64 μmol per liter]
Red cell distribution width (Coulter): 13 ± 1.5 percent
Sedimentation rate:
Westergren, <50 years of age:
Males: 0 to 15 mm/h
Females: 0 to 20 mm/h

Westergren, >50 years of age:
Males: 0 to 20 mm/h
Females: 0 to 30 mm/h
Wintrobe:
Males: 0 to 9 mm/h
Females: 0 to 20 mm/h
Sucrose hemolysis: negative

Leukocytes   See Table A-13.

Platelets and coagulation

Alpha₂ antiplasmin: 70 to 130 percent
Antithrombin III: 80 to 120 percent
Bleeding time:
Ivy method, 5-mm wound: <9 min
Duke method: <4 min
Simplate: <7 min
Clot retraction, qualitative: apparent in 60 min, complete <24 h, usually <6 h
Euglobulin lysis time: >2 h
Factor II: 60 to 100 percent
Factor V: 60 to 100 percent
Factor VII: 60 to 100 percent
Factor IX: 60 to 100 percent
Factor X: 60 to 100 percent
Factor XI: 60 to 100 percent
Factor XII: 60 to 100 percent
Factor XIII: clot stable in urea
Fibrinogen: 200 to 400 mg/dL
Fibrin split products: <10 μg/mL
Plasminogen: 2.4 to 4.4 CTA U/mL
Protein C (antigenic assay): 58 to 148 percent
Protein S (antigenic assay): 58 to 148 percent
Partial thromboplastin time (activated PTT): comparable to control
Prothrombin time (quick one-stage): control ± 1 s
Protamine paracoagulation (3P) test: negative
Platelets: 130,000 to 400,000 per cubic millimeter
Thrombin time: control ± 3 s
von Willebrand's antigen: 60 to 150 percent

Miscellaneous

Leukocyte alkaline phosphatase (LAP): 13 to 100
Lysozyme (muramidase), serum: 5 to 25 μg/dL
Lysozyme, urine: <2 μg/mL
Schilling test: excretion in urine of orally administered radioactive vitamin B₁₂: 7 to 40 percent
Viscosity, plasma: 1.7 to 2.1
Viscosity, serum: 1.4 to 1.8

STOOL

Bulk:
Wet weight: <197.5 (115 ± 41) g per day
Dry weight: <66.4 (34 ± 16) g per day
Alpha₁ antitrypsin: 0.98 (±0.17) mg per gram of dry weight stool
Coproporphyrin: 400 to 1000 μg in 24 h [610 to 1500 nmol per day]
Fat (on diet containing at least 50 g fat): <6.0 (4.0 ± 1.5) g per day when measured on a 3-day (or longer) collection
Percent of dry weight: <30.4 (13.3 ± 8.07)
Coefficient of fat absorption: >95 percent
Fatty acid:
Free: 1 to 10 percent of dry matter
Combined as soap: 0.5 to 12 percent of dry matter
Nitrogen: <1.7 (1.4 ± 0.2) g per day
Protein content: minimal
Urobilinogen: 40 to 280 mg in 24 h [67 to 470 μmol per day]
Water: approximately 65 percent

URINE

See also "Metabolic and Endocrine" under "Function Tests."

Acidity, titratable: 20 to 40 meq in 24 h [20 to 40 mmol per day]

α-Amino nitrogen: 0.4 to 1.0 g in 24 h [28 to 71 mmol per day]

Ammonia: 30 to 50 meq in 24 h [30 to 50 mmol per day]

Amylase: 35 to 260 Somogyi units per hour

Amylase/creatinine clearance ratio [$(Cl_{am}/Cl_{cr}) \times 100$]: 1 to 5

Bentiromide (pancreatic function): 50 percent excreted in 6 h as *p*-amino benzoic acid (PABA) after 500 mg oral bentiromide

Calcium (10 meq or 200-mg calcium diet): <7.5 meq in 24 h; <150 mg in 24 h [<3.8 mmol per day]

Catecholamines: <100 μg in 24 h

Copper: 0 to 25 μg in 24 h [0 to 0.4 μmol per day]

Coproporphyrins (types I and III): 100 to 300 μg in 24 h [150 to 460 nmol per day]

Creatine, as creatinine:

  Adult males: <50 mg in 24 h [<0.38 mmol per day]

  Adult females: <100 mg in 24 h [<0.76 mmol per day]

Creatinine: 1.0 to 1.6 g in 24 h [8.8 to 14 mmol per day]

Glucose, true (oxidase method): 50 to 300 mg in 24 h [0.3 to 1.7 mmol per day]

5-Hydroxyindoleacetic acid (5-HIAA): 2 to 9 mg in 24 h [10 to 47 μmol per day]

Ketones, total (mean $\pm$ 1 SD): 50.5 $\pm$ 30.7 mg in 24 h

Lactic dehydrogenase: 560 to 2050 units in 8-h urine

Lead: <0.08 μg/mL; <120 μg in 24 h [0.39 μmol per liter]

Protein: <150 mg in 24 h [<0.05 g per day]

Porphobilinogen: none

Potassium: 25 to 100 meq in 24 h (varies with intake) [25 to 100 mmol per day]

Sodium: 100 to 260 meq in 24 h (varies with intake) [100 to 260 mmol per day]

Urobilinogen: 1 to 3.5 mg in 24 h [1.7 to 5.9 μmol per day]

Vanillylmandelic acid (VMA): <8 mg per day [<40 μmol per day]

D-Xylose excretion: 5 to 8 g within 5 h after oral dose of 25 g [33 to 53 mmol in 5 h]

TABLE A-1 SI and other units

Quantity	Name of unit	Symbol for unit	Derivation of units
SI BASE UNITS			
Length	meter	m	
Mass	kilogram	kg	
Time	second	s	
Thermodynamic temperature	Kelvin	K	
Amount of substance	mole	mol	
SI DERIVED UNITS			
Force	newton	N	$(m \cdot kg)/s^2$
Pressure	pascal	Pa	$N \cdot m^2$
Work, energy	joule	J	$N \cdot m$
Celsius temperature	degree Celsius	°C	K
OTHER UNITS RETAINED FOR USE			
Time	minute	min	
	hour	h	
	day	d	
Volume	liter	L	

TABLE A-2 Radiation derived units

Quantity	Old unit	SI unit	Name for SI unit (and abbreviation)	Conversion
Activity	curie (Ci)	Disintegrations per second (dps)	becquerel (Bq)	1 Ci = 3.7 $\times 10^{10}$ Bq; 1 mCi = 37 mBq; 1 μCi = 0.037 MBq or 37 GBq; 1 Bq = 2.703 $\times$ 10^{-11} Ci
Absorbed dose	rad	joule per kilogram (J/kg)	gray (Gy)	1 Gy = 100 rad; 1 rad = 0.01 Gy; 1 mrad = 10^{-3} cGy
Exposure	roentgen (R)	coulomb per kilogram (C/kg)	—	1 C/kg = 3876 R; 1 R = 2.58 $\times 10^{-4}$ C/kg; 1 mR = 258 pC/kg
Dose equivalent	rem	joule per kilogam (J/kg)	sievert (Sv)	1 Sv = 100 rem; 1 rem = 0.01 Sv; 1 mrem = 10 μSv

TABLE A-3 SI prefixes and their symbols

Factor	Prefix	Symbol for prefix
10^9	giga	G
10^6	mega	M
10^3	kilo	k
10^2	hecto	h
10^1	deka	da
10^{-1}	deci	d
10^{-2}	centi	c
10^{-3}	milli	m
10^{-6}	micro	μ
10^{-9}	nano	n
10^{-12}	pico	p
10^{-15}	femto	f
10^{-18}	alto	a

TABLE A-4 Plasma lipid concentration in normal subjects*

Age	Total plasma cholesterol, mg/dL		Plasma LDL-cholesterol, mg/dL		Plasma HDL-cholesterol, mg/dL		Plasma triglyceride, mg/dL	
	Men	Women	Men	Women	Men	Women	Men	Women
19	113–197	120–203	62–130	59–137	30–63	35–74	37–148	39–132
29	133–244	130–229	70–165	71–164	31–63	37–83	46–249	40–172
39	146–270	141–245	81–189	75–172	29–62	34–82	54–321	41–194
49	158–276	152–268	98–202	79–186	30–64	34–87	58–327	47–228
59	156–276	169–294	88–203	89–210	28–71	37–91	58–286	56–257
69	158–274	171–297	98–210	92–221	30–78	35–98	57–267	60–241
70+	151–270	167–288	80–186	96–206	31–75	33–92	58–258	60–235

* 5th and 95th percentiles not ideal ranges for white men and women; data are too fragmentary to ascertain whether these values apply to other groups.
SOURCE: *The Lipid Research Clinics Population Studies Data Book, vol 1, The Prevalence Study, NIH Publication No 80-1529, Bethesda, National Institutes of Health, July 1980.*

TABLE A-5 Hemodynamic values

Pressures (mmHg):
- Systemic arterial:
  - Peak systolic/end-diastolic — 100–140/60–90
  - Mean — 70–105
- Left ventricle:
  - Peak systolic/end-diastolic — 100–140/3–12
- Left atrium (or pulmonary capillary wedge):
  - Mean — 2–12
  - *a* wave — 3–10
  - *v* wave — 3–15
- Pulmonary artery:
  - Peak systolic/end-diastolic — 15–30/4–14
  - Mean — 9–17
- Right ventricle:
  - Peak systolic/end-diastolic — 15–30/2–7
- Right atrium:
  - Mean — 2–6
  - *a* wave — 2–8
  - *v* wave — 2–7

Resistances [(dyn·s)/cm⁵]:
- Systemic vascular resistance — 700–1600
- Total pulmonary resistance — 100–300
- Pulmonary vascular resistance — 20–130

Flows:
- Cardiac index (liters per minute per square meter) — 2.4–3.8
- Stroke index (milliliters per beat per square meter) — 30–65

Oxygen consumption (liters per minute per square meter) — 110–150

Arteriovenous oxygen difference (milliliters per liter) — 30–50

TABLE A-7 Normal values of echocardiographic measurements in adults*

	Range, cm	Mean, cm	Number of subjects
Age (years)	13 to 54	26	134
Body surface area (m²)	1.45 to 2.22	1.8	130
RVD—flat	0.7 to 2.3	1.5	84
RVD—left lateral	0.9 to 2.6	1.7	83
LVID—flat	3.7 to 5.6	4.7	82
LVID—left lateral	3.5 to 5.7	4.7	81
Posterior LV wall thickness	0.6 to 1.1	0.9	137
Posterior LV wall amplitude	0.9 to 1.4	1.2	48
IVS wall thickness	0.6 to 1.1	0.9	137
Mid IVS amplitude	0.3 to 0.8	0.5	10
Apical IVS amplitude	0.5 to 1.2	0.7	38
Left atrial dimension	1.9 to 4.0	2.9	133
Aortic root dimension	2.0 to 3.7	2.7	121
Aortic cusps' separation	1.5 to 2.6	1.9	93
Percentage of fractional shortening†	34 to 44%	36%	20
Mean rate of circumferential shortening (Vcf)‡, or mean normalized shortening velocity	1.02 to 1.94 circ/s	1.3 circ/s	38

* RVD = right ventricular dimension; LVID = left ventricular internal dimension; d = end diastole; s = end systole; LV = left ventricle; IVS = interventricular septum.

$$\dagger \quad \frac{LVIDd - LVIDs}{LVIDd}$$

$$\ddagger \quad \frac{LVIDd - LVIDs}{LVIDd \times ejection\ time}$$

SOURCE: *From H Feigenbaum, Echocardiography, in Heart Disease—A Textbook of Cardiovascular Medicine, E Braunwald (ed), Philadelphia, Saunders, 1980.*

TABLE A-6 Systolic time intervals in normal individuals (in milliseconds)

Regression equation	SD of index
QS₂ (M) = −2.1 HR + 546	14
QS₂ (F) = −2.0 HR + 549	14
PEP (M) = −0.4 HR + 131	13
PEP (F) = −0.4 HR + 133	11
LVET (M) = −1.7 HR + 413	10
LVET (F) = −1.6 HR + 418	10

NOTE: *QS₂ = total electromechanical systole, PEP = preejection phase, LVET = left ventricular ejection time, HR = heart rate, M = male, F = female, SD = standard deviation of the systolic time interval index. Systolic ejection period = 220–320 ms per beat; diastolic filling period = 380–500 ms per beat.*
SOURCE: *AM Weissler, CL Garrard, Mod Concepts Cardiovasc Dis 40:1, 1971.*

TABLE A-8 Amplitude of Q, R, S, and T waves in scalar electrocardiogram of 100 normal adults*

	I	II	III	aVR	aVL	aVF	V₁	V₅	V₆
Patients with Q wave	38%	41%	50%	—	38%	40%	0%	60%	75%
Q amplitude:									
Mean	0.4	0.6	0.9	—	0.4	0.7	0	0.3	0.3
Range	0 to 0.10	0 to 1.6	0 to 2.3	—	0 to 1.1	0 to 1.7	0	0 to 1.8	0 to 1.8
R amplitude:									
Mean	5.6	8.9	4.5	1.3	3.4	6.0	1.9	12.6	10.2
Range	1.0 to 10.0	2.0 to 16.9	1.0 to 12.1	0 to 2.9	0 to 8.2	0 to 13.8	1.0 to 6.0	7.0 to 21.0	5.0 to 18.0
S amplitude:									
Mean	2.0	2.1	2.4	7.0	2.6	—	8.0	2.5	1.3
Range	0 to 5.0	0 to 3.7	0 to 6.4	2.2 to 11.8	0 to 5.8	—	3.0 to 13.0	0 to 5.0	0 to 2.0
T amplitude:									
Mean	1.9	2.3	1.0	—	0.3	1.7	1.0	3.3	1.0
Range	1.0 to 3.0	1.0 to 4.0	−2.0 to 2.0	—	−1.0 to 2.0	0 to 4.0	−2.0 to 2.0	2.0 to 7.0	1.0 to 4.0

* Values of Q, R, S, and T amplitudes are in millimeters (1 mm = 0.1 mv).
SOURCE: *From J D Cooksey et al, Clinical Vectorcardiography and Electrocardiography, 2d ed, Chicago, Year Book Medical Publishers, 1977. Used by permission.*

TABLE A-9 Summary of values useful in pulmonary physiology

	Symbol	Typical values Men	Women
PULMONARY MECHANICS			
Spirometry—volume-time curves:			
Forced vital capacity	FVC	≥4.0 liters	≥3.0 liters
Forced expiratory volume in 1 s	FEV_1	>3.0 liters	>2.0 liters
FEV_1/FVC	$FEV_1\%$	>60%	>70%
Maximal midexpiratory flow	MMF (FEF 25–27)	>2.0 liters per second	>1.6 liters per second
Maximal expiratory flow rate	MEFR (FEF 200–1200)	>3.5 liters per second	>3.0 liters per second
Spirometry—flow-volume curves:			
Maximal expiratory flow at 50% of expired vital capacity	$\dot{V}_{max}$ 50 (FEF 50%)	>2.5 liters per second	>2.0 liters per second
Maximal expiratory flow at 75% of expired vital capacity	$\dot{V}_{max}$ 75 (FEF 75%)	>1.5 liters per second	>1.0 liters per second
Resistance to airflow:			
Pulmonary resistance	RL (R_L)	<3.0 cmH_2O/s per liter	
Airway resistance	Raw	<2.5 cmH_2O/s per liter	
Specific conductance	SGaw	>0.13 cmH_2O/s	
Pulmonary compliance:			
Static recoil pressure at total lung capacity	Pst TLC	25 ± 5 cmH_2O	
Compliance of lungs (static)	CL	0.2 L/cmH_2O	
Compliance of lungs and thorax	C(L + T)	0.1 L/cmH_2O	
Dynamic compliance of 20 breaths per minute	C dyn 20	0.25 ± 0.05 liters per cmH_2O	
Maximal static respiratory pressures:			
Maximal inspiratory pressure	MIP	> 90 cmH_2O	> 50 cmH_2O
Maximal expiratory pressure	MEP	>150 cmH_2O	>120 cmH_2O
LUNG VOLUMES			
Total lung capacity	TLC	6–7 liters	5–6 liters
Functional residual capacity	FRC	2–3 liters	2–3 liters
Residual volume	RV	1–2 liters	1–2 liters
Inspiratory capacity	IC	2–4 liters	2–4 liters
Expiratory reserve volume	ERV	1–2 liters	1–2 liters
Vital capacity	VC	4–5 liters	3–4 liters
GAS EXCHANGE (SEA LEVEL)			
Arterial O_2 tension	Pa_{O_2}	95 ± 5 mmHg	
Arterial CO_2 tension	Pa_{CO_2}	40 ± 2 mmHg	
Arterial O_2 saturation	Sa_{O_2}	97 ± 2%	
Arterial blood pH	pH	7.40 ± 0.02	
Arterial bicarbonate	HCO_3^-	24 + 2 meq per liter	
Base excess	BE	0 ± 2 meq per liter	
Diffusing capacity for carbon monoxide (single breath)	DL_{CO}	25 mL CO/min/mmHg	
Dead space volume	V_D	50 ± 25 mL	
Physiologic dead space: dead space-tidal volume			
ratio (rest)	V_D/V_T	≤35% V_T	
(exercise)		≤20% V_T	
Alveolar-arterial difference for O_2	A-a D_{O_2}	≤20 mmHg	

TABLE A-10 Prediction equations for spirometric tests, lung volumes, and gas exchange in adults

Variable	Sex	Age (A)	Height (H)	Weight (W)	Constant (C)	Standard deviation (SD)
PULMONARY MECHANICS						
Spirometry—volume-time curves* (H in inches):						
FVC	M	−0.025	+0.148	—	−4.241	0.74
	F	−0.024	+0.115	—	−2.852	0.52
FEV$_1$	M	−0.032	+0.092	—	−1.260	0.55
	F	−0.025	+0.089	—	−1.932	0.47
MEFR	M	−0.047	+0.109	—	+2.010	1.66
(FEF 200–1200)	F	−0.036	+0.145	—	−2.532	1.19
MMF	M	−0.045	+0.047	—	+2.513	1.12
(FEF 25–75)	F	−0.030	+0.060	—	+0.551	0.80
Spirometry—flow-volume curves† (H in centimeters):						
$\dot{V}_{max}$ 50	M	−0.015	+0.069	—	−5.400	1.422
(FEF 50%)	F	−0.013	+0.035	—	−0.444	1.22
$\dot{V}_{max}$ 75	M	−0.012	+0.044	—	−4.143	1.026
(FEF 75%)	F	−0.014	—	—	+3.042	0.936
Lung volumes‡ (H in meters; W in kilograms):						
TLC	M	—	+6.92	−0.017	−4.30	0.67
	F	−0.015	+6.71	—	−5.77	0.48
FRC	M	+0.015	+5.30	−0.037	−3.89	0.56
	F	—	+5.13	−0.028	−4.50	0.41
RV	M	+0.022	+1.98	−0.015	−1.54	0.38
	F	+0.007	+2.68	—	−3.42	0.32
VC	M	−0.020	+4.81	—	−2.81	0.50
	F	−0.022	+4.04	—	−2.35	0.40
Gas exchange§ (H in meters; W in kilograms):						
DL$_{CO}$	M	−0.20	+32.5	—	−17.6	5.1
	F	−0.16	+21.2	—	−2.66	3.6

NOTE: *Answer = (A × age) + (H × height) + (W × weight) + C ± 2 SD. Example: The normal value and lower limit for the FEV$_1$ are sought in a man, age 40 years, height 183 cm, and weight 91 kg. The following equation gives the normal value:*

FEV$_1$ = (−0.032 × 40) + (0.092 × 72) + (−1.260) = 4.08 liters

The lower limit of normal:

4.08 − (2 × SD) = 4.08 − (2 × 0.55) = 2.98 liters

Only 2.5% of a normal population will fall below this value (2 SD below the mean).

For other abbreviations, see Table A-9.

* *Morris et al, Am Rev Respir Dis 103:57, 1971.*
† *Knudson et al, Am Rev Respir Dis 113:587, 1976.*
‡ *Grimby G, Söderholm B, Acta Med Scand 173:199, 1963.*
§ *Coates, JE, Lung Function and Application in Medicine, Davis, 1965.*

TABLE A-11 Differential nucleated cell counts of bone marrow

	Normal, mean%*	Range, %†
Myeloid:	56.7	
Neutrophilic series:	53.6	
Myeloblast	0.9	0.2–1.5
Promyelocyte	3.3	2.1–4.1
Myelocyte	12.7	8.2–15.7
Metamyelocyte	15.9	9.6–24.6
Band	12.4	9.5–15.3
Segmented		
Eosinophilic series	3.1	1.2–5.3
Basophilic series	<0.1	0–0.2
Erythroid:	25.6	
Pronormoblasts	0.6	0.2–1.3
Basophilic normoblasts	1.4	0.5–2.4
Polychromatophilic normo-blasts	21.6	17.9–29.2
Orthochromatic normoblasts	2.0	0.4–4.6
Megakaryocytes	<0.1	
Lymphoreticular:	17.8	
Lymphocytes	16.2	11.1–23.2
Plasma cells	2.3	0.4–3.9
Reticulum cells	0.3	0–0.9

* *Frm MM Wintrobe et al, Clinical Hematology, 8th ed, Philadelphia, Lea & Febiger, 1981.*
† *Range observed in 12 healthy men.*

TABLE A-12 Erythrocytes and hemoglobin: Normal values at various ages

Age	Red blood cell count,* millions/mm³	Hemoglobin,* g/dL	Vol. packed RBCs,* mL/dL	Corpuscular values MCV, fl	MCH, pg	MCHC, g/dL	MCD, μm
Days 1–13	5.1 ± 1.0	19.5 ± 5.0	54.0 ± 10.0	106–98	38–33	36–34	8.6
Days 14–60	4.7 ± 0.9	14.0 ± 3.3	42.0 ± 7.0	90	30	33	8.1
3 months to 10 years	4.5 ± 0.7	12.2 ± 2.3	36.0 ± 5.0	80	27	34	7.7
11–15 years	4.8	13.4	39.0	82	28	34	
Adults:							
Females	4.8 ± 0.6	14.0 ± 2.0	42.0 ± 5.0	90 ± 7	29 ± 2	34 ± 2	7.5 ± 0.3
Males	5.4 ± 0.9	16.0 ± 2.0	47.0 ± 5.0	90 ± 7	29 ± 2	34 ± 2	7.5 ± 0.3

* *The range of values represents almost the extremes of observed variations (93 percent or more) at sea level. The blood values of healthy persons should fall well within these mean ± SD figures.*
NOTE: *MCV = mean corpuscular volume, MCH = mean corpuscular hemoglobin, MCHC = mean corpuscular hemoglobin concentration, MCD = mean corpuscular diameter.*
SOURCE: *MM Wintrobe et al, Clinical Hematology, 8th ed, Philadelphia, Lea & Febiger, 1981.*

TABLE A-13 Normal leukocyte count, differential count, and hemoglobin concentration at various ages

Age	Leukocytes, total	Neutrophils Total	Band	Segmented	Eosinophils	Basophils	Lympho-cytes	Monocytes	Hemoglo-bin, g/dL blood
12 mo	11.4(6.0–17.5)	3.5(1.5–8.5)	0.35	3.2	0.3(0.05–0.7)	0.05(0–0.20)	7.0(4.0–10.5)	0.55(0.05–1.1)	11.6(9.0–14.6)
		_31_	_3.1_	_28_	_0.4_	_0.4_	_61_	_4.8_	
4 yr	9.1(5.5–15.5)	3.8(1.5–8.5)	0.27(0–1.0)	3.5(1.5–7.5)	0.25(0.02–0.65)	0.05(0–0.20)	4.5(2.0–8.0)	0.45(0–0.8)	12.6(9.6–15.5)
		_42_	_3.0_	_39_	_2.8_	_0.6_	_50_	_5.0_	
6 yr	4.3(1.5–8.0)	0.25(0–1.0)	4.0(1.5–7.0)	4.0(1.5–7.0)	0.23(0–0.65)	0.05(0–0.20)	3.5(1.5–7.0)	0.40(0–0.8)	12.7(10.0–15.5)
		_51_	_3.0_	_48_	_2.7_	_0.6_	_42_	_4.7_	
10 yr	8.1(4.5–13.5)	4.4(1.8–8.0)	0.24(0–1.0)	4.2(1.8–7.0)	0.20(0–0.60)	0.04(0–0.20)	3.1(1.5–6.5)	0.35(0–0.8)	13.0(10.7–15.5)
		_54_	_3.0_	_51_	_2.4_	_0.5_	_38_	_4.3_	
21 yr	7.4(4.5–11.0)	4.4(1.8–7.7)	0.22(0–0.7)	4.2(1.8–7.0)	0.20(0–0.45)	0.04(0–0.20)	2.5(1.0–4.8)	0.30(0–0.8)	♂15.8 (14.0–18.0)
		_59_	_3.0_	_56_	_2.7_	_0.5_	_34_	_4.0_	♀13.9 (11.5–16.0)

NOTE: *Values are expressed as "cells × 10³/μL." The numbers underlined are percentages.*
SOURCE: *WJ Williams et al (eds), Hematology, 3d ed, New York, McGraw-Hill, New York, 1983. By permission.*

INDEX

INDEX